DeLee, Drez, & Miller's

Orthopaedic Sports Medicine

Principles and Practice

MW01074110

FIFTH EDITION

DeLee, Drez, & Miller's

Orthopaedic Sports Medicine

Principles and Practice

Mark D. Miller, MD

S. Ward Casscells Professor of Orthopaedic Surgery
Head, Division of Sports Medicine
University of Virginia
Charlottesville, Virginia
Adjunctive Clinical Professor and Team Physician
James Madison University
Harrisonburg, Virginia

Stephen R. Thompson, MD, MEd, FRCSC

Associate Professor of Sports Medicine
Eastern Maine Medical Center
University of Maine
Bangor, Maine

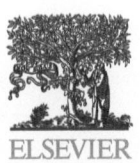

ELSEVIER

DELEE, DREZ, & MILLER'S ORTHOPAEDIC SPORTS MEDICINE, FIFTH EDITION

ISBN: 978-0-323-54473-3

Notices

Knowledge and best practice in this field are constantly changing. As new research and experience broaden our understanding, changes in research methods, professional practices, or medical treatment may become necessary.

Practitioners and researchers must always rely on their own experience and knowledge in evaluating and using any information, methods, compounds, or experiments described herein. In using such information or methods they should be mindful of their own safety and the safety of others, including parties for whom they have a professional responsibility.

With respect to any drug or pharmaceutical products identified, readers are advised to check the most current information provided (i) on procedures featured or (ii) by the manufacturer of each product to be administered, to verify the recommended dose or formula, the method and duration of administration, and contraindications. It is the responsibility of practitioners, relying on their own experience and knowledge of their patients, to make diagnoses, to determine dosages and the best treatment for each individual patient, and to take all appropriate safety precautions.

To the fullest extent of the law, neither the Publisher nor the authors, contributors, or editors, assume any liability for any injury and/or damage to persons or property as a matter of products liability, negligence or otherwise, or from any use or operation of any methods, products, instructions, or ideas contained in the material herein.

Previous editions copyrighted 2015, 2010, 2003, 1994.

International Standard Book Number: 978-0-323-54473-3

Senior Content Strategist: Kristine Jones
Senior Content Development Specialist: Joan Ryan
Publishing Services Manager: Catherine Jackson
Senior Project Manager: Amanda Mincher
Design Direction: Ryan Cook

Printed in the United States of America
Last digit is the print number: 9 8 7 6 5 4

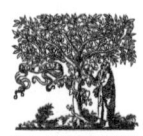
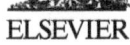

1600 John F. Kennedy Blvd.
Ste 1600
Philadelphia, PA 19103-2899

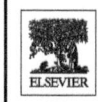

Working together
to grow libraries in
developing countries

www.elsevier.com • www.bookaid.org

To sports medicine professionals in every discipline and to athletes at every level and every sport. Without them there would be no sports medicine.

And to Drs. Jesse DeLee and David Drez. Thank you for entrusting us to keep your vision alive.

MARK D. MILLER

For Linden Ellis: You are too young to read this now, and you may choose never to read this later, but it is nonetheless still for you.

And, for Shannon. As always, thank you for everything you do, including enabling me to do what I do.

STEPHEN R. THOMPSON

SECTION EDITORS

Amiethab A. Aiyer, MD
Assistant Professor, Chief Foot and Ankle Service
Department of Orthopaedics
University of Miami, Miller School of Medicine
Miami, Florida
Leg, Ankle, and Foot

Asheesh Bedi, MD
Chief, Sports Medicine and Shoulder Surgery
Professor of Orthopaedics
Head Orthopaedic Team Physician
University of Michigan
Ann Arbor, Michigan
Basic Principles

Stephen F. Brockmeier, MD
Associate Professor
Department of Orthopaedic Surgery
Fellowship Director, University of Virginia Sports Medicine
Fellowship
University of Virginia School of Medicine
Charlottesville, Virginia
Shoulder

Rajwinder Deu, MD
Assistant Professor
Department of Orthopaedics
Johns Hopkins University
Baltimore, Maryland
Medical

F. Winston Gwathmey, Jr., MD
Associate Professor of Orthopaedic Surgery
University of Virginia School of Medicine
Charlottesville, Virginia
Pelvis, Hip, and Thigh

Joe M. Hart, PhD, ATC
Associate Professor
Department of Kinesiology
University of Virginia
Charlottesville, Virginia
Rehabilitation and Injury Prevention

Anish R. Kadakia, MD
Associate Professor of Orthopaedic Surgery
Northwestern Memorial Hospital
Northwestern University Feinberg School of Medicine
Chicago, Illinois
Leg, Ankle, and Foot

Sanjeev Kakar, MD, FAOA
Professor of Orthopaedic Surgery
Mayo Clinic
Rochester, Minnesota
Elbow, Wrist, and Hand

Morteza Khodaee, MD, MPH, FACSM, FAAFP
Associate Professor
University of Colorado School of Medicine
Department of Family Medicine and Orthopaedics
Denver, Colorado
Medical

Bryson Lesniak, MD
Associate Professor
University of Pittsburgh Medical Center
Rooney Sports Complex
Pittsburgh, Pennsylvania
Basic Principles

Eric C. McCarty, MD
Chief, Sports Medicine and Shoulder Surgery
Associate Professor
Department of Orthopaedics
University of Colorado School of Medicine
Director Sports Medicine, Head Team Physician
University of Colorado Department of Athletics
Associate Professor, Adjunct
Department of Integrative Physiology
University of Colorado
Boulder, Colorado
Knee

Matthew D. Milewski, MD
Assistant Professor
Division of Sports Medicine
Department of Orthopaedic Surgery
Boston Children's Hospital
Boston, Massachusetts
Pediatric Sports Medicine

Francis H. Shen, MD
Warren G. Stamp Endowed Professor
Division Head, Spine Division
Co-Director, Spine Center
Department of Orthopaedic Surgery
University of Virginia
Charlottesville, Virginia
Spine and Head

PREFACE

What's in a name? In developing and editing the fifth edition of DeLee, Drez, & Miller's Orthopaedic Sports Medicine: Principles and Practices, we considered removing "orthopaedic" from the title. In an effort to keep pace with the rapidly growing specialty of sports medicine that includes internal medicine, pediatrics, rehabilitation medicine, athletic training, as well as orthopedics and many other disciplines, it is essential to expand the book's focus beyond orthopedics and address a more all-inclusive vision of sports medicine. Regardless of how sports medicine touches your individual practice, this updated version of this classic textbook remains the most comprehensive in the field.

As sports medicine continues to evolve, the need to include additional topics is essential. For this fifth edition, one focus is addressing problems of revision surgery. Important new chapters have been added on revision shoulder instability, revision rotator cuff, and revision anterior cruciate ligament surgery. Additionally, we have fine-tuned the organization of chapters under the dutiful watch of section editors. The hand section has been revised to include more comprehensive chapters on sports-related injuries. The hip section has been updated to reflect the current thinking on the hottest new topics in sports medicine, including new chapters on posterior hip pain and peritrochanteric lesions.

And the non-operative sections have been extensively edited and expanded, to include new information on sports nutrition, psychological adjustment to athletic injury and genitourinary trauma in the athlete.

Incredibly, there are over 300 contributors to this new edition, many of whom are widely regarded as the foremost experts in their fields. To each of them, we extend heartfelt gratitude for their willingness to participate and share their knowledge. Similarly, we would be remiss if we did not thank our outstanding section editors: Drs. Bedi, Lesniak, Khodaee, Deu, Hart, Brockmeier, Kakar, Gwathmey, McCarty, Kadakia, Aiyer, Shen, and Milewski. They did the heavy lifting in the publishing process and we are deeply appreciative of their efforts.

It remains a distinct honor and pleasure to continue the tradition of Drs. Jesse DeLee and David Drez, who first produced this text in 1994. We hope it enables practitioners to remain on the cutting edge of sports medicine to the benefit of the widest possible spectrum of athletes and patients under our collective care.

Mark D. Miller
Stephen R. Thompson

Kathleen C. Abalos, MD
Department of Medicine
Beth Israel Deaconess Medical Center
Boston, Massachusetts

Jeffrey S. Abrams, MD
Clinical Professor
School of Graduate Medicine
Seton Hall University
South Orange, New Jersey
Clinical Associate Professor
Penn Medicine Princeton Medical Center
Princeton, New Jersey

Julie E. Adams, MD
Professor of Orthopedic Surgery
Mayo Clinic Health System
Austin, Minnesota and Rochester, Minnesota

Bayan Aghdasi, MD
Orthopaedic Surgery
University of Virginia
Charlottesville, Virginia

Amiethab A. Aiyer, MD
Assistant Professor, Chief Foot and Ankle
    Service
Department of Orthopaedics
University of Miami, Miller School of
    Medicine
Miami, Florida

Nourbakhsh Ali, MD
Spine Surgeon
Wellstar Atlanta Medical Center
Atlanta, Georgia

David W. Altchek, MD
Co-Chief Emeritus
Sports Medicine and Shoulder Service
Hospital for Special Surgery
New York, New York

Raj M. Amin, MD
Resident Physician
Department of Orthopaedic Surgery
The Johns Hopkins Hospital
Baltimore, Maryland

Kimberly K. Amrami, MD
Professor of Radiology
Chair, Division of Musculoskeletal Radiology
Mayo Clinic
Rochester, Minnesota

Christian N. Anderson, MD
Orthopaedic Surgeon
Tennessee Orthopaedic Alliance/The
    Lipscomb Clinic
Nashville, Tennessee

Lindsay M. Andras, MD
Assistant Professor of Orthopaedic Surgery
Children's Orthopedic Center
Children's Hospital Los Angeles
Los Angeles, California

James R. Andrews, MD
Medical Director
The Andrews Institute
Gulf Breeze, Florida
Medical Director
The American Sports Medicine Institute
Birmingham, Alabama

Michael Antonis, DO, RDMS, FACEP,
CAQSM
Emergency Medicine & Sports Medicine
Georgetown University
Washington, District of Columbia

Chad A. Asplund, MD, MPH
Director, Athletic Medicine
Associate Professor, Health and Kinesiology
Georgia Southern University
Statesboro, Georgia

Rachid Assina, MD, RPH
Assistant Professor
Department of Neurological Surgery
Rutgers–New Jersey Medical School
Newark, New Jersey

Ashley V. Austin, MD
Resident
Family Medicine and Physical Medicine and
    Rehabilitation
University of Virginia
Charlottesville, Virginia

Luke S. Austin, MD
Associate Professor of Orthopaedics
Rothman Institute
Egg Harbor Township, New Jersey

John T. Awowale, MD
Orthopedic Surgery
University of Wisconsin Hospitals and
    Clinics
University of Wisconsin
Madison, Wisconsin

Derek P. Axibal, MD
Department of Orthopedics
University of Colorado School of Medicine
Aurora, Colorado

Bernard R. Bach Jr., MD
The Claude Lambert-Helen Thompson
    Professor of Orthopedic Surgery
Rush University Medical Center
Chicago, Illinois

Aaron L. Baggish, MD
Director, Cardiovascular Performance
    Program
Massachusetts General Hospital
Boston, Massachusetts

Wajeeh Bakhsh, MD
Surgical Resident, Department of
    Orthopaedics
University of Rochester Medical Center
Rochester, New York

Christopher P. Bankhead, MD
Resident, Orthopaedic Surgery
University of New Mexico
Albuquerque, New Mexico

Michael G. Baraga, MD
Assistant Professor of Orthopaedics
UHealth Sports Medicine Institute
University of Miami, Miller School of
    Medicine
Miami, Florida

Jonathan Barlow, MD, MS
Mayo Clinic
Rochester, Minnesota

Robert W. Battle, MD
Team Cardiologist
Associate Professor of Medicine and
    Pediatrics
Department of Cardiology
University of Virginia Medical Center
Charlottesville, Virginia

Matthew Bessette, MD
Sports Medicine Fellow
The Cleveland Clinic Foundation
Cleveland, Ohio

Thomas M. Best, MD, PhD
Professor of Orthopaedics
Research Director of Sports Performance
    and Wellness Institute
University of Miami Sports Medicine Institute
Miami, Florida

Bruce Beynnon, PhD
McClure Professor of Musculoskeletal
  Research
Director of Research
Department of Orthopaedics and
  Rehabilitation
University of Vermont College of Medicine
McClure Musculoskeletal Research Center
Burlington, Vermont

Kieran Bhattacharya, BS
Research Assistant
Department of Orthopaedic Surgery
University of Virginia
Charlottesville, Virginia

Debdut Biswas, MD
Hinsdale Orthopaedics
Chicago, Illinois

Matthew H. Blake, MD
Assistant Director, Sports Medicine
Orthopaedic Sports Medicine
Avera McKennan Hospital and University
  Health Center
Sioux Falls, South Dakota

Liljiana Bogunovic
Assistant Professor
Department of Orthopaedic Surgery
Washington University School of Medicine
St. Louis, Missouri

Margaret Boushell, PhD
Department of Biomedical Engineering
Biomaterials and Interface Tissue
  Engineering Laboratory
Columbia University Medical Center
New York Presbyterian Hospital
New York, New York

James P. Bradley, MD
Clinical Professor
Orthopaedic Surgery
University of Pittsburgh Medical Center
Pittsburgh, Pennsylvania

William Brady, MD, FAAEM, FACEP
Professor of Medicine and Emergency
  Medicine
University of Virginia
Charlottesville, Virginia

Jonathan T. Bravman, MD
Assistant Professor
Director of Sports Medicine Research
CU Sports Medicine
Division of Sports Medicine and Shoulder
  Surgery
University of Colorado
Denver, Colorado

Stephen F. Brockmeier, MD
Associate Professor
Department of Orthopaedic Surgery
Fellowship Director, University of Virginia
  Sports Medicine Fellowship
University of Virginia School of Medicine
Charlottesville, Virginia

Jeffrey Brunelli, MD
Assistant Professor of Orthopaedic Surgery
  and Rehabilitation
Chief, Sports Medicine and Shoulder
  Surgery
University of Florida-Jacksonville College of
  Medicine
Jacksonville, Florida

Jackie Buell, PhD, RD, CSSD, LD, ATC
Assistant Professor, Clinical Health Sciences
  and Medical Dietetics
The Ohio State University
Columbus, Ohio

Alissa J. Burge, MD
Assistant Professor of Radiology
Weill Cornell Medicine
New York, New York

**Jessica L. Buschmann, MS, RD, CSSD,
LD**
Clinical Dietician—Board Certified
  Specialist in Sports Dietetics Sports
  Medicine
Nationwide Children's Hospital
Columbus, Ohio

Brian Busconi, MD
Associate Professor of Orthopaedic Surgery
Sports Medicine
University of Massachusetts
Worcester, Massachusetts

Charles A. Bush-Joseph, MD
Professor of Orthopaedic Surgery
Division of Sports Medicine
Rush University Medical Center
Chicago, Illinois

Kadir Buyukdogan, MD
Department of Orthopaedic Surgery
University of Virginia
Charlottesville, Virginia

E. Lyle Cain Jr., MD
Founding Partner
Andrews Sports Medicine and Orthopaedic
  Center
Fellowship Director
American Sports Medicine Institute
Birmingham, Alabama

Jon-Michael E. Caldwell, MD
Resident, Department of Orthopedic
  Surgery
Columbia University Medical Center
New York Presbyterian Hospital
New York, New York

Mary E. Caldwell, DO
Assistant Professor of Physical Medicine and
  Rehabilitation and Sports Medicine
Medical College of Virginia
Virginia Commonwealth University
Richmond, Virginia

Ryan P. Calfee, MD, MSc
Associate Professor of Orthopedics
Washington University School of Medicine
St. Louis, Missouri

Christopher L. Camp, MD
Assistant Professor of Orthopedics
Mayo Clinic
Rochester, Minnesota

John T. Campbell, MD
Attending Orthopaedic Surgeon
Institute for Foot and Ankle Reconstruction
Mercy Medical Center
Baltimore, Maryland

Kevin Caperton, MD
Department of Orthopedics and Sports
  Medicine
Georgetown Orthopedics
Georgetown, Texas

Robert M. Carlisle, MD
Resident, Orthopaedic Surgery
Greenville Health System
Greenville, South Carolina

Rebecca A. Cerrato, MD
Attending Orthopaedic Surgeon
Institute for Foot and Ankle Reconstruction
Baltimore, Maryland

Courtney Chaaban, PT, DPT, SCS
Doctoral Student
Sports Medicine Research Laboratory
Department of Exercise and Sport Science
University of North Carolina at Chapel Hill
Chapel Hill, North Carolina

Jorge Chahla, MD
Regenerative Sports Medicine Fellow
Center for Regenerative Sports Medicine
Steadman Philippon Research Institute
Vail, Colorado

Peter N. Chalmers, MD
Assistant Professor
University of Utah Department of
    Orthopaedic Surgery
Salt Lake City, Utah

Angela K. Chang, MD
Center for Outcomes-Based Orthopaedic
    Research
Steadman Philippon Research Institute
Vail, Colorado

Sonia Chaudhry, MD
Assistant Professor of Orthopaedic Surgery
University of Connecticut School of
    Medicine
Pediatric Orthopaedic, Hand, and
    Microvascular Surgery
Connecticut Children's Medical Center
Hartford, Connecticut

Austin W. Chen, MD
Hip Preservation and Sports Medicine
BoulderCentre for Orthopedics
Boulder, Colorado
Academic Faculty
American Hip Institute
Chicago, Illinois

Edward C. Cheung, MD
Resident Physician
Orthopaedic Surgery
University of California, Los Angeles
    Medical Center
Los Angeles, California

A. Bobby Chhabra, MD
Lillian T. Pratt Distinguished Professor and
    Chair
Orthopaedic Surgery
University of Virginia Health System
Charlottesville, Virginia

Woojin Cho, MD, PhD
Assistant Professor, Orthopaedic Surgery
Albert Einstein College of Medicine
Chief of Spine Surgery
Orthopaedic Surgery
Research Director
Multidisciplinary Spine Center
Montefiore Medical Center
New York, New York

Joseph N. Chorley, MD
Associate Professor of Pediatrics
Baylor College of Medicine
Houston, Texas

John Jared Christophel, MD, MPH
Assistant Professor of Otolaryngology—
    Head and Neck Surgery
University of Virginia
Charlottesville, Virginia

Philip Chuang, PhD
Department of Biomedical Engineering
Biomaterials and Interface Tissue
    Engineering Laboratory
Columbia University Medical Center
New York Presbyterian Hospital
New York, New York

Nicholas J. Clark, MD
Orthopedic Surgeon
Mayo Clinic
Rochester, Minnesota

John C. Clohisy, MD
Professor of Orthopaedic Surgery
Washington University School of Medicine
St. Louis, Missouri

Christopher Coleman, MD
Department of Radiology
University of Colorado
Aurora, Colorado

Francisco Contreras, MD
Department of Radiology
Jackson Memorial Hospital
University of Miami Hospital
Miami, Florida

Joseph D. Cooper, MD
Resident, Orthopaedic Surgery
University of Southern California
Los Angeles, California

Chris A. Cornett, MD, MPT
Associate Professor of Orthopaedic Surgery
University of Nebraska Medical Center
Department of Orthopaedic Surgery and
    Rehabilitation
Medical Director Physical/Occupational
    Therapy
Co-Medical Director, Spine Program
Nebraska Medicine
Omaha, Nebraska

Paul S. Corotto, MD
Chief Fellow
Department of Cardiology
University of Virginia Medical Center
Charlottesville, Virginia

Ryan P. Coughlin, MD, FRCSC
Department of Orthopaedic Surgery
Duke University
Durham, North Carolina

Jared A. Crasto, MD
Resident, Department of Orthopaedic
    Surgery
University of Pittsburgh Medical Center
Pittsburgh, Pennsylvania

Shannon David, PhD, ATC
Assistant Professor
Coordinator of Clinical Education
North Dakota State University
Fargo, North Dakota

Thomas M. DeBerardino, MD
Orthopaedic Surgeon
The Orthopaedic Institute
Medical Director
Burkhart Research Institute for
    Orthopaedics
The San Antonio Orthopaedic Group
Co-Director, Combined Baylor College of
    Medicine and The San Antonio
    Orthopaedic Group, Texas Sports
    Medicine Fellowship
Professor of Orthopaedic Surgery
Baylor College of Medicine
San Antonio, Texas

Richard E. Debski, PhD
Professor
Departments of Bioengineering and
    Orthopaedic Surgery
University of Pittsburgh
Pittsburgh, Pennsylvania

Marc M. DeHart, MD
Associate Professor of Orthopaedic Surgery
Chief of Adult Reconstruction
UT Health San Antonio
San Antonio, Texas

Arthur Jason De Luigi, DO, MHSA
Professor of Rehabilitation Medicine and
    Sports Medicine
Georgetown University School of Medicine
Washington, District of Columbia

Elizabeth R. Dennis, MD, MS
Resident, Department of Orthopedic
    Surgery
Columbia University Medical Center
New York Presbyterian Hospital
New York, New York

John J. Densmore, MD, PhD
Associate Professor of Clinical Medicine
Division of Hematology/Oncology
University of Virginia
Charlottesville, Virginia

Joshua S. Dines, MD
Sports Medicine and Shoulder Service
Hospital for Special Surgery
New York, New York

Benjamin G. Domb, MD
Founder
American Hip Institute
Chicago, Illinois

Jason Dragoo, MD
Associate Professor of Orthopaedic Surgery
Stanford University
Stanford, California

Jeffrey R. Dugas, MD
Surgeon
Andrews Sports Medicine and Orthopaedic
    Center
American Sports Medicine Institute
Birmingham, Alabama

Guillaume D. Dumont, MD
Assistant Professor of Orthopaedic Surgery
University of South Carolina School of
    Medicine
Columbia, South Carolina

Eric W. Edmonds, MD
Associate Professor of Clinical Orthopedic
    Surgery
University of California, San Diego
Director of Orthopedic Research and Sports
    Medicine
Division of Orthopedic Surgery
Rady Children's Hospital San Diego
San Diego, California

Karen P. Egan, PhD
Associate Sport Psychologist
Department of Athletics
University of Virginia
Charlottesville, Virginia

Bassem T. Elhassan, MD
Orthopedic Surgeon
Mayo Clinic
Rochester, Minnesota

Claire D. Eliasberg, MD
Resident, Orthopaedic Surgery
Hospital for Special Surgery
New York, New York

Fatih Ertem, MSc
Department of Biomechanics
Dokuz Eylul University Health Science
    Institute
Inciralti, Izmir, Turkey
Visiting Graduate Researcher
Department of Orthopaedics and
    Rehabilitation
McClure Musculoskeletal Research Center
Burlington, Vermont

Norman Espinosa Jr., MD
Head of Foot and Ankle Surgery
Institute for Foot and Ankle Reconstruction
FussInsitut Zurich
Zurich, Switzerland

Anthony Essilfie, MD
Resident Physician
Orthopaedic Surgery
University of Southern California
Los Angeles, California

Jack Farr, MD
Professor of Orthopedics
Indiana University School of Medicine
OrthoIndy Knee Preservation and Cartilage
    Restoration Center
Indianapolis, Indiana

Derek M. Fine, MD
Associate Professor of Medicine
Fellowship Director
Division of Nephrology
The Johns Hopkins University School of
    Medicine
Baltimore, Maryland

Jake A. Fox, BS
Research Assistant
Center for Outcomes-Based Orthopaedic
    Research
Steadman Philippon Research Institute
Vail, Colorado

Salvatore Frangiamore, MD, MS
Summa Health Orthopaedic and Sports
    Medicine
Akron, Ohio

Rachel M. Frank, MD
Department of Orthopaedic Surgery
Rush University
Chicago, Illinois

Heather Freeman, PT, DHS
Physical Therapist
Assistant Research Coordinator
University of Indianapolis, Krannert School
    of Physical Therapy
Indianapolis, Indiana

Jason Freeman, PhD
Sport Psychologist
Department of Athletics
University of Virginia
Charlottesville, Virginia

Nikhita Gadi, MD, MScBR
Internal Medicine Resident, PGY-1
Hackensack University Medical Center
Hackensack, New Jersey

Seth C. Gamradt, MD
Associate Clinical Professor
Director of Orthopaedic Athletic Medicine
Orthopaedic Surgery
University of Southern California
Los Angeles, California

J. Craig Garrison, PhD, PT, ATC, SCS
Director, Sports Medicine Research
Texas Health Sports Medicine
Texas Health
Fort Worth, Texas

R. Glenn Gaston, MD
Hand and Upper Extremity Surgeon
OrthoCarolina
Chief of Hand Surgery
Division of Orthopedics
Carolinas Medical Center
Charlotte, North Carolina

William B. Geissler, MD
Alan E. Freeland Chair of Hand Surgery
Professor and Chief
Division of Hand and Upper Extremity
    Surgery
Chief, Arthroscopic Surgery and Sports
    Medicine
Department of Orthopaedic Surgery and
    Rehabilitation
University of Mississippi Health Care
Jackson, Mississippi

Brandee Gentile, MS, ATC
Athletic Trainer
Department of Neurosurgery
Rutgers–New Jersey Medical School
Newark, New Jersey

J. Robert Giffin, MD, FRCSC, MBA
Professor of Orthopedic Surgery
Western University
London, Ontario, Canada

Todd M. Gilbert, MD
Department of Orthopaedic Surgery and
    Rehabilitation
University of Nebraska Medical Center
Omaha, Nebraska

G. Keith Gill, MD
Department of Orthopaedics
University of New Mexico Health Sciences
    Center
Albuquerque, New Mexico

Thomas J. Gill, MD
Professor of Orthopedic Surgery
Tufts Medical School
Chairman, Department of Orthopedic
    Surgery
St. Elizabeth's Medical Center/Steward
    Healthcare Network
Boston, Massachusetts

Jacob D. Gire, MD
Department of Orthopaedic Surgery
Stanford University
Palo Alto, California

Pau Golanó, MD
Professor of Human Anatomy
Laboratory of Arthroscopic and Surgical
    Anatomy
Human Anatomy and Embryology Unit
Department of Pathology and Experimental
    Therapeutics
University of Barcelona–Spain
Department of Orthopaedic Surgery
University of Pittsburgh School of Medicine
Pittsburgh, Pennsylvania

Jorge E. Gómez, MD, MS
Associate Professor of Adolescent Medicine
    and Sports Medicine
Baylor College of Medicine
Houston, Texas

Juan Gomez-Hoyos, MD
Baylor University Medical Center at Dallas
Hip Preservation Center
Dallas, Texas

Howard P. Goodkin, MD, PhD
The Shure Professor of Pediatric Neurology
Director
Division of Pediatric Neurology
Departments of Neurology and Pediatrics
University of Virginia
Charlottesville, Virginia

Gregory Grabowski, MD, FAOA
Associate Professor
University of South Carolina School of
    Medicine
Department of Orthopedic Surgery
Co-Medical Director
Palmetto Health USC Spine Center
Residency Program Director
Palmetto Health USC Orthopedic Center
Columbia, South Carolina

Tinker Gray, MA
The Shelbourne Knee Center at Community
    East Hospital
Indianapolis, Indiana

James R. Gregory, MD
Assistant Professor of Pediatric Orthopedic
    Surgery
Department of Orthopedic Surgery
University of Oklahoma College of
    Medicine
Oklahoma City, Oklahoma

Phillip Gribble, PhD
Professor of Rehabilitation Sciences
University of Kentucky
Lexington, Kentucky

Letha Y. Griffin, MD, PhD
Team Physician
Georgia State University
Atlanta, Georgia
Staff
Peachtree Orthopedics
Atlanta, Georgia

Warren C. Hammert, MD
Professor of Orthopaedic Surgery and
    Plastic Surgery
Chief, Hand Surgery
Department of Orthopaedics and
    Rehabilitation
University of Rochester Medical Center
Rochester, New York

Kyle E. Hammond, MD
Assistant Professor, Department of
    Orthopaedic Surgery
Emory Sports Medicine Center
Atlanta, Georgia

Joseph Hannon, PhD, PT, DPT, SCS,
CSCS
Research Physical Therapist
Texas Health Sports Medicine
Texas Health
Fort Worth, Texas

Colin B. Harris, MD
Assistant Professor
Department of Orthopaedics
Rutgers–New Jersey Medical School
Newark, New Jersey

Joshua D. Harris, MD
Orthopedic Surgeon
Associate Professor, Institute for Academic
    Medicine
Houston Methodist Orthopedics and Sports
    Medicine
Houston, Texas
Assistant Professor of Clinical Orthopedic
    Surgery
Weill Cornell Medical College
New York, New York

Andrew Haskell, MD
Chair, Department of Orthopedics
Geographic Medical Director for Surgical
    Services
Palo Alto Medical Foundation
Palo Alto, California
Associate Clinical Professor
Department of Orthopaedic Surgery
University of California, San Francisco
San Francisco, California

Hamid Hassanzadeh, MD
Assistant Professor
Department of Orthopaedic Surgery
University of Virginia
Charlottesville, Virginia

Michael R. Hausman, MD
Professor of Orthopaedic Surgery
Mount Sinai Medical Center
New York, New York

Stefan Hemmings, MBBS
Post-Doctorate Fellow
Division of Nephrology
The Johns Hopkins University School of
    Medicine
Baltimore, Maryland

R. Frank Henn III, MD
Associate Professor of Orthopaedics
University of Maryland School of Medicine
Baltimore, Maryland

Daniel Herman, MD, PhD
Assistant Professor
Department of Orthopedics and Rehabilitation
Divisions of Physical Medicine and
    Rehabilitation, Sports Medicine, and
    Research
University of Florida
Gainesville, Florida

Jay Hertel, PhD, ATC, FNATA
Joe H. Gieck Professor of Sports Medicine
Departments of Kinesiology and
    Orthopaedic Surgery
University of Virginia
Charlottesville, Virginia

Daniel E. Hess, MD
Department of Orthopaedic Surgery
University of Virginia
Charlottesville, Virginia

Carolyn M. Hettrich, MD
University of Iowa
Iowa City, Iowa

Benton E. Heyworth, MD
Assistant Professor of Orthopedic Surgery
Harvard Medical School
Attending Orthopedic Surgeon
Department of Orthopedic Surgery
Division of Sports Medicine
Boston Children's Hospital
Boston, Massachusetts

Ben Hickey, BM, MRCS, MSc, FRCS (Tr & Orth), MD
Consultant Orthopaedic Foot and Ankle
    Surgeon
Wrexham Maelor Hospital
Wrexham, Wales, United Kingdom

Michael Higgins, PhD, ATC, PT, CSCS
Professor, Kinesiology
University of Virginia
Charlottesville, Virginia

Betina B. Hinckel, MD, PhD
Department of Orthopaedic Surgery
Brigham and Women's Hospital
Harvard Medical School
Boston, Massachusetts

Gwendolyn Hoben, MD, PhD
Instructor
Plastic and Reconstructive Surgery
Medical College of Wisconsin
Milwaukee, Wisconsin

Christopher Hogrefe, MD, FACEP
Assistant Professor
Departments of Emergency Medicine,
    Medicine—Sports Medicine, and
    Orthopaedic Surgery—Sports Medicine
Northwestern Medicine
Northwestern University Feinberg School of
    Medicine
Chicago, Illinois

Jason A. Horowitz, BA
Research Fellow
Department of Orthopaedic Surgery
University of Virginia
Charlottesville, Virginia

Benjamin M. Howe, MD
Associate Professor of Radiology
Mayo Clinic
Rochester, Minnesota

Korin Hudson, MD, FACEP, CAQSM
Associate Professor of Emergency Medicine
Team Physician, Department of Athletics
Georgetown University
Washington, District of Columbia

Catherine Hui, MD, FRCSC
Associate Clinical Professor
Division of Orthopaedic Surgery
University of Alberta
Edmonton, Alberta, Canada

R. Tyler Huish, DO
First Choice Physician Partners
La Quinta, California

John V. Ingari, MD
Division Chair, Hand Surgery
Department of Orthopaedic Surgery
The Johns Hopkins Hospital
Baltimore, Maryland

Mary Lloyd Ireland, MD
Professor
Department of Orthopaedics
University of Kentucky
Lexington, Kentucky

Todd A. Irwin, MD
Director of Research
OrthoCarolina Foot and Ankle Institute
Associate Professor
Carolinas Medical Center
Charlotte, North Carolina

Nona M. Jiang, MD
Department of Medicine
University of Virginia
Charlottesville, Virginia

Darren L. Johnson, MD
Director of Sports Medicine
University of Kentucky
Lexington, Kentucky

Jared S. Johnson, MD
St. Luke's Clinic–Sports Medicine: Boise
Boise, Idaho

Grant L. Jones, MD
Associate Professor of Orthopaedic Surgery
The Ohio State University
Columbus, Ohio

Jean Jose, DO, MS
Associate Chief of Musculoskeletal
    Radiology
Associate Professor of Clinical Radiology
Division of Diagnostic Radiology
University of Miami Hospital
Miami, Florida

Scott G. Kaar, MD
Associate Professor of Orthopaedic Surgery
Saint Louis University
St. Louis, Missouri

Anish R. Kadakia, MD
Associate Professor of Orthopaedic Surgery
Northwestern Memorial Hospital
Northwestern University Feinberg School of
    Medicine
Chicago, Illinois

Samantha L. Kallenbach, BS
Steadman Philippon Research Institute
The Steadman Clinic
Vail, Colorado

Robin N. Kamal, MD
Assistant Professor of Orthopaedic Surgery
Chase Hand and Upper Limb Center
Stanford University
Palo Alto, California

Thomas Kaminski, PhD, ATC, FNATA
Professor of Kinesiology and Applied
    Physiology
University of Delaware
Newark, Delaware

Abdurrahman Kandil, MD
Stanford University
Stanford, California

Jonathan R. Kaplan, MD
Attending Orthopaedic Surgeon
Orthopaedic Specialty Institute
Orange, California

Christopher A. Keen, MD
Citrus Orthopedic and Joint Institute
Lecanto, Florida

Mick P. Kelly, MD
Resident, Department of Orthopaedic
    Surgery
Rush University Medical Center
Chicago, Illinois

A. Jay Khanna, MD, MBA
Professor and Vice Chair of Orthopaedic
    Surgery
Department of Orthopaedic Surgery
The Johns Hopkins University School of
    Medicine
Baltimore, Maryland

Anthony Nicholas Khoury
Baylor University Medical Center at Dallas
Hip Preservation Center
University of Texas at Arlington
Bioengineering Department
Dallas, Texas

Christopher Kim, MD
Instructor of Orthopaedic Surgery
Saint Louis University
St. Louis, Missouri

Lucas R. King, MD, BS
Sports Orthopedic Surgeon
Department of Orthopedic Surgery
Parkview Medical Center
Pueblo, Colorado

Susan E. Kirk, MD
Associate Professor of Internal Medicine
    and Obstetrics and Gynecology
Division of Endocrinology and Metabolism,
    Maternal–Fetal Medicine
Associate Dean, Graduate Medical
    Education
University of Virginia Health System
Charlottesville, Virginia

Georg Klammer, MD
Consultant
Institute for Foot and Ankle Reconstruction
FussInsitut Zurich
Zurich, Switzerland

Derrick M. Knapik, MD
Orthopaedic Surgery
University Hospitals
Cleveland Medical Center
Cleveland, Ohio

Lee M. Kneer, MD, CAQSM
Assistant Professor, Department of
    Orthopaedic Surgery
Assistant Professor, Department of Physical
    Medicine and Rehabilitation
Emory Sports Medicine Center
Atlanta, Georgia

Mininder S. Kocher, MD, MPH
Professor of Orthopaedic Surgery
Harvard Medical School
Associate Director
Division of Sports Medicine
Department of Orthopaedic Surgery
Boston Children's Hospital
Boston, Massachusetts

Gabrielle P. Konin, MD
Assistant Professor of Radiology
Weill Cornell Medicine
New York, New York

Matthew J. Kraeutler, MD
Department of Orthopaedic Surgery
Seton Hall-Hackensack Meridian School of
    Medicine
South Orange, New Jersey

Alexander B. Kreines, DO
Resident, Orthopaedic Surgery
Rowan University
Stratford, New Jersey

Vignesh Prasad Krishnamoorthy, MD
Section of Young Adult Hip Surgery
Division of Sports Medicine
Department of Orthopedic Surgery
Rush Medical College
Rush University Medical Center
Chicago, Illinois

Marshall A. Kuremsky, MD
Orthopaedic Surgeon
Hand and Upper Extremity Surgeon
Sports Medicine and Arthroscopic Surgeon
EmergeOrtho
Raleigh, North Carolina

Shawn M. Kutnik, MD
Orthopedic Surgeon
Archway Orthopedics and Hand Surgery
St. Louis, Missouri

Michael S. Laidlaw, MD
Department of Orthopaedic Surgery
University of Virginia
Charlottesville, Virginia

Joseph D. Lamplot
Chief Resident
Department of Orthopaedic Surgery
Washington University School of Medicine
St. Louis, Missouri

Drew Lansdown, MD
Section of Young Adult Hip Surgery
Division of Sports Medicine
Department of Orthopedic Surgery
Rush Medical College
Rush University Medical Center
Chicago, Illinois

Matthew D. LaPrade, BS
Steadman Philippon Research Institute
The Steadman Clinic
Vail, Colorado

Robert F. LaPrade, MD, PhD
Chief Medical Research Officer
Steadman Philippon Research Institute
The Steadman Clinic
Vail, Colorado

Christopher M. Larson, MD
Minnesota Orthopedic Sports Medicine
    Institute
Twin Cities Orthopedics
Edina, Minnesota

Evan P. Larson, MD
University of Nebraska Medical Center
Department of Orthopaedic Surgery and
    Rehabilitation
Omaha, Nebraska

Samuel J. Laurencin, MD, PhD
Department of Orthopaedic Surgery
University of Connecticut School of
    Medicine
Farmington, Connecticut

Peter Lawrence, MD
Wiley Barker Professor of Surgery
Chief, Division of Vascular and
    Endovascular Surgery
University of California, Los Angeles
Los Angeles, California

Adrian D.K. Le, MD
Department of Orthopedic Surgery
Stanford University
Stanford, California

Nicholas LeCursi, CO
Certified Orthotist
Vice President, Services
Chief Technology Officer
Becker Orthopedic
Troy, Michigan

Sonya B. Levine, BA
Department of Orthopedic Surgery
Columbia University Medical Center
New York Presbyterian Hospital
New York, New York

William N. Levine, MD, FAOA
Frank E. Stinchfield Professor and
    Chairman of Orthopedic Surgery
Columbia University Medical Center
New York Presbyterian Hospital
New York, New York

Xudong Joshua Li, MD, PhD
Associate Professor of Orthopaedic Surgery
    and Biomedical Engineering
University of Virginia
Charlottesville, Virginia

Gregory T. Lichtman, DO
Department of Orthopedic Surgery
Rowan University School of Osteopathic
    Medicine
Stratford, New Jersey

Christopher A. Looze, MD
Orthopaedic Surgeon
MedStar Franklin Square
Baltimore, Maryland

Gary M. Lourie, MD
Hand Surgeon
The Hand and Upper Extremity Center of
    Georgia
Atlanta, Georgia

Helen H. Lu, PhD
Professor of Biomedical Engineering
Vice Chair, Department of Biomedical
    Engineering
Columbia University Medical Center
New York Presbyterian Hospital
New York, New York

Timothy J. Luchetti, MD
Resident, Orthopedic Surgery
Rush University Medical Center
Chicago, Illinois

Jessica A. Lundgren, MD
Lecturer
Department of Internal Medicine
Division of Endocrinology and Metabolism
University of Virginia Health System
Charlottesville, Virginia

Travis G. Maak, MD
Associate Professor of Orthopaedic Surgery
University of Utah
Salt Lake City, Utah

John M. MacKnight, MD
Professor of Internal Medicine and
    Orthopaedic Surgery
Team Physician and Medical Director
UVA Sports Medicine
University of Virginia Health System
Charlottesville, Virginia

Nancy Major, MD
Department of Radiology
University of Colorado School of Medicine
Aurora, Colorado

Francesc Malagelada, MD
Foot and Ankle Unit
Department of Trauma and Orthopaedic
    Surgery
Royal London Hospital
Barts Health National Health Service Trust
London, England, United Kingdom

Michael A. Marchetti, MD
Assistant Attending, Dermatology Service
Department of Medicine
Memorial Sloan Kettering Cancer Center
New York, New York

Patrick G. Marinello, MD
Hand and Upper Extremity Surgeon
Capital Region Orthopaedic Group
Bone and Joint Center
Albany, New York

Hal David Martin, DO
Medical Director
Baylor University Medical Center at Dallas
Hip Preservation Center
Dallas, Texas

Scott D. Martin, MD
Director, MGH Joint Preservation Service
Director, Harvard/MGH Sports Medicine
    Fellowship Program
Associate Professor of Orthopaedic Surgery
Harvard Medical School
Department of Orthopaedic Surgery
Massachusetts General Hospital
Boston, Massachusetts

Rebecca Martinie, MD
Assistant Professor of Pediatrics
Baylor College of Medicine
Houston, Texas

Lyndon Mason, MB BCh, MRCS (Eng),
FRCS (Tr & Orth)
Trauma and Orthopaedic Consultant
Aintree University Hospital
Liverpool, England, United Kingdom

Augustus D. Mazzocca, MD
Department of Orthopaedic Surgery
University of Connecticut School of
    Medicine
Farmington, Connecticut

David R. McAllister, MD
Chief, Sports Medicine Service
Professor and Vice Chair
Department of Orthopaedic Surgery
David Geffen School of Medicine
University of California, Los Angeles
Los Angeles, California

Meagan McCarthy, MD
Fellowship Trained Orthopaedic Sports
    Medicine Surgeon
Reno Orthopaedic Clinic
Reno, Nevada

Eric C. McCarty, MD
Chief, Sports Medicine and Shoulder
    Surgery
Associate Professor
Department of Orthopaedics
University of Colorado School of Medicine
Director Sports Medicine, Head Team
    Physician
University of Colorado Department of
    Athletics
Associate Professor, Adjunct
Department of Integrative Physiology
University of Colorado
Boulder, Colorado

Sean McMillan, DO
Chief of Orthopedics
Director of Orthopedic Sports Medicine
    and Arthroscopy
Lourdes Medical Associates
Lourdes Medical Center at Burlington
Burlington, New Jersey

Heather Menzer, MD
Fellow, Orthopaedic Surgery
University of Virginia
Charlottesville, Virginia

Sean J. Meredith, MD
Resident Physician
Department of Orthopaedics
University of Maryland School of Medicine
Baltimore, Maryland

Dayne T. Mickelson, MD
Department of Orthopaedic Surgery
Duke University
Durham, North Carolina

Michael R. Mijares, MD
Department of Orthopaedics
Jackson Memorial Hospital
Jackson Health System
Miami, Florida

Matthew D. Milewski, MD
Assistant Professor
Division of Sports Medicine
Department of Orthopaedic Surgery
Boston Children's Hospital
Boston, Massachusetts

Mark D. Miller, MD
S. Ward Casscells Professor of Orthopaedic
    Surgery
Head, Division of Sports Medicine
University of Virginia
Charlottesville, Virginia
Adjunctive Clinical Professor and Team
    Physician
James Madison University
Harrisonburg, Virginia

Dilaawar J. Mistry, MD
Team Physician
Primary Care Sports Medicine
Western Orthopedics and Sports Medicine
Grand Junction, Colorado

Erik Mitchell, DO
Valley Health Orthopaedics Front Royal
Front Royal, Virginia

Andrew Molloy, MBChB, MRCS
Consultant Orthopaedic Surgeon
Trauma and Orthopaedics
University Hospital Aintree
Honorary Clinical Senior Lecturer
Department of Musculoskeletal Biology
University of Liverpool
Consultant Orthopaedic Surgeon
Spire Liverpool
Liverpool, England, United Kingdom

Timothy S. Mologne, MD
Sports Medicine Center
Appleton, Wisconsin

Scott R. Montgomery, MD
Franciscan Orthopedic Associates at St. Joseph
Tacoma, Washington

Amy M. Moore, MD, FACS
Associate Professor of Surgery
Plastic and Reconstructive Surgery
Washington University School of Medicine
St. Louis, Missouri

Claude T. Moorman III, MD
Professor of Orthopaedic Surgery
Duke Center for Integrated Medicine
Durham, North Carolina

Gina M. Mosich, MD
Resident Physician
Orthopaedic Surgery
University of California, Los Angeles
Los Angeles, California

Michael R. Moynagh, MBBCh
Assistant Professor of Radiology
Mayo Clinic
Rochester, Minnesota

Andrew C. Mundy, MD
Department of Orthopaedic Surgery
The Ohio State University
Columbus, Ohio

Colin P. Murphy, BA
Research Assistant
Center for Outcomes-Based Orthopaedic
    Research
Steadman Philippon Research Institute
Vail, Colorado

Volker Musahl, MD
Assistant Professor
Department of Orthopaedic Surgery
University of Pittsburgh Medical Center
Pittsburgh, Pennsylvania

Jeffrey J. Nepple, MD
Assistant Professor of Orthopaedic Surgery
Director
Young Athlete Center
Washington University School of Medicine
St. Louis, Missouri

Shane J. Nho, MD, MS
Assistant Professor
Head, Section of Young Adult Hip Surgery
Division of Sports Medicine
Department of Orthopedic Surgery
Rush Medical College
Rush University Medical Center
Chicago, Illinois

Carl W. Nissen, MD
Professor
Department of Orthopaedics
University of Connecticut
Elite Sports Medicine
Connecticut Children's Medical Center
Farmington, Connecticut

Blake R. Obrock, DO
Sports Medicine Fellow
Department of Orthopaedics
University of New Mexico
Albuquerque, New Mexico

James Onate, PhD, ATC, FNATA
Associate Professor
School of Health and Rehabilitation
    Sciences
The Ohio State University
Columbus, Ohio

Scott I. Otallah, MD
Carilion Children's Pediatric Neurology
Roanoke, Virginia

Brett D. Owens, MD
Professor of Orthopedics
Brown Alpert Medical School
Providence, Rhode Island

Gabrielle M. Paci, MD
Physician
Orthopaedic Surgery
Stanford University
Palo Alto, California

Richard D. Parker, MD
Department of Orthopaedic Surgery
The Cleveland Clinic Foundation
Cleveland, Ohio

Jonathan P. Parsons, MD
Professor of Internal Medicine
Department of Pulmonary, Critical Care,
    and Sleep Medicine
Wexner Medical Center
The Ohio State University
Columbus, Ohio

Neel K. Patel, MD
Department of Orthopaedic Surgery
University of Pittsburgh Medical Center
Pittsburgh, Pennsylvania

Thierry Pauyo, MD
Fellow
Department of Orthopaedic Surgery
University of Pittsburgh Medical Center
Pittsburgh, Pennsylvania

Evan Peck, MD
Section of Sports Health
Department of Orthopaedic Surgery
Cleveland Clinic Florida
Weston, Florida
Affiliate Assistant Professor of Clinical
    Biomedical Science
Charles E. Schmidt College of Medicine
Florida Atlantic University
Boca Raton, Florida

Liam Peebles, BA
Research Assistant
Center for Outcomes-Based Orthopaedic
    Research
Steadman Philippon Research Institute
Vail, Colorado

Andrew T. Pennock, MD
Associate Clinical Professor
Orthopedic Surgery
University of California, San Diego
San Diego, California

Anthony Perera, MBChB, MRCS,
MFSEM, PGDip Med Law, FRCS (Tr &
Orth)
Consultant, Orthopaedic Foot and Ankle
    Surgeon
University Hospital of Wales
Cardiff, Wales, United Kingdom

Jose Perez, BS
Research Fellow
Department of Orthopedics
Sports Medicine
Miami, Florida

William A. Petri Jr., MD, PhD
Chief, Division of Infectious Disease and
    International Health
Wade Hampton Frost Professor of
    Epidemiology
University of Virginia
Charlottesville, Virginia

Frank A. Petrigliano, MD
Assistant Professor of Orthopaedic Surgery
David Geffen School of Medicine
University of California, Los Angeles
Los Angeles, California

Adam M. Pickett, MD
Faculty, West Point Sports Medicine
    Fellowship
Department of Orthopaedic Surgery
United States Military Academy
West Point, New York

Matthew A. Posner, MD
Director, West Point Sports Medicine
  Fellowship
Department of Orthopaedic Surgery
United States Military Academy
West Point, New York

Tricia R. Prokop, PT, EdD, MS, CSCS
Assistant Professor of Physical Therapy
Department of Rehabilitation Sciences
University of Hartford
West Hartford, Connecticut

Matthew T. Provencher, MD, CAPT, MC,
USNR
Professor of Surgery and Orthopaedics
Uniformed Services University of the Health
  Services
Complex Shoulder, Knee, and Sports
  Surgeon
The Steadman Clinic
Vail, Colorado

Rabia Qureshi, MD
Research Fellow
Department of Orthopedic Surgery
University of Virginia
Charlottesville, Virginia

Fred Reifsteck, MD
Head Team Physician
University Health Center
University of Georgia
Athens, Georgia

David R. Richardson, MD
Associate Professor of Orthopaedic Surgery
University of Tennessee–Campbell Clinic
Memphis, Tennessee

Dustin Richter, MD
Assistant Professor, Sports Medicine
Sports Medicine Fellowship Assistant
  Director
Director of Orthopaedics Sports Medicine
  Research
University of New Mexico
Albuquerque, New Mexico

Andrew J. Riff, MD
Assistant Professor of Clinical Orthopaedic
  Surgery
Indiana University Health Orthopedics and
  Sports Medicine
Indianapolis, Indiana

Christopher J. Roach, MD
Chairman, Orthopaedic Surgery
San Antonio Military Medical Center
San Antonio, Texas

Eliott P. Robinson, MD
Orthopedic Surgeon
OrthoGeorgia Orthopaedic Specialists
Macon, Georgia

Scott A. Rodeo, MD
Professor of Orthopaedic Surgery
Weill Cornell Medical College
Co-Chief Emeritus, Sports Medicine and
  Shoulder Service
Attending Orthopaedic Surgeon
Hospital for Special Surgery
New York, New York

Anthony A. Romeo, MD
Department of Orthopaedic Surgery
Rush University
Chicago, Illinois

Kyle Rosen, MD
Dartmouth College
Hanover, New Hampshire

William H. Rossy, MD
Clinical Associate Professor
Penn Medicine Princeton Medical Center
Princeton, New Jersey

Paul Rothenberg, MD
Resident Physician
Department of Orthopaedics
University of Miami
Miami, Florida

Todd A. Rubin, MD
Orthopaedic Surgeon
Hughston Clinic Orthopaedics
Nashville, Tennessee

Robert D. Russell, MD
Orthopaedic Surgeon
OrthoTexas
Frisco, Texas

David A. Rush, MD
Department of Orthopaedic Surgery and
  Rehabilitation
University of Mississippi Medical Center
Jackson, Mississippi

Joseph J. Ruzbarsky, MD
Resident, Orthopedic Surgery
Department of Orthopaedics
Hospital for Special Surgery
New York, New York

Marc Safran, MD
Professor of Orthopedic Surgery
Associate Director
Department of Sports Medicine
Stanford University
Redwood City, California

Susan Saliba, PhD, ATC, MPT
Professor, Kinesiology
University of Virginia
Charlottesville, Virginia

Adil Samad, MD
Florida Orthopaedic Institute
Tampa, Florida

Anthony Sanchez, BS
Medical Doctor Candidate
Oregon Health and Science University
Portland, Oregon

Laura W. Scordino, MD
Orthopaedic Surgeon
OrthoNY
Albany, New York

Virgil P. Secasanu, MD
Clinical Instructor, Housestaff
Department of Pulmonary, Critical Care,
  and Sleep Medicine
Wexner Medical Center
The Ohio State University
Columbus, Ohio

Terrance Sgroi, PT
Sports Medicine and Shoulder Service
Hospital for Special Surgery
New York, New York

Jason T. Shearn, MD
Associate Professor
Department of Biomedical Engineering
University of Cincinnati
Cincinnati, Ohio

K. Donald Shelbourne, MD
The Shelbourne Knee Center at Community
  East Hospital
Indianapolis, Indiana

Seth L. Sherman, MD
Department of Orthopaedic Surgery
University of Missouri, Columbia
Columbia, Missouri

Ashley Matthews Shilling, MD
Associate Professor of Anesthesiology
University of Virginia Medical Center
Charlottesville, Virginia

Adam L. Shimer, MD
Assistant Professor of Orthopaedic Surgery
University of Virginia
Charlottesville, Virginia

Anuj Singla, MD
Instructor, Orthopaedics
University of Virginia
Charlottesville, Virginia

David L. Skaggs, MD, MMM
Professor of Orthopaedic Surgery
Keck School of Medicine of USC
University of Southern California
Chief, Orthopaedic Surgery
Children's Hospital Los Angeles
Los Angeles, California

Mia Smucny, MD
University of Washington
Seattle, Washington

Niall A. Smyth, MD
Resident, Orthopaedic Surgery
University of Miami, Miller School of
    Medicine
Miami, Florida

Frederick S. Song, MD
Clinical Associate Professor
Penn Medicine Princeton Medical Center
Princeton, New Jersey

Kurt Spindler, MD
Cleveland Clinic Foundation
Cleveland, Ohio

Chad Starkey, PhD, AT, FNATA
Professor
Division of Athletic Training
Ohio University
Athens, Ohio

Siobhan M. Statuta, MD
Associate Professor of Family Medicine and
    Physical Medicine and Rehabilitation
University of Virginia
Charlottesville, Virginia

Samuel R. H. Steiner, MD
Orthopedic Surgery
Orthopaedic Associates of Wisconsin
Pewaukee, Wisconsin

John W. Stelzer, MD, MS
Research Fellow
Department of Orthopaedic Surgery
Harvard Medical School
Massachusetts General Hospital
Boston, Massachusetts

Christopher L. Stockburger, MD
Department of Orthopedic Surgery
Washington University School of Medicine
St. Louis, Missouri

J. Andy Sullivan, MD
Clinical Professor of Pediatric Orthopedic
    Surgery
Department of Orthopedic Surgery
University of Oklahoma College of
    Medicine
Oklahoma City, Oklahoma

Eric Swanton, MBChB, FRACS (Orth)
Orthopaedic Consultant
Department of Orthopaedics
North Shore Hospital, Waitemata District
    Health Board
Auckland, New Zealand

Matthew A. Tao, MD
Assistant Professor
Orthopaedic Surgery
University of Nebraska Medical Center
Omaha, Nebraska

Sandip P. Tarpada, BS
Department of Orthopaedic Surgery
Montefiore Medical Center
Albert Einstein College of Medicine
New York, New York

Kenneth F. Taylor, MD
Department of Orthopaedics and
    Rehabilitation
The Pennsylvania State University
Milton S. Hershey Medical Center
Hershey, Pennsylvania

Michael Terry, MD
Professor
Department of Orthopaedic Surgery
Northwestern Medicine
Northwestern University Feinberg School of
    Medicine
Chicago, Illinois

Charles A. Thigpen, PhD, PT, ATC
Senior Director of Practice Innovation and
    Analytics
ATI Physical Therapy
Director, Program in Observational Clinical
    Research in Orthopedics
Center for Effectiveness in Orthopedic
    Research
Arnold School of Public Health
University of South Carolina
Greenville, South Carolina

Stavros Thomopoulos, PhD
Director, Carroll Laboratories for
    Orthopedic Surgery
Vice Chair, Basic Research in Orthopedic
    Surgery
Robert E. Carroll and Jane Chace Carroll
    Professor of Biomechanics (in
    Orthopedic Surgery and Biomedical
    Engineering)
Columbia University Medical Center
New York Presbyterian Hospital
New York, New York

Jason Thompson, MD
Orthopedic Surgery Resident, UT Health
    San Antonio
Adult Reconstructive Surgery Fellow
University of Western Ontario
London Health Sciences Centre
London, Ontario, Canada

Stephen R. Thompson, MD, MEd,
FRCSC
Associate Professor of Sports Medicine
Eastern Maine Medical Center
University of Maine
Bangor, Maine

Fotios P. Tjoumakaris, MD
Associate Professor
Department of Orthopedic Surgery
Sidney Kimmel College of Medicine
Thomas Jefferson University
Philadelphia, Pennsylvania

Drew Toftoy, MD
Sports Medicine Fellow
University of Colorado
Aurora, Colorado

John M. Tokish, MD, USAF MC
Orthopedic Surgery Residency Program
    Director
Tripler Army Medical Center
Honolulu, Hawaii

Gehron Treme, MD
Associate Professor, Orthopaedics
University of New Mexico
Albuquerque, New Mexico

Rachel Triche, MD
Attending Orthopaedic Surgeon
Santa Monica Orthopaedic and Sports
    Medicine Group
Santa Monica, California

David P. Trofa, MD
Resident, Department of Orthopaedic
    Surgery
Columbia University Medical Center
New York, New York

Gift Ukwuani, MD
Section of Young Adult Hip Surgery
Division of Sports Medicine
Department of Orthopedic Surgery
Rush Medical College
Rush University Medical Center
Chicago, Illinois

M. Farooq Usmani, MSc
Department of Orthopaedic Surgery
The Johns Hopkins University School of
    Medicine
Baltimore, Maryland

Ravi S. Vaswani, MD
Resident, Department of Orthopaedic
    Surgery
University of Pittsburgh Medical Center
Pittsburgh, Pennsylvania

Aaron J. Vaughan, MD
Family Physician
Sports Medicine Director
Mountain Area Health Education Center
Asheville, North Carolina

Jordi Vega, MD
Orthopaedic Surgeon
Etzelclinic
Pfäffikon, Schwyz, Switzerland

Evan E. Vellios, MD
Resident Physician
Department of Orthopedic Surgery
David Geffen School of Medicine
University of California, Los Angeles
Los Angeles, California

Armando F. Vidal, MD
Associate Professor
Department of Orthopedics
University of Colorado School of Medicine
Aurora, Colorado

Michael J. Vives, MD
Professor and Chief of Spine Surgery
Department of Orthopedics
Rutgers–New Jersey Medical School
Newark, New Jersey

James E. Voos, MD
Associate Professor of Orthopaedic Surgery
Division Chief, Sports Medicine
Medical Director, Sports Medicine Institute
University Hospitals
Cleveland Medical Center
Cleveland, Ohio

Dean Wang, MD
Fellow in Sports Medicine and Shoulder
    Surgery
Hospital for Special Surgery
New York, New York

Robert Westermann, MD
University of Iowa
Iowa City, Iowa

Barbara B. Wilson, MD
Associate Professor of Dermatology
University of Virginia
Charlottesville, Virginia

Benjamin R. Wilson, MD
Resident Physician
Orthopaedic Surgery and Sports Medicine
University of Kentucky
Lexington, Kentucky

Brian F. Wilson, MD
Director of Orthopaedic Surgery Stormont
    Vail Health
Washburn University Orthopaedic Sports
    Medicine
Topeka, Kansas

Jennifer Moriatis Wolf, MD
Professor
Department of Orthopaedic Surgery and
    Rehabilitation
University of Chicago Hospitals
Chicago, Illinois

Rick W. Wright, MD
Jerome J. Gilden Distinguished Professor
Executive Vice Chairman
Department of Orthopaedic Surgery
Washington University School of Medicine
St. Louis, Missouri

Frank B. Wydra, MD
Department of Orthopedics
University of Colorado School of Medicine
Aurora, Colorado

James Wylie, MD, MHS
Director of Orthopedic Research
Intermountain Healthcare
The Orthopedic Specialty Hospital
Murray, Utah

Robert W. Wysocki, MD
Rush University Medical Center
Chicago, Illinois

Haoming Xu, MD
Dermatology Service
Department of Medicine
Memorial Sloan Kettering Cancer Center
New York, New York

Kent T. Yamaguchi, MD
Resident Physician
Orthopaedic Surgery
University of California, Los Angeles
Los Angeles, California

Jeffrey Yao, MD
Associate Professor of Orthopedic Surgery
Stanford University Medical Center
Palo Alto, California

Yi-Meng Yen, MD, PhD
Assistant Professor, Harvard Medical School
Boston Children's Hospital
Department of Orthopaedic Surgery
Division of Sports Medicine
Boston, Massachusetts

Jane C. Yeoh, MD, FRCSC
Vancouver, British Columbia, Canada

M. Christopher Yonz, MD
Summit Orthopaedics
Southeast Georgia Health System
St. Marys, Georgia

Tracy Zaslow, MD, FAAP, CAQSM
Assistant Professor
University of Southern California, Los
    Angeles
Children's Orthopaedic Center (COC) at
    Children's Hospital–Los
Angeles
Medical Director
COC Sports Medicine and Concussion
    Program
Team Physician, LA Galaxy
Los Angeles, California

Andrew M. Zbojniewicz, MD
Department of Radiology
Michigan State University
College of Human Medicine
Advanced Radiology Services
Grand Rapids, Michigan
Division of Pediatric Radiology
Cincinnati Children's Hospital Medical
    Center
Cincinnati, Ohio

Connor G. Ziegler, MD
New England Orthopedic Surgeons
Springfield, Massachusetts

Mary L. Zupanc, MD
Professor and Division Chief
Neurology and Pediatrics
University of California, Irvine
Children's Hospital of Orange County
Orange, California

CONTENTS

Volume I

SECTION 1 Basic Principles
Asheesh Bedi, Bryson Lesniak

1. **Physiology and Pathophysiology of Musculoskeletal Tissues,** 2
   Dean Wang, Claire D. Eliasberg, Scott A. Rodeo
2. **Basic Concepts in Biomechanics,** 16
   Richard E. Debski, Neel K. Patel, Jason T. Shearn
3. **Basic Science of Graft Tissue in Sports Medicine,** 30
   Mia Smucny, Carolyn M. Hettrich, Robert Westermann, Kurt Spindler
4. **Basic Science of Implants in Sports Medicine,** 35
   Elizabeth R. Dennis, Jon-Michael E. Caldwell, Sonya B. Levine, Philip Chuang, Margaret Boushell, Stavros Thomopoulos, Helen H. Lu, William N. Levine
5. **Orthobiologics: Clinical Application of Platelet-Rich Plasma and Stem Cell Therapy,** 50
   Adrian D.K. Le, Jason Dragoo
6. **Exercise Physiology,** 62
   Thomas M. Best, Chad A. Asplund
7. **Imaging Overview,** 74
   Francisco Contreras, Jose Perez, Jean Jose
8. **Basic Arthroscopic Principles,** 105
   Michael R. Mijares, Michael G. Baraga
9. **Overview of Sport-Specific Injuries,** 114
   Jared A. Crasto, Ravi S. Vaswani, Thierry Pauyo, Volker Musahl
10. **Commonly Encountered Fractures in Sports Medicine,** 131
    Christopher Kim, Scott G. Kaar

SECTION 2 Medical
Rajwinder Deu, Morteza Khodaee

11. **Team Medical Coverage,** 144
    Daniel Herman, Nikhita Gadi, Evan Peck
12. **Comprehensive Cardiovascular Care and Evaluation of the Elite Athlete,** 158
    Paul S. Corotto, Aaron L. Baggish, Dilaawar J. Mistry, Robert W. Battle
13. **Exercise-Induced Bronchoconstriction,** 175
    Virgil P. Secasanu, Jonathan P. Parsons
14. **Deep Venous Thrombosis and Pulmonary Embolism,** 180
    Jason Thompson, Marc M. DeHart
15. **Gastrointestinal Medicine in the Athlete,** 189
    John M. MacKnight
16. **Hematologic Medicine in the Athlete,** 196
    John J. Densmore
17. **Infectious Diseases in the Athlete,** 201
    Nona M. Jiang, Kathleen C. Abalos, William A. Petri Jr.
18. **The Athlete With Diabetes,** 218
    Jessica A. Lundgren, Susan E. Kirk
19. **Renal Medicine and Genitourinary Trauma in the Athlete,** 227
    Stefan Hemmings, Derek M. Fine
20. **Sports and Epilepsy,** 230
    Mary L. Zupanc, Scott I. Otallah, Howard P. Goodkin
21. **Environmental Illness,** 235
    Jorge E. Gómez, Joseph N. Chorley, Rebecca Martinie
22. **Dermatologic Conditions,** 246
    Haoming Xu, Barbara B. Wilson, Michael A. Marchetti
23. **Facial, Eye, Nasal, and Dental Injuries,** 260
    John Jared Christophel
24. **Psychological Adjustment to Athletic Injury,** 272
    Karen P. Egan, Jason Freeman
25. **Sports Nutrition,** 277
    Jessica L. Buschmann, Jackie Buell
26. **Doping and Ergogenic Aids,** 283
    Siobhan M. Statuta, Aaron J. Vaughan, Ashley V. Austin
27. **The Female Athlete,** 294
    Letha Y. Griffin, Mary Lloyd Ireland, Fred Reifsteck, Matthew H. Blake, Benjamin R. Wilson
28. **The Para-Athlete,** 315
    Daniel Herman, Mary E. Caldwell, Arthur Jason De Luigi
29. **Anesthesia and Perioperative Medicine,** 325
    Ashley Matthews Shilling

SECTION 3 Rehabilitation and Injury Prevention
Joe M. Hart

30. **The Athletic Trainer,** 342
    Chad Starkey, Shannon David
31. **Principles of Orthopaedic Rehabilitation,** 347
    Courtney Chaaban, Charles A. Thigpen
32. **Modalities and Manual Techniques in Sports Medicine Rehabilitation,** 354
    Susan Saliba, Michael Higgins
33. **Basics of Taping and Orthotics,** 368
    Phillip Gribble
34. **Injury Prevention,** 376
    Jay Hertel, James Onate, Thomas Kaminski
35. **Return to Activity and Sport After Injury,** 385
    J. Craig Garrison, Joseph Hannon

SECTION 4 Shoulder
Stephen F. Brockmeier

36. **Shoulder Anatomy and Biomechanics,** 393
    Timothy S. Mologne
37. **Shoulder Diagnosis and Decision-Making,** 402
    Thomas J. Gill

38. **Glenohumeral Joint Imaging,** 408
Alissa J. Burge, Gabrielle P. Konin

39. **Shoulder Arthroscopy,** 433
Thomas M. DeBerardino, Laura W. Scordino

40. **Anterior Shoulder Instability,** 440
Stephen R. Thompson, Heather Menzer, Stephen F. Brockmeier

41. **Posterior Shoulder Instability,** 463
James Bradley, Fotios P. Tjoumakaris

42. **Multidirectional Instability of the Shoulder,** 476
Robert M. Carlisle, John M. Tokish

43. **Revision Shoulder Instability,** 489
Salvatore Frangiamore, Angela K. Chang, Jake A. Fox, Colin P. Murphy, Anthony Sanchez, Liam Peebles, Matthew T. Provencher

44. **Superior Labrum Anterior to Posterior Tears,** 502
Sean J. Meredith, R. Frank Henn III

45. **The Thrower's Shoulder,** 511
Matthew A. Tao, Christopher L. Camp, Terrance Sgroi, Joshua S. Dines, David W. Altchek

46. **Proximal Biceps Tendon Pathology,** 526
Samuel R.H. Steiner, John T. Awowale, Stephen F. Brockmeier

47. **Rotator Cuff and Impingement Lesions,** 540
Gina M. Mosich, Kent T. Yamaguchi, Frank A. Petrigliano

48. **Subscapularis Injury,** 556
William H. Rossy, Frederick S. Song, Jeffrey S. Abrams

49. **Revision Rotator Cuff Repair,** 567
Joseph D. Cooper, Anthony Essilfie, Seth C. Gamradt

50. **Other Muscle Injuries,** 574
James E. Voos, Derrick M. Knapik

51. **Stiff Shoulder,** 579
Jonathan Barlow, Andrew C. Mundy, Grant L. Jones

52. **Glenohumeral Arthritis in the Athlete,** 592
Jeffrey Brunelli, Jonathan T. Bravman, Kevin Caperton, Eric C. McCarty

53. **Scapulothoracic Disorders,** 609
G. Keith Gill, Gehron Treme, Dustin Richter

54. **Nerve Entrapment,** 621
Daniel E. Hess, Kenneth F. Taylor, A. Bobby Chhabra

55. **Vascular Problems and Thoracic Outlet Syndrome,** 632
Matthew A. Posner, Christopher J. Roach, Adam M. Pickett, Brett D. Owens

56. **Injury to the Acromioclavicular and Sternoclavicular Joints,** 645
Connor G. Ziegler, Samuel J. Laurencin, Rachel M. Frank, Matthew T. Provencher, Anthony A. Romeo, Augustus D. Mazzocca

SECTION 5 Elbow, Wrist, and Hand
Sanjeev Kakar

57. **Elbow Anatomy and Biomechanics,** 680
Marshall A. Kuremsky, E. Lyle Cain Jr., Jeffrey R. Dugas, James R. Andrews, Lucas R. King

58. **Elbow Diagnosis and Decision-Making,** 687
Nicholas J. Clark, Bassem T. Elhassan

59. **Elbow Imaging,** 697
Benjamin M. Howe, Michael R. Moynagh

60. **Elbow Arthroscopy,** 707
Todd A. Rubin, Shawn M. Kutnik, Michael R. Hausman

61. **Elbow Tendinopathies and Bursitis,** 720
Jennifer Moriatis Wolf

62. **Distal Biceps and Triceps Tendon Ruptures,** 731
James Bradley, Fotios P. Tjoumakaris, Gregory T. Lichtman, Luke S. Austin

63. **Entrapment Neuropathies of the Arm, Elbow, and Forearm,** 742
Wajeeh Bakhsh, Warren C. Hammert

64. **Elbow Throwing Injuries,** 757
Marshall A. Kuremsky, E. Lyle Cain Jr., Jeffrey R. Dugas, James R. Andrews, Christopher A. Looze

65. **Loss of Elbow Motion,** 772
Timothy J. Luchetti, Debdut Biswas, Robert W. Wysocki

66. **Anatomy and Biomechanics of the Hand and Wrist,** 785
Raj M. Amin, John V. Ingari

67. **Hand and Wrist Diagnosis and Decision-Making,** 793
Patrick G. Marinello, R. Glenn Gaston, Eliott P. Robinson, Gary M. Lourie

68. **Imaging of the Wrist and Hand,** 806
Kimberly K. Amrami

69. **Wrist Arthroscopy,** 817
William B. Geissler, David A. Rush, Christopher A. Keen

70. **Carpal Injuries,** 835
Gabrielle M. Paci, Jeffrey Yao

71. **Wrist Tendinopathies,** 857
Raj M. Amin, John V. Ingari

72. **Disorders of the Distal Radioulnar Joint,** 865
Julie E. Adams

73. **Tendon Injuries in the Hand,** 873
Robin N. Kamal, Jacob D. Gire

74. **Digit Fractures and Dislocations,** 883
Christopher L. Stockburger, Ryan P. Calfee

75. **Neuropathies of the Wrist and Hand,** 898
Gwendolyn Hoben, Amy M. Moore

Volume II

SECTION 6 Pelvis, Hip, and Thigh
F. Winston Gwathmey, Jr.

76. **Hip Anatomy and Biomechanics,** 907
Marc Safran, Abdurrahman Kandil

77. **Hip Diagnosis and Decision-Making,** 925
Austin W. Chen, Benjamin G. Domb

78. **Hip Imaging,** 935
Brian Busconi, R. Tyler Huish, Erik Mitchell, Sean McMillan

79. **Hip Arthroscopy,** 947
Joshua D. Harris

80. **Femoroacetabular Impingement in Athletes,** 957
Shane J. Nho, Vignesh Prasad Krishnamoorthy, Drew Lansdown, Gift Ukwuani

81. **Hip Dysplasia and Instability,** 971
Jeffrey J. Nepple, John C. Clohisy

82. **Iliopsoas Pathology**, 979
   Christian N. Anderson
83. **Peritrochanteric Disorders**, 990
   John W. Stelzer, Scott D. Martin
84. **Athletic Pubalgia/Core Muscle Injury and Adductor Pathology**, 1007
   Christopher M. Larson, Jeffrey J. Nepple
85. **Posterior Hip Pain**, 1018
   Hal David Martin, Anthony Nicholas Khoury, Juan Gomez-Hoyos
86. **Hamstring Injuries**, 1034
   Kyle E. Hammond, Lee M. Kneer
87. **Hip and Thigh Contusions and Strains**, 1043
   Blake R. Obrock, Christopher P. Bankhead, Dustin Richter
88. **Hip Arthritis in the Athlete**, 1053
   Guillaume D. Dumont, Robert D. Russell

SECTION 7 Knee
Eric C. McCarty

89. **Knee Anatomy and Biomechanics of the Knee**, 1062
   Matthew J. Kraeutler, Jorge Chahla, Francesc Malagelada, Jordi Vega, Pau Golanó, Bruce Beynnon, Fatih Ertem, Eric C. McCarty
90. **Knee Diagnosis and Decision-Making**, 1089
   Andrew J. Riff, Peter N. Chalmers, Bernard R. Bach Jr.
91. **Imaging of the Knee**, 1104
   Nancy Major, Christopher Coleman
92. **Basics of Knee Arthroscopy**, 1121
   Stephen R. Thompson, Mark D. Miller
93. **Arthroscopic Synovectomy of the Knee**, 1127
   Mick P. Kelly, Charles A. Bush-Joseph
94. **Meniscal Injuries**, 1132
   Joseph J. Ruzbarsky, Travis G. Maak, Scott A. Rodeo
95. **Meniscal Transplantation**, 1154
   Frank B. Wydra, Derek P. Axibal, Armando F. Vidal
96. **Articular Cartilage Lesions**, 1161
   Michael S. Laidlaw, Kadir Buyukdogan, Mark D. Miller
97. **Frontiers in Articular Cartilage Treatment**, 1178
   Rachel M. Frank, Armando F. Vidal, Eric C. McCarty
98. **Anterior Cruciate Ligament Injuries**, 1185
   Edward C. Cheung, David R. McAllister, Frank A. Petrigliano
99. **Revision Anterior Cruciate Ligament Injuries**, 1199
   Joseph D. Lamplot, Liljiana Bogunovic, Rick W. Wright
100. **Posterior Cruciate Ligament Injuries**, 1211
   Frank A. Petrigliano, Evan E. Vellios, Scott R. Montgomery, Jared S. Johnson, David R. McAllister
101. **Medial Collateral Ligament and Posterior Medial Corner Injuries**, 1231
   M. Christopher Yonz, Brian F. Wilson, Matthew H. Blake, Darren L. Johnson
102. **Lateral and Posterolateral Corner Injuries of the Knee**, 1244
   Ryan P. Coughlin, Dayne T. Mickelson, Claude T. Moorman III
103. **Multiligament Knee Injuries**, 1264
   Samantha L. Kallenbach, Matthew D. LaPrade, Robert F. LaPrade
104. **Knee Arthritis**, 1277
   Catherine Hui, Stephen R. Thompson, J. Robert Giffin

105. **Patellar Instability**, 1293
   Seth L. Sherman, Betina B. Hinckel, Jack Farr
106. **Patellofemoral Pain**, 1308
   Meagan McCarthy, Eric C. McCarty, Rachel M. Frank
107. **Extensor Mechanism Injuries**, 1318
   Matthew Bessette, Drew Toftoy, Richard D. Parker, Rachel M. Frank
108. **Loss of Knee Motion**, 1335
   K. Donald Shelbourne, Heather Freeman, Tinker Gray
109. **Vascular Problems of the Knee**, 1345
   Peter Lawrence, Kyle Rosen

SECTION 8 Leg, Ankle, and Foot
Amiethab A. Aiyer, Anish R. Kadakia

110. **Foot and Ankle Biomechanics**, 1359
   Andrew Haskell
111. **Leg, Ankle, and Foot Diagnosis and Decision-Making**, 1370
   Anish R. Kadakia, Amiethab A. Aiyer
112. **Imaging of the Foot and Ankle**, 1380
   Anish R. Kadakia, Amiethab A. Aiyer
113. **Leg Pain and Exertional Compartment Syndromes**, 1393
   Christopher Hogrefe, Michael Terry
114. **Peripheral Nerve Entrapment Around the Foot and Ankle**, 1402
   Norman Espinosa Jr., Georg Klammer
115. **Ankle Arthroscopy**, 1421
   Niall A. Smyth, Jonathan R. Kaplan, Amiethab A. Aiyer, John T. Campbell, Rachel Triche, Rebecca A. Cerrato
116. **Sports Shoes and Orthoses**, 1436
   Nicholas LeCursi
117. **Ligamentous Injuries of the Foot and Ankle**, 1444
   Paul Rothenberg, Eric Swanton, Andrew Molloy, Amiethab A. Aiyer, Jonathan R. Kaplan
118. **Tendon Injuries of the Foot and Ankle**, 1462
   Todd A. Irwin
119. **Articular Cartilage Injuries and Defects**, 1484
   David R. Richardson, Jane C. Yeoh
120. **Heel Pain and Plantar Fasciitis: Hindfoot Conditions**, 1504
   Anish R. Kadakia, Amiethab A. Aiyer
121. **Forefoot Problems in Sport**, 1515
   Ben Hickey, Lyndon Mason, Anthony Perera

SECTION 9 Spine and Head
Francis H. Shen

122. **Head and Spine Anatomy and Biomechanics**, 1528
   Colin B. Harris, Rachid Assina, Brandee Gentile, Michael J. Vives
123. **Head and Spine Diagnosis and Decision-Making**, 1538
   Rabia Qureshi, Jason A. Horowitz, Kieran Bhattacharya, Hamid Hassanzadeh
124. **Imaging of the Spine**, 1544
   Adil Samad, M. Farooq Usmani, A. Jay Khanna

125. **Emergency and Field-Side Management of the Spine-Injured Athlete,** 1553
     Korin Hudson, Michael Antonis, William Brady
126. **Concussion and Brain Injury,** 1562
     David P. Trofa, Jon-Michael E. Caldwell, Xudong Joshua Li
127. **Stingers,** 1570
     Sandip P. Tarpada, Woojin Cho
128. **Traumatic Injuries of the Cervical Spine in the Athlete,** 1578
     Adam L. Shimer, Bayan Aghdasi
129. **Traumatic Injuries of the Thoracolumbar Spine in the Athlete,** 1582
     Nourbakhsh Ali, Anuj Singla
130. **Degenerative Conditions of the Cervical and Thoracolumbar Spine,** 1593
     Gregory Grabowski, Todd M. Gilbert, Evan P. Larson, Chris A. Cornett

SECTION 10 Pediatric Sports Medicine
Matthew D. Milewski

131. **The Young Athlete,** 1606
     Benton E. Heyworth, Mininder S. Kocher
132. **Imaging Considerations in Skeletally Immature Athletes,** 1616
     Andrew M. Zbojniewicz

133. **Shoulder Injuries in the Young Athlete,** 1637
     Andrew T. Pennock, Eric W. Edmonds
134. **Elbow Injuries in Pediatric and Adolescent Athletes,** 1661
     James P. Bradley, Luke S. Austin, Alexander B. Kreines, Fotios P. Tjoumakaris
135. **Wrist and Hand Injuries in the Adolescent Athlete,** 1677
     Sonia Chaudhry
136. **Pediatric and Adolescent Hip Injuries,** 1688
     Yi-Meng Yen, Mininder S. Kocher
137. **Knee Injuries in Skeletally Immature Athletes,** 1697
     Matthew D. Milewski, James Wylie, Carl W. Nissen, Tricia R. Prokop
138. **Foot and Ankle Injuries in the Adolescent Athlete,** 1725
     J. Andy Sullivan, James R. Gregory
139. **Head Injuries in Skeletally Immature Athletes,** 1741
     Tracy Zaslow
140. **Spine Issues in Skeletally Immature Athletes,** 1749
     Lindsay M. Andras, David L. Skaggs

Index, I1

VIDEO TABLE OF CONTENTS

Chapter 1
Video 1.1 Physiology and Pathophysiology of Musculoskeletal Tissues—Dean Wang, Claire D. Eliasberg, and Scott A. Rodeo

Chapter 2
Video 2.1 Basic Concepts in Biomechanics—Richard E. Debski, Neel K. Patel, and Jason T. Shearn

Chapter 4
Video 4.1 Basic Science of Implants in Sports Medicine— Elizabeth R. Dennis, Jon-Michael Caldwell, Sonya B. Levine, Philip Chuang, Margaret Boushell, Stavros Thomopoulos, Helen H. Lu, and William N. Levine

Chapter 5
Video 5.1 Orthobiologics: Clinical Application of Platelet-Rich Plasma and Stem Cell Therapy—Adrian D.K. Le and Jason Dragoo

Chapter 7
Video 7.1 Imaging Overview—Francisco Contreras, Jose Perez, and Jean Jose

Chapter 8
Video 8.1 Basic Arthroscopic Principles—Michael R. Mijares and Michael G. Baraga

Chapter 9
Video 9.1 Overview of Sport-Specific Injuries—Jared A. Crasto, Ravi S. Vaswani, Thierry Pauyo, and Volker Musahl

Chapter 10
Video 10.1 Commonly Encountered Fractures in Sports Medicine—Christopher Kim and Scott G. Kaar

Chapter 11
Video 11.1 Team Medical Coverage—Daniel Herman, Nikhita Gadi, and Evan Peck

Chapter 12
Video 12.1 Comprehensive Cardiovascular Care and Evaluation of the Elite Athlete—Paul S. Corotto, Robert W. Battle, Dilaawar J. Mistry, and Aaron L. Baggish

Chapter 13
Video 13.1 Exercise-Induced Bronchoconstriction—Virgil P. Secasanu and Jonathan P. Parsons

Chapter 14
Video 14.1 Deep Venous Thrombosis and Pulmonary Embolism—Marc M. DeHart and Jason Thompson

Chapter 15
Video 15.1 Gastrointestinal Medicine in the Athlete—John M. MacKnight

Chapter 16
Video 16.1 Hematologic Medicine in the Athlete—John J. Densmore

Chapter 17
Video 17.1 Infectious Diseases in the Athlete—Nona M. Jiang, Kathleen C. Abalos, and William A. Petri Jr.

Chapter 18
Video 18.1 The Athlete with Diabetes—Jessica A. Lundgren and Susan E. Kirk

Chapter 19
Video 19.1 Renal Medicine and Genitourinary Trauma in the Athlete—Stefan Hemmings and Derek M. Fine

Chapter 22
Video 22.1 Dermatologic Conditions—Haoming Xu, Barbara B. Wilson, and Michael A. Marchetti

Chapter 23
Video 23.1 Facial, Eye, Nasal, and Dental Injuries—John Jared Christophel

Chapter 25
Video 25.1 Sports Nutrition—Jessica L. Buschmann and Jackie Buell

Chapter 26
Video 26.1 Doping and Ergogenic Aids—Siobhan M. Statuta, Aaron J. Vaughan, and Ashley V. Austin

Chapter 27
Video 27.1 The Female Athlete—Letha Y. Griffin, Mary Lloyd Ireland, Fred Reifsteck, Matthew H. Blake, and Benjamin R. Wilson
Video 27.2 The Female Athlete—Letha Y. Griffin, Mary Lloyd Ireland, Fred Reifsteck, Matthew H. Blake, and Benjamin R. Wilson

Chapter 28
Video 28.1 The Para-Athlete—Daniel Herman, Mary E. Caldwell, and Arthur Jason De Luigi

Chapter 30
Video 30.1 The Athletic Trainer—Chad Starkey and Shannon David

Chapter 31
Video 31.1   Principles of Orthopaedic Rehabilitation—Courtney Chaaban and Charles A. Thigpen

Chapter 32
Video 32.1   Modalities and Manual Techniques in Sports Medicine Rehabilitation—Susan Saliba and Michael Higgins

Chapter 38
Video 38.1   Glenohumeral Joint Imaging—Alissa J. Burge and Gabrielle P. Konin

Chapter 41
Video 41.1   Posterior Shoulder Instability—James Bradley and Fotios P. Tjoumakaris

Chapter 42
Video 42.1   Multidirectional Instability of the Shoulder—Robert M. Carlisle and John M. Tokish

Chapter 44
Video 44.1   SLAP Tears—Sean Meredith and R. Frank Henn III

Chapter 45
Video 45.1   The Thrower's Shoulder—Matthew A. Tao, Christopher L. Camp, Terrance Sgroi, Joshua S. Dines, and David W. Altchek

Chapter 46
Video 46.1   Proximal Biceps Tendon Pathology—Samuel R.H. Steiner, John T. Awowale, and Stephen F. Brockmeier

Chapter 47
Video 47.1   Rotator Cuff and Impingement Lesions—Gina M. Mosich, Kent T. Yamaguchi, and Frank A. Petrigliano

Chapter 48
Video 48.1   Subscapularis Injury—William H. Rossy, Frederick S. Song, and Jeffrey S. Abrams

Chapter 49
Video 49.1   Revision Rotator Cuff Repair—Joseph D. Cooper, Anthony Essilfie, and Seth C. Gamradt

Chapter 52
Video 52.1   Glenohumeral Arthritis in the Athlete—Jeffrey Brunelli, Jonathan T. Bravman, Kevin Caperton, and Eric C. McCarty

Chapter 53
Video 53.1   Scapulothoracic Disorders—G. Keith Gill, Gehron Treme, and Dustin Richter

Chapter 54
Video 54.1   Nerve Entrapment—Daniel E. Hess, Kenneth F. Taylor, and A. Bobby Chhabra

Chapter 55
Video 55.1   Vascular Problems and Thoracic Outlet Syndrome—Matthew A. Posner, Christopher J. Roach, Adam M. Pickett, and Brett D. Owens

Chapter 56
Video 56.1   Injury to the Acromioclavicular and Sternoclavicular Joints—Connor G. Ziegler, Samuel J. Laurencin, Rachel M. Frank, Matthew T. Provencher, Anthony A. Romeo, and Augustus D. Mazzocca

Chapter 57
Video 57.1   Elbow Anatomy and Biomechanics—Marshall A. Kuremsky, E. Lyle Cain Jr., Jeffrey R. Dugas, James R. Andrews, and Lucas R. King

Chapter 58
Video 58.1   Elbow Diagnosis and Decision-Making—Nicholas J. Clark and Bassem Elhassan

Chapter 59
Video 59.1   Elbow Imaging—Benjamin M. Howe and Michael R. Moynagh

Chapter 61
Video 61.1   Elbow Tendinopathies and Bursitis—Jennifer Moriatis Wolf

Chapter 62
Video 62.1   Distal Biceps and Triceps Tendon Ruptures—James Bradley, Fotios P. Tjoumakaris, Gregory T. Lichtman, and Luke S. Austin

Chapter 63
Video 63.1   Entrapment Neuropathies of the Arm, Elbow, and Forearm—Wajeeh Bakhsh and Warren C. Hammert

Chapter 64
Video 64.1   Elbow Throwing Injuries—Marshall A. Kuremsky, E. Lyle Cain Jr, Jeffrey R. Dugas, James R. Andrews, and Christopher A. Looze

Chapter 65
Video 65.1   Loss of Elbow Motion—Timothy J. Luchetti, Debdut Biswas, and Robert W. Wysocki

Chapter 66
Video 66.1   Anatomy and Biomechanics of the Hand and Wrist—Raj M. Amin and John V. Ingari

Chapter 67
Video 67.1   Hand and Wrist Diagnosis and Decision-Making—Patrick G. Marinello, R. Glenn Gaston, Eliott P. Robinson, and Gary M. Lourie

Chapter 68
Video 68.1   Imaging of the Wrist and Hand—Kimberly K. Amrami

Chapter 69
Video 69.1   Wrist Arthroscopy—William B. Geissler, David A. Rush, and Christopher A. Keen

Chapter 71
Video 71.1   Wrist Tendinopathies—Raj M. Amin and John V. Ingari

Chapter 72
Video 72.1   Disorders of the Distal Radioulnar Joint—Julie E. Adams

Chapter 73
Video 73.1   Tendon Injuries in the Hand—Robin N. Kamal and Jacob D. Gire

Chapter 74
Video 74.1   Digit Fractures and Dislocations—Christopher L. Stockburger amd Ryan P. Calfee

Chapter 75
Video 75.1   Neuropathies of the Wrist and Hand—Gwendolyn Hoben and Amy M. Moore

Chapter 76
Video 76.1   Hip Anatomy and Biomechanics—Marc Safran and Abdurrahman Kandil

Chapter 77
Video 77.1   Hip Diagnosis and Decision-Making—Benjamin G. Domb and Austin W. Chen

Chapter 78
Video 78.1   Hip Imaging—Brian Busconi, R. Tyler Huish, Erik Mitchell, and Sean McMillan

Chapter 79
Video 79.1   Hip Arthroscopy—Joshua D. Harris

Chapter 80
Video 80.1   Femoroacetabular Impingement in Athletes—Shane J. Nho, Vignesh Prasad Krishnamoorthy, Drew Lansdown, Gift Ukwuani

Chapter 82
Video 82.1   Iliopsoas Pathology—Christian N. Anderson

Chapter 83
Video 83.1   Peritrochanteric Disorders—John W. Stelzer and Scott D. Martin
Video 83.2   Peritrochanteric Disorders—John W. Stelzer and Scott D. Martin
Video 83.3   Peritrochanteric Disorders—John W. Stelzer and Scott D. Martin

Chapter 85
Video 85.1   Posterior Hip Pain—Hal David Martin, Anthony Nicholas Khoury, and Juan Gomez-Hoyos

Chapter 87
Video 87.1   Hip and Thigh Contusions and Strains—Blake R. Obrock, Christopher P. Bankhead, and Dustin Richter

Chapter 89
Video 89.1   Knee Anatomy and Biomechanics of the Knee—Matthew J. Kraeutler, Jorge Chahla, Francesc Malagelada, Jordi Vega, Pau Golanó, Bruce Beynnon, Fatih Ertem, and Eric C. McCarty

Chapter 90
Video 90.1   Knee Diagnosis and Decision-Making—Andrew J. Riff, Peter N. Chalmers, and Bernard R. Bach Jr.

Chapter 92
Video 92.1   Basics of Knee Arthroscopy—Stephen R. Thompson and Mark D. Miller

Chapter 94
Video 94.1   Meniscal Injuries—Joseph J. Ruzbarsky, Travis G. Maak, and Scott A. Rodeo

Chapter 96
Video 96.1   Articular Cartilage Lesions—Michael S. Laidlaw, Kadir Buyukdogan, and Mark D. Miller

Chapter 98
Video 98.1   Anterior Cruciate Ligament Injuries—Edward C. Cheung, David R. McAllister, and Frank A. Petrigliano

Chapter 99
Video 99.1   Revision Anterior Cruciate Ligament Injuries—Joseph D. Lamplot, Liljiana Bogunovic, and Rick W. Wright

Chapter 100
Video 100.1   Posterior Cruciate Ligament Injuries—Frank A. Petrigliano, Evan E. Vellios, Scott R. Montgomery, Jared S. Johnson, and David R. McAllister

Chapter 101
Video 101.1   Medial Collateral Ligament and Posterior Medial Corner Injuries—M. Christopher Yonz, Brian F. Wilson, Matthew H. Blake, and Darren L. Johnson

Chapter 102
Video 102.1   Lateral and Posterolateral Corner Injuries of the Knee—Ryan P. Coughlin, Dayne T. Mickelson, and Claude T. Moorman III

Chapter 103
Video 103.1   Multiligament Knee Injuries—Samantha L. Kallenbach, Matthew D. LaPrade, and Robert F. LaPrade

Chapter 108
Video 108.1   Loss of Knee Motion—K. Donald Shelbourne, Heather Freeman, and Tinker Gray

Chapter 110
Video 110.1 Foot and Ankle Biomechanics—Andrew Haskell

Chapter 115
Video 115.1 Ankle Arthroscopy—Niall A. Smyth, Jonathan R. Kaplan, Amiethab A. Aiyer, John T. Campbell, Rachel Triche, and Rebecca A. Cerrato

Chapter 117
Video 117.1 Ligamentous Injuries of the Foot and Ankle—Paul Rothenberg, Eric Swanton, Andrew Molloy, Amiethab A. Aiyer, and Jonathan R. Kaplan

Chapter 118
Video 118.1 Tendon Injuries of the Foot and Ankle—Todd A. Irwin

Chapter 119
Video 119.1 Articular Cartilage Injuries and Defects—David R. Richardson and Jane C. Yeoh

Chapter 121
Video 121.1 Forefoot Problems in Sport—Ben Hickey, Lyndon Mason, and Anthony Perera

Chapter 122
Video 122.1 Head and Spine Anatomy and Biomechanics—Colin B. Harris, Rachid Assina, Brandee Gentile, and Michael J. Vives

Chapter 123
Video 123.1 Head and Spine Diagnosis and Decision-Making—Rabia Qureshi, Jason A. Horowtiz, Kieran Bhattacharya, and Hamid Hassanzadeh

Chapter 124
Video 124.1 Imaging of the Spine—Adil Samad, M. Farooq Usmani, and A. Jay Khanna

Chapter 125
Video 125.1 Emergency and Field-Side Management of the Spine-Injured Athlete—Korin Hudson, Michael Antonis, and William Brady

Chapter 132
Video 132.1 Imaging Considerations in Skeletally Immature Athletes—Andrew M. Zbojniewicz

Chapter 133
Video 133.1 Shoulder Injuries in the Young Athlete—Andrew T. Pennock and Eric W. Edmonds

Chapter 134
Video 134.1 Elbow Injuries in Pediatric and Adolescent Athletes—James P. Bradley, Luke S. Austin, Alexander B. Kreines, and Fotios P. Tjoumakaris

Chapter 137
Video 137.1 Knee Injuries in Skeletally Immature Athletes—Matthew D. Milewski, James Wylie, Carl W. Nissen, and Tricia R. Prokop

Chapter 138
Video 138.1 Foot and Ankle Injuries in the Adolescent Athlete—J. Andy Sullivan and James R. Gregory

Chapter 139
Video 139.1 Head Injuries in Skeletally Immature Athletes—Tracy Zaslow

Basic Principles

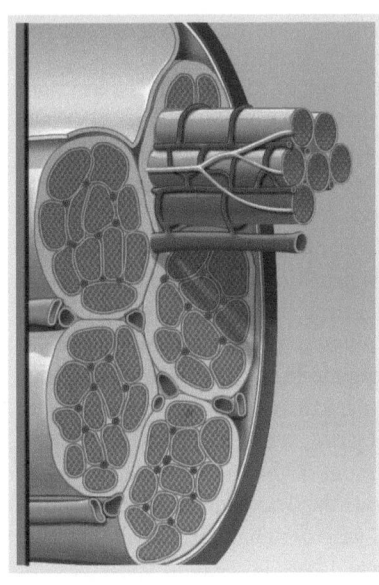

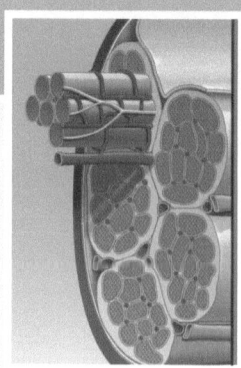

1

Physiology and Pathophysiology of Musculoskeletal Tissues

Dean Wang, Claire D. Eliasberg, Scott A. Rodeo

TENDON AND LIGAMENT

Structure

Tendons and ligaments are both dense, regularly arranged connective tissues. The surface of the tendon is enveloped in a white, glistening, synovial-like membrane, called the *epitenon*, which is continuous on its inner surface with the *endotenon*, a thin layer of connective tissue that binds collagen fibers and contains lymphatics, blood vessels, and nerves. In some tendons, the epitenon is surrounded by a loose areolar tissue called the *paratenon*, which functions as an elastic sheath through which the tendon can slide. In some tendons, the paratenon is replaced by a true synovial sheath or bursa consisting of two layers lined by synovial cells, called the *tenosynovium*, within which the mesotendon carries important blood vessels to the tendon.[1] In the absence of a synovial lining, the paratenon often is called a *tenovagina*. Together the epitenon and the paratenon compose the *peritenon* (Fig. 1.1). The blood supply to tendons has several sources, including the perimysium, periosteal attachments, and surrounding tissues. Blood supplied through the surrounding tissues reaches the tendon through the paratenon, mesotenon, or vincula. Vascular tendons are surrounded by a paratenon and receive vessels along their borders; these vessels then coalesce within the tendon. The relatively avascular tendons are contained within tendinous sheaths, and the mesotenons within these sheaths function as vascularized conduits called *vincula*. The muscle-tendon and tendon-bone junctions, along with the mesotenon, are the three types of vascular supply to the tendon inside the sheath. Other sources of nutrition[2] include diffusional pathways from the synovial fluid, which provide an important supply of nutrients for the flexor tendons of the hand, for example. The nervous supply to a tendon involves mechanoreceptors located near the musculotendinous junction, which provide proprioceptive feedback to the central nervous system.

Ligaments grossly appear as firm, white fibrous bands, sheets, or thickened strips of joint capsule securely anchored to bone. They consist of a proximal bone insertion, the substance of the ligament or the capsule, and a distal bone insertion. Because most insertions are no more than 1 mm thick, they contribute only a small amount to the volume and the length of the ligament. Bundles of collagen fibrils form the bulk of the ligament substance.[3–5] Some ligaments consist of more than one band of collagen fibril bundles. For example, the anterior cruciate ligament (ACL) has a continuum of fiber lengths; different fibers become taut throughout the range of motion.[6] The alignment of collagen fiber bundles within the ligament substance generally follows the lines of tension applied to the ligament. This is in contrast to the alignment of collagen fiber bundles within the tendon, which is generally parallel to its longitudinal axis. In addition, thinner collagen fibrils extend the entire length of the tendon. Light microscopic examination has shown that the collagen bundles have a wave or crimp pattern. The crimp pattern of matrix organization may allow slight elongation of the ligament without incurring damage to the tissue.[6] In some regions, the ligament cells align themselves in rows between collagen fiber bundles, but in other regions, the cells lack apparent orientation relative to the alignment of the matrix collagen fibers. Scattered blood vessels penetrate the ligament substance, forming small-diameter, longitudinal vascular channels that lie parallel to the collagen bundles. Nerve fibers lie next to some vessels, and, like tendon, nerve endings with the structure of mechanoreceptors have been found in some ligaments.[4,7,8]

Tendon and ligament insertions vary in size, strength, angle of the ligament collagen fiber bundles relative to the bone, and proportion of ligament collagen fibers that penetrate directly into bone.[4,5,9] Based on the angle between the collagen fibrils and the bone and the proportion of the collagen fibers that penetrate directly into bone, investigators group tendon and ligament insertions into two types: direct and indirect. Direction insertions typically occur at the apophysis or epiphysis of bone, often within or around a synovial joint, and consist of sharply defined regions where the collagen fibers appear to pass directly into the cortex of the bone.[9,10] Although the thin layer of superficial collagen fibers of direct insertions joins the fibrous layer of the periosteum, most of the tendon or ligament insertions consist of deeper fibers that directly penetrate the cortex, often at a right angle to the bone surface. The deeper collagen fibers pass through four zones with increasing stiffness: ligament substance, fibrocartilage, mineralized fibrocartilage, and bone.[9,10] This four-zone interface is known as the fibrocartilaginous enthesis.[11] Dissipation of force is achieved effectively through this gradual transition from tendon to fibrocartilage to bone. A larger area of fibrocartilage can be found on one side of the insertion, which is thought to be an adaptation to the compressive forces experienced by the tendon or ligament on that side.[12] Conversely, indirect or oblique insertions, such as the tibial insertion of the medial collateral ligament of the knee or the femoral insertion of the lateral collateral ligament, typically occur at the metaphysis

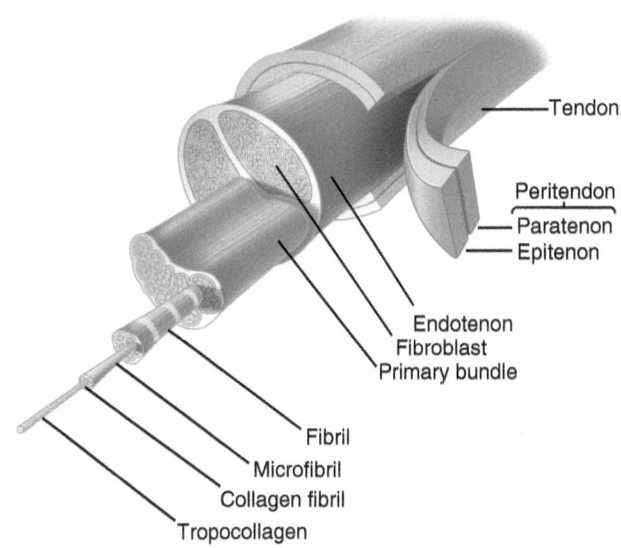

Fig. 1.1 Structural organization of tendon.

Tendon

Peritendon
Paratenon
Epitenon

Endotenon
Fibroblast
Primary bundle

Fibril
Microfibril
Collagen fibril
Tropocollagen

or diaphysis of bone without an intervening fibrocartilage zone. They usually cover more bone surface area than do direct insertions, and their boundaries cannot be easily defined because the collagen fibers pass obliquely along the bone surface rather than directly into the cortex.

Extracellular Matrix

Tendons and ligaments consist of relatively few cells and an abundant extracellular matrix primarily containing collagen, proteoglycans, and water. Tenocytes (tendon-specialized fibroblasts) are the dominant cell of tendons, whereas fibroblasts are the dominant cells of ligaments. Tenocytes and fibroblasts form and maintain the extracellular matrix. Within ligaments, fibroblasts vary in shape, activity, and density among regions of the same tissue and with the age of the tissue.[4,5,9,13] Both tenocytes and fibroblasts are spindle shaped, with fibroblasts being rounder, and extend between the collagen fibrils.[14] Endothelial cells of small vessels and nerve cell processes are also present.[4,5,9,13] Studies have shown that tendon and ligament contain a small population of resident stem cells which function to maintain tissue homeostasis during growth and repair.[15–17]

Type I collagen, which is the major component of the molecular framework, composes more than 90% of the collagen content of ligaments. Type III collagen constitutes approximately 10% of the collagen, and small amounts of other collagen types also may be present. Ligaments have a higher content of type III collagen than do tendons.[18] All types of collagen have in common a triple helical domain, which is combined differently with globular and nonhelical structural elements. The triple helix conformation of collagen is stabilized mainly by hydrogen bonds between glycine residues and between hydroxyl groups of hydroxyproline. This helical conformation is reinforced by hydroxyproline-forming and proline-forming hydrogen bonds to the other two chains. The physical properties of collagen and its resistance to enzymatic and chemical breakdown rely on covalent cross-links within and between the molecules.

Elastin is a protein that allows connective tissues to undergo large changes in geometry while expending little energy in the

process. Tendons of the extremities possess small amounts of this structural protein, whereas most ligaments have little elastin (usually less than 5%), although a few, such as the nuchal ligament and the ligamentum flavum, have high concentrations (up to 75%). In most tendons, elastin is found primarily at the fascicle surface,[19] comprising less than 1% of the tendon by dry weight, and it is responsible for the crimp pattern of the tendon when viewed by a light microscope. Elastin forms protein fibrils or sheets, but elastin fibrils lack the cross-banding pattern of fibrillar collagen and differ in amino acid composition, including two amino acids not found in collagen (desmosine and isodesmosine). In addition, unlike collagen, elastin amino acid chains form random coils when the molecules are unloaded. This conformation of the amino acid chains makes it possible for elastin to undergo some deformation without rupturing or tearing and then, when the load is removed, to return to its original size and shape.

Approximately 1% of the total dry weight of tendon and ligament is composed of ground substance, which consists of proteoglycans, glycosaminoglycans, structural glycoproteins, plasma proteins, and a variety of small molecules. Most ligaments have a higher concentration of glycosaminoglycans than do tendons, due to the functional need for more rapid adaptation.[18] Proteoglycans and glycosaminoglycans both have important roles in organizing the extracellular matrix and control the water content of the tissue.[4,20–23] Tendon and ligaments contain two known classes of proteoglycans. Larger proteoglycans contain *long* negatively charged chains of chondroitin and keratan sulfate. Smaller proteoglycans contain dermatan sulfate. Because of their long chains of negative charges, the large articular cartilage-type proteoglycans tend to expand to their maximal domain in solution until restrained by the collagen fibril network. As a result, they maintain water within the tissue and exert a swelling pressure, thereby contributing to the mechanical properties of the tissue and filling the regions between the collagen fibrils. The small leucine-rich proteoglycans usually lie directly on the surface of collagen fibrils and appear to affect formation, organization, and stability of the extracellular matrix, including collagen fibril formation and diameter. They may also control the activity of growth factors by direct association.[21,24]

Although noncollagenous proteins contribute only a small percentage of the dry weight of dense fibrous tissues, they appear to help organize and maintain the macromolecular framework of the collagen matrix, aid in the adherence of cells to the framework, and possibly influence cell function. One noncollagenous protein, fibronectin, has been identified in the extracellular matrix of ligaments and may be associated with several matrix component molecules and with blood vessels. Other noncollagenous proteins undoubtedly exist within the matrix, but their identity and their functions have not yet been defined. Many of the noncollagenous proteins also contain a few monosaccharides and oligosaccharides.[4,5]

Injury

Acute strains and tears to tendons and ligaments disrupt the matrix, damage blood vessels, and injure or kill cells. Damage to cells, matrices, and blood vessels and the resulting hemorrhage start a response that leads to a sequential process of inflammation, repair, and remodeling.[25,26] These events form a continuous sequence of cell, matrix, and vascular changes that begins with the release of inflammatory mediators and ends when remodeling ceases.[25] As with any injury to biologic tissue, acute inflammation lasts 48 to 72 hours after the injury and then gradually resolves as repair progresses. Some of the events that occur during inflammation, including the release of cytokines or growth factors, may help to stimulate tissue repair.[25] These mediators promote vascular dilation and increase vascular permeability, leading to exudation of fluid from vessels in the injured region, which causes tissue edema. Blood escaping from the damaged vessels forms a hematoma that temporarily fills the injured site. Fibrin accumulates within the hematoma, and platelets bind to fibrillar collagen, thereby achieving hemostasis and forming a clot consisting of fibrin, platelets, red cells, and cell and matrix debris. The clot provides a framework for vascular and fibroblast cell invasion. As they participate in clot formation, platelets release vasoactive mediators and various cytokines or growth factors (e.g., transforming growth factor-β [TGF-β] and platelet-derived growth factor). Polymorphonuclear leukocytes appear in the damaged tissue and the clot. Shortly thereafter, monocytes arrive and increase in number until they become the predominant cell type. Enzymes released from the inflammatory cells help to digest necrotic tissue, and monocytes phagocytose small particles of necrotic tissue and cell debris. Endothelial cells near the injury site begin to proliferate, creating new capillaries that grow toward the region of tissue damage. Release of chemotactic factors and cytokines from endothelial cells, monocytes, and other inflammatory cells helps to stimulate migration and proliferation of the fibroblasts that begin the repair process.[25]

Overuse tendon injury is one of the more common forms of musculoskeletal injury and clinical causes of pain, although controversy exists in the literature about a universal classification and the responsible pathologic entities. A classification of Achilles tendon disorders[27] provides a guide to the structural manifestations of overuse injury as follows: (1) peritendinitis, or inflammation of the peritenon; (2) tendinosis with peritendinitis; (3) tendinosis without peritendinitis; (4) partial rupture; and (5) total rupture. Other classifiers have added a sixth category, tendinitis, in which the primary site of injury is the tendon, with an associated reactive peritendinitis.[28] The classification is not universal because some tendons lack a paratenon and instead have synovial sheaths; furthermore, it is unclear if certain histopathologic conditions are actually separate entities. For instance, human biopsy studies have been unable to show histologic evidence of acute inflammation within the tendon substance.[29] Because of uncertainty regarding the histologic features of these conditions, several authors have suggested use of the term *tendinopathy* rather than *tendinitis*.[30,31]

Studies have shown that in cases of chronic tendinosis, the pathologic lesion is typical of a degenerative process rather than an inflammatory one and that this degeneration occurs in areas of diminished blood flow. Several authors have documented the existence of areas of marked degeneration without acute or chronic inflammatory cell accumulation in most of these cases.[32–34] These changes are separate and distinct from the site of rupture.

A review of patients with chronic tendinitis syndrome revealed similar findings of tendon degeneration.[27,35] Nirschl[35] described the pathology of chronic tendinitis as "angiofibroblastic hyperplasia." A characteristic pattern of fibroblasts and vascular, atypical, granulation-like tissue can be seen microscopically.[35,36] Cells characteristic of acute inflammation are virtually absent. These observations suggest that factors other than mechanical overuse play an important role in the pathogenesis of these tendon lesions.

In several studies, a correlation between age and the incidence of chronic tendinopathy has been identified.[37,38] In vitro studies have shown decreased proliferative and metabolic responses of aging tendon tissue.[39] Other causative factors include the lack of blood flow in certain areas (e.g., supraspinatus and Achilles tendon) that may predispose a tendon to rupture or may result in chronic tendinopathy.[40] Biopsy specimens of young patients with symptoms of chronic tendinopathy have revealed a change in the morphology of tenocytes adjacent to areas of collagen degeneration.[28]

Repair

Tendons and ligaments may possess both intrinsic and extrinsic capabilities for healing, and the contribution of each of these two mechanisms probably depends on the location, extent, and mechanism of injury and the rehabilitation program used after the injury. Several studies[2,41–46] have suggested that the inflammatory response is not essential to the healing process and that these tissues possess an intrinsic capacity for repair. Recent research has isolated intrinsic stem cells within tendon and ligament, although their in vivo identities, niche, and role in healing remain controversial.[17,47] Lindsay and Thomson[43] were the first to show that an experimental tendon suture zone can be isolated from the perisheath tissues and that healing progressed at the same rate as when the perisheath tissues were intact. Later, in isolated segments of profundus tendon in rabbits, these researchers found anabolic and catabolic enzymes, which showed that an active metabolic process existed in the isolated tendon segments.[44]

As in other areas in the body, tendon healing proceeds in three phases: (1) an inflammatory stage, (2) a reparative or collagen-producing stage, and (3) a remodeling phase.

Inflammatory Phase

Tendon and ligament healing begins with hematoma formation and an inflammatory reaction that includes an accumulation of fibrin and inflammatory cells. A clot forms between the two ends and is invaded by cells resembling fibroblasts and migratory capillary buds. Within 2 to 3 days of the injury, fibroblasts within the wound begin to proliferate rapidly and synthesize new matrix. They replace the clot and the necrotic tissue with a soft, loose fibrous matrix containing high concentrations of water, glycosaminoglycans, and type III collagen. Inflammatory cells and fibroblasts fill this initial repair tissue. Within 3 to 4 days, vascular buds from the surrounding tissue grow into the repair tissue and then canalize to allow blood flow to the injured tissue and across small tissue defects. This vascular granulation tissue fills the tissue defect and extends for a short distance into the surrounding tissue but has little tensile strength. The inflammatory phase is evident until the 8th to 10th day after injury.

Reparative Phase

As the repair progresses during the next several weeks, proliferating fibroblasts continue to produce fibrous tissue containing a high proportion of type III collagen. Collagen synthesis reaches its maximal level after approximately 4 weeks, and at 3 months, collagen synthesis continues at a rate 3 to 4 times that of normal tissue. Over time, water, glycosaminoglycan, and type III collagen concentrations decline, the inflammatory cells disappear, and the concentration of type I collagen increases. Newly synthesized collagen fibrils increase in size and begin to form tightly packed bundles, and the density of fibroblasts decreases. Matrix organization increases[48–51] as the fibrils begin to align along the lines of stress, the number of blood vessels decreases, and small amounts of elastin may appear within the site of injury. The tensile strength of the repair tissue increases as the collagen concentration increases.

Remodeling Phase

Repair of many tendon and ligament injuries results in an excessive volume of highly cellular tissue with limited mechanical properties and a poorly organized matrix. Remodeling reshapes and strengthens this tissue by removing, reorganizing, and replacing cells and matrix.[25] In most tendon and ligament injuries, evidence of remodeling appears within several weeks of injury as fibroblasts and macrophages decrease, fibroblast synthetic activity decreases, and fibroblasts and collagen fibrils assume a more organized appearance. As these changes occur in the repair tissue, collagen fibrils grow in diameter, the concentration of collagen and the ratio of type I to type III collagen increase, and the water and proteoglycan concentrations decline. During the months after the injury occurs, the matrix continues to align, presumably in response to loads applied to the repair tissue. The most apparent signs of remodeling disappear within 4 to 6 months of injury. However, removal, replacement, and reorganization of repair tissue continue to some extent for years.[50,52,53] The mechanical strength of the healing tendon and ligament increases as the collagen becomes stabilized by cross-links and the fibrils assemble into fibers.

Factors Affecting Healing

Among the most important variables that affect healing of tendon and ligament are the type of tendon or ligament, the size of the tissue defect, and the amount of load applied to the repair tissue. For example, injuries to capsular and extra-articular ligaments stimulate production of repair tissue that will fill most defects, but injuries to intra-articular ligaments, such as the ACL, often fail to produce a successful repair response. Treatments that achieve or maintain apposition of torn tissue and that stabilize the injury site decrease the volume of repair tissue necessary to heal the injury, which can benefit the healing process. Such treatments may also minimize scarring and help to provide near-normal tissue length. For these reasons, avoidance of wide separation of ruptured tendon or ligament ends and selection of treatments that maintain some stability at the injured site during the initial stages of repair are generally desirable.

Early excessive loading in the immediate postoperative period may have a deleterious effect on tendon and ligament healing by disrupting the repair tissue, leading to gap formation and ischemia, adverse changes in tendon matrix, and possible rupture.[4,25,54–56] However, controlled loading of tendon and ligament repair tissue can promote healing and enhance the mechanical and biologic characteristics of tendon-to-bone healing.[57] The optimal amount of tension necessary to promote an acceptable clinical response is currently not well understood and depends on the type of tissue and healing environment, but it is clear that remodeling of collagen scar tissue into mature tendon tissue depends on the presence of tensile forces.[58,59] The concept of immediate passive mobilization after flexor tendon repair in the hand was introduced by Kleinert and coworkers,[60] who showed that, during limited active extension, reciprocal relaxation of the flexor tendons occurs, allowing passive extension of the repaired tendon. This controlled passive motion was found to be effective experimentally and clinically in decreasing the tethering effect of adhesions and in improving the rates of tendon repair, gliding function, and strength of the tendon.

Methods for Augmentation of Tendon and Ligament Healing

A large body of research has demonstrated the potential for growth factors to improve tendon and ligament tissue healing by stimulation of cell proliferation, chemotaxis, matrix synthesis, and cell differentiation (summarized in Table 1.1). In addition to multifunctional cytokines such as TGF-β and platelet-derived growth factor, work has focused on recapitulating the cellular and molecular signals that are expressed during embryonic tendon development, such as scleraxis and TGF-β3.[61] However, challenges in the delivery of these growth factors, specifically regarding the optimal carrier vehicles and proper dosing regimen, to the desired site still remain.

Platelet-rich plasma (PRP), an autologous blood concentrate, can be used to locally deliver a high concentration "cocktail" of cytokines and has gained popularity as a treatment modality for tendon and ligament injuries. Recent studies have reported potentially promising results with the use of PRP to augment healing of rotator cuff repair[62–64] and patellar tendinopathy.[65] However, the results of PRP for augmentation of tendon and ligament healing have been variable, which can partially be attributed to the lack of understanding of the optimal PRP formulation for different tissues and pathologies, as well as the tremendous variability in the methods of PRP production among commercial systems.[66,67] To complicate matters further, within a given separation technique, there is a high degree of intersubject and intrasubject variability in the composition of PRP produced.[68]

Cell-based approaches appear promising for tendon and ligament tissue engineering and improvement of healing. Therapies using mesenchymal stem cells (MSCs) derived from adipose and bone marrow to augment tendon and ligament healing have garnered the most attention due to their multipotent potential and ability to exert a paracrine effect to modulate and control inflammation, stimulate endogenous cell repair and proliferation, inhibit apoptosis, and improve blood flow.[14,69] However, like PRP augmentation therapy, continued research is needed to identify the optimal cell source and the ideal treatment protocol needed to drive differentiation of these or neighboring

TABLE 1.1   Growth Factors in Soft Tissue Repair

Biologic Factor	Functions	Reference
TGF-β	Influx of mononuclear cells and fibroblasts Enhanced collagen deposition	Lee J et al: *Iowa Orthop J* 1998 Spindler KP et al: *J Orthop Res* 2002 Spindler KP et al: *J Orthop Res* 2003 Kashiwagi K et al: *Scand J Plast Reconstr Surg Hand Surg* 2004 Kim HJ et al: *Connect Tissue Res* 2007 Kim HM et al: *Connect Tissue Res* 2011 Manning CN et al: *J Orthop Res* 2011 Kovacevic D et al: *Am J Sports Med* 2011
GDF 5/6/7	Influx of mononuclear cells and fibroblasts Enhanced collagen deposition	Wolfman NM et al: *J Clin Invest* 1997 Aspenberg P et al: *Acta Orthop Scand* 1999 Rickert M et al: *Growth Factors* 2001 Forslund C et al: *J Orthop Res* 2003 Virchenko O et al: *Scand J Med Sci Sports* 2005 Fealy S et al: *Am J Sports Med* 2006 Dines JS et al: *J Shoulder Elbow Surg* 2007 Saiga K et al: *Biochem Biophys Res Commun* 2010 Date H et al: *J Orthop Res* 2010
IGF-1	Proliferation of fibroblasts Enhanced collagen deposition	Abrahamsson SO et al: *J Orthop Res* 1991 Abrahamsson SO et al: *J Orthop Res* 1996 Kurtz CA et al: *Am J Sports Med* 1999 Dahlgren LA et al: *J Orthop Res* 2002 Dahlgren LA et al: *J Orthop Res* 2005 Provenzano PP et al: *BMC Physiol* 2007
PDGF-B	Influx of mononuclear cells and fibroblasts Enhanced angiogenesis Enhanced collagen deposition	Lee J et al: *Iowa Orthop J* 1998 Hildebrand KA et al: *Am J Sports Med* 1998 Nakamura N et al: *Gene Ther* 1998 Kobayashi M et al: *J Shoulder Elbow Surg* 2006 Uggen C et al: *Arthroscopy* 2010 Hee CK et al: *Am J Sports Med* 2011
bFGF	Proliferation of fibroblasts Enhanced collagen deposition	Lee J et al: *Iowa Orthop J* 1998 Cool SM et al: *Knee Surg Sports Traumatol Arthrosc* 2004 Saiga K et al: *Biochem Biophys Res Commun* 2010 Date H et al: *J Orthop Res* 2010
HGF	Enhanced angiogenesis Enhanced collagen deposition	Ueshima K et al: *J Orthop Sci* 2011
PRP	Enhanced angiogenesis Enhanced collagen deposition	Murray MM et al: *J Orthop Res* 2006 Murray MM et al: *J Orthop Res* 2007 Joshi SM et al: *Am J Sports Med* 2009
VEGF	Enhanced angiogenesis Enhanced collagen deposition	Boyer MI et al: *J Orthop Res* 2001 Petersen W et al: *Arch Orthop Trauma Surg* 2003
BMP-12	Enhanced ossification Enhanced angiogenesis Enhanced collagen deposition	Aspenberg P et al: *Scand J Med Sci Sports* 2000 Lou J et al: *J Orthop Res* 2001 Seeherman HJ et al: *J Bone Joint Surg Am* 2008

bFGF, Basic fibroblast growth factor; *BMP-12,* bone morphogenetic protein-12; *GDF,* growth/differentiation factor; *HGF,* human growth factor; *IGF-1,* insulin-like growth factor-1; *PDGF-β,* platelet-derived growth factor-β; *PRP,* plasma-rich protein; *TGF-β,* transforming growth factor-β; *VEGF,* vascular endothelial growth factor.

cells into mature tenocytes and fibroblasts. Recent studies have identified resident tissue-specific stem cells in the perivascular regions of native tendon and ligament that detach from vessels in response to injury, migrate into the interstitial space, and deposit extracellular matrix,[70,71] although their precise potential for use in augmenting tendon and ligament healing remains to be elucidated.

Research has also investigated scaffold materials to augment tendon repair and ligament reconstruction. Porcine-derived small intestine submucosa has been used as a collagen scaffold to augment Achilles tendon and rotator cuff tendon repair. However, negative clinical results have been reported, including inflammatory/immunologic response to the small intestine submucosa material believed to be due to residual porcine DNA in the implant.[72,73] Various other allografts and xenografts, such as collagen allograft matrices and porcine dermal xenografts, are commercially available and differ from porcine small intestine submucosa in both biologic and mechanical composition.[74,75] Nanomaterials are promising for tendon and ligament tissue engineering because the microstructure of the material mimics

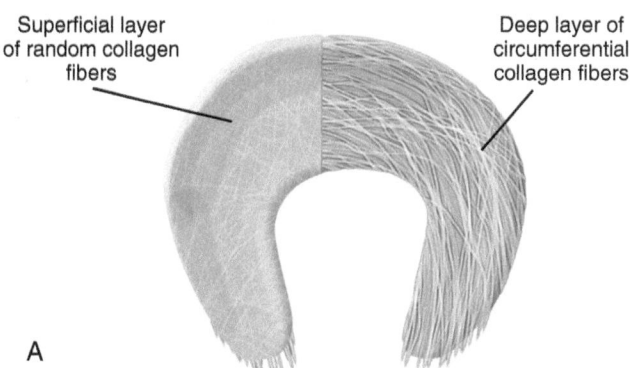

Superficial layer of random collagen fibers

Deep layer of circumferential collagen fibers

A

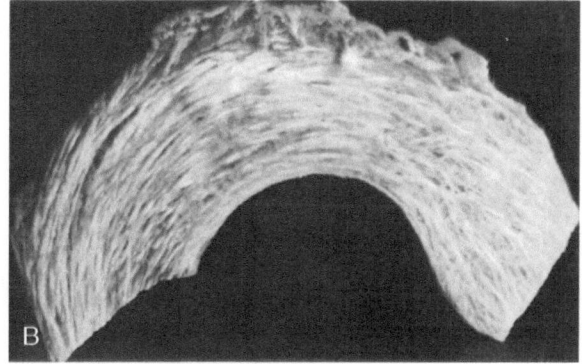

B

Fig. 1.2 (A) Diagram of collagen fiber architecture throughout the meniscus. Collagen fibers of the thin superficial sheet are randomly distributed in the plane of the surface and are predominantly arranged in a circumferential fashion deep in the substance of the tissue. (B) Macrophotograph of bovine medial meniscus with the surface layer removed, showing the large circumferentially arranged collagen bundles of the deep zone. ([A] Modified from Bullough PG, Munuera L, Murphy J, et al. The strength of the menisci of the knee as it relates to their fine structure. *J Bone Joint Surg Br.* 1970;52:564–570. [B] From Proctor CS, Schmidt MB, Whipple RR, et al. Material properties of the normal medial bovine meniscus. *J Orthop Res.* 1989;7:771–782.)

native extracellular matrix. Multiphasic scaffolds are being used to create bone-ligament composites.[76] In addition to various scaffold materials and cell types, it has become clear that mechanical stimulation of the neotissue is also critical to optimize the structure and composition of the tissue.[77] The specific scaffold can be modified in vitro by seeding marrow stromal cells on the scaffold and applying cyclic stretching to increase the alignment of cells, as well as to improve the production and orientation of collagen. When applied in vivo, such a tissue-engineered scaffold could serve to accelerate the healing process, ultimately helping to make a better neoligament or tendon.

MENISCUS

Structure

Human menisci are semilunar in shape[78] and consist of a sparse distribution of cells surrounded by an abundant extracellular matrix.[79–81] The meniscus functions to optimize force transmission and provide stability to the knee. The medial meniscus is the dominant secondary stabilizer in an ACL-deficient knee during the Lachman maneuver,[82] whereas the lateral meniscus is the dominant secondary stabilizer in an ACL-deficient knee during the pivot shift maneuver.[83] Within the meniscus lies an anisotropic, inhomogeneous, and highly ordered arrangement of collagen fibrils. The meniscal surface is composed of a randomly woven mesh of fine collagen type II fibrils that lie parallel to the surface. Below this surface layer, large, circumferentially arranged collagen fiber bundles (mostly type I) spread through the body of the tissue (Fig. 1.2).[84,85] These circumferential collagen bundles give menisci great tensile stiffness and strength parallel to their orientation.[85] The collagen bundles insert into the anterior and the posterior meniscal attachment sites on the tibial plateau, providing for rigid and strong attachment sites. Fig. 1.2A illustrates these large fiber bundles and the thin superficial surface layer. Fig. 1.2B is a photograph of a bovine medial meniscus with the surface layer removed, showing the large collagen bundles of the deep zone.

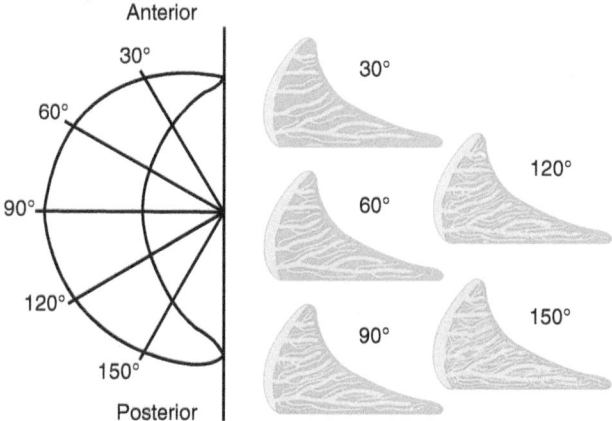

Anterior

30°
60°
90°
120°
150°

30°
60°
90°
120°
150°

Posterior

Fig. 1.3 Radial collagen fiber bundles of the meniscus. Radial tie fibers consisting of branching bundles of collagen fibrils extend from the periphery of the meniscus to the inner rim in every radial section throughout the meniscus. They are more abundant in the posterior sections and gradually diminish in number as the sections progress toward the anterior region of the meniscus. (Modified from Kelly MA, Fithian DC, Chern KY, et al. Structure and function of meniscus: basic and clinical implications. In: Mow VC, Ratcliffe A, Woo SL, eds. *Biomechanics of Diarthrodial Joints.* Vol 1. New York: Springer-Verlag; 1990.)

Radial sections of meniscus (Fig. 1.3) show radially oriented bundles of collagen fibrils, or "radial tie fibers," among the circumferential collagen fibril bundles, weaving from the periphery of the meniscus to the inner region.[85,86] These tie fibers help to increase the stiffness and the strength of the tissue in a radial direction, thereby resisting longitudinal splitting of the collagen framework. In cross section, these radial tie fibers appear to be more abundant in the posterior sections than in the anterior sections of the meniscus.[87]

Unlike articular cartilage, the peripheral 25% to 30% of the lateral meniscus and the peripheral 30% of the medial meniscus[78,88–90] have a blood supply, and the peripheral regions of the meniscus, especially the meniscal horns,[91,92] have a nerve supply as well. Branches from the geniculate arteries form a capillary plexus along the peripheral borders of the menisci, with the medial inferior geniculate artery supplying the peripheral medial meniscus and the lateral inferior geniculate artery supplying the peripheral lateral meniscus.[88,89] Small radial branches project from these circumferential parameniscal vessels into the meniscal substance.[90] The central aspects of the meniscus do not have a direct arterial supply and instead receive nutrients primarily through synovial fluid diffusion.

Extracellular Matrix

The mechanical functions of the menisci depend on a highly organized extracellular matrix consisting of fluid and a macromolecular framework formed of collagen (types I, II, III, V, and VI), proteoglycans, elastin, and noncollagenous proteins, along with the cells that maintain this matrix.

Based on morphologic characteristics, two major types of meniscal cells exist.[80,93] Near the surface, the cells have flattened ellipsoid or fusiform shapes and are considered more fibroblastic; in the deep zone, the cells are spherical or polygonal and considered more chondrocytic. The superficial and the deep meniscal cells appear to have different metabolic functions and perhaps different responses to loading.[94] Like most other mesenchymal cells, these cells lack cell-to-cell contacts. Because most of the cells lie at a distance from blood vessels, they rely on diffusion through the matrix for transport of nutrients and metabolites. The membranes of meniscal cells attach to matrix macromolecules through adhesion proteins (e.g., fibronectin, thrombospondin, and type VI collagen).[80] The matrix, particularly the pericellular region, protects the cells from damage due to physiologic loading of the tissue. Deformation of the macromolecular framework of the matrix causes fluid flow through the matrix[94,95] and influences meniscal cell function. Because meniscal tissue is more fibrous than is hyaline cartilage, some authors have proposed that meniscal cells be called fibrochondrocytes.[80,96]

Water comprises 65% to 75% of the total weight of the meniscus.[94,95,97] Some portion of this water may reside within the intrafibrillar space of the collagen fibers.[98,99] Most of the water is retained within the tissue in the solvent domains of the proteoglycans due to both their strong hydrophilic tendencies and the Donnan osmotic pressure exerted by the counter ions associated with the negative charge groups on the proteoglycans.[94,100,101] Because the pore size of the tissue is extremely small (<60 nm), very large hydraulic pressures are required to overcome the impact of frictional resistance when forcing fluid flow through the tissue. These interactions between water and the macromolecular framework of the matrix significantly influence the viscoelastic properties of the tissue.

Some meniscal regions have a proteoglycan concentration of up to 3% of their dry weight.[80,81,95,102] Like proteoglycans from other dense fibrous tissues, meniscal proteoglycans can be divided into two general types. The large, aggregating proteoglycans expand to fill large volumes of matrix and contribute to tissue hydration and the mechanical properties of the tissue. The smaller, nonaggregating proteoglycans usually have a close relationship with fibrillar collagen.[80,103,104] The large aggregating meniscal proteoglycans have the same structure as the large aggregating proteoglycans from articular cartilage.[81,104] The concentration

of large aggregating proteoglycans suggests that they probably contribute less to the properties of meniscus than to the properties of articular cartilage.[94,95] As with the quantitatively minor collagens, the smaller nonaggregating meniscal proteoglycans may help to organize and stabilize the matrix, but currently their exact function remains unknown.

Noncollagenous proteins also form part of the macromolecular framework of the meniscus and may contribute as much as 10% of the dry weight of the tissue in some regions.[80] Two specific noncollagenous proteins, link protein and fibronectin, have been identified in the meniscus.[80] Link protein is required for the formation of the stable proteoglycan aggregates that are capable of forming strong networks.[105,106] Fibronectin serves as an attachment protein for cells in the extracellular matrix.[107] Other noncollagenous proteins such as thrombospondin[108] may serve as adhesive proteins in the tissue, thus contributing to the structure and the mechanical strength of the matrix; however, the exact details of their composition and function in the meniscus remain largely unknown.

Finally, elastin contributes less than 1% of the dry weight of the meniscus.[80] The contribution of elastin to the mechanical properties of meniscal tissue is not well understood because the sparsely distributed elastic fibers are unlikely to play a significant role in the organization of the matrix or in determining the mechanical properties of the tissue.

Injury

Traumatic meniscal tears occur most frequently in young, active people. Tension, compression, or shear forces that exceed the strength of the meniscal matrix in any direction can lead to tissue failure. Acute traumatic injuries of normal meniscal substance usually produce longitudinal or transverse tears, although the morphology of these tears can be highly variable, including oblique, radial horizontal, bucket-handle, and complex tears. The configuration of tears due to overloading of normal meniscal tissue depends strongly on the direction of the load and the rate of stretch.[94] Unlike acute traumatic tears through apparently normal meniscal tissue, degenerative meniscal tears occur as a result of age-related changes in the tissue. These degenerative tears are most common in persons older than 40 years. Often, these persons do not recall a specific injury, or they recall only a minor load applied to the knee. Degenerative tears often have complex shapes or may appear as horizontal clefts or flaps, as though they were produced by shear failure. Multiple degenerative tears often occur within the same meniscus. These features of degenerative meniscal tears suggest that they result more from age-related changes in the collagen-proteoglycan solid matrix than from specific acute trauma.

The response of meniscal tissue to tears depends on whether the tear occurs through a vascular or an avascular portion of the meniscus.[89] The peripheral, vascular regions respond to injury as other vascularized, dense fibrous tissues do. The tissue damage initiates a sequence of cellular and vascular events including inflammation, repair, and remodeling[109] that can result in healing and restoration of tissue structure and function. Although tears through the vascular regions of the meniscus can typically heal, tears through the avascular regions do not typically heal spontaneously, resulting in tissue deficiency.[78,89] Therefore strategies for meniscal repair in the avascular zone are continuously being explored.[110]

Meniscal Repair
Factors Affecting Healing

Repair in vascular regions of the meniscus. Partial meniscal resection through the peripheral vascularized region or complete meniscal resection initiates production of repair tissue that can extend from the remaining peripheral tissue into the joint.[111–116] Although the repair cells usually fail to replicate normal meniscal tissue, many authors have referred to this phenomenon as *meniscal regeneration.*[114,116] Some repaired menisci grossly resemble normal menisci, but the functional capabilities and mechanical properties of this "regenerated" meniscal tissue have not been comprehensively studied. Surgeons have reported meniscal regeneration in many clinical situations. Investigators have also examined the tissue produced by meniscal regeneration in animals. Meniscal regeneration can occur repeatedly in the same knee[115] and occasionally occurs after total knee replacement.[114] In rabbits, meniscal regeneration occurs more frequently on the medial side of the knee than on the lateral side, and development of degenerative changes in articular cartilage after a meniscectomy is inversely correlated with the extent of meniscal regeneration.[111–113] Synovectomy appears to prevent meniscal regeneration, which suggests that synovial cells contribute to the formation of meniscal repair tissue. The mechanisms and conditions that promote this type of repair, its functional importance, and the factors related to the predictability and frequency of meniscal regeneration remain unknown.

Repair in avascular portions of the meniscus. The response of meniscal tissue to tears in the avascular portion resembles the response of articular cartilage to lacerations in many respects. Experimental studies show that a penetrating injury to the avascular region of the meniscus causes no apparent repair or inflammatory reaction. Meniscal cells in the injured region, like chondrocytes in the region of an injury limited to the articular cartilage, may proliferate and synthesize new matrix, but they appear to be incapable of migrating to the site of the defect or producing enough new matrix to fill it. The ineffective response of meniscal cells in the avascular region of the meniscus has led investigators to develop novel methods to stimulate repair. Some promising approaches include creation of a vascular access channel to the injury site and stimulation of cell migration to the avascular region using implantation of a fibrin clot, an artificial matrix, or growth factors.[117] Synovial abrasion has also been shown to stimulate proliferation of the synovial fringe into the meniscus and allows blood vessels to enter the avascular regions. Although early results appear promising, the quality of the repair tissue, its biomechanical properties, and the long-term results of these methods have not been evaluated.

Augmentation of Meniscus Healing

Given the well-established poor intrinsic healing potential of the meniscus, particularly in avascular regions, intense interest exists regarding methods to augment healing using cytokines, exogenous cells, and scaffolds. Fibroblast growth factor-2 and connective tissue growth factor have been evaluated in rabbit models,[118,119] and vascular endothelial growth factor has been tested in a sheep meniscus tear model.[120,121] Although these cytokines appear to have a positive effect on basic meniscal fibrochondrocyte biology, the challenge at this time is to identify the optimal carrier vehicles and dosage to translate these preclinical data to clinical trials. Although some studies have suggested that PRP, as a source of cytokines, may confer some benefit in meniscus healing,[122,123] other studies have demonstrated no differences in outcomes or reoperation rates.[124] In addition, in an animal model of meniscus injury, PRP treatment increased hypertrophic fibrous tissue rather than meniscal cartilage.[125] Thus further investigation is necessary to better elucidate the role of growth factors and PRP in meniscal healing.

Cell-based approaches have also been evaluated for augmentation of biologic healing mechanisms. Various sources of both autogenous[126] and allogeneic cells[127] have been evaluated using different carrier materials. Both differentiated cells, such as chondrocytes, and undifferentiated cells, such as MSCs,[128,129] have been tested in animal models. Few human studies investigating the role of MSCs for meniscal repair have been performed.[130–133] Although the authors suggest that MSCs may be effective in repairing meniscal tears, these studies are limited, and more rigorous, placebo-controlled trials are necessary.[134]

Scaffolds. The use of scaffold materials to replace a portion of the damaged meniscus or to replace the entire structure is an appealing option and has the theoretical benefit of providing mechanical stability to the injured site while allowing for cell attachment and proliferation.[135,136] A collagen-based scaffold (Collagen Meniscus Implant, Menaflex, ReGen Biologics, Glen Rock, NJ) and a resorbable porous polyurethane-based scaffold (Actifit, Orteq Sport Medicine, London, United Kingdom) have demonstrated satisfactory clinical outcome in up to 80% of cases at up to 10 years and 2 years of follow-up, respectively.[137,138] Both of these devices are designed for partial meniscus replacement. Although it remains unclear whether the use of such scaffolds can affect the long-term sequelae of meniscectomy, early results are promising and may represent a new horizon in the treatment of these complex injuries. Further optimization of these materials may occur by incorporating undifferentiated cells into the scaffold.

ARTICULAR CARTILAGE

Synovial joints allow the rapid controlled movements necessary to support joint motion and to participate in sports. Normal function of these complex diarthrodial structures depends on the structural integrity and macromolecular composition of articular cartilage. Sports-related traumatic disruptions of cartilage structure and alterations in the macromolecular composition or organization change the biomechanical properties of the tissue, compromise joint function, and can lead to progressive pain and disability.

The specialized composition and organization of hyaline articular cartilage impart its unique biomechanical properties that permit normal synovial joint function. In the joint, cartilage distributes the loads of articulation, thereby minimizing peak stresses acting on the subchondral bone. The tensile strength of the tissue provides its structural integrity under such loads. Alterations in the mechanical properties of cartilage due to injury, disease, or increasing age have not been well defined, but the available information shows that these properties change with age and loss of structural integrity. Cartilage from skeletally immature joints (open growth plates) is much stiffer than cartilage from skeletally mature joints (closed growth plates).[139] Older cartilage and fibrillated cartilage have much lower tensile stiffness and strength.[109] Participation in sports often subjects the articular cartilage to intense repetitive, compressive high-energy impact forces that can cause tissue injury. These abnormally large forces generate high shear stresses at the cartilage-subchondral bone junction, causing matrix disruption and death of the articular chondrocytes that may lead to early osteoarthritis.[140,141] Because cartilage is aneural, patients with pure chondral injuries can remain asymptomatic.

Structure and Composition of Articular Cartilage

Like the dense fibrous tissues and meniscus, articular cartilage consists of cells, matrix water, and a matrix macromolecular framework.[142] Unlike the most dense fibrous tissues, cartilage lacks nerves, blood vessels, and a lymphatic system. The composition, organization, and mechanical properties of the matrix of articular cartilage and the cell morphology and function vary according to the depth from the articular surface (Fig. 1.4).[143,144] Matrix composition, organization, and function also vary with

distance from the cell.[109] Morphologic changes in articular cartilage cells and matrix from the articular surface to the subchondral bone make it possible to identify four zones or layers of articular cartilage.

Zones of Articular Cartilage

Superficial zone. The thinnest zone, the superficial tangential zone, has two layers. A sheet of fine fibrils without cells covers the joint surface (see Fig. 1.4). On phase-contrast microscopy, it appears as a narrow bright line, the "lamina splendens." In the next layer of the superficial zone, flattened ellipsoid chondrocytes are arranged so that their major axes are parallel to the articular surface (see Fig. 1.4). They synthesize a matrix that has a high collagen concentration and a low proteoglycan concentration relative to the other cartilage zones. Water content is the highest in this zone, averaging 80%.[143] In addition, a specific protein, called lubricin (or PRG4) is also only produced in this zone. Lubricin plays an important role in joint lubrication and in allowing frictionless articulation.[145–147]

Transitional zone. The transitional (middle) zone has several times the volume of the superficial zone (see Fig. 1.4). The cells of this zone assume a spheroidal shape and synthesize a matrix with collagen fibrils of a larger diameter and a higher concentration of proteoglycans than is found in the superficial zone. In this zone, the proteoglycan concentration is higher than in the superficial zone, but the water and the collagen concentrations are lower.[148]

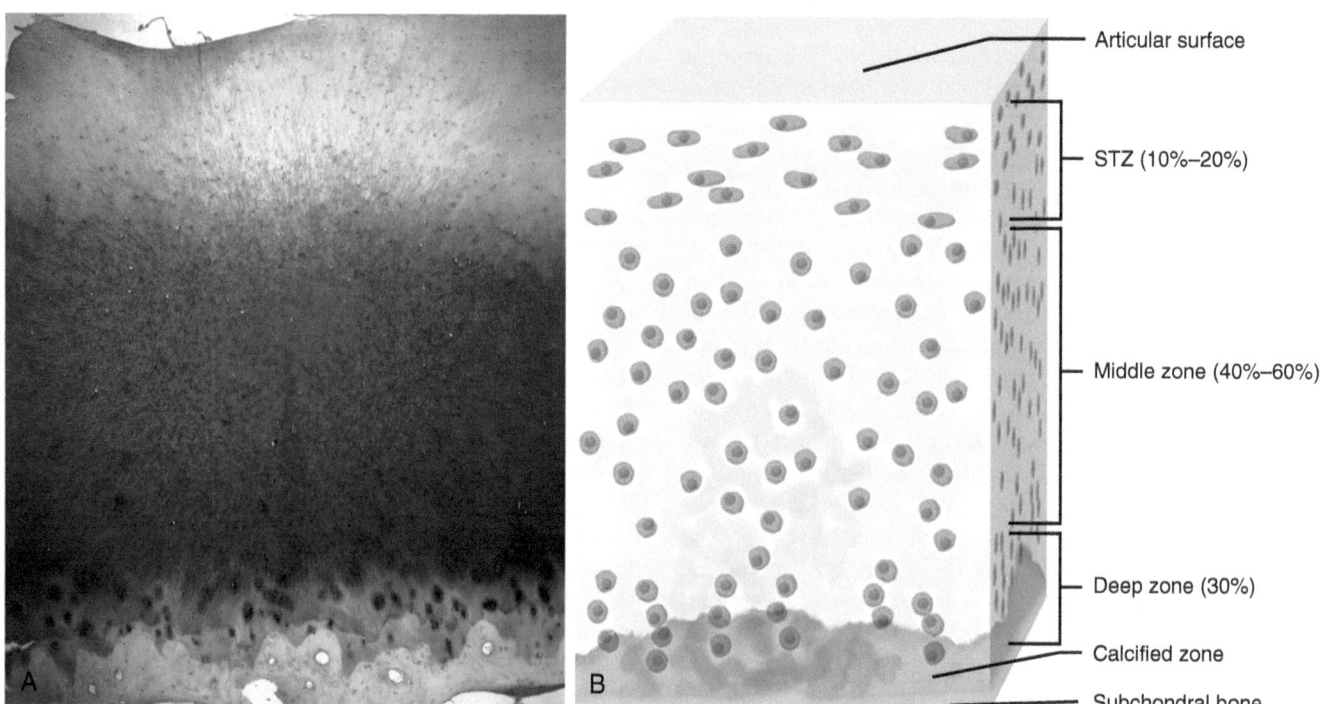

Fig. 1.4 Normal articular cartilage structure. Histologic (A) and schematic (B) views of a section of normal articular cartilage. The tissue consists of four zones: the superficial tangential zone *(STZ)*, the middle zone, the deep zone, and the calcified zone. Notice the differences in cell alignment among zones. The cells of the superficial zone have an ellipsoidal shape and lie with their long axes parallel to the articular surface. The cells of the other zones have a more spheroidal shape. In the deep zone, they tend to align themselves in columns perpendicular to the joint surface. (Schematic from Nordin M, Frankel VH. *Basic Biomechanics of the Musculoskeletal System.* 2nd ed. Philadelphia: Lea & Febiger; 1989.)

Deep zone. The chondrocytes in the deep zone resemble those of the middle zone, but they tend to align in columns perpendicular to the joint surface (see Fig. 1.4). This zone contains the collagen fibrils with the largest diameter, the highest concentration of proteoglycans, and the lowest concentration of water. The collagen fibers of this zone pass through the tidemark (a thin basophilic line seen on light microscopic sections that marks the boundary between calcified and uncalcified cartilage)[141] into the calcified zone.[149]

Calcified cartilage zone. A zone of calcified cartilage lies between the deep zone of uncalcified cartilage and the subchondral bone. The calcified layer plays an integral role in securing the cartilage to bone by anchoring the collagen fibrils of the deep zone to the subchondral bone. In this zone, the cell population is scarce and chondrocytes are hypertrophic. Type X collagen is present in the calcified cartilage.

Chondrocytes

The chondrocyte is the predominant cell in cartilage. Chondrocytes contribute only 5% or less to the total volume of cartilage. Like other mesenchymal cells, chondrocytes surround themselves with their extracellular matrix and rarely form cell-to-cell contacts. In normal cartilage, they are isolated. Because the tissue lacks blood vessels, the cells depend on diffusion through the matrix for their nutrition and rely primarily on anaerobic metabolism.

After completion of skeletal growth, chondrocytes rarely divide, but throughout life they synthesize and maintain the extracellular matrix that gives cartilage its essential material properties. Synthesis and turnover of proteoglycans are relatively fast, whereas collagen synthesis and turnover are very slow.[150,151] The limited potential for chondrocyte replication contributes to the limited inherent capacity of cartilage to regenerate or heal after injury.

Extracellular Matrix

Water contributes up to 80% of the wet weight of articular cartilage. The interaction of water with the matrix macromolecules, particularly the large aggregating proteoglycans, significantly influences the material properties of the articular cartilage.[109,143,152,153] This tissue fluid contains gases, small proteins, metabolites, and a high concentration of cations that balance the negatively charged proteoglycans.[152,154] The interaction between proteoglycans and tissue fluid significantly influences the compressive stiffness and resilience of articular cartilage.[139,152]

Collagens contribute approximately 60% of the dry weight of cartilage, proteoglycans contribute 25% to 35%, and the noncollagenous proteins and glycoproteins contribute 15% to 20%. Collagens are distributed relatively uniformly throughout the depth of the cartilage except in the collagen-rich region near the surface. The collagen fibrillar meshwork and cross-linking give cartilage its form and tensile strength.[139,155] Proteoglycans and noncollagenous proteins bind to the collagenous meshwork or become mechanically entrapped within it, and water fills this molecular framework. Proteoglycans give cartilage its stiffness in compression and its resilience. Some noncollagenous proteins organize and stabilize the matrix macromolecular framework, whereas others bind chondrocytes to the macromolecules of the matrix.

Cell-Matrix Interactions

Maintenance of cartilage depends on continual complex interactions between chondrocytes and the matrix they synthesize. Normal degradation of matrix macromolecules, especially proteoglycans, requires that the chondrocytes continually synthesize new molecules.[143,144] If the cells did not replace the lost proteoglycans, the tissue would deteriorate. Mechanical loading also affects cartilage homeostasis.[156,157]

Chondrocytes respond to changes in patterns of matrix deformation due to persistent changes in joint use. Both mechanical and physicochemical events during matrix deformation likely play significant roles. A chondrocyte embedded in the charged extracellular matrix may exist in either an undeformed state or a deformed state. Deformation during compression alters the charge density around the cells and induces a streaming potential throughout the tissue. These physicochemical effects vary according to proteoglycan concentration relative to depth from the surface in the different zones of the charged collagen-proteoglycan extracellular matrix[143,144] and are important in modulating chondrocyte proteoglycan biosynthesis.[152,158-161] In addition to these events, biochemical agents such as growth factors,[162] cytokines, and enzymes are also potent stimulators of chondrocytes. Altogether, studies addressing these important questions offer great challenges for the future.

Relevance for Articular Cartilage Repair

The typical tissue response of vascularized connective tissues to injury follows a cascade of inflammation, repair, and scar remodeling, which is facilitated by cells and other mediators brought in from the surrounding vasculature. However, because hyaline cartilage is avascular, this vital response cannot be generated, and the intrinsic reparative ability of cartilage is very low.[163-165] In healthy cartilage, a homeostasis of extracellular matrix metabolism balances the degradation of macromolecules with their replacement through newly synthesized products. Insult to the cartilage can lead to imbalance of this equilibrium and a shift toward degradation, leading to progression of the chondral defect and potentially, osteoarthritis. Factors associated with this physiologic imbalance and repair response include joint loading, depth of the defect, size of the defect, and patient age.

Joint Loading

Acute or repetitive direct blunt trauma or abnormal loading can cause a spectrum of cartilage injuries ranging from those isolated to microscopic matrix damage to those that lead to visible fissures causing matrix disruption and chondrocyte death. Abnormal loading can be caused by mechanical malalignment or concomitant ligament injury that leads to excessive focal stresses on the cartilage. Loss of proteoglycans typically occurs before other signs of tissue injury[166,167] and may be due to either increased degradation or altered synthesis of the molecules, including the collagen fibrils, thus increasing the vulnerability of the tissue to damage from further impact loading.[166-168] Disruption of the surface collagen matrix leads to increased hydration, fissuring in the cartilage, and thickening of subchondral bone. A study of the response of human articular cartilage to blunt trauma showed that impact loads exceeding 25 N/m^2 (25 megapascal [MPa]) caused chondrocyte death and cartilage fissures.[149]

Depth of the Defect

Articular cartilage defects are generally classified as chondral or osteochondral, depending on the depth. Chondral defects can be further classified into partial thickness or full thickness (i.e., down to subchondral bone). The repair response depends on whether the injury extends down to the subchondral vascular bone marrow. For partial-thickness chondral injuries, the local response depends entirely on chondrocytes near the injury site, which proliferate and increase the synthesis of matrix macromolecules.[109,169] However, the newly synthesized matrix and the proliferating chondrocytes are unable to fill the tissue defect, and soon after injury, the increased proliferative and synthetic activity ceases. Because chondrocytes cannot repair these matrix injuries, the fissures either remain unchanged or progress. Injuries that extend down into the subchondral bone marrow lead to migration of osteoprogenitor cells into the defect region and synthesis of a new fibrocartilaginous tissue. However, this repair tissue is biomechanically and structurally inferior to hyaline cartilage and thus prone to breakdown with time and loading.[170,171]

Size of the Defect

Smaller defects are less likely to affect the stress distribution on the subchondral bone and progress in size, whereas larger defects are more likely to progress due to increased rim stresses and an inadequate repair response. A study in horses revealed that defects less than 3 mm in diameter may lead to complete repair after 9 months, whereas those larger in size (up to 21 mm in diameter) failed to heal.[172]

Age

Articular cartilage undergoes significant structural, matrix composition, and mechanical changes with age.[104,139,173,174] As with most type of cells in the body, mitotic and synthetic activities of chondrocytes decline with age.[175] These changes are responsible for higher incidence of chondral lesions and development of osteoarthritis in older patients. As a result, any reparative response or ability to maintain extracellular matrix homeostasis decreases with older age. Animal studies in rabbits have demonstrated a better reparative response for chondral defects in younger animals compared with older ones.[176,177]

Clinical Relevance and Further Developments

Small, symptomatic chondral defects may be treated by marrow-stimulating techniques such as microfracture. However, the resultant fibrocartilage repair tissue after microfracture is histologically different and biomechanically inferior to native hyaline cartilage.[178] For larger lesions, a myriad of options is available, including osteochondral autografts or allografts, autologous chondrocyte implantation (ACI), or matrix-induced autologous chondrocyte implantation (MACI). Osteochondral grafts are able to treat defects that extend into the subchondral bone, whereas ACI and MACI require well-preserved bone stock at the base of the chondral defect. The use of particulated juvenile cartilage allograft, which may have increased proliferative and

restorative potential, has demonstrated promising early results for treatment of cartilage defects of the knee.[179,180] Future developments include improved scaffolds,[178,181] augmentation with therapeutic factors such as proteins or genes,[182] and the use of MSCs.[182,183] Furthermore, small molecules and activation of endogenous repair (homing of intrinsic progenitors/MSCs) are potential forthcoming therapeutic avenues.[184,185]

BONE

Types of Bone

Normal bone is lamellar and can be classified as cortical or cancellous. Immature bone and pathologic bone are woven and, in contrast to lamellar bone, have more random orientation with more osteocytes, increased turnover, and inferior integrity. Lamellar bone is stress oriented, whereas woven bone is not stress oriented.

Cortical bone (compact bone) (Fig. 1.5) makes up 80% of the skeleton and is composed of tightly packed osteons or haversian systems which are connected by haversian (or Volkmann) canals. These canals contain arterioles, venules, capillaries, nerves, and possibly lymphatic channels. Interstitial lamellae lie between the osteons. Fibrils frequently connect lamellae but do not cross cement lines. Cement lines define the outer border of an osteon and represent the area where bone resorption has stopped and new bone formation has begun. Nutrition occurs through the intraosseous circulation, which involves networks of canals and

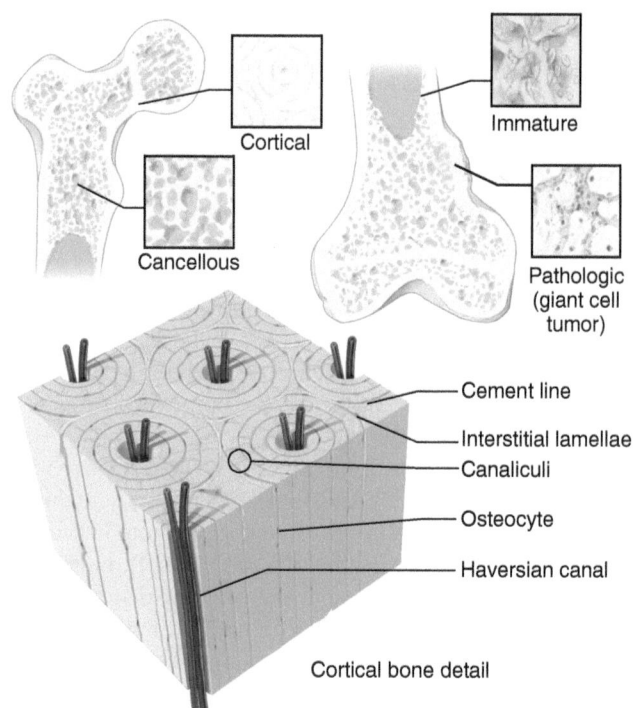

Fig. 1.5 Types of bone. Cortical bone consists of tightly packed osteons. Cancellous bone consists of a meshwork of trabeculae. In immature bone, unmineralized osteoid lines the immature trabeculae. In pathologic bone, atypical osteoblasts and architectural disorganization are seen. (From Brinker MR, Miller MD. *Fundamentals of Orthopaedics.* Philadelphia: WB Saunders; 1999.)

canaliculi. Radiating processes of bone osteocytes, also known as filopodia, project into the canaliculi and allow for osteocyte interaction.

Cortical bone is characterized by a slow turnover rate, a relatively high Young's modulus (E), and a high resistance to torsion and bending. Cancellous bone (spongy or trabecular bone) (see Fig. 1.5) is less dense than cortical bone and undergoes more remodeling according to lines of stress (Wolff's law). Cancellous bone has a higher turnover rate and a smaller Young's modulus and is more elastic than cortical bone.

Cellular Biology

Osteoblasts are responsible for bone formation and are derived from undifferentiated mesenchymal cells. More differentiated, metabolically active cells line bone surfaces, and less active cells in "resting regions" or entrapped cells maintain the ionic milieu of bone. Disruption of the lining cell layer activates these cells.

Osteocytes (see Fig. 1.5) make up 90% of the cells in the mature skeleton and serve to maintain bone. These cells consist of former osteoblasts that have been trapped within newly formed matrix, which they help to preserve. Osteocytes are not as active in matrix production as are osteoblasts.

Osteoclasts are responsible for bone resorption.[186] These multinucleated, irregularly shaped giant cells originate from hematopoietic tissues.[187] Bone resorption occurs in depressions known as Howship lacunae and is more rapid than bone formation; however, bone formation and resorption are linked ("coupled").

Osteoclasts have specific receptors for calcitonin, osteoprotegerin, and other molecules which allow them to directly regulate bone resorption. Interleukin-1 (IL-1) is a potent stimulator of osteoclastic bone resorption in nonphysiologic situations and has been found in the membranes surrounding loose total joint implants. IL-10 suppresses osteoclast formation.[188]

Bone Matrix

Bone matrix is composed of both organic and inorganic components. The organic components make up 40% of the dry weight of bone. Organic components include collagen (mainly type I) proteoglycans, noncollagenous matrix proteins (glycoproteins, phospholipids, and phosphoproteins), growth factors, and cytokines. Collagen is responsible for the tensile strength of bone.

Proteoglycans are partially responsible for the compressive strength of bone. Matrix proteins include osteocalcin,[189] osteonectin, osteopontin, and others. Growth factors and cytokines, which are present in small amounts in bone matrix, include TGF-β; insulin-like growth factor; interleukins (e.g., IL-1 and IL-6); and bone morphogenetic proteins. These proteins aid in bone cell differentiation, activation, growth, and turnover. The inorganic or mineral component of bone matrix makes up 60% of the dry weight of bone. Calcium hydroxyapatite $[Ca_{10}(PO_4)_6(OH)_2]$ is responsible for the compressive strength of bone. Calcium hydroxyapatite makes up most of the inorganic matrix and is responsible for matrix mineralization.

Bone Remodeling

Bone remodeling is affected by mechanical stress according to Wolff's law. Removal of external stresses can lead to significant bone loss, but this situation can be reversed to varying degrees on remobilization. In addition to remodeling in response to stress, bone remodels in response to piezoelectric charges. The compression side is electronegative, stimulating osteoblasts and bone formation; the tension side is electropositive, stimulating osteoclasts and bone resorption.

Both cortical bone and cancellous bone are continuously remodeled by osteoclastic and osteoblastic activity. Bone remodeling occurs in small packets of cells known as basic multicellular units. This bone remodeling is modulated by systemic hormones and local cytokines. Bone remodeling occurs throughout life. The Hueter-Volkmann law (i.e., compressive forces inhibit growth and tensile forces stimulate growth) suggests that mechanical factors can influence longitudinal growth, bone remodeling, and fracture repair. Cancellous bone remodels by osteoclastic resorption followed by osteoblastic bone formation.

Bone Circulation

As an organ system, bones receive 5% to 10% of the cardiac output. The long bones receive blood from three sources: the nutrient artery system, the metaphyseal-epiphyseal system, and the periosteal system. Bones with a tenuous blood supply include the scaphoid, the talus, the femoral head, and the odontoid.

The nutrient artery enters the diaphyseal cortex through the nutrient foramen and then enters the medullary canal. In the medullary canal, the nutrient artery branches into ascending and descending small arteries, which, in turn, branch into arterioles which penetrate the endosteal cortex to supply the inner two-thirds of mature diaphyseal cortex through vessels that traverse the haversian system. The metaphyseal-epiphyseal system arises from the periarticular vascular plexus. The periosteal system is composed primarily of capillaries that supply the outer one-third of the mature diaphyseal cortex. Although the nutrient artery system is a high-pressure system, the periosteal system is a low-pressure system.

At the site of bony injury, the initial response is decreased flow to a fracture as a result of disruption of the nutrient artery system at the fracture site.[190] However, within hours to days, bone blood flow increases (as part of the regional acceleratory phenomenon) and peaks at approximately 2 weeks. Blood flow returns to baseline between 3 and 5 months. The arterial system of bone has great potential for vasoconstriction (from the resting state) and much less potential for vasodilation. The vessels within bone possess a variety of vasoactive receptors, which may be useful in the future for pharmacologic treatment of bone diseases related to aberrant circulation (e.g., osteonecrosis and fracture nonunion).[191]

Tissue Surrounding Bone

The periosteum is the connective tissue membrane that covers bone. It is more highly developed in children because of its role in the deposition of cortical bone, which is responsible for growth in bone diameter. The inner, or cambium, layer of periosteum is loose and more vascular and contains cells that are capable of becoming osteoblasts. These cells are responsible for enlarging the diameter of bone during growth[192] and forming periosteal callus during fracture healing; the outer, fibrous layer is less cellular and is contiguous with joint capsules.

Bone marrow is the soft, gelatinous tissue within the interior of bones, which consists of both stromal and progenitor cells. Red marrow is more commonly found in flat bones, contains hematopoietic stems cells and MSCs, and slowly changes to yellow marrow with age. Yellow marrow is most commonly found in the long bones, contains primarily fat cells, and has a lower water content than red marrow.

Types of Bone Formation
Endochondral Bone Formation and Mineralization
In the process of endochondral bone formation, undifferentiated cells secrete cartilaginous matrix and differentiate into chondrocytes. This matrix mineralizes and is invaded by vascular buds that bring in osteoprogenitor cells. Osteoclasts then resorb calcified cartilage, and osteoblasts form bone. Bone replaces the cartilage model. Examples of endochondral bone formation include embryonic long-bone formation, longitudinal growth (physis), development of fracture callus, and the formation of bone via the use of demineralized bone matrix.

Intramembranous Bone Formation
Intramembranous bone formation occurs without a cartilage model. Undifferentiated mesenchymal cells aggregate into layers (or membranes). These cells differentiate into osteoblasts and deposit organic matrix that mineralizes to form bone. Examples of intramembranous bone formation include embryonic flat-bone formation (e.g., the pelvis, clavicle, and vault of the skull), bone formation during distraction osteogenesis, and blastema bone formation (which occurs in young children with amputations).

Appositional Ossification
In the process of appositional ossification, osteoblasts align themselves on an existing bone surface and lay down new bone. Examples of appositional ossification include periosteal bone enlargement (width) and the bone formation phase of bone remodeling.

Biology of Fracture Healing
Overview
Fracture healing involves a series of cellular events: inflammation, fibrous tissue formation, cartilage formation, and endochondral bone formation.[193] The cellular events of fracture healing are influenced by undifferentiated cells in the vicinity of the fracture, osteoinductive growth factors released into the fracture environment, and the mechanical loading environment.

Fracture Repair
The response of bone to injury can be thought of as a continuum of histologic processes, beginning with inflammation, proceeding through repair (soft callus followed by hard callus), and finally ending in remodeling. Fracture repair is unique in that healing is completed without the formation of a scar. Fracture healing may be influenced by a variety of biologic and mechanical factors.[194–196]

In the inflammation phase, bleeding from the fracture site and surrounding soft tissues creates a hematoma, which provides a source of hematopoietic cells capable of secreting growth factors. Subsequently, fibroblasts, mesenchymal cells, and osteoprogenitor cells accumulate at the fracture site, and fibrovascular tissue forms around the fracture ends. Osteoblasts from surrounding osteogenic precursor cells, fibroblasts, or both proliferate.

In the repair phase, primary callus response occurs within 2 weeks. If the bone ends are not in continuity, a bridging (soft) callus occurs. Fibrocartilage develops and stabilizes the bone ends. The soft callus (fibrocartilage) later is replaced by woven bone (hard callus) through the process of endochondral ossification. Another type of callus—medullary callus—supplements the bridging callus, although it forms more slowly and occurs later in the repair process. The amount and type of callus formation are dependent upon the method of treatment (Table 1.2).[197] Primary cortical healing, which resembles normal remodeling, occurs with rigid immobilization and anatomic (or near-anatomic) reduction with the bone ends in continuity. With rigidly fixed fractures (such as with a compression plate), direct osteonal or primary bone healing occurs without visible callus formation. In contrast, "endochondral healing," with periosteal bridging callus formation, occurs in the setting of nonrigid fixation.

The remodeling phase begins during the middle of the repair phase and continues long after the fracture has clinically healed (can be for several years). Remodeling allows the bone to assume its normal configuration and shape based on the stresses to which it is exposed (Wolff's law). Throughout the process, woven bone formed during the repair phase is replaced with lamellar bone. Fracture healing is complete when repopulation of the marrow space occurs.

TABLE 1.2 Type of Fracture Healing Based on Type of Stabilization

Type of Immobilization	Predominant Type of Healing	Comments
Cast (closed treatment)	Periosteal bridging callus	Enchondral ossification
Compression plate	Primary cortical healing (remodeling)	Cutting cone–type remodeling
Intramedullary nail	Early: periosteal bridging callus	Enchondral ossification
	Late: medullary callus	
	Dependent on extent of rigidity	
	Less rigid: periosteal bridging callus	
	More rigid: primary cortical healing	
Inadequate	Hypertrophic nonunion	Failed endochondral ossification; type II collagen predominates

From Brinker MR. Basic sciences. In: Miller MD, Brinker MR, eds. *Review of Orthopaedics.* 3rd ed. Philadelphia: WB Saunders; 2000.

TABLE 1.3 Factors Affecting Bone and Bone Healing

Factor	Example	Action	Clinical Comment
Growth factors	BMPs	Osteoinductive, induce metaplasia of mesenchymal cells into osteoblasts	Used clinically to stimulate bony healing in challenging injuries such as open tibial fractures[42] and nonunions
	TGF-β	Induces osteoblasts to synthesize collagen	
	IGF-I and IGF-II and IGFBPs 1–6	Regulate proliferation and differentiation of bone-forming osteoblasts	
	Platelet-derived growth factor	Attracts inflammatory cells to the fracture site	
Ultrasound	Low-intensity pulsed ultrasound	Accelerates fracture healing and increases the mechanical strength of callus, including torque and stiffness	Decreases consolidation time during distraction osteogenesis and stimulates healing of nonunions
Electricity	Direct current	Stimulates an inflammatory-like response	
	Alternating current	Affects collagen synthesis and calcification	
	Pulsed electromagnetic fields	Initiates calcification of fibrocartilage	Does not induce calcification of fibrous tissue

BMP, Bone morphogenetic protein; *IGF,* insulin-like growth factor; *IGFBP,* insulin-like growth factor–binding protein; *TGF-β,* transforming growth factor-β.

The different factors affecting bone are summarized in Table 1.3.

For a complete list of references, go to ExpertConsult.com.

SELECTED READINGS

Citation:

O'Keefe R, Jacobs JJ, Chu CR, et al, eds. *Orthopaedic Basic Science.* 4th ed. American Academy of Orthopaedics; 2013.

Level of Evidence:

V

Summary:

An excellent textbook covering all aspects of the basic science of musculoskeletal tissues.

Citation:

Andarawis-Puri N, Flatow EL, Soslowsky LJ. Tendon basic science: Development, repair, regeneration, and healing. *J Orthop Res.* 2015;33(6):780–784.

Level of Evidence:

V

Summary:

A review focusing on the challenges and important questions regarding tendinopathies and tendon healing.

Citation:

Proffen BL, Perrone GS, Roberts G, et al. Bridge-enhanced ACL repair: A review of the science and the pathway through FDA investigational device approval. *Ann Biomed Eng.* 2015;43(3):805–818.

Level of Evidence:

V

Summary:

A review of the approaches for bioenhanced ACL repair and the group's journey to carry their novel technology from bench to bedside.

Citation:

Eleftherios MA, Gomoll AH, Malizos KN, et al. Repair and tissue engineering techniques for articular cartilage. *Nat Rev Rheumatol.* 2015;11(1):21–34.

Level of Evidence:

V

Summary:

A comprehensive review of the biology of cartilage repair and the science supporting current reconstructive surgical techniques and future tissue engineering endeavors.

Citation:

Erggelet C, Mandelbaum B. *Principles of Cartilage Repair.* Heidelberg: Springer-Verlag; 2008.

Level of Evidence:

V

Summary:

Clinical overview of current techniques for cartilage repair with detailed descriptions and graphics.

Citation:

Einhorn TA, Gerstenfeld LC. Fracture healing: mechanisms and interventions. *Nat Rev Rheumatol.* 2015;11(1):45–54.

Level of Evidence:

V

Summary:

A comprehensive review of the biology of fracture healing at the tissue, cellular, and molecular levels.

2

Basic Concepts in Biomechanics

Richard E. Debski, Neel K. Patel, Jason T. Shearn

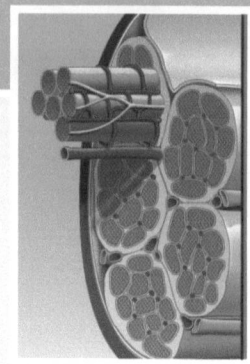

Biomechanics is an interdisciplinary field that uses the principles of mechanics to improve the human body through design, development, and analysis of equipment, systems, and therapies. This biomechanical knowledge can help in understanding the loading of the musculoskeletal system and its mechanical responses, which can be used to determine normal function, predict changes, and propose interventions. More specifically, basic biomechanics explores forces and moments required for movement and balance of the human body by muscle recruitment and the consequence of internal forces on loading of soft tissues. This chapter explores biomechanics in terms of four topics: statics, dynamics, mechanics of materials, and applications. Additionally, examples of these concepts are provided throughout the chapter to illustrate how they can be directly applied to sports medicine.

BASIC CONCEPTS

Units of Measure

Understanding the basic units of measure for biomechanics is important in describing the dimensional or spatial analyses. There are three primary dimensions—length, time, and mass—from which secondary dimensions are subsequently derived (Table 2.1). Metric unit measurements are commonly used in the field of biomechanics to describe such dimensions and are also used in this chapter. One measurement not described in Table 2.1 is that used for angular descriptions. The unit for angles is typically defined in terms of radians or degrees.

Scalars and Vectors

Most of the physical quantities encountered in mechanics are either scalars or vectors. Scalar quantities describe only the magnitude of an element and are used for concepts such as time, length, speed, mass, temperature, volume, work, power, and energy. In contrast, both a magnitude and a direction are associated with vector quantities. Examples of vector quantities are displacement, force, moment, velocity, and acceleration. The magnitude of an object's velocity is identical to its speed, but the velocity vector also contains information about the direction of motion. Graphically, a vector is represented as an arrow, with the orientation of the arrow indicating its line of action or direction. For example, the force of gravity is a vector quantity that can be represented by a downward arrow at an object's center of mass. Typically vectors are represented in a Cartesian coordinate system.

Coordinate Systems

A coordinate system is a frame of reference for a structure or system. Coordinate systems are spatial tools that are useful in describing body position and orientation and the directionality of all vector quantities. To apply mechanical principles to a system, all vector quantities must be expressed with respect to the same coordinate system. Several types of coordinate systems are available, but the most commonly used in sports medicine research is the Cartesian coordinate system. This system can be either two- or three-dimensional. All axes are perpendicular to one another (a condition known as orthogonality) and have both positive and negative components. A vector quantity contains a component in each dimension corresponding to the magnitude associated with each axis. In a two-dimensional system, the horizontal and vertical axes are typically labeled "x" and "y," respectively. In a three-dimensional system, the "z"-axis is added. This axis lies perpendicular to both the x- and y-axes, with its positive side determined by the right-hand rule. This rule states that if you align the index finger of your right hand with the positive x-axis and the middle finger with the positive y-axis, your thumb will be pointing in the positive direction of the z-axis. Similarly, the right-hand rule can be used to determine the positive and negative directions of angles and moments about a specified axis. While the thumb of your right hand is aligned with the rotational axis, your fingers will curl in the positive direction of rotation. These rules are very important in establishing the correct spatial quantities within a designated coordinate system.

Anatomic Coordinate System

An anatomic coordinate system is a Cartesian coordinate system with each axis representing anatomic directions such as superior-inferior, medial-lateral, and anterior-posterior. The corresponding rotations about these axes are represented by internal-external rotation, flexion-extension, and abduction-adduction, respectively. Researchers and clinicians use the anatomic coordinate system whenever possible because it is the most clinically relevant for diagnosis and treatment.

Degrees of Freedom

Degrees of freedom are the total number of independent movements needed to completely describe the position and orientation of a body in a given coordinate system. The musculoskeletal system has numerous degrees of freedom through which countless

TABLE 2.1 Dimensional Quantities and Corresponding Units in the International System of Units

Dimensions	SI Unit
Primary	
Length	Meter (m)
Time	Second (s)
Mass	Kilogram (kg)
Secondary	
Area	m^2
Volume	m^3
Velocity	m/s
Acceleration	m/s^2
Force	Newton (N) = kg • m/s^2
Pressure/stress	Pascal (Pa) = N/m^2
Moment/torque	N • m
Work/energy	Joule (J) = N • m
Power	J/s

SI, International System of Units.

TABLE 2.2 Newton's Laws of Motion Applied to Static and Dynamic Analyses

Law	Definition	Equation
First (inertia)	An object at rest tends to stay at rest and an object in motion tends to stay in motion with the same speed and in the same direction unless acted upon by an external unbalanced force.	$\Sigma F = 0$ $\Sigma M = 0$
Second (acceleration)	The rate of change of the moment of a body is directly proportional to the applied force and takes place in the direction in which the force acts.	$F_{NET} = m \cdot a$ $M_{NET} = I \cdot \alpha$
Third (action-reaction)	For every action there is an equal but opposite reaction.	

movements are accomplished. These movements can be performed in three-dimensional space through a set of translations and rotations and are typically described in an anatomic coordinate system. For example, the glenohumeral joint has a total of six degrees of freedom: three translations (superior-inferior, medial-lateral, and anterior-posterior), and three rotations (internal-external, abduction-adduction, and flexion-extension). However, depending on the analysis, the glenohumeral joint can be assumed to be a ball-and-socket joint, thus reducing the number of degrees of freedom to three rotations by constraining the translations. Similarly, the elbow only allows for one degree of freedom when it is considered a simple hinge joint.

Degrees of freedom are important to consider when describing body motion and position numerically. Joint motion may be constrained by the shape of the articular surfaces or by stabilizing ligaments, reducing the degrees of freedom and simplifying the description. However, some joints, such as the knee and ankle, also allow for small amounts of translation that are important to consider when interpreting a clinical examination. With an anterior cruciate ligament (ACL) injury, the knee will have an increased level of anterior translation, thereby altering the anterior degree of freedom. Using reduced degrees of freedom is strategic when modeling or characterizing joints of the body. For example, when a person picks up an object from the floor and subsequently returns to an erect posture, each vertebra moves in three-dimensional space to achieve the desired posture, representing a large number of degrees of freedom. To evaluate lower back injuries using modeling techniques, the degrees of freedom can be significantly reduced by only considering the L5–S1 joint and assuming that the motion occurs only in the sagittal plane, resulting in a two-dimensional analysis. Similarly, in assessing the tibiofemoral joint during a kicking motion, it could be assumed that the tibia moves in only two dimensions within the sagittal plane (Fig. 2.1A). These reductive assumptions often overestimate the translations, rotations, forces, and moments required to perform the motion.

Newton's Laws

Three basic rules of physics—Newton's laws of motion—are used to describe the relationship between the forces applied to the body and the consequences of those forces on human motion (Table 2.2).

Newton's First Law (Inertia)

Newton's first law states that an object at rest tends to stay at rest and an object in motion tends to stay in motion with the same speed and in the same direction (velocity) unless acted upon by an unbalanced force. This law is also commonly referred to as the *law of inertia*. Therefore a nonzero resultant force must act on a rigid body to change its velocity. For example, headrests are placed in cars to prevent whiplash injuries during rear-end collisions by stopping the motion of the head, which illustrates decreasing linear velocity and acceleration by application of an unbalanced force. Furthermore, if the resultant moments and forces are zero, then the body will also have no rotational or linear acceleration.

Newton's Second Law (Acceleration)

Newton's second law pertains to the behavior of objects for which all forces are not balanced. Therefore the resultant force is not equal to zero, and acceleration in the direction of the applied force will occur. The magnitude of the acceleration is proportional to the magnitude of the resultant forces or moments applied to the body. Thus, in essence, the first law is a special case of the second law:

$$\Sigma F = m \cdot a : \Sigma M = I \cdot \alpha$$

where "F" is the resultant force, "m" is the mass of the body being acted upon, "a" is the acceleration of the body due to the unbalanced external forces, "M" is the resultant moment, "I" is the mass moment of inertia (resistance of a body to rotation), and α is the angular acceleration.

Linear acceleration can exist as an extremity is sent through a range of motion (ROM) during a task (see Fig. 2.1F). In sports, an athlete frequently controls his or her mass moment of inertia or center of mass of the entire body by altering the positioning

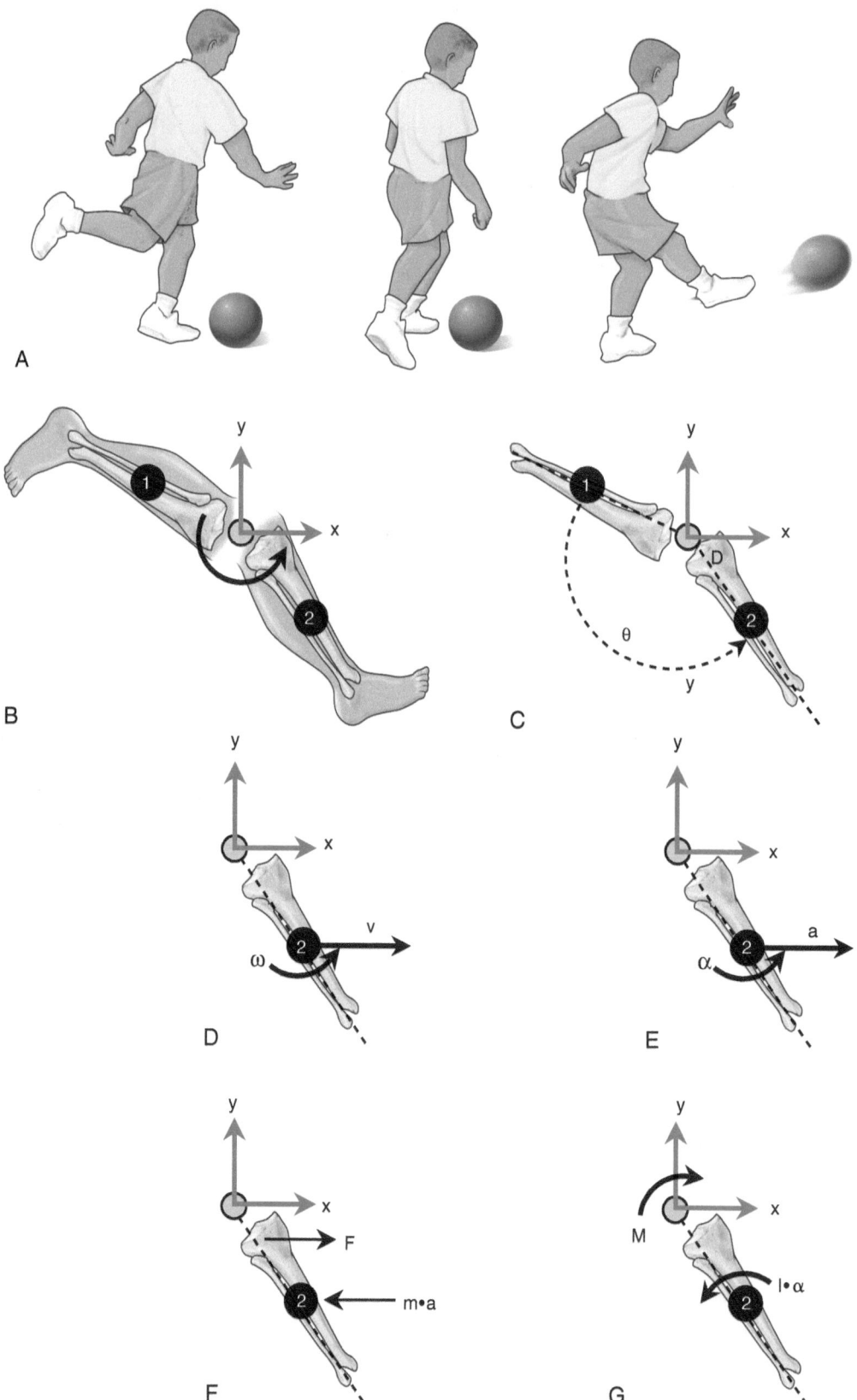

Fig. 2.1 (A) Sequence of leg positions while kicking a ball. (B) The motion of the leg in the acceleration phase of kicking in the sagittal plane at positions 1 and 2. (C) Displacement *(D)* and rotation *(θ)* of the tibia during the motion. (D) The linear *(v)* and angular *(ω)* velocity vectors. (E) The linear *(a)* and angular *(α)* acceleration vectors in the acceleration phase of kicking. (F) The linear and angular inertial forces, with the applied force *(F)* resisted by the inertial force *(m • a)*. (G) The applied moment *(M)* resisted by the angular inertia *(I • α)*.

of the individual body segments to achieve stability or a particular motion. Gymnasts and divers use this concept to achieve multiple somersaults while in the air by tucking in the head and limbs closer to the center of the body, which is an example of angular acceleration due to changes in angular inertia (see Fig. 2.1G).

Newton's Third Law (Action-Reaction)

Newton's third law states that for every action there is an equal but opposite reaction. This law explains the idea that if a person pushes against a wall, it will in essence push back. Forces of action and reaction are equal in magnitude, but in the opposite direction. This concept is important in examining the principle of equilibrium and when using tools that assess forces being applied to the body of interest. Reaction forces act to constrain motions by reacting to an applied force. A daily application of this concept is simple walking and running. Every time a person places a foot on the ground, a force is exerted from the foot on the ground throughout the gait cycle. Simultaneously, however, a force of equal magnitude is exerted in the opposite direction from the ground up to the foot, which is termed a *ground reaction force*. Ground reaction forces are the forces applied by the ground because of the weight of the body. Similarly, within joints, muscles and connective tissues are found that create a *joint reaction force* (Fig. 2.2). Both passive and active stabilizers maintain the humeral head within the glenoid fossa of the glenohumeral joint,[1] which has implications for surgical repair of Bankart lesions by changing the arc of the glenoid and tendon transfers in changing the line of muscle action. If these joint structure changes alter the natural forces and/or the direction of these forces, joint instability would result, potentially leading to long-term degenerative changes.

When a body is balanced by equal but opposite reactions for every action, the system is considered to be in a condition of equilibrium, which means that the net effect of the applied forces is zero as well as the net moment about any point. Although the sum of the force and moment vectors is zero, the body may still be moving at a constant velocity. Assuming a state of static

equilibrium with a set of known force vectors, it is possible to determine unknown forces within a system. To do so, each force vector can be resolved into its individual components, such as the vertical (Fy) and horizontal (Fx) components for a two-dimensional coordinate system (Figs. 2.3 and 2.4D). Therefore the resulting equations for force and moment equilibrium in three dimensions are:

$$\Sigma Fx = 0; \Sigma Mx = 0$$
$$\Sigma Fy = 0; \Sigma My = 0$$
$$\Sigma Fz = 0; \Sigma Mz = 0$$

For static equilibrium, no linear or rotational motion occurs.

STATICS

Using the aforementioned equations of static equilibrium, static analyses evaluate the external effects of forces on a rigid body at rest or during motion with a constant velocity. Applied to the body, static analyses are used to further determine the magnitude and direction of forces at joints and in the muscles. Forces provide both mobility and stability to the body but also introduce the potential to deform and injure the body. Typically, healthy tissues are able to withstand changes in their shape, but a tissue structure that has been injured by disease or trauma may not be able to adequately sustain the same loads required to perform activities of daily living. To perform static analyses, we must be able to

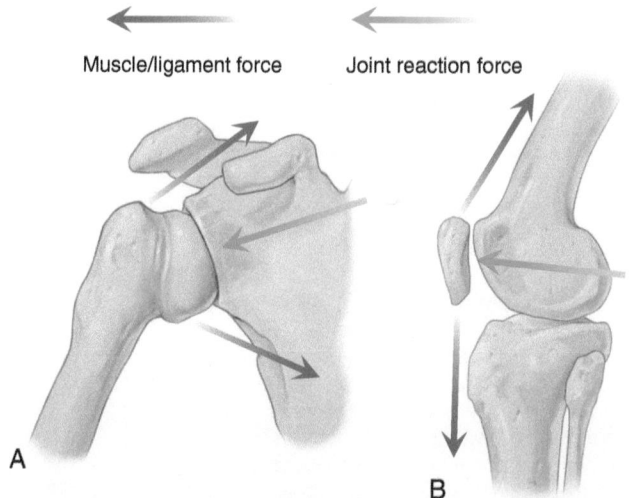

Fig. 2.2 Resulting joint reaction force at the glenohumeral (A) and patellofemoral (B) joints.

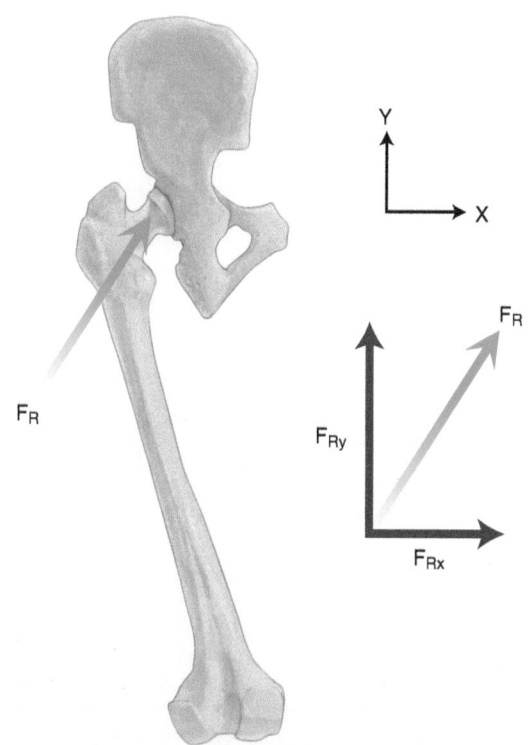

Fig. 2.3 Force vector *(F$_R$)* representing the joint reaction force between the femoral head and acetabulum, and F$_R$ resolved into its individual component forces *(F$_{Rx}$* and *F$_{Ry}$)* in the x and y directions.

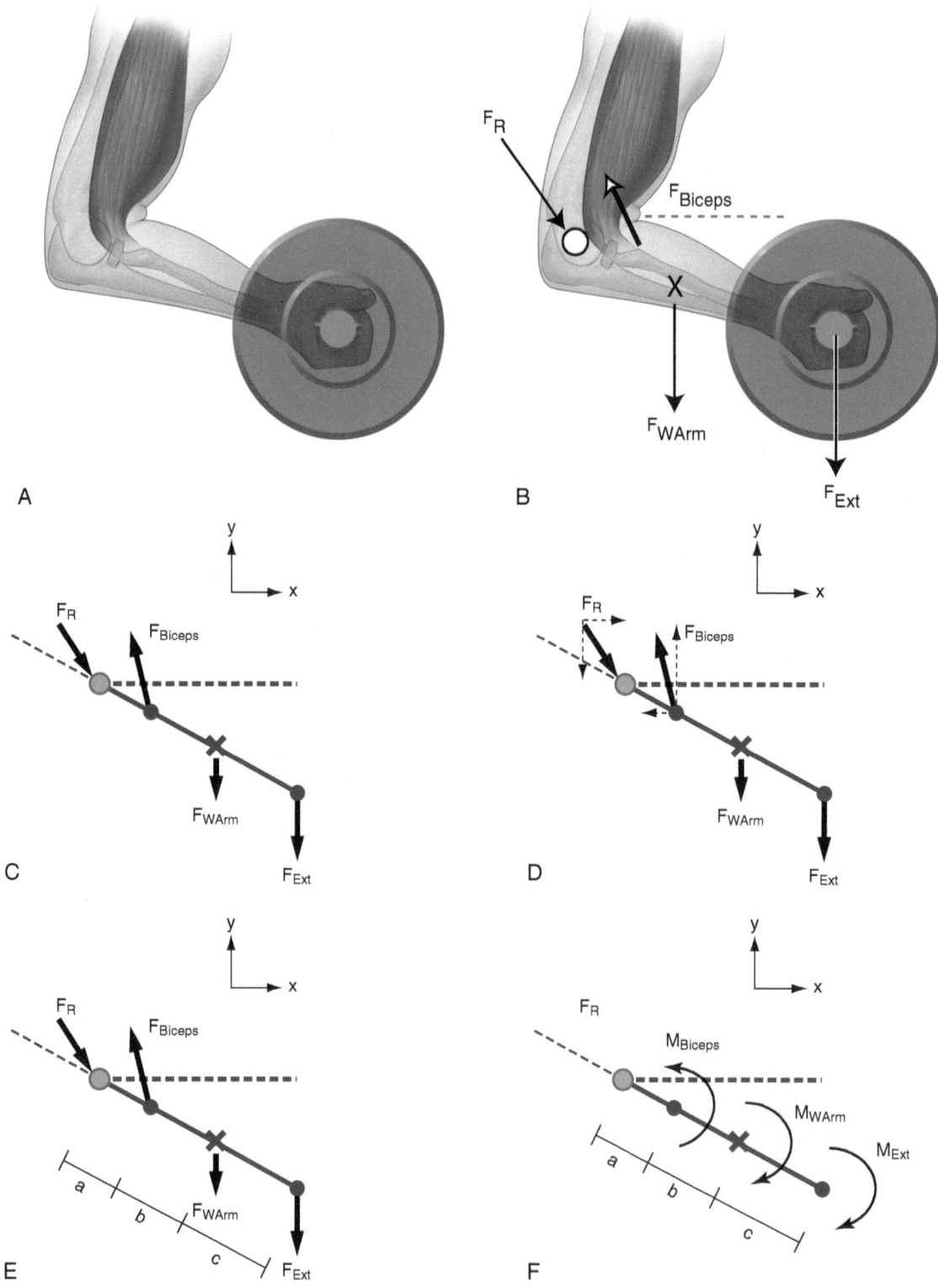

Fig. 2.4 (A) Simulation of a person performing a biceps curl. (B) The dumbbell applies an external force *(F_Ext)* downward in addition to the downward force due to the weight of the arm *(F_WArm)*. The biceps muscle generates a force *(F_Biceps)* to the forearm and causes a joint reaction force *(F_R)* at the elbow to keep the joint stabilized. (C) A free-body diagram of the forearm representing each force as an *arrow*, with the head of the *arrow* pointing in the direction of the applied force. (D) These forces are then decomposed into component vectors. (E) The varying moment arms for each force vector are identified with respect to the axis of rotation at the elbow. (F) The biceps muscle creates a counterclockwise moment *(M_Biceps)* to resist the clockwise moments due to the weight of the arm *(M_WArm)* and dumbbell *(M_Ext)*.

represent the complex interactions of forces and moments acting on a body through the use of vectors and free-body diagrams.

Force Vectors

The most common vector quantity in mechanical systems is a force. A force is applied on an object to create either a pushing or pulling response. Depending on the original state of the object, a force can cause a stationary object to move or alter the state of an object already in motion. Such forces can be either internal or external. Internal forces include those that hold a rigid body together, such as muscle tension generated within an extremity, whereas external forces are those applied to a rigid body. An example of an external force is the weight of an object being held in a person's hand. Forces can be further categorized into two subgroups: contact (tension, friction, external, and internal) and distance (gravitational and magnetic) forces. Distance forces act at a distance from the object or body with no direct physical contact. Additionally, forces can contain components acting in both the normal (perpendicular) and tangential (parallel) directions of the surface to which they are being applied.

Moment/Torque Vectors

Vector quantities can represent not only translational motions in response to an applied force but also the rotation, twisting, and bending of an object. A moment (or torque) is determined by the magnitude of the force acting about a point and the length of the shortest distance between the point and line of action of the force. This distance is known as the *moment* or *lever arm*. A larger moment arm requires less force to achieve equivalent angular motion about the axis of rotation, which means that if the force remains the same but the lever arm increases, the moment will be of greater magnitude. Although a moment can realistically be calculated about any point, typically it is calculated about a joint axis of rotation during biomechanical analyses. For example, when tension is generated in the biceps muscle during a biceps curl exercise, the tendon pulls on the forearm at a distance from the elbow axis of rotation (see Fig. 2.4). This tension from the biceps muscle generates a positive moment about the elbow that can either help maintain the posture of the elbow or increase the amount of flexion, depending on whether the biceps muscle force is equal to or greater than the applied external forces of the weight.

Free-Body Diagrams

To better evaluate a biomechanical system, such as forces being applied to a specified part of the body, free-body diagrams are an effective tool to simplify a complex analysis. Free-body diagrams allow for visualization and ease of calculation by properly identifying all the forces and moments acting on the body of interest in order to successfully achieve equilibrium. These diagrams are used by first drawing the body of interest and then isolating the body from its environment, only including the forces acting on the body. Again using the example of a biceps curl exercise to evaluate the elbow joint, the system should be drawn as only the forearm (with the radius and ulna combined as one), because this segment is the body segment of interest, with the elbow as the axis of rotation (see Fig. 2.4B). It is important to note the position and orientation of the object by defining a coordinate system.

Applied forces are then identified and considered. Arrows representing the force vectors are drawn at every point where two (or more) bodies interact or join (see Fig. 2.4C). Recalling that internal forces are those that hold a rigid body together, two examples within the human body are muscle contractions and bony contact at a joint line. Internal forces are further examined with the concept of stress, which is introduced in a later section of the chapter. External forces can be the weight of an object, friction, or gravity applied at the center of mass of a body segment. In a simplified situation, flexion of the elbow is counteracted by the weight of the forearm itself and the weight of the dumbbell. The point of application of the forearm weight is at the segment's center of gravity. Commonly this point is determined from anthropometric data. The point of application of the biceps force on the forearm is its tendon insertion. The remaining force is the result of contact with the distal end of the humerus and the proximal end of the forearm, whereby the point of contact is approximately at the joint surface of the bones. These forces can then be further resolved into their respective components along the previously identified x- and y-axes (see Fig. 2.4D).

In addition to forces, the forearm experiences various applied moments. Because the points of application for the forces are known, the distances of each force along the forearm from the axis of rotation—the elbow—is also known (see Fig. 2.4E). Using these distances as moment arm values, the next step is to identify moments created by each force. The direction of the moment is relative to the applied force and its relationship to the axis of rotation. No moments are generated by the forces at the elbow because their moment arms are zero (see Fig. 2.4F). Once all the forces and moments applied to the body or body segment of interest are identified, they can be summed to determine the resultant force and moment. When the body is in a state of static equilibrium, the resultant forces and moments sum to zero, according to Newton's third law of motion.

Ligament and Joint Contact Forces

These concepts of static analyses can be applied not only to whole-body analyses but also at the joint and tissue level. For the typical joint, forces can be related to compression and shear. For example, when a person is standing with the knee in full extension, the tibial plateau and femoral condyles experience compressive forces in the normal direction to each articular surface. However, an increased shear force is experienced during an anterior drawer test or when stopping quickly in a sporting event. Shear forces are experienced in the tangential direction along the tibial plateau. These forces are not only experienced between the bony structures but also transmitted through the soft tissue structures. During an anterior drawer test or quick stop, the ACL can become significantly loaded to resist anterior tibial translation and provide stability at the joint. The ACL becomes loaded as a result of a generated tensile force within the ligament to maintain equilibrium. However, after an injury such as an ACL rupture, opposing shear forces cannot be transferred through the ligament, and thus equilibrium cannot be maintained at the joint without excessive translation, resulting in anterior instability.

DYNAMICS

Based on the equations from Newton's second law of motion, dynamic analyses evaluate bodies in motion and can be divided into two subgroups: kinematics and kinetics. For dynamic systems, the forces and moments do not have a net value of zero, which violates the principle of equilibrium, and thus a different approach must be taken. Kinematics simply describes the motion of bodies, without regard to the factors that cause or affect the motion, by characterizing the geometric and time-dependent aspects of the motion. Conversely, kinetics is based on kinematics but includes the effects of forces and moments. Motion analyses and sports mechanics typically involve dynamic systems.

Kinematics

Simply stated, kinematics deals with motions without regard to forces and moments. These motions include translations and rotations. Translations are simply the linear motions in which all the parts of a rigid body move simultaneously in the same direction as every other point in that body and at the same velocity. Rotations are the angular motions of a rigid body along a circular path and about an axis of rotation. During passive knee flexion, the tibiofemoral joint undergoes both linear and angular motions. As the knee progresses through the ROM, the tibia experiences rotation in the sagittal plane, and simultaneously, the point of contact between the tibial and femoral articular surfaces translates in the posterior direction. Although flexion is the primary angular motion, internal tibial rotation also occurs, which exemplifies the complex motion that can occur at a single joint.

Linear and Angular Kinematics

The spatial components used to describe linear kinematics are position, distance, and displacement. Position is a vector that simply defines the location of the object in space relative to a reference frame, commonly the center of a joint or a point of contact. Once the initial position changes, the object has moved a specified distance and displacement. Distance is a scalar quantity that describes the length of the entire path traversed. Displacement is a vector quantity (d) defining the shortest distance (straight line) between the starting and ending positions of the object independent of the path taken (see Fig. 2.1C). Additionally, temporal descriptions of linear kinematics are speed, velocity, and acceleration. Velocity is a vector quantity (v) describing the rate of change of the position with respect to time, whereas speed is a scalar quantity equal to the magnitude of the velocity vector (see Fig. 2.1D). Furthermore, acceleration is also a vector quantity (a) that describes the rate of change of velocity with respect to time, but it is commonly used to express an increase or decrease in speed (see Fig. 2.1E).

Angular kinematics is experienced when a change in angular position occurs such that the body undergoes rotational motion about an axis of rotation. The angular distance through which the body moves is equal to the length of the angular path. Angular kinematics can describe rotatory motion for a body segment, such as the lower leg during a kick (see Fig. 2.1A), in addition to the body as a whole, such as for a gymnast swinging on the bar to perform a giant circle. Descriptors used for these motions with respect to time are angular position, displacement, distance, velocity, and acceleration. These terms are similar to those used for linear kinematics, but they apply to a rotatory motion (see Fig. 2.1C–E). The lower leg undergoes large changes in angular velocity (ω) and acceleration (α) throughout the ROM for activities such as running, swimming, or kicking a soccer ball. Most general movements in the body are a combination of both linear and angular motion. For example, during a normal gait cycle, the lower extremities translate and rotate. Similarly, during athletics, combined motions are clearly illustrated during pitching, as the glenohumeral joint creates an instantaneous axis of rotation when the ball is swung along an imaginary arc about the shoulder in addition to being propelled forward.

Relative Motion

When considering forces and moments applied to a body, it is important to know the relative relationship in terms of both position and orientation for the individual bodies to each other in addition to the overall environment. An illustration of this concept is that a moving object may appear to have a different motion for two different observers depending on their location to the moving object. Knowing relative relations allows for an accurate description of the system when solving for unknown forces by establishing a frame of reference, or coordinate system. If a frame of reference is not identified, the measurements become irrelevant. A frame of reference describes the position of one body with respect to another whereby a relative measurement can be performed. This measurement is made by comparing the change in position and orientation of the object to the reference frame. For example, the position and orientation of the femur can be defined relative to the pelvis when describing motions of the hip or of the tibia with respect to the femur during kicking (see Fig. 2.1B).

Joint Motions

Motion at an articular surface can be described in terms of three motions that exist as a result of convex surfaces moving on a concave surface (Fig. 2.5). A *rolling motion* occurs when the bone with the convex surface rotates to cause a change in the point of contact for both articular surfaces in addition to a corresponding linear motion. A ball experiences this type of motion when it is rolled across a smooth surface. A *sliding motion* is experienced when one articular surface translates across the other with no rotation and progressively changes the point of contact. Sliding occurs when a box is pushed across a smooth surface. A *spinning motion* occurs when there is a single point of contact on the fixed surface and the point of contact changes on the rotating surface that does not undergo any linear motion. Spinning can be experienced on an automobile tire when the tire is rotating but the automobile is not moving forward or backward because of ice on the road. For certain joints, a combination of two or all three of these motions occurs. The motion achieved at a joint is based on the shape of the articular surface.

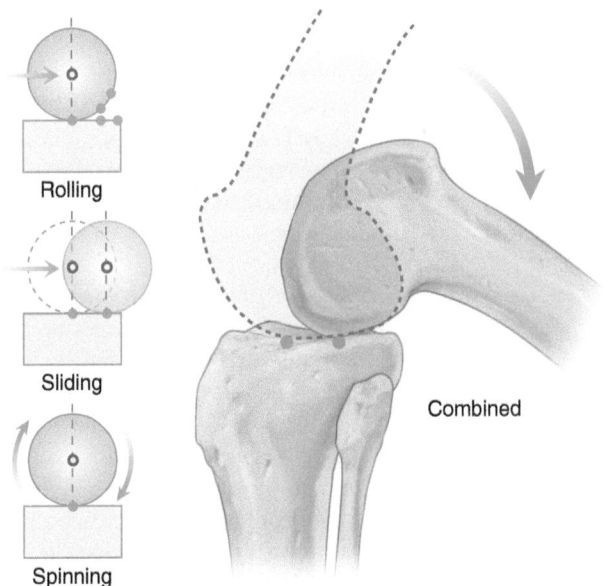

Fig. 2.5 Three fundamental motions that occur between articular surfaces. The point of contact changes on both articular surfaces during a rolling motion. The point of contact on the moving surface remains constant during a sliding motion. A single point of contact occurs on the fixed surface during a spinning motion. Some joints, such as the tibiofemoral joint, experience up to all three of these motions simultaneously.

For example, at the tibiofemoral joint during flexion, the knee experiences femoral condylar rollback on the tibial plateau. This phenomenon encompasses all three motions (rolling, sliding, and spinning) through flexion rotation, posterior translation, and external rotation, respectively, of the femur relative to the tibia. Although it is important and beneficial to understand the translations and rotations occurring at a joint, it can also be beneficial to understand the forces and moments associated with the observed translations and rotations, thus introducing the necessity of kinetic analyses.

Kinetics

Kinetics is the branch of mechanics that describes the effect of forces and moments on the body by utilizing Newton's second law of motion. More specifically, by using kinetics, it is possible to determine the forces and moments on a joint produced by mass, muscle tension, soft tissue loading, and externally applied loads. The appropriate range of joint loading that can be considered noninjurious can also be determined using kinetic analyses. Conversely, situations can be identified that produce excessively high moments and forces that exceed these limits, thus leading to musculoskeletal injuries. If an excessive valgus moment is experienced at the knee because of contact during a sport such as football, the medial collateral ligament may become overloaded and rupture in an attempt to maintain stability and resist the applied load. High forces can also be applied internally by overloading tendons as a result of extreme muscle tension.

CLASSES OF MECHANICS

Mechanics is the study of forces and their effects on motion. Depending on the system being studied, different branches of

mechanics may apply. When examining the behavior of solid bodies, such as the forces acting on human limbs and their motions, rigid body mechanics may apply. When examining the effects of a body moving through air or water, fluid mechanics are applicable.

Rigid Body Mechanics

In rigid body mechanics, it is assumed that any deformation caused by forces acting on a body is negligible. By assuming that a body is nondeformable—that the distance between any two points in the body will remain constant for any given translation or rotation—any changes in the shape of the body due to an applied force can be ignored, making kinematic analyses much simpler. No material in the human body can truly be considered a rigid body because all tissues undergo some degree of deformation, and thus it is important to note when the rigid body assumption is applicable. If the deformations experienced by a body are much smaller than the translations or rotations of that body, then the rigid-body principle can be applied. For example, when analyzing gait, the translations and rotations of the lower extremity will be much greater than any deformations experienced by the segments of the lower extremity, allowing each segment to be treated as a rigid body. Similarly, when using training equipment such as during weight lifting (see Fig. 2.4), the bar and limb segments of the upper extremity can be considered rigid bodies to allow for kinematic and kinetic analyses because any translations or rotations are much greater than any deformation in the equipment or limbs. Additionally, if one material is much stiffer than another, the stiffer material can be considered to be a rigid body that undergoes no deformation. For example, when performing mechanical testing of a joint complex, such as the femur–medial collateral ligament–tibia complex, the bones can be considered rigid bodies because they are much stiffer than the ligament tissue.

Fluid Mechanics

Fluid mechanics takes the concepts of statics and dynamics for solid bodies and applies them to fluids in order to study their behavior under applied forces and displacements. The term *fluid* refers to both gases and liquids and can be defined as a material that flows freely as the result of the application of a force and cannot support shear stresses. The most important parameter describing the behavior of a fluid is its viscosity (μ), a measure of how a fluid resists flow because of an applied force. Certain fluids, such as blood, have higher viscosities, whereas other fluids, such as air, have very low viscosities that can be considered to have negligible resistance. The viscosity of blood depends on its cellular content; when hematocrit levels rise above normal, blood viscosity rises and flow becomes more resistant to the forces pumping it through the body, leading to higher blood pressure as the heart works harder to pump blood through the body. During respiration, viscosity contributes to airflow patterns through the trachea and bronchi, relating to resistance of airflow. Although the viscosity of the air does not change, changes in the airway diameters due to disease can increase resistance to airflow, leading to respiratory pathology.

Additionally, movement of a solid object through fluid can result in the phenomenon of "drag," or fluid resistance, which reduces the velocity of the body. Drag is dependent on both the surface area exposed to the fluid in the direction of movement and on the velocity of the object: the greater the velocity and surface area, the greater the fluid resistance. At the whole-body level, water resists the movement of the body while swimming, and air resists the movement of sprinters traveling at high speeds. To reduce the effects of drag, athletes position their bodies during running or sprinting to reduce the surface area of their bodies perpendicular to the direction of motion.

Fluids can be considered to be either Newtonian or non-Newtonian. Newtonian fluids, such as water or air, exhibit a linear relationship between force applied to the fluid and the fluid deformation rate. Non-Newtonian fluids do not exhibit this relationship, an example being blood, as a result of its composition of particles (cells) suspended in aqueous plasma. The importance of Newtonian versus non-Newtonian flow relates to being able to accurately predict the behavior of fluids in the body, particularly blood. Depending on the size of the vessel, Newtonian blood flow may be assumed in some cases even if the fluid is non-Newtonian. The accurate prediction of blood flow patterns is important for understanding how abnormal blood flow can lead to atherosclerosis or low blood perfusion in tissues.

Viscoelasticity

A tissue is viscoelastic when it possesses to some degree both solid-like characteristics, such as elasticity and strength, and liquid-like characteristics, such as flow depending on temperature, time, rate, and amount of loading. Most tissues within the musculoskeletal system demonstrate at least some degree of viscoelasticity. After plotting the load-elongation results of a nondestructive tensile load, there remains a region between the loading and unloading curves that is known as hysteresis and clearly shows the time-dependent effects that viscoelasticity introduces (Fig. 2.6). Preconditioning with repeated loading and unloading of the tissue decreases this area of hysteresis and

maximizes elongation of the tissue, which is why athletes precondition the tissues in their bodies by completing repetitive stretching activities.

A viscoelastic material experiences the phenomena of creep and stress-relaxation. *Creep* describes a progressive increase in elongation of a material when exposed to a constant load over time (Fig. 2.7A). In simple terms, creep can be considered the tendency of a material to move or deform in response to a constant stress. Conversely, with stress-relaxation, a decrease in load occurs over time upon application of a constant elongation (see Fig. 2.7B). Stress-relaxation is the phenomenon that occurs in a material to relieve stress under a constant strain due to the liquid-like characteristic of viscoelasticity. After a period of time, for both creep and stress-relaxation, the tissue will reach an equilibrium state of elongation and load, respectively.

A practical use of both stress-relaxation and creep in the clinic is for initial graft tensioning of ligament or tendon reconstructions. Over time it is impractical to expect that the initial graft tension will be maintained after being fixed. The length of the graft will inevitably increase from its original length because of a creep response. Moreover, the rate of loading is important because a faster loading rate will result in greater stiffness. Viscoelasticity is also experienced in the articular cartilage of the knee. For example, as the rate of compressive loading increases, such as during running activities, the tissue becomes much stiffer.[2] This increase in stiffness allows for improved protection to the underlying bone while forces at the joint are high. Overall there is not a substantial strain rate dependency on tendons and ligaments; however, bones exhibit large changes in stiffness with increases in the rate of loading. In addition, bone has a greater compressive strength than tensile strength, which is advantageous during sporting activities when a sudden powerful blow may occur to a portion of the body.

BIOMECHANICAL METHODS

In traditional approaches to evaluating both static and dynamic systems, it is assumed that each object in the system is a rigid body. Biomechanics accounts for the biologic materials of the musculoskeletal system in a more realistic manner by considering that load is experienced at the tissue level and that these tissues are deformable. These biologic materials include both soft (articular cartilage, tendons, ligaments, capsular tissues) and hard (bone) tissues. Tissue structures that have been weakened by disease or trauma may not be able to adequately resist the loads that are applied.

Structural Properties

Structural properties are represented by the mechanics of a structure that may incorporate multiple materials or tissue types, including the response of this complex to tensile, shear, and compressive loading. For example, the structural properties of the femur-ACL-tibia complex can be determined in response to a tensile load to assess its load-elongation behavior. To do this, a tensile force (F) is applied to the bone-ligament-bone complex, causing the tissue to become stretched until the complex ruptures. While loading is applied, the corresponding increase of length

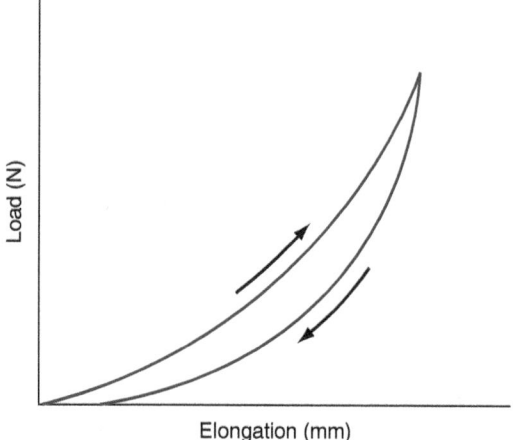

Fig. 2.6 Load-elongation curve of a biologic soft tissue in response to the application of a tensile load. The area between the loading and unloading curves represents the energy absorbed by the tissue during this loading regimen, or hysteresis.

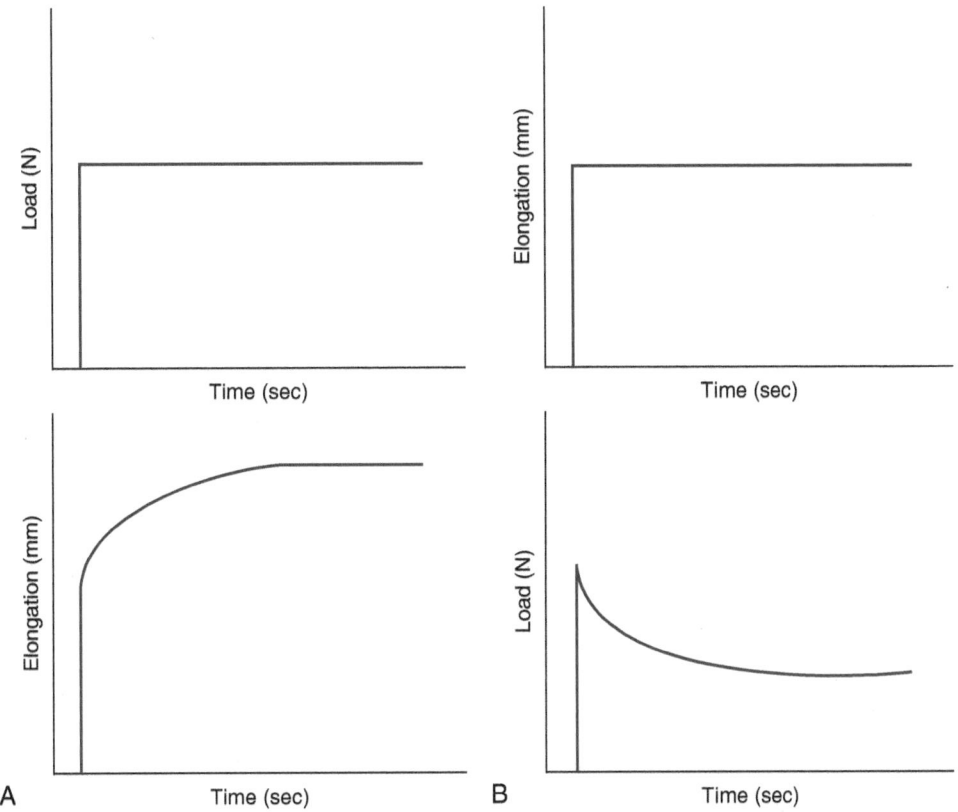

Fig. 2.7 Viscoelastic phenomena exhibited by biologic tissues include creep (A), that is, response due to a constant applied load, and stress-relaxation (B), that is, response due to a constant applied elongation over some time.

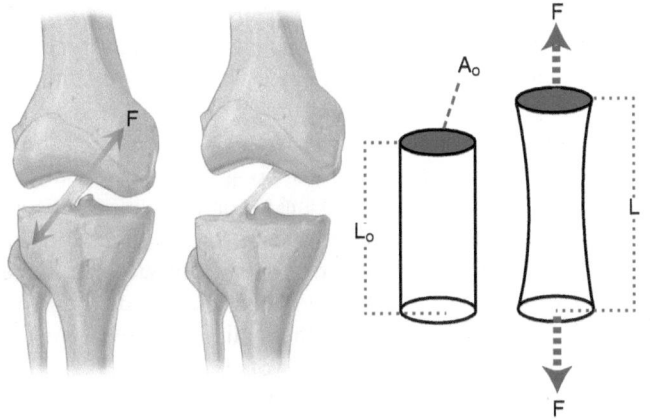

Fig. 2.8 Tensile loading along the longitudinal axis of the anterior cruciate ligament causes a change in length from its initial length (L_0) to an elongated state (L). A_0, Cross-sectional area; F, applied force.

is measured (Fig. 2.8). The resulting nonlinear load-elongation curve that is typical of biologic soft tissues consists of four primary regions (Fig. 2.9A). As the tensile load is first applied, the relationship between load and elongation is nonlinear and is referred to as the *toe* region. This level of loading is typically experienced during a clinical examination as normal fiber recruitment occurs. However, with increasing loads, the relationship becomes more linear and represents loading experienced during daily and sporting activities. The slope of this linear region of the curve is known as the *stiffness*. When the soft tissue begins to sustain more load than the structure can support, plastic deformation begins to occur. Finally, the entire structure approaches the failure region and completely ruptures. The point at which failure occurs is known as the *ultimate load*. Another structural property is the energy absorbed as a result of loading of the tissue, which is determined by the area under the load-elongation curve.

Mechanical Properties

It is also important to understand the mechanical response of an individual tissue or material, which is independent of specimen geometry, specifically of the cross-sectional area and initial length, by using normalized load and deformation parameters. Mechanical properties can be used to evaluate the quality of the tissue when making comparisons between normal, injured, and healing states and are represented by the stress-strain relationship. *Stress* is defined as the amount of force applied per unit area and is one of the most basic engineering principles. *Strain* can be considered a dimensionless measure of the degree of deformation and is defined as the change in length per unit length. Specimens with a greater length can withstand more total deformation, whereas specimens with a larger cross-sectional area can carry loads of greater magnitude. The mechanical properties can be derived from a plot of the stress and strain data and may include modulus, ultimate strength, ultimate strain, and strain energy density. Stress-strain relationships are obtained

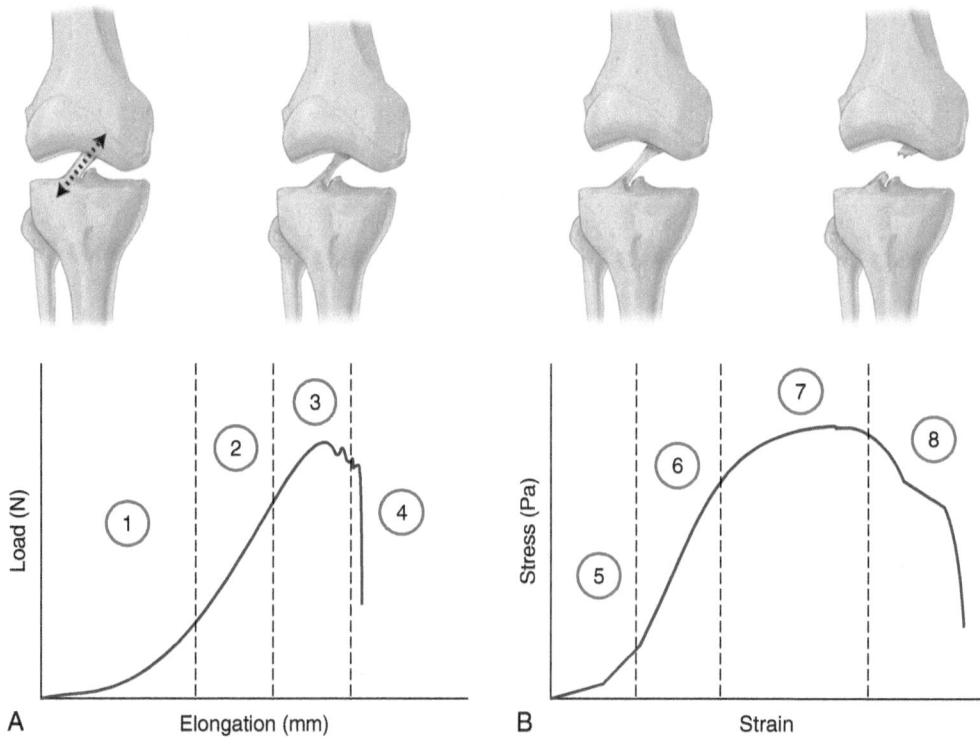

Fig. 2.9 (A) Load-elongation curve of a bone-ligament-bone complex in response to tensile loading characterizing its structural properties. Regions 1, 2, 3, and 4 correspond to the toe region, linear region, partial failure of the complex, and complete rupture of the complex, respectively. The loading of the tensile-bearing structure during activities of daily living will remain in regions 1 and 2. (B) Stress-strain curve of the ligament substance that characterizes its mechanical properties. Regions 5, 6, 7, and 8 correspond to the toe region, linear region, partial failure of the material, and complete rupture of the material, respectively. *Pa,* Pascal.

experimentally during tensile, compressive, or shear loading of the excised tissue.

There are four distinct regions along a stress-strain curve for biologic tissues (see Fig. 2.9B). A typical stress-strain curve begins with a nonlinear toe region (region 5). Stretching of the crimped collagen fibrils occurs within this region as the fibers are being drawn taut before significant tension can be measured. Strain becomes linearly proportional to stress in region 6, and the slope of the curve in this region can be calculated to determine the tangent modulus of the tissue. The area under the curve within this region can be referred to as the *strain energy density*. The tissue returns to its original length or shape once the stress is removed within this zone, which is usually reached during most daily activities. Furthermore, the energy used to deform the tissue is released when the applied stress is removed. When the tissue experiences extreme and abnormally large strain, the tissue undergoes only a marginal increase in corresponding stress (region 7). It is at this point that the tissue begins experiencing microscopic failures. The area under this region of the curve represents plastic deformation energy. Once the tissue undergoes this amount of deformation, the tissue does not recover and return to its original state in its entirety upon release of the deforming stress. If the tissue continues to deform, it will eventually experience complete failure (region 8). The mechanical properties of a tissue can be used to evaluate injured and healing states. When ligament repair is being evaluated, the medial collateral

ligament has much lower modulus and maximum stress mechanical properties during the healing process after rupture, although it shows some improvement over time without full recovery.[3]

To determine the mechanical properties of a knee cruciate ligament, a tensile load is applied along the long axis of the excised tissue sample after measuring the original cross-sectional area of the tissue (see Fig. 2.8). When a load is applied in the direction perpendicular to the tissue structure such that there is only a linear change in deformation, the load and deformation are considered to be axial stress and strain, respectively. As the load is applied along the long axis of the ACL in Fig. 2.8, a decrease in the cross-sectional area at the midsubstance occurs in response to an increase in the overall length (L) of the ligament from the initial length (L0). This response is important to consider in converting load data, a structural property, to stress data, a mechanical property, because the structure is changing dimensions throughout the testing. In calculating the mechanical properties, these changes are often ignored and the original, initial conditions are used. Compressive loading is commonly used to test bone or articular cartilage, whereas tensile and shear testing may be used for connective structures (e.g., tendons, ligaments, and capsular tissues).

Shear stress and strain act parallel to the surface of the tissue (Fig. 2.10), and the body is observed to deform into a rhomboid with sides equal to 1 if the body is originally a unit cube. Shear strain can be measured as the angular change (γ) at any point

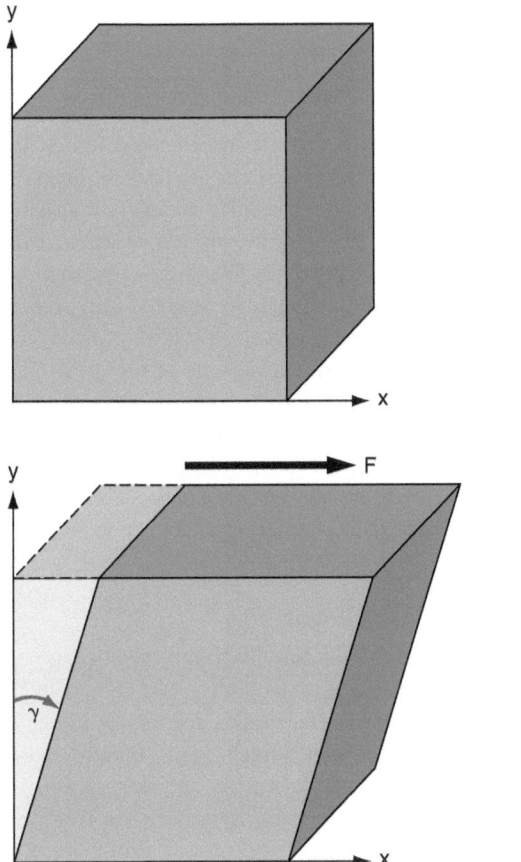

Fig. 2.10 Applying a shear force *(F)* to the top of a cube results in deformation from the *y*-axis through an angle, γ, in the direction of the load.

in the body owing to the applied shear force (F). Experimental shear loading of knee articular cartilage has shown that loading parallel to the articular cartilage surface may lead to the degeneration of cartilage and osteoarthritis.[4]

Factors Affecting Biomechanical Properties

Structural and mechanical properties can be significantly affected by both biologic and testing-related factors. The age and activity level of the person from whom the specimen was acquired are examples of biologic factors, and tissue storage and gripping are examples of testing-related factors. As a child or adolescent matures toward skeletal maturity, tendon and ligament tissue modulus increases slowly, but the maximum stiffness rapidly increases because of increasing tissue size.[5] In addition, the failure mode is predominantly through the bone attachment rather than in the midsubstance in growth and development.[6] However, after skeletal maturity, both modulus and maximum strain decrease two- and threefold, respectively, up to the age of 50 years, and the primary failure mode changes to midsubstance rupture. Beyond age 50 years, the primary failure mode is bony avulsion.[7] Donor activity level can have a significant biologic effect on the structural and mechanical properties. Tissue samples obtained from donors who have been immobilized or inactive for an extended period possess tissue stiffness and strength that is significantly less than that for control samples.[8,9] These factors

can influence the structural and mechanical properties and must be taken into account when performing an experiment.

Although testing-related factors can also influence the final structural and mechanical properties, these factors are controllable.

Tissue Storage

Improper tissue storage can significantly degrade the tissue's properties. To ensure that the tested tissue better represents the in vivo tissue, the tissue should be stored below −15°C for a minimal duration, and the number of freeze-thaw cycles should be kept at a minimum. These conditions help slow the release of proteinases from the cells, thus maintaining the extracellular matrix. The temperature at which the test is performed will also influence the structural and mechanical properties. Ligaments are stiffer at room temperature compared with body temperature.

Testing Rate

The rate at which the tissue is strained will alter the tissue's properties. Ligaments and tendons are mildly rate-sensitive, producing only a 10% to 15% increase in stiffness for a ×100 increase in strain rate.[10] By contrast, bone is more rate-sensitive, showing greater than 25% increase in stiffness for a ×100 increase in strain rate.[11]

Stiffness Versus Flexibility Testing

To examine the functional role of individual joint structures, researchers have used stiffness- and flexibility-based testing methods. For stiffness-based testing, a displacement (either translations, rotations, or a combination) is applied to the joint and the resulting forces and moments are recorded. The structure of interest is removed, and the same displacement is applied to the joint. The change in forces and moments is attributed to the structure that was removed. In flexibility-based testing, however, known forces, moments, or a combination are applied to the joint, and the resulting displacements are recorded. Once again, the structure of interest is removed, and the same force-moment profile is applied. The displacement change is attributed to the structure of interest. These two tests provide valuable information about the role of individual structures such as the forces and moments developed during activities of daily living (stiffness testing) or the structure responsible for restraining excessive motions (flexibility testing). A disadvantage of the flexibility testing method is that it is sequence-dependent, meaning that the role of each structure is influenced by the structures that have previously been cut. For the stiffness-based testing, the contribution of an individual structure can be overestimated if this structure physically interacts with adjacent tissues. An example is the wrapping of the ACL and posterior cruciate ligament as the knee extends. If the ACL is removed, the forces and moments provided by the posterior cruciate ligament also change because the constraint provided by the ACL is now gone. The change in forces and moments is greater than what is truly generated by the ACL.

Practical Application

The concepts presented throughout this chapter provide a way of understanding and quantifying how the human body operates to perform activities of daily living. This information can be used in orthopedic sports medicine to improve athletic performance, prevent injury, and develop surgical reconstruction techniques.

Improving Performance

Endurance is an important part of performance for any athletic activity. As activity is sustained over time, energy stores within the body are depleted, leading to fatigue. To postpone fatigue, energy expended in the activity should be minimized. For example, proper posture in cycling decreases the air resistance that must be overcome by the cyclist. Another example involves energy recuperation through the use of muscle and tendon elastic energy during running. As the foot of a runner strikes the ground, the force of the impact elastically elongates the muscles and tendons of the leg, allowing them to store energy to be released at toe-off. By properly preconditioning these tissues prior to activity, a greater proportion of impact energy can be stored, lessening the amount of active energy that must be expended by the runner's legs to achieve the same performance. Biomechanical analysis is also useful for maximizing force output, as in striking a baseball with a bat or throwing a football. As coaches and trainers are well aware, the relative positioning of each body segment is extremely important in generating the maximum moments between segments that will translate to physical power, or the rate of doing work.

Injury Prevention

Understanding the normal forces and moments or displacements applied to different structures surrounding joints—as well as their structural and mechanical properties—can be powerful in preventing injuries. In addition, analyses of tissue failure can allow clinicians and researchers to develop devices and training protocols to minimize injury risk. A high rate of collateral knee ligament injury among football linemen was a driver for the development of protective knee braces. Female athletes' greater risk of ACL rupture has led to the development of muscle training programs designed to provide better dynamic stabilization and to reduce the number of ACL ruptures. Additionally, normal biomechanical data are also useful during the creation of rehabilitation protocols. A rehabilitation protocol that maintains ROM and muscle strength is advantageous to the long-term healing of the patient. However, overaggressive rehabilitation can lead to failure of the repair. Knowledge of normal biomechanical properties can be used to design a regimen that maintains motion and muscle tone while also protecting the susceptible repair.

Surgical Reconstruction

The purpose of surgical reconstruction is to restore function by replacing nonfunctional tissue with a graft or other implant. However, to adequately restore function, it is important to understand the mechanics and biomechanical properties of the original tissues and whatever material is being used to replace them. Any materials being used to replace natural tissues, such as tendons or ligaments, must be able to function under the same ROM experienced by those connective tissues while also

maintaining adequate strength and stiffness. For example, the ACL is part of a complex loading environment experiencing both shear and longitudinal stresses during normal gait; it must resist anterior translation of the tibia with respect to the femur. The graft choice for ACL reconstruction must match the stiffness of the original tissue to sufficiently resist anterior translation of the tibia for the forces and moments experienced during gait. However, it must also be compliant enough to allow for the normal range of knee motion. Time-dependent viscoelastic properties of the graft must also be taken into account because any amount of creep occurring after the surgical reconstruction can result in increased translations at the joint. Similarly, for acromioclavicular joint reconstruction after shoulder separation, the structural properties of the graft construct must match the stiffness of the acromioclavicular and coracoclavicular ligaments to provide stability for the scapula without restricting normal ROM or failing under normal loading conditions for the shoulder.

Functional Tissue Engineering

Although researchers have developed novel tissue engineering therapies since the late 1980s, surgeons remain concerned about the fragility of tissue-engineered constructs (TECs) and their efficacy in patients after surgery.[12] In 2000, "functional tissue engineering" (FTE) was advanced, so that engineers, biologists, and surgeons might develop design criteria to judge potential TECs. Central to FTE was a set of core principles,[13,14] including the need to "establish in vivo load and deformation histories for native tissues under a wide range of activities of daily living (ADLs)," "establish safety factors and relevant biomechanical properties for native tissues," and compare the properties of repairs with similar histories for native tissues. FTE has been applied to the repair of numerous load-bearing tissues, including articular cartilage[15] and tendon.[16,17] Researchers have determined in vivo forces in the goat ACL and patellar tendon for numerous activities of daily living,[18] as well as in the rabbit flexor profundus tendon, patellar tendon, and Achilles tendon.[13,14,19–21] These studies revealed that although tendons can experience a range of in vivo forces up to 40% of failure force,[22] ligaments such as the ACL routinely never exceed 7% to 10% of failure force.[18] These studies established "functional" loading and deformation regions in which tissues normally reside for various ADLs.[23] Tissue engineers could thus provide a minimum set of design criteria for specific tissue applications by (1) knowing the peak in vivo forces for a tissue and adding a safety factor to account for still higher unexpected forces not normally experienced by the tissue and (2) knowing the tangent stiffness or slope of the force-deformation curve for the tissue during failure testing. Applying these two design criteria (exceeding peak in vivo forces with safety factor and matching tangent stiffness) has led to improved cell-collagen TECs through changes in cell and collagen density and through mechanical preconditioning of the constructs before surgery.[23–26] This strategy allows for rapid determination of whether a repair is acceptable by one or both criteria or requires redesign. Parallel in vitro studies using TECs that contain cells from the same animals as those for repair assessment have also permitted the establishment of positive correlations between in vitro stiffness and in vivo repair stiffness.[23] These correlations, in turn, have permitted optimization of the conditions that most enhance in vitro stiffness.[27] These new conditions can then be periodically evaluated to determine changes in repair outcome.

Additional studies in FTE are now under way to meet new challenges. Investigators will need to broaden their design criteria to include biologic and mechanical measures. This approach requires paradigms that focus on the factors (such as gene expression, protein synthesis, and collagen alignment) that greatly affect repair results. Furthermore, additional research is needed to more faithfully simulate ADLs for tissues that typically experience complex loading patterns (e.g., the cruciate ligaments).[28] Finally, the process of developing these cell-based therapies must be accelerated while controlling costs so that FTE can be used to treat patients in the near future.

CONCLUSIONS

This chapter introduced the basic terminology and concepts of statics, dynamics, and mechanics of materials using examples relevant to sports medicine. With these foundations, the reader should be able to communicate using common units of measure to describe various physical quantities. The chapter also presents concepts that illustrate how to approach both a static and dynamic system to calculate unknown forces and moments experienced on the body through use of a free-body diagram. A description of biologic materials within the musculoskeletal system is also presented. Although biomechanics has great depth and breadth, these concepts should allow the reader to begin making the link between sports medicine and biomechanics.

For a complete list of references, go to ExpertConsult.com.

SELECTED READINGS

Citation:

Abramowitch SD, Yagi M, Tsuda E, et al. The healing medial collateral ligament following a combined anterior cruciate and medial collateral ligament injury—a biomechanical study in a goat model. *J Orthop Res.* 2003;21:1124–1130.

Level of Evidence:

I

Summary:

Combined ACL reconstruction and MCL repair resulted in an ACL graft that lost force over time, overloading the MCL and producing an MCL with inferior biomechanical quality compared with an MCL after an isolated injury.

Citation:

Butler DL, Juncosa-Melvin N, Boivin GP, et al. Functional tissue engineering for tendon repair: a multidisciplinary strategy using mesenchymal stem cells, bioscaffolds, and mechanical stimulation. *J Orthop Res.* 2008;26:1–9.

Level of Evidence:

Review

Summary:

Through the principles of functional tissue engineering, tissue-engineered repairs have been created that produce tendon tissue that matched the normal tendon failure curve to 150% of the normal in vivo forces. During these studies, in vitro construct stiffness predicted final repair stiffness; however, additional biologic in vitro predictors of in vivo outcome are needed to continue advancing the field.

Citation:

Debski RE, Yamakawa S, Musahl V, et al. Use of robotic manipulators to study diarthrodial joint function. *J Biomech Eng.* 2017;139(2).

Level of Evidence:

Review

Summary:

An improved understanding of the structure and function of diarthrodial joints needs to be obtained to gain a better understanding of injury mechanisms and improve surgical procedures. Robotic testing systems have been developed to measure the resulting kinematics of diarthrodial joints as well as the in situ forces in ligaments and their replacement grafts in response to external loading conditions to achieve this purpose.

Citation:

Guilak F, Butler DL, Mooney D, et al. *Functional Tissue Engineering.* New York: Springer-Verlag; 2003:480.

Level of Evidence:

Book

Summary:

This book discusses the principles of functional tissue engineering and their application across different tissue systems.

Citation:

Nordin M, Frankel V, eds. *Basic Biomechanics of the Musculoskeletal System.* 2nd ed. Philadelphia: Lea & Febiger; 1989.

Level of Evidence:

Book

Summary:

This book provides a more in-depth discussion of biomechanics.

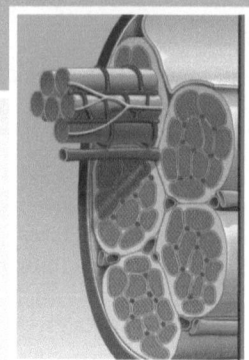

3

Basic Science of Graft Tissue in Sports Medicine

Mia Smucny, Carolyn M. Hettrich, Robert Westermann, Kurt Spindler

Graft tissue is widely used in sports medicine for soft tissue reconstruction and augmentation of ligaments and tendons. Understanding the physiology of fixation and incorporation of tendon and/or bone within the tunnels is important for the surgeon, because this knowledge can help guide postoperative rehabilitation and educate patients when they return to play. Many options exist for graft tissue, both as autografts and allografts, and for the processing of these grafts. The healing of such grafts has been most carefully studied in patients who have undergone anterior cruciate ligament (ACL) reconstruction, for whom a significantly increased rate of graft failure with allografts has been found clinically.[1,2]

AUTOGRAFT

Investigators have conducted numerous studies to examine graft incorporation and viability of autografts using the patellar tendon (PT) and semitendinosus (ST) in animal models. These grafts have been examined both individually and in comparison.

BONE-TENDON-BONE AUTOGRAFT

Several studies of patellar tendon autografts have been performed. A rabbit model of patellar tendon autografts by Amiel et al. demonstrated that PT autografts undergo a process of "ligamentization" and that cells responsible for this process were of extra-graft origin.[3] The investigators came to this conclusion because they found that the autografts were centrally acellular with a peripheral rim of cells at 2 weeks, progressed to having a central focal proliferation of cells at 3 weeks, and then progressed to cellular homogeneity by 4 weeks after surgery. Microscopically, the patellar tendon autografts gradually changed from having the properties of the patellar tendon to having those seen in the native ACL. By 30 weeks after surgery, an increase in type III collagen and glycosaminoglycan content was observed from the levels typically found in PTs to those found in native ACLs, and collagen-reducible cross-link analysis demonstrated that grafted tissue changed from the normal PT pattern of low dihydroxy-lysinonorleucine and high histidinohydroxymerodesmosine to the opposite pattern seen in the normal ACL.[3]

PT autograft healing was also studied in a goat model at 3 and 6 weeks postoperatively. The total anteroposterior (AP) translation significantly increased from 3 to 6 weeks, with in situ forces in the graft decreasing by as much as 22.2% at 6 weeks. At 3 weeks, the mode of failure was the graft pulling out of the tibial tunnel, which changed to a mix of midsubstance failures at 6 weeks. Histologic evaluations revealed progressive and complete incorporation of the bone block in the femoral tunnel but only partial incorporation of the tendinous part of the graft in the tibial tunnel. The investigators did not study any longer time points in this study.[4]

Lastly, in a rabbit model using medial one-third PT autografts, investigators concluded that on gross inspection the autografts did not resemble the control ACLs. Biomechanically, AP knee laxity was more than double that of the control knees at 52 weeks, and the strength of the PT autografts plateaued at 30 weeks, but the ultimate load to failure and stiffness never reached those of the control native ACLs. Histologically, the autografts progressed from being hypercellular with a random collagen fiber bundle organization to having a near normal cellularity with a more parallel collagen fiber bundle pattern.[5]

AUGMENTED AUTOGRAFT

In an attempt to augment the healing of bone-patellar tendon-bone (BPTB) autograft, Yasuda et al.[6] performed ACL reconstruction in the bilateral knees of 20 canines. The left knee either had a fibrin sealant with transforming growth factor–β and epidermal growth factor or fibrin sealant alone. The right knee served as a control, with no augmentation. These investigators found that the application of the growth factors increased the stiffness and maximum failure load of the femur-graft-tibia complex at 12 weeks, with no difference between the fibrin sealant alone and the control knees. A qualitative histologic analysis showed that most of the cells in the grafts treated with growth factors had spindle-shaped nuclei, whereas cells in the other grafts had round-shaped nuclei. The investigators concluded that these growth factors improved the structural properties.[6]

To examine the effect of collagen platelet composites and platelet concentration on BPTB autografts, Spindler et al.[7] placed a collagen-platelet composite around autologous PTs and compared these with goats that received the collagen scaffold only and their contralateral native knees. At 6 weeks after surgery, the average increase in AP laxity was 40% less in the collagen-platelet composite group than in the group that had collagen wrapped around their grafts alone at 30 degrees. Significant correlations were found between serum-platelet concentration and AP laxity, maximum load to failure, and graft stiffness. The authors concluded that use of a collagen-platelet composite with a BPTB autograft enhanced healing and that a higher serum-platelet count was inversely correlated with sagittal plane laxity and highly predictive of ACL reconstruction graft strength and stiffness at 6 weeks.[7]

SEMITENDINOSUS OR SOFT TISSUE AUTOGRAFT

Numerous studies have also been performed on ST autografts, with findings largely similar to those of the PT studies. In rabbits, bony fixation of the ST graft was complete by 26 weeks, but large differences persisted in the strength and stiffness of the graft compared with the native ACL and ST tendons at 52 weeks. By 52 weeks, the graft did not fail because of pullout from the tunnels, but rather by intrasubstance rupture.[8] In a study by Grana et al., it was found that failure of the graft occurred in the midsubstance rather than from pullout as early as 3 weeks postoperatively. The authors found that fixation occurs by an intertwining of graft and connective tissue, with anchoring to bone by collagenous fibers and bone formation in the tunnels that have the appearance of the Sharpey fibers seen in an indirect tendon insertion.[9] Papachristou et al.[10] examined the histologic changes that occurred between 3 and 12 weeks using ST tendons that were harvested without detachment from their tibial insertion and free ST autografts. They found that the ST tendon when harvested without detachment from the tibial insertion retained viability without graft necrosis, whereas the free tendon group did have necrosis of the graft 3 weeks after surgery, with progressive revascularization at 6 and 12 weeks postoperatively.[10]

Studies of ST autografts have also been performed in sheep models.[11,12] In one study it was found that the tendon graft was predominantly acellular at 2 weeks, with the core portion remaining necrotic even at 12 weeks. The area of necrosis had disappeared at 24 and 52 weeks. At all time points, the AP translation of the reconstructed knee remained significantly greater than that of the control subject, and the load to failure was still less than that of the control at 52 weeks.[12] In another study in sheep using ST autografts, the authors did not find evidence of any graft necrosis. They observed that the random collagen fiber orientation progressed to a longitudinal orientation from the peripheral to the central areas of the graft over the initial 12 weeks, with a uniform sinusoidal crimp pattern similar to that seen in the normal ACL in nearly half of each graft by 24 weeks, with further maturation at 52 weeks.[11]

The differences in healing between ST and BPTB autografts were studied in beagles. Soft tissue grafts were placed in the left knees, and BPTB grafts were placed in the right knee. The soft tissue graft was anchored to the tunnel wall with collagen fibers resembling Sharpey fibers by 12 weeks. In the BPTB graft, the bone plug was anchored with newly formed bone at 3 weeks, although osteocytes in the plug trabeculae were necrotic for 12 weeks. In load to failure testing of the soft tissue graft, the graft failed at the graft-bone interface at 3 weeks and then at the midsubstance by 6 weeks. In the BPTB graft, the graft failed at the graft-wall interface at 3 weeks and the proximal site in the

bone plug at 6 weeks. The ultimate failure load of the soft tissue graft was significantly inferior to that of the BPTB graft at 3 weeks, but a significant difference was not observed 6 weeks postoperatively.[13]

Marumo and colleagues evaluated the process of graft "ligamentization" in humans in the first study to address biochemical properties of autografts in living subjects after ACL reconstruction.[14] From a cohort of 50 patients who underwent "clinically effective" hamstring or BPTB reconstruction, biopsies of grafted tissue were collected at 4 to 6 months and 11 to 13 months postoperatively. These were compared with tissue samples from cadaveric native ACL, patellar tendon, and semitendinosus and gracilis tendons. The investigators found that the total collagen content and nonreducible/reducible crosslink ratios increased significantly during the postoperative period and closely resembled the native ACL by one year.[14]

ALLOGRAFT

Numerous studies also have been performed on allograft tendons in animal models. An important consideration in these studies is the processing of the allograft, which differs between the studies.

Freeze-dried BPTB allografts in a goat model were compared with contralateral controls. Allograft revascularization occurred within the first 12 weeks, and the grafts matured to resemble normal connective tissue within 26 weeks. Graft stiffness and maximum load to failure was 29% and 43% of the control values, respectively. The authors concluded that the results of freeze-dried PT allografts were biomechanically and biologically similar to the published results of PT autografts.[15]

Goertzen et al.[16] compared deep-frozen gamma-irradiated (2.5 mrad) BPTB allografts with argon gas protection to BPTB allografts without gamma irradiation in a canine model. At 12 months, the irradiated allografts had a load to failure that was 63.8% of the contralateral normal ACLs. The nonirradiated allografts had a load to failure of 69.1% of the load to failure of the control subjects. Histologic analysis demonstrated that the allografts appeared to be developing well-oriented collagen fibers compared with the normal ACL. A modified microangiographic technique demonstrated similar vascularity to normal ACL in the nonirradiated allograft, compared with slight hypervascularization in the irradiated group.[16]

Using a sheep model, Zimmerman et al.[17] compared frozen, untreated allografts to frozen grafts that were processed with a chloroform-methanol solvent extraction technique and another group of frozen tendons treated with a permeation-enhanced extraction technique. Two months after surgery, enhanced cellular repopulation was noted in both chemically treated allograft groups compared with the untreated grafts. Mechanical testing at 6 months after surgery showed statistically similar anterior drawer resistance in all grafted knees; however, the two chemically processed grafts had significantly decreased stiffness compared with the untreated grafts, and both treatment groups also tended to be weaker.[17]

Fromm et al.[18] investigated the revascularization and reinnervation of cryopreserved ACL allografts in a rabbit model. They found minimal immune response to the grafts, with considerable revascularization by the 24th postoperative week. Reinnervation was complete by 24 weeks.[18]

Arnoczky et al.[19] compared fresh and deep-frozen PT allografts in a dog model. Deep-frozen PT allografts appeared to undergo remodeling in a manner comparable with that observed in autogenous patellar-tendon grafts, with avascular necrosis followed by revascularization and cellular proliferation. At 1 year after reconstruction, the gross and histologic appearance of the deep-frozen patellar tendon allograft resembled that of a normal ACL. The fresh PT allografts incited a marked inflammatory and rejection response depicted by perivascular cuffing and lymphocyte invasion. The investigators concluded that the deep-frozen PT grafts were more likely to survive within the knee joint than the fresh allografts as a result of the absence of an obvious rejection response and the similarity of the remodeling process.[19]

Harris et al.[20] looked at tibial tunnel enlargement with allograft ACL reconstruction in a goat model. They found significant increases in tibial tunnel size within the first 6 weeks of healing. The increased tunnel size persisted up to 36 weeks with no further remodeling. Histologic analysis showed remodeling and incorporation of the bone plug in all cases by 18 weeks with fibrous attachment within the tunnel. All allografts had progressive ligamentization with tendon-to-tunnel wall biologic fixation with dense connective tissue. These investigators concluded that the tibial tunnel enlargement did not appear to affect the ultimate incorporation of the allograft on a histologic level.[20]

Freeze-dried bone-ACL-bone allografts were compared with control subjects that did not undergo surgery in a goat model. At 1 year after reconstruction, the reconstructed knees had a significantly greater total AP laxity than the control subjects. Stiffness was significantly less than in control subjects. The maximum load to failure was also significantly reduced in the allograft group. Histologic evaluation and microangiography of the allografts was similar to that of the native ACL.[21]

Jackson et al.[22] used deoxyribonucleic acid (DNA) probe analysis to determine the fate of donor cells in fresh BPTB allografts after transplantation in a goat model. They found that donor DNA was completely replaced by recipient DNA in the transplanted ligaments within a 4-week period.[22]

AUGMENTATION OF ALLOGRAFT

Because of decreased structural properties found in allografts, mesenchymal stem cells (MSCs) have been investigated as potential agents to enhance bone tunnel and tendon healing. In a study by Soon et al.,[23] bilateral ACL reconstructions were performed in a rabbit model using Achilles tendon allografts, with the graft on a single side being coated with autogenous MSCs in a fibrin glue carrier. These investigators found a significantly higher load to failure in the group treated with MSCs. Histologic analyses at 8 weeks showed mature scar tissue resembling Sharpey fibers in the control group and a mature zone of fibrocartilage blending from bone to the allograft in the MSC-treated group that resembled the normal ACL insertion.[23] Li et al.[24] also looked at modifying irradiated Achilles allografts in a rabbit model with autogenous MSCs or platelet-derived growth factor-β (PDGF-β) transfected MSCs. Bilateral ACL reconstructions were again

performed, with the left knee allograft being seeded with either MSCs or PDGF-β transfected MSCs. The right knee served as a control. Seeding the allograft with MSCs (auto or PGDF-β) was found to accelerate cellular infiltration and enhance collagen deposition.[24]

Fleming et al.[25] studied the effect of collagen-platelet composites on BPTB allografts in a porcine model. The collagen-platelet composite group was compared with animals receiving an allograft alone. After 15 weeks of healing, the AP laxity values of the reconstructed knees and the load to failure were superior in the collagen-platelet composite group compared with the group that received the allograft alone. In addition, no regions of necrosis were found in the collagen-platelet composite group, but regions of necrosis were found in the nonaugmented grafts.[25]

A BPTB allograft with synthetic polypropylene augmentation was compared with a fresh BPTB allograft and a cryopreserved BPTB allograft in a sheep model.[26] In this study, cryopreservation did not have any effect on graft characteristics. Gross and histologic examination did not reveal any significant differences between the augmented and nonaugmented groups at any of the time periods. The augmented group had significantly reduced AP translation at 52 weeks compared with the nonaugmented group. The ultimate tensile strength was significantly higher in the augmented group at 4 weeks, but at 52 weeks both groups had attained only 50% of the normal ACL strength.[26]

HEALING OF AUTOGRAFT VERSUS ALLOGRAFT

Three studies examining the difference between allografts and autografts have also been performed. All studies found a slower biologic incorporation for allografts, with decreased load to failure at 6- and 12-month time points. Jackson et al.[27] used similar-sized PT autografts and fresh-frozen allografts to reconstruct the ACL in goats. These autografts and allografts were evaluated at 6 weeks and 6 months postoperatively. The investigators found that whereas the structural and material properties of autografts and allografts at time zero were similar, differences in healing occurred during the first 6 months. The allografts demonstrated a greater decrease in their structural properties, a slower rate of biologic incorporation, and the prolonged presence of inflammatory cells. At 6 months the autograft had improved stability and increased strength to failure.[27] Dustmann et al.[28] and Scheffler et al.[29] found similar findings in sheep models when they compared soft tissue autografts with identical nonsterilized fresh-frozen allografts.[28,29] Revascularization and recellularization and reformation of the collagen crimp formation were significantly delayed at 6 and 12 weeks of healing compared with the autografts, but differences were less distinct at 52 weeks. At 52 weeks, the mechanical, structural, and AP laxity were worse in the allografts, but no difference was found in these qualities at early time points.[28,29]

Nikolaou et al.[30] found conflicting results in a dog model comparing autografts with cryopreserved allografts. They found no evidence that the cryopreservation had any effect on healing, with no difference between autografts and allografts in terms of their load to failure at 36 weeks. Revascularization approached normal by 24 weeks in both groups, and no evidence of structural degradation or immunological reaction was seen. These authors concluded that "a cryopreserved ACL allograft can provide the ideal material for ACL reconstruction."[30]

FUTURE DIRECTIONS

There has been renewed interest recently in the possibility of augmented native ACL repair. Murray and colleagues have developed a biologically enhanced acute primary repair that uses a whole blood-soaked collagen scaffold and suture stent to stabilize a provisional clot in the gap between the torn ACL ends.[31] Preclinical porcine studies have demonstrated a healed ACL repair with similar mechanical properties to an ACL reconstruction and less development of posttraumatic osteoarthritis.[32,33] The latter finding is subject to ongoing research on the underlying mechanism of cartilage protection—the complete interactions between collagen-platelet composites and the intra-articular tissues are yet unknown. The bio-enhanced repair technique has demonstrated safety in a small human feasibility study and has received Food and Drug Administration approval for a larger in-human clinical trial.[34]

SUMMARY

The intra-articular biologic and biomechanical behavior of both autografts and allografts for ACL reconstruction has been extensively researched. Several common features have emerged. First, a "ligamentization" of all these grafts occurs over months. Second, all the new cells populating the graft are derived from the recipient. Third, the weakest link in early time points (<4 weeks) for both BPTB and soft tissue grafts are the fixation points within tunnels, whereas after 6 weeks it is the failure of the grafts within joint or "midsubstance." Fourth, the bone heals more rapidly within the tunnels than soft tissue by "Sharpey-like fibers." Fifth, evidence shows that growth factor, collagen-platelet composite, and stem cells augment the biologic incorporation and enhance the structural properties of the grafts. Sixth, the majority of studies comparing autografts and allografts found that allografts have slower biologic incorporation and decreased structural properties. Finally, in animal models, freeze-dried BPTB, 2.5 mrad, and cryopreservation all were successful in ACL reconstructions; however, clinical results have not confirmed these observations.

For a complete list of references, go to ExpertConsult.com.

SELECTED READINGS

Citation:
Amiel D, Kleiner JB, Roux RD, et al. The phenomenon of "ligamentization": anterior cruciate ligament reconstruction with autogenous patellar tendon. *J Orthopaed Res.* 1986;4(2):162–172.

Level of Evidence:
Basic science

Summary:
A rabbit model of patellar tendon autografts demonstrated that patellar tendon autografts undergo a process of "ligamentization"

and that the cells responsible for this process were of extragraft origin.

Citation:
Arnoczky SP, Warren RF, Ashlock MA. Replacement of the anterior cruciate ligament using a patellar tendon allograft. An experimental study. *J Bone Joint Surg Am.* 1986;68(3):376–385.

Level of Evidence:
Basic science

Summary:
Comparison of fresh and deep-frozen patellar tendon (PT) allografts in a dog model showed that deep-frozen PT allografts appeared to undergo remodeling in a manner comparable with that observed in autogenous PT grafts, with avascular necrosis followed by revascularization and cellular proliferation. The fresh PT allografts incited a marked inflammatory and rejection response depicted by perivascular cuffing and lymphocyte invasion.

Citation:
Ballock RT, Woo SLY, Lyon RM, et al. Use of patellar tendon autograft for anterior cruciate ligament reconstruction in the rabbit—a long-term histologic and biomechanical study. *J Orthopaed Res.* 1989;7(4):474–485.

Level of Evidence:
Basic science

Summary:
This study used a rabbit model with patellar tendon (PT) autografts. The authors found that the anteroposterior knee laxity of the autografts was more than double that of the control knees at 52 weeks, and the strength of the PT autografts plateaued at 30 weeks, but the ultimate load to failure and stiffness never reached those of the control native anterior cruciate ligaments.

Citation:
Grana WA, Egle DM, Mahnken R, et al. An analysis of autograft fixation after anterior cruciate ligament reconstruction in a rabbit model. *Am J Sports Med.* 1994;22(3):344–351.

Level of Evidence:
Basic science

Summary:
This study of autografts in a rabbit model demonstrated that graft failure occurs in the midsubstance, not as a result of pullout as early as 3 weeks postoperatively, and that this fixation in the bone tunnels occurs by an intertwining of graft and connective tissue and anchoring to bone by collagenous fibers and bone formation in the tunnels that have the appearance of the Sharpey fibers seen in an indirect tendon insertion.

Citation:
Harris NL, Indelicato PA, Bloomberg MS, et al. Radiographic and histologic analysis of the tibial tunnel after allograft anterior cruciate ligament reconstruction in goats. *Am J Sports Med.* 2002;30(3):368–373.

Level of Evidence:
Basic science

Summary:
This study examined tibial tunnel enlargement with allograft anterior cruciate ligament reconstruction in a goat model. The

authors found significant increases in tibial tunnel size within the first 6 weeks of healing. The increased tunnel size persisted up to 36 weeks with no further remodeling.

Citation:

Jackson DW, Grood ES, Goldstein JD, et al. A comparison of patellar tendon autograft and allograft used for anterior cruciate ligament reconstruction in the goat model. *Am J Sports Med.* 1993;21(2):176–185.

Level of Evidence:

Basic science

Summary:

This study compared patellar tendon autografts and fresh-frozen allografts in a goat model. The structural and material properties of autografts and allografts at time zero were similar; however, the allografts demonstrated a greater decrease in their structural properties, a slower rate of biologic incorporation, and the prolonged presence of inflammatory cells. At 6 months the autograft had improved stability and increased strength to failure.

Citation:

Kaeding CC, Aros B, Pedroza A, et al. Allograft versus autograft anterior cruciate ligament reconstruction: predictors of failure from a MOON prospective longitudinal cohort. *Sports Health.* 2011;3(1):73–81.

Level of Evidence:

I

Summary:

This study of 1000 patients with 94% follow-up demonstrated that in 18-year-old patients, a failure rate of 20% occurred in patients who received allografts compared with a 6% failure rate in patients who received autografts. In 40-year-old patients, a failure rate of 3% occurred in patients who received autografts compared with a 1% failure rate in patients who received autografts. The number needed to harm from using allografts is seven for high school–aged patients.

Citation:

Marumo K, Saito M, Yamagishi T, et al. The "ligamentization" process in human anterior cruciate ligament reconstruction with autogenous patellar and hamstring tendons: a biochemical study. *Am J Sports Med.* 2005;33(8):1166–1173.

Level of Evidence:

II

Summary:

This study investigated the process of ligamentization of ACL autograft in living human specimens. They found that in a cohort of 50 subjects with either BTB or hamstring autograft, surgical biopsies at 1 year postoperatively confirmed that collagen content and nonreducible/reducible crosslink ratio more closely resembled that of the native ACL rather than patellar tendon or semitendinosus/gracilis tendon.

Citation:

Spindler KP, Murray MM, Carey JL, et al. The use of platelets to affect functional healing of an anterior cruciate ligament (ACL) autograft in a caprine ACL reconstruction model. *J Orthopaed Res.* 2009;27(5):631–638.

Level of Evidence:

Basic science

Summary:

The authors used bone-patellar tendon-bone autografts in a goat model and found that placing a collagen-platelet composite around an autologous patellar tendon resulted in an average increase in anteroposterior laxity that was 40% less in the collagen-platelet composite group than in the group that had collagen alone wrapped around their grafts.

Citation:

Tomita F, Yasuda K, Mikami S, et al. Comparisons of intraosseous graft healing between the doubled flexor tendon graft and the bone-patellar tendon-bone graft in anterior cruciate ligament reconstruction. *Arthroscopy.* 2001;17(5):461–476.

Level of Evidence:

Basic science

Summary:

The differences in healing between semitendinosus and bone-patellar tendon-bone (BPTB) autografts were studied in beagles. The soft tissue graft was anchored to the tunnel wall with collagen fibers resembling Sharpey fibers by 12 weeks. In the BPTB graft, the bone plug was anchored with newly formed bone at 3 weeks, although osteocytes in the plug trabeculae were necrotic for 12 weeks. In load to failure testing of the soft tissue graft, the graft failed at the graft-bone interface at 3 weeks and then at the midsubstance by 6 weeks. In the BPTB graft, the graft failed at the graft-wall interface at 3 weeks and the proximal site in the bone plug at 6 weeks.

Citation:

Zimmerman MC, Contiliano JH, Parsons JR, et al. The biomechanics and histopathology of chemically processed patellar tendon allografts for anterior cruciate ligament replacement. *Am J Sports Med.* 1994;22(3):378–386.

Level of Evidence:

Basic science

Summary:

This study compared frozen, untreated allografts with frozen grafts that were processed with a chloroform-methanol solvent extraction technique and another group of frozen tendons treated with a permeation-enhanced extraction technique. Mechanical testing 6 months after surgery showed statistically similar anterior drawer resistance in all grafted knees; however, the two chemically processed grafts had significantly decreased stiffness compared with the untreated grafts, and both treatment groups also tended to be weaker.

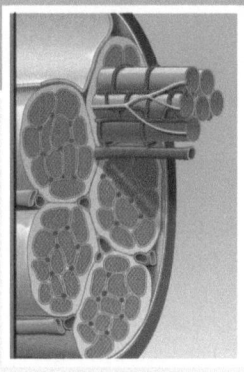

4

Basic Science of Implants in Sports Medicine

Elizabeth R. Dennis, Jon-Michael E. Caldwell, Sonya B. Levine,
Philip Chuang, Margaret Boushell, Stavros Thomopoulos,
Helen H. Lu, William N. Levine

Sports injuries in athletes are commonly associated with injury to soft tissues, specifically tendons, ligaments, menisci, and cartilage. Common tendon and ligament injuries in the physically active population include rotator cuff tears, Achilles tendinopathy, anterior cruciate ligament (ACL) tears, and lateral epicondylitis ("tennis elbow"). These injuries can be classified as either repetitive microtrauma, which is caused by overuse, or macrotrauma, which typically results from external physical impact.[1] Because each joint is a complex system that is made up of different types of tissue that work together, trauma or degeneration of one tissue often results in the injury to another tissue. For example, in the knee, a common sports-related injury such as an ACL tear is usually associated with subsequent damage to the meniscus and/or the neighboring articular cartilage. This in turn leads to a longer-term increased risk for osteoarthritis. Thus an understanding of tendons, ligaments, menisci, cartilage, and other joint soft tissues is essential for the clinical management of sports injuries.

Current options used to treat sports injuries in orthopedics include autografts, allografts, and tissue-engineered grafts. Autografts are harvested from the patient and remain the "gold standard" for reconstruction. However, they also have disadvantages, such as longer surgical time due to graft acquisition, along with the risk of donor-site morbidity. Allografts eliminate the need to harvest grafts on site and the risk of donor-site morbidity. Although they have been used successfully for musculoskeletal tissue reconstruction, they are not appropriate for every situation and have some limitations.[2-7] The major shortcomings of allografts are their limited availability, a lack of functional integration with the surrounding host tissue, and, although low, the potential risk of disease transmission or an immunologic response.[8]

To overcome the limitations of biologic grafts, synthetic grafts have been developed as an alternative to autografts and allografts for orthopedic applications. Because these implants are fabricated out of synthetic materials, naturally derived materials, or a combination of the two, the risk of disease transmission is either nonexistent (in the case of synthetics) or significantly reduced (in the case of naturally derived materials). For connective tissue repair, polymers (e.g., polyethylene, polylactic acid [PLA], and polycaprolactone) are commonly used to form the implants, many of which are already used in medical devices approved by the US Food and Drug Administration (FDA).[9-11] Examples of naturally derived biopolymers include collagen, chitosan, and alginate.[12-15] These materials have been tested for biocompatibility using in vitro culture models or in vivo animals models to reduce the risk of adverse responses when used clinically.[16-18] The versatility and sophistication of their properties can be fine-tuned by manipulating the materials to improve biocompatibility, bioactivity, mechanical properties, and integration with the host tissue.[19-23]

In addition to synthetic grafts, recent advances related to tissue engineering have promoted the development of cell-based and scaffold-based approaches to orthopedic tissue regeneration. Unlike permanent implants, scaffold systems work as temporary structures supporting tissue formation by cells. Early synthetic scaffold systems relied on host cells to infiltrate the scaffold at the repair site; in more advanced scaffolds, biologic molecules are preincorporated and/or cells are preseeded onto the scaffolds prior to implantation. For both cases the scaffold degrades away and the structural template is replaced completely by new tissue, which is achieved by maintaining a delicate balance in cell biosynthesis and scaffold degradation. Thus when designing these implants, the materials and implant morphology need to elicit a cell response favorable for formation of the site-specific tissue. The mechanical properties also need to match the native tissue to support loading while the cells deposit new tissue, and the scaffold needs to be designed to degrade at an appropriate rate. Currently many implants have been approved by the FDA for tendon augmentation and cartilage repair, with many more devices undergoing clinical trials and further research.

This chapter focuses on synthetic implants for the treatment of tendon, ligament, meniscus, and cartilage injuries, highlighting those that have either been approved by the FDA or have reached the clinical trial stage. For cases in which synthetic grafts are not yet available, tissue-engineered implants are discussed. Each section begins with a brief overview of the tissue of interest, followed by a discussion of current synthetic or tissue-engineered grafts. A brief summary is included at the end of each section.

IMPLANTS FOR TENDON REPAIR

The rotator cuff consists of four tendons that attach their respective muscles to the proximal humerus through direct tendon-to-bone insertions.[24] The rotator cuff acts to stabilize the glenohumeral joint and is prone to degeneration and injury, with cuff tears being the most common form of pathology afflicting the shoulder. Each year more than 250,000 rotator cuff repairs are performed in the United States alone.[25] The incidence of rotator cuff repair is also increasing because of an aging, yet active, population. Primary tendon-to-bone repair and healing are the goals of these surgical procedures. In some cases, augmentation with commercially available patches is performed, with the patch applied to the superficial tendon surface to enhance the repair. However, because of a variety of factors including graft degeneration, poor vascularization, muscle atrophy, and the lack of graft-to-bone integration after surgery,[26–30] failure rates between 20% and 94% have been reported after primary repair of chronic rotator cuff injuries.[31]

To improve healing, biologic or synthetic polymer-based tendon implants or augmentation devices have been developed to reconstruct large and massive rotator cuff tears.[32,33] To date, most biologic tendon grafts that are commonly used are derived from a decellularized allogeneic or xenogenic extracellular matrix (ECM).[34–37] Synthetic grafts are usually made of biocompatible and biodegradable polymers that break down into nontoxic metabolites in the body. There are several commercially available tendon grafts currently available, as well as several ongoing clinical trials testing new technology for these implants.

Most commercially available synthetic grafts are developed around biologic materials derived from ECM, such as small intestinal submucosa (SIS) and dermis. These patches provide a chemical and three-dimensional (3D) structural framework, native matrix composition, and residual remodeling biomolecules that direct repair and remodeling of the rotator cuff tendons by the host cells.[38] However, their clinical use, especially for SIS-based grafts, has been in question due to suboptimal or negative outcomes in human trials.[39,40] Several reported adverse outcomes have been reported, attributed either to immunologic issues, and/or a mismatch in mechanical properties between the graft and the host tissue; this has been particularly apparent in the demanding environment of the shoulder joint. A systematic comparison of four commercially available ECM patches (Restore, derived from porcine SIS; CuffPatch, derived from porcine SIS; GraftJacket, derived from human dermis; and TissueMend, derived from bovine dermis) was conducted using a canine model.[41] All four patches were inferior mechanically to the native tendon and underwent premature graft resorption.

The ineffective results using natural grafts motivate the search for appropriate synthetic grafts for tendon repair. However, synthetics grafts may also incite a local negative response due to local toxicity or acidity from graft degradation products. Examination of synthetic patches in canine and rat models[42,43] showed that both patches (X-Repair, made of poly-L-lactide, and Biomerix RCR Patch, made of polycarbonate polyurethane) were biocompatible with host cell responses and showed minimal inflammation response, supporting their use for tendon repair. Alternatively, hybrid rotator cuff patches are also available, synthesized with the aim of combining the benefits of both poly-L-lactide and polyurethane. However, very limited data are available for the performance of these scaffolds. Currently, Tornier BioFiber-CM, a patch made by adding bovine collagen I to poly-4-hydroxy-butyrate, is in clinical trials for full-thickness rotator cuff tear repair.[44]

Although rotator cuff patches are frequently used in surgery, systematic follow-up studies that evaluate performance of such scaffolds are sparse. Results from the limited number of follow-up studies available demonstrated a mixed performance of commercially available patches. Restore, an SIS-based scaffold, was the first implant on the market for tendon repair and was widely used. However, clinical outcomes for Restore have been mixed. An early study reported that, when compared with preoperative levels, shoulders repaired with the Restore patch improved in strength, motion, and function, with no increased risk of infection at 24 months.[45] Sclamberg et al.[40] performed a 6-month follow-up study of 11 patients (5 women and 6 men between the ages of 52 and 78 years) who underwent large rotator cuff repair augmented with the Restore implant and found that the repair failed in 10 of the 11 patients. Of even greater concern were the results reported by Iannotti et al.[39]: in a study of 15 patients (4 women and 11 men with mean age of 58 years), those treated with the Restore patch had a lower healing rate and a lower postoperative PENN score compared with members of the control group, who underwent repair without the patch. In a later study, Walton et al.[46] compared healing results of patients (5 women and 10 men with a mean age of 60.2 years) who had their rotator cuff repaired with or without the Restore implant.[46] It was observed that 2 years after surgery, patients who received the Restore implant reported higher rates of repeat tears, and their measured mechanical properties were significantly weaker. The patients also had more impingement and decreased levels of sports participation. In another study, Malcarney et al.[47] examined the postoperative responses of 25 patients who underwent rotator cuff repair augmented with the Restore implant and found that four of them experienced an acute inflammatory response shortly after surgery (a mean of 13 days). The inflammatory responses were nonspecific, and all four patients required implant removal. Based on these results, SIS-based scaffolds such as Restore are not recommended for use in rotator cuff repair.

The next generation of ECM-based implants focused on improving matrix mechanical properties to more closely match the mechanical properties of tendon. TissueMend is derived from fetal bovine dermis and is decellularized through a series of chemical processes. Magnussen et al.[48] used TissueMend to repair cadaveric Achilles tendons and tested the tendon mechanical properties under cyclic tensile loading. Results showed decreased gapping in the implant-augmented group, and the ultimate failure load increased significantly from a mean of 392 N to 821 N for the control group compared with the augmented group, respectively. Although currently the literature does not include any reports on the use of the TissueMend implant for rotator cuff repair, Seldes and Abramchayev[49] demonstrated, in a cadaver, the feasibility of using this implant to repair a massive rotator cuff tear.

Another implant available for rotator cuff repair is the Zimmer Collagen Repair Patch, which is derived from porcine dermis. In addition to being decellularized, this patch is cross-linked with hexamethylene diisocyanate to increase its strength and stability. The Zimmer Collagen Repair Patch also similarly showed inconsistent performance. Proper et al.[50] used the Zimmer patch to repair massive rotator cuff tears in 10 patients (5 women and 5 men between the ages of 46 and 80 years) and found that the implant caused no major postoperative complications and no adverse reactions. These investigators also found that the pain score and interval function score improved at 1 year after surgery; similarly, better range of movement and strength were reported. In the medium-term follow-up (a duration of 3 to 5 years), Badhe et al.[51] found that although two implants had detached after the original surgery, pain was reduced and abduction power and range of motion improved significantly, with no adverse effects reported. However, when Soler et al.[265] used the Zimmer patch to repair massive rotator cuff tears in four patients (three women and one man between the ages of 71 and 82 years), all four grafts failed between 3 and 6 months after surgery, leading to recurrent tears.

Compared with the SIS-based scaffold and Zimmer Collagen Repair Patch, published results evaluating GraftJacket have demonstrated more consistent results. In a prospective, randomized study, patients with a massive rotator cuff tear repaired with GraftJacket showed improved pain scores and a higher ratio of intact tendon at the 24-month follow-up compared with the patients with shoulders repaired without the graft.[52] In other studies, results demonstrated that augmentation with GraftJacket led to a lower retear rate, improved pain score, and increased shoulder functionality compared with the preoperative condition with no inflammatory response.[53-55] Currently, only one study is available reporting the performance of the synthetic Biomerix RCR Patch. In this study, patients showed improved pain scores, satisfactory range of shoulder movement at 6 and 12 months, a low retear rate (10%), and no adverse reactions.[56]

Barber et al. evaluated the mechanical properties of major commercial implants (Restore, Permacol, TissueMend, and GraftJacket) under tension.[57] These investigators found that products derived from human skin were the strongest, followed by porcine and bovine skins, with the small intestine submucosa–based implant being the weakest. This difference in mechanical properties could be the potential cause of the difference in performance of the implants in patients. Even with the limited number of follow-up studies performed, it is clear that despite a wide selection of commercial patches, very limited success has been found in early clinical trials. Surgical outcomes are also associated with other nonpatch factors such as age of the patient, size and severity of the tear, and surgical techniques used. Surgeons should therefore keep these factors in mind when evaluating the literature and be cautious when selecting an augmentation graft.

Because of the aforementioned challenges associated with ECM-derived implants for rotator cuff repair, a demand exists for new technologies to better meet the needs of functional tendon regeneration and soft tissue–to-bone integration. For integrative rotator cuff repair, the scaffold should match the mechanical properties of the native tendon, which is the major limitation of available biologic implants. The ideal implant should also mimic the ultrastructural organization of the native tendon. In addition, the implant should be biodegradable so it can be gradually replaced by new tissue while maintaining its physiologically relevant mechanical properties. Lastly, the graft must integrate with the host tendon and surrounding bone tissue by promoting the regeneration of the native tendon-to-bone interface. Several groups have explored synthetic grafts and tissue engineering methods for the development of tendon implants.[1,58-60] It is common to use scaffolds composed of nanofibers based on a variety of synthetic polymers, such as poly-L-lactic acid (PLLA), polylactide-co-glycolic acid (PLGA), polycarbonate polyurethane, and biologic materials, such as collagen and silk.[1,56,60-63] In addition to being biodegradable, both PLLA and PLGA are materials already used in FDA-approved devices. In a study by Baker et al.[64] using a canine model, 11 subjects underwent bilateral rotator cuff repair with one shoulder using a novel PLLA (human) fascia patch and then other without to assess whether these patches enhance the strength or likelihood of healing of the repair. At time 0 and at 12 weeks, the group compared repair retraction, cross-sectional area, biomechanical properties, and biocompatibility between the two sides. They found that at time 0 the patch side was able to withstand higher loads (296 N ± 130 N more) than the contralateral side; however, at 12 weeks, the augmented sides could withstand less (192 N ± 213 N) than the nonaugmented side and there was no difference in stiffness between the groups.[64] McCarron et al.[65] looked at cyclic gap formation and failure properties of a scaffold-augmented rotator cuff repair in human cadaveric shoulders. In nine paired cadaveric shoulders, the augmented and nonaugmented controls were loaded from 5 N to 180 N for 1000 cycles. They found that the augmented shoulder had a statistically significantly decreased gap at cycles 1, 10, 100, and 1000 compared with the nonaugmented repairs. Notably, all of the augmented repairs successfully completed the full cycling trials, whereas three of the nine nonaugmented repairs failed before completion. The gap remained less than 5 mm for the augmented group, whereas the nonaugmented group averaged a 7.3-mm gap. These studies are part of the ongoing body of work that will expand to include additional animal and eventually human studies to fully determine the efficacy of fascially augmented rotator cuff repairs.

The nanoscale architecture of the collagen-rich tendon matrix can be readily recapitulated with nanofiber scaffolds, which exhibit high surface area–to-volume ratio, low density, high porosity, variable pore size, and mechanical properties approximating those of the native tissues. Moffat et al.[21] first reported on the fabrication of PLGA nanofiber scaffolds with physiologically relevant structural and mechanical properties for rotator cuff repair. It was observed that human rotator cuff fibroblast morphology and growth on aligned and unaligned fiber matrices were dictated by fiber alignment, with distinct cell morphology and integrin expression profiles. Upregulation of $\alpha2$ integrin, a key mediator of cellular attachment to collagenous matrices, was observed when the fibroblasts were cultured on aligned fibers, and upon which types I and III collagen-rich matrices were deposited. More recently, Xie et al.[66] developed a continuous PLGA nanofiber scaffold that transitioned from aligned to random orientation, to examine the effects of this transitional region on rat tendon fibroblasts in vitro. After 1 week of culture, the cells proliferated on both aligned and random nanofiber orientations. Although a rounded morphology was found on unaligned nanofibers, cells cultured on aligned nanofibers appeared long and spindlelike and were aligned along the long axes of the fibers.

The biologic response to polymeric nanofibers may also be enhanced by additional surface modifications. For example, Rho et al.[67] electrospun aligned type I collagen nanofiber scaffolds with a mean fiber diameter of 460 nm and evaluated the response of human epidermal cells after coating the scaffolds with several adhesion proteins. It was found that cell proliferation was enhanced by coating the scaffolds with both type I collagen and laminin. Park et al.[68] applied a plasma treatment to polyglycolic acid (PGA), PLGA, and PLLA nanofibers and grafted a surface layer of hydrophilic acrylic on these scaffolds. It was found that NIH-3T3 fibroblasts seeded on these modified scaffolds spread and proliferated faster than those on unmodified control scaffolds. Nanofibers have also been used to improve existing scaffold design, resulting in a graft with a more biomimetic surface for eliciting desired cell responses. For example, Sahoo et al.[61] electrospun PLGA nanofibers directly onto a woven microfiber PLGA scaffold to increase cell seeding efficiency while maintaining a scaffold that was mechanically competent. The attachment, proliferation, and differentiation of porcine bone marrow stromal cells was evaluated on these scaffolds and, when compared with scaffolds seeded via a fibrin gel delivery, it was found that seeding the cells onto nanofiber-coated scaffolds enhanced proliferation and collagen production and upregulated the gene expression of several tendon-related markers, namely decorin, biglycan, and type I collagen.

In addition to being used as synthetic tissue–engineered implants, polymer fibers can be used to modify allogeneic non-tendon tissue and make it more suitable for rotator cuff augmentation. Aurora et al.[69] sutured PLLA and PLLA/PGA braids (diameter = 400 μm) to a human fascia patch to increase its suture retention properties. Results showed that all reinforced patches withstood 2500 cycles of 5 N to 150 N cyclic loading, with the PLLA/PGA patch withstanding 5000 cycles of loading. In addition, the suture retention properties and the maximum construct load of the reinforced patch were observed to be greater than those of human rotator cuff tendon, even after 3 months in vivo. Although more foreign body giant cells were seen in the reinforced patches, it is expected that this response will decrease after the polymer has fully degraded. These promising results suggest that the polymer fiber–reinforced tendon patch could be a more functional alternative for rotator cuff augmentation.

To address the challenge of regenerating the tendon-to-bone insertion site, several groups have evaluated the feasibility of integrating tendon implants with bone or biomaterials through the formation of anatomic insertion sites. Fujioka et al.[70] examined the effects of reattaching the bone and tendon in a rat model for Achilles tendon avulsion. After 4 weeks, surgical reattachment of tendon to bone increased type X collagen deposition and allowed tissue to maintain distinct regions of calcified and noncalcified fibrocartilage tissue. In addition, Inoue et al.[71] promoted supraspinatus tendon integration with a metallic implant using a bone marrow–infused bone graft. These early attempts demonstrate that the direct tendon-bone insertion may be regenerated. To this end, the ideal implant for tendon-to-bone interface tissue engineering must exhibit a gradient of structural and mechanical properties mimicking those of the multitissue insertion.[72] Thus a scaffold recapturing the nanoscale interface organization, with preferentially aligned nanofiber organization and region-dependent changes in mineral content, would be highly advantageous. Building on the functional PLGA nanofiber scaffold designed for tendon tissue engineering, Moffat et al.[73,74] designed a biphasic scaffold, with the top layer consisting of nanofibers of PLGA and the second layer consisting of composite nanofibers of PLGA and hydroxyapatite nanoparticles. The biphasic design is aimed at regenerating both the nonmineralized and mineralized fibrocartilage regions of the tendon-to-bone insertion site while promoting osteointegration with PLGA-HA nanofibers.[73] The responses of tendon fibroblasts, osteoblasts, and chondrocytes have been evaluated on these nanocomposite scaffolds, with promising results in vitro. When tested in vivo subcutaneously, as well as in a rat rotator cuff repair model, the biphasic scaffold supported regeneration of continuous noncalcified and calcified fibrocartilage regions, demonstrating the potential of a biodegradable nanofiber-based implant system for integrative tendon-to-bone repair.[73,74] Lastly, the efficacy of the biphasic scaffold to repair acute, full-thickness rotator cuff tears was confirmed in a sheep model. In an alternative approach, nanofiber PLGA scaffolds with gradients in mineral content were produced using electrospinning.[75–77] The gradients in mineral content resulted in gradients in mechanical properties and cellular responses, mimicking features of the natural tendon-to-bone attachment. These scaffolds showed some promise in a small animal model of rotator cuff repair.[78] Collectively, these results demonstrate the potential of the biomimetic, biphasic scaffold for integrative, tendon-bone repair.

In summary, commercially available, ECM-derived tendon grafts and augmentation devices have exhibited mixed outcomes in clinical studies. In general, tendon implants made from dermis performed better than implants made from other types of ECM, as reflected in the reported lower repeat tear rates and improved postoperative scores. Alternative treatment options such as synthetic and tissue-engineered grafts are being developed, with promising results for tendon regeneration and tendon-to-bone integration. However, several challenges remain to be overcome before the widespread clinical application of the tissue-engineered tendon implants can be realized. For example, one challenge is the scale-up of the tissue-engineered implants from small animal models to humans. Currently, most of the tissue-engineered implants are being evaluated in vitro and are prepared in small batches. High-throughput fabrication and delivery processes need to be developed for them to augment their commercial applicability. The other challenge is that the fabrication process of the tissue-engineered implants generally uses a variety of toxic solvents or several steps of chemical reactions to dissolve polymers, which may have undesired effects on biomolecules or cells once they are implanted in humans.

IMPLANTS FOR LIGAMENT RECONSTRUCTION

The ACL is one of the major ligaments that connect the femur and tibia, and it is the primary stabilizer in the knee. The ACL inserts into bone through a direct transition consisting of spatial variations in cell type and matrix composition, resulting in three distinct tissue regions of ligament, fibrocartilage, and bone.[79–81] Tearing of the ACL is among the most common knee injury afflicting the young and active population, with more than 100,000 ACL reconstructions performed annually in the United States alone.[82,83] Because of the inherent poor healing potential of the ligament, ACL reconstruction based largely on biologic grafts is required. Because of the relative scarcity and donor site morbidity of autografts, as well as the inherent risks associated with allografts, significant interest has been expressed regarding synthetic- and tissue-engineered alternatives for ACL reconstruction. In the late 1980s the FDA approved synthetic materials for use as an alternative implant for ACL reconstruction. However, because of significant complications and failures in humans, all of the synthetic implants were withdrawn from the market by the late 1990s, and at the present, only biologic grafts such as hamstring tendon or bone-patellar tendon-bone grafts are used clinically for ACL reconstruction.

One of the commercial implants tested for ACL reconstruction was the Gore-Tex implant, which is based on polytetrafluoroethylene (PTFE). This implant is composed of solid PTFE nodes interconnected by PTFE fibers at each end for bony attachment.[84] In 1987 Ahlfeld et al.[85] used the Gore-Tex implant to treat 30 patients with unstable knees. During the follow-up period (average 24 months), the group treated with the Gore-Tex implant showed improved satisfaction compared with patients who underwent reconstruction with a different material (ProPlast ligament) (83% satisfactory vs. 52%). Glousman et al.[86] used this implant in 82 patients (23 women and 59 men, ages 16 to 51 years) and at 18 months follow-up found that a number of patients had complications (15) and repeat operations (14). On the other hand, the subjective scores improved in all evaluation categories, including pain, swelling, giving way, locking, and stair climbing. Although the authors suggested that the results were positive, they also recommended longer-term follow-up before definitive conclusions could be determined. In another study, Indelicato et al.[87] reported that of 39 patients (12 women and 27 men whose ages ranged between 17 and 42 years) who received the Gore-Tex implant, 87% had satisfactory results 2 years postoperatively. However, in many of these studies, some complications were noticed, such as tears of the implant and sterile effusions. In addition to the failure of the implant itself, use of Gore-Tex led to other complications in the knee, including bone tunnel widening. Muren et al.[88] examined 17 patients at 13 to 15 years after they had ACL reconstruction with the Gore-Tex implant. It was found that six patients underwent revision surgery as a result of implant rupture and pain; moreover, 15 patients had tibia bone tunnel widening. In another study, surgery with the Gore-Tex implant was performed in 123 patients, and complete rupture of the graft was seen in 26 patients.[89] In addition, half of the patients exhibited graft loosening, 62% experienced osteoarthritic change, and bone tunnel osteolysis at both ends was identified in most cases. Consequently, the Gore-Tex implant was no longer recommended for ACL reconstruction and eventually was withdrawn from the market in 1993. Similarly, for other synthetic ACL implants such as the Ligament Advanced Reinforcement System (LARS; Surgical Implants and Devices,

Arc-sur-Tille, France) and Leeds-Keio ligament implants that were used in ACL reconstruction with short-term satisfactory results, many long-term complications were reported, including repeat rupture, bone tunnel widening, severe synovitis, and inflammatory responses. Therefore these implants were likewise withdrawn from the market, and currently no synthetic implants have been approved by the FDA for ACL reconstructions.

To overcome limitations of the failed synthetic implants and the inherent shortcoming of allografts currently in use, tissue-engineered implants have been investigated. Such implants involve implantation of a bioactive material that regenerates tissues with material properties that are comparable with those of the native ACL.[90] Similar to the requirement for tendon repair, the ACL implant should be biodegradable, match the mechanical properties of the native ACL, and mimic the ultrastructural organization of the native ACL. Finally, the implant must integrate with both the femoral and tibial bone tunnels to promote the regeneration of the native ligament-to-bone interface. To this end, most of the studies have investigated the use of synthetic polymers such as PLLA, PLGA, and polyurethane, as well as biologic materials, such as collagen and silk.[91–95]

Dunn et al.[96] were among the first investigators to evaluate a biomimetic ACL replacement in vivo. Studies were performed using a type I collagen fiber–based prosthesis with polymethylmethacrylate (PMMA) bone fixation plugs on the ends. Although neoligamentous tissue formation was reported, the majority of scaffolds were reported to have ruptured after 20 weeks in a rabbit model, demonstrating that, although it was biomimetic, this system was insufficient to support long-term knee stability.[96] A series of studies also were performed that focused on the development of a silk-based ACL replacement both in vitro and in vivo.[94,95,97–99] Specifically, a novel silk-fiber based scaffold was designed, and several studies were performed to assess the impact of chemical and mechanical stimulation on the differentiation of seeded mesenchymal stem cells (MSCs). It was demonstrated that individually, soluble chemical factors such as basic fibroblast growth factor, as well as tensile and torsional loading, could drive matrix elaboration and fibroblastic differentiation of MSCs on the silk scaffold.[94] In addition, chemical and mechanical stimulation, when applied concomitantly and controlled temporally, have been reported to enhance MSC response.[97,98] The system was implanted in vivo in a goat model, with promising results reported based on histologic and mechanical outcomes such as significantly increased knee stiffness and ultimate tensile strength after 12 months of implantation. This prosthesis is currently undergoing clinical trials.[99]

Also using a silk-based scaffold, Liu et al.[100] performed a series of studies to optimize a knitted graft combined with a microporous silk sponge for ACL reconstruction. This biphasic system was designed to mimic the ECM of native tissue and provide sufficient mechanical strength for ligament replacement. The scaffold was implanted in vivo using a rabbit model and later a pig model, with substantial ligament-like tissue observed on the scaffold after 24 weeks.[101,102] In addition, several in vitro studies were performed to further optimize the scaffold, including the use of silk cables to increase tensile strength, the incorporation of basic fibroblast growth factor–releasing PLGA and RADA16 peptide nanofibers to enhance cell biosynthesis, and the addition of a silk-based aligned nanofiber topography to direct cell orientation and matrix production.[62,103–105]

Progressing from single-phase systems, Cooper et al.[91,92,106] designed and optimized, both in vitro and in vivo, a braided, α-hydroxyester, microfiber-based scaffold for ligament engineering. The architecture and porosity was standardized in vitro using a braiding technique to recapitulate the native ligament mechanical properties and included a denser fiber arrangement at each end of the construct for bone formation.[106] Scaffold composition was also optimized based on in vitro degradation and cell response, with PLLA selected because of its ability to maintain structural integrity over the 8-week culturing duration.[92] Subsequently, the optimized scaffold was evaluated in vivo using a rabbit ACL reconstruction model. It was demonstrated that cell seeding of the implanted scaffold resulted in a marked improvement in functional outcomes, but scaffolds in both groups ruptured after 12 weeks of implantation.[91] In a follow-up study, Freeman et al.[107,108] evaluated the effect of both braiding and twisting on the mechanical properties of the PLLA microfiber system, demonstrating that twisting coupled with braiding could increase both ultimate tensile strength and the toe-region length of the graft. Barber et al.[109] reported on the development of a braided nanofiber–based scaffold for ACL replacement. Scaffold architecture was optimized by varying the number of braided bundles and evaluating mechanical properties, with minimal differences in toe-region or elastic modulus as a function of braid number. The scaffold was seeded with MSCs in vitro, and both cell viability and proliferation were observed.

Also in development are scaffold systems that target the regeneration of the ligament-to-bone interface, which is critical for biologic fixation of either biologic or synthetic grafts. Spalazzi et al.[110,111] reported on the design and evaluation of a triphasic scaffold for the regeneration of the ACL-to-bone interface both in vitro and in vivo. The scaffold consists of three distinct yet continuous phases, each engineered for a specific tissue region found at the interface: Phase A is designed with a PLGA mesh, phase B consists of PLGA microspheres, and phase C is composed of a sintered PLGA and 45S5 bioactive glass composite.[112] They are intended for ligament, interface, and bone formation, respectively. When this stratified scaffold was evaluated in a subcutaneous athymic rat model, abundant tissue formation was observed on phases A, B, and C. Cell migration and an increased matrix production were also observed in the interfacial region, and the phase-specific controlled matrix heterogeneity was maintained in vivo. Once ligament fibroblast, chondrocyte, and osteoblast triculture were established on their respective phase of the scaffold, the formation of both anatomic ligament-like and bonelike matrices was observed on the triphasic scaffold (phases A and C, respectively), as well as the deposition of a fibrocartilage-like tissue (phase B). At 2 months after implantation, the interface-like region consisted of chondrocyte-like cells embedded within a matrix containing collagen types I and II, as well as glycosaminoglycans, indicating the formation of interface-like tissue.

In addition to ACL reconstruction, a new approach emphasizing primary ACL repair has been developed in response to the issue that ACL reconstruction was not delaying premature onset of osteoarthritis in patients with ACL injury.[113–115] Through a series of in vitro and in vivo experiments, a proprietary scaffold that combines collagen-based implants with whole blood for ACL repair has been designed and optimized.[116] This system was first evaluated in an ACL central defect model, in which the collagen implant was augmented with platelet-rich plasma (PRP) was used only to fill in the defects, not to replace the ACL. In a canine model, Murray et al.[116,117] used collagen with or without PRP to repair an ACL central defect and evaluated histologic and mechanical properties of the repaired ACL over a period of 6 weeks. Results indicate that the collagen gel with PRP showed a significantly higher percentage of defect filling and strength compared with the control group. In addition, it was found that the PRP-augmented collagen resulted in regenerated tissue that had similar properties to those of the medial collateral ligament, which has a better healing ability than the ACL. This collagen-platelet composite (CPC) is also used as a supplement to the standard allograft reconstruction approach. In one study, Joshi et al.[118] performed unilateral ACL reconstruction procedures in pigs with a bone-patellar tendon-bone allograft with or without the addition of CPC at the surgery site, and outcomes were evaluated at 4 weeks, 6 weeks, and 3 months after surgery. Although at 6 weeks a temporary decrease in yield load and stiffness was seen in both groups, by 3 months the group that underwent repair with CPC had improvements in yield load and linear stiffness. In another study, using the same animal model, Fleming et al.[118] evaluated the effect of the addition of CPC over a period of 15 weeks. Results confirmed the previous findings that in the long term, yield and maximum failure load of CPC-supplemented groups were greater than that of the group that underwent standard ACL reconstruction. In addition, histologic analysis revealed that the graft structure properties were also improved by the addition of CPC. Furthermore, the composite can be used by itself as an implant to enhance the suture repair procedure on the ACL. Two studies were conducted to evaluate the individual effects of collagen or PRP in ACL regeneration in a porcine model, and it was found that neither improved the functional properties.[119,120] Mastrangelo et al.[121] combined collagen with PRP and used CPC with different PRP concentrations (×3 and ×5 of the baseline, respectively) to bridge the ACL stump and the femoral tunnel and evaluated the mechanical properties of the repaired ACL over 13 weeks. It was found that regardless of PRP concentration, CPC increased the mechanical properties of repaired ACL. Further in vitro work found that both platelets and plasma proteins were important in the healing process of the ACL cells, red blood cells aided with collagen production by fibroblasts, and white blood cells released anabolic growth factors.[122–127] This led to the determination that PRP was no better than whole blood in the augmentation of the collagen scaffold for enhanced ACL repair.[128,129] Therefore the ongoing trials testing the collagen scaffold in large animal models and humans used whole blood. In a large animal model, results at 6 and 12 months showed that ACL repair with the collagen scaffold and whole blood augment had similar mechanical properties to ACL reconstruction.[130,131] Importantly, they also noted that the porcine knee that underwent ACL repair with the collagen scaffold and whole blood had significantly less osteoarthritis at 1 year than the knee that underwent ACL reconstruction.[130] Based on these promising animal model studies, a first in human phase I FDA-approved trial of 20 patients was performed.[132] Ten patients underwent ACL repair with the collagen scaffold, whole blood, and a primary suture repair of the ACL, and 10 patients underwent reconstruction with a hamstring autograft. There were no significant inflammation or joint injections in either group, no difference in pain or effusion, and MRI at 3 months postoperative showed intact ACL or graft in all patients. Hamstring strength was significantly stronger in the ACL repair group.[132]

Murray et al.[133] is currently conducting an FDA-approved randomized controlled trial on 100 patients using the proprietary collagen scaffold to enhance repair of proximal femoral avulsion ACL injuries with promising early results.

In summary, because of the inherent poor healing potential of ligaments such as the ACL, implants are used for ligament reconstruction, with autografts and allografts being the most common. In the 1980s, synthetic ACL such as Gore-Tex, LARS ligament, and Leeds-Keio were popular and were used widely in ACL reconstruction surgeries. Although satisfactory short-term results were reported, long-term outcomes were poor and eventually resulted in most of the synthetic implants being extracted and withdrawn from the market. To address the unmet market demand for ligament grafts that were an alternative to biologic grafts, tissue engineering has arisen as a promising method by which to regenerate the ACL. A variety of polymeric materials were tested in vitro and in vivo; different methods such as incorporation of growth factors and active loading of the scaffolds were used to enhance graft performance. In addition, stratified implants were designed and showed promising results in vitro and in vivo for ligament-to-bone integration. Although they are promising, most of the tissue engineering options are still at the in vitro and small animal in vivo evaluation stages, and their true clinical potential remains to be demonstrated in clinical trials. One recent approach in clinical trials that uses natural scaffolding combined with whole blood may allow for primary ACL healing and has the potential to shift the care of these injuries from reconstruction to repair, which may be instrumental in delaying the onset of osteoarthritis after ACL injury.

IMPLANTS FOR MENISCUS REPAIR

The meniscus is a fibrocartilaginous tissue in the knee that functions to dissipate compressive and shear stresses during normal activity, as well as to distribute synovial fluid throughout the knee during loading and unloading.[134,135] With a high water content (78 weight percent), the meniscus is 80% avascular and is composed primarily of type I and II collagen, with other minor types of collagen, as well as proteoglycans.[136] Meniscal tears can either be traumatic or degenerative in nature. The current treatment options include nonoperative (e.g., physical therapy, nonsteroidal antiinflammatory medications, and cortisone injections) and operative procedures, which include meniscal repairs and partial meniscectomies.[137] Meniscal repairs, which consist of repairing a tear via suturing, are typically performed only for tears located in the vascular region of the meniscus that is associated with the meniscosynovial junction.[137] Because of the specific

nature of the types of injuries that can be repaired with this technique, partial meniscectomies are more common. In the United States alone, 690,000 partial meniscectomies were performed in 2006.[6] A partial meniscectomy consists of removing the damaged tissue from the meniscus while leaving behind as much normal meniscal tissue as possible. Because the removed tissue extends into the avascular region, the limited access to blood flow results in a low repair rate, resulting in a hole in the meniscus that leaves a loss of functionality.

Consequently, meniscal allografts and tissue-engineered implants have been researched extensively to restore functionality to the knee. Although allografts have been shown to decrease pain and improve knee function in patients in the short term, inherent shortcomings of allogeneic tissue include limited supply, potential disease transmission (such as human immunodeficiency virus or hepatitis), and risk of infection or an immunologic response. The grafts have also been shown to demonstrate some shrinkage via magnetic resonance imaging (MRI) and a reduction in mechanical strength, leading to tears and dysfunction of the allograft.[138] More recently, tissue-engineered meniscus implants have been developed as a viable alternative to allografts, as reviewed extensively by Brophy and Matava[6] and van Tienen et al.[139] The tissue-engineered graft serves as a scaffold structure at the defect site, which allows for cell infiltration from the surrounding native tissue into the structure. The cells are then able to regenerate new tissue while the scaffold structure sustains the mechanical loading and degrades away for eventual total replacement with regenerated, functional tissue filling the defect site.

This section will focus on three synthetic options for meniscal replacement: collagen meniscus implant (CMI), hydrogels, and polymer scaffolds. These implants have all undergone extensive in vitro and in vivo testing for biocompatibility, cell response, biodegradability, and mechanical properties.

The CMI is a purified type I collagen scaffold derived from bovine Achilles tendon, and glycosaminoglycans are added to the collagen, after which the structure is cast in a mold, lyophilized, and cross-linked in formaldehyde.[140] The implant requires a meniscal rim and intact anterior and posterior meniscal horns for attachment during surgery and is used to treat medial and lateral meniscus injuries.[140,141] Multiple clinical studies were conducted in which the CMI scaffold was implanted in patients with meniscal tears to evaluate the feasibility of the scaffold. In terms of the chondroprotective capabilities of the CMI, several studies have shown that the joint space and chondral surfaces were preserved after implantation.[141-145] MRI revealed that at 5 to 10 years after surgery, new meniscal tissue was formed and integrated well with host tissue. However, the neotissue differed in MRI signal from the surrounding native tissue, suggesting that the regenerated tissue did not completely match the native tissue in structure and composition.[144,146,147] In most cases the newly formed meniscus tissue was reduced in size compared with the host tissue, but based on patient scoring, these differences were not found to be clinically significant.[144,146,147] In addition, the defect filling was estimated to reach 70% in 1 year.[141,146] Mixed results on implant resorption have been reported, spanning from no observable resorption to complete implant degradation in 5 years; as such, in all cases, no inflammation or negative effects have been reported. To assess the efficacy of the CMI compared with a control group that underwent partial meniscectomy without use of a scaffold, Rodkey et al.[146] followed up on 311 patients (aged 18 to 60 years) who underwent either CMI implantation or a partial meniscectomy. Results showed that patients treated with CMI had an improvement in activity levels, as evaluated at 5 years using the Tegner index for activity, whereas Lysholm scores for pain were found to be the same for both procedures. Moreover, the number of revision surgeries required was reduced by 50% with the CMI.[146] A 10-year study was performed by Zaffagnini et al.[143] with 36 male patients (aged 24 to 60 years). Regardless of CMI implantation, two patients per group required revision surgery during the 10-year period. The improved activity level compared with the control group at 5 years as evaluated by the Tegner index was also observed here, with a similar activity level being maintained for over 10 years. In addition, patients implanted with the CMI showed either significant pain improvement at 10 years (when evaluated using a visual analog pain scale) or a similar pain score compared with the control group (when evaluated using the Lysholm score, as was found previously by Steadman and Rodkey[141]).[143] In a recent systematic review of 11 studies (396 patients) to compare clinical outcomes and complications of CMI by Grassi et al.,[148] Lysholm score and visual analogue scale (VAS) showed an improvement at 6 months up to 10 years. The Tegner activity level, although peaking at 12 months and declining at subsequent evaluations, was reported to be above the preoperative level. Overall, this review concluded that CMI could produce good and stable clinical results, particularly regarding knee function and pain, with low rates of complications and reoperations.[148] CMI obtained FDA approval in 2015.

Another class of meniscal implants is based on polymeric materials. Actifit is an aliphatic polyurethane implant developed for medial and lateral partial meniscus tears. The graft is composed of two types of degradable polymers with distinct mechanical properties: 80% of a mechanically soft polymer poly(ε-caprolactone) and 20% of a mechanically stiffer segment polyurethane.[149] This polymer blend was optimized through in vitro and in vivo testing for mechanical properties, degradation properties, and biocompatibility.[150–153] The scaffold exhibits a relatively slow degradation rate (it takes up to 5 years to fully degrade).[154] It has also been shown to improve contact area and pressure in a sheep cadaver model,[155] and in testing in the canine model, tissue ingrowth into the scaffold and capsule were noted at 6 months.[156] During clinical testing by Verdonk et al.,[157,158] of the 52 patients with partial meniscus defects, patients receiving the Actifit implant were compared with patients undergoing a standard partial meniscectomy. For one group treated with Actifit, tissue ingrowths of 85.7% were observed at 3 months, with 12-month biopsies showing cells with meniscus-like differentiation potential. All patients receiving the Actifit implant measured significant improvements in terms of International Knee Documentation Committee (IKDC) score, Knee Injury and Osteoarthritis Outcome score, and Lysholm knee scale, showing that in 2 years, the scaffold is capable of restoring a certain level of knee functionality. A recently published midterm follow-up report of the clinical and MRI results 4 years after Actifit showed

that sustained improvement of pain scores and knee function scores compared with baseline.[159] Review of MRI scans did not reveal any appreciable change in articular cartilage. Although Actifit does not yet have FDA approval, it is approved for use in Europe.

Recently, results have been published on a novel resorbable polymer fiber-reinforced meniscus reconstruction scaffolds.[160] Using an ovine model the integrity, tensile and compressive mechanics, cell phenotypes, matrix organization and content, and protection of the articular cartilage surfaces were studied over 1 year. Fibrocartilagenous repair with both types 1 and 2 collagen were observed, with areas of matrix organization and biochemical content similar to native tissue concluding that this resorbable fiber-reinforced meniscus scaffold may support the formation of functional "neomeniscus" tissue.

Another meniscal implant with potential is the NUsurface, a polycarbonate-urethane implant reinforced circumferentially with Kevlar fibers to mimic the functional properties of the meniscus.[161] These fibers are based on the native menisci's oriented collagen fiber network. Preliminary studies in a sheep model showed that the implant resisted wear and mild cartilage degeneration,[162] although the total osteoarthritis score was not affected.

Many other promising technologies are being investigated, although most have not yet reached the clinical testing stage. For example, biodegradable polycaprolactone nanofibers have been used to mimic the native fiber alignment of collagen found in the meniscus with promising results and potentially superior long-term biocompatibility.[163] In vivo testing of foam polycaprolactone scaffolds revealed the formation of meniscus-like tissue with initial mechanical properties approaching those of the native meniscus.[151,156,164] Hydrogel scaffolds (e.g., polyvinyl alcohol) for meniscus repair have also been evaluated in vivo and have been shown to be chondroprotective in addition to promoting meniscus-like tissue regeneration.[153,165–167] Although these tissue-engineered implants appear to be promising, clinical applications are pending based on preclinical and clinical outcomes. The most recent meniscal therapy approaches are incorporating MSCs in their approach.[168–171]

IMPLANTS FOR CARTILAGE AND OSTEOCHONDRAL REPAIR

Articular cartilage lines the surfaces of joints and enables near frictionless motion and load bearing. Composed of both liquid and solid phases, cartilage is a highly specialized tissue, with complex structure-function relationships.[172] It is largely avascular and aneural, and consequently, it has a limited capacity for self-repair.[173] Clinical treatments of cartilage defects include joint lavage, subchondral drilling, microfracture, and osteochondral transplantation (with autografts or allografts). However, poor long-term outcomes are associated with many of these techniques because of unwanted fibrocartilage formation and inadequate graft-to-bone integration.[174–176] Furthermore, although the use of osteochondral allograft has demonstrated positive results, risk of disease transmission and issues with graft availability, preservation, and storage remain.[177] Alternative techniques have been developed and studied, including the use of autologous chondrocyte implantation (ACI), use of particulated juvenile hyaline cartilage (DeNovo, Zimmer), and chondrogenesis using stem cells. There are many scaffold options available for ACI, as well as both a two-stage and one-stage technique, which will be reviewed next.

Brittberg et al.[178] published the first clinical report demonstrating the promise of ACI, a two-step procedure in which autologous chondrocytes are arthroscopically harvested from a healthy cartilage donor site (typically the intercondylar notch of the knee), expanded in vitro, and then reintroduced to the defect site through a second open procedure. In addition, an autologous periosteum flap is harvested from the patient and used to contain the cells within the defect site. This procedure was the first FDA-approved cell-based product for cartilage repair and served to bridge the gap between previously available techniques and total joint replacement, because this procedure eliminated issues of disease transmission, as well as graft availability, preservation, and storage. Although ACI results in satisfactory clinical outcomes,[179] several limitations are inherent to the procedure. Of note, the necessity of two surgical procedures increases cost and leads to extended recovery times.[180] Furthermore, cases of cartilage hypertrophy have been reported.[181] Finally, it is unclear if the cells recover completely from long-term monolayer culture, if they are homogeneously distributed within the repair tissue, and how many cells are actually retained within the defect site.[182]

To tackle the shortcomings of the ACI procedure, second- and third-generation techniques have been developed that use matrices that eliminate the need for periosteal harvest, support and retain the chondrocytes in a 3D matrix, and enable a homogeneous distribution of the cells within the defect. The matrices that have been developed are composed of a wide variety of materials, both natural and synthetic, and have shown great promise in initial trials. Natural matrices are attractive because they can be designed to closely mimic the native cartilage matrix. Matrix-assisted chondrocyte implantation (MACI) is a second-generation ACI technique in which a porcine-derived collagen I/III bilayer is seeded with autologous expanded chondrocytes. The use of a scaffold effectively eliminates the need for periosteal harvest. Bartlett et al.[183] conducted a randomized comparison of MACI and ACI-C (ACI with a collagen I/III flap used in place of periosteum) for treatment of chondral knee defects in 91 patients and found that the two treatments resulted in clinically comparable outcomes. More recently, MACI has been compared with microfracture by Basad et al.[184] in a study of 60 patients with isolated cartilage defects, and it was found that MACI was significantly more effective over time than microfracture according to three different scoring systems (the Tegner index, International Cartilage Repair Society–patient, and International Cartilage Repair Society–surgeon). Zheng et al.[185] performed histologic analysis on a cohort of 56 MACI-treated patients and found that this technique supported chondrocyte phenotype maintenance, which was determined by aggrecan, type II collagen, and S-100 expression. After 6 months, 75% hyaline cartilage regeneration was reported. Behrens et al.[186] and Ebert et al.[187] have both performed 5-year follow-up studies for 11 and 41 patients, respectively, and found high patient satisfaction and low failure rates. MACI received FDA approval in 2016.

The Cartilage Regeneration System (CaReS) also uses a collagen matrix for cell-based cartilage regeneration; however, CaReS is made from a rat-derived collagen type I matrix that is seeded with primary cells that have not been expanded in monolayer culture. This technique is based on the assumption that cells that have not been exposed to monolayer expansion are more effective for regenerating cartilage tissue. Flohé et al.[188] compared the CaReS system with the MACI procedure for repair of cartilage defects in the knees of 20 patients and found that both treatments resulted in improved clinical outcomes after 1 year, with no significant differences detected between treatments. In a multicenter clinical trial, Schneider et al.[189] followed up with 116 patients who received the CaReS implant between 2003 and 2008. The overall treatment satisfaction was judged as good or very good in 88% of the cases by the surgeon and in 80% of the cases by the patient. These observations are highly promising, but longer-term follow-up will be necessary to determine if the CaReS system has distinct advantages over other approaches.

Monolayer expansion of autologous chondrocytes is also avoided in the NeoCart system, in which chondrocytes are cultured on scaffolds made of bovine collagen type I in custom bioreactors that mimic the conditions of the knee through varying pressure and low oxygen tension. Crawford et al.[190] demonstrated the clinical safety of this system in a small trial in which eight patients received the NeoCart treatment. In this study, pain scores were significantly reduced after treatment, and none of the patients experienced hypertrophy or arthrofibrosis. More recently, the NeoCart implant was compared with microfracture in a randomized trial of 30 patients, and it was found that significantly more patients treated with NeoCart responded positively to the treatment at both 6 and 12 months, with the trend continuing at the 2-year follow-up.[191]

A more complex implant, ChondroMimetic, is composed of three natural materials and is designed to closely mimic the natural cartilage environment. This implant is a dual-layer porous plug composed of collagen, glycosaminoglycans, and calcium phosphate. The scaffold can be prehydrated with sterile fluids and autologous blood. Although ChondroMimetic is an acellular, off-the-shelf product, it can be used in conjunction with ChondroCelect, which is a cell-based technology that is offered by the same company, TiGenix. ChondroMimetic was launched in October 2010 in Europe; patient enrollment in an open-label extension study just commenced in July 2017.

In addition to collagenous implants, several hyaluronan-based matrices have been developed. Hyalograft C is a hyaluronic acid scaffold (HYAFF) that is combined with autologous chondrocytes. Hyalograft C can be used in both arthroscopic and open procedures, and satisfactory clinical outcomes have been reported after 7 years.[192] Improved clinical outcomes were reported for young patients in a prospective study of 70 patients with 3- and 4-year follow-up and in a study of 36 patients with 2- and 3-year follow-up analysis.[193,194] A study of 62 patients with 7-year follow-up found that, when compared with female patients, young active men had the best clinical outcomes when treated with Hyalograft C.[192] Nehrer et al.[195] reported that although Hyalograft C resulted in satisfactory repair for patients with a primary indication (e.g., young patients with a stable and healthy knee joint with an isolated chondral defect), it is a poor option for salvage procedures or for patients with osteoarthritis. Kon et al.[196] compared Hyalograft C with microfracture in 41 professional or semiprofessional soccer players and found that although microfracture allowed players to return to competition more quickly, repair with Hyalograft C may offer more durable clinical results. In addition, Hyalograft C was compared with MACI by Kon et al.[197] in a trial of 61 patients who were older than 40 years. A faster improvement in the IKDC subjective score was reported for the patients treated with Hyalograft C, whereas similar scores were reported at the 2-year follow-up.

A more recent product, BioCart II, combines recombinant hyaluronan with homologous human fibrin to form a macroporous sponge that is seeded with autologous chondrocytes that have been primed with a recombinant fibroblast growth factor 2 variant. A preliminary study by Nehrer et al.[198] reported good defect filling with the BioCart II system in a study of eight patients. Significant improvement in defect healing over time was subsequently reported by Eshed et al.[199] in a study that evaluated 31 patients at time points ranging from 6 to 49 months after BioCart II implantation.

Another scaffold based on a polymer derived from nature is BST-CarGel, which is an injectable chitosan-based scaffold that is used in conjunction with bone marrow stimulation to form a volume-stable clot that drives cartilage regeneration. BST-CarGel is injected into the defect in a single-step procedure and cross-linked in situ. Shive et al.[200] followed up with 33 patients treated with BST-CarGel and reported preliminary evidence suggesting that BST-CarGel has the potential for treatment of focal cartilage defects with varying etiology. In addition, alginate- and agarose-based scaffolds such as the Cartipatch system and a bead system have been investigated; however, few clinical reports of these approaches have been published.[201,202]

In addition to naturally derived products, several synthetic polymer-based scaffolds are currently on the market in Europe. BioSeed-C is a polyglycolic/PLA- and polydioxane-based material that is combined with culture-expanded autologous chondrocytes that are suspended in fibrin. Kreuz et al.[203] followed up on 19 patients with osteoarthritis who had received BioSeed-C treatment and reported good clinical outcomes 1 year after implantation. Moreover, BioSeed-C remained stable over the course of a period of 4 years, suggesting that it may be a promising treatment option for the repair of focal degenerative cartilage defects in the knee.[203] In a larger study of 52 patients with full-thickness defects by Kreuz et al.,[204] BioSeed-C treatment resulted in good clinical outcomes after 4 years despite a persisting deficit in mechanical strength. The authors suggest that this deficit may be addressed with a focus on muscular strength during rehabilitation.[204]

The Cartilage Autograft Implantation System (CAIS) is another polymer-based approach which consists of absorbable copolymer foam of 35% polycaprolactone and 65% PGA, reinforced with a polydioxanone (PDO) mesh (Advanced Technologies and Regenerative Medicine). In a one-step procedure, autologous cartilage is harvested, minced, and uniformly distributed within the scaffold using a fibrin sealant. The polymer foam is designed to keep the tissue fragments in place while the PDO mesh enables the foam to have adequate mechanical strength during implant handling. Cole et al.[205] compared CAIS treatment with microfracture in a randomized study of 29 patients at 1 and 2 weeks and periodically up to 2 years after surgery. It was found that CAIS resulted in significant increases in select subdomains in the Knee Injury and Osteoarthritis Outcome Score assessment tool, and it was concluded that CAIS is a safe, feasible, and effective method for treating patients with focal chondral defects that may improve long-term clinical outcomes.[205]

In addition to chondral grafts, several implant systems have been developed to address both chondral and osteochondral defects. Cartiva is a polyvinyl alcohol cryogel that has been used in patients since 2002 and consists of cylindrical gels that can be used to replace osteochondral grafts (either autografts or allografts). Falez and Sciarretta[206] performed a preliminary clinical study and concluded that the use of this type of treatment should be limited to precise indications: grade 3 and 4 chondral or osteochondral symptomatic defects, focal unicompartmental defects with 15-mm maximum extent, limitation of the patient's age to the fourth to seventh decade of life, or absence of angular deformities or articular instabilities. Although cases of failure and dislocation have been reported,[207] the synthetic cartilage resurfacing technique has the advantages of no donor defect, one short-step surgical procedure, and immediate weight-bearing ability.[206]

The TruFit CB plug is also a synthetic osteochondral implant that consists of a porous PLGA scaffold that is reinforced with PGA fibers and calcium sulfate mineral. Dhollander et al.[208] investigated the TruFit CB for osteochondral repair and observed modest outcomes. In a more recent study, Joshi et al.[209] reported that, although the TruFit CB system led to initial symptom relief in 10 patients with a median age of 33.3 years, a failure to regenerate subchondral bone over a 2-year period was observed, which in the long term could lead to implant failure and a repeat operation.

In a systematic review of the use of scaffolds in the repair of articular cartilage lesions by Filardo et al.,[210] nine approaches were identified using two-stage procedures and seven approaches were identified using single-stage procedures. It was noted that, although there are a multitude of cell/scaffold options available, well-designed studies exploring efficacy and long-term outcomes are lacking. Overall, a plethora of implants based on both natural and synthetic materials for cartilage and osteochondral repair are commercially available. Implants offer advantages over the ACI procedure because they circumvent the use of periosteal tissue, they address the challenge of homogenous cell distribution and retention within the defect site, and they can provide a 3D matrix that supports chondrocyte phenotype maintenance. Although most implants are engineered to regenerate cartilage tissue, osteochondral implants provide support for both bone and cartilage tissue regeneration. As mentioned previously, the next frontier in cartilage restoration will likely augment the aforementioned scaffolds with MSCs. Kon et al.[211] performed a systematic review of scaffold treatments with and without the use of cells and found that the majority of studies that incorporated cells found them superior to scaffold alone (71 of 89 articles). However, given the variety in scaffold products and types of cells used, it has proven difficult to fairly compare outcomes. Looking forward, approaches may focus on the recruitment of appropriate cells into acellular scaffolds, development of optimal scaffold microstructure, and integration of grafts with host tissue.[170]

SUTURES

Many of the synthetic implants discussed in this chapter require fixation via suturing at the site of implantation. Similar to the implants described previously, biocompatibility and the mechanical properties of the suture must be considered. In addition to sustaining physiologic loading, suture mechanical properties also need to withstand pressure from knot-tying techniques.[212] In this section, nonabsorbable versus absorbable sutures and monofilament versus braided sutures are discussed. Nonabsorbable sutures are fabricated from inert materials that do not degrade and are left at the repair site permanently or removed manually. Absorbable sutures degrade over time within the body; they are typically made of polymers that degrade by hydrolysis or enzymatically. Each type of suture has advantages for certain tissue repair procedures and can further be broken down into monofilament and braided sutures. Monofilament sutures are composed of a single fiber, whereas multifilament sutures are composed of multiple fibers, often encased in an outer sheath. Braided sutures are made up of multiple fibers and have the advantages of a grooved surface that prevents knots from loosening, improved handling, and low memory (i.e., a minimal tendency for the suture to recoil back to its original position). Sutures may be composed of single polymers or polymer blends, depending on the desired mechanical and degradation requirements.

Nonabsorbable sutures are made from inert materials such as nylon (e.g., Dermalon, Monosof, Surgilon, Nurolon, and Ethilon), polybutester (e.g., Novafil and Vascufil), polyester (e.g., Surgidac, Ti-cron, and Cottony II), polyethylene (e.g., MaxBraid, Mersilene, and Ethibond), and polypropylene (e.g., Surgipro, Deklene, and Prolene). These materials all elicit a low level of inflammatory response.[213] These nonabsorbable sutures are commonly used for deep tissue repair, where long-term support is required, or for skin closures, where they are manually removed after healing.[214] Although nonabsorbable sutures only risk causing a foreign body response upon implantation, absorbable sutures may elicit further responses from the body during degradation because of degradation products in the local environment.

Absorbable sutures are fabricated from biodegradable polymers. Although many sutures have been developed from materials that elicit minimal inflammatory responses during degradation, a few materials that are associated with moderate foreign responses are still commercially available. Common biodegradable polymers used in sutures include PGA (e.g., Dexon S), PLLA, PDO (e.g., Monodek and Ethicon), and poly-D, L-lactic acid and their copolymers.[212] These materials exhibit varied rates of degradation, with a higher lactic acid content corresponding to a slower resorption rate.[212] In terms of inflammatory response, studies have shown that polyglyconate (e.g., Maxon) and PDO sutures elicit less of a foreign body response than do materials such as PGA (e.g., Dexon) and polyglactin (e.g., Vicryl).[214–219] Cat gut and silk fibers have been shown to promote a moderate to intense inflammatory response and are commonly used for skin.[212] Other examples of commercially absorbable sutures,

which can include modifications that serve different purposes for varying knot-tying properties and tensile strengths, are PGA with a polycaprolactone:PGA coating (e.g., Bondek Plus), poliglecaprone 25 (e.g., Monocryl), polycaprolate (e.g., Dexon II), PDO with polyglactin 910 coating (e.g., Vicryl), and polyglytone (e.g., Caprosyn).

Monofilament sutures minimize foreign body response because of the low surface area that is exposed to the body.[220,221] This reduction in surface area also results in a lower hydrolysis rate, and thus these sutures maintain their mechanical properties longer than other sutures.[218,219] They are also more easily removed but have issues with high memory, which complicates handling of the suture during surgery because of the stiffness of the material, causing the suture to recoil back to its original shape. Braided sutures have unique advantages related to knot-tying capabilities.[222–225] The braided structure helps the suture to maintain the knot structure and minimizes the risk that the suture will come undone after surgery. Braided sutures also have low memory, making them much easier to handle than monofilament sutures. Further modifications have been made to these sutures to improve their knot-tying capabilities. For example, Ethibond is a braided polyester suture coated with polybutylate for a slicker surface that improves arthroscopic knot tying.[226,227] Tevdek and Polydek have PTFE coatings to improve their strength, whereas FiberWire was developed to combat the issue of suture breakage during arthroscopic knot tying. It is composed of ultra–high-molecular-weight polyethylene (UHMWPE) surrounded by a polyester braid.[213,214,225,228,229] Braided sutures composed entirely of UHMWPE have been developed more recently (e.g., ForceFiber, MagnumWire, Ultrabraid, and Hi-Fi). Orthocord is another UHMWPE suture with a PDO core, and it is coated with polyglactin 910, which makes the surface of the suture more frictionless to improve knot-tying characteristics. Thicker material such as FiberTape (Athrex) have been developed, and in studies compared with No. 2 suture in double row rotator cuff repair, the thicker FiberTape has shown threefold higher contact pressures at the footprint and 1.5 times higher load to failure.[230] However, despite these superior biomechanical properties, the difference in retear rates at 6 months postoperative (16% in the tape group and 17% in the suture group) was not statistically significant.[230]

Despite the benefits of the braided sutures for improved handling, the grooved formation introduces complications. Contamination is more prominent in braided sutures because of the structure of the fibers, specifically in the grooved areas where immunocompetent cells are unable to infiltrate.[223,224] Thus many sutures with antimicrobial coatings have been developed, with an example being the triclosan coating from Ethicon on the Vicryl, PDO, and Monocryl sutures.[222,231–234] The triclosan coating was found to inhibit the growth of the bacterium *Staphylococcus aureus* in vitro and in vivo in a guinea pig model over 48 hours.

Recent laboratory work has extended the function of sutures for growth factor delivery and improved mechanics. A number of studies have demonstrated the potential of sutures to deliver growth factors to the repair site for enhanced healing. For example, animal model work showed that the growth factor PDGF-BB, delivered from suture surfaces, improved tendon healing.[235,236] More recently, porous sutures were developed, allowing for dramatically higher levels of growth factor delivery without compromising the mechanical properties of the sutures.[237] To improve load transfer between sutures and the tissue they are grasping, adhesive-coated sutures were also developed.[238] In an example case of flexor tendon repair, such an approach could improve the repair strength by twelvefold.

SUTURE ANCHORS

Different sutures are used in combination with a variety of suture anchors, depending on the needs of the damaged tissue to be repaired. Suture anchors are widely used in orthopedic surgery, especially in shoulder procedures, such as rotator cuff[239,240] and glenoid labrum repair,[154,241] as well as in the elbow.[242,243] A typical suture anchor consists of the anchor, which is placed in bone during surgery, and its suture, which comes either preloaded by the manufacturer or loaded at the time of surgery through an eyelet on the anchor. Most sutures used in suture anchors are UHMWPE, which have a higher resistance to breakage but fail through slippage, making knot tying critical.[244,245] This section will focus on the design and performance of the anchor.

A typical suture anchor resembles a screw with an eyelet loaded with suture material. Details of the design parameters, such as the length and diameter of the screw, the number of threads on the screw, and the location of the eyelet on the screw, depend on the properties of the bone tissue where the anchor will be placed to reattach soft tissue to bone. For rotator cuff repair, the greater tuberosity of the humeral head is the targeted region for placement of suture anchors. In general, the cortical bone of the greater tuberosity is thin, and thus excessive decortications during bone surface preparation in surgery could compromise the pullout strength of anchors that rely on cortical or subcortical fixation. In addition, trabecular bone density of the greater tuberosity varies with location and pathologic states.[231,246] For example, in a torn rotator cuff, the bone density of the greater tuberosity decreases significantly because of decreased mechanical loading in the region.[110,212,247] Because the bone mineral density can affect anchor fixation and pullout strength, this factor should be considered when choosing a suture anchor.

Suture anchors can be divided into screw anchors and impaction anchors based on the way in which they are fixed to bone. As its name suggests, the screw anchors are threaded, which helps them to advance into bone and hold the anchor in place once implanted. The screw anchor has a major and a minor diameter; the major diameter is the entire width of the anchor, and the minor diameter is the width of the inner core of the anchor. On the other hand, impaction anchors are threadless. These anchors are placed into the bone through external impaction onto a cortical hole that has a slightly smaller diameter compared with that of the anchor. After placement in the bone, the anchor expands, which prevents it from pulling out. Compared with impaction anchors of similar size, threaded anchors displace less bone but provide an improved holding strength because of the increased contact surface area between anchor and bone, given the presence of threads.[248–250]

Based on how the sutures are tightened after reattaching soft tissue to the bone, suture anchors can be categorized as either normal or knotless anchors. Knotless anchors have a special eyelet-suture system that makes suture tying unnecessary. The knotless anchor design has become instrumental in the lateral row of double-row rotator cuff repair.[251–254]

Suture anchors can also be categorized on the basis of their material. Early suture anchors used for shoulder surgery were made with metals (primarily titanium and stainless steel). Before suture anchors came into use, metals were already widely used in orthopedic implants such as total hip prostheses and had been shown to provide rigid fixation. Metal anchors can be visualized on standard postoperative radiographs, which makes it possible to assess anchor migration and potential treatment failure. These anchors are also bioinert and have minimal osseous integration with the host bone tissue. For example, it was found that stainless steel anchors became encapsulated by a fibrous layer, whereas titanium anchors induced a minimal inflammatory response. However, obvious disadvantages were also associated with the metal anchors. The first disadvantage relates to postoperative imaging. MRI is the preferred imaging modality for evaluating glenohumeral pathology, but metal anchors can cause distortion of the scans. The second disadvantage is that if a revision surgery is required, the previously placed anchors could make placement of new anchors difficult because the former may not be easy to remove. In addition, complications with metal anchors, such as chondral damage caused by anchor loosening and fatigue, have been reported. Therefore demand remains for alternative materials for suture anchors.

To avoid compromising the anchor performance criteria while satisfying the need for an anchor that does not interfere with imaging or additional surgical procedures, bioabsorbable anchors were developed. These anchors are more biocompatible than metal anchors but provide the same initial fixation strength of soft tissue to bone. However, biodegradable anchors should be absorbed at appropriate rates (i.e., not so fast that the anchor degrades and fails to maintain its mechanical strength before the newly formed tissue regains mechanical integrity, but not so slow that the anchor stress shields the repair site and prevents healing). Furthermore, the bioabsorbable anchors should be made from biocompatible materials that elicit minimal toxicity, antigenicity, pyrogenicity, or carcinogenicity. Given these requirements, polymers have become the preferred material for suture anchors. Early bioabsorbable suture anchors were made from PGA because it was already used in other FDA-approved biomedical devices. However, its relatively fast degradation profile (3 to 4 months) was reported to be associated with early loss of fixation, osteolysis, loose body formation, and glenohumeral synovitis. Therefore PLA, which has a much slower degradation profile, was used in the next generation of suture anchors. Currently, most bioabsorbable suture anchors are made from PLA, copolymer of PLA and PGA (PLGA), or a combination of the two. Although they are developed to outperform metal anchors, bioabsorbable anchors still could lead to postoperative complications such as bone osteolysis, chondral damage, and significant patient morbidity. To bridge the gap from initial fixation strength to eventual bone formation at the anchor placement site, without inducing osteolysis or synovitis, biocomposite anchors were then developed. These anchors consist of a bioabsorbable polymer and an osteoconductive bioceramic such as β-tricalcium phosphate. As the anchor degrades, so does the ceramic, resulting in the release of calcium and phosphate substrates, providing an environment that promotes bone formation. Compared with anchors that are made from solely from bioabsorbable polymers, biocomposite anchors may accelerate new bone formation. As a result, few inflammatory reactions and complications have been reported with the use of these anchors.

Polyetheretherketone (PEEK) has been developed as an anchor material.[246] It is a nonbiodegradable, bioinert polymer that is radiolucent and resists chemical, thermal, and radiation-induced degradation. Because of these properties, suture anchors made from PEEK provide high initial repair strength, minimal bone ingrowth, minimal inflammatory responses, and good postoperative imaging. In addition, because it is a plastic, PEEK is soft enough to be drilled through, which makes revision surgeries possible. Thus although they were introduced relatively late compared with metal and biodegradable anchors, PEEK anchors have quickly gained popularity in the market.

Because of the functional requirements, the most important parameter used to evaluate suture anchor performance is pullout strength. Barber et al.[79,110,246,255-257] has routinely evaluated and compared the pullout strength of commercially available suture anchors on porcine femurs. Previously they used a single-pull destructive test to discern pullout strength[246,255,258,259]; however, more recent studies use cyclic loading to more realistically stimulate the postoperative setting.[260,261] In addition, the glenoid anchors are typically placed in dense cortical bone, whereas anchors for rotator cuff repair are placed in cancellous bone. In previous studies from 2003 through 2011, 66 types of commercial suture anchors were tested, and it was determined that the main failure mode of metal anchors was suture breakage, the main failure mode of bioabsorbable anchors was eyelet breakage, and for PEEK anchors, failure by anchor pullout was also observed in addition to eyelet breakage.[57,246,255,258,259] In the 2013 study by Barber et al., strong UHMWPE suture was used and suture breakage was not a factor.[256] Twenty-four cuff anchors and 13 glenoid anchors were trialed. Each anchor was tested 20 times, 10 samples in cortical bone and 10 in cancellous. All were loaded with UHMWPE suture. The samples underwent 200 cycles of a 10- N to 100-N load. After the 200 cycles were performed, destructive testing was performed. No difference was recorded for the rotator cuff anchors or the glenoid anchors placed in cortical versus cancellous bone. The rotator cuff anchors withstood greater loads than glenoid anchors. The rotator cuff anchors failed mostly by eyelet breakage, whereas the glenoid anchors failed most often by anchor pullout. Of note, the all-suture anchors that were tested performed comparably with the solid-body anchors.[256] In a study by Goschka et al.[254] comparing all-suture anchors in double-row rotator cuff repair to solid-body anchors, the biomechanical performance under cyclic loading was comparable.

A recent study by Postl et al.[262] showed that augmentation of suture anchors with bioabsorbable osteoconductive fiber-reinforced calcium phosphate such as PMMA enhanced failure load by 66.8%. This may be a useful tool in patients with significant subchondral cyst formation or osteoporosis.

All-suture anchors were recently developed for rotator cuff repair to decrease bone damage. A recent study by Nagra et al.[263] compared four commercially available all-suture anchors to traditional suture anchors with a cyclic loading model. The tensile strength was significantly higher for traditional anchors (181 N) compared with the all-suture anchor (133 N). The all-suture anchors failed predominantly by pullout, whereas the traditional failed by suture breakage.[263] However, of note, knotless suture tape repair of a quadriceps tendon showed biomechanical superiority when compared to transosseous tunnels or suture anchor repair.[264]

Over the years, the suture anchor has evolved to become an instrumental tool in orthopedic surgery, especially in arthroscopic rotator cuff and labral repair. As its design has improved and diversified, its utility has been realized in other surgical sites such as the elbow and patella. As suture strength continues to improve and advances in knotless suture anchor strength and all-suture anchors develop, optimized surgical technique and subsequent improvement in patient outcomes will be achieved.

■ SUMMARY

In this chapter, current synthetic and tissue-engineered graft repair options for soft tissues associated with sports injuries were reviewed, specifically for tendons, ligaments, menisci, and cartilage. Development and implementation of these implants have reached various stages of commercialization and clinical use. In the case of tendon repair, ECM-derived tendon grafts and augmentation devices have exhibited mixed outcomes in clinical studies. Alternative treatment options such as synthetic and tissue-engineered grafts are being developed, with promising results for tendon regeneration and tendon-to-bone integration. However, several challenges remain to be overcome before the widespread clinical application of the tissue-engineered tendon implants can be realized. For ACL injuries, autografts are still the gold standard of care because synthetic and tissue-engineered grafts have yet to demonstrate their long-term efficacy and are at the in vitro or in vivo evaluation stages, but new techniques for ACL repair with collagen scaffold augmentation show promising results in early clinical trials. CMI was recently FDA approved for use in meniscal implant, and many other promising technologies such as biodegradable polycaprolactone nanofibers, foam polycaprolactone scaffolds, and hydrogel scaffolds for meniscus repair are being investigated, although most have not yet reached the clinical testing stage. The new frontier in meniscal therapy is incorporating MSCs. Finally, for cartilage and osteochondral repair, a wide variety of commercially available synthetic and tissue-engineered implants are available in Europe. In 2016 the FDA approved MACI as the first autologous expanded chondrocyte augmented scaffold for cartilage restoration. In summary, given the ever-increasing knowledge base regarding the mechanisms of musculoskeletal tissue formation and repair, as well as the promising results from the many preclinical and clinical studies currently under way, it is anticipated that both synthetic and tissue-engineered grafts will be widely used clinically for the treatment of debilitating orthopaedic injuries and will ultimately help to improve the quality of life for numerous patients.

For a complete list of references, go to ExpertConsult.com.

SELECTED READINGS

Citation:

Barber FA, Herbert MA, Coons DA. Tendon augmentation grafts: biomechanical failure loads and failure patterns. *Arthroscopy.* 2006;22:534–538.

Level of Evidence:

II

Summary:

The purpose of this study was to determine the load to failure strengths and modes of failure of various commercially available tendon augmentation xenografts and allografts. GraftJacket, CuffPatch, Restore, Permacol, and TissueMend were tested. Failure modes differed significantly among the implant types. Understanding of the unique properties of each graft and suture placement requirements was the focus of this work rather than determining of superiority of one graft over another.

Citation:

Lu HH, Thomopoulos S. Functional attachment of soft tissues to bone: development, healing, and tissue engineering. *Annu Rev Biomed Eng.* 2013;15:201–226.

Level of Evidence:

IV, systematic review of Level I to IV studies

Summary:

This review describes the developmental processes and structure-function relationships between soft tissue and bone. It discusses the interface healing response, with a focus on the influence of mechanical loading and the role of cell-cell interactions. It also explores the current efforts in interface tissue engineering, highlighting key strategies for the regeneration of the soft tissue-to-bone interface, and concludes with a summary of challenges and future directions.

Citation:

Perrone GS, Proffen BL, Kiapour AM, et al. Bench-to-bedside: bridge-enhanced anterior cruciate ligament repair. *J Orthop Res.* 2017;doi:10.1002/jor.23632.

Level of Evidence:

III

Summary:

This review details the pathway of how a tissue-engineering strategy can be used to improve the healing of the anterior cruciate ligament (ACL) in preclinical studies and then translated to patients in an FDA-approved clinical study. It outlines the clinical importance of ACL injuries, history of primary repair, the pathology behind failure of the ACL to heal, preclinical studies, the FDA approval process for a high risk medical device, and the preliminary results from a first-in-human study.

Citation:

Grassi A, Zaffagnini S, Marcheggiani Muccioli GM, et al. Clinical outcomes and complications of a collagen meniscus implant: a systematic review. *Int Orthop.* 2014;38:1945–1953.

Level of Evidence:

IV, systematic review of Level I to IV studies

Summary:

This systematic review summarizes and evaluates the clinical outcomes of the collagen meniscus implant (CMI) and its complication and failure rates. Eleven studies were included, the pooled number of patients involved in CMI surgery were 396. The Lysholm score and VAS for pain showed an improvement at 6 months up to 10 years. The Tegner activity level reached its peak at 12 months after surgery and showed a progressive decrease through 5 and 10 years post CMI implantation, however always remaining above the preoperative level. Only a few knees were rated as "nearly abnormal" or "abnormal" at International Knee Documentation Committee grading at all follow-up evaluations. The authors concluded that CMI had good outcomes regarding knee function and pain, with low rates of complications and reoperations.

Citation:

LaPrade RF, Dragoo JL, Koh JL, et al. AAOS Research Symposium updates and consensus. *J Am Acad Orthop Surg.* 2016;24:e62–e78.

Level of Evidence:

IV, systematic review of Level I to IV studies

Summary:

The American Academy of Orthopaedic Surgeons hosted a research symposium in November 2015 to review the current state-of-the-art biologic treatments of articular cartilage, muscle, tendon, and bone injuries and identify knowledge gaps related to these emerging treatments. This review outlines the findings of the symposium and summarizes the consensus reached on how best to advance research on biologic treatment of orthopedic injuries.

Citation:

Filardo G, Kon E, Roffi A, et al. Scaffold-based repair for cartilage healing: a systematic review and technical note. *Arthroscopy.* 2013;29:174–186.

Level of Evidence:

IV, systematic review of Level I to IV studies

Summary:

This systematic review explored the treatment of chondral and osteochondral knee lesions through the use of scaffolds, by showing surgical options and results of this scaffold-based repair approach for the healing of the articular surface. The authors selected 51 articles, with 40 focusing on two-step procedures and 11 focusing on one-step procedures.

Citation:

Barber FA, Herbert MA. Cyclic loading biomechanical analysis of the pullout strengths of rotator cuff and glenoid anchors: 2013 update. *Arthroscopy.* 2013;29:832–844.

Level of Evidence:

II

Summary:

The purpose of this study was to evaluate the biomechanical and design characteristics of suture anchors under cyclic loading. More than 30 anchors were tested, including all-suture anchors and knotless anchors. Rotator cuff anchors showed greater failure loads than did glenoid anchors in metaphyseal bone and cancellous bone. Rotator cuff anchors failed principally by eyelet breaking, whereas glenoid anchors failed more often by anchor pullout than by any other mode. No differences in stiffness were observed across the different rotator cuff and glenoid anchors tested.

Citation:

Lu HH, Subramony SD, Boushell MK, et al. Tissue engineering strategies for the regeneration of orthopedic interfaces. *Ann Biomed Eng.* 2010;38(6):2142–2154.

Level of Evidence:

II

Summary:

One of the major challenges associated with tissue-engineered bone and soft tissue grafts is biologic fixation at the implant site. This article reviews current tissue engineering strategies for the regeneration of ligament-to-bone, tendon-to-bone, and cartilage-to-bone interfaces, which are critical for improving biologic fixation and enabling integrative repair of soft tissue with bone.

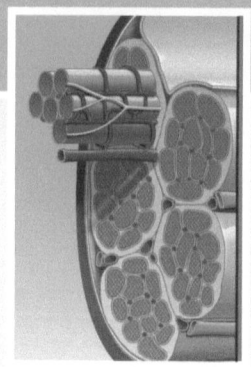

5

Orthobiologics: Clinical Application of Platelet-Rich Plasma and Stem Cell Therapy

Adrian D.K. Le, Jason Dragoo

The human body possesses a tremendous healing potential. However, despite its innate restorative capacity, in many instances the body's ability to heal is limited. Musculoskeletal tissues such as tendon, ligament, and cartilage present challenges to clinicians because these tissues tend to heal slowly because of their limited blood supply and slow cell turnover. Furthermore, conservative management or surgical intervention alone may not reliably recapitulate the normal architecture and function of the injured tissue. Therein lies the potential benefit of biologic therapy, in which the addition of growth factors and reparative cells may not only augment the normal body healing process but also restore normal form and function.

The use of biologic therapy or regenerative medicine has grown exponentially in the field of sports medicine in recent years. Although these emerging therapies may be based on solid preclinical evidence, these therapies are still in the stages of building clinical evidence before they are incorporated into standards of care. This chapter reviews the basic principles and best available clinical evidence on two growing categories of biologic therapy in sports medicine: platelet-rich plasma (PRP) and stem cell therapy.

PLATELET-RICH PLASMA AND SPORTS MEDICINE

The use of human blood concentrates to treat various tendon, ligament, and cartilage disorders and to augment surgical repairs continues to grow within sports medicine. The availability of PRP and its autologous nature allow for easy clinical application without the risk associated with allogenic products. As a result, PRP has been used in several clinical studies for the management of pathologic conditions of ligament, tendon, bone, and cartilage (Fig. 5.1). Although an extensive body of literature on PRP exists, a clear consensus for or against the use of PRP in the treatment of musculoskeletal diseases has not been achieved. What is clear is that not all PRP preparations are created equal,[1-4] and our understanding regarding the various components of PRP, along with its optimal composition, timing, and delivery, continues to be refined.

Definitions and Properties of Platelet-Rich Plasma

PRP is an autologous concentration of human platelets in a small volume of plasma produced from a patient's own centrifuged blood. The concentrated platelets contain increased amounts of growth and differentiation factors, which can then be delivered to an injury site to augment the body's natural healing process. The normal human platelet count ranges anywhere from 150,000 to 350,000 per μL. Improvements in bone and soft tissue healing properties have been demonstrated with concentrated platelets of 1,000,000 per μL, and thus it is this concentration of platelets in a 5-mL volume of plasma that has been suggested as one working definition of PRP.[5,6] A more modern definition of PRP is any plasma fraction that concentrates platelets greater than baseline. A resultant three- to fivefold increase in growth and differentiation factors can be expected with PRP compared with normal nonconcentrated whole blood. PRP preparations are typically further categorized into leukocyte-rich PRP (LR-PRP) preparations, defined as having a neutrophil concentration above baseline, and leukocyte-poor PRP (LP-PRP) preparations, defined as having a leukocyte (neutrophil) concentration below baseline.

Preparation and Composition

Currently more than 16 commercial PRP systems are available on the market, and hence quite a bit of variation exists in the PRP collection and preparation protocol depending on the commercial system being used (Table 5.1). Each commercial system has a different platelet capture efficiency that results in different whole-blood volume requirements to achieve the necessary final platelet concentration for PRP. The commercial systems may also differ in their isolation method (one- or two-step centrifugation), the speed of centrifugation, and the type of collection tube system and operation. In general, whole blood is usually collected and mixed with an anticoagulant factor, such as acid citrate dextrose, sodium citrate, or ethylene diamine tetraacetic acid. Centrifugation is then required to separate red blood cells (RBCs) from platelet-poor plasma (PPP) and the "buffy coat," which contains the concentrated platelets and ± leukocytes. The RBC and PPP layers may be discarded using various processing techniques to isolate the platelet-concentrated layer (Fig. 5.2). The platelets can then be directly injected into the patient or be "activated" via the addition of either calcium chloride or thrombin, which then causes the platelets to degranulate and release the growth and differentiation factors. Approximately 70% of the stored growth factors are released within the first 10 minutes of activation, and nearly 100% of the growth factors are released

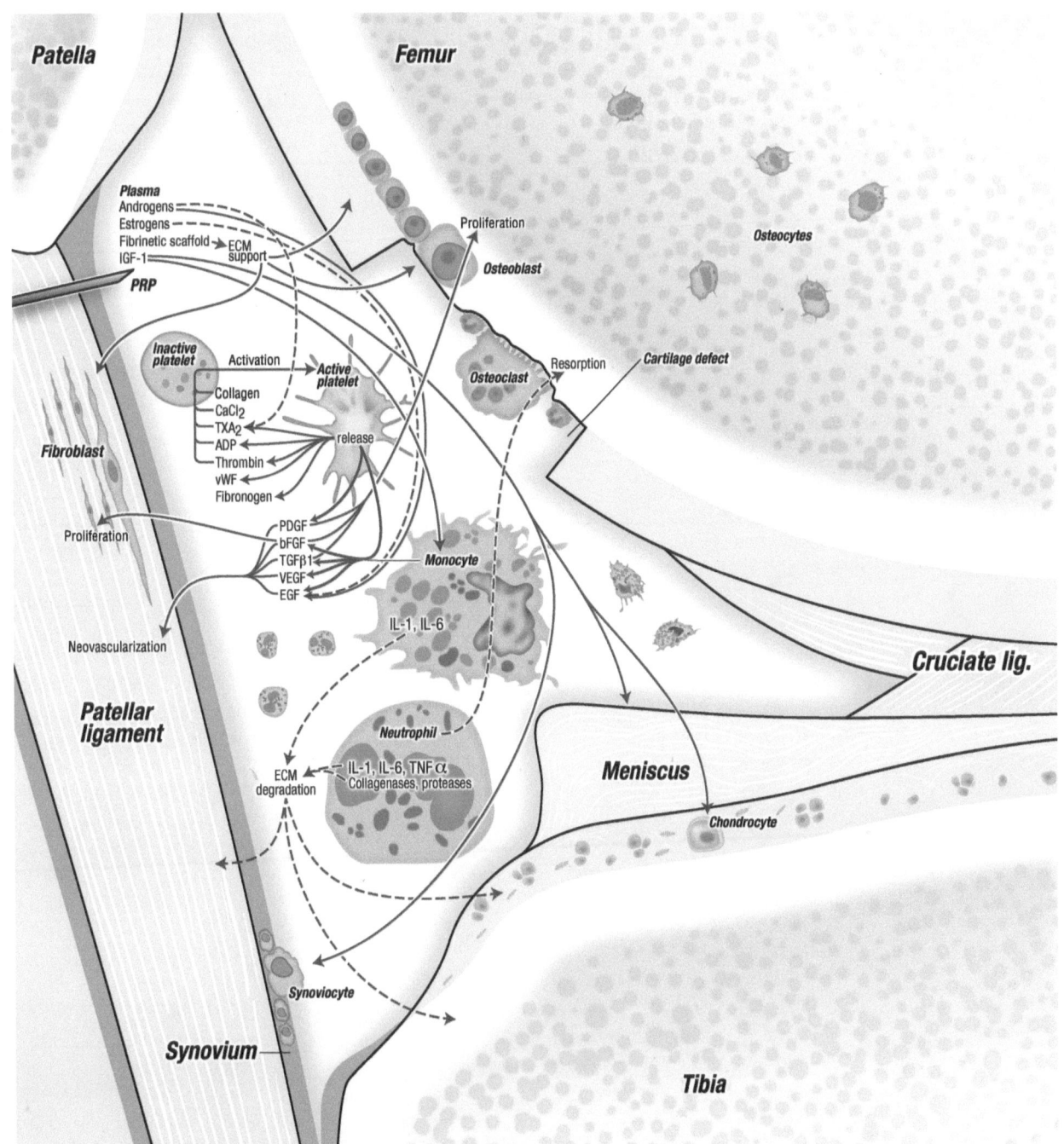

Fig. 5.1 The effect of various components of platelet-rich plasma on different types of tissues surrounding a joint. *ADP,* Adenosine diphosphate; *bFGF,* basic fibroblast growth factor; *CaCl₂,* calcium chloride; *ECM,* extracellular matrix; *EGF,* epidermal growth factor; *IGF,* insulin growth factor; *IL,* interleukin; *PDGF,* platelet-derived growth factor; *PRP,* platelet-rich plasma; *TGF-β1,* transforming growth factor-β1; *TNF,* tumor necrosis factor; *TXA₂,* thromboxane A₂; *VEGF,* vascular endothelial growth factor; *vWF,* von Willebrand factor. (From Boswell SG, Cole BJ, Sundman EA, et al. Platelet-rich plasma: a milieu of bioactive factors. *Arthroscopy.* 2012;28:429–439.)

within 1 hour of activation.[5,6] Small amounts of growth factors may continue to be produced by the platelet during the remainder of its life span (8 to 10 days).

Platelets contain a milieu of growth factors and mediators in their alpha granules (Table 5.2).[2,5] However, the specific composition of PRP likely varies not only from person to person but also when the isolation process is repeated in the same individual.[4]

Several elements are known to influence the specific makeup of PRP, which includes patient-specific factors and different commercial system preparation methods.[1,4,7] The variability in the cellular composition of PRP preparations creates challenges in interpretation of the literature regarding the clinical efficacy of PRP.

Our current understanding appears to suggest that PRP with elevated leukocyte content (i.e., LR-PRP) is associated with an

TABLE 5.1   Available Commercial Platelet-Rich Plasma Systems and Characteristics

System	Company	Blood Volume Required (mL)	Concentrated Volume Produced (mL)	Processing Time (min)	PPP Produced?	Gel Activator Available?	Increase in [Platelets] (Times Baseline)	Platelet Capture Efficiency (% Yield)
Leukocyte-Rich PRP								
Angel	Arthrex	52[137]	1–20[a]	17[137]	+		10[a]	56–75%[137]
GenesisCS	EmCyte	54[137]	6[137]	10[107]	+		4–7[137]	61 ± 12%[137]
GPS III	Biomet	54[137]	6[137]	15[137]	+	+	3–10[137]	70 ± 30%[137]
Magellan	Isto Biologics/ Arteriocyte	52[137]	3.5–7[137]	17[137]	+		3–15[137]	86 ± 41%[137]
SmartPReP 2	Harvest	54[137]	7[137]	14[137]	+		5–9[137]	94 ± 12%[137]
Leukocyte-Poor PRP								
Autologous Conditioned Plasma (ACP)	Arthrex	11[138]	4[138]	5[138]		+	1.3[138]	48 ± 7%[138]
Cascade	MTF	18[3]	7.5[3]	6[3]		+	1.6[3]	68 ± 4%[3]
Clear PRP	Harvest	54[a]	6.5[a]	18[a]	+		3–6[a]	62 ± 5%[a]
Pure PRP	EmCyte	50[a]	6.5[a]	8.5[a]	+		4–7[a]	76 ± 4%[a]

[a]Data obtained from manufacturers' promotional literature or internal studies.
PPP, Platelet-poor plasma; *PRP*, platelet-rich plasma.

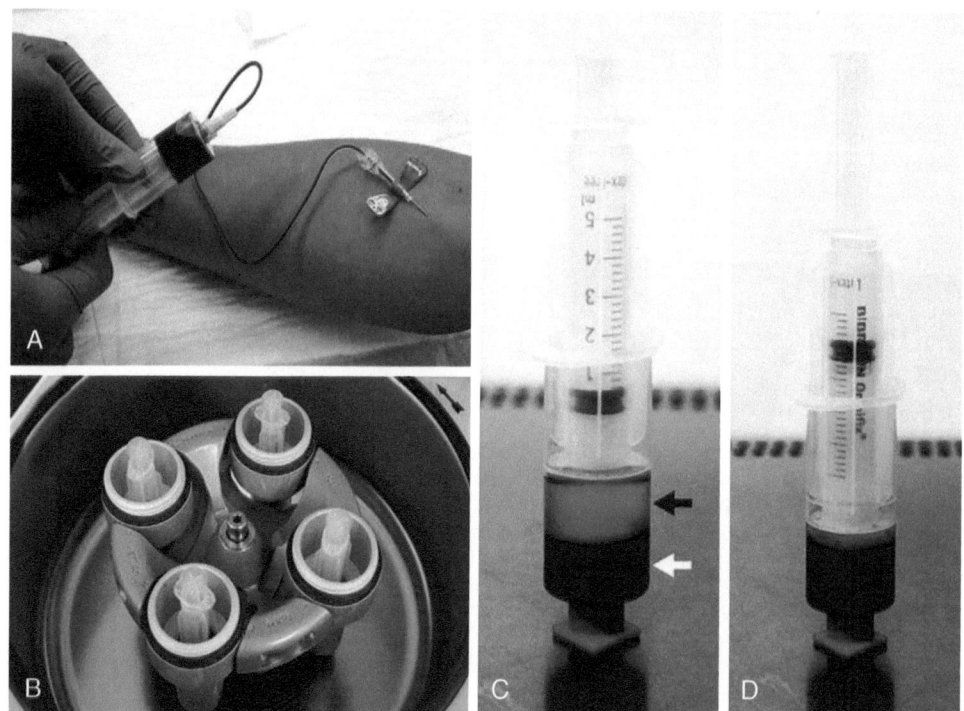

Fig. 5.2 Autologous platelet-rich plasma preparation using a single-step centrifugation system. (A) Autologous whole blood is aspirated in a double-syringe system. (B) The syringe is then placed in corresponding buckets of a desktop centrifuge and spun after balancing. (C) The serum fraction containing the clotting factors, white blood cells, and the platelets (buffy coat) *(black arrow)* is separated from the red blood cell fraction *(white arrow)*. (D) By pulling the stamp of the second syringe of the closed system, the serum fraction is extracted from the red blood cell fraction in a sterile manner for further use. (From Steinert AF, Middleton KK, Araujo PH, et al. Platelet-rich plasma in orthopaedic surgery and sports medicine: pearls, pitfalls, and new trends in research. *Oper Tech Orthop.* 2012;22:91–103.)

TABLE 5.2   Platelet-Rich Plasma Growth Factors and Their Physiologic Effects

Factor	Target Cell and Tissue	Function
PD-EGF	Epithelium, endothelial cells Fibroblasts, keratinocytes	Cell growth and recruitment Cell differentiation, skin closure Cytokine secretion

PDGF AB	Fibroblasts, smooth muscle cells, chondrocytes,
	   osteoblasts, mesenchymal stem cells
		Potent cell growth, recruitment
		Blood vessel growth, granulation
		Growth factor secretion; matrix formation with
		   BMPs (collagen and bone)

TGF-β1	Endothelial cells, keratinocytes Fibroblasts, lymphocytes, monocytes Osteoblasts	Blood vessel and collagen synthesis Growth inhibition, apoptosis (cell death) Differentiation, activation
IGF-I, II	Bone, blood vessel, skin, other tissues Fibroblasts	Cell growth, differentiation, recruitment Collagen synthesis with PDGF
bFGF	Endothelial cells, smooth muscle, skin Fibroblasts, keratinocytes	Cell growth Cell migration, blood vessel growth
VEGF, ECGF	Blood vessel cells	Cell growth, migration, new blood vessel growth Antiapoptosis

bFGF, Basic fibroblast growth factor; *BMP*, bone morphogenetic protein; *ECGF*, endothelial cell growth factor; *IGF*, insulin-like growth factor; *PD-EGF*, platelet-derived epidermal growth factor; *PDGF*, platelet-derived growth factor; *TGF*, transforming growth factor; *VEGF*, vascular endothelial growth factor.

acute inflammatory response. In an animal model, Dragoo et al.[1] demonstrated this large inflammatory response in vivo with increased cellularity and vascularity in rabbit tendons 5 days after treatment with LR-PRP, compared with LP-PRP. Elevated leukocyte (neutrophil) concentrations present in LR-PRP are also associated with elevated catabolic cytokines, such as interleukin-1β (IL-1β), tumor necrosis factor-α (TNF-α), and metalloproteinases,[7,8] which may antagonize the anabolic cytokines contained within platelets. The clinical ramifications and cellular effects of these different PRP preparations, including leukocyte content, are still currently being elucidated but have begun to allow for more customized PRP treatments to target specific indications.

PLATELET-RICH PLASMA IN TENDON- AND LIGAMENT-RELATED DISORDERS AND REPAIR

Tendon and Ligament Injuries

PRP has been most actively evaluated in the treatment of tendon and ligament injuries. Tendon and ligaments heal through a dynamic process with stages of inflammation, cellular proliferation, and subsequent tissue remodeling. Many of the cytokines found in PRP are involved in the signaling pathways that occur during this restorative process.[2,5] PRP may also promote neovascularization, which may not only increase the blood supply and nutrients needed for cells to regenerate the injured tissue but may also bring new cells and remove debris from damaged tissue. Both these mechanisms of action are particularly attractive in chronic tendinopathy conditions in which the biologic milieu may be unfavorable for tissue healing.

Clinical studies on the use of PRP for tendon and ligament injuries have mainly focused on the areas of the elbow, knee, and ankle. Studies on lateral epicondylitis suggest that LR-PRP may be effective and a reasonable option for patients who have failed to respond to a physical therapy regimen. In a prospective

cohort study, Mishra et al.[9] evaluated 230 patients who failed to respond to at least 3 months of conservative treatment for lateral epicondylitis. Patients were treated with LR-PRP and followed up for 24 weeks. At 24 weeks, the patients who received LR-PRP reported a 71.5% improvement in their pain scores compared with a 56.1% improvement in the control group ($P = .019$). The percentage of patients reporting significant residual elbow tenderness at 24 weeks was 29.1% in the patient group receiving PRP compared with 54.0% in the control group ($P = .009$). There was a clinically meaningful and significant improvement at 24 weeks in patients treated with LR-PRP versus active control.

In terms of the sustainability of treatment effect, PRP may provide longer continuous relief of symptoms for lateral epicondylitis than do corticosteroids. Peerbooms et al.[10] evaluated the efficacy of PRP versus corticosteroids in 100 patients who had a minimum 6-month history of recalcitrant chronic epicondylitis and had failed to respond to conservative management. Treatment success within this study was defined as, at minimum, a 25% reduction in the visual analog scale (VAS) score or Disabilities of Arm, Shoulder, and Hand score without a repeat intervention after 1 year. Although both groups improved in VAS scores from baseline, 73% (37 of 51 patients) in the PRP group versus 49% (24 of 49 patients) in the corticosteroid group were considered to have a successful response at 1 year ($P < .001$). Furthermore, 73% (37 of 51 patients) in the PRP group versus 51% (25 of 49 patients) in the corticosteroid group noted improved Disability of Arm, Shoulder, and Hand scores at 1 year ($P = .005$). Patients who received PRP also continued to report symptom relief 1 year after receiving the injection. In contrast, the short-term benefits of corticosteroids began to wane after 12 weeks. In a separate report, the improvement within this group of patients who received PRP continued to be noted 2 years after the PRP injection.[11]

In addition to the use of PRP to treat lateral epicondylitis, results from randomized controlled trials support the use of LR-PRP to treat chronic refractory patellar tendinopathy. Dragoo et al.[12] evaluated 23 patients with patellar tendinopathy on examination and magnetic resonance imaging (MRI) who had failed conservative management. Patients were randomized to receive ultrasound-guided dry needling alone or with injection of LR-PRP. Patients were followed for greater than 26 weeks. At 12 weeks, the PRP group had improved, as measured by Victorian Institute of Sport Assessment-Patella (VISA-P) score, significantly more than the dry needling group ($P = .02$). However, the difference was not significant at greater than 26 weeks ($P = .66$), suggesting that the benefit of PRP for patellar tendinopathy may be earlier improvement of symptoms. Vetrano et al.[13] also reported the benefit of PRP injections for treatment of chronic refractory patellar tendinopathy. Forty-six patients with ultrasound-confirmed chronic unilateral patellar tendinopathy were randomized to received two PRP injections over 2 weeks or 3 sessions of focused extracorporeal shock wave therapy (ECSWT). Although there was no significant difference between groups at 2-month follow-up, the PRP group showed statistically significant improvement, as measured by VISA-P and VAS, over ECSWT at 6-month and 12-month follow-up, and as measured by Blazina scale score at 12-month follow-up ($P < .05$ for all).

Compared with findings for lateral epicondylitis and patellar tendinopathy, the higher-level data with regard to the use of PRP in patients with Achilles tendinopathy have been less promising. In a prospective randomized trial, de Vos et al.[14,15] found no significant benefits with PRP versus a saline solution injection as an adjunct to eccentric exercises for mid-Achilles tendinosis. The authors reported no significant differences in Achilles tendon structure, the degree of neovascularization, and clinical outcome compared with the saline solution group. In a follow-up study on the same patients, de Jonge et al.[16] similarly reported no significant benefit in terms of pain reduction, activity level, and tendon appearance on ultrasound at 1 year after injection of PRP for chronic Achilles tendinopathy.

Rotator Cuff Repair

Most studies on the use of PRP products as an adjuvant to tendon repairs have focused on rotator cuff repairs. Some studies used a fibrin matrix as a carrier for the PRP,[17,18] whereas others injected PRP directly into the repair site.[19–21] In a randomized controlled study, Castricini et al.[17] reported outcomes based on Constant score and MRI-evaluated integrity of the repaired rotator cuff in 88 patients after 16 months follow-up. There was no significant benefit with PRP for small- (<1 cm) and medium-sized (1 to 3 cm) rotator cuff tear repairs. The authors found no significant differences between the PRP and the control group in terms of the Constant score, tendon thickness, and repeat rupture rate.[17] In another randomized controlled trial, Weber et al.[18] similarly reported no significant improvement using PRP in perioperative morbidity, clinical outcomes, or structural integrity. The study randomized 60 patients and found that structural results correlated with age and size of tear but did not differ between the PRP-treated group and control.

Randelli et al.[19] evaluated use of PRP in a randomized control study of 53 single-tendon rotator cuff repairs. Patients in the PRP-treated group reported short-term pain reduction and increased Simple Shoulder Test scores at early postoperative periods, with all clinical scores superior for PRP at 3 months after surgery ($P < .05$). In their subgroup analysis, patients who had undergone repairs of small-sized tears (grade 1 and 2 tears, with less retraction) had lower repeat tear rates (9 of 16 patients or 40% vs. 12 of 19 patients or 52%) and increased external rotation strength throughout the 24-month follow-up period ($P < .05$). Jo et al.[20] assessed the efficacy of PRP augmentation in a randomized controlled trial of 74 patients undergoing arthroscopic repair of medium to large rotator cuff tears. There was no difference between PRP and control in the Constant score at 3 months nor in VAS for pain, strength, or functional scores. However, the retear rate of the PRP group (3.0%) was significantly lower than the control group (20.0%) ($P = .032$) and the PRP group had a lower decrease in the cross-sectional area (CSA) of the supraspinatus muscle ($P = .014$), indicating an improved structural outcome. Finally, Pandey et al.[21] used an only moderately concentrated LP-PRP preparation in a randomized study of 102 patients undergoing repair of medium and large degenerative tears. VAS scores were significantly lower in the PRP group at 1, 3, and 6 months ($P = .0005$) but not later. Constant scores were significantly better in the PRP group at 12 and 24 months ($P < .01$) and UCLA scores were significantly higher at 6 and 12 months ($P = .002$). At 24 months, the retear rate in the PRP group was significantly lower than in the control group ($P = .01$), with subgroup analysis showing significance only for large tears ($P = .03$).

Achilles Tendon Repair

Data are limited on the use of PRP in the repair of acute Achilles tendon tears, and findings in the existing literature are conflicting. Schepull et al.[22] evaluated the use of PRP in Achilles tendon repair in a randomized study ($n = 30$). Although no differences were reported with regard to tendon elasticity and heel raise index between the PRP and control groups, the authors did note a lower Achilles Tendon Total Rupture score among the PRP group, which suggests a detrimental effect of PRP on subjective outcome after repair. However, Zou et al.[23] enrolled 36 patients with acute Achilles tendon rupture in a prospective randomized controlled study using intraoperative LR-PRP injection versus repair without PRP. Patients were followed for 24 months. Patients from the PRP group had better isokinetic muscle at 3 months and had higher SF-36 and Leppilahti scores at 6 and 12 months, respectively ($P < .05$ for all). Ankle range of motion (ROM) was also significantly better in the PRP group at all time points of 6-, 12-, and 24-months ($P < .001$).

Anterior Cruciate Ligament Surgery

The success of anterior cruciate ligament (ACL) surgery not only hinges on technical factors (e.g., graft tunnel placement and graft fixation) but also biologic healing of the ACL graft. Given its potential for improving tissue vascularity and ligament healing, PRP has been used to augment ACL graft maturation and graft–bone tunnel incorporation after reconstruction. Within the research literature, ACL graft maturation tends to be assessed with MRI. The assumption is that a low homogenous intensity signal on T2- and proton density–weighted MRI is likely indicative of a healthy maturing ACL graft. In terms of the effect of PRP on ACL graft maturation, some studies have demonstrated improved graft maturation with PRP,[24–27] whereas others reported a lack of significant differences.[28,29] Authors of a recent systematic review of 11 controlled trials, which included studies in which statistical significance was not reached, concluded that PRP likely improves ACL graft maturation, by up to 50%. The authors pointed to insufficient sample size as a potential rationale for lack of statistical significance despite MRI improvement in some metrics measuring ACL graft maturation.[30]

The other component to successful biologic healing of an ACL graft is graft–bone tunnel incorporation. The existing literature on the use of PRP to augment healing of the graft-bone interface is inconclusive at best. Vogrin et al.[29] evaluated the effects of PRP gel treatment for hamstring autograft ACL reconstruction in a controlled double-blinded study. MRI was used after the operation to assess vascularization along the ACL graft-bone interface. The authors reported evidence of improved vascularization along the interface at 3 months with use of PRP, but the observed benefit dissipated by 6 months after the surgical procedure. Other studies have similarly reported limited to no evidence to support the use of PRP to augment ACL graft–bone tunnel incorporation.[24,31] Of note is that nearly all of the studies used an LR-PRP formulation and LR-PRP formulations increase local tissue inflammation, which may delay or alter healing.[1]

One final point of consideration is whether any of the observed benefit of PRP on ACL graft maturation or graft-tunnel healing would translate into improved clinical results. The current best available evidence seems to suggest no significant benefit for functional outcome with use of PRP.[24,28,32] Ventura et al.[32] found no differences in Knee Injury and Osteoarthritis Outcome score (83 vs. 84 points), KT-1000 (0.8 mm vs. 1.2 mm), or Tegner scores (0.9 vs. 0.8 difference preoperative to postoperative) between the PRP-treated group and control subjects at 6 months despite reporting a significant difference in graft appearance. Orrego et al.[24] similarly noted no significant benefit in both Lysholm and International Knee Documentation Committee scores at 6 months after the operation despite identifying a positive effect of PRP on graft maturation. In summary, evidence from the current literature suggests that PRP may improve the rate at which ACL grafts achieve a low signal on MRI T2-weighted imaging but have little to no effect on graft-tunnel incorporation. A demonstrable benefit in patient outcome after use of PRP in patients undergoing ACL surgery is also lacking.

PLATELET-RICH PLASMA IN CARTILAGE RESTORATION

When considering biologic approaches to cartilage problems, it is important to understand that focal cartilage injuries differ from arthritis in terms of joint biology, homeostasis, and levels of metalloproteases and inflammatory cytokines.[33] Therefore PRP applications and clinical results for cartilage lesions and osteoarthritis may be quite different for either condition. The idea of using PRP for cartilage repair is based on in vitro basic science literature that growth factors released by the platelet

alpha granules may increase the synthetic capacity of chondrocytes through upregulation of gene expression, proteoglycan production, and deposition of type II collagen.[34–36]

Although very few clinical reports or trials have evaluated the use of PRP for treatment of focal cartilage lesions, Dhollander et al.[37] reported a pilot case series of five patients surgically treated with autologous matrix-induced autologous chondrocyte implantation (MACI) combined with a PRP gel. The authors reported that although VAS scores for pain decreased, the lesion was not filled after 12 and 24 months based on MRI evaluations, and intralesional osteophytes developed in three of the five patients.

Most clinical reports on the use of PRP for cartilage injury involve patients with osteoarthritis of the knee. A recent meta-analysis by Riboh et al.[38] compared LP-PRP and LR-PRP in the treatment of knee osteoarthritis and found that LP-PRP injections resulted in significantly improved WOMAC scores compared with hyaluronic acid (HA)[39,40] or placebo.[41,42] Patel et al.[41] performed a prospective randomized trial comparing single- or double-injection LP-PRP with saline solution in 78 patients with early osteoarthritis. They concluded that a single injection of PRP was as effective as a double injection. On the other hand, Filardo et al.[43] enrolled 192 patients in a randomized controlled study and found no difference between LR-PRP and HA, providing further evidence that LP-PRP may be an effective choice for treatment of osteoarthritis symptoms and LR-PRP appears not to be.[38] The biological basis for this may be in the relative level of inflammatory versus antiinflammatory mediators present in LR-PRP and LP-PRP. Inflammatory mediators TNF-α, IL-6, interferon-γ (IFN-γ), and IL-1β are increased significantly in the presence of LR-PRP,[7,44,45] whereas injection of LP-PRP increases IL-4 and IL-10, which are antiinflammatory mediators. IL-10 specifically was found to be helpful in the treatment of hip osteoarthritis[46] and may also suppress the release of the inflammatory mediators TNF-α, IL-6, and IL-1β, and block the inflammatory pathway by neutralizing nuclear factor–kB activity.[7,44,46] In addition to its deleterious effects on chondrocytes, LR-PRP may also fail to help treat osteoarthritis symptoms due to its effect on synoviocytes. Braun et al.[47] found that treatment of synovial cells with LR-PRP or erythrocytes resulted in significant proinflammatory mediator production and cell death.

PLATELET-RICH PLASMA IN MENISCAL REPAIR

The idea of augmenting meniscus repair with growth factors is not a recent one. In 1988 Arnoczky et al.[48] proposed the use of an exogenous fibrin clot to stimulate a reparative response in the avascular portion of the meniscus. In 1990 Henning et al.[49] reported that the failure rate for an isolated meniscus tear repair was 41% without a fibrin clot versus 8% with a fibrin clot. Bhargava et al.[50] demonstrated that platelet-derived growth factor increases the number of cells and tissue formation in a meniscus defect explant model. Several other in vitro and in vivo studies have demonstrated the potential for cytokines found in PRP to improve meniscal cell growth and meniscus repair healing.[51–55] Ishida et al.[53] performed a combined in vivo and in vitro study demonstrating that PRP led to improved meniscal repair in full-thickness 1.5-mm diameter defects in the avascular zone of the rabbit meniscus.

Augmenting meniscal repair with PRP is logical because it may deliver growth factors to the healing tissue, but a paucity of human clinical data exists. Pujol et al.[56] evaluated 34 young patients (age 13 to 40, median age 28) with symptomatic grade 2 or 3 horizontal meniscus tears in a case-control study. PRP was injected prior to skin closure in an open meniscal repair versus open meniscal repair alone. One year after surgery, KOOS scores for pain, symptoms, daily activities, sports, and quality of life were superior in the PRP-treated group, reaching statistical significance for pain and sports parameters ($P < .05$). Five out of the 17 cases in the PRP group had complete disappearance of any abnormal signal within the repaired meniscus on MRI, compared with none in the open repair alone group ($P < .01$).

PLATELET-RICH PLASMA FOR MUSCLE INJURIES

The use of PRP in the treatment of muscle injuries has attracted a significant amount of interest in recent years. Similar to tendon healing, the steps in muscle healing involve the initial inflammatory response, which is then followed by cell proliferation, differentiation, and tissue remodeling. Hamid et al.[57] conducted a single-blind randomized study of 28 patients with grade 2 hamstring muscle injuries comparing an injection of LR-PRP with a rehabilitation program versus rehabilitation alone. The group treated with LR-PRP was able to return to play (RTP) in a significantly shorter amount of time compared with control (mean time in days, 26.7 vs. 42.5, $P = .02$), but structural improvement was not achieved. In a double-blind randomized controlled trial, Reurink et al.[58] evaluated 80 patients comparing PRP injections to placebo saline injections, with all patients receiving standard rehabilitation. The patients were followed for 6 months and there were no significant differences in RTP time or with reinjury rate.

Although clinical studies have not found PRP to be efficacious in treating muscle injuries, advances in laboratory research may lead to improved understanding of treatment modalities. In vitro studies have found that PRP is capable of leading to myoblast proliferation but not to myoblast differentiation,[59] a requisite step in producing muscle tissue. Furthermore, growth factors contained in platelets, specifically myostatin (MSTN) and transforming growth factor-β1 (TGF-β1), are actually detrimental to muscle regeneration.[60,61] Miroshnychenko et al.[62] found in vitro that treatment with PPP or PRP with a second centrifugation step to remove the platelets induced myoblasts into muscle differentiation. This suggests that perhaps the most beneficial treatment of muscle injuries may be with PPP, although in vivo animal studies followed by human clinical trials will be necessary to further explore this treatment option in the future.

STEM-CELL–BASED THERAPY IN SPORTS MEDICINE

A fundamental limitation in healing of musculoskeletal tissue is the relative avascular nature of certain tissues, such as cartilage and tendon, which poses a barrier to mobilization of reparative cells and mediators to the site of injury or damage. Proinflammatory cytokines and mitogenic factors are sometimes unable to recruit progenitor cells in sufficient numbers to meet the regenerative needs of the tissue. In a way, this remains an inadequacy of PRP therapy in that the injection of autologous cytokines and growth factors may not achieve its full beneficial effect in stem cell–poor tissues, which may a contributing factor in the mixed efficacy of PRP and cellular therapy, depending upon the clinical indication. The advent of cell-based therapies has been seen as an intriguing advancement in meeting this deficiency in musculoskeletal tissue healing.[63]

Cell-based approaches may use cells that have already differentiated into a specific tissue type and function (such as autologous chondrocyte implantation [ACI] for cartilage repair) or undifferentiated multipotent stem cells, mesenchymal stem cells (MSCs),[64] that retain the capacity to adapt their form and function based on environmental cues. MSC populations were initially discovered in bone marrow but have been isolated from other mesenchymal tissues, including adipose tissue, skin, synovial fluid, periosteum, umbilical cord blood, placenta, and amniotic fluid.[65–67] MSCs are now known to originate as pericytes[68,69] and can differentiate into bone, cartilage, tendon, muscle, and adipose tissues.[70,71] Although MSCs can regenerate various mesenchymal tissues in vitro and some degree of direct engraftment into the repair tissue is suspected in vivo, the greatest therapeutic impact of MSCs in vivo are their trophic and immune-modulatory effects via paracrine mechanisms (Fig. 5.3).[67,72–74] MSCs secrete growth factors and chemokines to promote cell proliferation (such as TGF-α, TGF-β, hepatocyte growth factor [HGF], endothelial growth factor [EGF], fibroblast growth factor [FGF]-2, and insulin-like growth factor [IGF]-1)[75,76] and angiogenesis (vascular endothelial growth factor [VEGF], IGF-1, EGF, and angiopoietin-1),[77] as well as possessing antiapoptotic potential.[78–80] MSCs may also play a potent role in regenerative processes through their antiinflammatory effect through secretion of prostaglandin 2, HGF, stromal cell–derived factor 1 (SDF-1), nitrous oxide, indoleamine 2,3-dioxygenase (IDO), IL-4, IL-6, IL-10, IL-1 receptor antagonist, and soluble TNF-α receptor[81,82]; as well as through inhibition of inflammatory cells such as T cells, natural killer (NK) cells, B cells, and other immune cells.[83] Furthermore, it is believed that MSCs also possess antimicrobial properties through upregulation of IDO and secretion of LL-37 (a member of the cathelicidin peptide family)[84] in response to microbes.[85,86]

Definitions and Preparations of Stem Cell Therapy

In 2006 the International Society for Cellular Therapy established a minimum set of criteria for defining MSCs. According to their criteria, MSCs: (1) must be plastic adherent; (2) must express cell surface antigens CD105, CD73, and CD90; (3) must not express cell surface antigens CD45, CD34, CD14, CD11b, CD79α, CD19, or HLA-DR; and (4) must be capable of trilineage induction (osteoblasts, adipocytes, and chondroblasts) in vitro.[87] However, these criteria are based on characteristics of the cultured cells in vitro and may not reflect the native phenotype in vivo.[88,89] For this reason, among others, the criteria and strict definition of an MSC continue to evolve. Assays for MSC populations

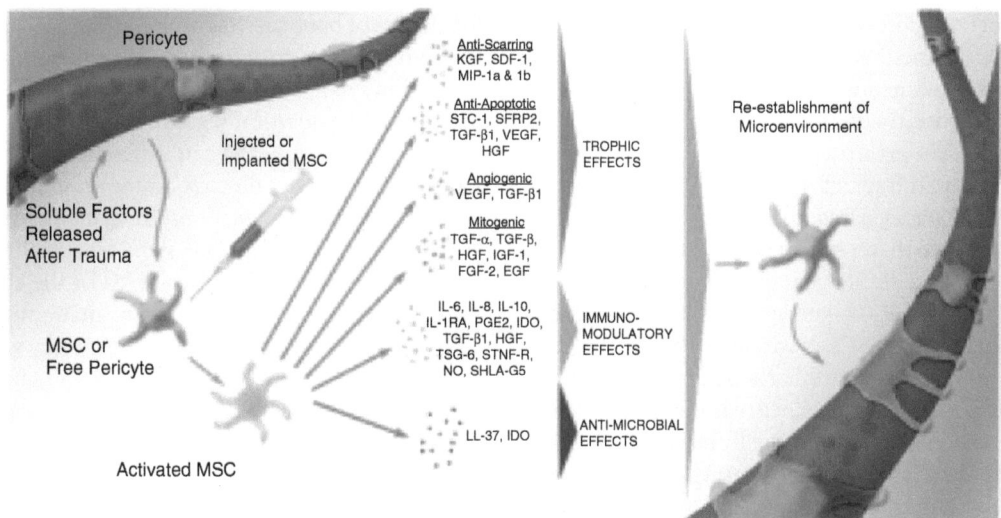

Fig. 5.3 Pericytes are stimulated by soluble growth factors and chemokines to become activated mesenchymal stem cells *(MSCs)*, which respond to the microenvironment by secreting trophic (mitogenic, angiogenic, antiapoptotic, or scar reduction), immunomodulatory, or antimicrobial factors. (From Murphy MB, Moncivais K, Caplan AI. Mesenchymal stem cells: environmentally responsive therapeutics for regenerative medicine. *Exp Mol Med*. 2013;45[11]:e54.)

measure their colony-forming capacity, or colony-forming unit (CFU), which is the number of single cells able to give rise in vitro to colonies of progeny cells.[90] Although the optimal method of autologous MSC preparation or isolation has yet to be determined,[89] current practices typically involve harvesting MSC-containing tissue from a source area of high yield and then concentrating the tissue to further isolate the MSCs before delivering them to the area of treatment. Stem cell therapy with MSCs for sports medicine indications most commonly uses MSCs isolated from bone marrow aspiration, or bone marrow aspirate concentrate (BMAC), or from adipose tissue, otherwise known as adipose-derived stem cells (ADSCs).[63]

In a BMAC preparation, bone marrow is percutaneously aspirated from a marrow harvest site and mixed with an anticoagulant such as heparin, then concentrated using centrifugation.[91] Several different marrow harvest sites have been used, such as the iliac crest, proximal tibia, proximal humerus, and calcaneus. Analyses have identified the iliac crest as the marrow harvest site with the greatest MSC yield,[92] with posterior iliac crest preferred over anterior iliac crest due to its superior safety profile (Fig. 5.4).[93] Various advances have sought to optimize aspiration technique and improve MSC yield. Muschler et al.[94] first looked at the effect of aspiration volume on the resulting MSC concentration. Their findings demonstrated that MSC concentration was maximized with aspirations of 2 mL and that aspirations larger than 4 mL had peripheral blood dilution.[94] Hernigou et al.[91] further examined technique using different sized syringes for bone marrow aspiration and determined that for a given marrow harvest volume; using 10 mL syringes resulted in a 300% higher MSC concentration than using 50 mL syringes. Further studies have suggested larger-volume aspirations are best performed from multiple harvest sites, through different harvest locations or through advancement of the aspiraction needle deeper below the cortex, instead of from a single location[95]; and rapid

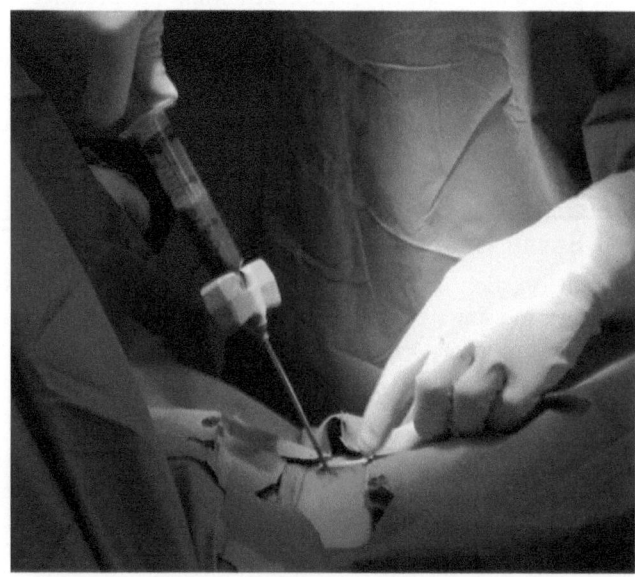

Fig. 5.4 Bone marrow aspirate is extracted from the iliac crest prior to concentration. (From Murawski CD, Duke GL, Deyer TW, Kennedy JG. Bone marrow aspirate concentrate [BMAC] as a biological adjunct to osteochondrallesions of the talus. *Tech Foot Ankle Surg*. 2011;10[1]:18–27.)

aspiration of the syringe increases MSC yield but increases patient discomfort.[96] Despite improved harvest techniques, MSCs still represent only a small fraction of the cells obtained from BMAC; of the $6-18 \times 10^6$ nucleated cells per mL of bone marrow aspirate obtained, only 0.001% to 0.01% are MSCs, whereas the remainder are various myelopoietic cells, erythropoietic cells, or peripheral blood cells, including platelets.[70,97]

In an ADSC preparation, adipose tissue is obtained through either a lipoaspiration technique or an operative tissue resection (open or arthroscopic).[98,99] The lipoaspiration harvesting technique typically involves percutaneous infiltration of subcutaneous fat (e.g., abdominal or gluteal) with a tumescent fluid, most often a mixture of local anesthetic and saline.[100] After the tumescent fluid is in the subcutaneous tissue and the area sufficiently anesthetized, the adipose tissue is aspirated using manual or mechanical suction.[99] The arthroscopic technique of harvesting adipose tissue from the infrapatellar fat pad was described by Dragoo et al.[101] [AJSM paper, Dragoo], whereby the fat pad is resected using a motorized shaver system which allows the adipose tissue to be collected in a sterile container. The mononuclear fraction of the adipose tissue, also known as the stromal vascular fraction (SVF), contains the MSCs, as well as endothelial precursor cells (EPCs), monocytes, and other vascular and immune cells.[102] Once the adipose tissue is obtained, whether by aspiration or arthroscopic resection, the tissue is usually mechanically fractionated, using either syringes using decreasing diameter Luer-Lok adapters or with proprietary systems, and then centrifuged in order to isolate the SVF from the majority of the adipocytes (Fig. 5.5).[103] Although adipose tissue contains fewer nucleated cells per milliliter of tissue (0.6–2.0×10^6 per mL of lipoaspirate),[104] MSCs make up a greater proportion of these cells (1% to 4%),[105] therefore making MSCs 100 to 1000 times more frequent in adipose tissue compared with bone marrow aspirate on a per volume basis.[105,106] However, while the presence of platelets and peripheral blood cells makes supplementation with PRP unnecessary for BMAC, ADSC on its own may lack some required growth factors. Therefore optimal treatment with ADSC may involve the addition of PRP to augment its regenerative potential.[107]

Challenges for Application of Cell-Based Therapies

Efficient isolation and delivery of MSCs remains one of the challenges in using stem-cell–based therapies as a point-of-care treatment in clinical scenarios. Hernigou et al.[108] suggested that

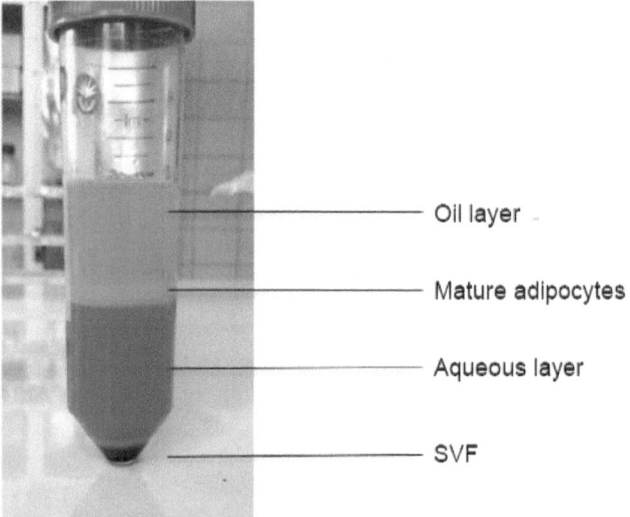

Fig. 5.5 Adipose-derived stem cell preparation with labels denoting the oil layer, mature adipocyte layer, aqueous layer, and mononuclear stromal vascular fraction layer *(SVF)*. (From Malec K, Goralska J, Hubalewska-Mazgaj M, et al. Effects of nanoporous anodic titanium oxide on human adipose derived stem cells. *Int J Nanomedicine.* 2016;11:5349–5360.)

the success of bone marrow aspirate grafting appears to be related to the number of progenitor cells in the aspirate. Several centrifugation systems are now commercially available to concentrate MSCs, but the question regarding the optimal number of cells needed to achieve healing in different musculoskeletal tissues remains. A significant obstacle for the optimization of cell therapy is related to federal regulations, particularly in the United States, governing use of autologous stem cells, including MSCs. Currently no method has been approved by the US Food and Drug Administration (FDA) to expand or manipulate MSCs, such as culture expansion or enzymatic digestion, which limits one's ability to optimize cell concentration and characteristics prior to implantation. The FDA regulates cell therapies primarily under sections 351 and 361, which are subject to different levels of regulation.[109] Products registered under section 351 require an investigational new drug exemption and biologics license application on file with the FDA, whereas products regulated under section 361 bypass the bulk of the requirements. To be eligible for regulation under section 361, cell preparations must be minimally manipulated, only used for homologous use, must not be combined with a drug or device, and must be used autologously.[110] For this reason, controversy exists around the potential use of allogeneic umbilical cord blood or amniotic sources of MSC therapy because currently no such product has been registered with the FDA under section 351.[111]

CELL-BASED THERAPY IN TENDON AND LIGAMENT HEALING AND REPAIR

Tendons and ligaments are relatively hypocellular and hypovascular connective tissues,[112] and this relative lack of cellular machinery and poor vascularity results in poor healing potential after acute or overuse injuries.[67] These tissues often heal by reactive scar formation rather than true regeneration, leading to altered function.[113] In response to this problem, biologic augmentation with use of cell-based therapy has been investigated. MSC therapy is thought to improve tendon and ligament healing through its immunomodulatory effects by reprogramming macrophages from a proinflammatory M1 phenotype to an antiinflammatory M2 phenotype.[114,115] Saether et al.[116] evaluated MSC therapy for enhancing MCL healing in rats, finding that treatment with a low dose of MSCs (1×10^6 cells) resulted in lower amounts of inflammatory cytokines (IL-1α, IL-12, and IFN-γ) and significant improvements in procollagen I, proliferating cells, and endothelialization. Mechanical testing also found improved strength and stiffness, thus demonstrating improved functional healing. Nixon et al.[117] evaluated the reparative properties of adipose-derived MSCs in an equine collagenase-induced tendon injury model. Compared with tendons treated with saline solution, the tendons injected with stem cells demonstrated decreased inflammation and significantly improved collagen fiber architecture and organization 6 weeks after MSC treatment.

Although clinical studies are limited, early data are promising for cell-based approaches to ligament and tendon disorders. Pascual-Garrido et al.[118] evaluated the use of autologous MSCs from BMAC for chronic patellar tendinopathy in eight patients. The authors were able to demonstrate both structural and symptom improvements in this small sample size. Although most of the gains were made in the first 12 months, the authors reported sustained benefit after injection of MSCs as long as 5 years. In a randomized controlled study, de Girolamo et al.[119] compared injection of ADSCs against injection of PRP in 56 patients with Achilles tendinopathy recalcitrant to conservative treatment. Both groups had significant improvements in VAS pain, VISA-A, and AOFAS scores ($P < .05$), with the ADSC group improving faster but with equivalent results between groups after 6 months. Lee et al.[120] examined the use of ADSCs from an allogeneic source in the treatment of lateral epicondylosis in 12 patients followed over 52 weeks. Throughout the entire follow-up period, all patients had improved VAS pain scores and elbow function scores, along with significant decrease in tendon defect areas as measured on ultrasound.

Clinical data are also limited with regard to use of MSCs for tendon repairs, which revolve around rotator cuff repairs, but have shown some encouraging preliminary results. Ellera Gomes et al.[121] evaluated 14 patients with complete rotator cuff tears (one to three tendon tears) who underwent a rotator cuff repair along with a single injection of BMAC. MRI analysis 12 months after surgery revealed good tendon integrity in all the subjects, with favorable clinical outcomes, although no control group was included in the study. In a case-control study, Hernigou et al.[122] followed 90 patients for 10 years after rotator cuff repair, with 45 patients receiving BMAC injection intraoperatively and 45 patients receiving single-row surgery alone. At 6-month follow-up, 100% of the patients receiving BMAC had healed versus 67% of the control group. At 10-year follow-up, 87% of the patients that received BMAC had intact tendons compared with only 44% of the control group. Among the patients receiving BMAC, the retear rate was inversely correlated to the concentration of MSCs delivered because patients with loss of tendon integrity received fewer MSCs compared with those that stayed intact. Although identifying a convenient localized source of MSCs during shoulder surgery could allow for easier augmentation of rotator cuff repairs, patients with symptomatic rotator cuff tears have decreased MSCs counts (30% to 70% less) at the greater tuberosity of the proximal humerus compared with those without rotator cuff injury.[123]

CELL-BASED THERAPY IN CARTILAGE REPAIR

Although no therapy or procedure has been shown to stop degenerative joint destruction in osteoarthritis, a significant cause of population-level morbidity, it is hoped that cell-based therapies can slow down or reverse articular cartilage damage through regenerative mechanisms. MSCs for chondrocyte differentiation can be derived from synovium, bone marrow, adipose, and muscle.[124] Stem cells for the treatment of osteoarthritis are primarily delivered via intra-articular injections, with or without accompanying surgical intervention.

Surgical delivery of MSCs with a scaffold is typically performed for focal articular cartilage lesions. Nejadnik et al.[125] reported their results comparing a cohort of 36 patients treated with ACI and a cohort of 36 patients treated with culture-expanded bone marrow–derived MSCs. The authors reported no statistically significant difference between the two treatments in functional evaluation. The authors also obtained biopsy specimens of seven patients (four in the MSC group and three in the ACI group) during second-look arthroscopy, which demonstrated hyaline-like cartilage in both.[125] Gobbi et al.[126] performed a comparative study on 37 patients with patellofemoral chondral lesions. Nineteen patients were treated with MACI and 18 with nonexpanded BMAC implantation, all with hyaluronan scaffold. After 3-year follow-up, both groups showed significant improvement ($P = 0.001$) with no significant difference between groups; 76% of MACI-treated patients showed complete filling of their lesion compared with 82% of BMAC-treated patients.[126] In a randomized controlled trial, Koh et al.[127] assessed the addition of ADSC injection with microfracture surgery versus microfracture surgery alone in 80 patients with femoral cartilage defect greater than 3 cm^2. The patients were followed for 24 months clinically and with MRI. The group treated with ADSC had significant improvement in KOOS pain score compared with control ($P = .034$). On MRI, 65% of ADSC-treated patients had complete cartilage coverage compared with 45% of control patients and significantly better signal intensity with 80% of ADSC-treated patients having normal or near-normal signal intensity compared with 72.5% of control.[127]

Clinical trials for intra-articular injections of MSCs for treating osteoarthritis have also been promising. Wong et al.[128] evaluated the use of intra-articular injections of culture-expanded BMAC in a randomized trial. Fifty-six patients with unicompartmental knee osteoarthritis and genu varum all underwent microfracture and medial opening-wedge high tibial osteotomy (HTO) surgery and were then randomized to receive an injection of cultured BMAC with hyaluronic acid versus hyaluronic acid alone 3 weeks after surgery. Although both treatment arms demonstrated clinical improvement, BMAC-treated patients had significantly better Tegner ($P = .021$), Lysholm ($P = .016$), and IKDC scores ($P = .001$) at 1-year postoperative. The BMAC group also had significant improvement by MRI evaluation ($P < .001$).[128] Koh et al.[129] looked at the intra-articular injection of ADSC plus PRP versus PRP alone in a randomized trial of patients undergoing HTO for genu varum. The group receiving ADSC injection with their treatment had significantly greater improvements in VAS pain ($P < .001$), KOOS pain ($P < .001$), and KOOS symptoms ($P = .006$) scores. Furthermore, ADSC-treated patients had significantly better cartilage healing ($P = .023$) on second-look arthroscopy.[129] Kim et al.[130] evaluated 41 patients (75 knees) with Kellgren-Lawrence grade 1 to 4 osteoarthritis of the knee. They underwent a single BMAC injection with adipose tissue scaffold and were followed for 1 year. At 12 months, there was significant improvement in clinical pain and function scores (as measured by VAS, KOOS, SF-36, IKDC, and Lysholm) compared with baseline and furthermore demonstrated that patients with more advanced Kellgren-Lawrence (K-L) grade had significantly poorer results ($P = .002$). In a randomized controlled study, Vega et al.[131] compared intra-articular injection of culture-expanded allogenic BMAC to hyaluronic acid in 30 patients with K-L grade II-IV knee osteoarthritis. The patients were followed for 12 months, and patients treated with MSCs had significant improvement in clinical pain scores and MRI cartilage improvement both in quantity and quality of articular cartilage. Michalek et al.[132] evaluated the use of ADSC with PRP in 1114 patients with knee or hip osteoarthritis in a multicenter case-controlled study. The patients were followed up for a mean of 17.2 months (range, 2.1 to 54.3 months) and measured modified KOOS/HOOS scores. At 12 months, 91% of patients treated with ADSC with PRP reported at least 50% improvement in symptoms, whereas less than 1% of patients were nonresponders, with four patients undergoing arthroplasty. In subgroup analysis, there was no difference in groups where the ADSC was treated with collagenase or not.

CELL-BASED THERAPY IN MENISCAL REPAIR

The potential of stimulating meniscus repair with use of bone marrow–derived cells has been described by Freedman et al.[133] by performing a microfracture adjacent to the PCL femoral origin to allow release of bone marrow elements into the joint. Meniscal repair performed with concomitant ACL reconstruction has historically demonstrated better healing rates, potentially as a result of the bone marrow elements in the joint due to drilling of the bone tunnels.[49] Several animal models have demonstrated the effectiveness of MSC augmentation in meniscal healing.[134,135] Although there is a great amount of available data from preclinical studies, the available evidence for use of stem cells in humans to augment meniscal repairs is much smaller. Vangsness et al.[136] performed the first randomized controlled trial assessing intra-articular injection of MSCs following partial meniscectomy. In this trial, 55 patients underwent a partial medial meniscectomy and were then randomized to receive low-dose allogenic MSCs, high-dose allogeneic MSCs, or hyaluronic acid (control). After 1-year follow-up, a significant increase in meniscal volume (defined as a 15% threshold) on MRI in 24% of patients in the low-dose MSC group and 6% of patients in the high-dose MSC group ($P = .022$), whereas no patients from control met this threshold. Furthermore, patients with underlying osteoarthritis who received the MSCs experienced a significant improvement in their symptoms (measured by VAS pain scores) compared with control ($P < .001$).

SUMMARY

The use of biologic augmentation, such as PRP and stem cell therapy, has great potential because it may help restore a tissue's form and function. Early clinical data demonstrate that the use of PRP and autologous stem cells for musculoskeletal treatment is safe; however, significant evidence of efficacy has yet to be shown. Certain biologic preparations appear to be more effective for certain indications, but the nuances of applying each therapy are still evolving. Interpreting existing literature has also been complicated because of a lack of standardization of the PRP or specific cell populations. Regulatory issues governing the use of stem cells and orthobiologics have continued to be a barrier in the development of these products. Despite these limitations, this technology has shown promise and will likely become an important component of the clinical treatment armamentarium in orthopedic and musculoskeletal medicine.

For a complete list of references, go to ExpertConsult.com.

SELECTED READINGS

Citation:

Mshra AK, Skrepnik NV, Edwards SG, et al. Efficacy of platelet-rich plasma for chronic tennis elbow: a double-blind, prospective, multicenter, randomized controlled trial of 230 patients. *Am J Sports Med.* 2014;42(2):463–471.

Level of Evidence:

II, randomized controlled study

Summary:

Leukocyte-rich PRP (LR-PRP) was evaluated against local injection of bupivacaine in 230 patients with lateral epicondylitis refractory to conservative therapy for at least 3 months. LR-PRP significantly improved symptoms at 24 weeks follow-up compared with active control.

Citation:

Jo CH, Shin JS, Shin WH, et al. Platelet-rich plasma for arthroscopic repair of medium to large rotator cuff tears: a randomized controlled trial. *Am J Sports Med.* 2015;43(9):2102–2110.

Level of Evidence:

I, randomized controlled study

Summary:

Seventy-four patients underwent arthroscopic repair of medium to large rotator cuff tears and were randomized to PRP-augmented repair or conventional repair. At 3 months follow-up, there was no significant in clinical symptom or function scores. However, at 1 year postoperatively, patients treated with PRP had a significantly decreased retear rate.

Citation:

Dragoo JL, Wasterlain AS, Braun HJ, et al. Platelet-rich plasma as a treatment for patellar tendinopathy: a double-blind, randomized controlled trial. *Am J Sports Med.* 2014;42(3):610–618.

Level of Evidence:

I, randomized controlled trial

Summary:

This randomized controlled trial evaluated dry needling with injection of LR-PRP for the treatment of patellar tendinopathy versus dry needling only. All patients were given standard eccentric exercises. Injection of LR-PRP significantly accelerated recovery from patellar tendinopathy. The benefit of PRP dissipated over time.

Citation:

Michalek J, Moster R, Lukac L, et al. Autologous adipose tissue-derived stromal vascular fraction cells application in patients with osteoarthritis. *Cell Transplant.* 2015.

Level of Evidence:

III, multicenter case controlled study

Summary:

Multicenter case control study involving 1114 patients with knee or hip osteoarthritis were injected with adipose tissue-derived stem cells (ADSCs) plus PRP and followed up for a median of 17.2 months. At 12 months of follow-up, 91% of patients had at least 50% improvement in symptoms and 63% of patients had at least 75% symptom improvement; 0.9% of patients were nonresponders.

Citation:

Patel S, Dhillon MS, Aggarwal S, et al. Treatment with platelet-rich plasma is more effective than placebo for knee osteoarthritis: a prospective, double-blind, randomized trial. *Am J Sports Med.* 2013;41:356–364.

Level of Evidence:

I, randomized controlled trial

Summary:

A total of 78 patients (156 knees) with bilateral osteoarthritis were divided randomly into three groups: group A received a single injection of PRP, group B received two injections of PRP 3 weeks apart, and group C received a single injection of normal saline solution. A single dose of white blood cell–filtered PRP (LP-PRP) in concentrations of 10 times the normal amount was as effective as two serial injections to alleviate symptoms in patients with the early presentation of knee osteoarthritis. However, the results deteriorated after 6 months.

6

Exercise Physiology

Thomas M. Best, Chad A. Asplund

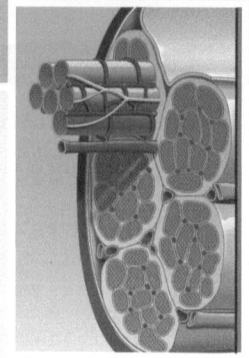

Exercise physiology is the identification and study of the physiologic mechanisms underlying physical activity and the body's response and adaptation to exercise. Most training programs used by athletes, whether they are for strength or endurance, aim to change the underlying physiology for the benefit of sport competition or fitness. This chapter discusses the major concepts of exercise physiology to provide a background that sports medicine practitioners can draw upon when treating or training athletes.

SKELETAL MUSCLE PHYSIOLOGY

The human body contains three types of muscle: smooth, cardiac, and skeletal. Training adaptations occur across all three types of muscle; however, this section focuses on skeletal muscle. Skeletal muscles support the body by working together to generate force across joints, leading to joint motion. Muscles also work to attenuate external forces in an effort to absorb shock and protect the joints.

Skeletal muscles are made up of different fiber types that have different properties, such as rate of contraction, force generation, and resistance to fatigue (Table 6.1). Skeletal muscle is made up of different fiber types. Fibers are currently classified by the myosin heavy chain isoform: one slow (type I) and three fast (IIA, IIB, and IIX). During the past several years, significant progress has been made in identifying signaling pathways that control the expression of muscle fiber types. With the recently discovered microribonucleic acids encoded within myosin genes that regulate muscle gene expression and performance,[1] a new individualized genetic differentiation may be possible.[2]

Muscle fibers are currently classified as types I, IIA, IIB, and IIX. In general type I muscle fibers operate at a slower twitch rate and are responsible for longer-term, endurance-type activities because of their ability to resist fatigue. Type IIA and IIB/X muscle fibers operate at a faster twitch rate and are responsible for high-force contractions, which dominate during explosive power maneuvers.

The true functional unit of the neuromuscular system is the motor unit. A motor unit is an alpha motoneuron (originating in the spinal cord) and all the muscle fibers that it innervates. Singular motoneurons innervate muscle fibers of the same contractile type in an all-or-none fashion. Although a muscle will contain more than one or all types of motor units, the percentage of each fiber type within a muscle contributes to its function and fatigability. Motor units can also be classified as either slow- or fast-twitch types, with the fast-twitch units divided into fatigue-resistant, fatigue-intermediate, and fatigable units. However, motor units can change in size in response to training and can also convert from one type to another.[3] This plasticity of both contractile and metabolic properties allows the skeletal muscle system to adapt to different functional demands.

Structure of a Skeletal Muscle

Bundles of fascicles encased in connective tissue (epimysium) make up skeletal muscles. Each fascicle is surrounded by a layer of connective tissue (perimysium), which contains multiple muscle fibers. The muscle fiber, itself an individual skeletal muscle cell, is cylindrical in shape, multinucleated, and composed of bundles of myofibrils surrounded by an endomysium (Fig. 6.1). These myofibrils contain thin and thick proteins that form repeating light and dark bands along the length of the myofibril, which give the muscle its striated appearance (Fig. 6.2); these repeating sections are called *sarcomeres* and are arranged end to end within each myofibril.

Sarcomeres are the functional, contractile units of skeletal muscle. Contractions are mediated through a dynamic interaction between actin and myosin, which are the contractile proteins. Spherical actin molecules in a helical arrangement form the thin protein structural lattice of the sarcomere. Each actin molecule contains a binding site protected by tropomyosin, a thread-like protein, and troponin, which acts as a stabilizing protein. Myosin molecules group together, each with a globular end, and form cross bridges, which are staggered toward opposite ends of the thick filament. These myosin molecules have a binding site with a high affinity for actin. This orientation of thick filaments at the center of the sarcomere provides the framework for sarcomere shortening and ultimately muscle contraction.

Physiology of Skeletal Muscle Contractions

Skeletal muscle contractions are a mechanical process driven by a neurochemical cascade. Several theories have been proposed about muscle contraction. The most widely accepted theory is the "sliding filament theory" proposed by Huxley and Hanson,[4] in which the active shortening of the sarcomere and the muscle results from actin and myosin "sliding" past one another while retaining their original length. An action potential from the motoneuron is propagated and acetylcholine is released from the axon at the neuromuscular junction, increasing permeability to sodium and potassium ions and causing an end-plate potential.

TABLE 6.1 Classification of Human Skeletal Muscle Fibers

	I	IIa	IIx	IIb
Contraction time	Slow	Medium fast	Fast	Very fast
Size of motor neuron	Small	Medium	Large	Very large
Resistance to fatigue	High	Fairly high	Intermediate	Low
Activity	Aerobic	Long-term anaerobic	Short-term anaerobic	Short-term anaerobic
Mitochondrial density	High	High	Medium	Low

Modified from McArdle WD, Katch FI, Katch VL. *Exercise Physiology: Nutrition, Energy, and Human Performance.* 7th ed. Philadelphia: Lippincott Williams & Wilkins; 2009.

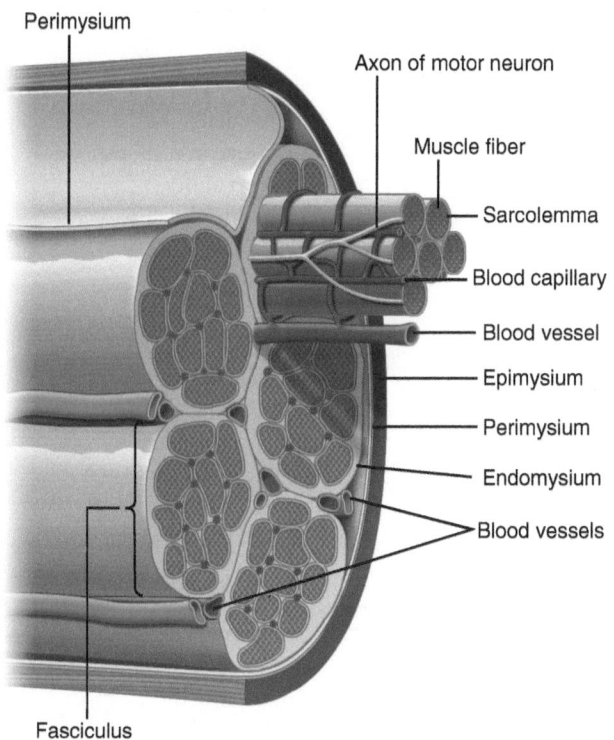

Fig. 6.1 Basic structure and organization of skeletal muscle with associated connective tissues, blood vessels, and motor neurons. (Modified from Palastanga NP, Field D, Soames R. *Anatomy and Human Movement—Structure and Function.* Edinburgh: Butterworth Heinemann; 2006.)

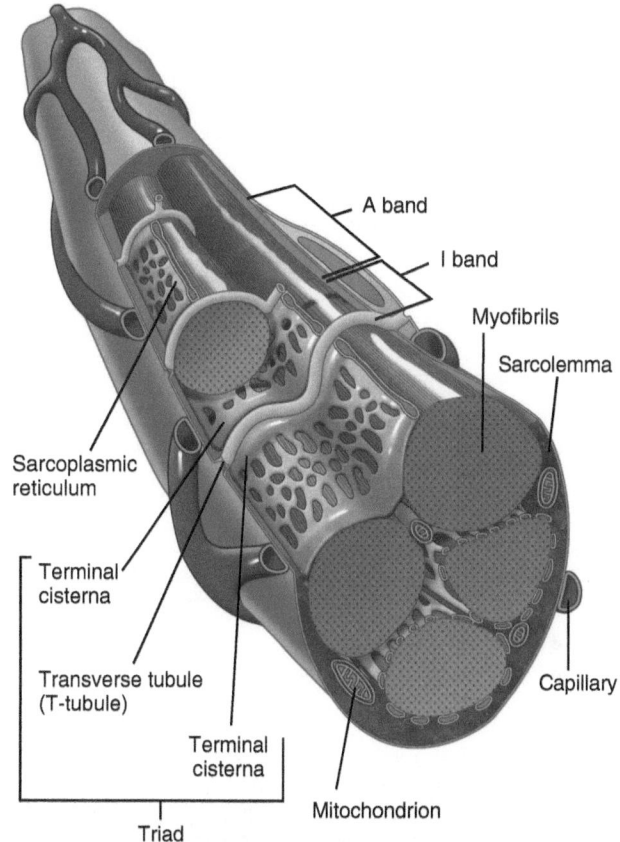

Fig. 6.2 Illustration of repeated sarcomere structure and organization within each individual muscle fiber. Each sarcomere contains thick (myosin) and thin (actin) contractile protein filaments that are responsible for sarcomere shortening. Alternating light and dark bands characterizing skeletal muscle are due to repeated bands of thick *(A band)* and thin *(I band)* filaments. The transverse (T)-tubule system is contiguous with the sarcoplasmic reticulum and sarcolemma. Once an action potential from a motor neuron is initiated, it propagates along the sarcolemma and is internalized to the myofibrils within a muscle fiber through the T-tubule system. (Modified from Seeley RR, Stephens TD, Tate P. *Anatomy and Physiology.* 3rd ed. St. Louis: Mosby; 1995.)

This potential travels along the muscle cell membrane through the transverse tubule system throughout all the myofibrils. Calcium ions released from the sarcoplasmic reticulum quickly bind to troponin molecules on the thin contractile filament, resulting in the binding of tropomyosin to the exposed binding sites on actin, which allows the myosin cross bridges to bind with actin, pulling the actin filaments toward the middle of the sarcomere (Fig. 6.3) and resulting in the filaments sliding past one another, causing muscle shortening and contraction. The collective shortening of myosin throughout the muscle is vital to force production and is termed the *power stroke.*

Calcium and adenosine triphosphate (ATP) are cofactors (nonprotein components of enzymes) required for the contraction of muscle cells. ATP supplies the energy, as previously described, but what does calcium do? Calcium is required by two proteins, troponin, and tropomyosin, that regulate muscle contraction by blocking the binding of myosin to filamentous actin. The power stroke requires the hydrolysis of ATP, which breaks a high-energy phosphate bond to release energy, leading to the release of the linkage between myosin and actin to prepare the myosin for another power stroke or for relaxation. If no new ATP is available, this linkage cannot separate, resulting in rigor mortis. Power-stroke cycles continue until the concentration of calcium is no longer sufficient to cause the binding of actin and myosin.

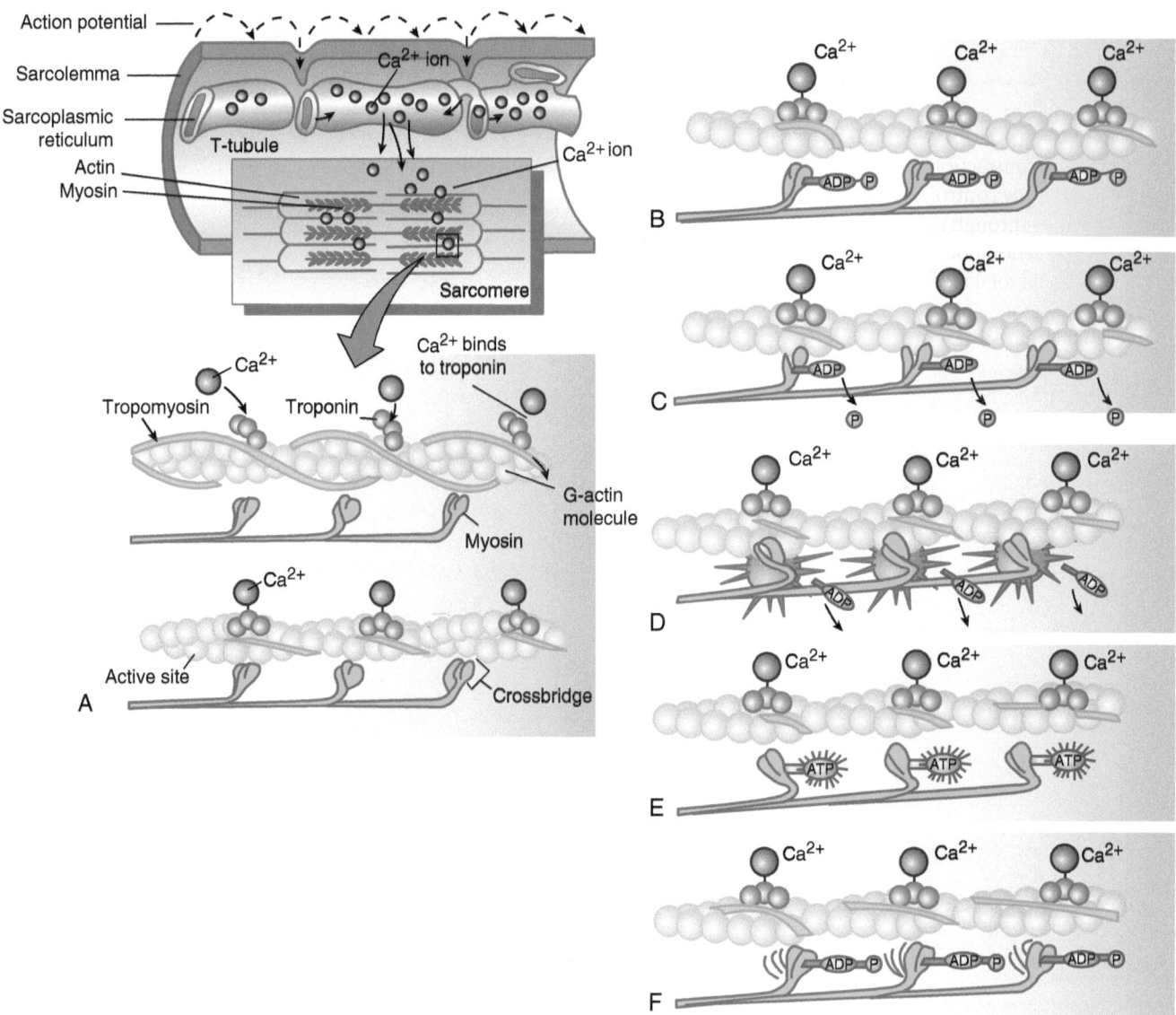

Fig. 6.3 Sequence of skeletal muscle contraction: sarcolemma depolarization causes calcium release from the sarcoplasmic reticulum. (A) Calcium binds with troponin and shifts tropomyosin molecules to expose myosin-binding sites on actin. Myosin cross bridges bind to actin, producing a "power stroke" of contraction. Adenosine triphosphate *(ATP)* is needed to break the link and prepare for the next cycle. Cycles (B to F) continue as long as sufficient calcium is present to inhibit the troponin-tropomyosin system from blocking actin-binding sites. *ADP,* Adenosine diphosphate; *P,* phosphate; *T-tubule,* transverse tubule. (Modified from Seeley RR, Stephens TD, Tate P. *Anatomy and Physiology.* 3rd ed. St. Louis: Mosby; 1995.)

Since the publication of the sliding filament theory by Huxley and Hanson in 1954,[4] new mechanisms have been proposed for muscle contractions. Several questions still remain, including enhancement of contractile force with stretch, depression of force with muscle contraction, and efficiency of force production during contraction. The winding filament model[5] and the sticky spring model[6] may both provide a means to assist in answering these questions by acknowledging the importance of the protein titin. Titin is activated by calcium influx and is wound upon the thin filaments by the cross bridges, which shorten but also rotate the thin filaments. Titin is also actively involved in force regulation of skeletal muscles, especially when muscles are stretched actively to long sarcomere lengths.[7] These new models account for force enhancement during stretch and force depression during shortening, but additional study is needed to further validate these theories.

Force Production of Muscle

Muscle force can be increased or decreased by the recruitment of more or fewer motor units. For any motor task, many possible combinations of motor units can be recruited, and it has been proposed that a simple rule, the "size principle,"[8] governs the selection of motor units recruited for different contractions. Motor units can be characterized by their different contractile, energetic, and fatigue properties, and it is important that the selection of motor units recruited for given movements allows units with the appropriate properties to be activated.[9] The structural presence of titin also plays a role in the force generated by muscle.[10]

Types of Muscle Contractions

Skeletal muscle contractions produce force and control joint movement and body control; they are capable of different activities and demands through different types of muscle contraction. Isometric contractions occur when force is generated but no apparent change in total muscle length occurs. Concentric muscle contractions generate a force that shortens the muscle. Eccentric muscle contractions occur when a force is generated as the muscle lengthens. Isotonic contractions produce muscle tension and joint movement against a constant load with a variable rate of movement. Isokinetic contractions have a constant rate of movement, which is maintained by varying the amount of muscle effort. Isokinetic efforts are rare in sport training but are utilized in the rehabilitation setting. In weight lifting or sport training, the two most common types of muscle contractions are the isometric, concentric activities, where muscles are shortened in a voluntary fashion to lift a constant load (weight), and the eccentric contractions, where the muscle lengthens against a constant load (negatives).

Although concentric muscle contractions are the contractions most people consider, eccentric contractions are probably more useful in the sports training and rehabilitation setting. During locomotion, eccentric contractions act to dissipate energy both as heat and as a shock absorber, reducing kinetic energy through a braking effect.[11] The energy absorbed within the stretched muscle-tendon can then be stored as potential energy and returned, allowing the muscle-tendon complex to act as a spring.[12] The muscle protein titin may be important in this spring-like property of the muscle.[13] Finally, the energy cost for eccentric contractions is unusually low,[14] whereas the magnitude of forces produced is very high. Therefore as a response to eccentric loading, muscles gain strength, which makes eccentric loading well suited for both strength training and as a rehabilitation tool.

Energy Metabolism of Skeletal Muscle

Exercise results in an increased rate of ATP demand. To sustain muscle contraction, ATP must be regenerated at a rate complementary to ATP demand. Three energy systems (phosphagen, glycolytic, and mitochondrial respiration) are available to synthesize ATP in muscle (Fig. 6.4). The three systems differ in the substrates they use, the products they generate, their maximal rate of ATP regeneration, and their capacity for ATP regeneration.

Phosphagen Energy System

The phosphagen system is important for exercises that require short-term singular muscle contractions or a limited number of intense, near-maximal muscle contractions. Within the phosphagen system, the creatine kinase and adenylate kinase reactions both produce ATP, but the creatine kinase reaction has a much higher capacity for ATP regeneration, given the large store of creatine phosphate (CrP) at rest. Another important feature is the adenylate kinase reaction, which produces adenosine monophosphate (AMP), which then activates two enzymes

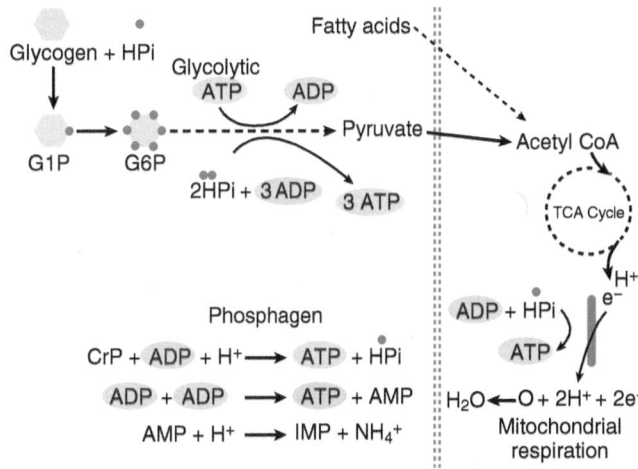

Fig. 6.4 Energy systems to synthesize adenosine triphosphate *(ATP)* in muscle. *ADP*, Adenosine diphosphate; *AMP*, adenosine monophosphate; *ATP*, adenosine triphosphate; *CrP*, creatine phosphate; *G1P*, glucose-1-phosphate; *G6P*, glucose-6-phosphate; *HPi*, hydrogen phosphate ion.

influential in glycolysis. AMP activates phosphorylase, which increases glycogenolysis and the rate of glucose-6-phosphate (G6P) production that becomes immediate fuel for glycolysis. AMP also activates phosphofructokinase, allowing an increase flux of G6P through glycolysis, which increases the rate of ATP regeneration.

It has been hypothesized that during the first 10 to 15 seconds of exercise, CrP is solely responsible for ATP regeneration.[15] Near-complete recovery of CrP may take from 5 to 15 minutes, depending on the extent of CrP depletion, severity of metabolic acidosis, and characteristics of the muscle fibers utilized.[16] Evidence is conflicting about the importance of oxygen during the resynthesis of CrP after high-intensity exercise. Some investigators suggest that CrP resynthesis is reliant on oxidative metabolism,[17] whereas others found that after high-intensity exercise under ischemic conditions, glycolytic flux remained elevated for a short period.[18] More recent work, however, supports the theory that glycolytic ATP production may contribute to CrP resynthesis during the initial fast phase of recovery after high-intensity exercise.[19]

Glycolytic Energy System

When exercise continues for longer than a few seconds, the energy to regenerate ATP is derived primarily from blood glucose and muscle glycogen stores. This prolonged exercise increases the production of AMP. This production, coupled with the increases in intramuscular calcium and inorganic phosphate levels, causes increases in the phosphorylase reaction and the increased uptake of glucose by active muscle. The increased rate of G6P production from glycogenolysis and the increased glucose uptake provide a rapid source of fuel for several pathways that degrade G6P to pyruvate within the glycolytic pathway.

Traditionally it was thought that CrP was the sole fuel used at the initiation of glycolysis, with glycogenolysis occurring only once the CrP levels began to fall. However, research suggests that ATP resynthesis from glycolysis during 30 seconds of maximal exercise begins almost immediately with exercise.[20,21] Maximal ATP regeneration capacity from glycolysis occurs when exercise at or above maximal oxygen uptake is performed for 2 to 3 minutes or as long as is sustainable by the athlete.[22]

Lactate. During higher-intensity exercise, an incomplete oxidation of glucose or glycogen occurs, with the excess pyruvate being converted to lactate via the lactate dehydrogenase reaction. For many years this leftover lactate was considered a waste product and a major cause of muscle fatigue or drop in performance.[23] However, starting in the 1970s and continuing with the recent work of Brooks,[24] this view has been challenged. It has now been shown that lactate is in fact beneficial during intense exercise. Production of lactate is essential in removing pyruvate to sustain glycolysis, and it is an oxidation-reduction process, reducing oxidized nicotinamide adenine dinucleotide (NAD+) to reduced nicotinamide adenine dinucleotide phosphate (NADPH), which allows glycolysis to continue to produce ATP. Without lactate this process would slow and the amount of ATP, and thus the energy available for muscles, would drop. Most of the lactate formed during steady-state exercise is removed by oxidation and only a small amount is converted to glucose. The lactate may also be "shuttled" from areas of high glycogenolysis to areas of high respiration via lactate shuttles.[25] Although production of lactate initially was thought to occur only when anaerobic work was performed, it has been demonstrated that lactate is a valuable fuel during oxidative metabolism as well.[26]

Mitochondrial Respiration (Oxidative System)

The connection between glycolysis and the mitochondria is complete when pyruvate and the electrons and protons from the reduction of NAD+ to NADH are transferred into the mitochondria as substrates for mitochondrial respiration. The resynthesis of ATP involves the combustion of fuel in the presence of sufficient oxygen and occurs in the mitochondria. The fuel can be obtained from within the muscles (free fatty acids and glycogen), outside the muscle (fats), and in the form of blood glucose (ingestion of carbohydrates or release from the liver).

Carbohydrates in the form of glucose are the major fuel of the body during exercise. Humans gain most of their glucose from their diet. In the resting state, glucose is stored in the form of glycogen in both the liver and in skeletal muscle. The main fatty acid utilized at rest and during muscle contractions is palmitate (a 16-carbon fatty acid). Because the inner mitochondrial membrane is impermeable to fatty acids larger than 15 carbons, the fatty acids are transported via the carnitine shuttle into the mitochondria. Finally, muscle has an ample supply of amino acids (free amino acids) that can be used in a catabolic state when carbohydrate supply is too low. However, if carbohydrate supply is inadequate, protein catabolism and amino acid oxidation must occur. Intense exercise also increases this amino acid oxidation. Carbohydrate oxidation is the most efficient fuel in the production of ATP.

The energy systems respond differently to the diverse demands of sporting exercise. The nonmitochondrial (anaerobic) system is capable of responding immediately and is able to support high-power output via extreme muscle force. The phosphagen system is utilized for explosive, maximal efforts, which are very short in duration. The glycolytic pathway is used for activities that require sustained, intense efforts but are not maximal. Unfortunately the anaerobic system is limited in its capacity, such that a reduction in power output will occur unless the demands can be supplemented by the aerobic system. The aerobic system is capable of responding quickly, yet it is incapable of meeting the initial high demands of intense exercise and is much better suited for longer efforts. The oxidative system is best for long-duration, low-intensity activities.

MUSCULAR RESPONSE TO TRAINING

Skeletal muscle exhibits superb plasticity in response to changes in functional demands. Chronic increases of skeletal muscle contractile activity, such as endurance exercise, lead to a variety of physiologic and biochemical adaptations in skeletal muscle, including mitochondrial biogenesis, angiogenesis, and fiber-type transformation. These mitochondrial adaptions can be increased through the use of high-intensity interval resistance training methods.[27] These adaptive changes are the basis for the improvement of physical performance and other health benefits.[28]

Muscles gain strength by getting larger (hypertrophy) and also by increasing skeletal muscle cell division (hyperplasia). The overload principle states that when a muscle is exposed to a stress or load that is greater than what it usually experiences, it will adapt so that it is able to handle the greater load.[29] A meta-analysis of 17 studies concluded that mechanical overload resulted in increases in muscle mass, muscle fiber area (hypertrophy), and muscle fiber number (hyperplasia).[30] Increases in fiber area were approximately twice as great as increases in fiber number.[31]

As a skeletal muscle hypertrophies, contractile proteins are synthesized, and the muscle is therefore capable of producing more force. In response to heavy resistance training, type IIA fibers exhibit the greatest growth, whereas types IIB and I exhibit the least amount of growth.[32] Muscle hypertrophy is more common in fast- than in slow-twitch muscles. Strength training leads to muscle hypertrophy, which increases muscle mass and typically occurs after weeks of such training. It appears that hyperplasia in skeletal muscle is greatest when certain types of mechanical overload, particularly stretch, are applied.

Muscle fibers within a motor unit have the same fiber type; however, skeletal muscles may contain several types of fibers based on demand of the muscle. This fiber type is genetically determined, but it may be altered with a training stimulus. Although the type of fiber cannot be changed, the amount of area taken up by a fiber type can be altered with training. Heavy resistance training causes increased type IIA and decreased type IIB fibers, whereas type I fiber composition in human skeletal muscle remains unchanged.[33] In bench studies, structural and genetic characteristics of muscle fiber types have been modulated with fiber-specific stimulation[34]; it is unclear if this modulation will translate to human skeletal muscle.

Many of the initially observed strength gains of a weight-lifting program are mostly due to neuromuscular adaptations.[32] As exercise intensity increases and muscles begin to fatigue, the nervous system recruits larger motor units with higher frequencies of stimulation to provide the force necessary to overcome the imposed resistance. Early strength gains and increased muscle tension production from training result from a more efficient neural recruitment process.[35,36]

In recent years, however, research has demonstrated that traditional strength training methods may be augmented through use of low-load resistance training with blood flow restriction (LL-BFR). The use of LL-BFR training with low loads has been found to yield hypertrophy responses comparable to those found with heavy-load resistance training.[37] It is hypothesized that an ischemic and hypoxic muscular environment is generated during blood flow restriction, which causes high levels of metabolic stress. This metabolic stress combined with the mechanical tension of training is theorized to activate factors associated with muscle growth. These factors may include systemic hormone production,[38] production of reactive oxygen species,[39] anabolic/catabolic signaling,[40] and/or increased fast-twitch muscle recruitment.[41] Currently, however, these factors are still only theorized and more research is needed to better elucidate the exact mechanisms.[42]

MUSCLE FATIGUE

Muscles that are used intensively show a progressive decline of performance that largely recovers after a period of rest; this reversible phenomenon is denoted as *muscle fatigue*. Many muscle properties change during fatigue, including the action potential, extracellular and intracellular ions, and many intracellular metabolites. Fatigue can be the result of peripheral causes, at the level of the skeletal muscle, or central causes.

Energy consumption of skeletal muscle increases dramatically with high-intensity exercise. The rate of energy need can exceed the aerobic capacity, forcing the muscles to rely on the anaerobic pathways for energy. Because high-intensity exercise leads to fatigue, it seems plausible that a relationship may exist between anaerobic exercise and fatigue. Anaerobic exercise leads to an accumulation of inorganic acids, mostly lactic acid, which dissociates into lactate and hydrogen ions.[43] As previously discussed, lactate is a muscle fuel and therefore is probably not a factor in muscle fatigue, but the increase in hydrogen ions may be an important cause of muscle fatigue. Studies supporting this theory have shown a good temporal correlation between the decline of muscle pH and the reduction of force or power production.[44] In addition, studies have demonstrated that acidification may reduce both the isometric force and the shortening velocity.[45]

Peripheral fatigue can be a result of a reduced level of calcium during contractions, or it may be related to the contractile proteins themselves. During exercise, muscles depend on an ATP pump to return calcium to the sarcoplasmic reticulum; as exercise continues and the level of ATP drops, the ability to return calcium back to the sarcoplasmic reticulum drops and peripheral fatigue results. Another mechanism of peripheral fatigue occurs at the level of the cross bridges. It has also been demonstrated that the initial fall in muscle force is due to a reduction of the force generated by the individual cross bridges, whereas as fatigue progresses, a decline in the total number of cross bridges actually occurs.[46]

Finally, when muscles are fatigued, fewer motor units are available; thus reduced motor unit activation is a cause of fatigue.[47]

Exercise performance is also dictated by the perception of effort of the brain and its inhibitory effects on central motor drive to the periphery. It is believed that these peripheral and central factors are closely linked, with the development of peripheral fatigue influencing the rate of development of "central" fatigue, operating through neural feedback pathways from working muscle to the motor control areas of the central nervous system.[48,49]

Differentiation between central versus peripheral etiologies of muscle fatigue can be investigated via electrical stimulation. Muscles can be stimulated in a nonfatigued state and then again while fatigued, and if the characteristics of the contraction are different before and after fatigue, the likely cause is peripheral. If the contraction is reduced before fatigue, then the cause may be more central.[50,51] Other etiologies of central fatigue are psychological and may be more difficult to determine. A major direction for future studies should be to identify the mechanisms that contribute to human fatigue in various activities and particularly during disease processes.

NEUROMUSCULAR ADAPTATION TO EXERCISE

Neuromuscular performance is determined not only by the quality and quantity of involved muscles but also by the ability of the nervous system to appropriately activate the muscles. These neural adaptive changes in response to training are referred to as neural adaptation. These neural factors are important for increases in strength early in resistance training, whereas muscular hypertrophy of trained muscles develops after prolonged resistance training.[52] In order for athletes to make performance gains, neuromuscular adaptation must occur.[36]

Resistance training–induced adaptations are supraspinal in nature and include increased excitation[53] and changes in the organization of the motor cortex.[54] Such adaptations can influence the manner in which muscles are recruited for functional tasks. Changes at the neuromuscular junction, which are associated with functional alterations in transmission, may lead to enhanced neuromuscular transmission. These adaptations can improve the activation of muscles and are likely the result of muscle training.[54] Increased levels of muscle activation and subsequent increase in force achieved by increases in individual firing at the motor unit leads to the recruitment of more motor units.[55]

In addition to these neural factors, the amount of force that a muscle can exert is influenced by the number and size of fibers and the fiber type. Heavy resistance exercise results in increases in strength and changes in both neuromuscular function and muscle morphology.[56,57] Finally, neural adaptations are found in the level of coactivation of antagonist muscles[58] and changes in the synergistic patters of muscle activations,[59] which could also contribute to maximization of force generation.

In contrast to resistance training, the neural response to endurance training involves strategies to improve efficiency, such as reducing the number of motor units needed to maintain force and increasing the activation of synergistic muscles.[60] Endurance training results in increased capillary density and decreased muscle cross-sectional area to facilitate oxygen delivery to tissues. In addition, endurance training leads to an increase in cellular mitochondrial content and oxidative enzyme activity as well as increased aerobic capacity. These changes require 8 to 12 weeks of training to be realized. The net results of long-term endurance training are increased metabolic capacity of muscle, increases in muscular force output, and muscle hypertrophy.

DELAYED-ONSET MUSCLE SORENESS

The demands of the training stimulus causes microdamage to muscles, and their ability to recover and regenerate is part of the training process. Muscle soreness may occur during this period, which peaks 24 to 48 hours after a strenuous bout of training and typically resolves by 96 hours. This phenomenon is known as *delayed-onset muscle soreness* (DOMS). DOMS is typically experienced by all persons regardless of fitness level and is a normal physiologic response to increased exertion and the introduction of unfamiliar physical activities. The resulting sensation of pain and discomfort can impair physical training and performance; thus the etiology and prevention of DOMS is of interest to athletes and trainers.

More muscle damage may occur with higher-intensity or unfamiliar exercises, predominantly eccentric loading exercises. Other factors that may be involved include muscle stiffness, contraction velocity, fatigue, and angle of contraction.[61] Some evidence indicates that fast-twitch muscle fibers are more susceptible to eccentric-induced injury.[62] The initial injury to the muscles is a mechanical disruption of the sarcomeres,[63] which proliferates a secondary inflammatory response[64] releasing prostaglandin E2 and leukotrienes, giving the sensation of pain and contributing to swelling as a result of increased vascular permeability. The initial injury pattern is sporadic throughout the muscle, and the damage to the sarcomeres does not extend to the length of the myofibril or across a whole muscle fiber.[62] Thus the muscle injury pattern of DOMS differs from that of an acute muscle strain, which occurs as an isolated disruption of the muscle-tendon junction extending across the fibers.[65]

Can the symptoms and functional consequences of DOMS be mitigated or prevented? It would seem reasonable that if DOMS is thought to be an inflammatory problem and is mediated by prostaglandins, the use of nonsteroidal antiinflammatory drugs (NSAIDs) or the application of ice would help to reduce or prevent DOMS. However, studies show mixed results with NSAIDs,[66,67] and because NSAIDs are not without risk, further data are needed to recommend the use of NSAIDs to treat DOMS. Ice offers an analgesic effect but little sustained benefit.[68] Muscle stretching does not appear to produce clinically important reductions in DOMS in healthy adults[69]; however, foam rolling may.[70] The ideal strategies (time, amount of pressure applied during foam rolling, etc.) are not known at this time.[71] Antioxidants are not effective and may actually delay muscle recovery.[61] However, studies do show that massage,[72–74] as well as massage plus the use of compressive clothing,[75] is of benefit in reducing the symptoms of DOMS. Finally, whole-body vibration prior to exercise may be effective for reducing DOMS.[76]

STRENGTH TRAINING IN YOUNG ATHLETES

Strength training in young athletes has been controversial. Some of the controversy originated from misconceptions about benefits of training and the risk to the skeletally immature. Previously it was thought that prepubertal athletes could not benefit from weight training because of their low levels of gonadal hormones[77]; it was also feared that youths might lose flexibility and range of motion with strength training.[78] Finally, it was thought that strength training would expose the growth plates of young athletes to excessive risk of injury.[77] Recently, however, research has demonstrated that well-designed resistance training programs can enhance the strength of children and adolescents beyond what is expected with normal maturation.[79] Many leading sports organizations now recognize the importance of muscular strength during childhood and adolescence[80–83] both to improve performance and for injury prevention.[84]

Strength gains of up to 75% can be observed in young athletes after an 8- to 12-week training program.[83] Lighter loads and a greater number of repetitions (10 to 15) are recommended to increase strength.[85,86] These training-induced changes in youths are predominately due to neural adaptations as opposed to the muscle hypertrophy seen in adults.[85] Strength training in the young also has the potential to offer other many health benefits. Improved bone health,[87] body composition, reduction of cardiovascular risk factors,[88] and decreased risk of sports injury[89] result from strength training. Therefore it would appear that the benefits outweigh the risks and that properly designed and supervised programs are safe and effective for young athletes.

EFFECTS OF AGING ON SKELETAL MUSCLE

Aging has been associated with loss of muscle mass, which is referred to as *sarcopenia*. This decrease begins around age 50 years but becomes more dramatic after 60 years.[90] Aging negatively affects power, strength, and endurance in skeletal muscles. Recently muscle power has been found to be a better predictor of functional performance than muscle strength.[91] Loss of power contributes to a decrease in short-term anaerobic performance and is directly related to the increase in falls among older people and impairment in the performance of daily activities.[91] The etiology of this loss of power is from both a loss of muscle mass and a slowing in the firing of motor neurons[92] and maximal shortening velocity.[93] The loss of strength is directly related to the loss of muscle mass. Sarcopenia accounts for more than 90% of age-related strength decrease.[94] Other factors involved in strength reduction are decreases in the tension of muscle tissue due to aged myofibrils[95] or a decrease in the number of functioning cross bridges.[96] Despite the negative effects of aging, strength training can improve power and strength, reversing some of the decrement and leading to improved functionality in older adults. Despite the loss of muscle mass, the addition of high-intensity interval training (HIIT) increases the mitochondrial content almost back to that of younger athletes.[97] High-velocity resistance training[98,99] and increasing lower extremity strength[100] have been shown to be the best way to achieve this goal.

TABLE 6.2 Hormonal Responses to Exercise

Hormone	Change	Function
Pituitary		
Growth hormone	Increases proportionally to exercise intensity	Stimulates metabolism
β-Endorphins	Increase with exercise above 60% VO$_2$ max	Analgesic, "natural high"
Antidiuretic hormone	Increases with exercise	Maintains hydration
Prolactin	Increases with exercise	Unclear
Adrenal		
Glucocorticoids, adrenocorticotropic hormone	Increase with exercise above 50% VO$_2$ max	Stimulate metabolism
Aldosterone	Increases proportionally to exercise intensity	Maintains hydration
Epinephrine and norepinephrine	Increase proportionally to exercise intensity[a]	Mediate cardiovascular responses
Pancreatic		
Insulin	Decreases proportionally to exercise duration (and blood glucose levels)[a]	Guards against hypoglycemia
Glucagon	Increases proportionally to exercise duration	Increases serum glucose levels
Gonadal		
Testosterone	Increases proportionally to exercise intensity[a]	Unclear
Estrogen and progesterone	Increase with exercise[a]	Unclear

[a]Basal levels also decrease with long-term endurance training.
VO$_2$ max, Maximum oxygen uptake.

CORE STRENGTH AND NEUROMUSCULAR TRAINING

Core stability is an important component in maximizing efficient athletic function as well as in preventing injury. Core stability can be defined as the "ability to control the position and motion of the trunk over the pelvis to allow optimum production, transfer and control of muscle activity."[101] The core consists of the muscles of the trunk and pelvis as well as the neural, osseous, and ligamentous elements. Its stability is dependent not only on muscular strength but also on proper sensory input that alerts the nervous system about interaction between the body and the environment, providing constant feedback and allowing for refinement in movement.[102] These proprioceptive abilities have a positive impact on reducing injuries,[103] and exercise programs targeting the enhancement of these abilities may prevent injuries.[104,105] Some evidence indicates that balance training or multifaceted training programs are effective in preventing lower limb injuries such as ankle sprains[106,107] and anterior cruciate ligament tears[108–110] among young adults when they participate in ball sports.[111] Finally, after injuries have occurred, rehabilitation of deficits may prevent future injuries.[112] To date, however, the most effective training program and the optimal frequency and duration of these sessions have yet to be determined, and more research is needed.[113]

HORMONAL ADAPTATION TO EXERCISE

Many changes that occur in response to exercise are mediated by hormones. Growth hormone (GH), endorphins, and antidiuretic hormone from the pituitary assist in the performance and recovery of muscles. Adrenal hormones such as catecholamines, glucocorticoids, and mineralocorticoids are responsible for most of the key changes needed in exercise, although many other hormones are also involved. Pancreatic and gonadal hormones also play a key role (Table 6.2).

Pituitary

GH is a peptide hormone that stimulates muscle growth, cell reproduction, and cell regeneration. GH also stimulates protein synthesis and promotes lipid metabolism, both of which conserve blood glucose levels during exercise to allow for sustainment of performance and contribute to muscle regeneration. GH levels are increased with resistance exercise.[114] The exact mechanism is not known, but afferent stimulation, lactate, or nitric oxide may play a role.[115] Both concentric and eccentric loading resistance training exercises lead to increased GH levels.[116,117] Endurance exercise training above the lactate threshold may amplify the pulsatile release of GH at rest, increasing 24-hour GH secretion; however, studies suggest that weight training may lead to a higher level of serum GH.[118] Another potent stimulator of GH is sleep,[119] which underscores the importance of sleep in recovery for athletes in training.

Administration of supraphysiologic doses of GH to athletes as a performance enhancer may increase lean body mass and improve athletic performance.[120] However, the model of acromegaly demonstrates that long-term GH excess does not ultimately improve performance and may be dangerous. Recently a systematic review failed to find any evidence to show that exogenous GH administration improves sports performance.[121] However, despite the lack of scientific evidence, GH is banned by most sporting agencies.

β-Endorphins are endogenous opioid peptides secreted by the pituitary in response to exercise. Exercise of sufficient intensity and duration has been demonstrated to increase circulating β-endorphin levels. β-Endorphins are active at opioid receptors, provide analgesic effects[122] and may be responsible for the "runner's high" experienced by persons who perform vigorous endurance exercise.[123]

Muscle activity and exercise cause perspiration, which leads to fluid loss and hemoconcentration of electrolytes as a result of the relative loss of water and sodium. This low plasma volume stimulates the posterior pituitary to release antidiuretic hormone to promote water concentration by increasing the permeability of the kidneys' water-collecting ducts, leading to less water being excreted and minimizing the risk of dehydration. Exercise also leads to increased prolactin secretion from the pituitary,[124] which is maximized after a hard anaerobic effort.[125] The exact role of prolactin in response to exercise is unclear, but it has been shown to stimulate the phagocytic activity of the immune system,[124] possibly in an early attempt to repair the exercise-damaged muscles or as an early precursor to DOMS.

Adrenal Hormones

Glucocorticoids, primarily cortisol, are released from the adrenal cortex in response to pituitary adrenocorticotropic hormone. Cortisol functions to stimulate liver gluconeogenesis, adipose lipolysis, and protein degradation in both liver and predominantly type II muscle fibers.

Levels of both adrenocorticotropic hormone and cortisol have been shown to rise in response to resistance and endurance training. The minimum intensity of exercise (i.e., threshold) necessary to produce a cortisol response is 60% of the maximum oxygen uptake (Vo_2 max). Above 60% Vo_2 max, a linear increase between the intensity of exercise and the increase in plasma cortisol concentrations is observed.[126] Cortisol levels may not increase at exercise below this intensity and may in fact decrease.[127] Other factors that modulate cortisol release include hypohydration, meals, and time of day. Hypohydration (up to 4.8% of body mass) amplifies the exercise-induced response of cortisol to exercise.[128] Cortisol response to exercise is significantly higher during evening exercise compared with morning exercise.[129]

Finally, enhanced activation of the sympathoadrenal system may occur in game or race situations and may be one of the key "driving forces" to performance improvement.[130]

Aldosterone functions in the kidney to prevent sodium and water loss. Aldosterone secretion is regulated by the kidneys and is driven by decreased renal blood flow accompanying hypohydration and shunting of blood peripherally to lower temperature during exercise. Aldosterone levels increase in a graded fashion with hypohydration, heat stress, and exercise intensity.[131] An additive effect of combined hypohydration and exercise intensity is also believed to exist, and these responses are closely coupled to plasma osmolality.[131] Response can be significant, with marathon runners having documented increases in aldosterone levels for almost a full day after completion of a race.[132,133] This prolonged elevation in aldosterone levels may be important to athletes who sustain an injury that requires surgery shortly after prolonged competition.

Catecholamine (epinephrine and norepinephrine) secretion from the adrenal medulla increases with exercise. These hormones have a range of effects that include increased heart rate (HR), respiratory stimulation to meet aerobic demands, and generalized vasoconstriction with vasodilatory effects on skeletal and cardiac muscles to promote profusion of active tissues. Catecholamines also stimulate the renin-angiotensin-aldosterone system to secrete aldosterone and thus to protect against hypohydration; they work in the pancreas to decrease insulin and increase glucagon to increase lipolysis and maintain blood glucose levels for working muscles. As in the case of the other adrenal hormones, increased secretion is directly related to exercise intensity. However, unlike many other hormones discussed thus far, basal levels of catecholamines do change with prolonged training.[134] Findings have reported a higher adrenaline response to exercise in endurance-trained compared with untrained subjects in response to intense exercise at the same relative intensity as all-out exercise. This phenomenon is referred to as the "sports adrenal medulla." This higher capacity to secrete adrenaline was observed both in response to physical exercise and to other stimuli such as hypoglycemia and hypoxia.[135] Long-term endurance training can enhance plasma catecholamine concentrations in response to supramaximal exercise.[134]

Gonadal Hormones

Testosterone is a male sex hormone produced in the testes; it has both androgenic and anabolic effects. Testosterone has an important role as a regulator of muscle protein synthesis and hypertrophy, so its importance for exercise is clear. Regulation of testicular production occurs via a negative feedback loop involving the anterior pituitary, hypothalamus, and testicles, referred to as the *hypothalamic-pituitary-testicular* (HPT) *axis*. High-intensity, near-maximal resistance training will increase systemic testosterone levels.[136] This increased testosterone level as a result of resistance training appears to become blunted in persons who are long-term weight lifters.[137] Short-term, moderate intensity and low-volume endurance training can also significantly increase testosterone concentration in previously untrained men.[138] Interestingly, prolonged endurance training may lead to decreased testosterone levels. The mechanism of this lowering is currently unclear but may be related to dysfunction within the HPT axis brought about by months or years of endurance training.

Estrogen and progesterone are the female sex steroid analogs produced in the ovary; they are also regulated via a negative feedback loop involving the pituitary, hypothalamus, and ovaries. Resistance exercise increases levels of both estrogen and progesterone,[138] which have been shown to increase muscular strength in women. Evidence indicates that estradiol working through estrogen receptors does not accomplish this increase in muscular strength by affecting muscle size but rather by improving the intrinsic quality of skeletal muscle, whereby fibers are enabled to generate more force.[139] Estrogen is also implicated in bone health, and estrogen's effects on bone would be enhanced if, in addition to the direct effects of the hormone on the skeleton, muscle contractions were more forceful and/or numerous, creating additional osteogenic stimuli. Although estrogen may have a beneficial effect with resistance training in women, prolonged endurance training in the face of calorie restriction may create an energy deficit, which then leads to a lowering of the estrogen level and a decreased protective effect on bone. Women with menstrual disturbances who have low estradiol and progesterone levels have an attenuated anabolic hormone response to exercise, suggesting that menstrual disorders may affect exercise-induced changes to strength and bone health in women.[140]

Pancreatic Hormones

Insulin and glucagon are secreted by the pancreas and interact with muscle, liver, and fat cells. Insulin causes muscles and the liver to take up glucose from the blood stream and store it as glycogen while inhibiting the use of fat as a fuel source by inhibiting the secretion of glucagon. Glucagon, meanwhile, acts to raise blood sugar levels by signaling the liver to break stored glycogen down into available glucose. Thus insulin and glucagon are part of a feedback system that regulates blood glucose levels and as such are important hormones for exercise.

During a bout of exercise, the working muscle rapidly increases its need for glucose. Therefore it does not result in hypoglycemia. This augmentation of glucose utilization must be accompanied by an almost synchronous and equivalent increase in glucose production.[141] Glucagon responds rapidly to meet this need; simultaneously, a decrease in plasma insulin levels during exercise occurs to maintain higher levels of blood glucose. Glucagon also plays a critical role in coupling the glycogenolysis response of the liver to the glucose demands of the working muscle.

A single bout of exercise increases skeletal muscle glucose uptake via an insulin-independent mechanism that bypasses the typical insulin signaling defects associated with these conditions. However, this "insulin sensitizing" effect is short-lived and disappears after approximately 48 hours. In contrast, some studies demonstrate that prolonged exercise training results in a persistent increase in insulin action in skeletal muscle.[142] Other studies, however, suggest that there is no attenuation period of insulin sensitivity in obese persons, implicating exercise as much more effective than diet in changing body composition among those who are obese.[143,144] Finally, it has been shown that insulin plays only a small role in actual muscle protein synthesis but may inhibit muscle protein breakdown, which, combined with the ingestion of small amounts of protein and carbohydrate, can transiently increase muscle protein buildup.[145] Because of insulin's ability to direct glucose into muscle tissue, it could be useful as an anabolic agent and thus may have the potential for abuse in an effort to maximize muscle gains from exercise or increase glycogen storage for prolonged endurance events.[146]

EXERCISE CAPACITY

Peak exercise capacity is the maximum ability of the cardiovascular system to deliver oxygen to exercising skeletal muscle and the exercising muscle's ability to extract oxygen from blood. Maximum oxygen uptake, or Vo_2 max, is generally used to provide an overall assessment of exercise capacity (Fig. 6.5). The Fick equation states that oxygen uptake (Vo_2) equals cardiac output (CO) times the arterial oxygen content minus the mixed venous oxygen content: $Vo_2 = CO \times (CaO_2 - CvO_2)$, where CO equals stroke volume (SV) times HR; therefore $Vo_2 = (SV \times HR) \times (CaO_2 - CvO_2)$. At maximal exercise, Vo_2 max is calculated as follows: $(SVmax \times HRmax) \times (CaO_2max - CvO_2 max)$, which reflects a person's ability to take in, transport, and utilize oxygen.

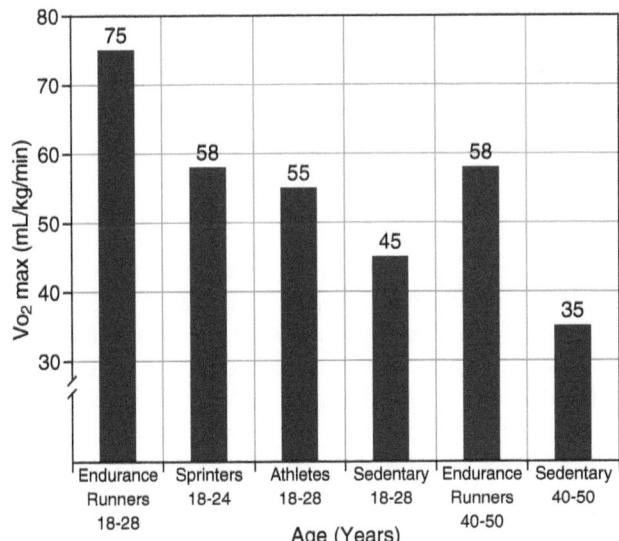

Fig. 6.5 Contrast of maximum oxygen uptake *(Vo_2 max)* among men of various ages and aerobic fitness levels. (Data from Pollock ML, Wilmore JH, Fox SM. *Health and Fitness Through Physical Activity*. New York: John Wiley and Sons; 1978.)

Vo_2 max has become the preferred laboratory measure of cardiorespiratory fitness and is the most important measurement during functional exercise testing. In healthy people, a Vo_2 plateau occurs at near-maximal exercise. This plateau in Vo_2 has traditionally been used as the best evidence of Vo_2 max.[146] It represents the maximal achievable level of oxidative metabolism involving large muscle groups. However, in clinical testing, a clear plateau may not be achieved before symptoms limit exercise. Consequently, peak Vo_2 is often used as an estimate of Vo_2 max.[96]

In healthy people, the Vo_2 max response to exercise is linear until Vo_2 max is achieved. Exercise training, however, will enable the person to increase his or her Vo_2 max. Training leads to a lower resting HR but does not significantly affect maximal HR. Initially the SV increases with exercise, but then the response is attenuated. Training increases resting SV and therefore SV at each level of work. Finally, the difference between the arterial and venous oxygen content widens with training. Thus although Vo_2 max increases with training, an age-related decline occurs. Aging is associated with a progressive decline in the capacity for physical activity, mainly as a result of this reduction in Vo_2 max. A reduction in muscle oxygen delivery, principally due to reduced CO, appears to play the dominant role up until late middle age. Mitochondrial dysfunction is the major factor in older age because skeletal muscle Vo_2 max declines by approximately 50% compared with younger muscle.[147]

The ventilator anaerobic threshold, formerly referred to as the anaerobic threshold, is another index used to estimate exercise capacity. During the aerobic phase of exercise (up to 60% of max Vo_2), ventilation increases linearly with Vo_2 and mirrors carbon dioxide produced aerobically in the muscles. No significant change in blood lactate levels occurs during this phase because muscle lactic acid production is minimal. As the intensity and duration of exercise continue, the oxygen supply can no longer keep up with the increasing metabolic requirements of the exercising muscles.

At this time, lactic acid and therefore blood lactate concentration increases. The V_{O_2} at the onset of this blood lactate spike is referred to as the *lactate threshold* or the *ventilator anaerobic threshold*. This threshold also denotes the point at which minute ventilation increases disproportionately relative to V_{O_2}, which generally occurs at 60% to 70% of V_{O_2} max.

Cardiorespiratory Response to Exercise

The cardiovascular system serves several important functions during exercise. It delivers oxygen to working muscles, oxygenates blood by returning it to the lungs, delivers nutrients and fuel to active muscles, transports hormones, and transports heat from the core to the skin. Exercise places an increased demand on the cardiovascular system. Oxygen demand by the muscles increases sharply, metabolic processes speed up, and more waste is created, more nutrients are utilized, and body temperature rises.[148] To perform efficiently and effectively, the cardiovascular system must regulate these changes to meet the body's increased demands.

Exercise CO is defined as HR multiplied by SV, with SV defined as the volume of blood ejected per ventricular contraction. Aerobic capacity is determined by the ability of the body to modify the CO in response to exercise, with approximately a fivefold increase in output during vigorous exercise. This increase in CO is primarily due to the increase in HR with exercise; to a lesser extent, it is due to an increase in SV. The resting HR is typically between 60 and 100 beats per minute and increases linearly with exercise intensity to a maximal HR of 200 beats per minute in the young adult (Fig. 6.6).[149] Individual maximal HR decreases with age and may be loosely approximated by 220 minus age (in years).

Endurance training is associated with an increased CO and volume load on the left and right ventricles, causing the endurance-trained heart to generate dilation of the left ventricle combined with a mild to moderate increase in left ventricular wall thickness. This training-induced increase in CO allows trained athletes to have a lower resting HR compared with persons who are not trained. Also, during exercise, the active muscles of the lower extremities require increased blood flow; therefore peripheral vascular resistance decreases to accommodate this need. To generate this large CO, athletes must increase their SV to counteract the decrease in HR and vascular resistance. Endurance athletes have larger increases in left ventricular end-diastolic volume compared with nonathletes, which allows them to generate the necessary larger SV. SV increases early in exercise, but unlike HR, it plateaus before maximal intensity at about 40% to 60% of V_{O_2} max.[150] Trained athletes have also demonstrated the ability of the heart to adapt to maintain CO. Training-related expansion of vascular volume is associated with decreased HR response to baroreceptor stimulation.[151] Levels of skeletal muscle blood flow increase up to 20 times resting value during exercise to maximize oxygen delivery.[152] Visceral vasoconstriction likewise aids in redistributing blood flow to the skeletal muscle (Table 6.3).

Respiratory Response

The lungs are critical in oxygenating blood and in their ability to maintain consistent arterial oxygen concentrations both at rest and with the increased demands of exercise. The ventilatory

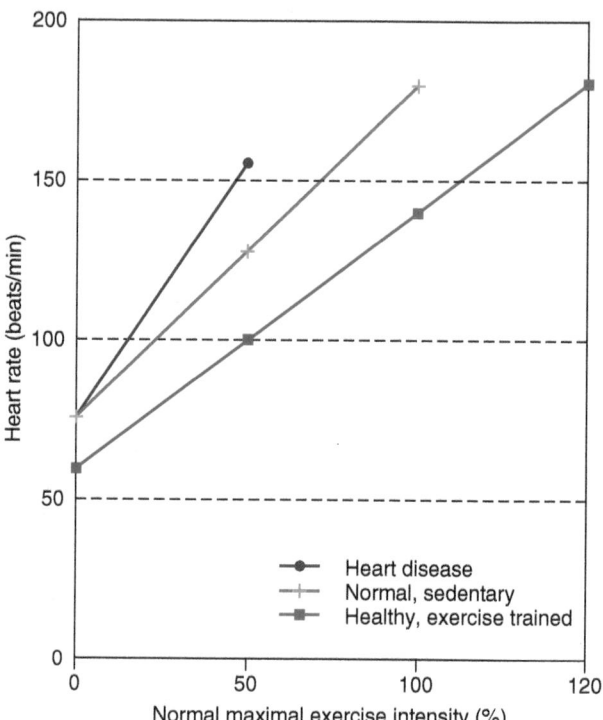

Fig. 6.6 Heart rate increase in proportion to exercise intensity among groups in various states of health. (Data from Hasson S. *Clinical Exercise Physiology*. St. Louis: Mosby; 1994.)

TABLE 6.3	**Cardiovascular Response to Exercise**
Function	**Response**
Cardiac output	Large increase
Heart rate	Large increase (primarily responsible for cardiac output increase)
Stroke volume	Modest increase
Systolic blood pressure	Modest increase
Pulse pressure	Modest increase
Mean blood pressure	Modest increase
Total peripheral resistance	Large decrease (massive skeletal muscle vasodilation dominates over visceral vasoconstriction)
Arteriovenous oxygen difference	Increase due to oxygen consumption

demands of vigorous exercise require airway flow rates that often exceed 10 times resting levels and tidal volumes that approach five times resting levels.

Basic to understanding this respiratory response is the importance of diffusion in the process of gas exchange between alveolar air and pulmonary capillary blood. For gas to be exchanged, concentration differences must be maintained by the ventilation of lung airway and the perfusion of pulmonary capillaries. This diffusion rate is directly rated to the concentration gradient of oxygen and the surface area of lung available for diffusion and is the most important factor for lung diffusion; therefore it is necessary to ensure that oxygen and carbon dioxide gradients are sufficiently steep to maximize diffusion.

It was long thought that the capacity of the healthy respiratory system is overbuilt for the demands placed on ventilation and gas exchange by exercise.[153] However, for endurance athletes, the pulmonary system may lag behind the exceptional cardiovascular and aerobic muscular adaptations.[154] This potential for ventilation-perfusion inequality during high-intensity exercise may compromise arterial saturation and the capacity for oxygen transport; it is termed "exercise-induced arterial hypoxemia." The exact etiology of these respiratory system limitations to exercise is unknown but may be due to the specific ability of training to increase the capacity of the muscles and heart for oxygen transport and utilization without significantly changing the structural or functional capacities of the lungs and airways.[155]

CONCLUSION

Exercise physiology—the study of the identification and study of physiologic mechanisms underlying physical activity and the body's response to exercise—provides the scientific basis for training that is used to maximize performance. A better understanding of the underlying mechanisms of muscle structure, function, and adaptation will aid providers in the evaluation and treatment of exercising athletes.

For a complete list of references, go to ExpertConsult.com.

SELECTED READINGS

Citation:
Brooks GA. Cell-cell and intracellular lactate shuttles. *J Physiol.* 2009;587(23):5591–5600.

Level of Evidence:
II

Summary:
This article contradicts previously held theory that lactate is a waste product in muscle metabolism, indicating that it is a viable substrate for muscle energy and that glycolytic and oxidative pathways work in concert rather than in competition.

Citation:
American College of Sports Medicine. *ACSM's Guidelines for Exercise Testing and Prescription.* 7th ed. Philadelphia: Lippincott, Williams & Wilkins; 2006:237–251.

Level of Evidence:
III

Summary:
A comprehensive guide to exercise testing and prescriptions for athletes of all ages and stages of their careers.

Citation:
Herzog W, Duvall M, Leonard TR. Molecular mechanisms of muscle force regulation: a role for titin? *Exerc Sport Sci Rev.* 2012;40(1):50–57.

Level of Evidence:
II

Summary:
The authors support their theory that in addition to the proteins actin and myosin discussed in the cross-bridge theory, a new protein may have a role in muscle force. They demonstrate that titin plays a major role in muscle force regulation, particularly for eccentric concentrations and at long muscle and sarcomere lengths.

Citation:
Reid KF, Callahan DM, Carabello RJ, et al. Muscle power failure in mobility limited older adults: preserved single fiber function despite lower whole muscle size, quality and neuromuscular activation. *Eur J Appl Physiol.* 2012;112(6):2289–2301.

Level of Evidence:
II

Summary:
This study contradicts the previously held theory that muscle fibers degenerate as we age. The authors find that in older adults, contractile properties of muscle fibers are preserved in an attempt to maintain overall muscle function.

Citation:
Yan Z, Okutsu M, Akhtar YN, et al. Regulation of exercise-induced fiber type transformation, mitochondrial biogenesis, and angiogenesis in skeletal muscle. *J Appl Physiol.* 2011;110:264–274.

Level of Evidence:
III

Summary:
This article summarizes the variety of physiologic and biochemical adaptions in skeletal muscle, which forms the basis for the improvement of physical performance and other health benefits.

7

Imaging Overview

Francisco Contreras, Jose Perez, Jean Jose

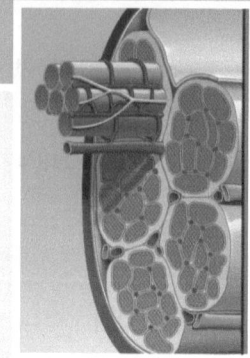

Imaging is important in the diagnosis and management of orthopedic disorders and sports-related injuries. Athletic injuries are common among all age groups. Patients are becoming more knowledgeable with respect to their injuries and the imaging modalities available to diagnose them. Meanwhile, physicians have become more adept at combining their clinical skills with imaging findings to affect better patient care. Subspecialization in the fields of sports medicine and musculoskeletal imaging provides a higher level of clinical service for patients and their primary health care providers. All of these factors have contributed to an increase in utilization of imaging.

Physicians must be aware that the imaging workup for clinical problems can often take a number of routes, ultimately leading to the correct diagnosis. In many instances there is no single "right or wrong" imaging algorithm. A number of factors should be taken into account in planning the optimal imaging strategy for a given clinical problem with respect to variable patient demographics. These factors include the desire to avoid ionizing radiation from computed tomography (CT) and scintigraphy in younger patients, regional geographic variations in the accessibility to magnetic resonance imaging (MRI), the relatively high costs of MRI and scintigraphy, and the availability of local expertise in musculoskeletal sonography. These factors must be balanced against the likelihood of establishing a diagnosis with various investigational imaging modalities in order to determine the optimal course of imaging.

In this chapter, basic imaging techniques are reviewed, encompassing radiography (including fluoroscopy and arthrography), ultrasonography, CT, nuclear medicine, and MRI. Technical concepts related to each modality are outlined, particularly with regard to variables that affect image quality. An overview of the advantages and disadvantages unique to each modality is also provided. Arthrography, fluoroscopy, and orthopedic interventional procedures are briefly discussed. An overview of radiation doses associated with common diagnostic procedures is presented.

IMAGING TECHNIQUES

Conventional Radiography

In 1895, Wilhelm Konrad Röntgen discovered the x-ray, which ultimately led to the field of medical imaging. In 1901, Röntgen received the Nobel Prize in physics for his discovery of the x-ray.

Technical Considerations

X-rays are a form of ionizing radiation composed of short-wavelength electromagnetic photons with variable penetration through different tissues in the body. A wire filament in an x-ray tube generates an electron beam that bombards a tungsten target, resulting in a stream of x-ray photons directed toward the patient. Upon reaching the patient, x-rays can be absorbed or scattered within the patient, or they may pass through the patient. The x-rays that pass through the patient strike x-ray–sensitive material positioned behind the patient (Fig. 7.1). Film-based radiographs have largely been supplanted by digital radiography in modern centers during the past two decades. In digital radiography, the x-rays that are transmitted through the area of interest interact with a digital detector system positioned behind the patient to create a radiographic image. The primary benefit of digital radiography is to implement a complete digital picture archiving and communication system (PACS) where images are stored digitally and are readily available through computer networks.

Two types of digital detector systems are currently available—computed radiography (CR) and direct radiography (DR)—each with its own advantages and disadvantages.[1] Both systems are currently required to provide a full complement of digital radiographic images in modern medical imaging facilities. CR systems can be integrated into older film-based radiographic equipment at a substantial cost savings compared with installation of a DR flat panel system, which comes with a high capital cost. CR technology utilizes a storage-phosphor image plate, which replaces film in older systems and requires a separate laser scanner readout step. DR systems convert x-rays into images through a direct readout process built into a detector unit, eliminating a separate image-processing step and resulting in the immediate production of an image. The need for a separate readout step in CR is similar to processing film in older systems and is inefficient, with relatively reduced patient throughput compared with DR systems. Furthermore, the use of cassettes in CR systems can lead to work-related chronic repetitive strain injuries in technologists. Work-related strain injuries are less common in DR systems because cassettes are not used. Current DR technology cannot be used for most portable radiographs and certain specialized views, such as an axillary projection of the shoulder or a skyline view of the patella. In these instances CR must be used, although DR capability in this area is currently in evolution. A greater

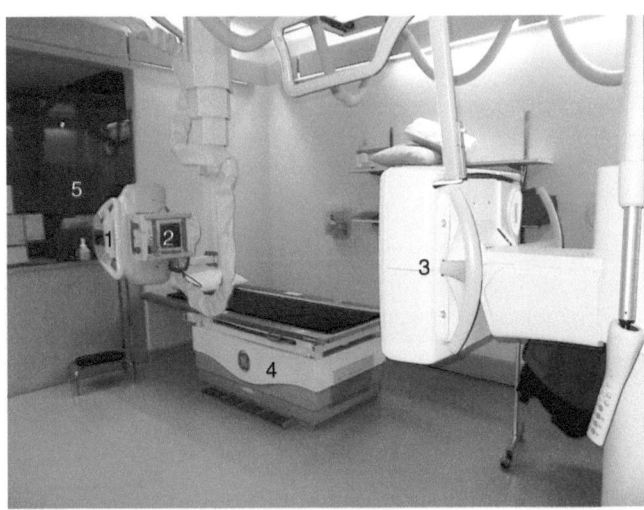

Fig. 7.1 Equipment in a general digital radiography room. *1*, X-ray tube; *2*, collimator; *3*, wall-mounted flat panel detector; *4*, table detector; *5*, operator console behind a glass screen.

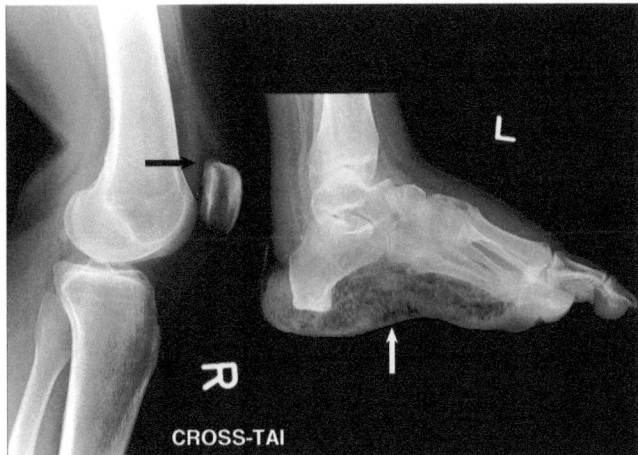

Fig. 7.2 Radiographic densities. A cross-table lateral radiograph of the knee *(left)* shows a fat-fluid level *(arrow)* associated with a lipohemarthrosis indicative of an intraarticular fracture corresponding to marrow fat that has escaped from the fracture into the joint space. The marrow fat layers superficially to the dependent red blood cells in the joint and appears more lucent than muscle in the soft tissues. A lateral radiograph of the foot *(right)* in a patient with diabetes shows extensive lucencies in the soft tissues of the plantar soft tissues of the foot *(arrow)* associated with a gas-forming infection. Bones and calcified structures have the greatest density on radiographs and appear white. Muscle tissue is light gray, fatty tissue is dark gray, and gas is black.

dynamic range may be obtained with both systems, potentially reducing the amount of radiation to which patients are exposed.

Several factors contribute to the optimization of radiographic images. Proper positioning of the patient and elimination of motion is essential. Optimal exposure of the film prior to the advent of digital imaging used to be crucial; however, greater latitude is now permitted in the range of exposure values while remaining diagnostic, because the brightness and contrast of an image can be manipulated and optimized at the physician's workstation. Exposure is controlled by altering the number and/or energy of the incident x-ray photons. The number of incident photons is determined by the strength of the current used to generate the electron beam, abbreviated as mA-s (milliampere-second). The energy of the x-ray photons is related to the strength of the voltage potential, abbreviated as kVp (kilovoltage potential), through which the electrons are accelerated before striking the tungsten target. Once x-rays are formed, their individual energy cannot be modified. However, filters that provide differential absorption can modify the quality of the x-ray beam. These filters function to remove low-energy x-rays that typically are randomly scattered within the patient and never reach the film, contributing to patient dose and not to image formation. As a general rule, thicker and denser structures generally require both a higher energy and a greater of quantity of x-ray photons for a diagnostic image. The converse is true for thinner and less dense anatomic locations.

Variable transmission of the x-ray photons through tissues of different composition results in the classic radiographic densities of bone, water/soft tissue, fat, and gas (Fig. 7.2).

Fluoroscopy

Fluoroscopy is a special type of x-ray technology that produces rapid images, thus allowing real-time visualization of structures. It is an essential tool for both the radiologist and the orthopedic surgeon. In fluoroscopy, x-rays penetrate the patient and are transformed into light photons upon striking a fluoroscopic screen. The fluoroscopic screen is coupled to an image intensifier

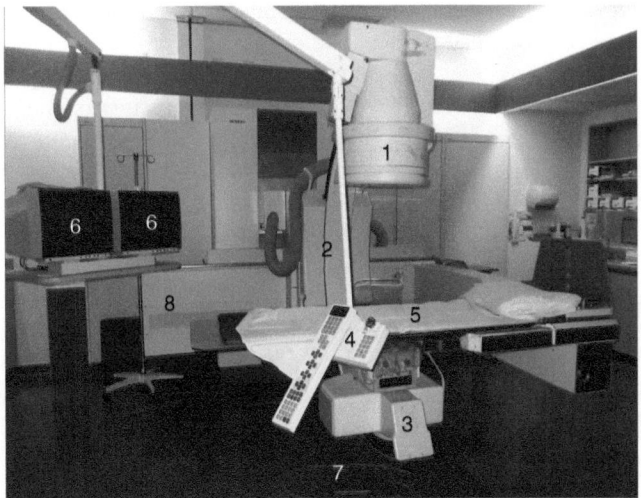

Fig. 7.3 Equipment in a fluoroscopy suite. *1*, Image intensifier; *2*, C-arm (to angle the x-ray beam); *3*, x-ray tube; *4*, remote control panel; *5*, patient table; *6*, image monitor; *7*, floor pedal; *8*, wall mount for C-arm.

and video camera, and the images are displayed on a monitor (Fig. 7.3). Image intensifiers are currently being replaced by flat-panel detector technology with improved spatial resolution and higher absorptive capability, potentially resulting in a dose reduction to the patient. A single static image mode or a rapid series of images in a video mode using frame rates of 30 to 35 images per second can be generated.[2] The spatial resolution of fluoroscopic images is inferior to that of radiographs because less radiation is used to form the image.

Radiologists often use fluoroscopy for needle guidance in musculoskeletal procedures such as arthrography, arthrocentesis, and administration of medication (Fig. 7.4). Non–image-guided

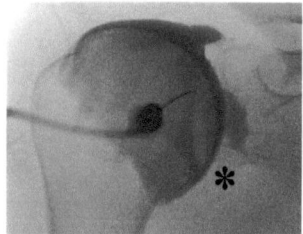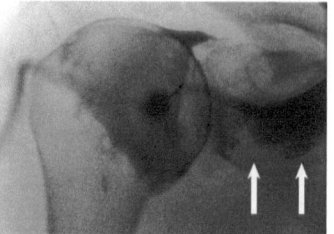

Fig. 7.4 A distension arthrogram for adhesive capsulitis. The initial fluoroscopic spot view *(left)* in a shoulder arthrogram for adhesive capsulitis shows restricted filling of the axillary *(asterisk)* and subscapularis recesses and early rupture of the capsule medially, which is consistent with the diagnosis. Further injection of contrast material *(right)* shows additional extraarticular extravasation into the soft tissues medially *(arrows)*.

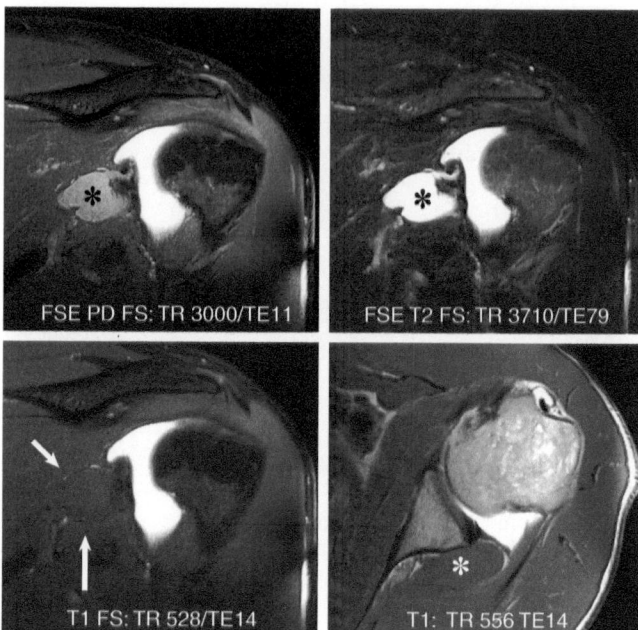

Fig. 7.5 A magnetic resonance (MR) arthrogram. Dilute gadolinium (1/200) is injected into the glenohumeral joint followed by MR imaging. The small amount of gadolinium is sufficient to create high T1 signal intensity in the joint fluid on both T1 with fat saturation *(T1FS; bottom left)* and T1 without fat saturation images *(T1; bottom right)*. The joint fluid is also bright on the proton density *(FSE PD FS)* and T2-weighted *(FSE T2 FS)* sequences *(top left* and *top right* images, respectively). A large paralabral cyst is present medial to the glenoid *(arrows* and *asterisk)*. The cyst fluid is isointense to muscle on both the T1-weighted images with and without fat saturation and is easily missed. T2-weighted images are required to visualize extraarticular pathology in MR arthrography.

joint injections and interventional spine procedures have failure rates up to 30%, even in large joints such as the shoulder.[3] Orthopedic surgeons routinely use intraoperative fluoroscopy for a variety of surgical procedures ranging from fracture reduction and fixation to joint replacement surgery. Video fluoroscopy can also play a role in the dynamic assessment of joints to evaluate them for instability.

Intraoperative fluoroscopy also assists orthopedic surgeons while performing total knee arthroplasties (TKAs) by allowing for precision of alignment in the coronal plane, using only a mean fluoroscopy time of 3 seconds. Patients operated on using this new technique had a lower risk of malalignment and a lower exposure to radiation, compared with the conventional technique.[4]

Different techniques to reduce radiation using intraoperative fluoroscopy have recently been studied. Double C-arm fluoroscopy, a technique using two C-arms instead of the conventional single C-arm, allows for assessment of screw placement in three dimensions and has a burgeoning role in the treatment of intertrochanteric fractures with intramedullary nails. This has been shown to significantly reduce surgical times and intraoperative radiation exposure.[5] In addition, different sizes of C-arms have been investigated in an effort to reduce radiation exposure to surgeons with studies indicating that mini C-arms may increase dosimeter absorption.[6]

Arthrography

Arthrographic procedures involve placing a fine-gauge needle (20 or 22 gauge) into a joint under fluoroscopic or ultrasound imaging guidance. These procedures are minimally invasive and relatively short in duration and are generally well tolerated by patients. Arthrography is often required for administration of medication such as steroids, local anesthetics, and viscose supplements, along with intraarticular contrast material for magnetic resonance (MR) and CT arthrography. In MR arthrography, a very dilute (1/200) mixture of gadolinium with saline solution and/or iodinated contrast media is injected into the joint before MRI is performed (Fig. 7.5). Use of a mixture of iodinated contrast material to dilute the gadolinium allows for continuous monitoring during the arthrographic procedure and provides the ability to switch to a CT arthrogram if the MRI is unsuccessful because of claustrophobia. In CT arthrography, an iodinated contrast agent is injected to produce a single-contrast CT

arthrogram (Fig. 7.6). Intraarticular air can be added after the iodinated contrast material is administered to produce a double-contrast CT arthrogram, although single-contrast studies are often preferred.[7] A small amount of epinephrine may be added to the injectate to constrict synovial vessels and prolong resorption of the contrast material.[8] The arthrogram must be coordinated with the booking of the CT or MR appointment, which should be scheduled so that imaging is carried out within 30 to 45 minutes after the injection, because rapid systemic absorption of contrast material through the synovium starts immediately after the joint injection. Given the logistics of trying to coordinate fluoroscopy and MR appointment bookings, MR and CT arthrographic examinations are more challenging to schedule. Patients may have longer wait times for the appointment compared with noncontrast studies, with the wait averaging up to 6 months in some institutions where MR resources are more limited per capita. Joints that typically are imaged with MR and CT arthrography examinations include the shoulder, hip, wrist, ankle, and knee. It is advisable to avoid the abbreviations *MRA* or *CTA* when requesting CT or MR arthrographic examinations because confusion with the request for an MR or CT *angiogram* may occur; the latter procedure corresponds to a completely different imaging technique in which intravenous contrast is administered to visualize vascular structures.

Diagnostic arthrography is helpful in pinpointing the source of nonspecific periarticular symptoms in patients. This technique

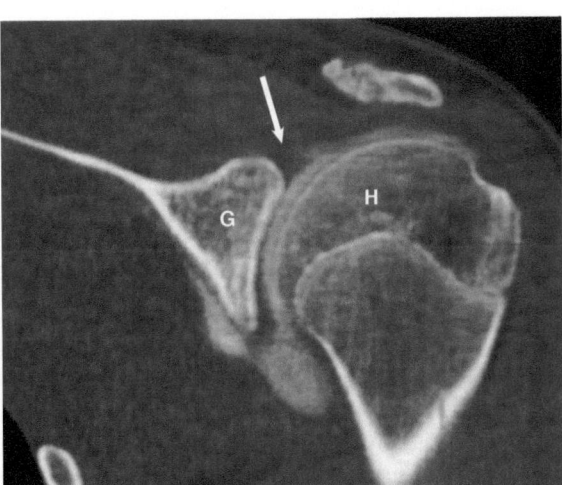

Fig. 7.6 A computed tomography (CT) shoulder arthrogram for a 16-year-old patient with clinical concern regarding a superior labral anterior to posterior (SLAP) tear. This study was originally arranged as a magnetic resonance (MR) arthrogram in which approximately 12.0 mL of 0.1 cc gadolinium diluted in 20 mL Isovue 300 was instilled into the joint. The patient was claustrophobic and unable to complete the MR arthrogram. A CT scan was immediately arranged to image the shoulder prior to systemic resorption of the contrast media. The small amount gadolinium in the joint fluid does not degrade the quality of the CT image. The superior labrum *(arrow)* is intact, without evidence of a SLAP tear or other abnormality. *G,* Glenoid; *H,* humeral head.

involves the injection of both short- and long-acting local anesthetics after establishing the intraarticular position of the needle with radiographic contrast material. The response of the patient's pain to the initial injection of anesthetic is documented immediately after the procedure, and the patient is then given a pain diary to monitor the effectiveness of the anesthetic for several hours after the procedure.

Arthrography is associated with small risks, the most significant of which is sepsis. Sepsis is reported to occur in less than 1 in 2000 cases.[9] Allergy to intraarticular contrast media is extremely rare compared with intravenously administered contrast media but can occur as a result of the slow systemic absorption of contrast material from the joint; the incidence of an allergic reaction is greatest in patients who have a known significant previous allergic reaction to contrast material, such as anaphylaxis. In patients with a history of a significant previous reaction to contrast material, alternative imaging or investigations should be sought. In patients who take anticoagulants, reversal is often required prior to the procedure to reduce the risk of bleeding. Pregnancy is a relative contraindication to fluoroscopy, although the radiation dose is minimal. These small risks should be carefully considered and balanced with the added information gained from arthrography compared with alternative noncontrast imaging options.

MR arthrography is generally preferred over CT arthrography because of the relatively higher diagnostic quality of the MR images, which is related to superior contrast discrimination and lack of ionizing radiation. CT arthrography images are often less optimal compared with MR arthrography images, particularly in the hip and shoulder joints, because of relatively thick surrounding soft tissues. These thick tissues cause scatter of the CT

x-rays, resulting in increased noise and overall image degradation. However, CT arthrography is an alternative option in patients who cannot undergo MR examinations because of claustrophobia or the presence of other MR-incompatible material.

CT arthrography also has added utility compared with MRI in the diagnosis of evaluation full thickness osteochondral lesions, specifically in the ankle. Only half of full thickness cartilage lesions found on CT arthrography were detected on MRI. Early detection of these lesions is especially important, as they may predispose patients to osteoarthritis. In addition, the evaluation of osteochondral defects is not only important in the preoperative but also the postoperative phase. Many of these patients have metallic hardware, which CT arthrography does a better job of suppressing. CT arthrography is also better than MRI in the detection of subchondral cysts or fissural defects which allow communication between intraarticular synovial fluid and cysts. This knowledge aids the surgeon in deciding whether to take an antegrade or retrograde approach.[10]

The diagnostic utility of CT arthrography is also optimal compared with MR arthrography in the evaluation of hyaline cartilage lesions within the shoulder.[11] Although CT arthrography is superior in the evaluation of shoulder cartilage, MR arthrography is excellent in evaluating labral tears and bony Bankart lesions; however, caution should be taken in the evaluation of glenohumeral ligament and rotator cuff tendon injury, as it is not as sensitive as conventional arthroscopy in the evaluation of these structures.[12] The position of the shoulder also influences the utility of MR arthrography, as studies have shown indirect MR arthrography of the shoulder in the abduction, external rotation view has a higher sensitivity in the detection of partial and full-thickness tears of the supraspinatus tendon[13] when compared with the neutral shoulder position.

Evaluation of partial/degenerative ligamentum teres tears of the hip is also aided by MR arthrogram, where it has better capability of detecting tears compared with conventional MRI. Limitations of conventional MRI in patients with chronic rotator cuff tears are likely secondary to fibrotic changes, simulating intact tendon.[14]

Advantages

Radiographs provide the basis for the initial evaluation of virtually all bone and joint pathology. They are essential in the diagnosis of bone and joint trauma because they provide a high degree of specificity in the setting of acute trauma. Plain radiographs are a valuable utility in the preoperative phase for bone pathology, while using a fraction of the radiation compared with CT.[15] Radiographs are inexpensive and widely available,[16] and recent studies have demonstrated they continue to provide clinical utility with a dose reduction of radiation without sacrificing radiographic details.[17,18]

Disadvantages

The projectional nature of radiographs can lead to underdiagnosis of dislocations and fractures, especially when fractures are minimally displaced, incomplete, or in a complex anatomic area. Fractures or dislocations identified on a single view may be difficult to appreciate on a second view. A minimum of two orthogonal views are required for assessment of underlying pathology (Fig. 7.7).[19] When there is a high degree of clinical suspicion for a fracture in the setting of normal radiographs, options for further workup include follow-up radiographs or additional imaging with CT, MR, or scintigraphy. False-negative radiographs are also common in the setting of early stages of osteolytic pathology, which is commonly associated with osteomyelitis and neoplastic pathology. At least 30% to 50% of the diameter of the bone must be destroyed to perceive underlying pathology (Fig. 7.8).[20] With the exception of calcified or ossified lesions, abnormalities of the soft tissues are not well demonstrated on radiographs because muscle, tendons, ligaments, fluid, and most soft tissue masses have a similar density. MRI and ultrasound are more optimal for demonstrating soft tissue pathology.

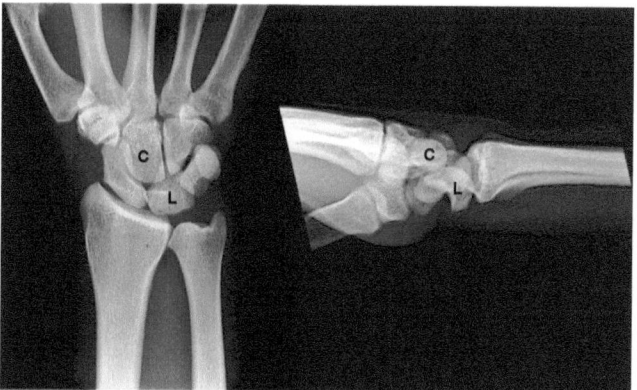

Fig. 7.7 A midcarpal dislocation shows the necessity for two orthogonal radiographic projections. The posteroanterior view of the wrist *(left)* shows subtle abnormalities consisting of a minor disruption of the proximal and midcarpal alignment and a triangular-shaped lunate *(L)*. The lateral view *(right)* confirms malalignment of the midcarpal joint with the capitate *(C)* situated dorsal to the lunate *(L)*.

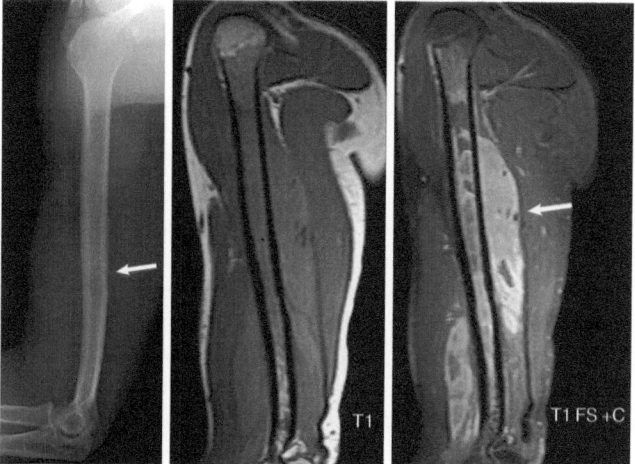

Fig. 7.8 False-negative radiographs in a patient with lymphoma of bone. A lateral radiograph of the humerus *(left)* shows a subtle small area of osteolysis in the mid diaphysis of the humerus *(arrow)*. A sagittal spin-echo T1-weighted image *(T1; middle)* shows replacement of virtually all of the visualized marrow cavity by tumor with intermediate signal intensity. A spin-echo T1-weighted image with fat saturation *(T1FS + C; right)* shows heterogeneous enhancement of the tumor both within the marrow and also in the posterior *(arrow)* and anterior soft tissues after administration of gadolinium contrast material.

Ultrasonography

The use of ultrasound in the evaluation of the musculoskeletal system has increased substantially during the past 20 years and provides an important adjunct to the repertoire of imaging modalities. Ultrasound is often used as a first-line investigation in the evaluation of tendon, muscle, and ligament injuries and soft tissue masses.

Technical Considerations

Ultrasound images are created by transmitting high-frequency sound waves above the audible range of human hearing into the body. The key component of the imaging system is the transducer, or probe, which is connected by a cable to a computer and an image screen. The technology is based on the piezoelectric physics principle in which a specialized piezoelectric transducer crystal can convert an electrical signal into a sound wave or vice versa.[21] The piezoelectric transducer crystal, which is housed in an ultrasound probe, vibrates when an electrical current is applied to it and emits sound waves. The sound waves interact with the body tissues. Some of the sound waves are reflected back toward the transducer at soft tissue interfaces that have significantly different impedances, whereas other sound waves are refracted or absorbed. The reflected sound waves are detected by the transducer, amplified, and subsequently converted back into an electric signal that is processed by the computer to generate a digital image.

When the ultrasound probe is placed on the skin overlying the area of interest, the sound waves are directed into the soft tissues located immediately beneath the probe, allowing visualization of structures encountering the sound waves. Manipulation of the ultrasound probe by the operator at the bedside determines how the structure of interest is viewed. For example, when imaging a tendon, the long axis of the probe is aligned parallel to the long axis of the tendon to produce a long axis view of the tendon. By turning the transducer 90 degrees perpendicular to the long axis of the tendon, a true short-axis view of the tendon is obtained. Slight rocking movements of the transducer from side to side provide further visualization of the medial-lateral or cranial-caudal extent of the structure of interest. If the structure of interest is larger than the footprint of the probe, the entire probe is repositioned over the area that was not previously imaged to view the additional area. Depending on how the transducer is angled, an infinite number of image planes can be obtained; however, standard axes include long-axis/sagittal and short-axis/transverse views, depending on the orientation of the structure of interest. During scanning, a rapid continuous series of images is generated, producing the appearance of a movie, termed *real-time* imaging. Typically, individual representative images are captured and stored as part of the examination record; however, video images or a series of images can be stored in a movie loop and occasionally are obtained to give other personnel the opportunity to view relevant aspects of the study after the examination is completed. It should be emphasized that no other imaging modality is more reliant on the operator performing the study at the bedside than is the case with sonography because this is where all of the pathology is initially observed during real time and documented. If the bedside operator cannot distinguish between normal and pathologic findings or does not scan the abnormal area, the examination will not document the underlying pathology. It also should be understood that the individual images stored to document the examination reflect a tiny, hopefully representative portion of the entire examination, which is akin to reviewing a few photographs compared with watching an entire movie.

A variety of configurations of ultrasound probes are available for musculoskeletal imaging with different contact surfaces or footprints, including linear and curved array configurations (Fig. 7.9). Linear array probes are most commonly used for evaluation of the musculoskeletal system. The sound waves are emitted from the probe in a parallel fashion, which is optimal for imaging the linear internal architecture of tendons, ligaments, and muscles. A water-based coupling gel is applied over the area to be scanned to improve the contact between the ultrasound probe and skin to facilitate sound transmission. The frequency of the sound waves used for evaluation of the musculoskeletal system is generally in the 10- to 15-MHz range. The transducer frequency is directly proportional to image resolution, with high-frequency transducers providing exquisite architectural detail of soft tissue structures. Unfortunately, the higher frequency transducers come with a penalty, because the depth of sound penetration is inversely proportional to the frequency. Thus the highest frequency transducers are only able to image very superficial structures a few centimeters deep to the skin.[21]

Ultrasound machines are equipped with several operator-controlled features that allow optimization of the image quality (Fig. 7.10). A depth control adjusts the amount of tissue imaged up to a maximum of several centimeters, determined by the frequency of the transducer. The focal zone should be adjusted to the area of concern to enhance resolution and simultaneously optimize the frame rate. The overall gain controls the signal amplification of the returning sound waves to either increase or decrease the desired level of brightness of the image. A Doppler mode can be applied, which uses the Doppler effect of moving blood to assess for the presence of blood flow in tissues. Both color and power color Doppler options, which are available on most machines, provide information on tissue vascularity. Color Doppler signal reflects the mean frequency shift of moving blood cells, providing information on velocity and direction of blood flow (Fig. 7.11). The direction of blood flow is encoded as either a red or blue color, depending on whether the blood flow is toward or away from the transducer. Power Doppler shows the total power of the Doppler shift, without regard for direction of flow or flow velocity, and is very sensitive to flow. The optimal Doppler mode for showing tissue vascularity in musculoskeletal sonography is controversial and likely related to individual features that are unique to the manufacturer. Recently many hospital-based imaging departments have introduced intravenously administered ultrasound contrast agents that serve as an alternative for selected patients who are not suitable candidates for use of contrast agents with MRI or CT; experience with the use of these contrast agents in musculoskeletal ultrasound applications is limited to date.

Musculoskeletal Ultrasound: Appearance of Normal and Pathologic Structures

The interaction of the sound waves at soft tissue interfaces determines the appearance of a structure on the ultrasound image. In areas where a significant difference in acoustic impedance exists, all of the sound waves are reflected back to the transducer, creating an area of increased echogenicity or hyperechoic focus. Because most of the sound waves are reflected back to the

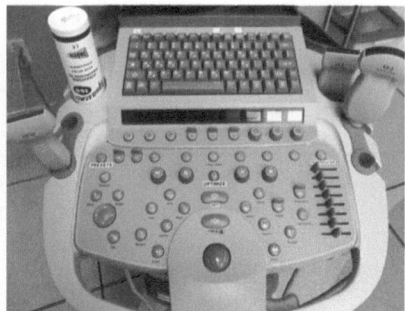

Fig. 7.10 A compact portable ultrasound machine. The machine is similar in size to a notebook computer *(left image)*. Fewer imaging options may be available with compact portable machines than with larger machines. A close-up view of the control panel of a slightly larger portable unit is shown *(right image)*. Physicians and technicians need to learn the functionality of the individual controls of the equipment used in their facility to optimize the image quality.

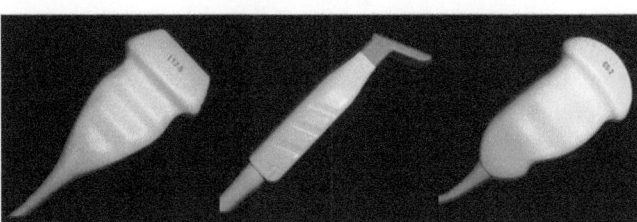

Fig. 7.9 Ultrasound probes for musculoskeletal imaging. A 17-5 MHz linear array probe *(left)* is used for general musculoskeletal examinations. A 15-7 MHz "hockey stick" probe *(middle)* is used for assessment of small superficial musculoskeletal abnormalities, allowing evaluation of structures less than 6.0 cm deep to the skin. A 5-2 MHz curved sector array *(right)* is available for evaluation of deep-seated musculoskeletal structures, enabling visualization of structures up to 30 cm deep to the skin.

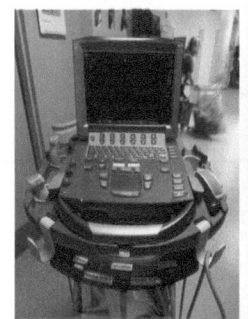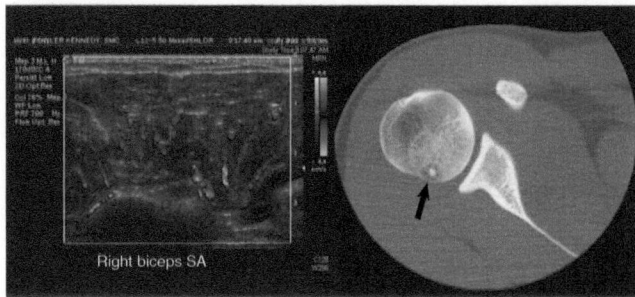

Fig. 7.11 Hyperemia on a color Doppler image. A 16-year-old male adolescent presented with shoulder pain, but the only abnormality evident on an initial shoulder ultrasound was prominent hyperemia in the deltoid muscle as seen on a color Doppler image *(left image)*. A computed tomography scan performed for further investigation revealed an osteoid osteoma *(arrow)*. *SA,* Short axis.

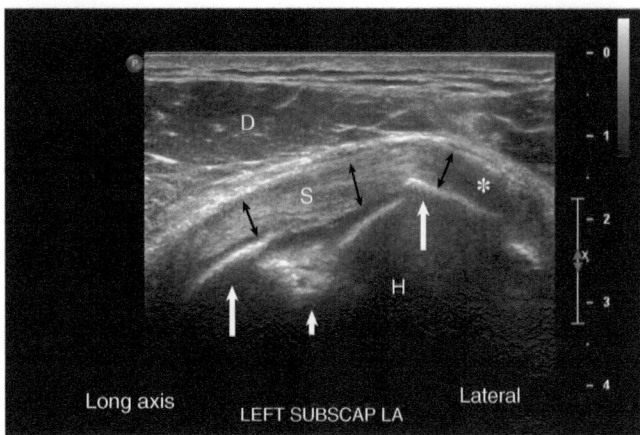

Fig. 7.12 A shoulder ultrasound image showing a Hill-Sachs fracture. A long-axis *(LA)* sonogram of the subscapularis *(subscap)* tendon *(S; black arrows)* was performed. The subscapularis tendon *(S)* appears normal, as manifested by an organized fibrillar appearance. A focal hypoechoic area is present at the tendon insertion laterally *(asterisk)* that is related to an anisotropic artifact at the curved insertion of the tendon where the orientation of the transducer is off the 90-degree axis relative to the long axis of the distal tendon. The cortical bone of the humeral head *(white arrows)* deep to the tendon is manifested by a hyperechoic line with pronounced acoustic shadowing due to attenuation of the sound waves by bone. The bone is irregular at the site of an impaction fracture *(short white arrow)*. The deltoid muscle *(D)* shows a normal appearance, manifested by hypoechoic tissue with fine hyperechoic linear septations. *H,* Humeral head.

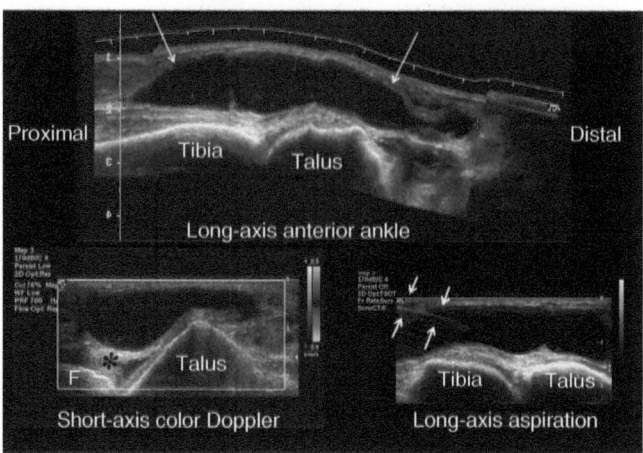

Fig. 7.13 Extensor digitorum longus tenosynovitis. A long-axis extended field of view image at the anterior aspect of the ankle *(top image)* shows an elongated fluid collection *(arrows)*. The collection is predominantly anechoic, containing a few low-level echoes. The short-axis color Doppler image *(bottom left)* shows that the posterior wall of the fluid collection is well defined. Increased through transmission of sound is evident posteriorly *(asterisk)*. No internal flow is evident on the color Doppler image. The findings confirm the diagnosis of a fluid collection. Ultrasound-guided aspiration of the fluid in the tendon sheath followed by injection of a steroid was performed *(bottom right)*. An 18-gauge needle *(arrows)* was used for the procedure. *F,* Fibula.

transducer, few sound waves travel further into the soft tissues deep to the reflective surface, producing an artifact manifested by focal loss of echogenicity, termed *acoustic shadowing* (Fig. 7.12). An example of this phenomenon occurs at soft tissue–bone or calcium interfaces. In areas where there are no soft tissue interfaces, no sound waves are reflected back to the transducer, as occurs with simple fluid collections. In this setting, the fluid appears black, or anechoic, often with transmission of more sound waves posterior to the structure, creating an artifact termed *increased through transmission*. Three criteria must be met to confirm the diagnosis of a simple fluid collection on ultrasound, including lack of internal echoes (i.e., anechoic), a well-defined posterior wall, and increased through transmission of the sound waves (Fig. 7.13). Soft tissue interfaces with similar interfaces and acoustic impedances show a similar degree of echogenicity and are termed *isoechoic* (Fig. 7.14).

The high resolution afforded by sonography enables the detailed internal architecture of tendons, superficial ligaments, and muscle tissue to be accurately assessed. Normal tendons appear as linear hyperechoic fibrillar structures in their long axis (Fig. 7.15). Tendinosis or microtearing typically manifests, as varying degrees of loss of the normal fibrillar pattern of the tendon replaced by hypoechoic areas and may become increased/hypertrophic or decreased/atrophic in thickness. Frank tendon tears manifest as focal areas of discontinuity of tendon fibers (see Figs. 7.15 and 7.16). While scanning tendons, it is imperative to align the ultrasound transducer perpendicular to the long axis of the structure of interest to prevent anisotropic artifact. Anisotropy is the artifactual apparent decrease in echogenicity in a structure when the angle of insonation relative to the

structure of interest is off the 90-degree perpendicular axis, potentially resulting in the misdiagnosis of tendinosis or tear (Fig. 7.17). Anisotropy is most problematic in anatomic areas where the structure of interest has a curved geometry, such as the insertion of the tendons of the rotator cuff (see Fig. 7.12). It also can affect the echogenicity of ligaments and muscles. Sonography has played a long-established role in the diagnosis of rotator cuff tears and has proven to be as accurate as non-contrast MRI (see Fig. 7.17).[22] Ligaments are typically thin hyperechoic structures that become thickened and hypoechoic or discontinuous when torn. Muscle tissue is hypoechoic, with fine linear areas of increased echogenicity corresponding to fibro-fatty perimysium surrounding the muscle fascicles (see Fig. 7.12). Subcutaneous fat, which is hypoechoic, contains small echogenic septations. Articular cartilage is near anechoic. Fibrocartilaginous structures such as the glenoid, meniscus, and acetabular labra are hyperechoic. Nerves appear as fascicular structures with variable echogenicity, depending on adjacent structures (Fig. 7.18). Assessment of large peripheral nerves is feasible with sonography and more efficient than MR, because a greater length of the nerves can be scanned without any restriction in coverage created by a local coil in MR.[23]

Ultrasound also frequently serves as a first line of investigation in the evaluation of soft tissue masses. Sonography can be used to confirm the presence of a clinically suspected lesion and at times can establish a definitive diagnosis. Ultrasound enables the differentiation of simple fluid-containing masses such as ganglia, bursae, and synovial cysts from solid lesions, eliminating the need for further imaging with MRI (see Fig. 7.13). However, differentiation of complex cystic fluid collections that contain proteinaceous or hemorrhagic fluid from solid masses is not always feasible with ultrasound (Figs. 7.19–7.21). The diagnosis

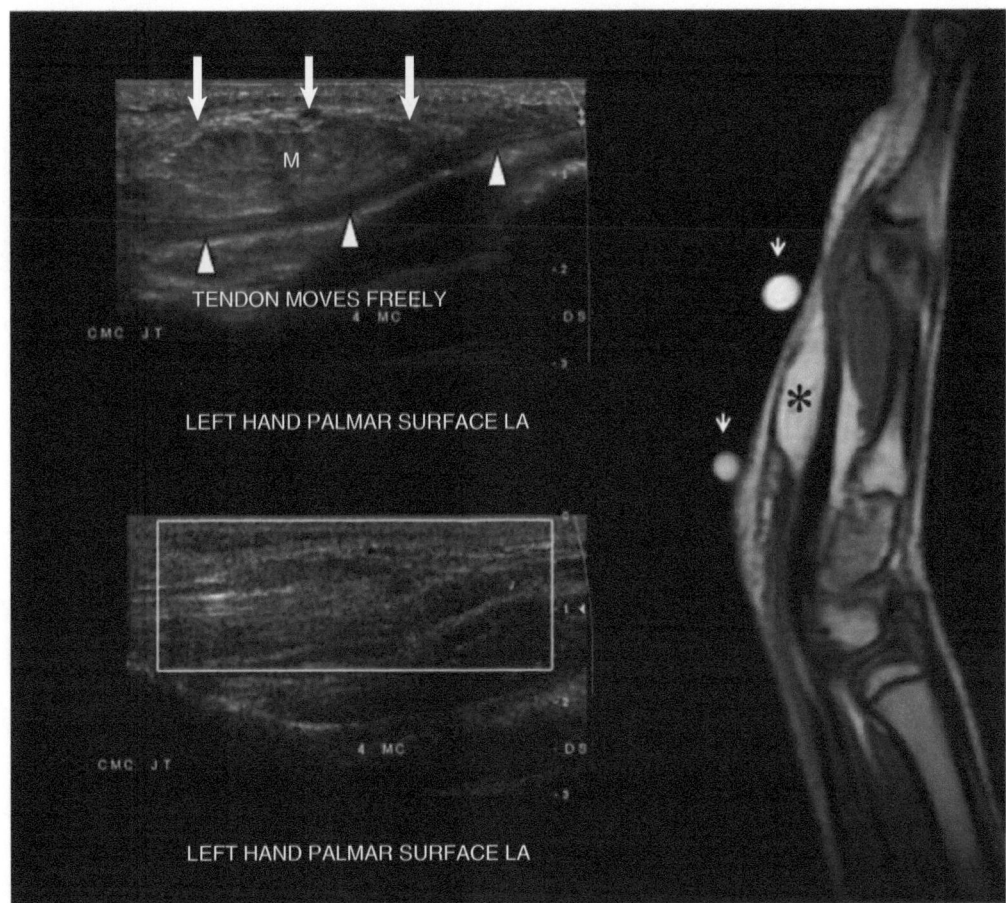

Fig. 7.14 An isoechoic mass without flow on a color Doppler image. A 13-year-old had a palpable mass on the palmar aspect of the hand. A long-axis *(LA)* sonogram *(top left)* shows a subtle isoechoic soft tissue mass *(M, arrows)* corresponding to the area of concern, causing slight displacement of the adjacent flexor tendon *(arrowheads)*. A color Doppler image *(bottom left)* shows no internal vascularity, confirming a hypovascular lesion. A sagittal T1-weighted spin-echo magnetic resonance image (MRI) *(right)* shows the lesion *(asterisk)* has a high-intensity signal, confirming the diagnosis of a lipoma. Markers were positioned over the area of clinical concern prior to the MRI scan *(small arrows)*.

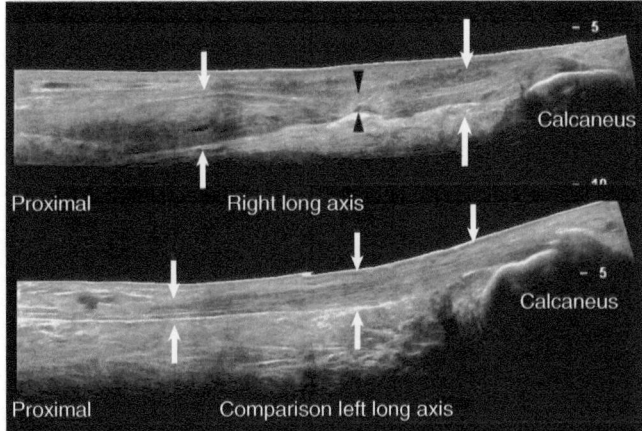

Fig. 7.15 The sonographic appearance of tendons. An extended field of view long-axis sonogram of a normal Achilles tendon *(bottom, arrows)* shows an organized fibrillar appearance. A long-axis view of a completely torn Achilles tendon *(top, arrows)* shows focal discontinuity of tendon fibers *(black arrowheads)* in the watershed zone several centimeters proximal to the calcaneal insertion. The proximal tendon is swollen and hypoechoic as a result of intrasubstance hemorrhage and edema. The distalmost aspect of the tendon is thickened and mildly hypoechoic, related to a background of tendinosis.

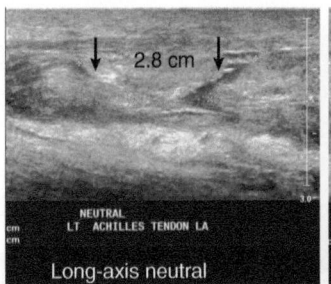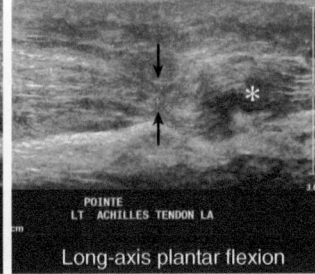

Fig. 7.16 A complete tear of the Achilles tendon is shown with dynamic imaging. The long-axis *(LA)* view of the Achilles tendon *(left image)* with the foot in a neutral position shows a 2.8-cm gap between the edges of the torn tendon fibers *(arrows)*. In plantar flexion *(right image)*, the tendon fibers co-apt *(arrows)*. An ill-defined hypoechoic area is now evident, corresponding to a refraction artifact *(asterisk)*.

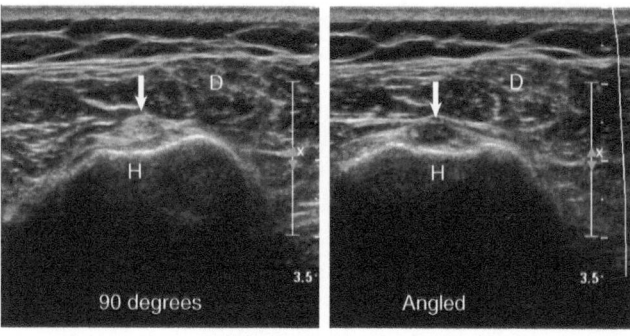

Fig. 7.17 Anisotropy. A short-axis view of the long head of the biceps tendon *(arrow, left)* shows the normal echogenic appearance of the tendon when the ultrasound probe is oriented 90 degrees to the long axis of the tendon. The tendon becomes artifactually hypoechoic as a result of anisotropy when the probe is angled off the 90-degree axis *(arrow; right)*. *D*, Deltoid; *H*, humeral head.

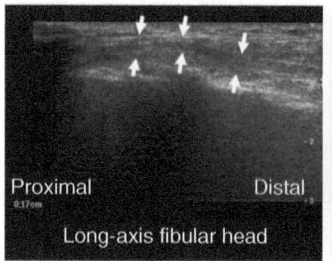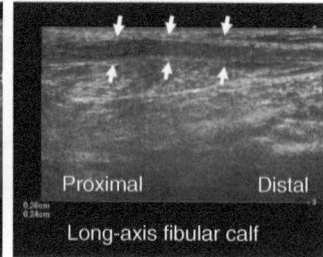

Fig. 7.18 Ultrasound images of the peroneal nerve. The long-axis view *(left)* of the common peroneal nerve just distal to the level of the fibular head shows a normal appearance of the nerve appearing as a fine fibrillar hypoechoic structure *(arrows)*. In the proximal calf *(right)*, the nerve becomes thickened but retains its fibrillar structure *(arrows)*.

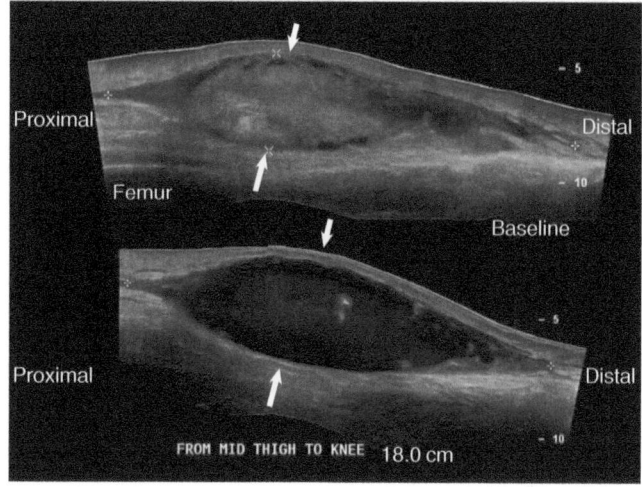

Fig. 7.19 Thigh hematoma illustrating overlap of the appearance of complex cystic fluid collections and solid lesions. An extended field of view long-axis sonogram of the anterior thigh *(top)* shows a large isoechoic mass corresponding to an acute hematoma *(arrows)*, which could be easily misconstrued as a solid soft tissue mass. A long-axis sonogram of the same area *(bottom)* 2 weeks later shows the normal evolution of a hematoma, now manifested as a complex fluid collection containing a few low-level echoes *(arrows)*.

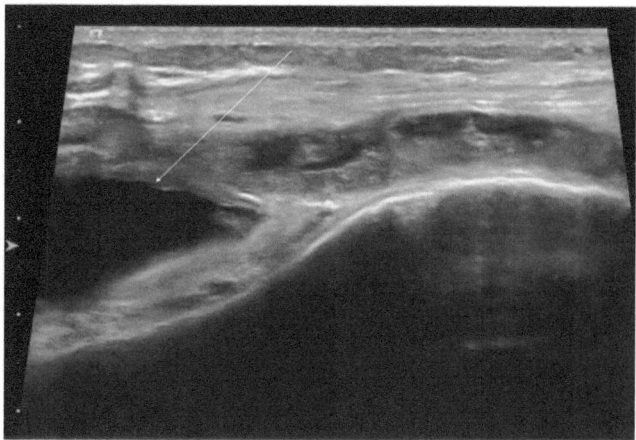

Fig. 7.21 Ultrasound at the level of the suprapatellar bursa demonstrates a heterogeneous, thick-walled effusion most compatible with complex suprapatellar synovitis.

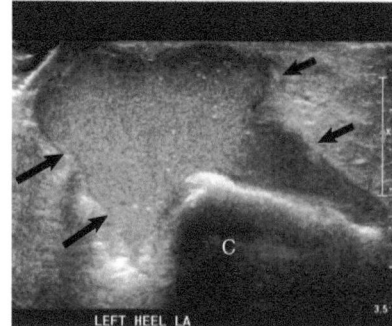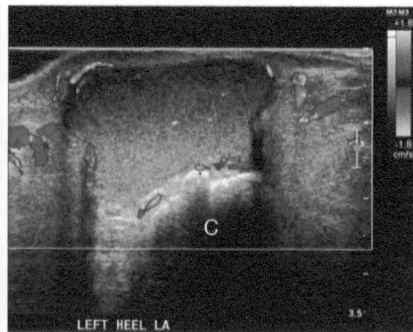

Fig. 7.20 A soft tissue abscess mimicking a solid mass lesion in a diabetic patient with a heel abscess. A long-axis *(LA)* sonogram *(left)* shows an irregular isoechoic mass *(arrows)* superficial to the calcaneus *(C)* with mobile internal echoes at real time (not shown). A long-axis color Doppler image of the lesion *(right)* shows peripheral hyperemia.

of a solid lesion is established when internal vascularity is demonstrated within a lesion with color Doppler imaging. However, occasionally solid hypovascular lesions may not reveal flow with Doppler imaging, because the signal from slow flow may be below the threshold sensitivity of the ultrasound probe (see Fig. 7.14). Detection of soft tissue calcifications associated with calcific tendinopathy, ossificans, and some tumors on ultrasound is superior to radiography, CT, and MR (Fig. 7.22).

Sonography can be used to guide interventional procedures, including biopsy of soft tissue masses, diagnostic and therapeutic aspiration of joint effusions and periarticular fluid collections, aspiration and lavage (barbotage) of calcium deposits for treatment of calcific tendinosis, and injection of a local anesthetic and steroids for diagnosis and therapy. In general, sonographic-guided procedures are more technically demanding than fluoroscopic procedures, because fewer radiologists have the expertise and training to perform the procedures. Sonography is an alternative

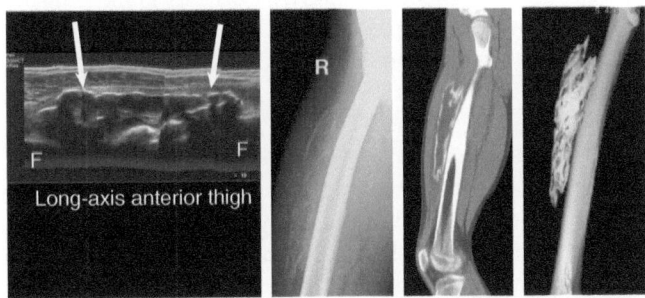

Fig. 7.22 Soft tissue calcifications on an ultrasound image. The patient has myositis ossificans. A long-axis sonogram of the anterior thigh *(left)* shows extensive calcification *(arrows; F,* femur). A lateral radiograph of the femur *(middle left)* confirms the presence of peripheral zonal calcification in the anterior soft tissues of the thigh. A sagittal multiplanar reformatted computed tomography (CT) scan *(middle right)* and three-dimensional CT reformat *(right)* confirm the diagnosis of myositis ossificans.

to fluoroscopic-guided arthrography, which often is reserved for patients who have contrast allergies or to reduce radiation exposure in young patients. The individual preference of the radiologist, the age of the patient, and the length of the waiting list for the appointment (if applicable) often determine whether sonographic or fluoroscopic guidance is preferred. Consultation with the radiologist performing such procedures is suggested. Ultrasound also plays an occasional role in foreign body localization.[24] Although metal and glass can usually be identified on radiographs, wood is infrequently detected because its attenuation is similar to that of soft tissues. Ultrasound enables detection of all three materials, confirming the presence of the foreign body and providing guidance to aid removal of the object.

Ultrasound Elastography

Ultrasound elastography is a relatively new technology, which primarily assesses the mechanical properties of tissue, such as tendons, ligaments, and muscles. There are multiple techniques to perform sonographic evaluation of the mechanical properties of tissues; however, the most common way is free hand strain (compression) elastography. Compression elastography is performed by manually applying stress with a handheld ultrasound probe, which in turn results in the displacement of soft tissues with varying tensile strengths. Based on these color-coded distribution maps, elastograms are created, which measure the elasticity of soft tissues relative to one another (Fig. 7.23).[25]

In sports medicine, sonographic elastography evaluation primarily focuses on the Achilles tendon and is able to quantify the elasticity value. It is based upon the hypothesis that mechanical stress upon soft tissues causes its appearance to change on sonographic evaluation. This principle is best used to examine degenerative and traumatic changes and has added utility in the ability to monitor the effectiveness of physical therapy on healthy and diseased musculotendinous tissue.

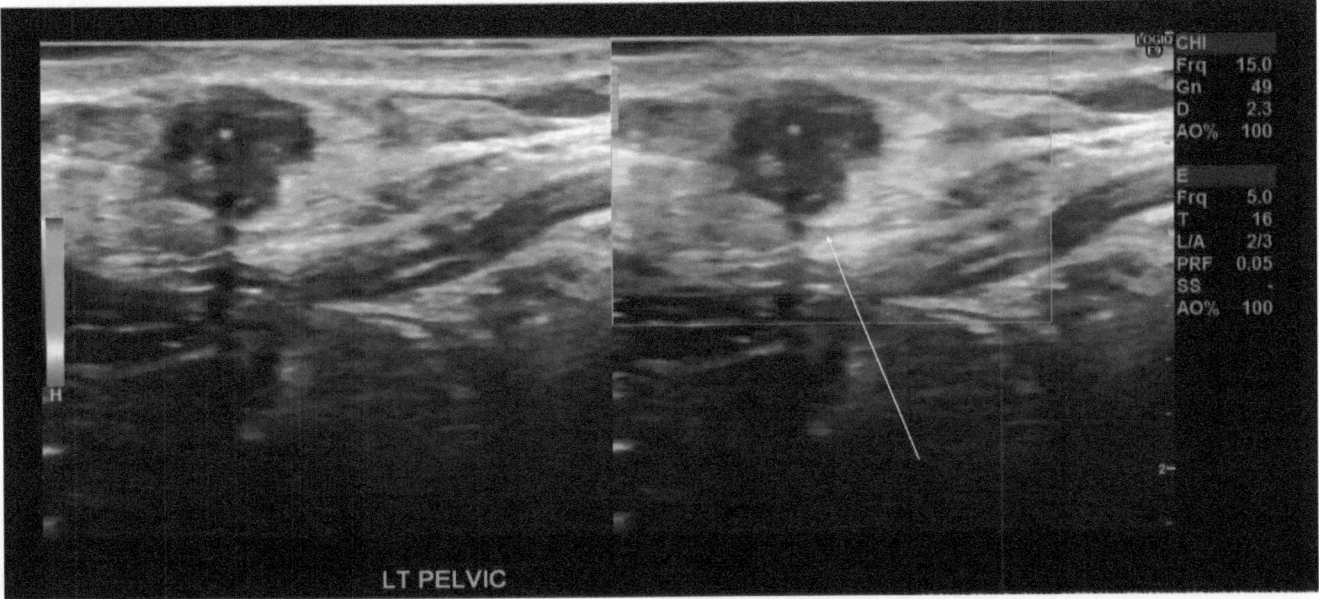

Fig. 7.23 Ultrasound elastography demonstrates a left groin mass that was biopsy proved to be an endometrioma. The color maps demonstrate different tensile strengths of the endometrioma and the musculature of the left groin.

Sonographic elastography of the Achilles tendon is most effective in the evaluation of Achilles tendinopathy by detecting alterations in tendon tensile strength, particularly in those with areas of softening. Future applications of elastography are aimed toward identifying patellar tendinopathy and rotator cuff tendinopathy.[26,27]

Ultrasound elastography also has a burgeoning role in rehabilitation of musculoskeletal injury and chronic myofascial pain, by measuring the mechanical properties of tissue, including muscle stiffness. It has also been found to assist in certain pain syndromes such as iliotibial syndrome, particularly in stretching prior to exercise.[28,29]

Dynamic Ultrasound

Dynamic ultrasound has proven to be of great utility in the evaluation of abnormalities of the ligamentous, tendinous, and muscular structures that can only be identified in a dynamic evaluation. Dynamic evaluation of the rotator cuff tendons can be of utility when determining the severity of shoulder impingement syndrome, specifically when there is moderate to severe impingement. In moderate impingement, there will be prominence of the subacromial/subdeltoid bursa or fluid lateral to the acromion process. In severe impingement, the humeral head migrates and the supraspinatus tendon will appear to be more prominent, as it is not able to glide smoothly underneath the acromial-acoustic shadow. In addition, ulnar neuropathies, which may otherwise go undetected using conventional ultrasound methods, may be better appreciated on dynamic ultrasound imaging, as the nerve enters the cubital tunnel (Fig. 7.24).

In addition, dislocation/subluxation of the long head of the biceps tendon may sometimes be transient and sit within the bicipital groove while the shoulder is in the neutral position. In these circumstances, dislocation/subluxation can only be identified on dynamic maneuver and external rotation will elicit the abnormality. The long head of the biceps tendon can dislocate anterior or deep in relation to the subscapularis tendon.

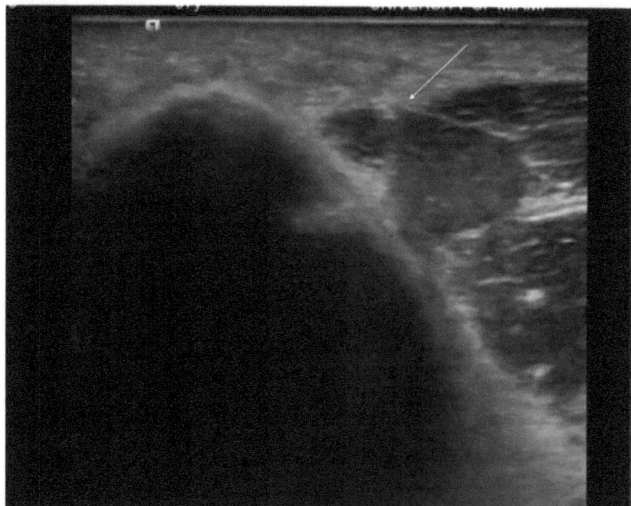

Fig. 7.24 Dynamic ultrasound of through the cubital tunnel demonstrates an enlarged and hypoechoic ulnar nerve, most compatible with ulnar neuritis.

Subluxation of the peroneus brevis and longus tendons can also be assessed using dynamic sonography. Diagnosis may be difficult to make using physical examination, and MRI may not reveal tendons that are transiently dislocated. This applies to tendons in the foot as well, as placing the foot in dorsiflexion and eversion of the ankle will reveal lateral displacement/dislocation of the perineal tendons in relation to the fibula.

In addition, subtle muscle tears may also only become apparent on dynamic sonographic evaluation. These tears may appear as areas of echogenic infiltration, a heterogeneous mass, or focal disruption of muscle fibers. These findings are also frequently accompanied by perifascial fluid. Dynamic sonography is also appropriate in the discrimination of a pseudo mass caused by a muscle tear, as during isometric muscle contraction the torn muscle appears as a focal bulge.[30]

Within the wrist, dynamic ultrasound provides a fairly rapid and cost-effective evaluation of the intrinsic and extrinsic ligaments. Dynamic ultrasound has also proven to be effective in the evaluation of rotator cuff injury, particularly in the evaluation of full-thickness tears. The diagnostic accuracy of shoulder ultrasound in the evaluation of partial and full thickness rotator cuff tears reaches approximately 91% to 100%.[31]

Advantages

Sonography has numerous advantages compared with other imaging modalities. Unlike radiography and CT, which subject the patient to small risks associated with the use of ionizing radiation, ultrasound has no known deleterious effects. Because ultrasound equipment is relatively inexpensive, the technology is widely available. Portable ultrasound equipment is commercially available, enabling immediate on-site point of care evaluation. Ultrasound images have relatively high spatial resolution compared with MR images. Dynamic evaluation of the musculoskeletal system is possible with sonography, unlike with MR and CT, with which only limited assessment is possible.[30] Vascular information from Doppler interrogation is available on virtually all ultrasound machines with the push of a button, unlike CT and some vascular pulse sequences in MRI that require the use of intravenous contrast material, subjecting patients to the small risk of an allergic reaction and adding to the cost of the examination.

Ultrasound has the added capability of adding reliability in diagnosis of cam-type femoroacetabular impingement (FAI) and can serve as an alternative or additional method in initial imaging.[32] New studies have demonstrated ultrasound also has an added benefit in the trauma setting in regard to contributing to the workup of acute coracoclavicular ligament injury,[33] as well as providing valuable information in regard to fracture healing.[34]

Disadvantages

Although musculoskeletal sonography is used widely in European and Canadian institutions, acceptance has been slow in many centers in the United States. Limitations include a relatively long learning curve and a high degree of operator dependence compared with other imaging modalities. To provide consistent and reliable results, technologists and physicians involved in musculoskeletal sonography should receive proper training.[35] The contact area or "footprint" of the ultrasound probe restricts the volume of tissue interrogated at any single site during the examination to a small area constrained to several centimeters, which makes it challenging for clinicians to grasp a complete perspective of the pathology, particularly when assessing large, soft tissue structures. Extended and dual-image/split-screen modes allow a larger area of tissue to be captured in a static image with a standard probe to alleviate this issue, and these options are currently available on most machines. These large field of view images are obtained when either the technologist or physician overseeing the study decides it would help illustrate the abnormality to provide a clearer understanding of the pathology (Fig. 7.25). Because bone reflects sound waves, evaluation of osseous structures is limited to their topography. The quality of ultrasound images is affected by the patient's body habitus, with poorer quality images in large patients because of the absorption of the sound waves. The challenge of assessing deep-seated anatomic regions is another limitation; because of the absorption of sound waves, lower frequency transducers are required to gain depth penetration, with a consequent reduction in spatial resolution. Musculoskeletal ultrasound typically is performed as a focused evaluation in an anatomic region or of a specific structure and is generally not performed as a survey technique, unlike CT and MRI.

Computed Tomography

CT has revolutionized medical imaging since its introduction as a clinical tool in 1974. Sir Godfrey Hounsfield received a Nobel Prize in 1979 for his contribution to the development of this technology. The original generation of scanners had extremely limited capacity to assess the musculoskeletal system; they were composed of single-detector configurations with longer acquisition times and low-resolution limited diagnostic quality image reformats. Since the introduction of spiral scanners in 1989 and multidetector scanners in 1992, CT has become an integral tool in the evaluation of the musculoskeletal system. Multidetector CT scanners have evolved rapidly from the earliest four-channel units to the latest generation commercially available 160-channel scanners.

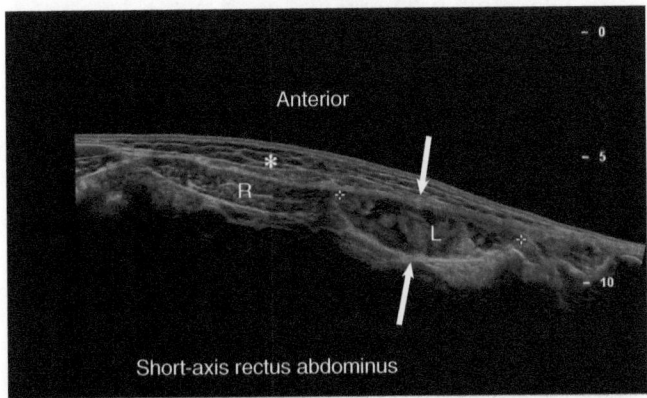

Fig. 7.25 Extended field of view ultrasound. The large field of view short-axis image of the anterior abdominal wall optimally displays enlargement and heterogeneous decreased echogenicity in the left rectus abdominis muscle (L; arrows) associated with a complete tear. The right rectus abdominis muscle (R) is normal in comparison. The asterisk denotes subcutaneous tissues.

Technical Considerations

CT is a tomographic technique that takes advantage of x-ray interaction with tissues in the body, similar to radiography. The technology differs from radiography in that the x-ray source and opposing detector array are housed in a gantry that rotates circumferentially around the patient. The patient is positioned supine on a moving table inside the opening in the gantry. The x-ray tube emits a narrow x-ray beam continuously during the circumferential rotation that passes through the patient and is received by the detector. The detector measures differences in x-ray absorption (attenuation) as the beam rotates around the patient, and the x-ray signal is then back-computed mathematically (using a Fourier transform), resulting in the creation of a raw projectional data set.

Early conventional CT images were acquired using a "step and shoot" technique in which a single slice was obtained with the patient lying on the CT table, which was incrementally moved a short distance. The second slice was acquired and the process was repeated many times, until the anatomic area of interest was imaged. This technique required a large amount of time for image acquisition and had the potential for significant image degradation due to motion artifact.

Advances in CT engineering led to continuous spiral (helical) CT technology.[36] In spiral CT, the x-ray tube and detector rotate continuously with the patient lying on the scanner table, which simultaneously moves through the gantry, resulting in a significant reduction in imaging time. Further technical developments led to multislice technology, in which multiple detectors formed in an array are used to acquire multiple slices with each rapid rotation of the gantry. The latest generation CT scanners have up to 160 detector arrays, which are capable of acquiring up to 160 slices with each 360-degree rotation of the tube. Multislice scanners have resulted in very fast acquisition times and ultrathin collimation, resulting in exquisitely detailed anatomic images, thus enabling reformatting in any plane with excellent resolution. Electron-beam CT scanners were introduced in the mid-1980s and use a different technique to obtain even faster imaging. In this technology, the x-ray tube is stationary and an electron beam is electronically swept around the patient. This technology has been developed primarily for imaging cardiac and other moving structures.

Each pixel of the CT image is assigned a Hounsfield unit (HU) value that reflects the attenuation of the x-ray beam. The attenuation values are potentially useful in characterizing tissues and can be measured by placing a region of interest cursor over the area in question. The density of water is set at 0 HU, and air is set at −1000 HU. The density of soft tissue typically ranges between 10 and 90 HU. Medullary bone ranges between 30 and 230 HU, and cortical bone typically measures between 230 and 1000 HU. Less dense tissues such as fat have a lower attenuation value of around −80 HU.[37] Similar to radiography, dense tissues appear bright/white and less dense tissues appear dark/black. A grayscale map corresponding to the HU value assigned to each pixel is applied, with the resultant CT image display reflecting underlying tissue composition. The image can be manipulated by selecting the range of HUs in which the grayscale map is applied, termed *window width*, and selecting the value that should be assigned to the middle of the grayscale map, termed *window level*. For optimal visualization of osseous structures, a *bone window* is used, consisting of a high window width of 1000 to 2000 HU and a window level of approximately 250 HU. For optimal soft tissue contrast, termed a *soft tissue window*, a narrower window width of 400 to 600 HU is used, with a window level of about 50 HU (Fig. 7.26). The window width and window levels can be adjusted at the PACs computer workstation using the x- and y-axes of the computer mouse. Both bone and soft tissue windows should be reviewed to provide a complete assessment of the images. Occasionally a hematoma or an incidental but clinically significant visceral neoplasm is detected on the soft tissue windows.

If information regarding vascular structures is required in the setting of trauma, an iodinated intravenous contrast agent can be administered, with the scanning timed to reflect the desired vascular phase (arterial or venous). Contraindications to the use of an iodinated intravenous contrast agent include renal failure and a previous allergic reaction to iodinated contrast media.

All multidetector CT scanners produce a preliminary raw projection data set in the transverse plane that is routinely converted into a volumetric data set of thin 0.625-mm transverse sections for musculoskeletal applications. Special reconstruction kernels (computer algorithms) are applied to the raw data set prior to generating reformatted images that optimize the structure of interest. In musculoskeletal imaging, these options include bone, soft tissue, and metal algorithms (Fig. 7.27).

The transverse volumetric thin-slice data set is postprocessed in a variety of ways and typically is carried out at a separate workstation as part of an automated program or is processed manually by a technologist or radiologist.[38,39] The generation of large sets of more than a thousand postprocessed images and the subsequent transmission of the images to PACs adds to the time required to complete the examination. For musculoskeletal applications, thin-slice multiplanar reformats are typically routinely reconstructed in the sagittal and coronal planes. Selected additional reformats are obtained when they are deemed to be

contributory by the radiologist or if they are specifically requested by the referring physician. Curved multiplanar reformats are useful in anatomic areas with curved geometry such as the clavicle, carpus, and tarsus. Additional three-dimensional (3D) postprocessing options include surface and volume rendered images (Fig. 7.28); 3D surface rendering produces grayscale images based on the surface anatomy, whereas 3D volume rendering generates images using the entire data set, including deeper anatomy, with a full color range where useful. 3D rendering is routinely used in musculoskeletal imaging and provides a global overview of

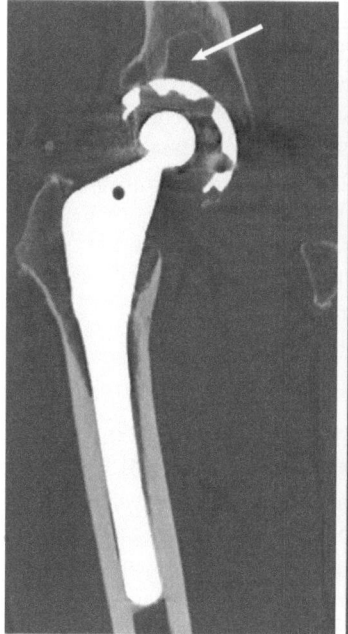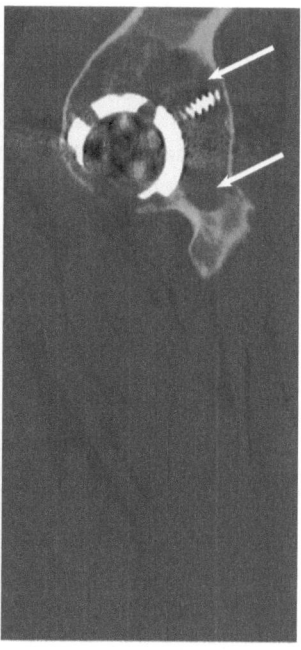

Fig. 7.27 A computed tomography image of a hip arthroplasty with a metal algorithm. Coronal *(left)* and sagittal *(right)* multiplanar reformats of the right hip show a cementless right total hip arthroplasty. A large irregular area of osteolysis is present in the periprosthetic acetabulum as a result of particle disease *(arrows).*

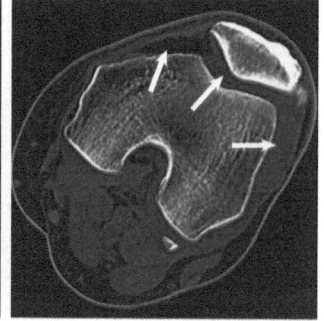

Fig. 7.26 The effect of windowing on the appearance of tissues on computed tomography. A transverse image of the knee was windowed to optimize assessment of the soft tissues *(left)* in a patient with a tibial plateau fracture. A moderate-sized suprapatellar effusion is present, revealing a hematocrit effect. Nondependent marrow fat is most superficial, blood serum (fluid) is in the middle, and slightly heavier blood cellular blood products are in a more dependent location *(arrows).* The same slice is windowed for evaluation of bone detail *(right).*

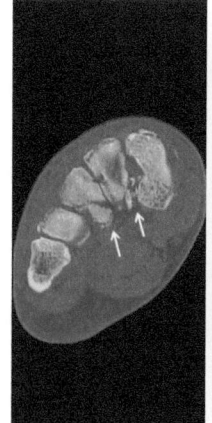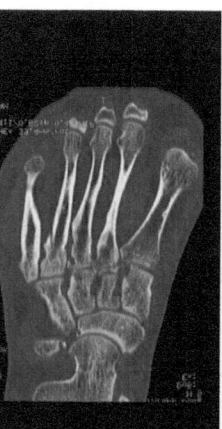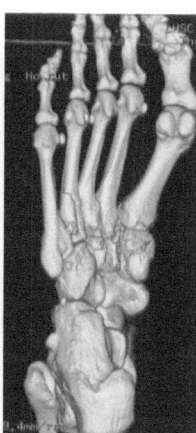

Fig. 7.28 Computed tomography (CT) reformats of second through fourth metatarsal fractures. Radiographs indicated a solitary fourth metatarsal fracture (not shown). A transverse CT image *(left)* through the midfoot with curved coronal multiplanar *(middle)* and three-dimensional volume-rendered *(right)* reformats confirm comminuted minimally displaced fractures involving the second and third metatarsal bases *(arrows).*

pathology. Segmentation is another postprocessing technique, whereby certain structures in the image can be cropped out, allowing a selective display of only the structure of interest. Segmentation is most useful in the setting of intraarticular fractures in which the articular surface of the affected bone is displayed in isolation to eliminate overlapping structures (Fig. 7.29).

CT arthrography is a technique in which a CT scan is obtained after the intraarticular administration of radiographic contrast. This technique has lower inherent soft tissue discrimination and has largely been supplanted by noncontrast MR or contrast MR arthrography; however, it occasionally is warranted in patients who have contraindications to MRI (Fig. 7.30).[40]

CT-guided biopsies are typically performed in lesions that are confined to bone. If a soft tissue mass is present in association with a bone lesion, ultrasound-guided biopsy is typically the preferred route because it is more efficient and prevents interruption of the workflow on CT. On some units, CT fluoroscopy is an option for guiding biopsies, but currently it is not widely utilized because of concerns regarding the high radiation dose delivered to both the patient and the radiologist.[41,42]

Advantages

CT images have superb spatial resolution that is typically greater than that of MR images. Multidetector array machines facilitate

ultrafast imaging, generating total body scans in several seconds; thus they reduce the potential for motion artifacts and eliminate the need for sedation in pediatric patients. High-resolution image reformats can be produced in multiple planes with use of a variety of postprocessing options from a single transverse data set.

CT serves as an adjunct to conventional radiographs in the evaluation of skeletal trauma; it provides a more detailed and diagnostically sensitive examination, which helps determine appropriate clinical management. CT plays an essential role in the diagnosis of radiographically occult fractures and in the evaluation of comminuted and/or intraarticular fractures, particularly in anatomically complex regions (Figs. 7.31 and 7.32).[43] Although MRI is the modality of choice in the evaluation of bone tumors, CT is used for problem solving in selected instances when cortical integrity is questioned and for the definitive assessment of matrix mineralization.[44] CT is often used to guide percutaneous biopsy of bone lesions when ultrasound guidance is not feasible (Fig. 7.33). In postoperative patients, CT can be used to assess arthroplasty or other hardware-related complications, along with bone graft and fracture healing (see Fig. 7.27).[45,46]

Disadvantages

Shortcomings of CT are mainly related to the radiation dose received by the patient, which occurs to the greatest extent in parts of the body where the soft tissues are thickest, particularly in the spine, pelvis, and chest, resulting in exposure of radiosensitive gonadal and breast tissue. The peripheral extremities

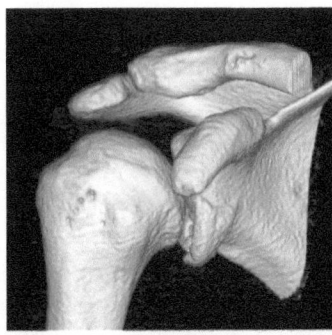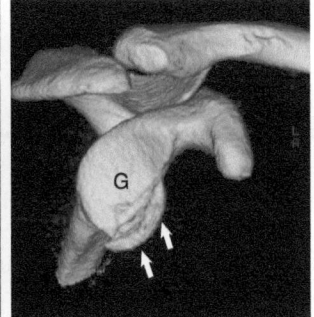

Fig. 7.29 Volume-rendered computed tomography reformats with segmentation. The entire right shoulder joint is displayed *(left)*. Using a segmentation technique *(right)*, the humeral head was removed and the image was rotated to show the glenoid *(G)* en face for better visualization of the Bankart fracture *(arrows)*.

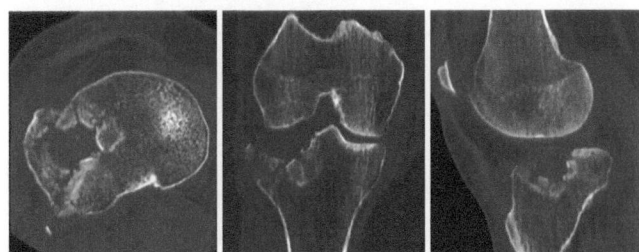

Fig. 7.31 A tibial plateau fracture. Transverse *(left)*, coronal *(middle)*, and sagittal *(right)* multiplanar reformats of the knee demonstrate a comminuted lateral tibial plateau fracture with significant depression of the articular surface.

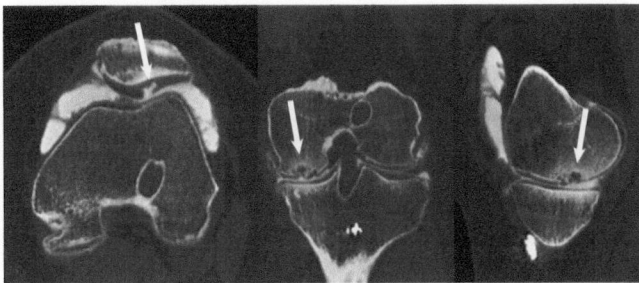

Fig. 7.30 A computed tomography (CT) arthrogram of the knee. CT images of the knee are shown after injection of iodinated contrast material. The patellofemoral cartilage is well visualized, with contrast outlining a large cartilage flap along the lateral patellar facet *(arrow)* on a transverse multiplanar reformat *(left)*. Sagittal *(right)* and coronal *(middle)* multiplanar reformats demonstrate areas of full-thickness cartilage loss along the posterior weight-bearing surface of the medial femoral condyle with subchondral sclerosis and cystic change *(arrows)*.

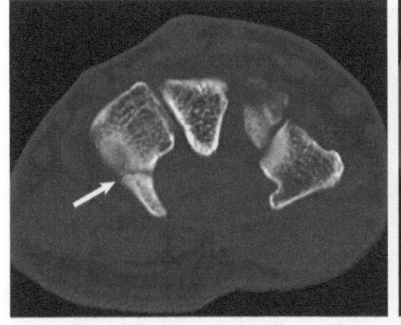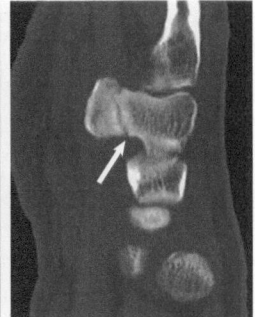

Fig. 7.32 A radiographically occult fracture of the hook of hamate on computed tomography. Transverse *(left)* and sagittal multiplanar reformat *(right)* views of the wrist demonstrate an undisplaced fracture at the base of the hook of hamate *(arrows)* that was not evident on radiographs of the wrist.

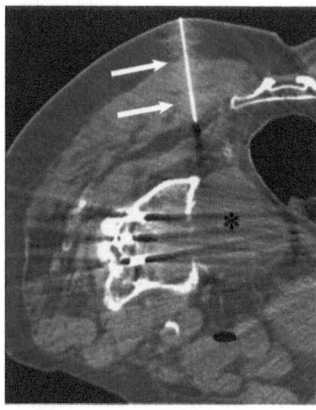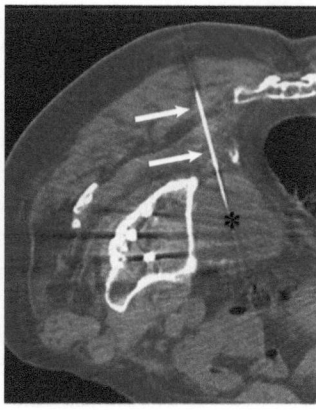

Fig. 7.33 A computed tomography–guided biopsy. Transverse images of the right hip show a large lytic lesion *(asterisk)* that has eroded through the medial aspect of the right acetabulum and extends into the right hemipelvis. A biopsy needle *(arrows)* is directed toward the lesion *(left)*. The needle was advanced into the lesion *(right)*. Aspiration revealed bloody synovial fluid related to particle disease from the right hip arthroplasty.

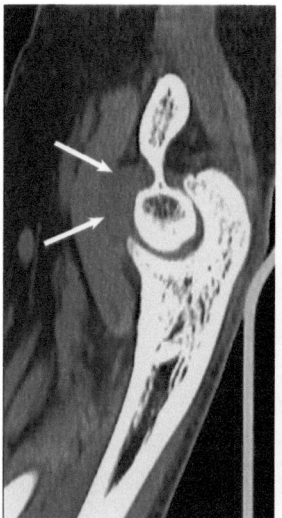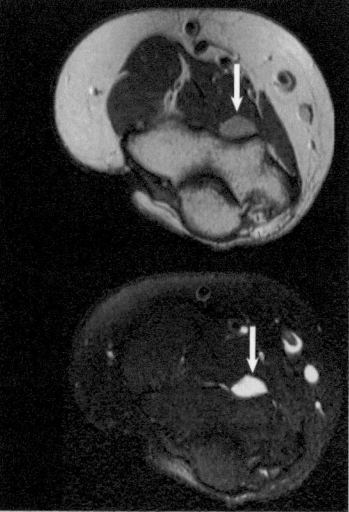

Fig. 7.34 Limited assessment of soft tissue structures with computed tomography (CT). The images are from a 24-year-old woman with a 2-year history of elbow pain. Results of the elbow CT scan, including a sagittal multiplanar reformatted CT image *(left)*, were reported as normal. In retrospect, a small mass is present anterior to the distal humerus *(arrows)* that is isodense to muscle. A transverse fast spin-echo proton density image *(top right)* shows a small, slightly hyperintense mass *(arrow)*, and a fast spin-echo T2-weighted image with fat saturation *(bottom right)* readily demonstrates a focal hyperintense soft tissue mass *(arrow)*. Pathologic findings confirmed that the lesion represented synovial sarcoma.

are not subjected to the same risks as the proximal extremities because the radiosensitive organs are outside of the field of scattered x-rays. Thus alternate imaging strategies should be considered when feasible in young patients, particularly when radiosensitive tissues are included in the scanning range.

Soft tissue contrast discrimination in CT is inferior compared with MRI, although limited assessment of larger soft tissue structures such as muscles, tendons, and some ligaments can be obtained (Fig. 7.34).

Nuclear Medicine

Nuclear medicine examinations involve the use of radioactive substances administered to patients. These studies are a common clinical tool in use since the 1950s. This modality has evolved considerably with respect to the number and variety of agents available for use and also in the development of hybrid imaging technologies, with the latter incorporating concurrent anatomic and morphologic information from CT and more recently MR. Nuclear medicine differs from other imaging modalities in that it provides information primarily related to disease processes based on cellular function and physiology, with limited inherent spatial resolution and anatomic information.

Technical Considerations

Unlike radiographs and CT examinations that depend on x-ray photons generated from a source external to the patient, nuclear medicine studies involve the administration of radioisotopes to patients. These radioisotopes then concentrate in the patient and emit gamma radiation, which is captured by an external camera. Radioisotopes are tagged to specific chemical substances (or ligands), forming radiopharmaceutical agents that target certain biologic processes in the body. Radiopharmaceutical agents are frequently administered intravenously, but they also may be given orally or subdermally, or they may be inhaled in different types of scans. Nuclear medicine provides images reflecting areas of clinical concern shown by areas of accumulation of radiotracer as a result of increased blood flow in the setting of inflammation, injury, and some neoplastic pathologies.

Planar, Single Photon Emission Computed Tomography, and Single Photon Emission Computed Tomography/ Computed Tomography Imaging

Scintigraphic images may be obtained in a planar or tomographic fashion (Fig. 7.35). In planar imaging, the images are displayed in a similar fashion as radiographs, with all data superimposed along the length of the image. Tomographic techniques, termed single photon emission computed tomography (SPECT), involve a 360-degree rotation of the gamma camera followed by multiplanar image reconstructions in the transverse, sagittal, and coronal planes similar to CT, leading to improved anatomic localization and diagnostic sensitivity.[47] SPECT images take longer to acquire than planar images, and as a result are more sensitive to patient motion.

A major advance in the field of nuclear medicine during the past decade has been the development of hybrid technology combining SPECT with CT, termed SPECT/CT, which provides even greater spatial resolution and diagnostic specificity. SPECT/ CT equipment incorporates variable resolution CT scanners, typically in the range of 4 to 16 detector units. Depending on the need for simple anatomic localization or higher resolution images for detailed morphologic assessment of the underlying pathology, the CT is programmed to adjust the radiation dose for either a low dose or standard scan, respectively (Fig. 7.36).

Bone Scans

Skeletal scintigraphic examinations, also termed *bone scans*, are an invaluable tool in the assessment of musculoskeletal conditions.

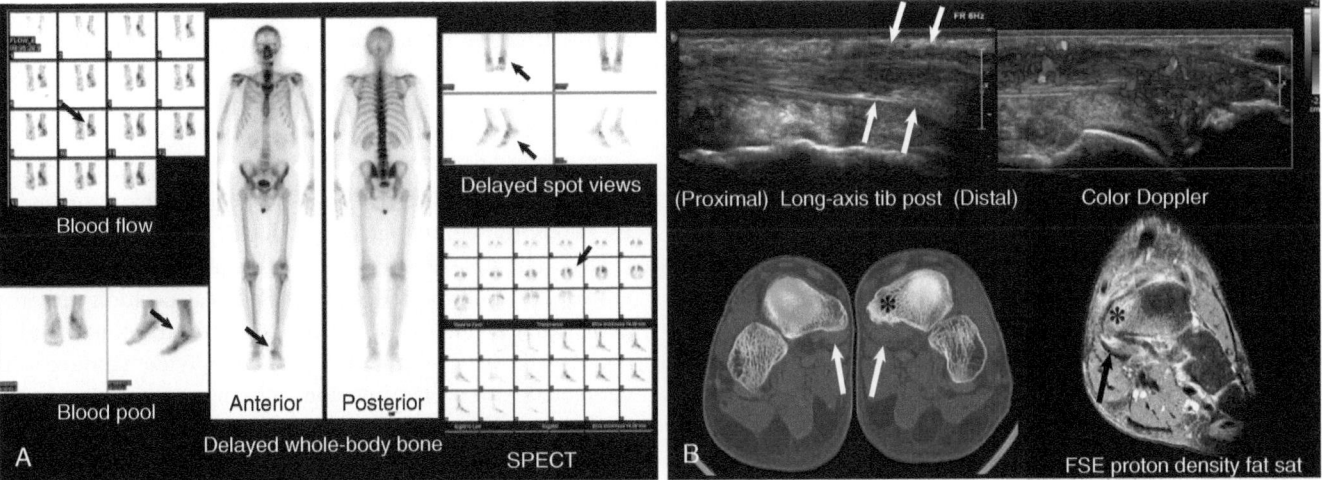

Fig. 7.35 (A) Nonspecific increased activity is shown on a bone scan image in a patient with navicular stress reaction from tibialis posterior tendinopathy. A bone scan was obtained because of clinical suspicion of a left navicular stress fracture. Radiographs (not shown) were reported as normal. Imaging including blood flow, blood pool, and whole body with spot and single photon emission computed tomography *(SPECT)* views show focal uptake in the region of the left navicular *(arrows)*. (B) Further investigation with computed tomography (CT), ultrasound, and magnetic resonance imaging (MRI) was carried out. A CT scan *(bottom left)* obtained for evaluation of a possible stress fracture after the bone scan was conducted shows mild cortical irregularity in the navicular tuberosity *(asterisk)* from tibialis posterior enthesopathy. The soft tissues show mild asymmetric thickening of the left tibialis posterior tendon *(arrows)*. A grayscale ultrasound image *(top left)* shows thickening and decreased echogenicity *(arrows)* in the distal tibialis posterior tendon *(arrows)*. A color Doppler image *(top right)* shows pronounced hyperemia. The ultrasound findings confirmed distal tibialis posterior tendinosis. An MRI image *(bottom right)* obtained after the ultrasound, CT, and bone scan were conducted shows all the findings in a single examination, including edema in the navicular tuberosity *(asterisk)* and thickening and increased signal in the distal tibialis posterior tendon *(arrow)*. MR would have established the diagnosis in the most cost-effective and efficient way if it had been performed as the initial investigation in this patient. *fat sat,* Fat saturated; *FSE,* fast spin-echo.

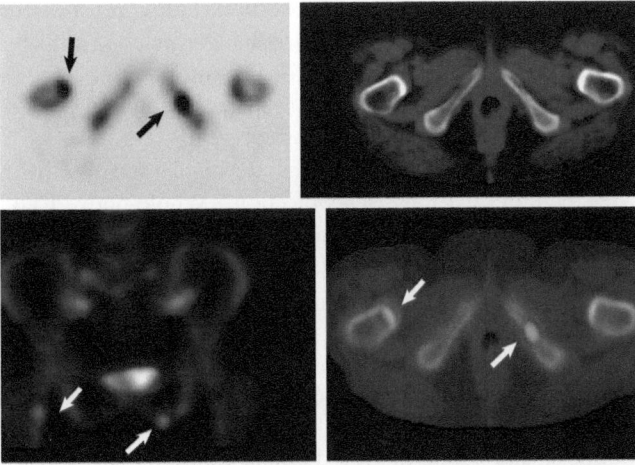

Fig. 7.36 Single photon emission computed tomography/computed tomography (SPECT/CT) images (from a 4-detector CT unit) of left ischiopubic ramus and right femoral neck fractures. A 70-year-old woman had atraumatic severe bilateral hip pain and negative radiographs (not shown). The planar anteroposterior spot view *(inverted image)* from a total body bone scan *(bottom left)* shows focal areas of uptake in the right medial femoral neck and left inferior ischiopubic ramus *(arrows)*. A transverse SPECT image *(top left)* shows focal uptake of radiotracer in the same regions *(arrows)*. A low-dose CT image from a 4-detector CT scan *(top right)* shows no obvious abnormality in the regions. The quality of the low-dose 4-slice scan is suboptimal compared with the image quality from a standard-dose 16- to 64-detector unit. A hybrid SPECT/CT image *(bottom right)* confirms the precise site of increased radiotracer uptake on the CT scan *(arrows)*.

These studies involve the intravenous administration of bone-seeking analogues of calcium, phosphate, or hydroxyl groups tagged to technetium-99. The ligands most commonly used for tagging technetium are phosphate analogues in the form of biphosphonate compounds such as methylene or hydroxymethylene diphosphonate. The biologic half-life of technetium diphosphonates is 24 hours. The radiopharmaceutical agents are incorporated into bone as hydroxyapatite crystals in inorganic matrix during the process of bone turnover.[48]

Because bone is a very dynamic tissue, incorporation of the radiotracer occurs rapidly, often 15 to 30 minutes after it is injected. However, unincorporated radiotracer within the soft tissues must be cleared systemically through the urinary tract prior to imaging to eliminate the potential for overlying artifact. Prolonged soft tissue clearance causing increased background soft tissue uptake occurs in patients with impaired renal function, potentially reducing the diagnostic quality of the examination. To facilitate clearing of the isotope from the background soft tissues, patients are instructed to drink plenty of fluids after the injection, with imaging typically performed 2 to 4 hours after the injection.

Labeled White Blood Cell Scans

Both MRI and labeled white blood cell scans are highly sensitive and specific in the diagnosis of osteomyelitis and are reported in the range of 75% to 100% and 80% to 90%, respectively.[49] The diagnosis of osteomyelitis and soft tissue infection can be established using autologous leukocytes labeled with either technetium-99m hexamethylpropylene amine oxine or indium-111 oxine.[50] White blood cell scans are generally performed in conjunction with a triple-phase bone scan to distinguish cellulitis from osteomyelitis and aid in the interpretation. When necessary, a sulfur colloid bone marrow scan also may be required as part of the investigation. The total radiation dose for this type of study is relatively high, which is related to the additive dose from the initial bone scan, the white blood cell scan, and the sulfur colloid scan when it is also is performed, although the dose from the latter scan is relatively small.

White blood cell uptake is not specific for infection and occurs in any condition associated with an inflammatory response.[51] Labeled white blood cell scans are a two-staged examination. The first component of the study takes approximately 1 to 2 hours and involves the withdrawal of blood from the patient, labeling of the white blood cells with the radioisotope, and injection of the cells back into the patient. The labeled leukocytes migrate to sites of inflammation and to areas of normal hematopoietic marrow in the axial and central appendicular skeleton. Technetium-labeled white blood cells are then imaged within 1 to 2 hours after injection, whereas indium-labeled white blood cells usually require a delay of approximately 24 hours. Spot views and SPECT reconstructions are often obtained as part of these examinations.

White blood cell scans rely on the presence of the radiolabeled functional white blood cells migrating to areas of inflammation as a result of infection. In the appropriate clinical context, an area of focally increased activity more intense than that of normal marrow activity indicates infection (Fig. 7.37). White blood cell scans are less sensitive in the assessment of chronic infections.

Gallium Scans

Gallium-67 is an isotope that behaves in a similar fashion to free iron in tissues, binding nonspecifically to rapidly dividing cells in inflammatory and neoplastic conditions. Gallium-67 can be used in the assessment of many pathologies, including sarcoidosis, neoplasms, infection, and other aseptic inflammatory conditions. The use of gallium in the evaluation of neoplastic and infectious conditions has been gradually replaced by MRI and positron emission tomography (PET), but it can be considered as a second-line investigation in instances in which the diagnosis is equivocal or the technology is not immediately accessible or is contraindicated (Fig. 7.38).[52] Similar to labeled white blood cell scans, a whole-body bone scan with spot views and SPECT tomographic reconstructions are often obtained as part of a gallium study to distinguish osteomyelitis from cellulitis and increase the accuracy of the interpretation.[53] Gallium-67 has a relatively long half-life of 78 hours, resulting in a relatively high radiation absorbed dose, which is additive to the technetium bone scan. Gallium-67 images are acquired 24 hours after injection and may require additional further delayed sequences to optimize target to nontarget soft tissue activity. For these reasons, labeled white blood cell scans are generally preferred for imaging of most inflammatory conditions because they are accurate, generate faster results, and are more convenient to use. However,

gallium-67 is much more sensitive than labeled white blood cells in the detection of infection in the spine and is the agent of choice in this regard (Fig. 7.39).[53]

Positron Emission Tomography/Computed Tomography Scans

PET is a more recent clinically available scintigraphic technique that uses a positron-emitting glucose analogue, 18F-fluorodeoxyglucose (FDG). The uptake of FDG in cells is directly proportional to glucose metabolism, which is increased in association with many pathologies, including neoplasms and infection. Because the half-life of FDG is 110 minutes, it is technically demanding to use compared with technetium and gallium.

Because FDG uptake is nonspecific, occurring in both normal physiologic and pathologic conditions, this technique is used in combination with CT to improve the accuracy of the examination. The PET and CT scanners function separately but often are housed together within a cover, creating the illusion of a single machine (Fig. 7.40). CT and PET images are obtained from the top of the patient's head to the knees. Multiplanar and maximum intensity projection reconstructions are performed from both the extended CT and PET data sets, generating thousands of images. The images are fused using computer software, providing both anatomic and physiologic data (see Fig. 7.38).[54]

Advantages

Bone scans are highly sensitive for osseous pathology. Uptake of radiotracer is related to increased bone turnover due to reparative change that can result from a number of entities, including trauma, infection, neoplasm, and arthritis. Bone scintigraphy has a high negative predictive value in excluding most osseous conditions. In addition, the entire skeleton is included in a single study, providing a rapid survey for polyostotic disease seen in association with conditions such as metastases, Langerhans cell histiocytosis, Paget disease, and osteomyelitis (Fig. 7.41).[55]

Labeled white blood cell scans are highly accurate in the assessment of musculoskeletal infection.[56] Whole-body PET/CT scans are highly sensitive to many neoplastic pathologies and are valuable in the diagnosis, staging, and follow-up assessment of tumors.

Disadvantages

The inherent specificity of skeletal scintigraphy is relatively low. Benign and malignant tumors, fractures, and inflammatory conditions all show focal increased uptake of radiopharmaceutical agents and can be difficult to differentiate without additional imaging modalities, even with the use of SPECT/CT. In the past decade, the use of scintigraphy for the evaluation of suspected local bone pathology has been increasingly replaced by CT and MR imaging. MRI in particular has relatively equivalent high sensitivity compared with bone scintigraphy but provides greater diagnostic specificity and anatomic detail.

Although bone scans are generally highly sensitive, false-negative scans can occasionally occur. Acute fractures may not manifest in elderly patients with osteoporosis because of generalized reduced bone turnover and may show diminished and delayed uptake at the site of a fracture, sometimes more than 72 hours

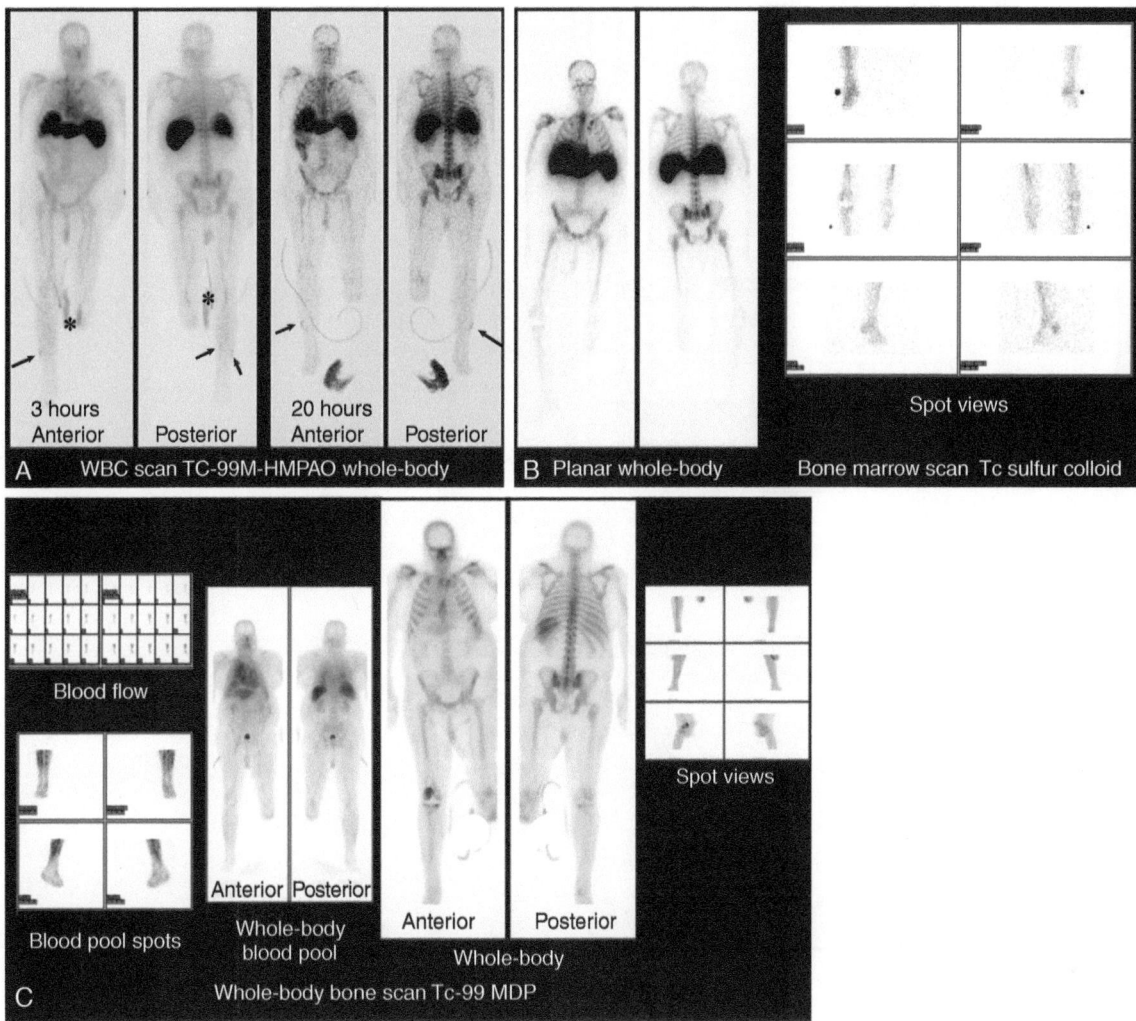

Fig. 7.37 (A) A labeled white blood cell scan to check for osteomyelitis in a 69-year-old patient with brittle diabetes who had cutaneous ulcers in the right lower extremity. The patient had a history of left below-knee amputation and failed right knee arthroplasty. A technetium-99m hexamethylpropylene amine oxine *(Tc-99m-HMPAO)* labeled whole-body white blood cell *(WBC)* scan shows two small superficial areas of faint uptake corresponding to the site of the ulcers on both the 3-hour *(left)* and 20-hour *(right)* scans *(arrows)*. No focal increased uptake of tracer is evident in the bone marrow to suggest osteomyelitis. Normal uptake of tracer is evident in the liver and spleen. A small amount of uptake is evident in the medial aspect of the left knee on the 3-hour scan corresponding to contamination from the urine *(asterisk)*. (B) A technetium *(Tc)* sulfur colloid bone marrow scan to check for osteomyelitis. The sulfur colloid study was performed in conjunction with the labeled WBC scan in the same patient as in A. The bone marrow scan shows a similar concordant distribution in both the whole-body *(left)* and spot views *(right)* compared with the WBC scan. The absence of increased WBC uptake relative to the bone marrow scan makes the diagnosis of osteomyelitis unlikely. The soft tissue uptake on the WBC scan most likely reflects cellulitis rather than osteomyelitis. Sulfur colloid scans may be required as part of a labeled WBC scan to provide a map of the normal regional variations in the distribution of bone marrow. (C) A bone scan to check for osteomyelitis. A technetium-99 methylene diphosphonate *(MDP)* skeletal scintigram in the same patient as in A and B was performed as part of a WBC scan for possible osteomyelitis in the left leg. Blood flow, blood pool, and delayed whole-body images show no increased activity in the right lower extremity, ruling out the diagnosis of osteomyelitis. Increased activity present in the right knee is related to patellofemoral osteoarthritis and recent removal of an arthroplasty prosthesis.

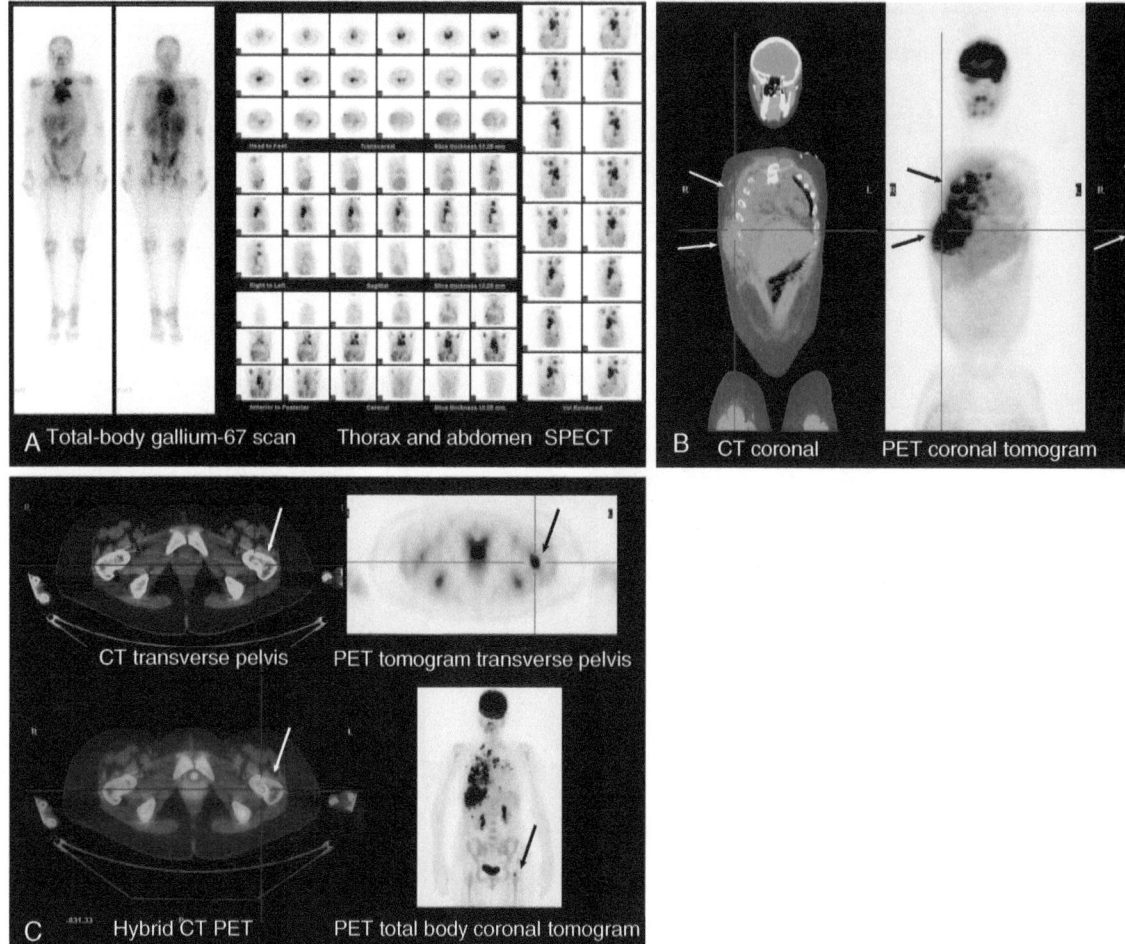

Fig. 7.38 (A) A gallium scan for tumor surveillance in a 17-year-old with relapse of Hodgkin lymphoma. Total-body *(left)* and single-photon emission computed tomography *(SPECT)* images through the thorax and abdomen in the transverse *(top center)*, sagittal *(middle center)*, and coronal *(lower center)* planes are shown (additional SPECT tomographic views were obtained but are not included in the figure). Volume-rendered maximum intensity projectional rotational projections *(right)* are also included. Focal areas of gallium uptake are present in the supraclavicular, perihilar, central mediastinum, and right paratracheal regions, confirming extensive recurrent lymphoma. (B) A positron emission tomography *(PET)* scan for tumor surveillance in the same patient. Multiplanar coronal reconstruction from a 16-slice multidetector computed tomography (CT) scan *(left)* shows a soft tissue mass in the right anterolateral chest wall and right lung *(arrows)*. A coronal whole-body PET tomogram *(middle)* in the same plane as the CT scan shows that the right chest wall mass and lung lesions are 18F-fluorodeoxyglucose (FDG) avid *(arrows)*, corresponding to recurrent lymphoma. A hybrid-fused coronal PET/CT image *(right)* shows that the FDG uptake corresponds precisely to the soft tissues on CT, facilitating precise anatomic localization and characterization. (C) CT/PET of a femoral lesion. An additional FDG-avid focus is present in the left femoral neck *(arrows)* on the PET axial and coronal body tomograms *(top and bottom right)*. A small sclerotic focus is present on the transverse image from the pelvic CT *(top left)* in the same area *(arrows)*. The hybrid image *(bottom left)* confirms that the two abnormalities correspond to a focus of recurrent lymphoma *(arrow)*.

after a trauma is sustained (Fig. 7.42A and B).[57] False-negative bone scans occur in 2% of patients with osseous metastases and have a greater propensity to occur in patients with multiple myeloma, renal cell carcinoma, thyroid carcinoma, neuroblastoma, and reticulum cell sarcoma.[20] In addition, pathology located near the epiphyseal plates in skeletally immature patients may be obscured by the increased uptake normally present in the physis.

Isotopes are often excreted via the urinary tract when scintigraphy is performed, with accumulation in the urinary bladder prior to voiding. This situation results in a radiation dose to the gonads regardless of the site of clinical concern.

Magnetic Resonance Imaging

MRI has revolutionized musculoskeletal imaging since its introduction as a clinical tool in 1977. Lauterbur and Mansfield received a Nobel Prize in 2003 for their contributions to the development of MRI. The technology plays an important role in the investigation of sports-related injuries and many other musculoskeletal

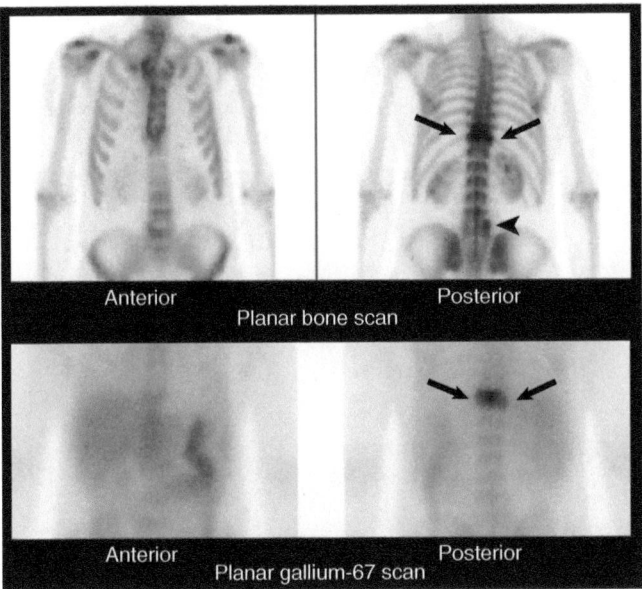

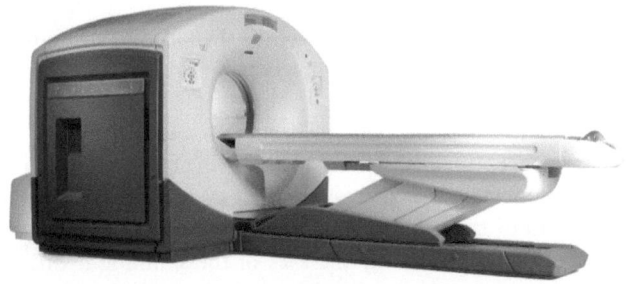

Fig. 7.39 A gallium scan for diskitis. A planar bone scan in the anterior and posterior projections *(upper images)* demonstrates focal uptake in the region of the T10-T11 vertebral interspace *(arrows)*. Mild focal uptake in the region of the right L4/L5 posterior elements *(arrowhead)* is likely secondary to L4/L5 right facet joint arthropathy. Gallium-67 planar images in the anterior and posterior projections *(lower images)* demonstrate intense uptake in the region of the T10-T11 vertebral interspace *(arrows)*, consistent with T10-T11 diskitis. (Courtesy Mark Bryanton.)

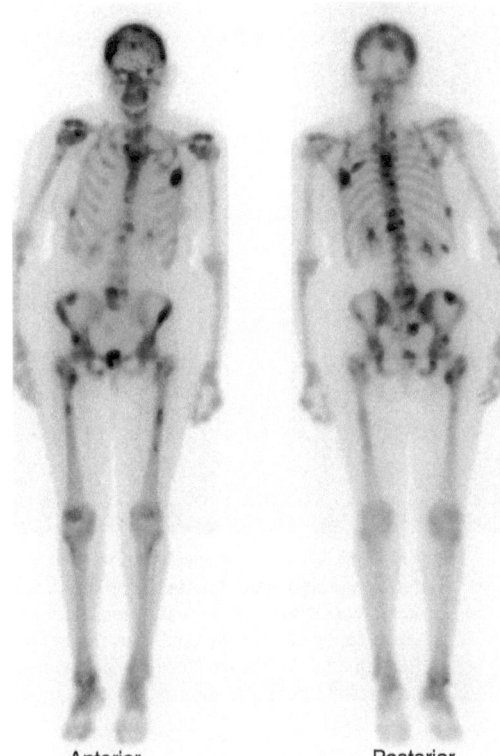

Anterior   Posterior

Fig. 7.41 A total body bone scan of a woman with metastatic breast carcinoma. Anterior and posterior whole-body skeletal scintigraphic images demonstrate multiple areas of abnormal radiotracer accumulation in the axial and proximal appendicular skeleton in a pattern consistent with extensive osseous metastatic disease.

Fig. 7.40 The General Electric Discovery positron emission tomography/computed tomography (PET/CT) 690 System. Both the CT and PET scanners are housed together in a single piece of equipment. (Courtesy General Electric, Milwaukee, WI; used with permission.)

pathologies. Ongoing developments in the hardware and software associated with this modality have occurred during the past three decades, including the more recent introduction of clinical high-field–strength magnets, leading to substantial improvement in image quality and reduction in scan times.

Technical Considerations

Imaging protocols. MR examinations are interpreted by synthesizing data from several image series. Each series is composed of a pulse sequence (e.g., spin echo, gradient echo, or inversion recovery [IR]), typically with T1, proton density, or T2 weighting (described later) in the sagittal, coronal, transverse, or oblique plane, resulting in multiple adjacent images. Fat saturation, 3D imaging, and use of gadolinium are options that can be added

to some pulse sequences (see the section on pulse sequences). The collection of image series comprises the MR protocol. For example, to assess for internal derangement of the knee, the protocol might consist of the following series: coronal spin-echo T1, coronal and sagittal spin-echo proton density with fat saturation, oblique sagittal fast spin-echo T2, and axial fast spin-echo proton density (Fig. 7.43). Unlike other cross-sectional imaging modalities such as CT, where essentially identical standardized imaging is routinely carried out at different institutions, MR protocols consist of a variety of imaging planes and pulse sequences that take advantage of an institution's particular MR hardware and software and, often to a greater extent, reflect the individual preferences of the physician responsible for the scan. However, routine protocols are usually consistent for a given clinical indication within an institution.

Moreover, different manufacturers have developed a huge number of minor proprietary variations on the basic MR pulse sequences, resulting in an explosion of vendor-specific nomenclature and acronyms. The vendor-specific variations on pulse sequences and corresponding acronyms, together with differing institutional and individual MR protocols, contribute to a great deal of confusion among clinicians who are attempting to understand MRI. A good strategy for physicians who wish to comprehend what they are looking at is to gain an understanding of the common pulse sequences for standard protocols used at their own institutions.

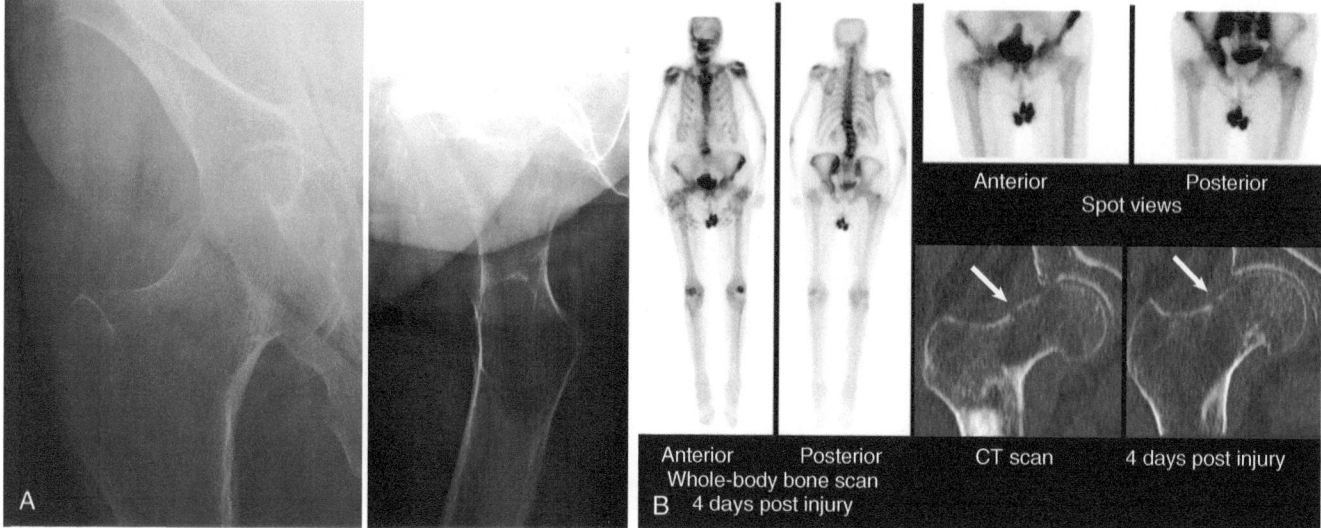

Fig. 7.42 (A) A false-negative bone scan in an 85-year-old with a radiographically occult fracture of the right femur. Angled anteroposterior and lateral radiographs of the right hip show no convincing fracture. (B) Scintigraphy performed 4 days after the trauma including whole-body *(left)* and spot views of the pelvis *(top right)* were reported as mild uptake in the right intertrochanteric region without definite fracture. A computed tomography *(CT)* scan *(bottom right)* obtained the same day as the bone scan confirms an undisplaced subcapital fracture of the right femur *(arrows).*

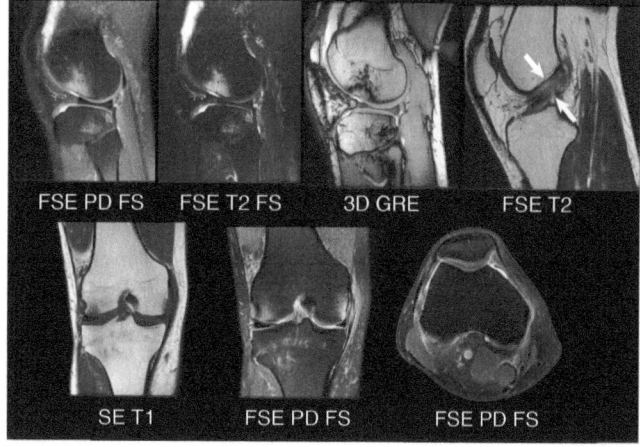

Fig. 7.43 Standard knee protocol for internal derangement. The protocol includes a sagittal fast spin-echo proton density scan and T2-weighted scan with fat saturation *(FSE PD FS and FSE T2 FS,* respectively), sagittal three-dimensional gradient echo *(3D GRE),* oblique sagittal fast spin-echo T2 along the plane of the anterior cruciate ligament *(FSE T2),* coronal spin-echo T1 *(SE T1),* coronal and axial fast spin-echo proton density with fat saturation *(FSE PD FS).* Each image plane and sequence contributes to the overall assessment. Specific protocols typically vary among institutions. A complete midsubstance tear of the anterior cruciate ligament *(arrow),* medial and lateral compartment bone contusions, a grade 2 tear of the medial collateral ligament, and discoid lateral meniscus is evident.

Image formation. The physics of MR image production is extremely complex and beyond the scope of this chapter. The background fundamental principles associated with MRI are reviewed in this section in an effort to aid clinicians in their understanding of the common terminology used in association with this modality.[58–60]

MRI involves the manipulation of hydrogen protons in the form of water that is abundant within the body, composing approximately 98% of human tissue. MRI is based on the electromagnetic activity of atomic nuclei that have an odd number of protons and neutrons. The odd number of particles results in an imbalance, causing the nucleus to spin on its own axis. The spinning hydrogen protons cause a small magnetic vector to develop along the axis of the spin, similar to a tiny bar magnet. In the presence of a strong external magnetic field, the interaction between the external magnetic field and the magnetic field of the proton causes the proton to wobble or precess at a frequency directly related to the strength of the external magnetic field, termed the *resonant frequency*. While precessing, the axes of the spinning hydrogen protons are randomly distributed across the magnetic field. In the presence of a strong external magnetic field, the protons align with the applied external magnetic field, creating a net magnetic vector directed along the axis of the external magnetic field.

Energy in the form of a radio wave at resonant frequency, termed a *radiofrequency excitation pulse*, is then temporarily applied to the area of interest, exciting some of the hydrogen protons to a higher energy level and simultaneously changing the direction of the proton's net magnetic vector away from the direction of the external magnetic field. The extent to which the direction of the magnetic vector of the excited protons is reoriented is termed the *flip angle*. The duration and amplitude of the radiofrequency pulse serves to control the flip angle. With a 90-degree flip angle, the net longitudinal magnetic vector is reoriented away from the external magnetic field 90 degrees into the transverse plane. Concurrent with the change in the direction of the proton's net longitudinal magnetic vector, the radiofrequency excitation pulse simultaneously causes the hydrogen protons to precess in unison, resulting in a net transverse component of the magnetic vector.

After the radio wave is turned off, the excited hydrogen protons undergo relaxation back to their original lower energy level. In the process of relaxation, the transverse magnetization precesses around a receiver coil and induces a current in the coil that is used to form a signal to create an image. For the maximum signal to be measured during the process of relaxation, of the protons must be rephased temporarily to synchronize the transverse magnetization vector using another 180-degree refocusing radiofrequency pulse, or magnetic gradient, termed a *gradient refocusing pulse.*

Tissue contrast: T1, T2, and proton density. The relaxation process of the protons can be broken down into two independent components that occur simultaneously. The longitudinal component of the relaxation process is termed *T1 relaxation* (or *spin lattice relaxation*), which is defined as the time for 63% of the hydrogen protons to return to their original resting state, as reflected by restoration of a substantial component of the net magnetic vector realigned with the external magnetic field. The transverse component of the relaxation process, termed *T2 relaxation* (or *spin-spin relaxation*), reflects the gradual loss of the synchronous spinning, or *dephasing,* of the protons back to their original random distribution. T2 relaxation time is defined as the amount of time it takes for 63% of the protons to return to their original random distribution of spins.[61]

The process of exciting hydrogen protons and allowing them to relax is repeated many, many times to obtain a single MR image. The time between successive radiofrequency excitation pulses is termed the *repetition time,* abbreviated as TR. The time between the radiofrequency excitation pulse and the detection of the radiofrequency wave emitted by the protons returning to their lower energy state is termed the *echo time,* abbreviated as TE.

The exact molecular environment of the hydrogen protons in water is related to the unique composition of healthy and pathologic tissues, which affect the MR signal generated during the relaxation process and the subsequent appearance of the images. The TR and TE can be adjusted to produce an image with contrast emphasizing either T1 or T2 relaxation or the number of hydrogen protons, the latter termed a *proton density* or a *balanced image* (neither T1 nor T2 weighted).[62]

An image that emphasizes tissue contrast related to T1 relaxation has a short TR and TE and is referred to as being *T1 weighted.* T1-weighted images can be recognized by the low to intermediate (dark to dark gray) signal intensity of water, high (white) signal intensity of fat, and intermediate (gray) signal intensity of muscle. Structures that contain very few mobile protons, such as cortical bone, tendons, and fibrous tissue, are manifested as low (dark) signal intensity on T1-, T2-, and proton density–weighted sequences. Although T1-weighted pulse sequences yield excellent anatomic detail, they are less sensitive to pathology. Pathology is often obscured on T1-weighted sequences because it is similar in signal intensity, *isointense,* to muscle (Fig. 7.44). T1-weighted fat-saturated sequences (see the later description of fat saturation) are used to maximize the effect of gadolinium contrast and typically show relatively low signal intensity of fat, muscle, and bone, with pathology frequently showing contrast enhancement manifested by high signal intensity.

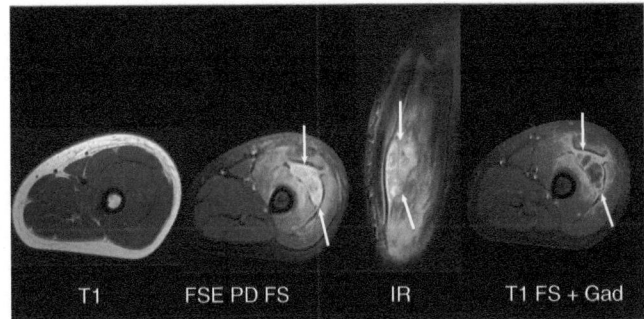

Fig. 7.44 A T1-weighted spin-echo sequence of an isointense lesion. A 7-year-old patient has an intramuscular abscess. An abscess and adjacent intramuscular inflammatory change in the quadriceps muscles is barely perceptible on the transverse T1-weighted spin-echo sequence *(left image).* On the axial fast spin-echo proton density with fat saturation *(FSD PD FS)* image *(center left),* which is at the same level as the T1-weighted image and sagittal inversion recovery *(IR; center right)* image, the pathology becomes very conspicuous, showing extensive edema in the quadriceps muscle. An area of slightly higher T2-weighted signal is present centrally, corresponding to loculated fluid in an abscess *(arrows).* On the fat-saturated postgadolinium spin-echo T1-weighted sequence *(T1 FS + Gad; right image),* the abscess shows rim enhancement *(arrows).* A moderate amount of enhancement is present in the quadriceps muscles surrounding the abscess.

An image that emphasizes tissue contrast related to T2 relaxation has a long TR and long TE and is referred to as being *T2 weighted.* Fatty tissue has intermediate signal intensity (i.e., it is light gray) on spin-echo T2-weighted sequences. Because both the background fat and pathology have a relatively high signal intensity, pathology can be difficult to appreciate. Therefore fat saturation is often applied as on option in a T2 sequence, which serves to darken the signal from fat and increases the conspicuity of high signal pathology (Fig. 7.45).

An image emphasizing tissue contrast related to the total number of hydrogen protons has a long TR and short TE and is termed *proton density–weighted.* On proton density–weighted images, fat tissue has a high (white) signal intensity and muscle and water have an intermediate (gray) signal intensity. Proton density images provide a good balance of contrast and signal to noise compared with T1- and T2-weighted sequences and are commonly used in the assessment of internal derangement of joints. However, because both pathology and fat are bright, proton density sequences are less sensitive to marrow and soft tissue pathology than are T1- and T2-weighted sequences. Proton density images are often obtained with fat saturation to null the signal from fat and increase the conspicuity of high signal pathology (see Fig. 7.45). Table 7.1 summarizes the appearance of musculoskeletal structures on T1-, T2-, and proton density–weighted sequences.

Pulse sequences. Technical adjustments that can be made during the manipulation of the hydrogen protons produce variations in the appearance of the MR images. The combination of specific technical parameters used to manipulate the protons a certain way is termed a *pulse sequence.* The adjustments can affect a number of factors, including image contrast, spatial resolution, signal to noise, or speed of image acquisition. Three

TABLE 7.1   Appearance of Musculoskeletal Structures on T1-Weighted, Proton Density, and T2-Weighted Sequences

	TR (ms)	TE (ms)	Water Signal	Fat Signal	Muscle Signal	Cortical Bone/ Fibrous Tissue Signal	Optimal Assessment
T1	Short (<500)	Short (<30)	Low to intermediate	High	Intermediate	Low	Anatomy
T2 proton	Long (>1000)	Long (>70)	High	Intermediate	Intermediate	Low	Pathology
density	Long (>1000)	Short (<30)	Intermediate	High	Intermediate	Low	Anatomy + pathology

TE, Echo time; *TR*, repetition time.

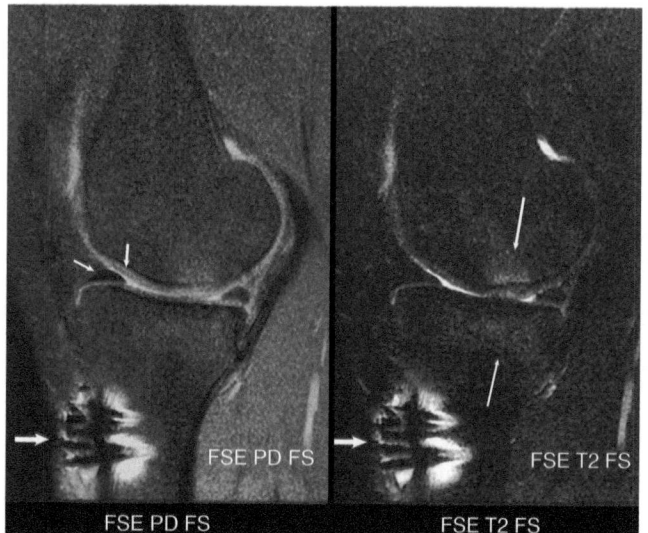

Fig. 7.45 A fast spin-echo proton density with fat saturation *(FSE PD FS)* image compared with a fast spin-echo T2 with fat saturation *(FSE T2 FS)* image. The proton density fat-saturated image *(left)* has slightly greater latitude and shows better detail in the meniscus and articular cartilage *(short arrows)* and overall poor signal to noise *(grainy appearance)*, although it is better than on the T2-weighted image. The T2-weighted image *(right)* has a narrower range of contrast, with the marrow edema in the medial tibial plateau and femoral condyle being slightly more conspicuous. The fat saturation is adversely affected by the indwelling tibial staples with artifact at the site of the staples *(block arrow)*.

basic types of pulse sequences are predominantly used in musculo-skeletal MRI: spin echo, gradient echo, and IR.[59]

Spin echo. A conventional spin-echo sequence is the most basic pulse sequence and is included in virtually all musculoskeletal imaging protocols. It begins with a radiofrequency excitation pulse applied to hydrogen protons, resulting in rotation of the net longitudinal magnetization 90 degrees into the transverse plane. The initial 90-degree pulse is followed by a 180-degree radiofrequency refocusing pulse that manipulates the transverse vector of the relaxing protons to produce an echo, or signal, detected by a coil. Spin-echo sequences can be T1-, T2-, or proton density weighted. T1-weighted spin-echo pulse sequences have a short TR of around 500 ms and a short TE that is less than 30 ms.

T2-weighted spin-echo sequences are characterized by a long TR of around 2000 ms and a long TE of around 70 ms. Because of the long TR, T2-weighted spin-echo sequences take more time to acquire compared with T1-weighted images. The longer

echo times in T2-weighted sequences results in a relative reduction in overall signal compared with a T1-weighted sequence, which is manifested by a grainy appearance and overall reduced quality of the images, referred to as a poor signal-to-noise ratio. Increased extracellular water associated with most pathologic processes is characterized by prolonged T2 relaxation, and as a result, fluid usually appears with a high (white) signal intensity (i.e., it is hyperintense) on T2-weighted images. Consequently, T2-weighted images are optimal for demonstrating pathology.

Proton density–weighted spin-echo images have a short TE that is less than 30 ms and a long TR of around 2000 ms. MRI technology is continuously advancing, and faster spin-echo pulse sequences have been developed, reducing acquisition times for imaging and the potential for motion artifact. The most common version of the faster sequences is termed *fast spin-echo* and uses multiple radiofrequency refocusing pulses, termed an *echo train*. Fast spin-echo has largely replaced conventional spin-echo sequences (Fig. 7.46).

Gradient echo. Gradient echo sequences are used selectively in musculoskeletal imaging protocols. These sequences differ from spin-echo sequences in that the flip angle induced by the radiofrequency excitation pulse is always less than 90 degrees. The other major difference is that a magnetic gradient is used to rephase the spinning protons to form an echo instead of the 180-degree radiofrequency refocusing pulse used in spin-echo sequences. Gradient echo sequences often have much shorter TR and TE values compared with spin-echo sequences, enabling faster image acquisition. The use of a magnetic gradient instead of a 180-degree refocusing radiofrequency pulse in gradient echo images can result in magnetic susceptibility, or blooming artifact.[63] This artifact results from local magnetic field inhomogeneity at the interface of any two substances with different magnetic susceptibilities (e.g., water/fat, calcium/soft tissue, and metal/soft tissue) and produces focal areas of prominent low signal intensity on an image. The amount of artifact is related to the quantity of indwelling metal or calcium and is more pronounced with metal. This artifact can be used to aid in the detection of intraarticular bodies, hemosiderin, or subtle matrix mineralization in bone lesions (Fig. 7.47). However, susceptibility artifact can be detrimental to image quality in patients with indwelling metallic hardware because structures adjacent to the hardware are obscured (Fig. 7.48). Gradient echo sequences are less sensitive to marrow pathology because susceptibility artifacts due to calcium in trabecular bone can override and obscure increased

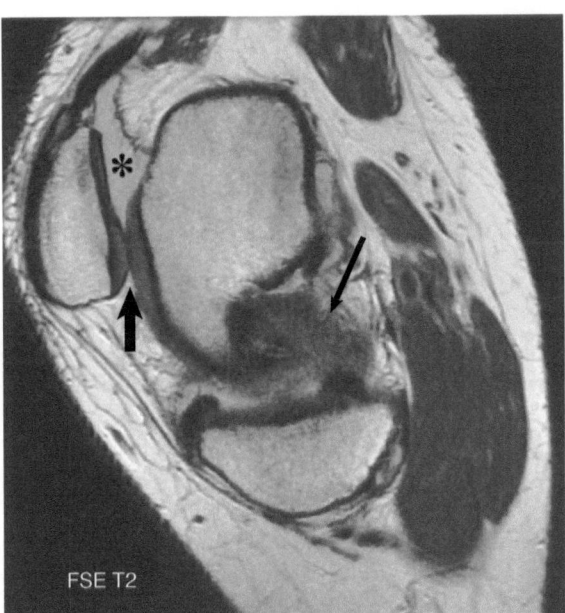

Fig. 7.46 A fast spin-echo T2 *(FSE T2)* sequence without fat saturation. Without the addition of fat saturation, the image appears similar to a T1-weighted sequence because of the bright white signal from subcutaneous and marrow fat. On T2-weighted sequences, the joint fluid in the suprapatellar bursa *(asterisk)* typically appears bright, unlike the signal of fluid on a T1-weighted image, which typically has low to intermediate signal intensity. The patellofemoral articular cartilage *(thick arrow)* also has intermediate signal intensity that is slightly higher than the normal low to intermediate signal intensity on spin-echo T1-weighted images. A tear of the posterior cruciate ligament is evident *(thin arrow)*, manifested by diffuse thickening and increased signal intensity.

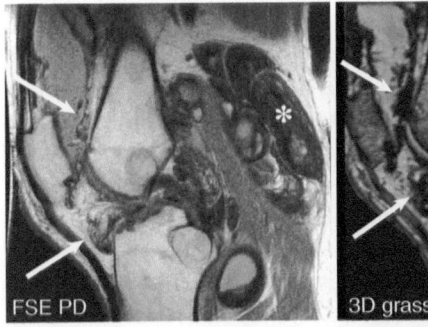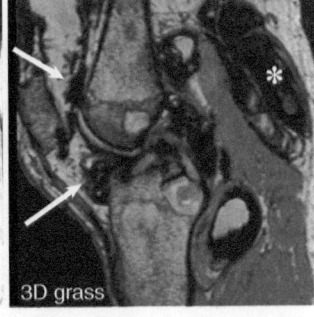

Fig. 7.47 Magnetic susceptibility artifact on gradient echo sequences is depicted. The patient has pigmented villonodular synovitis of the knee. A sagittal fast spin-echo proton density image *(FSE PD; left)* and sagittal three-dimensional gradient echo recalled in the steady-state image *(3D grass; right)* of the knee are shown. On the proton density image, prominent low signal intensity is distributed throughout the synovium and is most marked in a Baker's cyst in the popliteal fossa *(asterisk)*. On the 3D grass sequence, more pronounced darkening of the synovial signal is present, in keeping with magnetic susceptibility artifact. The artifact is more pronounced in areas where only a small amount of hemosiderin deposition is evident on the FSE PD sequence, in the suprapatellar bursa, and anterior aspect of the femoral-tibial joint *(arrows)*.

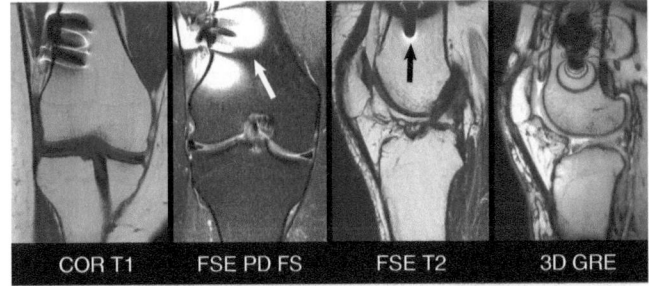

Fig. 7.48 Magnetic susceptibility artifact from indwelling metal hardware. Two metal staples present in the distal femur are related to a previous ACL reconstruction. On the coronal spin-echo T1-weighted image *(COR T1; left)*, low signal intensity from a femoral staple is mildly accentuated. On the fast spin-echo proton density with fat saturation *(FSE PD FS)* image *(center left image)*, the magnetic field is distorted, causing inhomogeneity in the appearance of the structures *(arrow)*. The fast spin-echo T2-weighted *(FSE T2)* image *(center right image)* shows a similar appearance as the spin-echo T1-weighted image with slight blooming artifact *(arrow)*. On the three-dimensional gradient echo *(3D GRE)* image *(right image)*, the artifact is much more pronounced.

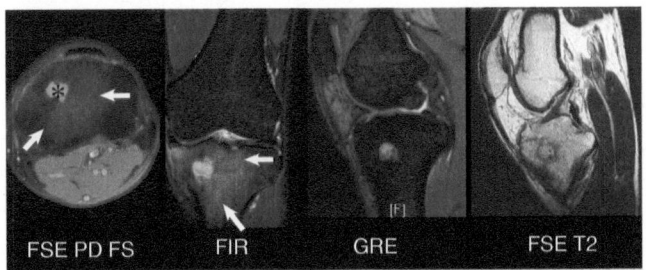

Fig. 7.49 Susceptibility artifact on a gradient echo sequence masking bone marrow edema. Transverse fast spin-echo proton density-weighted with fat saturation *(FSE PD FS; left)*, coronal fast inversion recovery *(FIR; center left)*, sagittal T2-weighted gradient echo *(GRE; center right)*, and oblique sagittal fast spin-echo T2-weighted *(FSE T2; right)* images are shown. Bone marrow edema from osteomyelitis is only seen on the FSE PD FS and FIR images *(arrows)* surrounding an intraosseous abscess *(asterisk)*. On the GRE image, a susceptibility artifact from trabecular bone obscures the edema. On the FSE T2 image without fat saturation, the marrow fat and edema are isointense, limiting visualization of the edema.

bone marrow signal associated with traumatic, infectious, or neoplastic pathology. Thus gradient echo sequences should always be combined with at least one spin-echo proton or T2 fat-saturated sequence (Fig. 7.49).

Inversion recovery. IR sequences are commonly used in musculoskeletal imaging. This pulse sequence is highly sensitive to the presence of increased free water associated with most pathology and is complementary to spin-echo sequences. IR pulse sequences begin with an excitation radiofrequency pulse that inverts the net magnetic vector of the protons 180 degrees from their original state aligned with the external magnetic field. The resultant 180-degree inversion of the protons is then followed by a second 90-degree radiofrequency pulse that reoriented the protons into the transverse plane after a specified time, termed the *inversion time*. Depending on what inversion time is programmed into the sequence, the signal from protons in certain tissues can be eliminated, which is termed *suppression* or *nulling*. This technique is commonly used to null signal that arises from fat. This latter form of IR sequence is termed *short tau inversion recovery* (STIR). The black background signal created by the nulled signal from fat increases the conspicuity of water associated with pathologic entities (see Figs. 7.44 and 7.49). The technique of eliminating signal from fat in an IR pulse sequence is more robust than the frequency selective fat saturation (see the section on fat saturation) used in spin-echo sequences and is particularly useful when imaging at the periphery of the bore of the magnet, as in the elbow or arm, where magnetic field inhomogeneity is problematic. Most IR sequences are currently modified to include fast spin-echo techniques using multiple 180-degree refocusing pulses to speed up acquisition time, commonly termed fast spin-echo inversion recovery.

Although IR sequences have excellent contrast discrimination between normal and pathologic tissue, the general quality of the images is often poorer compared with that of spin-echo sequences because of reduction in overall signal and motion artifact. Correlation with a similarly acquired T1 or proton density spin-echo sequence is often necessary to confirm the anatomic location and clarify the nature of the pathology that is evident on the IR images.

2D and 3D acquisitions. All pulse sequences can be T1, T2, or proton density weighted. Images are routinely acquired in a two-dimensional (2D) or individual sequential slice excitation mode. Some pulse sequences have the option for a 3D mode corresponding to a slab or "*volume*" excitation, in which the entire area to be imaged is excited and subsequently encoded into individual slices.[64] 3D sequences usually provide thinner slices with robust signal to noise compared with 2D acquisitions but require longer imaging times, increasing the potential for motion artifact and prolonged scan times. The thin slices obtained with 3D sequences provide the ability to generate a data set with isotropic voxels, potentially allowing reformatting in any plane while maintaining spatial resolution. This latter technique is routinely used in multidetector CT imaging. The high resolution of 3D imaging is most advantageous in the evaluation of articular cartilage. For many years, 3D sequences were only available with gradient echo pulse sequences; however, more recently a 3D option has become available with fast spin-echo (Fig. 7.50).

Fat suppression. Fat suppression is a common technique used in conjunction with pulse sequences to eliminate or null the bright signal from fat to make pathology more conspicuous. Fat suppression can be achieved with two different methods, including the STIR pulse sequence (previously described) and *frequency selective fat saturation.*[59]

Frequency selective fat saturation is a technique often added to spin-echo sequences in which a preliminary 90-degree radio-frequency excitation pulse matching the resonant frequency of protons in lipids excites the protons in fat, followed by a dephasing magnetic gradient to null their signal. Fat saturation is often applied to T2 fast spin-echo sequences because fat is typically bright on these sequences and the bright T2 signal of increased water associated with pathologic conditions may be more difficult to appreciate. The use of frequency selective fat saturation creates an image similar to a STIR image, but it generally has better signal to noise and anatomic resolution than a STIR image. Frequency-selective fat saturation is also commonly used with

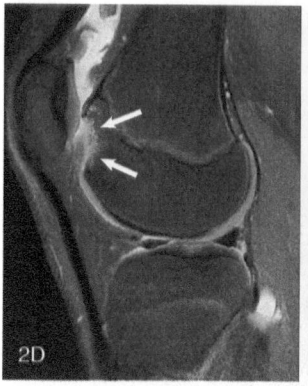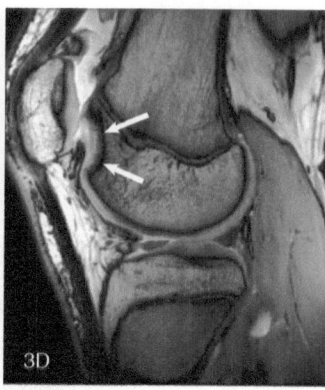

Fig. 7.50 A three-dimensional *(3D)* compared with a two-dimensional *(2D)* pulse sequence. 3D sequences enable thinner slices and have more robust signal to noise compared with 2D sequences. A 3D gradient echo COSMIC (Coherent Oscillatory State Acquisition for the Manipulation of Imaging Contrast) sequence *(right image)* obtained with 2.0 mm thick slices has excellent signal to noise compared with 4.0 mm thick slices from a 2D fast spin-echo with fat saturation sequence *(left image)*. A large area of osteochondritis dissecans *(arrows)* is evident in the femoral trochlea in a 15-year-old patient.

T1-weighted spin-echo sequences in conjunction with intravenous or intraarticular administration of a contrast agent (gadolinium; see Fig. 7.44). Fat-saturated gadolinium-enhanced T1-weighted images do not suppress the signal from gadolinium contrast because gadolinium is typically the only bright signal visible on the subsequent images (see Fig. 7.44).

Frequency selective fat saturation techniques do not always provide as uniform a level of fat suppression compared with *STIR* images because of the nature of the technique. Specifically, inherent local magnetic field variations slightly alter the resonant frequency of the precessing lipid protons, making uniform fat suppression with this technique less precise. Magnetic field inhomogeneity is more prominent in the periphery of the magnet and has the greatest impact on upper extremity imaging, including the shoulder and elbow joints (Fig. 7.51). In these anatomic locations, a STIR sequence is often a better choice instead of a spin-echo T2-weighted image with fat saturation. Although T2-weighted fast spin-echo fat-saturated images increase the conspicuity of soft tissue and marrow edema, the effect is typically less compared with *STIR* images. The elimination of fat signal from the images with either spin-echo or IR sequences leads to an overall reduction in the signal to noise and an image that generally is of inferior quality but nonetheless is diagnostic.

Magnetic resonance artifacts. Many artifacts are related to MR imaging. Common artifacts include motion, magnetic susceptibility (see the section on "Gradient Echo"), inhomogeneous fat saturation (see the section on "Fat Suppression"), and magic angle artifact. Magic angle artifact occurs in tendons and other structures that are oriented 55 degrees relative to the external magnetic field on short TE sequences, resulting in apparent increased signal intensity that can be misconstrued as pathology. Examples of short TE sequences include spin-echo T1- and proton density–weighted and all gradient echo sequences. This artifact is frequently encountered in shoulder MR examinations because of the orientation of the supraspinatus tendon. Magic angle

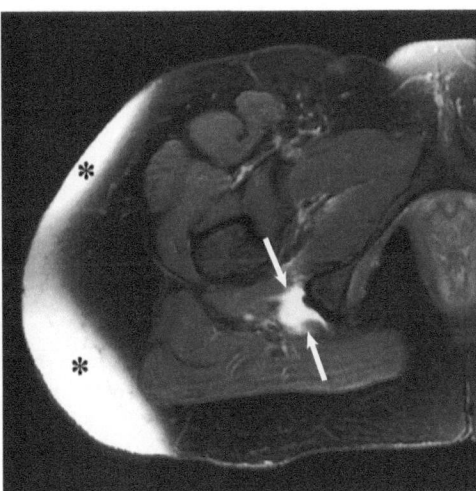

Fig. 7.51 Inhomogeneous fat suppression. An axial fast spin-echo proton density with fat suppression image shows bright signal intensity *(asterisk)* at the periphery of the image related to artifact from nonuniformity of the magnetic field at the periphery of the bore of the magnet. Inversion recovery sequences are more optimal for providing uniform fat suppression in this setting. An avulsion of the hamstring tendon origin is present *(arrows)*.

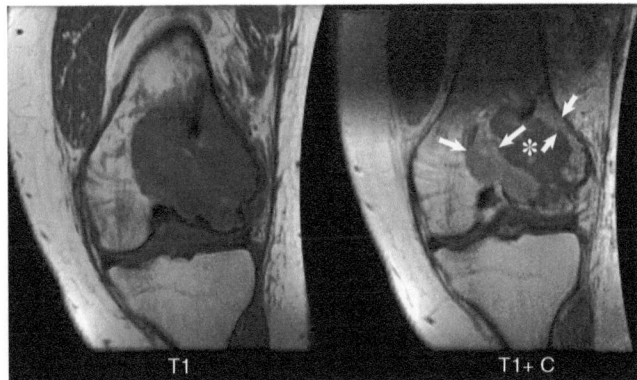

Fig. 7.52 Intravenous gadolinium enhancement in a giant cell tumor of bone. Precontrast coronal spin-echo T1-weighted *(left)* and postgadolinium coronal spin-echo T1-weighted *(right)* images show a thick irregular rind of enhancement *(arrows)*. A moderate-sized central nonenhancing area is present *(asterisk)*.

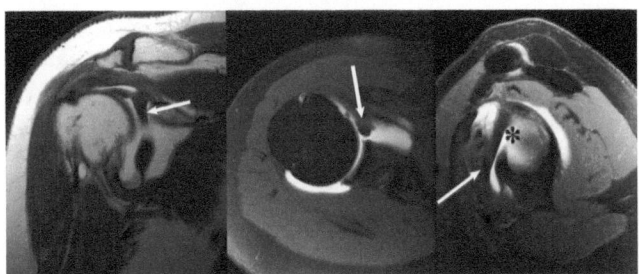

Fig. 7.53 A magnetic resonance shoulder arthrogram. Coronal spin-echo T1-weighted *(left)*, transverse *(middle)* and sagittal spin-echo T1-weighted with fat saturation *(right)* images show an absent anterior superior fibrocartilaginous glenoid labrum *(asterisk)* associated with a thickened middle glenohumeral ligament *(arrows)* in keeping with a Buford complex.

artifact can be distinguished from tendinosis or other real pathology because it disappears on long TE sequences such as spin-echo T2-weighted sequences.[65]

Magnetic resonance contrast agents. Although intravenous contrast agents are routinely used in a wide variety of MR examinations, these agents are used selectively for musculoskeletal studies. The most common contrast agent is a chelate of the rare–earth metal gadolinium. Gadolinium is paramagnetic and acts to reduce the T1 relaxation time, resulting in high signal intensity on T1-weighted sequences. The most widely used agents ultimately distribute nonspecifically from the vascular spaces into the extracellular space of tissues.[66] After administration of gadolinium, fat-saturated T1-weighted images are often obtained, providing excellent anatomic detail and contrast discrimination (see Fig. 7.43).

An intravenously administered contrast agent, which is used as a problem-solving tool, typically is required only for the evaluation of some mass lesions and synovial pathology. Occasionally, after an initial noncontrast imaging study has been performed, an unsuspected finding necessitates the return of the patient for further imaging with an intravenous contrast agent. Cystic and necrotic lesions lack gadolinium enhancement and continue to have low signal intensity (i.e., they are dark) on T1-weighted images. Solid lesions show internal enhancement, which is manifested as increased signal intensity (i.e., they are white) on T1-weighted images (Fig. 7.52).

MR arthrography involves the administration of contrast material, which provides high-resolution and high-contrast images of joints, facilitating the depiction of small cartilage tears. MR arthrography is most commonly used to evaluate the shoulder and hip joints but can be helpful in imaging other joints. Direct MR arthrography involves the administration of dilute gadolinium contrast material via a percutaneous route into the joint prior to imaging (Fig. 7.53). Indirect arthrography is a technique

in which intravenous contrast material is administered with subsequent indiscriminate diffusion into all joints, which is augmented by exercising the joint of interest prior to imaging. This technique is more commonly used in European centers and results in limited distention of the joint with contrast. Direct arthrography has the advantage of controlled filling and distension of the joint, forcing the contrast agent into cartilage tears and defects, which may be not be visualized in a nondistended joint. However, direct arthrography carries the small risk of septic arthritis as a complication of the procedure.

Magnetic field strength. The strength of the magnetic field affects the strength of the signal received, directly affecting the overall quality of the image. However, the image quality of lower field strength magnets can be improved to some extent with use of longer imaging times. Low-field strength magnets are less than 0.5 tesla (500 G, or about 500 times the earth's magnetic field), mid-field strength magnets are between 0.5 and 3.0 tesla, and high-field strength magnets are 3.0 tesla or greater (3.0 tesla is currently the highest field strength clinical magnet, but higher field strength units up to 7.0 tesla are available in research facilities). Most clinical magnets are 1.5 tesla.

Coils. A coil concealed within the main magnet housing surrounding the patient, termed the *body coil*, functions to transmit the radiofrequency waves for all examinations and receive the

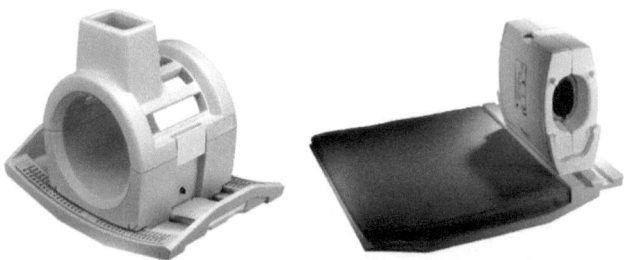

Fig. 7.54 Magnetic resonance coils. Extremity coils for evaluation of the foot, ankle, and knee *(left)* and wrist *(right)* are shown. The coils provide high-quality images at the expense of restricting imaging coverage to the confines of the coil. (Courtesy General Electric, Milwaukee, WI.)

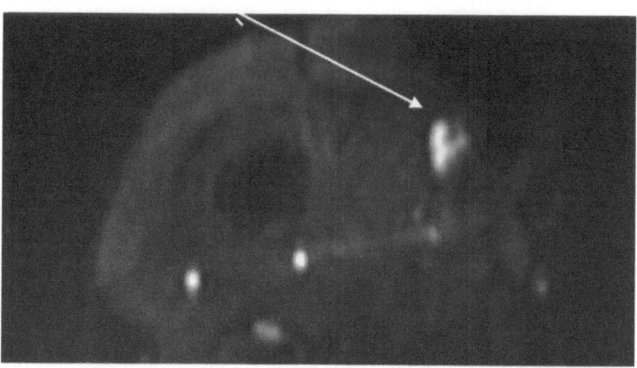

Fig. 7.55 Diffusion weighted imaging of the thigh demonstrates a restricting lesion *(arrow)* within the vastus medialis, representative of a partially sclerosed vascular anomaly.

signal for the imaging of larger body parts.[67] For imaging of smaller body parts, special additional smaller radiofrequency coils positioned directly over the area of interest and connected by cables to the main scanner are required to improve the image quality. The coils are configured differently depending on the anatomic area. Numerous types and models of coils are available for purchase by the imaging institution, including shoulder, extremity, ankle, wrist, spine, body, breast, and head coils (Fig. 7.54). Phased array coil technology, which was developed more than a decade ago, utilizes multiple receiver elements, leading to a further improvement in signal to noise and image quality. Although the use of a localized coil provides higher signal to noise that can be used to gain higher spatial resolution and improved image detail, the benefits are offset by restricted anatomic coverage that is limited to the length of the coil. This restricted coverage can be problematic when imaging structures such as nerves, muscles, and tendons over a long distance. In this situation, a coil with longer coverage may be selected, often with a reduction in image detail. Alternatively, the coil may be repositioned to provide additional coverage after imaging a portion of the area of concern is completed. However, this technique is best avoided because it effectively doubles the imaging time.

Image quality. More than with other cross-sectional imaging modalities, the quality of MR images can be variable and, at times, suboptimal. Because the imaging times are relatively long for MR, patient motion and image blurring can become an issue. Nonuniform signal related to magnetic field inhomogeneity can degrade the image quality when imaging joints at the periphery of the bore of the magnet, such as the shoulder or elbow, particularly in large patients (see Fig. 7.51). Other adjustable technical factors, including the image matrix, field of view, and number of excitations, also can affect the image quality, directly affecting on the signal-to-noise and contrast-to-noise ratios and spatial resolution. Typically, the major penalty related to adjusting technical parameters for optimization of images is increased imaging time. MR protocols are designed to balance parameters contributing to image quality (i.e., spatial and contrast resolution and signal to noise) with imaging times to produce the highest quality diagnostic images possible within the scheduled appointment time.

Diffusion Weighted Imaging

Diffusion weighted imaging (DWI) has proven to be useful in the characterization of neoplastic lesions and in assessing treatment response.[68] DWI can analyze the Brownian motion of water particles, which as a result yield information regarding the tissue's microstructure. In order to confirm findings on DWI, one must look at the Apparent Diffusion Coefficient images as well. This is because lesions may appear to be bright due to T2 shine through artifact, since DWI is a T2-weighted sequence. ADC mapping yields a dark signal in highly, cellular micro environments in which diffusion is restricted by the presence of cell membranes.

Assessment of musculoskeletal neoplasms using DWI is important as it is sometimes difficult to discriminate between peritumoral edema versus hyper intense tumor on fluid-sensitive sequences. In addition, it may be of utility in patients who are not able to receive intravenous contrast, such as patients in renal failure, pregnant patients, or patients with allergy to contrast material. In addition, partially embolized vascular anomalies can be identified on DWI (Fig. 7.55).

DWI has also been shown to better identify granulation tissue and scarring from residual tumor compared with contrast-enhanced imaging, where they have similar enhancement patterns. DWI, particularly single-shot fast spin-echo, has also been shown to assist in the differentiation of bone marrow disease in regard to osteoporosis versus malignant, vertebral compression fractures.[69] Furthermore, DWI has been shown to assist in the assessment of synovitis in patients with rheumatoid arthritis (RA) who cannot receive contrast due to renal impairment or allergies.[70]

Ultrashort Time to Echo Sequence

Ultrashort time to echo (TE) sequences have added another dimension to MRI evaluation of the musculoskeletal system. Ultrashort TE sequences allow for the morphologic evaluation of certain musculoskeletal tissues that were not readily evident on MRI. These include the deepest layers of the articular cartilage, cartilaginous endplates at the discovertebral junction, meniscus and the cortical bone. In general, the basic imaging principle is the more solid the material, the more short T2 properties that would be displayed. In particular, assessment of the calcified portion of the articular cartilage is now visualized with UTE imaging. Increased layers of calcified cartilage are seen with increased grades of degradation, which were not previously seen on conventional MRI.

Improved resolution of the cartilaginous endplate reveals a bilaminar intermediate to high-signal appearance with a thicker superficial and a thinner deep layer consistent with noncalcified and calcified cartilage layers, respectively. Ultrashort TE sequences can unmask the collagen infrastructure of the meniscus, and can also characterize calcifications within the meniscus. Normal cortical bone typically does not produce signal on T2-weighted imaging given its very short T2 time. UTE imaging has revealed collagen-methylene protons, collagen-bound water, and a broad peak consistent of pore water and lipid.[71]

Evaluation of other vital structures such as the osteochondral junction has also been shown in UTE imaging. Particularly, changes believed to be secondary to osteoarthritis have been found in the medial tibial osteochondral junction in patients aged 40 to 50.[72] Evaluation of Achilles tendons in healthy runners using UTE imaging have also found subclinical changes, specifically within the midportion of the Achilles tendon, likely secondary to adaptive changes within the micro architecture secondary to repetitive movements.[73]

Injuries to the cartilage and menisci, specifically in patients with history of anterior cruciate ligament (ACL) tear and reconstruction, which are sometimes not evident on conventional knee MRI until the degenerative changes, are irreversible. Studies have specifically found that UTE is sensitive to identifying changes within the deep tissue matrix of the medial meniscus, articular surface of the medial femoral condyle, and the medial tibial plateau. In addition, using a specific grading criteria, UTE may be more sensitive than arthroscopic surgery in detecting early degenerative changes of the aforementioned tissues. By using this information, there is promise as well as potential to identify cartilage and menisci at risk for rapid degenerative changes and to monitor potential new therapy, which may delay the irreversible osteoarthritis changes.[74]

dGEMRIC (Delayed Gadolinium)

Delayed gadolinium enhanced MRI of cartilage has also proven to be efficacious, particularly in the evaluation of focal cartilage defects. It is a relatively new technology that is aimed at monitoring early cartilage breakdown by detecting the amount of intraarticular gadolinium contrast. dGEMRIC is particularly effective in detecting cartilage changes prior to the time point when conventional MRI may detect these changes. Specifically the anionic charge of gadolinium is an indirect measure of areas of sparse glycosaminoglycan as it distributes inversely to the amount of glycosaminoglycan. Images are then acquired approximately 90 minutes following contrast administration to allow for sufficient diffusion of gadolinium into the intraarticular space. dGEMRIC is also used for the evaluation of determining the quality of articular cartilage prior to autologous transplantation, high tibial osteotomy, and matrix-assisted autologous chondrocyte implantation.[75]

This data are then analyzed and readily measured using color coding, as opposed to conventional MRI imaging, where a discrete tear has to be large enough to visualize. This advanced MRI technology has been specifically useful in examining assessment of cartilage changes within the knee prior to reconstructive surgery, femoroacetabular impingement prior to periacetabular osteotomy, following injury such as patellar dislocation and anterior cruciate

and posterior cruciate ligament tears, and suspected early osteoarthritis prior to its manifestation on plain films.

dGEMRIC has also been found to be of utility in sparing patients from major joint-preserving procedures with risk of complications. One such procedure is the Bernese periacetabular osteotomy in patients with symptomatic congruous acetabular dysplasia. Traditionally, standard anteroposterior and supine anteroposterior radiographs of the hip in maximum abduction and internal rotation were used for preoperative evaluation. However, with the advent of dGEMRIC, there has been improvement in the detection of early osteoarthritis in patients who would be poor candidates for periacetabular osteotomy.[76]

dGEMRIC has also been shown to be useful in monitoring glycosaminoglycan concentration within cartilage prior to repair of focal articular cartilage lesions. Focal cartilage defects are generally treated through microfracture or autologous chondrocyte implantation. dGEMRIC has shown a relationship between patient age and focal cartilage defect size influencing improvement of delayed gadolinium enhancement within the joint. The age of the patient and size of the focal cartilage defect have shown a direct relation to the overall improvement of delayed gadolinium enhancement within the articular cartilage of the knee, 12 months post surgery. Focal cartilage defects greater than 3 cm in size have also been found to show less improvement following surgery. It is postulated that younger patients are more likely to have better outcomes due to senescence of the cells and tissues due to the effects of aging.[75]

Dynamic Contrast Enhancement

Dynamic contrast enhancement (DCE), another relatively recent technological advancement, is primarily effective in the evaluation of musculoskeletal neoplastic processes. Three minutes following contrast administration, ultrafast T1-weighted images are acquired and postprocessing software is then utilized to extrapolate signal-intensity to time curves, which measure the uptake of contrast. Dynamic imaging has also been found to be useful in the assessment of measuring the initial chemotherapeutic response of tumors by comparison of the pre- and postcontrast enhancement curves prior to and following initial chemotherapy.[77]

Evaluation of treatment response in patients with RA has also been shown with the use of highly accelerated three-dimensional DCE wrist, specifically in adult patients undergoing treatment with Methotrexate or Methotrexate and antitumor necrosis factor therapy. Attention was specifically paid to perfusion patterns of the synovium as well as bone marrow edema within the intraarticular portions of the wrist.[25]

In addition, in patients who are status post double bundle anterior cruciate ligament reconstruction, there has been found to be correlation with knee pain secondary to poor neovascularization of the repair graft, on DCE imaging, which may be an early indicator of graft failure. The assessment of neovascularization was found to correlate better with knee pain compared with primary and secondary signs of ACL graft failure, respectively such as graft signal intensity, graft orientation and continuity, as well as cystic degeneration, anterior translation of the tibia, and arthrofibrosis. It is also believed that primary and secondary signs of ACL graft failure may not be as reliable due to the expected process of graft evolution following repair and due to the transplanted tendon not being as inherently strong as the patient's native tendon.[78]

In the pediatric population, DCE has also found a role in the evaluation of the perfusion patterns of the proximal femur. Precise evaluation of enhancement patterns within the proximal femur is of the utmost importance in discerning normal osseous development from pathologic processes. Contrast uptake within the metaphyseal spongiosa is very brisk and eventually declines, and within the periosteum increases with time and eventually plateaus. Given the brisk vascularity within the metaphyseal spongiosa, it is a fertile ground for osteomyelitis as well as metastases. Therefore a baseline understanding of these enhancement patterns is important to determine normal vascularity from pathologic processes.[79]

Prior to the advent of multi acquisition variable-resonance image combination (MAVRIC), postoperative radiographs were the gold standard avascular/osteonecrosis of the femoral head in patients status post fixation of femoral neck fractures. MRI was previously limited due to severe image distortion due to metallic hardware artifact; however, the advent of MAVRIC imaging has helped eliminate the presence of metallic hardware artifact and allows for detection of bone and soft tissue detail surrounding metallic implants. Subchondral collapse at 3 months was seen on 14% of patients, and at 12 months 35% of patients using MAVRIC weighed sequences, and was not seen on the same patient population using conventional radiography.[80]

Advantages

MRI has the highest soft tissue contrast discrimination compared with other modalities, thus providing the means to evaluate muscle, tendons, ligaments, cartilage, and bone marrow pathology with exquisite sensitivity. This technique uses a strong magnetic field and radiofrequency waves to generate images. Unlike CT and conventional radiography, no ionizing radiation is used, and consequently, MRI poses no known biologic risks to patients. Images can be obtained directly in any plane, allowing protocols to be tailored to a specific clinical concern. Allergy to gadolinium contrast agents used in MRI is relatively rare compared with the iodinated conventional radiographic contrast agents used in CT. No cross-reactivity to gadolinium-based contrast agents is known in patients with a history of allergy to conventional iodinated CT contrast agents.

Disadvantages

MRI is a relatively costly technology that is similar in cost to scintigraphy and is more expensive than CT, ultrasound, and plain films. Because of the large capital cost required for purchasing and siting the MR equipment and high routine maintenance expenses, MR technology is less widely available than other modalities.

Approximately 5% to 10% of patients experience claustrophobia, which compromises imaging with a standard magnet because of the narrow tunnel-like opening bore that accommodates the patient.[81] Newer magnet designs have been developed to shorten the length and widen the bore of the magnet in an effort to reduce claustrophobia. In patients with less severe

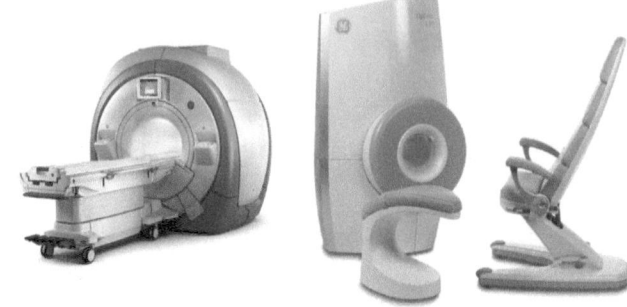

Fig. 7.56 Magnetic resonance imaging (MRI) machines. The General Electric (GE) Discovery 450 1.5-tesla MR machine *(left image)* has a newer design with a shorter length and wider diameter (70 cm) bore, which can accommodate larger patients and enhance patient comfort. The GE Optima 430S dedicated extremity 1.5-tesla MRI machine *(right image)* for wrist, knee, hand, or ankle imaging is an alternative option that can be used with claustrophobic patients. (Courtesy General Electric, Milwaukee, WI; used with permission.)

claustrophobia, short-acting sedatives may be effective when they are administered immediately prior to the scan. Open-configuration magnets (which are much scarcer than conventional units) and dedicated extremity magnets have become more available in the past decade, providing an alternative option to the problem of claustrophobia (Fig. 7.56).

MR studies consist of a number of imaging series that typically are composed of different pulse sequences and imaging planes. The acquisition time for each series is variable, often taking a few minutes. The cumulative examination time is considerably longer than that of CT, radiography, and ultrasound. The total scan time is variable depending on the body part and clinical indication, but on average it takes 30 minutes. Motion artifact can be problematic, especially in pediatric patients or in patients experiencing pain. Anesthesia with its consequent risks may be required in pediatric and claustrophobic patients.

Contraindications to Magnetic Resonance Imaging

Unlike ultrasound, CT, and radiography, MRI has a number of contraindications.[82] The MR institution is responsible for screening patients prior to imaging to ensure that no contraindications exist; however, the referring physician should have an understanding of the most common contraindications to avoid cancellation of the patient's appointment after his or her arrival at the imaging facility.

The strong external magnetic field used in most clinical MR units can affect the operation of implanted electrical, magnetic, or mechanically activated devices. The more commonly encountered contraindicated devices include cardiac pacemakers and defibrillators, neurostimulators, and cochlear implants. Some implanted ferromagnetic material is at risk of dislodgement or heating, resulting in a thermal injury. Metallic foreign bodies situated in the eye can dislodge and damage the globe, resulting in blindness. Welders or other patients at risk for harboring metallic orbital foreign bodies are routinely screened with orbital radiographs prior to imaging. Some intracranial aneurysm clips are ferromagnetic and are contraindicated for MR because of the risk of dislodgement and subsequent vascular injury resulting in stroke or death. Orthopedic hardware, including arthroplasty implants, is not typically composed of ferromagnetic material and is not at risk for dislodgement. To determine whether a patient can safely undergo MRI, the exact name and manufacturer of the implanted medical device (obtained from an operative report or clinic note) must be provided prior to the scan to determine whether the device is MR compatible.[83] Any concern regarding potential incompatibility of an indwelling device should be brought to the attention of the MR facility prior to the patient's appointment to determine whether MRI is safe.

Although the safety of MRI during pregnancy has not been proven definitively, no deleterious effects are known. MRI of pregnant patients should be undertaken only if no other non-ionizing imaging alternatives exist and the clinical concern warrants relatively urgent imaging that cannot be safely postponed until the postpartum period. Ideally, imaging should be avoided during the first trimester when the natural incidence of spontaneous abortion is relatively high (~30%).[84]

The use of gadolinium contrast agents in patients with impaired renal function and reduced glomerular filtration rates of less than 30 mL/min/1.73 m^2 is a relative major contraindication because of the risk of nephrogenic systemic fibrosis, a rare, potentially life-threatening condition.[85] Finally, MRI is contraindicated for some obese patients because of the mechanical load on the MR table and the risk of damage. The threshold weight for contraindication is unique to the individual MR machine. Older equipment often can handle patients weighing up to 350 lb. Newer machines have increased capacity that can be as high as 500 lb.

RADIATION EXPOSURE IN MEDICAL IMAGING

Increased utilization of medical radiation during the past two decades, mainly related to abdominal and thoracic CT scans, have exposed patients to cumulative high levels of ionizing radiation. Some scientists predict that the increased radiation exposure from CT scans will lead to thousands of radiation-induced cancers and cancer deaths in the future and potentially will be responsible for up to 1% to 2% of all future cancers in the United States.[86,87] Physicians should be cognizant of the risks and relative dose of radiation associated with imaging procedures. Careful consideration of the risks and benefits of an investigation and potential alternatives in the imaging algorithm for clinical conditions is essential. Imaging modalities that do not utilize ionizing radiation such as MR or ultrasound should be used where possible, especially in young patients.

The biologic effects of radiation exposure are categorized into stochastic (random) and deterministic (predictable) effects. Deterministic effects include cataracts and cutaneous burns and reflect predictable cell damage that is directly related to a threshold radiation dose. Deterministic effects are uncommonly associated with radiographic procedures because it is rare for the dose associated with an individual examination to exceed the threshold value above which damage occurs.

Stochastic effects include radiation-induced cancer and genetic mutations. With stochastic effects, the severity of the effect is not dose related. Although stochastic effects are more likely to

occur with larger radiation doses, *any* dose may cause a cell to mutate and result in cancer or a genetic defect.[88] The dose of radiation received from a radiographic procedure is variable and depends on multiple factors, including the patient's body habitus, intrinsic equipment factors, and parameters involved in setting up the particular examination. Assessment of individual radiation dose and consequent risk to a patient from an imaging procedure is generally the domain of physicists specializing in medical imaging.

Several methods can be used to quantify radiation exposure, but the various terminologies can be confusing to physicians. The simplest measure is radiation exposure, a measure of the amount of radiation-induced ionization in air, quantified in roentgens. It does not reflect the actual amount of energy absorbed by the irradiated tissue. Radiation absorbed dose is a measurement that quantifies the amount of energy absorbed by tissues from the ionizing radiation, measured in grays (international units) or rads (conventional units), with 1 gray equivalent to 100 rads. However, radiation absorbed dose does not reflect the location or the radiosensitivity of the individual tissues exposed. The effective dose is a weighted average of organ doses, taking into account the specific tissues in the body that have absorbed the radiation dose (recognizing that some tissues such as the breast, bone marrow and gonads have greater sensitivity to radiation and consequently a greater risk of undergoing mutation). The effective dose is measured in sieverts (international units) or rems (conventional units), with 1 sievert equivalent to 100 rems[2].

Humans are constantly exposed to naturally occurring background radiation that provides a reference with which to compare doses from medical imaging. Background radiation averages approximately 3 mSv per annum. Average radiation doses for a variety of imaging procedures are summarized in Table 7.2.

TABLE 7.2 Average Radiation Dose From Imaging Examinations

Examination	Effective Dose (mSv)
Chest (2 views)	0.1
Hand (1 view)	0.005
Lumbar spine (2 views)	1.5
Pelvis (1 view)	0.7
Hip (1 view)	0.8
CT pelvis	10.0
CT spine	6
CT chest (shoulder)	7
Bone scan (technetium-99 MDP)	4.2
PET CT (18-FDG)	14
Background radiation per annum	3.0
Fluoroscopy for hip pinning (hip)	0.7[62]
Fluoroscopy for myelogram	2.46[62]
Average skin dose during fluoroscopy	20–50 mGy/min

1 mSv = 0.1 rem.
CT, Computed tomography; *FDG*, 18F-fluoro-deoxy-D-glucose; *MDP*, methylene diphosphonate; *mSv*, millisievert; *PET*, positron emission tomography.
Modified from RadiologyInfo.org. Patient safety: radiation dose in x-ray and CT exams (website). http://www.radiologyinfo.org/en/safety/?pg=sfty_xray.

Further details regarding estimates of radiation dose from imaging examinations with comparative background radiation equivalents and additional lifetime risk of fatal cancer are available.[89]

KEY POINTS

The imaging workup for clinical problems can take a number of routes, ultimately leading to a correct diagnosis. In many instances no single "right or wrong" imaging algorithm exists. Several factors should be taken into consideration in determining the optimal strategy for imaging, which include the likelihood of achieving a specific diagnosis, the desire to avoid ionizing radiation in younger patients, the accessibility and the relative cost of the investigation, and the availability of local expertise in musculoskeletal sonography. Radiographs serve as a first-line investigation for most musculoskeletal pathologies, but they are often insensitive and nonspecific.

Ultrasound is highly operator dependent, but in experienced hands it is excellent for the evaluation of superficial muscle, ligament, and tendon injuries. It is useful as a first line of investigation for confirming and characterizing the presence of soft tissue lesions that contain fluid, such as ganglia and bursae. Point of care assessment is possible with small portable ultrasound units.

CT is an important adjunct to radiographs in the assessment of occult and complex osseous trauma. CT provides limited soft tissue assessment.

Bone scintigraphy is essential in the workup of polyostotic disease. The quality of the CT component of SPECT/CT is variable; it is used for localizing abnormalities in complex anatomic areas and not for characterizing pathology.

White blood cell scans are highly sensitive and specific in the assessment of osteomyelitis in areas other than the spine, where gallium is used. Both agents are typically interpreted in conjunction with a bone scan, adding to the expense and radiation dose of the examination. Definitive results often are unavailable for at least 24 hours.

PET/CT scans are currently limited to a few major centers. PET/CT is increasingly used in the diagnosis, staging, and monitoring of neoplastic pathology.

MRI is sensitive and often specific in the assessment of most soft tissue and osseous pathologies, but it is relatively expensive and not always immediately available. Clinicians should be aware of contraindications to MRI.

Increased utilization of CT scans during the past decade has raised concerns regarding risks related to the radiation dose that is associated with CT and scintigraphy.

Musculoskeletal imaging examinations ideally are performed and interpreted by subspecialty trained orthopaedic radiologists.

ACKNOWLEDGMENT

The authors and editors are grateful for the contributions of the previous author of this chapter, Alison Spouge.

For a complete list of references, go to ExpertConsult.com.

SELECTED READINGS

Citation:

Helms CA, Major NM, Andersen MW, et al. *Musculoskeletal MRI.* 2nd ed. Philadelphia: Saunders; 2008.

Level of Evidence:

VII

Summary:

This textbook reviews technical aspects related to magnetic resonance imaging and the appearance of common musculoskeletal conditions.

Citation:

Manaster BJ, May DA, Disler DG. *Musculoskeletal Imaging: The Requisites.* 3rd ed. Philadelphia: Mosby; 2007.

Level of Evidence:

VII

Summary:

This general textbook provides a comprehensive multimodality imaging review of common musculoskeletal conditions.

Citation:

Mettler FA, Guiberteau MJ. In: *Essentials of Nuclear Medicine Imaging.* 6th ed. Philadelphia: Saunders; 2012.

Level of Evidence:

VII

Summary:

A core radiology textbook covering all aspects of imaging in nuclear medicine, including scintigraphy of common musculoskeletal conditions.

Citation:

Jacobson JA. *Fundamentals of Musculoskeletal Ultrasound.* Philadelphia: Saunders; 2007.

Level of Evidence:

VII

Summary:

A concise but comprehensive textbook focusing on ultrasound technique and the interpretation of common soft tissue and joint-related pathologies as revealed by sonography.

Citation:

Dalrymple NC, Prasad SR, Freckleton MW, et al. Informatic in Radiology (*info*Rad). Introduction to the language of three-dimensional imaging with multidetector CT. *Radiographics.* 2005;25:1409–1428.

Level of Evidence:

V

Summary:

This general review article provides a detailed review of computed tomography image acquisition and three-dimensional postprocessing techniques.

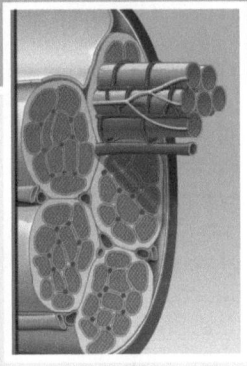

8

Basic Arthroscopic Principles

Michael R. Mijares, Michael G. Baraga

The first arthroscope was developed in 1920 with an optical cannula diameter of 7.3 mm by Dr. Kenji Takagi from Tokyo. His idea to look inside a closed knee with an instrument, a cystoscope, in 1918 came from his interest in the early diagnosis of tuberculous knees in Japan, which was a problematic disease at the time. Dr. Takagi is credited with being the first innovator and developer of arthroscopy. His successor, Dr. Masaki Watanabe, continued advancing Dr. Takagi's arthroscope design, which contributed largely to the popularization of arthroscopy. He also developed the concept of triangulation. Prior to Dr. Takagi, Dr. Nordentoft, a Danish surgeon, in 1912 published a manuscript at a meeting in Berlin, where he adapted the use of an endoscope to the knee joint and is credited as being the first to apply endoscopy to the knee, as well as the first to use the term "arthroscopy."[1]

Arthroscopy has revolutionized the treatment of intraarticular pathology. Arthroscopy has become the standard of care for many orthopedic problems and is currently the most common orthopedic procedure performed in the United States, with 1 million cases reported annually.[2] Arthroscopy in experienced hands has low morbidity and high diagnostic yield. The benefits of arthroscopic surgery include reduced morbidity, less postoperative inflammation, smaller incisions, improved diagnostic accuracy, lower complication rates, reduced hospital stay, and reduced cost.[3] The decision to use arthroscopy must involve consideration of the potential benefits of this method weighed against its limitations.

ARTHROSCOPIC APPLICATIONS

Advancements in arthroscopic technology have expanded its use in nearly every joint in the body, including those in the elbow, wrist, ankle, foot, and spine. Although results in some areas are superior to those of open surgery, such superiority has not been demonstrated for all arthroscopic procedures. The primary applications of arthroscopy are the diagnosis and treatment of intraarticular pathology. Arthroscopy is commonly used in the knee and shoulder for irrigation and débridement, synovectomy, removal of a foreign or loose body, débridement or repair of osteochondral lesions, and ligament reconstruction. Arthroscopy has also been applied to the hip for treatment of femoroacetabular impingement with repair or reconstruction of the labrum, cartilage, osseous deformity, and capsule.[4] Absolute contraindications to arthroscopy are skin infection over the operative site or at a remote site, with risk of seeding. Relative contraindications are ankylosis of the joint and major capsular disruptions that risk excessive extravasation of fluid and make joint distension difficult.

EQUIPMENT

Arthroscopy is performed in a standard surgical suite in a hospital or ambulatory surgical center. Arthroscopic equipment has become more streamlined, occupying less space in the operating room. Some operating rooms are now specifically made for use with arthroscopy and are fully equipped with mobile monitors and an arthroscopic tower attached to the ceiling along with the standard operating room lights (Fig. 8.1). The operating room must be large enough to accommodate the required equipment and should be staffed by operating room personnel experienced with arthroscopy.

Arthroscopic cables and equipment are sterilized mostly by steam sterilizing autoclaves. The word autoclave comes from Greek roots auto (self) and clave (key), which together means self-locking. Autoclaves have an automatic locking ability that allow temperatures to exceed 270°F and pressures of 15 psi, which are the recommended settings for steam sterilization, creating an environment that no organism can survive in. The arthroscopic sterilization process begins with a standard wash of all the instruments, which then get wrapped with a blue sterilization wrap and sterilization indicator tape. Along with the sterilization indicator tape, a steam chemical indicator strip is attached to each individual tray and a Bowie-Dick Plus Test Pack is placed alongside the entire load to be autoclaved to ensure complete sterilization. These indicators turn black once fully autoclaved. A biologic indicator is also placed with the autoclave set, then inserted into a steam incubator and compared against a control biologic indicator for 1 hour to ensure all organisms have been eliminated. A plus sign for the control indicator and minus sign for the autoclaved indicator are digitally displayed to ensure complete sterilization. These sterilization tests are all documented and kept on record by the OR staff. For temperature-sensitive instruments such as smaller cameras and plastics, alternate methods of sterilization are used such as gas sterilization with ethylene oxide, low-temperature sterilization using peracetic acid (Steris, Mentor, OH), and cold disinfection using activated glutaraldehyde (Civco, Kalona, IA).[5]

Arthroscope

Advances in technology have resulted in improved arthroscope design and function. The arthroscopes currently used have improved optics and field of view with smaller diameter lenses, and they use fiberoptic and digital technology to improve visualization. Modern camera systems have the ability to use ultra HD 4K technology. Most arthroscopy systems allow video recording and the ability to take pictures. Newer technology integrating the camera system with tablet computers for arthroscopic video recordings, pictures, and editing will allow for higher-quality presentations and improved media for educational purposes.

The arthroscope is designed to fit inside a cannula, which is inserted into the joint first with use of a blunt trocar. Modern cannulas allow the flow of irrigation fluid into the joint. The camera is housed within the arthroscope and connected to the digital monitor for direct visualization of the joint. The light source, which comes from the light projector in the form of a

fiberoptic cable, is attached to the arthroscope to allow visualization and minimizes the heat generated at the arthroscope.

Arthroscopes have different optical characteristics, with several options in terms of lens diameter, field of view, and angle of inclination. The diameter of the lens determines the size of the arthroscope and the field of view and can vary from 1.7 to 7 mm. The field of view is represented by the total angle visualized by the lens of the arthroscope, with a larger lens diameter allowing a greater field of view. The angle of inclination is defined as the angle between the long axis of the arthroscope and a line perpendicular to the lens and can vary typically from 0 to 70 degrees. The advantage of using angled arthroscopes is that they provide better control and allow a wider field of view with rotation of the arthroscope, but a central blind spot directly in front of the arthroscope is created with arthroscopes that have a higher angle (70 to 90 degrees) (Fig. 8.2). The degree of magnification of an object viewed with an arthroscope is determined by its distance from the lens. This characteristic makes judging arthroscopic distances and sizes difficult, but the use of an object of known size for comparison (such as a probe) can be of assistance.

The most commonly used arthroscope is 4 mm in diameter and has an angle of inclination of 25 to 30 degrees. Smaller joints can be accessed using arthroscopes with a smaller diameter (1.9 or 2.5 mm). Arthroscopes with increased angles of inclination (70 or 90 degrees) can be used to view difficult areas such as the posterior corners of the knee.

The fiberoptic light source and power console for shavers and drills are typically housed on an arthroscopic cart. Such a cart can be positioned easily in the operating room so it is close to the patient but does not obstruct personnel. Arthroscopy using modern equipment requires a light source capable of producing 300 to 350 watts, for which tungsten, halogen, LED, and xenon arc sources have been adapted. Fiberoptic cable uses bundled glass fibers to transmit light from the source to the

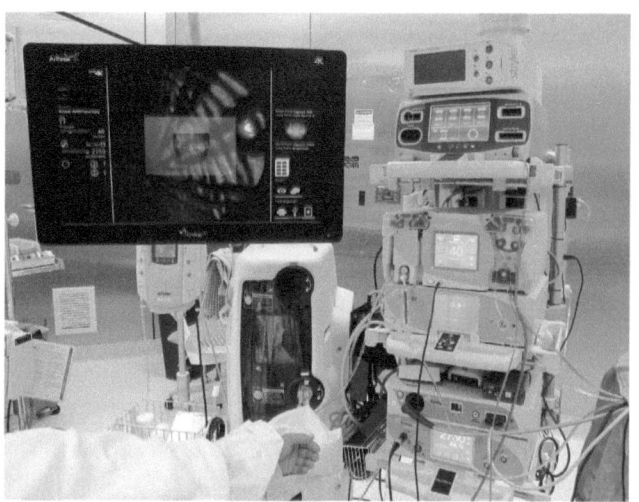

Fig. 8.1 The arthroscopic cart with camera, monitor, light source, power for shaver and handpieces, and pump.

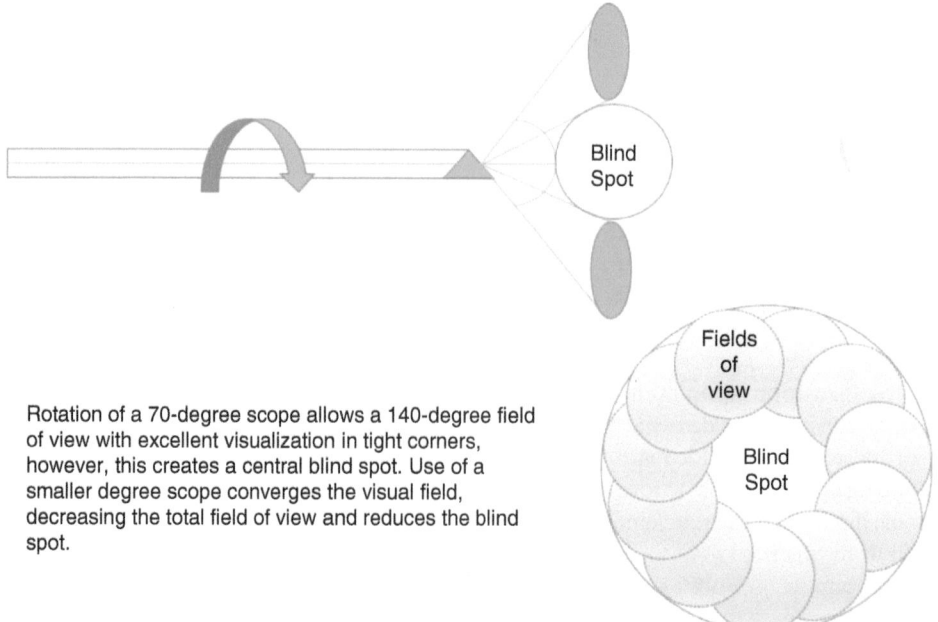

Rotation of a 70-degree scope allows a 140-degree field of view with excellent visualization in tight corners, however, this creates a central blind spot. Use of a smaller degree scope converges the visual field, decreasing the total field of view and reduces the blind spot.

Fig. 8.2 The angulation of each scope determines the field of view as well as the potential blind spot.

arthroscope. The intensity and quality of light are diminished by the length of cable or damage to it, although modern fiber-optic cables are more durable.

Reduction of camera size, improved camera resolution, digitization of the video signal, and the integration of high-definition technology have all contributed to considerable improvement in the quality of visualization obtained using arthroscopy.

Fluid Pump

Irrigation fluid is vital for arthroscopy because it is responsible for joint distension, removal of debris, and improvement of visualization. Joint distension is supplied by the hydrostatic pressure of the irrigation fluid, which can be maintained using gravity, mechanical pumps, or manual control of outflow usually by the scrub tech. Every foot of elevation of the irrigation solution above the joint results in approximately 22 mm Hg of pressure. The use of a fluid pump allows more precise control of the rate of flow and hydrostatic pressure in the joint and can be used to minimize extravasation of fluids into the tissues.

Fluid management in arthroscopy consists of balancing the flow of fluids in and out of the joint. This balance is vital to maintain appropriate distension of the joint without causing excessive fluid extravasation into the tissues, and it plays a role in the management of bleeding, visualization, and debris clearance. Imbalances between inflow and outflow can cause turbulence of the irrigation fluid, reducing visualization and thus increasing operative time. This can occur when the shaver is used without compensatory changes in inflow/outflow or when the manual outflow of fluid is not controlled appropriately. Control of intraarticular pressure is critical, especially when working with the shaver in the posterior aspect of the knee. A situation where flow is decreased secondary to overzealous suction through the shaver can potentially deliver the posterior capsule into the shaver inadvertently. To prevent this problem, the inflow rate can be increased, the outflow through the suction or arthroscope can be decreased (or closed to prevent back flow), or outflow through the shaver can be decreased manually or by ensuring that the shaver window is occupied with tissue to be cut. Development of automated inflow and outflow mechanical irrigation pumps have shown promising results with consistent flow, greater degree of joint distension, and improved visualization, leading to reduced operative times.[6] Modern irrigation systems also have functions that allow brief increases in pressure and flow to clear bleeding or debris, as well as functions to drain fluid such as at the end of the procedure.

A physiologic solution such as Ringer lactate or normal saline should be used for irrigation; the surgeon decides which solution to use. The addition of epinephrine to the irrigation fluid (1 mg/L) has been shown to shorten operating time and decrease bleeding, leading to improved visualization.[7,8] Recently, it was shown that norepinephrine added to irrigation fluid reduces the incidence of hypotensive/bradycardic events significantly compared with epinephrine and is as efficacious in controlling intraoperative bleeding, thus maintaining clarity of the visual field when used in shoulder arthroscopy.[9]

The temperature and osmolarity of the irrigation fluid used in shoulder arthroscopy has been a recent topic of discussion in the literature. Three randomized controlled studies evaluated the effect of warmed irrigation fluid versus room temperature irrigation fluid. One study did not demonstrate a significant difference in reducing perioperative hypothermia, whereas the other two showed that hypothermia occurred more often in the room temperature irrigation fluid group.[10,11] Kim et al. showed that age and the amount of irrigation used correlated with core body temperature when using room temperature fluid and that warmed irrigation fluid decreased perioperative hypothermia, especially in elderly patients.[12] The osmolarity of irrigation fluid may also be an important factor to consider when performing arthroscopy. An in vivo animal study was performed to evaluate the safety of using a hyperosmolar irrigation fluid (600 mOsm/L) compared with normal saline (300 mOsm/L) prior to designing a study on humans. They tested bilateral shoulders in dogs and found the mean percentage change in shoulder girth to be higher in the isotonic control group (13.3%) compared with the hyperosmolar group (10.4%). There were no detrimental effects on chondrocyte viability with either solution.[13] Future clinical studies on this topic may provide more information on ways to decrease fluid extravasation during prolonged arthroscopic procedures.

Instruments and Motorized Shavers

A variety of hand-operated instruments are used in arthroscopy. Many are generalized, but some instruments have been developed for particular joints or procedure-specific tasks. These instruments include various arthroscopic probes, graspers, baskets, scissors, knives, suture passers, and radiofrequency instruments. The actual instruments required for arthroscopy depend on surgeon preference, the joint involved, and the procedure being performed.

Arthroscopic Probe

The probe is the most important and used instrument in both diagnostic and therapeutic arthroscopy. Most probes are right angled at the working end, with a tip length of 4 mm that can be used to estimate intraarticular size, depth, and distance. Its primary purpose is palpation and identification of pathology, such as soft cartilage, loose bodies or cartilage flaps, meniscal tears, or insufficient tension of the anterior cruciate ligament. It is also a useful instrument for learning triangulation, planning surgical approaches, and positioning or retracting intraarticular structures or loose bodies. Care should be taken when palpating structures with the arthroscopic probe, because use of the tip may cause injury to tissues, and therefore use of the elbow for such activities is advisable.

Basket Forceps

Basket forceps are commonly used in procedures that involve the removal of intraarticular tissue, such as a meniscectomy. Basket forceps have a central opening and remove a portion of tissue that is then allowed to fall free into the joint, eliminating the need to remove the instrument from the joint to clear the basket each time (Fig. 8.3). These forceps typically range in size from 3 to 5 mm and are available in straight, left- or right-curved, and up- and down-angled varieties to facilitate work in different areas. Left- and right-curved varieties enable the surgeon to access

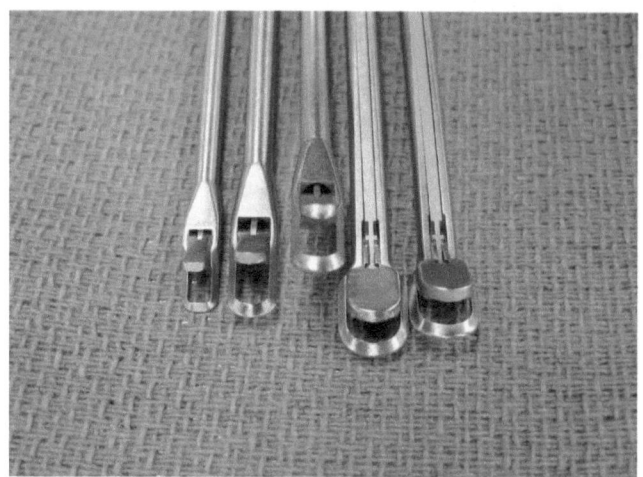

Fig. 8.3 Basket forceps for meniscal resection.

the anterior portion of the meniscus, whereas the up and down angled instruments permit trimming of the posterior meniscus around the femoral condyles. These instruments are also available in low-profile varieties for work in tight spaces, and some have hooked jaws that prevent tissue from slipping forward between the jaws when they are closed. Proper technique with these instruments is to use the jaws to remove small pieces of tissue because too large of a bite will strain the mechanical joints and may damage the instrument.

Grasping Forceps

Grasping forceps are used to securely hold, apply tension to, or retrieve intraarticular materials. These forceps are available in jaw configurations that include numerous serrated interdigitating teeth or with one or two sharp hooks at the distal end of the jaws. Configuration of the grasping jaws can also differ, in that varieties exist with both or only one mobile jaw. The graspers with forceps that have both jaws mobile are more suited to grasping and gripping larger intraarticular objects.

Scissors

Arthroscopic scissors are available in small and large sizes and with both straight and hooked blades to ensure an appropriate instrument for each situation. Hooked blades are easier to use compared with straight blades because they prevent the tissue from being pushed out from between the blades during the cutting motion. Curved and angled options, in which the shaft and blades are curved or the blades deviate from the shaft, respectively, are also available for difficult-to-reach resections.

Knives

Disposable arthroscopic knives are available in various shapes and sizes and should always be used with a cannula to protect the tissues during joint insertion and removal. Blade varieties include straight, curved, end cutting, and hooked, all of which allow the appropriate instrument for each situation. An important and useful characteristic of many arthroscopic knives is that the blades are magnetic to facilitate removal from the joint should it break.

Motorized Shavers

Motorized shavers consist of a pair of cylinders, one inside the other, each with a matching window. The inner cylinder spins within the outer and has an edge to both sides of its window that cuts tissue drawn into the outer cylinder by the attached suction. The removed tissue is then drawn down the inner cylinder, out of the joint, and into a suction trap. Commonly used motorized shavers range in diameter from 3 to 5.5 mm, but a 2-mm option is available for access to smaller or tight joints. Shavers with a larger diameter have larger windows and can expedite removal of tissue. Shavers also are available in various shapes and angles with different blades or burrs, all designed for specific purposes. Control of the motorized shaver is possible either by a hand or foot pedal and allows clockwise, counterclockwise, and alternating rotation to improve the efficiency of tissue cutting and allow clearing of the blade. Practically, when the motorized shaver is in use, the blades should be in the field of view to prevent unwanted damage to normal tissues.

Cannulas and Switching Sticks

Cannulas and switching sticks of numerous sizes are available to assist with the insertion and use of instruments during arthroscopic procedures; they are all designed for use in specific joints. Cannulas are used to maintain the integrity of a portal into the joint so that the intervening soft tissues do not interfere with activities such as knot tying. They also allow easy insertion of instruments without trauma to the tissues through which the portal is made. Switching sticks are used to ease the passage of the arthroscope and cannulas into the joint in question by holding the path through the soft tissues into the joint so that a cannula or arthroscopic sheath can be inserted into the joint over it. When working in joints that are deep from the surface, switching sticks are particularly useful in maintaining these paths.

Electrocautery and Radiofrequency Instruments

Electrocautery and radiofrequency instruments can be used for cutting and shrinking soft tissues and can play an important role in maintaining hemostasis. A variety of these instruments have been developed for use in specific joints or for specific purposes, including some with flexible tips. Electrocautery uses heat directly from the probe to effect tissue changes and has been adapted for intraarticular use with various irrigation solutions.[14]

Radiofrequency instruments generate a high-frequency electromagnetic current at their tip, causing heat to be generated by the resistance to current passage through tissue.[14] Monopolar and bipolar radiofrequency systems have been adapted for arthroscopic use. Monopolar systems allow current flow from the tip of the instrument to a grounding pad on the patient, using the path of least resistance, and generate heat at the tissue closest to the tip.[14] Bipolar devices permit passage of current between two electrodes at the tip of the instrument, heating the tissue between them. The primary difference between the two radiofrequency systems is that monopolar instruments require a grounding pad to allow energy to pass from the body, whereas bipolar instruments pass energy between electrodes at the intraarticular site of interest.

The specific effect of radiofrequency instruments on tissues depends on the amount of heat transferred. Low levels of heat transfer cause collagen, which is the major constituent of most soft tissues, to denature and shrink by as much as 50% of its length.[15] Higher levels of heat destroy collagen and are commonly used for tissue ablation and débridement.[14] Use of these instruments intraarticularly may cause high fluid temperatures leading to cartilage damage or chondrolysis. Cadaveric studies have been performed measuring the effect of radiofrequency devices on intraarticular fluid temperature and cartilage. Increased duration of application, decreased distance between the probe and soft tissue, and decreased fluid rate showed temperatures deleterious to articular cartilage chondrocytes (>50°C).[16,17] Irrigation-fluid flow is critical for maintaining low fluid temperatures rather than the continuous or intermittent use of the thermal device, because decreased flow rates significantly increase the temperature of the irrigation fluid.[18] The penetration depth and area affected are proportional to the power and temperature used.[14] A level I study evaluated a standard radiofrequency device compared with a new plasma radiofrequency device and found no significant difference between the two systems with respect to temperature generation or operative time.[19]

ARTHROSCOPIC PRINCIPLES

Surgical Technique

"Arthroscopy is an art that requires three dimensional thought and vision."

–Dr. Ronald Krinick, MD, New York, 2010

There are several skills required before one can successfully perform arthroscopy. The top four general skills are anatomic knowledge, tissue manipulation, spatial perception, and triangulation. The top two skills specific to arthroscopy are portal placement and triangulating the tip of the probe with a 30-degree scope.[20] Triangulation is the process by which your brain converts a two-dimensional arthroscopic image into a three-dimensional space, allowing your hands to manipulate an instrument entering from one portal in front of an arthroscopic camera with a specific degree of angulation from a separate portal. This is the most difficult aspect of arthroscopy initially and one that requires experience. Cadavers, arthroscopic computer simulators, and homemade arthroscopic simulators are great tools to have for acquiring these basic skills.[21]

Preoperative

It is important that the surgeon always meet the patient in the preoperative holding area prior to the patient being taken to the operating room. It is in this critical moment that the surgeon can have a clear discussion with the patient prior to any anxiolytic or narcotic medications on the correct procedure to be performed and to confirm the correct operative extremity. The operative extremity should be identified with confirmation by the patient and marked in the preoperative area with indelible ink, an ink that cannot be washed away, as recommended by the American Academy of Orthopaedic Surgeons.[22] Marking the extremity with indelible ink prior to sterile prepping and draping has not been

shown to increase infection.[23] Knee arthroscopy is the most frequent "wrong side" surgery in malpractice claims.[24]

A preoperative pause or "time out" should be enacted prior to the administration of anesthesia with the entire operative team present to confirm the correct patient, operative procedure, and operative site and to ensure that all required equipment is available. Discussing any concerns that members of the operative team may have regarding the case is also performed at that time.

Patient Positioning and Preparation

Patients undergoing arthroscopic surgery require careful positioning, especially during shoulder arthroscopy with the beach chair or lateral decubitus position (Fig. 8.4). Be cautious of the nonoperative extremities and ensure that they are secured. All bony prominences on the operative and nonoperative extremity should be well padded to avoid pressure on nerves that may result in a postoperative neuropraxia. If positioning the patient in the lateral decubitus position, an axillary roll should be placed three fingerbreadths distal to the axillary fold to avoid brachial plexus neuropraxia. Tourniquets are often used during knee arthroscopy. Zhang and Li performed a level one meta-analysis study to determine whether routine use of a tourniquet is beneficial in terms of arthroscopic visualization and operative time in knee arthroscopy. The study showed no significant difference in visualization or operative time between the tourniquet and nontourniquet group; however, multiple studies did suggest there were fewer visualization difficulties when a tourniquet was used during anterior cruciate ligament (ACL) surgery.[25] Tourniquets, if used, should be wide to distribute the compressive force over a larger surface area and should be limited to less than 90 minutes.[26] A tourniquet should be avoided if the patient has a history of thrombophlebitis, severe peripheral vascular disease, or endovascular stent placement which can be visualized on x-ray.

Surgical preparation and draping should be performed to ensure a sterile and sealed operative field. Surgical skin preparation is best performed with chlorhexidine and isopropyl alcohol because this combination has been shown to reduce bacterial

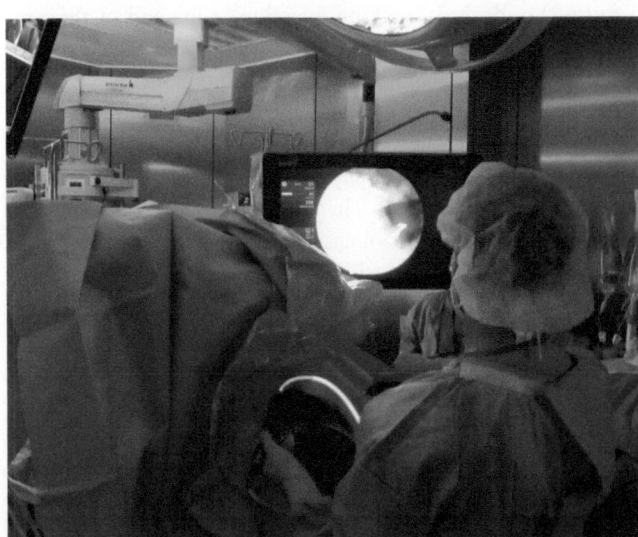

Fig. 8.4 Careful patient positioning and room setup for patient safety and clear visualization of the arthroscopic monitor.

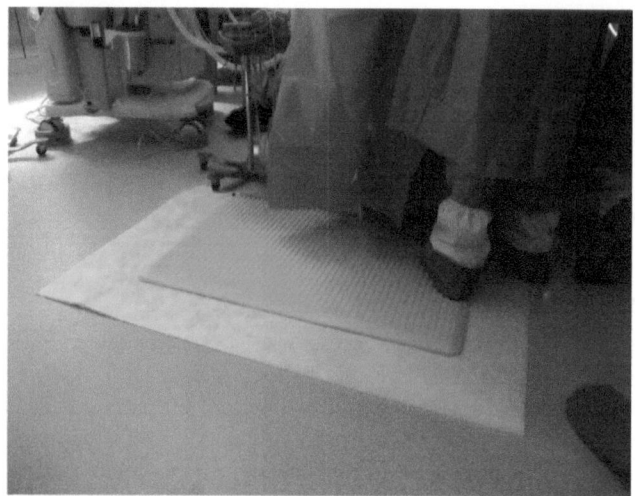

Fig. 8.5 The antislip irrigation collection mat prevents excess irrigation on the floor.

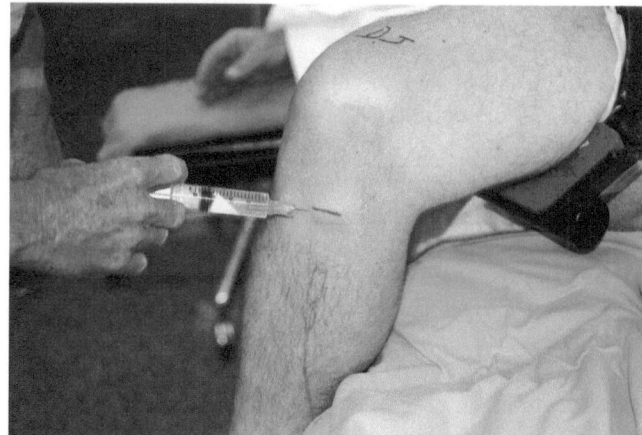

Fig. 8.6 The line of the incision is injected with local anesthetic before making the incision.

counts to a significantly greater degree than use of isopropyl alcohol, chlorhexidine, or povidone iodine alone.[27] Chlorhexidine has also been shown to have antimicrobial effects on the skin for up to 24 hours.[28] Benzoyl peroxide has been shown to be effective in the reduction of *Propionibacterium acnes,* lowering the risk of postoperative infection.[29] Sterile surgical draping technique will be determined by the joint undergoing arthroscopy and can be performed in many ways, according to the surgeon's preference. Prefabricated disposable draping is made specifically for a specific joint and has a fluid collection pouch to minimize fluid leakage onto the floor. There are also antislip mats with an integrated water collection system to assist with excess irrigation (Fig. 8.5).

Anesthesia

Local intraarticular anesthesia and injection of portal sites has been used alone for diagnostic arthroscopy,[30] although the use of a tourniquet or any bony procedures may not be tolerated in this setting. Recently, intraarticular Marcaine has also been shown to cause chondrolysis, making injection at the end of the procedure less favorable.[31] Regional or spinal anesthetics can be used but carry the risk of hematoma and femoral neuritis. Femoral blocks or adductor canal blocks (saphenous nerve) may be used for regional anesthesia. General anesthesia is used most commonly and can be combined with regional techniques to enhance postoperative pain control. The patient, the procedure, and the preferences of the anesthesiologist and orthopedic surgeon should all be considered when deciding on the method of anesthesia (Fig. 8.6).

After anesthesia is induced, an examination of the joint in question should be performed in every case and compared with the contralateral side.

Arthroscopic Portals

Portal placement is vital for safe and effective arthroscopy. Knowledge of surface anatomy is key to successful placement of portals. The portals used will depend on the joint undergoing arthroscopy, and their placement also may be varied slightly by the procedure

being performed. For diagnostic arthroscopy, a minimum of an arthroscopic portal and a working portal (for instruments such as the probe) are required. Depending on the procedure, additional accessory portals may be needed. The arthroscope sheath generally is inserted first using a blunt trocar, which is then replaced by the arthroscope. The blunt trocar also may be used to define additional portals prior to their use for the insertion of instruments.

Diagnostic Arthroscopy

One must routinely perform a systematic diagnostic arthroscopy prior to any therapeutic intervention. This allows visualization of the entire joint, giving you a thorough picture of what is normal and what is not. A systematic diagnostic arthroscopy has been described for each joint. This procedure provides confirmation of the preoperative diagnosis and surgical plan, while allowing the opportunity for any required modification. It also minimizes operative time and the incidence of incorrect procedures or missed pathology.

ARTHROSCOPIC COMPLICATIONS

Arthroscopic complications are rare and are usually minor, but they do occur and surgeons and patients should be aware of them. The most critical complication to avoid is wrong side surgery. Preoperative planning and communication with the patient is paramount prior to the operation. Evaluating the patient in the preoperative holding area and marking the correct extremity with patient confirmation can eliminate this error.[22] It is also helpful to have the radiographic images or magnetic resonance imaging available for review in the operating room, which also aids in confirming the correct extremity and planned performed. Careful positioning of the patient for arthroscopy, surgical technique, and a comprehensive knowledge of the anatomy are important to decrease inadvertent damage to extra- and intraarticular structures. A preoperative "time out" should always be performed to verify the correct patient, site of surgery, procedure to be performed, and equipment required and to identify and address any concerns.

Arthroscopic complications can be joint specific. A large cross-sectional study with data taken from the ABOS database looked at the complications and complication rates of knee arthroscopies. They noted 4305 complications out of 92,565 knee arthroscopies (4.7%) from 2003 to 2009. The most common complication was infection, at 0.84%. The highest complication rates at 20.1% and 9.0% were for posterior cruciate ligament (PCL) and ACL reconstructions, respectively. Complications for meniscectomy, meniscal repair, and chondroplasty were 2.8%, 7.6%, and 3.6%, respectively.[32]

In a review of elective shoulder arthroscopies, complications were noted in 93 of 9410 arthroscopies (0.99%). Of those 93 patients, 51 were considered a major morbidity (0.54%) and 42 considered a minor morbidity (0.44%). The most common complication was return to the operating room (29 cases, 0.31%). This was followed by superficial surgical site infection (15 cases, 0.16%), pulmonary embolism (6 cases, 0.06%), deep vein thrombosis (DVT) or thrombophlebitis (8 cases, 0.09%), peripheral nerve injury (1 case, 0.01%), and deep infections (1 case, 0.01%). The risk factors identified for complications included a history of chronic obstructive pulmonary disease (COPD), OR time greater than 1.5 hours, and an American Society of Anesthesiologists (ASA) class 3 or 4 compared with 1 or 2.[33]

Harris et al. performed a systematic review of 92 studies and more than 6000 patients, collecting every reported hip arthroscopy in the literature prior to 2012. There were 512 complications out of 6134 patients (8.3%). The rate of major and minor complications was 0.58% and 7.5%, respectively. Minor complications were attributed to surgeon experience. The most common complications were iatrogenic chondrolabral injury (4.8%) during portal placement and temporary neuropraxia, at less than 1.4% (most commonly pudendal nerve and lateral femoral cutaneous nerve) secondary to prolonged or excess traction. The overall reoperation rate was 6.3% at a mean of 16 months postoperatively for conversion to total hip arthroplasty.[34]

Intraoperative Complications

In general, the most common complication of arthroscopy is damage to intraarticular structures; however, this risk is lessened by the experience and care of the surgeon.[35] The cartilage surfaces of the joint undergoing arthroscopy are the intraarticular structures that are most at risk of complications, with damage being due to instruments or the arthroscope itself. Improper portal placement can also place intraarticular structures at risk during the insertion or removal of instruments or while working within the joint. If a poor portal is increasing the risk of complications, it is advisable to make a new properly placed portal. Working in tight joints or in areas of the joint that are difficult to reach will also place intraarticular structures at risk. The use of a different-angled scope, leverage, or traction to assist with opening the working area may decrease the risk of complications by ensuring appropriate room to manipulate the arthroscope and instruments. It is vital to maintain this working space until both the arthroscope and instruments are safely removed from the compartment in question to ensure that damage is avoided or minimized.

Extraarticular structures are also at risk during arthroscopy and can be a source of severe complications. Nerves and blood vessels are the primary extraarticular concern because they can be injured directly by portal placement or during arthroscopy as a result of their proximity to the work being performed. Similar to intraarticular complications, these complications also can be minimized with anatomic knowledge and appropriate exposure, being mindful of the location of extraarticular structures relative to the intraarticular work during arthroscopy, and using retractors for protection whenever possible. The use of the "nick and spread" method during portal placement will decrease the chance of injury. In this method, the skin alone is cut using a blade, and a hemostat is used to bluntly spread and create a path for insertion of arthroscopic instruments. Using blunt trocars to further define the portal prior to the insertion of instruments also may help protect neurovascular structures from injury. Appropriate articular distension and the avoidance of overly aggressive use of the motorized shaver near extraarticular structures will also minimize the chances of direct injury.

Indirect injury to extraarticular structures can occur as a result of pressure from the use of a tourniquet, fluid extravasation into surrounding tissues, or improper patient positioning. These structures also may be injured by traction that is required during arthroscopy of some joints. To avoid these complications, patients should be positioned with care and bony prominences should be padded, tourniquets should be applied properly and their use minimized (consider deflating them after 90 minutes), and traction should be used with care or avoided if possible. The use of gravity or low pump pressures may help minimize the extravasation of fluid into surrounding tissues, which can rarely cause a compartment syndrome if severe. Tourniquet paresis can be seen postoperatively but typically resolves spontaneously in days.

Instrument breakage can occur during arthroscopic procedures, particularly when instruments are older or used improperly. Small instruments are most likely to break, such as knife blades, or those with mobile parts, such as basket forceps. When an instrument breaks, intraarticular pieces must be removed. To remove the pieces, the outflow should be closed to stop turbulent flow and avoid movement of the broken piece, while maintaining distension of the joint. If the fragment moves and cannot be grasped before it becomes obscured in another part of the joint, radiographs may be useful for localization. For pieces that are difficult to grasp, suction or a magnet may be useful to remove or stabilize the piece so it can be grasped.

Postoperative Complications

The most common postoperative complication of arthroscopy is hemarthrosis,[36,37] although it usually is of little consequence. Although certain arthroscopic procedures are known to be associated with a greater risk for this complication, a persistent or progressive hemarthrosis may require further vascular investigations or clotting studies to determine the cause.

A worrisome and potentially dangerous postoperative complication of arthroscopy is thrombophlebitis. Fortunately, this complication has been shown to be extremely rare in the upper extremity after arthroscopy, and it is uncommon in the lower extremity.[36] Large retrospective studies have demonstrated that the incidence of venous thromboembolism (VTE) after knee arthroscopy is less than 1%.[38] Risk factors for DVT after arthroscopy remain controversial, but it is advisable to minimize both the tourniquet and operative times, mobilize patients postoperatively, and consider prophylaxis in patients who are known to be high risk or immobile.

Surgical infections are a rare but potentially devastating complication, and this is no different for arthroscopy. However, the rate of infection observed after arthroscopic surgery is a fraction of that seen in standard open procedures, likely because of many favorable patient and surgical factors. Arthroscopy typically is performed in young and healthy patients, using small incisions, with extensive irrigation for the majority of the short operative time. When postoperative infection is seen with arthroscopy, it is often in older patients who undergo complex procedures that require significant operative and tourniquet time, or it occurs as a result of breaks in sterile technique or instrument contamination.[39-41] Most infections following arthroscopy are remedied with antibiotics and rarely require irrigation and débridement.

Preoperative prophylactic antibiotic use in arthroscopy remains controversial, and several studies in the last decade have shed light on the subject. Inappropriate use of antibiotics has led to an increase in antibiotic resistance and a rise in *Clostridium difficile* infections. Antibiotic stewardship programs (ASPs) are being implemented nationwide to increase the efficient use of antibiotics. The ASP at NYU Hospital for Joint Diseases recommend that perioperative antimicrobial prophylaxis is not required for arthroscopic surgeries without the use of an implant in patients with any risk factors.[42] Multiple large studies have shown no association between the use of preoperative prophylactic antibiotics and postoperative deep or superficial infection rates.[43,44] However, it may be advisable to consider antibiotic prophylaxis in patients at high risk for infection, such as those with diabetes, immune insufficiency, or skin problems.

Synovial herniation or fistula are both uncommon postoperative complications of arthroscopy. Synovial herniation is due to soft tissue or synovium protruding through the arthroscopic portal. These herniations typically do not require anything more than conservative measures, but they can be excised and closed if they are persistent and symptomatic. A synovial fistula is rarely seen but is thought to result from inadequate or lost closure because of a stitch reaction or abscess. Fistulas are treated with 7 to 10 days of immobilization and are unlikely to cause infection (although antibiotics should be considered) or require an additional procedure for excision and closure.

For a complete list of references, go to ExpertConsult.com.

SELECTED READINGS

Citation:
Chierichini A, Frassanito L, Vergari A, et al. The effect of norepinephrine versus epinephrine in irrigation fluid on the incidence of hypotensive/bradycardic events during arthroscopic rotator cuff repair with interscalene block in the sitting position. *Arthroscopy.* 2015;31(5):800–806.

Level of Evidence:
I

Summary:
A double-blind, prospective, randomized controlled study of 120 patients comparing norepinephrine (0.66 mg/L) versus epinephrine (0.33 mg/L) use in shoulder arthroscopy irrigation fluid to assess the incidence of hypotensive/bradycardic events (HBEs) and efficacy in controlling intraoperative bleeding. Norepinephrine added to the irrigation fluid reduces the incidence of HBEs significantly compared with epinephrine and is as efficacious in controlling intraoperative bleeding thus maintaining clarity of the visual field.

Citation:
Hsiao M, Kusnezov N, Sieg RN, et al. Use of an irrigation pump system in arthroscopic procedures. *Orthopedics.* 2016;39(3):e474–e478.

Level of Evidence:
IV

Summary:
A review of arthroscopic irrigation systems and advancements in pump technology. The recent development of automated inflow and outflow mechanical irrigation pumps shows promising results with consistent flow, greater degree of joint distension, and improved visualization. Preliminary studies also show reduced operative times with automated systems secondary to improved visualization.

Citation:
Jackson RW. A history of arthroscopy. *Arthroscopy.* 2010;26(1):91–103.

Level of Evidence:
IV

Summary:
Professor Takaji from Tokyo is credited with being the first innovator and developer of arthroscopy. Other arthroscopy pioneers such as Dr. Bircher, Dr. Kreuscher, Dr. Burman, and Dr. Watanabe were integral in paving the road for arthroscopy. This paper gives a great historical recollection in the development of arthroscopy for the treatment orthopedic pathology.

Citation:
Kim YS, Lee JY, Yang SC, et al. Comparative study of the influence of room-temperature and warmed fluid irrigation on body temperature in arthroscopic shoulder surgery. *Arthroscopy.* 2009;25(1):24–29.

Level of Evidence:
I

Summary:
A prospective randomized study on 50 patients undergoing shoulder arthroscopy to determine the effect of room temperature versus warmed (37°C to 39°C) irrigation fluid on core body temperature. Hypothermia occurred more often in the room temperature fluid than the warmed fluid. Warmed irrigation fluid decreased perioperative hypothermia, especially in elderly patients.

Citation:
van Montfoort DO, van Kampen PM, Huijsmans PE. Epinephrine diluted saline—Irrigation fluid in arthroscopic shoulder surgery:

a significant improvement of clarity of visual field and shortening of total operation time. A randomized controlled trial. *Arthroscopy*. 2016;32(3):436–444.

Level of Evidence:

I

Summary:

A prospective, randomized, double-blind controlled trial evaluating the effect of epinephrine saline irrigation in shoulder arthroscopy procedures on clarity of view and operating time. Visual clarity was significantly better and total operating time was significantly shorter in the epinephrine group. No effect on the addition of epinephrine was seen on heart rate and blood pressure.

Citation:

Wyatt RWB, Maletis GB, Lyon LL, et al. Efficacy of prophylactic antibiotics in simple knee arthroscopy. *Arthroscopy*. 2017;33(1):157–162.

Level of Evidence:

IV

Summary:

A retrospective study of patients receiving simple knee arthroscopy between 2007 and 2012 to determine the association between the use of preoperative antibiotics and postoperative infection. Of the 40,810 simple arthroscopies, 80% received preoperative antibiotics and 20% did not. Deep infections accounted for 0.08% in the antibiotic group and 0.14% in the no-antibiotic group. Superficial infections accounted for 0.41% in the antibiotic group and 0.40% in the no-antibiotic group. There was no association between preoperative antibiotic use and postoperative deep or superficial infection rates.

Citation:

Zhang Y, Li L, Wang J, et al. Do patients benefit from tourniquet in arthroscopic surgeries of the knee? *Knee Surg Sports Traumatol Arthrosc*. 2013;21:1125–1130.

Level of Evidence:

I

Summary:

A meta-analysis of randomized controlled trials determining whether or not routine use of a tourniquet in knee arthroscopies is beneficial in terms of arthroscopic visualization and operative time. There was no significant difference in visualization or operative time between the tourniquet and nontourniquet group; however, multiple studies suggested that there was less visualization difficulties when a tourniquet was used with ACL surgery.

9

Overview of Sport-Specific Injuries

Jared A. Crasto, Ravi S. Vaswani, Thierry Pauyo, Volker Musahl

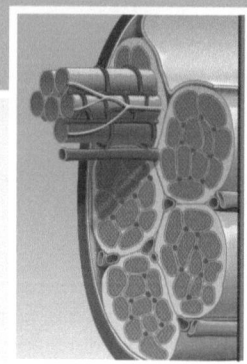

The intricacies of many sports result in patterns of injury that are different compared with those of the general athletic population. It is important that health care providers caring for professional and nonprofessional athletes are familiar with their specific needs to afford accurate recognition and swift treatment. Sports injuries have been well documented in high school and collegiate settings.[1] Overall, injury rates appear to be higher in competition than in practice. While non-time-loss injuries account for more than half of all injuries, the remainder can be devastating to the athlete and difficult to treat. Lower extremity injuries account for about half of all injuries at both the high school and collegiate levels.[1] Ankle sprains are the most common. Though anterior cruciate ligament (ACL) injuries are infrequent (3% of all lower extremity injuries), growing interest exists due to their cause for significant time loss from sport. Upper extremity injuries comprise about one quarter of all injuries at both levels, with shoulder injuries most common. Head and neck injuries are low, about 10% of all sporting-related injuries. Concussions represent 4% to 6% of all injuries, with men's wrestling, hockey, and football; and women's soccer, basketball, and lacrosse causing the vast majority.[1] Of the nearly 12,000 spinal cord injuries per year in the United States, 10% are related to athletic activity.[1] From 1982 to 2013, 2101 catastrophic spinal cord injuries occurred from athletic activity and more than 80% of these injuries occur in high school athletes as compared with collegiate athletes.[1]

Medical issues such as sudden cardiac arrest and death further plague athletes, with a reported incidence of 0.5 to 2.5/100,000 athlete-years.[2] Among collegiate athletes, sudden cardiac arrest was reported in 1:43,770 athletes per year, and 1:3000 athletes per year in African American Division 1 basketball players.[2] Though not commonplace in the United States, across Europe and elsewhere, electrocardiograms (ECGs) are gaining favor in preparticipation athletic evaluations, as it is estimated that over two-thirds of common causes of sudden cardiac death can be detected by ECG.[2]

The continued prevalence of injury and illness in the athletic population elucidates the need for team physicians to be knowledgeable of the issues, to provide the best care to athletes at all levels. This chapter will highlight the common injuries facing many sports in specific, and their potential causes based on each sport.

BASEBALL

Baseball is nicknamed "America's Pastime," which supports its status as the second-most commonly played team sport in the United States, with about 19 million people involved in playing every year.[3,4] It is a ball-and-bat sport played by two teams with nine players on each team. The goal is to score "runs" by hitting a thrown ball and advancing around four bases. The game is broken up into nine sections ("innings"), during which each team has an opportunity to play offense ("at bat") and defense (in the field). Players are categorized by the position they play in the field. The pitcher is the person who throws the ball for the batter from the opposing team to hit. The catcher is the person who receives the ball from the pitcher. Basemen can be first, second, or third basemen, and they predominately position themselves around these bases. The "shortstop" plays between the second and third basemen. Outfielders are deep in the field and play the farthest away from the pitcher. The batter is on the opposite team, and becomes a runner upon successfully hitting the ball and advancing to one of the three bases.

Most baseball injuries are by nonhuman contact (45%) or no contact at all (42%).[5] Contact injuries consist of collisions with high-velocity balls, bats, bases, outfield walls, and the ground. In addition, running, throwing, and pitching can cause acute and overuse injuries.

Pitchers tend to sustain more injuries than other players, with predictable predilection for the upper extremity of course due to their role.[6] The pitching motion is broken up into six phases: wind-up, stride, arm cocking, arm acceleration, arm deceleration, and follow-through.[7] Maximal forces occur in the arm acceleration phase.[8] Studies have demonstrated forces of up to 500 N at the lateral radiocapitellar joint, velocities as high as 7000 degrees per second during the late arm cocking and arm acceleration phases, and an estimated external rotation torque as high as 67 Nm.[9]

Shoulder Injuries

Injuries specific to the thrower's shoulder most commonly involve the labrum and undersurface of the rotator cuff.[9] These injuries can be brought on by tissue changes in both the anterior and posterior glenohumeral capsule, that alter shoulder kinematics.[9] Maximal stress to the rotator cuff is exerted during the follow-through phase of throwing, as the cuff musculature functions to decelerate the arm.[4] Since the superior labrum is the attachment site for the long head of the biceps tendon, repeated traction of the biceps tendon with overhead throwing can also lead to superior labrum anterior to posterior (SLAP) tears.[4]

Elbow Injuries

The throwing motion generates significant valgus stress on the elbow and rapid elbow extension. This combination places tension on the medial structures of the elbow, shear stress on the posterior structures, and compression forces on the lateral structures. The combination of this is described as valgus extension overload syndrome, and is responsible for the pathophysiology of most throwing elbow injuries.[10] Medial epicondylitis is one sequela from the syndrome, in addition to ulnar collateral ligament (UCL) sprain or tear from overuse.[10]

Lower Extremity Injuries

The lower extremity is the most frequently injured body part among fielders. Upper leg muscle and tendon strains are the most common lower extremity injury, with hamstring strains being the most common.[11] Knee ligamentous injuries and ankle and foot sprains make up the other large numbers of lower extremity injuries.[11] Most of these injuries occur during sudden sprints, while sliding, or while manipulating one's body to catch a ball.

Young Athlete Injuries

Almost 5 million children and adolescents participate in baseball every year in the United States.[3] Adolescent pitchers are at particular risk for overuse injuries from throwing.[9] Studies have demonstrated a steady increase in surgical rates for pitching-related injuries in immature throwers.[12] In one study, pitching more than 100 innings per year demonstrated a significantly increased risk of injury in the adolescent population.[12] The elbow is most commonly affected, with a spectrum of pathology that includes an apophysitis or avulsion of the medial epicondyle and osteochondritis desiccans of the capitellum or radial head.[10] In the shoulder, an epiphysiolysis of the proximal humerus may develop.[10] Collectively, these conditions are known as "little leaguer's elbow" and "little leaguer's shoulder." Consensus recommendations include avoiding pitching with arm fatigue/pain, avoiding 80 pitches or more per game (2500 pitches or more per year), avoiding competitive pitching for longer than 8 months per year, and exercising caution and restraint in pitching showcases.[13] In 2008, Little League Baseball guidelines disposed of inning restrictions for pitchers and moved to pitch counts, which were deemed more prognostic from their ongoing studies.[14] Maximum allowable pitch counts per game are as follows: 50 pitches (age 7 to 8), 75 pitches (age 9 to 10), 85 pitches (age 11 to 12), 95 pitches (age 13 to 16), and 105 pitches (age 17 to 18).[14] Depending on the amount of pitches thrown, mandatory rest is enforced as well. For example, if a pitcher aged 15 to 16 pitches 76 or more pitches in a single day, he must take four calendar days of rest before returning to pitching. The guidelines also suggest that youth pitchers take 4 months of rest per year, but this has not been mandated.[14]

Sliding Injuries

In the major league and collegiate levels, sliding injuries are low, accounting for less than 10% of all injuries.[5,6,15] In a study of five seasons of Major League Baseball (MLB) play, an injury occurred in about 3 per 1000 slides.[15] Average time loss was 12.3 days if no surgery was required, and 66.5 days if surgery was required, as was the case in 8.2% of injuries.[15] Interestingly, players were almost four times more likely to be sliding into second base for their injury as compared with any other base.[15] Feet-first slides most commonly caused ankle injury, and head-first slides most commonly caused injury to the hand, fingers, or thumb.[15] At the collegiate level, the overall injury rate from sliding was 9.5 per 1000 slides, with feet-first slides resulting in double the amount of injuries as head-first slides.[16] In stark contrast, sliding injuries may represent as many as 70% of all injuries sustained in recreational baseball and softball.[17] Presently, low-impact or breakaway bases are available, and have been shown to significantly reduce the amount of injury caused by sliding.[15]

BASKETBALL

Basketball is a game played with five players on each team. The object is to score by shooting the ball into a hoop that is mounted 10 feet above the playing surface. The team with the ball is on offense, and the team without the ball is on defense. It is similar to soccer and hockey in that the possession of the ball can change teams rapidly. To advance the ball down the court, it must be dribbled by hand or passed from player to player. The five playing members usually have defined roles: point guard, shooting guard, forward, and center.

Basketball is an inherently vertical sport requiring 35 to 46 jumping and landing activities per game, constant acceleration/decelerations that are multidirectional in nature, and direction changes almost every 2 to 3 seconds.[18,19] It's no surprise these contribute to its status as one of the leading sports causing injury, with an estimated half million physician visits per year.[20-25] Injury rates are reportedly between 7 and 10 per 100,000 athlete exposures.[26] The most commonly reported injuries include ankle sprains, finger sprains/fractures, knee traumatic and overuse injuries, facial lacerations, dental injury, and concussion.[26]

Ankle Sprains

Ankle sprains are the most common diagnosed injury in both male and female basketball players, accounting for 25% of all basketball injuries overall.[27,28] Neuromuscular training and external ankle supports were found effective in significantly reducing ankle sprain incidence.[29] One study estimates that seven basketball players need to undergo neuromuscular training (consisting of a 9 week balance training program) for it to effectively prevent one ankle injury.[30] Ankle braces work by reducing the weight-bearing and non-weight-bearing inversion range of motion (ROM) at the ankle, increasing muscle activation and excitability, and decreasing joint velocity.[31]

Knee Injuries

ACL injuries are common in basketball. Females are two to four times more likely to sustain ACL rupture as compared with males, with a 16% chance of occurring sometime during their career.[32] Neuromuscular training has failed to show any tangible benefit in ACL rupture prevention in the basketball population in specific.[33-35] ACL injury prevention programs are successful in other sports such as soccer, team handball, and volleyball.[34,36]

Tendinitis

The patellar and Achilles tendons are vulnerable to overuse tendinopathies from the repetitive eccentric loading involved in jumping. Patellar tendinitis ("jumper's knee") is the most common overuse injury in basketball.[37] In junior basketball, its prevalence is reported as high as 10%.[37] Risk factors include high jumping, deep knee flexion during landing, and valgus strain during eccentric load phase of landing.[37]

Finger/Hand

Injuries to the hand are very common in basketball.[23,38] Most hand injuries (>90%) involve sprains and volar plate injuries of the proximal interphalangeal (PIP) and metacarpophalangeal joints.[39] Dislocations at the PIP joint are common from direct ball contact with axial load. Players are also at risk for avulsion of the extensor digitorum when the ball creates an axial load through the fingertip ("mallet finger") and avulsion of the flexor digitorum profundus (FDP) when the finger is caught on an opponent's jersey or on the rim during a slam dunk ("jersey finger"). Boutonnière deformity can result from rupture of the extensor tendon central slip; early recognition of this condition is important. Gamekeepers' injuries to the thumb usually occur as a result of a fall to the floor or an extension load to the thumb while blocking an opponent.

Facial/Dental Injury

Facial injuries are more common in male basketball players as compared with female players.[23,38] Dental injuries are composed of fractures, avulsions, and oral lacerations. Ocular trauma is common from contact with opponents' fingers or elbows and can result in corneal abrasions, retinal detachments, hyphemas, lacerations, contusions, and fractures. Nasal fractures may occur, either from a blow by the opponent's elbow or from head-to-head contact.

Concussion

Concussion is common in basketball, particularly during the physical contact of rebounding a ball under the basket. As in other sports a prior history of concussion is a predictor for repeat injury and should be evaluated during preseason examination. Every concussion should be managed on site and have medical clearance before returning to play.[40] Consensus guidelines exist to guide medical staff on recognizing and appropriately managing players with suspected concussion.[40]

Sudden Death

Basketball is a high-intensity sport with moderate static and high dynamic cardiac demands. It is estimated that up to 35% of sudden deaths in sport occur in basketball. The majority of these deaths were classically thought to result from occult hypertrophic cardiomyopathy; however, more recent literature fails to prove this at time of autopsy.[41] Connective tissue disorders such as Marfan syndrome can also induce cardiac abnormalities. With a high preponderance of these disorders in tall people, and the predominantly tall basketball player population, it is important that adequate preparticipation screening with a cardiac-specific history is performed. Twelve-lead ECG and echocardiogram testing may prove useful in the correctly screened population and can potentially detect more than two-thirds of common causes of sudden cardiac death.[2,39]

BOXING

Boxing is one of the most antique Olympic sports dating back to the ancient Greece. It is an individual sport where two pugilists engage in a gloved-fist fight in an enclosed ring. Amateur boxing is an Olympic sport as opposed to professional boxing, which is regulated by four international organizations. A match is usually composed of 3 to 12 rounds that are 3 minutes long, supervised by a referee who ensures the athletes' safety as well as compliance with the rules of the match. The boxing match is won if an opponent is knocked down for a count of 10, if the referee disqualifies a boxer, if he judges that one of the opponent is incapable of protecting himself, or based on the decision of a panel of three judge after all rounds are completed.

Professional Versus Amateur

The majority of the epidemiological study in boxing is done in amateur boxing, where the majority of injuries involves the head and face.[42] Amateur and professional boxing generally share similar rules, including that boxers can only be struck in the face or body; however, the differences in these two types of boxing explain variations in the type of injuries. One of the most obvious differences stems from the protective equipment. Amateur boxers wear protective headgear that shields the head and face from lacerations and orbital fractures.[43] In addition, amateur boxers have limits on the amount of bandage and tape allowed under the boxing glove, which diminishes the weight and momentum of their punches.[44] In professional boxing, there is generally no limit on hand wrapping, and heavier, more protective gloves are worn, increasing the weight and momentum of their punches. There are typically more injuries in competition at both levels because of the desire to maximize the forces of punches.

Facial Injuries

In a retrospective cohort study of competitive amateur boxers, the overall incidence of injuries was 24 for every 100 fights.[42] Injuries including wounds and lacerations to the face and head represented 62% of injuries. In another study of professional boxers, the overall injury rate was 17 per 100 fights, with 51% of injuries involving wounds or lacerations to the face and head.[45] The other injuries evaluated where hand injury and eye and nose injuries. Injuries to the nose are very common often leading to epistaxis often impairing the boxers breathing during a match. The boxers with epistaxis should be evaluated for maxillofacial fractures, septal deviation, and possible septal hematoma.[42,45] Repetitive trauma to the face can also lead to injuries to the eyes and surrounding structures. Soft-tissue injuries to the eyelids can lead to the development of an expanding hematoma an effectively impair the sights of the boxer. Furthermore, direct impact to the eyes can lead to more serious conditions such as retinal detachment and orbital floor fractures. When suspecting a fracture, the evaluation of the athlete for impaired ocular movement, ptosis, and diplopia should be promptly completed.

Upper Extremity Injuries

Injuries to the hand and wrist are the most common musculoskeletal pathology encountered. Injuries to the hand represents 7% of all boxing injuries.[42] In a cohort study of professional boxers, injury rate for hand and wrist injuries in competition was 347 injuries per 1000 hours, while the estimated injury rate in training was less than 1 injuries per 1000 hours.[46] The most common hand injuries observed were carpometacarpal instability and boxer's knuckle (neck of the fifth metacarpal fracture). Other fractures readily seen in the hand are metacarpal shaft fracture, and first metacarpal base fracture (Bennet fracture). Soft-tissue injuries involving the hand and wrist typically involve the scapholunate joint and interphalangeal dislocation. Most of these injuries necessitate a surgical intervention for stabilization. Soft-tissue injuries such as ligament strains are more readily seen than fracture.

Neurologic Injuries

Concussion represents from 10% to 17% of injuries seen in boxing and is the most common neurologic injury encountered.[42] When a boxer is knocked down, there is a brief or prolonged loss of consciousness where the athlete is unable to stand or defend himself. In the majority of cases, the altered mental status lasts for a short period of time. There are cases of more severe trauma to the brain that can lead to death. Subdural hematoma are such cases and should be treated as emergencies.[42] While a boxer can receive more than 100 punches to the head during a boxing match, the repetitive blows to the head through a boxer's career can lead to traumatic encephalopathy. It has been shown that about 17% of boxers can have a central nervous system lesion, which may have been caused by the repeated blow. Other studies have found mid to late stage chronic traumatic encephalopathy in 17% and cerebral or cerebellar atrophy or ventricular enlargement in 50% to 60% of the professional boxers.[47]

AUTO RACING

Auto racing is a popular sport around the world that takes many different forms. In the United States, NASCAR is a popular sport where highly tuned stock cars are raced around an oval track at high speeds. In Europe and other parts of the world, auto racing takes the form of Formula 1, in which drivers of specialized racecars compete to go around a circuit track as quick as possible. Other forms of auto racing include rally car racing, stylistic driving competitions (e.g., drifting), and motorbike racing, each of which requires its own unique set of skills. In general, auto racing is considered a high-risk sport, as collisions can be morbid and fatal. While collisions are fairly common, safety standards have improved to decrease the injuries experienced from them.[48] Drivers also face a number of other injuries associated with the

sport.[49-51] Neck sprains and bruises are the most common injuries, presumably from the whiplash effect of the hard braking required in these sports and from the fact that the helmet increases the weight supported by the neck. Drivers may also experience wrist sprains, ankle sprains, tibia fractures, lumbar spine fractures, and abrasions around the body.[49-51]

FIGURE SKATING

Figure skating is a unique and highly technical sport involving jumps, spins, footwork, dancing, and even acrobatics all on ice skates.[52] There are four disciplines of the sport: singles skating, pair skating, ice dancing, and synchronized skating. The United States Figure Skating Association reports there are 680 skating clubs with more than 196,000 figure skating members in the nation.[53] The judging system tries to be as technical and objective as possible, and is composed of components such as speed of skating, transitions, performance/execution, choreography, amount of ice covered, and height of jumps.[52] Due to the technical demand, figure skaters are susceptible to a number of injuries. Most of these are injuries are due to overuse.[52,53]

Foot Injuries

Figure skates themselves consist of a stiff leather boot and a metal blade. The unique aspects include high heel of the boot—which places the foot into constant slight plantarflexion and the large toe pick on the front of the blade—which is used for some jump take-offs and jump-landings.[53] "Lace bite" is irritation of the tibialis anterior, extensor digitorum, or extensor hallucis longus tendons.[53] This occurs from excessive friction across the tendons, usually from improper placement of the tongue of the skate, and can be mitigated by ensuring proper tongue placement, or using boots with alternative lacing styles. "Pump bump" or Haglund's deformity is a protrusion of the lateral heel.[53] It is caused by an overly wide heel of the boot, allowing the skater's heel to move up and down, and can be mitigated by ensuring optimal boot heel fit. An accessory navicular is present in 4% to 21% of the normal population, excessive friction from a tight boot can make this a symptomatic process.[53] Treatment involves building up the arch of the skate, or having the area of the skate "punched out." Stress fractures can occur most commonly in the first and second metatarsals.[54] They are caused by the force from jump take-offs, especially when engaging the toe pick of the skate. Treatment involves rest, screening for nutritional deficiencies, and in some cases implementing a "jump count" similar to a pitch count for stress injuries to baseball pitchers.[53]

Ankle Injuries

Ankle injuries are the most common in all of figure skating.[55] They are usually sprains and in fact happen more commonly during "dry land" training as opposed to when on ice.[53] Malleolar bursitis can also occur from friction inside of the boot and is more common on the medial side.[53] Padding the affected malleolus or "punching out" the inside of the skate can mitigate the problem. Achilles tendinitis is common from overuse, thought to happen from the repetitive jumps, or compression from the rim of the boot.[53] Treatments include modifying the rim of the boot, rest, ice, stretching, and eccentric strengthening of the posterior leg musculature.

Knee and Hip/Pelvis Injuries

Patellofemoral pain syndrome and patellar tendinitis can occur from jumping. Repetitive falls while learning new jumps and routines can lead to contusions throughout the lower extremity. Meniscus, ligamentous, and fractures of the lower extremity (outside of the foot and ankle) are actually quite rare.[53]

Since many figure skaters will rotate in the same direction when performing jumps, they can develop an asymmetry in strength and flexibility.[53] Triple and quadruple jumps require a large amount of torque to achieve rotation speed commensurate with the jumps, and can lead to iliac crest apophysitis.[54] Since the iliac crest apophysis is one of the last to close (around age 16 in boys, and age 14 in girls), this can be an ongoing source of pain for teenagers.[56]

Back and Upper Extremity Injuries

Arching trunk extension is a common motion in figure skating and can lead to a myriad of back conditions such as spondylosis, spondylolisthesis, lumbar strain, and facet joint pain.[57]

Upper extremity injuries are rare, and occur more in pairs and dance skaters who have a higher risk of collision during practice and warm-ups compared with singles skaters. This can lead to lacerations, fractures, and even head injuries. These skaters also encounter shoulder and wrist problems resulting from the lifting and throwing elements in their discipline. Synchronized skating can be quite dangerous because of the number of skaters on the ice and the tight formations and maneuvers that they perform. A domino effect often occurs when one skater falls, creating a high risk for lacerations, finger amputations, fractures, and head injuries.[58]

AMERICAN FOOTBALL

American football is a sport played between two teams of 11 players (in the United States) or 12 players (in Canada). The objective is to score points by either advancing the ball into the "end zone" of the field or kicking the ball through two raised goal posts. The team with the ball is considered on offense and the team without the ball is on defense. In the United States, the offense has four opportunities to advance the ball at least 10 yards to gain a new set of "downs." In Canada, only three downs are allowed. The goal of the defense is to tackle the player with the ball and bring him to the ground to end a play (or "down"). Unlike basketball or soccer, players typically play only offensive or defensive positions. Each position is highly specialized, with a set of unique injuries that may occur.

American Football carries the highest injury rate of any team sport at all levels of play in the United States.[59] It is the most popular contact sport in North America, with more than 2 million athletes partaking in the sport in the United States alone.[60] Football players are susceptible to noncontact and repetitive stress injuries, and they are of course highly vulnerable to contact injuries. In some cases, as discussed below, football produces more contact-based mechanisms for injuries that in other sports

are commonly borne from noncontact mechanisms. A majority of injuries in football occur in the lower extremity, with a substantial portion of the remainder in the upper extremity. The most common types of injury are sprains and strains (40%), contusions (25%), fractures (10%), dislocations (15%), and concussions (5%).[61]

Head and Neck Injuries

Of most concern in this category are concussions. Concussions occur in an estimated 3 million youth athletes, 1.1 million high school athletes, and 100,000 college athletes each year; however, there is also an estimated 27:1 ratio of underreporting in college football, particularly among offensive linemen.[62] New consensus guidelines exist to guide physicians and other health care providers.[40] Specific guidelines on when to remove athletes from play are critical, as adolescent and young athletes not removed from play have almost a 10-times risk of prolonged recovery as compared with those removed from play.[63] Though our recognition and treatment of concussions have come a long way, the barriers remain underreporting of injury, premature return to play (RTP), and receiving routine rather than individualized treatment.[62]

Cervical spine injuries are uncommon, but a source of catastrophic injury in football. Due to recent rule changes modifying tackling and blocking techniques, the incidence has decreased—particularly the incidence of catastrophic injuries. Cervical spine injuries are composed of a spectrum of ligament and/or soft tissue damage, fractures, and neurologic impairment.[61] Mechanism of injury is typically an axial load applied to a flexed or extended cervical spine.[61] A "stinger" is neurapraxia of the brachial plexus or cervical spine nerve roots. It occurs in 50% to 60% of collegiate football players at some time in their careers.[64] The mechanism is either from neck hyperextension, lateral flexion, and axial load, or from a direct blow to the brachial plexus.[60]

Upper Extremity

Upper extremity injuries are common in football, comprising about 30% of all injuries, with the shoulder affected most commonly.[65] Quarterbacks are most susceptible to shoulder injuries from throwing (overuse) or resulting from tackles while throwing (traumatic).[66] Shoulder injuries include acromioclavicular (AC)/sternoclavicular joint separations, acute rotator cuff injuries, repetitive strain injuries, subluxations/dislocation, and fractures.[66] Wrist sprains are another common injury, resulting from the heavy trauma to the distal upper extremity during tackling, blocking, and maneuvering other players on both offense and defense.[67] Fractures of the forearm and wrist are an additional common injury, usually resulting from impact with the ground while being tackled or with other players.[67]

Lower Extremity

Lower extremity injuries are the most common type of injury in football. Starting in the thigh, muscle strains and contusions are extremely common. Contusions result from direct blows from the helmet, knee, or shoulder and can lead to bleeding within the musculature, swelling, pain, stiffness, and loss of muscle excursion limiting joint motion.[59] Muscle strains are common in muscles crossing two joints, as they experience higher stress during eccentric contraction, with the quadriceps and hamstrings at particular risk.[59]

Ligamentous injuries in the knee are the most common serious injury in football, and additionally the knee is the most common site of season-ending injury.[68,69] Players injure their ACL with a reported incidence of 11 to 18 per 100,000 athlete exposures with increasing incidence at higher levels of play.[70-72] Valgus collapse of the knee is the common mechanism in both contact and noncontact injuries, with a forceful blow causing the former, and usually a sudden deceleration prior to change in direction causing the latter.[73] Though in many sports noncontact ACL injuries are more common, in football contact ACL injuries are in fact more common (55% to 60%).[73] Injury to the medial collateral ligament (MCL) is the most common knee injury at all levels of play, with estimated incidence of 24.2 per 100,000 athlete exposures in high school.[74] In a study examining collegiate athletes presenting to the National Football League (NFL) combine, 23% of offensive linemen had a history of MCL injury.[75] The mechanism (especially in linemen) is thought to be from "chop blocks" and other players "rolling up" on the outside of their legs.[74] Patellar subluxations and dislocations occur in 4.1 per 100,000 athlete exposures in high school.[76] The mechanism is commonly from result of knee flexion with the tibia in a valgus position. Though in general sporting most are from noncontact mechanisms, a majority of football instances (63%) are due to contact, similar to ACL injuries in football players.[76]

Foot and ankle injuries have a reported incidence from 9% to 39%, with as many as 72% of all collegiate players presenting to the NFL combine having a history of foot and ankle injury, and 13% receiving prior surgical treatment.[77] Offensive and "skill position" players are particularly susceptible to foot and ankle injury from high levels of force and torque placed on the distal extremity during running, cutting, and tackling.[75] Lateral ankle sprain is the most common injury.[77] Turf toe is a hyperextension injury and plantar capsule-ligament sprain of the hallux metatarsophalangeal joint and is caused from increasing playing surface hardness and decreasing shoes stiffness.[77] Jones fracture is fracture of the fifth metatarsal at the metadiaphyseal junction, where there is a watershed area of decreased vascularity. The rising rate recently may be due to flexible, narrow cleats that don't provide enough stiffness and lateral support for the fifth metatarsal during running and cutting.[78] Also, lateral overload from baseline cavovarus foot posturing with possible metatarsus adductus and/or skewfoot contributes as well.[78] Most of these are surgically fixed due to a delayed union rate of 25% to 66%, nonunion rate of 7% to 28%, and re-fracture rate of 33% in high-level athletes.[79] Lisfranc injuries are bony or ligamentous damage to the tarsometatarsal joints and occurs commonly from axial loading to a fixed plantar-flexed foot.[77] Noncontact twisting injuries are more common among NFL players, resulting in a purely ligamentous injury.[77] Comparison of weight-bearing radiographs of both feet is crucial to accurate and timely diagnosis.[77]

GOLF

Golf is a sport in which an individual hits a small ball into a hole located hundreds of yards away with a club in as few strokes

as possible. A typical round of golf consists of 9 or 18 such holes of varying distances and topography. Each hole is graded on difficulty with a "par" number, which is the number of strokes it should take a skilled golfer to complete the course. Most holes fall between a 3 and 5 par. A sport requiring fine skill and concentration, golf is popular around the world and is played at all levels from friends engaging in a leisure activity to professional players competing in tournaments. Furthermore, as it is a light aerobic activity, people of nearly all ages can participate.[80]

Injuries in golf are relatively common, as up to 40% of amateur players can experience a golf related injury.[81-83] While golf is not considered a high impact sport, the golf swing is a complex motion that involves the whole body. It requires rapid contraction and coordination of many muscle groups in order to accelerate the club to high velocities.[84] Factors that lead to the majority of golf injuries include poor mechanics, inadequate warm-up,[83] the seasonality of the sport, and occasional trauma. Furthermore, the swing can be performed 50 times or more[84] during a round, and this repetitive motion can lead to a number of injuries commonly seen in golfers.

The most commonly injured areas are the lower back (18.3%), elbow/forearm (17.2%), foot/ankle (12.9%), and the shoulder/upper arm (11.8%). Other rare but serious injuries related to golf cart trauma and environmental exposure can occur.[82,85]

Lower Back Injuries

Low back pain is common among amateur and professional golfers. This can be primarily attributed to the biomechanics of the golf swing, which has evolved with changes in club technology to produce higher club head velocity at impact. The modern swing emphasizes greater rotation of the thorax through an arc of about 120 degrees. This places the vertebral column in a hyperextended position during the follow through phase of the swing and leads to large lateral flexion and anteroposterior forces on the lumbar spine.[84,85] In addition, microtrauma to the hip leads to joint contractures and loss of rotation. Therefore, in order to adequately rotate the pelvis and torso for the swing, many golfers need to rotate the lumbar spine past its native rotational capacity. This leads to repetitive microtrauma, which predisposes golfers to paraspinal muscular strains, intervertebral disc herniation, and facet joint arthropathy. In concordance with these findings, most golfers report low back pain primarily during the follow-through phase and radiographs show more degenerative changes in lumbar facets of golfers compared with controls.[81,82,84] Other contributors to low back pain can include carrying heavy bags and frequent bending on the course.[83,86] Finally, many golfers with low back pain can rely on other muscle groups, such as the abdominal musculature, to achieve the same rotation, which can predispose these areas to overuse injuries as well.[84]

Elbow/Forearm Injuries

Injuries to the elbow and forearm are the second most common in golfers after low back injuries.[80,82] "Golfer's elbow" is the term applied to medial epicondylitis, which typically occurs when the golf club strikes the ground forcefully during the downswing. This traumatic injury typically occurs in players with poor swing mechanics.[85,87] Lateral epicondylitis, on the other hand, is typically an overuse injury due to repetitive forceful forearm extension along with twisting and is actually five times more common than "golfer's elbow."[85,87] Other potential elbow injuries include ulnar neuritis and medial epicondyle avulsion fractures.[87]

Shoulder Injuries

The shoulder is next most common area of upper extremity injury. The lead shoulder (left in a right-handed golfer) is the most commonly affected side.[80,88] The rotator cuff is active with elevating the club above the head for the address phase of the swing, and players can experience symptoms of subacromial impingement with this activity. Pain from the AC joint can also manifest during this phase of the swing, especially during maximal cross body adduction when forces along the AC joint are greatest.[88] In order to generate more power during the downswing phase of the swing, many golfers will rotate their shoulder joint as much as possible, which can lead to microtrauma to the joint capsule and labrum, leading to symptoms of glenohumeral instability. Posterior instability is more common than anterior, and many golfers will have a positive load and shift test on exam. SLAP tears and biceps pathology are also possible, but less common than other true overhead sports.[80,84,85,88]

Wrist/Hand Injuries

Wrist and hand injuries can be traumatic or due to chronic overuse. Instability of the extensor carpi ulnaris tendon can result with forceful striking of the club into the ground during the downswing. Patients will complain of a snapping sensation on the ulnar side of their wrist. Hook of the hamate fractures can occur with traumatic strike of the club and typically occur in the lead hand. Patients will experience tenderness at the hook with gripping the club and may have ulnar paresthesia symptoms.[80,81,85,89] Chronic overuse injuries include triangular fibrocartilage complex (TFCC) tears, triquetro-hamate impingement, pisotriquetral arthritis, and ulnar styloid impingement. These injuries occur due to the excessive ulnar deviation and wrist extension during the golf swing. They can be difficult to differentiate without advanced imaging, as they all present with ulnar-sided wrist pain and tenderness and pain with gripping the golf club.[89]

GYMNASTICS

Gymnastics is an Olympic sport that has more than 5 million participants per year in the United States.[90] While more than 75% of participants are female, the men and women athletes participate in different events.[91] The women participate in four categories: vault, uneven parallel bars, floor, and beam performance. The men participate in six events: vault, parallel bars, high bar, ring, floor, and pommel horse. As in other sports discussed in this chapter, gymnasts are subjected to a higher frequency of injury in competition than in practice.[91] An observational study of collegiate athletes found that female gymnasts are twice more likely to sustain an injury during competition than in training.[90] Furthermore, the same study found that the majority of injuries were lower extremity injuries sustained during the vault or floor

exercises.[90] While events such as the vault are proponents of lower extremity injuries because of one acute landing following an acrobatic jumping maneuver, the floor exercise possess an increased risk with the sheer number of landings during a normal routine. Other events such as the parallel bar (uneven and even) and the rings place the upper extremities at risk with placing the shoulder in vulnerable position with swings, handstands, and isometric contractions; moreover, the constant release and regrasp of the bars adds to the complexity of the routine and increases exposure to injury. Of note, the majority of athletes participating in gymnastics are skeletally immature children and thus they are subject to injuries to their growth plates. The gymnast wrist is the most frequent injury encountered in the growing child. It entails an injury to the distal radial physis secondary to the repetitive stress from the axial loads to the hand and wrist. It has been reported that gymnast wrist has an incidence of 1.9 to 2.7 injuries per 100 participants per season.[92]

Lower Extremity Injuries

The most common injury encountered in gymnastics is during landing and therefore involves the lower extremity. This type of injury represents around 69% of all gymnastic injuries.[91] The technical complexity of landing, coupled with the high energy of an acute landing, place the lower extremity at high risk of injury. While ankle sprains are the most frequent injury encountered, injuries to the knee come second including those involving the anterior cruciate or collateral ligaments.[90] The repetitive bounding and landing place the foot at risk of overuse injuries such as calcaneal apophysitis, sesamoiditis, planter fasciitis, and stress fracture. Furthermore, the routines are executed barefoot, and that places the foot at risk for nerve entrapment syndrome.[90] The pathology of the knee is due to overuse and can lead to chronic injuries of the knee including patellofemoral syndrome, patellar tendonitis, and Osgood-Schlatter disease in addition to acute injuries of the cruciate and collateral ligaments.

Upper Extremity Injuries

Musculoskeletal injuries to the upper extremities are readily seen both in male and female gymnasts. In males they are the most common injury and more often involve the glenohumeral joint.[93] In females, the upper extremity is the second most common site of injury and most often involves the wrist and elbow.[93] The glenohumeral joint pathology includes dislocation and labral tearing from instability. These athletes are often hyperlax and vulnerable to shoulder instability. Other pathology in the shoulder are rotator cuff tendinosis from overuse and rotator cuff impingement.[90,93] The injuries to the wrist and elbow include fracture of the long bones, collateral ligament injuries, and overuse injuries to the apophysis and ligaments.

Back and Pelvis Injuries

Lastly, lumbar spine pathology is often encountered in gymnasts with the repetitive jumps and landing during the majority of the events. There is a prevalence of 25% to 85% of lower back pain ranging from strains, herniated discs, to spondylosis and stress fractures due to flexion and hyperextension of the back. The treating physician should be aware of stress fracture that may mimic an array of injuries and should investigate menses history and eating habits.

ICE HOCKEY

Ice hockey is a sport practiced on a sheet of ice, which is surrounded by a perimeter of boards and glass. It is a rectangular surface with rounder corners and its dimensions may vary depending the geographical location. In North America, the surface is smaller with dimensions of 200 ft × 85 ft (61 m × 26 m)[94] compared with the wider international dimensions of 200 ft × 98 ft (61 m × 30 m).[95] The game is played with each team having six players on the ice at a given time, which comprise of three forwards, two defensemen, and one goaltender. An ice hockey game is played with three 20-minute periods where players compete to shoot a rubber puck with a stick into the opponent's net in order to score points. A team typically has 20 players on the bench with forwards and defensemen alternating on ice play every minute and each team with goaltenders playing the entire game.

The game of hockey is played worldwide by youth and adults alike and is sanctioned as a Winter Olympic sport. The rules of ice hockey differ between males and females in that body checking is not permitted in women's hockey.[96] The age where body checking is allowed in men's hockey varies depending on regional regulation. A recent youth hockey study found a threefold increased risk of all game-related injuries in youth hockey where body checking was allowed.[97] The players wear full body protective equipment along with skates with metal blades, which enable them to glide on the ice surface. The protective equipment is similar across women's and men's hockey with the exception of facial protection. Females and under-18-year-old males must wear full-facial protection, but men over 18 can wear partial-facial protection or no facial protection in certain professional leagues.[98] The injuries encountered in ice hockey are predicated around the following: it is a contact sport, players can move as fast as 45 km per hour and shoot the puck as fast as 190 km per hour, and players use a metal composite stick while wearing skates with sharp metal blades.

Head Injuries

While players wear head protective gear, concussions are readily encountered in this fast-paced contact sport where players are often hit while in vulnerable positions. Concussions are the most common injury encountered, with head and neck injuries representing between 20% and 30% of all injuries.[99] Facial laceration, contusions, and maxillofacial injuries are seen when full-facial protective equipment is not mandated or when fighting is allowed.[100] The incidence of concussion ranges from 0.2/1000 to 6.5/1000 game-hours and 0.72/1000 to 1.81/1000 athlete-exposures, and is estimated at 0.1/1000 practice-hours.[101] The injury prevention efforts surrounding concussion has been the subject of many changes by the regulating bodies of ice hockey. To this effect, injury prevention efforts have been successful in focusing on improved and proper use of equipment,[102,103] changes of on-ice rules,[104,105] and educational prevention programs.[103,105] The injuries preventions education program has drastically affected the incidence of spinal injuries when body checking an opponent from behind is banned.[106] Furthermore, the risk of concussion was significantly lower if games were played on rinks with flexible boards and glass.[98]

Upper Extremity Injuries

The upper extremities injuries represent around 8% to 20% of all injuries, with the majority involving glenohumeral dislocation and AC dislocations.[107] Since ice hockey is performed with a hockey stick and is sometimes used to stop or prevent an opponent from progressing, it also inflicts a significant amount of trauma to the upper extremities. Fractures around the hand and wrist are inflicted either by contact with a stick or with a puck, even with adequate protection because of the high velocity generated. Lastly, players can sustain rib fractures and contusion from contact with the boards after receiving a body check from an opponent.

Lower Extremity Injuries

Injuries to the lower extremities represent between 20% and 30% of injuries in ice hockey.[107] There is a constellation of hip injuries that are specifically encountered in ice hockey.[108] These include extraarticular injuries such as hip adductor, flexor muscles strain, hip pointers, and also core muscle injury. Intraarticular injuries such as acetabular labral tears and femoral impingements are also prevalent in this athletic population.[108] Furthermore, fractures of the proximal femur or the long bone and contusion of large muscles groups are also encountered in light of the collision nature of the sport. The injuries involving the knee include the meniscus and most frequently the MCL. Lastly, high ankle sprain and fracture around the foot and ankles are often encountered from receiving a high velocity shot. The blade of the hockey skate can often inflict significant trauma to the blood vessels or traumatic laceration to the soft tissue such as the Achilles tendon. Furthermore, there are documented tracheal injuries from players receiving the puck in the neck area.

TEAM HANDBALL

Team handball is played on an indoor court with a layout similar to a soccer field. There are two goals, one on either end. Two teams compete, with seven on each team, composed of one goalie and six court players.[109] The object of the game is to score by throwing the ball into the goal of the opposing team. Players can dribble the ball or pass similar to basketball, and are only allowed to take three steps with the ball in hand otherwise.

Handball is one of the Olympic sports with the highest risk of injury.[110,111] The game is characterized by high playing tempo, rapid changes in movement, jumps with hard landings, frequent contact/collision between players, and repetitive knee and shoulder joint stress.[112] The overall incidence of injury is about 104 to 108 injuries per 1000 player-hours, or about 1.5 injuries per match.[113] In surveillance at the world championship in 2015, 27% of players suffered at least one injury.[113] A majority of injuries occur during match play. Also a majority are in the lower extremity (58%), as compared with the upper extremity (17%), head/face (13%), and torso (12%).[113] Most injuries were classified as contusions (39%)—especially to the face, thigh, knee, and lower back—followed by ligament sprains (24%), and muscle strains (13%), especially to the thigh and groin areas.[113] Most injuries were a result of contact between players (61%), with less occurring due to noncontact trauma (16%), or overuse (12%).[113]

Shoulder Injuries

Shoulder injuries comprise a substantial portion of all injuries in handball. Shoulder pain is most common in senior handball, with a prevalence estimated at 19% to 36% at season start, and a weekly prevalence of 28% during the season.[114] The prevalence in the elite adolescent population is lower (about 14%, or 1.4 per 1000 player-hours); however, 80% of these involve the dominant (throwing) arm.[115] A significant risk factor is a large increase in playing load of 60%, conferring a hazard ratio of 1.91 in this population versus those with a decrease or small-to-moderate increase in load.[115] This is also exacerbated by reduced shoulder external rotation strength and scapular dyskinesis.[115]

Facial/Dental Injuries

Facial trauma in handball is caused mainly by blows to the facial area with hands or elbows during collisions between players due to the high-speed and physical style of play.[116] In addition, some injuries are caused by being hit by the ball at close range.[117] Most nondental facial injuries are lacerations (19%), followed by nose injuries (18%), and eye and periorbital injuries (16%).[118] Dental injuries account for 22% of facial injuries, consisting mostly of socket bleeding, tooth fracture, tooth avulsion, and tooth luxation.[118] Dental injuries in handball carry a 76% complication rate, most commonly resulting in tooth color change, pulp necrosis or infection, and potentially culminating in tooth loss.[118] Mouthguards have been demonstrated to significantly reduce dental injuries and decrease jaw fracture risk.[118] Though the American Dental Association has classified handball as a sport requiring use of mouthguards, use is still rare.[119]

LACROSSE

Field lacrosse is played on an outdoor field setup similar to a hockey rink. There are two goals, one on either end, and space behind the goal is utilized as well. Two teams compete, with 10 on each team, composed of one goalie, three defensive players, three midfielders, and three offensive players. The offensive and defensive players from each team must remain in their respective areas, while the midfielders are allowed to freely traverse both sides of the field.[120] The object of the game is to score by launching the ball from the lacrosse stick into the goal. Players can advance the ball by passing it in the air or on the ground to their teammates, or can "cradle" the ball in their stick and run with it. The game is played for a set amount of time, after which the winner is the team with more points.

Men's and women's lacrosse are the two fastest growing contact sports in the United States.[121] The National Collegiate Athletic Association (NCAA) has noted a constant increase in varsity men's programs in the past decade from 211 schools and 7103 student-athletes in 2003 to 2004 to 350 schools and 13,165 student-athletes in 2014 to 2015.[122] The injury rate is 5.29 per 1000 athlete-exposures, just over half of which are time-loss injuries.[121] The lower extremity is most commonly injured (58%)—especially involving the knee.[121] The upper extremity is also commonly involved (21%)—with the arm/elbow causing the highest proportion of non–time-loss injuries.[121] The trunk (11%) and head/neck (9%) are less frequently involved.[121] The most common injury types are sprains (25%), strains (25%), and contusions (17%).[121] Contact-related mechanisms accounted for 50% of injuries, with noncontact (36%) and overuse (11%) contributing to a lesser extent.[121] The top three specific injuries include ankle sprains, knee internal derangement injuries, and concussions.[40,121,123]

Ankle Injuries

Ankle injuries are typically caused from noncontact cutting, dodging, or torsional activities.[124] Fortunately, these injuries are typically not very severe, and confer no significant time loss or complications in most cases. Prevention strategies are being developed; presently they include evaluation for preexisting ankle instability during the preparticipation examination, complete rehabilitation and recovery following injury, and taping/bracing to protect the athlete from further injury in addition to adequate rehabilitation.[124]

Knee Injuries

Knee internal derangements, specifically ACL injuries, are a common injury in lacrosse.[124] These injuries are typically caused from noncontact, cutting, and pivoting, causing indirect injury to the knee.[124] Since these injuries are often severe and result in significant time loss from sport, injury prevention strategies and programs are being developed. These incorporate balance training, plyometrics, strengthening, and feedback to alter biomechanical and neuromuscular contributing factors.[124,125]

Concussions

Lacrosse carries the fourth and third highest rates for concussions at the collegiate level in men's and women's sports, respectively.[126,127] Concussions are most commonly caused by player-to-player contact in men's games and from incidental contact with the lacrosse stick in women's games.[124] Management is comprehensive, and includes preseason planning, education, and initial evaluation. This is then compared with postconcussion assessment and disposition. From this, RTP decisions can be made more appropriately and accurately, to achieve an optimal long-term neurological outcome. Baseline assessments are becoming a crucial factor in the above protocol.[128] A study utilizing a nonhelmeted mastoid-patch accelerometer to collect head impact data demonstrated fortunately that a vast majority of head impacts in lacrosse do not result in concussion.[126] However, the authors note that the hypothesized short- and long-term detrimental effects of "subconcussion" on brain function and structure, coupled with their proposed role in increasing susceptibility to neurodegenerative disorders, suggest that quantification of "subconcussion" in sport may be more important in the future.[126]

ROWING

Rowing is a competitive sport that has been practiced for centuries and was one of the inaugural Olympic sports. It is practiced by amateurs and professionals, and is a popular collegiate sport as well. Rowing is an aerobic and anaerobic exercise with great cardiovascular benefits. Competitive rowing is divided into sculling, which is the use of two oars, and sweep rowing, in which athletes use one oar on opposite sides to propel the boat. Training is typically done on an ergometer, which is a stationary rowing machine.[129]

Understanding the rowing stroke is paramount to proper understanding of the injuries that can occur in this sport. The first phase is the drive in which the athlete is in the "catch position" where the arms are extended, and the trunk and the knees are flexed. As the oar is lowered into the water, force is applied through the body from the feet through extension of the knee and then extension of the trunk to drive the oar forward. This phase finishes with flexion of the arms to propel the boat forward. Next is the recovery phase, in which the oar is extracted from the water and rotated ("feathered") so it is parallel to the ground. In reverse order from the drive, arms extend, the trunk flexes, and the knees flex. Injuries typically occur from overuse and overtraining on the ergometer.[130]

Lumbar Spine Injuries

Low back pain is the most common musculoskeletal complaint among rowers with up to 53% of athletes with this complaint.[131,132] The rowing stroke requires lumbar spine hyperflexion and twisting forces with transmission of up to 4.6 times the rower's mass in compressive load. The repetitive nature of rowing combined with excessive training can lead to fatigue, impaired muscle contractility, impaired proprioception, and altered kinematics, all of which increase the risk of muscular or ligamentous strain in the lumbar spine.[130] Furthermore, the cyclical compressive loading can lead to disc herniation, facet capsule strain, and even end plate compression fractures. Studies have also shown a higher risk of lumbar spine spondylolysis among rowers compared with the general population, likely due to the rotational forces seen.[129,131]

Chest Injuries

Rib stress injuries are a relatively common injury with an incidence of up to 9% and are responsible for most of the missed time for athletes.[129,132] Ribs 5 to 9 are most commonly involved, and the mechanism is thought to be an imbalance between microtrauma from repetitive forceful muscle contraction and ability of the bone to remodel and heal in response to this stress. The exact mechanism is unknown, but several theories have been postulated, including opposing forces of the serratus anterior and external oblique muscles and ribcage compression during force transmission to the oar.[130] Costochondritis and intercostal muscular strains can also occur, typically due to the oar striking the thorax at the end of the stroke.[130]

Upper Extremity Injuries

Shoulder injuries occur from altered glenohumeral mechanics. The humeral head can be anteriorly shifted, the posterior capsule may be tight, the latissimus dorsi may be tight as well, and the rotator cuff muscles can become weak. The combination of these changes can lead to symptoms of impingement and instability. Sweep rowers experience unilateral shoulder pain on the lead side.[130] Wrist and forearm injuries typically arise from improper mechanics, excessive wrist motion during feathering the oar, tight grip, or use of the elbow rather than the shoulder to initiate drive phase of the stroke. Injuries include exertional compartment syndrome, De Quervain's tenosynovitis, intersection syndrome, and lateral epicondylitis. "Sculler's thumb" is a rowing specific injury in which improper feathering using the thumb leads to hypertrophy of the extensor pollicis brevis and abductor pollicis longus causing compression of the underlying radial extensor tendons.[129,130]

Knee Injuries

Knee pain is common complaint among rowers.[132] However, as rowing is not a weight-bearing activity and does not involve pivoting, acute ligamentous and meniscal injuries are typically not seen. Patellofemoral syndrome accounts for the majority of knee pain in this population. During the rowing stroke, the knee goes through the full ROM. The rower starts with the knee in full deep flexion when the patellofemoral joint experiences high compressive loads. As the knee is extended, patellar maltracking can occur due to valgus position of the knee during the drive phase. The combination of these two can lead to chronic patellofemoral pain.[130] Some rowers can experience lateral knee pain from iliotibial (IT) band syndrome as the IT band moves across the lateral femoral condyle in a repetitive fashion.[129,130]

RUGBY

Rugby is a form of football where two teams of 13 or 15 players attempt to score a touchdown by carrying or kicking the ball downfield. Players are able to pass the ball either sideways or backwards to each other. Positions include forwards, whose role it is to contest the ball, and backs, whose role it is to carry the ball and score touchdowns. A certain number of passes is allowed before the other team is granted the ball and a chance to score. The teams can fight over possession during a "scrum," which occurs after each play stoppage. After a tackle, teammates protect the ball by forming a platform, which the opposite team attempts to break. Unlike American football, players only wear shoulder and chest pads and scrum caps.[133]

Due to the large amount of collisions and relatively little protective gear, musculoskeletal injuries are relatively common in rugby. Most injuries are acute and occur in the lower extremity. Forwards also experience more injuries than backs. In the lower extremity, the knee is the most common location, and MCL sprains/tears are the most common. ACL tears represent a serious injury, causing players to miss a significant amount of time. Backs are at higher risk for hamstring injuries, as they need to sprint and stop quickly during the game.[134]

Shoulder injuries can occur from direct contact with other players, especially during a scrum. AC joint injuries are the most common, but some players can experience traumatic shoulder dislocations, which are more serious.[135-137]

During the scrum, players are at risk for spinal injuries. With their heads flexed, an axial load can lead to a cervical spine injury. The hooker is the player at the tip of the pyramid, a position that puts him at higher risk for cervical spine injuries. These players typically have their arms wrapped around other adjacent players in the scrum, so they are less able to shift their body and shield themselves from damaging their C spines. Lumbar spine injuries are also possible, but occur more in the training season as an overuse injury rather than an acute traumatic one.[133,134]

Head injuries are also seen in rugby players. Given the physical and sometimes violent nature of the sport, players put themselves at higher risk for closed head injuries. While headgear can protect against serious head injuries, they have not been shown to prevent the most common mild injuries.[138]

RUNNING

Running is a very common activity that has been shown to provide significant cardiovascular health benefits. Practiced at a wide variety of levels, running can be a leisurely activity or highly competitive sport. Running encompasses many different forms of activity, including endurance running in marathons, sprinting, and hurdling, each of which requires a different set of skills and has different associated injuries.[139] Lower extremity injuries, as expected, account for the grand majority of complaints in runners and are typically chronic overuse type injuries. Acute injuries can occur in runners, but are much less common than in other sports.[140] Running injuries are complex, and significant sex differences exist. Risk factors for injuries in runners include little running experience and running distances greater than 32 km/week.[141]

The knee is the most common site of injury, accounting for up to 50% of running injuries. Patellofemoral pain is the most common knee injury followed by IT band syndrome, and meniscal injuries. Females tend to have higher rates of patellofemoral knee pain, while males tend to have more meniscal injuries.[140,141]

Overuse injuries can occur below the knee as well and include Achilles tendinopathy, medial tibial stress syndrome, exertional compartment syndrome, and plantar fasciitis. Thin (BMI <21 kg/m^2) runners with poor nutrition can have metatarsal stress fractures as well. Blisters can also develop in areas of high friction.[139,140]

More serious injuries related to the environment can occur as well. Marathon runners can experience heatstroke and dehydration. Running in extreme cold temperatures can lead to frostbite or hypothermia.[139]

SKIING AND SNOWBOARDING

Skiing

Skiing is a popular sport and leisure activity across the world with an estimated 200 million skiers. Skiers place long thin boards on their feet to allow them to slide down a mountainside. Shifting the person's weight on the skis allows them to turn. They use poles to help keep balance and push off at the start. In the most common competition, downhill skiers attempt to navigate a course on the mountainside formed by poles in the least amount of time. Other forms exist as well, such as cross-country skiing and high jump. Advances in ski technology as well as course maintenance have allowed skiers to go faster and have increased the popularity of the sport, but also increased the resultant incidence of injury.[142]

Knee Injuries

Knee injuries account for a large proportion of all skiing injuries due to the high rates of speeds and failure of the boot bindings to release, leading to a rotational force on the knee.[143] Isolated MCL sprains are the most common injury, but ACL tears are the most significant. Downhill skiing has one of the highest rates of ACL tears, matching that of American football. Skiers can also have associated knee injuries along with ACL tears, including MCL and meniscal tears. Female skiers, as in other sports with high rates of ACL injuries, have significantly higher rates of ACL tears than males.[143] Prevention strategies have been implemented, such as improved equipment and educating skiers on the common mechanisms of ACL tears and how to position themselves appropriately in those situations. Other acute injuries can occur as well, such as isolated meniscal tears. PCL injuries and tibial plateau fractures are generally rare in skiing.[142,143]

Shoulder and Thumb Injuries

The most common upper extremity injury in skiing is "skier's thumb," which is a sprain of the thumb UCL at the metacarpophalangeal joint.[142] Shoulder injuries are also relatively common in skiing and occur primarily due to axial load from falling on to the extremity, but can also occur through direct trauma to the shoulder or from wrist straps on the poles, which can force the shoulder into abduction and external rotation. The commonly seen shoulder injuries include rotator cuff strains, glenohumeral dislocations, AC separations, and clavicular fractures.[144]

Other Skiing Injuries

The "boot top" fracture is a tibia/fibula fracture that is less common now with higher boots that have release bindings. Other sprains, fractures, and lacerations have been reported, but are less common in skiing.[142,144]

Snowboarding

Compared with skiing, snowboarding is a younger sport with a smaller but still sizable number of participants. Competition in snowboarding is similar to that in skiing, but snowboarders also participate in style events such as the halfpipe, in which aerobatic maneuvers are judged on execution and style. These events require high jumps and put snowboarders at elevated risk for higher energy mechanism injuries.[144]

Upper Extremity Injuries

In contrast to skiing, upper extremity injuries are more common in snowboarding. This is due to the fact that snowboarders tend to fall more often and without poles they then use their outstretched hands to break their fall.[145] Furthermore, the boots worn are fixed to the board and are nonreleasable, so there is less lower extremity movement than in skiing. Wrist injuries include distal radius fractures, carpal fractures, sprains, and contusions. Shoulder injuries include glenohumeral dislocations, clavicle fractures, AC separations, rotator cuff tears, and proximal humerus fractures.[142,144,145]

Lower Extremity Injuries

While lower extremity injuries are less common than upper extremity, there has been an increasing incidence of them due to advances in equipment and courses that allow snowboarders to go faster, thus leading to higher energy injuries. These injuries tend to occur more often in the lead extremity.[145] Ankle injuries are the most common, and fractures about the ankle are also the most common lower extremity fracture. An injury specific to snowboarding is the "snowboarder's ankle" or a fracture of the lateral process of the talus. These are relatively rare injuries but are important, as they are often missed on plain X-rays and often misdiagnosed as ankle sprains. Knee injuries are much less common in snowboarding compared with skiing and often occur when only one foot is attached to the board.[142,145]

Injuries in Both Skiing and Snowboarding

Experienced skiers and snowboarders may attempt to traverse steeper slopes and unchartered courses, which can put them at higher risk for head and spinal injuries, which are less common than other sports but are a cause of significant morbidity. Recent high-profile cases have shed light on the dangers of skiing at high speeds. Skiers and snowboarders can collide with various obstacles along the course such as trees, rocks, pylons, and lifts. Helmets are now commonplace on ski slopes. They may also fall onto their backs or necks leading to spinal injuries.[142]

SOCCER

The sport of soccer, also known as football for the rest of the world, is the most widely practiced sport worldwide. In Europe alone, there are more than 20 million licensed soccer players.[146] Both female and male players participate in this sport, which is sanctioned by the Olympic program. Soccer is played either indoors, or more traditionally, outdoors. The outdoors field dimensions range from 64 to 75 m long by 100 to 110 m wide, and at the adult level, it is played with a circular ball around 22 cm in diameter. The two opposing teams have 12 players on the field, including a goaltender on each end of the field. The game is played with two 45 minutes halves of running time where the opposing team competes to score the most goals by using any part of the body except the upper extremities. Soccer is classified as a collision sport; however, body checking is not permitted. The players are permitted to challenge the opponent while jumping for headers or by slide tackles targeted at the ball. During a professional soccer game, it is estimated that a player will run an average of 10 kilometers. While it is considered an aerobic sport, the frequent stop and go and sprints bring the average intensity of close to the anaerobic threshold with heart rate reaching 80% to 90% of its maximum.[147]

The incidence of soccer injuries has been widely studied in professional and nonprofessional athletes in virtually all continents of the world. In a cohort study of eleven professional clubs in five European countries, the mean injury incidence was 9.4 injuries per 1000 hours, with 30.5 injuries per 1000 match hours

and 5.8 injuries per 1000 training hours.[146] The risk of injury during matches can be eight times greater than in practice.[146,148] Men and women have the same incidence of injuries with an increased in injury rate with age.[148,149] Another variable that influences the incidence of injury is the type of surface of the soccer field. While earlier studies had shown an increased in injuries on artificial turf field, recent studies comparing newer artificial turf with natural turf have not shown any differences. The majority of injuries are traumatic in nature, where 41% are caused by contact and 59% are cause by noncontact mechanism.[150] Furthermore, 25% of injuries that occur during matches are directly caused by foul play.[146]

Lower Extremity Injuries

In soccer, the overall majority of injuries affect the lower extremity. In a cohort study of a professional European soccer team, Walden et al. found that 85% of injuries were located in the lower extremity, where the most common type of injury was thigh strain.[146] Hamstring strain was more prevalent than quadriceps strain, followed adductor muscles strain. About 50% of the ligament sprains were located in the ankle and 40% in the knee. The most common knee ligament injured was the MCL.[146] Other injuries encountered in the knee ACL tear, meniscus tear, and patellofemoral syndrome. ACL tears account for 14% of injuries in soccer.[151] There are differences in the rate of ACL injuries based on sex. Recent studies have estimated that women are six times more likely to sustain an ACL tear in a noncontract mechanism than men.[151] Since soccer is mainly played with the feet, there is a wide array of different mechanisms that create foot and ankle trauma. Low and high ankle sprains can occur when the foot is planted and subjected to axial load with external rotation, or while the player is landing from a header. While ankle strains are the most prevalent pathology of the foot and ankle, fractures and stress fractures are often encountered. Furthermore, overused tendinopathy of the Achilles tendon is also observed frequently.

Upper Extremity Injuries

Upper extremity injuries are more frequent in youths than in adults. These injuries can include fractures of the arm, wrist, hand, and clavicle. Specific to youth are the apophyseal disorders that can include Osgood-Schlatter disease; Sever disease; Sinding-Larsen-Johansson disease; and apophysitis of the anterior superior iliac spine, anterior inferior iliac spine, and iliac crest of the pelvis. Acute avulsion fractures to apophyses (anterior inferior iliac spine, tibial tuberosity, and lesser trochanter) can occur, along with growth plate fractures.

Concussions

Concussions can represent up to 9% of injuries and are caused by collisions between players while jumping for headers, or when the head strikes the ground or objects like the soccer ball or the goal post. The remaining head and neck injuries are typical of sports where accidental collision is frequently encountered. Maxillofacial injuries such as fracture, laceration, contusions, and abrasion are sustained due to the lack of facial protective equipment. The U.S. Soccer Federation released concussion guidelines in 2016 to reduce risk especially in the youth population. These guidelines prohibit heading the ball for children age 10 and younger, and limit the amount of heading permissible in practice for children between the ages of 11 and 13.[152]

Young Athlete Injuries

Youth soccer also involves specific type of injures. Fracture involving the growth plates, along with avulsion fractures of the apophysis, is encountered. Furthermore, overuse injuries can affect the youth soccer player with pathologies such as jumper's knee, Osgood-Schlatter, or patellofemoral chondrosis or low back pain from spondylolisthesis. As in other sports, educational injury prevention programs have been efficient in decreasing the incidence of injury. These programs often target neuromuscular training and functional dynamic strengthening of core muscle strength.[151] The Federation Internationale de Football Association (FIFA) 11+ is a program that was effective at reducing the incidence of ACLs per year in youth female soccer with neuromuscular training and strengthening exercises.[153]

SWIMMING

Swimming is a popular sport enjoyed by all generations and all levels, from recreation to fitness to competition. Though the buoyant effect of water seems to protect swimmers from impact-type injuries, injuries still occur from overuse, repetitive strain, and microtrauma mechanisms.[154] Competitive swimmers at a club level may swim about 10 km/week, whereas elite international competitors may swim upward of 100 km/week.[155] In a NCAA survey, elite swimmer injury rates were about 4 per 1000 hours of training.[156] The difference between swimming and most other sports is that the propulsion or advancement through the water is generated from the upper extremity more than the lower extremity.[155] Not surprisingly, the most common injury is to the upper extremity—specifically to the shoulder as the keystone of the upper extremity conveying the propulsive force.

Shoulder Injuries

Shoulder injuries are the most common swimming injury, with a reported prevalence of 40% to 91%.[157] Elite swimmers may swim more than 9 miles per day, which translates to more than 2500 shoulder revolutions.[155] "Swimmer's shoulder" was initially described as anterior shoulder pain during and after workouts, and its cause postulated to be from impingement of the rotator cuff tendons under the coracoacromial arch (outlet impingement).[158] However, it became evident that swimmers have multiple factors contributing to their shoulder pain, and "swimmer's shoulder" is now a catchall term for any shoulder pain in a swimmer. The mechanisms driving this shoulder pain include poor stroke biomechanics; overuse and fatigue of muscles of the shoulder, scapula, and upper back; and glenohumeral laxity with subsequent shoulder instability.[157]

Knee Injuries

Knee injuries are the second-most common injury in swimming. "Swimmer's knee" is an equally ambiguous term as "swimmer's shoulder," coined for any knee pain in a swimmer. Its reported prevalence ranges from 34% to 86%.[157] It also goes by "breaststroker's knee," indicating its high prevalence in this group; in fact breaststrokers are five times more likely to have "swimmer's knee" as compared with all other swimmers.[159] Breaststroke imparts a high valgus load to the knee secondary to an adducted hip position. The valgus strain placed on the MCL of the knee is further exacerbated during the "whip kick." Affected swimmers present with medial-sided knee pain, either along the length or insertions of the MCL or overlying the pes tendons and/or bursa. Of note, the "flutter kick" of the freestyle swimmers involves much less coronal plane strain, resulting in a 10-times lower risk of developing "swimmer's knee" as compared with breaststrokers.[159] However, the repetitive "flutter kick" can lead to increased patellofemoral contact stresses from the forceful and repetitive quadriceps contractions, resulting in anterior knee pain. The incidence of knee pain in freestyle swimmers is still low despite this.

Back Injuries

All swimming strokes maintain hyperextension of the lower back to achieve a streamlined position; this is exaggerated in the "undulating" style of breaststroke and butterfly, making these swimmers at high risk for spondylolysis and possible spondylolisthesis.[160] It is estimated that the prevalence of low back pain in breaststroke swimmers is 22% to 47% and in butterfly swimmers is 33% to 50%.[161]

TENNIS

Tennis is a sport in which a racket is used to hit a small ball across a net with the goal of keeping the ball within the court lines during back-and-forth rallies until either player hits the ball out of the court lines or into the net. It is the most popular racquet sport and is a very popular activity worldwide. It is practiced as a leisure activity as well as a professional sport. A tennis match can be contested either between two individuals ("singles") or between two groups of two athletes ("doubles").

Biomechanically, the racquet strokes in tennis involve muscles in the whole body, which allows the generation of high racquet head velocities. The serve is an important part of the game and can be thought of as a kinetic chain that starts from the feet and transmits force through the whole body into the racquet. Large loads are generated especially at the elbow and shoulder joints, which helps explain the pattern of injuries commonly seen.[162]

Injuries in tennis can be to either the lower or upper extremity. Lower extremity injuries tend to be more acute in nature, while upper extremity injuries tend to be chronic overuse injuries.[163]

Lower Extremity Injuries

Ankle injuries tend to be the most common in the lower extremity due to the rapid change of direction required during rallies. Different playing surfaces also likely place different strains on the ankle, but these differences have not been explored in the literature. Ankle ligament sprains resulting from inversion mechanisms are the most common acute injury.[162,163] Players may also develop peroneal subluxation, as the peroneal muscles are the primary restraint to ankle inversion and thus the tendon sheath can become weak with repetitive inversion forces. Other ankle injuries include anterior impingement, subtalar instability, and osteochondral lesions. Hip injuries can also occur as the serve and stroke require forceful hip rotation to generate sufficient power. Muscle and ligament strains are the most common, and other less common injuries include labrum tears and posterior impingement. Repetitive and forceful acceleration can lead to Achilles tendon, gastrocnemius, and hamstring tears. Common knee injuries include patellar tendinitis and patellofemoral syndrome. Other injuries include plantar fasciitis, stress fractures, and tennis toe (repetitive impact of second and third toes on the shoe).[162,163]

Upper Extremity Injuries

As tennis is an overhead racquet sport, upper extremity injuries are quite common. Lateral epicondylitis or "tennis elbow" occurs from the torque generated at the racquet, which leads to microtrauma at the extensor tendon insertion. Vibrations from the ball hitting the strings are also transmitted to the forearm and contribute to this microtrauma. Advances in technology have made racquets lighter, allowing higher velocities during the tennis swing and as a result higher torque and vibrations transmitted to the forearm.[162] Other common elbow injuries include flexor-pronator tendinitis, medial epicondylitis, ulnar neuritis, and posterior impingement. Shoulder injuries are also relatively common. The injuries with the highest incidence include glenohumeral internal rotation deficit (GIRD), rotator cuff tears, and SLAP tears.[163] Wrist injuries include extensor carpi ulnaris tendinitis and subluxation. Players often complain of ulnar-sided wrist pain.[164]

Low Back Injuries

Low back pain is a frequent complaint among tennis players. The lumbar spine is subjected to considerable axial load and torque during the tennis serve and swing. These repetitive motions can fatigue the ligaments and muscles around the lumbar spine, leading to sprains and tears. Rotational forces and hyperextension of the lumbar spine can also lead to intervertebral disk degeneration and degenerative disk disease.[162]

VOLLEYBALL

Volleyball is a sport that typically takes two forms: court and beach. In court volleyball, two teams of six players play on a court separated by a high center net. One player serves the ball from one end of the court over the net to the other team to start the rally. The goal is to keep the ball from hitting the ground and using only the player's arms/hands to propel the ball and create shots. Players on the receiving team may "bump" the ball over the net or "set" the ball up for a teammate with a high bounce so that he/she may "spike" the ball downward with increased force. Other ways to hit the ball are to "dig" the ball up just before it hits the floor and to "block" the ball at the net before it crosses over. The team that allows ball to hit the ground on their side of the net, hits the ball out of the court, or hits the ball more than three times loses the point.[165]

Beach volleyball has the same basic rules as the court variety, but is played on a sand court outdoors. The teams also consist of only two players. There also other rule differences between the two types of volleyball, but they share the same shots and the same point structure. Both beach and court volleyball are practiced at a variety of levels, including at high-level professional and Olympic events.[165]

The characteristics of volleyball play require high jumping and using the whole upper extremity in an arc motion to accelerate the ball to high velocities. Therefore injuries can be seen to both the upper and lower extremity in players.[165,166] While injuries in volleyball are less common than those in contact sports such as football, the incidence of injuries has been increasing, likely due to an increase in the number of amateur players.[167] Injury patterns differ between beach and court volleyball. Beach volleyball players experience more overuse injuries, whereas court volleyball players have a higher incidence of acute injuries.[165]

Ankle Injuries

Ankle sprains are the most common acute injury in volleyball players, with studies estimating an incidence of up to 40% of all injuries. Sprains typically occur when a player jumps and lands with his/her foot on the foot of another player, leading to an inversion injury. These injuries occur more frequently in court volleyball due to the higher number of players on the court and the hard surface they play on.[166-169] Prevention strategies that have been shown to decrease the incidence and recurrence of ankle sprains include rule changes, improved landing techniques, neuromuscular training, and the use of ankle braces and taping.[168,169]

The repetitive jumping and landing in volleyball can also lead to Achilles tendinitis in the acute setting and tendinosis, typically in older players as an overuse injury. Players will complain of tenderness and crepitus about the Achilles tendon.[165-167]

Knee Injuries

The most common knee injury seen is patellar tendinopathy, which results from the explosive jumping. Some studies have estimated the incidence of acute patellar tendinitis to be about 40%. Overuse tendinopathy or "jumper's knee" can occur due to the deep flexion angle of the knee that players experience while jumping and landing.[166,170,171] Beach volleyball players experience less patellar tendon pathology than court volleyball players, likely due to the differences in playing surfaces.[165]

ACL tears are less common in volleyball compared with other sports such as basketball, but are more serious than other injuries. The mechanism for ACL tears is similar to other sports. Players may land awkwardly or pivot while landing, which can lead to a large valgus moment and eccentric loading of the knee. In general, players with ACL tears are unable to continue playing and have to miss a significant amount of time to undergo ACL reconstruction. Many athletes are unable to return to their previous level of play.[165,168]

Finger/Wrist Injuries

The high velocity of the ball can lead to many acute and chronic injuries of the fingers and wrist, especially in blockers who attempt to stop the ball with their hands as it crosses the net. The axial and hyperextension load of the ball can lead to finger fractures and IP joint dislocations. Displaced fractures or irreducible dislocations require a referral to an orthopedic surgeon for evaluation. Soft tissue injuries can also occur including volar plate injuries, jersey fingers (distal interphalangeal [DIP] joint hyperextension leading to FDP injury), and ligamentous injury to the PIP joint. Thumb radial collateral and UCL damage can also occur when the thumb is forced into abduction during blocking or falling to the ground. Falling on the outstretched hand while attempting to perform a "dig" can lead to hook of the hamate fractures.[165,167,172]

While returning the serve, the ball repetitively hits the volar aspect of the wrist. This microtrauma can lead to De Quervain's tenosynovitis, inflammation of the first dorsal compartment of the wrist.[165]

Shoulder Injuries

The glenohumeral joint involves a large humeral head articulating with a relatively small glenoid. This gives it a large ROM, but also makes it an inherently unstable joint. The ligaments, rotator cuff muscles, and capsule of the shoulder work together to provide stability to the joint in normal daily activities. During the volleyball serve and spike, the shoulder is brought into the extremes of this ROM, and the resultant microtrauma with each swing leads to damage of these elements and resultant shoulder pain. The arm swing involves three phases: cocking, acceleration, and deceleration. The initial cocking phase places the arm in the extremes of external rotation and extension, which can lever the humeral head anteriorly.[167,171,173] The rotator cuff normally prevents subluxation or dislocation of the humeral head, but with repeated swings, overuse of the rotator cuff can lead to strains and tears of the cuff muscles and tendon. This position of the humeral head can also lead to tearing of the labrum or inferior glenohumeral ligament, or internal impingement. Shoulder dislocations can occur as well, typically when the player attempts a "dig" and lands on an outstretched hand.[165,172]

Suprascapular nerve palsy is also fairly common, with many volleyball players complaining of periscapular pain and weakness. Various theories exist as to the etiology. The nerve can become entrapped in the spinoglenoid notch by a ganglion, which can develop after a labral tear. Another theory postulates that the extreme ranges of motion cause traction on the nerve, and with the repeated swings, a nerve palsy develops.[165,167,170]

GIRD may also develop from repetitive arm swings. The posterior capsule becomes tightened in order to prevent anterior subluxation of the humeral head, restricting the ability of the glenohumeral joint to internally rotate.[165]

Back Pain

Low back pain can occur in volleyball players when the spine is repetitively flexed and rotated during the swing. The force is primarily transmitted through the pars interarticularis and stress reactions can occur. Players typically complain of back pain localized to the facet joints. Although not common, bilateral pars defects can lead to spondylolisthesis with possible neurologic deficits, which require a surgical consultation. Disc pathology is also less common, but can occur due to the repeated spine flexion.[165,166,172]

Concussion

Concussions are less common in volleyball compared with collision sport athletes, but have been reported in the pediatric age group. These injuries typically occur from collision of the player's head with the pole or ground. Preventative measures have not been studied in the literature.[165]

WRESTLING

Wrestling is the world's oldest sport, boasting hand-to-hand combat with the ultimate goal of pinning the opponent's back to the mat. Points are awarded for moves that gain control over the opponent, or bring him closer to being pinned on his back. Two main styles exist internationally: Freestyle and Greco-Roman. The main difference between these is that in Greco-Roman, attacks to the legs are prohibited, encouraging upper body maneuvers, such as headlocks, throws, and suplexes. In the United States, Folkstyle is the main style contested in the youth, high school, and collegiate levels. In Folkstyle there are no additional points awarded for throws as compared with traditional takedowns, additionally there are no points for quickly exposing the opponents back, only for holding the opponent on their back in a controlled fashion. These differences de-incentivize wrestlers to perform more dangerous moves allowed and rewarded in the international styles, which thus lessens the overall injury incidence in Folkstyle wrestling.[174] Nevertheless, injury rates in high school are reportedly 2.33 to 2.50 per 1000 athlete exposures.[175] Injury rates increase in college to 7.25 per 1000 athlete exposures.[174] In the 2008 Beijing Olympics, 9.3% of wrestlers participating in the event sustained an injury.[176] Since both wrestlers are on their feet and more mobile in the neutral position, the majority (39% to 42%) of injuries occur in this position.[174]

Musculoskeletal Injuries

The shoulder is the most commonly injured upper extremity joint, followed by the elbow and wrist. Shoulder injuries make up the most (18% to 24%) single joint injury in high school wrestlers.[174] Subluxation and dislocations are common and often precipitated by extreme forward flexion, abduction, and external rotation occurring either actively or passively.[174] These events can be associated with rotator cuff strain or labral tear, predisposing the wrestler to subsequent recurrent injury with less force. One study found that wrestlers with generalized ligamentous laxity experienced half the number of injury as those without, postulating that a "stiff" shoulder is injured more commonly than a lax shoulder.[177]

The elbow is commonly injured when a defensive wrestler is being returned to the mat from a standing position, falling onto an outstretched arm while catching himself. Dislocations in this setting are common, with most (80%) being posterior and having significant disruptions of supporting ligaments.[174]

Wrist and hand sprains are common with either the hand or wrist becoming caught on an opponent or the mat during various attack and evasive maneuvers. Finger dislocations are especially common.[174] If dislocated in the coronal plane, then one or both collaterals are damaged, and if in the sagittal plane, then the volar plate is likely injured.[178] The PIP joint is the most common finger joint to be dislocated.

The knee is the most commonly injured lower extremity joint, followed by the ankle. Sprains to collateral ligaments, especially the MCL are common. These are precipitated by various defensive maneuvers during takedown from neutral position, as well as self-imposed valgus loads to the knee when a defensive wrestler is slowly standing against an offensive wrestler's force. Meniscal injuries are also common, as significant force is often encountered across an unstable knee in a flexed position from driving into an opponent, or standing up against significant resistance. Pre-patellar bursitis can also develop from repetitive trauma of a wrestler striking their own knee on the mat during takedowns, and maneuvering defensive positions. A small percentage of these will go on to infectious bursitis and can cause time loss from sport. Ankle ligament sprains also occur frequently.

Cervical spine injury is usually noncatastrophic, and composed mainly of cervical strains and sprains, though fractures and other trauma can occur.[174] These are precipitated by defensive techniques and counter moves. Catastrophic injuries are rare, but tend to occur more so at the high school level.[179] Catastrophic injuries occur almost exclusively when wrestlers are in the neutral position, during takedown maneuvers.

Head injuries can result from collision with an opponent's head, knee, elbow, or the mat. Concussion is the primary form of head injuries seen in wrestlers. It should be recognized and treated as with other sports, with swift recognition and removal from further participation crucial and the responsibility of the covering health care provider.

Soft Tissue Injuries

Lacerations are common in wrestling from contact with opponents' head, elbow, knee, and/or fingers/nails. The eyebrow is a common site for laceration, and though different methods exist to quickly stop the bleeding to allow the match to continue, the best is to suture the area when time permits.[174]

Auricular hematoma (or "cauliflower ear") is very common in wrestlers. The process involves blunt trauma to the ear, causing an accumulation of blood in the subperichondrial space, resulting in hematoma formation.[180] This interrupts the blood supply to the cartilage, and if the hematoma is not removed, the cartilage will ultimately die. Subsequently, new abnormal cartilage forms with fibrosis, resulting in the typical "cauliflower" deformity.

Epistaxis is the most common cause of bleeding in wrestling. The dry winter air during the season makes nasal mucosa more friable and prone to bleeding. The most common site is Kies-selbach's plexus.[174] As with lacerations above, it is important for the bleeding to be controlled quickly to minimize match delay, which in some cases can lead to disqualification. Application of cotton rolls can keep pressure on the area during the match, and vasoconstrictive sprays are helpful after the match.

Skin Infections

Skin infections are the most common condition for wrestlers seeking medical attention, and the single condition accounting for the most time loss from practice and competition.[181] The primary risk factors are localized breakdown in the natural skin barrier from repetitive trauma and exposure to skin pathogens. Herpes simplex virus has a predilection for the head, neck, and face, which suggests that skin-to-skin contact between wrestlers is a major vehicle for transmission. In examining skin conditions preventing wrestlers from participating in competition, 45% were due to herpetic whitlow, 25% from bacterial infections, and 22% from fungal infections.[174] It is important to wrestlers frequently self-inspect as early detection can minimize time loss, spread to other wrestlers, and duration of infection.[174]

Weight-Loss-Related Issues

Wrestlers commonly reduce their weight to gain a strength advantage wrestling at a lower weight class. Wrestlers will not lose the weight and maintain throughout the season, however, but will instead cycle their weight 5 to 10 lbs. in a single week before competition.[182] Depending on the season, this could translate to gaining and losing that amount of weight 10 to 30 times per season. The common techniques utilized are sweating and fluid or caloric restriction. Sweating is induced by exercise in hot environments with excessive clothing or impermeable suits. Less commonly used methods include consumption of diuretics or laxatives, and self-induced vomiting. In the fall of 1997, three collegiate wrestlers died within a 5-week period from rapid intentional weight loss.[183] Since this unfortunate event, wrestling governing bodies have implemented regulations of weight loss to mitigate the growing problem. Wrestlers are prohibited from cutting weight below a level of 5% body fat in college or 7% body fat in high school. In addition, certification in the beginning of the season involves hydration testing and body fat calculations, if over the aforementioned minimums, wrestlers are allowed to reduce their weight by 1.5% per week to reach their final weight. In addition, weigh-ins are held usually within 1 hour of the start of competition, and not the night before competition.

For a complete list of references, go to ExpertConsult.com.

SELECTED READINGS

Citation:
McCrory P, Meeuwisse W, Dvorak J, et al. Consensus statement on concussion in sport–the 5th international conference on concussion in sport held in Berlin, October 2016. *Br J Sports Med.* 2017.

Level of Evidence:
V

Summary:
This article is the most recent consensus statement on the diagnosis and management of sports-related concussions. They cleverly institute 11 Rs to cover all aspects of the paper: Recognize, Remove, Re-evaluate, Rest, Rehabilitation, Refer, Recover, Return to sport, Reconsider, Residual effects and sequelae, Reduction.

Citation:
Kinsella SD, Thomas SJ, Huffman GR, et al. The thrower's shoulder. *Orthop Clin North Am.* 2014;45(3):387–401.

Level of Evidence:

I

Summary:

This article represents a concise review of the thrower's shoulder. Many aspects of shoulder pain in throwing athletes can be understood better from knowing about the phases of throwing, the different muscle groups involved, and where poor mechanics may start to cause pathology.

Citation:

Dines JS, Bedi A, Williams PN, et al. Tennis injuries: epidemiology, pathophysiology, and treatment. *J Am Acad Orthop Surg*. 2015;23(3):181–189.

Level of Evidence:

I

Summary:

This article reviews common injuries sustained by tennis players. The authors begin by discussing the tennis serve and stroke including the biomechanics and kinetic chain that are used as the basis to explain the mechanisms of injury. They also discuss the advances in equipment that have changed the patterns of injury seen. Each area of the body is then discussed and the epidemiology and mechanisms of injury are reviewed.

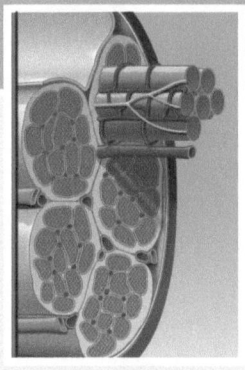

10

Commonly Encountered Fractures in Sports Medicine

Christopher Kim, Scott G. Kaar

Almost any type of fracture can occur during athletic activities. This is because of the many different types of sports and the corresponding situations in which athletes are found. All athletes undertake various fracture risks with participation. Many of these specific fractures are covered in detail in other chapters. This chapter focuses on certain specific fractures and their management, particularly on stress fractures in various bones in the extremities and spine. Also discussed are some of the more commonly seen acute fractures in sports, such as clavicular and rib fractures. Returning an injured athlete to practice and competition, whether a recreational or an organized sport, is an issue specific to athletes. Return to participation guidelines are addressed and guidance for practicing sports medicine clinicians is offered further on.

STRESS FRACTURES

Stress fractures are commonly seen in athletes and in the military, particularly in trainees. They are seen in as many as 20% of military trainees[1] and in up to 20% of individuals presenting to a sports medicine clinic.[2] History of a prior bone stress injury is the strongest predictor of a new injury.[3,4] Athletes are susceptible to developing stress fractures because they are often exposed to repetitive high-intensity, load-bearing activities in both training and competition. This overuse leads to microdamage to the involved bone that is not repaired by normal bone homeostasis. These microcracks accumulate and lead to fatigue failure and eventually a visible fracture line can be seen on imaging.[5] Stress injuries occur on a continuum from an asymptomatic stress reaction visible only on magnetic resonance imaging (MRI) as edema, to a symptomatic fracture line visible on imaging, to a chronic nonunion. Unfortunately physical exam including the use of a tuning fork and ultrasound are of little use for diagnosing a stress fractures.[6] Both bone scan and MRI are commonly used for imaging diagnosis, although MRI is more useful; it involves comparatively less radiation and testing time, fewer false positives, and better correlation with return to participation.[7,8] A recently proposed classification system (Table 10.1) has been found to have high intra- and interobserver reliability and was also found to be easily remembered.[9]

Certain bone locations are more susceptible to stress injuries. Slower bone remodeling occurs in cortical bone; therefore cortical regions are more likely to sustain stress fractures. On the other hand, cancellous bone has a higher turnover and is susceptible to altered homeostasis from poor bone quality (i.e., osteoporosis). Typically cancellous bone stress injuries occur in athletes with low bone mineral density (BMD). Furthermore, the location of the fracture within the bone can be predictive of healing potential. Injuries on the compression side of a bone are likely to do well with nonoperative management. Those that occur on the tension side of a bone are inherently unstable and may require surgery to heal.[5] Some specific bone locations, such as the fifth metatarsal and navicular, are also predisposed to stress injury due to poor vascularity. These watershed areas are likely less able to respond to mechanical stress with an appropriate and robust healing response.[10]

Female Athlete Triad

Female sex is the most important predictor of stress fracture in endurance athletes. Long-distance running, in particular, poses the highest risk; it can predispose to stress fractures by itself. However, associated nutrition and menstrual irregularities are likely major contributors to injury. Lower levels of estrogen in the amenorrheic female athlete may be due to lower levels of gonadotropins. A relative lack of estrogen disrupts the normal bone turnover response to repetitive stress.[5]

The female athlete triad involves low energy availability, menstrual dysfunction, and low BMD. Early intervention is important to prevent the development of eating disorders, amenorrhea, and osteoporosis. Cardiovascular health as well as endocrine, gastrointestinal, renal, and neuropsychiatric health can also be affected.[11] There is evidence that athletic performance may worsen in athletes with triad symptoms.[12] Athletes can be stratified as at low, moderate, and high risk based on specific criteria involving the presence of a dietary restriction, low body mass index (BMI), delayed onset of menarche, other menstrual abnormalities, low Z score on Dexa scan, and the presence of a bone stress injury.[11] Female athletes who fall into the moderate- and high-risk categories are two and four times more likely to develop a bone stress injury.[13]

Biomechanical Factors

Biomechanical factors may also be associated with stress fracture risk. Interestingly, ground reactive forces do not seem to be different between uninjured and injured athletes.[14] Increased lower body muscle mass may help to absorb forces during running. Athletes with smaller calf girth and less lower limb muscle mass have a higher risk of injury. Lower extremity limb alignment

Grade	Pain	Radiographic Findings (CT, MRI, Bone Scan, or Radiography)	Description
I	No	Imaging evidence of stress fracture, no fracture line	Asymptomatic stress reaction
II	Yes	Imaging evidence of stress fracture, no fracture line	Symptomatic stress reaction
III	Yes	Nondisplaced fracture line	Nondisplaced fracture
IV	Yes	Displaced fracture (≥ 2 mm)	Displaced fracture
V	Yes	Nonunion	Nonunion

TABLE 10.1   **Stress Fracture Classification System**

CT, Computed tomography; *MRI*, magnetic resonance imaging. From Kaeding CC, Miller T. The comprehensive description of stress fractures: a new classification system. *J Bone Joint Surg Am.* 2013;95:1214–1220.

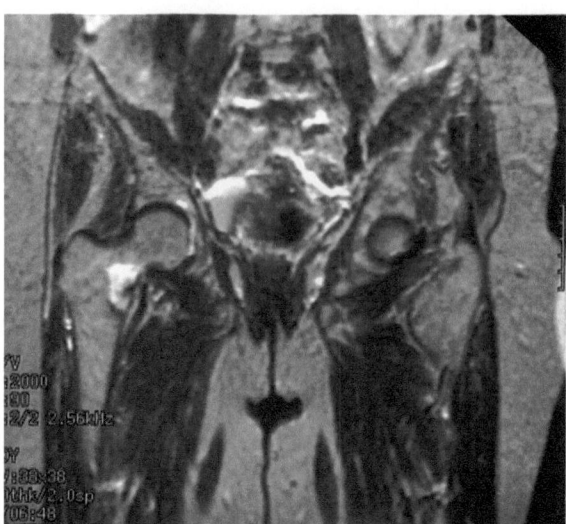

Fig. 10.1 A T2-weighted magnetic resonance image showing a medial femoral neck stress fracture. (From Canale ST, Beaty JH. *Campbell's Operative Orthopaedics.* Philadelphia: Mosby; 2008.)

may matter as well. A quadriceps angle greater than 15 degrees is related to a higher risk of stress fractures. Also, leg-length discrepancies are related to injury risk in runners.[5] There may be a training adaptation period during which an athlete or military recruit is at increased risk of stress fracture. After this period, the stress injury risk may decrease.[1]

Fatigue and Training Errors

There is some association between athlete fatigue and changes in loading patterns in the lower extremity. This may place a fatigued athlete at higher risk of fracture. Changes in training regimen, such as sudden increases in running mileage, are also risk factors for injury.[15] Running in a fatigued state may lead to greater lower extremity mechanical forces.[16-18]

Nutrition

Nutrition and diet influence the development of stress injuries. Higher dairy and calcium intake results in fewer stress fractures.[3,19,20] Also, a higher intake of calcium may have a protective effect when taken in doses of 1500 to 2000 mg/d.[5,20-23] Both vitamin D intake and vitamin D levels are lower in athletes who develop stress fractures and are inversely correlated with the risk of developing a stress fracture in both the adolescent and adult population.[24-27]

Genetic Factors

Some recent data support a genetic predisposition to the development of stress injuries. The RANK pathway has been implicated in distance athletes.[28] The androgen receptor gene CAG allele distribution is different among military recruits with bone stress injuries versus those without injury.[29] The *CALCR* and *VDR* genes may also confer a risk for stress fracture.[30] Other gene sequences have been implicated as well.[31,32] To date, however, no clear cause-and-effect relationship has been determined.

The following sections focus on the specific stress fractures most commonly seen in athletes. Risk factors for injury, recommended diagnostic workup, treatment strategies, and in some cases prevention are discussed.

Femoral Neck Stress Fractures

A femoral neck stress fracture can be devastating to an athlete and the long-term health of his or her hip. Care should be taken to avoid missing a rare presentation in children.[33] Fractures cause anterior groin pain of insidious onset that is worse with weight bearing. Fractures can be bilateral even with unilateral groin pain.[34] A missed stress fracture can lead to displacement and the development of femoral head avascular necrosis (AVN). These fractures are described in long-distance runners and military recruits, specifically those with lower levels of fitness at the start of training.[35] Internal forces in the femur are concentrated along the femoral neck with running,[36] and there may be a genetic predisposition to the development of femoral neck stress fractures.[31] Additionally there is an association of femoroacetabular impingement, specifically acetabular overcoverage or retroversion, with the development of femoral neck stress fractures.[37-39]

Athletes with groin pain should undergo a standard hip radiographic series. If no fracture is visualized on radiographs, then an MRI can serve to evaluate the femoral neck in more detail (Fig. 10.1). Most fractures are first diagnosed on MRI, and an abbreviated MRI sequence is effective.[40] A bone scan positive on all three phases also indicates a stress fracture, and a single photon emission computed tomography (SPECT) scan has improved diagnostic accuracy.[41] However, lack of anatomic detail limits its usefulness for treatment planning. Fractures can be classified based on whether they are nondisplaced or displaced, complete or incomplete, tension side or compression side. These characteristics have implications for recommended treatment.

Displaced fractures require urgent treatment, as they are typically seen in younger patients in their 20s and 30s. Open reduction and internal fixation is required, with a goal of restoring function and decreasing the chance of developing AVN and secondary osteoarthritis. Treatment of nondisplaced fractures depends on fracture location and the extent of involvement of the femoral neck. Fractures that are incomplete and involve only the compression side (medial aspect) of the femoral neck can be treated nonoperatively with an extended period of non–weight bearing (Fig. 10.2). Time to return to running for compression-sided injuries increases with the severity of injury as seen on MRI. This ranged from 7.5 weeks for low-grade injuries seen only as edema without a visible fracture line to 17.5 weeks when a fracture line is visible.[7]

Fractures that involve the tension side (lateral aspect) of the femoral neck are typically treated surgically (Fig. 10.3). Percutaneous internal fixation is achieved with cannulated screws to prevent varus displacement. Of note, there is no correlation between the femoral neck shaft angle and the outcome of femoral neck stress fracture treatment.[42] Postoperatively these patients

are also treated with an extended period of non–weight bearing. Both nonoperatively and operatively treated patients require an extended period of time for rehabilitation and return to running as well as other high-impact athletic activities. It is important to gradually increase loading during the rehabilitation process so as to be sure that the femoral neck is healed and able to handle the required stresses.

Tibia Stress Fractures

Tibia stress fractures are the most common stress injuries in endurance athletes.[43] Athletes place significantly more load on the tibia while running than while walking.[44,45] It is unclear if mechanical factors alone can account for tibia stress fractures; overall bone health along with other factors likely play an important role.[46] Running speed has been correlated with risk of tibial stress fracture.[47] Although such fractures are not as devastating as some other lower extremity stress injuries, they can lead to prolonged time off from running and impact activities.

Running athletes, including military trainees, who experience focal tibial pain with impact exercise should be evaluated for a tibial stress fracture. Patients who have such fractures are tender focally over the location of the fracture. Provocative maneuvers such as hopping on the injured leg and using the leg as a fulcrum may cause pain. A stress fracture can be distinguished from medial tibial stress syndrome (MTSS) by the focal nature of the fracture compared with the classic diffuse area of tenderness in MTSS.[43] Radiographs are often negative, although the presence of the "dreaded black line" is a poor prognostic indicator for fracture healing with nonoperative treatment. In most cases this represents a chronic fracture nonunion. Stress injuries not visible on radiographs can be imaged with MRI. Bone scan is used less commonly for reasons listed previously.

Tibial stress fractures are most commonly located posteromedially on the compression side of the proximal tibia. Fractures can also occur on the tension side, and these are seen along the anterior cortex of the midshaft of the tibia. Those fractures occurring on the compression side of the tibia can be treated

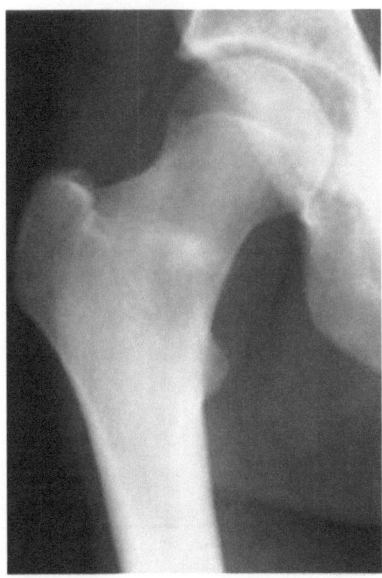

Fig. 10.2 An anteroposterior radiograph of the proximal femur showing a compression-side femoral neck fatigue fracture. Periosteal new bone formation is present in the inferior femoral neck, and healing endosteal callus formation is present in the inferior half of the femoral neck. (From Shin AY, Gillingham BL. Fatigue fractures of the femoral neck in athletes. *J Am Acad Orthop Surg.* 1997;5:293–302.)

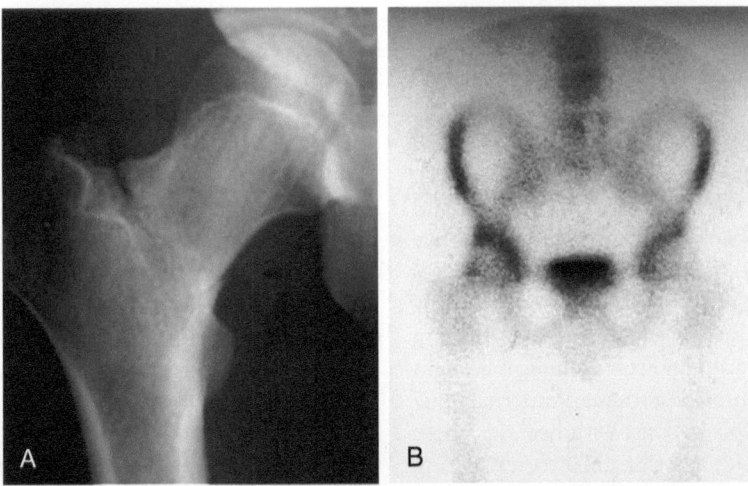

Fig. 10.3 (A) An anteroposterior radiograph with tension-side cortical disruption and propagation of the fracture across the femoral neck. (B) Magnetic resonance imaging with uptake on the superior (tension) side of the right femoral neck.

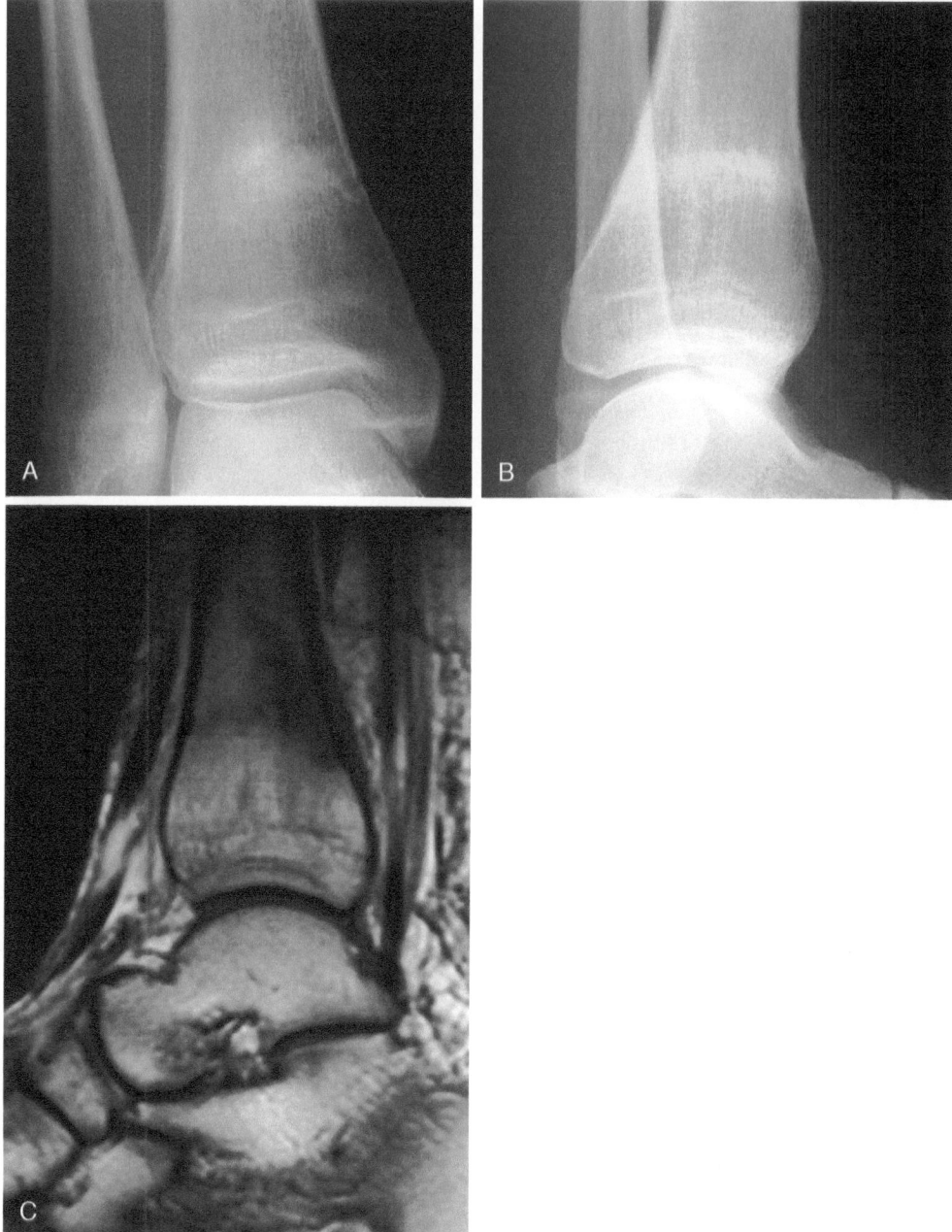

Fig. 10.4 (A and B) This tibial stress fracture is incomplete medial to lateral, but cortical disruption facilitates the diagnosis. (C) Magnetic resonance imaging demonstrates the lesion with high sensitivity. (Courtesy James W. Brodsky, MD.)

with a period of non–weight bearing and immobilization (Fig. 10.4). Fractures that occur on the tension side of the tibia and those that are visible on radiographs typically require operative intervention to heal (Fig. 10.5).[48] Traditionally these fractures were treated with an intramedullary nail. The intramedullary device promotes fracture healing by creating a load-sharing environment with the native tibia. Additionally, reaming is thought to stimulate bone marrow and provide a source of internal bone graft within the canal of the tibia to assist with healing. These fractures can also be treated with anterior tibial cortex plating with or without local bone grafting. The advantages of plating include placing the implant on the tension side of the fracture, allowing access for direct fracture débridement and bone

grafting, as well as not violating the knee joint. Such patients may experience less anterior knee pain, which is as high as 80% in some studies involving the use of an intramedullary nail to treat these injuries.[43] Drawbacks include plate prominence over a location of the tibia with minimal soft tissue coverage as well as the potential to devitalize the tibial cortex surrounding the fracture.[49,50]

Proximal Fifth Metatarsal Stress Fractures

The proximal aspect of the fifth metatarsal is also a common site for a stress fracture. Athletes of any running or marching sport are susceptible. Abnormal forefoot loading may contribute to these injuries, especially with minimalist shoe wear, which

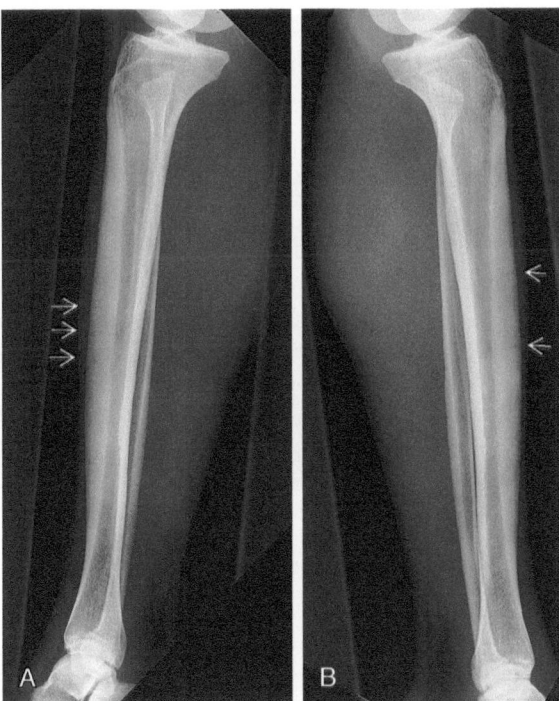

Fig. 10.5 (A and B) Radiographs of both tibiae showing multiple wedge-shaped fractures of the anterior cortex of the midtibia, the "dreaded black lines," indicating high-risk tension-side stress fractures *(arrows)*. (From Berger FH, de Jonge MC, Maas M. Stress fractures in the lower extremity: the importance of increasing awareness amongst radiologists. *Eur J Radiol.* 2007;62:16–26.)

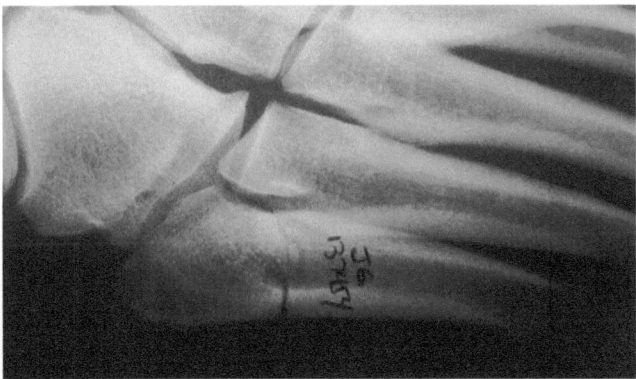

Fig. 10.6 An acute Jones fracture at the diaphyseal-metaphyseal junction of the fifth metatarsal. (Courtesy James W. Brodsky, MD.)

increase forefoot loading.[51] Athletes with a cavovarus hindfoot place additional stresses on the lateral border of the foot, predisposing them to injury. Additionally, the proximal metatarsal is a vascular supply watershed area, which perhaps leads to a poor regenerative response to repetitive injury. Also, toe grip weakness is correlated with an increased incidence of fifth metatarsal stress fractures.[52]

These injuries should be suspected in athletes with pain along the lateral border of the foot. The pain is often insidious and chronic, although the injury may also present with pain after a twisting type of injury. Stress fractures of the proximal fifth metatarsal should be distinguished from Jones fractures, which involve the fourth and fifth metatarsal articulation, as well as smaller, proximal avulsion type injuries. This distinction can be made on plain radiographs, where stress injuries are visible more distal at the proximal junction of the metatarsal shaft and metaphysis. These injuries can be seen as a lateral cortical thickening representing attempted healing in response to repetitive stress. They may also present with a visible fracture line that most often is incomplete and involves the lateral cortex. MRI and bone scan can be used for diagnosing injuries not seen on radiographs. Ultrasound has been proposed as a cheaper imaging option, although its sensitivity is not as high as that of MRI.[53]

When a fracture is visible on radiographs, most patients are treated with surgical stabilization (Fig. 10.6). Distinguishing a true Jones fracture from a diaphyseal fracture may not be important.[54] Nonoperative treatment has higher nonunion rates and longer time to sports and physical labor.[55] Typically surgical repair involves placing an intramedullary screw with sufficient screw threads past the fracture (Fig. 10.7). Intramedullary cortical thickening may make canal drilling difficult. Additionally, it is important not to penetrate the cortex distally with the drill or screw, thus creating a stress riser susceptible to fracture. There is debate over screw diameter, since larger screws are less susceptible to fatigue fracture.[56] For most patients a screw 5 mm to 50 mm in diameter, based on computed tomographic (CT) studies, is appropriate.[57] Some surgeons prefer a solid screw as opposed to a cannulated one to also help resist fatigue failure. Most commonly, exposing the fracture site to débride the fracture and place bone graft is not necessary for a first-time attempt at fixation, although it may be considered on a case-by-case basis and might be more likely in revision cases. Patients with incomplete fractures on radiographs and a plantar fracture gap less than 1 mm healed faster than those with a gap greater than 1 mm.[58] Patients with a cavovarus hindfoot might require a valgus-producing calcaneal osteotomy to unload the lateral aspect of the foot and create a more favorable mechanical environment.[59] This is especially important in athletes who sustain recurrent injuries.

Postoperatively an assessment should be made of the factors, in addition to patient-specific health characteristics, that may have contributed to the injury. These may include running style, training volume, running shoe quality and wear, as well as foot shape. Additionally, athletes with low vitamin D levels (<30 ng/mL) have a higher incidence of fifth metatarsal stress fracture and should therefore be treated with oral supplementation.[26,60] Adjusting each of these factors is important in order to minimize the chance of recurrence. Custom orthotics should be considered to ensure that stresses to the athlete's feet are properly distributed. Recurrence of injury after operative fixation is more likely in athletes who return to sports earlier, prior to complete healing.[61,62] This is also true for those with a higher BMI and a wider fourth-to-fifth intermetatarsal angle and curved fifth metatarsal head.[63]

Other Metatarsal Stress Fractures

Stress fractures involving the first to fourth metatarsals are also common, especially in running athletes and dancers.[64] The second metatarsal is subjected to the highest bending stresses and is therefore the most commonly involved of the metatarsals. This is followed by the third metatarsal.[65]

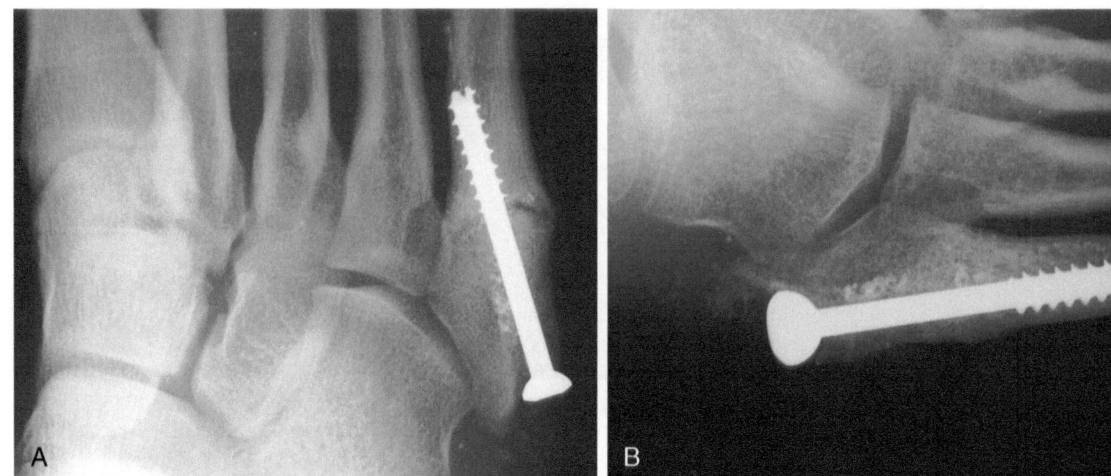

Fig. 10.7 Images of an 18-year-old collegiate soccer player with recurrent pain and nonunion of a Jones fracture after previous surgery. (A) Note the hypertrophic beaking and sclerosis at the fracture site. (B) Healing was achieved 10 weeks after revision intramedullary fixation and bone grafting. (Courtesy James W. Brodsky, MD.)

Fractures can occur anywhere along the metatarsal and maximal stress occurs 3 to 4 cm distal from the base of the bone.[65] Fractures that are more distal heal more predictably. In most cases, with a period of immobilization and limited weight bearing, treatment is successful. Once the foot pain has subsided, it is important to progress activities in a gradual process to allow for mechanical adaptation of the foot to increased loads. It is also important to address any factors involving the patient's systemic homeostasis as well as foot biomechanics and loading patterns. Achilles stretching, cross training, limiting mileage, regular shoe replacement, and custom orthotics are all treatment strategies that should be considered.

Forth metatarsal fractures can have delayed or incomplete healing with nonoperative treatment, especially in patients with metatarsus adductus.[66] Open reduction and plate fixation is an option in these injuries to hasten return to athletics.[67]

Navicular Stress Fractures

Navicular stress fractures, while uncommon, are challenging to diagnose and treat. Delay in diagnosis is the norm.[68] They are seen in sprinting and jumping sports such as basketball and, unlike most stress fractures, are more common in male athletes.[4,65] The central third of the bone is an area of high shear stress. The navicular is the keystone to the medial longitudinal arch and the link between the midfoot and hindfoot. It serves as an important structural support for both the longitudinal and transverse arches.[69] With weight bearing, forces are generated medially across the navicular from the first metatarsal through the medial cuneiform and the talus. Forces through the second metatarsal and middle cuneiform are not resisted in the same way, thereby generating shear forces. Additionally, the central third of the navicular is thought to be a relatively avascular zone, which limits its ability to resist changes in forces and subsequently its healing potential.[10,70] Recent data note that an avascular zone in the central navicular is present only 12% of the time. The majority of the time the navicular is well perfused from the dorsalis pedis and branches of the posterior tibial artery.[71]

Patients present with insidious dorsal foot pain, and diagnosis of a navicular stress injury can often be delayed. Tenderness is described over the navicular. Pain can be exacerbated by axially loading a plantarflexed foot such as standing on tiptoe or hopping on a single leg.[68] Radiographs may become positive only on a delayed basis owing to lack of involvement of the plantar surface.[65] Therefore MRI is more commonly used for fracture detection.

Once the fracture has been diagnosed, treatment requires an extended period of immobilization. When fractures are diagnosed in early stages, they can be treated successfully with casting for a minimum of 6 weeks. Non–weight bearing during this period is also important; allowing weight bearing too soon can lead to nonunion.[72,73] On average, these fractures result in about 4 months loss of athletic participation.[72] Pain with therapeutic ultrasound can be used to follow navicular healing and correlates with MRI findings.[74]

Athletes with fracture lines visible on radiographs or those hoping to return to participation sooner may be candidates for operative fixation. Operative treatment allows return to athletics at a mean of 16 weeks, compared with 22 weeks for conservative treatment.[48] In most cases two partially threaded screws placed perpendicular to the fracture line from lateral to medial suffice to generate compression and healing (Fig. 10.8). Postoperative limited weight bearing for 1 to 2 months is important. Repeat imaging to confirm fracture healing can be considered prior to release to return to sports participation. Outcomes of navicular stress fractures are not always optimal regardless of treatment. There is a high rate of persistent pain and disability and those patients are more likely to develop a nonunion.[75] With operative treatment there is a high rate of secondary osteoarthritis and need for reoperation.[76]

Pars Stress Fractures

Stress fractures of the lumbar spine are commonly seen in athletes who perform repetitive lumbar extension activities. Sports-related back pain in patients under the age of 18 years is due to a stress injury up to 40% of the time.[77,78] Although less

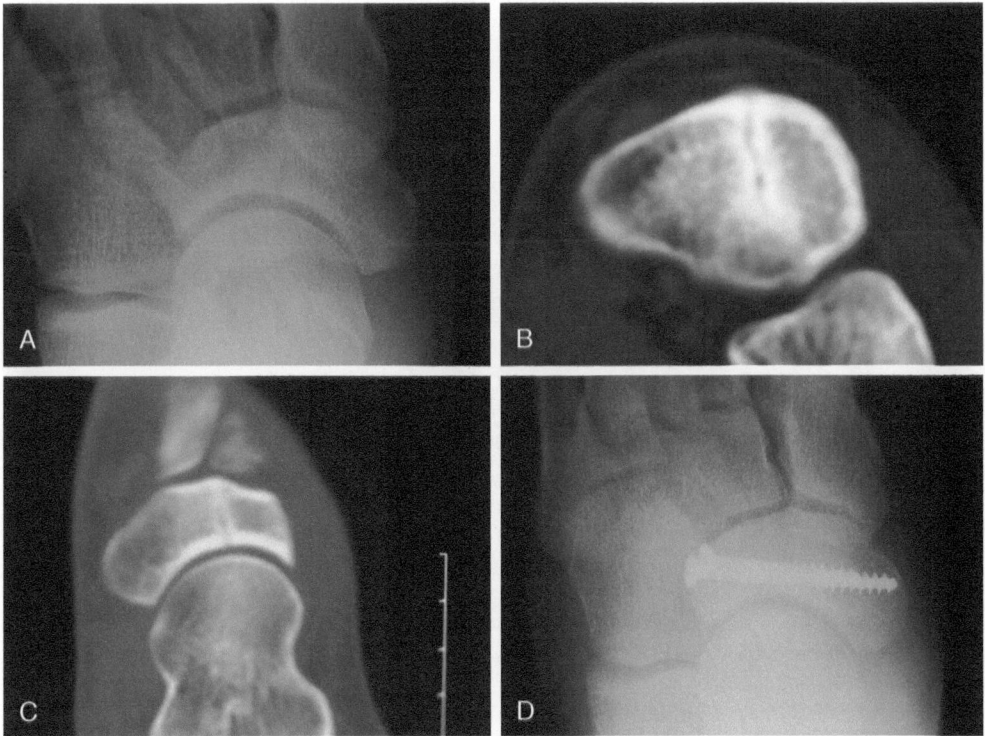

Fig. 10.8 A navicular stress fracture. (A) Subtle linear lucency in the navicular is seen on the radiograph. (B and C) Computed tomography confirmed the diagnosis. (D) The patient was treated with internal fixation and bone grafting. (Courtesy James W. Brodsky, MD.)

common, new-onset spondylolysis is also seen in adults.[79] Susceptible athletes include gymnasts and football linemen. Repetitive axial loading of the lumbar spine with spinal extension leads to stress injuries of the pars interarticularis, or spondylolysis. These injuries are usually bilateral, and most occur at L5, with L4 being the next most common location. Most patients with spondylolysis are asymptomatic, although the diagnosis of stress injury should be kept in mind with athletes presenting with chronic lumbar pain.[80]

Patients presenting with spondylolysis may have a stiff-legged gait with shortened stride length due to hamstring spasm, along with limited forward flexion. A palpable step-off may be present in patients with advanced spondylolisthesis. Lumbar nerve root radiculopathy may be present as well, from irritation due to the nearby inflamed pars defect. Plain radiography is part of the initial workup, and oblique views are more sensitive for diagnosis. Flexion-extension radiographs can document and grade instability in patients with spondylolisthesis. Advanced imaging with CT is used to best evaluate the bony architecture and MRI to evaluate the nerve roots and associated disk disease (Fig. 10.9). MRI has a high sensitivity as well for diagnosing spondylolysis and is likely comparable to CT.[81,82] SPECT bone scan is the most sensitive test for diagnosis.[80]

Patients with pars defects only and those with low-grade spondylolisthesis are typically treated with activity modification and extension bracing. Rehabilitation involving lumbopelvic flexibility and strengthening is important in the later stages of recovery and to foster return to participation. Additionally, stress injuries to the pars interarticularis are seen in patients with low vitamin D levels; therefore testing should be considered.[25] Most

patients will improve with nonoperative treatment; however, the union rate is low and only around 25% heal successfully.[83] Additionally, patients are susceptible to recurrence of symptoms as long as they remain involved in high-level athletics.[84] Patients unresponsive to extensive conservative treatment, those with neurologic deficits, and patients with unstable and high-grade spondylolisthesis may consider pars repair if the associated disks are nondegenerative. In patients with degenerative disk disease, a lumbar fusion of the involved levels is indicated. However, the outcomes data are limited for adult athletes who have failed nonoperative treatment. Surgical pars interarticularis repair is likely to bring improvements in pain, function, and eventual return to athletics.[85] Studies on return to play (RTP) after pars repair note that this often takes 1 year from the time of surgery, especially for contact sports, and is successful around 80% of the time.[86]

Rib Fractures

Rib fractures in athletes can be troublesome. They can either be traumatic or nontraumatic secondary to stress injury. Although traumatic injuries may be easier to diagnose, stress fractures of the ribs can be missed and present variably in athletes. It is important for the clinician to be familiar with the risks and causes of stress fractures and to have a high level of suspicion in the athlete presenting with atraumatic pain.

Traumatic injuries are typically easy to diagnose, since they are usually associated with a direct blow to the rib cage. There will be very localized pain at the fracture site, which is exacerbated with direct pressure or deep breaths. On examination, a deformity may be seen, with a hematoma or overlying bruising.

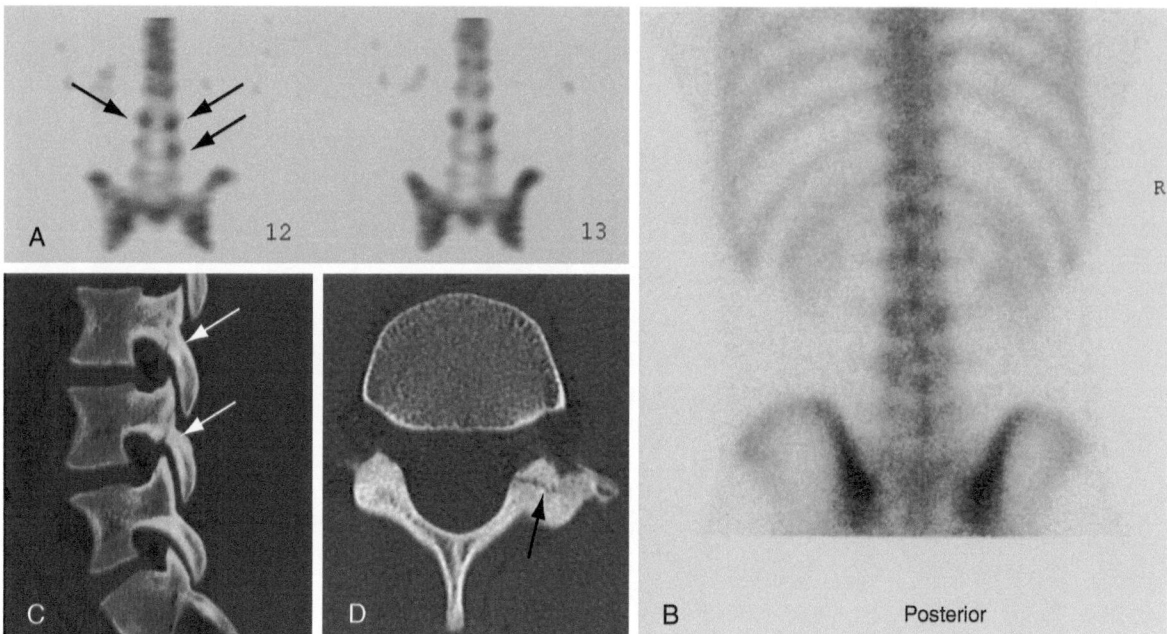

Fig. 10.9 A pars stress fracture. (A) Four-hour delayed bone single-photon emission computed tomography (CT) images of the lumbar spine demonstrating increased uptake in the bilateral L3 posterior elements and the right L4 posterior element corresponding to active pars interarticularis stress fractures *(black arrows)*. (B) The abnormalities are barely visible on the standard bone scan image of the lumbar spine. (C) A sagittal reformation CT image demonstrates linear lucencies in the right L3 and L4 pars interarticularis corresponding to areas of abnormal uptake *(white arrows)*. (D) An axial CT image demonstrates a left-sided pars defect at L3 *(black arrow)*.

The physician is typically able to localize the area of pain with palpation directly over the fracture. Deep breaths and any motions requiring contraction of the thoracic musculature will cause pain. Anteriorly, separation of the costochondral junction is possible with intense thoracic contraction and twisting motions. Such injuries are common in wrestlers, for example. With worse separations, the displacement at the costochondral junction can be seen and felt.

Stress fractures of the ribs are much less common, present variably, and can often be missed in the differential diagnosis. Symptom onset is usually insidious, and athletes will typically have pain only during the inciting activity. In the early stages they may complain of shoulder or abdominal pain, depending on the location of the fracture. The pain will worsen as the athlete continues with the causative activity without rest or modification. Rib stress fractures are primarily caused by repetitive tensile muscular forces, which are typically seen in sports requiring throwing and swinging of the upper extremities.[87-94] Common sports in which stress rib fractures occur include rowing, gymnastics, basketball, and baseball. The most common sites for stress fractures include the first rib anterolaterally, the fourth through ninth ribs posterolaterally, and the upper ribs posteromedially.[92] Generally first-rib fractures are seen in sports requiring repetitive overhead activities, such as baseball, basketball, and tennis.[88-90] Athletes may present with a vague history of pain in the posterior shoulder, midclavicular region, or upper back.[89] Lower-rib stress fractures are seen in sports requiring repetitive torsion of the body, such as rowing or golfing.[92,93]

Evaluation of the athlete with a rib fracture should include examination of the chest, heart, lungs, and abdomen. Particularly in the case of traumatic fractures, other associated organ injuries—involving the lungs, liver, spleen, or kidneys—should be ruled out. In atraumatic fractures, other potential nonmusculoskeletal causes of pain should be considered, as these patients may present variably.

Imaging studies typically begin with plain radiographs of the chest and ribs. Traumatic fractures should be visible, but imaging of the ribs can be challenging and requires careful examination of each rib. It is helpful to review the findings with a radiologist to ensure that all the fractures are noted. Stress fractures, on the other hand, are not always seen initially. Up to two-thirds of initial x-rays are negative and only become positive once healing has begun.[95]

Bone scans will show increased uptake in the area of the stress fracture with 100% sensitivity and allow for earlier diagnosis versus radiographs.[96] However, MRI is the modality of choice to diagnose stress fractures. It has the highest combined sensitivity and specificity and adds the benefit of evaluating for soft tissue abnormalities.[95,96]

Both traumatic and nontraumatic rib fractures in athletes can be treated nonoperatively. Rest, ice, analgesia, and cessation of the inciting activity are important while the fracture is given sufficient time to heal. As healing progresses, activities are modified and increasingly guided by symptom improvement. For severe pain, "rib strapping" or intercostal nerve blocks can be considered. Rehabilitation should include evaluation of mechanics and training regimens to prevent future fractures. Nonunions of rib fractures is rare.[87,91]

Clavicle Fractures

Clavicular fractures account for up to 10% of all sport-related fractures,[97,98] and 30% of all clavicular fractures occur during sports.[98] These are common fractures in the athlete, with midshaft fractures being the most common (Fig. 10.10). Midshaft fractures are displaced nearly 50% of the time and comminuted in 19%.[99,100] These injuries usually occur with direct blows to the shoulder, either from collisions with other players or falls onto the shoulder. A deformity may be seen, and the clinician should note any open wounds or skin tenting. A thorough neurovascular examination should be performed, and other concomitant injuries should be ruled out.

The treatment of clavicular fractures has been the topic of much discussion. Nondisplaced fractures can be treated successfully without surgery. However, midshaft clavicular fractures are often displaced,[99,100] and in such cases their optimal treatment has been much debated. Traditionally all clavicular fractures were treated nonoperatively.[101,102] However, recent reports suggest that conservative treatments may give suboptimal results, including unacceptable nonunion rates, increased return times to sports, and poor residual shoulder function.[103-106] Particularly in the athlete, where early RTP, optimal function, and early union are desirable, the findings from nonoperative treatment are unacceptable to most. Hence there has been a trend towards surgical fixation of displaced midshaft clavicular fractures, especially with studies suggesting lower rates of nonunion and malunion, earlier return to sports, and improved functional outcomes.[107-109]

Surgical treatment of displaced clavicular fractures in the pediatric population remains controversial. As children increasingly participate in sports, the optimal treatment has also been a topic of discussion for the same reasons as in the adult athlete. Because of the great remodeling potential, clavicular fractures in children have traditionally been treated nonoperatively. There are reports, however, of improved outcomes with plate fixation, particularly in adolescent patients.[110] In younger patients, however, surgical fixation becomes more controversial. The benefits of surgical fixation should always be weighed against the risks of surgery, including infection and neurovascular injury.

Clavicular stress fractures are rare but may occur in athletes participating in rowing, diving, baseball, weight lifting, and gymnastics.[88,91,111] These fractures are thought to occur due to a muscular imbalance of repetitive bending, shearing, and rotational forces across the clavicle.[91] As most stress fractures are undisplaced, treatment is typically nonsurgical.

Most patients will successfully return to sports after a clavicular fracture, with at least 80% of patients returning to their preinjury level of play.[109,112] The decision to return is multifactorial and begins with clinical and radiographic evidence of fracture healing. Patients should demonstrate full pain-free range of motion (ROM) with near full strength. An RTP training regimen should be started and gradually advanced before exposure to a real game situation. Sport-specific drills and functional exercises should be incorporated to make sure that the patient does not have pain and to give him or her an opportunity to regain confidence after a prolonged absence from playing. The timing of RTP is controversial and quite variably reported.[109,113] Generally, with nonoperative treatment, return to sports may take 6 to 12 weeks from the time of injury.[103,114,115] Surgical treatment may allow for earlier return to sport, with some reporting returns earlier than 6 weeks after surgery.[112,113] This is a minority, however, and it appears that average return times are 68 to 83 days after surgery.[112,113] Ultimately the decision to RTP will depend on the type of treatment, evidence of healing, and certainly by the level and type of sport (i.e., contact vs. noncontact) to which the athlete is returning. Return to sport is discussed in further detail in the next section.

RETURN TO SPORT

The decision of returning an athlete to sports participation can be complex and difficult, yet it remains a critical component of the clinician's treatment of the injured athlete. In today's competitive climate, the physician is burdened with questions of when an athlete will eventually RTP. These questions are unavoidable and come from the athlete, his or her parents, agents, coaches, and the media, to list a few. Despite being a hallmark of the clinician's treatment, the decision to RTP remains controversial and a topic of much debate. The complex nature of the decision-making process perhaps accounts for the scarcity of higher-level evidence in the literature providing a systematic and objective approach to returning an athlete to sports. The ultimate goal is to expedite the athlete's recovery and return to sports while making sure that the initial injury is healed and the risk of reinjury is minimal.

To help with the decision-making process, Creighton et al. presented a three-step model that outlines the factors to be

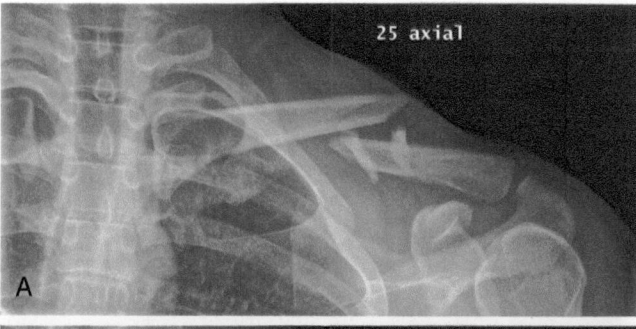
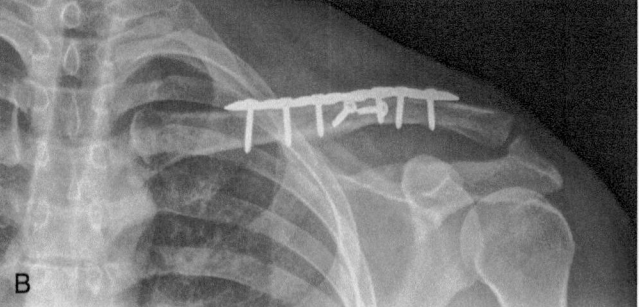

Fig. 10.10 Left comminuted midshaft clavicle. (A) Preoperative. (B) Postoperative.

Decision-Based RTP Model

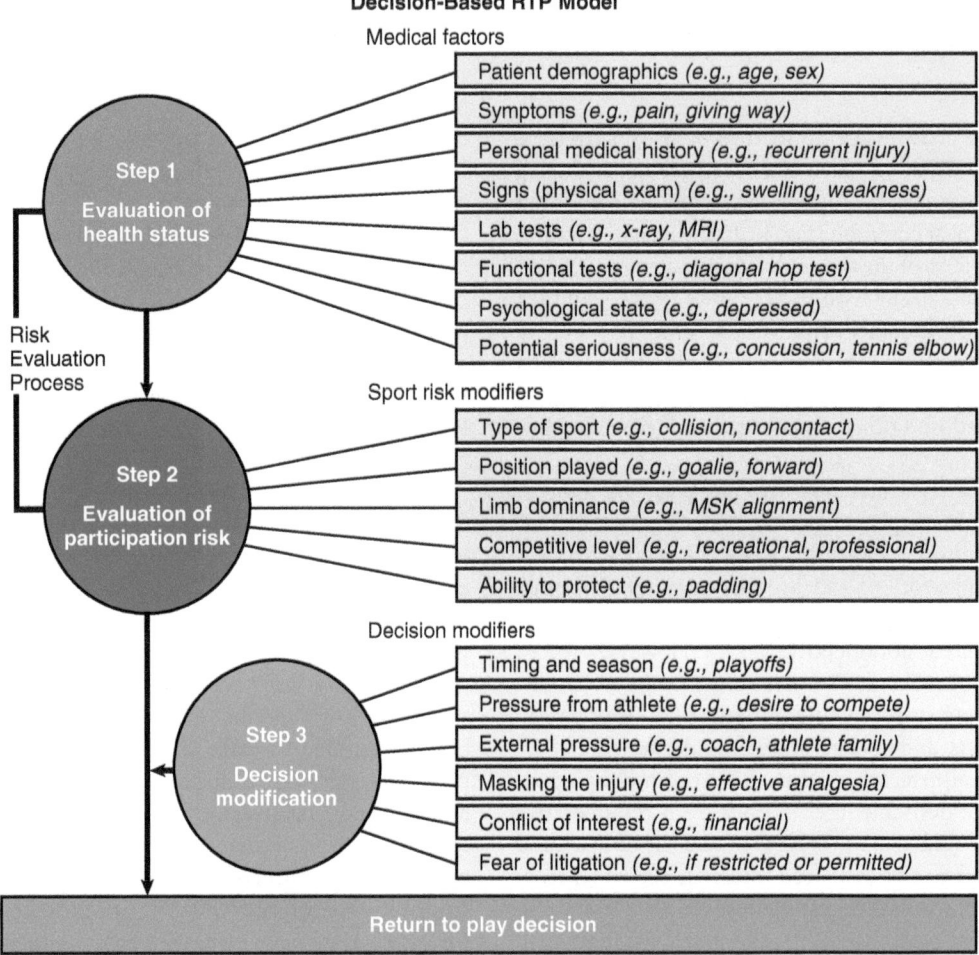

Medical factors

- Patient demographics *(e.g., age, sex)*
- Symptoms *(e.g., pain, giving way)*
- Personal medical history *(e.g., recurrent injury)*
- Signs (physical exam) *(e.g., swelling, weakness)*
- Lab tests *(e.g., x-ray, MRI)*
- Functional tests *(e.g., diagonal hop test)*
- Psychological state *(e.g., depressed)*
- Potential seriousness *(e.g., concussion, tennis elbow)*

Sport risk modifiers

- Type of sport *(e.g., collision, noncontact)*
- Position played *(e.g., goalie, forward)*
- Limb dominance *(e.g., MSK alignment)*
- Competitive level *(e.g., recreational, professional)*
- Ability to protect *(e.g., padding)*

Decision modifiers

- Timing and season *(e.g., playoffs)*
- Pressure from athlete *(e.g., desire to compete)*
- External pressure *(e.g., coach, athlete family)*
- Masking the injury *(e.g., effective analgesia)*
- Conflict of interest *(e.g., financial)*
- Fear of litigation *(e.g., if restricted or permitted)*

Step 1 — Evaluation of health status

Step 2 — Evaluation of participation risk

Step 3 — Decision modification

Risk Evaluation Process

Return to play decision

Fig. 10.11 A decision-based return to play *(RTP)* model. *MRI,* Magnetic resonance imaging; *MSK,* musculo-skeletal. (From Creighton DW, Shrier I, Shultz R, et al. Return-to-play in sport: a decision-based model. *Clin J Sport Med.* 2010;20[5]:379–385.)

considered before returning the athlete to play.[116] This model incorporates important factors that go beyond the medical status of the player's injury. It includes the evaluation of the health status, evaluation of participation risk, and includes modifiers that could affect the decision (Fig. 10.11).

The first step is an evaluation of the athlete's health status. This includes typical objective and subjective medical factors that the clinician usually considers before returning an athlete to play. Much of this evaluation is done in the clinic setting, and the physician must decide whether the initial injury has healed enough to tolerate the forces of the sporting activity. The patient should have resolution of symptoms such as pain and instability. Objective assessment includes examination for ROM, laxity, strength, and the presence of swelling and inflammation. These are typically compared with the contralateral extremity, and many have established specific measurable criteria to determine readiness.[117-119] A more dynamic and functional assessment is usually part of the decision-making process (e.g., the diagonal hop test) and includes tests to ensure adequate balance and proprioception. In many instances, these assessments are performed as part of the athlete's functional rehabilitation, with the report made available to the physician. In today's competitive sporting climate and increasing sports specialization involving young athletes, it is common to introduce sport-specific functional rehabilitation as part of the return-to-sport process. For example, ballet dancers place different demands on their knees compared with golfers or soccer players. Therefore functional assessments would also have to be sport-specific.

Traditionally, the decision to allow athletes to RTP exclusively involved step 1 of this model. Many RTP guidelines in the literature are in fact restricted to step 1 as well.[120] According to Creighton et al., the second step is to evaluate participation risk and consider sport risk modifiers.[116] These are factors such as the type of sport, the position played, and the competitive level of play. For example, swimming may put different demands on the knee compared with a full-contact sport such as football. A long-distance track-and-field runner with a shoulder injury may return sooner than a tennis player with the same injury. The position played also makes a difference, as a soccer goalkeeper may have different demands compared with a striker. The level of competition should also be a consideration. A weekend recreational athlete will have different demands than the professional elite athlete. Such factors should certainly come into consideration in determining an athlete's return to their sport.

The final step involves the consideration of decision modifiers and should not be taken lightly. These modifiers may be reason enough for the athlete to decide to forego surgery and continue playing through an injury or even to RTP early despite the risks of reinjury. These decision modifiers can change the decision to return if participation risk is considered alone. For example, athletes may injure themselves midseason of their high school senior year and may choose to play through the injury and delay surgery so that they may finish playing in their final year. Removing athletes from play at a critical time of the season may cause them to miss an opportunity for a college scholarship, again swaying the decision to return early. The physician may also encounter external pressure from the coach, media, and family to proceed with a certain type of treatment plan, while the athlete may also encounter the same pressures. Fear of litigation may also sway one's decision. If an athlete is not allowed to play, he may blame the physician for losing the opportunity for a bonus, scholarship, or position on a team. On the other hand, if the athlete returns to play and is reinjured, the physician may be blamed for clearing him too early. The consideration of step 3 of this model involves clear and open communication between the athlete and physician regarding appropriate expectations. The discussion may involve family, agents, coaches, and a sporting organization, but the physician must use caution when disclosing personal, medical, or other sensitive information to different parties. These "decision modifiers" can easily be ignored by the treating physician, but their consideration is paramount in the optimal treatment of today's athletes.

Despite the increasing discussion of RTP in the literature, there are few guidelines providing a standardized approach to these difficult decisions. Creighton et al. provided one such model[116]; however, even this was later modified to address limitations in its ability to be applied in all situations.[121] Some of the challenges were the model's ability to be applied to serious injuries such as concussions, or when there were multiple injuries and risks. The author proposes that these difficulties arose because the original model was a sociologic construct, whereas the decision to RTP involves biologic considerations. Therefore the Strategic Assessment of Risk and Risk Tolerance, or StARRT, framework was introduced (Fig. 10.12).[121] In short, the original model was modified to produce a better fit with the biological considerations when assessing RTP. The "medical factors" were modified to "tissue health," and the "sport risk modifiers" were changed to represent the stresses applied to the tissues. These again encompass steps 1 and 2, respectively, and represent the risk assessment process. Finally, the "decision modifiers" were changed to "risk tolerance modifiers." Ultimately, the decision to RTP is based on whether the risk tolerance exceeds the risk assessment. In other words, if the risk assessment is greater than the risk tolerance, the athlete should not RTP.

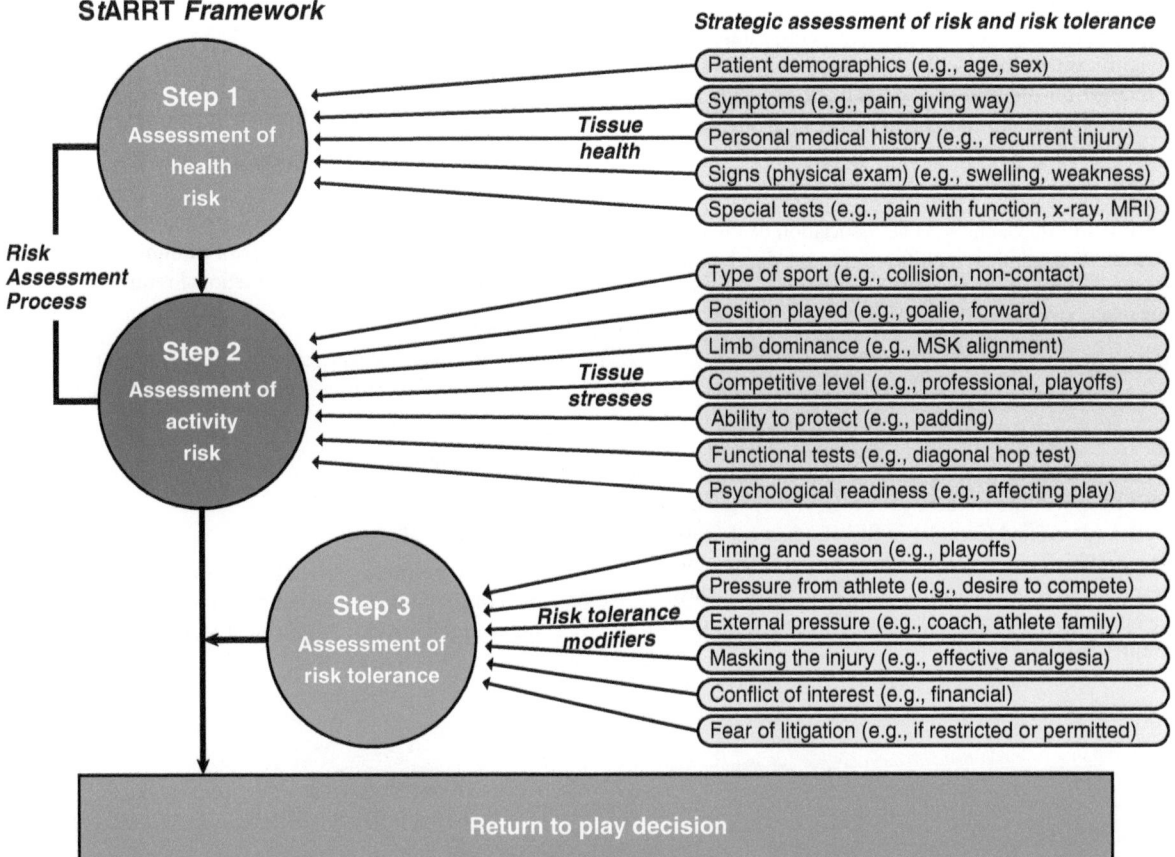

Fig. 10.12 The Strategic Assessment of Risk and Risk Tolerance *(StARRT)* framework for return to play. *MRI,* Magnetic resonance imaging; *MSK,* musculoskeletal. (From Shrier I. Strategic Assessment of Risk and Risk Tolerance [StARRT] framework for return-to-play decision-making. *Br J Sports Med.* 2015;49:1311–1315.)

Numerous factors are involved in the decision to return an athlete to play. Even for experienced team physicians, the decision can be complex and difficult. With the multitude of factors to be considered, however, there is still great variability among physicians with regard to the decision-making process.[122] Ultimately the decision to RTP should be made jointly between the physician and athlete, with appropriate communication also involving other parties such as therapist, family, coaches, and the sports organization. Too much communication and involvement of outside parties may complicate the decision-making process; on the other hand, it may also help the physician to consider the multiple factors involved in deciding to return an athlete to his or her sport.

For a complete list of references, go to ExpertConsult.com.

SELECTED READINGS

Citation:

Burgi AA, Gorham ED, Garland CF, et al. High serum 25-hydroxyvitamin D is associated with a low incidence of stress fractures. *J Bone Miner Res.* 2011;26(10):2371–2377.

Level of Evidence:

II

Summary:

In this study there was a monotonic inverse dose-response gradient between serum 25(OH)D and risk of stress fracture, indicating that there was double the risk of stress fractures of the tibia and fibula in women with serum 25(OH)D concentrations of less than 20 ng/mL versus those with concentrations of 40 ng/mL or greater. A target for prevention of stress fractures would be a serum 25(OH)D concentration of 40 ng/mL or greater, achievable with 4000 IU/d of vitamin D3 supplementation.

Citation:

Tenforde AS, Carlson JL, Chang A, et al. Association of the female athlete triad risk assessment stratification to the development of bone stress injuries in collegiate athletes. *Am J Sports Med.* 2017;45(2):302–310.

Level of Evidence:

III

Summary:

Using published guidelines, 29% of female collegiate athletes in this study were classified into moderate- or high-risk categories using the Female Athlete Triad Cumulative Risk Assessment Score. Moderate- and high-risk athletes were more likely (two and four times, respectively, compared with low risk) to subsequently sustain a bone stress injury (BSI); most BSIs were sustained by cross-country runners.

Citation:

Kaeding CC, Miller T. The comprehensive description of stress fractures: a new classification system. *J Bone Joint Surg Am.* 2013;95(13):1214–1220.

Level of Evidence:

III

Summary:

This paper proposes a five-tier stress fracture classification system based on imaging and symptoms; the system is clinically relevant, easily applied, generalizable, and has excellent interobserver and intraobserver reliability.

Citation:

Miller TL, Harris JD, Kaeding CC. Stress fractures of the ribs and upper extremities: causation, evaluation, and management. *Sports Med.* 2013;43:665–674.

Level of Evidence:

III

Summary:

This paper presents a review of the literature discussing upper extremity stress fractures, including their risk factors, clinical presentation, and treatment.

Citation:

McKee RC, Whelan DB, Schemitsch EH, et al. Operative versus nonoperative care of displaced midshaft clavicular fractures: a meta-analysis of randomized clinical trials. *J Bone Joint Surg Am.* 2012;94:675–684.

Level of Evidence:

I

Summary:

This paper presents a meta-analysis of clinical trials comparing operative and nonoperative treatment of displaced midshaft clavicular fractures. The report concludes that operative treatment results in lower rates of nonunion and symptomatic malunion as well as earlier functional return.

Citation:

Shrier I. Strategic assessment of risk and risk tolerance (StARRT) framework for return-to-play decision making. *Br J Sports Med.* 2015;49:1311–1315.

Level of Evidence:

IV

Summary:

This article presents a revised framework to guide RTP decision-making. It addresses limitations noted in the original three-step model presented by Creighton et al. in 2010.

SECTION 2

Medical

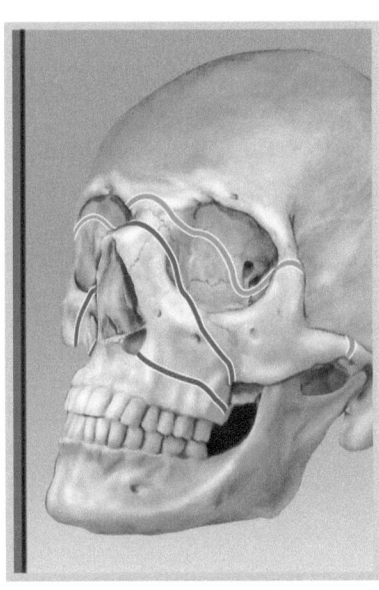

143

11

Team Medical Coverage

Daniel Herman, Nikhita Gadi, Evan Peck

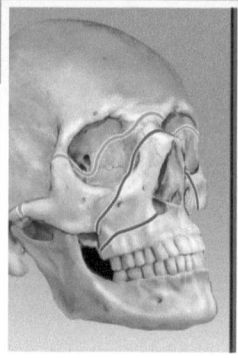

The roots of peak athletic performance are embedded in the optimal health of athletes. It is the responsibility of every member of the sports medicine team to provide consistent, thorough, evidence-based, and comprehensive care for each athlete. Team medical coverage has evolved rapidly and has become a pivotal component of athletics at all levels of competition. The ultimate responsibility for medical decisions regarding both prevention and treatment rests with a team of professionals, which includes the medical director, other team physicians, athletic trainers, and allied health care providers.[1] The minimum qualifications for the medical director and other team physicians include[1]:

1. Having a Doctor of Medicine (MD) or a Doctor of Osteopathy (DO) degree in good standing, with an unrestricted license to practice medicine.
2. Possessing a fundamental knowledge of emergency sport-related medical care.
3. Being trained in cardiopulmonary resuscitation (CPR) and the use of an automated external defibrillator (AED).
4. Having a working knowledge of musculoskeletal injuries, medical conditions, and psychological issues affecting athletes.

Duties of the medical team are numerous but primarily include: (1) effectively coordinating preparticipation evaluations, (2) managing on-field emergencies, and (3) navigating the ethical and medicolegal issues unique to sports medicine. These topics are discussed in detail in this chapter.

PREPARTICIPATION PHYSICAL EVALUATION

A mainstay of modern medicine is the idea of preventive health care. In the realm of organized athletics, the preparticipation physical evaluation (PPE) has historically served as the cornerstone of the prevention of unnecessary morbidity and mortality in sport. In May 2010, recommendations for the PPE were updated and published (PPE-4).[2] Based on expert consensus and a comprehensive review of the medical literature, the PPE-4 was developed with input from six medical societies and is endorsed as the "gold standard" for the PPE.[2] However, historically, PPE standards in the United States have been determined by individual state and local legislative authorities, with varying medical and legal guidelines and community resources. As a result, the implementation of the PPE nationally has been heterogeneous, with variable compliance by educational institutions and athletic associations. The lack of uniform application of the PPE has made it difficult to interpret outcome data for the few studies

that exist.[3] A review found no medium- or better-quality evidence that the PPE reduces morbidity or mortality.[4] Despite variation in the format and use of PPEs, it is held that, at the very least, the PPE allows for establishment of a "medical home," an immunization record, identification and management of acquired and congenital medical conditions, and proactive counseling related to medical conditions in sports and lifestyle risk factors.[5]

Goals and Objectives

Many sports governing bodies mandate a PPE not only to ensure the health and well-being of the participant but also to minimize legal liability for conditions that may occur or worsen with participation in sports.[5] The principal goal of the author societies who formulated the PPE-4 is the promotion of the health and safety of athletes.

Primary objectives of the PPE include[2]:
1. Screening for potential life-threatening or disabling conditions.
2. Screening for conditions that may predispose to injury or illness.

Secondary objectives that address general health care and prevention[2] include:
1. Determining general health.
2. Serving as an entry point to the health care system.
3. Providing an opportunity to initiate a discussion on health-related topics.

The PPE may be the only annual medical appointment that athletes have. It is thus important to take advantage of this valuable time to initiate a discussion on drug use, seat belt and helmet use, and safe sexual practices. Failure to limit risk-taking behaviors is more likely to cause harm in adolescents than is participation in sports.[6]

Timing, Setting, and Organization

Ideally, the PPE should take place at least 6 weeks before the start of organized practices. A small percentage of athletes may be conditionally withheld from participation pending further workup or consultation with a specialist, or they may have ongoing medical issues that need to be resolved. In general, more frequent evaluation is recommended for younger athletes because cardiac abnormalities may manifest during dynamic growth periods, despite normal results of earlier evaluations. At the secondary school level, comprehensive examinations should occur every 2 to 3 years, interspersed with problem-focused evaluations annually. For the collegiate age group, it is recommended that a comprehensive evaluation be performed prior to the first season and that shorter, more focused evaluations be performed annually thereafter. A new recommendation by the PPE-4 is for children (>6 years) and adolescents to undergo a PPE as part of their annual health maintenance examination. The authors of the PPE-4 reason that all children should be encouraged to be active, given recent trends in obesity and inactivity. Children who plan to be active in nonstructured sport settings are equally susceptible to injury and illness and thus should be offered a PPE.[2]

The two typical approaches to the PPE are (1) a primary care physician's office visit and (2) coordinated team examinations. A comparison of the two settings is outlined in Table 11.1. The PPE-4 recommends examinations at the primary care physician's office. During team examinations, the ultimate responsibility to clear athletes for sport participation is incumbent upon a physician with an unrestricted MD or DO license.[2] A standardized history questionnaire should be completed by the athlete prior to arrival, and parental guidance is advocated for minors. The PPE-4 consistently reinforces the adage that the history is the most important diagnostic tool. It has been shown that 75% or more of medical and orthopedic conditions are detected by history alone.[7-9] The PPE-4 History and Physical Exam forms are free and are available online.[10]

History and Physical Examination
Head, Ears, Eyes, Nose, and Throat

A detailed history of eye disorders, injuries, and the need for corrective or protective eyewear should be obtained. Visual acuity should be assessed via a standard Snellen eye chart. Poor visual acuity is one of the most frequently reported findings on PPEs, and appropriate consultation with a specialist should be facilitated.[11] Athletes whose visual acuity in the poorer eye is worse than 20/40 with optical correction should be classified as being "functionally one-eyed," and akin to persons missing an eye, they should wear protective eyewear when participating in sports with a high risk for eye injury. Furthermore, they should be restricted from participating in sports that feature intentional harm, such as full-contact martial arts, boxing, and wrestling.[2] A pupillary examination to document baseline anisocoria should be performed for reference in the event of a head injury. Odontogenic pathology such as oral ulcers, gingival atrophy, and decreased enamel may be a sign of an eating disorder.[2]

Cardiovascular System

Sudden cardiac death (SCD) is the most feared complication of sports participation. The annual incidence of SCD in the United States is approximately 1 in 80,000 high school athletes and 1 in 50,000 college athletes.[12] Box 11.1 outlines the most common causes of sudden death in young athletes in the United States. To reduce the risk of SCD during sports participation, the PPE-4 endorses the recommendations made by the 2007 American Heart Association (AHA) consensus statement on preparticipation cardiovascular screening.[13] According to multiple studies, the sensitivity of history taking and a physical examination for detecting cardiac disorders associated with SCD is 20%.[14,15] The author societies of PPE-4 admit that no outcome-based studies have demonstrated that the PPE is effective for preventing or detecting athletes at risk for SCD.[2] The PPE-4 questions used to evaluate cardiac history (personal and family) are listed in Fig. 11.1. These questions have been expanded in the PPE-4 to help identify ion channelopathies such as long QT and Wolff-Parkinson-White syndromes.

Current AHA guidelines recommend that the standard 11-point screening guideline and those of the PPE-4 are used by examiners as part of a comprehensive history and physical examination to detect cardiovascular abnormalities for high school and college athletes in the United States.[16] The physical examination recommended by the AHA includes[17] cardiac auscultation for heart murmurs,[18] palpation of radial and femoral pulses to assess for aortic coarctation[19] examination for physical stigmata of Marfan syndrome (MFS),[19] and brachial artery blood pressure taken in the seated position.[13] Cardiac auscultation should be performed with athletes seated and also with Valsalva maneuver and squatting. The murmur related to hypertrophic cardiomyopathy (HCM) will be accentuated by the Valsalva maneuver and decreased with squatting, whereas the murmur related to aortic stenosis would follow the opposite pattern. Soft early systolic murmurs are common in athletes and represent hyperdynamic flow rather than anatomic pathology.[2] Blood

---

TABLE 11.1 Comparison of Preparticipation Physical Evaluation Clinical Settings

Office Based	Coordinated Team
Pros	**Pros**
Better continuity of care	Time efficient
Established relationship	Reduced cost
Privacy	Available to athletes without a primary care provider
Access to medical records	Immediate access to specialists and athletic trainers
Allows time for counseling	
Cons	**Cons**
Time intensive	Lack of privacy
Potential need for specialist referral	Decreased time for counseling
Increased cost	Success is dependent on the ability of the athlete or parent to accurately complete a questionnaire

---

BOX 11.1 Common Causes of Sudden Death in Young Athletes

- Hypertrophic cardiomyopathy
- Commotio cordis
- Coronary anomalies
- Left ventricular hypertrophy of indeterminate cause
- Myocarditis
- Ruptured aortic aneurysm
- Arrhythmogenic right ventricular cardiomyopathy
- Heat stroke

Modified from Maron BJ. Sudden death in young athletes. *N Engl J Med.* 2003;349(11):1064–1075.

HEART HEALTH QUESTIONS ABOUT YOU	Yes	No
5. Have you ever passed out or nearly passed out DURING or AFTER exercise?		
6. Have you ever had discomfort, pain, tightness, or pressure in your chest during exercise?		
7. Does your heart ever race or skip beats (irregular beats) during exercise?		
8. Has a doctor ever told you that you have any heart problems? If so, check all that apply: ☐ High blood pressure ☐ A heart murmur ☐ High cholesterol ☐ A heart infection ☐ Kawasaki disease Other: _____		
9. Has a doctor ever ordered a test for your heart? (For example, ECG/EKG, echocardiogram)		
10. Do you get lightheaded or feel more short of breath than expected during exercise?		
11. Have you ever had an unexplained seizure?		
12. Do you get more tired or short of breath more quickly than your friends during exercise?		

HEART HEALTH QUESTIONS ABOUT YOUR FAMILY	Yes	No
13. Has any family member or relative died of heart problems or had an unexpected or unexplained sudden death before age 50 (including drowning, unexplained car accident, or sudden infant death syndrome)?		
14. Does anyone in your family have hypertrophic cardiomyopathy, Marfan syndrome, arrhythmogenic right ventricular cardiomyopathy, long QT syndrome, short QT syndrome, Brugada syndrome, or catecholaminergic polymorphic ventricular tachycardia?		
15. Does anyone in your family have a heart problem, pacemaker, or implanted defibrillator?		
16. Has anyone in your family had unexplained fainting, unexplained seizures, or near drowning?		

Fig. 11.1 Cardiac history screening. (From Bernhardt DT, Roberts WO, eds. *Preparticipation Physical Evaluation*, 4th ed. Elk Grove Village, IL: American Academy of Pediatrics; 2010.)

BOX 11.2   Phenotypic Features of Marfan Syndrome

Cardiac
- Aortic root dilation
- Mitral valve prolapse

Ocular
- Ectopia lentis
- Myopia

Musculoskeletal
- Tall stature (males taller than 183 cm [6 feet] and females taller than 178 cm [5 feet, 10 inches]); *Note: Tall stature is not formally considered a criterion of the revised Ghent nosology*
- Increased upper segment to lower segment ratio; increased arm span relative to height
- Arachnodactyly (wrist and thumb sign)
- Pectus carinatum/excavatum
- Hindfoot deformity or plain pes planus
- Protrusio acetabuli
- Scoliosis, kyphosis
- Reduced elbow extension

Facial Features
- Dolichocephaly
- Enophthalmos
- Downslanting palpebral fissures
- Malar hypoplasia, retrognathia

Other Systemic Features
- Pneumothorax
- Dural ectasia
- Skin striae

Modified from Loeys BL, Dietz HC, Braverman AC, et al. The revised Ghent nosology for the Marfan syndrome. *J Med Genet.* 2010;47(7):476–485; Giese EA, O'Connor FG, Brennan FH, Depenbrock PJ, Oriscello RG. The athletic preparticipation evaluation: cardiovascular assessment. *Am Fam Physician.* 2007;75(7):1008–1014.

pressure measurements should be made with an appropriately sized cuff. All athletes with hypertension require further workup and monitoring. Athletes with stage I hypertension (i.e., the 95th to 99th percentile plus 5 mm Hg in children and 140/90 to 160/100 mm Hg in adults) who do not have heart disease, end-organ damage, or left ventricular hypertrophy should not be restricted, except from sports that may make heavy use of the Valsalva maneuver, such as weightlifting. Athletes with stage II hypertension (i.e., >99th percentile plus 5 mm Hg in children and >160/100 mm Hg in adults) should initially be restricted from all participation pending a thorough workup and control of blood pressure.[20]

Special attention should be directed at excluding MFS (and related connective tissue disorders, such as Ehlers-Danlos and Loeys-Dietz syndromes), which all manifest genetic deficiencies of connective tissue proteins and thereby increase risk of dissection of the aorta and other smaller arteries. Clinical manifestations of MFS may also include the ocular, musculoskeletal, respiratory, neurologic, and integumentary systems (Box 11.2). For the diagnosis of MFS, revised Ghent criteria were published in 2010 and consequently are not referenced in the PPE-4.[21] The revised Ghent criteria have placed more weight on the three cardinal features of MFS[17]: aortic root enlargement,[18] ectopia lentis,[19] and FBN1 mutation to differentiate the manifestations of the cardiovascular, ocular, and skeletal organ systems. In the absence of family history, the presence of both aortic root changes and ectopia lentis[19] are sufficient to make the diagnosis. However, these two features are not easily assessed in the PPE setting, and thus clinicians should be vigilant to identify any possible physical stigmata of MFS, particularly in male athletes taller than 183 cm (6 feet) and female athletes taller than 178 cm (5 feet, 10 inches). Athletes with a family history of MFS or two or more of the aforementioned physical examination findings should be referred for cardiology consultation to comprehensively assess aortic morphology.[22] Given the greater emphasis on ectopia lentis in the revised criteria, a referral to ophthalmology for slit-lamp testing is also prudent.[21]

Significant debate exists regarding noninvasive cardiac screening during the PPE, and although comprehensive coverage of this subject is beyond the scope of this chapter, related controversies are discussed in detail elsewhere in this book. The current AHA guidelines limit the use of electrocardiography (ECG) screening to small cohorts of young people aged 12 to 25 years with suspected cardiovascular pathology based on history and physical examination, provided that close physician supervision and quality control are achieved.[16] The guidelines suggest that limitations of using a 12-lead ECG, including poor sensitivity and specificity, should be anticipated. Otherwise, current guidelines do not agree on systematic inclusion of ECG in preparticipation screening of athletes and nonathletes to identify congenital or other cardiovascular abnormalities.[16,23] These guidelines are in contradistinction with recommendations of the International Olympic Committee[24] and the European Society of Cardiology (ESC),[25] which recommend the use of a screening ECG during PPEs. Routine ECG screening is supported by Italian data showing a 90% decrease in SCD rate with the inclusion of ECG in PPE cardiovascular screening.[14] The dispute in recommendations among societies is largely based on studies performed in Italy[26-28] which demonstrated that an ECG had a 77% greater power to detect HCM than did a history and physical examination alone.[28]

There are important sex and race differences in SCD rates that may influence the decision to use the ECG as part of the PPE. It has been shown that there is an increased likelihood of obtaining abnormal ECGs with PPEs of older adolescent males and a decreased likelihood with females.[29] Male athletes have been shown to be at 5 to 6 times greater risk than female athletes for SCD.[30] In addition, the rate of SCD among black athletes has been shown to be 3 to 5 times higher in comparison with all other ethnic groups.[30]

A systematic approach to interpreting screening ECGs as part of the PPE are the Seattle Criteria.[31] These criteria were initially created to balance the sensitivity and specificity of ECG use, while maintaining a practical and concise checklist for physicians to use for ECG interpretation with athletes. The goal of the Seattle Criteria is to aid physicians in distinguishing ECG abnormalities that may be considered normal in athletes from abnormal ECG findings that are concerning for pathology. However, use of the Seattle Criteria has not been shown to decrease morbidity or reduce incidence of SCD among athletes.[31-33] The Refined Criteria published in 2014 for ECG interpretation have been shown to decrease the occurrence of false-positive and false-negative results.[33] Data suggest that the Refined Criteria outperform the ESC recommendations and Seattle Criteria by reducing false-positive rates of ECG interpretation in black athletes from 40.4% (ESC) and 18.4% (Seattle Criteria) to 11.5%, and in white athletes from 16.2% (ESC) and 7.1% (Seattle Criteria) to 5.3%.[33,34] These studies suggest that established criteria and standardized guidelines for ECG interpretation are useful to avoid false-positive interpretations and potentially costly and unnecessary additional workup. Recently, the American Medical Society for Sports Medicine (AMSSM) formed a task force to address the need for preparticipation cardiovascular screening in young competitive athletes. Although the AMSSM supported the position that the ECG increases early detection of cardiac disorders associated with SCD, the absence of clear outcome-based research precluded the endorsement of using the ECG as a universal cardiovascular

screening strategy.[15] If physicians choose to incorporate routine ECG screening into their PPEs, proficiency in accurate ECG interpretation and access to cardiology resources are of paramount importance to maximize its utility without unnecessary cost escalation. However, the use of ECG as a global cardiovascular preparticipation screening modality in athletes is limited by the low prevalence of SCD in athletes.

A newer area of debate is use of an echocardiogram as part of the routine PPE cardiac screening protocol. It has been demonstrated that ECGs have a higher rate of false-positives as a screening modality in comparison with echocardiogram for detection of causative risk factors for HCM.[17] This is in large part due to the similarities between ECG changes that are physiologic resulting from physical conditioning and the structural and electrical changes found in HCM. The increasing availability of portable ultrasound has led to the development of the Early Screening for Cardiac Abnormalities with Preparticipation Echocardiography (ESCAPE) protocol, which produced accuracy and reliability in diagnosing results indicative of HCM and aortic root dilation.[35] The protocol demonstrated that limited echocardiography measurements by noncardiologists were not statistically different from values obtained from cardiologists trained in echocardiography interpretation.[34,35] However, as with ECG interpretation, the ability of the team physician, not frequently a cardiologist, to accurately and efficiently interpret echocardiograms is paramount to this modality being as useful as is reported in the literature.

Reducing the incidence of SCD is a noble goal, but clinicians should be aware of the high false-positive rates associated with PPE ECGs, along with high costs, increased use of medical resources, potentially erroneous disqualification of athletes from participation, and the potential for lost "life-years" following needless sedentary lifestyle recommendations.[36] Therefore although controversial, at present there are insufficient data available to promote universal use of screening ECGs or echocardiograms in asymptomatic individuals for detecting cardiovascular disease. A rational decision to include ECG or echocardiography as part of the PPE could conceivably be made in the appropriate setting and with sufficient provider training and resources.

Pulmonary System

It is imperative that athletes be questioned regarding a personal or family history of asthma or exercise-induced bronchoconstriction (affecting 50% to 90% of athletes), asthma-like symptoms and their severity, use of bronchodilators, degree of asthma control, and the use of tobacco or exposure to secondhand smoke.[37] A thorough auscultation of the lung fields should be performed during the PPE. Proper diagnosis may require provocative pulmonary function testing, and in patients with exercise-induced bronchospasm, this is imperative to evaluate for undiagnosed asthma.[32] Because an athlete's symptoms may be related to the environment, these tests may need to be performed in environmental conditions that stimulate symptoms.[37] Athletes who are recovering from an asthma exacerbation and who are actively wheezing must be restricted from sports activity until stabilized.[32] Vocal cord dysfunction should be considered as a potential diagnosis in athletes with asthma-like symptoms who fail to respond to usual bronchodilator therapy. Athletes with stable asthma or exercise-induced bronchoconstriction can usually be cleared to participate in sports, unless they are recovering from a recent asthma exacerbation. It may be indicated for athletes with severe underlying asthma or pulmonary disease to have a rescue inhaler available as a condition for athletic participation.[32]

Gastrointestinal/Genitourinary System

The abdomen should be thoroughly examined for masses, tenderness, rigidity, or enlargement of the liver or spleen. The AMSSM, among other sports medicine professional organizations, recommends that a detailed genitourinary examination should be performed to assess for masses, testicular descent, tenderness, and hernias in male athletes.[2] Liver or spleen enlargement is a contraindication to participation in sports. The athlete with a solitary kidney or testicle may be cleared to participate in contact sports; however, each athlete should be counseled on an individual basis about the harmful consequences of injury, and appropriate protective gear should be mandated during practice and competition. Acute diarrheal illness is a contraindication to participation in sports unless symptoms are mild and the athlete remains well hydrated.[2]

Musculoskeletal System

The musculoskeletal history has a very high sensitivity (92%) for detecting abnormalities, and thus the physician should inquire about current injuries and a history of injuries requiring evaluation, casting, bracing, surgery, or missed participation.[5,38] Given the high sensitivity of the history, a screening musculoskeletal examination is sufficient but should be supplemented with a more in-depth joint-specific examination when pathology is suspected.[2] Box 11.3 reviews the 11-step general musculoskeletal screening examination. In general, literature suggests that generalized joint laxity, imbalance in strength ratios, excessive foot pronation or supination, level of physical maturity, multidirectional

---

BOX 11.3   General Musculoskeletal Screening Examination

The general musculoskeletal screening examination consists of the following: (1) inspection, athlete standing, facing toward examiner (symmetry of trunk, upper extremities); (2) forward flexion, extension, rotation, lateral flexion of neck (range of motion, cervical spine); (3) resisted shoulder shrug (strength, trapezius); (4) resisted shoulder abduction (strength, deltoid); (5) internal and external rotation of shoulder (range of motion, glenohumeral joint); (6) extension and flexion of elbow (range of motion, elbow); (7) pronation and supination of forearm or wrist (range of motion, elbow and wrist); (8) clench fist, then spread fingers (range of motion, hand and fingers); (9) inspection, athlete facing away from examiner (symmetry of trunk, upper extremities); (10) back extension, knees straight (spondylolysis/spondylolisthesis); (11) back flexion with knees straight, facing toward and away from examiner (range of motion, thoracic and lumbosacral spine; spine curvature; hamstring flexibility); (12) inspection of lower extremities, contraction of quadriceps muscles (alignment, symmetry); (13) "duck walk" 4 steps (motion of hip, knee, and ankle; strength; balance); (14) standing on toes, then on heels (symmetry, calf; strength; balance).

From Bernhardt DT, Roberts WO, eds. *Preparticipation Physical Evaluation.* ed 4. Elk Grove Village, IL: American Academy of Pediatrics; 2010.

---

balance, and body mass all may be predictive for risk of injury in the adolescent athlete population.[39,40] The PPE-4 recommends functional testing with the duck walk and single-leg hop as part of the musculoskeletal examination.[2] These physical examination tests are time-efficient, require no additional equipment, and may help clinicians to effectively assess multiple physical attributes during the PPE.

Clearance for sport participation is determined based on the degree and type of injury or condition, the ability of the injured athlete to compete safely, and the necessities of a given sport. In general, if the athlete has no tenderness to palpation, has normal range of motion (ROM) and normal strength in the affected area, and performs adequately on functional tests, clearance for sport participation can typically be given. Use of protective padding, taping, or bracing may also enable the athlete to participate in sports safely.[2]

Neurologic System

Physicians should inquire about prior concussions or head injuries, seizure disorders, frequent or exertional headaches, problems with recurrent burners or stingers (transient brachial plexopathy), or a prior transient quadriparesis or cervical cord neuropraxia.[2] A positive history demands a thorough neurologic examination, including assessment of cognition, cranial nerves, motor-sensory function, muscle tone, reflexes, coordination testing, and gait evaluation.[5] Athletes who have a history of multiple concussions or who have prolonged postconcussive symptoms should be counseled about risks and encouraged to discuss with their families the potential for harm, although not presently well understood, that may result from repeated concussions.[5] The Sport Concussion Assessment Tool (SCAT),[41] exercise testing such as the Buffalo Concussion Treadmill Test,[42] vestibuloocular system testing such as the Vestibular/Ocular Motor Screening Assessment,[43] vestibulospinal testing such as the Balance Error Scoring System,[32] and neuropsychological testing[44] may increase the sensitivity of detecting residual concussion symptoms. Athletes with persistent symptoms should be disqualified and cleared for participation only after they have successfully completed a graded return-to-sport protocol without recurrence of concussion-related signs or symptoms.[41] Likewise, after sustaining a single stinger, athletes must be asymptomatic with a normal neurologic examination prior to medical clearance, although further diagnostic testing may be necessary for persistent symptoms or recurrent injury.[45] Athletes who have had transient quadriparesis should have an MRI to evaluate for spinal stenosis.[46] For atypical, exercise-related headaches, advanced intracranial imaging may be necessary to evaluate for occult causes of secondary headaches.[47] Although a history of seizures does not preclude athletic participation, sports-specific modifications may be needed, particularly for persons involved in water sports.[2]

Hematologic and Infectious Disease

The risks of transmission of human immunodeficiency virus, hepatitis B, and hepatitis C during routine sports participation are considered minimal, and the presence of these infections is not considered a contraindication to participation.[48,49] However, guidelines from the National Hemophilia Foundation advise that athletes with bleeding disorders such as hemophilia be restricted from contact or collision sports. In addition, a diagnosis of infectious mononucleosis should preclude all sports participation for the first 3 weeks because of a significantly elevated risk of splenic rupture.[50] Light, noncontact activity may be recommended 3 weeks after diagnosis if the athlete is asymptomatic and without complications. Participation in full-contact sports should be deferred for at least 28 days from the start of symptoms or from clinical diagnosis if the symptom onset date is imprecise.[2] Febrile illness is also a contraindication to participation in sports because of increased susceptibility to heat illness and because it may occasionally accompany conditions such as myocarditis that may make sports participation unsafe.[2]

Sickle cell trait (SCT) is associated with 2% of deaths in National Collegiate Athletic Association (NCAA) football players.[51] Athletes should be questioned about a personal or family history of SCT or sickle cell disease (SCD). Phenotypic expression is varied, and thus medical clearance or exercise modifications should be made on an individual basis. To prevent exertional sickling collapse, athletes with SCT should avoid strenuous activity in extreme heat and high-altitude environments, especially when they are poorly acclimated.[52] Deaths from exertional sickling have reportedly been more common among football players as well.[53] In recognition of these risks, the NCAA in 2010 mandated that all Division I and II athletes be screened for SCT and that the status be established at the time of the PPE[32]; however, athletes may decline screening.[51] This requirement by the NCAA was extended to Division III competitors as of 2014.[54] If SCT is confirmed with screening, affected athletes are offered counseling on its implications to their health, athletics, and family planning.[55] Debate still exists on universally screening athletes for SCT. Some proponents have estimated that universal screening of NCAA Division I student athletes would save seven lives over 10 years.[54] Based on the available evidence, we recommend that all active individuals be screened for SCT with a 1-time hemoglobin electrophoresis test.

Endocrine System

Persons with types I and II diabetes mellitus can participate in sports without restriction but are encouraged to monitor blood glucose more frequently, maintain a balanced diet, adjust medications appropriately, and hydrate suitably.[2] Education regarding activities with relatively higher risk of cutaneous foot injury such as hiking, rock climbing, or surfing is also recommended. Obese patients should not be discouraged from participating in sports but should receive counseling on lifestyle changes such as dietary and activity modifications, as well as prevention of heat-related illness.[2] Athletes in weight-sensitive sports such as wrestling and boxing, and aesthetic sports such as diving and figure skating are at risk for eating disorders, particularly in females.[32] The female athlete triad consists of disordered eating, amenorrhea, and decreased bone mineral density. A history of stress fractures with prolonged healing in a female athlete should increase clinical suspicion for this treatable yet potentially deadly medical condition. These patients should undergo a multidisciplinary treatment program with further risk stratification before they return to sports. It is recommended that sports medicine professionals include female athlete triad risk assessment in the standard PPE and consider expanding the history to include full menstrual history, reasons for hormonal therapy use, and questions concerning eating disorders and eating irregularities.[56]

Dermatology

Athletes should be asked about a history of dermatologic pathology, with particular attention to highly communicable infections such as herpes or methicillin-resistant *Staphylococcus aureus*.[2] The athlete should be inspected for evidence of common cutaneous infections such as herpes gladiatorum, tinea gladiatorum, impetigo, molluscum contagiosum, warts, and community-acquired methicillin-resistant *S. aureus*.[2] Prevention of transmission is critical and may be achieved by covering the infected site, using prophylactic medications as indicated, refraining from sharing personal items, thoroughly cleaning athletic equipment, or ultimately restricting the athlete from participation for a specific period based on the characteristics of the sport, the type of microorganism involved, and governing body guidelines.[2]

Immunizations

Lack of immunizations does not inherently affect sports participation, but many states require them for school enrollment, and thus the PPE provides a good opportunity to discuss vaccinations.[2] Athletes traveling internationally for competition should be aware of local immunization guidelines recommended by the Centers for Disease Control and Prevention.[2]

Medications and Allergies

It is imperative that medical personnel are familiar with regulations established by drug-enforcing agencies such as the World Anti-Doping Agency. Some medications are strictly prohibited, whereas others, such as albuterol, may be used with therapeutic use exemption.[5] Over-the-counter drugs and supplements may contain banned substances and should also be thoroughly reviewed. The PPE provides a good opportunity to address the detrimental effects of illicit drug and alcohol use, particularly in the adolescent population. Medication, food, and environmental allergies should be documented in detail. Specifications should include the name of the allergen, the type of reaction, and whether athletes require an epinephrine autoinjector.[2] Four recommendations for persons with a history of anaphylaxis include:

1. All medical personnel and athletes with allergies who may potentially require treatment with an epinephrine autoinjector should be trained in how to use it.
2. All medical kits should be stocked with an epinephrine autoinjector and over-the-counter diphenhydramine.
3. Athletes with allergies should carry an epinephrine autoinjector in their backpacks, have an additional one in their homes or dormitory rooms, and have over-the-counter diphenhydramine readily available at all times.
4. An emergency action plan (EAP) should be detailed for athletes with allergies during the PPE.

Heat Illness

Athletes with a history of exertional heat illness (EHI) are at enhanced risk for recurrent heat illness.[57] Such athletes should be educated about preventive measures, including adequate hydration and gradual acclimatization over a period of 10 to 14 days. If possible, use of stimulant and antihistamine medications should be avoided during warm-weather activities.[5] Athletes who use stimulant medications (e.g., for attention-deficit/hyperactivity disorder) and team health care professionals should be informed about the possible deleterious effects of using these medications in hot environments.

The National Athletic Trainers' Association (NATA) has guidelines for athletes to help mitigate risks involved with EHI.[58] It is recommended that individuals are gradually acclimatized to heat over 7 to 14 days to prevent the risk of EHI. Athletes who are currently sick with any viral infection or fever or have a skin rash should be withheld from participation until the condition is resolved. It is recommended that players have access to fluids at all times. Athletes should consume sodium-containing food or fluids to help replace loss of sodium in sweat and/or urine. Monitoring proper fluid consumption and replacement can help to minimize body mass loss to 2% during activity participation, which should be measured before and after the activity. Athletes should also be encouraged to sleep a minimum of 7 hours per night in a cool environment, eat a balanced diet, and properly hydrate before, during, and after exercise. Of most importance, rest periods should consist of at least 3 hours for food, nutrients, and electrolytes to be properly digested and absorbed before the next practice or game. Cold-water or ice towels should be readily accessible for all patients because immediate whole-body cooling is essential to treat EHI.

Athletes With Special Needs

The PPE-4 includes a chapter that discusses athletes with special needs and a separate form to aid the provider with unique issues affecting this patient population. The history and physical examination should be similar to that used with athletes who do not have special needs but may need to focus on diseases more common in this population such as seizures, hearing loss, vision loss, congenital heart disease, and renal disease.[2] Athletes with Down syndrome should always be assessed for a history of atlantoaxial instability (AAI), and athletes with spinal cord injuries should be asked about difficulties with thermoregulation, autonomic dysreflexia, pressure ulcers, and use of urinary catheterization.[2] The physical examination should focus on the visual, cardiovascular, musculoskeletal, neurologic, and dermatologic systems. Congenital heart disease is present in up to half of all athletes with Down syndrome and may require a cardiology referral for further testing prior to participation in sports.[59]

The neurologic examination in athletes with Down syndrome should include evaluation for symptomatic AAI, which may present with upper motor neuron signs such as spasticity, hyperreflexia, clonus, and clumsiness. Persons with symptomatic AAI should undergo lateral cervical spine flexion and extension plain x-ray views to assess stability.[2] Wheelchair athletes should be evaluated for nerve entrapments, pressure ulcers, and overuse injuries of the shoulders, hands, and wrists.[2]

Conclusion

The PPE has continued to evolve, with updated recommendations to perform a PPE for all children in an office-based setting. Despite these broad recommendations, evidence showing that the PPE reduces morbidity and mortality is scarce.[4] The PPE-4 emphasizes that history, rather than physical examination, is most sensitive for gleaning information relevant to medical clearance for sports participation. Nonetheless, a thorough PPE using a systematic approach and current guidelines may help to identify those athletes who need additional investigation prior to safe athletic participation and may also aid in preparation by the sports medicine team and the athlete for any injuries or medical complications that may result from sports.

ON-FIELD EMERGENCIES

The preceding section outlined the limitations in preventing potentially life-threatening events. Although rare, medical emergencies in sports will inevitably occur despite thorough preventive measures. This section outlines the core components of managing sports-related emergencies, including development of an effective EAP, the general approach to the collapsed athlete, and select examples of medical emergencies encountered on the playing field.

Emergency Action Plan

Before hosting athletic events, every institution has a duty to formulate an EAP,[60] which should be developed and reviewed annually as a coordinated effort by the medical team, school administrators, local emergency medical services (EMS), and first responders. The key components of the EAP are (1) effective communication, (2) training personnel, (3) acquiring equipment, (4) emergency transportation, (5) practice and review, and (6) postevent guidelines.[61]

Effective communication with local EMS is a critical link in the chain of survival. Communication systems such as telephones or two-way radios should be tested before each game. An EAP coordinator should be identified at each institution, and all other potential first responders should receive training in EAP guidelines, as well as in CPR and AED use. Resuscitation equipment should be centrally located and well marked for easy access. Personnel trained in basic life support (BLS) should have quick access to barrier masks for rescue breathing and an on-site AED. Providers trained in advanced cardiac life support (ACLS) may consider having advanced airways, oxygen delivery systems, and cardiac medications available.[61] Other critical contents of a sideline physician's emergency kit are listed in Box 11.4. A plan for efficiently directing EMS to the field of play should be in place, and on-site ambulance coverage is ideal at particularly high-risk events. In the event that medical personnel must leave the playing field to tend to an injured athlete, a plan for continued event coverage should be established.[60] The EAP should be rehearsed on an annual basis, which will ensure a coordinated team effort, and the EAP should be evaluated frequently to ensure its durability. Lastly, a protocol for release of medical information should be established and an incident form should be available for documentation and evaluation purposes.[61]

BOX 11.4 Recommended Contents of the Sideline Physician's Emergency Bag

Medications
- Aspirin
- Beta-agonist inhaler
- Epinephrine
- Oral glucose solution

Wound Care
- Bandage scissors
- Bandage tape
- Sterile saline and sterile bowl (0.5–1 L)
- 60-mL syringe for irrigation
- Large-bore needles: 18 gauge or angiocatheter
- Antibacterial cleansing agent
- 1% lidocaine with and without epinephrine
- Lidocaine jelly (2%) or LET gel for abrasions
- Sterile scrub brush
- Povidone-iodine
- 5-mL syringes
- 25-gauge needles (1 Y2-in. long)
- Needle driver
- Tweezers

- Skin stapler
- Sterile drapes or towels
- Nylon sutures: 3-0, 4-0, 5-0, 6-0
- Polyglactin sutures: 3-0, 4-0, 5-0
- Liquid cyanoacrylate adhesive
- Compound benzoin tincture
- Bacitracin or triple antibiotic ointment
- Adhesive strips: Y4-, Y2-, and 1-in. wide
- Nonadherent pads
- Sterile gauze pads
- Sterile adhesive dressings in various sizes
- Hydrocolloid dressings
- Protective skin covering
- Aluminum chloride solution
- Athletic tape
- Latex and nonlatex (e.g., nitrile) gloves
- Aftercare instructions for patients

Airway Devices
- Pocket mouth-to-mouth mask
- Cutting tool for facemask loops

Modified from Daniels JM, Kary J, Lane JA. Optimizing the sideline medical bag preparing for school and community sports events. *Phys Sportsmed.* 2005;33(12):9–16; Bouchard M. Sideline care of abrasions and lacerations: preparation is key. *Phys Sportsmed.* 2005;33(2):21–29.

TABLE 11.2 Initial Approach to the Collapsed Athlete

Nontraumatic	Traumatic
BLS Assessment[49]	**ATLS Primary Survey**[41]
1. Check for responsiveness.	**A**irway maintenance with cervical spine control
2. Activate the emergency response system; obtain and activate the AED.	**B**reathing and ventilation
3. Check for breathing and a carotid pulse for 5–10 s. If no pulse is present, initiate CPR with chest compressions first and then rescue breathing. If a pulse is present, begin rescue breathing.	**C**irculation and hemorrhage control **D**isability/drugs: assessment of neurologic status **E**xposure: completely undress the patient but prevent hypothermia
4. Perform defibrillation with the AED when indicated.	
ACLS Primary Assessment[49]	**ATLS Secondary Survey**[41]
Airway: Maintain airway patency and use advanced airway management if needed.	History:
Breathing: Monitor ventilation and oxygenation and provide supplementary oxygen if needed.	**A**llergies **M**edications
Circulation: Monitor CPR quality; monitor for arrhythmias; provide defibrillation, cardioversion, and administer cardiac drugs when needed; obtain intravenous or intraosseous access and provide fluids if needed; monitor glucose, temperature, and perfusion.	**P**ast illness/**P**regnancy **L**ast meal **E**vents/**E**nvironment related to injury
Disability: Check neurologic function; check for responsiveness, levels of consciousness, and pupil dilation.	Physical examination: Thorough head-to-toe physical examination
Exposure: Remove clothing and observe for signs of trauma, bleeding, or medical alert bracelets.	

ACLS, Advanced cardiac life support; *AED,* automated external defibrillator; *ATLS,* advanced trauma life support; *BLS,* basic life support; *CPR,* cardiopulmonary resuscitation.

General Approach to the Collapsed Athlete

A pivotal duty of physicians is to be a keen observer of on-field emergencies, because the injury mechanism is often critical to the initial management of the athlete. For example, the clinical approach to a 65-year-old masters track athlete who clutches his chest before collapsing in the middle of a race will differ from the care of a 15-year-old football cornerback who collapses after "spear tackling" an opponent. In the first nontraumatic case, cardiac etiology would be suspected, and thus the BLS and ACLS assessments would be used (Table 11.2). Conversely, the approach to the trauma patient should follow the advanced trauma life support (ATLS) guidelines (see Table 11.2).[62] With ATLS, the rapid primary survey assesses vital functions with simultaneous stabilization of any life-threatening conditions. After stabilization, a thorough history and physical examination of the secondary survey should commence.[62] Physicians covering a sporting event may not always be able to determine the injury mechanism or extent of the injury, particularly when the patient remains unconscious or the inciting event was not witnessed.

In these situations, it should be assumed that the cervical spine is compromised, and physicians should follow appropriate precautions (outlined later in this chapter).

Head Injury

Head injuries account for 69% of fatalities in American football athletes.[63] The leading cause of death after a sports-related head injury is intracranial hemorrhage,[64] which may present as either an epidural, subdural, intracerebral, or subarachnoid hematoma. Epidural hematomas, which typically result from a tear of the middle meningeal artery as a complication of fracture of the temporal bone, are the most rapidly progressive intracranial hemorrhage and may cause death within 30 to 60 minutes.[64] In contrast, subdural hematomas evolve at a considerably slower rate, over a period of days to months, and yet they are the most common cause of fatal head injury in athletics.[63] Fortunately, most head injuries are less severe, with concussions being more common. A concussion is defined as a traumatic brain injury induced by direct or indirect biomechanical forces.[41] The sideline physician should be trained to recognize the symptoms of concussion, which vary greatly and include combinations of different symptoms including but not limited to headaches, nausea, dizziness, photophobia, and difficulties with concentration and memory.[65]

The approach to a collapsed athlete with a suspected head injury should always begin with the ATLS survey. An unconscious athlete should be assumed to have a cervical spine injury and should be appropriately stabilized. For conscious athletes, the primary survey should involve rapid assessment of circulation, airway, and breathing, followed by an assessment for spinal tenderness and neurologic assessment of the upper and lower limbs.[65] The athlete who remains unconscious for greater than 1 minute, has focal neurologic deficits, or has deteriorating mental status should be transferred emergently for advanced imaging to assess for intracranial hemorrhage. Stable athletes should be removed from play, and a thorough neurologic examination should be performed either on the sideline or in the locker room. The SCAT[41] provides a systematic approach to concussion evaluation both immediately on the field and for more extensive evaluation in the locker room, training room, or medical office. Following a potential head injury during athletic participation, serial examinations are essential because epidural hematomas frequently present with a lucid interval prior to rapid neurologic deterioration.[64] The concussed athlete should never return to play (RTP) the same day and should follow a gradual stepwise return-to-sport protocol, returning to play only after symptoms have resolved and medical clearance has occurred.[41] Current guidelines no longer allow for "rare exceptions" to be made with respect to same day RTP guidelines for elite adult athletes. We recommend that team physicians, in concert with athletic trainers and other medical personnel involved in the care of athletes, establish a written policy regarding concussion management. The policy should detail a stepwise algorithm to carefully assess clinical progress, cognitive function (using computerized testing when available), a graded return-to-sport protocol, and, as needed, a plan for specialist consultation.

Cervical Spine Injury

Approximately 12,000 new spinal cord injuries occur each year in the United States, with 8% resulting from sports participation.[66] The injury typically results from traumatic axial loading of the cervical spine, which creates transient, geometric changes in the spinal column with resultant injury to neural structures.[67]

The recommendations provided in this section are primarily based on the NATA position statement on prehospital management of the spine-injured athlete. At the time of press, the NATA was completing a position statement update process, and the recommendations herein are reflective of changes outlined in the corresponding executive summary; however, these updates had not been officially endorsed by the NATA and participating professional organizations. The authors encourage the reader to review the NATA website for updates (https://www.nata.org/news-publications/pressroom/statements/consensus).

The management of suspected cervical spine injury requires a coordinated team effort, and prior to each season, neck stabilization techniques, methods of transferring injured players, airway and equipment management, and immobilization techniques should be rehearsed carefully. EAPs should be developed and coordinated with local emergency responders prior to the season, and on-site sports medicine teams should perform a "time out" prior to competition to review EAPs. Considerations should include the personnel and equipment available for that event, stabilization and transportation plans, and the use of a hospital that can deliver immediate, definitive care for cervical spine injuries.[68]

In a collapsed athlete, symptoms and signs that raise the index of suspicion for severe traumatic cervical spine injury include (1) unconsciousness or an altered level of consciousness, (2) bilateral neurologic findings or complaints, (3) significant midline spine pain with or without palpation, and (4) obvious spinal column deformity.[69] An ATLS survey should commence immediately with special attention to cervical spine precautions. Moving the patient to a supine position with use of the log-roll maneuver may be obligatory if the athlete is found prone and the primary survey cannot be performed. The head and neck should be manually maintained in a neutral position without traction.[69] Airway patency and accessibility should be established, and rescue breathing should be initiated if necessary, which may entail the removal of a facemask or mouth guard. A cordless screwdriver is the initial equipment of choice for removal of a facemask because it induces less movement than other tools. However, an appropriate manual tool for cutting helmet loops should also be available at all times, and medical personnel should rehearse the use of these tools before the season begins. Helmet screws also should be routinely inspected and maintained throughout the season by equipment managers and/or athletic trainers. Removal of helmets and pads prior to transfer when appropriate should be done by three rescuers trained and experienced with equipment removal, or at the earliest possible time three such trained rescuers are available in order to have unhindered access to the athlete to facilitate delivery of care.[68,69] Manual stabilization should be augmented, but not replaced, by mechanical stabilization with use of a cervical collar. A full-body stabilization should be facilitated by transfer to a spine board. Supine athletes should be transferred via the "lift-and-slide" technique, whereas prone athletes should be transferred with use of the "log-roll" method. Head and neck stabilization should continue during transportation and until a destabilizing injury has been excluded. For an in-depth review, we recommend perusal of the NATA position statement[68] on acute management of the cervical spine–injured athlete.[69]

Cardiac Arrest

The most common cause of SCD in athletes younger than 35 years is congenital cardiac disease, and in athletes older than 35 years, the most frequent etiology is atherosclerotic heart disease.[70] The initial presenting feature of occult cardiac disease may be SCD, and thus the PPE is designed to screen for potential symptoms and signs that may be representative of underlying cardiac disease. In the event of a nontraumatic collapse of an athlete, a potential cardiac etiology should be strongly considered and a thorough evaluation and cardiology consultation are imperative before the athlete is allowed to resume participation. After cardiac arrest, the inclusive goal is to support and restore effective oxygenation, ventilation, and circulation with return of neurologic function.[71] Keys to ensuring successful resuscitation are (1) immediate recognition of cardiac arrest and activation of the emergency response system, (2) early initiation of CPR with an emphasis on high-quality chest compressions, (3) rapid defibrillation, (4) effective use of advanced life support measures, and (5) integrated post–cardiac arrest care.[71]

Initial evaluation should follow the BLS assessment and ACLS primary assessment (see Table 11.2). For unconscious athletes with cardiac or respiratory arrest, initial management should move to the ACLS primary assessment once the BLS assessment is completed. For conscious athletes, the ACLS primary assessment should be conducted first.[71] The 2015 AHA BLS guidelines recommend beginning CPR with chest compressions immediately, without a delay for administering rescue breaths first. Factors for effective CPR include a rate of 100 to 120 chest compressions per minute, adequate depth of compressions to 5 cm, allowing complete chest recoil after each compression, minimizing interruptions of chest compressions, avoiding excessive ventilation, and switching the CPR provider who is administering the chest compressions to avoid fatigue, ideally changing positions during cardiac rhythm interpretation by the AED, as applicable.[71] At a minimum, we recommend that all medical providers involved in the care of athletes maintain BLS certification, and ACLS certification for team physicians should be strongly considered.

Tension Pneumothorax

Pneumothorax (PTX) is the presence of air in the pleural space, which occurs spontaneously as a result of a traumatic tear of the pleura after a chest injury or may be iatrogenic as a result of a medical procedure.[72] Tension PTX is a rare form of PTX that may develop as a result of a chest wall defect or a displaced fracture, or as a progression of a simple PTX. The underlying mechanism is a "one-way valve" air leak that forms through a defect in the

lung or chest wall, which leads to a progressively enlarging PTX with each inspiration.[62] Typical symptoms include dyspnea and ipsilateral pleuritic chest pain. Physical examination may reveal tachycardia, tachypnea, hypotension, hyperresonance to percussion, unilateral absence of breath sounds, tracheal deviation, and distended neck veins.[72] Sideline diagnosis of this medical emergency is dependent on symptoms and signs noted with clinical evaluation, and clinicians should not await radiographic imaging to confirm this diagnosis.[62] Initial management entails immediate decompression via insertion of a large-caliber (11- to 16-gauge) needle into the affected hemithorax by way of the second intercostal space in the midclavicular line.[62] Definitive treatment involves emergent hospital transportation, tube thoracostomy, and supplementary administration of oxygen. RTP guidelines should be individualized, yet it is possible for athletes to resume participation 3 to 4 weeks after a traumatic PTX has occurred.[72] We recommend a thorough workup for occult connective tissue disorders (e.g., MFS) in athletes who experience a spontaneous PTX.

Anaphylaxis

Anaphylaxis is an acute, alarming, and accelerated life-threatening systemic reaction with varied mechanisms, clinical presentations, and severity that results from the abrupt systemic release of mediators from mast cells and basophils.[73] The overall incidence is estimated to be 1%–2% worldwide, and food and drugs are thought to be the most common causes.[74] Exercise-induced anaphylaxis is a well-described phenomenon in which exercise triggers symptoms, including extreme fatigue, warmth, flushing, pruritus, and urticaria, occasionally progressing to angioedema, wheezing, upper airway obstruction, and collapse.[73] The precise pathophysiology is ill defined, yet co-triggers such as nonsteroidal antiinflammatory drugs, pollen, or specific foods have been implicated and should be identified if possible.[75] Anaphylaxis as a result of insect stings is also a concern; symptoms are similar to those previously described but may also include a large, localized skin reaction.[73]

The circulation, airway, breathing, and level of consciousness of athletes with a possible anaphylactic reaction should be evaluated. EMS should be activated followed by the rapid administration of an age-appropriate dose of epinephrine intramuscularly into the anterolateral thigh. Epinephrine injections can be repeated every 5 minutes for protracted symptoms. It is important to note that epinephrine injections alone do not definitively treat anaphylaxis in all cases and further emergent care may still be indicated. Athletes should be placed in a supine position with their lower limbs elevated. Vital signs should be monitored diligently, and oxygen and intravenous fluids should be administered if available. An advanced airway may be necessary for persons with respiratory compromise. Other adjunctive medications include nebulized bronchodilators, antihistamines, and glucocorticoids. After stabilization, athletes should undergo a workup to identify possible triggers of anaphylaxis, and future prevention should include appropriate prophylactic medications and avoidance of triggers. An epinephrine autoinjector should be prescribed, and a personalized EAP should be developed (as detailed in the PPE section).[73]

Limb-Threatening Injuries

Knee Dislocation

Defined as complete disruption of the integrity of the tibiofemoral articulation, knee dislocation is typically accompanied by rupture of at least two of the four major knee ligaments.[76] Sports activities account for one-third of all cases of knee dislocation.[77] The most feared complication is potential limb amputation as a result of vascular compromise. Dislocations are classified according to tibial dislocation in relation to the femur. Anterior dislocation as a result of hyperextension is the most common type of dislocation.[78] Clinical signs may be subtle if the dislocation reduced spontaneously, yet hemarthrosis and severe multidirectional instability are suggestive of a possible dislocation. If the knee remains dislocated, closed reduction should be attempted emergently. Common fibular nerve and popliteal artery function and integrity should be tested and documented. Distal pulses may remain intact despite significant popliteal artery compromise, which necessitates more definitive evaluation with angiography.[79] The athlete should be emergently transported for orthopedic and vascular surgery consultation.

Traumatic Amputation

The primary clinical goals after a traumatic amputation occurs are hemorrhage control and digit/limb salvage. Even small digital amputations may result in significant bleeding. Pressure should be applied to the area, and the affected limb should be elevated. A tourniquet should be applied only if significant hemorrhaging continues. The residual limb should be rinsed with sterile saline solution and wrapped with sterile gauze. The amputated portion should be wrapped in moist sterile gauze, sealed in a plastic bag, placed in an ice bath, and sent with the athlete during emergency transport to the hospital.[80]

Acute Compartment Syndrome

Acute compartment syndrome (ACS) is caused by altered tissue homeostasis within a closed muscle compartment. Tissue pressure greater than vascular perfusion pressure reduces capillary blood flow and induces local tissue hypoxia and necrosis.[81] ACS can occur in any limb but is much more common in the lower limbs. Causes of ACS in sports include fractures and crush injuries. Symptoms typically present within a few hours of the initial injury and include progressive pain, paresis, and paresthesias.[81] Passive and active ROM worsen pain, and severe cases present with diminished pulses, pallor, and paralysis.[82] Clinical suspicion for ACS mandates rapid transportation to a hospital for an emergent fasciotomy.

Environmental Factors

Heat Illness

EHI includes heat cramps, heat exhaustion, and heat stroke. Exertional heat stroke (EHS), the most severe type of heat illness, is defined by a core temperature greater than 40.5°C (105°F) at collapse, accompanied by central nervous system changes.[83] EHS manifests when body organ temperature rises above critical levels, leading to cell membrane damage and cell energy disruption. Early symptoms of EHS include clumsiness, stumbling, headache, nausea, dizziness, apathy, confusion, and impairment of consciousness.[83] Risk factors include obesity, prior heat stroke, dehydration, certain medications, poor fitness, hot and humid environments, and lack of acclimatization.[83] Early recognition and treatment are fundamental to reducing morbidity and mortality. Circulation, airway, and breathing should be assessed, along with rectal temperature in athletes exhibiting signs of EHS. The goal is to lower core body temperature to less than 38.9°C (102.5°F) within 30 minutes of collapse. Confirmation of EHS should result in initiation of immediate cooling measures, ideally in the form of whole-body ice-water immersion, which should be performed *prior* to emergency transportation.[83,84] The water should be approximately 1.7°C (35°F) to 15°C (59°F) and stirred continuously to maximize cooling. The patient should be removed from cold water immersion once core body temperature reaches 38.9°C (102°F) to prevent overcooling. Establishing intravenous access with volume resuscitation may help to prevent cardiovascular collapse and end-organ damage. A rectal temperature should be obtained every 3 to 5 minutes, and cooling should continue until body temperature is less than 39°C.[85] All persons experiencing EHS should be transported to a medical facility for advanced care and monitoring.

Lightning

Injuries from lightning kill approximately 24,000 people annually worldwide.[85] Participants in outdoor recreational activities have the greatest risk of sustaining an injury from lightning.[62] Lightning can cause injuries via direct contact, contact with an object that is struck, or "side splash," which occurs when the electrical current jumps from an object to the victim.[85] The most common cause of fatality resulting from a lightning injury is cardiopulmonary arrest.[86] Other sequelae may include burns, fractures, and dislocations resulting from violent muscle contraction and neurologic conditions such as loss of consciousness, seizure, headache, paresthesia, confusion, memory loss, and transient paralysis.[85,86]

Initial management may require movement of the injured person if ongoing thunderstorms threaten the safety of first responders. It should be noted that after a lightning strike, the injured person does not retain an electrical charge, and thus treatment should not be delayed.[87] After the scene of the lightning strike is deemed secure, management should follow the ATLS primary and secondary surveys. A tenet of triage after lightning trauma dictates that the "apparently dead" should be resuscitated first. This tenet pertains to the unique pathophysiology of cardiopulmonary arrest in lightning strikes that necessitates immediate ventilatory support to prevent secondary hypoxic arrhythmias.[86]

Conclusion

Paramount to the management of on-field emergencies are the precepts of preparation and anticipation. Team physicians should coordinate EAPs and have them rehearsed annually by all staff involved in the care of athletes. In addition, the physician's kit should be restocked adequately on a periodic basis to help ensure effective and timely treatment. Physicians should remain alert on the sideline, monitoring play vigilantly so they can view injuries as they occur, which will facilitate optimal care.

Lastly, thorough assessment of injured and ill athletes can be enhanced by meticulous adherence to the BLS, ACLS, and ATLS guidelines.

ETHICAL AND LEGAL ISSUES IN SPORTS MEDICINE

Ancient Greeks were credited with the birth of both rational medicine and professional sports.[65] With Western medicine in its infancy, the physician's role in the sporting microcosm was neither well defined nor respected. Greek athletes sought advice from their trainers regarding their inclusive training methods, including diet and physiotherapy.[88] The awkward inception of medicine in the sporting arena was broadened by the sometimes contrasting goals of the athletes and physicians. Although the health of the athletes takes precedence for physicians, athletes often view victory as the ultimate goal.[88] Some persons believe that it is these opposing philosophies that lie beneath most ethical and legal issues in modern-day sports medicine. In addition, the evolution of the traditional dyad of the patient-physician relationship into a triad of patient-team-physician has been further recognized as a source of potential medicolegal conflict.[89] This section is intended to serve as a general guide for ethical and legal issues and should not be perceived as binding legal advice. For detailed advice regarding specific medicolegal issues, we recommend that legal counsel be obtained.

Confidentiality

Inherent to the integrity of any patient-physician relationship is the concept of trust. In modern medicine, a primary approach to maintain the trust of our patients is to preserve confidentiality. The following case example illustrates potential problems surrounding trust.

Case 1

A 21-year-old star running back cuts to the sideline during a midseason game. He hears a "pop" in his right knee, which is accompanied by immediate pain and swelling. As the team physician, you evaluate him, and examination reveals positive right knee Lachman and anterior drawer tests. Immediately following your examination, you are approached by the athletic trainer, the head coach, and a member of the media who ask for return-to-play prognosis. During this encounter, you have not asked the player for his consent to release medical information.

Question: Who can you talk to, and what can you tell them?

Many clinicians reflexively cite confidentiality guidelines outlined in the Health Information Portability and Accountability Act (HIPAA). Remarkably, the primary goal of HIPAA was not to enforce confidentiality but rather to improve the portability and continuity of health insurance coverage.[90] A section of HIPAA details the principles of patient confidentiality and subsequently had far-reaching effects on patient information when it was enacted in 2003. A key determinant to the enforcement of HIPAA guidelines depends on whether the information is "protected." These regulations apply only to clinical encounters for which physicians bill for their services, receive payments, or transmit claims to a health plan in an electronic form.[90] Regardless of the clinical scenario, revealing whether an athlete is "cleared" or "not cleared" is considered an exception to HIPAA.[90]

High School Athletics

At the high school level, with rare exception, sideline coverage is voluntary and does not involve any form of billing, and thus the information obtained during these encounters would not be considered under the jurisdiction of HIPAA. Theoretically, information could be shared with coaches and team administrators without fear of prosecution from the Department of Health and Human Services, which implements HIPAA. Although no legal precedent exists, some persons believe that HIPAA guidelines should be adhered to in high schools.[90] Regardless, if medical services are billed, for example, as an in-office follow-up visit, HIPAA guidelines are enforceable.

Collegiate Athletics

HIPAA guidelines are usually the rule in collegiate athletics. One particular exception is clinical scenarios that involve health information governed by the Federal Education Records Protection Act (FERPA). At private or public colleges and universities that receive federal educational funding, information obtained during clinical encounters may be covered by this act. Information governed by FERPA guidelines are exempt from HIPAA and enable health information to be released to administrators and coaches who have an educational interest in the athlete without formal consent by the patient.[90] School-based athletic training room records maintained by team physicians or certified athletic trainers are often considered to be governed by FERPA. Given the complex nature of FERPA and HIPAA regulations, it is advisable to review privacy policies with the institution's legal counsel.[2]

Professional Athletics

In the arena of professional athletics, athletes sign an employment contract with the team, and health information can be considered to be a part of the employment record. Thus health information gathered by a team physician may be shared with employers who have a vested interest in the athlete's health, such as coaches and administrators.[90] As previously illustrated, the issue of whether information can be divulged to coaches varies with the clinical situation. To avoid controversy when dealing with sensitive medical information, most professional teams have their athletes sign a preparticipation waiver that details with whom health information can be shared as needed. Thus consent for release of information does not have to be obtained repeatedly throughout the season. In the absence of such a waiver, if an athlete begins to reveal information to the team physician that could potentially restrict him or her from play, it is recommended that the physician preempt any further revelations by notifying the athlete that if further information is shared, he or she may need to share this information with the team's administration. At that juncture, the athlete can consent to the release of medical information or refuse to reveal additional information and request a referral to another provider.[91]

TABLE 11.3   Key Components of Informed Consent

Component	Description
Disclosure	Relevant information must be provided regarding the proposed treatment including potential risks, benefits, and alternatives.
Capacity	Athletes must have the ability to understand information and its relevance.
Voluntariness	Athletes must voluntarily express their wishes in a noncoercive environment.

Informed Consent

Informed consent is one of the primary means of ensuring patient autonomy when making nonemergent medical decisions.[92] Most physicians are familiar with the concept of informed consent in the context of preprocedure planning, but any medical decision affecting an athlete's health and future should involve three key components of informed consent: disclosure, capacity, and voluntariness (Table 11.3).[93] To illustrate the importance of informed consent, we provide the following case.

Case 2

A 20-year-old female middle distance runner reports recurrent right medial ankle pain and swelling consistent with a previous diagnosis of posterior tibial tendinopathy. She is scheduled to participate in a regional qualifying meet for the national championships in 1 week. She requests a steroid injection into the posterior tibial tendon sheath and states that a prior injection by her primary care physician allowed her to successfully obtain a national qualifying result last year.

Question: Should you proceed with the injection or opt for more conservative measures?

In this example, pressure from the coach and athlete to do whatever it takes to win may affect clinical judgment by the team physician. Further complicating the scenario is the fact that she had a prior injection in the past with good results, and as such, it is reasonable for the coach and athlete to expect similar treatment. Referring to the basic components of informed consent (see Table 11.3), it is imperative to reestablish the three criteria in the current scenario because it is unlikely that the athlete can still recite the potential risks, benefits, and alternatives. It is also incorrect to assume that informed consent was actually obtained prior to her last injection.

The short-term, antiinflammatory, and analgesic effects of the injection would need to be weighed with the short-term risks of acute rupture and long-term risk of chronic weakening and progression of posterior tibialis tendon dysfunction.[94] By educating the patient about the risks, benefits, and alternatives, the physician is fulfilling a protective role in medical decision-making. This scenario does not involve a life-threatening injury; accordingly, it is reasonable that if informed consent is obtained, an injection may be justified. Conversely, in rendering return-to-play decisions for potentially catastrophic injuries such as cervical spine instability, patient autonomy would be less important than

the principles of beneficence and nonmaleficence. In addition, when athletes join a sports team, they voluntarily sacrifice a certain degree of their autonomy by agreeing to abide with the decisions of team physicians.[93]

Another potential pitfall is the assumption that a signed consent form automatically fulfills the medicolegal criteria needed to substantiate informed consent. A legal precedent exists indicating that a signed consent form does not necessarily guarantee legal immunity. Medical jargon may be overly complicated, and the patient may not fully understand the potential risks of the procedure. It is recommended that if doubt exists about whether the patient fully understands the ramifications of a medical decision, the patient should write a letter in his or her own words detailing his or her understanding of the risks, benefits, and alternatives.[95]

Drug Use

A trend in modern sports is the use of performance-enhancing drugs. In opposing the use of performance-enhancing drugs, most physicians cite the potential harms and the unfairness for the spirit of competition and good sportsmanship. The practice of physicians supplying banned substances to athletes is entirely unacceptable, and yet numerous well-publicized examples of such practices exist.[96] Although condemnation of the distribution of performance-enhancing drugs by a physician is clear-cut, other potential scenarios may be unclear.

Case 3

You are the primary care physician for an 18-year-old male sprinter who is competing on the junior national track team. He presents to your clinic with a report of acne. Upon further questioning, he reveals that he has recently started taking anabolic steroids.

Questions: Should this information be kept confidential? Should you continue to treat the patient? Would your decision change if you were the national team physician?

The physician may believe that it is necessary to inform his patient's coaches and potentially an antidoping agency that governs the sport. However, in this case, the athlete has addressed his use of steroids during a clinic visit with his primary care physician, who does not have a legal obligation to disclose this information. Some persons have suggested that athletes who use performance-enhancing drugs should not be viewed any differently from those who abuse alcohol or tobacco,[96,97] because with the latter forms of abuse, physicians would provide counseling regarding potential adverse effects. Likewise, it is beneficial for physicians to advise athletes on the potential detrimental effects of performance-enhancing drugs, without overstating risks, to maintain their trust. In addition, psychosocial triggers that may have fueled drug use should be considered and addressed. On the other hand, in this scenario, if the physician was taking care of an athlete on the national team rather than serving as a primary care provider, an obligation to divulge information to administrators is logical. However, in most instances at the national level, the athlete will have signed an agreement acknowledging forfeiture from participation for use of performance-enhancing drugs.

Disagreements With Coaches

Sideline medical coverage can exemplify the potentially incompatible goals of physicians and coaches. Occasionally, coaches may disagree with medical assessments, as illustrated in the following case.

Case 4

A 16-year-old football cornerback tackles an opposing player in the second quarter of play. You witness him jog back to the huddle with his right arm held at his side. He reports having radiating pain down his arm. A preliminary examination reveals no neck tenderness and ⅗ shoulder abduction and elbow flexion strength. You instruct him not to RTP and tell him you plan to reexamine him in 10 minutes. The coach cannot understand why you have restricted play because the coach "used to play with stingers."

Questions: What should you tell the coach? Could this situation have been avoided?

The RTP guidelines with regard to transient brachial plexopathies (also known as stingers) were different in the past, and athletes often returned to play relatively soon. However, current guidelines clearly state that RTP is contraindicated in the presence of residual neurologic deficits.[45] Knowledge of current guidelines and education of athletes and coaches can be of great help to team physicians.[98] A thorough explanation of the potential immediate and long-term sequelae of premature RTP should suffice for most coaches. Perhaps a solution to avoid a power struggle with a coach on the sideline is to preemptively delineate duties as team physician in writing. This approach typically would not be feasible in a situation in which a team physician is at odds with an opposing team's coach, especially when only one physician is on site at a game. In this situation, the physician should arrive early, introduce himself or herself to the opposing team's athletic trainer(s) and coaching staff, and delineate his or her role during the contest. To make unbiased medical decisions on either sideline, it is recommended that team physicians avoid excessive emotional involvement with their team and maintain a sense of objectivity throughout the contest.[93]

Conclusion

The team physician encounters unique bioethical issues when interacting with coaches and athletes. Most of these issues stem from the nontraditional patient-doctor relationship and the dichotomous goals of "health first" versus "victory at all costs." Team physicians should rely on their knowledge of current medical guidelines and the basic principles of medical ethics.

In addition, it is recommended that physicians strictly adhere to the rule of "full disclosure" and notify all athletes of potential risks and conflicts of interest, which will facilitate autonomous and informed decision-making.[92]

ACKNOWLEDGMENT

The authors and editors are grateful for the contributions of the previous authors of this chapter, C. Joel Hess and Dilaawar J. Mistry.

For a complete list of references, go to ExpertConsult.com.

SELECTED READINGS

Citation:
Bernhardt DT, Roberts WO, eds. *Preparticipation Physical Evaluation.* 4th ed. Elk Grove Village, IL: American Academy of Pediatrics; 2010.

Level of Evidence:
V, expert opinion

Summary:
A product of six author societies, the fourth edition of the preparticipation physical evaluation guides the team physician through the intricacies of preseason screening for sport participation.

Citation:
McCrory P, Meeuwisse W, Dvorak J, et al. Consensus statement on concussion in sport – the 5th international conference on concussion in sport held in Berlin, October 2016. *Br J Sports Med.* 2017;[Epub ahead of print].

Level of Evidence:
V, expert opinion

Summary:
The most recent and widely accepted concussion management guideline, including in-depth discussion on RTP decisions.

Citation:
Swartz EE, Boden BP, Courson RW, et al. National athletic trainers' association position statement: acute management of the cervical spine-injured athlete. *J Athl Train.* 2009;44(3):306–331.

Level of Evidence:
V, expert opinion

Summary:
A consensus statement of the on-field management of the athlete with a cervical spine injury.

12

Comprehensive Cardiovascular Care and Evaluation of the Elite Athlete

Paul S. Corotto, Aaron L. Baggish, Dilaawar J. Mistry, Robert W. Battle

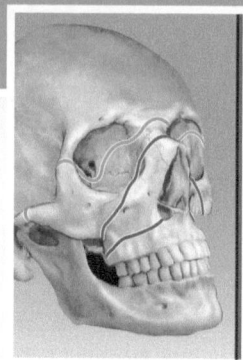

HISTORICAL PERSPECTIVE

The elite athlete has enjoyed a celebrated status within our culture since ancient times. The Olympic Games solidified that status as early as 776 BC, and it was amplified by Pheidippedes, who was a legendary Greek Olympic champion in 500 BC. Ten years later when the Persians arrived at the plains of Marathon and threatened to conquer Athens, Pheidippedes was dispatched from Athens to recruit the assistance of the Spartans. While remembered most for his 26-mile run from Marathon to Athens to announce the Greek victory, this run was only part of a remarkable triathlon of events for this remarkable Greek athlete. He began the first leg of his journey with a 145-mile run over mountains and plains that included swimming across the aquatic obstacles on his way to reach Sparta in only 2 days and without sleep. The second leg included travel by boat from Sparta to Marathon, where he joined in the victorious battle against the Persians. Only then did he embark upon his now infamous run back to Athens, where he proclaimed victory before dying suddenly in front of his fellow Greek citizens.[1] The remarkable athletic accomplishments of Pheidippedes emphatically etched the Marathon run into sports modernity and deeply engraved the tragic event of athletic sudden death (SD) into our cultural consciousness. The Oxford poet and scholar A. E. Housman captured the effect of sudden athletic death in the poem "To an Athlete Dying Young" (1896):

The time you won your town the race
We chaired you through the market place

The metaphor of the winning athlete on the shoulders of the townspeople is an image we have all witnessed in some form many times. With the unexpected death of the athlete, Housman brings the same metaphor full circle from celebration to sadness with athlete's coffin resting upon the shoulders of those same townspeople:

Shoulder-high we bring you home,
And set you at your threshold down,
Townsman of a stiller town.

Estimates of the incidence of athletic SD reassure us that this is a rare event.[2-4] The consequences of athletic SD, however, resound far beyond the individuals directly affected. The advent of continuous media coverage through television, radio, and the internet that is now further augmented by social media has created instant access to any adverse event involving a previously healthy and seemingly invincible athlete. Accordingly, a tragic athletic SD immediately affects family, friends, fellow athletes, students, coaches and administrators, and that effect can rapidly ripple into the minds of sports fans anywhere in the world. The sudden deaths on the soccer pitch of Marc Vivien Foe in 2003 (a Cameroon national player with hypertrophic cardiomyopathy) and Fabrice Muamba in 2012 (a player for Bolton in the English Premier league) illustrate the magnitude of the amplification of modern information. Disturbing videos of both events are widely available on the internet and have been viewed by millions of fans around the world.

The SD of Hank Gathers in 1990 had a seminal impact upon the landscape of sports cardiology in the United States. Gathers played Division I college basketball for Loyola Marymount on a team that had realistic aspirations for a national championship. The previous season, he had become the second player in NCAA history to lead the nation in scoring and rebounding. Gathers fainted on the court, and both sustained and nonsustained ventricular arrhythmias were documented most likely as a result of underlying myocarditis.[5] With the extraordinary success of this team from a small university, there was tremendous pressure for Gathers to continue to play. He ultimately returned to play later in the season and died tragically on the court during a tournament game. This case illustrates the entwined complexity inherent to any cardiovascular diagnosis in an elite athlete. Gathers was admittedly noncompliant with his propranolol. The reluctance to disqualify him under the circumstances was profound. The emotional cost to Gather's family, friends, teammates, and the Loyola Marymount community at large is beyond measure. There was also a profound financial impact, with judgments and settlements against the physician and the university.[6] Now that we are more than 25 years removed from this event, it is reasonable to assume that Loyola Marymount is still suffering beneath the dark cloud of this occurrence. Death during competition would intercede as "the most unwelcome spectator" (Jim Murray, *The Los Angeles Times*)[1] for other notable athletes as well, including Tom Simpson, an English cyclist who died on Mont Ventoux in the 1967 Tour de France (likely from amphetamines); Flo Hyman, an Olympic volleyball player who died of aortic dissection from the Marfan syndrome four years before Gathers; basketball players Pete Maravich (anomalous coronary artery), Reggie Lewis, and Jason Collier; Sergei Grinkov (ice-skating), Jiri Fischer (hockey), Thomas Herrion (football), and Fran Crippen (swimming). In addition to elite athletes with national and international notoriety,

SD has also had a profound impact in communities around the world coping with unexpected deaths of athletes of all ages and levels of ability. The amplification of athletic SD into our cultural consciousness has stimulated considerable research and medical practice interest into the causes of SD in athletes, potential preventive measures inclusive of screening, and the development of care and management guidelines for athletes with known cardiovascular abnormalities. In practice, the prevention of SD represents only a part of the comprehensive cardiovascular care of the elite athlete. In this chapter, we will discuss the current state of practice, controversy with regard to screening, and the detection and management of cardiovascular disorders, with particular emphasis on the normal physiologic cardiovascular remodeling that can occur with elite levels of training.

MEDICAL HOME OF THE ELITE ATHLETE

It is imperative that the elite athlete begin with a medical home composed of a multidisciplinary team, ideally led by a primary care sports medicine provider. Athletic trainers are a vital part of this medical home as well, and bring a rapidly evolving expertise involving the overall health and wellness of the athlete. Trainers are keenly aware of the importance of cardiovascular health and are now familiar with a wide array of useful technology and equipment including blood pressure cuffs, stethoscopes, automatic external defibrillators (AEDs), and electrocardiogram (ECG) machines. In addition, smartphone technology has greatly enhanced the ability of the sports trainer to assess their athletes in real time. Trainers at some Division 1 programs now use a digital application that provides immediate rhythm analysis for symptomatic athletes. It is very helpful when trainers can accompany athletes to subspecialty encounters, because they can reliably relay important information onto the practice and playing field and report back on the development of any important signs, symptoms, or physical findings that may place the athlete at risk.

There is increasing recognition that the medical home of an elite athlete should ideally include a dedicated cardiovascular specialist, with their scope of practice and depth of involvement depending on the specific needs of the individual. These cardiovascular specialists, often referred to as sports cardiologists, may be tasked with oversight of preparticipation screening as well as the evaluation and management of athletes with suspected or previously diagnosed cardiovascular disease. Given this evolving role of cardiovascular specialists in the care of elite athletes, both the European Society of Cardiology (ESC) and the American College of Cardiology (ACC) have dedicated resources to define specific skills and core competencies to guide the practice of sports cardiologists.[7]

Preparticipation Screening

The initial history and physical exam performed by the primary care sports medicine provider now includes the fourth edition of the Preparticipation Physical Evaluation (PPE-4)[9] and has evolved to include a somewhat more reliable detection process for familial cardiovascular abnormalities that might increase the risk of SD and were adopted by the American Heart Association consensus panel for preparticipation cardiovascular screening.[6]

However, the state of the current initial athlete evaluation suffers from significant limitations. There is a wide variation from state to state with regard to the type of provider performing the PPE-4 and the content of the PPE-4. In addition, the PPE-4 relies on self-reporting by the athletes themselves, which is inherently prone to error.[10] Furthermore, the PPE-4 has been demonstrated to have poor sensitivity for the detection of cardiovascular disorders. Indeed, in a retrospective look at SD in athletes who had participated in preparticipation screening, only 3% were thought to have potential cardiovascular abnormalities, and none were restricted from participation.[11] Following the PPE-4, referral of an athlete for more advanced cardiovascular care or evaluation occurs as a result of an abnormal physical finding, a family history of premature sudden death, or the development of new symptoms that elicit concern. Many of the most dangerous cardiovascular conditions that could threaten the athlete often are asymptomatic and have no physical finding that would trigger a referral. This includes conditions such as hypertrophic cardiomyopathy (HCM), arrhythmogenic right ventricular cardiomyopathy (ARVC), congenital Long QT and Brugada syndromes, Wolff-Parkinson-White (WPW), and the anomalous coronary artery. The absence of a positive family history for SD can be falsely reassuring in the autosomal dominant familial conditions (HCM, ARVC, Long QT, the Marfan syndrome), because up to 25% to 33% of affected individuals will have new spontaneous mutations with no previously affected family members.[12,13] Accordingly, the current state of evaluation of the elite athlete in the United States is unlikely to detect most threatening cardiovascular conditions. Furthermore, the normal physiologic adaptations of hypertrophy of the left ventricle to rigorous isometric training (often referred to as the "athlete's heart") can very closely mimic HCM, which is the most prevalent and dangerous cardiovascular disease in young athletes.[14] In addition, physiologic changes in left and right ventricular cavity size and systolic function can be difficult to distinguish from forms of dilated cardiomyopathy and ARVC. Perhaps nowhere in medicine does normalcy mimic disease as it does in this circumstance. As a result, further screening or evaluation of elite athletes requires a sophisticated and programmatic approach that is designed to avoid the pitfall of potentially life-changing false-positive results that will be the inherent weakness in the evaluation of large populations of athletes with a low prevalence of disease. Because of these inherent complexities, expert consensus in the United States, including the American College of Cardiology and American Heart Association (ACC/AHA), has not recommended routine evaluation of the athlete beyond the PPE-4. While this recommendation is well wrought and reasonable, evidence is lacking regarding the efficacy of the PPE-4 in prevention of morbidity and mortality in athletes.[10] In addition, this differs from other expert guidelines, including the ESC and the International Olympic Committee (IOC), which recommend the addition of ECG screening in order to improve the sensitivity of preparticipation screening. Current practice in the United States varies in regard to the inclusion of diagnostic screening tools beyond the PPE-4. As an example, more than one third of National Collegiate Athletic Association (NCAA) Division-1 athletes undergo additional screening with either an ECG or echocardiogram.[15]

Current recommendations have created an unanticipated consequence in the field of sports cardiology. There is a paucity of well trained and knowledgeable cardiovascular providers familiar with the nuances of the normal physiologic adaptations to elite training and how to differentiate normalcy from disease. Encounters with elite athletes are uncommon for most practicing cardiologists. Accordingly, athletes who undergo more extensive testing and evaluation by inexperienced providers are commonly sidelined unnecessarily, subjected to over testing, relegated to the emotional consequences of concern for survival, and temporary or permanent disqualification from sports altogether. The incorporation of cardiovascular care into the medical home of the athlete must be done very carefully with knowledgeable providers dedicated to understanding the complex world of the athlete.

CARDIOVASCULAR ADAPTATIONS AND REMODELING ASSOCIATED WITH RIGOROUS ATHLETIC TRAINING

The earliest recognition of the physiologic changes commonly referred to as the "athlete's heart" were astutely described in 1899 by a Swedish physician who detected cardiac enlargement in elite Nordic skiers utilizing remarkably accurate skills of auscultation and percussion. That same year, these findings were reinforced in a study of Harvard University rowers.[16] It is not surprising that the earliest descriptions of cardiac enlargement were made in Nordic skiers and elite rowers, because these disciplines include extreme combinations of endurance training (isotonic, dynamic, aerobic) and strength training (isometric, static, anaerobic) that lead to more striking combinations of both left ventricular (LV) cavity dilation and hypertrophy. A few years later, Paul Dudley White would strengthen the legacy of sports cardiology in Boston by observing pulses in endurance-trained runners participating in the Boston Marathon[17] and would later describe bradycardia associated with this level of endurance training.[18] The evolution of more sophisticated technology would allow for the complex assessment of the electrophysiologic and structural cardiovascular adaptations to varying degrees and types of athletic training.[19,20] Accordingly, any cardiovascular evaluation of an athlete inclusive of electrocardiography or any form of cardiovascular imaging must be undertaken with in-depth knowledge of the training-specific changes in cardiac structure and function. Pure endurance training involves prolonged activities with sustained increases in cardiac output without significant elevation in mean arterial pressure. This type of volume load can lead to dilation of all four chambers of the heart and to some degree the great vessels as well. Strength-training subjects the heart to more brief but dramatic increases in mean arterial pressure that in turn leads to an increase in myocardial muscle hypertrophy. Marathon running is a good example of pure endurance training, and weight lifting is an example of pure strength training. Most sports, however, will have varying degrees of both types of training that will also vary with the approach of the individual athlete. Therefore the heart of any athlete may manifest changes across a broad spectrum of physiologic adaptation.

Structural Adaptations to Rigorous Training
Left Ventricle

The effects of training on the LV are routinely detected on the ECG and increases in voltage have been documented for decades.[21] Endurance training that also incorporates increasing degrees of isometric/strength training (cycling, rowing, cross country skiing, canoeing) are more likely to demonstrate these manifestations on the resting ECG.[22] Transthoracic echocardiography (TTE) has been used extensively to document the spectrum of LV cavity dilation and increase in LV wall thickness/left ventricular hypertrophy (LVH) associated with rigorous training.[14,23-25] LV cavity size across a large variety of sports is larger than sedentary controls and ranges from 43 to 70 mm (mean 55 mm) in men and 38 to 66 mm (mean 48 mm) in women.[25] LV wall thickness is generally less than 13 mm in elite athletes,[23] but larger increases in wall thickness (1.3 to 1.5 mm) that stray into the "gray zone" with hypertrophic cardiomyopathy are more commonly seen in older elite athletes (rowers) who train with large degrees of static and dynamic exercise.[26] LV systolic function as measured by TTE is usually normal in elite athletes.[27-29] It is important to recognize, however, that LV systolic function can be low normal to mildly depressed (mimicking mild forms of dilated cardiomyopathy), as shown in some of the fittest athletes in the world participating in the Tour de France.[30] These adaptive changes in cavity dimension, wall thickness, and the associated increase in LV mass have also been demonstrated in magnetic resonance imaging (MRI) studies[31,32] and have been recently reviewed in depth.[33] LV diastolic function is usually normal in elite athletes and can be improved with endurance training, leading to more robust early diastolic filling.[26,34] Less is known about the effects of strength training on diastolic function, but there is evidence that diastolic function may be impaired, which could be an untoward long-term effect of hypertrophy that warrants further study.[20]

Right Ventricle

Sustained increases in cardiac output have a similar effect on the right ventricle (RV) as compared with the LV, particularly with regard to cavity dilation. Older M-mode and 2-D TTE studies in endurance-trained athletes showed symmetrical dilation in both the RV and the LV.[35,36] Due to the unique geometry of the RV, echocardiography has struggled to assess RV size and function, and cardiac MRI has greatly enhanced our ability to evaluate the RV. More recent MRI studies in elite endurance athletes have reinforced the balanced dilation of the RV and LV demonstrating increases in LV and RV mass, LV and RV diastolic volumes, and LV and RV stroke volumes.[31,32,37] Abnormalities in systolic function in endurance athletes can also be abnormal and generally seen in athletes with more extensive RV dilation.[38] The impact of strength training on the RV is less clear but likely to be a topic of future clarification utilizing TTE and cardiac MRI.

Atria

As expected, increased right and left atrial volumes and sizes are also seen in endurance athletes with more numerous studies evaluating the left atrium.[35,39-41] A large volume of data supports the physiologic effects of sustained endurance volume loading on all four cardiac chambers, including the atria. In the largest Italian series, 20% of athletes had left atrial dimensions of >40 mm measured by TTE, and supraventricular arrhythmias were not common in this group.[42]

Great Arteries and Veins

The great arteries and veins are subject to the physiologic effects of endurance training. The aorta is of particular interest with regard to strength training, as extraordinary increases in both systolic and diastolic blood pressure (480/350 mm Hg!) have been documented in weight lifters.[43] Studies have documented somewhat inconsistent aortic root dilation with regard to specific types of sports and training regimens. Strength-trained athletes have been shown to have larger dimensions of the aorta measured by TTE at the aortic annulus, the sinuses of Valsalva, sinotubular junction, and proximal aortic root when compared with controls, and this effect increased with the duration of training.[43,44] Aortic root size was greater in taller athletes and typically measured between 3.0 and 4.0 cm, and only rarely measured greater than 4.0 cm. While aortic regurgitation was found in none of the controls, 9% of the strength-trained athletes had mild ($n = 5$) or moderate ($n = 4$) aortic regurgitation.[44] Another large trial supported these findings comparing strength-trained with endurance-trained athletes.[45] In a large trial of a wide range of sports in Italy, the largest measurements were found in endurance-trained athletes, particularly in the disciplines of cycling and swimming.[46] This apparent inconsistency may be attributed the sustained combination of isometric and isotonic exercise associated with these sports. In totality, it is important to note that while athletic training in various disciplines may lead to increase in aortic root dimensions, these increases have not been shown to approach diameters typically concerning for pathologic dilatation. In this light, a meta-analysis investigating aortic root dimensions in athletes versus nonathlete controls found that elite athletes have a minor, and likely clinically insignificant, increase in aortic root dimensions.[47] The authors rightfully noted that marked aortic root dilatation likely represents a pathologic process rather than an adaptation to exercise.

The effects of training are also seen on a wide range of great vessels in endurance athletes and taller athletes, including larger caliber carotids, branch pulmonary arteries, superior and inferior vena cavae, and abdominal aorta as shown in cyclists, long-distance runners, and volleyball players.[48] It has been our observation in endurance-trained athletes that the inferior vena cava is routinely larger than normal, and that published estimates of RA pressure based upon vena cava size and inspiratory collapse do not apply to the elite athlete.

The Athlete's Electrocardiogram and Electrophysiologic Adaptations to Rigorous Training

Training-induced alterations in cardiac structure and autonomic regulation are reflected on the ECG of the athlete in many ways, and the resting ECG will have a range of well-documented variations as compared with normal controls in most cases.[18,49-51] Common training-related findings on the athlete's ECG include sinus bradycardia, first degree atrioventricular (AV) block, incomplete right bundle branch block (RBBB), early repolarization, and voltage criteria for LVH (Fig. 12.1). Electrophysiologic aberrations, like their structural counterparts, are more common in endurance sports that include a significant amount of strength training as well (cycling, rowing, canoeing, and cross-country skiing).[22]

GENDER, GENETICS, AND RACE

Gender, genetics, and race have a pronounced influence upon the structural and electrophysiologic adaptations to rigorous athletic training. Abnormal findings on the athlete's ECG are more common in males and in athletes of African or Caribbean descent.[22,52] Dramatic examples of LVH by voltage with markedly

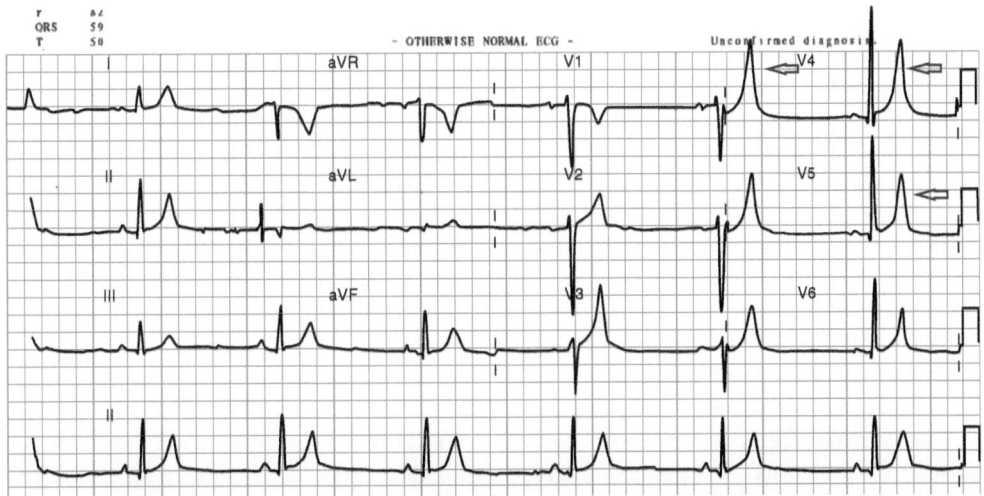

Fig. 12.1 The electrocardiogram (ECG) of a 17-year-old white freshman intercollegiate distance runner who had undergone several years of intense endurance training. The ECG shows a marked sinus bradycardia with a heart rate of 37 bpm at rest. Also note the diffuse, prominent, high-voltage T-waves *(red arrows)*.

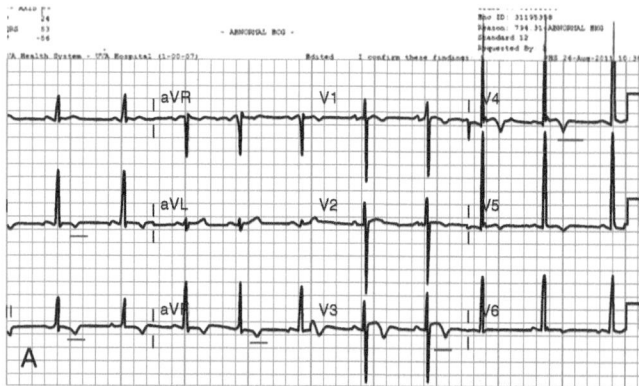

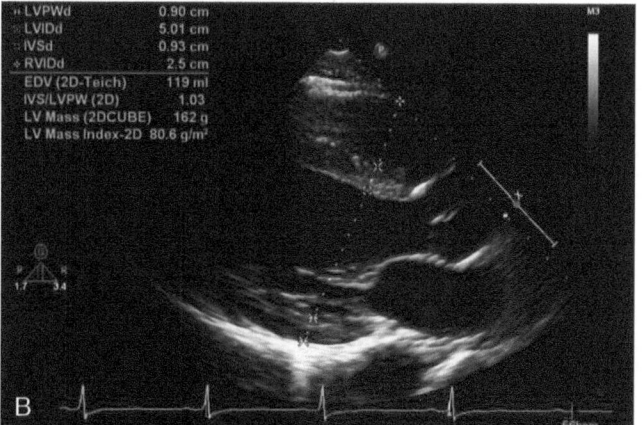

Fig. 12.2 (A) The resting electrocardiogram (ECG) of an intercollegiate 800-meter runner of Nigerian descent. Diffuse increased QRS voltage is present, particularly in leads V4 and V5, which is very common in endurance-trained athletes. This athlete has T-wave inversion in the inferior leads (red marker) and ST elevation with biphasic T-waves in the precordial leads (blue marker). These findings are uncommon in white athletes. (B) Transthoracic echocardiography showing the parasternal long-axis view in this same athlete. Left ventricular (LV) cavity size, wall thickness, and LV mass are all normal. This ECG is a normal variant for this athlete of African descent.

abnormal T-waves and repolarization abnormalities are commonly seen in elite African athletes (Fig. 12.2) and should not be mistaken for HCM. In 1962, these findings were described in the Bantu and Nilotic people of Africa, and in the case of an Olympic boxer, an ECG performed after prolonged detraining demonstrated complete regression of the ECG findings of LVH and T-wave abnormalities.[53] Gender and ethnicity have a similar impact upon imaging studies (TTE). A study of 600 elite female athletes undergoing TTE screening demonstrated a low incidence of LV cavity dilation, and not one female athlete had an LV wall thickness greater than 12 mm.[54] Black female athletes show a modest but more pronounced tendency toward hypertrophy with LV wall thickness measuring 6 mm greater when compared with Caucasian female athletes.[55] In a study of elite rowers, a familial genetic influence was suggested when Baggish et al. found that athletes with a family history of hypertension developed a more pronounced increase in LV mass when compared with rowers without a family history of hypertension. The pattern of hypertrophy was different as well, with concentric hypertrophy more commonly seen in rowers with a family history of hypertension and eccentric hypertrophy seen in controls.[56] In addition,

angiotensin converting enzyme gene polymorphisms have been shown to predispose athletes to more pronounced remodeling with increases in both LV mass and LV wall thickness.[57,58] These studies underscore the complexity of the process of training induced cardiac remodeling. This process is influenced by the type and duration of training, the gender, and the genetic heterogeneity of the individual athlete.

CARDIOVASCULAR SCREENING OF THE ATHLETE

Because of the devastating consequences of unexpected athletic SD, a wide array of approaches has been developed outside of recommended guidelines by individual universities, countries, and professional athletic teams to more reliably identify potential life-threatening and asymptomatic abnormalities that would not be detected on the PPE-4. The modern elite athlete stresses the cardiovascular system to remarkable levels of both strength and endurance. The examples of Pheidippedes and Fran Crippen, who died in a 10-kilometer open-water swim in extreme heat in 2010 in the United Arab Emirates, may both be examples of athletic SD occurring as a result of heroic athletic effort in the absence of any underlying cardiovascular abnormality. Accordingly, any undiagnosed cardiovascular abnormality could expose the athlete to distracting symptoms, impaired performance, and ultimately athletic SD. Landmark papers on the causes of SD in athletes under the age of 35 are well established.[11,59] In the United States, athletic SD occurs at a rate of approximately 125 per year, and a spectrum of underlying pathologies are implicated. It was previously thought that HCM accounted for more than one third of these tragic occurrences,[3] but recent data have challenged that assessment by demonstrating a lesser prevalence of autopsy-proven HCM in SCD cases across various countries, in age-matched noncompetitive athletes, and in US military personnel.[60-64] In this light, it has been demonstrated that more than 30% of NCAA athletes and 40% of US military recruits had structural normal hearts at autopsy, with a sudden arrhythmia presumed to be the etiology of their death.[65,66] In the most rigorous review of SCD in athletes to date, a British study of 357 consecutive cases of SCD demonstrated that HCM accounted for only 5% of cases.[67] In this study, pathologic analysis was performed by a dedicated cardiac pathologist, a crucial detail, as it has been shown that up to a 40% disparity in documented cause of death exists when standard autopsy results are compared with those performed by a pathologist specializing in cardiac disease.[68] When rigorous pathologic criteria for diagnosing HCM are applied, the percentage of SCD cases attributable to this disease state is significantly reduced as compared with earlier assessments.[67] In British athletes, sudden arrhythmic death accounted for 42% of cases with a strong predilection for younger athletes, whereas myocardial disease accounted for just under 40% and in contrast had a predilection for older athletes. However, it should also be noted that there may be an inherent referral bias in that straightforward cases, such as easily identified HCM, may be not be referred for autopsy. Other congenital cardiac anomalies comprise the majority of the other causes of athletic SD, including the anomalous coronary artery, congenital aortic stenosis, ARVC, and ruptured aorta from the Marfan syndrome or related vascular disorders. A much smaller percentage of athletic SD in young athletes results from acquired heart diseases like myocarditis and coronary artery disease.

In addition to serious cardiovascular disorders, there are many other less threatening congenital and acquired abnormalities that are often asymptomatic and may have subtle if any physical findings that could affect the future of the athlete's health, cause symptoms in the athlete, or impair performance (Box 12.1). Accordingly, any programmatic attempt to screen athletes for potential cardiovascular abnormalities beyond the PPE-4 will need a very sharp edge, an edge that can reliably distinguish training related remodeling from real disease, and an edge that is familiar with the congenital anomalies that will be found and can distinguish the benign from the more serious disorders. Screening must remain non-invasive and pose no risk to the athlete; therefore ECG and TTE are the most widely utilized modalities. Unless exercise-induced arrhythmias or coronary artery disease (CAD) are suspected, routine stress testing is of little value, while computed tomography (CT) and MRI expose the athlete to radiation (CT) and intravenous contrast (CT and MRI). These tests along with Holter monitoring, and genetic testing should be performed only when significant cardiovascular

---

BOX 12.1 Congenital and Acquired Cardiovascular Disorders Often Undetected in Childhood

1. Bicuspid aortic valve—functionally normal or mild valve disorder:
   - Fifty percent will have an associated abnormality of the ascending aorta (congenital aortopathy)
2. ASD/left to right shunts:
   - Secundum ASD, which includes atrial septal aneurysm with small or multiple ASD/patent foramen ovale
   - Venosus ASD
   - Coronary sinus ASD
   - Partial anomalous pulmonary venous return
3. Hypertrophic cardiomyopathy
4. Anomalous coronary arteries, coronary artery fistulae
5. Marfan syndrome and related disorders:
   - Ehlers-Danlos syndrome
   - Loeys-Dietz syndrome
   - Mitral valve prolapse, aortic root diameter at upper limits of normal for body size, stretch marks of the skin, and skeletal conditions similar to Marfan syndrome (MASS) phenotype
6. Wolff-Parkinson-White syndrome
7. Long QT syndrome
8. Brugada syndrome
9. Ventricular tachycardia, pathologic premature ventricular contractions
10. Arrhythmogenic right ventricular cardiomyopathy
11. Coarctation of the aorta (particularly milder forms)
12. Pulmonary hypertension (particularly mild to moderate forms)
13. Myocarditis (acute or with chronically impaired ventricular function)
14. Congenital cardiomyopathy (including congenital noncompaction)
15. Mitral valve prolapse

ASD, Atrial septal defect.
From Battle RW, Mistry DJ, Malhotra R. Cardiovascular screening and the elite athlete: advances, concepts, controversies, and a view of the future. *Clin Sports Med.* 2011;30:503–524.

---

disease is strongly suspected and interpreted by providers knowledgeable in sports cardiology.

Electrocardiogram Screening in Athletes

The ECG is a widely available screening tool that can provide valuable information regarding cardiac structure and function. Accordingly, ECG is the most frequently used diagnostic test to screen athletes above and beyond the PPE-4. Mandatory ECG screening has been in place in the Veneto region of Italy since the 1971. Mandated by the Medical Protection of Athletes Act, ECGs were performed on Italian athletes from ages 12 to 35. Corrado et al.[69] have published an extensive 25-year experience with athlete ECG screening in a variety of sports, and from the Italian perspective, this has been shown to be cost-effective.[70] Investigators argue that the data from Italy support ECG screening, and that has led to the disqualification of athletes at risk (particularly with HCM), thereby shifting the demographics of athletic SD in Italy away from HCM as the most common cause of SD and toward ARVC.[71] As a result of these findings, the IOC supported ECG screening of Olympic athletes in 2004,[72] and the following year a similar recommendation emerged from the European Society of Cardiology.[73] ECG screening has also been shown to more reliably identify college athletes with cardiovascular disorders in the in the United States, albeit with an increase in false-positive results,[74] but because of the inherent interpretive complexity of this process, there has been considerable controversy regarding the routine addition of the ECG to athletic screening. In support of the European approach, the use of ECG has been advocated in the United States,[75] while the complexity of cost and inherent limitation of widespread ECG screening have been elegantly argued,[76] even discouraged,[76,77] and thus it has not been endorsed by the US Olympic Committee, the American Heart Association, the American College of Cardiology, and has not been incorporated into the most recent Joint Conference on Eligibility Recommendations for Competitive Athletes with Cardiovascular Disorders.[78] As stated by the ESC, the goal of ECG screening is to "differentiate between physiologic adaptive ECG changes and pathologic ECG abnormalities, with the aim to prevent adaptive changes in the athlete being erroneously attributed to heart disease, or signs of life-threatening cardiovascular conditions being dismissed as normal variants of athlete's heart."[69] With this goal in mind, in recent years, both European and American researchers have made significant strides in improving ECG screening guidelines in an effort improve sensitivity as well as to decrease the rate of false-positive results.

In 2010, the ESC published recommendations for ECG interpretation in athletes, commonly referred to as the "European guidelines." These guidelines were the first to formally differentiate adaptive physiologic ECG patterns from those suggestive of underlying cardiovascular disease, a dichotomous approach that has subsequently become the standard of care. "Common and training-related" changes included sinus bradycardia, first-degree AV block, incomplete RBBB, early repolarization, and isolated QRS voltage criteria for LVH. "Uncommon or training-unrelated" changes included T-wave inversion, ST-segment depression, pathologic Q-waves, left atrial enlargement, left-axis deviation/left anterior hemiblock, right-axis deviation/left posterior hemiblock, right ventricular hypertrophy, ventricular pre-excitation, complete left bundle branch block (LBBB) or RBBB, long- or short-QT interval, or Brugada-like early repolarization (Figs. 12.3 and 12.4). When applied to a cohort of more than 1000 previously studied ECGs, it was demonstrated that greater than 70% of ECGs previously identified as being suggestive of cardiovascular disease could be reclassified as "physiologic" on the basis of either isolated voltage criteria for LVH or early repolarization.[22] Such a significant decrease in the rate of false-positives demonstrated the significant advantage of a formal dichotomous approach in ECG screening of athletes; however, further investigation demonstrated that the false-positive rate still remained between 10% and 20%.[79] In subsequent years, attempts were made to further improve the specificity of screening recommendations.

The "Seattle Criteria" added sinus arrhythmia, ectopic atrial rhythm, junctional escape rhythm, and Mobitz Type I (Wenckebach) secondary AV block to the benign ECG changes included in the European guidelines, while refining the specific electrocardiographic changes required to define pathologic changes in regards to RVH or right-axis deviation, intraventricular conduction delay, and isolated anterior T-wave inversion, along with an increase in QTc required to define a long QT-interval.[80] Subsequent analysis has shown that the Seattle criteria perform to a higher level of

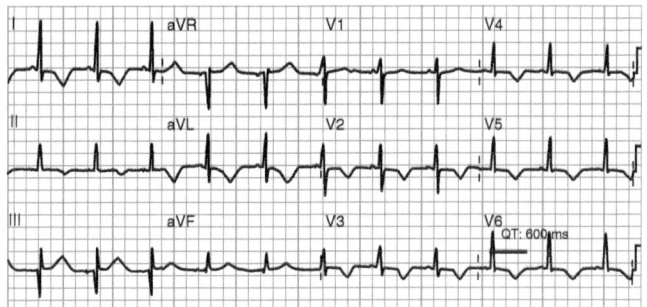

Fig. 12.3 An electrocardiogram at rest shows long QT in a patient with torsades des pointes. The QT interval indicated by the bar in V6 is prolonged to approximately 600 ms. (From Battle RW, Mistry DJ, Malhotra R. Cardiovascular screening and the elite athlete: advances, concepts, controversies, and a view of the future. *Clin Sports Med.* 2011;30:503–524, with permission.)

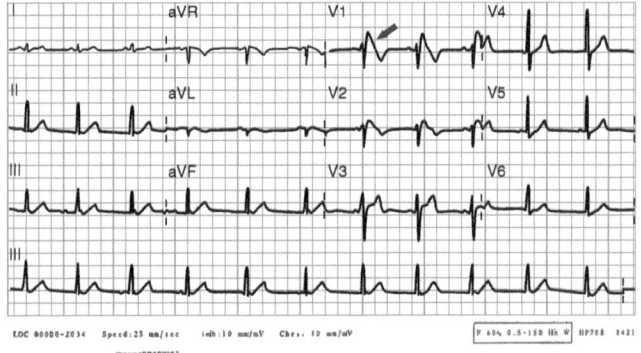

Fig. 12.4 An example of Brugada syndrome with "coved" type ST segment elevation >2 mm in V1 *(arrow)* followed by a negative/inverted T-wave. (From Battle RW, Mistry DJ, Malhotra R. Cardiovascular screening and the elite athlete: advances, concepts, controversies, and a view of the future. *Clin Sports Med.* 2011;30:503–524, with permission.)

specificity, and thus achieve a lower false-positive rate, primarily through this refinement in criteria to define an ECG change as pathologic.[81] Further studies attempted to enhance specificity to an even greater degree by evaluating the pathologic relevance of "borderline variants," including RVH, isolated axis deviation, and atrial enlargement specifically,[82,83] as well as the applicability in subpopulations of athletes of African or Caribbean decent. In this light, the "Refined Criteria" were published in 2014 and defined a scheme that distinguished borderline variants identified in isolation, previously defined as abnormal by the European guidelines and some by the Seattle criteria as not requiring further workup.[84] When applied to a cohort of both black and white athletes, the Refined Criteria improved specificity in white athletes from 73% to 84%, and even more substantially in black athletes from 40% to 80%. Further analysis has demonstrated that whereas the European guidelines, Seattle Criteria, and Refined Criteria were each 100% sensitive in identifying the case of HCM and WPW, the Refined Criteria greatly reduced the prevalence of ECGs identified as abnormal and significantly increased specificity across all ethnicities.[85]

In summary, we believe the ECG has considerable value particularly when applied with a comprehensive understanding of normal adaptations associated with training, the effects of race and gender, and when formally evaluated using newly defined criteria to distinguish normal adaptation from "uncommon and training unrelated ECG changes."[69] Use of the Refined Criteria specifically has been demonstrated to significantly reduce the rate of false-positive screenings while not compromising sensitivity in identifying pathology. In addition, these criteria can be used with confidence by providers who see larger volumes of athletes of African descent and thus will be exposed to a much wider range of repolarization abnormalities (ST elevation, biphasic T-waves) associated with dramatic increases in voltage as shown in Fig. 12.2 and Fig. 12.5A. When supplemented by available on-site high-quality TTE when necessary, these criteria can greatly reduce unnecessary withdrawal from participation.[74,76] While current AHA guidelines do not support a universal ECG screening program for athletes, it does support the concept of formal and standardized ECG screening programs when adequate cardiology resources are available for further investigation of pathologic variants when discovered.[86] While the controversy over the inclusion of ECG screening in preparticipation screening will undoubtedly continue, institutions and team physicians will be left to decide what is feasible, affordable, and what level of risk is acceptable within their particular circumstance.

Accordingly, incorporation of ECG screening alone in conjunction with the PPE-4 will likely lead to unnecessary sidelining of athletes, particularly athletes of African and Caribbean descent, while further testing is performed at the expense of the athlete in question. Therefore any consideration of the cost effectiveness of ECG screening alone must incorporate the added and often unnecessary cost of downstream imaging (TTE) generated by a false-positive screening ECG.

Transthoracic Echocardiography Screening in Athletes

TTE screening for athletic preparticipation has not been formerly included in any guidelines or recommendations in Europe or the

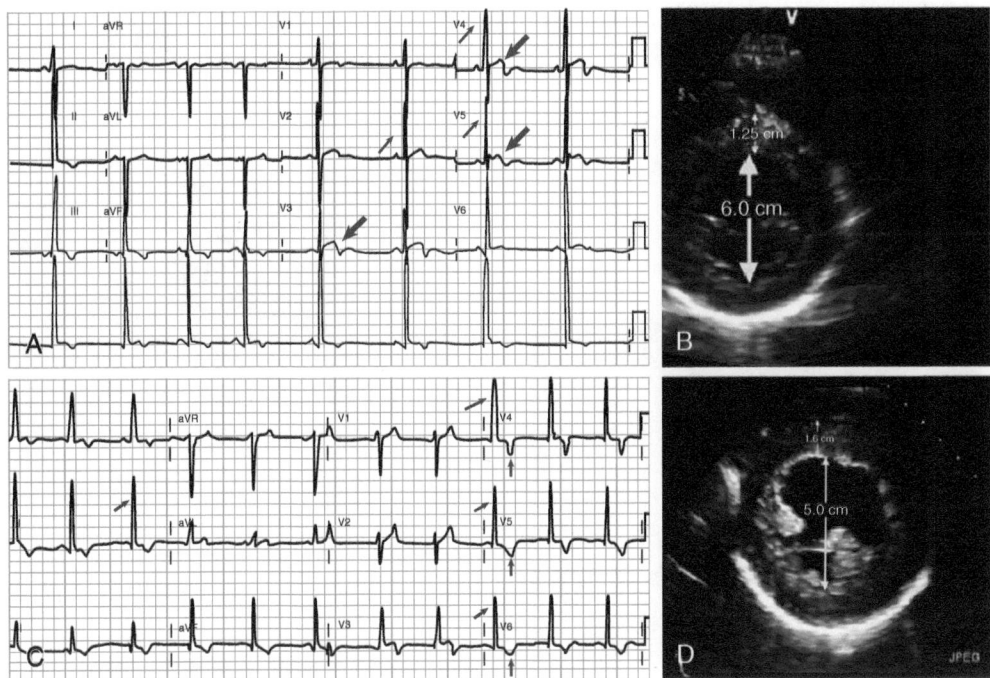

Fig. 12.5 Examples of athlete's hearts as shown by electrocardiogram (ECG) and transthoracic echocardiography (TTE). (A) The ECG of an African American Division I basketball player demonstrates diffusely increased QRS voltage without QRS widening *(narrow arrows)* and upwardly convex ST elevation followed by inverted T-waves *(broad arrows)*. This ECG shows more pronounced abnormalities of the athletic heart seen in African American athletes. (B) This same athlete's short-axis TTE image demonstrates a mild increase in septal wall thickness to 1.25 cm *(thin arrows)* with mild left ventricular (LV) cavity dilation of 6.0 cm *(broad arrows)* and a corresponding increase in LV mass. The image is a representative example of athlete's heart in an elite African American athlete. (C) An 18-year-old white high school football player with hypertrophic cardiomyopathy (HCM). The ECG reveals increased QRS voltage but with mild prolongation in QRS duration *(thin arrows)* and prominent T-wave inversion *(broad arrows)*. (D) A short-axis TTE image in an African American Division I basketball player with HCM and exertional angina. The septum is abnormally hypertrophied, measuring 1.6 cm *(thin arrows)*, and the LV cavity size is 5.0 cm *(broad arrows)*, which is considerably smaller than noted with the athletic heart. Stress echocardiography revealed complete systolic LV cavity obliteration. (From Battle RW, Mistry DJ, Malhotra R. Cardiovascular screening and the elite athlete: advances, concepts, controversies, and a view of the future. *Clin Sports Med*. 2011;30:503–524, with permission.)

United States, except when the abnormalities found during the PPE-4, screening ECG, or the development of new symptoms indicate the need for additional testing. TTE is far more expensive and logistically challenging than ECG, and it suffers from similar challenges with regard to the definition of acceptable limits of normal remodeling and the presence of true disease. Accordingly, inclusion of TTE also carries with it the important problem of false-positive results exceeding the detection of real disease states. Performance of TTE as a screening tool or as a consequence of concern for disease places the sports cardiologist in and around the "gray zone" defined by Maron as the overlap area between training related hypertrophy and HCM.[14] This presents a strong challenge, but there are, however, tools to sharpen our discerning edge that allow for more precise separation of the two.[14,23,87,88] The autosomal dominant mutation of the cardiac sarcomere known as HCM is a phenotypically very heterogeneous condition with LV wall thickness ranging from normal (<12 mm) to severe hypertrophy (30 to 50 mm); the hypertrophy can be focal or symmetric; obstruction may be present or absent at rest or with exercise; and symptoms are highly variable.[12,14,89] Training-related remodeling can induce

degrees of hypertrophy that frequently exceed the upper limit of normal and stray into the "gray zone" (13 to 15 mm) and occasionally beyond to mimic the most feared condition any athlete could have: HCM.[14] Features on TTE can help distinguish between athletic remodeling and HCM. LV end-diastolic cavity size tends to be larger in trained athletes and is often greater than 55 mm, whereas LV end-diastolic cavity size in HCM tends to be smaller. Examples of athletic remodeling and HCM are provided in Fig. 12.5. As discussed, abnormalities of diastolic Doppler indices are not typically seen in athletes and are more suggestive of HCM, as is systolic anterior motion of the mitral valve or evidence of left ventricular outflow tract obstruction. Focal hypertrophy of the septum or apex that is localized is also much more suggestive of HCM and can be missed by routine or screening TTE and is more readily detected by cardiac MRI (Fig. 12.6).[90,91] Late Gadolinium enhancement on MRI provides additional information with regard to the presence of early scar formation and fibrosis in HCM and may also be of prognostic value (Figs. 12.7 and 12.8).[92-94] In addition, improvements in the resolution of digitally analyzed TTE images have resulted in the increased recognition of left ventricular noncompaction

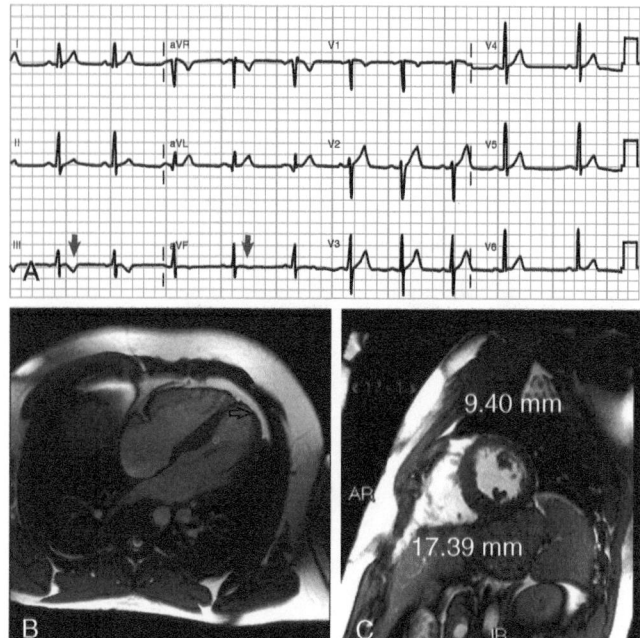

Fig. 12.6 Image of a division I football lineman with palpitations at peak exercise. (A) the resting electrocardiogram (ECG) is unremarkable except for nonspecific T-wave inversions in the inferior leads *(red arrows)*. Transthoracic echocardiography suggested left ventricular (LV) hypertrophy but was of poor quality due to the very large body surface area of the athlete. (B) A four-chamber view on a cardiac magnetic resonance imaging scan shows localized hypertrophy of the septum *(red arrow)* and a normal thin apex (outline of arrow). (C) A short-axis view of the LV shows severe septal hypertrophy (17 mm) beyond the "gray zone" and normal thickness of the anterolateral wall (9 mm). This athlete has closely coupled premature ventricular contractions with exercise, and as expected, detraining had no impact on his focal hypertrophy. This case is an example of hypertrophic cardiomyopathy (HCM) with a normal ECG, which occurs in 15% of patients with HCM; the large chest wall cavity in this football lineman likely contributed to the presentation.

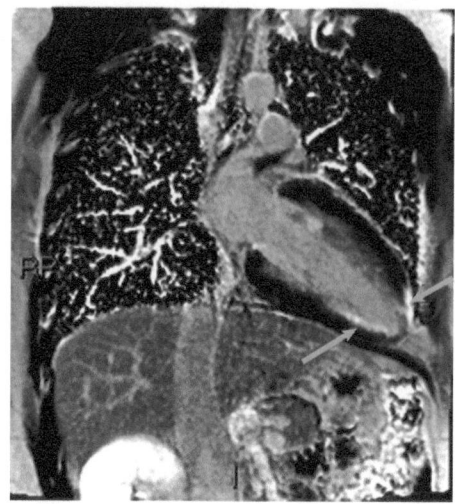

Fig. 12.7 A cardiac magnetic resonance imaging scan of an 18-year-old symptomatic high school football player with hypertrophic cardiomyopathy. (This athlete's electrocardiogram is shown in Fig. 12.5C.) Subendocardial late gadolinium enhancement involving the inferior wall is present in both the mid and apical part of the left ventricle, along with delayed transmural enhancement of the apex *(arrows)*. These findings are consistent with infarction and fibrosis. This athlete was also experiencing angina, which resolved with beta-blocker therapy. The athlete was restricted from competition, and cardioverter-defibrillator implantation was performed. (From Battle RW, Mistry DJ, Malhotra R. Cardiovascular screening and the elite athlete: advances, concepts, controversies, and a view of the future. *Clin Sports Med.* 2011;30:503–524, with permission.)

(LVNC), which can be pathologic and thus of a concern in elite athletes.[95] It has been demonstrated that nearly 20% of athletes may exhibit hypertrabeculation that meets current criteria for the diagnosis of LVNC, but this is felt to be due to physiologic adaptions of increased blood volume rather than an underlying cardiomyopathy.[96,97] This example demonstrates the importance of interpreting echocardiographic abnormalities in elite athletes within the appropriate context in order to avoid unnecessary disqualification from participation.

Application of TTE can be very useful in the diagnosis of a host of disorders that may not immediately threaten the athlete (see Box 12.1), but because of the "gray zone" mimicry of HCM in addition to previously discussed milder forms of dilated cardiomyopathy and ARVC, application of TTE is not for the faint-hearted.[88] Clearly there will be cases that challenge our diagnostic certainty and that may require more extensive testing or detraining. It is common practice to perform "limited" TTE in screening programs, often by fellows in training and without recording or digitally storing images. While we applaud the interest and the effort, we discourage this because once the screening process has been initiated, physicians assume liability related to accuracy of the test. "Limited" screening TTE that focuses primarily on

HCM is less likely to detect focal HCM, the anomalous coronary artery, or more subtle abnormalities of the ascending aorta (particularly those associated with the bicuspid aortic valve). Furthermore, limited TTE screening will be less discerning with regard to remodeling versus real disease, and could trigger unnecessary testing and anxiety over a false-positive diagnosis that is unnecessary and costly. For this reason, we recommend incorporation of high-quality and thorough TTE (we have found this can be done in the screening setting in <10 min) that ideally would include the knowledge of congenital anomalies to best serve the athlete at the initiation of the evaluation.[98]

STRUCTURAL/CONGENITAL DISEASE STATES IN ELITE ATHLETES

It is prudent for the sports cardiologist to proceed with great caution and a meticulous approach prior to establishing a concrete diagnosis of a structural abnormality in any elite athlete, particularly when the diagnosis overlaps with the previously discussed remodeling changes that mimic real disease. If a structural abnormality is diagnosed in an elite athlete, the most recent expert consensus from the joint conference provides us with general guidelines for management, particularly with regard to the eligibility for athletic participation.[78] Each athlete must be considered individually and thoroughly, and the sports cardiologist may be confounded by the overall lack of data that support any survival benefit derived from restriction from participation. Providers will also struggle to maintain equipoise during this

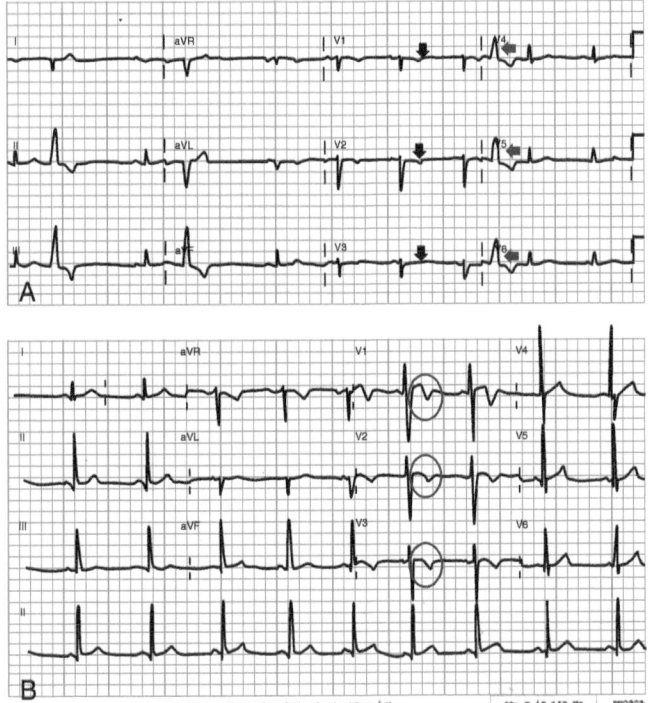

Fig. 12.8 (A) An electrocardiogram (ECG) in an athlete with arrhythmogenic right ventricular cardiomyopathy (ARVC). Consecutive T-wave inversions are seen in precordial leads V1–V3 *(black arrows)*. Premature ventricular contractions are emanating from the right ventricle in a left bundle branch block morphology suggestive of ARVC *(red arrows)*. (B) A 17-year-old asymptomatic intercollegiate 800-meter runner with T-wave inversions in V1 to V3 on a screening ECG (findings were circled during screening). Because the patient was of Italian descent and concern existed about the possibility of ARVC, transthoracic echocardiography and cardiac magnetic resonance imaging were performed, and findings were completely normal. The finding is a normal variant in young athletes.

process, with competing interests vying for influence, including the strong desire of the athlete to continue competing; pressure from parents, fans, administrators, teams, and schools; a shared loyalty to the athlete/patient and the institution or team that employs or consults the provider; the athlete seeking multiple opinions until a provider acquiesces to allowance of participation; and concern for adverse publicity or medical-legal repercussions[99] that can have a profound impact on any individual physician managing a celebrated athlete. The cases of basketball players Hank Gathers and Reggie Lewis are dramatic examples of the difficult and damaging nature of this process.[5]

HCM occurs in approximately 1/500 of the general population and has been considered the most common cause of athletic SD in the United States, although this assertion has been recently challenged.[3] Initially described in 1958 by a British pathologist in a very high risk family with dramatic asymmetric LVH,[100] HCM would be further evaluated in major referral centers, creating a significant referral bias exaggerating the true risk of sudden death faced by individuals with the diagnosis.[12,88,101] Indeed, we have more recently understood this to be a condition with a widely variable phenotypic expression ranging from significant risk of SD to a benign clinical course with unusual longevity. In

many ways, the only consistency with HCM is inconsistency. There are data suggesting an increased risk of athletic SD in HCM associated with race, young age, and vigorous physical activity[102,103]; however, excepting inference from the Italian experience, data supporting a survival benefit from sports participation withdrawal in athletes are lacking. Because the safest course of action is probably withdrawal of all athletes with the confirmed diagnosis of HCM from all but low intensity sports, this recommendation was adopted by the 36th Bethesda Conference[104] in 2005 and integrated again by expert consensus on HCM in 2011.[78] Disqualified athletes and sports cardiologists will both suffer from the lack of compelling data when complying with these guidelines, knowing that low-risk athletes will be unnecessarily sidelined from competition. Accordingly, individual cardiologists may decide to challenge these recommendations and allow participation. Division I college basketball player Monty Williams was diagnosed with HCM his sophomore year at Notre Dame in 1990, the same year of Hank Gathers death. He was initially disqualified and told he would never play basketball again. Two years later, he sought another opinion, and after a battery of tests he was cleared to compete by a controversial decision from his consulting cardiologist and went on to play in the NBA. Others have advocated for individualized participation for athletes with defibrillators (ICD),[105] but this is a very complex process. The effects of extreme motion and bodily contact could disrupt function of the ICD; thus managing physicians will be reliant upon the athlete to frequently check the device remotely and respond immediately to any alerts signaling malfunction. Nicholas Knapp, a 17-year-old high school senior who had accepted a basketball scholarship at Northwestern, arrested while playing informally, and ventricular fibrillation was documented.[106] He was resuscitated and recovered completely. He was subsequently found to have mild asymmetric LVH localized to the septum, with hyperdynamic LV systolic function and mild systolic anterior motion of the mitral valve and diffuse T-wave inversion on his resting ECG. He was diagnosed with HCM, and following a negative electrophysiology study, an implantable defibrillator was inserted. Knapp matriculated at Northwestern the following year and was declared medically ineligible but allowed to maintain his full scholarship. Despite the profile of serious risk established, Knapp pursued his right to participate in intercollegiate basketball in federal district court *(Knapp v. Northwestern University)*, arguing that restricting him was a violation of his rights established in the Rehabilitation Act of 1973.[107] The federal district court initially ruled in favor of Knapp, but this was overturned in the US Court of Appeals.

Athletes disqualified with suspected HCM within the "gray zone" should be subjected to a period of detraining and then re-evaluated. In an interesting case report, investigators describe a vigorously trained 17-year-old male swimmer (14 hours/week, 16 miles/week) who had LVH by voltage on his ECG, along with inverted and biphasic T-waves with LV wall thickness of 14 mm and end diastolic LV cavity size of 48 mm by TTE. The athlete was evaluated after 8 weeks of detraining, which revealed complete regression of all training-related remodeling on both the ECG and TTE.[107] Pelliccia et al. prospectively evaluated 40 elite Italian athletes with hypertrophy and cavity dilation following a more prolonged period of detraining (1 to 13 yrs) and found that LVH regressed to normal in all subjects, whereas LV cavity dilation persisted (>60 mm) in 22%.[108] Accordingly, detraining is particularly helpful in the circumstance of the "gray zone," and it would seem reasonable to re-evaluate after approximately 2 months and again at around 1 year. Genetic testing is problematic because only a positive test is helpful, while a negative test does not exclude a new and private mutation. Athletes who are referred for a family history of HCM, with no evidence by ECG, TTE, or symptoms that they are affected, may benefit greatly from genetic testing if the affected parent/relative can have the gene identified; the athlete can be subsequently tested for the presence of the same genotype.[109] Because the timing of phenotypic development of LVH in HCM is variable, a positive genetic test in the phenotypically negative athlete would stimulate frequent interval of follow-up and serial testing that should include yearly TTE and stress testing at a minimum, as well as consideration for disqualification depending on the risk profile of the family history and the individual athlete. For these reasons, current guidelines do not support restriction of the genotype positive but phenotypically negative athlete. In contrast, athletes with negative genetic testing would be free to participate and not subjected to frequent and expensive diagnostic testing.

The congenital anomalous coronary artery is the second most common cause of athletic SD in the United States.[2,3,11,59] The left coronary arising from the right sinus is more prevalent in cases of athletic SD than the right coronary arising from the left sinus;[110] however, both can be threatening. When an oblique orifice arising from the contrary sinus is subjected to aortic expansion from increased cardiac output with exercise, the slit-like narrowing can be accentuated, leading to acute ischemia and arrhythmic SD. This may be the most elusive and difficult anomaly for the sports cardiologist, because symptoms are often absent, and of the athletes who suffered SD and underwent screening, none (9/9) had an abnormal ECG, and of those who underwent stress testing, none had abnormal findings (6/6).[110] The only opportunity to make this diagnosis prior to an event would be on screening TTE, which can correctly identify the right and left coronary arteries in most elite athletes.[111] Imaging of coronary arteries, however, is not routinely done in standard adult TTE laboratories, whereas it is standard to assess coronary origin and course in congenital TTE laboratories, and this can also be done quite successfully in elite athletes.[112] Accordingly, any athlete undergoing TTE for screening, chest pain, or syncope with exertion imaging of the coronaries should be undertaken. Indeed, it is recommended to include coronary artery imaging into any TTE protocol involving elite athletes.[98] CT angiography is the best test for athletes suspected of this anomaly, and anatomy can be elegantly identified with this technique.[113] When detected, conventional wisdom dictates at least temporary disqualification and subsequent surgical repair of the anomalies noted previously, although there are no randomized data to support that recommendation. This recommendation is advisable and clearer in the symptomatic athlete. If incidentally found in the asymptomatic athlete, careful stratification of risk based upon the duration and nature of event-free participation and the structural appearance of the anomaly will be necessary to individualize any

recommendation about whether or not the athlete should be able to continue to participate or undergo surgery.

ARVC has historically been a difficult diagnostic challenge, and TTE and ECG have not been ideal for this diagnosis. As previously discussed, athletes may have training-related dilation and systolic dysfunction of the RV that can mimic the condition of ARVC.[31,32,35-37,94] Diagnostic criteria for ARVC have evolved with better RV imaging with MRI;[114] however, we urge caution with regard to this diagnosis, particularly in the asymptomatic athlete without documentation of ventricular arrhythmia. Precordial T-wave inversion of >2 mm in 2 or more adjacent leads (see Fig. 12.8) is uncommon in older athletes and may warrant further evaluation with MRI.[69,111,115] T-wave inversion in precordial leads V1 to V3 occurs in <3% of healthy individuals from age 19 to 45 (more common in children) and in 87% of patients with ARVC.[116] Therefore the diagnosis should only be made in the context of the individual patient based upon age and whether premature ventricular contractions (PVCs) or ventricular tachycardia (VT) of LBBB morphology are present. For suspected cases of ARVC, temporary disqualification is warranted and expert EP consultation should be sought. In confirmed cases, disqualification from all but low intensity sports may be permanent and a defibrillator required.

The most prevalent congenital cardiac anomaly is the bicuspid aortic valve (BAV), which is more common in males and occurs in up to 2% of the general population.[117] This prevalence is important for sports cardiologists, because a significant number of affected individuals will have functionally normal valves or only mild valve disease, and a significant percentage of those individuals will also have congenital dilation of the ascending aorta that could place them at risk.[117,118] The majority of affected individuals have fusion of the right and left coronary cusps, and this is the pattern more likely to be associated with functionally normal valve or mild valve disease.[119] This topic has been reviewed in depth,[108] with aortic root dilation noted in affected individuals as follows: sinuses of Valsalva—up to 78%, sinotubular junction—up to 79%, and above the sinotubular junction—up to 68%. If the athlete does not have an audible murmur, and because an isolated systolic ejection click is easily missed, it would seem likely that a significant number of elite athletes could escape detection during the physical exam and still have congenital aortic valve disease and significant abnormalities of the ascending aorta. At the University of Virginia (UVA), screening with a congenital focus on TTE has effectively identified these patients, and out of 175 incoming freshmen athletes, 2 males were found to have BAV: 1 with mild to moderate aortic regurgitation AR, and 1 with a functionally normal valve with mild dilation of the ascending aorta.[120] Indeed using both screening congenital TTE and general sports medical care, including the PPE-4 of 670 athletes at UVA, we have identified seven athletes with BAV; four have aortic root dilation, and 5 out of the 7 athletes have the more hemodynamically benign pattern of right and left coronary cusp commissural fusion. Not surprisingly, there is a high prevalence of the BAV among elite athletes that is >1% and thus five times more common than HCM. Examples of a familial BAV syndrome in two brothers that are Division I intercollegiate athletes are shown in Fig. 12.9. Both have right and left cusp fusion with mild to moderate aortic regurgitation, and one has mild aortic root dilation at the sinuses of Valsalva exceeding 40 mm. Both are followed every 6 to 12 months with TTE, and the athlete with aortic root dilation has been restricted from isometric weight training to avoid the impact of hypertension associated with rigorous isometric weight training.

The Marfan syndrome is another autosomal dominant cardiovascular disorder that was first meticulously described by Edgar Allan Poe in a short story ("A Tale of the Ragged Mountains"), written about his earlier experience at the University of Virginia.[121] The protagonist of this tale has all of the classic features of this syndrome, described by Poe more than 50 years before the first documented case in medical literature noted in Paris by Professor Antoine Marfan.[122] The PPE-4 has been adapted to better detect the family history, medical history, and physical findings that might suggest the Marfan syndrome or related disorders such as Ehlers-Danlos or Loeys-Dietz syndrome.[13,123] These syndromes all manifest genetic deficiencies of vital matrix proteins that can predispose the athlete to aortic dissection and, in the case of Ehlers-Danlos and Loeys-Dietz syndromes, to smaller arteries as well. In general, these athletes are restricted from all but low-intensity sports[104] and usually do not develop into elite athletes. Exceptions do occur, however, and athletes with the Marfan syndrome may gravitate toward sports that require taller athletes, as illustrated by Flo Hyman who was an Olympic volleyball player before she died tragically of aortic dissection in a professional game. Furthermore, due to inconsistencies in administration of the PPE-4, athletes may inadvertently be allowed to participate, like the college swimmer in Fig. 12.10 with Marfan syndrome who was prescribed losartan and suffered a type B dissection of the aorta during practice. In the event of a positive family history of one of these autosomal dominant disorders, it may be prudent, as we suggested with family histories of HCM, to have the affected parent/relative genetically tested, followed by genetic testing of the athlete in question if appropriate.

ACQUIRED CARDIOVASCULAR CONDITIONS IN THE ATHLETE

Myocarditis and myopericarditis should be considered in any athlete with new symptoms or evidence of arrhythmia, sustained chest pain, troponin elevation, or new findings of LV systolic dysfunction or ECG changes, particularly diffuse ST elevation and repolarization abnormalities. A Division I college basketball player with syncope and documented ventricular arrhythmia due to myocarditis is shown in Fig. 12.11. Previously difficult to diagnose in cases of preserved systolic function, this disorder is now readily detected utilizing gadolinium MRI with classic findings of sub-epicardial late gadolinium enhancement.[124] Because the clinical course of myocarditis, and the arrhythmias and ventricular systolic dysfunction that may accompany it, varies widely, withdrawal and treatment recommendations must be individualized. It is prudent, however, to temporarily restrict any athlete with confirmation of this diagnosis at least temporarily and until any documented arrhythmias or LV systolic abnormalities resolve.

CAD is a rare finding or cause of athletic SD in athletes <35 years old.[3] However, premature CAD cannot be ignored, as illustrated by the SD of the Russian Olympic and world champion pairs skater Sergie Grinkov while practicing on Lake Placid in 1995 at the age of only 28. Grinkov had a genetic predisposition to premature CAD due to the platelet antigen gene (PLA-2) and had a family history of premature death (father) from CAD.[125] Tobacco was a staple in the major league baseball dugout years ago, and the cardiologist and former major league baseball player and then president of the American League Bobby Brown recollected a player who recovered from a myocardial infarction and returned to pitch effectively in Major League Baseball.[126] There has been a dramatic culture shift in the awareness of health and nutrition among athletes since then; therefore it is logical to assume that CAD is a more important concern in older athletes who participate in a variety of sports some of which are highly competitive. Data from several studies have demonstrated that SD in the athlete over 35, CAD is the proximate cause in the vast majority (80%) of those cases.[59] Recent data from the Race Associated Cardiac Event Registry (RACER) analyzed 10.9 million athletes participating in marathon and half marathon races in the United States from 2000 to 2010.[127] In this group of older athletes (mean age 59), the RACER investigators found that the overall risk of SD was quite low (54/100,000 participants); SD was more common in males and was more likely to occur in full marathons and toward the end of the race. Accordingly, the risk of SD remains low in athletes as CAD becomes more prevalent in the population at risk, and the RACER results further illustrate the salutary effects of regular physical exercise in both men and women, reinforcing previous prospective data that habitual vigorous exercise reduces exercise-related SD.[128]

It is imperative that sports medicine providers and sports cardiologists address the finding of hypertension (HTN) when this is discovered. As discussed, familial hypertension has an important impact upon cardiovascular training adaptations in athletes[56] (particularly those engaging heavily in strength training), and this coupled with untreated hypertension could amplify unfavorable long-term physiologic alterations, thus negatively affecting the health and longevity of the athlete. Sports participation reduces the incidence of hypertension in athletes to approximately 50% of that seen in more sedentary controls,[129] yet athletes may still present early, and up to 10% of HTN will initially present between the ages 20 and 30.[130] Furthermore, of adolescent athletes found to have a blood pressure higher than 142/92 mm Hg at the PPE, 80% will go on to develop chronic hypertension at 1 year follow-up[131] and will thus be at significant risk for the development of hypertensive heart disease into adulthood. Multiple factors can contribute to hypertension in young athletes, including obesity, male sex, African race, oral contraceptive pills, alcohol binging, nonsteroidal anti-inflammatory drugs, diet with excessive salt and fat, supplements (containing ephedra, ma huang, and guarana), and performance-enhancing drugs (PED), including steroids and erythropoietin; in-depth reviews are available.[132] Athletes with hypertension should be evaluated according to published guidelines,[133] and treatment needs to be tailored to the individual athlete. Initially any environmental factors that are contributing to hypertension should be corrected and dietary recommendations high in fruits, vegetables, and potassium, and low in sodium DASH diet[134] should be implemented, initiating a nonpharmacologic program designed to reduce blood pressure.

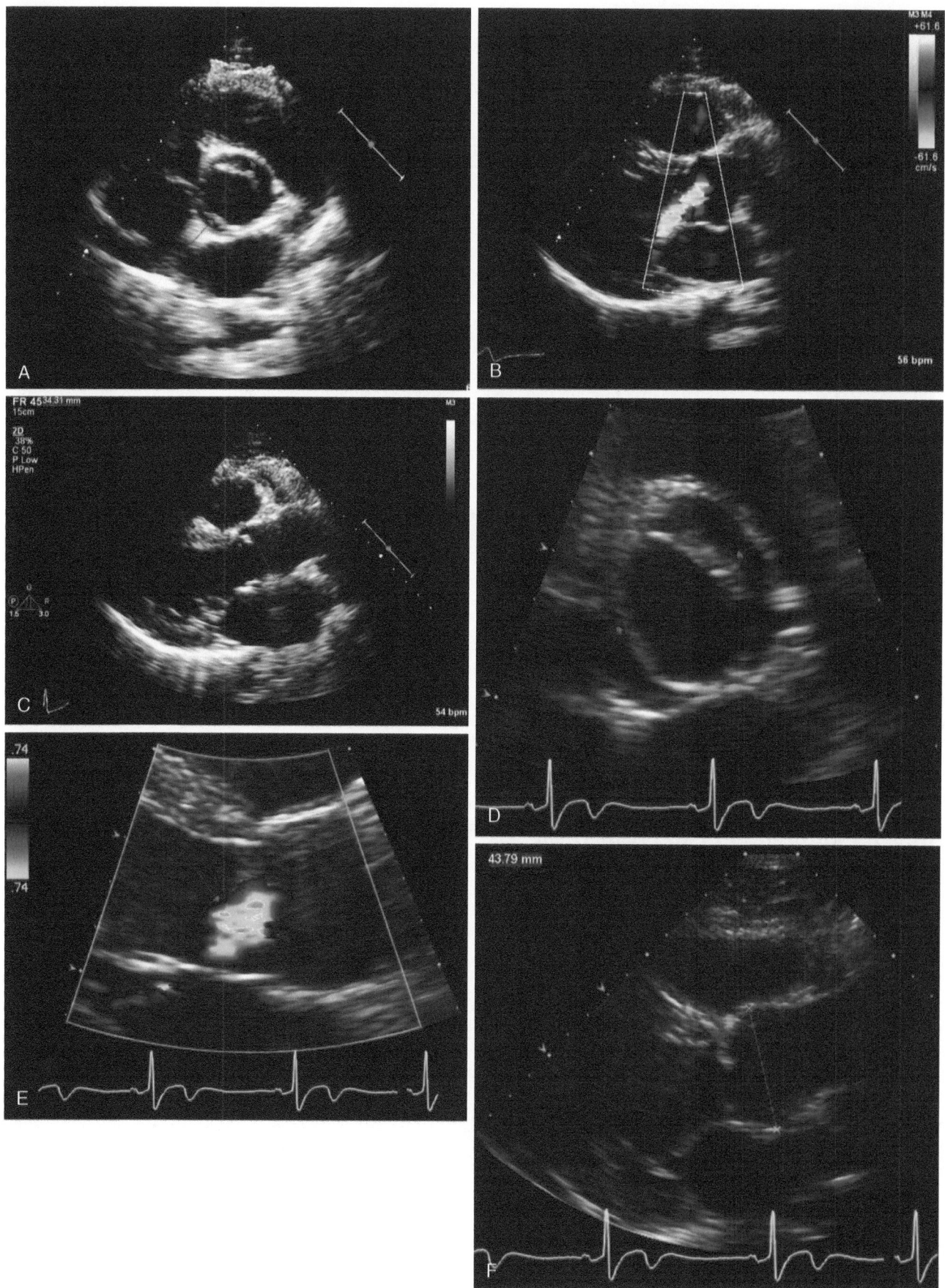

Continued on page 171

Fig. 12.9 Transthoracic echocardiogram (TTE) examples of a familial bicuspid valve syndrome in two brothers, both of whom are Division I lacrosse players; one brother has an associated congenital aortopathy. (A) A parasternal short-axis view of an 18-year-old athlete with a bicuspid aortic valve *(arrows)* with fusion of the right and left coronary cusps and a horizontally oblique aperture. (B) A parasternal long-axis view with color Doppler imaging demonstrating moderate aortic insufficiency oriented directly toward the anterior leaflet of the mitral valve *(arrow)*. This posterior orientation of aortic insufficiency is characteristic of prolapse of the anterior cusp. (C) A parasternal long-axis view showing the typical systolic doming of the aortic cusps *(arrow)* and measurement of the ascending aorta at the sinuses of Valsalva is normal for body-surface-area at 3.4 cm (red line). (D) A parasternal long-axis view of the previously described patient's 21-year-old brother with a near-identical valve with the same fusion pattern and aperture *(arrows)*. (E) A parasternal long-axis view shows a similar orientation of the aortic insufficiency by color Doppler imaging *(arrow)*. In this brother, the aortic insufficiency is mild to moderate. (F) A parasternal long-axis view demonstrating the presence of a congenital aortopathy in the older brother. Maximal dilation is mild to moderate at 4.4 cm when measured at the sinuses of Valsalva *(red line)*. Both brothers are eligible to play by current guidelines. Because of the hemodynamic effects of elite training that could accelerate either the aortic insufficiency or the aortopathy, both athletes are followed up by TTE every 6 months. (From Battle RW, Mistry DJ, Malhotra R. Cardiovascular screening and the elite athlete: advances, concepts, controversies, and a view of the future. *Clin Sports Med.* 2011;30:503–524, with permission.)

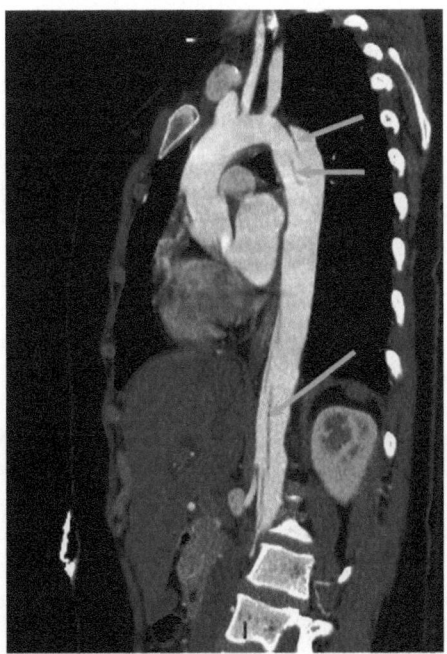

Fig. 12.10 A computed tomography scan with contrast material demonstrating a spiral type B dissection of the descending thoracic aorta *(arrows* indicate the intimal flap) in a female intercollegiate swimmer with Marfan syndrome. The dissection occurred during practice. The sinuses of Valsalva were only borderline abnormal with an eccentric posterior sinus. (From Battle RW, Mistry DJ, Malhotra R. Cardiovascular screening and the elite athlete: advances, concepts, controversies, and a view of the future. *Clin Sports Med.* 2011;30:503–524, with permission.)

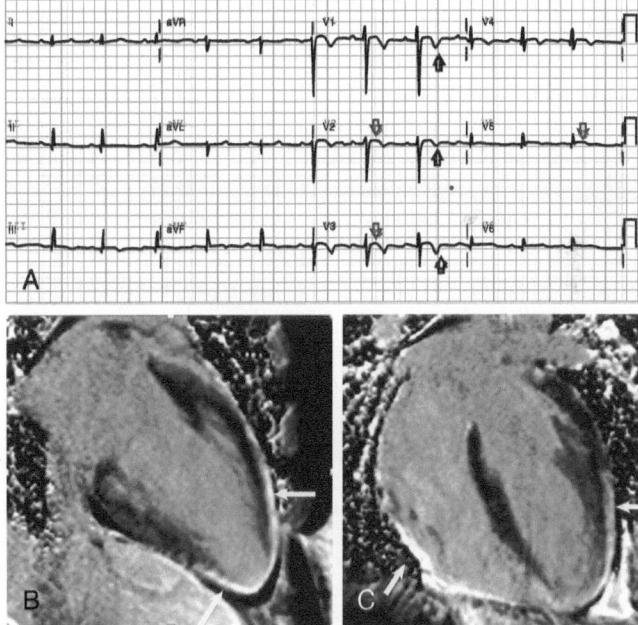

Fig. 12.11 A 21-year-old African-American Division I college basketball player with myocarditis. This athlete initially presented with syncope, and a second syncopal episode occurred five months later. (A) An electrocardiogram (ECG) reveals persistent diffuse ST-elevation *(red arrows)* followed by T-wave inversion *(black arrows)*. (B) A magnetic resonance image (MRI) shows late gadolinium enhancement (LGE) of the epicardial aspect of the anteroapex and inferoapex *(arrows)*. (C) Late epicardial enhancement of the right ventricular free wall is also noted *(leftward arrow)*. The ECG is suggestive of chronic pericarditis and myocarditis, and the typical MRI finding of epicardial LGE is characteristic of this disorder, compared with patchy LGE/fibrosis seen in persons with hypertrophic cardiomyopathy. An electrophysiologic study revealed easily inducible rapid ventricular tachycardia, and the athlete was restricted from competition. (From Battle RW, Mistry DJ, Malhotra R. Cardiovascular screening and the elite athlete: advances, concepts, controversies, and a view of the future. *Clin Sports Med.* 2011;30:503–524, with permission.)

If the initial approach is insufficient, a pharmacologic strategy may be required, and this is a complex process that has been reviewed previously.[132,135] Many of our standard choices will not apply to elite athletes. Diuretics cannot be taken by athletes who undergo drug testing, because these drugs can be used as effective masking agents, therefore concealing the use of PEDs. Furthermore, diuretics could promote dehydration in many types of activities and predispose to hypokalemia. Medications that affect the sinus node, including beta blockers and nondihydropyridine calcium channel blockers (verapamil and diltiazem), blunt the achievement of peak heart rate and can lead to impaired performance. Conversely, beta blockers are considered to enhance performance and may not be permitted in sports like archery, golf, and shooting, where controlling the heart rate may be an advantage. In general, angiotensin converting enzyme (ACE) inhibitors, angiotensin receptor blockers (ARBs), and the dihydropyridine calcium channel blockers (nifedipine XL, amlodipine, felodipine, and isradipine) are best suited for athletes. Endurance athletes, particularly those competing in ultra-marathons, may be subject to very high circulating creatine phosphokinase (CK) levels from muscle breakdown, and this, in combination with ACE inhibitors or ARBs and varying degrees of dehydration, could lead to serious acute kidney injury. Accordingly, it may be prudent to advise these athletes not to take these medications on days when extreme training or competition could put them at risk. Female athletes should always be advised of the potential for birth defects, and athletes of African descent (low renin) are more likely to respond to calcium antagonists than ACE inhibitors or ARBs. Most athletes with HTN can be managed and allowed to compete according to the guidelines established by the Hypertension Task Force at the 36th Bethesda Conference.[126] Athletes with more advanced stage 2 HTN (BP > 160/100 mm Hg) should be restricted from isometric training until the blood pressure is well controlled. All athletes with HTN should be closely followed so that ongoing counsel on diet and lifestyle is repeatedly provided, blood pressure is monitored, and the remodeling effects of training can be assessed when appropriate.

Hyperlipidemia (including familial hyperlipidemia [FH] in particular) poses a difficult problem for sports medicine providers. Statin therapy for hyperlipidemia in the elite athlete is problematic, because many athletes will develop muscle pain in the absence of CK elevation,[136] and in elite professional athletes, up to 80% will be intolerant to this class of drugs due to this side effect.[137] Accordingly, treatment of this condition is close to incompatible with the activities associated with vigorous training and will prove a difficult challenge for most athletes, excepting those participating in less vigorous sports. Data to guide us in this area are few, yet it is reasonable to recommend at the minimum nonpharmacologic treatment according to guidelines[138] and referral of any athlete with a family history of premature death from CAD with hyperlipidemia or FH to a lipid specialist, ensuring that, once retired from competition, this problem is readdressed.

Arrhythmias

As discussed, conduction abnormalities and bradyarrhythmias are common in the trained athlete, including sinus bradycardia (which can be profound in endurance-trained athletes, see Fig. 12.1), junctional bradycardia, first-degree AV block, and Mobitz type I second-degree AV block. Mobitz type II and third-degree (complete) heart block are uncommon and should be judged abnormal, warranting referral to an electrophysiologist.[139] Premature atrial and ventricular contractions and nonsustained ventricular tachycardia are also common in trained athletes and are typically overdriven and disappear at higher heart rates associated with exercise. In the absence of structural heart disease (normal resting ECG and TTE) and when suppressed by exercise, these findings are typically benign and do not have long-term implications.[140-142] Atrial fibrillation (AF) is more common in elite endurance-trained athletes than sedentary controls.[143-145] In athletes, AF may develop during training with high adrenergic tone (endurance athletes will suddenly feel a "power outage") or during sleep and periods of more predominant vagal tone when AF may be focally initiated by premature atrial contractions arising from the pulmonary veins. Evaluation should include exclusion of structural heart disease, hyperthyroidism, and the intake of any type of inciting stimulant or supplement. Treatment is once again compromised by the performance-compromising effects of beta blockers and calcium blockers, neither of which suppress AF and which only slow the ventricular rate. We have found the Class IC agents flecainide and propafenone to be the most useful in athletes. For infrequent episodes, the "pill and pocket" approach as a single dose can effectively convert AF successfully to sinus rhythm.[146] For athletes with a more significant clinical burden and/or impairment of performance during training or important competition, a daily dose of flecainide or propafenone may be required; and athletes with structurally normal hearts are also likely to respond favorably to radiofrequency ablation of the pulmonary veins. Following radiofrequency ablation, there is a required period of anticoagulation; therefore the timing of this procedure will have a temporary impact on participation depending upon the sport. WPW syndrome can be asymptomatic or cause symptomatic supraventricular re-entrant tachycardia (SVT); and in extreme cases, rapid atrial fibrillation with aberrant conduction that can degenerate into ventricular fibrillation. Accordingly, athletes with WPW should be referred to an electrophysiologist to discuss the risks and benefits of bypass tract ablation, which can be curative. Common forms of re-entrant SVT also occur frequently in athletes, and if event or Holter monitoring detects this in a symptomatic athlete, ablation can be curative in this circumstance as well.

Brugada syndrome and the congenital long QT channelopathies can be life-threatening and warrant electrophysiology referral, whether found incidentally or due to symptoms. Once again, the future will see the current guidelines challenged with regard to participation with these diagnoses. In a recent publication of the Mayo experience with congenital long QT 130, patients continued to participate in a variety of sports and 20 of those had ICDs.[147] Of that group, 25% participated in high school sports, with 6% participating at the college and professional levels. Only one case of ICD discharge was documented in a 9-year-old boy who received two shocks for ventricular fibrillation occurring during warm-ups in the setting of admitted beta-blocker noncompliance. Catecholamine polymorphic ventricular tachycardia (CPVT) is another genetic syndrome, with the triggering of VT/

VF occurring with exercise-induced surges in adrenalin, and symptomatic patients have a poor prognosis unless treated with ICD.[148] An example of an asymptomatic 17-year-old Division I pole-vaulter with CPVT detected on a screening ECG is shown in Fig. 12.12. Life-threatening arrhythmias will be one of the more difficult future challenges for the sports cardiologist. Athletes with ICDs and a strong inclination to participate are at the top of that list. These athletes will still be at risk for syncope with exercise and should be counseled with regard to risk of participation in sports and activities where syncope could be a threat to themselves, other athletes or spectators including but not restricted to: swimming, scuba diving, archery, shooting, race-car driving, sky diving, skiing, and snowboarding. Athletes and their families may focus on their own concerns and needs once limited or disqualified and not think about the emotional consequences an event such as aborted SD might have on teammates, coaches, friends, and spectators.

Syncope is common in athletes and is unrelated to structural heart disease in the vast majority of cases, and typically occurs during nonexertional activities or immediately after exercise (likely due to sudden decrease in venous return).[149] Accordingly, in this setting, neurocardiogenic syncope is the most likely cause; however, electrical and structural abnormalities should be excluded. Syncope with exercise should bring to mind more concerning diagnoses, including HCM, anomalous coronary artery, CPVT, and so on. Occasionally athletes with syncope at peak exercise will manifest recurrent vasodepressor (hypotension) and/or cardio-inhibitory (bradycardia) syncope, but this must be demonstrated during stress testing with reproduction of symptoms before the diagnosis can be reliably established. The presumed mechanism is the Bezhold-Jarish reflex mediated by hyperdynamic LV function stimulating receptors in the left ventricle, which in turn activate the dorsal medial nucleus of the vagal nerve.[150,151] Athletes who we have found to have unique problems in this area are the elite rowers. It is common during training for upward of 60 intercollegiate rowers to line up side by side, often in confining spaces

for erg training on rowing machines. These athletes are capable of extreme outputs under these circumstances, and coupled with the heat emanating from so many exercising athletes at this level in close proximity, syncope and presyncope with peak exertion can occur in the absence of structural or electrical abnormalities. Syncope while seated seems implausible, but this may in part be due to compromised return of inferior vena cava blood during the forward posture portion of the rowing stroke. Standard treadmill testing cannot reproduce this reliably, and erg testing on the portable rowing machine in the stress lab can simulate training and competition and thus be useful.

Postural orthostatic tachycardia syndrome (POTS) and other disorders of autonomic regulation may also affect elite athletes causing symptoms and impairing performance.[152] This condition has been a common cause for referral in our experience with university athletes, probably because of transmission of viral illnesses that can spread through large groups of athletes and may be responsible for many of these disorders. Affected athletes may have inappropriate increases in heart rate (sinus tachycardia), with upright posture and stress testing with varying degrees of postural hypotension. Most athletes will be reassured to know that compromised performance is physiologic and that patience and continued graduated training (usually to include isometric training) will be required. Many treatments have been proposed, but most, other than careful attention to proper hydration and perhaps salt tablets, have been disappointing.

Commotio cordis is emerging as an important cause of athletic SD in the absence of structural or electrical cardiovascular abnormalities. SD during sports following blunt impact of a projected object (baseball, lacrosse ball, hockey puck) is uncommon but well described in the literature as commotion cordis, albeit with the mechanism unknown.[153] In an elegant animal model, Link et al. demonstrated that a wooden object the size and weight of a regulation baseball projected into the chest of pigs at 30 miles per hour timed to 15 to 30 m/sec ahead of the T-wave induced VF in 9/10 impacts. This did not occur in any impacts at other times during the cardiac cycle.[154] Furthermore, commercially available chest wall protectors fail to protect against this rare but often fatal event.[155] A registry of commotio cordis has been established and has taught us that it more commonly affects children (mean age 12), presumably because of the underdeveloped thorax and that only 10% of individuals before 1999 survived the arrest.[156] This research has resulted in a widespread appreciation of commotio cordis among sports medicine physicians and trainers, particularly in the vulnerable sports like baseball, softball, lacrosse, and hockey. VF induced by blunt impact is a time-sensitive rhythm, and knowledge by providers and availability of AEDs may have a beneficial impact on this rare but tragic occurrence in the future.

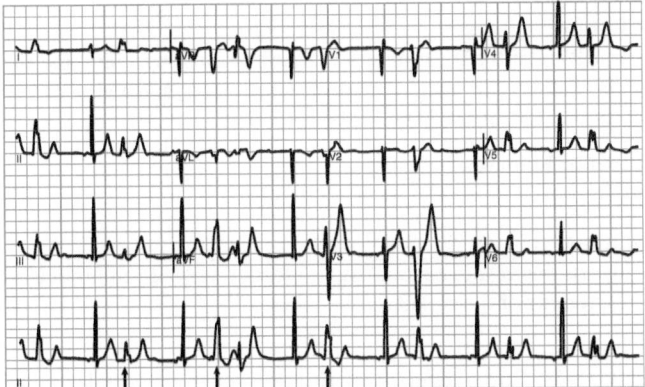

Fig. 12.12 A 17-year-old female Division I collegiate pole-vaulter with premature ventricular contractions on a screening electrocardiogram (ECG). Exercise treadmill test revealed polymorphic ventricular foci *(arrows)*. An epinephrine challenge corroborated the diagnosis of catecholaminergic polymorphic ventricular tachycardia. This athlete was disqualified and the arrhythmia was suppressed with a beta blocker. (From Battle RW, Mistry DJ, Malhotra R. Cardiovascular screening and the elite athlete: advances, concepts, controversies, and a view of the future. *Clin Sports Med.* 2011;30:503–524, with permission.)

CONCLUSIONS AND AN OPTIMISTIC VIEW OF THE FUTURE

Athletes who have suffered athletic SD have not done so in vain and are in large part responsible for many advances in this field. The feats of Pheidippides led to the reincarnation of the marathon race in Boston by the Boston Athletic Association in 1897. That race in turn would stimulate considerable interest in the cardiovascular adaptations to exercise and the diagnosis and evaluation of cardiovascular disease in those athletes. This sports cardiology tradition in Boston continues today and has gone well beyond its 100th year. Similar remarkable advances in basic science and the clinical spectrum of the athlete have come from around the world since the first description of the athlete's heart by Henschen in 1899.[157] We have optimism that this field will continue to grow beyond expert consensus and will bridge the gap between research and the clinical arena, and provide ample knowledgeable sports cardiologists to care for athletes of all ages in all locations. Incorporation of training in this discipline into standard cardiology fellowships should become routine rather than exceptional. Cardiologists entering this field will encounter complex relationships between athletes, their families, schools, teams, fans, and finally the media. It is also imperative that the role of the cardiologist within the medical home of the athlete continues to evolve within a shared decision-making framework alongside primary care sports medicine providers and athletic trainers. As stated by Dr. Andrew Krahn of the University of British Columbia in reference to the expanding role of specialized multidisciplinary clinics, "Shared decision-making supported by evidence-guided medical therapy and incremental interventions lays the foundation for a more permissive approach to not only allowing, but potentially encouraging participation in physical activity, including competitive sports."[158] Notably, the role of the physician in this complicated and often treacherous skein of relationships was thoughtfully and elegantly discussed by Harvard cardiologist Dr. Adolf Hutter Jr. in the keynote address prior to the 26th Bethesda Conference in 1994 and is mandatory reading for anyone entering this field.[159]

In closing, we emphasize the evolving improvements in the survival rate of athletic SD. The RACER investigators[127] showed that during athletic SD from 2000 to 2010, the mortality of athletes dropped to 71%, which is a marked decrease in previously published mortality for out-of-hospital cardiac arrest. Bystander CPR was identified as a predictor of survival. Recently released unpublished data from the European Society of Cardiology Congress from the fall of 2012 reinforces this finding, comparing out-of-hospital cardiac arrest during athletic and nonathletic circumstances. SD with exercise was associated with a 45% survival as compared with nonexercise survival of 15%.[160] None of the athletic survivors suffered significant cognitive brain damage. These advances in survival are likely due to heightened awareness, improved techniques of CPR, education and training of bystanders, accessibility of AEDs, and availability of sports medicine providers, all of which are more readily accessed at many sporting events. No example is more dramatic than the case of Fabrice Muamba, who arrested on the pitch during a soccer match and underwent CPR for 78 minutes, including multiple defibrillation attempts, directed by a bystanding cardiologist who was present as a fan. Sinus rhythm was restored only after admission to the hospital. Muamba survived, recovered, and received an ICD. Athletes, and the trainers, volunteers, and spectators who surround them, embody a culture of enthusiasm and accomplishment—a culture that will pursue success even under the most adverse circumstance. An inspirational example can be found in Grand Junction, Colorado, in response to the survival of a female with ARVC. The not-for-profit foundation "ARVD Heart for Hope" founded by her mother has partnered with Western Orthopedics and Sports Medicine and Community Hospital of Grand Junction to provide 54 AEDs for all local schools. This remarkable initiative in Grand Junction (a community of athletes) is the result of caring people making their community safer for athletes and, indeed, for all of us.

This chapter is dedicated to the memory of Fran Crippen (April 17, 1984, to October 23, 2010). Fran attended the University of Virginia, where he was an All-American swimmer and went on to earn six national titles. We honor and remember Fran as a student athlete whose character and commitment were commensurate to his remarkable athletic ability.

For a complete list of references, go to ExpertConsult.com.

SELECTED READINGS

Citation:
Williams RA. *The Athlete and Heart Disease: Diagnosis, Evaluation, and Management*. Philadelphia: Lippincott Williams and Wilkins; 1999.

Level of Evidence:
I

Summary:
An outstanding book on the entire subject that reviews the available data in depth.

Citation:
Baggish AL, Wood MJ. The athlete's heart and clinical cardiovascular care of the athletic patient: overview and scientific update. *Circulation*. 2011;123(23):2723–2735.

Level of Evidence:
I

Summary:
This article provides an excellent review of the athlete's heart and the care of the athlete.

Citation:
Battle RW, Mistry DJ, Malhotra R. Cardiovascular screening and the elite athlete: advances, concepts, controversies, and a view of the future. *Clin Sports Med*. 2011;30:503–524.

Level of Evidence:
I

Summary:
This article provides a recent and in-depth review of cardiovascular screening of the athlete

Citation:
Hutter AM. Cardiovascular abnormalities in the athlete: role of the physician. Keynote address: 26th Bethesda Conference. *J Am Coll Cardiol*. 1994;24:851–853.

Level of Evidence:
V

Summary:
This article addresses the complex role of the physician in dealing with cardiovascular abnormalities in the athlete.

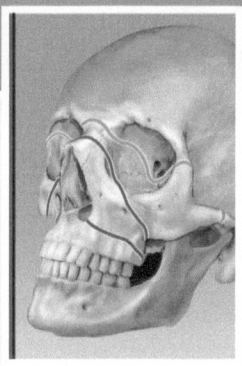

13

Exercise-Induced Bronchoconstriction

Virgil P. Secasanu, Jonathan P. Parsons

DEFINITION AND PREVALENCE

Exercise-induced bronchoconstriction (EIB) describes acute, transient airway narrowing that occurs during and after exercise. EIB is characterized by symptoms of cough, wheezing, or chest tightness during or after exercise. Exercise is one of the most common triggers of bronchoconstriction in asthmatic patients. Approximately 80% of individuals with chronic asthma have exercise-induced respiratory symptoms.[1] However, EIB can also occur in up to 10% of people who are not known to be atopic or asthmatic.[2] These patients do not have the typical features of chronic asthma (i.e., frequent daytime symptoms, nocturnal symptoms, impaired lung function), and exercise may be the only stimulus that causes respiratory symptoms.

The mechanism of EIB is characterized by the inspired volumes of relatively low-humidity air. Dry air leads to water loss from the airways, creating an osmotic change on the airway surface. The resultant hyperosmolar environment stimulates mast cell and eosinophil degranulation. The released mediators, predominantly leukotrienes, cause bronchoconstriction and airway inflammation. Inspiring cool air is thought to have a similar effect on the airways, albeit a less potent affect than hyperventilation with dry air.

EIB occurs commonly in athletes. The prevalence rates of exercise-related bronchoconstriction in athletes range from 11% to 50% (Table 13.1).[3] Holzer and colleagues[4] found 50% of a cohort of 50 elite summer athletes had EIB. Wilber and associates[5] found that 18% to 26% of Olympic winter sport athletes and 50% of cross-country skiers had EIB. The US Olympic Committee reported an 11.2% prevalence of EIB in all athletes who competed in the 1984 Summer Olympics.[6]

Despite numerous studies that investigate the prevalence of EIB in athletes, few studies have investigated the prevalence of EIB in cohorts of athletes without known history of asthma or EIB. Mannix and associates[7] found that 41 of 212 subjects (19%) in an urban fitness center, none of whom had a previous diagnosis of asthma, had EIB. Rupp and colleagues[8] evaluated 230 middle and high school student athletes and, after excluding those with known EIB, found that 29% had EIB. These studies suggest that EIB occurs commonly in subjects who are not known to be asthmatic and likely is underdiagnosed clinically.

The prevalence of EIB may be further underestimated because patients with asthma and EIB have been shown to be poor perceivers of symptoms of bronchoconstriction.[9,10] Specifically, athletes often suffer from lack of awareness of symptoms suggestive of EIB.[11,12] Health care providers and coaches also may not consider EIB as a possible explanation for respiratory symptoms occurring during exercise. Athletes are generally fit and healthy, and the presence of a significant medical problem often is not considered. The athlete is often considered to be "out of shape," and vague symptoms of chest discomfort, breathlessness, and fatigue are not interpreted as a manifestation of EIB. Athletes themselves are often not aware that they may have a physical problem. Furthermore, if they do recognize they have a medical problem, they often do not want to admit to health personnel that a problem exists because of fear of social stigma or losing playing time.

SPECIFIC ATHLETIC POPULATIONS AT RISK

Athletes who compete in high-ventilation or endurance sports may be more likely to experience symptoms of EIB than those who participate in low-ventilation sports[13]; however, EIB can occur in any setting. EIB is prevalent in endurance sports in which ventilation is increased for long periods of time during training and competition such as such as cross-country skiing, swimming, and long-distance running.[13] EIB also occurs commonly in winter sports athletes.[5] In addition, environmental triggers may predispose certain populations of athletes to an increased risk for development of EIB. Chlorine compounds in swimming pools[14] and chemicals related to ice-resurfacing machinery in ice rinks,[15] such as carbon monoxide and nitrogen dioxide, may put exposed athletic populations at additional risk. These environmental factors may act as triggers and exacerbate bronchoconstriction in athletes who are predisposed to EIB. Thus it is important for athletes, coaches, and athletic trainers supervising athletes in these sports to be aware of these important environmental issues.

CLINICAL PRESENTATION

The clinical manifestations of EIB are extremely variable and can range from mild impairment of performance to severe bronchoconstriction and respiratory failure. Common symptoms include coughing, wheezing, chest tightness, and dyspnea. More subtle evidence of EIB includes fatigue, symptoms that occur in specific environments (e.g., ice rinks or swimming pools), poor performance for conditioning level, and avoidance of activity (Box 13.1).

TABLE 13.1   Prevalence of Exercise-Induced Bronchoconstriction in Selected Studies

Reference No.	Athletes	EIB Prevalence (Bronchoprovocation Technique)
(5)	Winter Olympians	18%–26% (exercise)
(29)	Elite figure skaters	41% (EVH)
		31% (exercise)
(4)	Elite athletes	50% (EVH)
		18% (methacholine)
(11)	Collegiate athletes	39% (EVH)

EIB, Exercise-induced bronchoconstriction; *EVH*, eucapnic voluntary hyperventilation.

BOX 13.2   Mimics of Exercise-Induced Bronchoconstriction

- Vocal cord dysfunction
- Gastroesophageal reflux disease
- Allergic rhinitis
- Cardiac pathology (arrhythmias, cardiomyopathy, shunts)

BOX 13.1   Common Symptoms of Exercise-Induced Bronchoconstriction

- Dyspnea on exertion
- Chest tightness
- Wheezing
- Fatigue
- Poor performance for level of conditioning
- Avoidance of activity
- Symptoms in specific environments (e.g., ice rinks, swimming pools)

In general, exercise at a workload representing at least 80% of the maximal predicted oxygen consumption for 5 to 8 minutes is required to generate bronchoconstriction in most athletes.[16] Typically, athletes experience transient bronchodilation initially during exercise, and symptoms of EIB begin later or shortly after exercise. Symptoms often peak 5 to 10 minutes after exercise ceases and can remain significant for 30 minutes or longer if no bronchodilator therapy is provided.[17] However, some athletes spontaneously recover to baseline airflow within 60 minutes, even in the absence of intervention with bronchodilator therapy.[17] Unfortunately, it is currently impossible to predict which athletes will recover without treatment. Athletes who experience symptoms for extended periods often perform at suboptimal levels for significant portions of their competitive or recreational activities.

DIAGNOSIS

History and Differential Diagnosis

The presence of EIB can be challenging to recognize clinically because symptoms are often nonspecific. A complete history and physical examination should be performed on each athlete with respiratory complaints associated with exercise. However, despite the value of a comprehensive history of the athlete with exertional dyspnea, the diagnosis of EIB based on self-reported symptoms alone has been shown to be inaccurate. Hallstrand and colleagues[18] found that screening history identified subjects with symptoms or a previous diagnosis suggestive of EIB in 40% of the participants, but only 13% of these persons actually had EIB after objective testing. Similarly, Rundell and associates[12]

demonstrated that only 61% EIB-positive athletes reported symptoms of EIB, whereas 45% of athletes with normal objective testing reported symptoms. The poor predictive value of the history and physical examination in the evaluation of EIB strongly suggests that clinicians should perform objective diagnostic testing when there is a suspicion of EIB.

Other medical problems that can mimic EIB and should be considered in the initial evaluation of exertional dyspnea include vocal cord dysfunction, gastroesophageal reflux disease, and allergic rhinitis. Cardiac pathology such as arrhythmia, cardiomyopathy, and cardiac shunts are more rare, but these possibilities should also be considered (Box 13.2). A comprehensive history and examination is recommended to help rule out these confounding disorders, and specific testing such as echocardiography may be required. A history of specific symptoms in particular environments or during specific activities should be elicited. Timing of symptom onset in relation to exercise and recovery is also helpful. A thorough family and occupational history should be obtained because a family history of asthma increases the risk for other family members developing asthma.[19]

Objective Testing

Objective testing should begin with spirometry before and after inhaled bronchodilator therapy, which will help to identify athletes who have asthma. However, many people who experience EIB have normal baseline lung function.[20] In these patients, spirometry alone is not adequate to diagnose EIB. Significant numbers of false-negative results may occur if adequate exercise and environmental stress are not provided in the evaluation for EIB. In patients being evaluated for EIB who have a normal physical examination and normal spirometry, bronchoprovocation testing is recommended. A positive bronchoprovocation test indicates the need for treatment of EIB. Specific tests have varying positive values, but in general, a change (usually ≥10% decrease in forced expiratory volume in 1 second [FEV_1]) between pretest and posttest values is suggestive of EIB.[21] In a patient with persistent exercise-related symptoms and negative physical examination, spirometry, and bronchoprovocation testing, we recommend reconsidering alternative diagnoses.

Not all bronchoprovocation techniques are equally valuable or accurate in assessing EIB in athletes. The International Olympic Committee recommends eucapnic voluntary hyperventilation (EVH) challenge to document EIB in Olympians.[22] EVH involves hyperventilation of a gas mixture of 5% CO_2 and 21% O_2 at a target ventilation rate of 85% of the patient's maximal voluntary ventilation in 1 minute (MVV). The MVV is usually calculated as 30 times the baseline FEV_1. The patient continues to hyperventilate for 6 minutes, and assessment of FEV_1 occurs at specified intervals up to 20 minutes after the test. This challenge test has been shown to have a high specificity[23] for EIB. EVH has also been shown to be more sensitive for detecting EIB than lab- or field-based exercise testing.[23]

In the United States, lab-based exercise testing is widely available, although often less sensitive than EVH. Lab-based exercise testing measures serial lung function tests before and after an exercise challenge. In general, FEV_1 is measured because this value has shown good repeatability.[24] Subjects are first asked to perform spirometry before an exercise challenge to measure the baseline FEV_1 value. Subjects are then asked to exercise, and FEV_1 is measured serially at 5, 10, 15, and 30 minutes after exercise. EIB is diagnosed as a 10% or greater drop in preexercise FEV_1 measured during the 30-minute postexercise phase. Severity of EIB is characterized by the degree of reduction: mild (10% to 25% reduction), moderate (25% to 50% reduction), and severe (≥50% reduction).[25–28]

In contrast to lab-based testing, field-based exercise testing involves an athlete performing a sport and assessing FEV_1 after exercise. Similar to lab-base testing, field-based testing has been shown to be less sensitive than EVH.[29] Moreover, such field-based exercise testing allows for little protocol standardization. Pharmacologic challenge tests, such as the methacholine challenge test, have been shown to have a lower sensitivity than EVH for detection of EIB in athletes[4] and are also not recommended for first-line evaluation of EIB.

TREATMENT OPTIONS

Pharmacologic Therapy

Pharmacologic therapy for EIB (Table 13.2) has been studied extensively. The most common therapeutic recommendation to minimize or prevent symptoms of EIB is the prophylactic use of short-acting bronchodilators (selective β-adrenergic receptor agonists) such as albuterol shortly before exercise.[30] Treatment with two puffs of a short-acting β-agonist shortly before exercise (15 minutes) will provide peak bronchodilation in 15 to 60 minutes and protection from EIB for at least 3 hours in most patients.

Long-acting bronchodilators work in a similar manner pharmacologically as short-acting bronchodilators; however, the bronchoprotection afforded by long-acting β-agonists has been shown to last up to 12 hours, whereas that of short-acting agents is no longer significant by 4 hours.[31] Ferrari and associates[32] demonstrated inhalation of formoterol, a long-acting β-agonist, is effective in protecting asthmatic athletes as early as 15 minutes after dosing. However, tachyphylaxis also has been shown to occur after repeated use of long-acting β-agonists,[33] and they are not recommended in patients with normal or near-normal baseline lung function tests or as monotherapy.[28]

Inhaled corticosteroids are first-line controller therapy for patients who have chronic asthma and experience EIB.[30] Airway inflammation is also often present in athletes without asthma who have EIB[14,34]; therefore inhaled corticosteroids may be an effective medicine for treatment, but efficacy of corticosteroids in this cohort has not been studied. Inhaled corticosteroids are also valuable in athletes that train multiple times per day.

Leukotriene modifiers have also been shown to be effective in treating EIB.[35] Leff and colleagues[36] evaluated the ability of montelukast, a leukotriene receptor antagonist, to protect asthmatic patients against EIB. Montelukast therapy offered significantly greater protection against EIB than did placebo therapy and was also associated with a significant improvement in the maximal decrease in FEV_1 after exercise. In addition, tolerance to the medication and rebound worsening of lung function after discontinuation of treatment were not seen. In another study, daily zafirlukast treatment protected against EIB for at least 8 hours after regular dosing.[37] Leukotriene modifiers are an effective second line agent for treatment of EIB.

Mast cell stabilizers have been studied extensively for the prophylaxis of EIB. These medications prevent mast cell degranulation and subsequent histamine release. In a meta-analysis of the prevention of EIB in asthmatic patients, nedocromil sodium was found to improve FEV_1 by an average of 16% and to shorten the duration of EIB symptoms to less than 10 minutes.[38] Although these agents are effective and traditionally used to treat EIB, they are often used as a second line treatment because of their cost, lack of availability in the United States, and their decreased duration of action and efficacy compared with β2-agonists.[27]

Nonpharmacologic Therapy

Many athletes find that a period of precompetition warm-up reduces the symptoms of EIB that occur during their competitive activity. Athletes often draw this conclusion without any guidance from health care specialists. It has been shown by investigators that this refractory period does occur in some athletes with asthma and that athletes can be refractory to an exercise task performed within 2 hours of an exercise warm-up.[39,40] However, the refractory period has not been consistently proven across different athletic populations, and it is currently not possible to identify which athletes will experience this refractory period.[41]

Other nonpharmacologic strategies (see Table 13.2) can be used to help reduce the frequency and severity of symptoms of EIB. Breathing through the nose rather than the mouth will also help to ameliorate EIB[42] by warming, filtering, and humidifying the air, which subsequently reduces airway cooling and dehydration. Wearing a facemask during activity warms and humidifies inspired air when outdoor conditions are cold and dry. Facemasks are especially valuable to elite and recreational athletes who exercise in the winter.[43] In addition, people with knowledge of triggers (e.g., freshly cut grass) should attempt to avoid them if possible.[28]

TABLE 13.2 Treatment and Prevention of Exercise-Induced Bronchoconstriction	
Pharmacologic Therapy	**Nonpharmacologic Therapy**
Short-acting β-agonists	Adequate preexercise warm-up
Inhaled corticosteroids	Wearing a mask in cold environment
Long-acting β-agonists	Avoidance of triggers
Leukotriene modifiers	Nasal breathing
Cromolyn compounds	

Authors' Preferred Technique

Our preferred method for diagnosis and treatment of exercise-induced broncho-constriction (EIB) is shown in Fig. 13.1. The diagnosis of EIB based on symptoms alone is extremely inaccurate. Objective testing is necessary to make a confident diagnosis of EIB. We recommend using eucapnic voluntary hyperventilation (EVH) as the bronchoprovocation test of choice to document EIB; however, EVH may not be available to many health care providers. If EVH is not easily accessible, spirometry before and after an adequate exercise challenge is our second line recommendation. It is essential to ensure that the exercise challenge is strenuous enough to generate adequate ventilation rates in patients who have excellent physical fitness.

In our experience, both pharmacologic and nonpharmacologic approaches are essential to minimizing the adverse effects of EIB. We recommend that athletes who have clinical evidence of EIB be treated with short-acting bronchodilators before exercise and be counseled on the importance of adequate warm-up and avoidance of known triggers. This regimen will prevent significant EIB in more than 80% of athletes.[30] If symptoms persist, especially in athletes with asthma, we recommend adding corticosteroids as maintenance therapy. Although the efficacy of inhaled steroids in nonasthmatic athletes has not been evaluated, we recommend using them in nonasthmatic athletes whose symptoms are not completely controlled with short-acting bronchodilators. This recommendation is based on evidence of airway inflammation in subjects without known asthma as a result of hyperventilation and exercise.[14,34,44] Alternatively, leukotriene modi-fiers or cromolyn compounds can be used in athletes inadequately controlled with β_2-agonists.

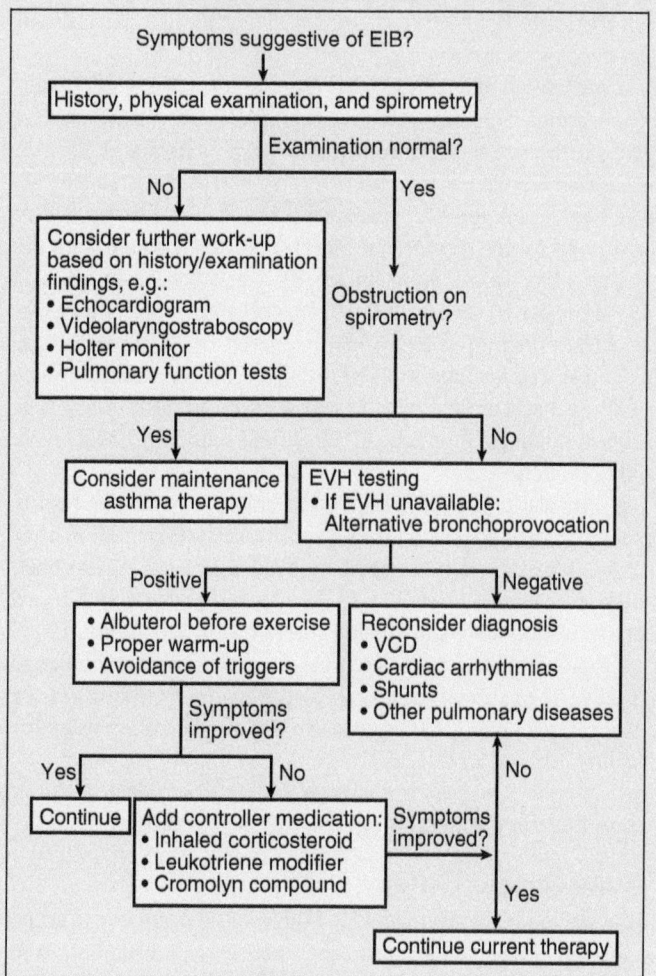

Fig. 13.1 Evaluation and management of exercise-induced broncho-constriction *(EIB)*. *EVH*, Eucapnic voluntary hyperventilation; *VCD*, vocal cord dysfunction. (Redrawn from Parsons JP, Mastronarde JG. Exercise-induced bronchoconstriction in athletes. *Chest*. 2005;128:3966–3974.)

SIDELINE MANAGEMENT

Acute, sideline management of EIB requires athletic trainers and coaches to be prepared to intervene if an athlete experiences an acute episode of EIB. All athletic trainers should have pulmonary function–measuring devices such as peak flow meters at all athletic events, including practices.[45] In addition, a rescue inhaler should be available during all games and practices. Spacers should be used with all rescue inhalers, and nebulizers should be readily available for emergencies in the event that inhalers are inadequate for control of acute symptoms.

On-field management of asthma begins with awareness of the signs and symptoms of respiratory distress (Box 13.3). Any athlete presenting with respiratory distress should be removed from competition and immediately evaluated by a physician. It is recommended that any athlete with a peak expiratory flow lower than 80% of "personal best" be removed from activity until their peak flow returns to at least 80% of "personal best."

BOX 13.3   Symptoms of Respiratory Distress

- Increase in wheezing or chest tightness
- Unable to speak in full sentences
- A respiratory rate greater than 25 breaths/min
- Persistent cough
- Breathing with nostril flaring
- Breathing with paradoxical abdominal movements

POTENTIAL COMPLICATIONS

The goals of treating an athlete with EIB are to optimize pulmonary function before starting athletic competition and to attempt to prevent significant episodes of EIB from occurring during exercise. Unfortunately, EIB often goes unrecognized, and consequences of unrecognized or inadequately treated EIB

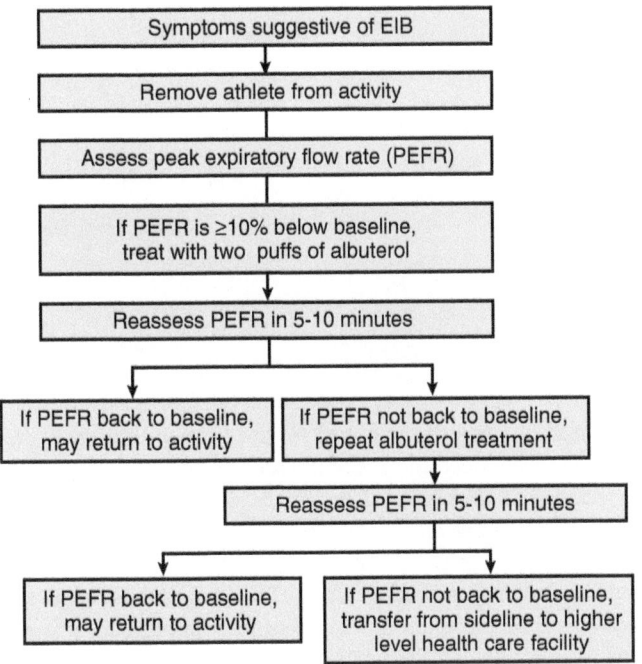

Fig. 13.2 Sideline management of exercise-induced bronchoconstriction *(EIB)* and criteria for return to play.

are significant. Becker and associates[46] identified 61 deaths secondary to asthma over a 7-year period occurring in close association with a sporting event or physical activity. Of these deaths, 81% occurred in subjects younger than 21 years and 57% occurred in subjects considered elite or competitive. Strikingly, almost 10% of deaths in this review occurred in subjects with no known history of asthma. Similarly, Amital and colleagues[47] found that asthma was the single greatest risk factor for unexplained death in a review of Israeli military recruits' data over a 30-year period. Results from these reviews suggest that all individuals involved in organized sports or physical activity should be cognizant of the risk for EIB. Coaches, athletic trainers, parents, and team physicians who care for competitive athletes who have asthma or EIB should be specifically trained in the recognition and treatment of EIB.

CRITERIA FOR RETURN TO PLAY

Criteria for safe return to play (RTP) after an acute episode of EIB are based on expert opinion only. Most experts agree that no athlete should RTP until lung function returns to baseline.[45] However, no consensus RTP protocol exists, and each athlete must be evaluated for returning to play after an acute episode of EIB. An algorithm outlining acute, sideline management of EIB and suggested criteria for RTP are shown in Fig. 13.2.

KEY POINTS

- Exercise-induced bronchoconstriction (EIB) occurs in athletes with and without chronic asthma.
- EIB occurs more commonly in athletes than the general population.
- The symptoms of EIB are often subtle and difficult to differentiate from normal manifestations of intense exercise.
- Diagnosis of EIB based on subjective symptoms alone is extremely inaccurate.
- Objective testing is strongly recommended to document a diagnosis of EIB.
- The consequences of unrecognized or inadequately treated EIB can be significant.
- Treatment of EIB with a short-acting bronchodilator before exercise is 80% effective.
- Coaches and athletic trainers should be prepared to manage an athlete with an acute episode of EIB at all practices and competitive events.

For a complete list of references, go to ExpertConsult.com.

SELECTED READINGS

Citation:
Anderson SD, Argyros GJ, Magnussen H, et al. Provocation by eucapnic voluntary hyperpnoea to identify exercise induced bronchoconstriction. *Br J Sports Med.* 2001;35:344–347.

Level of Evidence:
I

Summary:
This article describes eucapnic voluntary hyperventilation protocol.

Citation:
Parsons JP, Hallstrand TS, Mastronarde JG, et al; American Thoracic Society Subcommittee on Exercise-induced Bronchconstriction. An official American Thoracic Society Clinical Practice Guideline: exercise-induced bronchoconstriction. *Am J Respir Crit Care Med.* 2013;187:1013–1027.

Level of Evidence:
I

Summary:
Expert position statement on exercise-induced bronchoconstriction

Citation:
Parsons JP, Mastronarde JG. Exercise-induced bronchoconstriction in athletes. *Chest.* 2005;128:3966–3974.

Level of Evidence:
I

Summary:
Systematic review of EIB in athletes

14

Deep Venous Thrombosis and Pulmonary Embolism

Jason Thompson, Marc M. DeHart

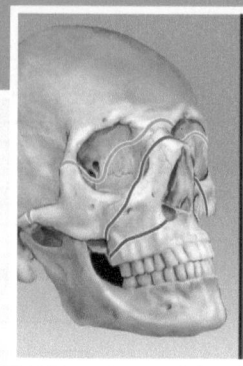

Bleeding in the athlete can result from injury or after orthopedic surgery. Hemostasis—the body's process to stop bleeding—prevents what can be a life-threatening hemorrhage. Immobilization and hypercoagulable states can also induce clotting at improper sites (thrombosis). If the resultant clot dislodges and migrates (thromboembolism), it can lead to devastating tissue damage and organ failure. The most feared complication of that cascade is a fatal pulmonary embolism (PE). Although rare, it can occur after minor orthopedic surgeries, including arthroscopic procedures. The majority of clots cause few symptoms and are not recognized clinically. A reduction in peak aerobic performance may be the only hint of a clot in the elite athlete.[1] Chemical thromboembolic prophylaxis with anticoagulation therapy helps reduce the risk of thromboembolic events in the postoperative patient, but the use of these medications comes with significant risks of its own, as well as an added expense. Controversy surrounds the balance between the morbidity and mortality associated with thromboembolic events and the risks and costs of chemical prophylaxis.

NORMAL PHYSIOLOGY AND VIRCHOW TRIAD

Hemostasis and thrombosis are physiologic mechanisms of the coagulation system, platelets, endothelial cells, and the vascular wall. Following an injury, hemostasis is our body's ability to form a blood clot and is usually followed by the dissolution of that clot as injured tissues repairs. Thrombosis can be considered "hemostasis in the wrong place and the wrong time."[2] When a clot emerges in the arterial system, the subsequent loss of oxygenated blood can lead to stroke, myocardial infarction, and peripheral extremity necrosis. Clot formation within the venous system leads to local tissue congestion and decreased venous return, most often in the lower extremities. When the final destination of an embolus within the venous system is the lungs (PE), complications related to pulmonary infarction, abnormal gas exchange, and cardiovascular compromise may result.

In honor of Rudolph Virchow, who is responsible for coining the term *embolus*, "Virchow triad" describes the three primary influences on thrombus formation. *Endothelial damage* exposes collagen and triggers the extrinsic clotting cascade by activating platelets to perform their three primary functions—adhesion (sticking to damage endothelium), secretion (releasing thrombotic chemicals), and aggregation (combining platelets into a group). (Fig. 14.1). *Stasis* permits the bonds of protein clotting factors

and platelets to assemble and results from immobility (from postoperative/postinjury pain, cast, limb paralysis, stroke), increased blood viscosity (from cancer, estrogens, polycythemia), decreased inflow (from intraoperative tourniquets, vascular disease),[3] and increased venous pressure (from venous scarring, varicose veins, heart failure).[4] *Hypercoagulability* is the result of activation of the catalytic system of plasma proteins known as the coagulation cascade, whose main product—thrombin—converts soluble fibrinogen to insoluble fibrin. The biologic goal of this network of interdependent enzyme-mediated reactions is to limit hemorrhage at sites where damage occurs by rapidly stabilizing the initial platelet plug with insoluble fibrin.

Once formed, a thrombus has the ability to (a) undergo *dissolution* by the fibrinolytic system, (b) remain stationary with subsequent incorporation into the vein wall *(organization and recanalization)*, (c) continue to grow *(propagation)*, and/or completely or incompletely break free to travel downstream to imbed in the pulmonary vessels *(embolization)*.[4] Ninety percent of thrombi form in lower extremity veins, where those that form distal to the popliteal space occur in smaller veins of the calf and pose essentially no clinical threat because these typically dissolve spontaneously. However, a thrombus formed in the larger-diameter veins within the pelvis and proximal thigh are associated with increased risk of embolism.

PREOPERATIVE THROMBOEMBOLIC RISK FACTORS

Thrombophilia is the predisposition to venous thromboembolism disease (VTE) and is caused by inherited (primary) and acquired (secondary) factors. Primary hypercoagulability is often a result of genetic mutations, which may lead to an abnormal quantity or quality of protein clotting factors. Screening for prothrombotic defects has not been shown to be effective in selecting a strategy for thromboembolic prophylaxis.[5] The quality and quantity of the protein clotting factors can be a consequence of either malproduction or autoimmune alteration or destruction of these important factors. Clinical factors of secondary hypercoagulability are commonly found in orthopedic patients and play a significant role in the perioperative management of thrombosis. These classic, sometimes modifiable, preoperative risk factors for VTE include, but are not limited to, previous VTE, malignancy, pregnancy, age older than 40 years, obesity, smoking, peripheral vascular disease, and oral contraceptive (and/or estrogen) use.

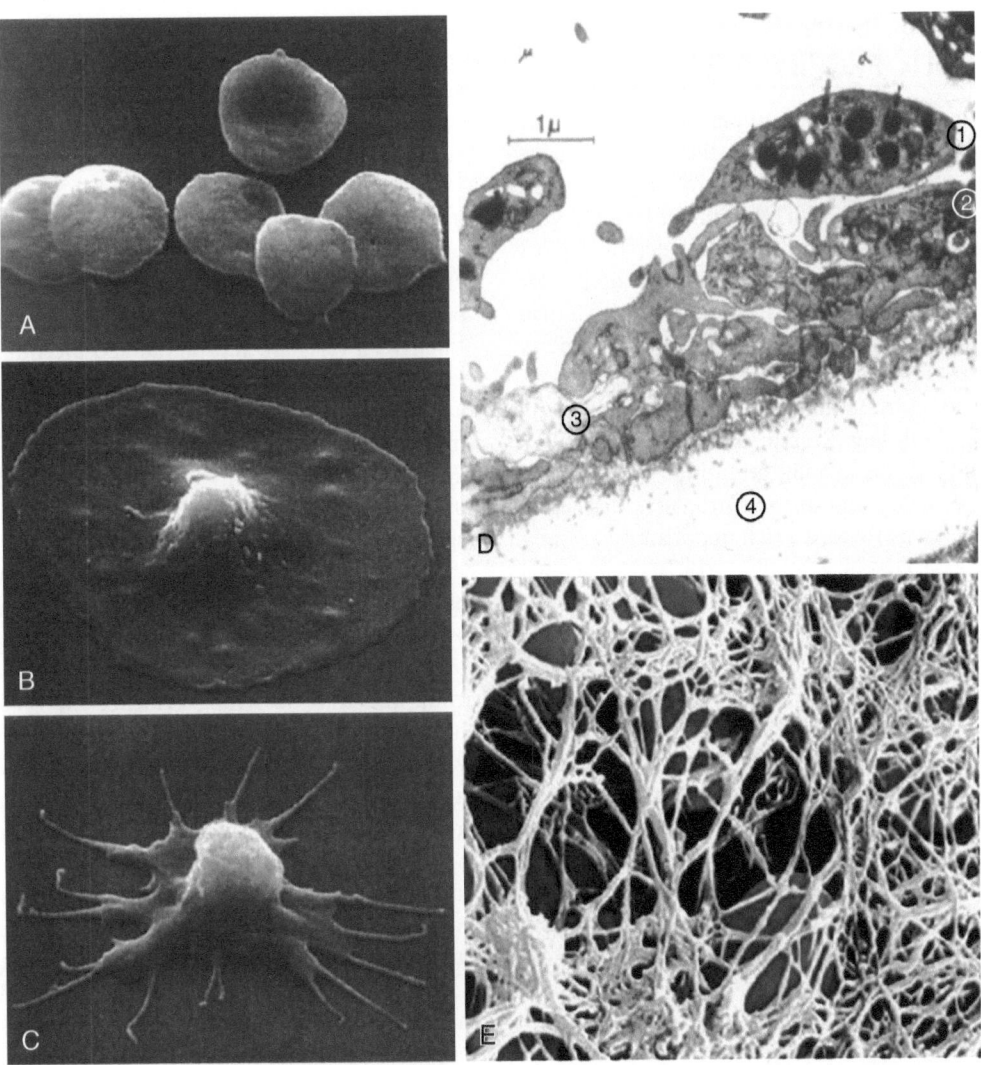

Fig. 14.1 (A) Scanning electron micrograph (SEM) of free platelets. (B) SEM of platelet adhesion. (C) SEM of platelet activation. (D) Transmission electron micrograph (TEM) of aggregating platelets. *1*, Platelet before secretion. *2* and *3*, Platelets secreting contents of granules. *4*, Collagen of endothelium. (E) SEM of fibrin mesh encasing colorized red blood cells. (Platelet EM courtesy James G. White, MD, Regents' Professor, Department of Laboratory Medicine and Pathology, University of Minnesota School of Medicine.)

Studies have found an association of high-altitude locations with a two to nine times greater rate of VTE in both young health populations and in autopsy records.[6-8] At high altitude, hypoxia, dehydration, hemoconcentration, low temperature, and use of constrictive clothing, as well as enforced stasis due to severe weather, would support the occurrence of thrombotic disorders.[9] Ascending from a low elevation to an elevated altitude (4000 feet above sea level) initially causes an acute hypoxic ventilation period, followed by a respiratory system response where the lungs increase ventilation (minutes to hours). Higher altitudes stimulate renal and hepatic erythropoietin production that then stimulates erythropoiesis with an increase in size and concentration of red cells. This erythropoietin process is most active 2 days after introduction to the elevation but usually returns to sea level measurements after approximately 3 weeks at higher elevation. Physiologic changes occur to acclimatize over the course of several years with sustained hyperventilation while at higher elevation. Changes occur to the oxygen-hemoglobin dissociation curve, pulmonary circulation, cardiac function, fluid hemostasis, and hematologic components.[10] The relative risk of VTE after knee arthroscopy in residents of areas 4000 feet above sea level is as high as 3.8 times that of similar patients residing in and having their operations in areas at sea level (but the risk is still very low, <.5%).[10]

Larger and longer operations on more proximal joints of the lower extremity have higher risks of clinically significant VTE. Careful individualized risk stratification may help identify patients at highest risk for VTE. Patients who have a history of VTEs and/or malignancy, or two or more of the classic risk factors, are at an increased risk of postoperative thromboembolic disease and may be considered for chemoprophylaxis for arthroscopy and distal procedures.[11]

PERIOPERATIVE DECISION OF THROMBOEMBOLIC PROPHYLAXIS

The necessity of prophylaxis is based on balancing the risks of developing venous thrombosis and PE against the cost and dangers of prophylaxis. Operative factors under control of the surgeon can alter the risk of developing a VTE by influencing the size, location, and frequency of thrombosis. These perioperative factors include duration of operative and tourniquet time, complexity of the surgery, extremity paralysis, and length of postoperative extremity immobilization. Sports medicine generally involves less invasive procedures on younger and healthier patients who are often motivated to return to function at an accelerated pace. Despite a population with low thromboembolic risk, fatal PEs can occur and command considerable attention.[12]

The large volume of hip and knee arthroplasty that share elevated risks of VTE have provided a rich opportunity to study thromboembolic disease. Despite averaging a risk of deep venous thrombosis (DVT) of approximately 40% to 50%, the incidence of symptomatic/fatal PE is so low it is impractical to measure, and no study has had sufficient power to demonstrate a significant decrease. To provide statistically significant results, studies measure distal and proximal DVTs ("total DVT") as efficacy end points for prophylaxis. Total DVT is a high-frequency surrogate outcome that is practical to objectively measure but may not be clinically relevant. Experts question whether adequate data are available to say whether DVTs cause all PEs.[13,14] The majority (79%) of studies on thromboprophylaxis after total joint arthroplasty were sponsored by industry, and evidence of potential bias exists.[15] However, these studies include some of the highest level of evidence available in orthopedic surgery and are used by panels that create clinical practice guidelines and review comparative effectiveness. Most studies are powered to show efficacy in reducing total DVT. It takes a much smaller study group to statistically demonstrate a decrease in a high-frequency *but less clinically relevant* event such as total DVT (risks ~40%) than to detect an increase of a clinically relevant, low-frequency event such as bleeding (risks ~1% to 5%).[13,16] Large prospective randomized trials frequently exclude patients who have increased bleeding risks, yet these patients suffer equally from arthritis and are often candidates for arthroplasty. Bleeding is a predictable complication of surgery and the most common complication of the use of anticoagulants. Higher rates of bleeding are seen when more effective prophylactic drugs are used and when drugs with more rapid onset of action are used closer to the time of surgery.[17] Potent anticoagulation is not associated with a reduced rate of PE[18] or mortality rate, nor is it associated with a reduction in the proportion of deaths related to PE.[19] Observational studies show higher infection rates (odds ratio [OR] 1.5) with strict compliance with the use of strong chemoprophylaxis.[20] Modern arthroplasty literature finds wound-related complications, bleeding, hematoma formation, persistent wound drainage, and periprosthetic joint infection are reduced with the use of aspirin when compared with more powerful anticoagulants.[14]

Clinical practice guidelines, comparative effectiveness research, and consensus opinions can serve as a convenient starting point for surgeons and hospitals to make daily care decisions based on current evidence. The orthopedic community has resisted a single standard regimen in favor of individualized judgments based on patient's clinical information. Understanding the recommendation guidelines creates opportunities for improved patient care (Table 14.1 Guidelines). Mechanical methods of prophylaxis have low bleeding risks and include aggressive range of motion, early weight-bearing activity, and the use of venous foot pumps and intermittent pneumatic compression hose.[21] Use of mechanical devices is encouraged in patients at high risk for bleeding and as adjuncts with other prophylactic techniques. When VTE risks are substantial and bleeding risks allow, chemoprophylaxis is supported for patients undergoing major orthopedic surgeries, including operative fixation of pelvic fractures, hip fractures, polytrauma, and joint replacement of the hip and knee. Common VTE prophylactic and treatment medications are listed in Table 14.2 with their mechanisms of action (see Table 14.2 Prophylaxis Drugs).

The vast majority of sports medicine procedures have minimal thromboembolic risk (Table 14.3 DVT Incidence). Literature reviews on routine VTE prophylaxis with stronger anticoagulants suggest adverse events are more common in the intervention group and find no strong evidence for DVT prophylaxis for routine patients undergoing arthroscopy.[22] Because the rates of symptomatic DVT and PE are so low following arthroscopic cases,[17,23] guidelines recommend against routine use of chemoprophylaxis with the exception of using mechanical prophylaxis in the form of early mobilization. Despite the frequent need for immobilization and/or casting, smaller procedures such as distal fractures, tendon ruptures, and foot and ankle surgeries do not raise concern for an increased risk of VTE in the average patient. A large study that examined clinically symptomatic VTE in more than 45,000 patients undergoing foot and ankle surgery found the rate of VTE was 1%.[24] In one of the rare adequately powered multicentered randomized controlled studies of symptomatic thromboembolic disease in patients undergoing knee arthroscopy and a similar study in patients using casts concluded prophylaxis for these patients was not effective.[25] For sports patients with multiple risk factors undergoing long or complicated procedures, chemoprophylaxis may be effective and can be used when bleeding risks allow.

DIAGNOSIS AND CLINICAL MANIFESTATIONS: IMAGING AND LABORATORY FINDINGS

Diagnosis of venous thrombosis relies on a patient's history because there is no single physical exam finding that is diagnostic. Although VTE can cause leg pain, tenderness, swelling, or a palpable cord, most are asymptomatic. Homans sign (calf pain with foot dorsiflexion when the knee is flexed) and Moses' sign (pain with calf compression against the tibia) are known as the "classic" physical exam tests for a DVT. However, venographic evidence of concurrent DVT is found in fewer than 50% of patients who are positive for these classic signs of DVT (Fig. 14.2, *upper panel*).[26] Even with venographic evidence of VTE, only 50% of those patients will display the classical clinic signs.[27] Most orthopedic patients with a PE are asymptomatic. When emboli create large occlusions of the pulmonary vasculature, it

---

TABLE 14.1   Guidelines on Prevention of Venous Thromboembolism Disease in Hip and Knee Arthroplasty

AAOS Guideline and Grade of Recommendation: !Strong, +Moderate, ~Weak, *Consensus, ?Inconclusive		Notes From Other Guidelines: [1]ACCP, [2]NICE, [3]AHRQ
!	No "screening" duplex US	
+	Hx normal risks of VTE and bleeding use drugs *and/or* IPC	
+	D/C platelet inhibitors preop (aspirin, clopidogrel, prasugrel)	Discuss with medical team, stop 1 week prior[2]
+	Neuraxial anesthesia to decrease bleeding (No effect on VTE)	Caution with drugs and neuraxial[1]
		Wait 12 h after drugs[2]
~	Ask history of previous VTE	
*	Hx of VTE get IPC *and* Drugs	DRUGS: LMWH, fondaparinux, dabigatran, rivaroxaban, VKA, aspirin[1]
*	Ask history of bleeding disorder (hemophilia) and active liver disease	
*	Hx of bleeding disorder (hemophilia or active liver disease) *only* IPC	If bleeding risk: IPC or nothing[1] If bleeding risk > clotting risk: IPC[2]
*	Discuss duration with patient	≥10 days, consider 35 days[1]
*	Early mobilization	
?	Assess other clotting risk factors	
?	Assess other bleeding risk factors	
?	No one technique optimal	Drugs and IPC[1,2] D/C drugs when TKA mobile[2]
?	IVC filter	If VTE risks high and contraindication to prophylaxis[2]

Guideline Title	**Source**
2011 AAOS Preventing Venous Thromboembolic Disease	http://www.aaos.org/research/guidelines
2012 ACCP Prevention of VTE in Orthopedic Surgery Patient	http://journal.publications.chestnet.org/
2012 AHRQ VTE Prophylaxis in Orthopedic Surgery, CER 49	http://effectivehealthcare.ahrq.gov/
2010 NICE Reducing the Risk of VTE in patients admitted to hospital	http://guidance.nice.org.uk/CG92/

D/C, Discontinue; *IPC* intermittent pneumatic compression; *IVC,* intra-vena caval; *US,* ultrasound; *VKA,* vitamin K antagonist; *VTE,* venous thromboembolism.
AAOS. Guideline on Preventing Venous Thromboembolic Disease in Patients Undergoing Elective Hip and Knee Arthroplasty. *AAOS Clinical Practice Guidelines (CPG)*; 2011. http://www.aaos.org/research/guidelines/VTE/VTE_guideline.asp/. Accessed June, 20, 2012.
AHRQ. Comparative Effectiveness Review, Number 49: Venous Thromboembolism Prophylaxis in Orthopedic Surgery; 2012. http://effectivehealthcare.ahrq.gov/ehc/products/186/992/CER-49_VTE_20120313.pdf/. Accessed July 20, 2012.
NICE. CG92 Venous thromboembolism—reducing the risk: NICE guideline; 2010. http://guidance.nice.org.uk/CG92/NICEGuidance/pdf/English/.

can lead to right heart failure and hypoxemia. Healthy individuals may remain asymptomatic if an occlusion obstructs less than 60% of the pulmonary circulation.[28] The most common presenting symptoms in patients diagnosed with PE on pulmonary angiogram are chest pain (typically pleuritic) and sudden onset of shortness of breath (dyspnea). Objective physical exam findings seen in greater than 50% of patients are tachypnea (>20 breaths/min) and crackles with lung auscultation.[28] Massive *saddle emboli* block all cardiopulmonary circulation and can cause immediate death.

The nonspecific nature of the signs and symptoms of VTE can be confused for other diagnoses or even easily dismissed, and therefore these complaints demand a high clinical suspicion in patients particularly at high risk. There is no ideal objective test for VTE, but contrast venography, duplex compression ultrasound, spiral computed tomography (CT) venography, CT pulmonary angiography, ventilation-perfusion (V/Q) scintigraphy, and D-dimer levels, usually used in combination, can be useful. Duplex ultrasound is the most practical diagnostic tool for lower extremity DVTs because it is inexpensive, noninvasive, and easily administered at the patient's bedside. Assessing blood flow and compressibility of the vein with real-time B-mode Doppler

ultrasound is more than 95% sensitive and specific for detecting proximal DVTs.[26] When a DVT is suspected, an urgent outpatient screening is indicated where duplex ultrasound serves as the best first line test in a stable patient (see Fig. 14.2, *lower panel*).[29] All guidelines agree that routine screening with duplex ultrasound at discharge from hospital is not cost effective and is not recommended.[16,30] If nearby wounds, burns, or the presence of a cast or when DVT of the pelvis or inferior vena cava vessels are suspected, CT and magnetic resonance venography have shown good sensitivity and specificity.[31]

A postoperative patient who presents with chest pain, dyspnea, or cardiovascular collapse raises the clinical suspicion of PE; the diagnostic workup, provided that the patient is stable, should include a chest radiograph, electrocardiogram (ECG), and determination of an arterial blood gas (ABG) value. The plain film of the chest will often have subtle and nonspecific findings, whereas the ECG findings in patients with a PE potentially show sinus tachycardia, T-wave inversion, and ST abnormalities; however, these are not diagnostic alone. The tachypnea of a PE causes hyperventilation, which is represented by hypocapnia (low serum carbon dioxide level) in the ABG.[32] D-dimer levels are often not helpful in the orthopedic setting because the trauma from

TABLE 14.2   Common Drugs for Venous Thromboembolism Disease Prophylaxis/Treatment

COMMON DRUGS FOR THROMBOEMBOLIC PROPHYLAXIS/TREATMENT

Drug	Mechanism of Action	Complications	Notes	Reversal
Aspirin[a]	Irreversibly blocks platelet COX-1 production of TXA_2	Bleeding & GI issues Rare allergies	Least effective chemical agent	None
Heparin[b]	Binds AT to inactivate Xa & II (thrombin) and IXa, XIa, XIIa	Bleeding HIT and osteoporosis	Must monitor: aPTT or anti-Xa activity	Protamine: 1 mg IV per 100 U UFH
LMWH[b]	Bind AT to inactivate Xa, & IIa (thrombin)	Bleeding Rare HIT	Monitor anti-Xa activity if: BMI >50 or CrCl <30	Protamine: 1 mg IV per 1 mg LMWH
Fondaparinux[c]	Binds AT to selectively inactivate only Xa	Bleeding	Avoid in: thin <50 kg, elderly >75, CRI: CrCl <30	No antidote
VKA[d] Coumadin	Blocks γ-carboxylation of: factors II, VII, IX, X	Bleeding Skin necrosis Fetal Warfarin syndrome	Oral good for long term therapy Multiple reactions: diet, drugs, disease	Vitamin K1 (phytonadione): FFP 8–10 mL/kg
Dabagitran[d]	Direct thrombin inhibitor	Bleeding	Oral	Idarucizumab (monoclonal Ab)[e]: 5 g IV
Rivaroxaban[d]	Direct factor Xa inhibitor	Bleeding	Oral Avoid if on antifungals or HIV	No antidote (Andexanet alfa in trials)[e]
Apixaban	Direct factor Xa inhibitor	Bleeding	Oral	No antidote (PER977 in trials)[5]
Edoxaban	Direct factor Xa inhibitor	Bleeding	Oral	No antidote (PER977 in trials)[e]

Original data from:

[a]Patrono C, Coller B, FitzGerald GA, et al. Platelet-active drugs: the relationships among dose, effectiveness, and side effects: the Seventh ACCP Conference on Antithrombotic and Thrombolytic Therapy. *Chest.* 2004;126(3_suppl):234S–264S.

[b]Hirsh J, Raschke R. Heparin and low-molecular-weight heparin: the Seventh ACCP Conference on Antithrombotic and Thrombolytic Therapy. *Chest.* 2004;126(3_suppl):188S–203S.

[c]Weitz JI, Hirsh J, Samama MM. New anticoagulant drugs: the Seventh ACCP Conference on Antithrombotic and Thrombolytic Therapy. *Chest.* 2004;126(3_suppl):265S–286S.

[d]Ageno W, Gallus AS, Wittkowsky A, et al. Oral anticoagulant therapy: Antithrombotic therapy and prevention of thrombosis, 9th ed: American College of Chest Physicians Evidence-Based Clinical Practice Guidelines. *CHEST.* 2012;141(2_suppl):e44S–e88S.

[e]Leitch J, van Vlymen J. Managing the perioperative patient on direct oral anticoagulants. *Can J Anaesth.* 2017;64(6):656–672.

fracture and surgery can cause prolonged elevations with or without thromboembolic disease. A negative D-dimer excludes DVT or PE in patients with low probability of thromboembolic disease.[33] The first-line test to confirm a diagnosis of an acute PE is a multidetector spiral (helical) CT pulmonary angiography, where PE causes an intravascular filling defect in a pulmonary artery that occludes all or part of the vessel (Fig. 14.3A). The helical CT's excellent sensitivities and specificities of greater than 95% have raised concerns about overdiagnosing clinically unimportant PEs. The growing use of spiral CT has been linked to an increase in both the diagnosis of PEs and bleeding complications but has not been associated with a decrease in overall mortality rate from PE.[34,35] Most recent guidelines recommend withholding anticoagulation for smaller subsegmental pulmonary embolisms (SSPE) with low risk for recurrent VTE.[36] Ventilation-perfusion scintigraphy scans (V/Q scans) lack the sensitivity and specificity of the spiral CT and are now a second line study. A negative, or low, probability excludes significant PE, but V/Q scans are best reserved for patients with contraindications to radiographic dye.[37]

THROMBOEMBOLIC DISEASE TREATMENT

Prompt treatment prevents progression of thrombosis and minimizes mortality from embolic disease. Hematologists and internal medicine specialists are often the most expert in the management

of VTE; however, knowledge of current guidelines can be helpful to provide reassurance to patients and to expedite care when needed (Table 14.4). Patients who sustain their first DVT provoked by surgery are treated with 3 months of anticoagulation therapy with novel oral anticoagulants (NOACs; examples: factor Xa inhibitors or direct thrombin inhibitors), vitamin K antagonists (VKA = warfarin), or low-molecular-weight heparin.[38] Early mobilization after the diagnosis of DVT is encouraged without fear of dislodging the thrombus and creating an embolism. Studies using VQ scans have demonstrated no decrease in PE when bed rest was used after DVT diagnosis. Pain and swelling resolves more quickly when early ambulation is encouraged.[39–41] Graded compression stockings (GCSs) may help with symptoms of leg swelling, but they do not relieve symptoms of pain better than placebo[42] and do not prevent postthrombotic syndrome after a first DVT.[43] Early discharge and home management is possible and is a cost-effective approach for many DVTs and PEs.[39,44] Intravenous vena cava filter use is generally discouraged but may play a role when there is a contraindication to or complication of anticoagulation therapy.[38,39] Finally, after experiencing a second separate episode of VTE, a patient may benefit from receiving anticoagulation for an indefinite period.

Isolated venous thrombosis of the calf veins is not an uncommon issue in orthopedic patients. As ultrasonographers develop better tools and skills, this far distal pathology of the smallest

TABLE 14.3 Rates of Symptomatic Thromboembolism in Sports Medicine

RATES OF SYMPTOMATIC THROMBOEMBOLISM		
Procedure	sDVT (%)	PE (%)
All hospital admission[a]	.048–.07	.023–.03
Major ortho: THA, TKA, HFS		
In 2 weeks no prophylaxis[b]	1.8	1
In 35 days no prophylaxis[b]	2.8	1.5
In hospital with prophylaxis[c]	.26–.8	.14–.35
In 35 days with prophylaxis[b]	.45	.20
Knee arthroscopy[d]	.25–9.9	.028–.17
ACL reconstruction[e]	.3	.8
Hip arthroscopy[f]	0–3.7	0
Shoulder arthroscopy[g]	.01–.26	.01–.21
Shoulder fracture[h]	0	.2
Shoulder arthroplasty[g]	.19–.2	.1–.4
Elbow arthroplasty[i]		.25
Foot and ankle surgery[j]	0–.22	.02–.15
Ankle fracture[k]	.05–2.5	.17–.47
Ankle arthroscopy[f]	0	0

Original data from:

[a]White RH. The epidemiology of venous thromboembolism. *Circulation.* 2003;107(90231):I-4-8.

[b]Falck-Ytter Y, Francis CW, Johanson NA, et al. Prevention of VTE in orthopedic surgery patients: Antithrombotic therapy and prevention of thrombosis, 9th ed: American College of Chest Physicians Evidence-Based Clinical Practice Guidelines. *Chest.* 2012;141(2_suppl):e278S–e325S.

[c]Januel J, Chen G, Ruffieux C, et al. Symptomatic in-hospital deep vein thrombosis and pulmonary embolism following hip and knee arthroplasty among patients receiving recommended prophylaxis: a systematic review. *JAMA.* 2012;307(3):294–303.

[d]Hetsroni I, Lyman S, Do H, et al. Symptomatic pulmonary embolism after outpatient arthroscopic procedures of the knee: the incidence and risk factors in 418,323 arthroscopies. *J Bone Joint Surg Br.* 2011;93(1):47–51.

[e]Jameson SS, Dowen D, James P, et al. Complications following anterior cruciate ligament reconstruction in the English NHS. *Knee.* 2012;19(1):14–19.

[f]Bushnell BD, Anz AW, Bert JM. Venous thromboembolism in lower extremity arthroscopy. *Arthroscopy.* 2008;24(5):604–611.

[g]Ojike NI, Bhadra AK, Giannoudis PV, et al. Venous thromboembolism in shoulder surgery: a systematic review. *Acta Orthop Belg.* 2011;77(3):281–289.

[h]Jameson SS, James P, Howcroft DW, et al. Venous thromboembolic events are rare after shoulder surgery: analysis of a national database. *J Shoulder Elbow Surg.* 2011;20(5):764–770.

[i]Duncan SF, Sperling JW, Morrey BF. Prevalence of pulmonary embolism after total elbow arthroplasty. *J Bone Joint Surg Am.* 2007;89(7):1452–1453.

[j]Jameson SS, Augustine A, James P, et al. Venous thromboembolic events following foot and ankle surgery in the English National Health Service. *J Bone Joint Surg Br.* 2011;93(4):490–497.

[k]SooHoo NF, Eagan M, Krenek L, et al. Incidence and factors predicting pulmonary embolism and deep venous thrombosis following surgical treatment of ankle fractures. *Foot Ankle Surg.* 2011;17(4):259–262.

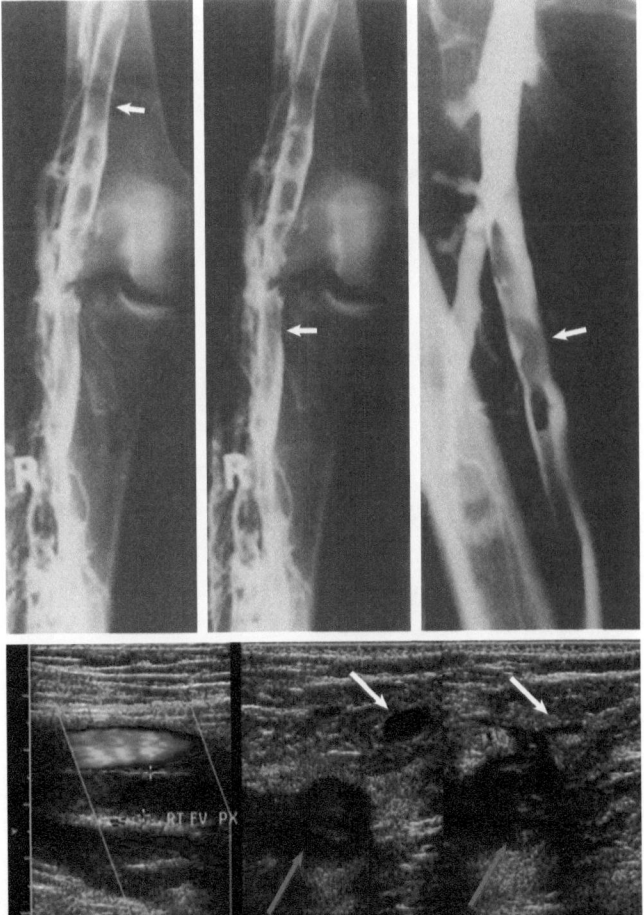

Fig. 14.2 *Upper panel,* The "gold standard" diagnosis for deep vein thrombosis: Intraluminal filling defects seen on two or more views of venogram. Left two images at the knee; right image at the hip. *Lower panel,* A color duplex ultrasound of femoral vessels with a venous clot in the deeper vessel. (B) demonstrates cross section ultrasound without compression and (C) demonstrates the same view with compression. *Red arrows* demonstrate deep vein with venous clot that fails to collapse with compression. *White arrows* demonstrate the normal more superficial vein collapses (no clot). (*Upper panel,* From Jackson JE, Hemingway AP. Principles, techniques and complications of angiography. In: Grainger RG, ed. *Grainger & Allison's Diagnostic Radiology: A Textbook of Medical Imaging.* 4th ed. Philadelphia: Churchill Livingstone, 2011. *Lower panel,* Original images courtesy Austin Radiological Association and Seton Family of Hospitals.)

leg veins is more easily diagnosed. Experts suggest that this can be managed with surveillance with repeat duplex ultrasound at 2 weeks to look for progression of the clot. Treatment may be warranted if the patient has severe symptoms, if the clot is large (>5 cm, involves multiple veins, or is >7 mm in diameter), or if the patient is considered high risk (unprovoked, history of prior VTE or cancer).[38]

SPORTS ISSUES, RETURN TO PLAY, AND TRAVEL

Spontaneous DVTs and PEs in athletes with and without thrombophilia can occur.[45–50] Comparison studies show a risk reduction

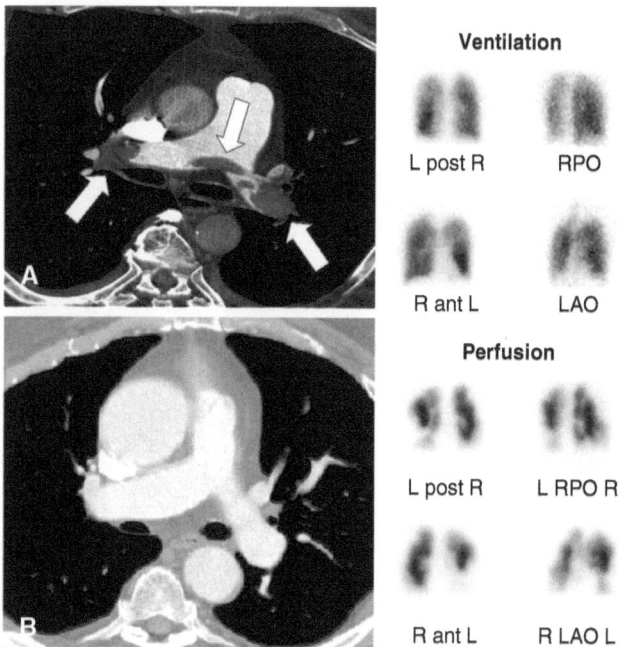

Ventilation

L post R   RPO

R ant L   LAO

Perfusion

L post R   L RPO R

R ant L   R LAO L

Fig. 14.3 *Left image,* Helical computed tomography pulmonary angiography. (A) Patient with symptoms of syncope and hypoxia. Large clots *(arrows)* are present at the bifurcation of the main pulmonary artery and extend into the left and right pulmonary arteries. (B) Normal scan in a different patient at same level. *Right image,* High-probability pulmonary V/Q scan: Ventilation scan above demonstrates full lung fields. Perfusion scan below shows multiple areas lacking tracer. (Original image courtesy Austin Radiological Association and Seton Family of Hospitals.)

in thromboembolic disease with activity[51] and sports participation.[52] Although DVTs usually affect athletes in the lower extremity, those who present with upper extremity pain, swelling, feeling of heaviness or dilated upper arm veins, the diagnosis of axillary-subclavian vein thrombosis or "effort thrombosis" (Paget-Schroetter syndrome) should be entertained.[53] Sports that involve shoulder abduction and extension (wrestling, gymnastics, weightlifting, throwing, and swimming) may have increased incidence in patients with anatomic abnormality of their thoracic outlet (cervical rib, congenital bands, hypertrophy of scalenus tendons, and/or abnormal insertion of the costoclavicular ligament). Upper extremity duplex ultrasound may help diagnosis, and thoracic outlet decompression may optimize their care.[54,55]

Athletes with DVT should be encouraged to start a gradual return to their usual daily activities when they begin anticoagulation therapy. A formal return-to-training program with progressively increasing intensity can be undertaken shortly thereafter, if the athlete is closely monitored for recurrence of VTE. Traditionally, athletes have been prohibited from contact or collision sports until anticoagulation therapy has been completed; however, the NOACs may allow protocols that allow earlier participation.[56,57]

Athletes involved in international competition may be at increased risk for "traveler's thrombosis" (also known as "economy-class syndrome" or "rail coach syndrome"[58]) when facing travel durations longer than 4 hours.[59] Young elite athletes who are at their peak physical condition are unlikely to experience significant health compromise; however, subclinical

thromboembolic disease could potentially jeopardize performance.[1,60] Multiple studies have made an association between taller individuals and increased risk of a first or recurrent venous thromboembolism.[61–64] Injuries during competition and their treatment may put athletes at increased risk on their return journey. Prolonged air travel before surgery may also increase the risk of perioperative VTE.[65–67] The risk of VTE is related to a person's risk factors and the duration of the flight. The cause of the increased risk is likely related to a decrease in vascular flow of immobility; however, dehydration, decreased cabin pressure, and relative hypoxia may also play a role. The absolute risk of fatal PE is very low (2.57 per 1 million flights that last longer than 8 hours),[68] but air travel lasting longer than 8 hours carries eight times the risk of fatal PE in nontravelers.[69,70] Most patients who experience travel-related thrombosis have one or more other risk factors. Potential ways to help reduce the risk of VTE are by avoiding constrictive clothing, staying adequately hydrated, performing calf-stretching exercises, and taking frequent walks in the cabin.

For a complete list of references, go to ExpertConsult.com.

SELECTED READINGS

Citation:

van Adrichem RA, Nemeth B, Algra A, et al. Thromboprophylaxis after knee arthroscopy and lower-leg casting. *N Engl J Med.* 2017;376(6):515–525.

Level of Evidence:

II

Summary:

A randomized controlled trial of patients important to sports medicine doctors looking at clinically relevant thromboembolic disease in both knee arthroscopy and cast immobilized patients. After studying more than 3000 patients, the conclusion is that chemical prophylaxis was not effective in preventing symptomatic VTE.

Citation:

Kahn SR, et al. Compression stockings to prevent post-thrombotic syndrome: a randomised placebo-controlled trial. *Lancet.* 2014;383(9920):880–888.

Level of Evidence:

II

Summary:.

A multicenter randomized placebo-controlled trial of active versus placebo elastic compression stockings used for 2 years to prevent postthrombotic syndrome (PTS) after a first proximal DVT. Elastic compression hose did not prevent PTS after DVT, and their routine use was not supported.

Citation:

Falck-Ytter Y, et al. Prevention of VTE in orthopedic surgery patients: antithrombotic therapy and prevention of thrombosis, 9th ed: American College of Chest Physicians Evidence-Based Clinical Practice Guidelines. *Chest.* 2012;141(suppl 2): e278S–e325S.

Level of Evidence:

II

TABLE 14.4 Treatment of Acute Venous Thromboembolism Disease

Phases of anticoagulation

Initial	Long-term	Extended
(0 to ~7 days)	(~7 days to ~3 months)	(~3 months to indefinite)

Parenteral — Xa inhibitors, Dabagitan or Vit K

Drug		Dose	Duration	Monitoring
Parenteral	IV heparin+	80 U/kg IV bolus 18 U/kg/h IV	≥5 days	aPTT:1.8–2.5 × control or Anti-Xa activity: 0.3–0.7 U/mL
	SC heparin+	333 U/kg SC then 250 U/kg SC BID	≥5 days	aPTT: 1.5–2.5 × control QAM 6 h after am dose
	LMWH–	1 mg/kg BID SC 2 mg/kg QD SC	≥5 days	None—unless RI or pregnancy Anti-Xa activity: 0.6–1.0 l U/mL
	Fondaparinux–	7.5 mg SC QD 5 mg if <50 kg 10 mg if >100 kg	3 mos+	None
Oral	Rivaroxaban–#	10 mg PO QD		
	Apixaban	5 mg PO BID	3 mos+	None
	Edoxaban	60 mg PO QD		
	Dabigatran	150 mg PO QD	3 mos+	None (aPTT/thrombin clotting time)
	VKA	5–10 mg PO QD Adjust dose	3 mos+	INR: 2–3 QAM

+ preferred for patients with severe renal impairment
– avoid in patients with marked renal impairment (<30 mL/min)
avoid in patients on azole (antifungals) and HIV protease inhibitors

Special Notes:
Bed rest: Not recommended, early mobilization for both DVT patients
Distal DVT: Repeat US in 2 weeks, only Rx if severe symptoms or ↑ risk: ≥5 cm long, ≥7 mm diameter, cancer, Hx of VTE, inpatient
Home DVT Rx: If home circumstances adequate (+phone, family or friends, near hospital)
Early PE D/C: If home circumstances adequate (+phone, family or friends, near hospital)
Subsegmental PE: If proximal LE veins duplex negative, clinical surveillance ok
GCS: Graded compression stockings *NOT* recommended for preventing VTE or postthrombotic syndrome
IVC filters: Only if contraindication to anticoagulation (May resume anticoagulation if bleeding risks resolve)
Superficial VT: If severe symptoms, then 45 days of prophylactic anticoagulation, if not serial duplex looking for extension
Upper extremity: Axillary or more proximal veins get anticoagulation (not GCS)
Controversial: In the postoperative arthroplasty situation, consider thrombectomy and embolectomy before thrombolytics

Duration of treatment: 3 mos use same drug.
DVT, Deep vein thrombosis; *GCS,* Graded compression stocking; *IVC,* intravena caval; *VKA,* vitamin K antagonists; *VTE,* venous thromboembolism disease.
Graphic modified from and original data from Kearon C, Akl EA, Comerota AJ, et al. Antithrombotic therapy for VTE disease: Antithrombotic therapy and prevention of thrombosis, 9th ed: American College of Chest Physicians Evidence-Based Clinical Practice Guidelines. *Chest.* 2012;141(2_suppl):e419S–e494S; Holbrook A, Schulman S, Witt DM, et al. Evidence-based management of anticoagulant therapy: Antithrombotic therapy and prevention of thrombosis, 9th ed: American College of Chest Physicians Evidence-Based Clinical Practice Guidelines. *Chest.* 2012;141(2_suppl):e152S–e184S; and Garcia DA, Baglin TP, Weitz JI, et al. Parenteral anticoagulants: Antithrombotic therapy and prevention of thrombosis, 9th ed: American College of Chest Physicians Evidence-Based Clinical Practice Guidelines. *Chest.* 2012;141(2_suppl):e24S–e43S.

Summary:

Chest physician's guidelines summarize a multispecialty consensus of the literature that is updated. This comprehensive guideline covers many topics rarely addressed in orthopedic literature. Optimal strategies for thromboprophylaxis after major orthopedic surgery include pharmacologic and mechanical approaches.

Citation:

Jacobs JJ, Mont MA, Bozic KJ, et al. Prevent venous thromboembolic disease in patients undergoing elective hip and knee arthroplasty: evidence-based guideline and evidence report; September 23, 2011. *AAOS Evidence-Based Clinical Practice Guidelines.*1-861. http://www.aaos.org/Research/guidelines/VTE/VTE_full _guideline.pdf.

Level of Evidence:

III

Summary:

Generated by an AAOS physician Work Group and experts in systemic reviews, this AAOS clinical practice guideline is based on an assessment of the highest-level research available and makes recommendations summarized in the chapter. The full guideline available online shares the research details in depth.

Citation:

Grabowski G, Whiteside WK, Kanwisher M. Venous thrombosis in athletes. *J Am Acad Orthop Surg.* 2013;21(2):108–117.

Level of Evidence:

V

Summary:

This excellent review article in the JAAOS specifically summarizes the current literature on venous thrombosis in athletes and walks the orthopedic surgeon from the basic science level of DVT and completes the story by reviewing the prevention and management of DVTs.

Citation:

Tornetta P, Bogdan Y. Pulmonary embolism in orthopaedic patients: diagnosis and management. *J Am Acad Orthop Surg.* 2012;20(9):586–595.

Level of Evidence:

V

Summary:

Orthopedic surgeons will have a patient present with signs and symptoms concerning for a pulmonary embolism at some point during their careers. This review article does a great job scanning and summarizing the current scientific data and practices of diagnosing and managing those patients with a pulmonary embolism.

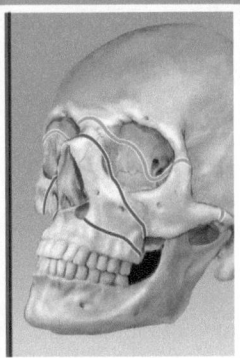

15

Gastrointestinal Medicine in the Athlete

John M. MacKnight

Gastrointestinal (GI) conditions in athletes and active individuals are common and are seen frequently by sports medicine care providers. Although there are many well-defined benefits that result from high-level physical activity, exercise places significant stress on the GI tract, which in turn may result in a number of characteristic GI disorders. Collectively, GI problems are perhaps the most common cause of underperformance in endurance sports and may also impact on subsequent recovery. The appreciation of this relationship is important for both care providers and athletes who must team together to minimize distressing GI symptoms and to prevent subsequent impairment in performance.

GI disorders in athletes often mimic those seen in the general population but may also present as unique entities seen primarily in those who exercise at a high level. This chapter will address a number of these common conditions, with a focus on their recognition and appropriate management in athletes.

PATHOPHYSIOLOGY

Frequent, high-intensity exercise may cause a number of undesirable GI symptoms, such as heartburn, chest pain, bloating, belching, nausea, vomiting, abdominal cramps, frequent urge to defecate, diarrhea, and GI bleeding. Historically, these symptoms have been reported by up to 50% of endurance athletes and are more common in women and younger athletes.[1] Body position and movement appear to play a role because the forward positioning of cyclists appears to protect them from GI tract issues as opposed to the higher-impact, jostling abdominal movements of runners.[2] Other suggested mechanisms for increased GI distress include a number of neuro-immuno-endocrine adaptations to exercise. Increased catecholamines and several GI peptides including gastrin, motilin, secretin, peptide histidine-methionine, and vasoactive intestinal peptide result in increased gut transit time with negative effects on digestion and absorption.[3–6]

Gastrointestinal Tract Ischemia

GI tract ischemia secondary to attenuated GI blood flow[4,7] is a well-defined exercise adaptation that results from the redirection of blood flow to active muscles and the pulmonary vasculature. Vigorous exertion, hyperthermia, dehydration, hypoglycemia, mental stress, and fatigue all increase sympathetic nervous system activity, which in turn shunts blood away from the GI viscera to provide increased blood and oxygen supply to working muscles. Exercising moderately at up to 70% of maximum oxygen uptake

($VO_{2\,max}$) reduces blood flow to the GI tract by 60% to 70%, and higher-intensity exercise may result in GI blood flow reductions exceeding 80%.[5] Subsequent impairment in oxygen delivery to GI tract structures may result in mucosal injury, increased gut mucosal permeability, increased risk for occult blood loss, translocation of protective bacterial flora, and generation of endotoxins.[4,8] These changes contribute to ischemia-associated GI symptoms, including nausea, vomiting, abdominal pain, and bloody diarrhea.[9] It has been postulated that GI complaints relating to gut ischemia are the result of a reperfusion injury after exercise has ceased. Reperfusion after ischemia may result in a number of chemical and vascular changes that result in "leaky mucosa." When this occurs, the GI tract partially loses its barrier ability to protect itself from inherently irritating intraluminal substances such as endotoxins, food antigens, digestive enzymes, and bile.[10]

Impact of Nutrition and Hydration

The overall fluid status of athletes has been shown to play an important role in the relative GI toxicity of high-level activity. Dehydration contributes significantly to GI tract dysfunction because it further accentuates the intrinsic blood flow changes associated with exercise, as noted previously. Research has shown that 80% of runners who lose at least 4% of their body weight from fluid losses during exercise experience lower GI tract symptoms.[2] Exercise-related fluid and electrolyte shifts result in intracellular electrolyte imbalances and cell dysfunction, which may lead to colonic smooth muscle and mucosal irritation.[11] In runners with restricted water intake, GI symptoms are more likely to arise due to increases in upper GI tract and intestinal permeability relative to resting individuals.[12] In a study of nutritional intake patterns in endurance athletes,[13] it was shown that high rates of carbohydrate intake (up to 90 g/h) were associated with an increased risk for nausea and flatulence. In contrast, ingestion of a lower-carbohydrate liquid meal before exercise is generally well tolerated, may help to maintain GI tract perfusion,[14] and may prevent gut ischemia related to decreased splanchnic blood flow.

UPPER GASTROINTESTINAL TRACT CONDITIONS

Upper GI tract complaints are experienced by 30% to 70% of athletes,[10,15,16] with the prevailing conditions being gastroesophageal reflux disease (GERD) and dyspepsia.[17,18] When assessing the pathophysiology behind the high rate of upper GI tract symptoms in athletes, three primary mechanisms have been postulated: (1) mechanical forces, (2) alterations in GI tract blood flow, as noted previously, and (3) neuroendocrine changes that influence overall GI tract function. Mechanical forces include increased abdominal pressure from straining in high-exertion activities such as weightlifting, mechanical trauma to the GI tract from repetitive motion of the abdomen during exercise, and the impact of body position during exercise such as the flexed/compressed position of cyclists.[19] GI mucosal activity and alterations in absorption may result from mechanical factors or neuroendocrine changes. Neural activity changes, as referenced previously, have all been documented to negatively influence GI tract function in athletes.[5]

Exercise also greatly affects esophageal motility. Relaxation of the lower esophageal sphincter (LES), increased pressure gradient between the stomach and esophagus, and decreased esophageal clearance of food all have been associated with high-level physical exertion, and all appear to be potentially important in the development of GERD symptoms.[20] As exercise intensity reaches peak levels exceeding 90% of $VO_{2\,max}$, the frequency and duration of esophageal reflux episodes increase.[21,22] Exercise type also influences esophageal motility. Running has been found to decrease upper GI tract motility more than cycling,[23] and the highest rate of heartburn and esophageal reflux has been seen in weightlifters, with correspondingly lower rates found in runners and cyclists.[24]

Gastroesophageal Reflux Disease

GERD is the most common cause of upper GI tract symptoms in athletes and results from the irritating effects of acidic gastric secretions as they reflux up into the esophagus due to loss of competence of the LES. The incidence of GERD increases with intensity of exercise, is more common in endurance sports, and is exacerbated by postprandial exercise. Runners demonstrate a threefold increase in GERD symptoms when running 45 minutes after completing a meal as compared with running in a fasting state.[24] Activities with large increases in intra-abdominal pressure, most notably weightlifting and cycling when in the "aero" position, contribute to higher rates of symptomatic GERD as the LES is overwhelmed by the external pressure applied to the stomach.

Cardinal features of GERD include heartburn, retrosternal burning, and regurgitation with a sense of refluxed gastric contents arising into the mouth or hypopharynx.[25] The majority of athletes with true exertional GERD actually have GERD at rest as well[26]; thus the greatest risk factor for GERD symptoms during exercise is the presence of GERD symptoms at rest.

Gastroesophageal Reflux Disease Pathophysiology

Although precise GERD mechanisms are not well defined, suggested mechanisms include inappropriate relaxation of the LES,[4] gastric dysmotility, enhanced pressure gradient between the stomach and esophagus in sports such as football, weightlifting, and cycling, gastric distension, delayed gastric emptying, and increased mechanical stress by bouncing of organs.[4]

Normal peristaltic motions of the esophagus, which aid in ensuring that the acidic contents of the stomach remain in the stomach and do not migrate superiorly into the neutral environment of the esophagus, decrease in the setting of higher levels of activity. Thus any food or fluid intake that fails to pass through the stomach prior to exercise predisposes the athlete to reflux. Food choice is important because high-fat foods (fried foods, creamy sauces, and gravy), coffee, caffeine, chocolate, peppermint, alcohol, acidic foods such as tomatoes and onions, and tobacco products are well known to decrease LES pressure. In exercising individuals, the widespread use of nonsteroidal antiinflammatory drugs (NSAIDs) may also impact negatively on the proximal GI tract due to inherent GI tract irritation from suppression of protective prostaglandins.

Gastroesophageal Reflux Disease, Asthma, and Other Related Conditions

GERD may present with a number of less typical symptoms, including cough, sore throat, hoarseness, asthma, bronchitis, recurrent pneumonia, intermittent choking, or chest pain. Athletes presenting with any of these symptoms or complaints should be considered potential GERD sufferers. Many of these individuals have "silent" reflux that fails to generate classic GI manifestations. GERD can provoke or exacerbate asthma by either silent aspiration into the tracheobronchial tree or by stimulating an acid-mediated esophagobronchial reflex that provokes dyspnea and wheezing.[27] It is estimated that up to 90% of asthmatics have GERD and that up to 40% of asthmatics have esophagitis.[28] However, to date only those with nocturnal GERD symptoms have demonstrated improvements in their asthma from aggressive GERD treatment.[29] It is always important to consider GERD as the potential primary pathology in an athlete who has new or unusual asthmatic symptoms.

Several clinical variants of GERD are also recognized. Laryngopharyngeal reflux disease (LPRD) is typically manifest by hoarseness, voice change, and chronic cough. It is believed to result from an esophageal reflux mechanism with secondary inflammation and damage of the proximal airway and laryngeal area. Duodenogastroesophageal reflux (DGER) results from reflux of duodenal, rather than gastric, contents, including biliary secretions, pancreatic enzymes, and bicarbonate. DGER is often responsible for refractory GERD symptoms despite appropriate management with maximal dose medications.[30] Finally, a number of proposed extraesophageal manifestations of GERD include recurrent pharyngitis, otitis media, sinusitis, and pulmonary fibrosis.

Gastroesophageal Reflux Disease Treatment

The importance of proper GERD management cannot be overstated, not only to prevent acute symptoms and their impact on sport performance but also to decrease the risk of long-term complications including peptic strictures and Barrett esophagus with its potential for malignant transformation. Successful GERD management includes lifestyle modifications, medications, or both. Lifestyle modifications should always be the first line treatment in athletes who have GERD. These include sleeping on two pillows or elevating the head of the bed to enhance gravity-associated esophageal clearance, avoidance of laying down to sleep within 4 hours of the evening meal, avoiding postprandial exercise, and limiting consumption of foods known to relax the LES, as noted previously. Athletes should also avoid solid food, high carbohydrate drinks, caffeine and alcohol prior to strenuous activity.[19] Rather, they should consume liquid meals with lower carbohydrate content and ensure adequate hydration. Sports drinks containing up to a maximum of 10% glucose are believed to be the optimal calorie-containing beverages for training because of their low tendency to cause upper GI tract symptoms.[26]

If these interventions fail to improve symptoms, pharmacologic therapy should be considered. The two primary classes of medications used to treat GERD include proton pump inhibitors (PPIs; e.g., omeprazole, lansoprazole, pantoprazole, esomeprazole) and H2-receptor antagonists (e.g., ranitidine, famotidine). Initially, a 2-week trial of a once-daily PPI such as 20-mg omeprazole or 30-mg lansoprazole, taken prior to a meal, should be instituted. If once-daily therapy is inadequate, PPI dosing should be doubled. If initially effective, completion of an 8-week course is generally appropriate and effective for long-term benefit, particularly if combined with lifestyle measures. For GERD symptoms limited to discreet competitive times, it has been shown that markers of exercise-induced gastroesophageal reflux—percentage reflux time and number of reflux episodes—can be effectively reduced by pretreatment with an H2-receptor antagonist (i.e., 300 mg ranitidine) 1 hour prior to activity.[31] Rapid onset of benefit with H2 blockers makes them the preferred therapies for such acute indications.

If symptoms recur within 3 months, additional evaluation to confirm the diagnosis is generally warranted to determine the appropriateness of ongoing therapy. Upper endoscopy is the evaluation tool of choice for diagnosis confirmation and is also indicated for more concerning clinical presentations, including failure of empiric therapy, need for continuous therapy, presence of atypical symptoms such as odynophagia, dysphagia, weight loss, bleeding, or anemia, or if symptoms are long-standing. Additional workup should include *Helicobacter pylori* testing to exclude its potential role in non-GERD syndromes such as peptic ulcer disease and nonulcer dyspepsia. Confirmation of *H. pylori* infection is most effectively achieved via gastric mucosal biopsy at the time of upper endoscopy or via serologic, breath, or stool antigen testing. If such testing is positive, a 2-week triple-drug antibiotic/acid suppressive combination treatment course should be pursued. Such combination therapies include PPI + clarithromycin + amoxicillin or metronidazole, or PPI + a bismuth compound + metronidazole + a tetracycline.

Functional Heartburn

Studies reveal that up to 60% of individuals presenting with signs and symptoms compatible with GERD but who fail aggressive PPI therapy have a syndrome referred to as "functional heartburn." This disorder is also known as "esophageal hypersensitivity" and bears resemblance to other common functional GI disorders that include a pattern of visceral hyperalgesia such as irritable bowel syndrome (IBS).[17] The Rome III diagnostic criteria for functional heartburn include burning retrosternal discomfort or pain, absence of evidence that GERD is the cause

of the symptom, absence of an esophageal motility disorder, and symptom onset of at least 6 months.[18] As such, this diagnosis can be made only following formal referral to a gastroenterologist with completion of an appropriate diagnostic workup.

Management is challenging and many sufferers continue to have symptoms despite therapy. Biofeedback to modify nervous system input to the GI tract is the treatment of choice. Tricyclic antidepressants and prokinetic agents also have potential value, but their significant side effect profiles are generally incompatible with sport participation.

Dyspepsia

Dyspepsia refers to a spectrum of vague GI symptoms, including gnawing or burning epigastric pain, nausea, vomiting, eructation, bloating, indigestion, generalized abdominal discomfort, and early satiety. The three most common causes of dyspepsia in athletes include GERD, gastritis, and peptic ulcer disease. In addition, many drugs are associated with dyspepsia, including NSAIDs, antibiotics, and estrogens. In fact, most drugs have a potential to cause dyspepsia in at least some patients.

Regardless of the cause of dyspepsia, the common pathologic feature is mucosal inflammation and damage of the upper GI tract. Gut mucosal injury in athletes may be multifactorial from mucosal ischemia, dehydration, stress of competition, use of NSAIDs or a variety of medications, alcohol, caffeine products, or dietary supplements. These same factors increase the risk for upper GI tract bleeding and ulcer disease in athletes. Upper GI evaluations in professional long-distance runners revealed at least one GI mucosal lesion in approximately 90% of runners even in the absence of symptoms.[32]

Dyspepsia management focuses on the limitation or elimination of the provocative factors mentioned previously. Should those interventions provide inadequate benefit, acid suppressive therapy with H2 blockers or PPIs is the pharmacologic treatment of choice. For those individuals who suffer from chronic dyspepsia or who have had frank GI bleeding with heavy exercise, consistent use of a H2 blocker or PPI is prudent to prevent symptoms or complications from upper GI tract damage. Data from ultramarathon runners have shown that regular use of a PPI significantly decreased their incidence of GI tract bleeding.[33]

Impact of Aspirin and Nonsteroidal Antiinflammatory Drugs

Aspirin and NSAID use places the GI tract at risk due to the blockade of cyclooxygenase and the subsequent loss of production of protective gastric prostaglandins. Although clearly linked to a risk of gastritis and peptic ulcer disease with prolonged use, NSAIDs have yet to be shown to correlate with risk for GI bleeding in endurance athletes.[34] Whenever feasible, it is advisable to have athletes minimize the use of NSAIDs; however, the need for pain and inflammation management in highly active individuals makes complete avoidance of NSAIDs unrealistic. For those who require NSAIDs, it is prudent to add a daily PPI for GI tract protection, particularly if they have a previous history of ulceration or bleeding. Special note should be made of the NSAID ketorolac. Although it possesses analgesic properties equivalent to opioid therapy, ketorolac carries a high risk of GI bleeding with long-term use. Present dosing guidelines mandate discontinuation of ketorolac therapy after a maximum of 5 days of use.

Pill Esophagitis

Pill esophagitis results from the local irritating effects of certain medications if they remain in the esophagus for a prolonged amount of time. In athletes, NSAIDs are the classic family of medications with greatest risk. The tetracycline antibiotic family, often used in athletes chronically for acne or in shorter-term courses for tick-borne illness, and the antimalarial mefloquine are notoriously problematic for this condition as well. Prevention is best achieved by taking medication in the morning with food or a moderate volume of liquid, remaining upright for at least 30 minutes after pill ingestion, and avoiding bedtime dosing. It is always important to educate athletes about a medication's potential risk for GI toxicity as well.

Dysphagia

Dysphagia is a condition characterized by difficulties with swallowing, which are typically driven by alterations in either nerve or muscle function. Sport-associated dysphagia is most commonly caused by the irritative effects of GERD, although any intrinsic esophageal disorder may be responsible. Clinically, dysphagia is divided into two subtypes based on anatomic location and pathologic mechanism. Oropharyngeal dysphagia (OD) typically presents with greater difficulty swallowing liquids than solids and is characterized by repeated attempts to swallow due to a sensation of choking or incomplete swallowing. OD occurs within the first second of the initiation of swallowing and presents with discomfort or pain that localizes to the neck. Other characteristics may include a change in dietary habits, dehydration, regurgitation, or unexplained weight loss. In contrast, esophageal dysphagia (ED) presents with difficulty swallowing both solids and liquids, occurs several seconds after the initiation of swallowing, and is characterized by discomfort or pain that localizes to the substernal area. Dysphagia management focuses on addressing presumptive GERD or identifying and managing other underlying conditions.

Nausea and Vomiting

Nausea and vomiting may be experienced by athletes in association with strenuous or prolonged exercise.[15] Although the etiology is not always clear and thus may create a challenge for prevention and management, nausea and vomiting are most often associated with postprandial exercise. Reflux of stomach contents coupled with changes in esophageal motility, sphincter tone, and GI ischemia contributes to the increased incidence of nausea and vomiting associated with exercise. Nevertheless, athletes may have these manifestations even when relatively inactive, a phenomenon supported by research in runners who actually demonstrated a higher incidence of bloating and vomiting when not training.[35] Although the reasoning is unclear, this is likely a function of the chronic irritative effects of running on the GI tract.

Prevention of nausea and vomiting focuses on prudent dietary and fluid choices to minimize gastric irritation or altered GI absorption. In keeping with general intake guidelines, for events lasting less than 1 hour, optimal energy supplementation to minimize GI effects is provided by sports drinks with carbohydrate concentrations of 6% to 8%. For longer duration activities, carbohydrate intake of 30 to 60 g/h should be well tolerated and effective.[36] Athletes should also avoid solid food within 3 hours of an athletic event. Finally, because NSAID use has been shown to increase nausea and vomiting in endurance runners,[37] caution should be exercised in their use around the time of athletic participation even for activities of shorter duration.

The primary treatment for nausea and vomiting associated with exercise is the prompt cessation of physical activity. However, in athletes with protracted nausea and vomiting, evaluation for complications of dehydration and electrolyte disturbances should be pursued. In addition, other causes such as peptic ulcer disease and biliary pain should be considered. If nausea is associated with prominent heartburn during activity, a trial of H2 blocker or PPI may be warranted. Studies have shown that H2 blockers and PPIs, as well as antinausea therapies such as ondansetron, can be helpful for exercise-related nausea, and the sports medicine provider should have a low threshold to treat affected athletes when they are participating in activities that are likely to provoke symptoms.[38]

LOWER GASTROINTESTINAL TRACT CONDITIONS

As with upper GI disorders, issues relating to the small intestines and colon are common in sport, with nearly two-thirds of endurance athletes reporting lower GI symptoms at some point in their training or competition.[39] Conditions such as diarrhea and rectal bleeding are often directly related to intensity of activity, whereas functional disorders, as seen frequently in the general population, are often exacerbated by the physical demands of exercise. Although the typical athlete presents with the conditions discussed next, the differential is broad and must be considered individually for each case (Table 15.1).

Diarrhea

Diarrhea results from excessive fluid content of stool that overwhelms the colon's absorptive ability and results in loose or frankly watery bowel movements. Diarrhea is a common concern in athletes, with approximately 25% of marathon runners reporting diarrhea and more than half reporting fecal urgency with running. As expected, the severity of diarrhea is directly proportional to training mileage or training intensity, with women affected more commonly than men.[11,39] Although generally benign, prominent diarrhea in athletes may be associated with dehydration and subsequent risk for heat injury, rhabdomyolysis, and acute tubular necrosis.

The etiology of exercise-related diarrhea is often multifactorial. Increased sympathetic nervous system stimulation with exercise decreases gut tone and resistance, accelerates transit of colonic contents into the rectum, and increases the urge to defecate.[40] Gastroenteropancreatic hormone secretion of gastrin and motilin with high-level exercise may further contribute to the development of diarrhea.[41] Nutritional factors may cause diarrhea relative to their ability to increase stool water content. More highly

TABLE 15.1 Differential Diagnosis of Lower Gastrointestinal Symptoms in Athletes

Nutritional Factors
- Dietary fiber
- High glycemic index foods
- High carbohydrate concentration sports drinks or gels
- Food allergies and intolerances

Irritable Bowel Syndrome

Malabsorption Syndromes
- Lactose intolerance
- Celiac disease

Medications, Herbals, Supplements
- Laxatives and cathartics
- H2 blockers and antacids
- Nonabsorbable sugars (e.g., mannitol, sorbitol)
- Antibiotics
- Caffeine
- Alcohol
- NSAIDs

Infectious Diarrhea
- Bacterial
- Parasitic
- Viral

Toxic Diarrhea
- Pseudomembranous enterocolitis (*Clostridium difficile*)
- Staphylococcal toxin

Inflammatory Bowel Disease
- Crohn disease
- Ulcerative colitis

Ischemic Bowel Disease
- Acute arterial mesenteric infarction
- Chronic mesenteric ischemia
- Mesenteric venous thrombosis
- Colonic ischemia

Hepatic, Biliary, and Pancreatic Diseases

Lower GI Tract Lesions
- Ulcerations
- Polyps
- Arteriovenous malformations
- Anorectal hemorrhoids, fissures, or fistulae

Colon Cancer and Other Neoplastic Processes

GI, Gastrointestinal; *NSAIDs,* nonsteroidal antiinflammatory drugs. From Ho GWK. Lower gastrointestinal distress in endurance athletes. *Curr Sports Med Rep.* 2009;8(2):85–91.

carbohydrates such as glucose and fructose, gastrointestinal symptoms seem to be reduced compared with the consumption of the same amount of a single carbohydrate. Foods with high glycemic index and/or high fiber content may also contribute to osmotic "dumping," whereas caffeine may produce diarrhea directly through its laxative properties.

Runner's Diarrhea ("Runner's Trots")

Although all athletes may be at increased risk for diarrhea, runners are at particular risk for a specific running-related diarrheal condition often referred to colloquially as "runner's trots." This condition is classically encountered in distance runners, but its exact pathophysiology is still largely unknown. Conjectured mechanisms include impairment in GI tract function as a result of the repetitive jarring associated with lengthy stints of running, fluid and electrolyte shifts associated with prolonged exercise, and relative ischemia of the GI tract. It is clear that unique intrinsic factors also may play a role in this condition because some endurance athletes rarely suffer with it whereas others are chronically affected. Clinically, athletes experience an urgent need to defecate mid-run with stools that may be loose or essentially normal. Management focuses on prevention, as noted next.

Diarrhea Management

Management centers on training and lifestyle modification to allow the gut to perform optimally in the face of high levels of exertion. Modifying physical stress through reduction of training intensity, duration, and/or distance for 1 to 2 weeks may lead to symptom resolution.[5] The athlete should then transition to cross-training for several weeks, followed by resumption of running at progressively higher levels. Adequate hydration is always a crucial part of lifestyle management, and avoidance of NSAIDs, aspirin, antibiotics, and caffeine may also be helpful. Dietary modification to include a low-residue, low-fiber diet with avoidance of sports drinks and/or gels with carbohydrate concentrations greater than 8% should be recommended. Avoiding solid food at least 2 hours prior to exercise may help, as may adherence to an antidiarrheal diet such as the BRAT (bananas, rice, applesauce, toast) diet. Making an effort to have a bowel movement before exercise can greatly minimize the likelihood of midactivity GI distress.

In general, anticholinergic medication use for exercise-associated diarrhea is discouraged because the side effect profile and physiologic properties of these medications have a negative impact on sweat rate and thermoregulation. Opiate- and atropine-based preparations should also be avoided. Loperamide (Imodium) may be considered in athletes with nonbloody diarrhea who are at risk for dehydration and associated heat illness but are otherwise clinically well. Similarly, antispasmodic agents such as dicyclomine or hyoscamine may be considered for severe symptoms, but their use must be weighed against the risk of anticholinergic side effects.

Stool studies should be obtained in athletes with "alarm" features, including gross hematochezia, profound diarrhea associated with dehydration, persistent diarrhea greater than 48 hours, fever, severe abdominal pain, recent travel, or possible exposure to infectious diarrheal pathogens. Consideration

concentrated fluids (>7% to 10%) present a solute load to the GI tract, which produces an osmotic drive for fluid to remain in the GI tract rather than being absorbed. This shift toward fluid deposition into the gut produces a "dumping syndrome" that overwhelms the colon's absorptive abilities and results in diarrhea. For endurance athletes, it has been noted that when a beverage is consumed that contains multiple transportable should also be given to studies in immunocompromised patients or older athletes,[42] especially if they have comorbid medical conditions.

Lower Gastrointestinal Bleeding

Microscopic heme-positive stools, rectal bleeding, or frank bloody diarrhea may be seen commonly with high-level training or competition particularly marathoning, ultramarathoning, or high-mileage cycling. Occult rectal bleeding has been demonstrated in approximately 25% of recreational triathletes, 20% of marathon runners, and almost 90% of 100-mile ultramarathoners.[34] More dramatically, frankly bloody stools have been reported in up to 6% of postmarathon runners.[43] As described earlier, long-duration events create prolonged ischemia in the GI tract, which compromises mucosal integrity, resulting in varying degrees of lower GI tract bleeding. This condition is generally benign and self-limited in the absence of underlying GI tract diseases. Pronounced or protracted rectal bleeding may predispose to anemia and may be a marker of a more worrisome underlying GI issue.

Ischemic Conditions

There are four distinct ischemic syndromes seen in the GI tract.[9] Although primarily seen in patients with vascular comorbidities such as hypertension, diabetes mellitus, or tobacco abuse, they must be considered by the sports medicine practitioner in light of the breadth and variable health characteristics of the exercising population.

Colonic ischemia is the most common form of ischemic bowel disease. Crampy left lower quadrant abdominal pain and bowel movements of stool mixed with frank blood are the common presenting clinical features. Colonoscopy should be performed acutely in the setting of rectal bleeding to make a definitive diagnosis. Mucosal changes of ischemia, typically manifest by congestive and hemorrhagic vascular lesions, are the classic findings. This condition is self-limited and the associated colonic changes will typically resolve in 1 week, thus limiting the yield of diagnostic testing performed at that time or beyond.

The less common ischemic syndromes include acute arterial mesenteric infarction (AAMI), chronic arterial mesenteric ischemia (CAMI), and mesenteric venous thrombosis. Although a discussion of these entities is beyond the scope of this text, it is important to consider them for older athletes presenting with severe abdominal pain and lower GI bleeding.

Although some risk for GI ischemia is unavoidable in the most intense of activities, aggressive hydration and heat management remain the key means of attempting to prevent or minimize lower GI bleeding.

Irritable Bowel Syndrome

A functional GI disorder without evidence of structural, biomechanical, radiologic, or laboratory abnormalities, IBS affects up to 15% of the general population.[44] Two forms have been described—"diarrhea predominant" and "constipation predominant"—although the classic pattern typically involves alternating manifestations of both. IBS is twice as common in women and typically presents in the second or third decade of life.

Approximately 50% of patients who have IBS have comorbid psychiatric illnesses, most commonly depression and anxiety. Proposed mechanisms for IBS include increased GI sensitivity to various stimuli including stress, food, cholecystokinin secretion, impaired transit of bowel gas, visceral hypersensitivity, autonomic dysfunction, and altered immune activation.[45]

The clinical presentation of IBS is variable, with the most common symptoms including cramping abdominal pain relieved by defecation, altered stool frequency, altered stool form (watery, mucus, loose, hard), altered stool passage (urgency, strain), a sense of incomplete evacuation, and abdominal distention especially following meals. Athletes with IBS rarely have nocturnal symptoms and do not manifest features of systemic illness or gross GI bleeding. The diagnosis is generally made clinically based on presentation and lack of evidence of other GI disorders. Current evidence does not support the routine use of laboratory studies or imaging to exclude organic GI disorders in patients who have typical IBS symptoms and are lacking "alarm" features such as significant abdominal pain, fevers, GI bleeding, or weight loss.[44]

Primary management strategies focus on lifestyle measures including high-fiber diet, adequate hydration, and stress reduction techniques. For ongoing symptoms, drug treatment of IBS is based on the athletes' predominant symptoms. For diarrhea-predominant IBS, antidiarrheal (loperamide) or antispasmodic (dicyclomine, hyoscamine) medicines used as needed are typically efficacious. Constipation-predominant IBS is generally managed with an increase in the lifestyle measures noted previously coupled with nonstimulant laxatives such as polyethylene glycol (Miralax) or psyllium-containing products. Adequate hydration is particularly important in constipation-prone athletes.

Celiac Disease

Celiac disease is a hereditary autoimmune disorder resulting in malabsorption in the GI tract. Hypersensitivity of the immune system to gluten- or gliadin-containing foods is the primary pathophysiologic mechanism. Gluten protein found in wheat, barley, and rye results in an immunologic reaction in the intestinal mucosa that causes villous atrophy and subsequent impairment in absorption of important nutrients. Increasingly, celiac disease is being recognized and diagnosed in the general population and, as such, is also being more commonly encountered in athletes and active individuals. Although its primary pathology is found in the GI tract, celiac disease may also have effects on blood, bone, brain, nervous system, and skin.[46] Iron deficiency anemia has been reported in up to 70% of patients with newly diagnosed celiac disease,[47] and calcium and vitamin D deficiencies are also common, which may increase the risk of stress fractures and osteopenia.[48]

The diagnosis of celiac disease is often delayed many months or even years because the presenting symptoms may be suggestive of other more common entities or may be sufficiently mild as to be largely ignored by the athlete. Signs and symptoms of classic celiac disease include chronic diarrhea, abdominal bloating/cramping/pain, malnutrition, fatigue, vomiting, anemia, myalgia/arthralgia, osteopenia/osteoporosis, menstrual irregularities, irritability, constipation, short stature, and dermatitis herpetiformis.[49] Initial serologic testing is traditionally via serum tissue transglutaminase (tTG) antibody levels. More specialized studies are available but are beyond the scope of our discussion. The "gold standard" for definitive diagnosis of celiac disease is tissue biopsy of small intestinal mucosa demonstrating classic blunted villi.

Eating a strict gluten-free diet is the only effective management of celiac disease, and this can be challenging on many levels for the competitive athlete. The elimination of all sources of wheat, rye, and barley requires that the athlete find ample alternative sources of carbohydrate to meet the recommended carbohydrate intake of 6 to 10 g/kg body weight. Beans, rice, corn meal, corn flour, nuts, potatoes, tapioca, and quinoa are excellent sources of gluten-free carbohydrates, along with fresh fruits and vegetables. Travel and team meals can be particular challenges for athletes with celiac disease who must ensure appropriate food choices to adequately meet their healthy fat, protein, and carbohydrate intake goals and to provide sufficient energy for maximum performance. In recent years, it has become increasingly popular for nonceliac athletes to consume a gluten-free diet because of perceived GI or general health benefits. However, research into the effects of gluten-free food intake in this group demonstrated no overall effect on performance, GI symptoms, well-being, indicators of intestinal injury, or inflammatory markers.[50]

For a complete list of references, go to ExpertConsult.com.

SELECTED READINGS

Casey E, Mistry DJ, MacKnight JM. Training room management of medical conditions: sports gastroenterology. *Clin Sports Med.* 2005;24:525–540. [Level of Evidence III, Systematic Review].

Cronin O, Molloy MG, Shanahan F. Exercise, fitness, and the gut. *Curr Opin Gastroenterol.* 2016;32(2):67–73. [Level of Evidence III, Systematic Review].

de Oliveira EP, Burini RC, Jeukendrup A. Gastrointestinal complaints during exercise: prevalence, etiology, and nutritional recommendations. *Sports Medicine.* 2014;44(suppl 1):79–85. [Level of Evidence III, Systematic Review].

Ho GWK. Lower gastrointestinal distress in endurance athletes. *Curr Sports Med Rep.* 2009;8(2):85–91. [Level of Evidence III, Systematic Review].

Leggit JC. Evaluation and treatment of GERD and upper GI complaints in athletes. *Curr Sports Med Rep.* 2011;10(2):109–114. [Level of Evidence I, Systematic Review].

Pfeiffer B, Stellingwerff T, Hodgson AB, et al. Nutritional intake and gastrointestinal problems during competitive endurance events. *Med Sci Sports Exerc.* 2012;44(2):344–351. [Level of Evidence III, Comparative Study].

Viola TA. Evaluation of the athlete with exertional abdominal pain. *Curr Sports Med Rep.* 2010;9:106–110. [Level of Evidence V, Expert Opinion].

Waterman JJ, Kapur R. Upper gastrointestinal issues in athletes. *Curr Sports Med Rep.* 2012;11(2):99–104. [Level of Evidence I, Systematic Review].

16

Hematologic Medicine in the Athlete

John J. Densmore

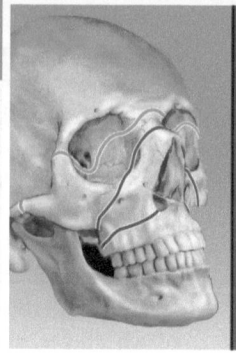

Athletic performance depends on proper functioning of the blood. From problems with the oxygen-carrying function of red blood cells to the prevention of bleeding by the hemostatic system, many hematologic issues can affect athletes adversely. These hematologic issues include both acquired and inherited disorders that can affect athletes of all ages. This chapter reviews many of the hematologic issues that may arise in caring for athletes, focusing on those relating to red blood cells and the hemostatic system.

DISORDERS OF RED BLOOD CELLS

Definition

Anemia is defined as a reduction of red blood cells below the normal range, with the normal range differing for men and women. Hemoglobin and hematocrit are commonly used to identify the red blood cell concentration in the blood. Mild anemia can be asymptomatic, although compared with more sedentary persons, athletes generally notice it much earlier because of its effects on their performance. It is important to identify the underlying cause of the anemia, which can be due to decreased red cell production or increased red cell destruction.

Hemoglobin is the oxygen-carrying protein in red blood cells. Normal hemoglobin (hemoglobin A) consists of two alpha chains and two beta chains.[1] Inherited disorders of hemoglobin are referred to as *hemoglobinopathies* or *thalassemia*. A number of hemoglobinopathies have been identified that result from mutations in the alpha or beta chains and have varying degrees of anemia and symptoms. The most common hemoglobin mutation in the United States is hemoglobin S, which causes sickle cell disease in persons with two copies of the mutated gene. *Thalassemia* refers to decreased production of normal alpha or beta chains and can be clinically silent or markedly symptomatic.[2] Thalassemias are referred to as alpha or beta, depending on which chain is affected. Thalassemias increase in clinical severity as the number of genes affected increases. In general, persons with one or two mutations are asymptomatic, a condition referred to as *thalassemia minor*.

It also appears that some athletes have anemia that is caused by mechanisms not seen in nonathletes, including dilutional "pseudoanemia" and exercise-related intravascular hemolysis. Pseudoanemia refers to a temporary condition that occurs as a result of training-related expansion of the plasma volume.[3] The degree of volume expansion relates to the duration and intensity of exercise and can result in a dilutional drop in the hemoglobin concentration.[4] Intravascular hemolysis is also common in athletes. Initially referred to as *march hemoglobinuria* or *foot-strike hemoglobinuria,* the mechanism for hemolysis was thought to be induced by mechanical damage to red cells with each foot strike.[5] However, others suggest that the effects of contracting muscles on red cells may contribute to hemolysis and the development of anemia in athletes.[6]

Epidemiology

Anemia is a condition commonly experienced by persons in the United States. Rates are highest in children and adult women, largely because of iron deficiency. The most recent National Health and Nutrition Examination Surveys (2003–2012) estimate that 3.5% of men and 7.6% of women in the United States are anemic, with the highest rates among menstruating women.[7] Iron deficiency is the most common cause of anemia in the United States and is the most common nutritional deficiency worldwide.[8] A recent retrospective study evaluated the results of iron-related testing in 2749 individuals at a National Collegiate Athletic Association (NCAA) Division 1 institution.[9] In women, 2.2% had iron deficiency anemia and another 30.9% had iron deficiency without anemia. The incidence for men was much lower, 1.2% with iron deficiency anemia and 2.9% with iron deficiency without anemia.

Hemoglobin S is the most common inherited blood disorder in the United States. It is estimated that 1 in 12 African Americans carries one copy of the mutated gene, a condition referred to as *sickle cell trait.*[10] The thalassemias are also common and are considered the most prevalent genetic mutation worldwide.[2] Incidence varies geographically; alpha thalassemia is frequent in Southeast Asia and western Africa, whereas beta thalassemia is more common in the Mediterranean region of Europe.

Pathophysiology

As previously stated, anemia is caused by either decreased production or increased destruction of red blood cells. Red blood cell production problems (Table 16.1) can be due to a vitamin or mineral deficiency, inflammation, erythropoietin deficiency, or a primary bone marrow disorder. Iron deficiency is the most common cause and is most often the result of chronic blood loss. Menstruation or chronic gastrointestinal blood loss will lead to iron deficiency if oral absorption is not able to balance iron loss. Other avenues for iron loss in athletes are hemolysis leading to hemoglobinuria and increased sweat production.[10]

TABLE 16.1	Types of Anemia in Athletes and Treatment Recommendations			
Condition	Frequency	Hemoglobin	Ferritin	Treatment Required
Dilutional pseudoanemia	Common	Normal to mild decrease	Normal	No
Iron deficiency without anemia	Common	Normal	Decreased	Controversial
Iron deficiency anemia	Less common	Decreased	Decreased	Iron replacement indicated
Thalassemia minor	Less common	Normal to mild decrease	Normal to elevated	No

Another potential cause of iron deficiency in athletes is celiac disease, which results in iron malabsorption and can occur even in the absence of the gastrointestinal symptoms that are suggestive of celiac disease.[11]

Iron deficiency occurs in three stages.[8] Stage I, also known as prelatent iron deficiency, is associated with an isolated decrease in serum ferritin. At this stage, stainable iron is not present in the bone marrow, but hemoglobin levels remain normal. Stage II is latent iron deficiency; at this stage, the ferritin drops further, serum iron and transferrin saturation decrease, and total iron-binding capacity rises. As in stage I, hemoglobin levels remain normal during stage II, although the mean corpuscular volume (MCV) of the red cells may start to decrease. However, in stage III, with progressive depletion of iron stores, an overt microcytic and hypochromic iron-deficiency anemia develops.

Inflammatory conditions have long been known to lead to decreased red cell production, but only recently has the pathophysiology been understood fully. Hepcidin, a protein produced by the liver in response to infection or inflammation, inhibits iron absorption and its release from storage sites for use by developing red blood cell precursors.[12] Although significant data are lacking in athletes, it appears that chronic inflammation from training can result in elevated hepcidin levels, contributing to disordered iron metabolism and resultant anemia.

Erythropoietin is an important hormone that promotes red blood cell production.[1] It is produced by the kidney but is also manufactured as a pharmaceutical agent for use in persons with kidney failure and some primary bone marrow disorders. Deficiency in an athlete would be unusual unless significant renal insufficiency was also present. Similarly, primary bone marrow disorders such as leukemia or multiple myeloma often cause significant anemia, but these disorders are rare in athletes.

Hemoglobin S in red blood cells protects against malaria and has been shown to reduce mortality from the disease compared with hemoglobin A.[13] Sickle cell trait has long been believed to be a benign condition, but evidence is increasing that carriers experience an increased number of adverse events.[14] Exertional sickling, which was first reported in military recruits more than 25 years ago, has been associated with sudden death during exercise.[15] Causes of sudden death include metabolic acidosis, rhabdomyolysis, renal failure, and cardiac arrhythmia. Risk for adverse events is increased by conditions that can promote sickling of red blood cells, including intense exercise, particularly at a high altitude or in extreme heat. In a recent review of NCAA athletes who died suddenly, it was determined that the relative risk for sudden death is 37 times higher for an athlete with sickle cell trait.[16]

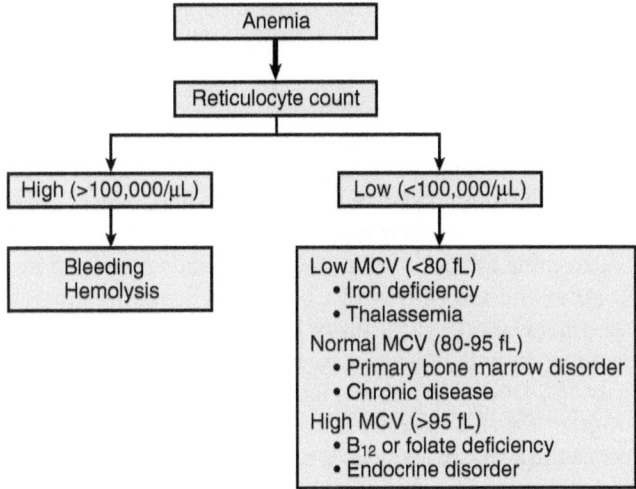

Fig. 16.1 An approach to the patient with anemia, based on reticulocyte count at presentation. *MCV,* Mean corpuscular volume.

Compared with athletes who have sickle cell trait, athletes with thalassemia have a much lower risk for sudden death. Athletes with either alpha or beta thalassemia minor often have a very mild anemia due to decreased production of hemoglobin A. Athletes with more significant disease will have significant anemia and may also have splenomegaly and skeletal abnormalities, which would likely preclude participation in competitive athletics.

Diagnosis

The diagnostic approach to the athlete with anemia is aimed at isolating the exact etiology in order to determine the appropriate therapy. A complete blood cell count (CBC) can be a useful guide to the initial evaluation. Significant abnormalities of white blood cells and platelets signal an occult, potentially serious bone marrow disorder that requires referral to a hematologist. However, an isolated anemia is much more common, and the workup can be guided by the CBC and reticulocyte count. Reticulocytes are immature red blood cells and are produced in higher numbers in the presence of bleeding or hemolysis. A high reticulocyte level indicates an appropriate bone marrow response to anemia and is not indicative of a bone marrow problem. Conversely, a low reticulocyte count is suggestive of anemia resulting from decreased red blood cell production (Fig. 16.1).

For disorders associated with decreased red blood cell production, evaluation of the size of red blood cells is pivotal in determining etiology. Microcytosis (MCV <80 fL) is most commonly associated with iron deficiency and thalassemia. Macrocytosis

(MCV >95 fL) may indicate deficiencies of either vitamin B_{12} or folic acid as well as various endocrine or primary bone marrow disorders. Normocytic anemias (MCV 80–95 fL) can be induced by inflammation, bone marrow disorders, and early vitamin or mineral deficiency.

Iron deficiency is generally evaluated using a series of tests, including hemoglobin, hematocrit, MCV, serum iron, total iron-binding capacity, transferrin saturation, and serum ferritin. Although a bone marrow biopsy with Prussian blue staining for iron is generally regarded as the gold standard for diagnosing iron deficiency, serum ferritin is an excellent surrogate marker for iron stores in most patients. A serum ferritin level less than 10 to 15 ng/mL is nearly always suggestive of iron deficiency.[17] However, higher ferritin values may also be suggestive of occult iron deficiency because a number of underlying inflammatory or malignant conditions can stimulate a threefold elevation in serum ferritin. The combination of low ferritin and decreased transferrin saturation is strongly suggestive of true iron deficiency.[18]

Screening for sickle cell disease is currently mandated in all 50 states and the District of Columbia.[19] Screening programs use either isoelectric focusing or high-performance liquid chromatography, both of which have very high sensitivity and specificity. In 2010, the NCAA announced a sickle cell trait screening program for all Division 1 athletes.[20] This has been expanded to include all NCAA athletes despite concerns from many professional groups.[21]

A diagnosis of thalassemia minor can often be made by evaluating a CBC and family history. Thalassemia minor generally presents with severe microcytosis (MCV <70 fL) and mild or borderline anemia. Iron studies typically do not reveal iron deficiency, although some persons may have combined abnormalities. Hemoglobin electrophoresis is used to diagnose beta thalassemia, but results are normal in persons with alpha thalassemia, which is diagnosed by genetic testing.

For normocytic or macrocytic anemias, further testing should include assessment of levels of vitamin B_{12}, folate, and thyroid-stimulating hormone. Because of their larger size, a significant increase in reticulocytes can cause an increase in the MCV. Any athlete with an MCV greater than 110 fL should be referred to a hematologist.

Treatment

An adequate understanding of the various causes of anemia and related laboratory data is pivotal for adequate treatment of anemia in athletes (see Table 16.1). Athletes with iron deficiency anemia commonly present with the gradual onset of fatigue and decreased performance or exercise tolerance. A detailed history—including queries about gastrointestinal or urinary bleeding, menstruation, and nutritional practices—should be obtained. Characteristic laboratory findings include a microcytic hypochromic anemia; decreased serum ferritin, iron, and transferrin saturation levels; and elevated total iron-binding capacity. Additional testing to determine the etiology of iron deficiency (e.g., evaluation of the gastrointestinal tract) may be advised if necessary.

The replacement of iron in nonanemic iron-deficient athletes is controversial, although a recent review suggests that iron replacement improves the aerobic capacity of endurance athletes with iron deficiency.[22] One reasonable approach would be to first ensure that the athlete's diet included sufficient amounts of iron in the form of iron-rich foods such as lean meats, poultry, fish, grains, and vegetables. Dietary sources of heme iron have a higher bioavailability than do foods containing nonheme iron, and coingestion of foods containing ascorbic acid may enhance intestinal iron absorption. If dietary changes fail to improve the athlete's iron status, a therapeutic trial of oral iron supplementation may be useful.

Athletes with documented iron deficiency anemia should be treated with iron replacement therapy, typically with oral ferrous sulfate. Gastrointestinal adverse effects such as nausea or constipation may be dose limiting. Within 2 to 3 weeks, an increase in reticulocytes and MCV should be noted. Improvement in hemoglobin and ferritin levels may take several weeks. A minimum of 6 to 12 months of therapy is usually required, although some athletes may need more extended treatment depending on the underlying cause and severity of the anemia. Athletes who fail to respond to oral iron supplements or experience intolerable adverse effects with medication should be referred to a hematologist for consideration of alternative forms of iron replacement therapy.

The approach to athletes with sickle cell trait is controversial. The literature in this area largely consists of case reports or series; no prospective studies in athletes are available to guide the assessment of risk-reduction strategies. The American Heart Association and American College of Cardiology have issued a consensus statement on sickle cell trait and the athlete, which concludes that athletes should not be kept from participating, but preventative strategies and emergency response preparation are recommended.[23] Additionally, there are published guidelines for preventing sudden death in college and secondary school athletes that focus on risk reduction, gradual acclimatization to conditioning activities, and medical supervision.[24,25] Because individuals with sickle cell trait may be more prone to exertional heat illness, recommendations for future research have focused on heat exposure, exercise intensity, and hydration as primary risk factors.[23]

Return-to-Play Guidelines

Anemia generally does not preclude athletic participation. Athletes typically notice a decrement in athletic performance before they present with a severe anemia. For athletes with additional hematologic abnormalities, such as leukopenia or thrombocytopenia, referral to a hematologist is suggested before the athlete returns to full activity. For athletes with sickle cell trait, education and risk reduction are important components of safe participation in all athletics.[18] Following these guidelines while closely monitoring the athlete for signs of difficulty should permit full participation.

DISORDERS OF HEMOSTASIS

Definition

Hemostasis is the process of blood clot formation at the site of an injured vessel. It is a complex interaction of platelets, von Willebrand factor (vWF), and a multitude of coagulation factors.[26]

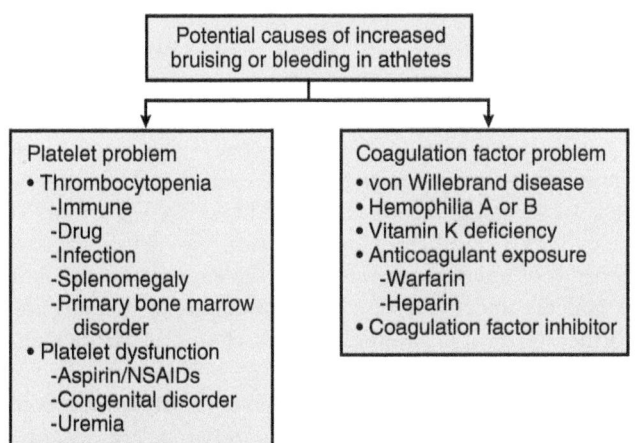

Fig. 16.2 Causes of increased bruising and bleeding in athletes. *NSAIDs,* Nonsteroidal antiinflammatory drugs.

Disorders of hemostasis can be acquired or congenital and can lead to spontaneous bleeding or increased bruising at the site of an injury (Fig. 16.2). Platelets are a critical part of the hemostatic plug that forms to stop bleeding acutely. Thrombocytopenia is defined by a platelet count of below 150,000/µL, and although it can be congenital, it is more often acquired. The risk of spontaneous bleeding does not increase significantly until the platelet count is less than 20,000/µL or the individual takes aspirin or nonsteroidal antiinflammatory drugs, both of which can inactivate platelets and enhance bleeding risk.

von Willebrand disease (vWD) is a congenital bleeding disorder that occurs as a result of reduced levels of vWF.[27] vWF has two important roles in hemostasis. First, it binds factor VIII in the blood, prolonging its half-life, and second, it forms a bridge between the endothelium of blood vessels and platelets to initiate hemostasis. Persons can bleed to varying degrees based on their levels of vWF. Persons with moderate or severe deficiency usually present with bleeding complications during childhood, whereas persons with mild deficiency may either have no symptoms or only mildly increased bleeding at mucosal sites.

Deficiencies of the many coagulation factors can occur and lead to increased bleeding. Two of the more common inherited deficiencies are hemophilia A and hemophilia B, which result from decreased production of factor VIII and factor IX, respectively.[28] As with vWD, moderate and severe deficiencies result in serious bleeding early in childhood, whereas persons with mild deficiencies may not have severe bleeding unless they undergo surgery or experience trauma.

Epidemiology

Disorders of hemostasis are uncommon among athletes, both because these disorders are relatively rare in the US population and because when they do occur, many are severe enough to prevent meaningful athletic participation. The incidence of idiopathic thrombocytopenic purpura (ITP) is 2 to 4 per 100,000 adults.[29] ITP can occur in both children and adults, and it is more common in women than in men. Drug-induced thrombocytopenia is also rare but can occur with exposure to many classes of drugs, including sulfa, antibiotics, and quinine.[30] The most common drug-induced thrombocytopenia is related to

heparin exposure, which would most likely occur either in the postoperative or perioperative setting.

vWD is the most common inherited bleeding disorder, affecting up to 1% of the population.[27] Persons with severe disease will generally present with bleeding in childhood, whereas milder disease may not be diagnosed until adulthood. Because the hemophilias are X-linked recessive traits, most cases present in males.[28] Hemophilia A occurs in about 1 in 5000 male births; hemophilia B is less common and presents in 1 in 30,000 male births. As with vWD, persons with severe disease present with bleeding very early in life, whereas persons with milder disease usually present much later in life due to a lack of spontaneous bleeding.[31]

Pathophysiology

The various etiologies of thrombocytopenia have different mechanisms. ITP is thought to be induced by autoantibodies that bind platelets, with subsequent removal from the circulation by the spleen.[32] The antibodies cannot be detected clinically, and therefore the diagnosis of ITP is generally made by a process of exclusion. The antibodies can be induced by drug exposure or can be generated spontaneously, as with an autoimmune disorder. Drugs can also trigger decreased production of platelets, a mechanism that is dissimilar from the peripheral destruction of platelets observed in persons with ITP. Splenic enlargement (hypersplenism), in addition to other cytopenias, can also cause thrombocytopenia.[33] Chronic infections may also lead to thrombocytopenia, which is commonly noted in persons with human immunodeficiency virus and hepatitis C infection.[34-36] In general, low platelets lead to increased bruising, mucosal bleeding, and, very rarely, spontaneous intracranial hemorrhage due to the loss of one of the primary mediators of hemostasis.

Bleeding from vWD is due to either decreased binding of platelets to damaged endothelium or the lack of vWF, which can cause decreased levels of factor VIII.[27] Bleeding is most often mucosal and typically presents as epistaxis or menorrhagia. The degree of bleeding is generally related to the levels of vWF, although other factors likely also contribute to a person's predisposition to bleeding.[37]

Bleeding in persons with hemophilia is a result of decreased activity of either factor VIII or IX, each of which is critical for the integrity of the intrinsic clotting system. Patients with severe hemophilia (<1% of normal levels) have significant difficulty with spontaneous hemorrhage, most often in joints or muscles.[17] Persons with milder deficiencies may not have spontaneous bleeding but will be at risk for significant hemorrhage with trauma or surgery.

Diagnosis

Initial evaluation of an athlete with increased bruising or bleeding should include a CBC, partial thromboplastin time (PTT), and prothrombin time (PT). The CBC will indicate the level of platelets, which may be extremely low in persons with ITP. The PTT is often prolonged in persons with vWD and is significantly prolonged in cases of hemophilia. To mitigate risk for significant bleeding, any athlete with significant abnormalities of platelets, PT, or PTT should be advised to refrain from all physical activity until a thorough evaluation has been conducted by a hematologist.

Isolated thrombocytopenia on a CBC may be induced by a variety of hematologic abnormalities. Occasionally platelets may clump as a result of anticoagulant in the blood sample, thus repeating a CBC is an appropriate first step.[32] A history of other autoimmune diseases should increase suspicion for ITP. Because several drugs can cause thrombocytopenia, a detailed review of exposure to prescription drugs, over-the-counter medications, and supplement use is essential.[29,30] Thrombocytopenia is also relatively common during pregnancy, which must be ruled out in a premenopausal woman. Athletes with more serious diseases, such as thrombotic thrombocytopenic purpura or leukemia, would likely have other symptoms and laboratory abnormalities, yet these diseases should be considered in the differential diagnosis.

Conditions that cause prolongations of the PT and PTT are also relatively common. Vitamin K deficiency and treatment with warfarin are common causes of prolonged PT, and vitamin K deficiency and heparin exposure can prolong PTT. Last, although the situation occurs very rarely, persons can acquire inhibitors to any of the coagulation factors, with factor VIII inhibitors being the most common.

Treatment

Conditions that affect the hemostatic system should be treated as directed after consultation with a hematologist. First-line treatment for ITP is systemic steroids—usually either prednisone or dexamethasone.[29] Most persons respond favorably with an increase in their platelet count, but many experience a relapse after discontinuing steroids, or a relapse may occur spontaneously several months later. If drug-induced ITP is suspected, the first step is to discontinue use of the drug and monitor platelet counts vigilantly. For persons who fail to respond to steroids or withdrawal of the offending drug, a bone marrow biopsy may be necessary to elucidate the etiology.

vWD can be treated with desmopressin, which stimulates release of vWD and factor VIII from storage pools in the body.[27] Patients undergo "desmopressin challenge," and for those who respond, desmopressin is prescribed for use as needed for excessive bleeding. Potential adverse effects of desmopressin include hyponatremia, flushing, alterations in blood pressure, and headache.

The hemophilias are treated with replacement therapy. Both factors VIII and IX are available as recombinant factors that can be administered either for bleeding or prophylaxis against bleeding.[38,39] Patients using replacement therapy should be followed up closely by a hematologist and should be evaluated emergently for either significant hemorrhage or lack of response to treatment at home.

Return-to-Play Guidelines

Decisions about returning to activity should be directed by the degree of hemostatic abnormality and the inherent "sport-specific" risk. A runner who does not have a substantial risk for contact may return to activity with a platelet count below 50,000/μL. This approach is obviously not suitable for persons engaging in contact sports, and evaluation by a hematologist before clearance for participation is critical. It is also crucial that platelet levels be monitored closely, because conditions such as ITP are prone to relapse. A similar algorithm should be adhered to for athletes with either vWD or hemophilia. The degree of deficiency, characteristics of any recent injury, and the amount of contact in the athlete's sport are all vital considerations that facilitate informed medical decisions about return to play by the hematologist and sports medicine staff.

For a complete list of references, go to ExpertConsult.com.

SELECTED READINGS

Citation:

Naik RP, Haywood C. Sickle Cell Trait diagnosis: clinical and social implications. *Hematology Am Soc Hematol Educ Program.* 2015;2015:160–167.

Level of Evidence:

VII

Summary:

This review provides an excellent overview of the current state of knowledge of sickle cell trait, implications of testing and the areas of greatest need for research.

Citation:

Burden RJ, Morton K, Richards T, et al. Is iron treatment beneficial in, iron-deficient but non-anemic (IDNA) endurance athletes? A systematic review and meta-analysis. *Br J Sports Med.* 2015;49:1389–1397.

Level of Evidence:

I

Summary:

This article provides a thorough review of potential benefits of treating of iron deficiency without anemia in athletes.

Citation:

Maron BJ, Harris KM, Thompson PD, et al. Eligibility and disqualification recommendations for competitive athletes with cardiovascular abnormalities: Task Force 14: Sickle Cell Trait: A scientific statement from the American Heart Association and American College of Cardiology. *J Am Coll Cardiol.* 2015;66:2444–2446.

Level of Evidence:

VII

Summary:

This report from a task force from the American College of Cardiology and American Heart Association provides recommendations for athletes with sickle cell trait.

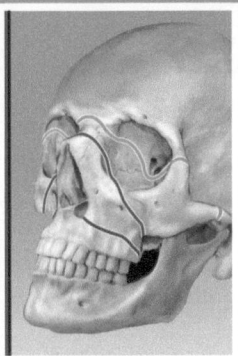

17

Infectious Diseases in the Athlete

Nona M. Jiang, Kathleen C. Abalos, William A. Petri Jr.

Athletic activities and the competitive sports environment present the athlete with unique exposures and risks for infectious diseases. Infectious diseases are responsible for up to 50% of visits in high school and college training rooms. Infections in athletes pose a significant public health concern because of a high frequency of close social and physical contact with teammates, coaches, support staff, and spectators, especially in organized sports at the high school, college, and professional levels. In most cases, the morbidity associated with infectious diseases is mild in this generally healthy population. However, in some rare cases, significant morbidity or even death may occur. Moreover, infectious diseases can disrupt the performance of an individual athlete or a team in competition.[1]

EPIDEMIOLOGY

In sports, the three general modes of transmission of infection are (1) direct person-to-person contact (i.e. through skin), (2) indirect contact (e.g. respiratory, blood-borne, or fecal-oral), and (3) via a common source (e.g. shared water coolers, athletic equipment, locker rooms, whirlpools, swimming pools, and contaminated freshwater venues).[2] Athletes may be more susceptible to infection than the general population for several reasons. They come into close physical contact with each other and may share personal items and equipment. Furthermore, athletes often live in dormitories or hotel rooms while traveling and come into close contact with one another in these settings. Several studies suggest that athletes may be more likely than the general population to engage in risky behaviors.[3] For example, fewer athletes practice safe sex, and athletes are more likely to use illicit drugs, alcohol, and injectable substances such as steroids and hormones, placing them at higher risk for intravenous needle exposures.[3] Last, the growing popularity of adventure sports and ecotourism places participants at risk for exotic illnesses.

Turbeville and colleagues[2] performed a systematic review of the literature characterizing infectious disease outbreaks among athletes that occurred between 1966 and 2005. The skin was the most common site of infection, representing 56% of reported infectious disease outbreaks. Direct, person-to-person (skin-to-skin) contact was the most common mode of transmission. As might be expected, the majority of outbreaks occurred in high-contact sports such as football (34%), wrestling (32%), and rugby (17%). Outbreaks were also reported in soccer, adventure races, swimming, triathlon, track and field, gymnastics, basketball, and

fencing. The most common pathogens are as follows: herpes simplex virus (HSV) (22%), *Staphylococcus aureus* (22%), enteroviruses (19%), tinea (14%), *Streptococcus pyogenes* (7%), hepatitis A and B viruses (7%), measles virus (5%), leptospira (3%), and *Neisseria meningitides* (3%). Norwalk virus, rickettsia, chlamydia, and pseudomonas infections were also reported. Similarly, in a review of infectious disease outbreaks in competitive sports from 2005 to 2010, skin and soft tissue were the most common sites of infection (71%). In this study, methicillin-resistant *S. aureus* (MRSA) (33%) and tinea (29%) were the most common pathogens.[4] It is important to note that nonoutbreak infections also occur and that infections common in the general population are also common in athletes.

EXERCISE AND THE IMMUNE SYSTEM

Physical exercise is known to have important effects on the human immune system that may affect an athlete's risk of infection. The human immune system consists of the innate immune system and the adaptive or acquired immune system. The innate immune system is set up to fight infection regardless of whether a person has been previously exposed. The innate system comprises physical and functional barriers including the skin, mucous membranes, nasal hairs, areas of extreme temperature and pH, and debris removal systems such as the gastrointestinal tract and the mucociliary elevator.[5] The innate immune system also fights infection through natural killer (NK) cells, phagocytes, and proteins such as tumor necrosis factor, cytokines, and the complement system.[5] The acquired immune system is activated by exposure to specific antigens and provides long-lasting protection against anything it has previously encountered, but it does not immediately begin to fight new pathogens. It comprises T and B lymphocytes and their products, immunoglobulins (Ig), and cytokines. The acquired immune system produces IgM about 7 days after exposure to a new pathogen and IgG about 7 days later.[5] Secretory IgA resides in mucous membranes and acts as a first line of defense against infection.

The relationship between the intensity and duration of exercise and the incidence of upper respiratory tract infections (URTIs) tends to follow a J-shaped curve, as illustrated in Fig. 17.1.[6] It is thought that other infectious diseases may follow a similar pattern. Persons who exercise at moderate intensity have the lowest incidence of URTIs. Sedentary persons have a higher incidence of URTIs, whereas extreme exercisers have the highest

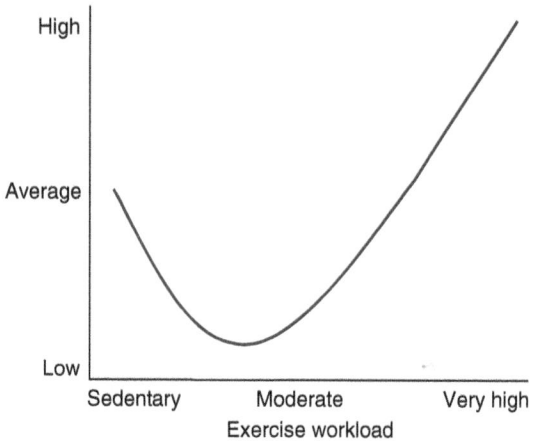

Fig. 17.1 The relationship between exercise duration/intensity and incidence of upper respiratory tract infections/infection risk (J curve). (Modified from Nieman DC. Current perspective on exercise immunology. *Curr Sports Med Rep.* 2003;82:239–242.)

risk. Moderate exercise, defined as exercise for 5 to 60 minutes within a range of 40% to 60% of the maximum heart rate, enhances the immune system by increasing neutrophil and NK counts as well as salivary IgA concentrations.[5] On the other hand, intense exercise, defined as 5 to 60 minutes of exercise at 70% to 80% of maximal heart rate, and prolonged exercise, that is, lasting more than 60 minutes, has detrimental effects on the immune system. An increased requirement for oxygen necessitates transition from nose breathing to mouth breathing during intense exercise.[5] In addition to bypassing the nasal hairs and turbulent flow that normally protects the lungs from exposure to pathogens, inhaling larger volumes of colder and drier hair also thickens mucus and disrupts the mucociliary elevator.[5] Thus greater quantities of foreign particles reach the lungs, and the body's natural defenses are impaired in their ability to clear them. With intense exercise, NK cell, lymphocyte, and neutrophil cell numbers fall, B-cell function decreases, and secretory IgA and serum IgG1, IgG2, and IgE concentrations decline.[5] Levels of cortisol, prolactin, adrenaline, and growth hormone increase, thereby impairing cell immunity.[5] A decrease in salivary lactoferrin and lysozyme concentrations impairs mucosal immunity.[5] All of these factors contribute to a relative immunosuppression that may increase the risk of infection after intense exercise.

PREVENTION

Preventive efforts should focus on primary prevention—that is, avoiding infection before it occurs. Primary prevention includes immunization and good personal hygiene. Secondary prevention consists of infection control measures aimed at preventing the spread of disease to others or recurrence in the source patient, which may include isolation of infected persons or, in some cases, postexposure prophylaxis.

Immunization

Active immunization stimulates an immune response to protect against future exposure to an infectious organism by administering all or part of a microorganism or a modified product of the microorganism such as antigens or proteins. Most vaccines are more than 90% effective, but they are not guaranteed to provide immune protection.[3] Before participation in organized sports, a physician should verify that the athlete has received appropriate immunizations and administer "catch-up immunization" if necessary. Athletes traveling abroad should consider the diseases endemic in the geographic area to which they are traveling. Ideally, immunizations should be planned at least 4 months in advance to ensure adequate time for administration.

Hygiene

Good personal hygiene can help reduce the transmission of infectious agents among athletes. The following general measures are advisable[3]:

- Use universal body fluid precautions; wash hands frequently, and always use disposable gloves when coming into contact with bodily fluids, the oral cavity, or wounds.
- Avoid sharing personal items (e.g., soap, towels, and water bottles), food, and water.
- Routinely clean shared equipment; bleach diluted with tap water in a 1:10 ratio is an effective cleanser.
- Any athlete with skin lesions that are weeping or leaking blood or serous fluid should be excluded from play until the area has dried and can be securely covered with occlusive bandages or dressings.
- Athletes should be instructed to report all illnesses or skin lesions promptly.

Return-to-Play Guidelines

Appropriate and timely guidelines are pivotal for prevention. The decision about whether an athlete may return to play (RTP) after experiencing an infectious illness is based on a number of factors, including the judgment of physicians, coaches, and individual athletes. The first consideration is the effect of athletic activity on the health and safety of the individual athlete. Another important consideration is preventing the transmission of infectious diseases to teammates, support staff, coaches, and spectators. Frequent close contacts during practice, in locker rooms, and in shared living spaces as well as in sharing equipment and facilities create abundant opportunities for spreading and acquiring illness.

Exercise may prolong or intensify the disease course or cause dangerous complications. Fever inhibits fluid and temperature regulation while also impairing coordination, concentration, muscle strength, aerobic power, and endurance.[5] Viral illnesses contribute to tissue wasting, muscle catabolism, and negative nitrogen balance.[5] Drugs used to treat infectious diseases may also have considerable effects on the athlete. For example, quinolone antibiotics carry a risk of tendon rupture. The use of compounds that contain ephedrine, which is banned by many sports organizations, may lead to the disqualification of an athlete. Finally, illness may limit an athlete's performance in competitive sports. Pain, discomfort, and other symptoms of infection can be distracting during play.

A good rule of thumb traditionally used in sports medicine is Eichner's "neck check."[7] Athletes should not work out while experiencing systemic symptoms (e.g., fever or myalgias) or symptoms below the neck (such as a hacking cough, vomiting, or diarrhea). If symptoms are limited to above the neck, such as a runny nose, watery eyes, or sore throat, the athlete can attempt a "test drive." The athlete exercises at "half speed," and if he or she feels better after 10 minutes, it should be safe to complete the workout at a tolerated intensity. Where specific RTP guidelines exist, they are discussed in their corresponding sections.

SKIN AND SOFT TISSUE INFECTIONS

Skin and soft tissue infections comprise most common infectious disease outbreaks in athletes, representing anywhere from 56% to 71% of outbreaks.[2,4] Participants in contact sports such as wrestling, football, and rugby are at highest risk for acquiring such an infection. Frequent skin trauma, moist environments, and direct contact with equipment and other players are all factors that make athletes particularly vulnerable to these infections. The most common causative agents are *S. aureus* and HSV, each constituting 22% of reported infectious disease outbreaks.[2] During the past decade, MRSA has emerged as a common cause of superficial skin infections in the community and has been known to affect a significant number of athletes at the high school and collegiate level. Although most skin infections resolve without complication, they are highly contagious and can result in significant loss of playing time; thus they warrant prompt recognition and treatment. The Centers for Disease Control and Prevention[8] and the American College of Sports Medicine[9] recommend the following preventive measures:

- Practice good personal hygiene: minimize contact, wash hands frequently, shower with soap and hot water after all practices and competitions, and wear sandals in public showering facilities.
- Avoid sharing items that come in contact with the skin (e.g., razors, clothing, linens, and towels).
- Discourage body shaving, which increases the risk of trauma and predisposes to infection.
- Cover wounds (including abrasions, blisters, and lacerations) until they have healed. When wounds cannot be properly covered (by a securely attached bandage that will contain all drainage and remain intact throughout the activity), athletes should be excluded from play.
- Immediately inform coaches of any skin lesions.
- Athletes with active infections or open wounds should avoid common-use water facilities such as swimming pools.
- Thoroughly clean high-touch surfaces (i.e., surfaces that come in frequent contact with people's bare skin each day), including counters, doorknobs, bathtubs, and toilet seats.

When an athlete is diagnosed with a skin infection, care should be taken to appropriately document the diagnosis and treatment to ensure adequate treatment and guarantee meeting return-to-play guidelines. Documentation should include the diagnosis, culture results, date and time of initiation of therapy, and exact names of medications used.[10]

Bacterial Skin Infections
Definition
Superficial bacterial skin infections are most often caused by *Streptococcus* or *Staphylococcus* species.[11] The prevalence of MRSA

has risen dramatically in the community during the past decade. MRSA is a type of staphylococcal bacteria that is resistant to traditional penicillin-based antibiotics and has historically affected patients in health care settings.

Epidemiology
Open or broken skin is the biggest risk factor for bacterial skin infection. Close skin-to-skin contact, contact with contaminated items and surfaces, crowded living conditions, and poor hygiene also place a person at risk for bacterial skin infection.[12] Whereas 25% to 30% of people are colonized in the nose with *Staphylococcus,* fewer than 2% are colonized with MRSA.[13] *S. aureus* and HSV are the most common causes of infectious disease outbreaks in athletes, with each responsible for 22% of outbreaks.[2]

Pathobiology
Bacterial skin infections have a variety of clinical presentations. *S. aureus* and MRSA commonly present as folliculitis, furuncles or "boils" (abscessed hair follicles), carbuncles (coalesced masses of furuncles), and abscesses. Impetigo describes a weepy skin lesion with a honey-colored crust. Erysipelas (a superficial infection of the skin with well-demarcated borders) and cellulitis (subcutaneous involvement with possible systemic symptoms) are most commonly caused by group A *Streptococcus* and *Staphylococcus* species in the athletic population.[12] More virulent strains of *Staphylococcus*, including MRSA, can cause osteomyelitis, sepsis, toxic shock syndrome, and necrotizing pneumonia.[9]

Diagnosis
The hallmarks of a bacterial skin and soft tissue infection include redness, swelling, warmth, and pain/tenderness. MRSA should be considered in the differential diagnosis of any such skin lesions. Cellulitis and abscesses are both considered to be types of superficial wound infections. Cellulitis demonstrates features of both skin erythema and increased warmth and can be more diffuse in nature (Fig. 17.2). An abscess, on the other hand, involves a localized collection of purulent material (Fig. 17.3).[1] MRSA

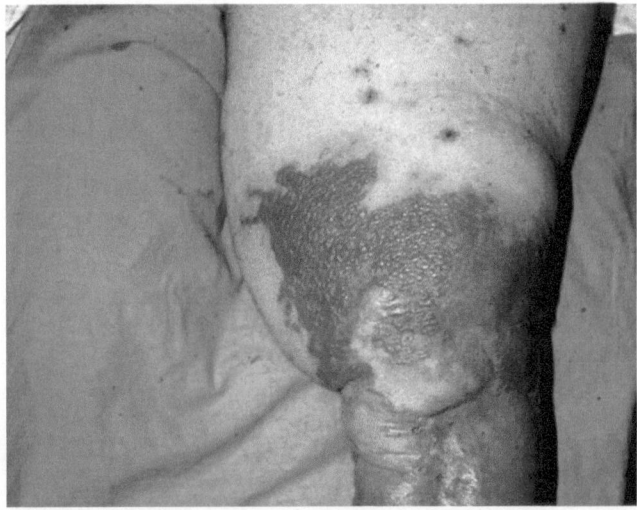

Fig. 17.2 Orthopedic cellulitis. (Courtesy University of Virginia Department of Dermatology, Kenneth Greer, MD, Chairman.)

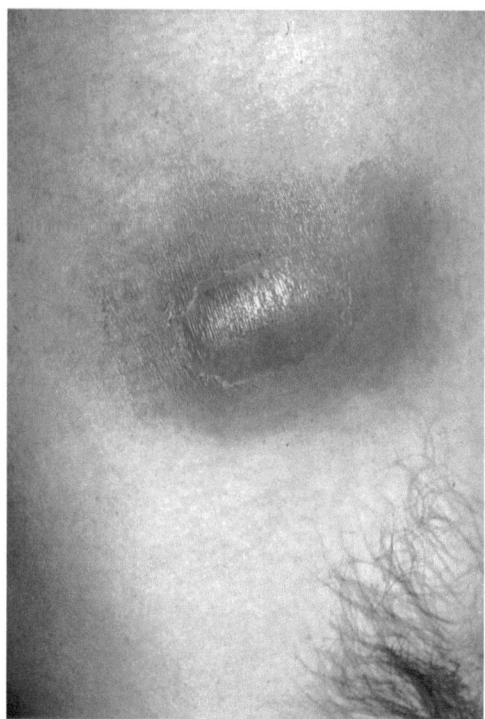

Fig. 17.3 An abscess. (Courtesy University of Virginia Department of Dermatology, Kenneth Greer, MD, Chairman.)

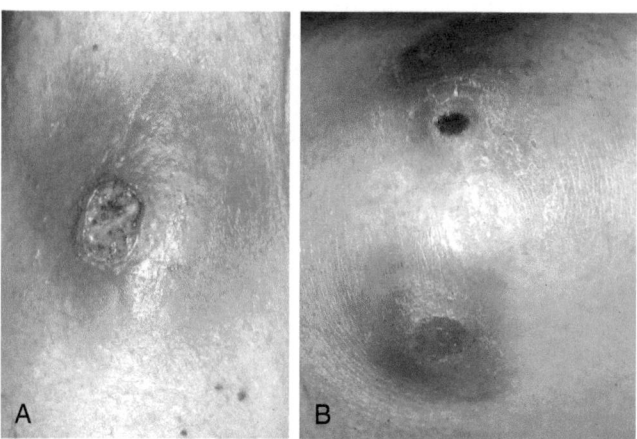

Fig. 17.4 (A and B) Examples of community-acquired methicillin-resistant *Staphylococcus aureus* (MRSA) infections of the skin. Lesions that have signs of necrosis, resemble spider bites, or have pain and erythema out of proportion to visual inspection are highly suggestive of community-acquired MRSA. (Courtesy University of Virginia Department of Dermatology, Kenneth Greer, MD, Chairman.)

infections are commonly mistaken for spider bites. On physical examination, lesions suspicious for MRSA are purulent, exhibiting fluctuance (i.e., a palpable, movable, compressible fluid-filled cavity), a yellow or white center, and a central point or head (Fig. 17.4A and B).[1] They are commonly found at sites of visible skin trauma and areas of the body covered by hair. Nonpurulent cellulitis or erysipelas strongly suggests *Streptococcus* as the causative agent. Bacterial skin infections may resemble insect bites, trauma, superficial burns, contact dermatitis, acne, tinea, dermatophytes, or HSV.[14] A gram stain may elucidate the diagnosis in uncertain cases. A culture of the skin lesion may be useful in

cases of recurrent or persistent infection, antibiotic failure, or advanced or aggressive infections.

Treatment and Prevention

In 2011, the Infectious Diseases Society of America released evidence-based guidelines for the empiric treatment of bacterial skin infections based on clinical features.[15] Simple infections presenting as impetigo, simple abscesses, furuncles, and carbuncles may resolve by applying moist heat and/or applying mupirocin topically twice daily for 10 days. Incision and drainage is the mainstay therapy for simple infections that do not resolve when treated with moist heat and mupirocin. Drainage fluid should be sent for culture and susceptibility testing to direct antibiotic therapy. In addition to incision and drainage, empiric antimicrobial therapy with coverage for MRSA should be considered if the lesion is severe or extensive (e.g., involving multiple sites, associated with cellulitis, or having signs and symptoms of systemic illness), located in an area that is difficult to drain (such as the face, hand, and genitalia), or fails to respond to incision and drainage alone after 48 hours, or if the patient is immunosuppressed or at the extremes of ages. Five to 10 days of therapy is recommended. If cellulitis is present without evidence of purulence or abscess, the causative organism is more likely to be *Streptococcus* and can be treated with a β-lactam antibiotic (e.g., first-generation cephalosporin). If it fails to improve or the patient experiences systemic symptoms, treating physicians should strongly consider the possibility of community-associated MRSA. The treatment of purulent cellulitis warrants empiric treatment for MRSA with trimethoprim-sulfamethoxazole, doxycycline, clindamycin, linezolid, or minocycline.

No clear evidence exists for the effectiveness of decolonization therapy for recurrent MRSA skin and soft tissue infections. However, decolonization may be considered if (1) the patient experiences recurrent skin and soft tissue infections despite optimizing hygiene and wound care or (2) ongoing transmission is occurring among close contacts despite optimization of hygiene and wound care. Decolonization methods include use of nasal mupirocin, skin antiseptic solution (e.g., chlorhexidine), or dilute bleach baths. Oral antimicrobial therapy is recommended only for the treatment of active infection. An oral agent in combination with rifampin may be considered for decolonization if infections recur despite use of the aforementioned methods.

Return-to-Play Guidelines

RTP guidelines for all bacterial skin infections (e.g., furuncles, carbuncles, folliculitis, impetigo, cellulitis, erysipelas, staphylococcal disease, and community-acquired MRSA) are grouped together. As published in the National Collegiate Athletic Association (NCAA) guidelines for wrestling, the following criteria apply before returning to play[10]:

- The athlete must have no new skin lesions for 48 hours before participating in a tournament or practice.
- The athlete must have completed 72 hours of oral antibiotic therapy (the National Federation of High Schools requires oral antibiotic therapy for 48 hours).
- The athlete must have no moist, exudative, or draining lesions while participating in a tournament or practice.

Although no specific guidelines are outlined for other sports, the guidelines for wrestling should be followed for other contact sports (such as football and rugby), sports with shared equipment or facility use (such as gymnastics or aquatic sports), and noncontact sports on a case-by-case basis. All dry lesions should be covered during play.

Herpes Simplex Virus

Definition

HSV can cause primary or recurrent infections and is highly contagious. HSV infections are exceedingly common in the general population and sufficiently prevalent in the athletic population that special terms have been coined to describe outbreaks in sports medicine: *Herpes gladiatorum* was originally used to describe HSV infection in wrestlers, and *scrumpox* to describe HSV in rugby players.[16,17]

Epidemiology

HSV is responsible for 22% of infectious disease outbreaks in athletes, making it and HSV the most common pathogens encountered. One survey reported that the annual incidence of HSV lesions was 7.6% among college wrestlers and 2.6% among high school wrestlers.[8] Transmission can occur by direct skin-to-skin contact or bodily fluids including saliva, semen, and vaginal secretions. It is estimated that the likelihood of contracting herpes when sparring with an infected partner during an active outbreak is 32.7%.[8]

Pathobiology

HSV-1 is the most common cause of herpes labialis (affecting the lips), and HSV-2 is the most common cause of urogenital herpes. Primary infection occurs after an incubation period of 2 to 20 days and may be accompanied by systemic symptoms including fever, adenopathy, malaise, myalgias, and headache. HSV remains latent in the neural ganglia, and reactivation may occur in the setting of reexposure, autoinoculation, physical or emotional stress, poor nutrition, ultraviolet radiation, fever, coexisting infection, or immunosuppression. Reactivation of skin lesions is typically preceded by a prodromal phase of neuralgia, tingling, or burning sensations.[16] Systemic symptoms are typically absent in reactivation. Lesions are most commonly present on the lips, head, extremities, and trunk but can also affect the eyes.

Diagnosis

Diagnosis is typically made on the basis of the characteristic clinical appearance of the lesions. Herpetic lesions form a cluster of vesicles on an erythematous base. Vesicles may ulcerate and leave a shallow painful ulcer with surrounding erythema. Lesions subsequently crust or scab while healing, and complete resolution may take up to 2 to 3 weeks. Laboratory testing can be performed to confirm questionable diagnoses but is not required. Viral isolation from tissue culture is the test of choice.[9] A Tzanck test of fluid from a vesicle reveals characteristic multinucleated giant cells.

Treatment

Oral systemic antiviral medication for 5 days is the standard treatment for HSV outbreaks to reduce the duration of the outbreak and time to complete lesion healing. Medications are effective if taken within the first 48 hours of the appearance of any lesion. Acyclovir, valacyclovir, and famciclovir are commonly used. Athletes with a history of recurrent herpes labialis or herpes gladiatorum should be considered for season-long suppressive therapy. Ocular herpes requires an urgent ophthalmologic referral.

Return-to-Play Guidelines

Athletes engaged in contact sports should refrain from playing until all lesions are dry with a firm adherent crust and until the athletes have been taking an appropriate dose of systemic antiviral therapy for at least 120 hours. The NCAA guidelines for RTP for wrestlers after HSV infection are summarized in Table 17.1.[10] Although no official guidelines are available for other sports, these same guidelines can be used to guide RTP for all other contact sports.

Fungal Skin Infections

Definition

Superficial fungal skin infections are caused by dermatophytes, and nomenclature is based on the location of lesions on the body. Tinea capitis refers to infection of the skin and hair on

---

TABLE 17.1 National Collegiate Athletic Association Guidelines for Return to Play After Herpes Simplex Virus Infection

Nature of Infection	Guidelines
Primary	Free of systemic symptoms (e.g., fever and malaise)
	No new blisters for 72 h before practice or tournament
	No moist lesions; must be dried and surrounded by a firm adherent crust
	Must have been taking an appropriate dose of a systemic antiviral therapy for at least 120 h before and at the time of practice or play in a tournament
	Active herpetic infections shall not be covered to allow participation
Recurrent	No moist lesions; must be dried and surrounded by a firm adherent crust
	Must have been taking an appropriate dose of systemic antiviral therapy for at least 120 h before and at the time of practice or play in a tournament
	Active herpetic infections shall not be covered to allow participation
Questionable cases	Tzanck preparation and/or herpes simplex virus antigen assay
	Participation deferred until Tzanck prep and/or herpes simplex virus antigen assay results complete

Modified from National Collegiate Athletic Association Rules Committee. Skin infections in wrestling (Appendix C). In *2017–2018 and 2018–2019 NCAA Wrestling Rules Book*. Indianapolis, IN: National Collegiate Athletic Association; 2017.

the scalp. Tinea corporis, also known as ringworm, refers to infections on the body. Tinea cruris, or jock itch, is the term used to describe groin infections. Foot infections are called tinea pedis or athlete's foot. Tinea gladiatorum describes fungal infections of the skin or scalp in athletes.

Epidemiology

Fungal infections affect between 10% and 20% of the population worldwide, with tinea pedis being the most common clinical manifestation; 70% of adults experience tinea pedis in their lifetimes.[16] Tinea pedis is common in athletes, with an infection rate of about 35%; it is especially common in swimming pool users and marathon runners.[16]

Pathobiology

The causative agents of fungal skin infections are dermatophytes. The major genera of dermatophytes are *Trichophyton, Microsporum,* and *Epidermophyton.* Dermatophytes are transmitted by direct person-to-person contact, animal-to-human contact, contact with fomites, or directly from the soil. Dermatophytes infect the stratum corneum layer of the skin. The host responds by increasing proliferation of the basal cell layer, resulting in epidermal thickening and scale formation. The characteristic tinea corporis lesion is a singular, well-defined, erythematous plaque with an expanding red, raised ring and a central clearing, often accompanied by flaking and pruritus. Tinea corporis in athletes most commonly affects the head, neck, trunk, and upper extremities. Tinea capitis is characterized by an annular patch of hair loss and a gray hyperkeratotic plaque. Tinea cruris affects the pubic area, inguinal folds, and medial thighs. Tinea pedis can present as the interdigital type, with red, weeping, macerated skin and fissures in the web space between toes; the moccasin type, with plaques on the sole and sides of the foot; or the bullous type, with vesicles or bullae filled with clear fluid.

Diagnosis

Dermatophyte infection may be diagnosed clinically based on the characteristic appearance of the skin lesions. Questionable cases may be confirmed by direct microscopy of a potassium hydroxide (KOH) preparation demonstrating septated hyphae. A fungal culture using Sabouraud dextrose agar may be performed if lesions are suspicious but the KOH preparation is negative. Tinea capitis can be distinguished from other causes of localized alopecia by its characteristic gray hyperkeratotic plaque. Tinea corporis and tinea cruris may be distinguished from impetigo, psoriasis, lichen planus, seborrheic dermatitis, pityriasis rosea, and secondary or tertiary syphilis with use of a KOH preparation or fungal culture. Erythrasma, a *Corynebacterium* infection, may resemble tinea cruris, but examination under a Wood light reveals a coral-red color.

Treatment and Prevention

Topical or oral medications may be used to treat cutaneous fungal infections. For the general population, topical therapy is the first-line treatment for tinea corporis and tinea cruris. Oral medications can have significant adverse effects and are thus reserved for extensive or disabling disease, patients for whom topical therapy has failed, and patients who are immunosuppressed. However, tinea capitis requires treatment with an oral agent. When possible, wrestlers and participants in contact sports should also be treated with oral fungicidal medications.[16] Topical agents include imidazoles, allylamines, and napthiomates. The standard duration of treatment is 2 to 4 weeks, and common regimens include terbinafine 1% cream one to two times daily, ketoconazole 2% cream once daily, or Clotrimazole 1% one to two times daily. Oral agents include fungicidal drugs such as allylamines and fungistatic drugs such as imidazoles and griseofulvin. Fungicidal drugs are often preferred because they require shorter courses of therapy.[16] Showering daily after practice or play, drying thoroughly, and wearing cotton socks and underwear can help reduce the incidence of fungal rashes.

Return-to-Play Guidelines

As with other skin infections, athletes with active tinea lesions should refrain from participating in contact sports until the infection has cleared and been adequately treated to avoid transmission to other athletes. The affected athlete should have completed a minimum of 72 hours of topical therapy for skin lesions and a minimum of 2 weeks of systemic antifungal therapy for scalp lesions.[10] Resolution of treated lesions can be evaluated by KOH preparation or review of the therapeutic regimen. All lesions should be covered with a gas-permeable dressing. If lesions are extensive and cannot be adequately covered, the athlete should refrain from play.

UPPER RESPIRATORY TRACT INFECTIONS

Epidemiology

A URTI, or the common cold, is the most common acute illness in the general population. It affects every healthy adult one to six times each year, especially during the fall and winter seasons, and thus is also the most common infection seen among athletes. Respiratory tract infections were found to be among the most common causes of cough in the athletic population.[18] Transmission occurs through (1) direct contact, when secretions are transferred from hand to hand, then from hand to mucus membranes of the nose or eyes, or (2) respiratory transmission via small-particle aerosols and large-particle droplets. Athletes have an elevated risk of exposure because of the high frequency of close contact while practicing and traveling together.

Pathobiology

The vast majority of URTIs have a viral etiology: rhinoviruses (40%), coronaviruses (20%), respiratory syncytial virus (10%), influenza virus, parainfluenza virus, and adenovirus.[19] Two to 3 days after exposure a patient typically experiences rhinorrhea, cough, and fever. URTIs are generally self-limiting and last 5 to 14 days. Complications may include acute sinusitis, lower respiratory tract infection, otitis media, and asthma exacerbation. URTIs are a common trigger for asthma attacks and are estimated to be responsible for 40% of asthma attacks.[19]

Inflammation of the paranasal sinuses, especially maxillary and frontal sinuses, are caused by the same viruses that cause URTIs, and approximately 2.5% of adult patients experience acute bacterial sinusitis as a complication after a URTI.[5] Acute bacterial sinusitis is most commonly caused by *Streptococcus pneumoniae, Haemophilus influenzae, Moraxella catarrhalis, S. aureus,* and anaerobes. Athletes who participate in swimming, diving, water polo, and surfing seem to have a higher incidence of sinusitis.

Diagnosis

Laboratory testing is not routinely needed for URTIs; the diagnosis is clinical and treatment is based on symptoms. Acute bacterial sinusitis should be suspected in patients whose URTI symptoms are accompanied by purulent nasal discharge and maxillary or facial pain and who demonstrate a poor response to decongestants or abnormal transillumination.[19] Sinus aspirate culture is the gold standard for diagnosing sinusitis, but it is rarely performed because of its invasive nature. Imaging studies such as a computed tomography (CT) scan or magnetic resonance imaging (MRI) may be used if disease persists despite optimal therapy.

Treatment and Prevention

URTIs are treated symptomatically with oral decongestants and antihistamines or nasal decongestant sprays, analgesics, and antipyretic agents. The use of compounds that contain ephedrine, including many oral decongestants, is banned by many sports organizations and may lead to disqualification of an athlete. Athletes should take care to remain adequately hydrated. If the URTI is caused by an influenza virus, a neuraminidase inhibitor such as zanamivir or oseltamivir may decrease the severity and duration of symptoms if it is initiated within 48 hours of exposure.[3] Antibiotics are not beneficial for simple URTIs but may be useful for acute bacterial sinusitis if symptoms worsen over 5 to 7 days or fail to improve after 10 days. Empiric treatment for acute bacterial sinusitis is amoxicillin for 10 to 14 days.[19] Influenza vaccine has an efficacy of 70% to 90%; thus athletes without contraindications should be vaccinated annually.[5]

Return-to-Play Guidelines

In the case of a simple URTI, RTP generally depends on the athlete. It can be expected that athletic performance may be adversely affected during illness, but exercise does not seem to alter the course of the illness. Sedentary subjects who exercised after getting a URTI did not experience an effect on symptoms or duration of illness.[20,21] The "neck check" principle applies; as long as the patient is afebrile and symptoms described are "above the neck," an athlete may continue physical activity as tolerated.

Infectious Mononucleosis
Definition

Infectious mononucleosis (IM), a common medical condition caused by Epstein-Barr virus (EBV), warrants special mention for two reasons: (1) epidemiologically, it is most clinically significant in the adolescent and young adult age group, which is the primary age group engaged in athletic activity, and (2) the most feared complication of IM, splenic rupture, raises important questions for sports medicine physicians making decisions for suitability of an athlete to RTP.

Epidemiology

The prevalence of IM in the general population is 45 cases for every 100,000 people.[22] Antibodies to EBV eventually develop in approximately 95% of adults, indicating prior infection.[22] The peak incidence of IM occurs in 15- to 25-year-olds, and this age group is also most likely to experience acute symptomatic infection. Symptoms rarely develop in adults older than 35 years or in children younger than 15 years.

Pathobiology

EBV is a DNA herpesvirus that is transmitted via oropharyngeal secretions; it is thus referred to as the "kissing disease." It may be acquired through sharing drinks or eating utensils and through aerosolized secretions from sneezing and coughing. EBV enters squamous epithelial cells of the oropharynx and has also been isolated from epithelial cells of the cervix and semen. It is often difficult to identify the source because EBV has a very long incubation period of 30 to 50 days before the onset of symptoms. The classic triad of IM is fever, sore throat, and lymphadenopathy. Patients often experience a prodrome of malaise, headache, and high fever that can last up to 3 weeks. Splenomegaly occurs in 50% to 100% of patients. A rash on the trunk and upper arms occurs in 10% to 40% of patients and is more common in persons treated with ampicillin or amoxicillin.[23]

Whereas most cases of IM are moderate in severity and resolve without complication, complications have the potential to be severe. Reported but rare complications include Guillain-Barré syndrome, meningitis, neuritis, hemolytic uremic syndrome, disseminated intravascular coagulation, and aplastic anemia. In the athletic population, three complications are of particular concern:
1. Severe tonsillar enlargement leading to acute respiratory compromise
2. Prolonged fatigue limiting return to the preillness level of activity for up to 3 months
3. Splenic rupture, which, although extremely rare, usually occurs within the first 3 weeks of symptomatic illness[22]

It is thought that lymphocytic infiltration of the spleen disrupts its normal anatomy, weakening supporting structures and increasing splenic fragility. Rupture can be caused by trauma in the setting of a sudden increase in portal venous pressure from a Valsalva maneuver or compression from external trauma. The occurrence of spontaneous rupture in the absence of trauma has been reported in only a handful of cases.[24]

Diagnosis

Clinical assessment remains the predominant method of diagnosing IM. The differential diagnosis should include viral or bacterial pharyngitis, *Streptococcus, Gonococcus,* human immunodeficiency virus (HIV), and cytomegalovirus. It is particularly important to test for *Streptococcus,* with which an estimated 30% of patients with IM are coinfected.[22] Untreated group A, β-hemolytic streptococcal infections may result in glomerulonephritis or rheumatic fever.

On physical examination, fever is often high and can be greater than 104°F. Exudative tonsillar pharyngitis is present and may be accompanied by palatal petechiae. Lymphadenopathy is typically painful and most commonly affects the posterior cervical chain. Axillary and inguinal involvement may help to differentiate IM from other forms of viral or bacterial pharyngitis. Laboratory findings of leukocytosis in the range of 12,000 to 18,000 white blood cells with greater than 50% lymphocytes and at least 10% atypical lymphocytes on a peripheral blood smear are highly suggestive of IM. The monospot test for heterophile antibodies is specific but not sensitive, especially early on in the disease course. The false-negative rate is 25% in the first week but drops to 5% in the third week. In children younger than 10 years, the monospot test detects fewer than 50% of EBV infections.[22] In a small minority of patients, a seropositivity for heterophile antibodies will never develop.[9] When the monospot test is negative and IM is strongly suspected, EBV titers can be obtained. Specific antibody tests for EBV include viral capsid antigen (VCA), IgG, and IgM antibodies, along with antibody to Epstein-Barr nuclear antigen. VCA IgM appears early in infection and disappears after 4 to 6 weeks. VCA IgG peaks at 2 to 4 weeks after onset and then declines slightly and persists for life. Epstein-Barr nuclear antigen antibody appears after 2 to 4 months and persists for life.[22]

Splenomegaly is almost universal, but no gold standard exists for its diagnosis. The utility of bedside examination to detect splenomegaly is limited. Both palpation and percussion are recommended, but they have a sensitivity of 46% and a specificity of 97%.[22] Physical examination may further be limited by the rigid abdominal musculature of athletes. Few data exist to support the use of diagnostic imaging to evaluate for splenic size. When evaluating for splenomegaly, serial measurement by ultrasound is preferred rather than CT because of its lower cost and the avoidance of radiation exposure. Although the spleen can be accurately sized, spleen size varies greatly between persons, and no normative data are available. Without knowing a baseline spleen size, one cannot determine whether a patient has splenomegaly, but serial studies may be helpful. If splenic injury is suspected, CT or MRI is preferable to ultrasound to acquire higher-resolution images.

Treatment and Prevention

IM is generally self-resolving and thus the mainstay of treatment is symptomatic relief and supportive care: fever control, analgesia for pharyngitis, rest, and hydration. Antiviral medications have not been shown to diminish the severity or duration of symptoms.[9] All patients should be evaluated for coexisting streptococcal pharyngitis. If present, it should be treated with antibiotics other than amoxicillin and ampicillin, which may provoke rashes in patients with IM. Oral corticosteroids may be helpful if the course is complicated by hepatitis, myocarditis, hemolytic uremic syndrome, neurologic complications, or airway obstruction. Patients should be advised to avoid consumption of excessive alcohol, acetaminophen, and other liver toxins. Athletes should be advised that EBV is present in oropharyngeal secretions. Avoiding contact with secretions through the sharing of food, eating utensils, water bottles, and kissing may decrease the risk of transmission.

Return-to-Play Guidelines

The decision about when an athlete can RTP after an IM infection is difficult because the risk of splenic rupture is not well characterized. The consensus statement by the American College of Sports Medicine states that light, noncontact activity may gradually be introduced as tolerated 3 weeks after illness onset provided that the patient is afebrile, has good energy levels, and has no other complications.[9] Although splenic rupture can occur with trauma, most ruptures are atraumatic and occur in the first 3 weeks of illness. During this time, athletes should be advised to avoid chest or abdominal trauma, significant exertion, or Valsalva activities including weightlifting and rowing.

The American College of Sports Medicine recommends avoiding contact or collision sports until 4 weeks after the onset of illness.[9] However, it is important to remember that splenic rupture has been reported to occur up to 7 weeks after the onset of illness.[22] Athletes should be aware that the risk of splenic rupture decreases with time but is never zero. Many persons advocate that the athlete should have a "normal"-sized spleen before returning to play, with the thought that risk of rupture may be highest when the spleen is enlarging. In reality, the relationship between splenomegaly and rupture is unclear. Because of the limitations previously discussed, it is not standard practice to determine splenic size using diagnostic imaging. Serial ultrasonography may be useful in cases where the patient becomes clinically asymptomatic early and is considering early RTP.[22] Prolonged fatigue may limit full performance status for as long as 3 months.[22]

Measles
Definition and Epidemiology

Measles, or rubeola, is an acute, highly contagious viral illness. Airborne measles outbreaks have been known to occur in indoor sports among gymnasts, wrestlers, basketball players, and spectators in crowded and humid gymnasiums and sports domes.[20] Measles is still endemic in many countries worldwide and results in an estimated 800,000 deaths per year. In the United States, between 1996 and 2000, the incidence of measles was less than 1 case per million.[25] Approximately 62% of cases were internationally imported, but a number of cases had an unknown source. The majority of infections occur in unvaccinated patients (46%) and in patients in whom vaccination status was unknown (27%), but 27% of cases in the year 2000 occurred in patients with a documented history of measles vaccination.[25]

Pathobiology

Measles is primarily transmitted directly via respiratory droplets traveling over short distances and less commonly via small-particle aerosols that persist in the air for a long time.[26] During the incubation period of 10 to 14 days, the measles virus replicates initially in the epithelial cells of the upper respiratory tract and then spreads to local lymphatic tissue, the blood, and many organs including the lymph nodes, skin, kidney, gastrointestinal tract, and liver. The host cellular immune response at the sites of replication produces signs and symptoms. Persons with impaired cellular immunity may have absent or delayed presentation of symptoms. The prodromal phase of measles presents with fever, cough, coryza, and conjunctivitis. Koplik spots, which are small white lesions on the buccal mucosa during the prodromal phase, are diagnostic for measles. Several days before the onset of rash, prodromal symptoms intensify. The characteristic rash is an erythematous macropapular eruption beginning on the face and then spreading to the trunk and extremities, which lasts for 3 to 5 days. Patients are infectious for several days before and after the onset of the rash.[26]

In uncomplicated cases of measles, resolution begins shortly after the appearance of the rash. However, after infection with measles, persons have depressed immunity as a result of delayed-type hypersensitivity and are thus more susceptible to secondary bacterial or viral infection.[26] Consequently approximately 40% of cases are followed by complications, including pneumonia, laryngotracheobronchitis, keratoconjunctivitis, stomatitis, and diarrhea. Rare but serious central nervous system (CNS) complications may occur 2 weeks to several years after infection, including postmeasles encephalomyelitis, measles inclusion body encephalitis, and subacute sclerosing panencephalitis.

Diagnosis

Measles should be suspected in any patient who presents with fever and a generalized rash. The differential diagnosis includes other viral exanthems such as rubella. Koplik spots are diagnostic of measles prior to the appearance of a rash. A physical examination should include investigation for secondary viral or bacterial infections. The diagnosis of acute measles can be confirmed with serology. The most common test is detection of measles virus–specific IgM in serum or oral secretions, but it may not be detectable for 4 days after rash onset and disappears within 4 to 8 weeks of infection. Levels of measles virus–specific IgG four times greater than convalescent levels may also be diagnostic of an acute infection.[26]

Treatment

The World Health Organization recommends administration of vitamin A, 200,000 international units daily for 2 consecutive days, for all patients older than 12 months to treat measles and reduce morbidity and mortality.[26] No specific antiviral agents are indicated for treatment of measles, but ribavirin, interferon-β, and other antiviral drugs are used in persons with severe infections. Antibiotics may be required if the patient is coinfected with bacteria. *S. pneumoniae* and *H. influenzae b* are common pathogens. The attenuated vaccine is the best available method of primary prevention.

Return-to-Play Guidelines

Athletes with suspected measles should be isolated from other players expediently. All cases of measles should be reported to public health authorities so that appropriate infection control measures can be administered.

LOWER RESPIRATORY TRACT INFECTIONS

Lower respiratory tract infections have two main clinical presentations: acute bronchitis and acute pneumonia.

Acute Bronchitis
Definition
Acute bronchitis is inflammation of the bronchial tree with cough lasting about 3 weeks, with or without sputum production.[5] Acute bronchitis is usually of viral origin, with the most common pathogens being influenza A and B, parainfluenza viruses, coronaviruses, rhinoviruses, and adenoviruses.

Diagnosis
Acute bronchitis is usually diagnosed clinically. Patients present with a dry cough for no more than 3 weeks. On physical examination, coarse breath sounds or wheezes are occasionally heard on auscultation. Chest radiographs are not routinely needed.

Treatment
Acute bronchitis is usually a self-limiting illness that resolves after 3 weeks; thus treatment is symptomatic. Antibiotics are rarely indicated because most cases are of viral etiology. Bronchodilators may be useful to improve respiratory flow dynamics.[5]

Return-to-Play Guidelines
No specific guidelines exist for RTP after an episode of acute bronchitis. Athletes can resume activity as long as they are afebrile, lack other systemic symptoms, and pass the "neck check" described previously.

Acute Pneumonia
Definition
Pneumonia, an infection of the lung, is viral in 30% to 50% of cases. Other pathogens include *S. pneumoniae, Legionella,* and *Chlamydia.*

Pathobiology
Patients present with a cough productive of purulent sputum, shortness of breath, chest pain, malaise, anorexia, fevers, and chills. Symptoms usually improve within 3 days. Fever lasts 3 days and dyspnea may last for 6 days, whereas cough and fatigue last approximately 2 weeks.[27] Of particular concern to the athletic population is that acute pneumonia may be complicated by reactive airway disease, a transient airway obstruction, and hyper-responsiveness, which may take up to 2 months to resolve and thus significantly delay RTP.[27]

Diagnosis
On physical examination, the patient may demonstrate abnormal vital signs including fever, tachycardia, tachypnea, hypoxemia, and hypotension. A chest examination may reveal dullness to percussion, crackles, rales, bronchial breath sounds, tactile fremitus, or egophony. Diagnosis of pneumonia in the context of the clinical picture requires visualization of an infiltrate on a chest radiograph.[28] Investigation for specific pathogens should be performed based on clinical and epidemiologic data if it would significantly alter management from standard empiric treatment. If the patient presents with gastrointestinal symptoms such as nausea, vomiting, or diarrhea in addition to the classic symptoms of pneumonia, *Legionella* is the likely culprit. A blood culture, sputum culture, and urine antigens for *S. pneumoniae or Legionella* may be performed.

Treatment
The first consideration in treating acute pneumonia is whether the patient requires inpatient or outpatient management. To

guide this decision, two severity indices are commonly used in combination with psychosocial factors: (1) the pneumonia severity index, based on patient demographics, comorbidities, examination, and laboratory or radiologic findings,[5] and (2) the CURB-65 (*C*onfusion, *U*remia [>20 mg/dL], *R*espiratory rate [>30 breaths/min], low *B*lood pressure [<90/60 mm Hg], age *65* years or older).[28] Each factor is assigned a point. Recommendations for scoring include the following:

- 0–1: Outpatient treatment
- 2–3: Consider hospitalization versus outpatient treatment with close observation
- 3–5: Inpatient treatment (consider intensive care unit admission on an individual basis)

The Infectious Disease Society of America has published guidelines for empiric antibiotic therapy of community-acquired pneumonia.[28] For previously healthy patients treated as outpatients, macrolides are the first-line treatment. Patients with comorbidities, immunosuppression, or use of antimicrobial agents within the previous 3 months should be treated with a respiratory fluoroquinolone or a β-lactam agent plus a macrolide drug. With regard to duration of therapy, patients should be treated for a minimum of 5 days, be afebrile for 48 to 72 hours, and have stable vital signs.[28] A short-term inhaled bronchodilator may be used if the course is complicated by reactive airway disease.[27]

Return-to-Play Guidelines

As with other respiratory tract infections, athletes can gradually resume activity as long as they are afebrile, lack other systemic symptoms, and pass the "neck check."

BLOOD-BORNE INFECTIONS

It is important to understand and communicate the risk that blood-borne pathogens pose to athletes, how they are transmitted, and how they can be avoided. This section focuses on hepatitis B virus (HBV), hepatitis C virus (HCV), and HIV. Rare reports have been made of sports-related transmission, but it must be emphasized that the vast majority of infections are acquired from off-field behavior. High-risk behaviors include unsafe sexual practices and use of contaminated needles for blood doping and illicit injectable recreational and performance-enhancing drugs. Athletes at greatest risk for sports-related transmission are those who sustain bleeding injuries, have close contact with other players, and play in high-prevalence regions.

It is not recommended that athletes undergo mandatory testing, disclosure, or removal based on their blood-borne pathogen-infected status.[29] The following prevention strategies, published by the American Academy of Pediatrics, should be used to minimize the risk of transmission of blood-borne infections in the athletic setting[30]:

- Adhere to universal precautions when managing bleeding injuries: wear gloves when coming into contact with bodily fluids, remove and dispose of gloves immediately in appropriate containers, and then wash hands thoroughly with soap and water.
- Vaccinate all athletes and support staff coming into contact with injured athletes against HBV.

- Properly cover any wounds or damaged skin.
- Practice good personal hygiene and avoid sharing personal items such as razors, toothbrushes, and nail clippers that may be contaminated with blood.
- Educate athletes regarding the risks of acquiring blood-borne infections on and off the field.

Hepatitis B Virus

Among the blood-borne pathogens, HBV poses the greatest risk of transmission in the athletic setting. HBV is thought to be 100 times more transmissible than HIV and 10 times more transmissible than HCV.[30] HBV infections may clear spontaneously, but in some persons chronic infections develop, and they often have high viral loads. Fortunately a safe and effective HBV vaccine is available, and it is recommended that all athletes and support staff coming into contact with injured athletes be vaccinated.

HBV is highly prevalent in some regions of the world where perinatal transmission is common. The most efficient modes of transmission are through sexual intercourse and parenteral exposure. Mucosal contact with infected blood products can also occur, but to a lesser degree. Sports-related transmission has been reported in high-prevalence regions of the world when chronic carriers engaged in high-contact activities with uncovered wounds. Various professional athletic organizations publish specific guidelines regarding prevention strategies. The NCAA recommends considering the removal of athletes with acute HBV from participation in close-contact sports until they are negative for hepatitis B surface antigen and removal of chronic carriers from close-contact sports.[31] The International Olympic Committee, on the other hand, does not recommend barring athletes based on blood-borne pathogen-infected status.[30]

Hepatitis C Virus

Approximately 1.6% of the US population is infected with HCV.[30] Transmission is predominantly parenteral; most persons acquire the infection through intravenous drug injection. Perinatal and sexual transmission may also occur, but to a much lesser degree. No documented cases of sports-related transmission have been reported, but transmission has been reported in athletes during use of performance-enhancing drugs.[30]

Human Immunodeficiency Virus

The risk of transmission of HIV during athletic activity appears to be extremely low. To date, sports-related HIV transmission has not been reported. Evidence from health care workers suggests that the risk from mucocutaneous exposure is approximately 0.1%. The greatest risks to athletes remain high-risk off-field sexual behaviors and intravenous drug use.[30]

WATERBORNE DISEASES AND RECREATIONAL WATER-RELATED ILLNESS

Waterborne diseases can be transmitted through contaminated drinking water or participation in water-based sports in recreational water facilities. Participation in water-based sports and recreational activities presents a unique set of infectious disease concerns. Epidemiologically, swimmers have higher rates of illness than do nonswimmers, especially gastrointestinal, respiratory, eye-ear-nose, and skin symptoms.[32] Recreational water-related illnesses (RWIs) are associated with swimming in contaminated water venues including swimming pools, hot tubs, rivers, lakes, and oceans. Although most RWIs are self-limited, some infections may be life-threatening or progress to serious chronic conditions.

RWIs peak in the summer months, when recreational water facilities are most heavily used. The majority of waterborne disease outbreaks occur in treated water venues, resulting in 90.7% of cases of waterborne illness.[33] Inadequate treatment, bad hygiene, or equipment failures are responsible for most outbreaks. Higher rates of infection occur among children than among adults because of a naive immune system and behavioral factors such as poor hygiene and ingestion of recreational water. Infections are also more likely to be severe in children, who are more prone to dehydration because of their small size.

The spectrum of illnesses transmitted through recreational swimming from most to least common includes gastrointestinal (48%); skin (21%); respiratory (11%); and ear, eye, neurologic, and wound infections.[33] Diarrheal illnesses are the most commonly reported RWIs, caused by *Cryptosporidium, Giardia, Shigella, Escherichia coli* O157:H7, and norovirus. In treated water venues, *Cryptosporidium* is responsible for 66% of outbreaks. *E. coli* O157:H7 and *Shigella* spp. are responsible for 12% of outbreaks.[34] In freshwater venues, *E. coli* O157:H7 and *Shigella* spp. are the most common pathogens.[34]

Many cases of RWIs are linked to fecal contamination of water. Nonfecal shedding in the form of vomit, mucus, saliva, and skin also occurs. Disease may also spread through contact with contaminated surfaces, biofilms, and free-living organisms in pools, natural spas, hot tubs, and their components—heating, ventilation, and air conditioning—as well as other wet surfaces in recreational facilities. In recreational water facilities, chlorination is the primary defense against infectious disease. In such disinfected settings, disease may result from (1) poor maintenance of disinfectant levels (<1 ppm chlorine, equipment failure, inadequate or improper use of hydrogen peroxide and/or ultraviolet light), (2) chlorine resistance in waterborne pathogens, and (3) failure to practice healthy swimming habits.[32] Although the majority of infections occur in treated water facilities, the increasing popularity of ecotourism and adventure sports has given rise to a number of rare, serious infections including leptospirosis, *Naegleria* infection, and schistosomiasis.

The following general preventive measures are recommended to reduce the risk of waterborne infections:
- Persons with diarrhea should refrain from swimming while symptomatic and for 2 weeks after cessation of diarrhea (especially if diagnosed with cryptosporidium or *Giardia*).[35]
- Shower with soap and water before and after swimming.
- Wash hands with soap and water for at least 20 seconds after using a toilet or after changing diapers and before eating or drinking.
- Avoid swallowing pool water.
- Avoid urinating in pools and prevent direct animal access to recreational waters when possible.

- Take care not to overload facilities; shallow, heavily populated water carries a higher risk of infection.
- Avoid sharing water bottles, ice buckets, and eating utensils.

Fecally-Derived Recreational Water–Related Illnesses

Fecal contamination of water can occur through (1) accidental fecal release by humans, (2) residual fecal material on swimmers' bodies, or (3) direct animal contamination in outdoor pools.[35] Poor personal hygiene is a significant concern because an average of 0.14 g of feces is found on the perianal surface. Children can have up to 10 g of feces on the perianal surface.[34]

Cryptosporidiosis
Definition and Epidemiology

Cryptosporidium is a parasite that causes the diarrheal disease cryptosporidiosis. "Crypto" is a common term referring to both the parasite and the disease. *Cryptosporidium*, transmitted through both drinking and recreational water, is one of the most frequent causes of waterborne illness among humans in the United States. It is responsible for 66% of outbreaks in treated water facilities.[34] *Cryptosporidium* parasites are found worldwide and in every region of the United States. An estimated 748,000 cases of cryptosporidiosis occur in the United States annually.[35]

Pathobiology

Parasites are shed in the stool of persons infected with *Cryptosporidium*. Transmission is via the fecal-oral route and may occur if a person swallows recreational water contaminated with *Cryptosporidium* or ingests food or water that has come in contact with infected stool or contaminated surfaces. Numerous factors contribute to the high transmissibility of this parasite in recreational water facilities. The oocyst form of *Cryptosporidium* is highly resistant to environmental stress and disinfectants. The levels of chlorine required to kill *Cryptosporidium* oocysts are in excess of 30 mg/L, a level prohibitive to swimming. At standard chlorine levels, disinfection requires additional methods such as ozonation, ultraviolet radiation, or filtration. Infected hosts shed a high concentration of parasites, around 10^6 oocysts per gram of stool, and the infectious dose is relatively low; 132 oocysts infects 50% of persons.[32] Hosts may continue to shed oocysts for weeks after cessation of diarrhea.[32] After human ingestion of the oocysts, a 4- to 9-day incubation period occurs, after which the host experiences prolonged diarrhea, vomiting, and abdominal cramps. Gastrointestinal symptoms are usually self-limiting, resolving after 1 to 3 weeks. Some persons may experience a recurrence of symptoms after a brief period of recovery, and symptoms can come and go for up to 30 days.[35] Persons with weakened immune systems, such as those with HIV or those taking immunosuppressive medications, may experience chronic, severe, life-threatening illness.

Diagnosis

The differential diagnosis includes other parasitic, viral, and bacterial gastrointestinal infections. Cryptosporidiosis should be suspected especially if the diarrhea is prolonged, lasting longer than 48 hours. Diagnosis may be made by microscopically visualizing oocysts in the stool using acid-fast staining, direct fluorescent antibody, and/or enzyme immunoassays for *Cryptosporidium* spp. antigens. Detection may be difficult and require several stool samples. Molecular methods such as the polymerase chain reaction (PCR) also may be used.[35]

Treatment

For most persons with healthy immune systems, cryptosporidiosis is a self-limited, self-resolving illness. Preventing dehydration by drinking plenty of fluids is the most important management principle. Young children and pregnant women are especially susceptible to dehydration. Nitazoxanide, 500 mg by mouth twice daily for 3 days, is approved by the US Food and Drug Administration for treatment of diarrhea caused by *Cryptosporidium* in patients with healthy immune systems age 12 years and older, but it may have limited efficacy in immunocompromised persons.[35]

Return-to-Play Guidelines

Persons should refrain from swimming while they are experiencing diarrhea. Those diagnosed with cryptosporidiosis should avoid, swimming for at least 2 weeks after the diarrhea stops. Good personal hygiene should always be practiced: washing hands before preparing or eating food, showering before entering the water, and avoiding swallowing of recreational water.[35]

Infectious Diarrhea

Cryptosporidium is the most common cause of infectious diarrhea acquired through recreational water sports because of its unique resistance to chlorine. Gastrointestinal infections constitute the vast majority of RWIs and may be caused by a number of parasites, bacteria, and viruses. Other causes of infectious diarrhea—which may be transmitted through recreational water, drinking water, or food—are discussed here.

Epidemiology and Pathobiology

High school and college athletes are at risk for gastrointestinal infections because of exposure to common sources of food, water, the environment, person-to-person contact, and the dormitory lifestyle, in which students share bathrooms, living areas, and snack foods. Swimming is an independent risk factor for *Giardia* infection. *Giardia*, like *Cryptosporidium*, is a parasite with a cyst form that is resistant to harsh environmental conditions. However, *Giardia* is much more sensitive to chlorine and is inactivated by standard disinfectant levels. Giardiasis presents with diarrhea, cramps, loss of appetite, fatigue, and vomiting usually lasting 7 to 10 days.[36]

The most common causes of bacterial infectious diarrhea are *E. coli* O157:H7 and *Shigella* spp. Both bacteria are susceptible to chlorine, but failure to maintain disinfection levels may result in infection. *E. coli* O157:H7 initially presents as a nonbloody diarrhea but may have serious complications. Infection can progress to hemorrhagic colitis, and 5% to 10% of persons infected with *E. coli* experience hemolytic uremic syndrome. Patients with hemolytic uremic syndrome present with hemolytic anemia and acute renal failure, often accompanied by vomiting and fever. *E. coli* diarrhea usually resolves in 1 week but the organism may be shed in the stool for 7 to 13 days. *Shigella* infections present with diarrhea, fever, and nausea. *Shigella* is typically a self-limiting infection lasting 4 to 7 days, but the organism may be shed in the stool for 30 days.[36]

Viruses cannot multiply in water, but they may be present in recreational water as a result of shedding by a person during and after infection. In the past 2 decades, an increase in viral outbreaks has occurred, with a preponderance occurring in treated water venues. Sinclair and colleagues[32] have reported that among all known waterborne disease outbreaks between 1951 and 2006, 49% occurred in treated water and 40% occurred in freshwater venues such as lakes and rivers. Inadequate disinfection was linked to 69% of cases involving treated water venues. Six types of viruses are shed after an infection: rotavirus, norovirus, adenovirus, astrovirus, enterovirus, and hepatitis A virus.[32] The most common viral pathogens are noroviruses (45%), adenovirus (24%), echovirus (18%), hepatitis A virus (7%), and Coxsackieviruses (5%).[32] Norovirus is the most common cause of gastroenteritis in adults. Within 48 hours of exposure, patients present with 24 hours of diarrhea, nausea, vomiting, and fever. Viral shedding can occur for up to 5 days after the onset of symptoms. Norovirus may be somewhat chlorine-resistant. Many fecally-derived viruses also cause extraintestinal symptoms; these viruses are discussed separately.

Diagnosis

Most cases of infectious diarrhea are self-limiting, and thus laboratory tests are not routinely needed. In severe or recalcitrant cases, multiple diagnostic tests are available to identify the infectious pathogen. These tests include but are not limited to fecal leukocyte determination, stool culture for enteric pathogens and parasites, stool PCR, *Clostridium difficile* toxin testing, and endoscopy. Laboratory testing may be indicated if the patient has grossly bloody stools, profuse diarrhea with dehydration, duration of illness longer than 48 hours, fever, severe abdominal pain, or diarrhea in immune-compromised or elderly persons.

Treatment

The mainstay of therapy for most cases of infectious diarrhea is supportive treatment and adequate hydration. Treatment of more severe or prolonged cases of infectious diarrhea should be guided by laboratory testing and diagnosis of the specific causative agent.

Return-to-Play Guidelines

Persons should refrain from swimming while experiencing diarrhea and generally for 2 weeks after cessation of symptoms.

Other Fecally-Derived Waterborne Diseases

1. *Adenovirus* may be transmitted both fecally and nonfecally and can present with gastrointestinal infection or pharyngoconjunctival fever.
2. *Hepatitis A* is transmitted through the fecal-oral route and presents with anorexia, nausea, vomiting, and jaundice after an incubation of 15 to 50 days. Infected persons may shed virus prior to the onset of symptoms.
3. *Aseptic meningitis* caused by enteroviruses has occurred in the high school football setting and during an international

soccer tournament in Belgium.[37] The most common pathogens are echoviruses (5, 9, 16, and 24) and Coxsackie viruses (B1, B2, B4, and B5). Infections peak during the summer months. Transmission through sharing of water bottles or drinking cups, ice buckets, and water coolers have been responsible for outbreaks in the athletic setting. Athletes should be discouraged from sharing drinking vessels and ice buckets and encouraged to wash their hands frequently. Echovirus meningitis has also been associated with recreational water use.[32]

NONFECALLY-DERIVED WATERBORNE DISEASES

Pseudomonas Infections

Pseudomonas infections acquired in the setting of recreational water sports have two main clinical manifestations: (1) acute otitis externa (swimmer's ear), commonly acquired in swimming pools, and (2) hot tub folliculitis, acquired in hot tubs and spas.

Pathobiology

Pseudomonas is ubiquitous in water, vegetation, and soil, with a preference for warm, moist environments. *Pseudomonas* bacteria are shed by bathers in pools and hot tubs and on surrounding wet surfaces; they can also accumulate in biofilms in filters. In hot tubs, high temperatures and turbulence promote perspiration and desquamation or shedding of epithelial cells. The increased organic load in the water both provides nutrients for bacterial growth and decreases residual disinfectant levels. *Pseudomonas* is chlorine-sensitive; thus all outbreaks have occurred as a result of inadequate disinfection. Patient risk factors for infection include communal use of an athletic spa, increased duration of exposure, and the presence of skin trauma, such as turf burns and abrasion due to body shaving.[36]

Hot Tub Folliculitis

Hot tub folliculitis is an infection of hair follicles caused by the bacterium *P. aeruginosa*. When bathers use a hot tub, the warm water supersaturates the epidermis, dilating dermal pores and facilitating bacterial invasion. Extracellular enzymes produced by *Pseudomonas* damage the skin. A pustular rash appears anywhere between 8 hours to 5 days after exposure and usually resolves spontaneously within 5 days. The rash is generally more severe in areas that bathing suits cover because swimwear traps the bacteria. Some people report other symptoms such as headache, muscle ache, burning eyes, and fever.[12] This self-limiting infection generally does not require treatment.

Acute Otitis Externa
Definition and Epidemiology

Acute otitis externa (AOE), also known as "swimmer's ear" or "tropical ear," is defined as generalized inflammation of the external ear canal, which may also involve the pinna or tympanic membrane. AOE is a very common infection. The annual incidence of AOE is between 1:100 and 1:250 of the general population, and the lifetime incidence is up to 10%.[38] AOE is more common in regions with warmer climates and increased humidity

and with increased water exposure from swimming. Patient risk factors are increased amounts of time spent in water, age less than 19 years, and a history of previous ear infections.

Pathobiology

In North America, nearly all cases of AOE (98%) are caused by bacteria. The most common pathogens are *P. aeruginosa* (20% to 60%) and *S. aureus* (10% to 70%). Gram-negative bacteria other than *P. aeruginosa* are implicated in 2% to 3%, and polymicrobial infections are common. Fungal involvement is uncommon in primary AOE but may be found in persons with chronic otitis externa or after treatment of AOE with topical antimicrobial agents.[38] Cerumen, with a slightly acidic pH, helps to inhibit infection. Repeated water exposure removes the protective wax coating of the external ear canal. Other behaviors that alter this natural barrier—including removal of cerumen by cleaning of the ear canal, leaving soapy deposits, or use of alkaline eardrops—may increase a person's risk for AOE. Other factors are local trauma, sweating, allergy, and stress.

Diagnosis

The classic presentation of diffuse AOE is tenderness of the tragus (when pushed) and/or pinna (when pulled up and back) that is intense and disproportionate to what might be expected based on visual appearance. Diagnosis is made on the basis of the following clinical criteria[38]:
1. Rapid onset, within 48 hours, in the past 3 weeks AND
2. Symptoms of ear canal inflammation including otalgia, itching, or fullness WITH OR WITHOUT hearing loss or jaw pain AND
3. Signs of ear canal inflammation that include tenderness of the tragus, pinna, or both OR diffuse ear canal edema, erythema, or both, WITH OR WITHOUT otorrhea, regional lymphadenitis, tympanic membrane erythema, or cellulitis of the pinna and adjacent skin.

Alternative diagnoses to consider are acute otitis media, furunculosis (localized AOE usually caused by *S. aureus*), otomycosis, herpes zoster oticus, and contact dermatitis. Unlike the case with acute otitis media, the tympanic membrane should demonstrate normal tympanic mobility in persons with AOE.

Treatment

The clinical practice guidelines released by the American Academy of Otolaryngology–Head and Neck Surgery Foundation in 2006[38] include the following key points:
1. Assess for pain and recommend appropriate analgesic treatment.
2. Use topical preparations for initial therapy of diffuse, uncomplicated AOE. Appropriate topical treatments include acetic acid, boric acid, aluminum acetate, silver nitrate, and *N*-chlorotaurine. A topical steroid is effective as a single agent or in combination with acetic acid. Symptoms should improve or resolve in 48 to 72 hours.
3. Systemic antimicrobial therapy should be used only if there is extension outside of the ear canal or for specific host factors such as diabetes, an immunocompromised state, or a history of radiotherapy.

Prevention strategies attempt to limit water accumulation and retention in the external auditory canal and to maintain a healthy skin barrier. The following measures may help to reduce the risk of AOE: (1) remove obstructing cerumen; (2) use acidifying ear drops shortly before swimming, after swimming, or at bedtime; (3) use a hair dryer to dry the ear canal; (4) use ear plugs while swimming or showering; and (5) avoidance of trauma to the external auditory canal.[38]

Return-to-Play Guidelines

It is recommended that patients with AOE refrain from water sports for 7 to 10 days during treatment. Competitive swimmers may sometimes return to competition with well-fitted earplugs 2 to 3 days after treatment or after the pain has resolved.

NEUROLOGIC INFECTIONS

Meningitis and Encephalitis

Definition and Classification

Acute meningitis is a medical emergency that requires prompt recognition and treatment. Delay in treatment can result in significant morbidity or death. Meningitis is defined as inflammation of the meninges—that is, the membranes lining the brain and spinal cord. Encephalitis is inflammation of the brain parenchyma. The term "meningoencephalitis" refers to a combination of these two processes and the disease usually has a viral etiology.

Meningitis is often classified as either septic (bacterial) meningitis or aseptic (usually viral) meningitis. Septic meningitis is most commonly caused by associated *N. meningitides* (meningococcus) and *S. pneumoniae* (pneumococcus). Aseptic meningitis, usually of viral etiology, is much more common and refers to a clinical syndrome of meningitis with negative Gram stain and bacterial culture of the cerebrospinal fluid (CSF). Meningitis is also classified according to its disease course. Acute meningitis presents within 1 day of onset of symptoms, subacute meningitis occurs within 1 to 7 days of onset, and chronic meningitis persists for 4 or more weeks.

Epidemiology

N. meningitidis outbreaks have been reported among soccer and rugby players.[2] Additionally, multiple reported outbreaks of acute viral meningitis occurred in high school football teams in the United States between 1960 and 1993. This population may be at elevated risk over the general population for several reasons, including repeated close physical contact, close living quarters, and the practice of sharing water bottles. Enteroviruses are usually transmitted via the fecal-oral route but may also be transmitted via respiratory secretions. Finally, the US football season coincides with the peak enteroviral season (late summer and autumn).[39]

Pathobiology

Acute aseptic meningitis is the most common form of meningitis and is usually caused by viruses. Other causes include Lyme disease, tuberculosis, and rickettsia.[40] The most common causes of septic meningitis are *S. pneumoniae* and *N. meningitidis*.

Listeria monocytogenes and group B streptococcus also cause septic meningitis. Cases of *H. influenza* meningitis have declined considerably since the initiation of universal vaccination.

Diagnosis

Management of a patient with suspected meningitis is driven by a critical fact—that a delay in the initiation of therapy significantly increases the already high risk of morbidity and mortality. The practice guidelines published by the Infectious Diseases Society of America present an algorithm for pursuing diagnostic testing in a manner that does not compromise the timely delivery of antimicrobial and adjuvant therapy.[41]

The hallmark symptoms of meningitis are fever, headache, and meningismus (stiff neck). Patients may also have nausea, vomiting, photophobia, malaise, and drowsiness. Altered consciousness is highly suggestive of encephalitis. Septic meningitis is a medical emergency that usually presents with more severe symptoms than aseptic meningitis but may be clinically indistinguishable. All cases of suspected meningitis should be presumed septic until proven otherwise. Initial assessment should determine airway status, respiratory effort and rate, and circulation.

The physical examination should focus on the following goals: (1) detecting signs to support the diagnosis of meningitis, (2) signs that may help identify the offending pathogen, and (3) signs of cerebral edema prior to performing a lumbar puncture. The examiner should check for other signs that may explain symptoms, such as trauma, conjunctivitis, intraocular hemorrhage, or papilledema. The patient is then evaluated for nuchal rigidity, or a decrease in neck suppleness, a sign of meningeal irritation due to infection or hemorrhage. With the patient relaxed, the examiner should first move the head in all planes to assess for resistance to motion. While the patient is supine and passively flexing the neck forward, the examiner should observe the hips and knees. Two signs of meningeal irritation are as follows: (1) flexion of the hips and knees with neck flexion represents a positive Brudzinski sign and (2) pain or resistance to flexion of the hip to 90 degrees with the knee extended represents a positive Kernig sign. A bilateral positive Kernig sign may distinguish meningeal irritation from lumbrosacral nerve root compression, which is usually unilateral. A complete neurologic examination should be performed, including cranial nerve, strength, sensation, and cerebellar testing. Focal neurologic deficits are unusual for most types of acute meningitis and may suggest a mass effect or an atypical infection.

For clues regarding the specific etiology of meningitis, the examiner should perform a skin examination with full exposure. Hemorrhagic skin lesions such as petechiae or purpura are associated with meningococcal meningitis, especially noted most commonly on the limbs. A rash in a stocking-glove distribution is suggestive of a rickettsial infection. Herpetic lesions may implicate HSV.[39]

Lumbar puncture and analysis of the CSF is important for diagnosing meningitis. Although it may reduce the sensitivity of CSF analysis, empiric antibiotic therapy should not be delayed while attempting to perform a lumbar puncture or other testing. Cerebral herniation is a feared complication of lumbar puncture. If the patient is immunocompromised and has a history of CNS disease, papilledema, or focal neurologic deficits, blood cultures should be drawn, empiric antimicrobial therapy should be initiated, and a CT scan should be obtained before a lumbar puncture is performed.[41] Gram stain and culture of CSF should be obtained, but their sensitivity may be reduced by antimicrobial therapy. In persons with aseptic meningitis, the CSF classically demonstrates mononuclear pleocytosis with less than 1000 white blood cells/mm³ and a normal or mildly decreased glucose level. Persons with septic meningitis have a neutrophil-predominant pleocytosis with more than 1000 white blood cells, a low glucose level, and a high protein level. PCR of CSF can detect enterovirus or HSV. Enterovirus can also be detected in the stool or oral mucous membranes.

Treatment and Prevention

For persons with acute meningitis, the primary management goal is early empiric antibiotic treatment in an inpatient setting, preferably with ready access to intensive care. Empiric antimicrobial therapy should be initiated once bacterial meningitis is diagnosed by CSF analysis or upon high clinical suspicion if there is a delay in lumbar puncture.[41] For adults and children between the ages of 2 to 50 years, empiric therapy includes vancomycin plus a third-generation cephalosporin.[41] The spectrum of antibiotic coverage should be narrowed as soon as possible on the basis of CSF culture and susceptibility results. Empiric treatment with intravenous acyclovir is also recommended if the clinical picture suggests HSV infection. Adjunctive dexamethasone is recommended for adults with pneumococcal meningitis.[41]

Routine vaccination with meningococcal vaccine is recommended for college freshmen living in dormitories and other populations at increased risk.[3] For secondary prevention, persons with "high risk" exposure after a confirmed case of meningococcal meningitis should receive chemoprophylaxis with ceftriaxone, rifampin, ciprofloxacin, or passive immunization. The American Academy of Pediatrics Infectious Disease Committee defines "high risk" contacts as household contacts, child care contacts, and anyone with direct exposure to the index patient's secretions through kissing or sharing toothbrushes or eating utensils during the 7 days before the onset of illness.[39]

Return-to-Play Guidelines

Infected players should be isolated from the rest of the team as soon as possible. To date, no evidence-based guidelines exist for RTP from meningitis. As with any other infection, the athlete should be afebrile and have no constitutional signs, and it would be prudent to refrain from play until all symptoms have resolved. A careful neurologic examination should be performed, including a hearing test, and any changes should be noted before RTP. Viral shedding may occur for several weeks after resolution of symptoms; therefore athletes should be counseled on adequate hand hygiene, advised to avoid sharing ice buckets or drinking vessels, and dissuaded from refilling receptacles by dipping them in team coolers. School and local public health authorities should be informed when an outbreak occurs on an athletic team to address risk to close contacts and the community at large.

UNUSUAL INFECTIONS

The increasing popularity of adventure sports and ecotourism, such as triathlons and kayaking, have fostered some rare yet potentially life-threatening infections that are discussed in this section.

Leptospirosis
Definition and Epidemiology

The bacterium *Leptospira interrogans* causes the disease leptospirosis, also known as swineherd's disease, Stuttgart disease, and Weil syndrome. Several outbreaks of leptospirosis have occurred among triathletes and outdoor adventure participants since the 1980s.[42] Leptospirosis occurs worldwide but is more prevalent in temperate or tropical climates. Swimming, wading, kayaking, and rafting in freshwater contaminated with animal urine are associated with leptospirosis.

Pathobiology

Many animals carry *L. interrogans*, including cattle, pigs, horses, dogs, and rodents. Humans can become infected via direct contact with urine from infected animals or contact with water, soil, or food contaminated with the urine of infected animals. Bacteria enter the body through skin cuts and abrasions as well as mucosal surfaces of the mouth, nose, and conjunctiva. Measures should be taken to prevent direct animal access to recreational water. The majority of cases occur in bodies of freshwater such as rivers and lakes or unchlorinated swimming pools. However, *L. interrogans* is susceptible to standard disinfection and has a low resistance to harsh physical conditions.[36] Upon exposure to the bacteria, there is an incubation period of 2 days to 4 weeks. Illness usually begins abruptly with fever, chills, headache, muscle aches, vomiting, or diarrhea. After a period of recovery, a second phase of illness may occur in some patients. The second phase, also called Weil disease, is a severe and potentially fatal condition associated with liver and kidney failure, hemorrhagic jaundice, and aseptic meningitis.[43]

Diagnosis and Treatment

The most sensitive laboratory test early in infection is an IgM enzyme-linked immunosorbent assay for *Leptospira* antibodies. Leptospirosis is treated with doxycycline. More severe infections may require administration of intravenous antibiotics. Persons traveling to areas where leptospirosis is endemic or epidemic and participating in high-risk exposure activities such as swimming or kayaking in freshwater may be benefit from preexposure chemoprophylaxis. Several studies have demonstrated the efficacy of preexposure oral doxycycline 200 mg orally, weekly, begun 1–2 days before and continuing through the period of exposure in reducing clinical symptoms and mortality rate.[43]

Naegleria fowleri
Definition and Epidemiology

Naegleria fowleri, a free-living amoeba that causes a very rare but usually fatal illness in humans called primary amebic meningoencephalitis, is found around the world in soil and bodies of warm freshwater such as lakes, rivers, and hot springs. *N. fowleri* prefers warm water and can reproduce in temperatures up to 46°C.[36] Most infections in the United States have occurred in the southern states. From 2001–2010, a total of 32 infections were reported in the United States; 30 people were infected by contaminated recreational water and 2 were infected from a geothermal drinking water source.[44]

Pathobiology

Infection occurs through forceful inhalation or splashing of contaminated water into the olfactory epithelium, which can occur through diving, jumping, underwater swimming, or nasal irrigation. The amoebae then move into the brain and CNS. After an incubation period of 7 to 10 days, the patient presents with symptoms and signs resembling bacterial meningitis, including headache, high fever, stiff neck, nausea, vomiting, seizures, and hallucinations. Death usually occurs 3 to 10 days after the onset of symptoms.[12]

Treatment

No known treatment exists for *N. fowleri*, and almost all infections are fatal. The only definite way to prevent infection is to refrain from water-related activities in warm, untreated, or poorly treated water. Measures that may reduce risk of infection include the following:

1. Avoidance of water-related activities in warm freshwater during periods of high water temperature and low water levels
2. Holding the nose shut or using nose clips during water-related activities
3. Avoidance of digging or stirring the sediment while swimming in warm freshwater areas
4. Using only water that has been distilled, sterilized, or boiled to irrigate the sinuses

Schistosomiasis

Definition and Epidemiology

Schistosomiasis, a parasitic disease caused by *Schistosoma haematobium, S. japonicum,* and *S. mansoni,* affects approximately 300 million people worldwide. The parasite lives in freshwater in most African countries and some parts of South America, the Caribbean, the Middle East, and Asia. The highest prevalence and parasite load occurs in children aged 5 to 15 years. The emergence of ecotourism and adventure tourism has resulted in a number of imported cases since the 1980s.[45]

Pathobiology

Eggs are excreted in the feces or urine of infected hosts. Snails act as intermediate hosts, releasing cercariae, the infective form. Humans are infected by swimming in contaminated freshwater, when cercariae swim and penetrate the skin. In the human host, the parasite migrates through several tissues and stages before settling in the mesenteric venules. *S. japonicum* and *S. mansoni* usually occupy the superior mesenteric veins draining the small and large intestines, causing gastrointestinal and hepatosplenic schistosomiasis, whereas *S. haematobium* often resides in the venous plexus of the bladder, causing urinary schistosomiasis.[46]

Most infections are asymptomatic and often overlooked. Contact with the penetrating cercariae may cause "swimmer's itch" or "cercarial dermatitis," a micropapular dermatitis that disappears within 48 hours after contact with contaminated water. Katayama fever may occur 3 to 6 weeks after heavy exposure and is an acute toxemic syndrome that affects a varying percentage of exposed persons. Hallmark clinical features include fever, malaise, and eosinophilia. Less commonly hepatosplenomegaly, diarrhea, urticaria, and edema can occur.[45]

Left untreated, transient symptoms disappear and infection progresses to a chronic phase. *S. haematobium* typically causes urinary schistosomiasis, with hematuria, proteinuria, leukocyturia, dysuria, and nocturia. Patients with chronic urinary schistosomiasis experience obstructive uropathy, hydronephrosis, and calcified fibrotic bladder and/or ureter. *S. mansoni, S. japonicum, S. mekongi, and S. malayi* typically cause gastrointestinal and hepatosplenic schistosomiasis. Patients initially present with bloody diarrhea, followed by the development of chronic colitis with possible colonic polyps. Severe, long-standing infections may lead to portal hypertension caused by fibrosis induced by retained eggs. CNS involvement may occur after embolization of eggs from the portal mesenteric system.[45]

Diagnosis

Diagnosis is usually made on clinical and epidemiologic grounds. Eggs may not be detectable in the stool during the acute phase because of a low parasitic load. Serologic confirmation of the diagnosis based on antigen detection is possible 5 to 6 weeks after the acute infection. Tissue biopsy or ultrasonography may also aid in diagnosis.

Treatment

Praziquantel at a dose of 40 mg/kg per day orally in two divided doses for 1 day is effective against all *Schistosoma* spp., but it kills only the adult worm. *S. japonicum* requires a higher dose of 60 mg/kg per day orally in three divided doses for 1 day. If treatment is started during the initial phase of illness, a second dose is required once all worms have reached the adult stage. The drugs trichlorfon and oxamniquine are also used in areas where a single species exists. Corticosteroids are helpful in reducing the immunologic reaction in Katayama fever, but with the use of corticosteroids, praziquantel dosing must to be increased to 20 mg/kg every 12 hours for 3 days.

For a complete list of references, go to ExpertConsult.com.

SELECTED READINGS

Citation:
Turbeville SD, Cowan LD, Greenfield RA. Infectious disease outbreaks in competitive sports. *Am J Sports Med.* 2006;34:1860–1865.

Level of Evidence:
IV

Summary:
An epidemiologic study reviewing the medical literature for reported outbreaks of infectious diseases in competitive athletes from 1966 through May 2005.

Citation:
Sedgwick PE, Dexter WW, Smith CT. Bacterial dermatoses in sports. *Clin Sports Med.* 2007;26:383–396.

Level of Evidence:
IV

Summary:
An expert review of clinical presentation, diagnosis, treatment, and return-to-play guidelines for the most common bacterial dermatoses in athletes.

Citation:
Pleacher MD, Dexter WW. Cutaneous fungal and viral infections in athletes. *Clin Sports Med*. 2007;26:397–411.

Level of Evidence:
IV

Summary:
An expert review of the clinical presentation, diagnosis, treatment, and return-to-play guidelines for the most common fungal and viral dermatoses in athletes.

Citation:
Boulet LP, Turmel J, Irwin RS, et al. Cough in the athlete: CHEST guideline and expert panel report. *Chest*. 2017;151(2):441–454.

Level of Evidence:
IV

Summary:
This systematic review examines the main causes of acute and recurrent cough, how cough is assessed, and how cough in treated in athletes.

Citation:
American Medical Society for Sports Medicine, American Orthopedic Society for Sports Medicine. Human immunodeficiency virus and other blood-borne pathogens in sports. (Joint position statement). *Clin J Sport Med*. 1995;5:199–204.

Level of Evidence:
IV

Summary:
A concise summary of blood-borne illnesses and safe practices in competitive sports.

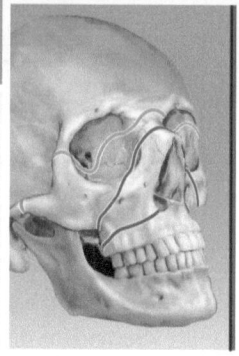

18

The Athlete With Diabetes

Jessica A. Lundgren, Susan E. Kirk

DEFINITION

Diabetes mellitus is a disorder of glucose metabolism that affects millions of athletes of all types around the world. It is caused by either an absolute (type 1 diabetes) or relative (type 2 diabetes) deficiency in insulin, the principal hormone that regulates carbohydrate and fat metabolism. Diabetes mellitus is one of the most common chronic medical illnesses to be encountered by sports medicine specialists, coaches, and athletic trainers who work with adolescent and young adult athletes. Two other classifications of diabetes, *gestational* and *overt,* are both associated with pregnancy and are also caused by a relative insulin deficiency. In the former, glucose metabolism is normal at the time of conception and early in pregnancy. However, as the pregnancy progresses, glucose intolerance develops as a result of placental hormones that induce insulin resistance in the mother. The latter category is a recent classification which reflects that in women at high risk for diabetes, glucose intolerance or frank diabetes likely existed at the time of conception or early in pregnancy but had been undetected or undiagnosed.[1] Although women with gestational or overt diabetes may represent only a small fraction of the athletes competing with underlying diabetes, good control of blood glucose, in part achieved by regular physical activity, is especially important to protect the health of the mother and the fetus.

Exercise and athletic activity, together with medication and diet, have long been cornerstones in the treatment of diabetes and the subsequent prevention of long-term complications that affect the eyes, kidneys, cardiovascular, and nervous systems. However, the alterations in metabolism that occur during athletic activity—specifically those related to the control of blood glucose—can often present a significant challenge for the athlete with diabetes, along with his or her coaches and care providers. Athletic activity, if not properly managed, can increase the risk for the short-term complications of hypoglycemia or significant hyperglycemia, especially in athletes with type 1 diabetes. Both of these metabolic disturbances can have a negative impact on athletic performance. Athletes with diabetes must commit to understanding their illness, and they must expend considerable effort to record and analyze the impact of different activities on their blood glucose levels. In addition, all persons involved in the care of an athlete with diabetes need to have a basic understanding of the metabolic changes that accompany the disorder, how they are influenced by exercise, and methods of testing and treating diabetes so they can promote both good health and ideal performance.

EPIDEMIOLOGY

The prevalence of diabetes in American adults has increased markedly in recent decades, from 0.2% in the 1980s, 3.5% in 1990, 7.9% in 2008, and 8.3% in 2012.[2] Recent data published by the Centers for Disease Control and Prevention also show alarming incidence in children and young adults in the United States.[3] As of 2012, 29.1 million children and adults, or 9.3% of the total population, had either type 1 or type 2 diabetes. Eight million of these persons were living with undiagnosed diabetes. Furthermore, 37% of US citizens aged 20 or older have "prediabetes," determined by a fasting glucose or hemoglobin A1c that is elevated but not yet diagnostic for diabetes. Many of these 86 million people are at risk for developing type 2 diabetes; importantly, lifestyle modifications, and in particular exercise, can substantially lower this risk.

The prevalence of diabetes in children and young adults is also striking: nearly 1 in every 400 has diabetes, representing 0.25% of this population.[3] In 2008–09, more than 18,000 people aged 20 or younger in the United States were diagnosed with type 1 diabetes and more than 5000 aged 20 or younger were diagnosed with type 2 diabetes. Children of African-American, Hispanic/Latino, Native American, Asian, and Pacific Islander descent are more likely to be diagnosed with type 2 rather than type 1 diabetes. Type 1 diabetes is diagnosed at the highest rate in non-Hispanic white children. Because of the substantial increase in the number of children, adolescents, and young adults with diabetes, it is quite likely that persons involved in the management of sports will encounter, with increasing frequency, athletes who have diabetes.

DIAGNOSIS

Most athletes with diabetes are already aware of their disease when they enroll in athletic activity. However, because the incidence in children, adolescents, and young adults is considerable, it is important that coaches and athletic trainers be aware of the symptoms of hyperglycemia. When an athlete experiences a significant (>180 mg/dL) and persistent elevation of blood glucose levels, the resultant osmotic diuresis leads to dehydration and a hyperosmolar state. Symptoms of hyperglycemia include blurry vision, polyuria, nocturia, and polydipsia. Coaches and athletic trainers associated with the athlete are more likely to first notice subtle signs of hyperglycemia, such as easy fatigability or malaise. A thorough evaluation and the initiation of treatment at that time may help prevent the more serious complications of hyperosmolar coma or diabetic ketoacidosis. Although it would be difficult for an athlete to continue to practice or play regularly in the setting of serious metabolic disturbance, these critical states will eventually develop in the absence of treatment.

In the presence of any of the symptoms of hyperglycemia, a random glucose level of greater than 200 mg/dL is diagnostic of diabetes mellitus.[4] Both a fasting plasma glucose greater than 126 mg/dL (repeated once for confirmation) or a 2-hour glucose value of greater than 200 mg/dL after a 75-g oral glucose load are also diagnostic. However, a more convenient method is the measurement of a hemoglobin A1c level, a blood test that calculates the average blood glucose level over the previous 2 to 3 months. Values of ≥6.5% convey the diagnosis of diabetes,[5] although one recent report suggested that hemoglobin A1c levels may differ depending on race and should be interpreted with caution in certain groups.[6] These tests establish only the diagnosis of diabetes and do not distinguish between type 1 and type 2. The distinction is generally determined by clinical characteristics or response to medications. Patients with type 1 diabetes generally are lean and active and usually have few or no other family members with the disease. They may have or be at risk for other autoimmune disorders. Patients with type 2 diabetes are generally obese and sedentary, have a strong positive family history of diabetes, and are often members of a high-risk ethnic group, such as African American, Asian, Asian American, Latino, or Pacific Islander. In past decades, patients with type 1 diabetes were generally younger at the time of diagnosis and those with type 2 diabetes were generally middle-aged or older, but this distinction has been blurred considerably in recent years. It is now recognized that patients with type 1 diabetes can be diagnosed as older adults. In addition, in some regions of the United States, a child with newly diagnosed diabetes is more likely to have type 2 than type 1 diabetes.

Monitoring After Diagnosis

Monitoring technology allows athletes with diabetes to know the value of their blood glucose levels in real time. The most widely used method employs a handheld device (a glucose meter) that measures capillary glucose, which is obtained by lancing the skin. The meters are thought to be highly accurate except when measuring values in the extreme ranges of hypoglycemia or hyperglycemia. The main disadvantages for athletes is that a single measurement does not show the rate or direction of change of glucose over time and that most athletic activity must be stopped to perform a measurement. Over the past decade, a second type of technology, continuous glucose monitoring (CGM), has been extensively developed. An enzyme-coated filament is placed under the skin, where it reacts with tissue glucose levels. The results are wirelessly communicated every few minutes to either a separate handheld device, smartphone, or an insulin pump. This method is clearly superior to a traditional glucose meter because the athlete does not have to stop athletic activity

for a measurement to be obtained. Moreover, the rate of change in glucose levels, including risk for impending hypoglycemia can be calculated and portrayed on the receiving device's screen. Several organizations, including the Endocrine Society, have endorsed CGM as the "gold standard" of monitoring for people with type 1 diabetes.[7] With advances in technology, CGM data now can inform automated pump processes. In 2016 the US Food and Drug Administration (FDA) approved the Medtronic MiniMed 530G, a pump with a low-glucose threshold suspend feature, meaning that when glucose is sensed below a set threshold, insulin infusion halts. In early 2017 the first CGM to communicate with an insulin pump to control the rate of infusion of insulin became commercially available (see *Treatment*, later).

In addition to its use as a diagnostic test, hemoglobin A1c levels can be followed to determine the degree of maintenance of blood glucose levels within a target range. In general, a hemoglobin A1c level of 6.5% or less is considered to represent good control, with control becoming increasingly poor as the level increases. When good control is maintained, athletes should be able to exercise or compete safely without concern for sudden deterioration of glucose control or ketone production, which is especially relevant for athletes with type 1 diabetes. Each athlete should consult with his or her health care provider to determine if exercising or competing is safe when glucose values are elevated.

Urine ketone testing is recommended when glucose values are consistently elevated (>250 mg/dL), or before an athletic event of significant intensity or endurance when the production of ketones may be expected. It is carried out with a reactive strip dipped into a fresh urine sample and uses a reaction of alkali and nitroprusside, which provides a semiquantitative measurement of the ketone acetoacetate.[8] Any athlete with ketones present in urine prior to training or intense competition should suspend athletic activity until the ketonuria is resolved.

TREATMENT

An in-depth discussion of all the treatment modalities used for persons with diabetes mellitus is beyond the scope of this chapter; however, each person involved in the care or performance of an athlete with diabetes should be familiar with the basic families of medications and the expected actions and potential problems with their use during athletic competition.

Medical Nutrition Therapy

Part of the triad of treatment for patients with type 1 and type 2 diabetes involves careful attention to diet and regular exercise. Patients with diabetes are at risk for cardiovascular disease, and most patients with type 2 diabetes are overweight or obese. Therefore medical nutrition therapy is recommended not only to help normalize blood glucose levels but also to help achieve targets for blood pressure and lipids.[9] Patients with type 1 diabetes generally focus on balancing the amount of carbohydrate in meals and snacks with administered insulin, but persons with type 2 diabetes are often prescribed a lower-calorie diet to enhance weight loss. Ideally, athletes with diabetes will consult with a registered dietician to discuss individualized dietary plans accounting for their goals and personal food preferences. Specific recommendations for carbohydrate consumption include choosing from a wide variety of fruits, vegetables, legumes, and whole grains and avoiding excess intake of carbohydrate sources that contain added sugar, fat, or sodium. Fiber intake from food sources is recommended at 25 g/day for women and 38 g/day for men. Intake of sugar-sweetened beverages should be limited; with the commercial availability of low calorie or zero calorie electrolyte replacement beverages, this is now easier than it had been during athletic competition. Protein and total fat intake goals should be individualized because there is no clear evidence supporting specific targets for these macronutrients. Saturated fats should comprise less than 10% of total calories, cholesterol intake should be less than 300 mg/day, and trans fat intake should be avoided. For people with diabetes, as in the general population, there is no evidence supporting use of vitamin or mineral supplements in the absence of diagnosed deficiencies.

Oral Hypoglycemic Agents

Several types of oral hypoglycemic agents (OHAs) are available in the United States. Most are not useful in the treatment of type 1 diabetes because some endogenous insulin secretion is necessary for them to be clinically effective in this population.

- *Sulfonylureas* are insulin secretagogues. They increase endogenous insulin levels in the absence of food intake and can cause hypoglycemia, especially if taken prior to exercise. Glucose levels should be carefully monitored during training and competition so the athlete can decide whether reducing or withholding their use is necessary to prevent hypoglycemia.
- *Metformin* is a member of the biguanide family and is an insulin sensitizer. Although it does not lead to an increase in endogenous insulin levels, like sulfonylurea agents, its effect should be carefully monitored in athletes with type 2 diabetes to determine if it should be reduced or withheld during training and competition.
- *Alpha-glucosidase inhibitors* alter the absorption of starch from the gut. This effect leads to a slower and smaller increase in postmeal glucose excursion. Patients have had difficulty tolerating these agents because of the adverse effects of flatulence and diarrhea.
- *Thiazolidinediones* are peroxisome proliferator-activated γ-receptor agonists that enhance insulin sensitivity. Because of a number of adverse effects, their use has been restricted in the United States. The common adverse effects of weight gain and edema make their use particularly unattractive in athletes with diabetes.
- *Meglitinides* lead to an increase in insulin synthesis within pancreatic cells. Insulin is then released when it is triggered naturally by food intake. Although the theoretic risk for hypoglycemia is less than that seen with sulfonylureas, the same care should be given to individualize their use in athletes with type 2 diabetes after careful testing has been performed during training.
- *Dipeptidyl peptase-IV (DPP-4) inhibitors* are oral agents that utilize the incretin pathway (see later) to lower blood glucose levels after meals by indirectly increasing insulin secretion and suppressing glucagon release. DPP-4 agents are not believed to cause hypoglycemia, but their data regarding their use in athletes are limited.
- *Sodium glucose cotransporter 2 (SLGT2) inhibitors:* The SGLT receptors (1 and 2) promote reabsorption of glucose through the proximal tubules of the kidney.[10] When this receptor is blocked, glucose is excreted in the urine, rather than reabsorbed into the bloodstream, resulting in lower serum glucose levels. Genital and urinary tract infections are the main side effects experienced with the three available agents (canagliflozin, dapagliflozin, and empagliflozin). However, there are no published reports of the use of these agents in the setting of intense exercise. Because other effects (positive and negative) also include osmotic diuresis, natriuresis, and a lowering of blood pressure, it is the authors' opinion that these agents should be used with caution, if at all, until data support their safe use in athletes.

Ideally, as patients with type 2 diabetes lose weight, become better conditioned with exercise, and experience an increase in insulin sensitivity, they can reduce or eliminate the need for OHAs from their regimen.

Insulin and Insulin Analogs

Many patients with type 2 diabetes use insulin in addition to or in the place of OHAs to control their blood glucose levels, but patients with type 1 diabetes are dependent on exogenous insulin to live. Several types of recombinant human insulin and insulin analogs are available in the United States. Most regimens use a combination of long-acting (basal) and short-acting (bolus) injected insulin to approximate the secretory patterns found in normal islet call physiology. Subcutaneous continuous insulin infusion (SCII or insulin pump therapy) has the capacity to deliver insulin in much smaller increments in either a basal (continuous) pattern or as a bolus designed to cover mealtime excursions in blood glucose. Pumps infuse only short-acting insulin analogs, which might be an issue for athletes who want or need to suspend pump therapy for an extended period. Active efforts are underway to develop and commercialize several artificial pancreas systems, using "closed-loop" technology to sense blood glucose levels and respond with appropriate insulin doses without need for human intervention. The FDA-approved low-glucose threshold suspend system was described previously in the section on monitoring. In addition, the first closed-loop system to receive FDA approval was the Medtronic MiniMed 670G System in September 2016.[11]

The pharmacokinetics of the various insulins and their durations of action can be found in Table 18.1. Because many patients with type 2 diabetes have insulin resistance that requires large (>200 units) daily doses of insulin, regular insulin can also be prescribed in 5× and 2× concentrations to reduce the volume of insulin injected.

It is important for athletes, coaches, and trainers to be aware that insulin, as an anabolic agent, is included on the prohibited substances list of the World Anti-Doping Agency (WADA). For elite athletes requiring insulin for diabetes management, therapeutic use exemption (TUE) must be obtained. Information related to this process can be found at wada-ama.org.

TABLE 18.1 Pharmacokinetics of Insulin Preparations			
Insulin Preparations	Onset	Peak	Duration
Aspart (Novolog→)	5–15 min	45–90 min	3–4 h
Glulisine (Apidra→)	5–15 min	45–90 min	3–4 h
Lispro (Humalog→)	5–15 min	45–90 min	3–4 h
Regular[a]	30–60 min	2–4 h	5–6 h
Neutral protamine Hagedorn	1–3 h	4–6 h	8–12 h
Detemir (Levemir→)	1 h	6–8 h	12–24 h
Glargine (Lantus, Basaglar→)	1 h	—	24 h

[a]Regular insulin is also available in 5× (U-500) and 2× (U-200) concentrations.

Incretin and Amylin Analog Therapy

Incretins are peptides found in the gastrointestinal tract that act to lower glucose by pathways that are independent of the insulin receptor. The two currently recognized forms are glucagon-like peptide-1 (GLP-1) and gastric inhibitory peptide. GLP-1 agonists are injectable agents that lower blood glucose by delaying gastric emptying, inhibiting glucagon secretion, and increasing insulin secretion after a meal. DPP-4 is an endogenous enzyme that inactivates the incretins. Adverse effects of GLP-1 agonists include hypoglycemia, and therefore they should be used with caution before or during exercise. Amylin is a peptide that is normally cosecreted with insulin from the pancreas and which usually antagonizes its action. The amylin analog pramlintide is available as an injectable agent and is approved by the FDA for use in type 1 and type 2 diabetes. Its method of action is very similar to that of incretin therapy, and the risk of hypoglycemia with exercise is also a concern.

PHYSIOLOGIC CHANGES OF EXERCISE IN HEALTHY ATHLETES AND IN ATHLETES WITH DIABETES

A comprehensive review of the very complex changes that occur during exercise in healthy persons can be found elsewhere.[12] However, because critical changes occur in glucose metabolism during exercise and recovery, it is important that persons who are managing athletes with diabetes have a basic understanding of what occurs during both aerobic and anaerobic metabolism.

Glucose Regulation During Exercise in Athletes With Type 1 Diabetes Mellitus

Soon after the discovery of insulin and its use in patients with type 1 diabetes, it was observed that physical activity could reduce insulin requirements. In addition, it was recognized that the decrease in blood glucose after an insulin injection was magnified by subsequent exercise.[13] Exercise increases blood flow to muscles and skin, leading to an increased rate of insulin absorption in the athlete with type 1 diabetes (Figs. 18.1 and 18.2).[14] This effect is most pronounced when insulin is administered less than 60 minutes before exercise. Because insulin is given exogenously in persons with type 1 diabetes, the body cannot

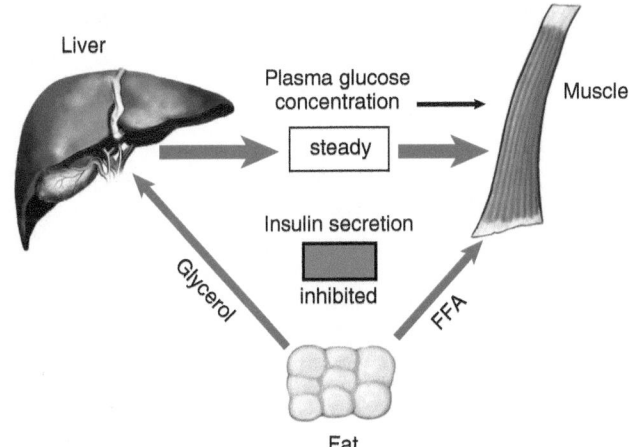

Fig. 18.1 The response to exercise in healthy persons and in insulin-dependent diabetic patients. When plasma insulin is normal or slightly diminished, hepatic glucose production increases markedly, as does skeletal muscle usage of glucose, whereas blood glucose remains unchanged. *FFA*, Free fatty acids. (From Ekoe JM. Overview of diabetes mellitus and exercise. *Med Sci Sports Exerc.* 1989;21:353–368. Copyright The American College of Sports Medicine.)

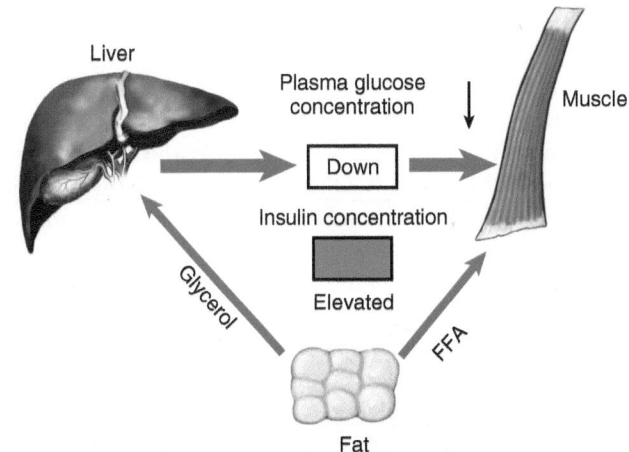

Fig. 18.2 The response to exercise in hyperinsulinemic insulin-dependent diabetic patients. When plasma insulin is increased, skeletal muscle use of glucose during exercise increases markedly, but the increase in hepatic glucose production is smaller than normal: blood glucose levels decrease. *FFA*, Free fatty acids. (From Ekoe JM. Overview of diabetes mellitus and exercise. *Med Sci Sports Exerc.* 1989;21:353–368. Copyright The American College of Sports Medicine.)

decrease its release of insulin, and increased serum insulin levels inhibit hepatic glucose production and peripheral lipolysis. At the same time, continued insulin-independent glucose uptake by exercising muscles depletes energy stores. In type 1 diabetes, glucagon secretion in response to hypoglycemia is usually lost approximately 5 years after diagnosis; the epinephrine response to hypoglycemia is also attenuated in these persons.[15] Deficiencies of these counterregulatory hormones further limit fuel availability during exertion (Table 18.2). The balance between energy supply and demand is often disrupted in the diabetic athlete by an excessive or inadequate insulin effect.

TABLE 18.2   Actions of Major Counterregulatory Hormones

Hormone	Mechanism of Hyperglycemic Effect
Glucagon[a]	Activates hepatic glycogenolysis and gluconeogenesis
Epinephrine[a]	Stimulates hepatic glucose production, limits peripheral glucose use, and suppresses insulin secretion
Growth hormone	After initial glucose-lowering effect, limits glucose transport into cells, mobilizes fat, and provides gluconeogenic substrate (glycerol)
Cortisol	Initially inhibits glucose use; with time, mobilizes substrate (amino acids and glycerol) for gluconeogenesis

[a]Hormones important in recovery from acute hypoglycemia.

Pathophysiologic Responses to Exercise in Persons With Diabetes Mellitus

Data are inconclusive with regard to whether athletes with diabetes mellitus have inherently impaired exercise performance. It is possible that the associated epiphenomena of diabetes, such as acute hypoglycemia or chronic hyperglycemia, diminish the capacity of the athlete to perform at his or her highest capacity. In the setting of obesity or chronic illness, exercise performance is undeniably diminished, but in fit athletes with diabetes, particularly lean athletes with type 1 diabetes, this question remains unanswered. Therefore it is worth exploring the available literature so that both care and expectations can be managed accordingly.

In a study that compared adolescent girls who had either type 1 or type 2 diabetes with either obese or normal-weight girls without diabetes, it was found that female adolescents with type 2 diabetes have reduced aerobic capacity and reduced heart rate response to maximal exercise.[16] Moreover, investigators found that subjects with either type 1 or type 2 diabetes had a blunted stroke volume response compared with nondiabetic control subjects. However, subjects with either type 1 or type 2 diabetes had evidence of poor glucose control at baseline (hemoglobin A1c level = 8.8% and 8.2%, respectively). Moreover, no determinations of baseline activity levels were made. Therefore it is possible that the subjects with either type 1 or type 2 diabetes were more sedentary than their matched nondiabetic control subjects. This concept is supported by another study comparing aerobic capacity and pulmonary function in athletes with type 1 diabetes and both matched, nondiabetic control subjects and nonexercising, diabetic control subjects.[17] In this instance, the glycemic control of the athletes with diabetes was much better than that of the nonathletes with type 1 diabetes (mean hemoglobin A1c = 7.5% vs. 9.0%), but the average glucose level was still much higher than that of the athletes without diabetes (mean hemoglobin A1c level = 4.4%). In addition, the type and duration of programmed exercise was not described. Nevertheless, aerobic capacity (as measured by $VO_{2\,max}$) was found to be similar in athletes both with and without diabetes and was higher in both groups than in nonathletes with diabetes. Of note, both forced expiratory volume in 1 second and anaerobic threshold (as measured by nonlinear increases of pulmonary ventilation and peak CO_2 production compared with O_2 consumption) were lower in athletes with diabetes compared with nondiabetic athletes. Because aerobic capacity was normal, the authors speculated that other factors besides ventilation were adversely lowering the anaerobic threshold. They hypothesized that elastin and collagen abnormalities may negatively affect bronchial adaptation to air flow. With average glucose values significantly higher in the diabetic versus nondiabetic athlete subjects in this study (an average difference of greater than 80 mg/dL according to hemoglobin A1c levels), it is difficult to exclude the effect of chronic hyperglycemia alone on exercise performance in study subjects. In that regard, Wheatley et al.[18] reported that the diffusing capacity for carbon monoxide and the membrane diffusing capacity were lower in athletes with uncontrolled type 1 diabetes compared with athletes with better glycemic control. However, an inverse relationship between glycemic control and pulmonary function was less clear after the investigators found that arterial oxygen saturation was lower in the subjects with well-controlled diabetes.

Other investigators have used additional technologies to observe athletes with diabetes. Peltonen et al. used near-infrared spectroscopy to study local tissue deoxygenation rates during cycling in men with type 1 diabetes (mean hemoglobin A1c 7.7 ± 0.7%) and healthy control men, who were matched for age, body measurements, and baseline reported physical activity.[19] Despite similar reported baseline physical activity, the men with type 1 diabetes were found to have lower aerobic capacity ($VO_{2\,peak}$). As a novel finding in this population, the men with diabetes had more rapid leg muscle deoxygenation at submaximal workloads. Because there was no difference in arterial oxygen saturation in the two groups of men, the authors noted that impaired alveolar gas transfer was an unlikely contributor to this observation. The investigators suggested that this finding instead could indicate inadequacy in circulatory capacity to amplify oxygen delivery to meet increasing tissue demand.

Baldi et al. attempted to directly address the issue of glycemic status on exercise response in endurance athletes with type 1 diabetes.[20] They reported no difference between aerobic capacity or cardiopulmonary exercise response between athletes with type 1 diabetes compared with subjects who did not have diabetes. However, significant differences were found between athletes with diabetes when the group was stratified into those with good glycemic control (hemoglobin A1c level <7%, mean = 6.5%) and those with poor glycemic control (hemoglobin A1c level >7%, mean = 7.8%), despite a similar time spent exercising per week. Multiple indicators of cardiopulmonary fitness were altered in the group with poorer glycemic control, including a lower resting cardiac output and higher systemic vascular resistance. In addition, the group with poor glycemic control had a 24% lower workload during peak exercise, a 10% lower $VO_{2\,max}$, and a 25% lower calculated cardiac output. All measured parameters of pulmonary function were lower in the group with poor glycemic control. When interpreting these findings, it is important to note that in most clinical settings, a hemoglobin A1c level of 7.0% to 7.8% would indicate glycemic control that was only minimally above target.[5]

Finally, Nguyen et al. studied children with and without type 1 diabetes to assess fitness levels in the setting of poor glycemic control (hemoglobin A1c ≥9.0% for the 9 months prior to the study period) versus good glycemic control (hemoglobin A1c ≤7.5% over the 9 months prior).[21] The investigators assessed the children's grip strength, short-term muscle power during cycling, aerobic capacity while cycling, and physical activity while wearing an accelerometer for 7 days. They found no significant differences between groups for grip strength or short-term muscle power but identified lower $VO_{2\,peak}$ in the children with poorly controlled diabetes as compared with the controls or children with well-controlled diabetes. The groups of children had no significant differences in physical activity by minutes of activity per day or by activity intensity level.

If poor glycemic control has a direct negative effect on exercise performance, several potential explanations exist. First, even acute elevations in blood glucose levels are known to diminish autoregulation of capillary blood flow, leading to diminished oxygen consumption.[22] In addition, chronic hyperglycemia is associated with neuropathic changes, both autonomic and peripheral. Veves et al. noted reduced aerobic capacity and diminished heart rate in subjects with type 1 diabetes and neuropathy compared with subjects without neuropathy.[23] As the distinction between exercise performance in athletes with good glycemic control compared with poor glycemic control becomes better defined, it is expected that additional mechanisms that might explain these differences will be determined.

MANAGEMENT OF ATHLETES WITH DIABETES DURING TRAINING AND COMPETITION

Despite the fact that exercise is strongly recommended as a mainstay of therapy for persons with diabetes mellitus and that chronic athletic conditioning evokes positive metabolic changes, studies have shown a lack of improvement in hemoglobin A1c levels in patients with type 1 diabetes.[24] Several possible explanations exist for this finding. First, exercise introduces variables of glucose utilization and insulin sensitivity that may cause difficulty in keeping glucose levels consistent, especially if exercise is not performed regularly. Perhaps more important is the justifiable concern of hypoglycemia both during but especially after competition. Anecdotally, concern for developing hypoglycemia leads many recreational, high school, and even collegiate athletes to induce hyperglycemia prior to training or competition either by consuming an excessive amount of simple carbohydrates or by underdosing insulin. The resultant hyperglycemia can offset any positive effects of athletic activity on long-term glycemic control. Therefore perhaps the most important advice for helping athletes manage their blood glucose levels is to encourage each athlete to meticulously record glucose levels and the conditions that are present during different types of training or competition. As an adjunct to capillary glucose values, the use of CGM may help to inform a more complete understanding of an athlete's glucose trends before, during, and following exercise; importantly, CGM also can help to reduce athletes' fear of developing exercise-induced hypoglycemia.

Altogether, glycemic data help the athlete and his or her care provider recognize patterns of glucose control and implement nutritional or pharmacologic strategies during athletic activities to prevent hypoglycemia or hyperglycemia. A prototype glucose log for this purpose is shown in Fig. 18.3. In addition, multiple apps and websites are available to help athletes with diabetes. A particularly useful site is *Excarbs*, developed by a University of Toronto team led by professor Michael Riddell. Recreational athletes can enter values for current glucose and the time and dose of last insulin bolus taken, and the app will recommend either additional carbohydrates or reduction in insulin to prevent hypoglycemia.[25]

Training Versus Competition

It has long been known that different intensities of athletic activity lead to different compensatory hormonal responses,[26] including those of the counterregulatory hormones epinephrine, cortisol, and growth hormone. Shetty et al. studied nine adolescents and young adults with type 1 diabetes at four different exercise intensities on 4 separate days.[27] At low-to-moderate exercise intensities, they observed that exogenous glucose was necessary to maintain euglycemia, whereas at high exercise intensities ($VO_{2\,peak}$ >80%) exogenous glucose requirements were absent. Furthermore, athletes at every level of competition have anecdotally reported that insulin requirements and postevent glucose excursions are generally higher on days of actual competition compared with days of training, despite the fact that the same activity is performed for the same interval of time. Little information exists in the scientific literature to explain this phenomenon. Indeed, it would be difficult to test in a clinical laboratory setting. Even if the intensity or duration of athletic activity was closely replicated, it would be challenging to control for the emotional response or other psychological elements that accompany actual competition. It is important for athletes to be aware of this phenomenon, and with regular sporting activity, to make adjustments for it as they learn their own responses.

Glycemic Log for Athletic Events

Date/Time	Event and Duration		Basal insulin adjustment	Last insulin bolus/amount	Timing/CHO (g) last meal	Timing/CHO (g) during event	Glucose			Conditions (Temp, Altitude)	Performance Outcome
	Training	Competition					Before	During	After		

Fig. 18.3 A proposed log that athletes with diabetes can use to record parameters affecting glycemic control and athletic performance. *CHO*, Carbohydrate.

Management of Type 1 Diabetes

Although the American Diabetes Association has a position statement regarding exercise and diabetes management,[28] no single guideline or source of recommendations is available that athletes with type 1 diabetes can follow for management of their disease during training or athletic competition. As one elite athlete commented, it is an "independent disease," and each athlete must know how his or her body will respond during different types of athletic conditions.[29] However, some basic treatment principles and monitoring strategies can be used.

- *Glucose target:* Although the target glucose value must be determined for each individual athlete, a general recommendation would be to attempt to keep glucose levels between 100 and 180 mg/dL during training and competition. Values less than 100 mg/dL may place the athlete at risk for hypoglycemia during activity, and values greater than 180 mg/dL are above the renal threshold for glucose. The resultant osmotic diuresis may lead to additional loss of fluids and electrolytes. Most athletes believe that they compete best when their glucose values are in the middle-to-upper portion of this target range, which allows a gradual decrease to occur without significant risk for hypoglycemia during activity. Note that athletes who use a low-glucose suspend insulin pump may be able to set their target glucoses considerably lower because their theoretic risk for hypoglycemic should be reduced or eliminated. However, data regarding this outcome are limited only to clinical trials at this time.

- *Glucose monitoring:* For athletes not utilizing CGM, capillary glucose levels should be checked before, during, and after training or competition. Until patterns are recognized, it is advisable to check at 15-minute intervals prior to exercising to determine the rate of change of blood glucose. This is especially important if the athlete has injected an insulin bolus for a meal or snack within the previous 3 hours. If possible, athletes should also check their glucose levels during exercise or competition to determine its effect. This task will clearly be less practical during actual competition, although sports such as tennis or golf that have breaks between play or team sports with scheduled breaks or the ability to substitute players make this task more feasible. Athletes competing in individual sports, especially endurance sports such as running, cycling, or swimming, may have more difficulty with this recommendation and should use the help of others to assist with monitoring at various points in the competition. Although CGM devices should provide a superior option, these devices may not perform as well during exercise as they do at rest.[30] However, a study comparing accuracy of one sensor (Dexcom G4 Platinum) during moderate versus intermittent high-intensity exercise found that, despite significant differences in mean glucose, lactate, and pH levels, the sensor was comparably accurate at both levels of activity.[31] For persons who do not want or are unable to obtain a CGM device, one can be prescribed by their health care provider for a 72-hour to 7-day diagnostic period. The device captures glucose levels every 5 minutes during this period, and a graphic printout is provided at its completion. Ideally the athlete would wear the device during both a training session and competition to maximize its utility in determining patterns of glucose levels. Finally, it is important for athletes to recognize when they are most at risk for hypoglycemia after exercise. Typically the period of highest risk occurs 6 to 15 hours following exercise, when glycogen stores are repleted.[32] By regularly checking glucose levels during this period, the athlete can know whether insulin administration should be reduced or additional carbohydrates should be consumed in the postexercise period.

- *Insulin administration:* Athletes must consider the level of insulin in their system and its duration of action when planning athletic activity. Unless a sufficient amount of carbohydrate is consumed before or during activity, it is generally ill advised to take a bolus of insulin directly prior to training or competition. The duration of action for the short-acting insulin analogs is approximately 3 hours, and the risk of hypoglycemia should be reduced if athletic activity is performed outside of this time frame. In addition, one must consider that once it is injected or infused, insulin will be bound to its receptor and biologically active for approximately 30 minutes. Therefore athletes should avoid reducing or suspending insulin pump basal rates immediately before an athletic event but rather should do so approximately 30 minutes beforehand. For new athletes or athletes beginning a new activity, basal insulin might be reduced by 50% before and during the activity until glucose patterns can be determined and a more tailored adjustment can be made. This should help prevent hypoglycemia during the event and help the athlete to avoid finishing the event with significant hyperglycemia. This objective is more easily accomplished with an insulin pump, and particularly so with sensor augmentation, meaning that when low-range glucoses are detected, the pump automatically suspends insulin infusion. Glycemic management is anticipated to be increasingly automated and safer with the emergence of closed-loop artificial pancreas systems. In research settings, artificial pancreas systems are being adapted to include mechanisms for detection of exercise. In a recent clinical trial, closed-loop systems integrated with heart rate detection appeared to improve adolescents' glycemic management during exercise, specifically by reducing the amount of exercise time with glucose levels less than 70 mg/dL.[33] As the exercise detection mechanisms and functional algorithms for artificial pancreas systems are optimized, the artificial pancreas is anticipated ultimately to become the standard of care for athletes with insulin-dependent diabetes. Particularly, it should benefit those with a propensity to become hypoglycemic or hyperglycemic during and after activity.

Comparatively, with injections of long-acting insulins such as insulin glargine or neutral protamine Hagedorn (NPH), additional carbohydrates may need to be consumed to counterbalance the effect of exogenous insulin (see the next section). As mentioned previously, glucose levels during and after intense competition are likely to be higher than those encountered during training, but use of additional basal insulin should be considered only after the athlete is confident of his or her individual glucose patterns during these times.

- *Carbohydrate consumption:* In the authors' experience in working with athletes who have diabetes, carbohydrate consumption is the area of most personal variability between individuals. Some athletes make adjustments to their insulin and will not require any additional carbohydrates before or during competition. Others will consume a small snack immediately prior to activity: in a survey of 91 adult endurance athletes with type 1 diabetes, 37% reported consuming preexercise carbohydrate snacks most or all of the time.[34] Still others will use fast-acting glucose in the form of tablets, gels, or sports drinks at regular intervals while training or competing. In general, carbohydrates should be consumed shortly after exercise to prevent early postactivity hypoglycemia.[35] Athletes should record both the type and amount of carbohydrate consumed to determine its effect on glucose levels during and after athletic activity. Of note, one study demonstrated that more carbohydrates should be consumed on the day after exercise to prevent hypoglycemia.[36] Because this is beyond the expected period of glycogen repletion, it suggests that any increase in insulin sensitivity gained from exercise can be prolonged. Finally, the combination of CGM and an individualized algorithm for carbohydrate intake was shown to be effective in preventing hypoglycemia in children and adolescents involved in athletic activities at a summer camp.[37] It is possible that strategies for athletic activity can be optimized by utilizing several treatment modalities at once (both for monitoring and adjusting glucose).
- *Monitoring ketones:* In most situations, ketones do not need to be routinely monitored by athletes with diabetes. However, because athletic activity can worsen ketoacidosis in persons with very poor glycemic control, a general recommendation is to check urine ketones if capillary blood glucose is 250 mg/dL or greater. If ketones are present, athletic activity should be postponed until glucose levels are lowered and ketonuria is resolved.

For additional recommendations on managing athletes with type 1 diabetes from the viewpoint of the athletic trainer, see the comprehensive review by Jimenez et al.[38]

Management of Type 2 Diabetes

Although patients with type 2 diabetes are generally sedentary and obese, they are occasionally both fit and athletic. It is the relative lack of insulin that leads to hyperglycemia, and this condition can occur with any body habitus. For patients with type 2 diabetes who are embarking on a new exercise program or athletic activity, several points should be kept in mind.

- *Risk of hypoglycemia:* Although athletes with type 2 diabetes are more resistant to the effects of insulin than those with type 1 diabetes, any oral agent that increases endogenous insulin secretion or exogenous insulin injections can increase the risk for hypoglycemia if not properly managed. Therefore athletes with type 2 diabetes, especially those who are already at their ideal body weight, should use the same strategies previously listed for patients with type 1 diabetes. They should also log glucose levels and conditions and regularly analyze the recorded results to determine if and when nutritional or

pharmacologic therapies need to be modified in the setting of athletic activity.
- *Screening for cardiovascular disease:* Patients with type 2 diabetes and those with type 1 diabetes who have long-standing disease (>20 years) or microvascular complications are at increased risk for undiagnosed cardiovascular disease. Before the start of any new exercise or athletic activity, a complete medical evaluation should be performed and formal graded exercise testing should be considered for persons initiating more intense activities.[39] Athletes with diabetes may take statins for primary cardiovascular risk reduction or in the setting of known cardiovascular disease. These athletes should not be discouraged from using an indicated statin or be restricted in appropriately planned exercise. For athletes engaging in training that gradually increases in intensity, muscular metabolic adaptation appears to reduce the risk of statin-induced muscle injury.[40] Statin users who engage in vigorous exercise without appropriate training may be at heightened risk of rhabdomyolysis.[41]
- *Weight loss:* For athletes who weigh more than their ideal body weight, regular exercise should promote weight loss. Gradual modifications to the athlete's pharmacologic and nutritional regimen may be needed to prevent hypoglycemia as the athlete becomes more insulin sensitive. In some cases, pharmacologic treatment may be discontinued altogether.

Additional Considerations for Elite Athletic Competition in Persons With Type 1 Diabetes

In the authors' experience, most athletes with type 1 diabetes who are engaged in recreational, high school, or collegiate sports are most concerned about becoming hypoglycemic during competition. The most common strategy is to allow or induce hyperglycemia, either by consuming extra carbohydrates with no insulin coverage or by reducing or withholding insulin. Experiencing a hypoglycemic event in the midst of competition would no doubt diminish performance. However, for the elite or professional athlete, significant or modest hyperglycemia could also be detrimental during athletic competition. Moreover, when an elite level of competition demands the most perfect of conditions, even mild hyperglycemia could negatively impact performance. There remains a notable lack of scientific investigation and clinical guidelines for glucose management during elite competition in athletes with diabetes. Individual elite athletes, often with teams of nutritionists, personal trainers, and exercise physiologists, are primarily responsible for determining the balance of insulin and nutrition that allows them to optimally train, compete, and recover from competition.

SUMMARY

Athletes with diabetes mellitus face several challenges when training for and competing in athletic activity. To avoid hypoglycemia and hyperglycemia, many variables must be considered and adjusted to keep glucose levels in an optimal range, which is especially important because exercise itself significantly affects glucose levels. All persons involved with an athlete who has diabetes, including health care providers, coaches, athletic trainers, and most importantly, the athlete, must understand the basic principles of exercise physiology and the different types of medications used in the treatment of diabetes. This understanding is especially important as more children, adolescents, and young adults are diagnosed with diabetes. Despite significant challenges encountered during training and competition, performing well in athletic activity is very possible for athletes with diabetes. It is hoped that with continued technologic advancement, both in the arena of CGM and in the delivery of insulin, including the long-anticipated development of an artificial pancreas,[42] the challenges faced by athletes with diabetes will continue to diminish.

ACKNOWLEDGMENT

The authors thank their patients who have shared their many experiences with exercise and athletic competition over the years.
For a complete list of references, go to ExpertConsult.com.

SELECTED READINGS

Citation:
Baldi JC, Cassuto NA, Foxx-Lupo WT, et al. Glycemic status affects cardiopulmonary exercise response in athletes with type 1 diabetes. *Med Sci Sports Exerc.* 2010;42:1454–1459.

Level of Evidence:
V

Summary:
This study is an important investigation into whether the underlying condition of diabetes negatively affects athletic performance or whether the degree of glycemic control is more responsible for aberrations in exercise physiology.

Citation:
Jimenez CC, Corcoran MH, Crawley JT, et al. National Athletic Trainers' Association position statement: management of the athlete with type 1 diabetes mellitus. *J Athl Train.* 2007;42:536–545.

Level of Evidence:
V

Summary:
This article includes useful recommendations for the athletic trainer who works with patients with type 1 diabetes. In addition to providing practical suggestions regarding supplies to carry and guidelines for travel, the recommendations focus on unique management issues for athletes with type 1 diabetes such as preparticipation physicals and healing of injuries.

Citation:
Blauw H, Keith-Hynes P, Koops R, et al. A review of safety and design requirements of the artificial pancreas. *Ann Biomed Eng.* 2016;44:3158–3172.

Level of Evidence:
V

Summary:
This article provides an updated and comprehensive review of the history, ongoing investigation, and expected future use of the technologies being applied to the development of a closed-loop system in the management of blood glucose.

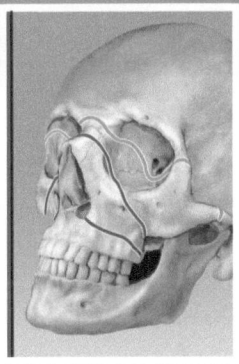

19

Renal Medicine and Genitourinary Trauma in the Athlete

Stefan Hemmings, Derek M. Fine

Trauma to the genitourinary (GU) tract is relatively uncommon because of the anatomic location of key internal GU organs, the kidneys and bladder. However, prompt recognition of the signs and symptoms associated with GU trauma will allow the clinician to order appropriate imaging tests and implement therapeutic plans that can save organs and even a person's life.

DEFINITION (CLASSIFICATIONS)

Table 19.1 summarizes the classification of kidney trauma injuries according to severity. This classification correlates with the need for surgical intervention.[1]

EPIDEMIOLOGY

Of all the GU organs, the external genitalia (penis, scrotum, and vulva) are most likely to be injured. Of the internal GU organs, the kidneys are the most likely to be injured after a patient experiences abdominal trauma.[2]

Overall, the most common sport causing abdominal injury is cycling. Football, rugby, gymnastics, horseback riding, wrestling, martial arts, and hockey are a few of the sports that include activities capable of causing significant abdominal and consequent GU organ injury; the use of exercise equipment can do so as well.[3,4]

The overall incidence of renal injury as a result of trauma ranges from 1.4% to 3.25%.[5] Sports-related trauma to the kidney is uncommon and is reported to constitute only 15% to 20% of all traumatic renal injuries.[6] Most cases of renal trauma are the result of blunt trauma specifically relating to motor vehicle accidents and falls.[5] Kidney injuries are particularly common when a person is subjected to rapid deceleration forces. One analysis shows that of the 23,666 sports-related injuries among high school–age varsity athletes, only 18 kidney injuries were reported, none of which was serious.[4] In an analysis of more than 653,000 trauma cases from the National Trauma Data Bank, 16,585 were identified as trauma from bicycle injuries.[7] Only 2% of the patients in these cases experienced a GU tract injury, with the kidneys being the organ most likely affected (in 75% of cases), followed by the bladder and urethra (in 15% of cases) and the penis and scrotum (in 10% of cases). Sixty percent of the patients with GU injuries had evidence of concomitant fractures of the spine or pelvis, suggesting that isolated GU trauma is uncommon.[7] Compared with renal injuries, testicular injuries in sports occur at a much lower rate. A review of a trauma registry of all cases of renal and testes injuries (1.4% of all injuries) showed that 92% involved the kidneys and 8% the testes.[8] It is estimated that more than half of injuries to the testes occur during sporting events.[9]

PATHOBIOLOGY/PATHOPHYSIOLOGY

The kidneys are located in the retroperitoneal space and are surrounded by visceral fat and the Gerota fascia. The kidneys lie on either side of the spinal column in front of the psoas muscle and medial to the quadratus lumborum muscle. The hepatic flexure of the colon on the right and the spleen and the splenic flexure on the left cover the kidneys anteriorly. Because the kidneys are protected by surrounding structures, traumatic kidney injuries during sporting activities occur mainly in association with major forces and are usually associated with injury to other organs.

Injuries to the renal parenchyma constitute the vast majority of cases. Preexisting renal abnormalities such as hydronephrosis, renal cysts, or an abnormal renal anatomic position increase the likelihood of renal injury during trauma and are reported in 4% to 19% of adults and 12% to 35% of children.[5,10--12] These subjects have more severe symptoms and are more likely to require surgical intervention.[10–12] Vascular injuries of the kidneys occur during deceleration forces and result from damage to the renal pedicle. These cases may present with thrombosis or rupture of the vasculature.

Bladder injuries also occur as a consequence of blunt force trauma to the abdomen. The bladder's anatomic location deep in the anterior bony pelvis makes it less frequently injured by trauma. However, the weakest part of the bladder is the dome, which is mobile and susceptible to injury when the bladder is full.

The testes are particularly vulnerable to trauma because of their external location and lack of anatomic protection when blunt trauma forces the scrotum against the pelvic bone. Testicular rupture, scrotal wall hematoma, or intrascrotal hematocele are possible.[13]

DIAGNOSIS

Obtaining a thorough history is imperative. The initial evaluation of patients should include attention to vital signs recorded on the field and upon arrival at the hospital. The lowest recorded

TABLE 19.1   Organ Injury Severity Scale for the Kidney (American Association for the Surgery of Trauma)

Grade	Type	Description
I	Contusion	Microscopic or gross hematuria; urologic studies normal
	Hematoma	Subcapsular and nonexpanding without parenchymal laceration
II	Hematoma	Nonexpanding perirenal hematoma confined to the renal retroperitoneum
	Laceration	Less than 1 cm parenchymal depth of renal cortex without urinary extravasation
III	Laceration	Greater than 1 cm parenchymal depth of renal cortex without collecting system rupture or urinary extravasation
IV	Laceration	Parenchymal laceration extending through the renal cortex, medulla, and collecting system
	Vascular	Main renal artery or vein injury with contained hemorrhage
V	Laceration	Completely shattered kidney
	Vascular	Avulsion of the renal hilum, devascularizing the kidney

From Santucci RA, McAninch JW, Safir M, et al. Validation of the American Association for the Surgery of Trauma organ injury severity scale for the kidney. *J Trauma.* 2001;50:195–200.

systolic blood pressure may indicate the need for radiologic assessment of subjects for a kidney injury. Careful examination of the abdomen, chest, and back is critical. Patients with evidence of abdominal or flank tenderness or hematoma, rib fractures, and penetrating injuries to the low thorax or flank may have sustained an injury to the kidney and require further assessment. Pelvic fractures in trauma may alert the physician to the potential of bladder injury. Increasing abdominal girth with "ascites" without hemodynamic instability and without a drop in hemoglobin levels should be cause for suspicion, as the diagnosis can be delayed.[14] Persons with a testicular injury usually present with swelling, tenderness, and ecchymosis. Rupture of the testis is associated with immediate severe pain.[13]

Laboratory Findings

Hematuria, either microscopic or gross, is the best indicator of injury to the urinary tract after trauma. Although hematuria is seen in 80% to 90% of cases of kidney trauma, lack of hematuria does not eliminate the possibility; therefore a high degree of clinical suspicion should be maintained if the mechanism of injury suggests renal trauma. In addition, the degree of hematuria may not correlate with the degree of injury. However, in general, gross hematuria associated with blunt trauma increases the likelihood of major injury.

A rising serum creatinine in the absence of anuria/oliguria, especially in the context of ascites, could indicate bladder injury with intraperitoneal/intraabdominal urinary leak, as urinary ascites is resorbed across the peritoneum.

Imaging

Imaging studies specifically focused on the GU tract are required for all patients with rapid deceleration as the mechanism of blunt trauma (e.g., a motor vehicle accident or fall from a height), patients with hypotension, adults with gross hematuria, and children with microscopic hematuria.[15] Hemodynamically stable patients with only microscopic hematuria may not require further imaging but should undergo a thorough follow-up evaluation for potentially harmful delayed effects of trauma.[16]

An abdominal computed tomography (CT) scan with use of intravenous contrast is the imaging modality of choice in patients with trauma to the GU tract. In one series, the most common findings on CT were perirenal hematoma (29.4%), intrarenal hematoma (24.7%), and parenchymal disruption (17.6%).[17] Measurement of serum electrolytes and serum creatinine is useful in guiding diagnostic and treatment plans. Contrast should be avoided in those with severely reduced renal function, although emergent situations may necessitate its use.

For suspected bladder injury, CT and plain retrograde cystography are equivalent imaging modalities that would demonstrate extravasation of contrast.[18] Early diagnosis is essential for testicular salvage when there is trauma to the scrotum, the likelihood of which decreases with time. Scrotal ultrasonography is a safe, noninvasive, and valuable tool for rapid detection of testicular rupture, hematocele, hematoma, or traumatic torsion.[13]

Differential Diagnosis

Exercise-induced hematuria is a relatively common, benign finding among athletes. The incidence ranges between 50% and 80%, with the highest incidence reported among swimmers, track athletes, and lacrosse players.[19] A thorough medication history is critical, particularly for use of nonsteroidal inflammatory drugs (NSAIDs). In one study, more than half of the athletes with idiopathic hematuria regularly used NSAIDs.[20] Preexisting glomerular or cystic kidney disease may be the source of microscopic hematuria and must be differentiated from trauma-induced hematuria. The presence of proteinuria may suggest a preexisting glomerular lesion.

TREATMENT

A detailed discussion of specific surgical management is beyond the scope of this chapter. However, awareness of the following therapeutic considerations is important:

1. Surgical exploration of the kidney is required in cases with severe, persistent, or life-threatening renal hemorrhage, pedicle avulsion, or an expanding retroperitoneal hematoma.[5]
2. A nephrectomy may be required in persons who have sustained severe trauma and in unstable patients. However, patients who are more stable, especially those with a solitary kidney or with bilateral injuries, may be candidates for renovascular repair and reconstruction or the angioembolization of bleeding vessels.[5]
3. Hemodynamically stable patients who do not have hematuria and even patients with microscopic hematuria can be managed conservatively with careful monitoring.

4. Vigorous hydration to dilute gross hematuria will facilitate the avoidance of clot formation and the potential for urinary obstruction.

5. Immediate surgical exploration is suggested for patients with testicular trauma when testicular rupture is suspected.[13]

6. Surgical intervention is recommended for complicated intra- or extraperitoneal bladder injury and conservative management with Foley catheter drainage for uncomplicated extraperitoneal injuries.[18]

RETURN-TO-PLAY GUIDELINES

No specific guidelines are available to dictate the timing for a return to maximal activity after GU trauma; thus prudent decisions should take into account the severity of the injury and the required recovery period. Contact sport activities such as football should be avoided for a longer period during recovery, and specific protective padding to shield the flank regions may be indicated.

Recommendations for safe athletic participation in special populations have been controversial. For example, athletes with either a single kidney or those who have undergone a kidney transplant are intuitively considered at higher risk for the effects of GU trauma. However, the American Academy of Pediatrics recommends a "qualified yes" for participation in contact/collision sports by athletes with a single kidney.[21]

Despite this recommendation, most physicians continue to discourage participation in contact/collision sports for patients with a single kidney.[22]

Patients who have had a renal transplant are also believed to be at higher risk for trauma to the allograft because of the unique location of the allograft in the preperitoneal space. Despite the potential for increased risk of trauma to the allograft, few actual reports of such trauma have surfaced, and the medical literature does not include any reports of allograft loss due to trauma.[23,24] Given the risk of severe consequences with allograft trauma, the general consensus is that contact sports should be avoided altogether by patients who have undergone renal transplantation.[24] Individual decisions should be made for other sports that have a theoretical reduced risk of injury, such as basketball, mountain biking, and other sports.

METABOLIC PROBLEMS IN RENAL SPORTS MEDICINE

Acute Kidney Injury, Hyponatremia, and Rhabdomyolysis

Acute kidney injury (AKI) is not an infrequent occurrence in endurance sports. In one study, 83.6% of 28 ultramarathon runners developed AKI with elevations in serum creatinine levels after the race concluded, but recovery of renal function was quick, within 24 hours. Dehydration and rhabdomyolysis are notable risk factors for AKI in endurance events.[25]

Acute hyponatremia (serum sodium <135 mEq/L) can be seen when there is excessive ingestion of water in endurance sports or water drinking challenges. This can lead to severe or critical hyponatremia, leading to encephalopathy, seizures, pulmonary edema, and death.[26,27] Hyponatremia is not infrequently seen in marathon runners and triathletes and has even been reported in a training camp for rowers that lasted for several weeks.[28–30] The mechanism is dilutional, due to inadequate solutes in fluids ingested, solute loss in sweat, and inappropriate release of arginine vasopressin (antidiuretic hormone) preventing free water loss by the kidney. The therapeutic approach in symptomatic patients is an infusion of hypertonic 3% normal saline.[26]

Exertional rhabdomyolysis (ER) is relatively uncommon and often goes unrecognized. However, ER can have significant morbidity and mortality if it is severe and not managed appropriately. In such instances, inpatient hospitalization is required for intravenous hydration and serial laboratory monitoring of renal function and electrolytes. Consultation with a nephrologist should be sought in the case of athletes who have muscle enzymes that are continuing to rise. The administration of diuretics is not indicated, as this can worsen kidney function. There are no evidence-based guidelines for return to play after an episode of ER.[31]

For a complete list of references, go to ExpertConsult.com.

SELECTED READINGS

Citation:

Dane B, Baxgter AB, Bernstein MP. Imaging genitourinary trauma. *Radiol Clin N Amer.* 2017;55(2):321–335.

Level of Evidence:

V

Summary:

Article gives great overview of types of imaging modalities best suited for patients with trauma to the genitourinary tract in appropriate clinical scenarios.

Citation:

Bjurlin MA, Fantus RJ, Fantus RJ, et al. Comparison of nonoperative and surgical management of renal trauma: Can we predict when nonoperative management fails? *J Trauma Acute Care Surg.* 2017;88(2):356–362.

Level of Evidence:

II

Summary:

A retrospective cohort study analyzing risk factors that determine the success of salvage and failure of nonoperative management of renal trauma.

Citation:

Chiron P, Hornez E, Boddaert GM, et al. Grade IV renal trauma management. A revision of the AAST renal injury grading scale is mandatory. *Eur J Trauma Emerg Surg.* 2016;42(2):237–241.

Level of Evidence:

I

Summary:

Systematic review of existing literature on outcomes of Grade IV renal trauma based on imaging and risk factor stratification with recommendations for management.

20

Sports and Epilepsy

Mary L. Zupanc, Scott I. Otallah, Howard P. Goodkin

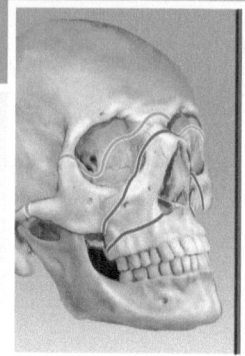

Epilepsy is a common clinical condition characterized by recurrent, unprovoked seizures. It affects approximately 1% of the general US population, with the highest incidence in infancy and childhood.[1,2] Although previous recommendations precluded sports participation for persons with epilepsy,[3–5] it is now recognized that exercise is part of a comprehensive treatment plan for epilepsy and that participation in sports and exercise should be encouraged.[6,7]

TERMINOLOGY AND CLASSIFICATION

Seizure

An epileptic seizure is the clinical manifestation of an abnormal, hypersynchronous discharge of a group of neurons in the cerebral cortex. The clinical manifestations are determined by the seizure's anatomic focus within the brain and can include an altered state of awareness, stereotyped or repetitive movements, loss of muscle tone (atonic), tonic or clonic movements, sensory (e.g., visual) or psychic experiences, or autonomic dysfunction.

Seizures are classified as either generalized or focal. A generalized seizure is the result of rapid activation of bilaterally distributed networks, which include both cortical and subcortical structures. Generalized seizures can be either convulsive (e.g., tonic, clonic, tonic-clonic, myoclonic, or atonic) or nonconvulsive (e.g., absence). Focal seizures, previously classified as partial seizures,[8] involve a limited network of neurons localized to a region of the brain. Although seizures traditionally have been subdivided into simple focal or complex focal categories, based on altered (simple) or impaired (complex) consciousness, it has been proposed[9] that the traditional terminology be replaced with a description of the elemental features of the seizures and the sequence of occurrence.[10,11]

Simple focal seizures can include motor, sensory, autonomic, and psychic phenomena. These seizures, often referred to as an "aura," can transform into a complex focal seizure as the seizure focus expands to involve other regions of the cortex that mediate awareness. A seizure that starts in the temporal lobe may initially begin as a simple focal seizure (aura) of a rising gastric sensation followed by staring, diminished responsiveness, and stereotypic automatisms including repetitive swallowing or lip smacking (a complex focal seizure). Focal seizures can evolve into a generalized tonic-clonic seizure, an event referred to as "secondary generalization."

Epilepsy

Epilepsy, which is defined as a condition of unprovoked, recurrent seizures, can be either inherited or acquired. Inherited or genetic forms of epilepsy (previously called "idiopathic" epilepsy) are often channelopathies, that is, disorders that alter the excitability of the neurons, resulting in epilepsy. Examples include sodium channelopathies and potassium channelopathies. Other types are "symptomatic," implying an underlying central nervous system lesion/abnormality, such as encephalomalacia due to trauma, stroke, infection, or cortical dysplasia. Symptomatic epilepsies are generally difficult to treat and usually do not go into remission.

An epilepsy syndrome is defined by the seizure type(s), age of seizure onset, developmental and family history, electroencephalogram (EEG) and neuroimaging results, neurologic examination, and medication response. Examples of epilepsy syndromes include childhood absence epilepsy, juvenile myoclonic epilepsy, and benign rolandic epilepsy.

The epilepsy syndromes were previously subdivided into two major categories: generalized epilepsy syndromes and localization-related (or focal) epilepsy syndromes.[12] However, an expanding knowledge of epilepsy recommends excluding the prior classification system in favor of a system that separates the manifestations of epilepsy from the pathogenesis. In the newly proposed system,[9] syndromes are subdivided into pure electroclinical syndromes, constellations, structural/metabolic epilepsies, and epilepsies of unknown causes.

DIAGNOSIS AND EVALUATION

The diagnosis of epilepsy is based on clinical history. A single seizure can be provoked by electrolyte imbalances, dehydration, infection, or trauma. Other conditions should also be considered in persons presenting with a paroxysmal event, including cardiac arrhythmias, prolonged QT syndrome, syncope, complicated migraine, paroxysmal movement disorders, and psychogenic events. Although an outpatient EEG is an indispensable tool in clinical diagnosis, clinical history is the most critical determinant. Of all persons with epilepsy, 17% have normal interictal EEG findings (when they are not having an overt seizure). In addition, abnormal EEG findings do not guarantee that a seizure has occurred.[13–15] Lastly, following the diagnosis of epilepsy, a head imaging study—preferably a magnetic resonance imaging scan of the head—should be obtained. Exceptions to this rule may include a child or an adult diagnosed with childhood absence epilepsy, juvenile absence epilepsy, or juvenile myoclonic epilepsy.[16]

TREATMENT

Therapy with an antiepileptic drug (AED) is not typical after a single seizure because recurrence risk after a first unprovoked seizure is only 30% to 40%. Risk for additional seizures increases to approximately 75% after a second unprovoked seizure.[17–19] After this second seizure, an AED is usually prescribed. Occasionally, an AED is started after a first unprovoked seizure if the EEG demonstrates epileptiform discharges (spike or sharp waves) in the temporal region or generalized spike and slow wave discharges. The chance of recurrence in these situations may be closer to 90%.

Approximately 30 AEDs are used to treat epilepsy. The choice of AED is based on seizure type and epilepsy syndrome. The following general principles relate to the choice of AED:

1. Monotherapy is effective and avoids unpleasant drug interactions. About 60% of patients will experience control of their epilepsy with an appropriate first AED. An additional 10% will respond to a second AED. Unfortunately, chances of a subsequent medication trial succeeding when the first two AEDs have failed are less than 5%.[20,21] Thus 30% of patients will most likely be refractory to therapy. For these patients, alternative therapies including vagus nerve stimulation, diet therapies (e.g., a ketogenic diet), and epilepsy surgery need to be considered.
2. If possible, AEDs should be titrated slowly and only to the point of seizure control.
3. Seizure control should not be achieved at the expense of adverse effects. An alternative medication should be chosen if a person experiences adverse effects.
4. Drug compliance is enhanced when medication is administered once or twice daily. When available, a sustained-release medication should be considered.
5. Therapeutic blood levels are not absolute; they are formulated based on trough levels and represent a statistical range of efficacy.

Persons caring for patients with epilepsy should be cognizant of AED adverse effects that may impair sports participation. For example, some AEDs at high doses can produce cognitive or behavioral changes, diplopia, dizziness, and general fatigue. Phenytoin, carbamazepine, valproate, and lamotrigine can induce tremors or dyskinesias.[22,23] Topiramate and zonisamide can cause oligohydrosis.[24,25] Thus patients should be advised to maintain hydration, carry a spray bottle of cool water, and monitor for overheating when participating in sports. Carbamazepine and oxcarbazepine can cause hyponatremia.[26] Additionally, valproate can cause weight gain and topiramate can induce weight loss.[27–29]

Several AEDs can affect bone health by decreasing bone mineral density in adults and children.[30] One study demonstrated that as a group, people with epilepsy had lower overall bone density than did the general population.[31] Furthermore, the bone density of persons for whom an enzyme-inducing AED was prescribed was lower than that of persons for whom a nonenzyme-inducing agent was prescribed. Therefore monitoring bone health is critical in patients with epilepsy, especially those using phenytoin, phenobarbital, or carbamazepine. Both the patient and health care provider should be aware of the risk of bone fractures as a result of sports participation.

EXERCISE AND SEIZURES

In 1960, Dr. William G. Lennox, an early leader of pediatric epileptology, wrote: "Epilepsy prefers to attack when the person is off guard, sleeping, resting, idling. This is easily demonstrable in persons who experience very frequent petits [absence seizures], which may be almost absent during skating, swimming, or running, and abundant while sewing, eating, or just sitting. Parents picture their child as stopping or falling in a seizure and being run over while attempting to cross a busy street. I have never known this to happen, and I can remember only a few instances of a person having an attack while running or swimming."[32] Based on these observations, Lennox labeled activity as an *antagonist of seizures.*

Most human and translational animal studies completed in the interim support Dr. Lennox's empirical conclusion that exercise may, in fact, be protective against seizures and that it is rare for seizures to occur during activity. However, it is reasonable to expect that physical activity may induce seizures because strenuous exercise can result in hyperventilation, and in the EEG laboratory, hyperventilation is used to provoke seizures. However, the net effects of hyperventilation at rest and during exercise are different. At rest, hyperventilation triggers a decrease in carbon dioxide (respiratory alkalosis). The ensuing drop in cerebral blood flow and hypoxia results in network excitability and seizures. During exercise, however, hyperventilation is a compensatory mechanism that avoids hypercapnia and meets increased oxygen demands, thus the respiratory alkalosis required to induce a seizure does not occur.[33]

In addition, the most common provoking factors for seizures include stress, mental strain, and physical fatigue,[34] all of which can occur with intense physical exercise and competition. Stress may activate seizures through sympathetic stimulation,[35] and fatigue may cause seizures because of a chronically drowsy state.[36] Metabolic disturbances during prolonged, strenuous exercise, such as hyponatremia, dehydration, and overhydration, can theoretically aggravate an underlying propensity for seizures. However, the literature includes only a few cases of clear exertion-induced seizures,[37–40] and larger studies have not documented exercise-induced seizures, even during contact sports.[41]

Several studies and observations bear mention. In a single-center study of more than 15,000 patients with epilepsy, not a single case of exercise-induced seizures was reported.[42] In a second observational study of 400 patients, only two patients reported seizures during exercise.[43] Nakken[44] has reported that 10% of 204 patients with epilepsy had minor injuries during exercise because of a seizure. Additionally, 36% reported injuries during exercise that were unrelated to seizures and 36% reported that seizure frequency was reduced as the result of exercise. Conversely, Ablah and colleagues[45] reported a higher frequency of seizures related to exercise. However, only 53% of the 18% who reported seizures around the time of exercise had a seizure while exercising.

Experimental intervention studies have found that exercise either leads to fewer seizures or does not change seizure frequency. A study examining physical activity in women with intractable epilepsy found that average seizure frequency decreased from 2.9 to 1.7 per week with exercise.[46] In contrast, Nakken and colleagues demonstrated that a 4-week training program did not alter seizure frequency.[47] In addition, a longer 12-week study found no significant impact on seizure frequency, but did demonstrate improved vigor, as well as decreased anxiety and depression.[48] Although these studies do not provide evidence for exercise as a prophylaxis for seizures, the data do not demonstrate that exercise triggers seizures.

The mechanism by which exercise may serve as an antagonist to seizures is not known. Studies that have found a decrease in the frequency of epileptiform discharges on EEGs during exercise[49–52] suggest that exercise affects the cerebral mechanisms responsible for generating these discharges. During exercise, persons are typically more vigilant, alert, and attentive. Epileptiform discharges can be activated with drowsiness, and studies have documented a decrease in epileptiform discharges when patients with epilepsy are engaged in an interesting task or activity.[53] Exercise can also reduce stress and increase endorphin levels.[54] Stress is a known precipitant for seizures in persons with epilepsy,[43] and β-endorphins have been shown to reduce epileptiform discharges.[52]

Lastly, studies using animal models of epilepsy to investigate the effects of exercise on seizure threshold[55,56] have suggested other protective effects through mechanisms such as insulin growth factor 1 pathways[57] or the prevention of oxidative free radical mechanisms.[58]

Although seizure risk with exercise appears to be low, AED compliance is critical because a decrease in serum drug levels increases the risk for seizures in any setting. Variations in drug metabolism could theoretically increase seizure risk (increased metabolism) or increase adverse effects (decreased metabolism). However, changes in drug metabolism have not been observed in studies that have evaluated drug levels during exercise.[47,48]

ACUTE MANAGEMENT OF SEIZURES

Persons with well-controlled epilepsy may have a seizure during exercise. The first tenet of acute seizure management is to stay calm, because a seizure is almost always a self-limited event that requires minimal intervention. It is important to protect the person from self-injury. Objects close to the person, particularly during a convulsive seizure, should be removed. Restricting equipment or uniforms should be loosened. A tongue blade or other object should never be inserted between the teeth because a person will not swallow his or her tongue. Instead, the person may bite and break the object or injure the care provider. If a mouthpiece is present, it should be removed only if removal can be accomplished safely.

If the seizure does not terminate within 5 minutes, emergency medical services should be activated. Rectal diazepam is often prescribed for persons prone to prolonged seizures. The person administering diazepam should be aware of the potential for decreased respiratory drive. However, the benefit of stopping the seizure generally outweighs the risk of respiratory suppression.[59]

When the seizure is over, the person may be tired and confused. He or she may be allowed to lie down, but because vomiting may occur during the postictal period, he or she should be turned sideways to prevent aspiration. This position is not imperative if the seizure was nonconvulsive (e.g., a focal seizure with alteration of awareness with stereotypic or bizarre behaviors).

After acute management of a seizure, it is important to consider the person's emotional needs. The embarrassment that may be felt should be acknowledged, and it is important to recognize that although some persons may wish to speak about their experience, others may not. A simple "How are you feeling?" is often appreciated. The same approach applies to persons who witness the seizure. Given the many misperceptions about epilepsy,[60] the witnesses need to know that self-limited seizures are often not harmful, that these persons usually recover, and that most persons lead fulfilling lives with only rare or zero breakthrough seizures.

RETURN-TO-ACTIVITY GUIDELINES

No clear guidelines exist for safe return to activity after a seizure. Activity should be restricted if the person is either lethargic or confused. However, not all seizures result in a prolonged period of postictal symptoms (e.g., absence seizures), and thus return-to-activity decisions should be made on an individual basis.

Although a single self-limited seizure is not harmful, seizures can potentially result in injuries. The most common seizure-related injuries include fractures of the humeral neck, femur, clavicle, and ankle; chipped teeth; and shoulder and hip dislocations.[44] However, in a study that spanned more than 16 years, Aisenson et al. documented that the accident rate in patients with epilepsy was similar to that of their control patients without epilepsy.[61] In a more recent study by Fischer and Daute, it also was found that during exercise, no difference in accident rates existed in children with or without epilepsy.[44]

Safety Considerations Regarding Participation in Sports

A few factors should be considered to determine eligibility for sports or exercise participation, including (1) seizure types and frequency, (2) seizure precipitants, and (3) the activity in which the person wishes to participate. In general, sports participation should be allowed because restricting participation may have a substantial detrimental impact on a person's health and quality of life. Also, psychological and social responses to epilepsy may induce anxiety, depression, low self-esteem, and peer isolation. Exercise is known to reduce these symptoms.[62–64]

Participation also should be encouraged because persons with epilepsy may tend to be less active and physically fit. Patients with epilepsy who participate in exercise generally perform the exercise at less intense levels than control subjects, which is well documented in two studies.[65,66] In addition, the epilepsy group tended to be overweight.[66]

For most people with good seizure control, few restrictions are recommended. However, notable exceptions exist for persons with frequent or semifrequent atonic (drop) seizures and those who experience frequent or prolonged seizures. For persons recently diagnosed, participation in sports and exercise may need to be delayed until therapy and control of seizures are established.

Sport-specific restrictions are detailed in Box 20.1. Participation in extremely high-risk activities is typically discouraged because even a single seizure during these activities could have dire consequences. For example, a seizure during participation in gymnastics or stunts while cheerleading may significantly predispose a person to injury. Correspondingly, a seizure while climbing monkey bars or trees could have a similar result. In these circumstances, a confident and able "spotter" should be used. In addition, any person prone to seizures should avoid standing near a cliff's edge or placing themselves in any situation that could cause a fall from a height.

Helmets should always be encouraged for persons who choose to participate in "speed activities" such as bicycling, horseback riding, skateboarding, waterskiing, and snow skiing. With many of these activities, extra supervision is recommended. For persons who choose to participate in motor sports, state laws that guide the "right to drive" need to be considered.[67] It is important to be aware that sanctioned competitive driving options are also available for children. For this group of children, a frank discussion with the family of the risks versus the benefits, as well as compliance with state laws, is recommended.

Concerns that participation in contact sports, such as football, can exacerbate epilepsy because of repeated head trauma are valid. However, currently no published studies prove that chronic head trauma either increases the frequency of seizures or worsens the epileptic condition.[60,68–71] In one of the most notable studies previously mentioned, Livingston and Berman[42] reported their experience with 15,000 young children spanning 36 years. Hundreds of their patients participated in all types of sports, including contact sports such as lacrosse, wrestling, and soccer. Not a single instance of recurrence or aggravation of epilepsy related to head injury occurred in their cohort. Furthermore, it is important to recognize that many athletes with epilepsy have successfully competed at the highest levels of competition, including current NFL players Samari Rolle[72] and Jason Snelling,[73] and professional soccer player Leon Legge.[74] Nevertheless, as is the case with participation in other sports, the decision to participate in contact sports should be made prudently. The characteristics of the individual's epilepsy need to be considered because even a single seizure during an inopportune moment could have grave consequences.

Precautions are undeniably necessary during swimming because of an increased risk of drowning.[75–77] Diekema and colleagues[77] documented a relative risk of 23.4 for a child (0 to 19 years of age) with epilepsy drowning in a pool. Other studies[78] have suggested that the risk of drowning for a child with epilepsy is four times that of normal control populations. Nonetheless,

---

BOX 20.1 Risk of Selected Sports or Recreational Events

High Risk
Bungee jumping
Gymnastics (selected events)
Hang gliding
Motor racing
Mountain or rock climbing
Scuba diving
Skydiving
Stunting
Surfing

Moderate Risk
Bicycling[a,b]
Horseback riding[a,b]
Ice skating[a,b]
Rollerblading[a,b]
Skateboarding[a,b]
Sailing/canoeing[b,c]
Swimming[c]
Waterskiing/wakeboarding/wakesurfing[a,c]

Low or No Risk
Aerobics
Bowling
Cross-country running or skiing[b]
Dancing
Field hockey
Golf
Hiking
Track

Contact Sports With No Known Risk
Baseball
Basketball
Football[a]
Soccer

[a]A helmet should be worn.
[b]The activity should be performed with a partner.
[c]Someone with lifeguard training should be present and aware that the person has epilepsy, a life jacket should be worn, and the activity should not be performed in the ocean or in murky lakes.

---

these findings do not suggest that persons with epilepsy should not be allowed to swim. With proper precautions, including good seizure control with a stable medication regimen, most persons concur that swimming in a pool or a clear-bottom lake is permitted if the person is well supervised by someone who is trained in rescue and resuscitation and aware of the person's epilepsy.[76,79–81] Conversely, swimming in oceans and lakes with murky water is dangerous because in such venues it may be difficult to locate a person who is drowning. Therefore swimming in these environments is discouraged, and if persons choose to swim in murky water, it is essential that a life preserver/vest be used. Additionally, with very few exceptions, scuba diving and competitive diving should be prohibited.[82,83]

Interestingly, several studies have shown that taking a bath presents a more serious risk for drowning than does swimming.[76,78,79,84] In a study by Diekema et al.,[77] children with epilepsy had a high relative risk of 96 for drowning in a bathtub. In fact, older adolescents and adults run the highest risk because they tend to bathe alone, whereas younger children are usually supervised closely by a parent while bathing.

SUMMARY

Epilepsy does not automatically exclude a person from exercising or participating in sports. However, in making this decision, a balance must always be found between the patient's medical condition and his or her perceived need to participate. Frequently, the health and quality-of-life benefits such as an improved feeling of self-worth, decreased depression, and reduced stress will outweigh the risk of injury resulting from a seizure.

For a complete list of references, go to ExpertConsult.com.

SELECTED READINGS

Citation:
Nakken KO, et al. Effect of physical training on aerobic capacity, seizure occurrence, and serum levels of anti-epileptic drugs in adults with epilepsy. *Epilepsia*. 1990;31:88–94.

Level of Evidence:
IV

Summary:
The study of 21 patients with medically intractable epilepsy demonstrated a largely stable or decreased seizure frequency and stable drug levels during an intensive 4-week training program.

Citation:
Steinhoff B, Neusiiss K, Thegeder H, et al. Leisure time activity and physical fitness in patients with epilepsy. *Epilepsia*. 1996;37(12):1221–1227.

Level of Evidence:
IV

Summary:
This study assessed 136 patients with epilepsy, 145 controls based on a questionnaire, and 35 patients and controls based on standardized clinical tests of physical fitness. The authors concluded that patients with epilepsy show a considerable lack of physical fitness that might have an important impact on their general health and quality of life.

Citation:
Commission of Pediatrics of the ILAE. Restrictions for children with epilepsy. *Epilepsia*. 1997;38(9):1054–1056.

Level of Evidence:
II

Summary:
This is the most recently published guideline by a national medical organization regarding the subject of epilepsy and sports participation. It emphasizes the importance of considering positive effects of activities, such as exercise, before applying restrictions to children with epilepsy.

Citation:
Berg AT, et al. Revised terminology and concepts for organization of seizures and epilepsies: report of the ILAE Commission on Classification and Terminology, 2005–2009. *Epilepsia*. 2010;51(4):676–685.

Level of Evidence:
II

Summary:
These are the most up-to-date recommendations for classifying seizures and epilepsy from the International League Against Epilepsy.

Citation:
Nakken KO. Physical exercise in outpatients with epilepsy. *Epilepsia*. 1999;40(5):643–651.

Level of Evidence:
II

Summary:
This is a survey-based study of 204 adult patients with epilepsy who were compared with the average Norwegian's lifestyle. The authors concluded that for most of the patients, physical exercise had no adverse effects, and for more than one-third, it may have contributed to better seizure control.

Citation:
McAuley JW, et al. A prospective evaluation of the effects of a 12-week outpatient exercise program on clinical and behavioral outcomes in patients with epilepsy. *Epilepsy Behav*. 2001;2:592–600.

Level of Evidence:
II

Summary:
This is a randomized, controlled trial of moderate exercise in 23 patients with epilepsy that demonstrated a positive influence on behavior outcomes with no impact on seizure frequency.

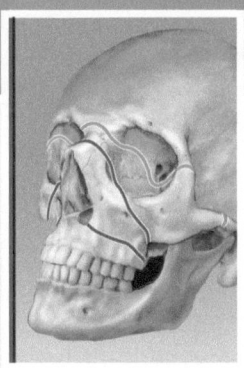

21

Environmental Illness

Jorge E. Gómez, Joseph N. Chorley, Rebecca Martinie

EPIDEMIOLOGY

Emergency department visits in the United States for exertional heat illness (EHI) increased 133% during the period 1997–2006.[1] Cases of EHI consisted of heat exhaustion (72.7%), heat syncope (9.7%), heat cramps (5.4%), and heat stroke (1.8%). Patients younger than 19 years (47.6%) and males (71.9%) accounted for a disproportionate percentage of EHI cases. The highest incidence of exercise-related heat illness in the United States occurs in August.[2,3,4] From 1990 to 2010, there were 49 heat-related deaths in high school and college football, more than any other sport.[5] Of these fatalities, 86% were lineman.

DEFINITION

EHI represents a spectrum varying from mild symptoms to medical emergencies. Environmental heat stress is best estimated by using the wet bulb globe temperature (WBGT), which takes into account radiant heat from the sun, ambient temperature, and relative humidity.[6] However, heat stress is more commonly reported as the more intuitively understood heat index (see http://www.nws.noaa.gov/om/heat/index.shtml).

Exercising muscle is relatively inefficient, converting ATP into muscular work with less than 25% efficiency, resulting in marked heat production, the amount of which increases with exercise intensity.[7] The initial responses to increasing core temperature include increased sweat, cardiac output, vasodilation, and redistribution of blood to the muscles and skin.[8] Heat dissipation during exercise is accomplished primarily by evaporation of sweat off the skin. High humidity will impede sweat evaporation. Dehydration (loss of 1% to 2% of body weight) is sufficient to impair effective sweat production.[9]

Forms of EHI can be subdivided by the presence of elevated body temperature. Elevated temperature EHI includes heat exhaustion and heat stroke. Normal body temperature EHI includes exercise-associated muscle cramps, heat syncope, exertional rhabdomyolysis, exertional sickle crisis, and exercise-associated hyponatremia.

EXERTIONAL HEAT EXHAUSTION

Pathophysiology

Exertional heat exhaustion (EHE) is likely due to a combination of dehydration, central nervous system fatigue, depletion of muscle energy stores, and in some cases, electrolyte imbalance.[7,10] Heat exhaustion typically occurs in high-temperature environments but may also occur in moderate- to low-temperature environments with high humidity.

Diagnosis

The diagnosis of EHE is made clinically. Symptoms include fatigue, dizziness, muscle cramps, headache, and nausea. Mild mental status changes may be observed (mild confusion, irritability, and emotional lability). Common physical signs include pallor and weakness. Vital signs will show elevated heart rate and body temperature (<39.5°C) with normal to low blood pressure.

Laboratory Findings

Laboratory testing is of little value except in cases of suspected hyponatremia (described later). Elevated urine-specific gravity and hemoconcentration reflect dehydration.

Differential Diagnosis

Other conditions that may resemble EHE include concussion, hypothermia, viral illness, alcohol or other drug use, and cardiac problems.

Treatment

The athlete should rest in a cool place. Oral rehydration is the initial treatment of choice, with the goal of replacing 1.5 L of fluid for every kilogram of body weight lost.[11] If body weight is unknown, adequate rehydration is evidenced by improved vital signs, ability to urinate, less orthostasis, and generally "feeling better." Cooled fluids containing less than 8% carbohydrate are absorbed more rapidly than plain water.[12-15] Rehydration fluids containing sodium appear to restore total body water levels more completely than water alone.[16,17] Intravenous (IV) hydration may be required for vomiting or significant orthostatic issues. Recommended IV solutions are normal saline (NS) and 5% dextrose in NS (D5NS).[18] The authors prefer D5NS to help limit the depletion of glycogen stores in the post-exercise hypermetabolic state. The infusion of IV fluids in heat exhaustion patients does not improve dehydration quicker than oral fluid, and IV infusions are prohibited by the World Anti-Doping Agency for athletes who are able to drink.[19,20]

Return to Play

No evidence-based guidelines have been developed for return to play (RTP) after heat exhaustion. Our recommendations are

---

BOX 21.1   Return-to-Play Criteria After Heat Exhaustion

- Minimum of 24–48 h of rest before returning to activity
- No headache, gastrointestinal symptoms, or muscle soreness
- Normal tolerance of orally ingested food and fluids
- Normal serum electrolytes (if the athlete was known to have an electrolyte disturbance)
- Normal-appearing urine

BOX 21.2   Return-to-Play Criteria After Heat Stroke

- Demonstration of normal mental status
- Return to normal dietary and elimination habits
- Normal variation in daily body temperature
- Normal complete blood cell count, blood urea nitrogen/creatinine, anion gap, liver enzymes, creatine phosphokinase, and urinalysis, including specific gravity
- Normal echocardiogram
- Persons with complicated heat stroke (i.e., significant organ failure and extensive rhabdomyolysis) should refrain from exercise for 1 month
- Persons with uncomplicated heat stroke (i.e., a brief emergency department or hospital stay) should refrain from exercise for 1 week
- Begin exercise in a cool environment, gradually increasing the duration, intensity, and heat exposure
- Athletes who demonstrate heat tolerance after 2–4 weeks of training may return to competition

---

listed in Box 21.1. RTP should address risk factors including deconditioning, chronic dehydration, habitual fatigue, and excess body weight.

Prevention

Several sports organizations recommend modifying outdoor physical activity when heat index values are in the "extreme caution" or "danger" zones.[21-23] Modifications include reducing the number of practices, scheduling practices during cooler times of the day, shedding equipment, and increasing access to water. These recommendations pertain especially to North American football, which is responsible for more cases of heat-related illness and deaths than any other sport.[24-26] In addition, athletes should be educated about gauging hydration status based on urine color; urine the color of apple juice reflects dehydration, whereas lemonade-colored urine reflects adequate hydration.

Acclimatization to hot environments occurs by a number of physiologic adaptations, including initiation of sweating at a lower core temperature and thirst at a lower serum osmolality, increased sweat rate, increased sodium absorption from sweat and urine, and expanded plasma volume.[7,18,27] The time required for acclimatization depends on age, baseline level of conditioning, practice and equipment requirements, and environmental factors. College athletes have been shown to acclimatize in as few as 12 days of practice.[28] Younger athletes typically require a longer period of acclimatization.[29,30]

EXERTIONAL HEAT STROKE

Exertional heat stroke (EHS) occurs when the body is not able to compensate for environmental heat stress combined with body heat produced by exercise. EHS is defined as an elevated core temperature (usually >40°C [104°F]) associated with signs of organ system failure. Central nervous system changes (altered mental status) are often the first markers of EHS.[31] EHS usually occurs in otherwise healthy, fit persons participating in high-intensity exercise in the heat.

Once homeostatic mechanisms fail to maintain a stable core temperature, continued heat stress will increase the shunting of blood flow from the core to the periphery, leading to organ hypoxia and acidosis. Resulting anaerobic metabolism depletes carbohydrate stores, which compounds organ damage.[8,32] Organ damage, particularly to the gastrointestinal tract, allows endotoxins to enter the circulation, resulting in hypotension, and the release of inflammatory cytokines results in decreased cerebral blood flow and neuronal injury.[8] Muscle injury results in increased serum [Ca] and [K]. Death usually occurs as a result of shock.

Diagnosis

The person with EHS may start out as dizzy, nauseated, and confused, but lethargy, obtundation, or unresponsiveness indicate more advanced, critical EHS. Physical examination typically reveals hot, sweaty skin, rapid pulse, and low blood pressure. Body temperature is above 40°C (104°F). Rectal temperature measurement is the most reliable method of monitoring core body temperature in the exercising athlete.[26]

Treatment

The keys to a favorable outcome for a person with EHS are (1) early recognition and (2) a minimal delay in initiating cooling.[33] Cooling should never wait for rectal temperature measurement in an athlete suspected of having EHS. The first responder should initiate basic cardiopulmonary resuscitation if necessary and activate EMS. Clothing and equipment should be removed immediately. Immersion should occur first if removing cumbersome equipment would delay treatment.[34] Immersion of the entire body in cold water is the treatment of choice.[35] Alternatives include pouring cold ice water continuously over the entire body, placing ice bags on the scalp, neck, axillae, groin, and popliteal fossae, and performing ice massage of large muscles.[36] Cooling continues until the rectal temperature reaches 38.6°C (101.4°F) to prevent overcooling.[37]

Return to Play

Recommendations for RTP criteria are summarized in Box 21.2.[38,39] No validated tests are available to measure responses to graded exercise in the heat to assist in making return-to-play decisions.[40]

EXERCISE-ASSOCIATED MUSCLE CRAMPS

Pathophysiology

Exercise-associated muscle cramps (EAMC), commonly known as *heat cramps*, are involuntary, painful muscular contractions during exercise. Several hypotheses have been proposed to explain EAMC, including excessive sodium losses, muscle fatigue, and central nervous system fatigue.[41-43] Prospective studies have failed to correlate sodium losses with the onset of EAMC.[41] Fatigue causes an increased firing rate of type Ia and II (excitatory) muscle spindle afferents and a decrease in afferent activity from the Golgi tendon organ (inhibitory) that results in sustained alpha motor neuron firing.[43] Poor conditioning may be result in premature fatigue.

Diagnosis

EAMC are usually self-evident. The athlete who has been exercising vigorously experiences painful cramping and is unable to function normally.

Laboratory Findings

In the majority of cases, electrolytes, pH, and muscle creatine phosphokinase (CPK) levels are within normal limits.

Differential Diagnosis

It is important to exclude drug effects as a cause of muscle tetany, including the use of lipid lowering and antihypertensive drugs, beta-agonists, oral contraceptives, insulin, and creatine.[44]

Treatment

The most effective treatment for EAMC appears to be passive stretching, which presumably increases the inhibitory activity of the Golgi tendon organ.[41,43] Cooling the muscles with ice massage may provide additional relief. Little evidence indicates that ingestion of an electrolyte solution or pickle juice consistently resolves EAMC.

Prevention

Athletes who are prone to cramping should be encouraged to consume more than normal amounts of salt in their diet and to use oral hydration fluids that contain sodium during and after practice. Adequate conditioning and improved rest may also help prevent EAMC.[43,44]

Return to Play

Athletes may return to the field of play after the resolution of muscle cramps if they are able to perform sports-specific drills without recurrence of EAMC.

HEAT SYNCOPE/EXERCISE ASSOCIATED COLLAPSE

Pathophysiology

Heat syncope (HS) and exercise-associated collapse (EAC) occur immediately following the stress of heat exposure and/or exercise. Upon cessation of exercise (i.e., the finish line of a marathon), the absence of rhythmic muscular contraction combined with dehydration limits, venous return, and thus cerebral perfusion pressure, results in syncope in susceptible individuals.[45] Syncope may occur similarly after prolonged standing in the heat or sudden rising from a sitting or lying position after exercise.

Diagnosis

Syncope that occurs upon stopping prolonged exercise in the absence of any other cause of syncope is EAC. Likewise, syncope in the heat after prolonged standing or sudden postural changes is likely HS. Orthostatic blood pressure changes may be present.

Laboratory Findings

Laboratory findings should be normal.

Differential Diagnosis

When syncope occurs during or immediately after exercise, a cardiac etiology must be assumed until proven otherwise. Seizure with postictal confusion can look very similar to HS and EAC. EHS must also be considered in EAC but in HS/EAC, the core temperature will be normal and individuals will respond to positional support. Hypoglycemia associated with diabetes must also be considered in the syncopal athlete not responding to supportive care.

Treatment

Supportive care to restore normal perfusion of the brain is essential. Placing patients in the Trendelenburg position for 15 to 30 minutes will help to restore cerebral blood flow. Squeezing crossed legs together and making a strong fist have been useful in increasing venous return and reestablishing adequate perfusion.[46]

Prevention

Adequate hydration with sufficient salt intake is important to maintaining normal fluid volume. Continuing to walk after completing a running race can minimize the risk for EAC. Moving or contracting the muscles of the legs during prolonged standing in the heat can help to maintain adequate perfusion.

Return to Play

Athletes may RTP after resolution of symptoms as long as they have reestablished normal blood pressure without orthostasis and have no signs of dehydration.

EXERTIONAL RHABDOMYOLYSIS

Pathophysiology

Exertional rhabdomyolysis (ER) is characterized by the breakdown of skeletal muscle during and after exercise that exceeds the working ability of the muscles.[47]

Excessive exercise will result in elevated intracellular free ionized calcium (Ca) especially in the mitochondria, compounded by depletion of ATP causing dysfunction in the Ca-ATPase pump.[48] This elevated calcium results in the activation of proteases and oxygen free radicals that cause myocyte death. Muscle injury causes intense muscular pain, weakness, swelling and elevated levels of serum CPK at least five times the upper limit of normal.[49] Risk factors for ER include dehydration, acidosis, excess ambient temperature, and hypoxia. In persons with ER, large amounts of myoglobin, proteases, and inflammatory mediators enter the circulation. Filtration of myoglobin results in glomerular injury, and proteases damage the respiratory epithelium, which may lead to respiratory distress. Rarely, inborn errors of metabolism may present with ER in apparently healthy persons.[48,50]

Diagnosis

Affected persons typically present with severe muscle pain especially those muscles involved in the extreme exercise. The muscles are tender to palpation and may be swollen. Severely affected patients may present with tachypnea and edema. Severe consequences include renal failure, disseminated intravascular coagulopathy, and acidosis.

Laboratory Findings

CPK levels usually exceed 20,000 IU/L or five times the upper limit of normal. Myoglobinuria may portend renal injury, but has also been report in asymptomatic endurance athletes.[51] Severe cases can have elevated serum potassium, positive D-dimer, elevated blood urea nitrogen (BUN), and creatinine.[52]

Differential Diagnosis

ER must be distinguished from compartment syndrome and pyomyositis. *Exertional myositis* refers to moderately elevated CPK levels (≤20,000 IU/L) in an athlete experiencing mild-to-moderate muscle pain and weakness without evidence of renal or metabolic injury.[51,53]

Treatment

Treatment usually requires hospitalization for the correction of acidosis, careful hydration to aid in the clearance of myoglobin without inducing fluid overload, monitoring renal function, and supporting cardiac and pulmonary function. If CPK does not improve after 72 hours, renal consultation should be considered. Persons who meet the following criteria may be treated as outpatients with close follow-up: (1) CPK less than 15,000 IU/L; (2) normal renal function *and* mild dehydration; and (3) the absence of sickle cell trait, infectious disease, or an underlying metabolic syndrome.[54] These persons should be encouraged to recover in a cool environment, refrain from exercise, and drink plenty of fluids.

Return to Play

Our RTP criteria are listed in Box 21.3.[38,54,55]

Prevention

ER can be prevented by gradually increasing training intensity and volume, and by ensuring adequate hydration and recovery between exercise bouts. ER has occurred in persons involved in activities, such as physical education, band, cheerleading, drill team, and Reserve Officers' Training Corps, especially when excessive exercise is used as a reprimand. Persons involved in these activities should be provided free access to water and sufficient rest during exercise, and they should be educated about symptoms and signs of heat illness and muscle injury.

EXERTIONAL SICKLING COLLAPSE

Pathophysiology

Sickle cell trait (SCT) is defined as the presence of 30% to 40% hemoglobin-S. Persons with SCT are normally asymptomatic. SCT occurs in 7% to 10% of African Americans and is common in persons of Mediterranean ancestry. Football players with SCT

BOX 21.3 Return-to-Play Criteria After Exertional Rhabdomyolysis

- Absence of muscle soreness or tenderness
- Normal strength
- Creatine phosphokinase less than five times the upper limit of normal
- Normal urinalysis, blood urea nitrogen/creatinine
- Persons with severe rhabdomyolysis (i.e., significant cardiac, pulmonary, and renal dysfunction) should not participate in any activity for 2–4 weeks after hospital discharge
- Persons with mild rhabdomyolysis may return to light activity when the aforementioned criteria are met
- Follow-up medical examination after 1 week
- May return to competition after tolerating 2–3 weeks of gradually increasing activity and demonstration of normal creatine phosphokinase values

Data from George M, Delgaudio A, Salhanick SD. Exertional rhabdomyolysis—when should we start worrying? Case reports and literature review. *Pediatr Emerg Care.* 2010;26:864–866; and O'Connor FG, Brennan FH, Campbell W, et al. Return to physical activity after exertional rhabdomyolysis. *Curr Sports Med Rep.* 2008;7(6):328–331.

TABLE 21.1 Exertional Sickling Collapse Versus Exercise-Associated Muscle Cramps

Feature	Exertional Sickling Collapse	Exercise-Associated Muscle Cramps
Muscles	Weakness > pain No spasm (tetany)	Cramping pain ≥ weakness, spasm
Behavior	Alert, may become listless, rapid breathing	Listless, irritable, may become combative
Temperature	Normal	Normal or elevated
Timing in exercise	Often occurs early in training session	Nearly always occurs late in training session

See references 57, 58.

---

have a 37 to 67 times higher risk of exertion-related death compared with non-SCT athletes.[5,56]

Heat stress, dehydration, and intense exercise especially at high altitude can cause severe hypoxemia, acidosis, hyperthermia, and red cell dehydration, which may induce sickling of red blood cells, leading to ESC.[57,58] Persons with SCT appear to be at greatest risk when they perform short bursts of repetitive, high-intensity activity (e.g., sprints), especially during the preseason when they be deconditioned.

Diagnosis

Athletes who experience ESC have sudden onset of extreme weakness and may collapse on the field, appearing anxious, and tachypneic. Features that help distinguish an athlete with ESC from an athlete with exercise-associated muscle cramps are outlined in Table 21.1.[58]

Laboratory Findings

The presence and percentage of sickle hemoglobin (HgbS) is determined by hemoglobin electrophoresis. In the acutely ill athlete, a complete blood cell count reveals anemia, and a blood smear reveals classic sickled red blood cells. Acutely, arterial blood gas findings reveal a partially compensated metabolic acidosis (low carbon dioxide, high pH, and increased anion gap). Muscle CPK is elevated and may continue to rise, akin to elevations observed in persons with ER.

Differential Diagnosis

Conditions that may mimic ESC include collapse from cardiac abnormalities (conduction or structural), asthma, heat exhaustion, or EHS. Cardiac arrest or heat stroke are unconscious or obtunded, whereas an athlete who collapses with ESC is usually lucid.[58]

Treatment

An athlete with suspected SCT-associated ER should not be allowed to perform any further exercise that day. EMS should be summoned and the athlete's condition should be treated as a "medical emergency." On-field measures should include oral rehydration, removal of the athlete to a cool environment, and the expeditious use of supplemental oxygen and IV fluids if available.

Return to Play

For general guidelines, medical staff may refer to the guidelines for RTP after ER (see Box 21.3).[38,54,55]

Prevention

The sickle trait status should be known in all athletes born in states that mandate determination of hemoglobin status as part of the newborn metabolic screen. Universal screening for sports beyond the newborn period is controversial.[58] Currently, the NCAA mandates screening of all athletes entering collegiate programs.[56] In other settings, selective screening of high-risk groups, particularly African Americans, may be warranted. Athletes with SCT should be counseled to set their own pace, slowly build-up training with longer recovery between exercise bouts, maintain good hydration, avoid extreme performance tests, and to stop exercising immediately if they experience unusual muscle pain or weakness.[58] The authors feel these guidelines should apply to all athletes regardless of whether their sickle trait status is known.

EXERCISE-ASSOCIATED HYPONATREMIA

Pathophysiology

Exercise-associated hyponatremia (EAH) is defined as the serum sodium (Na) below normal reference values (usually 135 mmol/L) during or 24 hours following physical activity.[59] EAH has been most frequently reported in endurance athletes, but has also been reported in the soldiers, hikers, and football players.[60-63] EAH has a spectrum of severity from mild cases complaining of nausea, dizziness, and "not feeling right" to vomiting, headaches, and confusion, and ultimately to coma, seizures, pulmonary edema, and death. The most common etiology of EAH is exercising while over hydrating, which may be related to lack of education about proper hydration or attempts to treat EAMC.[64,65] The syndrome of inappropriate antidiuretic hormone secretion (SIADH) will cause fluid retention when diuresis is needed. Tightly regulated osmotic control of body fluids can be overridden by nonosmotic stimuli, including nausea/vomiting, pain, exercise, elevated body temperature.[66-70] Much less frequently, EAH can be related to excessive sweat sodium losses with relatively normal fluid replacement with hypotonic fluid.[59]

Diagnosis

Increased body weight with decreased production of urine in an endurance athlete with the symptoms described above, especially with adequate water consumption, should raise suspicion of EAH.

Laboratory Findings

Clinical suspicion of EAH should prompt evaluation of a basic metabolic panel. Mild or asymptomatic cases usually have a serum Na between 130 to 135 mmol/L while more severe cases are ≤129 mmol/L. Associated elevation urine osmolality indicates SIADH.

Differential Diagnosis

Altered mental status associated with exercise may be caused alternatively by EHS, HS, or EAC, head trauma, seizure, drug ingestion, and diabetic ketoacidosis.

Treatment

In mild cases, fluid restriction with free access to salty snacks and broth will prevent the progression to more severe hyponatremia. Reestablishment of the body's homeostatic mechanisms is indicated with improving serum Na and the production of dilute urine. In severe cases with significantly altered mental status, an IV bolus of 100 mL 3% hypertonic saline should be given and can be repeated twice at 10-minute intervals for lack of clinical improvement.[67] Rapid correction of serum Na in EAH poses minimal risk for central pontine myelinolysis, which is seen with rapid correction of chronic hyponatremia.[59]

Return to Play

The athlete with EAH may return to activity when asymptomatic, the serum Na is normal, and urine production is normal. Proper hydration practices must be instituted and exercise should be done at a moderate intensity and duration, at least during the initial 1 to 2 weeks, avoiding extreme environmental conditions.

Prevention

Proper hydration is the best prevention and intervention. While some advocate drinking to thirst, replacing sweat loss using an individualized objective strategy will help novice athletes especially who may have difficulty in distinguishing thirst from fatigue. The sweat rate should be measured under different environmental conditions (Box 21.4). Secondary prevention can be achieved by measuring body weight before and after an event. Those who fail to lose weight during a marathon are seven times more likely to develop exercise-associated hyponatremia.[65,70] Medical and

---

BOX 21.4   Sweat Rate Measurement

1. Go to the bathroom and urinate/defecate if needed.
2. Towel off any sweat if needed.
3. Measure weight in minimal clothes/naked (PREWEIGHT).
4. Get dressed.
5. Perform planned exercise/practice for 1 hour with access to water in a container marked for volume.
6. Towel off any sweat.
7. Measure weight in minimal clothes/naked (POSTWEIGHT).
8. Measure the amount of fluid consumed (FLUID).

SWEAT RATE FOR 1 HOUR = PREWEIGHT − POSTWEIGHT + FLUID

---

emergency response personnel should be educated about the possibility of EAH.

COLD INJURY

Individuals participating in winter sports performed for a long periods at high levels of exertion are at an increased risk for cold injury, primarily hypothermia and frostbite.[71-74]

HYPOTHERMIA

Pathophysiology

Hypothermia, defined as a core body temperature of less than 35°C (95°F), is the most common cause of weather-related death, with individuals 65 years and older being at greatest risk.[75-79] Mortality increases proportionately with the severity of the hypothermia.[80] Dropping the core temperature results in nerve conduction delay, which leads to mental status changes, global depression of function, ataxia, and muscle stiffness. As hypothermia is neuroprotective, full neurologic recovery can occur even at remarkably low core temperatures.[81-84] Hypothermia results in electrocardiogram (ECG) changes, including abnormal repolarization, atrial fibrillation, and the J wave (a positive deflection at the QRS and ST-segment junction).[85,86] With dropping core temperature, there is sequential prolongation of the PR, QRS, and QT intervals.[79] Vasoconstriction causes a relative hypervolemia, and leads to the "cold diuresis" that may in turn result in hypovolemia.

Heat Balance

To avoid functional impairment in cold environments, core temperature must be maintained within a 4°C range by increasing heat production and decreasing heat loss.

Body heat production, or thermogenesis, is achieved in four major ways.[87] The resting (or basal) metabolic rate refers to energy expenditure at rest in a thermoneutral environment. During exercise 75% of muscle metabolic energy is released as heat, and 25% is converted to work. The absorption, breakdown, and storage of ingested food produce heat, called the "thermic effect," and provides a minimal proportion of total body heat production.[87] "Thermoregulatory thermogenesis" refers to shivering that can increase the metabolic rate up to five times the resting state.[87-89] The amount of shivering is proportional to the amount of cold stress experienced, but can be maintained only

as long as glycogen stores are available.[88] Shivering ceases at a core temperature of 30°C.[82,84]

About 90% of heat loss is through the skin, which is controlled by vasoconstriction. About 10% is lost through the lungs, which varies depending on the type and intensity of activity. Heat loss increases when an athlete is wet.[85] Radiation accounts for about 60% of total heat loss.[75] Radiation losses in children are higher due to their greater surface area-to-mass ratio.[90]

Other Factors Contributing to Thermal Balance

Certain medical conditions such as hypothyroidism, hypoadrenalism, hypopituitarism, and diabetes can impair the body's ability to produce heat.[75,79,88] Altered heat balance occurs in the elderly, and in individuals with multiple sclerosis, Parkinson disease, certain skin conditions, and those taking certain drugs.[75,91] Ethanol, the substance most commonly associated with hypothermia, leads to heat loss through peripheral vasodilation.[75,91-93] Phenothiazine drugs impair shivering thermogenesis.[94] Medications, such as benzodiazepines, barbiturates, and tricyclic antidepressants, decrease centrally mediated thermoregulation.[95]

Diagnosis

The diagnosis of hypothermia requires an accurate and reliable measurement of the core temperature. An esophageal probe placed in the lower one-third of the esophagus is preferred if there is a secure airway. If an esophageal probe is not available or if the airway is not secured, an epitympanic probe is recommended, although these can give falsely low measurements in the field. Rectal or bladder thermometers should not be used until the patient is in a warm environment.[82,84] Oral or axillary probes do not reliably reflect core temperature.

In mild hypothermia (32°C to 35°C or 90°F to 95°F), the extremities are cool and pale, and performing fine movements of the hands is difficult. Shivering is evident. Neurologic exam reveals listlessness, confusion, disorientation, dysarthria, and ataxia. The person with moderate hypothermia (28°C to 32°C or 82°F to 90°F) exhibits markedly altered mental status, dysarthria, apathy, and amnesia. The mental status may deteriorate into stupor and coma. Deep tendon reflexes diminish and become absent. Vital signs become unstable; hypotension and bradycardia emerge. Shivering slows and ceases. Death will ensue without treatment.[82,96] The person with severe hypothermia (<28°C or 82°F) is often comatose and may appear dead. The pupils may be fixed and dilated. Hypotension and bradycardia are severe; the respiratory rate decreases, and the vital signs may be difficult to obtain. Ventricular fibrillation and asystole are common. The muscles become rigid, and oliguria occurs. Persons with severe hypothermia have the highest mortality rate. Some investigators include a fourth category, profound hypothermia, which is defined as a core temperature less than 24°C or 20°C.[82]

Laboratory Findings

ECG is helpful in diagnosing cardiac manifestations. Laboratory evaluation should include serum electrolytes (e.g., calcium, magnesium), amylase, and lipase, and blood glucose, arterial blood gas, a complete blood cell count, BUN, creatinine, prothrombin time/international normalized ratio, partial thromboplastin time, and fibrinogen.[95]

Treatment

Treatment depends on the severity of the hypothermia and the treatment setting. Rewarming is the primary treatment for hypothermia. Persons with mild hypothermia may be treated with passive rewarming, consisting of insulating the patient and allowing thermogenesis to increase the core temperature. All wet clothes should be immediately replaced with dry garments.[82,84] Persons with moderate hypothermia require active external rewarming with care to avoid burns to the skin. Rewarming the trunk before the limbs is recommended to avoid *afterdrop*, in which core temperature drops precipitously because of shunting of cold blood away from the periphery to the core. Examples of methods for active external rewarming include blankets or electrical, chemical, or forced air heat packs.[97] A bath or a hot shower should not be used for rewarming as these can lead to cardiovascular collapse.[82,84] The clothing of persons with a markedly altered mental status should not be removed; rather, warm blankets should be placed over them.[85] Care should be observed when moving patients with severe hypothermia to prevent the precipitation of ventricular fibrillation.

Patients with severe hypothermia require active internal rewarming using warmed IV fluids (38°C to 42°C) and warmed fluids instilled into the gastrointestinal tract. In severe hypothermia, extracorporeal rewarming appears to increase survival.[83,97]

Extracorporeal rewarming refers specifically to shunting blood from the body, usually by cardiopulmonary bypass or venoarterial or venovenous shunt (extracorporeal membrane oxygenation [ECMO]), to a machine that rewarms the blood and returns it to the body. Extracorporeal rewarming is highly invasive and should be carried out only in centers with experience in these techniques. Patients with severe hypothermia can have profound bradycardia; carotid pulses should be checked for 60 seconds and cardiopulmonary resuscitation should begin if the pulse is absent.[82,84] Intensive care monitoring is essential in cases of moderate to severe hypothermia.

Prevention

Athletes should know the weather conditions and dress appropriately. Inner layers ideally are composed of materials that wick moisture from the skin. Outer layers should allow moisture to transfer to the air, where it can evaporate without significant heat loss.[88] Head covering can diminish heat loss up to 50%.[98] Thick, loose socks are essential; socks should be changed frequently during prolonged exposure so the feet stay dry.[88] Athletes undertaking long training routes in remote areas should both train with a partner and carry a cell phone. Athletes participating in winter sports must pay close attention to energy stores; increased intake of carbohydrates is recommended. Adequate hydration is important to avoid hypovolemia from cold diuresis. Athletes participating in winter sports should be aware of the warning signs of hypothermia, and if they find themselves lost in the cold, they should remember that their chances for survival are better if they take temporary shelter and conserve heat than if they continue to trek in the cold.

FROSTBITE

Pathophysiology

The military and mountaineering have traditionally been the groups with higher risk of frostbite.[99] In frostbite, tissues of an extremity or appendage (nose, ears, penis) become frozen.[79] Frostbite progresses through four pathologic phases.[100,101] In the prefreeze phase, vasoconstriction occurs as heat is lost in an effort to shunt blood to the core. Vasodilation will intermittently relieve this vasoconstriction approximately every 5 to 7 minutes in a phenomenon known as *cold-induced vasodilation*.[102,103] At the freeze–thaw phase, ice crystals form intracellularly, altering the protein structure and causing cell dehydration and shrinkage. Inflammatory mediators are released and accumulate. Vascular stasis occurs and endothelial damage occurs, causing blood leakage and thrombus formation. Affected tissues undergo progressive ischemia leading to cell death.[100,101] With continued exposure to the cold environment, frostbite progresses from distal to proximal and from superficial to deep.[104]

Diagnosis

Frostbite patients present with a cold and sometimes frozen extremity with numbness and paresthesias. Frostbite has been classified into four degrees of injury.[101,105,106] In first-degree injury, the affected area becomes firm and yellow to white, with significant edema. Second-degree frostbite will additionally exhibit characteristic clear to milky-appearing blisters. In third-degree injury, smaller hemorrhagic blisters indicate damage to the deeper dermis. Fourth-degree frostbite includes damage to the bone and muscle with gangrene and mummification likely.

Laboratory

Technetium (Tc) bone scanning within the first 5 days following rewarming reliably predicts which persons with frostbite would eventually require amputation and the extent of that amputation.[107,108]

Treatment

Treatment of hypothermia should be the first priority.[79,100,101] The mainstay of treatment of frostbite is rewarming, which will lead to significant pain, marked edema, and hyperemia. Rewarming should not be initiated in the field if refreezing is a possibility, because refreezing can cause more extensive tissue injury. If conditions in the field and during transport are such that the risk of refreezing is minimal, then the thawing process should be undertaken.[101] Rapid rewarming is performed in warm water with a temperature in the range of 37°C to 42°C (98.6°F to 107.6°F) with added antiseptic solution.[101,105] Care must be taken to ensure that the water temperature remains constant, which can be facilitated by keeping the water continually circulating. Rewarming should proceed until the extremity becomes red–purple and the skin is pliable, which typically occurs in 30 to 45 minutes. The affected tissue is often quite fragile; care must be taken to avoid having the extremity touch the sides of the water vessel to prevent tissue damage.[101] The injured extremity should be gently cleaned and allowed to air dry. Dry bulky dressings help to minimize any further tissue trauma, and the extremity should be elevated. Optimal management of blisters is controversial.[101,105,106] Blisters should not be débrided in the field. Once in the hospital setting, needle aspiration may be performed on any clear blisters but not on hemorrhagic blisters. Topical aloe vera, a thromboxane inhibitor, in cream or gel form, is a recommended adjunctive treatment.[101,105]

The rewarming process is extremely painful, and opioid analgesics are required for pain control.[101,105] Ibuprofen, 12 mg/kg per day in two divided doses to a maximum of 2400 mg/day, should be given to inhibit inflammation.[101] Tetanus prophylaxis should be administered per standard guidelines. Prophylactic antibiotics are not recommended. Antibiotics should only be given if signs or symptoms of infection/sepsis develop.[101]

Because part of the pathophysiology of frostbite involves microthrombi formation, thrombolytic therapy can be instituted in severe cases of frostbite. The use of an IV or intra-arterial tissue plasminogen activator within 24 hours of thawing has been shown to be of potential benefit in salvaging tissue at risk for necrosis.[109,110] However, treatment with a tissue plasminogen activator has significant potential risks, and should only be undertaken at a medical facility with intensive care monitoring and experience in using it in cases of frostbite. Vasodilators have been used for the treatment of frostbite. The use of IV iloprost is recommended, but this medication is currently not available in the United States.[105,109]

Surgical intervention with amputation should not be undertaken too early in the course of frostbite. Necrotic tissue demarcation can take up to 3 months. Most experts recommend early amputation only in cases of sepsis due to frostbitten tissue.[101,107,108] Pain, burning, and electric shock-like sensations are the result of an ischemic neuritis and can persist for weeks to months. Long-term sensory deficits occur in virtually all persons with frostbite.[100]

Prevention

Measures to prevent frostbite are the same as for preventing hypothermia.[79,100,101,104,105] In addition, in extremely cold weather, mittens should be worn instead of gloves. People exercising in the cold should know the signs and symptoms of frostbite and check for them frequently. They should move to a sheltered environment at the earliest signs of frostbite.

HIGH-ALTITUDE ILLNESS

High-altitude illness (HAI) usually occurs at levels of 2500 m or greater, although susceptible individuals may develop symptoms as low as 2000 m. At high altitudes, athletes are subject to lower oxygen tension and air resistance, greater exposure to ultraviolet radiation, drier air, and colder temperatures. The rate of ascent is more strongly associated with the risk of HAI than absolute altitude. Although no precise definition of "rapid ascent" exists, an ascent to greater than 2400 m in the first day, or greater than 600 m/day above 2400 m, would be rapid enough to induce HAI.[111]

The use of hypoxia or altitude as a training modification to improve athletic performance is beyond the scope of this chapter, but has been covered in recent reviews.[112-114]

Physiologic Adaptations to Altitude

At altitude, hypoxia induces cerebral arterial dilatation and venous occlusion, resulting in increased cerebral perfusion pressure, which stimulates hyperventilation, resulting in respiratory alkalosis.[115-119] Pulmonary vasoconstriction increases pulmonary perfusion pressure. The affinity of hemoglobin for oxygen decreases, favoring increased oxygen delivery to the tissues. Within 48 hours the kidneys increase bicarbonate excretion (in response to the alkalosis) and increase erythropoietin production.[115]

HIGH-ALTITUDE HEADACHE, ACUTE MOUNTAIN SICKNESS, HIGH-ALTITUDE CEREBRAL EDEMA

Pathophysiology

High-altitude headache (HAH) is a common isolated finding in unacclimatized individuals ascending to altitude, and is likely due to mild cerebral edema.[120,121] Increased pulmonary vascular pressure may trigger a mismatch in ventilation to perfusion, resulting in the mild dyspnea, whereas both dyspnea and hypoxia likely disrupt normal sleep.[122,123]

Diagnosis

Acute mountain sickness (AMS) is defined as HAH accompanied by at least one other symptom: nausea, vomiting, shortness of breath, lethargy, sleep disturbance, and anorexia.[121,124] The Lake Louise Consensus Scoring System has been widely used in the clinical diagnosis of AMS in adults (Box 21.5).[125-127] A Children's Lake Louise Score has been developed for young children.[128] A Lake Louise score of 3 or greater is consistent with a diagnosis of AMS. High-altitude cerebral edema (HACE), a potentially fatal global encephalopathy, is the end stage of AMS. HACE is diagnosed clinically in persons who ascend rapidly to a high altitude and consequently experience headache, mental status changes (e.g., confusion, difficulty concentrating, stupor, and drowsiness), and ataxia. Clinicians should be vigilant regarding persons with apparent AMS who continue to worsen, because deterioration from mild AMS to HACE may be swift. Patients with HACE typically present a nonfocal neurologic exam, although hemiparesis, hemiplegia, papilledema, retinal hemorrhage, and cranial nerve deficits have been reported.[129-131] A suggested simple test for subtle ataxia is to have the patient heel-toe walking in a straight line followed by a 90-degree turn; look for any unsteadiness.[131]

Risk factors for AMS include a history of AMS, a history of migraine, the use of alcohol, increased body mass index, elevated blood pressure, psychological stress, and inexperience with high altitudes.[132-134] Greater physical fitness is not protective, and vigorous activity increases the risk for AMS.[135-138] Lower arterial oxygen saturation with exercise at low altitude, and arterial desaturation in response to hypoxic exercise (hypoxic ventilatory response [HVR]), appear to be markers for susceptibility to AMS.[132,137,139-141]

Laboratory Tests

Patients with altered mental status or ataxia should have magnetic resonance imaging (MRI) of the brain, but treatment of HACE

BOX 21.5 Lake Louise Consensus Scoring System for Acute Mountain Sickness

Self-Reported Symptoms

Headache
0 = None
1 = Mild
2 = Moderate
3 = Severe, incapacitating

Gastrointestinal Symptoms
0 = Good appetite
1 = Poor appetite or nausea
2 = Moderate nausea and/or vomiting
3 = Severe nausea and/or vomiting

Fatigue and/or Weakness
0 = None
1 = Mild
2 = Moderate
3 = Severe

Dizziness or Light-Headedness
0 = None
1 = Mild
2 = Moderate
3 = Severe, incapacitating

Difficulty Sleeping
0 = Slept as well as usual
1 = Did not sleep as well as usual
2 = Woke many times; poor night's sleep
3 = Could not sleep at all

Clinical Findings

Changes in Mental Status
0 = No change
1 = Lethargy/lassitude
2 = Disorientation/confusion
3 = Stupor/semiconsciousness
4 = Coma

Ataxia
0 = None
1 = Use of balancing movements
2 = Steps off the line
3 = Falls down
4 = Unable to stand
TOTAL SCORE

See references 115, 127.

should not be delayed waiting for imaging. Brain MRI reveals vasogenic cerebral edema that may involve both gray and white matter, especially the splenium of the corpus callosum, and microhemorrhages.[119,142,143]

Differential Diagnosis

HAH is easily distinguished from migraine by its rapid resolution with supplemental oxygen.[130] Ailments that may resemble AMS include viral illness, a hangover, dehydration, exhaustion, hypothermia, or adverse effects of medication. Other conditions that may mimic HACE include hypoglycemia, stroke, transient ischemic attack, hypothermia, central nervous system infection, carbon monoxide poisoning, drug or alcohol use, complex migraine, and diabetic ketoacidosis.

Treatment

Most cases of HAH and AMS can be treated symptomatically with supportive measures including rest, oxygen, avoidance of exertion, attention to hydration, and analgesics for headache. Treatment guidelines for AMS are detailed in Table 21.2.[116,117,120,137,139,144,145] The most effective treatment for all types of HAI, including AMS, is immediate descent to lower altitudes. The urgency for descent will depend on the severity of illness. Individuals with HACE and high-altitude pulmonary edema (HAPE) should descend immediately.

Acetazolamide is the mainstay of pharmacologic treatment of AMS for both adults and children. Acetazolamide is contraindicated for individuals allergic to sulfonamides. Dexamethasone, alone or in combination with acetazolamide, is also effective in treating moderate AMS and HACE. Currently, there are insufficient data to recommend other medications, including antioxidants, magnesium, ginkgo biloba, sildenafil, and spironolactone, for the treatment of HAI.[146-149] Temazepam, zolpidem, or zaleplon may be used as an adjunct to therapy in persons with AMS and significant sleep disturbance.[150]

Return to Play

It is essential that the athlete be entirely symptom-free before resuming training or play at altitude.[117,145] Regimens for graded ascent are suggested in recent reviews.[111,144,151] Medication prophylaxis for susceptible persons should include acetazolamide, 125 to 250 mg twice a day, beginning 24 hours prior to ascent, and continuing for 2 to 4 days upon arrival at high altitude. Dexamethasone, 2 mg every 6 hours or 4 mg every 12 hours, can be used alone or in combination with acetazolamide and continued for the duration of the ascent to avoid rebound symptoms.[117] Persons with permanent neurologic sequelae following HACE should never return to a high altitude.

HIGH-ALTITUDE PULMONARY EDEMA

Pathophysiology

HAPE presents within 2 to 5 days after arrival at a high altitude with dyspnea, exercise intolerance, and a persistent dry cough.[152] Tissue changes with HAPE include patchy pulmonary vasoconstriction that results in elevated capillary pressure, damage to pulmonary capillaries with resultant leakage, which may induce inflammation, and hypoxia as a result of ventilation/perfusion mismatch.[115,116,153]

Diagnosis

Production of pink, frothy sputum, although classically described, is not common.[154] Auscultation reveals rales. Peripheral cyanosis and edema may be present in severe cases. Fifty percent of persons with HAPE also have AMS, and up to 14% have HACE.[115] HAPE accounts for the majority of deaths from high-altitude illness.[115]

TABLE 21.2	Treatment of High-Altitude Illness			
Intervention	AMS—mild (LLS < 5)	AMS—moderate to severe (LLS ≥5)	HACE	HAPE
Supportive	Rest, hydration, analgesics	Rest, hydration, analgesics	Rest, hydration, analgesics	Rest, hydration, analgesics
Descent	Usually not necessary; consider descent 500–1000 m if symptoms fail to improve after 24 h of treatment	Immediately descent 500–1000 m	Descend as soon as possible to lowest possible altitude at which symptoms improve	Descend as soon as possible to lowest possible altitude at which symptoms improve
Oxygen	May be administered to alleviate symptoms	Low-flow O_2 (1–2 L/min) or utilize portable hyperbaric chamber if descent not possible	2–4 L/min to maintain O_2sat[a] >90%	2–6 L/min to maintain O_2sat >90%
Medications	Acetazolamide 125–250 mg PO every 12 h Anti-emetics if necessary	Acetazolamide 250 mg every 12 h AND Dexamethasone 4 mg by PO, IV, or IM every 6 h	Dexamethasone, load with 8 mg PO, IV, or IM, then 4 mg every 6 h If descent is delayed, add Acetazolamide 250 mg every 12 h	Nifedipine 10 mg by mouth initial dose, then 30 mg extended-release every 12 h Consider Salmeterol inhaled 125 µg every 12 h Consider dexamethasone if symptoms suggest HACE

See references 116, 117, 120, 137, 139, 144, 145.

[a]Arterial oxygen saturation.

AMS, Acute mountain sickness; *HACE*, high-altitude cerebral edema; *HAPE*, high-altitude pulmonary edema; *IM*, intramuscular; *IV*, intravenous; *LLS*, Lake Louis Score; O_2, oxygen; *PO*, per os (by mouth).

Laboratory Findings

Arterial oxygen (O_2) saturation less than 90% is characteristic of HAPE. Chest x-ray reveals engorgement of the pulmonary arteries and patchy infiltrates, although diffuse lung involvement may be seen in more severe cases. Arterial blood gas analysis reveals severe hypoxemia (30 to 40 mm Hg) and respiratory alkalosis.[152] ECG may reveal right ventricular strain (e.g., right-axis deviation and p-wave abnormalities) and a right bundle branch block.[115]

Differential Diagnosis

Other causes of respiratory distress that may resemble HAPE include asthma, bronchitis, pneumonia, heart failure, myocardial infarction, and pulmonary embolus.

Treatment

Treatment guidelines for HAPE are summarized in Table 21.2. Patients whose O_2 saturation either fails to improve to 90% or greater who have evidence of HACE should descend immediately. Adding nifedipine, 30 mg by mouth twice a day, may be useful when either descent is not possible or oxygen is not available.[152,155] The administration of high-dose salmeterol, five puffs (125 µg) twice a day may improve oxygenation.[156]

Return to Play

Guidelines for RTP after AMS are applicable to persons with HAPE. Prophylaxis with dexamethasone, 8 mg twice a day, should commence 24 hours prior to ascent.[157] Tadalafil, 10 mg by mouth twice a day, begun 24 hours prior to ascent, is almost as effective as dexamethasone in preventing HAPE.[158] In a randomized controlled trial, nifedipine 30 mg twice a day afforded greater reduction in HAPE recurrence than inhaled salmeterol 125 µg twice a day.[156]

Advice for the Team Physician Traveling to Altitude

The physician accompanying a team to altitude for training or competition can implement measures to both minimize performance decrements and the risk of HAI. The team physicians and athletic training staff should review symptoms of HAI before traveling and regularly remind players to report symptoms, particularly headache, immediately.[159]

The strongest predictor of performance decrement at altitude is the HVR, a measure of how well the individual's respiratory apparatus compensates for lower oxygen tension. Measuring the HVR could identify athletes who may require individualized acclimatization, but doing so requires special equipment, which is not always readily available.

Athletes with positive risk factors for HAI, including a prior history of HAI, a history of migraine, a history of anemia or low iron stores, an increased BMI, and elevated blood pressure, should receive prophylaxis. Prophylaxis and treatment of HAI must be chosen with consideration of applicable antidoping regulations. Both dexamethasone and acetazolamide are on the World Anti-Doping Agency (WADA) banned drug list.[160] An acceptable prophylactic regimen is ibuprofen 600 mg by mouth 3 times/day begun 1 to 2 days before ascent for AMS.[161] The authors recommend the coadministration of omeprazole 20 mg by mouth once daily to avoid gastritis. Prophylaxis of HAPE may consist of nifedipine or tadalafil. WADA allows a maximum daily dose of salmeterol of 200 µg, which also may be used for HAPE prophylaxis, equivalent to four puffs twice a day (which is 20% less than the recommended dose for prophylaxis).[144,160] The team physician should always contemporaneously consult the latest applicable banned drug list.

The ideal approach to guard against the effects of altitude would be to acclimatize. The use of techniques, such as intermittent hypoxemic exposure (IHE), intermittent hypoxemic training (IHT), and live high, train low (LHTL), have been shown to improve the HVR, but require hypobaric or hypoxemia chambers that are not readily available to most teams.[162] Recommended graded ascent acclimatization to altitudes above 3000 m consists of increasing sleep altitude by no more than 500 m to 600 m per day, and a day of rest for each additional 1000 m if possible.[163]

Augmenting carbohydrates, such as pushing a carbohydrate-containing sport drink instead of water, may help to prevent performance decrements and dehydration.[164-167] Individuals with a history of anemia or low iron stores should have their iron status rechecked several weeks prior to travel to altitude and should begin supplemental iron accordingly. Reducing the intensity of workouts and increasing recovery periods in the first 1 to 2 days at altitude may allow partial acclimatization.

For a complete list of references, go to ExpertConsult.com.

SELECTED READINGS

Citation:
Casa DJ, DeMartini JK, Bergeron MF, et al. National Athletic Trainer's Association position statement: exertional heat illness. *J Athl Train*. 2015;59(9):986–1000.

Level of Evidence:
III

Summary:
Evidence-based, best-practice recommendations for the prevention, recognition, and treatment of exertional heat illnesses (EHIs) and description of the relevant physiology of thermoregulation.

Citation:
Bergeron MF, Devore C, Rice SG. Council on Sports Medicine & Fitness and Council on School Health. Policy statement—climatic heat stress and exercising children and adolescents. *Pediatrics*. 2011;128(3):e741–e747.

Level of Evidence:
III

Summary:
Evidence-based summary of differences in response to exercise heat stress between child and adult athletes, with specific recommendations for avoiding heat illness for child athletes.

Citation:
Paal P, Gordon L, Strapazzon G, et al. Accidental hypothermia—an update: the content of this review is endorsed by the International Commission for Mountain Emergency Medicine (ICAR MEDCOM). *Scan J Traum Rescuc Emerg Med*. 2016;24(1):111.

Level of Evidence:
III

Summary:
This paper provides an up-to-date review of the management and outcome of accidental hypothermia patients with and without cardiac arrest.

Citation:
McIntosh SE, Dow J, Hackett PH, et al. Wilderness Medical Society. Wilderness Medical Society practice guidelines for the prevention and treatment of frostbite: 2014 update. *Wilderness Environ Med*. 2014;25(suppl 4):S43–S54.

Level of Evidence:
III

Summary:
Evidence-based guidelines from an expert panel convened by The Wilderness Medical Society on the prevention and treatment of frostbite. The paper reviews pertinent pathophysiology, and discusses primary and secondary prevention measures and therapeutic management.

Citation:
Luks AM, McIntosh SE, Grissom CK, et al. Wilderness Medical Society practice guidelines for the prevention and treatment of acute altitude illness: 2014 update. *Wilderness Environ Med*. 2014;25:S4–S14.

Level of Evidence:
III

Summary:
Best practices guidelines from an expert panel convened by the Wilderness Medical Society for the prevention and treatment of acute mountain sickness, high-altitude cerebral edema, and high-altitude pulmonary edema. These guidelines present the main prophylactic and therapeutic modalities for each disorder and provide recommendations about their role in disease management. Recommendations are graded based on the quality of supporting evidence.

Citation:
Bärtsch P, Swenson ER. Clinical practice: acute high-altitude illnesses. *N Engl J Med*. 2013;368:2294–2302.

Level of Evidence:
III

Summary:
An evidence-based clinical guideline on high-altitude illness, including a review of formal guidelines, as well as authors' expert recommendations.

22

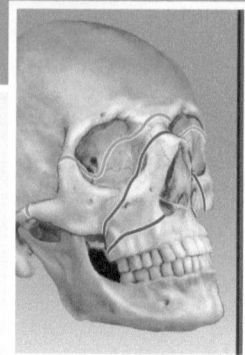

Dermatologic Conditions

Haoming Xu, Barbara B. Wilson, Michael A. Marchetti

The skin and its appendages constitute a complicated and highly regulated organ known as the integumentary system. Its functions are diverse and include protecting the body from an array of external insults by means of physical and immunologic mechanisms, regulating temperature homeostasis, providing sensory receptors for interactions with the environment, preventing water loss, and initiating vitamin D synthesis. As such, optimal athletic performance relies on the proper health and function of the integumentary system. It is therefore crucial that health care providers be able to recognize and effectively treat dermatologic disorders affecting the athlete. This chapter introduces disorders affecting athletes and focuses on providing a framework to evaluate the skin and effectively establish a diagnosis.

CUTANEOUS INFECTIONS

Cutaneous infections are among the most common dermatologic disorders that affect athletes. Making an accurate diagnosis is critical because infections may result in morbidity and lead to missed practices or game ineligibility. Familiarity with return-to-play guidelines is essential. Readers are encouraged to consult published guidelines, such as the *2014–2015 NCAA Sports Medicine Handbook,* which is emphasized in this chapter.[1] Guidelines for skin infections are primarily for athletes in contact sports, particularly wrestlers, because they are at highest risk for acquisition and transmission of cutaneous infections.

Bacterial Infections
Folliculocentric Infections: Bacterial Folliculitis, Furuncles, and Carbuncles

Bacterial folliculitis, furuncles, and carbuncles are infections that begin within hair follicles and can be conceptualized as a disease continuum. All of these infections are common among athletes, and one study documented that 25% of a high school's varsity athletes experienced an episode of furunculosis over 1 year.[2] Bacterial folliculitis presents as tender, follicular-based pustules, whereas a furuncle is a deeper inflammatory nodule. Furuncles often, but not invariably, arise from folliculitis (Fig. 22.1). Carbuncles are more extensive, deeper, communicating masses that arise when multiple, closely set furuncles coalesce (Fig. 22.2). Patients with carbuncles often are ill and present with fever and malaise. All are most commonly caused by *Staphylococcus aureus* and can evolve into an abscess or a pus-filled cavity. These infections typically arise in hair-bearing sites, particularly in areas subject to friction,

occlusion, and perspiration, such as the neck, face, scalp, axillae, groin, extremities, and buttocks. Shaving of hair may promote infection, and any injury that disrupts skin integrity may lead to increased risk of infection. Diagnosis is made clinically, and if pus is obtainable, a bacterial culture should be submitted for organism identification and antibiotic sensitivity.

The initial therapy for bacterial folliculitis includes washing the affected area daily with an antibacterial soap (e.g., a chlorhexidine gluconate 2% to 4% solution or a benzoyl peroxide 10% wash) and applying a topical antibiotic, such as mupirocin 2% ointment, two to three times daily. In resistant cases, short courses of oral antibiotics can be used as directed by culture results. Nonfluctuant furuncles can be treated with warm compresses to promote drainage. Fluctuant furuncles and carbuncles that have evolved into abscesses require incision, drainage, and culture. Oral antibiotic therapy has traditionally been considered on a case-by-case basis (e.g., suspicion for community-acquired methicillin resistant *S. aureus* [MRSA], severe or extensive disease, rapid progression, associated cellulitis, systemic illness, and/or the presence of comorbidities or immunosuppression). However, multicenter, prospective, double-blind, placebo-controlled, randomized trials in 2016 and 2017 have demonstrated that the use of clindamycin or trimethoprim-sulfamethoxazole in conjunction with incision and drainage improves short-term outcomes, including cure rate, in patients with uncomplicated, simple abscesses.[3,4]

Patients with recurrent disease should be evaluated for chronic nasal carriage of *S. aureus*, which may serve as a reservoir for infection. Eradication measures include intranasal application of mupirocin 2% ointment twice daily for 5 to 10 days, washing the skin and in particular the axillae and groin daily with chlorhexidine gluconate 2% to 4% solution, and use of dilute sodium hypochlorite (i.e., bleach) baths ($\frac{1}{4}$ cup bleach per $\frac{1}{4}$ tub or 13 gallons of water). Oral antibiotic therapy is not routinely recommended for decolonization.[5]

National Collegiate Athletic Association (NCAA) wrestling guidelines require that wrestlers must be without any new skin lesions for 48 hours before competition, must have completed 72 hours of antibiotic therapy, must have no moist, exudative, or purulent lesions, and must not cover active purulent lesions, to allow for participation.[1]

Impetigo

Impetigo is a superficial bacterial infection of the skin. Both *S. aureus* and Group A *Streptococcus* can produce impetigo, but *S.*

246

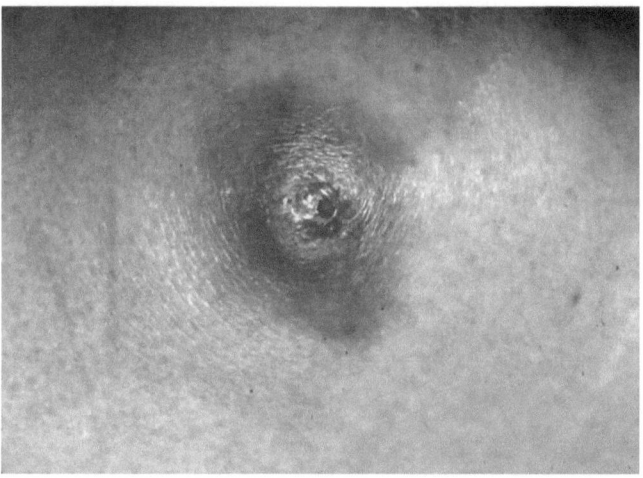

Fig. 22.1 A methicillin-resistant *Staphylococcus aureus* furuncle. (Courtesy Kenneth E. Greer.)

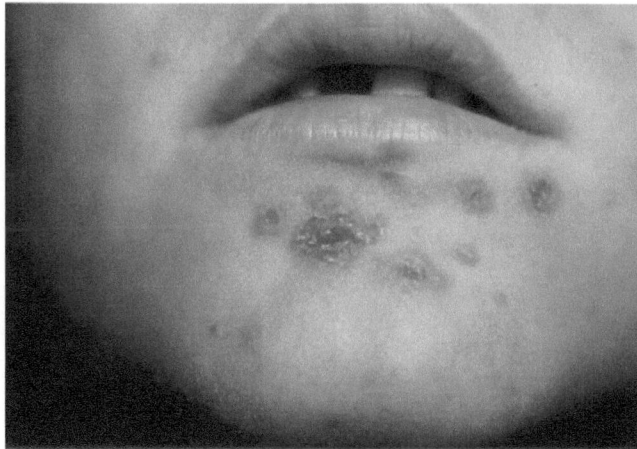

Fig. 22.3 Nonbullous impetigo on the chin with golden crusting. (Courtesy Kenneth E. Greer.)

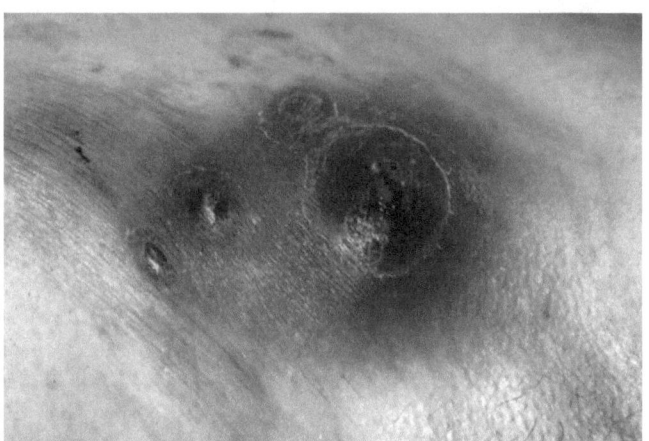

Fig. 22.2 Multiple furuncles coalescing to form a carbuncle. (Courtesy Kenneth E. Greer.)

aureus is the more common etiology in industrialized nations. Athletes who engage in contact sports are at higher risk for acquisition of disease via trauma and disruption of skin integrity.

Two presentations are recognized: bullous and nonbullous impetigo. Nonbullous impetigo typically begins as a transient vesicle or pustule that evolves into a honey-colored crusted plaque with surrounding erythema (Fig. 22.3). Infection is most common on the central face. The differential diagnosis includes herpes simplex, contact dermatitis, and atopic dermatitis. Bullous impetigo is characterized by superficial vesicles and bullae that rupture after 1 to 2 days, leading to weeping erosions that eventually heal over. Contact dermatitis, herpes simplex, bullous arthropod bites, drug rash, burns, and erythema multiforme should be ruled out.

Diagnosis is usually suspected based on the clinical appearance, but bacterial culture is recommended for diagnostic confirmation and antibiotic sensitivity, given the increasing prevalence of community-acquired MRSA infections. Initial treatment should include local wound care with soap and water and use of topical mupirocin 2% ointment three times daily. For widespread infections, penicillinase-resistant antistaphylococcal antibiotics (cephalexin or dicloxacillin) can be considered, pending antibiotic

sensitivity results. Empiric MRSA coverage can be considered in areas with high prevalence of infection. Impetigo is contagious, particularly in its bullous form, and may spread among athletes practicing contact sports. Affected individuals should be advised against sharing towels or soap. Return-to-play (RTP) guidelines are identical to those for bacterial folliculitis (described in the previous section).

Cellulitis/Erysipelas

Cellulitis and erysipelas are common infections of the skin in athletes, usually caused by *S. aureus* and Group A *Streptococcus*. Cellulitis is defined as an infection of the dermis and subcutaneous fat, whereas erysipelas is a more superficial variant affecting the upper dermis and lymphatic vessels. Less common causative organisms include *Haemophilus influenzae*, groups B and G *Streptococcus*, enteric gram-negative rods, coagulase-negative *Staphylococcus*, and *Streptococcus pneumoniae*.[6-10] Risk factors for the development of cellulitis include any injury or trauma to the skin that allows for bacterial entry, such as cuts and/or scrapes, which are more prevalent in athletes participating in direct contact sports.

Cellulitis classically presents as a unilateral erythematous, warm, tender, indurated, and edematous plaque with indistinct margins. Erysipelas is similar in appearance but tends to be more sharply defined with a bright red color (Fig. 22.4). Occasionally cellulitis may undergo bullae formation with necrosis, resulting in localized skin sloughing and ulcer formation. Systemic symptoms are variable, with fever, chills, malaise, and regional lymphadenopathy being the most common. The absence of pain or pain out of proportion to the clinical appearance should prompt consideration of a deeper infection, such as necrotizing fasciitis or myonecrosis. Other clinical red flags for necrotizing fasciitis or myonecrosis include erythema evolving into a dusky gray color, malodorous watery discharge, and crepitus in the soft tissues.

Diagnosis is primarily clinical, based on the history and clinical presentation. Culture studies of the leading edge of cellulitic plaques are not indicated in routine, uncomplicated cellulitis or erysipelas because of their low yield, but they should be obtained in the presence of open, fluctuant, or bullous lesions.

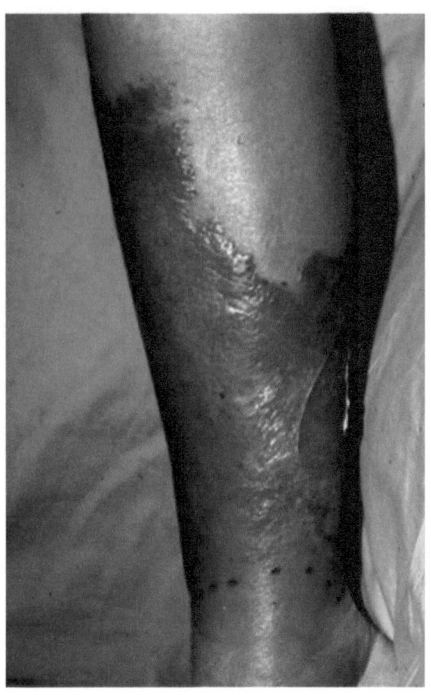

Fig. 22.4 Erysipelas with bulla formation and subsequent erosion. Note the sharply defined border, which can help distinguish erysipelas from cellulitis. (Courtesy Kenneth E. Greer.)

The differential diagnosis is extensive and includes deep venous thrombosis, superficial thrombophlebitis, Sweet syndrome, contact dermatitis, stasis dermatitis, arthropod bites, panniculitides, necrotizing soft tissue infections, and erythema migrans.

Treatment depends on the severity of infection, with more severe cases necessitating hospitalization and parenteral antibiotics. Routine, uncomplicated, and non-purulent cellulitis can be treated in the outpatient setting with β-lactam antibiotics (e.g., dicloxacillin and cephalexin) as empiric first-choice therapy. Studies have consistently shown that empiric β-lactam antibiotics continue to be the most cost-effective choice with fewer adverse events in the treatment of uncomplicated cellulitis.[11,12] Furthermore, in a 2017 multicenter, double-blind, randomized, superiority trial among patients with uncomplicated, nonpurulent cellulitis, the use of cephalexin plus trimethoprim-sulfamethoxazole compared to cephalexin alone did not result in higher rates of clinical resolution of cellulitis.[13]

Simple measures including bed rest and elevation of the involved site should be routinely emphasized, but warm compresses should be avoided because they predispose the skin to vesicle formation. Empiric MRSA coverage (e.g., clindamycin, trimethoprim-sulfamethoxazole, and tetracyclines) should be reserved for patients with purulent cellulitis, systemic symptoms (i.e., fever, hypotension, tachycardia), a history of MRSA infection or colonization, a lack of clinical response to an antibiotic regimen that does not cover MRSA, risk factor(s) for MRSA infection (recent hospitalization or surgery, hemodialysis, and human immunodeficiency virus infection), or proximity of cellulitis to indwelling medical device (e.g., prosthetic joint or vascular graft).[14] RTP guidelines are identical to those for bacterial folliculitis (described in the section "Folliculocentric Infections: Bacterial Folliculitis, Furuncles, and Carbuncles").

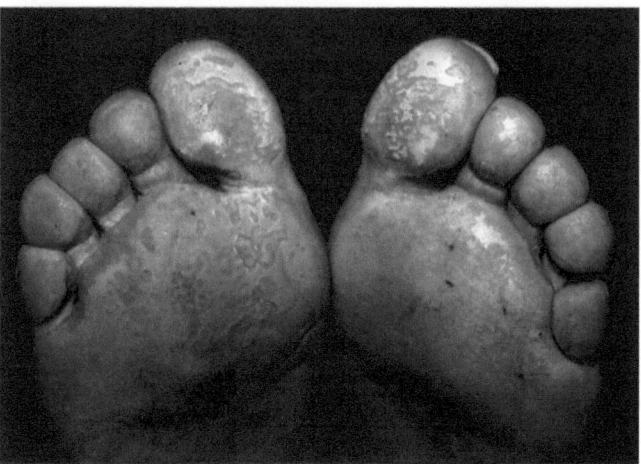

Fig. 22.5 Pitted keratolysis. (Courtesy Kenneth E. Greer.)

Pitted Keratolysis

Pitted keratolysis is a superficial bacterial infection of the feet caused by bacteria of the *Corynebacterium* genus, particularly *Kytococcus sedentarius*.[15,16] Numerous small crateriform punched-out pits are seen predominantly on the thickest areas of the plantar surface and may coalesce to form large, irregular, scalloped lesions (Fig. 22.5). Less commonly, the toe web spaces are affected. Infection usually occurs in younger males with sweaty feet, but it can affect all ages and sexes. Patients note a distinctive malodor, and some may describe a slimy sensation. Moisture, occlusion, and tropical climates are predisposing factors. The clinical appearance is distinctive, but the differential diagnosis of interdigital involvement includes tinea pedis and erythrasma. Therapeutic options include thorough cleansing combined with use of a clindamycin 1% solution or a benzoyl peroxide 10% wash or 5% gel. Dilute sodium hypochlorite (bleach) soaks may speed resolution. Adjunctive and preventative measures aim at reducing moisture and include keeping feet dry by changing socks frequently, using absorptive foot powders (e.g., microporous cellulose and talc powder), and applying antiperspirants topically (e.g., aluminum chloride 20% solution nightly). Footwear should be replaced as indicated.

Erythrasma

Erythrasma is an underdiagnosed superficial bacterial skin infection caused by *Corynebacterium minutissimum* that is commonly confused with dermatophyte infections. The condition is most common in warm, temperate climates and leads to clinical disease, particularly in folds of the skin, such as the inguinal creases, axillae, or interdigital toe web spaces. Lesions are often pinkish-tan, scaly patches, and unlike dermatophyte infections, they do not demonstrate an active, raised advancing border (Fig. 22.6). Erythrasma can be asymptomatic or mildly pruritic.

The diagnosis can be confirmed by demonstrating coral-red fluorescence with Wood's lamp (ultraviolet A [UVA]) examination. Of note, this finding may be absent in patients who have recently washed the involved area. Potassium hydroxide (KOH) preparations of skin scrapings will be negative. The differential diagnosis often includes other intertriginous eruptions, such as

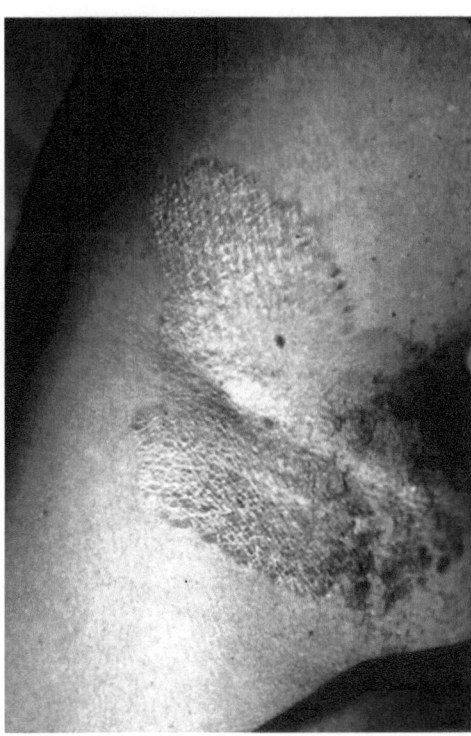

Fig. 22.6 Erythrasma affecting the axilla. (Courtesy Kenneth E. Greer.)

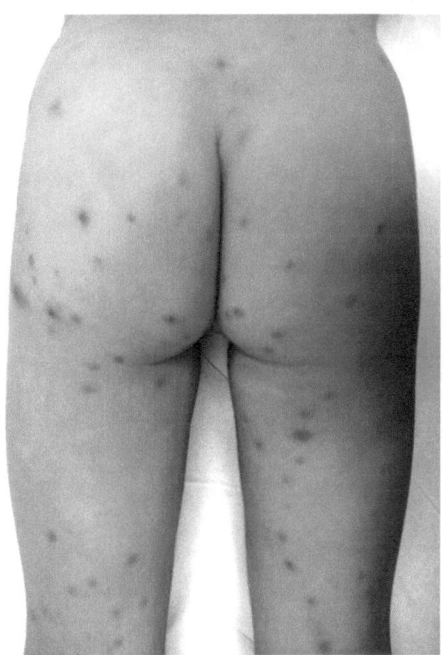

Fig. 22.7 A child with pseudomonas folliculitis after bathing in a hot tub.

dermatophytoses (e.g., tinea cruris or tinea pedis), candidiasis, seborrheic dermatitis, contact dermatitis, and inverse psoriasis. First-line treatment is with topical erythromycin 2% solution, clindamycin 1% solution, or benzoyl peroxide 5% gel. Oral doses of clindamycin and erythromycin are also effective.

Pseudomonal Folliculitis (Hot Tub Folliculitis)

Use of hot tubs, whirlpools, or swimming pools can lead to the development of a self-limited folliculitis caused by *Pseudomonas aeruginosa*. Lesions present as pruritic, follicular-based papules and pustules that develop 1 to 5 days after the use of bathing facilities (Fig. 22.7). Occasionally patients may experience fever, chills, and lymphadenopathy. Lesions may be generalized over the body, may appear underneath clothing, or may be localized if only a certain body site is immersed. The differential diagnosis includes staphylococcal folliculitis, Pityrosporum folliculitis, and arthropod bites. Bacterial culture of pustule contents can be performed to confirm the diagnosis. In immunocompetent persons without systemic involvement, the infection is self-limited and no treatment is necessary. For athletes who require treatment, ciprofloxacin, 250 mg by mouth twice daily for 7 days, is recommended. Suspected water sources should be inspected for adequate pH levels and chlorine content. RTP guidelines are identical to those for bacterial folliculitis (described in the section "Folliculocentric Infections: Bacterial Folliculitis, Furuncles, and Carbuncles").

Fungal Infections

Dermatophytoses

The three fungal genera *Trichophyton*, *Microsporum*, and *Epidermophyton* comprise more than 40 species and are collectively referred to as "dermatophytes." These fungi can be found living in soil and on the skin of animals and humans. Common infections in humans are colloquially referred to as "jock itch" (tinea cruris), "athlete's foot" (tinea pedis), and "ringworm" (tinea corporis). Dermatophytes can infect any superficial skin surface, including appendageal structures, such as hair follicles and nails, but they cannot penetrate into the dermis or infect mucous membranes. Athletes are at higher risk for infection, because perspiration and trauma facilitate growth and penetration of dermatophytes on the skin. Additionally, fungi are transmitted via skin-to-skin contact and the use of shared facilities and items (such as locker rooms and towels). Wrestlers in particular are at risk for tinea corporis.

Dermatophyte infections of the skin—no matter the location— typically demonstrate a red, scaly, raised, advancing border, which is the most useful diagnostic clue on physical examination. Lesions on the body variably show an annular or ring-shaped appearance. Tinea cruris favors the inguinal folds and advances onto the thighs (Fig. 22.8). As opposed to candidiasis, tinea cruris almost never involves the scrotum. Tinea pedis classically presents with scaling, maceration, and erythema in the interdigital toe web spaces (particularly the fourth) but can involve the entire foot (Fig. 22.9). Tinea capitis is most common in children and presents as red, scaly patches of alopecia.

The differential diagnosis is location dependent and extensive but most commonly includes seborrheic dermatitis, eczema, or alopecia areata in the scalp; contact dermatitis, atopic dermatitis, psoriasis, tinea versicolor, pityriasis rosea, or subacute cutaneous lupus erythematosus on the body; candidiasis, erythrasma, seborrheic dermatitis, psoriasis, or contact dermatitis in the groin; and dyshidrotic eczema, contact dermatitis, psoriasis, candidiasis, and scabies on the feet. Diagnosis can be suspected on clinical examination but should be confirmed with a diagnostic test. Scraping the advancing edge of a lesion for microscopic examination with 10% KOH is an in-office procedure that is easy to

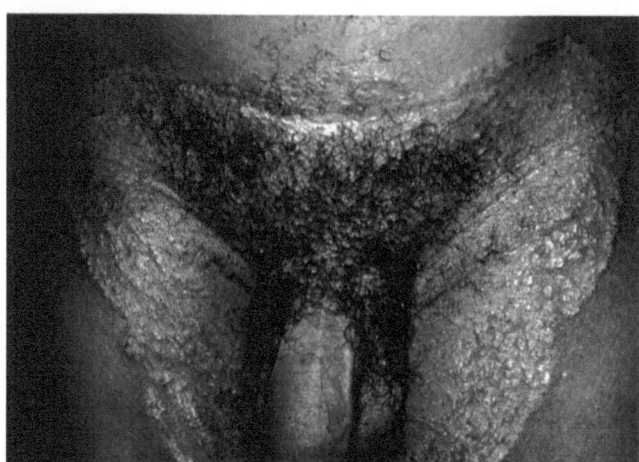

Fig. 22.8 Tinea cruris with characteristic sparing of the penis and scrotum. Note the active, advancing border typical of dermatophyte infections. (Courtesy Kenneth E. Greer.)

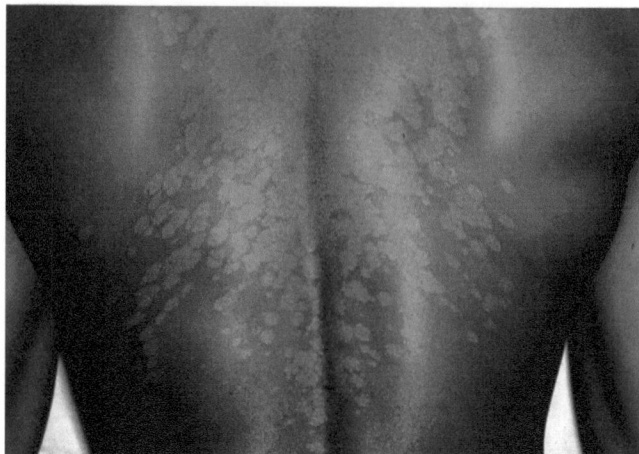

Fig. 22.10 Hypopigmented tinea versicolor. (Courtesy Kenneth E. Greer.)

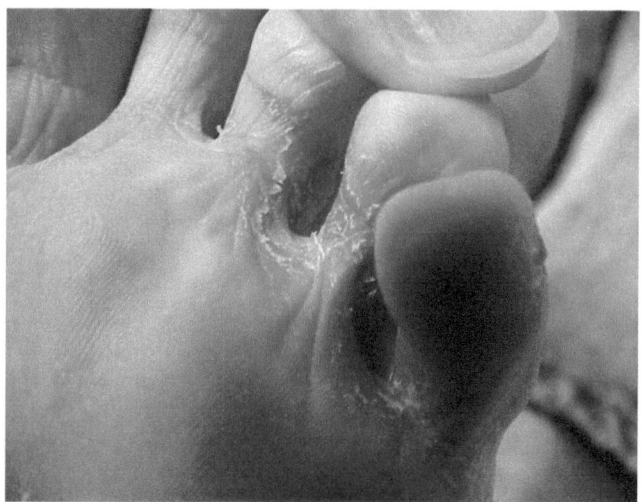

Fig. 22.9 Interdigital tinea pedis. (Courtesy D. Stulberg.)

perform. The presence of septate, branching hyphae is diagnostic. Alternatively, hair shafts, skin scrapings, or swabs taken from the scalp can be submitted for fungal culture.

Multiple systemic and topical antifungal agents are available to treat dermatophyte infections of skin, hair, and nails. Most cases of tinea corporis, cruris, and pedis can be successfully treated with topical therapy alone. Terbinafine 1% cream or ketoconazole 2% cream applied twice daily for several weeks are good first-line treatments. Consideration of an oral antifungal agent, such as fluconazole, 200 mg by mouth weekly for 2 to 4 weeks, or terbinafine, 250 mg by mouth daily for 1 to 2 weeks, can be considered in widespread, inflammatory, or refractory cases. Treatment of tinea capitis always requires systemic therapy, with griseofulvin ultramicrosized capsules, 15 mg/kg/day in divided doses for 8 weeks, remaining first-line treatment. Consultation with a dermatologist is recommended in severe cases, after treatment failure, and when the diagnosis is unclear.

NCAA guidelines mandate that for wrestlers to return to competition, a minimum of 72 hours of topical therapy is required for skin lesions and two weeks of oral antifungal therapy is required

for scalp lesions. Wrestlers with extensive and active lesions may be disqualified, with infection determined by KOH preparation or a review of the therapeutic regimen.[1]

Malassezia

The fungal genus *Malassezia* (formerly *Pityrosporum*) includes several species of lipophilic yeasts that form part of the normal skin flora and flourish in warm, moist, sebum-rich body areas. Under certain circumstances, proliferation of the yeast can produce the skin conditions tinea versicolor and Pityrosporum folliculitis. By the nature of their physical activity, young athletes are at higher risk for the development of these infections.

Tinea versicolor presents as finely scaling macules that coalesce, forming irregularly shaped patches of pigment alteration. Lesions may be tan to brown or white to pink in color and are most commonly located on the back, chest, abdomen, proximal upper extremities, and neck (Fig. 22.10). A clue to the diagnosis includes the extensive dust-like scaling that can be produced by scratching the lesions. On microscopic examination with 10% KOH, the scale will show clusters of oval, budding yeast cells and short, septate hyphae. The differential diagnosis usually includes tinea corporis, pityriasis rosea, and progressive macular hypomelanosis. Tinea versicolor is neither transmissible nor caused by poor hygiene. Pityrosporum folliculitis presents as follicular, erythematous, 2- to 3-mm papules and pustules on the chest and back and is due to *Malassezia* yeast proliferating within the hair follicle (Fig. 22.11). The diagnosis is often confused with bacterial folliculitis and acne vulgaris.

Both conditions are treated with topical antifungal agents, such as ketoconazole 2% shampoo and selenium sulfide 2.5% lotion, which are lathered onto the skin for 10 minutes and rinsed off. Patients should perform this treatment daily for at least 10 days, with tapering of frequency to weekly use thereafter for 1 to 2 months for prevention. Occasionally, oral antifungal drugs are used in persons with resistant disease.

Viral Infections
Herpes Simplex

Infection by human herpesvirus 1 (HSV-1) and human herpesvirus 2 (HSV-2) is common in both the general population and

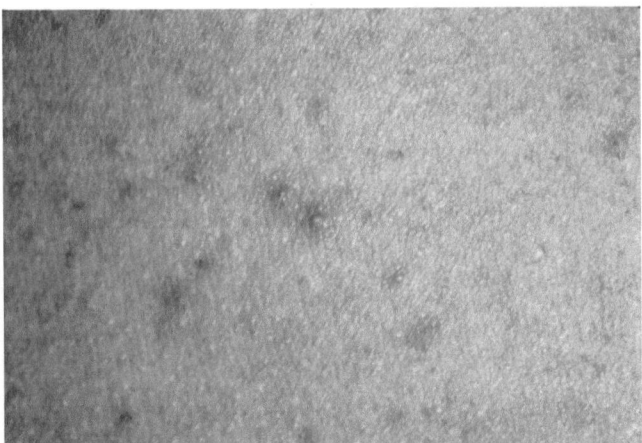

Fig. 22.11 Pityrosporum folliculitis. (Courtesy Kenneth E. Greer.)

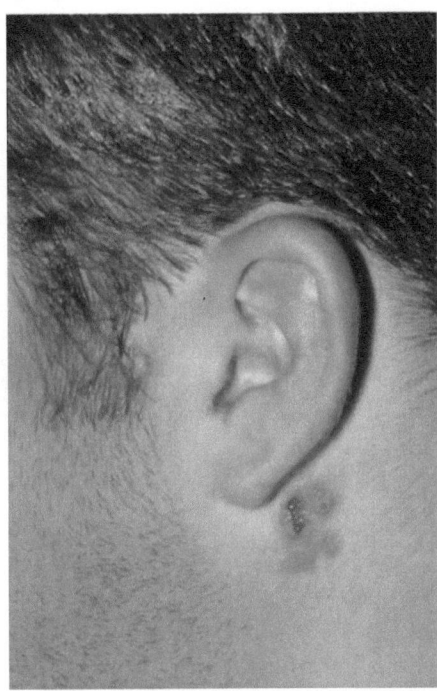

Fig. 22.12 Herpes gladiatorum. (Courtesy Kenneth E. Greer.)

among athletes, with herpes labialis and genital herpes being the most familiar clinical presentations. After primary acquisition of the virus from direct skin contact, the virus replicates at the site of inoculation, with variable production of a primary skin lesion. The virus spreads to infect sensory nerve terminals and travels by retrograde axonal transport to neuronal nuclei in regional sensory ganglia, where it establishes latent, lifelong infection. The virus will subsequently reactivate with anterograde axonal transport to the original site of primary infection.

Contact sports place athletes at higher risk for both acquisition and transmission of the virus, whereas excessive UV radiation exposure (e.g., among skiers) may place certain athletes at risk for reactivation. HSV outbreaks are well described among wrestlers ("herpes gladiatorum") and rugby players ("scrum pox"). HSV lesions are divided into primary and recurrent infection. Either may begin with a prodromal phase (marked by pain, burning, stinging, and itching), before development of erythema and edematous red papules, which subsequently become vesicles. Systemic symptoms (e.g., fever and malaise) are most common in primary infections. Classic skin lesions are small (2 to 5 mm) grouped vesicles on an erythematous base. Confluent vesicles may produce a scalloped border. Lesions soon ulcerate, develop an adherent crust, and eventually resolve within 5 to 14 days. Among wrestlers, the most common locations are the head and neck (Fig. 22.12), but they can occur anywhere, including the trunk and extremities.[17] It is critical to note that the majority of patients with HSV are asymptomatic but can transmit the virus via asymptomatic shedding.

The differential diagnosis of HSV is site-specific. Aphthous ulcers, syphilis, herpangina and erythema multiforme, or epidermal necrolysis may simulate orolabial HSV. On the trunk and extremities, contact dermatitis, herpes zoster, and impetigo should be considered. One study demonstrated that HSV in wrestlers is often misdiagnosed, with impetigo, tinea corporis, or eczema being the most common misdiagnoses.[18] Clinical clues to the diagnosis include recurrences of disease at the same location, prodromal symptoms, and grouping of individual small vesicles. The definitive diagnosis of HSV can be made with an appropriate laboratory test. Viral culture of the vesicle fluid or ulcer base has been the gold standard for many years, but newer

diagnostic modalities are available, including polymerase chain reaction and direct fluorescent antibody tests.

Treatment, if indicated, is with oral antiviral medications such as acyclovir and valacyclovir, which may shorten lesion duration if they are begun soon enough. Numerous acceptable dosing regimens exist and are dependent on the site of infection and whether infection is primary or recurrent. Daily suppressive therapy can be considered in athletes who are prone to recurrences.

The NCAA has developed stringent guidelines for wrestlers with HSV infections. In order to participate with a recent primary infection, the wrestler must be free of systemic symptoms, have developed no new vesicles in the last 72 hours, have all lesions covered by a firm, dried adherent crust, be taking appropriate oral antiviral therapy at least 120 hours before the time of participation, and not cover lesions to allow participation. Wrestlers with recurrent infection must meet the last three requirements before returning to event participation.[1] The authors recommend caution for athletes in contact sports returning to competition with any lesions suspicious for HSV, because the infection is commonly misdiagnosed and can lead to widespread outbreaks.

Verruca vulgaris (Common Warts)

Warts are one of the most common infections in humans and are particularly prevalent among children and young adults. They are caused by human papillomavirus, which infects epithelial cells. Disruption of the epithelial barrier by maceration and/or physical trauma and increased direct skin-to-skin contact places athletes at higher risk for infection. Warts typically present as rough, velvety, hyperkeratotic papules, plaques, and nodules with disruption of normal skin markings (Fig. 22.13). The hands, feet, fingers, toes, and periungual and subungual skin are particularly affected, but lesions can occur anywhere on the skin surface. The diagnosis is clinical, and the differential diagnosis

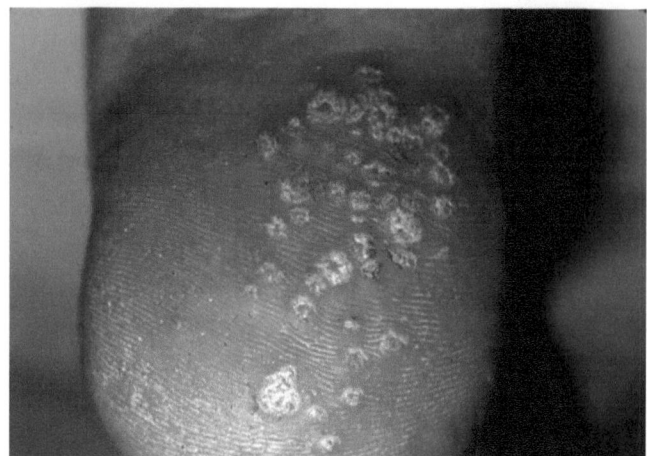

Fig. 22.13 Plantar warts. Note the disruption of normal skin markings. (Courtesy Kenneth E. Greer.)

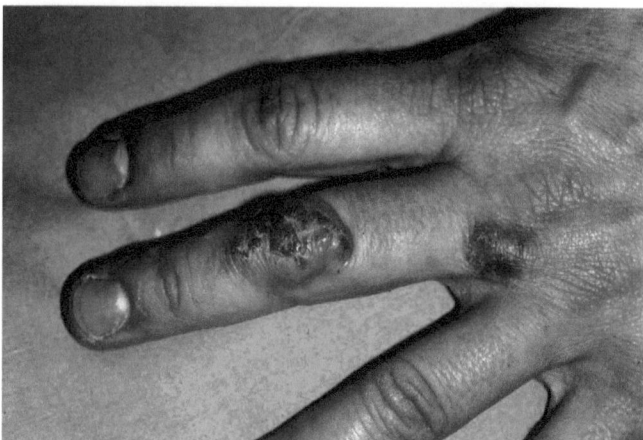

Fig. 22.15 *Mycobacterium marinum.* (Courtesy Kenneth E. Greer.)

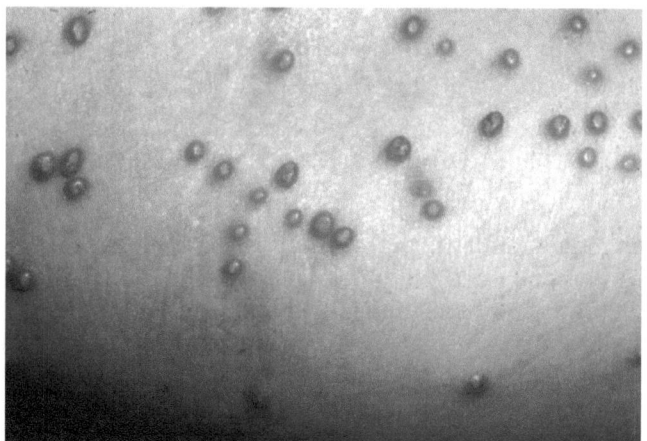

Fig. 22.14 Molluscum contagiosum. (Courtesy Kenneth E. Greer.)

on the palms and soles most commonly includes corns and calluses. Punctate black dots that represent thrombosed capillaries after paring are a useful diagnostic clue. Warts will often spontaneously regress after months to years. If treatment is desired, physical modalities, such as liquid nitrogen cryotherapy and daily use of over-the-counter salicylic acid 40% plasters, are most effective. Warts resistant to these therapies should be referred to a dermatologist for consideration of laser treatment, immunotherapy, or topical/intralesional chemotherapeutic agents.

NCAA wrestling guidelines require that warts on the face be treated or covered by a mask and that other warts be adequately covered.[1]

Molluscum Contagiosum

Infection with the poxvirus, molluscum contagiosum virus, results in a viral infection restricted to the skin. Transmission occurs mainly through direct skin contact; as a result, persons in close-contact sports are at higher risk. Furthermore, the use of school swimming pools and shared bathing fomites (i.e., sponges and towels) has been reported to increase the risk of infection.[19,20] The virus most commonly affects children, but it can be a sexually transmitted infection in adults. Lesions present as small, dome-shaped, pink to flesh-colored papules with central dell or umbilication (Fig. 22.14). Patients typically have numerous lesions

on the body. The differential diagnosis includes common warts and, in immunocompromised patients, dimorphic fungal infections *(Cryptococcus or Histoplasma)*. Treatment is not always necessary because the infection will eventually spontaneously resolve (in months to years), but if required, liquid nitrogen cryotherapy, topical cantharidin 0.7% liquid, and/or curettage are most effective.

NCAA guidelines require that lesions on wrestlers must be curetted or removed before competition but that solitary or localized, clustered lesions can be covered with a gas-impermeable membrane, followed by application of tape that is appropriately anchored and cannot be dislodged.[1]

Mycobacterial Infections
Mycobacterium marinum (Swimming Pool or Fish Tank Granuloma)

Mycobacterium marinum is an atypical mycobacterium that can infect persons exposed to freshwater and saltwater, including swimming pools, lakes, fish tanks, and ocean water. One epidemic involving a single swimming pool infected 290 individuals.[21] Risk factors include immunosuppression and skin trauma. Skin lesions present as violaceous papules that evolve into granulomatous nodules and/or verrucous plaques (Fig. 22.15). Ulceration may be noted, and occasionally spread along lymphatic channels may produce a sporotrichoid pattern. In some cases, *M. marinum* infections can cause deeper infections including tenosynovitis, septic arthritis, and osteomyelitis. Skin biopsy with tissue culture establishes the diagnosis. Other mycobacterial infections, dimorphic fungal infections, and *Nocardia* can present with similar clinical findings.

Consultation with a dermatologist and/or infectious disease expert is recommended for diagnosis, treatment, and return-to-play guidelines on an individual case basis.

Parasitic Infections
Pediculosis Capitis

Pediculosis capitis results from infestation by the head louse, *Pediculus humanus capitis*. Transmission occurs by direct head-to-head contact or via fomites such as hair care products, pillows, helmets, or other protective headgear. The most common presentation is the presence of eggs firmly attached to scalp hairs, which can be readily seen by the naked eye. Less commonly, adult lice and erythematous macules and papules corresponding to bites may be found. Often, secondary changes from scratching predominate, including excoriations, erythema, and scaling. Patients may report pruritus, regional lymphadenopathy, or low-grade fever. The differential diagnosis includes dandruff, pseudonits (from hair casts or hair spray), psoriasis, and eczema. First-line therapy includes daily wet combing with a fine-toothed comb to physically remove eggs and the use of over-the-counter shampoos such as permethrin 1%, or synergized pyrethrins, or dimethicone 4% lotion.

NCAA guidelines recommend that wrestlers be treated with an appropriate pediculicide and be reexamined for completeness of response before return to competition.[1]

Scabies

Infestation by the mite *Sarcoptes scabiei* is common and produces a diffuse, pruritic eruption that is seen worldwide. Patients typically experience severe pruritus 4 to 6 weeks after initial infestation, although subsequent infections can present sooner. Scaly papules and plaques preferentially affect the interdigital web spaces, fingers, volar wrists, lateral palms, axillae, scrotum, penis, labia, and areolae (Fig. 22.16). Thin, thread-like burrows less than 1 cm in length are pathognomonic. Although the infection can be suspected clinically, diagnosis can be confirmed with microscopic confirmation of skin scrapings demonstrating scabies mites, eggs, or fecal pellets (scybala) or with use of a dermatoscope. The condition is commonly misdiagnosed, and the differential diagnosis includes atopic dermatitis, dyshidrotic eczema, contact dermatitis, insect bites, and other conditions characterized by pruritus. Treatment is with permethrin 5% cream applied

topically to all areas of the body from the neck down and washed off after 8 to 14 hours, or with a single dose of ivermectin, 200 μg/kg orally. Both treatments should be repeated in 2 weeks.[22] All cohabitants and close contacts must be simultaneously treated and living environments need to be thoroughly cleaned. Symptoms typically rapidly improve, but rash and pruritus may persist for up to 4 weeks or longer.

NCAA recommendations for wrestlers include documenting negative scabies prep (i.e., microscopic examination of skin scrapings) at meet or tournament time.[1]

Cutaneous Larva Migrans

Animal hookworms, particularly *Ancylostoma braziliense* and *A. caninum*, can infect athletes playing barefoot on sand or soil contaminated by animal feces.[23] Lesions are characteristically erythematous raised serpiginous burrows that are 3 mm wide and several centimeters long and are intensely pruritic (Fig. 22.17). Occasionally, lesions may be vesicular. Burrows expand by several centimeters daily and are most commonly found on the feet and buttocks. Infection is most prevalent in tropical and subtropical climates.[24] The clinical context of barefoot sand or soil exposure with serpiginous lesions on examination is diagnostic. Phytophotodermatitis or jellyfish stings may produce similar-appearing serpiginous inflammatory lesions. Treatment is a single oral dose of ivermectin, 200 μg/kg or albendazole, 400 to 800 mg by mouth daily for 3 days.[25] Footwear use can prevent infection. Cutaneous larva migrans is not transmissible.

MECHANICAL DERMATOSES

Abrasions/Lacerations

Abrasions and lacerations result from physical trauma to the skin but differ in their depth of involvement. Abrasions are superficial wounds that disrupt the epidermis and typically result from shearing forces, such as when an athlete falls on a turf field or road. Lacerations are deeper wounds that penetrate the epidermis and involve the dermis. Both forms of injury can result in bleeding and put athletes at risk for secondary infection or acquisition and/or transmission of blood-borne pathogens. Tetanus status

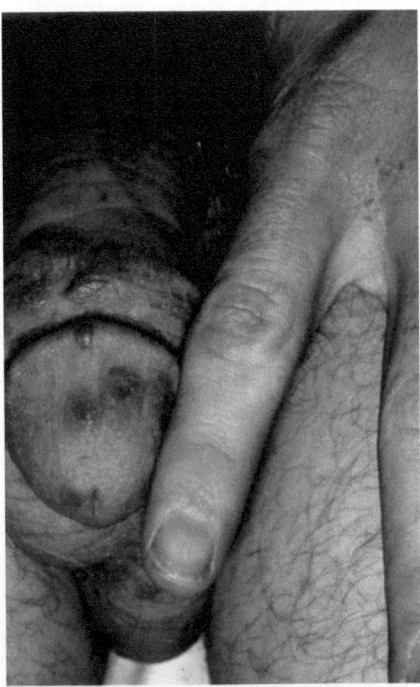

Fig. 22.16 Scabies affecting the penis, scrotum, and interdigital web space. (Courtesy Kenneth E. Greer.)

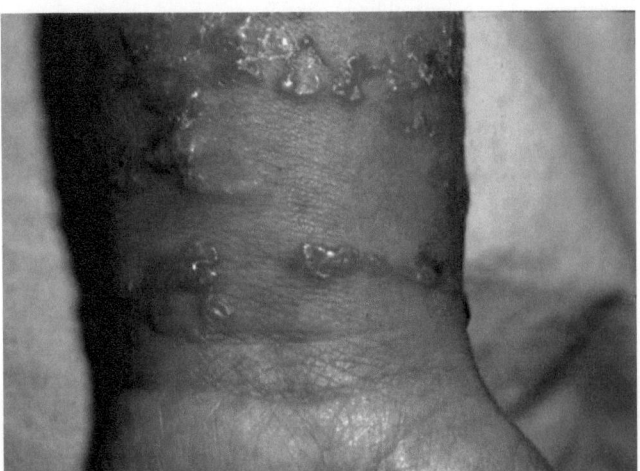

Fig. 22.17 Cutaneous larva migrans on the wrist. (Courtesy Kenneth E. Greer.)

should be assessed with all forms of injury, and if necessary, a tetanus booster should be administered. Wounds should be generously irrigated with saline solution and all foreign material should be removed. Minor abrasions can be cleaned with antibacterial soap and covered with antibiotic ointment and an occlusive hydrocolloid dressing before returning to play. Lacerations may require local anesthesia for comfort of the athlete and closure of the defect with sutures, staples, or cyanoacrylate glues.

Friction Blisters

Blisters are a common occurrence in athletes that result from repetitive shearing forces. Mechanical trauma leads to a split within the epidermis, with fluid collection resulting in tender vesicles and bullae. Blisters occur most commonly on thick skin of the palms and soles, and moisture increases the risk of development. Prevention includes the use of properly fitting footwear and keeping the skin dry. If excessive sweating is noted, therapies that reduce perspiration can be pursued, such as topical aluminum chloride 20% solution, and absorbent cellulose and talc powders. Treatment includes puncture of the blister edge to release fluid but leaving the blister roof intact to act as a biologic dressing. Additional protective bandages can be applied to encourage epithelization and provide cushioning.[26] Excessive and dramatic blistering among multiple family members should raise suspicion for a genetically inherited trait, such as epidermolysis bullosa simplex.

Athletes can resume competition if bleeding is stopped and wounds are firmly covered by occlusive dressings that are able to withstand the demands of activity.

Calluses and Corns

Calluses and corns are common dermatologic conditions that result from prolonged mechanical shear, friction, and/or pressure placed on the skin. They are characterized by scaly papules and plaques and occur most commonly on the hands and feet. Athletes are at particular risk because of the forces applied during training and competition, and lesions can result in significant pain. If mechanical forces are applied over a broad skin surface, a callus forms. However, when forces are applied to a focused location, such as a bony prominence, a corn develops and is characterized by a central hard core. Warts should be considered in the differential diagnosis and can be differentiated by the loss of normal skin markings and the presence of punctate black dots that become evident after paring. Therapeutic options include paring and padding of lesions and topical use of keratolytics such as salicylic acid 40% plaster or urea 40% cream. Properly fitting footwear and the use of donut-shaped pads can help offset the pressure placed on corns, which often leads to improvement and/or their disappearance.

Hemorrhage

Mechanical trauma to the skin can result in damage to small capillaries in the dermis with local hemorrhage. Several characteristic presentations occur in athletes, including subungual hemorrhage, talon noir, and subperichondrial hematomas. Subungual hemorrhage is a frequent occurrence among athletes, presenting with brown-black discoloration underneath the toenail.

An acute, painful subungual hematoma may need to be evacuated with electrocautery through the nail for pain relief. The differential diagnosis includes acral lentiginous melanoma. If uncertainty exists, referral to a dermatologist is prudent for a possible biopsy. Talon noir presents as pinpoint, blue-black dots on the posterior heel and represents an accumulation of red blood cells in the stratum corneum (Fig. 22.18). The differential diagnosis again includes melanocytic neoplasms, including melanoma. However, with paring of the skin, the lesion disappears. Trauma to the anterior ear sustained during contact sports such as wrestling, boxing, or rugby can lead to hemorrhage beneath the perichondrium. If recognized, the hematoma should be drained immediately with needle incision to prevent necrosis of the perichondrium with resulting fibrosis leading to deformity and a "cauliflower" appearance (Fig. 22.19).

Striae

Striae (stretch marks) are common in the general population, especially during pregnancy and puberty. Their development among athletes is typically associated with intense training periods with rapid muscle growth and weight gain. Lesions are violaceous, linear atrophic streaks and favor the upper arms and thighs (Fig. 22.20). The sudden appearance of striae in athletes should prompt some consideration of the use of anabolic steroids, especially when coupled with other signs of anabolic steroid use (e.g., acne, male-pattern balding, deepened voice, personality change, and gynecomastia). Striae tend to improve in appearance with time. Treatment, which is usually not particularly effective, includes topical retinoids and the pulsed dye laser for vascular lesions.

Acne Mechanica

Acne mechanica is a variant of acne precipitated by any combination of pressure, friction, occlusion, rubbing, and heat.[27] It is characterized by the appearance of inflammatory red papules and pustules in areas covered by clothing, uniforms or other protective equipment (Fig. 22.21). Lesions result from blockage of the pilosebaceous unit with comedo formation and eventual inflammation. The differential diagnosis includes acne vulgaris (i.e., typical teenage acne), acneiform drug reactions, Pityrosporum folliculitis, and anabolic steroid use. Acne mechanica is

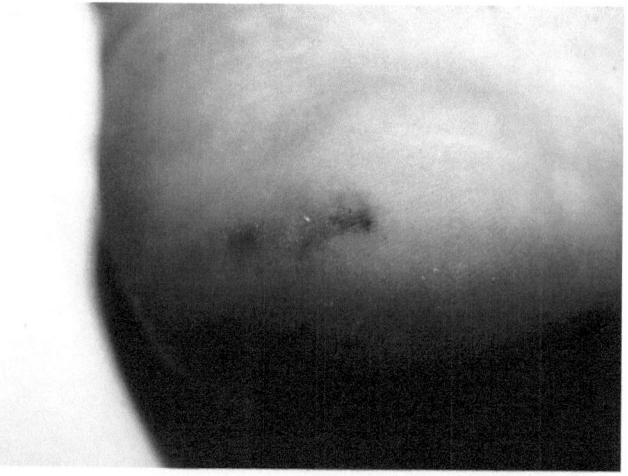

Fig. 22.18 Talon noir. (Courtesy Kenneth E. Greer.)

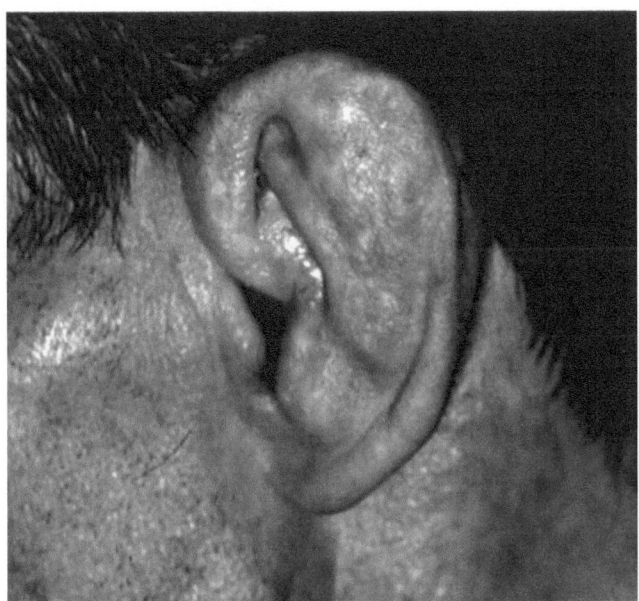

Fig. 22.19 End-stage fibrosis from repeated subperichondrial hematomas in a wrestler, resulting in a "cauliflower ear." (Courtesy Kenneth E. Greer.)

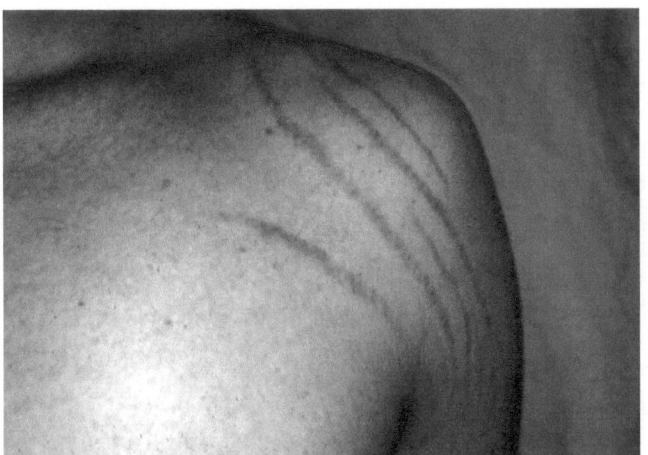

Fig. 22.20 Striae. (Courtesy Kenneth E. Greer.)

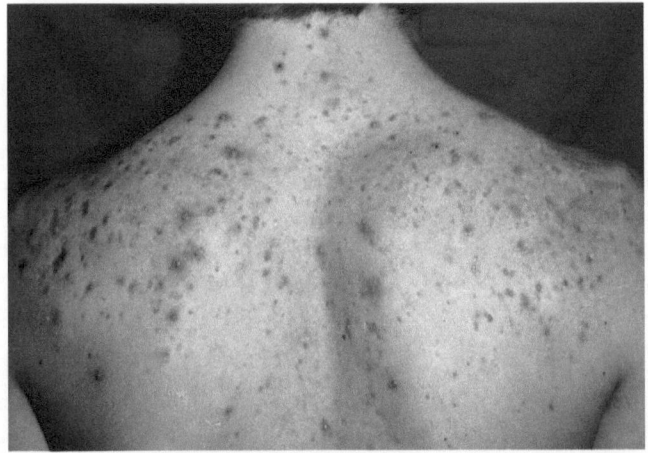

Fig. 22.21 Acne vulgaris aggravated by acne mechanica as a result of the use of athletic shoulder pads.

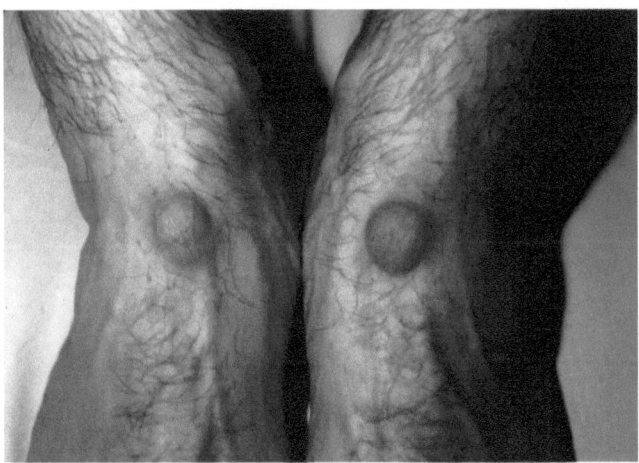

Fig. 22.22 Athlete's nodules on the dorsal feet in a runner. (Courtesy Kenneth E. Greer.)

often challenging to treat. Simple therapy includes the use of cotton undershirts to minimize direct skin contact with occlusive equipment and immediate showers after practice with the use of benzoyl peroxide or sulfur-based washes (e.g., selenium sulfide 2.5% lotion).[26] More severe presentations may require use of topical comedolytics at night (e.g., tretinoin 0.05% cream), topical antibiotic therapy (e.g., clindamycin 1% lotion or solution) and/or oral antibiotic therapy (e.g., a doxycycline hyclate capsule, 100 mg by mouth twice daily; cephalexin, 500 mg by mouth twice daily; or a trimethoprim-sulfamethoxazole double-strength tablet by mouth twice daily). Athletes taking doxycycline should be counseled regarding potential sun sensitivity. Cessation of the precipitating etiology will lead to spontaneous resolution in the off-season.

Athlete's Nodules (Collagenomas)

Athlete's nodules are benign, nonpainful, reactive flesh-colored papules, plaques, or nodules that occur in areas exposed to long-term friction and trauma (Fig. 22.22). They have been found on the tibial tuberosities of surfers ("surfer's nodules"), dorsal feet of runners ("Nike nodules"), knuckles of boxers ("knuckle pads"), and shins of hockey players ("skate bites").[26,28] These reactive growths have also been reported to develop in marbles players, skiers, soccer players, karate enthusiasts, and football players.[28–30] Histopathology reveals reactive fibrosis with thickened and irregular collagen bundles.[28] The differential diagnosis includes hypertrophic scar, callus, dermatofibroma, foreign-body reaction, verrucae, granuloma annulare, and other neoplastic growths. They can be distinguished from sports-related callosities by their failure to resolve after discontinuation of athletic activity. The clinical appearance and history are diagnostic. Treatment is unsatisfactory and is not required in the absence of symptoms; cessation of activity may lead to a decrease in size, but excision is usually required for definitive therapy.

Hidradenitis Suppurativa

Hidradenitis suppurativa is a common, debilitating, chronic disorder of uncertain etiology that is under-recognized and often misdiagnosed.[31] Sites rich in apocrine glands are preferentially

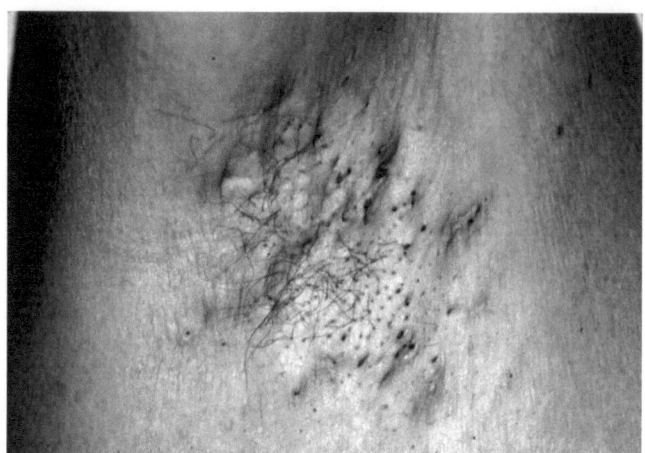

Fig. 22.23 Hidradenitis suppurativa in the axillae with scarring and fibrosis. (Courtesy Kenneth E. Greer.)

affected, such as the axillae, perineum, and inframammary folds. Females are more likely to experience the disease, and smoking and obesity are known exacerbating factors.[32] Lesions present after puberty in the second to third decade of life and begin as painful papules or nodules that evolve into sterile draining abscesses, scars, sinus tracts, and fistulae (Fig. 22.23). The restriction to intertriginous areas and disease chronicity are helpful diagnostic clues. Although bacteria are sometimes cultured from draining lesions, the role of bacterial infection in hidradenitis suppurativa is uncertain, and their presence most likely represents secondary colonization rather than primary infection.[32] The differential diagnosis is extensive but most commonly includes bacterial infections and cutaneous Crohn disease. Patients are often treated for furunculosis for years before the disease is recognized.

Consultation with a dermatologist is recommended. The NCAA states that a wrestler will be disqualified if extensive or purulent draining lesions are present and that lesions shall not be covered to allow participation.[1]

ENVIRONMENTAL DERMATOSES

Photodermatoses

Sunburn

Acute exposure to UV radiation leads to sunburn, which is clinically visible as skin erythema but may progress to vesicles and bullae with associated warmth, pain, and swelling. The health risks of sunburn with respect to melanoma development cannot be overemphasized. One or more blistering sunburns in childhood or adolescence more than doubles a person's chances of developing melanoma,[33] and a person's risk for melanoma doubles with more than five sunburns at any age.[34] Protection from sunburns includes avoidance of peak hours of UV radiation (10 a.m. to 3 p.m.), wearing sun-protective clothing including hats and sunglasses, and the regular use of broad-spectrum, water-resistant sunscreen that protects against UVA and UVB wavelengths with at least a sun protection factor 15 rating. Fair-skinned athletes who spend significant time outdoors may benefit from use of oral polypodium leucotomos extract, which has been shown to have molecular and photobiologic protective effects

against UVB radiation.[35] Treatment of sunburn is symptomatic with use of cool compresses, oral antiinflammatory medications (e.g., acetaminophen or ibuprofen), and bland emollients.

Skin Cancer

Athletes who train and compete outdoors must be educated regarding an increased risk of skin cancer. UV radiation has been demonstrated to be one of the most important risk factors in the development of both malignant melanoma and nonmelanoma skin cancer. Particular efforts should be aimed at sun protection in young athletes, because tanning may be desired in this age group. Extreme UV radiation exposure has been documented among skiers, mountaineers, cyclists, and triathletes.[36] In an age- and sex-matched study of 210 marathon runners, these athletes were found to have an increased risk for malignant melanoma and nonmelanoma skin cancer.[37] Furthermore, sweating has been shown to potentially contribute to skin cancer development by lowering the sunburn threshold.[38] Athletes should be counseled to avoid training and competition at peak hours of UV radiation, to wear adequate sun-protective clothing, and to consistently and repeatedly apply a broad-spectrum water-resistant sunscreen that protects against UVA and UVB wavelengths.

Aquatic Dermatoses

Swimmer's Itch and Seabather's Eruption

Swimmer's itch results when miracidia of several species of *Schistosoma cercariae* penetrate the skin during fresh or saltwater activity. Lesions predominate in uncovered skin and are typically red papules and vesicles that are intensely itchy and painful. There is no risk of systemic infection because the organisms die in the superficial dermis. Treatment is symptomatic and includes the use of topical corticosteroids, antihistamines, and antipruritic lotions. Prevention is challenging but includes wearing protective clothing and coating the skin with emollients.

Seabather's eruption is caused by minute stings of coelenterate larvae of jellyfish and sea anemone, which become trapped underneath clothing during saltwater activity. Itchy papules or wheals are characteristically confined to areas covered by swimwear (Fig. 22.24). Treatment is symptomatic and includes the use of topical corticosteroids, antihistamines, and antipruritic lotions.

Hair Discoloration

Competitive swimmers may present with hair discoloration. A peculiar greenish discoloration occurs in persons with natural or tinted blond, gray, or white hair, and is caused by copper ions in the water.[39] Treatment includes use of a hydrogen peroxide 2% to 3% solution or commercial chelating shampoos. In addition, discoloration of dark hair has been reported in Japan, with affected persons having golden hair. Electron microscopy has demonstrated cuticle damage, allowing hypochlorous acid to penetrate the hair cortex, leading to oxidation and the degeneration of melanosomes.[40]

Irritant Contact Dermatitis

Irritant contact dermatitis is a nonimmunologic, inflammatory reaction of the skin that requires no previous sensitization and

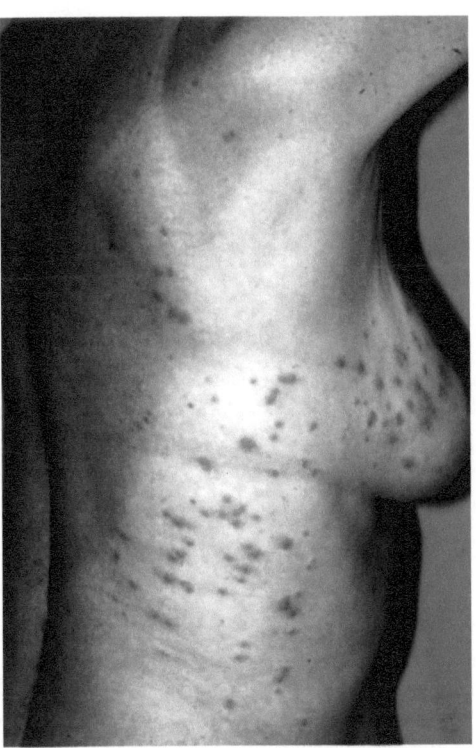

Fig. 22.24 Seabather's eruption. Note that the lesions are confined to bathing suit distribution. (Courtesy Kenneth E. Greer.)

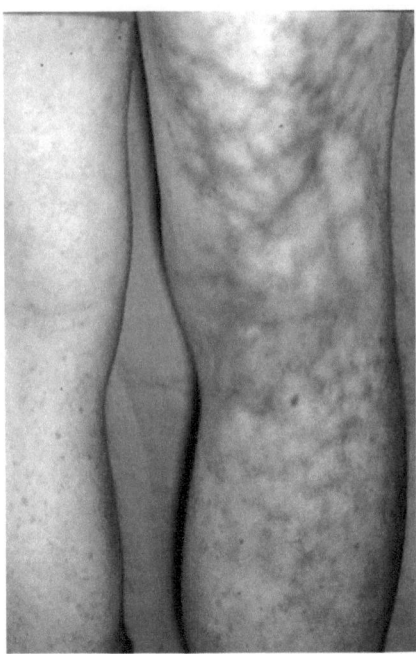

Fig. 22.25 Erythema ab igne from chronic heating pad use for knee pain. (Courtesy Kenneth E. Greer.)

represents the majority of cases of contact dermatitis. Any chemical or physical insult that damages the integrity of the skin can lead to irritant contact dermatitis. Clinical presentations vary based on the acuity of disease and the specific etiologic agent, but can include vesicles and bullae, red and scaly plaques, cracks and fissures, hives, pustules, and acneiform papules. Etiologies specific to athletes include fiberglass used in hockey sticks, shin guards among soccer players, abrasive outdoor basketballs with a pebbled surface, alkaline lime used in field markings, chemicals in swimming pools, and seaweed, corals, sea cucumbers, sea mosses, and plants encountered by saltwater enthusiasts.[41] Both surfers and runners can experience nipple dermatitis from chronic friction with surfboards or shirts, respectively, and swimmers can experience "swimmer's shoulder" from an unshaven beard that repeatedly rubs the shoulder.[41] Treatment centers on identification and avoidance of irritants and protection of the skin barrier with bland emollients.

Thermal Damage

Athletes often use heat or ice packs to treat injuries, which can result in specific skin reactions. Inappropriate use of ice packs can result in frostbite with erythema and bullae. Rarely, panniculitis (i.e., inflammation of subcutaneous fat) can present as painful, firm, violaceous, indurated nodules 1 to 3 days after pronged cold exposure. Chronic use of heating pads on the skin surface may result in a rare condition called erythema ab igne (Fig. 22.25). A red–brown, nonblanchable, netlike discoloration of the skin occurs. It should be distinguished from livedo reticularis, which is violaceous and blanchable. The pigmentary changes are long lasting but eventually fade. Further use of heat should be avoided.

Chilblains (perniosis) are localized inflammatory lesions induced by prolonged exposure to cold and damp weather, and occur primarily on the fingers and toes. Lesions are nonblanching, erythematous-to-purple macules and papules that may be pruritic, burning, or painful (Fig. 22.26). Lesions are often misdiagnosed as vasculitis. Treatment is symptomatic with rewarming the area and using topical antipruritic agents.

URTICARIA, ANAPHYLAXIS, AND IMMUNOLOGIC DISORDERS

Urticaria

Urticaria is one of the most common skin disorders confronted by physicians across all specialties. Allergies, autoimmune conditions, medications, and infections are among the most common causes of urticaria in the general population. Specific subsets of urticaria, including cholinergic, solar, aquagenic, and cold urticaria may develop during athletic activity. Cholinergic urticaria presents as hives within a few minutes of sweat-inducing stimuli, such as physical exertion, hot baths, or sudden emotional stress. The lesions are typically small (2 to 3 mm) monomorphic wheals; they favor the upper half of the body and are surrounded by an obvious red flare (Fig. 22.27). Solar and aquagenic urticaria are defined by wheals and/or pruritus occurring within minutes of exposure to UV radiation, or visible light and water, respectively. Exposure to a cold stimulus results in cold urticaria. Management of these specific subsets of urticaria includes avoidance or protection from the inciting stimulus, and the use of oral antihistamines.

Exercise-Induced Anaphylaxis

Anaphylaxis provoked by exercise is divided into exercise-induced anaphylaxis and food-dependent exercise-induced anaphylaxis.

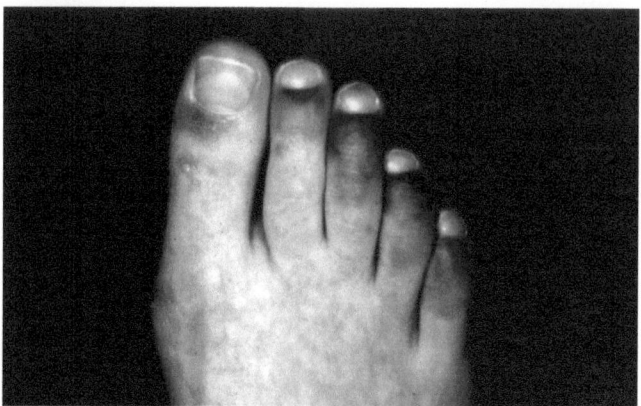

Fig. 22.26 Chilblains (perniosis). (Courtesy Kenneth E. Greer.)

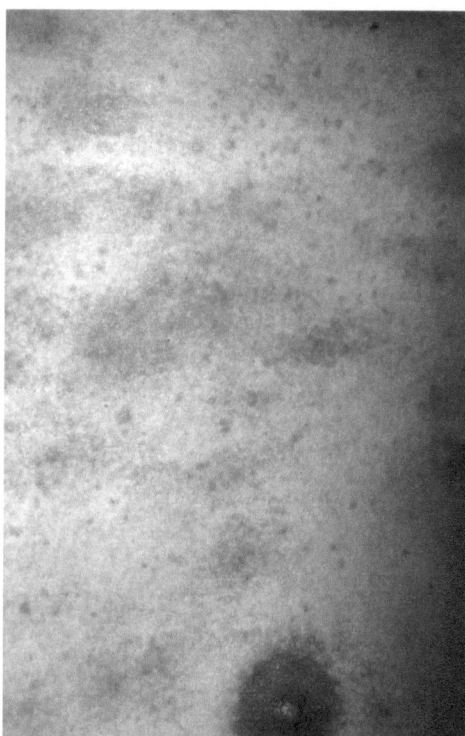

Fig. 22.27 Cholinergic urticaria. Note the distinctive erythematous flare surrounding each wheal.

The pathophysiology of either subset is not fully understood, but in food-dependent exercise-induced anaphylaxis, the ingestion of certain foods is required. Patients experience anaphylactic symptoms with hives and/or angioedema associated with exercise. The differential diagnosis includes anaphylaxis secondary to other etiologies (e.g., medications), cholinergic urticaria, exercise-induced asthma, mastocytoses, and hereditary angioedema. The diagnosis is clinical and acute management is identical to other forms of anaphylaxis.

Allergic Contact Dermatitis

Allergic contact dermatitis is an immunologically mediated delayed-type hypersensitivity response to a specific allergen. Lesions are usually localized to sites of skin contact but can generalize and present as itchy, red, scaly plaques. Sources of contact allergens common to athletes include adhesives used in athletic tape, topical medications (e.g., anesthetics, antiseptics, and antibiotics), plus rubbers and rubber accelerators found in shoes, knee pads/guards, wet suits, and swimming goggles.[41] The diagnosis is suspected based on the location and morphology of the rash and can be confirmed by the use of specialized patch testing. Treatment includes avoidance of the specific allergen and the use of topical corticosteroids.

For a complete list of references, go to ExpertConsult.com.

SELECTED READINGS

Citation:
Daum RS, et al. A placebo-controlled trial of antibiotics for smaller skin abscesses. *N Engl J Med.* 2017;376(26):2545–2555.

Level of Evidence:
I

Summary:
In this multicenter, prospective, double-blind, placebo-controlled trial involving outpatient adults and children with simple abscesses, cure rates at day 10 were higher in patients receiving incision and drainage with clindamycin (83.1%), or incision and drainage with trimethoprim and sulfamethoxazole (81.7%) compared to incision and drainage with placebo [(68.9%), P < .001 for both comparisons].

Citation:
Moran GJ, et al. Effect of cephalexin plus trimethoprim-sulfamethoxazole vs. cephalexin alone or clinical cure of uncomplicated cellulitis: a randomized clinical trial. *JAMA.* 2017;317(20):2088–2096.

Level of Evidence:
I

Summary:
In this multicenter, prospective, double-blind, placebo-controlled trial of patients older than 12 years with uncomplicated cellulitis, there was no difference in clinical cure among participants receiving cephalexin plus trimethoprim-sulfamethoxazole (83.5%) compared to cephalexin plus placebo [(85.5%), P = .50].

Citation:
National Collegiate Athletic Association (NCAA): 2014-2015 NCAA Sports Medicine Handbook. Retrieved February 5, 2017, from http://www.ncaapublications.com/DownloadPublication.aspx?download=MD15.pdf: Accessed February 8, 2017.

Level of Evidence:
V

Summary:
This publication is a useful reference for NCAA sports medicine guidelines, including eligibility and return-to-play guidelines for skin infections.

Citation:
Cordoro KM, Ganz JE. Training room management of medical conditions: sports dermatology. *Clin Sports Med.* 2005;24:565–598.

Level of Evidence:
V

Summary:
An excellent review article of the most relevant sports-related dermatoses with numerous representative clinical images.

Citation:
Kockentiet B, Adams BB. Contact dermatitis in athletes. *J Am Acad Dermatol.* 2007;56(6):1048–1055.

Level of Evidence:
V

Summary:
This review article examines the published literature of contact dermatitis in athletes and provides a comprehensive resource of specific allergic and irritant contactants unique to athletes.

Citation:
Adams BB. Dermatologic disorders of the athlete. *Sports Med.* 2002;32(5):309–321.

Level of Evidence:
V

Summary:
A well-organized general review of skin conditions seen in athletes.

23

Facial, Eye, Nasal, and Dental Injuries

John Jared Christophel

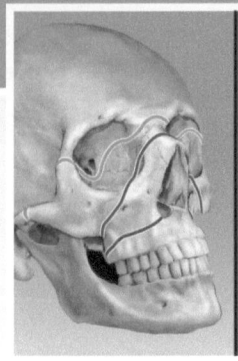

Despite advances in protective gear for the face, facial trauma remains a common injury treated by sports medicine physicians. The face is a rather "high rent" district with sole proprietorship of four out of five senses (vision, hearing, taste, and smell) and 10 out of 12 cranial nerves (all but the vagus and spinal accessory cranial nerves). In addition, the face plays a large role in a person's appearance, and his or her ability to communicate and eat. Injuries in this area carry a higher risk of detriment to an athlete's quality of life.[1] Given the central role of the face in a person's functioning, even simple lacerations are often treated with greater care than a similar injury elsewhere on the body. This chapter addresses the most common sports injuries to the face, focusing on injuries that need to be referred to a specialist, and treatment of injuries that typically do not require referral.

SOFT TISSUE INJURIES TO THE FACE
General Considerations
Timing of Repair
It is not necessary to repair facial wounds immediately. However, when possible, most wounds should be closed within 4 to 6 hours. The rate of infection in facial lacerations does rise significantly until after 24 hours, but the progressive tissue edema makes meticulous closure more difficult and therefore should be performed sooner rather than later.[2] In the case of significantly contaminated wounds, it is appropriate to perform "delayed primary" closure after extensive débridement and a period of packing/cleansing over 24 to 72 hours to lessen the chance of infection. This procedure is usually only undertaken for extensive contaminated wounds that require closure in the operating room.

Healing by secondary intention is less than ideal for soft tissue injuries on the face unless significant tissue loss has occurred; the scar from primary closure of a laceration is significantly better than that of a similar wound left to heal on its own.

Anesthesia
Simple lacerations that are not full thickness through the epidermis will, at a minimum, require cleaning prior to treatment; thus a topical anesthetic cream can be considered. Topical anesthetic creams include a eutectic mixture of local anesthetics (EMLA): tetracaine, liposome-encapsulated tetracaine, and liposome-encapsulated lidocaine.[3] However, most patients will require injection of a local anesthetic prior to definitive treatment of their wounds, and prior application of a topical anesthetic

can deaden the pain of needle insertion to a small degree. This factor is probably most important in pediatric patients who have very little tolerance for pain before they become frightened, with a resultant need for sedation.

In most adults, local anesthetic injections are well tolerated without prior application of topical anesthetic cream and allow the wound to be treated in the most expeditious manner. The pain from local anesthetic injection evolves from both the acidity in the commercially prepared anesthetic (to prolong shelf life) and the dermal distension from the volume of the anesthetic. The buffering of local anesthetic with sodium bicarbonate in a 10% volume to volume can significantly reduce the perception of pain.[4] However, even if buffered anesthetic is used, poor injection technique will result in significant pain.[5] Local anesthetic solution should be injected with a 27-gauge or smaller needle. Experienced practitioners often do not let patients see the needle to be used, and recent studies have shown that visualizing the needle increases the perception of pain.[6] The plane of injection should be in the subcutaneous tissue immediately beneath the dermis. The most common mistake is to inject anesthetic intradermally, which will be exquisitely painful as the pain receptors in the dermis distend. Whenever possible, the subcutaneous plane should be entered through an existing laceration, because pain is experienced when the needle enters through intact skin.

The use of an anesthetic combined with epinephrine is helpful both for increasing the duration of the anesthesia and for decreasing bleeding during wound repair. Epinephrine as dilute as 1:200,000 g/mL is as efficacious as more concentrated solutions in providing vasoconstriction.[7] The onset of anesthesia after infiltration is rather rapid (<1 minute), but the vasoconstrictive effect is maximal after 20 minutes. Use of an anesthetic that contains epinephrine is safe in all areas of the face, including the ear and nose. The practitioner should not be concerned about ischemia of the tissue because the blood supply in the face is very robust.

Cleaning
All traumatic soft tissue wounds should be considered contaminated and require some degree of cleansing prior to treatment, the degree of which is determined by the extent of the wound. In partial-thickness wounds, copious irrigation is not required and a simple cleaning with moist gauze will suffice prior to bandaging or applying superficial sutures in a sterile fashion. In full-thickness skin lacerations, tap water has shown to be as

effective as sterile solutions.[8] Because the irrigation of wounds can be painful, an anesthetic should be infiltrated beforehand, which also provides time (a maximum of 20 minutes) for the vasoconstrictive effect of epinephrine.[9] In extensive soft tissue injuries, pulsed irrigation provides the best treatment. The content of the irrigant is not as important as the pulsed method of delivery. In fact, the use of more concentrated antiseptics, such as hydrogen peroxide, can inhibit early fibroblasts, which are important in wound healing.

Choice of Closure

Wounds closed "primarily" result in better scars than those allowed to heal by secondary intention, because the opposed wound edges allow for direct healing. Although individual variations exist in the way a wound heals, there are clear distinctions between well-approximated wounds and those that are closed poorly. To obtain the finest scar, wound edges must be closed with minimal tension, edge eversion, and edge height match.

Partial-thickness lacerations (i.e., lacerations with at least a portion of the dermis still intact) have already met the criteria for primary wound healing; that is, the dermis is already opposed, has matched height, and will heal under no tension. Therefore sutures are not required and an occlusive dressing can be applied with excellent results. For full-thickness lacerations, a physical force is required to hold the wound edges in opposition. Because the dermis is the strength layer of the skin, classically it was thought that it needed to be held together with sutures. However, tissue glues, such as Dermabond, which only hold the more superficial epidermis together, have similar wound outcomes when compared with suture closure of simple lacerations.[10]

As mentioned, simple lacerations can be closed with tissue glues. However, many practitioners are hesitant to use tissue glues for any wounds other than simple lacerations, because it provides a limited amount of control in managing the wound edges. When tissue glue is used, care must be taken not to apply pressure with the applicator (to prevent spread of the wound edges), which could allow glue to enter the space between the wound edges, resulting in delayed healing and a wider scar.[11] Suturing of simple linear lacerations can be achieved with a single layer of sutures, as long as the sutures include both epidermal and dermal portions of the skin. However, a single layer of sutures means that the tension-bearing strength layer (the dermis) is included in the same suture throw as the edge height match and eversion layer (epidermis). If concern exists about proper wound approximation, it is easier to use two separate layers of suture: a deeper dermal layer to bear the strength of the closure and a more superficial layer to match the height and provide eversion of the epidermis.

Complex lacerations should be closed with two layers of sutures for the aforementioned reasons. The suture choice varies widely. For single-layer closure, permanent sutures should be used and removed at the appropriate time (discussed in the Postclosure Wound Care section). The use of 6-0 suture is preferred on the face, and no larger than 5-0 suture should be used. If a two-layer suture technique is to be used, a 4-0 or 5-0 absorbable suture such as Vicryl or PDS should be used for the deep layer.

Antibiotics

Traumatic lacerations anywhere on the body have an infection rate of 3.5%. Those on the head and neck have a significantly lower risk (1%), which is thought to be due to the robust blood supply in these areas.[12] Factors that increase the rate of infection include the presence of diabetes mellitus, a wide laceration, and the presence of a foreign body. Given the low risk of infection, prophylactic antibiotics are not required for most small lacerations. However, after repair of soft tissue injuries, most plastic surgeons will prescribe a short course (5 to 7 days) of antibiotics that cover skin flora (e.g., cephalexin or clindamycin).[13] However, there is a likely selection bias because plastic surgeons typically are consulted to treat larger wounds.

Postclosure Wound Care

If tissue glue has been used to close a wound, nothing should be applied to the hardened glue, because water or petroleum will cause the glue to fall off the wound sooner than the expected (7 to 10 days). If sutures have been used to close the wound, a significant improvement in the scar outcome can be achieved by the constant application of petroleum-based ointments for the first 2 weeks. If preferred, an emollient that contains an antibiotic, such as Bacitracin, can be used for the first week after closure but no longer, because a small percentage of patients will experience a reactive dermatitis. If permanent sutures were used to close the wound, they can be removed as early as postclosure day 5 in areas under minimal tension. They should stay no longer than 7 days because "railroad" tracks tend to form with longer duration. However, sutures or staples used in the hair-bearing scalp should stay for 10 to 14 days because more time is needed in this thicker skinned area for healing, and "railroad" tracks will not be as visible (unless patient has the potential for future hair loss in the region).

After suture removal followed by a week of petroleum emollient application (for a total of 2 weeks), some further improvement in the ultimate outcome can be obtained with 2 months of silicone treatment (Fig. 23.1).[14] Silicone therapy can be applied either as sheeting (at night) or as a gel (during the day). To some patients, the added burden of silicone therapy may not be worth the small return. However, for most patients the ability to affect even a slight change in the appearance of their scar gives them a sense of control over something that has otherwise been out of their control. More recently, the application of paper tape over a scar has been shown to result in equal improvement in scar healing as in silicone therapy.[15] However, silicone therapy remains the standard of care for managing scars.

In addition to silicone therapy, patients should be counseled regarding exposing newly formed scars to the sun. Beginning 2 weeks after repair or after full epithelialization of the wound, patients should apply sunscreen daily to prevent darkening of the scar. After this time, makeup also can be applied if desired. Sun protection is especially important on facial scars because they receive regular sunlight during routine activities.

A scar takes 6 months to fully mature, and patients should be counseled that the scar will evolve through a red, raised, indurated phase with telangiectatic vessel ingrowth that will

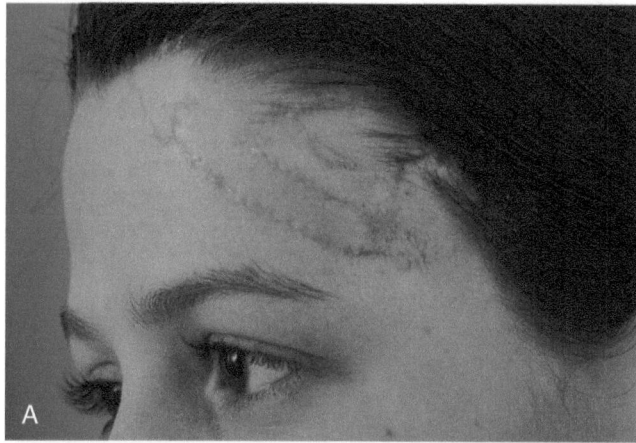

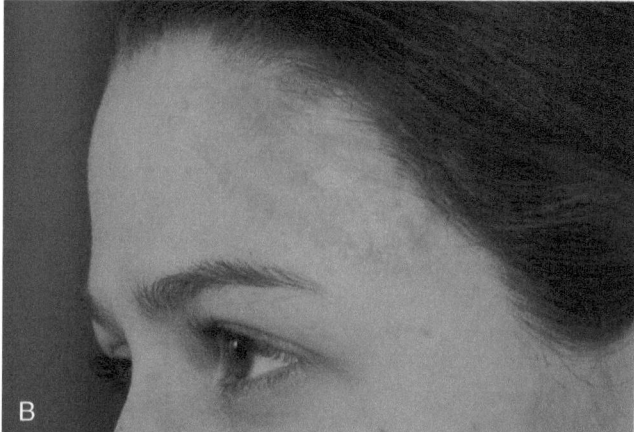

Fig. 23.1 (A) A traumatic soft tissue injury to the temple 6 weeks after injury. (B) The same injury as in part A after 2 months of silicone sheeting.

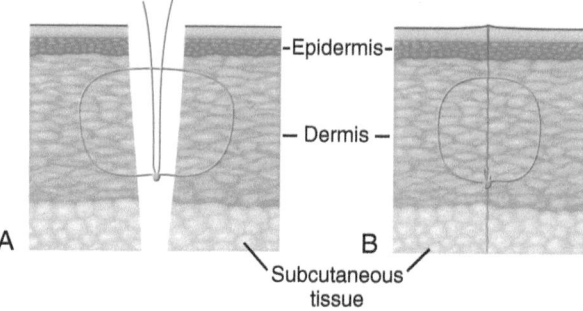

Fig. 23.2 (A) Placement of a deep buried suture must enter and exit the same levels of the dermis on opposing wound edges. One must be careful not to include the overlying epidermis. (B) A well-placed deep suture will help create epidermal wound edge eversion.

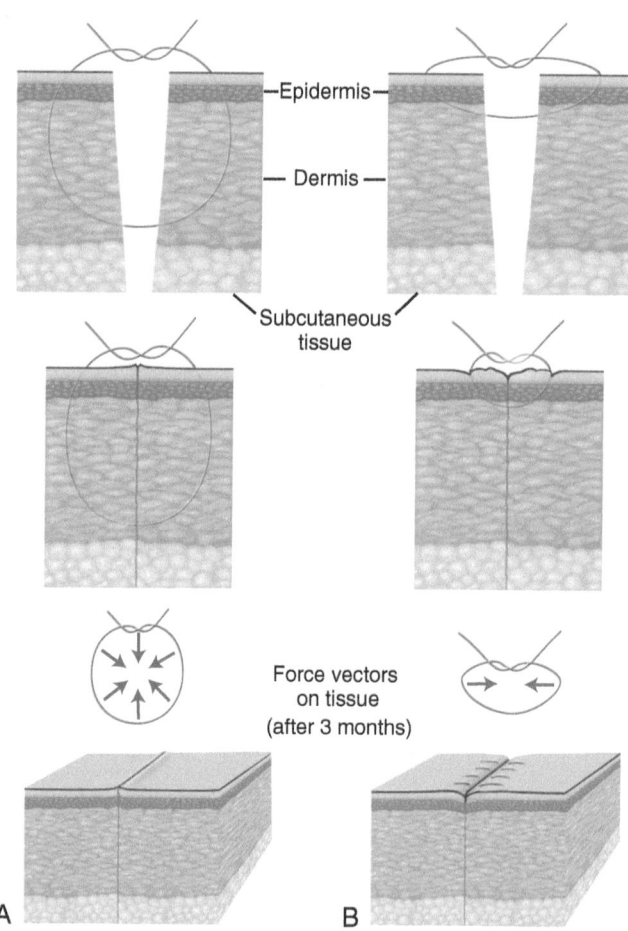

Fig. 23.3 (A) Proper placement of a cutaneous suture showing equal distribution of tension along the entire vertical height of the wound. Everted edges provide a better aesthetic result. (B) Improper placement of cutaneous suture farther from the skin edge with a superficial bite. Force vectors are more horizontal and create edge inversion. In addition, "train tracks" form where pressure necrosis of skin occurred.

progress to a softer, paler, less noticeable scar.[16] In the case of hypertrophic or keloid scar formation, the patient should be referred to a specialist for possible early intervention.

Specific Injury Management
Simple Lacerations

Simple lacerations can be closed by using one of many suture methods. The use of deep dermal sutures should be considered for simple lacerations with any diastasis of the dermis. Dermal sutures will minimize wound tension, reduce dead space, and, if placed properly, help with edge eversion. When placing deep dermal sutures, every effort should be made to start and end at a point farthest from the surface of the skin. Care must be taken to match the entry and exit points of the suture on both sides of the wound (Fig. 23.2).

Cutaneous closure can be performed with the use of tissue glue or various methods of cutaneous suture techniques. When using a cutaneous (epidermal) suture technique, the practitioner must take care to properly place the suture with equal distribution of wound edge tension and create everted wound edges (Fig. 23.3). In time, an everted wound edge will deflate, leaving a flat scar. If a wound is closed with no eversion, contractile forces will result in a depressed or widened scar (Fig. 23.4). A common mistake is the placement of cutaneous sutures too far from the wound edge, which results in telltale suture marks (train tracks) from pressure necrosis.

Complex Lacerations

Any laceration that is more complicated than a simple linear cut is considered complex. The practitioner must maintain the same goals of minimizing tension, everting wound edges, and matching the edge height. These goals can be more difficult

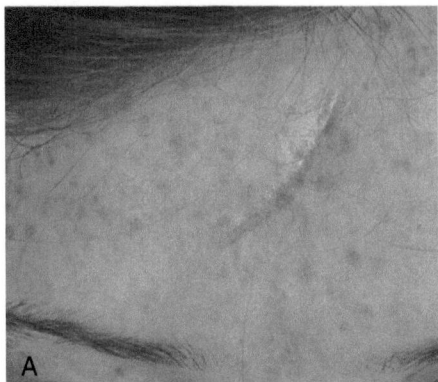 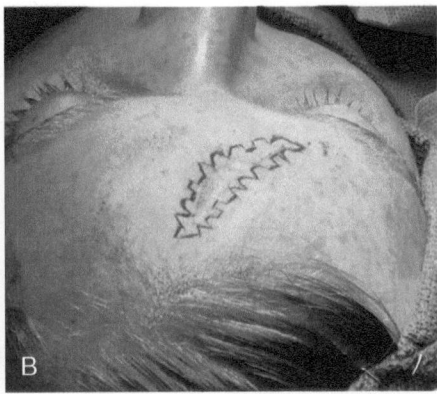 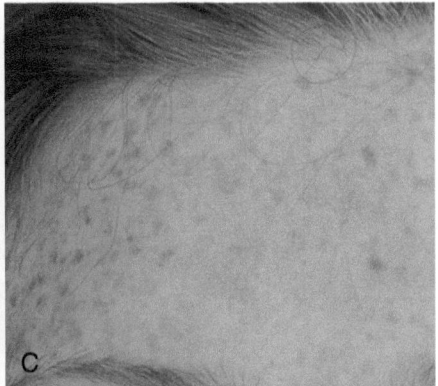

Fig. 23.4 (A) A widened and depressed scar on the forehead that was not closed in layers. (B) A geometric broken line scar revision. (C) A 3-month postoperative photo.

when the edges converge, akin to pieces of a puzzle, instead of being two parallel lines. In these cases, using the "known to unknown" principle can work well. Often a jagged edge can be matched to its sister portion of the wound. Once a few "known" areas are worked together, the final result can be enhanced to a degree better than expected (Fig. 23.5). The practitioner must resist the urge and tendency to prune any edges of the laceration that may not seem viable. Most skin attached to the patient will survive, and if it loses its viability, it can always be trimmed later.

Many traumatic lacerations can occur at oblique angles to the skin surface, causing a skive-type laceration. These lacerations can be difficult to repair well because differing amounts of dermis and epidermis are present on the opposing edges of the laceration. In this type of laceration, the use of a single cutaneous layer of suture may be best to ensure that the edges match appropriately. Placing deep dermal sutures will often result in superficial edge mismatch, which is difficult to correct with the superficial layer.

Lip Lacerations

Repairing a lip laceration can be a challenging task. The lip is vital in speech, food intake, and appearance. A detailed discussion on the aesthetics of the lips is beyond the scope of this chapter, but it is important to understand the fundamentals. The lips are separated into the white lip and the red lip. The red lip is further divided into the dry and wet portions, with the separation being where the lips make contact. The junction of the white and dry red lip is referred to as the anterior vermilion border, and the junction of the dry and wet red lip is referred to as the posterior vermilion border (Fig. 23.6). The anterior vermilion border is the most important landmark to reestablish during closure because a 1-mm discrepancy in edge match will be noticeable at a normal talking distance. Edge eversion is also important in lip closure because the mobile lips tend to form depressed scars if they are closed without eversion. If muscle is involved, referral to a plastic surgeon is recommended.

Intraoral/Tongue

Tongue lacerations are common in sports and can cause a significant amount of bleeding as a result of the tongue's abundant vascularity. Immediate first aid includes controlling bleeding through the application of compression with moist gauze inside the mouth. Vicryl sutures are preferred for the tongue. Simple suture repair will often tear through the tissue because the tongue is predominantly muscle, and hence the use of either vertical mattress or horizontal mattress sutures is preferred. If the laceration is deep, referral to a specialist is often warranted.

Lacerations of the intraoral mucosa, such as the inner lip or cheek, are treated identically as external facial lacerations with regard to anesthetization, cleansing, and closure. A soft absorbable suture is preferred for patient comfort and obviously will not require removal.

Lateral Face Lacerations

A physician treating any deep laceration lateral to the lateral canthus needs to ensure function of the facial nerve. Any injury to the facial nerve in this area is possibly treatable with early surgery (within 3 days) to reanastomose the nerve (Fig. 23.7).

Soft Tissue Ear Injuries

Most injuries to the ear are simple lacerations that do not involve the underlying cartilage and can be sutured in a single layer. If the underlying cartilage is involved, it is important to reapproximate the cut edges. A nonbraided absorbable suture such as PDS or Monocryl is the most effective suture to use for the ear.

An auricular hematoma is another common injury of the ear. Untreated, it can lead to formation of a "cauliflower ear," which is commonly seen in wrestlers. This complication occurs because the blood supply to the cartilage is dependent upon the overlying perichondrium. A hematoma develops as a result of a shearing injury that separates the perichondrium from the cartilage, with the cartilage subsequently resorbing over time. To prevent this phenomenon, the hematoma needs to be drained and the perichondrium needs to be held fast to the cartilage for a week with use of a pressure bolster. These injuries are best treated by a specialist because of the risk of recurrence.

Periorbital Lacerations

Any wound deeper than a superficial eyelid laceration is best treated by either a plastic surgeon (a face specialist) or an ophthalmologist. The many lamellae and muscles of the eyelids require precise, layered closure of the lid structures.

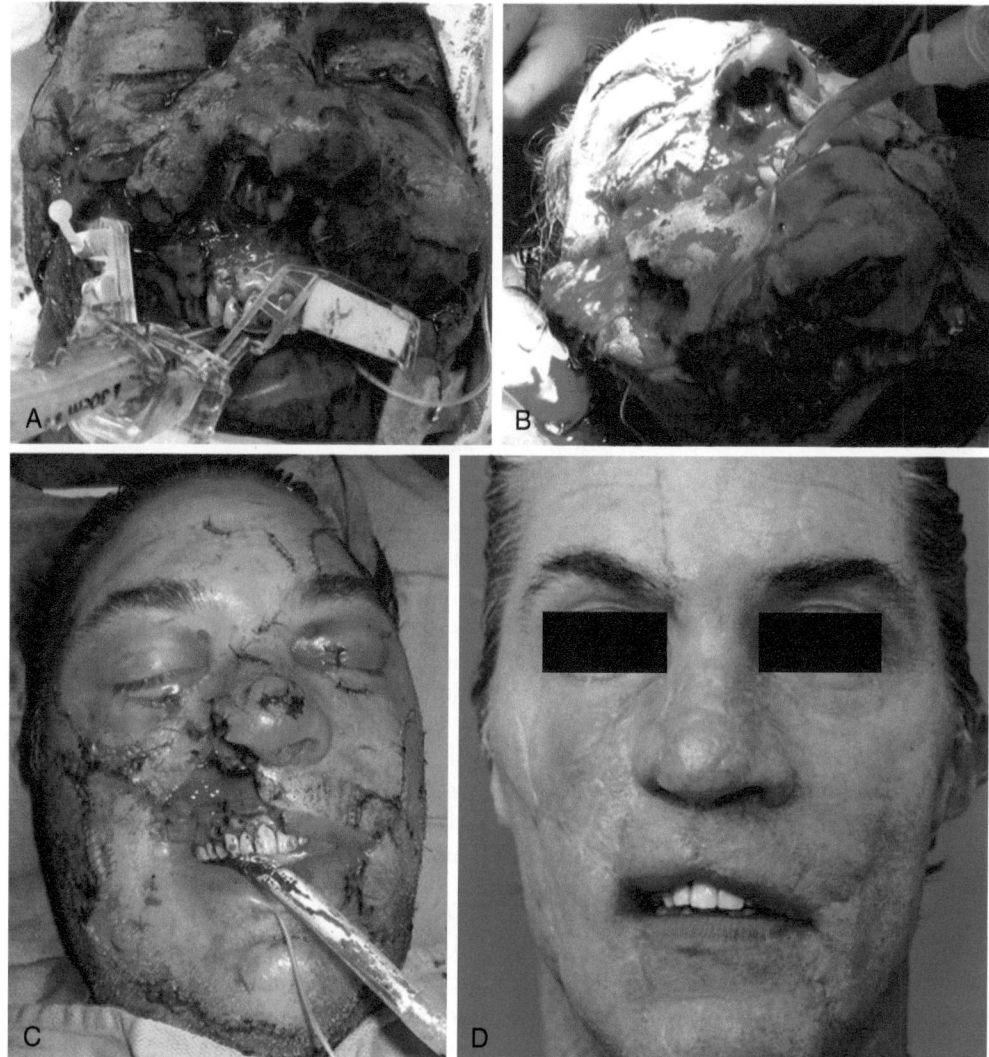

Fig. 23.5 (A and B) Complex lacerations resulting from a dog mauling. The patient was also missing his right upper lip and right nasal ala. (C) After closure of complex lacerations using the "known to unknown" principle. (D) The patient after reconstructive surgery on the right upper lip and right nasal ala using a lip-switch procedure and forehead flap.

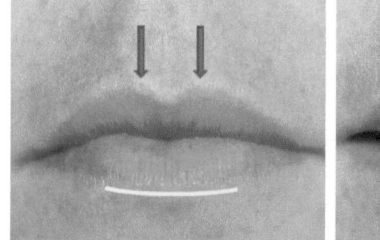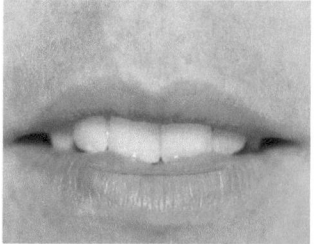

Fig. 23.6 Cutaneous lip landmarks. The *yellow line* marks the anterior vermilion border of the lower lip. Note the smooth anterior vermilion border on the lower lip, whereas the upper lip is punctuated by peaks of cupid's bow *(red arrows)*. The posterior vermilion border *(green line)* is where dry vermilion meets wet vermilion. This is the area where the upper and lower lips meet when in repose.

FACIAL FRACTURES

Facial fractures in the athlete are a common reason for referral to a facial traumatologist. A characteristic of facial fractures sustained during athletics is the focused nature of the fracture. Unlike fractures sustained in automobile accidents or as a result of interpersonal violence where massive force or repeated blows are the norm, facial fractures in athletes tend to occur as a result of a single blow from an inadvertent limb or a stray ball and thus are usually limited in extent. However, the evaluating physician must be aware of signs of life-threatening injuries.

Evaluation

After the ABCs of trauma are assessed (i.e., airway, breathing, and circulation), a rapid primary survey should be performed to assess for any other bodily injuries. Once the patient is deemed

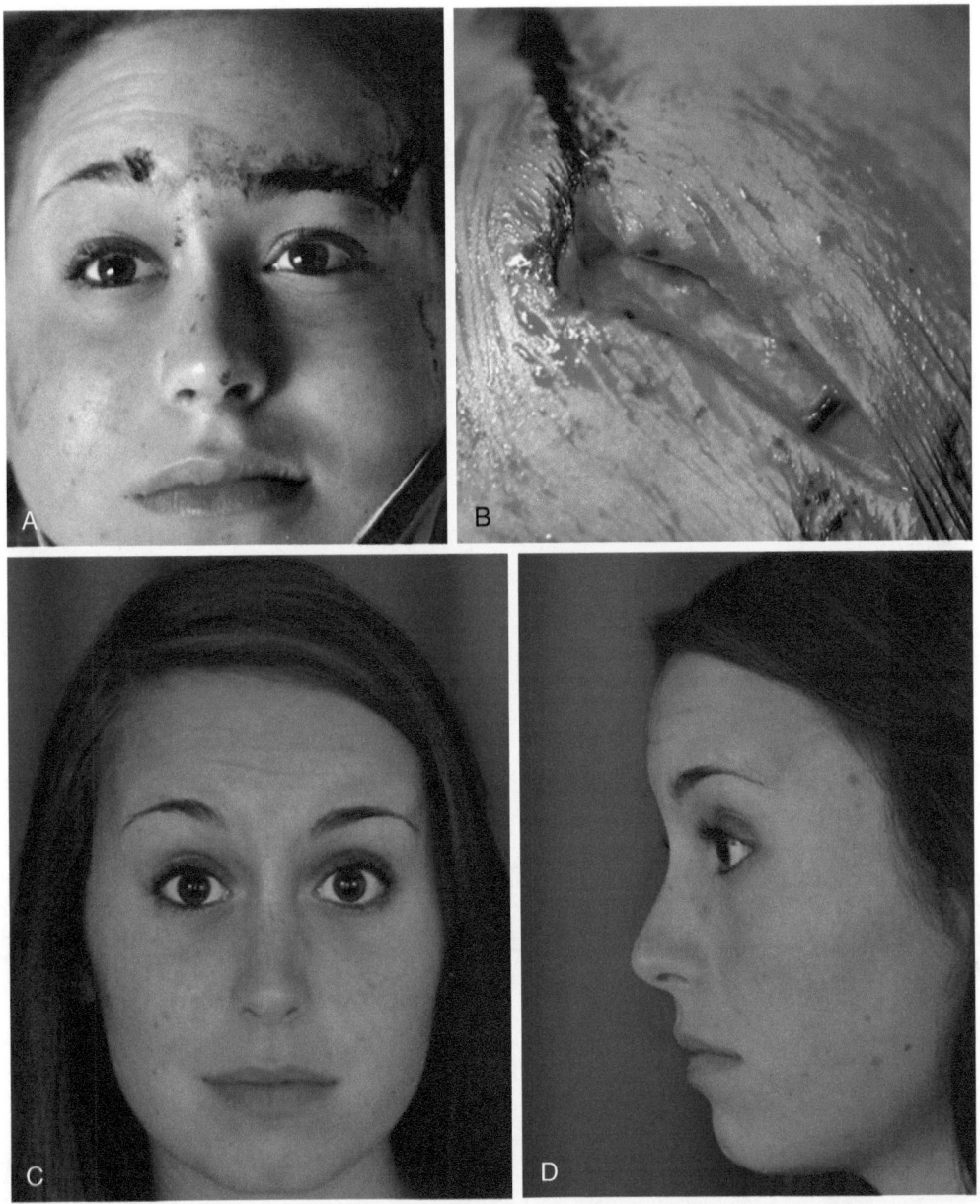

Fig. 23.7 (A) A patient with a deep laceration to the left temple region. Note the lack of frontalis motion on the left, indicating injury to the left temporal branch of the facial nerve. (B) A close-up view reveals a laceration through the temporoparietal fascia, sparing the sentinel vein of the forehead. (C and D) Six months after microscopic approximation of nerve fibers and wound closure.

stable, a focused examination of the head and neck should be performed. A facial trauma checklist can be used to guide the evaluation (Box 23.1). This examination does not need to be completed in any particular order; however, by beginning with the craniofacial skeleton and transitioning to the sensory organs, the practitioner will have completed the cranial nerve examination without the need to do so separately.

The facial skeletal examination should commence by palpating the facial buttresses, including the frontal bar, orbital rims, malar eminences, zygomatic arches, and mandible. Any focal area that elicits pain should raise concern for a fracture. Symmetrical sensation in the V_1 to V_3 dermatomes can be assessed when palpating the facial skeleton. Next, the oral cavity should be assessed, including tooth occlusion (how the teeth unite); the patient should

be asked if his or her bite feels normal. Any hematoma around the gingiva or floor of mouth is pathognomonic of a mandible fracture. Grasp the palate with one hand, hold the forehead with the other, and assess for any anterior/posterior mobility, as well as any lateral mobility. Any Le Fort–type fracture will induce mobility, crepitus, and pain with manipulation. Next, examine the nose, including the nasal bones and septum. The auricles should be examined for any sign of hematoma and for any bleeding or fluid from the ear canal. An ear canal laceration raises concern for a mandible fracture (transmitted via the mandibular condyle) or a skull base fracture. Bruising around the mastoid cavity is known as the Battle sign and is also a concern for a skull base fracture. A temporal bone fracture often results in blood in the middle ear. A tuning fork is an easy way to perform an initial

BOX 23.1   Facial Trauma Examination Checklist

Glasgow Coma Score =

Neck
C-spine?
Crepitus?
Ecchymoses?
Palpable landmarks?
Voice?

Facial Skeleton
The midface is stable?
Bony step offs?
Pain?

Soft Tissue
Lacerations?
Damage to salivary structures?
Foreign bodies in wounds?

Cranial Nerve Examination
Cranial nerve V injury?
Cranial nerve VII injury?

Eyes
Afferent System
Visual acuity?
Visual fields?

Pupillary Reactivity? Orbital Evaluation
Pupils are: Right? Left?
Extraocular motion deficits?
Vertical/horizontal dystopia?

Axial Displacement
  Proptosis?
  Pulsating exophthalmos?
  Enophthalmos?
Eyelid abnormalities?
Ptosis (medial reflex distance)?
Canthal position (telecanthus?)
Intercanthal distance =
Interpupillary distance =

Nose
Septal hematoma?
Nasal fracture?

Oral Cavity
Dentition is _____
Occlusion is _____
Lacerations?

Ears
Tympanic membranes are _____
Hemotympanum?
Otorrhea?
Tuning fork examination?
Auricular hematoma?

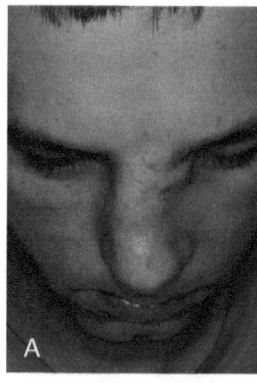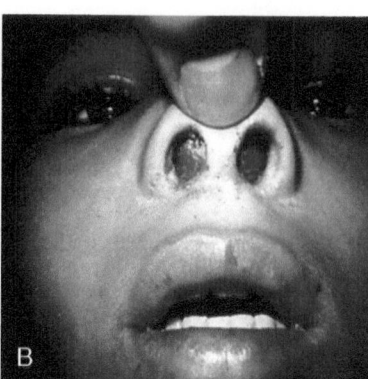

Fig. 23.8 (A) A nasal bone fracture. Note the obvious deviation of the nasal bones to the patient's right. (B) A pediatric patient with a septal hematoma. Note that the septal mucosa is bulging and fills both nasal cavities. This area of bulge is exquisitely painful to the touch.

hearing assessment and to determine whether any hearing loss is conductive or sensorineural.

The facial trauma examination concludes with an inspection of the eye and visual function. A basic eye examination should be performed by assessing the external eye, including the eyelids, palpebral fissure (look for widening), vertical or horizontal dystopia (worm's-eye view), and interpupillary and intercanthal distance. Visual acuity in the absence of a Snellen chart can be assessed through use of confrontation and by examining one eye at a time. Check extraocular motions and assess for any diplopia. Assess pupillary function by using the mnemonic PERRLA (**P**upils **E**qual **R**ound **R**eactive to **L**ight, **A**ccommodation). The swinging flashlight test is the best field method for accomplishing this assessment.

Fine-cut computed tomography of the face is the gold standard for imaging the facial skeleton. An orthopantogram (Panorex) can be helpful in assessing injury to the teeth.

Nasal Fractures

The nasal bones are the most commonly fractured bones in the face. Signs that a patient may have experienced a nasal bone fracture include an obvious deviation of the nasal skeleton and epistaxis (Fig. 23.8A). If epistaxis is the presenting symptom, it can be difficult to control. Most cases of epistaxis after nasal trauma are self-limiting but occasionally necessitate intervention by a physician. A helpful measure in the field is the use of nasal packs. Many commercially available nasal packs work well, including Rapid Rhino, Epistat, Rhino Rocket, and Merocel sponges. These products usually temporarily control significant bleeding until the patient can be transferred to an emergency department.

It is helpful to think of nasal fractures as having both a nasal bone and a nasal septal component. Any significant fracture of the nasal bones is likely to have fractured the intranasal septum, which can result in a septal hematoma (see Fig. 23.8B). Although they are rare, septal hematomas require more urgent intervention than an isolated nasal bone fracture. The sequelae of nasal fractures are both cosmetic and functional (nasal obstruction). Most nasal bone fractures are amenable to closed reduction within the first 10 days. When the initial 3 to 6 hours has passed after the fracture occurs, the edema in and around the nose precludes a proper reduction, and thus most facial traumatologists prefer to see the patient approximately 5 days after the trauma occurs. In the interim, elevation of the head and application of ice can hasten the resolution of the edema and minimize pain.

Although naso-orbitoethmoid fractures are rare in athletic injuries and are more common in high-speed accidents, they

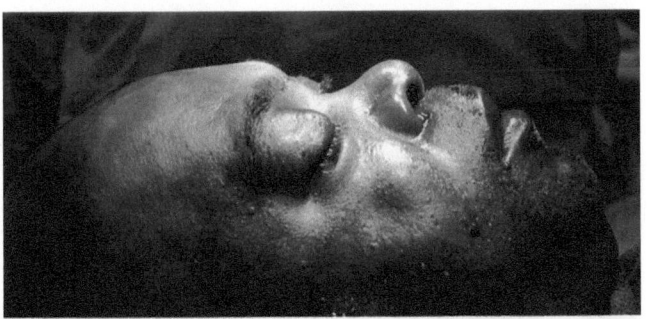
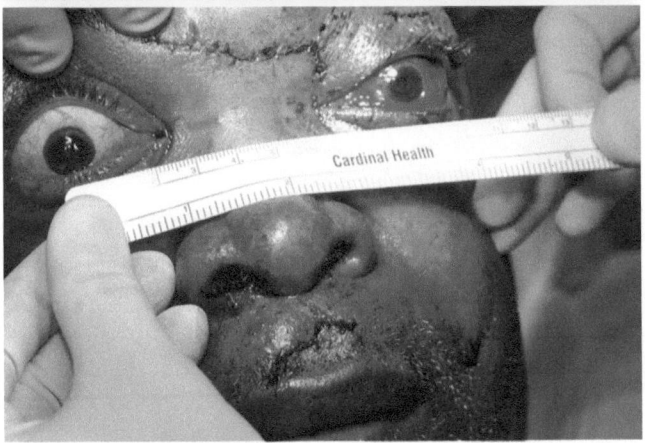

Fig. 23.9 A nasoorbitoethmoid fracture. Note the depressed nasal dorsum in the upper photo. The lower photo shows traumatic hypertelorism.

are a more serious form of isolated nasal bone fractures and require more urgent evaluation. These fractures have added perceptible signs on examination, including a significantly depressed nasal dorsum, widening of the palpebral fissures, and widening of the intercanthal distance (Fig. 23.9).

Mandible Fractures

The mandible is the second most common bone fractured in the facial skeleton.[17] Signs of a mandible fracture include pain, malocclusion, intraoral hematoma, hypesthesia of the affected mental nerve, and mobility across the fracture line. Any fracture that involves the tooth-bearing portions of the mandible is considered open and at a higher risk of infection. Mandible fractures require urgent referral because most centers prefer to treat the fracture within 72 hours. However, recent reports have shown similar outcomes for fractures treated in a delayed fashion.[18] If referral to a treatment center will be delayed, a Barton-type bandage can be placed around the chin to splint the mandible and prevent mobility (Fig. 23.10A).

Midface Fractures

Zygomatic (or malar bone) fractures are almost as common as mandible fractures. Although classically they have been described as "tripod" fractures because of the three obvious connections to the malar bone, they are in reality a quadrapod, or four-point fracture. These fractures include zygomaticotemporal, zygomaticofrontal, zygomaticomaxillary, and zygomaticosphenoid components. Fractures can vary greatly in severity and displacement and range from an isolated fracture of the zygomatic arch to comminuted fractures with significant bone loss. Hence the preferred term for a fracture in the region is a zygomaticomaxillary complex fracture.

Fractures can vary significantly in their severity and presenting signs. Cheek hypoesthesia is one of the more common signs

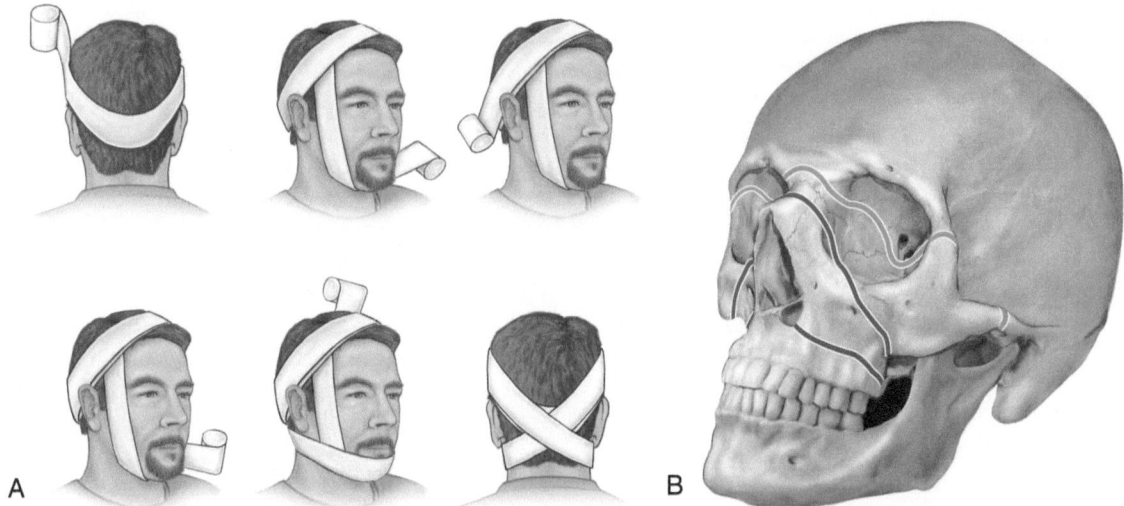

Fig. 23.10 (A) A diagram of a Barton bandage. This bandage was developed by John Rhea Barton, an orthopedic surgeon in Pennsylvania in the 1800s. (B) A drawing of a Le Fort-type pattern of fractures. The red line denotes a Le Fort I fracture; the blue line is a Le Fort II fracture; and the green line is a Le Fort III fracture.

and is the result of disruption of either the infraorbital nerve or the zygomaticofacial nerve. A degree of cheek asymmetry is usually also present as viewed from a "worm's-eye" view, noting the malar height. Often a "step off" can be felt on the inferior orbital rim as well.

Definitive treatment of these fractures is not as urgent as mandible fractures, because they are not usually "open fractures." However, evaluation should be performed urgently to rule out more serious associated fractures, including a 1 in 20 chance of a cervical spine injury.[17]

Although zygomaticomaxillary complex fractures often result from a side or angled blow to the midface, a frontal blow will more often result in a Le Fort-type fracture. These fractures are named after the French surgeon, Rene Le Fort, who found reproducible fracture patterns in cadaver skulls after the application of blunt force. The essential but not sufficient component of a Le Fort fracture is a fracture of the pterygoid plates (PP). A fracture of the PP plus a pyriform aperture creates a Le Fort I fracture; a fracture of the PP plus the infraorbital rims creates a Le Fort II fracture; and a fracture of the PP plus the zygomatic arch creates a Le Fort III fracture (see Fig. 23.10B). All persons with a Le Fort fracture will have a mobile palate or midface upon manipulation of the maxillary arch with a gloved hand. All midface fractures should be evaluated by a facial traumatologist.

Frontal Sinus Fractures

The frontal bar is the strongest buttress of the facial skeleton. It takes a force of 2000 Newtons to fracture the frontal sinus, which is designed to protect the globes and the brain.[19] The frontal sinus is composed of an anterior table that creates the forehead, and a posterior table that abuts the dura of the frontal lobe. The anterior table is much thicker (approximately 4 mm) than the posterior table (which is 1 to 2 mm thick). Between 20% and 30% of patients with a frontal sinus fracture will have a cerebrospinal fluid leak. Additionally, the force required to fracture the frontal sinus is often enough to produce, at a minimum, a concussion, or more serious cases of cerebral trauma or hemorrhage. Patients with a frontal sinus fracture will have forehead swelling, pain, and hypoesthesia on examination.

The management of frontal sinus fractures has evolved significantly during the past several decades, with many more of these fractures being treated conservatively with the advent of computed tomography scanning for monitoring. The main indications for operative intervention include significant cosmetic deformity and persistent cerebrospinal fluid leak. Regardless of the severity, any patient with a frontal sinus fracture should be evaluated by a facial traumatologist.

Orbital Fractures

The seven bones of the orbit serve to protect the globes and visual apparatus. The orbit can be visualized as a pyramid, with the thicker orbital rims as the base, and the thin orbital walls convening at the orbital apex. Blows to the periorbital region can result in fractures of the thin orbital walls by transmission of force through the globe (Fig. 23.11). The orbital floor and medial wall are most commonly fractured because they are

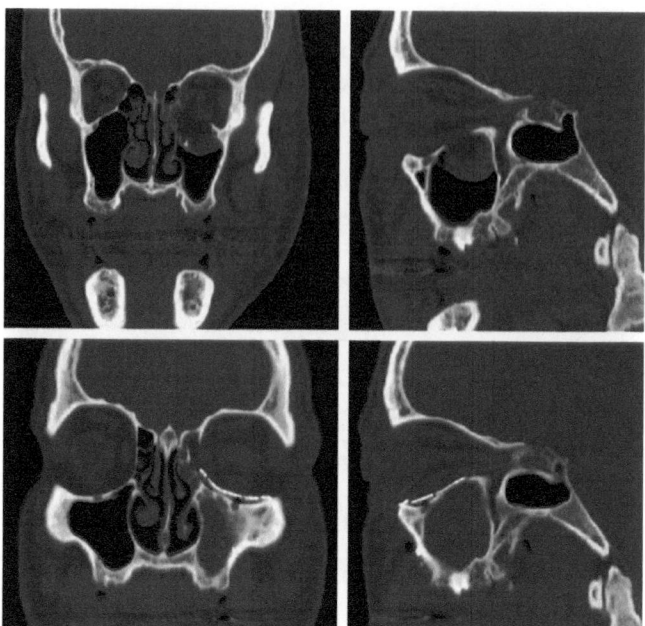

Fig. 23.11 A left orbital floor fracture. The upper photos reveal coronal and sagittal views of herniated contents of the left orbit. The lower photos are of the same patient after placement of a titanium orbital floor plate. Orbital fat and muscles are reduced, but the maxillary sinus remains filled with blood.

opposed only by air of the maxillary antrum and the ethmoid sinuses, respectively. Herniation of the contents of the orbit into fractures of the orbital floor can result in serious functional or cosmetic problems. Damage to the inferior rectus or medial rectus muscles is common and often results in diplopia.

Examination of patients with orbital floor fractures often reveals significant injury to the periorbital region. Rather rapidly occurring periorbital edema and chemosis often are present. In addition, injury to the extraocular muscles can result in gaze restriction and diplopia. The position of the globe also can be altered, with notable vertical and horizontal dystopia.

In children, the bone of the orbital walls is less ossified, and the bone tends to "greenstick" as it does in other areas of the body. A greenstick fracture can allow the orbital fat and muscle to herniate through the fracture, and then the bone can snap back and entrap the muscle. In children, this phenomenon can present as a "white-eyed blowout fracture"; the external orbit has no obvious signs of injury, but the gaze will be restricted in the affected eye. This type of fracture can also stimulate the oculocardiac reflex and cause persistent nausea and vomiting, bradycardia, and hypotension. The sports medicine physician must consider this diagnosis in a child with a periorbital injury who either cannot walk because of "dizziness" or has nausea and vomiting.

Orbital fractures require prompt evaluation by an ophthalmologist and facial traumatologist, because muscle entrapment or a persistent oculocardiac reflex requires urgent intervention. Many fractures of the orbital floor do not require surgery, but a thorough ophthalmologic examination must be performed so any injury to the globe can be monitored.

EYE INJURIES

Approximately 3% of all emergency department visits in the United States involve ocular trauma.[20] Injuries to the eye can be divided into those caused by physical trauma, foreign bodies, and chemical injury. The sports medicine physician is more likely to encounter injuries caused by blunt physical trauma and the occasional impacted foreign body. One-third of eye injuries occurring in children and adolescents are sports related.[21] Water sports, basketball, racquet sports, wrestling, martial arts, and archery are the sports most commonly implicated.

Injuries to the eye in which the globe remains intact are referred to as nonpenetrating trauma. Injuries to the surrounding bony structures of the orbit were discussed earlier in this chapter, in the "Facial Fractures" section. Blunt injuries can also affect the globe with or without associated bony trauma.

Corneal Abrasion

Corneal abrasions result from trauma to the surface of the eye. These abrasions can result from either blunt trauma (e.g., from a finger or a ball) or from small pieces of dirt/foreign bodies that are subsequently rubbed into the eye. Symptoms of a corneal abrasion include pain (which is often severe), a sensation of a foreign body in the eye, excessive squinting, and excessive tear production. On examination, patients may have gross epithelial defects and edema, scleral injection, mydriasis, and an anterior-chamber reaction. Visual acuity may be decreased because of corneal edema or excessive tear production.

Some corneal abrasions may be visible with a portable ophthalmoscope, but examination by an ophthalmologist with a slit lamp microscope and the use of a fluorescein stain is considered standard.

Most corneal abrasions will heal spontaneously as long as the offending foreign body has been removed. Water from a clean source should be used to clean the eye; washing the eye under a tap or plunging open eyes into a filled sink are effective measures. Over-the-counter artificial tears and lubricants and acetaminophen can help with discomfort. The use of topical antibiotic eye drops and antiinflammatory drops may be prescribed by an ophthalmologist. Patching the eye has recently been criticized because some studies have shown delayed healing.[22] More recently, "bandage contact lenses" are being used to aid healing.[23] Topical anesthetics should not to be used because they can reduce healing and cause secondary keratitis.

Hyphema

Hyphema is the presence of blood in the anterior chamber of the eye after a trauma. Patients may have partial vision loss as a result of the blockage of light. On examination, a visible pooling of blood in the anterior chamber is usually observed. Treatment is generally conservative but should be managed by an ophthalmologist.

Iridodialysis

Also known as coredialysis, iridodialysis is a localized separation of the iris from its attachment to the ciliary body. It can be caused by trauma to the eye and has been noted after injuries sustained by boxing, air bag deployments, water jets, bungee cords, water balloons, and various types of balls.[20] Patients with iridodialysis may have no symptoms, but increasing severity of the injury will present increasing symptoms. On examination, the typically smooth outer rim of the iris will have a lentiform defect where it has detached from the ciliary body. Iridodialysis needs to be evaluated by an ophthalmologist.

Retinal Detachment

Retinal detachment occurs when the retina peels away from the underlying support layer. Initially the area of detachment may be small, but it can progress. Risk factors for retinal detachment include high-force blunt trauma to the eye. Patients can have a dense shadow in a specific area of their vision or the sensation of a curtain being drawn over their vision. They also may note that straight lines may suddenly appear curved. Retinal detachment is a medical emergency and requires prompt referral to an ophthalmologist.

Ruptured Globe

If trauma to the globe has been severe, the integrity of the outer membranes can be disrupted. This disruption can occur as a result of blunt or penetrating trauma. Globe rupture from blunt trauma is most common at sites where the sclera is thinnest; for example, at the insertions of the extraocular muscles, at the limbus, and at the site of previous intraocular surgery.[20] Patients will present with varied degrees of symptoms, from pain to complete vision loss. Globe rupture is often "occult"; clinical examination initially may be benign, and therefore the practitioner needs to maintain a high index of suspicion.

DENTAL INJURIES

Differentiating Between Primary and Permanent Teeth

Dental trauma management depends on whether the injury involves primary or permanent teeth. Children maintain their primary teeth until they are approximately 6 years old, at which point permanent teeth begin to replace primary dentition. This process occurs until the age of approximately 14 years, when most children will have all their permanent dentition. In the case of mixed dentition, the following guidelines can help differentiate between primary and permanent teeth. Primary teeth (Fig. 23.12A) are smaller than permanent teeth, very white, have bulbous crowns, and often have worn, flat edges. Permanent teeth (see Fig. 23.12B) are larger, creamier in color, and have more jagged edges. This distinction is important because primary teeth are never repositioned, splinted, or reinserted.

The goals of treatment of dental injuries are to retain the tooth in the dental arch, maintain the viability of the pulp, and prevent root resorption—all of which are aimed at restoring the form and function of the teeth. Most dental injuries will require treatment by a dentist, but recognizing which ones are serious and require referral often falls to the sports medicine physician.

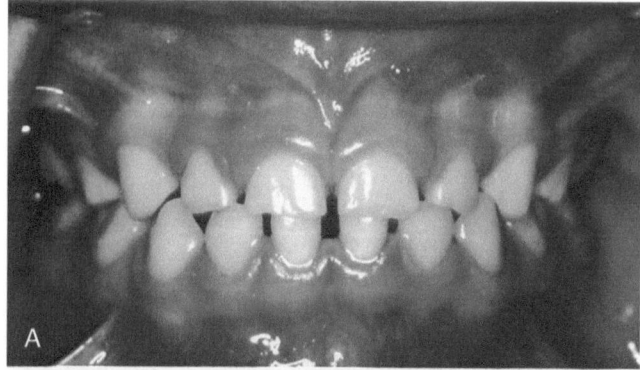

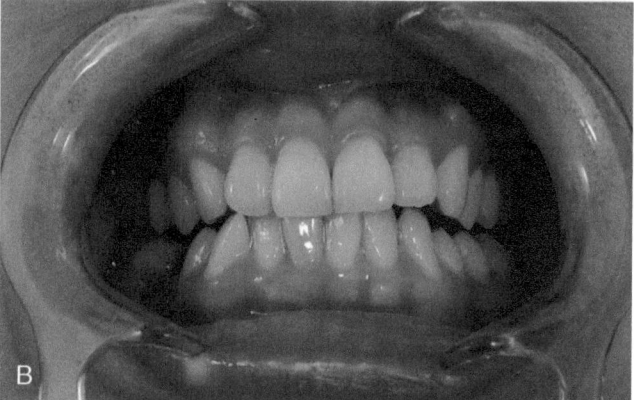

Fig. 23.12 (A) Primary teeth. The teeth are small, very white, and have worn flat edges and bulbous crowns. (B) Permanent teeth. The teeth are larger, cream in color, and have jagged edges.

Periodontal/Displacement Injuries (Loose Teeth)

A concussion injury to the tooth will cause the tooth to be tender yet firm to the touch. If the tooth remains firm and occlusion remains normal, the teeth can be reexamined at a later date by the patient's local dentist. If the tooth is tender and loose or if blood is present around the gum line, subluxation of the tooth may have occurred, and splinting by a dentist may be required. If the tooth is displaced in any direction, it will generally require repositioning and splinting by a dentist. If the tooth has been completely avulsed, it is important to distinguish between a primary and a permanent tooth, because a primary tooth is never reinserted. However, a permanent tooth can be successfully reinserted. To achieve the best chance of reinsertion, the tooth should have a "dry time" of less than 60 minutes. The preferred method of keeping the tooth viable is to reinsert it in the socket and have the patient hold it in place by biting on a piece of gauze. If that technique cannot be used, the tooth can be placed in "tooth saver" or milk until the patient can be evaluated by a dentist.

Importantly, if the tooth is "missing," it is important to ensure that a complete intrusion injury has not occurred in which the tooth is pushed into the alveolus. In such cases a radiograph is required for thorough assessment.

Intrusive displacement is the most common type of dental injury in young children with primary dentition.[24] Even if complete intrusion has not occurred, the teeth will likely require extraction because the impacted roots will affect the eruption of the permanent dentition.

Fractured Teeth

The most common sports injury to occur to permanent teeth is a crown fracture.[25] For teeth that are fractured, it is again vital to distinguish between primary and permanent teeth. In either case, if the injury is only through enamel (which is white) or dentin (which is yellow), the patient can be examined within a few weeks by his or her primary dentist. If the fracture is deeper and involves the pulp (which is pink), a primary tooth will likely require extraction, whereas with a permanent tooth, the tooth fragments can potentially be reattached. The pieces of a permanent tooth should be preserved in tooth saver or milk until the patient can be evaluated by a dentist.

If just the outer enamel of the tooth is fractured, the tooth often can be fixed by dental smoothing and contouring at a later date. In fact, many of these minor dental injuries are not noticed until the athlete has a formal dental examination.

If the enamel and deeper dentin are fractured, painful sensations will be felt when the tooth is exposed to touch, air, or cold drinks.[26] In these cases, attempts to locate the fractured segment should be made because they can potentially be bonded to the remaining tooth. If the fractured segment cannot be located and the athlete is experiencing significant pain, on-site management can be performed with use of a pulp-protecting agent. These agents, which include calcium hydroxide paste or zinc oxide mixed with eugenol,[26] will reduce sensitivity until the athlete can be seen by a dentist, who eventually will perform a functional restoration.

In the case of enamel/dentin/pulp fractures, the status of the dental pulp determines the method of treatment.[27] The root can be vital or nonvital, and the root apex can be closed or open. Combinations of these conditions determine whether an aesthetic restoration can be performed (with a possible intermediate root closure procedure) or whether a root canal is needed. Again, immediate evaluation by a dentist is required for a crown fracture, in which the pink of the dentin is visible. Bleeding from the pulp will often occur as well, and this later sign should make the severity of the fracture more clear.

For a complete list of references, go to ExpertConsult.com.

SELECTED READINGS

Citation:
Eidelman A, Weiss JM, Lau J, et al. Topical anesthetics for dermal instrumentation: a systematic review of randomized, controlled trials. *Ann Emerg Med.* 2005;46:343–351.

Level of Evidence:
I

Summary:
Administration of eutectic mixture of local anesthetics (EMLA) is an effective, noninvasive means of analgesia before dermal procedures. However, at least three other topical anesthetics are at least as efficacious: tetracaine, liposome-encapsulated tetracaine, and liposome-encapsulated lidocaine.

Citation:
Scarfone RJ, Jasani M, Gracely EJ. Pain of local anesthetics: rate of administration and buffering. *Ann Emerg Med.* 1998;31:36–40.

Level of Evidence:

I

Summary:

Slow administration of a local anesthetic (over 30 seconds) does more for pain with injection than does buffering with sodium bicarbonate.

Citation:

Fernandez R, Griffiths R. Water for wound cleansing. *Cochrane Database Syst Rev.* 2012;(2):CD003861.

Level of Evidence:

I

Summary:

No evidence exists to indicate that the use of tap water to cleanse acute wounds in adults increases infection, and some evidence indicates that it reduces infection. However, strong evidence has not been found that cleansing wounds, per se, increases healing or reduces infection. In the absence of potable tap water, boiled and cooled water or distilled water can be used as wound-cleansing agents.

Citation:

Farion K, Osmond MH, Hartling L, et al. Tissue adhesives for traumatic lacerations in children and adults. *Cochrane Database Syst Rev.* 2002;(3):CD003326.

Level of Evidence:

I

Summary:

Tissue adhesives are an acceptable alternative to standard wound closure in the repair of simple traumatic lacerations. No significant difference in cosmetic outcome has been found between tissue adhesives and standard wound closure or between different tissue adhesives. Tissue adhesives offer the benefit of decreased procedure time and less pain compared with standard wound closure. A small but statistically significant increased rate of dehiscence with tissue adhesives must be considered when choosing the closure method (number needed to treat to cause harm to an individual = 25).

Citation:

Mulligan RP, Mahabir RC. The prevalence of cervical spine injury, head injury, or both with isolated and multiple craniomaxillofacial fractures. *Plast Reconstr Surg.* 2010;126:1647–1651.

Level of Evidence:

II

Summary:

In the setting of an isolated mandible, nasal, orbital floor, malar/maxilla, or frontal/parietal bone fracture, cervical spine injury ranged from 4.9% to 8.0%, head injury ranged from 28.7% to 79.9%, and concomitant cervical spine and head injury was present in 2.8% to 5.8% of patients. In the setting of two or more facial fractures, the prevalence of cervical spine injury ranged from 7.0% to 10.8%. The prevalence of head injury ranged from 65.5% to 88.7%, and the prevalence of concomitant cervical spine and head injury ranged from 5.8% to 10.1%.

24

Psychological Adjustment to Athletic Injury

Karen P. Egan, Jason Freeman

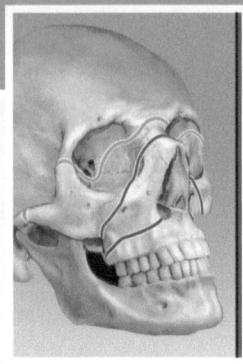

Participation in athletics involves physical risk that can result in limited ability or inability to continue sports play. Medical advances have led to the improved diagnosis of athletic injury and formulation of rehabilitative treatment plans. Psychological variables influence how individuals cope with physical injury; therefore understanding and effectively managing the psychological reaction to injury can enhance recovery from injury, facilitate return to play (RTP), and aid athletes in adapting to changing roles.

The number of persons participating in sports continues to grow. High school student participation has increased by more than 130% over the last 30 years according to the National Federation of High School Sports (NFHS), with over 7.8 million participants in 2014–2015.[1] These figures, importantly, only account for those playing scholastically, as club participation across youth sports has been estimated to be above 44 million annually.[2] Overall injury rates in high school sports were at 2.32 per 1000 athlete exposures, roughly 1.4 million for the 2015–2016 school year.[3] From the 2005–2006 school year through the 2013–2014 school year, 6.0% of the 59,862 total injuries tracked among high school athletes were career or season-ending injuries.[4] Sports-related injuries accounted for up to 1 in 5 of all emergency department (ED) visits in those under the age of 18,[5] and 19% of visits to the pediatrician's office.[6]

In a study that estimated average injury data for all 25 NCAA sports over a 5-year period from the 2009–2010 school year through the 2013–2014 school year, there were an estimated average of 210,674 total injuries per year from 28,860,299 practices and 6,472,952 competitions each year.[7] About one-fifth of these injuries required 7 days or more away from full participation in sport as part of the recovery process.[7] Among male student-athletes, football accounted for the largest number of estimated injuries per year while men's wrestling had the highest overall injury rate.[7] Among female student-athletes, soccer accounted for the largest number of estimated injuries per year while gymnastics had the highest overall injury rate.[7]

While it is common for athletes to experience athletic injury, there are many potential impacts on an athlete's emotions, thoughts, behaviors, and overall well-being. Common emotional responses include stress and anxiety,[8,9] such as fear of reinjury,[10] fear of not being able to perform at the same preinjury level, and/or to improve performance after injury,[11] sadness, depressive symptoms, loss,[12-15] isolation,[16] anger,[12,13,17] and decreased self-esteem.[13] Such negative emotions have been associated with a longer rehabilitation process,[11] decreased motivation to attend rehabilitation appointments,[12] and an increased risk of reinjury.[18]

Although many athletes are impacted in negative ways by athletic injury, each athlete may respond differently. Some athletes do not experience much disruption.[8] Some athletes are able to interpret their athletic injury as a challenge and focus on learning from the experience.[13,19] Providing support to athletes in order to increase their likelihood of experiencing these positive outcomes is critical to athlete well-being and to athletic success.

In addition, the age of the participant, the level of competition (youth, high school, club, collegiate, professional, weekend warrior), the severity of injury, and the degree of investment in the athlete identity by the participant are important factors in how the psychological response to injury is conceptualized. This chapter does not provide a comprehensive review of the developmental conceptualizations of the psychological impact of athletic injury or a comprehensive discussion of how competition level influences psychological variables. Rather, the psychology of injury is discussed more broadly, reviewing some of the general paradigms for understanding how injury psychologically impacts athletes and the literature on utilization of psychological principles to enhance recovery. Specific application of these efforts are also presented through discussion of pre-participation screening, the referral process, the value of multi-disciplinary treatment teams, and the importance of continuing to support injured athletes beyond the initial return to sport.

HISTORICAL PERSPECTIVE AND EVOLUTION

Psychological models of injury were initially divided into two categories: Stage Models and Cognitive Models.[20] Stage Models were largely adapted from examining psychological reactions to terminal illnesses. Injury is conceptualized as triggering grief and loss, because of the resulting perceived loss of an aspect of the self.[21] Commonly applied models of the stages of grief are adapted from Kubler-Ross.[22] Limitations included the reduced ability to incorporate the variety of athletes' perceptions of injury and the contextual differences that influence the psychological consequence of the injury. These limitations gave rise to Cognitive Models, which borrowed significantly from the stress and coping theory. Rather than stages, the interpretations of the injury itself are the focal point. These include cognitive attributions for injury, self-perceptions following injury, methods of coping, and perceived benefits of injury.[20] Subsequently, these models have been integrated to include biopsychosocial influences[23] and updated to reflect the bidirectional relationship between an individual athlete's coping tendencies and contextual factors.[18,20] See *The Handbook of Sport Psychology* for a more detailed review of this history.[24]

Some of the most widely supported models include the Stress and Injury Model, the Self-Determination Model, and the Wiese-Bjornstal Integrated Model of Psychological Response to the Sport Injury and Rehabilitation Process. The Stress and Injury Model[18] posits that heightened distress associated with the fear of reinjury saps available attention resources and peripheral vision, leading to increased muscular fatigue and reduced timing and coordination. Building off Ryan and Deci's[25] initial formulations of the Self-Determination Model, other researchers have emphasized the importance of meeting three psychological needs during the return to sport process in accordance with Self-Determination Theory: competence, or trust in one's own ability, autonomy, or a belief that one can influence their own outcomes, and relatedness, or a sense of connection to others.[26-28] The Wiese-Bjornstal Integrated Model of Psychological Response to the Sport Injury and Rehabilitation Process extends Lazarus and Folkman's 1984 cognitive appraisal theory of stress and coping and argues that preinjury variables (personality, history of stressors, coping resources, etc.), injury variables (injury history, severity of injury, etc.), and postinjury variables (cognitive appraisals made by an athlete, etc.) influence an athlete's response to athletic injury.[20,29]

PREPARTICIPATION SCREENING

Assessing for potential mental health concerns upon entry of an athlete to a club team, a collegiate program, or a professional team allows services to be provided proactively to support athletes who may be at-risk of developing mental health concerns in the future, who have already sought care in the past and wish to continue, and/or who are interested in proactively establishing support prior to experiencing stressors such as athletic injury. Some early-stage research suggests that identifying individuals who experience preseason anxiety and connecting them to support to reduce symptoms may also help reduce rates of athletic injury.[30]

When preparticipation physicals are conducted, brief screening measures can be used to assess for potential mental health concerns and/or measure well-being to enable referrals to licensed mental health providers. The NCAA Mental Health Best Practices document encourages the use of preparticipation screening measures to assess alcohol and cannabis use, depressive symptoms, anxiety, disordered eating behavior/eating disorders, sleep, and attention-deficit/hyperactivity disorder among student-athletes.[31] Upon experiencing an athletic injury, additional assessment of mental health and well-being symptoms can be undertaken and compared to these baseline values to help inform treatment decisions. If screenings are conducted, it is critical to have a plan in place to protect confidentiality, to ensure timely follow-up, and to know when and how to refer to a licensed mental health provider for the athlete's care (see Authors' Preferred Technique for more information).

DECISION-MAKING PRINCIPLES

For all front-line sports injury professionals, it is important to recognize potential mental health concerns. Rather than treating these issues as taboo, open discussion among all providers in the training room setting can validate the importance of psychological issues, the active role each provider can take in directly intervening, and the importance of referring to other resources when available. Taking an active role in supporting athletes directly makes a difference in their recovery. Professionals can also address pressures to return to sport (direct or indirect) from coaches, parents, teammates, administration, and athletes themselves to shape the influence of these assets and to enhance a healthy recovery process.

Caring for the injured athlete ideally involves collaboration between many potential resources. These include the athlete him/herself, sports physicians, Certified Athletic Trainers (ATCs), sports nutritionists, sports psychologists and/or licensed mental health providers, administration, coaches, teammates, family members, professors, academic coordinators, and other potential support systems. Integrating these potential resources into a multi-disciplinary team with well-defined roles and recognition of role limitations can be invaluable in addressing the complete biopsychosocial needs of the recovering athlete.

It is important to note that only licensed mental health providers are qualified to focus on mental health concerns while a qualified sport psychology consultant can focus on skill-building for sports performance while the athlete is returning from athletic injury. A qualified licensed mental health provider with training and experience working with athletes can fluidly work on both mental health concerns and skill-building for performance during the return-to-sport process. While it is ideal that all injured athletes have access to properly trained and credentialed professionals serving these roles, such resources do not exist at all levels across the breadth of athletics. However, consultations and/or referrals to these providers through access to school resources not specific to the athletics department and/or in the surrounding community can also be a great fit.

There are a number of potential challenges that can prevent athletes from seeking care with a mental health provider, such as the role of stigma or the belief that seeking care would be a sign of "weakness," not wanting to express emotions, lack of time to seek care, being unsure how to access a provider who is competent in working with athletes, and/or the belief that treatment may not help.[32] The role of sports medicine personnel is critical in helping athletes overcome these barriers. When referring to a mental health provider, it is often helpful to meet with an athlete individually, to use "I" statements, to focus on observed behaviors/events, to ask the athlete how they are doing and listen before moving to problem-solving, to emphasize the athlete's value to the team despite the athletic injury, to be clear about how to contact the mental health provider and what the treatment may look like, to talk about the confidentiality of available mental health services, and to follow-up after making the referral to see if the athlete was able to get connected to a mental health provider.

Authors' Preferred Technique

Treatment Options

A number of options exist for supporting athletes' psychological needs in their return-to-sport process, including techniques that focus on building skills for sport performance, strategies that focus on mental health concerns, and approaches that address both concerns. Techniques that focus on sport performance when an athlete is recovering from athletic injury often include goal-setting, the use of imagery or visualization exercises, teaching the athlete about self-talk, improving confidence in current and future athletic capabilities, and reframing the injury as an opportunity to learn and develop a new relationship with sport that can be positive. In a study conducted with 1283 athletes from the United States, the United Kingdom, and Finland, only 27% of athletes (*n* = 346) reported using mental skills during injury rehabilitation, but of those who used these skills, 72% (*n* = 249) said they believed the mental skills helped them rehabilitate faster.[33] The top four skills these athletes reported using included goal setting (46.8%), positive self-talk (33.2%), imagery (31.8%), and relaxation (24.3%).[33]

A positive relationship has been found between goal setting and adherence to rehabilitation exercises during the recovery process.[34] When setting goals, use of the SMARTS principle[35] is a pragmatic approach that can be used by many different members of the athlete's multi-disciplinary team. An injured athlete's attention is directed to *S*pecific, *M*easurable, *A*ction-oriented, *R*ealistic, *T*ime-based, and *S*elf-determined indicators of progress to enhance perceptions of competence and facilitate a healthy and efficient return to sport process. When goals do not meet the SMARTS criteria, the normal anxiety and fear experienced by the injured athlete may undermine adherence to treatment and lengthen the rehabilitation process. Again, having an established consultation relationship with a licensed mental health provider can be invaluable when an athlete experiences significant changes in anxiety or depression over the course of recovery.

Techniques that focus on mental health concerns or both mental health and athletic performance concerns at the same time often target anxiety symptoms (including pre-performance anxiety, fear of reinjury, and worry about not being able to perform at preinjury levels); depressive symptoms and feelings of loss; feelings of isolation, anger, relationship conflicts that emerged as a result of the injury and/or removal from sport participation; changes in eating behavior; changes in sleep; addressing problematic coping strategies such as substance abuse; and fostering the use of positive coping strategies. Exploration of identity outside of sport also can be critical for the athlete's well-being, both for those who are temporarily removed from athletic participation and for those whose have suffered career-ending athletic injuries. Podlog et al.[28] highlight the importance of promoting a perspective shift from active sport participation as the sole basis for team membership. Affiliation can be redefined through work with a licensed mental health provider in the context of reexamining the intrinsic value of sport participation, redefining competence as a contributing teammate, exploring the notion that active sport participation is only one facet of the athlete's identity (i.e., what else is part of who you are?), and supporting an athlete in identifying "transferrable skills" from sport to other elements of their identity. In some instances, this can also be supported through actions by sports medicine staff, coaches, and teammates, such as creating a new interim or permanent role on the team (e.g., volunteer coach, training partner) and through building relationships with other injured athletes through a formal venue (e.g., a support group) or through informal exchanges with others who have been through this experience before.[28]

While the strategies focusing on mental health concerns should only be practiced by an appropriately trained and licensed mental health provider, having all treatment team members know how to speak to an injured athlete about options for care and about what treatment may entail can help to ensure a successful referral and allow holistic support to be provided to the athlete throughout the return-to-sport process. There are a number of different theoretical approaches that mental health providers may use, which can be beneficial for injured athletes, including cognitive-behavioral therapy (CBT), interpersonal therapy (IPT),[36] positive psychology, mindfulness-based stress reduction (MBSR), acceptance and commitment therapy (ACT), humanistic therapy, and more. For example, a cognitive-behavioral therapist may work with an athlete on ways to identify automatic negative thoughts that emerge related to athletic injury and the return-to-sport process, and teach the athlete how to use thought-challenging techniques to determine an alternative thought that can be associated with a different and more desired emotional response.[37] Stress inoculation training has also been proposed as an intervention using cognitive restructuring, thought control, imagery, and simulation.[38] Athletes who were randomly assigned to a similar intervention, Cognitive Behavioral Stress Management, who received education on CBT techniques and relaxation strategies had significantly fewer illness and injury days compared to the control group of athletes. Therefore the proactive use of these strategies may also reduce the risk for injury and/or teach athletes a set of skills they can build upon should they experience athletic injury in the future.[39]

A therapist using acceptance and commitment therapy may focus on the goal of accepting both positive and negative thoughts and emotions without needing to change them, and may also use mindfulness techniques.[40] Positive psychology work can be integrated by focusing on the athlete's strengths and how these can be helpful during the recovery process.[41] Many athletes excel at being goal-oriented, open to feedback/coaching, maintaining motivation, being able to push through physical pain to enhance athletic performance, and managing time efficiently. Each of these skills can be invaluable during the recovery process, but may need to be adapted in new ways that are less familiar to the athlete. Treatment team providers who remind athletes of their strengths will help recovering athletes direct their attention from the deficits resulting from the athletic injury and removal from sport participation to the opportunities to facilitate their own recovery process and to minimize challenges.

In addition, interventions that modify physiological arousal following injury are thought to reduce the attentional disruption associated with a stress response to injury and improve focus. These benefits have been explored in using progressive muscle relaxation (PMR), meditation, autogenic training, and diaphragmatic breathing exercises.[42] They have been shown to enhance concentration and decrease distractibility during the recovery process.[43]

It has also been proposed that improving social support, teaching coping skills by training injured athletes and coaches, and building confidence will increase resilience to athletic injury.[44] Evidence is growing in other related recovery areas that argues for the benefit of combining biological and psychosocial approaches—areas as diverse as behavioral research in oncology[45] as well as premorbid[46] and comorbid[47] psychological contributions to mild traumatic brain injury. Despite the existence of social support, which shows great value in the psychological recovery from sports injury,[17,48,49] it may not be perceived as available.[50] Ensuring that education and information are not only available, but also perceived as available is key in managing sports injury recovery. In addition, different types of injuries may be associated with different levels of satisfaction with social support. While athletes who experienced orthopedic injuries and concussion injuries reported similar sources of social support, those who experienced orthopedic injury expressed more satisfaction with their support than the group who experienced concussion.[49] It may be that some of these social support systems lack knowledge of typical symptoms of concussion or are unsure of how to support someone experiencing concussion symptoms. The invisibility of concussion injuries also may allow social support systems to "forget" that the need for support exists, or can result in greater stigma for an athlete who is removed from sport participation without a visible wound, brace, or crutches. Sports medicine personnel can offer social support by keeping the injured athlete involved in the team by including supportive medical providers, friends, or family members in the rehabilitation process and through collaborative goal-setting with the athlete throughout the rehabilitation process.[51] In addition, providing frequent communication and education about why a particular rehabilitation process is used supports injured athlete autonomy. Updates about measured progress (SMARTS goals) and offering an injured athlete regular choices about the rehabilitation plan can reduce pressure and enhance the perception of an internal locus of control.

POSTINJURY MANAGEMENT AND OUTCOME

Continuing to support injured athletes after their initial return to sport is important in providing them with coping strategies for their worry about experiencing another athletic injury and their concerns about their current and future level of play. Athletes who have experienced an injury that required more time away from sport, and/or repeated athletic injuries, often need additional support. Athletes who have experienced a severe injury express more fear of returning to sport and more fear of reinjury.[52] Athletes who experienced anxiety about potential reinjury more frequently and more strongly were also more likely to decrease the time and effort they put into their rehabilitation exercises and treatment plan.[53] This can then increase their likelihood of experiencing reinjury and/or add additional stressors to their return to sport experience (e.g., limited range of motion, decreased flexibility, and/or lower athletic performance). Therefore there is a need for continued collaboration and involvement between a qualified sport psychologist or licensed mental health provider and the athlete after his/her physical return to sport.

When athletes were asked to define what a "successful" return to sport meant to them, answers included a number of performance measurements (e.g., a return to preinjury athletic performance and having realistic athletic goals postinjury), psychological measurements (e.g., "staying on the right path" of believing that one could still achieve long-term success postinjury, and feeling the "self-satisfaction" of meeting their own internal standards of success), and physical measurements (e.g., remaining uninjured and feeling confident that the injured body part is fully recovered).[26] A focus group conducted with injured athletes reported three aspects of psychological readiness to return to sport: feeling confident returning to sport, having realistic expectations about their current athletic capabilities, and being motivated to achieve performance standards that they had previously obtained prior to athletic injury.[54] These findings also highlight the important roles that sports medicine staff have in continuing to support the athlete after the initial RTP, as these athletes reported that trust in their rehabilitation providers, the achievement of physical outcomes/measurement points, goal setting, and reducing boredom during the rehabilitation process were important contributors to these three aspects of readiness to return to sport.[54]

COMPLICATIONS

Despite the efforts of athletes, coaches, and treatment team members to reduce complications throughout the return-to-sport process, real or imagined time pressure can influence the psychological and physical response to injury.[28] Athletes may perceive direct pressure from coaches, teammates, and/or family members; may perceive indirect pressure on their coaches from others; and/or may project their own desire for a rapid RTP onto their coaches. This places athletes in a vulnerable position to rush their RTP timeline ineffectively and dangerously. Coaches themselves may directly or indirectly convey perceived time pressure (from administrations, team owners, parents, boosters, or even the press) to have their athletes ready for the next competition.

These pressures can exacerbate an athlete's fears of losing their abilities, "losing ground" relative to others who are not injured, losing a spot on the team, and losing "right of membership" on the team. Pressures, expectations, and cognitions regarding the past (i.e., what my abilities were and who I was) and the future (i.e., who I was on track to be, who I am supposed to be, who I "have" to be) lead to maladaptive arousal that detracts from the body's performance of recovery in the present moment. For the injured athlete, rest, recovery, refueling, and rehabilitation often take precedence over testing their new limits of strength and fitness. If an injured athlete is externally guided or internally compelled to push beyond the body's capabilities in the present, recovery is jeopardized. These pressures may push the athlete to rush the return-to-sport timeline, and paradoxically extend the return-to-athletics participation process[55] as the athlete may experience reinjury, illness, and/or perform poorly due to an incomplete recovery that continues to limit physical and psychological performance. Reducing return-to-sport pressures by talking openly to injured athletes, coaches, and family members about the expected return-to-sport timeline—and the reasons for this timeline—will allow everyone to be on the same page about the anticipated return and the expectations of the return-to-sport process.

FUTURE CONSIDERATIONS

Medical providers are often the staff members who interact with injured athletes earliest after their experience of athletic injury and most frequently throughout the rehabilitation and return-to-sport process. Therefore the sports medicine team (consisting of ATCs, team physicians, specialists, and other medical providers) is in a key position for establishing a multidisciplinary team that can holistically support the injured athlete during and beyond his or her return-to-sport process. Consulting with and referring to other providers as needed throughout the process, including a licensed mental health provider or qualified sport psychologist, can help reduce the negative impacts of athletic injury, and to facilitate a successful and timely return to sport. It is important to identify the gaps in your care model that leave unmet needs for injured athletes so you can determine appropriate solutions.

While this is not a new concept, and despite increased sport participation across all competence levels, there are too few resources aimed at easing the psychological impact of sports-related injuries. We hope that chapters such as this increase awareness of the importance of this issue, and encourage all those working with athletes at all levels to incorporate such conceptual understanding into their practice.

For a complete list of references, go to ExpertConsult.com.

SELECTED READINGS

Citation:
Singer RN, Hausenblas HA, Janelle CM, eds. *Handbook of Sport Psychology.* Wiley; New York: 2000.

Level of Evidence:
I/II

Summary:

Chapter 30 Psychology of Injury Risk and Prevention (Jean M. Williams). Revised version of the stress and injury model (Williams and Anderson, 1998).

Chapter 31 Psychology of Sport Injury Rehabilitation (Britton W. Brewer). Presents the biopsychosocial model of sport injury rehabilitation (Brewer, Andersen, and Van Raalte).

Citation:

Weiss MR. Psychological aspects of sport-injury rehabilitation: a developmental perspective. *J Athl Train*. 2003;38:172–175.

Level of Evidence:

III

Summary:

Brief review of developmental factors in sport injury. Provides a brief background of developmental perspective, as well as an overview of research design, sampling procedures, and measurement/statistical issues in sport injury rehab. Recommends more research in this area, especially given the widespread nature of this type of injury.

Citation:

Yang J, Peek-Asa C, Lowe JB, et al. Social support patterns of collegiate athletes before and after injury. *J Athl Train*. 2010;45:372–379.

Level of Evidence:

I/II

Summary:

Prospective study that examined pre/post injury social support among male/female collegiate athletes.

Citation:

Podlog L, Dimmock J, Miller J. A review of return to sport concerns following injury rehabilitation: practitioner strategies for enhancing recovery outcomes. *Phys Ther Sport*. 2011;12:36–42.

Level of Evidence:

II

Summary:

Review of psychosocial stresses in returning athletes. Their review suggests that athletes returning to sports from injury may have difficulty with sense of competence, autonomy, and relatedness (Self-Determination Theory).

Citation:

Putukian M. The psychological response to injury in student athletes: a narrative review with a focus on mental health. *Br J Sports Med*. 2016;50:145–148.

Level of Evidence:

III

Summary:

Reviews trends in mental health concerns postinjury and barriers for student-athletes in seeking care, plus the importance of educating medical staff to recognize mental health concerns, including through preparticipation screening, and referring to mental health resources.

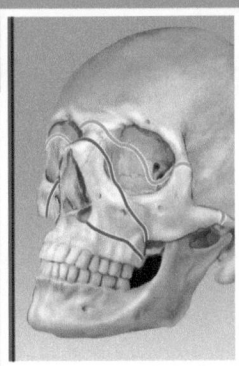

25

Sports Nutrition

Jessica L. Buschmann, Jackie Buell

Proper nutrition is often an undervalued facet of athletic competition. However, in recent years sports nutrition has gained popularity and has secured recognition as a key piece of the training regimen. Within the past decade there has been a notable increase in sports nutrition original research publications. It is undoubtedly an emerging area of science and practice that continues to thrive and progress. Proper fueling techniques equip an athlete with adequate energy to train and compete, enhance recovery post workout, manage optimal body composition, prevent and/or facilitate injury healing, strengthen the immune system, and reduce or delay the onset of fatigue. Athletes interested in seeking an individualized nutrition plan are encouraged to seek a Board Certified Specialist in Sports Dietetics (RDN, CSSD) by visiting the Sports, Cardiovascular, and Wellness Nutrition Practice Group (SCAN) website: http://www.scandpg.org/search-rd/.[1]

ENERGY BALANCE

Energy balance is the primary nutritional consideration for athletes' health and performance, especially for those trying to manipulate body weight (BW) and/or composition. Losing BW requires an athlete to eat fewer calories than expended, while gaining weight requires a small overconsumption of calories. Intentional energy imbalance should be within 300 to 500 calories of the energy needs to avoid losing lean mass in weight loss programs[2] or gaining fat in weight gain programs (unless the athlete is indifferent to the composition of the weight gain). Getting the energy balance fine-tuned to help the athlete reach performance and body goals is likely the trickiest piece of nutritional counseling.[3] Equations are often used to estimate resting metabolic rate, and then are adjusted for the amount of physical activity.[4] When using generic values, the growth status, body size, and volume and intensity of training will influence the predicted energy needs. In general, female athletes of an average body size will need between 2000 and 2400 calories per day. Growing male athletes may need upwards of 3500 to 4500 calories, while average size adult males (such as collegiate athletes) may be more reasonable at 3200 to 3600 calories. The current paradigm used to look at energy balance in athletes is the energy availability (EA) equation, which requires the practitioner to know both the body composition and the energy expenditure of exercise.[5] The ideal EA for athletes is greater than 45 kcal/kg lean mass while less than 30 is currently the definition of inadequate EA.[2] Low EA is the likely genesis of the Female Athlete Triad[6] and is now part of a larger energy insufficiency paradigm, coined "relative energy deficiency in sport" (RED-s).[2] Again, there are a lot of factors to consider in the estimation of energy needs, and this is a good space for a sports dietitian to help your practice.

MACRONUTRIENTS: CARBOHYDRATE, PROTEIN, AND FAT

The macronutrient profile of the performance diet should also match the athlete's sport, position or event, and the desired body changes. Prolonged high-intensity exercise requires carbohydrate (CHO) as the primary fuel for muscle contraction, and glycogen is the storage form of CHO in the muscle.[4] Athletes who require "high gear" should consume a diet adequate in CHO to keep muscle glycogen reserves maximized in preparation for performance.[2] The literature also suggests that CHO adequacy will support the immune system and help athletes avoid overtraining syndrome.[3] CHO needs can vary widely by sport, intensity, and volume of exercise (Table 25.1). Dairy products, fruits, and grains are the primary CHO sources for the training diet.

The defined protein needs for athletes has steadily increased with additional research, and current recommendations may be justified as high as 2.2 g/kg BW to optimize lean mass accretion in male resistance-trained athletes.[7] Most athletes would benefit from a protein intake in the range of 1.2 to 1.7 g/kg BW.[3] While it is suggested in the literature that males need more protein than females, there is no demonstrated harm for slight overconsumption of protein for an athlete with healthy liver and kidneys, and the extra protein may benefit body composition.[8] Optimizing protein intake is important to ensure muscle recovery and training adaptations as well as hormonal health. Meats, dairy, and beans are among the good protein sources for the training diet.

How much fat to feed athletes is a source of constant contention among practitioners, and is typically expressed as a percentage of calories in the training diet. Within an eating pattern where all food groups are included, most sports nutrition guidelines agree that 20% to 35% of the calories should come from a variety of fat-containing foods for good health and muscle performance.[3] Athletes restricting CHO as part of a well-formulated ketogenic or metabolic optimizing program will likely consume a much higher amount of dietary fat.[10] Fats have long been held as the culprit in heart disease and obesity, and this has led to fear of consuming fats. Athletes need to understand

TABLE 25.1	Macronutrient Needs for Athletes			
	Endurance	**Strength**	**High Intensity**	**Recreational**
CHO needs (g/kg/day)	6–12	3–7	5–7	3–5
Protein needs (g/kg/day)	1.2–1.7	1.6–2.4	1.4–2.2	1.2–1.7
Special population concerns	Bone health with low EA Iron status	Third-party approval of PES if used	Pre-event and recovery fueling important	Over-fueling leads to weight gain

Endurance: Sports or events performed at submaximal effort over longer periods of time.
Strength: Athletes trying to increase lean mass and strength in a periodized program.
High Intensity: Sports that require multiple bursts of high-intensity performance (most team sports).
Recreational: Usual workout is less than 1 hour once per day, and performance not a priority.
CHO, carbohydrate; *EA*, energy availability; *PES*, performance-enhancing supplements.
Values have been adapted from references 9, 27, and 29 position statements.

that periods of low intensity exercise rely on fat oxidation[4] and the intramuscular triglyceride (IMTG) pool is an important source of muscle energy.[11] Foods such as oils, nuts/seeds, avocados, and salad dressings should be included in a balanced diet.

Appropriate to age, the practitioner should remember to query the athlete on the nonessential macronutrient: alcohol. Athletes often use alcohol for relaxation and social enjoyment, and alcohol can decrease performance as well as negatively impact body composition and increase calorie intake. Alcohol after exercise also impedes glycogen recovery.[12] The intentional macronutrient composition of the athlete's diet can make or break their performance and health goals. Table 25.1 provides the current sports nutrition macronutrient guidelines adjusted for the type of sport.

HYDRATION

Adequate hydration practices are critical for optimal performance and safety standards for athletes. Water makes up approximately 70% of tissue—including muscle tissue—within the body. Adequate hydration helps maintain countless functions within the human body, including food absorption, digestion, transporting nutrients, body temperature regulation, joint lubrication, waste removal, and the protection of organs. The hydration needs of athletes vary greatly based on individual preference, sweat rate, acclimation to the environment, characteristics of the sport, and the duration and intensity of exercise.[13] Three common concerns surrounding hydration status include dehydration, exercise-associated hyponatremia (EAH), and exercise associated skeletal muscle cramps (EAMC). If athletes drink when thirsty, have access to free clean water, and implement a hydration plan, he or she should be able to maintain a euhydrated state.[13,14]

Hydration Considerations

Many athletes struggle with under-hydrating when preparing for or participating in competitions. A key consequence of dehydration is an increase in the body's core temperature during physical activity, causing impaired skin blood flow and altered sweat responses. Body temperature has the ability to rise 0.15°C to 0.20°C for every 1% weight lost secondary to sweating during physical activity.[13] Early signs of dehydration include thirst, general discomfort and complaints; more severe signs soon follow, including flushed skin, cramps, dizziness, headache, vomiting, nausea,

heat sensations on the head or neck, chills, decreased performance, and dyspnea.

Conversely, the risk for overhydration should not be underestimated. EAH is commonly observed in recreational or novice athletes participating in endurance events such as half marathons, sprint triathlons, and military training events. EAH commonly stems from overconsumption of water or other hypotonic beverages in events lasting more than 4 hours. EAH is defined by a blood sodium concentration below the normal reference range, which for most laboratories is a value below 135 mmol/L.[15] Signs and symptoms of EAH may occur during or up to 24 hours after physical activity and may include vomiting, headache, confusion, delirium, seizures, respiratory distress, and loss of consciousness. Without immediate medical attention, EAH can result in severe consequences, including death.

Despite the commonality of muscle cramping with exercise, etiology is often multifactorial and overall is not well understood. Despite popular belief, dehydration and electrolyte imbalances are not evidence-based causes of EAMC.[16–18] Strong mounting evidence shows that EAMC is likely linked to a neuromuscular control abnormality and muscle fatigue. Athletes prone to cramping are advised to focus on sound nutrition principles, regular stretching routines, appropriate hydration, and the prevention of muscle damage by tapering and maintaining proper conditioning.

Monitoring Hydration

Hydration status can be monitored in several ways, such as observing weight changes pre/post exercise, subjective feelings, urine color, and thirst sensation. Studies show maintaining a hydration schedule versus ad libitum drinking helps maintain and/or improve performance. However, it is advisable for athletes to listen to their bodies and adjust the plan if needed, particularly if an individual experiences significant weight fluctuations during exercise.[14] If an athlete has historic concern for maintaining weight during exercise, thirst alone may not be enough to promote a euhydrated state.[19] Current guidelines suggest limiting loss of fluids to less than 2% of total BW compared to their precompetition weight. Athletes with an observed fluid loss greater than 2% may experience impaired cognitive function and exercise performance, especially in hot weather.[13,14] Despite this recommendation, a recent study observed that ultra-endurance runners with greater than 3% weight loss did not experience an adverse effect during their performance.[20] In addition, athletes with a high sweat rate and elevated sweat sodium concentration ("salty sweater") present a greater risk for developing muscle cramps secondary to electrolyte imbalances and hypohydration.[14] Athletes not acclimatized to heat and the surrounding environment are particularly susceptible.[21] Therefore a calculated sweat rate for athletes who have challenges with hydration, have exercise-associated muscle cramps, or who perform at an elite level is encouraged. While there is weak evidence to support formal recommendations, Table 25.2 offers suggestions for the timing of fluid intake before, during, and after exercise.

VITAMINS AND MINERALS

Many athletes chose to take a "more is better" approach to supplementation versus ensuring consumption of a diet rich in a variety of wholesome, natural food. It is well recognized that diets low in certain vitamins and minerals may lead to health and performance side effects. However, athletes who consume above the tolerable upper intake level limit may also result in undesired adverse reactions. Athletes are therefore encouraged to focus on consuming adequate amounts of vitamins and minerals, which is ideal for absorption and metabolic functions throughout the body.

Iron

Iron plays a critical role in helping athletes achieve peak performance, namely in terms of aerobic endurance and muscular function. Iron is responsible for oxygen transport, energy metabolism, erythropoiesis (red blood cell production), immune system maintenance, and thyroid hormone function.[4] Hemoglobin and myoglobin bind oxygen by means of the porphyrin ring of heme.[22] Hemoglobin in red blood cells carries oxygen to the exercising skeletal muscles, whereas myoglobin is responsible for oxygen transfer from erythrocytes to muscle cells—more specifically, the mitochondria. Within the mitochondria, iron is a part of the cytochrome system for oxidative phosphorylation, along with other oxidative enzymes responsible for the generation of energy available to the body.[4] Therefore an athlete with iron deficiency will experience reduced endurance capacity secondary to impaired ATP production.[22] Low iron stores can result from insufficient consumption of iron-rich food sources, periods of rapid growth, training at high altitudes, menstrual blood loss, foot-strike hemolysis, blood donation, or injury.[23] Athletes at the greatest risk for

developing low iron levels include females, distance runners, and plant-based athletes.

Dietary sources of iron vary based on type. Heme iron is found in animal sources including red meat, pork, seafood, and dark cuts of poultry. Nonheme iron sources are plant-based and are not absorbed as readily compared to their heme iron counterparts. The absorption of heme iron is enhanced when consumed alongside a vitamin C source such as dark green leafy vegetables, peppers, broccoli, melons, tomatoes, berries, and citrus fruits. Conversely, several food items are known to lead to impaired absorption of iron including calcium-enriched products, oxalates (spinach, beets, nuts, fresh herbs), polyphenols (black tea, coffee, cocoa, berries), and phytates (soy protein, fiber, lentils, whole grains). If an athlete intends to ingest a food item containing one of the above, it is recommended to delay consumption of an iron-rich food item for 2 hours.[24]

Calcium

Calcium is an important mineral required for bone health including growth, maintenance, repair, and structure. In addition, calcium is also required for muscle contraction, nerve transmission, and blood clotting. Deficiency can lead to weak bones, increased risk for fracture or stress fracture, and blood pressure disturbances. Dietary sources of calcium include dairy products, leafy green vegetables (when cooked), fortified food items (juice, cereal), alternative milks (soy, almond), and legumes. Leafy greens can be cooked (typically blanched) in order to reduce the amount of oxalate in the vegetable, therefore improving the delivery potential for calcium to the body.

Vitamin D

Vitamin D has a significant impact on maintenance of adequate bone density, muscle strength, immune system function, possession of antiinflammatory properties, and hormonal regulation. Vitamin D2 is found in some plants consumed in the diet; it is produced commercially by the irradiation of yeast, and is fortified in some food products. Vitamin D3 (the active form) is manufactured in the skin in response to ultraviolet B (UBV) rays from sunlight; additionally, dietary or animal sources, such as deep sea fatty fish, egg yolks, or liver, also can provide this vitamin. Supplements of Vitamin D3 also may be taken when needed for plant-based athletes given food sources that are animal based.

Another potential benefit of vitamin D is linked to its potential antiinflammatory properties. Intense exercise, overtraining, and

TABLE 25.2	Hydration Timing Techniques			
Exercise	Fluid Goals	Timing	Additional Goals
Pre-exercise	17–20 ounces / 7–10 ounces	2–3 h pre-exercise / 10–20 min pre-exercise	• Have a little salt with meal or snack to promote water retention
During exercise	7–10 ounces	Every 10–20 min during activity if able or tolerated	• Be mindful of acceptable individual preferences and sweat rates • Sweat rates vary amongst athletes • Find a sports drink palatable to the athlete
Postexercise	19–23 ounces fluid per pound lost	After exercise; ideally within 2 h post exercise	• Replace fluid losses completely especially if going into another exercise session • Discourage alcohol intake

Values adapted from References 13 and 14.

other sports-related injuries are known to elevate levels of pro-inflammatory cytokines. Vitamin D has been shown to reduce the production of these cytokines while increasing the production of antiinflammatory cytokines.[25] This suggests that an adequate supply of vitamin D may reduce inflammation and muscle soreness, and promote quicker recovery after intense exercise. Athletes with a history of stress fracture, bone or joint injury, signs of overtraining, muscle pain or weakness, and a lifestyle involving low exposure to UVB rays may benefit from lab work to determine if an individualized vitamin D supplementation protocol is required.[21]

NUTRIENT TIMING

Proper nutrient timing should be a fundamental part of an athlete's fueling plan. A well-balanced nutrition plan should not only contribute to performance enhancement, but also to an athlete's psychological and gastrointestinal comfort. Avoidance of dehydration, electrolyte imbalances, glycogen depletion, hypoglycemia, and acid-base disturbances are also notable considerations.[32] Nutrient timing and strategies vary greatly based on duration of activity, type of sport, and time between preceding or upcoming events. Food availability and an athlete's personal food preferences are also important considerations. Table 25.3

provides basic strategies to help an athlete fuel before, during, and after exercise.

SPORTS SUPPLEMENTATION

Many athletes feel the need to use dietary supplements. It is important to emphasize to an athlete that these "Performance Enhancing Supplements" (PES) are meant to *supplement* a strong training diet. Dietary supplements are poorly regulated and athletes consuming tainted products are at risk for disqualification regardless of how the illegal ingredient got into their body.[33] This must be taught and emphasized to high-level athletes from a young age to avoid mishaps leading to the stripping of a coveted championship and a tarnished reputation. The National Collegiate Athletic Association, International Olympic Committee (IOC), and other sports organizations and federations usually provide a published list of banned substances with a championship drug testing process to ensure a level playing field. Researching the safety, purity, and efficacy of products reveals a complex and daunting process.[33] Table 25.4 provides current commonly consumed PES with the purported benefits and usual protocols. This information is provided for professional guidance, not to encourage use.

For a complete list of references, go to ExpertConsult.com.

TABLE 25.3   Nutrient Timing Strategies

Timing Recommendations	Goals

Pre-exercise
>60 min before activity
	• Timing, amount and type of food and drink should match the practical needs of the event and the individual preferences
	• Foods higher in fat, protein, or fiber may cause gastrointestinal issues during activity
	• Carbohydrate goals:
	  • Light: low intensity or skilled-based activity
	    • 3–5 g/kg/day
	  • Moderate: 1 h exercise program per day
	    • Carbohydrate 5–7 g/kg/day
	  • High: 1–3 h/day moderate/high intensity
	    • 6–10 g/kg/day
	  • Very high: extreme >4–5 h/day moderate/high intensity
	    • 8–12 g/kg/day

During exercise	• *Brief:* <45 min
	  • Nothing needed
	• *Prolonged high intensity:* 45–75 min
	  • Small amounts if needed per individual preference
	• *Endurance:* 1–2.5 h
	  • 30–60 g carbohydrate
	  • Example: 8 oz. sports drink
	  • Example: (3) Clif Shot Bloks
	• *Ultra-endurance:* >2.5 h
	  • Up to 90 g of carbohydrate per hour

Post exercise
Aim for 45–60 min after activity
	• Focus on carbohydrate and protein food pairings
	  • Carbohydrate: Replenishing glycogen stores and limiting cortisol-induced muscle damage during exercise
	    • Recommendation: 1 g/kg
	  • Protein: crucial to muscle protein synthesis and repair
	    • Recommendation: 20 g of high-quality protein
	  • Meal examples:
	    • Example: 8 oz. chocolate milk with turkey sandwich (2 slices of whole grain bread & 3 oz. turkey)
	    • Example: 1 cup ready-to-eat cereal (i.e., Cheerios) with 1 cup skim milk and 1 medium banana

Values adapted from reference 27, 29, 31, and 32.

TABLE 25.4 Common Performance Enhancing Substances

Substance	Purported Benefit	Usual Dose and Timing to Event	Comments
Creatine	Increased muscle ATP allowing higher workload	3–5 g/day, not necessarily important when taken[33]	Muscle will hold more water and increase weight of athlete
Nitrates (e.g., beetroot juice)	Precursor to nitric oxide (vasodilator) thus improving tissue oxygenation and metabolism	0.1 mmol/kg/day or 5–6 mmol/day over 5–6 days or more[34]	Complex pathway of conversion to nitric oxide in the body
Beta alanine	Precursor to muscle carnosine thus improves muscle buffering allowing higher workload	Small doses multiple times per day, 4–6 g/day in total for at least 4 weeks[7]	May cause tingling or paresthesia (thought to be harmless)
Caffeine	Decreases perception of fatigue centrally, or peripheral mechanism	3–6 mg/kg 1 h prior to event 1–2 mg/kg during later endurance tasks[33]	
Pre-workouts	Help athlete increase arousal	No set research numbers	Ensure third-party verification to help avoid illegal ingredients such as stimulants
Mass gainers	Help athlete gain lean mass	No set research numbers	Consider the extra calories in overall diet; ensure third-party verification to help avoid illegal ingredients such as anabolic agents

SELECTED READINGS

Citation:

American College of Sports M, Sawka MN, Burke LM, et al. American College of Sports Medicine position stand. Exercise and fluid replacement. *Med Sci Sports Exerc.* 2007;39(2):377–390.

Level of Evidence:

Various topics defined by position statement

Summary:

The American College of Sports Medicine on exercise and fluid replacement for athletes provides a review of current recommendations and strategies to optimize fluid-replacement practices of athletes.

Citation:

Thomas DT, Erdman KA, Burke LM. Position of the Academy of Nutrition and Dietetics, Dietitians of Canada, and the American College of Sports Medicine: Nutrition and Athletic Performance. *J Acad Nutr Diet.* 2016;116(3):501–528.

Level of Evidence:

Various topics defined by position statement

Summary:

The Academy of Nutrition and Dietetics, Dietitians of Canada, and the American College of Sports Medicine merged to create a Position Statement regarding Nutrition and Athletic Performance. These organizations provide guidelines for the appropriate type, amount, and timing of intake of food, fluids, and supplements to promote optimal health and performance across different scenarios of training and competitive sport.

Citation:

Buell JL, Franks R, Ransone J, et al. National Athletic Trainers' Association. National athletic trainers' association position statement: evaluation of dietary supplements for performance nutrition. *J Athl Train.* 2013;48(1).

Level of Evidence:

Various topics defined by position statement

Summary:

The National Athletic Trainer's Position Statement on the evaluation of dietary supplements for performance nutrition promoting a "food-first" philosophy to support health and performance; to understand federal and sport governing body rules and regulations regarding dietary supplements and banned substances; and to become familiar with reliable resources for evaluating the safety, purity, and efficacy of dietary supplements.

Citation:

Meeusen R, Duclos M, Foster C, et al. Prevention, diagnosis, and treatment of the overtraining syndrome: joint consensus statement of the European College of Sport Science and the American College of Sports Medicine. *Med Sci Sports Exerc.* 2013;45(1):186–205.

Level of Evidence:

Various topics defined by position statement

Summary

Within this consensus statement between the American College of Sports Medicine and European College of Sport Science the current state of knowledge on overtraining syndrome (OTS) including definition, diagnosis, treatment and prevention is discussed.

Citation:

Mountjoy M, Sundgot-Borgen J, Burke L, et al. The IOC consensus statement: beyond the Female Athlete Triad–Relative Energy Deficiency in Sport (RED-S). *Br J Sports Med.* 2014;48(7):491–497.

Level of Evidence:

Various topics defined by position statement

Summary:

This Consensus Statement replaces the previous and provides guidelines to guide risk assessment, treatment, and return-to-play decisions. The IOC expert working group introduces a broader, more comprehensive term for the condition previously known as *Female Athlete Triad*. This Consensus Statement also recommends practical clinical models for the management of affected athletes. The "Sport Risk Assessment and Return to Play Model" categorizes the syndrome into three groups and translates these classifications into clinical recommendations.

Citation:
IOC consensus statement on sports nutrition 2010. *J Sports Sci.* 2011;29(suppl 1):S3–S4.

Level of Evidence:
Various topics defined by position statement

Summary:
A practical guide to eating for health and performance prepared by the Nutrition Working Group of the International Olympic Committee.

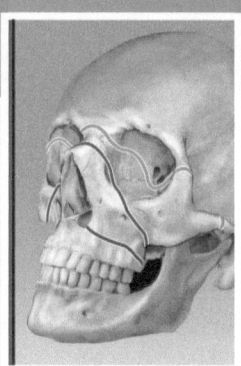

26

Doping and Ergogenic Aids

Siobhan M. Statuta, Aaron J. Vaughan, Ashley V. Austin

SPORTS PHARMACOLOGY: ERGOGENIC DRUGS IN SPORT

There is no room for second place. There is only one place in my game, and that's first place.

Vince Lombardi[1]

In this day and age, it is common for athletes to be scrutinized for using prohibited performance-enhancing drugs and methods. Our society places a high value on winning and rewards athletes who perform well. As a result, competitors are often motivated to do "whatever it takes" to perform at a higher level and thus improve in their sport. The word *ergogenic* is derived from the Greek *éaargon*, "to work," and *gennan*, "to produce"; it literally means "increasing the ability to do work." Athletes have sought ways to improve their performance for thousands of years. Athletes at the first Greek Olympics ate substances that they thought would give them a competitive advantage, including dried figs, mushrooms, large amounts of meat, and strychnine (a known poison). These ancient Greek athletes were willing to risk taking a potentially deadly substance in the hope of winning. History does repeat itself, because this trend continues today and has escalated to incomprehensible levels. The ensuing battle to weed out athletes who engage in unfair practices is a challenge to organizations that believe in the concepts of "an even playing field" and fairness in sport.

The desire to win at all costs was confirmed by a poll of Olympic athletes conducted by Mirkin[2] in the 1980s. The question was, "If you could take a pill that would guarantee you the Olympic gold medal but would kill you within a year, would you take it?" The shocking result was that more than 50% of the athletes would take the pill.

Goldman[3] subsequently conducted a modified poll in the 1990s and asked 198 aspiring Olympians, all elite athletes, two questions:

1. If you were offered a banned performance-enhancing substance that guaranteed that you would win an Olympic medal and you could not be caught, would you take it?
2. If you were guaranteed that you would not be caught, would you take a banned performance-enhancing drug that would allow you to win every competition for the next 5 years but would then cause you to die from the side effects of the substance?

Of 198 athletes, 195 answered yes to the first question; in response to the second question, more than 50% of the athletes said they would take the substance.

The results of these two polls reveal that a high percentage of athletes are willing to use substances that are potentially fatal if they believe that those substances will help them win. Athletes want to win *now* and may not consider or even be concerned about the future consequences of taking a performance-enhancing substance.

Testosterone: Historical Perspectives

In the 1950s it was discovered that Olympic weight lifters were gaining immense strength by injecting testosterone, a male hormone. An American physician, John Bosley Ziegler, saw the potential benefits, and in an effort to minimize the adverse androgenic effects that the weight lifters were experiencing, he developed the derivative methandrostenolone.[4] Although it was initially considered a superior ergogenic drug compared with testosterone, it had its own adverse effects related to its potent androgenic properties. Since then many scientists have attempted and failed to develop a pure anabolic agent without androgenic features. To underscore the important point that derivatives of testosterone have anabolic and androgenic properties, we categorize all ergogenic derivatives of testosterone in this chapter as anabolic-androgenic steroids (AASs). Hundreds of ergogenic variants of testosterone are now being used by athletes.

One of the first scientists to promote the ergogenic properties of testosterone was the prominent French physiologist Brown-Séquard.[5] Although largely remembered in the medical world today for his description of a spinal cord syndrome, Brown-Séquard played an important role in the history of AASs. In June 1889, at the Société de Biologie meeting in Paris, the 72-year-old Brown-Séquard announced that he had found a "rejuvenating compound" that had reversed many of his physical and mental ailments related to aging. He reported that he had injected himself with a liquid extract made from the testicles of dogs and guinea pigs and that these injections had dramatically increased his strength, improved his mental acumen, relieved his constipation, and increased the arc of his urinary stream. Brown-Séquard's findings were viewed with disdain, yet he had made an important discovery with enormous implications for the medical and athletic worlds. Brown-Séquard's discovery of the positive properties of the testicular extract was based on the earlier work of Berthold, who had proposed that the implantation of testicles in the abdomen of roosters reversed the effects of castration.[6]

Scientists continued the work of these two scientists, and several important discoveries were made that contributed to a better understanding of the properties of the testicular hormone. The Dutch scientist David and his colleagues first isolated testosterone in 1935.[7] Soon thereafter, German scientists published an article describing the synthesis of testosterone from cholesterol.[8] Subsequently, physicians and veterinarians started using testosterone and its intermediaries clinically,[9] and testosterone was first used medically in humans to help chronically ill patients recover muscle mass.[10] Testosterone was found to have positive effects on almost every organ of the body, and 60 years after Brown-Séquard announced his discovery, testosterone was promoted once again as a rejuvenation compound. In 1939 Boje[10] suggested that male sex hormones might improve athletic performance. In 1941, after a racehorse dramatically improved its performance following injections of testosterone,[11] human competitors who were looking for an advantage during competition started experimenting with testosterone use.[12]

The first systematic use of testosterone in sports was by Soviet Olympic athletes in the 1950s; by the 1960s, use of AASs was increasingly prevalent.[13] During that time, no sanctions against the use of ergogenic drugs existed, and many athletes believed that it was necessary to use drugs to be able to remain competitive. By the 1968 Olympics, the use of AASs was pervasive across various disciplines of sport, including both strength and aerobic events. New drugs claiming to have superior anabolic qualities were being marketed openly, and male athletes in large numbers from other sports such as American football soon began taking AASs either knowingly or allegedly as "vitamins."[14] It was estimated that 40% to 90% of professional football players were using AASs by the 1980s,[15] and soon thereafter, college football players followed suit.[15]

Female athletes began experimenting with the drugs to improve their own performance abilities. Before long, it was discovered that women who took AASs experienced increased muscular strength. In addition, the androgenic properties of AASs also induced masculinizing effects, including deepening of the voice, amplification of body hair, loss of breast tissue, and clitoral enlargement. The masculinization of female athletes from the Soviet Bloc nations was so dramatic that gender tests and chromosomal analyses were performed at the 1967 European Championships to ensure that male athletes were not masquerading as female athletes.

Women in Western nations have been suspected of using ergogenic drugs. Florence Griffith Joyner became one of the most famous athletes in the world when she reappeared on the world stage after coming out of semiretirement and achieved tremendous success at the 1988 Olympic Games. Joyner had progressed from a good runner to a world champion whose record in the 100-m run was unsurpassed for 10 years. Her muscular physique, combined with her newfound athletic success, led to speculation that her athletic superiority was a result of the use of performance-enhancing drugs—a charge she vehemently denied.[16] Joyner instead insisted that her athletic prowess was the result of a relentless training program supervised by her husband, Olympian Al Joyner. When Florence Griffith Joyner died in her sleep at the young age of 38 years, speculation that her death may have been related to adverse effects from taking ergogenic drugs was rampant. To date, it has not been verified that Joyner used ergogenic aids or that her death was related to the use of drugs, and her death has been attributed to a seizure.

Many young athletes believe that the use of ergogenic drugs is a worthwhile risk. An eye-opening study by Buckley and colleagues[17] revealed that 6.6% of high school seniors had, at some point, used anabolic steroids. Of these, 30% of users were nonathletes using ergogenic drugs to improve their appearance rather than their athletic performance. Evidence indicates that ergogenic drug abuse commences in middle school. The 2013 survey by the Partnership for Drug-Free Kids revealed that 11% of high school teens had tried synthetic human growth hormone (GH) at least once without a prescription—an increase of 5% in just 1 year![18] Furthermore, Yesalis and Bahrke[19] found that the percentage of 14- to 18-year-old *girls* using anabolic steroids had almost doubled in 7 years, as many considered the use an effective means of obtaining college athletic scholarships.[20]

When a Danish cyclist died at the 1960 Olympics after ingesting a combination of nicotinic acid and amphetamines, concerns were raised regarding both fairness and safety, and a plan of action to address these issues was formulated. One of the first steps was to define the problem, and in 1963, the Council of Europe established a definition of doping as "the administration or use of substances in any form alien to the body or of physiologic substances in abnormal amounts and with abnormal methods by healthy persons with the exclusive aim of attaining an artificial and unfair increase in performance in competition."[18]

Anabolic-Androgenic Steroids
Physiologic Considerations

The three main steroids in the human body are androgens, estrogens, and corticosteroids. The androgens are responsible for the development of male characteristics, whereas the estrogens express female characteristics. Corticosteroids—both glucocorticoids and mineralocorticoids—are responsible for a wide variety of essential body functions involving the immune, cardiovascular, metabolic, and hemostatic systems.

Females produce small amounts of androgens in the ovary and adrenal gland, and males produce small amounts of estrogen, but it is the production of androgens that makes males "masculine" and the production of estrogen that makes females "feminine." The most abundant androgen in males is testosterone, which is produced primarily in the testes. In many target cells of the body, testosterone is reduced at the 5α position to dihydrotestosterone, which serves as the intracellular mediator of the actions of testosterone.[21] Dihydrotestosterone exhibits a greater affinity for androgen receptors compared with testosterone and is thus the more stable and potent androgen. Precursors in the metabolic pathway to testosterone, dehydroepiandrosterone (DHEA) and androstenedione, bind less strongly to the androgen receptors and are known as weak androgens. Other weak androgens that are metabolites of testosterone include etiocholanolone and androsterone. Although they are weak, these androgens can induce significant anabolic effects.

In males, testosterone production peaks at three distinct phases of life. The first peak occurs during the fetal period, in the second trimester, and directs male fetal development. Subsequently, a smaller surge occurs during the first year of life and the largest surge occurs during puberty, resulting in several visible changes. Androgens cause laryngeal enlargement, thus deepening the voice; genital maturity; spermatogenesis in the testicles; and bone and muscle growth, with a relative decrease in body fat. The skin becomes thicker and oilier, and body hair on the face and in the axillae and groin grows to adult levels.

On the cellular level, testosterone, or its more active metabolite, dihydrotestosterone, works by binding to an intracellular androgen receptor in the cytoplasm. The steroid–androgen receptor complex is transported to the nucleus, where it attaches to a specific hormone regulatory complex on nuclear chromosomes. Here the complex stimulates the synthesis of specific ribonucleic acids and proteins. The ribonucleic acid compounds are transported through the bloodstream to act on target organs and stimulate spermatogenesis, effect sexual differentiation, and increase protein synthesis in muscle tissues. The androgenic message is received and processed in all organs that have androgenic receptors.

The metabolism of testosterone and its products occurs rapidly in the liver. Oral testosterone is absorbed immediately and metabolized so rapidly that it becomes ineffective. Scientists have therefore developed methods of altering the basic structure of the molecule to delay its metabolism and increase its half-life in the plasma. Alkylation at the 17α position with a methyl or ethyl group allows oral agents to be degraded slowly. Similarly, esterification of the 17β position allows parenteral agents to resist degradation. Testosterone esters, such as cypionate and enanthate esters, are more potent than testosterone. These compounds must be injected intramuscularly, usually at 1- to 3-week intervals. Newer preparations of testosterone can be administered transdermally.[22] These preparations were originally applied to the scrotum, but new transdermal patches and creams can be applied to other parts of the body.

In addition to promoting muscle development, androgens cause the skin to become unusually oily, which can lead to acne, increase body hair, and induce male pattern baldness, with hairline recession and thinning and loss of central scalp hair. The skin effects are crucial clues for physicians who suspect anabolic steroid use. The extent of the acne can be profound, and the back is often significantly affected. Lastly, the distinctive odor caused by the effects of anabolic steroids on the sebaceous glands is inimitable.

Athletic Performance Considerations

Despite the perceptions of athletes, scientific data regarding the effects of anabolic steroids on athletic performance are varied. When used at therapeutic doses, neither strength nor performance gains are expected, because in a homeostatic state, hormonal levels are maintained within a narrow window. After a therapeutic dose of a hormone is administered, the body halts its own endogenous hormone production to maintain constant levels. Athletes who are cognizant of this fact have taken doses 50 to 100 times the therapeutic dose, which shuts down endogenous production of AASs. But does taking such high doses improve athletic performance?

In the world of athletics, several popular theories foster steroid abuse. The first theory is that "In combination with training, AASs increase lean body mass and decrease body fat." Early studies that evaluated this theory showed equivocal results.[23] More recent studies have shown an increase in body weight and lean body mass but no significant decrease in the percentage of body fat.[24]

Another theory suggests that "AASs increase muscle strength." Early studies in which mostly low-dose AASs were evaluated were inconclusive.[25] Later, in 1996, Bhasin and colleagues[26] studied the effect of supraphysiologic doses of testosterone on healthy men; this was the first prospective randomized study that looked at the effect of "super dosing" of AASs. In this study of 43 healthy men, the group that received steroids had definite increases in strength and muscle size compared with the placebo group. Notably, no significant adverse effects were observed in the steroid group; however, the study had limitations, including a short term (6 weeks) and inadequate follow-up. However, this study was the first to provide scientific evidence for the theory that athletes believed for decades—that steroids do work, especially at the amplified doses that are popular in athletics. Other investigations have shown distinct advantages for muscle, with both expansion in cross-sectional diameter and proliferation of new fibers. The upper regions of the body are more susceptible to gains from AASs because of the relatively larger number of androgen receptors in these areas. AASs, however, do not appear to improve athletic endurance.[24]

AASs work on several different levels in the body. They stimulate not only protein synthesis but also the production of GH, a potent ergogenic agent. Furthermore, AASs display some anticatabolic features because they delay the effects of cortisol, a stress hormone. Cortisol is released in response to physical and psychological stress and causes protein degradation and muscle atrophy.[27] Testosterone slows this catabolism by displacing the corticosteroids from receptor sites.[28] Additionally, AASs may increase oxygen uptake, cardiac output, and stroke volume.[29] They are thought to improve athletic performance by increasing aggressive behaviors; however, the data on the relationship between testosterone levels and aggressive behavior remain inconclusive.[30,31]

Adverse Effects

The use of anabolic steroids may result in several less than desirable side effects. Oily skin, acne, small testicles, gynecomastia, and changes in hair patterns are the most common. Small doses of androgens increase sebaceous gland secretions, leading to the changes in the skin and the development of acne.[32] Enlargement of the male breast (gynecomastia) is characterized by the presence of firm glandular tissue and is usually associated with an increased production of estrogens or decreased levels of androgens. The specific pathophysiology of gynecomastia in men taking AASs remains unclear. One theory suggests that the body homeostatically shuts down the production of endogenous androgens. Once the user stops using AASs, an increase occurs in the relative level of estrogens, leading to the development of breast tissue. Gynecomastia is irreversible once levels of androgens return to normal. A means of offsetting the estrogen-related adverse effects of AASs is to take an antiestrogenic drug such as clomiphene citrate (Clomid). Clomid blocks the effects of increased estrogen in persons using AASs by binding and thus blocking estrogen receptors.

Small testicles often also develop in men who use AASs. The testicles atrophy and shrink, which is a response to the homeostatic effect triggered by high exogenous AASs. Often the testicles remain smaller after discontinuation of the AASs. Other adverse effects on the male reproductive system include oligospermia (a decreased number of sperm) and azoospermia (the absence of sperm).[33] Moreover, taking exogenous AASs decreases not only levels of endogenous testosterone but also the circulation of follicle-stimulating hormone and luteinizing hormone, which can lead to male infertility. Testosterone-dependent prostate enlargement and accelerated growth of prostate cancer have been documented.[34] Women who take AASs experience virilization effects, including deepening of the voice, an increased amount of body hair, loss of breast tissue, and enlargement of the clitoris. Irregularities in the menstrual cycle as well as infertility or early menopause may result, and many of these adverse effects in women are irreversible.[35]

Musculoskeletal. The musculoskeletal system may be affected adversely, especially in prepubertal athletes who take AASs. Although bone growth is stimulated immediately after the use of AASs, the growth plates of long bones may close prematurely. The resultant short stature is permanent.[36] Disproportionate changes in strength of the muscle-tendon unit (greater) than tendon strength (lesser) increases the susceptibility to tendon rupture.[37]

Cardiovascular. Numerous adverse changes occur in the heart of a person who takes AASs. Androgens are modulators of serum lipoprotein, thus increasing plasma levels of low-density lipoproteins ("bad" lipids) and decreasing levels of high-density lipoproteins ("good" lipids). Oral and synthetic AASs have more pronounced negative effects on lipid metabolism than do injectable or natural AASs.[38] An altered lipid pattern may lead to atherosclerotic heart disease. Male and female users of AASs show similar adverse changes in lipid metabolism.[39]

Animal studies have suggested that AASs may cause myocardial damage.[40] A study that investigated the relationship among resistance training, anabolic steroid use, and left ventricular function in elite bodybuilders showed concentric left ventricular hypertrophy. However, no effect on cardiac function was observed, which suggests that the heart may enlarge as a physiologic adaptation to the intensive training potentiated by use of AASs.[41] In a set of bodybuilding twins, one twin used AASs for more than 15 years whereas the other abstained. No significant difference in cardiac function was found between the twins.[42] However, noteworthy changes in cardiac function after the use of AASs have been reported in other cases, such as myocardial infarction and death in young athletes.[43] These case reports are no doubt worrisome yet do not provide scientific "proof" that the use of AASs directly leads to myocardial infarction or death. Nevertheless, cardiac pathology was evident upon postmortem examination in more than one-third of 34 persons (aged 20 to 45 years) who had used AASs and died as a result of accidents, suicides, and homicides.[44] Cardiac abnormalities may not resolve after

the use of AASs is stopped. A study of former users of AASs showed that many years after discontinuing their use, strength athletes showed persistent left ventricular hypertrophy compared with strength athletes who had not used AASs.[45]

Hepatic. Most AAS metabolism occurs in the liver, which is thus prone to liver damage. Athletes with preexisting liver dysfunction are at greatest risk for androgen-induced damage. Temporary liver disturbances are common in athletes who use oral androgens, although function appears to return to normal after discontinuation of the drugs.[46,47] Several investigators believe that AAS-induced hepatotoxicity is overstated, attributing resultant transaminitis to skeletal rather than liver damage.[48] A study of the effect of AASs on rats showed definite cellular damage to hep atocytes,[49] yet long-term studies on the effect of AASs on the liver in human subjects have not been conducted; until we have scientific data, hepatotoxicity should remain a potential concern.

Hepatotoxicity may manifest as peliosis hepatis, that is, the formation of blood-filled cysts in the liver. Enlarged liver cells block venous and lymphatic flow, producing cholestasis, necrosis, and peliosis cysts, which can rupture and may be life threatening. In contrast to most adverse effects of AASs, peliosis hepatitis does not appear to be dose related and can occur at any time after the use of AASs is started.[50] Pathogenesis is speculated to be from AAS-mediated hepatocyte hyperplasia.[51]

Last, although there is no definite evidence to support a causal relationship between hepatocellular carcinoma and steroid abuse, there have been multiple reports of the development of hepatocellular carcinoma after AAS use.[52]

Psychiatric. The most commonly associated psychiatric effect of AASs is an increase in aggressive behaviors, although only a few well-conducted prospective randomized studies confirm this observation. In fact, most studies using therapeutic doses of exogenous testosterone showed no adverse effects, and a short-term study of supratherapeutic dosing of AASs in athletes revealed no significant psychiatric effects.[53] However, some studies have reported positive effects on mood.[54] In Brown-Séquard's 19th-century study of the self-administration of testicular substrates, one of the reported positive effects was improvement in mood, which was accompanied by an enhancement of his physical stature.[5] Subsequently, benefits of AASs on mood and other psychiatric maladies were further evaluated by physicians following the advent of synthetic testosterone derivatives in the 1930s.[55,56] AASs were being researched during their use to treat a variety of conditions ranging from depression to psychoses, and although results were varied, some small studies revealed an increase in aggression, thought to be linked to other personality disorders such as antisocial, borderline, and histrionic personalities.[57]

Additional research suggests an association with AAS use and psychiatric disturbances. A study of 41 athletes using supratherapeutic doses of AASs for an average of 45 weeks revealed that 34% experienced symptoms of major mood disorders such as severe depression or mania. AAS users are also more likely to abuse alcohol, tobacco, and illicit drugs,[58] and data suggest that AAS users tend to meet criteria for substance dependence disorder more commonly than nonusers.[59]

Disorders of body image have also been reported after use of AASs. Many weight lifters who may appear muscular compared with the average athlete consider themselves small or weak. This dysmorphic disorder is similar to that of women with anorexia nervosa who, despite being much thinner than the average woman, erroneously perceive themselves as fat.

Steroid Supplements

In 1994, the US Congress passed legislation affecting all persons involved in the care of athletes—the Dietary Supplement Health and Education Act. This law permits numerous substances to be sold without prior approval from the US Food and Drug Administration (FDA) as long as they are sold as dietary supplements and not as "drugs."

The Dietary Supplement Health and Education Act also established a formal definition of a dietary supplement using several criteria. A dietary supplement is a product (other than tobacco) that is intended to enhance the diet. It bears or contains one or a combination of dietary ingredients, such as a vitamin, mineral, herb, or other botanical product. Products have included approved new drugs, certified antibiotics, or licensed biologic agents that were marketed as dietary supplements or food before approval, verification, or licensure. These products are not recommended for use as a conventional meal or diet and are labeled as a dietary supplement. Subsequent to this bill's passage, several synthetic AASs have become commercially available as dietary supplements; as such they do not have to pass the safety requirements of the FDA and are not held to strict quality control standards.[60] Claims regarding their effectiveness need not be substantiated by scientific proof as long as a disclaimer is listed on the product.

Dehydroepiandrosterone

DHEA is a naturally occurring hormone produced in the adrenal glands of the human body. Its synthetic form, isolated from soy and wild yams, is marketed as a supplement[61] and has become popular for its antiaging properties, fat-burning properties, and enhancement of muscle mass, strength, and energy. DHEA is a weak androgen, but it is the most abundant steroid in the body serving as a precursor to testosterone, estrogen, progesterone, and corticosterone. Levels are high in the prenatal period as well as in puberty, gradually decreasing as an individual ages. Some studies performed on patients older than 50 years (when DHEA levels have dropped significantly) showed beneficial results after DHEA supplementation.[62] Conversely, other studies have revealed inconsistent improvements in strength.[63]

Many athletes use DHEA for its androgenic and anticatabolic effects. With its use come some undesired effects of feminization, as DHEA is a precursor to estrogen. Athletes attempt to combat this outcome by using clomiphene citrate (Clomid), an antiestrogenic drug, while taking DHEA. Little evidence exists to support claims for DHEA, either as a potent anabolic agent or as an antiaging drug.[64,65] Furthermore, no studies of the long-term effects of taking DHEA have been published, particularly regarding the large doses used by athletes.[66]

Androstenedione

Androstenedione, originally touted as the "secret weapon of the East Germans," was first used in the 1970s, and its reputation as an effective anabolic agent encouraged worldwide use. In March 2004, the US Department of Health and Human Services announced that the FDA had asked manufacturers to stop distribution of androstenedione. By October 2004, President Bush signed into law the Anabolic Steroid Control Act, which added androstenedione to the list of banned nonprescription steroid-based drugs. Currently Major League Baseball, the National Football League, the Olympics, and the National Collegiate Athletics Association (NCAA) prohibit its use. Androstenedione received tremendous exposure in the media during the 1998 baseball season when St. Louis Cardinals slugger Mark McGwire was discovered to be using the supplement, albeit legally at the time, after which sales of androstenedione rose dramatically.[67]

Androstenedione is a potent AAS produced endogenously in the adrenal glands and gonads. In the liver, androstenedione is metabolized to testosterone. Similar to DHEA, during transformation it can be converted to testosterone and estrogen. As a result, a male athlete taking androstenedione can have elevated estrogen levels. One study observed that male subjects taking androstenedione experienced elevated estradiol levels equal to the estradiol levels seen in women during the follicular phase of the menstrual cycle, when levels are at their highest.[68] Additionally, as a testosterone precursor, it can lead to decreases in high-density lipoprotein cholesterol and enhance cardiac risk. Priapism has been described in an otherwise healthy young man using androstenedione who had no other precipitating factors; other concerns such as prostatic enlargement and cancer exist. Notably, significant ergogenic improvement after androstenedione supplementation has not been proved in the medical literature.

Doping
Historical Perspectives

The word *doping* originates from the Dutch word *dop*, an opium mixture used to enhance the racing capacity of horses. In 1967, the International Olympic Committee (IOC) published a medical code that included a list of banned drugs to "protect the health of athletes and to ensure respect for the ethical concepts implicit in Fair Play, the Olympic Spirit, and medical practice."[69] The World Anti-Doping Agency (WADA) was established from this committee in 1999. Through its affiliation with various international, national, and private governing bodies, WADA has helped to establish strategies to tackle organized doping schemes, trafficking, and detection. It also publishes an annual listing of banned substances—an invaluable resource for athletes and medical providers.[70]

Erythropoietin

WADA defines blood doping as "the misuse of certain techniques and/or substances to increase one's red blood cell mass."[70] Bonsdorff and Jalavisto[71] were the first to discover and name the blood-stimulating hormone now commonly referred to as erythropoietin (EPO). Scientists later discovered its molecular structure, which served as a base for the development of recombinant human EPO (rhEPO). The first experiments with enhanced red blood cell mass and exercise showed that blood transfusion decreases submaximal heart rate for several weeks, predicting performance enhancement.[72] Subsequent studies replicated the performance-enhancing effects of transfusion, including those of Berglund and Ekblom who showed a 17% increase in the time to exhaustion among male athletes after 6 weeks of EPO administration.[73,74] The IOC eventually banned blood transfusion for the 1988 Olympics.[75] In 1990, EPO was added to the IOC list of prohibited substances, and it has been on WADA's prohibited list since the organization's inception.

Mechanism of Action

Essential to athleticism and performance is how well trained or "conditioned" the athlete is. Basic physiology reminds us that muscle cells require oxygen to function optimally and that oxygen is transported throughout the body by erythrocytes. EPO is a hormone that stimulates the production of these erythrocytes in the range of 2.5×10^{11} erythrocytes per day, each of which has a life span of approximately 120 days.

Nearly 90% of EPO is produced in the peritubular renal cells, with the remainder being produced in the liver and brain. EPO production is triggered in response to hypoxia and stimulates an increase in erythrocyte production, leading to enhanced tissue oxygenation. Both epoetins and their synthetic analogues (erythropoiesis stimulating agents, or ESAs) have the ability to induce erythropoiesis by binding to EPO receptors on target cells.

Testing

WADA publishes an annual summary of prohibited substances and doping methods, the most recent having been released on January 1, 2017.[76] This list is commonly referred to as the Prohibited List, comprising a total of 10 different classes of banned substances (S0–S9), three different groups of prohibited methods (M1–M3), and two classes of drugs (P1 and P2) that are banned from selected sports only. The traceability of EPO abuse has been a complex issue, laborious and time-consuming, and frequently challenged by athletes. Drug testing in athletes is riddled with many hurdles, including cost. The inception of new ergogenic aids and novel masking agents has made the detection of illegal doping a challenge.[77] Allocation of innumerable research resources has been invested in improving analytical approaches as well as eliminating technical issues in detection. Given the negative ramifications of a positive drug test, it is critically important that the chain of custody be maintained and that testing protocols be updated and followed precisely to ensure the accuracy of sampling.

Detection of rhEPO includes both direct detection of recombinant isoforms and indirect approaches via the measurement of markers of enhanced erythropoiesis.[78] In the 1990s, the International Cycling Union introduced random blood tests to detect abnormalities in biologic parameters as a screening test for subsequent urinary detection of rhEPO. Although this technique was successful in preventing heavy use of rhEPO, it proved unable to discriminate against athletes with naturally elevated blood parameters. Individual reference ranges were introduced in 2007 in the form of "biologic transport," or the method of tracking each athlete's own blood numbers, known as the Athlete Biologic Passport hematologic evaluation. Markers that are currently tracked include hematocrit, hemoglobin, red blood cell count, reticulocyte percentage, reticulocyte number, mean corpuscular volume, mean corpuscular hemoglobin, and mean corpuscular

hemoglobin concentration, among others. Blood results are then processed by a model that identifies any abnormal blood parameters as compared with the athlete's individual baseline. These operating guidelines, in accordance with the WADA code, were implemented in 2009.

Newer generations of these models have since been employed to include advances in electrophoresis techniques—isoelectric separation, Western blot analysis, antibody detection, and mass spectrometry—to help distinguish between physiologic EPO versus rhEPO. Although there is still a lack of total understanding, research continues in an attempt to further develop new testing methods, decrease false positives, and improve the sensitivity of the current testing measures. What is clear is that the combination of an athlete's biologic passport (based on individual profiling) and urine tests targeting rhEPO has undoubtedly made it more challenging for athletes to compete illegally.[79]

Side Effects

To some athletes, the benefits of using performance-enhancing agents clearly outweigh any risk. EPO and its synthetic analogues are known to increase red blood cell mass. Physiologic benefits include normalization of cardiac output and enhanced immune function, leading to improved exercise tolerance, reduced fatigue, and subjective improved quality of life. EPO excess has been associated with hazardous adverse effects, including increased blood viscosity. This hyperviscosity, in turn, can lead to headache, hypertension, congestive heart failure, venous thromboses, pulmonary emboli, encephalopathy, and stroke. There have been some reports that rhEPO administration leading to excessive erythropoiesis may result in reduced thickness of cortical bone, trending toward osteoporosis and theoretically increased fracture risk.[80]

Creatine
Historical Perspectives

Creatine is one of the most popular supplements currently used by athletes. It is a compound synthesized within the body and also absorbed exogenously from fish and meats. In 1992, creatine was manufactured as a supplement to potentially improve muscular performance. Shortly thereafter, it was touted as a supplement that delayed fatigue and enhanced athletic performance.[81]

Physiology

Creatine has a fundamental role in the structure and function of adenosine triphosphate, the body's prime energy source. It is synthesized largely in the liver from amino acids and subsequently transported to skeletal muscles, the heart, and the brain, where it is absorbed. Intracellularly, creatine is phosphorylated into creatine phosphate, and in this state it serves as an energy substrate that contributes to the resynthesis of adenosine triphosphate for energy.[82] Creatine is also proposed to serve as a buffer to lactic acid produced during exercise. Lactic acid is a byproduct of intense exercise caused by the accumulation of H+ molecules. In excess, it limits exercise. Creatine binds these molecules, delays fatigue, and lengthens exercise duration. Creatine may also help athletic performance by promoting protein synthesis, thereby increasing muscle mass.[81] Additionally, when combined with a high-carbohydrate diet, creatine enhances glycogen stores, which is advantageous during long-duration, high-intensity exercise.[83]

Creatine may benefit athletes who engage in sports that emphasize short bursts of intense anaerobic activity, such as football, soccer, lacrosse, hockey, basketball, and powerlifting. Short-term creatine supplementation has been shown to enhance the ability to maintain muscular forces during jumping,[84] intense cycling,[85] and weight lifting.[81] It is important to note, however, that not all athletes appear to benefit from creatine supplementation.[83,86] Some individuals are "responders" while others are "nonresponders" to creatine.[87] It is estimated that about 30% of athletes are "nonresponders" because they already naturally possess a maximal amount of creatine—as much as can be stored by their muscle cells. Muscle creatine content is measured only by muscle biopsy, making it necessary for an athlete to use the supplement on a "trial and error" basis to determine if it will be beneficial.

Early studies emphasized the importance of a loading phase with creatine. Athletes would use large doses (20 g/day of creatine for 5 days) before reaching a maintenance dose (2 g/day).[88] More recent evidence has shown that loading is unnecessary and that a low-dose regimen of 3 g/day is just as effective, although it may take longer to for benefits to be noted.[89,90]

Adverse Effects

An increase in body mass of up to 2 kg occurs frequently and is believed to be the result of water retention.[83,91] According to some recommendations, creatine should not be consumed either before or during intense exercise.[92] Case reports of gastrointestinal distress (diarrhea) are common, but a direct cause-and-effect relationship has not been defined. Concerns regarding nephrotoxicity have been raised, but creatine supplementation does not appear to negatively affect renal function in healthy persons without a previous history of renal disorder if they adhere to recommended dosing.[93]

Thus the use of creatine in athletes is popular because it is considered a legal means of improving performance. Despite findings from a few controversial studies, supplementation with creatine can increase fat-free mass and strength. Creatine may also be of benefit to athletes who engage in high-intensity sprints or endurance training, but these benefits seem to diminish with prolonged exercise.[83]

Growth Hormone
Historical Perspectives

One of the most popular ergogenic drugs used by athletes, human GH, was discovered in the 1920s, when researchers noted that after an injection of ox pituitary glands, normal rats grew abnormally large. Animal breeders later used these injections to increase muscle mass and decrease body fat in their breeds.[94] In the 1950s, GH extracted from the brains of cadavers from Africa and Asia was administered to children whose growth was stunted by absence of this hormone.[95] Thousands of short-statured children were successfully treated with human GH. However, as a result of treatment with cadaver extracts, Creutzfeldt-Jakob disease developed in many of these children. This disease causes progressive dementia, loss of muscle control, and death.[96] By the early 1990s,

the FDA had stopped distribution of GH, yet there was a need to treat children who had short stature induced by low levels of GH. The Genentech Company used recombinant deoxyribonucleic acid technology to manufacture a biosynthetic GH, somatrem (Protropin), enabling GH to be safely provided to children in need. However, the use of human GH as a supplement is universally illegal.

GH affects almost every cell in the body. Because human GH levels dip with advancing age, it has been endorsed as an antiaging product. Human GH secretion can be stimulated throughout life by either sleep or exercise; thus combining exercise with rest may be beneficial. Currently long-term studies on the effectiveness of human GH are lacking.

Mechanism of Action

Human GH is a polypeptide produced and stored in the anterior pituitary gland. Its secretion is high during puberty and it continues to be secreted throughout life. Secretion occurs daily in a pulsatile fashion, with the highest levels observed shortly after sleep initiation.[94] Human GH works in two ways: first, by binding on target cells, it exerts its effects on adipocytes, which, in turn, break down triglycerides and prevent lipid accumulation; second, after reaching the liver, human GH is rapidly converted into insulin-like growth factor-1 and thus exerts its growth-promoting effects throughout the body.

Athletes have used human GH and insulin-like growth factor-1 as ergogenic supplements. Human GH is an appealing supplement for athletes because it stimulates protein metabolism. It is also a potent regulator of carbohydrate metabolism by decreasing insulin sensitivity and cellular uptake of glucose. In addition, human GH stimulates the catabolism of lipids, making free fatty acids available for quick energy use and sparing muscle glycogen.[97] Human GH also stimulates bone growth, which is crucial for growth in prepubertal youths.

Adverse Effects

Most notably, excess GH may cause problems with bone growth in adults. In adults, growth plates have fused but continue to enlarge in the presence of high levels of GH, resulting in dysmorphic, acromegalic features, particularly of the face, hands, and feet. Other problems include a predisposition to diabetes (attributed to decreased insulin sensitivity), cardiomyopathy, and congestive heart failure.[97] Correlations have been noted between human GH and the enlargement of intracranial lesions, amplification of intracranial hypertension, and leukemia in patients treated with recombinant human GH.[98]

No scientific studies have been conducted to show improved athletic performance with use of human GH. Nevertheless, human GH has been widely used by athletes. Limitations of human GH include poor quality (because much of it is supplied from international sources), exorbitant cost (about $1000 per month), and availability only in the parenteral form (increasing risk of infection). Nonetheless, human GH is used frequently, especially because few solid testing methods exist aside from two tests performed within a few days of dosing. The isoform test detects the presence of synthetic human GH and is effective for detection of use within 12 to 72 hours of administration. The second test, called the "biomarker test," evaluates the presence of chemicals produced by the body after human GH use[99]; it may be used alone or in conjunction with the isoform test.

Caffeine
Historical Perspectives

Caffeine is the most widely used legal ergogenic drug, with billions of people using it. The United States Olympic Committee (USOC) had previously placed caffeine in a restricted status, allowing no more than 12 µg/mL in urine; however, because of highly variable excretion rates, this restriction has been eliminated. Doses between 5 and 10 mg/kg 1 hour before an athletic contest are commonly used. Caffeine is not included on the 2017 Prohibited List of substances, having been removed since 2004. The drug is part of WADA's monitoring program, a program that includes substances not prohibited from sport but monitored to detect misuse in sport. Since 2010, caffeine use among athletes has increased, although there have been no global indications of misuse.[75]

Mechanism of Action

Caffeine has historically been used to enhance physical and mental performance. It employs its ergogenic effects both centrally and peripherally. Once in the bloodstream, caffeine is rapidly absorbed, leading to the stimulation of excitatory neurotransmitters. At a central location, caffeine increases perception of physical effort and improves neural activation of muscle transport. Peripherally, caffeine leads to the release of free fatty acids from adipose tissue, sparing muscle glycogen and maintaining blood glucose levels. It also stimulates potassium transport into tissue, maintaining muscle cell membrane excitability and decreasing muscle cell reaction time after neural stimulus, while reducing muscle fatigue.

Side Effects

Evidence indicates that caffeine ingestion helps with endurance while providing performance enhancement.[100] Beneficial effects occur at modest doses of about 1 to 3 mg/kg 1 hour prior to exercise without noticeable dose dependency, although higher doses (>6 to 9 mg/kg) tend to incur adverse side effects. The most common detrimental effects include anxiety, restlessness, panic attacks, gastritis, reflux, and heart palpitations.[101] Chronic users may experience withdrawal, including headache and fatigue with abrupt cessation of use. Acute caffeine intake is known to increase urinary loss of fluid, although a recent review proposes that there is little evidence that the drug affects overall fluid status.[102] Doses of caffeine within the ergogenic range do not alter sweat rates, urinary losses, or indices of hydration status.[103]

The majority of studies highlighting caffeine use and athletic performance concern endurance sports. In long-distance cycling competitions, time to exhaustion at VO_2 max was significantly improved.[104] In another cycling study, a 7% increase in distance covered in 2 hours was noted.[105] There is also evidence that caffeine can enhance performance in sustained, high-intensity activities. In one particular study, 1500-meter swim time was significantly improved in trained athletes.[106] There is a strong need to educate athletes regarding the responsible intake of caffeine

to appropriately balance and maximize benefit without eliciting the negative side effects of use.

Summary

For centuries, athletes have been willing to risk death in an attempt to improve their ability to compete in sports. What can persons entrusted with the health of athletes do to protect athletes from themselves? The first step is "meaningful education" as reflected by an important tenet in medicine—"you only recognize what you know." Most medical personnel receive very little education about doping and ergogenic aids during their schooling. To stay abreast with the practices of athletes, lifelong learning is essential. Health care professionals should be able to communicate openly with athletes regarding the health risks and legality of ergogenic aids and the importance of healthy nutrition and honest training as a viable and preferred alternative for promoting athletic superiority. Second, the medical community should conduct scientific controlled studies on athletes who are using ergogenic drugs. Obviously such studies would be difficult to conduct because many of these drugs are illegal, many ergogenic agents have significant adverse effects, and research oversight committees are often reluctant to approve studies using drugs with known or suspected adverse effects. Third, effective drug testing and stringent penalties for athletes, coaches, teams, and nations who use banned substances are imperative.

SPORTS PHARMACOLOGY: RECREATIONAL DRUG USE

Substance use among students and young adults continues to be a leading cause of morbidity and mortality. The Monitoring the Future Survey is an ongoing study of the behaviors, attitudes, and values of American secondary school students, college students, and young adults.[107] The 2016 updated survey shows that nearly 50% of young Americans have used some type of illicit substance between grades 8 and 12, with nearly 25% having used such a substance in the past 12 months. Cigarette smoking and alcohol use have continued to decline and are at all-time lows. Even so, vaping (the inhalation of vapors such as e-cigarettes), alcohol, and marijuana remain the most consistently abused substances. Consistent with prior studies, there appears to be little difference in the prevalence of recreational drug use in athletes and nonathletes. Clinicians need to be aware of the effects of these drugs in order to appropriately educate their athletes on the risk of these substances not only on performance measures but, more importantly, also on general health and wellness.

Alcohol
Epidemiology

Alcohol continues to be one of the most frequently abused substances in collegiate, professional, and Olympic sports.[108] The use of alcohol has declined since 1980, yet despite this fact, the National Institute of Drug Abuse reports that in 2016, approximately 33% of high school seniors acknowledged having consumed alcohol in the previous month.[109] According to the Harvard School of Public Health Alcohol Study, 80% of college students consume alcohol. Compared with nonathletes, collegiate athletes exhibit a higher rate of binge drinking; they also experience more alcohol-related complications including academic problems, driving under the influence, gambling, illicit drug use, and sexual promiscuity.[110,111]

Pathophysiology and Adverse Effects

Ethanol is the primary psychoactive constituent in alcoholic beverages; it exerts its effect on the central nervous system (CNS) via its action on gamma-aminobutyric acid receptors. It also interacts with acetylcholine, serotonin, and N-methyl-D-aspartate receptors. It is oxidized by the liver at a constant rate rather than having an elimination half-life. Systemic ethanol levels are typically quantified by the blood alcohol content (BAC). Adverse effects of ingestion often correlate with BAC levels; however, persons lacking effective forms of metabolizing enzymes may experience more severe symptoms, whereas those who have acquired tolerance may metabolize alcohol more rapidly. In general, persons with a low BAC level (0.05%) experience euphoria, talkativeness, and relaxation. BAC levels of 0.1% or higher frequently induce CNS depression, compromise motor and sensory function, and impair cognition. Levels in excess of 0.3% may lead to unconsciousness, with levels surpassing 0.4% placing individuals at risk of death.

In 1982, the American College of Sports Medicine issued a position statement regarding alcohol and its effect on sports performance.[112] The main points of the position statement are as follows:

1. Alcohol adversely affects coordination, balance, and accuracy.
2. Alcohol does not improve athletic performance.
3. Alcohol will not improve muscle work performance and negatively affects the ability to perform.
4. Alcohol may impair temperature regulation during prolonged exercise in a cold environment.

Other Considerations

In recognition of the epidemic of alcohol abuse among young Americans, the Surgeon General's Office released its Call to Action against Underage Drinking in 2007. This document identified the following six goals to help lower the incidence of alcohol abuse and associated morbidity and mortality.[113]

1. Foster changes in society that facilitate healthy adolescent development and that help prevent and reduce underage drinking.
2. Engage parents, schools, communities, all levels of government, all social systems that interface with youths, and youths themselves in a coordinated national effort to prevent and reduce underage drinking and its consequences.
3. Promote an understanding of underage alcohol consumption in the context of human development and maturation that takes into account individual adolescent characteristics, along with environmental, ethnic, cultural, and gender differences.
4. Conduct additional research on adolescent alcohol use and its relationship to development.
5. Work to improve public health surveillance on underage drinking and on population-based risk factors for this behavior.

6. Work to ensure that policies at all levels are consistent with the national goal of preventing and reducing underage alcohol consumption.

Despite campaigns to decrease binge drinking by athletes, excessive drinking is a reality. Team physicians should work closely with coaching staffs and athletic departments to develop prevention programs and an action plan for penalties for alcohol-related infractions of established rules.

Marijuana
Epidemiology

Marijuana is the second most commonly abused drug by athletes and the most commonly used illicit drug, with nearly 1 in 15 high school seniors reporting daily or nearly daily use.[114,115] According to the most recent National Survey on Drug Use and Health released by the CDC in 2015, an estimated 22.2 million Americans aged 12 years or older are current users. Though this is not an increase, use in individuals age 18 or older is on the rise. Despite legalization across several states, the NCAA continues its stance in considering this a banned substance. Nevertheless, the use of marijuana is still pervasive and persisting among student athletes.

Pathophysiology and Adverse Effects

All forms of cannabis are mind-altering (psychoactive) drugs. The main active chemical derivative, Δ-9-tetrahydrocannabinol, affects cannabinoid receptors found in the brain and peripheral tissues and also indirectly enhances dopamine release, producing its psychotropic influences. Marijuana is absorbed readily and has effects throughout the body, most predominantly in the CNS, the respiratory system, and the cardiovascular system.

Short-term effects of marijuana use include distorted perception, difficulty in thinking and problem solving, and loss of coordination. The psychotropic effects of cannabis include general euphoria and a mild release from inhibitions, drowsiness, stimulated appetite, and freedom from anxiety. Other persons experience an altered sense of consciousness.[116] Long-term use may be linked to behavioral changes similar to those caused by traumatic injury.

Recent studies document a spectrum of cardiorespiratory ailments associated with the smoking of marijuana. A large epidemiologic study suggests that marijuana smoke can cause the same types of respiratory damage as tobacco smoke.[117] The acute physiologic effects of marijuana on the cardiovascular system include a substantial dose-dependent increase in heart rate, a mild increase in blood pressure, and occasionally orthostatic hypotension. Athletic performance is affected, as marijuana use has been shown to decrease exercise test duration in maximal exercise tests, with premature achievement of maximal oxygen uptake.[118]

Other Considerations

Discussions with athletes should not only emphasize the negative effects of marijuana on athletic performance but also stress the often forgotten fact that marijuana continues to be a Schedule I drug despite legalization in many states. Moreover, more potent and dangerous synthetic derivatives have been developed and are increasingly popular in attempts to bypass screening tests. These products, such as "Spice" or "K-2," are herbal mixtures infused with chemicals to give effects similar to those of marijuana by their ability to bind to cannabinoid receptors throughout the body. Their popularity stems from the "marijuana-like high" and easy availability at retail outlets and via the Internet. Numerous reports of serious adverse effects—including convulsions, anxiety attacks, tachycardia, vomiting, psychosis, and disorientation—have necessitated their emergency classification in March 2011 as a Schedule I substance.[119]

Tobacco
Epidemiology

Smoking remains the most preventable cause of death in developed countries. The World Health Organization reports that tobacco use is responsible for more than 7 million deaths annually worldwide.[120] The use of tobacco by adolescents has declined since the peak levels of the mid-1990s; however, 15% of individuals in the United States continue to smoke. In addition to cigarette smoking, other forms of tobacco use include smokeless tobacco, pipes, cigars, chewing tobacco, snuff, and, most recently, the e-cigarette. In 2014, sales of e-cigarettes surpassed those of traditional cigarettes. In a recent press release regarding the e-cigarette epidemic, the Surgeon General reported that 1 out of every 6 high school students in the United States has used e-cigarettes in the previous month.[121] Although cigarette smoking is less of a problem in athletes than in nonathletes, use of smokeless or "spit" tobacco remains prevalent, particularly in the realms of baseball, football, and golf.

Pathophysiology and Adverse Effects

Nicotine is both a stimulant and a depressant. As nicotine enters the body, it crosses the blood-brain barrier within 10 to 20 seconds and exerts its effects by binding to nicotinic acetylcholine receptors, increasing levels of dopamine. Via this mechanism, tobacco is believed to have an addictive potential comparable to that of alcohol, cocaine, and morphine.[122]

The detrimental health consequences of tobacco use are well known. Smokeless tobacco users have an increased risk for oral cancer, including cancer of the lip, tongue, cheeks, gums, and the floor and roof of the mouth. Through its release of various chemical messengers—including acetylcholine, epinephrine, norepinephrine, serotonin, and dopamine, among others—nicotine appears to enhance concentration, memory, and alertness while decreasing appetite and promoting relaxation. Nicotine is considered a mood- and behavior-altering drug, often helping athletes to deal with stressful situations. Other effects, due to nicotine's vasoactive properties, include increases in pulse rate by 10 to 20 beats/min and blood pressure by 5 to 10 mm Hg. Nicotine also stimulates platelet aggregation, which may increase the risk for blood clots.

Other Considerations

In an effort to curtail tobacco use, both professional baseball (minor leagues) and junior hockey (Western Hockey League) have banned the use of spit tobacco by players, coaches, and officials. Similarly, the NCAA bans the use of spit tobacco by players, coaches, and officials during NCAA-sanctioned events. Dental screening, which can often detect precancerous lesions that may be caused by nicotine, is highly recommended for all athletes. Last, nicotine addiction is difficult to overcome. Epidemiologic studies indicate that the likelihood of addiction increases when cigarette smoking commences during adolescence. Thus addressing the dangers of nicotine in youth sports and its potential for refractory addiction is critical for prevention.

Cocaine
Epidemiology

The Monitoring the Future Survey documented that in 2006, 8.5% of 12th graders had used cocaine.[123] Since then, use has dropped to a historical low of 3.7% among this same cohort.[123] Cocaine abuse can lead to physical dependence. It is a controlled substance (Schedule II) and is banned in sport, with the IOC testing athletes routinely.

Pathophysiology and Adverse Effects

Cocaine is a naturally occurring alkaloid that is present in the leaves of *Erythroxylon coca*. It is commercially available and can be applied to mucous membranes of the oral, laryngeal, and nasal cavities for use as a topical anesthetic; however, it is most known for its abuse potential via its various processed forms. Cocaine exerts its adverse effects as a result of excessive sympathetic activity. Unlike other local anesthetics, cocaine affects the nervous system by potentiating catecholamines and leads to increased energy levels. It also results in the inhibition of presynaptic reuptake of norepinephrine, dopamine, and serotonin.

Cocaine causes an acute dopamine release and inhibits synaptic dopamine reuptake, which produces euphoria, reduced fatigue, elevated sexual desire, and increased mental ability as well as sociability. At higher doses, tremors and tonic-clonic convulsions may occur. Long-term use of cocaine can result in nasal congestion, rhinitis, chronic sinusitis, and increased risk for upper respiratory infection. CNS toxicity is extremely common with cocaine use, including agitation, anxiety, apprehension, confusion, headache, dizziness, emotional lability, euphoria, excitement, hallucinations, seizures, and psychosis.

Effects on Athletic Performance

The significant morbidity and mortality in athletes is a result of the effects of cocaine on the cardiovascular system. Through its sympathomimetic effects, cocaine augments ventricular contractility, blood pressure, heart rate, and myocardial oxygen demand. Myocardial ischemia is induced by coronary vasoconstriction, platelet aggregation, and accelerated atherosclerosis. The ensuing supply-demand deficit may manifest as angina, and cocaine-induced coronary spasm may lead to acute myocardial infarction and death. Cocaine is markedly pyrogenic because it induces muscular activity, augments heat production, and potentiates vasoconstriction—all of which can enhance the risk for heat stroke and death. Cocaine dependence is a significant problem in our society; it is associated not only with the outlined spectrum of medical complications but also with crime and violence. Educational programs regarding the hazards of cocaine use and addiction are highly recommended for all athletes.

Inhalants
Epidemiology and Classification

Inhalant use is the deliberate inhalation of volatile substances to induce a mind-altering effect. Purchase and possession are legal, and inhalants are cheap and easily accessible. National surveys of adolescents in the United States have reported that second to marijuana, inhalants are the most widely used class of illicit drugs among 8th and 10th graders. Fortunately, their use has continued to decrease. The American Academy of Pediatrics has taken the initiative to educate clinicians, parents, and children of the dangers of inhalant abuse.[124] Inhalants are divided into three groups on the basis of the inhalant pharmacology, as follows:

1. Type I agents include volatile solvents such as paint thinner, acetone, glue, rubber cement, butane, aerosols, hair spray, and gasoline.
2. Type II agents are nitrous oxide and whipping cream aerosols, which contain nitrous oxide.
3. Type III agents include volatile alkyl nitrites known as "poppers," "snappers," "boppers," and "Amys."

Inhalant agents are abused through a variety of methods. Glue or solids are emptied into a bag, held close to the nose, and inhaled either through the nose *(snorting or sniffing)* or through the mouth *(huffing)*. Other methods include placing one's entire head into a bag *(bagging)* and inhalation of either air fresheners (e.g., Glade, referred to as *glading*), or computer cleaning aerosols *(dusting)*.

Pathophysiology and Adverse Effects

Inhalants contain different solvents, each with its own unique toxicity, but all inhalants induce CNS depression, likely involving a γ-aminobutyric acid agonist or altered neuronal membrane function.[125] Death can occur as a result of the use of inhalant agents because of cardiac complications that occur as a result of asphyxia, ventricular fibrillation, or cardiac arrhythmia. Cerebral death may occur as a result of asphyxia, edema, and hyperpyrexia.[125]

Inhalants do not augment or improve athletic performance; in fact, their use can lead to serious health consequences. Some glues are metabolized and may cause peripheral neuropathy, characterized by muscle weakness and wasting. Inhalants have also been known to sensitize and potentiate the myocardium to epinephrine, which, during exercise, may increase an athlete's risk of an acute, fatal arrhythmia. No specific antidotes exist for inhalant toxicity, and treatment is rooted in prevention.

Conclusion

The use of recreational drugs and their potential for deadly consequences are a realities for athletes and our society. Most treatment entails meaningful educational programs. Athletes who are well informed about the potential dangers of using recreational drugs may be best able to avoid the temptation to "try" these drugs, which are readily available. Additionally, coaches should be involved in the education process; they should stress the importance of sobriety and healthy habits as core requirements for optimal health and the development of a successful team. The ongoing Monitoring the Future surveys have clearly demonstrated that all the drugs discussed in this chapter are used by many youth at very young ages, often in middle or elementary school. It is therefore imperative that the education of athletes, coaches, and parents commence in the earliest recreational leagues.

For a complete list of references, go to ExpertConsult.com.

SELECTED READINGS

Citation:

Cooper R, Naclerio F, Allgrove J, et al. Creatine supplementation with specific view to exercise/sports performance: an update. *J Int Soc Sports Nutr.* 2012;9:33.

Level of Evidence:

II

Summary:

More and more information is being discovered about the use of creatine, particularly with regard to its relevance in improving sports performance. This article reviews recent advances in understanding the science relating to creatine use and the methods of supplementation to make cellular and subcellular changes.

Citation:

Green GA, Uryasz FD, Petr TA, et al. NCAA study of substance use and abuse habits of college student-athletes: clinical investigations. *Clin J Sport Med.* 2001;11(1):51–56.

Level of Evidence:

III

Summary:

Monitoring the Future is an ongoing study that entails the administration of a series of annual surveys among representative samples of secondary school students throughout the United States, using a standard set of questions to determine usage levels of various substances. Cigarettes/e-cigarettes, alcohol, and marijuana continue to be the most frequently abused substances among adolescents, with synthetic marijuana recently falling under the Drug Enforcement Administration's list of prohibited substances.

Citation:

World Anti-Doping Agency. The 2012 Prohibited List. Available at: http://www.wada-ama.org/Documents/World_Anti-Doping_Program/WADP-Prohibited-list/2012/WADA_Prohibited_List_2017. Accessed June 12, 2017.

Level of Evidence:

V

Summary:

The World Anti-Doping Agency annually updates its list of prohibited substances among athletes. A review of and familiarity with the list is critical for providers so they can comply with up-to-date guidelines.

27

The Female Athlete

Letha Y. Griffin, Mary Lloyd Ireland, Fred Reifsteck,
Matthew H. Blake, Benjamin R. Wilson

THE GROWING IMPORTANCE AND RECOGNITION OF THE FEMALE ATHLETE

Over the past several decades there has been a rapid development of competitive sporting events for women, and parallel to this, an emergence of increasing numbers of excellent competitive women athletes.

Before the 1970s, few women participated in organized sport. However, the passage of Title IX of the Educational Assistance Act of 1972[1] required institutions receiving federal money to offer equal opportunities to both males and females in all programs including athletics. This sparked a rapid growth not only in collegiate women's sport opportunities, but also in those sport opportunities available to high school and recreational female athletes (Table 27.1).

The female athlete market is now a major target for businesses as exemplified by women's clothing. Women's sporting gear before the 1980s was difficult to find. However, with increased opportunities in sports for women following the passage of Title IX, the demand for female-specific sport clothes and equipment has increased. Prior to this time, female athletes often wore men's shoes (a practice that was associated with an increase in foot problems), men's warm-ups, and sport protection equipment (shin guards in soccer, eye protection in racket sports, mouth guards, etc.). However, in the 1990s the business of women's sport gear—including warm-ups, shorts, skirts, shirts, sports bras, protective pads, and shoes—grew rapidly. Women traditionally spend more money on all clothing needs compared to men, and sport wear has become a fashion statement for women. Sized to the women's figure, braces and other protective sport gear now have a more comfortable fit. Lightweight clothing that wicks away perspiration is prevalent and comes in pinks, purples, and other bright colors for stylish looks. Shoes made for women are now a more comfortable "fit," which has resulted in fewer calluses, corns, and other foot issues.

Before 1970, rarely were the results of women's sports contests found in newspapers or within the pages of *Sports Illustrated* or on nightly TV news or radio; however, this trend is changing.

Women's golf and tennis events are now aired on primetime television. The Women's National Basketball Association (WNBA) aired 45 regular season games in 2017. Fox reports that 6 of the top 10 searches of 2016 Olympic Athletes were for females.[5]

Parallel and (perhaps one could argue) secondary to the increased emphasis on women's sport participation, there has been an improvement in women's sport performance in swimming and running events, and the speed of basketball, soccer, tennis, and volleyball games has increased with the improvement in women's skills and overall athleticism.

Not only have the numbers and recognition of highly competitive female athletes increased over the last 50 years, but also the prevalence of women of all ages participating in recreational athletics has skyrocketed, making it essential that those caring for the female athlete appreciate her uniqueness as gender-based differences are important when developing novel approaches to prevention, diagnosis, and treatment of injury and illness.[6] The term "sexual dimorphism" is defined as: "The condition in which the two sexes of the same species exhibit different characteristics beyond the differences of their sexual organs."[7] In humans, these differences are related to the expression of genes on the X and Y chromosomes. These differences form the basis of this chapter and include not only anatomic and physiologic differences (Table 27.2) but also certain aspects of illnesses and injuries unique to the female athlete.

GENERAL CONSIDERATIONS

Conditioning

Conditioning has been defined as "a process in which stimuli are created by an exercise program performed by the athlete to produce a higher level of function."[9] A properly constructed conditioning program should maximize performance and minimize the chance of injury. There have been ongoing debates as to whether conditioning techniques used for males are appropriate for females. Little boys start out wishing to do weights with their fathers or older brothers or friends. This is infrequently true in girls. Hence, in the mid to late teenage years, boys are typically familiar with weight workouts and have already incorporated strengthening programs into their sport conditioning programs. At this time, girls most likely are just beginning to learn that a weight strengthening program is a needed part of a well-constructed conditioning program. Some theorize that girls and young women may be leery of participating in a weight training program for fear of developing bulky muscles. They should be reassured that strength training does not necessarily have to involve lifting heavier and heavier weights and is associated with not only better performance but also a decrease in injury.[9,10]

Static and dynamic balance are vital for maximizing sport performance as well as enhancing injury prevention.[11] Articles

TABLE 27.1   Growth in Women's Sports[2-4]

Participation Level	NUMBER OF WOMEN PARTICIPATING			
	1971–1972	2000–2001	2010–2011	2015–2016
High school	294,015	2,784,154	3,173,549	3,324,326
Collegiate	29,972	150,916	190,000	216,286
Olympic	1264 (17.5% of Olympians)	4935 (37.5% of Olympians)	5091 (42.4% of Olympians)	5800 (43.5% of Olympians)

www.nfhs.org; www.ncaa.org; www.olympic.org.

TABLE 27.2   Anatomic and Physiologic Gender Differences[8,a]

Parameter	Postpubertal Girls	Postpubertal Boys	Impact
Oxygen pulse (efficiency of cardiorespiratory system	Lower	Higher	Higher oxygen pulse provides boys an advantage in aerobic activity.
$VO_{2\,max}$ (reflects level of aerobic fitness)	Lower	Higher	Boys have greater aerobic capacity.
Metabolism (basal metabolic rate [BMR])	6%–10% lower (when related to body surface area)	6%–10% higher (when related to body surface area)	Girls need fewer calories to sustain the same activity level as boys.
Thermoregulation	Equals boys	Equals girls	They have equal ability to adequately sweat in a hot environment to decrease core body temperature.
Endocrine System			
Testosterone	Lower	Higher	Boys have increased muscle size, strength, and aggressiveness.
Estrogen	Higher	Lower	Unknown if it is related to increase in ligamentous laxity or in rate of ACL injuries.
Height	64.5 inches	68.5 inches	The increased height and weight in boys give them structural advantages.
Weight	56.8 kg	70.0 kg	
Limb length	Shorter	Longer	Boys can achieve a greater force for hitting and kicking.
Articular surface	Smaller	Larger	May provide boys with greater joint stability; boys have greater surface area to dissipate impact force.
Body shape	Narrower shoulders Wider hips Legs 51.2% of height More fat in lower body	Wider shoulders Narrower hips Legs 52% of height More fat in upper body	Girls have lower center of gravity and therefore greater balance ability; girls have increased valgus angle at the knee that increases knee injuries; boys and girls have different running gaits.
%Muscle/total	–36%	–44.8%	Boys have greater strength and greater body weight[a] speed.
%Fat/total body weight	–22% to 26%	–13% to 16%	Girls are more buoyant and better insulated; they may be able to convert fatty acid to metabolism more rapidly.
Age at skeletal maturation	17–19 years	21–22 years	Girls develop adult body shape/form sooner than boys.
Cardiovascular system			Stroke volume in girls is less, necessitating an increased
Heart size	Smaller	Larger	heart rate for a given submaximal cardiac output;
Heart volume	Smaller	Larger	cardiac output in girls is 30% less than in boys; the
Systolic blood pressure	Lower	Higher	risk of hypertension may be less in girls.
Hemoglobin		10%–15% > per 100 mL blood	The oxygen carrying capacity of blood is greater in boys.
Pulmonary System			
Chest size	Smaller	Larger	Total lung capacity in boys is greater than in girls.
Lung size	Smaller	Larger	
Vital capacity	Smaller	Larger	
Residual volume	Smaller	Larger	

[a]There are no appreciable differences in these parameters prior to puberty; therefore prepubertal boys and girls can compete on a fairly equal basis.

ACL, Anterior cruciate ligament.

From Yurko-Griffin LY, Harris S. Female athlete. In: Sullivan JA, Anderson SJ, editors. *Care of the Young Athlete*. Rosemont, IL: American Academy of Orthopaedic Surgery; 2000:138–148 with permission.

have been written and comments made in scientific meetings regarding the need, or the lack of need, to alter training and conditioning in several women's sports such as soccer, softball, basketball, volleyball, and lacrosse.[12] Suggestions have been made for players to incorporate more agility and balance exercises to try to decrease the frequency of noncontact anterior cruciate ligament (ACL) injuries in these sports.[13-15] The adage "stronger is better," is now being modified since strong muscles that fire at inappropriate times can cause harm rather than ensure protection from injury during an athletic event. Programs for women's sports where ACL risks are high are adopting training and conditioning routines that emphasize not only the traditional strength, flexibility, and aerobic conditioning exercises, but also they have drills aimed to enhance balance and agility.[14,16-20] Incorporating plyometric drills appears to be appropriate in both male and female sport programs. (See section on ACL injuries in women in this chapter.)

Greater emphasis on core strengthening may also be appropriate for females who have been reported to have more anterior pelvic tilt than men, a trait that is linked with patellofemoral pain syndrome.[13] Medial quadriceps exercises are recommended for females with laterally tracking patellae especially those with increased Q ankle, increased tibial tubercle to tibial groove distance, and those with increased knee valgus.[21] These exercises should commence during the prepubescent age and continue through the pubertal years and into post pubertal maturation. By building strength in the vastus medialis, hopefully the patella will sit more centrally in the trochlear groove decreasing patellofemoral pain by balancing patellar trochlear forces.

Since postpubertal females are reported to have increased flexibility compared to males, strengthening scapular stabilizers and the muscles of the rotator cuff to prevent shoulder instability issues is recommended in swimmers; in volleyball, lacrosse, and softball players; and in those playing racket sports.[22] Prevention rather than "cure" should be the norm and has been proven to be beneficial. Following puberty, training and conditioning programs should also account for inherent gender-based, physical, and physiologic differences (see Table 27.2). Males are more fully developed in the upper body with a narrow pelvis and hence, a higher center of gravity; whereas females have narrower shoulders compared to males, but proportionally a wider pelvis resulting in a lower center of gravity, but they have a more difficult time achieving the upper body strength of their male counterparts. Males have more muscle mass per body weight; whereas female athletes, even those who are considered to be well conditioned, have greater body fat than males (18% to 20% females vs. 10% to 15% males). Moreover, males have a greater thoracic capacity and hence, a greater VO$_2$ max than do females. Overall aerobic capacity in females is less than that of males following puberty. Hence, one notes that although female athletes have improved significantly over the last 10 years, their times in anaerobic and aerobic running events are still not equal to those of males (Table 27.3). A few "conditioning tips" for female athletes are listed in Table 27.4.

In the last decade there has been an emphasis on screening athletes at all levels of play from those who exercise for health and fitness to recreational players to highly trained competitive

TABLE 27.3 Improvements in Women's Anaerobic and Aerobic Running Events[23]

Collegiate Track	1972	1998	2012	2017
800 m	2:04:7	2:06:30	2:03:34	2:02.36
3200 m	10:51:0	10:25:99	10:08:11	10:00.13
10,000 m	33:36:51	32:56:63	32:41:63	32:38.57
Boston Marathon	1972	1996	2011	2017
	3:10:26	2:27:12	2:22:36	2:21:52

www.ncaa.org; www.baa.org.

TABLE 27.4 Conditioning Tips for Recreational Athletes[24,25]

Emphasize core strength to minimize stress on lower extremities.
Emphasize strengthening of scapular stabilizers and muscles involved in dynamic stabilization of the glenohumeral joint to minimize laxity issues of the shoulder joint.[a]
Emphasize vastus medialis obliques (VMO) strength when doing lower extremity strengthening exercises to improve patellar tracking.[b]
Minimize loading the patellofemoral joint in a fully flexed knee position, that is, consider short arc extension and leg press exercises in place of squats, lunges, and full arc extension exercises.[b]
Perform upper extremity strengthening exercises at shoulder height and below to minimize stress on the rotator cuff (pull downs, overhead dumbbell press, etc.).

[a]Kibler WB, Sciascia AD, Uhl TL, Tambay N, Cunningham T. Electromyographic analysis of specific exercises for the scapular control in early phases of shoulder rehabilitation. *Am J Sports Med.* 2008;36:1789.
[b]www.healthline.com/health/fitness-exercises/vastus-medialis-exercises.

athletes for functional movement skills and balance to detect deficits that could predispose the athlete to injury. Exercises to correct these deficits can then be incorporated into the athlete's exercise program not only to improve physical performance parameters (e.g., increased aerobic power, strength, speed, agility, and balance), but also to prevent injury. Such programs have proven to be very highly effective in achieving both of these goals.[11,26-30]

Nutrition and Hydration

Sports nutrition is currently recognized as one of the most important aspects of improving sports performance. Inadequate nutritional intake has been reported to be more common in female than male athletes. Both the content and timing of optimal nutrition may significantly impact the female athlete's performance. In individuals, dietary needs depend on not only sex, but also size, weight, and energy demands of the sport. A 5-foot female dancer may not require as high a caloric intake as a 6-foot female basketball player. Please see the chapter on nutrition for a more complete discussion of the nutritional needs in athletes in general. This section will focus on vitamin D, calcium, iron, and hydration—areas of particular concern for the female athlete.

Adequate consumption of carbohydrates, protein, fat, and other macronutrients, are critical to replace glycogen stores, and repair exercise-induced tissue damage. On average, an energy intake of less than 1800 kcal per day in a female athlete can result in a persistent state of negative energy balance and diminish sports performance.

Vitamin D is an emerging micronutrient with deficiency being linked to low bone mineral density (BMD), cancer, heart disease, autoimmune problems, and infections.[31] Vitamin D is needed for the absorption of calcium, which is critical to bone health. Vitamin D is also important in nervous system and skeletal muscle development and function.[32] Female athletes living in northern latitudes who participate in indoor sport are at risk for vitamin D deficiency. Indoor sport athletes are nearly twice as likely as outdoor athletes to be vitamin D deficient.[31] While sun exposure is important for vitamin D levels, low dietary intake may also lead to deficiency. Vitamin D can be obtained by one of two methods. Endogenous vitamin D is synthesized in the skin following direct sun exposure; exogenous vitamin D is ingested in foods or can be obtained as a supplement. A recent very interesting observation related to vitamin D is the risk of upper respiratory tract infections due to a lowered immune system response in patients with low vitamin D levels.[31] Respiratory infections are a leading medical cause of lost time for the female athlete. At-risk athletes, especially athletes aged 19 to 49, may benefit from 200 IU of vitamin D supplementation per day.[32] Female athletes with the female athlete triad or risk factors for osteoporosis may need 400 to 800 IU per day. (See sections on the Female Athlete Triad and Osteoporosis and Osteopenia in this chapter.)

Adequate calcium intake is essential for proper bone mineralization. Females may be more at risk than males for low calcium intake as females more frequently restrict caloric intake and often shun dairy products feeling they are too high in calories. However, this is not the case since we now have options such as low-fat milk, low-fat cottage cheese, low-fat yogurt, and low-fat string cheese that are high in calcium but low in calories. Table 27.5 lists the required daily calcium needs for women of various age ranges. Three servings of daily calcium products typically provide the needed daily requirements. Female athletes should be encouraged to drink low-fat milk for breakfast and eat two servings of low-fat yogurt or string cheese daily to fulfill their calcium needs. Table 27.6 lists the calcium present in some commonly consumed foods.

Iron is a mineral that has long been known to affect athletic performance in the female athlete. Iron deficiency has been shown to limit endurance training and sports performance.[35]

TABLE 27.6 Sources of Calcium

Food	Milligrams (mg)	
	Per Serving	Percent DV[a]
Yogurt, plain, low fat, 8 oz	415	42
Mozzarella, part skim, 1.5 oz	333	33
Sardines, canned in oil, with bones, 3 oz	325	33
Yogurt, fruit, low fat, 8 oz	313–384	31–38
Cheddar cheese, 1.5 oz	307	31
Milk, nonfat, 8 oz[b]	299	30
Soy milk, calcium fortified 8 oz	299	30
Milk, reduced fat (2% milk fat) 8 oz	293	29
Milk, buttermilk, low fat, 8 oz	284	28
Milk, whole (3.25% milk fat), 8 oz	276	28
Orange juice, calcium fortified, 6 oz	261	26
Tofu, firm, made with calcium sulfate, ½ cup[c]	253	25
Salmon, pink, canned, solids with bone, 3 oz	181	18
Cottage cheese, 1% milk fat, 1 cup	138	14
Tofu, soft, made with calcium sulfate, ½ cup[c]	138	14
Ready-to-eat cereal, calcium fortified, 1 cup	100–1000	10–100
Frozen yogurt, vanilla, soft serve, ½ cup	103	10
Turnip greens, fresh, boiled, ½ cup	99	10
Kale, fresh, cooked, 1 cup	94	9
Ice cream, vanilla, ½ cup	84	8
Chinese cabbage, bok choy, raw, shredded, 1 cup	74	7
Bread, white, 1 slice	73	7
Pudding, chocolate, ready-to-eat, refrigerated, 4 oz	55	6
Tortilla, corn, ready-to-bake/fry, one 6″ diameter	46	5
Tortilla, flour, ready-to-bake/fry, one 6″ diameter	32	3
Sour cream, reduced fat, cultured, 2 tablespoons	31	3
Bread, whole wheat, 1 slice	30	3
Kale, raw, chopped, 1 cup	24	2
Broccoli, raw, ½ cup	21	2
Cheese, cream, regular, 1 tablespoon	14	1

[a]DVs were developed by the US Food and Drug Administration to help compare the nutrient content within the context of a total daily diet.
[b]Calcium content varies slightly by fat content; the more fat, the less calcium the food contains.
[c]Calcium content is for tofu processed with a calcium salt. Tofu processed with other salts does not provide significant amounts of calcium.
DV, Daily value.
https://ods.od.nih.gov/factsheets/Calcium-HealthProfessional/#h2.

TABLE 27.5 Required Daily Calcium Needs for Women[33,34,a]

Age Group (years)	Suggested Intake (mg/day)
1–3	700
4–8	1000
9–18	1300
19–50	1000
51–70	1000
>70	1200
Amenorrhoeic athletes[b] (all ages)	1500
Pregnant/lactating women	1500
14–18	1300
19–50	1000

[a]Recommendation of National Osteoporosis Foundation (www.NOF.org)
[b]https://ods.od.nih.gov/factsheets/calcium-HealthProfessional.

Iron is required in hemoglobin and myoglobin production. Since hemoglobin is responsible for carrying oxygen to muscles, adequate levels are vital during exercise, especially for endurance sports. Female athletes are especially at risk for iron deficiency due to menstrual blood loss monthly and poor dietary intake. Vegetarian athletes especially are at risk since red meats are an excellent source of iron. Training at high altitudes, losses of iron in sweat, feces, urine, foot strike hemolysis, and intravascular hemolysis can contribute to iron loss and subsequent deficiency. The female athlete's *iron* is best screened by measuring serum ferritin. The complete blood count is used to screen for *anemia* by measurement of the hemoglobin. The female athlete can have iron deficiency anemia where both the ferritin and hemoglobin are decreased.

Replenishing iron in those who are significantly iron deficient can take 3 to 6 months of dietary changes and supplementation. Therefore diagnosing the deficiency early or identifying at-risk athletes is important in decreasing the potential of loss of performance. Increasing iron by supplementation in the deficient athlete results in increased work capacity by enabling increased oxygen uptake, decreasing lactate concentration, and reducing heart rate during exercise.[32] Current recommendations for dietary iron intake are 15 mg/day for girls 14 to 18 years of age and 18 mg/day for women 19 to 50 years of age. The bioavailability of dietary iron can be enhanced by ascorbic acid and fermented foods, and the inclusion of lean meat, chicken, and fish into the diet. Heme iron (type of iron found in animal protein) is better absorbed than nonheme iron, which is particularly important in counseling vegetarian athletes. Examples of iron-rich foods are listed in Table 27.7.

Athletes who are minimally dehydrated can experience increased core temperatures.[36,37] Females have a higher thermoregulatory threshold than males and begin sweating at a higher core temperature than males. This may make it harder for females to cool during times of intense training.[38] Nonreplaced sweat loss of 1% to 2% of body mass can impair performance. One can measure the degree of an individual's hydration by urine-specific gravity or by computing differences between pre- and postexercise weight.[39] Water is adequate replacement for fluid losses unless excessive sweat losses occur as in endurance events. In these instances, adding electrolytes to water or supplying a sport drink with electrolytes is recommended for females just as it is for males.

A sport medicine provider along with a sports' nutritionist can serve as a valuable resource for the female athlete in helping her plan her nutritional needs.

Female Athlete Triad

The female athlete triad is a complex medical syndrome of three interrelated entities: low energy availability (with or without disordered eating), menstrual dysfunction, and low BMD. The latter two entities can be linked to dysfunction secondary to low energy availability (Fig. 27.1).[40-42] The female athlete triad appears to be most common in sports where the "lean look" is valued (e.g., running, gymnastics, figure skating, and ballet) but can occur in any physically active female. A female athlete may present with one or more of the three components of the triad and may be mildly to severely affected in any of the three. However, up to 15.9% of athletes with the triad are reported to present severely affected in all three components.[43]

Energy availability is the term that refers to the total energy needed by a female athlete to perform all of her daily physiologic functions, including athletic activities. Energy availability is defined as energy intake (kcal) minus exercise energy expenditure (kcal) divided by kilograms of fat-free mass or lean body mass.[43] Functional hypothalamic amenorrhea can be divided into primary amenorrhea, secondary amenorrhea, or oligomenorrhea. Primary amenorrhea is defined as the absence of menarche by 15 years of age. Secondary amenorrhea is defined as a previously menstruating female having no menstruation for three consecutive menstrual cycles. Oligomenorrhea is a menstrual cycle length greater than 35 days, or less than nine cycles per year. The Z-score measures BMD in premenopausal women. Low BMD (osteopenia) is a Z-score between −1.0 and −2.5, and osteoporosis is a Z-score of less than −2.5 with one or more secondary conditions resulting from low BMD (e.g., stress fractures).

It may be difficult to recognize an athlete with the triad. Presenting symptoms can include disordered eating, hair loss, dry skin, fatigue, weight loss, increased healing time for injuries, increased incidence of stress fractures, and absent menses. The most important screening factors for the triad suggested by the 2014 Athlete Triad Coalition Consensus Statement on Treatment

TABLE 27.7	Examples of Iron-Rich Foods

- Liver
- Lean red meats, including beef, pork, lamb
- Seafood, such as oysters, clams, tuna, salmon, and shrimp, etc.
- Beans, including kidney, lima, navy, black, pinto, soy beans, and lentils
- Iron-fortified whole grains, including cereals, breads, rice, and pasta
- Greens, including collard greens, kale, mustard greens, spinach, and turnip greens
- Vegetables, including broccoli, swiss chard, asparagus, parsley, watercress and Brussels sprout
- Chicken and turkey
- Blackstrap molasses
- Nuts
- Egg yolks
- Dried fruits, such as raisins, prunes, dates, and apricots
- Curry powder, paprika, thyme

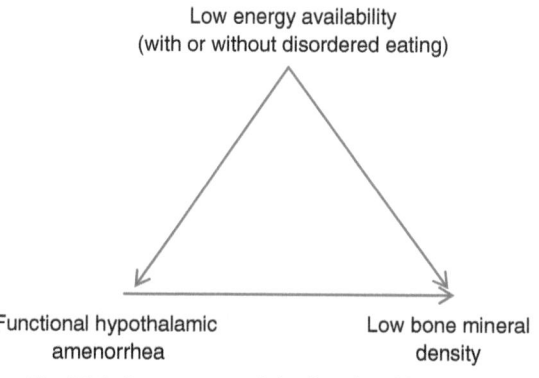

Fig. 27.1 Components of the female athlete triad.

TABLE 27.8 Suggested Screen Questions for Diagnosing the Triad[a]

Have you ever had a menstrual period?
How old were you when you had your first menstrual period?
When was your most recent menstrual period?
How many periods have you had in the past 12 months?
Are you presently taking any female hormones (estrogen, progesterone, birth control pills)?
Do you worry about your weight?

[a]Committee on Obstetric Practice. Physical Activity and Exercise During Pregnancy and the Postpartum Period. No. 650. Washington, DC: The American College of Obstetricians and Gynecologists; 2015:135–142.
DeSouza MJ, Nattiv A, Joy E, et al. 2014 female athlete coalition consensus statement on treatment and return to play of the female athlete triad: 1st international conference held in San Francisco, California, May 2012 and 2nd international conference held in Indianapolis, Indiana, May 2013. Br J Sports Med. 2014;48:289–309.

TABLE 27.9 Triad Coalition Panel Recommendations for Dual Energy X-Ray Absorptiometry Scanning

Who Should Get DEXA Scans for BMD Testing
"High risk" triad risk factors: (need 1)
  History of a DSM-V diagnosed ED
  BMI ≤17./5 kg/m², <85% estimated weight, OR recent weight loss of ≥10% in 1 month
  Menarche ≥16 years of age
  Current or history of <6 menses over 12 months
  Two prior stress reactions/fractures, one high-risk stress reaction/fracture or a low-energy nontraumatic fracture
  Prior Z-score of <–2.0 (after at least 1 year from baseline DEXA)
OR
"Moderate risk" triad risk factors: (need 2)
  Current or history of DE for 6 months or greater
  BMI between 17.5 and 18.5, <90% estimated weight, OR recent weight loss of 5%–10% in 1 month
  Menarche between ages 15 and 16 years
  Current or history of 6–8 menses over 12 months
  One prior stress reaction/fracture
  Prior Z-score between –1.0 and –2.0 (after at least a 1-year interval from baseline DEXA)

BMI, Body mass index; DE, disordered eating; DSM-V, diagnostic and statistical manual of mental disorders; ED, eating disorders.
Joy E, Kussman A, Nattiv A. 2016 update on eating disorders in athletes: a comprehensive narrative review with a focus on clinical assessment and management. Br J Sports Med. 2016;50:154–162.

and Return to Play of the Female Athlete Triad expert panel are listed in Table 27.8.[41] Psychologic characteristics that may be present in those with the triad include low self-esteem, depression, and anxiety disorders.[42,44] Physical findings on exam include anemia, orthostatic hypotension, electrical irregularities, vaginal atrophy, and bradycardia.[41,45]

The diagnosis of low energy availability can be difficult to make because there is no single test to make this diagnosis. It is recommended that a body mass index (BMI) rather than merely a weight of athlete should be obtained. If the BMI is less than 17.5 kg/m², the state of low energy availability is likely present. Low energy availability has been said to be less than 45 kcal/kg of lean body mass per day. Treatment for low energy availability focuses on a well-designed nutritional plan to attempt to reverse weight loss, achieve a BMI of ≥18.5 kg/m² or 90% of predicted weight, and have a minimum energy intake of 2000 kcal/day.[41] The diet needs to contain a balance of carbohydrates, fats, and proteins. Some athletes have low energy availability not because of inadequate energy intake but because of excessive exercise.

In making the diagnosis of amenorrhea (now known as functional hypothalamic amenorrhea), one must first rule out pregnancy and/or other metabolic or hormonal conditions that can lead to amenorrhea. Some of these conditions include thyroid disorders, hyperprolactinemia, primary ovarian dysfunction, polycystic ovary syndrome, and hypothalamic or pituitary disorders. In the female athlete with primary amenorrhea, physical examination of the female genitalia is mandatory to rule out anatomic abnormalities. Additional testing with blood work and/or hormonal challenges may reveal a correctable metabolic or hormonal irregularity. The treatment for amenorrhea or the menstrual irregularity of the triad is oral contraceptives; however, this is not just to regulate a girl's period but rather to resolve the major issue, which is energy imbalance.

Low BMD can be diagnosed through dual energy x-ray absorptiometry (DEXA) scans. The indications for DEXA scanning include a history of eating disorders, low BMI (≤17.5 kg/m²), low body weight, menarche ≥16 years of age, decreased number of menses over the previous year, history of stress fractures, and

a history of low Z-scores.[43] Screening is also indicated if the athlete has two or more moderate risk factors, which are similar to the high risk factors but less extreme; for example, menarche between the ages of 15 and 16 or a BMI of 17.5 and 18.5 or perhaps just one past stress fracture (Table 27.9). Treatment of low BMD should start with increasing energy availability and supplementing with calcium and vitamin D. The use of bisphosphonates, commonly used in postmenopausal females to increase bone density, is controversial and, in fact, is not US Food and Drug Administration approved for the young athlete nor are other medications presently used in treating low BMD in postmenopausal females.

Evaluation and treatment of the female athlete triad is a complex issue and should be determined by a multispecialty treatment team. At present there are no standard guidelines as far as returning the athlete to full participation. One needs to monitor carefully: caloric intake, weight gain, and resumption of menses. Sustained low energy availability can impair health and have associated with it cardiovascular, endocrine, reproductive, skeletal, gastrointestinal, renal, and central nervous system issues. Therefore early recognition and intervention in the female athlete with the triad is essential.

Osteoporosis and Osteopenia

Many women enjoy continuing their athletic careers as they age. There are senior or masters level competitions in a variety of sports. These female athletes exercise and train at a high level of intensity to maintain their sports participation. One of the

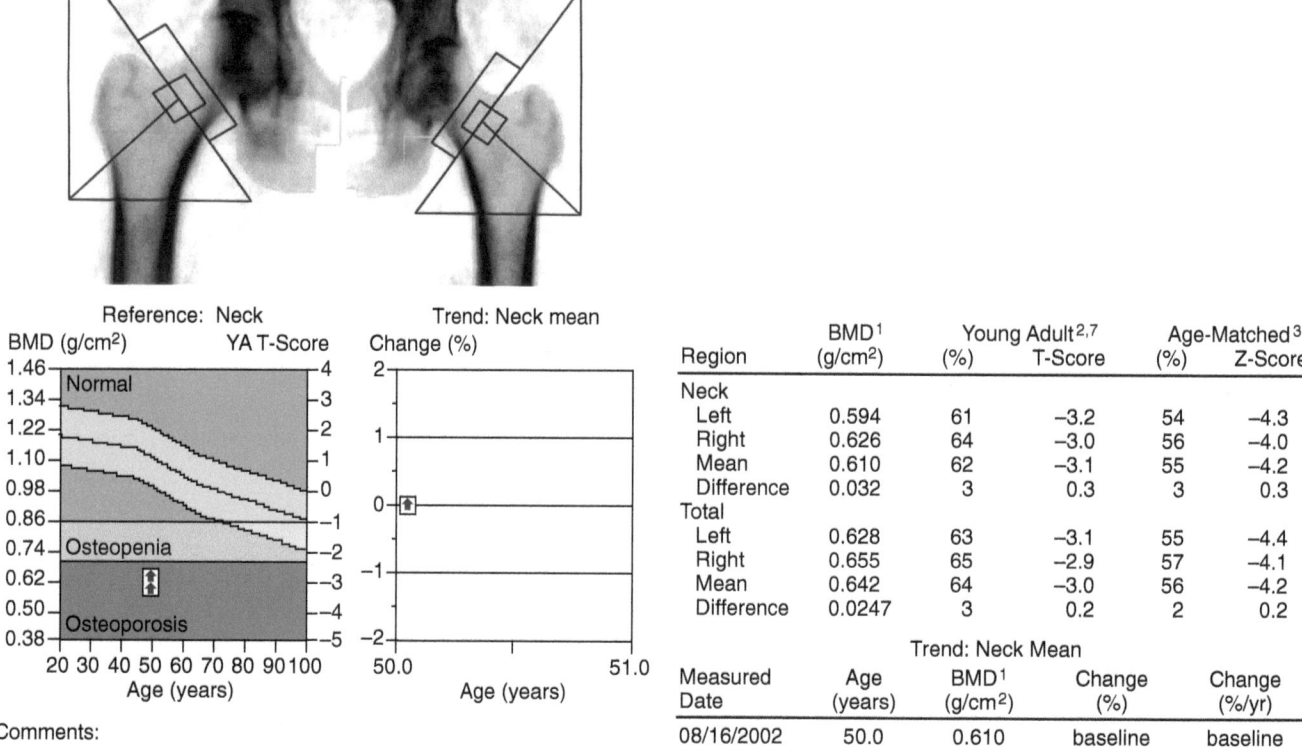

Fig. 27.2 Example of a DEXA scan.

Region	BMD[1] (g/cm²)	Young Adult[2,7] (%)	T-Score	Age-Matched[3] (%)	Z-Score
Neck					
Left	0.594	61	−3.2	54	−4.3
Right	0.626	64	−3.0	56	−4.0
Mean	0.610	62	−3.1	55	−4.2
Difference	0.032	3	0.3	3	0.3
Total					
Left	0.628	63	−3.1	55	−4.4
Right	0.655	65	−2.9	57	−4.1
Mean	0.642	64	−3.0	56	−4.2
Difference	0.0247	3	0.2	2	0.2

Trend: Neck Mean

Measured Date	Age (years)	BMD[1] (g/cm²)	Change (%)	Change (%/yr)
08/16/2002	50.0	0.610	baseline	baseline

TABLE 27.10   Defining Osteoporosis and Osteopenia Using the WHO "T-Score"

Normal BMD	BMD within 1 SD (T-score: +1 or −1) of the young adult mean
Osteopenia	BMD between 1 and 2.5 SD below the young adult mean (T-score: −1 to −2.5 SD)
Osteoporosis	BMD 2.5 SD or more below the young adult mean (T-score: −2.5 SD or lower)

BMD, Bone mineral density; *SD*, standard deviation; *WHO*, World Health Organization.
www.nof.org.

consequences of menopause in a female is a decrease in bone density secondary to decreasing estrogen levels, which results in an increased risk of fractures. As noted previously in the Female Athlete Triad section, BMD is most reliably measured by DEXA scanning (Fig. 27.2). Scores obtained are compared with a healthy, average, young adult population to yield a *T-score* rather than a *Z-score*, which is most frequently used in a younger population to compare the athlete's bone density to someone of like age. According to the World Health Organization, osteopenia is defined as a *T-score* of −1.0 to −2.5 standard deviation (SD) below normal average age-matched BMD, and osteoporosis is a *T-score* lower than −2.5 SD below average age-matched BMD, as measured by the DEXA scan Table 27.10.

There are specific indications for DEXA testing in the postmenopausal female: females over the age of 65, or females who are 50 to 65 who have a suspected secondary cause of osteoporosis such as hyperthyroidism, inflammatory bowel disease, chemotherapy, and hyperparathyroidism. Females 60 to 64 should be screened if they have a history of alcoholism, tobacco use, low weight (<125 pounds), sedentary lifestyle, or estrogen deficiency from a premature menopause either natural or as a result of hysterectomy and oophorectomy. Other risk factors that may merit early DEXA testing are first-degree relatives with osteoporotic fractures, previous history of fracture over 40 years of age, Caucasian or Asian heritage, and an anovulatory state for more than 5 years on no estrogen replacement.

Treatment for bone loss should start early in the osteopenia phase, if not before, to potentially slow the rate of the loss. Treatments for osteopenia and osteoporosis are both nonpharmacologic and pharmacologic. The primary nonpharmacologic treatment is weight-bearing exercise. Females should also stop smoking and avoid excessive weight loss. BMD is higher in postmenopausal females who exercise.[46] It has been shown that athletes (runners) who performed weight-bearing exercise had a higher BMD than athletes (swimmers) who did non-weight-bearing exercise. The athletes in this study had a higher BMD of the femoral neck than sedentary women.[46] Pharmacologic treatment includes 1000 to 1500 mg of calcium and 400 to 800 IU of vitamin D supplementation for at-risk females. The most controversial treatment may be hormone replacement therapy. The US Preventive Services Task Force (USPSTF)[47] along with the American Academy of Family Physicians (AAFP), and other groups, recommend against menopausal hormone therapy to prevent chronic conditions.

This includes a combination of estrogen and progestin, or estrogen therapy alone.[47] The best treatment for the female athlete with osteopenia and osteoporosis is not clear. It is known that weight-bearing exercise, calcium and vitamin D supplementation and smoking cessation are important. Athletes should consult their health care provider to make an informed decision as to what may be best for them.

Birth Control

There are many contraceptive choices available to women. Between 2006 and 2008, 7.3% of women who were at risk for an unintended pregnancy were not using a contraceptive method.[49] The female athlete, if sexually active, should have a yearly gynecologic examination and review contraceptive choices with her physician. Multiple alternatives for contraceptive use are available and include: intrauterine devices, spermicidal products, diaphragms, cervical caps, female condoms, male condoms, injectable progestin, vaginal ring (NuvaRing), implantable hormonal inserts, and oral contraceptives (Table 27.11). See Table 27.12 for a review of major risks and benefits of each of these methods of contraception.

At present, the most popular form of contraception is the oral contraceptive pill (OCP). Two types of OCPs are the progestin-only pill and the combination estrogen and progestin pill. The OCPs are 91% to 99% effective in preventing pregnancy. Their mechanism of action is the exogenous hormone in the pill, which suppresses the pituitary to decrease production of follicle-stimulating hormones and luteinizing hormones and thus suppresses ovulation. Female athletes who suffer from heavy or painful menstrual cycles may get decreased flow and pain relief from the OCP. This use may be the most important

noncontraceptive use for the OCP. Contraindications to the use of the OCP include personal history of blood clots, abnormal liver functions, breast cancer, migraines, and certain cardiac conditions. Many female athletes prefer not to take the OCP out of fear of weight gain. Several excellent studies have shown that OCPs are not responsible for weight gain, and in a study on runners compared to nonathletic controls, OCPs had neither an increase of weight, nor an increase of fat mass or body fat compared to nonathletic controls.[50,51]

A female's choice to start contraception and the method used should solely be hers. The goal of the sports medicine provider should be to provide accurate information about each method and to address concerns or questions to help the female athlete find a safe and effective method of birth control that does not interfere with her athletic lifestyle or put her health at risk.

Pregnancy

Many of the early exercise guidelines during pregnancy were based on supposition rather than well-executed scientific studies. Previous concerns that exercise might result in preterm labor are unproven.[52] It is currently recognized that mild to moderate exercise during pregnancy is not only safe but advantageous.[53] In 2015, the International Olympic Committee organized a meeting of 15 experts on the physiologic effects of exercise during pregnancy. Consensus from this meeting was that while pregnant women should be encouraged to "maintain an active lifestyle, i.e. do mild to moderate exercise, the limits and intensity of highly strenuous exercise on the fetus has not been thoroughly researched."[54]

Benefits of regular exercise include: improving self-image, avoiding excessive weight gain during pregnancy, aiding in the management of gestational diabetes, decreasing musculoskeletal complaints of pregnancy (i.e., an increase in core strength can result in fewer complaints of low back pain). In order to ensure safety, the pregnant female should undergo a preexercise program evaluation with her obstetric provider to review her desired program in terms of both the actual activities and intensity, and the length of the workout. Contraindications to exercise during pregnancy are listed in Table 27.13. Sports that are safe for the pregnant athlete and sports to avoid during pregnancy are listed

TABLE 27.11 Classes of Contraceptive Methods	
IUD	Progestin
Spermicidal products	Vaginal ring
Condoms	Implantable hormones
Diaphragms	Oral contraceptives

IUD, Intrauterine device.

TABLE 27.12 Risk and Benefits of Popular Contraceptive Methods		
Contraceptive Method	Risks	Benefits
Intrauterine device	Perforation of the uterus	Length of time it can be used
Spermicidal products	Used alone, low effectiveness	Improves effectiveness in preventing pregnancy when used with diaphragm, cap, condoms
Diaphragm	Low effectiveness, user error	Nonhormone contraception
Cervical cap	Low effectiveness, user error	Nonhormonal contraceptive
Condoms (male/female)	Allergic reaction to latex	Low cost, may reduce incidence of STI
Injectable progestin	Variation of menstrual bleeding Injection site reaction	Only has to be administered every 3 months
Vaginal ring	Blood clots from hormone	Does not need to be taken or changed daily
Implantable hormonal inserts	Skin infection at insertion site	Long-term use (3 years)
Oral contraceptives	Blood clots, migraines	Most effective method if used correctly

STI, Sexually transmitted infection.

TABLE 27.13 Contraindications to Exercise During Pregnancy[55,a]

Relative
Poorly controlled maternal hypertension
Poorly controlled maternal diabetes
Previous spontaneous abortion
Severe anemia
Underweight or maternal eating disorder

Absolute
Preeclampsia/eclampsia
Premature rupture of membranes
Placenta previa
Persistent 2nd or 3rd trimester bleeding
Preterm labor
Incompetent cervix
Growth restricted fetus

Committee on Obstetric Practice. *Physical Activity and Exercise During Pregnancy and the Postpartum Period. No 650.* Washington, DC: The American College of Obstetricians and gynecologists; 2015:135–142.

TABLE 27.14 Safe Sports and Sports to Avoid When Pregnant

Safe Sports During Pregnancy[a]

Walk	Aerobics
Swim	Pilates
Cycle	Yoga
Run	

Sports to Avoid During Pregnancy
Contact sports can potentially cause harm to the unborn fetus.
Downhill skiing includes the risk of fall and altitude sickness.
Scuba diving has the potential for decompression sickness.

[a]Always check with your physician first.

in Table 27.14 A healthy pregnancy and delivery should be the ultimate goal, and a well-structured exercise program can help attain that goal.

Several exercise precautions are recommended. The pregnant female needs to avoid substantial or sudden increases in temperature, as an increase in core body temperature greater than 103°F can result in neural tube defects during the development of the neural tube.[56] Pregnant females should avoid exercise in extreme heat and humidity, and should workout early in the morning or later in the day when temperatures are cooler, decrease the intensity of training (especially in hot environments), and ensure adequate fluid intake.

Postural changes (progressive lumbar lordosis and anterior rotation of the pelvis), which result from the pregnant uterus moving the center gravity forward, can combine with increased size and weight of breast tissue to necessitate significant balance adaptations to avoid injury while exercising. Signs that cause the pregnant mother to refrain from or discontinue exercise instantly including vaginal bleeding, amniotic fluid leakage, decreased fetal movement, chest pain, shortness of breath (before and during exercise), and dizziness.

The National Collegiate Athletic Association (NCAA) has guidelines for the pregnant student athlete that focus on the athlete's safety, and the safety of the unborn fetus.[57] The athlete can be granted a 1-year extension of the 5-year period of eligibility to account for lost time during the pregnancy. The NCAA guideline on pregnancy states that the team physician and the student's health care provider should work together to help the pregnant student athlete safely continue her sport participation. In any differences of opinion regarding the pregnant student athlete's medical care, the team physician should defer to the student athlete's health care provider.[57] The institution does not dictate the medical care.

Strenuous exercise can be started 6 to 8 weeks after delivery. Exercise does not have an adverse effect on lactation, and neither the volume nor composition of breast milk.[58] Thus a new mother can continue or resume her exercise program without worry and breastfeed without fear of negatively affecting the numerous benefits of breastfeeding.

Psychological Issues in the Female Athlete

It is important to encourage adolescent girls to participate in sport since it has been shown to increase self-esteem and decrease the incidence of depression.[59] Sport-active teenage girls are less likely to get pregnant and are more likely to graduate from high school.[59] They are also less likely to take drugs during their teenage years. The Women's Sport Foundation also emphasizes that sport participation in women will decrease shyness, increase social skills, decrease social anxiety, and help young females cope better with success and failure. Father/daughter bonding frequently develops through sport participation.[59-65]

Opinions are varied regarding the development of muscular bodies in females who exercise, from a perception of "increased sexuality" to "less feminine."[61,64] Years ago Goffman wrote that body image is a combination of many factors including the selection of clothing, the manner of carriage, and speech.[66] As females pursue characteristics associated with successful sporting performances (e.g., competitiveness and independence), and as they develop bodies that are stronger and more muscular, they may have difficulty accepting these characteristics that were once thought to be "feminine-threatening" characteristics. Over the last 30 years, the muscular body of the exercising female has become more desirable. The antithesis to the sports where the "thicker" muscular physique is desirable are sports where the lean look is favored (e.g., cross country, figure skating, and ballet). Girls involved in these activities are at risk for eating disorders as they may have an altered body image and perceive themselves as always being "too heavy."[67] Those involved in women's sports must recognize and be sensitive to these body image dilemmas that the young athletic female may face.

Moreover, most coaches of junior high, high school, or collegiate sports will tell you that coaching women necessitates a different approach than that used when coaching men. Although admittedly a generality, male players usually will respond to intimidation and encouragement to demolish the opposition whereas these tactics are typically not effective for female athletes. It is more effective to appeal to a female's emotions and encourage her to work harder out of loyalty to her team and coaches.

Boys and young men believe that proof of masculinity is rooted in sport participation; while girls and young women typically receive little such secondary gain from sports. In fact, girls—even if they are superb players—have been known to drop out of a sport to explore other activities. Coaches and parents may find this sport "burn out" or change of activity focus challenging to accept. The young athlete may find it difficult to explain to parents and her coach that she no longer wishes to participate in her sport and may find it more "socially acceptable" to have an "injury" that sidelines her. In this scenario, it is the health care provider's responsibility to be cognizant of the fact that an injury may merely be the superficial expression of a deeper issue, and they can help the young athlete and her family to recognize this reality. To retain female players during the teenage years, coaches often must be creative to make their sport enjoyable as well as competitive. As females progress through higher levels of sports their desire and motivation become more similar to their male counterparts.

Degenerative Arthritis and the Female Athlete

An important question frequently posed by the athletic female is, "Will exercise improve symptoms of osteoarthritis or does regular exercise enhance the risk of osteoarthritis?" In the United States, 27 million individuals are reported to have osteoarthritis and in the population older than 45 years of age, osteoarthritis is more common in females than males.[68] Osteoarthritis occurs both in athletic individuals and in those who are sedentary. Genetics is the largest risk factor for osteoarthritis and in those with knee arthritis (the most frequent presentation of osteoarthritis), obesity is the second greatest risk factor, and being female is the third largest risk factor, ranking higher than prior trauma.[69]

In the past, when athletes developed arthritis, they were often discouraged from exercising. On the contrary, the recommendation of Healthy People 2010 included educating individuals with arthritis about their disease process, the significance of obesity as a risk factor for osteoarthritis, and the value of maintenance of an exercise program.[68,70] Recommendations for exercise include strengthening programs, stretching, and balance and agility drills. In some individuals with significant degenerative changes in lower extremity joints, decreasing weight-bearing exercise while increasing non-weight-bearing exercise (swimming, water exercise, biking, use of the elliptical machine, or using light weights with multiple repetitions) is recommended.[70,71] Water exercise is effective in those with severe arthritis who find impact activity painful, but many with significant arthritis of the spine and lower extremities can do land exercise to increase mobility and decrease the pain of arthritis while also improving balance and agility.[72] The premise is that strong muscles help protect arthritic joints, which is especially true with lower extremity osteoarthritis where a strong core and strong lower extremity muscles can help to unload an arthritic joint.

Moreover, exercise has been found to improve self-esteem and decrease depression.[73,74] Flexibility exercises decrease stiffness. The combination of enhancing balance and decreasing stiffness helps to minimize the chance of falls in the arthritic population.[75] Furthermore, Kushi reported an association between increased physical activity and decreased risk of mortality.[76]

Exercise also helps to maintain or decrease weight. Since obesity is associated with an increased risk of developing arthritis, controlling weight helps decrease the incidence of osteoarthritis.[77] Curl reported that the risk of cardiovascular disease across all age groups in females decreased as a result of increased fitness.[74]

Moreover, studies by Hannan and Panush as well as Chakravarty have demonstrated that the incidence of osteoarthritis is not increased in an exercising population when compared to age-matched controls.[78-80] Although sports that subject joints to repetitive high levels of impact and horizontal loading may increase the risk of articular cartilage degeneration, moderate exercise has not been found to increase the risk of osteoarthritis.[80,81]

Concussions

A concussion is defined as a traumatic brain injury resulting in a transient disturbance of brain function. The injury results when linear and/or rotational forces affect the brain. The process involves a complex pathophysiologic process, which involves both ionic and metabolic components at the microscopic axonal level.[82] Research continues to study changes that occur in brain function acutely and the effects that such changes have on the long-term function of the brain. The hope is to potentially improve outcome by lowering the risk for progressive and degenerative changes seen in athletes who have suffered multiple concussions.

The female athlete with a suspected concussion needs to be evaluated acutely and carefully in a controlled setting. Depending on the mechanism of injury, cervical spine injuries need to be excluded. The female athlete should not be allowed to return to play (RTP) on the day of their injury. Components of the concussion evaluation need to include obtaining subjective symptoms, evaluating the physical signs, the behavioral changes, and any cognitive impairment.[83] The severity of subjective symptoms, such as headache, feeling in a fog, and emotional symptoms, needs to be obtained. Included in the initial evaluation is the determination of the loss of consciousness and amnesia, both anterograde amnesia and retrograde amnesia. Anterograde amnesia involves memories after the injury and retrograde involves loss of memories before the injury. Numerous quick, concise, and organized sideline assessment tools have been developed to assist with evaluation at the time of the injury. The SCAT 5[84] sideline assessment tool, and its variations, is commonly used for sideline evaluation, but other tools do exist.[83] The best tool is the one the clinician feels the most competent using. A more complete evaluation in a training room, medical office, or emergency room needs to be completed after the initial assessment. This includes a comprehensive physical exam including a comprehensive neurologic exam with attention paid to motor, sensory, balance, and cognitive components. If there is a concern for an intracranial hemorrhage an emergent noncontrast computed tomography scan is ordered.

Once the acute assessment has been completed the management and treatment phase begins. It is widely accepted that physical and mental rest is the most important initial phase of the treatment. Neuropsychological testing are objective tests used to assess cognitive impairment. The tests may be administered with paper and pencil or by a computerized version. The best type of test and the timing of the test have not been

TABLE 27.15   Example of Return-to-Play Protocol Following a Concussion

The athlete must perform each activity without symptoms before progressing to the next phase
No activity, physical and mental rest
Light aerobic activity
Sport-specific exercise
Noncontact training drills
Full contact practice
Return to game play

clearly determined. It is widely accepted that the tests need to be interpreted by trained individuals, such as a neuropsychologist, with experience using the testing tool. Some clinicians utilize neuropsychological testing during various stages in the athlete's RTP protocol. When the athlete becomes asymptomatic they may start a RTP protocol, which initially begins with light aerobic exercise eventually progressing to a full contact practice. If the female athlete progresses through each phase without a return of symptoms they can be returned to full play (Table 27.15).[83]

Concussions affect males and females differently, and evidence indicates that female athletes may be at greater risk for concussions than male athletes. Analyses of injury data from the NCAA databank reveal that compared to males, female athletes sustain more concussion in games than in practice.[85] Female soccer players have the most concussions followed by female basketball, lacrosse, softball, and gymnasts. Female soccer and basketball players sustain significantly more concussion than their male counterparts in their respective sports.[85] This trend was recently confirmed in a study involving high school athletes. In gender comparable sports (soccer, basketball, and baseball/softball), high school girls had higher rates of concussions (new and recurrent concussions) compared to high school boys and concussion represented a greater proportion of all injuries.[86,87] Concussions in high school girls are more frequent from contact with playing surfaces compared to boys, whose concussions occur following player to player contact.[86]

In addition to a higher number of concussions in certain sports, concussions in female athletes tend to be more severe. A meta-analysis review concluded that traumatic brain injury results in more somatic symptoms in females than in males, including poor memory, dizziness, fatigue, irritability in response to light and noise, impaired concentration, headache, anxiety, and depression.[88] Additionally, concussed female athletes are reported to be more cognitively impaired than males and have demonstrated significantly lower visual memory composite scores compared to males.[88] Without the use of helmets, female athletes are twice as likely than males to experience cognitive impairment following concussions.[89]

A recent study has also suggested that female athletes may take 6 days longer to begin their RTP protocol after a concussion compared to age-matched male controls.[90] In a study of US collegiate athletes' neuropsychological testing, it was found that female athletes performed significantly better on verbal memory compared to male athletes, whereas male athletes performed significantly better on baseline visual memory.[91]

Compared to new concussions, recurrent concussions tend to be more serious with delayed symptom resolution and "lost athletic time." Recurrent concussions also have the potential for unfavorable long-term aftermaths. In the high school population involved in "gender comparable sports," although girls had higher rates of recurrent concussions, the number was not statistically significant, which may indicate that, in this age group, gender differences equalize after the initial concussion.[86] Some concussed athletes suffer from lingering postconcussive symptoms including chronic headaches. Female athletes report a greater incidence of symptoms from postconcussion syndrome and depression than male athletes.[89]

Various theories have been proposed to explain the differences between female and male concussions. Suggested mechanisms include biomechanical differences in head and neck acceleration forces, hormonal variances, or a perception that boys are "tougher" than girls and continue to play through injury.[86]

ORTHOPAEDIC INJURIES IN THE FEMALE ATHLETE
Epidemiology of Sports Injuries

Much has been written on the epidemiology of sports injury. When one understands the incidence of sports injuries, one can then investigate the risk factors for the most common injuries or injuries associated with the greatest time loss from sport, and by decreasing these risks, can then increase the safety of sport. Although the majority of articles on the differences in sports injuries between males and females limit their discussion to a single sport, some articles do discuss differences between injuries in male and female athletes across a variety of sports often for a single age group (pediatric, adolescent, collegiate, or postcollegiate age athlete).

An epidemiologic study on pediatric sport injuries concluded that in young males the injuries differ by injury type, diagnosis, and body area from those of young females. A retrospective chart review of a 5% random sampling of medical records of children aged 5 to 17 years seen over a 10-year period in a sports medicine clinic in a large academic pediatric hospital (Boston Children's) concluded that female athletes had a higher percentage of overuse injuries compared to traumatic injuries (62.5% vs. 37.5%), whereas male athletes had a higher percentage of acute injuries (58.2% vs. 41.9%). Females sustained more injuries to the lower extremity (65.8% vs. 53.7%) and spine (11.3% vs. 8.2%), and males sustained a higher percentage of upper extremity injuries than females (29.8% vs. 15.1%). With regard to hip and pelvis areas, females had more overuse and soft tissue injuries and males had the greater number of traumatic bony injuries. Anterior (patellofemoral) knee pain was reported to be three times greater in the female pediatric population than in the male population. Notable also in this group was that ACL injuries were almost equal in the pediatric female and male populations.[92]

In a 20-year study of multisport middle school injuries, girls exhibited a higher rate for all injuries and a higher rate for time loss than boys in matched sport. Girls had a higher injury rate during practices than during games for all sports. Practice and game injury rates were nearly identical for boys in all sports. In this study, injuries to middle school athletes in this study were less frequent and less severe than those reported for secondary school and college athletes.[93]

A study from Kaiser Permanente in California compared the pattern of injuries in male versus female athletes in seven college sports (basketball, cross country, soccer, swimming, tennis, track and field, and water polo) in a Division III college during the years 1980 to 1995. A total of 1874 sport-related injuries occurred during this period, 856 (45.7%) in females and 1018 (54.3%) in males. Female swimmers had more back/neck, shoulder, hip, knee, and foot injuries than their male counterparts, and female water polo players reported more shoulder injuries. In summarizing injuries in all sports, females reported a higher rate of hip, lower leg, and shoulder injuries while males reported a higher rate of thigh injuries. However, on the whole, the authors stated that their data suggest very little difference in the pattern of injuries between males and females competing in comparable sports.[94]

A study of 573 Division I athletes participating in 16 sports over three seasons identified 1317 reported injuries. Female athletes had a lower acute injury rate than male athletes (38.6 vs. 49.8 per 1000 athletic exposures). Males had less overuse injuries than did females (13.2 vs. 24.6 per 1000 athletic exposures).[95] In a study of 16 collegiate sports over 6 years and 14 high school sports over 7 years, Roos et al. also reported a higher rate of overuse injuries in females compared to males in sex comparable sports at both the high school and collegiate level.[96] In an analysis of injury rates for time loss and non-time-loss injuries among college student athletes Powell and Dompier found that non-time-loss injury rates were 3.5 times the time-loss injury rate for males and 5.1 times the time-loss injury rate for females.[97]

Foot and Ankle Injuries

Lateral ankle sprains are common injures in both male and female athletes. However, minor ankle sprains are 25% more common in female basketball players than in male basketball players although the incidences of severe ankle injuries appear to be equally divided between males and females.[98] The increased ankle ligamentous laxity in females has been implicated as a risk factor for the disparity of minor ankle injuries in the female.[99] Interestingly, in pro basketball athletes, males and females have similar rates of injury.[100,101] However, a study of cadets at the United States Military Academy revealed that male cadets had a greater risk of medial ankle sprains than female cadets. Although the risk of syndesmotic sprains was not statistically different for male or female cadets, females with syndesmotic sprains of their ankle had a higher time loss to injury.[102]

Achilles tendon traumatic ruptures have been reported to be more common in males, and males are reported to have better outcomes at 1 year than females regardless of the treatment method.[103,104] Posterior tibial tendon dysfunction is, in general, more common in older female athletes than in all male athletes, but the risk factors that make this overuse entity more common in females have not been clearly identified, with the exception of obesity.[105] Shin splints appear to be more common in females

TABLE 27.16	Foot Conditions More Common in Females Than Males
Bunions	Hammer toes
Bunionettes	Digital neuromas
Plantar fasciitis	Metatarsal stress fractures

perhaps related to the greater incidence of pronation in the female.[106]

Perceived functional limitation from foot pain is more common in female than male athletes and nonathletes.[107] Females are more commonly affected by bunions, bunionettes, plantar fasciitis, hammer toes, digital neuromas, and stress fractures of the metatarsals (Table 27.16). Even in young females (less than 18 years old) foot pain is common (9%) although not as common as in older females where the incidence of foot pain is reported to be 75%.[108]

The shape of a woman's foot and the proportion of foot size and shape to body size and shape is different in females than in males.[109] Males have a greater foot length compared to body height than do females.[110] Moreover, females have a 20% to 25% lower volume and lower surface area in their subtalar ankle joints with thinner cartilage in these areas as well.[111] Females have a narrower heel compared to forefoot width than do males. In fact, overall, the female foot is smaller than the male foot compared to body height.[109] Therefore a woman's shoe, especially her athletic shoe, should be made not as a "smaller male shoe" but rather different from a man's shoe in all the parameters noted above.[109]

Females' feet differ from males not only anatomically but also functionally. For example, females pronate more than males, which may be related to women's greater tendency to increased joint laxity.[106] Also, female runners have been found to be predominately midfoot strikers,[106,112,113] have greater foot abduction with running and greater rear foot motion than male runners.[113]

Since the rate of foot problems in populations that do not wear shoes has been historically reported to be low,[114] shoes have been implicated as the cause of many of the foot ailments in females including bunions, bunionettes, corns, and hammer toes. Indeed, it has been reported that 8% of females wear shoes smaller than their feet and that this trend starts with adolescence.

Moreover, as females age, their feet become stiffer and flatter. Shoe size increases. Proper shoe fit is essential for avoiding foot issues. It has been suggested that females should buy shoes later in the day as feet often swell during the day, especially with prolonged standing. Girls and women should remember that athletic shoes should "fit" when they are purchased. Buying smaller, improperly fitted shoes and hoping the shoes will "stretch out" over time is highly discouraged as such a practice can lead to foot issues. Remember the adage, "If the shoe fits wear it!" or in this case, if the shoe doesn't fit, don't buy it!

Treatment of most forefoot abnormalities in female athletes is initially conservative care with taping, pads, creams, moleskin, foot and toe exercises, and shoe modification. Surgery should be approached with great caution as secondary biomechanical problems can result. Fig. 27.3 is a radiograph of a young cross-country runner who had bunion surgery and then developed stress fractures in the second and third metatarsals from altered mechanical forces resulting from a shorter first metatarsal.

Patellofemoral Pain Syndrome

Patellofemoral syndrome (PFS) is one of the most common causes of anterior knee pain with symptoms affecting nearly 30% of the adolescent population.[115,116] The incidence of PFS is estimated at 22/1000 persons per year.[117,118] The prevalence of PFS in adolescent athletes is 20% with females affected at a rate of 2 to 10 times higher than their male counterparts.[119-121]

Patellofemoral pain syndrome (PFPS) manifests as diffuse pain in the anterior aspect of the knee, which is increased by squatting, kneeling, running, and ascending or descending stairs. The onset is insidious and is provoked by overuse or underlying malalignment. New exercises or increases in frequency, intensity, or duration of sports activities are historical facts that suggest an overuse etiology. Exercises, such as squats, lunges, or leg extensions, can increase forces up to three to four times the body weight across the patellofemoral joint,[122-124] and are commonly an inciting factor.

The patella lies proximal to the trochlea when the knee is in full extension and will engage the articulation as knee flexion

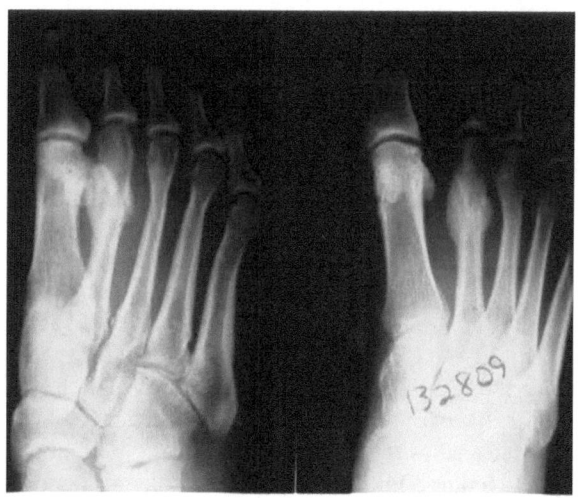

Fig. 27.3 Stress fracture of the second metatarsal in a cross-country runner following bunion surgery.

approaches 20 degrees, the patella is constrained within the trochlea, by the interaction of bony and soft tissue restrictions. Soft tissue restraints are most important in early flexion, yet as knee flexion increases, the congruency of the bony articulation becomes more pivotal as the patella is steered into the trochlea. Soft tissue constraints primarily consist of the quadriceps and patellar tendon, medial patellofemoral ligament, medial patellar retinaculum, and medial patellomeniscal ligament. Insertions of the vastus lateralis and vastus medialis oblique (VMO) are particularly important because contraction of these muscles can vary the "line of pull" on the patella. Deconditioning, altered activation, or tightness of these anatomic constructs can lead to an alteration in patellofemoral joint mechanics, ultimately resulting in abnormal patellar tracking and the development of pain.

Anterior knee pain is a common presenting symptom, and before making a diagnosis of PFPS patients should be evaluated thoroughly for other underlying pathology, such as patellar instability, osteochondral deficits, plica, and overuse injuries to the extensor mechanism, as all of these can cause pain in the anterior aspect of the knee (Table 27.17). Inciting and alleviating factors, a history of trauma, sports participation, medical history, and previous treatment are important to note. A history of patellar dislocations can help differentiate pain from instability and abnormal patellar tracking. Recurrent effusions, mechanical symptoms, and grinding should be documented and are more likely to indicate an underlying cartilage problem. Physical examination should focus on the entire lower extremity and not solely on the knee joint. Lower extremity alignment, quadriceps (Q) angle, femoral anteversion, tuberosulcus angle, and heel alignment should be assessed. Gait abnormalities, such as in-toeing, hip abductor weakness, hip and knee external rotation, and contractures of the hip abductors should be noted. The Q angle should be examined in full extension and 30 degrees of flexion because a laterally deviated patella in full knee extension can falsely decrease the Q angle. Quadriceps atrophy, especially of the VMO, is common in persons with chronic PFPS. Patellar mobility, tilt, and subluxation should be assessed both medially and laterally. A sensation of "catching" with patellar mobilization against the trochlea is suggestive of cartilage defects. The J sign suggests attenuations of the medial soft tissues and is performed by having a patient slowly extend the knee from full flexion. A positive sign is verified by lateral patellar subluxation as the knee

TABLE 27.17	Differential Diagnoses of Anterior Knee Pain	
Skeletally Immature Patients	**Skeletally Mature Patients**	**All Patients**
Osgood-Schlatter disease	Patellofemoral osteoarthritis	Patellar instability
Sinding-Larsen-Johansson syndrome	Posttraumatic arthritis	Articular cartilage injury
Distal femoral bone tumor	Patellar stress fractures	Chondromalacia patella
Osteochondritis dissecans	Quadriceps tendinopathy/rupture	Loose bodies
Symptomatic bipartite patella	Patellar tendinopathy/rupture	Inflammatory arthritis
Referred pain (Legg-Calvé-Perthes/	Referred pain (hip arthritis/lumbar spine pathology)	Infectious arthritis/bursitis
Slipped capital femoral epiphysis)	Hoffa disease	Complex regional pain syndrome
		Iliotibial band syndrome
		Bursitis (pes anserine/prepatellar)
		Plica syndrome

approaches extension and leaves the constraints of the trochlear groove.

In the absence of structural disorders, the development of patellofemoral pain is multifactorial. In a systematic review, Lankhorst et al. pooled data from 47 studies and examined 523 variables.[125] Compared with control subjects, persons with PFPS demonstrated larger Q angles, less hip abduction strength, lower knee extension peak torque, and less hip external rotation strength.[126] Alterations in neuromuscular activation patterns have also been reported. Electromyography studies have found delayed activation of the VMO compared with the vastus lateralis in patients with PFPS.[127,128] Multiple retrospective studies have reported that PFPS is associated with weak hip abduction. However, these conclusions have been called into question. The retrospective nature of the studies begs the question whether muscle weakness is a cause or an effect of PFPS. Three recent prospective studies suggest that female athletes with greater hip abduction strength may be at an increased risk for the development of PFPS.[129-131] Increased cartilage stress may play a role in the development of PFPS. Farrokhi et al. examined patellofemoral biomechanical factors and found that compared with pain-free control subjects, women with patellofemoral pain demonstrated elevated hydrostatic pressure and shear stress across the patellofemoral joint.[132] Carlson et al. evaluated patellar tracking in female athletes and found that rigorous athletic training might not be adequate to produce PFPS in female adolescents; rather, it may be caused by a combination of physical activity and pathologic kinematics.[133]

Treatment for PFPS is conservative and revolves around physical therapy. The goal of physical therapy is to restore soft tissue muscular and capsuloligamentous balance of the patellofemoral articulation. Rehabilitative exercises should include a quadriceps, hamstrings, and iliotibial band stretching regimen to restore flexibility, as well as patellar mobilizations to relax contracted lateral capsular structures, quadriceps, and the patellar tendon. A strengthening program that involves the hip abductors and external rotators as well as the quadriceps should be instituted. It is important to protect patellofemoral articulation from high stress by focusing on isometric and short arc closed chain concentric and eccentric muscle strengthening and avoiding open chain exercises and deep flexion weight-bearing activities. McConnell patellar taping, kinesio-taping or patellar bracing to centralize the patella also may be useful during sports participation.

Anterior Cruciate Ligament Injuries

With an exponential rise in the number of females participating in organized athletics, physicians are treating an increasing number of ACL tears in this population. Several studies have demonstrated an injury rate of 1 to 3 per 10,000 athletic exposures in females,[134-137] which is two to six times the rate seen in males.[100,135,138-140,142] Most of these ruptures occur during pivoting, cutting, changing directions, and jumping.[136,138,143-148] This disproportionate injury rate has been the driving force for numerous studies on noncontact ACL injuries in females including risk factors and prevention programs for vulnerable athletes.[136,138,139,142,149-154]

Risk Factors for Noncontact Anterior Cruciate Ligament Injury

Sex differences in the rate of noncontact ACL injury are multifactorial. Any factor that either increases the load placed on the ligament, or lowers the ligament's ultimate load to failure will increase the rate of rupture.[150] Potential risk factors can be grouped into anatomic, hormonal, environmental, and neuromuscular factors (Table 27.18).

Anatomic risk factors for ACL injury in female athletes are body mass, ligament size and mechanical properties, bony morphology, and limb alignment. A high BMI has been postulated to decrease core stability, resulting in excessive trunk motion and an increase in valgus load on the knee. For these reasons, BMI is associated with increased the ACL tear risk.[140,213] The cross-sectional area of the ACL has been shown to be significantly smaller in women,[165,169,214] and is related more to the height of the patient than the weight.[169] In addition, female ligaments show different mechanical properties, including lower stress and strain at failure, and a lower modulus of elasticity, even when size is accounted for.[168] This difference in ligament biomechanical properties can be explained by hormonal factors and differences in collagen genotypes. The AA genotype of the COL12A1 was shown to be associated with ACL injury,[215] while the CC genotype of COL5A1, and the TT genotype of COL1A1 have been shown to be protective.[216,217] Increased Q angle is proposed to be a risk factor because a lateral tug on the quadriceps increases medial knee stress.[218] Hip varus and knee valgus can lead to increased loading of the knee, especially when landing from a jump.[183] Femoral notch measurements have been associated with ACL rupture; however, there is no sex difference in notch size.[164,165,167,170] This injury risk seems to be related more to the size of the ligament, as notch volume has been shown to correlate with ligament size.[169] A larger femoral condyle offset ratio in combination with a larger lateral tibial slope is thought to increase anterior tibial translation and internal rotation, both of which increase strain.[150,214,219,220] Despite these reports, no single specific anatomic risk factor has conclusively been noted to be a reliable predictor of noncontact ACL injury.

Hormonal influences as risk factors for noncontact ACL injury are a topic of continual debate. This group represents one of the more obvious sex differences, due to elevated serum levels of hormones such as estrogen, progesterone, and relaxin in females. Physiologic levels of the hormones estradiol and relaxin have been shown to decrease ligament strength and enhance soft tissue relaxation. Although ligament tissue contains hormone receptors, suggesting a potential role of hormonal fluctuations on tear rates,[153,221] estrogen does not appear to have any negative effects on ligamentous mechanical properties.[171] Relaxin, on the other hand, has been shown to increase protein expression responsible for collagen degradation, and decreased collagen synthesis, thus potentially lowering the ultimate stress to failure of the ligament.[172] In addition, several proteins, such as agracan and fibromodulin, have been found to be upregulated in torn ligament tissue at the time of reconstruction.[222] It has also been suggested that hormonal influences on injury may be a result of neuromuscular changes during the menstrual cycle rather

TABLE 27.18   Summary of Risk Factors for Anterior Cruciate Ligament Injury

Anatomic

- Quadriceps angle,[155] knee valgus,[136,156-158] and increased foot pronation,[159-162] have been associated with increased risk of anterior cruciate ligament (ACL) tear in some studies.
- The role of body mass index is not clear,[163,164] but higher indices seems to be associated with injury risk.[132]
- Femoral notch indices,[165-167] ligament geometry,[140,164,165,167,168] and tibial measurements are not definitively associated with increased risk of ACL tear; however, the smaller femoral notch in females, even when normalized to body weight, seems to be more associated with risk of injury.[140,169,170]

Hormonal

- Sex hormones affect knee ligament laxity, but the overall effect is not clear.[171,172]
- Injury rates have been noted to vary with the phase of the menstrual cycle.[162,173-177]
- No evidence exists to recommend activity modification or restriction with respect to the phase of menstrual cycle to prevent ACL injury.

Environmental

- Harder ground, resulting from high evaporation and low rainfall, may increase the shoe traction interface.[178]
- Increasing the shoe-surface coefficient may increase risk of injury (direct) and alter movement (indirect).[179-181]

Biomechanical

- The ACL has different mechanical properties in women.[168]
- Neuromuscular factors appear to be the most critical difference between adult men and women and are modifiable.[182]
- The knee is part of a kinetic chain and as such is influenced by motion of the trunk, core, hips, and ankle.[183-189]
- Awkward landing, inability to recover from perturbed gait, and difficulty changing directions have been associated with increased risk of ACL injury.[190-192]
- Women exhibit less knee and hip flexion, increased knee valgus, increased internal rotation of the hip, and increased external rotation of the tibia when landing from a jump or changing direction.[190-199]
- Quadriceps-dominant activation patterns during deceleration, landing, and cutting have been noted in females.[190,194,195,199,200-203]
- Decreased quadriceps stiffness and strength and decreased knee stiffness in females are thought to be associated with increased risk.[176,204-206]
- Fatigue is associated with loss of dynamic control of the lower extremity.[207-211]
- Imbalance in strength, flexibility, and coordination is thought to be associated with increased risk of ACL injury.[134,158,209,212]

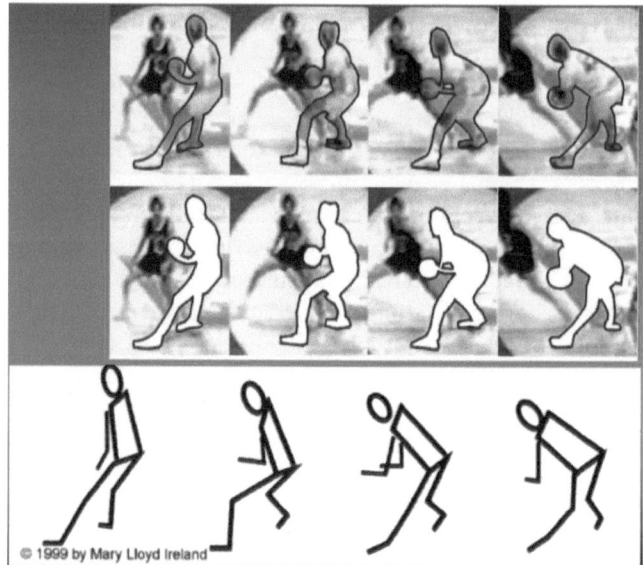

© 1999 by Mary Lloyd Ireland

Fig. 27.4 Mechanism of noncontact anterior cruciate ligament injuries: female basketball player at the time of anterior cruciate ligament injury.

Modifiable environmental risk factors include shoes, surfaces, and shoe-surface dynamics. There has been much research regarding the interaction of the playing surface with the athlete's footwear.[178-181,224-226] Playing surface material,[179,181,226,227] as well as the environmental condition,[178] can influence the tear rate. Specifically, surfaces and conditions that provide higher traction have been shown to increase the risk of injury.[179,180,225] However, researchers have yet to find the ideal shoe-surface combination that provides adequate traction for performance without increasing the risk of knee injury.[224] Furthermore, the variation of athletic movement required in different sports combined with individual differences in style of play precludes the development of a single "perfect" shoe-surface combination that can be generalized to a wide range of athletic events.[225,228]

Research on neuromuscular risk factors has revealed some of the most promising data on factors associated with ACL injuries; for example, 75% to 85% of noncontact injuries occur when landing from a jump, abruptly stopping, or pivoting to change direction with the knee in near full extension (Fig. 27.4).[136,138,143-148,221,229] Muscle strength, coordination, recruitment patterns, endurance, and knee stiffness are all important variables for maintaining knee joint stability. Compared with men and normalized to body weight, women have significantly weaker quadriceps and hamstrings and have a diminished ability to produce adequate muscle stiffness across the knee.[176,190,207] Additionally, elite female athletes tend to have quadriceps-dominant knees and forceful quadriceps contraction without appropriate hamstring co-contraction in response to the anterior tibial translation that increases ligament strain.[182,221] Female athletes who sustain ACL injuries also have significantly greater peak valgus angles and moments around the knee.[230] This observation has been validated by "drop jump" studies, which showed that in contrast to males, females achieved maximal hip adduction, knee valgus, and ankle eversion earlier in the stance phase and had less hip external rotation during landing; in addition, the

than a direct effect on knee ligaments.[156,221,223] Using urine and salivary hormone levels, as well as patient reported timelines, studies have shown that ACL tears are more likely to occur during preovulatory stages.[151,173-175] However, during this time period the ACL demonstrates less laxity and increased stiffness, contradicting the theory that estrogen increases ligament laxity and enhances the risk for rupture.[151] Hormonal intervention or activity modification based on the phase of the menstrual cycle is not recommended.

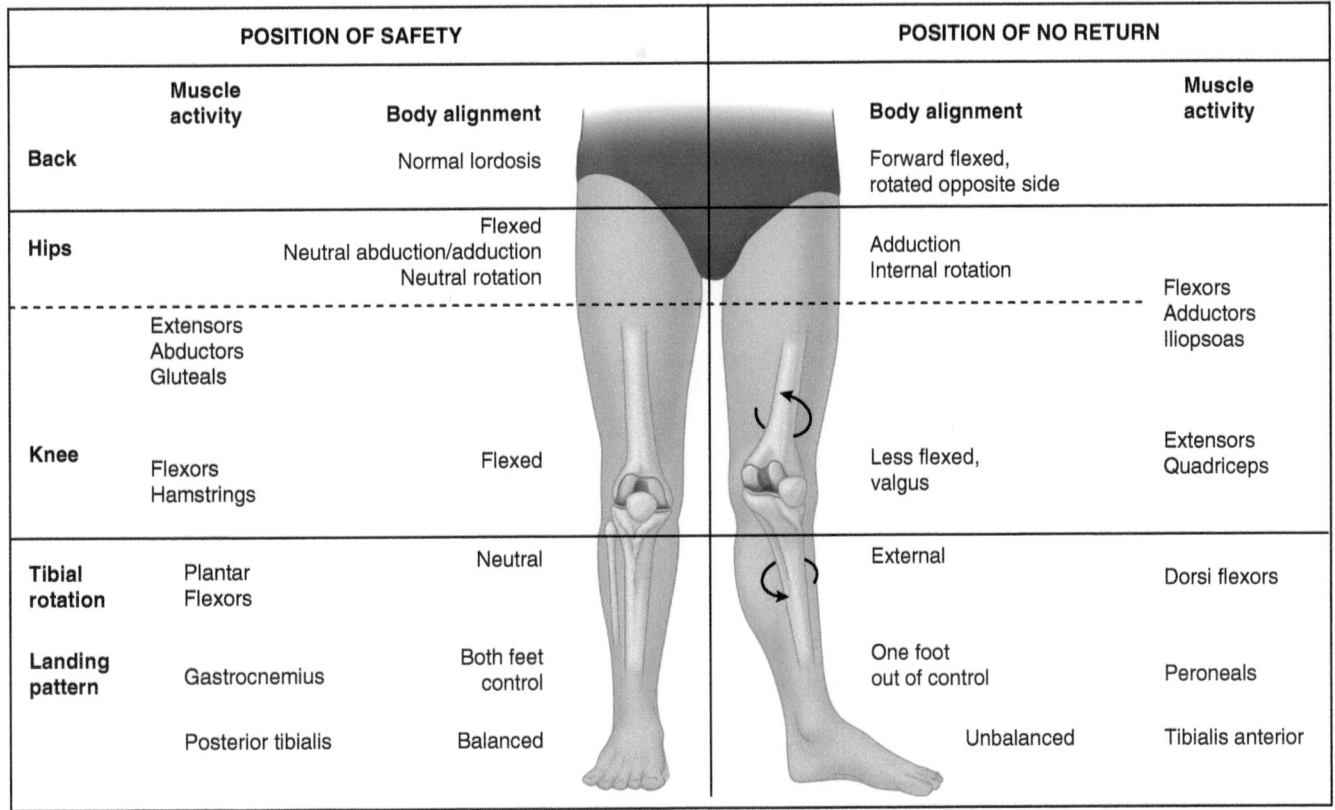

POSITION OF SAFETY				POSITION OF NO RETURN		
	Muscle activity	Body alignment			Body alignment	Muscle activity
Back		Normal lordosis			Forward flexed, rotated opposite side	
Hips		Flexed Neutral abduction/adduction Neutral rotation			Adduction Internal rotation	Flexors Adductors Iliopsoas
	Extensors Abductors Gluteals					
Knee	Flexors Hamstrings	Flexed			Less flexed, valgus	Extensors Quadriceps
Tibial rotation	Plantar Flexors	Neutral			External	Dorsi flexors
Landing pattern	Gastrocnemius	Both feet control			One foot out of control	Peroneals
	Posterior tibialis	Balanced			Unbalanced	Tibialis anterior

Fig. 27.5 Comparison of the position of safety with the position of no return that places the athlete at risk for anterior cruciate ligament injury.

angular velocity of knee valgus was nearly double.[230] The center of gravity, postural adjustment, and motion patterns of the lower extremity kinetic chain affect loading at the knee.[183-189,231] ACL load determinants include ground reaction force, body weight, muscle loading, knee stiffness, and the material properties of the ligament such as size, shape, and modulus.[231] Poor postural adjustment,[189,192,193] combined with knee extension,[190,191,193-195,232] valgus,[190,191,193-195,232] and internal rotation,[191-193] increases the load placed on the knee (Fig. 27.5). To make matters worse, neuromuscular control is reduced in fatigued states,[207-211] with less time to prepare for a cutting or landing movement.[189,200,233,234] Numerous tests have been developed to identify those athletes with poor neuromuscular control.[186,235-238] One such test, the single leg step-down test asks subjects to perform a series of controlled mini-squats. Athletes with poor performance on the test show some of the same kinematics seen at the time of ligament rupture (Fig. 27.6).[239] Although more research is necessary, it is apparent that the combination of dynamic neuromuscular control patterns and inherent mechanical properties of the ACL are the principal contributing factors for increased injury rates in females.

Prevention of Noncontact Anterior Cruciate Ligament Injury

Identification of modifiable neuromuscular risk factors for non-contact ACL injury has fostered the development of successful, specific, preventative training programs to decrease knee loading and to improve protective movements in the lower extremity

TABLE 27.19 Measured Benefits of Anterior Cruciate Ligament Prevention Programs

- Decreased landing forces
- Decreased dynamic knee valgus
- Decreased varus and valgus movements of the lower extremity
- Increased muscular activation
- Improved movement patterns

kinetic chain (Table 27.19). Several studies have shown that these neuromuscular training regimens can reduce the risk of tear in specific patient groups.[134,153,154,240-244] Many of these programs incorporate sport-specific drills to help athletes safely respond to unanticipated movement while emphasizing stretching, strengthening, aerobic exercise, agility drills, plyometrics, and risk awareness.[224] Recent adjuncts to prevention programs include core, hamstring, and quadriceps strengthening exercises to decrease fatigue, and the education of athletes on appropriate landing and cutting techniques.[183] By training female athletes to alter their techniques and mechanics, these programs have demonstrated increased muscle activation and decreased landing forces, dynamic knee valgus, and varus and valgus moments.[153,244] Although the long-term effectiveness of these programs is continually being evaluated, the early data and outcomes have shown immense promise, and some form of neuromuscular training is recommended for all at-risk individuals.

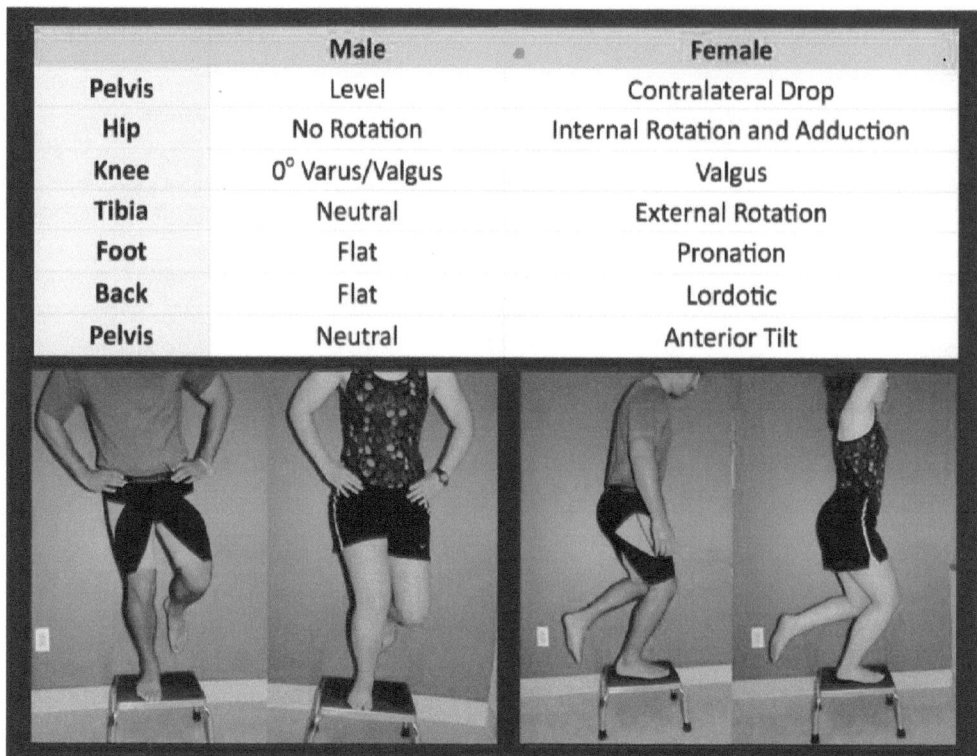

	Male	Female
Pelvis	Level	Contralateral Drop
Hip	No Rotation	Internal Rotation and Adduction
Knee	0° Varus/Valgus	Valgus
Tibia	Neutral	External Rotation
Foot	Flat	Pronation
Back	Flat	Lordotic
Pelvis	Neutral	Anterior Tilt

Fig. 27.6 Comparison of male and female strategies while performing a single leg squat.

Anterior Cruciate Ligament Reconstruction

Treatment guidelines for female athletes that sustain ACL tears are the same as those of their male counterparts, as overall results are similar between sexes.[245-250] Regardless of the type of graft used, studies have demonstrated that women report improved knee function and less instability after reconstruction.[245-249,251-259] Although previous studies have cautioned the use of hamstring grafts in women,[248,251,252,256] more recent studies have shown similar outcomes between graft type,[249,259,260] with lower surgical morbidity and improved pain with hamstring grafts.[255,258,259] The degree of postoperative anterior knee pain is variable, but less pain appears to occur after hamstring reconstruction in both men and women.[255] Graft fixation, surgical technique, and postoperative rehabilitation are not sex specific.

After surgery, female athletes may struggle to return to their active lifestyles. In a retrospective analysis of soccer players, Brophy et al. found that after reconstruction, females were less likely to RTP, and more likely to have future ACL surgery than their male counterparts.[261] Unfortunately, ligament reconstruction also has not been shown to prevent posttraumatic osteoarthritis.[262,263] Lohmander et al. evaluated female soccer players 12 years after an ACL injury.[262] Of the 84 women who answered questionnaires, 75% had knee-related symptoms that affected their quality of life and 51% had radiographic changes consistent with osteoarthritis. However, the development of posttraumatic osteoarthritis does not appear to be sex specific. After radiographic analysis of the MOON cohort, female sex was not identified as a risk factor for joint space loss at 2 or 6 years after surgery.[264,265] In addition, in a large retrospective cohort study of patients with ACL tears, no sex differences were found in the long-term results

of reconstruction compared with nonoperative management. However, regardless of gender, surgery decreased the need for subsequent procedures and was associated with fewer meniscal and chondral lesions.[266] Despite failing to prevent arthritis, ACL reconstruction provides stability and function, and decreases further intra-articular injury.

Frozen Shoulder/Adhesive Capsulitis

Idiopathic adhesive capsulitis (AC), also known as frozen shoulder, is a common condition that presents with pain and progressive loss of active and passive shoulder motion in the absence of a known intrinsic disorder.[267] AC occurs more frequently in women between 40 and 60 years of age and is associated with diabetes, cardiovascular disease, thyroid disorder, Dupuytren contracture, as well as in those who have undergone breast cancer treatment.[268-272] AC is rare in females under 40 years of age unless they are diabetic. The nondominant shoulder is most commonly affected,[273] with the contralateral shoulder affected in 20% to 30% of patients. There is an increased incidence of bilateral shoulder AC occurring in diabetics. This often occurs months to years after the original AC has resolved.[274] AC is also less common in individuals who perform manual labor than those who have sedentary vocations.[275]

The prevalence of AC has been estimated to be between 2% and 5% with up to 70% of those patients being female.[276,277] The rationale that explains gender disparity is ambiguous, and theories have been investigated, including hormonal fluctuations, autoimmune factors, genetic predisposition, and a causal associated with HSL-B27, have been inconclusive.[278-280]

Patients usually present with an insidious onset of vague pain at the deltoid insertion following minor or no trauma with restricted external rotation and forward elevation. Older female athletes often present with several months of symptoms after the onset of pain and decreased motion begins to limit performance in their sport. On physical exam, there is not one specific nidus of pain; however, patients usually feel global shoulder pain. A decrease in the passive range of motion (ROM) in multiple planes in comparison to the contralateral shoulder is the hallmark of AC. This is initially best appreciated with external ROM with the elbow at its side and then with shoulder abduction with the scapula stabilized.

Radiographs are typically normal but important to obtain to rule out other pathology such as glenohumeral joint arthritis, calcific tendinopathy, or an unrecognized shoulder dislocation (particularly posterior dislocation). Magnetic resonance imaging (MRI) is often normal; however, it may show coracohumeral ligament thickening, rotator interval infiltration, or axillary recess thickening with edema.[281]

The pathophysiology of AC is only partly comprehended. Histologic studies have shown inflammation of the subsynovial capsular layer. This inflammation leads to capsular thickening, fibrosis, and glenohumeral joint capsule tightening, with adhesion of the axillary pouch to itself and to the anatomic humeral neck.[282] Joint capsule inflammation also causes pain that is exacerbated by movement. Capsular biopsy reveals a chronic inflammatory infiltrate, an absence of synovial lining, and a moderate to extensive subsynovial fibrosis. Perivascular lymphocytic reactions also are seen.[283]

Synovial biomarkers also reveal that chronic inflammation is present in the shoulder joint. Kim et al. found elevated levels of intercellular adhesion molecule 1 (ICAM-1), a cytokine for leukocyte activation, proliferation, adhesion, and migration.[284] Rodeo et al. found an increased presence of transforming growth factor-β (TGF-β) and TNF-α, two markers of chronic inflammation, in synovial fluid in patients with AC.[285]

There are four stages of AC. Stage 1 is the preadhesive stage where there is an inflammatory synovitic reaction without adhesive formation. During this stage the patient will have near full ROM of the shoulder; however, it is painful, especially at night. Stage 2 is the proliferation stage associated with early adhesion formation with increased loss of ROM. Stage 3 is characterized by decreased synovitis; however, more fibrosis occurs. It is in this stage that the axillary pouch is obliterated and adhered. Pain is usually less but the ROM is significantly decreased. In stage 4, the adhesions start to resolve and motion improves. Biopsies throughout these stages reveal a progression from mononuclear inflammatory infiltrates at stage 1 to reactive capsular fibrosis at stage 3 with resolution to normal capsule at the end of stage 4 (Table 27.20).[270,286]

The natural history of AC is gradual symptomatic improvement. The time of progression through each stage is variable and the entire process can take 1 to 4 years for complete resolution.[287] Conservative treatment has resulted in a patient satisfaction rate of 90% in one clinical study. In another study 50% of patients reported continued pain with 60% with motion deficits with conservative treatment.[288,289]

Initial treatment of AC is nonoperative. No gender-related differences have been found in treatment or outcomes; however,

TABLE 27.20		Stages of Frozen Shoulder Syndrome		
Stage	Phase	Timing (Months)	Presentation	Treatment
1		0–3	Pain, decreased motion	NSAIDs, PT ± injection
2	Freezing	3–9	Pain (more chronic), increasing loss of motion	NSAIDs, PT ± injection
3	Frozen	9–15	Pain lessening, significant motion loss	NSAIDs, PT ± injection, Possible surgery
4	Thawing	15–24	Resolving	Resolving

NSAIDs, Nonsteroidal antiinflammatory drugs.

compared with men, women initially tend to present with poorer external and internal rotation.[290] The initial goal of treatment is analgesia and promotion of ROM. Gentle passive ROM with physical therapy or a home exercise program is the mainstay of treatment for AC. Formal physical therapy (PT) has not been shown to be superior to a home exercise program.[287] Nonsteroidal antiinflammatory drugs have not been shown to improve pain or function compared to placebo for this condition. However, corticosteroids have demonstrated short-term analgesic efficacy with enhanced ROM.[291]

Intra-articular corticosteroid injections have been found effective in providing short-term pain analgesia and improving the patient's tolerance of a stretching program.[292] It has been shown that a single intra-articular corticosteroid injection combined with a home exercise stretching protocol was effective in improving pain and ROM in patients with AC.[293] In a prospective randomized trial, a corticosteroid injection applied before the beginning of a physical therapy program accelerated pain relief and recovery of function faster than an oral steroid alone.[294] Three prospective randomized trials revealed no difference in pain relief or ROM between patients who received a glenohumeral or subacromial injection.[295-297] While studies of corticosteroid injection have found significant short-term pain reduction and restoration of mobility, they have failed to find benefit of steroid injections past 24 weeks compared to control groups.[296,298,299] A recent clinical study found that an ultrasound-guided extra-articular collagenase clostridium histolyticum injection with home exercise program has greater efficacy than a home exercise program alone in the treatment of AC. However, the use of collagenase may risk injury to other collagen-containing structures surrounding the shoulder.[300]

However, operative intervention should be reserved for patients who do not improve with PT or a home exercise program and in whom symptoms have been present for 6 months to 1 year. There is no consensus regarding the timing of a surgical procedure for AC other than patients should not be in the inflammatory phase of their disease. There is no evidence that early surgical intervention can shorten the recovery time of this disease.[301] Surgical treatments include capsular brismont, manipulation under anesthesia, arthroscopic capsular release, or open capsular release. Brismont is performed by injection 60 cc of saline into the joint to create distension and rupture of the capsule.[302] Manipulation under anesthesia has an increased risk of iatrogenic fracture and has a greater efficacy in individuals who do not have diabetes.[303,304] Arthroscopic capsular release is more controlled; however, meticulous dissection must be performed as the axillary nerve traverses close to the inferior aspect of the glenoid near the contracted axillary pouch. Manipulation is often performed after an adequate arthroscopic lysis of adhesions has been performed.[305,306] A recent systematic review failed to show significant differences in outcome after manipulation under anesthesia versus arthroscopic capsular release.[307] Open capsular release is rarely performed since the advent of arthroscopic techniques, and is usually only performed in patients with post-traumatic frozen shoulder who have retained hardware.

Shoulder Instability

The shoulder joint has a high functional ROM with a lack of inherent bony constraint. Glenohumeral joint stability is thus achieved through the interplay between the dynamic stabilizers (rotator cuff and deltoid muscles), static stabilizers (the labrum, glenohumeral ligaments, and joint capsule), and scapular kinesis. The shoulder has an inherent laxity, which is variable between individuals and allows for its normal physiologic motion.[308] Female athletes with increased shoulder laxity are not predisposed to develop symptomatic shoulder instability.[309,310]

"Laxity" is defined as increased normal physiologic motion of the glenohumeral joint, but it is not a pathologic entity.[311] Shoulder instability is an abnormal or painful subluxation or dislocation of the glenohumeral joint. Shoulder instability has been described as voluntary, traumatic, or multidirectional instability (MDI). It has also been described in terms of the direction of instability such as anterior, posterior, or MDI. Neer described MDI as symptomatic laxity of the shoulder in two or more directions—one of which is inferior.[312] MDI encompasses less than 10% of all patients with shoulder instability.[313,314] Half of the patients diagnosed with MDI are female with no history of trauma.[315-317] Half of those females with MDI also have generalized ligamentous laxity based on the Beighton scale.[318,319] Increased laxity has not been directly correlated with concomitant multidirectional shoulder instability.[320]

MDI has been described in overhead athletes such as baseball players, tennis players, swimmers, and gymnasts.[313,317,321,322] Atraumatic MDI is more common in the female athlete. A meta-analysis of shoulder instability in athletes revealed that 22% of unidirectional anterior instability, 27% of unidirectional posterior instability, and 35% of multidirectional instability were females.[323]

It has been proposed, but is debatable, that hormonal influences and decreased upper extremity muscle mass may predispose female athletes to MDI.[308,324-326] It is now believed that MDI often occurs through micro-trauma to the shoulder capsule–ligamentous complex causing plastic deformation to the capsule and subsequent instability.[308,312,327,328] Patients with MDI have significant imbalance of shoulder muscular control as well as alterations in shoulder kinematics and muscle activation during active ROM.[329,330] Loss of shoulder proprioception as well as the loss of reflexive muscular protection against excessive humeral head translation is also seen in female athletes with MDI.[328,331-333]

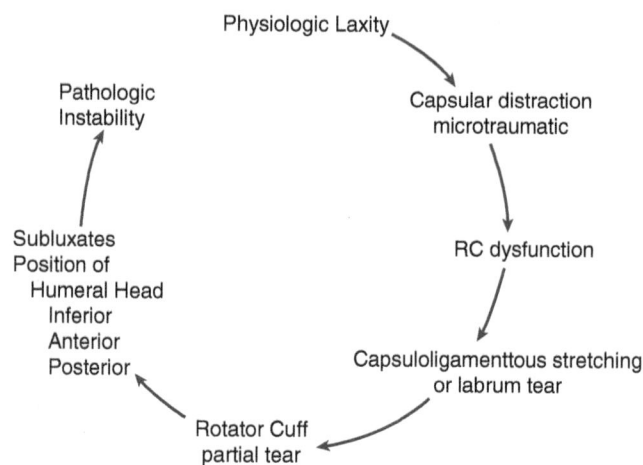

Fig. 27.7 Cycle of multidirectional instability in a shoulder.

Patients with MDI often have scapulothoracic dysfunction. Ideally, the scapula should move conjointly to keep the glenoid cornered underneath the humeral head. However, the scapula, in patients with MDI, droops laterally, increasing the inferior translation of the humeral head and increasing humeral head internal rotation leading to further instability (Fig. 27.7).[334,335]

MDI often occurs during the second to third decades of life. The athlete will describe decreased strength with deteriorating athletic performance. They may also complain of fatigue, aching, pain at night, looseness, slipping, and sensory symptoms.[336] Implicated sports include swimming (butterfly or backstroke), gymnastics, and overhead throwing sports.[322,323,337] Patients often learn compensatory shoulder movements to avoid inciting activities.[338]

On physical exam, an anterior as well as posterior load and shift test should be performed. The amount of translation should be evaluated on a scale of 1 to 3 and documented.[339] The sulcus test also should be performed with and without external rotation to evaluate the rotator interval (see Fig. 27.5). In addition, an anterior and posterior apprehension and relocation test should be performed. These tests are only positive if the test reproduces instability symptoms.[324]

It is important to obtain radiographs to identify any bony abnormalities of the shoulder, such as Hill-Sachs and bony Bankart lesions, glenoid version, dysplasia, hypoplasia and bone loss. However, x-rays are typically normal in patients with MDI. MRI arthrogram often reveals a normal labrum, biceps, rotator cuff, glenoid, and humeral head; however, a patulous capsule. MRI performed in the abduction external rotation (ABER) position may show the crescent sign or triangle sign secondary to a patulous capsule.[340]

Physical therapy for neuromuscular control, periscapular stabilization with strengthening, and rotator cuff strengthening are the primary treatments for MDI. The static stabilizers remain unchanged but improved muscle tone and proprioception leads to improvement in symptoms.[341] Burkhead reported good or excellent results in 83% of MDI patients treated with muscle-strengthening exercises.[341] More recently Misamore reported on a cohort of young athletic patients with MDI in which 52% had poor results and 25% had excellent results with physical therapy.[342] Despite these findings, a physical therapy program followed by maintenance therapy is felt to be essential to maximize long-term outcomes in patients with MDI. Physical therapy should focus on improving the dynamic positioning of the humerus in the glenoid, instituting a proprioceptive exercise program, and improving the efficiency of the dynamic glenohumeral stabilizers. Rotator cuff strengthening can also improve active compression of the humeral head in the glenoid. The result is less shear force across the glenohumeral joint with improved centering of the humeral head in the glenoid.[343]

Those who fail at least a 3- to 6-month course of formal physical therapy may be offered surgical correction. Neer reported a 97% success rate of patients undergoing an open anterior inferior capsular shift with only one of 36 patients experiencing a resubluxation event after surgery.[312] Baker reported a 2-year follow-up of 93% of good to excellent outcomes after an arthroscopic anterior inferior capsular shift with 86% of patients returning to sport.[338] Thermal capsulorrhaphy, which once was popular, is no longer performed due to the increased risk of failure, chondrolysis, and thermal nerve injury.[344,345]

Advances have been made in the diagnosis and treatment of MDI. Rehabilitation of the dynamic shoulder stabilizers is the gold standard of initial nonsurgical management. If this fails then surgical options can be used. Satisfactory outcomes have been obtained with either an open or an arthroscopic capsular shift. Treatment of patients with MDI can yield favorable results when there is careful examination, diagnosis, rehabilitation, and—when needed—appropriate surgical treatment.

Acetabular Labral Injuries and Femoroacetabular Impingement

There are many documented hip and groin injuries, which commonly affect athletes. Although in the past these injuries were often overlooked, improvements in diagnostic modalities including hip arthroscopy have led to improved identification of intra-articular hip pathology. Conditions, such as acetabular labral tears, capsular injuries, and intra-articular cartilage damage as a result of femoroacetabular impingement (FAI) and hip instability, have been increasingly recognized in athletes.[346-351]

Just as our understanding of the complexity of shoulder pathology was enhanced by the ability to view the shoulder dynamically during arthroscopy, so has the development of better hip arthroscopic techniques resulted in a ballooning of our knowledge of hip pathology especially FAI. FAI is caused by abnormal hip mechanics, which result in abnormal contact of the femoral head within the acetabulum. Pincer impingement results from an excessive prominence of the anterolateral rim of the acetabulum, which in hip flexion "impinges" the labrum of the hip against the neck of the femur. This prominence of the anterolateral rim of the acetabulum can result from overgrowth of the anterior edge of the acetabulum or retroversion of the acetabulum. Repetitive impingement of the labrum injures the labrum with secondary injury to the cartilage of the adjacent acetabulum. Some report that pincer impingement is equally as common in males and females presenting in middle-aged adults (4th and 5th decades).[352,353] However, a recent (2017) article by Shibata reported that in elite athletes pincer impingement was more common in females than males.[354]

Cam impingement occurs when a nonspherical femoral head, such as that which results from a prominence at the anterior superior head and neck junction of the proximal femur, rotates within the anterior superior acetabulum resulting in an injury to the articular cartilage at this location with secondary failure of the labrum. Cam impingement is more common in adolescent males than females (3:1 predilection).[352] Combined impingement can occur and, in elite athletes, was reported to be more common in males who also demonstrated greater acetabular cartilage damage secondary to this type of impingement. Bilateral symptomatic FAI is more common in males.[253]

Females have more issues with hypermobility of their hips than males and female ballet dancers have a greater incidence of hip dysplasia than do male ballet dancers.[355] This dysplasia results in wonderful turnout, a positive for the dancer, but it can lead to FAI and early arthritis.

A relatively high incidence of dysplasia (21% of 126 hips) was also reported by Kapron et al. in collegiate females participating in a variety of sports with an additional 46% of female collegiate track and field, soccer, and volleyball athletes exhibiting borderline dysplasia.[356]

FAI typically presents similarly in males and females with the insidious onset of groin pain, which may be preceded by minor trauma, although many will report no history of a precipitating event. The pain is usually intermittent and exacerbated by physical activity and exercise. Although nonspecific, mechanical symptoms, such as locking and catching, also may be reported. Treatment of FAI, if the symptoms are stable, is nonoperative in females as in males. One must identify the offending activities and modify these. Squats often advocated in the weight room for obtaining strength should be avoided in these athletes as they can exacerbate symptoms. Strengthening of the muscles of the core may be helpful. If symptoms do not resolve, arthroscopic treatment of FAI is recommended. A recent study by Shibata and associates on elite athletes demonstrated the rate of highly competitive athletes returning to their former level of competitive sport participation after hip arthroscopy was similar for female and male athletes (84.2% of female athletes and 83.3% of male athletes).[354]

Idiopathic Scoliosis

Idiopathic scoliosis refers to the occurrence of a spinal curvature in the absence of congenital or neurologic abnormalities and is the most prevalent type of scoliosis accounting for approximately 70% of cases. Idiopathic scoliosis is further classified based upon on the age of appearance. Infantile scoliosis has an onset before 3 years of age; juvenile scoliosis has an onset between 3 and 10 years of age, and adolescent idiopathic scoliosis (AIS) occurs between age 10 and skeletal maturity. The adolescent form of this disease is most common and accounts for the majority of cases of idiopathic scoliosis. Although spinal deformities are concerning to both male and female athletes, AIS is of particular concern for females due to the 10:1 female to male predominance and the higher likelihood of progression in the female.[357]

The prevalence of AIS is reported to be between 2% and 3% in the general population.[358] Although the etiology is largely unknown, current theories suggest a complex interplay of genetic,[359,360] biochemical signaling,[361] and neuromuscular control pathways.[362] A possible link between circulating levels of estrogen,[363,364] life-style factors, such as nutrition and exercise level,[365] and BMI[366,367] also have been reported but more evidence is needed.

AIS has been reported to be more prevalent in female-dominated sports such as gymnastics, ballet, and swimming. Many athletes now begin vigorous training in childhood. Wojtys et al., found a correlation between the amount of exposure to intense athletic training and spinal curvatures in the immature spine.[368] The authors felt that increased spinal curvature was associated with cumulative hours expended in training, and that overexposure to biomechanical stresses may play a role in progression.[368]

Warren et al. reported the incidence of idiopathic scoliosis to be 24% in ballet dancers.[369] This was correlated to small body habitus and delayed menarche suggesting that hypoestrogenism and prolonged intervals of amenorrhea may predispose ballet dancers to scoliosis.[369] A 10-fold higher incidence of scoliosis in rhythmic gymnastics trainees has also been reported, which was related to asymmetric loading, delayed menarche, and ligamentous laxity.[370] Burwell et al. reported on the association of delayed puberty and scoliosis in rhythmic gymnasts and ballet dancers; however, they felt that the differing curve progressions were related to the type of training, suggesting the notion of sports-associated scoliosis.[371] Similarly, Becker found a 6.9% incidence of idiopathic scoliosis and a 16% incidence of mild curves in a study involving junior Olympic swimmers. The authors noted that curves were toward the swimmers dominant breathing side suggesting muscle imbalance as a possible contributor.[372]

Similar in female and male athletes, the diagnosis of AIS should be made after a thorough history and physical examination. The Adam's forward bend test is a common test used for screening. During this test the patient bends forward to touch the toes enhancing the spinal curve and demonstrating rib cage asymmetry. Particular attention should be given to the neurologic exam. Secondary sex characteristics should be assessed and the skin should be examined for café au lait spots, which are suggestive of neurofibromatosis. If significant deformity is present during screening, a radiographic evaluation, including a long AP and lateral film of the torso, should be performed. Routine MRI is typically not recommended; however, the presence of neurologic abnormalities or back pain that does not respond to several weeks of conservative care may warrant MRI evaluation.[373]

Stress Fractures

Studies in the 1970s and 1980s—the majority of which were done on the military population—reported that women have a higher incidence of stress fractures than men.[374-378] In contrast, several recent studies in the athletic populations have shown a modest increased risk or no increased risk of stress fractures in women compared with men.[379-383] However, in 2004, following their survey of 5900 Division I collegiate athletes, Hame et al. found that although the incidence of all fractures was similar for men and women (0.0438 and 0.0461, respectively), the incidence of stress fractures was double for women and stress fractures were most common in track and field athletes.[384] More recently Changstrom et al. reported that in a high school population girls sustained more stress fractures (63.3%) than boys (36.7%).[385]

Most agree that female athletes with menstrual irregularities have a higher incidence of stress fractures than female athletes with regular menstrual cycles.[386-390] The reason for the relationship between abnormal menses and the increased incidence of stress fractures in athletic women is not well understood, nor is the literature consistent on the relationship between low BMD in amenorrhoeic athletes and stress fractures. Although one study in athletes with similar training schedules reported that athletes with stress fractures were more likely to have lower femoral neck and spine bone density, others report no association between the incidence of stress fractures and low BMD.[391-393] Both scenarios are reasonable since, in addition to hormonal variation, other variables that might influence the difference in the incidence of stress fractures between male and female athletes include bone geometric differences, the higher level of adipose tissue compared with lean body mass in females, and static and dynamic biomechanical differences between the sexes.[394]

As previously discussed in this chapter, a relationship has been defined between amenorrhea (loss of normal menstrual periods for over 3 months), low BMD and low energy availability—the so-called female athlete triad. Those with the triad have been reported to have an increased risk of stress fractures.[43,395,396]

Treatment of the female athlete with a stress fracture should include, in addition to treatment of her fracture, an investigation into potential predisposing factors for stress injury. Overachieving (training errors), lack of sleep, and biomechanical considerations, and—more recently—vitamin D deficiency, have been linked to stress fractures in males. However, in females one must not only analyze the athlete's training schedules, sleep habits, vitamin D levels, shoe wear, lower extremity alignment, and other biomechanical considerations, but also her eating habits and menstrual cycle irregularities.[43] Is the athlete getting enough calcium, iron, and sufficient calories in her diet to support the energy needs of her sport? Does she have regular menstrual periods? If her menstrual periods are irregular, as often they are, referral to a sports gynecologist or to a family physician or internist skilled in the evaluation of menstrual dysfunction in athletes is appropriate. In females with recurrent stress fractures or stress reactions, an evaluation of BMD is recommended even in the absence of reported menstrual abnormalities.

For a complete list of references, go to ExpertConsult.com.

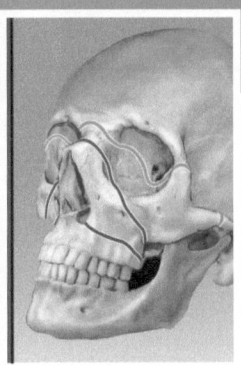

28

The Para-Athlete

Daniel Herman, Mary E. Caldwell, Arthur Jason De Luigi

Participation in sports and physical activity by persons with different abilities continues to grow within the general athlete population and within the adaptive sports community.[1-4] Sports participation provides these athletes with benefits in terms of their general state of health, functionality, life skills, self-esteem, and overall quality of life.[1-4] Given the increase in participation, performance, and injuries among the adaptive athlete, the American College of Sports Medicine (ACSM) encourages managing exercise in patients with disabilities like the general population.[5-7] It is incumbent upon medical providers to promote activity among this patient population but also to be knowledgeable and proficient regarding common complications of exercise to maximize their patients' safety and health.

This chapter provides clinicians with a broad overview of athletes with disabilities and important considerations regarding their optimal care. A brief overview of athlete competition classification systems and a discussion of the most common types of adaptive athletes are included, as well as any unique physiologic characteristics, medical needs, and adaptive equipment. Participation in the Paralympics is the pinnacle achievement of an adaptive athlete and is the primary context and framework for this discussion. However, the information and principles presented may be applied to nonelite athletes over a broad range of competition levels and sporting activities.

CLASSIFICATION

Athletes with disabilities are an inherently heterogeneous group with highly variable profiles of athletic capacity depending on the type, location, and severity of their inherent disability. Akin to the weight classes used in boxing and wrestling, the global governing body, the International Paralympic Committee (IPC), has developed classification systems. These classification systems maintain a measure of fairness in competition and most often apply to high-level athletes.[8] The common purpose of the classifications systems in summary is to (1) define eligibility for participation and meet minimum disability criteria to participate, (2) ensure the athlete is competing against a class of athletes with impairments that cause a similar amount of activity limitation, and (3) ultimately allow for skill and fitness to determine success.[8,9]

To be eligible for Paralympic sports, an athlete must have 1 of 10 eligible impairments (physical or structural): hypertonia, ataxia, athetosis, leg length difference, loss of muscle strength, loss of passive range of movement, limb deficiency, short stature, visual impairment, or intellectual impairment.

Athletes must then meet the minimum eligibility criteria determined by each sport as defined by the regulations of the sport's governing body. For example, athletes with visual impairment do not meet the criteria to compete in Paralympic wheelchair tennis, whereas they do meet minimum criteria for multiple track and field sports, as well as many other sports.[9]

Lastly, athletes undergo a sports class allocation (SCA). SCA allows athletes with similar activity limitations to compete together, meaning the impairments of the athletes competing can often be different within a class. The sporting event greatly influences the classification process because different types and severities of disability affect performance to different levels in different sports. Therefore, depending on the sport and locale, designations may be condensed into fewer classes based on a wider range of disability. For example, within track and field, the disciplines and classes include: running and jumping (16 classes), wheelchair racing (7 classes), standing throws (15 classes), and seated throwing sports (11 classes). Meanwhile there are sports which may have one SCA, such as para powerlifting or wheelchair curling, in which once an athlete meets minimal eligibility criteria they are either sports class eligible or noneligible.[9] Of note, team sports such as wheelchair basketball often incorporate a wide range of disability in direct competition via the use of point systems, in which athletes with less disadvantageous levels of disability are assigned higher point values, with the team not permitted to exceed a given total point value for its players in the game.

Direct observation of the athlete during play or competition is also a characteristic of some sports that are able to use more objective measures, such as perception and field of view in the visual impairment category.

Of the athletes who compete, there are six main major disability categories of athletes: amputees/limb deficient, wheelchair (typically spinal cord injury), cerebral palsy, visual impaired, the intellectually disabled, and "Les Autres." These athletes must meet 1 of the 10 eligibility requirements. Les Autres is a French term meaning "the others" and is made up of athletes with a variety of impairments and disabilities. Major disability category rather than IPC impairment-based classification will be used going forward to discuss differences in athletes with regard to exercise physiology, medical considerations, and adaptive sports equipment.

ATHLETES WITH LIMB DEFICIENCY/ AMPUTEE ATHLETES

Limb deficiency may be congenital, illness related, or traumatic and may involve the upper and/or lower extremities. The athlete with limb deficiency may compete as a standing or seated competitor depending on the sport and the participant's level of limb loss. Given the variance of the location and length of the congenitally abnormal or surgically amputated extremity, these athletes have a wide range of functionality.

Upper extremity limb deficiency is most commonly from amputation caused by trauma, followed by cancer, and then vascular disease.[10] In 2005 it was estimated that almost 41,000 were living with upper extremity limb loss.[11] The level of amputation is key in upper extremities for function and range of motion (ROM), as the preservation of movement in both the elbow and forearm is essential for positioning the hand in space and therefore performance of function.[12] The most common level of upper extremity amputation is transradial.[10]

Lower extremity limb deficiency is often secondary to amputation from peripheral vascular disease (82%), followed by trauma (16%), malignancy (0.9%), and lastly congenital deformity (0.8%).[13] The vast majority of lower limb amputations are at the transtibial and transfemoral levels.[10,13]

Given that the most common limb-deficient athlete is an amputee, amputee literature will be predominately referenced going forward.

Exercise Physiology

It is presumed that the cardiopulmonary physiology of amputee athletes with traumatic amputations or with vascular disease (dysvascular amputations) is similar to that of able-bodied athletes. Some exceptions may exist for persons who have had an amputation for congenital reasons when a cardiac abnormality may be a component of a syndrome.

The amputation of a lower extremity does however significantly affect the "energy expenditure" used during ambulation. Various measurements have been used to quantify the "expenditure" of ambulation in persons with limb loss, and these calculations can be expressed in functions of distance, rate, and velocity. Persons with limb loss typically walk slower than nonamputees to maintain a similar oxygen consumption rate. Therefore in athletic competition the amputee athlete will need to increase his or her rate of oxygen consumption to maintain a similar velocity of a nonamputee athlete. This energy use also differs between vascular versus nonvascular amputees of the same level of amputation (Table 28.1).[10]

Athletes with amputations or congenital limb abnormalities can compete in a variety of sports with various permissions for adaptive equipment, which may allow the use of a prosthesis, or the athlete can compete in certain wheelchair sports.[14]

Medical Considerations
Musculoskeletal Injuries

Injury patterns among amputee athletes are similar to those for athletes without disabilities; however, the severity and location of the missing limb dictates the frequency and type of injury.

TABLE 28.1	Energy Expenditure of Ambulation		
Level of Amputation	Etiology	Unilateral/ Bilateral	% of Energy Increase per Unit of Distance
Transtibial	Traumatic	Unilateral	25% (short: 40%; long: 10%)
		Bilateral	41%
	Dysvascular	Unilateral	40%
Transfemoral	Traumatic	Unilateral	60%–70%
	Dysvascular	Unilateral	100%
Transfemoral + transtibial		Bilateral	118%

From Uustal H, Baerga E, Joki J. Prosthetics and orthotics. In: Cuccurullo SJ, ed. *Physical Medicine and Rehabilitation Board Review*. Demos Medical; 2015.

Lower extremity amputees are at risk for injuries in both intact and residual limbs. The distal residual limb is often the site of skin trauma due to the prosthesis. Altered biomechanics, because of the asymmetric need for power and propulsion, may predispose athletes to knee, hip, sacroiliac, and lumbar spine pain.[15–17] Alternatively, an amputee may rely too heavily on the intact limb, which can increase the risk for overuse injuries and osteoarthritis.[18–21]

Similarly, in upper extremity amputees, altered use and load patterns of the intact limb can result in pain and injury to either limb or axial structures. Overuse injuries such as shoulder impingement, rotator cuff tears, epicondylitis, and peripheral nerve entrapments are common in the intact limb of upper extremity amputees.[22–24] Differences in weight and swing excursion between the upper extremities, as well as the need to compensate at the shoulder for loss of distal joint function, may cause significant asymmetry in the demands of the thoracic and cervical spines and paraspinal and parascapular musculature, resulting in pain and dysfunction.[25,26] Treatment for many of these conditions is identical to that for nonamputees. In addition, however, precise fitting of prostheses in this population is a critical aspect of beneficial treatment.

Dermatologic Conditions

After amputation of the limb and subsequent fitting of a prosthesis, the skin of the distal portion of the residual limb becomes a weight-bearing surface and as a result is at increased risk for skin disorders. Although studies can vary, studies range from 40% to 73.9% of amputees with at least one skin problem.[27–29] Risk factors that have been identified are male sex, older age, and amputation from diabetes or peripheral vascular disease.[28]

Rashes are frequently observed in persons who use prostheses. A noninfectious allergic rash should trigger examination of the type of liner used, with the goal of incorporating material that is less irritating and that promotes greater perfusion of sweat away from the skin. An allergen (including detergents, lotions, or the liner material) has been the cause in up to 43% of patients with dermatitis.[27] Cleaning the residual limb and prosthesis regularly can prevent rashes. Prevention of infections is a key priority and often a source of concern. Folliculitis, boils, and abscesses should be treated appropriately, along with keeping the skin dry and clean. As such, a break from the prosthesis may be warranted.[10] Keep in mind that the rash could also be fungal, which is commonly seen in excessive sweating. The rash would need to be treated, but long-term solutions to decrease the sweating by using an antiperspirant can be considered.[10]

Verrucous hyperplasia is a wartlike lesion that may develop at the distal end of the residual limb. It may occur as a result of untreated proximal residual limb constriction (choke syndrome) from a socket or wrap that has caused decreased pressure in the distal residual limb. Edema formation occurs and over time will result in wartlike skin overgrowth. The reversal and treatment of verrucous hyperplasia consists of equal distribution of pressure through the residual limb by relieving proximal constriction and reestablishing total contact within the socket.[10]

Blisters and sores are very common and can occur as a result of friction between skin of the residual limb and the prosthesis. Skin breakdown may also occur when pressure is applied disproportionately to a pressure-sensitive area of skin on the residual limb, such as the tibial tubercle in a transtibial amputee.[10] The risk may be compounded by impaired sensation in the residual limb or sweating with athletic activity, which may increase moisture at the skin-socket interface and heighten the risk for skin breakdown. A properly fitting socket will normally prevent blisters and sores, and it is important to maintain a good socket fit by adding and removing socks throughout the day to adjust for volume reduction,

Heterotopic Ossification

The formation of bone in tissues that are not normally ossified, heterotopic ossification (HO), usually evolves after traumatic brain injury, spinal cord injury, burns, and total arthroplasty. Recently, HO has been reported to develop frequently in injured tissue of residual limbs in traumatic amputees,[30] which may increase risk of skin breakdown or stimulate pain with weight bearing. HO is also more likely to develop around joints and muscle adjacent to trauma and typically develops within the first 6 months to a year after amputation. The development of HO typically occurs during the time an amputee is beginning prosthetic training. Thus the majority of persons with HO are diagnosed prior to engaging in athletic competition, which facilitates modifications in design of the socket and vigilance for signs of skin breakdown. Treatments for HO can include ROM, physical therapy, radiation, surgery, and medications.[31] Treatment options vary with location of the HO and medical comorbidities of the patient; therefore treatment should be tailored to each patient specifically.

Bone Spurs

Bone spurs and overgrowth can occur in cases where the periosteum of the bone is stripped during surgery or from trauma. The bone grows faster than the overlying skin. Bone spurs are more common in kids with acquired amputation and in young adults with traumatic amputations.[10]

Neuroma

Neuromas form at the distal end of transected nerves in the residual limbs of amputees. The development of a neuroma in a weight-bearing structure or in its vicinity can cause severe pain with ambulation and weight bearing and limit an athlete's ability to train and compete. Treatments include prosthetic modification to relieve pressure; oral medications, including antiepileptic agents and tricyclic antidepressant drugs (neuropathic medications); injections of corticosteroids and local anesthetics into the neuroma; and radiofrequency ablation of neuromas.[32–34] Many common medications that are used to treat neuropathic pain may be restricted in competition by the World Anti-Doping Agency (WADA), and clear knowledge regarding these limitations is vital for medical practitioners. We encourage medical practitioners who are caring for athletes with disabilities to visit WADA's website to review approved and restricted medications "in and out of competition."[35] Surgical excision, which can improve pain and patient quality of life, may ultimately be necessary if conservative treatments fail.[36–38]

Adaptive Sports Equipment

Numerous sporting events incorporate adaptive sports equipment for amputees. It is beyond the scope of this chapter to discuss the numerous prosthetic modifications and other adaptive equipment for several sports and recreational activities. However, medical practitioners should consider several pertinent facts when they prescribe adaptive equipment. Compared with common prosthetic devices, a range of modifications should be considered in this population.[39] Of particular importance is the prosthetic weight, particularly in sports in which increased weight may negatively affect speed. Occasionally, use of a conventional prosthesis may be advantageous compared with a technologically advanced prosthesis. The clinician should also consider alignment, prosthetic foot dynamics, shock absorption, and the possible need for transverse rotation.

Remember, not all athletes with limb deficiency will need or use a prosthesis to compete in their sport. For example, in para table tennis, athletes may use tape to hold their paddle in place on their limb. Athletes with limb deficiency can also use wheelchairs or Lofstrand crutches, depending on the sport.

WHEELCHAIR ATHLETES

Wheelchair athletes may have spinal cord injuries, amputations, or neurologic disorders such as polio, spina bifida, and cerebral palsy. The majority of wheelchair athletes have spinal cord injuries; hence discussion in this section is limited to the nuances of athletic participation of athletes with spinal cord injuries.

Exercise Physiology

The exercise capacity and physiologic responses to exercise of wheelchair athletes are different from that of able-bodied athletes. Furthermore, inherent physiologic differences among wheelchair athletes are observed. Based on the level and severity of their injury, their maximal exercise capacity may range from being comparable with either able-bodied athletes or sedentary able-bodied persons.

Spinal cord injuries and other neurologic pathologies induce a varying degree of paralysis of voluntary muscles, with a resultant decrease in muscle mass available for exercise. Diminished muscle mass also has a negative impact on performance via impaired supporting dynamic restraints (such as core musculature) and impaired hand and arm function in tetraplegic athletes. These phenomena can reduce the efficiency of energy transfer from the athlete to the chair and other objects. However, these differences in muscle mass only partly explain differences in exercise capacity, because the arteriovenous oxygen difference in submaximal exercise is typically altered in wheelchair athletes compared with able-bodied athletes.[40] This difference may be indicative of different levels of muscle recruitment to achieve a given work rate, as well as impairments in local and regional blood flow in response to exercise. In general, the lower the spinal level of the lesion, the more muscle mass is available for exercise, which translates to improved vasomotor regulation. Thus power output is inversely related to the level of the spinal lesion. Of note, in this population, high values of aerobic and anaerobic output which normally correlate with performance, may not correlate in this population.[41] For example, wheelchair tennis players with low-level spinal cord injuries have been able to reach physiologic thresholds for exercise intensity similar to able-bodied tennis players,[42] but these parameters (peak oxygen uptake) did not correlate to rank and performance.[43]

Cardiovascular responses to exercise are also altered in comparison with able-bodied athletes and demonstrate significant differences between wheelchair athletes with higher and lower level lesions. The loss of vasomotor regulation and active muscle pumping action below the level of the lesion results in impaired venous return, thus restricting central blood volume. Impaired sympathetic innervation to the heart, which is absent in persons with complete spinal cord lesions above the T1 level and reduced in persons with complete spinal cord lesions above the T6 level, results in a blunted cardiac response, and maximal heart rate is limited to 110 and 130 beats per minute via intrinsic sinoatrial activity.[41,44,45] Spinal cord athletes with cervical level injuries also demonstrate attenuated cardiac size and left ventricular hypertrophy compared with those with lower level injuries.[46] These factors lead to impaired cardiac performance, with reductions in cardiac output and stroke volume up to approximately 30% in persons with motor-complete cervical spinal cord injuries.[47,48] Although complete motor cervical spinal cord injuries should have no intact sympathetic nervous system, there may be a degree remaining, and this can vary between athletes. A 2013 study demonstrated in wheelchair rugby athletes with motor complete cervical injury who had partial preservation of descending sympathetic response (demonstrated by skin sympathetic response [SSR]), SSR correlated to heart rate peak and the degree of preservation further correlated to performance.[49]

With regard to heart rate response to exercise to measure fitness, it is likely more reliable to compare ratings of perceived exertion to monitor training and fitness improvements in SCI athletes.[50] For example, cerebral palsy athletes participating in power soccer had a significantly higher (>12 beats/min) heart rate response compared with spinal cord athletes. Furthermore, 22 athletes with cerebral palsy and 5 with muscular dystrophy had heart rates that exceeded 55% of the estimated maximum heart rate for at least 30 minutes of competing, compared with only 1 in the spinal cord injury group.[51]

Pulmonary function is also often impaired and influenced by the level of the lesion. These deficits occur primarily via paralysis of the expiratory muscles; however, persons with cervical lesions may also have paralysis of inspiratory musculature, resulting in significant impairments in ventilation relative to paraplegic persons.[52] Compared with able-bodied persons, the forced expiratory volume in 1 second, forced vital capacity, and tidal volume are approximately 90% in paraplegic patients and 60% in tetraplegic patients.[53]

Medical Considerations
Musculoskeletal Injuries

Wheelchair athletes are at risk for routine musculoskeletal injuries, such as muscle strains, at rates comparable with those of able-bodied athletes. Injuries in this population may affect participation and performance to a disproportionately high degree compared with able-bodied athletes, depending on the sport.

Upper extremity injuries are more common than lower extremity injuries in wheelchair athletes. The adaptive sport literature suggests that injuries most commonly involve the shoulder, ranging between 15% and 72%.[6,54] Arm and wrist injuries follow with the most likely diagnosis being muscle strains, tendinopathy, bursitis, and contusions.[55,56]

A history of shoulder pain is reported in more than 90% of selected wheelchair athlete populations, with an increasing prevalence in proportion to the amount of trunk and upper extremity disability.[54,57,58] Shoulder impingement syndrome is the most common injury; bicipital and rotator cuff tendinopathy and tears are also common.[59] Wheelchair athletes often have a protracted scapular position with dynamic scapular dyskinesis, resulting in loss of subacromial space and impingement.[60] In addition, the humeral head is often elevated as a result of relative muscle strength imbalance, favoring shoulder abduction strength over adduction and rotational strength. This risk can potentially be modifiable by alterations in trunk inclination, backrest height, and the position of the wheelchair axle relative to the shoulder. Physical therapy should improve shoulder flexibility, correct scapular kinematics, and address shoulder muscle imbalances.[61,62] Much attention has reviewed the "lack of the kinetic chain" and its impact on shoulder injuries. It appears this may be sport dependent, and, most importantly, the lack of kinetic chain should not be assumed to be the reason for pathology.[63,64]

Lower extremity injuries are also seen in this population, although they are less frequent than in ambulatory athletes.[65] Lower extremity fractures are more common in high-speed adaptive sports with collision, such as wheelchair basketball, rugby, and softball.[66] Compared with upper extremity injuries caused by overuse, these injuries are usually acute and posttraumatic. There are high rates of osteoporosis observed in lower extremities in the spinal cord–injured population. Thus clinicians should be vigilant because even minor trauma may result in fractures, and any resulting deformity or angulation after healing may adversely affect available seating positions, increase the risk for pressure sores, and alter functional status.

Peripheral Nerve Entrapment

Peripheral nerve entrapments are commonly encountered in wheelchair athletes. Significant entrapment neuropathies include median neuropathy at the wrist, ulnar neuropathy at the elbow, and radial neuropathy, likely partly secondary to the biomechanics required for wheelchair use.[67–69] Shoulder muscle imbalance and scapular dyskinesis may also result in suprascapular neuropathy at either the suprascapular or spinoglenoid notches.[70] In addition to standard therapies, protection of the wrist and elbow with padded gloves and sleeves, use of a wheelchair that has been properly fit to the athlete, and use of an adequate ROM and proper techniques during propulsion may help with prevention and treatment.[67,71]

Thermoregulation

Altered sympathetic, vasomotor, and sudomotor responses and diminished rates of venous return from the loss of muscle-pumping action result in a diminished ability to sense and respond to thermal imbalance.[72,73] The loss of skeletal muscle and function also impairs the response to negative thermal imbalances because of a reduced capacity for shivering.[70] These factors increase the risk for hypothermia and exertional heat illness, especially in persons with spinal cord lesions above the T6 level.[74]

Pressure Sores/Ulcers

Pressure sores are common among wheelchair athletes, particularly those with a spinal cord injury. Prolonged pressure, typically over bony prominences such as the sacrum and ischial tuberosities, combined with insensate skin that is moist from activity, increase compressive and shears forces, resulting in local tissue ischemia and injury. Wheelchair athletes with altered trunk stability often maintain a flexed lower extremity posture at the hips and knees that further distributes the athlete's weight to "at-risk sites."[70] Vigilance is mandatory for pressure sore prevention, including skin checks, shifting of weight every 15 to 20 minutes to relieve pressure, the use of appropriately fit seat cushions, and maintenance of a dry environment.

Spasticity

Spasticity is common in wheelchair athletes who have spinal cord injuries and is manifested by involuntary muscle contraction, hyperreflexia, and velocity-dependent increases in tone. Synergistic muscle activation patterning may inhibit performance by altering positioning within the wheelchair, item control/accuracy, and propulsion. However, it is important to note that in some cases, spasticity may be beneficial for these functions when other voluntary muscle action is insufficient. It is important for the sports physician to remember that spasticity is primarily a velocity-dependent increase in tone, and thus a routine bedside examination may not be conducive to a thorough appreciation of the detrimental effects of spasticity unless sports activities are entirely replicated.

Spasticity is usually treated with oral medications, physical therapy that emphasizes ROM, and tone-reducing orthoses. In more advanced cases or in cases in which the athlete cannot tolerate the sedative effects of antispasticity medications, Botox injections can focally reduce high levels of spasticity in a dose-dependent fashion. Surgical approaches such as muscle/tendon lengthening, tendon transfers, and selective dorsal rhizotomy may be considered in refractory cases.

Neurogenic Bladder and Bowel

Bladder dysfunction is common in wheelchair athletes who have spinal cord injuries and spina bifida. This dysfunction can result in urinary retention, often necessitating indwelling, suprapubic, or intermittent catheterization and resulting in increased rates of urinary tract infections and stone formation. Clinical presentation may include fever, fatigue, a general sense of unease, discomfort in the area of the bladder and kidneys, autonomic dysreflexia (AD), incontinence, and an increased level of muscle spasticity.

Bowel dysfunction is also common in persons with spinal cord injuries and spina bifida. Injuries above the S2-S4 spinal cord segments results in a "reflexic" neurogenic bowel, whereas injuries distal to these segments or involving the destruction of anterior horn cells (at these levels) result in an "areflexic" bowel. In addition to using other methods of facilitation, these persons are counseled to initiate regular bowel programs at the same time of day to condition the bowel to achieve effective defecation and avoid incontinence.

In the sports setting, the athlete may not adhere to appropriate frequency or technique of clean intermittent catheterization or appropriate timing of their bowel program because of an over focus on training, which may propagate infection, reduce vigilance of hydration status, and increase the risk of incontinence. Clinicians should counsel athletes on the importance of bowel and bladder management, which has significant performance and practical implications. Athletes should also be counseled to undergo slow alterations in bowel management to best accommodate their expected competition schedule at upcoming events and to always be cognizant regarding the available facilities for bowel and bladder management at each venue.

Heterotopic Ossification

HO may occur in up to 53% of patients with spinal cord injuries.[75] The development of HO is most common in the first 2 to 3 weeks after spinal cord injury. HO most commonly affects the hips but may also affect the knees, shoulders, and elbows.[75] HO may limit function and performance by restricting ROM for different seating positions, propulsion, and other tasks; it also may increase the risk for pressure sores and nerve entrapments.

Autonomic Dysreflexia

AD is a medical emergency usually seen in persons with complete spinal cord injuries involving or above the T6 segment. Noxious stimuli below the level of injury can cause reflexive sympathetic activity that cannot be modulated by supraspinal centers of control, resulting in high levels of sympathetic activity below the level of injury and incomplete parasympathetic compensation above the level of injury.[76]

During an episode of AD, persons typically experience hypertension and headache due to vasoconstriction below the level of injury, along with skin flushing, piloerection, diaphoresis, and bradycardia above the level of injury. Although mortality is rare, significant morbidity may result, including cerebral hemorrhage, seizures, and myocardial infarction. Treatment should include sitting the person upright, removing restrictive clothing, and searching for the source of the noxious stimulus, which is commonly a distended bladder or impacted colon, pressure sores, or another injury.[77] Systolic pressures of 150 mm Hg should be treated with short-onset and half-life antihypertensive medications. Transdermal nitro paste is highly effective and can be removed easily after resolution of the episode of AD to avoid subsequent hypotension.

An unsettling trend among wheelchair athletes is the intentional use of AD to improve performance during competition, a phenomenon known as "boosting."[78,79] Athletes will create a self-induced noxious stimulus via methods such as kinking a bladder catheter, sitting on ball-bearings, fracturing a toe, or excessively tightening legs straps to induce AD.[79] This strategy may lead to improvements in peak heart rate, peak oxygen consumption, and blood pressure and has been shown to enhance performance by 7% to 10%.[78,80,81] For obvious health and safety reasons and to promote fairness during competition, the IPC has banned the use of induced AD from competition and has begun testing athletes prior to competition at Paralympic events.[82]

Adaptive Equipment

Wheelchairs used in sporting endeavors are typically designed specifically for the particular demands of the sport involved, such as speed and endurance for racing, rigidity and stability for throwing, or agility and ruggedness for wheelchair basketball and rugby. Several variables can be manipulated to meet these needs: axle position (horizontally and vertically), wheels (number, size, and camber), hand rim size, seat back height and angle, seat cushioning, footplate (height and angle), the location and types of belts, and other fixations. For example, an elevated seat height may be advantageous for sports events such as wheelchair basketball, whereas a lower seat may be advantageous for sports requiring extra stability. The particular needs of the athlete and his or her disability level must be considered, including the level of truck support, altered location of the center of mass, and impaired hand function. These considerations are not only important to maximize performance but also to reduce the risk of injury and medical complications. Consultation with physical and occupational therapists and with prosthetists may be necessary depending on the needs and goals of the athlete.

ATHLETES WITH CEREBRAL PALSY

Cerebral palsy is defined as a group of disorders of the development of movement and posture that cause activity limitation and are attributed to nonprogressive disturbances that occurred in the developing fetal or infant brain.[83] Cerebral palsy is often accompanied by disturbances of sensation, cognition, communication, perception, and/or behavior, along with seizure disorder.[83] Patients with cerebral palsy are clinically classified on the basis of the type of movement disorder and the anatomic distribution. Cerebral palsy often shares clinical patterns similar

to those that occur with stroke and traumatic brain injuries. Consequently, athletes with impairments resulting from stroke or traumatic brain injury are often competing against cerebral palsy athletes.

Exercise Physiology

Studies assessing cardiorespiratory endurance, as measured by peak oxygen consumption during arm or leg ergometry, have consistently shown lower values for persons with cerebral palsy when compared with able-bodied control subjects.[84–90] Similarly, compared with able-bodied control subjects, a cerebral palsy group showed significantly lower muscular endurance measured with a hand grip dynamometer.[91] Muscular strength also appears to be decreased in persons with cerebral palsy when measuring force production in the lower extremities.[91,92] Of note, a 2015 study did demonstrate similar fatigue in elite cerebral palsy athletes compared with able body athletes, despite a significant difference in power.[93] This may suggest that previous studies not performed in the elite cerebral palsy population must be taken with that limitation in mind.

Factors that may cause decreased muscular strength and endurance include desynchronization of agonist/antagonist muscle groups, hypersensitive tonic stretch reflexes, an increase in the ratio of type I versus type II muscle fibers, and reduced muscle volume.[90,94] These factors may also account for the increased cost of energy and higher physical strain observed during ambulation in persons with cerebral palsy compared to able-bodied controls.[88,95] An equivalent cost of energy has been shown in persons with acquired traumatic brain injury and survivors of a stroke.[96,97]

The ACSM guidelines for persons with disabilities, including cerebral palsy and persons with similar chronic disorders, are detailed in Box 28.1.[98] Some authors believe that persons with cerebral palsy need to maintain higher levels of physical fitness than the general population to offset the decline in function that occurs as a result of aging, including changes related to their condition.[90] It has been shown that persons with cerebral

> **BOX 28.1 American College of Sports Medicine Exercise Recommendations for Persons With Chronic Diseases and Disabilities Such as Cerebral Palsy**
>
> 1. Professionals trained in strength and conditioning should supervise training exercise.
> 2. If there are significant movement limitations, obtaining moderate to vigorous exercise may be difficult, and reducing sedentary behaviors may be more reasonable.
> 3. For persons with mild to moderate impairment, aerobic capacity training is recommended in form of walking over ground or treadmill, or using ergometer or bicycle.
> 4. Perform single joint movements during training, one side at a time, and train these muscles within their available active range of motion.
> 5. Train the movement, prior to weight training and train power within the muscles available range.
> 6. Using a 1RM max calculator via the 10-repetition maximum is most feasible.

palsy respond well to resistance training and are capable of attaining normal strength.[99] It is also important to note that most studies in cerebral palsy persons in wheelchairs (that focus on physical activity and fitness interventions) indicate exercise is safe and promotes health, fitness, and well-being.[100] However, there are many types of exercise these patients can participate in and various sports may impact the success of exercise. The Cerebral Palsy International Sports and Recreation Association (CP-IRSA) is therefore helping to lead the world of research for exercise in cerebral palsy and related conditions, by studying the impact of training techniques, equipment, and impairment classifications in individual sports.

Medical Considerations
Medications
In persons who have had a traumatic brain injury, neurostimulants such as modafinil may increase susceptibility to either arrhythmia or heat exhaustion. Anticholinergic medications, which are used frequently by this population for the treatment of neurogenic bladder, can also increase susceptibility to heat exhaustion.[101] Medications used commonly in this population may be banned by WADA and require therapeutic use exemption forms. Individuals and clinicians can obtain therapeutic use exemption forms at the WADA website.[35]

Musculoskeletal Injuries
Musculoskeletal injuries are frequent in persons with cerebral palsy. Muscle strains and soft tissue injuries are most common.[24] The most frequent location includes the knee, followed by injuries to the shoulder.[102] Muscular imbalances and spasticity produce increased tension across the knee that can trigger patellofemoral pain syndrome, chondromalacia, and chronic knee pain. Hip development is typically poor in persons with cerebral palsy and can cause acetabular dysplasia and hip subluxation.[103] Authors have suggested that tone, which may limit power production, may lead to increased joint stability.[14,93]

Wheelchairs are used by approximately half of all athletes with cerebral palsy, which can lead to a high prevalence of shoulder injuries.[24,103] Injuries resulting from wheelchair use have been reviewed in the "Wheelchair Athlete" section of this chapter. Musculoskeletal rehabilitation in athletes with cerebral palsy should follow the same general principles used in able-bodied persons but with a special emphasis on the recognition of muscular imbalances that make this population more susceptible to injury.[41]

Epilepsy/Seizures
Epilepsy affects approximately half of all patients with cerebral palsy and has numerous ramifications.[104] Exercise in epileptic patients improves aerobic performance and sense of well-being, reduces sleep disorders and fatigue, and decreases seizure occurrence.[105] It is very important to support exercise, rather than restrict it, whenever deemed safe. The International League against Epilepsy reports that individuals who are seizure-free for 1 year should be cleared for most activities.[105] With regard to collision and contact sports, with appropriate protection, patients with epilepsy should not be restricted. With regard to water sports (except deep diving), athletes with good control can participate with direct supervision. Hang gliding, parachuting, and free climbing should be restricted due to the risk a seizure and subsequent fall poses. Gymnastics may be considered with direct supervision.[105]

Antiepileptic drugs may have a sedating effect in persons with cerebral palsy, traumatic brain injury, or stroke because they already have an inherent risk for diminished arousal and concentration. Furthermore, antiepileptic drugs may contribute to the risk for thermoregulatory impairment, impaired vision, and decreased bone mineral density. In addition to antiepileptic drugs, a lack of mobility, poor feeding, and nutritional deficiencies can contribute to osteopenia. Seventy-seven percent of persons with moderate to severe cerebral palsy are found to have reduced bone mineral density, as measured in the femur.[106] As a result of a higher risk of fractures with osteopenia, athletes with cerebral palsy should have their bone mineral density assessed, especially before commencing participation in a contact sport.[107]

Spasticity
Spasticity is common in the cerebral palsy population. The "Wheelchair Athlete" section of this chapter includes information regarding the recognition and treatment of spasticity. It is important to recognize that using certain medications can change an athlete's classification but are not banned from competition when needed. Spasticity can either improve or impair performance.[14]

Adaptive Equipment
As previously mentioned, wheelchair use is conspicuous among athletes with cerebral palsy. The "Wheelchair Athlete" section of this chapter includes a detailed discussion of the use of wheelchairs by paraplegic athletes. Most stroke survivors and many patients with cerebral palsy or a traumatic brain injury are hemiplegic rather than paraplegic. Depending on the sport, hemiplegic athletes may benefit from an ultra-lightweight chair that is lower to the ground than the typical wheelchair, with the footrest of the unaffected side eliminated to allow for steering and propulsion with the unaffected lower limb. In persons with severe motor deficits who need greater trunk control, adaptive power chairs, seating, and pelvic restraints are essential to facilitate athletic participation. There are also restrictions such as that wheelchairs during racing may not have any mechanical gears or levers.[14] Ambulatory athletes with cerebral palsy may benefit from wearing ankle-foot orthotics, which have been shown to normalize ankle kinematics in stance, increase stride length, decrease cadence, and decrease the energy cost of walking.[108] When prescribing ankle-foot orthotics, the suitable fit of an orthosis in specialized athletic shoes (e.g., track spikes or soccer cleats) should be considered. Because ataxia, seizures, and delayed reaction times are common in patients with cerebral palsy, helmets and mouth guards should be supplied to athletes at risk for trauma from falls or an impact from other players or sports implements.[105]

INTELLECTUALLY DISABLED ATHLETES
The intellectually disabled athlete may include athletes with a wide array of underlying conditions. The current literature

predominantly pertains to persons with Down syndrome, but conditions such as fragile X syndrome and autism spectrum disorders are also common. To qualify as intellectually disabled for the Paralympic Games, a person must meet the following criteria[109]:

1. Have an IQ score of 75 or lower, adaptive behavior, and age of onset younger than 18 years of age
2. Verification process of the evidence from #1 above
3. Reduced number of tests to measure IQ as a part of #1 above

Once an athlete meets the disability criteria, they will undergo on-site verification of sport-specific eligibility with a battery of tests and possibly sports-specific performance as well.[9,109]

Criteria for participation with other organizations for the intellectually disabled have similar but more inclusive criteria to allow for increased participation by nonelite athletes. For example, the Special Olympics requires the participant to be at least 8 years old and possess an intellectual disability, cognitive delay, or developmental disability that results in functional limitations in general learning and adaptive skills, regardless of severity, as documented by an agency or professional.[110]

Exercise Physiology

Although responses to training are typically similar, differences in magnitude of response and overall capacity may exist. Persons with Down syndrome typically have lower peak oxygen uptake, maximum heart rate, and maximum ventilation compared with nondisabled control subjects and intellectually disabled persons without Down syndrome.[111-113] Acute cardiac response and recovery from exercise also appear to be impaired in persons with this syndrome.[114,115] Similarly, peak heart rate has been found to be approximately 85% that of the age-predicted maximum.[110] Chronotropic incompetence and sympathetic dysfunction are often cited as being the main contributory factors to these effects.[116-119] Abnormalities of the atrioventricular node may also be associated with dysrhythmias and heart block of variable degrees. Pulmonary capacity and air flow dynamics may also be affected, because pulmonary dysplasia and relative upper airway obstruction have been described in this population.[110] In contrast to persons with Down syndrome, persons with fragile X syndrome may possess relatively increased levels of autonomic tone with possible consequences on heart rate during exercise and the recovery period. However, the effect that this characteristic has on exercise and performance is unclear.[120-122]

Medical Considerations
Musculoskeletal Injuries

Common musculoskeletal conditions in persons with Down syndrome or fragile X syndrome include strains, sprains, contusions, poor muscle tone, generalized joint laxity, and a variety of malalignments, including scoliosis, pes planus/cavus, hallux varus/valgus, and hip instability.[110,123-127] Although good data on injury rates and types of injuries are lacking, these conditions likely increase the risk of injuries such as patellofemoral pain syndrome, patellofemoral dislocation, spine pain, slipped capital femoral epiphysis, tendinopathies, and osteoarthritis.[110,123,124] Knee injuries are most common, with track and field accounting for

the most sport-related injuries in total at state, national, and international events.[110]

Injury rates for 1000 participant-hours have been reported at 0.4 for Special Olympics and 2.0 for special education high school students.[110] Special Olympics athletes in Texas with Down syndrome had a relative risk of injury or illness 3.2 times greater than other athletes.[128]

An issue that demands attention is the presence of atlantoaxial instability in athletes with Down syndrome. These athletes are at risk of spontaneous or traumatic subluxation of the cervical spine and are required by most organizations to undergo a physical examination and flexion/extension radiographs of the cervical spine. Although a large majority of persons with Down syndrome who have radiographic instability (>4 to 5 mm of odontoid-atlas separation) are asymptomatic, all such athletes should be restricted from participation in sports activities that pose a risk for neck injury or inherently require excessive neck flexion/extension. Sports and events with high risk include, but are not limited to, pentathlon, diving, butterfly swim (and no flip turns no matter the stroke), high jump, gymnastics, soccer, judo, snowboarding, and alpine skiing.[110] Atlantoaxial instability (AAI) can progress until skeletal maturity, and repeat evaluations throughout skeletal maturity may be necessary.[110]

Visual Impairment

Ocular and visual impairments are common in athletes with intellectual disabilities, with up to 50% afflicted by blepharitis, astigmatism, nystagmus, strabismus, lens opacities, and refractive errors.[129] Incorrect or delayed diagnosis and management of visual impairments may decrease coordination and motor skills, impair performance, and increase risk for injury.[130] The use of approved protective eyewear is strongly recommended, particularly during participation in high-risk sports and in those athletes with one functional eye.[131,132] Further details are discussed in the Visually Impaired Athletes section of this chapter.

Epilepsy/Seizures

Epilepsy has been found to occur in persons with several conditions that are common in this category, including Down syndrome (up to 13%), autism disorders (20%), and fragile X syndrome.[133-135] Further details are discussed in the Athletes with Cerebral Palsy section of this chapter.

Cardiac Abnormalities

Approximately half of all persons with Down syndrome have congenital heart problems, most often an endocardial cushion defect, followed by isolated septal defects.[110] Stenosis in surgically corrected valves or subaortic stenosis may complicate prior repair of an atrioventricular canal defect, and mitral and aortic regurgitation may present primarily without prior congenital heart problems. As a result of flawed connective tissue, persons with fragile X syndrome may have mitral valve prolapse and aortic root dilatation, which particularly occur in mature individuals. Although not well described in this population, these heart conditions have exercise implications similar to those in persons with Marfan or Ehlers-Danlos syndromes. Clinicians should obtain a detailed history to screen for significant cardiovascular problems, including syncope, lightheadedness, and dyspnea. Furthermore, a thorough clinical examination to evaluate for the presence of aortic regurgitation and mitral valve prolapse is critical. Lastly, detailed cardiac testing including stress testing and echocardiography may be necessary.

Adaptive Equipment

Intellectually disabled athletes may benefit from simple variations of standard equipment; for example, balance beams may be wider than standard size to accommodate impaired visual acuity and balance, balls may be larger and softer, and equipment may have straps and larger handles to help with grip. The athletes may benefit from assistance from other persons as well, such as with the use of tethers for alpine skiing.

VISUALLY IMPAIRED ATHLETES

Visually impaired athletes may possess a number of different conditions that limit visual acuity. In the Paralympics, these athletes are separated into categories based on visual acuity for some events, or they may compete directly against each other regardless of their amount of remaining sight. In the latter case, athletes are often required to wear "black-out" masks to reduce any possible competitive advantage based on sight.[9]

Exercise Physiology

Cardiopulmonary physiology of visually impaired athletes is similar to that of able-bodied athletes.[136] However, other associated syndromes, as previously described in various groups, may increase risk of cardiopulmonary abnormalities.

Medical Considerations
Musculoskeletal Injuries

Athletes with visual impairments may be particularly prone to acute injuries of the distal lower extremities such as ankle sprains and bruises. These injuries result from collisions and falls during competition in unfamiliar environments wherein adequate guidance is lacking.[102] Visually impaired athletes also may be at risk for chronic overuse injuries due to altered biomechanics, induced by poor proprioception, and loss of the visual component of balance.[70]

Flight Dysrhythmia

The visual input of light is an exogenous time cue for the body and for adjustments to the circadian rhythm that governs the sleep-wake cycle, core temperature, and other key aspects of bodily adjustment. Rapid desynchronization of the circadian rhythm, as noted with transmeridian travel, may result in flight dysrhythmia, commonly known as "jet lag." This may affect sleep characteristics, cognition, athletic performance, and risk of heat-related illness.[137] Loss of light as an exogenous cue in persons with visual impairment may result in a diminished physiologic response to flight dysrhythmia.[138] This diminished response may have a negative impact on athletes who are visually impaired as they plan for international travel in an effort to allow for time for synchronization to improve performance and reduce risk for injury.

Adaptive Equipment

Although some sports such as judo require minimal interventions, some events may make use of companions as guides. For example, during track events, some companions may provide auditory cues or tap when athletes are in danger of a lane violation. In other events such as goalball, companions may use a sound-based modification in which the ball has internal bells, requiring all participants, coaches, and spectators to remain quiet to allow for auditory tracking of the ball. Other modifications may include the use of bright light, course and equipment colors with high levels of contrast, heavily padded ropes and boundaries, and guide rails.

LES AUTRES

Athletes in the Les Autres group do not fit into one of the other five categories. This category encompasses a wide range of different medical conditions of at least some familiarity to most clinicians, including multiple sclerosis, osteogenesis imperfecta, muscular dystrophy, and dwarfism. However, this group potentially includes an enormous range of conditions and syndromes, with 1 of the 10 types of permanent impairments, listed in the "Classification" section of this chapter.

It is imperative that the clinician be familiar with other features of a given syndrome that may affect sports performance, safety, and overall health. Although an in-depth discussion of the various conditions is beyond the scope of this chapter, the clinician may draw upon some of the principles presented in the prior sections of this chapter. For example, aspects that warrant assessment include but are not limited to cardiopulmonary, thermoregulatory, cognitive, restricted ROM or motor functions, seizure risk, and adaptive equipment. A clinician may then draw upon this assessment and other knowledge of the person's condition to make informed recommendations regarding the choice of sport, safety, and precompetition planning.

SUMMARY

Medical conditions that affect athletes with special needs are numerous and diverse in clinical presentation, enhance risk for injury and illness, and can affect peak athletic performance. Yet given the plethora of benefits from regular physical activity, increased participation in competition, and the exploration and expansion of boundaries of sport in this population, it is important for clinicians to be familiar with the different "athlete classes" and their clinical characteristics. It is only then that clinicians will be able to perform comprehensive preparticipation physical examinations, provide quality care, match patients to appropriate sports, counsel on risk reduction for injury and illness, and appropriately refer athletes to consultants and allied health professionals to provide the best medical care.

ACKNOWLEDGMENT

The authors and editors gratefully acknowledge the contributions of the previous authors, C. Joel Hess and Dilaawar J. Mistry.

For a complete list of references, go to ExpertConsult.com.

SELECTED READINGS

Citation:
Slocum C, Blauwet C, Allen JA. Sports medicine considerations for the Paralympic athlete. *Curr Phys Med Rehabil Rep.* 2015;3(1):25–35.

Level of Evidence:
V

Summary:
A brief overview of the common athlete classifications and injuries seen in the para-athlete.

Citation:
Webborn N, Van de Vliet P. Paralympic medicine. *Lancet.* 2012;380(9836):65–71.

Level of Evidence:
V

Summary:
A brief evidence-based review of the Paralympic sports, impairment ratings, medical needs, equipment, event medical services, and antidoping issues.

Citation:
Patel DR, Greydanus DE. The pediatric athlete with disabilities. *Pediatr Clin North Am.* 2002;49(4):803–827.

Level of Evidence:
V

Summary:
A brief evidence-based review of the issues contained in this chapter, as well as psychosocial and assessment considerations as they specifically pertain to the pediatric disabled athlete population.

Citation:
Burkett B. Technology in Paralympic sport: performance enhancement or essential for performance? *Br J Sports Med.* 2010;44(3):215–220.

Level of Evidence:
IV

Summary:
A systematic review of technological requirements and considerations in the Paralympic athlete population.

Citation:
Lynch JH. The athlete with intellectual disabilities. In: O'Connor FG, ed. *ACSM's Sports Medicine: A Comprehensive Review.* Wolters Kluwer, Lippincott Williams and Wilkins; 2013.

Level of Evidence:
V

Summary:
A chapter within a highly used sports medicine textbook, with a brief summary of key points for the medical provider when caring for the intellectually disabled athlete.

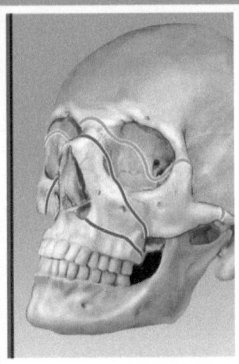

29

Anesthesia and Perioperative Medicine

Ashley Matthews Shilling

The term *athlete*, derived from the Greek word *athlon* meaning "prize" or "contest," conjures images of a healthy, fit person. Although athletes possess physical speed, strength, and talents, they also have a repertoire of medical problems as well as a number of sports-related injuries leading them to the operating room. This chapter discusses common medical problems in the sports patient within the context of surgical and anesthetic implications. Perioperative athletic concerns are also discussed, including preparation of the sports medicine patient for surgery, anesthetic choices, pain management, and common postoperative complications and concerns.

PREOPERATIVE CARE AND CONCERNS: COMMON MEDICAL ISSUES FOUND IN ATHLETES

Respiratory Considerations

Asthma

A common pulmonary disorder in athletes, asthma is marked by restriction of airflow in the lungs, narrowing of the airways, and inflammation of the bronchi. Bronchoconstriction and inflammation induce shortness of breath, wheezing, coughing, and chest tightness. The prevalence of exercise-induced bronchospasm is 8% to 12% in the general population but may be as high as 50% in elite athletes and those competing in cold-weather sports.[1] Several high-profile athletes with asthma, including Billy Jean King, Dennis Rodman, Jackie Joyner-Kersee, and Amy Van Dyken, have performed at the highest level with adequate treatment.

Triggers include smoking, environmental, respiratory viruses, odors, and exercise. The specifics of diagnosis and therapy for persons with asthma are detailed in a separate chapter in this book. Asthma can be diagnosed with a thorough history and physical examination and various provocative tests. Although multiple options are available to treat asthma, an important tenet is prevention by avoidance of triggering agents and maintenance therapy. Common strategies for maintenance and treatment of exacerbations include β_2 agonists (with albuterol being the most commonly used), inhaled corticosteroids, systemic corticosteroids, anticholinergic drugs, leukotriene-receptor antagonists, and methylxanthine agents. Drugs may be administered by nebulizer, metered-dose inhaler, orally, or intravenously in emergency situations. Before a patient undergoes elective surgery, it is important that asthma be optimally controlled. Despite the bronchodilating properties of most anesthetics, asthmatics are more prone to bronchospasm after airway manipulation under anesthesia. Avoidance of general anesthesia and endotracheal intubation may be beneficial. When a general anesthetic is needed, a laryngeal mask airway has been shown to cause less airway reactivity than an endotracheal tube.[2]

Obstructive Sleep Apnea

Obstructive sleep apnea (OSA) is defined by periods of hypoventilation or apnea caused by airway obstruction during sleep. The severity of disease can be determined by the number of obstructive episodes, degree of oxygen desaturation, number of microarousal episodes, and number of arrhythmias per unit of time. Up to 90% of individuals with moderate to severe sleep apnea may remain undiagnosed.[3-5]

OSA may be more common in athletes than originally thought.[5] A study of eight randomly selected NFL teams and 302 players demonstrated a 14% incidence of sleep apnea with a 34% incidence in linemen.[6] Dr. Archie Roberts, a retired heart surgeon who has teamed with the Mayo Clinic to screen retired NFL players, has noted an alarming incidence of OSA. The incidence of sleep-disordered breathing was present in 52.3% of the former football players.[7] Furthermore, a study of sumo wrestlers in Tokyo found that 11 of 23 wrestlers had significant sleep-disordered breathing.[8] Clearly, OSA is a problem that entails clinical vigilance, even in athletes who are presumed to be healthy.

Obstruction of the upper airway during sleep or sedation occurs from a decrease in oropharyngeal and laryngopharyngeal tone and leads to partial or complete airway obstruction.[9] An increase in airway resistance, hypoxia, and hypercarbia ensue, resulting in an increase in sympathetic tone and subsequent patient arousal. Complications of OSA include chronic hypoxia, hypoxemia, and hypercarbia leading to pulmonary hypertension, right heart failure, and sudden death. Less obvious associations between OSA and long-term sequelae include depression, hypertension, coronary artery disease, and stroke.

OSA is a significant problem in the postoperative period. Sedatives, narcotic drugs, hypnotic agents, and muscle relaxants can exacerbate symptoms. Because of pain and the inherent stress of surgery, patients experience disturbances in rapid eye movement sleep patterns for several days after the immediate postoperative period. The increased risk of obstruction and other complications should be considered when planning intraoperative and postoperative care. Limiting narcotics, benzodiazepines, and general anesthesia (GA) in addition to educating patients about the risks of OSA may be helpful.

A thorough clinical history and appropriate screening may suggest a diagnosis of OSA. Symptoms of OSA include daytime sleepiness, snoring, witnessed apnea, poor concentration, morning headaches, moodiness, and irritability. Males who have hypertension, are overweight, smoke, and have a larger neck circumference are more likely to have OSA. Fig. 29.1 shows the STOP-BANG questionnaire. Because many risk factors for OSA are well known, various screening tools to help identify patients with OSA are used extensively and include the most validated STOP-Bang scoring system, P-SAP screening tool, Berlin screening tool, and American Society of Anesthesiologists (ASA) checklist.[5,10,11]

Diagnosis of OSA can be made with polysomnography and a multiple sleep latency test. The mainstay of treatment is the use of a continuous positive airway pressure (CPAP) machine, which opens the upper airway and prevents obstruction. Oral or nasal masks are custom-fit for ease of use and comfort, but can still be obtrusive for some patients, leading to noncompliance. Other treatments for OSA include weight loss, dental devices, uvulopalatopharyngoplasty, tonsillectomy and/or adenoidectomy, craniofacial advancement techniques, somnoplasties, and nasal surgeries. OSA has been implicated in both inpatient and outpatient deaths and is exacerbated by many factors that occur in the perioperative period.

In 2016, guidelines and recommendations from the Society of Anesthesia and Sleep Medicine (SASM) were released. There is a moderate level of evidence that OSA increases patients' risk for perioperative complications. While it is generally recommended that adult patients be screened for OSA before surgery, there is little evidence to support benefits of preoperative screening. Despite this, there is consensus that identifying patients with or likely to have OSA allows providers to utilize multi-modal analgesic techniques and avoid general anesthesia when possible. Patients with OSA should be screened for other systemic diseases and all co-morbidities should be optimized prior to proceeding with elective surgery.[4]

STOP-BANG Scoring Method
Every Yes answer = 1 point

Snoring: Do you snore loudly (loud enough to be heard through closed doors)? ☐ Yes ☐ No
Tired: Do you often feel tired, fatigued, or sleepy during daytime? ☐ Yes ☐ No
Observed: Has anyone observed you stop breathing during your sleep? ☐ Yes ☐ No
Blood **P**ressure: Do you have or are you being treated for high blood pressure? ☐ Yes ☐ No
BMI more than 35? ☐ Yes ☐ No
Age older than 50 years? ☐ Yes ☐ No
Neck circumference greater than 40 cm? ☐ Yes ☐ No
Gender male? ☐ Yes ☐ No

Fig. 29.1 The STOP-BANG questionnaire is a tool that can be used to screen patients for obstructive sleep apnea. *BMI*, Body mass index. (From Chung F, Yegneswaran B, Liao P, et al. STOP questionnaire: a tool to screen patients for obstructive sleep apnea. *Anesthesiology.* 2008;108:812–821.)

Cardiac Considerations

Cardiac issues in athletes are discussed in detail elsewhere in this book, but two entities, the athletic heart syndrome (AHS) and hypertrophic cardiomyopathy (HCM), are discussed here.

Athletic Heart Syndrome

AHS is an adaptive physiologic condition manifested by enlargement of the heart in response to vigorous and frequent exercise, enhanced efficiency, and bradycardia (as low as 30 to 40 beats per minute). First described in 1899 by the Swedish physician Henschen, AHS was discovered by percussing hearts and comparing the heart sizes of cross-country skiers and sedentary patients.[12] The heart increases in size in response to recurrent systemic oxygen deficits, resulting in increased muscle mass and increased ventricular chamber size, which facilitates cardiac output during exercise. AHS is benign yet vital to recognize, because bradycardia and cardiac hypertrophy can be a concern for clinicians and can be confused with life-threatening HCM. Diagnosis is made with electrocardiogram, a chest radiograph, or a transthoracic echocardiogram. Although AHS is not a health concern, a low resting heart rate may predispose athletes to vasovagal reactions manifested by diaphoresis, nausea, and syncope.

Hypertrophic Cardiomyopathy

Also known as *hypertrophic obstructive cardiomyopathy*, HCM is a disease process that must be expeditiously diagnosed and treated to prevent significant morbidity and mortality. HCM is the most common cause of sudden cardiac death and has led to the untimely death of many well-known athletes.[13] Notable athletes who succumbed to HCM include Gaines Adams of the Chicago Bears, who died at age 26 years; Ryan Shay, a 28-year-old marathoner who died 5.5 miles into a race; and Marc-Vivin Foe, the brilliant Cameroon midfielder, who died at age 28 years during a semifinal soccer match. None of these athletes was diagnosed with HCM prior to their deaths.

HCM is a genetic disorder that leads to asymmetric thickening of the myocardium that can induce life-threatening arrhythmias. Whereas most forms of HCM are inherited, others are caused by sporadic mutations. The prevalence is thought to be as high as 1 in 500 people in the 23- to 35-year age group.[14] Although myocardial hypertrophy usually occurs in the ventricular septum, hypertrophy can occur in various locations, which can lead to outflow obstruction, particularly during vigorous exercise or during states of hypotension or dehydration.

For persons with HCM, it is imperative that medical clearance for participation in athletics be withheld pending consultation with a cardiologist. Obtaining a thorough personal and family history is critical because symptoms and signs typically do not present until teenage years. Common symptoms and signs include chest pain (which may present in the post-exercise period), shortness of breath, arrhythmias or palpitations, syncope, dizziness, and sudden death. Unfortunately, 1% of patients with HCM present with sudden death. In a study of 158 sudden deaths in athletes between the ages of 12 and 40 years in a 10-year period, it was found that 90% of all sudden deaths occurred during or immediately after competition.[15] Postmortem examinations and toxicologic data suggested that 134 of these deaths were related to cardiac pathology, of which 36% were the result of HCM. Physical examination in asymptomatic athletes who have occult HCM may be normal or may reveal a fourth heart sound and/or a left ventricular lift (nonspecific). In persons with a significant obstruction, a harsh crescendo-decrescendo systolic murmur may be heard that begins shortly after S1, is typically best auscultated at the apex and lower left sternal border, and may radiate to the axilla and base, yet not usually into the neck. As a result of increased obstruction, the murmur may increase with an assumption of an upright posture from a supine, sitting, or squatting position or after the Valsalva maneuver.

It is beyond the scope of this chapter to detail various diagnostic and therapeutic tools or to discuss the controversies of screening athletes for HCM. Pre-participation screening for HCM is an ardently debated subject, with conflicting recommendations from varying organizations. The American Heart Association has indicated that a thorough pre-participation history and physical examination may be adequate to detect underlying pathology in many cases and that more detailed testing (to improve sensitivity), including an electrocardiogram and transthoracic echocardiogram, be reserved for cases with features that raise concern on clinical examination.[16] Conversely, in Italy, pre-participation screening for athletes includes a detailed patient and family history, physical examination, and electrocardiogram (with additional cardiac testing as needed).[17] After institution of the mandated nationwide systematic screening program, the incidence of sudden cardiovascular death in young competitive athletes between 1979 and 2004 significantly decreased in the Veneto region of Italy. Therapeutic interventions included medications (β- or calcium channel blockers and antiarrhythmic agents), pacemakers and/or defibrillators, and/or invasive, surgical management (i.e., a myomectomy or ablation of the cardiac septum).

Diabetes Mellitus

Diabetes mellitus (DM) is prevalent in athletes. Although athletes of different ages may have either type 1 or type 2 DM, type 1 DM occurs more commonly in athletes, and it is estimated that about 215 000 people in the United States who are younger than 20 years have some form of diabetes.[18] Long-term complications of diabetes include cardiovascular disease, cerebrovascular disease, peripheral neuropathy, retinopathy, and nephropathy. Diagnostic tests include fasting plasma glucose level, oral glucose tolerance, or random plasma glucose level tests. Fasting glucose levels should be less than 100 mg/dL; levels between 100 and 125 mg/dL reflect impaired glucose tolerance, and levels greater than 200 mg/dL raise concern for diabetes.

Treatment of diabetes consists of maintaining normal or near-normal glucose levels and preventing hypoglycemia. Although hypoglycemia rarely occurs in persons with type 2 DM, it can lead to significant morbidity and mortality in persons with type 1 DM. Severe hypoglycemia can lead to seizures and irreversible brain damage due to the brain's need of glucose for normal metabolic activity. Hypoglycemia should be immediately treated by administration of glucose in the form of carbohydrates, glucose tablets, or IV dextrose. In the perioperative period, hypoglycemia may be missed in sedated or anesthetized patients, and hyperglycemia may lead to an increased number of wound infections and poor wound healing.

INTRAOPERATIVE CARE AND CONSIDERATIONS OF THE SPORTS MEDICINE PATIENT

Orthopaedic Surgeries and Pain

A study of ambulatory surgeries showed that orthopedic patients have the highest incidence of postoperative pain.[19] Inadequately treated pain can significantly affect recovery time, rehabilitation, patient satisfaction, and may increase readmission rates. When choosing the anesthetic, various factors should be considered, including the precise location of surgical intervention, extent of bone manipulation, instrumentation, osteotomies, ligamentous involvement, expected or planned nerve manipulation, use of bone or tendon autografts, size of incisions, the use of intraoperative tourniquets, and the requirements for postoperative physical therapy and range-of-motion (ROM) exercises. These perioperative factors will help the health care providers predict the level of postoperative pain, determine if a regional technique is indicated, and determine the needed duration of effect.

A peripheral nerve block (PNB) may provide excellent analgesia postoperatively, but may not be sufficient to cover the entire surgical field or for intraoperative retraction and manipulation. The necessary positioning for surgery can induce non-operative discomfort and can be a limiting factor in using a regional technique as the primary anesthetic. Pain induced by use of a tourniquet can be a source of substantial discomfort for a patient who is awake. Occlusion times more than 45 to 60 minutes may lead to break-through ischemic pain and may be intolerable despite the use of a PNB. Finally, certain surgical procedures put the patient at high risk for nerve injury or compartment syndrome and the surgeon may wish to identify this risk early in the postoperative course. In this setting, a regional technique may confound the postoperative examination for the first 24 hours or may mask a compartment syndrome.

Patient Characteristics

Several clinical features, including the aforementioned medical comorbidities, play an important role in shaping the anesthetic plan. In the younger athletic population, cardiovascular risk factors are fortunately rare, as GA is known to increase the risk of significant cardiac events in persons with certain cardiac risk factors.[20] For persons with OSA, the use of non-narcotic means of analgesia and avoidance of GA is recommended to reduce the risk of perioperative complications.[21-25] If a patient has a history of difficult intubation, it may be beneficial to avoid airway instrumentation to prevent potential airway complications. Patients with increased risk of aspiration as a result of preexisting esophageal or gastric pathology, or more commonly as a result of gastroesophageal reflux disease, may also benefit from the avoidance of GA. Patient psychological factors may play a prominent role in the anesthetic choice. Promising young athletes may fear a protracted nerve injury after undergoing a regional technique.

Regional Anesthesia

The term regional anesthesia implies analgesia and immobility of a region of the body. Regional anesthesia techniques may be further subdivided into those that target segmental spinal levels (i.e., central or neuraxial blocks such as spinal or epidural blocks), peripheral nerves (e.g., PNBs and plexus blocks), or extremities via IV regional block (i.e., Bier block). Neuraxial blocks and PNBs are achieved with the use of local anesthetic agents, narcotics, and other adjuvant medication. Field blocks typically describe the more superficial injection of local anesthetics. Both neuraxial nerve blocks and PNBs can be modified by the insertion of a catheter to continuously infuse medication during surgery, as well as for postoperative analgesia. Peripheral nerve catheters can be used in an inpatient or outpatient setting with proper patient selection and education. PNBs and neuraxial anesthetic agents may be used as the primary anesthetic or as an adjuvant to GA.

Contraindications to Regional Anesthesia

Absolute and relative contraindications to regional anesthesia typically vary by the type of planned intervention and the patient. Patient refusal, the inability to lie still during administration of a block, infection at the site of injection, recent use of thrombolytic agents, and operator inexperience for the proposed regional technique are perhaps the only shared absolute contraindications. Increased intracranial pressure may lead to brainstem herniation, which precludes use of neuraxial procedures. Other relative contraindications include evidence of systemic infection, preexisting neurologic disease, coagulopathy attributable to intrinsic disease or medication, or aberrant anatomy. All risks and benefits should be weighed thoroughly before proceeding with regional anesthesia.

Complications of Regional Anesthesia

The incidence of infection associated with neuraxial techniques is approximately 1 in 40,000.[26,27] The risk of PNB infection has yet to be clearly defined, but appears to be greater with the use of continuous, indwelling catheters in the axillary or femoral areas for more than 48 hours.[28,29] Skin contaminants either by colonization or local infection, systemic infection via seeding of catheter sites, or immune suppression enhance risk.[30] Spinal hematomas may form after induction of spinal or epidural anesthesia in patients with underlying coagulopathy.[31] Detailed recommendations for management are well described in the American Society of Regional Anesthesia 2010 Practice Advisory.[32] Although the data are less instructive for PNBs, the literature includes rare case reports of a hematoma causing nerve injury, which seems to be more prevalent with use of deeper techniques such as lumbar plexus block. Nerve injuries are a major concern for both the orthopedic surgeon and anesthesiologist, yet the overall risk of peripheral nerve injury (PNI) is fortunately small. A meta-analysis in 2007 showed rates of permanent nerve injury between 0 and 7.6 per 10,000 for neuraxial procedures and approximately 1 in 15,000 for PNBs.[33] Recent studies of PNI demonstrate long-term neurologic findings widely ranging from 0.029% to 0.2%, largely due to study methodology.[34-40] Most commonly, the incidence of neurologic findings after PNB are quoted between 2 and 4/10,000.[41] The incidence of short-term paresthesias or dysesthesias is thought to be much higher at 1% to 3%, with the highest incidence following interscalene brachial plexus blocks.[33]

The American Society of Regional Anesthesia (ASRA) published a practice advisory in 2016 with a specific focus on neurologic injury following regional techniques. In addition to reviewing the incidence, causes, and risks for neurologic injury following regional techniques, the advisory also reviews risks of PNI after common orthopedic procedures and describes treatment algorithms following PNI.[41]

Benefits of Regional Anesthesia in the Sports Medicine Patient

The benefits of regional anesthesia are abundant. Compared with narcotic analgesic agents, postoperative pain control is notably improved with peripheral nerve and neuraxial blocks.[42-45] As expected, these studies also demonstrate less nausea, vomiting, ileus, pruritus, and sedation because of the opiate-sparing effects. It is also well established that the use of regional anesthesia improves functional recovery in select patients. Peripheral nerve catheters resulted in earlier ambulation, shorter hospital stays, and shorter rehabilitation periods after discharge, as well as improved ROM and mobilization after knee surgery.[46-48] Epidural catheters also offer similar analgesic benefits when compared with peripheral nerve catheters, although hypotension and nausea are more common.[49] In the ambulatory setting, orthopedic procedures can account for a significant percentage of unplanned readmissions for pain control.[50] Use of outpatient perineural catheters resulted in fewer unplanned admissions after discharge in patients undergoing anterior cruciate ligament (ACL) surgery.[51]

Regional anesthesia may also benefit patients in measures that transcend pain control and its associated secondary gains. Operative blood loss may be decreased through decreased arterial and venous pressure and blockade of sympathetic tone in the affected extremity.[46] The incidence of deep venous thrombosis (DVT) and pulmonary embolism (PE) may be lower with neuraxial anesthesia because of increased blood flow, decreased viscosity, and modification of inflammatory mediators.[52,53] Neuraxial anesthesia may also reduce the risk of infections at surgical sites, possibly through modulation of inflammation and immune responses.[54] Furthermore, the avoidance of GA in high-risk patient populations is an immeasurable benefit.

Tourniquets

A precious commodity during orthopedic procedures, tourniquets provide a bloodless field for surgery. However, complications associated with tourniquet placement are not uncommon. Pain with resulting hypertension and tachycardia, "sickling" in sickle cell disease, nerve injury, and tissue damage may result.[55] Nerve injury can result from ischemia, pressure, or shearing at the edges of the tourniquet. The pain is typically dull and begins with inflation. Progressive symptoms may include tingling, numbness, paresthesia, and a change in quality of pain. Pain typically begins at 20 minutes and can become severe at approximately

40 minutes.[56] No duration of tourniquet use is guaranteed to be safe, yet most experts consider 2 hours to be the "maximum ischemic time."[57] At the conclusion of procedures, release of the tourniquet can lead to hypotension and metabolic acidosis as metabolites from an ischemic limb are released into the circulation.[58] In patients with congestive heart failure, a sudden increase in circulating volume can lead to volume overload and acute heart failure. Occluding venous blood flow distal to the tourniquet predisposes a patient to thrombi formation. Systemic release of the thrombi after tourniquet deflation may lead to stroke and PE.[58]

Positioning

Although many orthopedic surgeries may be performed in a supine intraoperative position, some operations require more complicated positions and padding. Proper positioning and padding is essential to minimize complications.

Beach Chair Position

The beach chair position has become the chosen intraoperative position for many orthopedic surgeons who perform procedures on the shoulder. This position is favored for many reasons, including better exposure of the shoulder joint, avoidance of the lateral position, decreased risk for brachial plexus injuries, and reduced bleeding in the joint. Nonetheless, the beach chair position has multiple physiologic consequences, including a decrease in mean arterial blood pressure, central venous pressure, stroke volume, cardiac output, and arterial oxygen content. Additional concerns include venous pooling, increased risk for air embolus, and poor access to the airway. Reports of fluid extravasation from the shoulder joint into soft tissue have led to airway compromise.

An important concern is the discrepancy that can exist between cerebral perfusion and the site of blood pressure measurement. This issue is especially vital in the hypertensive patient who may have a rightward shift of the cerebral autoregulatory curve and needs higher mean arterial blood pressure to maintain adequate perfusion. Blood pressure should be measured in the arm at the brachial artery, and the distance between the heart and external auditory meatus should be calculated. The hydrostatic gradient can be determined using the conversion of 0.77 mm Hg decrease for every centimeter height difference between the brain and the site of blood pressure measurement.[59] Additionally, placing a blood pressure cuff on the ankle (which could be as much as 150 cm below the brain) has been implicated in providing the anesthesiologist and surgeon with a false sense of increased cerebral perfusion pressures. Serious neurologic injury, presumably due to inadequate cerebral perfusion during beach chair positioning, has been documented in four patients.[60]

SPECIFIC REGIONAL ANESTHESIA TECHNIQUES
Neuraxial Anesthesia

Epidural, caudal, and spinal blocks are collectively referred to as neuraxial anesthetics. Spinal block also may be referred to as an intrathecal or subarachnoid block. Neuraxial techniques can be used for surgical anesthesia for any lower extremity, hip, or pelvic procedure. Most commonly, a mix of a local anesthetic (with or without a narcotic) is used, but other adjuncts exist to enhance block quality and duration. Placement of a catheter, which is most commonly used with epidural blockade, facilitates the ability to augment or lengthen the duration of the block intraoperatively or provide ongoing postoperative analgesia. The chief difference between epidural and spinal blockade is the location of drug administration. Whereas a spinal block requires puncture of the dura mater and injection of the drug into the cerebrospinal fluid, an epidural block requires injection of drug past the ligamentum flavum, outside the dura mater. Because of varying anatomy within the epidural space and the presence of vasculature, fat, and potential septations, an epidural block can occasionally result in a patchy or unilateral block quality when compared with a spinal block.

The most common adverse effects encountered with neuraxial blocks are hypotension, pruritus, nausea, sedation, and urinary retention. Hemodynamic effects, including hypotension and bradycardia, are more noticeable with a spinal block, which is due to rapid onset of sympathectomy, as well as blockade of cardioaccelerator fibers in the upper thoracic spinal levels. Pruritus and nausea are more pronounced with use of a narcotic in the neuraxial mixture. Postdural puncture headache is another complication of neuraxial anesthesia. Believed to occur from an alteration in cerebrospinal fluid dynamics due to dural puncture, the incidence is fortunately low (0% to 2%) with spinal anesthesia when performed by an experienced provider with a small-gauge, noncutting needle.[61-63] Typically, an epidural block should not interrupt the dura mater, yet an accidental puncture can occur. A "wet tap" or cerebrospinal fluid return during epidural placement with a large 17-gauge Tuohy needle can induce a headache in a significant number of patients. In such cases, definitive treatment with an epidural blood patch is highly effective. The use of certain local anesthetic agents and traumatic needle placement may increase this risk. Major complications such as "high spinal," local anesthetic toxicity, infection, neurologically significant bleeding, and permanent nerve damage are extremely rare.

Practically, for outpatient sports medicine procedures, neuraxial blocks can be used to limit risks and costs associated with GA and subsequent recovery. In the setting of outpatient procedures such as knee arthroscopy, comparisons between GA and epidural, spinal, or PNBs have yielded conflicting results regarding speed, cost, and complications.[64-68] Although discharge readiness may be expedited for neuraxial anesthetics when considering pain control, mental status, and nausea, other factors, such as urinary retention and time for spinal to regress, may ultimately delay discharge.

Peripheral Nerve Blocks
Overview
Surgical anesthesia, immobility, and analgesia can be achieved with the precise deposition of local anesthetics and adjuvants near peripheral nerves. This can be accomplished by using surface landmarks, nerve stimulation, and ultrasound-guided techniques. The duration of the block may be manipulated by altering the type of local anesthetic or adjuvant or by placement of a perineural catheter. Localization of the nerves to be blocked may

involve several techniques. Incorporating knowledge of the surface anatomy along with palpation of vessels and bony structures can help identify the location for blockade. PNBs were initially performed by provoking paresthesias in the desired nerve distribution with needle advancement. For nerve stimulation, an insulated needle is used to apply a low-level current at the tip, which can elicit a twitch in a corresponding muscle group supplied by a target nerve. Alternatively, "real-time" ultrasonography may be used to visualize the peripheral nerves and needle, which enables anesthesiologists to administer medications with great anatomic specificity. Thus far, no one technique has been shown to decrease neurologic complications.[41] There is mounting evidence that ultrasound can decrease local anesthetic toxicity by allowing visualization of the spread of local anesthetics and also by decreasing the total amount of local anesthetic needed to provide an adequate block.[37,69-72] Ultrasound-guided blocks have numerous advantages, including a faster onset of action, improved quality, decreased volume of local anesthetic used, and a decrease in accidental vascular puncture rates.[72-74]

Upper Extremity Innervation and the Brachial Plexus

The brachial plexus forms from the ventral rami of spinal nerves C5 to T1, with occasional contribution from C4 and T2. Fig. 29.2 shows the brachial plexus. The plexus exits between the anterior and middle scalene muscles of the neck, courses over the first rib and under the clavicle, surrounds the axillary artery, and divides into peripheral nerves that supply motor and sensory innervation to the upper extremity. A fascial sheath surrounds the plexus from the intervertebral foramina to the upper arm and can serve both to compartmentalize injected medication and provide a safe barrier to this approach. Several techniques can be used to block the brachial plexus, each of which differs in coverage of the plexus and adverse effect profiles. Fig. 29.2 demonstrates the different approaches used to block the brachial plexus.

Shoulder and Upper Arm Procedures
Interscalene Block

An interscalene block provides excellent anesthesia to the upper brachial plexus C5-C7, including the entire glenohumeral joint, rotator cuff, the lateral two thirds of the clavicle, and the proximal humerus. It frequently spares blockage of C8-T1, thus often does not provide block to the medial brachial cutaneous nerve and ulnar hand distribution. Interscalene block is therefore most useful for shoulder, upper arm, and forearm procedures. It is possible to perform shoulder surgery with an interscalene block and avoid GA. Many surgeons prefer this approach because it facilitates continuous neurologic assessment for the patient in the beach chair position. As previously mentioned, an anesthetized patient in this position can experience hypotension, leading to cardiovascular and cerebrovascular complications. The interscalene block is the most commonly performed regional technique for shoulder surgery since it blocks both the axillary and suprascapular nerves. A 2015 meta-analysis showed improved pain control up to six hours during movement and eight hours at rest as well as a reduction in opioid use up to 24 hours postoperatively in patients who received an interscalene

PNB.[75] Continuous catheter techniques have been shown to extend these benefits with improvements in sleep and patient satisfaction as well.[75]

The interscalene block is performed in the anterolateral neck in close proximity to the exiting nerve roots adjacent to the scalene muscles (Fig. 29.3). The proximity to the cervical plexus, the phrenic and recurrent laryngeal nerves, stellate ganglion, and other nerves of the head and neck can lead to side effects of the block. Blockade of the ipsilateral phrenic nerve almost always occurs, so this block is relatively contraindicated for persons with severe lung disease or a contralateral diaphragmatic paralysis. However, in the vast majority of healthy patients, a phrenic nerve block causes few or no symptoms and seldom requires treatment other than reassurance. Hoarseness and Horner syndrome are also possible, but usually pose only a minor inconvenience. Fortunately, all these effects typically resolve as the block wanes. More serious complications, such as vertebral artery injection, high spinal, and accidental spinal cord injection, have been documented but are rare.

Suprascapular Block

A suprascapular block can be used alone or in conjunction with an axillary nerve block for patients with contraindications to the interscalene block and phrenic nerve paresis.[76] The nerve supplies the muscles of the rotator cuff (except for the subscapularis), the glenoid, most of the joint capsule, the posterior scapula, part of the acromion and acromioclavicular joint, as well as the skin of the neck and most of the superior shoulder. The nerve is typically blocked via a posterior approach from the suprascapular notch either with nerve stimulation or ultrasound. The risk of inducing a pneumothorax is very low with this technique. A study comparing the interscalene, supraclavicular, and suprascapular block in patients undergoing shoulder surgery demonstrated the suprascapular block to have significantly less effect in mean vital capacity reduction. There was no significant difference in mean pain scores and 24-hour opioid consumption for the three different block approaches.[77]

Elbow, Forearm, and Hand Procedures
Supraclavicular Block

Performed at the level of the trunks and divisions of the brachial plexus in the supraclavicular fossa, the supraclavicular block provides coverage throughout most of the arm. It spares the upper shoulder proximally and the T2 distribution of the medial arm. The intercostobrachial nerve, a cutaneous nerve derived from the T2 intercostal nerve, provides sensation to the medial upper arm and is typically spared by brachial plexus approaches. Therefore a subcutaneous band of local anesthetic high in the axilla is used to block this nerve when an upper arm tourniquet is used.[78] Historically the supraclavicular block was avoided by many practitioners who feared a pneumothorax or puncture of the subclavian artery. However, the use of ultrasound and the ability to visualize the first rib and pleura have made this block one of the most popular upper extremity PNBs. The block evolves rapidly because of the dense concentration of nerves at this level. Insertion of a perineural catheter with this approach has been described for prolonged analgesia.[79] The supraclavicular block

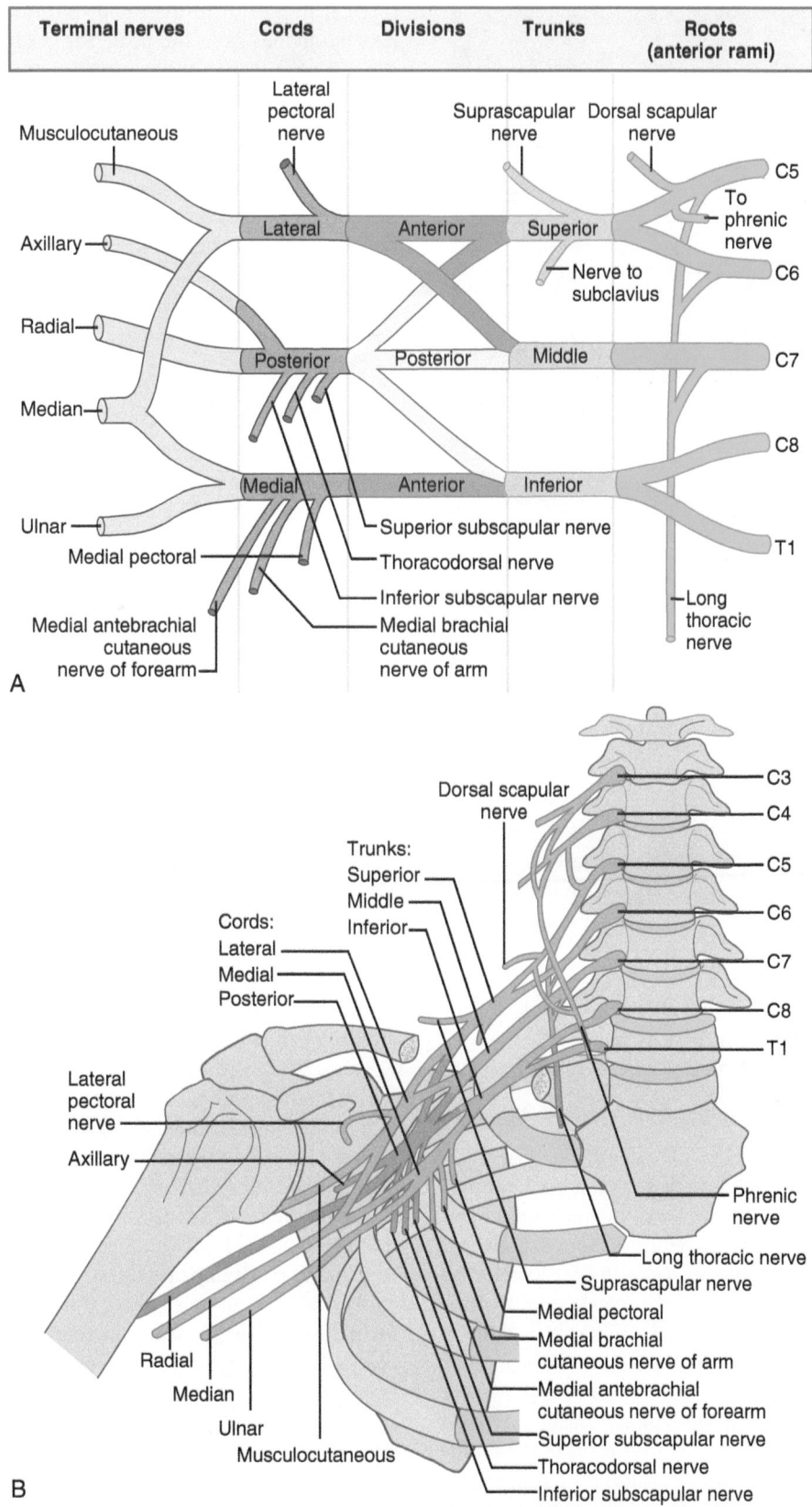

Fig. 29.2 (A) A schematic representation of the brachial plexus. (B) The brachial plexus in situ. (From Bogart BI, Ort VH. *Elsevier's Integrated Anatomy and Embryology.* Philadelphia: Mosby; 2007.)

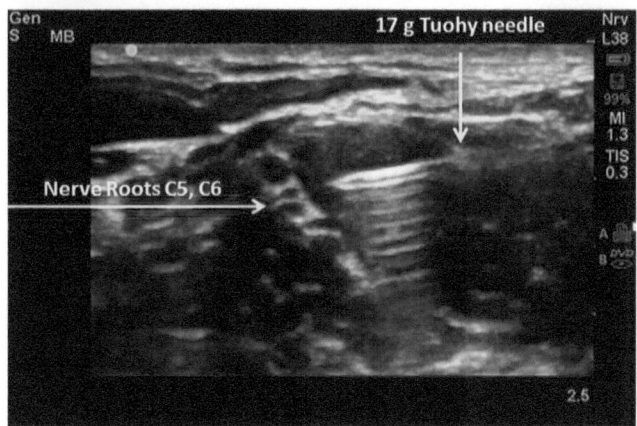

Fig. 29.3 An ultrasound image of the interscalene approach to the brachial plexus.

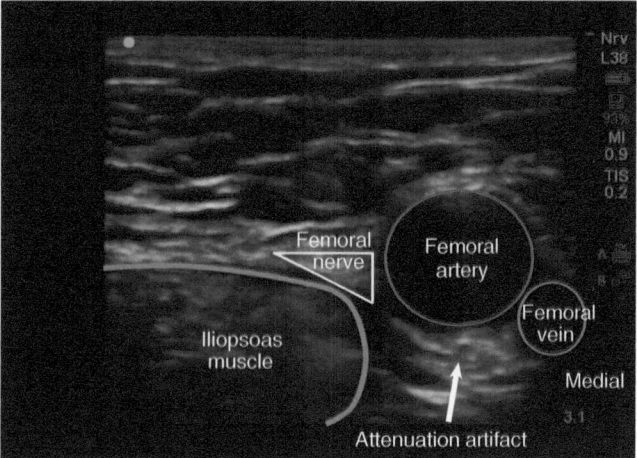

Fig. 29.4 An ultrasound image of the supraclavicular approach to the brachial plexus.

has potential adverse effects akin to the interscalene block, including phrenic nerve involvement (40% to 60%).[80]

Fig. 29.4 shows ultrasound images of the supraclavicular approach to the brachial plexus.

Infraclavicular Block

The infraclavicular block provides coverage similar to the supraclavicular block with a much lower risk of pneumothorax and phrenic nerve involvement, and therefore is more suitable for persons with lung disease. At this level, the deeper location of the nerves beneath the pectoralis muscles can make needle placement more challenging. Ultrasound visualization may be difficult in obese or very muscular patients. The block is performed inferior to the clavicle and slightly medial to the coracoid process where the lateral, posterior, and medial cords of the plexus surround the axillary artery. Speed of block onset is slower than the supraclavicular approach, but this approach is ideal for a continuous catheter due to the deeper target nerves with more tissue in which the catheter can anchor.

Axillary Brachial Plexus Block

The axillary block targets the plexus as it divides into the terminal peripheral nerves. Contrary to its name, the axillary nerve was often spared prior to the use of ultrasound because the nerve usually divides from the posterior cord of the brachial plexus more cephalad. The axillary block provides excellent coverage for forearm and hand procedures. This approach has fewer adverse effects and complications compared to interscalene or supraclavicular blocks because it is performed outside of the thorax, avoiding the lungs and numerous nerves and vessels of the neck. Additionally, this block is ideal for patients with coagulopathies because it is superficial and blood vessels may be compressed against the humerus. Many approaches and techniques for this block have been described, including use of simple landmarks and palpation of the axillary artery, nerve stimulation, and ultrasound.

Lower Extremity Innervation

The lower extremity peripheral nerves are formed by the lumbar and sacral plexuses and are supplied by anterior rami of spinal nerves L1-L4 and L4-S3, respectively. For complete anesthesia at these levels, many practitioners would choose a neuraxial block rather than plexus blocks because of its simplicity in covering multiple nerves with one procedure. In addition to other terminal peripheral branches, the lumbar plexus gives rise to the lateral femoral cutaneous, femoral, and obturator nerves, whereas the sacral plexus forms the sciatic nerve and the posterior femoral cutaneous nerve. As a result, many of these lower extremity peripheral nerves can be blocked outside the pelvis. Because of the complexity of innervation, complete anesthesia for many procedures requires combination blocks.

Hip, Femur, Anterior Thigh, and Knee Procedures
Femoral Nerve Block

The hip and ligaments of the knee are common sites of surgery in the orthopedic sports population. While ligament repairs of the knee have been performed as an outpatient procedure for decades, hip arthroscopies are newer to the outpatient arena and lend their own challenges. Pain can be significant and studies demonstrate postoperative pain scores ranging from seven to ten on the 10-point visual analogue scale (VAS).[81,82] Unfortunately, due to the complex innervation of the hip and involvement of both the lumbar and sacral plexus, performing regional anesthetic techniques can be challenging.

Several small studies have examined intra-articular local anesthetic and portal local anesthetic injection with some evidence to suggest benefit in pain scores, though data is limited by small study size.[83-85] A number of regional techniques have been performed in hip arthroscopy patients including femoral nerve blocks, fascia iliaca blocks (with target nerves of the femoral and lateral femoral cutaneous nerves), and lumbar plexus blocks. Insufficient data exists to perform a meta-analysis, but there is evidence that femoral nerve blocks and lumbar plexus blocks offer pain benefits when compared to intravenous pain medications.[86,87] There is less compelling evidence to show benefits of fascia iliaca blocks.[86]

The femoral nerve block is common in outpatient surgery and is used most frequently for knee procedures, though more recently the adductor canal has largely replaced the femoral nerve block due to favorable motor-sparing benefits. A femoral

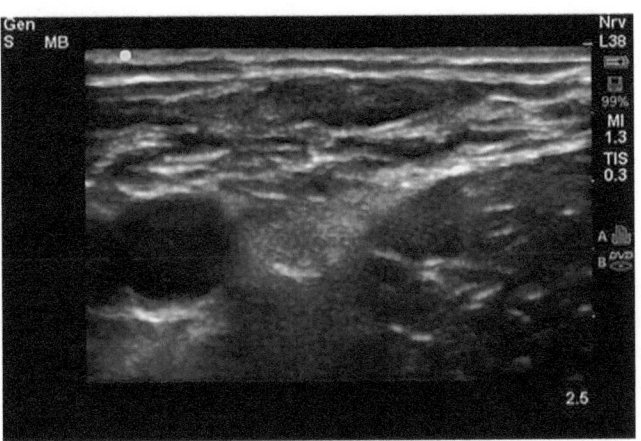

Fig. 29.5 An ultrasound image of the femoral nerve, artery, and vein.

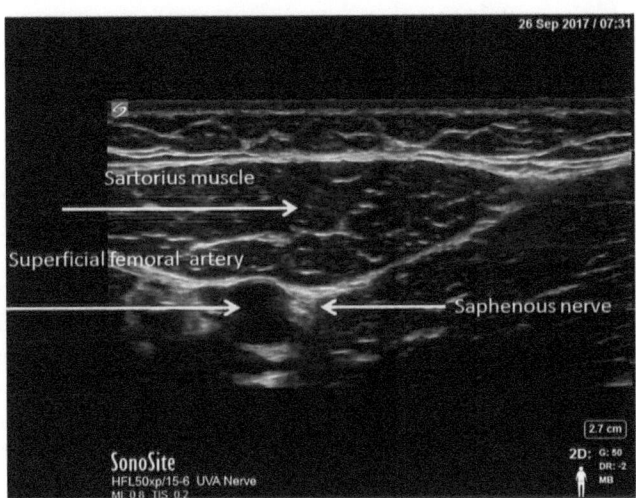

Fig. 29.6 An ultrasound image of the adductor canal block.

nerve block can be performed with relative ease using landmark, nerve stimulation, and ultrasound techniques because of the relatively shallow location of the nerve distal to the inguinal ligament and the predictable location relative to the femoral pulse. Blockade results in anesthesia of the anterior thigh and knee, quadriceps, anterior joint capsule, and the medial calf (via the saphenous nerve). ACL reconstruction surgery is one of the more commonly performed orthopedic surgeries and a procedure that may lead to significant pain. Intra-articular injections have not been shown to be as effective as regional techniques.[88,89] Data show that patients receiving femoral nerve blocks have decreased pain scores, decreased opioid consumption, decreased PACU stay, and decreased risks for unplanned admissions, with the addition of the sciatic block adding additional benefits over a femoral block alone.[90,91]

Catheter placement is simple, and significant improvements in postoperative pain have been described when a femoral block is used for outpatient ACL repair.[92] The risks of the femoral block are minimal, but may include intravascular injection, hematoma, and infection (after use of a catheter). Fig. 29.5 demonstrates an ultrasound examination of the femoral nerve.

Adductor Canal Nerve Block

The adductor canal block has largely replaced the femoral nerve block for procedures of the knee. Due to blockade of the quadriceps muscles with a femoral nerve block, many anesthesiologists are now performing a more distal block in hopes of sparing motor effects but still providing sensory block. The adductor canal houses the saphenous nerve, nerve to the vastus medialis, and branches of the anterior obturator nerve. A meta-analysis comparing adductor canal block versus femoral canal block for total knee arthroplasty showed no significant differences in pain scores in patients receiving adductor canal versus femoral nerve blocks and also demonstrated that the adductor canal block had significant improvement of quadriceps strength over the femoral nerve block.[93] Limitations of this meta-analysis are that only six studies and 408 patients were included and that the studies showed variability in how they defined the site of an adductor canal block. In the orthopedic sports medicine population, the adductor canal block provided noninferior analgesia and superior quadriceps strength compared with femoral nerve block in ACL

reconstruction.[94] While reports of falls due to motor weakness are rare, motor-sparing techniques facilitate early ambulation and may decrease falls in at-risk patients. Additionally, an injury incurred from the block is less likely to involve motor weakness as a complication. Fig. 29.6 shows an ultrasound image of the adductor canal block.

Lower Leg, Ankle, and Foot Procedures
Sciatic Nerve Block

There are a number of approaches to the sciatic nerve, beginning at the sciatic notch and extending down to the popliteal fossa where it divides into the tibial and common peroneal nerves. Nerve stimulation or ultrasound guidance is usually required for the deeper approaches. Analgesia of the leg below the knee can be completely achieved with a combination of sciatic plus saphenous nerve block. Blockade of the large sciatic nerve is more involved and takes longer to establish but may last longer than other PNBs. Catheters may be inserted via popliteal or subgluteal approaches with equal analgesia for foot surgery.[95] Studies combining sciatic with femoral catheters for knee arthroplasty have shown improved analgesia. However, no clear benefit is seen on functional measures, and early postoperative rehabilitation may be impaired by weakness when a sciatic nerve block is added to the femoral.[96]

Saphenous Nerve

The selective saphenous nerve block is used in conjunction with a popliteal block for complete anesthesia below the knee. It can be performed either above the knee in the adductor canal as noted above or below the knee using a field block. The former approach is associated with a higher degree of success.[97]

Ankle Block

The five terminal branches of the sciatic and femoral nerves can be individually blocked at the ankle to provide anesthesia and analgesia for foot procedures, provided no tourniquet is used above the ankle. If bone surgery is planned above the midfoot, this technique may be inadequate and a popliteal/saphenous approach should be used. The block can be executed entirely with landmarks alone, yet latency to onset is prolonged and patient discomfort is greater because of the need for multiple injections. Ultrasound has enhanced this block in clinical practice.

Intravenous Regional Anesthesia (Bier Block)

The Bier block is one of the older methods of providing regional anesthesia. Intravenous injection of a local anesthetic with a tourniquet creates a high venous pressure gradient that encourages the flow of the anesthetic to the smaller nerve endings of the extremity. The Bier block is best suited for short procedures that last less than 60 minutes, because pain from the tourniquet will develop. This block is most frequently used for upper extremity procedures, but it may be used for lower extremity surgery. A larger volume of medication is necessary for a lower limb block, which increases the risk for the most common complication of this block—local anesthetic toxicity. The risk of toxicity can be minimized by ensuring excellent tourniquet occlusion for a minimal time interval. With a lidocaine Bier block, 45 minutes is recommended for a sufficient amount of the drug to bind to tissues, which ensures safe serum levels prior to cuff release.[98] Soft tissue procedures, tendon repairs, and minor joint repairs are all acceptable applications.

Continuous Catheter Techniques

It is estimated that 50% to 70% of surgeries are being performed in the ambulatory setting; thus more complex sports and orthopedic procedures are occurring on an outpatient basis.[99] Total shoulder arthroplasty, unicondylar and total knee replacements, and multi-ligament knee surgeries are now standard procedures in ambulatory surgical centers. Management of pain with continuous catheter techniques has become standard of practice. Continuous brachial plexus catheters for shoulder, elbow and hand surgeries, popliteal catheters for foot and ankle surgeries, and femoral or adductor catheters for knee procedures have been shown to benefit patients and improve numerous outcomes. In addition to prolonging analgesic effects of a nerve block, lower doses of local anesthetics can be used, which can result in less motor block as well as a decrease in diaphragmatic paresis.[100]

Continuous nerve catheters have been shown to improve pain scores, decrease narcotic needs, and improve sleep in patients undergoing orthopedic procedures.[43] Additionally, outpatient continuous nerve catheters are safe if appropriate patient screening and education is performed.[101] Clinicians must carefully select appropriate catheter patients with attention to patient resources and understanding of the management of a continuous catheter. Relative exclusions for sending a patient home with a continuous nerve catheter include: patient lacks understanding or comfort managing or removing catheter; patient without caregiver present to monitor for signs of toxicity; patients without a means to communicate any problems or concerns; and patient lives far from medical facility to receive help if needed.

Local Anesthetic Agents

Classified into two chemical groups (amides and esters), local anesthetic agents impede transmission of nerve impulses by blocking voltage-gated sodium channels. Amide local anesthetic drugs include bupivacaine, ropivacaine, lidocaine, and mepivacaine.

Ester local anesthetic agents include procaine, chloroprocaine, tetracaine, and benzocaine. Amide local anesthetic drugs are degraded in the liver, and ester local anesthetic drugs are degraded by enzymes in the plasma. Compared with the amide group, ester anesthetic agents are more likely to induce allergic reactions as a result of para-aminobenzoic acid (PABA), a metabolite of ester anesthetics.[102]

Local anesthetic drugs differ in potency, speed of onset, duration of action, and toxicity.[103] The most commonly used local anesthetic drugs in clinical practice include bupivacaine, ropivacaine, lidocaine, and mepivacaine. Bupivacaine is the longest acting and most potent drug, but it has the highest degree of cardiotoxicity of any anesthetic agent, and thus a maximum dose of 2.5 mg/kg is typically recommended. Ropivacaine is less potent than bupivacaine and is less cardiotoxic; the maximum recommended dose is 3 mg/kg. Lidocaine, although less potent and shorter acting than either bupivacaine or ropivacaine, has a very stable toxicity profile. The maximum dose is 4.5 mg/kg without epinephrine and 7 mg/kg with added epinephrine.[104] Mepivacaine has a rapid onset of action and a longer duration than lidocaine, but it has a shorter duration than either bupivacaine or ropivacaine. Mepivacaine is a very useful anesthetic for regional blocks for patients who desire a primary regional anesthetic but do not want a prolonged nerve block postoperatively. The maximum dose is 300 mg without epinephrine and 500 mg with epinephrine. Adding epinephrine to a local anesthetic at a concentration of 1:200 000 increases the duration of analgesia by approximately 200%.[105] The addition of more concentrated epinephrine does not provide added duration benefits and can induce tachycardia and hypertension. Other adjuvants used in local anesthetic agents that can help improve the quality and duration of PNBs include clonidine, dexamethasone, dexmedetomidine, and buprenorphine.

Local Anesthetic Systemic Toxicity

Adverse events from local anesthetic drugs range from mild symptoms to severe neurologic and cardiovascular symptoms caused by systemic absorption and unintentional intravascular injection. Symptoms often begin with tinnitus, a metallic taste, dizziness, and lightheadedness and rapidly progress to seizures and ultimately to cardiovascular collapse.[106] Seizures, agitation, and loss of consciousness are the most common signs of neurologic symptoms. Central nervous system (CNS) symptoms can be treated with benzodiazepines such as midazolam, lorazepam, or diazepam. In addition, managing the airway becomes imperative because hypoventilation and respiratory acidosis can prolong and worsen the effects of local anesthetic toxicity.[107]

In high doses, local anesthetic drugs delay cardiac conduction and depress contractility, and bupivacaine has a particularly high affinity for cardiac sodium channels.[108,109] Randomized controlled trials to study local anesthetic systemic toxicity are needed, and although local anesthetic systemic toxicity is a rare event, it was traditionally thought to occur in up to 1 in 1000 PNBs.[110] From retrospective studies, it is known that half of all cases of toxicity are seen within 50 seconds of injecting a local anesthetic but that signs can be observed up to 60 minutes after the injection.[110]

Arrhythmias are the most common cardiac signs of toxicity. However, asystole can occur in 12% of patients. These findings do not apply if a local anesthetic is injected directly into the vertebral arteries or the carotid artery, after which a seizure can occur with a small dose of a local anesthetic.[110]

Treatment depends on the extent of the symptoms. Minor CNS effects do not require intervention and will typically resolve if no additional local anesthetic is injected. For major reactions, including CNS symptoms and cardiovascular collapse, lipid emulsion therapy has shown promise as a "first-line" treatment. Marketed under the trademark name Intralipid, lipid emulsion therapy is thought to function as a "lipid sink" that extracts hydrophobic drugs, such as bupivacaine, from cardiac tissue. Additionally, it is thought that Intralipid (Baxter Healthcare, Deerfield, IL) may stabilize myocardium and act as an energy substrate to cardiac myocytes.

It is administered intravenously as a bolus of 1.5 mL/kg, followed by an infusion of 0.25 mL/kg/minute, and is continued for 10 minutes after hemodynamic stabilization.[110] The nearest medical facility with the capability for cardiopulmonary bypass should be notified in case of complete cardiopulmonary collapse.[111] Algorithms have been published that guide the clinician through treating a patient with LAST. Table 29.1 shows the treatment of LAST.

PERIOPERATIVE PHARMACOLOGY

Perioperative Pain Management

Effective pain management can be challenging, particularly in the ambulatory setting, where patients must be discharged home with safe and effective medications. Ineffective pain control is a major cause of unanticipated hospital admissions after outpatient surgery. Narcotics have been the mainstay of acute postoperative pain control, yet they are associated with adverse effects, some of which can be lethal in a subset of patients (i.e., persons with OSA or significant respiratory disease). This section reviews the various options for perioperative analgesia. Prescription and nonprescription opioids have gained significant worldwide attention, as the opioid epidemic is now noted to be the worst drug crisis in the history of our country, with 91 Americans dying every day from opioid overdose.[112] While initially thought to be low risk, more recent studies demonstrate that patients prescribed short-term opioids following surgery are at increased risk of chronic opioid use as compared to patients who have never used opioids.[113] Currently, there is little data on optimal doses of narcotics after orthopedic-specific procedures, though more studies are being performed to examine best practice and help guide clinicians on prescribing parameters.[113–115,133]

The most commonly overdosed prescription drugs include methadone, oxycodone, and hydrocodone.[112] The American Pain Society released clinical practice guidelines for postsurgical pain management in February of 2016 in *The Journal of Pain*.[116] These guidelines included 32 recommendations for optimal pain management in surgical patients. Table 29.2 lists the recommendations. STRONG, high-quality EVIDENCE recommendations were made for four interventions. Three of the four *strong recommendations with high quality of evidence* to support

TABLE 29.1 Treatment of Local Anesthetic Systemic Toxicity Checklist for Treatment of Local Anesthetic Systemic Toxicity

The pharmacologic treatment of local anesthetic systemic toxicity (LAST) is different from other cardiac arrest scenarios
- Get help
- Initial focus:
  - Airway management: ventilate with 100% oxygen
  - Seizure suppression: benzodiazepines are preferred; AVOID propofol in patients having signs of cardiovascular instability
  - Alert the nearest facility having cardiopulmonary bypass capability
- Management of cardiac arrhythmias:
  - Basic and advanced cardiac life support (ACLS) will require adjustment of medications and perhaps prolonged effort
  - AVOID vasopressin, calcium channel blockers, beta blockers, or local anesthetic
  - REDUCE individual epinephrine doses to <1 μg/kg
- Lipid emulsion (20%) therapy (values in parentheses are for 70 kg patient):
  - Bolus 1.5 mL/kg (lean body mass) intravenously over 1 minute (~100 mL)
  - Continuous infusion 0.25 mL/kg/min (~18 mL/min; adjust by roller clamp)
  - Repeat bolus once or twice for persistent cardiovascular collapse
  - Double the infusion rate to 0.5 mL/kg/min if blood pressure remains low
  - Continue infusion for at least 10 minutes after attaining circulatory stability
  - Recommended upper limit: Approximately 10 mL/kg lipid emulsion over the first 30 minutes
- Post LAST events at www.lipidrescue.org and report use of lipid to www.lipidregistry.org

From Neal JM, Bernards CM, Butterworth JF, et al. ASRA practice advisory on local anesthetic systemic toxicity. *Reg Anesth Pain Med.* 2010;35(2):151–161.

that are pertinent to orthopedic sports patients include the use of multi-modal analgesics, the use of acetaminophen, with or without non-steroidal antiinflammatory drugs (NSAIDs), and the use of regional techniques as a consideration. The recommendations stress increased awareness of multi-modal analgesia and the treatment of pain by targeting various receptors of pain modulation in addition to opioid receptors. Attention to Enhanced Recovery After Surgery (ERAS) protocols has prompted a number of perioperative interventions that occur before surgery and continue throughout the days and weeks after surgery. ERAS began in the 1990s by Professor Henrik Kehlet with the goal of providing evidence-based, multi-modal, multi-disciplinary perioperative care pathways designed for early recovery after surgical procedures.[117] This begins before surgery with patient education and nutrition and continues throughout the perioperative period. Common components of ERAS protocols include close attention to multi-modal analgesia, fluid management, and early mobilization. Data is accumulating to show improved outcomes including earlier discharge, fast-tracking patients, decreased cost, and improved quality of care of surgical patients when ERAS protocols are implemented.

TABLE 29.2   Management of Postoperative Pain: A Clinical Practice Guideline From the American Pain Society, the American Society of Regional Anesthesia and Pain Medicine, and the American Society of Anesthesiologists' Committee on Regional Anesthesia, Executive Committee, and Administrative Council[a]

Recommendation 1	The panel recommends that clinicians provide patient and family-centered, individually tailored education to the patient (and/or responsible caregiver), including information on treatment options for management of postoperative pain, and document the plan and goals for postoperative pain management (strong recommendation, low-quality evidence).
Recommendation 2	The panel recommends that the parents (or other adult caregivers) of children who undergo surgery receive instruction in developmentally appropriate methods for assessing pain as well as counseling on appropriate administration of analgesics and modalities (strong recommendation, low-quality evidence).
Recommendation 3	The panel recommends that clinicians conduct a preoperative evaluation including assessment of medical and psychiatric comorbidities, concomitant medications, history of chronic pain, substance abuse, and previous postoperative treatment regimens and responses, to guide the perioperative pain management plan (strong recommendation, low-quality evidence).
Recommendation 4	The panel recommends that clinicians adjust the pain management plan on the basis of adequacy of pain relief and presence of adverse events (strong recommendation, low-quality evidence).
Recommendation 5	The panel recommends that clinicians use a validated pain assessment tool to track responses to postoperative pain treatments and adjust treatment plans accordingly (strong recommendation, low-quality evidence).
Recommendation 6	The panel recommends that clinicians offer multi-modal analgesia, or the use of a variety of analgesic medications and techniques combined with nonpharmacologic interventions, for the treatment of postoperative pain in children and adults (strong recommendation, high-quality evidence).
Recommendation 7	The panel recommends that clinicians consider TENS as an adjunct to other postoperative pain treatments (weak recommendation, moderate-quality evidence).
Recommendation 8	The panel can neither recommend nor discourage acupuncture, massage, or cold therapy as adjuncts to other postoperative pain treatments (insufficient evidence).
Recommendation 9	The panel recommends that clinicians consider the use of cognitive-behavioral modalities in adults as part of a multi-modal approach (weak recommendation, moderate-quality evidence).
Recommendation 10	The panel recommends oral over IV administration of opioids for postoperative analgesia in patients who can use the oral route (strong recommendation, moderate quality evidence).
Recommendation 11	The panel recommends that clinicians avoid using the intramuscular route for the administration of analgesics for management of postoperative pain (strong recommendation, moderate-quality evidence).
Recommendation 12	The panel recommends that IV PCA be used for postoperative systemic analgesia when the parenteral route is needed (strong recommendation, moderate-quality evidence).
Recommendation 13	The panel recommends against routine basal infusion of opioids with IV PCA in opioid-naive adults (strong recommendation, moderate-quality evidence).
Recommendation 14	The panel recommends that clinicians provide appropriate monitoring of sedation, respiratory status, and other adverse events in patients who receive systemic opioids for postoperative analgesia (strong recommendation, low-quality evidence).
Recommendation 15	The panel recommends that clinicians provide adults and children with acetaminophen and/or NSAIDs as part of multi-modal analgesia for management of postoperative pain in patients without contraindications (strong recommendation, high-quality evidence).
Recommendation 16	The panel recommends that clinicians consider giving a preoperative dose of oral celecoxib in adult patients without contraindications (strong recommendation, moderate-quality evidence).
Recommendation 17	The panel recommends that clinicians consider use of gabapentin or pregabalin as a component of multi-modal analgesia (strong recommendation, moderate-quality evidence).
Recommendation 18	The panel recommends that clinicians consider IV ketamine as a component of multi-modal analgesia in adults (weak recommendation, moderate-quality evidence).
Recommendation 19	The panel recommends that clinicians consider IV lidocaine infusions in adults who undergo open and laparoscopic abdominal surgery who do not have contraindications (weak recommendation, moderate-quality evidence).
Recommendation 20	The panel recommends that clinicians consider surgical site-specific local anesthetic infiltration for surgical procedures with evidence indicating efficacy (weak recommendation, moderate-quality evidence).
Recommendation 21	The panel recommends that clinicians use topical local anesthetics in combination with nerve blocks before circumcision (strong recommendation, moderate-quality evidence).
Recommendation 22	The panel does not recommend intrapleural analgesia with local anesthetics for pain control after thoracic surgery (strong recommendation, moderate-quality evidence).
Recommendation 23	The panel recommends that clinicians consider surgical site-specific peripheral regional anesthetic techniques in adults and children for procedures with evidence indicating efficacy (strong recommendation, high-quality evidence).
Recommendation 24	The panel recommends that clinicians use continuous, local anesthetic-based peripheral regional analgesic techniques when the need for analgesia is likely to exceed the duration of effect of a single injection (strong recommendation, moderate-quality evidence).
Recommendation 25	The panel recommends that clinicians consider the addition of clonidine as an adjuvant for prolongation of analgesia with a single-injection peripheral neural blockade (weak recommendation, moderate-quality evidence).
Recommendation 26	The panel recommends that clinicians offer neuraxial analgesia for major thoracic and abdominal procedures, particularly in patients at risk for cardiac complications, pulmonary complications, or prolonged ileus (strong recommendation, high-quality evidence).

TABLE 29.2 Management of Postoperative Pain: A Clinical Practice Guideline From the American Pain Society, the American Society of Regional Anesthesia and Pain Medicine, and the American Society of Anesthesiologists' Committee on Regional Anesthesia, Executive Committee, and Administrative Council—cont'd

Recommendation 27	The panel recommends that clinicians avoid the neuraxial administration of magnesium, benzodiazepines, neostigmine, tramadol, and ketamine in the treatment of postoperative pain (strong recommendation, moderate-quality evidence).
Recommendation 28	The panel recommends that clinicians provide appropriate monitoring of patients who have received neuraxial interventions for perioperative analgesia (strong recommendation, low-quality evidence).
Recommendation 29	The panel recommends that facilities in which surgery is performed have an organizational structure in place to develop and refine policies and processes for safe and effective delivery of postoperative pain control (strong recommendation, low-quality evidence).
Recommendation 30	The panel recommends that facilities in which surgery is performed provide clinicians with access to consultation with a pain specialist for patients with inadequately controlled postoperative pain or at high risk of inadequately controlled postoperative pain (e.g., opioid-tolerant, history of substance abuse) (strong recommendation, low-quality evidence).
Recommendation 31	The panel recommends that facilities in which neuraxial analgesia and continuous peripheral blocks are performed have policies and procedures to support their safe delivery and trained individuals to manage these procedures (strong recommendation, low-quality evidence).
Recommendation 32	The panel recommends that clinicians provide education to all patients (adult and children) and primary caregivers on the pain treatment plan, including tapering of analgesics after hospital discharge (strong recommendation, low-quality evidence).

ªRecommendations based on systematic review.
IV, Intravenous; *NSAIDs,* nonsteroidal anti-inflammatory drugs; *PCA,* patient-controlled analgesia; *TENS,* transcutaneous electrical nerve stimulation.

Opioids

Opioids, which are classified as natural (i.e., morphine) or synthetic (e.g., fentanyl, sufentanil, and remifentanil), have been the cornerstone of perioperative analgesia. However, unfavorable adverse effects include ventilatory depression, sedation, PONV, ileus, pruritus, and difficulty voiding. These problems can lead to unforeseen hospital admissions in the ambulatory surgery setting. Notwithstanding, opioids are the most commonly used perioperative pain medication. A significant advantage of opioids in the ambulatory setting is availability in parenteral form for use during procedures and in oral preparations for use at home.

The most commonly used IV opioids are morphine, hydromorphone, and fentanyl. Morphine, often considered the "gold standard opioid," has a duration of action of 4 to 5 hours, is metabolized by the liver, and is cleared by the kidneys. Because it is converted by the liver into an active metabolite, it must be used with caution in patients with renal failure or insufficiency. Hydromorphone is five times as potent as morphine. Analgesia is achieved within 5 minutes, and compared with morphine, its duration of action is shorter.[118] It is a better choice in patients with renal failure. Fentanyl is 100 times more potent than morphine, and onset of analgesia is within 3 to 7 minutes. Because of its short duration of action, fentanyl is a drug that must be administered more frequently. Additionally, it is safe to use in patients with renal failure.

Many commonly prescribed oral opioids are used in combination with acetaminophen, including a combination of hydrocodone and acetaminophen. Hydrocodone has a half-life of 2.5 to 4 hours and is thought to be a prodrug that requires the enzyme CYP2D6 to process and achieve analgesia. Patients lacking this enzyme may not have the expected pain relief from hydrocodone. Oxycodone is not a prodrug; it has a half-life of 2.5 to 4 hours, and it provides consistent pain relief.

Methadone

When caring for patients with chronic pain, a formal pain consultation can help guide pain management. Drugs such as methadone and buprenorphine can make acute surgical pain management in chronic pain patients extremely difficult. Methadone is a mu-receptor agonist and N-methyl-D-aspartate receptor antagonist that was developed in the 1930s as an alternative to addictive opioids. Methadone is used primarily for analgesia and for treatment from opioid addiction. Because of its antagonistic effects on NMDA receptors, it is a good drug for neuropathic pain. Other benefits include the longest half-life of opioids and low cost. Methadone can be administered orally, sublingually, or parenterally. Side effects include those of other opioids as well as prolonged QT and the potential for arrhythmias. Methadone has been used in the perioperative period in a number of orthopedic patients, most commonly spinal fusions.[119-122] Care must be taken when caring for patients on methadone and determining how to manage additional analgesics safely.

Buprenorphine

Buprenorphine was made available in the United States in the 1970s, with the initial use for outpatient opioid detoxification and addiction therapy. Buprenorphine is an agonist at the mu receptor and an antagonist at the kappa and delta receptors. Several different variants have been approved, including oral tablets, sublingual tablets, buccal films, and skin implants. Several contain the opioid antagonist naloxone to help prevent intravenous abuse of the drug. Commonly used brands include Suboxone (buprenorphine/naloxone sublingual tablet) and Subutex (buprenorphine sublingual tablet). Buprenorphine is a semi-synthetic opioid that is classified as a partial opioid agonist. Benefits of this drug include a decreased potential for abuse and fewer characteristics of euphoria, thus less potential for dependence. While the effects of buprenorphine increase with increasing doses, this effect reaches a plateau, thus called the ceiling effect. Other safety benefits include less respiratory depression as well as a reduction of opioid cravings. While advantages of this drug are clear, in the acute pain phase, patients on buprenorphine provide challenges. Patients on buprenorphine are resistant to traditional opioid analgesic effects and debates continue about whether patients should continue or stop buprenorphine prior to surgical procedures. Discontinuing 72 hours prior to surgery may be necessary with a bridge of oral analgesics.[123]

Acetaminophen

Acetaminophen (Tylenol) is an excellent analgesic with minimal adverse effects at therapeutic doses. It works both centrally and peripherally by activating serotonergic, cholinergic, noradrenergic, cannabinoid, and N-methyl-D-aspartate receptors. It has few gastrointestinal adverse effects and little effect on platelet function. Hepatotoxicity is the most concerning adverse effect. Fortunately, it is extremely rare and is easily minimized by limiting a daily dose to 4 g.[124] Liver function is unaffected after therapeutic dosing in persons with stable liver disease. In patients with severe liver disease and chronic alcohol abuse, reducing the dose to 1 g three times a day is safe.[124] Typical dosing is 500 to 1000 mg every 6 hours. Acetaminophen can be administered orally, rectally, or intravenously with benefits to each of the different routes. While oral acetaminophen is susceptible to first-pass hepatic metabolism and absorption may be negatively affected by opioids, it is economically the best choice and can be administered preoperatively for peak effect prior to emergence from anesthesia. IV acetaminophen can be notably beneficial in patients who cannot tolerate oral administration. Marketed in the United States under the trademark name Ofirmev, therapeutic concentrations are achieved within 20 minutes and last for 2 hours.[124] The addition of IV acetaminophen in one study reduced postoperative morphine consumption by 20% in the first 24 hours.[125] Postoperative nausea and vomiting (PONV) was reduced by 30% and sedation by 29% in other studies, and data from 14 placebo-controlled randomized controlled trials with 1464 patients showed improved analgesia with IV acetaminophen.[125] Pain intensity scores over 24 hours were improved in patients undergoing joint replacement, as was time until rescue opioids, rescue medication consumption, and administration of opioids when acetaminophen was given.[126]

Nonsteroidal Antiinflammatory Drugs

NSAIDs have antiinflammatory, antipyretic, and analgesic properties; they block the synthesis of the enzyme cyclooxygenase and slow the acute inflammatory response peripherally and hyperalgesia centrally. In persons undergoing ambulatory surgery, NSAIDs decrease opioid requirements and potentially reduce opioid-related adverse effects.[127] NSAIDs may be administered either orally or intravenously with similar benefit. NSAIDs have been shown to improve dynamic pain control. Selective and nonselective NSAIDs are used commonly with selective COX2 activity decreasing some of the side effects. Diclofenac and Celecoxib have been shown to be significantly more selective to COX2 with Ketorolac being nonselective. Despite this, Ketorolac is frequently used by anesthesiologists in the perioperative period and can be administered intravenously, intramuscularly, or orally. Ketorolac reduces postoperative pain with minimal incidence of PONV and has been shown to decrease time to discharge.[128] The optimal dose is 15 to 30 mg every 6 hours for a maximum of 5 days. The concern exists that ketorolac may increase microvascular bleeding, worsen renal function, and impair bone healing, though studies in humans are inconclusive on the effects on bone healing. However, for most sports medicine procedures, NSAIDs such as ketorolac are excellent opioid-sparing adjuvants for pain relief.

Ketamine

Ketamine is a unique anesthetic drug with significant analgesic properties. It works as an antagonist at the N-methyl-D-aspartate receptor. At small doses, ketamine has analgesic properties that extend 24 to 48 hours into the postoperative period even though the plasma half-life is 17 minutes. This effect is due to reduction of "wind-up," a hyper-excitable state of CNS sensitization. Preoperative administration of ketamine may reduce the requirement for narcotics by 40% to 60%.[129] Ketamine has been shown in multiple studies to reduce opioid tolerance and to reduce opioid-induced hyperalgesia. A single dose of intraoperative ketamine has a 50% morphine-sparing effect in the first 48 hours after surgery.[130] Disturbing hallucinations and acute psychosis-like symptoms have been described in patients receiving ketamine, though usually at doses higher than those used for analgesia.[131] Consequently, midazolam may be co-administered if ketamine is administered in doses greater than 1 mg/kg in a patient who is awake. Ketamine can also lead to tachycardia and hypertension.

Propofol

Propofol was first discovered in the 1970s and has since become the mainstay of induction agents in anesthesia. It is also used for sedation, typically in the form of an infusion. Its site of action is primarily on the GABA A receptor and has the clinical benefit of being very short-acting due to rapid redistribution. A single bolus has effects lasting only minutes. Two major benefits of propofol are its amnestic effects and anti-emetic effects. Side effects include pain on injection, hypotension, and apnea. Propofol decreases cerebral blood flow and also intracranial pressure. Propofol is the drug commonly used for a total intravenous anesthetic (TIVA) in patients with malignant hyperthermia.

Dexmedetomidine

Dexmedetomidine was approved as a sedative in the United States in 1999 and offers unique properties. As an alpha-2 receptor agonist, its site of action on presynaptic neurons decreases norepinephrine release with inhibition of postsynaptic activation. The effect on the central nervous system, particularly the locus ceruleus, leads to the intended effect of sedation with preservation of patient cooperation. Unique to dexmedetomidine, the sedation resembles nonrapid eye movement (REM) sleep.[132] Dexmedetomidine also provides a myriad of benefits, including analgesia without significant respiratory effects. Upper airway tone is preserved and respiratory drive is maintained, thus making it a nice choice in patients with respiratory co-morbidities and OSA.[133] Initially used as a sedative in mechanically ventilated patients, dexmedetomidine has become widely used in the perioperative setting for sedation, and as an adjunct to general anesthesia to reduce opioid and other anesthetic requirements. Side effects of dexmedetomidine include, most commonly, hypotension and bradycardia.

Sedation in the Orthopedic Patient

When providing sedation to patients undergoing minimally invasive orthopedic procedures such as reducing a fracture or superficial procedures using local anesthetics, it is critical to understand the recommendations of the ASA for standards of care. The ASA has published guidelines that define levels of sedation and standards for these four various levels of sedation.[134] These were approved by the ASA House of Delegates in 1999 and most recently amended in October of 2014. The four different levels of anesthesia, which are a continuum and can change throughout the procedure, are defined in Table 29.3. The ASA Task Force provides a number of recommendations based on the level of sedation and these include (1) presedation patient evaluation; (2) preprocedure preparation; (3) monitoring; (4) record keeping; (5) availability of an individual who is dedicated to patient monitoring and safety; (6) education of clinician providing sedation; (7) availability of rescue medications, airway devices, and oxygen; (8) appropriate use of sedative medications; and (9) aspects of recovery.[134]

TABLE 29.3 The American Society of Anesthesiologists Definitions of Sedation

Minimal sedation (anxiolysis) is a drug-induced state during which patients respond normally to verbal commands. Although cognitive function and physical coordination may be impaired, airway reflexes and ventilatory and cardiovascular functions are unaffected.

Moderate sedation/analgesia ("conscious sedation") is a drug-induced depression of consciousness during which patients respond purposefully[a] to verbal commands, either alone or accompanied by light tactile stimulation. No interventions are required to maintain a patent airway, and spontaneous ventilation is adequate. Cardiovascular function is usually maintained.

Deep sedation/analgesia is a drug-induced depression of consciousness during which patient cannot be easily aroused but respond purposefully*[a] following repeated or painful stimulation. The ability to independently maintain ventilatory function may be impaired. Patients may require assistance in maintaining a patent airway, and spontaneous ventilation may be inadequate. Cardiovascular function is usually maintained.

General anesthesia is a drug-induced loss of consciousness during which patients are not arousable, even by painful stimulation. The ability to independently maintain ventilatory function is often impaired. Patients often require assistance in maintaining a patent airway, and positive pressure ventilation may be required because of depressed spontaneous ventilation or drug-induced depression of neuromuscular function. Cardiovascular function may be impaired.

[a]Reflex withdrawal from a painful stimulus is NOT considered a purposeful response.
From www.asahq.org/quality-and-practice-management/standards-guidelines-and-related-resources.

PERIOPERATIVE COMPLICATIONS IN THE SPORTS MEDICINE PATIENT

Allergic Reactions

Intraoperative anaphylaxis can occur in otherwise healthy patients. It results from the release of various chemical mediators of inflammation from basophils and mast cells with resultant dysfunction of skin, mucous membranes, gastrointestinal, cardiovascular, and pulmonary systems. Its accurate incidence in the United States is unknown but is estimated at approximately 1:10,000 to 1:20,000 patients.[135,136] The most common agents include muscle relaxants, latex, and antibiotics. Less common causes include opioid drugs, local anesthetic agents, chlorhexidine, colloid drugs, and hypnotic agents such as propofol.[137] Very small quantities of the inciting substance are required to initiate the pathophysiologic cascade of anaphylaxis, and signs can be observed within a few seconds after the administration of drugs. Signs include hypotension, tachycardia, bronchospasm, angioedema, arrhythmias, cardiovascular collapse, and cardiac arrest. Immediate treatment is pivotal to sustaining life. The suspected drug should be discontinued promptly; the airway should be maintained with 100% oxygen supplementation; epinephrine, antihistamine drugs, and corticosteroid agents should be administered without delay; the patient should be placed in a Trendelenburg position; and surgery should be aborted until the patient is stabilized.

Parsonage-Turner Syndrome

Also known as *brachial plexus neuritis* or *neuralgic amyotrophy*, Parsonage-Turner syndrome (PTS) is a rare syndrome that can affect athletes in the perioperative period or may arise extraneous to a surgical event. Although it occurs infrequently (1.64 cases per 100,000 people), it is a disease process that has an atypical presentation and may be confusing to the orthopedic surgeon.[138] PTS was first described in 1897 by Feinburg, but it was not until the mid 1900s that Parsonage and Turner described more than 100 cases of this condition.[139,140] The syndrome usually involves the proximal brachial plexus and can affect many lower motor neurons of the plexus. Many reports have been made of isolated nerve findings, with weakness of the anterior interosseous nerve being a common presentation. The syndrome is more prevalent in males than females and can affect persons of all ages; approximately one fourth of all cases of PTS follow a systemic illness, and patients typically present with pain in the brachial plexus (mostly in the shoulder region) followed by motor weakness.[141]

PTS has been linked to a number of inciting events. Etiologies include surgery, trauma, PNB, viral and bacterial infections, vaccinations, and systemic illnesses. PTS can occur after surgery and can be difficult to differentiate from a surgical or anesthesia-related injury. PTS is a diagnosis of exclusion and is mostly clinically based. Nerve conduction studies and electromyography may be helpful in locating the lesion and ruling out unrelated nerve compression or injury. Encouragingly, most patients recover spontaneously and require only supportive care. A review of 99 patients revealed that complete recovery from PTS has been noted in approximately 90% of patients, but that recovery may be slow and can take up to 3 years. These data contradict another smaller study that showed that 50% of patients had residual, long-term deficits.[142]

For a complete list of references, go to ExpertConsult.com.

SELECTED READINGS

Citation:

Neal J. ASRA practice advisory on local anesthetic systemic toxicity. *Reg Anesth Pain Med*. 2010;35(2):151–161.

Level of Evidence:

II, systematic review of Level II studies

Summary:

Local anesthetic systemic toxicity (LAST) is a rare but potentially devastating clinical entity after use of local anesthetic agents. This practice advisory reviews the most current information known about the epidemiology, prevention, and treatment of LAST.

Citation:

Gersh BJ, Maron BJ, Bonow RO, et al. 2011 ACCF/AHA guidelines for the diagnosis and treatment of hypertrophic cardiomyopathy: executive summary: a report of the American College of Cardiology Foundation/American Heart Association task force on practice guidelines. *Circulation*. 2011;124:2761–2796.

Level of Evidence:

I, systematic review of Level I studies

Summary:

Hypertrophic obstructive cardiomyopathy is the most common cardiovascular cause of sudden cardiac death in young athletes. This excellent review outlines and grades the latest evidence and makes expert recommendations regarding management of patients with this complex condition.

Citation:

Antonakakis JG, Ting PH, Sites B. Ultrasound-guided regional anesthesia for peripheral nerve blocks: an evidence-based outcome review. *Anesthesiol Clin*. 2011;29(2):179–191.

Level of Evidence:

I, systematic review of Level I studies

Summary:

Regional anesthesia has become a mainstay of many orthopedic procedures, and interest in using ultrasound to provide regional anesthesia is explosive. This article provides an excellent review of current data, mostly consisting of randomized controlled trials, that compare ultrasound-guided nerve blocks with the traditional approach to nerve blocks.

Citation:

Neal JM, Barrington MJ, Brull R, et al. The second ASRA practice advisory on neurologic complications associated with regional anesthesia and pain medicine executive summary. *Reg Anesth Pain Med*. 2015;40:401–430.

Level of Evidence:

Ranges from II-IV

Summary:

This article defines the incidence of neurologic complications associated with peripheral nerve blocks, with a focus on the pathophysiology of mechanical, ischemic, and neurotoxic causes. Additionally, there is focus on neurologic complications associated with common orthopedic procedures. The advisory discusses modifiable risks for peripheral nerve injury. Additionally, the paper reviews the diagnosis and treatment of peripheral nerve injury and the level of evidence for these.

Rehabilitation and Injury Prevention

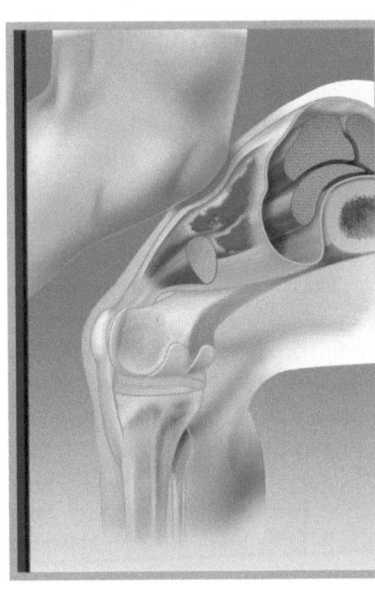

30

The Athletic Trainer

Chad Starkey, Shannon David

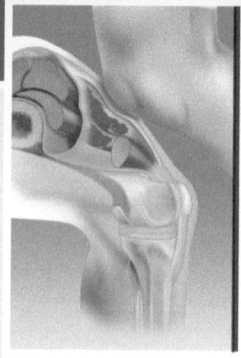

The name *athletic trainer* (AT) implies that ATs coach and train athletes to improve baseline performance. This title and the euphemism "trainer" create ambiguity regarding the AT's knowledge, skills, and abilities. ATs are multiskilled health care clinical professionals who deliver services in cooperation with and under the direction of physicians to provide optimal patient care. The AT's education and scope of practice encompass the areas of injury prevention and risk management, clinical examination and diagnosis, emergency care, therapeutic intervention (i.e., therapeutic modalities and rehabilitation), and health care administration (Box 30.1).

Although they are most visible when working with high school, collegiate, and professional sports teams, ATs are employed in a variety of settings, including physicians' offices, clinics, hospitals, performing arts, and the military.[1] ATs tend to work with a highly motivated, physically active population.

ATs can obtain third-party reimbursement in many settings. However, an advantage of ATs employed by high schools and intercollegiate athletics is the provision of capitated health care services. In the case of high schools located in poor and medically underserved areas, the presence of an AT is a cost-effective approach to the health care of these students. They often serve as the first point of medical contact for the community at large.

The knowledge, skills, and abilities that an AT possesses are found in other health care professions; however, the specific combination of skills is unique to AT. Because ATs have their roots in athletics, with a reasonable sense of urgency to return patients to competition, ATs have developed a philosophy of aggressive intervention that benefits both "athletic" and "nonathletic" patients. The AT skillset is applied according to the AT philosophy of an aggressive, yet safe, return to activity. This approach is based on the diagnostic principles and patient's intervention strategies and goals established by the World Health Organization's International Classification of Functioning, Disability, and Health.[2] The role of AT in the overall health care community is often misunderstood because of the overlap of skills with other professions, portrayals in movies and television (see "The Knute Rockne Story" and "The Water Boy"), the lack of understanding of the AT philosophy of care, and the misleading name, "athletic training" (K. K. Knight, C. Starkey, and D. Fandel, unpublished manuscript, 2009).

BRIEF HISTORY OF ATHLETIC TRAINING

The origin of athletic training can be traced back to the ancient Olympics, when paleotribes (loosely translated to "boy rubber") assisted athletes with their health care. In the United States the roots of athletic training emerged in the early 1900s, when individuals began to assist coaches and physicians in caring for the medical needs of athletes. In 1950, the National Athletic Trainers' Association was formed to help guide the practice of athletic training, which at the time was primarily limited to collegiate and professional teams.[3]

Similar to physical therapy and occupational therapy, the first athletic training academic programs have their roots in physical education. During the past 25 years, athletic training has progressed through an academic major to a formal degree and is currently transitioning to a professional (entry-level) master's degree to be eligible to practice as an AT. The focus of classroom and clinical education was once singularly focused on athletes. However, advancements in medicine and health care have extended the age of people participating in athletics and other forms of strenuous physical activity. Improved health care has also decreased the number of conditions that can disqualify a person from competitive athletics. In response, ATs have increased their knowledge of the unique challenges faced by people who have underlying medical or physical limitations throughout the life span.

Although the "traditional" athletic population remains a central theme of education, ATs have evolved to develop expertise in the care of a broad segment of the physically active population. This expanded educational base has changed the employment patterns of ATs, extending well beyond high school, collegiate, and professional team sports medicine venues to include industrial, military, the National Aeronautics and Space Administration (NASA), physician's practices, among others.

In just over half a century, ATs have evolved from the locker room to become a health care provider recognized by the American Medical Association. Contemporary ATs incorporate current evidence and best practices to treat a physically active patient base to ensure physical readiness to return to their desired level of function after injury (Box 30.2).[4-12]

EDUCATION

ATs must graduate from a professional bachelor's or master's degree program accredited by the Commission on Accreditation

BOX 30.1   Core Educational Competencies

- Evidence-based practice
- Interprofessional education and collaborative practice
- Quality improvement
- Health care informatics
- Professionalism
- Patient-centered care

BOX 30.2   Athletic Training's Research Contributions

The emergence of academic degree programs has resulted in the development of scholars who contribute to the sports medicine knowledge base. Athletic trainers are at the forefront of research regarding the prevention and diagnosis of conditions affecting athletes and others engaged in strenuous physical activity. Athletic training researchers were among the first to question the long-term consequences of athletic-related concussions and to question the efficacy of the clinical examination techniques used to identify these conditions.[4-12] Other researchers have added to the evidence base for orthopaedic diagnostic techniques, therapeutic interventions, and immediate care of musculoskeletal injuries.

Based on a strong, multidisciplinary evidence base, The National Athletic Trainers' Association has developed position statements regarding topics such as prevention of heat illness and sudden death, the management of concussions, athletes with cervical spine injuries, and athletes with type 1 diabetes, disordered eating, and asthma. Athletic trainers also have worked with other medical organizations on consensus statements regarding heat acclimation, the prehospital care of athletes with a spine injury, and athletes with sickle cell trait. For more information, see http://www.nata.org/membership/membership-benefits/athletic-training-publications.

Clinicians have the obligation to remain up-to-date regarding the current standard of care and best practices (via position statements) described in the prior paragraph. In addition, athletic trainers are required to obtain 10 hours of evidence-based practice continuing education every 2 years.

TABLE 30.1   Required Prerequisite and Foundational Knowledge

Prerequisite Coursework	Foundational Knowledge
Biology	Statistics and research design
Chemistry	Epidemiology
Physics	Pathophysiology
Psychology	Biomechanics and pathomechanics
Human anatomy	Exercise physiology
Human physiology	Nutrition
	Human anatomy
	Pharmacology
	Public health
	Health care delivery and payor systems

Note:

Prerequisite coursework is required prior to entering the professional program.

Foundational knowledge may be prerequisite coursework or incorporated into the professional program.

---

of Athletic Training Education (CAATE). By 2022, professional education will occur at the master's degree level. The educational content of an AT program is defined by the CAATE accreditation Standards,[13] whereas the Role Delineation Study[14] defines base entry-level practice. Box 30.1 presents the content area required in the professional preparation of ATs. Table 30.1 presents the prerequisite and foundational knowledge required in educational programs.

Professional coursework spans a range of musculoskeletal, neurologic, and metabolic conditions seen across the life span and focuses on the continuum of integrated prevention, care, and return to activity. The minimum program requirement is 2 years of classroom and clinical education with a proportion being in an interprofessional environment. A sampling of categories of professional education include:

- Developing emergency action plans (EAPs)
- Injury prevention including preparticipation examinations
- Clinical diagnosis and emergent care and appropriate referral
- Developing a plan of care for patients with conditions involving multiple systems
- Diagnostic testing (imaging, blood work, urinalysis, electrocardiography) to facilitate clinical diagnosis, referral, and plan of care

- Passive, active, and manual intervention to restore function (e.g., therapeutic modalities, therapeutic exercise, manual therapies)
- Knowledge of pharmacologic agents
- Concussion management and education
- Behavioral health conditions
- Durable medical equipment, orthotics, bracing, protective padding
- Mitigation of risk for long-term health conditions
- Environmental conditions
- Drug use/abuse education

These domains are tied together through the use of evidence-based practice. Many ATs are world-class scholars who have emerged as leaders in the diagnosis and management of concussion,[15] heat illness,[16] cervical spine trauma,[17] and therapeutic interventions.[12] ATs also consume research produced by physicians, physical therapists, and other professions who address the needs of persons who are physically active.

More than 70% of ATs possess advanced degrees, including accredited postprofessional programs (master's and doctoral degree programs and residencies).[18] Many currently credentialed ATs are dual credentialed, most often in conjunction with the fields of physical therapy, physician's assistant, and/or strength and conditioning/performance enhancement.

Regulation

Graduation from an accredited professional program is a requisite to sit for the Board of Certification, Inc. (BOC) examination as an entry-level AT. The "ATC" designation indicates that a person has passed the BOC examination, which serves as the common examination for individual states that issue the practice credential, typically "LAT" or "AT."[19] Although most states have licensure for professional practice, some states regulate practice via Registration or State Certification (Table 30.2). As of 2017 California is the only state that does not have any sort of state regulation of AT practice. Although the language of these practice acts is broad, a commonality is that ATs work collaboratively with and/or under a physician's direction.

TABLE 30.2   State Regulation of Athletic Trainers

Type	Description
Licensure	Licensure restricts practice to persons who have meet the licensing board's requirements. The practice act describes the athletic trainer's scope of practice. Unlicensed persons are prohibited from practicing athletic training.
Certification	Similar to state licensure, persons must meet minimum educational requirements and pass a state examination (the Board of Certification, Inc., examination is often recognized for this purpose). However, state certification only provides title protection; it does not limit uncertified persons from practicing.
Registration	Registration may or may not have educational or examination requirements. By registering with the state, title protection is granted.
Exemption	Exemption excludes a person from the standards of other licensed professions (e.g., physician assistant, physical therapy, or nursing).

Modified from Ray RR, Konin J. *Management Strategies in Athletic Training*. Champaign, IL: Human Kinetics Publishers; 2011.

PHYSICIAN/ATHLETIC TRAINER WORKING RELATIONSHIP

Regardless of the workplace setting, ATs function to extend the physician's services, serving as the physician's eyes, hands, and ears. The AT frequently is the point of first contact for injured/ill individuals. This role is unique because ATs often perform the first examination of an injury, usually minutes after its onset. This role triages the referral process, expediting those patients who need immediate medical assistance and preventing the physician's and patient's time loss in the event of needless referrals. In addition, this relationship has been shown to improve patient care and save the physician time.[20] Physicians have also reported better quality of life when they incorporate ATs in their practice.[21]

ATHLETIC TRAINER SCOPE OF PRACTICE

A unique aspect of athletic training is that, in many instances, ATs follow their patient throughout the continuum of care, from preinjury (prevention) through the diagnostic and intervention stages to the return-to-activity decision. The actual scope of practice within each state may differ from the description provided in this section. Physicians who direct AT practice should consult the state's AT practice act for applicable regulations. Specific scope of practice questions should be directed to the state practice board (http://www.bocatc.org/athletic-trainers#state-regulation). The following is a brief description of skills an AT practices on a daily basis.

Injury Prevention and Health Promotion

The basis of injury prevention and risk management is ensuring the individual's physical readiness to participate in strenuous activity, ensuring a safe playing/work environment, and developing and implementing EAPs. Another form of injury prevention is ensuring the safe return to activity after an injury has been sustained. Lastly, ATs spend significant time educating patients before, during, and after injury and illness.

Using both written health questionnaire and physical examination, the preparticipation physical examination identifies a person's physical readiness to engage in selected activities. During a routine preparticipation physical examination, the patient's and patient's family medical history are analyzed, and a review of systems and regional examinations are performed. In addition, baseline testing such as concussion testing and strength and range of motion (ROM) assessments may be conducted.

ATs work with physicians, administrators, and attorneys to develop EAPs. The EAP describes the standard of care and the procedures to follow in the event of foreseeable emergent situations (e.g., cardiac arrest, cervical spine injury), inclement weather (e.g., heat or lightning), or other possible venue-specific contingencies.

Patient education is the most encompassing method of injury prevention and risk management. When working with high school–aged patients (or younger), patient education also includes the athlete's parent(s) or legal guardian. The AT is often the primary source for information regarding concussions, heat illness, sickle cell trait, and nutritional and hydration needs. This role also extends to bridging the gap between the patient, the patient's family, and the physician regarding the potential outcomes of surgery or other interventions for an injury or illness (and, likewise, the possible consequences of not following the physician's advice). Because ATs tend to see their patients on a frequent (sometimes daily) basis, they serve as a valuable resource for answering questions that may arise during the patient's treatment.

Clinical Diagnosis and Immediate Care

The immediate (on-field) examination first rules out life- or limb-threatening conditions, fractures, or dislocations. The on-field examination ultimately culminates in the decision about how to remove the athlete from the playing field (e.g., assisted or unassisted) and whether the condition requires that the patient be immediately transported to a hospital for emergency care.

The clinical examination relies on obtaining a medical history and performing a functional assessment, inspection, palpation, and assessment of joint and muscle function to form a differential diagnosis. Joint-specific stress tests, selective tissue tests, and, when applicable, neurologic and vascular tests are used to rule in or rule out various pathologies, resulting in a working clinical diagnosis. The AT triages the patient and determines if a referral is indicated. Once a diagnosis has been established, the AT may consult with the physician to determine the appropriate course of care (Fig. 30.1).

Immediate and Emergent Care

In cases in which the findings of the acute (i.e., immediately following the injury) clinical examination and diagnosis indicate that the patient requires emergent care and/or direct transportation to a medical facility, the AT leads (or provides assistance during) the process.[22,23] The scheme of the on-field examination follows the principle of ruling out life-threatening conditions

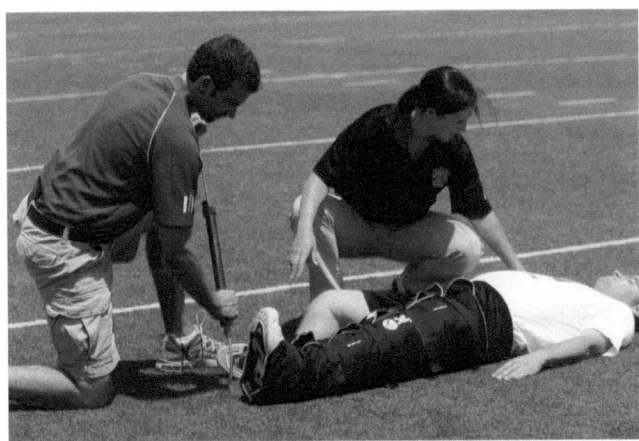

Fig. 30.1 Athletic trainers possess a range of skills that include clinical examination and diagnosis, immediate and emergent care, therapeutic interventions, and administrative skills.

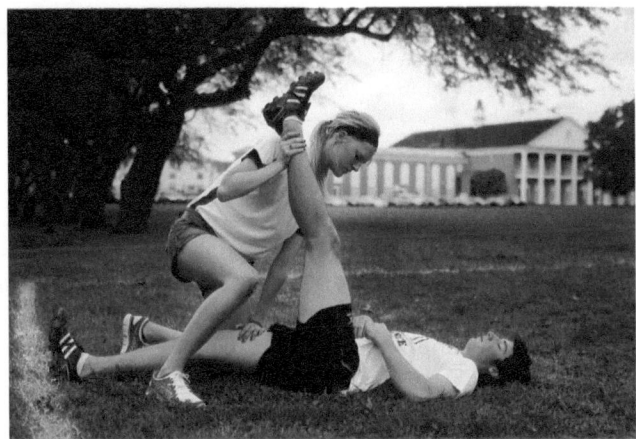

Fig. 30.2 Athletic trainers work clinically and in the field.

and conditions that jeopardize the integrity of the extremity and then performing a more finite musculoskeletal examination. In equipment-intensive sports such as football and hockey, the player's protective equipment may hinder the examination process.

Even before arriving at the scene, the AT begins the triage (i.e., the primary assessment of airway, breathing, and circulation, shock, severe bleeding, and spinal injury). If the athlete is experiencing cardiorespiratory compromise, life support is begun. If this initial screen is negative, the athlete's level of consciousness is ascertained. If the athlete is unconscious (or if a cervical spine injury is indicated), the AT stabilizes the cervical spine and leads the process of immobilizing the patient on a spine board. The AT is often the only person on site to make the return-to-play (RTP) determination, which is particularly important in the case of concussion management. ATs are well educated in the diagnosis and management of concussion, along with RTP criteria.

The on-field orthopaedic examination is more rote than a clinical examination. Although its underlying purpose is to determine if assistance is needed to transport the athlete to the sideline or directly to a medical facility (and, if so, the transportation method required), it is also the best opportunity to identify joint stability before a muscle spasm sets in. The focus is on the immediate history of the injury (primarily the mechanism), inspection and palpation for gross deformity, and determination of active ROM. Although exceptions occur, in general only uniplanar stress tests are performed on the field; selective tissue tests are reserved for a more controlled examination environment.

ATs are well educated regarding transportation techniques, ranging from spine boarding to manually assisted transport. When appropriate, the AT will apply an appropriate protective device and/or fit the patient with crutches to ensure safe ambulation.

Therapeutic Interventions

Therapeutic intervention includes therapeutic modalities, manual therapy, and therapeutic exercise to return the patient to the desired level of function. In a more athletic population, the primary emphasis is on reducing participation restrictions. However, the athletic training philosophy tends to yield

interventions that are more aggressive than those used with the general population. Although the protocols used are aggressive, the goal is to return the patient to activity safely and in the shortest time possible. Identification of the relative and absolute contraindications and precautions to intervention techniques is embedded in the patient examination.

Some therapeutic modalities, such as ice, moist heat, electrical stimulation, and therapeutic ultrasound, are passive devices used to regulate the physiologic response to trauma. Other modalities such as traction or compression are used to cause physical changes in the tissues. Typically, therapeutic modalities are used to allow active exercise or manual therapy to be performed.

Manual therapies include massage, myofascial release, augmented soft tissue mobilization, and joint mobilization (Fig. 30.2). These therapies are augmented by passive, active-assisted, active, and resisted ROM exercises. Once strength and ROM are restored, a functional progression relative to the body part that involves appropriate strengthening, proprioceptive activities, and activity-specific skills is implemented.

Prescription, over-the-counter, and herbal supplements are commonly used by athletes and other physically active persons. ATs understand the influence of pharmacologic approaches in the management of acute and chronic injury and disease and recognize the potential ramifications for patient care.

Psychosocial Strategies and Referral

Although the focus of athletic health care often focuses on physical injury and disease states, emphasis is growing on the mental and emotional components. Conditions such as drug use/abuse, disordered eating, and the female athlete triad have received substantial attention in professional journals and the lay press, and more recent attention has been placed on depression, anxiety, and stress. High school and collegiate student-athletes often turn to the AT as the point of first contact in seeking assistance. The AT does not presume to diagnose these conditions but rather intervenes on behalf of the individual to refer the patient to the proper provider for appropriate assistance.[24]

During the rehabilitation process, ATs also use social support[25] and motivational techniques such as imagery, mental rehearsal, and goal setting to maximize the patient's progression through the intervention program. These techniques often counter the sense of depression and isolation that some athletes experience after sustaining a significant injury.

Health Care Administration

Many athletic injuries require coordinated care involving physicians, surgeons, institutional and individual insurance providers, outpatient facilities, and billing departments. In many instances, the AT assumes the role of a case manager, acting as the liaison between the various medical personnel involved in the patient's care. Blending administration and education, the AT coordinates communication between the patient's parents, the coaching staff, and the media regarding the patient's disposition.

SUMMARY

ATs are state-regulated health care providers who extend the services of a physician. The AT's multidisciplinary educational background incorporates knowledge, skills, and abilities that include injury prevention, clinical diagnosis, emergency care, therapeutic intervention, and RTP decisions. The AT is an invaluable asset in the health care of athletes and other physically active persons.

For a complete list of references, go to ExpertConsult.com.

SELECTED READINGS

Citation:
Schmidt JD, Register-Mihalik JK, Mihalik JP, et al. Identifying impairments after concussion: normative data versus individualized baselines. *Med Sci Sports Exerc.* 2012;44(9):1621–1628.

Level of Evidence:
I

Summary:
In the absence of individualized baseline tests, normative data may be used for neurocognitive testing, postural control, and graded symptom checklists when diagnosing a concussion.

Citation:
Herring SA, Cantu RC, Guskiewicz KM, et al. American College of Sports Medicine. Concussion (mild traumatic brain injury) and the team physician: a consensus statement—2011 update. *Med Sci Sports Exerc.* 2011;43(12):2412–2422.

Level of Evidence:
V

Summary:
This document is a revision of the 2006 Team Physician Statement regarding the diagnosis and management of concussions. This statement reinforces the recommendation of not returning to play the same day as the concussion, describes the role and limitations of neuropsychologic testing, and supports the need for "cognitive rest."

Citation:
Hoch MC, Andreatta RD, Mullineaux DR, et al. Two-week joint mobilization intervention improves self-reported function, range of motion, and dynamic balance in those with chronic ankle instability. *J Orthop Res.* 2012;30(11):1798–1804.

Level of Evidence:
III

Summary:
In this study, the outcomes of Maitland grade III anterior/posterior joint mobilization treatments on ROM, star excursion balance test, and self-reported outcomes scales were compared in 12 subjects. The researchers concluded that the intervention resulted in improved scores for all measures.

Citation:
National Athletic Trainers' Association. *Athletic Training Education Competencies.* 5th ed. http://www.nata.org/education/competencies. Accessed July 19, 2013.

Level of Evidence:
V

Summary:
A multidisciplinary panel identified the knowledge, skills, and abilities that are required to be taught in an accredited professional (entry-level) athletic training program.

Citation:
Podlog L, Eklund RC. Return to sport after serious injury: a retrospective examination of motivation and psychological outcomes. *J Sport Rehabil.* 2005;14:20–34.

Level of Evidence:
II

Summary:
This article describes the effect of internal and external motivation factors in an athlete's return to participation after injury. The researchers found that intrinsic motivation led to more positive outcomes than did extrinsic motivation.

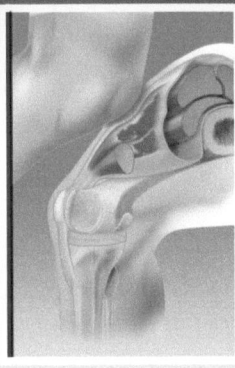

31

Principles of Orthopaedic Rehabilitation

Courtney Chaaban, Charles A. Thigpen

The purpose of this chapter is to describe the principles of orthopaedic rehabilitation. Orthopaedic rehabilitation should balance the load on tissues to stimulate adaptation but not so much to disrupt the healing process. This chapter will describe how loading models can be applied to the rehabilitation process and contrast how this loading is understood to effect different tissues. This paradigm will then be used to identify the key components to designing optimal rehabilitation protocols and pathways while differentiating key interventions and criteria in the context of important patient modifiers. Upon completion of this chapter, orthopaedic specialists will be equipped to develop and implement nonoperative and postoperative protocols or pathways that appropriately balance load and maximize the potential to return patients to their optimal level of function. This chapter will provide an overview of the key concepts and drivers of orthopaedic rehabilitation. The chapter will emphasize the importance of appropriate tissue loading throughout the rehabilitation process.

INTRODUCTION

Envelope of Function

Tissue response to loading has been described as the result of the magnitude and frequency of loading.[1] When load and frequency are matched appropriately, the individual is functioning in his or her "zone of homeostasis," which is loading that does not result in tissue adaptation or tissue failure (Fig. 31.1). When the magnitude or frequency of loading exceeds the tissue's physiologic tolerance, the individual begins to function outside of his or her "envelope of function." This results in supraphysiologic (i.e., stress that is greater than the normal stress of a given person) overload that is positive when the tissues can adapt. For example, when muscle experiences supraphysiologic load over time this results in hypertrophy and neural adaptation. However, when the load exceeds the maximum tissue tolerance threshold, either in magnitude or frequency, the result is structural failure. Following an injury or surgery, tissues are injured as depicted in the figure. This means that activities that were once within the envelope of function are now shifted outside of it. For example, prior to an anterior cruciate ligament (ACL) injury and reconstruction, walking 2 miles was likely within a patient's zone of homeostasis. However, in the weeks immediately following injury and surgery, this task would likely fall outside of the envelope of function. Thus at the beginning of a rehabilitation period,

the tissues involved should be considered when establishing the loading and motion limitations to set the boundaries of the rehabilitation.

Acute: Chronic Workload Ratio

Workload represents all of the stress a given structure experiences (Fig. 31.2). For example, femoral articular cartilage following a "bone bruise" would undergo stress not only from the rehabilitation exercises but also normal activities of daily living such as walking, going up/down stairs, and squatting to sit down/ get up from a chair. Acute workload is most often defined as the workload over the 7 days, and chronic workload over the past 28 days. The relationship between the acute (what is currently imparted on tissues) versus the chronic workload (what stress the tissue has been able to adapt to) plays a critical role in the appropriate progression of individuals as they return to sport.[2,3] Injury risk has been shown to be a function of the acute to chronic workload ratio, whereby higher ratios increase the likelihood of injury. Simply, acute dramatic increases in load compared with what the body is conditioned to respond to appears to increase injury risk.

The acute load is the load the individual has had over the past week, whereas the chronic load is the load the individual has had over the past 4 weeks. A load that had maintained a steady increase of 10% to 15% per week over time results in a "sweet spot" of the acute to chronic load ratio of approximately 1.3, which is an overall 30% greater load in the past 7 days compared with the past 28 days. In contrast, a recent spike in load, such as an increase of 30% in 1 week (increasing from 45 minutes running to 90 minutes, would result in an acute to chronic workload ratio of 2.0, which has been shown to increase an individual's risk of injury, which increases rapidly as the ratio increases.

This is important to consider in the rehabilitation process because workload should be increased gradually to allow tissue adaptation and decrease risk of injury. Throughout the rehabilitation process, this risk of injury can also be equated to risk of symptoms. If a patient has an acute spike in loading during rehabilitation, he or she may not have an injury but may return to the clinic with an increase in pain and swelling or a decrease in range of motion (ROM). These symptoms can be predictable based on which tissues are stressed.

Often athletes are injured in the first few months after return to sport, which may be due in part to too large a spike in acute workload relative to their chronic workload during the

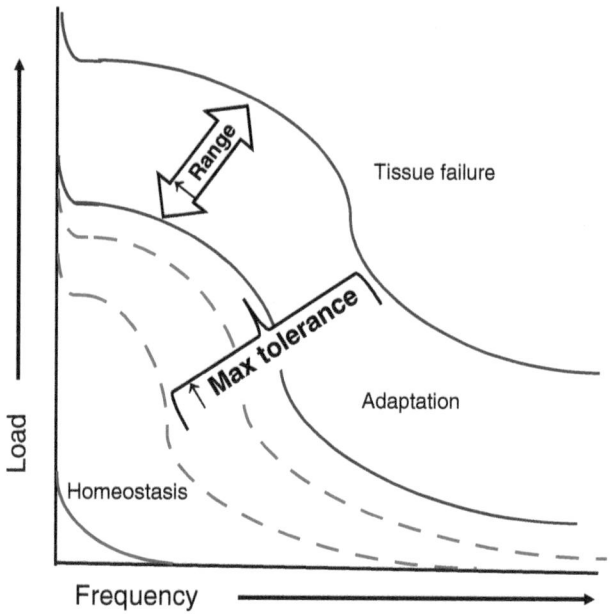

Fig. 31.1 Rehabilitation programs should increase tissue tolerance to the magnitude and frequency of loading, as well as increase the adaption range of that tissue.

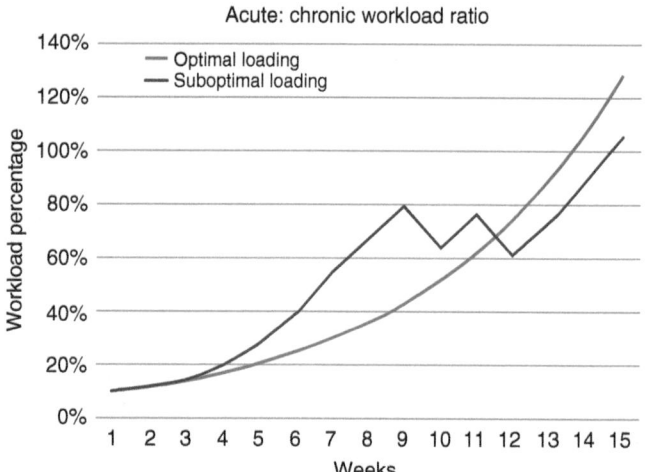

Fig. 31.2 Optimal loading results in the quickest path to return to prior level of function as a period of rest and/or decreased loading is not required to reach loading levels required to return to function.

0	Extremely easy
1	
2	Easy
3	
4	Somewhat easy
5	
6	Somewhat hard
7	
8	Hard
9	
10	Extremely Hard

Fig. 31.3 The OMNI rating of perceived exertion provides a meaningful way to document and manage response to a training load. (From Colado JC, Garcia-Masso X, Triplett NT, et al. Construct and concurrent validation of a new resistance intensity scale for exercise with thera-band(R) elastic bands. *J Sports Sci Med*. 2014;13[4]:758-766.)

External load should be increased systematically and gradually, based on bath knowledge of tissue healing, as well as tissue response to loading. If a patient arrives to a rehabilitation session having lost 5 degrees of knee extension ROM with an increase in pain and swelling after jogging last session, this may suggest the internal load is too high, with tissues giving clean warning signs of external overload. This patient's external load should be decreased until the symptoms of internal load decrease. Clinically, simple methods to measure internal load of the patient include pain, ROM, and rating of perceived exertion (RPE) (Fig. 31.3). The Borg RPE scales are the most commonly used and have been shown to reflect heart rate, breathlessness, and muscle fatigue following exercise.[4-6]

Tissue Healing Considerations

To prescribe the proper loading plan, understanding the basic tissue biomechanical properties is at the core of forming an effective plan of care in rehabilitation, whether nonoperative, preoperative, or postoperative. Tissues differ in both their ability to heal following injury and in their response to loading. A rehabilitation provider is equipped with the knowledge of these healing capacities and loading responses. This allows them to both unload tissue to the degree required to allow maximal healing while minimizing deleterious effects as well as load the tissue to the degree required for optimal return of function. An understanding of healing capacity and loading response dictates the degree to which specific tissues should be subject to forces across the continuum of loading based on both injury and surgery. Proper communication between a surgeon and rehabilitation provider regarding tissue pathology and surgical procedure allows the rehabilitation provider to incorporate this information into a patient's plan of care so they are loaded and progressed appropriately at an adaptive level through their course of rehabilitation.

Tissue healing is an important consideration in the development of time-based guidelines in a protocol. Some tissues affected during surgery require a period of immobilization for healing, whereas others can withstand immediate ROM. Likewise, some tissues benefit from limited or no weight bearing for a period of time, whereas others both withstand and benefit from immediate full weight bearing. There are additional patient-specific factors that may influence the timeline for postoperative

rehabilitation process. Optimal rehabilitation should progress load gradually from surgery through to full return to activity, with coordination between all providers.

Matched Dosing of Internal and External Load

With those models illustrated, it is important to consider how to apply load, how tissue responds, and how these changes lead to clinical decision-making. External load is what is typically thought of in rehabilitation, encompassed by the sets, reps, and resistance people use to perform an exercise or daily activities. Internal load is the tissue's response to an external load and can be viewed based on symptoms, including pain, swelling, change in ROM, etc. Matched dosing is a concept that is critical to successful rehabilitation, meaning that the external load should be matched based on the internal load with which a patient presents.

restrictions, some of which are patient health, tissue quality, comorbidities, etc. A rehabilitation provider will expect instruction from a patient's surgeon regarding any limitations he or she may have postoperative for tissue healing, including the amount and time frame, regarding weight bearing, immobilization and ROM, and muscle activation. This information should be included in an established postoperative protocol, as well as the patient's postoperative referral to a rehabilitation provider if any modifications from the established protocol are made.

Key Tissue-Specific Considerations

Tendon

Tendon repairs generally require a period of immobilization in a shortened position followed by a gradual increase in ROM and load across the tendon. Healthy tendon responds well to linear loads and eccentric exercises when ready.[7,8] However, damaged or less healthy tendons (degenerative rotator cuff or Achilles) may not respond as well as acute tendon injuries and are impacted by overall health such has smoking and hypercholeseterolemia.[9-13]

Ligament

Initially, ligamentous reconstructions are typically weakness at the interface between the bone and fixation device, thus restrictions should be based on the strength here. As the ligament graft undergoes "ligamentization," there is a time during which the cellular structure in the graft is disorganized and weaker, and restrictions on activity should be based on the strength of the graft.[14,15] In contrast, ligamentous repairs are weakest at the site of the repair, which is more tenuous, dictating that immediate postoperative care may be more conservative with a period of immobilization.[16,17]

Labral/Meniscal

Labral and meniscal tissue can vary in their blood supply based on location of injury and thus can vary in their ability to heal. In general, more vascular areas are more likely to heal, whereas areas with poor blood supply are limited in their capacity to heal.[18] This variance in ability to heal often dictates surgical procedure. In a labral or meniscal débridement, there is no structural healing of repaired tissue postoperatively because the tissue was débrided. As such, postoperative restrictions would be based around the remaining tissue's tolerance to loading. In the lower extremity, the forces distributed across articular cartilage will increase, and loading should be progressive to allow tissue to adapt to this new demand. In a labral or meniscal repair, the tissue should be protected from loading initially with the goal of allowing structural healing to take place to the extent possible while protecting the interface of any fixation. This tissue responds well to compression but not to shear forces, so typical postoperative protocols allow some compressive forces while minimizing shear.

Articular Cartilage

Articular cartilage is also limited in its ability to heal, in part due to lack of blood supply here.[19] Surgical procedures to improve articular cartilage are either aimed at stimulating a healing response or through transplanting other cartilage to the area. Due to this, there is typically a prolonged period of non–weight bearing if the lesion is on a weight-bearing surface. However, recent animal models show gradual loading and motion aid in healing.[20-22] This poses a critical challenge for the surgeon and rehabilitation team in designing effective rehabilitation programs following articular cartilage injury. Surgeons may also impose restrictions regarding the degree of motion the joint is allowed based on where in the ROM the lesion would engage.

Bone

Bone responds well to compressive loads and is the most predictable, and radiographs can be used to easily to monitor healing.[23,24] Injuries due to repetitive stress (fifth metatarsal fractures) are not as predictable and should receive special consideration. However, generally 6 weeks of immobilization provides adequate healing time to begin loading.

Patient Modifiers

There are many additional patient-specific factors that put into context tissue considerations. These include established risk factors for delayed healing, such as smoking, diabetes, obesity, nutritional status, and current exercise tolerance.[25,26] If a patient possesses some of these risk factors, a surgeon may dictate that postoperative rehabilitation progresses at a delayed pace relative to a normal protocol. For example, diabetes is a well-established risk factor for postoperative stiffness in shoulder and knee surgery, likely requiring a modification of the typical postoperative plan.[27-29] If a patient possesses some of these risk factors, the surgeon may dictate that rehabilitation to restore ROM progress at an accelerated pace relative to the normal protocol. These patient modifiers are very important in allowing for a successful postoperative rehabilitation.

MAINTENANCE AND RESTORATION OF MOTION

One goal of rehabilitation following surgery will be to restore normal motion at a rate that is dictated by the surgical procedure and what structures need to be protected.

Range of Motion

ROM is a joint's ability to achieve excursion in any given direction. ROM can be either passive or active. Passive ROM should be attained before the patient is able to achieve active control over motion, and thus passive ROM goals should come prior to active ROM goals in criterion-based protocols. In addition, passive ROM may be indicated prior to beginning active ROM in cases where muscle/tendon/bone interfaces require time to heal and muscle activation would be detrimental to healing. One example of such is the protected phase following rotator cuff repair where passive ROM is allowed prior to active ROM. Depending on involved tissue, passive and/or active ROM in specific directions may be indicated prior to ROM in other directions to protect healing tissue. For example, a subscapularis repair would have restrictions on passive external rotation to limit overstretching, as well as restrictions on active internal rotation to limit stress from muscle activation.

Patients can experience decreased ROM for several reasons, and rehabilitation providers work to determine the cause of that restriction, as well as interventions to address it so that functional ROM can be obtained. Some reasons for decreased ROM are decreased flexibility and decreased joint mobility.

Immobilization

There are cases in which immobilization for a period of time is recommended to allow healing from surgical procedure. This would include situations with tenuous repairs, such as an Achilles repair, when the surgeon requires the patient to be casted in plantarflexion to allow protection and healing. A surgeon, with knowledge of the structures he or she wishes to protect, will dictate the period of time, as well as the position of immobilization. This is balanced with the concerns for stiffness. However, it should be noted that for some surgeries, such as rotator cuff repair, stiffness is transient and resolves within 6 months to 1 year following surgery.[30,31] In contrast, stiffness following total knee arthroplasty (TKA) often requires manipulation or further surgery.[32] Therefore the risk of revision surgery, failed tissue repair, and stiffness must be weighed when choosing immobilization strategies.

When to Begin "Passive" and "Active" Motion

Based on the balance in restoring ROM and protection, timelines for initiation of passive and active ROM are established. In cases that require protection of contractile tissue, patients will generally begin passive ROM prior to beginning active ROM. Passive ROM is the ability to move through an ROM without to use of contractile tissue (such as a rehabilitation provider moving a shoulder into external rotation while the patient is relaxed). Passive motion is intended to protect the repair interface of the contractile tissue, no matter which portion of the muscle-tendon-bone. It is important to note that no passive motion is completely passive without some muscle contraction. Most "passive" exercises exhibit 10% to 20% of a muscles maximum contraction during these exercises.[33-35] In addition, when the joint is lengthened opposite the direction of the tissues under protection, the passive elements of the muscle will increase tensile forces. For this reason, passive ROM opposite the repaired muscle unit's action is generally limited for a period of time and progressed per surgeon direction. Active ROM generally follows passive ROM in these situations, particularly active in the direction of the muscle's line of action. Active ROM for a period of time based on healing properties of the repaired tissue.

In cases of cartilage lesions, the surgeon may restrict the patient from engaging these surfaces for a period of time. This may influence not only weight bearing but the portion of the joint's available motion that can be used. For example, following trochlear microfracture, knee flexion angle may be limited for a period of time based on the location of the lesion. The same is generally true for meniscal repairs, typically limiting end range flexion for 4 to 6 weeks. However, there is some evidence that continuous passive motion aids in healing cartilage and recovery following cartilage procedures.[20,36] This concept is based on regular joint motion stimulating synovial fluid production and bathing the tissues with the required micronutrients and lubrication.[21] Our experience suggests regular, easy motion (continuous passive motion, stationary bike) provides good relief from stiffness and promotes the joint towards a "steady state" or normal following injury or surgery.

Joint Mobility

Joint mobility is the capacity of a joint to move prior to restriction from the soft tissues surrounding it, including the bony articulation, capsuloligamentous structures, and muscle/tendon structures. Often following surgery, due to immobilization, limited ROM, or an inflammatory response, patients can experience a decrease in their joint mobility that limits their available ROM. This is often related to a decrease in capsular volume or mobility, and rehabilitation providers will use techniques to improve the joint mobility so that functional ROM may be attained.

Flexibility

Flexibility is a muscle's ability to lengthen to allow normal motion. Impairments in flexibility are commonly seen after surgical procedures, even those which do not have muscular involvement. Immobilization or limited ROM about a joint for protection following surgery often dictates that muscles surrounding the joint are not able to be stretched through their full excursion, and over time, these muscles lose flexibility. As ROM is allowed, rehabilitation providers will also work to restore normal flexibility of surrounding musculature. If decreased flexibility is the limiting factors in restoring ROM, rehabilitation providers will develop focused programs to improve flexibility through stretching and manual therapy techniques.

RESTORATION OF MUSCLE PERFORMANCE

Another goal following surgery will be to restore muscle performance at the rate that allows for congruency and healing of tissue structures.

Inhibition/Activation

Some muscle groups tend to be inhibited following surgery or injury, which can result in aberrant activation of muscle groups about a joint. One such example is the quadriceps, which tends to be inhibited following knee trauma or surgery due to pain and swelling, as well as spinal and cortical level changes.[37,38] Following most knee surgeries, a primary goal in early postoperative rehabilitation is to improve the activation of the quadriceps. Examples of techniques are neuromuscular electrical stimulation (NMES), biofeedback, transcranial stimulation as well as careful monitoring of swelling and pain at the knee.[39-42]

Hypertrophy Versus Motor Learning

One large component of postoperative rehabilitation is strengthening. There are many different ways to consider strength, which are outlined later in "Muscle Performance." When we consider strengthening in postoperative rehabilitation, it is important to note that early changes are largely due to improvement in the efficiency and effectiveness of motor unit firing.[43,44] It takes much longer (at least 6 to 8 weeks) to see changes due to muscle hypertrophy, or growth of the size of the muscle. Early postoperative rehabilitation should focus motor learning and improving the ability of muscle groups to fire appropriately, where later rehabilitation should focus on hypertrophy, or increasing the muscle's size.[45,46]

PRINCIPLES OF CRITERION BASED PROGRESSION

Progression in rehabilitation should be both time and criterion based. *Time-based criteria are based on setting* anatomic stoplights and provide the guideposts for rehabilitation programs. These timelines are aimed to protect tissue from loading that could disrupt or slow healing following surgery. These timelines are tissue specific and are limited because they are only estimates based mostly on animal studies and normal variation in individual patient healing. *Criterion-based progression* requires specific criteria to be achieved to move forward to the next phase of rehabilitation. These criteria are aimed at ensuring specific impairments are resolved along the recovery path. This optimizes the patient's ability to match their activities to allow a safe progression back to their desired level of functional. Therefore the time-based criterion guide the fastest that a patient could safely progress through rehabilitation, whereas the criterion-based progression may require longer and is patient specific.

Key Criteria for Rehabilitation Protocols and Progressions
Outcome Measures
There are many patient-reported outcome (PRO) measures which are used to assess patients' perception on some combination of their pain, function, and satisfaction. These measures can be specific to a joint, such as the PENN Shoulder Score[47] or International Knee Disability Committee (IKDC).[48] They can also be broad to capture a patient's overall health views, such as the Veterans Rand 12-item Health Survey (VR-12).[48] The American Academy of Orthopaedic Surgeons Quality Outcomes Data (QOD) Work Group on Patient Reported Outcome Measures has recommended specific PROs for general health and each body region.[49,50] These PROs were recommended based on the following criteria[51]:
1. PROs
2. Validated scores
3. Good psychometrics
4. Ease of use for the patient (i.e., brief)
5. Ease of scoring and understanding for physician
6. Standardized use nationally
7. Consideration for cost

Specifically, selected PROs should demonstrate good psychometrics including reliability, validity, and minimal clinically important differences (MCIDs) for the population in question. Individual patient progression compared with population norms at regular intervals throughout the recovery process can aid discharge planning and long-term prognosis.[51,52]

Pain
Postoperative pain is expected and normal in association with many procedures. Adequate pain control is requisite for progression through rehabilitation. If pain is not controlled, progression to more demanding activities will likely exacerbate pain. As pain is known to have an inhibitory effect on certain muscle groups, pain control is also essential for proper muscle performance and progression through muscle performance activities. Pain levels, generally through a Numeric Pain Rating Scale (NPRS) or visual analog scale (VAS) should be assessed regularly and monitored, and an increase in pain may signal a need to decrease demands of rehabilitation or modify activities accordingly. In general, minimal to no pain should be experienced both within and between rehabilitation sessions prior to progressing a patient to the next phase of rehabilitation. There are some surgical procedures and postoperative rehabilitation protocols which can be associated with increased pain, and patients should be educated accordingly for matched expectations of their progress.

Range of Motion
ROM can be measured passively as well as actively. In general, passive ROM should be attained before active ROM, as dictated by protecting healing tissue. Time-based parameters should be established for when passive and active ROM are allowed and to what extent. Criteria should be established for what amount of passive ROM and active ROM are required prior to progressing within a protocol.

Muscle Performance
There are many different measures of muscle performance. *Strength* refers to the maximal force output of a muscle group to a load. It is commonly measured in the physical therapy setting through the use of a dynamometer for a quantifiable measure or through the use of manual muscle testing when dynamometers are not available. Strength should be a component of any criterion-based protocol, with discharge criteria generally being set as attaining at least 90% strength relative to the contralateral limb.[53-55] Many protocols also cite a balance of strength between muscle groups, such as external rotation/internal rotation strength ratio of the shoulder in throwers, or quadriceps to hamstrings strength ratio on lower extremity athletes.[56,57] *Power* is defined as a muscle group's ability to produce work over a period of time and is often termed "rate of force development" in recent literature.[58,59] Power is proportional to the speed at which one can produce a force. There are many different ways to measure power, and in general, these tests are performed in patients whose activity level demand explosive movements, such as those who perform sprinting or jumping. *Endurance* is another measure of muscle performance, and it relates to a muscle group's ability to maintain strength over a period of time while under load.[60] Patients may use compensatory muscular or movement patterns when fatigued that increase their susceptibility to subsequent injury. There are many ways to measure endurance and fatigue, and these measures relate to placing patients in the fatiguing activity they would be performing, to assess their ability to

sustain a level of performance and how they are able to perform when fatigued.

Balance

Balance refers to one's ability to maintain their center of mass over their base of support without losing stability. Balance is a common impairment seen in patients following lower extremity surgery, especially amongst those who have compromised tissue that would otherwise contribute to congruency or proprioception. There are many ways to measure balance. In general, a measure of balance is commonly cited in criterion-based protocols in order to progress from assistive devices with gait activities. A measure of balance should also be cited prior to discharge to ensure adequate stability for a patient's full return to function. The Star Excursion Balance Test (SEBT) and modified SEBT are commonly used (Fig. 31.4).[61,62]

Movement Quality

Movement quality refers to a patient's ability to perform movements against a normative standard of movement. Deficits in movement quality, including "faulty movement patterns," have been identified as risk factors for future injury. Movement quality is assessed throughout rehabilitation, with movement retraining integrated as necessary in care. Examples of movement quality tests include scapula dyskinesis during arm elevation, the Landing Error Scoring System (LESS) for jumping landing mechanics, or the Functional Movement Screen for squatting.[63-66]

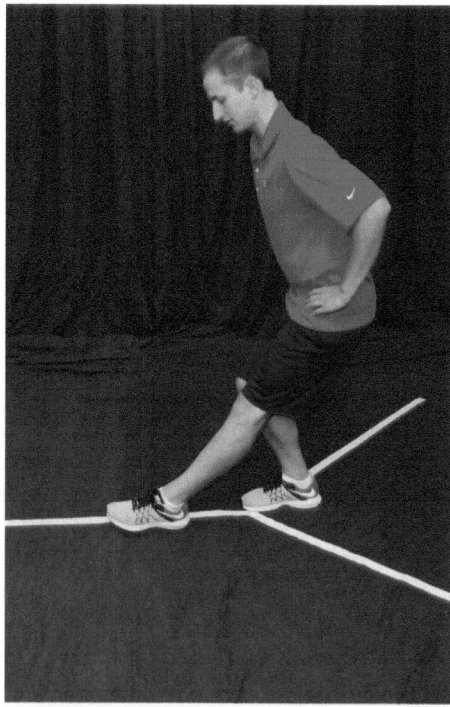

Fig. 31.4 The anterior direction of the modified Star Excursion Balance Test.

Return-to-Sport Considerations

The decision regarding when to return an athlete to sport is complex. There should be both time and criterion-based considerations based on both anatomic healing and functional performance. This allows the athlete to return at a point which optimizes the balance between minimizing time loss and maximizing function and ability to return safely without subsequent injury. This requires a team effort because the surgeon is best equipped to decide if the tissues have appropriately healed and the rehabilitation provider can assess the athlete's ability to function and the constructs associated with successful return to sport. It is the responsibility of the rehabilitation providers to communicate their assessment of the athlete's functional capabilities and readiness to return to sport to the athlete's surgeon. Recent evidence shows that those who return too soon (<7 months following ACL reconstruction) or do not meet the return-to-sport criteria are at significant risk for subsequent injury.

In addition to the factors referenced previously (pain, ROM, muscle performance, and outcome measures), there are additional functional measures that should be assessed when determining an athlete's readiness to return to sport.[67-71]

KEYS TO SUCCESSFUL REHABILITATION

Role of Preoperative Rehabilitation

Preoperative rehabilitation should be included as a portion of a patient's comprehensive surgical care. In our experience, preoperative rehabilitation has many benefits.[72-81]

- A preoperative visit allows a rehabilitation provide to establish baseline values for a patient's pain, ROM, and strength, along with other measures deemed appropriate.
- It allows patients to learn more about their postoperative rehabilitation process prior to surgery, when they are not dealing with postoperative pain and impaired cognition from postoperative medications. Patients learn what they can expect to feel and do during each phase of their postoperative case, as well as an estimated timeline on their duration of care to reach their functional goals. Having this conversation prior to surgery allows the patient time to plan accordingly so that they go into surgery with clear postoperative expectations for rehabilitation.
- It allows the rehabilitation provider an opportunity to provide recommendations that would be helpful prior to surgery to decrease pain and swelling, restore ROM, and restore muscle performance as appropriate in a safe manner. Many studies illustrate a relationship because preoperative function and postoperative function, so this allows patients to optimize their preoperative function so that they may have a more successful postoperative outcome.
- It allows patients an opportunity to receive training and education on any postoperative equipment they will be using, including assistive devices and protective devices such as slings or braces. This allows them the opportunity to practice prior to surgery.

Communication

Surgical protocols and referrals are used to detail the expected postoperative progression based on the surgery performed. These protocols are guidelines used by rehabilitation providers to progress patients accordingly. They may differ from surgeon to surgeon, but in general, their key is their ability to match dosing of load to allow the patient to heal, progress safely, and return to their activities with a minimized risk of future injury. The protocols combined with a detailed referral are the keystones of matching expectations. The surgeon should provide a detailed referral to guide the rehabilitation provider to deliver the care expected by the surgeon. The referral should at minimum include:

- *Diagnosis:* Postoperative referrals should detail the patient diagnosis, including what tissue damage was identified preoperatively and intraoperatively.
- *Operative details:* The postoperative referrals should outline any surgical procedures performed, including location and size of repairs or removal of tissue.
- *Patient modifiers:* As discussed regarding patient modifiers, a surgeon may wish to alter an established protocol based on patient-specific factors, whether specific tissue factors in the surgery, such as poor bone quality in a rotator cuff repair, or patient-specific factors, such as a metabolic concern for altered healing response. These modifications should be outlined on a postoperative referral if they deviate from the established protocol. If the surgeon wishes to modify a protocol based on patient presentation at a time point following surgery after a follow-up visit, this should be communicated to the patient's rehabilitation provider as well.

Matching Expectations

From the diagnosis through return to sport or activity, setting expectations for a patient will aid in smoothing through the difficult process. This begins with the preoperative visit and outlines for the patient the general timeline in which they can expect to progress following surgery. This way, patients can plan for expected time to use assistive devices or braces and to return to activities, including, driving, work, sports, etc. The protocol then establishes when progression is safe and expected for a standard surgical procedure. This allows rehabilitation providers and surgeons to be consistent in their message delivered to patients to minimize any confusion and create a positive patient experience.

Timing of Communication and Follow-Up

Surgeons vary in the amount and frequency of communication they expect from rehabilitation providers. In general, rehabilitation providers should communicate patient progress to surgeons prior to each of the patient's appointments with the surgeon. They should also communicate with the surgeon if they have concerns, including a new injury or failure to progress as expected, even if the patient does not have an upcoming appointment with the surgeon in the near future. They should never progress faster than a protocol timeline allows, without communication from the surgeon to do so. Following these principles will optimize communication and ultimate outcome for patients following surgery.

For a complete list of references, go to ExpertConsult.com.

32

Modalities and Manual Techniques in Sports Medicine Rehabilitation

Susan Saliba, Michael Higgins

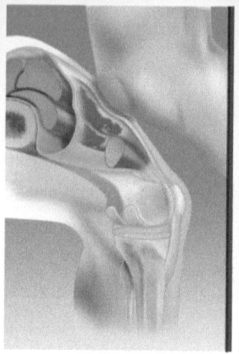

MODALITIES AND MANUAL THERAPY

Modalities, physical agents, and manual therapies (MTs) are commonly applied interventions for sports-related injuries and are designed to facilitate the rehabilitation process. These treatments are often associated with pain modulation techniques that can allow an earlier implementation of therapeutic exercise. Modalities such as ice and electrical stimulation can often reduce pain, and MT techniques similarly modulate the neuromuscular system so that the focus can remain on restoring function. New methods and devices are continually marketed and purported to alleviate symptoms and treat inflammatory conditions. Clinicians must stay vigilant to address the patient's impairments and then design and implement treatments that meet specific treatment goals. Using evidence, applying the treatments properly, and measuring results are imperative throughout the process.

Modalities

Modalities such as cryotherapy (ice), electrical stimulation, heat, ultrasound, and laser are commonly applied to the body to affect the inflammatory cascade and to reduce pain. Ice is probably the most commonly applied treatment and is part of the standard of care. For most acute injuries the acronym POLICE (*Protect, Optimal loading, Ice, Compression, Elevation*) should be followed (Fig. 32.1).[1] Electrical stimulation has been used in rehabilitation for thousands of years and dates back to the ancient Olympic Games in Greece when clinicians used electrical eels to treat athletes' injuries. Today electrical currents are applied as either transcutaneous electrical nerve stimulation (TENS) or as neuromuscular electrical nerve stimulation (NMES) to reduce pain or stimulate a muscle contraction. Newer forms of electrotherapy, such as patterned electrical nerve stimulation (PENS), have additional application in muscle activation and recruitment. Ultrasound and laser are often termed biostimulators since they use mechanical (acoustical energy) or light energy to stimulate cellular processes within the tissues. Thus the types of energies and equipment available for clinical use are continually expanding.

Literature that supports the use of therapeutic modalities varies and researchers often try to identify physiologic mechanisms or responses when these agents are applied. Studies on healthy individuals, as is often the case with cryotherapy studies, confound the literature since the neuromuscular changes induced with ice application would be different without pathology. Garnering evidence to support the use of modalities is difficult combined with the fact that clinical trials are difficult to control. For example, to study whether TENS enhances pain modulation in a specific injury, the researcher would need to control all other therapies including ice, oral analgesics, and activity. Typically, once a patient feels improvement, he or she increases their activity level, which can, in turn, result in more discomfort. The use of patient-reported outcome scales, physical measures of edema, range of motion (ROM), strength, and data from activity monitors can help provide evidence for specific treatments. Furthermore, modalities all have parameters that affect the dosage, which should be consistently applied and modified when appropriate. For example, electrical currents have a variety of waveforms, phase durations, pulse frequencies, and recommended intensities to elicit the desired response. Ultrasound can vary in frequency, duty cycle, and intensity; and lasers vary in wavelength, intensity, and possibly duty cycle. The area treated, the amount of tissues exposed, and how often the treatment is delivered can also affect the outcome. Thus the clinician is expected to understand the parameters and adjust them properly according to the desired outcome. Since modalities often apply thermal, electrical, acoustical, or light energy to the body, precautions include cardiac pacemakers (or implanted electromagnetic devices), sensory loss (especially to temperature changes), and peripheral artery disease that affects normal physiology in the extremities. Specific precautions should always be applied regarding the specific technique.

Manual Therapy

Similar to modalities, MT is a passive, nonsurgical type of conservative management that involves skilled movements applied by clinicians to the patient's body that directly or indirectly targets a variety of anatomical structures or systems.[2] MT is used to assess, diagnose, and treat a variety of symptoms and conditions that are intended to modulate pain; improve tissue extensibility; increase ROM; induce relaxation; mobilize or manipulate soft tissue and joints; and reduce soft tissue swelling, inflammation, or restriction.[2] Health care practitioners implement MT when the examination findings, diagnosis, and prognosis indicate the use of these techniques to decrease edema, pain, spasm, or swelling; enhance health, wellness, and fitness; improve or maintain physical performance; increase the ability to move; or prevent or remediate impairment in body functions and structures, activity limitations, or participation restrictions to improve physical

P	Protect	Minimizes stress to the injured structure
OL	Optimal loading	Soft tissues respond well to graded and controlled stress
I	Ice	Reduces local metabolism & pain
C	Compression	Reduces and controls edema
E	Elevation	Reduces and controls edema

Fig. 32.1 *POLICE* to treat acute injuries. (From Bleakley CM, Glasgow P, MacAuley DC. PRICE needs updating, should we call the POLICE? *Br J Sports Med.* 2012;46[4]:220–221. doi:10.1136/bjsports-2011-090297.)

function. Precautions, and contraindications for MT include joint pain with the technique, joint effusion, unknown pathology, auto-immune diseases, fracture, tumor, infection and osteoporosis. MT should be avoided with nerve and vascular pathologies where movement and pressure can exacerbate the condition. Although these techniques can be helpful and useful, there is no evidence that any one of them is the only way or even the best way to treat a particular condition.

There are many MT techniques with different names and uses. There are even types that offer practitioners certifications in a particular technique. You may see these listed as trigger point release (TPR), proprioceptive neuromuscular facilitation (PNF), muscle energy technique (MET), strain-counterstrain, active release technique (ART), cranio-sacral therapy, myofascial release, positional release therapy, and others. Most of these MT techniques may be categorized into four major groups: (1) manipulation (high velocity low amplitude—HVLA), (2) mobilization (nonthrust manipulation), (3) stretching, and (4) muscle-modifying techniques.

Collectively, the process of interventions with either modalities or MT is grounded on clinical reasoning to enhance patient management for musculoskeletal pain by influencing factors from a multidimensional perspective that have potential to positively impact clinical outcomes. The influence of biomechanical, neurophysiologic, psychological, and nonspecific patient factors as treatment mediators and/or moderators provides additional information related to the process and potential mechanisms by which the treatment may be effective. Additionally, the definition and purpose of MT varies across health care professionals. As health care delivery advances toward personalized approaches, there is a crucial need to advance our understanding of the underlying mechanisms associated with MT and modality effectiveness.

Modalities have been shown to be effective when applied in a variety of ways to various pathologies. MT has been shown to be effective for increasing function and pain reduction in the treatment of musculoskeletal disorders including low back pain,[3,4] carpal tunnel syndrome,[5,6] knee osteoarthritis,[7] and hip osteoarthritis.[8] Moreover, recent studies have provided even stronger evidence when participants are classified into sub-groups.[4,9] Refer to Table 32.1 for a summary. Despite the literature supporting its effectiveness, the mechanisms of these treatments are not well established.

IMPAIRMENT-BASED REHABILITATION PROGRAMS

Evidence-based practice describes a clinical paradigm that prescribes certain interventions when there is evidence, based on either research or empiricism, to support that intervention. Each treatment, whether it is a modality or a MT, should be applied with a specific goal in mind. A systematic evaluation of the injury, including biomechanical assessment should be conducted. That evaluation will reveal the presence of any impairment. For example, when evaluating an acute ankle injury, the clinician may find edema, localized pain on the lateral ankle, limited ROM, and pain with weight bearing. Those findings become the impairment list and only treatments with evidence to resolve a specific impairment should be administered (Fig. 32.2).[45] Evidence-based practice describes a clinical paradigm that prescribes certain interventions when there is evidence, based on either research or empiricism, to support that intervention. Each treatment, whether that is a modality or MT, should be applied with a specific goal in mind. A systematic evaluation of the injury, including biomechanical assessment should be conducted. That evaluation will reveal the presence of any impairment. For example, when evaluating an acute ankle injury, the clinician may find edema, localized pain on the lateral ankle, limited ROM, and pain with weight bearing. Those findings become the impairment list and only treatments with evidence to resolve a specific impairment should be administered. Clinicians who measure outcomes will develop their own evidence to support the continued use of an intervention or have the justification to cease the treatment. Thus the treatments and the rehabilitation program continually evolve. This chapter is not inclusive of all therapies that can or should be applied to facilitate the rehabilitation program. However, we aim to present the information in a style that might help direct a clinician to an appropriate therapy based on the results of the clinical evaluation and treatment goals.

Sports and orthopaedic injuries and pathologies cannot be resolved by these interventions alone. Time, resolution of the inflammation, and healing must occur and should be within the context of surgical repairs or reconstructions and immobilization. Tissues must be protected as they heal and the goal of both postoperative and conservative management is to restore or replace neuromuscular pathways and to provide strength and dynamic stability. Many chronic pain syndromes develop altered neural pathways that result in the inhibition of muscle function, decreased strength, and restriction of movement. Different treatments should be applied for those impairments. Sports medicine is all about returning the patient to function as quickly as possible. If an intervention might hasten the healing process by allowing earlier exercise, increasing ROM, or restoring more confidence while performing functional exercise, then best practice would suggest that the therapy should be used. Most of these treatments are safe, but keeping therapies aligned with the impairment contains costs and prevents unnecessary treatments.

TABLE 32.1   Effectiveness of Manual Therapy for Body Region

Region	Effectiveness of Manual Therapy (Associated With Improvements in Pain, Function, and Disability in Individuals With the Following Conditions)	Effectiveness of Modalities
Shoulder	• Shoulder impingement syndrome[10] • Adhesive capsulitis[11]	• Calcific tendonitis[12]
Elbow	• Lateral epicondylalgia[13,14]	• Lateral epicondylalgia[15]
Wrist	• Lateral epicondylalgia[16] • Carpal tunnel syndrome[17]	• Carpal tunnel[18]
Hip	• Hip osteoarthritis[19]	• Osteoarthritis[20] • Hip arthroplasty[21] • Hip pain[22]
Knee	• Knee osteoarthritis[19] • Limited evidence for PFP[23]	• Knee osteoarthritis,[24] patellofemoral pain[25] • ACL reconstruction[26,27]
Ankle[107]	• Ankle sprains[28,29] • Plantar heel pain[30] • Cuboid syndrome[31] • Symptomatic hallux abducto valgus[32]	• Ankle sprains[1,33]
Cervical spine	• Mechanical neck pain[34] • Cervical radiculopathy[35] • Whiplash associated disorder[36] • Cervicogenic headache[36] • Nonspecific shoulder pain[37] • Lateral epicondylalgia[38]	• Nonspecific neck & trigger point pain[39]
Thoracic spine	• Mechanical neck pain[40] • Cervical radiculopathy[35,40] • Shoulder pain[37]	
Lumbar spine	• Nonspecific low back pain[41,42] • Lumbar spinal stenosis[108] • Lumbosacral radiculopathy[43]	• Low back pain[44]

Pathology

Impairment

Pain
- Massage
- Myofascial release
- Trigger point therapy
- Cryothraphy
- TENS

Edema/Inflammation
- Electrical stim (HVS)
- Ultrasound
- Phonophoresis
- Iontophoresis
- Laser
- Intermittent compression

Loss of Motion:
- Superficial heat
- Thermal ultrasound
- Mobilization manipulation
- Mobilization with movement

Muscle Dysfunction:
- Cyrotherapy
- NMES
- PENS
- MET
- Myofascial & trigger
- Point therapy

Functional
Limitations

Fig. 32.2 Impairments and treatments in sports medicine conditions. (Modified from Vela and Denegar.) (From Iverson CA, Sutlive TG, Crowell MS, et al. Lumbopelvic manipulation for the treatment of patients with patellofemoral pain syndrome: development of a clinical prediction rule. *Orthop Sports Phys Ther.* 2008;38[6]:297–309; discussion 309–312. doi: 10.2519/jospt.2008.2669.)

Pain Modulation

Pain is perhaps the most common factor in any sports injury or orthopaedic condition and is involved with the inflammatory process. Pain is useful since it alerts the patient that there is a problem, but it can begin a cascade of factors that can change motor function that is designed to protect the injured body part. For example, friction in the glenohumeral joint of a swimmer may begin with some pain. Unknown to the swimmer, the supraspinatus muscle becomes inhibited. Although there is discomfort, the swimmer continues his workout and the poor motor function prevents adequate stabilization and depression of the humeral head. Minor adjustments in the scapular position permit another 20,000 to 30,000 strokes with no real change in the ability to perform. However, the change in mechanics may result in bursitis, tendinopathy, and impingement. Resolving the pain in this case is imperative to restoring the mechanical function of the supraspinatus.

Pain is a complex neurophysiologic phenomenon and methods to treat pain include medications as well as physical agents and MT. Medications typically act on the chemical cascade of the inflammatory process, and include non-steroidal antiinflammatory drugs (NSAIDs) and steroids. Various other analgesics, both narcotic and nonnarcotic, act on the chemical neurotransmitters throughout the nervous system. Physical agents and manual therapies act by stimulating various sensory systems to elicit endogenous neurotransmitters or by creating alternative sensory input that reduces the painful input. Regardless of the method used for analgesia, it is important to restore normal stimulus to the muscle system. Returning to the swimmer, when pain is reduced, the supraspinatus needs to be retrained to stabilize and depress the humeral head during the overhead motion. Just relieving pain without proper attention to the inhibited muscle group would only provide a temporary solution.

To simplify pain modulation for the purposes of this chapter, three manners of pain modulation will be presented. Sensory, rhythmical, and noxious mechanisms can explain the majority of pain modulation from common therapies (Table 32.2). Then, various treatments within each theory can be presented.

TREATMENTS FOR PAIN

Manual Therapy

The pain-modulating effects of most MT techniques has been suggested to be mainly neurophysiologic in origin, and may be mediated by the descending modulatory mechanisms (rhythmical and noxious). Current research suggests that this neurophysiologic response to MT is responsible for clinically significant decreases in pain.[50] It appears that different types of MT may work through different mechanisms (Table 32.3). Understanding the mechanisms may help clinicians choose which therapy is most appropriate for each patient, and may lead to more effective therapies in the future.

In a recent study investigating the effect of four MT techniques (manipulation/mobilization, muscle energy, massage, strain-counterstrain) performed on subjects with sites of muscle hypertonicity, tenderness, and joint restriction revealed that blood levels of β-endorphin and N-palmitoylethanolamide were elevated after treatment when compared to baseline. The greatest biomarker alteration was experienced in subjects with chronic low back pain.[51]

TABLE 32.2 Pain Modulation Mechanisms

Pain Modulation Theory	Examples of Therapy
Sensory Pain Modulation[47] Sensory pain modulation describes Melzack and Wall's classic Gate Theory. Pain is propagated on smaller myelinated axons (A delta) and unmyelinated fibers (c fibers) and synapses in the spinal cord to ascend to the thalamus and then the sensory cortex where pain is processed. Stimulation of large diameter sensory fibers (light touch, vibration, etc.) in the painful area can inhibit the transmission of pain sensation at the spinal cord. Thus mechanical stimulation of the skin and surrounding tissues can "close the gate" at the spinal cord, minimizing the pain signal as long as the stimulation continues.	• TENS • Massage • Intermittent compression
Rhythmical Pain Modulation[48] Rhythmical pain modulation is associated with a descending mechanism that elicits the production of endogenous opiates such as beta endorphin. This powerful analgesic method typically requires significant sensory input in a rhythmical fashion. Runner's high is one example of this type of pain modulation. The mechanical stimulation, which may include a muscle contraction, stimulates areas within the brain such as the Raphe nucleus and reticular formation to send signals to the pituitary to release beta lipotropin and adrenocorticotropic hormone (ACTH). The beta lipotropin will form endorphin and the ACTH results in cortisol production at the adrenal glands. Each neurochemical can produce long-lasting pain modulation.	• Rhythmical TENS • Myofascial release • Joint mobilization • Mobilization with movement • Muscle energy technique
Noxious Pain Modulation[49] Noxious pain modulation is the same as "central biasing" and descending noxious inhibitory control. This type of therapy requires a painful stimulus (c fiber stimulation) that elicits a cascade of neural factors in the midbrain and spinal cord to minimize pain. The periaqueductal gray is primarily responsible for producing enkephalins and serotonin when stimulated in this manner. This method can be combined with a rhythmical pattern for an added benefit.	• Instrumented soft tissue mobilization • Ice • Deep tissue massage • Trigger point therapy

Modified from Denegar CR, Saliba E, Saliba S. *Therapeutic Modalities for Musculoskeletal Injuries.* 4th ed. Champaign: Human Kinetics; 2015.[46]
TENS, Transcutaneous electrical nerve stimulation.

TABLE 32.3	**Manual Therapy Application Guidelines**
Myofascial release	Gentle sustained elongating pressure applied to the fascia for a minimum of 90–180 s
	May be repeated until no further progress has been made
Muscle energy	Isometric contraction:
	Take joint into resistance (barrier)
	Have patient contract 20%–50%
	Hold for 7–10 s
	Fully relax muscle
	Take to next barrier, repeat until no further progress is being made (3–5 times)
Mobilizations	Depending on grade (3 and 4) the joint is placed at or into the first tissue stop
	1–2 oscillations per second for 30–90 s
	Reassess:
	Take joint further into restriction
	Repeat usually 3–5 times
Manipulation (HVLA)	Patient is placed into the restricted movement until tension in felt
	Patient should be relaxed
	Practitioner imparts an HVLA into the restricted motion. (Cavitation may occur)
Mobilization with movement	Usually performed weight bearing
	Force directed in joint treatment plane
	Should be minimal pain or pain free
	Patient performs movement into the restriction while practitioner applies a force to help guide the motion
	Repeat for 3–5 cycles of 5–10×
TPR	Find active TP:
	Apply firm pressure to point
	Stretch area so TP becomes more taught
	Hold position until you feel the TP release (less taught and tender)
	Stretch tissue further unit TP becomes taught
	Repeat process (usually 3–5 times)

HVLA, High velocity low amplitude; *TPR*, trigger point release.

Cryotherapy

Ice is the mantra for clinicians as the first line of defense for pain. Ice application is an effective analgesic and can control pain for several hours after an activity. Cooling the temperature of an inflamed area will also diminish the metabolic activity in the area, slow the production of inflammatory cells and potentially decrease the need for oxygen in the tissues. Following an acute injury, ice is combined with compression and elevation to help control swelling, and as mentioned previously, it should be combined with protection of the structure and controlled or optimal loading. This treatment can be used conveniently at home and can be administered several times per day.

Ice has been shown to be an effective modulator of pain in the treatment of soft tissue injuries.[52-54] Many clinicians believe that the cold application results in the spinal gate mechanism to diminish pain response from the focal area. However, the application of cryotherapy is typically noxious, with the patient perceiving cold, burning, aching, and then numbness. The mechanism for pain reduction is likely to be associated with a more complex neurologic pathway that stimulates smaller diameter nerve fibers, as described in the noxious pain modulation theory.[54] Ice has been shown to slow nerve conduction velocity and increase pain threshold.[1] Research evaluating pain relief is often confounded by increases in physical activity. Any positive change in activity should be interpreted as a reduction in discomfort that often limits function.

With the recent attention to elite athletes receiving treatment with cold baths or cold-water immersion following exercise, ice has been examined as a postrecovery modality. Again, few data support the use of cold therapy as a mechanism to prevent the inflammatory effects of exhaustive exercise or to minimize the effects on subsequent performance.[55-58] However, cold water immersion has been shown to help regulate core temperature when exercising in the heat.[54] Similar to other studies, methods to examine appropriate temperature, and the time and timing of the treatment are inconsistent, particularly when used as a recovery modality. Guidelines for temperature should be followed, since extreme cold temperatures have been associated with increasing the inflammatory process.[59] Temperatures below 50°F should not be used, despite the habituation to cold therapy, particularly with cold water immersion.[60]

There are numerous methods to apply ice or cryotherapy. An plastic bag filled with crushed ice is a convenient and inexpensive ice pack. Air insulates as an interface, so crushed ice is optimal, especially since cubes may be uncomfortable since they may increase pressure. Ice penetrates up to 4 cm, so it can be used to decrease the temperature of many superficial joints. However, adipose insulates against cooling, and longer treatment times are required depending on the treatment area. Icing a large muscle group, such as the quads, hamstrings, or hip, may require 40 minutes or more of treatment time, while the ankles and knees may require only 10 to 15 minutes of cooling for a therapeutic effect. Generally, the more adipose present over the treatment site the longer the treatment required for adequate cooling.

Compression is often used in conjunction with ice and may be a confounder when investigating the therapeutic effects of cooling, since both may affect the development of edema.[3] Plastic wraps are often used to secure ice bags to the body so that sitting during the treatment is not necessary. Caution should be used with compressive wraps since a tourniquet effect can occur. Additionally, pressure with the cold can result in damage to superficial nerves, such as the ulnar nerve when treating the elbow, or the fibular nerve when treating the knee.

Electrical Stimulation

Electrical stimulation is characteristically applied for pain relief. There are numerous waveforms with specific parameters that permit a clinician to adjust intensity (amplitude), phase duration, and pulse frequency, or there are clinical units that select combinations of parameters with the push of a button. Most units for therapeutic electrical stimulation can be classified as TENS units since they are applied superficially, passing a current through the skin to affect an intact nervous system. Subclassifications of stimulators are used to distinguish the goal of the treatment (either for pain relief or for facilitation of motor function) or the waveform of the stimulator (high voltage, biphasic, interferential, etc.). For the purposes of this chapter, sensory TENS units will be distinguished from neuromuscular stimulators (NMES) since the goal of the treatments are different. The sensory stimulators are primarily used for pain relief and are capable of eliciting a motor response, but the purpose is not to facilitate the muscle function. NMES units, conversely, are designed to stimulate a motor nerve to elicit a muscular response that may be used during rehabilitation to improve the ability to contract a specific muscle.

Transcutaneous Electrical Nerve Stimulation

TENS operates by stimulating afferent nerves (sensory) to promote pain modulation. There are several proposed mechanisms for pain modulation, and the stimulation parameters associated with each mechanism are designed to enhance the effectiveness of that neuromodulation mechanism. For example, in the gate theory, large diameter sensory nerves are targeted to result in an inhibitory effect of the smaller pain fibers in the spinal cord. "Sensory" TENS is applied to target those large diameter nerve fibers to close the "gate" to modulate pain. Thus the parameters associated with "sensory" TENS are designed to maximize the stimulation of those large diameter nerves. Since the neuromodulation techniques are complicated, many modality companies have simplified the design of stimulators so the clinician can select the type of stimulation they want and the parameters will be packaged appropriately. However, in order for clinical trials to evaluate the usefulness of TENS, the parameter selection should be specified so that appropriate comparisons can be made, particularly with systematic reviews.

For the purposes of this chapter, the pain modulation mechanisms are categorized as (1) sensory TENS, (2) motor TENS, and (3) noxious TENS. These are common methods of applying electrical stimulation for pain relief and have application for injury management. The sensory TENS mechanism, as previously mentioned, is based on the gate theory and inhibits pain in the spinal cord. It is often used with acute injuries since the stimulation is comfortable, but the analgesic effect is short lived. This treatment is appropriate for use prior to therapeutic exercise or after activity for pain management. The motor TENS mechanism is sometimes a misnomer, since an electrically produced muscle contraction is not required for this mechanism. Many times, there is a rhythmical muscle contraction and therefore it is not used as frequently for acute injuries. The neural mechanism is associated with a descending analgesic pathway, meaning that the pain is first perceived by the cortex. Then, specific brain centers, such as the pituitary gland, are signaled to produce precursors to the endogenous opioid, endorphin. Similarly, precursors are released that signal the adrenal glands to produce the hormone cortisol. This neural mechanism is elicited by rhythmical stimulation of A delta fibers, which are the larger of the pain fibers (but smaller than A beta fibers). Finally, noxious TENS, as its name implies, produces a strong, uncomfortable stimulation, similar to a bee sting. Theoretically, that type of stimulation targets the smallest pain fibers to alert specific brain centers to release enkephalin (another endogenous opiate), and serotonin, which both have powerful analgesic qualities. The parameter selection in the stimulator is based on the attempt to preferentially stimulate the target nerve in each of these pain modulation schemes.

Edema/Inflammation

Interventions that may have an effect on edema and the inflammatory reaction include some ice, electrical stimulation methods, and bioenergies such as nonthermal ultrasound and laser. Mechanical methods of edema resolution include massage, compression, and any device that promotes muscle pumping, such as electrical stimulation. Ice traditionally has been thought to decrease blood flow to the cooled region, thereby diminishing the potential for edema formation. However, a recent study to determine the microperfusion effects of cold on skeletal muscle indicated that blood flow is not diminished at rest with therapeutic cooling.[56] Perhaps ice has the potential effect of attenuating the increased vascularity associated with an inflammatory event, although there is no strong evidence that ice alone reduces or minimizes edema.[61-63] Ice at extremely low temperatures has been shown to increase edema associated with rabbit tibial fractures, and caution should be used with low temperature ice or slush baths below 50°F.[60] Since ice has such strong effects on pain reduction, the treatment remains indicated as the standard of care in acute injuries.

Electrical stimulation has also been proposed for edema resolution. Although there is some evidence that high voltage stimulation can facilitate wound healing, it is difficult to ascertain whether high voltage can minimize or reduce soft tissue edema.[64]

Ultrasound

Therapeutic ultrasound uses high-frequency acoustic energy to produce thermal and nonthermal (mechanical) effects in the tissues. The frequency of therapeutic ultrasound is clinically applied at either 1 MHz or 3 MHz with the higher frequency units directed to more superficial pathologies. Ultrasound is commonly prescribed for pain and for tissue healing, or for the thermal benefits of increasing ROM or a reduction in muscle spasm. Similar to other modalities, the evidence for its use in improving outcomes in musculoskeletal pathologies remains equivocal.

NONTHERMAL ULTRASOUND TREATMENTS

The nonthermal effects of ultrasound are most often associated with lower intensities and the pulsed mode of treatment. However, nonthermal effects occur with higher doses of ultrasound, but the effects are overshadowed by the thermal result. In pulsed ultrasound, the emission of acoustic energy is interrupted systematically to decrease the overall output and to allow time for thermal dissipation, which occurs with continuous wave application. Most commercial units have options of either 50% or 20% duty cycles, although many units are produced that allow the clinician more options.

The nonthermal effects of ultrasound, particularly pain relief and wound healing, are desirable in the acute phase of injury treatment since additional heating in an actively inflamed are may have detrimental results. The nonthermal effects, specifically cavitation and acoustical streaming are created by the mechanical pressure energy of ultrasound. Cavitation is the compression and expansion of gas bubbles that are present in the blood or tissues. This vibration causes mechanical and chemical alterations in the tissues. Although cavitation has been associated with negative tissue effects, it also has been associated with ion diffusion across cell membranes.[65] This process of applying low level mechanical energy to the tissues may affect fibroblastic activity in the inflammatory process, stimulate mitosis, and contribute to wound healing.[66] Acoustical microstreaming is associated with a "pro-inflammatory" effect. The acute processes, particularly the degranulation of mast cells, are accelerated slightly, which can result in a faster resolution of the initial phase of inflammation. This hypothesis has not been confirmed with controlled clinical trials, but pulsed ultrasound at low intensities may lead to faster resolution of injury when applied early.

Stress Fracture Healing

Nonthermal ultrasound has been suggested to treat stress fractures. Low-intensity ultrasound (less than 3 mW) has been proposed as a treatment for nonunions and is currently FDA approved for these conditions. The application of either of these low-intensity mechanical or electromagnetic energies is proposed to stimulate the production of osteoblasts. Therefore there are bone stimulator units that deliver either ultrasound (acoustic) or electromagnetic (electrical field) energies, both of which have been used off-label for stress fracture management. Currently, there are few data on stress fracture healing to substantiate the use of these units. However, in the interest of trying any method of accelerating the healing phase for elite athletes, there are empirical observations of these treatments contributing to stress fracture management.

A specific device must be used to apply ultrasound for fracture healing, and the treatment cannot be reproduced on a standard therapeutic ultrasound machine, since the intensity is 1000 times lower. The units are designed for home treatment for nonunion fracture healing; therefore the units are preprogrammed with the appropriate dosage. The device provides a stationary treatment for a set treatment time at a given intensity. Because the intensity is so low (approximately 0.003 W/cm^2), there is little consequence to the stationary treatment. The treatment can be applied daily, and more frequent treatments are *not* suggested to improve outcomes. Therefore when these units are used for stress fracture healing, they are more likely to have the treatment applied in a clinic visit to prevent a coach or athlete from abusing the treatment. Empirically, these units have been used in conjunction with activity modification for stress reactions and stress fractures. One issue with conducting a randomized control trial is the subject's willingness to potentially receive the sham treatment. When the device is available, many runners decline the possibility of being randomized into the control condition.

Phonophoresis

Cavitation has been associated with phonophoresis, which is the transfer of medications through intact skin using ultrasound. Phonophoresis—similar to iontophoresis (which uses electricity to transfer ions into the skin)—is used to administer medications locally to theoretically maximize the effect at the injured area. There are several conflicting studies that have investigated phonophoresis using lidocaine or antiinflammatory drugs, including steroids in clinical trials.[46,67-69] The cavitation of ultrasound may change the structure of the stratum corneum, which is the barrier to transdermal delivery. Although phonophoresis increases the penetration of many medications through the skin, there are no specific guidelines on the best clinical method. Furthermore, some medications may block the transmission of ultrasound.[70] The variety of parameter choice and application method in clinical practice may explain the inconsistent research results. The best practice methods indicate the use of a drug that has good ultrasound transmission must be applied, and lower frequencies are more optimal for phonophoresis. The lower frequencies are recommended despite evidence that the higher frequencies concentrate the energy at the skin. Drugs should also be at a consistent concentration (not diluted with ultrasound gel) and may need to be in place longer than the typical 5-minute treatment.[71] The suggested clinical approach would be to apply the drug directly to the skin and apply an occlusive or hydrogel dressing to hydrate the skin and prevent dilution of the drug. A lower frequency of ultrasound should be used while the remaining parameters of ultrasound are based on the energy dosage desired. Pulsed ultrasound with a low intensity is used for more acute pathologies while continuous ultrasound and higher intensities are used for subacute conditions. Longer treatment times with lower doses of ultrasound may not affect drug absorption; therefore the drug absorption is not necessarily associated with thermal effects of ultrasound.[72] Drugs that have shown beneficial effects with phonophoresis are lidocaine, dexamethasone, and ketoprofen, while hydrocortisone has not produced positive effects (Fig. 32.3).

Iontophoresis

Iontophoresis is the transdermal administration of a medication with electrical current. The solution is placed in the active

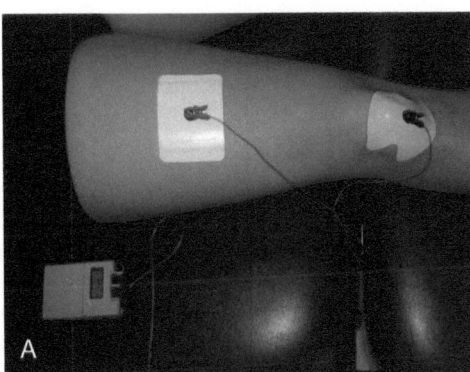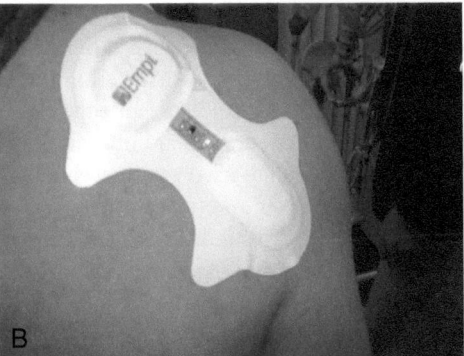

Fig. 32.3 Iontophoresis.

electrode and applied over the injured area, which is generally a focused point such as a tendon, bursa, or ligament. Iontophoresis requires galvanic or DC current, a monophasic waveform with an unlimited phase duration. The current "drives" ions of the same charge as the active electrode; therefore it is imperative that the polarity of the medication is known. This electrical propulsion is from like charges repelling; therefore a negatively charged ion should be placed in the negative electrode and a positively charged ion should be placed in the positive electrode. A second electrode (the dispersive) is placed at another location to complete the circuit. Similar to phonophoresis, the technique theoretically improves the transmission of a medication to a particular location and minimizes the effects of oral medication or undesired effects of an injection. Although there is evidence that iontophoresis increases the absorption of specific medications, clinical trials have not conclusively demonstrated an adequate effect using this technique.

There are many drugs that have been applied with iontophoresis (e.g., lidocaine), many corticosteroids, and botulinum for hyperhidrosis. NSAIDs, such as diclofenac and ketorolac, also have been used.[73] There are commercial devices that are marketed specifically for iontophoresis, and those units can be programmed to deliver a set amount of current over time (milliamp minutes). The current should be set to patient comfort and the duration of the treatment is automatically adjusted so that the total dosage, either 40 or 80 mA/min is applied. Shorter durations with higher amplitudes are not recommended since this does not affect the drug absorption.[74] State practice Acts may regulate the use of even topically administered medications by physical therapists or athletic trainers, so clinicians should be aware of the local regulations prior to use.

Laser

Light therapy has been used for centuries and laser is concentrated light at a specific wavelength. Laser is an acronym for Light Amplification of Stimulated Emission of Radiation and was invented in the 1960s. Now, lasers are used in industry, entertainment, medicine, and all aspects of technology. Laser therapy, often called low-level laser therapy (LLLT) has recently been approved by the US Food and Drug Administration for the treatment of some musculoskeletal conditions such as carpal tunnel or cervical spine pain. There are several types of LLLT

available for clinicians as well as many parameters to be manipulated to achieve the desired treatment outcome. More research is needed to expand the capabilities of this modality in providing potential benefits to the patient.

Therapeutic lasers are often difficult to discriminate between liquid crystal diodes (LCDs) light and it is important to read the product literature to understand the total power of the laser being used. Many companies combine a single laser with multiple LCDs, and the incorrect implication may be that all the lights are emitting similar energy. Lasers have unique properties—a single wavelength—and are able to penetrate into the skin and tissues better than other types of light. The biological effects of the laser are associated with the absorption of energy and the resultant production of ATP, an energy source to a cell. The cells respond by accelerating their normal activity and can thus facilitate the inflammatory response. LLLT has also been used effectively for pain; however, the mechanism for pain modulation is unknown.

Parameter selection is perhaps the most difficult aspect of LLLT since there are so many variables that must be considered.[75] There are few tested guidelines of dosing for specific pathologic entities and determining the amount of energy to be applied is often vague. Patient considerations include the type and condition of the tissue, and acute or chronic condition; even pigmentation may have an impact on the laser treatment outcome. Laser parameters that must be considered include wavelength, output power, average power, power density (intensity), and energy density (dosage). Many of the LLLT therapy devices marketed are menu driven, so selecting the tissue type and chronicity of the injury provides a specific treatment dosage. The total energy often is clinically determined by the treatment time. For example, once the unit has been purchased, the wavelength, power, and density are set, and the clinician determines the dosage by increasing or decreasing the treatment time. Each area should be treated for that time period, so units with more than one laser diode are more efficient, particularly when treating larger areas.

One of the problems with evaluating the evidence of LLLT is that laser treatment is often poorly documented in the literature. Different laser types were used and dosages were varied or not reported. Laser research should report the methodology and describe all factors of the clinical unit so that outcome-based evidence can be evaluated.

LLLT has been proposed for many conditions, such as pain and wound healing, and inflammatory conditions such as bursitis, tenosynovitis, or acute musculoskeletal traumas. Since LLLT is only currently approved for specific pathologies, an off-label treatment would be necessary. Higher energies are often more desirable, since many inconclusive studies used very low energy levels.[76,77] The treatment time to deliver an effective treatment increases the total amount of energy delivered. Treatment doses range from 4 to 50 J and it has been suggested that no more than 50 J should be applied to adults and no more than 25 J should be applied to children under the age of 14.[75]

MT is often used to mechanically affect edema. Once the injury has stabilized and there is hemostasis, light massage in the direction of lymphatic flow can facilitate the resolution of edema. Deeper massage and soft tissue techniques can be used to mobilize more brawny or pitting edema.

Compression: Intermittent Compression

In an attempt to provide this mechanical stimulation to reduce edema, devices have been manufactured to apply compression to the extremities. Various agents use intermittent compression therapy and newer units have sequential pressure chambers to increase pressure in the extremities from distal to proximal. The mechanical pressure provides a sensory stimulation, which often can reduce pain or facilitate recovery after exercise.[78] Most of the evidence to support the intermittent compression devices and tissue oscillation therapy are empirically based (Fig. 32.4).

Range of Motion

Improving ROM is an important therapeutic goal and attention should be made to have the patient actively use or move the joint after efforts to improve the range. When passive techniques, such as superficial heat, thermal ultrasound, or joint or soft tissue mobilization, are combined with active exercise, the patient learns to contract the muscle in the new range. Muscle inhibition often accompanies joint or soft-tissue tightness. Although "warming up" the area dynamically or with a passive intervention prepares the

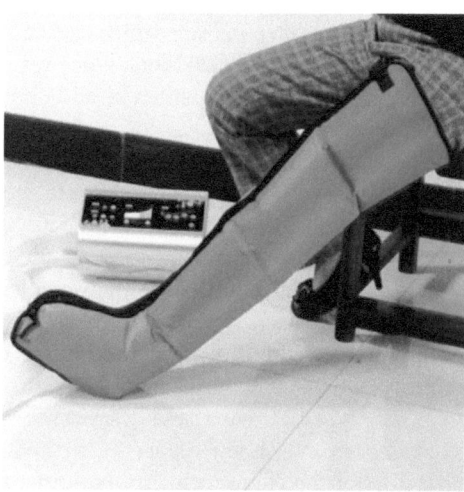

Fig. 32.4 Intermittent compression.

site, it is essential to do muscle re-education techniques directly following the initial treatment.

Superficial Heat

Superficial heat in the form of a moist heating pad may be used to help warm the body part up or to prepare for exercise. Heat should not be used if there is swelling or pain, but it can be very effective several days after a significant hamstring strain, for example, when there is ecchymosis and blood accumulated in the tissues. The increased vascularity helps mobilize and breakdown the fibrous hematoma. Like any other modality, the application of the agent in isolation does little to change the state of the condition. Therefore superficial heat, even with a hot tub or warm shower, should be followed closely with stretching, focused exercise to address the problem, or with MT techniques.

When superficial heat is applied, skin receptors detect the increased temperature, and there is a vasodilatory response in the skin and subcutaneous tissues. This protective mechanism helps to preserve core temperature and to dissipate the local increased temperature to prevent burns. If there is a vascular compromise, heat should not be used, and the addition of compression may prevent the appropriate dissipation of heat. Thus sitting on hot packs is not recommended since this might result in a local ischemic response associated with pressure. Because of the vascular response of the skin, there is very poor transmission of superficial heat deep into muscle. Intramuscular thermistors show only a 1 cm penetration that is affected by the superficial adipose layer.[79] Therefore if the goal is to provide heat and increased vascularity to a muscle, active exercise is the best choice rather than a hot pack. Superficial heat will penetrate many joints, such as the knee, wrist, or ankle, and may be effective prior to joint mobilization. Deeper tissues such as the hip, facet joints of the spine, and perhaps the shoulder may not respond, except through a cutaneous mechanism. There is some evidence that superficial heat may elicit a reflex action to underlying musculature, despite the lack of temperature increase in the muscle.

Heat often has a relaxing, sedating effect; therefore it is commonly used with muscle spasm.[80] Caution should be used because of a commonly documented phenomenon called heat hyperreflexia. The patient uses heat to relax the tissues and generally has good results during the application. Then, several minutes or hours after the treatment, there is an increase in pain, which is often associated with an exacerbation of muscle spasm. Focused heating with directed exercise while the tissues are heated may prevent this occurrence; however, superficial heat should be used judiciously with overuse injuries. Many times, spinal injuries are treated with heat, even in the acute phase, to promote relaxation. However, the evaluation should determine the phase of inflammation and the amount of activity that also results in heating of the tissues. Generally, if the condition is "tight," then heat can be used effectively. However, if the ROM is limited by "pain," then cold may improve the outcome.

Heat can theoretically affect the compliance of connective tissue by influencing the viscoelastic ground substance. Once the tissues are heated to an effective temperature of 40°C (104°F), there is less stress needed to change tissue length. Therefore if the goal is to improve ROM or joint mobility, heating prior to stretching or joint mobilization techniques may be effective. Higher tissue temperatures result in the denaturization of proteins, and burns result. Because of the limitation of superficial heating agents in increasing tissue temperatures beyond the skin, deep heating agents are often used. Stretching or joint mobility techniques should be done while the tissues are heated.[79,81] Simultaneous heat and stretch may accomplish this goal. Patent positioning with the appropriate tissues heated are essential in this technique. A common mistake is to place a hotpack over the top of a shoulder, for example, when the tight structures are generally in the axilla. Thus far, data that demonstrate a clinical benefit of using superficial heat on the ROM are sparse.[82,83] Furthermore, if increasing muscle temperature is the goal, active exercise is the best method. Activity improves blood flow and intramuscular temperature more effectively than hot packs or deep heating agents such as ultrasound.

Superficial heat has many therapeutic forms. For a home program, a moist towel can be heated in the microwave and applied to the body. The towel can be placed in an open zip-lock bag. Extreme caution should be used since burns are likely with this technique. Dry towels should cover the area completely. Likewise, cooked rice or a boiled egg holds heat for 20 to 30 minutes and can be used to apply heat to a focal area. Hot tubs, baths, and heating pads also can be used, but the patient should be directed to use short durations and then stretch or perform their stabilization exercises immediately. Hot tub temperatures should not exceed 100°F, although the extremities can tolerate temperatures of 104 to 107°F. Hot tubs potentially stress the thermoregulatory effects and should not be used after exercise.

THERMAL EFFECTS OF ULTRASOUND

Therapeutic ultrasound is most commonly applied as a deep heating modality. The acoustic energy penetrates well through superficial tissues, such as adipose, and the mechanical, vibrational energy is converted to thermal energy when absorbed by the tissues. Tissues that absorb ultrasound energy are those with high protein content, such as muscle, tendon, and nerve. Ultrasound does not penetrate through bone; therefore the energy reflects off bone and potentially magnifies the effect at the bone/muscle interface. Because the temperature changes occur in tissues other than the skin where there are no thermal receptors, there is little perception of heating other than mild warmth associated with the treatment. Likewise, since the energy is selectively absorbed, reflected, and refracted, the recommended doses of ultrasound are difficult to determine. Patients, particularly athletes, often request ultrasound treatments and since there is little perception of energy emitted, it is difficult to examine the effects of the treatment. However, tissue temperatures can increase substantially, and energy is selectively absorbed in the muscle, tendon, and nerve, and periosteal burns may result from higher doses. Indiscriminate use or self-prescribed treatments should never be condoned.

Ultrasound dosage is specified by the frequency, intensity, duration, and duty cycle. As stated previously, the lower intensities and lower duty cycles reduce the possibility of a thermal effect and are often prescribed for nonthermal mechanisms. A lack of a duty cycle, or continuous wave ultrasound (100%) is generally used for thermal effects. The frequency and intensity are inter-related, although each has specific effects. The frequency affects the depth of penetration, with higher frequencies concentrating the energy more superficially. A 3 MHz ultrasound will generally have a depth of penetration of approximately 1 to 3 cm, while a 1 MHz ultrasound will have a depth of penetration of 3 to 8 cm. However, the depth depends on the absorption of energy within the tissues. For example, if the energy is preferentially absorbed by tissues with a high protein content, such as tendon, then there is less energy to transmit; thus the depth of penetration is affected. Generally, when applying ultrasound for thermal effects in deep tissues such as a muscle belly, the lower frequencies are used, and when there is superficial bone the higher frequency is used. Thermal energy can also transmit via conduction, so the science in determining a specific frequency and intensity for a specific thermal effect is inexact.

Thermal ultrasound is commonly used to help break down scar tissue, to promote the alignment of collagen tissue in the remodeling phase, and to increase ROM when combined with stretching or mobilization techniques. Currently, there are no data to support the use of thermal ultrasound to affect blood flow to tissues other than subcutaneous structures. When attempting to increase ROM, it is important to stretch the connective tissue either during the ultrasound treatment or immediately afterward while the temperature remains elevated. Ultrasound treatments without the concomitant therapeutic exercise or MT technique have poor results.

MOBILIZATION/MANIPULATION

An MT technique comprising a continuum of skilled passive movements to the joints and/or soft tissues is applied at varying speeds and amplitudes, including a small amplitude/high velocity therapeutic movement.[2] Research has shown that mobilization used as a therapy can produce significant mechanical and neurophysiologic effects.[50,84,85] The explanations of these effects—the mechanism of mobilization—is still relatively unknown, especially in regards to the spine, and is subject to further research.[86] However, several theories have been established in accordance with effects seen, including the effects of pain relief, increasing ROM and the influence on the autonomic nervous system.

Multiple reviews have investigated the pain-modulating mechanisms of spinal manipulation[87,88] and agree that the analgesic origins are neurophysiologic in nature, occurring through some type of descending pain modulation circuit. However, the exact circuit is not fully understood, but is becoming clearer through the work of Bialosky et al.[50] and it appears that different types of spinal manipulations—namely the velocity with which and the location at which they are performed—may elicit different neurochemical responses indicative of different descending pain modulation mechanisms. Please refer to Figs. 32.5 to 32.9 for examples of common mobilization/manipulation techniques.

MOBILIZATIONS WITH MOVEMENT

The concept of mobilizations with movement (MWM) of the extremities and sustained natural apophyseal glides (SNAGS)

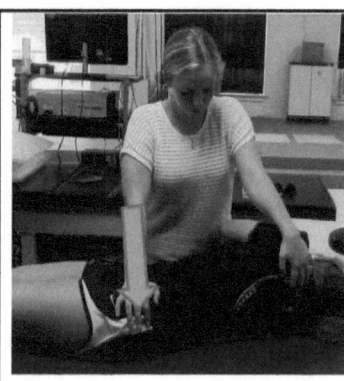

Patient Position:
- The patient lays supine, their hips aligned with the edge of the table and the side to receive treatment away from the clinician. Have the patient interlock their fingers and place their hands behind their neck and as far down the back of their neck as possible, or fold them across their chest.

Clinician Position:
- Stand on the opposite side of the patient to receive treatment.
- Set the patient up by maximally side-bending their lower extremities and trunk away (C shape).
- The patient's leg can be crossed over their opposite leg at the ankles to help maintain this side-bent position.
- The upper trunk is stabilized with the clinician's forearm over the patient's shoulder and their hand over the patient's scapular region.

Mobilization:
- Standing upright, the arm stabilizing the upper trunk is rotated toward the clinician while maintaining the patient in a side-bent position.
- The clinician's distal hand is placed on the patient's anterior superior iliac spine (ASIS) as it raises from table due to the rotation.
- Ensure that the hip has not risen off the table and apply pressure through palm of hand in an anterior-posterior direction.
- Once available motion is taken up, and the segment locked into position, apply a high velocity, low amplitude (HVLA thrust in the same direction (caudal and posterior directed).

Fig. 32.5 Lumbopelvic manipulation. *HVLA*, High velocity, low amplitude.

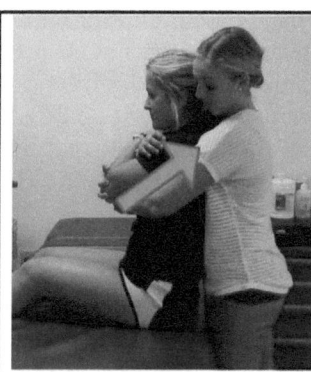

Patient Position:
- Seated at the middle of the treatment table with their legs hanging over the side. They should scoot back until their back is flush with the edge of the table behind them.
- The table should be high enough so that the clinician does not have to lean, bend down, or reach up to perform the technique. There should be a little room to stand up from the original position when performing the thrust portion of the manipulation.
- The patient crosses the arms over the chest ("hug yourself") and grasps the opposite shoulders.

Clinician Position:
- Standing directly behind the patient.
- Place your arms around the patient (hug) with your hands clasped together and resting on the patient's flexed elbows.
- Support the patient by providing compression at the rib cage through your forearms and a posterior-directed stabilization force through the patient's elbows.

Fig. 32.6 Mid-thoracic manipulation.

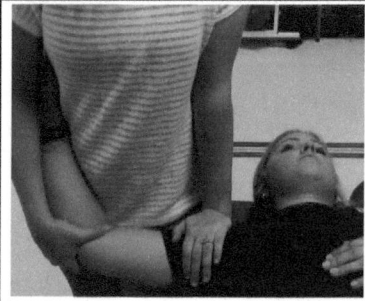

Patient Position:
- Laying supine with arm to receive treatment in shoulder abduction off the table and elbow flexion (range is relative to the specific effect the clinician prefers).

Clinician Position:
- Stabilizing hand: Grasp the patient's distal humerus and elbow; hold patient's forearm against yours.
- Mobilizing hand: Heel of hand placed against anterior humeral head with elbow locked out and perpendicular to the axis of the humerus.

Mobilization:
- A graded mobilization is applied in an anterior to posterior direction. The force should come from the body/trunk of the clinician down through the locked-out elbow and through the mobilizing hand to glide the humeral head in a posterior direction.
- The mobilization may be performed in varying degrees of progressive glenohumeral abduction.

Fig. 32.7 Superior–inferior glenohumeral mobilization (into joint resistance).

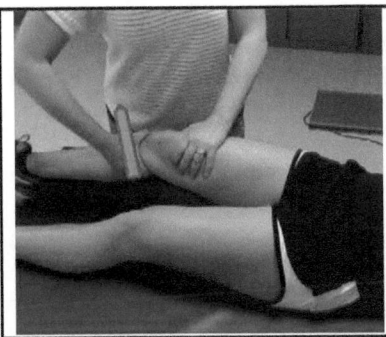

Patient Position:
- Supine with the knee placed into a comfortable position depending on the condition.

Clinician Position:
- Standing on the side of the injured knee.
- Stabilizing hand is placed just superior to the patella on the femur.
- Mobilizing hand is placed on the proximal aspect of the posterior tibia.

Mobilization:
- The tibia is pulled anteriorly in an graded oscillatory manner in the angel of the tibial plateaus (similar to a Lachman's test).

Fig. 32.8 Tibiofemoral posterior–anterior (mobilization).

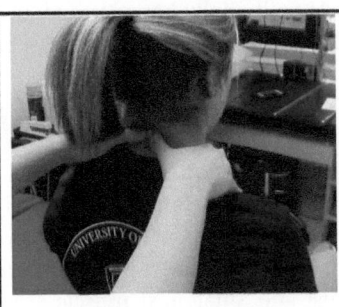

Patient Position:
- Seated looking straight ahead.

Clinician Position:
- Standing behind patient.
- Both thumbs place on distal spinous process of dysfunctional vertebral level with fingers gently resting on the patient's upper shoulders.

Mobilization:
- An upward gliding force is applied to the spinous process by the clinician.
- The patient extends their head as far as possible in the pain free range and then returns to the starting position.
- This is repeated until for 3-6 repetitions.

Fig. 32.9 Extension SNAG (cervical spine). Indications: facet joint dysfunction, cervical pain with extension, *SNAG*, Sustained natural apophyseal glides.

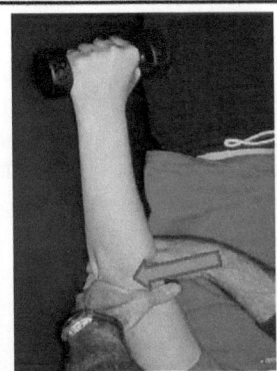

Patient Position:
- Patient is in supine with their arm by their side, elbow extended and forearm pronated.

Clinician Position:
- Standing on the involved of the patient.

Mobilization:
- A lateral glide is applied to the radius and ulna with the therapist's hands.
- The patient then either grips or extends the wrist against resistance as long as this is now pain-free.
- 6-10 repetitions are performed in a single treatment session.

Fig. 32.10 Mobilization with movement for lateral epicondylalgia.

of the spine were first coined by Brian R. Mulligan.[89] MWM is the concurrent application of sustained accessory mobilization applied by a therapist and an active physiologic movement to end range applied by the patient. Passive end-of-range overpressure, or stretching, is delivered without pain as a barrier.[89] Research has shown that MWM can be beneficial from increasing ROM and decreasing pain; however, the mechanisms by which it affects the musculoskeletal system, whether mechanical or physiologic, has not been fully determined. Common MWM for the spine are SNAGS (Fig. 32.10), which have been shown to decrease pain, disability, and headache; increase ROM and patient satisfaction; and be as effective as manipulation and other forms of mobilization. However, there is no evidence that these techniques resolve the biomechanics of the facet joint.[90,91] Several placebo-controlled studies[92,93] and a case series[94] have demonstrated that a single application of the MWM for upper extremity results in an immediate increase in pain-free grip force (strength).

MUSCLE DYSFUNCTION

Muscle dysfunction commonly accompanies orthopaedic injury, and stiffness, spasm, and muscle tightness may create more symptoms than a joint pathology. Articular receptors create neuroreflexive responses, making muscle inhibition (arthrogenic muscle inhibition), reducing muscle activation, and triggering points a consequence of joint injury. Interventions designed to reduce muscle inhibition, to reduce tension and spasm, and to improve timing and activation are appropriate therapies. Various treatments, such as cryotherapy on the joint, NMES and PENS, MET, PNF, and trigger point therapy (TrPT) are effective to change muscle function. Similar to all passive treatments, responses to the therapy should be measured, and therapeutic exercise should be initiated following the intervention.

JOINT CRYOTHERAPY TO COMBAT MUSCLE INHIBITION

The studies on muscle activation describe the usefulness of combining modality treatment with rehabilitation, rather than passively applying the treatment.[95] Ice is applied in time intervals where the joint is cooled, then exercise is conducted within the pain limits and the joint is re-cooled. This procedure is known as cryokinetics and is used to promote joint mobility and muscle function in the acute stage of healing.[96,97] Ice should be applied in the acute phase several times a day, if possible. However, there are currently no guidelines on the number of times per day, how long each treatment should last, or how frequent the treatments should be, based on clinical trials or outcome studies. Therefore treatments should be prescribed with pain as a guide for acute injuries. For example, during the early phase when pain is a problem, more frequent treatments are necessary. However, as the acute pain resolves, ice treatments should be used before and after therapeutic exercise to facilitate the muscle and to monitor postexercise inflammation.

Cryotherapy has been receiving attention as a complement to therapeutic exercise with its effect on muscle activation. Arthrogenic muscle inhibition (AMI) is a condition that often follows joint injury where the muscles surrounding that joint are reflexively inhibited. AMI exists despite rehabilitation efforts, and may result in abhorrent forces through a joint over time.[98] Focal application of cryotherapy over a joint has been shown to decrease AMI.[99] Using ice before therapeutic exercise as a mechanism to improve muscle activation could improve the outcomes of rehabilitation.

NEUROMUSCULAR ELECTRICAL STIMULATION

A different approach to electrical stimulation is to use it to stimulate the motor nerve to improve or facilitate muscle contractions. Since the treatment is directed at the motor nerve (α-motoneuron), the treatment is labeled neuromuscular electrical stimulation or NMES. This treatment should not be confused with Motor TENS, which is for pain relief. NMES is used to retrain a muscle to function, to overcome arthrogenic inhibition, or to permit exercise when there is an intact motor nerve. NMES can be used to improve the strength and coordination of motor units when used in conjunction with voluntary exercise, but the device has not been shown to strengthen or reduce adipose with passive use. The treatment has been shown to improve some outcomes in anterior cruciate ligament rehabilitation when used in conjunction with exercise therapy.[100]

NMES can be used when a specific muscle cannot be exercised volitionally. An effusion can result in a reflex inhibition of muscles that surround a joint and it is difficult to elicit a good contraction. The electrodes are placed over the muscle, generally with one electrode over the superficial aspect of the nerve to the muscle and one electrode over the motor point. The phase

duration should be between 200 and 400 µs, on the higher end of the TENS range because the targeted nerve is relatively deep. The amplitude should increase so that a tolerable and visible contraction is noted. The pulse rate should be at tetany, which is 35 to 50 pps.

Clinically, NMES is commonly used for quadriceps contractions and retraining following a knee injury or surgery. It is also effective in promoting lower trapezius function during shoulder and scapular exercise. The treatment also can be used to help retrain muscle function after a tendon transfer or following a nerve injury when the muscle is innervated, but the function is limited. Again, fatigue is common and overworking those muscles can further deteriorate function. Generally, once the ability to exercise the muscle volitionally has returned, the usefulness of this modality is limited, since active exercise is preferred.

PATTERNED ELECTRICAL NERVE STIMULATION

PENS is a different form of electrical stimulation based on electromyographic activity during functional tasks. The purpose of PENS is to replicate the normal firing pattern through a muscle re-education technique that delivers precisely timed stimulation of both the agonist and antagonist muscle groups. PENS has been applied to a variety of populations with improved results including knee osteoarthritis[101] and patellofemoral pain (Fig. 32.11).[25,102]

MUSCLE ENERGY TECHNIQUE

MET is a MT and involves the voluntary contraction of a muscle in a precisely controlled direction at varying levels of intensity against a distinct counterforce applied by the operator.[103] The five basic elements of MET are patient-active muscle contraction, controlled joint position, muscle contraction in a specific

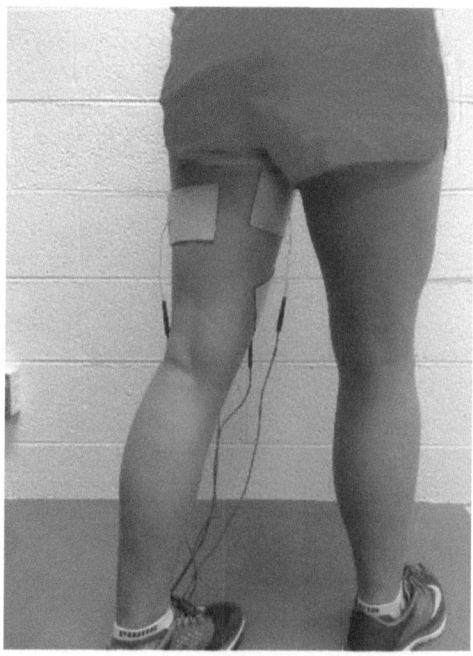

Fig. 32.11 Patterned electrical nerve stimulation.

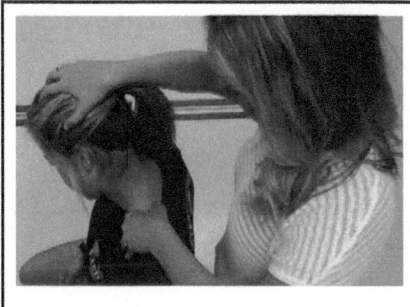

Patient Position: • Seated looking straight ahead. Clinician Position: • Standing behind patient. • One thumb placed on upper trapezius trigger point. Treatment: • One hand place on patient's head imparting sidebending and rotation away from the side of pain. • This position is held until the trigger point releases (~60-90 seconds). • The clinician places the head further into sidebending and rotation until the tension is felt under the clinician's thumb. • Repeat process until no further movement can occur. • Vapocoolant spray may also be used with this technique.

Fig. 32.12 Trigger point hold and release for upper trapezius.

direction, operator-applied counterforce, and controlled contraction intensity. Postisometric relaxation (autogenic inhibition) and reciprocal inhibition are the two neurophysiologic principles on which MET is based. There are three contractions that are utilized in MET: isometric, isotonic, and isolytic (eccentric). MET has been shown to decrease pain[104] and segmental dysfunction by increasing the pain threshold and increasing joint ROM and muscle mobility with effects that can be last for 1 week.[105]

MYOFASCIAL RELEASE/TRIGGER POINT THERAPY

These MT techniques are being discussed together because of the similarities with signs and symptoms and treatment, but they can be divided into two separate and distinct therapies. Myofascial release and TrPT are specialized MT techniques that attempt to effectively release fascial tension and restrictions. Fascia can become dysfunctional through any type of stressor (e.g., trauma, illness, postural dysfunction, psychological stress).

When fascia becomes problematic it causes pain, tenderness, and trigger points in local tissues. Trigger points are defined as areas of tenderness and hyperirritation, exhibition taut bands, proprioceptive changes, and a consistent pain referral pattern.[106] An example of TrPT for an upper trapezius trigger point is shown in Fig. 32.12.

CONCLUSION

There are numerous devices in the arsenal to facilitate rehabilitation techniques, particularly in a patient population with expectations of high activity levels. However, it is important to understand the limitations of physical agents and MT and to put their use in context with specific therapeutic goals. Physical agents can diminish the inflammatory response and are often effective in managing pain, but modality use in isolation is not recommended. The combination of therapeutic modalities and MT gives the clinician the best chance for successful outcomes.

For a complete list of references, go to ExpertConsult.com.

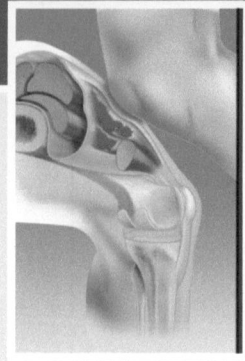

33

Basics of Taping and Orthotics

Phillip Gribble

TAPING

During physical activity, the integrity of a joint and its associated structures can be compromised, especially during high-risk activities that may introduce injurious mechanisms. Sports medicine clinicians can supplement mechanical support to a joint through a variety of taping techniques using elastic and nonelastic materials. Guidelines have been established that define taping procedures as standard interventions for domains such as "prevention" and "immediate care."[1]

Taping techniques are utilized extensively by athletic trainers and other sports medicine professionals to prevent excessive joint movements, especially in sports known to have a high risk for particular injuries. For example, an individual is at an increased risk for a lateral ankle sprain during participation in the sport of basketball, compared with the sport of baseball.[2,3] Therefore providing additional support to the ankle complex of a basketball player in order to restrict motions outside the anatomical limits is a common preventative measure performed to reduce the risk of an injury to the joint structures. A variety of taping techniques designed for prevention exist that are designed to limit unwanted joint motion or provide biomechanical support to a joint to alleviate discomfort during movement. In addition, a clinician, after evaluating the structures that may have suffered an injurious mechanism during participation in an activity, may determine that the individual can return back to participation with immediate care of supplementing joint stability with a taping technique.

Taping interventions may be employed with either elastic or nonelastic tape using several techniques. Taping materials are available from multiple manufacturers and come in a range of widths and lengths. Elastic tape, which is typically made in widths between 1 and 4 inches (2.5 to 10.2 cm), is used to provide some additional stability while still allowing a large freedom of movement, to secure pads or other protective implements to a body part, or to provide compression. Nonelastic tape can provide more joint support than elastic tape using applications intended to restrict excessive movements, and comes in typical widths between 1 and 2 inches (2.5 to 5.1 cm). Tape may be applied directly to skin that has been shaved or devoid of hair (i.e., sole of the foot), or if the patient does not wish to shave the area that will be taped, a thin layer of foam, called prewrap, may be wrapped around and over the skin surface to be taped.

A newer material used frequently in clinical practice is self-adherent tape and prewrap. This material will adhere to itself, but does not stick to the skin. In addition, it is a very pliable material, with high tensile properties, meaning it can be molded very easily to a body part and still provide a level of mechanical stiffness. The theoretical advantage is that it can provide less skin irritation compared to traditional nonelastic and elastic adhesive tape materials. In addition, the self-adherent prewrap is believed to contribute to the mechanical strength of the taping technique, while regular prewrap does not.

Prophylactic taping techniques can be applied to any part of the body, and there are many variations on the techniques used to apply the nonelastic and elastic materials. Because lower extremity injuries are more prevalent in sports, and these injuries are more likely to be preventable through taping techniques than upper extremity injuries, this overview will focus on some common techniques and associated outcomes related to foot, ankle, and knee taping. It should also be noted that any taping technique may, and often is, modified by a clinician to meet the preventative and treatment needs and comfort of the patient. Therefore the following descriptions are suggested guidelines for some of the more common taping techniques used in sports medicine settings.

FOOT TAPING TECHNIQUES

Plantar Fascia/Arch Taping

Plantar fasciitis or fasciosis is estimated to affect more than 10% of the general population.[4] The most common causes of this pathology relate to a high body mass index, and increased pronation of the midfoot with subsequent flattening of the medial longitudinal arch.[5] Pain persisting along the midfoot extending to the insertion of the plantar fascia at the calcaneus, especially with the first few steps after a period of non-weight-bearing, may benefit from added support to the midfoot. Low-dye and other forms of arch support taping techniques are intended to supplement the structural support of the medial longitudinal arch and the plantar fascia that creates a windlass mechanism needed for normal ambulation.[6]

These taping techniques involve strips of tape that initiate over the insertion of the plantar fascia at the calcaneus or encircle the heel and then extend to the base of each metatarsal head. Elastic or nonelastic tape can be used, with ½ inch widths typically employed. The strips will slightly overlap each other, with

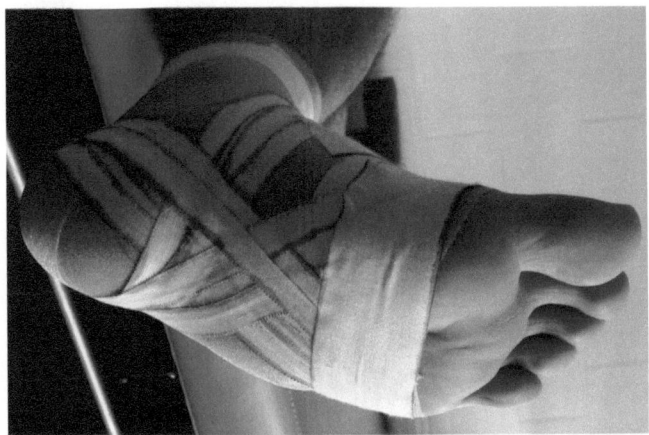

Fig. 33.1 Low-dye taping for foot pain.

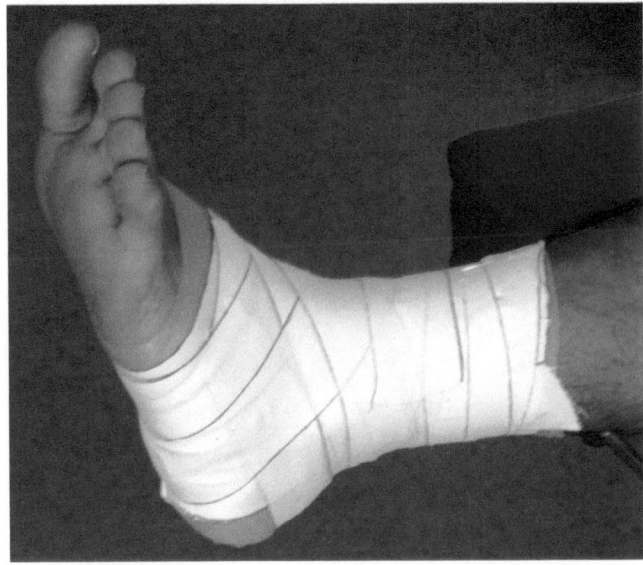

Fig. 33.2 Closed basket weave ankle taping technique.

a strip that secures the tape under the metatarsal heads. Versions of low-dye taping typically involve continuing a strip of tape under the medial longitudinal arch, and pulling up toward the lateral surface of the shank, effectively pulling the foot out of a pronated position (Fig. 33.1). Additional strips of elastic tape may be wrapped around the midfoot to support the fan shaped collection of strips supporting the arch of the foot.

In a systematic review, van de Water and Speksnijder[7] examined the short-term effects of taping techniques on treating pain and disability associated with plantar fasciosis. The limited evidence reviewed showed a positive short-term effect (<1 week) on pain reduction with taping techniques compared with control conditions and other interventions, but the evidence was inconclusive on the impact on patient disability. Similar positive short-term effects of taping on stiffness were observed by in combination with iontophoresis, with continued benefits observed after 4 weeks of continued treatment.[8] Relief of pain and symptoms through external support of the foot beyond a week may require additional interventions, such as orthotics, which is discussed later in this chapter.

Toe Taping

Sprains to the first metatarsophalangeal (MTP) joint are common in field sports and can be quite debilitating. "Turf toe," as it is commonly called, can result from a hyperextension or hyperflexion mechanism to the great toe (first MTP joint), which limits dorsiflexion of the great toe and restricts the ability of the patient to push off during ambulation. A taping technique may be employed to resist the painful motion of the MTP joint by looping ½ inch strips of tape to pull the toe into flexion or extension. Additional strips are wrapped around the midfoot to anchor the strips and complete the technique.

Ankle Taping Techniques

The most common anatomical injury among the physically active is to the ankle.[2,3] Subsequently, taping of the ankle for preventive and immediate treatment purposes is the most common technique used in clinical practice. Due to anatomical and biomechanical principles, the lateral ligaments are the most commonly affected structures of the ankle complex. The purpose of a typical ankle taping technique is to limit plantar flexion and inversion

of the ankle complex, which are injurious movements associated with a lateral ankle sprain.

The most common technique for providing support to the lateral ankle complex is called the "closed basket weave." Typically performed with 1.5 inch nonelastic tape, the strips of tape are applied as "anchors," "stirrups," and "heel-locks," which will cover the ankle complex from the midshank distally to the tarsals (Fig. 33.2). The combination of strips will position the ankle complex into a dorsiflexed and slightly inverted position. The strips of nonelastic tape may be applied either to skin that has been shaved or over a layer prewrap. In addition, thin square foam pads with petroleum jelly may be placed over the insertion of the Achilles tendon on the calcaneus and over the talus, to reduce friction over these skin areas that may suffer irritation from the crossing of the applied strips of tape.

To provide mild stability and compression to an acutely injured ankle, a clinician may utilize an "open basket weave" taping technique. The sequence of application of the anchor and stirrup strips of nonelastic tape is similar to the closed basket weave technique, but the crisscrossing heel locks are not applied with nonelastic tape, leaving the dorsum of the foot exposed (Fig. 33.3). The heel locks are applied with elastic tape under small amounts of tension, or with an elastic bandage. This technique allows some support to ankle complex with the primary purpose to provide comfortable compression to help minimize the early stages of the inflammatory process.

Knee Taping Techniques
Knee Stability

There are many forms of external prophylactic support for the knee, with rigid braces being the choice most clinicians use for long-term wear and prevention. However, there are taping techniques that can be applied to provide stability to the knee joint during physical activity. Most available knee braces are designed to supplement the cruciate and/or collateral ligaments of the knee. Taping techniques can be applied to mimic or supplement the limitations to knee movement these rigid braces are intended to create.

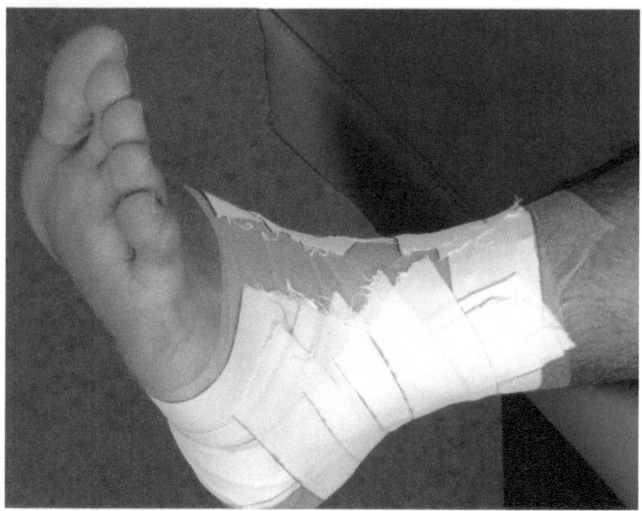

Fig. 33.3 Open basket weave ankle taping technique.

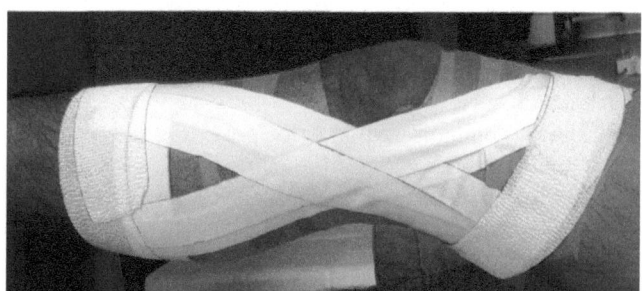

Fig. 33.4 Knee collateral ligament taping technique.

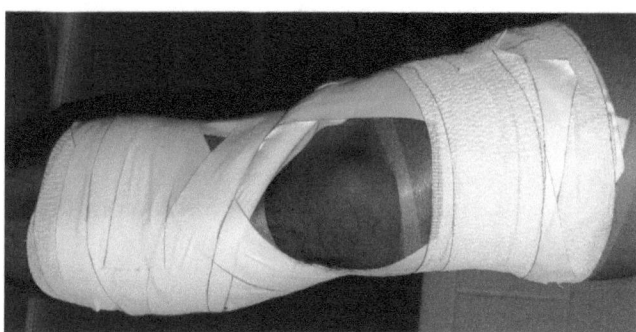

Fig. 33.5 Knee stability taping technique.

Protection against excessive valgus or varus forces that may threaten the medial and lateral collateral ligaments can be achieved by crisscrossing strips of tape over the medial or lateral surfaces of the knee joint and securing them proximally and distally to the thigh and shank (Fig. 33.4). Additional support can be provided to the cruciate ligaments with this technique by wrapping these crisscrossed strips around the anterior and posterior aspects of the thigh and shank (Fig. 33.5). The angle of each strip is varied in order to comprehensively support the knee joint complex.

Patellofemoral Pain

Patellofemoral pain syndrome (PFPS) is a classification of pathology that presents with anterior knee pain or retropatellar pain. The etiology of PFPS has multiple origins, with many attributed

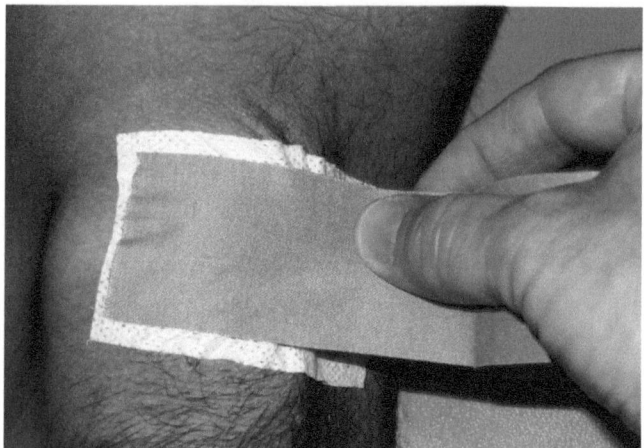

Fig. 33.6 McConnell medial patellar glide taping technique.

to malalignment and poor tracking of the patella in relation to the femoral groove, resulting in pain. One of the many treatments proposed to alleviate the symptoms of PFPS are taping techniques to reposition the patella statically and dynamically. A systematic review by Aminaka and Gribble[9] concluded that patellar corrective taping techniques have positive outcomes for alleviating pain and improving function, but the explanatory mechanisms are not well established by the existing literature. This is likely a result of the complexity and variability of the pathology, which also helps explain why there are so many variations on patellar taping techniques.

A basic tenet of patellar taping techniques is to determine what form of malalignment and maltracking the patient is suffering from (i.e., patella alta, medial rotation, etc.), and then attempt to pull and reposition the patella, using specialized tape, into the opposite direction or combination of directions. The specialized tape is then used to maintain the corrected position, in order to alleviate excessive pressures between the posterior surface of the patella and the trochlear groove of the femur. One popular collection of these techniques was developed by McConnell,[10] but many variations on these techniques exist and may be successful for individual patient needs.[9] In general, these applications are intended to be worn for longer periods of time (days or weeks; see the section below), as the symptoms may persist beyond physical activity into activities of daily living. Subsequently, specialized, and often more expensive, taping materials are utilized. A common technique is to draw the patella medially, using the tape to hold the position statically, and encourage a new movement pattern during dynamic positioning that prevents lateral patellar displacement during a strong contraction of the quadriceps muscle group (Fig. 33.6). Additional adjustments in the tilt, rotation, and vertical placement of the patella can be made with the taping technique.[9,10]

Length of Wear/Length of Effectiveness

The materials used for most athletic taping techniques are not designed for long-term wear. These materials provide a significant amount of stability and movement limitation immediately after application, with most of the published evidence focused on ankle taping techniques.[11–17] However, because they are cloth-based products, exposure to moisture, heat, and tension will quickly reduce the biomechanical stiffness properties of the materials, in as little as 10 minutes after application.[17–20] One study suggests that while both elastic and nonelastic cloth-based tapes will lose tensile strength after 30 minutes of exercise, elastic tape may not lose as much tension as nonelastic tape, and may be more comfortable.[20] Limited investigation on the amount of joint restriction after application and participation in exercise on the newer category of self-adherent tape materials suggests these newer materials may provide more sustainable stability to the ankle, specifically in restricting inversion movement, compared with nonelastic cloth tape.[17] More research is needed to determine how to improve the restrictive properties of taping materials to maximize their effectiveness.

Evidence on the optimal time period of lasting strength of taping materials used in treating foot and knee conditions discussed in this chapter is quite limited. One can only project that the properties of taping materials that have been studied related to ankle taping would apply to the materials if they are used on other joints of the lower extremity and are subjected to similar demands of physical activity. In most cases, taping techniques are designed for short-term wear (a few hours) before being removed. While a taping technique may be applied every day for many weeks or months (i.e., the length of a sport competition season), some techniques, like the Low-Dye and arch support techniques for plantar fasciitis, are typically applied as an intermediary until a more permanent orthotic can be obtained for the patient.

The exception to this are the materials used for patellofemoral corrective taping. These are applied with the intent of the patient wearing the material on the skin potentially for several days in order to receive a benefit of the repositioned patella during all forms of physical and daily living activities. These materials are constructed of more robust material that resists moisture and maintains its mechanical stiffness. The cost of these materials, such as Leukotape (Beiersdorf, Inc., Wilton, CT), is much higher per roll than cloth-based elastic and nonelastic tapes, and would severely limit joint movement, which explains why clinicians may choose not to use these materials in the daily application of most of the taping techniques that have been described in this chapter.

Injury Prevention

There is an ongoing debate in the literature and in clinical practice as to what is the most effective and cost-efficient prophylactic support for reducing injury in the lower extremity. Typically the comparisons are between taping and bracing of the joints of the lower extremity. While taping is a staple among sports medicine clinicians, there is a relatively limited amount of investigation into the efficacy of taping techniques for the prevention of injury, with the majority of this literature focused on ankle injuries.

Ankle Sprains

In general, ankle taping has been shown in clinical studies to reduce the rate of ankle sprain. In an early study, Garrick and Requa[21] reported that taping produced a twofold decrease in ankle sprains in intramural basketball players with a history of an ankle sprain, and a threefold decrease in players who had no history of ankle sprains. The literature continues to suggest that this intervention is effective at reducing ankle injury rates during physical activity and sport participation compared with not wearing a prophylactic support.[22–25] Similarly, a large amount of research supports the use of prophylactic ankle braces for the reduction of ankle sprain incidence.[22–26] However, the existing evidence does not seem to support a difference in the effectiveness of ankle taping versus ankle bracing, meaning both forms of prevention are useful in reducing ankle sprain incidence.[22–25,27] Short- and long-term cost of materials may be an important deciding factor, which will be discussed later in the chapter.

Plantar Fasciitis/Fasciosis

While low-dye and other taping techniques are used successfully in clinical practice to alleviate excessive pronation and plantar fasciitis and fasciosis symptoms, the published evidence is quite limited. Typically this treatment is used initially to alleviate symptoms, but long-term use commonly is avoided in favor of other forms of mechanical correction and support to the foot through orthotics and other forms of tissue treatment to reduce inflammation and irritation. Supporting the clinical use of this technique, a systematic review concluded that taping techniques are a short-term effective treatment for pain associated with plantar fasciitis/fasciosis, but the evidence is inconclusive for supporting these techniques to improve disability.[7] Similarly, a more recent investigation stated that low-dye taping was able to decrease patient-reported pain during walking and jogging immediately after application, but long-term effects were not assessed.[28] Therefore it appears that these taping techniques can provide an immediate and short-term resolution of pain in patients with plantar fasciitis.

Patellofemoral Pain

Taping techniques for PFPS continue to be a popular intervention in clinical practice. The repositioning of the patella may be able to change the movement patterns of the lower extremity, but the primary outcome variable that has been studied is alleviation of pain. Previous systematic reviews of the literature support the use of patellofemoral repositioning taping techniques to alleviate pain in short- and long-term periods,[9,29] while another review suggests the literature is too inconclusive to make a clinical recommendation.[30] While continued work is needed to verify how this category of taping technique is able to alleviate symptoms of patellofemoral pain, it appears it may represent a viable intervention for patients suffering this pathology.

Criticisms of Taping Techniques

One criticism of taping techniques that is often raised is that the applications will limit performance during physical activity. Cordova et al.[31] concluded in a meta-analysis that external ankle supports, including taping, do not significantly hinder most measures of physical performance. Most patients will be cognizant of the taping application immediately upon application, due to the intended restrictive or supportive nature of the technique. This may be a positive effect, as these techniques are likely providing stimulation to cutaneous receptors, which may be supplementing the neuromuscular control systems that will provide dynamic stability to the joint.[32,33]

Length of Effectiveness

As mentioned previously in this chapter, the materials used in athletic taping techniques do not maintain structural stiffness for very long after application.[11,12,16,18,19] While this is a legitimate criticism of these materials, the evidence shows that the use of taping techniques can reduce injury rates[22–25,27] and reduce pathology associated pain.[7–9,28] Therefore in spite of a precluion to lose mechanical stiffness, taping techniques are an effective intervention. A likely explanation is the increased afferent signaling that taping applied to the skin generates.[32,33] An increase in proprioceptive information may be generating feedforward responses in the central nervous system that contribute to improved muscle reaction and dynamic stability, and subsequently a decreased in injurious positions and alleviation of pain.

Cost Effectiveness

Most of the existing literature supports the effectiveness of all forms of ankle prophylactic support for the prevention of ankle sprains. However, the cost of materials and the time to apply them must be considered by clinicians. Olmsted et al.[24] showed that ankle taping and bracing were effective at reducing ankle sprains, especially in athletes with a history of ankle instability. However, during a full athletic competition season, taping an ankle is three times more expensive than bracing an ankle.[24] Similarly, Mickel et al.[27] found ankle taping and bracing to be equally effective at reducing ankle sprains in high school football players, but taping an ankle every day for an entire season would cost more than providing a brace that could be applied every day. In addition, taping requires substantially more time by the clinician to administer the taping techniques every day.[24]

Taping Summary

Athletic taping techniques are utilized commonly by sports medicine clinicians as an effective intervention to provide joint stability and relieve painful symptoms associated with lower extremity pathologies. While some limitations are associated with these techniques, the evidence supports the use of these materials and techniques, especially in prevention of injuries. Clinicians need to consider the cost and needs of the patient in selecting the most appropriate techniques and materials to meet the goals of injury prevention and initial treatment these interventions can provide.

ORTHOTICS

Participation in physical activity, such as running, increases the chance of lower extremity overuse injuries throughout the kinetic chain of the ankle, knee, hip, and low back. Many of these ailments can be attributed to malalignments and improper biomechanics of the foot. Intrinsic, structural abnormalities in the medial longitudinal arch (pes planus, pes cavus), as well as leg length discrepancies, may impact the static alignment of the lower extremity and low back, which can translate into inefficient force transmission during physical activity. Examining the alignment of the forefoot, midfoot, and rearfoot with the entire lower extremity kinetic chain may help elucidate the onset of static and dynamic abnormalities throughout the lower extremity. Foot structural malalignments may be creating problems elsewhere in the kinetic chain, or may be an adaptation to a biomechanical or neuromuscular problem proximal to the foot. A common and effective intervention is to correct malalignments of the foot with the use of an orthotic shoe insert to optimize force transmission from the foot into the leg and back during contact with the ground.[34–36] It is imperative that the clinician considers individual patient needs to ensure the selection of the most appropriate orthotic.

Evaluating the Foot

The primary goal of an orthotic is to create an optimal and comfortable orientation between the three areas of the foot (forefoot, midfoot, and rearfoot) in order to efficiently attenuate forces experienced during contact with the ground. Much of the attention of creating an optimal foot position centers on creating a subtalar neutral position, which means the talus is positioned in a neutral position within the ankle mortise and in relation to the calcaneus, while optimizing the integrity of medial longitudinal arch.

Examining the foot structure should involve observation of the orientation of forefoot, midfoot, and rearfoot in relation to each other in weight-bearing and non-weight-bearing, and how any changes in these foot positions affect the orientations of the lower leg, thigh, and pelvis. Root et al.[37] originally described a procedure to prescribe orthotics based on examining the static orientation of the rearfoot and finding a position of subtalar neutral. Later, Landorf et al. showed that prescription and construction of orthotics varies significantly among clinicians.[38] More recent approaches to prescribing orthotics suggest a much more comprehensive evaluation of the entire lower limb during static and dynamic assessments to determine the needs of the patient and how an orthotic may be able to help correct alignment issues and reduce pain.[36,39,40] Once the evaluation is complete, the clinician can decide what factors will be needed in the orthotic (i.e., motion control, cushioning, medial vs. lateral support, etc.) and which category of orthotic will be best for the patient's needs.

While multiple diagnoses may emerge from an evaluation of the possible foot and lower limb orientations, two of the more common categories of general foot malalignments, or foot types, are pes planus, or excessive pronation/flat arch, and pes cavus, or excessive supination/high arch. Pes planus typically presents with rearfoot and forefoot varus, causing the medial longitudinal arch to flatten excessively to the ground during weight acceptance. This foot type may benefit from more support on the medial side of the foot. Conversely, a pes cavus foot commonly will have contributions of rearfoot and forefoot valgus, limiting the ability of the medial longitudinal arch to flatten normally during gait. This condition may benefit from more orthotic support under the lateral surface of the foot. While this describes these conditions and approaches to orthotic intervention in general, it is important for a trained clinician to examine the foot thoroughly to determine the individual needs of the patient.

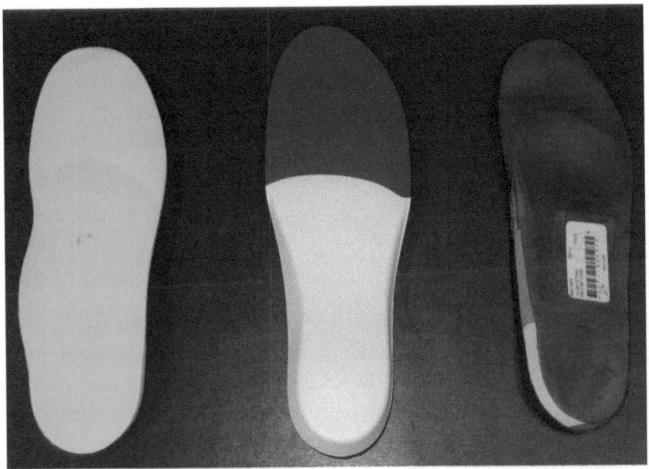

Fig. 33.7 Soft, semi-rigid, and rigid full-length orthotics *(bottom view)*.

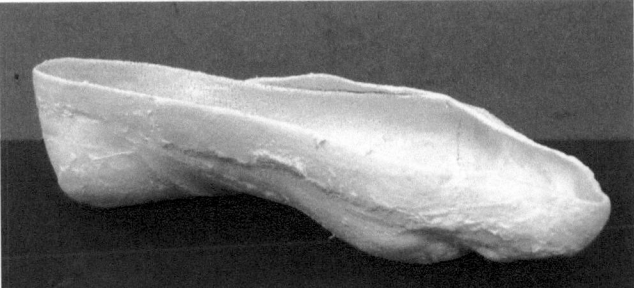

Fig. 33.8 Orthotic mold cast for creation of rigid orthotic.

Types of Orthotics and Materials

Foot orthotics can be constructed from a variety of soft, semi-rigid, and rigid materials, and may be categorized as molded, or custom-made, or nonmolded, or over-the-counter (Fig. 33.7). As emphasized previously, the selection of materials is specific to the needs of the patient, as determined by the evaluation of the clinician. In general, softer materials provide more cushioning, whereas rigid materials provide more stability and control of motion. Semirigid orthotics are intended to provide a combination of cushioning and motion control. Rigid orthotics are moldable and are custom-made to the meet the specifications of the patient's foot, whereas the soft orthotics are not designed to be altered, and can be used "off the shelf" immediately by the patient without having to wait for custom modifications. Semirigid orthotics provide an option that is off the shelf, and can be utilized as is, but also may be altered through minor customization by a clinician. Soft orthotics have a much shorter lifespan than rigid and semirigid orthotics because the inherent thickness and stiffness of the material in soft orthotics is much less. Subsequently, rigid and semirigid orthotics have higher associated costs because of more robust material and the added expense of professional construction and/or modification of the product.

If a decision is made by the evaluating clinician that the patient needs corrective orthotics to provide foot stability and/or motion control, either a semirigid or rigid orthotic will be selected and constructed. Treating basic foot abnormalities such as an excessive pes planus or pes cavus foot may be successful with a semirigid orthotic. These are constructed of material that provides shock absorption and motion control. Semirigid orthotics are manufactured in standard shoe sizes and may be worn as is by the patient, but are designed to allow a clinician to attach additional support, or "posting," with foam or thermoplastic materials to create more medial or lateral stability as needed. Semirigid orthotics offer a good solution for a customizable motion control orthotic, but depending on the demands and the degree of foot malalignment, the patient may benefit from a rigid, custom-made orthotic.

Rigid orthotics are designed to provide the greatest amount of motion control and stability. Constructed of acrylic plastics

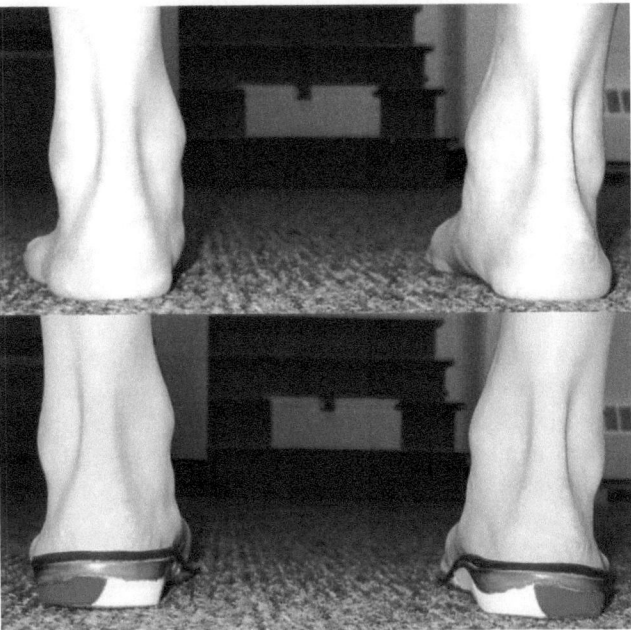

Fig. 33.9 Correction of pes planus with custom-made rigid orthotic.

and other composite materials, these orthotics require a lengthier process to produce. First, the clinician will make a cast impression of the patient's foot after positioning the patient in subtalar neutral and midtarsal joint stabilized against the rearfoot (Fig. 33.8). As stated earlier, the methods for determining the optimal alignment of the foot differ among clinicians,[36–40] and a comprehensive discussion of the methods utilized in clinical practice is outside the scope of this chapter. Nonetheless, once a cast of the foot is made, the cast is used to make a positive mold of an orthotic with the rigid materials. While the construction of the orthotic may be performed in a clinic, often the clinic will utilize a service that receives the cast mold, manufactures the orthotic, and sends the orthotic back to the clinic for distribution to the patient (Fig. 33.9).

Outcomes for Common Overuse Issues

Orthotics continue to be prescribed in the treatment of lower extremity musculoskeletal pathologies because they have a good rate of successful outcome. In controlled laboratory studies, orthotics are able to improve balance in subjects with cavus feet[41] and after suffering a lateral ankle sprain.[42,43] In addition, it is suggested orthotics are able to treat excessive pronation by decreasing eversion excursion and velocity during walking[44] and running.[45]

Running is an activity associated with a high rate of overuse injuries, and orthotics have been associated with successful reductions in a variety of injuries, including anterior knee pain, plantar fasciitis, and Achilles tendonitis.[46,47] One review of literature concluded that with an orthotic, 64% to 95% of runners will experience moderate to full alleviation of pain caused by running.[48] More recently, a systematic review reported that custom-made orthotics were very effective at reducing pain associated with pes cavus, and moderately effective at reducing pain associated with hallux valgus and in juvenile idiopathic arthritis.[49] Finally, a meta-analysis concluded that orthotics are successful at reducing pain and improving function in patients with plantar fasciitis.[50]

Unlike the taping techniques described earlier in this chapter, orthotics are typically used as a treatment, rather than as a preventative measure. A recent randomized-controlled trial showed that among military cadets in Finland, orthotics did not prevent overuse injuries during 8 weeks of military training compared with a control condition.[51] In a contrasting randomized-controlled trial, military cadets in the United Kingdom who were randomly given orthotics experienced fewer lower extremity overuse injuries during 7 weeks of military training compared with cadets who did not receive preventative orthotics.[52] With the limited evidence that exists, there seems to be potential for orthotics to prevent lower extremity injuries, but it is difficult to make definitive conclusions, especially for application among populations of varying levels of physical activity.

While most of the research suggests that orthotics are an effective intervention for correcting skeletal malalignments, it is also suggested that orthotics may enhance the role of cutaneous receptors,[35,53] leading to improvements in balance and function. In addition, clinicians should not ignore the importance of patient comfort when utilizing these interventions.[35] Vicenzino et al.[36,40] advocate that simply correcting the foot position does not necessarily alleviate the biomechanical problem in the lower limb; and an orthotic based only on the foot position may not result in the most comfortable orthotic for the patient. Therefore outcomes with orthotic intervention are likely to be improved by considering a comprehensive lower extremity evaluation and the comfort of the patient.

SUMMARY

Orthotics are an effective intervention for treating a variety of lower extremity musculoskeletal overuse injuries by correcting the position of the foot during standing and ambulation. Providing support and/or cushioning to the rearfoot, midfoot, and forefoot may lead to changes in the biomechanical orientation of the entire lower extremity, leading to an alleviation of pain in the feet, knees, and hips. It is important for a trained clinician to conduct a thorough biomechanical evaluation of the feet and the lower extremity kinetic chain to determine the most appropriate form of orthotic to provide comfortable relief.

For a complete list of references, go to ExpertConsult.com.

SELECTED READINGS

Citation:
Aminaka N, Gribble P. A systematic review of the effects of therapeutic taping on patellofemoral pain syndrome. *J Athl Train*. 2005;40(4):341–351.

Level of Evidence:
Ia

Summary:
This systematic review investigated the efficacy of patellar taping on pain control, patellar alignment, and neuromuscular control (i.e., vastus medialis oblique activation, knee extensor moment, etc.) in subjects with patellofemoral pain syndrome. Although patellar taping seems to reduce pain and improve function in people with patellofemoral pain syndrome during activities of daily living and rehabilitation exercise, strong evidence to identify the underlying mechanisms is still not available.

Citation:
Dizon J, Reyes J. A systematic review on the effectiveness of external supports in the prevention of inversion ankle sprains among elite and recreational players. *J Sci Med Sport*. 2010;13:309–317.

Level of Evidence:
Ia

Summary:
This study was conducted to evaluate the effectiveness of external ankle supports in the prevention of inversion ankle sprains and identify which type of ankle support was superior to the other. The main significant finding was the reduction of ankle sprain by 69% with the use of ankle brace and reduction of ankle sprain by 71% with the use of ankle tape among previously injured athletes.

Citation:
Vicenzino B, Collins N, Cleland J, et al. A clinical prediction rule for identifying patients with patellofemoral pain who are likely to benefit from foot orthoses: a preliminary determination. *Br J Sports Med*. 2010;44:862–866.

Level of Evidence:
Ib

Summary:
This post-hoc analysis of a RCT intended to develop a clinical prediction rule to identify patients with patellofemoral pain (PFP) who are more likely to benefit from foot orthoses. Age, height, pain severity, and midfoot morphometry were identified as possible predictors of successful treatment of PEP with foot orthoses, thereby providing practitioners with information for utilizing foot orthoses in patients with PFP.

Citation:
Hawke F, Burns J, Radford J, et al. Custom-made orthoses for the treatment of foot pain. *Cochrane Database Syst Rev*. 2008;(3):CD006801.

Level of Evidence:
Ia

Summary:
This systematic review from the Cochrane library evaluated the effectiveness of custom foot orthoses for different types of foot pain. There was strong evidence in support of using orthoses in

the treatment of painful pes cavus feet, and moderate evidence in treating juvenile idiopathic arthritis, rheumatoid arthritis, plantar fasciitis, and hallux valgus.

Citation:

Franklyn-Miller A, Wilson C, Bilzon J, et al. Foot orthoses in the prevention of injury in initial military training: a randomized controlled trial. *Am J Sports Med*. 2011;39(1):30–37.

Level of Evidence:

Ib

Summary:

Custom-made foot orthoses were found to be an effective preventative intervention to reduce overuse lower limb injury rates in an "at risk'" military trainee population.

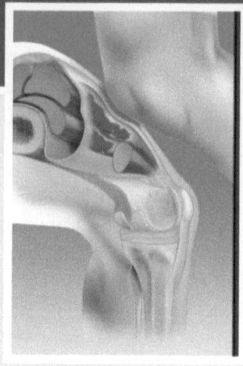

34

Injury Prevention

Jay Hertel, James Onate, Thomas Kaminski

Prevention of injuries is a critical, but often overlooked, component of the clinical practice of sports medicine. Incorporating injury prevention initiatives into an individual athlete's or team's training regimens requires forethought, planning, and persistence to maximize prophylactic benefits. To maximize these benefits, prevention initiatives must be targeted at known intrinsic or extrinsic injury risk factors, and targeted at athletes who are most susceptible to incurring the specific injuries being targeted for prevention. In this chapter, we highlight injury prevention initiatives aimed at three common lower extremity injuries: hamstring muscle strains, anterior cruciate ligament (ACL) ruptures, and ankle ligament sprains.

PREVENTION OF HAMSTRING MUSCLE STRAINS

Strains to the hamstring muscles are common occurrences in sports that involve maximal sprints and acceleration. Among sprinters, hamstring strains represent approximately one third of all acute injuries,[1] while they are also the first or second most common injury in soccer,[2–5] Australian rules football,[6,7] rugby,[8,9] and American football.[10,11] Hamstring strain injuries are also common in sports where the muscles may be stretched past the usual range of movement, such as in dancing and water-skiing.[13] There is evidence from American collegiate soccer that males are at a 64% increased risk of incurring hamstring strains than females.[14] Approximately 13% of all hamstring strains are recurrent injuries.[15]

CAUSES

Injury Mechanisms

The hamstring muscle group is composed of three muscles—semimembranosus, semitendinosus, and biceps femoris. All of them, except the short head of the biceps femoris, originate at the ischial tuberosity the pelvis. The two medial muscles, semimembranosus and semitendinosus, insert on the medial aspect of the proximal tibia, whereas the biceps femoris inserts onto the head of the fibula. The muscle group is biarticular, and its concentric actions are to extend the hip joint and flex the knee joint. However, it must be noted that the muscle group's eccentric actions in slowing hip flexion and knee extension are equally important.

Hamstring strains occur most often during maximal sprints. It is difficult to document exactly at what time injuries occur during the running cycle,[16] but the muscle group is thought to be vulnerable to strain injury in the late swing phase immediately before heel strike.[17,18] At this time point, the hamstring muscles work eccentrically.

RISK FACTORS

A number of risk factors have been proposed for hamstring strains, with the most prominent being the following four internal factors: reduced hip range of motion (ROM), poor hamstring strength, history of previous injury, and age.[19] In theory, limited ROM for hip flexion could mean that muscle tension is at its maximum when the muscle is vulnerable, at close to maximum length. However, this hypothesis has yet to be confirmed, because several studies involving soccer players suggest that hamstring flexibility is not a risk factor for strains.[20,21] However, other studies pertaining to soccer and Australian Rules football have shown that low quadriceps flexibility represents a risk factor not only for hamstrings[22] but also for quadriceps strains.[23]

Decreased hamstring strength would mean that the forces necessary to resist knee flexion and initiate hip extension during maximal sprints could surpass the tolerance of the muscle-tendon unit. Hamstring strength is often expressed relative to quadriceps strength as the hamstrings/quadriceps ratio, because it is the relationship between the ability of the quadriceps to generate speed and the capacity of the hamstrings to resist the resulting forces that is believed to be critical. Several studies show that players with decreased hamstrings/quadriceps ratios or side-to-side strength imbalances may be at increased risk of injury,[19] although the association has also been recently described as being of weak clinical importance.[24] Interestingly, reduced hamstring strength has been more strongly associated with increased risk of recurrent hamstring strains.[25]

A history of previous hamstring strains greatly increases injury risk.[19,26,27] Injury can cause scar tissue to form in the musculature, resulting in a less compliant area with increased risk of injury. A previous injury can also lead to reduced ROM or reduced strength, thereby indirectly affecting injury risk. Inadequate restoration of hamstring strength and endurance has been hypothesized as the primary reason for re-injury risk.[28]

Older players are at increased risk for hamstring strains, and although older players are more likely to have a previous injury, increased age is also an independent risk factor for injury.[21,27] Recent research has also provided preliminary evidence linking

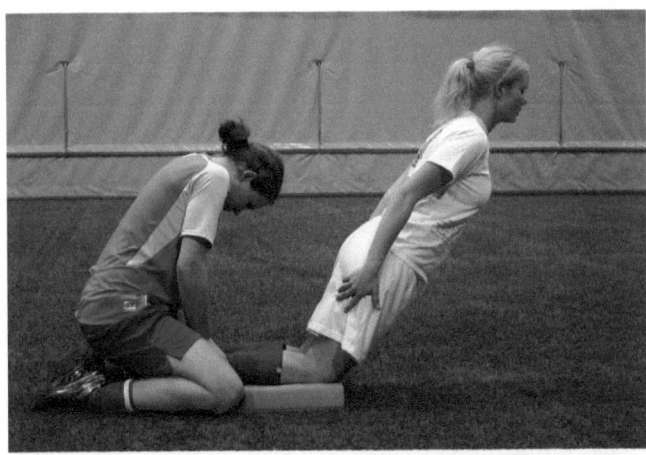

Fig. 34.1 The Nordic hamstring exercise. Subjects are instructed to let themselves fall forward, and then resist the fall against the ground as long as possible by using their hamstrings. (Copyright Oslo Sports Trauma Research Center.)

Week	Sessions/Week	Sets and Repetitions
1	1	2 × 5
2	2	2 × 6
3	3	3 × 6–8
4	3	3 × 8–10
5–10	3	3 sets, 12–10–8 repetitions

TABLE 34.1 Training Protocol for Nordic Hamstring Group

an increased volume of high velocity sprinting with increased hamstring injury risk[29] and the congestion of multiple competitions in a short time period with overall injury risk.[30]

METHODS FOR PREVENTING HAMSTRING STRAINS

Research on injury prevention methods for hamstring strains is limited, and the evidence available has mainly been collected from observational studies. None of the prevention methods described here have been tested in large-scale randomized clinical trials with hamstring strains as the main end point. Studies to date have examined intervention methods targeting the key risk factors for hamstring strains: hamstring strength, hamstring flexibility, and previous injury.

The use of the Nordic hamstring exercise, emphasizing eccentric strengthening, has been shown to reduce the risk of hamstring strains.[2,31] This simple exercise is performed with a partner (Fig. 34.1) and starts with the athlete upright with their knees on the ground. While their partner holds the athlete's lower leg and feet in place, the athlete very slowly moves into bilateral knee extension as they lower their head, arms, and trunk to the ground. Surprisingly few sets and repetitions are needed to stimulate both a strengthening response and an injury prevention response.[2,8,31–34]

Because the Nordic hamstring lowers are easily implemented in a team setting, this exercise is recommended as a specific tool to prevent hamstring injuries. However, to avoid delayed-onset muscle soreness, it is important to follow the recommended exercise prescription with a gradual increase in training load when introducing a program of Nordic hamstring lowers (see Table 34.1).

The consistent finding that a history of previous injury leads to a several fold increase in the risk for new strains has led to the suggestion that this finding is at least partly due to inadequate rehabilitation and early return to sport. A study pertaining to Swedish soccer[34] has documented that a coach-controlled rehabilitation program consisting of information about risk factors

for reinjury, implementation of rehabilitation principles, and use of a 10-step progressive rehabilitation program, including return-to-play (RTP) criteria, reduced the re-injury risk by 75% for lower limb injuries in general. Although the specific effect on hamstring strains could not be assessed in this study, it seems reasonable to recommend the use of functional and specific rehabilitation programs and careful screening of players before RTP.

No intervention studies on the preventive effect of flexibility training on hamstring strains in elite athletes have been performed. However, one study involving military basic trainees indicated a reduced number of lower limb overuse injuries after a period of hamstring stretching,[35] whereas another military-based study found no effect of stretching.[36] It should be noted that these studies were designed to examine the effect of general stretching on lower limb injuries in general, not the effect of a specific hamstring program on hamstring strain risk. Questionnaire-based data on flexibility training methods collected from 30 English professional football clubs, where the stretching practices of the teams were correlated to their hamstrings strain rates, indicate that using a standard stretching protocol reduces injury risk.[37] Also, in one study from Australian Rules football, a reduction in the incidence of hamstring strains was observed with a three-component prevention program, with stretching while fatigued being one of the components.[38] The other factors in the program were sport-specific training drills and high-intensity anaerobic interval training. Because the program included three components, it is not possible to determine which of these factors are responsible for the observed effect.

In conclusion, the best evidence for hamstring injury prevention is available for programs designed to increase hamstring strength, particularly eccentric hamstring strength.

PREVENTION OF ANTERIOR CRUCIATE LIGAMENT TEARS IN THE FEMALE ATHLETE

One of the most debilitating types of lower extremity injuries is a rupture of the ACL. Surgical reconstruction costs, length of rehabilitation time, and risk for future long-term disability have generated significant interest for prevention programs aimed at reducing ACL injury risk. The number of ACL injury prevention programs has proliferated during the past 2 decades, with several research-investigated and clinically initiated programs being instituted worldwide.[39–58] The essential component of most of these programs is a multivariate approach aimed at creating adaptations in movement technique, neuromuscular control, fatigue resistance, injury awareness, and mobility/stability concepts aimed at altering high-risk movement patterns.[59-65] Most prevention programs institute components of injury risk awareness, strengthening of the lower extremity and trunk, enhancement of whole-body proprioception, increase in neuromuscular coordination, improvement of balance, and correction of potentially at-risk movement patterns through technique instruction and motor learning feedback systems in isolation or combination. Two recent position statements by US- and German-based groups reiterated the main programmatic paradigms for ACL injury prevention programs.[64,65] A 2018 position statement by the National Athletic Trainers' Association on Prevention of Anterior Cruciate Ligament Injury stated that a multicomponent ACL prevention program should at the minimum include three of the following exercise types: strength, plyometrics, agility, balance, and flexibility.[64] A 2018 report from the German Knee Society stressed the importance of screening, identification, and correction of endangering movement patterns as the first crucial steps to preventing ACL injuries.[65]

Implementation of an ACL injury prevention program is ultimately the responsibility of the entire sports medicine team, including the player, coach, parent, athletic trainer, physician, strength and conditioning specialist, physical therapist, and other persons as necessary.[59] The success of the program depends on an integration of roles for all persons involved and requires careful planning, execution, and review to evaluate the potential success of the program. Ideally, ACL prevention programs should be considered as primary injury prevention plans that are modifiable as the situation demands because of the clinical considerations of individuals/teams, given that various components of each program need to be personalized (e.g., soccer-specific vs. basketball-specific). Another consideration is the age of the participants for inducing biomechanical changes. A recent study from a Stanford University research group demonstrated that prevention programs created more significant biomechanical changes in preadolescent participants (aged 10 to 12) as compared with adolescent-aged (14 to 18) participants.[66] Long-term retention of proper movement patterns is an important component of ACL prevention programs and needs to be a critical consideration of all preventative efforts.[67] Careful planning and use of the Finch model of translating research into injury prevention practice should also be considered a cornerstone in evaluating the effectiveness of any ACL injury prevention program.[68]

Effective ACL injury prevention programs implement off-season, preseason, and in-season phases[43,50,52,58,59] to enhance and maintain individual gains. Most of the promising programs with increased compliance have a similar schedule, including sport-specific warm-up two to four times per week during the off-season, training two or three times per week during the preseason, and training one time per week during in-season practice.[39-59] The fundamental components of the most successful programs are dynamic warm-up, strengthening exercises, plyometrics, balance, sport-specific agilities, and motor learning focused feedback concerning proper movement techniques. An example of one program is the Federation International de Football Association Medical Assessment and Research Center (F-MARC) 11+ program (Figs. 34.2 and 34.3).[41] The F-MARC program requires

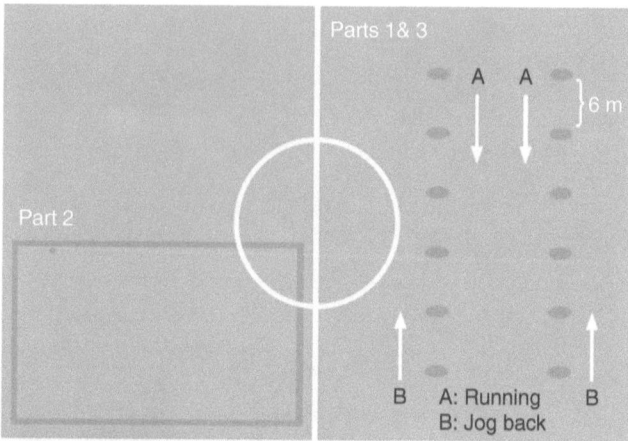

! FIELD SET UP

The course is made up of 6 pairs of parallel cones, approx. 5-6 m apart.
Two players start at the same time from the first pair of cones, jog along the inside of the cones, and do the various exercises on the way. After the last cone, they run back along the outside. On the way back, speed can be increased progressively as players warm up.

Fig. 34.2 Field setup. (From the Federation International de Football Association Medical Assessment and Research Center. More information is available at www.f-marc.com/11plus.)

minimal training and equipment (only a soccer ball required), making it an attractive alternative for persons with limited budgets and time. Three studies in which the F-MARC 11+ program was used with male and female adolescents demonstrated a reduction in injuries ranging between 21% and 71%.[46,56] The specificity of the 11+ soccer-focused training program can be performed in different sports by emphasizing the key components of the program and making the sport movement tasks match the desired activity. Similar training programs have been reported to produce a 49% reduction in lower extremity injury risk[46] and a 94% reduction in ACL injury risk[49] in Norwegian handball players.

Demonstration of program efficacy is essential before wide implementation. One of the main limitations to proving efficacy is that the "number needed to treat" to demonstrate a prophylactic effect as a result of training is relatively large. For pooled number needed to treat estimates, 89 persons (95% confidence intervals: 66 to 136) need to participate in the training program to prevent ACL injury during the course of a competitive athletic season.[62] This finding indicates that a typical youth recreational soccer program with a team of 20 participants would require approximately four teams to participate in the training program to prevent ACL injury. The cost/benefit of time and compliance aspects of programs must be considered when implementing a prevention training program. It is difficult to generalize findings from the various programs to different sports (e.g., soccer vs. team handball programs), different levels of play (e.g., youth vs. collegiate), varying program components (e.g., time of season, length of program, and amount of time per week), type of program (e.g., strength, balance, and feedback), and consistent integration across all levels of disciplines (e.g., strength and conditioning specialists, rehabilitation specialists, medical physicians, and sport-specific coaches).

FIFA 11+

PART 1 RUNNING EXERCISES · 8 MINUTES

1 RUNNING STRAIGHT AHEAD
The course is made up of 6 to 10 pairs of parallel cones, approx. 5-6 metres apart. Two players start at the same time from the first pair of cones. Jog together all the way to the last pair of cones. On the way back, you can increase your speed progressively as you warm up. 2 sets

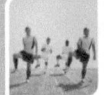
2 RUNNING HIP OUT
Walk or jog easily, stopping at each pair of cones to lift your knee and rotate your hip outwards. Alternate between left and right legs at successive cones. 2 sets.

3 RUNNING HIP IN
Walk or jog easily, stopping at each pair of cones to lift your knee and rotate your hip inwards. Alternate between left and right legs at successive cones. 2 sets.

4 RUNNING CIRCLING PARTNER
Run forwards as a pair to the first set of cones. Shuffle sideways by 90 degrees to meet in the middle. Shuffle an entire circle around one other and then return back to the cones. Repeat for each pair of cones. Remember to stay on your toes and keep your centre of gravity low by bending your hips and knees. 2 sets.

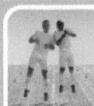
5 RUNNING SHOULDER CONTACT
Run forwards in pairs to the first pair of cones. Shuffle sideways by 90 degrees to meet in the middle then jump sideways towards each other to make shoulder-to-shoulder contact.
Note: Make sure you land on both feet with your hips and knees bent. Do not let your knees buckle inwards. Make it a full jump and synchronize your timing with your team-mate as you jump and land. 2 sets

6 RUNNING QUICK FORWARDS & BACKWARDS
As a pair, run quickly to the second set of cones then run backwards quickly to the first pair of cones keeping your hips and knees slightly bent. Keep repeating the drill, running two cones forwards and one cone backwards. Remember to take small, quick steps. 2 sets

PART 2 STRENGTH · PLYOMETRICS · BALANCE · 10 MINUTES

LEVEL 1

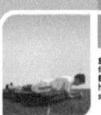
7 THE BENCH STATIC
Starting position: Lie on your front, supporting yourself on your forearms and feet. Your elbows should be directly under your shoulders.
Exercise: Lift your body up, supported on your forearms, pull your stomach in, and hold the position for 20-30 sec. Your body should be in a straight line. Try not to sway or arch your back. 3 sets.

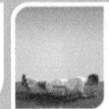
8 SIDEWAYS BENCH STATIC
Starting position: Lie on your side with the knee of your lowermost leg bent to 90 degrees. Support your upper body by resting on your forearm and knee. The elbow of your supporting arm should be directly under your shoulder.
Exercise: Lift your uppermost leg and hips until your shoulder, hip and knee are in a straight line. Hold the position for 20-30 sec. Take a short break, change sides and repeat. 3 sets on each side.

9 HAMSTRINGS BEGINNER
Starting position: Kneel on a soft surface. Ask your partner to hold your ankles down firmly.
Exercise: Your body should be completely straight from the shoulder to the knee throughout the exercise. Lean forward as far as you can, controlling the movement with your hamstrings and your gluteal muscles. When you can no longer hold the position, gently take your weight on your hands, falling into a push-up position. Complete a minimum of 3-5 repetitions and/or 60 sec. 1 set.

10 SINGLE-LEG STANCE HOLD THE BALL
Starting position: Stand on one leg.
Exercise: Balance on one leg whilst holding the ball with both hands. Keep your body weight on the ball of your foot. Remember: try not to let your knees buckle inwards. Hold for 30 sec. The exercise can be made more difficult by passing the ball around your waist and/or under your other knee. 2 sets.

11 SQUATS WITH TOE RAISE
Starting position: Stand with your feet hip-width apart. Place your hands on your hips if you like.
Exercise: Imagine that you are about to sit down on a chair. Perform squats by bending your hips and knees to 90 degrees. Do not let your knees buckle inwards. Descend slowly then straighten up more quickly. When your legs are completely straight, stand up on your toes then slowly lower down again. Repeat the exercise for 30 sec. 2 sets.

12 JUMPING VERTICAL JUMPS
Starting position: Stand with your feet hip-width apart. Place your hands on your hips if you like.
Exercise: Imagine that you are about to sit down on a chair. Bend your legs slowly until your knees are flexed to approx 90 degrees, and hold for 2 sec. Do not let your knees buckle inwards. From the squat position, jump up as high as you can. Land softly on the balls of your feet with your hips and knees slightly bent. Repeat the exercise for 30 sec. 2 sets.

LEVEL 2

7 THE BENCH ALTERNATE LEGS
Starting position: Lie on your front, supporting yourself on your forearms and feet. Your elbows should be directly under your shoulders.
Exercise: Lift your body up, supported on your forearms, and pull your stomach in. Lift each leg in turn, holding for a count of 2 sec. Continue for 40-60 sec. Your body should be in a straight line. Try not to sway or arch your back. 3 sets.

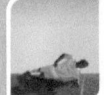
8 SIDEWAYS BENCH RAISE & LOWER HIP
Starting position: Lie on your side with both legs straight. Lean on your forearm and the side of your foot so that your body is in a straight line from shoulder to foot. The elbow of your supporting arm should be directly beneath your shoulder.
Exercise: Lower your hip to the ground and raise it back up again. Repeat for 20-30 sec. Take a short break, change sides and repeat. 3 sets on each side.

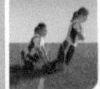
9 HAMSTRINGS INTERMEDIATE
Starting position: Kneel on a soft surface. Ask your partner to hold your ankles down firmly.
Exercise: Your body should be completely straight from the shoulder to the knee throughout the exercise. Lean forward as far as you can, controlling the movement with your hamstrings and your gluteal muscles. When you can no longer hold the position, gently take your weight on your hands, falling into a push-up position. Complete a minimum of 7-10 repetitions and/or 60 sec. 1 set.

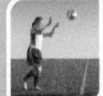
10 SINGLE-LEG STANCE THROWING BALL WITH PARTNER
Starting position: Stand 2-3 m apart from your partner, with each of you standing on one leg.
Exercise: Keeping your balance, and with your stomach held in, throw the ball to one another. Keep your weight on the ball of your foot. Remember: keep your knee just slightly flexed and try not to let it buckle inwards. Keep going for 30 sec. Change legs and repeat. 2 sets.

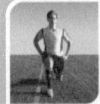
11 SQUATS WALKING LUNGES
Starting position: Stand with your feet hip-width apart. Place your hands on your hips if you like.
Exercise: Lunge forward slowly at an even pace. As you lunge, bend your leading leg until your hip and knee are flexed to 90 degrees. Do not let your knee buckle inwards. Try to keep your upper body and hips steady. Lunge your way across the pitch (approx. 10 times on each leg) and then jog back. 2 sets.

12 JUMPING LATERAL JUMPS
Starting position: Stand on one leg with your upper body bent slightly forwards from the waist, with knees and hips slightly bent.
Exercise: Jump approx. 1 m sideways from the supporting leg on to the free leg. Land gently on the ball of your foot. Bend your hips and knees slightly as you land and do not let your knee buckle inward. Maintain your balance with each jump. Repeat the exercise for 30 sec. 2 sets.

LEVEL 3

7 THE BENCH ONE LEG LIFT AND HOLD
Starting position: Lie on your front, supporting yourself on your forearms and feet. Your elbows should be directly under your shoulders.
Exercise: Lift your body up, supported on your forearms, and pull your stomach in. Lift one leg about 10-15 centimetres off the ground, and hold the position for 20-30 sec. Your body should be straight. Do not let your opposite hip dip down and do not sway or arch your lower back. Take a short break, change legs and repeat. 3 sets.

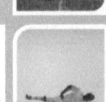
8 SIDEWAYS BENCH WITH LEG LIFT
Starting position: Lie on your side with both legs straight. Lean on your forearm and the side of your foot so that your body is in a straight line from shoulder to foot. The elbow of your supporting arm should be directly beneath your shoulder.
Exercise: Lift your uppermost leg up and slowly lower it down again. Repeat for 20-30 sec. Take a short break, change sides and repeat. 3 sets on each side.

9 HAMSTRINGS ADVANCED
Starting position: Kneel on a soft surface. Ask your partner to hold your ankles down firmly.
Exercise: Your body should be completely straight from the shoulder to the knee throughout the exercise. Lean forward as far as you can, controlling the movement with your hamstrings and your gluteal muscles. When you can no longer hold the position, gently take your weight on your hands, falling into a push-up position. Complete a minimum of 12-15 repetitions and/or 60 sec. 1 set.

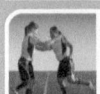
10 SINGLE-LEG STANCE TEST YOUR PARTNER
Starting position: Stand on one leg opposite your partner and at arm's' length apart.
Exercise: Whilst you both try to keep your balance, each of you in turn tries to push the other off balance in different directions. Try to keep your weight on the ball of your foot and prevent your knee from buckling inwards. Continue for 30 sec. Change legs. 2 sets.

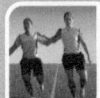
11 SQUATS ONE-LEG SQUATS
Starting position: Stand on one leg, loosely holding onto your partner.
Exercise: Slowly bend your knee as far as you can manage. Concentrate on preventing the knee from buckling inwards. Bend your knee slowly then straighten it slightly more quickly, keeping your hips and upper body in line. Repeat the exercise 10 times on each leg. 2 sets.

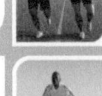
12 JUMPING BOX JUMPS
Starting position: Stand with your feet hip-width apart. Imagine that there is a cross marked on the ground and you are standing in the middle of it.
Exercise: Alternate between jumping forwards and backwards, from side to side, and diagonally across the cross. Jump as quickly and explosively as possible. Your knees and hips should be slightly bent. Land softly on the balls of your feet. Do not let your knees buckle inwards. Repeat the exercise for 30 sec. 2 sets.

PART 3 RUNNING EXERCISES · 2 MINUTES

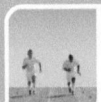
13 RUNNING ACROSS THE PITCH
Run across the pitch, from one side to the other, at 75-80% maximum pace. 2 sets.

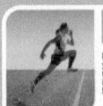
14 RUNNING BOUNDING
Run with high bounding steps with a high knee lift, landing gently on the ball of your foot. Use an exaggerated arm swing for each step (opposite arm and leg). Try not to let your leading leg cross the midline of your body or let your knees buckle inwards. Repeat the exercise until you reach the other side of the pitch, then jog back to recover. 2 sets.

15 RUNNING PLANT & CUT
Jog 4-5 steps, then plant on the outside leg and cut to change direction. Accelerate and sprint 5-7 steps at high speed (80-90% maximum pace) before you decelerate and do a new plant & cut. Do not let your knee buckle inwards. Repeat the exercise until you reach the other side, then jog back. 2 sets.

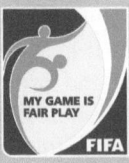
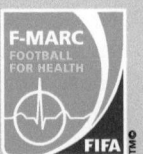

Fig. 34.3 Federation International de Football Association (FIFA) Medical Assessment and Research Center 11 + program. (From the Federation International de Football Association Medical Assessment and Research Center. More information is available at www.f-marc.com/11plus.)

Most evidence demonstrates a moderate to strong level of evidence exists to support the implementation of ACL injury prevention programs to reduce the risk of ACL injuries.[60,61,63] A 2012 systematic review of the literature on the effectiveness of ACL injury prevention training programs[60] found that several studies[39,42,44,48,53–55] met their inclusion criteria for evaluating the effectiveness of ACL injury prevention programs. Most of these programs are directed at the young female athletic population, which is considered to be at the greatest risk for ACL injury. The investigators found that the pooled risk ratio was 0.38 (95% confidence interval [CI], 0.20 to 0.72) for the eight programs evaluated, resulting in a significant reduction in the risk of ACL rupture in the prevention group ($P = .003$), with a risk reduction of 52% in female athletes and 85% in male athletes.[60] A meta-analysis conducted by Donnell-Fink et al.[69] found 24 studies focused on knee and ACL injury prevention that consisted of 1093 participants across a time span consisting from 1996 to 2014. After the training interventions focused on neuromuscular and proprioceptive training exercises, the incidence ratio for knee injury was 0.731, and ACL injury was 0.493, thus indicating that a link existed between training programs and injury reduction. Even though therapeutic level II evidence moderately to strongly supports the effectiveness of ACL injury prevention training programs, caution is warranted because two sets of the studies (Mandelbaum et al.[48] and Gilchrist et al.[42]; Peterson et al.[53] and Peterson et al.[54]) report on essentially the same prevention programs at two different time frames. Nonetheless, the evidence in support of the effectiveness of ACL injury prevention programs is promising, with more research needed to confirm their effectiveness in various types of populations.

The possible use of a screening process to evaluate whether individual athletes truly need to be involved in an ACL injury prevention program should be considered, in addition to the evaluation of an individual athlete's post-ACL injury to ensure that he or she has undergone adequate progression to a safe stage of rehabilitation to tolerate such an intervention program. In addition, the retention aspects of movement pattern changes after intervention programs have yet to be conclusively validated; however, an initial report shows that a longer duration (9-month) program results in greater retention of movement pattern changes compared with a program of shorter duration (3 months).[52] Future research needs to focus on clinical screening tools to evaluate persons most in need of an intervention, program dosage, and retention effects of the intervention.

Attention to ACL injury prevention has grown steadily. The development and implementation of ACL injury prevention programs require a systematic methodologic approach. The bridging of the research-clinical gap to aid persons at risk for injury requires a multidisciplinary team using an evidence-based approach. Future randomized controlled trials and clinically based ACL injury prevention programs require a standardized database. Critical questions remain: specific biomechanical factors associated with increased ACL injury risk, modifiable factors related to increased ACL injury risk, vital components of ACL injury prevention programs, clinical approaches to accommodate for implementation of research-based evidence, and behavioral change models for organizational implementation need to be considered.

KEY POINTS TO CONSIDER FOR AN ANTERIOR CRUCIATE LIGAMENT INJURY PREVENTION PROGRAM

1. Because risk factors are multifactorial, the prevention strategies that need to be used are most likely multifactorial.
2. Prevention programs need to be tailored to meet the demands of the task and individual requirements.
3. More evidence is needed on prevention program implementation factors (e.g., supervision, time frame, and long-term motor learning effects).
4. No single program is best for all; a plan for prevention encompassing baseline screening and intervention must be developed by all members of the sports medicine team.
5. All solutions for ACL injury prevention have not been answered, but current evidence seems to show moderate effectiveness for several ACL injury prevention programs with minimal evidence showing detrimental effects of programs.

PREVENTION OF ANKLE SPRAINS

Ankle sprains are not only a public health burden; they also constitute the most common injury in sport. Fong et al. have suggested that the sports having the highest incidence of ankle sprains include field hockey, volleyball, football, cheerleading, ice hockey, lacrosse, soccer, gymnastics, softball, and track and field.[70] Prevention of ankle sprains both in those having sprain reoccurrences and in those who have never sprained is of importance to the clinician from both a time lost and cost standpoint. An evidence-based approach to injury prevention seems appropriate to guide the clinician in their efforts. In light of this, two recent peer-reviewed clinical guidelines[71,72] issued on the treatment of lateral ankle sprains in the athletic population will be used as a foundation for this section of the chapter on injury prevention.

There is no one single intervention that provides the best ankle sprain protection; instead it is wise for the clinician to adopt a multi-intervention strategy. The two facets of lateral ankle sprain prevention with the best evidence for use include the practice of taping and bracing, as well as a focused balance and neuromuscular control program.

Taping and Bracing

Both lace-up and semirigid ankle braces, along with traditional ankle taping, are effective in preventing ankle sprains and reducing the rate of reoccurrence in athletic populations. Although the mechanism of prevention is unclear, it is likely that taping and bracing provide mechanical stability and proprioceptive enhancement to the ankle joint. Interestingly, it does not appear that one is more effective than the other. Clinicians should therefore be guided by personal preference, practicality, and cost effectiveness. A recent report focusing on the benefits of both ankle taping and bracing suggests that bracing may be the best cost affordable alternative.[73] Despite being more than 40 years old, Garrick and Requa[74] present some of the best evidence available supporting the use of ankle taping to prevent ankle sprains; this was especially true in those with previous ankle injuries. There are numerous reports showing the effectiveness of ankle braces in reducing the incidence of ankle sprains in the athletic population.[75–78] Perhaps the most compelling case for ankle bracing comes from a recent tightly controlled randomized clinical trial by McGuine and colleagues,[78] who reported a significant reduction in ankle injuries among high school basketball players, regardless of previous injury. There is no evidence to support the notion that ankle taping and bracing increases the risk for injuries in other joints of the lower extremity kinetic chain (i.e., knee or hip). Furthermore, despite a recent recommendation in the clinical guideline released by the BJSM (2012) that recommends the use of taping and bracing be phased out over time, there is no evidence available to support this position.[71]

Balance and Coordination Training

Clinicians working with athletes should perform a multi-intervention prevention program, lasting at least 3 months, and one that is focused on balance and neuromuscular control to reduce the risk of ankle injury. This is especially true in those who have suffered previous ankle injuries. There is good support that enhancing and/or improving neuromuscular control translates into ankle joint injury reduction.[79] Of importance to the clinician is that there appears to be evidence that suggests both supervised and unsupervised balance coordination programs are successful in preventing ankle sprains.[80,81] This means that athletes do not necessarily have to receive supervised care in sports medicine facilities (clinics, athletic training rooms) to benefit from these types of intervention programs. Programs should include tasks involving single leg stance balance activities, balance training with perturbations (wobble board, balance mat), balance raining with simultaneous upper extremity movement, as well as dynamic jumping activities that incorporate balance and coordination. McKeon and colleagues[79] offer an excellent series of progressing balance and coordination activities that can be easily implemented in a clinic or at-home environment (Fig. 34.4).

Strength Training

Adequate muscle strength remains at the core of most successful athletic maneuvers and a cornerstone in ankle sprain rehabilitation. However, there is no direct evidence to suggest that strengthening in and of itself prevent ankle sprains. Intuitively, most clinicians would agree that strength in the musculotendinous structures in and around the ankle joint are necessary and play a role in providing both mechanical and dynamic stability to the ankle during athletic performance. Although the exact mechanism for this remains unclear, it is widely postulated that having an appropriate level of muscle strength helps correct imbalances that may put the foot/ankle into vulnerable positions relative to one's center of mass during athletic movements. Therefore interventions that serve to strengthen the lower leg (evertor, invertor, plantar flexors, and dorsiflexors) as well as the hip extensors and abductors should be an integral part of ankle sprain injury prevention protocols.

Dorsiflexion Range of Motion

Although there is no direct evidence supporting the use dorsiflexion ROM activities in ankle sprain prevention strategies, no one would argue against the need for appropriate ankle joint flexibility needed for athletes in all sport endeavors to function. Reductions in dorsiflexion ROM can lead to tightness of the gastroc/soleus complex and produce capsular adhesions that limit arthrokinematic motions in the ankle. There are reports of dorsiflexion deficits during dynamic jumping tasks[82] as well as during gait maneuvers[83] in populations with unstable ankles. The most appropriate theory is that the deficits prohibit the foot from attaining its full closed packed position (one of most support) during the stance phase of gait and in addition move the toes closer to the ground during the swing phase, placing the foot/ankle in a vulnerable position to roll over and sprain. With this in mind, it is prudent for the clinician to appropriately address dorsiflexion ROM deficits with interventions aimed at restoring the flexibility needed to carry out both activities of daily living, as well as sporting activities. These techniques should involve stretching exercises for the lower leg muscles and manual joint mobilization interventions that enhance ankle joint arthrokinematics.

Hypomobility Issues

Hypomobility at any joint in the lower extremity kinetic chain can challenge the motor-control mechanisms of the athlete and lead to joint instabilities.[84] It has been suggested that hypomobility occurs in the subtalar, talocrural, and the distal and proximal tibiofibular joints following ankle sprains. One might argue that considerations addressing the mobility of these joints prophylactically before a sprain event may be wise as well. Although there is no direct evidence supporting this type of clinical intervention strategy, clinicians should be aware of any signs of hypomobility and address them appropriately using joint mobilization techniques.[85]

Education of Risk

Educating athletes about the inherent risks of sport activities as well as vulnerable positions that may produce ankle sprains is an important role that all clinicians must take seriously. Athletes should be made aware of high-risk activities that may place the foot and ankle in a position of vulnerability and injury predisposition. Although there is no evidence supporting the practice of educating athletes concerning the risk for ankle sprain injury, it seems logical that this concept be used as a prevention strategy.

In summary, there is considerable support in the existing literature for the use of taping/bracing, as well as a multidimensional balance and coordination program to prevent lateral ankle sprains in the athletic population. Lesser support has been provided for interventions involving strength training, dorsiflexion ROM deficits, and risk education, although these should remain an integral part of an overall injury prevention program.

The Basics:

6 Categories of Exercises

1. Single-Limb Balance
2. Balance with Ball Toss
3. Balance and Reach
4. Fast Hopping
5. Hop to Stabilization
6. Hop to Stabilization and Reach

Progressions:
There are specific criteria for progression in each category
Progressions increase challenge of exercises in various ways, such as:
- Changing surface (firm to foam)
- Increasing duration of activity
- Increasing intensity of activity

Frequency of Training
3 times per week for 4 weeks
All sessions supervised by school ATC

Exercise 1: Single-Limb Balance
Objective: Stand as still as possible while standing on the involved limb.
Duration: 3 repetitions   *Duration:* 3 repetitions
Progression:

Eyes Open	Eyes Closed
• Arms out for 15 seconds on firm surface	• Arms out on firm surface for 15 seconds
• Arms across chest for 15 seconds on firm surface	• Arms across chest on firm surface for 15 seconds
• Arms out for 30 seconds on firm surface	• Arms out on firm surface for 30 seconds
• Arms across chest for 30 seconds on firm surface	• Arms across chest on firm surface for 30 seconds
• Arms out for 15 seconds on foam surface	• Arms out on foam surface for 15 seconds
• Arms across chest for 15 seconds on foam surface	• Arms across chest for 15 seconds on foam surface
• Arms out for 30 seconds on foam surface	• Arms out for 30 seconds on foam surface
• Arms across chest for 30 seconds on foam surface	• Arms across chest for 30 seconds on foam surface
• Arms out for 60 seconds on foam surface	• Arms out for 60 seconds on foam surface
• Arms across chest for 60 seconds on foam surface	• Arms across chest for 60 seconds on foam surface

*All foam surface tasks will be performed on Airex pads.

Subjects cannot advance to next level in each category until they demonstrate 3 repetitions error free. Errors include:
1. Touching down with opposite limb
2. Excessive trunk motion (>30° lateral flexion)
3. Bracing the non-stance limb against the stance limb
4. Moving the stance foot from its starting position on the ground
5. Removal of arms from across chest during specified activities

Exercise 2: Balance with Ball Toss
Object: Maintain prescribed stance while playing 2-handed catch with a 6-pound medicine ball.
Duration: 3 repetitions
Progression: Bipedal stance performed only until first stage of single-limb stance can be started.

Double-Limb Stance	Single-Limb Stance
5 throws in bipedal stance on firm surface (~20 seconds)	5 throws in unipedal stance on firm surface (~20 seconds)
10 throws in bipedal stance on firm surface (~40 seconds)	10 throws in unipedal stance on firm surface (~40 seconds)
15 throws in bipedal stance on firm surface (~60 seconds)	15 throws in unipedal stance on firm surface (~60 seconds)
5 throws in bipedal stance on foam surface (~20 seconds)	5 throws in unipedal stance on foam surface (~20 seconds)
10 throws in bipedal stance on foam surface (~40 seconds)	10 throws in unipedal stance on foam surface (~40 seconds)
15 throws in bipedal stance on foam surface (~60 seconds)	15 throws in unipedal stance on foam surface (~60 seconds)

Subjects cannot advance to next level in each category until they demonstrate 3 repetitions error free. Errors include:
1. Moving the stance foot (feet) from starting position on the ground
2. Excessive trunk motion (>30° lateral flexion)
3. Bracing the non-stance limb against the stance limb in single-limb stance
4. Failure to catch and throw the ball accurately back to clinician

Exercise 3: Balance and Reach
Object: Reach the specified distance in the prescribed direction with the uninvolved limb while maintaining balance on the involved limb. (Same principle as Star Excursion Balance Test – controlled movements).
Duration: 15 repetitions in each of 8 directions
Progression:

For each direction:
18″ allowed to use arms on firm surface
18″ hands on hips on firm surface
27″ allowed to use arms on firm surface
27″ hands on hips on firm surface
36″ allowed to use arms on firm surface
36″ hands on hips on firm surface
18″ allowed to use arms on foam surface
18″ hands on hips on foam surface
27″ allowed to use arms on foam surface
27″ hands on hips on foam surface
36″ allowed to use arms on foam surface
36″ hands on hips on foam surface

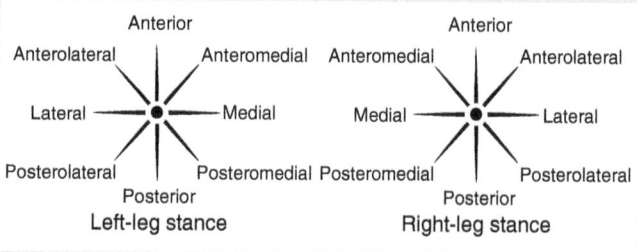

*Directions are named based on direction of reach in relation to the stance limb.

Subjects cannot advance to next level in each category until they demonstrate 20 repetitions error free. Errors include:
1. Touching down with reach limb other than at the intended target
2. Using the reach leg for a substantial amount of support during touchdown at end of reach
3. Moving the stance foot from its starting position on the ground
4. Bracing the reach limb against the stance limb
5. Removal of hands from hips during hands-on-hips activities

Exercise 4: Fast Hopping
Object: Hop in the prescribed direction, immediately hop back to the starting point, immediately repeat. Perform as quickly as possible. Involved limb only.
Duration: 3 sets of 5 repetitions in each of 4 directions (A/P, M/L, AM/PL, AL/PM)
Progression:

For each direction:
Hop across a 2″ line
Hop across a 4″ line
Hop across a 6″ line
Hop across a 9″ line
Hop across a 12″ line
Hop across a 6″ line and over 3″ high barrier
Hop across a 9″ line and over 3″ high barrier
Hop across a 9″ line and over 3″ high barrier

Subjects cannot advance to next level in each category until they demonstrate 3 sets of repetitions, all error free. Errors include:
1. Touching down with opposite limb
2. Not performing all hops continuously (i.e., prolonged stance)
3. Failing to jump completely across line or over barrier

Fig. 34.4 Balance intervention exercises. *ATC,* Certified athletic trainer. (Modified from McKeon PO, Ingersoll CD, Kerrigan DC, et al. Balance training improves function and postural control in those with chronic ankle instability. *Med Sci Sports Exerc.* 2008;40[10]:1810–1819.)

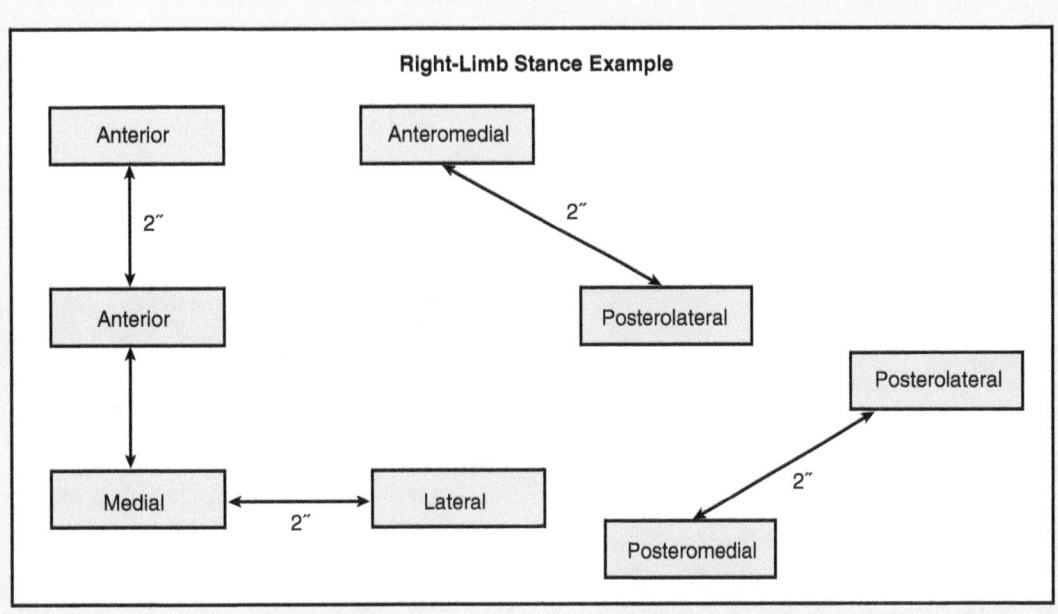

Right-Limb Stance Example

Exercise 5: Hop to Stabilization

Object: Hop to the target landing on the involved limb, stabilize and maintain balance in single-limb stance for 3 seconds, hop back to the starting point, again landing and stabilizing on involved limb for 3 seconds, repeat.

Duration: 3 sets of 5 repetitions in each of 4 directions (A/P, M/L, AM/PL, AL/PM)

Progression:

For each direction:
12″ hop allowed to use arms on firm surface
12″ hop hands on hips on firm surface
18″ hop allowed to use arms on firm surface
18″ hop hands on hips on firm surface
27″ hop allowed to use arms on firm surface
27″ hop hands on hips on firm surface
36″ hop allowed to use arms on firm surface
36″ hop hands on hips on firm surface
12″ hop allowed to use arms on foam surface
12″ hop hands on hips on foam surface
18″ hop allowed to use arms on foam surface
18″ hop hands on hips on foam surface
27″ hop allowed to use arms on foam surface
27″ hop hands on hips on foam surface
36″ hop allowed to use arms on foam surface
36″ hop hands on hips on foam surface

Subjects cannot advance to next level in each category until they demonstrate 3 sets of repetitions all error free. Errors include:
1. Touching down with non-stance limb
2. Bracing the non-stance limb against the stance limb
3. Excessive trunk motion (>30° lateral flexion)
4. Missing the target
5. Moving the stance foot from its landing position during stabilization
6. Removal of hands from hips during hands on hips activities

Exercise 6: Hop to Stabilization and Reach

Object: Hop to the target landing on the involved limb, stabilize yourself while maintaining balance in single-limb stance, reach with non-stance limb back to starting point (as in Exercise 3). Hop back to the starting point, again landing and stabilizing on involved limb, reach with non-stance limb back to previous target, repeat.

Duration: 3 sets of 5 repetitions in each of 4 directions (A/P, M/L, AM/PL, AL/PM)

Progression:

For each direction:
12″ allowed to use arms on firm surface
12″ hands on hips on firm surface
18″ allowed to use arms on firm surface
18″ hands on hips on firm surface
27″ allowed to use arms on firm surface
27″ hands on hips on firm surface
36″ allowed to use arms on firm surface
36″ hands on hips on firm surface
12″ allowed to use arms on foam surface
12″ hands on hips on foam surface
18″ allowed to use arms on foam surface
18″ hands on hips on foam surface
27″ allowed to use arms on foam surface
27″ hands on hips on foam surface
36″ allowed to use arms on foam surface
36″ hands on hips on foam surface

Subjects cannot advance to next level in each category until they demonstrate 3 sets of repetitions all error free. Errors include:
1. Touching down with reach limb other than for the prescribed reach
2. Bracing the non-stance limb against the stance limb
3. Excessive trunk motion (>30° lateral flexion)
4. Missing the target
5. Moving the stance foot from its landing position during stabilization
6. Removal of hands from hips during hands-on-hips activities

Fig. 34.4, cont'd

CONCLUSION

This chapter has highlighted the best practices for prevention of hamstring strains, ACL injuries in female athletes, and ankle sprains. Clinicians must use their best judgment when determining the need for implementing injury prevention initiatives with specific athletes and teams. It is critical that the sports medicine team consult with coaches and athletes about the best ways to incorporate injury prevention interventions into existing training programs to achieve maximum "buy-in" from all stakeholders.

ACKNOWLEDGMENT

We acknowledge the scholarly work of Roald Bahr and Adam Shimer, who were coauthors on a chapter on "Injury Prevention" that appeared in a previous edition of this book and served as a foundation for the current chapter.

For a complete list of references, go to ExpertConsult.com.

SELECTED READINGS

Citation:
Goode AP, Reiman MP, Harris L, et al. Eccentric training for prevention of hamstring injuries may depend on intervention compliance: a systematic review and meta-analysis. *Br J Sports Med.* 2015;49(6):349–356.

Level of Evidence:
I

Summary:
This meta-analysis of clinical trials concluded that eccentric strengthening, with good compliance, was successful in prevention of hamstring injury.

Citation:
Kaminski TW, Hertel J, Amendola N, et al. National athletic trainers' association position statement: conservative management and prevention of ankle sprains in athletes. *J Athl Train.* 2013;48(4):528–545.

Level of Evidence:
I

Summary:
This expert consensus statement concluded that both lace-up and semirigid ankle braces and traditional ankle taping are effective in reducing the rate of recurrent ankle sprains in athletes, and that injury-prevention programs lasting at least 3 months focusing on balance and neuromuscular control reduce the risk of ankle injury in athletes.

Citation:
Padua DA, DiStefano LJ, Hewett TE, et al. National Athletic Trainers' Association position statement: prevention of anterior cruciate ligament injury. *J Athl Train.* 2018;53(1):5–19.

Level of Evidence:
I

Summary:
This expert consensus statement concluded that multicomponent injury-prevention training programs consisting of strength, plyometrics, agility, balance, and flexibility exercises are recommended for reducing noncontact and indirect-contact ACL injuries, as well as other knee injuries during physical activity.

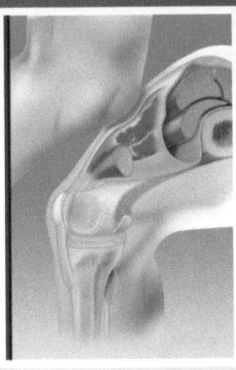

35

Return to Activity and Sport After Injury

J. Craig Garrison, Joseph Hannon

With sports participation comes an inherent risk of injury. In 2017, a summary report on the National High School Sports-Related Injury Surveillance Study for the school year of 2016–17 estimated that 7.9 million students participated in high school sports, with approximately 1.16 million injuries across the United States.[1] Based on this report, the overall injury rate in all high school sports combined was 2.09 injuries per 1000 athlete exposures. Similarly, according to a National Institute of Arthritis and Musculoskeletal and Skin Diseases report, there were more than 2.6 million children younger than 19 years of age who were treated in emergency departments for musculoskeletal injuries due to sport participation.[2,3] In the collegiate setting, Kay et al.[4] reported the number of severe (missing >3 weeks of participation) injuries across 25 National Collegiate Athletic Association (NCAA) sports from 2009 through 2015 to be as high as 3183 injuries over this time, which resulted in an injury rate of 0.66 per 1000 athletic exposures. These statistics help describe the current risk athletes face when participating in sports. While risk exists with sports participation, there are also many physical and psychological benefits that come from sports participation.[5,6] However, previous injuries have been shown over and over again to be a risk factor for future injuries.[7] This creates a challenging situation for sports medicine providers, as safely and successfully returning athletes to sports is generally the long-term goal for patients and providers.

The following chapter is meant to provide a brief overview of the current literature regarding return to sports (RTS) following injury.

Arguably one of the most researched orthopaedic injuries is the anterior cruciate ligament (ACL) injury. In the past 5 years there have been almost 600 review articles published on the topic of ACL injuries, and 50 specifically on the topic of RTS following ACL injury. Despite the plethora of research on the topic, the success of returning to sport following this injury is fair at best. There are variations on what is considered a successful RTS, as the definition of "success" varies among reports. These variations help explain the wide range of data reported in the literature, which currently ranges from 33% to 92% of individuals returning to sport following ACL injury.[8–12] In a systematic review and meta-analysis, Ardern and colleagues[13] reviewed 48 studies with a total subject pool of 5770. They reported that at an average of 3.5 years following ACL reconstruction (ACL-R), 82% of participants returned to some sports participation, 63% had returned to their pre-injury level of participation, and 44%

had returned to competitive sport at an average final follow-up of 41.5 months. One of the contributing factors to the current return-to-sport data is the high rate of re-injury associated with returning to sport following ACL injury. A systematic review by Wiggins et al.[14] reported on the risk of secondary injury following primary ACL injury in young athletes. Nineteen studies were included in the review, with a total number of 72,054 subjects pooled across the studies. Overall, the total second ACL re-injury rate was 15%, with an ipsilateral re-injury rate of 7%, and contralateral injury rate of 8%. The secondary ACL injury rate (ipsilateral and contralateral) for patients younger than 25 years was 21%, and the secondary ACL injury rate for athletes who returned to a sport was 20%. Combining these risk factors, athletes younger than 25 years who returned to sport had a secondary ACL injury rate of 23%.[14] Similarly, Webster et al.[15] examined the second injury risk in those patients less than 20 years of age and found a 29% injury rate (ipsilateral + contralateral) within 5 years following primary ACL reconstruction.

As a result of the high risk of re-injury in the ACL population, there is a need for a comprehensive overview of principles that help guide the clinician's decision-making process for returning an athlete to sport. For the purposes of this review, the ACL rehabilitation model will be used as an example of specific guidelines and criteria that require consideration when determining an athlete's readiness for RTS. Once the athlete is able to demonstrate foundational strength of the lower extremity (quadriceps, hamstrings, gluteals, gastrocnemius-soleus complex, etc.), normalized joint ranges of motion at the hip, knee, and ankle, core stability,[16] and the ability to jog/run without noticeable deviations,[17,18] multifactorial functional testing should be administered. Key factors for consideration include a functional testing algorithm (FTA)[17] or test battery[18] involving strength,[19–21] power,[20,21] balance or proprioception,[22,23] movement quality during athletic movements,[24,25] fear of reinjury assessment,[26–28] patient-reported outcomes,[19,29] and limb symmetry indices (LSI).[30]

First, restoration of range of motion (ROM) is imperative. This includes hip, knee, and ankle ROM, as all have been examined in a variety of lower extremity injuries. For example, decreased ankle dorsiflexion (Fig. 35.1) has been associated with increased knee valgus position during landing, which can contribute to a variety of knee injuries.[31,32] In particular, the lack of ankle dorsiflexion may alter lower extremity movement patterns[33] and has been demonstrated to have a relationship with ACL tears.[34] Restoration of knee extension ROM is considered to be important

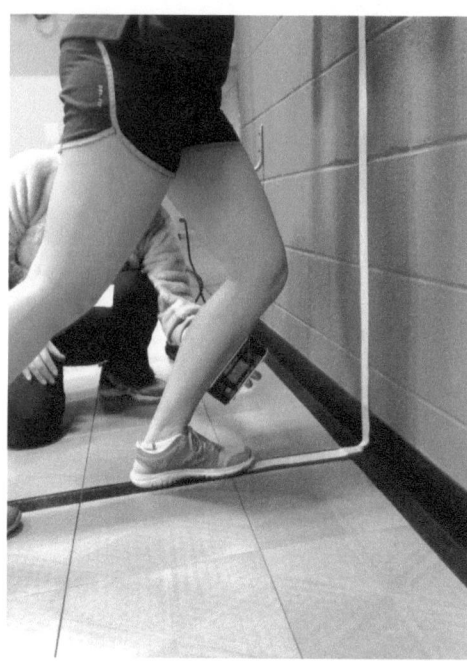

Fig. 35.1 Measurement of ankle dorsiflexion range of motion. The ankle is placed in a subtalar neutral position and the foot is aligned with a line marked on the floor. The line on the floor will be continuous with a line marked on the wall. The participant is instructed to bring the testing knee toward the line on the wall until he or she feels the ankle no longer goes into dorsiflexion without lifting the heel off the ground. The investigator places the top of the long base of the inclinometer on the tibial tuberosity to read the angle from the vertical line. The angle between the tibia and the vertical line is recorded.

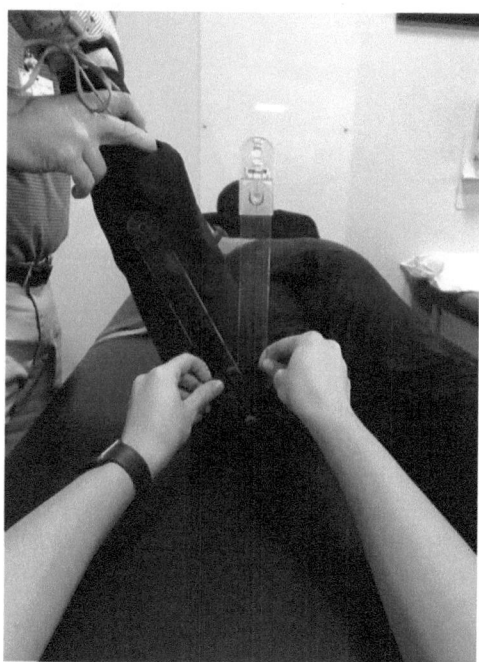

Fig. 35.2 Measurement of hip range of motion (ROM). Participant lays prone on the table with the knee flexed to 90 degrees while the investigator stabilizes the hip and passively moves the lower extremity through full internal and external ROM stopping just prior to movement at the hip.

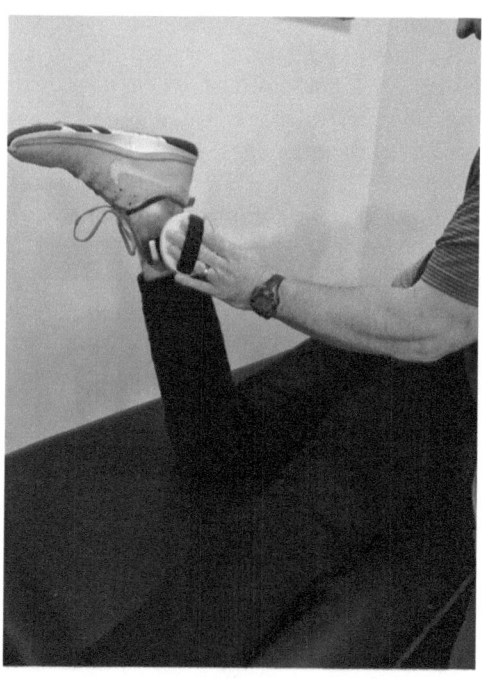

Fig. 35.3 Measurement of hip external rotator strength using a handheld dynamometer. Participant lays prone on the table with the knee flexed to 90 degrees while the investigator stabilizes the hip and places the dynamometer just superior to the medial malleolus. The participant is instructed to rotate the lower leg toward the midline of his or her body with maximal effort while the investigator meets the resistance of the moving lower leg.

following ACL-R in both the early and late stages of the rehabilitation process.[35,36] Decreased knee extension ROM following ACL injuries has been found to be a contributing factor to re-injury and to the development of osteoarthritis at a 20-year follow-up.[37] Decreased hip ROM (Fig. 35.2) has been found to correlate with hip, knee, and low back pain,[38–40] and may be associated with ACL injury.[41–43] In summary, restoration of ROM of the entire lower extremity to be equal to or similar to the uninvolved side should be an expectation prior to return-to-sports clearance.

In addition to ROM, restoration of lower extremity strength is considered a staple in return-to-sports testing. Deficits in gluteals, quadriceps, and hamstrings muscle strength have been shown to be correlated with changes in lower extremity kinematics and in some cases may be attributed as risk factors for both initial injury and re-injury.[44–48] The use of handheld dynamometry (Fig. 35.3) and isokinetic testing (Fig. 35.4) provides a more accurate means of muscle strength testing and should be encouraged over manual muscle testing when available. A 90% quadriceps and hamstrings limb symmetry index (LSI = involved limb/uninvolved limb × 100) at the time of RTS has been suggested as the minimal acceptable cutoff as a passing score for RTS, while some suggest a symmetry of 100% as an acceptable cutoff.[17,21] In addition to normalizing strength LSI, normalizing agonist and antagonist muscle function around the joint should also be considered. In the context of the ACL, this is typically looked at in the framework of quadriceps to hamstrings ratios. Literature recommends a ratio greater than 55% for females and greater than 62.5% for males as a minimum passing score for

RTS.[49,50] While the current review is using the ACL as a framework for this discussion, this concept can be extrapolated to the shoulder, where maintaining adequate shoulder external rotator to internal rotator cuff strength (66% to 75% ratio) may help minimize injury and/or re-injury risk.[51]

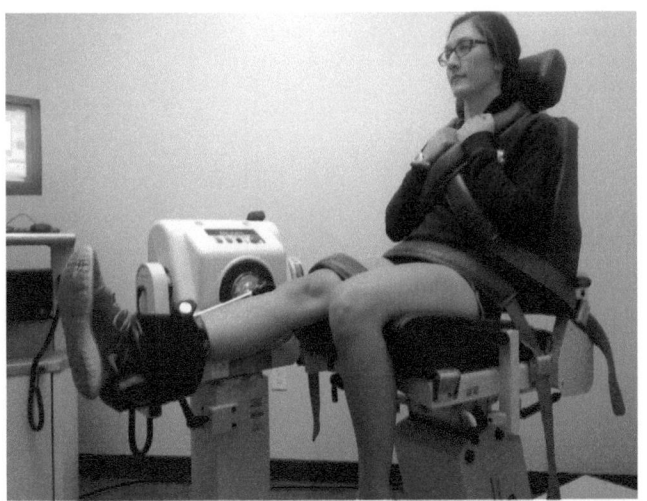

Fig. 35.4 Isokinetic strength testing. The participant is seated on the isokinetic dynamometer and secured with padded straps around the thigh, pelvis, and torso to minimize accessory and compensatory movements during testing. The participant is instructed to either push (knee extension) or pull (knee flexion) against the arm of the dynamometer with maximal effort for a total of five repetitions. Isokinetic testing is often ordered at 60 degrees/s and 180 degrees/s for both the quadriceps and hamstrings. A symmetry index of 90% or greater (involved limb/uninvolved limb) is considered acceptable for return to sport. In addition, the time to peak torque should be examined as this is a measure of how long it takes for each limb to produce the highest peak value during the test. If the peak torque value is similar or the same between limbs, but the involved limb takes twice as long to produce that force, this should be noted as an inability for the participant to produce force quickly, which is needed for dynamic athletic movements.

In conjunction with lower extremity ROM and strength, it is important to assess a patient's ability to produce power. This is especially important in sports that require quick and explosive movements. Assessing power has historically been done through the use of hop testing. Numerous jump tests are utilized throughout the literature including single hop,[52–54] triple hop,[52,54,55] crossover hop,[54,56,57] and timed hop.[54,55,57] Overall, a 90% LSI between limbs is considered to be acceptable and may be used as criteria for RTS.[56,58–60] There are many limitations to these tests, including the lack of assessment for movement quality and potential compensation strategies that patients may utilize as a means to complete the test; however, these tests (Fig. 35.5) are well supported in the literature and should be incorporated as part of a comprehensive evaluation when considering return to sport following ACL-R.[21]

Beyond the aforementioned criteria for RTS, movement quality should be considered, as numerous studies support the notion that poor lower extremity balance and movement patterns are associated with primary and secondary injury.[24,61–65] For example, performance on the Y-Balance Test has been shown to be an accurate screening tool for injury in numerous populations.[65–67] A cutoff of 94% composite score is considered the minimal acceptable threshold for passing this test, as scores below this threshold have been associated with increased injury risk.[65] Furthermore, anterior reach asymmetry on the Y-Balance Test (Fig. 35.6) has been shown to be correlated with performance during return to sport testing,[23] and a side-to-side asymmetry greater than 4 cm is considered a higher risk for lower extremity injury.[67]

In the ACL-R population at time of RTS, participants have previously demonstrated an anterior reach (ANT) of 97% LSI with individual components of 65% of leg length (LL) for ANT, 99% LL for posteromedial (PM), and 94% LL for posterolateral (PL).[22] Beyond the Y-Balance Test, additional screening tools should be applied for assessment of movement quality during dynamic activities. The jump-landing task has been used as a lower extremity screening tool, and performance on this task is associated with primary and secondary injury.[24] The most commonly used assessment of the jump-landing task is through the use of the Landing Error Scoring System (LESS).[24] This test is commonly utilized in the literature as a screening tool for lower extremity injury and is well supported as both an injury risk screen and return-to-sports test.[24,68,69] Deficits of decreased knee flexion, increased knee valgus positioning, and decreased trunk control during this task have been associated with primary and secondary ACL injury.[24,68,69] Overall, demonstration of asymmetry between limbs during dynamic movements could be harmful and should be given consideration.

As sporting movements tend to require the athlete to move in multiple directions, an assessment of movement in multiple planes is warranted. The Vail Sport Test assesses dynamic movements in multiple planes of motion and requires the athlete to move through both the frontal and sagittal planes while continuing to demonstrate vertical excursions.[25] Four components comprise the Vail Sport Test, and include single leg squat for 3 minutes, lateral bounding for 90 seconds, and forward/backward jogging for 2 minutes each. After each component, the participant is given 2.5 minutes of rest prior to proceeding to the next task.[25] Finally, the Vail Sport Test also incorporates external perturbation to the athlete during the testing procedure through the use of sport cord resistance. This test has been shown to be reliable and is recommended as part of a return-to-sport test battery with a passing score of at least 46/54.[25] Likewise, if a clinician has the capabilities for assessment of dynamic movement using 3D motion capture (Fig. 35.7) at time of return to sport, this information may provide in-depth analysis of an athlete's potential movement strategies that may be compensatory in nature and contribute to future injury.[64,70,71] Previous research has demonstrated that deficits in core stability,[72] high knee abduction angles and moments,[64,73] and low knee flexion angles[73] may place one at a greater risk for ACL injury. The use of 3D motion capture has previously been used at 6 months postoperative ACL-R and time of RTS, and findings of decreased knee flexion angles during gait,[74] running,[75] and landing[76] have been demonstrated. Furthermore, ACL-R individuals who were tested at time of RTS and demonstrated increased knee valgus, deficits in hip external rotation muscle torque, and asymmetries in knee moments during landing activities were at a significantly higher risk for a second ACL injury.[64] As such, the use of 3D motion capture can be a useful tool in determining an athlete's readiness for return to sport following ACL-R.

In addition to the previously mentioned objective measurements of physical performance, assessment of the athlete on a cognitive level is also warranted. Successfully returning to sport following ACL injury at 12 months postsurgery has been linked to a positive psychological state.[26] Prior research has established that psychological readiness to return to sport and recreation

Diagrammatic representation of the series of 4 hop tests: single hop for distance, 6-m timed hop, triple hop for distance, and crossover hop for distance.

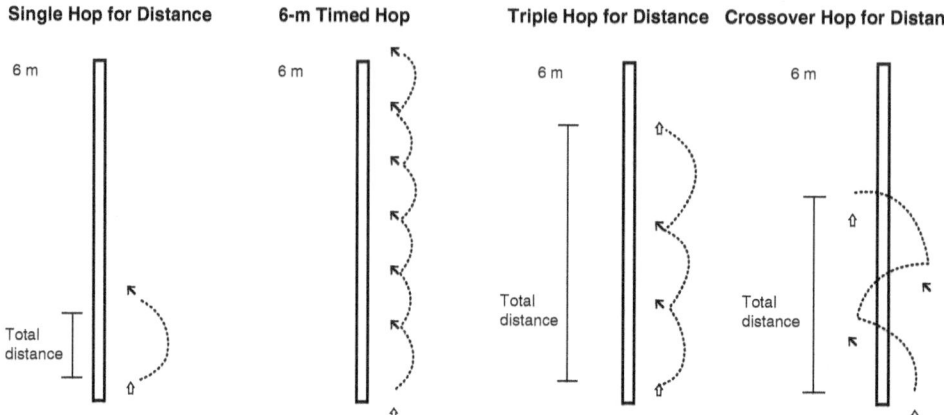

Physical Therapy
Journal of the American Physical Therapy Association

Fig. 35.5 Hop tests. *Single hop for distance*—The participant is instructed to stand on the limb to be tested and to hop off that limb with maximal effort while landing on the same limb. *6-m timed hop*—The participant is instructed to stand on the limb to be tested and to hop off that limb while performing repeated hops for the total distance as quickly as possible. *Triple hop for distance*—The participant is instructed to stand on the limb to be tested and to hop off that limb with maximal effort for three consecutive hops. *Crossover hop for distance*—The participant is instructed to stand on the limb to be tested and to hop off that limb with maximal effort for three consecutive hops while alternating crossing over a mark on the floor. For each hop test, the total distance covered during the hopping motion is recorded while the time taken to cover the 6 m is recorded for the timed hop. (Reid A, Birmingham TB, Stratford PW, Alcock GK, Giffin JR. Hop testing provides a reliable and valid outcome measure during rehabilitation after anterior cruciate ligament reconstruction. *Phys Ther.* 2007;87[3]:337–349.)

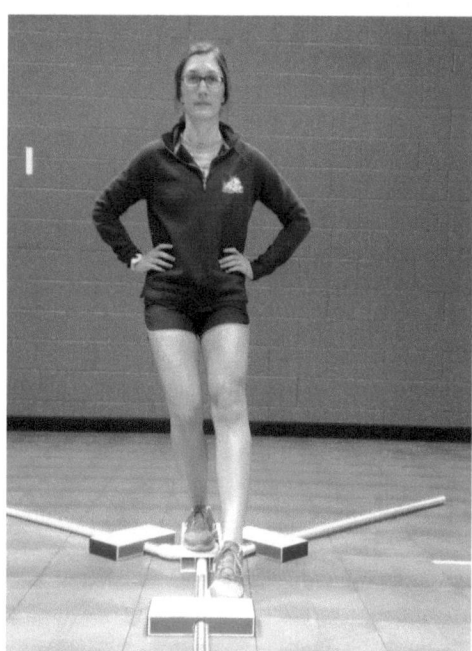

Fig. 35.6 Y-balance test anterior reach. The participant is instructed to perform a single limb stance on the extremity being tested while reaching outside their base of support with the uninvolved limb to push a reach indicator box along the measurement pipe.

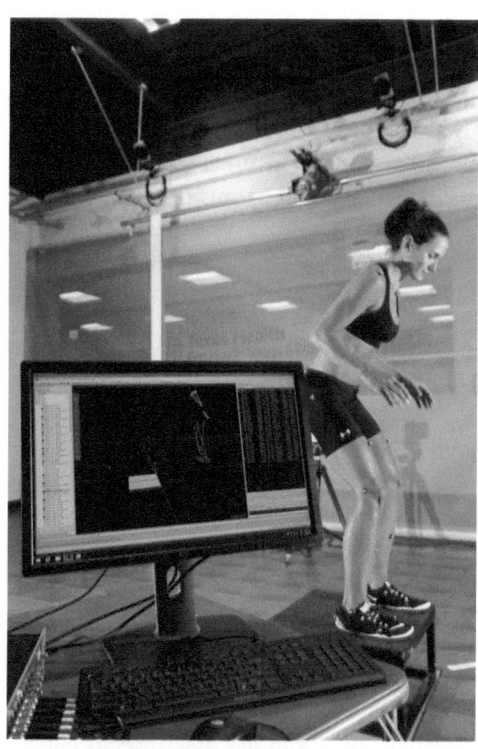

Fig. 35.7 3D motion capture of dynamic movement. Dynamic movements that replicate athletic movements seen on the field or court of play can be tested in the motion capture lab. Tasks such as box drop jump landings, forward hops, lateral hops, and cutting maneuvers can all be tested to determine a participant's quality of movement. Key indicators of faulty movement patterns include increased knee valgus angles and joint moments, decreased knee flexion angles, and overall asymmetry between limbs during the landing phase of the movement.

was the factor most strongly associated with returning to the preinjury activity.[77] One scale that is used to measure an athlete's psychological state at time of RTS following ACL-R is the ACL-Return to Sport After Injury (ACL-RSI) scale.[28,60] The ACL-RSI has been shown to be reliable and valid in a population of athletes considering a return to sport following ACL-R. The scale may be effective in discriminating between general confidence in returning to the sport and confidence in the injured knee with returning to sport.[28] Similarly, the ACL-RSI has demonstrated utility in predicting capabilities of returning to sport following ACL-R from a psychological perspective with those scoring greater than 76 returning at a higher rate.[78] These studies indicate that patient perception and patient self-rating may play a large role in achieving successful outcomes. The International Knee Documentation Committee short form (IKDC) is used throughout the literature as a patient reported outcome following injury.[60] The possible score of the IKDC ranges from 0 to 100, with a higher score indicating a higher level of functioning. The IKDC has been shown to be correlated with functional outcome measures such as quadriceps strength,[19,79,80] hop tests,[81,82] and has also been shown to have good psychometric properties, making it an ideal patient-reported outcome.[83–85] Furthermore, the IKDC has been shown to discriminate between successful and nonsuccessful performance on return-to-sport testing, with scores greater than 90 having more success.[29,86]

The final consideration that needs to be made when faced with the challenge of returning an athlete to sport is the principle of progressive loading. This basic principle is founded in physical training and at its simplest requires a gradual increase in volume, intensity, frequency, or time in order to achieve the targeted goal.[87] In the context of returning to sport, these principles must be balanced across rehabilitation, strength and conditioning,

practices and games to maintain a progressive overall load until a successful return has been achieved.[88,89] The concept of acute load (all physical activity done in a 1 week time frame) should be balanced with the chronic load (all physical activity done over the past 4 weeks). When spikes in acute load occur above what the chronic load has been, the risk of injury significantly increases (Fig. 35.8).[88] This concept of load needs to be considered by all members of the sports medicine team, and proper communication between disciplines is paramount to correctly managing load as an athlete prepares for return to sport. In general, an acute to chronic training load that falls between 0.8 and 1.3 (i.e., loads are approximately equal) carries a relatively low risk of injury.[88,90] When the training load exceeds 1.5, then athletes may be at a greater risk of suffering injury (Fig. 35.9).

CONCLUSION

The previous discussion outlines a thorough overview of components that need to be considered from a physical and psychological standpoint when considering return to activity following injury (Table 35.1). While this discussion focused on ACL injury, the principles of assessing ROM, strength, power, movement quality, and psychological readiness can and should be extrapolated to any athlete returning to activity/sport following injury.

For a complete list of references, go to ExpertConsult.com.

SELECTED READINGS

Citation:
Davies GJ, McCarty E, Provencher M, et al. ACL return to sport guidelines and criteria. *Curr Rev Musculoskelet Med.* 2017;10(7):307–314.

TABLE 35.1 Return to Sport Considerations Following Anterior Cruciate Ligament Reconstruction

ROM	• ROM of hip, knee, and ankle equal to or similar to the uninvolved side. Goal of side to side symmetry
• Hip	• Decreased hip IR associated with ACL injury[41–43]
• Knee	• ≤5 degrees side-to-side difference in knee extension[35,36]
• Ankle	• Ankle DF deficits alter lower extremity movement patterns and are associated with ACL injury[33,34]
Strength	• 90% or greater LSI of quadriceps and hamstrings at time of RTS[17,21]
• Quadriceps	• Quadriceps to Hamstrings ratio at time of RTS: >55% for females, and >62.5% for males[49,50]
• Hamstrings	• 90% or greater LSI of gluteals at time of RTS
• Gluteals	
Power	• 90% or greater LSI at time of RTS[56,58,59]
• Hop Tests	
Movement Quality	• <94% Y-Balance Test composite score related to increase risk of lower extremity injury[64]
• Y-Balance Test	• Y-Balance Test side to side anterior reach >4 cm related to increase risk of lower extremity injury[64,66]
• LESS	• Y-Balance Test anterior reach LSI of 97% with 65% of LL for anterior, 99% of LL for posteromedial, and 94% of LL for posterolateral[22]
• Vail Sport Test	• LESS score >6 = poor; LESS score ≤4 = excellent[24]
• 3D Motion Capture	• 46/54 passing score for RTS[25]
	• Assessment of increased knee valgus angles and moments,[63,72] and decreased knee flexion angles[72–75] during dynamic activities that may lead to increased risk of injury or re-injury

This table provides objective measurements for the clinician to consider prior to making a decision about the participant's ability to return to sport. These factors should be considered within the context of other variables such as patient-reported outcomes (IKDC, ACL-RSI) and acute to chronic workload ratio.
ACL, Anterior cruciate ligament; *IR,* internal rotation; *LL,* leg length; *LESS,* landing error scoring system; *LSI,* limb symmetry indices; *ROM,* range of motion; *RSI,* Return to Sport After Injury.

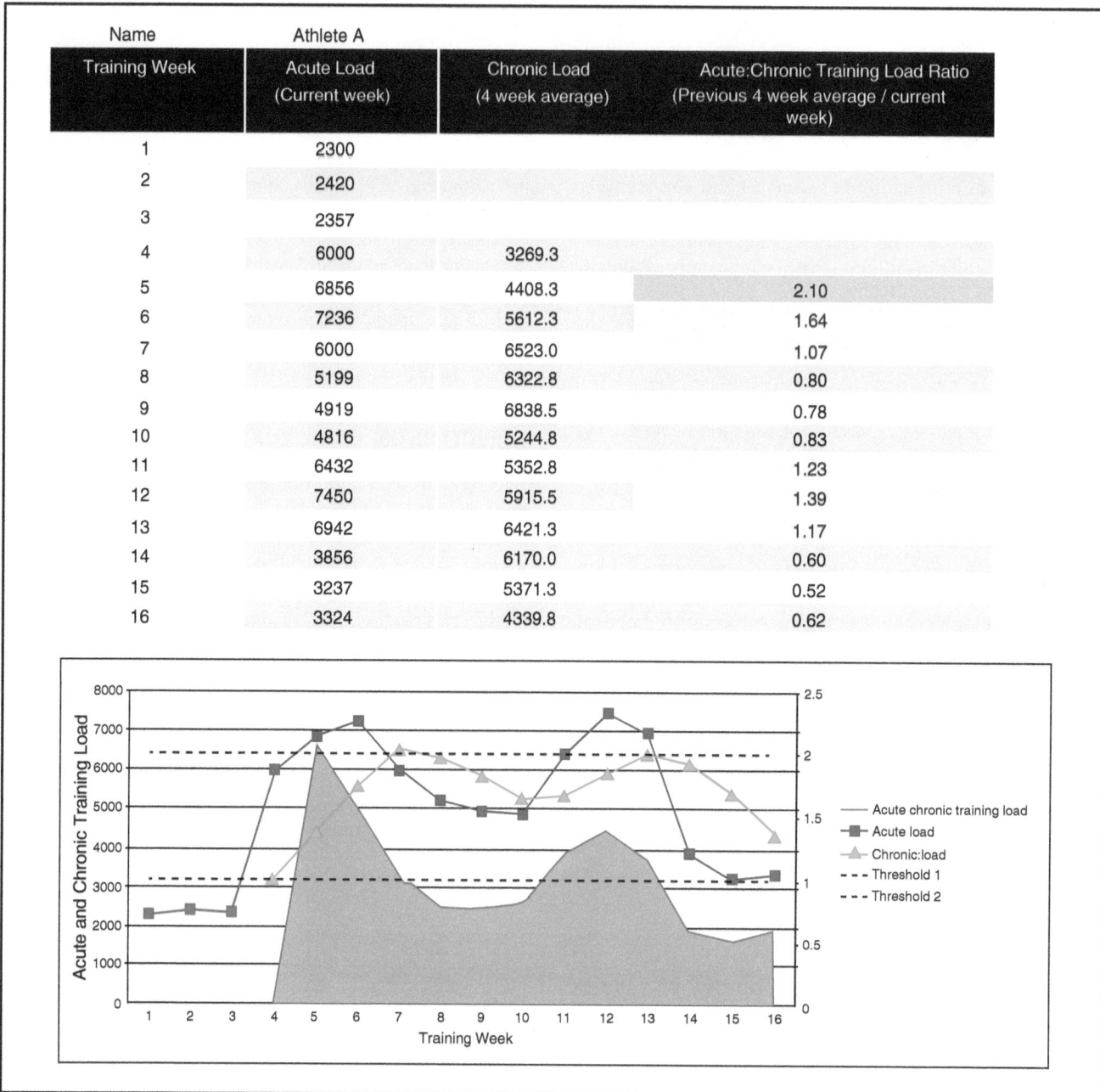

Name	Athlete A		
Training Week	Acute Load (Current week)	Chronic Load (4 week average)	Acute:Chronic Training Load Ratio (Previous 4 week average / current week)
1	2300		
2	2420		
3	2357		
4	6000	3269.3	
5	6856	4408.3	2.10
6	7236	5612.3	1.64
7	6000	6523.0	1.07
8	5199	6322.8	0.80
9	4919	6838.5	0.78
10	4816	5244.8	0.83
11	6432	5352.8	1.23
12	7450	5915.5	1.39
13	6942	6421.3	1.17
14	3856	6170.0	0.60
15	3237	5371.3	0.52
16	3324	4339.8	0.62

Fig. 35.8 Acute versus chronic training load. This table represents an example of a 16-week training load schedule for both the Acute (current week) and Chronic (4 weeks average) phases. The training load is calculated by multiplying the number of minutes in which participation in the activity occurred (internal load) and/or the external load (i.e., distance covered, balls thrown or hit, jumps, etc.) by the rating of perceived exertion (RPE) of the participant during the activity. This calculation provides the weekly value for total training load. The acute to chronic workload ratio can be calculated by dividing the current week's training load by the previous 4 weeks' training load average (acute load/chronic load).

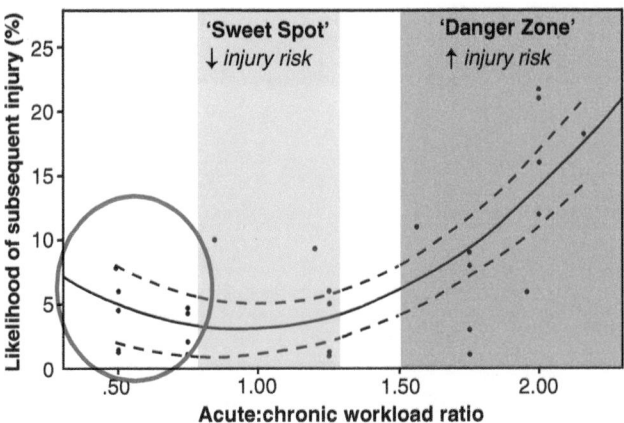

Fig. 35.9 Acute to chronic workload ratio. In general, this ratio should be close to 1.0. An acute to chronic training load that falls between 0.8 and 1.3 (i.e., loads are approximately equal) carries a relatively low risk of injury, while a training load that exceeds 1.5 may represent a greater risk of suffering injury.

Level of Evidence:

V

Summary:

This article provides functional clinical insight into evidence-based criteria that can be used to identify when an individual is ready to return to sport following anterior cruciate ligament reconstruction. An overview of functional tests is framed within an algorithm that helps clinicians qualitatively and quantitatively make clinical decisions.

Citation:

Ardern CL, Webster KE, Taylor NF, et al. Return to sport following anterior cruciate ligament reconstruction surgery: a systematic review and meta-analysis of the state of play. *Br J Sports Med.* 2011;45(7):596–606.

Level of Evidence:

I

Summary:

This meta-analysis and systematic review describes key factors that determine readiness for return to sport following anterior cruciate ligament reconstruction. These findings are based on objective data from more than 5500 participants who were attempting a return to sport. In addition, the results suggest that return-to-sport levels are not as successful as one might believe, and one of the factors that is lacking might involve a psychological component.

Citation:

Welling W, Benjaminse A, Seil R, et al. Low rates of patients meeting return to sport criteria 9 months after anterior cruciate ligament reconstruction: a prospective longitudinal study. *Knee Surg Sports Traumatol Arthrosc.* 2018. doi:10.1007/s00167-018-4916-4.

Level of Evidence:

III

Summary:

An overview of objective and subjective changes that occur in individuals from 6 to 9 months following anterior cruciate ligament reconstruction suggests that time may play an important factor in successful return to sport. This article highlights the lack of readiness of return to sport in patients who have undergone anterior cruciate ligament reconstruction secondary to deficits in quadriceps strength and patient-reported perception of function.

Shoulder

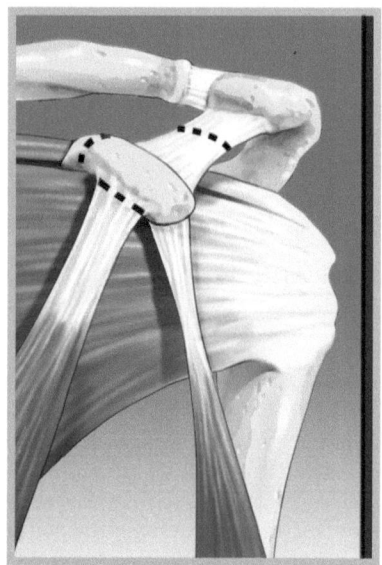

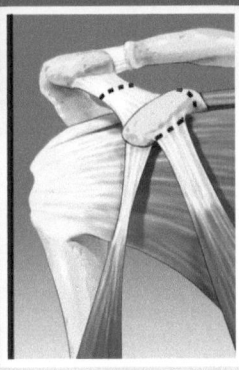

36

Shoulder Anatomy and Biomechanics

Timothy S. Mologne

The shoulder can really be considered a complex (Fig. 36.1), consisting of four joints or articulations (all with important stabilizing ligaments), two spaces, and more than 30 muscles and their respective tendons. The shoulder complex is an intricate structure that requires synchronized/orchestral-type motions/movements to function properly. A thorough understanding of the anatomy and complex biomechanics of the shoulder is helpful to clinicians in diagnosing disorders, applying appropriate surgical procedures, and implementing proper rehabilitation protocols.

PERTINENT BONY ANATOMY

The proximal humerus consists of the humeral head and articular surface, the greater and lesser tuberosities, which are the attachment sites for the rotator cuff muscles, and the humeral shaft. Between the tuberosities is the bicipital groove, the location of the tendon of the long head of the biceps brachii muscle, as it exits the glenohumeral joint. The articular cartilage on the humeral head has been shown to vary from 0.2 to 2.0 mm and is thickest in the central portion of the humeral head.[1] Multiple anatomic and radiologic studies have been performed in an attempt to better define the relationships and geometry of the various parts of the proximal humerus, glenoid, and glenohumeral joint.[2–8] Different measuring techniques and reference points make comparisons between the studies difficult. The inclination of the humeral head articular surface, as referenced to the humeral canal, varies from 30 to 55 degrees.[3,6–8] The mean radius of curvature of the humeral head is 24 ± 1.2 mm but can be as much as 30 mm.[4] The superior-most portion of the humeral head is a mean of 8 mm higher than the greater tuberosity. This relationship varies between men and woman but is proportional to the radius of curvature of the articular surface.[4] Retroversion of the humeral head, in reference to the center of the humeral canal, has been shown to be quite variable, ranging from 0 to 55 degrees (Fig. 36.2).[6,7,9] Medial and posterior offset of the humeral head is variable with reference to the humeral shaft.[3,6–8,10]

The scapula is a relatively flat, triangular-shaped bone that is positioned on the posterolateral aspect of the thorax at the level of the second and seventh ribs. The scapula has three angles—superior, inferior, and lateral. The lateral angle, formed by the superior and lateral borders of the scapula, gives rise to the glenoid. Anatomic variants at the superior angle are sometimes the cause of snapping scapula syndrome.[11] The scapular spine divides the dorsal aspect into the supraspinatus and infraspinatus fossa. The subscapularis fossa is located on the ventral or anterior portion of the scapular body. Several muscles originate on the scapula, namely the supraspinatus, infraspinatus, subscapularis, teres major and minor, triceps, and deltoid muscles. Several other important muscles insert on the scapula: the serratus anterior, levator scapulae, rhomboid major and minor, trapezius, pectoralis minor, short head of the biceps brachii, and coracobrachialis muscles.

The scapula has two processes or projections: the coracoid and the acromion. The coracoid projects from the superior and lateral aspect and projects anteriorly and laterally. The mean distance from the coracoid tip to the anterior border of the coracoclavicular ligament can vary from 22 to 28 mm.[12,13] The mean width of the coracoid is 15.9 mm, and the mean thickness is 10.4 mm.[13] The use of the coracoid as an extension of the glenoid for shoulder stabilization procedures is well described[14,15] and has, once again, become a treatment option for patients with glenohumeral instability and bone deficiencies. The acromion process is the lateral and anterior extension of the scapular spine. The anteroinferior aspect of the acromion serves as the attachment site for the coracoacromial ligament (Fig. 36.3). The morphology of the acromion has been studied, and some correlations have been made between aggressive anterior acromial hooks/spurs and rotator cuff tears.[16–20] Some evidence indicates that the coracoacromial ligament helps provide superior stability to the glenohumeral joint.[21,22] The lateral portion of the coracoacromial ligament has been found to have decreased mechanical properties, is shorter in length, and has a larger cross-sectional area in patients with rotator cuff tears.[19] Resection of the coracoacromial ligament can lead to anterosuperior humeral head escape in patients with massive rotator cuff tears. Biomechanical studies have shown that the rotator cuff becomes closest to the undersurface of the acromion between 60 and 120 degrees.[23] The subacromial bursa is located in the anterior portion of the subacromial space and is under the coracoacromial arch and deltoid. The bursa helps reduce friction between the coracoacromial arch and the rotator cuff when the arm is elevated but can be impinged under the acromion in certain conditions. The bursa has significant nerve endings, including Ruffini endings, Pacinian corpuscles, and free nerve endings,[24,25] and is a source of pain in the subacromial space.

Just medial to the coracoid and anterior to the supraspinatus fossa is the suprascapular notch of the scapula. As the suprascapular nerve travels from the upper trunk of the brachial plexus,

Shoulder

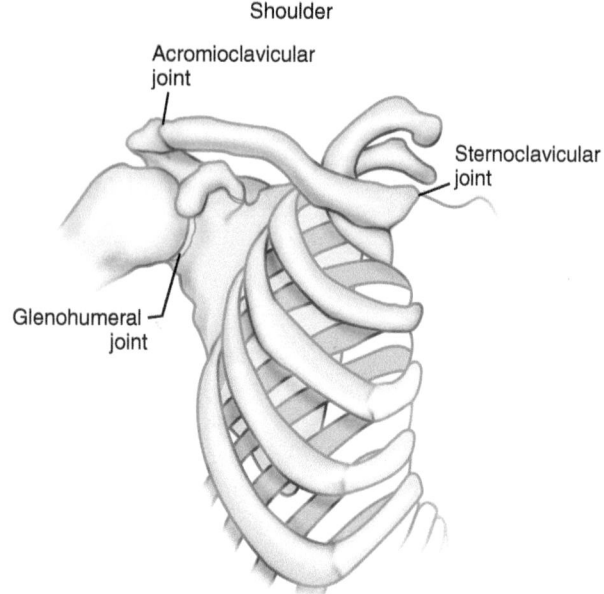

Fig. 36.1 The shoulder complex consists of the glenohumeral, acromioclavicular, and sternoclavicular joints, along with the scapulothoracic articulation.

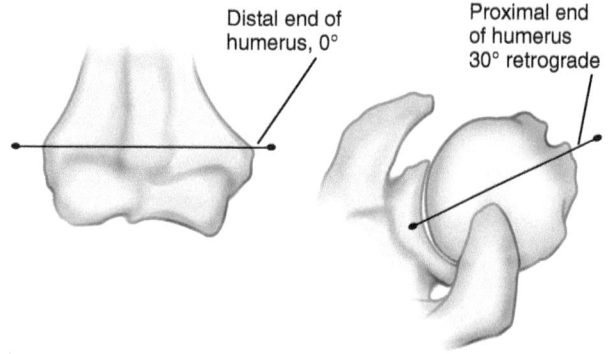

Fig. 36.2 With respect to the epicondylar axis of the distal humerus, the humeral head articular surface is retroverted from 0 to 55 degrees, averaging 30 degrees.

Acromioclavicular joint

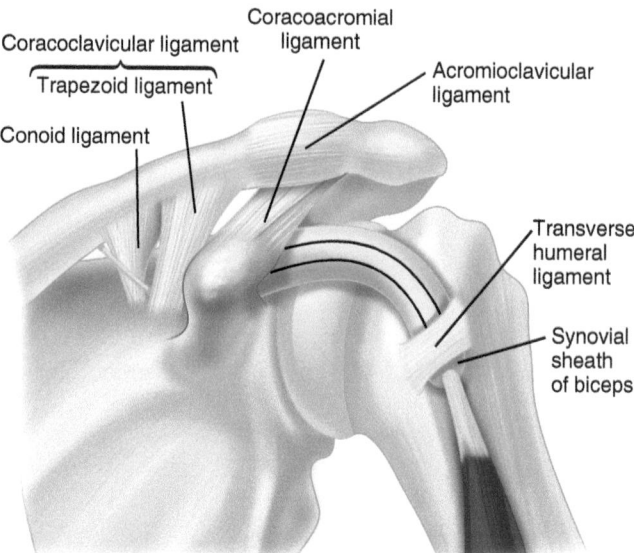

Fig. 36.3 An anterior view of the shoulder demonstrating the coracoclavicular ligaments, acromioclavicular joint, coracoacromial ligament, and transverse humeral ligament.

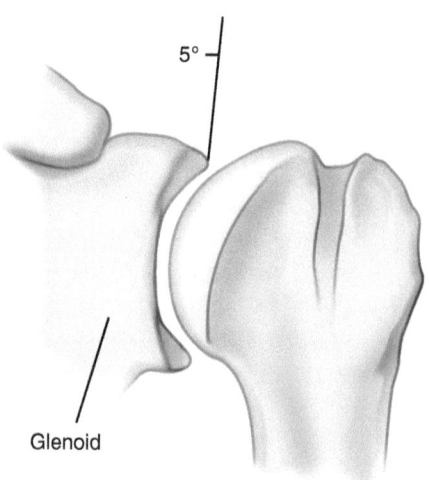

Fig. 36.4 Relative to the plane of the scapula, the fossa is angled slightly inferior and posterior, offering little bony support to inferior instability with the arm at the side.

it enters this notch prior to innervating the supraspinatus. The nerve branches to innervate the supraspinatus within 1 cm of the notch.[26] The superior transverse scapular ligament is the roof of the suprascapular notch. Anatomic studies have shown that the notch is U-shaped in three-fourths of specimens. The superior transverse scapular ligament can be partially or completely ossified in some people.[27]

The lateral angle of the scapula is the location of the glenoid. The glenoid has an average of 5 degrees of superior tilt, referencing the scapula (Fig. 36.4).[28] The superior slope to the glenoid plays a role in preventing inferior subluxation of the humerus. The glenoid is also retroverted with respect to the transverse axis of the scapula. Measurements vary depending on the imaging study used to perform the measurements. However, most studies have shown that the glenoid has 1 to 3 degrees of retroversion[29,30]; however, retroversion can vary from 14 degrees of anteversion to 12 degrees of retroversion in normal shoulders.[31] Retroversion may be overestimated on plain axillary radiographs and

is probably more accurately measured by computed tomography.[30] The scapula is anteroverted approximately 30 degrees to the coronal plane. The glenoid is shaped like a pear; it is wider inferiorly. The average superior-inferior length of the glenoid is 39 mm, and the anteroposterior width in the lower half averages 29 mm.[4,32] The glenoid has a bare spot, which has been shown to be in the center of the lower portion on the glenoid. The bare spot can be used as a reference in measuring anteroinferior glenoid bone loss.[33] The radius of curvature of the glenoid is, on average, 2.3 mm more than the humeral head.[4] Unlike the humeral head, where the articular cartilage is thickest in the center, the articular cartilage is thickest on the periphery of the glenoid and thinnest in the center.

The spinoglenoid notch is an indentation at the confluence of the lateral edge of the base of the scapular spine and glenoid neck. This notch connects the supraspinatus and infraspinatus fossae. The suprascapular nerve and vessels travel through this notch prior to the nerve innervating the infraspinatus. On average, the suprascapular nerve is 1.5 cm medial to the posterior glenoid rim.[26] Knowledge of the location of this nerve is important when one is directly dissecting in the posterior aspect of the shoulder and when placing screws from anterior to posterior across the glenoid.[34] Compression of the suprascapular nerve in this location can result in isolated weakness of the infraspinatus muscle. The spinoglenoid notch can have a ligament across it. This ligament is present in 14% to 61% of people.[27,35]

The clavicle is an **S**-shaped or double-curved bone that connects the shoulder complex to the axial skeleton via the sternoclavicular joint. It is formed by membranous bone but does have a physis at the medial aspect. As a strut from the sternum to the shoulder, it is important in maintaining proper scapular positioning and kinematics during shoulder movement. Shortening of the clavicle, as is seen in some clavicular fracture malunions, leads to significant changes in shoulder posture and scapular positioning during shoulder motions.[36,37] In addition to its role in shoulder kinematics, the clavicle protects vascular structures to the upper extremities and the brachial plexus. The clavicle is the site of origin of a portion of the deltoid and pectoralis major muscles, as well as the insertion site of a portion of the trapezius muscle; all these muscles influence shoulder motion.

JOINTS AND ARTICULATIONS OF THE SHOULDER COMPLEX

Glenohumeral Joint

The glenohumeral joint is the most mobile joint in the body. The joint has 6 degrees of freedom, allowing for glenohumeral joint translations and rotations. Shoulder joint rotations occur in the coronal plane and are commonly referred to as abduction and adduction. Rotations in the sagittal plane are called flexion and extension. Rotations relative to the long axis of the humerus are called internal and external rotation (Fig. 36.5). The normal shoulder has substantial translational motion, with as much as 8 to 14 mm of translation anterior, posterior, and inferior with manual clinical testing.[38,39] Examinations with use of an anesthetic have documented even greater laxity, with subluxation over the glenoid anteriorly in 81.6% of subjects and posteriorly in 57.5% of subjects.[40] Given the mobility and wide range of motion, it is really not surprising that the shoulder is also the most unstable joint in the body. Shoulder stability is achieved through a combination of inherent joint characteristics, static stabilizers, and muscular or dynamic stabilizers.

The shoulder is afforded some stability from the inherent negative intraarticular pressure. This negative articular pressure is due to the glenoid concavity's "plunger" effect on the humeral head. The loss of the intra-articular vacuum as a result of an opening in the joint capsule results in less shoulder stability.[41,42] Some inherent stability is also achieved as a result of an adhesion-cohesion effect that occurs when two wet surfaces come in contact. Concavity-compression is another mechanism that has been

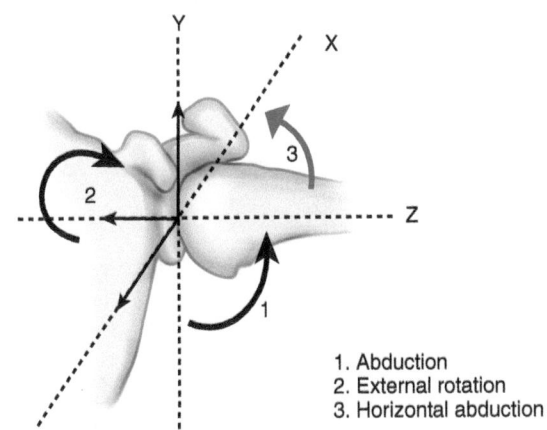

1. Abduction
2. External rotation
3. Horizontal abduction

Fig. 36.5 Shoulder motions are rotations along an axis. Rotations along the *X* axis or coronal plane are referred to as abduction and adduction. Rotations along the long axis of the humerus, when the arm is at the side, occur through the *Y* axis and are referred to as internal and external rotation. Rotations in the sagittal plane or *Z* axis (when the arm is at the side) are referred to as flexion and extension.

found to play a role in glenohumeral stability.[43] A compressive load provided by the rotator cuff forces the convex humeral head into the concave glenoid.

Static stability of the glenohumeral joint is provided by the glenoid labrum, glenohumeral ligaments, and joint capsule. The glenoid labrum is a fibrocartilaginous structure that is attached along the periphery of the glenoid. The labrum is wedge shaped, which increases the effective depth of the glenoid by approximately 50%.[44] Increasing the concavity of the glenoid contributes to overall shoulder stability because of the concavity-compression and the suction effect as a result of the intraarticular vacuum that occurs. The labrum contributes to glenohumeral stability by providing a bumper effect to prevent abnormal translations of the humeral head. The morphology and attachment of the labrum varies in the different quadrants of the shoulder. Inferiorly, the labrum is well attached to the glenoid, becoming an extension of the articular cartilage.[45] The firm attachment in the anteroinferior quadrant increases the diameter of the glenoid and increases the contact surface area. Removal of the anteroinferior labrum results in up to a 15% loss in glenohumeral contact area.[46] In the superior and anterosuperior quadrant, the labrum is less well adhered to the glenoid. In some incidences, the labrum has the appearance of a knee meniscus. The glenoid labrum in the anterosuperior quadrant can be quite variable, with sublabral foramen common. Absence of the anterosuperior labrum, in conjunction with a cordlike middle glenohumeral ligament, has been described as a Buford complex.[47,48] The labrum is the insertion of the glenohumeral ligaments and capsule. It is also the origin of the tendon of the long head of the biceps brachii muscle along the superior aspect.

The glenohumeral joint capsule has several areas of thickening that are called glenohumeral ligaments (Fig. 36.6). The inferior glenohumeral ligament is a hammocklike structure, with bands extending both anteriorly and posteriorly along the inferior aspect of the glenohumeral joint. The ligament originates along the inferior aspect of the humeral metaphysis and inserts onto the

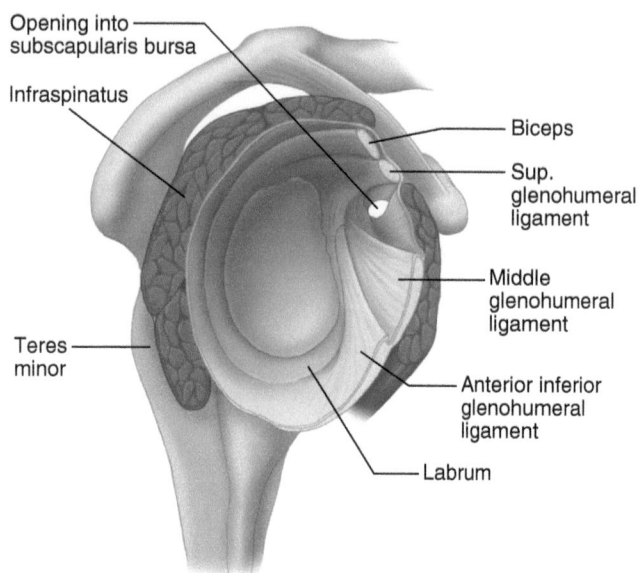

Fig. 36.6 A sagittal view of the glenohumeral joint showing the gleno-humeral ligament, glenoid labrum, and biceps tendon. *Sup.,* Superior.

anteroinferior and posteroinferior glenoid labrum. The inferior glenohumeral ligament is considered one of the most important stabilizing structures in the abducted, externally rotated shoulder.[49–51] The glenoid insertion site of the anterior band of the inferior glenohumeral ligament consists of two attachments, one to the glenoid labrum and the other directly to the anterior neck of the glenoid.[52]

The middle glenohumeral ligament is the most variable of the glenohumeral ligaments and has been shown to be absent in up to 36% of persons.[53] It can vary from a thin fold of capsule to a thick cordlike structure. The middle glenohumeral ligament originates from the anterosuperior labrum or glenoid rim and crosses over the deep portion of the subscapularis prior to inserting onto the anatomic neck of the humerus. Although its presence and morphology vary, it has been shown to be important for anterior stability with the shoulder in 45 degrees of abduction.[54]

The superior glenohumeral ligament (SGHL) arises from the anterosuperior labrum, runs parallel to the biceps tendon in the rotator interval, and inserts onto the lesser tuberosity.[55] Fibers of the SGHL help create the biceps pulley, which stabilizes the biceps in the bicipital groove. The function of the SGHL has generated considerable debate, with one study reporting that the SGHL was the most important stabilizer for inferior transla-tion.[56] Other investigators have concluded that the coracohumeral ligament is a more important stabilizer for inferior translation.[57] Yet other investigators have concluded that the inferior gleno-humeral ligament is the most important stabilizer for inferior translation of the adducted shoulder.[58]

The rotator interval is a triangular space that is bordered inferiorly by the subscapularis tendon, anteriorly by the supra-spinatus tendon, and medially by the glenoid. The rotator interval has been associated with shoulder instability, adhesive capsulitis, and isolated defects and tears. The rotator interval contains the coracohumeral ligament, which is a trapezoidal structure that originates on the lateral coracoid, traveling in two bands as it

inserts onto the lesser and greater tuberosities and over the bicipital groove. It also contains the SGHL, which arises from the superior labrum and supraglenoid tubercle, travels over the medial portion of the rotator interval, and blends with the cora-cohumeral ligament prior to inserting into the lesser tuberosity. The rotator interval also contains the joint capsule, which can be quite thin and variable. The rotator interval capsule can be as thin as 0.06 mm, and congenital defects are found in up to 75% of specimens.[59]

Sectioning of the coracohumeral ligament has been shown to result in increased inferior and posterior translation of the humerus, and imbrication and tightening of the coracohumeral ligament has been shown to decrease inferior and posterior translation.[60] During the past 15 years, as arthroscopic shoulder stabilizations have become more common, rotator interval clo-sures have been advocated as an adjunctive procedure to help with postoperative stability, particularly when the instability is inferior and posterior. However, arthroscopic rotator interval closures have not been shown to be of benefit in adding posterior or inferior stability in a cadaveric model.[61]

Glenohumeral Joint Capsule

The glenohumeral joint capsule is important in maintaining the intra-articular vacuum that helps to stabilize the joint. The joint capsule varies from 1.3 to 4.5 mm. It is thickest in the antero-inferior quadrant, which accounts for the anterior band of the glenohumeral ligament, and it is thinnest in the rotator interval and posterior quadrant.[62,63] A complex arrangement of the col-lagen fibers is present in the capsule, with a pattern of cross-linking in the superior capsule and a crossing pattern of spirals in the anterior and inferior capsule. The fibers in the ligamentous reinforcements radiate obliquely from the glenoid but vary greatly in orientation.[64] The inferior humeral attachment of the capsule may extend well below the articular surface. The inferior capsule has distinct internal and external folds.[65] Contracture of the glenohumeral joint capsule affects glenohumeral motion, which ultimately affect shoulder mechanics. This mechanism is com-monly seen in patients with adhesive capsulitis. Another example is posterior capsular contractures, a diagnosis commonly seen in overhead throwers. Posterior capsular contracture results in a loss of internal rotation of the shoulder. The contracture and loss of internal rotation force the humeral head into a postero-superior position as opposed to the normal posteroinferior posi-tion found in a normal shoulder when externally rotating in the cocking phase.[66] Ruffini end organs and Pacinian corpuscles are found in the inferior, middle, and SGHLs.[25] It is possible that these mechanoreceptors signal the dynamic muscle stabilizers when the capsule is stretched in the abducted-external rotated position.

The tendon of the long head of the biceps brachii originates from the superior labrum and supraglenoid tubercle (see Fig. 36.6). Anatomic variations of the biceps origin have been described, including a bifid origin,[67] an extraarticular origin,[68] and origin from the rotator cable.[69] The biceps tendon has been shown to be an additional dynamic stabilizer of the shoulder. Loading the biceps tendon has been shown to decrease both anterior-posterior and superior-inferior translation[70–72] and also has been shown to increase torsional rigidity against rotation force, limiting both external and internal rotation.[72,73] The biceps tendon travels out of the glenohumeral joint in the rotator interval prior to traveling distally in the bicipital groove of the proximal humerus. The tendon is stabilized in the proximal portion of the groove by the biceps pulley. The biceps pulley is a capsulo-ligamentous complex that is composed of fibers from the SGHL, the coracohumeral ligament, and the distal portions of the sub-scapularis tendon. More distally in the bicipital groove, the tendon is stabilized by the transverse humeral ligament. Recent evidence has suggested that the transverse humeral ligament is an exten-sion of the subscapularis tendon (see Fig. 36.3).[74]

Acromioclavicular Joint

The articulation between the distal end of the clavicle and acro-mion is called the acromioclavicular joint (see Fig. 36.3). The acromioclavicular joint is a synovial joint that consists of the articular facet of the acromion, the distal end of the clavicle, an intra-articular disk, and a joint capsule with thickening called the acromioclavicular ligaments. When viewed from the anterior position, the acromioclavicular joint is usually slightly medially or vertically oriented. With respect to the shaft of the clavicle, the inclination averages 12 degrees.[75] The joint is stabilized by the bony articulation but also by the acromioclavicular and coracoclavicular ligaments.[76] Several anatomic studies have assessed the location of the acromioclavicular ligaments and capsule.[75,77,78] Measurements in these studies are different, but one must be aware that the superior acromioclavicular ligament begins to insert as close as 2.3 mm from the lateral end of the clavicle.[78] The ligament does blend with the periosteum along the superior clavicle, and fibers of the ligament can be seen as far as 12 mm from the distal clavicle.[77]

It is generally accepted that superior-inferior stability of the acromioclavicular joint is due to the trapezoid and conoid liga-ments, commonly referred to as the coracoclavicular ligaments (see Fig. 36.3). The lateral of the two, the trapezoid ligament, originates from the base of the coracoid, anterior and lateral to the conoid ligament. It has a broad insertion on the undersurface of the clavicle. The trapezoid ligament helps to reduce axial compression forces at the acromioclavicular joint.[79] The cone-shaped conoid ligament originates from the posteromedial aspect of the base of the coracoid and inserts on the conoid tubercle of the clavicle.[80] The conoid ligament is the most important ligament for superior-inferior stability of the acromioclavicular joint.[79] Anterior-posterior stability is also due to the coracocla-vicular ligaments and the acromioclavicular ligaments. The trapezoidal ligament has been shown to provide the majority of restraint to the posterior translation of the clavicle.[76,81]

Some motion occurs at the acromioclavicular joint, but the motion is relatively small. Joint compression and translation occur as a result of protraction, retraction, and tilting of the acromion with overhead motion. Some clavicular rotation also occurs during abduction and adduction of the shoulder. Inner-vation of the acromioclavicular joint is from sensory branches from the suprascapular nerve.[82]

Distal clavicle resections are commonly performed, and this procedure can result in acromioclavicular joint instability.

Arthroscopic distal clavicle resection has been shown to increase acromioclavicular joint motion with a posterior applied force.[83] The acromioclavicular joint capsule is thickest superiorly and posteriorly. Preserving the superior and posterior acromiocla-vicular ligaments has been shown to be important in preserving joint stability when a distal clavicle resection is performed.[84] This preservation can usually be accomplished if less than 8 mm of bone is resected from the distal clavicle in men[78]; however, it is necessary to confirm that ligamentous tissue is present superiorly at the end of the procedure.

Sternoclavicular Joint

The sternoclavicular joint is truly the only connection of the shoulder complex to the axial skeleton. The proximal end of the clavicle has an irregular surface, being concave in the antero-posterior plane and convex superiorly. The articular surface along the sternum is small and not congruent to the end of the clavicle. Like the acromioclavicular joint, the sternoclavicular joint also has an intra-articular disk. As a result of the joint incongruity, the articular surfaces offer no significant stability to this joint. The stability of the sternoclavicular joint is therefore due to its surrounding capsular and ligamentous support (Fig. 36.7). The capsular ligament covers the anterosuperior and posterior aspects of the joint and helps to stabilize the clavicle against abnormal translations. The posterior capsule is the main stabilizer of the sternoclavicular joint against anterior and posterior translations. The costoclavicular and interclavicular ligaments do not seem to have a significant anteroposterior stabilizing effect on the joint,[85] although the interclavicular ligament does help to stabilize the joint to superior translations. Most of the motion of the clavicle occurs at the sternoclavicular joint. Motion analysis has shown that the ligamentous support allows for up to 15 degrees of elevation, 30 degrees of retraction, and 30 degrees of rotation along the long axis of the clavicle with active arm elevation.[86,87] The medial end of the clavicle does have a physis, which is the last physis in the body to fuse. In one radiographic study, the earliest observation of complete fusion was at 26 years of age.[88]

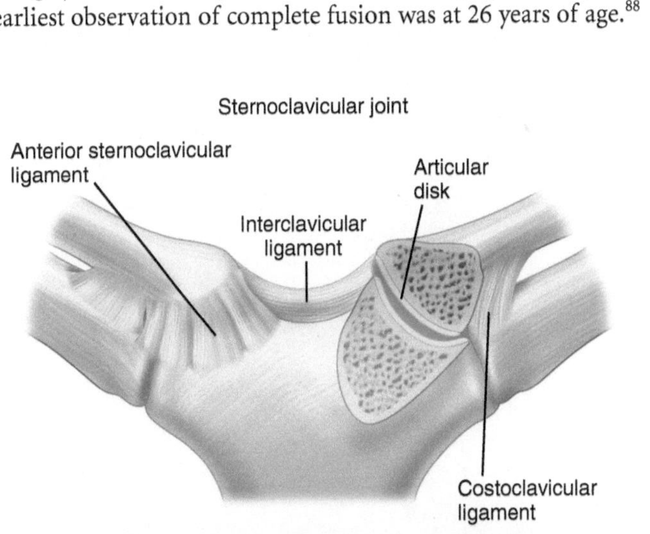

Fig. 36.7 A view of the sternoclavicular joint showing the anterior and posterior capsular ligaments, interclavicular ligament, articular disk, and costoclavicular ligament. The posterior capsular ligament provides the most stability against anterior and posterior translation of the sternocla-vicular joint.

Scapulothoracic Articulation

The scapular motion along the thoracic rib cage is referred to as the scapulothoracic articulation. Motion of the scapula is a result of the various stabilizing muscles that insert on it. The serratus anterior is an important stabilizing muscle because it holds the medial scapula to the thorax. It also helps to rotate and elevate the scapula in normal shoulder motions. The serratus anterior, along with the trapezius muscle, have the most muscle activity during arm abduction.[89] Smooth scapulothoracic motion is critical for normal shoulder kinematics. Alterations in scapular mechanics can lead to problems with glenohumeral instability and rotator cuff dysfunction. The biomechanics of normal shoulder motion, including scapular mechanics, will be discussed in more detail later in this chapter.

SHOULDER MUSCLES

Rotator Cuff

The rotator cuff consists of four muscles—the supraspinatus, infraspinatus, teres minor, and subscapularis (Fig. 36.8). The supraspinatus muscle originates in the supraspinatus fossa of the superior aspect of the scapula, passes in an anterolateral direction under the coracoacromial arch, and inserts on the greater tuberosity of the proximal humerus. The mean insertion footprint width of the supraspinatus is 14.7 mm, with the tendon insertion less than 1 mm lateral to the articular surface of the humeral head.[90] The supraspinatus muscle is innervated by the suprascapular nerve. The supraspinatus muscle is one of the main abductors of the humerus, accounting for 50% of the power to abduct in the scapular plane.[91] Other investigators have shown that paralysis of the supraspinatus and infraspinatus muscles results in a loss of 75% of abduction strength.[92] The anterior portion of the supraspinatus muscle contributes to internal rotation in adduction and works as an external rotator as the shoulder is abducted.[93] Macroscopically the tendons of the rotator cuff interdigitate to form a common insertion on the humerus. The supraspinatus muscle, along with the infraspinatus and teres minor muscles, have an area of insertion on the greater tuberosity of 6.24 cm^2.[90] The attachment site consists of a complex arrangement of collagen fibers capable of distributing tensile loads in various shoulder positions.[94] The cuff tendons have several layers, including a layer of tendon fibers that are both parallel and densely packed and another layer with obliquely oriented and loosely packed tendon fibers. The tendons also have layers composed of capsular and ligamentous tissue.[95]

The supraspinatus tendon has been shown to have a hypovascular area near the insertion,[96–98] which may play a factor in the pathogenesis of tears of the rotator cuff. Histologic sections from surgical specimens of patients with bursal-sided tears have been shown to be avascular, with no evidence of reparative tissue.[99] The articular side of the rotator cuff is subjected to and is more vulnerable to tensile forces, which might help to explain why partial rotator cuff tears occur more on the articular side compared with the bursal side.[100]

The main external rotators of the glenohumeral joint, the infraspinatus and teres minor muscles, originate on the posterior aspect of the scapula, with the infraspinatus muscle arising from the infraspinatus fossa (see Fig. 36.8). These muscles are inferior to the scapular spine and travel laterally to insert on the posterior aspect of the greater tuberosity. The infraspinatus muscle is innervated by the suprascapular nerve as it travels through the spinoglenoid notch. The teres minor muscle is innervated by the axillary nerve. The greater tuberosity has a small tubercle posteroinferiorly that is the site of the teres minor insertion. The infraspinatus muscle accounts for approximately 70% of the external rotation strength but also contributes approximately 45% of the abduction strength.[92] Clinically, the infraspinatus

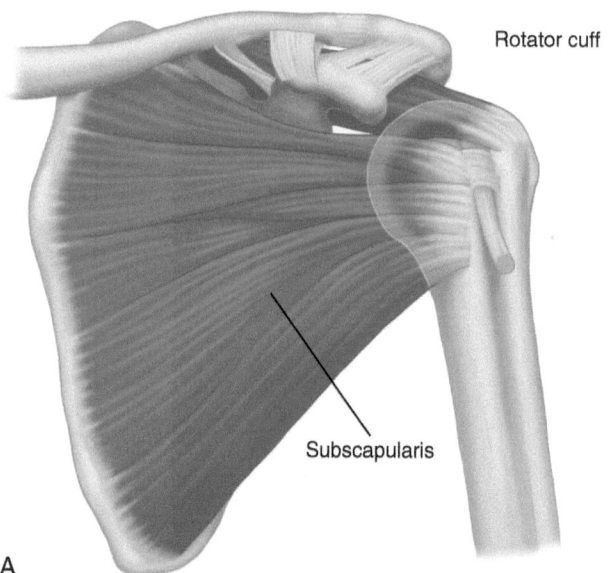

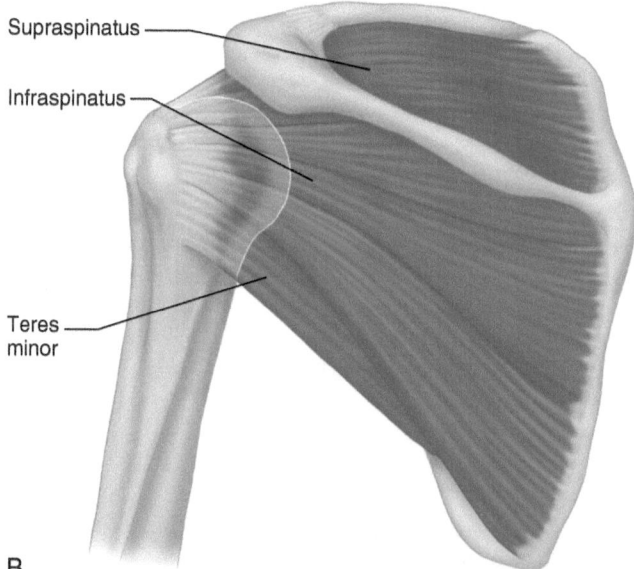

A   B

Fig. 36.8 Anterior (A) and posterior (B) views of the shoulder showing the subscapularis muscle and tendon anteriorly and the infraspinatus and teres minor muscles and tendons posteriorly. The supraspinatus is seen in the supraspinatus fossa. It travels anterolaterally to insert onto the greater tuberosity.

muscle is more functional at lower levels of abduction and elevation, whereas the teres minor muscle contributes more to external rotation power at higher levels of abduction and elevation.

The subscapularis is the anterior-most muscle of the rotator cuff; it originates from the ventral surface of the scapula and inserts on the lesser tuberosity. The lesser tuberosity insertion is trapezoidal in shape, with a broad insertion in the proximal portion. The upper 60% of the insertion site has a mean width of 2.5 cm.[101] As the subscapularis muscle travels laterally to insert, it passes under the coracoid process and the conjoined tendon of the short head of the biceps brachii and coracobrachialis. Narrowing of the distance from the lesser tuberosity to the coracoid may lead to subcoracoid impingement, which can lead to tearing of the subscapularis muscle.[102] The subscapularis muscle internally rotates and helps to adduct the humerus and is innervated by the upper and lower subscapular nerves. The subscapularis muscle has been shown to help provide stability to the shoulder from 0 to 45 degrees of abduction.[54]

The function of the rotator cuff, as its name implies, is to rotate the humerus. The rotator cuff also functions to maintain the center of rotation of the humeral head in the glenoid. The cuff muscles are important dynamic stabilizers of the glenohumeral joint. A 50% reduction in rotator cuff force has been shown to significantly increase anterior and posterior translation of shoulder specimens subjected to applied loads.[103]

Because of its orientation and vector of force, the rotator cuff also functions as a humeral head depressor. The head depressor effect is mainly due to the effect of the subscapularis and the external rotators. The supraspinatus muscle does not appear to have an effect on humeral head depression when it is studied biomechanically.[104] Although tears of the supraspinatus muscle can and do result in abnormal shoulder function, relatively normal kinematics can occur with active overhead motion with a balanced force couple of the subscapularis and infraspinatus/teres minor muscles.[105]

Scapular Muscles

The scapular muscles are important to shoulder function because they ensure proper positioning of the scapula in conjunction with glenohumeral joint motion. The scapula, through its connections to the axial skeleton, is an important structure that is needed to help transfer energy from the lower extremities and lower torso to the upper extremities. The transfer of lower body energy to the shoulder is referred to as the "kinetic chain."[106]

The scapular muscles stabilize the scapula, providing a stable base for shoulder movement. The scapular muscles include the serratus anterior, trapezius, levator scapulae, rhomboids, and pectoralis minor. Although all of these muscles have an important role, the serratus anterior and trapezius muscles appear to be most responsible for proper scapulothoracic motion.

The serratus anterior muscle originates from the upper thorax, along the ribs. It has a broad insertion along the anterior portion of the medial border of the scapula and is innervated by the long thoracic nerve (C5-C6-C7). The main function of the serratus anterior muscle is to protract the scapula laterally along the thorax with overhead motion of the shoulder. The serratus anterior muscle also works together with the upper and lower portions of the trapezius muscle to rotate the scapula upward with overhead activities. The serratus anterior and upper and lower trapezius muscles have the most electromyographic-documented activity of the scapular muscles with arm elevation.[89]

The trapezius is a posterior muscle along the posterosuperior aspect of the scapula. It has three functional sections—the upper, middle, and lower trapezius. The superior trapezius originates from the occiput and inserts on the posterior portion of the lateral clavicle. The upper trapezius functions to help support the weight on the upper extremity. The middle portion originates from the spinous process of C7 to T3. The fibers of the middle portion insert onto the medial acromion and posteriorly along the medial portion of the scapular spine. The inferior trapezius originates from the spinous processes of T4 to T12 and travels superior and laterally to insert on the medial aspect of the scapular spine. The main function of the upper and lower trapezius is to upwardly rotate the scapula during overhead activity. The upper and lower trapezius also work with the middle trapezius to help retract the scapula. The trapezius muscle is innervated by the spinal accessory nerve, as well as the third and fourth cervical nerves.

The levator scapulae muscle originates from the transverse processes of the cervical vertebra (C1-C4). It inserts on the superior angle of the scapula and helps to rotate the interior angle of the scapula medially. The levator scapulae muscle works with the rhomboids and pectoralis minor to rotate the medial scapula downward. It is innervated by the third and fourth cervical nerves.

The rhomboid major and minor muscles originate from the spinous processes of the thoracic vertebra from T2 to T5 and insert on the medial border of the scapula. The rhomboid muscles are innervated by the dorsal scapula nerve, which arises from C5. The main function of the rhomboid muscles is to help stabilize the scapula along the thorax. The rhomboid muscles help to retract the scapula and, as such, are antagonists to the serratus anterior. The rhomboid muscles work with the levator scapulae muscle to elevate the medial scapula and rotate the scapula downward.

The pectoralis minor muscle originates from the anterosuperior aspects of the anterior portions of ribs three through five. The muscle travels laterally to insert on the medial aspect of the coracoid. The main function of the pectoralis minor muscle is to pull the scapula inferiorly and medially. It is innervated by the medial pectoral nerve.

Other Muscles of the Shoulder Complex

The deltoid is the most superficial muscle covering the glenohumeral joint. It originates from the clavicle, acromion, and scapular spine and inserts on the deltoid tubercle on the lateral aspect of the midhumerus. The deltoid muscle provides a significant contribution to abduction of the humerus[91]; this function is provided by the anterior and middle portions of the muscle. The anterior portion of the deltoid muscle helps to flex the humerus, whereas the posterior portion of the deltoid muscle helps to adduct and extend the humerus. The deltoid muscle is innervated by the axillary nerve as it travels out of the quadrilateral space (the space bordered by the teres minor muscle superiorly, the teres major muscle inferiorly, the long head of the triceps brachii medially, and the humeral shaft laterally). The posterior humeral circumflex artery also travels in this space. The axillary nerve travels around the lateral aspect of the shoulder as it innervates the deltoid muscle. The distance from the lateral acromion to the axillary nerve averages 5 cm but can be as little as 3 cm. The distance decreases with shoulder abduction.[107] Surgical dissections through the deltoid muscle can injure the nerve if the deltoid muscle is split too far distally.

The teres major muscle, along with the latissimus dorsi muscle, helps to extend, internally rotate, and adduct the humerus. The teres major muscle takes its origin from the inferior angle of the scapula and inserts on the medial aspect of bicipital groove. The latissimus dorsi muscle inserts on the medial aspect of the bicipital groove, just anterior to the teres minor muscle.

The latissimus dorsi muscle originates from the spinous processes of T7 to L5, the thoracolumbar fascia, the posterior iliac crest, and the inferior angle of the scapula. The muscle fibers travel superiorly, laterally, and anteriorly to insert on the medial aspect of the floor of the bicipital groove. Is some persons, a conjoined tendon insertion with the teres major muscle occurs. The latissimus dorsi muscle helps to extend, adduct, and internally rotate the shoulder. It is innervated by the thoracodorsal nerve.

The pectoralis major muscle originates from the medial portion of the clavicle (clavicular head), the anterior surface of the sternum, the upper ribs, and the aponeurosis of the abdominal external oblique muscle (sternal head). The fibers from the clavicular head travel inferiorly and laterally. The sternal head fibers travel laterally. The two heads converge to form a common tendon that inserts onto the lateral aspect of the bicipital groove. The pectoralis major muscle is innervated by the lateral and medial pectoral nerves. The pectoralis major muscle helps to internally rotate, adduct, and flex the humerus.

The short head of the biceps brachii muscle and the coracobrachialis muscle originate from a common tendon at the tip of the coracoid. They are innervated by the musculocutaneous nerve, which pierces the muscles, on average, 5 cm distal to the coracoid. However, small branches of the nerve have been shown to innervate the muscle as close as 17 mm from the coracoid.[108] An appreciation of the neural anatomy and the variations is important to potentially avoid nerve injury during surgeries that retract the conjoined tendon or osteotomize the coracoid.

BIOMECHANICS AND KINETICS OF NORMAL SHOULDER MOTION

Normal glenohumeral and scapulothoracic biomechanics are prerequisites for achieving optimal shoulder function. Normal shoulder motion consists of a coordinated pattern of scapulothoracic and glenohumeral motion. The acromioclavicular and sternoclavicular joints also play a role in normal shoulder motion by guiding and limited scapular motion. The scapula has to move in conjunction with the humerus to maintain the humeral center of rotation in the various glenohumeral positions. In the normal shoulder, the center of rotation of the humeral head varies little with elevation or flexion/extension in the horizontal plane.

Coordinated scapular motion requires the scapula to protract and retract with elevation and lowering of the arm. Historically, glenohumeral to scapulothoracic motion has been described as being a 2:1 ratio after the initial 30 degrees of elevation.[109] More accurate three-dimensional motion analyses have been performed to better define the normal scapulohumeral motion.[86,87,110–116] Recent evidence would suggest that the ratio of glenohumeral elevation to scapular upward rotation is 2.3:1 during elevation and 2.7:1 when lowering the arm from overhead. Scapula upward rotation and posterior tilting increase until maximum elevation.[111] Posterior tilting is needed to clear the acromion from the rotator cuff to avoid impingement with overhead activity. Motion during humeral elevation includes clavicle elevation, retraction, and posterior rotation; scapular upward rotation, internal rotation, and posterior tilting; and glenohumeral elevation with humeral external rotation.[87] The largest amount of scapular rotation occurs between 80 and 140 degrees of arm abduction.[117] Obligatory humeral external rotation occurs as the arm is elevated at or anterior to the scapular plane, partly because of the geometry of the humeral head and glenoid.[87,110,118] Internal rotation is required from maximum elevation posterior to the scapular plane.[110] Therefore one can easily see how capsular contractions that prevent rotation can adversely affect elevation and overall motion. Scapular dyskinesia is common in patients with shoulder instability and rotator cuff impingement syndrome.[119–120] In fact, alternations in shoulder biomechanics can result from abnormalities in the scapular muscles, alterations in cervical and thoracic posture, abnormalities in joint mobility (such as seen in arthrosis or instability), and fractures of the scapula or clavicle that affect the position of the scapula or the length of the clavicle.

▌ SUMMARY

The shoulder is a complex arrangement of four bones, four articulations, and several muscles, tendons, and ligaments. The shoulder complex requires healthy and ligamentously stable joints and numerous muscles working in synergy to allow the upper extremity to be placed in various positions and to perform activities that subject it to extremes of force and torque. The various articulations and muscles are kinetically linked, and abnormalities in any of the joints or muscles can result in pain, dysfunction, and possibly injury to other structures. An appreciation of the anatomy and biomechanics of the shoulder complex will be beneficial to clinicians in making diagnoses, applying safe and appropriate surgical procedures, and implementing appropriate rehabilitation protocols.

For a complete list of references, go to ExpertConsult.com.

SELECTED READINGS

Citation:

Boileau P, Walch G. The three-dimensional geometry of the proximal humerus. Implications for surgical treatment and prosthetic design. *J Bone Joint Surg Br.* 1997;79B(5):857–865.

Level of Evidence:

V, basic science study

Summary:

In this cadaveric study, the authors showed that the articular surface of the proximal humerus varies with respect to the inclination, retroversion, size, and medial and posterior offset. Findings from this study have influenced design features of newer shoulder prostheses, which now allow surgeons to reproducibly replicate the native anatomy.

Citation:

Gerber C, Blumenthal S, Curt A. Effect of selective experimental suprascapular nerve block on abduction and external rotation strength of the shoulder. *J Shoulder Elbow Surg.* 2007;16(6): 815–820.

Level of Evidence:

I, prognostic study

Summary:

In this well-designed and well-performed study, the authors showed that the infraspinatus muscle is responsible for 70% of the external rotation strength of the shoulder and that it also contributes to abduction strength. The authors also showed that the supraspinatus and infraspinatus muscles were responsible for 75% of the abduction strength in healthy volunteers.

Citation:

Matsumura N, Ikegami H, Nakamichi N. Effect of shortening deformity of the clavicle on scapular kinematics: a cadaveric study. *Am J Sports Med.* 2010;38(5):1000–1006.

Level of Evidence:

V, basic science study

Summary:

In this cadaveric study, the authors showed that shortening of the clavicle by 10% of the original length had adverse effects on shoulder kinematics.

Citation:

O'Brien S, Schwartz R, Warren R. Capsular restraints to anterior-posterior motion of the abducted shoulder: a biomechanical study. *J Shoulder Elbow Surg.* 1995;4(4):298–308.

Level of Evidence:

V, basic science study

Summary:

In this cadaveric study, the authors demonstrated that the primary restraint to anterior and posterior translation of the abducted shoulder is the inferior glenohumeral ligament complex.

Citation:

Turkel S, Panio M, Marshall J. Stabilizing mechanisms preventing anterior dislocation of the glenohumeral joint. *J Bone Joint Surg Am.* 1981;63A(8):1208–1217.

Level of Evidence:

V, basic science study

Summary:

In this cadaveric study, the authors showed that the subscapularis muscle provides anterior stability to the adducted shoulder, the middle glenohumeral ligament provides stability at 45 degrees of abduction, and the inferior glenohumeral ligament provides anterior stability as the shoulder approaches 90 degrees of abduction.

Citation:

Kibler WB. The role of the scapula in athletic shoulder function. *Am J Sports Med.* 1998;26(2):325–337.

Level of Evidence:

V, review article/expert opinion

Summary:

In this review article, the author thoroughly reviews the role of the scapula in normal shoulder biomechanics and in athletics involving overhead actions. The author introduces the concept of the kinetic chain (i.e., the transfer of lower extremity energy to the upper extremity) and reinforces the importance of the scapula in the kinetic chain.

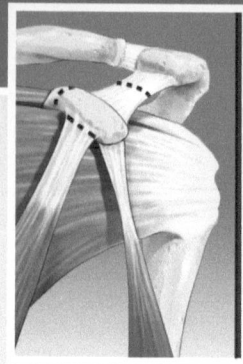

37

Shoulder Diagnosis and Decision-Making

Thomas J. Gill

Perhaps more than any other joint in the body, the shoulder can present a complex diagnostic challenge to the examining physician. There are a variety of anatomic and clinical reasons for this challenge. First, the "shoulder" is actually a functional complex of four distinct and separate articulations: the sternoclavicular joint, acromioclavicular joint, glenohumeral joint, and scapulothoracic joint. These joints all function together to allow a strong, stable platform with a wide arc of motion through multiple geometric planes. Thus it is not uncommon for patients to present with periscapular pain, for instance, which is actually secondary to a primary glenohumeral problem such as adhesive capsulitis or a large rotator cuff tear.

"Shoulder pain" can also be due to referred pain from the neck. Cervical radiculopathies, paracervical muscle strains, "whiplash," and other neck-related pathologies can all cause patients to present to the clinician with a subjective feeling of pain in their "shoulder." There are also vascular etiologies for shoulder pain, peripheral neuropathies and nerve entrapments, intrathoracic pathologies, and malignancies whose presenting symptoms are often shoulder pain or instability.

As a result of the diagnostic challenge presented by patients with shoulder-related symptoms, it is important to take a detailed history, perform a truly regimented and comprehensive physical examination, order and review appropriate diagnostic imaging, and carefully correlate all relevant findings prior to arriving at a final "diagnosis." In some instances, the selective use of injections can often confirm the etiology of the patient's pain much more accurately than high-cost advanced imaging techniques. The clinician cannot simply "get an MRI" (magnetic resonance imaging) to arrive at the correct source of the patient's symptoms, as might be done with other types of musculoskeletal pathologies. In fact, a shoulder MRI may show four or five structural "abnormalities," none of which have anything to do with the cause of the patient's presenting symptoms. No part of the diagnostic workup can be taken in isolation. It is only after careful consideration of all the clinical data that a diagnosis and treatment plan can be decided.

The goal of this chapter is to present a practical approach to the patient with shoulder-related symptoms. It will present the diagnostic clues that can be obtained from taking a focused, detailed history, the specific parts of the physical examination that lead to a specific diagnosis, the indications for advanced imaging techniques, the use of selective diagnostic and therapeutic injections that can confirm the etiology of the patient's shoulder complaints, and how these decisions can be made.

For most patients with shoulder complaints, it is helpful to divide the possible etiologies and diagnoses into the most likely diagnostic categories. These include (1) referred pain from the cervical spine, (2) acromioclavicular (AC) joint pathology, (3) rotator cuff–related pathology, (4) biceps-related pathology, (5) glenohumeral instability, and (6) glenohumeral arthritis. Although pathologies such as occult tumors, traumatic fractures, vascular disease, and peripheral nerve entrapments can also cause shoulder symptoms, they are not the primary focus of this chapter.

HISTORY

The most important parts of a patient's history are the patient's age and whether or not there was a specific trauma or incident involved in the onset of symptoms. For patients younger than 25 years of age, the most likely diagnosis is glenohumeral instability or AC joint–related pain. For patients older than 40 years, rotator cuff–related pathology, with or without biceps tendon involvement, is most common.

The next part of the history should be a precise determination of the patient's chief complaint. Is the reason for the patient's visit pain, instability, loss of motion, or weakness? Patients can often tell the clinician their own diagnosis if proper questioning is performed in this manner. Loss of motion indicates adhesive capsulitis, large rotator cuff tears, or glenohumeral arthrosis. Weakness is typically due to rotator cuff tears or, less likely, suprascapular nerve entrapment. Instability symptoms are typically related to glenohumeral labral tears or capsular redundancy. "Pain" is less specific but is most commonly due to subacromial impingement (specifically bursitis, rotator cuff tendinitis), biceps tendinitis, partial- or full-thickness rotator cuff tears, and AC joint arthritis. Glenohumeral instability can also present as pain, which is when the patient's age should also be considered.

If "pain" is the chief complaint, the question of referred pain must be considered. It is helpful to ask the patient to "put one finger where it hurts the most." If the patient points to his or her AC joint, the diagnosis is typically made. If specific localization is made to the biceps groove, then biceps pathology with or without rotator cuff involvement is common. Pointing to the lateral shoulder near the insertion of the lateral deltoid is indicative of rotator cuff–related pain. However, if the patient cannot "localize" the pain, the question of referred pain should be considered. When asked to localize the "shoulder" pain that is actually being referred from a cervical spine etiology, patients cannot use one specific finger to localize the pain. Instead, they use their palm to rub over their trapezius and upper arm. As a general rule, truly shoulder-related pain does not radiate below the elbow. If the patient indicates that symptoms travel below the elbow into the hand, then cervical stenosis or cervical disc herniation should be considered.

After the chief complaint is ascertained, the patient should be questioned about any history of trauma or inciting event. If there is no history of trauma, repetitive overuse injuries, tendinopathies and AC joint or glenohumeral arthrosis are most common. If there is a history of trauma, the question of fracture, labral tear, or rotator cuff tear becomes more important. It is helpful to then ask what position the patient's arm was in when the trauma occurred. If the patient fell with his or her arm at his or her side, an AC joint or clavicular injury is most common. In contrast, falling on an outstretched arm can lead to rotator cuff tears, superior labral tears, and traumatic glenohumeral instability episodes.

Patients should then be asked what position of their arm brings on their symptoms or worsens their pain. Symptoms that worsen when reaching overhead or at night indicate rotator cuff and/or bursal inflammation. Abduction and external rotation worsens symptoms of anterior instability, whereas pain reaching out to the side is often an indicator of biceps-related pain. If reaching across the body is problematic, AC joint arthritis should be considered.

PHYSICAL EXAMINATION

When assessing a patient with "shoulder pain," the examination should begin with a focused evaluation of the cervical spine to rule out an etiology of referred pain from the neck. First, the patient should be asked to fully flex, extend, and rotate his or her neck from side to side. Restrictions in motion may indicate the presence of cervical spondylosis. The presence of any tenderness along the cervical midline, paraspinal muscles, and trapezius should be assessed. Next, the "Lhermitte sign"[1] is tested, in which there is a generalized electric shock sensation associated with axial compression of the cervical spine. The "Spurling test"[2] is the most sensitive examination maneuver, in which radicular pain is exacerbated by extension and lateral bending of the neck toward the side of the lesion, which causes further neuroforaminal compromise. A detailed neurologic examination should also be performed to rule out a focal cervical radiculopathy.

The assessment of the shoulder itself is then performed. The patient's shirt must be removed to permit a thorough inspection of the entire affected shoulder girdle and to compare it with the opposite side. The evaluation begins by inspecting the sternoclavicular joint, clavicle, and acromioclavicular joint for evidence of prominence, swelling, deformity, or discoloration. Previous surgical incisions should be noted, as well as traumatic skin lesions, bruising, and muscular asymmetry. The pectoralis major muscles should be assessed for any asymmetry in their contours, which could indicate a rupture. The biceps muscle is inspected

for any evidence of a Popeye deformity, indicating a torn long head of biceps tendon. Next, any evidence of atrophy in the deltoid muscle is noted, which could indicate a C5 radiculopathy or axillary neuropathy.

It is important to also inspect the posterior aspect of the shoulder girdle. The presence of any atrophy in the supraspinatus and infraspinatus fossae can be diagnostic. For example, if there is evidence of muscle atrophy in the supraspinatus fossa alone, it may indicate the presence of a chronic tear of the supraspinatus tendon. If there is atrophy in both the supraspinatus and infraspinatus fossae, it could indicate a chronic tear of both the supraspinatus and infraspinatus tendons or entrapment of the suprascapular nerve at the level of the suprascapular notch. Isolated atrophy is in the infraspinatus fossa alone can indicate entrapment of the suprascapular nerve at the spinoglenoid notch, often from a paralabral cyst.[3]

Periscapular pathology is best assessed by asking the patient to actively raise his or her arms overhead while observing from behind. Evidence of scapular dyskinesis should be noted, as should evidence of scapular winging.[4] If the medial border of the scapula becomes prominent with either forward elevation or doing a "push up against the wall," the examiner should consider an injury to the spinal accessory nerve. Such an injury typically occurs during cervical lymph node biopsies. If the inferior border becomes prominent, injury to the long thoracic nerve is considered. Scapular winging can also contribute to symptoms of glenohumeral pain and instability. The examiner can confirm the contribution of the scapular dyskinesis to the patient's presenting symptoms by compressing/stabilizing the scapula against the chest wall and asking the patient to again elevate the arm. If this maneuver diminishes the patient's symptoms or improves active motion, it confirms the scapula as an etiology in the patient's diagnosis.

Next, palpation of the shoulder girdle should be performed in a systematic manner. The sternoclavicular joint should be palpated for evidence of tenderness or dislocation, followed by the clavicle and acromioclavicular joint. The biceps groove is then palpated just distal to the coracoid process with the arm in neutral rotation. The presence of tenderness typically indicates pathology of the long head of the biceps tendon or attachment of the subscapularis tendon to the lesser tuberosity. Posterior periscapular tenderness can be associated with muscle spasm ("trigger points") and occasionally cervical radiculopathy. Medial periscapular and trapezial spasms are not uncommon in patients with large rotator cuff tears, adhesive capsulitis, glenohumeral arthrosis, and instability for whom scapulothoracic motion is often used to achieve forward elevation of the arm. Crepitance at the superomedial border of the scapula during active shoulder elevation is seen with scapulothoracic bursitis.

An assessment of the patient's active and passive range of motion (ROM) is then performed. Specifically, notation should be made of forward elevation, internal rotation, and external rotation. In throwing athletes, it is important to check external rotation at both 90 degrees of glenohumeral abduction, as well as adduction. The "total arc of motion" should then be compared with the opposite shoulder, noting the presence of deficits in elevation or rotation.

Differences between active and passive motion can also indicate a potential diagnosis. If the patient has full passive motion but limited active motion, the presence of a large rotator cuff tear should be considered. If there is limited active and passive motion with a "firm end point," adhesive capsulitis is often the etiology. If there is limited active and passive motion in the presence of glenohumeral crepitus or a "gear shifting" sensation, glenohumeral arthrosis is typically present. Excess passive external rotation is seen when there is a rupture of the subscapularis tendon.

Strength testing is the next step in the examination of the shoulder. It is used to investigate the integrity of the rotator cuff or the presence of neurologic pathology. The neurologic motor examination of the upper extremity should be completed during the assessment of the cervical spine. At this stage, the supraspinatus muscle function is isolated by performing the "Jobe test" or "empty can" test.[5] The shoulder is tested in the scapular plane with the elbow extended and with the shoulder in a position of 90 degrees abduction, 30 degrees flexion, and full internal rotation. The patient is asked to resist downward pressure on the forearm by the examiner. Especially in athletes, it is helpful to assess both arms at the same time to identify often subtle differences in strength. The more posterior rotator cuff muscles are tested by resisted external rotation with the arm adducted and in neutral rotation. Weakness in this position is often present with injury to the infraspinatus, whereas weakness in external rotation with the shoulder abducted and externally rotated indicates injury to the teres minor.

It is important not to forget to examine the subscapularis while examining the rotator cuff and its strength. This is performed by the "lift-off," "belly-press," and "bear-hug" tests.[6] The lift-off test is performed by placing the dorsum of the patient's hand on his or her back and asking him or her to "lift it off." The result can be difficult to interpret because patients will often use their triceps to perform this task. It can be more reliable for the examiner to lift the hand/arm away from the patient's back instead, and ask the patient to hold it in that position. The belly-press test is performed by having patients place their hand on their abdomen, wrists in neutral position, and instructing the patients to keep their elbows forward as they press against their abdomen. Gentle pressure can be applied to the elbows to further assess strength. With this maneuver, the latissimus dorsi can substitute for the subscapularis function. The bear-hug test was developed to help isolate testing of the subscapularis.[7] In this maneuver, patients are asked to place their hand on their opposite shoulder and resist the examiner as he or she starts to pull the elbow anteriorly. When the elbow is lowered, the upper subscapularis is tested. When the elbow is initially elevated, the lower subscapularis is tested.

Lag signs were initially described by Hertel et al.[8] They are used to help quantify the degree of rotator cuff tearing or dysfunction. The "external rotation lag sign" is performed by asking patients to maintain their arm in a position of maximal passive external rotation with their arm by their side. Any change in position of the arm after it is released by the examiner is then noted and typically indicates a large tear or atrophy of the infraspinatus. The same test is then performed with the shoulder in a position of 90 degrees of abduction. This is called "hornblower's sign" and is used to assess injury to the teres minor.[9] The lift-off test is also considered a lag sign when testing the subscapularis.

After strength has been tested, specialty tests are performed to narrow the diagnosis further. It is helpful to group the exam maneuvers by shoulder pathology. First, the subacromial space and rotator cuff are further assessed by the "Neer" and "Hawkins" impingement signs. The Neer test[10] is performed by forward flexing the patient's arm with the elbow extending and hand pronated. The presence of pain at maximal forward elevation is a sign of subacromial impingement, as seen with bursitis and rotator cuff tendinopathy. Hawkins test[11] is sensitive for the presence of subacromial impingement and is tested by the examiner internally rotating the arm after placing it in 90 degrees of glenohumeral and elbow flexion.

Shoulder instability is the next diagnostic category to be considered. The examiner needs to perform multiple specialty tests when evaluating for shoulder instability, given the large spectrum of pathology that can be present in patients with an unstable shoulder. Perhaps the most sensitive and pathognomonic test for anterior shoulder instability is the "apprehension test." This test is best performed with the patient lying supine. In this position, patients tend to be less tense and relax their shoulder musculature to a greater extent. Once supine, the patient's arm is abducted to 90 degrees and slowly externally rotated while the examiner also exerts a gentle and steady anteriorly directed pressure on the posterior aspect of the shoulder. A positive test is when the patient indicates a feeling of "apprehension" that his or her shoulder may dislocate if external rotation and anterior pressure continues. It is important to differentiate between an expression of true "apprehension" versus "pain," because pain can be experienced in this position with other shoulder pathologies besides shoulder instability alone. The apprehension test is one of the most specific tests around the shoulder. It is difficult to assign a diagnosis of anterior instability in the absence of a positive apprehension sign. The "relocation test" can support the diagnosis of anterior instability. In this test, the examiner applies a posteriorly directed "relocation/reduction" pressure to the anterior aspect of the shoulder, which decreases the patient's apprehension and often allows the arm to be further rotated without issue.

The "posterior apprehension test" is performed with the patient supine or seated. The arm is forward flexed to 90 degrees and maximally adducted while the examiner applies a slight posteriorly directed axial load. The test is positive if the patient describes apprehension that the shoulder will dislocated. However, unlike the anterior apprehension test, the posterior apprehension test is much less sensitive for the presence of posterior instability. Because most patients with posterior instability seldom actually dislocate their shoulders posteriorly, there is typically not a learned "apprehensive" response to this position as is seen in anterior instability. Instead, a posterior "jerk test" is more sensitive to identify the presence of posterior instability. The examiner applies a posteriorly directed axial load to the arm in 90 degrees of flexion and full internal rotation while the arm is steadily adducted. A positive test is noted if the humeral head slides or "jerks" over the posterior glenoid rim. A jerk can also be noted upon reduction of the subluxated humeral head.

The "load and shift test" is used to assess and describe both anterior and posterior humeral head translation in the glenoid fossa. The examiner should note whether the humeral head can be translated to the anterior glenoid rim or over the glenoid rim with the patient supine and the arm at 90 degrees of abduction. The test should be repeated with the arm at both 45 and 90 degrees of abduction. The examiner should then apply a posterior load and note the degree of posterior translation. It is important that the load and shift test also be performed on the contralateral shoulder, because findings can be subtle and difficult to interpret in isolation.

The "sulcus sign" is performed to assess the degree of inferior instability and the integrity of the superior glenohumeral ligament and rotator interval. The examiner exerts an inferiorly directed pull on the arm with it placed at the patient's side. The presence and size of a dimple or "sulcus" at the edge of the acromion is then noted. The sulcus should be eliminated when the test is repeated with the arm in a position of adduction and external rotation. A persistent sulcus indicates a greater degree of shoulder laxity, especially in the rotator interval.

The presence and extent of labral tearing is further assessed by examining for injuries to the superior labrum. Although multiple tests have been described, the active compression test ("O'Brien test") is typically regarded as the most sensitive and specific for a torn superior labrum.[12] In this maneuver, the arm is placed in a position of 90 degrees forward flexion, 10 degrees adduction, maximum internal rotation, and elbow extension. The examiner exerts a downward pressure on the patient's arm, and the presence of pain and/or weakness is assessed. The test is repeated with the hand and forearm maximally supinated. The test is positive if the patient describes feeling a "deep" pain that is relieved or eliminated when the hand is supinated. If pain persists with the hand fully supinated, it often is a sign of AC joint arthritis. AC joint pain can be confirmed by performing a "cross-body adduction test" in which the arm is then maximally adducted across the body and pain is elicited at the AC joint.

The biceps tendon itself is tested by the "Speed test" and "Yergason test."[13] The Speed test is performed when the examiner exerts a downward pressure with the patient's arm extended in 90 degrees of forward flexion and fully supinated. A painful response is indicative of pathology in the biceps groove. Less commonly, it can be positive in the setting of a superior labral tear. The Yergason test is performed with the patient's arm by his or her side, the elbow flexed 90 degrees, and the forearm pronated. The patient is then asked to supinate the arm against resistance. Although this test is more sensitive for biceps pathology at the elbow, it can elicit pain in the biceps groove for patients with long head biceps tendon pathology as well.

DECISION-MAKING

Referred Pain From the Neck

The most common source of referred pain to the shoulder is cervical spine pathology. Of the various different anatomic diagnoses, the most commonly encountered are cervical strains, whiplash, cervical stenosis/spondylosis, cervical disc herniation, and "burners/stingers."

Cervical Strain

Cervical strains are typically the result of repetitive overuse or mild trauma. The patient can present with "shoulder pain," which, upon further questioning, localizes to the trapezius and paracervical area posteriorly. The mechanism of injury is generally a forced motion or trauma that causes an eccentric contraction of the neck, such as a sudden twist or turn. Important to the history is a lack of true radicular or arm symptoms. On physical examination, there is tenderness over the paraspinal muscles and trapezius and an absence of positive provocative neurologic tests such as the Lhermitte sign or Spurling test. Diagnostic testing should include plain x-rays if there is a significant trauma, including lateral flexion/extension views. There is often a loss of cervical lordosis in the acute stage from paracervical spasm. MRI is seldom indicated in the absence of true radicular complaints, and symptomatic treatment can progress as tolerated.

Whiplash

A whiplash injury is a subset of cervical strains. The patient typically complains of posterior shoulder and neck pain but no arm pain. There is a history of forced flexion and extension of the cervical spine, typically following a motor vehicle accident. In this situation, a careful neurologic examination should be performed to rule out an acute radiculopathy from a herniated cervical disc or instability. Lateral flexion/extension views of the cervical spine should be obtained to rule out ligamentous instability. If present, advanced imaging including an MRI is indicated.

Cervical Spondylosis/Stenosis

Degenerative changes of the cervical spine can lead to symptoms of shoulder pain. There is seldom a recent history of trauma, although one may exist in the distant past. Unlike cervical strain injuries, patients with spondylosis often complain of both neck/shoulder pain and radicular complaints that are worse with extremes of neck motion. On physical examination, the patient will have pain with cervical extension. There can be a positive Lhermitte sign, often with a generalized electric shock sensation associated with axial compression of the cervical spine. The Spurling test is the most sensitive examination maneuver, in which radicular pain is exacerbated by extension and lateral bending of the neck toward the side of the lesion, which causes further neuroforaminal compromise. A detailed neurologic examination should be performed, looking for dermatomal loss of sensation or motor weakness; and decreased biceps, triceps, or brachioradialis reflexes. Plain x-rays show hypertrophy of facet joints that cause central stenosis or foraminal encroachment. MRI is indicated when localizing neurologic signs are obtained on exam, such as dermatomal loss of sensation and weakness in the setting of radicular complaints.

Cervical Disc Herniation

Acute cervical disc herniations presenting as "shoulder pain" are relatively uncommon but do exist. The patient typically presents with a history of trauma that caused an acute hyperflexion of the cervical spine, followed by true radicular complaints. Less commonly, the disc herniation can cause a feeling of posterior shoulder pain and muscle spasm. Both the Lhermitte sign and Spurling test are generally positive, and an MRI is indicated for further treatment decision analysis.

Burners/Stingers

A burner is an upper cervical root neurapraxia (reduction or block of conduction across a segment of nerve with conservation of underlying nerve function) most common at C5/C6. In sports such as football, the diagnosis of a burner or stinger often leads to the chief complaint of shoulder pain and weakness. The player's head is forced to one side (lateral bend), and the contralateral shoulder is forced downwards; it is also seen with falls from a height. The player will give a history that "my arm went dead." On examination, there is often weakness of shoulder abduction due to axillary nerve involvement at C5 and, less commonly, biceps or triceps weakness. What differentiates this injury from a disc herniation is that the symptoms typically clear after several seconds to minutes, with a complete return of sensation and strength. Plain x-rays are recommended to rule out fracture or instability. MRI is not usually indicated acutely, unless motor weakness does not improve after 24 hours.

Referred Pain From an Intrathoracic Source

A rare but serious source of "shoulder pain" can be due to an intrathoracic etiology such as a hemothorax or pleural effusion. In this setting, there is irritation of the phrenic nerve, which has contributions from C3, C4, and C5 nerve roots. The C3 dermatome is located on the superior aspect of the shoulder. As a result, these patients can present with acute "shoulder pain."

COMMON SHOULDER PATHOLOGIES

Acromioclavicular Joint Pathology

Patients with shoulder pain due to AC joint pathology present with a typical history and physical examination. The history should include whether or not there was a history of trauma, and if so, how did it occur? The AC joint is typically injured by a direct blow to the lateral aspect of the shoulder. The patient should then be asked to "place one finger where you feel the pain the most." The patient will almost invariably point directly to the AC joint. On physical examination, there is tenderness at the AC joint, and pain can be elicited by cross-body adduction. If there is any question about whether the AC is the cause of the pain, a selective injection to the AC joint can be performed. Plain films are indicated in the presence of a traumatic injury to rule out fracture, AC joint widening, or dislocation. Weighted stress views are not typically needed. The x-rays will also help to classify an AC joint dislocation, which will have a direct effect on management decisions.[14] Rockwood type 1 and 2 injuries are usually managed nonoperatively. Types 4, 5, and 6 are indications for surgery, whereas type 3 management can be operative or nonoperative. If the type of AC dislocation cannot be made on plain x-ray alone, a computed tomography (CT) scan may be considered.

Rotator Cuff Pathology
Impingement Syndrome

Impingement syndrome is one of the most common causes of shoulder pain. Anatomically, impingement syndrome includes pain caused by rotator cuff tendinitis, subacromial bursitis, and biceps tendinitis. Acromioclavicular arthritis also can contribute to symptoms of impingement in the presence of hypertrophic bone spurs. When considering the diagnosis of impingement syndrome, the most important question to ask the patient is their age. Primary impingement is seldom seen in patients less than 30 years of age. The patient should be asked if they have pain at night or with overhead activity, the primary complaints of patients with rotator cuff–related pain. There is usually a history of repetitive overhead activity; such as seen with throwers, tennis players, swimmers, painters, or electricians. On physical examination, there is a positive Neer sign and Hawkins sign. The patient may or may not have weakness on the "empty can test."

In this situation, an injection test is helpful to differentiate between simple impingement syndrome and a full-thickness rotator cuff tear. An injection test can be performed using a 25-gauge, 1.5″ needle with 9 cc 1% lidocaine and with or without 1 cc steroid. A posterior approach is recommended, approximately 2 cm distal to posterolateral corner of the acromion. If the patient had pain and weakness prior to the injection but no pain or weakness afterwards, then there is not likely to be a torn rotator cuff. Plain x-rays alone are indicated to rule out arthritis or calcific tendinitis. On the other hand, if the patient's pain is gone but he or she still has weakness, then an MRI is indicated to investigate a torn rotator cuff.

Rotator Cuff Tear

Continuing along the spectrum of rotator cuff pathology are rotator cuff tears. The tear can be partial thickness or full thickness, with size and chronicity of the tear playing a major role in the decision-making of the clinician. Classically, the patient has a history of pain at night and with overhead use. There is often a history of trauma but not always. On physical examination, Neer and Hawkins impingement signs are usually positive and there is weakness with supraspinatus ("empty can") or external rotation resistance. There is a discrepancy between active and passive ROM for large and massive tears. In this setting, plain x-rays and an MRI are indicated. The MRI in particular is useful to help differentiate between partial- and full-thickness tears, labral tears, the presence of associated biceps lesions, the size of the tear, and whether any fatty atrophy of the rotator cuff is present. MRI also allows visualization of the subscapularis, which is often overlooked when evaluating patients with shoulder pain and weakness.

Shoulder instability. Shoulder instability is most commonly seen in patients younger than 25 years of age. It can result from both traumatic and atraumatic etiologies. Patients may present with a history of a single instability episode following an injury, or multiple subluxation events from a positional or even voluntary etiology. Shoulder instability occurs along a spectrum of severity. In fact, chief complaints of shoulder "pain" are more common than "instability." To help make the diagnosis of shoulder instability, several specific questions are helpful. For example, "Does your shoulder feel loose?" or "Have you ever dislocated your shoulder?" can lead to an immediate diagnosis. In addition, "Do you avoid placing your arm in certain positions?" and "Do you have difficulty reaching behind you, throwing, or pushing open a heavy door?" can also help to determine if anterior or posterior instability is present. "Is it difficult to lift a heavy bag or suitcase?" also indicates whether an inferior or multidirectional component are present.

On physical examination, the apprehension test is pathognomonic for anterior instability. The relocation test, in which the aforementioned apprehensive sensation is eliminated with posteriorly directed pressure on the joint by the examiner, helps to confirm the diagnosis. An anterior and posterior load test is similar to the Lachman test in the knee, in which a manual attempt to translate joint is performed. This test can be difficult to interpret, and a comparison to the contralateral shoulder can be helpful. Lastly, a "sulcus sign" can be performed.

Imaging tests are mandatory when considering the diagnosis of shoulder instability. Plain radiographs are first performed to assess for osseous lesions of the humeral head and glenoid and to confirm that the joint is reduced following a trauma. Specific x-ray views should be considered. First, actual reduction of the glenohumeral joint can only be confirmed by obtaining an axillary view or transscapular Y-view. An anteroposterior (AP) view alone is not acceptable. A Stryker notch view will help to assess for the presence of a Hill-Sachs deformity, whereas a West Point view will identify a bony Bankart lesion. MRI is useful to identify labral tears, capsular tears, or subscapularis tears that are contributing to the instability problem. If bony lesions are present, the physician may consider a CT scan with or without three-dimensional reconstructions to help determine whether an arthroscopic versus open approach to a shoulder stabilization is optimal.

Adhesive capsulitis. Adhesive capsulitis is most commonly seen in diabetic patients. Typically, there is an insidious onset of motion loss following a period of pain or "tendonitis." Patients have a chief complaint of pain and restricted motion. Early in its course, the pain is often more severe than that seen in patients with rotator cuff tears, arthritis, or simple impingement. The natural history is typically 18 to 24 months to restore motion and decrease pain, if untreated. On physical examination, patients have restricted active and passive motion, as opposed to patients with a torn rotator cuff who have restricted active motion but full passive motion. A true AP x-ray and axillary view should be obtained to rule out osteoarthritis and calcific tendinitis.

Superior Labrum, Anterior to Posterior tears. Superior Labrum, Anterior to Posterior (SLAP) tears typically occur after a history of an eccentric contraction of the biceps muscle. This mechanism is typically caused by a fall on an outstretched arm, or during the deceleration phase of throwing. Patients will present with a history of either anterior or posterior shoulder pain, "rotator cuff symptoms" such as pain at night and with overhead activity, and classically pain when reaching out to the side. There are multiple tests that have been described to test for a SLAP tear, but the active compression test (O'Brien test) is the most sensitive.[15] MRI with or without contrast helps to confirm the diagnosis, while ruling out confounding pathology such as a torn rotator cuff.

Glenohumeral arthritis. The shoulder is typically not a "weight-bearing joint." Therefore shoulder arthritis is not as common as hip or knee arthritis. Patients with glenohumeral arthritis typically present with complaints of posterior shoulder pain, limited motion, and difficulty sleeping. On physical examination, patients have glenohumeral crepitus, with limited ROM. The diagnosis is confirmed by plain radiographs. Specifically, a true AP x-ray of the glenohumeral joint ("Grashey view") is important, and an axillary view helps to confirm the diagnosis and assess for joint subluxation.

"Shoulder pain" can be a complex complaint to evaluate. It should be remembered that shoulder pathologies can be present in tandem, with a multifactorial basis for the patient's presenting complaints of pain and disability. An accurate diagnosis following injury to the shoulder requires a careful, focused history, a comprehensive physical examination, and judicious use of appropriate imaging modalities.

For a complete list of references, go to ExpertConsult.com.

SELECTED READINGS

Citation:
Neer CS. Impingement lesions. *Clin Orthop Relat Res.* 1983;173:70–77.

Level of Evidence:
IV

Summary:
Classic article describing the clinical and anatomic basis for impingement syndrome.

Citation:
Hertel R, Ballmer FT, Lombert SM, et al. Lag signs in the diagnosis of rotator cuff rupture. *J Shoulder Elbow Surg.* 1996;5(4):307–313.

Level of Evidence:
V

Summary:
Original description of lag signs in the diagnosis of rotator cuff tears.

Citation:
Lee S, Savin DD, Shah NR, et al. Scapular winging: evaluation and treatment: AAOS exhibit selection. *J Bone Joint Surg Am.* 2015;21(97):1708–1716.

Level of Evidence:
V

Summary:
Reviews the evaluation of different types of scapular winging and their treatment options.

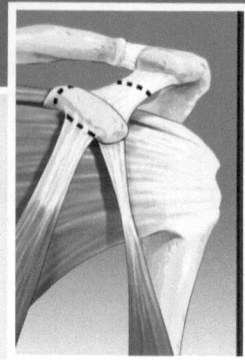

38

Glenohumeral Joint Imaging

Alissa J. Burge, Gabrielle P. Konin

CONVENTIONAL RADIOGRAPHY

Conventional radiography is and should be the initial imaging examination performed for a patient presenting with shoulder pain. Although radiographs provide limited evaluation of the rotator cuff and glenoid labrum, they can offer important information about the source of the patient's symptoms. Radiographs depict an assortment of osseous abnormalities, including fracture, arthritis, soft tissue calcifications, postsurgical changes, and tumor, and they are frequently complementary to more advanced imaging modalities, such as computed tomography (CT) and magnetic resonance imaging (MRI). A wide variety of radiographic views are available to aid in the evaluation of the glenohumeral joint. Knowledge about the advantages and disadvantages of each view will assist in optimizing imaging protocols, depending on the clinical presentation (Box 38.1).[1-3]

Anteroposterior View

The anteroposterior (AP) view (Fig. 38.1A) is obtained with the patient in either the upright or the supine position. The beam is directed in a true AP direction relative to the body. The glenoid rim is normally tilted anteriorly about 40 degrees, which results in overlap of the humeral head and glenoid rim in the AP view. This view can be obtained with the humeral head in the neutral position, internal rotation, or external rotation. When compared with other radiographic views of the shoulder, the AP view provides the best overview of the osseous structures of the shoulder girdle because the projection allows for relatively uniform distribution of soft tissue density across the entire shoulder. As a result, one or more of the AP views is nearly always included in the standard radiographic evaluation of the shoulder. These projections allow for adequate evaluation of the humeral head, glenoid, and body of the scapula, as well as the acromioclavicular (AC) joint and coracoid process. The AP projection is very helpful in the evaluation after acute trauma for evidence of fracture or dislocation and is also of value in assessing the cause of chronic pain from arthritis, impingement, calcific tendinitis/bursitis, tumor, or infection.

Grashey View

The Grashey view is a true or neutral AP view (see Fig. 38.1B), and differs from the standard AP view in that the patient is rotated posteriorly 35 to 40 degrees, thus providing a tangential view of the glenohumeral joint. The advantage of the Grashey

view is that it provides a superior evaluation of the glenohumeral joint. This view can demonstrate subtle subluxation in the superior or inferior direction and will show subtle joint space narrowing associated with glenohumeral arthritis. The disadvantage of this view is that a rapid change in soft tissue density occurs from medial to lateral, and as a result, the lateral aspect of the shoulder, including the acromion and AC joint, is difficult to evaluate because of a rapid change in density on the radiograph and loss of anatomic detail laterally. This loss can be decreased with use of a boomerang-shaped filter draped along the lateral shoulder.

Axillary Lateral View

Variations of the axillary lateral view exist, but the projection is most commonly obtained with the patient supine and with the arm abducted 90 degrees (see Fig. 38.1C). The beam is then directed from distal to proximal while tilted 15 to 30 degrees toward the spine. This projection is best suited for evaluation of the joint space as well as anterior or posterior subluxation or dislocation. Bankart fractures of the anterior glenoid rim may also be detected. Numerous variations of this projection have been developed, some with the goal of decreasing movement of the arm in the setting of acute trauma (Velpeau view), and others with the intention of accentuating certain anatomic features. The West Point view is a variation of the axillary view developed to optimize visualization of an osseous Bankart lesion. It is obtained by placing the patient in the prone position on the x-ray table with the arm abducted 90 degrees from the long axis of the body and with the forearm draped over the edge of the top of the table. The beam is directed 15 to 20 degrees in an inferior-to-superior direction and tilted 25 degrees toward the spine. This projection improves the detection of osseous Bankart lesions but is very difficult to obtain in the setting of acute trauma and is best reserved for the patient in the setting of subacute or chronic instability.[4]

Scapular Y View

The scapular Y view is easily obtained in the setting of acute trauma because it can be obtained with the arm immobilized by the side, and little or no movement of the arm is required (see Fig. 38.1D). This view can be very helpful in the setting of acute trauma to evaluate for anterior or posterior dislocation. The projection is obtained with the patient upright or prone and rotated approximately 30 to 45 degrees toward the cassette.

The beam is directed down the body of the scapula and results in a projection in which the body of the scapula is seen in tangent and the glenoid fossa en face as a Y-shaped intersection of the scapular body, coracoid process, and acromion process. It is also the projection commonly used when classifying the acromial morphology.

Stryker Notch View

The Stryker notch view is best suited for viewing the postero-lateral aspect of the humeral head and is an excellent radiographic

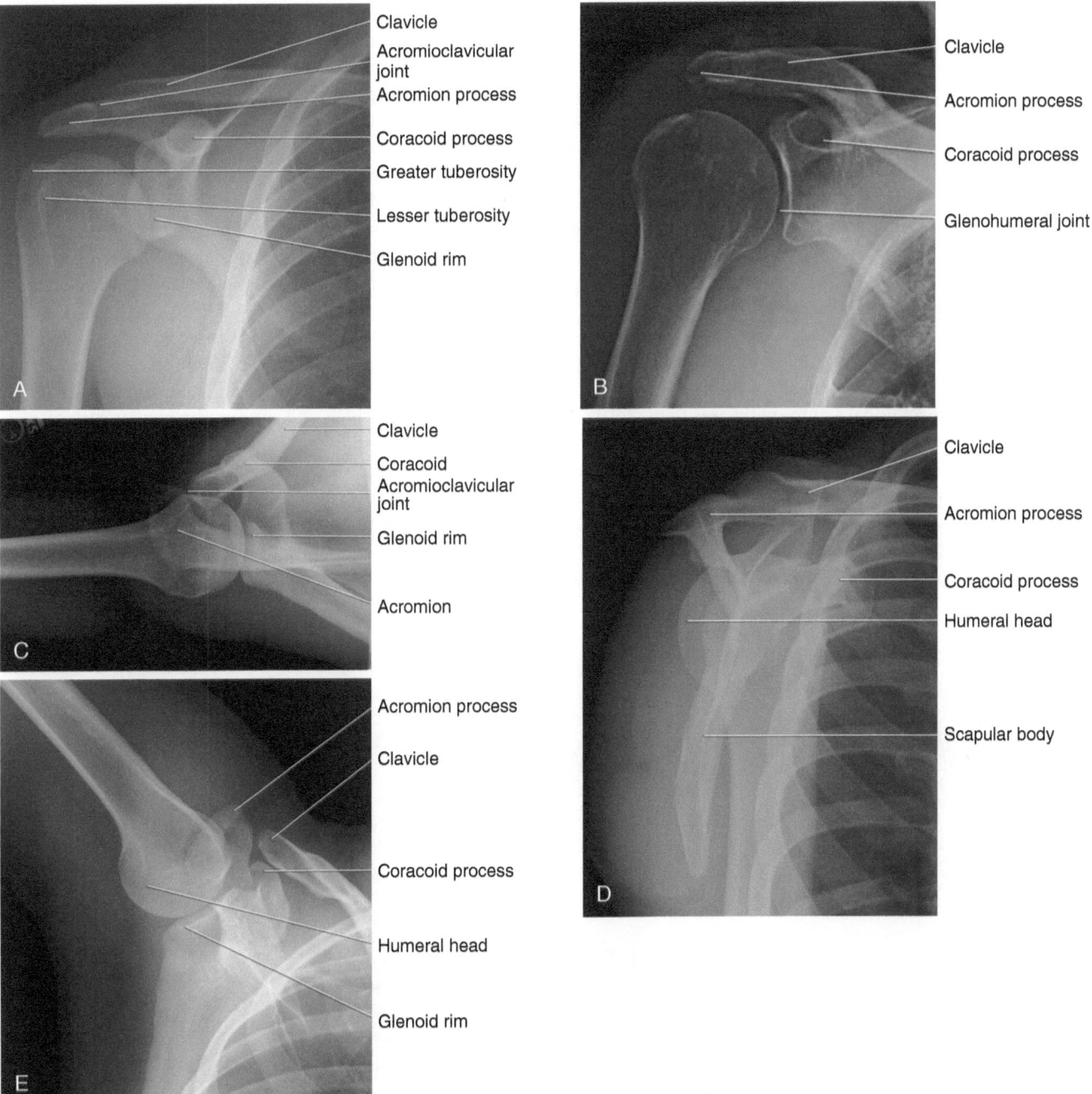

Fig. 38.1 (A) An anteroposterior (AP) view of the shoulder in external rotation. (B) An AP view of the gleno-humeral joint (Grashey view). (C) An axillary view of the shoulder. (D) A scapular Y view of the shoulder. (E) A Stryker notch view of the shoulder.

view for detecting a Hill-Sach's defects when the patient has sustained a translational event (see Fig. 38.1E). However, it is very limited in its evaluation of the glenoid rim for osseous Bankart lesions. The Stryker notch view is obtained with the patient in either the upright or supine position. The arm is positioned vertically overhead with the elbow flexed and the hand supported on the back of the head. The beam is directed toward the mid axilla and is tilted about 10 degrees cephalad.

Acromioclavicular Articulation Views

AC pathology is best evaluated with the patient either sitting or standing with the back flat against the cassette. The arms are usually freely hanging by the sides of the body. A Zanca view is the most accurate view to look at the AC joint, which is obtained by tilting the beam 10 to 15 degrees cephalad and centered over the AC joint with 50% of the standard shoulder AP penetration strength.[5] The standard axial radiographic view of the shoulder is valuable to assess for a type III versus a type IV AC joint separation. The patient is infrequently asked to hold weights or sandbags to accentuate AC joint separation, and the value of this measure is questioned.[6] Comparison with the contralateral AC joint can be helpful in detecting subtle abnormalities.

SHOULDER ARTHROGRAPHY

Historically, conventional arthrography of the shoulder (Fig. 38.2) was considered the gold standard for diagnosis of tears of the rotator cuff.[7] Conventional arthrography was then replaced with CT arthrography (CTA) and this technique provided a tool for assessing labral injuries associated with instability as well as cuff tears to a limited degree. Subsequently, CTA was largely replaced by MRI and magnetic resonance arthrography (MRA).

The primary factors contributing to the shift from conventional arthrography and CTA to MRI/MRA are the superb soft tissue contrast, multiplanar capabilities provided by MRI, and lack of exposure to ionizing radiation. MRI allows a global assessment of the painful shoulder, including the rotator cuff, labrum and capsular structures, osseous outlet, acromion, and articular surfaces. Bone marrow and muscle quality are readily evaluated with MRI without exposure to ionizing radiation. However, CTA is an effective alternative for patients who have contraindications to MRI.[8-14]

Arthrography Technique

Although many variations in technique exist, a method for performing arthrography prior to MRI or CT begins with a review of prior radiographs and/or scout films to ensure identification of pertinent abnormalities. The patient is then placed supine on the fluoroscopic table with the arm positioned next to the body in slight external rotation and a point is chosen with fluoroscopic guidance overlying the lower third of the humeral head about 0.5 cm lateral to the medial cortex of the humeral head. An alternative anterior approach is through the rotator interval[15] or a posterior approach.[16] Knowledge of all three approaches allows for tailored techniques based on the clinical situation; for example, a posterior approach may permit more consistent visualization of the anterior capsular structures. The skin is prepared and draped in sterile fashion and the subcutaneous tissues are anesthetized with 1% lidocaine (Xylocaine) using a 25-gauge needle, which can be advanced into the joint. Rarely, a 22-gauge, 3.5-inch spinal needle is required in order to access the joint. A small amount of radiopaque contrast material is initially injected, which will outline the medial surface of the humeral head and spill into the subscapularis recess and axillary pouch (see Fig. 38.2B). A total injection volume of 12 to 14 mL provides adequate distention of the shoulder joint without undue discomfort. Most practices use an iodinated contrast agent for CTA and a dilute gadolinium solution for MRA. The contrast agent can be mixed with 0.1 to 0.3 mL of 1:1000 epinephrine

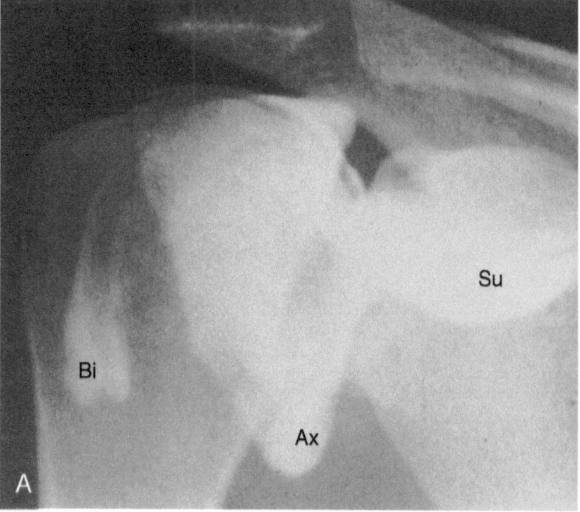
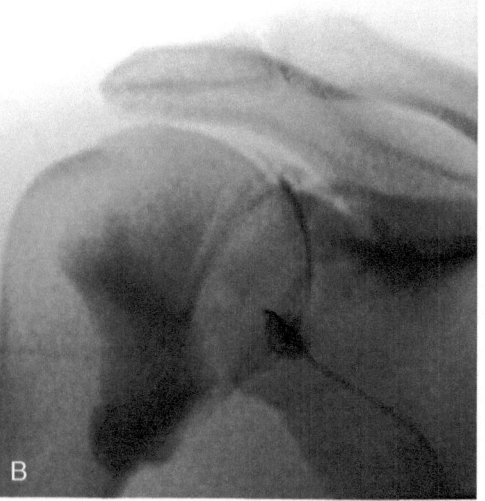

Fig. 38.2 Normal shoulder arthrography. (A) Contrast material is seen within the glenohumeral joint. (B) Early contrast filling in a joint during an arthrogram. Note the absence of contrast material near the needle tip and the normal contour of the axillary pouch. This procedure was performed from an anterior approach over the lower third of the joint. *Ax,* Axillary recess; *Bi,* bicipital tendon sleeve; *Su,* subscapularis recess.

to prolong retention of the contrast agent within the joint, thus allowing adequate time for transportation of the patient to the CT or MRI scanner and for imaging, which should be performed as soon as possible.

COMPUTED TOMOGRAPHY

CT imaging of the shoulder is performed primarily as a means of evaluating the osseous structures after trauma. Multidetector CT utilizing isotropic data sets and post-processing techniques can accurately detect the extent of displacement and angulation of fracture fragments involving the humeral head and neck. The scapula is a complex anatomic structure composed of the body, coracoid and acromion processes, and the glenoid with its articular surface. Following a glenohumeral translational event, CT and three-dimensional volume rendered imaging are useful for pre-surgical planning in order to accurately depict the extent of glenoid bone loss of an osseous Bankart and the magnitude of a Hill–Sachs defect (Fig. 38.3).[17–20]

ULTRASONOGRAPHY

Sonography of the shoulder (Fig. 38.4) is a noninvasive, accurate and cost-effective method for a dynamic evaluation of the

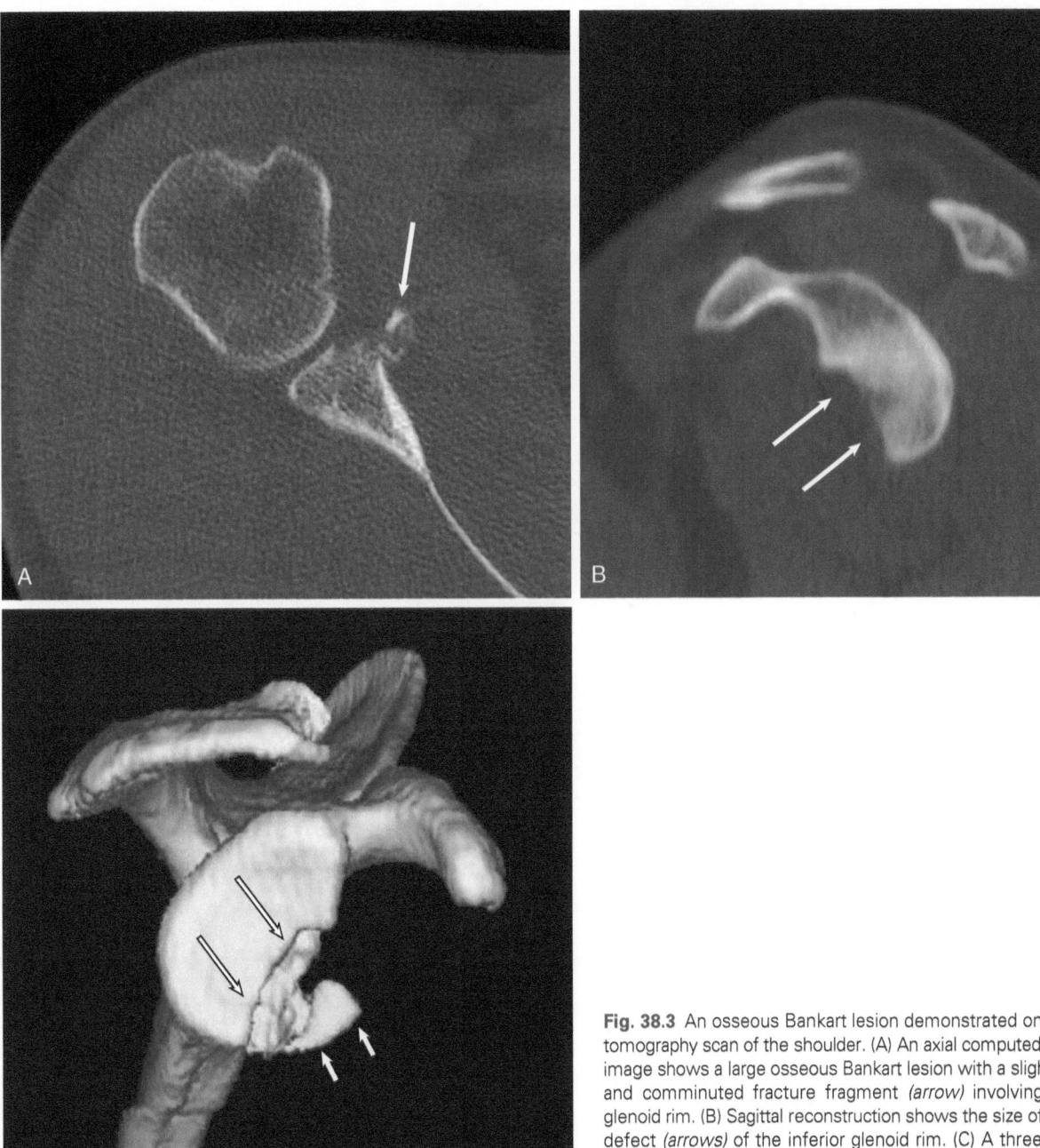

Fig. 38.3 An osseous Bankart lesion demonstrated on a computed tomography scan of the shoulder. (A) An axial computed tomographic image shows a large osseous Bankart lesion with a slightly displaced and comminuted fracture fragment *(arrow)* involving the inferior glenoid rim. (B) Sagittal reconstruction shows the size of the osseous defect *(arrows)* of the inferior glenoid rim. (C) A three-dimensional reconstruction shows the relationship of the fracture fragment *(short arrows)* with the glenoid rim osseous defect *(long arrows)*.

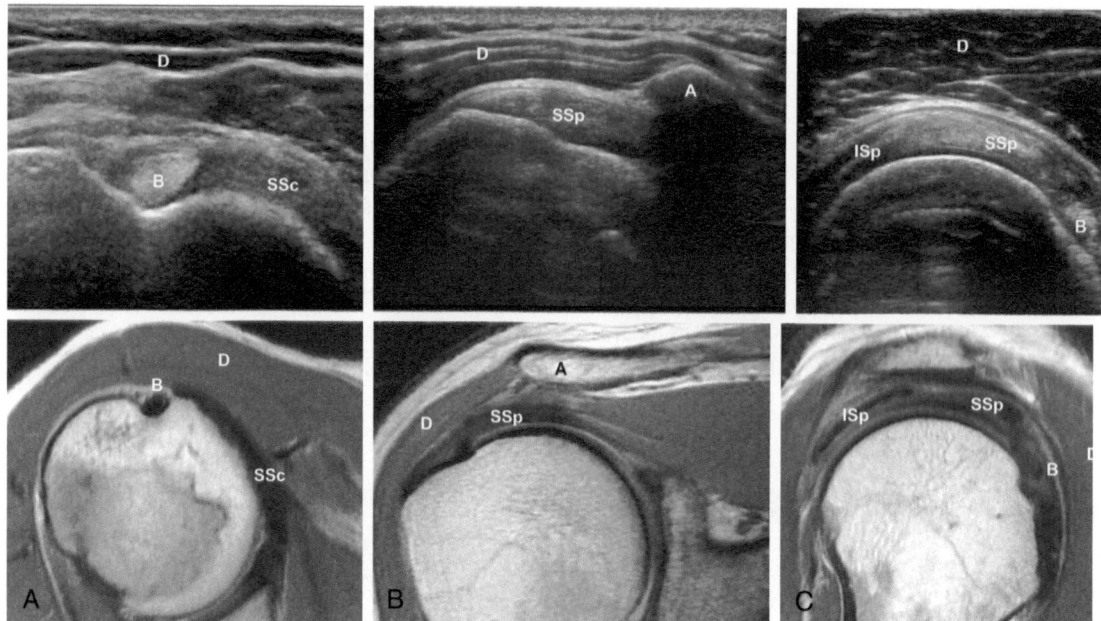

Fig. 38.4 Paired ultrasound and magnetic resonance images. (A) A short axis ultrasound image of the normal long head of the biceps tendon *(B)* and subscapularis tendon *(SSc)* with corresponding axial fast spin echo (FSE) image. (B) A long axis ultrasound image of the supraspinatus tendon *(SSp)* and acromion *(A)* with corresponding oblique coronal FSE image. (C) A short axis ultrasound image in the sagittal plane depicting the infraspinatus *(Isp)*, supraspinatus and biceps tendons with corresponding oblique sagittal FSE image. *D,* Deltoid.

rotator cuff and is a superb means for guided injections about the shoulder.[21–25] Ultrasound examination of the shoulder requires a high-resolution linear transducer (6 to 15 MHz) and is performed with the patient in the sitting position. The tendons of the rotator cuff and the long head of the biceps should be evaluated in both the long and short axes.

The examination begins with the arm positioned by the side and externally rotated for evaluation of the biceps long head tendon. In this position, the subscapularis can be evaluated with the elbow flexed 90 degrees and externally rotated. The infraspinatus is imaged with the arm adducted and the hand on the opposite shoulder. For evaluation of the supraspinatus, the shoulder is rotated internally, and the arm is placed behind the back, which allows the critical portion of the supraspinatus tendon to glide from beneath the acromion, allowing maximal visualization of this portion of the rotator cuff.[26] The normal rotator cuff is sharp and uniform in its fibrillar echotexture. It measures 4 to 6 mm in thickness anteriorly, and is normally somewhat thinner posteriorly.[22] A thin echogenic band paralleling the upper surface of the cuff reflects the subacromial–subdeltoid bursa. The overlying deltoid is characterized by the typical striated/marbled echogenicity of muscle that is distinct from the normal overlying tendons (Table 38.1).

Although sonography of the rotator cuff has been shown to be as accurate as MRI in the evaluation of the rotator cuff tendons,[27–29] sonographic evaluation of the shoulder has a steep learning curve and is operator dependent.[30] MRI has, in its favor, a more global evaluation of the shoulder, including the labrum and osseous structures, which has led to the use of MRI in most practices.

TABLE 38.1   Sonographic Imaging Signs of Rotator Cuff Disease

Type of Disease	Imaging Signs
Tendinosis	Heterogeneous echogenicity of the tendon with loss of fibrillar architecture; may be thickened or thinned
Partial-thickness tear	Difficult, but may see focal thinning of tendon
Full-thickness tear	Focal full-thickness discontinuity/absence of the cuff
Subacromial subdeltoid bursitis	Band of anechoic/hypoechoic fluid superficial to cuff ± power Doppler hyperemia

MAGNETIC RESONANCE IMAGING

MRI provides comprehensive evaluation of the shoulder, combining superior soft tissue depiction with the ability to simultaneously evaluate osseous pathology. MRI of the shoulder is best performed at 1.5 or 3.0 Tesla (T) utilizing a dedicated surface coil, and images are typically obtained in the axial, oblique coronal, and oblique sagittal planes relative to the anatomic axis of the shoulder (Fig. 38.5). Specific protocols vary by institution, but optimally should include a combination of pulse sequences allowing for both sensitive detection of mobile water and high-resolution evaluation of anatomy. At the authors' institution, routine shoulder imaging sequences consist of a single oblique coronal fat suppressed image (inversion recovery [IR] or T2 with fat saturation), followed by oblique coronal, axial, and oblique sagittal moderate echo time fast spin echo (FSE) images in the axial, oblique coronal, and oblique sagittal planes (Table 38.2).

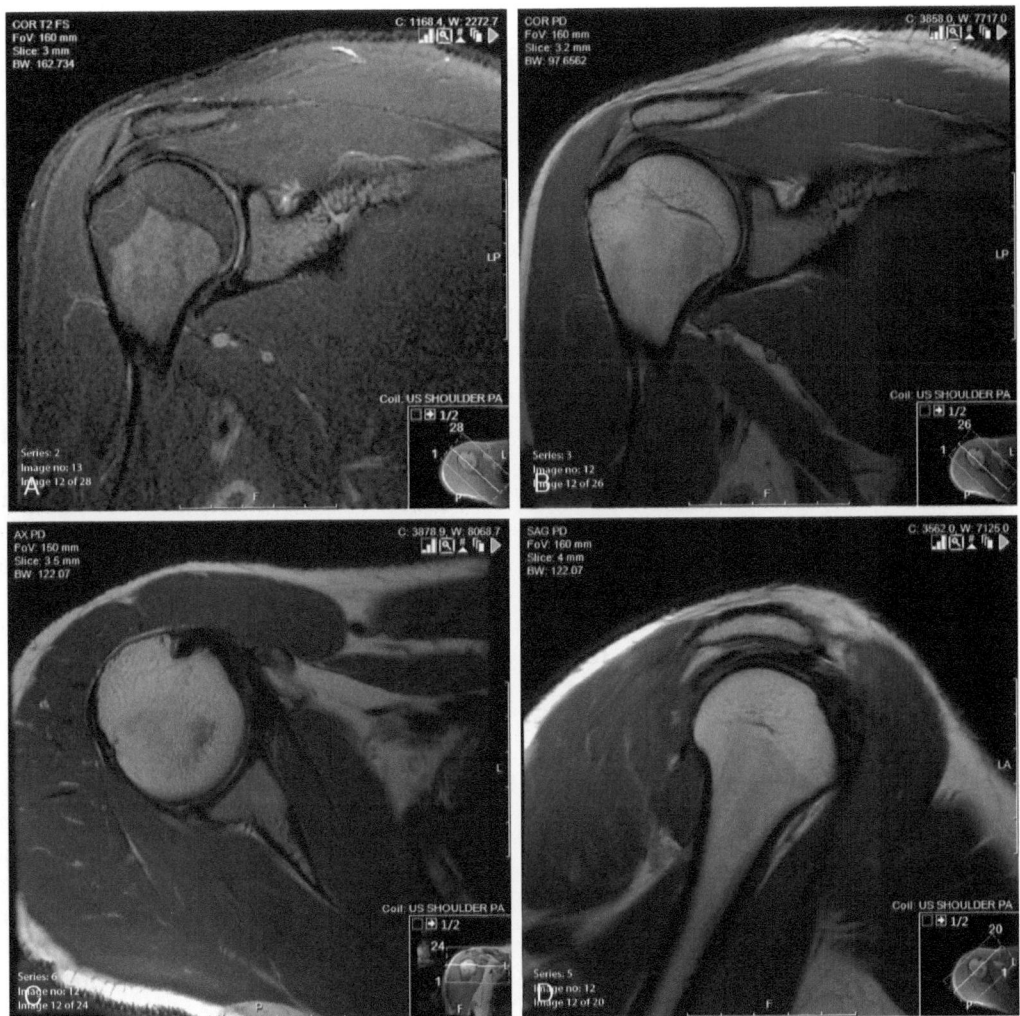

Fig. 38.5 Sample routine shoulder magnetic resonance imaging protocol, consisting of (A) oblique coronal T2 with fat saturation, (B) oblique coronal proton density, (C) axial proton density, and (D) oblique sagittal proton density.

Parameter	Coronal Fast IR	Oblique Coronal FSE	Oblique Sagittal FSE	Axial FSE
TABLE 38.2 **Sample Acquisition Parameters for Routine Clinical Imaging of the Shoulder at 1.5 Tesla**				
TR (ms)	5000	4000	4000	4000
TE (ms)	17	34	34	34
TI (ms)	150	na	na	na
BW (kHz)	31.25	31.25	31.25	31.25
ETL	7	10	10	9
NEX	2	2	2	2
FOV (cm)	16	16	16	15
Matrix	256 × 192	512 × 3S4	512 × 224	512 × 384
Slice/gap (mm)	3/D	3/0	4/0.5	3.5/0
NPW	Yes	Yes	Yes	Yes
Frequency	R/L	R/L	A/P	R/L

A/P, Anterior to posterior; *BW,* receiver bandwidth; *ETL,* echo train length; *FOV,* field of view; *FSE,* fast spin echo; *IR,* inversion recovery; *na,* not applicable; *NEX,* number of excitations; *NPW,* no phase wrap; *R/L,* right to left; *TE,* echo time; *TI,* time to inversion; *TR,* repetition time.

Specialized MRI techniques may be useful for certain applications. For reduction of motion artifact in patients who are unable to remain still during pulse acquisition, the periodically rotated overlapping parallel lines with enhanced reconstruction (PROPELLER) pulse sequence, utilizing radial sampling of parallel data lines rotating about the center of K space, reduces the severity of motion artifact, thereby improving image quality and diagnostic yield.[31]

MRI of the postoperative shoulder requires knowledge of the surgical intervention performed, in order to allow the implementation of proper pulse parameter modifications if necessary, such as in the presence of extensive metallic hardware. When utilizing conventional pulse sequences in the presence of metal, techniques that may be used to decrease artifact include widening the receiver bandwidth, aligning the frequency encoding axis along the long axis of the implant, and oversampling in the frequency direction. Additional improvement in image quality may be obtained by decreasing the voxel size and increasing the number of excitations. Because the artifact generated by a particular metal implant increases with field strength, imaging at higher field strengths, such as 3.0T, should be avoided. Additionally, frequency selective fat suppression methods should be avoided in favor of methods that are less frequency dependent (e.g., short tau inversion recovery [STIR]) and therefore more robust in the presence of field inhomogeneities that occur in the vicinity of metal hardware.[32,33]

In the setting of large metallic implants, specialized pulse sequences designed to significantly reduce metal artifact may be employed. These include multiple acquisition variable resonance image combination (MAVRIC) and slice encoding metal artifact correction (SEMAC). MAVRIC utilizes multiple acquisitions at varying off-resonance spectral frequency bins, which are subsequently postprocessed to create images with significantly reduced susceptibility artifact. SEMAC utilizes view angle tilting plus the addition of a phase encoding step in the Z axis, resulting in extremely robust spatial encoding which diminishes the amount of artifact.[32,34]

Evaluation of early chondral degeneration may be performed using quantitative parametric MRI techniques, which have been demonstrated to correlate to early changes in chondral matrix elements, including proteoglycan and collagen, prior to the development of gross morphologic changes visible on routine conventional imaging sequences. These techniques include T2 mapping, which is sensitive to changes in collagen orientation and free water content, and spin lattice relaxation in the rotating frame (T1 rho), which is sensitive to depletion of proteoglycan. Delayed gadolinium enhanced MRI of cartilage (dGEMRIC) is an additional biomarker for proteoglycan depletion, though requires the intravenous administration of gadolinium-based contrast material.[35,36]

While CT remains the gold standard for high resolution evaluation of mineralized bone, newer "silent" magnetic resonance (MR) techniques, such as zero TE imaging, allow evaluation of bone with CT-like contrast concurrently with the acquisition of routine clinical MR sequences, obviating the need for a separate imaging study and a dose of ionizing radiation, though these sequences are not yet in widespread clinical use.[37]

MRA: While some authors have described an advantage in detecting chondral and labral pathology following the intraarticular administration of gadolinium contrast material, others have achieved statistically equivalent or superior sensitivity and specificity utilizing optimized high resolution noncontrast techniques.[38] The accuracy of MRA versus noncontrast MRI depends largely upon the experience and preference of the interpreting radiologist, and therefore the viewpoint of which technique is optimal in a given situation will often depend on the convention of a particular institution. At the authors' institution, high resolution noncontrast imaging is preferred, given its ability to reliably detect chondral and labral lesions while simultaneously allowing direct visualization of the synovium and evaluation of chondral signal changes in the setting of early degeneration without a frank chondral defect.

IMAGING OF SPECIFIC SHOULDER ABNORMALITIES

Interpretation of a shoulder MRI examination requires the evaluation of images obtained in several imaging planes and with various pulse sequences. The following sections provide a systematic approach for MRI evaluation as the imaging basis for recognizing common pathologic processes; when appropriate, complementary imaging modalities are discussed. The important structures that must be thoroughly evaluated on each MRI examination include the osseous structures (outlet and acromion), the rotator cuff muscles and tendons, the biceps tendon and rotator interval, and the labrum (capsular structures and articular surfaces).

Osseous Outlet and Acromion

The clinical syndrome of shoulder impingement refers to a painful compression of the soft tissues of the anterior shoulder (i.e., the rotator cuff, subacromial bursa, and bicipital tendon) between the humeral head and the coracoacromial arch (i.e., the coracoid process, acromion, coracoacromial ligament and AC joint).[39–41] Pain occurs when the arm is elevated forward and internally rotated or placed in the position of abduction and external rotation.[40]

In the normal shoulder, the upward pull of the deltoid on the proximal humerus is resisted by an intact rotator cuff so that the humeral head remains centered on the glenoid in all ranges of motion. If this stabilizing mechanism becomes weakened as a result of trauma, overuse or age, the humeral head is pulled upward under the structures of the coracoacromial arch. Impingement is initially followed by subacromial bursitis and rotator cuff tendinopathy. Over time, irreversible cuff trauma occurs with fibrosis and degeneration. In the latter stages, subacromial enthesophyte tends to form at the anteroinferior margin of the acromion where the coracoacromial ligament attaches (Fig. 38.6). Tears of the rotator cuff are frequent in this stage, undoubtedly in part because of direct cuff trauma from the spur. After massive tears of the rotator cuff, the humeral head typically migrates anterosuperiorly and chronic impaction with the undersurface of the anterior acromion results in sclerosis and proliferative changes—acetabularization.

Neer (1983) introduced the term *impingement syndrome* and described three stages with the rotator cuff disorder.[41] The

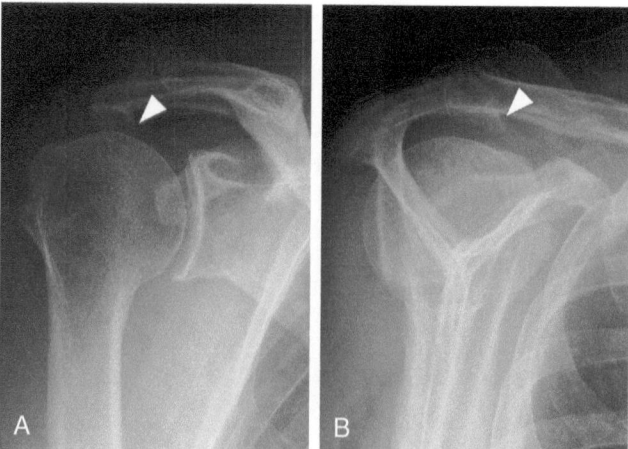

Fig. 38.6 Subacromial spur. (A) Grashey and (B) scapular Y views of the shoulder. The arrowheads point to the spur emanating off the anteroinferior acromion.

diagnosis of impingement syndrome is usually made clinically on the basis of appropriate historical and physical examination findings. A thorough history and physical examination by an experienced physician have an 84% to 90% sensitivity and a 75% to 95% specificity for diagnosis of a tear of the rotator cuff.[42–44] Many imaging modalities are available to assist in the evaluation of the progressively painful shoulder, and their role is both to assess the extent of abnormality of the rotator cuff and to identify configurations of the osseous outlet that may predispose to rotator cuff impingement.

The osseous changes that occur with impingement are seen late and thus offer little in establishing an early diagnosis and preventing progression of the associated soft tissue injuries. The following osseous abnormalities may be associated with the clinical syndrome of impingement[40,45–47]:

- Enthesophyte formation on the anteroinferior aspect of the acromion
- A long anterior portion of the acromion with downward sloping of the acromion
- An os acromiale that is not fused
- AC joint arthrosis with hypertrophy

Optimal conventional radiographic views have been described for identifying these variations of the osseous outlet.[48,49] The AP radiograph at a 30-degree caudal angle is helpful in visualizing the anterior aspect of the acromion and in detecting inferiorly directed enthesophytes. A modified transcapular lateral view obtained with 10 to 15 degrees of caudal angulation (the supraspinatus outlet view) helps further identify the anteroinferior aspect of the acromion (see Fig. 38.6). A high-riding humeral head with remodeling of the undersurface of the acromion and sclerosis of the greater tuberosity are conventional radiographic findings (Fig. 38.7) that are pathognomonic of a chronic rotator cuff insufficiency.

Magnetic Resonance Imaging of the Osseous Outlet and Acromion

The multiplanar capabilities of MRI and its ability to demonstrate the relationship of the entire osseous outlet to the underlying rotator cuff allow excellent assessment of the outlet. Bigliani[45] described three different radiographic acromial shapes (Fig. 38.8) and related the configuration of the undersurface of the acromion to the presence of rotator cuff tears. A type I acromion (see Fig. 38.8A) has a flat undersurface, a type II acromion (see Fig. 38.8B) has a curved undersurface, and a type III acromion (see Fig. 38.8C) has an anterior hook. The acromial types II and III have an increased association with rotator cuff tears.[45,47] A type IV acromion with a convex undersurface has been described, but no definite correlation has been shown to exist between type IV acromion and impingement (see Fig. 38.8D).[50] On MRI, the shape of the acromion is best assessed on the oblique sagittal view just lateral to the AC joint. However, one study suggests poor correlation of acromial arch shape between conventional radiography and MRI.[51] Another study found no association between rotator cuff tears and the acromial structure.[52] A third study reported poor interobserver agreement between radiographs and MRI scans at the categorization of the acromial shape.[53]

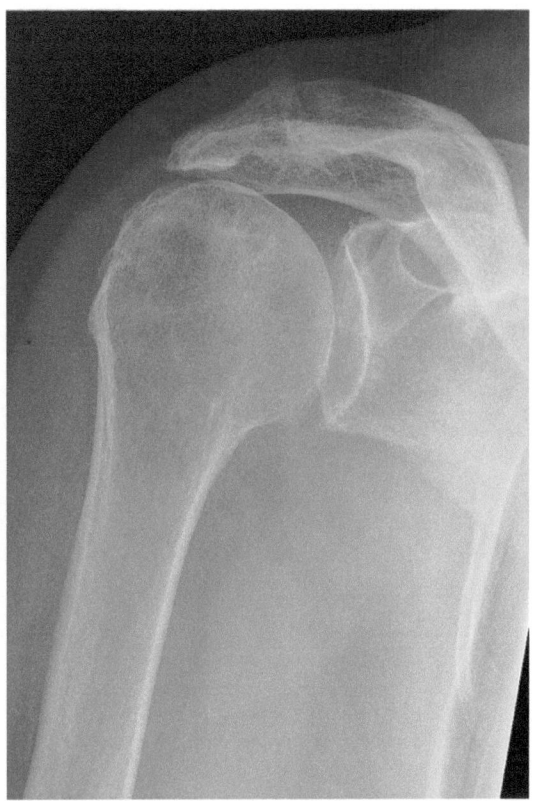

Fig. 38.7 Acromiohumeral interval. Frontal radiograph demonstrates superior migration of the humeral head and loss of the acromiohumeral interval with early acetabularization of the acromion indicating rotator cuff insufficiency. Mild glenohumeral osteoarthritis is evident.

Downward sloping of the acromion can also narrow the supraspinatus outlet and potentially result in impingement,[54,55] and is best seen on the oblique coronal images (Fig. 38.9). An enthesophyte (Fig. 38.10) extending off the anteroinferior aspect of the acromion also can be clearly demonstrated on MRI. It typically appears as a marrow-containing osseous excrescence. Potential pitfalls include the attachment of the coracoacromial ligament and the anterolateral acromial attachment of the deltoid (see Fig. 38.10). These structures may mimic an osseous excrescence, but they can be differentiated from enthesophytes by correlating with concurrent radiographs and because they lack marrow signal and appear dark on all pulse sequences. The acromion should also be evaluated for an os acromiale, which is an accessory ossification center along the outer edge of the anterior acromion. It is normally fused by 25 years of age. An association exists between persistent os acromiale and impingement of the rotator cuff.[56–59] The deltoid muscle attaches to the inferior aspect of the accessory ossicle, and contraction of the deltoid results in a downward motion of the unstable segment, potentially leading to impingement of the underlying rotator cuff (Fig. 38.11). Os acromiale are demonstrated best on axial MR images.[60] MRI signs of instability of the os acromiale include fluid signal within the synchondrosis as well as sclerosis, cystic change, and marrow edema on either side of the synchondrosis (Box 38.2).

Hypertrophic changes of the AC joint capsule and inferiorly directed osteophyte formation (Fig. 38.12) can also be associated with impingement.[40] MRI is useful to evaluate for mass effect

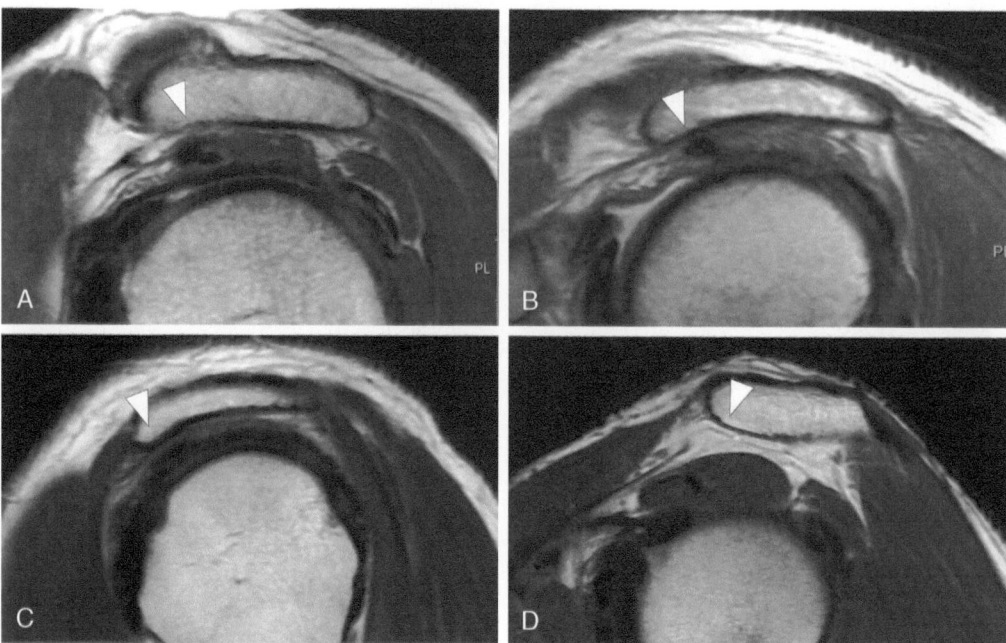

Fig. 38.8 Acromial morphology. Oblique sagittal fast spin echo images of the acromion lateral to the acromioclavicular joint. (A) A type I acromion demonstrates a flat undersurface *(arrow)*. (B) A type II acromion has a gentle curvature to the undersurface of the acromion *(arrows)*. (C) A type III acromion demonstrates a hook *(arrow)* extending off the anterior aspect of the acromion. (D) A type IV acromion demonstrates a curved acromial undersurface *(arrow)*.

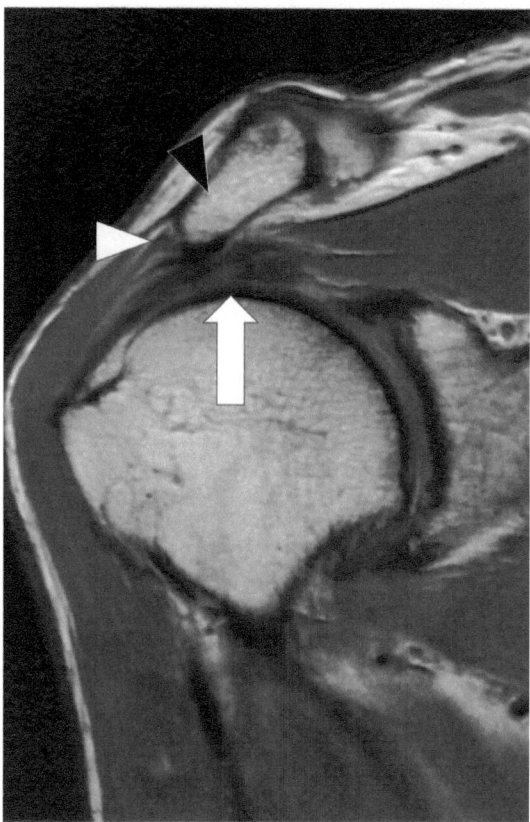

Fig. 38.9 Acromial downward sloping. An oblique coronal fast spin echo image demonstrates anterolateral downward sloping of the acromion *(black arrowhead)* resulting in mild mass effect upon the underlying supraspinatus muscle *(arrow)*, which shows mild increased signal intensity. Anterolateral acromial origin of the deltoid *(white arrowhead)*.

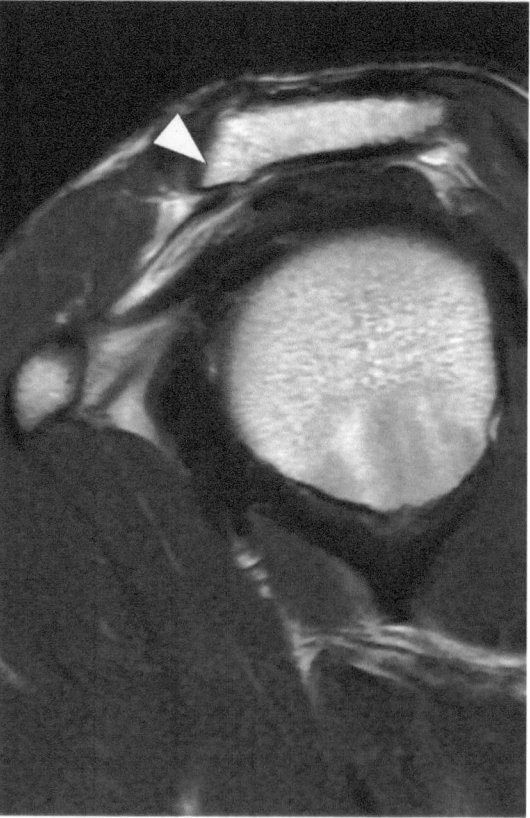

Fig. 38.10 Subacromial enthesophyte. Sagittal oblique fast spin echo (FSE) image demonstrates a marrow containing osseous excrescence extending off the anterior acromion *(arrowhead)*. Note that an enthesophyte contains marrow signal that is high to intermediate in signal on FSE images, which differs from the coracoacromial ligament attachment, which is of low signal intensity on all pulse sequences.

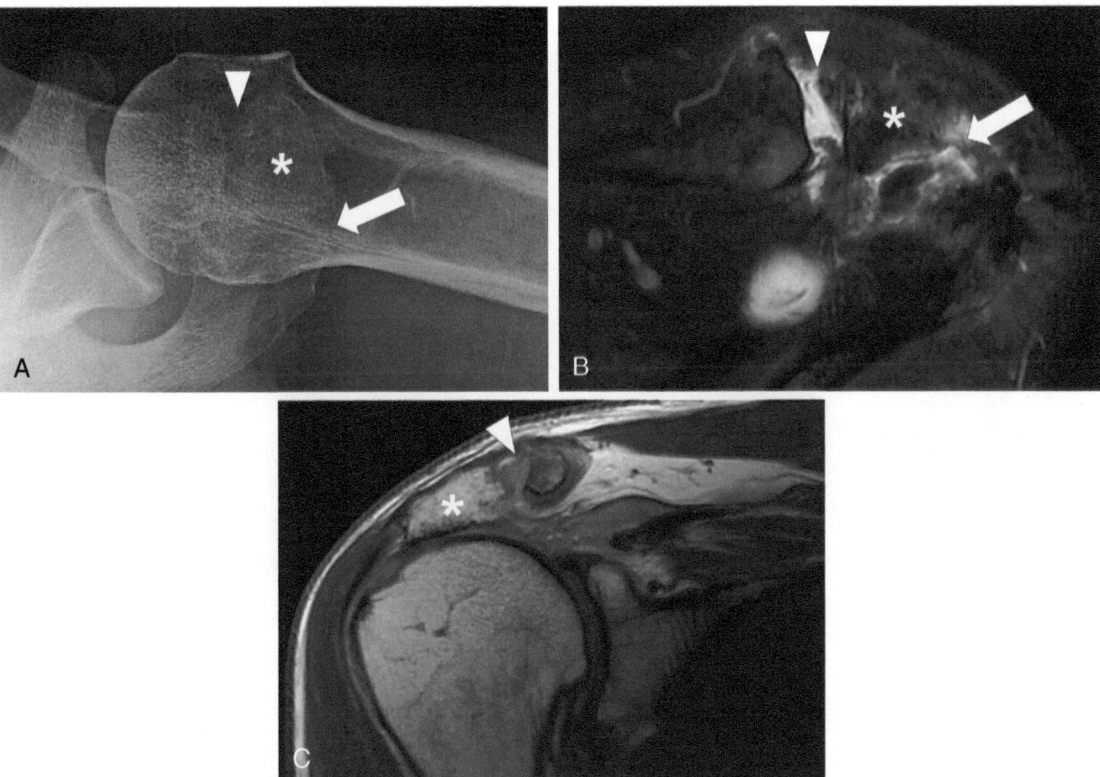

Fig. 38.11 (A) Axillary radiograph depicts an os acromiale and its synchondrosis with the acromion. (B) Axial fat-suppressed T2-weighted image demonstrates an os acromiale with degeneration at the synchondrosis and increased signal on either side of the synchondrosis suggesting instability. Note the chondral denudation over the acromioclavicular (AC) joint and effusion. (C) Oblique coronal fast spin echo image shows severe narrowing of the acromiohumeral interval and a chronic full-thickness supraspinatus tendon tear with retraction of the tendon medial to the glenoid. Os acromiale *(*)*, synchondrosis *(arrows)*, AC joint *(arrowheads)*.

BOX 38.2   Magnetic Resonance Imaging Findings of the Acromion Associated With Extrinsic Impingement

Acromion type—assessed on the oblique sagittal sequences on the image immediately lateral to the acromioclavicular joint:
- Type I: Flat undersurface
- Type II: Curved undersurface
- Type III: Anterior hook
- Type IV: Convex undersurface

Downward sloping—assessed on sagittal and coronal oblique sequences

Acromial spur—assessed on sagittal and coronal oblique fast spin echo sequences (fatty marrow signal within the bony excrescence differentiates a spur from the deltoid tendon slip or coracoacromial ligament)

Unfused os acromiale—best assessed on axial images (fluid signal within the synchondrosis suggests instability)

---

on the underlying rotator cuff. The coracoacromial ligament (Fig. 38.13), a soft tissue structure that forms part of the coracoacromial arch extends from the coracoid to the acromion and is well seen on oblique sagittal MR images. It normally measures less than 2 mm in thickness and extends across the rotator interval and anterior aspect of the supraspinatus tendon. The role of the coracoacromial ligament in impingement remains controversial; some believe that thickening or ossification of the ligament may

be a potential cause of impingement, whereas others believe that thickening results from impingement.[61,62]

Coracohumeral impingement, also referred to as subcoracoid or coracoid impingement, is an uncommon cause of extrinsic impingement that results from a narrowed distance between the coracoid process and the underlying humeral head (Fig. 38.14). Lo and Burkhart[63] suggested using an interval less than 6 mm to make the diagnosis at arthroscopy. On axial images, the normal interval is approximately 10 mm. A narrowed coracohumeral distance may result in entrapment of the subscapularis tendon between the coracoid process and the humeral head, and can lead to isolated tendinosis and disruption of the subscapularis tendon. Abnormalities isolated to the subscapularis tendon should prompt an investigation of the coracohumeral distance and consideration of this diagnosis.[64,65] However, after reporting on a small series of patients with subcoracoid impingement at arthroscopy and control subjects, Giaroli et al.[65] concluded that subcoracoid impingement is primarily a clinical diagnosis that may be supported with imaging.

Rotator Cuff

The rotator cuff is composed of four tendons: the supraspinatus superiorly, the subscapularis anteriorly, and the infraspinatus and teres minor posteriorly. These tendons are important dynamic stabilizers of the glenohumeral joint. Most cuff failures originate

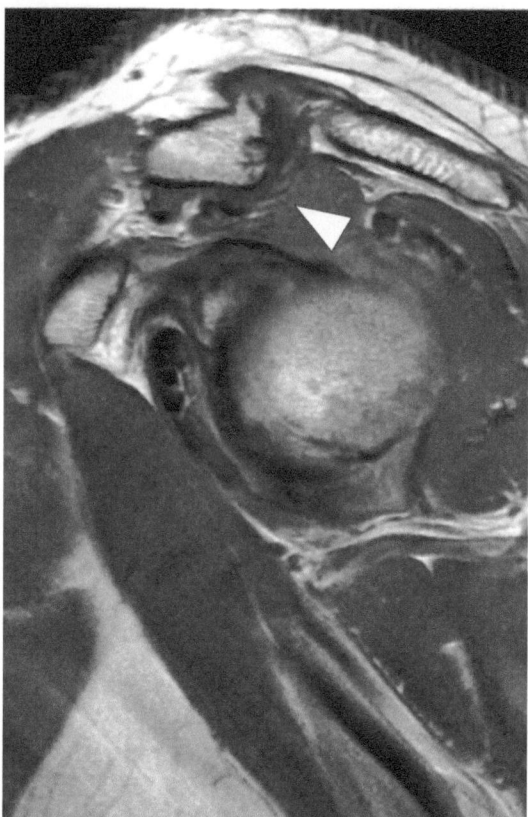

Fig. 38.12 Osteoarthritis of the acromioclavicular joint. A sagittal oblique fast spin echo image shows bony and capsular hypertrophy with an inferiorly directed spur resulting in mass effect upon the supraspinatus muscle tendon junction *(arrowhead)*.

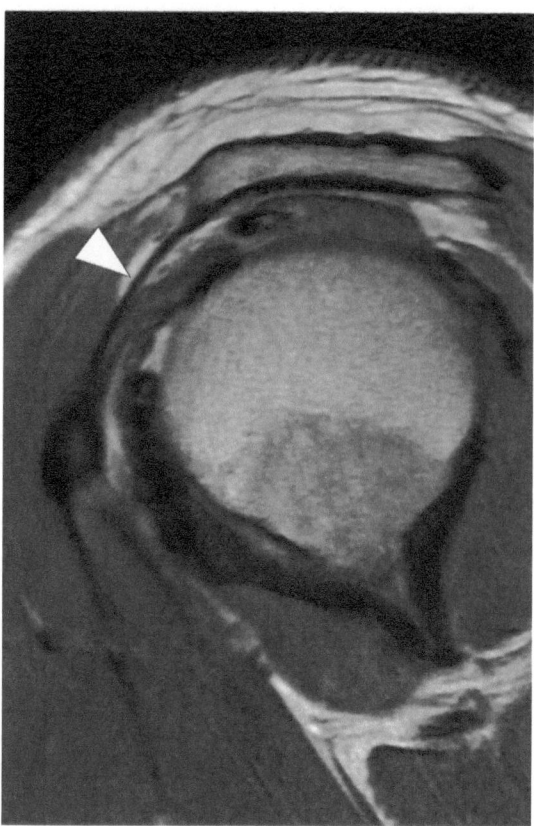

Fig. 38.13 Coracoacromial ligament. An oblique sagittal fast spin echo image demonstrates a normal coracoacromial ligament *(arrowhead)* extending from the coracoid process to the anterior acromion. The normal ligament measures less than 2 mm in thickness.

in the supraspinatus tendon at or near its insertion onto the greater tuberosity of the humeral head. The supraspinatus tendon receives its arterial supply from the anterior humeral circumflex, subscapular, suprascapular, and posterior humeral circumflex arteries.[66–68] A zone of relative avascularity has been described in the tendon proximal to its attachment site and may represent a "critical zone" for cuff failure.[66,67] Other authors have found this zone to be vascularized by anastomosing vessels from the tendon and humeral tuberosity.[69] Arterial filling of the cuff vessels in the critical zone depends on the position of the arm; poor filling is present when the arm is adducted.[67] A high correlation also has been shown to exist between rotator cuff tears and subacromial impingement.[41] It is probably a combination of avascularity and subacromial impingement that leads to most rotator cuff abnormalities originating in the critical zone of the supraspinatus tendon.

Conventional radiography only plays a limited role in the direct evaluation of the rotator cuff, although it is frequently the initial imaging study performed for patients with the clinical syndrome of impingement. Radiographs allow identification of associated pathologic change, especially of the osseous outlet and acromion. Conventional radiography findings associated with cuff pathology include the following[3,70]:

- Enthesopathic changes at the cuff footprint on the humeral head
- Calcific tendinopathy/bursitis

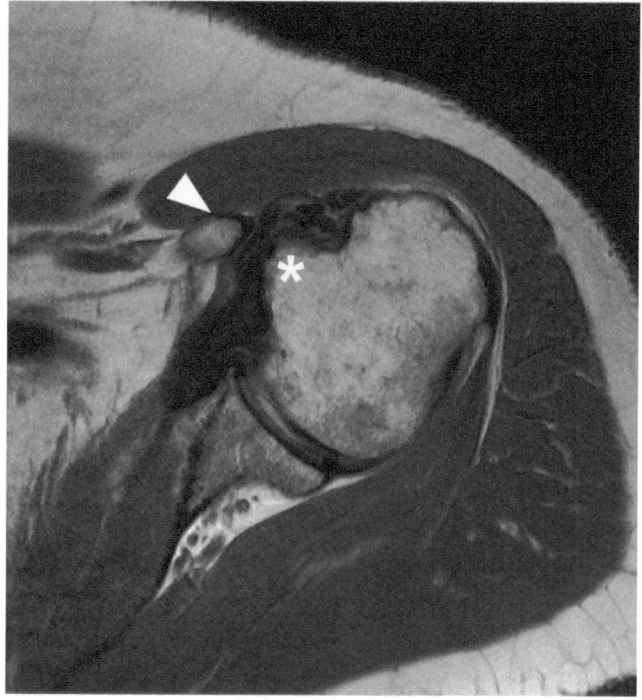

Fig. 38.14 Subcoracoid impingement. An axial fast spin echo image at the level of the coracoid process *(white arrowhead)* demonstrates narrowing of the coracohumeral interval with attenuation of the superior fibers of the subscapularis. Lesser tuberosity *(*)*.

- A high-riding humeral head with an acromiohumeral interval less than 7 mm is associated with rotator cuff insufficiency
- Remodeling of the acromial undersurface to frank acetabularization

Magnetic Resonance Evaluation of the Rotator Cuff

The normal anatomy of the rotator cuff is accurately depicted with MRI. The subscapularis is located anteriorly and has multiple tendon slips. It has a broad origin along the anterior aspect of the scapula and attaches to the lesser tuberosity on the anterior aspect of the humeral head. An extension of the subscapularis tendon known as the transverse ligament extends across the intertubercular groove and helps to stabilize the long head of the biceps tendon within the intertubercular groove. The subscapularis muscle and tendon are best evaluated on axial and oblique sagittal MRI. The supraspinatus muscle originates along the posterosuperior portion of the scapula above the level of the scapular spine. A single tendon arises out of the muscle and extends superiorly above the humeral head to insert onto the greater tuberosity of the humeral head. The supraspinatus tendon is best evaluated in the oblique coronal and oblique sagittal MRI planes. The infraspinatus is located posterosuperiorly and has a broad origin along the posterior aspect of the scapula inferior to the scapular spine. The teres minor is located posteroinferiorly, below the level of the infraspinatus, originating along the axillary surface of the scapula and inserting on the most inferior aspect of the greater tuberosity of the humeral head. The infraspinatus and teres minor are best evaluated on oblique coronal and oblique sagittal images.

The normal tendons demonstrate a uniformly dark signal intensity on all pulse sequences; increased signal on FSE sequences is a nonspecific finding that may represent a wide array of conditions ranging from artifact to a complete tear. T2-weighted images with fat suppression have a lower signal/noise ratio and provide less anatomic detail, but they are both sensitive and specific for depicting the full range of rotator cuff abnormalities.

When increased signal is identified on FSE images, the morphologic features of the tendon and the T2-weighted images should be evaluated.[42] A normal appearance of the tendon and normal signal intensity on T2-weighted images suggest that the tendon is probably normal. It is important to be aware of the magic angle effect, an MRI artifact likely to occur in the critical zone of the supraspinatus tendon, occasionally causing confusion about the tendon integrity. This MRI artifact results in increased signal in normal tendons that are angled 55 degrees relative to the direction of the main magnetic field. It occurs primarily on short TE sequences (proton density, T1 and GRE), and as echo time lengthens with T2 weighting, the signal intensity decreases. A wide spectrum of rotator cuff pathology can be accurately depicted on MRI, ranging from tendinosis to a full-thickness tear of the rotator cuff (Table 38.3). Tendinosis is noted as intermediate to high signal on FSE sequences, which does not reach the same brightness as fluid signal (Fig. 38.15). The tendon may demonstrate attritional wear or diffuse or focal thickening, but no evidence of tendon disruption will be seen. Tendinosis represents a degenerative process of the tendon, which histologically represents a combination of inflammation

TABLE 38.3 Magnetic Resonance Imaging Appearance of Rotator Cuff Pathology

Cuff Pathology	Magnetic Resonance Imaging Appearance
Normal tendon	Low signal on all pulse sequences
Tendinopathy	Intermediate signal on fast spin echo sequences
	Thickening or attenuation of the tendon
Calcific tendinosis	Globular low signal on all pulse sequences within the tendon
	Surrounding edema signal
Partial-thickness tear	Fluid signal extending partially through the thickness of the tendon
	Intramuscular cyst
Full-thickness tear	Fluid signal extending completely through tendon superior to inferior
	Discontinuity of the tendon, often with a gap and retraction of the tendon
Musculotendinous retraction	Measured as the length of the medial-to-lateral tendon gap
Fatty atrophy	Graded as mild, moderate, or severe
	Streaks of high signal on fast spin echo sequences and low signal on fat suppressed images: irreversible
	Loss of muscle bulk: reversible

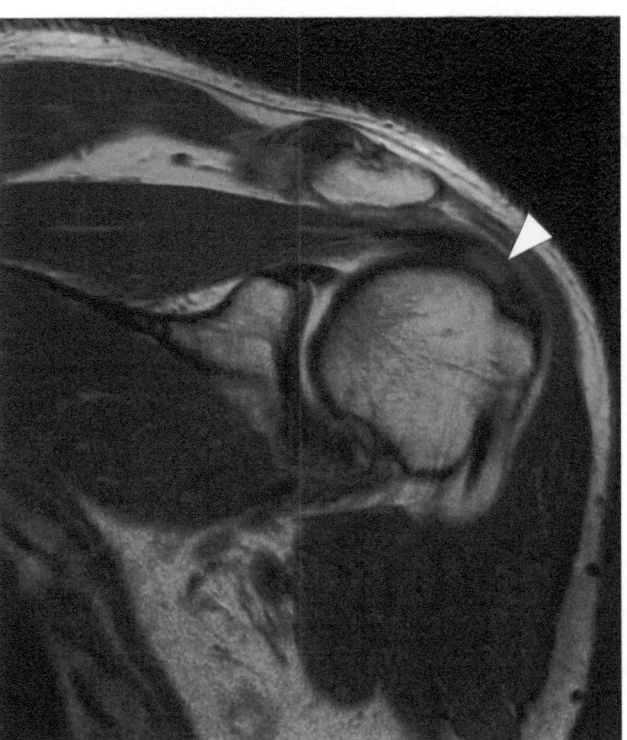

Fig. 38.15 Supraspinatus tendinosis. An oblique coronal fast spin echo image reveals mild thickening of the supraspinatus tendon, as well as increased signal intensity *(arrowhead)* arising from the tendon adjacent to its attachment site on the greater tuberosity, but without fluid signal intensity.

and mucoid degeneration.[71] On arthroscopic examination, the tendon may appear to be edematous and hyperemic, with occasional fraying, roughening, or degeneration of the surface of the tendon. At times, it may be difficult to differentiate tendinosis from early partial-thickness tearing both at arthroscopy and on MRI; however, with quality improvements in image acquisition protocols and scanners, the performance of detecting rotator cuff injuries by radiologists is improved.[72]

Partial-thickness tears (Figs. 38.16–38.18) can occur on either the articular or bursal surface or within the substance of the tendon. A partial-thickness tear is seen on MRI as fluid signal intensity, which extends only partially through the thickness of the tendon from superior to inferior. Tendon tears may partially heal with granulation tissue resulting in scar continuity, making them difficult to distinguish from tendinosis on MRI as they demonstrate intermediate to high signal as opposed to fluid signal. It has been suggested that the detection of partial-thickness articular-sided tears can be improved by adding an abduction external rotation view.[73]

Articular surface tears are the most common type to occur (see Fig. 38.16). A partial articular-sided supraspinatus tendon avulsion lesion is a subset of partial-thickness tears (PASTA).[74] The tear represents a partial-thickness articular-sided avulsion of the supraspinatus tendon, typically at its most anterior attachment site and deserves special attention as one study demonstrated the progression of this type of tear in 80% of the patients, suggesting that early surgical treatment should be considered.[75,76]

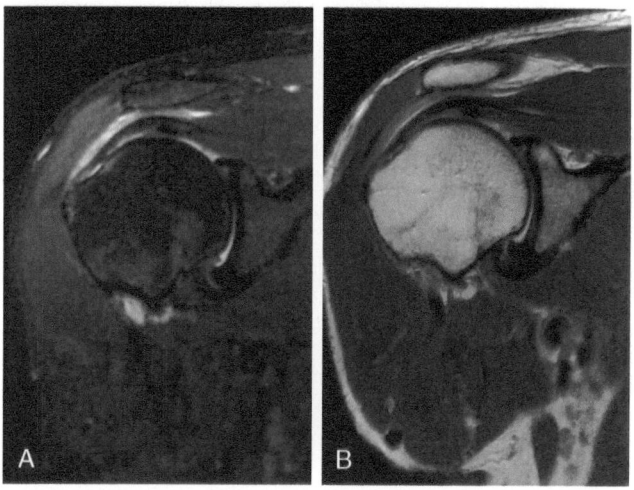

Fig. 38.16 Articular-sided tear. (A) Coronal oblique T2-weighted fat-suppressed and (B) coronal oblique fast spin echo images demonstrate a high-grade partial-thickness, articular-sided supraspinatus tendon tear with mild retraction of tendon slips. Overlying subacromial bursitis is present.

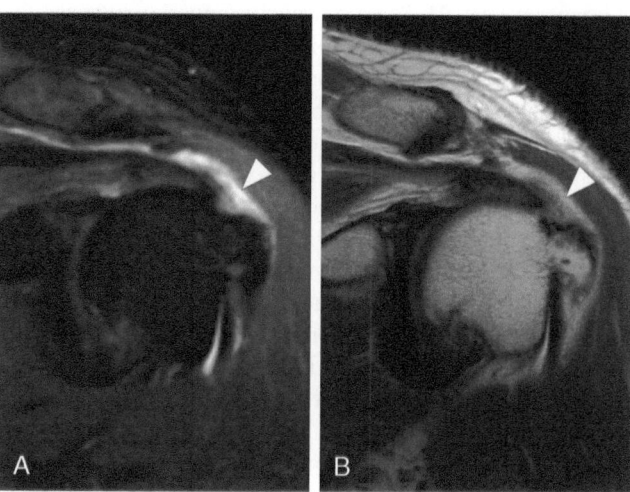

Fig. 38.17 Bursal-sided tear. (A) Coronal oblique T2-weighted fat-suppressed and (B) coronal oblique fast spin echo images show a bursal-sided, partial-thickness tear involving the superficial fibers of the supraspinatus tendon (arrowhead).

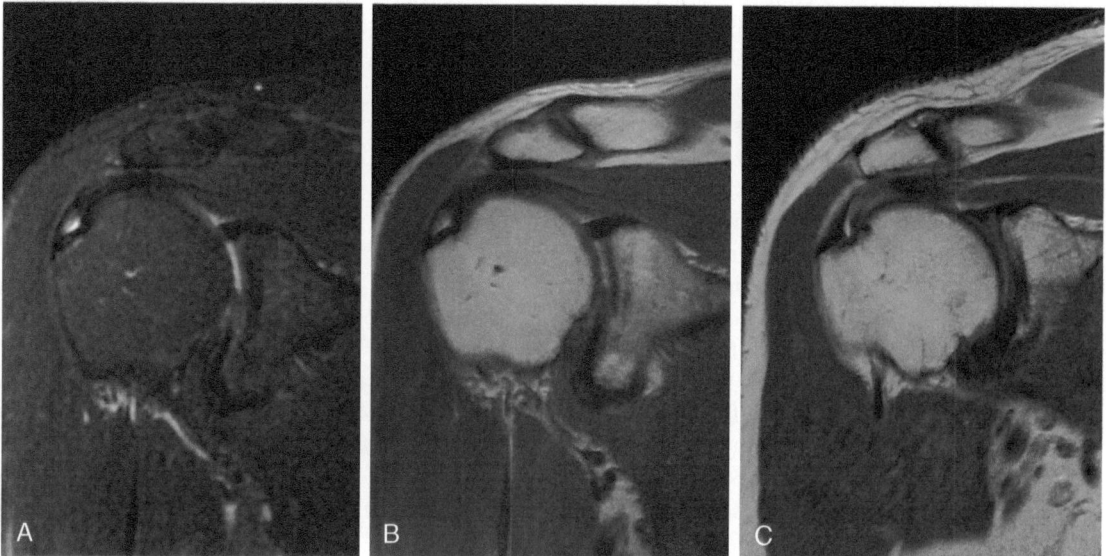

Fig. 38.18 Intrasubstance tear. (A) and (B) Coronal oblique T2-weighted fat-suppressed and fast spin echo (FSE) images show a small fluid signal partial interstitial attachment tear in the supraspinatus tendon. (C) Coronal oblique FSE image in a different patient demonstrates medial delamination of a small intrasubstance tear. Note that both the articular- and bursal-sided fibers are intact in both patients.

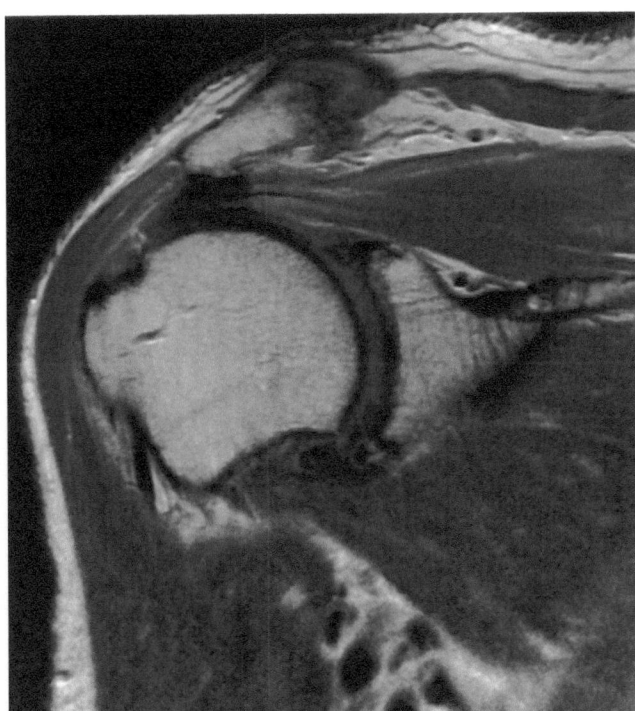

Fig. 38.19 Full-thickness tear. A coronal oblique fast spin echo image shows a full-thickness supraspinatus tendon tear at the critical zone with a stump of tendon remaining attached to the greater tuberosity and without medial retraction of the torn fibers. Note also the prominent subacromial spur with thickening of the coracoacromial ligament attachment (low in signal intensity) and a lateral downslope of the acromion.

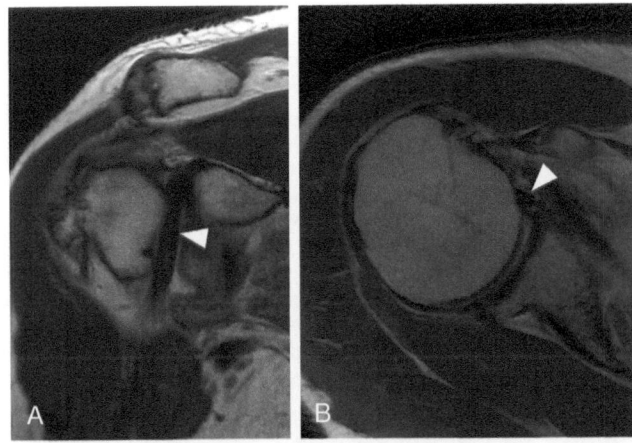

Fig. 38.20 Full-thickness tear. (A) Coronal fast spin echo and (B) axial fast spin echo images demonstrate a full-thickness tear of the subscapularis tendon allowing for medial intra-articular destabilization of the long head of the biceps tendon *(arrowhead)*.

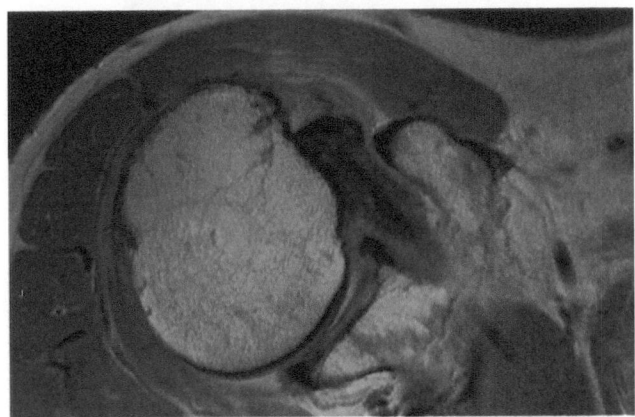

Fig. 38.21 Intrasubstance tear. Axial fast spin echo image demonstrates an intrasubstance tear of the subscapularis tendon allowing for medial destabilization of the biceps tendon into the substance of the subscapularis.

On MRI, an articular-sided avulsion is seen as fluid signal at the footprint with extension along the articular surface of the supraspinatus tendon. Bursal tears affect the superficial fibers of the tendon (see Fig. 38.17). Intrasubstance tears of the rotator cuff do not involve the bursal or the articular surface (see Fig. 38.18) and appear as a linear fluid signal contained within the substance of the tendon, which typically occurs at the footprint.

A full-thickness tear of the rotator cuff tendon is defined as a tear that extends through the complete thickness of the tendon from superior to inferior. This tear allows communication between the joint space and the subacromial-subdeltoid bursa. MRI criteria for establishing the diagnosis of a full-thickness tear include high signal to fluid signal completely traversing the tendon from superior to inferior on FSE images, a gap or absence of the tendon, and retraction of the musculotendinous junction (Fig. 38.19).

Many cuff tears originate in the supraspinatus tendon and large tears may extend into either the infraspinatus or subscapularis tendon. An isolated tear of the infraspinatus tendon is usually associated with the internal impingement syndrome (discussed further in the section on glenohumeral instability). An isolated tear of the subscapularis (Fig. 38.20 and Fig. 38.21) tendon may result from shoulder dislocation or in association with coracohumeral impingement,[77] and is best demonstrated on axial MRI as high signal traversing the tendon with medial retraction of the tendon from the lesser tuberosity. An extension of the subscapularis tendon, known as the transverse ligament, holds the long head of the biceps tendon in the intertubercular groove;

disruption of these fibers can lead to medial destabilization of the long head of the biceps tendon.[78] Depending on the type of subscapularis tendon tear, the biceps tendon may be displaced superficial to, deep to, or within the substance of the tendon.

An intramuscular cyst within the rotator cuff (Fig. 38.22) has been described as a finding associated with small full-thickness or partial-thickness tears of the rotator cuff.[79] Intramuscular cysts are similar to paralabral cysts of the shoulder or meniscal cysts of the knee. Fluid leaks through a defect in the cuff and tracks in a delaminating fashion along the fibers of the tendon, resulting in a fluid collection contained within either the muscle or fascia of the rotator cuff. They appear as lobulated fluid collections within the rotator cuff and should prompt a thorough search for a small associated cuff tear.

Calcific tendinitis (hydroxyapatite crystal deposition disease) can be diagnosed with MRI (Fig. 38.23). The crystalline deposits are typically within the critical zone of the rotator cuff and appear as areas of low signal intensity on all MR pulse sequences. Calcific deposits within the rotator cuff may be difficult to identify on MRI because both the tendon and the calcific deposit appear

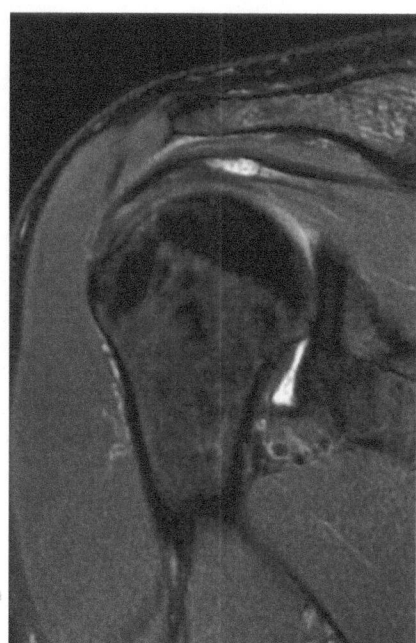

Fig. 38.22 Intramuscular cyst. Coronal oblique T2-weighted fat-suppressed image demonstrates a small intramuscular cyst, which has dissected medially into the muscle tendon junction of the infraspinatus. These intramuscular cysts typically indicate a prior delaminating tendon tear, which may not always be identified due to interval healing.

dark on all pulse sequences. Ancillary MRI findings that may aid in the identification of calcific tendinitis include globular thickening of the involved tendon, and high signal within the tendon and surrounding tissues as a result of associated inflammation. Gradient-echo imaging, although infrequently performed, may improve conspicuity of the deposits as a result of the "blooming" artifact associated with local magnetic field heterogeneity. More often, correlation with conventional radiographs will improve the likelihood of detecting calcific tendinitis.

Rotator cuff muscles can undergo atrophy after tendon tears or denervation. Denervation results in muscle edema followed by progressive fatty infiltration. Chronic rotator cuff tendon tears also result in muscle atrophy even if no nerve injury is present. The terminology with regard to atrophy of the rotator cuff musculature is confusing. The term *fatty infiltration* is typically used to describe actual fatty infiltration or replacement of the muscle, whereas *muscle atrophy* is used to describe a loss of muscle bulk. Muscle atrophy is seen on MRI as loss of muscle bulk, whereas fatty infiltration is seen as streaks of high signal within the substance of the muscle (Fig. 38.24). Goutallier and colleagues reported a system for grading fatty infiltration of the cuff musculature on the basis of CT imaging,[80] and is frequently adapted for use with MRI, as it is at our institution. Fatty infiltration is typically graded as mild, moderate, or severe based on the extent of fatty infiltration (high signal on FSE sequences and low signal on sequences with fat suppression) within the belly of the muscle. Muscle atrophy can be graded separately as mild, moderate, or severe on the basis of muscle bulk depicted on sagittal images at the level of the supraspinatus fossa.[81] At times, the muscle tendon junction will be retracted far medially

and the degree of atrophy will be overestimated. It is therefore important to confirm the degree of atrophy with another imaging plane. Regardless of the terms used to describe muscle atrophy and fatty infiltration, they are associated with poor functional outcomes after rotator cuff tendon repair and increased risk of a recurrent tear[81]; therefore assessment of preoperative MRI scans should include the degree of muscle atrophy and fatty infiltration.

Denervation of a rotator cuff muscle can result from either a compressive neuropathy or an acute traumatic injury of a nerve. Compressive neuropathies most commonly result from a paralabral cyst associated with a labral tear, but they also can be caused by fractures or other masses in the area of the shoulder. Paralabral cysts (Fig. 38.25) most commonly arise in association with a superior labrum, anterior, and posterior (SLAP) tear or a posterior labral tear. These cysts may extend into either the spinoglenoid or suprascapular notches and can result in entrapment of the suprascapular nerve, which innervates the supraspinatus and infraspinatus muscles.[82] Paralabral cysts arising from an anteroinferior labral tear are less common, but they may compress the axillary nerve as it traverses the quadrilateral space.[83] Compression of the axillary nerve can also result from adhesive bands in the quadrilateral space in athletes, such as pitchers, who participate in repetitive overhead activities.[84] The axillary nerve innervates both the teres minor and deltoid muscles. Anterior dislocation can result in a stretching injury of the axillary nerve and give rise to a temporary or permanent denervation of the teres minor and deltoid muscles and can occasionally mimic a rotator cuff tear on clinical examination in a person with previous anterior dislocation. Parsonage Turner syndrome, also referred to as idiopathic brachial plexopathy or neuralgic amyotrophy, remains elusive in etiology (various etiologies reported in the literature include postoperative, post-infectious, posttraumatic and post-vaccination) and demonstrates a characteristic diffuse denervation edema pattern (Fig. 38.26).[85]

On MRI, subacute denervation edema signal appears as homogeneous high signal on all pulse sequences within the affected muscle and is associated with reversible muscle atrophy (see Fig. 38.25). The more chronic and irreversible form of fatty atrophy appears as decreased muscle bulk and hyperintense streaks (representing the fat) within the muscles on FSE sequences (see Fig. 38.26) and low signal on fat suppressed images.

Rotator Interval, Biceps, and the Biceps Pulley

The rotator cuff interval is the gap between the supraspinatus and infraspinatus tendons at the anterior aspect of the shoulder, which is traversed by multiple structures, including the biceps tendon, coracohumeral ligament (CHL), and superior glenohumeral ligament (SGHL) (Box 38.3). Formed largely by contributions from the coracohumeral and SGHLs, with lesser contributions from the supraspinatus and subscapularis tendons, the biceps pulley is a sling-like confluence of predominantly ligamentous structures that supports the distal aspect of the proximal biceps tendon as it exits the joint (Fig. 38.27).[86–88] The biceps pulley may be conceptualized as two functional units: (1) a medial unit located along the inferomedial aspect of the biceps tendon and composed of fibers arising from the SGHL, capsule, and CHL;

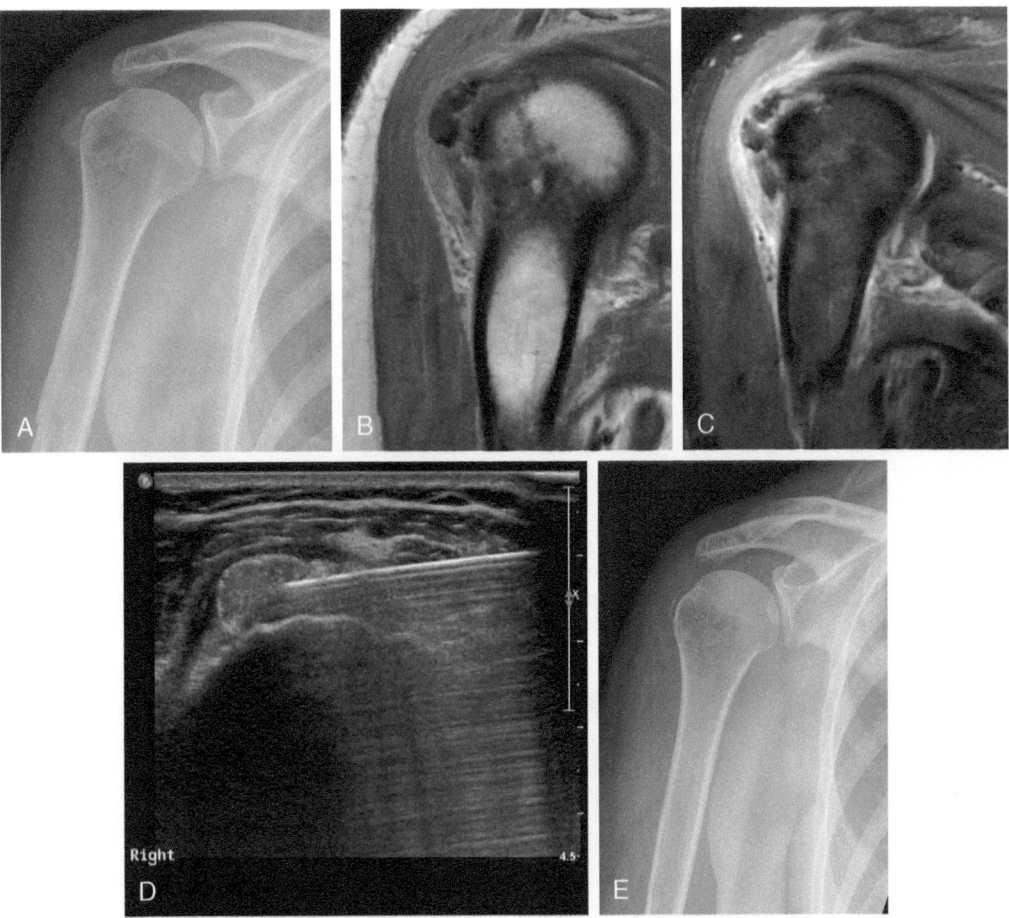

Fig. 38.23 Calcific tendinosis. (A) A globular focus of hydroxyapatite is seen within the infraspinatus bursal fibers/overlying bursa on this frontal radiograph. (B) Coronal oblique fast spin echo and (C) coronal oblique T2-weighted fat-suppressed images show the low signal intensity foci of calcium within the bursal fibers of the infraspinatus tendon and overlying bursa. Extensive edema signal is seen within the regional soft tissues representing associated inflammation. (D) Ultrasound-guided lavage aspiration of the calcium, and (E) a follow-up radiograph demonstrating near complete resolution of the calcium.

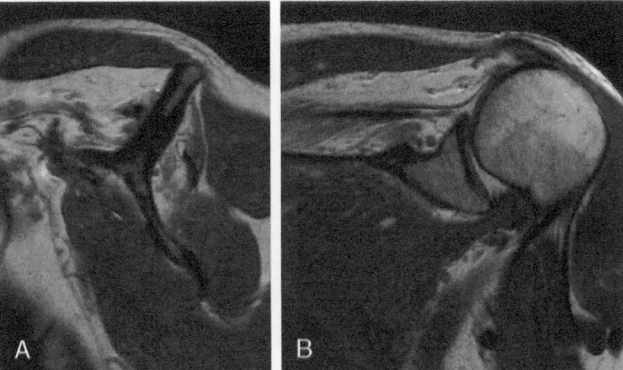

Fig. 38.24 Fatty infiltration. (A) Sagittal oblique and (B) coronal oblique fast spin echo images demonstrate severe fatty infiltration of the chronically torn and retracted supraspinatus and superior infraspinatus. It is important to triangulate with an additional view to confirm the degree of fatty infiltration, as medial retraction on the sagittal view may be misleading.

BOX 38.3   Rotator Interval: Anatomy, Function, and Pathologic Entities

Normal Anatomy

A gap within the rotator cuff formed by the interposition of the coracoid process

Superior border—anterior margin of the supraspinatus tendon

Inferior border—superior leading edge of subscapularis tendon

Roof—coracohumeral ligament (bursal surface); superior glenohumeral ligament (articular surface)

Contains the long head of the biceps tendon

Function

Limits excessive external rotation of the humeral head

Prevents superior migration of the humeral head

Pathologic Conditions

Traumatic disruption

Inflammatory arthritis

Adhesive capsulitis

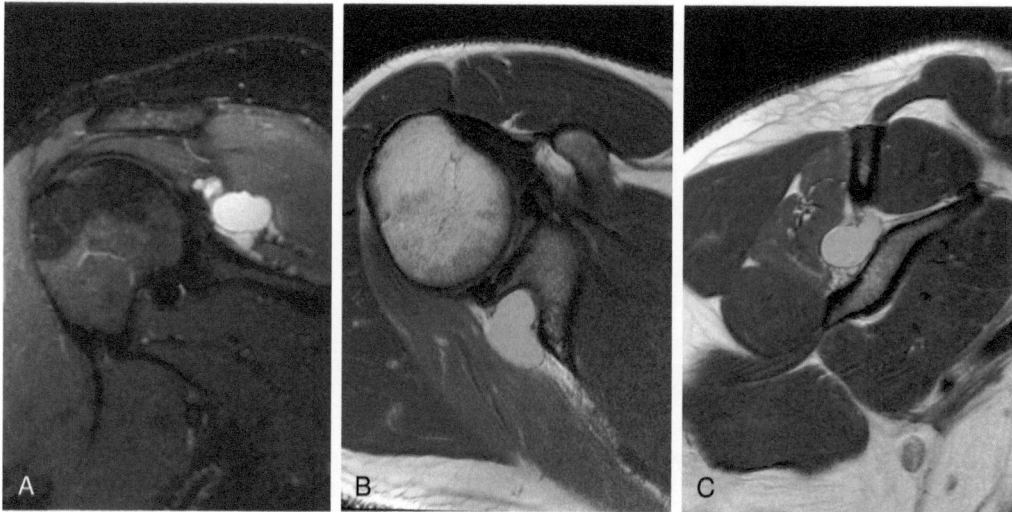

Fig. 38.25 Paralabral cyst. (A) Coronal oblique T2-weighted fat suppressed (B) axial fast spin echo and (C) oblique sagittal fast spin echo images demonstrate a lobulated paralabral cyst arising from a torn posterosuperior labrum, which extends into the spinoglenoid notch. There is mild homogenous increased signal within the infraspinatus indicating denervation.

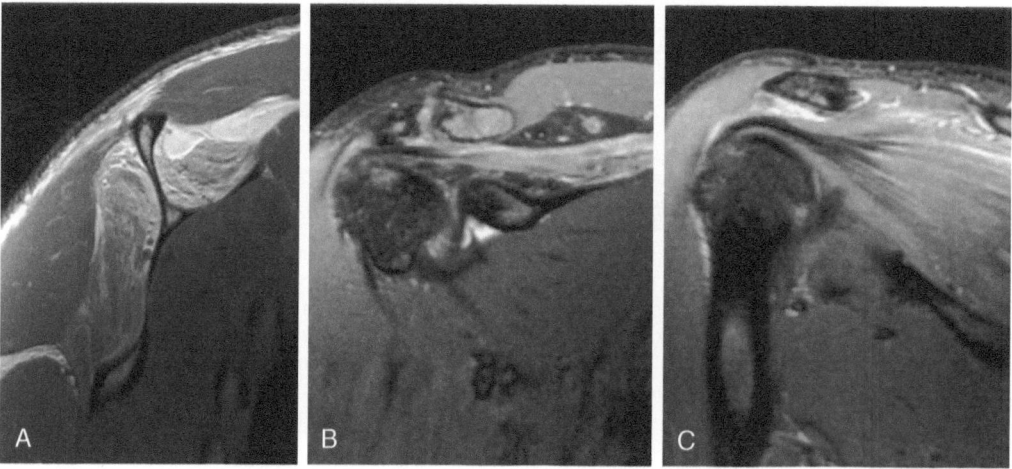

Fig. 38.26 Parsonage Turner syndrome. (A) Oblique sagittal fast spin echo and (B) and (C) coronal oblique fat-suppressed T2-weighted images demonstrates fatty infiltration as well as high-signal intensity within the supraspinatus and infraspinatus tendons, along with loss of supraspinatus muscle bulk.

and (2) a lateral unit, with contributions from the CHL, rotator cuff, and SGHL.[87]

Disruption of the structures within the rotator interval may contribute to instability of the long head of the biceps tendon; however, injury to the pulley structures may be difficult if not impossible to visualize directly, both at arthroscopy and on imaging studies.[86] Ancillary signs of pulley injury may be more easily visualized; these include tears of the superior subscapularis and anterior supraspinatus tendons, focal chondral wear adjacent to the bicipital groove, and medial subluxation of the biceps tendon (Fig. 38.28).[87,89,90]

Adhesive Capsulitis

Adhesive capsulitis is an idiopathic condition characterized by inflammation and subsequent fibrosis involving the soft tissues about the glenohumeral joint; in particular, the capsule and rotator interval (Box 38.4). Clinically, onset is typically insidious,

with progressive pain and limited range of motion (ROM), most commonly affecting women over the age of 40. The imaging characteristics of adhesive capsulitis evolve with the clinical stage of the disease; capsular hyperintensity and thickening tends to be most pronounced in the earlier inflammatory stages (particularly stage 2), while later fibrotic stages demonstrate less overt inflammation. Features observed at all stages include some degree of capsular thickening, scarring of the rotator interval, and decompression of synovitis into extracapsular recesses such as the biceps tendon sheath and the subscapularis recess. Autodecompression of synovitis may also result in a degree of local extracapsular edema (Fig. 38.29).[91]

Long Head of the Biceps Tendon

The long head of the biceps tendon takes origin at the superior aspect of the glenoid and labrum, with variation in the degree to which it originates from osseous versus labral tissue. The labral origin of the long head of the biceps tendon is referred to as the biceps anchor or biceps labral complex (Figs. 38.27 and 38.30). The tendon origin may vary in terms of both the anterior-posterior location of the tendon origin upon the superior labrum, as well as in the morphology of the attachment of the biceps-labral complex to the subjacent glenoid rim.[92,93] Accessory tendon origins have also been described; these arise most commonly from the anterior margin of the supraspinatus.[87,94]

The biceps tendon enters the biceps tendon sheath within the bicipital groove of the humerus upon exiting the glenohumeral joint (see Figs. 38.27 and 38.30). A structure that has been referred to as the transverse humeral ligament forms the soft tissue roof of the osseous groove, though this structure is thought to represent not a distinct ligament, but a confluence of fibers

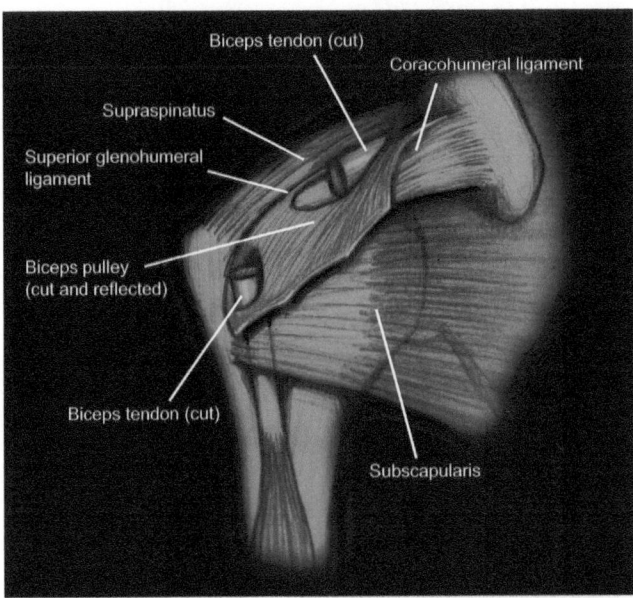

Fig. 38.27 Anatomy of the rotator interval and biceps pulley.

BOX 38.4   Adhesive Capsulitis: Clinical and Imaging Findings

Risk Factors
Female 40 to 70 years of age
Minor trauma
Rheumatologic disorders
Diabetes

Clinical Presentation
Insidious onset pain, stiffness
Decreased range of motion
Misdiagnosed as impingement

Arthrography
Decreased joint volume (<10 mL)
Contracted axillary pouch

Magnetic Resonance Imaging
Thickened capsule in axillary recess (>4 mm)
Pericapsular edema and enhancement
Synovitis in rotator interval
Thickened coracohumeral ligament

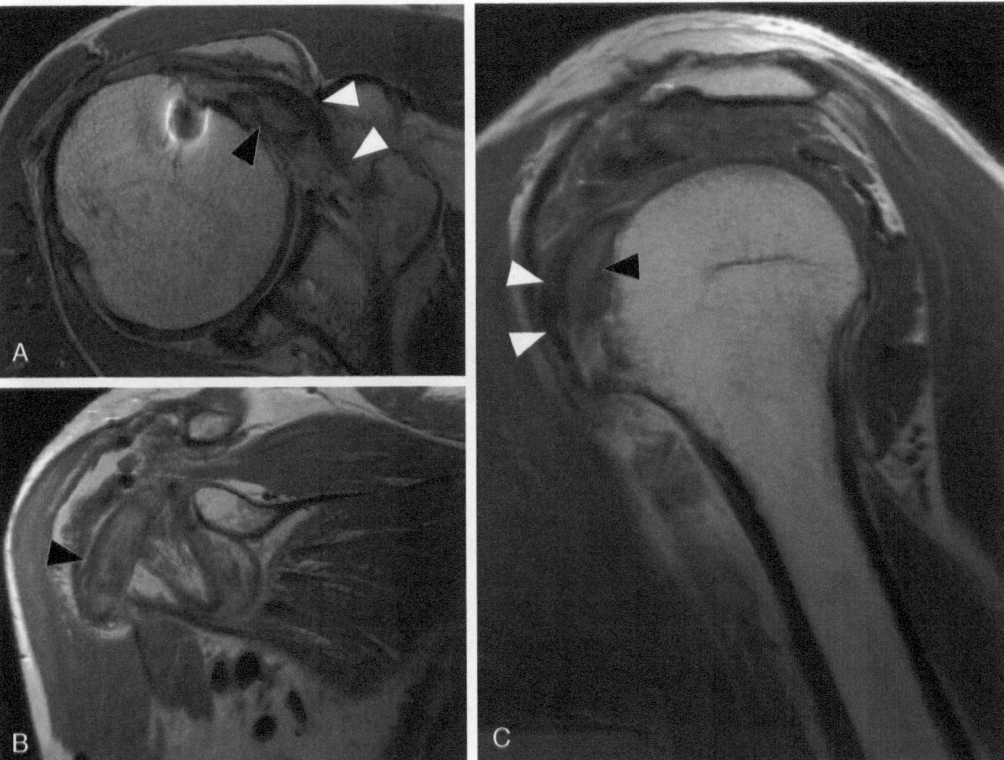

Fig. 38.28 Axial (A), oblique coronal (B), and oblique sagittal (C) fast spin echo proton density images of the shoulder demonstrate an intrasubstance tear of the subscapularis *(white arrowheads)* allowing for medial subluxation of the degenerated and chronically torn biceps tendon *(black arrowheads)*.

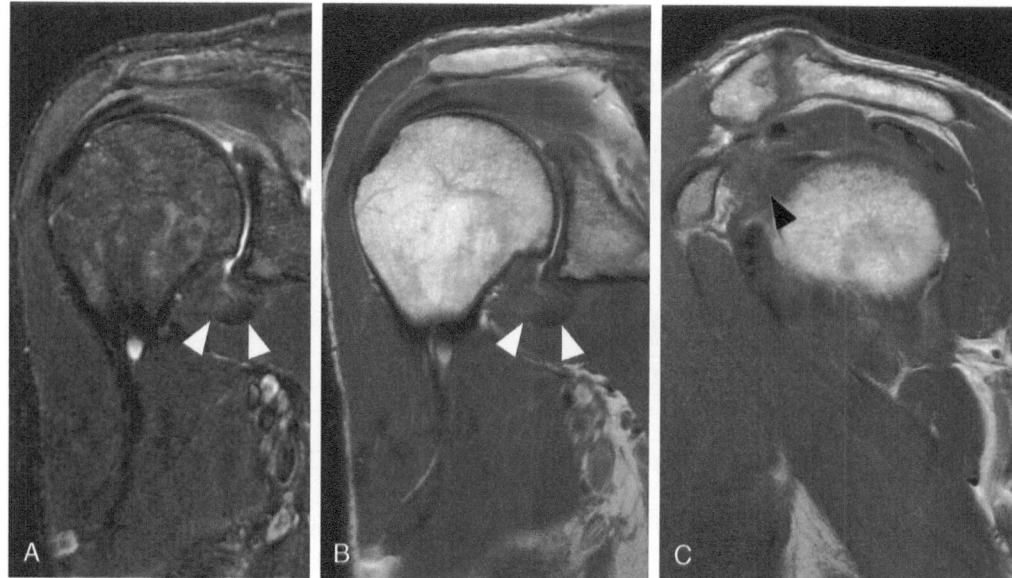

Fig. 38.29 Coronal inversion recovery (A) and fast spin echo (FSE) proton density (PD) (B) images demonstrate hyperintensity and thickening of the joint capsule *(white arrowheads)*, and (C) infiltration of the rotator interval *(black arrowhead)* on sagittal FSE PD image, in a patient with adhesive capsulitis.

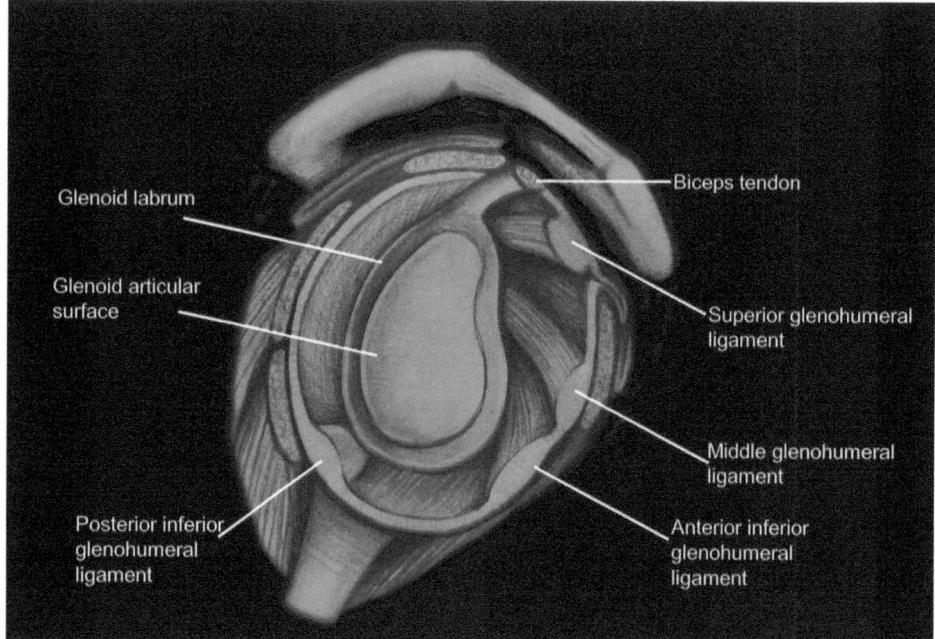

Fig. 38.30 Anatomy of the glenoid, labrum, and capsule.

arising from multiple structures, including the supraspinatus and infraspinatus tendons, with a possible fascial contribution from the pectoralis major tendon.[87] A small synovial band termed the vincula may be present within the biceps tendon sheath, traversing the interval between the anterior aspect of the tendon to the tendon sheath. Because the biceps tendon sheath communicates with the glenohumeral joint space, synovial fluid from the joint may decompress into the tendon sheath.

Given the complex course of the proximal biceps tendon, it is best evaluated in multiple planes, though axial images provide cross-sectional evaluation of a majority of the more distal tendon.

On most routine clinical MR sequences, tendinosis manifests as hyperintensity and thickening of tendon fibers; ancillary findings of impingement or tendon instability may also be observed.[87] Tendinosis may predispose the biceps tendon to partial tears, which often manifest as longitudinal splits, or to complete tendon rupture (Fig. 38.31). Spontaneous proximal biceps rupture occurs most commonly in the setting of a chronically degenerated tendon in an older patient, manifesting as discontinuity of the tendon, often with distal retraction of the torn tendon yielding a gap, with an empty tendon sheath more proximally. Fluid distention of the biceps tendon sheath may result from decompression of

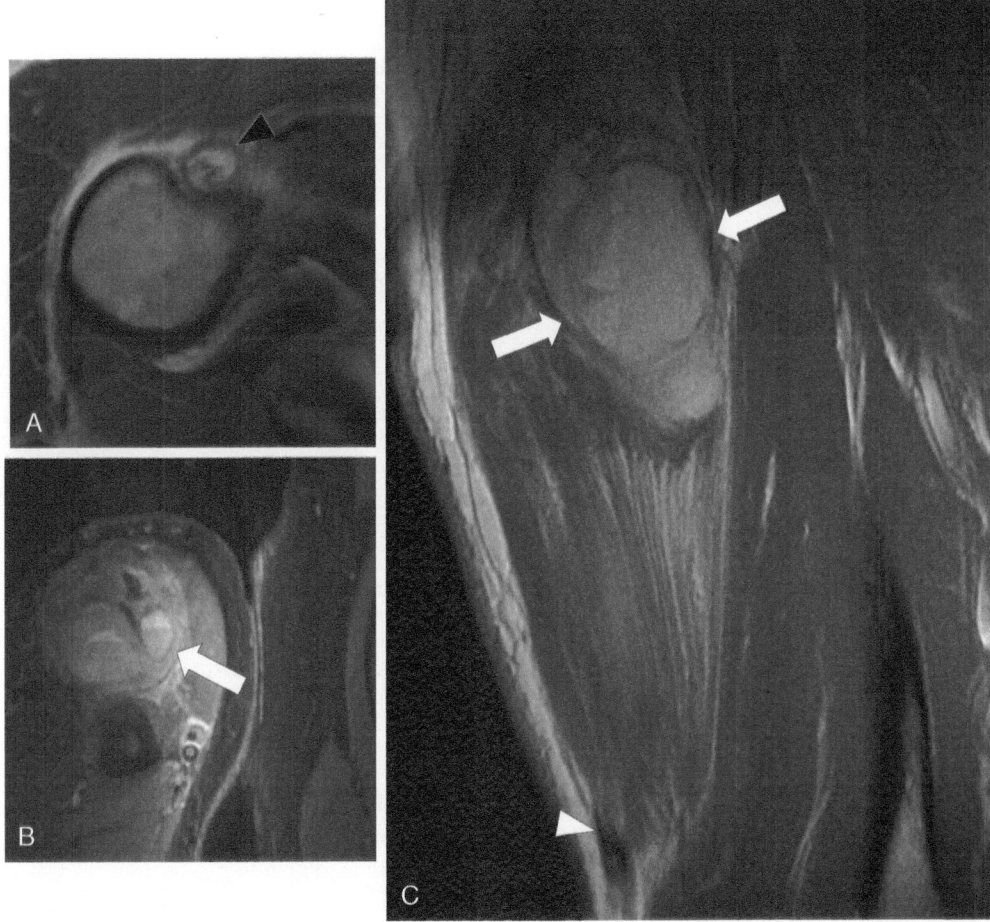

Fig. 38.31 Axial fast spin echo (FSE) proton density (PD) (A), inversion recovery (B) and sagittal FSE PD (C) images of the shoulder and upper arm demonstrate complete proximal biceps rupture, as manifest by empty biceps tendon sheath proximally *(black arrowhead)*, with prominent intramuscular hemorrhage *(white arrows)*, and retraction of the distal tendon stump *(white arrowhead)*.

synovial fluid from the glenohumeral joint, though it may also be related to tenosynovitis. Longstanding inflammation may result in associated tenosynovial adhesions. Hydroxyapatite depositional disease (HADD), also known as calcific tendonitis, may involve the biceps tendon, and, as with HADD involving the rotator cuff, is amenable to ultrasound-guided lavage (Fig. 38.32).

Labrum and Capsular Structures
Anatomy
The rather shallow osseous articulation between the glenoid and humeral head allows a relatively large ROM, with a great deal of the stability of the joint being conferred by peri-articular soft tissue structures. The glenoid labrum and capsular structures act as static stabilizers, whereas the rotator cuff provides dynamic stabilization of the glenohumeral joint.

The glenoid labrum is a rim of fibrous and fibrocartilaginous tissue that extends along the circumference of the glenoid, adding depth to the glenoid fossa, thereby augmenting joint stability, as well as serving as a point of attachment for the glenohumeral ligaments and biceps tendon. Normal labral tissue is uniformly dark on routine clinical MRI sequences, being composed of fibrous tissue and fibrocartilage, and the normal labrum is

typically roughly triangular in cross section. Location of labral pathology is often described in terms of clock position, with 12:00 being superior and 3:00 being anterior, as imaged in the sagittal plane. Alternately, the various portions of the labrum may be described simply by their relative anatomic position: direct superior, anterosuperior, anteroinferior, direct inferior, posteroinferior, and posterosuperior (see Fig. 38.30).[95] Anatomic variants are commonly described within the labrum, with variants most commonly involving the anterosuperior portion of the labrum. Common labral variants include the sublabral foramen and sublabral sulcus, focal defects confined to the anterosuperior labrum, as well as the Buford complex, which refers to a hypoplastic anterosuperior labrum with compensatory thickening of the middle glenohumeral ligament (MGHL). These labral variants may be mistaken for tears, and familiarity with their appearance may help prevent their being misinterpreted as pathology.[92,93]

Three glenohumeral ligaments, which represent thickenings of the capsule, also serve to improve stability of the shoulder. The inferior glenohumeral ligament (see Fig. 38.30) is the most important of the three thickenings and functions primarily to improve glenohumeral stability with the arm in abduction and external rotation.[96]

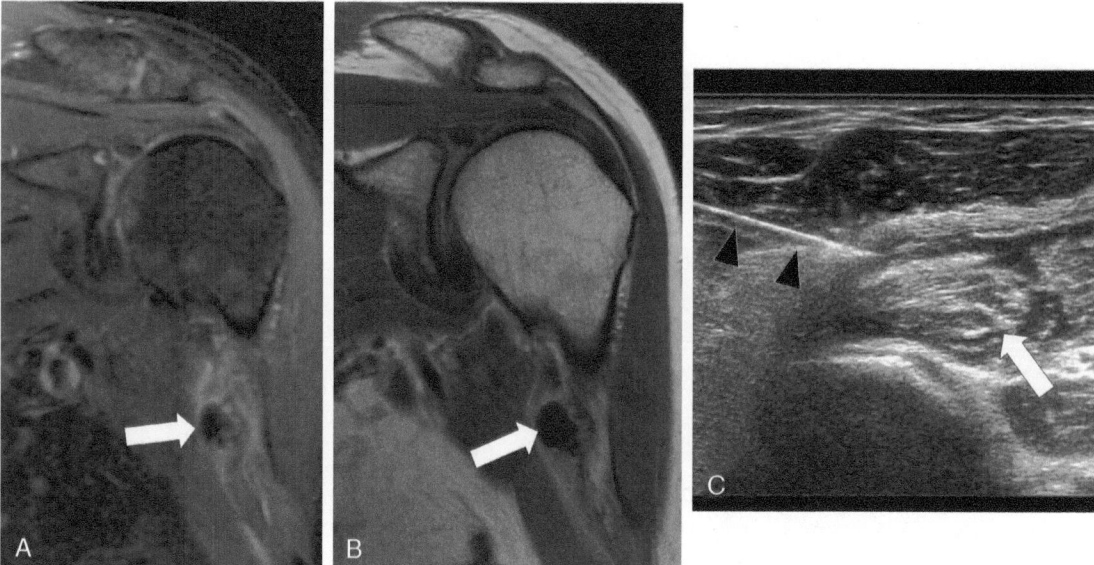

Fig. 38.32 Coronal inversion recovery (A) and fast spin echo proton density (B) images of the shoulder demonstrate a large focus of mineralization *(white arrows)* within the biceps tendon sheath, consistent with hydroxyapatite deposition. Long axis ultrasound images (C) re-demonstrate the mineralized focus *(white arrow)*, with subsequent ultrasound-guided lavage performed *(black arrowheads* indicate needle).

It is composed of three separate components: the anterior band, the posterior band, and the axillary pouch.[97,98] The origin of the inferior glenohumeral ligament is somewhat variable; it arises from either the inferior glenoid labrum or adjacent osseous glenoid. It then inserts in a collar-like fashion along the medial aspect of the humeral neck. It is lax when the arm is in the neutral position and appears redundant when the arm is imaged in the standard planes on MRI (see Fig. 38.30). The MGHL (see Fig. 38.30) is less important as a stabilizer, but it is responsible for preventing external rotation of the arm during abduction between 60 and 90 degrees.[99] In terms of size, it is the most variable of the three ligaments, ranging from a thick cordlike ligament to complete absence.[100] It arises from the superior glenoid tubercle adjacent to the origin of the biceps tendon and the SGHL, and then courses obliquely in an inferolateral direction to merge with the deep fibers of the subscapularis tendon just before attaching to the humeral neck. It is typically seen on axial MRI deep to the subscapularis muscle and superficial to the anterior labrum, occasionally mimicking an avulsed fragment of the anterior labrum.

The SGHL (see Fig. 38.30) contributes to shoulder stability, although a report suggests that it provides some degree of restraint, preventing inferior subluxation of the humeral head when the arm is in 0 degrees of abduction.[101,102] It arises from the superior glenoid tubercle adjacent to the attachment of the biceps tendon and then courses obliquely and anteriorly to merge with the CHL before its attachment on the humeral head. The SGHL forms the floor of the rotator interval and also plays a role in stability of the long head of the biceps tendon, merging with the CHL to form the biceps pulley.[103–105] It is consistently visualized on axial MRA images as a thick band-like structure arising from the glenoid tubercle and paralleling the coracoid process.[98]

Instability

The anatomic configuration, which permits a wide ROM at the glenohumeral joint, also predisposes the articulation to a degree of instability, with the potential for subluxation and dislocation. While radiographs are often the first line of imaging in instability, with specific views allowing the visualization of osseous pathology, such as Hills-Sachs and osseous Bankart lesions, injury tends to largely involve the periarticular soft tissue stabilizers; therefore MRI is often the main modality for definitive assessment of the degree and extent of injury in the setting of instability.

Anterior

The humeral head most commonly dislocates anteroinferiorly relative to the glenoid, often as a result of a fall on an outstretched hand or traumatic stress while the extremity is in the abducted externally rotated position. In younger patients, this results in a classic constellation of findings, including a Hill–Sachs lesion of the humeral head plus some degree of capsulolabral injury, commonly a Bankart lesion or variant. Capsular injury may occur at various attachment sites, often resulting in stripping along the scapula, or the classically described humeral avulsion of the glenohumeral ligaments (HAGL) lesion, which tends to warrant a change in the surgical approach.[106–108]

Hill–Sachs and osseous Bankart lesions are typically visible on radiographs, with MR evaluation in the acute setting demonstrating associated local marrow edema along the humeral head and anteroinferior glenoid impaction sites. Nonosseous Bankart lesions manifest as a tear of the anteroinferior labrum, which may be displaced or nondisplaced, and which may manifest as a discrete defect through the substance of the labrum, or as an irregular/amorphous appearance. A variety of Bankart variants have been described, with the configuration of the Bankart lesion having potential therapeutic implications in terms of surgical planning. A Perthes lesion is a nondisplaced Bankart in which the medial scapular periosteum remains intact, tethering the torn labrum to the glenoid, such that the tear may be difficult to visualize both on imaging and at arthroscopy. A displaced variant of the Perthes lesion is termed an anterior labral periosteal sleeve avulsion (ALPSA), with an anteroinferior labral tear and stripping of the medial scapular periosteum, allowing for medial displacement of the torn labrum, which may scar down in this abnormal medialized position if not properly reduced. In an osseous Bankart lesion, impaction results in some degree of anteroinferior glenoid rim fracture, yielding an ossific fragment with attached labral tissue. The size of this fragment is important in terms of treatment planning, with large fragments warranting surgical fixation. Excessive loss of glenoid bone stock may require some type of osseous augmentation, such as coracoid transfer. In older patients with rotator cuff pathology, anterior glenohumeral dislocation often results in a different constellation of imaging findings, including rotator cuff tears and avulsion fractures of the greater tuberosity (Figs. 38.33–38.36).[106–108]

Posterior

Posterior glenohumeral dislocation is much less common than anterior dislocation, and tends to occur in the setting of activities that result in specific injury patterns; for example, football linemen who incur repetitive forceful posteriorly directed forces at the glenohumeral joint. Certain anatomic anomalies, such as glenoid dysplasia, also contribute to a predisposition for posterior dislocation. Imaging findings in the setting of posterior dislocation are analogous to those observed in anterior dislocation, with reverse Hill-Sachs lesions occurring along the anterior aspect of the humeral head, and reverse Bankart lesions and variants occurring along the posterior glenoid (Box 38.5). Posterior HAGL lesions may also occur along the posterior capsular attachments at the humerus (Fig. 38.37).[107,108]

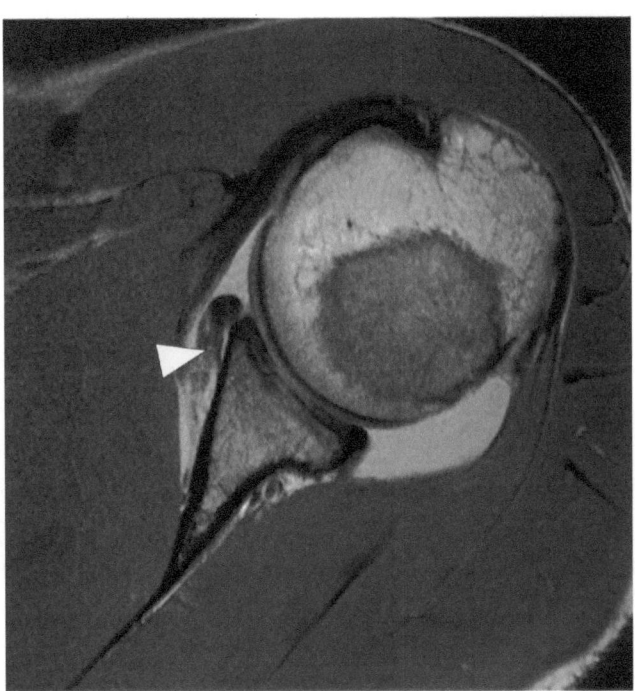

Fig. 38.34 Axial fast spin echo proton density image in a patient status post recent glenohumeral dislocation demonstrates anterior labral periosteal sleeve avulsion lesion, with anteroinferior labral tear, which is slightly medially retracted and tethered to a band of stripped periosteum *(white arrowhead)*.

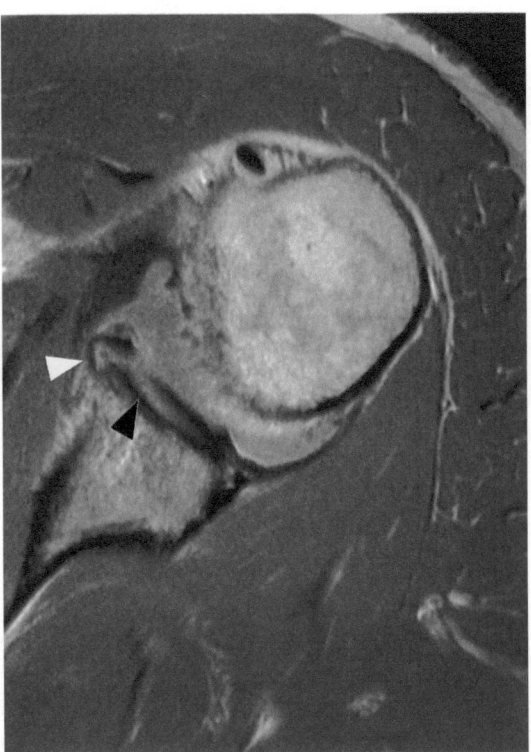

Fig. 38.35 Axial fast spin echo proton density image demonstrates anteroinferior labral tear *(white arrowhead)*, with adjacent focal area of chondral loss *(black arrowhead)*, consistent with glenoid labral articular defect lesion.

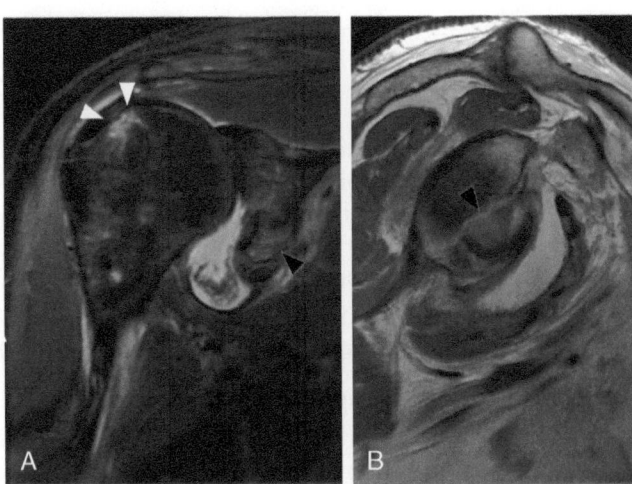

Fig. 38.33 Coronal inversion recovery (A) and sagittal fast spin echo proton density (B) images in a patient status post recent anterior glenohumeral dislocation demonstrates acute Hill-Sachs lesion *(white arrowheads)* and osseous Bankart lesion *(black arrowheads)*.

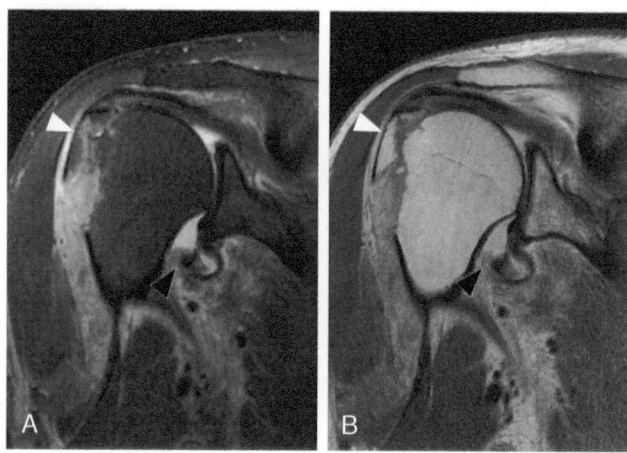

Fig. 38.36 Coronal inversion recovery (A) and fast spin echo proton density (B) images in an older patient status post glenohumeral dislocation demonstrates avulsion fracture of the greater tuberosity *(white arrowheads)* and humeral avulsion of the glenohumeral ligaments *(black arrowheads)*.

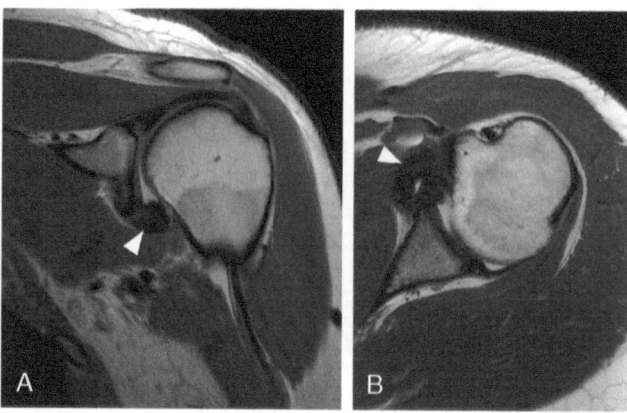

Fig. 38.38 Oblique coronal (A) and axial (B) fast spin echo proton density images demonstrate pronounced capsular remodeling with marked thickening anteriorly *(white arrowheads)* in a swimmer with multidirectional instability.

BOX 38.5 Posterior Shoulder Dislocation: Radiographic Findings

Positive rim sign (widening of glenohumeral joint >6 mm)
Humeral head appears in same position on internal and external rotation anteroposterior views
"Trough line," or reverse Hill-Sachs defect
Reverse Bankart lesion
Fracture of lesser tuberosity

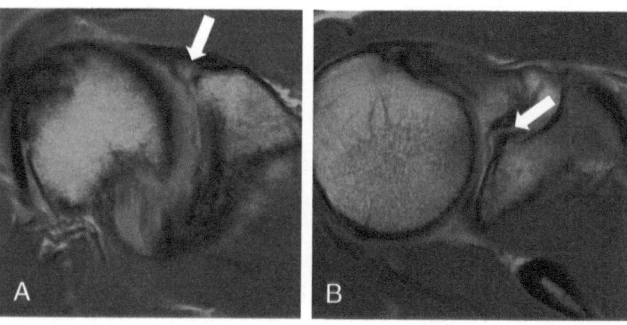

Fig. 38.39 Oblique coronal (A) and axial (B) fast spin echo images of the shoulder demonstrate a tear across the base of the superior labrum *(white arrow, A)*, extending to the anterosuperior labrum *(white arrow, B)*.

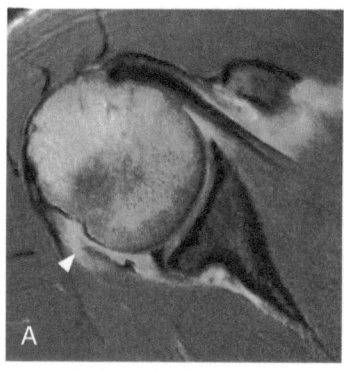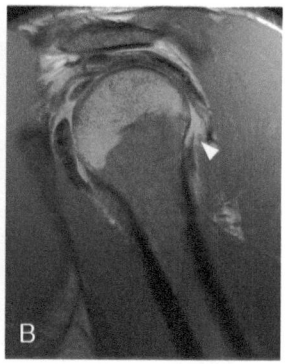

Fig. 38.37 Axial (A) and oblique sagittal (B) fast spin echo proton density images demonstrate posterior humeral avulsion of the glenohumeral ligaments *(white arrowheads)* in a patient status post recent posterior glenohumeral dislocation.

Multidirectional

Multidirectional instability occurs in the setting of generalized capsular laxity, which predisposes patients to subluxations and dislocations in at least two directions. This entity is often atraumatic, though it may develop in athletes with recurrent injuries and/or repetitive strain. Imaging findings in these patients may be nonspecific, though they may include a remodeled, patulous joint capsule as well as sequelae of recurrent dislocations (Fig. 38.38).[107,108]

Superior Labrum, Anterior, and Posterior Tears

The term *SLAP tear* refers to any superior labral tear that propagates anteroposteriorly to some degree, and which may also propagate along various adjacent structures.

Originally described in throwing athletes by Andrews et al. (1985),[109] with the term "SLAP" coined and the original four tear subtypes described by Snyder et al. (1990),[110] the initial classification of these tears has been expanded to include at least 10 types (Table 38.4).

A type I SLAP tear is described as superior labral fraying without involvement of the biceps tendon, and appears as intrasubstance signal hyperintensity without a defined intrasubstance tear on MRI. The remainder of SLAP injuries involve defined superior labral tears, manifesting as intrasubstance linear signal hyperintensity and/or labral detachment, with variable degrees and directions of extension. Type II SLAP tears are reportedly the most common, consisting of a superior labral tear with involvement of the biceps (Fig. 38.39).[111]

Classification of SLAP tears may provide insight into the type of injury, the probable mechanism, and the therapeutic options; however, precise classification of these lesions may not always be possible, and the classification system cannot be assumed to be universally known or accepted. Therefore when reporting these types of injuries, rather than providing a numeric classification,

TABLE 38.4 Classification of Superior Labrum, Anterior and Posterior (SLAP) Tears

SLAP	Location	Description		Management
I	11-1	Superior labral fraying with intact biceps tendon	Associated with repetitive overhead motion, also seen in the setting of degeneration	Conservative vs. débridement
II	11-1	Superior labral tear with involvement of biceps tendon	Associated with repetitive overhead motion; may have extension anteriorly, posteriorly, or both Most common type	Débridement and repair
III	11-1	Bucket handle tear of superior labrum with intact biceps	Associated with fall on outstretched hand	Excision of bucket handle fragment
IV	11-1	Bucket handle tear of superior labrum with involvement of biceps	Associated with fall on outstretched hand	Excision of bucket handle fragment, repair of biceps
V	11-5	Bankart lesion with extension to superior labrum and involvement of biceps tendon	Associated with anterior glenohumeral dislocation	Labral repair and biceps tenodesis
VI	11-1	Anterior or posterior superior labral flap tear with involvement of biceps	Associated with fall on outstretched hand	Labral repair and biceps tenodesis
VII	11-3	Superior labral tear with involvement of biceps tendon and middle glenohumeral ligament	Associated with anterior glenohumeral dislocation	Labral repair, biceps tenodesis, middle glenohumeral ligament repair
VIII	7-1	Superior labral tear with posteroinferior extension	Associated with posterior shoulder dislocation	Capsulolabral reconstruction
IX	7-5	Superior labral tear with extensive anterior and posterior extension	Typically associated with severe trauma.	Labral débridement and glenohumeral stabilization
X	11-1	Superior labral tear with extension to rotator interval	Typically associated with severe trauma	Labral débridement and glenohumeral stabilization

it is generally more important to provide an accurate description of the injury, including location and extent, the involvement of adjacent structures, the morphology of the tear including displacement, and any associated injuries.[95]

Posterior Impingement, Glenohumeral Internal Rotational Deficit

Athletes who perform repetitive overhead motions in the abducted externally rotated position, such as pitchers, are at risk for the development of impingement of the structures along the posterosuperior aspect of the glenohumeral joint, including the rotator cuff tendons and labrum. These athletes often develop a characteristic articular-sided tear centered along the junction of the supraspinatus and infraspinatus tendons, as well as degeneration and/or tearing of the posterosuperior labrum. Skeletally immature patients may develop chronic remodeling of the posterosuperior glenoid due to repetitive impaction in this region, resulting in relative glenoid retroversion. Remodeling of the joint capsule may also occur, with patulous anterior capsule and contracted posterior capsule resulting in a relative loss of internal rotation, a clinical condition referred to as glenohumeral internal rotational deficit (GIRD).[112]

Articular Surfaces

Normal hyaline articular cartilage consists of multiple layers, and therefore has a consistent laminar appearance on high resolution cartilage-sensitive imaging sequences. The deepest layer of articular cartilage, the tidemark, is mineralized and therefore is uniformly hypointense on typical clinical sequences. The next

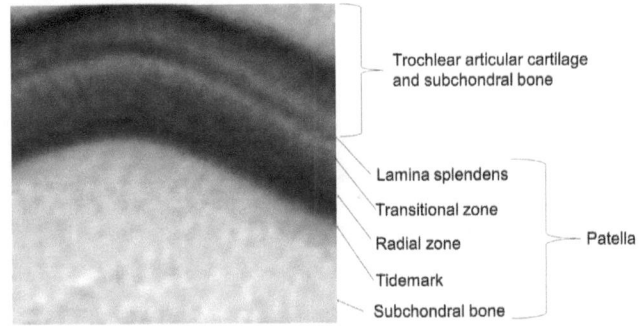

Fig. 38.40 Fast spin echo proton density image demonstrating the normal layered appearance of hyaline articular cartilage (the patella is shown for ease of visualization), with the tidemark being the deepest layer of cartilage, and the lamina splendens the most superficial.

deepest layer consists largely of radially oriented collagen fibers, conferring a shortened T2 relaxation time relative to adjacent superficial layer, in which the collagen fibers are organized in arcades. The most superficial layer, the lamina splendens, is a thin layer consisting of parallel horizontally oriented fibers, and is therefore hypointense (Fig. 38.40).

Early chondral wear is often evident as a loss of typical greyscale stratification, chondral hyperintensity, and surface fibrillation, often involving the medial aspect of the humeral head. As wear progresses, cartilage may delaminate and form flaps (Fig. 38.41). While typical osteoarthritis often first affects the superomedial humeral head, patients who develop osteoarthritis secondary to rotator cuff pathology often display a characteristic pattern of chondral wear, typically affecting the anterosuperior glenoid, in

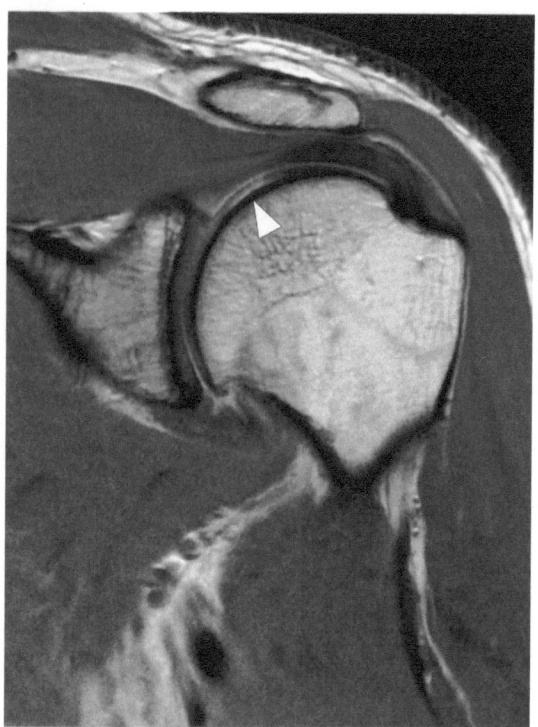

Fig. 38.41 Oblique coronal fast spin echo proton density image demonstrates chondral delamination and flap formation *(white arrowhead)* over the superomedial humeral head.

the setting of massive rotator cuff tear and resultant superior migration of the humeral head (Fig. 38.42).[113]

For a complete list of references, go to ExpertConsult.com.

SELECTED READING

Citation:
Dunham KS, Bencardino JT, Rokito AS. Anatomic variants and pitfalls of the labrum, glenoid cartilage, and glenohumeral ligaments. *Magn Reson Imaging Clin North Am.* 2012;20(2):213–228.

Level of Evidence:
V, expert opinion

Summary:
The authors of this review article discuss normal anatomy and variants in the shoulder labrum, glenohumeral ligaments, and cartilage.

Citation:
Fitzpatrick D, Walz DM. Shoulder MR imaging normal variants and imaging artifacts. *Magn Reson Imaging Clin North Am.* 2012;18(4):615–632.

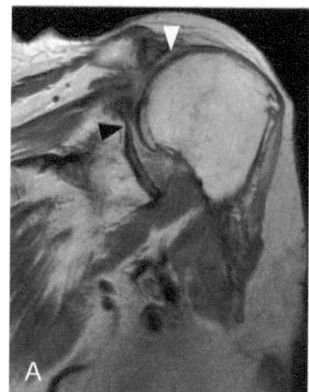 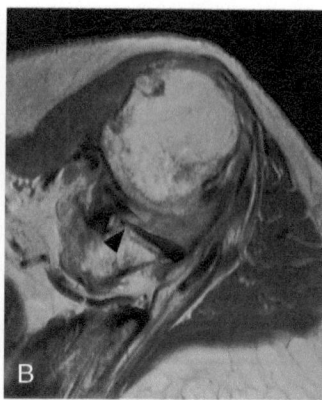

Fig. 38.42 Oblique coronal (A) and axial (B) fast spin echo proton density images demonstrate features of rotator cuff arthropathy, with superior migration of the humeral head in the setting of massive rotator cuff tear *(white arrowhead)*, and associated arthrosis preferentially affecting the anterosuperior aspect of the glenoid *(black arrowheads)*.

Level of Evidence:
V, expert opinion

Summary:
This article covers imaging artifacts and normal variations that can affect interpretation of shoulder magnetic resonance images.

Citation:
Sanders TG, Jersey SL. Conventional radiography of the shoulder. *Semin Roentgenol.* 2005;40(3):207–222.

Level of Evidence:
V, expert opinion

Summary:
This article covers conventional radiography of the shoulder. Views are discussed along with their strengths and role in diagnosing sources of shoulder pain.

Citation:
Sanders TG, Miller MD. Systematic approach to magnetic resonance imaging interpretation of sports medicine injuries of the shoulder. *Am J Sports Med.* 2005;33:1088–1105.

Level of Evidence:
V, expert opinion

Summary:
The authors of this article present a systematic approach to reading shoulder magnetic resonance imaging examinations.

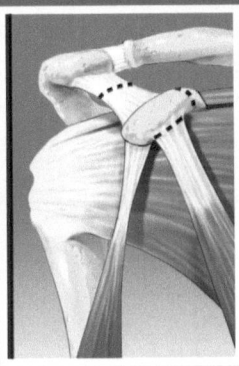

39

Shoulder Arthroscopy

Thomas M. DeBerardino, Laura W. Scordino

BACKGROUND

Shoulder arthroscopy was first described in the 1930s by Burman,[1] who learned how to perform arthroscopy on cadaveric joints. Remarkably, shoulder arthroscopy has been used regularly only for the past 30 years. The use of shoulder arthroscopy has continued to grow, and today it is one of the most commonly performed orthopedic procedures. It is the second most common procedure performed by persons taking Part II of the American Board of Orthopaedic Surgery certification examination.[2]

INDICATIONS AND CONTRAINDICATIONS

Shoulder arthroscopy allows excellent visualization of the glenohumeral joint, periarticular structures, and subacromial space, and thus facilitates both the diagnosis and treatment of intra-articular and periarticular pathology of the shoulder joint. Shoulder arthroscopy is indicated for, but not limited to, rotator cuff repair, revision rotator cuff repair, glenohumeral instability,[3] labral repair or débridement, removal of loose bodies, synovectomy or synovial biopsy, irrigation and débridement of a septic shoulder, repair of a glenoid fracture, bicep tenodesis or tenotomy, subacromial decompression, and distal clavicle excision. Contraindications include medical problems that preclude a patient from undergoing elective surgery, and infection of the shoulder joint or overlying tissue if surgery is being performed for a reason other than to eradicate the infection.

In a 2003 survey of 908 members of the Arthroscopy Association of North America, of the 700 members who responded, 24% stated that they repair rotator cuff injuries via an all-arthroscopic technique; however, 5 years earlier, only 5% reported using an all-arthroscopic technique.[4] Only 2 years later, in 2005, an electronic poll of 167 orthopedic surgeons attending the annual American Academy of Orthopaedic Surgeons meeting showed that 67% would fix a mobile, 3-cm rotator cuff tear.[5] The percentage of surgeons performing arthroscopic rotator cuff repairs continues to grow, and surgeons today not only feel confident about using arthroscopy for massive rotator cuff repairs, but also have even had good results for revision rotator cuff repairs.[6]

ARTHROSCOPIC VERSUS OPEN PROCEDURES

Reported benefits of shoulder arthroscopy compared with open shoulder procedures include limited damage to the surrounding structures, particularly the deltoid muscle and the area of insertion. Furthermore, with regard to rotator cuff repair, some surgeons believe that arthroscopy provides a more complete evaluation of both intra-articular and bursal anatomy. Many surgeons believe that arthroscopy allows easier mobilization of potential retracted cuff musculature. The main downside to arthroscopy is its large learning curve, which can result in longer operative times, iatrogenic injuries during the learning process, and potentially inferior repair compared with open techniques.

With regard to rotator cuff repair, many studies have shown that all-arthroscopic compared with mini-open rotator cuff repair has yielded comparable short-term and mid-term results.[7-10] Other studies have shown that pain, strength, motion, and strength may be improved with all-arthroscopic repair.

PREOPERATIVE IMAGING

In our practice we obtain a standard set of four radiographs preoperatively, including a true anteroposterior radiograph of the shoulder, the supraspinatus outlet view (SOV), an axillary view, and a bilateral Zanca view. These images allow us to evaluate a large number of pathologic shoulder conditions and to make preoperative plans. The SOV provides a look at the acromion for classification according to the system proposed by Bigliani and colleagues[11]: type 1, flat acromion; type 2, gently curved acromion; and type 3, "beaked" or sharp, inferiorly pointed acromion. The SOV radiograph also allows us to determine the amount of acromion that needs to be taken down if we are planning a subacromial decompression, based on how thick it is, and to confirm that there is no os acromiale, which may result in pain and instability if a decompression is performed. The Zanca view allows for evaluation of the acromioclavicular joints for pathology.[12]

Magnetic resonance imaging (MRI) without contrast provides visualization of the rotator cuff musculature. MRI with an arthrogram is an excellent imaging modality for patients with instability or when concern exists about the possibility of labral pathology, because intra-articular anatomy is more clearly defined with this procedure.

Many institutions and surgeons use ultrasound for the evaluation of shoulder joint pathology. This method of evaluation has proven to be both sensitive and specific for the radiologists and orthopedic surgeons who use ultrasound in their own office.[13-15] In direct comparison with arthroscopy as the standard, MRI and ultrasound have shown no significant difference in diagnostic accuracy.[15] Ultrasound also has the benefit of providing a dynamic evaluation. However, this imaging modality relies heavily on the experience of the person performing the examination.[15]

PATIENT POSITIONING

As depicted in Fig. 39.1, two main options exist for patient positioning: lateral decubitus and beach chair. Positioning is based on surgeon preference. Advantages and disadvantages of each position are described in this section.

Lateral positioning of the patient occurs after the patient is intubated while supine on a standard operating room table with the bean bag already underneath him/her, but uninflated (see Fig. 39.1A). The patient is then turned to the lateral position with the operative arm up and the torso posteriorly tilted approximately 20 degrees to position the glenoid parallel with the floor. An axillary roll is placed and the legs are positioned with adequate pillows and cushioning to protect bony prominences and the peroneal nerve as it passes around the fibular neck. The bean bag is then inflated, warm blankets are placed over the patient, and a belt is secured over as opposed to under the blankets so it is always clear that the belt is in place. The arm undergoing surgery is then positioned in approximately 70 degrees of abduction and 20 degrees of forward flexion. One cadaveric study showed that positioning the arm in 45 degrees of flexion with arm abduction of either 0 or 90 degrees allowed for the best visualization with the least amount of strain placed on the brachial plexus.[16] To distend the joint, 10 to 15 lb of traction is applied to a device set up at the foot of the bed. The arm is prepared and draped so that the entire shoulder and part of the arm is sterile and the distal extent of the arm that is hooked up to traction is not sterile and is draped out of the field. Some surgeons believe that the lateral position allows better visualization of the joint because of the traction. Lateral positioning has been reported to have a 10% rate of neurapraxia; most cases resolve in 48 hours. The neurapraxia is thought to be a result

of traction on the brachial plexus, with biomechanical studies showing a 100% incidence of abnormal somatosensory evoked potentials in the musculoskeletal nerve.[17,18]

Beach chair positioning often entails the use of a specialized operating table that bends to create a semiseated, or beach chair, position (see Fig. 39.1B). The patient is anesthetized while supine and then positioned. The anesthesiologist stabilizes the head while the surgeon and assistant move the patient cephalad on the table and the head holder attachment is positioned on the bed. A padded face mask is placed over the patient's face to hold the head against the head rest. A padded side post is placed on each side of the patient to hold him or her in position on the middle of the bed, and a pillow is placed under the knees to prop the patient up and prevent him or her from sliding down the beach chair. The heels are padded. Unlike with the lateral position, no traction is necessary when the beach chair position is used. The entire operative arm is prepped and draped so it is free for manipulation and movement throughout the operation. Some surgeons find it helpful to use a device that holds the operative arm in various adjustable positions, to free up the hands of their assistants so they can help with the case. The beach chair position facilitates an easy transition to an open procedure because the patient is already in a suitable position for an open procedure. Risks relating to head position do accompany the use of the beach chair position, and neurapraxia of cutaneous nerves in the cervical plexus related to the headrest itself has been reported, and thus a padded head rest should be carefully positioned and neck flexion should be avoided.[18] Also unique to beach chair positioning is the risk of hypoperfusion to the brain. Although the use of hypotensive anesthetic has been well supported in the literature for patients in the supine or lateral decubitus position to decrease operative blood loss and to improve visualization, concern exists about relative hypotension to the brain as a result of hydrostatic pressure. The literature includes rare case reports of patients who have sustained ischemic brain and spinal cord injury while receiving hypotensive anesthesia in the beach chair position.[18] Therefore it has been recommended that blood pressure

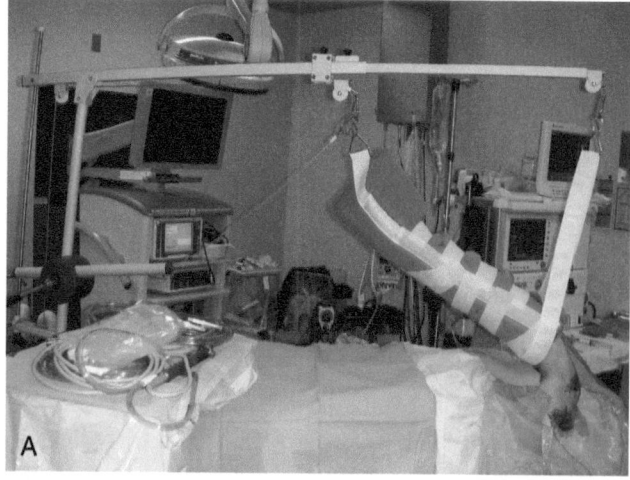
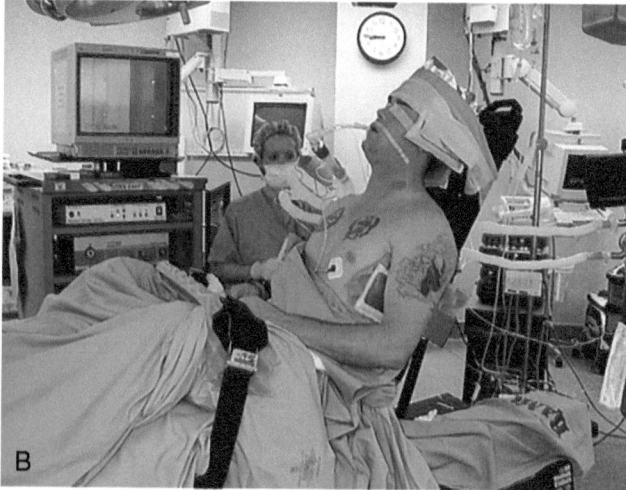

Fig. 39.1 (A) A patient with the right shoulder prepped in the lateral decubitus position with a distal forearm holder and longitudinal traction in place. (B) A patient with the left shoulder prepped in the beach chair position.

be measured in the contralateral arm and that attempts be made to keep systolic blood pressure and subacromial pressure (pump pressure) within 49 mm Hg of each other.[17,18]

ARTHROSCOPY SETUP

Arthroscopy is an equipment-intensive procedure. It involves the use of an arthroscope, which is a small fiber-optic camera that is usually 4 mm in size when used for the shoulder. The arthroscope projects images onto a television that can be seen by all the surgical team members. Arthroscopes come with varying degrees of angulation of the lens, but most commonly the 30-degree arthroscope is used for shoulder arthroscopy. It is advisable to have both 30- and 70-degree scopes available because each scope allows improved visualization depending on the procedure to be performed.

Arthroscopy involves the inflow of fluid through the joint both to distend the joint and to decrease bleeding. The best fluid to use with arthroscopy is a topic of debate. Some studies have shown that epinephrine allows better visualization, likely by decreasing bleeding without associated cardiovascular adverse effects[19]; however, other in vitro studies have suggested that epinephrine may damage articular cartilage.[20] Therefore we prefer to use the most diluted epinephrine in saline solution for our irrigation fluid. Surgeon preference also determines the use of gravity versus a pressure-controlled pump to manage irrigation inflow.

Outflow of fluid from the shoulder joint occurs through suction tubing attached to the motorized burr, which is a rotating blade within a smooth sheath. The suction of fluid through the burr allows debris and other tissue to be sucked into the shaver and removed from the joint.

Thermal heat in the form of monopolar devices are used for anticoagulation. Cartilage is sensitive to heat, with chondrocyte death being shown to occur with exposure to temperatures as low as 45°C, whereas devices provide heat at temperatures greater than 100°C.[21,22] Furthermore, previous use of thermal heat for capsulorrhaphy resulted in multiple complications, including chondrolysis, which will be discussed later. Therefore intra-articular devices providing thermal heat are used sparingly for débridement and mainly for anticoagulation to provide good visualization.

OPTIMIZING VISUALIZATION

One of the potentially limiting factors of arthroscopy is bleeding that compromises the ability to visualize pathology. Burkhart and Lo[23] describe four main factors to consider when attempting to control bleeding. First, the patient's systolic blood pressure should be kept between 90 and 100 mm Hg in the absence of medical contraindications. Second, arthroscopic pump pressure should be kept at around 60 mm Hg, with intermittent increases to 75 mm Hg as needed for visualization (for only 10 to 15 minutes at a time). If the pump pressure is not regulated and is too high, the shoulder will swell, which compromises the surgical technique. Third, if possible, a separate 8-mm inflow cannula should be used to maximize fluid flow. Surgical instrumentation

through this portal should be limited because it may increase turbulence. Finally, turbulence within the system must be minimized. Turbulence occurs as a result of rapid flow of fluid out of the shoulder, such as through a skin portal without a cannula. As Burkhart and Lo[23] indicate, the Bernoulli effect creates forces at right angles of the many capillaries in the subacromial space, increasing the bleeding into the operative field. Digital pressure over skin portals can obstruct the outflow of fluid and in effect decrease turbulence.[24]

ANATOMY AND PORTAL PLACEMENT

Having a thorough understanding of basic shoulder anatomy is essential to developing good shoulder arthroscopic technique. We will first address the superficial anatomy, which is the guide to adequate portal placement and thus facilitates maneuverability about the shoulder joint (Fig. 39.2). We start by palpating the bony anatomy. It is important to mark not only the superficial edge of the bone but also the depth of the bone because trocar placement must be directed inferior to the edge of the bone. The clavicle and the anterolateral and posterolateral acromion are outlined. A soft triangle that is often palpable just medial to the acromion serves as a guide. Anteriorly the clavicle can be palpated, moving laterally to where it meets the acromion at the acromioclavicular joint. The coracoid is another important anterior landmark that can be palpated and should be drawn out as well. The posterolateral acromion is a key landmark that can be felt even in larger patients.

Once the superficial anatomy is appreciated for each individual patient, portal placement sites are marked on the skin. We start with the posterior portal first. This portal is made 2 cm inferior and 1 to 2 cm medial to the posterolateral edge of the acromion. A sharp scalpel is used to make a deep incision. The trocar is then slowly advanced; it is aimed superior, anterior, and medial, toward the coracoid process anteriorly. The trocar is advanced through soft tissue, and often a soft gap can be gently appreciated between the glenoid and humeral head. In addition, the arm can be internally or externally rotated, and if this movement is felt with the trocar, it is on the humeral head and should be directed to a greater degree medially. If no movement is felt, the trocar may be on the glenoid and needs to be directed to a greater degree laterally. The trocar is advanced until it is felt to "pop" through the capsule of the glenohumeral joint. One way to tell if the trocar is in the shoulder joint instead of the subacromial space is to judge the ease of movement of the trocar superiorly and inferiorly, as would be suggested by the proper location in the shoulder joint. Furthermore, if synovial fluid drips out of the cannula when the trocar is removed, proper placement in the glenohumeral joint is likely. The camera is then introduced into this portal, and one can either proceed with a diagnostic examination or place the anterior portal. We prefer to evaluate the rotator interval and then place the anterior portal as the next step.

The anterior portal is ideally placed lateral to the coracoid process through the rotator interval. The portal should never be placed in a position that is inferior or medial to the coracoid process because that would place neurovascular structures at

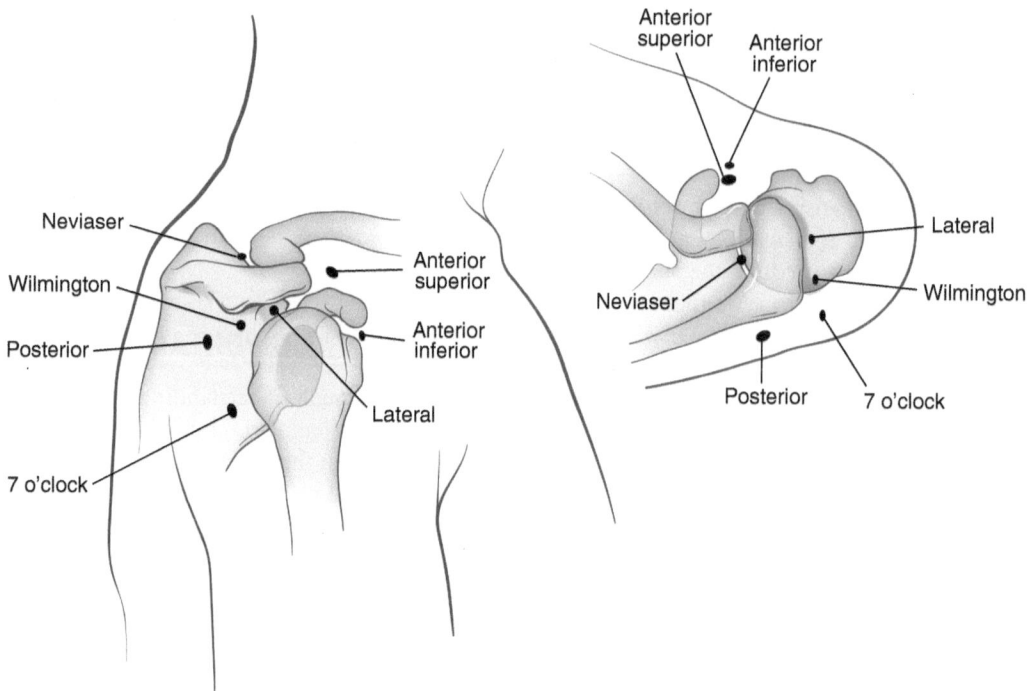

Fig. 39.2 A right shoulder demonstrating portal positions for the more standard posterior, anterior superior, anterior inferior, and lateral portals. Other common accessory portals shown include the Neviaser portal, the portal of Wilmington, and the 7 o'clock portal. (From Thompson S, Choi L, Brockmeier S, Miller MD. Shoulder and arm. In: Miller M, Cdhhabra A, Park J, Shen F, Weiss D, Browne J, eds. *Orthopaedic Surgical Approaches.* 2nd ed. Philadelphia: Elsevier Saunders; 2015:41, figure 2-52.)

risk. We prefer to visualize the anterior portal as it is placed from an outside-in technique. Therefore the arthroscope is kept in the posterior portal and moved anteriorly to view the rotator interval between the biceps tendon and the subscapularis tendon. A finger depresses the skin from the anterior side and is viewed on the arthroscope to be within the rotator interval. A spinal needle is then advanced into this area. If we are satisfied with this position for the anterior portal, a superficial skin incision is made (a deeper incision may create bleeding that will obscure visualization). The anterior portal is used mainly for instruments, but often surgeons alternate between portals depending on the procedure being performed.

To access the subacromial space, the same initial posterior portal is used, but the trocar is directed more superiorly. The trocar and cannula are advanced so that they hit the acromion and slide just inferior to it. The surgeon's other hand is used to palpate the anterior acromion and the trocar is advanced until it too can be palpated interiorly just inferior to the acromion. Often the coracoacromial ligament can be palpated with the trocar anteriorly, giving a good indication that the trocar is in the subacromial space. Medial to lateral movement of the trocar clears off some of the bursa that is often found with chronic impingement and is often located more posteriorly. Next, a lateral portal is established. This portal is made just inferior to the lateral border of the acromion, at the anterior third to middle third of the acromion, often 1 to 2 cm posterior to the antero-lateral border of the acromion. We like to use a spinal needle to judge our position before creating the portal because we try to

position the portal so it is as parallel to the acromion as possible to make the decompression easier.

Accessory portals can be made depending on the procedure to be performed. Often additional portals are useful for instability procedures for anchor placement.

DIAGNOSTIC EXAMINATION

We perform a standard diagnostic examination for each patient regardless of the planned procedure or diagnosis to ensure that no possible lesions are overlooked. We start with the arthroscope in the posterior portal and orient our position with the glenoid and humeral head in an upright position to go along with the patient in a beach chair position (Fig. 39.3A–D). The glenoid and humeral head are evaluated for signs of cartilage damage or the presence of osteoarthritis. The superior labrum–biceps tendon complex is a good landmark to find early because the biceps is seen traversing the glenohumeral joint from the labrum to its exit out of the glenohumeral joint. The labrum is evaluated for tears or degenerative fraying (Fig. 39.4). A probe can be used to check the stability of the labrum by pulling it away from the glenoid. Having a small foramen between the anterior–superior labrum and the glenoid is a normal variant that is often associated with a cordlike middle glenohumeral ligament.[22] The biceps is followed out to where it exits the glenohumeral joint, and a probe can be used to pull the biceps into the joint to look for signs of inflammation. The superior glenohumeral ligament is seen within the rotator interval, between the biceps tendon and

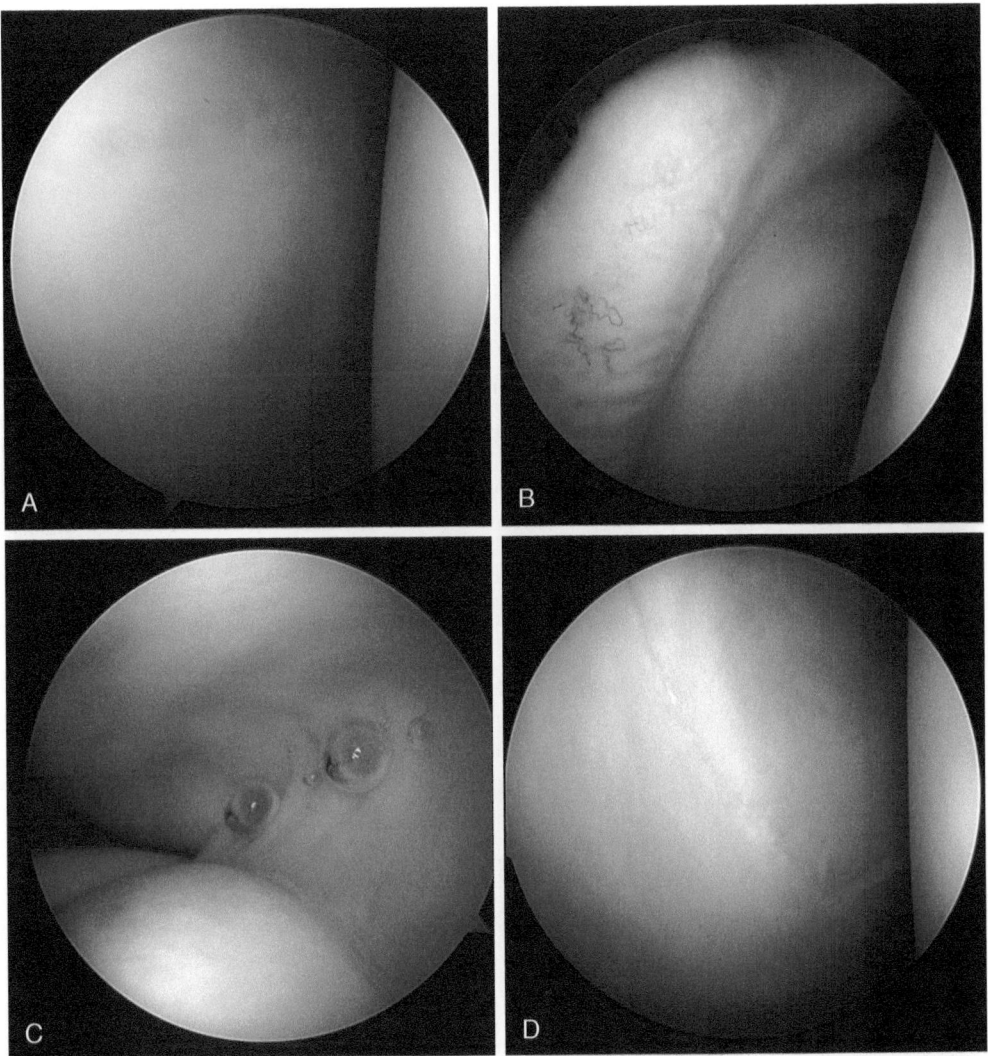

Fig. 39.3 A diagnostic shoulder scope. (A) The initial view of the glenohumeral joint viewed from the posterior portal. The glenoid is on the left and the humeral head is on the right. The labrum can be faintly visualized around the periphery of the glenoid. (B) Looking slightly superior, the insertion of the long head of the biceps into the superior labrum and superior glenoid can be visualized at the upper right. Again, the glenoid is on the left and the humeral head is on the right. (C) The biceps is followed from the mid-left portion of the picture as it exits the glenohumeral joint. An intact supraspinatus is visualized as it inserts at the articular margin of the humeral head at the middle to right portion of this figure. (D) An intact inferior labrum and glenohumeral ligament are visualized at the inferior portion of this figure. The glenoid is on the left and the humeral head is on the right.

subscapularis, and can be evaluated for thickening associated with frozen shoulder or looseness associated with laxity. If the arthroscope is turned inferiorly, the superior border of the subscapularis tendon can be visualized and followed laterally to its insertion onto the lesser tuberosity of the humerus. The anterior labrum is evaluated, and moving more inferiorly, the anterior and posterior labrum and glenohumeral ligaments are evaluated. The anterior-inferior glenohumeral ligament and labral complex makes up the classic Bankart lesion that is seen in anterior shoulder instability (Fig. 39.5).

To evaluate posterior portions of the rotator cuff, the anterior edge of the supraspinatus is visualized just lateral to the biceps tendon exit point and can be evaluated throughout its tendinous portion, moving posteriorly both by moving the camera posteriorly and by abducting the arm and externally rotating the arm. Posteriorly the supraspinatus insertion on the greater tuberosity ends and a bare area is seen because a gap exists between the edge of the articular surface and the infraspinatus insertion. Pitting is commonly seen in this area and represents vascular channels. Continuing posteriorly, the posterolateral humeral head can be seen, and the presence or absence of a Hill-Sachs lesion is confirmed. Moving more inferiorly, the axillary pouch is examined to ensure that no loose bodies are present.[25]

Finally, the posterior labrum and capsule are examined by slowly backing the arthroscope out of the posterior portal until they come into view, taking care not to pull the scope out completely. The posterior anatomy can be evaluated further by switching the arthroscope to the anterior portal as well.[25]

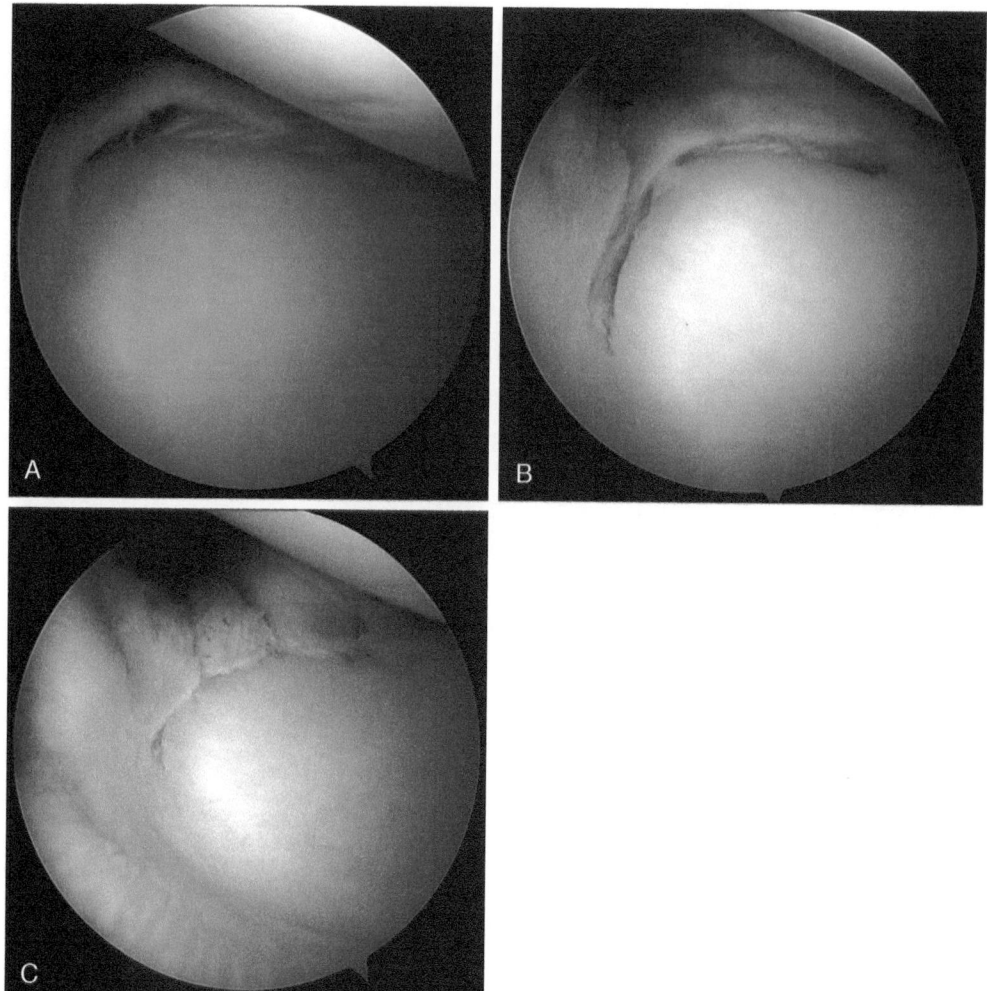

Fig. 39.4 A superior labral anterior to posterior (SLAP) tear. (A) Fraying of the superior glenoid labrum, a SLAP lesion. (B) A SLAP lesion as it is being prepared for repair. It has been separated from the glenoid, and the glenoid surface has been roughened to prepare a good healing bed for repair. (C) A SLAP lesion after repair with three suture anchors (which cannot be seen) and sutures passing around the superior labrum.

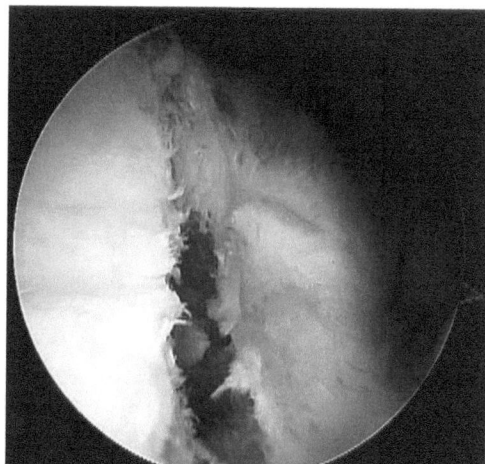

Fig. 39.5 A Bankart lesion. A traumatic Bankart lesion can be visualized with separation of the inferior glenohumeral ligament/labral complex from the anterior inferior glenoid. This lesion was repaired in a similar manner as the superior labral anterior to posterior lesion in Fig. 39.4, with glenoid bone preparation for a good healing bed, and then suture anchor placement and sutures to hold the Bankart complex down (not shown).

Often a diagnostic scope of the subacromial space also should be performed. The camera is inserted as previously described, with management of bursal tissue being the key to good visualization. To begin the examination, the anterior acromion and coracoacromial ligament are evaluated for impingement. The subacromial space also can be used to evaluate the bursal side of the rotator cuff. To evaluate the rotator cuff, the scope is then turned to look inferiorly so that the top or bursal side of the rotator cuff can be evaluated. Signs of impingement are suggested by the presence of fraying, inflammation, or partial bursal-sided rotator cuff tears. If partial-thickness articular-sided tears of the rotator cuff are suspected, a Prolene suture can be passed from the joint side through the rotator cuff and evaluated as it exits the cuff on the subacromial side. If a rent is visualized at the point where the suture comes through, then the tear is actually full thickness.

COMPLICATIONS

As with all surgeries, shoulder arthroscopy is not without risk, which includes bleeding, although this is minimal, and infection, which can be both superficial and deep.

As mentioned in the "Patient Positioning" section, neurapraxia is also a risk with shoulder arthroscopy, and patient positioning must be performed diligently to avoid this complication in both the beach chair and the lateral decubitus positions.

Although the risk of deep venous thrombosis (DVT) and pulmonary embolism is very low (a 0.08% risk of DVT with shoulder arthroscopy, which is only one-tenth of the risk of developing DVT after shoulder arthroplasty), the risk still exists, and no definitive recommendation is provided in the literature for postoperative anticoagulation.[26] For our patients, we prescribe enteric coated aspirin, 325 mg for 2 weeks after surgery.

Chondrolysis is a complication of shoulder arthroscopy that is characterized by the dissolution of the articular cartilage of the humeral head and glenoid. It presents with the onset of pain and loss of range of motion weeks to months after surgery, and joint space narrowing and subchondral cysts in the absence of osteophytes are noted on imaging.[27-32] Chondrolysis has been reported after use of intra-articular thermal energy, after intra-articular injection of radiopaque contrast medium, and most notably, after intra-articular postoperative infusion of a local anesthetic.[27-33] In one retrospective review of 375 shoulder arthroscopies, a 13% incidence of chondrolysis was found. It was more common in young patients when one or more suture anchors were used in the glenoid, and in each case a postoperative infusion of local anesthetic was used.[27] It is recommended that a postoperative infusion of local anesthetic not be administered to avoid this devastating complication.

CONCLUSION

Shoulder arthroscopy is commonly performed and has many potential indications. It is an equipment-intense procedure that involves two main patient positioning options, each of which has its own advantages and disadvantages. A systematic diagnostic examination should be performed at the start of each procedure so that pathology is not missed.

For a complete list of references, go to ExpertConsult.com.

SELECTED READINGS

Citation:

Youm T, Murray DH, Kubiak EN, et al. Arthroscopic versus mini-open rotator cuff repair: a comparison of clinical outcomes and patient satisfaction. *J Shoulder Elbow Surg.* 2005;14:455–459.

Level of Evidence:

III

Summary:

In this study, the outcomes of at least 2 years were compared for 40 patients who underwent arthroscopic rotator cuff repair and 40 patients who underwent mini-open rotator cuff repair. Results suggested similar outcomes and patient satisfaction scores for small-, medium-, and massive-sized cuff tears.

Citation:

Sauerbrey AM, Getz CL, Piancastelli M, et al. Arthroscopic versus mini-open rotator cuff repair: a comparison of clinical outcome. *Arthroscopy.* 2005;21:1415–1420.

Level of Evidence:

III

Summary:

In this retrospective review, the outcomes 53 patients who had either an arthroscopic or mini-open rotator cuff repair were examined. Patients were followed up for an average of 19 months (for the arthroscopic procedure) or 33 months (for the mini-open procedure), and results were similar for function and patient reported outcomes.

Citation:

Verma NN, Dunn W, Alder RS, et al. All-arthroscopic versus mini-open rotator cuff repair: a retrospective review with minimum 2-year follow-up. *Arthroscopy.* 2006;22:587–594.

Level of Evidence:

III

Summary:

In this retrospective review, the outcomes of 71 patients who were treated with either an arthroscopic or mini-open rotator cuff repair were examined. Patients were followed up for an average of 2 years with ultrasound to evaluate the repair. Results for function and patient-reported outcomes were similar, and patients had similar rates of rerupture, which was seven times more likely if the original tear was greater than 3 cm.

Citation:

Pearsall AW, Ibrahim KA. Madanagopal SG. The results of arthroscopic versus mini-open repair for rotator cuff tears at mid-term follow-up. *J Orthop Surg.* 2007;2:1–8.

Level of Evidence:

III

Summary:

In this study, 52 patients were treated with either a mini-open or arthroscopic rotator cuff repair for a small to large full-thickness rotator cuff tear. Results were similar for both function and patient reported outcomes, suggesting that either treatment option is acceptable at midterm follow-up.

Citation:

Teefey SA, Rubin DA, Middleton WD, et al. Detection and quantification of rotator cuff tears: comparison of ultrasonographic, magnetic resonance imaging, and arthroscopic findings in seventy-one consecutive cases. *J Bone Joint Surg Am.* 2004;86:708–716.

Level of Evidence:

Diagnostic study

Summary:

Seventy-four patients underwent ultrasound and magnetic resonance imaging (MRI) of their partial- or full-thickness rotator cuff, and then arthroscopy was used for a gold standard comparison. Ultrasonography and MRI had comparable accuracy rates in the identification and measurement of full- and partial-thickness rotator cuff tears.

40

Anterior Shoulder Instability

Stephen R. Thompson, Heather Menzer, Stephen F. Brockmeier

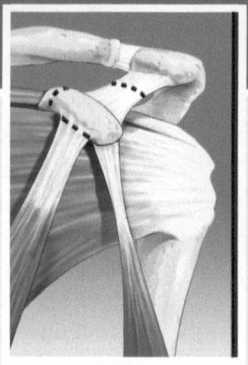

Anterior shoulder instability is the most common type of shoulder instability. It is typically the result of a traumatic event with dislocation of the glenohumeral joint. However, instability also may present as subluxation, a condition in which the joint symptomatically translates but does not completely dislocate.

The estimated incidence of shoulder dislocations in the United States in 23.9 per 100,000.[1] Patients of any age may sustain a shoulder dislocation; however, 48% of the patients reported were between the ages of 20 and 29 years. The prevalence of shoulder dislocations in high and collegiate school athletes is reported to be 2.04 and 2.58 respectively per 100,000 athletic exposures.[2] Football was reported to have the highest shoulder dislocation rate compared with other sports at each competition level. Dislocation occurred more frequently in competition than in practice, and direct contact was the most common mechanism. Ice hockey, wrestling, and basketball all had higher rates of dislocation compared with other sports, though soccer and baseball had increased rates of noncontact injury.

This chapter discusses the anatomy, clinical features, and treatment of anterior shoulder instability. Posterior and multidirectional instability may involve a component of anterior patholaxity; these topics are addressed separately in subsequent chapters. This chapter first reviews the anatomy and pathoanatomy of shoulder instability. The "History and Physical Examination" sections provide an evidence-based approach and assume a general knowledge of shoulder examination. The "Decision-Making Principles and Treatment Options" sections discuss acute shoulder reduction and immobilization, timing of surgery, arthroscopic versus open surgery, unique clinical scenarios, and the approach to bone loss. Our preferred technique for the treatment of shoulder instability is arthroscopic Bankart repair. For revision situations, or in cases of significant bone loss, we prefer the Latarjet procedure. Methods for both of these scenarios are outlined, along with postoperative management. Lastly, the results of treatment and complications are discussed, along with future directions of research.

ANATOMY

The glenohumeral joint is a unique diarthrodial joint. More than any other joint in the body, it must carefully balance function and stability. Because of its role in positioning the arm in space, it has 6 degrees of freedom and is the most mobile of the diarthrodial joints. However, to achieve this range of motion (ROM), stability is sacrificed.

When discussing the stabilizing anatomy of the shoulder, it has become common to dichotomize the stabilizers as static or dynamic. We recognize that this approach is an oversimplification[3] and that the entire system functions in a coordinated fashion, but we believe it serves as a useful pedagogic instrument, and thus we will retain it for the purposes of this discussion. Static stabilizers of the shoulder may be considered as the structures that provide a unidirectional limitation to translation. The three principle groups of static stabilizers are bony, ligamentous, and labral. Dynamic stabilizers are primarily musculotendinous and include the rotator cuff, biceps, deltoid, pectoralis major, and latissimus dorsi.

The bony anatomy of the glenohumeral joint has been compared with a golf ball on a tee. The humeral head is significantly larger than the overall size of the glenoid, with only 25% to 30% of the humeral head in contact with the glenoid at any given anatomic position. The bony glenoid concavity is quite shallow, with a depth of only a few millimeters. To confer some degree of stability, the glenoid concavity is deepened by the articular cartilage and the labrum. The articular cartilage is thinner in the center of the glenoid and progressively thickens toward the periphery, thus increasing the functional depth of the glenoid (Fig. 40.1). Loss of the articular cartilage has been found to decrease stability by nearly 50%.[4]

The glenoid labrum is a critical structure for the stability of the glenohumeral joint. It encircles the glenoid to both increase the depth of the glenoid concavity and the overall surface area of the glenoid in contact with the humeral head by approximately 50%.[5] Although it is commonly referred to as a fibrocartilaginous structure, anatomic studies have demonstrated that the glenoid labrum has a structure similar to a tendon, with dense fibrous connective tissue that is devoid of chondrocytes.[6-8] The labrum has a predominantly triangular cross-sectional shape and, consequently, functions as a "chock block" that prevents translation of the humeral head outside the articular surface of the glenoid. However, the stabilizing mechanism of the labrum is much more complex than this simple mechanical function.

The labrum has a complex anatomic structure and attachment to the glenoid. It is typically more adherent in the inferior half of the glenoid and quite variably attached in the anterior superior quadrant. The labrum serves as an attachment site for the glenohumeral joint capsule and the long head of the biceps tendon,

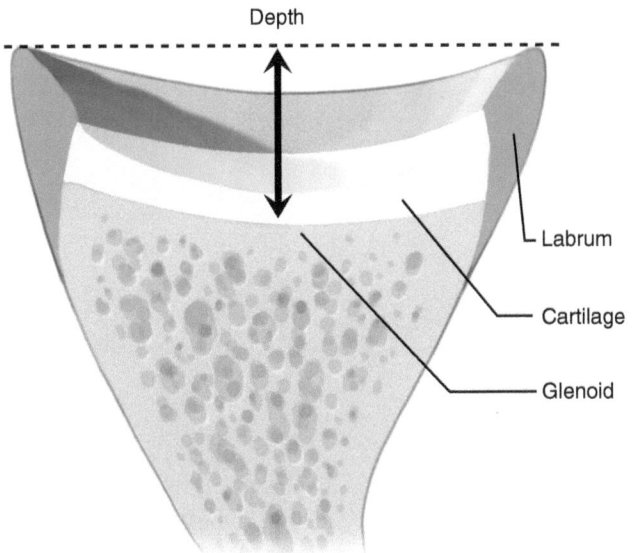

Fig. 40.1 Glenoid concavity is deepened by both the articular cartilage and labrum.

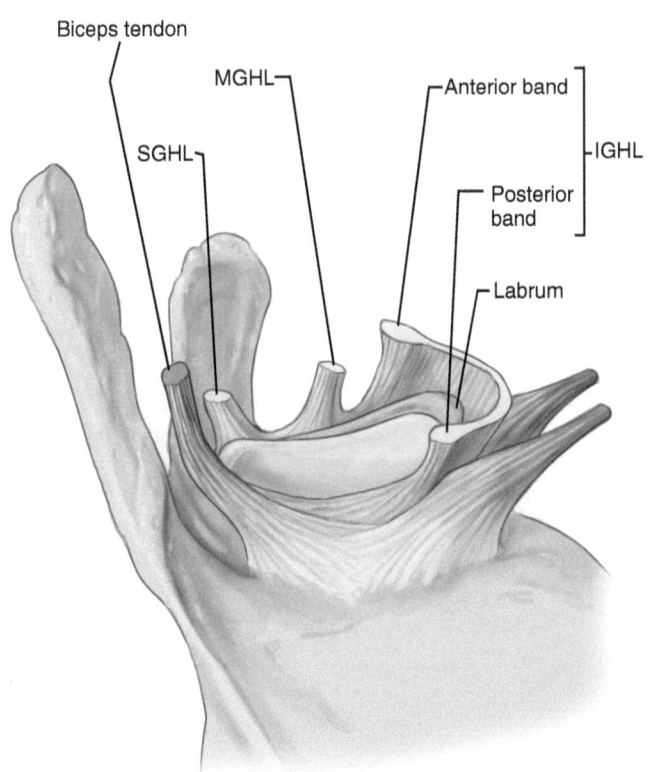

Fig. 40.2 Anatomy of the glenohumeral ligaments: superior glenohumeral ligament *(SGHL)*, middle glenohumeral ligament *(MGHL)*, and inferior glenohumeral ligament *(IGHL)*. The view is from the posterior aspect, as traditionally seen in lateral-position arthroscopy.

which helps create a suction seal that leads to a negative intraarticular pressure and aids in the creation of the concavity-compression effect of glenohumeral stability.

The glenohumeral capsule that attaches to the glenoid labrum has four distinct thickenings that have been termed the glenohumeral ligaments (GHLs): the superior, middle, and anterior band of the inferior and the posterior band of the inferior (Fig. 40.2). Of these ligaments, the inferior glenohumeral ligament (IGHL) is the most important for providing stability to the shoulder. The GHLs are not as strong as the knee ligaments; for example, the IGHL possesses an ultimate stress capability that is only 15% of that reported for the anterior cruciate ligament.[9] This characteristic underscores the importance of the entire relationship between the static and dynamic components that provide stability to the glenohumeral joint.

The IGHL should be considered a complex rather than an individual structure. Within the IGHL structure, an anterior band originates at the 3-o'clock position of the glenoid, a posterior band originates at the 8-o'clock position of the glenoid, and an intervening capsule exists that is termed the "axillary pouch." This complex is likened to a hammock. When the arm is brought into the "apprehension position" of abduction and external rotation, the axillary pouch becomes more taut as the anterior band is placed under tension from being pulled superiorly and anteriorly to span the midportion of the glenohumeral joint (Fig. 40.3).[10] In this position, the anterior band of the IGHL functions to prevent anterior translation of the humeral head while the taut axillary pouch prevents anteroinferior translation.

If the arm is brought into 45 degrees of abduction, the middle GHL becomes taut and prevents anterior displacement.[11] In 0 degrees of abduction, the superior GHL has a minor function in preventing anterior displacement and an accessory role in preventing inferior displacement along with the supraspinatus, deltoid, and coracohumeral ligament.[10,12]

The dynamic stabilizers of the shoulder provide stability by providing compression of the humeral head into the glenoid and coracoacromial arch concavities, which is termed the "concavity-compression effect."[13] The deltoid and the rotator cuff function to dynamically compress and center the humeral head within these concavities during shoulder motion, thereby enhancing (or perhaps providing primary restraint to)[14] glenohumeral stability.

In a review of anatomy relating to anterior shoulder instability, it is important to note two relatively common anatomic variants that should not be mistaken for pathology. The anterosuperior aspect of the capsulolabral complex is the most variable in the shoulder. A sublabral foramen (or sublabral hole) is the complete separation or absence of the labrum from the glenoid. It is the most common variant, with an incidence between 3% and 18%.[15–17] A Buford complex[18] is the combination of an absent anterosuperior labrum with an associated "cordlike" middle GHL that attaches to the superior labrum near the base of the biceps tendon. The incidence varies between 1.5% and 6%.[15–17] Other less common variants exist as well. Overall, recognition of variant anatomy both on magnetic resonance imaging (MRI) and at arthroscopy is vital to avoid inappropriate diagnosis or treatment.

PATHOANATOMY

When A. S. Blundell Bankart described the pathology and treatment of recurrent dislocation of the shoulder, he emphasized

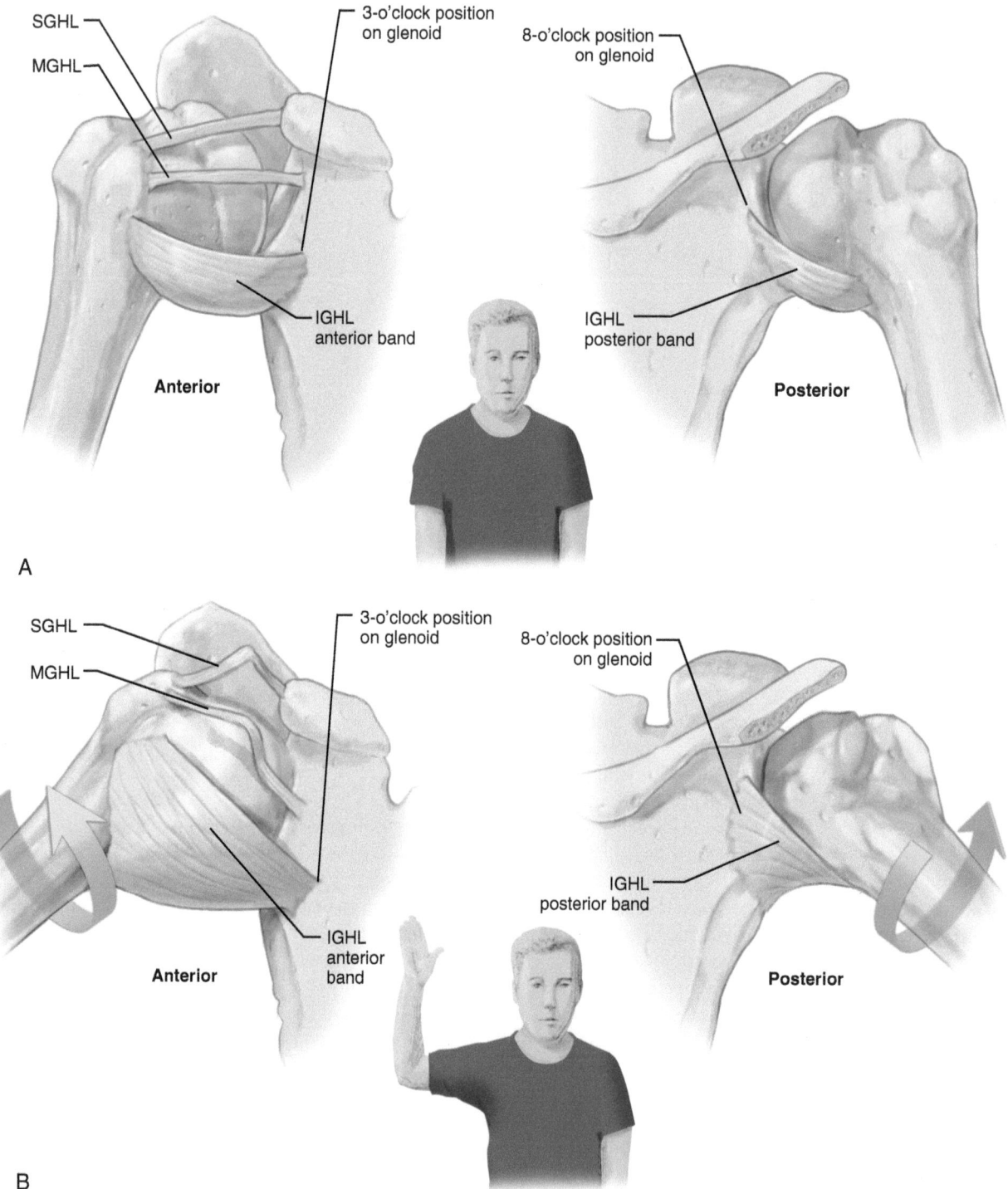

Fig. 40.3 The glenohumeral ligaments are dynamic structures. (A) In 0 degree of abduction, the superior glenohumeral ligament *(SGHL)* is taut. (B) As the arm is brought into the "apprehension position" of abduction and external rotation, the anterior band of the inferior glenohumeral ligament *(IGHL)* is pulled superiorly and anteriorly to span the midportion of the glenohumeral joint, thus providing anterior stability. *MGHL,* Middle glenohumeral ligament.

the importance of understanding the pathoanatomy to guide treatment. To him, the "essential lesion" occurred when the "[humeral] head shears off the fibrous or fibrocartilaginous glenoid ligament from its attachment to the bone."[19,20] His original description was based on his work with only four patients, and

his subsequent description 15 years later was based on work with a further 23 patients. Bankart believed that the essential lesion occurred in 100% of cases and that "no one who has ever seen this typical lesion exposed at operation could possibly doubt that the only rational treatment is to reattach the

TABLE 40.1 Capsulolabral Lesions

Lesion	Description
Associated With Anterior Instability	
Perthes	Avulsion of the anterior-inferior glenolabral complex with preservation of the medial scapular neck periosteum
Bankart	Complete avulsion of the anterior-inferior glenolabral complex along with a piece of scapular neck periosteum
Bony Bankart	Osseous avulsion fracture of the anterior-inferior glenolabral complex
ALSPA	Avulsion of the anterior-inferior glenolabral complex with stripping of the medial scapular neck periosteum but preservation of a medial hinge; the loose fragment subsequently scars medially down the scapular neck
HAGL	Avulsion of the glenohumeral ligaments from their humeral-sided attachment
Not Associated With Instability	
Glenolabral articular disruption[162]	A superficial tear of the anterior-inferior labrum with associated cartilage injury but preservation of the anterior-inferior glenolabral complex; presents with a painful shoulder but is not a cause of shoulder instability
SLAP[163]	Disruption of the superior labrum, originally described to stop at the midglenoid notch; recent descriptions have associated SLAP tears with Bankart lesions, but SLAP lesions alone are not a cause of shoulder instability

ALSPA, Anterior labroligamentous periosteal sleeve avulsion; *HAGL,* humeral avulsion of the glenohumeral ligaments; *SLAP,* superior labrum anterior posterior.

Pathogenesis of Bankart lesion

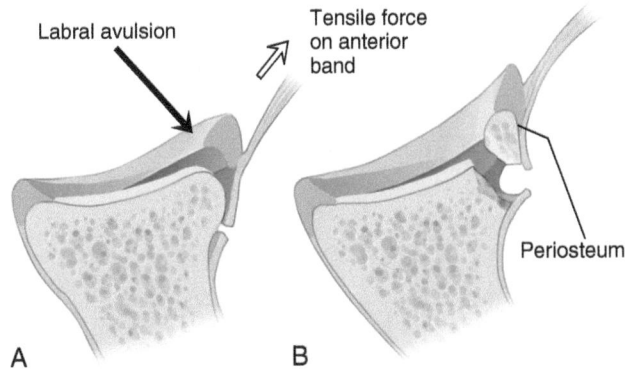

Fig. 40.4 (A) A Bankart lesion, which is defined as avulsion of the anterior-inferior capsulolabral complex with extension into the scapular periosteum and rupture of the periosteal tissue. (B) A bony Bankart lesion occurs when the capsulolabral complex is avulsed along with a variably sized fragment of bone.

glenoid ligament (or the capsule) to the bone from which it has been torn."[20]

Since Bankart provided this description, a more nuanced understanding of the pathoanatomy of recurrent anterior shoulder instability has been developed. Fundamentally, the pathoanatomy can be capsulolabral, osseous, or both. The capsulolabral lesions are typically related to the glenoid labrum and the anterior band of the IGHL. The nomenclature of these lesions has evolved into a mixture of eponymous terms and acronyms that can confuse even the most experienced clinician. The nomenclature includes the Perthes lesion, Bankart lesion (or "anterior labral tear"), bony Bankart lesion, anterior labroligamentous periosteal sleeve avulsion (ALPSA) lesion, and humeral avulsion of the glenohumeral ligaments (HAGL) lesion (Table 40.1).

Despite this confusing jargon, the Bankart lesion remains an "essential lesion" and has been found to occur in approximately 90% of patients with recurrent anterior instability.[21,22] A Bankart lesion can be arbitrarily defined as an avulsion of the anterior-inferior capsulolabral complex with extension into the scapular periosteum and rupture of the periosteal tissue (Fig. 40.4A). Acutely, the avulsed tissue is free to move about the shoulder. As such, the stabilizing function of the labrum is lost and the anterior band of the IGHL can no longer resist anterior translation in abduction and external rotation.[23] A bony Bankart lesion occurs when the capsulolabral complex is avulsed along with a variably sized fragment of bone (see Fig. 40.4B), which can create a significant osseous injury that can contribute to the

pathogenesis of shoulder instability in a manner more severe than that of a soft-tissue Bankart lesion (discussed later).

A Perthes lesion and an ALPSA lesion are variants of the Bankart lesion (Fig. 40.5). A Perthes lesion[24] can be thought of as representing the initial stages of a Bankart lesion. The capsulolabral complex is avulsed from the anterior-inferior aspect of the glenoid, but the medial scapular periosteum remains intact. In essence, it is a nondisplaced Bankart lesion. An ALPSA lesion[25] occurs when the capsulolabral complex is avulsed and the medial scapular periosteum is stripped (but not detached as in a Bankart lesion) and subsequently displaced down the denuded anterior glenoid neck. In essence, it can be conceptualized as a medialized Bankart lesion. In either lesion, the capsulolabral function is lost and recurrent instability ensues.

Although the most common site of injury relating to anterior instability is at the glenoid, rupture of the GHLs can also occur on the humeral side. This rupture has been termed an HAGL lesion and has an incidence between 1% and 9%.[26] Similar to that which occurs on the glenoid, the rupture of the humeral insertion, along with a bony avulsion, is coined a *bony HAGL* or B-HAGL (pronounced "bagel") lesion. Although loss of the GHL tension mechanism results in either case, it is important to recognize this lesion and thus perform the correct surgery.

In addition to capsulolabral injury, some degree of bony injury occurs in virtually every patient with anterior shoulder instability. Osseous glenoid lesions are thought to occur as the humeral head either passes over the glenoid rim or as the posterior superior aspect of the humeral head has an impact on the anterior glenoid rim upon dislocation. Conversely, osseous injury to the posterior superior humeral head occurs via an impression-impaction fracture of the soft humeral head bone against the less giving, sclerotic anterior rim of the glenoid when subluxation or dislocation occurs. The existence of this lesion was popularized by two radiologists, Hill and Sachs, in 1940 and has since been termed a *Hill-Sachs* lesion.[27,28]

Glenoid bone injury is common and predominantly occurs in two configurations. A visible bone fragment with its attached

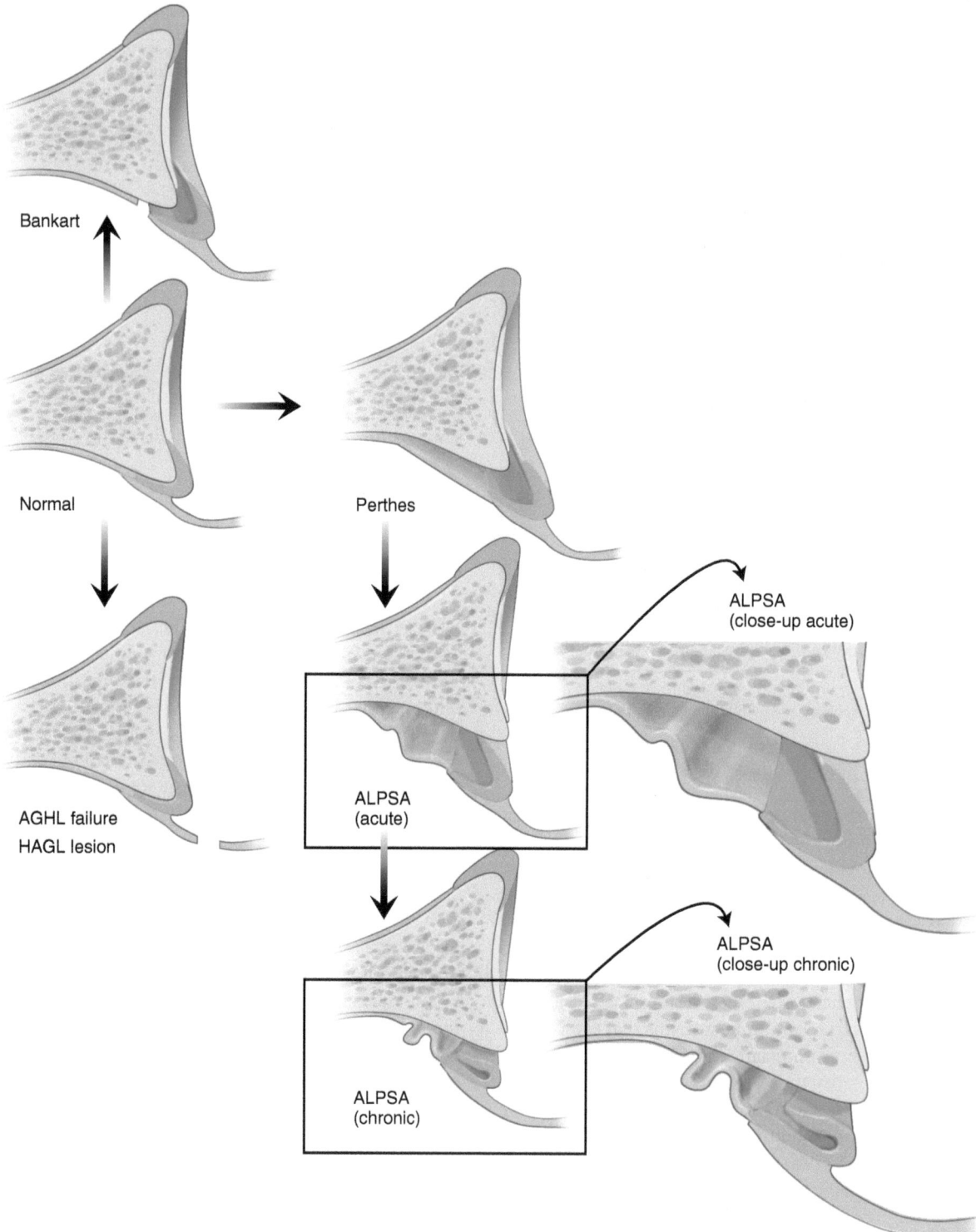

Fig. 40.5 Variants of the Bankart lesion. A Perthes lesion represents avulsion of the capsulolabral complex, but the scapular periosteum remains intact. An anterior labroligamentous periosteal sleeve avulsion *(ALPSA)* lesion occurs when the periosteum is stripped and displaced down the anterior glenoid neck. Failure of the glenohumeral ligaments on the humeral side is termed a humeral avulsion of the glenohumeral ligaments *(HAGL)* lesion. *AGHL,* Anterior glenohumeral ligaments.

capsulolabral structures may fracture from the anterior glenoid rim and is termed a bony Bankart lesion. Alternatively, the anterior glenoid rim may be impacted or eroded from the force of the humeral head during subluxation or dislocation. In a three-dimensional (3D) computed tomography (CT) scan of 100 consecutive shoulders with recurrent anterior instability, only 10% were found to have normal glenoid morphology[29]; 50% of patients had some degree of bony fragment, and 40% presented with erosion or a compression fracture of the glenoid. A subsequent CT study found similar results, with 40% of persons with first-time dislocations and 85% of persons with recurrent dislocations sustaining a degree of glenoid bone loss.[30] These noninvasive studies corroborate Rowe's observations that 73% of his patients undergoing open Bankart surgery had glenoid rim damage.[31]

Hill-Sachs lesions are common, but until recently, they were less regarded in the pathogenesis of recurrent instability. These lesions occur in approximately 40% of patients with recurrent subluxation but no dislocation, in 70% to 90% of patients with a single dislocation, and in virtually 100% of patients with recurrent dislocations.[32–35] The majority of these lesions are small, and in general, they are clinically insignificant. However, a minority have been termed "engaging," which means the Hill-Sachs lesion is oriented in such a manner that placing the shoulder in abduction and external rotation results in the humeral head losing contact with the glenoid and subsequent subluxation or dislocation of the glenohumeral joint.[36]

If we return to the analogy of the glenohumeral joint as a golf ball on a tee, it becomes apparent that if either the tee (glenoid) or golf ball (humeral head) is damaged, the stability is altered or even lost. But what degree of injury will result in instability? It is easiest to first consider the glenoid.

In a classic biomechanical study by Itoi and colleagues,[37] a series of glenoid osteotomies were performed to determine the effect of glenoid bone loss on the glenoid concavity mechanism of shoulder stability. Using the stability ratio,[38] these investigators found a significant loss of stability after the creation of a 6-mm defect, which is roughly equivalent to 28% of the total glenoid width. Practically speaking, however, it is difficult to measure the total glenoid width because this bone may be lost due to impaction or erosion. The glenoid length, defined as the superior to inferior distance of the glenoid (i.e., from 12 o'clock to 6 o'clock), can be used as a surrogate if some geometric assumptions and transformations are used. Accordingly, this critical defect size corresponded to 20% of the glenoid length. When the study was repeated with the soft tissue structures retained, the authors confirmed their original findings but also demonstrated that repair of the Bankart lesion failed to confer added stability. Stability was restored only after a coracoid bone graft was placed.

Clinically, these results have been supported by numerous studies that have found significant bone loss to be a risk factor for failure after a Bankart repair.[39–41] Burkhart and De Beer[36] described their clinical experience with bony glenoid loss. If the glenoid is viewed *en face,* it has an appearance similar to that of a pear. When anterior glenoid bone loss occurs, Burkhart and De Beer indicated that the glenoid has an "inverted pear"

appearance and hypothesized that this arthroscopically viewable appearance is an indicator of clinically significant bone loss. When patients were dichotomized into a normal glenoid or inverted pear glenoid group, the recurrent dislocation rate after arthroscopic Bankart repair was 4% for the normal glenoid group but 61% for the inverted pear glenoid group. Lo, Parten, and Burkhart then reexamined these data and compared them with a cadaveric model, demonstrating that approximately 6.5 mm of glenoid bone loss (or 29% of the glenoid width) was necessary to achieve an inverted pear glenoid configuration.[42] This led to a common acceptance that glenoid bone loss of 20% to 27% was "critical" bone loss and the surgeon should consider performing an open bone grafting procedure, such as a Latarjet, in these patients. However, a recent cohort study by Shaha and colleagues[43] of military recruits has questioned this dogma. In their population with high levels of mandatory activity, they found glenoid bone loss of 13.5% was associated with worse patient reported outcomes and higher failure rates following arthroscopic Bankart repair. In those patients with bone loss less than 13.5%, the failure rate was 5% compared with 22% in the group with more than 13.5% bone loss. A subsequent biomechanical study has supported this, finding that glenoid bone loss more than 15% resulted in an inability of a soft tissue procedure to restore stability.[44]

The significance of humeral bone loss via Hill-Sachs lesions has been more difficult to characterize. Numerous authors have proposed classification schemes in an attempt to guide clinical decision-making. They have variably defined the size according to length and depth,[45] percentage of humeral head involvement at arthroscopy,[33] percentage of humeral head involvement on a Notch View radiograph,[46] and circular degree involvement and location on axillary MRI.[47] Regardless of classification, it has been recognized that persons with *large* Hill-Sachs lesions are at risk for recurrent dislocation.[36,45] *Small* lesions have conversely been viewed as clinically insignificant. *Intermediate* lesions have represented something of a management quandary. Due to the multiple variables associated with Hill-Sachs lesions, many of these classification schemes are not useful. Recent interest in how both glenoid and humeral osseous defects can contribute to the pathogenesis of instability has increased and resulted in the concept of the "glenoid track."[48] This concept has been gaining significant traction in the classification and treatment paradigm of shoulder instability.

The glenoid track is defined as the zone of contact between the glenoid and the humeral head when the humerus is in maximal external rotation and horizontal extension and the arm is elevated and depressed (Fig. 40.6A). If a Hill-Sachs lesion is entirely contained by the glenoid track, regardless of its length, depth, or percentage of the humeral head, then it never has the ability to engage the glenoid and dislocate (see Fig. 40.6B). If the Hill-Sachs lesion does not engage with the glenoid defect, it is considered an "on-track" lesion.[49] Conversely, a small and shallow Hill-Sachs lesion can become an "off-track" symptomatic defect if its location is medial to the glenoid track (see Fig. 40.6C). It is also vital to understand that, by definition, any glenoid-side bone loss will decrease the width of the glenoid track (see Fig. 40.6D).

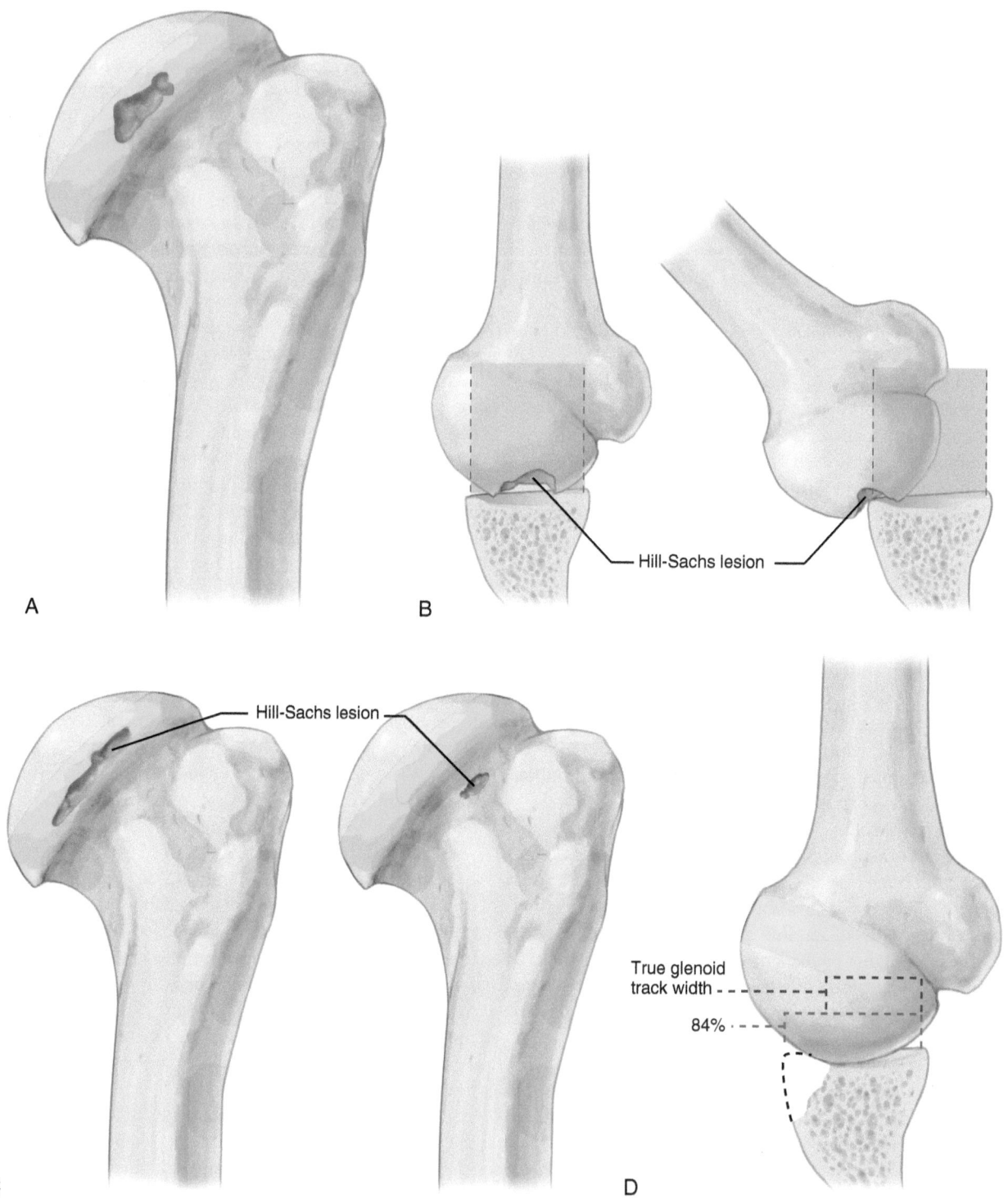

Fig. 40.6 Glenoid track. (A) The glenoid track is defined as the zone of contact between the glenoid and the humeral head when the humerus is in maximal external rotation and horizontal extension and the arm is elevated and depressed. (B) If the Hill-Sachs lesion is entirely within the glenoid track, then it will not dislocate. (C) A lesion outside the glenoid track can result in instability, even if it is small. (D) Any glenoid bone loss functionally decreases the width of the glenoid track.

Although the glenoid track is a recently proposed concept, its application was reported superior at predicting postoperative stability in a cohort of patients who underwent arthroscopic Bankart reconstruction.[50] It provides an excellent framework for considering the interaction and importance of both glenoid and humeral bone loss in the pathogenesis of shoulder instability. Given the high incidence of osseous injury in persons with either acute or recurrent anterior instability, it is vital for the clinical evaluation to account for potential osseous causes of instability to avoid the risk of treatment failure.[50]

HISTORY

The purpose of the history is both to establish the diagnosis of shoulder instability and to obtain information that will guide treatment. Often the diagnosis of shoulder instability is not in question after a traumatic dislocation and a physician-assisted reduction. Conversely, some persons present with more subtle forms of instability and require differentiation from patients with posterior or multidirectional instability. Information to guide treatment must include data that will allow the surgeon to identify the risk of recurrence, the risk of failure of arthroscopic surgery, and the risk of associated pathology.

When first approaching a patient who reports shoulder instability, it is useful to classify the patient as either having sustained or not having sustained a dislocation. If the patient has experienced a dislocation, the details should be ascertained, including the mechanism of injury, the use of radiographs, the need for reduction (as well as who performed the required reduction), and the length of disability resulting from the dislocation. What arm position aggravates the sense of instability? If the patient has experienced multiple dislocations, it is useful to proceed in chronologic order to evaluate how the mechanism of injury may have evolved. Are the dislocations becoming more frequent? Are they occurring with less traumatic force? Lastly, it is vital to document the age of the patient when the first dislocation occurred and his or her age at the time of subsequent dislocations, because age is a significant prognostic indicator for recurrence.

Symptoms of shoulder subluxation without dislocation are vague, difficult to evaluate, and difficult to distinguish from the symptoms of patients with multidirectional instability.[51] Typically the symptoms have an insidious onset and include a sense of looseness, shoulder achiness, and possibly transient neurologic deficits. The activities causing symptoms are often random and, in contrast to the cases of patients with traumatic instability, may occur with activities of daily living.

To distinguish patients with anterior instability from patients with posterior and multidirectional instability, identifying the arm position that aggravates symptoms is occasionally useful. Classically, anterior instability presents with discomfort when the shoulder is abducted and externally rotated (such as when throwing a ball). Posterior instability presents with discomfort when the shoulder is internally rotated, adducted, and forward elevated, such as when pushing a door open. Multidirectional instability presents with symptoms in a variety of positions, but by definition, symptomatic inferior translation is part of the spectrum of complaints.

Once the history of the present illness is concluded, a comprehensive social history is obtained. In which sport (or sports) does the patient participate? Are these sports competitive or recreational? Is the activity a contact sport? Which way does the patient typically shoot, throw, or swing? What is the patient's occupation? Does the patient's occupation require forced overhead activity? This vital information will guide treatment.

A small number of patients present with the ability to voluntarily dislocate their shoulder. A classic study by Rowe and colleagues[52] found that a substantial proportion of patients who could voluntarily dislocate their shoulder had an associated psychiatric condition and did very poorly after surgical stabilization. However, these investigators acknowledged that the majority of persons who could voluntarily dislocate their shoulder had no cognitive disturbance. Nevertheless, the association between persons who can voluntarily dislocate their shoulder and psychopathology has persisted. The astute clinician should screen for psychopathology but recall that the majority of these patients warrant more than cognitive and physical therapy. It is important to differentiate "voluntary" from positional instability. "Voluntary" suggests a muscular contraction and a volitional component, whereas patients with positional instability (commonly posterior) can reproduce the instability by positioning their hand in space. It is very common for patients with posterior instability to demonstrate their instability in forward elevation.

From the history alone, it is possible to estimate the risk for the presence and size of a glenoid bony defect. Milano and colleagues[53] demonstrated that the presence of a defect was significantly associated with multiple dislocations, male gender, and type of sport. The size of the defect was significantly associated with recurrent dislocation, an increasing number of dislocations, timing from first dislocation, and manual labor. Presence of a 20% defect of the glenoid width was significantly associated with the number of dislocations and age at first dislocation.

PHYSICAL EXAMINATION

As with the history, the physical examination must be goal directed. Goals of the examination are to:

- Either narrow the differential diagnosis or confirm the suspected diagnosis after the history is taken
- Rule out possible associated pathology
- Obtain information that will influence management

The standard systematic orthopedic approach of "look, feel, move," which was popularized by A. Graham Apley, should be used on a routine basis. First, a general impression of the patient is obtained. For example, unlike a 15-year-old underweight swimmer, a 22-year-old muscular football player is likely to have anterior instability. If the patient is older than 40 years, a rotator cuff tear should be considered, whereas if the patient is older than 60 years, a rotator cuff tear, axillary nerve injury, or brachial plexus palsy should be considered.

After inspection, palpation, and ROM testing, the examination proceeds to strength testing (see Chapter 43). All components of the rotator cuff musculature should be evaluated with great care. Massive subscapularis ruptures may manifest as anterior instability, whereas associated supraspinatus tears are not uncommon in older patients after shoulder dislocations.[54]

Once a generalized appreciation of both shoulders has been obtained, special tests are performed to confirm the diagnosis of anterior shoulder instability. It is important to note that instability is a subjective complaint of the patient and not a physical examination finding. By definition, instability is "symptomatic translation," not merely the presence of larger magnitudes of translation upon physical examination.

A multitude of tests has been described for instability, but within the literature, the most accurate test is the apprehension-relocation test.[55] To perform this test, the patient is placed supine at the edge of the examination table and the affected shoulder is brought into an abducted/externally rotated position. This arm position is considered to be the apprehension position because it maximizes the tension on the IGHL. If the patient has anterior instability with an incompetent IGHL, the restraints to anterior translation are lost and the patient feels a sense of apprehension that the shoulder will dislocate. The patient may alternatively experience pain, but pain is considered to be a less accurate criterion for a positive apprehension sign.[56] The relocation test, or Fowler sign, is a continuation of the apprehension test that entails placing a posterior force on the arm to relieve the symptoms of apprehension (Fig. 40.7). Without warning, the examiner may remove his or her hand, thus reproducing the symptoms of the apprehension test. This maneuver is termed the *surprise test* or *anterior release test*. The sensitivity of these tests is moderate, but they have high associated specificities, and the positive likelihood ratios for these examinations vary between 6 and 20.[56–58]

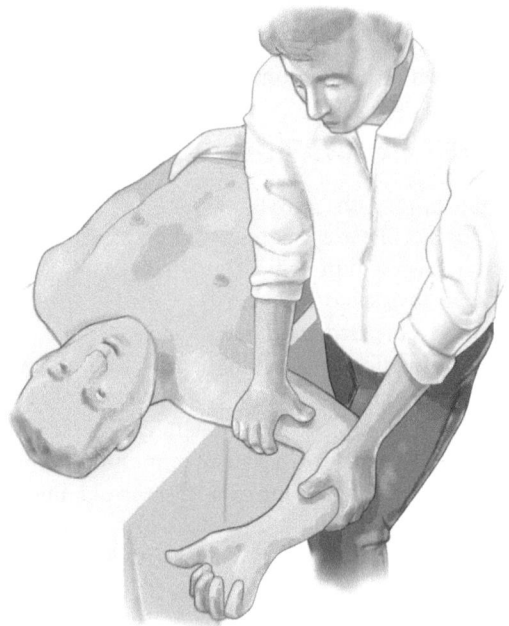

Fig. 40.7 The relocation test, or Fowler sign, is a continuation of the apprehension test, in which the examiner places a posterior force on the arm to relieve the symptoms of apprehension. It is useful to use a small stool on which the left leg is rested to provide stability to the elbow.

After the apprehension tests are used to diagnose anterior shoulder instability,[59] the examination turns to ruling out associated pathology. The most important concomitant pathology is a rotator cuff tear, which should have been detected with muscle strength testing. The belly-press test and lift-off test can be used to diagnose subscapularis insufficiency, the Jobe empty can test evaluates supraspinatus integrity, and massive cuff tears can be identified with the dropping sign and horn blower's sign *(signe de Clarion)*.[60] Other commonly associated lesions include superior labral anterior to posterior (SLAP) tears, posterior or circumferential labral tears, and incompetence of the rotator interval. SLAP tears are notoriously difficult to diagnose with physical examination.[61] Anecdotally, we have found that O'Brien's test works best to diagnose SLAP tears when combined pathology is present, but the significance of concomitant SLAP lesions is unclear. Posterior labral pathology can be detected with the posterior apprehension test and jerk test. Competency of the rotator interval can be evaluated by performing the sulcus test in 30 degrees of external rotation.

Lastly, but very certainly not of least importance, is the evaluation of laxity. Several tests are used to gain comprehensive knowledge of the various ligamentous structures. Anterior shoulder laxity is determined by performing external rotation with the arm at the side (Fig. 40.8A). More than 85 degrees of external rotation is considered to be lax. Inferior hyperlaxity is evaluated with the Gagey hyperabduction test, which is performed with the patient in the seated position and the examiner standing behind the patient. The examiner's arm is forcefully placed on the shoulder to prevent scapular movement (see Fig. 40.8B). The shoulder is passively abducted and the amount of glenohumeral abduction, prior to the initiation of scapulothoracic movement, is noted. More than 105 degrees of abduction is consistent with inferior laxity. The examination is concluded with an assessment of generalized ligamentous laxity, using the Beighton criteria (see Fig. 40.8C).

IMAGING

Imaging is vital in the diagnostic process of anterior shoulder instability. Imaging is obtained for several purposes; the foremost reason is to ensure that the joint is not currently dislocated. Imaging also allows for determination of glenoid or humeral bone loss, identification of the pathoanatomy, and detection of associated pathology. Plain radiographs, CT, and MRI all have a role in diagnosing anterior shoulder instability.

Plain radiographs are obtained initially and should include anteroposterior (AP) shoulder views in internal and external rotation, a true AP Grashey view, and an axillary view. The AP view in internal rotation allows for a generalized assessment of the joint and surrounding structures. Unexpected pathology, such as abnormal calcifications and tumors, can be detected with radiographs. Radiographs also should be carefully inspected for the presence of a Hill-Sachs lesion. The external rotation AP view is also examined for presence of a Hill-Sachs lesion, because only large lesions are typically visualized with this view. The Grashey view is used to assess the glenohumeral joint and the presence of subtle subluxation or joint space narrowing consistent

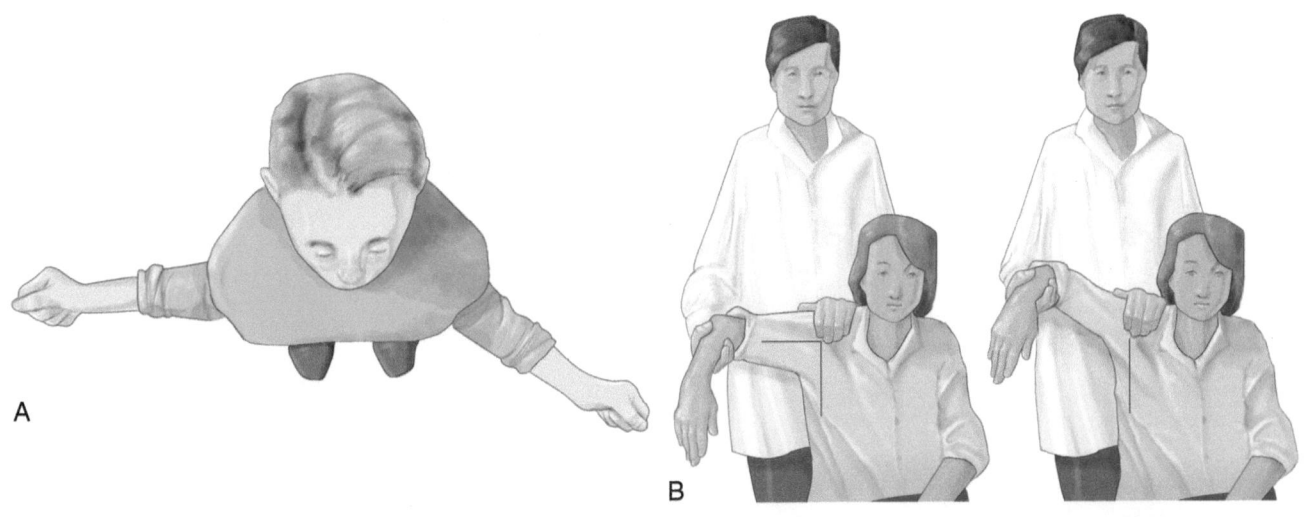

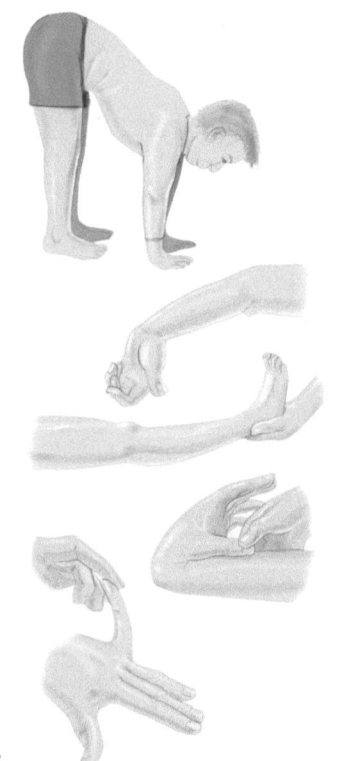

Joint	Finding	Points
Left little (fifth) finger	Passive dorsiflexion beyond 90°	1
	Passive dorsiflexion ≤90°	0
Right little (fifth) finger	Passive dorsiflexion beyond 90°	1
	Passive dorsiflexion ≤90°	0
Left thumb	Passive dorsiflexion to the flexor aspect of the forearm	1
	Cannot passively dorsiflex thumb to flexor aspect of the forearm	0
Right thumb	Passive dorsiflexion to the flexor aspect of the forearm	1
	Cannot passively dorsiflex thumb to flexor aspect of the forearm	0
Left elbow	Hyperextends beyond 10°	1
	Extends ≤10°	0
Right elbow	Hyperextends beyond 10°	1
	Extends ≤10°	0
Left knee	Hyperextends beyond 10°	1
	Extends ≤10°	0
Right knee	Hyperextends beyond 10°	1
	Extends ≤10°	0
Forward flexion of trunk with knees full extended	Palms and hands can rest flat on the floor	1
	Palms and hands cannot rest flat on the floor	0

Fig. 40.8 Evaluation of laxity. (A) Anterior shoulder laxity is determined by performing external rotation with the arm at the side. More than 85 degrees of rotation (for the patient's right arm) is considered lax. (B) The Gagey hyperabduction test. More than 105 degrees of glenohumeral abduction prior to initiation of scapulothoracic movement is considered abnormal. (C) Beighton criteria of generalized ligamentous laxity.

with a cartilage defect or dislocation arthropathy. The axillary view is key in detecting dislocation of the joint and can also be used to visualize a Hill-Sachs lesion. All patients should have an axillary radiograph performed before leaving an emergency department setting to confirm glenohumeral reduction.

Standard views are extremely helpful, but because of the anatomy of the shoulder, overlap of the humeral head and the glenoid on other structures is often significant. As such, a specialized view should be obtained to examine for the presence and severity of glenoid and humeral bone loss. Glenoid bone

loss can be detected using the West Point view or Bernageau view. Hill-Sachs lesions are easily identified with use of the Stryker Notch view or Didiée view. The apical oblique view (Garth view) is useful, as it adequately visualizes both glenoid bone loss and Hill-Sachs lesions with minimal patient positioning (Fig. 40.9).

Advanced imaging is dictated by the history, physical examination, and radiographic findings. CT is commonly used for the determination of bony anatomy, whereas MRI is more often used to detect occult soft tissue pathology. Recent studies show that glenoid bone loss can be accurately measured on MRI alone,

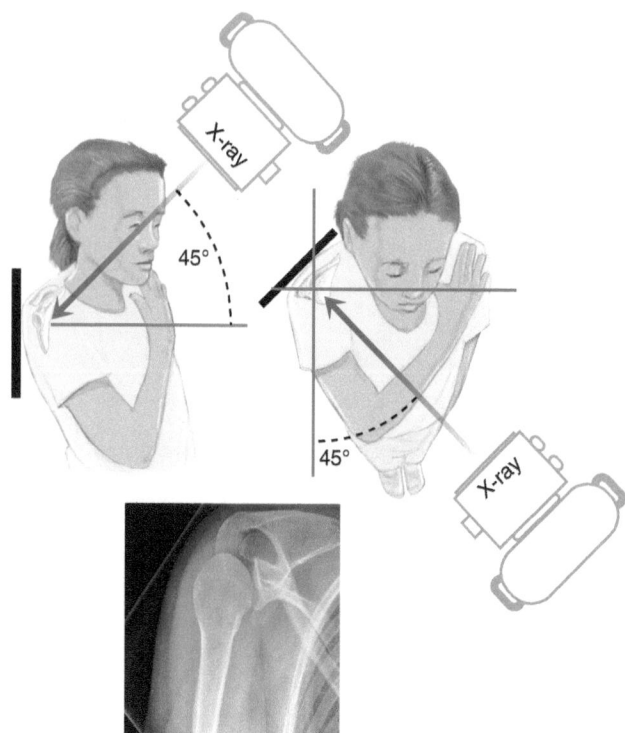

Fig. 40.9 Garth's apical oblique view adequately visualizes both glenoid bone loss and a Hill-Sachs lesion.

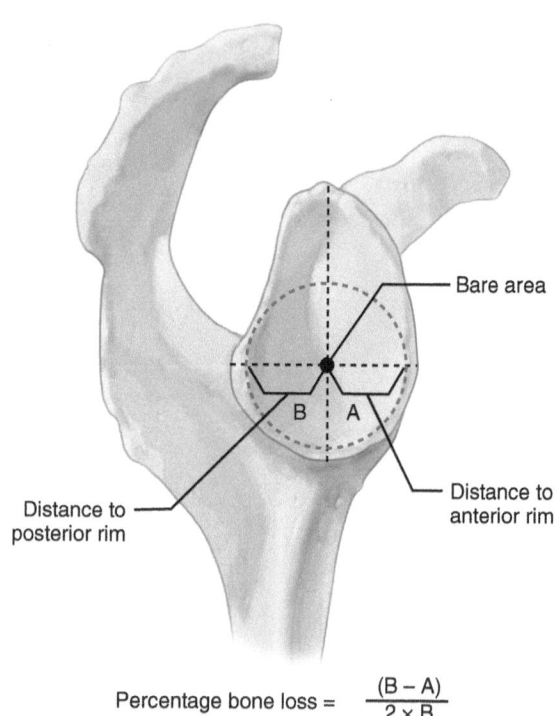

$$\text{Percentage bone loss} = \frac{(B - A)}{2 \times B}$$

Fig. 40.10 Determining glenoid bone loss using the anteroposterior distance from bare area method.

thereby avoiding the need for a CT scan, although the accuracy of the measurement correlates with level of experience and training of the persons reading the study.[62] Either scan can be performed in association with arthrography to increase the overall sensitivity of the examination. Detection of bony pathology is important prior to standard arthroscopic stabilization. Indications for obtaining advanced imaging include multiple dislocations, increasing ease of dislocations and/or reductions, apprehension on physical examination with the arm in less than 75 degrees of abduction, and radiographic evidence of glenoid bone loss.

Quantitative evaluation of glenoid bone loss is best performed using 3D CT.[63] Use of this imaging modality permits the humerus to be subtracted and the glenoid to be viewed en face. Numerous methods have been described to quantify bone loss, and currently no standard has been agreed upon. Perhaps the most straightforward technique is based on the observation that the inferior aspect of the glenoid is a true circle, with the bare spot located in the exact center.[64] As such, the simple mathematical principle that the diameter of the circle is twice the radius can be used to determine the percentage of bone loss.

This quantification method has been termed the *perfect circle technique*[50] in the literature (Fig. 40.10). To quantify bone loss, the 3D CT scan is used with the humerus subtracted. The first goal is to estimate the bare area. To do so, a vertical line from the supraglenoid tubercle at the most superior aspect is drawn. Next, a horizontal line at the widest AP distance is drawn. At the intersection of these two lines is the approximated bare area. The next goal is to draw a best-fit circle, which is centered about the bare area. The distance from the bare area to the posterior

glenoid rim is measured. The distance from the bare area to the remaining anterior glenoid rim is also measured. The percentage of bone loss can be calculated as [(posterior distance) − (anterior distance)]/(2 × posterior distance).[63,65] Significant instability that is not amenable to standard arthroscopic techniques has been described as low as 13.5% of glenoid width loss.[44]

If the diagnosis of shoulder instability is in question or an associated rotator cuff tear is suspected, an MR arthrogram is obtained. MRI is able to accurately detect a variety of soft tissue pathologies, but sensitivity is approximately 70%. Intraarticular injection of gadolinium contrast dye results in distention of the joint, thus enabling better anatomic resolution, as well as permitting T1 imaging with a higher signal-to-noise ratio compared with T2 imaging. This use of contrast dye improves the sensitivity into the mid-90% range.[66] In addition, placing the arm into the abducted and externally rotated position results in increased tension on the IGHL and can accentuate subtle pathology, thus further improving sensitivity.[67] The various soft tissue pathologies are demonstrated in Fig. 40.11. MRI is also accurate in identifying the HAGL lesion (Fig. 40.12), which has traditionally been treated in an open fashion and, as such, is key to identifying preoperatively if arthroscopic repair is typically performed.[68] Recent literature has suggested that CT arthrography is equal, if not superior, to MR arthrography in identifying HAGL lesions.[69]

DECISION-MAKING PRINCIPLES

Fundamentally, the most important decision in patients with anterior shoulder instability is operative versus nonoperative management. If surgical treatment is elected, the type of procedure must be determined. Options include open or arthroscopic

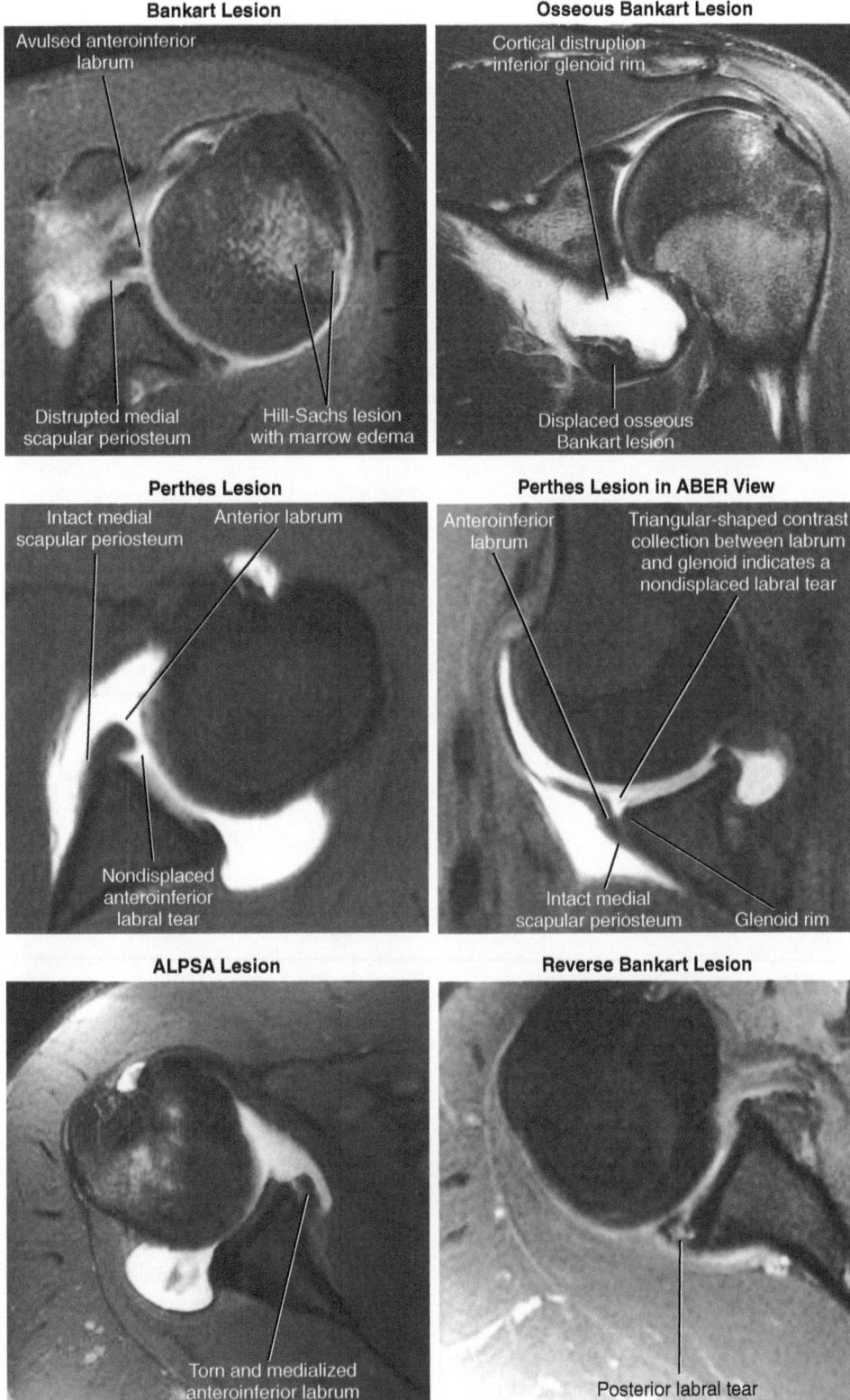

Fig. 40.11 Magnetic resonance imaging appearance of the various soft tissue pathologies associated with shoulder instability. *ABER*, Abduction external rotation; *ALPSA*, anterior labroligamentous periosteal sleeve avulsion. (Modified from Morrison WB, Sanders TG. *Problem Solving in Musculoskeletal Imaging.* St Louis: Elsevier; 2008.)

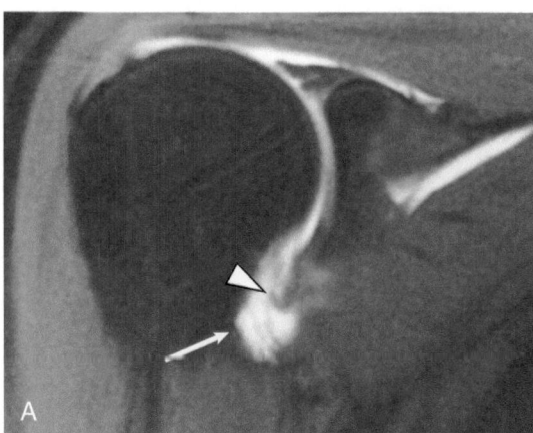
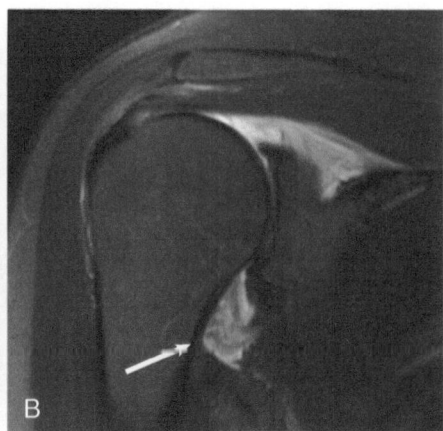

Fig. 40.12 Magnetic resonance imaging appearance of a humeral avulsion of the glenohumeral ligaments lesion. A coronal magnetic resonance T1-weighted (A) arthrogram anterior to a T2-weighted (B) image shows the humeral avulsion of the anterior band of the inferior glenohumeral ligament *(arrowhead)*. The attachment of the axillary recess capsule to the humerus is too distal, the so-called J sign *(arrows)*. (Modified from Pope TL, Bloem HL, Beltran J, et al. *Imaging of the Musculoskeletal System*. Philadelphia: Elsevier; 2008.)

stabilization or the Latarjet (coracoid transfer) procedure. The goals of treatment, regardless of method, are to provide the patient with a stable, durable shoulder that permits the patient to perform his or her desired activities without a loss in quality of life. To achieve these goals, a variety of factors are important to consider when making this decision. These factors include age at initial dislocation, first-time versus recurrent instability, in-season versus off-season with regard to sports activity, sporting activity level, and associated injuries.

Age at Initial Dislocation

Age at the time of the initial dislocation is the single most important factor for predicting recurrent instability. McLaughlin and Cavallaro[70] first discovered that the incidence of recurrence is approximately 90% in patients younger than 20 years and that the incidence of recurrence decreases to only 10% in persons older than 40 years. In a study spanning 20 years of admissions to the Massachusetts General Hospital, Rowe[71] observed an 83% recurrence rate in persons younger than 20 years. The largest prospective study with a 25-year follow-up was published in 2008 by Hovelius and colleagues.[72] They also found that age was the most important predictive factor, with a 72% recurrence rate in patients younger than 20 years. Recurrence decreased with age, with a 56% rate of recurrence in persons aged 23 to 29 years and a 27% rate in persons between 30 and 40 years of age.

Investigators have also examined recurrence rates in groups of patients on either end of the age spectrum. Marans and colleagues[73] found a 100% recurrence rate in children with open physes at the time of initial dislocation with a mean time to redislocation of 8 months. A systematic review by Olds et al.[74] observed an overall 73% rate of recurrent instability in children 18 years and under. Pooled data from this study reported a 94% recurrent in children with a closed proximal humerus physis, compared with 61% recurrence with an open physis, suggesting a child with a closed physis is 14 times more likely to experience recurrent instability. In addition, males were found to be 3.4 times more likely for recurrent episodes than females. The rate

of recurrence does not decrease to a negligible level in elderly patients, however. Gumina and Postacchini[75] found a recurrence rate of 22% in patients older than 60 years.

Many other studies have been published that have indirectly found associations between age and recurrent instability.[74,76–80] The results of these studies can be broadly summarized as observing a high rate in young patients and a lower rate in older patients. Recurrence occurs in 70% to 95% of persons younger than 20 years, 60% to 80% in persons aged 20 to 30 years, and 15% to 20% in persons older than 40 years at the time of the initial dislocation.

Age may also play a role in recurrent instability after arthroscopic stabilization procedures.[81–84] Voos and colleagues[81] reported an 18% rate of recurrent instability following arthroscopic stabilization. Patients under the age of 25 with ligamentous laxity and large Hill-Sachs lesions were at greatest risk for recurrent instability. Cho et al.[83] performed open stabilization after recurrent instability following arthroscopic treatment in 26 patients with a mean age of 24 years. Identifying age as a predictor of recurrence instability helps council patients and facilitates discussion about risk for revision procedures, including open stabilization.[81]

First-Time Versus Recurrent Instability

The decision to proceed with surgical stabilization after a first-time shoulder dislocation is controversial.[85,86] Four randomized controlled trials[87–90] and two meta-analyses[91,92] have been published to guide this decision. Three of the four randomized trials compare arthroscopic Bankart repair with conservative care, whereas the fourth compared open Bankart repair with use of a sling.

The meta-analyses of these studies demonstrate that Bankart repair results in a significant reduction in the risk of recurrent instability over a 2- to 10-year period compared with the use of a sling or arthroscopic lavage. Furthermore, with the use of the Western Ontario Shoulder Instability Index[93] as a disease-specific quality of life measurement tool, Bankart repair is associated with improved quality of life over a 2- to 5-year period. However, global patient satisfaction was no different between conservative treatment and operative groups.

These trials and meta-analyses have significant limitations that render the conclusions somewhat speculative. Two of the four studies use operative techniques that are no longer performed. Activity levels were poorly defined, different rehabilitation protocols were used, and the length of follow-up was highly variable.

The present literature supports use of the Bankart repair in young persons with a first-time dislocation as a method of reducing recurrent dislocation and improving quality of life. Two recent Markov decision models have further supported this claim.[94,95] A retrospective analysis comparing the results of repair after initial dislocation with repair after recurrent instability also supports surgical intervention for first-time dislocators.[96] Further primary research is required to better substantiate these claims.

In-Season Management

Anterior shoulder instability frequently occurs in athletes, with most traumatic events occurring during competition.[97] Approximately half of instability events lead to more than 10 days lost to sport,[97,98] despite the typical pressure on the athlete to return as quickly as possible. As such, the management of anterior shoulder instability during the sporting season is difficult. Ultimately, the goals of treatment remain the same, but in the competitive athlete, additional goals include minimizing time away from sport, preventing additional injury and ensuring the safe return to full activity.[99]

In a study of 30 athletes who sustained an in-season dislocation across a variety of sports, 90% were able to return to their sport in the same season using a supervised physical therapy program and no period of immobilization.[98] Seventy-five percent of patients returned to sport wearing either a Duke Wyre or Sully brace, and 37% had recurrent in-season instability episodes. Ultimately, 53% of all patients underwent surgical stabilization.

A multicenter trial at the military academies followed 45 contact intercollegiate athletes for two seasons who had sustained an in-season dislocation or subluxation.[100,101] Following a standardized rehabilitation protocol, 73% of individuals were able to return to play (RTP) that same season with a mean time to return of 5 days.[100] However, only 27% completed the season without further instability episodes. In a subsequent study following this same cohort into the following season, 74% of patients had elected arthroscopic Bankart repair while 26% continued with rehabilitation.[101] The operative group had a 90% successful completion of the subsequent season, while the rehabilitation group had only a 40% success rate.

These results suggest that that a highly competitive athlete who sustains an in-season shoulder instability event has the potential to be treated nonoperatively, but that surgical intervention should also be strongly considered. The algorithm developed by Owens and colleagues[99] is particularly helpful in identifying patients who are appropriate for a trial of nonoperative management and early return to sport. After a complete physical examination and radiographic evaluation, players with an initial instability episode who do not have significant osseous defects of the glenoid or humeral head and are at the beginning of the season with time to appropriately rehabilitate are most suitable for physical therapy and sport-specific training. Criteria for RTP include full ROM and normal strength. A brace should be used RTP when possible.

Athletes in Contact Sports

Athletes who compete in contact sports are particularly prone to anterior shoulder instability. Achieving return to sport is much more difficult for them, as evidenced by a study of professional rugby players whose mean absence from competition after a shoulder dislocation was 81 days.[102] In this cohort of athletes, the decision to proceed with surgical stabilization is typically not difficult. However, deciding between an open or arthroscopic technique can be problematic.

Athletes in contact sports have typically been treated with an open Bankart stabilization, based on its historical gold standard status[103] and early reports of increased failure rates after arthroscopic stabilization.[104,105] Pagnani and Dome[106] reported no postoperative dislocations and 3% postoperative subluxation in American football players after open Bankart stabilization, whereas Uhorchak and colleagues[107] reported a 3% recurrent dislocation rate and a 19% subluxation rate in contact athletes after open Bankart stabilization and anterior capsulorrhaphy. Despite the low rates of recurrence after open Bankart stabilization, more sophisticated arthroscopic techniques have recently been developed, and arthroscopic stabilization is being increasingly recommended to avoid the morbidity associated with open Bankart stabilization.[99,108] Recent reports of long-term outcome at 13-year follow-up after arthroscopic stabilization are comparable to reported results after open Bankart repair.[109] In addition, in National Collegiate Athletic Association (NCAA) Division I football, the RTP following arthroscopic Bankart repair has been demonstrated to be as high as 90%.[110] Open stabilization using the Latarjet technique has also been reported in rugby players. Neyton and colleagues[111] reported no postoperative dislocations or subluxations with a mean 12-year follow-up. Considering these results, in our clinical practice, we recommend the Latarjet procedure or arthroscopic Bankart repair for athletes participating in contact sports.

Associated Injuries

A variety of associated injuries may occur after an anterior shoulder dislocation, including rotator cuff tear, greater tuberosity fracture, brachial plexus palsy, axillary nerve palsy, and axillary artery injury. Associated injuries occur predominately in the older population, with 40% sustaining some form of injury after dislocation.[112] Dislocation with associated greater tuberosity fracture is most common and occurs in approximately 15% of older patients. Rotator cuff tears, which are the second most common associated injury, occur in 10% of older patients. Neurologic deficit, primarily involving the axillary nerve, occurs in 5% of older patients.

Identifying these associated injuries is critically important because they can significantly influence management. Patients with an associated greater tuberosity fracture are generally viewed as having a better prognosis than patients who have an associated rotator cuff tear. Associated greater tuberosity fracture decreased the odds of recurrent instability by 3.8 times after nonsurgical management of shoulder dislocation.[113] Hovelius and colleagues[114] found a 32% rate of redislocation in patients with isolated anterior dislocation but no redislocations in patients with an associated greater tuberosity fracture. Few studies have been performed to guide parameters for operative fixation of associated greater tuberosity fractures, but given the biomechanical disadvantage of small amounts of displacement of the greater tuberosity, the current consensus in the literature is fixation of fractures with more than 5 mm of displacement.[115,116]

Rotator cuff function must be carefully evaluated in the older patient. It is not uncommon for rotator cuff dysfunction to be confused with axillary nerve palsy,[117] and any patient with suspected axillary nerve palsy after anterior dislocation should undergo ultrasonographic or MRI evaluation to rule out a rotator cuff tear. Furthermore, given the prevalence of rotator cuff tears in the older population, any history of preexisting shoulder dysfunction should be obtained. As with greater tuberosity fractures, few studies are available in the literature to support management.[118] Older patients who sustain an anterior shoulder dislocation should be carefully monitored. Patients who experience significant dysfunction or pain should be considered for operative management.

When diagnostic imaging shows that patients with suspected axillary nerve palsies do not have rotator cuff tears, electrodiagnostic studies may be obtained. The prognosis for recovery is excellent, with one study demonstrating a 100% recovery rate.[75]

Synthesis

Should surgery be elected, the aforementioned considerations must be synthesized into a comprehensive view of the patient. Balg and Boileau[119] have developed the Instability Severity Index Score (ISIS) as a way to determine which patients would ultimately benefit most from arthroscopic Bankart repair or the Latarjet procedure. In a prospective case-control study, these investigators identified six risk factors that, when combined as a scoring system, resulted in unacceptably high rates of failure after arthroscopic stabilization (Table 40.2). Patients with more than 6 points had a recurrence risk of 70%, whereas patients with a score of 6 or less had a recurrence risk of 10%. Accordingly, patients with an ISIS greater than 6 should undergo an open Latarjet procedure, whereas patients with 6 points or fewer are acceptable candidates for arthroscopic Bankart repair.[120] A similar case-control study had a similar failure risk of 70% if ISIS was 4 or greater compared with 4% if ISIS was less than 4.[121] Currently, competitive athletes younger than 20 years who are involved in a contact or forced overhead sport should be counseled regarding the risks, benefits, and alternatives regarding Latarjet and arthroscopic Bankart reconstruction.

TREATMENT OPTIONS

Treatment options may be categorized into acute reduction on the field, reduction in the emergency department, nonoperative sling immobilization and rehabilitation, and surgery.

TABLE 40.2   Instability Severity Index Score

Prognostic Factor	Points/Type of Procedure
Age at Surgery (year)	
≤20	2
>20	0
Preoperative Sport Participation	
Competitive	2
Recreational or none	0
Preoperative Sporting Activity	
Contact or forced overhead	1
Other	0
Shoulder Hyperlaxity	
Anterior or inferior	1
Normal laxity	0
Hill-Sachs on Anteroposterior Radiograph	
Visible in external rotation	2
Not visible in external rotation	0
Glenoid Loss of Contour on Anteroposterior Radiograph	
Loss of contour	2
No lesion	0
Total Score	
≤4	Arthroscopic Bankart procedure
4–6	Current research suggests open procedure, but not definitive
>6	Open Latarjet procedure

From Balg F, Boileau P. The instability severity index score. A simple pre-operative score to select patients for arthroscopic or open shoulder stabilisation. *J Bone Joint Sur Br.* 2007;89:1470–1477.

On-Field Management

Despite the frequency with which traumatic shoulder dislocation occurs during sporting activity, surprisingly little literature exists to guide initial treatment. Fundamentally, on-field management can be dichotomized into an attempted reduction or direct transfer to an emergency department.

Based on experience, a brief window of time exists during which significant pain is associated with the dislocation but muscular spasm has not yet occurred. In this scenario and assuming a compliant and willing patient, on-field reduction is attempted. A focused neurovascular examination is performed prior to the reduction attempt. A single reduction attempt is performed. Reduction is accomplished via longitudinal traction with gentle forward elevation. If an immediate on-field reduction could not be performed with ease, the athlete can be escorted to the training room and placed in a prone position, with the shoulder hanging at approximately 90 degrees of forward flexion. A weight can be held by the athlete, if available. Gentle traction with slight external rotation of the arm and scapular manipulation is often a successful reduction technique without use of sedatives or analgesics.[122] If reduction is achieved, pain relief can be dramatic and the patient can be referred to the team physician for subacute radiographs to rule out bony injury. If reduction cannot be achieved, the patient should be transported to the emergency department.

Management in the Emergency Department

Patients who present to the emergency department with suspected anterior shoulder dislocation must undergo a comprehensive evaluation, including a history, complete physical examination, and radiographs, prior to any reduction attempt. Radiographs must include orthogonal views and should include an AP and axillary view. A scapular Y view is insufficient to diagnose a located shoulder. If the patient is unable to tolerate an axillary view, a modified axillary view, termed a *Velpeau view*, should be obtained.[123] This view does not require abduction of the injured shoulder and can be obtained in any patient without a spine injury. After radiographic documentation of an anterior shoulder dislocation is performed, the clinician must decide on the analgesia/sedation to be administered and the reduction technique.

Options for analgesia/sedation include no analgesia or sedation,[124] intraarticular injection of 20 mL of 1% lidocaine, or intravenous analgesics with or without sedatives. A Cochrane review suggests no difference between intraarticular injection of lidocaine and intravenous sedation with regard to the success rate of reduction, pain during reduction, or postprocedural pain.[125] The use of intraarticular lidocaine may require fewer resources, be more cost effective, and result in a faster discharge from the emergency department.[126]

A multitude of reduction maneuvers have been described for anterior shoulder dislocation. Despite reports, no one technique is 100% effective, and as such, it is important for the clinician to be familiar with several different maneuvers to ensure rapid reduction.[127] Recently, several nonrandomized and randomized trials from multiple institutions have demonstrated improved rates of success and time to achieve reduction with the use of the Milch technique.[128,129] Importantly, the Milch technique does not require any form of sedation or intraarticular injection, and as such, it is our preferred initial technique for shoulder reduction.[130] This technique is performed by slowly abducting and externally rotating the shoulder over a period of 5 to 15 minutes. Once the arm has reached 90 degrees of abduction and 90 degrees of external rotation, the joint has usually spontaneously reduced. If it has not spontaneously reduced, a modification of the maneuver can be performed that involves pulling gentle longitudinal traction in line with the humerus using one hand and manipulating the humeral head laterally and superiorly with the other to effect reduction.[124]

Nonoperative Sling Immobilization and Rehabilitation

Traditionally, after reduction, the shoulder is immobilized for a period and a course of physiotherapy may be prescribed. However, this basic principle of nonoperative management has recently come into question because of a wide range of recommendations on the duration of immobilization but seemingly similar rates of recurrence. To date, five level I studies and one level II study have been performed to investigate the duration of immobilization and the rate of recurrent instability.[131] A cohort of Swedish patients

in a study by Hovelius and colleagues has been followed up for 25 years and constitutes four of the five level I studies.[72,114,132,133] When comparing patients who were immobilized for 1 week or less with those who were immobilized for 3 to 4 weeks, no statistically significant effect could be detected on the rate of recurrent dislocation or the need for surgery at any of the four analyzed time points. Similar conclusions have been drawn in the remaining studies.[77,134]

The position of immobilization has also been challenged, based on findings of MRI[135] and cadaveric[136] studies that demonstrate a decreased degree of displacement and increased contact force between the Bankart lesion and glenoid with the arm in external rotation. Itoi and colleagues[137] were the first to report results of a randomized controlled trial comparing immobilization in internal rotation to external rotation; they found reduced rates of recurrent instability in patients immobilized 3 weeks in external rotation. However, this study had many limitations, and a larger trial was later conducted. Again, Itoi and colleagues[138] were able to demonstrate a reduced rate of recurrent instability using an intention-to-treat analysis. Compliance with treatment in external rotation was notably and significantly worse. An independent but smaller study also investigated the same question with patients who were 100% compliant with treatment.[139] Recurrence rates were not significantly different at a mean follow-up of 30 months. Abduction of the shoulder with 30 degrees external rotation during immobilization improves reduction of a Bankart lesion on MRI evaluation, which may help reduce recurrence rate after initial dislocation.[140] Meta-analysis of these data has failed to demonstrate a significant difference between immobilization in internal and external rotation.[141] Currently, at our clinic, we opt for simple immobilization in a sling for approximately 1 week or until the patient is comfortable using the shoulder again.

Surgical Management

Should surgical intervention be elected, a variety of options exist; indeed, more than 300 different techniques have been described. Although the vast majority of these techniques are now historic in nature, many are still in use. Options include open, arthroscopic, and adjunctive techniques, salvage operations, and techniques used in a revision setting (Box 40.1).

Open anatomic repair of the detached capsulolabral complex to the anterior glenoid rim, known as the Bankart procedure,[19] is considered the historic gold standard. However, the procedure is technically demanding and violates the subscapularis, and rehabilitation proceeds slowly. Arthroscopic techniques of the Bankart procedure have been refined over the years, and with the introduction of suture anchors to fixate the repair to the glenoid, the arthroscopic technique is becoming recognized as equivalent to open surgical repair.[142–144]

A number of treatment options are available to address Hill-Sachs, including benign neglect, arthroscopic remplissage, retrograde disimpaction, and placement of an osteochondral allograft.[145,146] Wolf and colleagues discuss remplissage as the arthroscopic treatment to engaging defects.[147] Increased stability is achieved by performing a posterior capsulodesis and infraspinatus tenodesis into the bony defect to increase. Aside from

BOX 40.1   Surgical Options for Anterior Shoulder Instability

Open
Bankart Repair[19]
- A Bankart repair is performed to reattach the labrum to the anterior articular margin of the glenoid.
- This repair is often combined with a capsular shift (Neer capsulorrhaphy) to restore tension to the capsulolabral complex.[164]

Coracoid Transfer
- A coracoid transfer procedure is performed to transfer a portion of the coracoid, along with the conjoint tendon, to the anterior glenoid neck. They are secured to the glenoid with one or two screws.

Bristow[165]
- The Bristow procedure is performed to transfer the most distal 1 cm of coracoid.
- The CA ligament is preserved.
- The coracoid is secured to the glenoid with one screw.

Latarjet[149] (with Patte modification)[150]
- The Latarjet procedure is performed to transfer the distal 2–3 cm of coracoid.
- The CA ligament is divided with a 1-cm stump.
- The inferior portion of coracoid is secured to the glenoid with two screws.
- The CA ligament is attached to the anterior glenohumeral capsule.

Latarjet (with congruent-arc modification)[36]
- The Latarjet procedure is performed to transfer the distal 2–3 cm of coracoid.
- The medial portion of the coracoid is secured to the glenoid with two screws.
- The CA ligament is not reattached.

Anterior Capsulolabral Reconstruction[166]
- Anterior capsulolabral reconstruction was designed by Jobe to address instability in athletes who frequently use overhead maneuvers.
- Anterior capsulolabral reconstruction is a glenoid-based capsular shift.
- Anterior capsulolabral reconstruction may be performed as an adjunct to Bankart repair.[167]

Arthroscopic
Bankart Repair
- A Bankart repair is performed to reattach the labrum to the anterior articular margin of the glenoid with the use of suture anchors.[168]
- Arthroscopic use of tacks or transglenoid sutures (known as the Caspari technique) is no longer considered modern practice because of high failure rates.[169]

Coracoid Transfer
- When a coracoid transfer is performed, highly specialized instruments are used to transfer the distal 2–3 cm of coracoid.[170]
- The CA ligament is not reattached.
- The coracoid transfer procedure can be combined with a Bankart repair.[171]

Anterior Capsular Plication[172]
- Anterior capsular plication is the arthroscopic version of an anterior capsulolabral reconstruction.

Supplementary Procedures
Remplissage[173]
- Remplissage means "to fill" in French.
- Remplissage is performed in patients with a large Hill-Sachs lesion.
- The infraspinatus and posterior capsule are fixated into the Hill-Sachs lesion arthroscopically using suture anchors.

Humeral Head Allograft[174]
- A humeral head allograft is performed in patients with a large Hill-Sachs lesion.
- An osteoarticular allograft is inserted into the lesion to prevent engagement.
- A humeral head allograft is typically performed with an open technique, but arthroscopic techniques have been developed.

Partial Humeral Head Resurfacing[175]
- Partial humeral head resurfacing is performed in patients with a large Hill-Sachs lesion.
- Partial humeral head resurfacing is an alternative to a humeral head allograft.
- A cobalt-chrome articular component is inserted into the Hill-Sachs lesion.
- Reported techniques are performed in conjunction with a Latarjet procedure.

Rotator Interval Closure[176]
- Rotator interval closure provides superior capsular shift of the MGHL to the SGHL.
- Rotator interval closure can be performed open or arthroscopically to limit external rotation.

Revision or Salvage Procedures
Iliac Crest Bone Grafting of the Glenoid[41]
- Iliac crest bone grafting of the glenoid is performed in patients with severe anterior glenoid bone loss.
- An autogenous iliac crest bone graft is contoured to match the concavity of the glenoid and secured with cannulated screws.

Humeral Hemiarthroplasty[177]
- Humeral hemiarthroplasty traditionally has been indicated for older patients with more than 45% of humeral head bone loss and preexisting degenerative arthritis.
- The humeral component must be retroverted up to 50 degrees to achieve stability.

Rotational Humeral Osteotomy[178]
- A rotational humeral osteotomy is performed in patients with severe Hill-Sachs lesions.
- A subcapital external rotational osteotomy of the humerus is performed to rotate the Hill-Sachs lesion outside of the glenoid track.

Allograft Anterior Capsulolabral Reconstruction[179]
- Allograft anterior capsulolabral reconstruction is performed in patients with severe capsular deficiency as a result of systemic soft tissue disorders, electrothermal capsular necrosis, or repeated surgical procedures without bone loss.
- Allograft anterior capsulolabral reconstruction is performed via an open technique; allograft tendon is used to reconstruct the anterior band of the IGHL and MGHL, with bioabsorbable screws used in the humerus and suture fixation performed in the glenoid.

CA, Coracoacromial; *IGHL*, inferior glenohumeral ligament; *MGHL*, middle glenohumeral ligament; *SGHL*, superior glenohumeral ligament.

recurrent traumatic dislocation in 4% of the included patients, there were no other complications at the 2- to 10-year follow-up. Many studies support remplissage and an arthroscopic solution to engaging defects.[146,148]

Coracoid bone block transfers represent an alternative to the anatomic reconstruction of the Bankart procedure. The most commonly used coracoid bone block transfer is the Latarjet.[149] Originally described in 1954, it has subsequently been modified by Patte[150] into the procedure performed today. Although transferring a block of bone is advantageous in cases of bony glenoid deficiency, Patte recognized that the so-called bone block effect only partially contributes to the efficacy of the Latarjet procedure to prevent recurrent instability. He described the mechanism as a triple effect: (1) a sling effect of the conjoint tendon that supplements the anteroinferior capsule and inferior aspect of the subscapularis tendon, particularly in abduction and external rotation; (2) a bony effect that increases the overall dimension of the glenoid; and (3) a ligamentous effect of the repaired anterior capsule to the stump of the coracoacromial ligament.[151]

Two viewpoints exist regarding the utility of the Latarjet procedure.[152] In the English-speaking world, it is primarily used as a revision procedure or a procedure that is used when significant bony glenoid loss is detected preoperatively.[36] In the French-speaking world, however, the Latarjet procedure is used as a primary procedure, even in the absence of glenoid bony loss.[153]

Allograft glenoid augmentation is another consideration for stabilization in patients with large glenoid defects or in revision cases (see Chapter 43).

🔖 Authors' Preferred Technique

Arthroscopic Bankart Repair (Fig. 40.13)

Patient Positioning and Setup

- The patient is anesthetized and an examination is performed.
- The patient is placed in the lateral decubitus position.
- A commercially available shoulder distraction device with lateral overhead distraction is used. The arm holder is angled at 45 degrees of abduction and 15 degrees of forward elevation, and 5 to 7 lb of longitudinal traction and 5 lb of lateral traction are used.
- The bed is rotated approximately 50 degrees to allow better access to the anterior shoulder.
- Osseous landmarks are drawn on the shoulder.

Portal Placement and Diagnostic Arthroscopy

- A standard posterior viewing portal is established. The portal is created blindly using the "Romeo three-finger-shuck"[154] to identify the soft spot that corresponds to the interval between the infraspinatus and teres minor. The joint line can then be palpated using a shucking maneuver. It is critical to be in line with the joint.
- The arthroscope is introduced into the joint and the rotator interval is immediately identified. With assistance from the transillumination of the arthroscope, an 18-gauge spinal needle is inserted and its obturator is removed. The needle is used both for outflow and as a probe.
- Diagnostic arthroscopy is undertaken, first evaluating the biceps anchor. The biceps is followed up into its grove and, using the needle, is pulled into the joint to examine for pathology. The arthroscope is then directed toward the insertion site of the supraspinatus, followed by the infraspinatus and posterolateral humeral head. A Hill-Sachs lesion may be identified at this point. Next, the inferior axillary recess is examined for the presence of a HAGL lesion or any loose bodies. The 5-o'clock position of the glenoid can often be examined at this juncture, and the glenolabral junction is followed posteriorly and superiorly. The articular cartilage of the glenoid and humeral head are next inspected. Finally, the arthroscope is advanced into the anterior aspect of the joint where the anterior labrum is identified, often detached or scarred as observed in an ALPSA lesion. Inspection of the subscapularis tendon completes the diagnostic evaluation.
- Once the Bankart lesion is identified, two portals are established with use of an outside-in technique. A 5.5-mm threaded cannula is placed at the most superior aspect of the rotator interval. It is also slightly medialized. An 8.5-mm threaded cannula is placed immediately off the rolled edge of the superior border of the subscapularis tendon. This cannula is slightly lateralized to permit the proper angle for anchor insertion.

Glenolabral Preparation

- With use of a knife-rasp instrument inserted from the high interval portal, the labrum is freed from the glenoid neck. This maneuver can make up a significant portion of the procedure and is vital to a successful operation. Alternatively, if a significantly scarred ALPSA lesion is encountered, a hook cautery probe can be used, but only with extreme caution.
- It can be difficult to ascertain when the labrum is sufficiently mobilized. A useful test is to insert the shaver into the joint, open the window, and turn the suction on. If the labrum floats up to an anatomic position, mobilization is complete.
- Next, the shaver is placed against the glenoid neck and used to roughen the bone and create a bleeding surface.

Anchor Insertion

- The tear configuration is carefully evaluated, and a plan is established for suture anchor placement. Typically a three- or four-anchor configuration is used.
- Using the insertion technique specific to the anchor being used, a single-loaded suture anchor is placed through the low-interval cannula at approximately the 5-o'clock position. It should be placed at a 45-degree angle to the glenoid face and just up on the glenoid face.
- The anterior suture limb (i.e., the limb closest to the labrum) is identified, and using a claw grasper inserted from the high-interval portal, the suture is grasped to shuttle it out through the portal.

Labral Repair

- A suture-relay technique with creation of a simple suture is used to achieve labral repair.
- An arthroscopic suture passer, such as the Spectrum suture hook (ConMed Linvatec, Largo, FL), is loaded with a 90-cm-long No. 0 polydioxanone (PDS) suture and inserted into the low-interval cannula.
- The claw grasper is inserted into the high-interval portal.
- The claw grasper is used to grasp the labrum and advance it superiorly. The Spectrum then penetrates the capsulolabral tissue 5- to 10-mm inferior to the level of the suture anchor and 1 cm lateral to the labral edge. The PDS suture is then advanced into the joint. The claw grasper is released and then used to retrieve the PDS suture out through the high-interval portal.
- Once the PDS suture is out of the cannula, an incomplete simple knot is tied. Through the open loop, the docked anterior suture limb is passed, and then the simple knot is completed. The Spectrum suture passer is rotated to

Continued

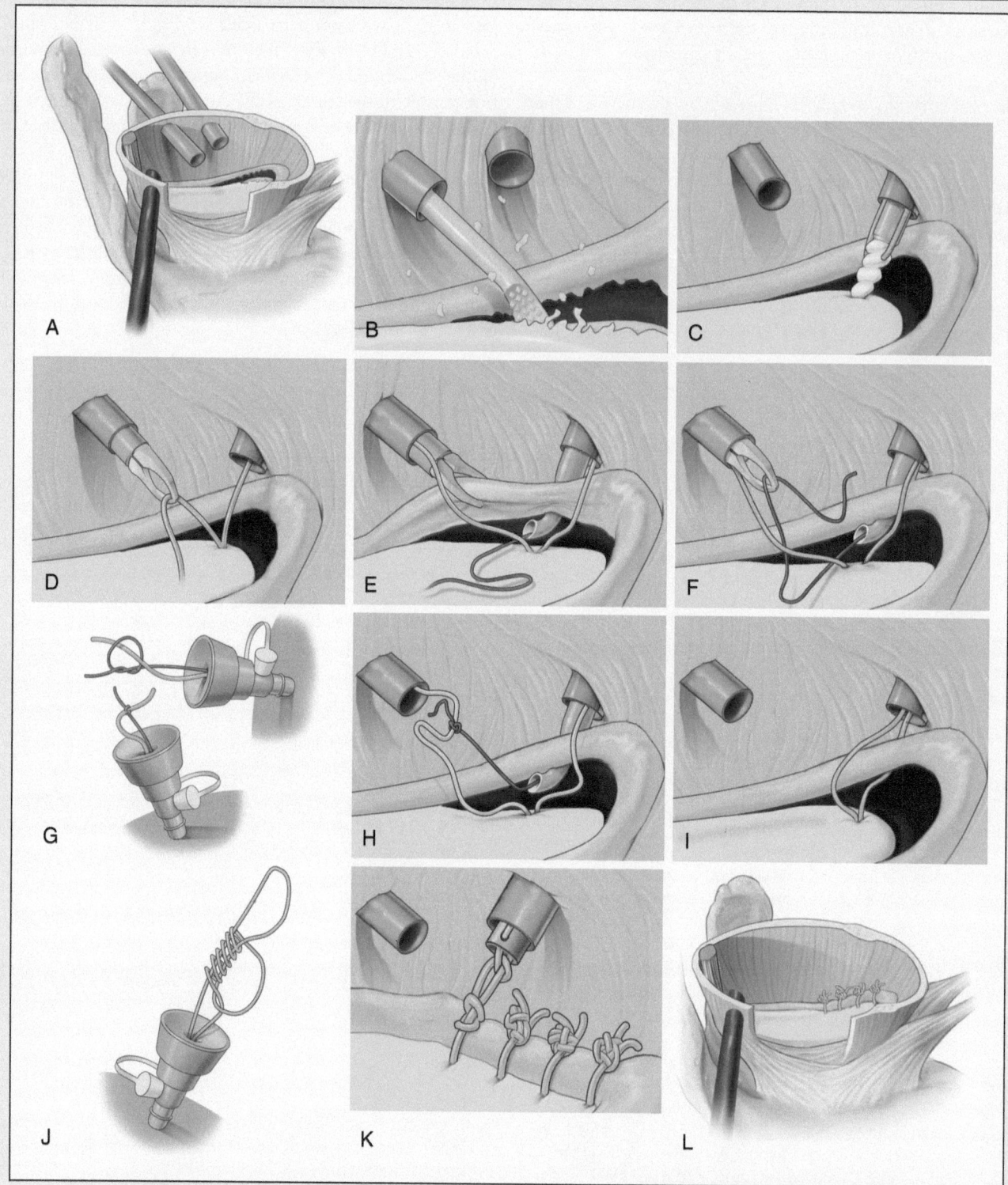

Fig. 40.13 Arthroscopic Bankart repair. (A) The patient is placed in the lateral decubitus position. "High" and "low" portals are established in the rotator interval. (B) A knife-rasp is used to free the labrum from the glenoid neck. (C) A suture anchor is inserted at a 45-degree angle to the glenoid face. (D) The anterior suture limb is identified and, using a claw grasper, is docked in the high portal. (E) An arthroscopic suture passer is used to penetrate the capsulolabral tissue while the claw grasper advances the labrum superiorly. A polydioxanone (PDS) suture is passed into the joint. (F) The PDS suture is retrieved out the high portal. (G) An incomplete knot is tied and the anterior suture limb is placed through to perform a suture relay. (H) The suture passer is withdrawn to accomplish the suture relay. (I) The suture relay is complete, and the passed suture is now the postsuture. (J) A sliding Duncan loop is tied and passed with the use of a knot pusher. (K) Sequential anchors are placed to create a three- to four-anchor configuration construct. (L) The repair is now complete.

Authors' Preferred Technique

Arthroscopic Bankart Repair (Fig. 40.13)—cont'd

disengage from the labral tissue, and the Spectrum suture passer is pulled out of the low-interval cannula, along with the PDS suture. The remaining PDS is pulled out through the low-interval cannula, thus completing the suture relay.

Knot Tying
- The passed suture is now the postsuture to ensure the knot is tied away from the articular surface. We prefer to use a sliding Duncan loop arthroscopic knot, but any arthroscopic knot can be used.
- The Duncan loop is tied, dressed, and passed with the use of a knot pusher. An assistant can use the claw grasper through the high-interval portal to aid in accurate placement of the knot. Four additional alternating post half-hitches are then tied to secure the knot. The sutures are then cut with an arthroscopic suture cutter.

Complete the Repair
- Following the plan established prior to the first anchor insertion, sequential anchors are placed in identical fashion.
- The capsulolabral tissue should be continually advanced superiorly to retension the capsulolabral complex.

Closure
- The completed repair is carefully evaluated with use of a hook probe.
- Additional procedures such as remplissage or rotator interval closure may be performed, if desired.
- The cannulae are removed from the shoulder.
- Portals are closed with interrupted 3-0 absorbable monofilament suture.
- Twenty milliliters of bupivacaine with epinephrine is injected around the portals.
- The arm is placed into a sling with a bolster.

ALPSA, Anterior labroligamentous periosteal sleeve avulsion; HAGL, humeral avulsion of the glenohumeral ligaments.

Authors' Preferred Technique

Latarjet-Patte Coracoid Transfer (Fig. 40.14)

Patient Positioning and Setup
- A towel is placed behind the scapula to make the coracoid process more prominent.
- The patient is placed into a 30-degree modified beach chair position.
- The patient is anesthetized, and an examination is performed.
- The arm is draped free and placed into a pneumatic arm positioner.

Initial Exposure
- Landmarks for surgery include the coracoid process and axillary fold.
- A 5-cm incision is made from the coracoid, directed inferiorly toward the axillary fold.
- A deltopectoral approach is used.
- The plane between the deltoid and pectoralis major is identified by the cephalic vein. The cephalic vein is typically retracted laterally with the deltoid using a Taylor retractor and dissection is continued medially. A Richardson retractor is used medially.
- Typically a crossing vein from the cephalic vein can be identified at the superior pole of the incision. This vein should be suture ligated to prevent a postoperative hematoma.
- The conjoint tendon is identified, and a Hohmann retractor is inserted immediately above the coracoid to provide superior retraction.
- The arm is placed into 45-degree of external rotation and 30 degrees of abduction to aid in the visualization of the coracoacromial ligament (CI).

Coracoid Mobilization
- The lateral aspect of the conjoint tendon is sharply dissected.
- The CI is divided 1 cm lateral to its insertion into the coracoid. This ligament is tagged for later repair.
- The arm is then brought into a neutral position.
- The insertion of the pectoralis minor into the coracoid is identified and sharply removed.

Coracoid Osteotomy
- A forked retractor or Darrach retractor is used to retract the pectoralis minor and expose the base of the coracoid.

- A 90-degree angled microsagittal saw is used to osteotomize the base of the coracoid, which is identified as the elbow, approximately 2 cm posterior to the coracoid tip, in a medial to lateral fashion.
- The coracohumeral ligament is released at the lateral base of the coracoid.
- The coracoid should now be completely mobile, and it is brought out of the wound inferiorly. It is placed onto a Darrach retractor overlying the skin.

Coracoid Preparation
- The CI stump is identified and protected by placing an Allis clamp on the stump. A towel clip is placed around the coracoid.
- The undersurface of the coracoid is decorticated using a high-speed burr.
- The 3.5-mm drill from the small fragment set is used to make drill holes in the coracoid. The drill should be angled in such a way that the drill holes are angled a few degrees away from the joint once the coracoid has been positioned against the glenoid.
- The coracoid is then returned to the wound and tucked into the medial aspect of the incision.

Glenoid Exposure
- The subscapularis is identified and split horizontally in line with its fibers at the midportion of the muscle belly.
- The subscapularis is elevated from the anterior scapula by packing a sponge in a superior direction into the subscapularis fossa.
- A large Steinmann pin is inserted into the superior aspect of the scapular neck to provide retraction of the superior portion of subscapularis.
- A 1-cm vertical capsulotomy is performed adjacent to the glenoid rim.
- A humeral head retractor may then be inserted through the capsulotomy to retract the humerus.
- Medially, an anterior glenoid neck retractor is inserted for further visualization.
- The anterior inferior capsule and labrum are excised, and the periosteum of the anterior inferior glenoid neck is elevated. An osteotome may be required to remove a loose bony fragment.

Coracoid Transfer
- The anterior inferior glenoid neck is decorticated with an osteotome in preparation for the coracoid transfer.

Continued

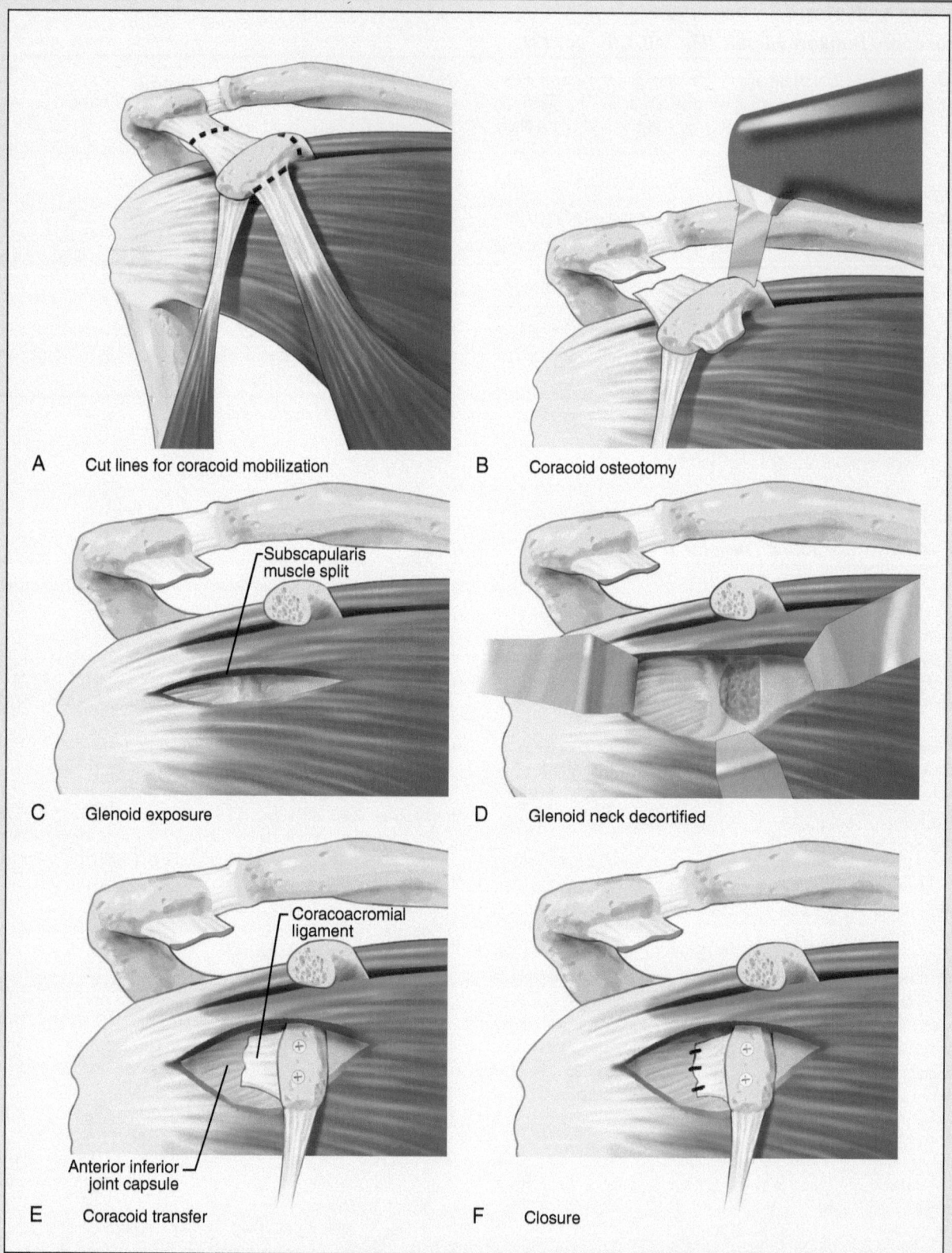

Fig. 40.14 Latarjet-Patte coracoid transfer technique. (A) Following a modified deltopectoral approach, the coracoacromial ligament is divided 1 cm lateral to its insertion into the coracoid. The insertion of pectoralis major is sharply released along the coracoid. (B) A 90-degree angled microsagittal saw is used to osteotomize the base of the coracoid, approximately 2 cm posterior to the coracoid tip. (C) The subscapularis is split horizontally. (D) After a vertical capsulotomy is performed, the anterior inferior capsule and labrum are excised and the periosteum of the anterior inferior glenoid neck is elevated to expose bone. (E) The coracoid is transferred and screwed into place with 4.0-mm cannulated screws. (F) The retained stump of the coracoacromial ligament is attached to the anterior inferior joint capsule.

Latarjet-Patte Coracoid Transfer (Fig. 40.14)—cont'd

- The coracoid is retrieved from the wound. A 30-mm-long 4.0-mm cannulated screw is placed into the superior hole of the coracoid only. This screw acts as a joystick to allow reduction of the coracoid onto the glenoid neck. The proposed placement is carefully evaluated to ensure it is neither too far medial nor too far lateral, resulting in coracoid overhang.
- A 1.25-mm guidewire is then inserted through the inferior hole of the coracoid to hold the reduction. This wire should be inserted approximately 10 degrees away from the joint to avoid intraarticular penetration. However, excessive medial angulation will displace the graft and put the suprascapular nerve at risk.
- The reduction is evaluated. If it is acceptable, a second 1.25-mm guidewire is then inserted through the cannulated screw in the superior hole. The reduction is again evaluated. If it is acceptable, the superior cannulated screw is removed.

- The 2.7-mm cannulated drill bit is then used to drill bicortical holes in the glenoid.
- The 30-mm cannulated screw is typically reused in the superior hole. The inferior hole is measured for length, and a length-appropriate 4.0-mm cannulated screw is inserted.

Closure
- The arm is placed into external rotation. The CI is reattached to the anterior inferior joint capsule, and the remaining CI stump with No. 1 Vicryl.
- A horizontal capsulotomy will allow for a north–south capsular shift if one is desired, but this procedure is not normally done.
- The subscapularis split is not repaired.
- The remainder of the wound is closed in a layered fashion.

Postoperative Management

Arthroscopic Bankart repair. The patient is discharged home with a sling and bolster to be worn at all times. Immediate goals after surgery are primarily to protect the repair, initiate gentle passive and active assisted ROM, and achieve pain control. Active external rotation, extension, and abduction are avoided in the first 2 weeks. ROM goals are flexion to 90 degrees, abduction to 90 degrees, and external rotation to 15 degrees by 3 to 4 weeks.

At 4 weeks, use of the sling is typically discontinued for daytime use, but it may continue to be used while sleeping if concerns exist. Gentle ROM is continued with progression to flexion of 130 degrees and external rotation to 30 degrees. Stretching exercises and proprioceptive activities may begin, along with scapular strengthening.

By 8 to 10 weeks, ROM should progress to full ROM, and strengthening activities may begin. At 4 months, strengthening continues and sport-specific physiotherapy is initiated.

RTP criteria include full ROM, satisfactory muscular strength and endurance, and absence of subjective and objective instability. In general, noncontact athletes may return to sport at 4 months, whereas contact athletes are permitted to resume play at 6 months.

Latarjet-Patte coracoid transfer. Rehabilitation after the Latarjet-Patte procedure is considerably different from that after a Bankart repair.[153] The patient is discharged home with his or her arm in a simple sling. The sling is used for the first 2 weeks continuously. After 2 weeks, the use of the shoulder, out of the sling, is permitted for all typical activities of daily living. At 1 month, ROM exercises, without limitation, are initiated. Return to sport criteria are the same as for Bankart repair, but also include radiographic evidence of healing of the coracoid graft. Athletes participating in contact sports are typically permitted to return at the 3-month mark.

Results

Based on the results of several systematic reviews and meta-analyses, the best available current evidence suggests the following:

- Duration of sling immobilization after primary anterior shoulder dislocation does not influence the rate of recurrent instability.[131]
- Immobilization of the arm in internal or external rotation does not influence the rate of recurrent instability.[131]
- Arthroscopic Bankart repair after primary anterior shoulder dislocation reduces the rate of recurrent instability compared with sling immobilization and may improve short-term quality of life.[91]
- Arthroscopic Bankart repair after recurrent anterior shoulder instability demonstrates equivalent rates of recurrent instability, return to work, and function outcomes compared with open Bankart repair.[143,155,156]
- Arthroscopic Bankart repair after recurrent anterior shoulder instability results in slightly improved ROM compared with open Bankart repair.[155,156]

Complications

Recurrent instability is the most common complication after surgical management. The rate of recurrent instability is difficult to estimate, however, based on many different definitions in the literature.[156] Preoperative risk factors also make instability difficult to predict. Aboalata and colleagues[109] reported overall redislocation rate of 18% after arthroscopic stabilization at 13-year follow-up. Marshall et al.[157] reported postoperative instability in 29% of patients treated after first-time dislocation and 62% of patients treated after multiples episodes at 51 months. A systematic review reported redislocation rates in collision athletes between 5.9% and 38.5% compared with 0% and 18.5% in noncollision athletes.[158] Infection and nerve palsy are less common but may occur.

After coracoid bone block surgery, specific risks include hardware breakage or pain as a result of the hardware.[159] The coracoid graft may achieve a fibrous union, may fail to unite, or may migrate. Coracoid graft osteolysis is also being increasingly recognized.[160]

FUTURE CONSIDERATIONS

Despite the multiple studies investigating the many facets of anterior shoulder instability, high-level evidence remains scarce.

Further research must continue to define the best imaging modality for diagnosis and as a guide for management.[161] The question of position of immobilization has not been fully answered because of less than ideal trial design. The contentious question of whether to offer surgery to a patient with a first-time shoulder dislocation requires a rigorous randomized controlled trial using modern suture-anchor fixation, standardized physiotherapy, and stratification of age and gender. Similarly, open versus arthroscopic management, particularly in athletes who participate in contact sports, has yet to be defined.

For a complete list of references, go to ExpertConsult.com.

SELECTED READINGS

Citation:

Yamamoto N, Itoi E, Abe H, et al. Contact between the glenoid and the humeral head in abduction, external rotation, and horizontal extension: a new concept of glenoid track. *J Shoulder Elbow Surg.* 2007;16(5):649.

Level of Evidence:

Biomechanical study

Summary:

This article introduces the concept of the "glenoid track," which informs the discussion of how to manage glenoid and humeral bone loss.

Citation:

Kirkley A, Griffin S, Richards C, et al. Prospective randomized clinical trial comparing the effectiveness of immediate arthroscopic stabilization versus immobilization and rehabilitation in first traumatic anterior dislocations of the shoulder. *Arthroscopy.* 1999;15(5):507.

Level of Evidence:

I

Summary:

In this study, patients with first-time dislocations were randomly assigned to arthroscopic stabilization or sling immobilization. A significant improvement in Western Ontario Shoulder Instability Index Score and a reduction in redislocation risk were demonstrated.

Citation:

Balg F, Boileau P. The Instability Severity Index Score. A simple pre-operative score to select patients for arthroscopic or open shoulder stabilisation. *J Bone Joint Surg Br.* 2007;89B(11):1470.

Level of Evidence:

III

Summary:

In this prospective case-control study, important risk factors for failure of arthroscopic Bankart repair were identified. A simple score was devised to determine which patients would benefit from the Latarjet versus the arthroscopic Bankart procedure.

Citation:

Burkhart SS, De Beer JF. Traumatic glenohumeral bone defects and their relationship to failure of arthroscopic Bankart repairs: significance of the inverted-pear glenoid and the humeral engaging Hill-Sachs lesion. *Arthroscopy.* 2000;16(7):677.

Level of Evidence:

IV

Summary:

In this retrospective study, causes of failure of arthroscopic Bankart repair were examined. Burkhart and De Beer recognized that significant bony defects were associated with a high rate of failure.

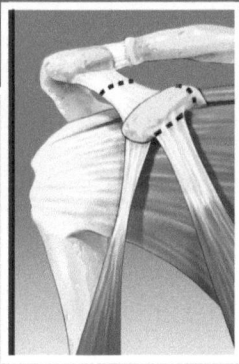

41

Posterior Shoulder Instability

James Bradley, Fotios P. Tjoumakaris

Posterior shoulder instability is a unique condition that not only represents a spectrum of instability, but can also be difficult to diagnose and technically challenging to treat. Although less common than anterior shoulder instability, accounting for only 2% to 10% of cases, this condition is becoming increasingly recognized in the athletic population.[1-4] Mclaughlin et al. first recognized the wide clinical spectrum of posterior shoulder instability ranging from the locked posterior shoulder dislocation to recurrent posterior subluxation (RPS).[2] The causes are multifactorial and include acute traumatic injury, repetitive microtrauma, and atraumatic or ligamentous laxity.[5] In the general population, seizures and electrocution are rare causes of posterior shoulder dislocation. More commonly in the traumatic setting, a posterior direct blow to an adducted, internally rotated and forward flexed upper extremity such as a fall on an outstretched arm is the mechanism of injury.[6] In the athletic population, however, instability results from repetitive microtrauma, which can occur in a variety of loading conditions and multiple arm positions.[2,7] Management of patients with posterior shoulder instability is challenging in recognition of the diagnosis and underlying pathology. Treatment includes both conservative and operative management. Surgeries for posterior instability include both open and arthroscopic procedures, with arthroscopic procedures recently gaining more popularity with advances in surgical techniques and decreased morbidity.

Background

RPS has been observed in overhead athletes, baseball hitters, golfers, tennis players, butterfly and freestyle swimmers, weightlifters, rugby players, and football linemen.[8-10] Other activities where RPS may be present include archery, riflery, and wheelchair use.[11] Distinct from the acute traumatic dislocation, the etiology of RPS is due to repetitive microtrauma to the posterior capsule leading to capsular attenuation and labral tears. In the overhead athlete, adaptive and structural changes in combination with the high forces across the glenohumeral joint result in posterior capsular contracture and posterosuperior labral tear, which is a distinct mechanism from other entities.

Diagnosis and workup of athletes with RPS is often challenging when determining the underlying pathology. These patients present with complaints of vague and diffuse shoulder pain and fatigue without a specific injury. A thorough history and physical and examination in combination with specific imaging studies are required to determine the pathogenesis and treatment for patients with RPS. Provocative clinical examination tests in addition to advanced imaging such as the MR arthrogram have aided in identifying RPS in the athletic population. A thorough history should include the mechanism of injury, which can consist of a true posterior shoulder dislocation, repetitive microtrauma, acute, or chronic subluxation. Specific direction of instability, meaning posterosuperior, directly posterior, posteroinferior as well as pattern of instability, including unidirectional or multidirectional, should be identified. All of these factors should be documented and considered, as they will ultimately affect treatment and outcome.[12] Structural abnormalities of the shoulder, to include any combination of the labrum, capsule, supporting ligaments, or rotator cuff, also must be taken in account to maximize optimal treatment outcome.

Posterior glenohumeral stabilization has evolved from various open procedures to an all arthroscopic approach.[13] This has allowed for enhanced identification of repair of intra-articular pathology.[14] As outcomes have been improving, clinical and biomechanical studies continue to refine our approach to RPS.

Pathogenesis

The posterior labrum, capsule, and posterior band of the inferior glenohumeral ligament (IGHL) are the primary stabilizers to posterior translation of the humeral head between 45 and 90 degrees of abduction.[15] The posterior capsule is identified by the area between the intra-articular potion of the biceps tendon and the posterior band of the IGHL. This area is the thinnest segment of the shoulder capsule and also does not contain any supporting ligamentous structures, making it susceptible to attenuation from repetitive stresses.[16]

The pathogenesis of RPS shares a direct relationship to the specific repetitive stresses placed onto the glenohumeral joint. This differs from the pathogenesis in a traumatic setting where the patient may sustain an acute capsulolabral detachment or reverse Bankart tear (Figs. 41.1 and 41.2).[17] In RPS, specific activities such as the tennis backhand, golf or baseball backswing, follow-through phase of throwing, and pull-through phase in swimming all can result in RPS. Activities such as push-ups, bench press, and blocking in football also place a direct posterior stress on the posterior capsulolabral complex of the shoulder. Due to the various positions athletes use in contact and noncontact sport, many other mechanisms likely exist that are continuously being identified.

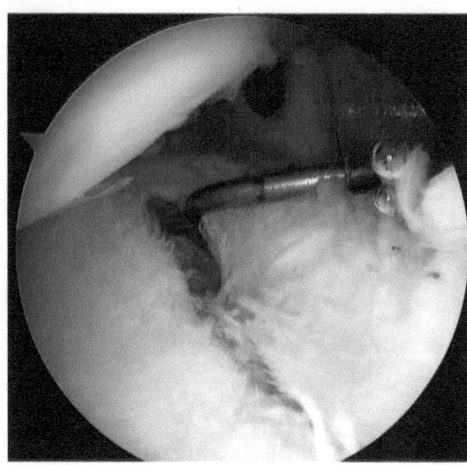

Fig. 41.1 A posterior labral tear from the glenoid (right shoulder, viewed from the anterior portal).

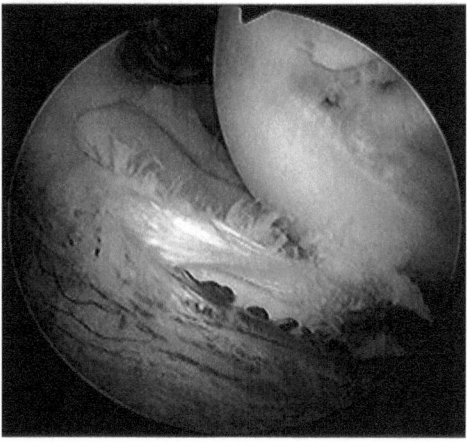

Fig. 41.2 Posterior labral splitting and tear (right shoulder, viewed from the posterior portal). Placing the patient in the lateral decubitus position facilitates posterior labral visualization and repair.

One proposed mechanism of RPS in overhead athletes, throwers, and swimmers is due to the progressive laxity of the posterior capsule and fatigue of static and dynamic stabilizers.[18] RPS can lead to deformation of the posterior capsule, resulting in a patulous posteroinferior capsular pouch that can be seen on both magnetic resonance arthrogram (MRA) and arthroscopically.

Cadaveric studies have examined position and applied force in relation to posterior instability. Pagnani et al. placed the arm into the position of flexion and internal rotation and found that transection of the infraspinatus, teres minor, and entire posterior capsule was sufficient to produce a dislocation.[16] When the anterosuperior capsule and superior glenohumeral ligament (SHGL) were transected, a posterior dislocation would occur. These studies validated the "circle concept," where a dislocation in one direction would require capsular damage on both the same and opposite side of the joint. A different study by Cole et al. found that with the arm in an adducted position, the rotator interval and SGHL provided static glenohumeral stability limiting inferior and posterior joint translations.[19] Wellmann et al. found in their cadaveric study that a lesion of the rotator interval contributes to increased glenohumeral translation.[20] However,

Provencher and colleagues demonstrated that rotator interval closure, while causing loss of external rotation, did not have an effect on reducing posterior instability.[21] Other anatomic studies have questioned the concept of injury to anterior structures, including the rotator interval in a posteriorly dislocated shoulder altogether.[22,23] This work, alongside others, suggests that in an overhead athlete, interval closure may not be clinically indicated and may in fact have an undesired effect on throwing athletes who function with their arm in the abduction and external rotation (ABER) position.

The muscles around the shoulder also significantly contribute to the dynamic cavity compression effect of the humeral head within the glenoid.[24] Of the rotator cuff muscles, the subscapularis provides the most resistance to posterior translation, acting as a dynamic supporter of the action of the posterior band of the IGHL.[25,26] In one cadaveric study, decreased subscapularis muscle strength in the late cocking phase of throwing motion resulted in increased maximum glenohumeral external rotation and increased glenohumeral contact pressure.[27] Therefore overhead throwers with subscapularis fatigue would be more susceptible to these forces, resulting in a type II superior labral anterior posterior (SLAP) tear. In some instances these tears can propagate posteroinferiorly around the glenoid resulting in type VIII SLAP tear and symptomatic RPS.[27,28] From an anatomic standpoint, the humeral head possesses an oblong shape. In the ABER position the anterior band of the IGHL becomes taut as it is draped over the anteroinferior aspect of the eccentrically positioned humeral head, providing a check-rein against excessive external rotation.[29,30]

Pitchers that have increased external rotation at the expense of internal rotation will have more rapid internal humeral rotation in their follow through and pitch velocity. Chronic use of the shoulder in this manner will result in a posterior capsular contracture and glenohumeral rotation deficit. Burkhart suggested that the oblong (cam) effect of the humerus is counteracted by the development of posterior capsular tightness, thus shifting the rotational fulcrum posterosuperiorly.[30] This shift allows the shoulder to clear the anteroinferior labroligamentous restraints while leading them to be susceptible to posterior and posterosuperior microtrauma events.[4,18,31] This occurs during the follow-through phase with the shoulder in a flexed, adducted, and internally rotated position.

The posteroinferior capsular thickening associated with glenohumeral internal rotation deficit (GIRD) has been visualized on magnetic resonance imaging (MRIs) of throwing athletes.[32] Dynamic MRA with the arm in the ABER position has shown a phenomenon known as posterosuperior labral "peel-back." On MRA with the arm in the ABER position, the detached posterosuperior labral tissue separates and moves medially toward the glenoid rim. This can also be visualized arthroscopically (Fig. 41.3).[28]

It has been observed that some adaptive changes can occur in the shoulder without negative consequence, whereas other athletes may go on to become symptomatic. Studies have demonstrated that after approximately 25 degrees of GIRD, the posterosuperior shift in the glenohumeral center of rotation progresses from adaptive to pathologic shearing forces on the

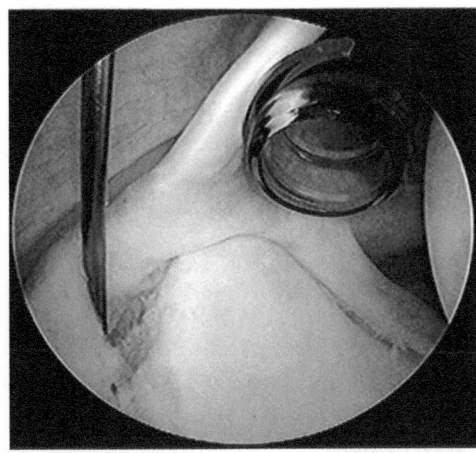

Fig. 41.3 Complete detachment of the posterosuperior labrum from the glenoid in an overhead thrower, as localized by the spinal needle (right shoulder, viewed from the posterior portal).

posterosuperior labrum and rotator cuff.[33] Excessive external rotation in the ABER position exposes the posterosuperior labrum, longhead of the biceps tendon, and undersurface rotator cuff tendons to excessive rotary forces resulting in peel-back phenomenon.[34] Posterior shift of the humeral head in the ABER position also results in a relative redundancy of the anteroinferior capsuloligamentous complex due to a decreased cam effect. Although not the primary pathology of a tight posteroinferior capsule, this secondary anterior pseudolaxity may have clinical implications in the pathophysiology of the disabled throwing shoulder.

The presentation of a posterosuperior labral tear in combination with posteroinferior capsular contracture in throwing athletes differs from the spectrum of pathology in lifters, offensive lineman, and athletes who receive repetitive high loads with the arm in the forward flexed and adducted position.[9] The pathogenesis of these conditions is important because initial treatment may differ based on the underlying etiology. Initial treatment in overhead athletes with GIRD and RPS is conservative with posteroinferior capsular contracture stretching, "sleeper stretches" is a more appropriate initial treatment.[30,35] Subscapularis treatment may also play a role. If the thrower remains symptomatic, arthroscopic posterior labral repair with optional capsular release can then be performed.

"Batter's shoulder" is another cause of RPS in baseball hitters where this syndrome affects the lead shoulder during the baseball swing.[36,37] As the dynamic pulling forces approach 500 Newtons, a posterior labral tear results. It has been inferred that golfers may experience a similar mechanism of injury along with any athlete with a similar follow through type motion during swinging.

Identification and treatment of scapular dyskinesia is also of importance when identifying the pathogenesis of RPS. Scapular winging can act as a compensatory mechanism to prevent posterior subluxation of the humeral head. In other patients, winging is thought to be the primary etiology of subluxation.[4] A study in golfers with posterior shoulder instability found that fatigue developed in the serratus anterior muscle.[38] This possibly contributing to scapulothoracic asynchrony and the combination

of posterior shoulder instability and subacromial impingement. An initial treatment in these patients should include a periscapular muscle strengthening program, which should be incorporated into the physical therapy protocol.

HISTORY

Patients with RPS often have vague and nonspecific complaints and symptoms that make clinical diagnosis difficult to elucidate. Symptoms can include any combination of activity related pain, crepitus, perceived weakness, and episodes of intermittent subluxation. If capsular contracture has developed, a complaint of loss of motion may also be present. One study by Pollock et al. noted that two-thirds of athletes who ultimately required surgery presented with difficulty using the shoulder outside of sports with use of the arm above the horizontal.[39] Another study found that 90% of patients with RPS note clicking or crepitation with motion.

PHYSICAL EXAMINATION

A thorough physical examination of the shoulder includes initial inspection focusing on shoulder asymmetry, muscular atrophy, or scapular dysrhythmia. A skin dimple over the posteromedial deltoid of both shoulders has been found to be 62% sensitive and 92% specific in correlating with posterior instability.[40]

On palpation, tenderness is assessed at the posterior glenohumeral joint line, greater tuberosity, and biceps tendon. In patients with RPS, posterior joint line tenderness is likely a result of posterior synovitis or posterior rotator cuff tendinosis secondary to multiple episodes of instability.[39]

Shoulder range of motion (ROM) should also be assessed in both shoulders. Record measurements of forward elevation, abduction in the scapular plane, external rotation with the arm at the side, and internal rotation with the hand behind the back to the highest vertebral level. Shoulder measurements while the patient is in the supine position should also be recorded. While supine, the arm is abducted 90 degrees, the scapula is stabilized, and glenohumeral external and internal rotation are measured. Total arc of rotation is calculated by adding total external plus total internal rotation, and GIRD is assessed by assessing the side to side difference in internal rotation. Crepitus can oftentimes be reproduced during ROM examination as well.

Strength testing is performed bilaterally, with a focus on the rotator cuff. Grading is performed on a five-point scale (Table 41.1). The majority of athletes with RPS will demonstrate grade 4 or 5 strength. Supraspinatus strength is tested with a downward force while the arm is abducted 90 degrees in the scapular plane, otherwise known as the "empty can" test. Infraspinatus and teres minor muscles are assessed with resisted external rotation, with the arm adducted and the elbow flexed 90 degrees. If the posterior cuff has been damaged, subtle differences can be detected. Subscapularis strength testing is performed with the lumbar lift-off, belly press, and bear hug tests.[41–43]

Glenohumeral stability is assessed in both shoulders with the patient supine. The load and shift maneuver is performed with the arm held in 90 degrees of abduction and neutral rotation.

TABLE 41.1   Muscle Grading Scale

0	No muscle contraction is detectable
1	A contraction can be seen or palpated but strength is insufficient to move the joint at all
2	The muscle can move the joint if the limb is oriented so that the force of gravity is eliminated
3	The muscle can move the joint against the force of gravity, but not against any additional applied force
4	The muscle can move the joint against the force of gravity and additional applied force but is not believed to be normal
5	The muscle strength is considered normal

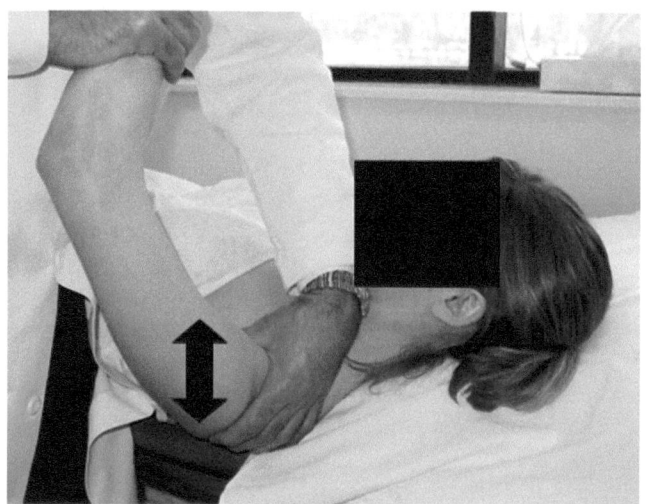

Fig. 41.4 The load-and-shift test is performed to assess anterior and posterior glenohumeral stability.

TABLE 41.2   Grading of Anterior and Posterior Laxity

0	A humeral head that does not translate to the glenoid rim
1+	A humeral head that translates to but does not translate over the glenoid rim
2+	A humeral head that translates over the glenoid rim but spontaneously reduces
3+	A humeral head that translates over the glenoid rim and does not spontaneously reduce

TABLE 41.3   Sulcus Test

1+	Acromiohumeral distance <1 cm
2+	Acromiohumeral distance between 1 and 2 cm
3+	Acromiohumeral distance >2 cm

A 3+ sulcus sign that remains 2+ or greater in 30 degrees of external rotation is considered pathognomonic for multidirectional instability.

TABLE 41.4   Beighton Score for Joint Hypermobility (9 Points)

Joint	Negative	Unilateral	Bilateral
Ability to hyperextend the elbows beyond 10 degrees	0	1	2
Ability to passively touch the thumb to the adjacent forearm with the wrist in flexion	0	1	2
Ability to passively hyperextend the small finger metacarpophalyngeal joint more than 90 degrees	0	1	2
Ability to hyperextend the knees beyond 10 degrees	0	1	2
Ability to touch the palms to the floor with feet together	0	1	1

Patients who score 5 points or more on the Beighton scale are considered ligamentously lax.[44]

Axial load is applied to the glenohumeral joint with an anterior-directed force applied then a posterior directed force (Fig. 41.4). Translation of the humeral head over the anterior glenoid rim is quantified from 0 to 3+ (Table 41.2).

The sulcus test is performed to asses for excessive IGHL and SGHL laxity. With the patient in a seated position, longitudinal traction is applied with the arm adducted and in neutral rotation. The test is repeated in 30 degrees of external rotation. Laxity is quantified based on the acromial humeral distance (Table 41.3). A sulcus sign that remains 2+ or greater in 30 degrees of external rotation is considered pathognomonic for multidirectional instability (MDI). Patients who present with RPS and concomitant MDI may need to have the rotator interval addressed at the time of surgery, in addition to the posterior capsulolabral complex for successful stabilization.

Generalized ligamentous laxity is also important to examine, as this may contribute to MDI. The Beighton scale assesses the spectrum of ligamentous laxity based on a 9-point scale (Table 41.4).[44] Patients with a score of 5 or more are considered ligamentously lax.

Special tests have also been applied to further identify capsulolabral pathology in the shoulder. The jerk test is used to assess posterior instability while in the seated position. The medial border of the scapula is stabilized with one hand while the other hand applies a posterior directed force to the 90 degree forward flexed, adducted, and internally rotated arm. The test is positive if posterior subluxation, dislocation, or pain and apprehension are present.[7,45]

The Kim test assesses posteroinferior shoulder instability.[46] With the patient seated, the arm is placed into 90 degrees of abduction in the scapular plane and an axial load is applied. The arm is then forward elevated an additional 45 degrees, and a posteroinferior vector is placed across the glenohumeral joint. A sudden onset of posterior subluxation with pain is positive, with 97% sensitivity in eliciting a posteroinferior labral lesion.[46]

The circumduction test is performed to assess patients with higher grades of chronic posterior instability. With the elbow in full extension, the arm is placed into 90 degrees of forward elevation and slight adduction. A posterior load is then applied, which subluxes or possibly dislocates the humeral head posteriorly. The arm is then circumducted with a combination of abduction and extension until the head reduces in the glenoid. A palpable clunk as the head reduces into the glenoid is significant for a positive test. In patients with chronic posterior instability, this test can often be performed without pain or guarding.

In some cases of RPS, and primarily involving overhead throwers, a posterior labral tear is seen in combination with a superior labral tear resulting in a type VIII SLAP tear.[28] The active compression (O'Brien) test for superior labral pathology should also be performed. With the patient seated, the arm is forward elevated 90 degrees, adducted 10 degrees, and internally rotated with the elbow extended; a downward force is placed on the arm. A positive test is when deep pain within the shoulder joint is elicited when the arm is in this position compared with when the arm is externally rotated and the same force is applied. It is important to note that deep pain in the shoulder joint is suggestive of superior labral pathology, and is different than pain at the acromioclavicular joint, which can result in a false positive result.

Impingement signs may also be present on physical examination. This impingement is typically due to underlying scapular dyskinesia. Stress-related changes in the posterior rotator cuff can manifest as a secondary impingement syndrome.

IMAGING

Initial radiographs of the shoulder should be obtained in the workup of RPS. Radiographs should consist of an anteroposterior view in the plane of the scapula, an axillary view, and a scapular Y lateral view. In most patients with RPS, these radiographic images are normal. In some cases, a posterior glenoid lesion or impaction of the anterior humeral head (reverse Hill-Sachs lesion) can be seen.[44,45] The axillary view is particularly useful in assessing glenoid version. A West Point radiographic view can be useful detecting fractures of the glenoid rim or subtle ectopic bone formation around the glenoid.[47,48] CT Scan can also be useful in providing osseous detail in posttraumatic or chronic cases.

MRA is the most sensitive diagnostic test for identifying lesions of the posterior labrum and capsule.[49] MRA findings indicative of posterior shoulder instability include posterior translation of the humeral head relative to the glenoid, posterior labrocapsular avulsion, posterior labral tear or splitting, discrete posterior capsular tears or rents, reverse humeral avulsion of the glenohumeral ligaments, posterior labrum periosteal sleeve avulsion, and subscapularis tendon avulsion (Fig. 41.5).[50,51] The Kim classification is used to describe posterior labral tear morphology (Figs. 41.6–41.8; Table 41.5).[52] Arthroscopically the Kim lesion appears as a crack at the junction of the posteroinferior glenoid articular cartilage and labrum through which a complete detachment of the deeper labrum from the glenoid rim can be identified. MRA can also be used to identify chondrolabral and glenoid version.[53] Kim examined 33 shoulders with atraumatic posterior instability, and when compared with age matched controls, the affected shoulders were found to have a glenoid that was more shallow and also had more osseous and chondrolabral retroversion present in the middle and inferior glenoid (Fig. 41.9).[53] Studies performed by Bradley and colleagues have also found in athletes with RPS higher chondrolabral retroversion and glenoid bony retroversion when compared with controls.[8,54] Another study by Tung et al. found 24 patients with RPS had MRA findings of

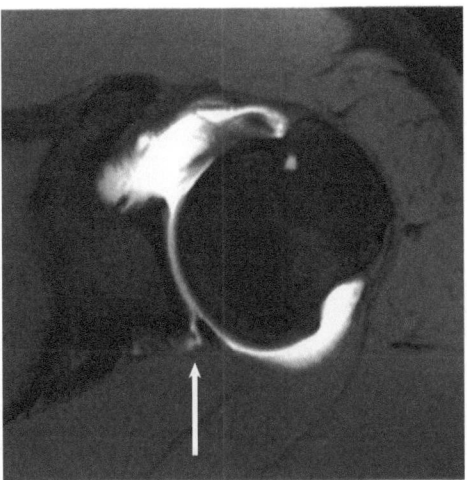

Fig. 41.5 An axial magnetic resonance imaging arthrogram image (left shoulder) demonstrating a posterior capsulolabral avulsion from the glenoid with associated posterior translation of the humeral head relative to the glenoid *(arrow)*.

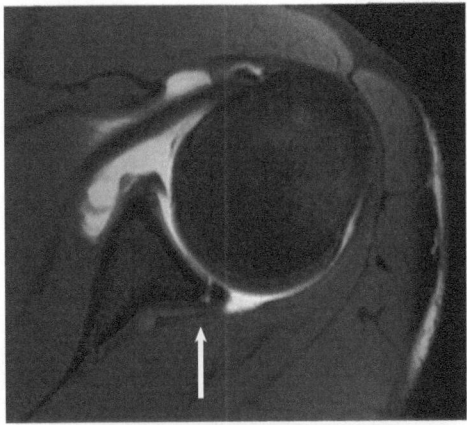

Fig. 41.6 An axial magnetic resonance imaging arthrogram image (left shoulder) demonstrating a type I Kim lesion: a posterior chondrolabral fissure without displacement *(arrow)*.

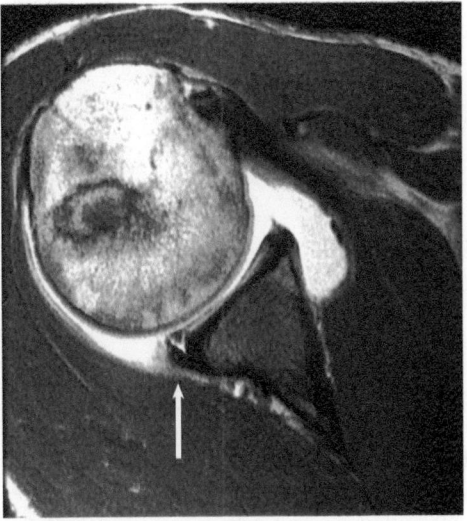

Fig. 41.7 An axial magnetic resonance imaging arthrogram image (right shoulder) demonstrating a type II Kim lesion: a concealed complete detachment of the posterior labrum from the glenoid *(arrow)*.

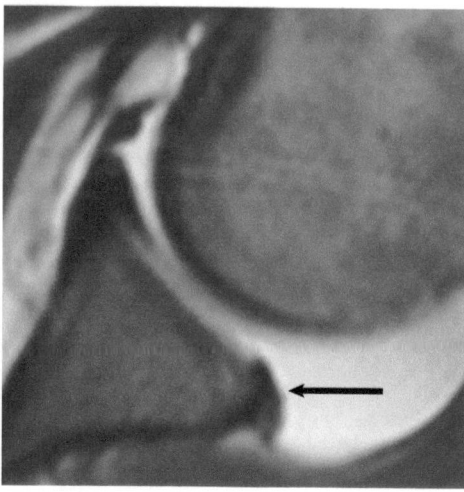

Fig. 41.8 An axial magnetic resonance imaging arthrogram image (left shoulder) demonstrating a type III Kim lesion: posterior chondrolabral erosion with loss of contour *(arrow)*.

TABLE 41.5	Kim Classification of Posterior Labral Tear Morphology
Type I	Incomplete detachment (Fig. 41.6)
Type II (Kim Lesion)	Concealed complete detachment (Fig. 41.7)
Type III	Chondrolabral erosion (Fig. 41.8)
Type IV	Flap tear of the posteroinferior labrum

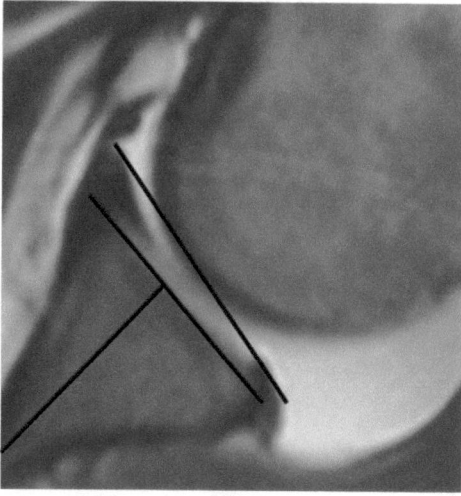

Fig. 41.9 An axial magnetic resonance imaging arthrogram image (left shoulder) demonstrating the technique used to measure the degree of chondrolabral retroversion, which can be increased in patients with recurrent posterior subluxation (RPS) of the shoulder.

more posterior humeral head translation, posterior labral tears, and posterior labrocapsular avulsions compared with healthier controls.[49] Dynamic MRA can also be performed to evaluate for the peel back phenomenon, which is consistent with a posterosuperior labral tear.[55] The use of CT is limited to cases in which a significant amount of bony glenoid retroversion is suspected.

DECISION-MAKING PRINCIPLES

Thorough knowledge of an athlete's sport, position, and training regimen is critical in determining the pathogenesis and specific pathology associated with their shoulder instability. Rehabilitation with an emphasis on strengthening the rotator cuff, posterior deltoid, periscapular muscles is commonly the first line of treatment.[7,31,39,56–59] It is recommended that this physical therapy protocol be maintained for a minimum of 6 months to decrease an athlete's functional disability. A total of 70% of athletes with this protocol can return to sport. Although the RPS is not eliminated, the functional disability is improved for the athlete to participate in play. Therapy has been traditionally more effective in patients with atraumatic RPS, as opposed to those with generalized ligamentous laxity or a discreet traumatic event.[31,57] For patients that fail therapy and are not able to return to preinjury levels of competition, surgery should be considered. Treatment options may ultimately include labral débridement, labral repair, posterior capsular release, posterior capsular plication, or a combination of these procedures.

TREATMENT OPTIONS

Many operative procedures have been described for the treatment of posterior instability, including both open and arthroscopic procedures. There has been a general trend in the transition from open procedures to arthroscopic repair, and from nonanatomic to an anatomic reconstruction. Open procedures included a reverse Putti-Platt procedure, biceps tendon transfer, subscapularis transfer, infraspinatus advancement, posterior opening glenoid wedge osteotomy, proximal humeral rotational osteotomy, bone block augmentation of the posterior glenoid or acromion, posterior staple capsulorrhaphy, allograft reconstruction, capsulolabral reconstruction, and open capsular shift.[2,7,17,18,31,59–62]

Posterior bone block repair has been found to have good outcomes, with one study by Scapinelli reporting 100% success at 9.5 year follow-up.[63] However, a separate biomechanical study has shown that posterior bone block capsulorrhaphy overcorrects posterior translation and does not restore inferior glenohumeral stability.[64] Notable soft tissue tightening procedures include the reverse Putti-Platt and Boyd and Sisk procedures (rerouting the longhead of the biceps tendon to the posterior glenoid).[3,65] In 1980 Neer and Foster reported good results in their laterally based posterior capsular shift to tighten a patulous posteroinferior capsule.[66] Other studies have attempted a medially based posterior capsular shift for posterior capsular tightening.[18,31,59] Misamore et al. reported on 14 patients with traumatic unidirectional posterior instability who were treated with an open posterior capsulorrhaphy. They found excellent results, with 12 of 14 returning to preinjury level of play.[59] Other studies by Rhee presented a review of 33 shoulders for which open, deltoid saving posterior capsulolabral reconstruction was performed and reported that at 25 month follow-up, four patients had recurrent instability.[67] Another study by Wolf and colleagues presented similar findings in a retrospective review of 44 shoulders after open posterior glenohumeral stabilization.[17] The recurrence rate was 19%, poor results in patients older than 37 years, and in those with chondral damage.[17]

Arthroscopic techniques for the treatment of shoulder instability have been implemented and become increasingly popular. Historically, arthroscopic thermal capsulorrhaphy was performed, but results have been fair at best. One study by Bisson presented 14 shoulders without labral detachment who underwent thermal capsulorrhaphy with 2-year follow-up.[68] They found that treatment failed in 3 of their 14 patients (21%). In another study, D'Alessandro found that 37% of patients who underwent thermal capsulorrhaphy for anterior, anteroinferior, or multidirectional shoulder instability had unsatisfactory results with American Shoulder and Elbow Surgeons (ASES) scores at 2- to 5-year follow-up.[69] Other studies by Miniaci reported 47% recurrent instability in patients being treated for MDI at 9 months post op.[70] Due to the variable response patients have demonstrated, thermal capsulorrhaphy for treatment of RPS is not recommended.

Arthroscopic capsulolabral repair has evolved over time, providing a minimally invasive approach with less morbidity and faster recovery.[13] With advances in arthroscopic techniques, the all-arthroscopic approach to posterior stabilization has the ability to treat a wide array of pathology. With open techniques, anterior pathology of the shoulder (labrum tearing, subscapularis disruption), in addition to superior pathology (supraspinatus, biceps tendon, and superior labrum tearing), is near impossible to address through the same exposure. The arthroscopic approach allows for clear visualization of the entire labrum, rotator cuff, and other pain-generating pathology around the glenohumeral joint, which also allows for adequate treatment. In addition, arthroscopic management of posterior instability allows for complete labrum repair, in addition to capsular plication in an "around the world" fashion. Recent studies evaluating postoperative outcomes of the arthroscopic approach have also surpassed those of open techniques, making the arthroscopic modality the current standard of care for the majority of patients.

Indications

Patients are candidates for arthroscopic posterior stabilization if they present with prior episodes of posterior dislocation or RPS of the glenohumeral joint that has not responded favorably to conservative management. After an initial posterior dislocation occurs, a closed reduction is performed and instability is assessed. Once a pain-free shoulder with full ROM is restored, patients are gradually returned to regular activity. If resultant instability or pain persists and physiotherapy is not ameliorative, then the patient is counseled regarding surgical intervention.

Patients with RPS may not report an initial traumatic event; however, they may have an insidious course with deep shoulder pain, reduced athletic participation (inability to throw long ball, loss of velocity and control), and pain with cross body and adducted shoulder movements. An initial course of physical therapy can be initiated in addition to a throwing regimen for overhead-throwing athletes. If pain subsides, gradual return to play (RTP) is begun and the patient can be assessed for recurrence of symptoms.

If pain or subluxation returns, a MRA can be obtained to confirm the diagnosis. Once confirmed, the specific anatomical considerations can be evaluated and the patient can be counseled regarding the need for surgical intervention. Primary indications for surgery include a history consistent with prior dislocation or RPS; physical examination that is positive for any or all of the provocative tests, including the Kim test, Jerk test, posterior load and shift, and pain with cross body adduction with reproduction of symptoms; diagnostic imaging (MRA) demonstrating a patulous posterior capsule, posterior labrum tear, capsular tear or concealed crack ("Kim" lesion); reverse humeral avulsion of the glenohumeral ligaments, reverse Hill-Sachs impaction fracture, reverse osseous Bankart lesion, relative increase in glenoid retroversion with hypoplastic labrum, and chondrolabral retroversion greater than 10 degrees; and patients who failed conservative treatment with a stretching and strengthening rotator cuff rehabilitation program and an inability to return to sport or activity at a preinjury level.

Contraindications

As arthroscopic techniques have evolved, so have the relative contraindications to an arthroscopic approach. Contraindications to arthroscopic surgery may include large glenoid (>25%) or reverse Hill-Sachs (>30%) lesions that may be better managed with an open bone grafting technique, capsular tearing with loss of capsular tissue (from prior surgery or thermal modification), excessive glenoid retroversion (type C glenoid), significant osteoarthritis or chondral erosion, neuromuscular abnormality resulting in motor deficit, and patients who have failed a prior arthroscopic procedure (relative contraindication). Patients unable to comply with a postoperative regimen that consists of a brief period of immobilization followed by a structured therapy protocol are not suitable candidates for surgical intervention.

Goals of the Procedure

The main purpose of arthroscopic posterior stabilization is to prevent recurrent macro (dislocation) or micro (RPS) posterior instability of the glenohumeral joint. Traditional techniques focused on open capsular plication with labrum repair, bone block, or wedge osteotomy to prevent recurrent posterior instability. Evolving techniques have allowed for better access to the glenohumeral joint with an arthroscopic approach with accompanying superior clinical outcomes in recent years.[13] The ultimate goal of arthroscopic management is to restore normal glenohumeral mechanics, prevent recurrent instability or subluxation, and allow for return to normal physiologic function of the joint and athletic participation. The arthroscopic method is also aimed at improving short-term ROM goals and preventing disruption of the deltoid or scapular musculature, which can delay postoperative rehabilitation and may accompany an open technique.

POSTOPERATIVE MANAGEMENT

At the completion of the surgery, the shoulder is placed in a shoulder abduction sling, which immobilizes the shoulder in 30 degrees of abduction and prevents internal rotation. An optional cryotherapy device may be used for the first 3 postoperative days to minimize swelling and pain. During the initial postoperative

🔖 Authors' Preferred Technique
Arthroscopic Posterior Shoulder Stabilization

Preoperative Preparation and Positioning
Preoperative Preparation

Prior to surgery, the magnetic resonance arthrogram (MRA) is evaluated for degree of glenoid retroversion, significance of any osseous pathology, and the degree of labrum pathology. Routine radiographs (AP, scapular Y, and axillary view) are also typically obtained prior to MRA to exclude the presence of fracture, subluxation, or frank dislocation. Understanding the needs of each patient is critical to achieving success with this technique. For instance, patients who engage in high-risk contact sports are more likely to have significant labral pathology and require added capsular plication. Patients who are overhead-throwing athletes will have difficulty returning to sports if excessive plication is performed, causing a decrease in ROM and capsular tightness. Patients are given information regarding the risks of surgery, which may include stiffness, infection, neurovascular injury, and recurrence of instability. On the date of the surgery, an interscalene nerve block is routinely used with general anesthesia for both intraoperative muscle relaxation and postoperative pain control.

Positioning

A lateral decubitus position is preferred; however, a beach-chair position can be utilized for this technique. The lateral decubitus position offers excellent access to the posterior joint and capsule without the use of accessory traction by an assistant. A beanbag positioner is typically used with an axillary roll to protect the nonoperative extremity. The down leg is padded over the peroneal nerve, fibular head, and lateral malleolus. The operative arm is placed in 10 to 15 lbs of balanced arm traction in 45 degrees of abduction and 20 degrees of forward flexion. When the posterior, inferior aspect of the labrum is approached arthroscopically, forward flexion can be increased to gain better exposure. The bed should be angled 45 degrees away from anesthesia, and the visualization tower should be placed across the surgical field and at eye level to the surgeon.

Operative Technique

Portal Placement

All bony landmarks are marked with a marking pen (the acromion, coracoid process and acromioclavicular joint). The anterior portal is typically placed in the rotator interval in a trajectory that is diagonal from the coracoid process to the anterolateral edge of the acromion. The posterior portal is created slightly lateral to a traditional posterior arthroscopy portal to allow tangential access to the posterior glenoid for anchor placement. The posterior portal is created first after insufflation of the joint with 30 cc of normal saline. This facilitates safe insertion of the arthroscope cannula and blunt trochar. The anterior portal is created in the rotator interval either using an "inside out" technique with a switching stick, or an "outside in" technique with a spinal needle. Once portals are created, a clear cannula is placed in the anterior portal using a traditional dilation technique. Either a 5.75 mm or 8.25 mm clear cannula (distally threaded) can be used for the anterior portal.

Diagnostic Arthroscopy

A 30-degree arthroscope placed through a posterior viewing portal is used to perform an initial diagnostic arthroscopy (see Figs. 41.2, 41.3). The joint is assessed for concomitant pathology such as superior labral tears, rotator cuff tears, and osteochondral injury. Débridement of the joint can be carried out with a 4.5 mm shaver through the anterior portal as needed. Following an initial diagnostic arthroscopy, the camera is placed into the anterior cannula, and inflow is placed on the side port on the cannula. A switching stick is placed in the posterior portal, and this portal is dilated to 8 mm. An 8.25-mm cannula (Arthrex, Naples, FL) is then placed in the posterior portal. The arthroscope can be switched to a 70-degree arthroscope, which allows better visualization of the posterior and inferior capsule and posterior inferior band of the inferior glenohumeral ligament.

Typical pathology associated with posterior instability includes posterior labral fraying and splitting, posterior labral detachment from the glenoid rim, a patulous posterior capsule, a discrete posterior capsular tear, undersurface partial-thickness rotator cuff tears, and widening of the rotator interval (Fig. 41.10). The surgeon also must be cognizant of the subtle Kim lesion—that is, a concealed incomplete detachment of the posterior labrum.[52]

Glenoid and Labrum Preparation

A meticulous glenoid preparation is critical to achieving success of the repair. An elevator is initially placed through the posterior portal, and the labrum is sharply elevated off the glenoid (Fig. 41.11). The labrum is mobilized until the underside of the capsule edge of the glenoid rim is visualized. Care is taken during labral elevation and mobilization to not transect the labrum. Adequate trajectory through the posterior portal is critical in achieving this goal. If the angle is difficult, the elevator can be brought in through the anterior portal and the labrum visualized posteriorly. Once adequate mobilization is achieved, a hooded burr is used to prepare the glenoid rim (Fig. 41.12). Great care should be used to ensure the labrum is protected during the bony débridement. A shaver is then used to remove any remaining soft tissue debris from the glenoid rim

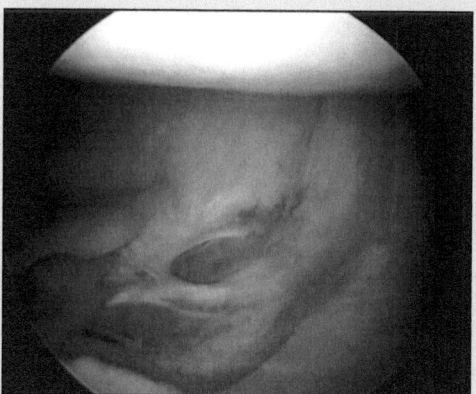

Fig. 41.10 A discrete posterior capsular tear in an athlete with recurrent posterior subluxation of the shoulder (right shoulder, viewed from the anterior portal).

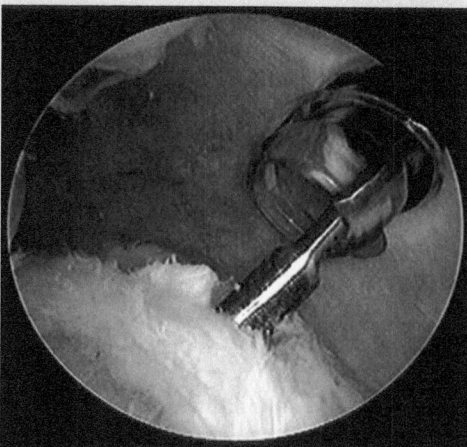

Fig. 41.11 An arthroscopic chisel used to elevate the torn labrum, which is scarred medially, away from the glenoid rim. In this case, a split in the labrum is used to access the scarred tissue (right shoulder, viewed from the anterior portal).

Authors' Preferred Technique
Arthroscopic Posterior Shoulder Stabilization—cont'd

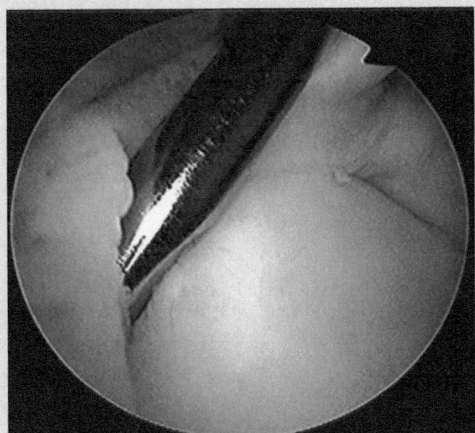

Fig. 41.12 A motorized shaver is used at the posterosuperior extent of the labral tear to decorticate the glenoid rim and abrade the labral undersurface (right shoulder, viewed from the posterior portal). To complete the abrasion posteroinferiorly, the shaver is switched to the posterior portal and the arthroscope is placed in the anterior portal.

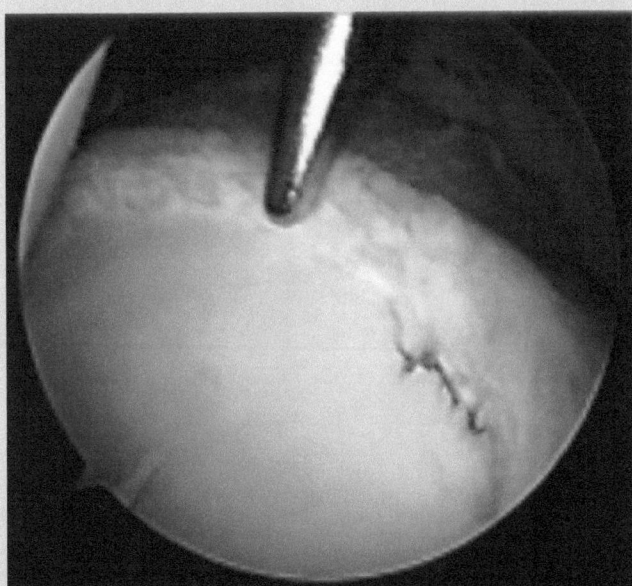

Fig. 41.13 Arthroscopic view from the posterior portal looking inferiorly along the glenoid after labrum mobilization and glenoid preparation is complete.

followed by rasping to create a fresh, bleeding surface conducive to soft tissue healing (Fig. 41.13).

Suture Passing and Labral Repair
A knotless anchor system is employed (2.4 mm biocomposite short PushLock anchors [Arthrex, Naples, FL] for patients with smaller glenoids [subequatorial width <25 mm] or 2.9 mm short PushLock anchors for patients with normal or large glenoid widths) with 1.3 mm Suture Tape (Arthrex, Naples, FL) as our primary fixation method. Knotless fixation superior to the equator of the glenoid may minimize the risk of humeral head chondral injury, as well as articular-sided rotator cuff knot abrasion. Furthermore, the suture tape has a low profile, which

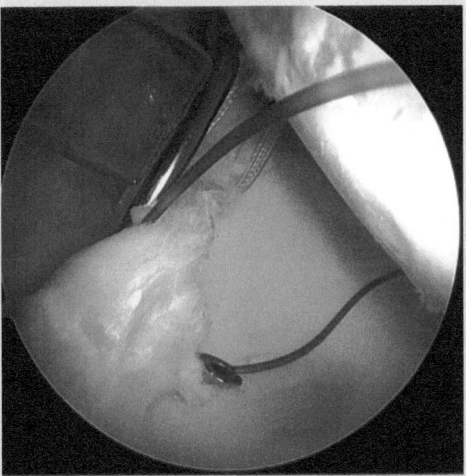

Fig. 41.14 A suture hook device is first used to shuttle a monofilament suture around the labrum for later suture tape passage.

allows it to lay flat against the labrum minimizing tear-through and provides excellent reduction without humeral abrasion. The first step in labral repair is predicated on the surgeon understanding the specific pathology and demands of the patient. Patients presenting with symptoms consistent with RPS and insidious shoulder pain without gross macro-instability (i.e., throwers) may benefit from a primary labral repair without significant capsular plication/advancement. Patients with macro-instability or dislocation and who participate in high-demand contact sports (i.e., offensive lineman) may require labral repair with plication of the posterior capsule.

For the standard posterior labral repair, we prefer to place anchors from approximately 6-o'clock to the 11-o'clock position on the glenoid. To achieve positioning of the inferior most anchor, an accessory posterior portal may need to be created 45 degrees tangential to the glenoid. This portal is typically created slightly inferior and lateral to the posterior working portal. While viewing from the anterior portal, a spinal needle is used to localize the correct site of entry for the accessory posterior portal. Once the correct location and trajectory are identified for anchor placement, an accessory 5 mm cannula is introduced into the joint using Seldinger technique. Great care should be taken to avoid damage to the axillary nerve on cannula introduction, as it lies at risk in this area. The anchors are all placed from inferior to superior after suture passage.

A curved suture hook (Spectrum, Linvatec, Edison, NJ, or ReelPass Suture Lasso, Arthrex, Naples, FL) loaded with a 0 monofilament suture is placed through the posterior working cannula while the arthroscope is placed in the anterior cannula. A bite of capsulolabral tissue is taken slightly inferior and lateral to the level of desired anchor location (to achieve capsular plication and advancement) and the suture is delivered through the labrum against the glenoid articular margin (Fig. 41.14). The monofilament suture is then shuttled through the posterior working cannula, and a loop of Suture Tape is placed in a knot of the monofilament suture. The goal is to create a "cinch" stitch akin to a luggage tag that will reduce the labrum and provide optimum suture security around the tissue. The loop of Suture Tape is then shuttled back through the posterior working cannula, and the tail ends of the suture are delivered through the loop created in the Suture Tape. The two tails of the Suture Tape are then pulled, and the cinch stitch is reduced to the labrum. A knot pusher can be used to help reduce the knot to the labral tissue if needed when there is concern that the tissue is of poor quality. This creates 2.6 mm of Suture Tape, as the tape is essentially doubled over to create a stable fixation construct around the labrum and capsular

Continued

Authors' Preferred Technique

Arthroscopic Posterior Shoulder Stabilization—cont'd

complex. The Suture Tape ends are then delivered through the accessory cannula for anchor placement. The drill guide is then placed through the accessory posterior cannula and a pilot hole drilled in the desired location. The suture ends are then shuttled through the eyelet of the knotless anchor and the anchor is then slid to the level of the glenoid and slight tension is applied to the limbs to reduce the labrum (Fig. 41.15). The anchor is then impacted into place within the pilot hole and the labrum, and capsule is reduced to the glenoid margin (Fig. 41.16). Additional anchors can be placed in an identical fashion as needed. Anchors in the 8-o'clock to 11-o'clock position are generally placed through the standard posterior portal, which provides a better angle of approach in this zone.

Posterior Portal Closure

The posterior portal is then closed using a No. 1 Polydioxanone (PDS) suture. The cannula is withdrawn to a level just external to the capsule. A suture passer is then used to pierce the capsule adjacent to the portal, and the PDS suture is introduced into the joint. A penetrating suture grasper is then used to pierce the capsule on the opposite side of the portal, and the suture is retrieved. A sliding Weston knot is then used to close down the capsule. Additional sutures can be placed in a wider fashion if additional plication is required based on the patient's predetermined needs from the preoperative plan.

Technical Considerations

- Positioning—The lateral decubitus position offers excellent exposure with minimal assistance to access the posterior joint capsule.
- Portal Placement—Placement of the posterior portal slightly lateral to the standard portal allows for easier placement of the anchors when utilizing a single portal technique.
- Anchor Placement—Anchors should be placed nearly perpendicular to the glenoid or at a tangent of 45 degrees to avoid chondral injury and "skiving."
- Repair—The repair should be tailored to the precise pathology of the patient as determined by history, examination, and diagnostic imaging. Knotless techniques can help avoid knot abrasion against the rotator cuff and scuffing against articular cartilage (Fig. 41.17).

What to Avoid

- Avoid placement of anchors too close to one another, as this could cause fragmentation of the glenoid bone and a "postage stamp" style fracture.
- Avoid transecting the posterior labrum during labrum preparation. Use of a periosteal elevator should be done from the portal that allows for the most mobilization of tissue without iatrogenic injury.
- Avoid over-tightening overhead-throwing athletes, as this could compromise their ability to RTP.

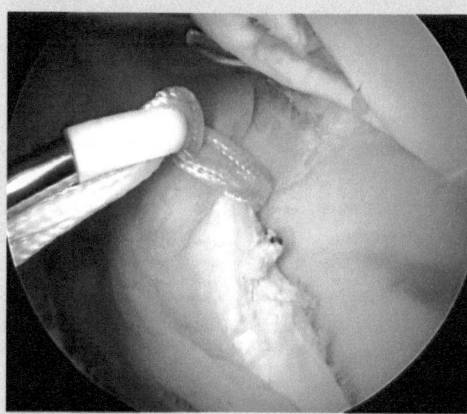

Fig. 41.15 A luggage tag or "cinch" stitch has been placed around the labrum and capsule and is delivered through the eyelet of the anchor for glenoid placement. Note the osteochondral injury present in this patient on the posterior aspect of the humeral head.

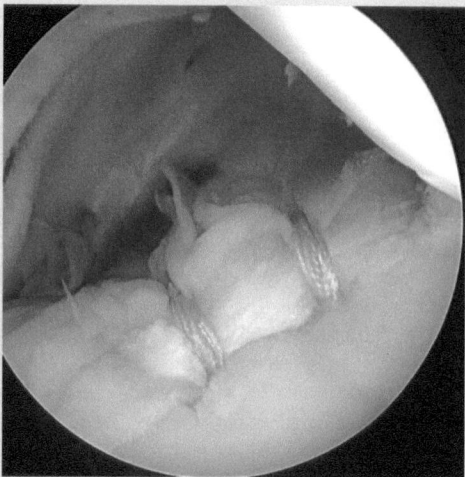

Fig. 41.16 Arthroscopic view from the posterior portal looking inferiorly at the completed labrum and capsular repair.

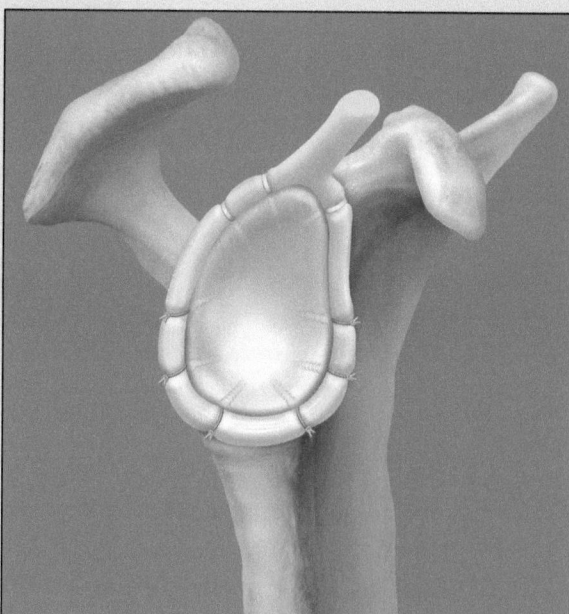

Fig. 41.17 Knotless anchors used for labral repair above the horizontal equator of the glenoid (right shoulder), with traditional suture anchors used below. (Courtesy of Arthrex Inc., Naples, FL.)

period, patients begin active ROM of the elbow, wrist, and fingers. At 1 week after surgery, formal physical therapy for the shoulder is initiated, beginning with passive forward flexion and abduction in the scapular plane to 90 degrees. During the subsequent 5 weeks, full passive ROM is achieved. At 6 weeks after surgery, use of the sling is discontinued and active-assisted ROM begins, progressing to full active ROM according to the patient's ability. Most patients are progressed to full active ROM by 8 to 12 weeks. Strengthening of the rotator cuff, deltoid, and periscapular muscles begins at 3 months after surgery.

Once patients are able to achieve 80% of the strength of their contralateral shoulders as measured by isokinetic testing, a sport-specific rehabilitation protocol is initiated that typically takes place between 4 and 6 months after surgery. Athletes are cleared to return to sport when they demonstrate full ROM and strength, along with restoration of glenohumeral stability, typically between 6 and 9 months after surgery.

Throwing athletes require special consideration and follow a specific protocol designed to monitor their throwing distance and speed, which is slowly advanced over 2 to 3 months. Initially, at 6 months after surgery, an easy tossing program is begun at a distance of 20 ft, without a windup. Before each session, stretching is performed and heat is applied to increase circulation and improve ROM. At 7 months, light throwing with an easy windup at a distance of 30 ft is allowed 2 to 3 days per week for 10 minutes per session. Easy throws from 150 to 200 ft are permitted 9 months after surgery, and stronger throws from the same distance are allowed at 10 months. Pitchers can throw at half to three-quarters speed from the mound, with an emphasis on accuracy and technique, at 11 months. At 12 months, pitchers can throw at three-quarters to full speed. Throwers are allowed to return to full competition when they are able to throw at full speed without discomfort for 2 weeks, typically between 9 and 12 months after surgery.

RESULTS

With expanding interest in minimally invasive surgical techniques, the first successful accounts of arthroscopic posterior glenohumeral stabilization were produced in the 1990s.[71–73] In 1998, Wolf et al. reported on 14 patients who had arthroscopic posterior capsular plication for unidirectional posterior instability; at 33-month follow-up, 86% had good or excellent results and 93% had restoration of stability.[73] With improvement in arthroscopic techniques and surgical implants, research has led to the evolution of suture-anchor–based arthroscopic posterior glenohumeral stabilization. Numerous recent studies have revealed that good or excellent results have been achieved in a majority of cases, driving further interest in these methods.

Arthroscopic stabilization for unidirectional posterior glenohumeral instability has been of particular interest. Williams et al. retrospectively reported on 27 shoulders with symptomatic posterior capsulolabral complex detachment from the posterior glenoid rim, with minimal posterior capsular laxity, after a distinct traumatic event.[14] Isolated arthroscopic posterior capsulolabral repair was performed with bioabsorbable tack fixation in all patients.[14] Subjective instability and pain were eliminated in 92% of patients, with all patients returning to unlimited athletic activity by 6 months. Kim prospectively reported on 27 athletes with traumatic unidirectional RPS who were treated with arthroscopic posterior labral repair and capsular shift; all patients had a labral lesion, and 81% also had stretching of the posterior band of the IGHL.[52] The posterior capsule was shifted superiorly in all cases. All complete labral lesions were repaired directly, and incomplete labral lesions were converted to complete tears and then repaired. The mean ASES scores improved from 51.2 to 96.5. All patients except for one experienced restoration of stability and were able to return to their previous athletic activities with few or no limitations.

Multiple additional studies involving between 12 and 34 shoulders have revealed similar successful results for arthroscopic posterior stabilization, with recurrence rates between 0% and 12% and a minimum mean follow-up of 3 years.[6,8,36,74–77] In 2008, Radkowski et al. reported on arthroscopic capsulolabral repair for posterior shoulder instability in throwing athletes compared with nonthrowing athletes.[74] At 27-month mean follow-up, no differences were found in the ASES score or scores for stability, ROM, strength, pain, and function between the 27 throwing shoulders and the 80 nonthrowing shoulders, with both groups showing significant improvement in all categories. Excellent or good results were achieved in 89% of throwers and 93% of nonthrowers. However, throwing athletes were less likely to return to the preinjury level of sport (55%) compared with nonthrowing athletes (71%).[74] Due to the relatively small patient population in this study, the reason for the lower rate of return to sport in throwers was difficult to identify. Interestingly, all of the three throwers in whom the procedure failed underwent capsulolabral repair without suture anchors. Based on the findings of this study, the authors presently advocate repair with suture anchors uniformly. In addition, within the thrower group more athletes were unable to return to their previous levels of sport compared with those for whom the procedure failed based on the subjective instability scale, which suggests that some of these athletes might have had lower levels of subjective instability but enough to keep them from returning to the same high level of competition and meeting the unique demands required from the shoulder during throwing activities.

In 2008, Savoie et al. reported a 97% success rate for the treatment of 92 shoulders with posterior instability using arthroscopic techniques.[78] The mean age of the patients was 26 years, and mean follow-up was 28 months. Pathology discovered at the time of surgery was an isolated reverse Bankart lesion in 51%, a stretched posterior capsule in 67%, and a combination of a reverse Bankart lesion and capsular stretching in 16%. The rotator interval was determined to be damaged in 61% and was closed in all but five patients (95%). One patient had recurrent gross subluxation, and one had recurrent dislocation.

Lenart et al. reported 100% return to previous level of athletic activity for 34 shoulders for which arthroscopic repair for posterior shoulder instability was performed.[77] The majority (78%) had sustained a traumatic event, but only two (6%) entailed a frank dislocation, consistent with a population of RPS. Suture anchor repair was performed in 30 patients (88%), and capsular plication to an intact labrum was performed in four patients (12%).

Wanich and colleagues also presented the results of arthroscopic treatment of posterior capsulolabral lesions in persons with batter's shoulder, defined as posterior subluxation of the lead shoulder during a baseball swing.[36] Eleven of 12 patients treated with surgery (92%) returned to their previous level of batting at an average of 5.9 months after surgery, with no detectable ROM deficit compared with before surgery.

Arner et al. evaluated 56 consecutive American football players with posterior shoulder instability who underwent an arthroscopic posterior capsulolabral repair with or without suture anchors.[79] At a mean follow-up of 44.7 months, 93% returned to sport and 79% returned to the same level of play. Statistically significant improvements were seen in ASES scores, as well as scores of stability, ROM, strength, pain, and function. Excellent or good results (ASES score >60; stability <6) were achieved in 96.5% of athletes, and 96% were satisfied with their surgery.[79]

In 2006, Bradley presented a larger prospective study that included 91 athletes (100 shoulders) treated with arthroscopic capsulolabral reconstruction for posterior instability.[8] He expanded upon this initial study to include 183 athletes (200 shoulders) in 2013, which is the largest patient cohort to date.[80] Included in the study were 99 athletes involved in contact sports and 101 athletes involved in noncontact sports. All patients had unidirectional posterior instability, and a course of nonoperative management had failed. Arthroscopy with suture anchor repair was the most common procedure performed ($n = 119$), followed by suture-only repair without anchors ($n = 44$) and suture anchor repair with supplementary plication sutures ($n = 37$). In his follow-up study at a mean of 36 months postoperatively, the mean ASES scores improved from 45.9 to 85.1, with 90% return to sport and 64% returning to their same level as before surgery. Potential reasons elucidated for the failures included undiagnosed MDI, inadequate capsular shift because of unappreciated capsular laxity, inadequate recognition of poor capsular tissue quality in patients referred after thermal capsulorrhaphy, and capsular plication performed in an isolated fashion without suture anchors.[8,80] The authors also concluded that the incorporation of bone suture-anchors in capsulolabral reconstruction led to higher ASES scores and rate of RTP.[80]

COMPLICATIONS

The most likely complication resulting from arthroscopic posterior stabilization is recurrent instability (<10%). The majority of patients, however, will achieve a successful outcome with proper technique and adherence to a strict protocol-driven rehabilitation program. Postoperative stiffness is relatively uncommon but can be encountered in patients that underwent concomitant posterior capsular plication. Early posterior capsular stretching can help avoid this complication, and in those patients where ROM is not restored, posterior capsulotomy can be performed if deemed necessary.

Various intraoperative complications may occur during arthroscopic posterior stabilization. Erroneous placement of the 7-o'clock posterior portal may result in damage to the posterior humeral circumflex artery or the suprascapular nerve and artery,

which lie on average 39 mm and 29 mm away, respectively.[81] The axillary nerve is also at risk during arthroscopic repair of the posteroinferior shoulder capsule, particularly with placement of the most inferior suture anchor. In a cadaveric study, Price et al. performed a microsurgical dissection through the IGHL from within the joint capsule to examine the relationship of the axillary nerve as it traversed the quadrangular space.[82] In each dissection, the teres minor branch was the closest to the glenoid rim. The closest point between the axillary nerve and the glenoid rim was at the 6-o'clock position on the inferior glenoid rim. At this position, the average distance between the axillary nerve and the glenoid rim was 12.4 mm. The axillary nerve lay, throughout its course, at an average of 2.5 mm from the IGHL. Thus when performing arthroscopic plication on the inferior glenohumeral joint capsule, care must be taken to avoid overpenetration with the suture passer, which could injure the adjacent axillary nerve. Further, the use of a thermal device for inferior capsular shrinkage should be avoided, because axillary nerve injury has been reported with that surgical technique.[83]

Perioperative complications can also occur as result of the implants selected for arthroscopic stabilization. Metallic anchors were first produced and used in soft tissue fixation around the shoulder. However, their use resulted in some reported complications, including articular surface damage from migrating implants and distortion, and artifact production in postoperative MRI.[84] Bioabsorbable anchors were developed to avoid these problems and have proved to have pull-out strength equal to that of metallic anchors, with a reported lower complication rate.[84] This finding led to a major shift away from metallic anchors toward bioabsorbable anchors. However, the use of some bioabsorbable suture anchors in the shoulder—in particular, those composed of polylactic acid—have resulted in notable complications. Rare cases of premature absorption, osteolysis, glenohumeral synovitis, cyst formation, soft tissue inflammation, and release of implant fragments into the joint space have been reported.[85–89] These results have been thought to be due specifically to the biologic properties of these early-generation implants. Thus patients who experience postoperative pain, stiffness, or mechanical symptoms or fail to progress as expected should be examined for these potential implant-related complications. Recent improvements in bioabsorbable suture-anchor materials, namely concerning their mechanical and resorptive properties, have potentially led to a decrease in these biocompatibility issues; further study is warranted to confirm these observed trends. In addition, newer materials, such as biocomposites and polyetheretherketone (PEEK), have recently been introduced. These materials may address concerns of biocompatibility and material strength, but additional rigorous in vitro and in vivo trials need to be conducted before their use becomes widespread.[88]

Iatrogenic glenoid chondral damage is a risk during arthroscopic posterior labral repair and typically occurs with a low, tangential drilling angle (<30 degrees) during anchor placement. This complication can be avoided with proper placement of the posterior portal, which allows a higher angle (>30 degrees) of approach to the glenoid rim. Transection of the labrum during preparation can occur and compromise the ability to achieve an anatomic repair. In instances where this occurs, the posterior capsule can be used utilizing an extracapsular technique to repair the capsule to the posterior glenoid margin. In addition to chondral or labral damage, malposition of the anchors can also lead to pain, decreased ROM, and failure of the repair.[90]

Venous thromboembolism (VTE) events are rare, but not unheard of, after shoulder arthroscopy. In a recent analysis of more than 65,000 arthroscopic procedures, Jameson et al. found the rate of deep venous thrombosis, pulmonary embolism, and mortality rates to be less than 0.01%, 0.01%, and 0.03%, respectively.[91] The authors concluded that thromboprophylaxis for VTE events may not be required, even in high-risk patients, because the 2007 National Institute for Health and Clinical Excellence guidelines did not affect VTE event rates.

▉ SUMMARY

Posterior shoulder instability poses a significant challenge to the orthopedist, both diagnostically and therapeutically. It is a broad clinical entity, ranging from RPS to locked posterior dislocations. Pathogenesis also varies tremendously and is based on the stress placed on the involved shoulder. As opposed to a singular traumatic event, athletes with RPS typically experience chronic, repetitive microtrauma that leads to a posterior labral tear, posterior capsular laxity, and symptoms. Overhead throwers are a unique patient population, often with a varied presentation that can include posterior capsular contracture and the type VIII SLAP tear. Extensive basic science and clinical research is ongoing to elucidate a biomechanical explanation of the pathogenesis of RPS in throwers. Increased clinical awareness, as well as advances in imaging and physical examination techniques, have improved diagnosis in athletes and patients from wide demographic presentations. Multiple distinct pathologic lesions can be identified on MRA in patients with RPS; these lesions should be sought carefully during the workup of symptomatic patients. Specific provocative physical examination tests have been found to be useful in making the diagnosis of posterior shoulder instability.

Successful outcomes can be achieved with physical therapy, although many patients still require surgical intervention to alleviate symptoms and return to sport at their preinjury level. The transition from open to arthroscopic surgical techniques has facilitated more comprehensive identification and treatment of coexisting structural pathologies in persons with RPS. For patients with unidirectional posterior instability, an arthroscopic repair of the capsulolabral complex is recommended. When a patulous posterior capsule or a posteroinferior component of instability is also present, an arthroscopic superiorly directed capsular shift and capsular plication are added. In throwing athletes with RPS and a posterior labral tear, we advocate repairing the posterior labrum only and initially treating excessive GIRD, if present, with preoperative sleeper stretches and, if it is recalcitrant, with a limited posterior capsular release at the time of surgery. With regard to addressing capsular pathology, we generally tend toward overtightening in athletes in contact sports and in persons with significant capsular laxity and undertightening in overhead throwers.

FUTURE CONSIDERATIONS

Success rates between 90% and 100% have been achieved with arthroscopic repair techniques, with generally lower results in throwing athletes. With midterm results demonstrating favorable results, longer term studies are necessary to evaluate the durability of arthroscopic techniques in the treatment of posterior glenohumeral instability. Further work is also needed to elucidate the complex mechanics of the elite thrower's shoulder and the best path to alleviating the symptoms of RPS while simultaneously allowing return to sport at the preinjury level.

For a complete list of references, go to ExpertConsult.com.

SELECTED READINGS

Citation:

DeLong JM, Jiang K, Bradley JP. Posterior instability of the shoulder: a systematic review and meta-analysis of clinical outcomes. *Am J Sports Med.* 2015;43(7):1805–1817, 2015.

Level of Evidence:

IV

Summary:

This systematic review and meta-analysis reviews the literature regarding clinical outcomes for arthroscopic and open treatment of unidirectional posterior instability of the shoulder. Fifty-three unique publications were included. Despite overall similar results in the overall athletic population, throwing athletes are less likely to return to preinjury level of play. Literature suggests arthroscopic treatment has improvement in outcomes in regard to recurrence of instability, patient satisfaction, return to sport and preinjury level of play.

Citation:

Kim SH, Ha KI, Park JH, et al. Arthroscopic posterior labral repair and capsular shift for traumatic unidirectional recurrent posterior subluxation of the shoulder. *J Bone Joint Surg Am.* 2003;85A(8): 1479–1487.

Level of Evidence:

II

Summary:

This clinical study features the Kim classification for describing posterior labral tear morphology, including the "Kim lesion," and a report on the overall successful arthroscopic management of unilateral recurrent posterior subluxation in 37 patients.

Citation:

Song DJ, Cook JB, Krul KP, et al. High frequency of posterior and combined shoulder instability in young active patients. *J Shoulder Elbow Surg.* 2015;24(2):186–190.

Level of Evidence:

III

Summary:

This retrospective review of 231 consecutive patients evaluated the frequency of posterior and combined shoulder instability in patients that underwent operative stabilization procedures. Secondarily this study assessed preoperative magnetic resonance imaging reports to determine their accuracy in identifying pathology that was addressed at the time of surgery.

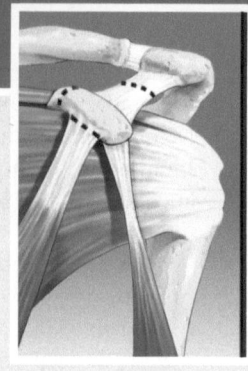

42

Multidirectional Instability of the Shoulder

Robert M. Carlisle, John M. Tokish

The shoulder is unique in that it is the most mobile joint in the human body. It serves primarily to position the hand in space and thus requires a delicate balance of stability and flexibility to accomplish its function. The inherent complexity of the glenohumeral joint requires contributions from both dynamic and static stabilizers to achieve this balance. Further, whereas some activities, such as swimming, place a premium on flexibility, others, such as lifting a weight overhead, value stability more highly. Shoulder instability is a spectrum of pathologic conditions in which the humeral head exceeds the functional or physiologic limit of the confines of the glenoid labral complex, resulting in a sensation that is troubling to the patient.

Instability of the shoulder can be in any cardinal direction or in a combination of directions. In 1980 Neer and Foster[1] introduced the term *multidirectional instability* (MDI), which refers to anterior and posterior instability associated with involuntary inferior subluxation or dislocation. Matsen[2] subsequently categorized shoulder instability into two general types: (1) traumatic and unidirectional with a Bankart lesion treated surgically, and (2) atraumatic, multidirectional, and bilateral, responds to rehabilitation, and may require an inferior capsular shift for surgical treatment. Although these categories are helpful for general classification, one must be careful not to oversimplify MDI. Patients with MDI can certainly present with unilateral symptoms, and although it is less common, they may present only after a traumatic event. As a result, both Neer's description of MDI and Matsen's description of the second general type have been modified to reflect our increasing understanding of the multidirectionally unstable shoulder.

It is important to consider the contributions of both normal anatomy and functional demands to more fully understand MDI.[3] Laxity is highly variable within the shoulder and thus, in and of itself, is not equal to instability. Many patients use an increase in laxity to optimize performance; for example, laxity provides elite swimmers with a competitive advantage. These athletes rely on a dynamic stability provided by the shoulder and periscapular musculature to allow extreme ranges of motion without pathologic instability.[4] Thus physical signs of laxity, such as the sulcus sign, or the ability of a patient to demonstrate subluxation, should not be equated with shoulder instability.[5,6] Without a precise definition of MDI, it is critically important to use all the tools available to the treating physician, including history, physical examination, imaging, examination while the patient is anesthetized, and diagnostic arthroscopy, to ensure that the appropriate anatomic deficiency of patients with MDI is addressed.

Glenohumeral stability results from a complex interplay of static and dynamic stabilizers. Static stabilization of the glenohumeral joint is controlled by such factors as the native depth of the glenoid and surrounding labral complex, as well as the length and stiffness of the shoulder capsule and supporting ligaments. Although the depth of the glenoid has been shown to provide a small restraint to glenohumeral translation, and patients with MDI demonstrate glenoid cavities that are more shallow than those of age-matched control subjects,[7-9] the characteristic pathologic entity in persons with MDI is increased capsular redundancy.[1,10,11] This redundancy may be congenital and associated with a systemic disease, such as Ehlers-Danlos syndrome,[12] osteogenesis imperfecta,[13] Marfan syndrome,[14] benign joint hypermobility syndrome, and fascioscapulohumeral dystrophy, or it can be acquired from repeated minor injuries (microtrauma) or repetitive use during exercises that stretch the capsuloligamentous restraints. Different parts of the capsule have been shown to be responsible for glenohumeral stability because the position of the shoulder and the direction of opposing forces are varied. The anterior and posterior bands of the inferior glenohumeral ligament act as a hammock to balance the humeral head on the glenoid.[15-17] The most significant restraint to inferior subluxation of the humeral head is the rotator interval complex, consisting of the superior glenohumeral ligament and coracohumeral ligament together with the inferior glenohumeral ligament complex.[18,19]

The shoulder is also dynamically stabilized by the rotator cuff, deltoid, and long head of the biceps, which collectively serve to compress the humeral head into the glenoid in a phenomenon coined *concavity compression*. One study demonstrated that the shoulder could resist translational loads equal to 60% of the compressive load applied.[20] In addition, the periscapular musculature can affect the position of the scapula, effectively altering glenoid version and inclination. Although the role of these dynamic stabilizers is more difficult to study, abnormal scapular kinematics and muscle activation patterns have been demonstrated in patients with MDI compared with asymptomatic control subjects.[9,21-23] One explanation of the etiology of MDI is the combination of baseline hyperlaxity and acquired scapular muscle dysfunction. This theory may explain why some swimmers present with impingement syndrome, why some baseball pitchers experience internal impingement, and why other patients with hyperlaxity present with pain as their chief complaint.

HISTORY

MDI can be very challenging to diagnose correctly. Patients usually do not report instability but rather vague pain of insidious onset, and thus the chief complaint is often not suggestive of the diagnosis. Further, although patients usually present with hyperlaxity, it is often not significantly different from their asymptomatic other side, and thus discerning between normal laxity versus instability in a particular patient can be confusing. Nevertheless, the history and physical examination are the critical steps in making an accurate diagnosis, and maintaining a high level of clinical suspicion is essential given the variety of presenting complaints.

Most patients with MDI present with a chief complaint of activity-related pain, but they may also report decreased strength or athletic performance. It is important to identify which activities are causative, because MDI is more common in overhead throwing sports, and the offending activity gives insight into both the focus of treatment and the patient's expectations for return. Reports of pain when carrying a heavy object, such as a suitcase, should raise suspicion. Cofield and Irving[24] stressed four questions in the workup of MDI: (1) What is the relationship to trauma? (2) Does the patient intentionally cause the instability? (3) What is the degree of instability? (4) What is the direction of instability? Regarding the first question, most patients with MDI have an atraumatic onset, whereas a single inciting event can be responsible for tipping the patient from hyperlaxity to instability. If one loosens the definition of "trauma" to include repetitive use or conditions that compromise the dynamic stabilizers, one can gain a much deeper understanding of the source of the patient's complaints and a rational approach to addressing them. The second question about volitional instability by Cofield and Irving is also critical. Since publication of the classic article by Rowe and colleagues,[25] it has become a tenet that patients with willful dislocation should be approached cautiously. However, as pointed out by Mallon and Speer,[10] it should be remembered that not all patients who have the ability to dislocate the shoulder have a psychological pathologic condition, which is an important differentiator in the treatment algorithm.

The degree of instability is another important component of the history. Patients with MDI may undergo either recurrent subluxation or dislocation, although the former is more common,[10] and an understanding of the degree of instability may help determine the aggressiveness of the treatment program. When patients report that their joint "slips" out in the absence of trauma or during sleep, clinical suspicion should be heightened. Finally, the question of the primary direction of instability in patients with MDI is critical to making a complete and accurate assessment and correctly designing an approach to treatment. Most patients do not have true global instability, and distinguishing between true MDI and unidirectional instability with multidirectional laxity is one of the critical steps guiding treatment.[3] Finally, it is critical to understand the diagnosis in the context of the patient. The type of activity the patient expects to resume and within what time frame, as well as the management of the individual patient's expectations about rehabilitation and return, are essential in guiding successful treatment.

PHYSICAL EXAMINATION

Foster[26] has noted that the most useful tool for making the diagnosis of MDI is the physical examination. Because patients with MDI often have vague complaints, it is essential to perform a thorough physical examination. Generalized ligamentous laxity has long been considered a hallmark of MDI and should be evaluated in each patient. Beighton et al.[27] reported on five physical signs of joint hyperlaxity (Table 42.1), which add up to a potential of nine points. Knee, elbow, thumb, and metacarpophalangeal hyperextension are all given a point for each side, along with the patient's ability to place his or her hands flat on the floor with straight knees from a standing position. Any score greater than 3 is considered good evidence of generalized ligamentous laxity and should alert the examiner to the presence of this condition. Other classification systems have been reported for collagen disorders, including the Villefranche nosology[28] system for Ehlers-Danlos syndrome subtypes and the Ghent criteria defining Marfan syndrome.[29] It is important to recognize these connective tissue disorders, because they have been associated with poorer results after surgical stabilization.[30] Finally, hyperelasticity and scarring in skin folds, as well as keloid formation or widening of scars, are also suggestive of a collagen disorder.[31] The presence of generalized ligamentous laxity is not sufficient for the diagnosis of instability because a wide spectrum of asymptomatic laxities exists in all cardinal directions.[32–34]

Since the original description by Neer and Foster,[1] the sulcus sign has been considered the *sine qua non* of MDI (Fig. 42.1).[35] This test is performed by placing axial traction on the arm in its resting position at the patient's side and can be evaluated with rotation, as well as at varying degrees of abduction. This action should produce a visible and palpable sulcus underneath the acromion as the humerus translates inferiorly. Although Harryman et al.[36] noted significant variation in what a "normal"

TABLE 42.1 Beighton Scale for Multidirectional Laxity	
Characteristic	**Score**
Passive dorsiflexion of the little finger beyond 90 degrees	1 point for each hand
Passive apposition of the thumb to the ipsilateral forearm	1 point for each hand
Active hyperextension of the elbow beyond 10 degrees	1 point for each hand
Active hyperextension of the knee beyond 10 degrees	1 point for each hand
Forward flexion of the trunk with extended knees so that the palms of the hands rest flat on the floor	1 point

A score greater than 3 out of a possible 9 points is diagnostic of hyperlaxity.

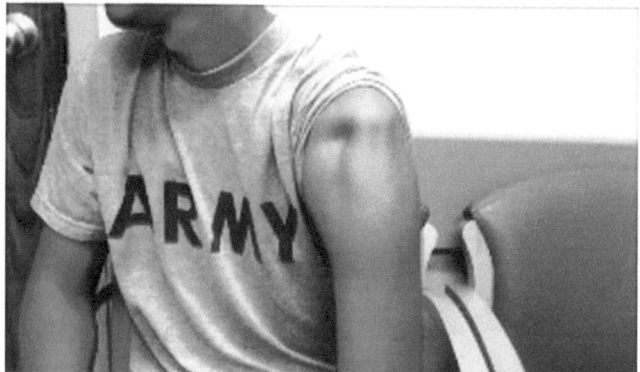

Fig. 42.1 The sulcus sign.

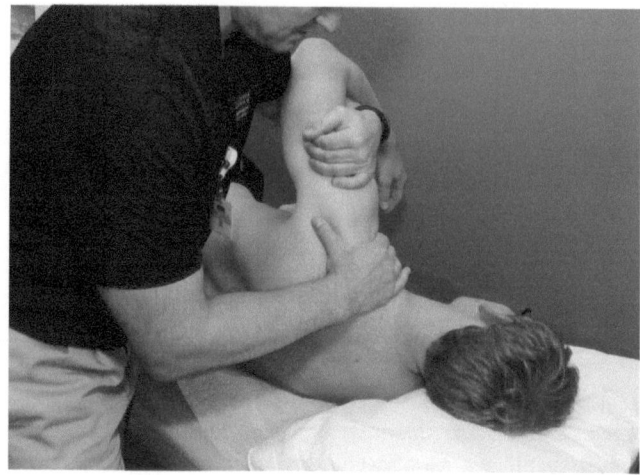

Fig. 42.2 The abducted anterior load-and-shift test. This test can be performed in the lateral decubitus position in a patient who is awake or anesthetized. This position allows the examiner to stabilize the scapula with one hand and translate the humerus with the other.

sulcus is, in a healthy control group, the sulcus measured approximately 11 mm upon testing. Humeral head displacement of more than 2 cm from the acromion, as well as the presence of a sulcus sign with 90 degrees abduction, is indicative of considerable inferior capsular laxity.[1,7,37] It is again important to heed Matsen's caution that to make the diagnosis of MDI, the sulcus sign must reproduce the patient's symptoms.[38]

The hyperabduction test as described by Gagey and Gagey[39] is another test for inferior glenohumeral laxity in which patients are evaluated for comparative glenohumeral abduction. In asymptomatic volunteers, abduction averages greater than 90 degrees, and a positive test is indicated by passive abduction greater than 105 degrees. Although MDI was an exclusion criterion in the study, Balg and Boileau[40] found shoulder hyperlaxity anteriorly or inferiorly, as defined by excessive external rotation and a positive hyperabduction test, respectively, to be an independent variable for recurrent instability after an arthroscopic Bankart procedure.

In addition to inferior instability, it is important to examine any patient with suspected MDI for anterior and posterior instability. With the common finding of generalized laxity, it is important that these provocative maneuvers result in the reproduction of the patient's symptoms. The apprehension test[41] is a workhorse test for anterior instability that is performed with the patient either seated or supine. With this test, the examiner takes the patient's arm into maximal external rotation with the shoulder at 90 degrees of abduction. Reproduction of the patient's symptoms here is a reliable indicator of anterior instability.[42] Another common method of assessment for instability is the abducted anterior load-and-shift test. This test is performed with the patient either in the seated, supine, or lateral decubitus position (Fig. 42.2). This latter position is particularly helpful because the scapula can be controlled with one hand while the humerus is translated with the other. The humeral head is loaded axially to ensure it is centered and then translated forward. The test is graded on the basis of how far the humeral head travels in relation to the glenoid (Table 42.2)[43]: Grade 0, little to no movement of the humeral head; grade 1, the humeral head rides up to the glenoid labrum; grade 2, the humeral head is shifted off the glenoid but spontaneously reduces when pressure is removed; and grade 3, the humeral head is shifted off the glenoid and remains dislocated once the pressure is removed.

TABLE 42.2 Grading System for Load and Shift for Instability

Grade	Characteristic Glenoid Position
1	Little to no movement of the humeral head
2	The humeral head rides up to the glenoid labrum
3	The humeral head is shifted off the glenoid but spontaneously reduces when pressure is removed
4	The humeral head is shifted off the glenoid and remains dislocated once the pressure is removed

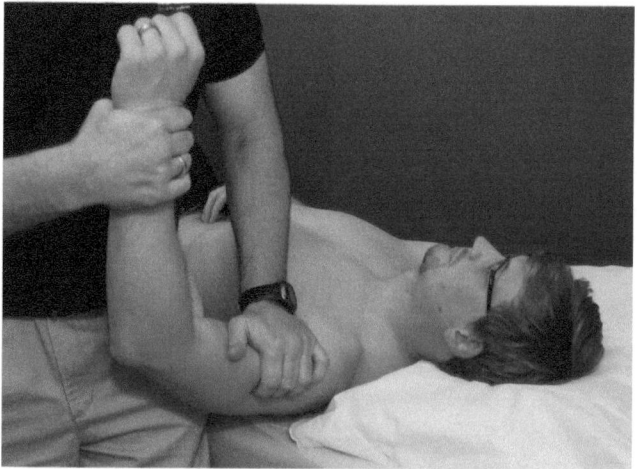

Fig. 42.3 The push–pull test performed with an anesthetized patient. This test can also be performed reliably in a patient who is awake.

For posterior instability, a similar load and shift maneuver can be performed. We have found that a modification of this test, the push-pull test,[44] is most effective in controlling posterior translation (Fig. 42.3). The push-pull test is performed with the patient supine; the arm is placed at 90 degrees abduction in neutral rotation and 30 degrees horizontal adduction. The examiner grasps around the patient's wrist with one hand (the pull) and posteriorly loads the humerus (the push), which places a fulcrum on the shoulder and enhances the examiner's ability to control subluxation. The evaluation of instability in all three directions is essential to determine the most effective treatment regimen for the patient.

It must be remembered that MDI is a combination of static and dynamic restraints, and therefore the physical examination of any patient with suspected MDI must include a thorough evaluation of the patient's musculature. This evaluation begins with visualization of the patient's scapular musculature and kinematics. Patients should be evaluated for atrophy, winging, and scapular motion. Deltoid and rotator cuff strength should be assessed and compared with the opposite side, with particular attention directed to scapular rhythm as the arm moves, specifically through the motion that causes the patient's symptoms. Symptoms can be far better explained by asymmetries in the musculature than by shoulder laxity.

IMAGING

Although MDI is primarily diagnosed clinically, imaging can enhance the work-up in many patients. Radiographs should be evaluated for abnormal glenoid version, dysplasia, or hypoplasia, and humeral head abnormalities also occasionally can be detected on radiographs. Magnetic resonance imaging provides a clearer picture of the soft tissue anatomy in the shoulder and is often combined with magnetic resonance arthrography to give perhaps the gold standard of anatomic evaluation for MDI. Although labral pathology can certainly be present in patients with MDI, the classic finding is increased capsular volume and a patulous capsule (Fig. 42.4).[45] Schaeffeler et al.[46] correlated the clinical diagnosis of atraumatic MDI with redundancy signs on magnetic resonance arthrography with high sensitivity and specificity. The finding of an increase in the rotator interval dimension of patients with MDI has been mixed.[47,48] A large retrospective review by Lee et al.[49] demonstrated larger rotator interval and capsular dimensions in MDI shoulders compared to controls. More recent research by Lim et al.[50] looked at labrocapsular distances on magnetic resonance arthrography and found

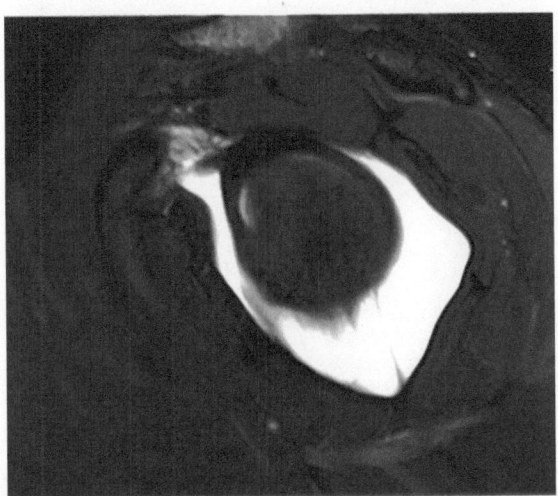

Fig. 42.4 Magnetic resonance imaging scan of a patulous capsule.

the inferior labrocapsular distance to have a high specificity and sensitivity of detecting clinical MDI.

DECISION-MAKING PRINCIPLES

The most important principle of treatment in patients with MDI or any shoulder pathology is an understanding of the activities performed by the patient. Especially in the athlete, a fine line often exists between the advantage of laxity and the limitations of instability. As noted earlier in the history section, understanding how the patient uses the shoulder and the expectations of the patient are essential to guide proper treatment.

In the absence of trauma, MDI usually results when a patient's dynamic stabilizers fail to compensate for a baseline lax joint. Consider a swimmer who presents with a chief complaint of pain after ramping up her training volume in preparation for a league championship, or a baseball pitcher who begins experiencing decreased control in the late innings of a game. In both cases, fatigue of the dynamic stabilizers results in their failure to restrain the baseline laxity, resulting in symptoms. Both scenarios illustrate the point that MDI has a significant dynamic muscular component, and that failure to recognize and treat this component will likely result in an unsatisfied patient. For this reason, conservative rehabilitation remains the mainstay of any initial treatment program of MDI.

Several studies have noted that in young patients with hypermobility, instability symptoms decrease as patients reach skeletal maturity, and thus a prolonged program of physical therapy is strongly recommended.[51-53] Kronberg et al.[54] found significant imbalances in muscular control in patients with generalized ligamentous laxity. These investigators noted that muscle-strengthening and scapular rhythm regimens may be more effective than soft tissue reconstructions in these patients. Such a treatment regimen improves tone and proprioceptive control of the deltoid and rotator cuff musculature and should focus on progressive resistance exercises that target the rotator cuff and deltoid muscles.[55] This targeting results in a substantial increase in rotator cuff activation, which functionally reduces instability.[56] In addition, scapulothoracic mechanics should be carefully evaluated, and any dyskinesia should be a major focus of the rehabilitation program. The synchronous firing of the serratus anterior, trapezii, rhomboids, and subscapularis position the scapular platform in space and can affect version and inclination, forming a stable base for the functioning of the glenohumeral joint. It is important to stress to the patient that these strengthening programs are a significant commitment, beginning with 6 months to 1 year of therapy, followed by a chronic maintenance program.[1,7,56]

In a classic study applying these principles, Burkhead and Rockwood[55] evaluated the results of a rehabilitation program to treat patients with instability. In patients with atraumatic instability, 83% of patients obtained a good or an excellent result with muscle strengthening, and nearly 90% of those with MDI obtained a similar result. However, other reports have been less favorable. Kiss et al.[57] evaluated a similar group and found good or excellent results in only 61% of their patients; they noted that patients with a work-related injury or psychological problems were less likely to benefit from the rehabilitation program. Misamore et al.[58] performed a careful longitudinal study of 64 patients with MDI who underwent physical therapy as their initial treatment. These investigators found that at 2-year follow-up, 66% of patients had either required operative stabilization or reported only fair or poor shoulder outcomes. More discouraging, at a final follow-up of 8 years, only 30% of the cohort had avoided surgical intervention and rated their shoulder as good or excellent, with only eight patients free of pain or instability complaints. In a study by Nyiri et al.[59] it was found that kinematic parameters and muscle activity patterns can be normalized after surgery and physical therapy, but not with physical therapy alone. Thus although rehabilitation remains a mainstay of treatment for patients with MDI, this condition represents a significant therapeutic challenge and may fail to result in long-term patient satisfaction and return to activity.

TREATMENT OPTIONS

Surgical treatment for MDI should be considered after failure of a long-term rehabilitation program and a frank discussion with the patient about expectations and the need for a postoperative commitment to rehabilitation. The primary pathologic condition in MDI is a loose, redundant capsule, especially inferiorly, and thus the aim of surgical intervention is to reduce the redundancy and effectively shorten the static stabilizers, especially in the primary direction of instability. Techniques, such as capsular shifts, thermal capsulorrhaphy, capsulolabral augmentation, supplementary support, and arthroscopic plication, have been used to accomplish this goal.

Open Inferior Capsular Shift

The open inferior capsular shift was the original operative procedure described by Neer and Foster,[1] in which they performed a humeral-based shift to eliminate capsular redundancy (Fig. 42.5). This procedure could be performed anteriorly or posteriorly or even combined in rare cases to address global capsular redundancy. Patients are positioned in a beach chair-type position, and a standard deltopectoral approach is used. The subscapularis is taken down and the rotator interval between the superior and middle glenohumeral ligaments is closed. A T-shaped humeral-based incision is then made, creating an inferior and superior flap of the anterior capsule, which is elevated from the humeral neck. From here, intra-articular pathology can be identified and addressed. The magnitude of the capsular shift remains an art, balancing the stability gained by reducing the volume of the capsule with expectations of postoperative range of motion (ROM). The inferior capsule is advanced superiorly, and the superior capsule is attached over the top to reinforce this shift. The subscapularis is then reattached separately in its original position, and the procedure is complete after examination reveals appropriate motion without undue stress on the repair. Several investigators have demonstrated that this technique results in high satisfaction rates with low rates of recurrence.[1,5,6,60–66] However, more modern evaluations of success, including return to sporting activities, have been less enthusiastic.[63,64,67] Since the

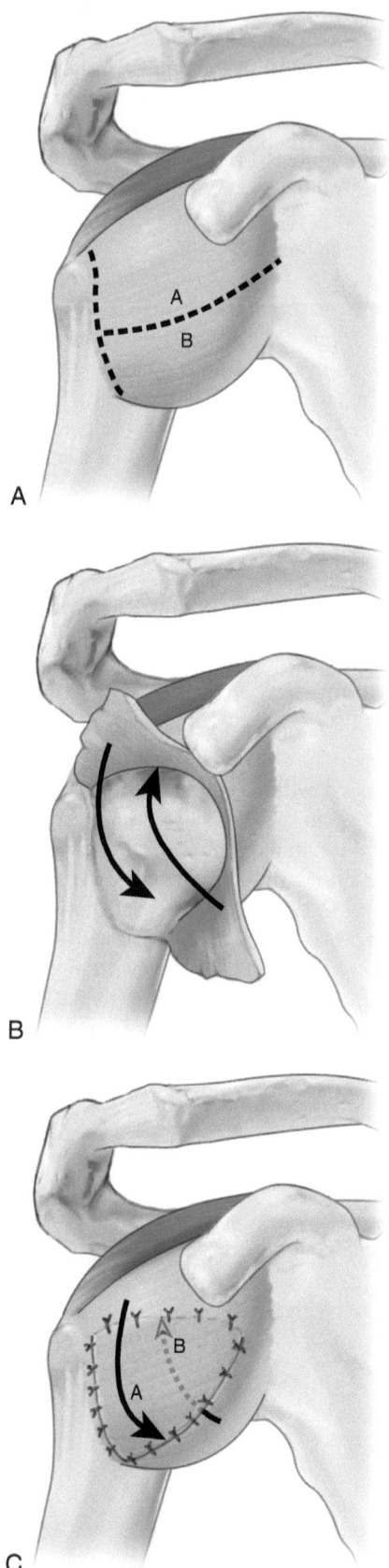

Fig. 42.5 Inferior capsular shift. (A) A T-shaped humeral-based incision is made in the anterior capsule, creating an inferior and superior flap. (B) These flaps are elevated off the humeral neck so they can be shifted. (C) The inferior capsule is advanced superiorly, and the superior capsule is then attached over the top to reinforce the shift.

original description, several modifications to this technique have been reported, including a subscapularis-sparing technique[5] and a glenoid-based shift.[67–69]

Arthroscopic Plication

The development of advanced arthroscopic techniques has provided increased visualization of the glenohumeral joint and the ability to approach the pathology on both sides of the glenoid through a single approach, without violating the subscapularis attachment. This technique is especially well suited for patients with posteroinferior MDI, in whom a lack of posterior labral height can decrease resistance to posterior shear stress and contribute to instability in some patients,[8,70] or for patients with both a posterior and anterior component, for whom traditionally a second approach would be required. Standard posterior and posterolateral portals, along with anterosuperior and midglenoid portals, suffice to address all aspects of instability.

Arthroscopic capsular plication can be performed in either the beach chair or lateral decubitus position. The history and physical examination (previously detailed), as well as an examination while the patient is anesthetized, can help determine the primary direction of instability, which should be addressed first. Wichman and Snyder[71] described an arthroscopic technique for addressing capsular redundancy through plication. After biologic preparation of the capsule with rasping or light débridement, a suture hook loaded with a suture shuttle relay is used to create a pinch stitch inferiorly within the capsule. This stitch is then advanced superiorly and medially through the labrum, creating an overlap that effectively shortens and thickens the capsule. A nonabsorbable suture is then passed in a retrograde fashion, creating the plication stitch. The opposite end can be passed in a similar fashion to create a mattress stitch, if desired. Additional sutures can be placed anteriorly and posteriorly, progressing superiorly until the desired amount of plication is achieved. Several authors have compared the ability of an arthroscopic capsular shift to reduce volume in the shoulder.[72–74] Ponce et al.[73] demonstrated that each plication stitch reduces the volume of the joint by 10% in a linear relationship, and five such stitches equals the volume reduction of a lateral-based open inferior capsular shift. These findings suggest that arthroscopic multiple-pleat plication may be as effective as an open inferior capsular shift for eliminating capsular redundancy.

Sutures can be passed through the capsular tissue and sutured directly to the labrum, or a suture anchor can be used. Provencher et al.[75] demonstrated that although the strengths of the constructs were similar, plication without suture anchors resulted in more displacement at the labrum and may be preferable. Anchor-based plication was shown to be better biomechanically than suture capsulorrhaphy in a biomechanical study by Kersten et al.[76]

Several authors have investigated these techniques in the clinical setting. Raynor et al.[77] followed 45 shoulders after arthroscopic pancapsulorrhaphy with suture anchors for a mean of 3.3 years. Kaplan-Meier survivorship at 1 year was 100% and 87% at 3 years. The recurrent instability rate was just under 17%, very similar to prior literature. Comparable results were reported by Alpert et al.[78] in their review of MDI patients with 270 degrees labral tears. While these two studies only utilized suture anchors, Gartsman et al.[79] followed up with 47 patients for 35 months

after arthroscopic suture and/or anchor-based plication for MDI. These investigators found good or excellent results in 94% of their patients, with a 2% recurrence rate, and noted that 85% of their patients were able to return to their desired level of sports. Several others have found success with a combination of suture anchors and/or plication sutures with similar results.[64,74–82]

Thermal capsulorrhaphy was advanced as an alternative to suture methods and provided the advantage of a simple and quick arthroscopic approach to address MDI. The theory was that heating the capsule disrupted the cross-linking of the collagen, allowing it to "crimp" and shorten. Despite early reported success,[89] other authors have reported high failure rates and the potential for chondrolysis and nerve injury with this technique,[90–92] and it has largely been abandoned. However, a recent multicenter, randomized, clinical trial by Mohtadi et al.[93] compared electrothermal arthroscopic capsulorrhaphy (ETAC) to open inferior capsular shift in patients with MDI. The group found nearly equivalent recurrence rates (1%) and outcomes in The Western Ontario Shoulder Instability Index (WOSI), American Shoulder and Elbow Surgeons (ASES) assessment form, and Constant scores at the 2-year follow-up.

Rotator interval closure remains a staple of the open procedure but is more controversial in the arthroscopic setting. Neer and Foster[1] routinely performed this adjunct at the beginning of their approach, and Harryman and colleagues[94] elegantly demonstrated that an open medial to lateral imbrication of the coracohumeral ligament greatly reduced inferior and posterior translation. The work by Harryman et al.[94] is often cited as justification for rotator interval closure in all settings. Other authors have been unable to replicate these findings[95] using a similar technique. In the arthroscopic setting, a rotator interval closure is most often performed in a superior to inferior fashion. However, cadaveric models have failed to demonstrate that this technique assists in reducing inferior translation,[96,97] instead, these models have shown that it results in a restriction of external rotation. As rotator interval closure continues to be debated, it should be applied judiciously with an understanding of its limitations.

It should be noted that most of the operative outcomes studies for MDI have short-term follow-up periods and that results may deteriorate over time.[10] Authors from Rowe et al.[25] to Krishnan et al.[98] have recommended a combination of procedures to address the true collagenopathy. Biceps augmentation, allograft reconstruction, and glenoid osteotomy have all been attempted to control stability in patients with collagen abnormalities and MDI, but few studies are available to evaluate clinical outcomes with these alternative approaches.[10,98] Nonetheless, new techniques are continually being developed to address the problem.[99]

POSTOPERATIVE MANAGEMENT

In general, the risk of recurrence after MDI is higher than the risk of stiffness, and therefore a cautious approach is best. The shoulder is placed in neutral rotation for 6 weeks using an immobilizer with a slight abduction pillow. One of the most critical points of the postoperative program is to understand that immobilization does not mean neglect. Patients are encouraged to begin using the hand, wrist, and elbow immediately after surgery. Further, although shoulder motion is limited for this period, we

🔖 Authors' Preferred Technique

Multidirectional Instability

- Understanding each individual patient's condition and expectations is critical in our treatment decision process.
- As previously expressed, making the diagnosis of multidirectional instability versus multidirectional laxity can be difficult, but it is vital for the appropriate treatment.
- In our experience, not all "therapy" is equal, and good communication among the surgeon, patient, and therapist to ensure the proper emphasis on strength and balance can result in excellent outcomes without operative intervention.
- For patients in which conservative management fails, an arthroscopic approach is preferred for its ability to address circumferential pathology and to allow more aggressive reengagement of the shoulder musculature postoperatively.
- We prefer an arthroscopic approach in the lateral position as it offers improved visualization in our experience.

Portals

- Preoperative examination under anesthesia is critical in our assessment of the patient's stability; you must have a baseline.
- All aspects of the glenoid labrum and capsule can be approached through standard posterior, anterosuperior, and midglenoid portals.[100]
- We will use a modified posterolateral portal for the proper angle of attack posteriorly and inferiorly as previously described in the literature.[100]

Plication Strategy

- After a thorough diagnostic arthroscopy, all identified associated pathology is addressed before the capsular plication. In our experience, it is common to have labral and other pathology in addition to capsular laxity.
- It is critical to biologically prepare the capsule for plication, using either a rasp or a shaver without suction to optimize postoperative healing.
- The plication begins inferiorly and advances superior using each stitch as a reference for the next.
- Capsular redundancy is eliminated with a pinch–tuck technique (Fig. 42.6) while suture anchors are used on the glenoid.
- The anterior and posterior insertions of the inferior glenohumeral cardinal ligament are grasped on either side using double-loaded suture anchors at the 5:30 and 7:30 positions.
- A full-thickness capsular bite is taken with each suture. We are cautious not to get overzealous with the inferior plication stitches as thicker bites increase the risk of axillary nerve injury.
- The amount of plication is approximately 1 cm, but it is dependent on multiple factors, including the examination while the patient is anesthetized, hand dominance, and goal activities.
- As the case proceeds superiorly, either simple or mattress sutures and a combination of suture anchor or plication stitches are utilized, depending on the quality of the glenoid labrum.

Rotator Interval

- We do not routinely perform a rotator interval closure except in revision cases and in patients with known collagen disorders, and when doing so we usually only perform this closure on a patient's nondominant side.
- We have not found plication stitches near the biceps anchor to be helpful and therefore we do not plicate superiorly.

Closure

- Using the preoperative examination under anesthesia as the baseline, the stability exam is repeated upon completion of the plication (Fig. 42.7).
- The portals are closed, dressed sterilely, and a shoulder immobilizer with abduction pillow is applied.

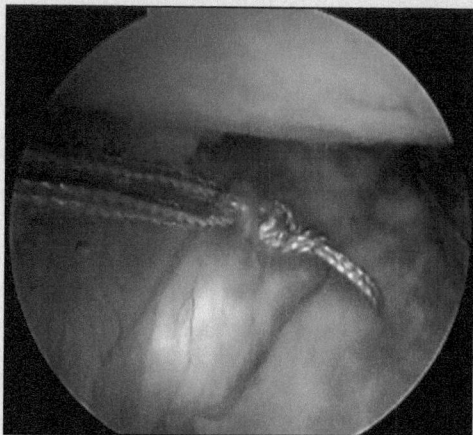

Fig. 42.6 Arthroscopic plication.

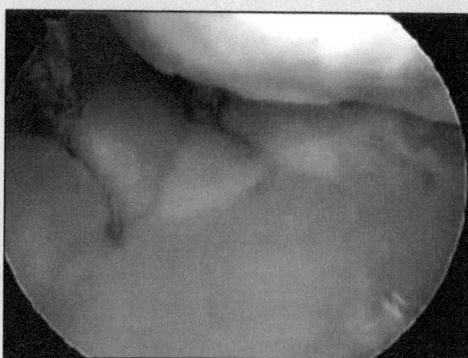

Fig. 42.7 Finished plication. At the completion of capsular plication, the glenoid bumper is restored and the capsular redundancy is diminished.

strongly believe that the rotator cuff and periscapular musculature should be dynamically reengaged as soon as possible after surgery. The arthroscopic and open approaches are similar, except that after arthroscopic capsular plication, the subscapularis is reengaged sooner than after an open repair. In our experience, it is rare for stiffness to develop in a patient with MDI, but atrophy of the dynamic stabilizers often persists after surgical intervention without a specific postoperative regimen to simultaneously protect the reconstruction and reactivate these muscle groups. Given the key role that the musculature plays in dynamic stability in persons with MDI specifically, 6 weeks of disuse atrophy must

be avoided. In one study, muscle strength decreased 54% after 7 weeks of immobilization and was only partially regained after remobilization.[101] Several authors have demonstrated that postoperative protocols can successfully restore normal muscle activation and motion patterns after capsular shift.[56,102] Thus early scapular mobilization (Fig. 42.8) is demonstrated to the patient preoperatively, along with isometric strengthening of the rotator cuff and periscapular musculature. Patients are encouraged to begin the exercises on postoperative day 1. In addition, because the shoulder works within a kinetic chain, core strengthening is an essential part of the perioperative strengthening program

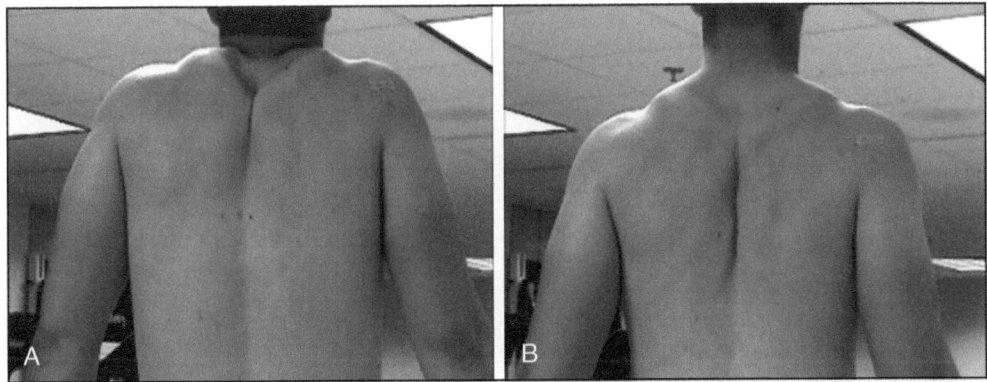

Fig. 42.8 Scapular mobilization. Early mobilization of the scapular musculature is performed to actively reengage the dynamic stabilizers of the shoulder. Here, scapular retraction and elevation are shown in (A) and (B), respectively, and protraction, depression, and rotation are emphasized.

and is actually taught in prehabilitation and is encouraged throughout the postoperative course.

At 6 weeks, the patient is evaluated for stiffness of the shoulder and maintenance of muscle rhythm and strength. At this point, the patient generally is allowed to stop using the sling and progress toward postoperative motion goals. These goals are tailored to the patient's expected needs. The chosen activity, arm dominance, and time frame of the ultimate return to sport are all considerations when making decisions about how quickly to proceed. Muscle strengthening is continued, and if the patient is on track, it is advanced. By 3 months, the patient should have reasonable humeroscapular rhythm with minimal scapular winging or substitution during elevation and abduction. Most of the patient's ROM is generally expected to have returned by this point.

Months 3 to 6 are devoted to fine tuning the desired ROM, and emphasis is placed on functional strength progression. Progression of loads is from low to high; speeds, from slow to fast; and direction, from unidirectional to multidirectional. Finally, the stability of the platform of these exercises can be perturbated to force dynamic co-contraction of the shoulder girdle. The physical therapist or corrective exercise specialist should be given the freedom to vary each of these parameters until the patient is confident and exhibits high performance in each of these aspects. At this point, usually around 6 months after surgery, the patient is cleared to progress to full activity, with emphasis on continued training with endurance activities so that fatigue won't precipitate decompensation of the dynamic stabilizers and compromise the result.

In the case of athletes, return-to-play (RTP) decisions should be made as a team. The surgeon must be confident that the reconstruction is healed and that the patient has achieved the necessary dynamic protection of the shoulder that was surgically repaired. The therapist or corrective exercise specialist is perhaps the most important decision maker for return to sport. This team member spends the most time with the athlete and learns to recognize how the athlete compensates or demonstrates poor dynamic control of the shoulder. It is the job of the therapist not only to help the patient regain strength in the shoulder girdle but also to ensure that this activity is placed well within an effective kinetic chain so that return to sport will not result in reinjury. The athlete also has an important role in the RTP decision. A patient's confidence in the stability of his or her shoulder, as well as open communication of any signs of trouble, are critical elements of the decision to return to activity that the patient alone can provide.

RESULTS

The results of the operative treatment of MDI are summarized in Table 42.3. Neer and Foster[1] originally reported a 97% satisfactory rate with the open inferior capsular shift, and this finding has been repeatedly borne out in the literature. However, patients with voluntary instability and an underlying psychiatric diagnosis are poor candidates for any operative approach.[1,10,25] It is also important to note that most of the reported series are relatively short term, and recurrence rates may increase with longer term follow-up.[10] Finally, the definition of MDI continues to be inconsistently applied. For example, the series by Altchek and colleagues[67] did not include any patients with generalized ligamentous laxity, yet it was described as a population of patients with MDI. The series by Kim and colleagues[70] consisted of patients with posteroinferior instability, and it was noted that all patients had a labral lesion, which is inconsistent with the definition provided by others.[31] A traumatic etiology has been frequently reported,[60] which is not a classic presentation in persons with MDI as defined by other authors.[2] Thus comparing findings across series is difficult, and surgeons should be careful not to oversimplify the diagnosis of MDI.

The arthroscopic approach to MDI has shown similar success rates to that of the classic open inferior capsular shift. In a systematic review of the MDI literature, Longo et al.[103] concluded that arthroscopic capsular plication and open capsular shift were the best procedures for MDI treatment after failed conservative management, and the results between the two modalities were comparable. The largest known meta-analysis of the literature by Chen et al.[104] found no difference between recurrent instability rates between open capsular shifts and arthroscopic capsular plications. However, Chen and colleagues did find a difference in postoperative stiffness between the two groups.

TABLE 42.3   Results for Operative Treatment of Multidirectional Instability

	Author	Follow-Up	Technique Details	Outcome Measure	Success Rate	Complications/Notes
Open inferior capsular shift	Neer and Foster[1]	<2 years	Open inferior capsular shift	Recurrence	98% satisfactory	None
	Pollock et al.[63]	5.1 years	Open inferior capsular shift	Satisfaction/recurrence	94% good/excellent; 4% recurrence	
	Cooper and Brems[6]	3.3 years	Open inferior capsular shift	Satisfaction/recurrence	86% improved; 10% recurrence	15% believed their shoulder deteriorated with longer term follow-up
	Lebar and Alexander[62]	2.3 years	Open inferior capsular shift	Satisfaction/recurrence	All improved; 10% recurrence	Military population
	Hamada et al.[61]	8.3 years	Open capsular shift	Rowe/recurrence	59% good/excellent; 26% recurrence	Mixed population of MDI and anteroinferior instability
	Choi and Ogilvie-Harris[60]	3.5 years	Open inferior capsular shift	ASES/recurrence	92% success for anterior repairs (8% recurrence); 81% success for posterior repairs (12% recurrence)	>75% of contact athletes returned to sport except those with bilateral repairs, of whom 17% returned to sport
	Bak et al.[5]	4.5 years	Open inferior capsular shift	UCLA/Rowe/recurrence	88% good/excellent; 8% recurrence	Return to sport rate of 84%, including 76% in overhead throwing athletes
	Vavken et al.[64]	7.5 years	Open inferior capsular shift	ASES/QuickDASH/recurrence	87% satisfied/very satisfied; 47% recurrence	Five Ehlers Danlos patients; one perioperative reflex sympathetic dystrophy; rotator interval closure did not affect stability, satisfaction, return to sport, or recurrence
	Bigliani et al.[65]	4 years	Open inferior capsular shift	Patient reported based on pain, stability, range of motion, and return to sport/recurrence	94% good/excellent; 3% recurrence	Anterior-inferior instability; one transient musculocutaneous neuropraxia
	van Tankeren et al.[66]	3.3 years	Open inferior capsular shift	Rowe/Constant/12 item Dawson questionnaire/satisfaction/recurrence	82% excellent Rowe scores; 88% satisfied; 24% recurrence	53% concomitant labral pathology
	Mohtadi et al.[93]	2 years	ETAC vs open inferior capsular shift	WOSI/ASES/Constant/range of motion/recurrence	7% recurrence for ETAC and 14% for open inferior capsular shift (no statistical difference)	Included MDI and MDL with primary anterior inferior instability; three post-op adhesive capsulitis/stiff shoulders; (one ETAC, two open inferior capsular shift)
	Altchek et al.[67]	3 years	T-plasty modification of inferior capsular shift	Satisfaction/recurrence	95% satisfied; 10% recurrence	Only half had general ligament laxity; throwers did not return to sport reliably
	Marquardt et al.[68a]	7.4 years	T-plasty modification of inferior capsular shift with suture anchors	Rowe/recurrence	89% good/excellent; 10% recurrence	Anterior-inferior instability
Arthroscopic capsular plication	Lyons et al.[89]	2.3 years	Laser-assisted arthroscopic plication	Neer criteria/stability	96% stable and asymptomatic	Added plication stitches to interval in many patients
	Duncan and Savoie[83]	1–3 years	Arthroscopic inferior capsular shift	Neer criteria/stability	All patients satisfactory, 90 on Bankart score	10 patients

TABLE 42.3 Results for Operative Treatment of Multidirectional Instability—cont'd

	Author	Follow-Up	Technique Details	Outcome Measure	Success Rate	Complications/Notes
Arthroscopic capsular plication	Gartsman et al.[79]	2.9 years	Arthroscopic plication	ASES/Constant/Rowe/UCLA	94% good/excellent; 2% recurrence ASES/Constant/UCLA all improved significantly	
	Baker et al.[82]	2.8 years	Arthroscopic capsular plication	ASES/WOSI	ASES: 94; WOSI: 91% normal	
	Treacy et al.[85]	5 years	Arthroscopic plication Caspari technique	Rowe/recurrence	88% satisfactory	Two patients with persistent pain from posterior knots
	McIntyre et al.[84]	2.8 years	Arthroscopic multiple suture technique	Rowe/recurrence	94% good/excellent; 5% recurrence	One transient musculocutaneous sensory neurapraxia
	Kim et al.[70]	4.3 years	Arthroscopic suture plication	Rowe/recurrence	94% good/excellent results; 3% recurrence	Patients had posteroinferior MDI, all with a labral lesion
	Witney-Lagen et al.[86]	5.1 years	Arthroscopic suture plication with purse stringing	OIS/recurrence	95% good/excellent; 4% recurrence	Rotator interval closure included in 10% of patients; one postop stiffness; one superficial wound infection
	Ma et al.[87]	3 years	Arthroscopic pancapsular plication with sutures	ASES/Constant/Rowe/VAS/recurrence	100% good/excellent; no recurrence	All patients had bilateral laxity; rotator interval closures performed in all patients
	Raynor et al.[77]	3.3 years	Pancapsular capsulorrhaphy with labral repair using suture anchors	ASES/QuickDASH/SF-12 PCS/SANE/recurrence	Kaplan–Meier survivorship 100% at 1 year and 87% at 3 years; 17% recurrence	29% of shoulders had rotator interval closures; SLAP and Bankart repairs were also included
	Buess et al.[80]	2.3 years	Arthroscopic repair with anchors and/or capsular plication	Constant/SST/Rowe Score Westpoint-Modification/VAS/recurrence	Significant improvement in Rowe score in all patients; 14% recurrence	Four instability groups with seven patients classified as predominantly posterior multidirectional instability
	Voigt et al.[81]	3.3 years	Arthroscopic anteropostero-inferior capsular plication with sutures/anchors and interval closure	SST/Constant/Rowe/VAS/recurrence	77% good/excellent Rowe scores at final follow up, 33% required reoperation	Eight patients; all patients were MDI with hyperlaxity (Gerber B5)
	Alpert et al.[78]	4.7 years	Arthroscopic capsular plication with suture anchors	WOSI/ASES/SST/VAS/satisfaction/recurrence	85% mostly/completely satisfied; 15% recurrence	All patients had a minimum of 270 degrees arthroscopic labral repair; Rotator interval closed in 38% of patients
	Hewitt et al.[88]	4.8 years	Arthroscopic pancapsular plication with sutures	ASES/Constant/Rowe/UCLA/WOSI/satisfaction/recurrence	97% mostly/extremely satisfied; 83% good/excellent Rowe scores	Three post-op traumatic dislocations

[a]Includes data from Steinbeck J, Jerosch J. Surgery for atraumatic anterior-inferior shoulder instability. A modified capsular shift evaluated in 20 patients followed for 3 years. *Acta Orthop Scand.* 1997;68(5):447–450.

ASES, American Shoulder and Elbow Surgeons; *DASH*, disabilities of the arm, shoulder, hand; *ETAC*, electrothermal arthroscopic capsulorrhaphy; *MDI*, multidirectional instability; *MDL*, multidirectional laxity; *OIS*, Oxford Instability Score; *SANE*, single assessment numeric evaluation; *SF-12 PCS*, short form-12 physical component summary; *SLAP*, superior labrum anterior to posterior; *SST*, simple shoulder test; *UCLA*, University of California–Los Angeles; *VAS*, visual analog scale; *WOSI*, Western Ontario Shoulder Instability.

On average, patients lost 5 degrees more of external rotation after an open capsular shift compared to an arthroscopic capsular plication. They also recommended against thermal capsular shrinkage in the treatment of MDI secondary to high failure rates.[104]

Return to Sport

Several studies have reported return to sports as a specific outcome measure after the surgical treatment of MDI (Table 42.4). The reported success rate varies from 17% to 97% and reflects variation in inclusion criteria and specific sport requirements.

TABLE 42.4   Return to Sport After Operative Treatment of Multidirectional Instability

Author	Technique	Outcome Measure	Success Rate
Bak et al.[5]	Open inferior capsular shift	Return to previous level of sport	Return to sport 84%, including 76% in overhead throwing athletes
Choi and Ogilvie-Harris[60]	Open inferior capsular shift	Return to previous level of sport	Anterior: 82%; posterior: 75%; bilateral: 17%
Vavken et al.[64]	Open inferior capsular shift	Return to previous level of sport	69% returned to sport; 38% returned to previous level of sport
Bigliani et al.[65]	Open inferior capsular shift	Return to previous level of sport	92% returned to sport; 75% returned to previous level of sport
Altchek et al.[67]	T-plasty modification of inferior capsular shift	Return to sport	83% returned to sport, but all throwers had decreased velocity
Marquardt et al.[68]	T-plasty modification of inferior capsular shift with suture anchors	Return to previous level of sport	72% including elite athletes
Lyons et al.[89]	Laser-assisted capsular plication	Return to previous level of sport	86%
Gartsman et al.[79]	Arthroscopic inferior capsular shift	Return to previous level of sport	85%
Baker et al.[82]	Arthroscopic inferior capsular shift	Return to sport with little or no limitation	86%
McIntyre et al.[84]	Arthroscopic inferior capsular shift	Return to previous level of sport	95% return to previous level, but no elite throwers
Witney-Lagen et al.[86]	Arthroscopic suture plication with purse stringing	Return to previous level of sport	90% return to previous level, but no professional athletes
Hewitt et al.[88]	Arthroscopic pancapsular plication with sutures	Return to sport	97% returned to sport with 20% at a reduced level
Ma et al.[87]	Arthroscopic pancapsular plication	Return to previous level of sport	22%; study included professional/amateur overhead athletes
Raynor et al.[77]	Pancapsular capsulorrhaphy with labral repair using suture anchors	Return to previous level of sport	77% returned to or slightly below their preoperative level of sport
Voigt et al.[81]	Arthroscopic anteropostero-inferior capsular plication with interval closure	Return to previous level of sport	78% returned to sport; 44% returned to previous level of sport

McIntyre et al.[84] reported a 95% return to sport after arthroscopic treatment for MDI, but these authors were careful to point out that their series did not contain elite throwers. A Ma et al.[87] study on professional and amateur overhead athletes noted a 100% RTP, but only 22% returned to their previous preoperative level. Bak et al.[5] also reported on overhead throwing athletes and found that only 76% resumed throwing. Direction and approach also seem to affect return to athletics. Choi and Ogilvie-Harris[60] reported an 82% return to sport for patients with an anterior approach, but contrasted this finding with a 17% return with a bilateral approach. It is likely that patients with a true collagen disorder may self-limit their activities long before presentation for surgical consideration, and thus the favorable results reported in the literature should be carefully applied to patients who had previously been able to achieve active sport participation.

Complications

Although the reported complication rates after the operative treatment of MDI remain low, several types of complications have been reported—the most feared of which is neurologic injury, although reported rates are uncommon and generally self-limiting throughout the literature. A thorough understanding of the proximity of neurologic structures is essential to minimize the risk of this postoperative complication. McFarland et al.[105] reported on the proximity of the applicable neurovascular structures for instability surgery. These investigators found the plexus to be as close as 5 mm from the glenoid rim. They also noted that retractors placed superficial to the subscapularis muscle or used along the scapular neck make contact with the brachial plexus in all positions. Other authors[106,107] have noted that the axillary nerve position averages 3.2 mm from the capsule of the inferior glenoid. Applicable to the posterior approach, the suprascapular nerve has been shown to be an average of 18 mm from the midportion of the posterior glenoid rim.[108]

Clinically, a total of seven axillary nerve injuries have been reported after treatment for MDI. Neer and Foster[1] reported three transient axillary neurapraxias in their original series of open inferior capsular shifts, and Miniaci and McBirnie[92] reported on four patients with transient neurapraxia after arthroscopic thermal capsulorrhaphy, including one patient with deltoid weakness. In both series, symptoms resolved for all patients without further intervention. Several authors have also reported transient neurapraxia of the musculocutaneous nerve, without persistence of symptoms,[60,65,67,79] and one median nerve neurapraxia has been reported.[63] Vavken et al.[64] had one case of reflex sympathetic dystrophy in their series of patients undergoing open inferior capsular shift. A meticulous anatomic understanding, along with the judicious use of retractors, is perhaps the best defense against these complications.[105]

Although postoperative stiffness is generally not a significant issue in patients with MDI, overaggressive plication can result in motion loss, especially in external rotation,[95,97,109] and several cases of adhesive capsulitis has been reported after arthroscopic treatment with thermal capsulorrhaphy for MDI.[92,93,110]

Recurrent instability is a far more common negative outcome than postoperative stiffness after treatment for MDI. When surgical intervention fails, it is generally accompanied by persistence or recurrence of capsular laxity. Zabinski et al.[111] evaluated 20 patients with MDI who underwent revision stabilization. At the time of the revision, the primary lesion was capsular laxity in all patients. At the 5-year follow-up, only 45% of patients had a good or excellent result, despite multiple reoperations.[111] Levine et al.[112] also reported on a series of revision surgeries for failed anterior stabilizations. Twenty-two percent had an unsatisfactory result, and atraumatic causes of failure, voluntary dislocations, and unaddressed capsular laxity—all signs of MDI—were noted risk factors associated with poorer results. A case series from Dewing et al.[113] analyzed revision patient outcomes after anterior capsulolabral reconstruction with tibialis anterior or hamstring allograft for recurrent shoulder instability. Although the patient population was not homogeneous, it included 13 patients with the diagnosis of MDI. At 3.8 years mean follow-up, 45% of shoulders remained completely stable. Some revision surgery series have been more successful when thermal capsulorrhaphy was the primary surgery. Massoud et al.[114] treated a small series of these patients with an open inferior capsular shift procedure and demonstrated improved outcome scores in all their MDI patients.

FUTURE CONSIDERATIONS

The treatment of MDI remains a challenging proposition. Although the reported success rates in the literature are consistently favorable for the operative treatment of MDI, expert opinion from experienced surgeons often reflects more cautious optimism. The lack of a comprehensive classification system hinders the ability to compare data across studies and would be an excellent future direction. Such a classification has been suggested by several authors,[3,31,115] but none has gained universal traction. Another future direction that would be of great benefit is a more complete evaluation of nonoperative management for MDI. All authors recommend a trial of physical therapy, but the length of program, specific recommendations, and results are mixed. Comparative studies to more clearly define how long a nonoperative trial should last and the risk factors for failure would go a long way in assisting the clinician in management decisions.

As previously mentioned, literature reviews have shown similar outcomes between arthroscopic and open treatment methods for MDI. However, there still is no direct comparison of arthroscopic versus open management. Furthermore, long-term clinical studies regarding suture material and anchors are lacking, specifically, knotless versus knotted plication sutures. Although studies have included return to sport as an outcome measure, further research is needed to clarify inclusion criteria and specific sport requirements. A long-term comprehensive return to sport and/or activity study would be very beneficial in the treatment of high-level athletes as well as the "weekend warriors." Defining the amount of stability required while

maintaining an acceptable ROM should also be an area of future research.

Finally, very few studies address the patient with recurrent or persistent MDI. MDI gets much of its infamous reputation from surgeons who have been challenged by patients with MDI for whom multiple surgical attempts at stabilization have failed, and it is somewhat surprising to contrast the near-uniform good and excellent results reported in the literature given the number of failed surgeries experienced by many patients with MDI. Risk factors for failure and definitive reconstructive treatments in the revision setting are an excellent future goal of research. Although allograft reconstructions have been described in the revision setting, further research on this topic may provide surgeons with another tool in their armamentarium for treating MDI.

For a complete list of references, go to ExpertConsult.com.

SELECTED READINGS

Citation:

Neer CS II, Foster CR. Inferior capsular shift for involuntary inferior and multidirectional instability of the shoulder. A preliminary report. *J Bone Joint Surg Am.* 1980;62(6):897–908.

Level of Evidence:

IV, retrospective case series

Summary:

This article reviews the initial results of 36 patients treated for multidirectional instability of the shoulder with an open inferior capsular shift, which was designed to decrease the overall volume of the shoulder joint. Only one of the patients had recurrent subluxation. This article defined the gold standard for treatment of this condition, and it remains the gold standard today.

Citation:

Burkhead WZ Jr, Rockwood CA Jr. Treatment of instability of the shoulder with an exercise program. *J Bone Joint Surg Am.* 1992;74A(6):890–896.

Level of Evidence:

IV, retrospective case review

Summary:

This article investigated results for 140 shoulders with instability that were treated with a specific exercise program. The authors found that only 16% of patients with a traumatic etiology had a good or excellent result, whereas 80% of patients with an atraumatic etiology had a good or excellent result. The authors concluded that every effort should be made to define the etiology of the instability, and if the etiology is atraumatic, the case should be managed conservatively.

Citation:

Gartsman GM, Roddey TS, Hammerman SM. Arthroscopic treatment of multidirectional glenohumeral instability: 2- to 5-year follow-up. *Arthroscopy.* 2001;17(3):236–243.

Level of Evidence:

IV, prospective case series without control

Summary:

This article reports the first arthroscopic treatment of multidirectional instability (MDI). The authors evaluated 47 patients with MDI, reporting 94% good and excellent results at 35 months follow-up. Functional scores improved: the constant from 60 to 92, the Rowe score from 14 to 92, and the University of California–Los Angeles score from 17 to 33.

Citation:

Harryman DT II, Sidles JA, Harris SL, et al. The role of the rotator interval capsule in passive motion and stability of the shoulder. *J Bone Joint Surg Am.* 1992;74A(1):53–56.

Level of Evidence:

Controlled laboratory study

Summary:

This study evaluated the effect of alteration of the rotator interval on translation of the shoulder. The authors found that the shoulder capsule in the region of the rotator interval played a significant role in the range of motion and stability of the shoulder. Release of the interval improved flexion and external rotation, and imbrication resulted in decreased posterior and inferior translation.

Citation:

Misamore GW, Sallay PI, Didelot W. A longitudinal study of patients with multidirectional instability of the shoulder with seven- to ten-year follow-up. *J Shoulder Elbow Surg.* 2005;14(5): 466–470.

Level of Evidence:

IV, retrospective consecutive case series

Summary:

This article reports on 64 consecutive patients diagnosed with multidirectional instability (MDI) of the shoulder who were followed up at both 2 and 8 years after completing a conservative physical therapy program. The authors reported that treatment was considered to have failed for 19 of 36 patients; only 14% of patients were free of pain and instability at final follow-up; and the results of this treatment deteriorated between the 2- and 7-year follow-up. The authors questioned the effectiveness of a nonoperative management program to successfully treat MDI.

Citation:

Warner JJ, Deng XH, Warren RF, et al. Static capsuloligamentous restraints to superior-inferior translation of the glenohumeral joint. *Am J Sports Med.* 1992;20(6):675–685.

Level of Evidence:

Controlled laboratory study

Summary:

The authors performed a cadaveric study evaluating the superior–inferior translation of the humerus after selected capsuloligamentous releases. They noted that the primary restraint to inferior translation is the superior glenohumeral ligament and that progressive abduction of the glenohumeral joint results in transfer of the main static restraints to lower in the capsule. The anterior glenohumeral ligament is most critical at 45 degrees of abduction, whereas the posterior portion was more dominant at 90 degrees of abduction in neutral rotation.

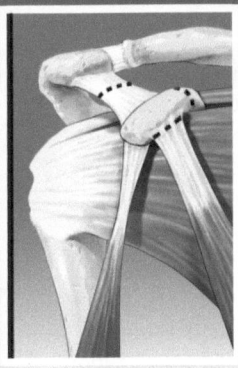

43

Revision Shoulder Instability

Salvatore Frangiamore, Angela K. Chang, Jake A. Fox, Colin P. Murphy,
Anthony Sanchez, Liam Peebles, Matthew T. Provencher

The recurrence of anterior glenohumeral instability is not uncommon following primary surgical repair with reported rates of 15% to 30%.[1–4] Optimal management for recurrent shoulder instability remains controversial; as many acceptable surgical options exist, and the decision-making process is heavily case dependent. Numerous level one studies have looked at risk factors for recurrent instability, consistently reporting a young age and arm position at the time of initial dislocation and repair, being of male gender, a history of multiple preoperative dislocations and instability events, hyperlaxity, and participation in competitive contact/overhead sports as the most common risk factors for recurrence following primary repair.[1,3,5–12] Furthermore, technical errors and failure to address concomitant shoulder pathologies during index surgery can place a patient at risk for recurrence.[3,9] Perhaps the most important predisposing risk factor in recurrent anterior glenohumeral instability is the presence of glenoid bone loss, as recurrence can be seen in as high as 90% to 100% of untreated cases.[11,13] The surgeon should consider individual risk factors for revision surgery that may affect outcomes such as patient age, activity level, and presence of coexisting shoulder injuries. Patients with recurrent glenohumeral instability can benefit from either arthroscopic or open treatment.[14–19]

With patients experiencing recurrent instability, it is crucial to address any bone loss or concomitant injuries in the context of recurrent instability to ensure that the best preoperative decision is made. The goal of treatment is to restore the anatomy and biomechanics of the shoulder and prevent further instability and damage to the joint. This chapter describes the diagnosis, our preferred surgical technique, and the outcomes following revision surgery for patients with chronic/recurrent anterior-inferior shoulder instability that have failed primary repair.

HISTORY

A thorough medical history is an integral component of the preoperative workup. A timeline with details about the patient's initial dislocation (including age at initial dislocation), history of instability events, type of instability (subluxation or dislocation), presence or absence of mechanical catching, previous surgical care and treatment thus far, and any history indicative of concomitant shoulder or connective tissue pathologies should be obtained.[13] Questions with an emphasis on injury mechanics, especially direction of instability (anterior, posterior, or multi-directional), magnitude of trauma required for instability, and ease of reduction (self vs. assisted) are essential for diagnosis of the type and severity of shoulder instability and its management.

The diagnosis of glenoid bone loss in the context of failed shoulder stabilization surgery should be suspected when patients describe a high energy mechanism of injury at initial dislocation, particularly with the arm in abduction ≥70 degrees and external rotation ≥30 degrees. Symptomatic bone loss from patient history may be reported as instability events occurring primarily during mid ranges of motion (20 to 60 degrees of abduction).[11] Patients with glenoid bone loss often notice that dislocation/subluxation of the glenohumeral joint has progressively become easier with a prolonged history of instability symptoms. Instability can present with variable symptoms. Some may report feelings of impending instability or pain at extreme ranges of motion. Others will experience subluxation or obvious dislocation with certain shoulder positions, specifically abduction and external rotation, or overhead activities. In some instances, patients may experience recurrent transient paresthesia and weakness stemming from recurrent subluxation.

Emphasis should be placed on diagnosis of instability and assessment of the bony deficit, but the treating surgeon should consider other pathologies, particularly in patients over the age of 40, who may have concomitant rotator cuff, labral, and cartilage injuries. These injuries, such as superior labrum anterior to posterior (SLAP) tear and rotator cuff tear, are important to diagnose in an initial history, because delaying surgery can lead to tissue of lesser quality and an inferior healing environment.[20] It is also pertinent to obtain information regarding patient activity level and participation in contact/overhead sports while determining realistic treatment goals.

PHYSICAL EXAM

Achieving the right diagnosis in a patient with recurrent instability may be difficult; therefore it is important to assess for other shoulder pathologies along with the standard shoulder exam. Physical exam should begin with inspection to identify for obvious deformity (associated with a history of traumatic instability), rotator cuff atrophy (in patients greater than 40 years of age) and scapular dyskinesia (a history suggestive of a rotator cuff pathology or prolonged instability). Then a careful neurovascular evaluation of the entire upper extremity, assessment of passive and active range of motion (ROM), and rotator cuff integrity and strength should be performed by the examiner.

Patients can have normal findings upon inspection, palpation, ROM and axillary nerve testing with preserved shoulder girdle and parascapular muscle strength. Patients may report feelings of shoulder instability and/or pain with overhead motion. Some may have limited abduction and external rotation because of discomfort and/or pain secondary to instability of the humeral head on the anterior glenoid rim. A comprehensive evaluation of the musculature of the rotator cuff and scapula is important as they comprise the dynamic relationship between the glenoid and humeral head and contribute to shoulder stability. The magnitude and direction of shoulder instability should be documented.

Provocative tests specific to assessing anterior shoulder integrity should be performed. These exams are most reliable when the patient is relaxed. Apprehension, rather than pain, should be used as the diagnostic criterion for a positive finding. Patients with recurrent instability may also have significant guarding during special maneuvers such as load and shift test, drawer test and apprehension sign/augmentation test, Jobe's relocation test,[21] and Gagey hyper abduction test.[22] These tests are highly predictive for instability when performed correctly. The shoulder of interest should be compared to the contralateral side for the reproduction of a sense of instability. Grading of instability during the movement of the humerus into an abducted and externally rotated position helps to guide the treatment plan (Fig. 43.1).

During evaluation, it is imperative to assess for a Hill–Sachs lesion, a SLAP lesion, a Bankart lesion, a humeral avulsion of the inferior glenohumeral ligament (HAGL) lesion, and other capsular injuries. For example, if the humerus begins to dislocate at mid ranges of abduction with external rotation, this may be indicative of an engaging Hill–Sachs lesion or, significant glenoid or humeral head bone loss, and warrants further evaluation.[23] An anterior-inferior labral tear may present with positive load and shift, modified load and apprehension relocation testing, and a sulcus sign. Performing an O'Brien test can be helpful for assessing the superior labral attachment. In a patient with recurrent instability over 40 years of age, the surgeon should evaluate for a rotator cuff tear.

It is important to distinguish asymptomatic laxity from instability and the perception of laxity by patients during a subluxation or dislocation event.[24] Boileau et al. described the difficulty in distinguishing between laxity and instability on young hyperlax overhead athletes who experienced reproducible pain upon anterior apprehension, which relieved upon relocation but had no true instability.[25] Generalized ligamentous laxity can be assessed using the Beighton Hypermobility Criteria: metacarpophalangeal hyperextension, thumb to forearm sign, elbow or knee recurvatum, and the ability to forward flex the trunk with knee in full extension and palm resting on the floor.[26]

The examiner should assess for glenoid bone loss as part of a comprehensive shoulder exam. Reproducible anterior translation of the humeral head over the glenoid rim is indicative of glenoid bone deficit. While patients with glenoid bone loss usually have a positive apprehension test at 90 degrees of abduction and at 90 degrees of external rotation, some may have positive signs at lesser degrees of abduction and external rotation, between 30 and 90 degrees.[11] This is largely in part due to concomitant injuries leading to disproportionately placed forces causing the feeling of apprehension. Performing shoulder apprehension test in various degrees of shoulder abduction and external rotation may provide additional insight on the extent of bone loss. Patients with positive findings of instability and signs of glenoid bone loss require diagnostic investigation with advanced imaging studies.

IMAGING

Appropriate imaging work up is critical to guiding the clinical decision-making process for the type of revision operative procedure to perform. First, routine radiographs should be obtained, true oblique anteroposterior (AP) view (Grashey view), axillary, lateral, and scapular Y.[27–29] The true AP view allows assessment of the glenohumeral joint for degenerative joint changes. The scapular Y view allows assessment for glenohumeral joint alignment. Further specialized radiographic imaging of the glenoid rim may be warranted in patients with recurrent instability to assess for bony defects of the anteroinferior glenoid rim: apical oblique,[30,31] West Point view,[32] or Didiee views.[33] In the context of acute traumatic dislocation, a West Point view or its alternative an apical oblique radiograph allows enhanced visualization of the anteroinferior glenoid to detect for an osseous Bankart lesion.[32] The addition of a Stryker Notch view and a true AP view with internal rotation allows the surgeon to visualize humeral head defects like Hill–Sachs lesions. While initial assessment should begin with radiographs, they often fail to detect or accurately quantify the degree of glenoid bone loss. Up to 60% of bony lesions can be missed upon radiographs alone[34,35]; therefore evaluation with magnetic resonance imaging (MRI) and computed

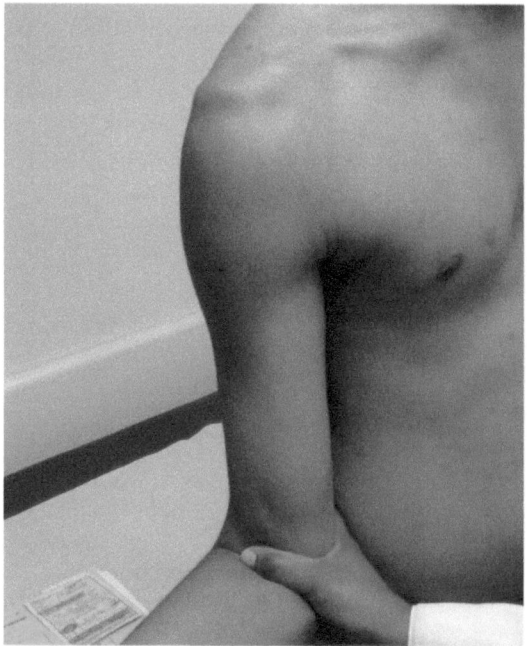

Fig. 43.1 Preoperative evaluation for recurrent shoulder instability should be comprehensive and include inspection, a careful neurovascular evaluation, assessment of passive and active range of motion, rotator cuff integrity and strength, and provocative tests specific for anterior shoulder instability. The involved shoulder is placed in abduction and external rotation, demonstrating symptomatic sulcus.

tomography (CT) is warranted for potential revision cases to determine the integrity of the surrounding soft tissue and bony structures, respectively.[36] CT with contrast is an especially effective method because it allows enhanced detection of the exact degree and location of osseous defects in comparison with a standard CT scan.[37]

High failure rates following surgery and recurrence of instability are known to be associated with soft tissue incompetence and bony deficiencies.[1,38–40] Preoperative diagnostic MRI with intra-articular gadolinium can identify any concomitant pathologies of the labrum, biceps anchor and pulley, glenohumeral (GH) ligaments and rotator cuff. The most common pathologic finding associated with instability is an avulsion of the glenohumeral ligament labral complex from its attachment to the anterior-inferior glenoid. Bony Bankart lesions are reported between 4% and 70% of anterior glenohumeral instability cases.[19,38–41] Perhaps the most reliable modality for obtaining detailed shoulder pathologies is a three-dimensional (3D) CT scan as these images are highly correlated with arthroscopic findings.[42–46] While two-dimensional (2D) CT and sagittal oblique MRI (also 2D) can aid to visualize glenoid bone loss and newly formed glenoid fragments,[13] they are unable to adjust for patient-specific glenoid topography and version. An MRI requires reasonable resolution to differentiate a glenoid bone injury from a soft tissue injury, while 2D CT affects the gantry angle. Furthermore, even with additional MRI slices and views, these images may still underestimate glenoid bone loss.[11]

The most accurate method for measuring the magnitude of glenoid bone loss and for assessing the humeral head for a Hill–Sachs lesion is a 3D CT scan with digital subtraction of the humeral head on sagittal oblique imaging (Fig. 43.2). Software for 3D CT allows digital subtraction of the humeral head from

the glenohumeral complex resulting in a precise *en face* view of the glenoid surface and vault and visualization of the scapula. Not only can 3D CT provide information about the extent of glenoid bone injury but also the type of injury (i.e., acute fracture, partial attritional bone loss, or complete attritional bone loss) (Figs. 43.3–43.5). As glenoid bone stock loss usually occurs along a line parallel to the long axis of the glenoid from 12 o'clock to 6 o'clock,[47] several studies have utilized this information to geometrically quantify bone loss from 3D CT images.[36,48–50] The inferior aspect of the glenoid on an *en face* view has been described as a shape of a true circle,[50] with the circle drawn with the center point roughly at the glenoid bare spot in the inferior two-thirds of the glenoid.[36,48] The glenoid bare spot can be identified upon CT as the area of cartilaginous thinning and increased subchondral density over the tubercle of Assaki.[50] The location of the bare spot is at the intersection between the longitudinal axis and the widest AP diameter of the glenoid. Using this point as the center, a circle is drawn and the radius is determined. The distance from the bare spot to the anterior edge is then measured. One method is to use the ratio of the radius to the previous distance in order to quantify the percentage of glenoid bone loss.[11] A simpler method also relies on the bare spot and quantifies bone loss as the difference between distance from the bare spot to the anterior edge from the bare spot to the posterior edge over twice the distance of the bare spot to the posterior edge.[51,52] Another important factor of instability is the length of the bony defect; it has been reported that defects greater than half the widest AP diameter results in 70% or less resistance to dislocation.[49] Perhaps the simplest technique of all for determining glenoid bone loss is a linear measurement in millimeters of the defect from the circle.[53]

Furthermore, 3D CT imaging provides information about glenoid inversion, inclination, and the relationship between the glenoid and humeral head (engaging or nonengaging, on-track or off-track).[23,27,39,45,46,54,55] Burkhart and DeBeer were the first to define an engaging Hill–Sachs lesion as the humeral head coming

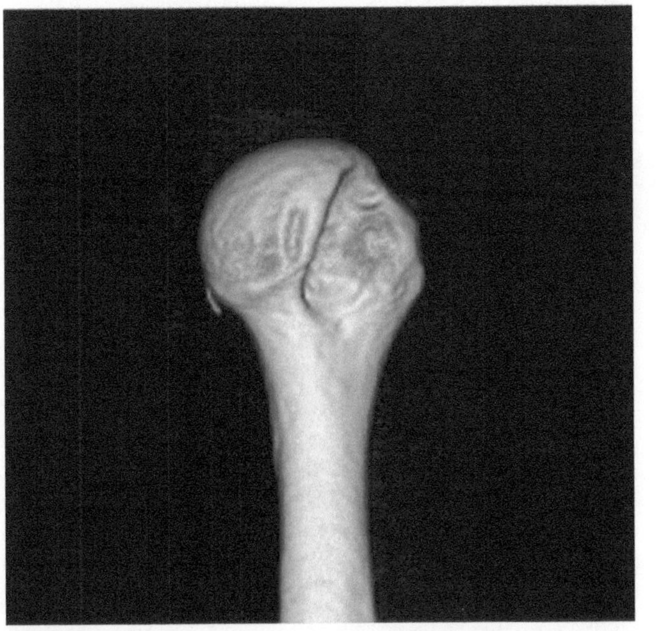

Fig. 43.2 A humeral head with Hill-Sachs lesion is shown here. Preoperative three-dimensional computed tomography imaging of the humeral head may help to guide the treatment plan. It is important to quantify bone loss and to determine location in relation to the glenoid track.

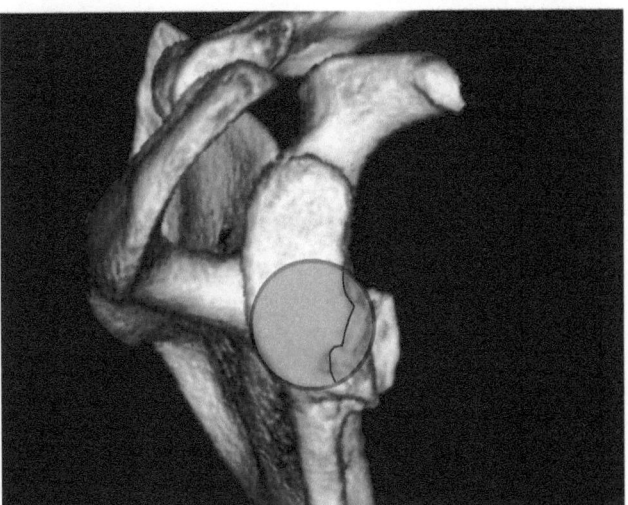

Fig. 43.3 *En face* view three-dimensional computed tomography image demonstrating the perfect circle technique to evaluate for glenoid bone loss. With this technique, a circle is drawn in the inferior glenoid with the bare spot at the center.

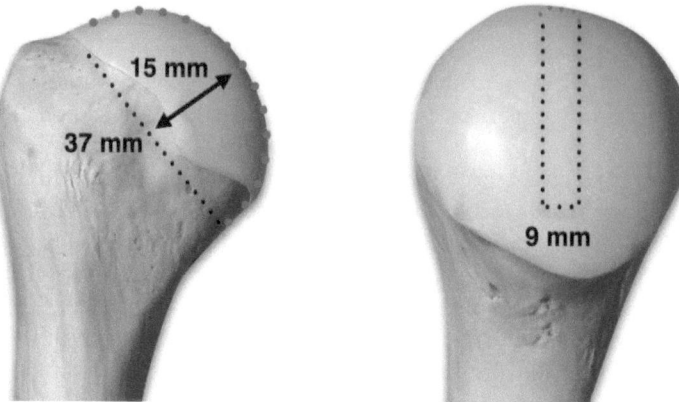

Fig. 43.4 Assessment of Hill-Sachs lesions begins with determining the dimensions of the humeral head, then determining the location and size of the humeral head defect. The risk of engagement can be determined using glenoid tract measurements.

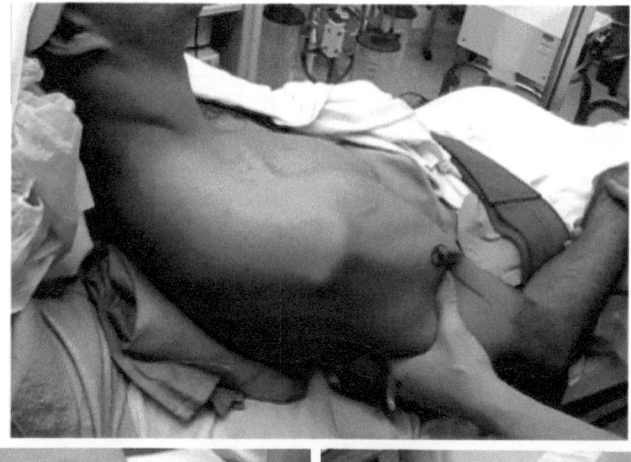

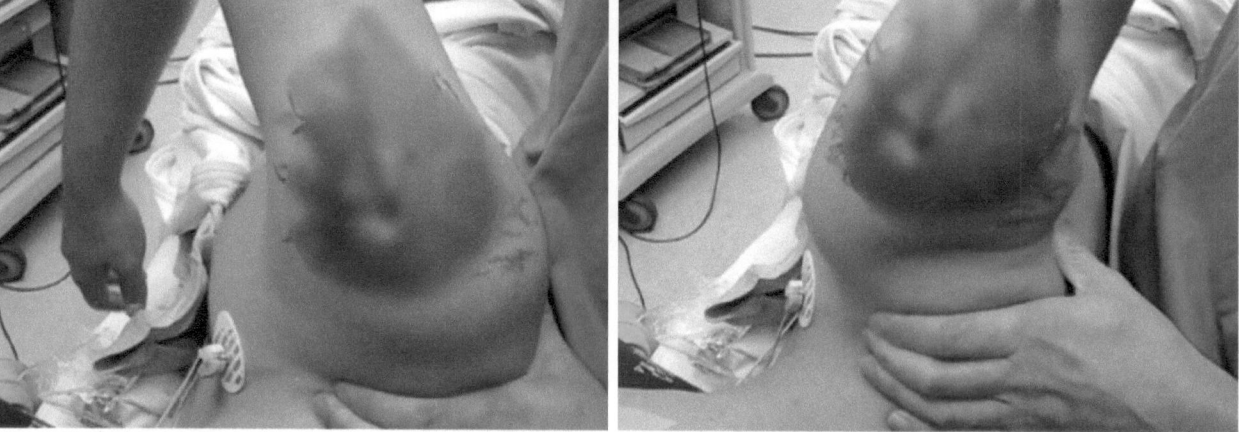

Fig. 43.5 Physical exam under anesthesia confirming anterior instability with anterior load and shift test.

into contact with the rim of the anterior glenoid during 90 degrees of abduction with external rotation between 0 and 135 degrees. In their study of 101 athletes undergoing surgical repair for traumatic anterior-inferior instability, a Hill–Sachs lesion was significant only if it was classified as engaging.[23] In the study, they utilized arthroscopic viewing portals to determine the "engagement" status of the Hill–Sachs lesion. After an average follow-up of 27 months (range, 14 to 79 months), they reported

that 100% of patients with engaging Hill–Sachs lesions experienced recurrent shoulder instability[23] and that soft tissue repair alone was sufficient without the presence of a concomitant engaging Hill–Sachs lesion. Later studies have also reported that engagement of a Hill–Sachs lesion, rather than the size, has been a greater predictor of recurrent instability.[56–58] True engagement occurs when the lesion extends over the medial margin of the glenoid track, whereas a nonengaging lesion will pass diagonally across the anterior glenoid,[54,58] allowing it to make continuous contact with the articular surface of the glenohumeral joint and prevent bone to bone contact.[23] Engagement can be determined either by a CT scan or via arthroscopy while the arm is in abduction-external rotation. An MRI study conducted by Gyftopolous et al. demonstrated that the on-track off-track method was an excellent way to predict engagement, as they found it 84.2% accurate.[57]

DECISION-MAKING PRINCIPLES

When selecting treatment options for recurrent shoulder instability, the most important factors to consider are the magnitude of glenoid bone loss or injury, the patient's expectations for outcomes, and their anticipated postoperative level of activity. The management of recurrent instability following failed stabilization procedure(s) is heavily reliant on clinical assessment and imaging findings. A thorough preoperative evaluation including a clear surgical history with information regarding patient age, sports participation (overhead/contact) if any, lifestyle/activity level, any medical conditions (smoking, current medications), or any voluntary component that may affect the patient's surgery or ability to follow through with rehabilitation can help set reasonable expectations for treatment outcomes. Other important prognostic factors include capsulolabral integrity, concomitant shoulder pathologies, poor tissue quality, and any osseous loss of the glenoid or humeral head.[11]

Nonoperative management can be acceptable for patients with less than 20 degrees of glenoid bone loss, low activity demands, greater age and higher surgical risk, or a history of voluntary glenohumeral dislocation.[11] However, it is imperative to rule out glenoid bone loss as a contributing factor for recurrent instability in these patients with a history of failed shoulder stabilization surgery.

Both open and arthroscopic surgery can provide acceptable options for soft tissue or bony repair in revision instability cases when managed appropriately.[14-19] Although the optimal treatment for glenoid bone loss is not well defined, current literature suggests recurrent instability with less than or equal to around 5 to 7 mm of glenoid bone loss (0% to 20% and up to 25% in some cases) may benefit from soft tissue arthroscopic stabilization with multiple suture anchors and a posterior repair.[11,18] In these patients with minimal bone loss, studies have reported excellent postoperative outcomes with the incorporation of a Bankart fragment should the operating surgeon choose to do so.[18,59] Studies with large cohorts of greater than 50 patients comparing the efficacy of open and arthroscopic Bankart repair techniques in preventing recurrent instability demonstrated no significant differences in postoperative shoulder stability outcome scores.[14,15] While one study noted a significantly higher ($P = .017$) ROM in the arthroscopic group[15]; there is a lack of well-defined outcome scoring systems to quantify the success of either surgical approach. Open stabilization is preferred for patients at a higher risk of recurrent instability, while arthroscopy is acceptable for patients with a lower risk.[60] In general arthroscopy is a less invasive procedure that may allow a greater degree of return of ROM, but the operating surgeon's level of expertise

and comfort level with either surgical techniques should be considered.

Bone loss is the most common reason for a failed stabilization surgery.[23,34,38] Though it varies in the literature, recurrence of instability can occur with as little as 15% to 20% glenoid bone loss.[1,23,40] One study suggested that 13.5% glenoid bone loss might even render surgical intervention with bony reconstruction.[61] To successfully correct instability, bony augmentation of the anteroinferior glenoid rim allows restoration of the anatomical arc of glenohumeral motion. While bony fragment fixation with open capsulolabral repair is considered the gold standard, arthroscopic repair is also acceptable.[19] A 20% to 25% bone stock loss correlates to approximately 6 to 8 mm of the glenoid from anterior to posterior.[62] The bare spot of the glenoid provides a reference point for measuring bone loss, and varies between 23 and 30 mm with the majority of shoulders ranging from 24 to 26 mm.[50] Five percent of glenoid bone loss correlates to approximately 1 to 2 mm of bone, further emphasizing that only a relatively small amount of bony injury is needed for clinical relevance.[11] It is also important for the surgeon to consider attritional bone loss of the remaining fragment in the setting of glenoid defects. McNeil et al. showed that 91.4% of patients exhibited moderate to severe attritional bone loss independent of the initial glenoid bone loss, implying that this fragment is insufficient to reconstitute the glenoid bone stock. Of note, this attritional loss was more pronounced in patients with a longer duration of instability symptoms, which may help further guide the surgeon's decision-making.[63]

Recurrent instability with 25% to 30% glenoid bone loss (~6 to 8 mm) should be treated with open repair with bone augmentation to reconstitute the glenoid arc. Generally, anteroinferior glenoid defect of this size cannot be managed through soft tissue repair alone due to the deficit in articular arc. Furthermore, patients with chronic instability may have attritional bone loss secondary to resorption of the previous osseous Bankart fragment. During the discussion of treatment, patients' expectations and postoperative desires should be thoroughly addressed in situation of increased glenoid bone loss as recurrence of instability is greater with arthroscopic than open repair.[13,23,64] These reconstruction techniques include Bristow[65] and Latarjet.[66] While coracoid transfer has been the standard for over 50 years with excellent postoperative stability and function, there are concerns regarding eventual postoperative arthrosis and limitations in shoulder motion, especially after nonanatomical coracoid reconstruction.[67,68] When using a different bone block to address the glenoid defect, graft options include autogenous iliac crest graft[69] and various frozen (femoral head and humeral head) and fresh osteochondral allografts (distal tibial plafond).[70] While the most logical reconstruction is to replace the missing glenoid bone with similar bone, glenoid allograft specimens are less commonly available, have been associated with contamination, and do not present proper curvature.[70] Iliac crest autograft may be preferred over a distal tibia allograft (DTA) when an extensive defect is present as it allows a more adequate supply of bone for reconstruction.[71,72]

Not only should the treating surgeon quantify the amount of glenoid bone loss, but he or she should also assess for the presence of an engaging Hill–Sachs lesion, capsular tissue quality, and associated defects or other soft tissue (rotator cuff, bicep tendon) pathologies.[28] Addressing an engaging Hill–Sachs lesion can prevent extensive stressing of a revision repair on the capsuloligamentous labral complex during abduction and external rotation.[54] A dynamic evaluation of shoulder abduction and external rotation under direct visualization during arthroscopy can provide the most direct view of engaging lesions, and help guide definitive management. When an engaging Hill–Sachs lesion is present, surgical intervention is warranted. The preferred methods for humeral head lesions include direct auto- or allograft transfer, remplissage, disimpaction, and prosthesis replacement. All these techniques increase the bony surface area of the humeral head to prevent further engagement and instability.

When it comes to deciding if a patient is a candidate for humeral head prosthesis (i.e., humeral head hemiarthroplasty), the size of the Hill–Sachs lesion is the most influential factor. Hill–Sachs lesions involving greater than 40% of the humeral head surface are generally managed with prosthetic replacement.[73] Both hemiarthroplasty and total arthroplasty are associated with failure rates, especially in the younger and active patient. Patients greater than 65 years of age may benefit from hemiarthroplasty or total shoulder arthroplasty at a lower percentage of bone loss due to the low physical demands placed upon their glenohumeral joint. The procedure can also be indicated in young patients with chronic defects and significant cartilage degeneration.[74]

Hill–Sachs lesions are especially clinically relevant in the setting of glenoid bone loss, as there is an increased likelihood of the humeral head engaging the glenoid. When determining treatment of combined lesions, the concept of the "glenoid track" is a prognostic indicator of surgical success. Metzger et al. found that the glenoid track could help predict engagement, as 84.5% of patients with lesions out of the track showed clinical engagement compared to the 12.4% of patients with lesions inside the track that had functionally engaging lesions ($P < .001$). Thus the glenoid track can identify lesions at high risk for engagement and help guide treatment options, especially when considering bone augmentation.[75] Prior to the study executed by Shaha et al., most advanced knowledge about the glenoid track was the algorithm developed by Di Giacomo et al., which could predict the track mathematically.[54] The algorithm reads as follows: glenoid track width = .83D − d (D as the diameter of the glenoid and d as the amount of glenoid bone loss [posterior radius–anterior radius]).[54] Shaha et al. found that out of the 49 patients in their cohort that were classified as on-track, only 4 (8%) of the patients experienced any form of instability recurrence. Eight patients were noted to be off-track, and of those patients 6 (75%) were documented to sustain recurrent dislocations due to engagement. They also found the negative predictive value of the study to be 92%, meaning that when the shoulder was on track, arthroscopy failed a mere 8% of the time (Fig. 43.6).[61]

Overall, surgical decision-making is dependent on the extent of glenoid and humeral osseous deficiency, surgeon experience, and training with specific reconstruction techniques and patient-specific factors (occupational and athletic demands). The surgeon must carefully consider the type of procedure and graft

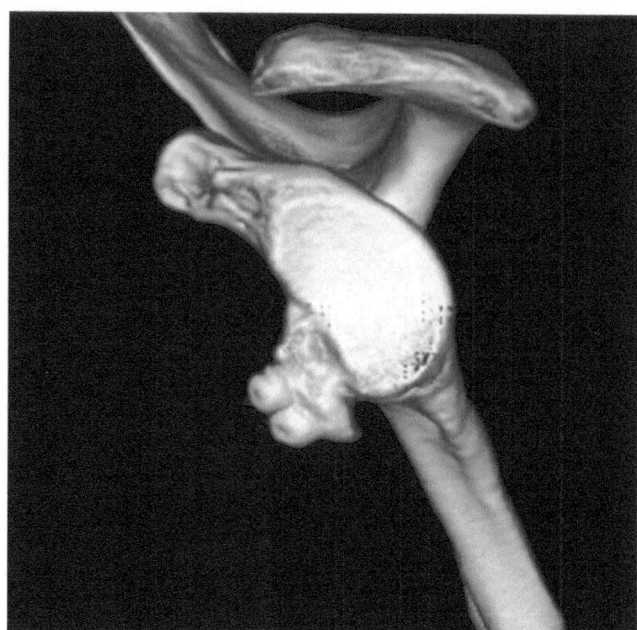

Fig. 43.6 Sagittal oblique three-dimensional computed tomography image following failed Latarjet bony reconstruction.

if indicated that would be of the most benefit to the patient, and treat concomitant pathologic conditions.

TREATMENT OPTIONS

Optimal treatment should be guided by the extent of glenoid bone loss and anticipated patient activity levels. Several surgical options can be considered in revision cases for anterior shoulder instability as both bony and capsuloligamentous pathologies may be present. The goal of a revision stabilization procedure is to restore the anatomy and ROM, and to repair the labrum with appropriate tensioning while preventing further complications (chondral damage, neurovascular injury). Glenoid bone deficit is most commonly addressed with two different methods: a Latarjet or Bristow procedure, or allograft augmentation. Restoration of the surface area can be achieved with an allograft of the iliac crest (bony implant) or distal tibia (bony and articular implant). With the option of utilizing either an autograft or an allograft comes the strategy of deciding which choice is optimal for the patient. Autografts are advantageous because they offer beneficial properties such as being osteoinductive, osteoconductive, and immunogenic. Allografts offer the advantage that they avoid causing donor harvest site morbidity and do not cause pain or sensory disturbance, unlike autograft harvesting.[76] It is imperative to adequately replace the glenoid bony stock, whether it be autograft or allograft, for the success of the revision repair. However, in cases when a graft is insufficient, a hemiarthroplasty or a total shoulder arthroplasty should be considered. Patients may benefit more from a prosthesis in the context of humeral head deficiency or significant glenoid bone loss. Further stabilization in patients with capsular laxity can be achieved through closure of the rotator interval; however, this results in decreased external rotation in adduction and increased potential for posterior inferior translation for some patients.

Removal of symptomatic hardware or osteophytes may improve pain in some cases of arthropathy. Lysis of adhesions should be performed for patients with stiffness secondary to adhesions. Repair of the rotator cuff and débridement of diseased soft tissue may be necessary in some cases of recurrent instability. Revision surgery can be successful with either open or arthroscopic surgery; however, arthroscopic repair requires a higher level of expertise and is preferred for isolated capsuloligamentous repair. An open repair approach better addresses glenoid bone loss,[77] humeral head lesions (Hill-Sachs), subscapularis deficiency, and large capsular defects.

PREFERRED SURGICAL TECHNIQUE

In our experience, an arthroscopic revision shoulder stabilization procedure is best to correct shoulders with inappropriately or untreated capsular laxity/injury and labral injury. An open revision shoulder stabilization procedure, such as a Latarjet or an allograft bony augmentation procedure, is indicated for patients with severe glenoid bone loss, Hill–Sachs lesion or a severe subscapularis deficiency.

While the arthroscopic stabilization can be performed in the beach chair or lateral decubitus position, a lower recurrence rate is seen following surgery with the patient in lateral decubitus.[78,79] The lateral decubitus position allows the surgeon to obtain circumferential access to the glenoid rim to better addresses the inferior component of anterior glenoid instability.[78,79] However, arthroscopy in lateral decubitus is technically challenging as the shoulder is in nonanatomic orientation and is at risk for traction-related injury or axillary and musculocutaneous nerve injury during anteroinferior portal placement.

Our preferred arthroscopic soft tissue stabilization is a Bankart repair with an added posterolateral portal for optimal visualization of and access to the anteroinferior glenoid.[28,78,80,81] Following interscalene block and general anesthesia, the patient is placed in the lateral decubitus position and the operative arm positioned in place with a beanbag and padded arm holder. The arm is suspended in gentle traction in slight abduction and forward flexion. Posterolateral, posterior and anterosuperior portals are created. The posterolateral portal is created 4 cm off the posterolateral acromion with the posterior viewing portal 2 cm inferior to the posterolateral corner of the acromion. An anterosuperior portal is created just anterior to the biceps, proximal in the rotator interval. Diagnostic arthroscopy is performed using a 30-degree arthroscopic through the anterosuperior viewing portal. The Bankart lesion and any concomitant injury to the glenohumeral complex, including the long head of the biceps tendon, rotator cuff, humeral head, and glenoid bone stock are identified. The anterosuperior portal allows for optimal viewing of the glenoid. A rasp or burr can be utilized to create glenoid bleeding. The posterolateral portal is used for percutaneous anchor placement to the inferior glenoid through an inside-out technique that follows the trajectory of the posterior border of the clavicle through the teres minor and capsule. This technique allows the trocar to be placed 1 to 2 mm from the glenoid rim and minimizes the risk for movement with drilling and skiving across the cartilage of the glenoid. Sutures are gently pulled to

ensure capture prior to trocar removal, and are retained in the posterolateral portal for suture management and knot tying. After successful anchor placement, the posterior portal is cannulated and the anterior capsule is grasped anterior to the anchor to avoid axillary nerve, closest to the 6 o'clock position,[28] and the labrum is brought to the inferior glenoid to enhance plication of the capsular pouch.

The degree of plication is based on clinical exam or exam under anesthesia (see Fig. 43.5). The labrum is repaired anteriorly through the anteroinferior portal and the sutures are shuttled with a single hoop suture configuration as it best allows appropriate tensioning. A sliding knot and alternating half stitches placed away from the articular surface recreates the inferior glenoid bumper. At least three suture anchors between the 3 o'clock and 6 o'clock position should be utilized to recreate the glenoid labrum and appropriate capsular tensioning.[3] The addition of a rotator interval closure can improve anterior instability but not inferior instability specifically.[82–84] While potentially beneficial for some patients, rotator interval closure can result in a significant loss of external rotation in neutral and abducted arm positions.[82,83,85]

Arthroscopic stabilization with bony augmentation should begin with quantification of glenoid bone loss using either a 2 o'clock or 3 o'clock posterior portal. Using the inferior two-thirds of the glenoid cavity as a circle, the glenoid bare spot is the marked center point in order for there to be a consistent radius in the anterior, posterior, and inferior directions.[50,86] This method of quantification is best for assessing the extent of lesions parallel to the long axis of the glenoid; if the defect occurs at a 45-degree angle relative to the long axis, the bare spot method overestimates the amount of true bone loss.[47] Note that the glenoid bare spot may not be identifiable in all shoulders and therefore findings from preoperative 3D CT may guide the surgical approach.

For smaller glenoid defects (<20% to 25%), a Bankart fragment may be repaired with arthroscopic techniques utilizing various suture anchors and suture constructs if adequate capsulabral tensioning can be achieved.[52,87] Suture anchor fixation of a Bankart lesion is performed through the use of the posterolateral, transubscapularis, and mid-glenoid portals. The posterolateral portal more readily allows access to the inferior-most aspect of glenoid, especially when the patient is placed in lateral decubitus position. For patients experiencing recurrent instability in the setting of revision surgery, our preferred surgical approach is the Latarjet procedure. The standard Latarjet and its variations have been described in literature with few studies addressing optimal graft orientation and placement. A biomechanical study evaluating the contact pressures and areas of a Latarjet graft demonstrated that the bone block should be oriented with the inferior aspect of the coracoid congruent to the glenoid arc to reconstruct the mean reconstructed glenoid diameter.[88] While some advocate for limited capsular and labral repair, suture anchors can be utilized on the anterior-most aspect of the native glenoid at the coracoid–glenoid interface. Two 3.5 mm metal screws fix the coracoid as flush as possible into position. The previously dissected native capsule from the glenoid neck is repaired with suture anchors and bone tunnels with the coracoid extraarticular. The locally harvested coracoid autograft is positioned to act as an extra-articular extension of the glenoid arc. The addition of an osseous block extends the glenoid rim and allows there to be more articular surface area for the humeral head to make contact with, limiting the opportunity for dislocation. The conjoined tendon acts as a sling to prevent anterohumeral translation when the arm in abduction and external rotation. Both the transferred coracoid process and conjoined tendon over the lower subscapularis tendon reinforce the anteroinferior aspect of the capsule, having an effect like that of a tenodesis.[23]

While the gold standard for glenoid bone augmentation is the Latarjet coracoid transfer procedure, we recommend the use of an articular allograft to reconstruct the glenoid when there is greater than 25% bone loss. The Latarjet procedure has low reported long-term instability rates, but there is a concern of graft resorption and early development of glenohumeral arthritis in the high-demand athletic patient population (Fig. 43.6).[89] The preferred technique for open reconstruction of the anterior glenoid rim begins with the patients placed in beach chair with the head elevated to 40 degrees and the operative arm in an arm holder. A modified deltopectoral exposure and subscapular splitting is performed to access the glenohumeral joint, then the joint and viable labral tissue are elevated to expose anterior glenoid. A combination of high speed burr or rasp and an arthroscopic bone cutting shaver (<3.5 mm diameter) is utilized to create a bleeding surface on the anterior glenoid for the incorporation of the allograft. Preparation of the native glenoid and osseous surfaces are key to successful incorporation of the graft and repair. Adequate preparation of the anterior aspect of the glenoid neck is determined when the posterior subscapular fibers can be visualized through the elevated capsule off the glenoid. Recently developed arthroscopic instruments, such as sharp penetrators, suture hooks, or curved suture devices, may be used in conjunction with standard arthroscopic repair devices to punch through bone (Fig. 43.7).

The allograft of choice is a fresh DTA, specifically of the lateral third portion.[89] The lateral aspect of the plafond provides a near anatomical match of the radius of the curvature and articular thickness with dense corticocancellous bone. DTA is readily available from allograft distributors and can be customized to the patient's shoulder. A deltopectoral approach with the subscapularis split longitudinally allows exposure of the capsule. Subperiosteal dissection is performed as medially as possible and tagged with No. 2 nonabsorbable suture. With the glenohumeral joint exposed, the amount of glenoid bone loss is determined. The glenoid is prepared to receive the allograft. Occasionally there is attrition of the labral tissue and it cannot be repaired in these patients. A high speed burr can be used to create a uniform glenoid graft bed that is perpendicular to the articular surface of the glenoid. The DTA is prepared on the back table with a 0.5 inch sagittal saw under continuous irrigation to prevent thermal necrosis. The graft should be secured with pointed reduction clamps or towel clips (Figs. 43.8–43.10). Using a template from a 3D CT scan, the allograft should be measured and cut from superior to inferior (~20 to 25 mm) and then anterior to posterior (~6 to 10 mm). The graft should be approximately 1 cm deep to match the dimensions of the prepped anterior glenoid defect with sufficient subchondral bone for eventual placement of 2 to 3.5 mm screws. The corners of the graft are rounded with pointed the sagittal saw to match the native glenoid morphology. The DTA is then transferred to the operative field and temporarily fixed with two 1.6 mm Kirschner wires at 45 degrees to the articular surface (Fig. 43.11). Washers with 2 to

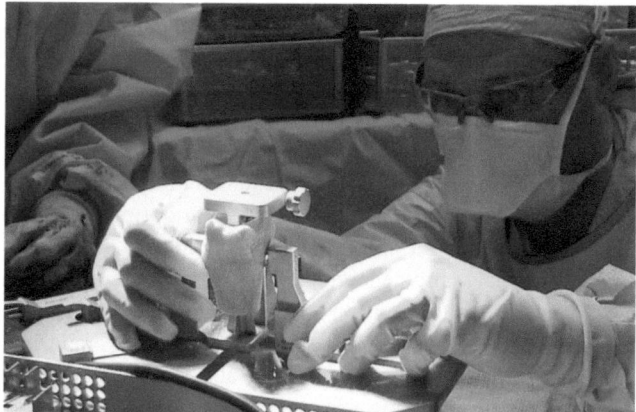

Fig. 43.8 Intraoperative preparation of lateral one-third of the distal tibia allograft on the back table using allograft fixation platform.

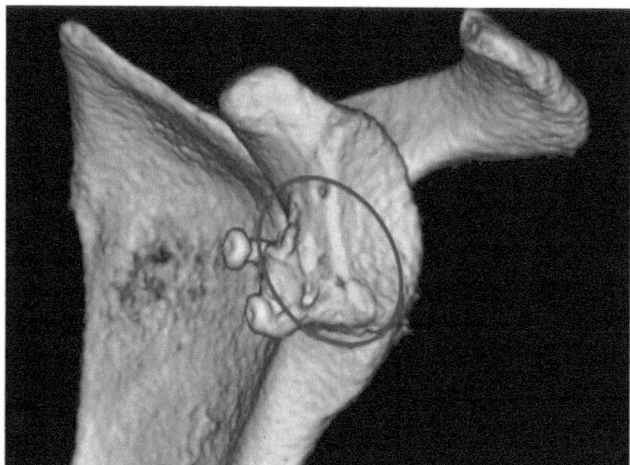

Fig. 43.7 Three-dimensional computed tomography image demonstrating fixation of a coracoid graft placed at the anteroinferior glenoid rim. Proper, medial position of the coracoid is highlighted. Some resorption is also evident.

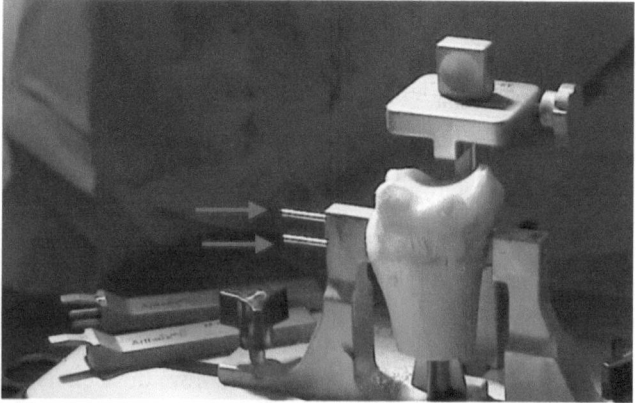

Fig. 43.9 Preparation of distal tibia allograft with fixation platform and cutting guide set. *Arrows* identify two smooth 1.6 mm Kirschner wires used to fix the graft on the platform.

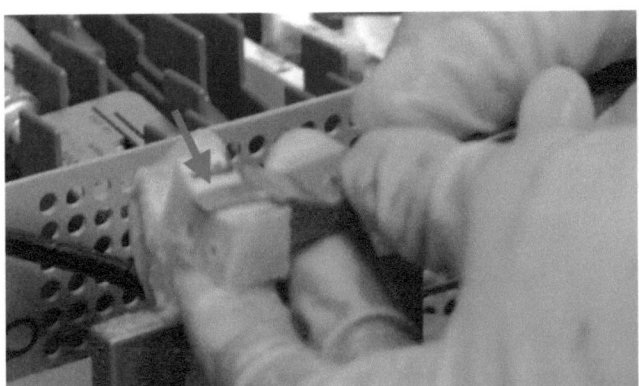

Fig. 43.10 Preparation of the distal tibial allograft. As indicated with a red arrow, a custom distal tibia allograft cutting device is used to achieve the desired graft dimensions for bony augmentation. The graft is secured with the distal cartilage surface facing up. Cuts are made to the lateral aspect of the bone to provide a better congruency with the humeral head. Several trials of intervening microadjustments are often necessary to match the contours of the glenoid rim. Constant saline irrigation is necessary throughout graft preparation to prevent thermal necrosis.

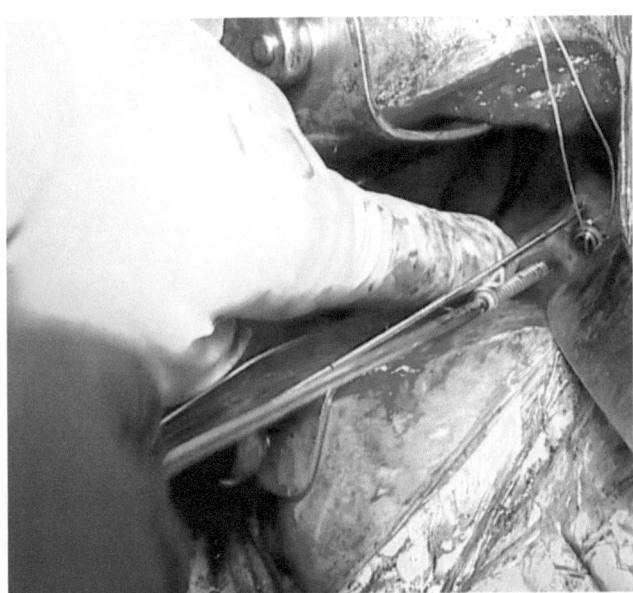

Fig. 43.12 Distal tibia allograft secured with two 3.5 mm fully threaded, noncannulated cortical screws and a suture washer.

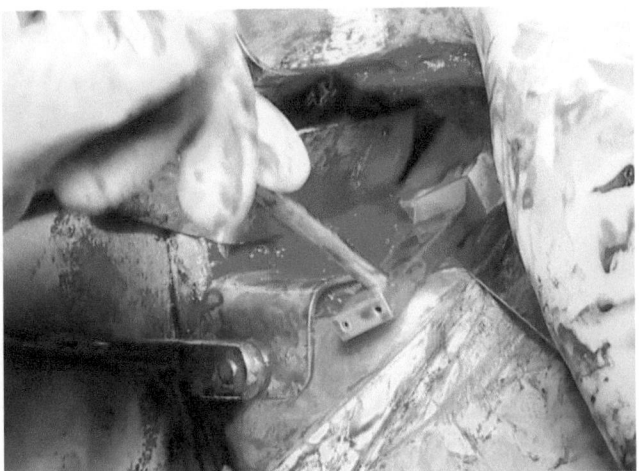

Fig. 43.11 Placement of the distal tibia allograft onto the anterior glenoid following preparation of the anterior glenoid rim.

3.5 mm fully threaded, noncannulated biocortical interference screws are used with the lag technique to achieve adequate graft compression against the anterior glenoid (Fig. 43.12). Capsular and labral repair with sutures attached to screw heads with or without washers may be necessary prior to final tightening of the graft. Prior to final screw tightening, sutures that were used to repair the capsular and labral tissue can be passed under the screwhead and washer for secure fixation. The capsule, subscapularis split, superficial soft tissues, and skin are closed in a standard fashion (Figs. 43.13 and 43.14).

Treatment of other concomitant pathologies is imperative in all revision cases to avoid recurrent instability after revision shoulder stabilization and is possible in multiple surgical approaches. Common pathologic findings include rotator cuff tears (partial and complete), acromioclavicular joint pain, extensive labral tear, SLAP lesion (with possible bicep lesion), anterior labroligamentous periosteal sleeve avulsion (ALPSA) lesion, HAGL lesion and Hill-Sachs lesion. Rotator cuff tear, extensive labral tear, and SLAP lesion require direct repair. Bicep tendon disease may be

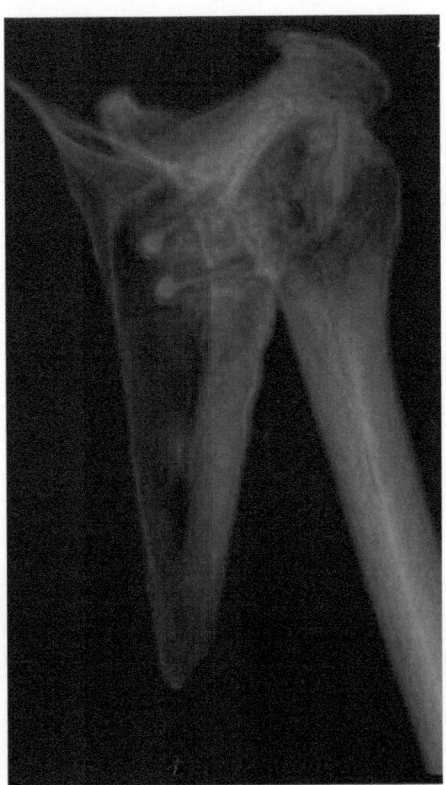

Fig. 43.13 Postoperative computed tomography image demonstrating screw fixation into the glenoid and humerus with anatomic reconstruction of the shoulder joint.

addressed with débridement and tenodesis. Acromioclavicular joint pain may be alleviated with a distal clavicle excision or a preoperative acromioclavicular joint injection. Important considerations for ALPSA lesion repair are that the labrum and scapular periosteal sleeve are detached medially and inferiorly on the glenoid, and the tear can occur in the anterior band of the inferior glenohumeral ligament. An HAGL lesion may be visualized in the posterior portal with a 30-degree scope in the

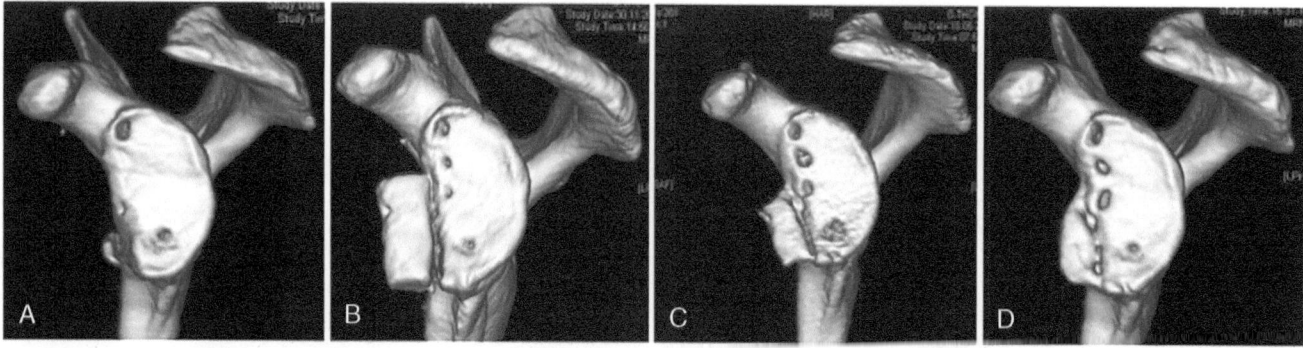

Fig. 43.14 Three-dimensional computed tomography images demonstrating glenoid bone loss (A), placement of graft (B), and progression of integration/osteolysis of the graft (C and D).

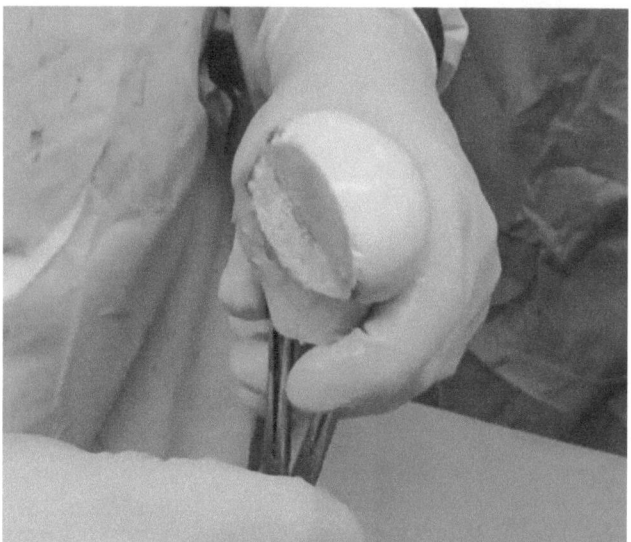

Fig. 43.15 Preparation of humeral head allograft. The dimensions of the implanted humeral head allograft are determined using preoperative three-dimensional computed tomography studies.

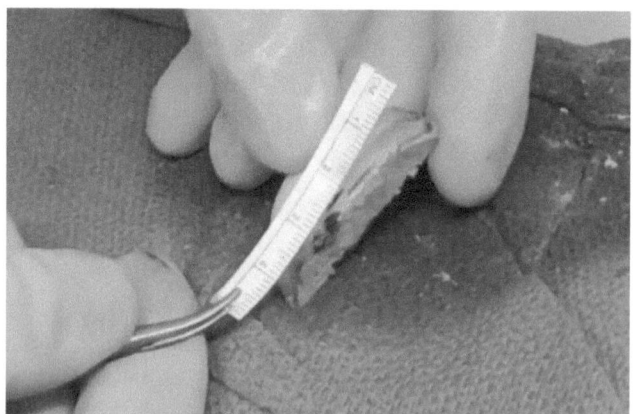

Fig. 43.16 It is important to prepare the humeral head allograft as precisely as possible in order to ensure the appropriate fit into the defect.

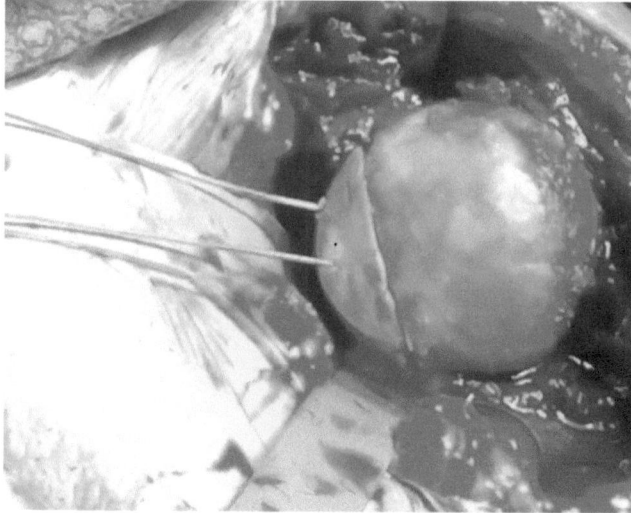

Fig. 43.17 Placement of humeral head allograft to repair a Hill-Sachs lesion, fixed with headless compression screws.

POSTOPERATIVE MANAGEMENT

Rehabilitation plays an important role in patient recovery. Patients are provided a standard abduction sling for arm support during the first 4 to 6 week postoperative period to allow healing of the osseous injury and capsular repair. Early mobilization with gentle passive exercises is encouraged to begin the process of regaining shoulder joint mobility. At 2 to 4 weeks, pendulum exercises and passive ROM exercises in the scapular plane can begin. Patients who underwent a rotator cuff repair may benefit from performing pendulum ROM exercises while supine to maintain scapular stabilization. At 4 weeks, the patient can begin active assisted exercises in flexion, external rotation, and elevation with a goal to gradually achieve full or the patient's normal external rotation in neutral (30 to 40 degrees), 120 to 140 degrees in flexion, and abduction of approximately 45 degrees. Usually around 6 to 8 weeks, the patient can begin strengthening exercises. Patients should not begin strengthening or resistance exercises until their ROM has significantly improved. If a subscapularis split was used, patients may be more aggressive with internal rotation strengthening with less protection of external rotation. Full return to activity is expected around 4 to 6 months postoperatively. Patients who desire to return to competitive contact/overhead sports or

axillary pouch when the surgical arm is placed in external and internal rotation. An HAGL lesion should be repaired inferiorly to superiorly, and medially to laterally. If engaging, a Hill-Sachs lesion may benefit from remplissage or bone augmentation (Figs. 43.15–43.18).

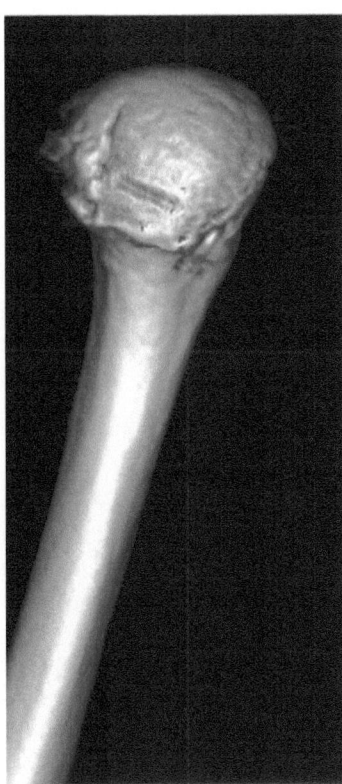

Fig. 43.18 Postoperative three-dimensional computed tomography image of a repaired Hill-Sachs lesion. The improved contour of the humeral head can be appreciated.

occupational activities that frequently places their shoulder in positions of instability, abduction, and external rotation, may benefit from waiting until at least 6 months postoperatively prior to full return of their activities. Patients should be educated on joint protection, such as forceful stretching or manipulation of the shoulder and heavy lifting above shoulder height, until the rehabilitation protocol has been completed.

RESULTS

The goal in managing revision shoulder stabilization is to reconstruct the anatomy through the correction of bony deficits and ligamentous laxity with a secure fixation. Biomechanical and clinical studies have demonstrated that the more anatomical the repair, the better the outcomes in terms of stability and motion.[90,91] Favorable clinical outcomes have been reported following both arthroscopic and open stabilization repair.[2,4,14,16,18,19,87,91–98]

Arthroscopic stabilization with suture anchors is an acceptable revision procedure for anterior shoulder instability.[99–104] One study reported that patients who underwent arthroscopic stabilization compared to those who underwent open repair have a greater return of external rotation in abduction, 90 degrees and 80 degrees, respectively.[17] Another study on active duty military patients reported a lower failed surgical rate with arthroscopic Bankart repair than with open repair.[105]

Proper treatment for glenoid bone loss is important for the success of revision shoulder stabilization, and a higher recurrence rate of glenohumeral instability is associated with uncorrected glenoid bone loss of 15% to 20%.[4,23,38] Glenoid defects less than

21% (mean of 6.8 mm bony loss) may benefit from capsular repair alone[90]; however, patients with greater than 21% bony loss who undergo capsular repair alone report persistent instability and limited external rotation from inadequate capsular restraints.[23,90,102] Arthroscopic repair with a glenoid bone loss between 20% and 25% can be successful with the use of small bony fragments to recreate a more normal anatomy.[87,106,107] The outcomes are less predictable if there is significant bone loss with this repair method. One study comparing arthroscopic revisions in either beach chair or lateral decubitus show no statistically significant difference in two postoperative outcome scores: Rowe and Constant-Murley.[79] The primary finding of the study was that performing the repair with the patient in lateral decubitus resulted in a lower recurrence rate than in beach chair; however, the overall recurrence rate was 12%.

Large anteroinferior glenoid defects can be addressed with a Latarjet procedure or bone graft fixation. Allograft augmentation is emerging as a viable option with large glenoid defects, especially in the setting of failed Latarjet. One study reported excellent stability upon clinical exam, minimal graft absorption, and excellent clinical outcomes based on American Shoulder and Elbow Society scores, Western Ontario Shoulder Instability Index, and single numerical assessment evaluation following DTA glenoid reconstruction at an average follow-up of 45 months.[89] A cadaveric study showed the distal tibia's articular surface radial curvature is similar to that of the glenoid, which allows recreation of the full arch ranges of motion intrinsic to the shoulder joint. Furthermore, the DTA is corticocancellous bone that allows for screw fixation. Reconstruction with DTA recreates the anatomy of the glenoid rim better than an iliac crest bone graft or a coracoid process via Latarjet procedure, with a good healing rate and a low lysis rate.[89,108,109] Replenishing the glenoid bone stock is imperative to the success of revision instability repairs. Mixed long-term outcomes have been reported following a Latarjet procedure. A retrospective review of 58 shoulder Latarjet stabilizations noted excellent results with no recurrence in dislocations at an average of 14.3 years follow-up.[110] Another study reported 25 shoulders having grade I changes out of 118 treated with a Bristow/Latarjet repair at an average follow up of 15.2 years.[111] While their patients reported an overall satisfaction rate of 98%, a follow up radiographic study for the same cohort found moderate to severe dislocation arthropathy in 14% of the patients.[112] One study on 49 patients treated with a modified Bristow procedure reported nearly a 70% rate of good to excellent results, but 15% of the shoulders had a recurrence of instability at a mean time of 7 years post-repair.

COMPLICATIONS

Postoperative complications include recurrence of instability, stiffness, pain, nerve injury, chondrolysis, subscapularis dysfunction, and infection.[113] Inadequate restoration of the glenoid concavity and defect can result in a recurrence of instability. This can be minimized through proper graft choice and avoiding excessive anteroinferior capsular tightening in overhead athletes. Proper tensioning of the capsule can help prevent joint stiffness and shearing of the posterior humeral head on the glenoid surface. Patients may experience pain following revision stabilization. Prolonged pain following surgery has been associated with the use of bioabsorbable tacks.[114,115] Pain may also be indicative of chondrolysis; however, this is mostly historical and more commonly associated with thermal capsulorrhaphy or the use of an intra-articular pain pump.[116–119] Hardware failure has been associated with the use of bioabsorbable tacks and improper placement of suture anchors. Three or more anchors should be placed firmly on the subchondral bone below the articular margin under the 3 o'clock position. Should more than three sutures be necessary, the first additional suture anchor should be placed at the 5:30 position and 45 degrees to the articular surface. The use of suture anchors is associated with a risk of glenoid rim fracture, osteolysis, infection, damage of the glenoid articular cartilage and the enlargement of drill holes.[6] Subscapularis dysfunction or insufficiency can occur after open procedures that utilize a subscapularis tendon and capsule incising technique. Tenderness to palpation in the anterior shoulder and pain associated with decreased internal rotation strength or excessive external rotation may be indicative of subscapular dysfunction.[120,121] Infection is a potential but rare complication following revision repair, particularly with indolent organisms such as *Propionibacterium acnes*. Joint infection with *P. acnes* is difficult to diagnose as it may present with nonspecific symptoms, such as generalized pain, up to 2 years following surgery.[122,123] *P. acnes* infection has a reported incidence between 0% and 6% after open stabilization and between 0.04% and 0.23% after arthroscopic stabilization.[124,125] There is a potential risk of damage to the axillary nerve, musculocutaneous nerve, the suprascapular nerve and artery, and the cephalic vein during exposure for arthroscopic stabilization; however, this risk is minimized by using the established portal locations described in our preferred surgical technique.[64,78,81,126–131] Careful placement of the humeral head to avoid excessive flexion–extension and distraction along with a strong knowledge of shoulder anatomy can further prevent this injury. The axillary nerve is located approximately 1 to 1.5 cm below the inferior aspect of the glenohumeral capsule and the musculocutaneous nerve sits approximately 5 to 8 cm inferior to the coracoid.

FUTURE CONSIDERATIONS

Various techniques have been described that adequately correct recurrent anterior shoulder instability. Diagnosis and management for patients with chronic instability following failed stabilization procedures continue to evolve. Studies reporting long-term outcomes following these surgical methods are necessary to elucidate which technique will allow the patient the greatest chance of full return to activity while minimizing the risk of recurrence (Fig. 43.19).

For a complete list of references, go to ExpertConsult.com.

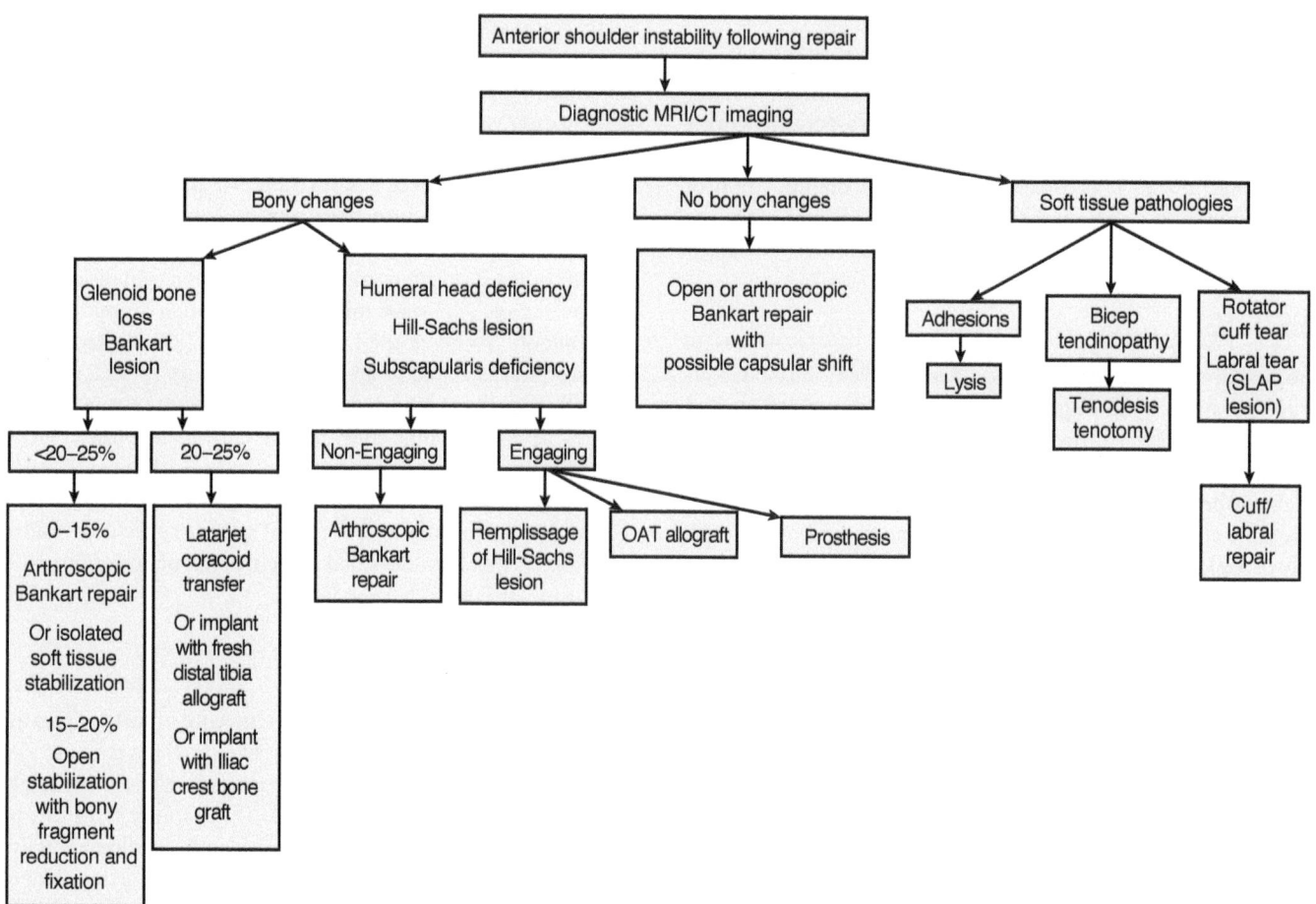

Fig. 43.19 Treatment algorithm and decision-making. *CT*, Computed tomography; *MRI*, computed tomography.

SELECTED READINGS

Citation:

Frank RM, Romeo AA, Provencher MT. Glenoid reconstruction with distal tibia allograft for recurrent anterior shoulder instability. *Orthopedics*. 2017;40(1):e199–e205.

Level of Evidence:

IV

Summary:

This article aims to assess the clinical and radiographic outcomes of patients experiencing recurrent anterior shoulder instability that were treated with fresh distal tibia allograft (DTA) for reconstruction. The study included patients that had a minimum of 15% anterior glenoid bone loss with recurrent shoulder instability. To test the efficacy of the DTA, the study used the American Shoulder and Elbow Society score, the Western Ontario shoulder instability index, and single numerical assessment evaluation score at a minimum of a 2-year follow-up. They found that DTA reconstruction leads to a stable glenohumeral joint, optimal clinical outcomes, and minimal graft resorption.

Citation:

Provencher MT, Bhatia S, Ghodadra NS, et al. Recurrent shoulder instability: current concepts in for evaluation and management of glenoid bone loss. *J Bone Joint Surg Am*. 2010;92(suppl 2): 133–151.

Level of Evidence:

I

Summary:

This article provides current concepts for diagnosis and management of recurrent instability with glenoid bone loss. It helps update the reader on the most advanced way to conduct a physical exam, inquire about history, and run an imaging protocol specific to the individual patient situation. The article details a surgeon's appropriate preoperative surgical decisions and when each unique procedure becomes relevant. It is also informative with regard to the different usages of arthroscopy and open procedures. They conclude that glenoid bone loss is a serious issue and must be suspected or considered in each patient presenting glenohumeral instability.

Citation:

Cvetanovich GL, McCormick F, Erickson BJ, et al. The posterolateral portal: optimizing anchor placement and labral repair at the inferior glenoid. *Arthrosc Tech*. 2013;2(3):e201–e204.

Level of Evidence:

I

Summary:

This article details the surgical technique for arthroscopic shoulder stabilization of a Bankart lesion with an additional posterolateral portal. They utilize the lateral decubitus position as it offers the superior viewing angle of the entire capsulolabral complex. The three different viewing portals used are posterior, anterosuperior, and posterolateral. They conclude that with the advances in arthroscopic techniques it is becoming more common and appropriate to shift away from open procedures when correcting shoulder instability.

Citation:

Frank RM, Saccomanno MF, McDonald LS, et al. Outcomes of arthroscopic anterior shoulder instability in the beach chair versus lateral decubitus position: a systematic review and meta-regression analysis. *Arthroscopy*. 2014;30(10):1349–1365.

Level of Evidence:

IV

Summary:

This article is a systematic review spanning the time frame from 1990 to 2013, and it includes 64 studies (38 beach chair position, 26 lateral decubitus) that comprise a total of 3668 shoulders. The purpose of the study was to discuss the advantages and disadvantages of performing arthroscopic stabilization with the patient in the lateral decubitus or the beach chair position. The postoperative details that the study used to test efficacy were percentage of recurrence, range of motion, and Rowe score. They found excellent clinical outcomes and low recurrence rates for both methods; however, the recurrence rate in the lateral decubitus position was lower. They conclude that there is a need for additional studies to determine the potential advantages and disadvantages of each position.

Citation:

Piasecki DP, Verma NN, Romeo AA, et al. Glenoid bone deficiency in recurrent anterior shoulder instability: diagnosis and Management. *J Am Acad Orthop Surg*. 2009;17(8):482–493.

Level of Evidence:

I

Summary:

This article offers a review of the diagnosis and management of recurrent shoulder instability, with specific focus on the issue of glenoid bone loss. It provides a detailed description of surgical treatment options for primary and revision surgery. It also discusses extracurricular activities that can influence the preoperative surgical decision.

Citation:

Bhatia S, Frank RM, Ghodadra NS, et al. The outcomes and surgical techniques of the Latarjet procedure. *Arthroscopy*. 2014;30(2):227–235.

Level of Evidence:

IV

Summary:

This study is a systematic review that includes a retrospective group of 10 different studies including patients that underwent a Latarjet procedure. This study goes in depth on the technique of the Latarjet including the glenoid exposure, anchor placement, and placement of coracoid process. This article also talks about the outcomes of the procedures and the various recurrence rates that came from grouping the studies.

44

Superior Labrum Anterior to Posterior Tears

Sean J. Meredith, R. Frank Henn III

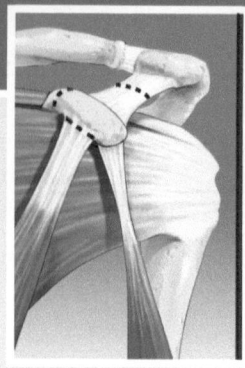

Superior labrum anterior to posterior (SLAP) lesions have been recognized as a cause of shoulder pain since the mid-1980s.[1] Controversy regarding normal variant labral anatomy versus truly pathologic lesions causing consistent clinical symptoms surfaced almost immediately thereafter.[2] Snyder and colleagues[3] described the pathologic anatomy of four types of SLAP lesions and the implications for treatment (Figs. 44.1 and 44.2). Other authors have described additional tear patterns.[4–6] Although the true incidence of SLAP lesions is unknown, in the initial study by Snyder and colleagues, the percentage of SLAP repairs as a function of their overall surgical cases was quite low (3.3%). This percentage increased slightly to 4.7% in a follow-up study in 1995.[7] Rates have varied slightly from these low numbers in other series.[4,8,9]

While the published literature consistently suggests that SLAP lesions are relatively uncommon, disproportionate enthusiasm for operative intervention for this diagnosis has been noted. A review of two statewide databases[10] found that SLAP repair volume increased 238% from 2002 to 2009 and 20% from 2005 to 2009, compared to an overall orthopedic case volume increase of 125% and decrease of 14%, respectively. This may be related to the high incidence of false-positive radiologic interpretations of magnetic resonance imaging (MRI) scans. An investigation performed by Weber and Kauffman[11] showed that up to 35% of community-read MRI scans were interpreted as either a labral tear or a "possible labral tear." Superior labral tears diagnosed on MRI in middle-aged and older patients are likely to actually be normal age-related changes as evidenced by Schwartzberg et al.,[12] which showed rates of labral tear in asymptomatic 45- to 60-year-old individuals of 55% and 72% as read by two fellowship-trained musculoskeletal radiologists.

Clinical findings upon examining the shoulders of patients with SLAP lesions are also inconsistent. Although a number of tests and clinical examination maneuvers have been suggested, all have proved to be difficult to validate (Table 44.1).[5,8,13–26] These issues create problems for the surgeon in the diagnosis of SLAP lesions preoperatively. The interpretation of intraoperative findings is also difficult, and even experienced surgeons disagree regarding which findings represent a normal variant, such as a sublabral recess (Fig. 44.3) that requires no treatment, and which findings are pathologic.[27] Electing for operative intervention involves carefully assessing the history, physical examination, and imaging findings, and then critically condensing the results into a patient-specific treatment plan.

HISTORY

SLAP lesions can be degenerative or traumatic. Maffett et al.[4] suggested that traction on the overhead or abducted arm is a common traumatic mechanism. Snyder et al.[7] described the injury as being due to compression from a fall on the outstretched arm. Throwers are at high risk from attritional superior labrum lesions. Burkhart and Morgan[14] described the "peel-back" mechanism where abduction and external rotation shoulder position places a torsional force on the posterior superior labrum and biceps anchor, causing the detachment of the anchor and a SLAP tear. Overuse symptoms created by activities performed below the shoulder generally do not cause labral pathology, and positive MRI scans obtained in this subset of patients should be viewed with suspicion. Because natural degeneration of the labrum occurs with age,[15] other shoulder pathology is more relevant in older patients, and the SLAP lesion can be incidental. Most persons with symptomatic SLAP lesions present with posterior pain, typically with overhead activities.[30] Night pain and pain at rest are atypical. Mechanical popping, catching, or grinding can suggest on unstable flap. Isolated SLAP lesions are uncommon,[31] and thus many of the symptoms may be masked by other diagnoses such as impingement, bicipital tendonitis, and acromioclavicular pain. Patients presenting with shoulder instability often have extension of the labral damage into the superior labrum,[4] and a high index of suspicion is necessary in this subset of patients. However, for the most part, the history will be nonspecific, and recognizing the appropriate demographic in which SLAP lesions occur remains the most important part of the history.

PHYSICAL EXAMINATION

Identifying symptomatic SLAP lesions on physical examination remains challenging because significant clinical findings upon examination of the shoulders of patients with SLAP lesions are inconsistent. The physical exam can be suggestive of a SLAP tear, but it is rarely conclusive. The O'Brien active compression test is one of the more common provocative maneuvers.[24] For this test, the shoulder is positioned in 90 degrees of flexion, internal rotation, and slight horizontal adduction. The test is positive when resisted shoulder flexion causes deep shoulder pain that is relieved with repeat exam of resisted shoulder flexion in external rotation. Although a number of other tests and clinical examination maneuvers have been suggested, they have all proved to be

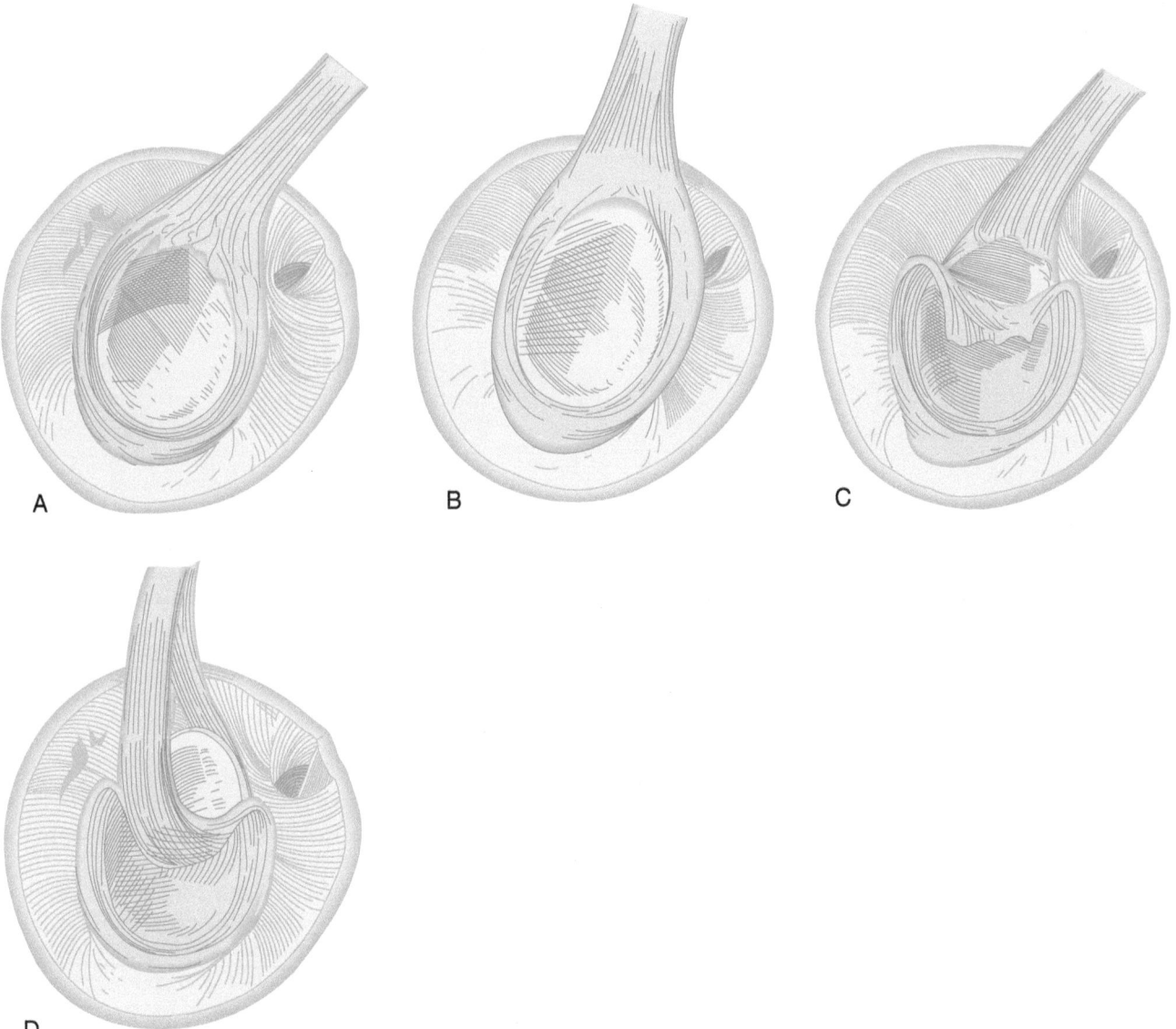

Fig. 44.1 The original Snyder classification of superior labrum anterior to posterior lesions. (A) Type I has degenerative superior labrum tearing but attached biceps. (B) Type II has detachment of the superior labrum–biceps tendon complex from the superior glenoid. (C) Type III has a bucket handle tear of a meniscoid superior labrum but attached biceps. (D) Type IV has tearing of the superior labrum up into the biceps tendon. Variable amounts of the biceps are left attached. (Modified from Snyder SJ, Karzel RP, Del Pizzo W, et al. SLAP lesions of the shoulder. *Arthroscopy*. 1990;6:274–279.)

difficult to validate.[5,8,13–26] The only test Weber and Kauffman found to have reasonable sensitivity was the apprehension test, but this was still poor.[11] The inability of other surgeons to reproduce the sensitivities and specificities described by the physician who originally performed the test led Kim and McFarland to state, "… our findings question the diagnostic value of the clinical assessment of SLAP lesions."[18] Snyder and colleagues[7] continue to make the argument that "there is no physical finding specific for SLAP lesion of the shoulder." Walsworth et al.[32] noted that even combining tests did not improve the results of physical examination testing. Consistent with the history, the presence of other pathology can render the identification of SLAP pathology difficult. SLAP lesions are difficult to diagnose clinically, and

tests must be performed in the context of the clinical history and the appropriate patient demographic.

IMAGING

Radiographic evaluation, including true anterior-posterior (AP) shoulder (Grashey view), axillary lateral, and scapular Y views, is used to identify other potential sources of shoulder pain. MRI is the mainstay of preoperative imaging. Noncontrast MRI remains the most common tool used to diagnose labral pathology. However, radiologic review of these studies remains highly variable. Kauffman and Weber[11] showed that up to 35% of community-read MRI scans were interpreted as either a labral

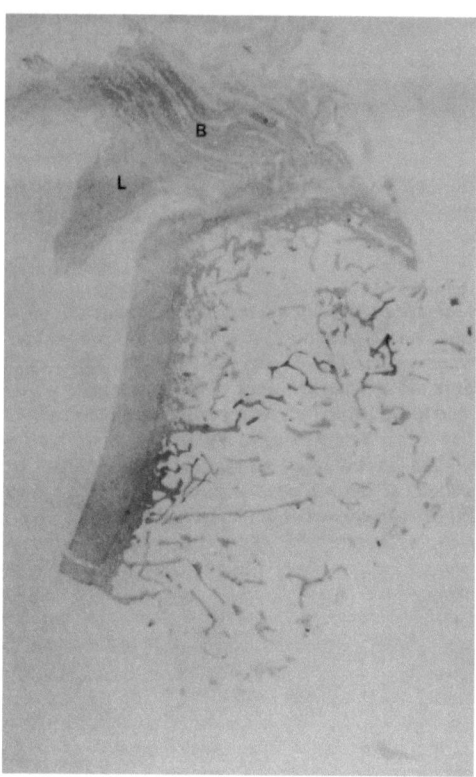

Fig. 44.2 A histologic picture of a cross section of the superior labrum (L), the glenoid, and the biceps tendon (B). This photomicrograph demonstrates primary attachment of the superior labrum to the biceps tendon before it inserts onto the supraglenoid tubercle. Note the lack of firm attachment of the superior labrum to the glenoid itself. (From Cooper DE, Arnoczky SP, O'Brien SJ, et al. Anatomy, histology, and vascularity of the glenoid labrum: an anatomical study. *J Bone Joint Surg Am.* 1992;74:46–52.)

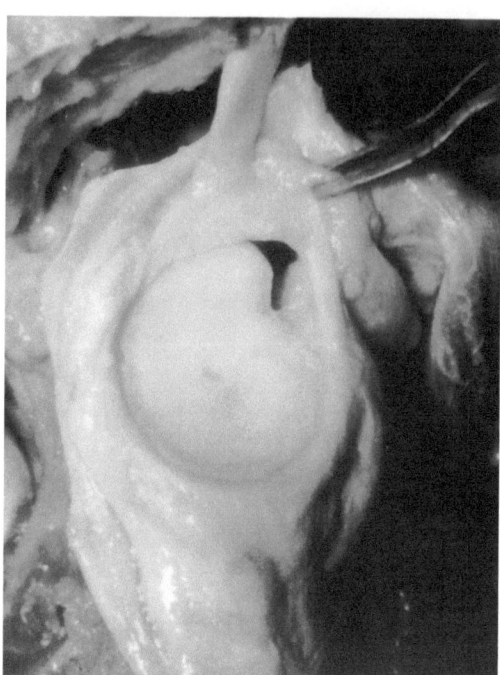

Fig. 44.3 An anterosuperior sublabral foramina. This cadaveric specimen demonstrates a normal sublabral foramina under the anterosuperior labrum. (From Cooper DE, Arnoczky SP, O'Brien SJ, et al. Anatomy, histology, and vascularity of the glenoid labrum: an anatomical study. *J Bone Joint Surg Am.* 1992;74:46–52.)

tear or a "possible labral tear," which is a worrisome statistic when the true incidence is probably between 3% and 5%.[7] Clearly the orthopedist will need to become confident in interpreting MRI images of the labrum if the study is to be useful. Higgins and Weber found that only 5 of 64 patients with surgically confirmed SLAP lesions were correctly diagnosed by the preoperative radiologist reading[9]; however, the use of contrast material may improve these results (Fig. 44.4). Overall, Belanger and Green[13] noted that "MRI was non-specific in identifying SLAP lesions," and Mileski and Snyder[22] stated that "diagnostic arthroscopy remains the only definitive way to diagnose SLAP lesions of the shoulder." A less common but important finding on MRI is a paralabral cyst, which is usually pathognomic of a labral tear. A paralabral cyst extending to the spinoglenoid notch from a posterosuperior labral tear can compress the suprascapular nerve and cause painful infraspinatus dysfunction (Fig. 44.5). In a large series of spinoglenoid notch cysts causing suprascapular nerve entrapment by Moore et al.,[33] 20 out of 22 spinoglenoid notch cysts were identified on preoperative MRI. Of those patients who underwent arthroscopy, 10 out of 11 cysts were associated with superior labral tears. Clearly, orthopedists who treat the shoulder will need to become facile in interpreting MRI scans of the shoulder, especially because numerous normal anatomic variants, such as sublabral recesses, can confound the interpretation of the scan. Despite advances in the performance and interpretation of MRI of the shoulder, surgeons need to be prepared to diagnose and treat SLAP lesions as they present at surgery. Arthroscopy is still the gold standard in the diagnosis of labral tears, and the surgeon should be prepared to address these lesions.

TABLE 44.1	Clinical Examination Tests for SLAP Lesions With Subsequent Studies Attempting to Validate the Original Authors' Results	
Clinical Test	Works Inconsistently	Failure to Validate
Snyder biceps compression test[7]		Weber and Higgins[9]; Kim and McFarland[18]
Jobe relocation test	Weber and Higgins,[9] 70% sensitivity Guanche and Jones,[28] 73% sensitivity	Mileski and Snyder[22]
Kibler anterior slide test[17]		Kim et al.[19]
Liu crank test[21]		Guanche and Jones[28] Stetson[25]
O'Brien active compression test	Guanche and Jones[28] Morgan and Burkhart[5]	Ottl et al.[29] Kim and McFarland[18]
Speed test	Holtby and Razmjou[16]	

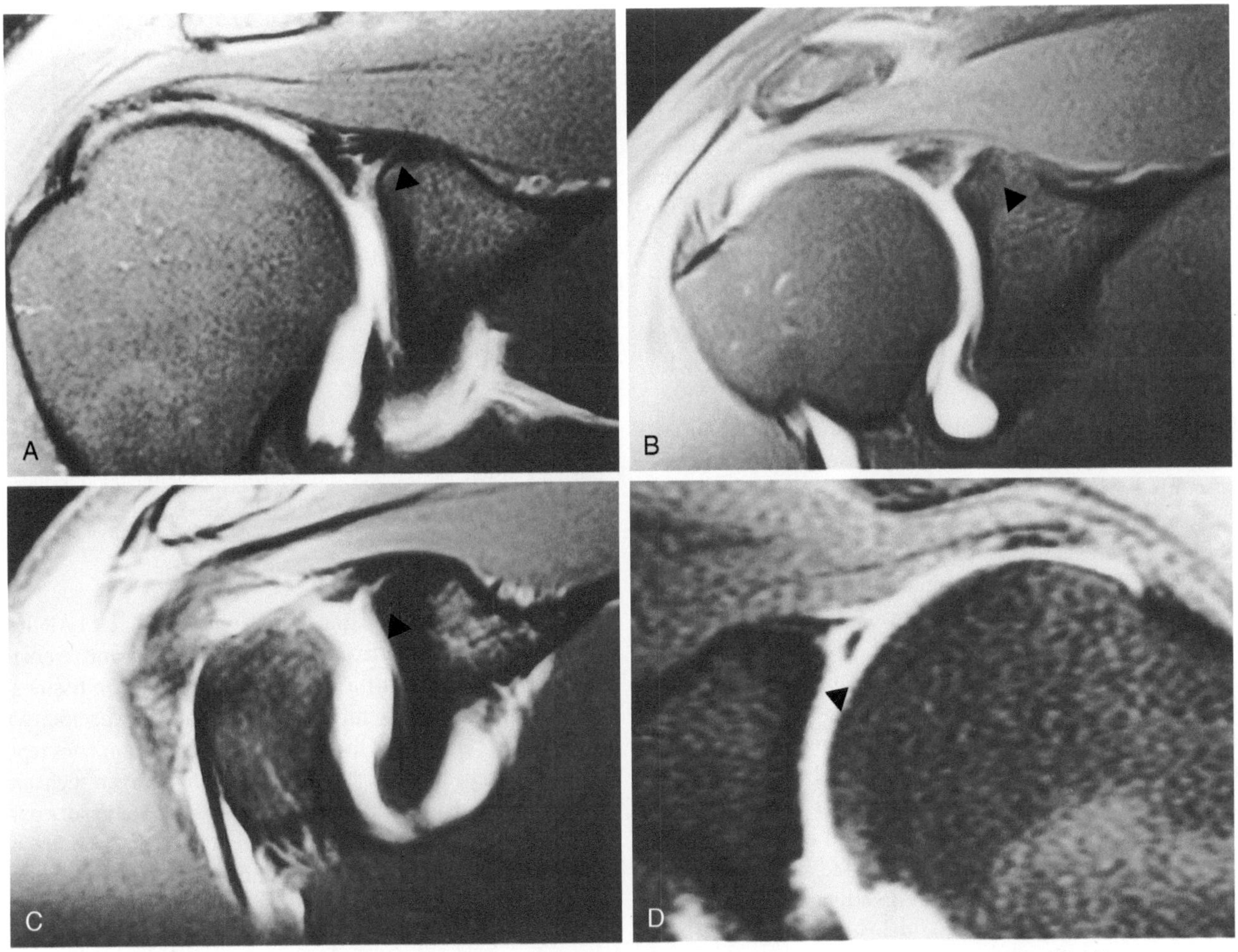

Fig. 44.4 Gadolinium-enhanced magnetic resonance images of superior labrum anterior to posterior (SLAP) lesions. Note the leakage of the dye under the biceps tendon insertion in four separate cases *(arrowheads)*. (A) Contrast dye extending lateral in the superior labrum, classically diagnostic of superior labral tear. (B) Complete extension of dye through the labrum superiorly. (C) Complex pattern with dye extending medial and intermediate signal extending lateral through the tissue of the labrum. (D) Contrast extending laterally with separation of labral tissue and irregular border of remaining labrum. These images can be diagnostic of a type II SLAP lesion.

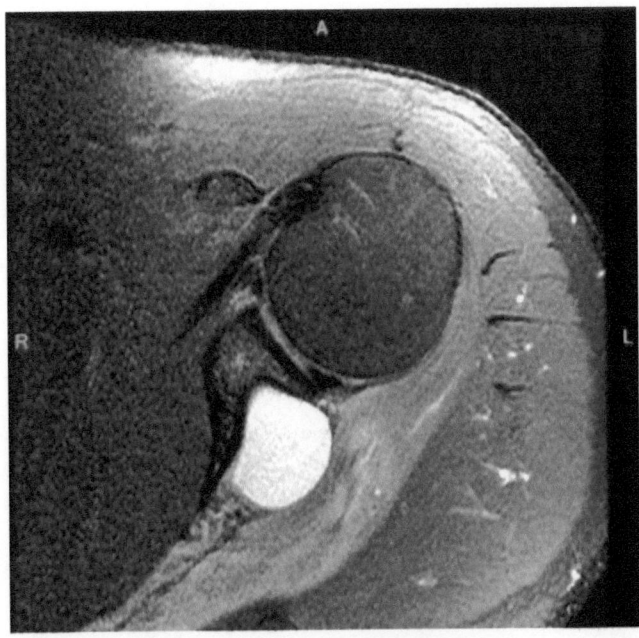

Fig. 44.5 A spinoglenoid notch cyst.

DECISION-MAKING PRINCIPALS

Decision-making with regard to the treatment of patients who may have SLAP pathology remains difficult. As previously indicated, the diagnosis will rarely be made by a clear-cut history, physical examination, or imaging study. The clinical information that is available with regard to this complicated problem is straightforward on one subject: SLAP lesions are relatively rare. True incidence rates are not available, but a number of studies have suggested that the percentage of SLAP lesions as a function of the total number of cases remains fairly low. Snyder et al.[3] had a percentage rate of 3% of their total shoulder cases, which increased to 5.9% in a subsequent follow-up study.[7] Subsequent studies have shown varying rates from 2% to 12%.[4,8,9] A review of American Board of Orthopaedic Surgery (ABOS) II data from 2003 to 2008 has shown a significant increase in the actual number and percentage of SLAP repairs among candidates, at 10% of shoulder cases.[34] However, another review[10] of the ABOS database from 2003 to 2010 show no statistically significant increase in the likelihood of performing SLAP repair among those candidates performing at least 1 SLAP repair. Candid assessment of the percentage of SLAP lesions performed by each surgeon may allow one to assess the indications selected for repair.

Another important factor is age. Numerous authors have suggested that patients older than 40 years may be better served by arthroscopic biceps tenodesis than SLAP repair.[15,34–37] The reasons are probably multifactorial, but again, labral degeneration is more common with age, and age-related biceps changes may make SLAP repair impractical. Erickson et al.[38] conducted a systematic review of SLAP repairs in patients 40 years of age and older and found significantly higher failure rates compared to those under 40 years old. They noted decreased patient satisfaction, increased re-operation rates, and increased postoperative stiffness with increasing age.

Older patients often have substantial additional pathology, the correction of which may further increase the morbidity of the procedure.[15] Multiple studies[39–42] have investigated concomitant rotator cuff tears. Franceschi et al.[39] conducted a randomized trial of SLAP repair versus bicep tenotomy for patients over age 50 with type II SLAP tear undergoing concomitant rotator cuff repair and showed no benefit with regard to clinical outcome score or range of motion (ROM) with SLAP repair. Abbot and Busconi[41] showed improved outcomes scores and pain relief with simple débridement of the type II SLAP tear with concomitant rotator cuff repair when compared to SLAP repair in patients over age 45. Oh et al.[42] compared débridement, biceps tenotomy, and biceps tenodesis with concomitant rotator cuff repair and all groups showed improved pain, ROM, and outcome scores. The biceps tenotomy group showed decreased bicipital groove tenderness but lower forearm supination strength compared to tenodesis and debridement. Simple débridement showed the least "Popeye" deformity. Most of the evidence to date supports one of these alternatives, débridement, biceps tenotomy, or biceps tenodesis, rather than SLAP repair with concomitant rotator cuff repair. Initial nonoperative treatment of a suspected SLAP lesion remains the primary choice for virtually all patients. Blaine et al.[43] showed a high rate of success with this approach. Whether the MRI diagnosis was a false-positive or the SLAP lesion healed is difficult to determine; nonetheless, the success rate was high. Jang et al.[44] found demand for overhead activities, a history of trauma, or mechanical symptoms predicted failure of their nonoperative treatment. Careful observation and differential injection can further define additional treatment that may be needed, given that SLAP lesions rarely occur in isolation.[3,4,9] Clearly a radiologic report of a "possible SLAP lesion" is not in itself an indication for surgery. Assuming that the history, physical examination, imaging study findings, and demographic category of the patient fit the diagnosis of a SLAP lesion and nonoperative treatment fails, then diagnostic arthroscopy can be undertaken to identify if in fact a symptomatic SLAP lesion is the cause of the symptoms.

Even when diagnostic arthroscopy is performed, the decision-making can be difficult. Numerous studies have shown that even experienced surgeons vary widely in their determination of which lesions are pathologic.[27] Whereas special assessments, such as the sulcus score of Mihata et al.,[45] may prove useful, even a visual diagnosis of SLAP lesions at surgery remains controversial. Although the diagnosis of type III and IV lesions is relatively

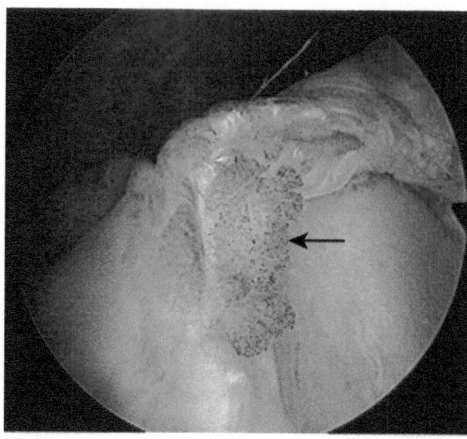

Fig. 44.6 A superior labrum with a type II superior labrum anterior to posterior lesion. Note the area of synovitis posterosuperiorly, indicating evidence of trauma *(arrow)*. Granulation tissue is an important finding to indicate a pathologic labral condition and not a normal variant.

straightforward, the diagnosis of type I and II SLAP lesions remains elusive. Data from both Snyder et al.[3] and Weber and Higgins[9] suggests that the presence of granulation tissue at the base of the labral attachment indicates a high specificity for a SLAP lesion (Fig. 44.6). Given the high complication rates reported with SLAP repair,[15,31,34,35,46–51] the decision to perform such a repair should not be made lightly. As previously suggested, older patients and those with concomitant rotator cuff tears may be better served by a biceps tenodesis or tenotomy.

A good indication for SLAP repair is spinoglenoid notch cyst with symptoms of suprascapular nerve compression. Shon et al.[52] showed good to excellent results in 90% of patients with intra-articular decompression of the cyst and superior labral repair. All patients who had postoperative MRI at 6 months had complete resolution of the cyst and neurogenic infraspinatus muscle edema. Kim et al.[53] showed similarly good results with their technique of subacromial decompression of the spinoglenoid notch cyst and SLAP repair. However, it is not clear if cyst decompression is required in this setting. In a prospective cohort study by Kim et al.,[54] 28 patients were treated with either SLAP repair and cyst decompression or SLAP repair alone. There was no significant difference between groups with regard to outcomes or cyst resolution, and 25 of 28 showed total resolution of the spinoglenoid cyst. This provides further evidence that SLAP repair is effective management of a SLAP tear with a spinoglenoid notch cyst.

TREATMENT OPTIONS

A variety of treatment options exist for symptomatic SLAP lesions. Simple débridement, as originally reported,[1] has been shown to have a high rate of failure in the athletic population,[55] but it is usually appropriate for some type I (Fig. 44.7) and type III SLAP lesions. Biceps tenotomy has also had its advocates[15] and remains a simple, quick procedure for patients with lower demands on the shoulder, although cramping and deformity can occur, and appropriate preoperative informed consent is required.[15] For the most part, treatment options center around repair or tenodesis. As previously discussed, tenodesis may be the appropriate choice

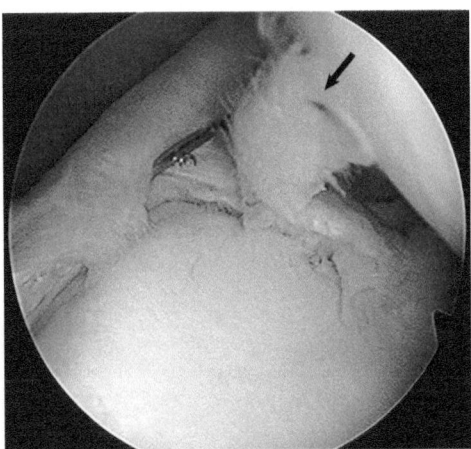

Fig. 44.7 A flap-type superior labrum anterior to posterior lesion. As viewed from the posterior portal, the posterior-based unstable superior labral flap *(arrow)* can be noted.

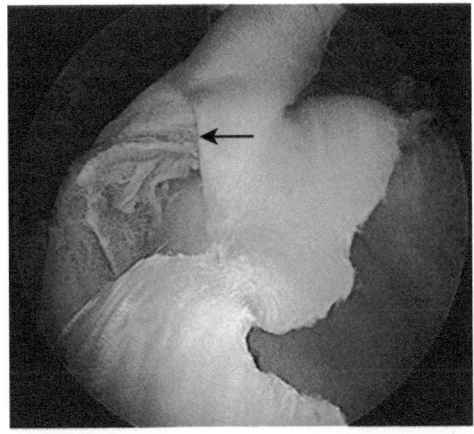

Fig. 44.8 A type IV superior labrum anterior to posterior lesion. The extension of the tear into the substance of the biceps tendon can be seen *(arrow)*.

for older patients,[15,34–37] in a revision situation,[15,35,51] or for a type IV SLAP lesion (Fig. 44.8). Both proximal arthroscopic and distal mini-open subpectoral techniques have been proposed. Kauffman et al.[37] and Sekiya et al.[56] have had success with proximal tenodesis techniques, which have shown good results with low revision rates, even at long-term follow-up.[37]

SLAP repair is a reasonable treatment for younger, active patients with a symptomatic SLAP lesion. Although the use of tacks was initially proposed, these techniques have been largely abandoned because of high complication rates.[15,35,46–48,50,51] Currently the standard of care is suture anchor repair. Biomechanical studies[57–60] have shown varying results of load to failure when comparing the simple versus the mattress suture technique, as well as a number of anchors and configuration. Suture anchor

placement anterior to the biceps has been shown in a biomechanical study[61] to decrease shoulder external rotation, which may be detrimental to the overhead athlete. No prospective, high-level studies have been performed to analyze the type of repair and number of anchors to be used. Recent anecdotal reports of knot "squeaking" have led some surgeons to revert to the use of bioabsorbable sutures for repair, especially as a result of articular cartilage injury.[35,51] Knotless anchors may have some technical advantages, but Sileo et al.[62] showed decreased load to gap formation at the repair site in a cadaver model compared to knotted anchors. The choice of anchors, configuration, simple versus mattress sutures, and knotted versus knotless anchors are all up to the preference of the surgeon, given the lack of prospective, comparative data.

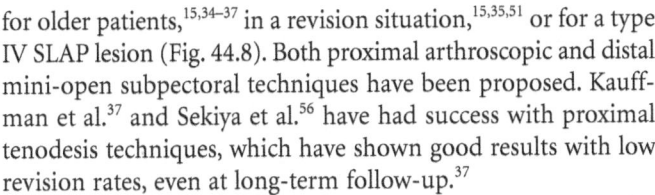
🔖 Authors' Preferred Technique

SLAP Lesions

The technique used by the authors is based on preference rather than on data from solid studies. Nonoperative treatment of all suspected SLAP lesions is preferred initial management for the reasons previously discussed, with the exception of spinoglenoid notch cysts compressing the suprascapular nerve and mechanical symptoms associated with an unstable flap (type III). When nonoperative treatment fails and a symptomatic SLAP lesion is suspected, diagnostic arthroscopy is indicated. If the clinical, imaging, and surgical findings support the presence of an isolated, symptomatic, unstable type II SLAP lesion without a paralabral cyst, we prefer to manage this with subpectoral biceps tenodesis in younger, high-demand patients, and biceps tenotomy in older low-demand patients. We perform SLAP repair and decompression of the cyst for patients with spinoglenoid notch cyst, and we perform SLAP repair in the setting of combined anterior and/or posterior labral repair. We prefer to use biocomposite labral anchors (2.9 mm) loaded with #2 polyethylene suture for both SLAP repair and biceps tenodesis.

The step-by-step procedure that we use for SLAP repair is as follows:
- Standard posterior viewing portal and anterosuperior working portal are created.
- The superior glenoid is prepared down to bone using a shaver from an anterior portal (Fig. 44.9).
- The portal of Wilmington is localized with a spinal needle 1 cm anterior and lateral to the posterolateral corner of the acromion.[5] The drill guide for the

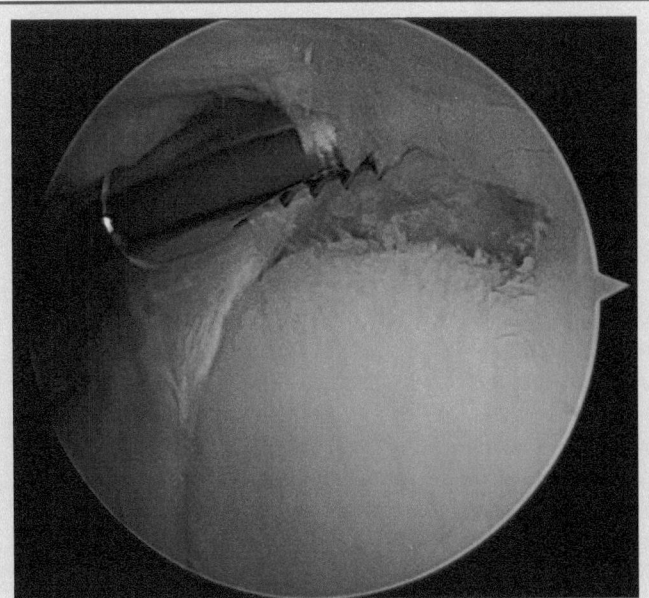

Fig. 44.9 Superior labrum anterior to posterior tear.

Continued

📌 Authors' Preferred Technique

SLAP Lesions—cont'd

anchor is passed percutaneously through the muscular portion of the infra-spinatus into the joint.

- One or two suture anchors are placed posterior to the biceps anchor through the portal of Wilmington depending on the posterior extent of the tear. A suture passer is used to shuttle one strand of suture around the superior labrum for a simple suture for each anchor.

- The sutures are then tied using standard knot-tying techniques (Fig. 44.10). For subpectoral biceps tenodesis, we use the same technique described by Dr. Warner. The bicep tendon is secured to the bone deep to the pectoralis major tendon with a single 2.9 mm double-loaded suture anchor.

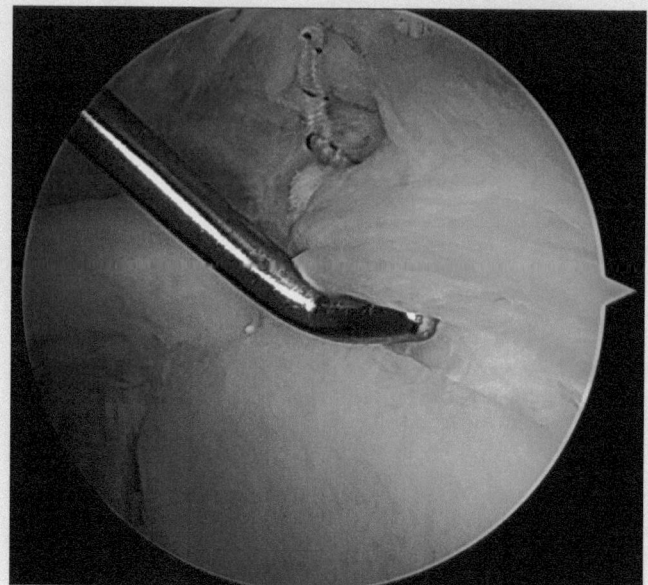

Fig. 44.10 Repair.

Postoperative Management

SLAP repair or biceps tenodesis are both managed similarly postoperatively. Cryotherapy is used postoperatively, and sling protection is utilized for 4 weeks. Pendulum exercises and passive external rotation start the day following surgery. Active-assisted and passive exercises are started at 2 weeks postoperatively. Active exercises are progressed at 4 weeks after surgery with goal of maximizing the ROM. Progressive strengthening begins at 6 weeks with the goal of clearance to return to sport by 4 months for biceps tenodesis and 6 months for SLAP repair postoperatively. Appropriate preoperative counseling regarding rehabilitation is necessary to provide reasonable expectations postoperatively.

Results

The results of SLAP repairs have generally been reported to be good, based on short-term level IV studies.[1,3–5,7,14,63] A prospective analysis by Provencher et al.[64] of 179 isolated type II SLAP repairs showed significant improvements in clinical outcome scores, but also a 37% failure rate and a 28% revision rate. They defined failure as a mean ASES score less than 70, the inability to return to sports or work duties, or undergoing a revision surgery. Age greater than 36 years was the only factor significantly associated with failure (relative risk of 3.45). A review by Weber et al.[34] of the outcomes of ABOS part II candidates with this procedure also showed more modest outcomes, with half of the patients older than 40 years, which is a worrisome statistic given the previous discussion of indications for SLAP lesions. Pain was absent in only 26.3% of patients at follow-up, and function was normal in only 13.1%. Only 40.1% of applicants self-reported their patients as having an excellent result

in short-term follow-up. The self-reported complication rate was 4.4%.

Burkhart and Morgan[65] reported an 87% rate of return to sports after SLAP repair in their study. Other follow-up studies specifically directed at return to play (RTP) have found lower rates. In a systematic review, Sayde et al.[66] reported "good-to-excellent" patient satisfaction rate of 83%. However, overall athlete return to previous level of play was 73%, and only 63% among overhead athletes. Fedoriw et al.[67] found a RTP rate of 48% among a series of 27 professional baseball pitchers and 85% for a series of 13 position players. Analyzing more closely the return to previous level of performance based on statistics, they found a return to previous performance rate of only 7% among pitchers and 54% among position players. Although SLAP repairs tend have good results in patients who place a lower demand on their shoulder as measured by standard shoulder outcome scores, return to sport remains problematic in most studies in which this parameter is carefully evaluated.

Superior labral repair versus biceps tenodesis for isolated type II SLAP tears has been a subject of debate, and there is increasing evidence supporting tenodesis as an alternative to repair for many patients. In a retrospective cohort study, Ek et al.[68] showed no difference in ASES scores, patient satisfaction, and return to sports between SLAP repair versus biceps tenodesis. Analysis of their indications showed younger, more active patients with healthy-appearing labral tissue were more commonly repaired, whereas older patients with degenerative or frayed labral tissue underwent biceps tenodesis. Patients were allowed to return to sports faster in the tenodesis group, and there was a trend towards higher RTP rate. Similarly, Boileau et al.[36] found a higher return to sport after tenodesis compared to SLAP repair for type II SLAP lesions. Most recently, Schroder et al.[69] conducted a blinded, randomized, sham-controlled trial of 118 patients with isolated type II SLAP tears indicated for surgical intervention. They found no significant difference in Rowe scores, Western Ontario Shoulder Instability Index, patient satisfaction, or pain scores between labral repair, biceps tenodesis, and sham surgery. They concluded that their data did not support labral repair or biceps tenodesis in this patient population. However, they did not include enough patients to perform a subgroup analysis by age, and the mean age was 40 years.

Complications

Complications associated with SLAP repair include persistent discomfort,[46] loose hardware or loss of fixation,[30,47] persistent rotator cuff defects at the site of transtendon portals,[46] articular cartilage injuries,[35,48] stiffness,[51] persistent synovitis,[48] and suprascapular nerve injury.[70] Two studies specifically looked at complications of SLAP repair. Weber[51] showed that 2 of 24 patients treated for failed SLAP repair had severe arthritis, and 14 of 24 had articular cartilage injury. Out of 24 patients, 10 presented with postoperative stiffness, and 6 presented with loose hardware, 4 of which were tacks. Mean University of California, Los Angeles (UCLA) scores were only 29.2, representing a fair result, and show that surgical treatment of the failed SLAP repair did not generally have a good outcome. The other study evaluating complications of SLAP repair was performed by Katz et al.[35] Similar to Weber's study,[51] postoperative stiffness was common, involving 78% of their patients. Nineteen percent had loose or prominent hardware, and only 68% were satisfied with their revision surgery. In a review of a single surgeon's shoulder arthroscopy series over a 5-year period, Byram et al.[71] found humeral head abrasion under the articulating portion of the biceps tendon in 13 out of 18 failed SLAP repairs. They postulated this was due to increased biceps-humeral head contact pressure from overtensioning of the biceps-labrum complex. Self-reported complications in ABOS part II applicants were 4.4%, even in short-term follow-up, and included both medical and surgical complications, such as implant failure, infection, nerve injury, dislocation, wound dehiscence, tendon injury, and implant failure.[34]

Complications after biceps tenodesis include stiffness, infection, nerve injury, and humerus fracture. Nho et al.[72] reported a complication rate of 2% after 353 subpectoral tenodesis procedures, including 2 with persistent pain, 2 with loss of fixation, 1 deep infection, and 1 musculocutaneous neuropathy. Rhee et al.[73] reported four cases of brachial plexus injuries after subpectoral tenodesis. Sears et al.[74] reported two cases of humeral fracture after tenodesis.

FUTURE CONSIDERATIONS

More research regarding the treatment of SLAP lesions is needed. Perhaps the greatest contribution would be a natural history study because even experts often disagree about what constitutes a pathologic SLAP lesion.[27] High-level, prospective, randomized studies are also needed to sort out which techniques or treatments work best and in which patient populations. The role of alternative treatments to SLAP repair, such as biceps tenotomy and tenodesis, needs to be clearly defined through prospective studies. Until then, understanding that SLAP lesions are real, but rare, and maintaining a healthy respect for the magnitude of the procedure and the possibility of complications is necessary.

ACKNOWLEDGMENT

The authors and editors are grateful for the contributions of the previous author of this chapter, Stephen C. Weber.

For a complete list of references, go to ExpertConsult.com.

SELECTED READINGS

Citation:
Burns JP, Bank M, Snyder SJ. Superior labral tears: repair versus tenodesis. *J Shoulder Elbow Surg*. 2011;20(2):S2–S8.

Level of Evidence:
IV

Summary:
This article provides an excellent summary by the experts in the area of current concepts of surgical treatment of superior labral anterior to posterior tears.

Citation:
Snyder SJ, Karzel RP, Delpizzo W, et al. SLAP lesions of the shoulder. *Arthroscopy*. 1990;6:274–279.

Level of Evidence:
IV

Summary:
This classic article describes the structural types of superior labral anterior to posterior lesions.

Citation:
Weber SC, Martin DF, Seiler JG, et al. Superior labral (SLAP) lesions of the shoulder: incidence rates, complications, and outcomes as reported by ABOS Part II candidates. *Am J Sports Med*. 2012;10(7):1538–1543.

Level of Evidence:
III, cross-sectional design

Summary:
This article describes the reported experience of American Board of Orthopaedic Surgery part II candidates, showing that patients had a mean age of 40 years and that 10% of shoulder surgeries performed were to repair SLAP lesions.

Citation:
Schroder CP, Skare O, Reikeras O, et al. Sham surgery versus labral repair or biceps tenodesis for type II SLAP lesions of the shoulder: a three-armed randomized clinical trial. *Br J Sports Med*. 2017;0:1–8.

Level of Evidence:
I, randomized, controlled clinical trial

Summary:
The authors found no significant difference in Rowe scores, Western Ontario Shoulder Instability Index, patient satisfaction, or pain scores between labral repair, biceps tenodesis, and sham surgery.

Citation:

Sayde WM, Cohen SB, Ciccotti MG, et al. Return to play after type II superior labral anterior-posterior lesion repairs in athletes: a systematic review. *Clin Orthop Relat Res.* 2012;470(6):1595–1600.

Level of Evidence:

IV

Summary:

This article is a systematic review of the literature, which identified 14 studies of type II SLAP tears undergoing repair with 2-year follow-up data on return to play. Overhead athletes returned to play at a rate of 63%, lower than some previously noted.

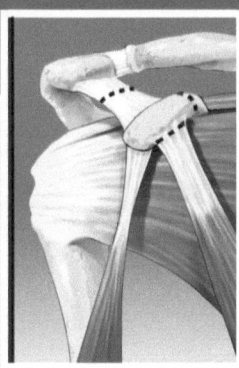

45

The Thrower's Shoulder

*Matthew A. Tao, Christopher L. Camp, Terrance Sgroi,
Joshua S. Dines, David W. Altchek*

The thrower's shoulder is a unique and challenging subset of sports medicine given the extreme demands placed on the glenohumeral joint and surrounding soft tissue structures. For purposes of discussion, we will mainly focus on medical issues as they relate to baseball players; however, we certainly acknowledge that many other sports (volleyball, tennis, handball) and positions (quarterbacks) have overlapping demands and injury patterns and will draw on literature based in those disciplines as well.

Generally, these are complex conditions that can present several difficulties in both diagnosis and treatment. The ability to throw a baseball at velocities exceeding 90 miles/h is the result of a complex transfer of energy from the lower extremity through the trunk, shoulder, elbow, and hand. The stresses placed on the individual links of the kinetic chain during throwing can lead to failure of and injury to these structures. The repetitive acceleration and deceleration of the arm during the throwing motion subjects the shoulder to extreme positions and stresses, which can lead to chronic overuse-type as well as acute shoulder injuries.

The thrower's shoulder endures supraphysiologic forces as professional pitchers have demonstrated the ability to generate up to 92 Nm of humeral rotation torque, which is greater than the torsional failure limit found in cadavers.[1] The shoulder experiences forces nearly half of body weight during the late cocking phase and distraction forces of nearly the entire body weight during the deceleration phase with peak angular velocities of 7250 degrees/s.[2,3] To perform such supraphysiologic feats, the shoulder makes key adaptations over time, which will be discussed further. However, the magnitude and repetition of such stresses placed on the shoulder can lead to injuries to important structures.

Sports medicine physicians who treat overhead athletes must be familiar with the subtle changes in their performance to recognize an injury to the shoulder. Differing from the general population, pitchers may not report pain or weakness, but instead complain of decreased velocity or accuracy. A thorough understanding of the anatomy and adaptive changes that occur in the thrower's shoulder along with the physiology of throwing is necessary to provide treatment in these complicated cases. In addition, a systematic approach to evaluating the shoulder is critical as many injuries are multifactorial due to mechanical, technical, training-related, and structural factors.

ADAPTATIONS TO THE THROWING SHOULDER

Over time, overhead athletes develop well-described adaptations in response to the stresses placed on the shoulder as a result of throwing. These changes likely begin in early childhood as the athlete begins throwing regularly. Both soft tissue and bony adaptations occur, and while sometimes subtle, they are imperative to the thrower's ability to function at a high level under otherwise nonphysiologic conditions.

One of the primary physiologic changes in the thrower's shoulder is seen in range of motion (ROM). Most throwers exhibit a difference in the amount of external rotation (ER) and internal rotation (IR) between their throwing and non-throwing shoulders, generally with an increase in ER and decrease in IR on their dominant side (Fig. 45.1).[2] A comparative loss of IR greater than 20 to 25 degrees has been termed glenohumeral internal rotation deficit (GIRD) although the pathologic nature of this change has been called into question more recently.

Brown et al.[4] reported that professional pitchers had a mean shoulder ER of 141 degrees with the arm at 90 degrees of abduction, which was 9 degrees more than their nondominant arm and also 9 degrees more than the throwing shoulders of position players. Although the magnitude of IR and ER seen in the dominant and nondominant arm differ, the total arc of motion is usually similar. Wilk et al.[5] reported a mean ROM arc of 176 degrees (both sides) and that the total motion in the throwing shoulder was within 7 degrees of the contralateral side. GIRD has classically been felt to be a maladaptive change, and indeed, some modern literature does support increased injury risk with GIRD.[6,7] However, total arc of motion[6–8] and even ER deficits[9] are increasingly recognized as perhaps more problematic and significant risk factors for injury.

Certainly, soft tissue accommodations occur over time in the static and dynamic stabilizers surrounding the shoulder, but bony adaptations have also been well documented. Several authors have demonstrated a 10- to 17-degree increase in humeral retroversion in the dominant arms of throwers relative to the contralateral side, which allows for increased external rotation.[10–12] Yamamoto et al.[13] assert that the repetitive throwing motion does not directly increase the retroversion of the humeral head but rather restricts the natural, physiologic derotation of the humeral head during growth. And while it is unclear at what age these bony changes begin to occur, they certainly appear to represent adaptive growth over time.

Soft tissue adaptations are also seen as a result of the large rotational and distractive forces acting upon the glenohumeral joint, resulting in posterior capsular tightness and anterior capsular laxity.[14–17] The term microinstability has been used to describe the acquired capsular laxity that allows increased humeral head translation and rotation. While a variety of theories exist, the cause of this microinstability is believed to be repetitive tensile loading as a result of scapular protraction or repetitive ER, particularly as it relates to the deceleration phase of throwing.[15–18] But despite the restrictive posterior soft tissue envelope, pitchers appear to have increased overall laxity of the shoulder compared with athletes who play other positions. Bigliani et al.[14] found a sulcus sign in 61% of dominant shoulders in professional pitchers compared to only 47% in position players. While there is likely a congenital component that self-selects for shoulders able to tolerate repetitive overhead motion, these capsular changes appear to be a necessary (as opposed to pathologic) adaptation to throwing as increased anterior–posterior humeral head translation has been demonstrated in both symptomatic and asymptomatic pitchers.[15,19]

BIOMECHANICS OF THROWING

To fully understand the spectrum of injuries, the stresses placed on the shoulder during the action of throwing must be

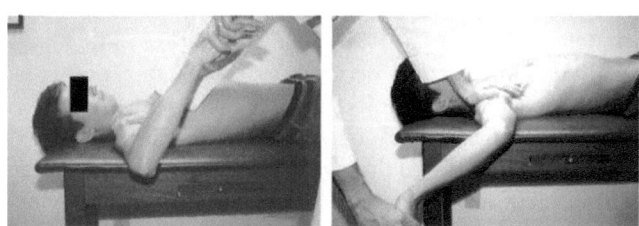

Fig. 45.1 An overhead throwing athlete wth asymmetric loss of internal rotation. The throwing shoulder shows an increase in external rotation, leading the average arc of motion of the arms to be similar. (From Burkhart SS, Morgan CD, Kibler WB. The disabled throwing shoulder: spectrum of pathology I: pathoanatomy and biomechanics. *Arthroscopy.* 2003;19:404–420.)

understood. The overhead throwing motion can be broken down into six discrete phases: wind-up, early cocking, late cocking, acceleration, deceleration, and follow-through (Fig. 45.2).[2,17,20,21] The entire motion takes approximately 2 seconds although 75% of that time occurs during the pre-acceleration phases.[21–23]

During the first phase of throwing (wind-up), the body rises over the center of gravity and the shoulder is placed in slight abduction and IR. At this point in the pitching motion, no stress is placed on the upper extremity.[24–26]

Early cocking is the second phase where the arm is placed into abduction and ER, and the arm rotates behind the body axis approximately 15 degrees. Once the arm reaches the top of its motion and stops moving backward, this is the onset of the late cocking phase.

The third phase is late cocking, which begins as the lead leg contacts the ground and ends when the arm reaches maximal ER of nearly 180 degrees. During this phase, the scapula retracts to provide a stable glenoid surface for the humeral head to compress against. The upper arm is maintained in 90 degrees to 100 degrees of abduction, and the elbow moves even with the plane of the torso. The humerus progresses into ER, and the humeral head translates posteriorly on the glenoid because of the increasing tightness of the anterior structures. The infraspinatus and teres minor muscles are active early in the late cocking phase, leading to the ER of the humerus. The subscapularis becomes active late in this phase as IR begins. The result is that the rotator cuff as a whole compresses the humeral head against the glenoid with significant force.[2]

The acceleration phase begins as the humerus internally rotates and ends when the ball is released. Although significant angular velocity is developed by the muscular forces around the shoulder during this phase, little stress is noted in the shoulder.[27] The triceps becomes active early in the acceleration phase, followed by the pectoralis major and the latissimus dorsi muscles later.[28]

The fifth phase (deceleration) begins just after the ball is released and ends when humeral IR ceases. This phase leads to tremendous stresses generated by the rotator cuff muscles as the arm is brought to an abrupt halt. Eccentric loads on the posterior cuff reach 1000 N as the muscle dissipates the kinetic energy generated in the earlier phases of the throw.[28,29]

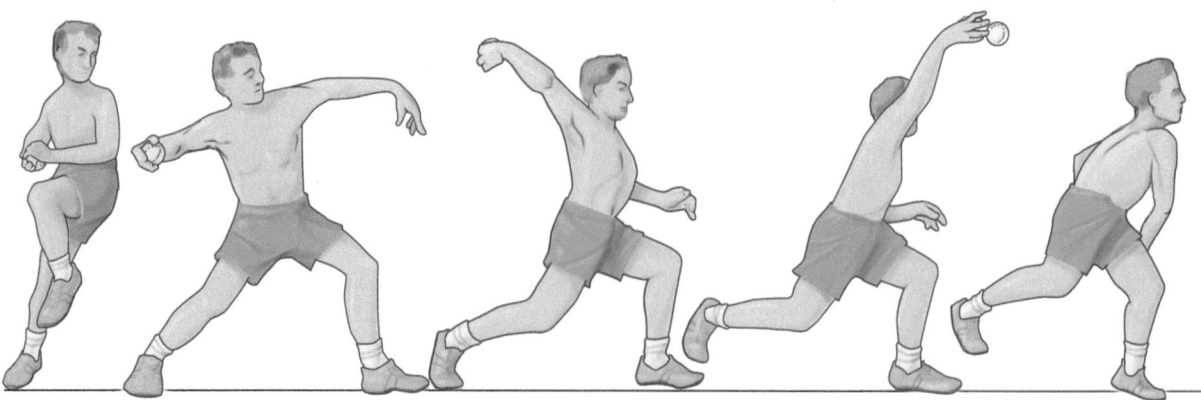

Fig. 45.2 Stages of the throwing motion.

The final phase of the throwing motion is the follow-through. It is at this point of the pitch that the body regains balance and stability. The muscles cease to fire and the compressive forces across the glenohumeral joint drop significantly.

PATHOPHYSIOLOGY

Internal Impingement

In 1992, Walch et al.[30] initially reported on contact that occurs between the supraspinatus tendon and the posterosuperior edge of the glenoid cavity in tennis players and coined the term internal impingement. It represents a collection of injuries characterized by pathologic contact between the rotator cuff (posterior supraspinatus and anterior infraspinatus) and the greater tuberosity with the posterosuperior glenoid and labrum leading to articular-sided rotator cuff tears and posterosuperior labral tears (Fig. 45.3).[31] This contact is only possible by placing the shoulder in the supraphysiologic position of extreme ER and anterior translation seen while throwing. While the concept of internal impingement endures, no clear etiology has been established, and multiple theories exist.

The theory of microinstability centers on the idea of hyperangulation—that as the humeral shaft moves posteriorly out of the plane of the scapula, the accompanying weakness allows the humeral head to drift anteriorly and subsequently produces a lengthening of the anterior capsule, which leads to a subtle form of anterior instability.[32] Jobe and Pink believed that the repetitive and forceful overhead activity causes a gradual stretching out of anteroinferior capsuloligamentous structures, leading to subclinical instability and impingement.[33] Indeed, throwers often have an element of hyperlaxity as previously discussed, and some would posit that tipping the scale from laxity to instability is the catalyst for developing internal impingement.[34]

Burkhart and Morgan[32] proposed that the pathology is a result of a hypertwisting mechanism with large shear stresses leading to fatigue failure of both the rotator cuff and the biceps tendon insertion point of the labrum. These lesions result from an acquired posterosuperior instability that is caused by posteroinferior

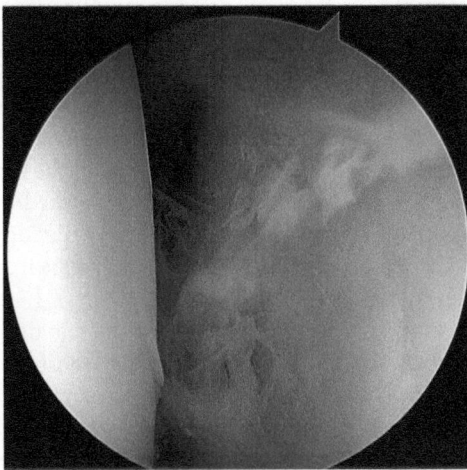

Fig. 45.3 An arthroscopic view of the superior labrum contacting the posterior aspect of the supraspinatus. These findings are consistent with internal impingement.

capsular tightness, which they termed the peel-back mechanism. They reasoned that the posterior capsule must withstand tensile forces of up to 750 N during the deceleration and follow-through phases of throwing. The posterior tensile forces placed on the shoulder during these actions are offset by the eccentric contraction of infraspinatus and the posteroinferior capsule, including the posterior band of the inferior glenohumeral ligament. The posterior contraction is believed to shift the center of rotation of the shoulder to a more posterosuperior location, creating instability with the shoulder in abduction and ER.

Muscle fatigue and imbalance may also play a role in the development of internal impingement by altering the mechanics of the shoulder. Fatigue-related humeral hyperextension can occur during the late cocking phase when the rotator cuff muscles cannot completely resist the large acceleration forces generated while pitching.[35] Progressive delamination of the posterior capsulolabral structures and the rotator cuff may occur as the violent deceleration of the arm during follow-through may cause an abrasive degeneration of the rotator cuff on the posterosuperior aspect of the glenoid.[36] Whether it is the driving force or simply a result of the process, scapular dyskinesis is also often seen with internal impingement.[37]

Although a range of theories have been proposed regarding the pathophysiologic etiology of internal impingement, it seems clear that the causes of disability in the shoulder used for throwing are multifactorial and require an equally multicentric approach to care.

Dynamic Shoulder and Scapular Stability

Particularly in overhead athletes, focal weakness and muscle imbalance play a role in the development of shoulder pain. Multiple studies have demonstrated the protective effect of maintaining shoulder strength (especially ER strength) as a means of preventing injuries.[6,8,38] Any muscle imbalance alters the anterior–posterior force couple that stabilizes the glenohumeral joint and increases the compression forces in the joint.[39,40] Disrupting the agonist–antagonist balance impairs a pitcher's ability to appropriately accelerate and decelerate while throwing.

Although often neglected, the scapula is the critical link in the kinetic chain of energy transfer from the trunk to the humerus.[41,42] The scapula provides a stable base upon which the rotator cuff muscles activate, and it coordinates scapulohumeral rhythm, the coupled movement between the scapula and the arm allowing for placement of the upper extremity in space. Scapular movement combines three motions (upward–downward rotation, internal–external rotation, and anterior–posterior tilt) with two sliding translations (up–down and anterior–posterior). It is commonly believed that scapular malposition can also be a cause of shoulder problems in throwers.[27,43]

Kibler and Thomas[44] described dyskinesis as an alteration of static scapular position or dynamic scapular motion in coordination with arm motion. The resulting protracted, downward rotated and anteriorly tilted scapula is caused by abnormal muscular imbalances.[45,46] The protracted scapula is almost universally unfavorable for shoulder function as it decreases the subacromial space and effectiveness of the rotator cuff while also increasing impingement and strain on the static glenohumeral ligaments and dynamic shoulder stabilizers.[41,47] Accordingly, most goals of management center on regaining functional retraction. And while dyskinesis may itself be the source of a thrower's dysfunction, it can also merely be the byproduct of underlying pathology. Recognition by the physician is key, but high-quality rehabilitation by a thoughtful physical therapist is the cornerstone of treatment for dyskinesis with the possibility of operative intervention if concomitant surgical pathology exists.

The mnemonic SICK scapula was originally coined by Burkhart and colleagues in 2003 and is a subset of dyskinesis relating exclusively to overhead athletes.[15] It represents scapular malposition, inferior medial border prominence, coracoid pain, and dyskinesis. The hallmark feature is a "dropped" scapula with asymmetry in the throwing shoulder where the scapula sits lower than the nondominant side. This static asymmetry is compounded by a dynamic dyskinesis as the athlete goes through the throwing motion. The physical exam should consist of static scapular measurements with the patient standing, a meticulous coracoid exam (as the anterior pain can mimic labral pathology), and pain-free forward flexion while performing the scapular retraction test. These changes in scapular position lead to external impingement as a result of anterior tilt, internal impingement, decreased rotator cuff strength, and anterior capsular strain.[2,3,18,31,46,48–52] Altered static and dynamic scapular mechanics arise from overuse and weakness of scapular stabilizers and posterior rotator cuff muscles.[53] Thus SICK scapula is a nonoperative condition that improves with diligent rehabilitation; however, success hinges on athlete compliance and the ability to get the scapula back to a symmetric position with the contralateral side and keep it there.[15]

Glenohumeral Internal Rotation Deficit

Bony and soft tissue adaptations over time allow pitchers to develop a relative increase in ER and loss of IR compared to their nondominant side as well as the general population. As discussed, GIRD has classically been felt to be a maladaptive state with an increased injury risk, but this has been called into question more recently. Posterior capsule tightness has been shown to result in multiple kinematic alterations such as increased ER but decreased IR, horizontal adduction, and flexion.[54,55] It has been associated with multiple injuries including external (subacromial) impingement, internal impingement, and superior labral from anterior to posterior (SLAP) tears.[6,7,16,28,37,56] More recently, the importance of total arc of motion as opposed to GIRD[6–8] and the importance of ER deficits over IR deficits[9] as it relates to injury risk has been established. Further investigation may help to parse out whether GIRD is truly pathologic or merely a necessary adaptation to repetitive throwing.

HISTORY

The etiology of a shoulder injury in an overhead throwing athlete is best determined by taking a thorough history, and thus a familiarity with not only the sport but also position-specific demands is required. Pitchers, for instance, frequently describe feelings of heaviness/sluggishness, stiffness, fatigue, weakness, and the inability to "bring it."[44] These subjective complaints are often accompanied by objective findings of decreased velocity on fastballs, lack of movement on breaking balls, and decreased accuracy. While acute injuries do occur in overhead throwing athletes, it is much more common for injuries to be a result of overuse and fatigue. The timing of the onset of symptoms, current and previous treatment modalities, and a history of a previous injury to the shoulder should be determined. The athlete should also be asked specific pitching-related questions including any recent change in mechanics, development of a new pitch, increased pitch count, alteration to training regimen, in what phase of the throwing the pain occurs, and if any other part of the body has been injured that could be changing the throwing mechanics. The role of the hip, core, and lumbar spine are also critical as injuries to these areas can lead to compensatory alterations in throwing mechanics and increased stress on the shoulder.

Typical symptoms in an overhead throwing athlete with pain include anterosuperior or posterosuperior shoulder pain in the late cocking phase. Labral tears specifically may lead to mechanical symptoms such as popping, locking, or snapping. Although the details are beyond the scope of this chapter, questioning the athlete about symptoms related to the cervical spine or thoracic outlet syndrome is also critical to rule out pathology masquerading as shoulder pain.

PHYSICAL EXAMINATION

A thorough and systematic physical examination should be performed for all throwers who present with shoulder pain. The aid of a physical therapist and/or athletic trainer with a solid understanding of throwing mechanics can also be helpful to isolate dynamic issues less familiar to clinicians. The examination should focus not just on the upper extremity but also on the entire kinetic chain, including the lower extremities and trunk. The athlete's natural posture may be evaluated while he or she walks into the room and during history taking. The overall alignment, shoulder height and position, pelvic tilt and rotation, lower extremity alignment, head and neck position, and arm position must be evaluated. Functional movements should be assessed to determine hip and trunk control, muscle imbalance, and inflexibilities, which can be accomplished by having the patient balance on one leg and do a single leg squat. While performing these maneuvers, the patient should be observed for compensatory movements such as pelvic tilt or rotation. Ankle flexibility, lumbar and thoracic spine, and shoulder girdle mobility can be assessed by having the patient perform a full squat with heels on the ground and arms overhead. Flexibility of the hamstrings and the thoracic and lumbar spine can be assessed by having the patient perform a straight-leg toe touch. While supine, both hips should be evaluated for ROM and to determine if any femoroacetabular impingement is present.

Once a comprehensive examination of the remainder of the kinetic chain is completed, a focused evaluation of the affected shoulder is performed. The entire shoulder complex must be visualized. Male patients are asked to remove their shirts, and female athletes should be asked to wear a tank top or sports bra. First, the shoulder is inspected visually to evaluate for muscular atrophy or scapular winging. The position of the scapula at rest should be noted, including asymmetry of scapular tilt, rotation, and elevation or depression. After visual inspection, the shoulder should be systematically palpated to identify areas of pain. All bony prominences are palpated, including the bicipital groove, greater tuberosity, coracoid, and acromioclavicular (AC) joint.

Shoulder ROM, both active and passive, should be assessed in both standing and supine positions with special attention given to glenohumeral and scapulothoracic motion. Glenohumeral joint passive ROM is assessed for ER and IR at 90 degrees of abduction and for ER at 45 degrees of abduction in the scapular plane. Increased ER with the arm at the side with the patient in the supine position can be reflective of rotator interval laxity. Increased ER in the abducted and externally rotated position reflects anteroinferior capsular laxity and/or humeral retroversion. In addition to ER and IR, passive and active forward flexion and abduction need to be recorded. Palpation of the shoulder during ROM can uncover crepitus, which may indicate bursal thickening, labral tear, or rotator cuff pathology. Subacromial impingement is assessed using the Hawkins-Kennedy and Neer tests.

Muscle strength should be evaluated after shoulder ROM is determined. Careful manual muscle strength testing should aim to isolate the muscle being tested and compare to the contralateral, uninjured side.

Several tests are helpful to examine the labrum of the throwing athlete. The O'Brien active compression test is frequently used to evaluate for SLAP tears.[57] Although the sensitivity has been reported at 100% with 97% to 99% specificity in the general population, the reliability markedly decreases in athletes (78% sensitivity, 11% specificity).[58] The passive distraction test is performed supine with the shoulder flexed to 150 degrees and the forearm is passively pronated to elicit increased biceps tension.[59] Deep pain or a pop with passive pronation is suggestive of a superior labral injury. Speeds test, commonly used for biceps pathology, has shown variable sensitivity and specificity in identifying SLAP tears in the literature.[60,61] The Crank test evaluates the anterior glenoid labrum although the sensitivity ranges widely in the literature from 13% to 91%.[62,63] The posterior labrum is evaluated with the labral shear, jerk, and Kim tests. Differentiating biceps pathology can be particularly challenging; however, the "3-pack" exam (O'Brien sign + throwing test + bicipital tunnel palpation) described by Taylor et al. has demonstrated excellent sensitivity in diagnosing both intra- and extra-articular injuries to the biceps labral complex.[64] The shoulder should also be evaluated for frank instability by testing the integrity of the anterior and posterior labrum as well as testing for a sulcus sign.

An important but often underemphasized part of the shoulder exam is evaluation of the scapulothoracic joint. Many injured throwers demonstrate loss of ER control and elevation and posterior tilt of the scapula, which are manifested as medial scapular border winging.[65] Both scapulas should be visualized with the arms at the sides; note is made of any asymmetry of tilt, rotation, elevation, or depression. As discussed, the SICK scapula presents with a static "dropped" appearance along with dynamic dyskinesis.[15] Evaluation of scapular movement and scapulohumeral rhythm in comparison to the contralateral side is important. When evaluating dyskinesis, the scapular assistance test (assisted upward rotation and posterior tilt) and scapular

retraction test (manually placing the scapula in a retracted position) are diagnostic by improving pain and increasing motion and strength respectively.[42]

In summary, examination of the painful throwing shoulder must be complete and systematic as these can be complex, subtle injuries. The examiner must develop a routine to avoid missing important findings. Additionally, the examiner must avoid focusing only on the shoulder and instead perform an assessment of the entire kinetic chain. The input of a physical therapist and/or athletic trainer well versed in overhead athletes also provides tremendous benefit.

IMAGING

Complete evaluation of the shoulder in an overhead throwing athlete should include the standard radiographic views of the shoulder consisting of anteroposterior, axillary, and outlet views. These images allow visualization of the glenohumeral articulation, as well as acromial morphology and visualization of the inferior glenoid. Other useful views may include the Stryker notch and West Point views depending on the situation.

After obtaining plain radiographs, the next step is generally magnetic resonance imaging (MRI). In overhead throwing athletes, the most common lesions are partial-thickness rotator cuff tears and glenoid labral pathology. MRI arthrograms (MRA) involve the use of intra-articular contrast material and can be helpful in delineating rotator cuff (particularly partial-thickness tears) and labral pathology with some studies demonstrating increased accuracy over plain MRI.[66,67] However, the difference is not dramatic[67] so our bias has generally been against the routine use of MRA for the reason that it adds a relatively large volume of fluid into the joint and distorts normal anatomy and potentially distracts from other pathology. The use of MRI alone requires modern protocols on high-quality (3-T) scanners and partnering with a trusted set of radiologists; in doing so, we have found this to be far preferable. Beyond the traditional sequences, throwers often warrant placing the arm in the abducted ER position (ABER) to delineate more subtle labral and articular-sided rotator cuff pathology (Fig. 45.4).[68] In the setting of internal impingement pathology, MRI findings include articular-sided degeneration and tearing at the junction of the posterior supraspinatus and anterior infraspinatus tendons with associated degeneration and tearing of the posterosuperior labrum. Subcortical cysts and chondral lesions may also be seen in the posterosuperior glenoid and humerus as a result of repetitive impaction.

Given that pitching is a repetitive, supraphysiologic exercise, caution must also be used when interpreting MRI imaging on throwers as there is a high rate of asymptomatic pathology. Connor et al.[69] reported that 40% of dominant shoulders in asymptomatic overhead throwing athletes had partial- or full-thickness rotator cuff tears in their throwing arm compared with no tears in the nondominant shoulders. Similarly, Halbrecht et al.[70] demonstrated a 30% rate of labral tears and 40% cuff tendinosis with dominant-arm MRIs performed in the ABER position compared with the contralateral side. Because MRI findings are often abnormal, particularly in elite athletes, the

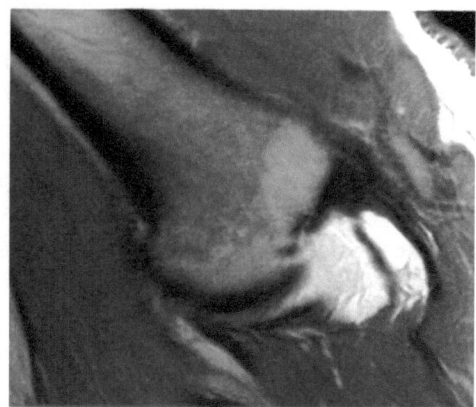

Fig. 45.4 A coronal image of a partial rotator cuff tear with the arm in the abducted and externally rotated position. Significant intrasubstance delamination of the tissue is seen in addition to a partial rotator cuff tear.

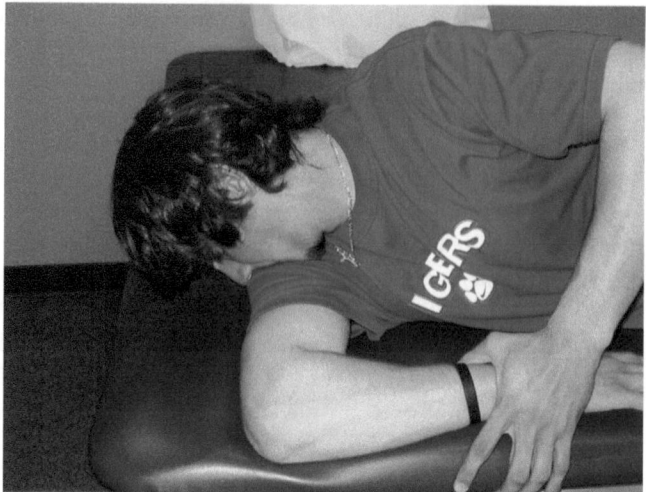

Fig. 45.5 In the sleeper's stretch, the patient lies on his or her side and stabilizes his or her scapula against the wall. Both the shoulder and the elbow are flexed 90 degrees. The nonaffected arm applies internal rotation to the affected arm. (From Kibler WB, Kuhn JE, Wilk K, et al. The disabled throwing shoulder: spectrum of pathology—10-year update. *Arthroscopy.* 2013;29:141–161.)

history and physical exam are critical to help delineate the source of the pathology and must be used in conjunction with imaging.

Computed tomography (CT) is less commonly used in the setting of the painful throwing shoulder. However, it remains the gold standard for evaluation of bony anatomy and measuring both humeral and glenoid version.[71]

DECISION-MAKING PRINCIPLES

Decision-making in the management of the throwing shoulder ideally follows an algorithmic approach based on available findings and evidence-based treatments. In general, the initial management of most shoulder injuries in overhead athletes is nonoperative, consisting of a period of rest, activity modification, and rehabilitation. Corrective efforts are directed not only at the shoulder but also at abnormalities of the entire kinetic chain. The younger the athlete, the more conservative our approach and the more willing we are to remove them completely from sports for a period of time. However, elite and professional athletes constitute a unique population in which relative rest and targeted therapy may be done to maintain fitness and certain skills while rehabbing. As discussed, the role of a thoughtful physical therapist who understands the demands on that specific athlete cannot be overstated, and communication between patient, physician, therapist, and team is critical.

Wilk and colleagues[72] have described several phases of rehabilitation for overhead throwers with shoulder pain, including the acute phase, intermediate phase, strengthening phase, and return to throwing phase. In the acute phase, local therapeutic modalities focus on reducing pain and inflammation. Nonsteroidal antiinflammatory drugs, injections, ice, and iontophoresis may be used to accomplish this goal. A key to this phase is discontinuation of all activity to allow the shoulder to rest and the modalities to take effect. Shoulder motion must be addressed during this phase of rehabilitation. Stretches such as the sleeper's stretch (Fig. 45.5) are used to treat posterior capsule tightness. A major focus of the first phase of rehabilitation is improving the strength and muscle balance. Focus is therefore placed on

returning strength to the external rotators, scapular, and lower extremity muscles.

The goals of the intermediate phase are to progress with strengthening and enhanced flexibility of the shoulder. More aggressive isotonic strengthening activities are used as focus is placed on strengthening the external rotators, scapular retractors, protractors, and depressor muscles. Wilk prefers side-lying ER and prone rowing into ER. Strengthening of the lumbopelvic region and core are also a focus of the intermediate phase of rehabilitation. Jogging and sprinting are integrated into this phase as well to improve lower extremity strengthening and endurance. Upper extremity stretching exercises are also continued.

During the third phase of rehabilitation, the goals are to enhance power and endurance, perform functional drills, and gradually initiate throwing activities. Plyometric drills are also initiated during this phase. These drills are used to enhance dynamic stability, enhance proprioception, and gradually increase the functional stresses placed on the shoulder joint. Dynamic stabilization drills are also performed to enhance proprioception and neuromuscular control. During this phase, an interval throwing program is started. The interval throwing program is started once the athlete has a satisfactory clinical examination, nonpainful ROM, reliable kinetic chain movements, satisfactory isokinetic test results, and appropriate progress in his or her overall rehabilitation program.

Return to throwing is the fourth and final phase of the rehabilitation protocol. This phase typically involves progression of the throwing program. Although a number of approaches for this phase have been described with some variation, the general principles emphasize a strategic progression, often over a period of 6 to 12 weeks, during which the athlete progresses from the initial phase, consisting of short throwing over a limited duration to long toss and subsequently to position-specific throwing and/or throwing from the mound. Each step is taken in a careful fashion, and any increase in symptoms prompts a short period of rest combined with a retreat to the prior phase to allow for resolution of symptoms. Once the athlete has accomplished the final phase of position-specific throwing, the decision can be made to return to competition. A judicious return to play (RTP) is recommended with careful monitoring of activity, innings, pitch count, and periods of rest aimed at limiting the risk of symptomatic recurrence.

Surgical options should be reserved for cases when nonoperative treatment fails and in the setting of certain acute injuries. The surgical procedure is determined by the shoulder pathology that is present; however, the approach in this population is patient-specific. All surgical pathology must be considered and managed systematically for optimal recovery of the athlete, which may require several concomitant surgical interventions such as SLAP repair and articular-sided rotator cuff débridement in the example of recalcitrant internal impingement.

TREATMENT OPTIONS

Aside from acute, operative injuries, the timing of surgery may depend on the relationship to the season of play. An athlete who is currently in-season may attempt to manage a structural shoulder injury conservatively to get through the season before undergoing surgery. This again emphasizes the importance of communication with all of the involved parties and allowing the athlete to participate in shared decision-making. How aggressive the timing and nature of the treatment are also depends on the age of the athlete and his or her level of play.

Internal Impingement

One of the challenges with internal impingement is differentiating normal adaptations from pathologic degeneration. We believe that many of the changes seen on imaging and even at the time of surgery are normal adaptations to the repetitive loads over time in throwers—in order to attain the supraphysiologic motions and forces necessary to throw, impingement must occur. Consequently, some level of change is also seen to the undersurface of the rotator cuff as well as the labrum, creating a so-called "thrower's footprint." Parsing out typical impingement findings from a pathologic process is challenging and underscores the need for a comprehensive nonoperative regimen.

Internal impingement is associated with a spectrum of pathology and lends itself to multiple treatment options.[73] Those in the early states of impingement tend to have poorly localized pain and may have accompanying stiffness. Starting with a period of rest and nonsteroidal antiinflammatories is reasonable in this setting. For those throwers with more localized posterior shoulder pain, a prolonged period of rest (4 to 6 weeks) is in order along with formal physical therapy.[35] Therapy has been shown to be acutely therapeutic as well as protective against future injuries.[5,15,28] The rehabilitation regimen is mainly directed at posterior capsular stretching, correcting scapular dyskinesis, and core strengthening. Given that one theory behind the pathogenesis of internal impingement is microinstability, anterior capsular stretching is generally avoided. Proper throwing mechanics should also be reviewed.

Only after clear failure of high-quality nonoperative treatment of appropriate duration should surgical intervention be considered. Throwers place tremendous demand on the shoulder and should generally give one pause prior to proceeding with surgery; however, internal impingement is a particularly challenging diagnosis to solve operatively.[74] Similar to the algorithm laid out by Heyworth and Williams,[75] we advocate for an approach dictated by the pathology. Exam under anesthesia (EUA) of both shoulders provides a sense of asymmetric laxity, which may be addressed with labral repair ± capsulorrhaphy. Rotator cuff tears in the setting of internal impingement are generally treated with débridement with the exception of high-grade tears, which will be discussed in the following section. Similarly, tears of the posterosuperior labrum can be débrided or repaired depending on the significance of the pathology.

Partial-Thickness Rotator Cuff Tears

The treatment of partial-thickness rotator cuff tears depends on several factors, including the depth and location of the tear, the quality of the tissue, and the athlete's age and playing position. Surgical options include débridement, tear completion and subsequent full-thickness repair, transtendinous repair, and intratendinous repair constructs. However, operative intervention on the rotator cuff of a thrower should be the absolute last resort. Our preference is for a comprehensive course of nonoperative management, and the athlete must definitively fail this conservative treatment by demonstrating persistent inability to throw prior to consideration for surgery.

In the general population, the conventional rule-of-thumb is that a tear involving less than 50% of the tendon insertion is débrided, whereas tears greater than 50% are more suitable for repair. These guidelines were initially adopted by several authors for overhead throwing athletes.[76–79] However, Rudzki and Shaffer[80] contend that the demands of overhead athletes are different than the average individual and they have concerns about the integrity of a repair withstanding the high forces that will be placed on it. As such, they advocate for a 75% tear threshold prior to repair.

Articular-sided partial-thickness tears represent the most common rotator cuff injuries in throwers, and as such, the vast majority of our surgical management centers around simple débridement back to healthy, stable tendon. For the select few tears involving 80% to 90% thickness, we favor tear completion and anatomic repair. This general rule is particularly relevant for tears involving the anterior or posterior margins of the supraspinatus, which represent the attachment points of the rotator cable; we are less concerned about tears in the mid-portion of the supraspinatus.

Superior Labral From Anterior to Posterior Tears

Injury to the superior labrum in overhead throwing athletes can occur in conjunction with other pathologies or in isolation. Understanding the normal anatomic variants of the superior labrum and biceps insertion is critical to recognizing pathologic changes to the structures. Although the utilization of SLAP repair in the general population is decreasing, it still has a viable role in throwers. Similar to our treatment of partial-thickness rotator cuff tears, a thrower with a SLAP tear must fail extensive nonoperative management and be unable to throw prior to consideration for surgery. In the setting of true pathology to the superior labrum, the stability of the SLAP tear dictates its treatment. Type I SLAP lesions are characterized by fraying of the central labrum without detachment of the biceps anchors and are treated with débridement. Type II lesions consist of isolated detachment of the superior labrum and biceps anchor either anteriorly (II-A), posteriorly (II-B), or involving the entire biceps anchor (II-C); these are typically treated with repair as the tear is believed to be unstable. A bucket-handle tear is present in type III lesions; these tears are treated with débridement and removal of the bucket-handle tissue. Type IV tears involve a bucket-handle component that extends up into the biceps tendon itself, and treatment involves repair of the SLAP ± biceps tenodesis as described in the next section.

Biceps Tenodesis

The popularity of biceps tenodesis is increasing dramatically[81]; however, there has been understandable trepidation to perform this procedure in overhead athletes.[82] Generally, we have avoided tenodesis in throwers if at all possible given historically poor outcomes; however, in a very selective population, we have had success even with professional pitchers. Type IV SLAP tears that involve a significant portion of the biceps tendon (>30%), such that it is unstable, are candidates. The other role for biceps tenodesis is in the setting of so-called biceps chondromalacia on the humeral head assuming this is consistent with history and physical exam as the etiology of the athlete's symptoms.[51,83–85]

Posterior Capsular Contracture and Glenohumeral Internal Rotation Deficit

Posterior capsular contractures have generally responded well to conservative treatment. The "sleeper stretch" is typically the first-line treatment with historical failure rates being exceedingly low, especially in younger pitchers.[15,28,53] There are some conflicting reports in more recent literature, though. A randomized, controlled trial of college-level overhead athletes found significant improvement of both IR and adduction with the sleeper stretch.[86] However, a systematic review attributed no benefit to the sleeper stretch and instead found cross-body adduction to be more efficacious.[87] Stretching certainly has limitations based on athlete compliance, and it can only be expected to overcome soft-tissue contracture with the understanding that certain bony adaptations may exist that inherently limit the motion of the shoulder. Still, nonoperative management is overwhelmingly the front-line treatment for posterior capsular tightness.

✦ Authors' Preferred Technique

The surgical bar should be set very high when discussing the dominant shoulder of a thrower, and aside from acute traumatic injuries, we advocate that athletes complete comprehensive conservative management prior to operative intervention. It must also be emphasized that our discussion centers around general algorithms that should be individually tailored to the clinically relevant pathology of each athlete. When approaching surgery on a throwing athlete, it is important to understand the spectrum of injuries that are commonly seen, as outlined above, and to be prepared to address all intraoperative possibilities. We have found that utilizing a consistent team from nursing to surgical technician to anesthesiologist provides high-level, efficient care for this unique subset of patients.

Regional anesthesia provides tremendous benefit in shoulder surgery over traditional methods with regards to both intra- and postoperative courses[88]; particularly with the advent of ultrasound guidance, we have found interscalene and supraclavicular blocks to be safe and effective in general practice. However, as it relates to the narrow population of elite and professional athletes, we generally avoid the use of neuraxial blocks given the risk, albeit small, of nerve injury and lasting dysfunction postoperatively. It is important to discuss this prior to surgery with the team as well as the patient to ensure a uniform understanding of the plan.

In terms of positioning, patients are placed in a modified beach chair that is fairly vertical such that the acromion is parallel to the floor. A beanbag is utilized and placed at the medial border of the scapula, which allows for maximal clearance as well as customized support and elevation of the ipsilateral trunk. An articulated arm holder is used for arm positioning throughout the procedure. Prophylactic antibiotics are always given. The skin is cleaned the evening prior and morning of surgery with chlorhexidine as well as formal surgical scrub prior to draping, also with chlorhexidine.

Internal Impingement
As discussed, internal impingement is a spectrum that envelops multiple injuries (Fig. 45.6), and treatment for each condition will be detailed in subsequent

sections. Internal impingement remains incompletely understood; however, we have found the theory of anterior micro-instability to be cogent at times. In our hands, anterior capsular procedures are only performed if we feel clear that instability is the primary source of pain as these patients will almost universally have a positive relocation test. One overriding principle in treatment is to take special care to avoid overtightening the anterior soft tissue envelope, which would limit the ER required to remain a competitive overhead thrower.

For anterior capsular plication, we prefer to capture capsule and labrum and repair it as one to the glenoid via knotless anchors instead of a capsule-to-capsule plication. While viewing posteriorly, we utilize a low anterior working portal directly above the superior border of the subscapularis tendon and a high

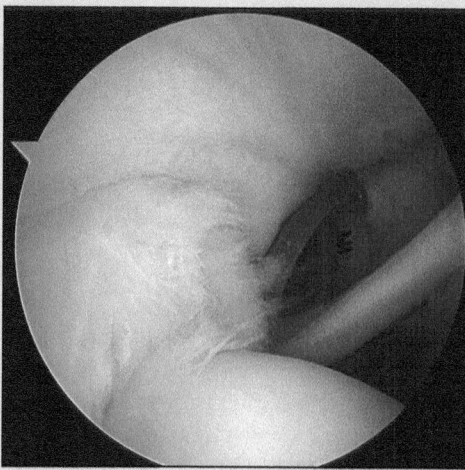

Fig. 45.6 An arthroscopic view from the posterior portal of an arm that is in abduction and external rotation. From this view, the rotator cuff can be seen encroaching on the superior labrum.

🔖 Authors' Preferred Technique—cont'd

anterolateral portal at the leading edge of the supraspinatus. Cannulas are placed in both portals for ease of suture passage and anchor placement. The arm is forward flexed and adducted over a large, sterile bump high in the axilla. This bump is a critical portion of the technique as it causes glenohumeral distraction and allows for excellent visualization and the necessary working space to pass instruments.

Many repair techniques are present in the literature, but our preference in throwers is unequivocally for a horizontal mattress configuration in knotless fashion. Both simple sutures and knots, even when tied away from the joint surface, have the potential to articulate with the humeral head given the extreme motions and forces that are applied to a thrower's shoulder. High-tensile strength, nonabsorbable #2 sutures are passed through the anterior capulolabral tissue in horizontal mattress fashion with care to avoid capturing too much capsule as this pathology differs from gross, traumatic instability. Anchors are placed slightly onto the glenoid face to repair the tissue back to its anatomic position, but prior to final fixation, the arm is placed in a late-cocking position (ABER) to avoid overtightening. In our experience, 2-anchor fixation is generally sufficient for symptomatic anterior microinstability.

Rotator Cuff Tears

Following diagnostic arthroscopy, special attention is paid to the articular side of the cuff. If the pathology is clearly either low-grade or full-thickness, we then proceed with débridement or repair, respectively. But if the degree of tearing is not readily visualized, a spinal needle with a monofilament suture is passed through the tear via the subacromial space, and the area of concern is then visualized from the subacromial space.

The vast majority of rotator cuff tears in throwers are articular-sided and partial-thickness in nature (Fig. 45.7). As such, the bulk of our surgical management involves simple but thoughtful débridement with a shaver back to healthy, stable tendon. If at all possible, we favor débridement alone as the historical results of rotator cuff repair in pitchers have been poor.

For those tears involving more than 80% of the tendon thickness, we favor tear completion and restoration of the native anatomy via a lateralized footprint repair (Fig. 45.8).[89] Although intra- and transtendinous repair techniques exist, we have not found these to be predictable in overhead athletes. And while we believe that a broad footprint is important for repair, over-medialization negatively alters the native length–tension relationship, which can have devastating effects

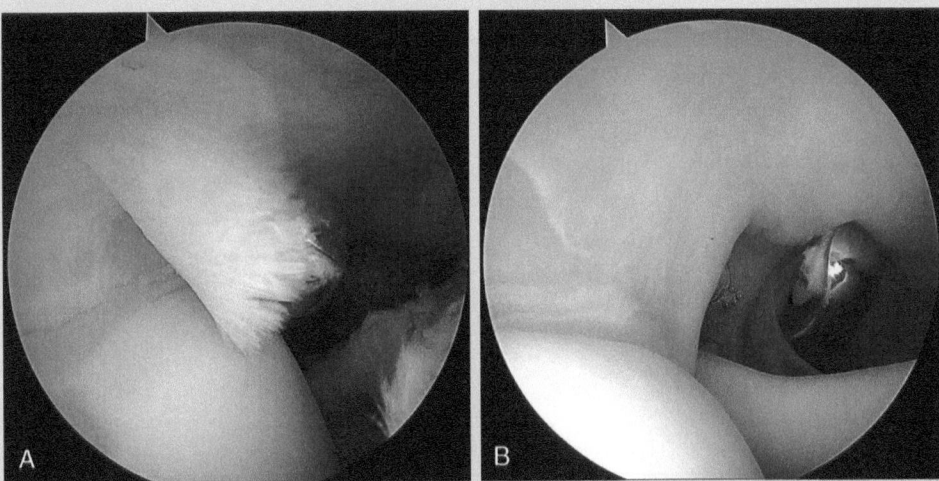

Fig. 45.7 (A) An arthroscopic view from the posterior portal looking at the articular side of the rotator cuff. A partial delaminated tear of the undersurface of the posterior rotator cuff is seen. (B) The frayed tissue is débrided, allowing evaluation of the true thickness of the tear.

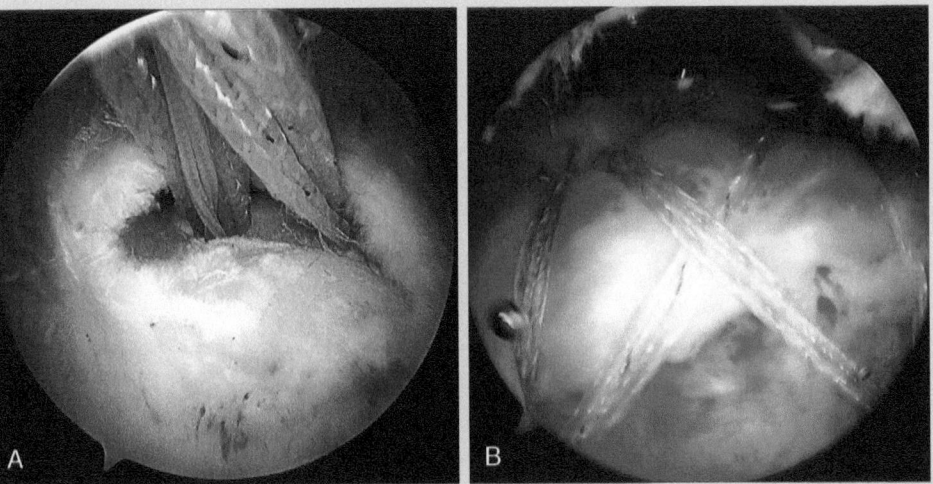

Fig. 45.8 (A) A crescent-shaped full-thickness tear of the supraspinatus with two double-loaded anchors placed at the articular margin. (B) Suture bridge repair of the full-thickness tear. Two medial and two lateral anchors were used for the repair.

Continued

📌 Authors' Preferred Technique—cont'd

in a high-level thrower.[90,91] The anatomy of the supraspinatus is readily visible and quite familiar to most sports surgeons as it begins at the articular margin and extends laterally. However, the infraspinatus has a more varied insertion as it begins superiorly at the articular margin but moves laterally as much as 16 mm at the inferior inerstion.[92] Precision in restoring a lateralized footprint is particularly relevant in an overhead throwing population where the goal is to recreate the "thrower's footprint" and avoid the potential for even small changes to motion or strength that can have amplified consequences in terms of function.

Prior to rotator cuff repair, a thorough subacromial bursectomy is performed to improve visualization. An acromioplasty is only performed if the presence of an impingement lesion is noted, which is uncommon in this population. The greater tuberosity is lightly abraded with a shaver in the region of the desired repair to enhance healing potential. A transosseus-equivalent, double-row construct is used in suture bridge fashion. Medial row anchor placement is critical in recreating native anatomy and preventing postoperative motion loss. The anterior supraspinatus anchor is placed immediately adjacent to the articular margin, which replicates the anatomic attachment of the rotator cable. Posteriorly, the infraspinatus anchor is placed 10 to 15 mm lateral to the articular margin. Medial row sutures are never tied as the knots can remain prominent and lead to irritation and a mechanical sensation during the throwing motion. The sutures are then brought down in crossing fashion to lateral row anchors just off the edge of the greater tuberosity. The number of anchors is dictated by the size of the tear although generally two medial and two lateral row anchors is sufficient in this population. We then critically assess the repair from both the subacromial and glenohumeral sides to ensure it restores the native footprint.

Superior Labral From Anterior to Posterior Tears

After diagnostic arthroscopy, particular attention is given to the "kissing lesion" (Fig. 45.9) between the posterosuperior labrum and undersurface of the posterior rotator cuff. While the circumferential labrum must be inspected carefully, the SLAP region should be of particular interest (Fig. 45.10). There are several normal anatomic variants, such as a sublabral foramen, Buford complex, and meniscoid labrum, which should be recognized and distinguished from true pathology. A close eye to hemorrhage or granulation tissue beneath the biceps-labral complex can help to distinguish pathology from a normal variant. The SLAP type and location must be identified as it will dictate accessory portal placement and ultimately treatment.

The type II-B (posterior) SLAP lesion is most common in throwers, so a portal of Wilmington is typically established under direct visualization using a spinal needle, and the trajectory of the needle should mimic that of the anchor. One

of the tenants of labral surgery that is often overlooked is adequate preparation of the labrum and the glenoid. While it is tempting to identify the tear and quickly begin the repair, inadequate preparation is a mistake that can compromise the healing potential of an already tenuous area. We take great care to fully mobilize the labrum with an arthroscopic elevator. This requires being slightly more medial on the glenoid but not undermining anteriorly to further destabilize the biceps anchor. Preparation of the glenoid bone bed deep is also critical to remove soft tissue and scar and provide a bleeding cancellous surface for healing; we favor the judicious use of shaver for this task. We will then assess the mobility of the labrum and its relation to the potential anchor site prior to proceeding with the repair.

High-tensile strength, nonabsorbable #2 sutures are passed through the posterior labrum in horizontal mattress fashion. Both suture limbs are grasped and placed over the template anchor position to ensure adequate position and tensioning. An anchor is then placed just barely onto the glenoid face, and the labrum is transfixed in knotless fashion. Most commonly, two anchors are required posterior to the biceps, and unless the tear truly extends anterior to the biceps anchor (type II-A/C), we avoid placing anchors anterior given concern for overconstraint. If there is anterior tear extension, the repair is conducted in identical fashion but with care to avoid the middle glenohumeral ligament.

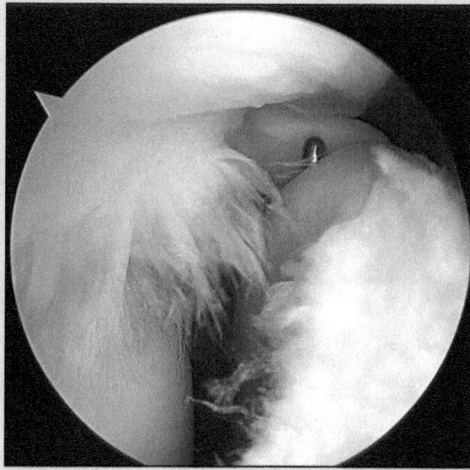

Fig. 45.9 Portals used for repair of a superior labral anterior to posterior tear. The high interval portal is commonly used.

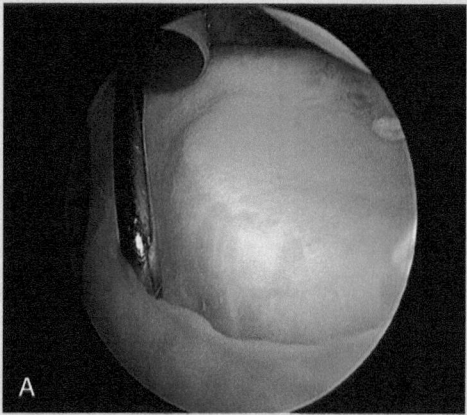 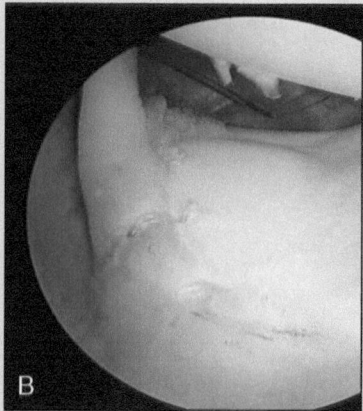

Fig. 45.10 (A) An arthroscopic view of a superior labral anterior to posterior tear. (B) This is repaired in knotless, horizontal mattress fashion.

Authors' Preferred Technique—cont'd

Biceps Tenodesis

Biceps tenodesis comes as a last resort in throwers, but our limited experience has been positive when adhering to the aforementioned indications. We advocate for a minimally invasive subpectoral technique with secure fixation through limited violation of the humeral diaphysis. Subpectoral tenodesis has the advantage of fully decompressing the intra- and extra-articular portions of the bicipital tunnel and allowing for cortically based fixation. The advent of a unicortical button has been a tremendous innovation as it improved cyclic loading over standard interference screw fixation, and the 3.2 mm drill hole minimizes the fracture risk for subpectoral tenodesis.[93]

After arthroscopic tenotomy and addressing the necessary intra-articular pathology, we move to the open subpectoral portion. The beach chair position is altered from nearly vertical to closer to 45 degrees, and the arm is placed in slight abduction and ER to allow the surgeon to stand in the axilla. A small vertical incision is made just proximal to the axillary fold and centered over the inferior border of the pectoralis tendon. Our incision is more medial than sometimes described, and while it is closer to the brachial plexus, it allows for easy access to the humerus without requiring vigorous retraction on either the tendon or medial soft tissue structures. After incising through skin, the clavipectoral fascia is split with a needle-tip bovie electrocautery, which provides tremendous precision. We then bluntly finger-dissect through the soft tissue and under the pectoralis tendon. A lateral retractor is placed momentarily to allow the biceps to be identified and pulled out of the wound; the tendon is then whip-stitched starting at the musculotendinous junction. The lateral retractor is again placed along with a gently held blunt retractor on the medial border of the humeral shaft. A 3.2 mm hole is drilled unicortically, and the tendon is secured to the diaphysis via a unicortical metal button. The suture limbs are then tied over top of the tendon for additional security.

The most important tips to avoid neurologic injury are to identify the correct incision and surgical plane and avoid prolonged or aggressive medial retraction. We have been very pleased with this technique in the general population as well as overhead athletes and have not had any fractures, which are a concern in throwers given the tremendous force and torque applied to the humerus. The most important principle, though, is not the technique but a very stringent patient selection process.

POSTOPERATIVE MANAGEMENT

A well-defined and thoughtful rehabilitation program is a critical component of a successful recovery and should be specific to the procedure performed. As is true preoperatively, a skilled physical therapist and athletic trainer play a vital role in the outcome as they are in much more frequent contact with the athlete, and open lines of communication between all parties are key. We have found that early cryotherapy in conjunction with scheduled oral antiinflammatory medications provides reasonable comfort and ability to participate in rehabilitation with only minimal narcotic usage. An exhaustive list of postoperative protocols is not practical, but we have listed below our approach to the most commonly addressed pathology in throwers. Our protocol follows five basic phases: acute postoperative, protection, intermediate stretching and strengthening, advanced stretching and strengthening, and RTP.

Following débridement of SLAP and rotator cuff tears, we initiate a fairly aggressive protocol (although the size and location of the tears must be considered). In the immediate postoperative period, we focus on controlling pain and inflammation while maintaining passive motion and scapular stability. We begin early active motion with progressive strengthening. Once the athlete demonstrates full motion and good manual muscle testing in all planes, he may focus on regaining and improving functional strength and normalizing scapular kinematics. Proprioceptive training and core, trunk, and lower extremity strength and endurance training are initiated. If all progresses well, the athlete is prepared to begin throwing in about 6 weeks. Our return to throwing protocol is detailed in Tables 45.1 and 45.2.

In cases involving repair of the SLAP and rotator cuff and possibly capsular plication, the rehabilitation protocol is slowed significantly to allow for healing. The athlete is maintained in an abduction sling during phases 1 and 2 except while doing therapy exercises. The goals of phase 1 (days 1 to 14) are to maintain the repair, minimize pain and inflammation, gradually increase passive motion, and practice dynamic stabilization to prevent muscular atrophy. In phase 2, we begin strengthening and proprioceptive drills between weeks 3 and 4 in those undergoing capsular or labral surgery; this is delayed until 6 weeks following rotator cuff repair. Phase 3 focuses on restoration of full passive motion, supine active motion, and reestablishing dynamic shoulder stability. As dynamic strength improves, the athlete enters phase 4, and our return to throwing protocol is initiated and continued for approximately 3 months. Overhead throwing typically begins at 5 to 6 months postoperatively.

The issue of RTP is addressed following completion of the throwing program. We typically utilize the Kerlan Jobe Orthopedic Clinic Shoulder and Elbow Score and expect a score greater than 85 for consideration of RTP. High-speed (240 frames per second) video analysis from both the front and side perspectives is also done for high-level throwers. Ultimately, the decision for final RTP must be made in conjunction with the player, trainer, and therapist.

RESULTS

Overall, the results following operative intervention on the shoulders of overhead athletes are sobering and should give surgeons pause when considering the treatment plan. A recent systematic review investigating collegiate and professional pitchers undergoing all forms of shoulder surgery found only a 68% RTP at 1 year, and while performance tended to improve from the preoperative state, most players did not achieve return to prior performance (RPP).[94] No doubt a major factor in this equation is the tremendous force across the glenohumeral joint and surrounding soft tissue structures in high-level throwers. Pitchers, in particular, require a finely tuned environment to function at an optimal level, and even small alterations to the balance within

TABLE 45.1   Interval Throwing Program

Distance	Number of Throws	Rest (Min)	Distance	Number of Throws	Rest (Min)
Phase 1 (50% Effort)			**Phase 9 (75%)**		
30'	20	5	90'	20	5
30'	20	10	90'	20	10
45'	10		120'	10	
Phase 2 (50%)			**Phase 10 (75%)**		
30'	20	5	90'	20	5
30'	20	10	90'	20	10
45'	20		120'	20	
Phase 3 (50%)			**Phase 11 (100%)**		
45'	20	5	120'	20	10
45'	20	10	120'	20	
60'	10				
Phase 4 (50%)			**Phase 12 (100%)**		
45'	20	5	120'	20	10
45'	20	10	120'	20	10
60'	20		120'	20	
Phase 5 (50%)			**Phase 13* (Optional)**		
60'	20	5	150'	20	5
60'	20	10	150'	20	
75'	10				
Phase 6 (50%)			**Phase 14* (Optional)**		
60'	20	5	150'	20	10
60'	20	5	150'	20	10
75'	20		150'	20	
Phase 7 (75%)			**Phase 15* (Optional)**		
75'	20	5	180'	20	10
75'	20	10	180'	20	
90'	10				
Phase 8 (75%)			**Phase 16* (Optional)**		
75'	20	5	180'	20	10
75'	20	10	180'	20	10
90'	20		180'	20	

*Our progressive program is designed to minimize re-injury risk and can be adapted for pitchers and position players. For phases 1–12, advance only 1 phase every 3 days with 2 days of rest following each workout. Beyond phase 12, ok to advance 1 phase every other day with 1 day of rest in between. Advancement is only allowed under pain-free conditions; dull pain and soreness often occur, however an athlete shoulder never throw through sharp pain. Of note, players should continue to work through their training program simultaneously to maintain flexibility, strength, and endurance.

the shoulder can precipitate a significant deterioration in function. Surgeons should allow these historical results to serve as a background for their approach and provide a basis for discussion with the athletes when setting expectations.

Rotator Cuff Débridement

Rotator cuff débridement remains our preference for partial-thickness tears of less than 80% thickness in part due to the poor results of repair; however, débridement is certainly not a guarantee to return to preinjury levels. A review of débridement in athletes demonstrated variable outcomes with success (as defined by the authors) ranging from 50% to 89% although

generally less favorable in high-level baseball players.[95] Payne et al.[96] provided an analysis of 43 athletes with partial, articular-sided rotator cuff tears treated with débridement and subacromial decompression. At 2 years, there was only a 66% satisfaction rate with 45% RPP in overhead athletes, which was notably lower than the 86% satisfaction rate and 64% RPP in their non-overhead counterparts. Subgroup analysis revealed that the athletes with the best results from débridement were those with isolated rotator cuff pathology without labral tearing, instability, or subacromial bursitis. Reynolds et al.[95] reported on 67 professional pitchers who underwent débridement alone for small partial-thickness tears with a high rate of RTP at 76% but only 55%

TABLE 45.2   Pitching Program

Distance	Number of Throws	Rest (Min)	Number of Throws	Rest (Min)
Phase 1: Winding Up Off Flat Ground (75%)			**Phase 9**	
60'6" (Warm-up throws)	20	5	Warm-up throws—20 fastballs at 50%	5
60'6"	20	5	20 Fastballs at 75%	5
60'6"	20		20 Fastballs at 75%	5
			20 Fastballs at 100%	5
Phase 2 (75%–100%)			15 Fastballs at 100%	
60'6" (Warm-up throws)	20	5		
60'6"	20	5	**Phase 10**	
60'6"	20	5	Warm-up throws—20 fastballs at 50%	10
60'6"	20		20 Fastballs at 100%	10
			15 Breaking balls and changeups	10
Number of Throws		**Rest (Min)**	20 Fastballs at 100%	10
Phase 3: Off the Mound (100%)			15 Fastballs at 100%	
Warm-up throws—20 fastballs at 50% intensity		5		
20 Fastballs at 50%			**Phase 11**	
			Warm-up throws—20 fastballs at 75%	5
Phase 4			20 Fastballs at 100%	10
Warm-up throws—20 fastballs at 50%		5	6 Breaking balls and changeups	10
20 Fastballs at 50%		5	20 Fastballs at 100%, 6 breaking balls and changeups	
20 Fastballs at 50%				
			Phase 12	
Phase 5			Warm-up throws—20 fastballs at 75%	5
Warm-up throws—20 fastballs at 50%		5	20 Fastballs at 100%	
20 Fastballs at 50%		5	10 Breaking balls and changeups	10
20 Fastballs at 50%		5	15 Fastballs at 100%	
20 Fastballs at 50%			10 Breaking balls and changeups	10
			15 Fastballs at 100%	
Phase 6			10 Breaking balls and changeups	
Warm-up throws—20 fastballs at 50%		5		
20 Fastballs at 50%		5	**Phase 13**	
15 Fastballs at 75%		5	Warm-up throws—20 fastballs at 75%	
15 Fastballs at 75%			20 Breaking balls and changeups	
			Batting practice—50–60 pitches	
Phase 7				
Warm-up throws—20 fastballs at 50%		5	**Phase 14**	
20 Fastballs at 50%		5	Warm-up throws—15 fastballs at 75%	
20 Fastballs at 75%		5	15 Breaking balls and changeups	
20 Fastballs at 75%			Batting practice—70–80 pitches	
Phase 8			**Phase 15**	
Warm-up throws—20 fastballs at 50%		5	Simulated game[a]	
20 Fastballs at 75%		5		
20 Fastballs at 75%		5		
20 Fastballs at 75%		5		
15 Fastballs at 100%				

[a]The simulated game is to be designed specifically for each individual pitcher.
Following phase 16 of the Interval Throwing Program, pitchers will progress to this program.

RPP. Maximum velocity also decreased from 94.2 to 90.1 miles/h. These results again underscore the difficulty obtaining predictable results when operating on elite throwers.

Rotator Cuff Repair

The results of rotator cuff repair have traditionally been poor in this population and are part of the driving force behind débridement for partial-thickness tears. Tibone et al.[97] conducted open acromioplasty and repair in overhead athletes with a 41%

RTP overall. RTP for pitchers was 40% but none were able to attain RPP. Mazoué and Andrews[98] reported on a small series of professional baseball players who underwent mini-open technique for full-thickness repair. Pitchers did poorly as only 8% were able to RTP; however, position players fared better with 75% RTP, particularly when the surgery involved their nondominant arm.

Although no direct comparison exists in overhead athletes between transtendinous repair and tear completion with subsequent repair, a randomized trial in the general population did not demonstrate any statistical difference between the two techniques although there was a nonsignificant relative increase in power for the tear completion and repair group.[99] In a similar comparison, Shin[100] found equal satisfaction rating in each group but quicker recovery of motion and less pain in the initial postoperative period following repair after tear completion.

Ide[52] initially reported the transtendinous technique in 6 throwers with an 83% RTP rate but only 40% RPP. Conway[101] described his initial experience with intratendinous repair in 9 professional baseball players although this was a mixed cohort as all athletes had SLAP tears and half had anterior instability. Regardless, he demonstrated excellent results with 89% RPP at 1 year.

Our lateralized full-thickness repair in a series of 6 professional pitchers has allowed for 100% RTP and 83% RPP for at least one season.[89] We feel that this is the optimal technique and provides the highest likelihood of success in the face of a difficult injury. However, this high rate of return should be tempered by the fact that pitching productivity generally did not return to preinjury levels. Athletes played for an average of 3.3 seasons following surgery, but the mean number of innings pitched decreased from 1806.5 to 183.7 and performance (ERA) decreased slightly for two-thirds of players.

Superior Labral From Anterior to Posterior Tear Débridement

Early in the treatment of SLAP tears in throwers, suture anchors were not available, and thus débridement was the only option, but the results of unstable SLAP débridement were poor and deteriorated over time. Cordasco et al.[102] evaluated 52 consecutive patients who underwent labral débridement and reported 78% excellent pain relief at 1 year, which decreased to 63% by 2 years. Only 45% of throwers whose SLAP tears were treated with débridement were able to return to their preinjury level of throwing. Altchek et al.[103] reported follow-up findings for 40 patients who underwent débridement for unstable SLAP tears. At an average follow-up of 43 months, 70% had moderate pain and 23% had severe pain. Only 1 out of 40 throwers was able to return to preinjury level of throwing. Alternatively, Tomlinson and Glousman[104] reported 75% of professional baseball players were able to RTP with mild or no pain following labral débridement; however, it should be noted their cohort included all labral tears, not specifically SLAPs. These results underscore the importance of an intact superior labrum and the need to carefully scrutinize the stability of the tear pattern.

Superior Labral From Anterior to Posterior Tear Repair

With improvement in technology and introduction of suture anchors, repair becomes a viable option. However, the results over the past 15 years have been inconsistent, with overhead athletes generally having the worst outcomes. Early on, Conway[101] described an 89% RPP at 1 year following SLAP repair in a small cohort of baseball players. In a slightly larger series of type II SLAP repairs in overhead throwing athletes, Ide et al.[105] reported 90% RTP at 3 years. Of pitchers specifically, there was a 95% RTP rate but only 63% RPP.

Recent systematic reviews of type II SLAP repairs demonstrate positive but inconsistent results. One report denotes 88% good to excellent results in overhead athletes with more modern anchor repair but still only 63% RTP.[106] Another revealed good to excellent results ranging from 40% to 90% depending on the study.[107] They found that throwers had the most modest results, though, with 22% to 64% RTP rates in baseball players.

Finally, a recent case series of SLAP tears by Fedoriw et al.[108] involving a professional baseball organization highlights the difficult nature of this injury in throwers and particularly pitchers. Following a nonoperative algorithm, results were fairly similar with pitchers able to RTP at 40% with 22% RPP compared with 39% RTP and 26% RPP for position players. However, after SLAP repair, position players were much more likely to RTP at 85% with RPP of 54%, whereas pitchers had only a 48% RTP rate and 7% RPP.

Biceps Tenodesis

Although discussed, there is currently no literature on the results of biceps tenodesis in an isolated overhead athlete population.[82]

COMPLICATIONS

Overall, shoulder arthroscopy is quite safe with a low incidence of complications. A recent analysis of 30-day morbidity of more than 9000 elective cases revealed a 0.99% complication rate with major morbidity of 0.54%.[109] The most common incident was return to the operating room (without specified reason) at 0.31%. Infection, albeit rare, did occur with 0.16% superficial and 0.01% deep rates. Thromboembolic events were equally uncommon with occurrence rates of 0.09% deep vein thrombosis and 0.06% pulmonary embolus. Only a 0.01% rate of peripheral nerve injury was noted. On multivariate analysis, risk factors included smoking history, chronic obstructive pulmonary disease, operative time greater than 1.5 hours, and American Society of Anesthesia class 3 to 4.

Fortunately, the overhead athletic population tends to be young and healthy and on the lower end of the risk spectrum. Care should always be taken to minimize complications, but fortunately, shoulder arthroscopy is a fairly safe procedure with minimal morbidity. From our perspective, though, the greatest risk is not postoperative complications as discussed above but rather failure to return to the supraphysiologic level of function required for throwing. Limitations in motion and persistent alterations in kinematics are always a possibility when performing any shoulder surgery on an overhead athlete, and even when seemingly minor, these changes can have dramatic effects on downstream function.

SUMMARY AND FUTURE CONSIDERATIONS

Overhead athletes are a high-demand but rewarding patient population, and physicians should approach their care with a solid knowledge base, realistic expectations, and stringent surgical criteria. Quite the opposite of elbow operations,[110] the rate of shoulder surgery in throwers is decreasing both in our practice as well as nationally.[111,112] As discussed, early postoperative outcomes for a variety of conditions have been modest, and while results continue to improve, there should be trepidation prior to considering surgery. Conservative care should be the mainstay of treatment for most shoulder-related issues in this population with operative intervention truly being a last resort.

Several questions, such as the role for biceps tenodesis in throwers, remain unanswered but are certainly of interest around the world. The future of the field will likely focus on more specific treatment guidelines and operative indications, surgical techniques specific to this population, and evidence-based rehabilitation protocols and RTP guidelines.

For a complete list of references, go to ExpertConsult.com.

SELECTED READINGS

Citation:

Burkhart SS, Morgan CD, Kibler WB. The disabled throwing shoulder: spectrum of pathology part I: pathoanatomy and biomechanics. *Arthroscopy*. 2003;19(4):404–420.

Level of Evidence:

IV

Summary:

This three-part series of articles covers all aspects of the disabled shoulder in detailed fashion.

Citation:

Sewick A, Kelly JD, Rubin B. Physical examination of the overhead athlete's shoulder. *Sports Med Arthrosc Rev*. 2012;20(1):11–15.

Level of Evidence:

V

Summary:

Succinct guide to examining the shoulder of an overhead athlete.

Citation:

Kibler BW, Sciascia A, Wilkes T. Scapular dyskinesis and its relation to shoulder injury. *J Am Acad Orthop Surg*. 2012;20(6):364–372.

Level of Evidence:

V

Summary:

Scapular dyskinesis is a common clinical entity relating to the general population in addition to throwers, and it is often poorly recognized and not well understood. This provides a review of the salient points.

Citation:

Kibler WB, Thomas SJ. Pathomechanics of the throwing shoulder. *Sports Med Arthrosc Rev*. 2012;20(1):22–29.

Level of Evidence:

V

Summary:

Analysis of the pathology seen within the throwing shoulder. This provides a comprehensive evaluation of how throwing mechanics are altered in the setting of injury.

Citation:

Corpus KT, Camp CL, Dines DM, et al. Evaluation and treatment of internal impingement of the shoulder in overhead athletes. *World J Orthop*. 2016;7(12):776.

Level of Evidence:

IV

Summary:

A current review on the pathogenesis, evaluation, and treatment of internal impingement.

Citation:

Thorsness R, Alland JA, McCulloch CB, et al. Return to play after shoulder surgery in throwers. *Clin Sports Med*. 2016;35(4):563–575.

Level of Evidence:

V

Summary:

Specific focus on the data and challenges faced with getting throwers back to competition.

46

Proximal Biceps Tendon Pathology

Samuel R.H. Steiner, John T. Awowale, Stephen F. Brockmeier

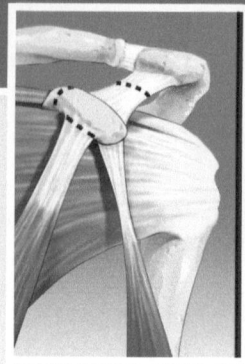

INTRODUCTION

Pathology to the proximal aspect of the long head of the biceps tendon (LHBT) has long been recognized as a source of shoulder pain and dysfunction.[1-3] Referred by some as the biceps-labral complex,[4] the proximal biceps tendon includes its origin on the superior labrum, the intra-articular tendon, and the tendon as it courses its way through its stabilizing pulley down the bicipital tunnel to the biceps brachii muscle belly. For lesser abnormalities of the biceps tendon, such as tendinopathy, conservative treatment modalities are often successful. In the setting of superior labral pathology, partial LHBT tears, or instability of the biceps tendon in the bicipital groove, surgical intervention is an accepted treatment option after a conservative algorithm has failed. This chapter focuses on identifying proximal LHBT pathology based on a thorough history and physical examination in conjunction with imaging, and from there selecting the proper treatment. This chapter also reviews the current surgical techniques.

HISTORY

The structure of the glenohumeral joint makes diagnoses of LHBT pathology challenging. Other disease processes localized to the shoulder, such as rotator cuff disease, superior labral from anterior to posterior (SLAP) tears, glenohumeral joint arthritis, subacromial impingement, or acromial clavicular (AC) joint arthrosis, can complicate the differential diagnosis. Thus a thorough history and physical examination is needed to correctly diagnose LHBT disease.

Patients with suspected pathology of the long head of the biceps will present with progressive anterior shoulder pain and declining function as a result of chronic overuse. In many cases, this occurs from repetitive overhead activities. Patients who participate in baseball, softball, or volleyball may report ongoing clicking or snapping sensations with throwing or spiking motions. Alternatively, an isolated event may also be identified such as catching a heavy object with a flexed arm, resulting in an eccentric force causing an acute rupture. This is often described as an audible "pop" resulting in swelling of the arm, and ecchymosis with or without a visible defect commonly referred to as the "Popeye sign." Pain is most commonly reported down the anteromedial aspect of the shoulder around the bicipital groove, sometimes traveling distally into the biceps muscle belly. In older patients with long head of the biceps pathology there is often

an associate rotator cuff tear present that is felt as pain along the anterolateral shoulder region.[5]

PHYSICAL EXAMINATION

The long head of the biceps originates at the supraglenoid tubercle and the superior glenoid labrum. It inserts distally along with the short head of the biceps on the bicipital tuberosity of the radius. The tendon is extrasynovial spanning the glenohumeral joint within the rotator interval (region anterior to the supraspinatus tendon and superior to the subscapularis tendon). The tendon sits in the bicipital groove, which is defined as the region between the greater and lesser humeral tuberosities. The bony anatomy and soft tissue structures help to maintain the long head of the biceps within the bicipital groove. As the tendon exits the bicipital groove it travels under the pectoralis major insertion, eventually combining with the short head of the biceps. The main blood supply to the long head of the biceps is provided by the branches of the anterior circumflex humeral artery.[6]

There are over 180 physical examination tests described for diagnosing pathology of the shoulder.[7] As discussed earlier, proximal biceps tendon pathology is difficult to isolate on physical exam as many examination findings are not specific to proximal biceps tendon dysfunction alone (Table 46.1). The presence of the "Popeye sign" indicates a rupture of the long head of the biceps thus solving the diagnostic dilemma; however, this sign is often not present, necessitating the correct execution of physical examination maneuvers and interpretation of results to diagnose other proximal tendon pathology. Furthermore, patients with concomitant rotator cuff tears can make diagnosis of biceps tendon pathology via physical examination even more difficult.[8] One of the most common findings is tenderness over the intertubercular groove of the proximal humerus showing up to 90% sensitivity in some studies for detecting long head of the biceps pathology.[9] During this exam the practitioner palpates the bicipital groove along the anterior proximal humerus approximately 5 to 7 cm below the acromion with the arm internally rotated 10 degrees. The diagnosis of tendon pathology is more likely if pain during palpation moves laterally with continued palpation and external rotation (ER) of the arm. The asymptomatic contralateral arm should also be tested for comparison, as a normal biceps tendon also may be tender to deep palpation. Pathology of the biceps tendon under the proximal aspect of the pectoralis major muscle can be tested using the subpectoral bicep tendon

TABLE 46.1 Typical Physical Examination Tests for the Long Head Biceps Tendon and Concomitant Pathology

Pathology	Test	Specific Site	Examination	Positive
LHBT	Biceps instability[65]	LHBT within the groove	Full abduction, external rotation; palpate bicipital groove	Palpable "click"
	Point tenderness[66]	LHBT within the groove	Palpate the bicipital groove 3–6 cm below the acromion; internally rotate the arm 10 degrees	Reproducible pain; dynamic evaluation shows groove tenderness laterally as the arm is externally rotated
	Speed[67]	LHBT within the groove; SLAP	Elbow extended, forearm supinated, arm elevated to 90 degrees	Pain localized within the bicipital groove
	Yergason[68]	LHBT	With the elbow flexed and the forearm pronated, the examiner holds the arm at the wrist and the patient actively supinates against resistance	Bicipital groove pain
	Gerber's lift-off test[65]	Subscapularis LHBT	The patient stands with his/her hand behind the back and the dorsum of the hand resting on the midlumbar spine; the patient attempts to raise his/her hand off the back by maintaining or increasing internal rotation of the humerus and extension of the shoulder	Inability to move the dorsum of the hand off the back
Concomitant RC	Belly press[65]	Subscapularis	The hand is on the abdomen and attempts are made to move it anteriorly	Difficulty moving the elbow forward
	Neer impingement[69]	AC joint	The arm is maximally passively elevated forward, with internal rotation with the scapula stabilized	Pain/weakness in the subacromial space/edge of the acromion of the biceps region
	Kennedy-Hawkins[58]	Impingement of the greater tuberosity and CH ligament	The arm is forward-flexed 90 degrees, then quickly rotated internally	Pain/weakness in deltoid or anterior shoulder
	Empty can[70]	Supraspinatus	The arm is forward-flexed 90 degrees, with full internal rotation 90 degrees; downward force is resisted	Pain/weakness deep in the shoulder
Concomitant labrum	Compression rotation[71]	Labrum	The patient lies supine; the affected arm is elevated 90 degrees and the arm is rotated while an axial load is applied	Pain or clicking deep in the shoulder
	O'Brien's active compression[72]	AC joint superior labrum	The patient stands with the arm adducted 15 degrees and forward-flexed 90 degrees with the elbow fully extended; the arm is maximally internally rotated and elevated with the palm up and the thumb pointing down against resistance	Pain in the AC joint and pain or a deep "click" in the GH joint
	Anterior slide[73]	Labrum	The patient stands with a hand on the hip of the affected side while the examiner applies an axial load along the humerus	Pain or a "click" is produced

AC, Acromioclavicular; CH, coracohumeral; GH, glenohumeral; LHBT, long head of the biceps tendon; RC, rotator cuff; SLAP, superior labral anterior to posterior.

test. The proximal biceps tendon is palpated underneath the pectoralis muscle just medial to its insertion. The arm is then internally rotated against resistance with pain indicating a positive test. Again, the contralateral normal shoulder also should be evaluated. A more painful response on the affected side validates the test result.[10]

Several other traditional physical examination techniques have been described to evaluate long head of the biceps. The Speed test is performed with forward flexion of the shoulder to 90 degrees with the forearm supinated and the elbow fully extended; pain with resisted shoulder flexion in this position is

a positive result. This test may also be positive in patients with SLAP lesions. The Yergason test is positive with pain to palpation over the bicipital groove during resisted supination of the forearm as the elbow is flexed at 90 degrees.[5] Both the Speed and the Yergason tests have been shown to be less sensitive 27% to 40%, though more specific 80% to 100%.[9] A less specific test, although more sensitive, is the O'Brien active compression test, which may indicate either long head of the biceps tendonitis, SLAP lesions, or AC joint arthrosis.[9] This test is performed with the arm adducted 10 to 15 degrees across the body with the elbow extended. Pain with resisted forward flexion of the arm in this position with the forearm pronated indicates a SLAP tear; however, pain with resisted forward flexion in this position with both pronation and supination indicates potential AC joint pathology.[5] Newer tests for evaluating long head of the biceps pathology have also been developed, such as the "upper cut" maneuver.[11] This is performed with the involved shoulder at in neutral position with the elbow flexed to 90 degrees, forearm supinated, and the patient's hand making a fist. The patient then attempts to forward flex the shoulder and elbow towards the chin in a punching-like maneuver as the practitioner holds the patient's fist, resisting the motion. A positive test is seen with pain along the anterior shoulder during the resisted movement. The 3-Pack examination is also a newer test for evaluating for proximal biceps pathology (Fig. 46.1). The maneuvers that comprise the 3-Pack exam are the active compression test (O'Brien sign), the resisted throwing test, and the bicipital tunnel palpation. The 3-Pack examination demonstrated a higher sensitivity but lower specificity when compared to more traditional exam maneuvers such as the Speed test, Yergason test, full can test, and the empty can test.[12]

The biceps tendon is held within the bicipital groove by a tendoligamentous sling or pulley made up of the supraspinatus tendon, coracohumeral ligament, superior glenohumeral ligament, and notably the subscapularis tendon. Medial biceps tendon subluxations or dislocations occur when this pulley mechanism has been disrupted, most commonly with partial or complete tearing of the subscapularis tendon. On physical examination, medial biceps instability can be detected by a palpable click or tenderness to palpation of the biceps tendon on full abduction and ER of the affected arm. When the tendon is fully dislocated it can be palpated anterior to the lesser tuberosity and rolled under the examiner's finger, eliciting tenderness.[5]

Selective injections about the shoulder are a good way to distinguish various pathology as they can be used therapeutically and diagnositically.[13] A subacromial space injection will alleviate pain with impingement. Pain relief with an injection into the area of the bicipital groove may be indicative of long head of the biceps tendonitis.[9] Intra-articular glenohumeral joint injections are useful when evaluating a potential SLAP lesion.[5]

IMAGING

The diagnosis of biceps tendon pathology is often aided via imaging modalities. Plain radiographs with orthogonal views (AP, lateral, and axillary) should be obtained initially. Although pathology of the biceps tendon will usually not be apparent on plain radiographs, they are useful in ruling out other shoulder pathology such as glenohumeral joint degeneration or rotator cuff calcific tendonitis. To further evaluate the bicipital groove radiographically, a Fisk view can be obtained. This may show bicipital groove osteophytes or narrowing. The view is obtained with the patient supine with their arm at their side with the hand fully supinated, the cassette is placed on the top of their shoulder and the x-ray is directed cephalad down the bicipital groove.[14] In certain patients for whom magnetic resonance imaging (MRI) is contraindicated, a plain arthrogram or computed tomography (CT) arthrogram could be helpful. In these cases, a visible sharp outline of the tendon sheath suggests no significant biceps inflammation; however, a negative arthrogram has been reported in up to 30% of cases with biceps pathology.[15,16]

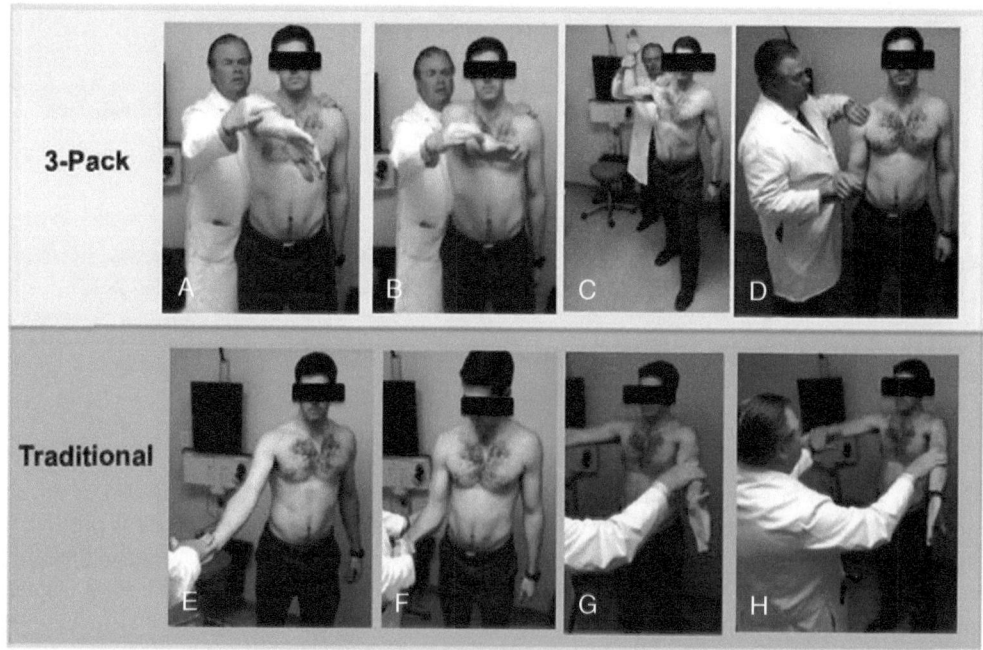

Fig. 46.1 The 3-pack examination includes (A) the active compression test with resisted elevation of the arm in pronation and (B) repeated again in supination, (C) resisted throwing maneuver, and (D) bicipital groove tenderness. Traditional examinations include (E) Speed test, (F) Yergason sign, (G) full can, and (H) empty can. (Modified from O'Brien's article: Taylor SA, Newman AM, Dawson C, et al. The "3-Pack" examination is critical for comprehensive evaluation of the biceps-labrum complex and the bicipital tunnel: a prospective study. *Arthroscopy.* 2017;33[1]:28–38.)

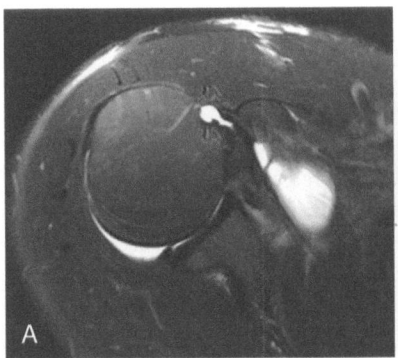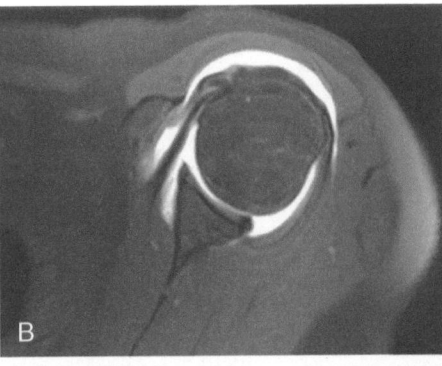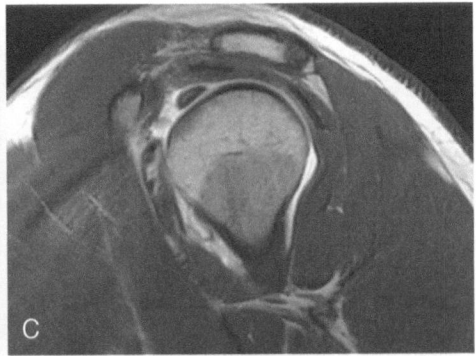

Fig. 46.2 Magnetic resonance imaging of the proximal biceps. (A) High-grade partial, near complete rupture of the long head biceps tendon at the groove entrance (axial image). (B) Biceps tendon subluxation into an upper third split in the subscapularis tendon (axial image). (C) Intrasubstance degeneration of the proximal biceps tendon within the joint (hourglass lesion) (sagittal image).

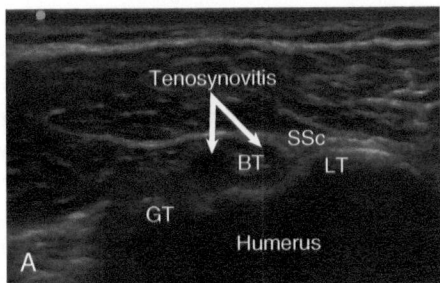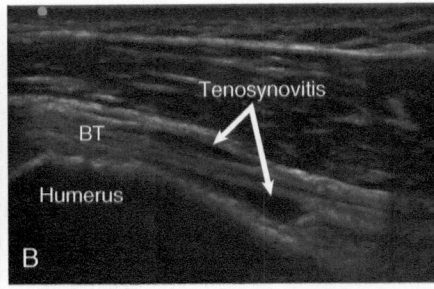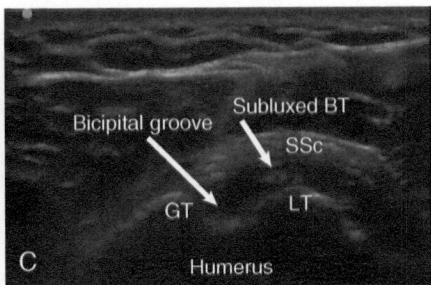

Fig. 46.3 Ultrasound images. (A) An axial view of long head biceps tenosynovitis. (B) An ultrasound longitudinal view of long head biceps tenosynovitis. (C) An ultrasound axial view of a subluxed long head biceps tendon and subscapularis tear. *BT*, Biceps tendon; *GT*, greater tuberosity; *LT*, lesser tuberosity; *SSc*, subscapularis.

MRI is the modality of choice for imaging of the biceps tendon and surrounding soft tissues structures within the shoulder (Fig. 46.2). MRI provides visualization of the biceps tendon, bicipital groove, bony osteophytes, and fluid. The biceps tendon is best visualized on the axial and sagittal oblique views. Although more sensitive then noncontrast MRIs, MRI arthrograms still show a poor concordance with arthroscopic findings concerning biceps pathology with rates of concordance reported at 34.9%.[17] Complete proximal biceps ruptures are readily apparent. More subtle pathology, such as partial-thickness tears, tendinitis, and tendinopathy, are more difficult to assess. Other studies have reported sensitivity and specificity rates at 27% and 86%, respectively, regarding the ability of MRI to detect partial biceps tendon tears when compared to arthroscopy.[18] MRI arthrography enhances the sensitivity and specificity in the diagnosis of biceps pathology and is the image modality of choice for evaluating SLAP tears.[19] On MRI arthrography, the long head of the biceps is normally surrounded by contrast fluid and has the shape of a kidney bean on the axial view. If a subscapularis partial or full-thickness tear is suspected, the axial and sagittal oblique views should be scrutinized for potential long head of the biceps subluxation or dislocation.[20]

Ultrasound is becoming increasingly popular in the diagnosis of musculoskeletal pathology (Fig. 46.3). Although inexpensive, it is highly operator dependent. Regarding the shoulder, ultrasound is accurate at detecting full-thickness rotator cuff tears, bicipital instability, and bicipital tendon rupture; however, it has low sensitivity (49%) when detecting partial-thickness biceps

tendon tears, and the modality is unable to assess tendon inflammation.[21] Ultrasound has also been used for selective shoulder injections improving the accuracy of the injections specifically when injecting the bicipital tendon sheath.[13]

DECISION-MAKING PRINCIPLES

When treating any disorder, patient factors should be considered and proximal biceps tendon pathology is no different. The practitioner should consider the patient's age, activity level, body habitus/body mass index, occupation, sporting activities, comorbidities, and overall functional expectations. As discussed previously, the close proximity of potentially pathologic structures in the shoulder, such as the rotator cuff, AC joint, superior labrum, and anterior capsule, makes diagnosing and treating proximal biceps disorders challenging. A successful patient outcome necessitates the correct diagnosis of not only the proximal biceps tendon pathology but also any concomitant pathology.

Surgical-intervention is reserved for cases of failed nonsurgical management consisting of rest, rehabilitation, physical therapy, nonsteroidal antiinflammatory drugs, and/or selective corticosteroid injections. Generally agreed upon indications for surgery include partial long head of the biceps tendon tears and biceps tendon subluxation with or without concomitant subscapularis tear. Relative indications include type IV SLAP tears, symptomatic type II SLAP tears in patients over the age of 35 to 40, failed SLAP repair, and chronic anterior shoulder pain from bicipital tendonitis.[22]

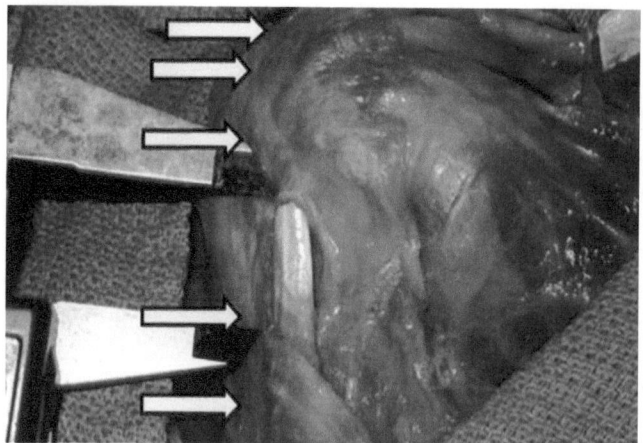

Fig. 46.4 Various tenodesis locations *(arrows)* of the proximal long head biceps tendon.

Biceps tenodesis is a well-described technique and can be performed arthroscopically, in conjunction with an open procedure, or stand alone as a mini open procedure. Many different techniques have been described for fixation of the tendon distally including the use of bone tunnels, keyholes, suture to decorticated bone, interference screws, and suture anchors. Interference screws have been shown to have the highest load to failure compared to suture anchors.[23,24]

Controversy still remains over the location of the tenodesis, which includes above or in the bicipital groove, below the groove just above the superior margin of the pectoralis major tendon (suprapectoral), or in the subpectoral region just above the inferior margin of the pectoralis major tendon (Fig. 46.4). Proponents of more distal fixation (supra- or subpectoral) theorize that removing the tendon from the groove removes residual tenosynovitis potentially found within the tendon sheath.[6,25]

TREATMENT OPTIONS

Nonoperative Management

Unless the patient has a complete tendon rupture or a high-grade partial tear at risk for complete rupture, treatment for proximal biceps tendon pathology begins with a conservative (nonoperative) management algorithm for at least 6 to 12 weeks.[26] A trial of rest, activity modification, oral antiinflammatory medications, and physical therapy can often lead to improvement if not resolution of symptoms.[10,14,26] It is important that physical therapy be focused on underlying scapular disorders and concomitant shoulder pathology often seen in conjunction with biceps pathology. If pain persists, a local anesthetic combined with corticosteroid can be injected either into the glenohumeral joint or bicipital sheath, depending on the location of pathology and clinician preference (Fig. 46.5). For either location, it is imperative that the medication reach its intended location. Fluoroscopy and ultrasound are typically employed for glenohumeral joint and bicipital sheath injections, respectively, and improve both diagnostic and therapeutic accuracy, ensuring accurate placement of the injection. The success rate for biceps tendon sheath

ultrasound-guided injections has been reported at 87% compared to a 27% unguided success rate.[27]

Surgical Management
Indications

Surgical intervention is considered in patients who have failed a conservative management algorithm. Effective surgical options are available for the management of pathologies to any portion of the LHBT. This includes SLAP lesions, partial tendon tearing greater than 25% to 50%, rupture, subluxation, or pulley lesions.[22] Additional intraoperative findings that would warrant addressing the biceps tendon surgically would include a hyperemic tenosynovium, hypertrophied tendon (hourglass deformity),[28,29] superior subscapularis tearing, or biceps chondromalacia to the humeral head.[30,31]

Optimal surgical management of pathologies involving the LHBT remains controversial, with biceps tenotomy and tenodesis being the two most commonly performed procedures. Biceps tenotomy has the advantages of being technically less demanding to perform and does not require postoperative restrictions or immobilization. Disadvantages include cosmetic deformity (Popeye sign)[32-34] secondary to distalization of the muscle belly, muscle cramping, and fatigue discomfort with repetitive use.[35-41] Biceps tenodesis is typically advocated by surgeons who favor the procedure in laborers, active patients, younger persons, and those concerned with cosmetic appearance.[42] Tenodesis preserves muscle tone and prevents distal migration of the biceps, thus preserving the contour of the muscle and avoiding a cosmetic deformity.[14,43,44] Strength and function, especially during elbow flexion and forearm supination, are maintained.[44-47] While muscle cramping and spasms following tenodesis have been reported, they occur at a significantly lower rate than tenotomy.[44,48] Disadvantages of tenodesis compared to tenotomy include a higher technical demand on the surgeon, longer postoperative restrictions and rehabilitation, and a risk of fixation failure.[49] While a traditional approach is to perform a tenotomy on patients older than 60 years of age,[50] newer studies have pointed to patient-specific preferences, such as cosmesis, need for hardware, and postoperative restrictions, as the main determinates when choosing between tenotomy and tenodesis.[51]

Systematic reviews have failed to demonstrate a difference in outcomes between biceps tenodesis and tenotomy.[36,37,39,50,52] This may be due to the fact that some of these articles did not differentiate between the varying types of tenodesis, or it may be due nonrandomization and patient selection. It also may be due to addressing associated shoulder pathologies, such as rotator cuff tears or external impingement, at the time of surgery.

Despite the lack of evidence showing superior outcomes of tenodesis over tenotomy, there has been an increase in the number of biceps tenodesis procedures being performed. In a recent study by Werner et al., there was a reported 1.7-fold increase in biceps tenodesis over tenotomy in the United States from 2008 to 2011, with an increase in the incidence of arthroscopic biceps tenodesis significantly outpacing the increase in open tenodesis.[53] They speculate that a portion of the overall increase in tenodesis may reflect patients with failed SLAP repairs or surgeons who

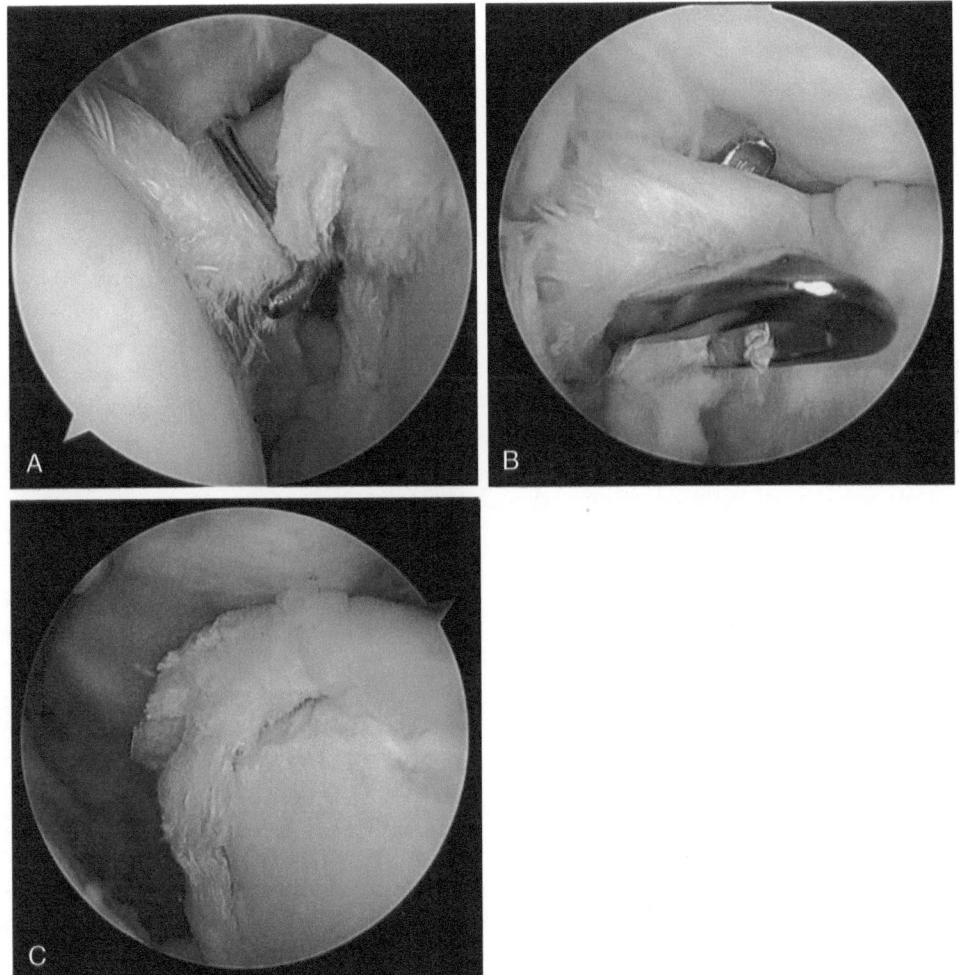

Fig. 46.5 Arthroscopic biceps tenotomy. (A) A 72-year-old male with a degenerative biceps tendon with longitudinal high-grade tearing. (B) Biceps tendon release at the superior labral attachment with a punch biter. (C) Completed biceps tenotomy.

prefer biceps tenodesis as a primary procedure for SLAP lesions based on trends in current literature.[54-57] Additionally, it may be due to surgeons gaining an understanding and comfort level with performing newer techniques.

Diagnostic Arthroscopy and Biceps Tenotomy

Arthroscopic tenotomy can be performed with the patient in the lateral decubitus or beach chair position, depending on surgeon preference and concomitant procedures required. The arthroscope is introduced through a standard posterior portal. Under direct arthroscopic visualization, a spinal needle is used to localize proper placement of an anterior portal in the rotator interval. Once the anterior portal is established, a probe is inserted, and a thorough diagnostic arthroscopy of the glenohumeral joint is performed.

The LHBT is evaluated first at its attachment. The probe is used to lift the superior labrum to evaluate for a SLAP lesion. From there the biceps tendon is evaluated distally. The intraarticular tendon is inspected for tearing and tenosynovitis. The probe is used to evaluate for instability of the LHBT by attempting to displace the tendon from its groove and sling.[58] Intraarticular findings indicating possible biceps instability include

superior subscapularis tearing, anterior supraspinatus tearing, or antero–superior humeral head chondromalacia.[30,31] The probe is further utilized to pull the biceps tendon into the joint. Forward shoulder elevation and elbow flexion can provide further excursion of the biceps tendon.[59,60] The distal tendon is inspected for inflammation, tearing, or hypertrophy (hourglass deformity).[29] The biceps pulley, a capsuloligamentous complex formed by a coalescence of fibers form the coracohumeral ligament, superior glenohumeral ligament, and portions of the subscapularis and supraspinatus tendons, functioning to stabilize the LHBT within the proximal portion of the groove,[4] is inspected for pathology. To aid in arthroscopic evaluation, some advocate the use of a 30-degree scope via the lateral portal or a 70-degree scope via the posterior portal.[61]

After a diagnostic arthroscopy the biceps tenotomy can be performed. Viewing from the posterior portal, the biceps is tenotomized using a punch biter or electrocautery device via the anterior portal to separate the tendon from its attachment to the superior labrum and supraglenoid tubercle (see Fig. 46.5). Careful attention is made not to violate the labrum. Any residual stump is gently débrided using a shaver. The elbow can be extended and the biceps tendon observed as it retracts. If the biceps tendon does not retract into the bicipital groove, it may be due to hypertrophied proximal tendon. This will need to be excised. If it still does not retract, the bicipital sheath may need to be released arthroscopically, depending on biceps pathology observed during diagnostic arthroscopy and the location of the patient's pain prior to surgery.

Biceps Tenodesis

Tenodesis of the LHBT can be performed in a variety of ways that include arthroscopic[28,33,45,62,63] or open[10,44,55,64] technique and can be positioned high at the entrance of the bicipital groove at the chondral junction,[49,61,65] in the suprapectoral location just proximal to the pectoralis major tendon,[42,44,45] in a subpectoral location at, or distal to, the pectoralis major tendon,[10,44,55,64] or in other positions, including the conjoint tendon or soft tissue tenodesis sites.[26,66,67] Regardless of location, there is an increasing recognition that restoration of the anatomic length-tension relationship of the LHBT is a critical aspect of the tenodesis procedure.[42,63,68,69]

Arthroscopic Biceps Tenodesis

Biceps tenodesis can be performed entirely arthroscopically without the need for a separate larger incision. This minimizes the risk of infection, which is a concern with open subpectoral tenodesis that uses an incision near the axillary fold. A disadvantage of arthroscopic compared to open subpectoral tenodesis is an increased risk of postoperative stiffness.[70] Arthroscopic biceps tenodesis can be performed in the beach-chair or lateral decubitus positions. After a diagnostic arthroscopy and prior to release from its superior labral attachment, the tendon is typically tagged percutaneously to prevent retraction and preserve the length-tension relationship.[42,44,68,69,71]

Two main locations for arthroscopic tenodesis include a high intertubercular groove entrance site at the chondral junction, and a low suprapectoral site just proximal to the pectoralis major tendon. Advocates for tenodesis at the chondral junction note that the interference screw can be incorporated as a suture anchor during rotator cuff repair, a procedure commonly performed in conjunction with biceps tenodesis.[61] It also leaves a substantial amount of tendon proximal to the pectoralis major, which allows for revision tenodesis should it be necessary. In some studies, this location results in a low surgical revision rate of 0.4%, a low rate of residual pain, and a significant improvement in outcome scores.[65] However, there are those who feel that a tenodesis performed at the chondral junction does not address bicipital tunnel disease, which can be a source of residual groove pain, and instead advocate for a suprapectoral tenodesis site.[33,63] This location places the tenodesis tunnel distal to the bicipital groove, which allays concerns about the groove as a source of pain after tenodesis.[62]

Arthroscopic tenodesis fixation, regardless of location, can be performed with a variety of methods, most commonly with an interference screw[33,45,61,72] or suture anchor.[47,73,74] In a biomechanical study by Richards and Burkhart,[75] a biceps tenodesis with interference screw provided greater fixation strength than the same procedure performed with a double suture anchor technique.

Open Biceps Tenodesis

Open biceps tenodesis is typically performed at the subpectoral location. The procedure is less technically demanding than arthroscopic tenodesis and removes the majority of the LHBT and associated tenosynovium from within the groove, thus eliminating a potential source for postoperative pain.[44,60,64] In a biomechanical study using matched cadavers, open subpectoral tenodesis had a significantly increased ultimate load to failure when compared with an arthroscopic suprapectoral technique using an interference screw.[76] Disadvantages of the open subpectoral technique include the need to make an incision near the axilla, which has the potential for wound issues, as well as the removal of the majority of the LHBT, which leaves little usable tendon should a revision be necessary.

Open biceps tenodesis can be performed in the lateral decubitus or beach-chair position depending on surgeon preference. Diagnostic arthroscopy is performed first. Prior to tenotomy, a tag suture is typically placed in the biceps tendon to prevent overretraction and to aid in tendon identification. After tenotomy, the open portion of the case is begun. A 3 cm longitudinal incision is made at the inferior border of the pectoralis major tendon near the axillary fold on the anteromedial aspect of the upper arm. The tendon is retrieved through the wound and whipstitched. Either an interference screw,[10] cortical button, or bone tunnel[32] is typically used for fixation. Compared with suprapectoral biceps tenodesis with interference screw, subpectoral tenodesis with interference screw may have an increased risk of proximal humerus fracture through the humeral socket for the screw.[77,78]

Other Techniques

Soft tissue tenodesis, as described by Sekiya et al., involves securing the biceps tendon to the soft tissues in the rotator interval.[59] In this technique, a spinal needle is percutaneously placed through the lateral aspect of the rotator interval and through the biceps tendon approximately 1 to 2 cm distal to its origin on the superior labrum. Suture is shuttled through and retrieved through the anterior portal. The process is repeated, passing suture distal to the first but proximal to the bicipital groove. The scope is introduced into the subacromial space and the suture ends retrieved through a cannula and tied. Tendon proximal to the tenodesis site is then excised.

Originally described by Froimson, the keyhole technique involves first performing a proximal tenotomy.[79] The tendon is then retrieved through an open suprapectoral approach and the proximal end balled-up. In the bicipital groove a bone tunnel with distal trough (keyhole) is created. The balled-up portion of the tendon is inserted into the bone tunnel. The distal, tubular portion of the tendon is slide distally in the trough and is secured in place by the balled-up tendon that is deep in the canal and too wide for the trough.[80,81]

Another less commonly used procedure includes the arthroscopic transfer of the LHBT to the conjoint tendon.[26,67] With this technique, the LHBT is released from its origin, transferred to the subdeltoid space and sutures to the conjoint tendon in a side-to-side manner with nonabsorbable sutures.

✎ Authors' Preferred Techniques

Arthroscopic Suprapectoral Biceps Tenodesis

The biceps tendon is tagged while viewing arthroscopically by percutaneously inserting a spinal needle just lateral to the anterior portal and piercing the biceps tendon (Fig. 46.6). The arthroscope is placed in the subacromial space via the posterior portal. Using a spinal needle and outside-in technique, a standard lateral portal is established. A combination of a shaver and radiofrequency ablator are used to remove the subacromial bursa in order to aid in visualization.

The arthroscope is then moved to the lateral portal. With the radiofrequency ablator in the anterior portal, the arm is forward flexed to approximately 80 degrees and slightly externally rotated while dissection is continued anterior and distal to identify the biceps tendon in between the distal margin of the subscapularis tendon and proximal margin of the pectoralis major tendon.[25] Starting lateral and working medial, the biceps tendon is liberated from its sheath. Once mobilized, a spinal needle is used to localize for a distal anterolateral portal directly over the biceps tendon and just proximal to the pectoralis major tendon. We have found that identifying a point distal and equidistant to the anterior and lateral portals creates an equilateral triangle and is a typical location for creating an anterolateral portal.

After needle localization and establishment of an anterolateral portal, a cannula is introduced. A suture-passing device is introduced through the cannula and used to pass a heavy, nonabsorbable suture in luggage-tag fashion. Each limb is additionally passed through the tendon, one immediately proximal and the other distal to the first suture pass. At the site where the tendon is sutured, a guide pin is placed perpendicular to the humerus and in the bicipital groove. The near cortex is then reamed with a cannulated reamer to the appropriate diameter given the size of the tendon and desired interference screw. We most commonly ream to the same size of the interference screw (line to line), which is typically 4.5–7 mm in diameter. It is important to ensure that the reamed depth is enough to accommodate the screw. A radiofrequency ablator is used to tenotomize the tendon just proximal to the suture. The suture limbs are passed through the fork-tipped interference screw and the tendon is guided into the bone socket and screwed into place. Care is taken not to countersink the screw as this can result in reduced fixation. The suture is subsequently sewn over the top to reinforce the fixation. The arthroscope is then reinserted into the glenohumeral joint and the residual biceps tendon is tenotomized at its origin and removed with a traumatic grasper.

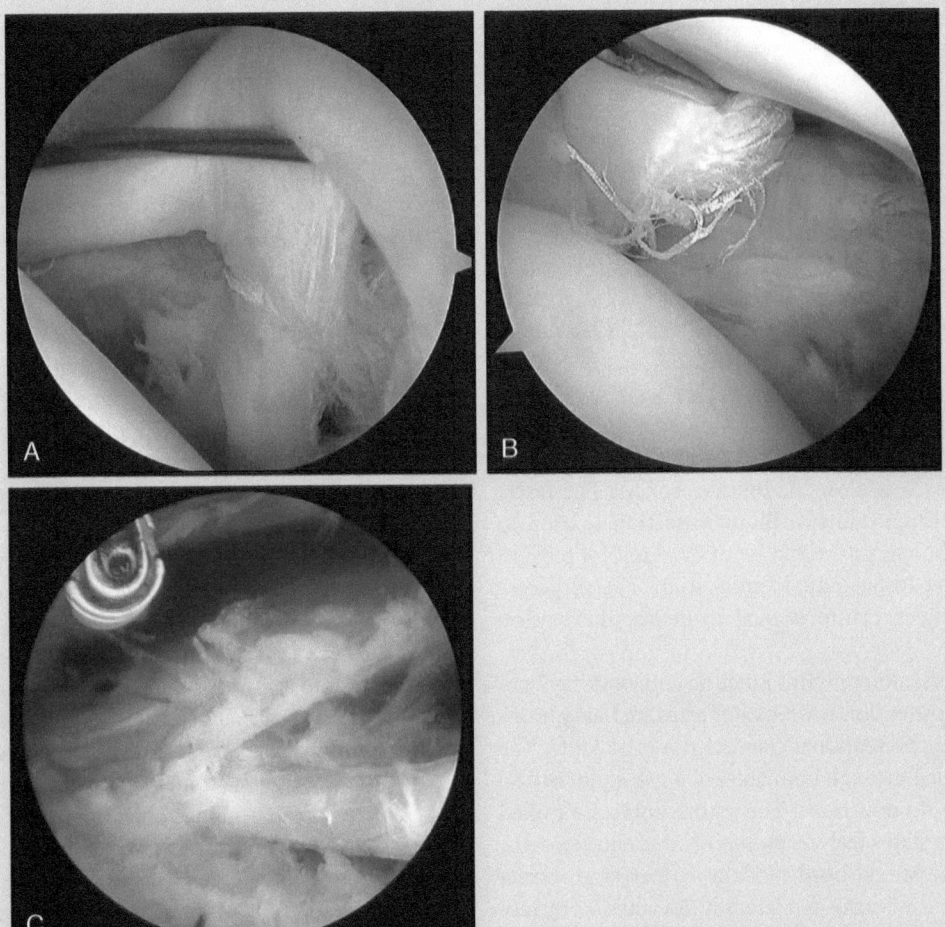

Fig. 46.6 Arthroscopic suprapectoral biceps tenodesis. (A and B) A 56-year-old male with a type 2 superior labral from anterior to posterior tear and a high-grade partial long head of the biceps tendon (*LHBT*) tear at the groove entrance. (C) Identification of the LHBT at the upper border of the pectoralis major tendon (viewing from direct lateral portal, working from low anterior "tenodesis" portal.

Continued

⚡ Authors' Preferred Technique—cont'd

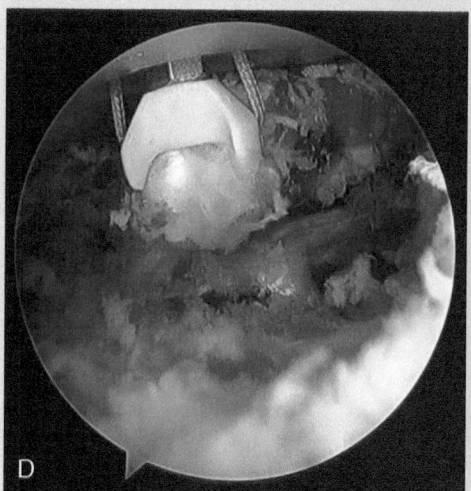 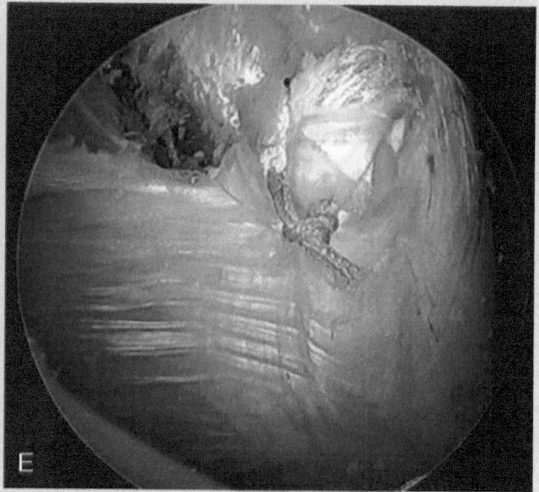

Fig. 46.6, cont'd (D) LHBT has been secured with a suture and then tenotomized at the planned location for tensioning; the humeral tunnel has been prepared; and the tendon is attached to an interference screw for tenodesis. (E) Final tenodesis at the upper border of the pectoralis major tendon, secured with an interference screw and suture back-up.

Open Subpectoral Biceps Tenodesis

After a diagnostic shoulder arthroscopy, a tag suture is placed into the biceps tendon under arthroscopic visualization and a tenotomy is performed (Fig. 46.7). Subpectoral tenodesis is performed in an open fashion through a longitudinal incision at the lower border of the pectoralis major muscle as described by Mazzocca et al.[10] An ~3 cm vertical incision is made just lateral to the axillary fold, with 1 cm over the pectoralis major tendon and 2 cm distal to the inferior border. The skin is incised sharply and blunt dissection is used to identify the fascia overlying the biceps brachii. The pectoralis major tendon can be palpated to ensure the approach is along its inferior border. The fascia is carefully incised longitudinally. Blunt dissection is used to locate the LHBT. The tag suture can be utilized to pull tension on the biceps tendon to facilitate identification. The surgeon's finger or a right-angled clamp is used to deliver the tendon from the wound.

Starting at the musculotendinous junction and working 2 cm proximally, the biceps tendon is whipstitched using heavy, nonabsorbable suture. Excess tendon is transected using a knife. The suture limbs are passed through both holes of a two-hole cortical button but in opposite directions. The suture limbs are pulled to ensure the button slides feely. A pointed Hohmann retractor is placed around the lateral border of the humerus to retract the pectoralis major superiorly and laterally. A Chandler retractor is placed around the medial aspect of the humerus to retract the coracobrachialis and short head of the biceps medially while at the same time protecting the neurovascular structures. In a cadaveric study, it was reported that the average distance of the musculocutaneous nerve to the musculotendinous junction of the long head of the biceps is 2.6 cm. Controlled retraction with the Chandler retractor should be employed to prevent traction injuries to surrounding nerves. The bicipital groove should be able to be visualized and palpated. If further retraction is needed, a Sauerbruch or Army-Navy retractor can be used to pull the inferior border of the pectoralis major proximally.

The osseous bed is prepared with a periosteal elevator. A spade-tip drill bit specific to the cortical button implant is drilled unicortically, centered in the groove and approximately 3 cm proximal to the inferior border of the pectoralis major insertion. The button is deployed within the humeral canal and flipped by toggling the suture limbs. The length-tension relationship of the biceps is checked. A free needle is used to pass one suture limb through the proximal tendon and the suture limbs are tied.

POSTOPERATIVE MANAGEMENT

Biceps Tenotomy Rehabilitation Protocol

The goals of rehabilitation following biceps tenotomy are to control pain and inflammation in the acute phase while attempting to restore range of motion (ROM) and function. Patients are placed into a simple sling for comfort following surgery and are instructed to discontinue it within the first 1 to 2 weeks. Rotator cuff isometrics and scapular exercises are initiated immediately after surgery without any limitation to ROM. After 2 weeks patients can begin isotonic rotator cuff and scapulothoracic strengthening and advance as tolerated. Starting 6 weeks after surgery, patients can begin conventional weight lifting with machine weights and progress slowly to free weights. If the patient is free of pain and has reached their baseline strength and motion, they can return to sport or activity.

Biceps Tenodesis Rehabilitation Protocol

Whether the biceps tenodesis was performed arthroscopically or open, the rehabilitation protocol is the same. It is imperative that the biceps tendon be protected to allow bone-tendon healing.[64,82] Biceps loading is not allowed for the first 12 weeks

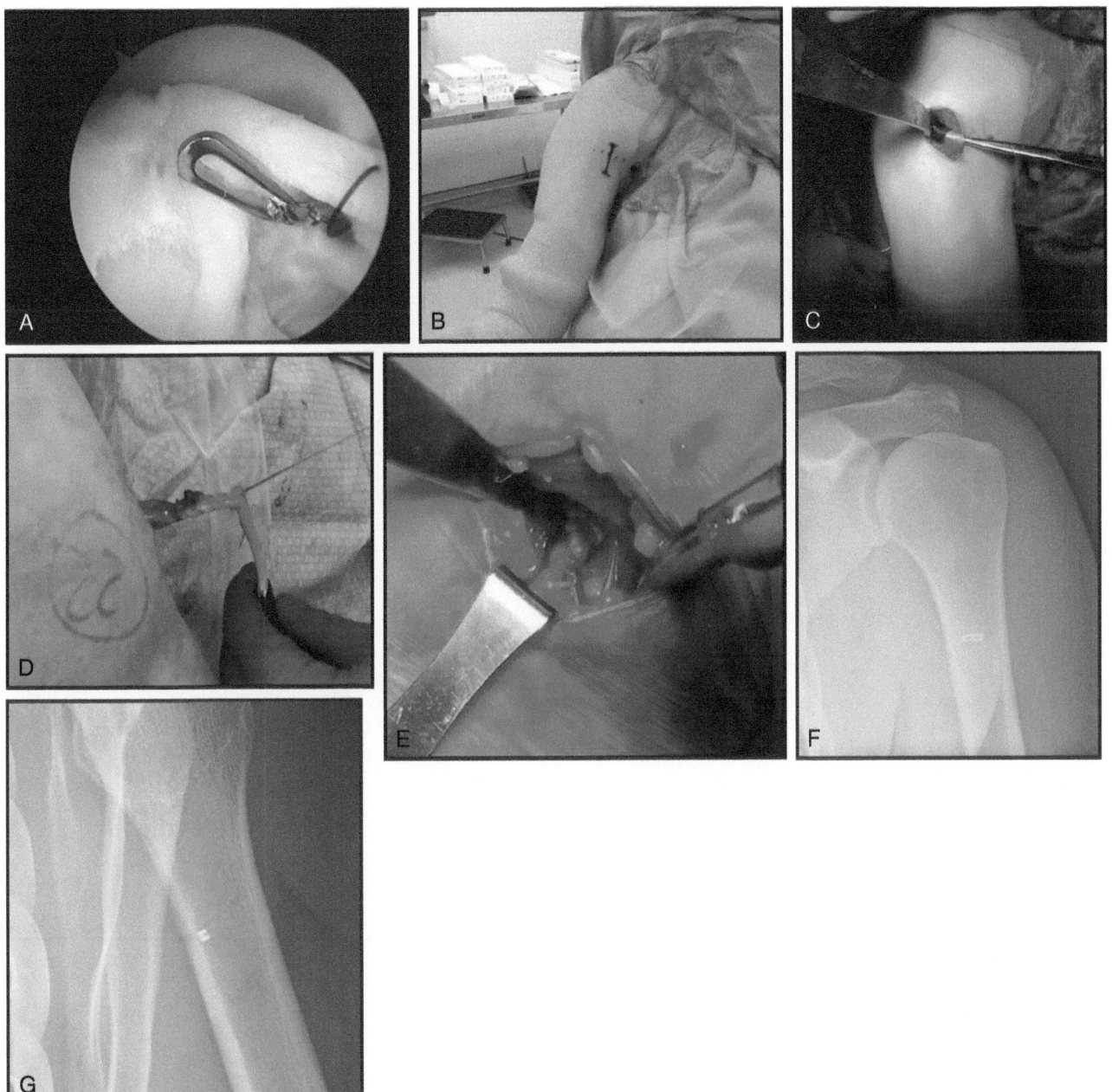

Fig. 46.7 Open subpectoral biceps tenodesis. (A) In a 43-year-old male with a type 2 superior labral from anterior to posterior lesion, the long head of the biceps tendon (*LHBT*) has been tagged with polydioxanone suture and is tenotomized. (B) Typical incision for an open subpectoral biceps tenodesis positioned lateral to the axilla with one-third above the lower edge of the pectoralis major tendon, two-thirds below. (C) LHBT is secured in the subpectoral region and externalized. (D) A tendon-grasping stitch has been placed securing the tendon along the 20 mm segment above the muscle/tendon junction. (E) The tenodesis is completed with the tendon secured to the anterior humerus using a unicortical button fixation. (F and G) Final radiographs of an open subpectoral biceps tenodesis.

following surgery. Throwing or overhead sports are not allowed until week 20.

Phase I: Protective Phase (Day 1 to Week 6)

The goals of phase I are to control pain, swelling, and inflammation, and to restore ROM. The arm is placed into an ultrasling for the first 6 weeks. Immediately after surgery, passive and gentle active assisted ROM exercises are initiated under the guidance of a physical therapist and are limited to flexion and scaption to 90 degrees, ER to 30 degrees, and internal rotation (IR) to 45 degrees for the first 4 weeks. Starting week 5, ROM is increased with flexion and scaption to full, ER to 50 degrees, and IR to 60 degrees.

Phase II: Moderate Protection Phase (Weeks 7 to 12)

The goals of phase II are to initiate active ROM and increase muscle endurance. The sling is discontinued. Both active and

TABLE 46.2   Clinical Outcomes of Proximal Long Head Biceps Tenodesis

Procedure Type	Authors	Study Design	Patients	LHBT Condition	Concomitant Procedures
Arthroscopic/ anchor	Checchia et al. (2005)[46]	Level IV retrospective case series	n = 15; mean age, 62 years; range, 41–80 years	Subluxated, 13% (2/15); dislocated, 40% (6/15); preruptured, 47% (7/15)	RCT, 100% (15/15); acromioplasty, 67% (10/15); SLAP, 7% (1/15)
Arthroscopic/ suture anchor through subclavian portal	Nord et al. (2005)[47]	Level IV prospective case series	n = 10; mean age 60 years; range 41–77 years	NR	RCT (all intra-articular) and/or labral tears 100% (10/10); acromioplasty 40% (4/10); impingement syndrome 100% (10/10)
Arthroscopic/ suture anchor	Franceschi et al. (2007)[52]	Level IV retrospective case series	n = 22; mean age, 60 years; range, 40–81 years	Subluxated, 32% (7/22); dislocated, 32% (7/22); preruptured, 36% (8/22)	RCT 100% (22/22); other concomitant repairs NR
Arthroscopic/ interference screw	Boileau et al. (2002)[45]	Level III prospective, nonrandomized case series	n = 43; mean age, 63 years; range, 25–78 years	Subluxated, 26% (11/43); dislocated, 30% (13/43); preruptured, 35% (15/43); tenosynovitis, 9% (4/43)	RCT, 86% (37/43); SLAP, 14% (6/43)
Arthroscopic/ interference screw	Koh et al. (2010)[90]	Level II cohort study	n = 43; mean age, 61 years; range, 55–77 years	Subluxated/dislocated, 9% (4/43); preruptured, 12% (5/43); severe tenosynovitis, 7% (3/43)	RCT, 79% (34/43); SLAP, 44% (19/43); SAD, 5% (2/43); DCE, 12% (5/43)
Open/suture anchor	Warner et al. (2001)[91]	Level IV retrospective case series	n = 19; mean age, 58 years; range, 36–72 years	Subluxated, 100% (19/19); preruptured, 74% (14/19)	RCT, 100% (19/19); acromioplasty, 79% (15/19)
Mini open/ interference screw	Mazzocca et al. (2008)[64]	Level IV retrospective case series (single surgeon)	n = 41; mean age, 50 years; range, NR	NR	RCT, 59% (24/41); Bankart w/ anterior capsulorrhaphy, 5% (1/41); SAD, 20% (8/41); DCE, 10% (4/41); acromioplasty, 5% (2/41); SLAP, 5% (2/41); lipoma excision, 5% (1/41)
Open/ interference screw and suture anchor	Millett et al. (2008)[86]	Level IV retrospective case series (2 surgeons)	n = 88; interference screw 34, suture anchor 54; mean age, 51 years; range, 22–77 years	Subluxated (NR)	RCT, 73% (64/88); DCE, 14% (12/88); acromioplasty, 47% (41/88); capsular reconstruction, 9% (8/88)
Open/ interference screw	Nho et al. (2010)[85]	Level IV retrospective case series	n = 13; mean age, 52 years; range, 32–65 years	Subluxated, 100% (13/13)	RCT, 100% (13/13); acromioplasty, 100% (13/13); DCE, 31% (4/13)

ASES, American Shoulder and Elbow Surgeons; *CM,* Constant Murley Functional Assessment of the Shoulder; *DCE,* distal clavicle excision; *LHBT,* long head of the biceps tendon; *MC,* modified CM; *MRI,* magnetic resonance imaging; *NR,* not reported; *RC,* rotator cuff; *RCT,* randomized controlled trial; *ROM,* range of motion; *SAD,* subacromial decompression; *SANE,* single assessment numeric evaluation; *SLAP,* superior labral anterior to posterior; *SST,* simple shoulder test; *UCLA,* University of California–Los Angeles; *VAS,* visual analogue scale.

Follow-Up	Outcome Measures	Positive (Excellent/ Good Outcome)	Negative (Fair/Poor Outcome)	Overall Results
Mean, 32 months; range, 20–67 months	UCLA; ROM	93% (14/15); improved scores; improved ROM	7% (1/15); weakness and residual pain; MRI revealed severe atrophic RC muscles, but RC suture and tenodesis were intact	Concomitant repair revealed satisfactory results with no significant complications
Mean, 24 months; range, NR	UCLA	90% (9/10); improved scores	10% (1/10); 1 patient had an adhesive capsulitis postoperative complication at 2-year follow-up	Suture anchor placement slightly proximal to bicipital groove was effective for LHBT tenodesis with concomitant intra-articular RCTs
Mean, 47 months; range, 36–59 months	UCLA; ROM	100% (22/22); improved scores; improved ROM	0%	No patients rated surgery as unsuccessful; no patients had bicipital pain, Popeye sign, or daily activity limitations
Mean, 17 months; range, 12–34 months	CM; ROM strength	95% (41/43); improved scores; no loss of elbow movement, and biceps strength was 90% of the other side	5% (2/43); rupture of tenodesis; MRI revealed tight fixation of the biceps tendon in the humeral socket	Good clinical results with isolated pathologic biceps tendon or cuff repair; very thin, fragile, almost ruptured biceps tendon is the technical limit to the arthroscopic approach
Mean, 28 months; range, 24–35 months	Patient satisfaction; ASES; CM	84% (36/43); improved scores	16% (7/43); 2 patients complained of arm pain at resisted flexion; 4 patients had Popeye deformity	Suture anchor tenodesis of LHBT is associated with <10% incidence of Popeye deformity
Mean, 40 months; range, 24–75 months	Patient satisfaction; MC	42% (8/19); improved scores	58% (11/19)	Although prior surgery did not directly correlate with Constant score, delayed repair of more than 6 months of symptoms resulted in negative outcomes; 9/19 patients had prior failed RC surgeries, which may have resulted in less favorable outcomes
Complete follow-up at minimum 1 year after surgery (mean, 29 months; range, 12–49 months)	Rowe; ASES; SST; CM; SANE	100% (41/41); improved scores	0%	All clinical outcome measures (Rowe, ASES, SST, CM, SANE scores) demonstrated a statistically significant improvement at follow-up when compared with preoperative scores for all 41 patients; 1 failure was due to pull-out of tendon from bone tunnel resulting in Popeye deformity; patients with coexistent RC lesions had less favorable outcomes (lower ASES, SST scores)
Mean, 13 months; range, 3–25 months	Patient satisfaction; SES; VAS; MC	87% (48/55) (subjective outcome only collected for n = 55); mean scores improved (scores collected for all n = 88)	5% (4/88); 1 patient indicated shoulder was worse after surgery and 1 patient did not return to normal activities	No failures of fixation; no complications after surgery; 5 patients reported persistent groove tenderness; 2 patients reported persistent spasm
Mean, 35 months; range, 14–52 months)	Patient satisfaction; ASES; SST; VAS	100% (13/13); improved scores	0%	Arthroscopic repair of anterosuperior RC tears with open biceps tenodesis significantly improved clinical outcomes scores, pain relief, and shoulder function

passive ROM are increased with a goal of full motion by week 10. Starting week 10, submaximal isometrics and active ROM are initiated. The patient may also begin more aggressive exercises for rotator cuff and scapulothoracic musculature.

Phase III: Minimum Protection Phase (Weeks 13 to 20)

The goals of phase III are for full, nonpainful active and passive ROM, restoration of muscle strength, power and endurance, and gradual initiation of functional activities. Isotonic elbow flexion and forearm supination are initiated along with light plyometric activities.

Phase IV: Advanced Strengthening Phase (Weeks 21 to 26)

The goals of phase IV are to increase functional activities and return to sport. Overhead athletes may slowly begin their sport specific activities.

RESULTS

Regardless of technique, most articles demonstrate good to excellent outcomes following biceps tenodesis with relief of pain and return of function (Table 46.2).[22,53,60,64,83,84]

There is sufficient evidence in the literature to support performing open subpectoral biceps tenodesis for the treatment of pathology to the LHBT. Mazzocca et al. evaluated outcomes after open subpectoral biceps tenodesis with an interference screw. They reported improved patient reported outcomes in 41 patients at an average follow-up of 29 months.[64] In a similar study, Nho et al. obtained outcomes of open subpectoral tenodesis with interference screw in concomitant arthroscopic rotator cuff repairs and found that all 13 patients had significant clinical improvement in outcome scores at 1 year after surgery.[85] Millet et al. also reported successful results in a study comparing open subpectoral tenodesis fixation with interference screw to suture anchor. Both groups demonstrated significant improvement in outcomes scores at 13 months postoperatively, but a higher rate of bicipital groove pain in the suture anchor subset compared with the interference screw subset.[86]

Clinical outcomes of arthroscopic biceps tenodesis are not as well reported as those of open subpectoral tenodesis. However, a reasonable amount of current literature demonstrates improved outcomes and patient satisfaction. Boileau et al. reported on 43 patients who underwent arthroscopic biceps tenodesis with interference screw. They reported a significant improvement in postoperative Constant scores.[45]

Current literature also demonstrates comparable results after arthroscopic tenodesis to open subpectoral biceps tenodesis. In a study comparing arthroscopic suprapectoral and open subpectoral biceps tenodesis, Werner et al. showed that arthroscopic tenodesis had a higher rate of stiffness.[70] However, in a follow-up study comparing 2-year results, that stiffness resolved as both arthroscopic suprapectoral and open subpectoral tenodesis demonstrated no significant differences in clinical and functional outcomes, including ROM, between techniques.[87]

COMPLICATIONS

There is a low incidence of complications following biceps tenodesis. These complications include hematoma, seroma, wound infection, humeral fracture, persistent bicipital pain, shoulder stiffness, fixation failure, cosmetic deformity, and neurovascular injury, with the latter being less common in arthroscopy due to the close proximity of the open approach to neurovascular structures.[84,88,89] In a review of 353 patients who underwent open subpectoral biceps tenodesis with interference screw fixation, there were seven reported complications (2.0%). These included persistent bicipital pain, failed fixation, wound infection, musculocutaneous neuropathy, proximal humerus fracture, and complex regional pain syndrome.[84]

Biceps tenotomy is not without complications. These include persistent bicipital pain, cosmetic deformity, muscle cramping, and fatigue discomfort with repetitive use.[35-41]

FUTURE CONSIDERATIONS

Recognition of optimal location for tenodesis, whether at the articular margin, suprapectoral, or subpectoral regions, is an important area for future clinical investigation. Biceps tenodesis is commonly performed in conjunction with rotator cuff repair, which has a confounding effect when comparing outcomes after surgery. To date, there are no randomized trials collecting prospective data comparing isolated tenodesis at these locations. As we still try to gain an overall understanding of the function of the LHBT as it relates to the mechanics of the glenohumeral joint, we will perhaps develop new techniques for tendon restoration in the setting of tendon pathology.

For a complete list of references, go to ExpertConsult.com.

SELECTED READINGS

Citation:
Werner BC, Burrus MT, Miller MD, et al. Tenodesis of the long head of the biceps: a review of indications, techniques, and outcomes. *JBJS Rev.* 2014;2(12).

Level of Evidence:
Basic science review, operative technique

Summary:
This article gives a comprehensive review of arthroscopic and open, suprapectoral and subpectoral biceps tenodesis. It discusses outcomes and provides a review of the current literature.

Citation:
Mazzocca AD, Cote MP, Arciero CL, et al. Clinical outcomes after subpectoral biceps tenodesis with an interference screw. *Am J Sports Med.* 2008;36(10):1922–1929.

Level of Evidence:
IV, retrospective case series

Summary:
Clinical outcomes were reported to be good to excellent in all 41 patients undergoing subpectoral biceps tenodesis. Patients with coexisting rotator cuff lesions had less favorable outcomes.

Citation:

Nho SJ, Reiff SN, Verma NN, et al. Complications associated with subpectoral biceps tenodesis: low rates of incidence following surgery. *J Shoulder Elbow Surg.* 2010;19(5):764–768.

Level of Evidence:

IV, case series, treatment study

Summary:

Outcomes in 373 patients undergoing open subpectoral biceps tenodesis by two fellowship-trained orthopaedic surgeons at a single institution.

Citation:

Nho SJ, Strauss EJ, Lenart BA, et al. Long head of the biceps tendinopathy: diagnosis and management. *J Am Acad Orthop Surg.* 2010;18:645–656.

Level of Evidence:

Basic science review, operative technique

Summary:

This article provides a comprehensive review of biceps tendinopathy, starting with anatomy, pathophysiology, and clinical diagnosis before discussing techniques and results for tenotomy, open and arthroscopic tenodesis.

Citation:

Brady PC, Narbona P, Adams CR, et al. Arthroscopic proximal biceps tenodesis at the articular margin: evaluation of outcomes, complications, and revision rate. *Arthroscopy.* 2015;31:470–476.

Level of Evidence:

IV, therapeutic case series

Summary:

This article retrospectively reviews 1083 patients who underwent an arthroscopic biceps tenodesis at the articular margin by interference screw fixation.

Citation:

Elser F, Braun S, Dewing CB, et al. Anatomy, function, injuries, and treatment of the long head of the biceps brachii tendon. *Arthroscopy.* 2011;27(4):581–592.

Level of Evidence:

V

Summary:

Current review of the anatomy and biomechanical properties of the long head of the biceps tendon and evidence-based approach to current treatment strategies for disorders to the biceps tendon.

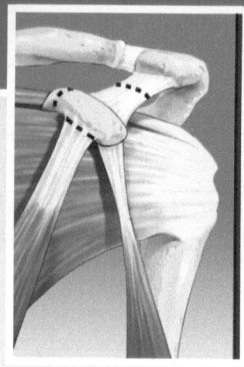

47

Rotator Cuff and Impingement Lesions

Gina M. Mosich, Kent T. Yamaguchi, Frank A. Petrigliano

HISTORICAL PERSPECTIVE

A description of rotator cuff pathology is found in the earliest surgical text, the Edwin Smith Papyrus (c.1500 BCE). Subsequently, throughout ancient and modern history, multiple authors have written about the rotator cuff, its disease, and its nonoperative and operative treatment. Monro penned the first modern case report and illustration of a rotator cuff tear in 1788 in his treatise, *A Description of All the Bursae Mucosae of the Human Body*. John Gregory Smith reported the first cases series of seven rotator cuff tears in a letter to the editor of the *London Medical Gazette*, and Muller described a rotator cuff repair in 1889. However, it was the publication of Ernest Amory Codman's landmark book, *The Shoulder*, in 1934 that ushered the rotator cuff, its pathology, and its treatment into mainstream medical discourse and consciousness. Codman was a Boston general surgeon who dedicated a tremendous amount of his energy, talent, skill, and clinical practice to the study of the shoulder and its maladies. The foundation of contemporary care of rotator cuff disease—and arguably the care of surgical patients in general—can be traced to the principles described in this book. Although Codman's book and the works of other authors have shed light on the subject, many questions regarding the care of the rotator cuff remain, and nowhere is this more relevant than in the rotator cuff of the athlete.

The years following the publication of Codman's book saw a rapid proliferation of active study of the shoulder by authors such as Harrison McLaughlin, Carter Rowe, and Charles Neer. The pioneering work of Charles Neer set the stage for the contemporary discussion and debate of how to best care for the rotator cuff. Neer expanded on the concept of outlet impingement first elucidated by Meyer in 1937.[1] Neer vigorously investigated subacromial outlet impingement and argued that impingement was the basis of a spectrum of disease, encompassing most disorders involving the rotator cuff.

Neer proposed three stages of impingement. Initially, in stage I, there is inflammation and edema within the cuff. This is followed by the fibrosis and tendinitis seen in stage II. Finally, there is partial or complete tearing of the rotator cuff in stage III.[2,3] Neer eventually came to argue that a vast majority, if not all, lesions of the rotator cuff were due to subacromial impingement. This argument generated vigorous and vocal opposition from other surgeons who argued that the etiology of rotator cuff disease is more degenerative in nature. The debate of extrinsic impingement versus intrinsic degeneration as the etiology of rotator cuff tears continues to this day. In reality, rotator cuff tears are likely the result of a multifactorial combination of these two sources.

ANATOMY

The glenohumeral joint is the most mobile in the body, allowing for precise positioning of the hand in space. The glenohumeral joint also acts as a fulcrum for the upper extremity, absorbing the majority of forces in activities that require propulsive action. Vitally linked to these motions in terms of precision, propulsion, and stability is the rotator cuff. The cuff is composed of the confluent tendons of the supraspinatus, infraspinatus, subscapularis, and teres minor muscles,[4] which originate from the anterior and posterior aspects of the scapula and insert as a composite onto the greater and lesser tuberosities of the humerus. The cuff envelops and blends with the glenohumeral capsule on all sides except at the redundant inferior pouch.

The biceps tendon originates at the supraglenoid tubercle and traverses the glenohumeral joint as an intra-articular but extrasynovial structure. The biceps passes deep to the interval between the supraspinatus and subscapularis (the "rotator interval") and exits the joint in the intertubercular sulcus, which is bound by the coracohumeral (CH) ligament superiorly and the confluence of the superior tendinous slip of the subscapularis and superior glenohumeral ligament (SGHL) inferiorly. These ligaments, along with the tendinous slip of the subscapularis, form a pulley for the biceps tendon as it enters the intertubercular groove.[5,6] The groove has a variable shape and depth, and the bony anatomy of the supratubercular region has been implicated in degenerative lesions of the biceps tendon.[7-10]

The rotator interval is an anatomic space defined by the inferior edge of the supraspinatus tendon and the superior edge of the subscapularis tendon.[11-13] The superficial roof of the rotator interval is the CH ligament and the floor of the interval is the SGHL. The biceps tendon occupies this interval as it enters the shoulder joint, with the CH ligament and SGHL forming a pulley for the biceps tendon (Fig. 47.1). The rotator interval functions, biomechanically, as a suspensory structure for the humeral head. Lesions of the rotator interval have been recognized as an important pathology in the genesis of shoulder pain.[4,14]

The vascular supply of the biceps and rotator cuff has been studied extensively.[15-18] Anatomic studies have demonstrated that the vascular supply of the rotator cuff comes from six branches

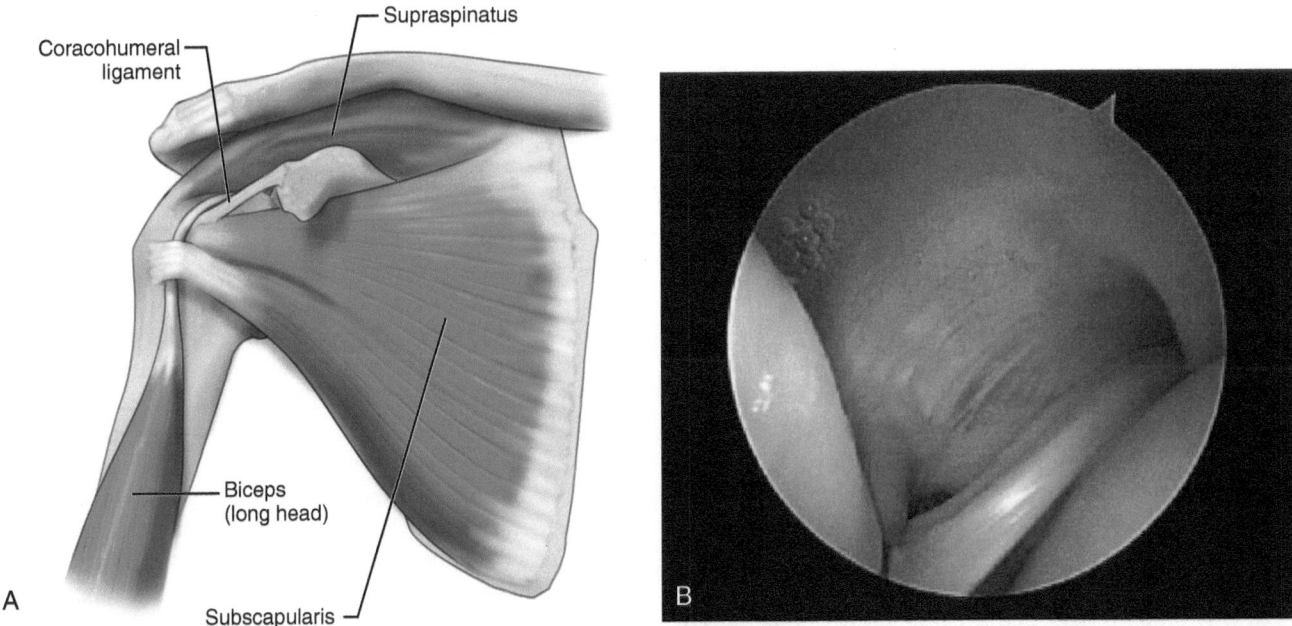

Fig. 47.1 (A) Anterior cuff structures with biceps tendon entering the rotator interval. (B) Arthroscopic view from within the glenohumeral joint. The biceps tendon is seen entering the joint.

of the axillary artery, with the largest contributions arising from the suprascapular and the anterior and posterior humeral circumflex arteries.[18] Previous belief held that there is an area of relatively poor vascularity known as the "critical zone." This area lies within the supraspinatus tendon immediately proximal to its insertion onto the greater tuberosity,[19] where most degenerative changes and degenerative rotator cuff tearing begin.[20–22] However, recent intraoperative Doppler flowmetry studies failed to show a critical zone of decreased vascularity in normal supraspinatus tendons,[23] although there is a demonstrated decrease in overall tendon vascularity with increasing age.[24] The biceps tendon also demonstrates an area of hypovascularity in its intra-articular portion related to tension or pressure from the humeral head when the tendon is in the anatomic position. With arm abduction, these areas demonstrate complete vascular filling.[19]

Superficial to the rotator cuff is the deltoid and coracoacromial (CA) arch. The acromion is an extension of the spine of the scapula and has a variable shape and slope that form the posterolateral bony roof of the arch.[25] The acromion serves as the origin of the deltoid laterally and articulates with the clavicle anteriorly and medially, its undersurface creating a finite space for the rotator cuff tendons superior to the humeral head. The CA ligament extends from the outer edge of the coracoid and widens to insert on the anteromedial aspect and undersurface of the acromion. The CA ligament encompasses the anterior extent of the CA arch and, with the anteroinferior edge of the acromion and the coracoid process, is implicated in classical extrinsic impingement of the rotator cuff.[26,27] Some authors have suggested that the shape and slope of the acromion may be related to extrinsic rotator cuff pathology.[26,27] However, whether the variability in acromial shape is the result or the cause of the underlying cuff degeneration remains controversial (Fig. 47.2).[28]

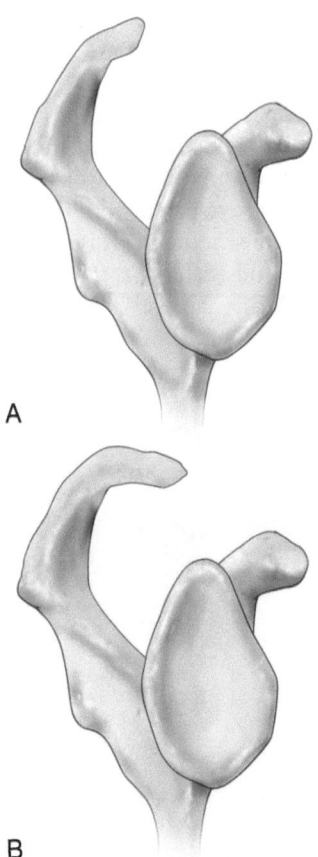

Fig. 47.2 Variability in acromial morphology. Lateral views of a normal acromion (A) and a more hooked acromion associated with impingement (B).

Deep to the CA arch lies the subacromial bursa. It is a filmy synovium-lined sac that attaches at its base to the greater tuberosity with its roof fixed to the undersurface of the acromion and CA ligament.[29] The remaining superior and inferior surfaces of the bursa articulate loosely with the deltoid and rotator cuff, respectively. The roof and base of the bursa are separated by a thin interface of synovial fluid that allows relatively frictionless motion between the cuff and the overlying deltoid and CA arch.

BIOMECHANICS

The biomechanics of the shoulder involve a complex interaction between several "joints," including the scapulothoracic, glenohumeral, acromioclavicular, and sternoclavicular articulations. The most relevant to this topic are the scapulothoracic and glenohumeral articulations.

Rotator Cuff Function

Because the glenohumeral joint lacks inherent bony stability, it relies heavily on both static and dynamic soft tissue stabilizers for its stability and function.[30,31] The muscles of the rotator cuff contribute to glenohumeral motion. But much more importantly, they help maintain a stable fulcrum at the glenohumeral joint around which the other muscles of the shoulder girdle can effectively act on the humerus.

Although previously believed to initiate abduction, the supraspinatus is currently considered to function primarily as a stabilizer of the glenohumeral joint. Its orientation 70 degrees from the plane of the glenoid means it provides a compressive force driving together the humeral head and the glenoid cavity (Fig. 47.3).[32] By maintaining the articular congruity through concavity compression, a stable fulcrum is created for the more powerful muscles of the shoulder girdle. The powerful deltoid, for example, requires this stability at the glenohumeral joint to function effectively. Without the stabilizing, synergistic action of the supraspinatus the humeral head would displace superiorly

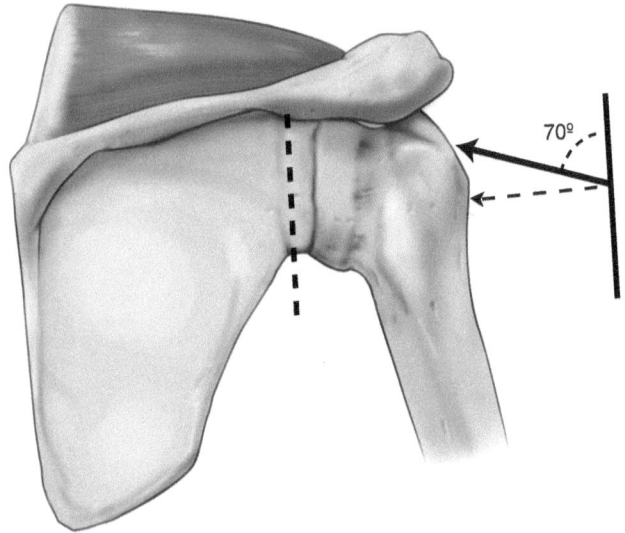

Fig. 47.3 Angle of pull of the supraspinatus with a direct line of force (*solid arrow*) and the compressive component of the force (*dashed arrow*).

as the deltoid contracts, resulting in impingement of the rotator cuff between the humeral head and the undersurface of the acromion.[32,33]

By virtue of their orientation, the action of the infraspinatus and teres minor muscles is external rotation of the arm and depression of the humeral head,[33] with the infraspinatus being the primary depressor. The subscapularis muscle also depresses the humeral head and acts as an internal rotator of the arm. The infraspinatus and subscapularis act as a "force couple," stabilizing the glenohumeral joint, especially during eccentric contraction and overhead activity.[34] The rotator cuff provides stability through eccentric contraction, whereas the large superficial muscles around the glenohumeral joint (such as the deltoid, trapezius, latissimus dorsi, and pectoralis major) provide the propulsion for movements of the shoulder by their powerful concentric contractions.

With concentric muscular contraction producing motion in one direction, there is a concomitant eccentric muscular contraction on the opposite side of the joint that produces stability. These eccentric contractions are provided by the muscles of the rotator cuff and point to their essential role in shoulder stability. For example, with external rotation of the arm, the infraspinatus contracts concentrically while the subscapularis shows significant electromyographic (EMG) activity as it contracts eccentrically.[34–41] In this case, the infraspinatus produces the propulsive power on one side of the joint while the subscapularis produces a counteracting, stabilizing force on the opposite side of the joint. This balance is biomechanically important for fine-tuning the movements in the athlete's shoulder.

Biceps Function

The long head of the biceps, long thought of as a humeral head depressor, is most likely a passive player during most shoulder motions (Fig. 47.4).[31,42] Yamaguchi and colleagues[43] used electromyography to assess the activity of the long head of the biceps with shoulder-related activity. They controlled elbow function with the use of a brace that locked the elbow at 100 degrees of flexion and neutral forearm rotation. With elbow motion thus eliminated, they demonstrated that the long head of the biceps is essentially inactive during shoulder-related activities in normal shoulders. Furthermore, they showed that the presence of a rotator cuff tear results in the same lack of activity. Rodosky et al.[44] demonstrated in an in vitro cadaveric model that the long head of the biceps may passively contribute to anterior stability of the glenohumeral joint in the abducted and externally rotated position by increasing the resistance of the shoulder to torsional forces.[44] More recent studies have shown a complex interaction between the shoulder and the elbow, including the biceps tendon. Loading of the biceps tendon and changes in elbow position lead to changes in shoulder motion and shoulder muscle recruitment.[45,46]

Static Stabilizers

The static structures of the shoulder, such as the glenohumeral ligaments and labrum, are important for stability but also may be implicated in the internal impingement phenomenon.[12] For example, tight posterior structures cause greater anterior translation of the humeral head with forward elevation and may

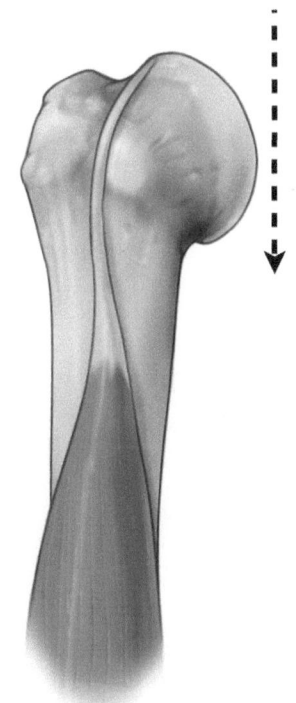

Fig. 47.4 By virtue of its location, the biceps tendon can resist superior translation of the humeral head in situations in which normal restraints have failed.

contribute to secondary impingement.[47] Similarly, anterior laxity and subluxation may result in compromise of the available subacromial space leading to classical outlet impingement,[48] or may result in increased hyperangulation of the humeral head in the abduction/external rotation position, leading to posterosuperior glenoid or "internal" impingement.[49,50]

Scapular Function

Biomechanically, the scapula plays an intimate role in shoulder function. It is the origin of the rotator cuff musculature as well as the deltoid and acts as a base for the motions of the glenohumeral joint. Many pathologic situations such as impingement and various instabilities result in subtle winging through dysfunction of the scapula as it moves on the chest wall, termed *scapular dyskinesia*. Fatigue of the scapular rotators on the chest wall leads to inability of the scapula to rotate properly and prevents the acromion from getting out of the way when the arm is elevated. This situation, termed *scapular lag*, may result in secondary impingement.[51–53] Recent work related to treatment of patients with scapular dyskinesia has shown improvement in the biomechanics of the rotator cuff, acromial humeral distance, and impingement-related symptoms with improved scapular stabilization,[54–57] emphasizing the importance of the scapulothoracic articulation, specifically the scapula-stabilizing musculature, regarding rotator cuff function and subacromial impingement.

HISTORY

A thoughtful, concise history and physical examination remain the most important components in establishing the diagnosis

in an individual with shoulder symptoms. Treating the shoulder can be significantly complex; imaging studies, examination under anesthesia (EUA), and arthroscopy can sometimes be used to help clarify the clinical picture and make an accurate diagnosis. Such studies, however, should only be a supplement to a good history and physical exam.

The history can begin by questioning the patient. What bothers you about your shoulder? How did it start bothering you? When did it start? Do you have pain? Does your shoulder feel unstable? Is there a history of trauma? What specific activities exacerbate the pain or exacerbate the difficulties with your shoulder? If the shoulder is painful during a throwing motion or other type of athletic motion, at what phase of the motion does the pain occur? What specific modalities or activities alleviate or exacerbate what is bothering you? Is there a history of previous shoulder surgery? It is also important to exclude other diagnoses such as cervical radiculopathy. Pain that stems from a cervical origin may often radiate distal to the elbow and into the hand, and consequently, the patient should be asked about such symptoms. These questions, coupled with a standard medical history, can help point the surgeon toward the diagnosis.

PHYSICAL EXAMINATION

Because shoulder pathology can be complex, the specific physical exam tests that may elicit these symptoms can be specific and quite subtle, even when positive. As such, it is not useful to apply the "shotgun" approach to diagnosis, in which every test described for the shoulder is performed on every shoulder. The differential-directed approach, as in the history-taking part of the examination, helps direct the physical exam toward the tests that will either confirm or refute the tentative diagnosis. The physical examination should nonetheless be organized and thorough.

At the start of the physical exam, an initial impression is taken regarding the athlete's age, overall health, and level of specific distress related to the shoulder problem. Inspection, palpation, range of motion (ROM), strength testing, and neurologic and vascular stability assessment constitute an orderly sequence.[35,36,52,53,58–70]

Inspection considers symmetry (taking into account that overhead athletes may have unilateral drooping of the dominant shoulder) or deformities such as old acromioclavicular injuries and muscle wasting, which is most often located in the infraspinatus fossa with a rotator cuff tear (Fig. 47.5). A proximally ruptured biceps tendon shows the characteristic bulging distally with muscle contraction or "Popeye" sign (Fig. 47.6).

The location and degree of tenderness found on palpation often provide a reliable physical sign leading to an accurate diagnosis. Tenderness in the bicipital groove (2 to 5 cm distal to the anterior acromion and midway between the axilla and the lateral deltoid with the arm in the anatomic position) is a reliable sign of bicipital tendonitis (Fig. 47.7). Tenderness in this region with palpation and passive external rotation of the arm (rolling the bicipital groove under the examiner's fingers) is another reliable sign of bicipital pathology.[63] The supraspinatus insertion (Codman's point) is palpated through the deltoid just distal to the anterolateral border of the acromion with the shoulder extended

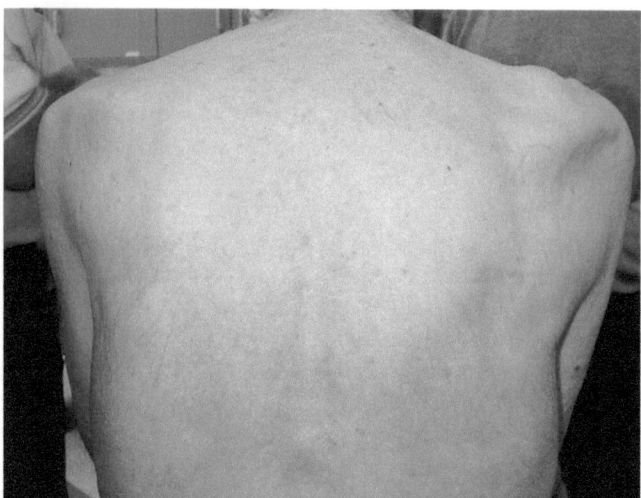

Fig. 47.5 A patient with prominent infraspinatus wasting in the right shoulder.

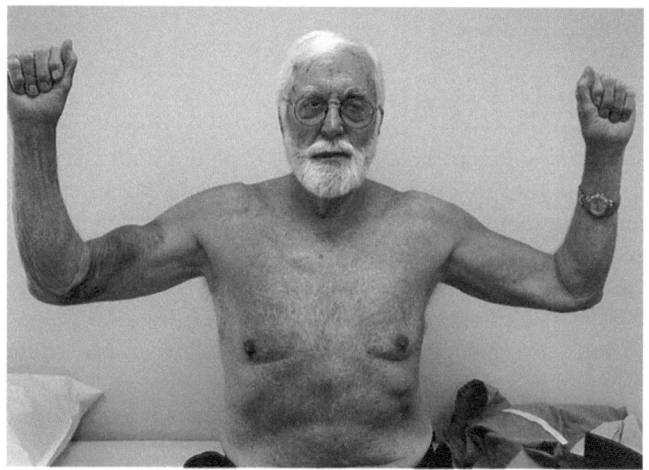

Fig. 47.6 A patient with a ruptured long head of the biceps tendon in the right arm with ecchymosis and a "Popeye" deformity.

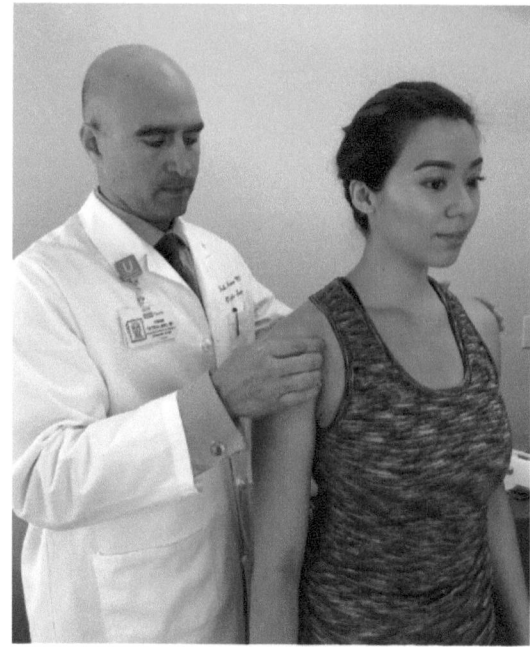

Fig. 47.7 Palpation of the bicipital groove can elicit pain in cases of biceps pathology.

and internally rotated.[21] Maximal tenderness over the acromioclavicular joint may also indicate specific pathology.

Active and passive ROM should be documented in all planes. This includes elevation in the scapular plane and external rotation with the arm at the side, which can be recorded in degrees. It is also important, especially in athletes, to document external rotation (particularly passively) in the 90-degree abducted position in the coronal plane. This position represents a more functional measure of external rotation.[63] Internal rotation can be recorded as the most cephalad vertebral level obtainable by the "hitchhiking thumb" or index finger (Fig. 47.8).

Strength is considered along with ROM. Although assessment of strength is part of the neurologic examination, it is particularly important in patients with rotator cuff pathology. Objective weakness beyond that which can be attributed to pain or a neurologic deficit is a highly specific sign of rotator cuff deficiency. The remainder of the neurologic examination helps rule out pathology such as a cervical root, brachial plexus, or peripheral nerve lesion.

Examination of the regional vascular supply is necessary as a baseline and also to evaluate for conditions such as thoracic outlet syndrome.

Finally, a number of special tests should be considered. The signs of impingement are characteristic of rotator cuff tendinitis and tears. These include a painful arc of abduction between 60 and 120 degrees, pain on forced forward flexion in which the greater tuberosity is forced against the anterior acromion (Neer's sign), and pain on forcible internal rotation of the 90-degree forward flexed arm (Hawkins' sign, or the impingement reinforcement test) (Figs. 47.9 and 47.10).[2,71] The latter maneuver causes impingement of the anterosuperior rotator cuff and biceps against the coracoid and CA ligament. Biceps tendon involvement is demonstrated by Speed's test, in which pain is reproduced on resisted forward elevation of the humerus against an extended elbow. The lift-off test assesses for subscapularis pathology and involves bringing the patient's hand to the lumbar spine region with the palm facing outward. An inability to lift the hand away from the back in this internally rotated position indicates subscapularis pathology (Fig. 47.11). Another method of isolating the subscapularis muscle involves internally rotating the arm across the patient's chest and testing strength (Fig. 47.12). Jobe's test for supraspinatus weakness or impingement involves abducting the patient's arm to 90-degrees, angling forward 30-degrees (thereby bringing the arm into the scapular plane), and internally rotating so the thumb points to the floor (Fig. 47.13). Pain with the Jobe's test indicates supraspinatus tendinopathy, whereas gross weakness likely indicates a supraspinatus tear. The examiner then presses down on the arm while the patient resists movement. Any elicited pain or weakness indicates supraspinatus pathology. Assessment of the infraspinatus muscle is performed by testing external rotation strength with the arm in neutral abduction/adduction (Fig. 47.14). Yergason's test is performed

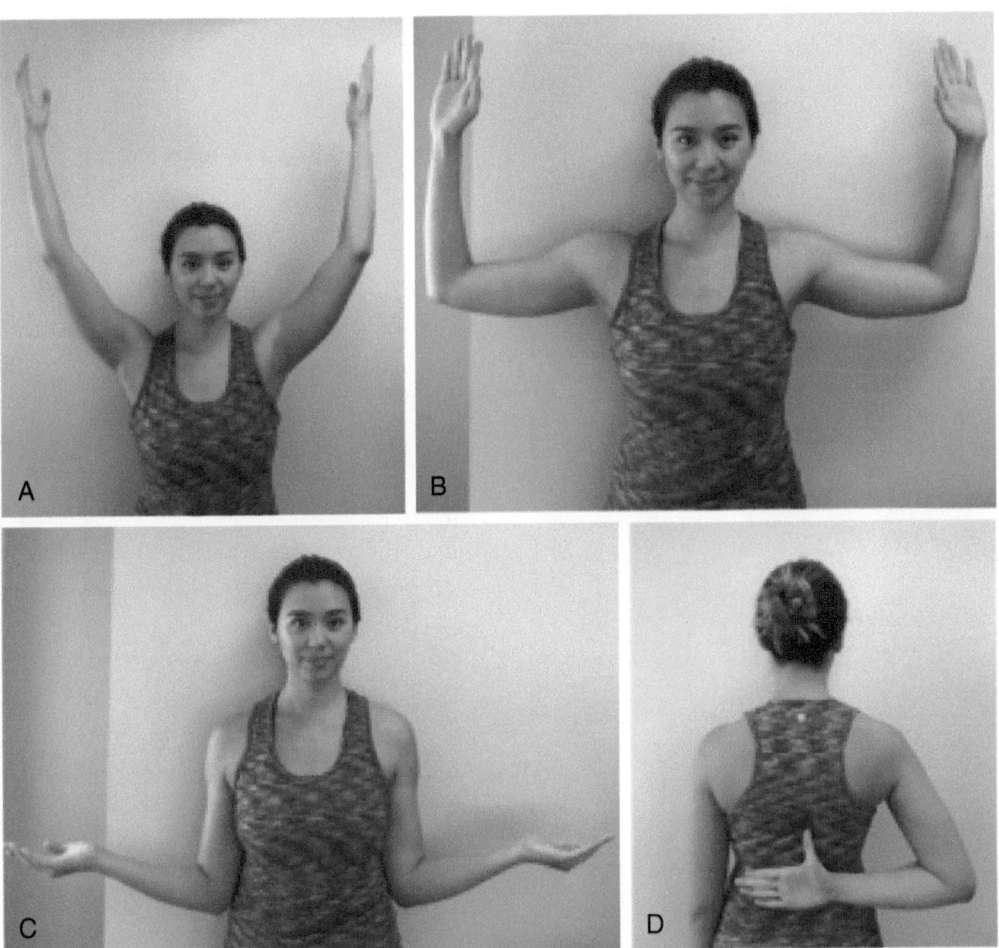

Fig. 47.8 (A–D) Active range of motion is tested for absolute range as well as symmetry.

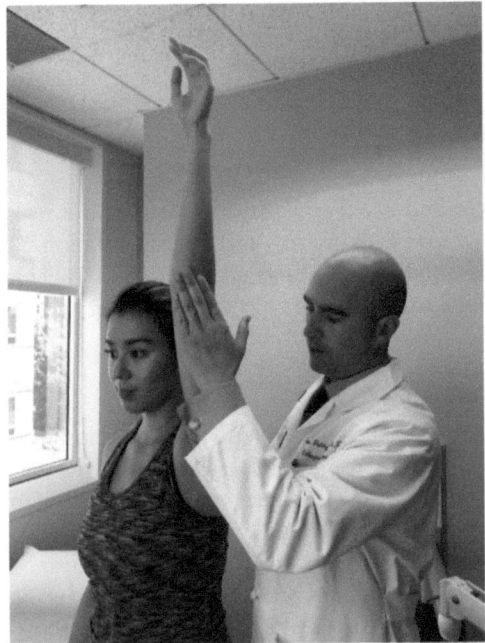

Fig. 47.9 Neer's sign suggests classic impingement when this maneuver elicits pain.

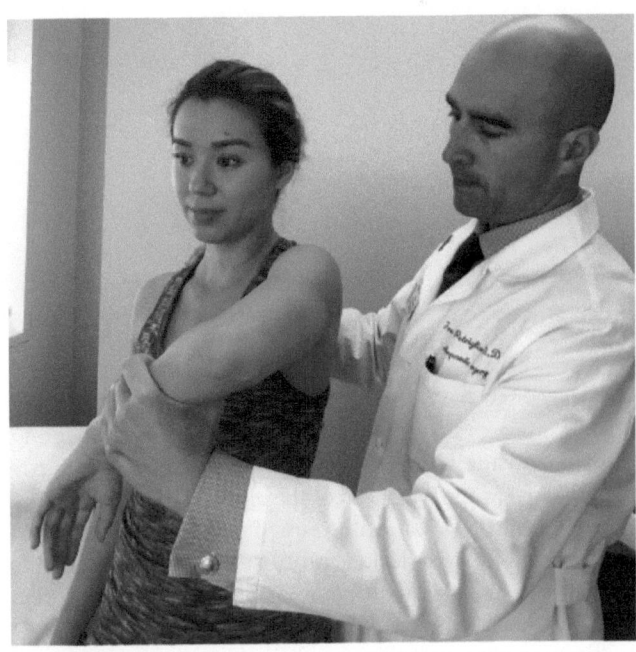

Fig. 47.10 Hawkins' sign may elicit pain with anterosuperior cuff impingement.

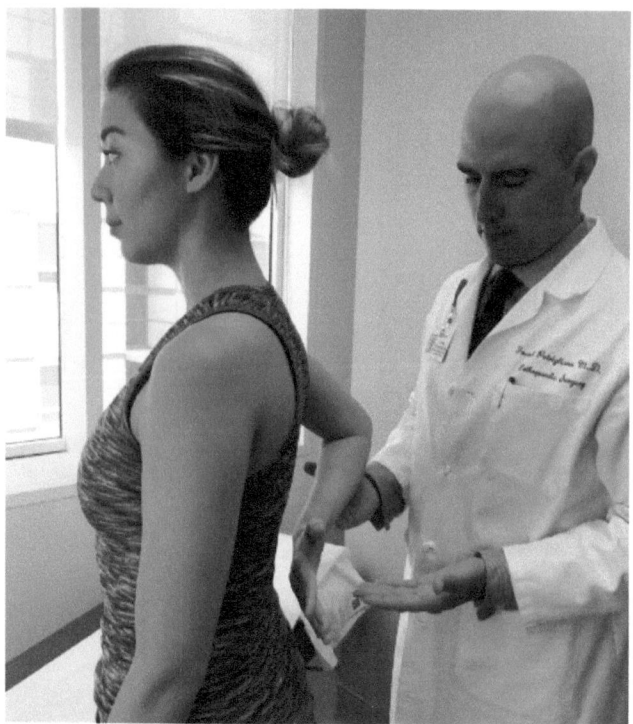

Fig. 47.11 Lift-off test for subscapularis pathology.

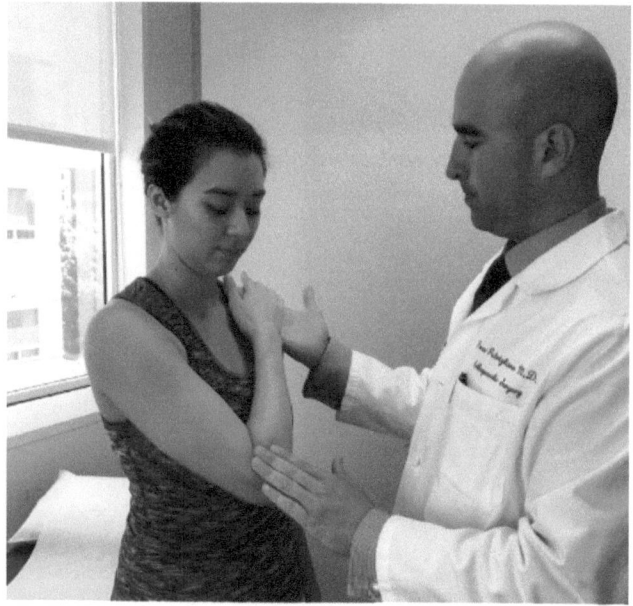

Fig. 47.12 Isolation of subscapularis to assess for weakness and/or pain.

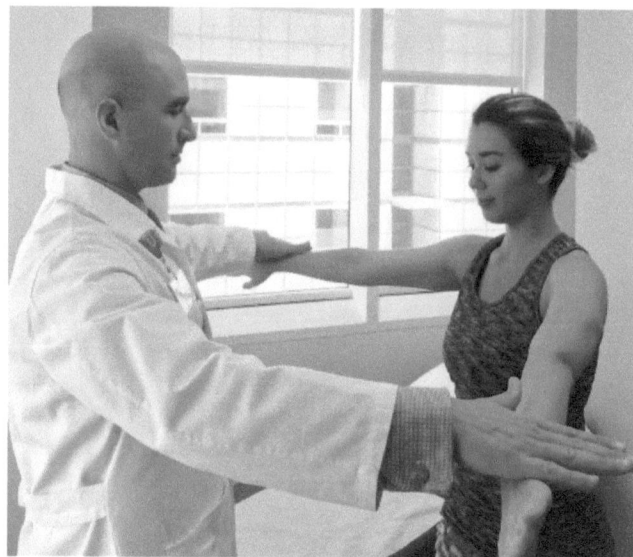

Fig. 47.13 Jobe's test for supraspinatus weakness or impingement.

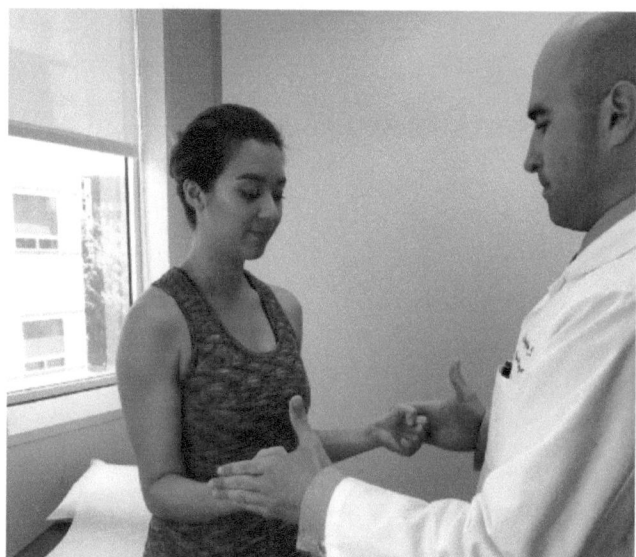

Fig. 47.14 External rotation strength testing to assess for infraspinatus or teres minor weakness.

with the elbow flexed to 90 degrees and the forearm pronated.[72] The examiner grasps the wrist and resists active supination by the patient. Pain in the area of the bicipital groove is suggestive of pathology in the long head of the biceps. The active compression test (O'Brien's test, with resisted elevation and the arm at 90 degrees of forward flexion and 10 to 15 degrees of adduction) may also be positive with pathology of the long head of the biceps without a superior labral-anterior posterior (SLAP) lesion.[73]

Biceps tendon instability (medial subluxation or dislocation) can be determined by passively abducting the shoulder to 80 to 90 degrees and eliciting a palpable snap in the region of the bicipital groove with internal and external rotation.[9,74–77] This is a rare presentation as an isolated entity and usually indicates a lesion to the superior fibers of the subscapularis tendon and/or the SGHL.

Impingement Test

This test, as described by Neer, involves injection of local anesthetic into the subacromial region after a positive Neer's sign.[2,3,78] The injection is performed under sterile conditions with insertion of the needle from the anterior, lateral, or posterior direction into the subacromial space. After the injection, impingement signs should be sought as previously described. Subjective relief or significant diminution of the previously present painful with impingement testing demonstrates impingement to be at least a component of the patient's underlying problem. Nevertheless, it should be emphasized that this is a nonspecific test and can be misleading since it may be positive in those with primary impingement as well as those with secondary impingement due to instability.[79,80]

Although not strictly an impingement test, injection of local anesthetic into the acromioclavicular joint or the bicipital groove can supply additional information about the source of the pain. Subacromial anesthetic can mask or minimize the symptoms from these two areas. The clinical examination is critical in guiding the selections and order of the injection sites. Ultrasound may be useful for improving the accurate delivery of local anesthetic for diagnostic testing and therapeutic effect.

In summary, a concise history and physical examination are essential to reach an accurate diagnosis. Furthermore, an appropriate diagnosis is required to generate both a nonoperative and operative treatment algorithm that includes addressing not only the rotator cuff lesion, but also associated pathologies including biceps or acromioclavicular disease.

IMAGING

Diagnostic imaging for rotator cuff lesions has advanced significantly in recent years. The most commonly used methods to evaluate the cuff are detailed here.

Plain Radiographs

Standard plain radiographs should include an anteroposterior film at right angles to the scapular plane, a lateral film in the scapular plane with the beam tilted 10 degrees to evaluate acromial shape and slope, and an axillary view. Mild rotator cuff disease is often evidenced by mild cystic changes or the presence of small spurs in and around the greater tuberosity. The characteristic changes of advanced rotator cuff disease include sclerosis and cystic changes in the greater tuberosity, osteophyte formation on the acromion, and cephalad migration of the humeral head. This has been described as acetabularization of the acromion and femoralization of the proximal humerus. There can be a more pronounced notch between the greater tuberosity and the articular surface, changes in the shape of the acromion and, in the presence of a massive rotator cuff tear, a narrowed acromiohumeral distance of less than 6 mm can be seen. There may be osteophyte formation on the inferior surface of the acromioclavicular joint as part of chronic rotator cuff disease. Although plain radiographs are often normal, they are nonetheless invaluable because they help rule out other conditions that may present with shoulder pain, such as glenohumeral arthritis, calcific tendinitis, or even neoplasm.

Ultrasonography

Diagnostic ultrasound is a noninvasive form of examination of the rotator cuff.[57,81,82] It allows comparison with the contralateral side and can provide good anatomic detail. It has a reported 91% sensitivity and specificity, with a 100% positive predictive value when it shows nonvisualization or focal thinning.[83,84] It has also been reported to be useful in diagnosing bicipital pathology and is helpful in patients who have previously undergone a rotator cuff repair. However, the results are related to the operator's

experience, and the technique has inherent limitations because of the surrounding bony anatomy. Ultrasound may be best utilized in cases where the suspicion for a rotator cuff tear is high, and the presence of associated pathology such as labral tears or mild arthritis is less likely as ultrasound may be less useful for diagnosis in these settings.[85,86]

Magnetic Resonance Imaging

Magnetic resonance imaging (MRI) has become the gold standard for the assessment of rotator cuff pathology, with sensitivity and specificity exceeding 90% in most current series (Fig. 47.15).[57,83,84,87–90] MRI can demonstrate the size, location, and characteristics of the cuff pathology—and whether full thickness, partial thickness, or intratendinous. Furthermore, MRI allows for the assessment of rotator cuff muscle atrophy, fat infiltration, and the presence of concomitant pathology such as acromioclavicular arthrosis or biceps tenosynovitis. The evaluation of muscle quality is essential as this may allow the physician to more accurately counsel the patient as to the reparability of the rotator cuff and expected outcomes.[91–93] There are drawbacks to MRI, however. Patients are occasionally unable to tolerate the exam because of claustrophobia or inability to remain still for the period necessary to obtain a useful scan. The presence of metallic implants may interfere with image acquisition, and other implants such as pacemakers or recently placed vascular clips may preclude MRI evaluation.

DECISION-MAKING PRINCIPLES

The key principle in treating a patient with a rotator cuff injury is the judicious correlation of a patient's history, physical

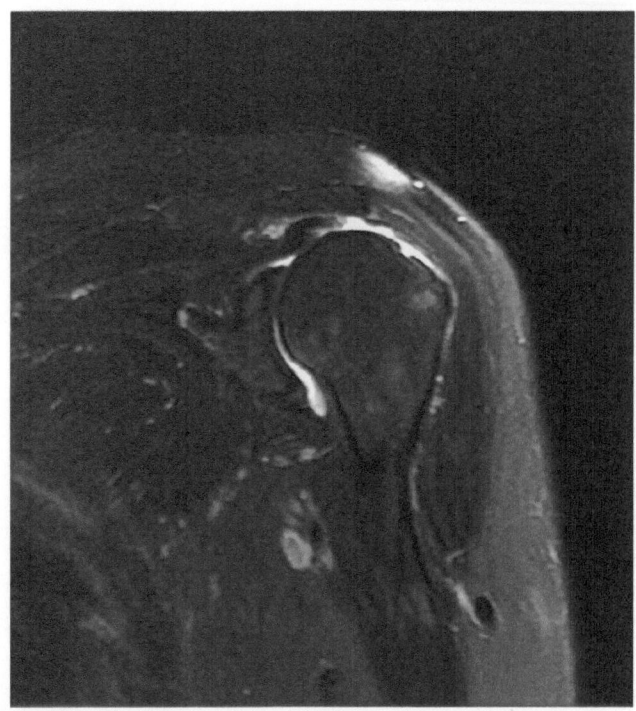

Fig. 47.15 Coronal magnetic resonance image of a supraspinatus tear.

examination, imaging studies, and, if necessary, intraoperative findings to make an accurate diagnosis of the etiology of the patient's complaint. When an accurate diagnosis has been made, the surgeon and patient can have an informed discussion of treatment options and determine the most effective way to help the patient achieve the patient's goals.

First and most important in the management of any individual with a rotator cuff, impingement, or biceps problem is establishing the correct diagnosis. We place strong emphasis on a careful history, thorough physical examination, plain radiographs, and the judicious use of diagnostic injections. Further investigation (usually in the form of MRI) is reserved for individuals with an atypical presentation, those who are older, those with a significant traumatic episode, and those in whom a lesion requiring surgery is suspected.

The diagnosis and treatment of the rotator cuff or biceps injury is based on the etiology, as outlined below. The type of management used follows from the etiologic classification. Of note, the focus of treatment is nonoperative in the great majority of individuals.

Subacromial Impingement and Biceps Tenosynovitis

Patients with primary impingement more commonly present at an older age. This diagnosis implies an anatomic narrowing of the subacromial space, and in some cases, a partial or intrasubstance tear of the rotator cuff or a biceps lesion. The emphasis is on strengthening of the rotator cuff and periscapular musculature. If pain is substantial, a corticosteroid injection into the subacromial space or biceps tendon sheath can be considered. Only after extensive nonoperative management has been attempted for a prolonged period and failed is surgical management pursued. This usually is in the form of a bursectomy, subacromial decompression and biceps tenodesis or tenotomy. Although most small partial-thickness articular-sided rotator cuff tears can be treated with débridement, serious consideration should be made to repairing a high-grade partial-thickness articular-sided tear or bursal-sided tear in this setting.

Acute Rotator Cuff Trauma

In younger patients (<40) rotator cuff tears are uncommon even in the setting of acute trauma. Eccentric loading or a direct blow to the upper extremity may result in a strain of the rotator cuff musculotendinous unit. These injuries require rest until the symptoms have subsided, and while pain may be significant in this setting, immobilization should be avoided. Antiinflammatory agents are often helpful and should be coupled with organized rehabilitation and physical therapy to strengthen the rotator cuff and periscapular musculature. In an older individual (>40 years) acute trauma is more likely to result in a disruption of the rotator cuff tendon. This should be initially treated with rest to allow sufficient healing to take place followed by ROM and rehabilitation. Persistent pain or weakness in a patient of any age requires further investigation to rule out a full-thickness tear of the rotator cuff. Surgical repair should be considered early (within 2 months) to minimize the long-term effects of such an injury.

Chronic Rotator Cuff Disease

In general, patients with shoulder pain and a rotator cuff tear may benefit from a trial of nonoperative management. Our exceptions for surgical intervention include an acute tear or a large tear (>1 cm) in a young patient (<50 to 60 years). For these patients, early surgical intervention is warranted to prevent tear progression and restore preinjury function.[94–97] Small tears in young patients can be followed with ultrasound or MRI for progression. If symptoms do not abate, then surgical intervention should be pursued.

In regard to management of the biceps tendon, we typically reserve biceps tenodesis for younger, active patients or manual laborers with significant fraying, degeneration, or positive response to diagnostic injection. In older sedentary individuals, biceps tenotomy is preferred for its technical ease and predictable outcomes in this population.[7,98]

TREATMENT OPTIONS

In the majority of patients, treatment of a rotator cuff or biceps tendon problem is nonoperative. Three important items to be considered are the etiology of the condition, as previously discussed; activity level and sport involvement; and the severity of the problem.

Types of Treatment

Treatment options can be divided into three general categories: (1) preventive, (2) nonoperative, and (3) operative.

Preventive Treatment

When dealing with shoulder pathology, the paramount concern to the sports medicine physician, surgeon, trainer, therapist, or coach should be prevention of injury.[16,96,99–115] Prevention is of particular importance in relation to the shoulder, in which many of the injuries are related to overuse, particularly in athletes. Intense training and practice may be detrimental to the athlete when poor technique or improper training methods are used. The underlying principle of prevention is applied common sense. A musculotendinous unit is capable of resisting only as much as it has been prepared to resist. The basis of prevention is preparation.[16] This involves overall body conditioning, flexibility, strengthening, and careful attention to technique while recognizing the stresses that both training and competition present.

The influence of shoulder flexibility has been demonstrated in swimmers.[116,117] Published reports have demonstrated a clear correlation between anterior shoulder inflexibility and shoulder pain. It follows that stretching is an important preventive measure. The particular goal in stretching is to try to maintain internal rotation and adduction (Fig. 47.16). It is not necessarily the intention to normalize internal rotation compared with the opposite side. The intention is to avoid posterior capsular contractures and maladaptive loss of internal rotation and adduction. Stretching is as important in older athletes, in whom the potential for stiffness is greater.

A strong, well-balanced shoulder is critically important in the prevention of overuse injuries.[18,52,53,60,62–64,68] This balance

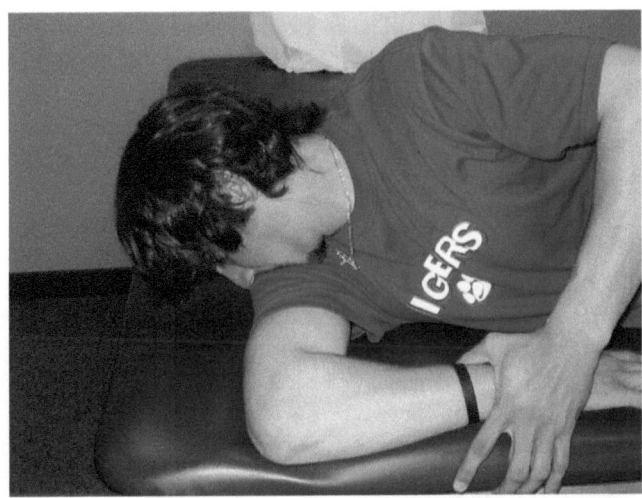

Fig. 47.16 "Sleeper" stretch for stretching of the posterior capsule. (From Kibler WB, Kuhn JE, Wilk K, et al. The disabled throwing shoulder: spectrum of pathology—10-year update. *Arthroscopy.* 2013;29:141–161.)

with the scapular platform and periscapular stabilizing muscles. Both the periscapular stabilizers and the rotator cuff can be strengthened with the use of many aids, such as free weights, Thera-Bands, and surgical tubing. Isokinetic machines are also recommended. Any strengthening program must be well controlled, particularly in the young athlete. In addition, the use of some isokinetic equipment does not allow eccentric muscle contraction. This may be of considerable importance given the pathophysiology of rotator cuff lesions, which is that of eccentric overload.[118–122]

Nonoperative Treatment

Nonoperative treatment is in essence an extension of preventive management with the addition of specific measures dealing with the injury.[52,68] It can be divided into four components: (1) modification of activity, (2) local and systemic measures to reduce and relieve the symptoms, (3) stretching and strengthening exercises, and (4) reevaluation and maintenance treatment.

Modification of activity. In the patient with mild symptoms, modification of activity means reducing the frequency and duration of the specific activity that causes pain. It also involves activity substitution, or what is sometimes called *active rest.* In a tennis player, avoiding the service action but still hitting groundstrokes may be all that is required. In a baseball pitcher, cutting back on the daily number of pitches and decreasing velocity may be helpful. A swimmer should decrease yardage or use a kickboard. Other methods of treatment involve specific changes in technique, such as throwing side-arm for a pitcher or using a higher arm entry for a freestyle swimmer. Changing equipment may also be of benefit. For less active patients, avoiding overhead lifting of heavy weight or sleeping with a pillow to avoid stress of the painful shoulder may be useful. With time these patients usually improve, but return to activity is a longer-term goal and more involved treatment may be necessary.

Local and systemic methods. Although the patient experiencing pain with activity that is not disabling may be manageable with various methods of modified activity, most patients have a more involved problem and require more advanced therapies. The use of nonsteroidal antiinflammatory drugs (NSAIDs) is

ubiquitous. They do provide symptomatic relief; however, the essential problem (whether acute or due to overuse) is tissue injury, and the inflammatory response to this injury is a normal part of the healing mechanism. There is also evidence that in chronic overuse type injuries, the surgical pathologic tissue is noninflammatory. The value of these medications lies in the initial treatment given to decrease pain and allow rehabilitation. Ice treatment is also a recognized local treatment modality with the action of reducing vascularity, diminishing the pain, and possibly reducing swelling and inflammation. Ice is particularly useful after an acute episode or injury. It is commonly advocated after overuse activity to minimize the pain and lessen the immediate postactivity inflammatory response.

Therapeutic ultrasound may be helpful in the treatment of rotator cuff and biceps tendinopathies because it is believed to increase the local vascular response to the injured tissue.[123] This, in turn, allows the egress of the products of injury and the ingress of the reparative cells needed for repair. Other modalities include high-voltage electrical stimulation, transcutaneous nerve stimulation, electromagnetic field therapy, and the use of lasers. The specific benefits of some of these modalities are not clear, yet many patients seem to gain relief with few side effects.[124–129]

The use of local corticosteroid injections is a more invasive form of therapy. The deleterious effects of steroid injections have been documented. Critical analysis of the literature cannot lead to the conclusion that they are of any long-term benefit. Their use is still advocated and may be of value in a patient with an acutely painful lesion to halt the vicious circle of pain related to overuse. This would then allow earlier institution of corrective rehabilitation.[130] Repetitive or long-term local steroid administration is not advocated.

A growing method of nonoperative treatment and area of research is the use of biologics to improve healing of the rotator cuff. The most widely studied intervention is the injection of platelet-rich plasma (PRP) for the treatment of partial rotator cuff tears as well as for adjuvant therapy after rotator cuff repair. Currently there are conflicting reports as to the effectiveness of PRP in reducing symptoms or reducing retear rates after repair with most meta-analyses demonstrating no significant benefit and calling for more studies.[131–137] Other biologics such as mesenchymal stem cells, growth factors, and the use of scaffolds are showing great promise in augmenting healing and enhancing biologic repair; however more clinical studies are needed to truly assess the benefit of these interventions.[138–140]

Stretching, strengthening, and conditioning. Stretching exercises are both therapeutic and quite clearly preventive and provide the basis for maintenance treatment.[16,68] The warm-up, including stretching, helps the patient improve timing and control and also allows the muscles to function efficiently. Stretching increases muscle blood supply and improves contractility. Lack of flexibility has been associated with a higher incidence of shoulder problems in swimmers. An increased range of external rotation compared with internal rotation is also associated with shoulder problems, especially in throwers. These factors in the patient with a painful shoulder require specific attention to the treatment regimen.[141] Stretching should be generalized but should focus on internal rotation and adduction across the chest[142] and internal rotation and extension behind the back. These exercises should be performed before activity in addition to the usual routine.

Strengthening is the mainstay of treatment for the majority of individuals with rotator cuff or biceps tendon problems.[39,68,143-148] Whether the problem is due to an acute direct injury, eccentric overload, or chronic degeneration, the patient is left with a compromised, weakened musculotendinous unit. This unit is usually contracted either primarily as a result of muscular imbalance or secondarily due to the injury mechanism. A complete tear or disruption of the tendons obviously needs to be addressed through therapy or be repaired through surgery before active use can resume to the preinjury level.

Strengthening of the cuff should emphasize the external rotators.[68] The use of rubber tubing is simple and effective for both prophylaxis and treatment. Initially, the exercises need to be performed with the arm at the side until pain has been relieved. When pain is present, the 90-degree abducted position should be avoided with resisted rotational strengthening. The arm can be brought into the abducted position gradually, initially to 45 degrees until the pain has completely disappeared and then to the functional range. Most recreational and nonthrowing athletes do not require strengthening at 90 degrees of abduction.

If scapular dyskinesia is a primary cause of shoulder dysfunction, nonoperative physical therapy aimed at retraining and restrengthening the scapular stabilizers can be curative.[55,149] When scapular dyskinesia is the result of other forms of shoulder pathology, physical therapy may be necessary—even after the primary lesion is addressed—to return the shoulder to normal.

In addition to the specific components of shoulder strengthening, it is important to understand that the shoulder cannot be viewed in isolation. Kibler and associates[150] have described the importance of "core stability" and the "kinetic chain" to athletic performance. Equal concern should be paid to the associated joints and muscles to ensure that appropriate body mechanics are used in the rehabilitation of the athlete.

Reevaluation and maintenance. During reevaluation, the treatment phase blends into prevention of further injury. Throughout the process of treatment, the patient, physical therapist, and physician should be part of an educational program. This involves education about the clinical problem, its course, and its ultimate prognosis. Most patients are willing to perform a daily routine of exercises if it means participating in the activities they enjoy. Unfortunately, compliance with this routine is more likely *after* rather than *before* an injury.

Operative Treatment

Nonoperative treatment must be emphasized over surgical management in many patients with rotator cuff pathology. The great majority of patients will recover, modify their activities, or even give up painful activity before undergoing surgery. However, in young patients or in those who have failed a prolonged course of nonoperative management, surgical intervention is often indicated.

Surgical techniques.

Subacromial decompression and rotator cuff repair. Arthroscopic evaluation is now the standard of care for patients with rotator cuff and impingement lesions. Diagnostic arthroscopy allows confirmation of the diagnosis. Intra-articular structures are visualized, and evidence of articular damage is documented. The undersurface of the cuff is carefully examined.

Full-thickness tears of the rotator cuff should be repaired at arthroscopy due to the high rate of tear progression, especially in the high-demand population.[151] Partial-thickness tears should be examined and evaluated for the appropriateness of repair.[152] Snyder and Ellman[153,154] have both proposed classifications for the arthroscopic evaluation of rotator cuff tears. A spinal needle and/or a marker suture can be placed through the articular surface partial tear for later bursal surface identification and evaluation. Most authors currently recommend débridement and subacromial decompression if the partial tear involves less than 50% of the cuff based on the medial-lateral dimensions of the footprint.[94,95,155-159] If the tear involves more than 50% of the cuff, repair and decompression are indicated.[94-97,151,152,160,161] If there is degeneration of the biceps tendon, or grossly positive biceps exam maneuvers, then biceps tenotomy or tenodesis is recommended.

🏃 Authors' Preferred Technique

Surgical Management

The primary indication for surgery is the failure of an adequate, nonoperative management program. An adequate nonoperative program should be carefully coordinated with good patient compliance, and the patient should be followed for at least 3 to 6 months (depending on the athlete and the sport) before surgery is considered. Inherent in establishing failure of this nonoperative program is significant pain and disability warranting intervention.

With an acute traumatic injury, especially in an older athlete, the possibility of a full-thickness rotator cuff tear must be considered. MRI is the gold standard in providing a diagnosis in this situation. If a full-thickness tear of the rotator cuff is present, surgical repair is performed. Another situation in which surgery may be considered early is the presence of obvious primary impingement due to bony overgrowth of the acromion or an abnormally angled acromion (usually in an older athlete). In both these situations, the obvious anatomic abnormality causing the patient's symptoms necessitates surgical correction.

Overall, the choice of surgical procedure depends on a number of factors, including the underlying etiology and the extent of the abnormality.[161] If a full-thickness tear of the rotator cuff is present, open or arthroscopic repair can be performed. The basic principles for successful repair are the same in both open and arthroscopic rotator cuff repair and should not be compromised regardless of the technique selected. The decision on how these basic principles are fulfilled (whether with an open or arthroscopic technique) is then individualized to the surgeon.

Partial-Thickness Rotator Cuff Tears and Internal Impingement Lesions

With regard to partial-thickness cuff tears, we currently perform only a débridement of the cuff if the tear involves less than 50% of the tendon. If the tear involves more than 50% of the tendon, we consider excision of the damaged

Authors' Preferred Technique

Surgical Management—cont'd

tissue and formal repair to bone. In either case, subacromial decompression can be performed arthroscopically as deemed necessary.

Postoperatively, passive assisted motion and stretching are started immediately. The patient progresses rapidly to active and resisted motion as tolerated. The nonoperative routine is then instituted to build strength and regain function.

For athletes with internal impingement, we débride and/or repair both the posterosuperior labral lesion and the corresponding cuff lesion. We use the physical examination and EUA to determine whether subtle but pathologic differential anterior laxity and posterior contracture are present and perform and manage appropriately. It should be emphasized again that this is a very difficult population of patients to diagnose and treat, and the surgeon should be certain of the appropriate treatment before proceeding with any surgical management that might result in postoperative failure to regain external rotation in the overhead athlete.

Full-Thickness Rotator Cuff Tears
Arthroscopic Surgical Technique
Anesthesia

We prefer regional brachial plexus blockade with an indwelling perineural catheter for all procedures with the addition of general or sedative anesthesia for most rotator cuff repairs. This allows for excellent intraoperative and postoperative pain control. Furthermore, improved hypotensive blood pressure control may be achieved with regional anesthesia as compared to the use of general anesthesia in beach chair cases. This improved blood pressure control may diminish the likelihood of intraoperative hypotension (reducing cerebral perfusion) or hypertension (reducing surgical visualization).

Setup

Our preferred treatment technique is arthroscopic repair performed in a 70-degree beach chair position. Positioning precautions are observed as with any operative procedure, taking care to pad and protect areas of potential pressure. The patient's head and neck are positioned in neutral flexion. The blood pressure is monitored during positioning to avoid hypotension. The operative arm is examined to evaluate ROM and then routinely examined under anesthesia prior to draping. If a mild adhesive capsulitis is noted, a gentle manipulation under anesthesia is performed.

The patient is then prepped and draped and a sterile articulated arm holder is used to aid in arm positioning throughout the procedure (Fig. 47.17). The importance of arm positioning is that, as the arm is manipulated, the various compartments of the shoulder are differentially accessed. Appropriate arm positioning can therefore make an already technically demanding surgery easier. Conversely, inappropriate arm positioning can make it much more difficult.

Arm Positioning

Although subtle adjustments to obtain the optimal view and access must be performed intraoperatively, some general principles of arm positioning should be kept in mind. These principles may seem obvious but are discussed here briefly because proper arm positioning is often overlooked.

When working within the glenohumeral joint, the arm is best placed in slight abduction, slight flexion, and approximately 30 degrees of external rotation in line with the scapular plane. In this position, tension is removed from the supraspinatus and the glenohumeral joint is easily distracted. As the arm is abducted and internally rotated, the cuff attachments are also brought medially and into the field of view.

When working in the subacromial space, position of the arm depends on what structures are to be visualized. Bringing the arm into a more adducted position allows traction to be applied to the arm to distract the humeral head inferiorly and away from the acromion. This improves access to the inferior aspect of the

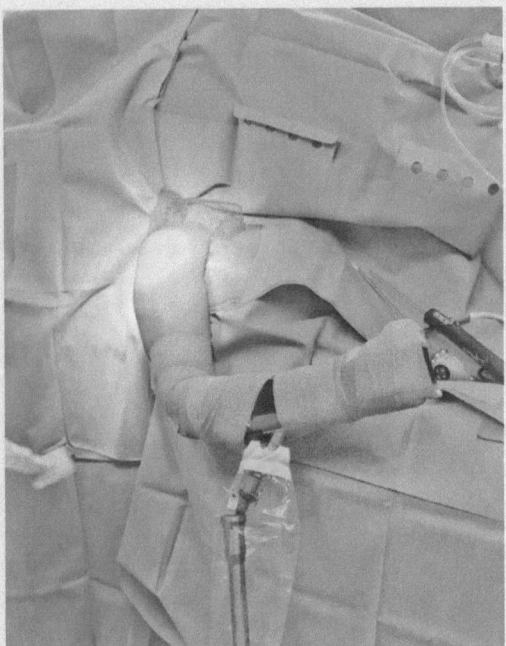
Fig. 47.17 Patient in standard beach chair position with a sterile arm holder.

acromion, which may be useful during arthroscopic subacromial decompression. At the same time, however, adducting the arm collapses the subdeltoid space, making it more difficult to visualize the rotator cuff. To visualize the cuff, it is necessary to relax the deltoid by flexing and abducting the arm, or externally rotating the arm for anterior tears.

Portals

Ultimately, portals are intended to provide safe optimal visualization and access. Three main portals are classically described for arthroscopic access to the shoulder, namely a posterior, a lateral, and an anterior portal (Fig. 47.18). These three "standard" portals are routinely drawn as shown in the figure and employed in each case. It is important to note that effective rotator cuff visualization and repair should not be limited by the "standard" portal positions. Accessory anterolateral and posterolateral portals are made as needed on a case-by-case basis. The portals are anesthetized with local anesthetic with epinephrine to reduce bleeding. The posterior portal is established by placing it within the palpable sulcus just inferior to the posterolateral acromion and superior to the humeral head as it slopes inferiorly and medially to the glenoid. This results in an entry point on the skin that is roughly 2 cm inferior and 2 cm medial to the posterolateral corner of the acromion, but may be slightly more superior and lateral for optimal rotator cuff visualization. The lateral portal is made at the "50-yard-line" of the acromion under direct visualization. The anterior portal is located at the midpoint between the coracoid and the anterolateral corner of the acromion. This puts it roughly in line with the acromioclavicular (AC) joint. Its trajectory should result in the anterior portal entering the glenohumeral joint through the rotator interval. To help establish this trajectory, a spinal needle may be placed first as a rough guide. In general, the arthroscope is placed in the posterior portal and the lateral and anterior portals are used as working portals (Fig. 47.19).

Arthroscopy

The glenohumeral joint is entered through the posterior portal and the arthroscope is introduced. The arm is immediately positioned in slight abduction, slight

Continued

Authors' Preferred Technique
Surgical Management—cont'd

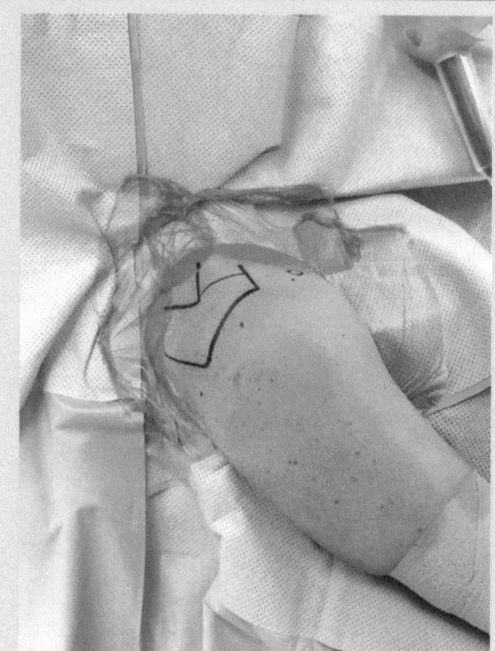

Fig. 47.18 Right shoulder marked with the authors' preferred portals for rotator cuff repair.

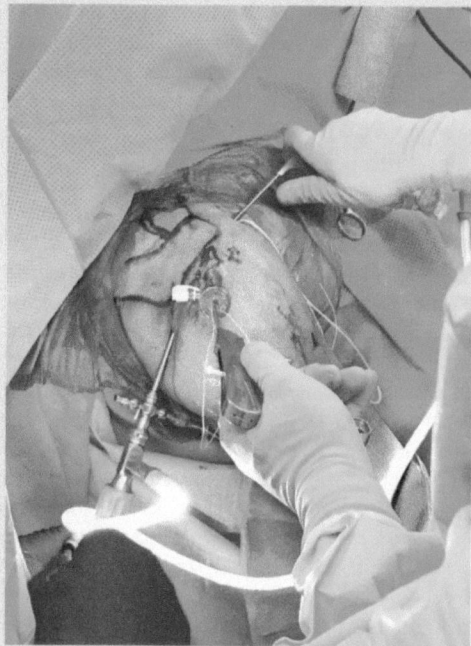

Fig. 47.19 For repair of the cuff, the arthroscope is in the posterior portal. The lateral and anterior portals are used as working portals.

flexion, and external rotation to allow glenohumeral work. The lateral portal is then established under direct needle visualization in line with the midpoint of the tear in the anteroposterior dimension of a full-thickness tear. A routine diagnostic arthroscopy is then performed. The purpose of the diagnostic arthroscopy is to identify alternative or associated pathology. The biceps tendon and

its intertubercular portion are drawn into the joint and evaluated. If the biceps tendon is implicated as a contributing factor, synovitis and partial tearing can be débrided. If significant, an arthroscopic biceps tenodesis or biceps tenotomy can be performed depending on the demands of the patient. The rotator cuff attachment can be easily visualized by internal and external rotation of the arm. If desired, a marker suture introduced through a spinal needle may be placed to mark the location of a partial tear of the rotator cuff tear if there are concerns it will not be easily visible from the subacromial space. Instruments can be introduced through the anterior cannula as needed. A shaver is typically introduced through either the anterior or lateral portal and any labral fraying is resected to a stable rim.

After the intraarticular work is completed, the subacromial space is then entered through the posterior portal. Through the previously established skin incision, an arthroscopic trocar is used to feel the posterior border of the acromion. The trocar is then slid just underneath it and into the subacromial space. The trocar is advanced to the anterolateral aspect of the subacromial space. The trocar is swept medially and laterally to clear the bursal tissue and the camera is introduced to visualize the "room with a view." The rotator cuff, CA ligament, and investing interior deltoid fascia should be well visualized.

Bursectomy
A bursectomy is then performed with a shaver through the posterior portal. Care is taken to resect any adhesions of the posterior cuff to the deltoid as well as any adhesions of the anterior cuff to the coracoid. The rotator cuff tear is identified at this point from the bursal side. Medially, and far posteriorly, care is taken to avoid small vessels that may bleed with aggressive shaving. We prefer the use of radiofrequency ablation in these areas to reduce iatrogenic bleeding and loss of visualization.

Rotator Cuff Repair
The arthroscope is then placed in the posterior portal and an 8.5-mm cannula is placed in the lateral portal. For most of the rotator cuff repair, the high posterolateral portal is the viewing portal; the anterior and lateral portals are the working portals. However, visualization through the lateral portal may be utilized for characterizing a tear, placing suture anchors, or passing sutures through the rotator cuff.

The goal of the rotator cuff repair is to recreate normal rotator cuff anatomy. To this end, various techniques, instrumentation, and suture configurations have been proposed. The tendon edges are débrided with a shaver or biter. The bony bed of the repair is prepared with a burr to expose bleeding bone. The cuff is mobilized by releasing the cuff off the superior glenoid, releasing any adhesions to the scapular spine or the coracoid, including the CH ligament. The CA ligament is released converting a type 2 or 3 acromion to a type 1 acromion. In general, small tears less than 1 cm in anteroposterior extension are treated with a single row technique. Moderate to large tears between 1 cm and 3 cm in anteroposterior dimension with good mobility are treated with a double row transosseous equivalent technique. Tears greater than 3 cm with limited mobility are advanced to the medial rotator cuff footprint with a single row technique and margin convergence as needed.

A spinal needle is inserted anterolaterally to determine the proper angle for the suture anchor placement. A small stab incision is typically made just off the lateral acromion and an awl is introduced and malleted at a 45-degree angle into the bony bed of the rotator cuff. For a double row technique, the medial row is established just lateral to the articular margin. A triple loaded suture anchor is then twisted into the bone and the inserter gently retracted, revealing 3 color-coded suture pairs. One strand is taken out through the lateral portal and loaded onto an anterograde suture-passing device and passed through the

Authors' Preferred Technique
Surgical Management—cont'd

rotator cuff exiting medially in the cuff. A grasper is introduced through the anterior cuff and takes the suture anteriorly after the suture is passed through the rotator cuff under direct visualization. The next two suture pairs are passed in a horizontal mattress fashion using the suture-passing device from the lateral portal and a grasper from the anterior portal. In order to pass the suture in a horizontal mattress fashion, one strand is passed posteromedially in the cuff, and the next strand more anteromedially. The suture strands are grasped and taken out the lateral portal and are then tied using an arthroscopic knot-tying device. The simple fashion suture ends are also taken out the lateral portal and tied using a standard sliding-knot technique. The sutures are tied in order to compress the cuff down to its footprint medially. The remaining suture strands are secured into the lateral tuberosity with a knotless impaction type anchor device. This step effectively pulls the cuff laterally into an anatomic position with excellent footprint compression.

Open Surgical Technique

If open rotator cuff repair is chosen after diagnostic arthroscopy, the shoulder is re-prepped to decrease the risk of infection before the open incision. The incision is then made starting from the posterior aspect of the acromioclavicular joint and extending to the anterolateral corner of the acromion and extending down the deltoid a few centimeters. The subcutaneous plane is developed with a bovie, and the AC joint, acromion, deltoid, and deltoid raphe between the anterior and middle deltoid are identified. A No. 15 blade is used to first incise obliquely across the AC joint, taking advantage of the thick tissue here. This is extended as a single incision to the anterolateral corner of the acromion and down the deltoid raphe. Care is taken to avoid distal extension beyond 5 cm, where the axillary nerve could be in jeopardy. Subperiosteal flaps are elevated using the No. 15 blade, exposing the anterior acromion. In the process of completely exposing the anterior acromion, the CA ligament is released from its attachment to the undersurface of the acromion. The AC joint is likewise exposed. It is important to maintain this as a thick, single flap, taking the tissue right off the bone so that a solid repair can be performed at the end of the procedure. With adequate exposure, distal clavicle excision and subacromial decompression can easily be performed through this exposure. Attention is then turned to the rotator cuff. Bursectomy can be performed with Mayo scissors and releases performed, including release of CH ligament. The cuff should now be mobilized. Just as with the arthroscopic procedure, the footprint is prepared with a burr, and a repair with the same configuration of anchors and sutures as described above can be performed. Alternatively, the medial row of anchors can be combined with a lateral transosseous passage of the same sutures to achieve the biomechanically strongest repair of the cuff attachment.[162] Heavy absorbable suture is then used to repair the subperiosteally raised flaps and the deltoid raphe, and the overlying skin is closed.

Postoperative management. Postoperatively, a shoulder immobilizer with a small pillow is used to keep the arm in approximately 20 to 30 degrees of abduction and to take tension off the repair. This sling is worn for 4 to 6 weeks after surgery and removed only for showering and performing twice daily prescribed home exercises. Passive assisted motion is started immediately in most cases.[60,163] For the first 1 to 2 weeks postoperatively the patient is instructed to perform passive supine elevation of the arm to 90 degrees using the opposite hand as well as passive external rotation to neutral. Active ROM of the hand, wrist, and elbow is reinforced. A detailed physical therapy prescription is provided to each patient. The patient progresses to active motion at approximately 6 weeks depending on the extent of the tear.[66,68,164] Active motion is combined with terminal stretching, and resistive motion is added according to each individual's progress, usually at the 10-week mark.[65] The remaining postoperative regimen includes the components outlined in the nonoperative section.

Results. Results of open and arthroscopic procedures for treatment of rotator cuff and biceps pathology have generally been positive.[29,53,102,145,153–156,158,165–177] Historically, the procedures designed to correct these problems have involved various forms of cuff repair and biceps tenodesis using a variety of approaches, including acromionectomy. Today, three main procedures for subacromial-based pathology are typically used in the general population: subacromial decompression (and variants such as débridement), rotator cuff repair, and biceps tenodesis. Patient factors predisposing to repair failure include older age, larger tear size, poor muscle quality, osteoporosis, diabetes, and hypercholesterolemia.[178,179] Double row repairs are biomechanically stronger and demonstrate better healing rates than single row repairs as evidenced by time zero testing.[180] Performing open or mini-open versus arthroscopic procedures to accomplish these goals produces largely equivalent outcomes.[173,181–184]

Open techniques. Most authors recommend early surgical repair for full-thickness cuff tears that are symptomatic.[49,68,94–96,152,185–188] Studies evaluating the natural history of rotator cuff tears also support this recommendation.[151,189] In an athlete with higher demands, a prediction of full return to premorbid levels of play is not possible based on a current review of the literature.[190] This caution applies both to decompression of the cuff and to rotator cuff repair, regardless of the methods used. A symptomatic full-thickness tear without surgery yields predictably poor results, with larger tears (>3 cm) having a poor functional recovery even with surgery.[105,166,171,187,191]

Arthroscopic techniques. The treatment of full-thickness rotator cuff tears at the time of arthroscopy is widely accepted; however, concurrent acromioplasty remains controversial.[192]

The results of subacromial decompression in 24 patients active in sports who had a diagnosis of primary impingement revealed that 87.5% returned to active participation.[185] The overall success rate in another heterogeneous series (including both sport- and nonsport-related etiologies) was 88%.[170]

The treatment of partial-thickness tears remains somewhat controversial regarding the technique. Good results have been published with takedown of the lesion and repair as well as transtendon repair using various suture configurations.[159,193–199] Past work has demonstrated that partial tears may significantly predispose to the development of a full-thickness tear.[10] Hence, some have advocated repair for all partial-thickness tears, although this clearly remains controversial, especially in the athletic population.

The complications of arthroscopic procedures are relatively few in all reported series.[200,201]

Complications

Complications after operative management of rotator cuff tears can include stiffness, failure of the rotator cuff to heal, and persistent pain.[200,202] Less common issues can include infection, nerve injury, and issues related to patient positioning in the lateral or beach chair positions.[200,203,204] In general, arthroscopic and open rotator cuff repair are quite safe.[200]

FUTURE CONSIDERATIONS

Many refinements and expansions have been made to the body of knowledge on the rotator cuff and its disease since Codman's monumental text, but multiple mysteries remain unsolved. Among the questions that remain include the following: (1) What is the etiology of rotator cuff tears? (2) When a rotator cuff tear has formed, what is the natural history of this tear? (3) When viewed in terms of the natural history of cuff tears, what rotator cuff tears can be treated nonoperatively, and what tears require surgical repair? (4) For rotator cuff tears that require surgery, what is the optimal surgical technique and repair construct? (5) What biologic approaches can be used to improve rotator cuff repair? Answers to each of these questions could easily fill their own volumes, but a brief review is presented here.

A precise unifying description of the etiology and natural history of rotator cuff tears has not yet been written, but contemporary literature has defined certain principles. Classically, the debate over the etiology of rotator cuff tears has hinged on the question of intrinsic degeneration[155,205–207] versus extrinsic impingement/wear.[2,27,208,209] The more accurate description is likely that the etiology of rotator cuff tears is multifactorial, with intrinsic degeneration, external impingement/wear, and microtrauma and macrotrauma to the cuff all playing a contributing role. Regardless of the etiology of a rotator cuff tear, recent literature is shedding light regarding the population in whom these tears develop. In addition, the natural history of rotator cuff tears is being more accurately described, although many questions remain.[151] Rotator cuff tears are most commonly found in patients in the fifth decade of life and beyond.[210] Without a traumatic event, rotator cuff tears are rare in patients younger than 40 years.[211] The incidence of rotator cuff tears—either symptomatic or asymptomatic—increases with age. In addition, in patients with a symptomatic rotator cuff tear in one shoulder, there is a high probability of an asymptomatic tear in the contralateral shoulder. Also, symptomatic cuff tears are more likely to progress in size than are asymptomatic tears.[82,85,86,191,210,212–216] As rotator cuff tears increase in size, cuff musculature atrophies and fatty infiltration progresses.[217–221] At some critical point as the infiltration progresses, the tear becomes irreparable.[222,223] The surgeon faces the clinical challenge of placing a patient within this incomplete natural history and discerning the optimal nonoperative or operative treatment.

For rotator cuff tears that require surgery, a recent debate in the literature has occurred regarding the optimal technique—open versus mini-open versus arthroscopic—for rotator cuff repair. Classically, open repair has been considered the gold standard for the treatment of rotator cuff tears. However, contemporary series of arthroscopic rotator cuff repair have shown the results of arthroscopic repair to be equivalent to open repair, quieting the controversy over open versus arthroscopic. Out of the denouement of the open versus arthroscopic debate has arisen a new line of inquiry regarding the optimal arthroscopic rotator cuff repair construct. The question currently posed is which is the superior repair construct: single-row versus double-row versus transosseous equivalent? Double-row constructs have proven to be biomechanically superior to single-row constructs.[180,224–231] In addition, transosseous equivalent double-row repairs have been shown to more accurately restore the anatomic footprint of the rotator cuff.[232–234] Despite the theoretical and biomechanical advantages, clinical results have not yet definitively shown the superiority of these techniques. Nevertheless, researchers still advocate the use of double-row constructs in arthroscopic rotator cuff repair.[235]

Recently many studies have evaluated the role for potential biologic therapies in improving the outcomes of rotator cuff repair. Examples of these biologics range from mesenchymal stem cell therapies to growth factor injections, to superior capsular reconstruction and the use of biologic patches and scaffolds. The most popularized biologic adjuvant is PRP, which is theorized to bring essential growth factors to the rotator cuff and promote healing. Currently there are conflicting reports as to the effectiveness of PRP.[131–137] A potentially more promising adjuvant therapy may be mesenchymal stem cell derivatives, which are sorted for their expected regenerative properties prior to injection and therefore may have more predictable results in diminishing muscle fibrosis and degeneration making repair more successful. Animal studies have demonstrated decreased muscle atrophy after rotator cuff injury with lipoaspirate derived perivascular stem cell treatment.[139] As the properties of native cells within the rotator cuff are better understood, improved biologic therapies to target muscle atrophy and fibrosis are expected to develop.

Scaffolds are also being developed that may serve as a delivery system for mesenchymal stem cells or growth factors to promote healing.[236] Bioinductive patches have been developed to decrease retear rates and improve outcomes of massive rotator cuff tears or tears with poor tissue quality.[237,238] Patch augmentation can deliver cells with regenerative properties while decreasing tension on the repair site.[238] The use of scaffolds and biologic graft patches are showing great promise in augmenting healing and enhancing biologic repair; however more clinical studies are needed to truly assess the benefit of these interventions.[138–140,239]

For a complete list of references, please go to ExpertConsult.com.

SELECTED READINGS

Citation:

Millett PJ, Warth RJ. Posterosuperior rotator cuff tears: classification, pattern recognition, and treatment. *J Am Acad Orthop Surg.* 2014;22(8):521–534.

Level of Evidence:

V

Summary:

This is a valuable comprehensive review of the most common rotator cuff tear patterns, classifications, and management strategies.

Citation:

Burkhart SS, Lo IK. Arthroscopic rotator cuff repair. *J Am Acad Orthop Surg.* 2006;14(6):333–346.

Level of Evidence:

V

Summary:

This is a quality review of the principles, techniques, and biomechanics of arthroscopic rotator cuff repair.

Citation:

Depres-Tremblay G, Chevrier A, Snow M, et al. Rotator cuff repair: a review of surgical techniques, animal models, and new technologies under development. *J Shoulder Elbow Surg.* 2016;25(12):2078–2085.

Level of Evidence:

V

Summary:

This is a quality current review of the surgical techniques and new technologies employed in rotator cuff repair surgery.

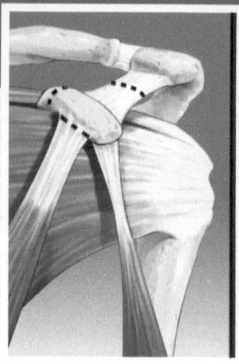

48

Subscapularis Injury

William H. Rossy, Frederick S. Song, Jeffrey S. Abrams

The subscapularis represents the anterior portion of the rotator cuff and is an important stabilizer and internal rotator for the glenohumeral joint.[1,2] The first reported case documenting a subscapularis tendon tear was by Smith in 1834,[3,4] with the first reported repair described by Hauser in 1954.[5] Despite these reports, operative management of subscapularis pathology remained relatively neglected until Gerber et al. described their management of 16 patients with isolated subscapularis tears in 1991.[6]

Subscapularis injury can be an isolated injury or be found in combination with other rotator cuff tendons. It may also include injury to the long head of the biceps. A missed subscapularis injury can lead to prolonged disability including pain, weakness, and poor function.[7] More recent studies have demonstrated higher rates than expected of subscapularis pathology. Bennett reported a 27% rate of subscapularis pathology in a series of 165 arthroscopically treated shoulder patients, with subscapularis tearing involved in 35% of all rotator cuff pathology.[8] Other authors have corroborated these findings with similar or even higher rates of incidence ranging up to 49%.[9–11]

Different age groups will often present with different injuries to the subscapularis. The adolescent athlete may injure the lesser tuberosity physis (i.e., a Salter II fracture) or avulse the subscapularis in combination with a humeral capsular avulsion (HAGL lesion) while playing sports (Fig. 48.1).[12–14] Tuberosity displacement along with the attached subscapularis can be a challenge diagnostically and surgically. The middle-age athlete may sustain a traumatic isolated subscapularis tear or an anterosuperior cuff tear, which can range from articular-sided partial tears with destabilization of the long head of the biceps, to a large tear combined with pain and stiffness (Fig. 48.2).[15–17] The elderly patient may present with a massive tear, often the result of an acute extension of a prior minimally symptomatic chronic tear leading to instability and possible anterior escape (Fig. 48.3).[18] Many patients have found a way to continue participating with a small supraspinatus tear; however, when tears extend into the subscapularis and infraspinatus, the stabilization effect of the cuff can be compromised and create significant problems. During open surgical repair, tear extension can be undetected, leading to persistent symptoms.[19]

ANATOMY

The subscapularis muscle is the largest and most powerful of the four rotator cuff muscles. In isolation, it provides approximately 50% of the rotator cuff force.[20] The muscle originates from the anterior surface of the scapula and is typically split up into the upper two-thirds and the lower third. The upper two-thirds has a tendinous insertion on the lesser tuberosity, with the lower third demonstrating a muscular insertion onto the humeral metaphysis as described by Hinton et al.[21] It has also been found that the musculotendinous junction was fully formed approximately 2 cm from the lesser tuberosity. The upper tendinous portion is what can be visualized arthroscopically. Wright et al., in their cadaveric study of six shoulders, demonstrated that the superior 44% of the subscapularis could be visualized arthroscopically.[22] This study also found the course of the axillary nerve passed immediately caudal to the lower border of the subscapularis—approximately 32.8 ± 6.0 mm caudal to its arthroscopically visualized superior tendinous border. More recent cadaveric studies have demonstrated the width of the subscapularis insertion to range from 16 to 20 mm with its length ranging from 25 to 40.[23,24] The upper portion of the subscapularis tendon interdigitates with the anterior fibers of the supraspinatus tendon to contribute to the rotator interval structure, as well as the transverse humeral ligaments. This interval is important to the athletic shoulder, providing stability in the overhead athlete. Articular blending of fibers is significant in biceps pulley stability. Extra-articular structures of the interval include the coracoid and coracohumeral ligament.

The upper and lower subscapular nerves provide the innervation to the subscapularis muscle. The majority of the muscle is innervated by the upper subscapularis nerve originating from the C5-C6 nerve roots off of the posterior cord of the brachial plexus. The lower subscapularis nerve innervates the axillary portion of the subscapularis as well as the teres major. In a common variation of the nervous supply, the axillary nerve can give off one or two small branches and supply innervation to the axillary portion of the subscapularis.[25] The majority of the blood supply to the subscapularis muscle is derived from the subscapular artery. The subscapular artery, the largest branch of the axillary artery, arises at the lower border of the subscapularis, which it follows to the inferior angle of the scapula.

Several cadaveric studies have shown that the superior portion of the footprint on the lesser tuberosity represents the widest portion of the insertion.[9,24,26–28] The insertion is trapezoidal in geometry, with the widest portion being superior, tapering in width at the distal attachment. Based on these studies, it has been thought that the most superior attachment of the subscapularis

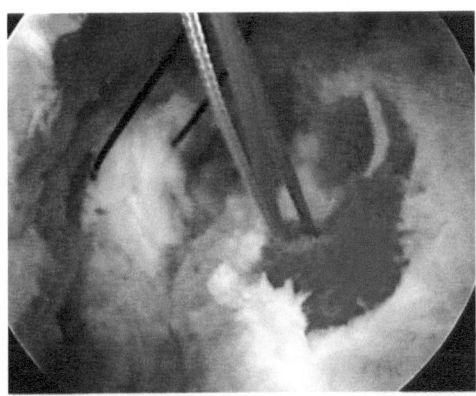

Fig. 48.1 Bursal view of retracted subscapularis tear with lesser tuberosity. A traction stitch has been placed on the subscapularis.

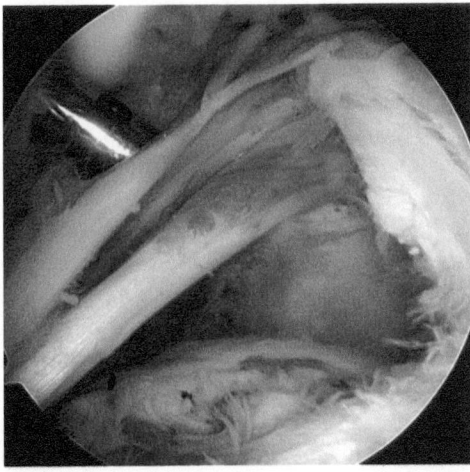

Fig. 48.2 Anterosuperior tear, including subscapularis and supraspinatus tendons.

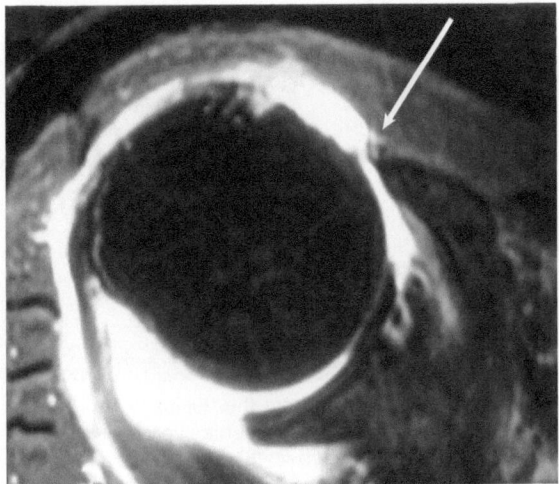

Fig. 48.3 MRI study of unstable shoulder with anterior subluxation due to massive rotator cuff tear. The arrow indicates the torn subscapularis tendon that is retracted medially from the lesser tuberosity.

is the strongest, and is the location where tears initiate and progress.[9,27]

FUNCTION

The primary function of the subscapularis muscle, along with the pectoralis major, the latissimus dorsi, and teres major muscles, is to internally rotate the shoulder. Favre et al.[29] described the cranial and middle segments of the subscapularis muscle as internal rotators with the arm in an adducted position. The muscle also acts as a force couple along with the posterior rotator cuff (infraspinatus and teres minor).[2,30] In concert, these muscles provide a stable fulcrum for motion—contributing to the dynamic stability required of the glenohumeral joint. The subscapularis also opposes the action of the deltoid to allow humeral elevation and abduction by the supraspinatus.[2,18] Given its anterior location with relation to the glenohumeral joint, the subscapularis contributes to humeral head stability opposing anterior subluxation/dislocation.[17,21]

MECHANISM OF INJURY

There seems to be a bimodal distribution when it comes to subscapularis injuries. In the traumatic setting, typically injuries are sustained to the subscapularis with the arm in hyperextension and external rotation.[3-5] Gerber and Krushnell described 16 patients who sustained isolated subscapularis tendon tears with a forced external rotation in an adducted arm.[6] Deutsch et al. evaluated a cohort of 14 shoulders with subscapularis injuries.[31] All but three patients sustained a traumatic injury of hyperextension or external rotation of the abducted arm. The average age of their patient population was 39 years, with all of the patients being male.

There has also been an association with anterior glenohumeral dislocation in the older patient population and subscapularis failures.[32,33] Neviaser and Neviaser described a series of 11 patients with traumatic, recurrent anterior instability of the glenohumeral joint leading to subscapularis insufficiency. The average patient age in their series was 62.7, and in all cases, stability was restored with repair of the anterior capsule and subscapularis. In skeletally immature patients, lesser tuberosity avulsion has been described.[12,13] A missed diagnosis and subsequent missed repair can lead to significant morbidity (see Fig. 48.1).

The majority of acute subscapularis tears occur in conjunction with supraspinatus tears termed "anterosuperior lesions of the rotator cuff." With more degenerative tears of the subscapularis, coracoid impingement has been implicated. Lo and Burkhart have described the "roller-wringer effect," which can occur when the coracohumeral interval is less than 6 mm.[34] In this phenomenon, the tip of the coracoid impinges upon the subscapularis tendon, creating tensile forces on the articular surface leading to tensile undersurface fiber failure (TUFF) lesions. Forward elevation, internal rotation, and cross-body adduction may cause impingement of the subscapularis tendon between the tip of the coracoid and lesser tuberosity.

A common associated pathology found concomitantly with subscapularis injuries is biceps injuries. Several studies have demonstrated medial biceps subluxation or frank tearing resulting from subscapularis insufficiency.[7,16,17,19,31,35] Concomitant injuries have been studied by Burkhart et al., and described arthroscopically as the "comma sign"—signifying scarring of the disrupted medial biceps sling to the torn subscapularis tendon.[36] Arai et al. reviewed 435 consecutive arthroscopies and found that in all cases where there was biceps instability, there was associated subscapularis tearing.[9] In fact, biceps symptoms and pathology often lead to the diagnosis of subscapularis insufficiency. A likely phenomenon for this association is that the superior border of the subscapularis contributes to the pulley mechanism that retains the biceps tendon groove.

It is less common, but the biceps can dislocate with an intact subscapularis. Here, the lateral pulley is disrupted and the biceps dislocates superficially to the intact medial pulley and subscapularis. In these patients, lateral pulley and supraspinatus tears can lead to this form of biceps instability.

CLASSIFICATION

There have been several proposed classification systems for subscapularis tendon tears. In general, tears are classified as partial thickness, full thickness with no retraction, and full thickness with retraction. Pfirrman et al.[37] classified tears according to three grades. Grade I: involvement of less than 25% superior to inferior length of the tendon. Grade II: greater than 25% of the tendon. Grade III: complete, full-thickness tears. LaFosse et al.[10] classified the subscapularis tendon tears based on intraoperative evaluation and preoperative computed tomography (CT) scan into five types: type I, partial lesion of superior one-third; type II, complete lesion of superior one-third; type III, complete lesion of superior two-thirds; type IV, complete tendon lesion with centered head and fatty degeneration less than or equal to stage 3; and type V, complete lesion with eccentric head and coracoid impingement as well as fatty degeneration greater than stage 3.

More recently, Yoo et al. studied the three-dimensional anatomic footprint of the subscapularis tendon in order to describe a new classification system based on the four facets of the tendon's insertional anatomy. They then confirmed their cadaveric findings arthroscopically and devised a classification system based

on five different categories: type I, fraying or longitudinal split of the subscapularis tendon; type IIA, less than 50% subscapularis detachment of the first facet; type IIB, greater than 50% detachment without complete disruption of the lateral hood (approximately one-third of footprint); type III, entire first facet with complete-thickness tear (lateral hood tear); type IV, first and second facets are exposed with much medial retraction of the tendon (approximately two-third of footprint); and type V, complete subscapularis tendon tear involving the muscular portion.[38]

HISTORY AND PHYSICAL EXAM

The clinical presentation for ruptures of the subscapularis can be extremely varied, especially if the injury is an acute and traumatic versus a degenerative process. Younger patients with an acute, traumatic injury typically have acute onset shoulder pain with limited motion. Even if they did not sustain a frank dislocation, their symptoms may mimic those of a dislocation. Pain may also be related to concomitant biceps pathology. Patients with degenerative subscapularis tendon tears typically present like those degenerative superior and posterior rotator cuff tears. They have gradual, progressing symptoms, usually in the anterior shoulder region. Once again, biceps pain is quite common in this setting and can be disabling.

During the physical exam, it is important to be able to visualize and inspect both shoulders to compare for symmetry. Tenderness in the anterior shoulder region over the bicipital groove and lesser tuberosity is common. If pain is limited, patients can demonstrate exaggerated passive external rotation compared to the contralateral side. Weakness in internal rotation is common, but in chronic tears, patients often use the other internal rotators (latissimus, pectoralis major, and teres major) to compensate for their lack of subscapularis, which can cloud this physical exam finding.

There are three described accepted specialty tests that isolate the subscapularis muscle (Fig. 48.4). The *lift-off test* and *belly press test* have been described by Gerber et al.,[6,39] while the more recently described *bear-hug test* has been demonstrated by Barth et al.[40] to accurately diagnose subscapularis tears. A prerequisite

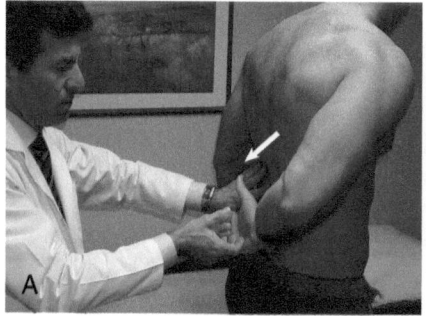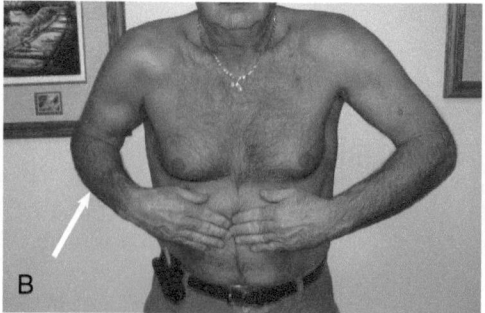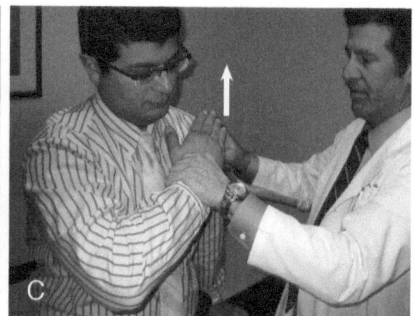

Fig. 48.4 Clinical tests for subscapularis injury. (A) Lift-off test: Placing the arm away from the trunk and asking the patient to maintain the separation. A positive test means he or she cannot maintain the separation. Note the force vector of the patient attempting to lift his hand off of his back *(arrow)*. (B) Belly-press sign: Have the patient press hands against abdomen with the elbows projected forward. Weak internal rotation forces elbow to collapse next to torso *(arrow)*. (C) Bear-hug sign: Have the patient place hand on opposite shoulder in forward flexion. Examiner tries to lift hand up and away, and the patient cannot maintain this position. Note the force applied by the examiner when an attempt is made to pull the patient's hand off the opposite shoulder *(arrow)*.

for the lift-off test is for the patient to have minimal pain with motion and to be able to internally rotate the shoulder without pain. In this test, the patient internally rotates the hand behind his or her back and initially rests the dorsum of the hand on the mid-lumbar region. A positive test occurs when the patient is unable to lift or maintain the hand away from the back. Clinicians have made comparisons to the accuracy and validity of these examination techniques.[41–43]

The *belly-press test* is easier for a patient with more limited, painful motion to perform compared with the *lift-off test*. In this test, the patient places the palms of both hands around the level of his or her umbilicus with wrists in a neutral position. A positive test occurs when the patient is forced to volar flex his or her wrist in an attempt to maintain a forward position of the elbow, while the elbow actually falls posteriorly. A decrease in his or her ability to maintain a forward position of the elbow compared to the contralateral side also indicates subscapularis insufficiency. A prerequisite for this test is normal passive range of motion (ROM). Loss of passive internal rotation will lead to false positive testing.

The *bear-hug test* involves the patient placing the palm of the hand on the tested side upon the opposite shoulder with fingers extended. The patient then attempts to resist an external force trying to pull the hand away from the shoulder in a perpendicular fashion. A positive test occurs when the patient is unable to maintain the hand on the opposite shoulder or shows weakness compared to the contralateral side.

Electromyographic (EMG) testing has demonstrated that the subscapularis muscle activity is proportionally greater than the other internal rotators of the arm in the lift-off test with the hand at the midlumbar level. In addition, Tokish et al., using EMG validation and comparison, demonstrated the belly-press test was found to preferentially activate the upper subscapularis, whereas the lift-off test preferentially activated the lower subscapularis muscle.[42] Another EMG study evaluated arm position while performing the bear-hug, belly-press, and lift-off tests.[43] Their conclusions indicated that all three tests were successful at significantly isolating subscapularis function and that there was no difference in activation at different arm angles.

IMAGING

The initial diagnostic workup includes radiographs of the shoulder including an anteroposterior view in external rotation, transscapular outlet view, and an axillary lateral view. Preservation of the glenohumeral joint, the acromiohumeral interval, and anatomy of adjacent structures including the acromion and acromioclavicular joint can be determined. In acute subscapularis ruptures, there can sometimes be a small segment of the lesser tuberosity avulsed that can be appreciated on radiographs.

Additional studies to evaluate the soft tissue are also necessary, including magnetic resonance imaging (MRI), contrast CT, or ultrasound. Ultrasound has the added benefit of a dynamic imaging study, although it is operator dependent. These studies can help evaluate tear retraction, but MRI and CT studies are better indicators for muscular atrophy and fatty infiltration. The presence of muscle atrophy and extensive fatty infiltration has been correlated to poor healing after repair.[44–46] MRI provides

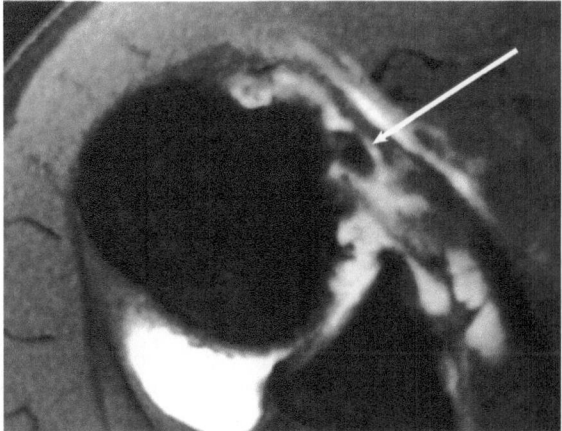

Fig. 48.5 MRI image of subscapularis insertion tear and biceps dislocation out of groove *(arrow)*.

the added benefit of evaluating common concomitant pathology such as labral tears and biceps injuries (Fig. 48.5).

The accuracy of MRI imaging in the detection of subscapularis lesions has been called into question in the literature. Adams et al. retrospectively reviewed 120 patients who underwent arthroscopic rotator cuff repair and correlated their arthroscopic findings to their MRI findings with respect to subscapularis tears.[47] All 16 patients with a subscapularis tear identified on preoperative MRI imaging had confirmed tears at arthroscopy, giving a specificity of 100%. However, only these 16 tears were identified on MRI imaging while a total of 44 tears were found at the time of arthroscopy, yielding a sensitivity of only 36%. A more recent study performed by Foad et al.[48] confirmed the aforementioned findings, even when MRI arthrography was implemented. In their study, 40 shoulders had subscapularis tears identified at the time of arthroscopy. Only 15 of these shoulders had an identified lesion on their preoperative MRI study. Interestingly, the sensitivity of noncontrast MRI versus MRI arthrography was 40% versus 36%, indicating that the accuracy of identifying subscapularis tears does not dramatically differ even when arthrography is utilized.

The dynamic nature of ultrasound is one major advantage over traditional MRI. Farin et al.[49] utilized ultrasound to evaluate 17 patients with confirmed subscapularis tears at the time of arthroscopy. In their study, 14 of 17 tears (82%) were accurately determined preoperatively using ultrasound.

DECISION-MAKING PRINCIPLES

Different surgical approaches have been recommended for different presentations when determining surgical repair. When considering an arthroscopic repair, posterior tear extension in multiple tendon tears and destabilizing the pulleys of the biceps should be appreciated when planning the steps of surgical repair. The surgical access to the subscapularis is limited, and swelling can make it difficult. The initial repair of the subscapularis can avoid problems with access, and can be followed with repair of the adjacent structures.

Open and arthroscopic approaches have been described for repairing cuff tears that include the subscapularis.[16,17,50–54]

Arthrotomy and repair of an isolated subscapularis tear can be performed through a deltopectoral approach. Tears may extend posteriorly through the supraspinatus, and potentially the infraspinatus, and this may require an additional deltoid split to avoid extensive traction on the deltoid.[16] A single skin incision can allow access to the deltopectoral interval and the deltoid split for the posterior extension. Arthroscopic expansion with saline may dissect along the chest wall and base of the neck. Anesthesiologists should be informed preoperatively, since this may impact their decision on intubation, patient positioning, etc.

The timing of surgical repair and delay in treatment can be detrimental to outcome.[16,39,55,56] The anterosuperior cuff tear is often the result of a traumatic event, and has been shown to lead to significant stiffness at the time of presentation.[17] This may be due to rotator interval and biceps proximity. Initiating ROM preoperatively, followed by planned repair, would be recommended to optimize the recovery from this injury.

Tendon mobilization is performed through a series of releases from the articular and bursal surfaces. The articular releases include portions of the middle glenohumeral ligament. The bursal releases can be performed along the lateral border of the coracoid, with the addition of a decompressive coracoplasty. There are thickened capsule structures along the superior border of the subscapularis that comprise the medial pulley to the biceps and the coracohumeral ligament. Preservation of these structures will assist in reduction of the leading edge of the supraspinatus tendon. Interval releases medial to these structures can be performed and assist in visualization of the superior portion of the subscapularis repair.

There are two different philosophies on arthroscopic repair of the subscapularis, and this involves the portal to visualize the repair. Some choose to visualize the repair from the posterior articular portal. The superior border tears, either partial or complete, have easy access through working portals in the rotator interval. Significantly retracted tears that require additional bursal releases may utilize a bursal view. Surgeons who prefer this view from either a lateral or anterosuperior portal can mobilize tears that have retracted. It is prudent to understand both viewing portals to maximize the approach on the more complex retracted tears.

TREATMENT OPTIONS

There are several approaches to patients following a subscapularis injury, ranging from nonoperative to surgical repair.[7] Due to the importance of shoulder internal rotation strength and the potential for developing chronic anterior instability, the recommendation of repair often follows an acute event.

Nonoperative management can have variable results. There are few anecdotes that have suggested benign neglect in patients who are otherwise debilitated or have multiple morbidities. Certain patients may have a thin or deficient subscapularis following prior surgical arthrotomies, z-plasties, or releases. Fortunately, there are other muscles extending from the thorax that can assist with internal humeral rotation. A concern is the possible development of anterior instability, which can present at varying degrees of severity, ranging from episodic subluxation to a fixed

anterior deformity (see Fig. 48.3). These are complex problems on which to attempt reconstruction, and therefore earlier management of the subscapularis tear is recommended in most patients following injury to this structure.

The surgical repair of a torn subscapularis has traditionally been an open approach. Through a deltopectoral anterior approach, muscle detachment is not necessary. From a bursal perspective, the biceps and brachialis attachment to the coracoid can be protected, and the shoulder can be positioned with moderate external rotation to create easier exposure of the lesser tuberosity. Finger palpation of the musculocutaneous nerve and axillary nerve will permit mobilization of the subscapularis tendon in patients with retraction following a tear. In most cases, the biceps is tenodesed by a variety of techniques during the open repair. The main disadvantages of an open repair include potential difficulty managing portions of the rotator cuff tear that extend posteriorly and superiorly. By internally rotating the humerus and extending the arm, a limited view of the anterior portion of the supraspinatus can be visualized; however, this posture often tensions this structure, making mobilization and repair to the greater tuberosity challenging. In cases where surgeons choose an open approach, the addition of a deltoid split, posterior to the junction of the anterior and middle thirds of the deltoid, would make the exposure of the greater tuberosity easier to obtain, with less deltoid retraction.

In massive anterior rotator cuff tears of the subscapularis tendon, anterosuperior escape of the humerus can lead to loss of the anterior force coupling and significant disability. In these instances, if significant fatty infiltration of the subscapularis muscle is seen on MRI, tendon transfers have been advocated for reconstruction. Both pectoralis transfers and latissimus dorsi transfers (+/− Teres major transfer) have been described.[57–60] Elhassan has recently described his preferred technique of latissimus transfer through a deltopectoral approach for irreparable subscapularis tears. Once the latissimus is identified and released subperiostally from its insertion on the humerus, Krackow stitches are placed, and the tendon is transferred and secured to the lesser tuberosity, recreating the anterior coupling force.[61]

More recently, arthroscopic approaches to repairing subscapularis and rotator cuff tears have increased in popularity. The advantages of the arthroscopic approaches include complete articular examination, visualizing articular and bursal releases, avoidance of detachment or mobilization of the deltoid, the potential management of articular and bursal coexistent pathologies, and the reduction of certain complications (i.e., infection due to the nature of arthroscopic irrigation).

Arthroscopic techniques to repair the subscapularis can be performed with either articular or bursal viewing portals. Proficiency with both techniques allows the surgeon multiple options for large retracted tears (Fig. 48.6).

When patients present with large and massive tears, the arthroscopic repair of the subscapularis often precedes the supraspinatus and infraspinatus repairs. This is done for a number of reasons. First, there is saline extravasation that may limit visualization in longer cases. The working area is limited and should be dealt with prior to extensive swelling. Second, the reduction of the subscapularis will assist in the reduction of the

Arthroscopic Repair of Subscapularis Tear
(bursal view)

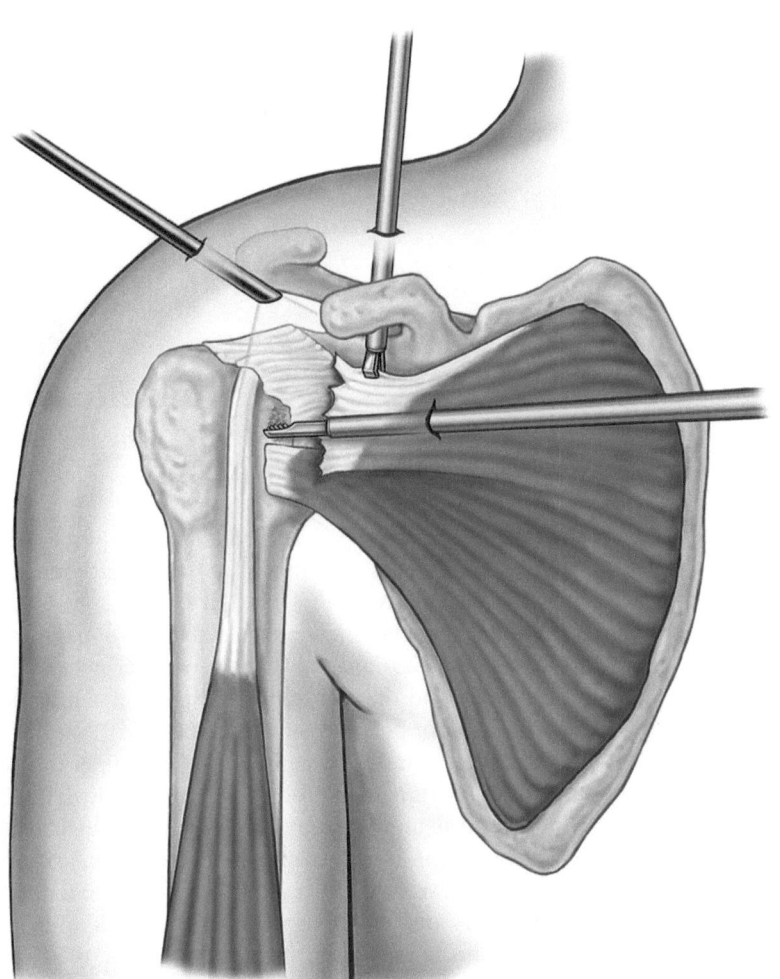

A Lesser tuberosity preparation

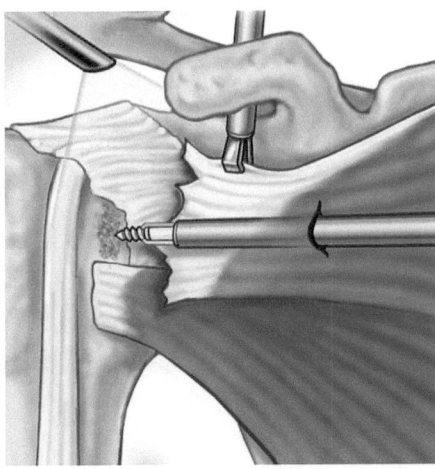

B Anchor placement

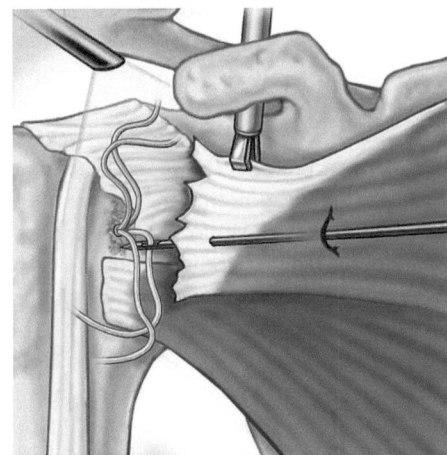

C Pointed piercing suture retriever

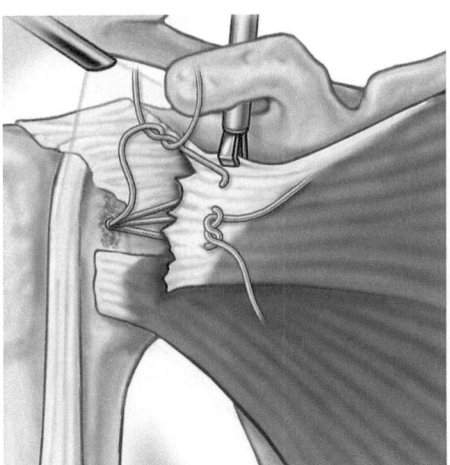

D Mattress suture (yellow)
   Superior, simple suture (blue)

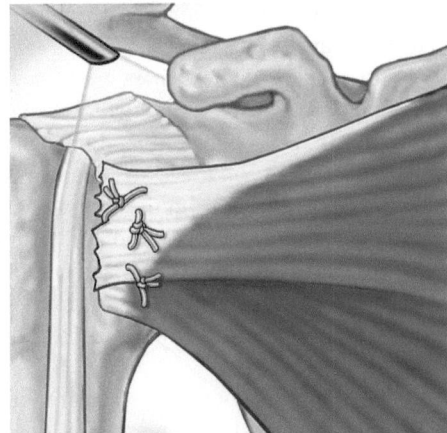

E Completed repair with inferior
   and superior anchors

Fig. 48.6 Arthroscopic technique to repair a subscapularis tear. (A) Orientation of suture portals. (B) Subscapularis view from the posterior viewing portal. (C) Suture anchor placement along the superior border of the lesser tuberosity. (D) Sutures are passed through the free edge of the tear in a mattress and simple suture configuration. (E) Repaired subscapularis tendon.

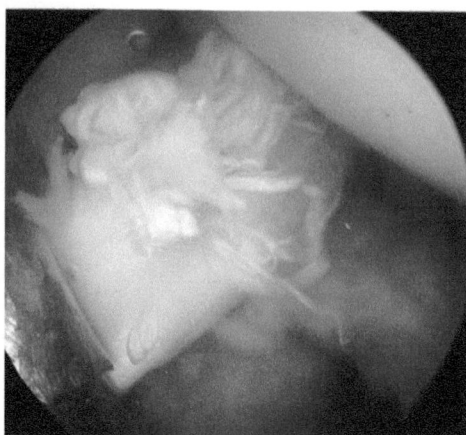

Fig. 48.7 View of subluxed biceps tendon with subscapularis tear.

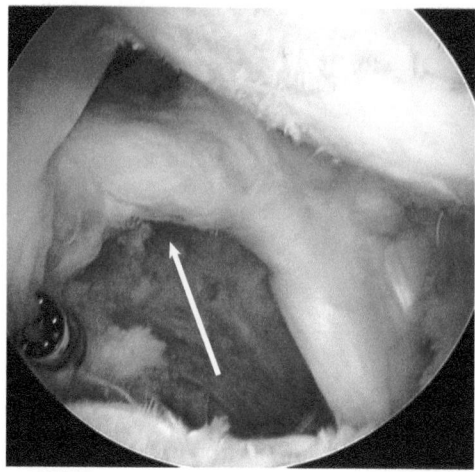

Fig. 48.8 Medial retraction of torn subscapularis with detachment of medial biceps pulley—called the comma sign *(arrow)*.

supraspinatus due to attachments to the pulley system adjacent to the rotator intervals. Third, it is easier to judge tissue tension and avoid "dog-ear" deformity when approaching tears from their margins and working toward the central defect when performing release and repair on significantly retracted tears.

The subscapularis is repaired to the lesser tuberosity. The critical zone of repair is the superior, tendinous portion of the subscapularis. The superior margin rests on the long head of the biceps and serves as the attachment of the medial pulley. A biceps tenodesis is generally performed in patients who demonstrate medial instability or intrinsic damage to the biceps.

An arthroscopic approach begins with the articular view of the subscapularis and biceps (Fig. 48.7). The capsular structures cause some obstruction to visualizing the middle and inferior subscapularis. Some tears may appear as a thin attenuated subscapularis tendon. Gentle humeral rotation while visualizing this structure will demonstrate the deficient attachment to the lesser tuberosity. Medialization of this tissue is significant since it represents loss of proper tension of this structure.

There are less severe tears that occupy the articular surface of the subscapularis. These tears are best visualized with the articular posterior portal. With internal rotation of the humerus, combined with a posterior humeral drawer, the damaged subscapularis as it inserts on the lesser tuberosity footprint becomes apparent. A small shaver from the interval can remove remnants of the tissue to allow for evaluation of this tear. A bursal view of this problem may be misleading since these fibers are not disrupted. This has been referred to as a "hidden lesion" and should be evaluated on any rotator cuff tear that articulates with the rotator interval.

The superior border of the subscapularis is an important structure to support the medial support to the long head of the biceps. Injury to the subscapularis can destabilize the biceps, allowing for medial subluxation (see Fig. 48.7). The subscapularis superior border is the tendinous support to the medial pulley.[13] As the tendon attachment is disrupted, the medial subscapularis retraction displaces ligamentous structures within the rotator interval. This is generally a combination of medial pulley, coracohumeral ligament, and interval capsule. The resultant curved band of tissue has been referred to as a "comma sign" (Fig. 48.8).[30,52] This

structure can be incorporated as additional support to reparative stitches and serves as a landmark for the superior medial repair of the subscapularis repair.

Opening the rotator interval medial to these structures allows for bursal visualization even with an articular portal. The coracoid process and the coracohumeral interval can be débrided using an anterior portal. Alternating a 30- and 70-degree arthroscope can assist in the visualization of the superior border of the subscapularis tendon. Placing the scope through this interval window and aligning the light cord superiorly provides an excellent view of the bursal aspect of the subscapularis. A gentle posterior drawer will increase this space. Combining small amounts of bone resection with soft tissue débridement can help with tissue mobilization and visualization of the repair.

The bursal view for repair is created with the arthroscope being placed in an anterolateral portal (see Fig. 48.1). This can provide additional exposure to tendons that have retracted medially and inferiorly. Sharp and motorized dissection laterally can provide excellent exposure to the lesser tuberosity. Those surgeons choosing medial and lateral anchors (i.e., double-row fixation) will prefer this approach. Be aware of the biceps and brachialis attachment to the coracoid. This can become entangled with stitches used to lateralize the subscapularis tendon. Gentle humeral rotation throughout the procedure will often distinguish the cuff from these structures.

Bursal-viewed repairs of the subscapularis can allow additional releases to the coracohumeral ligament. This will assist with the supraspinatus mobilization to the greater tuberosity. As the superior border of the subscapularis is repaired, the interval tissues often reduce the supraspinatus from a medially retracted position.

Postoperative Rehab

The postoperative program for a subscapularis repair begins in a supportive sling with a small pillow that reduces the internal rotation. Patients are permitted to perform elbow flexion and extension, grip strength, shoulder shrugs, and pendulum exercises. After 1 week, the skin portals are examined and patients are instructed on passive external rotation to 20 degrees. These

Authors' Preferred Technique

Identify any restriction in elevation or rotation, and apply a gentle manipulation to determine if the limited motion is due to soft tissue or potentially degenerative joint changes. The patient is positioned in the lateral decubitus position, slightly favoring a posterior tilted position. This allows the best visualization of the anterolateral aspect of the humerus. The arm is positioned with approximately 30 degrees of abduction and 20 degrees of forward flexion. The arm generally maintains an internally-rotated resting position and can be gently rotated throughout the procedure. The portals are marked on the skin, and joint inflation begins with a spinal needle placed in the posterior "soft spot," inflating the joint space with normal saline. A small stab incision is made approximately 2 cm from the posterior junction of the acromion with the spine of the scapula. The articular examination is performed visualizing the biceps entrance and attachment to the superior labrum, pulleys, and superolateral insertion of the subscapularis. Gentle internal rotation and a posterior drawer will help identify subtle defects of the subscapularis insertion.

An anterior portal is developed inferior to the acromioclavicular joint. A window of capsule can be removed to better visualize the superior border of the subscapularis tendon from both articular and bursal perspectives. If there is significant medial retraction, then this portal can be developed lateral to the "comma," opening the interval and visualizing the lesser tuberosity prior to tissue mobilization. Place the scope in the anterior portal to complete the joint exam and visualize the medial border of the subscapularis as it traverses along the glenoid neck. A bursal exam follows, and an appreciation of the posterior extent of the rotator cuff tear is determined.

Return the scope to the posterior viewing portal and evaluate the biceps tendon. Tagging and releasing the biceps can be performed if there may be further use during the supraspinatus repair. Débridement of the lesser tuberosity footprint is completed from the anterior portal. If coracoplasty is anticipated, this would be best completed prior to repair. Soft tissue between the coracoid and the subscapularis is carefully resected.

Tissue mobilization begins with an articular view. Place an anterior switching stick and elevate the retracted comma tissue to best visualize the subscapularis tendon. A traction suture can be placed and percutaneously retrieved, clamping it adjacent to the skin (Fig. 48.9). Using the anterior portal, a shaver or punch is introduced to divide the superior border of the capsule to visualize the more inferior aspect of the tendon. The scope is then passed through the interval window, and bursal tissue is removed lateral to the coracoid and coracobrachialis tendons to improve tendon mobility.

Using a needle to localize the best angulation for suture anchor insertion, a small puncture in the skin is created. Begin the repair along the inferior aspect of the tear, and providing external humeral rotation, a suture anchor is placed along the medial footprint (Fig. 48.10). Sutures are passed through the inferior part of the tear using either an antegrade instrument that pushes a needle through or via a retrograde device that shuttles or directly picks up suture ends and places them through the tendon. Sutures can be simple sutures, since the tissue is often muscular with a short tendon inferiorly.

A suture anchor is placed at the superior margin of the medial lesser tuberosity. This tendinous portion is very strong, and mattress sutures tension the subscapularis against the prepared footprint. A suture configuration is a mattress suture through the superior border of the tendon and the second arm through the interval medial to the pulley or "comma" tissue. As this stitch is tied, there is excellent fixation of the superior third of the subscapularis (Figs. 48.11 and 48.12). If one prefers a lateral fixation in addition to the medial repair, leave the mattress sutures tied and uncut. After the supraspinatus repair is completed, the multiple suture arms can be collected and fixed with a knotless anchor lateral to the rotator interval (Fig. 48.13).

The scope is switched to the lateral bursal portal, and the infraspinatus and supraspinatus tears are repaired. Adhesions are released and the repair is confirmed visualizing the sutures with humeral rotation.

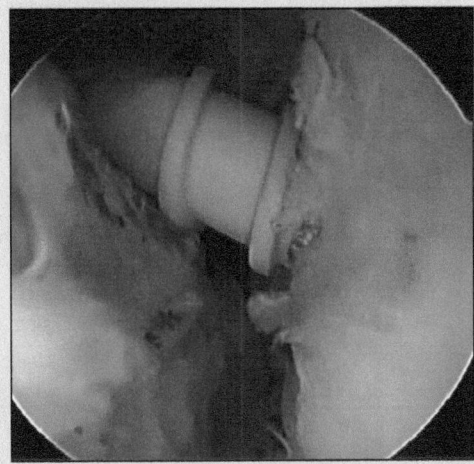

Fig. 48.10 Suture anchor placement into the superior border of the lesser tuberosity.

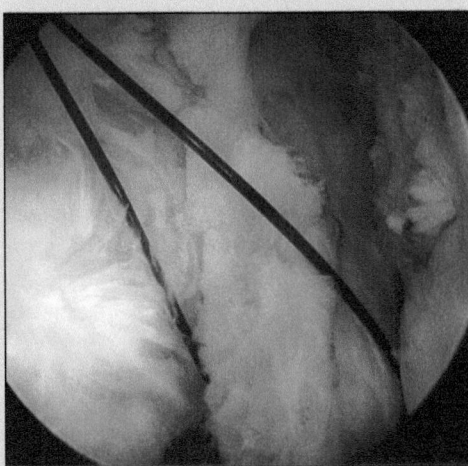

Fig. 48.9 Articular view of a traction stitch assisting reduction of a retracted subscapularis tear.

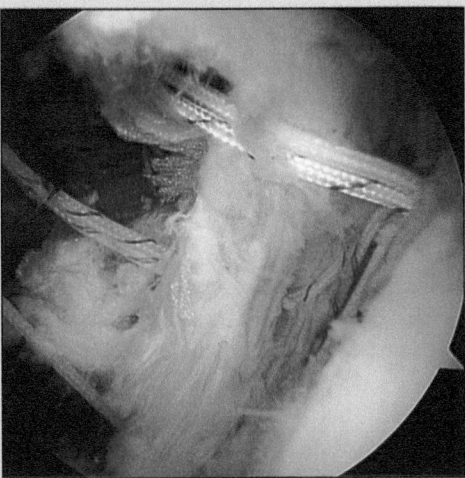

Fig. 48.11 Suture passes through the superior border of the subscapularis, including a combination of mattress and simple sutures.

Continued

Authors' Preferred Technique—cont'd

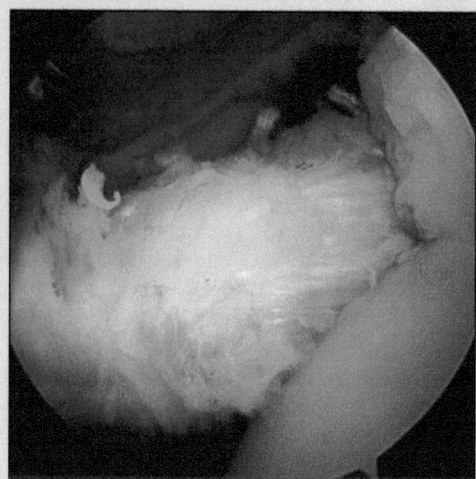

Fig. 48.12 Posterior view through interval window of articular and bursal reduction of torn subscapularis tendon.

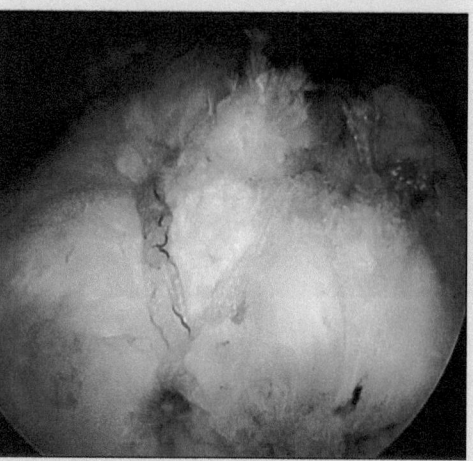

Fig. 48.13 Bursal view of a repaired supraspinatus and subscapularis tendon with double-row stabilization across the biceps groove.

In select cases, the anterior or lateral portals are used to view the mobilization and fixation of the subscapularis. If a lateral portal is chosen, this is usually placed more anteriorly than the portal used to perform an acromioplasty. Mattress

or simple suture techniques can be utilized. Since many tears are continuous with structures posterior to the rotator interval, this perspective assists with reduction of a displaced supraspinatus tear.

exercises are performed two to three times per day for four additional weeks. Avoid forward flexion and internal rotation behind the torso during this critical healing period.

After week 5, the sling is removed and physical therapy is started. Table slides, supine passive shoulder flexion, and scapular stabilization are begun. Gentle external rotation stretches are increased to 30 degrees. Cross-chest stretching can begin, and internal rotation stretches usually begin at 8 to 9 weeks. These stretches are gradual and should be carefully applied, since tendons may internally impinge on the glenoid.

Resistance exercises are started between 10 and 12 weeks. The quality of the tendon and security of the repair determine when active exercises progress to resistive exercises. Additional stretches will include elevation and external rotation. Return to sports and activities will vary between 4 and 6 months. Reestablishing comfort, normal ROM, and moderate strength gains should be achieved before physical activity is anticipated. In young athletes who require significant internal rotation strength, sports participation should be delayed until strength gains have been confirmed.

Results

The literature has several studies on both open and arthroscopic treatment to patients with subscapularis injuries. The isolated subscapularis tear is a relatively uncommon injury and more commonly is an extension of the supraspinatus tear.[62] Delays in diagnosis have been problematic and are due to less familiarity with the injury and findings, muscular changes and retraction, and imaging studies that may not clearly define the problem. With increased awareness of this entity and its physical findings, early diagnosis and repair have shown to produce improvement in pain, strength, function, and patient satisfaction.[6,31,54,55,63]

Open surgical repair by Gerber produced 13 of 16 good and excellent results.[39] Two-thirds reversed their positive lift-off signs and many returned to work. Deutsch et al. had a younger series, and 10 of 14 had significant pain relief and improvement in strength, and 12 returned to sports and work.[31] Edwards had reported a large, multicenter study of 84 patients, ranging in age between 23 and 77 years old. He found that biceps tenodesis or tenotomy reduced pain and improved function.[54] As with Warner's studies, he found that delay in diagnosis and advanced fatty infiltration negatively influenced results, and complications following open repairs were not uncommon. Some of these problems improved with additional therapy, while others required additional surgery.[16] More recently, Di Schino et al. reported long-term outcomes of open repairs and demonstrated durable functional improvement with limited degenerative changes 4 to 10 years out from open repair. Constant scores were noted to improve from 63 preoperatively to 76 postoperatively in this series.[64]

Arthroscopic repair of these injuries has recently increased in popularity. Burkhart and Tehrany reported significant gains in constant score, UCLA score, and good-to-excellent results in 92% of their operated patients.[52] LaFosse reported on 17 patients with isolated subscapularis tears and reported improvement in pain, function, and 15 of 17 were intact by postoperative imaging. He showed reduction in stiffness following surgical repair in contrast to an open repair noted by others.[10]

A recent series of 33 patients with isolated subscapularis tears treated arthroscopically with a single anchor repair demonstrated improved function with decreased pain and high patient satisfaction at a minimum of 2 years' follow up. Full thickness tears were noted to have more favorable outcomes than high-grade partial tears.[65] Although long-term outcome studies of isolated subscapularis tears treated arthroscopically are sparse in the literature, Seppel et al. recently reported on 17 patients with a minimum of 8 years' follow-up following arthroscopically repaired isolated injuries. Significant clinical improvement and long-term tendon integrity was noted on MRI, although decreased strength of the subscapularis on final follow-up was notable. Despite the loss of strength compared to the uninjured side, overall patient satisfaction was greater than 88%.[63]

Overall pain relief following subscapularis repair ranged from 43% to 94%, and patient satisfaction from 88% to 94%. Early diagnosis and repair has the best chance of success with repair integrity, functional gain, and return of strength. The age of the patient continues to be a factor in rotator cuff healing. Chronicity of the tear and biologic limitations can be a challenging aspect when deciding on patient options.[18]

In a personal series (2009) that included both isolated subscapularis and combined tears, the results were favorable for pain relief, strength gains, and return to sport and work.[17] Eight patients with preoperative adhesive capsulitis could be repaired with combined releases and repair. None of the patients developed anterior instability or anterosuperior escape, and patient satisfaction was 89%. It was uncommon for patients to identify weakness as a problem, but some satisfied patients had persistence of the lift-off and belly-press signs.

Complications

Complications of treating patients with subscapularis injuries include missed diagnosis, failure of repair, and injury or adhesions to local structures. Physical findings are a very important aspect of making a diagnosis. Younger patients with a history consistent with anterior instability should raise suspicion when combined with internal rotator weakness. Imaging techniques are very good at identifying full-thickness retracted tears. In patients with inferior subscapularis injuries, partial-thickness tears or prior surgery can be difficult to visualize.

Retearing a subscapularis repair, or failure to heal, are potential complications. The relative risk of rotator tendon repair failure has been reported to be high with multiple tendon tears. Risk factors include the patient's age; however, this repair can be immobilized with less tension in internal rotation. Additional risk factors include lack of compliance with immobilization and vitamin D deficiency; osteopenia can play a role in disrupting a repair. Securing the superior interval ligaments (i.e., the comma sign) is helpful in positioning and securing the subscapularis tendon to the lesser tuberosity. Muscular atrophy and fatty infiltration may play a role in determining the quality of the repair and the mobility of the tendon. The subscapularis plays a role in anterior glenohumeral stability, and an intact tenodesis effect is still beneficial even if the internal rotation strength is diminished. Late attempts at repair have shown tissue retraction and muscle changes as a poor prognosis.[6,16,54] Grafting the repair site with allograft, or performing tendon transfer using the pectoralis major or latissimus, as described above, may be necessary in patients where repair is not possible.

Stiffness is less common with the arthroscopic repair when compared to open surgery.[10,17] Medially placed suture anchors in the lesser tuberosity and utilizing the full length of the avulsed tendon can minimize this loss. Complete intraoperative release on three sides of the mobilized tendon is needed to provide adequate mobility for repair. Additional adhesions to the coracoid and short head of the biceps and brachialis can also restrict terminal rotation. It is easier and safer to create releases during the repair, rather than performing as a second-stage procedure. Those who require releases should have a healed repair and will not require immobilization following additional surgery. The musculocutaneous nerve is located approximately 2 cm inferior to the coracoid process, although variations have been found. Dissection in this area is slow and proceeds from superiorly to inferiorly.

Biceps complications can occur in both isolated subscapularis injuries and combined anterosuperior tears. The medial pulley and supportive superior border of the subscapularis is disrupted. In many cases, the tendon is unstable and can injure the repaired subscapularis with continued instability. It is often safer to perform a biceps tenodesis or tenotomy at the time of index surgery. In a young patient, restoring the medial pulley in a patient with a stable biceps tendon within the groove can be considered. Most older patients would be better treated with release or tenodesis to avoid problems with pain or delayed instability.

Hardware complications are uncommon due to the large size of the subscapularis footprint. Older female patients with osteoporosis may be at risk for hardware migration when repairing a chronic tear. Immobilization with internal rotation and delay of rehabilitation is prudent when soft tissue and bone are deficient. Sutures that secure capsular ligaments along with the subscapularis tendon may provide additional strength the repair.

Neurologic structures are adjacent to the surgical repair site. The axillary nerve rests along the inferior border of the subscapularis muscle, and tendon mobilization needs to be cautious due to its adjacent location. Blunt dissection is safest, and use of motorized instruments and suction can cause injury to this structure. The musculocutaneous nerve passes inferiorly to the coracoid and can be in potential danger during tissue mobilization. Using blunt dissection to liberate the tendons inserted on the coracoid tip can provide a safe window for tissue mobilization. Be aware of cautery in this area. Other plexus structures and the axillary artery can be exposed as dissection is carried medial and inferior to the coracoid. Fortunately for most patients with subscapularis tears, the tendon edge rarely retracts medial to the glenoid articular margin. It is safer to grasp the edge of the tendon, apply a traction suture, and release the tendon while placing gentle laterally directed traction (see Fig. 48.1). Both articular and bursal releases can be performed.

FUTURE CONSIDERATIONS

Early recognition and treatment of subscapularis tears improve the prognosis following repair. Younger patients, less degree of tissue retraction, and less fatty infiltration are promising aspects of returning patients to greater strength and function. Biologic augmentation is a consideration for patients with complex tears or delayed recognition. Tendon transfer is an option for irreparable tears, but the results will not surpass a primary repair. Although a pectoralis major transfer has been popularized, Elhassan has recently introduced the latissimus transfer for late reconstruction. Reverse shoulder arthroplasty becomes an option in an older patient, but use in middle-aged patients is a concern.

Protection of the repair, followed by limited mobilization, allows muscular weakness to continue in favor of tissue healing to the tuberosity. Earlier active stimulation to the repaired cuff may reduce recovery and improve overall strength. Subscapularis weakness can follow delayed treatment of a traumatic tear, as well as commonly performed anterior approaches to the glenohumeral articulation. Minimizing these deficits will likely improve outcomes for our patients.

For a complete list of references, go to ExpertConsult.com.

SELECTED READINGS

Eduardo TB, Walch G, Nove-Josserand L, et al. Anterior superior rotator cuff tears: repairable and irreparable tears. In: Warner JJP, Ianotti JP, Flatow EL, eds. *Complex Revision Problems in Shoulder Surgery*. 2nd ed. Philadelphia: Lippincott, Williams, Wilkinson; 2005:107–128.

Lyons RP, Green A. Subscapularis tendon tears. *J Am Acad Orthop Surg*. 2005;13:353–363.

Nove-Josserand L, Gerber C, Walch G. Lesions of the anterosuperior rotator cuff. In: Warner JJP, Ianotti JP, Gerber C, eds. *Complex and Revision Problems in Shoulder Surgery*. Philadelphia: Lippincott-Raven; 1997:165–176.

Srikumaeran U, Monica JT, Kuye IO, et al. Subscapularis tears. In: Maffulli N, Furia JP, eds. *Rotator Cuff Disorders: Basic Science and Clinical Medicine*. London: JP Medical Publishers; 2012:107–115, [chapter 12].

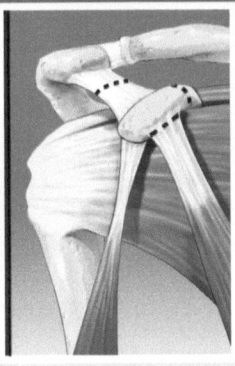

49

Revision Rotator Cuff Repair

Joseph D. Cooper, Anthony Essilfie, Seth C. Gamradt

Primary rotator cuff repair frequently leads to successful subjective results with decreased pain and increased function, but incomplete healing or retearing is known to commonly occur.[1-5] Retear rates following repair of small to medium tears have been reported as high as 40%, and up to 94% following massive, chronic cuff tears.[6,7] Despite retear, many patients can maintain pain relief and improved functional outcome.[8] However, patients who do not heal, on average, tend to have worse satisfaction, clinical outcomes, and decreased function compared to those with an intact repair.[9,10] Of those patients with retear who are unsatisfied and have continued symptoms, 6% to 8% will require revision rotator cuff repair.[11,12] This chapter provides an approach to patient evaluation after unsatisfactory rotator cuff repair and details surgical options for this difficult problem.

HISTORY

A careful history is critical in understanding the etiology of rotator cuff repair failure and to understand the patient's expectations. Typically, patients with failed rotator cuff repairs present with shoulder pain and weakness. It is important to ascertain the onset, location, characterization, intensity of the pain, and the patient's physical demands for both work and recreation. Furthermore, it is important to elucidate whether any specific motions or activities elicit the pain. The surgeon should ask if there was a period of improvement after the primary surgery or if the symptoms continued to persist since the index procedure. The indication for most revision rotator cuff repairs is usually to manage persistent pain and weakness since the initial surgery.[13,14] All previous surgeries should be discussed with the patient; obtaining previous medical records, operative reports, preoperative imaging, and arthroscopic pictures are helpful in assisting with treatment decisions.

When considering a revision procedure, the most important factor to ascertain from the history is the possible cause of failure—the exact cause of which is often multifactorial. Factors causing rotator cuff nonhealing or retear can be classified into three broad categories: biologic, technical, and traumatic. Injured tendons develop a fibrovascular scar at the tendon bone interface, which is altered from the native tissue with decreased vascularity and decreased healing potential.[15] This biologically inferior milieu predisposes a repaired tendon to retearing.

Biologic

This category of risk factors includes both the biology and the nature of the cuff tear itself, as well as the patient as a whole. Patient factors, such as increased age, nicotine use, and diabetes, have all been consistently reported to lead to decreased healing rates and poor clinical outcomes.[7,15-19] Preoperative factors related to the cuff tear itself, including tear size, degree of retraction, and muscle atrophy, have all been shown to correlate with increased failure rates.[16,20] As the cuff ages, and the longer the tear has persisted, there is an increased level of fatty infiltration with decreased muscle in the cuff. Studies have shown that fatty infiltration and cuff atrophy can lead to increased tension on the repair and increased failure rates.[21,22]

Infection is an uncommon cause of cuff repair failure; however, it must be ruled out. Patients who have persistent postoperative pain with no period of relief, who have compromised immune systems, a history of fevers, redness, or problems with their incision should undergo an infection work-up consistent with white blood cell count, erythrocyte sedimentation rate blood test, c-reactive protein test, joint aspiration for cell count, and culture.

Technical Factors

Identifying potential surgical errors as a cause of failure can be essential when planning a revision. These factors can include knot failure, inadequate recognition of tear size or pattern, poorly fixed or positioned anchors, and over-tensioning the repair. One of the most common modes of failure for rotator cuff repair is when sutures cutout through poor quality tendon[23,24] Suture configurations, such as double row, single row, transosseous, and transosseous equivalent repairs, have been described to address this problem. Biomechanical data support double row fixation and/or transosseous equivalent repair,[25-29] but clinical data have not consistently shown improved outcomes over a single row repair.[30-32] Surgeon familiarity with the chosen technique is likely most essential, as low surgeon volume has been shown to be an independent risk factor for reoperation.[18]

Failure to address other pain generators in the shoulder can also lead to persistent pain and decreased function, which can be incorrectly attributed to a failed repair. Failure to address biceps tendon pathology, prominent acromial spurs, or a symptomatic

TABLE 49.1   Noncuff Tear Etiologies of Residual Shoulder Pain

Extrinsic Pain Generators
- Cervical radiculopathy
- Referred pain from intrathoracic or intra-abdominal pathology
- Suprascapular neuropathy

Intrinsic Pain Generators
- Os acromiale
- Instability
- Biceps tendinopathy
- Acromioclavicular joint pain
- Labral tear
- Adhesive capsulitis
- Subacromial impingement
- Glenohumeral arthritis

acromioclavicular joint at the index surgery can contribute to a persistently symptomatic shoulder after rotator cuff repair. Other noncuff tear etiologies of shoulder pain are shown in Table 49.1.

Traumatic

Traumatic tearing can be defined as early (before tendon healing has occur) or late (after healing has occurred). Early tears usually occur between 6 and 26 weeks postoperatively[33] and can be a result of overly aggressive physical therapy in the acute recovery period. Late traumatic retears usually have a history of improved or return to normal shoulder function, followed by an identifiable trauma or injury that led to onset of new symptoms.

PHYSICAL EXAMINATION

The physical exam is paramount in identifying the cause of a failed rotator cuff repair and also the suitability of the patient for a second surgery. We start our evaluation with a cervical spine examination. Many patients with cervical spine disease have associated shoulder pain. They usually have limited cervical range of motion (ROM) particularly with hyperextension. It is important to note if there is any decreased sensation in a particular dermatome. A Spurling test should be performed to evaluate for radicular symptoms.

Examination of the shoulder begins with inspection of the shoulder by looking for evidence of supraspinatus or infraspinatus atrophy. Also assessing previous portals or incisions should be noted for healing, contracture, or signs of infection. The surgeon should palpate the glenohumeral joint, rotator cuff insertion, biceps groove, and acromioclavicular joint. Active and passive ROM of the shoulder should be evaluated and compared to the contralateral shoulder. Often passive ROM is greater than active ROM in the setting of a rotator cuff tear. Patients that have equal loss of passive and active ROM (true stiffness) without deficits in strength may have postoperative adhesions, glenohumeral arthritis, or capsular contracture. The strength of each rotator cuff tendon should be evaluated systematically. Having the patient internally rotate the arm and elevate it 90 degrees

in the scapular plane against resistance tests the supraspinatus. The infraspinatus is tested with resisted external rotation with the arm at the side and elbow with 90 degrees of flexion. The lift-off test and belly press test are done to assess the strength of the subscapularis. The subscapularis also can be assessed with a bear hug test where the patient places the ipsilateral hand on the contralateral shoulder and the elbow positioned anterior to the body. The patient then actively resists the examiner's attempt externally rotate the forearm. If the patient is unable to keep his hand on his shoulder or weakness is detected, the test is positive.[34]

Neer and Hawkins signs are used to evaluate for subacromial impingement. A hornblower sign is representative of significant deficit in the posterior rotator cuff (infraspinatus and teres minor). These patients commonly abduct the arm when trying to bring their hand to their face with their arm at the side. The cross-body adduction test is used to evaluate for AC joint pathology. Yergason and Speed test assess for biceps pathology.

When it is difficult to discern between cervical radiculopathy versus true shoulder pain, a diagnostic injection in the subacromial space can be helpful.

IMAGING

Standard radiographs of the shoulder including the anteroposterior, Grashey, scapular Y, and axillary views of the shoulder should be taken. When evaluating the radiographs, it is critical to evaluate the glenohumeral joint for degenerative changes or evidence of superior migration of the humeral head as these radiographic changes are most often contraindications to revision rotator cuff repair.

Magnetic resonance imaging (MRI) is probably most important in the work-up of symptomatic patients after a previous rotator cuff repair. It has been shown that MRI is accurate in diagnosing recurrent full thickness rotator cuff tears but is inaccurate in defining tear size.[35] MRI has a reported 85.5% sensitivity and 90.4% specificity for all tears.[36] There is conflicting evidence assessing whether there is any benefit of a magnetic resonance arthrogram (MRA) versus a noncontrast MRI.[37-39] Additionally, there is a report of high false-positive results with MRA when used for evaluation for retears.[40] In the event that a patient has a contraindication for an MRI, computed tomography arthrography is a viable substitute.

Ultrasonography, when performed by an experienced technician, is comparable to MRI in diagnosing and assessing tear size and retraction of primary rotator cuff tears.[41] Ultrasonography has a high sensitivity of 91%, specificity of 86%, and accuracy of 89% for detecting rotator cuff tears postoperatively.[42] However, MRI is often more useful to surgeons than ultrasound since it allows the ability to assess the shoulder in three planes. When assessing the reparability of a tear, it is important to look at the degree of retraction on the coronal view and the degree of muscle atrophy on the sagittal view.

DECISION-MAKING PRINCIPLES

Factors to consider when determining treatment options of these patients include tear size, degree of retraction, quality of the rotator cuff muscle, the presence or absence of glenohumeral arthritis, and patient function. Rotator cuff repairs are most likely to fail when the tendon has Goutallier grade 3 or grade 4 fatty degeneration[43]; muscle atrophy that is greater than grade 3 is a relative contraindication to revision.[44]

An extensive trial of nonoperative management should be exhausted before considering revision repair, as even in the setting of a failed repair radiographically, acceptable clinical and subjective patient outcomes can be achieved with therapy.[12]

Management of asymptomatic patients with a known retear on imaging is challenging. Jost et al.[45] followed 20 patients that were found to have a rerupture on MRI. These patients were evaluated on average at 3.2 years and again at 7.6 years after the index procedure. Despite retears seen on MRI, there was no significant decrease in Constant score, and the size of the tears did not significantly increase between the two follow-up time points. However, there was significant progression of fatty infiltration of the infraspinatus and the acromiohumeral distance, making future surgeries, if required, significantly less likely to be successful when treated in this delayed fashion. Further research in this cohort is needed to identify factors that lead to symptomatic tears.

Previous literature has shown that ideal candidates for revision rotator cuff repair have an intact deltoid origin, with preoperative active elevation of 90 degrees and forward flexion of 120 degrees.[4] There should be good tissue quality, adequate bone stock, and the apex of the tendon should not have retracted beyond the glenohumeral joint. There should be no signs of active infection, glenohumeral arthritis, or cuff tear arthropathy (Fig. 49.1).

Prior to considering revision surgery there should be a candid discussion and understanding between patient and surgeon regarding the reason for revision and the expected outcomes (Table 49.2).

TREATMENT OPTIONS

Nonoperative

As discussed in the previous section, a trial of physical therapy and nonoperative management should be exhausted before revision surgery in most patients. The only exception being physiologically young active patients with an acute traumatic retear. These cases should be fixed acutely. Therapy focusing on periscapular strengthening and the anterior deltoid has been shown to be most effective at helping restore the force couple of a failed rotator cuff.[46]

Débridement Alone

In elderly, low-demand patients with persistent pain, but preserved ROM, arthroscopic débridement with a biceps tenotomy or tenodesis can be considered.[1] The biceps tendon is a pain generator and can be released without loss of shoulder function. Short-term outcomes have shown that débridement alone can successfully relieve pain in shoulders with massive cuff tears but no significant arthritis.[47,48]

TABLE 49.2 Decision-Making Prior to Revision Cuff Repair

Is This Patient a Candidate?
- Patient factors:
  - Age
  - Function/demand level
  - Overall health status
  - Number of prior surgeries
  - Pain level
- Cuff/shoulder factors:
  - Preoperative range of motion
  - Status of the deltoid
  - Level of fatty degeneration
  - Tendon retraction
  - Other pain generators causing problems
  - Arthritis

Has There Been Sufficient Nonoperative Management?
- Duration of therapy
- Adherence to prescribed therapy program
- Effectiveness of prescribed therapy program (anterior deltoid focused)
- Nonsteroidal antiinflammatory drugs

Does the Patient Have Appropriate Expectations/ Understanding?
- Patient should understand:
  - Revision surgery is primarily for pain relief
  - Functional improvements cannot be promised
  - Retearing (again) is common
  - Will not result in a "normal" shoulder

Revision Repair

Once it is determined that the patient is a candidate for revision cuff repair, planning the revision procedure begins with evaluation of the failed procedure. Open versus arthroscopic repair options are based on surgeon familiarity and preference, with current repair trends largely biasing arthroscopic repair.

In modern rotator cuff repair, biologically absorbable screws are frequently used. If metal anchors were used these should only be removed if prominent, because removal causes bony defects that weaken the greater tuberosity or fixation.[1] New anchors should be tapped to prevent damaging them on retained hardware. When possible, oversized hardware should be used at prior hardware sites to avoid further bone disruption. An alternative is to perform a transosseous repair and avoid new anchor placement.[1]

In revision rotator cuff repair the tendons are often retracted and scarred, requiring various mobilization techniques and soft tissue releases to free the tissues from adhesions and allow a tension-free anatomic repair. Multiple interval slide techniques have been described for open surgery[49-54] and have been adapted for arthroscopic use. An anterior interval slide, oriented towards the base of the coracoid releasing the interval between the supraspinatus and the rotator interval, can achieve 1 to 2 cm of lateral excursion.[55] A posterior interval slide releases between the supraspinatus and the infraspinatus and provides 1 to 2 cm of lateral excursion; however, the suprascapular nerve is at risk with this

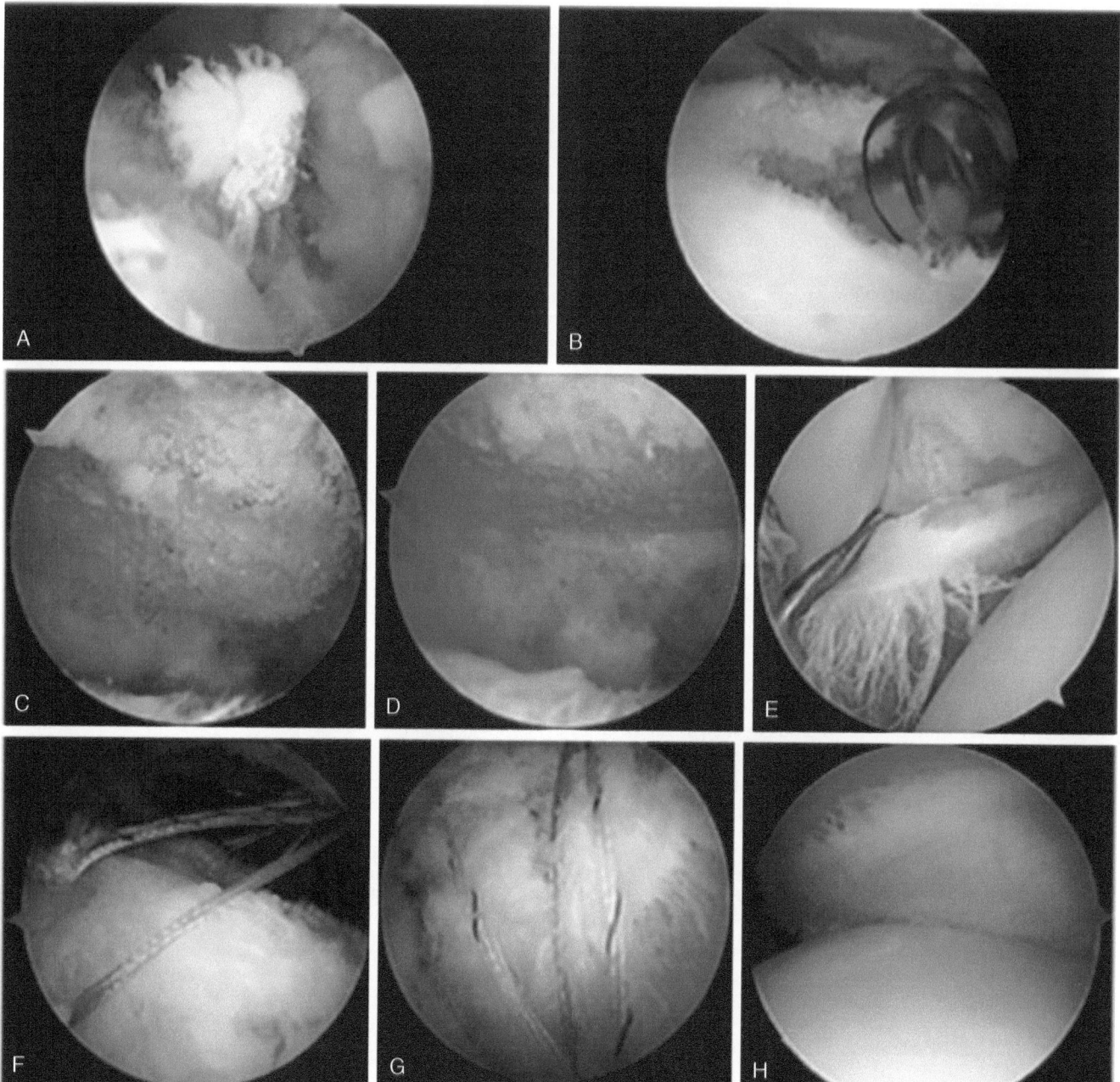

Fig. 49.1 Arthroscopic images demonstrate concomitant pathology in revision rotator cuff repair in a 55-year-old man who is a surfer. (A) View shows simple sutures pulled through the lateral cuff. (B) Views show a 2×2 cm supraspinatus tear following débridement of suture material and nonviable rotator cuff. (C) View shows residual acromial spur. (D) View obtained following acromioplasty. (E) View shows biceps tear and severe tendinitis that necessitated biceps tenodesis. (F) View of medial row sutures. (G) Subacromial view of a double-row revision repair. (H) Intra-articular view of completed rotator cuff repair. (Reproduced with permission from Johnson BC, Dunphy TR, Gamradt SC. Revision Rotator Cuff Repair. In: Gamradt SC, Sperling, JW, Galatz LM, eds. *Let's Discuss Revision Shoulder*. Rosemont, IL: AAOS; 2015:23–41.)

release. These procedures can be combined in a double interval slide and achieve up to 5 cm of additional laterality for a tension-free repair.[55]

When the tendons are mobilized sufficiently to reach the tuberosity they can be fixed to the humerus with anchors. As previously mentioned, double row and transosseous-equivalent repairs have been shown to be biomechanically superior to a single row in multiple studies[25-29]; however, no study has yet shown a clinically significant difference in outcomes following primary rotator cuff repair (RTC) repairs.[30-32] This has not been specifically studied in revision procedures. However, in the revision setting with compromised tissue the theoretical benefit of a stronger repair is likely warranted, and a double row repair should be used when possible.

Burkhart[56] described a partial RTC repair technique for irreparable tears when the tendon cannot be fully mobilized to the tuberosities. This technique restores the force couple of the RTC by repairing the inferior half of the infraspinatous and the whole subscapularis. Multiple modifications of this technique have since been described.[57] These techniques have up to a 41.7% retear rate and in the modern treatment of failed RTCs have largely given way to reverse total shoulder arthroplasty or other biologic repair techniques such as patch augmentation.

Repair With Biologic Augmentation

Poor patient biology is a frequent cause for primary RTC failure, whether that be muscle atrophy, tendon or bone quality, or tendon retraction. In the revision setting, surgeons frequently look to augment the biologic milieu of the shoulder to aid in healing. The use of growth factors, stem cell therapy, gene therapy, and bioimplants have all been described, although currently mostly in animal models.[58] The most frequently used technique involves stimulating marrow elements from the humeral head with a microfracture technique with or without the application of a biologic patch based on the integrity of the tissue. Marrow elements provide polymorphonuclear cells, macrophages, and a fibrin clot (acts as a temporary scaffold), as well as growth factors and platelets to aid in cuff healing.[59] Multiple patch types have been described including degradable or nondegradable, synthetic grafts, xenografts, and extracellular-matrix-based patches.[60-64] The patch can be used as an additional support for tendons with poor quality, and sewn over the repair.[64,65]

Superior capsular reconstruction has been described by Mihata and colleagues for massive irreparable rotator cuff tears.[66] This technique uses a graft that spans from the superior glenoid to the greater tuberosity. Early outcomes in primary RTC repairs have shown it to reliably decrease pain and to provide some return of shoulder function.[67] This technique has not been specifically evaluated in regard to revision RTC procedures, but it may be an option for patients with minimal arthritis trying to avoid reverse total shoulder arthroplasty.

Other biologic additives have also been described and are used with anecdotal success; however, their outcomes have not been clinically proven in the literature.[58]

For Tears That Cannot Be Repaired

Massive revision cuff tears that cannot be mobilized enough to restore the RTC tendons to their native position have to be repaired by alternative means. Patients with preserved joint space but limited ROM are candidates for tendon transfers. Both latissimus dorsi and trapezius transfers have been described.[68,69] These procedures can successfully restore joint motion and are a reasonable option for the young patient who does not want to undergo shoulder arthroplasty. Reverse total shoulder arthroplasty is the treatment of choice for elderly patients with tears that cannot be repaired and who have significant glenohumeral arthritis.

POSTOPERATIVE MANAGEMENT

Patient immobilization is based on tear size and quality. Large tears are fully immobilized for 4 weeks postoperatively. In smaller tears we allow shoulder shrugs, passive external rotation to neutral, and passive forward elevation to 90 degrees. No large studies have evaluated the optimal rehabilitation strategies after revision rotator cuff repair, and management is largely based on surgeon preference and experience. We advise patients that pain and functional improvement can continue for 1 year or longer.

RESULTS AND COMPLICATIONS

Revision rotator cuff surgery can result in reduced pain with improved shoulder function and patient satisfaction.[3] Multiple studies have now supported this and are summarized in Table 49.3.

While revision RTC repair does generally lead to pain relief and improved function, it does have a higher complication rate and higher failure rate than primary repair. The retear rate

---

🖈 Authors' Preferred Technique

We offer revision RTC repair to patients with acceptable tissue quality on MRI, no pseudoparalysis, a functioning deltoid, and only one previous repair. Patients are counseled preoperatively that retearing is common, pain relief and restoration of function may not be complete, and the durability and long-term results of revision rotator cuff repair are not well studied.

We use only arthroscopic techniques for revision cuff repair. This avoids the risks associated with splitting the deltoid or other deltoid takedown techniques required for an open approach. The patient is positioned in the beach chair position with the arm in a pneumatic arm holder that facilitates subacromial distraction and allows rotational positioning of the arm. Epinephrine in the arthroscopy fluid at of 1 mL of 1:1000 per 3000 mL of saline improves hemostasis and visualization.

Arthroscopic portals from the initial procedure should not influence portal placement for the revision procedure. We start with a posterior viewing portal placed at 1 cm inferior and 1 cm medial to the posterolateral acromion (slightly more superolateral than is standard). This position is not ideal for glenohumeral access but provides better visualization of the subacromial space. Anterior and lateral portals are placed under direct vision based on access to required working

sites. Tear mobilization for a tension-free repair is frequently required. Articular sided mobilization is performed with radiofrequency ablation by releasing adhesions between the cuff and the labrum. This release is limited to 2 cm medial to the glenoid to avoid suprascapular nerve injury. A bursal-sided release can be carried anteriorly to the coracoid and as far posteriorly as necessary, often to the scapular spine. During revision bursectomy, scarring can make differentiation of the cuff tissue from bursa difficult; the cuff can be protected by starting from normal tissue anteriorly and carrying the bursectomy posteriorly with the shaver aimed cephalad. In anterosuperior cuff tears, an anterior interval slide, or a release of the thickened medial sling between the subscapularis and the supraspinatus can be performed without affecting the failure rates.[70]

Vessels are frequently encountered during the posteromedial release and bleeding can lead to a "redout" situation obscuring the camera. This can be managed by keeping the site of bleeding directly in the camera field of vision using the pressure of the water to slow the bleeding then moving the cautery device to the arthroscope and cauterizing the source.

Repairs are performed using bioabsorbable anchors in a double row formation when possible (Fig. 49.2).

Continued

Authors' Preferred Technique—cont'd

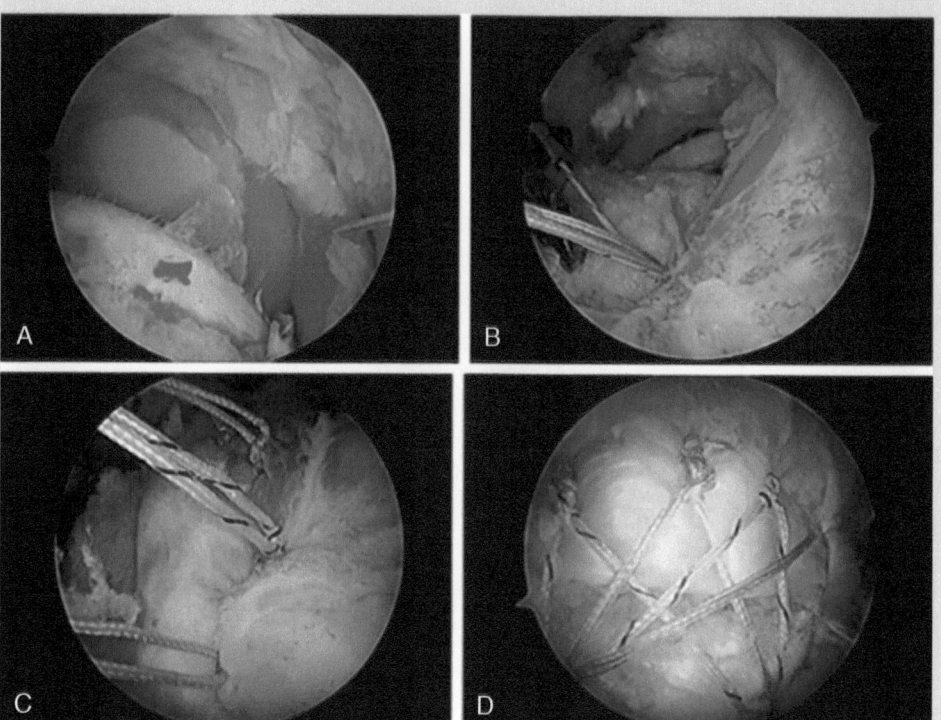

Fig. 49.2 Arthroscopic views of the shoulder in a 62-year-old man who is a dock worker, with weakness 6 months after rotator cuff repair who underwent revision of a massive tear with grade 2 atrophy seen on MRI. (A) View obtained from the lateral portal before mobilization. (B) View obtained from the posterior portal following bursal and articular release. (C) View shows medial-row sutures. (D) View of completed double-row revision repair. *MRI*, Magnetic resonance imaging. (Reproduced with permission from Johnson BC, Dunphy TR, Gamradt SC. Revision Rotator Cuff Repair. In: Gamradt SC, Sperling, JW, Galatz LM, eds. *Let's Discuss Revision Shoulder*. Rosemont, IL: AAOS; 2015:23–41.)

TABLE 49.3   Revision Rotator Cuff Repair Studies

Authors	Year of Publication	No. of Shoulders	Mean Age (Years)	Average Follow-Up in Months	Massive Tears (% of Total)	Design
A. Outcomes						
Mora et al.[72]	2017	51	60	25	59%	Retrospective review of prospective data
Shamsudin et al.[71]	2015	50	63	35	NA	Retrospective review of prospective data
Chuang et al.[73]	2014	32	69	70	59%	Retrospective case series
Parnes et al.[2]	2013	94	58	No average reported, minimum 12	54%	Retrospective case series
Lädermann et al.[74]	2012	74	61	59	72%	Retrospective case series
Keener et al.[13]	2010	21	56	36	NA	Retrospective case series
Piasecki et al.[75]	2010	54	55	31	7%	Retrospective case series

TABLE 49.3   Revision Rotator Cuff Repair Studies—cont'd

Authors	Active Postop Elevation (Gain)	Clinical Outcomes (Gain)	Retear Rate	Complications/Revisions (%)
B. Outcomes				
Mora et al.[72]	135.6° (39)	CS: 69.1 (26.4) SST: 7.58 (3.6) VAS: 6.49 (3.2) Unsatisfactory outcome: 27%	60%	15.7% revision rate
Shamsudin et al.[71]	NA (2)	4 Newton increase in abduction strength, no improvement in lift-off strength	40% at 2 years	12% revision rate
Chuang et al.[73]	156° (9)	ASES: 87 (NA) UCLA: 30 (14) VAS: 0.9 (3.7)	NA	NA
Parnes et al.[2]	NA	NA	NA	Failure to heal: 10.6% Stiffness: 7.4% Infection: 2.1% Nerve injury: 1%
Lädermann et al.[74]	152° (16)	ASES: 77 (26) UCLA: 27 (9) VAS: 2 (3) Pt satisfaction: 78%	NA	8% Revision rate
Keener et al.[13]	146° (NA)	ASES: 74 (NA) SST: 8.9 (3.5) VAS: 2.7 (NA)	52%	0% Surgical complication
Piasecki et al.[75]	136° (15)	ASES: 68 (24) SST: 7.5 (4) VAS: 2.7 (2.4)	NA	11.1%

ASES, American Shoulder and Elbow Surgeons; *CS*, constant score; *NA*, not available; *SST*, simple shoulder test; *UCLA*, University of California Los Angeles; *VAS*, visual analogue scale.

following revision RTC surgery has been reported as high as 53% at the 2-year follow-up.[44] When it does occur, retearing has been shown to have a poor prognosis with regard to patient function and pain relief.[71] These rates are the reason that patient selection and proper preoperative counseling are imperative for revision cuff repair. The failure of a revision cuff repair should be approached with extreme caution as an increased number of surgeries have been shown to directly correlate with an increased rate of complications and failures.[2]

FUTURE CONSIDERATIONS

Further investigation into biologic augmentation methods will have the greatest effect on the future of revision cuff surgery. Gene therapy and stem cell therapy could have a tremendous effect on optimizing the biology of the degenerating shoulder and help to prevent primary cuff failure and to improve the outcome of revisions.

For a complete list of references, go to ExpertConsult.com.

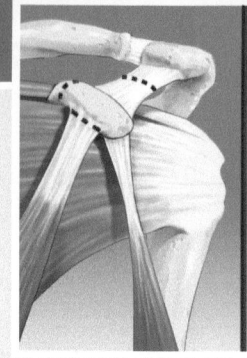

50

Other Muscle Injuries

James E. Voos, Derrick M. Knapik

Muscle injuries about the shoulder are increasingly common in active individuals, with the prevalence of upper extremity muscle sprains, strains, and ruptures rising as more athletes join gyms and engage in recreational and professional strength training and weight lifting.[1-3] However, these injuries remain inadequately described and defined despite their ability to cause significant functional disability, pain, and time lost from sport.[1]

PECTORALIS MAJOR

Injuries to the pectoralis major muscle occur primarily in males 20 to 40 years of age, with 75% of cases being secondary to sporting activities.[4] Weight lifting has been shown to be responsible for approximately 50% of reported cases in the literature,[5,6] with injuries also being reported in athletes participating in wrestling, jujitsu, American football, and gymnastics.[5-8] Although the vast majority of patients are young males, injuries in females have been reported.[9,10] Injuries are typically sustained secondary to violent, eccentric muscle contractions,[2] with operative repair yielding significantly improved outcomes and restoration of preinjury strength and activity level as compared with nonoperative management.[11]

Anatomy

The pectoralis major muscle covers the anterior chest wall and is composed of two separate heads (clavicular and sternal) that serve to adduct, internally rotate, and flex the shoulder.[4] The muscle originates as a broad sheet from the clavicle, sternum, ribs, and external oblique fascia, with the two heads converging and inserting over a 5-cm area on the lateral lip of the bicipital groove of the humerus.[2] The tendons are hypothesized to twist 90 degrees,[11] 180 degrees,[12] or simply to overlap at their insertion,[13] resulting in the inferior (sternal) segment inserting proximal to the more distal insertion of the superior (clavicular) segment on the humerus.[2,4] Because of this configuration, the fibers of the sternal segment experience increased excursion with the arm in 0 to 30 degrees of extension, as experienced during bench press, resulting in maximal stretching of the tendon fibers and increasing the risk for rupture.[4,11,14] The pectoralis major muscle is innervated by the medial (lower sternocostal segments) and lateral (clavicular segments) pectoral nerves arising from the C5 to T1 nerve roots.[15]

Mechanisms

The majority of injuries to the pectoralis major are secondary to substantial contraction applied to the distal tendon while it is maximally stretched,[2] with direct trauma to the shoulder and arm being less common.[6,11,16] Multiple studies have found that the most common mechanism of injury was the bench press,[3,17,18] in which the abducted, extended, and externally rotated arm is eccentrically contracted, placing the pectoralis tendon under maximal tension.[2,4] Owing to the anatomic configuration of the tendons distally, application of maximal load results in a significant mechanical disadvantage to the fibers of the inferior sternal segment of the pectoralis major, thus often causing them to rupture and accounting for the high incidence of sternal head ruptures.[11,17] Although partial ruptures are more common, up to 65% of complete ruptures have been reported to occur at the humeral insertion, with up to 29% occurring at the musculotendinous junction.[5,6] Moreover, distal tendon injuries are more likely to be complete ruptures.[2] Injuries to the muscle belly or the clavicular and sternal origins of the pectoralis major are less common and usually result from direct trauma.[1]

Other mechanisms—including direct trauma sustained during American football and rugby[3] along with other sporting activities associated with a risk of rapid, forceful shoulder abduction, such as rodeo, windsurfing, sailing, handball, wrestling, hockey, and artistic gymnastics[19-23]—have been described. In addition, injuries have also been described in individuals attempting to break a fall in which the force of impaction on the ground on the contracted muscles results in injury.[1,2]

Abuse of anabolic steroids has been tied to an increased risk for tendon ruptures.[24,25] Pochini et al.[3] have reported that in 60 patients with complete ruptures, more than 90% endorsed anabolic steroid use, whereas Aarimaa et al.[19] point to a 36% rate of abuse in their case series of 33 patients. Other authors have proposed that steroids weaken and stiffen the tendon fibers secondary to tendinopathy.[3,19,24] Concomitant with disproportionate gains in muscle mass and force,[3,6,8,9,19] the weakened tendon is overwhelmed, resulting in rupture with continued stress placed across the tendon with weight lifting.

Classification

Injuries to the pectoralis major are generally classified using the classification system proposed by Tietjen et al.,[26] which describes the site of the lesion without accounting for the severity (partial versus complete), timing (acute versus chronic), or segments of involvement (sternal versus clavicular head).[3,4] A recent meta-analysis by El Maraghy and Devereaux[5] proposed a new classification scale focusing on lesion acuity (acute or chronic), the qualitative degree of tendon involvement (incomplete versus complete), and the location of the rupture (muscle, musculotendinous junction, or humerus).

Physical Examination

In addition to a thorough history, a comprehensive physical examination is essential for diagnosis and to ensure proper clinical decision-making while ruling out concomitant injuries in and around the shoulder. Acute ruptures to the distal tendons present with edema, ecchymosis, and hematoma to the lateral chest and proximal arm, while injuries to the sternal or clavicular origins are isolated over the anterior chest wall. Patient typically report hearing or feeling a popping or tearing sensation at the time of injury, accompanied by pain in the chest wall, axilla, or down the arm.[4,27] Examination will demonstrate weakness with concomitant discomfort with resisted adduction, forward flexion, and internal rotation, along with tenderness at the axilla and humeral insertion.[1,4,28] Further inspection may reveal an asymmetric prominence from hematoma or from retraction of the muscle belly near the axilla.[4] As swelling subsides, examination of the axillary fold may demonstrate a palpable defect in the anterior axilla, accompanied by thinning, hollowing, or loss of the fold accentuated with isometric contraction with adduction as the patient presses the hands against one another in the front of the chest.[8,11] Patients may also demonstrate a visibly retracted stump within the anterior axillary fold on lateral inspection of the arm during forward flexion, known as the "S" sign.[4] Asymmetric webbing of the axilla is commonly reported to describe the loss of musculature from the anterior wall of the axilla.[10] Whereas some authors describe the ability to differentiate full-thickness tears from partial tears by the presence of a distinct gap or defect,[4] lack of a palpable defect in the axilla has not been shown to be a reliable indicator of pectoralis continuity.[1] In cases of chronic tendon injuries, patients may develop a prominent skin fold, known as cicatricial fibrosis, along with webbing and prominence of the distal deltoid insertion.[7,11] Retraction of the tendon and muscle with appreciable asymmetry is more pronounced as compared with the intact contralateral side in chronic tears as well.

Imaging

In the setting of suspected injury to the pectoralis major, plain radiographs are of limited use; however, they are essential to assess for bony abnormalities and avulsions, which are reported to occur in 2% to 5% of cases.[5,6,10] Furthermore, radiographs allow for assessment of the glenohumeral joint, as concomitant dislocations of the shoulder have been reported.[29] Magnetic resonance imaging (MRI) is the modality of choice for assessing the site (muscle belly, tendon, or myotendinous junction) and degree of tendon injury,[6,12,25,30] with axial oblique and coronal views offering the best visualization.[2] Acute tears can be distinguished from chronic tears on MRI by high signal intensity at

the musculotendinous junction on T2-weighed images owing to hemorrhage and edema with visualization of tendon and muscle retraction or tendon-bone discontinuity.[25,30] Chronic tears demonstrate low signal intensity and muscle retraction, suggestive of fibrosis and scarring.[30] Studies reporting on the correlation of findings on MRI with those of surgery have found excellent correlations based on the extent and location of injury.[2,12,31] MRI of the chest wall instead of the shoulder along with external rotation of the arm may improve visualization and aid in proper diagnosis.[4,32] However, investigations have found that MRI may not successfully identify or allow for complete differentiation of the affected portions of the pectoralis muscle or tendon.[12,25] Therefore advanced imaging modalities should serve only to complement the clinical examination.

Treatment

The treatment of pectoralis injuries depends on the extent and location of tearing as well as the activity level of the patient. Conservative management is recommended for strains, contusions, muscle belly ruptures, and partial tears as well as complete tears in low-demand sedentary individuals.[4,6] Treatment involves rest, ice, pain control, and sling immobilization with the arm adducted and internally rotated.[8,33] Patients treated conservatively have demonstrated good functional outcomes with the ability to perform activities of daily living and no significant limitations.[11,17,34] Reported complications include hematoma, abscess formation, incision breakdown, and myositis ossifans as well as cosmetic defects or persistent deficits in strength, especially in younger patients.[33,35]

Surgery is reserved for young, active individuals suffering complete tears, including those to the sternal head/posterior lamina,[9] tears at the myotendinous junction, intratendinous tears, or those at the tendon insertion.[4] Surgery is recommended to allow for restoration of normal strength, allowing active athletes to successfully return to sport at preinjury levels.[2,6,20] Multiple techniques for fixation in the acute period have been reported, including suturing tendon to periosteum[17] or remaining tendon[16] in addition to bony fixation using drill holes through the humerus fixed with anchors,[36] screws, and washers[7] or endosteal buttons (Fig. 50.1). Studies have found that young, active patients treated surgically experience significantly better excellent/good functional outcome scores,[2,6,7] improvement in strength,[11,37] and patient satisfaction,[23] cosmesis, pain control, and return to sport as compared with those treated nonoperatively.[3,6,7,11,27,33,37] Reported complications following operative management include postoperative stiffness, hypertrophic scarring, infection, and recurrent tearing.[2,11,18,38]

The timing from injury to repair has been shown to influence the ease of repair and subsequent outcomes, with authors recommending surgical treatment as soon as possible.[3] Currently, no consensus exists on the definition in timing for acute tears, with multiple studies citing 2 weeks,[23] 3 weeks, 6 weeks,[19,39,40] and up to 8 weeks.[6] Compared with outcomes following operative management of chronic tears, authors have cited statistically better outcomes with treatment occurring soon after injury in the acute phase.[3,6,19,39] This is because the repair of chronic injuries requires increased surgical exposure and dissection owing to

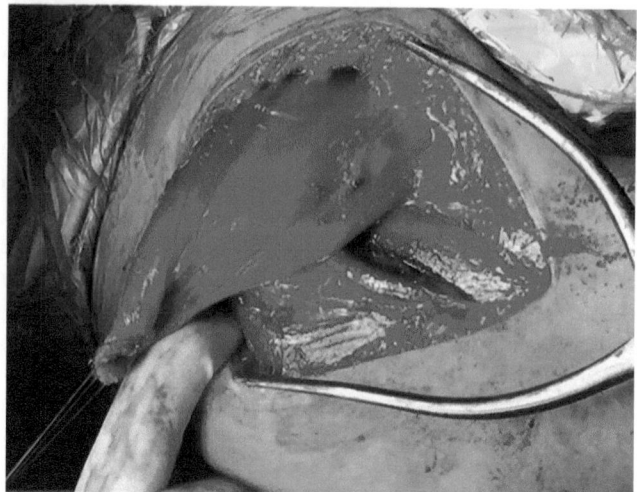

Fig. 50.1 Intraoperative photo demonstrating fixation of acute pectoralis major tearing using suture fixation to the distal tendon.

muscle retraction and fibrosis.[5] Moreover, direct repair can be difficult or impossible, necessitating reconstruction using allograft or autograft augmentation.[4] Reconstruction has been described using human- and animal-derived patches, hamstring augmentation,[7] Achilles tendon allograft,[41] fascia lata allograft,[42] flexor tendon grafts,[43] and bone patellar tendon autograft.[44]

LATISSIMUS DORSI

Injuries to the latissimus dorsi are rarely reported; they are limited to case reports, small case series, and retrospective analyses. Ruptures have been noted to occur in baseball pitchers, golfers, and participants in rodeos, tennis matches, wrestling, water skiing, and rock climbing.[45–53] Complete tendon ruptures are generally season-ending injuries with lengthy rehabilitation and the potential for significant disability.[53]

Anatomy

The latissimus dorsi is a large triangular muscle originating from the spinous processes and supraspinous ligaments of T7-T12 along with the lumbar and sacral vertebrae, lumbar fascia, posterior third of the iliac crest, four most caudal ribs, and inferior angle of the scapula. The muscle spans across the posterior thoracolumbar region, converging into a thick fasciculus transitioning into a tendon that inserts on the floor of the bicipital (intertubercular) groove of the humerus via a conjoint tendon with the teres major.[54] The latissimus dorsi functions to adduct, extend, and internally rotate the humerus in addition to lifting the trunk forward and upward during climbing. Innervation is provided by the thoracodorsal nerve coming off of the posterior cord of the brachial plexus, which runs with the thoracodorsal artery, innervating the muscle on its anteroinferior surface approximately 2 cm medial to its muscular border.[55] Pearle et al. reported that the thoracodorsal pedicle, consisting of the artery and nerve, inserted on the anterior part of the latissimus dorsi muscle belly an average of 13.1 cm (range, 11.0 to 15.3 cm) medial to its humeral insertion.[56]

Mechanisms

Strains, tears, and ruptures to the latissimus are generally sustained from a sudden power extension or hyperabduction force applied to the arm or shoulder.[49] The majority of reported cases have occurred in baseball pitchers,[45,53] in whom the latissimus dorsi has been shown to be active during several phases of the pitching cycle, especially during late cocking and serving. These movements are among the most powerful generators of force during the acceleration phase.[57] The role of the latissimus during pitching effectively places an eccentric force across the distal tendon attachment, increasing the risk of injury and rupture.[53] Moreover, a number of pitchers report sensing the injury and most of the pain during the follow-through phase, accounting for the continued role of the latissimus during the deceleration phase of pitching.[53] Activation of the latissimus during the pitching cycle has been noted to be higher among professional pitchers versus amateur pitchers.[58] Athletes generally report a "popping" or tearing sensation to the posterior aspect of the shoulder; however, evolving tightness and fatigue to the posterior shoulder have also been reported.[53]

Classification

Because of the rarity of the injury, no classification system in the literature has been proposed to date.

Physical Examination

Athletes generally seek medical attention as a result of loss of power with pain in the shoulder that limits athletic and overhead activities. Athletes may also complain of a burning pain to the superior aspect of the triceps area, along with ecchymosis.[52] The most significant deficit in strength has been reported in shoulder extension.[48] In addition, individuals will possess decreased strength with both isometric internal rotation and adduction of the arm; however, athletes may maintain excellent strength with these movements secondary to the recruitment of adjacent muscles.[52] A palpable mass, indicative of a retracted latissimus muscle belly or hematoma, may be appreciated to the posterolateral aspect of the chest and shoulder girdle[52] (Fig. 50.2A and B), while the asymmetry is more pronounced with the arms abducted on the hips or with adduction and internal rotation of the shoulder against resistance.[49,52] Such individuals are generally without any neurologic deficits.

Imaging

No investigation has reported on the benefit of plain radiographs in the diagnosis of latissimus dorsi ruptures; however, ruling out fracture and dislocation is critical. Multiple studies have reported MRI as the most reliable modality to confirm diagnosis while also demonstrating the extent of injury along with ruling out concomitant lesions to the shoulder girdle (Fig. 50.3A–C).[49,53,59,60] Ultrasound in trained hands has also been reported to enable detection of muscle lesions.[59,60]

Treatment

Successful management of latissimus dorsi injuries has been reported with both operative[49,54,61] and nonoperative treatment.[46,52,53]

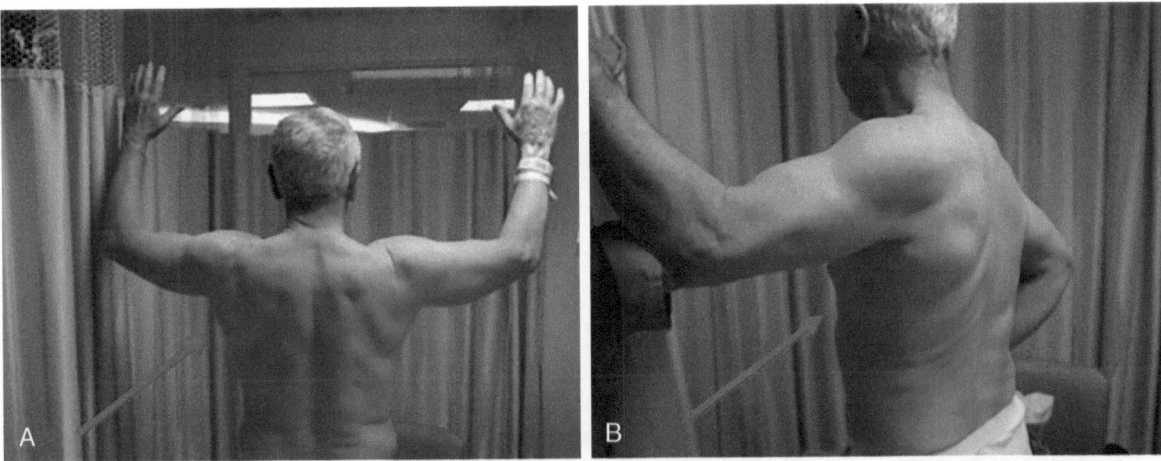

Fig. 50.2 Physical examination findings showing a palpable mass *(red arrows)* along the posterolateral aspect of the shoulder girdle as seen from the posterior and lateral views, indicative of a retracted latissimus dorsi rupture.

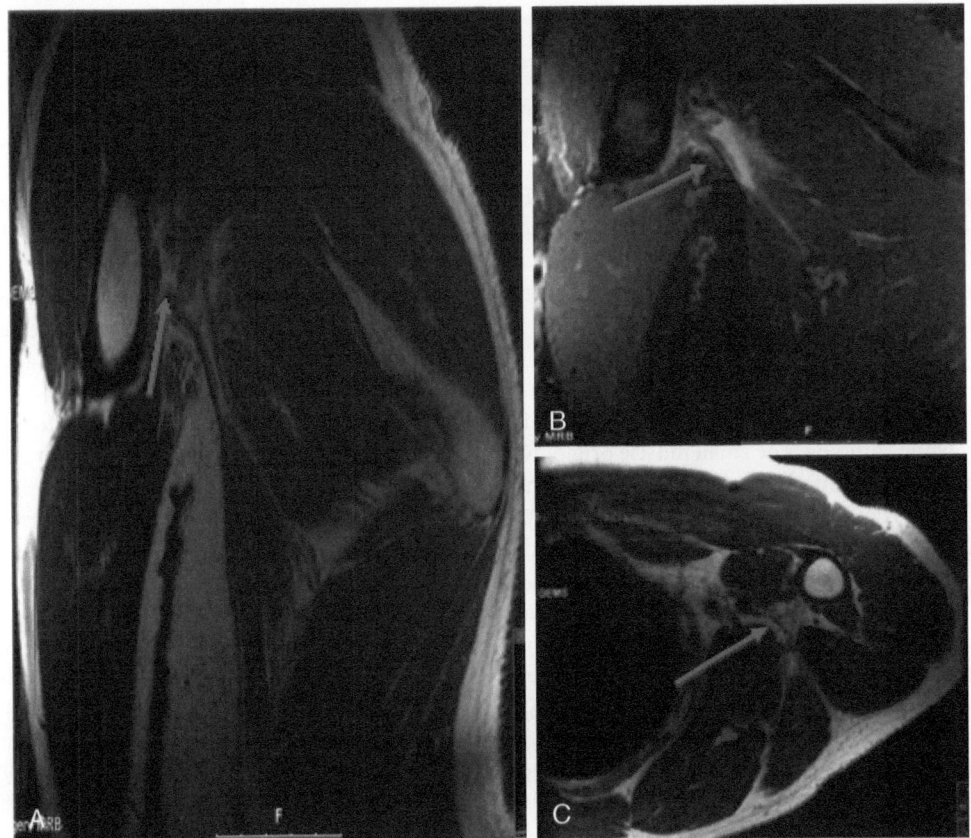

Fig. 50.3 Magnetic resonance imaging demonstrating complete rupture of the latissimus dorsi tendon *(red arrows)* in the sagittal (A), coronal (B), and axial (C) planes.

However, owing to the infrequency of reported cases, there is no consensus on the standard of care for these injuries or whether surgical intervention provides any advantages as compared with conservative management. In their treatment of 10 professional baseball pitchers including 3 with tendon avulsions and 7 with strains, Nagda et al.[53] reported that all but one athlete returned to the same or a higher level of play following rest for up to 28 days in addition to rehabilitation with advancement to a supervised throwing program. Athletes sustaining strains were reported to return to play (RTP) after 12 weeks and those with avulsions after 16 weeks. The authors did note, however, that avulsions were season-ending injuries and that the three pitchers who began throwing soonest experienced setbacks that prolonged the delay in their return to sport. Advocates of surgical intervention cite the restoration of preinjury strength and function in high-level athletes[48,51,62] with repairs becoming technically more challenging 2 or months following injury.[63] Operative techniques included repair of the tendon to the humeral footprint utilizing

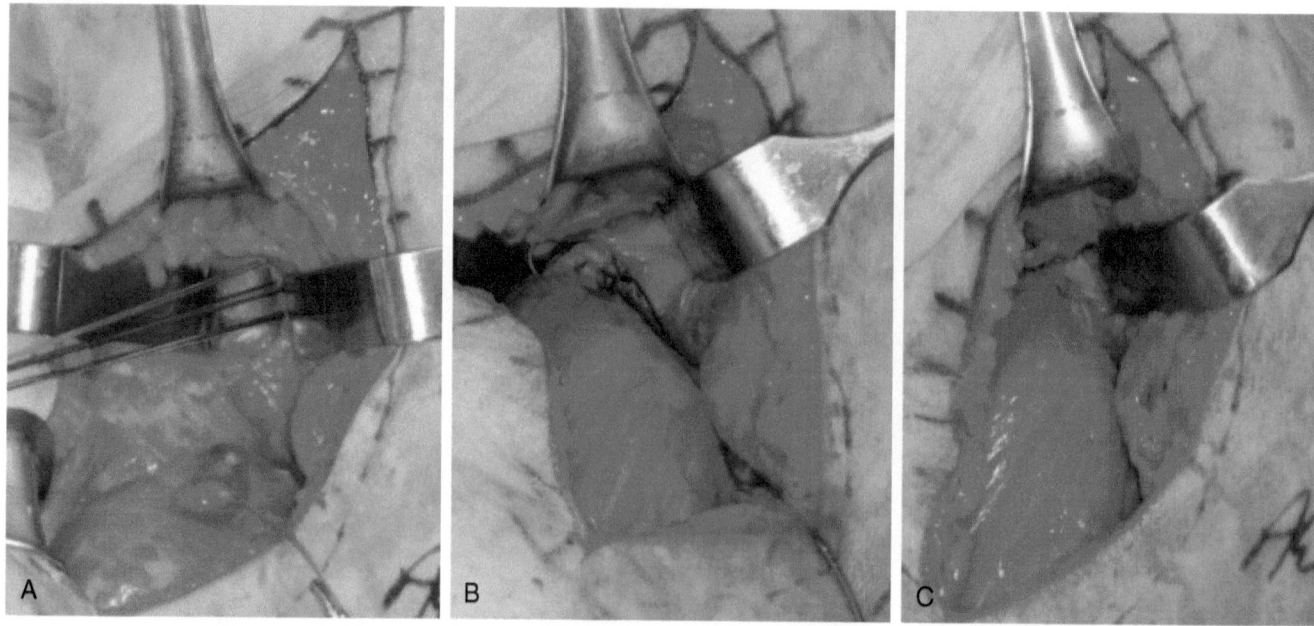

Fig. 50.4 Intraoperative photo demonstrating (A) placement of suture within the torn distal aspect of the latissimus dorsi followed by (B) placement of free suture ends through suture anchors to recreate the spiral anatomy of the tendon insertion with (C) final repair.

transosseous tunnels[47,51,63] or suture anchors (Fig. 50.4A–C).[62,63] In the limited studies reported in the literature, operative management has demonstrated good functional outcomes and restoration of strength in athletes,[46,49] with RTP usually reported 5 to 6 months following repair.

Teres Major

The teres major functions in pulling objects toward the body and lifting the body while climbing. The small muscle originates from the dorsal surface off the inferior angle of the scapula and inserts on the bicipital groove of the humerus via a conjoint tendon with the latissimus.[54] The largest series of cases, by Nagda et al.,[53] comprised 11 pitchers, among whom isolated injuries to the teres major were found in 6 (three avulsions and three strains), a combined latissimus/teres major avulsion in 1, and combined latissimus dorsi/teres major strains in 4. All were treated nonoperatively, with only one athlete not returning to play following arthroscopic superior labrum anterior and posterior (SLAP) repair. Other reported injuries to the teres major in the athletic population include an avulsion in a baseball pitcher[64,65] and another in a water skier who sustained an isolated tear caused by the arm being forced forward from a tow rope.[66] Although the teres major has been speculated to serve a function similar to that of the latissimus dorsi during the pitching cycle, no study examining the exact contribution of the teres major has been performed.[53] MRI is used to differentiate between injuries to the teres major versus latissimus dorsi, as individual discrimination on physical examination is difficult.[65] Although no consensus regarding optimal treatment has been presented in the literature, all reported cases in baseball pitchers have been treated nonoperatively with rest, rehabilitation, and gradual return to sport without any reported complications.

For a complete list of references, go to ExpertConsult.com.

SELECTED READINGS

de Castro Pochini A, Andreoli CV, Belangero PS, et al. Clinical considerations for the surgical treatment of pectoralis major muscle ruptures based on 60 cases: a prospective study and literature review. *Am J Sports Med.* 2014;42:95–102.

Bak K, Cameron EA, Henderson IJ. Rupture of the pectoralis major: a meta-analysis of 112 cases. *Knee Surg Sports Traumatol Arthrosc.* 2000;8:113–119.

Petilon J, Carr DR, Sekiya JK, et al. Pectoralis major muscle injuries: evaluation and management. *J Am Acad Orthop Surg.* 2005;13:59–68.

Butterwick DJ, Mohtadi NG, Meeuwisse WH, et al. Rupture of latissimus dorsi in an athlete. *Clin J Sport Med.* 2003;13:189–191.

Nagda SH, Cohen SB, Noonan TJ, et al. Management and outcomes of latissimus dorsi and teres major injuries in professional baseball pitchers. *Am J Sports Med.* 2011;39:2181–2186.

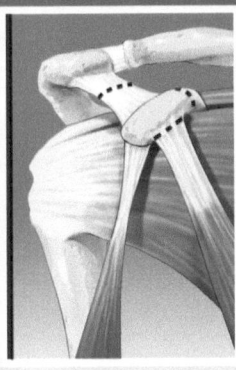

51

Stiff Shoulder

Jonathan Barlow, Andrew C. Mundy, Grant L. Jones

The structural anatomy of the glenohumeral articulation affords considerable range of motion (ROM) to the shoulder. The osseous and soft tissue structures provide limited yet sufficient static and dynamic restraints to allow significant motion not only for activities of daily living but also for high-level athletic endeavors. At one end of the motion spectrum is shoulder instability, a pathologic and symptomatic condition in which the humeral head is unable to stay seated on the glenoid. At the other end of the continuum is the stiff shoulder. A vast range of clinical encounters and diagnoses encompass the stiff shoulder, both traumatic and atraumatic.

Patients with a stiff shoulder may present with a brief or long-standing persistent loss of motion. The shoulder may be stiff and/or painful. The treating physician may be the first to evaluate and manage these patients. However, many patients have already seen several clinicians and have undergone both nonoperative and operative treatments that have either been unsuccessful or only partially successful. It is not uncommon to encounter a frustrated and discouraged patient. It is also not uncommon to see patients who are unaware that they are stiff and whose perception of the primary issue is pain and, less commonly, motion loss. Thus the stiff shoulder is a commonly encountered diagnostic and therapeutic challenge. This chapter discusses the framework for evaluation, management, and outcomes of patients with a stiff shoulder.

HISTORY

The ability to obtain an accurate history is a key component of establishing a correct diagnosis. Obtaining an accurate history requires not only asking specific questions pertinent to a chief complaint but also *actively* listening and responding with successive adaptive questions related to the patient's responses. The treating physician must recognize that the presence of pathology on advanced imaging (radiographs and magnetic resonance imaging [MRI]) is quite common in asymptomatic patients. Conversely, patients with minimal MRI changes may have severe clinical diseases, especially in the setting of frozen shoulder. Thus the history and physical examination are *the only way* to determine if patients' complaints are concurrent with imaging findings ("treat the patient and not the MRI").

Often the history of a present illness can all but definitively lead to a diagnosis before the patient is even examined or images are reviewed when assessing a stiff shoulder. Characterization of the principal symptoms attributable to the chief complaint should describe seven entities[1]: location, quality, severity, timing (i.e., onset, duration, and frequency), setting, exacerbating and relieving factors, and associated manifestations. Patient demographics and epidemiology also must not be overlooked, especially age and gender, because these factors play a significant role in evaluating the stiff shoulder. More than two thirds of patients with a frozen shoulder are female.[2] Rotator cuff tears are an age-related phenomenon, along with the risk of stiffness associated with their operative or nonoperative management.[3]

Pain

Pain is usually the patient's chief presenting complaint. Patients less often report stiffness, although the two frequently coexist. To understand how a painful, stiff shoulder is affecting one's daily life, several descriptors of pain must be established with explicit questioning adapted to each response given by the patient (Box 51.1). Pain is a difficult parameter to analyze because it is a wholly subjective complaint that, despite numerical scales, cannot be compared between individuals. It is the physician's perception of the patient's pain that often guides management. The two most common reasons that pain drives a patient to seek medical attention are severity and timing (Box 51.2).

Severe pain brought on acutely by trauma generally mandates medical care soon after the injury occurs. Underlying differential diagnoses include fracture, dislocation, rotator cuff tear, biceps tendon (long head or distal/elbow) tear, pectoralis major tear, and labral tear. Further examination with or without imaging can typically lead to an accurate diagnosis in this situation. The pain attributed to adhesive capsulitis is usually minimal at rest but can become severely disabling at the end extremes of arc of motion (the freezing stage). With time, this pain usually minimizes to being present at just the extremes of motion while stiffness prevails in the frozen stage. However, by this point, many patients have been dealing with this for some time, and have grown frustrated. Intermittent severe pain is also common with compressive joint loads in persons with osteoarthritis and with calcific tendonitis (which is sometimes even referred to as the "kidney stone of the shoulder"). Patients who sustain an injury with minimal pain may not seek care for several weeks to months, if at all. Some patients do not even recall a clearly identifiable event that precipitated pain. However, in this situation, mild pain may lead to unappreciated chronic disuse or underuse of the extremity ("pseudoimmobilization" of the shoulder) and possibly incite a

BOX 51.1 Pain Descriptors to Be Evaluated

- Location (anterior, posterior, lateral, neck, back, arm, chest wall, or axilla)
- Radiation (neck, arm, below elbow, into hand)
- Quality (sharp, dull, achy, throbbing, or stabbing)
- Severity (mild, moderate, severe, or on a scale of 1–10)
- Timing
- Onset (acute, subacute, chronic, acute on chronic, insidious, traumatic, or atraumatic)
- Duration (days, weeks, months, years)
- Frequency (constant, once daily, weekly, monthly)
- Setting (at rest, at night, with activity, with throwing, when reaching behind the back, when lifting overhead)
- Exacerbating factors (activity, arm position, day/night)
- Relieving factors (activity, arm position, day/night, medications, therapy, injection, surgery)
- Associated conditions (weakness, numbness/paresthesias, crepitus, instability)

BOX 51.2 Unique Pain Descriptors

Severe Pain
Trauma (fracture, dislocation, tendon tear)
Adhesive capsulitis
Calcific tendonitis
Postsurgical

Night Pain
Malignancy
Infection
Rotator cuff/impingement
Adhesive capsulitis
Shoulder arthrosis (glenohumeral, acromioclavicular)
Posterior capsule tightness/glenohumeral internal rotation deficit

Chronic Pain
Adhesive capsulitis
Rotator cuff/impingement
Shoulder arthrosis
Posttraumatic
Cervical spine

Location
Lateral arm/deltoid insertion (rotator cuff/impingement)
Neck/posterior periscapular (cervical spine, trapezius, adhesive capsulitis, scapular dyskinesis)
Anterior (long head biceps tendon)
"Top of the shoulder" (acromioclavicular joint, cervical spine)
"Deep in the shoulder" (infection, arthrosis, avascular necrosis)
Radiating distal to elbow (cervical radiculopathy)

stiffness response that may eventually warrant medical attention (e.g., rotator cuff tear and impingement).

Night Pain

Pain that awakens the patient from sleep (night pain) often compels the patient to seek care. Differential diagnoses in this situation include malignancy or infection but more commonly entail rotator cuff pathology, impingement, adhesive capsulitis, and shoulder arthrosis (glenohumeral or acromioclavicular arthritis). Pain may not only awaken the patient from sleep but also preclude sleep. Pain associated with adhesive capsulitis typically prevents a person from sleeping on the affected side. Pain that is present while lying on the unaffected side may be due to the across-body position of stretching the posterior capsule.

Chronic Pain

Patients with adhesive capsulitis often present with pain of an insidious onset that is localized to the joint line or around the deltoid insertion; the pain is gradually progressive and is associated with usually underappreciated degrees of shoulder stiffness. Often the pain may not be severe enough to warrant evaluation until it and the associated stiffness preclude performance of activities of daily living (e.g., reaching into the back pocket for a wallet, combing one's hair, getting dressed, and fastening a brassiere). Although patients with inflammatory shoulder arthropathies (e.g., rheumatoid arthritis) may have severe destructive radiographic disease, they have dealt with the pain and loss of function for such a long time that their description of chronic pain is typically inconsistent with their imaging. In these situations, it is important for the clinician to remember to treat the patient and not the radiograph. Patients with rotator cuff pathology who do not have acute tears often report chronic, dull, boring pain without a discrete time of onset. Often the pain is related to overhead activities or is aggravated by lifting the arm out with an extended elbow (increased moment arm).

Pain Localization

The location of pain is an important component in clinical diagnosis. In the shoulder, however, localization is poor, because the patient's perception of the location of pain often does not coincide with the actual source of pathology. Pain related to the neck (e.g., cervical radiculopathy) may begin proximal to the ear, jaw, or neck and radiate down the trapezius into the posterior periscapular region. True radiculopathy, however, radiates distal to the shoulder, usually to the hand into the appropriate dermatomal distribution. True intrinsic shoulder pathology typically does not radiate distal to the elbow. Posterior periscapular pain may also be noted in pathology related to glenohumeral joint stiffness (e.g., adhesive capsulitis) because it invokes greater use of the scapulothoracic articulation. Glenohumeral joint pathology is perceived down the arm around the deltoid insertion (e.g., rotator cuff and subacromial bursitis). Pain that is poorly localized or felt "deep in the shoulder" may be ascribed to glenohumeral osteoarthritis, rheumatoid arthritis, avascular necrosis, malignancy, or infection. Anterior shoulder pain may be attributable to long head biceps tendon pathology along the bicipital groove. Pain localized to "on top of the shoulder" is often related to the acromioclavicular joint, with radiation anteriorly and/or medially.

Exacerbating and Relieving Factors

Situational circumstances that aggravate a painful sensation often provide a clue to the diagnosis. Patients with adhesive capsulitis often have sudden worsening of severe pain at the end points of the arc of motion. Overhead motion and lifting with an extended arm worsens pain related to the rotator cuff or sub-acromial space (impingement). In athletes with glenohumeral internal rotation deficit (GIRD) whose sport entails throwing, the loss of internal rotation motion is related to timing during the season: dynamic GIRD early in the season (primarily a muscle spasm) can develop into a posteroinferior capsule contracture later in the season (as a result of repetitive microtrauma from early acceleration through deceleration during the throwing cycle). This pathology tends to manifest as tightness, discomfort, and loss of velocity that becomes greater in severity as the season progresses. Repetitive activity tends to exacerbate intraarticular pathology (e.g., arthrosis). Factors that relieve pain include motions, medications, and procedures. Persons with some condi-tions (e.g., adhesive capsulitis) report that nothing relieves pain. Patients with rotator cuff tendon pathology often find relief at night by sleeping with their arm over their head, which takes the tensile stress off the rotator cuff. Patients with cervical radicu-lopathy experience similar relief by reproducing the shoulder abduction relief test. An injection of local anesthetic also may help to localize a pain source depending on the pain relief response to the injection. This technique is especially valuable for the subacromial space and acromioclavicular joint. The response to injection may replicate the response to a surgical intervention, and this possibility should be adequately conveyed to the patient.

Other Findings (Stiffness, Weakness, Crepitus)

When pain is mild, other factors that limit function are usually stiffness, weakness, or crunching/grinding at the shoulder. Weak-ness is a common symptom in patients with a rotator cuff tear and neuromuscular dysfunction (e.g., cerebrovascular disease, a cervical spine disorder, Parsonage-Turner syndrome, a burner/stinger, and myasthenia gravis). Crepitus is commonly reported after surgery (especially after rotator cuff repair) and with rotator cuff tendonitis, subacromial bursitis, snapping scapula (i.e., scapulothoracic bursitis, a space-occupying mass, or dyskinesis), arthrosis, and instability.

One of the primary goals in diagnosing the stiff shoulder is determining the direction of motion loss. This determination allows the location of the pathologic process that is responsible for the motion deficit to be deduced, thereby pointing to the methods necessary to treat it. For example, global loss of both active and passive motion reflects idiopathic adhesive capsulitis. Early in the disease process, loss of external rotation in the adducted arm is attributable to rotator interval contracture.[4] The shoulder of an athlete whose sport involves throwing may lose internal rotation with the arm abducted (GIRD), which is attributable to tightness of the posterior capsule.[5] The latter two conditions are only two among many shoulder and non–shoulder-related pathologies contributing to a stiff shoulder (Box 51.3).

Primary/Idiopathic Adhesive Capsulitis

In 1934, Codman[6] described a clinical condition of glenohumeral stiffness that he called "frozen shoulder." The term *idiopathic adhesive capsulitis* was then coined by Neviaser[7] in 1945 to describe pathologic conditions in stiff shoulder capsules. Neviaser described findings of fibrosis, chronic inflammation, and capsular con-tracture that were responsible for the pathologic loss of motion.

BOX 51.3   Pathologies Causing a Stiff Shoulder

Primary/Idiopathic
Idiopathic adhesive capsulitis
Type I and II diabetes mellitus
Endocrinopathy, including thyroid disorders
Autoimmune disease

Secondary/Acquired
Postoperative stiffness
Posttraumatic
Rotator cuff tear
Glenohumeral arthrosis
Glenoid labral tear
Fracture malunion
Thrower's shoulder (glenohumeral internal rotation deficit)

The terms *frozen shoulder* and *adhesive capsulitis* are used inter-changeably, leading to confusion and ambiguity in shoulder stiffness nomenclature literature. Inconsistencies in disease clas-sification, diagnosis, staging, and treatment have led to further uncertainty in the literature. Although the disease is commonly believed to be self-limiting, the true natural history is not defini-tively known.[8] Adhesive capsulitis may affect up to 5% of the population, with a greater preponderance in women.[9] The con-dition tends to affect middle-aged patients[10] in their nondominant arm[2] with a variable history of minor trauma (up to 30%). A link between adhesive capsulitis and lower body mass index and positive family history has also been described.[11] Development of adhesive capsulitis in the contralateral shoulder will occur in approximately one third of patients.[9] The disease does not seem to recur in the same shoulder.[2]

Adhesive capsulitis has been associated with other systemic conditions that have an apparent lack of innate relation to the shoulder. The most commonly associated systemic disease is diabetes mellitus.[11–14] In a large retrospective review of diabetics with adhesive capsulitis, Yian et al.[15] showed a correlation between adhesive capsulitis and the use of insulin or oral glycemic agents, suggesting that diabetics requiring more aggressive glycemic management tend to be predisposed to an increased risk of adhesive capsulitis; however, hemoglobin (Hgb)A1c, in and of itself, did not appear to have a direct correlation. Importantly, patients with adhesive capsulitis and diabetes tend to be more difficult to manage, with less clinical improvement and higher rates of recurrence, especially in patients with peripheral neu-ropathy, patients who have had a longer duration of time since the diagnosis of diabetes, and older patients.[16] Both hypothyroid-ism[17,18] and hyperthyroidism[19] have also been observed with adhesive capsulitis, with some suggestion that higher thyroid stimulating hormone (TSH) levels may be independently linked with bilateral and more severe cases.[18] Dupuytren contracture, an inherited condition of the hand characterized by digital flexion contracture and adhesions, has also been associated with adhesive capsulitis.[20] Although autoimmune disease has been suggested to be an associated condition,[21] autoimmune serology testing has proved to be inconclusive.[10,22]

The true cause of adhesive capsulitis remains unknown. Nevertheless, a progression of stages (freezing, frozen, and thawed stages) has been cited and is often used in the literature.[23] Initially the instigation of a fibrinous hypervascular, hypertrophic synovitis leads to capsular scarring and loss of the axillary fold (the freezing stage). The precipitating factor may be related to a fibrotic cascade involving inflammatory cytokines, including transforming growth factor-β,[24] tumor necrosis factor α, interleukins, or cyclooxygenase 1 or 2.[25] These various cytokines have been found to be markedly elevated in the subacromial space and capsular tissue in patients with adhesive capsulitis.[25]

Pain is often moderate to severe, especially at night.[23] Once resolution of the synovitis occurs, a dense hypercellular collagenous fibrotic capsule remains, which exhibits significant stiffness (frozen stage). Pain is improved and is generally present only at the ends of motion and at night.[23] Adhesions and stiffness variably persist, both in severity and in duration. Pain eventually minimizes or resolves completely (thawed stage).[10] Despite the lack of a well-defined natural history, Grey[26] reported that 96% of patients with a minimum of 2 years of follow-up had normal function with reassurance and use of oral pain medication. At 4-year follow-up, Miller et al.[14] reported that 100% of patients had normal function and minimal pain with home-based therapy and use of oral antiinflammatory medications. In contrast, O'Kane et al.[27] reported that up to 40% of patients could not lift an 8-lb object onto a shelf or a 20-lb object at their side at 2-year follow-up. Further, Binder et al.[9] reported on 16 patients with residual mild to severe limited motion at 3.5-year follow-up. At longer follow-up (more than 4 years), residual pain and lost motion has also been reported in up to half of patients.[2,28]

Secondary/Acquired Causes of Shoulder Stiffness

Postoperative loss of motion is the most common acquired cause of shoulder stiffness. The incidence of stiffness after arthroscopic and open-shoulder surgery is variable but nonetheless is an ever-present risk that must be discussed with patients before undertaking elective shoulder surgery. Intraarticular arthroscopic shoulder surgery (e.g., labral repair for instability or superior labral anterior to posterior [SLAP] repair) generally leads to intraarticular adhesions and capsular contracture, but not extraarticular contracture.[29] Rotator cuff repair (both open and arthroscopic) and fracture fixation may result in subacromial adhesions in addition to capsular contracture.[29] Huberty et al.[30] reported that after arthroscopic rotator cuff repair, patient dissatisfaction due to stiffness was observed in 4.9% of nearly 500 repairs. Further, patients with Workers' Compensation status (9%) and who were younger than 50 years (9%) were more likely to be dissatisfied as a result of stiffness.[30] A systematic review by Denard et al.[31] reported stiffness outcomes after arthroscopic rotator cuff repair for seven Level I through IV evidence studies. In this review it was found that the incidence of transient stiffness that was responsive to nonoperative treatment and resistant stiffness requiring surgical release was 10% and 3.3%, respectively. Further, the outcomes of patients requiring a repeat operation were successful in that their motion improved to a level comparable with that of the persons who did not require a repeat operation. Stiffness after instability surgery (anterior[32–34] and posterior[33,35]) is also common, especially

in cases that involve loss of external rotation, although to some degree, this is the goal of the surgery: to prevent instability. This treatment requires a balance of safe immobilization for healing but early enough motion to prevent stiffness. Nevertheless, if postoperative immobilization is continued for too long or the capsule is overtightened intraoperatively, patients are at risk for stiffness. After SLAP repair, stiffness is a common cause of pain and dissatisfaction.[32,36,37]

Patients with shoulder arthrosis (e.g., primary glenohumeral arthritis or rheumatoid arthritis) also have a tendency toward stiffness. Joint capsule thickening, especially anteriorly and in the rotator interval in persons with osteoarthritis, correlates to motion loss, especially with external rotation.[38] In addition, early findings in persons with primary glenohumeral osteoarthritis include loss of internal rotation as a result of posterior capsular contracture. In these situations, stiffness often leads to unsatisfied patients who are experiencing pain. In patients with osteoarthritis who underwent arthroplasty (total shoulder and hemiarthroplasty) in four randomized clinical trials, stiffness improved significantly at final follow-up, with a greater degree of motion improvement, especially forward elevation, in patients who underwent total shoulder arthroplasty.[38] In a subset of patients with shoulder stiffness after arthroplasty, it must be ascertained whether loss of motion is due to true adhesion formation or component malpositioning. In patients with component malpositioning, stiffness surgery is likely to be unsuccessful unless the underlying reason, the malaligned prosthesis, is addressed.

Patients undergoing surgical intervention for subacromial impingement and acromioclavicular joint arthritis have also been shown to develop secondary stiff shoulder.[39] Evans et al.[39] found an ~5% risk of developing adhesive capsulitis postoperatively in patients who have had an isolated subacromial decompression or in conjunction with arthroscopic distal clavicle excision. Additionally, it was found that history of contralateral adhesive capsulitis and an age between 46 and 60 years old were independent risk factors for developing secondary stiff shoulder.

In patients who have subacromial impingement without a rotator cuff may have significant posterior capsule tightness (correlating with loss of internal rotation) in their dominant arms and a more global capsule tightness (correlating with loss of internal and external rotation) in their nondominant arms.[40] Athletes with internal impingement whose sport involves throwing have also been shown to have significant GIRD and posterior shoulder tightness.[41] The shoulder used in throwing is an amazing example of adaptation of a joint to the repetitive high forces generated during the throwing motion. The motion disparity (excessive external rotation and loss of internal rotation) has been theorized to be due to both bony (humeral head retroversion) and soft tissue (static capsule and dynamic muscular tightness) adaptations.[42] Further, throwers with GIRD have a higher risk of shoulder injury and need for shoulder surgery, which emphasizes the need for preemptive therapy to increase motion early when minor motion discrepancies are detected.[42] In patients with internal impingement that is treated with physical therapy (posterior capsule stretching), symptom resolution is thought to be related to correction of posterior shoulder tightness (measured via cross-body adduction) but not GIRD correction.[43] For further information regarding this topic, the reader is referred to Chapter 45, which pertains to throwing injuries.

PHYSICAL EXAMINATION

The physical examination for a person with a stiff shoulder—as with the physical examination of all shoulders—should be comprehensive and systematic, which allows for consistency and reproducibility while permitting the clinician to consider different causes. As with the questioning involved in obtaining a comprehensive history, the physical examination should be adaptive. When a thorough history indicates that a patient has a stiff, painful, or weak shoulder, the physical examination techniques performed should focus on these subjective symptoms. Physical assessment of any joint requires visual inspection (with men disrobed and women gowned to maintain modesty), palpation, motion, strength, and special testing (e.g., relating to instability, the rotator cuff, and the biceps tendon). To ascertain whether pathology exists in the involved shoulder, the clinician must also thoroughly examine the contralateral shoulder. Extensions of the physical examination of the shoulder may require examination of the cervical spine and elbow, wrist, and hand.

Physical Examination of the Stiff Shoulder

The key physical examination finding to distinguish adhesive capsulitis from other causes of shoulder stiffness is a similar loss of both active and passive ROM. As discussed in the History section, loss of external rotation commonly results from anterior shoulder tightness (attributed to the anterior capsule, rotator interval, anteroinferior capsule, and glenohumeral ligaments). The most common diagnoses related to the anterior shoulder tightness include adhesive capsulitis, glenohumeral osteoarthritis, postanterior instability surgery stiffness, and postimmobilization (effectively shortening the anterior structures). Stiffness with internal rotation movements are experienced while trying to reach behind the back, toward the back pocket of one's trousers, and occasionally across the body. Motion loss here may be attributed to the posterior capsule and often the shoulder capsule as a whole. The most common diagnoses related to the latter pathology include adhesive capsulitis, articular-sided partial rotator cuff tears, posterior capsule tightness, and glenohumeral internal rotation deficit. In addition to pathology that is primarily related to the shoulder, stiffness may be present from non-shoulder etiologies including axillary node dissection (especially with perioperative radiation therapy), cervical node dissection, elbow or arm conditions (especially if immobilization is required), and systemic conditions (e.g., diabetes, thyroid, cardiopulmonary, and neuromuscular disease).

Inspection

Thorough inspection of the shoulder requires observation of the entire upper extremity, neck, and upper thorax. Simultaneous inspection of both shoulders allows immediate comparison for signs of trauma (e.g., ecchymosis, abrasion, laceration, deformity, and bony prominence), atrophy (e.g., the deltoid or rotator cuff) (Fig. 51.1), infection (e.g., erythema), and prior surgical incisions. Often patients may not recall the timing or number

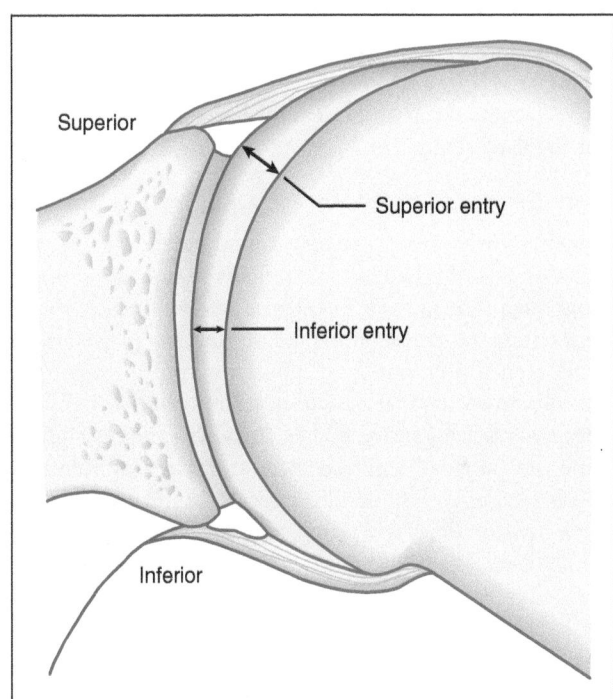

Fig. 51.1 Posterior view of bilateral atrophy of the infraspinous fossa related to infraspinatus atrophy. (From Lippitt SB, Rockwood Jr CA, Matsen III FA, et al. *The Shoulder.* 4th ed. Vol 1. Philadelphia: Elsevier; 2009.)

of prior surgical procedures (or even their existence, in some situations), but observation of an anterior deltopectoral approach for remote shoulder dislocations may provide a clue to the examiner regarding the open procedure performed. Further, although the patient may not recall why the procedure was performed, a superior shoulder saber incision (relating to the rotator cuff or acromioclavicular joint), an axillary incision (for node dissection), a cervical spine incision (relating to cranial nerve XI or a spinal accessory nerve injury leading to lateral scapular winging), or a chest wall incision/laceration (pertaining to a long thoracic nerve injury leading to medial scapular winging) may assist in evaluation. A prominent acromioclavicular joint may indicate arthrosis. The appearance of a superior fluid bulge may indicate subacromial effusion extension as a sign of a chronic massive rotator cuff tear. Static or dynamic scapular winging may indicate a neurologic injury or dysfunctional muscular coordination. Often the appearance of an atraumatic stiff shoulder without prior shoulder conditions may reveal no obvious pathology.

Palpation

All joints, bony surfaces and prominences, and soft tissue structures are palpated for tenderness, crepitus, deformity, or any asymmetry. The sternoclavicular and acromioclavicular joints, anterior and posterior glenohumeral joint lines, and elbow and wrist joints are inspected. Bony prominences that are palpated include the cervical spinous processes, the clavicle, the scapular spine, the acromion, the coracoid, the greater and lesser tuberosities, and the humerus. Soft tissue structures that are palpated include the paraspinal, trapezius, and periscapular muscles, the deltoid, the supraspinous and infraspinous fossae, the supraspinatus insertion, the long head biceps tendon, and the muscles and tendons of the arm and forearm. Although primary adhesive capsulitis may demonstrate diffuse, nonspecific, poorly localized tenderness, secondary/acquired causes may easily be ascertained with palpation of involved structures.

Motion, Strength, and Special Testing

Assessment of motion and strength around the shoulder requires examination of *both* shoulders in both passive and active motion. Although each clinician may have his or her own specific routine for performing the examination and minimizing patient movement between sitting, standing, supine, and prone positions, it is important to ensure that a complete examination is performed and documented for every patient. It is also often helpful to examine the "normal" uninvolved shoulder before examining the involved shoulder. In addition, cervical spine motion (e.g., flexion/extension, lateral bending, and axial rotation) must be assessed. The cardinal planes of motion evaluated include scapular plane (30 degrees off the coronal plane of the body) elevation, external rotation in the adducted arm, and internal rotation behind the back using a spinal column reference. Other planes commonly assessed include elevation in the sagittal plane, internal and external rotation at 90-degree abduction, and abduction in the coronal plane. Total shoulder motion is assessed because it is not possible to isolate the individual (glenohumeral, acromioclavicular, sternoclavicular, and scapulothoracic) articulations around the shoulder. Stabilization of the scapula posteriorly helps reduce the scapulothoracic contribution to shoulder motion (which is possible by having the patient lie on the examination table supine), thus illustrating a greater proportion of glenohumeral motion. As previously discussed, the key physical examination finding (and sometimes the only finding) for diagnosis of primary adhesive capsulitis is the equal loss of both active and passive motion. This fundamental characteristic helps distinguish primary adhesive capsulitis from rotator cuff pathology (e.g., pseudoparalysis). Further, the contracted capsule in a person with adhesive capsulitis often gives a tethered end point sense at the end of motion, which is different from the loss of motion limited by pain.

Assessment of muscle strength is performed using a common grading system (Box 51.4). Deltoid testing should assess the

anterior, middle, and posterior fibers anteriorly in the sagittal plane, abducted in the coronal plane, and posteriorly in the sagittal plane, respectively. Rotator cuff strength may be tested with a combination of special tests. Rotator cuff strength is usually normal in patients with primary adhesive capsulitis, although it may be limited by pain. Similarly, long head biceps tendon and superior labral pathology may be assessed using the Yergason, Speed, and O'Brien tests, although pain from adhesive capsulitis may limit the utility of these tests in severe cases. Scapular dyskinesis special testing is also warranted as indicated by other parts of the history and physical examination. These tests include simple observation posteriorly of repetitive arm elevation (looking for dysfunctional muscle activation, which is often apparent as winging), the scapular assist test, the scapular stabilization test, and the wall push-up test. Patients with a tight glenohumeral joint often exhibit proportionally increased scapulothoracic compensatory motion, which may induce dyskinesis and scapulothoracic crepitus. Special testing of the cervical spine includes the Spurling maneuver and shoulder abduction relief test to identify cervical radicular signs. The Adson maneuver to assess for thoracic outlet syndrome is also performed as indicated. Thorough neurovascular testing requires bilateral assessment of pulses, reflexes, and dermatomal distribution sensation. Findings of a neurovascular examination in persons with primary adhesive capsulitis is often normal.

IMAGING

Imaging findings for a person with a stiff shoulder often are not helpful in evaluating the idiopathic frozen shoulder. Although plain radiographs do not reveal pathognomonic findings for adhesive capsulitis, they are helpful in identifying and ruling out other common causes of the stiff shoulder, such as primary glenohumeral and acromioclavicular osteoarthritis, cuff tear arthropathy, pathology after a trauma (e.g., a nonoperative or operative fracture), postdislocation arthropathy (if anchors have been placed in the glenoid), postarthroscopic glenohumeral chondrolysis, and calcific tendonitis.

Other imaging modalities include MRI and ultrasound. Some MRI changes have been described in patients with frozen shoulder. The presence of edema in the axillary recess may be associated with pain intensity and the degree of capsular thickness is more robust in early stages of adhesive capsulitis.[44] Carbone et al.[45] described the presence of a high intensity signal in the subscapular recess on T2-weighted images as having a high degree of specificity (0.96 to 0.98) and sensitivity (0.91) for adhesive capsulitis. The same locations of capsular thickening visualized in persons with adhesive capsulitis on ultrasound are also reliably visualized on MRI/magnetic resonance arthrography (MRA) with the added benefit of diagnosing other potential intra- and extraarticular causes of shoulder stiffness (e.g., a rotator cuff tear or degenerative changes). Interestingly, however, in patients with severe global motion loss (<100 degrees of forward flexion, <10 degrees of external rotation, and less than L5 internal rotation), the risk of substantial rotator cuff pathology is extremely low. In a study by Ueda et al., there were no full thickness rotator cuff tears in this patient group.[46] For this reason, in the setting

---

BOX 51.4   Manual Muscle Strength Grading System

Grade 0: Complete paralysis, absent fasciculations
Grade 1: Visible or palpable contraction, although too weak to move even without gravity
Grade 2: Contraction able to move joint without gravity, but unable to move joint against gravity
Grade 3: Strength adequate to move against gravity, but unable to move joint against manual resistance
Grade 4: Strength adequate to range joint against resistance, but less than on the uninvolved contralateral side
Grade 5: Normal full strength equal to the contralateral side

Modified from Table 4.3 from Lippitt SB, Rockwood Jr CA, Matsen III FA, et al. *The Shoulder.* 4th ed. Vol 1. Philadelphia: Elsevier; 2009.

of classic adhesive capsulitis, we defer MRI imaging for failure to respond to nonoperative management.

Even though ultrasound is operator dependent, it may be useful in measuring rotator interval thickness (e.g., the coracohumeral ligament) and inferior capsule/axillary pouch thickness, which is suggestive of adhesive capsulitis. Dynamic ultrasound can be used to diagnose subacromial gliding limitation of the supraspinatus tendon, which strongly correlates with MRA features and maximum intraarticular injection volume.[47]

DECISION-MAKING PRINCIPLES

Once the inciting factor(s) involved in the pathogenesis of the stiff shoulder is/are determined, treatment is instituted. Given the lack of clarity that is often present in the diagnosis and natural history, it is not surprising that numerous treatments are described with variable success. The principles of management include evaluation of the severity of the patient's pain, stiffness, loss of function, and the effect on activities of daily living, employment, and recreation. Mild stiffness with minimal pain may not require any other treatment than oral antiinflammatory medications and gentle physical therapy encouraging maintenance of ROM and pain-relieving modalities. High-risk groups (e.g., diabetics), those suffering with severe chronic stiffness and pain, or with bilateral involvement, may warrant early surgical management.[48] However, most patients do not necessitate such aggressive management. The presence of pain that prevents sleep or awakens the patient from sleep is often a key ingredient in the pursuit of the next step in treatment. An initial escalation in treatment may involve an intraarticular injection (with or without a subacromial injection) of a corticosteroid or hyaluronate. This treatment can be followed by use of oral antiinflammatory medication (steroid and nonsteroidal) with therapy. Failure to improve after several months may warrant the next escalation to a discussion of surgical interventions. The risks, benefits, alternatives, and expected outcomes of operative management should be thoroughly discussed with the patient.

TREATMENT OPTIONS

The available evidence supports active treatment of adhesive capsulitis as opposed to "benign neglect." Treatment options include physical therapy, use of oral medications (e.g., nonsteroidal antiinflammatory drugs, steroids, and analgesics), intraarticular and subacromial injections, joint hydrodilatation and capsular rupture, suprascapular nerve blockade, and manipulation with the patient anesthetized with or without arthroscopic or open lysis of adhesions. A nonoperative course should be attempted initially, combining physical therapy modalities with use of oral medications and intraarticular injections. These modalities are generally successful, with reconstitution of motion, relief of pain, and improved function.[28,49-51]

Russell et al.[52] compared group physical therapy, individual physical therapy, and a home exercise programs in treatment of patients with adhesive capsulitis. The group and individual therapies had significantly improved pain and ROM, but the group-based therapy had the most significant gains at a 12-month follow-up.

Oral antiinflammatories may yield modest benefit, but a single corticosteroid injection often provides improved short-term relief.[53,54] Shin et al.[54] demonstrated superior short-term relief in patients receiving one corticosteroid injection regardless of subacromial or intraarticular location when compared to no injection. Additional modalities, such as hydrodilatation, have also been used to treat acute pain and improve ROM. In a prospective study by Yoon et al.,[55] patients were randomized to a subacromial injection, intraarticular injection, or hydrodilatation group. The hydrodilatation group had improved pain at 1 month with better functional outcomes at the 1- and 3-month follow-up when compared to the other injection groups. Despite these findings, there were no differences between groups at the final 6-month follow-up. Similar results were presented by Mun et al.,[56] which demonstrated improved short-term ROM and pain in patients undergoing hydrodilatation with joint manipulation versus intraarticular injection alone. Any early benefit was not appreciated at 12 months. A recent level II evidence systematic review by Griesser et al.[49] involving eight studies and 409 shoulders demonstrated significantly greater improvements ($P < .05$) in shoulder-specific outcome scores, pain, and motion at early follow-up after intraarticular glenohumeral joint injection versus other nonsurgical treatments for adhesive capsulitis. However, these differences were transient, with equalization of outcomes by 1 year after treatment onset.

A new novel form of therapy utilizing collagenase clostridium histolyticum injections has recently been described.[57] Badalamente et al.[57] were able to demonstrate that serial collagenase injections of 0.58 mg/1 mL or 0.58 mg/2 mL have superior outcomes to therapy alone and ultrasound allows for safe extraarticular placement. Although early studies have been promising, US Food and Drug Administration (FDA) approval has yet to be granted.

The lack of sustained effectiveness of the aforementioned nonoperative modalities, in conjunction with the prolonged course of adhesive capsulitis, tends to push both the patient and the treating physician toward a more aggressive means for treatment. In persons wishing to avoid surgery, manipulation under anesthesia (MUA) has been shown to be an effective option with lasting, long-term pain relief and retained motion.[58] Optimal timing is largely unknown, but Vastamaki et al. demonstrated improved pain and ROM when MUA was performed 6 to 9 months after onset of symptoms.[59] Arthroscopic intervention can be successfully used to treat adhesive capsulitis that is refractory to nonoperative treatment or MUA (indications and contraindications are provided in Box 51.5). Arthroscopic release allows visualization and the ability to address both intra- and extraarticular adhesions without subscapularis detachment. Successful results can be achieved and maintained at long-term follow-up after arthroscopy. At a mean of 7 years (range, 5 to 13 years) after arthroscopic capsular release, Le Lievre and Murrell[60] reported that 43 patients had significant improvements in pain, function, stiffness, and performance of activities of daily living. Motion had returned to the same level as that of the contralateral shoulder without any complications or repeat operations. Of note, a large systematic review by Grant et al.[61] did not demonstrate any discernible difference between MUA and capsular release as treatment options for adhesive capsulitis.

POSTOPERATIVE MANAGMENT

We favor a preemptive pain protocol to help patients maintain the gains in motion obtained in the operating room. Most patients receive a one-time interscalene long-acting local anesthetic block or a continuously infused anesthetic catheter to reduce postoperative pain. This allows for better compliance with early postoperative motion during physical therapy. Intraarticular local anesthetic pain pumps are not used to avoid possible glenohumeral chondrolysis. Intraarticular injections are avoided because they immediately extravasate from the joint, and efficacy is lost.

We believe it is important to demonstrate to the patient that full motion was obtained in the operating room. Although this objective can be achieved with use of intraoperative photographs, performing this demonstration postoperatively, while the patient is awake and alert (but while the block is still active) is most effective. This demonstration reinforces the concept that motion is possible and that success depends upon early compliance with exercises. After arthroscopic treatment, no restrictions are placed on shoulder motion or weight bearing.

Authors' Preferred Technique

Before a patient is taken to the operating room, a local anesthetic interscalene block (or temporary interscalene catheterization) is performed by a well-trained anesthesiologist. Administration of a successful block/catheter is imperative so the patient may begin early and frequent motion/therapy immediately after surgery. Once the patient is supine on the operating table, inducement of muscle relaxation in addition to administration of the anesthetic of choice is essential to prevent undue osseous stress (thus reducing the risk of iatrogenic fracture). Manipulation of the shoulder while the patient is anesthetized should proceed, with motion using short lever arms to reduce the risk of fracture. Contracted shoulders that are amenable to manipulation should move with relatively gentle applied force. Forward elevation, which should be applied first, helps to "opens up the joint."

Following manipulation under anesthesia, we prefer an arthroscopic release of remaining contracted tissues. Standard arthroscopic portals are utilized. Arthroscopic entry to the joint requires care in trocar placement to avoid iatrogenic damage, because the joint volume is reduced and the capsule is thick and fibrotic. The entry point should be slightly superior, because the joint is widest here (Fig. 51.2). The rotator interval (Figs. 51.3 and 51.4) and anterior capsular releases are performed first (Fig. 51.5), followed by releases of the posterior (Figs. 51.6 and 51.7) and inferior (Fig. 51.8) capsules, if these releases are performed arthroscopically rather than via manipulation. Because of axillary pouch contracture, posterior and posteroinferior release is performed prior to inferior release. Subacromial space inspection and a bursectomy are typically performed as well (Fig. 51.9). Acromioplasty may increase the risk of the formation of recurrent subacromial adhesions and thus should be avoided. After capsular release, a rotational torque may be applied. In abduction, external rotation is applied first, followed by internal rotation. These motions are followed by across-the-body adduction and behind-the-back internal rotation.

Other acceptable and successful sequences include arthroscopic release first, followed by manipulation. Proponents of this sequence believe that less torque is necessary to perform the manipulation after the arthroscopic release has been

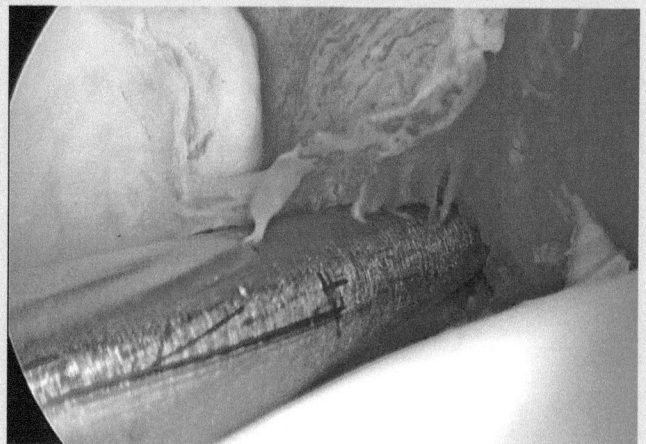

Fig. 51.2 Entering the joint from a slightly higher position allows easier access to the joint.

performed. We believe that by avoiding an inferior release with arthroscopic instrumentation, the risk of iatrogenic axillary nerve injury is reduced.

Using this approach of gentle manipulation, followed by arthroscopic capsular release, we feel that motion can be restored, and complications can be minimized.[12,49,62] Without direct visualization via arthroscopy or arthrotomy, the possibility of an incomplete release exists. In addition, the forceful manipulation may induce fracture, dislocation, or unintended soft tissue or neurovascular injury. Immediate postoperative care includes active and passive motion to prevent the reformation of scar tissue.

This procedure may be safely accomplished with reliable improvement in short-term motion (within 3 to 6 months)[63] in all planes, and with sustained long-term

📌 Authors' Preferred Technique—cont'd

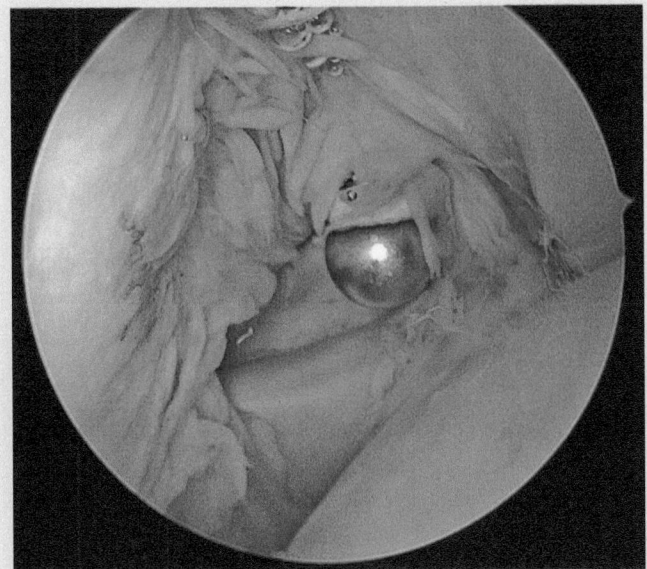

Fig. 51.3 Contracted rotator interval, with synovitis and thickening.

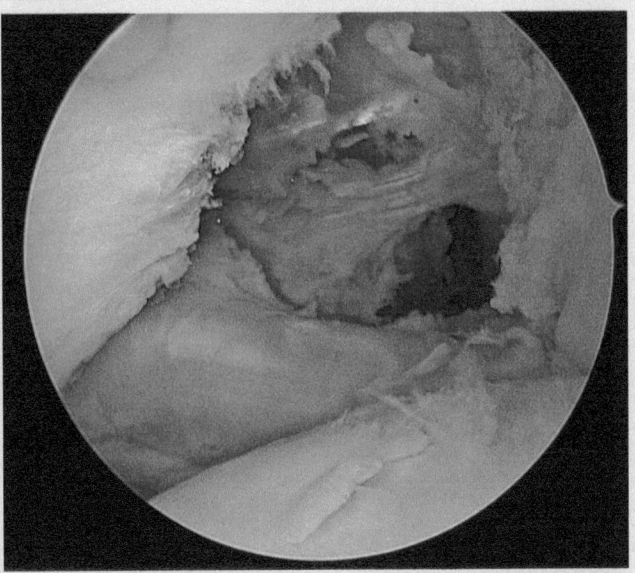

Fig. 51.4 Following complete rotator interval release, fibers of the deltoid, coracoacromial (CA) ligament, and conjoint tendon should be visualized.

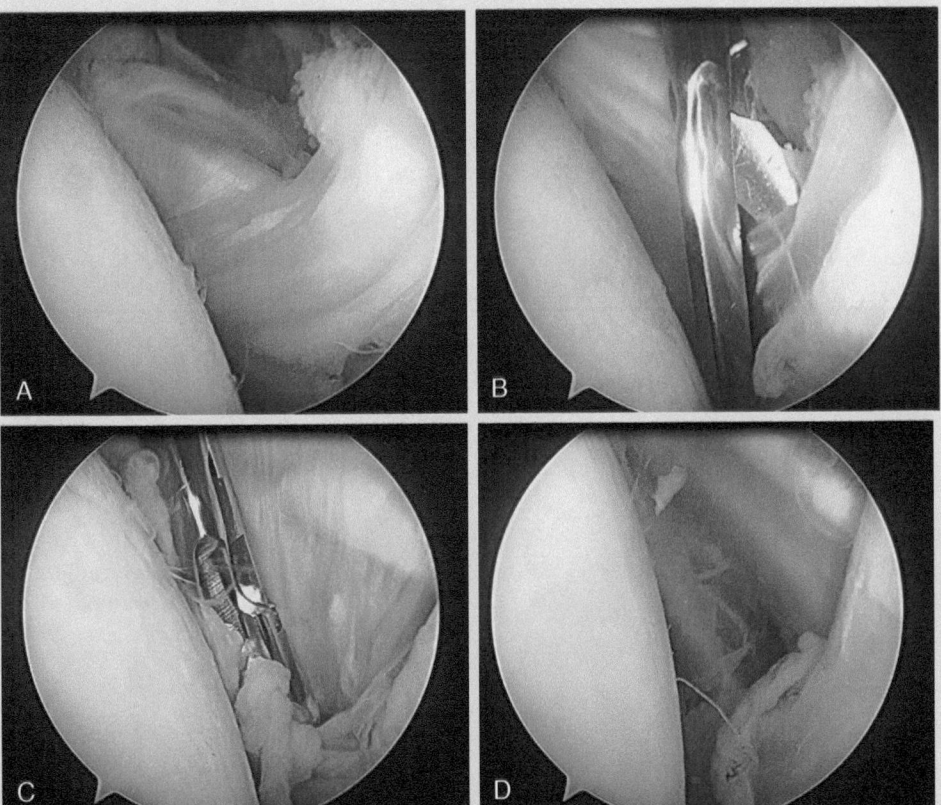

Fig. 51.5 Arthroscopic view (A) of the anterior middle and anterior inferior glenohumeral ligaments. Release (B) of the anterior middle glenohumeral ligament. Release (C) of the anterior inferior glenohumeral ligament. Status post release (D) of the anterior ligaments with full visualization of the subscapularis tendon and muscle belly.

Continued

📌 Authors' Preferred Technique—cont'd

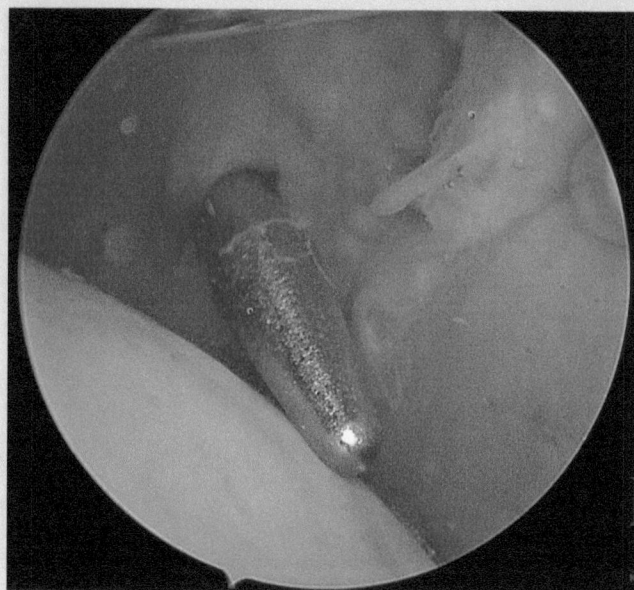

Fig. 51.6 Viewing from the anterior portal, the thickened posterior capsule can be easily visualized. Entry point just lateral to the labrum will allow safe circumferential release.

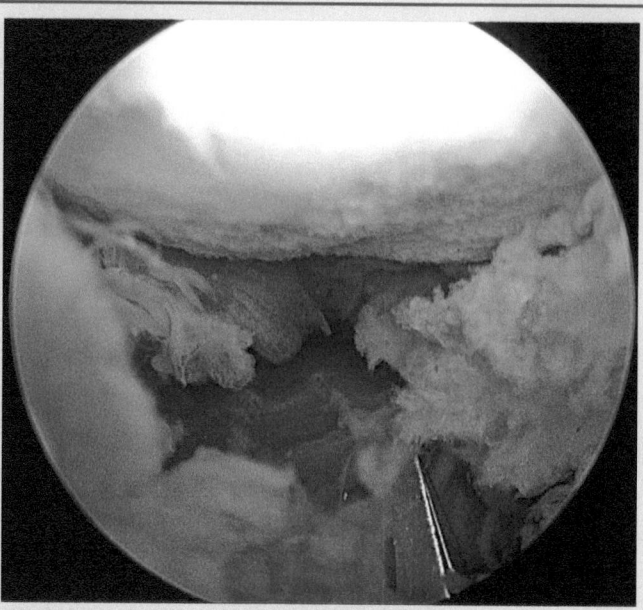

Fig. 51.8 If desired, the inferior capsule can be released, by using a low posterior accessory portal. Using an arthroscopic scissors allows dissection of the capsule from the underlying muscle and axillary nerve.

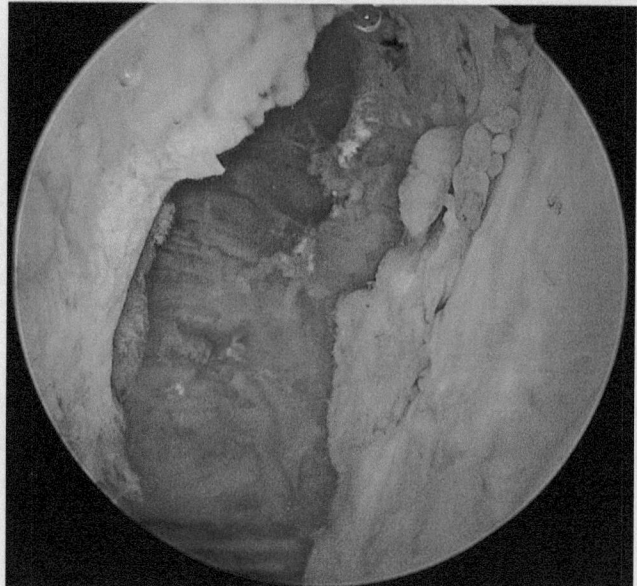

Fig. 51.7 Following complete release of the posterior capsule, muscle fibers of the infraspinatus can be visualized.

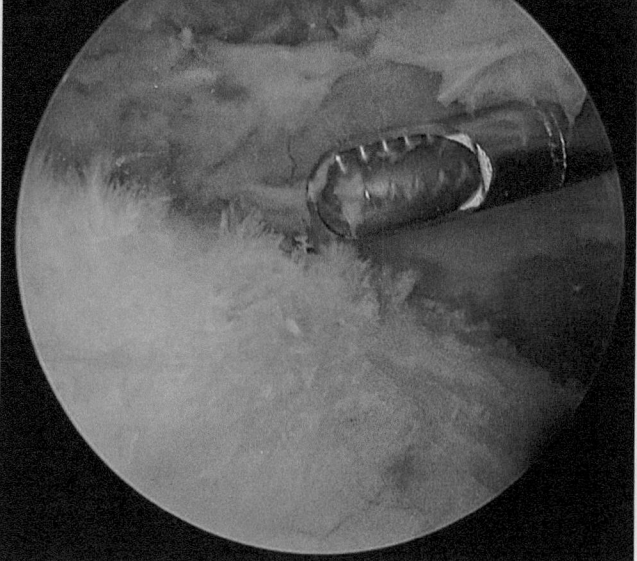

Fig. 51.9 Completed subacromial bursectomy and adhesion release.

improvements (up to 7.5 years)[64] in pain, motion, and function. Ogilvie-Harris et al.[12] compared pain and motion in patients undergoing isolated manipulation versus arthroscopic release. Similar gains in ROM were observed; however, the arthroscopic group had significantly improved relief of pain and function. Improvements in arthroscopic management of the stiff shoulder have led to a reduction

in the indications for and performance of open capsular release. However, if shoulder anatomy is distorted enough to preclude safe arthroscopic release, then open capsular release is indicated. The key technical aspects of successful open release include lysis of subdeltoid adhesions, release of the rotator interval, and release or lengthening of the subscapularis, with or without inferior capsular release.[65–68]

In patients who have severely restricted motion or those who may not be compliant with exercises or who have limited physical therapy visits with their health insurance, we consider utilization of shoulder continuous passive-motion machines. We encourage supervised physical therapy at least three to four times per week for a minimum of the first 2 postoperative weeks in addition to home exercises. We then recommend supervised physical therapy two to three times per week for the next 4 to 6 weeks. Pulleys and dowels are recommended to assist with maintenance of full passive and active-assisted forward elevation and external rotations.

RESULTS

A recent systematic review of randomized trials (31 studies) investigating all treatments for stiff shoulders revealed that limited evidence exists regarding the effectiveness of definitive treatment.[69] Because of the heterogeneity in participants, interventions, and outcome measures, a meta-analysis could not be performed.[69] Nevertheless, based on the outcomes of that review, intraarticular corticosteroid therapy combined with physiotherapy was the only treatment that showed a statistically and clinically significant beneficial treatment effect compared with placebo for short-term pain relief. Further, cost-effective analysis within the review concluded that intraarticular steroid therapy alone may be more cost-effective than steroid therapy plus physiotherapy or physiotherapy alone. De Carli et al.[70] compared shoulder manipulation and arthroscopic arthrolysis versus intraarticular glenohumeral joint corticosteroid injection in patients with idiopathic adhesive capsulitis. The results of that randomized trial revealed satisfactory motion in both groups and significant improvements in Constant, University of California–Los Angeles, American Shoulder and Elbow Surgeons, and Simple Shoulder Test evaluations. The only difference was an earlier improvement in the surgical group (6 vs. 12 weeks). Outcomes of MUA without arthroscopy have demonstrated significantly improved outcomes including pain, motion, and function (Table 51.1).[58,71–73] Outcomes of arthroscopic capsular release and lysis of adhesions with and without manipulation for stiff shoulders are presented in Table 51.1.[60,74–78] Patients undergoing arthroscopic release for postsurgical stiffness improve significantly after surgery (based on pain, motion, subjective shoulder value, and Constant scores), but not to the same degree as patents with idiopathic and posttraumatic stiffness.[78] The same difference was observed by Wang et al.,[73] who reported fewer improvements in postoperative stiff shoulders than in idiopathic and posttraumatic shoulders. Open glenohumeral capsular release has also demonstrated sustained significant improvements in pain, motion, and function (see Table 51.1).[65,79,80] Despite successful outcomes after open release, most surgeons choose arthroscopic means because of 360-degree joint access, avoidance of subscapularis transection, and avoidance of larger skin, subcutaneous, and capsular incisions and dissection.

COMPLICATIONS

Complications arising in the nonoperative and surgical treatment of stiff shoulders are possible but may be avoided with

TABLE 51.1 Selected Recent Outcomes of Arthroscopic and Open Release for Adhesive Capsulitis

Study	Outcomes
Arthroscopic	
De Carli et al.[70]	1-year follow-up, 44 shoulders, randomized trial
	Significant improvement in motion and in Constant, ASES, SST, and UCLA scores
	Earlier improvement (6 vs. 12 weeks) in arthroscopy vs. nonoperative group
Le Lievre and Murrell[60]	7-year follow-up, 49 shoulders
	Significantly improved pain, function, stiffness, ADLs
Lafosse et al.[74]	3.5-year follow-up, 10 shoulders
	Significantly improved Constant score, motion, pain, satisfaction
Jerosch[75]	2-year follow-up, 28 shoulders
	Significantly improved Constant score, motion
Diwan and Murrell[76]	2-year follow-up, 40 shoulders
	Significant early improvements in pain, motion
Snow et al.[77]	5-month follow-up, 48 shoulders
	Significantly improved motion, satisfaction, Constant score
Elhassan et al.[78]	4-year follow-up, 115 shoulders
	Significantly improved pain, motion, Constant score, SSV
Open	
Eid[79]	3-year follow-up, 19 shoulders
	Significantly improved pain, motion, Constant score
Omari and Bunker[80]	1.5-year follow-up, 25 shoulders
	Significantly improved pain, motion, function
Ozaki et al.[65]	7-year follow-up, 17 shoulders
	Significantly improved pain and motion
Manipulation Under Anesthesia	
Thomas et al.[71]	3.5-year follow-up, 246 shoulders, + corticosteroid injection
	Significantly improved Oxford Shoulder Score
Ng et al.[72]	6-week follow-up, 86 shoulders
	Significantly improved pain, motion, DASH score
Wang et al.[73]	7-year follow-up, 49 shoulders
	Significantly improved pain, motion, Constant score

ADL, Activity of daily living; *ASES,* American Shoulder and Elbow Surgeons; *DASH,* Disability of the Arm, Shoulder, and Hand; *SST,* Simple Shoulder Test; *SSV,* subjective shoulder value; *UCLA,* University of California, Los Angeles.

appropriate measures. In nonsurgical management, corticosteroid injection has the potential to elevate serum blood glucose levels, potentially exacerbating hyperglycemia and leading to diabetic ketoacidosis. The risk of infection, although low, is increased in patients receiving multiple injections. In patients undergoing arthroscopy, capsular thickness makes trocar advancement into the glenohumeral joint difficult, potentially increasing the risk of iatrogenic articular cartilage or bone injury. Further, the reduced joint volume makes navigation difficult without collateral damage to the articular cartilage until the release has commenced to permit greater freedom of arthroscopic instrumentation. If thermal electrocautery devices are used without vigilance regarding suction and the temperature of irrigation fluid, then the potential exists to cause chondrolysis. Because the intraarticular arthroscopic perspective does not allow easy visualization of the axillary nerve, extreme care must be taken to perform inferior release as near as possible to the inferior glenoid labrum to avoid injury to the axillary nerve. Given the force required to manipulate the stiff shoulder, even with the patient anesthetized and with excellent muscle relaxation, the potential exists to fracture the humerus, dislocate the humeral head, cause rotator cuff and labral tears, and cause temporary nerve injuries to the brachial plexus.

Despite the known risks, the actual number of reported complications are relatively low. Lafosse et al.[74] reported on 10 patients with recalcitrant stiff shoulder for whom nonsurgical treatment had failed and who underwent arthroscopic arthrolysis; no complications such as axillary nerve injury, fracture, or infection occurred. In addition, no complications were reported by Jerosch,[75] who performed 360-degree arthroscopic release for idiopathic adhesive capsulitis. Recurrence of stiffness after standard 155-degree arthroscopic anteroinferior capsular release was observed by Diwan and Murrell.[76] In the latter investigation, in a separate cohort of subjects, an extension of the release 65-degree posteriorly preserved the motion and function gains, and none of these patients had a recurrence of stiffness. Similarly, Snow et al.[77] compared patients who underwent a standard arthroscopic anteroinferior release with a group that underwent an additional posterior release and found that both groups had significantly improved motion and Constant and satisfaction scores with no difference between groups and no recurrence of stiffness in either group.[77] In both the studies by Diwan and Murrell[76] and Snow et al.,[77] no complications were observed in relation to the addition of the posterior release.[76,77] No significant complications have been reported after mini-open[79] or open[65,80] release in the treatment of stiff shoulders. Despite success with open surgery, inherent risks of infection, subscapularis transection, and neurovascular injury (axillary nerve) still exist.[66,67]

FUTURE CONSIDERATIONS

Treatment has not evolved significantly over the past several years, and the above-discussed treatment options remain the mainstay. In more recent investigations, though, markers such as inflammatory cytokines (IC, COX, and MMPs) have been shown to be elevated in patients with adhesive capsulitis. So, in the future, we may be able to obtain serologies that measure these factors and help us diagnose adhesive capsulitis in an earlier phase before significant motion loss. Furthermore, we may be able to prescribe medications to inhibit these factors and prevent the onset of adhesive capsulitis. Finally, other nonsurgical options such as collagenase injections,[57] hyaluronic acid injections,[81] and transcatheter embolization to reverse the abnormal neovasculature seen in the rotator interval in adhesive capsulitis patients[82] have also shown some promise and may be incorporated into the treatment algorithm in the future if further studies show they are efficacious.

ACKNOWLEDGMENT

We thank Gary M. Gartsman, Matthew D. Williams, Joshua Harris, and Michael Griesser, the authors of this chapter in previous editions of this book.

For a complete list of references, go to ExpertConsult.com.

SELECTED READINGS

Citation:
Miller MD, Wirth MA, Rockwood CA Jr. Thawing the frozen shoulder: the "patient" patient. *Orthopedics.* 1996;19(10):849–853.

Level of Evidence:
IV

Summary:
This retrospective review demonstrated that at a 4-year mean follow-up, after 50 patients who had adhesive capsulitis were treated with moist heat and oral antiinflammatory medications, all patients regained a significant amount of motion and returned to activities of daily living without pain.

Citation:
Hand C, et al. Long-term outcome of frozen shoulder. *J Shoulder Elbow Surg.* 2008;17(2):231–236.

Level of Evidence:
IV

Summary:
This retrospective review of 269 shoulders with adhesive capsulitis at 4.4-year mean follow-up after both nonoperative and operative treatment demonstrated that 41% of patients were still symptomatic (based on the Oxford Shoulder Score). Symptoms reported were generally mild pain; however, persons with the most severe symptoms at onset reported the worst long-term prognosis.

Citation:
Shaffer B, Tibone JE, Kerlan RK. Frozen shoulder. A long-term follow-up. *J Bone Joint Surg Am.* 1992;74A(5):738–746.

Level of Evidence:
IV

Summary:
Seven years after nonoperative treatment of 68 shoulders with adhesive capsulitis, subjective and objective findings at follow-up showed that 50% of patients either had pain, stiffness, or both. A strong association existed between functional limitation and the presence of symptoms.

Citation:
Griggs SM, Ahn A, Green A. Idiopathic adhesive capsulitis. A prospective functional outcome study of nonoperative treatment. *J Bone Joint Surg Am.* 2000;82A(10):1398–1407.

Level of Evidence:
IV

Summary:
At 2-year follow-up using Disability of the Arm, Shoulder, and Hand and Short Form–36 scores after nonoperative management of 77 shoulders with adhesive capsulitis, 90% of patients achieved a

satisfactory outcome using a structured shoulder stretching program. Nevertheless, significant differences in pain and motion of the involved shoulder versus the uninvolved shoulder were still found.

Citation:
Harryman DT 2nd, Matsen FA 3rd, Sidles JA. Arthroscopic management of refractory shoulder stiffness. *Arthroscopy*. 1997;13(2):133–147.

Level of Evidence:
IV

Summary:
After failed nonoperative management of 30 shoulders with adhesive capsulitis at 3-year follow-up, motion averaged 93% compared with the contralateral side with significant improvements in pain and function (per American Shoulder and Elbow Surgeons and Simple Shoulder Test scores) after arthroscopic release of capsular contractures. Three patients had recurrent stiffness after surgery with no other long-term complications.

52

Glenohumeral Arthritis in the Athlete

Jeffrey Brunelli, Jonathan T. Bravman, Kevin Caperton, Eric C. McCarty

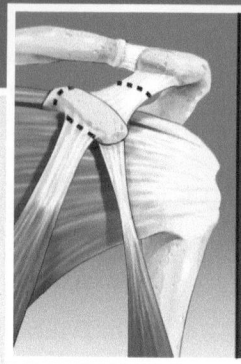

Arthritis or degenerative joint disease (DJD) of the shoulder in young athletes is a disabling condition that often limits sports participation and is extremely challenging to treat. Shoulder arthritis, defined as a degeneration of the articular cartilage of either the humeral head or glenoid, is caused by multiple etiologies, including primary osteoarthritis and secondary causes such as trauma, iatrogenic disease, and rheumatoid disease. Although each subtype has a unique set of considerations and treatment options, all have the same end goal of providing a functional, pain-free shoulder that has the durability to withstand the forces of daily and recreational activities for the duration of the athlete's life—a particularly important and challenging consideration in this young, active, population.

Shoulder DJD begins with loss of mobility and the inability to maintain function because of contracture and pain in and around the shoulder. This condition eventually leads to difficulty in continuing recreational activities, which is a substantial hurdle for individuals who wish to lead an active lifestyle. A wide spectrum of disease can be present, from focal cartilaginous softening to diffuse, full-thickness lesions of both the glenoid and humeral head.

EPIDEMIOLOGY

In the United States the overall incidence of glenohumeral chondral lesions and their natural history are largely unknown. These lesions are often found incidentally at the time of arthroscopy for other pathologies. The causes of these lesions range from idiopathic to specific underlying pathologies that eventually lead to osteoarthritis. Chondrolysis, a specific form of osteoarthritis, has been studied in national registries and has an incidence of 5.5 per 10 million person-years. It has an increased incidence in persons with diabetes and in those who have undergone an orthopedic procedure.[1] Nakagawa et al.[2] studied primary osteoarthritis, specifically excluding patients with rheumatoid disease and those with rotator cuff arthropathy, and found an incidence of 0.4% in persons with orthopedic problems versus 4.6% in those with shoulder disease presentation.

Primary osteoarthritis is typically found in persons older than 60 years.[2–4] In the young, healthy, and active population, the incidence is expected to be much lower, although specific data are lacking in the current literature. Cadaveric studies have shown an increased incidence of chondral lesions associated with rotator cuff tears, with glenoid defects in 32% and humeral defects found in 36% compared with rates of 6% and 7%, respectively, in shoulders without rotator cuff tears.[5]

Posttraumatic osteoarthritis, specifically those related to shoulder dislocations, have been studied extensively to look at chondral injuries. In 1997 Taylor and Arciero[6] reported that 57 of 63 patients had a Hill-Sachs lesion after anterior dislocation; 40% were chondral lesions, and 60% were osteochondral lesions. Furthermore, arthroscopic evaluation of 212 patients demonstrated a 23% incidence of glenoid defects and an 8% incidence of humeral head defects in persons who had one dislocation, whereas persons who reported more than two dislocations had a significantly increased incidence of arthritic lesions (27% and 36%, respectively).[7]

CLASSIFICATION

Primary Osteoarthritis

Primary shoulder osteoarthritis is a rare phenomenon in the young athlete; this disease occurs mostly in patients 60 years and older, and its etiology is unknown. It begins with glenohumeral joint stiffness, followed by joint space narrowing and humeral head and inferior glenoid osteophytes, which is considered the classic finding, with an intact rotator cuff.[8] Samilson and Prieto[9] first described radiographic parameters for glenohumeral arthritis in 1983. Since then, the classification has been revised, and in 2002 Guyette et al.[10] further refined this classification, with radiographs evaluated for humeral osteophytes, glenoid changes, and loss of joint space, collectively.

Walch et al.[11] have further noted that fixed posterior humeral head subluxation may precede the development of osteoarthritic changes and may be the first sign of primary glenohumeral arthritis, and Ropars et al. indicated that a spinoglenoid cyst is an even earlier sign of glenohumeral degeneration.[12] Patients often have anterior capsular tightness that causes a static subluxation of the humeral head in relation to the glenoid. As arthritis progresses beyond the 55% humeral subluxation index, described by Kidder,[13] further osteophyte formation develops, including progressive central loss of cartilage on both the glenoid and humeral head.

Instability Arthropathy

Although the rates of shoulder arthritis have been demonstrated to be higher in patients who have sustained a shoulder dislocation (so-called *dislocation arthropathy*) and in patients who have had that dislocation treated surgically (so-called *capsulorrhaphy arthropathy*), we believe that these entities, although deserving of discrete consideration, may have significant overlap and are various points on a spectrum of the same disease process. However, to date, the literature has separated these processes into two distinct entities.

Dislocation Arthropathy

Impaction and shear across the glenohumeral joint causes an articular cartilage lesion during shoulder dislocation, with an incidence of chondral and osteochondral lesions of 47% and 46%, respectively.[6,14] Initially described by Neer et al. in 1982, Samilson and Prieto classified the condition in 1983.[9,15] This form of arthritis is associated with increasing age at the initial event, direction of dislocation (with posterior causing more changes than anterior), and associated glenoid fractures.[16–18] However, the number of dislocations and prior stabilization procedures were not associated with development of shoulder arthritis.[9] Interestingly, Matsoukis et al.[19] reported no difference between patients treated with and without surgery in regard to the severity of arthritis, and the overall incidence of arthritis after shoulder dislocation in patients treated nonoperatively ranges from 10% to 20%.[16–18] Most recently, 25-year follow-up data, reported by Hovelius and Saeboe[20] in 257 shoulders that sustained primary anterior dislocation, show that shoulders were radiographically normal in only 44% of patients at 25 years and the arthrosis development was related to age at primary dislocation (>25 years), recurrence of instability, participation in high-energy sports causing injury, and an alcohol abuse history. Although the rate of moderate to severe arthritis was 18% in shoulders without a recurrence compared with 26% with surgically stabilized shoulders, the rate of arthrosis in these surgically stabilized shoulders was less than in shoulders that were reported to have "stabilized over time," raising a significant question regarding the role of recurrent instability in the future development of arthrosis.

Capsulorrhaphy Arthropathy

Capsulorrhaphy arthropathy, as coined by Matsen and Wirth,[21] is described as arthrosis that is attributed to overtightening of the capsular structures which results in abnormal translation of the humeral head opposite the direction of capsulorrhaphy. Found in male patients at a mean age of 45, it has been linked to length of time since follow-up, amount of external rotation contracture, and the age at initial trauma.[16,22] Biomechanical testing of selective capsular plication has shown that this mechanism causes alterations in humeral head translation.[23–26] These translational differences lead to nonanatomic biomechanics, asymmetric cartilage wear, and ultimately arthritis (Fig. 52.1).

Surgical options have evolved as we have come to better understand the effects of biomechanics on shoulder articulation. Surgical options can now be divided into anatomic and nonanatomic procedures. Most nonanatomic repairs have been abandoned, including the Putti-Platt[27] and Magnuson-Stack methods[28]; however, the Bristow-Latarjet method[29,30] (although modified from its original description)[31] has continued to be a mainstay of treatment in cases of anterior instability in the setting of bony glenoid deficiency.

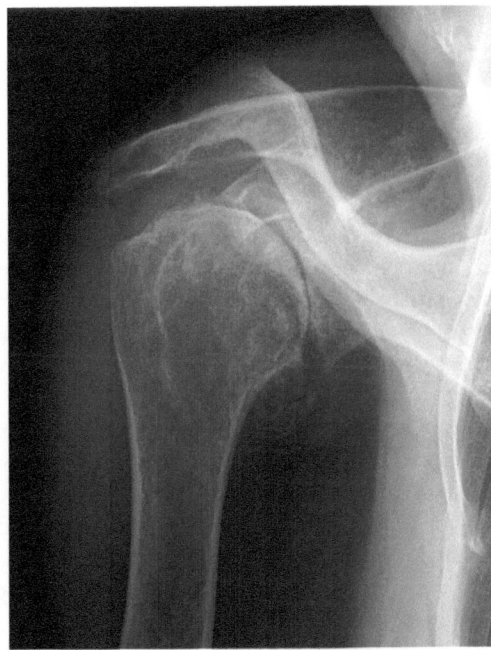

Fig. 52.1 An anteroposterior radiograph of capsulorrhaphy arthropathy after anterior stabilization.

In contrast to most nonanatomic repairs, anatomic procedures including Bankart repair[32] and capsulorrhaphy[33] have become the mainstay of treatment and have evolved significantly with use of arthroscopic techniques for primary and revision instability repairs; some persons argue that these procedures are the current standard of care. However, this paradigm shift from primarily open to arthroscopic techniques leaves unanswered questions about the long-term outcomes of open versus arthroscopic procedures, especially with regard to arthritis.

Long-term data indicate the presence of degenerative changes after the Putti-Platt procedure in 30% to 61% of patients at 9 to 26 years of follow-up.[34–36] These results have led to the abandonment of this procedure; however, the Bristow-Latarjet reconstruction remains part of the current treatment algorithm even though it has a reported incidence of arthritis of as high as 49% at 14 years.[16,37,38] It may be argued that several technical details in the techniques used in these procedures (specifically, complete subscapularis takedown) are not currently performed, which may greatly affect outcomes, although few studies refuting this high rate of arthrosis have been reported. However, a more recent study has demonstrated that, despite an overall incidence of arthrosis in 34% of patients, moderate or severe arthrosis was present in only 6% (which correlated with worse outcomes), whereas the patients with only mild arthrosis had no degradation of outcomes from joint damage after the Bristow-Latarjet procedure.[38] These studies have shown that the development of arthrosis may be more closely related to graft malposition than other factors previously thought to be responsible.[38,39]

Chondrolysis

Chondrolysis of the glenohumeral joint is a devastating problem that has proven to be one of the most vexing diagnoses faced by shoulder surgeons during the past decade. It has many associated (although not well proven) causes and is characterized by unexpected pain and loss of joint mobility for weeks to months, typically after arthroscopic shoulder surgery. Global dissolution of cartilage occurs on both the glenoid and humeral head, with the characteristic findings of joint space narrowing, periarticular bone edema, and subchondral cystic changes, although without osteophyte formation.[40–43] Although this condition has been associated with the use of radiofrequency energy in the shoulder, low-grade infection, intra-articular injection of contrast medium, use of bioabsorbable suture anchors, and postoperative pain pump infusion, small case series and case reports have led to difficulty in extrapolating meaningful data with regard to the true etiology of this condition.[41,44–46]

Recently, 375 patients who underwent an arthroscopic intra-articular shoulder procedure by an individual community orthopedic surgeon were evaluated specifically with regard to chondrolysis.[47] This cohort demonstrated a 13% incidence of chondrolysis, with all cases associated with an intra-articular postarthroscopic infusion of local anesthetic (bupivacaine or lidocaine); chondrolysis did not develop in any patients who underwent arthroscopy without a postoperative anesthetic infusion and is not present following an intra-articular steroid injection.[48] In addition, Bankart repair, arthroscopic débridement, suture anchor placement in the glenoid, and operative time were associated with this finding. This finding of the association between a postoperative anesthetic infusion and chondrolysis has been further supported by the results of a recent systematic review of 100 cases of chondrolysis in the literature, with this situation demonstrated in 59% of the cases reviewed.[49]

In addition, it has been demonstrated that the development of chondrolysis after a postoperative anesthetic infusion may be a dose-related phenomenon, which has been demonstrated in several basic science studies[50,51] and supported in a recent clinical cohort. When a high-flow pain pump was used postoperatively, chondrolysis developed in 16 out of 32 patients, whereas it developed in only 2 out of 12 patients with a low-flow pump containing bupivacaine, epinephrine, and infusate.[52]

With regard to low-grade infection as a causative agent, in their systematic review of 100 cases, Scheffel et al.[49] reported that of 91 patients who underwent revision surgery, 41 had microbiologic cultures taken at the time of revision surgery. Growth was reported for only 3 of these 41 cases, with *Propionibacterium acnes* reported in all 3 cases and no finding of any other positive cultures mentioned.[49]

The possibility that bioabsorbable suture anchors are an etiologic agent has also recently been analyzed; Dhawan et al. performed an evaluation of the 1,072,000 bioabsorbable anchors placed about the shoulder in 2008.[53] Of these cases, 10 suture anchor–related complications were reported to the US Food and Drug Administration, all of which were thought to be related to anchor malposition and typically demonstrated geographic rather than global cartilage loss. This finding was viewed as a best-case scenario, in that many cases of complications may not be reported; however, the authors still concluded that use of bioabsorbable anchors remains a safe practice when they are implanted properly based on the available literature.

Unfortunately, a reliable treatment algorithm or diagnostic modality to definitively identify patients with chondrolysis does not currently exist. Chondrolysis remains largely a diagnosis of exclusion, although surgeons need a high index of suspicion in the setting of failed previous surgery with early, progressive, and advanced arthritic changes of the glenohumeral joint. The outcomes of further definitive treatment of these patients have also been disappointing, and chondrolysis thus remains a major challenge for shoulder surgeons.

Rheumatoid Arthritis

Rheumatoid arthritis is an inflammatory arthritic condition that affects the synovial linings of both small and large joints. Although other inflammatory arthritides may affect the young athletic population (particularly psoriatic arthritis, spondyloarthropathy, and reactive arthritis), most is known about rheumatoid disease in this setting. The inflammatory nature of the disease leads to a disabling secondary erosive arthritis. It most commonly affects the small joints of the body but is found in the shoulder in 90% of patients with chronic rheumatoid disease.[54] Rheumatoid disease in the shoulder is progressive in nature, with early symptoms of pain, swelling, and decreasing shoulder motion. With disease progression, extra-articular structures become involved, including the subacromial bursa, acromioclavicular (AC) joint, and rotator cuff.[55] Radiographic progression begins with medial migration of the humeral head into the glenoid with characteristic central erosion of the articular surface (Fig. 52.2). Bone quality is typically osteopenic with periarticular erosions involving the superior and medial humeral head. Cystic formation may occur at the rotator cuff insertion, which, coupled with intrinsic degeneration of the rotator cuff, may lead to functional rotator cuff deficiency, static superior migration, and uneven joint erosion. Late sequelae of the rheumatoid shoulder leads to painful joint destruction, loss of

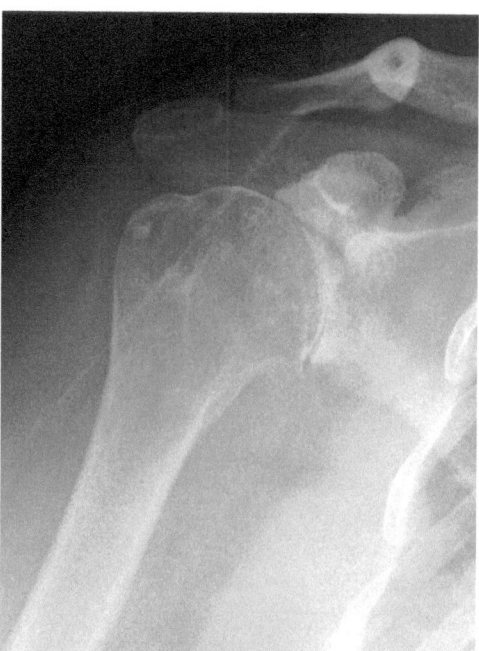

Fig. 52.2 An anteroposterior radiograph of central erosion seen in persons with rheumatoid arthritis.

bone stock (which has significant implications for reconstructive options), rotator cuff compromise, and poor overall function.[55,56] Further evaluation, especially in the preoperative setting, of all patients with rheumatoid arthritis should also include flexion and extension lateral views of the cervical spine to check for cervical instability and further causes of rheumatologic problems that may affect the shoulder joint concomitantly.

Osteonecrosis

Osteonecrosis (also known as avascular necrosis [AVN]) is another form of progressive glenohumeral arthritis that may be encountered during evaluation of the shoulder of a young athlete with arthritic disease. Osteonecrosis is characterized by the development of avascular regions of periarticular bone, resulting in infarction, necrosis, and ultimately collapse of the bony architecture of the subchondral plate with resultant deformity and arthrosis as a result of incongruity. Early workup of this disease should include testing for sickle cell anemia, particularly in the African-American population. Also to be considered etiologically are protein C and S deficiency, factor V Leiden, and hyperlipidemia.

Although many causes of osteonecrosis have been described, including dysbarism, hemoglobinopathies, coagulopathies, Gaucher disease, and connective tissue disorders, steroid use and alcohol abuse predominate clinically.[57,58] If radiographs reveal a crescent sign and collapse, the contralateral shoulder should be imaged to rule out asymptomatic bilateral disease, and use of the aggravating agent (if identified) should be stopped to prevent further progression of the disease. Collapse of the articular surface is secondary to fractures in weak subchondral bone, and pain is often the most common complaint, specifically with difficulty sleeping and pain interfering with activities of daily living. Pain is usually present with flexed and abducted shoulder positions because of the incongruous central superior position of the humeral head contacting the glenoid in this position.

Classification of osteonecrosis of the humeral head has been described by Cruess (Table 52.1).[59] Osteonecrosis has six stages based on radiograph and magnetic resonance imaging (MRI); these stages are largely based on and parallel the original description in the femoral head by Arlet and Ficat.[60] Indeed, osteonecrosis of the humeral head is similar to that in the femoral head, first with edema visible only on MRI, followed by sclerosis and then development of the crescent sign, with further collapse of the

articular surface and finally degeneration on both sides of the joint (Fig. 52.3).

PATIENT EVALUATION

Presentation and History

Glenohumeral arthritis has no classic or pathognomonic history but typically presents as a progressive loss of shoulder rotary mobility coupled with pain. Some persons report noise, grinding, crepitus, and a feeling of a point of "clunking with release." Another suggestive history includes instability without a history of dislocation, with the incongruent articular surfaces having a mechanical catch. In addition, patients may report morning stiffness that improves throughout the day, along with pain during sleeping.

Primary glenohumeral arthritis in the young population (i.e., younger than 50 years) is exceedingly rare and warrants an exhaustive history to identify the underlying primary diagnosis. History should include prior episodes of trauma, current and previous medications, family history, prior surgical procedures, and recreational and social factors. In addition, the patient's desired activity level should be taken into consideration. We have found that the desired activity level is a critical aspect of the evaluation of these patients because outcomes from certain procedures can be perceived as "catastrophic" if patients are not counseled about the longevity and limitations of implants and their ability to meet patients' expectations.

Physical Examination

Examination of the shoulder starts with evaluation of the cervical spine, with notation of deficits in range of motion (ROM) and reproduction of pain with provocative maneuvers, such as the Spurling test. Referred pain from the cervical spine is common; patients with cervical spine pathology are often more comfortable

TABLE 52.1	Stages of Humeral Head Osteonecrosis (Cruess Classification)
Stage	Description
I	Normal radiograph; changes on magnetic resonance imaging
II	Sclerosis (wedged, mottled), osteopenia
III	Crescent sign indicating a subchondral fracture
IV	Flattening and collapse
V	Degenerative changes extend to glenoid

From Cruess RL. Experience with steroid-induced avascular necrosis of the shoulder and etiologic considerations regarding osteonecrosis of the hip. *Clin Orthop Relat Res*. 1978;130:86–93.

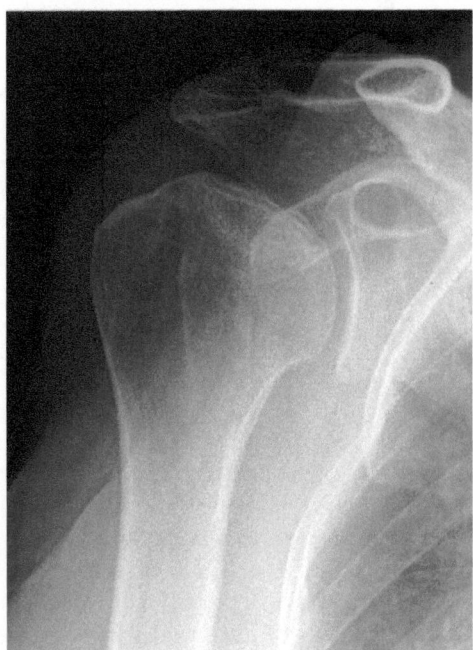

Fig. 52.3 Humeral head collapse in a patient with stage IV osteonecrosis.

with their hand draped over their head. Although referred pain and findings of cervical spine pathology do not exclude shoulder pain, patients suspected of having cervical pathology should be referred for proper care and the possibility excluded from the differential diagnosis.

The shoulder examination begins with visual inspection for symmetry, muscle atrophy, and previous surgical incisions. It is critical that the entire shoulder be visualized, including the entirety of the scapula, to ensure that the patient is examined for subtle but significant pathology, including scapular winging. Next, palpation of the posterior capsule, AC joint, greater tuberosity, and biceps groove helps to delineate and isolate glenohumeral pathology. Further evaluation includes both passive and active mobility with careful delineation of the painful arc of motion, while looking for the typical finding of an equal limitation of active and passive ROM in all planes. Motion is evaluated in forward flexion, abduction (controlling for scapulothoracic motion), external rotation at zero and 90 degrees of abduction, and internal rotation with regard to the vertebral level reached by the hand behind the back. Findings should be compared with the contralateral (presumably unaffected) side. Decreased rotational movements and mid ROM pain should alert the examiner to the presence of an arthritic process, whereas terminal ROM pain is more typically indicative of impingement, osteophytes, and capsular contraction.

Strength testing and impingement signs aid in the evaluation of rotator cuff pathology. Each tendon of the rotator cuff must be evaluated independently. The supraspinatus is evaluated using the champagne toast test,[61] whereas infraspinatus testing is accomplished via external rotation strength with the arm adducted at the side.[62] Lag signs must be elicited if they are present, and the Hornblower sign (external rotation with the shoulder abducted 90 degrees) tests the integrity of the teres minor.[63] In this patient population, we have found that it is critical to evaluate the integrity of the subscapularis, especially in the setting of capsulorrhaphy arthropathy after an open anterior instability procedure, where we have noticed a high rate of this finding.[64–66] Subscapularis tear is typically characterized by asymmetric hyperexternal rotation with the arm in adduction with a positive belly press (a test for the upper subscapularis) and lift-off (a test for the lower subscapularis).[67] The implications of these findings are critical because they may play a significant role in surgical decision-making; for example, consideration of procedures such as a concomitant pectoralis major transfer in the setting of subscapularis insufficiency with arthroplasty may be necessary.

Evaluation of Prior Operative Notes and Arthroscopic Images

A complete evaluation of the dates of individual surgeries, prior imaging, and arthroscopic images should also be undertaken for each patient. Such an evaluation can help differentiate between existing pathology and a new diagnosis. Particular attention to results after prior procedures is imperative to understand if recurrent pathology is present or if further problems have developed. Arthroscopic images help provide a firsthand view of the cartilage surfaces and the previously treated pathology. Previous MRI scans and radiographs can help put together a picture to further understand previous and new pathology. A review of the operative report of previous surgeries can help the surgeon understand the exact surgical procedures and difficulties affecting the surgical outcomes. Patients often understand that they have a problem in their shoulder but do not effectively communicate exact pathologies that may help guide future considerations.

Careful examination of the detailed operative note should include notation of implants, intraoperative findings, and difficulties with the previous procedures. Prior implants could limit the ability to access the canal if, for example, a biotenodesis screw has been previously placed for a biceps tenodesis. Placement of metal suture anchors into the glenoid and greater tuberosity also could be limiting. These anchors may scratch sensitive metal and polyethylene components that would lead to early failure of further implants, without removal of the previous anchors. In addition, certain glenoid anchors have been thought to cause cyst formation, which may make it difficult to place a stable glenoid component on the subchondral surface.

Imaging

Evaluation of all types of arthritis starts with plain film radiographs. X-ray views should include at a minimum a Grashey anteroposterior view, an axillary lateral view at 45 degrees of abduction, and a scapular Y view (Fig. 52.4). These three views are able to document the position of the humeral head in relation to the glenoid, the presence of osteophytes, bone quality, the glenohumeral joint space, and glenoid bone loss. They should be evaluated for humeral head posterior subluxation, which may be the earliest sign of arthritis found on radiographs.[11]

Further evaluation includes advanced modalities such as computed tomography (CT) and MRI. CT arthrography is extremely helpful in evaluating joints, especially in the setting of prior hardware placement. Glenoid morphology, bone stock and quality, and the status of the cartilage and rotator cuff can be well evaluated with a CT arthrography scan. A glenoid version can be further assessed by the techniques described by Friedman and colleagues (Fig. 52.5).[68] Walch et al.[11,69] further described the bony anatomy of posterior glenoid wear in the anteroposterior plane, specifically evaluating for biconcavity, which is best evaluated by CT (Fig. 52.6). MRI is especially helpful in evaluating changes to the subchondral bone and associated soft tissue comorbidities.[70,71] However, the sensitivity and specificity of evaluating chondral lesions is generally regarded as poor; up to 45% of grade IV chondral lesions may be missed.[72,73] Newer evaluations with 1.5T and 3.0T MRIs have been found to detect glenoid and humeral lesions at 84% and 78%, respectively, with lower-grade lesions often missed.[74]

TREATMENT OPTIONS

Treatment goals for the younger athletes with glenohumeral arthritis are resolution of symptoms and restoration of function and mobility. However, patient expectations must be matched to the durability and longevity of the specific treatment chosen. In fact, in 2008 McCarty et al.[75] demonstrated that the most common reason this population pursued treatment was to attempt to return to their previous level of sporting activity. Although

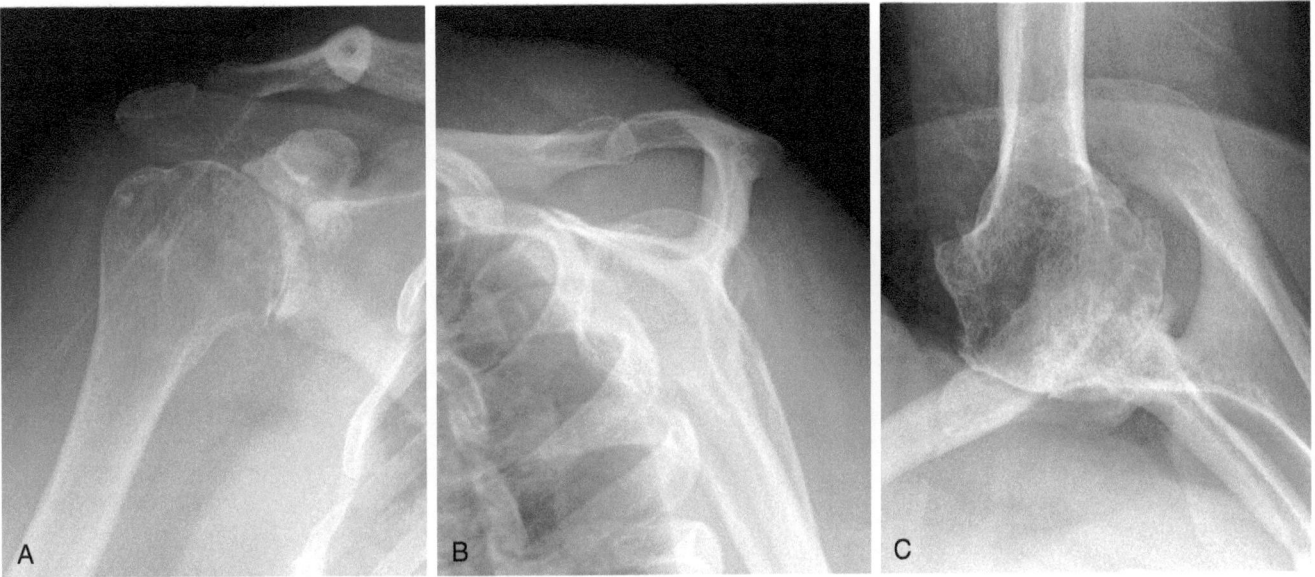

Fig. 52.4 A standard radiograph series. (A) Anteroposterior. (B) Scapular Y. (C) Axillary lateral.

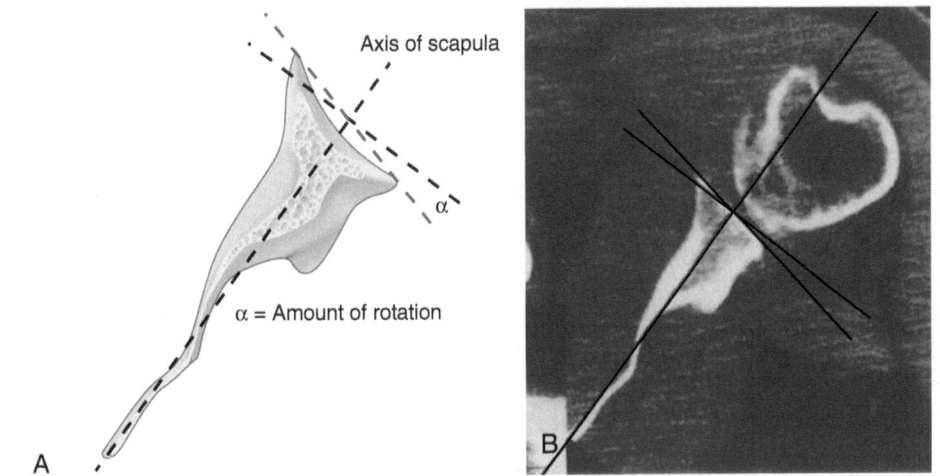

Fig. 52.5 The method of measuring the glenoid version as described by Friedman et al. (From Friedman RJ, Hawthorne KB, Genez BM. The use of computed tomography in the measurement of glenoid version. *J Bone Joint Surg Am*. 1992;74:1032–1037.)

older patients have reliable outcomes with shoulder replacement, young glenohumeral arthritis patients have worse arthroplasty outcomes,[76] and their treating surgeons have difficult decisions to make with regards to implant survivability. The Neer-type total shoulder arthroplasty (TSA) implants have demonstrated an 84% survival rate at 15 years,[77] although revision surgery in the area of the shoulder is extremely complex and few implants have been able to compensate for the glenoid bone loss frequently encountered in revision settings. In young patients, nonoperative treatments should be thoroughly pursued and exhausted before surgical interventions are contemplated. The mainstay of successful outcomes, whether surgical or nonsurgical, is related to patient education that clearly outlines the natural history and functional process that is present, along with the provision of acute and chronic pain management.

Nonoperative Treatment

The initial treatment of symptomatic glenohumeral osteoarthritis involves recommendation of activity modification, supervised physical therapy, and a trial of oral nonsteroidal antiinflammatory medications. Physical therapy should include a daily regimen of exercise with a focus on strengthening periscapular, deltoid, and rotator cuff musculature. Stretching the joint with manual manipulation helps to improve ROM, which counteracts restrictions caused by cartilage damage and resultant capsular contracture. In addition to these modalities, image-guided or blind injection into the glenohumeral joint with a mixture of corticosteroid and lidocaine is an excellent diagnostic and therapeutic tool. However, such an injection may not provide long-term relief for athletic patients engaging in high-demand sports who

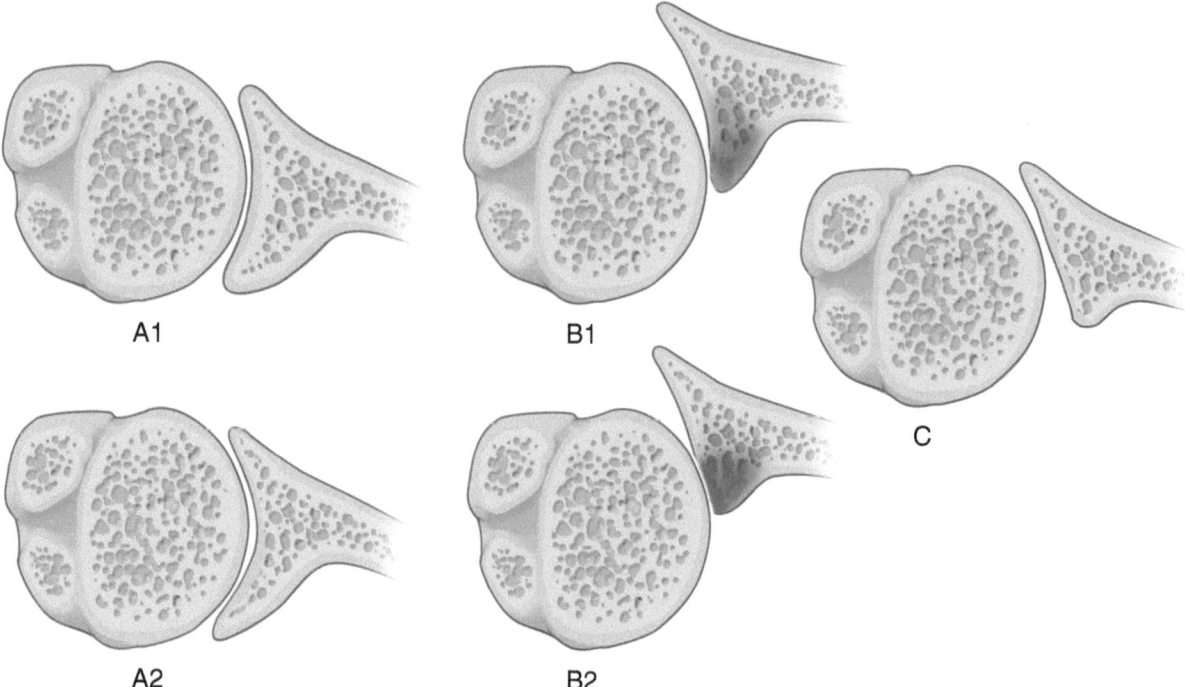

A1   B1

                                              C

A2   B2

Fig. 52.6 The classification of glenohumeral morphology as described by Walch et al. (From Walch G, Badet R, Boulahia A, et al. Morphologic study of the glenoid in primary glenohumeral osteoarthritis. *J Arthroplasty.* 1999;14[6]:756–760.)

continue to participate in athletic endeavors, because their symptoms often return with continued activity.[78] In addition, off-label use of viscosupplementation with hyaluronic acid injections has been shown to provide partial symptom relief[79] but has not been shown to provide statistically improved outcomes over saline injections.[80] The relief experienced often involves improvement in overall pain and has been effective in allowing patients to sleep through the night with minimal shoulder pain after treatment.

Operative Treatment
Joint-Sparing Techniques

Arthroscopic débridement. The diagnosis of glenohumeral arthritis is often made incidentally at the time of arthroscopic intervention aimed at other pathology, unless radiographic changes or underlying conditions are present.[81–83] However, arthroscopy provides a minimally invasive means to evaluate and treat chondral lesions and concomitant pathology in the shoulder, allowing for early rehabilitation and return to activity in symptomatic patients who have not responded to nonoperative measures.[84] Unfortunately, arthroscopy in this setting remains a temporizing measure that does not alter the underlying disease process; however, it can provide pain relief and functional improvement for a considerable amount of time.[73,85–87]

Several authors have reported successful results of arthroscopic débridement for glenohumeral arthritis and isolated cartilage lesions in patients younger than 55 years, and several prominent themes have emerged from this work.[73,86,88,89] Results have been reliable and have correlated with the extent of disease in those younger than 50 years.[90] Risk factors for failure are chondral lesions larger than 2 cm², grade IV bipolar lesions, residual joint space less than 2 mm, the presence of large osteophytes, and Walch B2, C glenoids.[90] Weinstein et al.[86] reported that pain relief and maintenance of function was sustained for 76% of patients at 34-month follow-up, and it was sustained in 88% of patients at 2-year follow-up in the series by Cameron et al.[73] Conversion to arthroplasty was required in 22% of patients at an average of 10.1 months after débridement in one series[89] and in 15% of patients at 20 months in another series.[88]

Several concomitant procedures were performed in the aforementioned series, including bicep tenotomy/tenodesis, distal clavicle resection, subacromial decompression, microfracture, loose body/osteophyte removal, and capsular release. We have found that capsular release is extremely useful, and it has been recommended that capsular release be included in arthroscopic treatment if rotation is limited by greater than 15 degrees in any plane of motion.[73] Significant attention must be given to these aforementioned concomitant pain generators in the setting of arthritic disease, and furthermore, failure to address these pathologies has been demonstrated to produce worse postoperative results.[91–95]

Microfracture. In addition to débridement, it has been recommended that full-thickness cartilage lesions be managed with use of microfracture, similar to that described in the knee (Fig. 52.7).[96] In 2009 Millett et al.[97] reported on 31 patients (average age: 43 years) with full-thickness cartilage lesions in the glenohumeral joint who underwent treatment using microfracture. At a mean follow-up of 47 months, the patients demonstrated significant improvement in the visual analog scale score, American Shoulder and Elbow Surgeons (ASES) score, and painless use

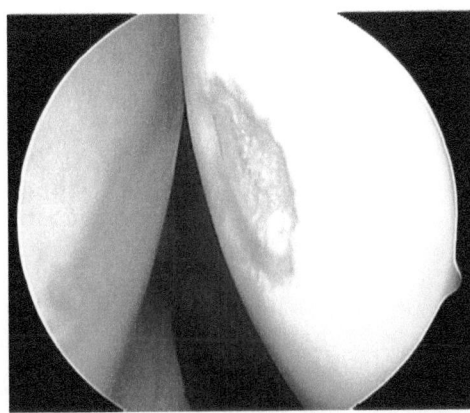

Fig. 52.7 An incidentally encountered isolated humeral head osteochondral lesion in a young patient undergoing arthroscopy for labral repair.

of the arm, as well as improvement in patients' ability to work, perform activities of daily living, and participate in sports activity, with failure in 19% of patients, who required additional procedures. These investigators demonstrated the greatest improvement in patients with smaller, isolated humeral head lesions and the worst results in patients with bipolar lesions.

More recently, Frank et al.[98] published their experience with a similar cohort of 15 shoulders in 14 patients (average age: 37 years) who underwent glenohumeral microfracture and demonstrated similar results. At an average follow-up of 28 months, these investigators showed significant improvements in the visual analog scale, simple shoulder test, and ASES scores, with 92% of patients stating that they would have the procedure again.[98] The procedure was considered a failure in three patients in this series (20%), who required further operative intervention during the study period.

Glenoidplasty and osteocapsular arthroplasty. In concordance with the concept of posterior subluxation and nonconcentric posterior glenoid wear, the technique of glenoidplasty was developed in an effort to restore glenoid morphology from a biconcavity to a single concave surface. Restoration of uniform concavity theoretically reduces posterior humeral head subluxation and increases the effective joint surface, thus reducing point loading while increasing stability. This technique is performed by using an arthroscopic burr where the anterior glenoid (or "high side") is resected until it is flush with the posterior joint.[99] Recommendations for this procedure are aimed at pain relief; however, it has been demonstrated that patients with pain in their mid-arc ROM do not fare as favorably after surgery as those who have end–ROM pain, pain at rest, and painless crepitus. Also associated with favorable results are the radiographic findings of a biconcave glenoid with posterior humeral subluxation and the presence of osteophytes and loose bodies. Contraindications to this procedure are glenoids without biconcavity and patients with severe pain in mid-arc motion, because these findings have been associated with severe arthritis and patients with these findings have not done well after glenoidplasty.

Osteocapsular arthroplasty involves removal of humeral osteophytes with release of capsular contractures. Complete capsular release from the rotator interval to the posterior-inferior capsular

recess should be performed to gain maximal mobility. In a cohort with an average age of 50 years who were treated with this procedure, Kelly et al.[100] demonstrated that more than 85% of patients reported improvement in both pain and ROM at an average 3-year follow-up. Elser et al.[101] have briefly presented their data on 27 young patients who underwent a similar procedure that they have termed *comprehensive arthroscopic management*, which includes débridement, capsular release, and humeral osteoplasty. One-year follow-up demonstrated a patient satisfaction rate of 8.5/10 with the procedure, with only one patient progressing to arthroplasty in that period.[101] In another series Millet et al. reported 76% 5-year survival of a comprehensive arthroscopic management (CAM) procedure, including débridement of degenerative labrum, biceps tenodesis, burring of inferior humeral head osteophytes, and occasional axillary nerve decompression. ASES and Single Assessment Numerical Evaluation (SANE) scores indicating improved pain score and function with work, activities of daily living, recreation, sleep, and use of the arms all significantly improved.

Arthroscopy for rheumatoid arthritis and osteonecrosis. Arthroscopy has also proven useful in the early treatment of both rheumatoid arthritis and osteonecrosis. The hypertrophic synovium of rheumatoid disease leads to bony destruction, and thus a synovectomy may help slow the disease progression. Synovectomy results in increased motion and decreased pain in 80% of patients; however, this procedure is only useful early in the disease process, and when radiographic signs of disease are present, synovectomy is no longer a viable option.[102–105] Concomitant procedures should be performed as indicated, including subacromial decompression and rotator cuff repair, and the synovium may reproliferate, requiring a repeat synovectomy.

Patients with osteonecrosis have also benefited from arthroscopy and core decompression early in their disease process, and results have been shown to correlate to the severity of humeral head involvement.[106,107] This technique was first described in 1993 by Mont et al.[108] and has been shown to be successful in 94% and 88% of patients with stage I and II disease, respectively. These results decline to 70% and 14% success in patients with stage III and IV disease, respectively. Core decompression may delay the time until arthroplasty in persons with stage III disease, although indications are controversial and this procedure is contraindicated in persons with stage IV and V disease.

Joint Resurfacing Techniques

Humeral head resurfacing, biologic resurfacing, and osteochondral grafting. Secondary treatment options include humeral head resurfacing, biologic resurfacing of the glenoid, and osteochondral allograft or autograft of the humeral head or glenoid. These techniques are used along the spectrum depending on the amount and chronicity of injury to the articular surfaces. Also involved is the level of instability present as a result of underlying pathology. Osteochondral allografts have been suggested as a means for reconstructing defects in both the glenoid and humeral head in cases of instability of the shoulder, particularly in the setting of large Hill-Sachs lesions (i.e., >45% of articular surface). In the chronic setting, or when larger humeral defects are present, a structural allograft can be used as a biologic means of extending the range of contact with the glenoid surface in external rotation.[109] Algorithms for treating humeral head defects have been well described.[110] For older patients with more than 45% of the humeral head affected, a prosthetic replacement is recommended. For younger patients with greater than a 45% structural defect, an osteochondral allograft should be considered (Fig. 52.8). Evaluation of outcomes has largely relied on case reports demonstrating success at 2-year follow-up.[111,112] Given the rarity of these cases and limited reports, each patient should be approached individually and treatment should be determined on a case-by-case basis. Allograft reconstruction techniques isolated to the glenoid have been shown to be beneficial at 5- to 7-year follow-up.

Humeral head resurfacing has been reviewed as a further consideration for patients who are young and active. Since its inception in 1979, this treatment has undergone numerous changes, including the addition of hydroxyapatite coating in 1993. Current techniques including the "ream and run," designed to promote articular congruity, were first studied by Matsen et al.[113] in a canine model and demonstrated fibrocartilage formation on the glenoid at 6 months. This model was then transitioned into a human population, and results were reported in 2007.[114] They demonstrated equivalent subjective shoulder test values at 3-year follow-up when compared with TSA. An important note regarding this technique is that the glenoid should be normalized in morphology, and if posterior subluxation is present, the physician should not perform a posterior release and the inferior glenohumeral ligament should be left intact.

Bailie et al.[115] in 2008 and Tibone et al.[116] in 2015 again looked at results after isolated humeral resurfacing and found that patients uniformly had improved outcome scores at 3-year follow-up. Bailie et al.[115] looked at a subset of patients younger than 50 years, which suggests that resurfacing is an acceptable treatment option for patients younger than 50 years who would like to maintain an active lifestyle. Levy and Copeland[117] also looked at a subset of patients younger than 50 years and concluded at an average follow-up of 8.2 years that ROM and Constant scores were equal to the outcomes of TSA. These studies provide

validated outcome measures that give the treating surgeon an alternative to traditional shoulder replacement in the younger population without concern for glenoid component loosening.

Biologic resurfacing that focuses on glenoid "coverage," combined with a humeral-sided hemiarthroplasty or resurfacing, has also been proposed as a solution to glenoid longevity and ultimate implant survival in the young, active population. Several glenoid resurfacing techniques have been proposed and studied, including use of a fascia lata autograft, the anterior shoulder capsule, an Achilles allograft, a meniscal allograft, and xenograft tissue (Fig. 52.9).[118-121] However, the results of these techniques have been mixed. Although the techniques engendered much early enthusiasm because of the initial reports by Nowinski[120] demonstrating that 81% of patients had good or excellent results, with 21 of 26 patients returning to predisease activities (including heavy lifting and manual labor), more recent reports have demonstrated conflicting results. A longer-term follow-up study by Krishnan et al.[122] showed excellent results in 18 of 36 patients (50%), satisfactory results in 13 of 36 patients (36%), and unsatisfactory

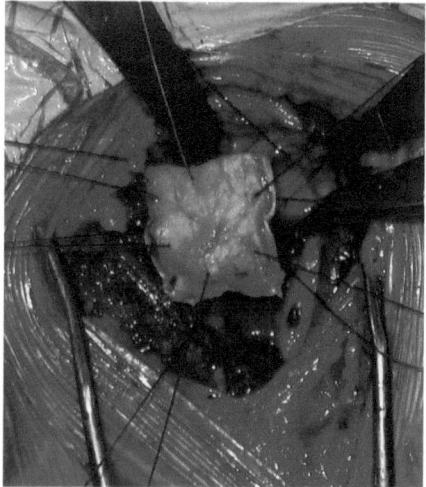

Fig. 52.9 Fascia lata autograft biologic glenoid resurfacing.

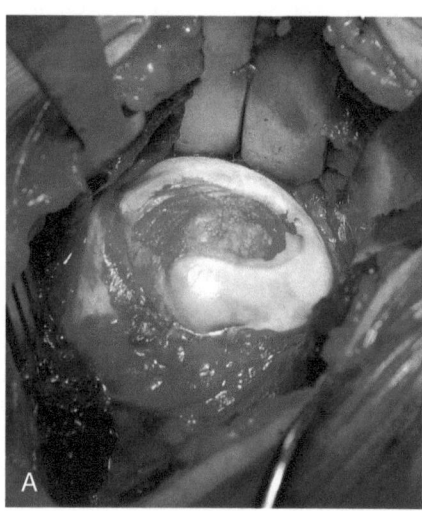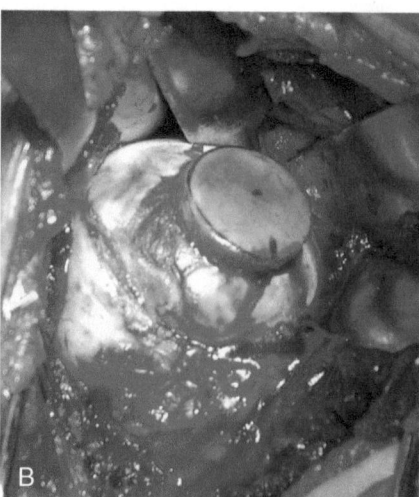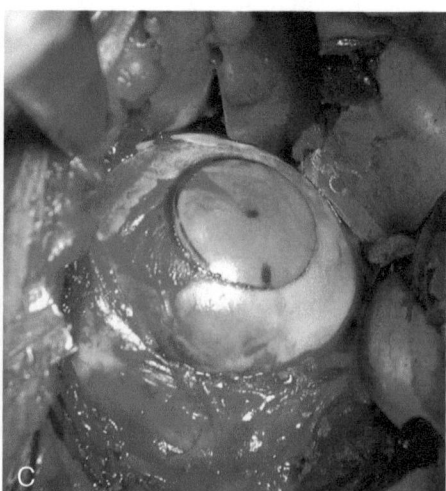

Fig. 52.8 (A) A large osteochondral lesion of the humeral head in a young patient. (B) Matched osteochondral allograft preparation. (C) Completed allograft osteochondral resurfacing.

results in 5 of 36 patients (14%) at 2- to 15-year follow-up with use of an anterior capsule, fascia lata, or Achilles allograft. These investigators concluded that use of capsular tissue was an independent predictor of failure, and thus they recommend use of an Achilles allograft in this setting. Similarly, Wirth[123] reported on 27 patients who underwent resurfacing with a lateral meniscal allograft and demonstrated significant improvements in pain relief and function at an average of 3 years of follow-up, with a 70% survivorship at 8 years.[124] However, this group demonstrated uniform progression of joint space narrowing, which calls into concern the long-term functional outcome in this cohort. These mostly positive results must be contrasted with results reported by Elhassan et al.,[125] Romeo et al.,[126,127] and Gobezie et al.[128] regarding reoperation rates. Ten of 13, 12 of 21 patients, and 7 of 16 patients, respectively, required revision TSA. These studies give validated, yet conflicting results as a surgical option that is attractive because it allows younger, more active patients to return to their previous level of activity, including weightlifting and manual labor, without concern for eccentric glenoid wear, although the long-term results may be unpredictable.

Glenohumeral arthroplasty. Shoulder arthroplasty pioneered by Neer in the 1950s, with a persistent evolution of prosthetic design and surgical technique, has continued to improve function in patients undergoing shoulder arthroplasty. Patients with primary osteoarthritis, posttraumatic arthritis, inflammatory arthritis, osteonecrosis, capsulorrhaphy, and dislocation arthropathy can be effectively treated with shoulder arthroplasty. Pain that has failed to respond to other interventions is the most common indication for arthroplasty; however, patients often obtain statistical improvement with regard to ROM, strength, and function as well. The status of the soft tissues, bony structures, and underlying etiology must be taken into account when counseling patients about expected results and when planning the details of operative intervention.

Primary osteoarthritis of the glenohumeral joint that is unresponsive to nonoperative or joint-preserving techniques is a well-supported indication for shoulder arthroplasty (Fig. 52.10). Godeneche et al.[129] reported excellent results in a series of 268 patients. Objective outcomes improved based on Constant scores, with 77% good or excellent results, motion gains were seen with 50-degree improvements in elevation, and subjective scores demonstrated 94% satisfaction rates.[129] In a large multicenter study of more than 600 patients, Edwards et al.[3] showed clinically and statistically significant improvements for all variables in patients undergoing total and hemiarthroplasty of the shoulder, including Constant scores, pain, ROM, activity, and strength. Khan et al., in a 10-year prospective evaluation of patients who underwent TSA, found a mean improvement of 41 points in Constant scores and a 65-degree improvement in forward elevation for patients with primary osteoarthritis. Component survival was found to be 100% for the humeral component and 92% for the glenoid.[130] Raiss et al.[131] evaluated younger patients with mean age of 55 years who underwent TSA for primary osteoarthritis and found a 40-point increase in Constant scores, 95% satisfaction rates, and 100% component survival at a minimum 5-year follow-up. These results are consistent with the results of other series on arthroplasty for

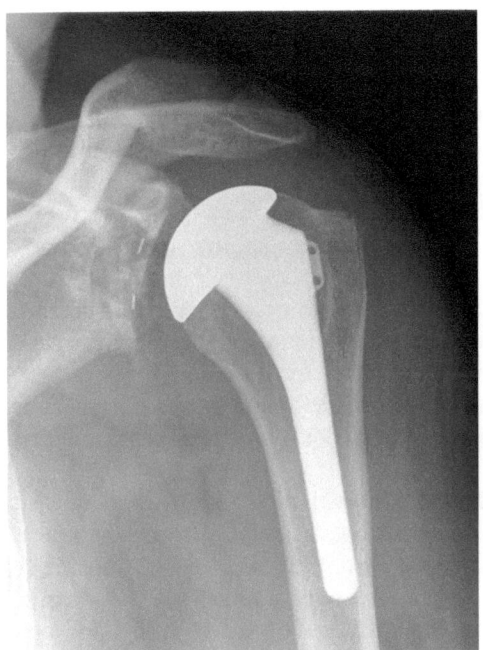

Fig. 52.10 An anteroposterior radiograph of total shoulder arthroplasty for primary osteoarthritis.

primary osteoarthritis and demonstrate predictable and reproducible improvements in all parameters evaluated, providing thorough evidence when counseling patients.

Both preoperative and intraoperative factors can affect results of shoulder arthroplasty for glenohumeral joint degeneration. Preoperative factors include underlying etiology, rotator cuff tears, fatty degeneration of rotator cuff musculature, and glenoid morphology. Fatty degeneration of the rotator cuff musculature may result in less favorable postoperative outcomes in patients with Goutallier grade 2 or higher infiltration in the infraspinatus and subscapularis, resulting in decreased forward elevation and strength.[129] Small tears of the supraspinatus have little effect on outcomes after arthroplasty.[132] However, larger tears negatively affect active ROM and strength and have a more important effect on component biomechanics. Larger tears can make it difficult for the rotator cuff to maintain the center of rotation, which allows superior migration of the humeral head in relation to the glenoid. In the setting of TSA, this phenomenon can have profound effects on glenoid component survival, due to elevation of the center of rotation, with subsequent asymmetric contact mechanics of the glenoid component. This situation results in the "rocking horse" effect in the cephalocaudal plane from point loading of the superior aspect of the glenoid component, which has been demonstrated to be a significant factor in early glenoid component loosening and failure.[133]

Posterior humeral subluxation and posterior glenoid wear are associated with primary glenohumeral osteoarthritis, resulting in altered glenoid morphology, and must be taken into account when considering arthroplasty for degeneration of the glenohumeral joint.[8,134] Native glenoid morphology, as well as changes resulting from glenohumeral degeneration, may affect operative planning and decision-making regarding the type of implant. Hoenecke et al.[134] classified glenoid morphology, including neutral, biconcave, worn, dysplastic, displaced, and angled. In this report, as well as in studies by Gerber et al.[135] and Walch et al.,[136] the glenoid version was not associated with humeral head subluxation. Humeral head posterior subluxation is associated with a biconcave glenoid, and authors have recommended caution when attempting to correct the glenoid version if the goal is to address humeral head subluxation, using soft tissue balancing through capsular releases for implant stability instead of relying on bony correction alone. Indeed, Levine et al.[137] demonstrated that outcomes of hemiarthroplasty were most closely correlated to the status and extent of posterior glenoid wear. An individual approach should be used for glenoid preparation, with cautious correction of glenoid deformity and version while maximizing preservation of glenoid bone stock and glenoid component fixation.

Both hemiarthroplasty and TSA provide pain relief, but TSA has been shown to be statistically superior. Early reports revealed improved results with TSA compared with hemiarthroplasty; however, sample sizes were too small to show statistical significance until a meta-analysis by Kirkley et al.[138] and a multicenter study by Edwards et al.[3] confirmed superiority in nearly all outcome measures. TSA outperformed hemiarthroplasty with regard to Constant scores, pain, motion, strength, activity scores, active forward elevation, and external rotation. Humeral head replacement alone has been reported to have poorer results for pain and function, as well as increased revision rates, compared with TSA.[139] In addition, TSA was reported by Mather et al.[140] to be a cost-effective procedure, of greater utility to the patient, and of lower overall cost to the payer compared with humeral head replacement alone.

Although TSA and hemiarthroplasty alone have had predictable and satisfactory results in older patients, the results in younger patients have been less favorable in some reports. Sperling et al.[77] reviewed 78 Neer hemiarthroplasties and 36 Neer total shoulder replacements in patients younger than 55 years and found 36 unsatisfactory results (46%) in the hemiarthroplasty group and 14 unsatisfactory results (38%) in the total shoulder replacement group, underscoring the challenges of treating glenohumeral arthritis in the younger patient. However, Rais et al.[131] reported a 95% satisfaction rate with no revisions in patients with an average age of 55 years and 5- to 9-year follow-up, and Burroughs et al.[141] found an 86% satisfaction rate and a 9% revision rate at midterm follow-up in patients younger than 50 years. Saltzman and colleagues[142] evaluated patients undergoing shoulder arthroplasty before and after age 50 years and found a much larger proportion of patients requiring arthroplasty for reasons other than primary osteoarthritis, with the most common reason being capsulorrhaphy arthropathy. It was also reported that the pathoanatomy associated with the younger patient group complicated the surgery, rehabilitation, and outcome after shoulder arthroplasty.[142] Arthroplasty for chondrolysis has had similar results at 2-year outcomes with reoperation rates of 25%.[143] Considering that the majority of articles confirm the challenges of performing shoulder arthroplasty in younger patients, caution should be taken and alternative treatments should be considered and exhausted before making the recommendation to proceed with arthroplasty.

Given the complex nature of arthritis in the young patient and inconsistent results with TSA, hemiarthroplasty, and biologic resurfacing, and given the fact that the most common complication after TSA is failure of the glenoid component, the ream-and-run technique has been described as an alternative to potentially avoid some of these issues. This technique involves concentric reaming of the glenoid while leaving the labrum intact, allowing correction of glenoid deformity and denervating the glenoid articular surface. Preliminary results of this technique in all age groups demonstrated significant improvements in both pain and function.[144] Saltzman et al.[142] also evaluated this technique in patients younger than 55 and found significant improvement in pain and function with a low revision rate and little progression of glenoid erosion. Clinton et al.[145] confirmed satisfactory results using this technique, reporting similar self-assessed outcomes with ream and run compared with TSA; however, recovery time was slightly longer in the ream and run group.

Arthroplasty for inflammatory arthritis. Shoulder arthroplasty has shown consistent improvements in pain, function, and quality of life in patients with inflammatory arthritis. Most studies have favored TSA over hemiarthroplasty for functional outcomes; however, this conclusion is controversial, with several studies reporting no difference or improved outcomes with hemiarthroplasty compared with TSA in this patient population.[139,146–151] Arthroplasty can be considered for inflammatory arthritis of the glenohumeral joint, with the most favorable outcomes in patients with an intact or repairable rotator cuff and adequate glenoid bone stock.[152] Late tears of the rotator cuff from the underlying disease process are not uncommon after a successful TSA, and therefore patients should be followed up yearly to monitor for and prevent early failure from rotator cuff insufficiency.

Arthroplasty for instability arthropathy. Approximately 9% of patients who have undergone shoulder arthroplasty have a history of shoulder instability.[153] Marx et al.[154] demonstrated that the likelihood of experiencing glenohumeral arthritis is 10 times higher in patients with a history of shoulder dislocation and that, after surgical treatment of the instability, the probability increased 20-fold. Neer et al.[15] first reported on the results of shoulder arthroplasty for osteoarthritis after instability surgery with satisfactory to excellent results. Shoulder arthroplasty for arthritis after instability has shown favorable results with high satisfaction rates and marked improvements in pain, mobility (specifically external rotation and abduction), and quality of life; however, complication rates, including revision rates, are clearly higher than with primary osteoarthritis.[76,155,156] Complications such as continued instability, loosening, and decreased ROM are more common than in primary osteoarthritis, with some reports of up to 40% complication rates, and revision rates in the literature range from 20% to 40%.[153]

Given the less consistent results in this patient population, arthroplasty must be approached with greater caution, taking into account the younger patient age and associated pathoanatomy in the setting of dislocation arthropathy. Prior operations can alter the native anatomy and should be addressed at the time of the arthroplasty; for example, nonanatomic stabilization procedures can cause internal rotation contractures and require that an anterior release be performed to address the loss of external rotation. Prior procedures can also alter the native biomechanics of the glenohumeral joint and likely are the most significant factors responsible for less favorable results after shoulder arthroplasty for instability arthropathy compared with primary osteoarthritis.[153] Glenoid defects may require bone restoration, and soft tissue balancing is critical to prevent eccentric loading of the glenoid component, which may cause abrasive wear and early failure. Internal rotation contracture is the most common soft tissue abnormality found and may require extensive anterior capsular release. Subscapularis lengthening should be considered in more severe cases. However, subscapularis lengthening procedures can cause internal rotation weakness and may increase the likelihood of ultimate subscapularis failure. A preoperative CT scan is critical when a patient has evidence of glenoid defects, and the surgeon's index of suspicion must be high when evaluating patients with instability arthropathy. Determination of the extent and location of glenoid defects should be made preoperatively so appropriate plans can be made to address bony defects at the time of arthroplasty. Despite higher complication rates and increased surgical complexity, patients with instability and postcapsulorrhaphy arthropathy[173] can have acceptable outcomes after shoulder arthroplasty, with predictable improvements in pain and function.

An additional specific patient population that warrants separate consideration consists of patients undergoing TSA after the development of chondrolysis. There have been two case series addressing this issue in the literature, Levy et al.[41] and Sperling et al.[157] Levy demonstrated good to excellent results in 10 of 11 patients, whereas Sperling experienced a 25% reoperation rate at 2 years. These investigators demonstrated an opportunity for improvements in both pain and function but cautioned that progressive glenoid lucencies may develop, thus highlighting the difficulty surrounding definitive care of these patients and the still unanswered questions with regard to optimal management of this complex problem.

Arthrodesis. Glenohumeral arthrodesis is considered an end-stage salvage procedure indicated in the setting of shoulder pain, weakness, and instability that is not suitable for soft tissue or prosthetic reconstruction.[158] Some situations may arise in the younger active population for which glenohumeral arthrodesis is an option, given the limitations with regard to the potential durability and longevity of arthroplasty solutions. Arthrodesis is a reliable procedure in which bony fusion is obtained in nearly all patients. The optimal position of arthrodesis is 20 degrees forward flexion, 20 degrees abduction, and 40 degrees internal rotation. Most patients report pain relief after this surgery, although few are completely pain free.[159,160] The functional results of arthrodesis unfortunately lag behind improvements in pain. Few patients are able to return to any type of overhead work, although many patients find their fusion functionally beneficial from their preoperative state and can typically reach their mouths and hair, cross the midline for dressing, and reach their back pocket on the affected side.[161] Obviously, given the mobility restrictions after this procedure, return to sporting activities is limited; however, in the salvage situation, it may be an option and can be later reversed to shoulder arthroplasty when implant

longevity becomes an option.[162] This particular outcome has not been well studied in the younger active population.

DECISION-MAKING PRINCIPLES

In general, in our practice, young, active patients who are diagnosed with glenohumeral arthritis are individually evaluated, specifically with regard to determining the disease etiology, pathology severity, and their personal functional demands and goals. Determination of the etiologic cause of the disease is often critical because first line treatment in these patients is often directed at treatment of the underlying or inciting disease process (e.g., infection, inflammatory arthritis, or instability).

Initially we prescribe a formal course of nonoperative treatment, including supervised physical therapy, activity modification, and nonsteroidal antiinflammatory drugs, and injections as necessary. All concomitant pathology is evaluated, and treatment is directed at these entities, specifically focusing on identified concomitant bicep and AC disease. Our threshold for using image guidance for these injections is low, and we commonly use such guidance because the osseous anatomy of these patients is often distorted, and routine office-based injection techniques are technically more challenging and less successful. Initial treatment with an intra-articular corticosteroid injection is attempted, and based on the clinical response, these injections are continued sparingly as needed, or glenohumeral viscosupplementation is considered. When patients fail these modalities, they are considered candidates for operative intervention.

Operative decision-making depends on the pathology, disease severity, and functional demands of the patient. As previously mentioned, selective injections are used both as a diagnostic and therapeutic tool, especially when planning treatment of the AC joint and long head of the biceps tendon. In patients who have pain in these areas and respond positively to injection, distal clavicle resection and biceps treatment (tenodesis vs. tenotomy) is indicated, respectively, with subpectoral tenodesis preferred. We prefer this approach in younger patients who have bicep groove pain, because it has been our experience that tenotomy or tenodesis above the transverse ligament has led to unacceptable rates of residual pain, and this approach has been supported by a recent report in the literature.[163] An arthroscopic approach is typically entertained first, especially if the patient demonstrates a well-centered glenohumeral joint with a congruent humeral head and glenoid articulation and greater than 2 mm of joint space. If capsular contracture greater than 15 degrees is present, we perform capsular release in a controlled manner with a radiofrequency device under direct visualization. Cartilage lesions are initially considered for treatment with microfracture or débridement. This decision is made on the basis of a combination of factors, although data to support firm cutoffs based on the size of the lesion are currently lacking. However, we do not perform microfracture in the setting of diffuse, uncontained cartilage loss, bipolar or "kissing" lesions geographically, and untreated instability.

Failure of arthroscopic débridement and the aforementioned techniques, including 6 months of postoperative rehabilitation, may be an indication for consideration of osteoarticular allograft filling or partial metallic resurfacing of residual humeral head cartilage defects with a Hemicap device (Hemicap, Arthrosurface Inc., Franklin, MA). Focal lesions of the glenoid are treated similarly with regard to débridement and microfracture; however, resurfacing options are limited.

Diffuse lesions or bipolar disease in the setting of advanced DJD, osteonecrosis, inflammatory arthritis, or capsulorrhaphy arthropathy are treated with humeral head resurfacing or hemiarthroplasty and individualized glenoid treatment. We have used the ream-and-run technique successfully, especially in the setting of an incongruous glenoid surface such as when a Bristow-Latarjet procedure that has failed. Decision-making regarding resurfacing versus stemmed humeral components is based on the need for glenoid exposure and visualization and the quality of the metaphyseal bone support (as in AVN), with stemmed components favored if a concern about fixation exists, especially in older persons.

Additional consideration is given to the status of the periarticular soft tissue, particularly in the setting of failed open anterior capsulorrhaphy and subscapularis deficiency. These patients demonstrate hyperexternal rotation from loss of the static restraint to external rotation and a positive belly press/lift-off sign. We have treated these patients concomitantly with a split pectoralis major tendon transfer, based on the recent anatomic study by Fung et al.[164]; in our experience it has functioned well in the setting of future arthroplasty.

We have used an arbitrary age of 40 years old for patients for whom we will typically perform a traditional TSA with a cemented glenoid component because of a perceived long-term survival benefit, extrapolated from older populations that have been studied, because data in this particular population are lacking. However, this decision is highly individualized, and when patients wish to continue with heavy-lifting activities or concerns of early glenoid loosening predominate, glenoid component implantation is avoided.

Authors' Preferred Technique
Glenohumeral Arthritis

In the setting of the athlete with glenohumeral arthritis, our preferred surgical technique greatly depends on the individual demands and severity of the disease. In the setting of a focal full-thickness cartilage defect, arthroscopic treatment is preferred. This treatment focuses on microfracture as appropriate, débridement, capsular release (if contracture is greater than 15 degrees), and treatment of concomitant acromioclavicular and bicep disease with a preference for biceps tenodesis if the patient has biceps groove pain. Arthroscopic treatment is also the initial surgical treatment of choice in the setting of diffuse disease, although only when a round humeral head, greater than 2 mm of joint space, and well-centered glenohumeral articulation are present. Upon treatment failure of this approach or in the presence of diffuse cartilage disease, our preference has been humeral head resurfacing with individualized glenoid treatment, using either a "ream-and-run" technique or formal pegged glenoid component implantation. If there is any question of the support for a resurfacing component, such as in the setting of avascular necrosis, a standard stemmed arthroplasty is performed. Figs. 52.11 and 52.12 provide a more detailed outline of our preferred surgical treatment.

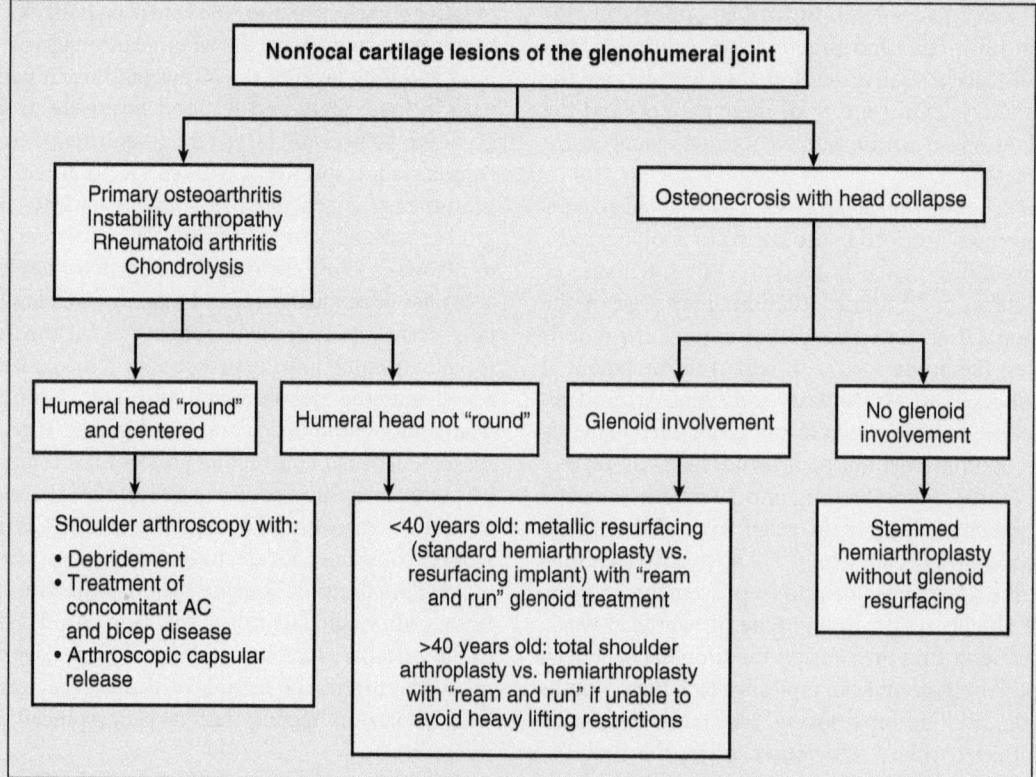

Fig. 52.11 The authors' preferred treatment of nonfocal cartilage lesions of the glenohumeral joint. *AC,* Acromioclavicular.

Authors' Preferred Technique
Glenohumeral Arthritis—cont'd

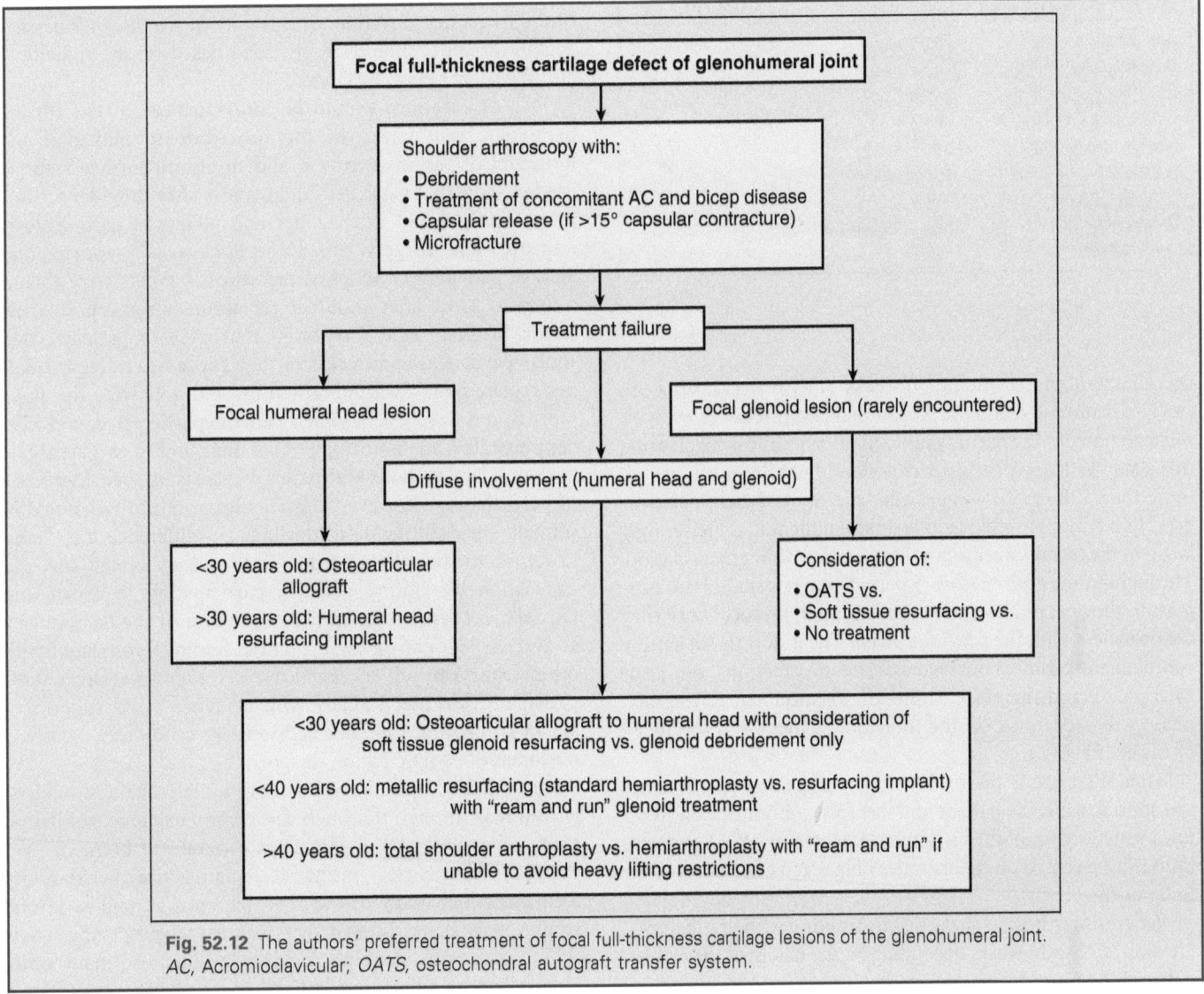

Fig. 52.12 The authors' preferred treatment of focal full-thickness cartilage lesions of the glenohumeral joint. *AC*, Acromioclavicular; *OATS*, osteochondral autograft transfer system.

POSTOPERATIVE MANAGEMENT

Postoperative Rehabilitation

Rehabilitation after arthroscopic intervention of the arthritic shoulder in the athlete is aimed at restoration and maintenance of functional ROM. Within 3 to 5 days, a regimen involving active, active assisted, and gentle passive ROM exercises is begun. Initially the goal is control of pain and edema. After this goal is achieved, ROM is emphasized. Strengthening is initiated after acceptable motion is achieved. This timing will often vary based on the extent of the patient's disease and preoperative ROM. This regimen may be performed with the assistance of a physical therapist or with a home exercise program in the case of a patient who is motivated and well educated on the proper regimen.

The surgical procedure (arthroscopic or open), the type of prosthesis used, and associated procedures performed determine the type of orthosis used and the length of time its use is required in the postoperative period. Table 52.2 provides common orthosis protocols.

All patients, irrespective of the type of procedure, begin elbow, wrist, and hand mobility exercises daily, beginning on the first postoperative day.

Rehabilitation After Arthroplasty

The initial 6 weeks of the postoperative period consist of pain and edema control and prevention of excessive stiffness, while protecting the subscapularis repair. Irrespective of exposure technique, via subscapularis tenotomy or osteotomy, a sling should generally be worn for the first 6 weeks, removing it only for light deskwork, sedentary periods, bathing, or hygiene. A daily home program should be provided by the patient's therapist and performed two to three times per day. External rotation past 20 degrees and active internal rotation should be avoided to protect

TABLE 52.2 Postoperative Orthosis Protocols/Duration of Treatment

Procedure Performed	Orthosis	Duration (Weeks)
Arthroscopic procedure	Simple sling	1–2 as needed
Hemiarthroplasty or TSA	Simple sling	6
Resurfacing arthroplasty	Simple sling	6
Osteochondral grafting or partial resurfacing	Simple sling	6
Arthroplasty plus posterior capsulorrhaphy	Neutral rotation sling	6
Reverse total shoulder arthroplasty	Sling and abduction pillow	6

the subscapularis for the first 6 weeks. After 6 weeks, sling use can be discontinued and the patient may begin active ROM with reintegration of the extremity into activities of daily living. During this point in the recovery, patients should not lift, push, or pull more than 1 lb until 10 weeks after surgery but then may progress to 2.5 lbs per week. Isometric strengthening exercises may begin in the second week, with the exception of internal rotation. Throughout the entire recovery period, patients should not progress to the next phase of their rehabilitation protocol until they are proficient with the previous phase. The goal is to not simply complete the protocol but to maximize the functional results of each phase, and therefore timing of advancement to the next phase will vary based on the individual patient and the speed of his or her gains.

After sling use is discontinued, strengthening exercises are introduced, while the patient and therapist concentrate on ROM until functional mobility is achieved. However, ROM expectations must be based on preoperative ranges and often are unlikely to be normal.

Patients may begin sport-specific training with gradual progression at 12 to 16 weeks depending on the nature of the pathology and the procedure performed.

Return to Sport/Work

Activities of daily living generally resume by 6 weeks after surgical intervention for glenohumeral arthritis. Patients should be instructed to resume their normal activities gradually. This reintegration of the operated extremity into routine tasks serves to increase ROM, strength, and stamina with minimal risks. However, routine daily tasks may need to be specifically defined so athletes do not advance their activities beyond the protocol prescribed.

All patients are encouraged to pursue their preoperative activities and sports; however, we recommend strongly that patients avoid contact sports after a TSA. Before patients begin return to play (RTP) without restriction, we recommend completion of the rehabilitation protocol, as well as gradual progression of sport-specific activities and exercises, which helps facilitate the transition to RTP to prevent setbacks or reinjury. In a series of 75 patients evaluating RTP after shoulder replacement, McCarty et al.[75] reported that patients had a mean time to partial return

to sport of 3.6 months and a full return at 5.8 months. Weightlifting for maintenance of muscle tone is encouraged, but powerlifting exercises are discouraged. Recommendations for alteration of the frequency, duration, or intensity of the patient's desired activity or sport should be provided based on the individual and the sport being considered.

RTP expectations should be individualized to the athlete, pathology, and nature of the procedure to maximize the longevity of the intervention and minimize further trauma. Studies show that participation in sports after shoulder arthroplasty is high, and often a person's ability to participate is improved after surgery. Jensen and Rockwood[165] reported that 96% of patients in a series of recreational golfers were able to return to sport after shoulder replacement surgery. In their series, McCarty et al.[75] reported that 64% of patients cited sports participation as a reason they chose to undergo shoulder replacement. Swimming, tennis, and golf were the three most common sports in which patients participated, and 71% demonstrated an improvement in their ability to participate in their sport, with 50% of patients increasing their frequency of participation. However, a lower rate of return was noted in softball, weightlifting, and bowling. No difference was found in return to sport between hemiarthroplasty versus TSA. No association was found between participation in sports and requirement for further surgery or failure of the components at average 3.7-year follow-up. These findings, consistent with other reports of athletic participation after shoulder arthroplasty, provide practitioners with evidence-based support to aid in counseling shoulder arthroplasty candidates regarding postoperative participation in sport.[166]

In addition, optimization of the kinetic chain should be encouraged through thorough completion of the rehabilitation protocol, as well as a maintenance program of home or gym exercises. Patients can continue to remain active after shoulder reconstruction; many of our own patients, as well as several studies, have demonstrated that a return to golf, tennis, snow skiing, mountain climbing, jogging, cycling, and many other physically demanding sports is possible.[75,165,166] Patients have been able to return to work with hemiarthroplasty 69% of the time, with moderate intensity return to work of 50%. Patients have a higher risk of failure with higher upper extremity demand in sports such as softball, baseball, and basketball.[167] In Gulotta et al., 97% of TSA were able to return to sport versus 65% for HA at 2 years postoperative, with an average RTS at 5 months postoperative. These included swimming, baseball, softball, and basketball.[168]

Complications

Complications in the treatment of glenohumeral arthritis depend on use of arthroscopic versus open techniques. Arthroscopic treatment has few complications, but complication rates of open procedures have been reported to be as high as 20% to 40%. Although many different problems may arise, they can often be avoided and solved by meticulous preoperative planning, careful surgical technique, and close attention to postoperative care. Tables 52.3 and 52.4 describe common complications and treatments for those complications in this setting.

TABLE 52.3 Common Intraoperative Complications and Treatment

Location	Complication	Treatment
Humerus	Diaphyseal fracture	Long-stemmed prosthesis Allograft struts and cables
Humerus	Greater tuberosity fracture	Suture fixation Postoperative modifications
Glenoid	Glenoid fracture	Rim—no treatment necessary Body—bone grafting/staged reconstruction
Rotator cuff	Supraspinatus/infraspinatus rupture	Repair may require reverse prosthesis if irreparable
Neurovascular injury	Axillary and musculocutaneous	Avoid overzealous retraction—observation
Vascular injury		Emergent vascular consultation for repair

TABLE 52.4 Common Postoperative Complications and Treatment

Location/Diagnosis	Complication	Treatment
Wound	Hematoma Dehiscence	Irrigation and débridement if >7 days Local wound care
Humerus	Component loosening	Infection workup

	Periprosthetic fracture	A. Revision longer stem
		B. Loose stem revision longer stem with allograft
		   Well-fixed stem ORIF with allograft
		C. Loose stem—revision long stem component
		   Well-fixed stem—trial nonoperative

Infection	Early, <6 weeks	Irrigation and débridement 6 weeks of IV antibiotics Attempt at component retention
	Late, >6 weeks	Staged procedure Removal of components 6 weeks of IV antibiotics
Instability	Anterior	Pectoralis major transfer Achilles tendon allograft Revision to reverse TSA
Instability	Posterior	Correction of humeral retroversion Increasing humerus head thickness
Glenoid	Loosening	Revision to pegged glenoid ± bone graft

FUTURE CONSIDERATIONS

Several novel ideas have been presented that may ultimately have applicability for the young, active patient with glenohumeral arthritis. The use of platelet-rich plasma is gaining in notoriety and popularity as several recent studies have begun to demonstrate the potential efficacy with regard to treatment of joint arthrosis.[169,170] To our knowledge, the use of platelet-rich plasma has not yet been studied in the shoulder, although it may develop into a viable treatment option with further examination. Furthermore, advances in technique with regard to arthroscopic-based resurfacing techniques have recently been presented[171] and may represent an alternative or adjunct to current resurfacing options. Further studies into implant longevity based on design, specifically with regard to glenoid fixation, are also ongoing and may contribute to a significant long-term outcome benefit in this patient population. Another consideration is matrix-induced autologous chondrocyte implantation (MACI) for the shoulder. This has been provisionally studied in rabbits and has indicated results poorer to microfracture.[172]

For a complete list of references, go to ExpertConsult.com.

SELECTED READINGS

Citation:

Edwards TB, et al. A comparison of hemiarthroplasty and total shoulder arthroplasty in the treatment of primary glenohumeral osteoarthritis: results of a multicenter study. *J Shoulder Elbow Surg.* 2003;12(3):207–213.

Level of Evidence:

III

Summary:

This study of 601 patients who underwent total shoulder arthroplasty (TSA) versus 89 patients who underwent hemiarthroplasty demonstrated the superiority of TSA with regard to pain, mobility, functional scores, and activity in persons with primary osteoarthritis.

Citation:

Samilson RL, Prieto V. Dislocation arthropathy of the shoulder. *J Bone Joint Surg Am.* 1983;65A(4):456–460.

Level of Evidence:

IV

Summary:

This article reports on a case series demonstrating high rates of arthrosis in unstable shoulders; the arthrosis was demonstrated to be worse in the setting of delay of diagnosis, nonoperative treatment, and posterior instability.

Citation:

Hovelius L, Saeboe M. Neer Award 2008: arthropathy after primary anterior shoulder dislocation—223 shoulders prospectively followed up for twenty-five years. *J Shoulder Elbow Surg.* 2009;18(3):339–347.

Level of Evidence:

IV

Summary:

This 25-year radiographic follow-up study of patients with primary anterior shoulder dislocation demonstrates that age at time of dislocation (25 years), recurrence of instability, participation in high-energy sports, and alcohol abuse are associated with greater risk of the development and severity of resultant arthropathy.

Citation:

Warner JP, et al. Glenohumeral arthritis in the young patient. *J Shoulder Elbow Surg.* 2011;20(6):s30–S40.

Level of Evidence:

IV

Summary:

This systematic review of the literature on the arthroscopic and open treatment options for early glenohumeral osteoarthritis reviews multiple treatment options and their outcomes.

Citation:

McCarty EC, et al. Sports participation after shoulder replacement surgery. *Am J Sports Med*. 2008;36(8):1577–1581.

Level of Evidence:

IV

Summary:

In this case series of 75 patients (average age, 65 years) who were followed up for 2 years, 64% reported "participation in sports" as a reason they decided to have surgery, with 71% reporting improvement in their ability to play their sport and 50% reporting increased frequency of participation. The most favorable sports for RTP were swimming, tennis, and golf, with softball demonstrating the lowest return (20%). The mean time to return to these activities was 3.6 months.

Citation:

Elser F, et al. Glenohumeral joint preservation: current options for managing articular cartilage lesions in young, active patients. *Arthroscopy*. 2010;26(5):685–696.

Level of Evidence:

V

Summary:

This article provides a comprehensive review of joint-preservation techniques for the shoulder, including a surgical decision-making guide for arthroscopy, microfracture, osteochondral autograft transfer system, autologous chondrocyte implantation, allograft, and biologic resurfacing.

Citation:

Levine WN, et al. Hemiarthroplasty for glenohumeral osteoarthritis: results correlated to degree of glenoid wear. *J Shoulder Elbow Surg*. 1997;6(5):449–454.

Level of Evidence:

IV

Summary:

This retrospective review of 31 patients who had undergone hemiarthroplasty for glenohumeral osteoarthritis demonstrates a satisfactory result in 74% of patients, which correlated directly with the amount of posterior glenoid wear. In patients with type I glenoids, 86% achieved satisfactory results, compared with 63% in patients with a type II glenoid, although similar pain relief was achieved in both groups, with the greatest deficits in forward elevation and external rotation.

Citation:

Saltzman MD, et al. Comparison of patients undergoing primary shoulder arthroplasty before and after the age of fifty. *J Bone Joint Surg Am*. 2013;95A(1):562–569.

Level of Evidence:

IV

Summary:

This instructional course lecture of the AAOS reviews possible complications of a TSA. In reviewing the complications, it also gives treatment options and intraoperative suggestions when dealing with particularly difficult situations that may prevent future complications.

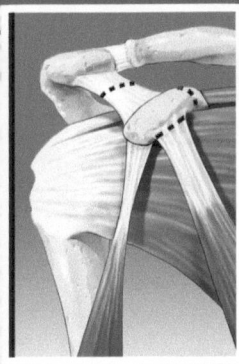

53

Scapulothoracic Disorders

G. Keith Gill, Gehron Treme, Dustin Richter

The scapula connects the upper extremity to the thorax and allows for complex movements about the shoulder. Although there are minimal bony connections to the axial skeleton, the scapula plays an integral role in the function of the upper extremity and especially in the throwing mechanism. In total there are 17 muscles that have their origin or insertion on the scapula (Table 53.1[1] and Fig. 53.1), which acts to collect forces passing through the trunk and transfer them to the arm. These muscles provide intrinsic, extrinsic, and stabilization/rotational functions of the shoulder. Scapular motion is critical to the phases of throwing, with protraction and retraction required from cocking to deceleration. Errors in timing are critical because the glenoid and humeral head must remain centered to allow maximum efficiency during this activity. Altered strength and mechanics of the scapula can have detrimental effects on the throwing shoulder.

Scapulothoracic (ST) disorders can be broken down into three main categories: scapular bursitis and crepitus, scapular winging, and scapular dyskinesis or SICK scapula. These disorders are seldomly found in isolation but frequently are associated with scapular malposition and tracking disorders, as well as structural injuries, including labral and rotator cuff tears. Often, successful treatment and rehabilitation of the painful shoulder depend heavily on recognizing scapular disorders. This chapter provides an overview of ST disorders, focusing on accurate diagnosis and successful treatment.

SCAPULAR BURSITIS AND CREPITUS

The shoulder has three major and several minor described bursae (Table 53.2 and Fig. 53.2), although significant variability exists among individuals. In addition, some of the minor bursae may be absent all together. The term "snapping scapula" has been used when the scapular bursitis and crepitus becomes symptomatic. These symptoms can result from numerous etiologies (Box 53.1).[2–6]

SCAPULAR WINGING

Scapular winging is defined as abnormal motion of the scapula and may result from a number of anatomic disorders (Table 53.3).[7–18] Primary winging is a neurologic or muscular disorder that affects the scapular stabilizers and is described as medial or lateral. Medial winging is the result of a dysfunctional serratus anterior muscle secondary to long thoracic nerve pathology. In contrast, lateral winging is the result of a dysfunctional spinal accessory nerve (cranial nerve XI) affecting the trapezius muscle or dysfunction in the dorsal scapular nerve (C5) affecting the rhomboid muscles (Fig. 53.3). Secondary scapular winging occurs in conjunction with glenohumeral pathology and involves alteration of the normal scapular rhythm. Addressing the glenohumeral pathology and instituting a rehabilitation plan that targets the scapular dynamics will typically resolve the winging.

SCAPULAR DYSKINESIS

Scapular dyskinesia has become synonymous with the term "SICK scapula," which was coined by Burkhart and colleagues[19] in 2003. This acronym describes a common constellation of findings in this disorder, including Scapular malposition, Inferior medial border prominence, Coracoid pain and malposition, and dysKinesis of scapular movement. In the disabled thrower, abnormal muscle activation leads to alteration in the resting position of the scapula and SICK and may be a precursor to intra-articular injuries. Scapular dyskinesis has been divided into three types, with various associated structural issues identified with each type. Type I involves prominence of the inferior medial angle of the scapula, whereas type II involves medial border prominence. Both types I and II are associated with labral pathology. Type III involves prominence of the superior medial border and is associated with shoulder impingement and rotator cuff tears.

HISTORY

ST disorders are common in patients who perform repetitive overhead activities as a result of their occupation or choice of sport.[2,20] These disorders may be underrecognized in the office setting, which can lead to delay in diagnosis and treatment. Repetitive microtrauma is theorized to lead to soft tissue inflammation underlying the scapula and, if allowed to progress, to development of chronic ST bursitis.[1,3] Scarring and fibrosis ensue, and the thickened fibrotic tissue occupies excessive space within the ST compartment leading to impingement and maltracking.

ST dysfunction often starts insidiously, although on occasion, the onset of symptoms is preceded by a minor traumatic event.[3,21] Motion of the ST joint becomes extremely painful and is usually exacerbated by overhead activities. Patients often report crepitus in the posterior aspect of the shoulder, with or without pain.[3,4]

TABLE 53.1 Scapula Muscular Attachments

Region	Muscle	Scapular Attachments	Action
Rotator cuff	Infraspinatus	Infraspinous fossa	Rotates arm laterally
	Subscapularis	Medial two-thirds of subscapular fossa	Adducts and rotates arm medially
	Supraspinatus	Supraspinous fossa	Abducts arm
	Teres minor	Upper portion of lateral border of scapula	Rotates arm laterally
Scapulohumeral	Biceps brachii	Short head—coracoid process; long head—supraglenoid tubercle of scapula	Flexes arm and forearm, supinates forearm
	Coracobrachialis	Apex of coracoid process	Flexes and adducts arm
	Deltoid	Spine of scapula, acromion, lateral third of clavicle	Abducts, adducts, flexes, extends, rotates arm medially and laterally
	Teres major	Dorsal surface of inferior angle of scapula	Adducts and rotates arm medially
	Triceps brachii (long head)	Infraglenoid tubercle of scapula	Extends forearm at elbow joint; accessory adductor and extensor of the arm
Scapulothoracic	Latissimus dorsi	Attaches as it crosses the inferior angle of scapula	Adducts, extends, and rotates arm medially; retraction and downward rotation of scapula
	Levator scapulae	Medial border of scapula	Elevates scapula, rotates glenoid cavity
	Omohyoid	Inferior belly from medial lip of suprascapular notch and suprascapular ligament	Depresses and retracts hyoid and larynx
	Pectoralis minor	Coracoid process of scapula (medial border and upper surface)	Depresses and protracts scapula; elevates ribs
	Rhomboid major	Medial border of scapula	Adducts scapula
	Rhomboid minor	Root of spine of scapula	Adducts scapula
	Serratus anterior	Costal surface of medial border of scapula	Protraction and rotation of scapula, keeps medial border and inferior angle of scapula opposed to thoracic wall
	Trapezius	Spine of scapula, acromion	Adducts, rotates, elevates, and depresses scapula

From Moore KL. *Clinically Oriented Anatomy*. 6th ed. Baltimore: Lippincott Williams & Wilkins; 2010.

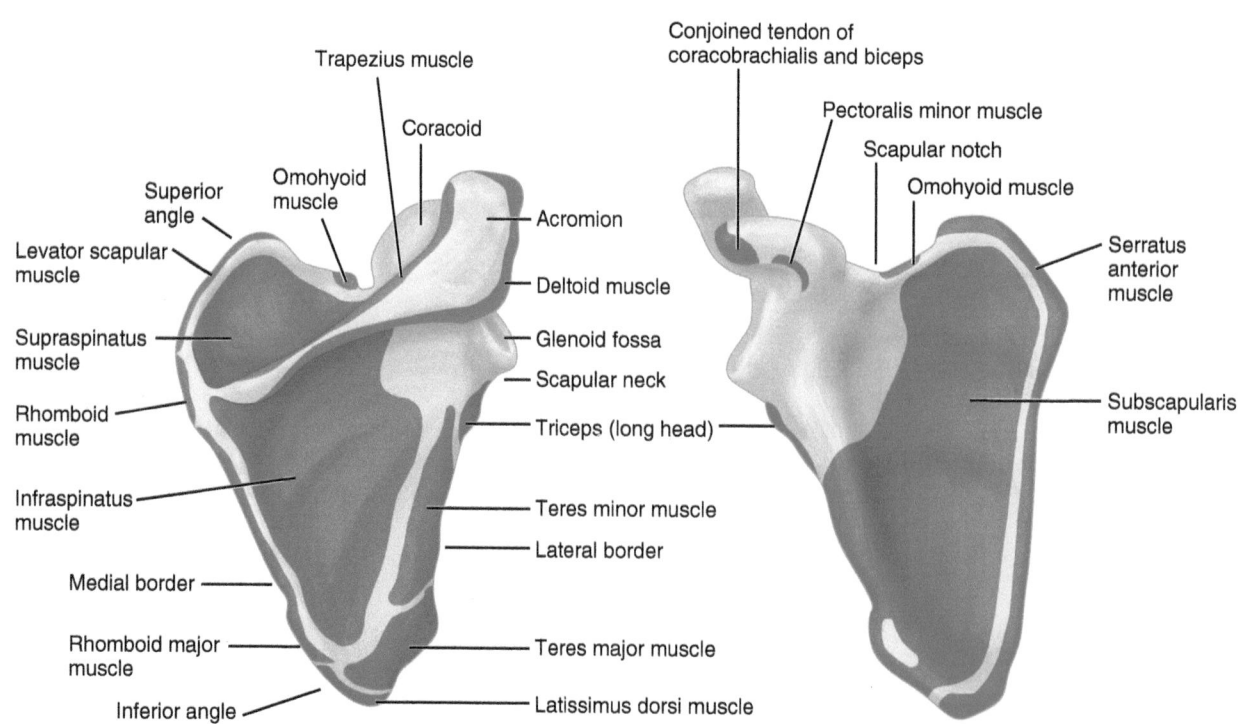

Fig. 53.1 Scapular muscular attachments.

Throwing athletes with SICK scapula may report a "dead arm feeling" with resultant loss of maximum velocity and control. Pain may be variable, with some patients describing it anteriorly, posteriorly over the scapula, or even laterally and often radiating into the neck or the affected extremity. Pain anteriorly adjacent to the coracoid is a common presenting complaint. The patient should be questioned about prior surgery, including minor procedures near the long thoracic nerve, such as a lymph node biopsy.

PHYSICAL EXAMINATION

Inspection

As always, a good physical examination begins with inspection. It is imperative that the patient disrobe to allow both scapulae to be revealed simultaneously so that any signs of asymmetry in position or during motion can be observed (Fig. 53.4). The superior and inferior medial angles of the scapulae should align symmetrically, and the scapular borders should be equidistance

TABLE 53.2	Bursae Types	
Bursa	**Location**	
Major (anatomic)	Infraserratus	Between serratus anterior and chest wall
	Supraserratus	Between subscapularis and serratus anterior
	Scapulotrapezial	Between superomedial scapular angle and trapezius (contains spinal accessory nerve)
Minor (adventitial)	Infraserratus (superior)	Superomedial scapular angle
	Infraserratus (inferior)	Inferior scapular angle
	Supraserratus	Superomedial scapular angle
	Trapezoid	Medial base of spine of scapula underlying the trapezius

BOX 53.1 Differential Diagnosis/Pathogenesis of Bursitis

- Soft tissue lesions such as atrophied muscle[2,3]
- Fibrotic muscle[2,4]
- Anomalous muscle insertions[2,3]
- Masses such as an elastofibroma (a rare benign soft tissue tumor on the chest wall elevating the scapula) or an osteochondroma (arising from under the scapular surface or posterior aspect of the ribs)[2]
- Luschka tubercle (a prominent bone with an excessive "hook" at the superomedial aspect of the scapula)[2]
- Malunited fractures of the scapula or ribs can lead to crepitus[2,5]
- Reactive bone spurs (can form repetitive microtrauma of the periscapular musculature)[2,5]
- Incongruity of the articulation leading to altered biomechanics (may exist as a result of scoliosis or thoracic kyphosis)[3,6]
- Rule out unrelated disorders such as cervical spondylosis and radiculopathy, glenohumeral pathology, and periscapular muscle strain[3,6]

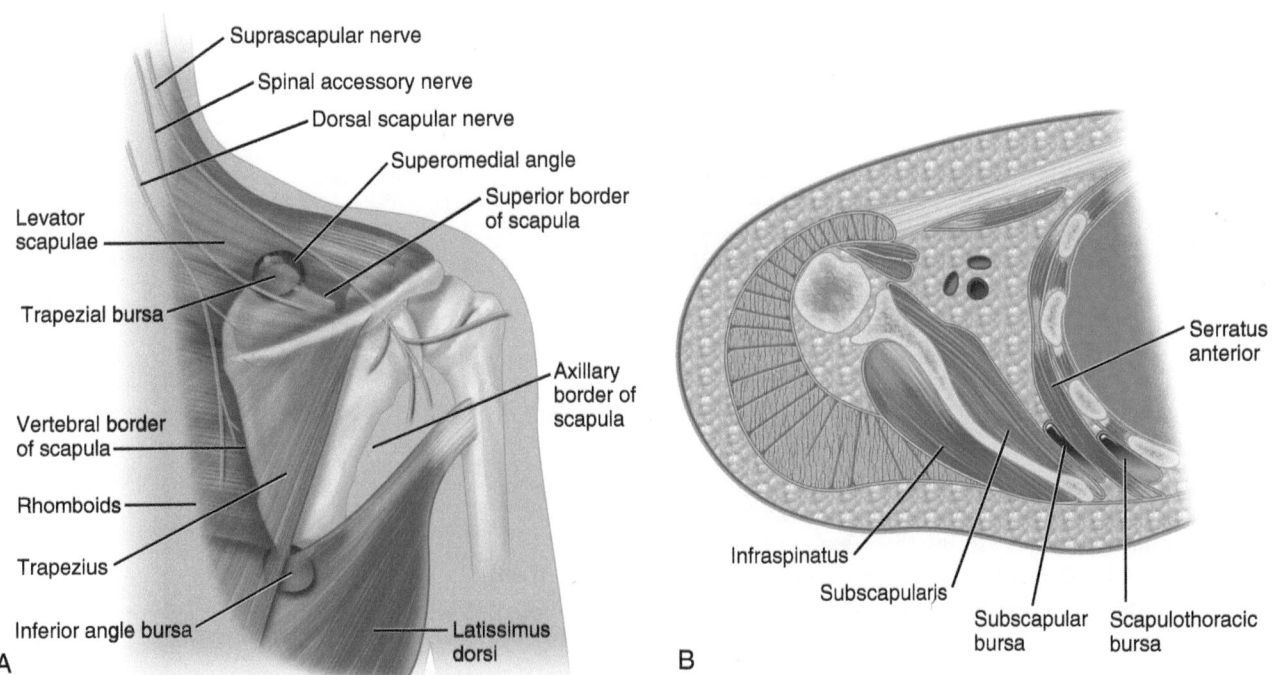

Fig. 53.2 (A) Trapezial bursa at the superior medial angle and inferior angle bursa. (B) Subscapularis (supraserratus bursa) shown just anterior to the subscapularis muscle and scapular body.

TABLE 53.3   Causes of Scapular Winging

Etiology	Type	Injury	Causes
First degree	Medial winging	Serratus anterior palsy—long thoracic nerve (C5-C7)	Most common cause of medial winging Damage to nerve from pressure lesions or neuritis (inflammation) Enlarged subcoracoid or subscapular bursa[7] Nerve is vulnerable to injury because of the torturous route from the neck to the serratus anterior muscle
	Lateral winging	Trapezius palsy—spinal accessory nerve (C3-C4)	Isolated loss of trapezius function is rare The most common cause is iatrogenic resulting from cervical lymph node or tumor removal[8–12] Due to the superficial course of nerve[8,12,13]
		Rhomboid palsy—dorsal scapular nerve (C5)	Primarily neurogenic in nature Entrapment in the middle scalene muscle is the most common[14] Anterior shoulder dislocation[15] C5 radiculopathy[16] Overhead motion muscle strain injuries[17]
Second degree	Medial and lateral winging	Loss of scapular suspensory mechanism	Usually affects overhead-throwing athletes; causes abnormal scapula rhythm and produces scapular winging with overhead maneuvers Dislocation of the AC joint or fracture of the outer third of the clavicle causing rupture of the CC ligaments
		Myopathies; weakness of the scapular stabilizers	Brachial plexus injury Muscular dystrophies, most commonly FSHD Peripheral nerve disease[18] Parsonage-Turner syndrome (brachial neuritis)

AC, Acromioclavicular; *CC,* coracoclavicular; *FSHD,* fascioscapulohumeral dystrophy.

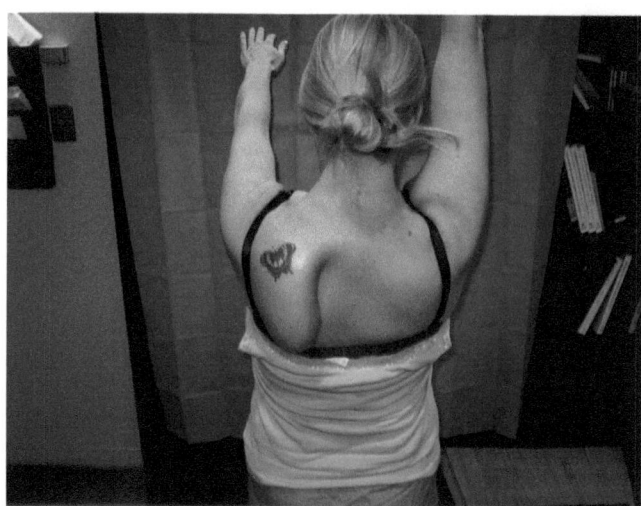

Fig. 53.3 Lateral winging of the scapula.

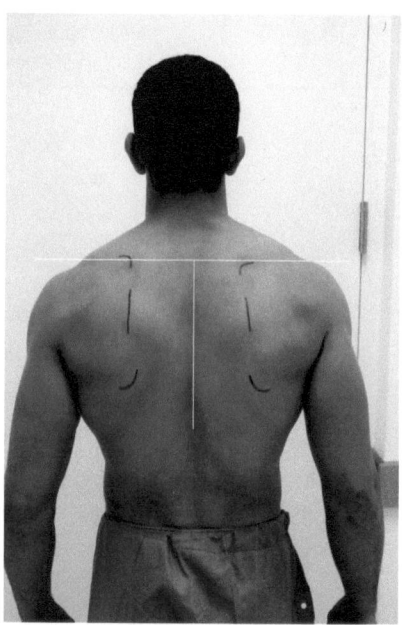

Fig. 53.4 A throwing athlete with type II scapular dyskinesia of the left shoulder. Note the difference in shoulder height, the distance and angle of the medial border from midline, and the location of scapular prominence.

from a vertical line connecting the spinous processes. The examiner should always note whether the superior angle, inferior angle, or medial border of the scapula is most prominent.

Although less common, asymmetry may result from other causes such as scoliosis, pelvic obliquity, and scapular winging. The exam should include measuring shoulder and hip height, and the spine should be inspected for scoliotic deformity. Often, the injured shoulder will appear lower on inspection from behind because the scapula moves laterally, tilts forward, and drops inferiorly (Fig. 53.5). Pseudowinging is periscapular fullness that is biomechanical compensation as a result of painful bursitis.[3,4]

Palpation

Palpation of the entire scapula allows localization of symptomatic areas and masses. Patients often experience tenderness over the superior medial angle of the scapula, and in some occasions, a palpable mass may be present.[4] In addition, the inferior medial angle is a common location for point tenderness. Patients with positive palpation at this location should raise suspicion for labral pathology, most commonly superior labrum anterior and posterior (SLAP) lesions, and should be tested for their presence. Palpable crepitus can often be detected by placing one hand over the medial aspect of the scapula while grasping the patient's symptomatic arm and performing range of motion (ROM) testing.

Ipsilateral coracoid tenderness is common in those patients with SICK scapula syndrome. The pathophysiology is likely from scapular tilt and lateral positioning of the coracoid, which lead to tightness in the pectoralis minor and conjoint tendons. Palpation over the insertion of the levator scapulae can also elicit tenderness as it becomes lengthened due to tilting away from its normal position.

Range of Motion

On examination, shoulder ROM is often diminished as a result of pain around the scapula or in the subacromial space. Scapular

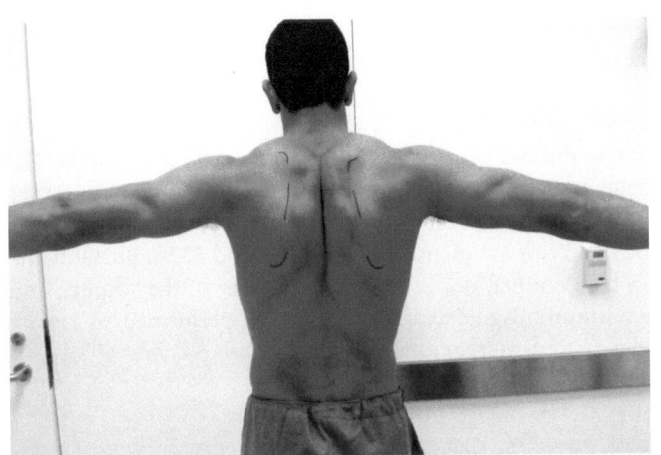

Fig. 53.5 Marking the scapular landmarks improves diagnostic accuracy.

stabilizers lose ability to properly rotate the scapula due to subacromial bursitis causing subacromial impingement with overhead activities.

Patients with scapular dyskinesia will often have limited forward shoulder flexion, both passively and actively. Forward flexion limitations can often be alleviated by manual repositioning the scapula.

Examining scapular motion is paramount, and the examiner should look for asymmetric movement of the scapula during elevation of the shoulder. Measuring and marking of the scapular borders and comparing with the contralateral side improves ease of diagnosis (see Fig. 53.5). In examining for winging of the scapula, the examiner stands behind the patient and asks the patient to slowly raise both arms overhead. Primary winging is due to neurologic abnormalities described previously, whereas secondary winging occurs in the setting of normal trapezius (lateral) and serratus anterior (medial) function and represents a painful response to glenohumeral pathology and not neurologic pathology.[4]

Strength

Loss of strength in the shoulder from ST disorders is proportional to the severity of the subacromial symptoms present. Strength may vary from breakaway weakness to full strength. The patient should be asked to perform a shoulder shrug against resistance to test the strength of the scapular elevators. A rolling shrug should then be performed while the examiner palpates the superior medial angle of the scapula for crepitus; this is then repeated for the inferior medial angle.

Testing
Wall Push-Up
Subtle winging can be detected by having the patient perform a wall push-up, carefully noting the direction of winging (Fig. 53.6).

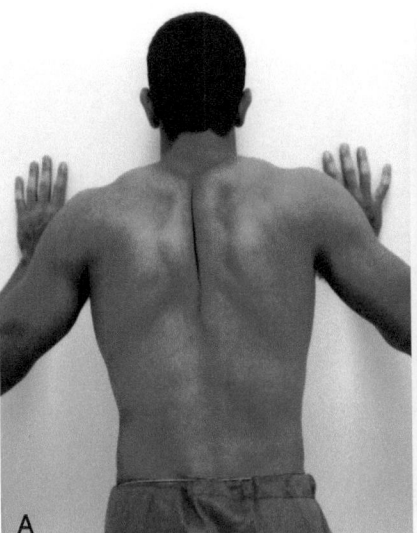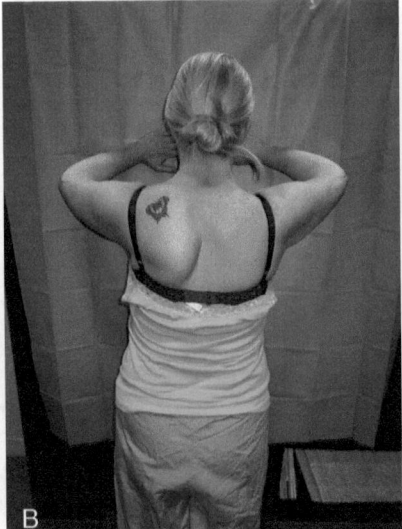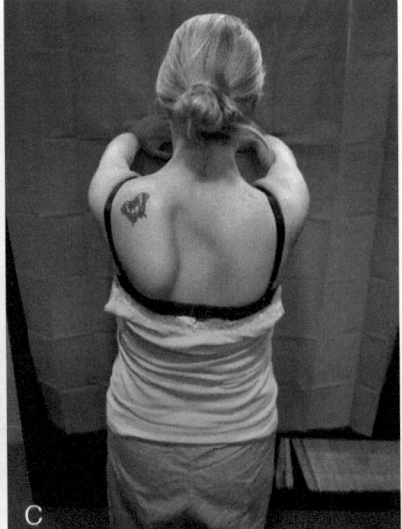

Fig. 53.6 (A–C) The patient is asked to perform a wall push-up to accentuate scapular winging if present. Symmetry of scapular tracking, prominences, and musculature should be apparent.

Scapular Retraction Test

To perform the scapular retraction test, an examiner performs passive ROM from behind the patient while palpating the coracoid. A positive test is defined as coracoid tenderness with diminished forward flexion that improves or resolves with manual repositioning of the scapula medially and inferiorly, symmetric to the contralateral scapula.

Impingement Examination

Impingement examination is generally positive because the acromion is malpositioned, reducing subacromial space. Failure of the scapula to rotate out of the way during forward elevation leads to impingement of the rotator cuff. Frequently used examination maneuvers for impingement including those described by Neer and Hawkins may be useful. The empty can test or Jobe test also can be helpful. This test is performed by asking the patient to actively abduct both arms to 90 degrees in the scapular plane and rotate their arms internally until the thumbs point down at the floor. Standing behind the patient, the examiner places their hands on the patient's forearm and asks the patient to resist downward pressure. Increased pain in the shoulder indicates a positive test (Fig. 53.7).

IMAGING

Radiographs

A shoulder series of radiographs with tangential views of the scapula should be obtained to rule out associated bony abnormalities or neoplastic lesions. Although radiographs are not truly necessary for diagnosis, they are encouraged for completeness.[2,4]

Computed Tomography Scan

A computed tomography scan should be obtained when bony abnormalities are identified on plain radiographs because the bony anatomy of the scapula makes complete visualization of some bone lesions challenging. Bone lesions, such as osteochondromas, can be the etiology behind ST crepitus and pain and can be more thoroughly defined by computed tomography

modalities. Computed tomography in the setting of normal radiographs has not been shown to be beneficial.[22,23]

Magnetic Resonance Imaging Scan

A magnetic resonance imaging (MRI) scan may show increased signal and fluid accumulation as a result of bursal inflammation.[2,4] The films should be ordered and viewed in consultation with a trained musculoskeletal radiologist because this area is often not heavily scrutinized and in some cases is not well visualized during normal interpretation of a shoulder MRI. The presence of palpable crepitus is enough to confirm the diagnosis of ST bursitis, and the use of MRI, especially with the use of an intravenous contrast medium, is probably best reserved for cases in which a palpable mass raises the concern for neoplasia. In addition, because secondary ST disorders may be a result of more common shoulder pathology, MRI represents an important tool to fully diagnose the cause of the ST symptoms.

Electromyography

Electromyography should be obtained in cases of scapular winging to evaluate injury to the long thoracic or spinal accessory nerves.[2]

Ultrasound

Ultrasound can be used to evaluate inflamed bursal tissue. The probe is placed over the medial border of the scapula, either perpendicular or parallel to the medial border, and the scapular body and ribs are identified (Figs. 53.8 and 53.9). Bursal tissue can be identified under the medial border of the scapula, and an ultrasound-guided injection can be performed to ensure delivery to the target tissues (Fig. 53.10).

DECISION-MAKING PRINCIPLES

Pain and/or Crepitus

Crepitus without pain can be considered normal and is present in up to 35% of otherwise asymptomatic shoulders.[24] Surgery should be considered only in those patients with crepitus

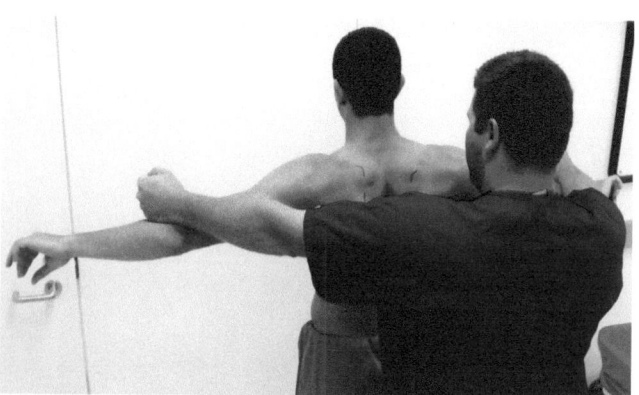

Fig. 53.7 The empty can test is performed by having the patient abduct the shoulder in the scapular plane to 90 degrees, internally rotate both arms until the thumbs point at the floor, and resist downward pressure. A positive test indicates an inflamed subacromial space.

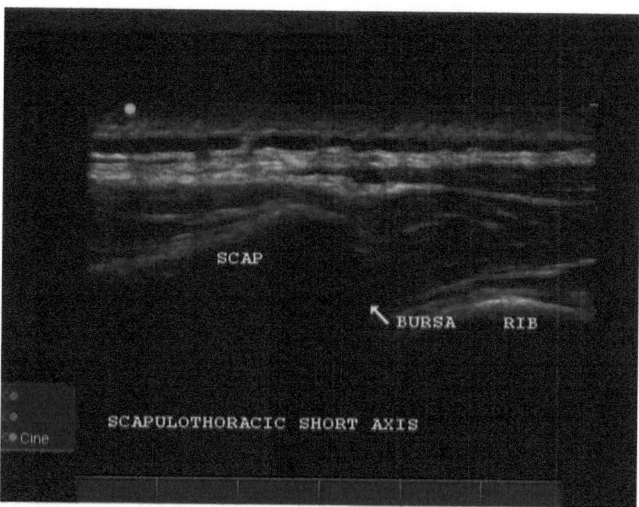

Fig. 53.8 An ultrasound image of scapular bursa *(white arrow)* visualized below the scapular body *(SCAP)*. (Courtesy Alan Hirahara, MD.)

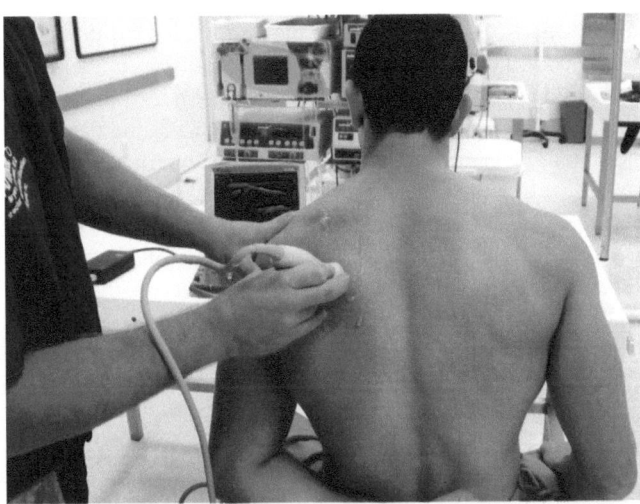

Fig. 53.9 Positioning of the patient for an ultrasound examination.

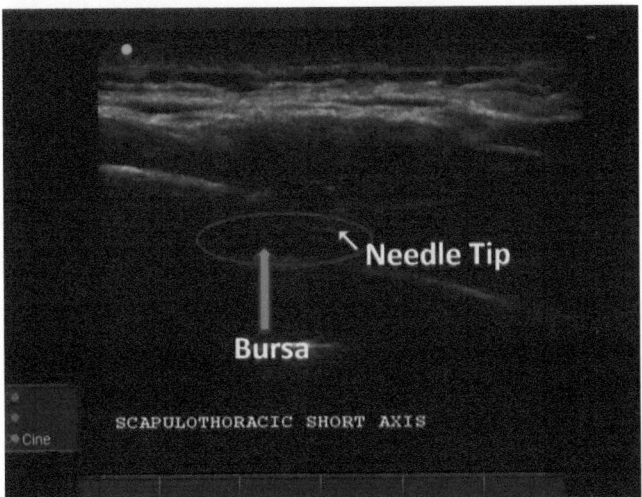

Fig. 53.10 An image of an ultrasound-guided injection into the subscapular bursa. The needle tip (white arrow) is visualized, and fluid can be observed entering the bursa in real time. (Courtesy Alan Hirahara, MD.)

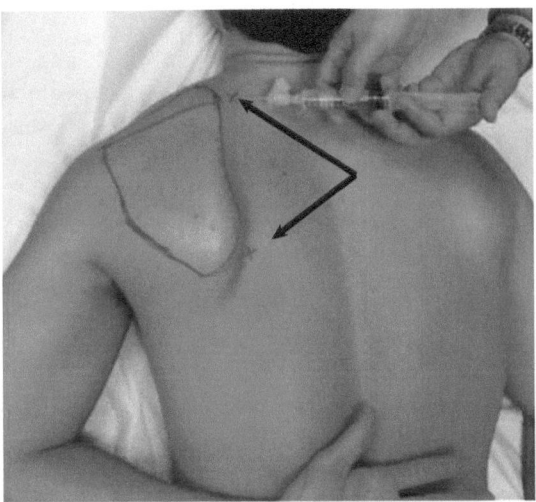

Fig. 53.11 The injection technique begins with marking out the scapula, palpating the areas of greatest crepitus, and marking the injection sites (arrows) before administering a local anesthetic. (Courtesy Reuben Gobezie, MD.)

When surgical intervention is being considered, patients with pain localized to the superior or inferior medial angles have the best postoperative prognosis and are good surgical candidates. In contrast, surgery should be avoided in patients with global pain or documented nerve deficits.

Response to Injection

Patients who experience no improvement from an appropriately placed corticosteroid injection containing a local anesthetic (Fig. 53.11) are less likely to benefit from surgical débridement or intervention of that area. Patients experiencing improvement after an injection, including immediately after administration of a local anesthetic, are most likely to have beneficial outcomes and relief of symptoms after arthroscopic bursal resection.

TREATMENT OPTIONS

Nonoperative

Nonoperative treatment consisting of rest, activity modification, analgesics, nonsteroidal antiinflammatory drugs, and physical therapy are the mainstay of treatments and should be prescribed initially.[2,4,20] The goals of therapy are to improve scapular posture, stretch and strengthen the subscapularis and serratus anterior muscles, and elevate the scapula from the chest wall.[4,25] Strengthening the serratus anterior reduces forward tilt of the scapula and allows subsidence of bursal irritation.[4]

Corticosteroid injections into the area of maximal tenderness can be effective in reducing pain and symptoms as well. Injections in this area are relatively safe, but care must be taken during the injection because too steep an angle can lead to a pneumothorax. The scapular spine and superior and inferior angles should be marked prior to performing the injection, being sure to approach just anterior to the scapular body. Positioning the patient prone with the shoulder in full internal rotation and the hand on the lower back, as used for a lift-off examination, increases the space between the scapula and the thorax and

combined with another symptom, such as pain, dyskinesia, or winging.

Prior Treatment

Surgery should be considered only in patients with concomitant pathology or in persons for whom 6 months of physical therapy with a dedicated scapular stabilization protocol has failed. Patients who have not had a dedicated trial of conservative treatment should be referred for therapy.

Associated Pathology and Location of Pain

Surgery should be considered in patients with confirmed glenohumeral or rotator cuff pathology or in whom bony pathology has been verified. It has been theorized that scapular dyskinesia may be a prodrome in the development of SLAP tears and early correction may prevent future labral injury. Prior to the development of structural pathology, treatment is nonoperative and should focus on scapular muscle rehabilitation, ST kinematics, glenohumeral motion, and core strengthening.

facilitates the procedure. It is also recommended to mark injection sites before a local anesthetic is administered (see Fig. 53.11, black arrow). Ultrasound guidance can be a useful tool to help confirm location of the needle in the correct plane, which may improve results and reduce risk of inadvertent penetration into the thoracic cavity.

For patients with scapular dyskinesia, all throwing activities should be discontinued immediately, and a course of physical therapy should be undertaken (Table 53.4). An interval throwing program should be initiated when the patient is completely asymptomatic and scapular position has returned to near normal. For dedicated patients who perform rehabilitation exercises three times daily, scapular position will dramatically improve in 2 to 3 weeks and a period of 3 months is typically required to return to normal.

Operative Treatment
Scapular Bursitis/Crepitus

Open technique. Historically, a superior medial scapular resection and open bursectomy at either the superior medial angle or inferior pole has been performed to relieve chronic bursitis. The downside of these procedures is that they require a large exposure and significant subperiosteal dissection of the medial musculature.[4,25-28]

The surgical technique for the resection of the superomedial angle of the scapula begins with the patient in the prone position. An incision following Langer lines is made just lateral to the medial border of the scapula, from the superior angle to 3 cm below the scapular spine. The soft tissue is dissected down to the spine of the scapula (Fig. 53.12). The periosteum over the spine is incised, and a plane is developed between the superficial trapezius and the underlying scapula. Next, a plane is developed between the supraspinatus and the rhomboids and

the levator scapulae muscles along the medial border of the scapula, starting at the spine of the scapula. The supraspinatus is elevated in a subperiosteal plane from the supraspinatus fossa. The medial ST muscles are dissected from the medial border of the scapula, and the dissection in this subperiosteal plane is carried around the medial border and to the subscapularis fossa, elevating the serratus and subscapularis with the rhomboids and levator (Fig. 53.13). The superomedial angle of the scapula is resected with an oscillating saw (Fig. 53.14). Because the resection is carried laterally, caution is warranted to avoid injury to the dorsal scapular artery and the suprascapular nerve in the suprascapular notch. After resecting the bone, the reflected muscles fall back into place, and the medial border of the supraspinatus is repaired to the rhomboid-levator flap. Inferiorly, the periosteum is repaired back to the spine of the scapula using suture passed

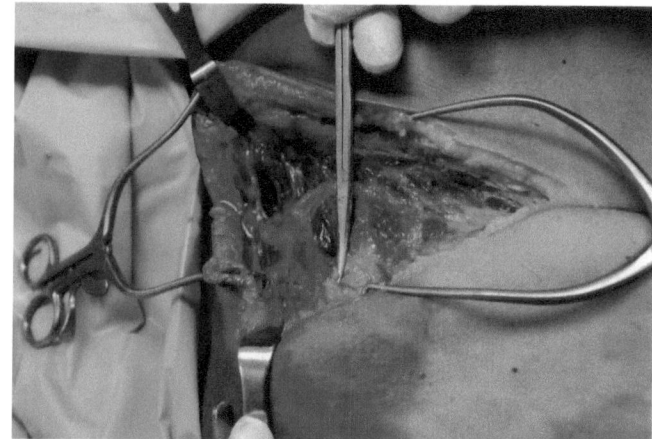

Fig. 53.12 The scapular spine is palpated (scissors), and the periosteum is incised over the spine.

Phase	Timeline	Focus	Goals
TABLE 53.4	**Scapular Dyskinesia Rehabilitation Guidelines**		
I	0–3 weeks	Scapular base	Initiate soft tissue mobilization
			Stretching via passive, active assisted, active, and proprioceptive neuromuscular to improve internal rotation, horizontal adduction, and scapular posture
			Initiate closed kinetic chain scapular motion exercises to regain scapular strength and control[19]
			Protraction
			Retraction
			Elevation and retraction
			Depression and retraction
			Internal rotation and elevation
			External rotation and depression
II	3–8 weeks	Rotator cuff	Progression of strengthening and flexibility exercises
			Restore muscle balance
			Enhance dynamic stability via open chain cable exercises with forward/lateral lunges with diagonal pulls
			Initiate rotator cuff strengthening once a stable scapular base has been restored[19]
III	8–12 weeks	Sport-specific training	Continue flexibility exercises
			Aggressive strengthening, power, and endurance
			Progressive neuromuscular control
			Initiate light throwing activities at short distances and progress to competitive throwing
			Exercises that promote effective energy transfer through the kinetic chain
			Return to sport/activity

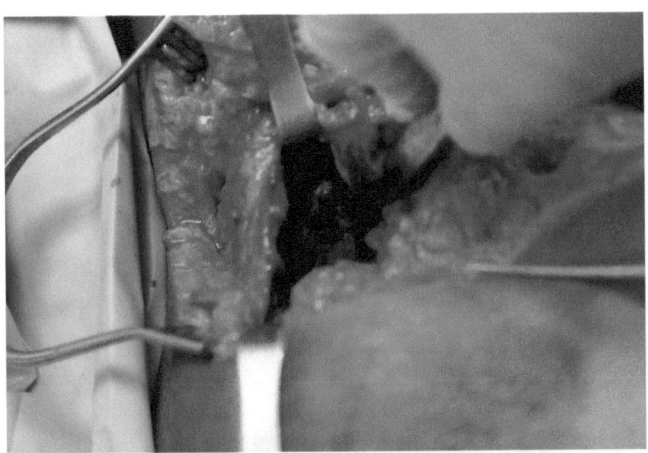

Fig. 53.13 The soft tissue attachments above the spine are elevated to skeletonize and expose the superior medial angle.

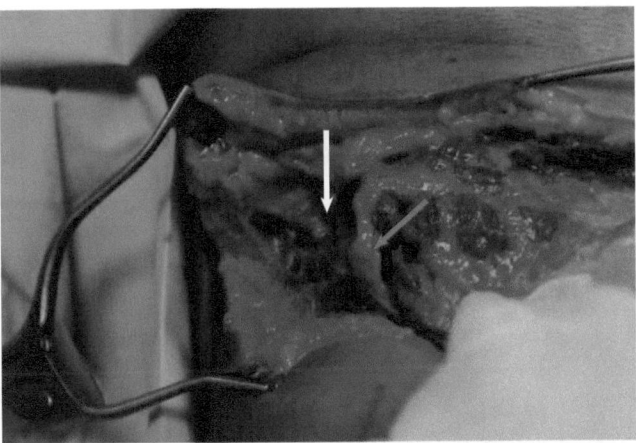

Fig. 53.15 The previously elevated soft tissues *(white arrow)* are brought back down to the spine of the scapula and are sutured to it, using three drill holes in the spine *(blue arrow)*.

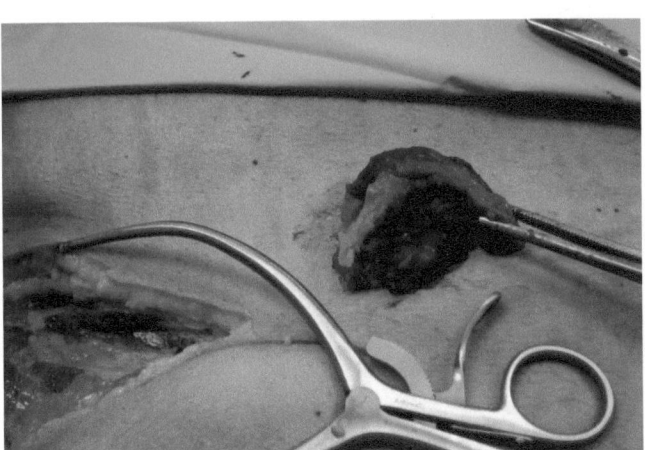

Fig. 53.14 Resected superior medial scapula.

through drill holes (Fig. 53.15). Postoperatively, the patient uses a sling and begins passive motion immediately. Active motion is begun after 6 weeks, and resistance exercises follow after 8 to 12 weeks.

Complications associated with partial scapulectomy include pneumothorax and postoperative hematoma; in younger patients, bone may try to reform, but this process rarely produces symptoms.

The reported results for this procedure are generally good.[17,29-33] However, it must be remembered that because athletes typically do not require surgical intervention, the literature includes little data regarding the effect of superomedial angle resection of the scapula on athletic performance. It is also important to note that the bone resected is not pathologic and appears normal histologically, which has prompted some surgeons to perform bursectomies and avoid a partial scapulectomy.[31,34]

Authors' Preferred Technique

Arthroscopic Bursal Resection

In the current age of advanced arthroscopic techniques and expertise, bursal resection can be safely accomplished arthroscopically without detaching muscle insertions, thus minimizing morbidity from the surgical exposure. The arthroscopic approach facilitates earlier rehabilitation and return to sport.[4,26,27] Arthroscopy is our preferred technique in symptomatic patients for whom conservative treatment has failed. Our preference is positioning the patient prone. Due to difficulty in identifying landmarks, with the exception of the ribs (Fig. 53.16), which can be exposed by inadvertent resection of the overlying serratus anterior musculature, we recommend tracing out the borders of the scapula and believe it also helps with arthroscopic orientation. Most surgeons believe that the prone position aids in triangulation. Portals should be positioned 2–3 cm medial to the scapular border to avoid the dorsal scapular nerve and artery (Fig. 53.17). The superior medial angle is usually localized with a spinal needle, taking care not to plunge into the thoracic cavity. In addition, working medial to lateral is preferred to avoid the neurovascular structures and smooth cannulas should also be used to protect vital structures.

The middle portal is created first, midway between the scapular spine and inferior angle. In practice, this portal is 4–5 cm below the scapular spine. After

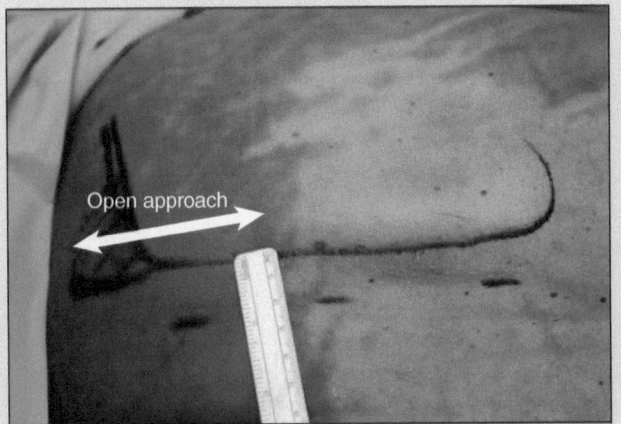

Fig. 53.16 Open and arthroscopic incisions are shown for a right scapula. The incision for the open resection of the superior medial scapula is placed just lateral to the medial border of the scapula and extended from the superior border to 3 cm distal to the spine.

Continued

Authors' Preferred Technique

Arthroscopic Bursal Resection—cont'd

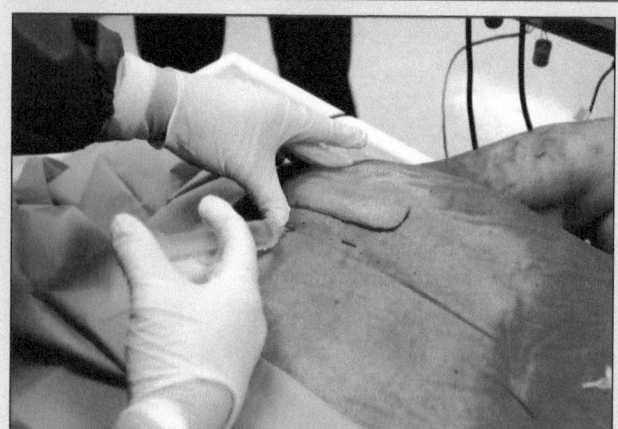

Fig. 53.17 Thirty milliliters of saline solution is injected into a portal 4 to 5 cm below and 2 cm medial to the scapular spine to distend the bursa.

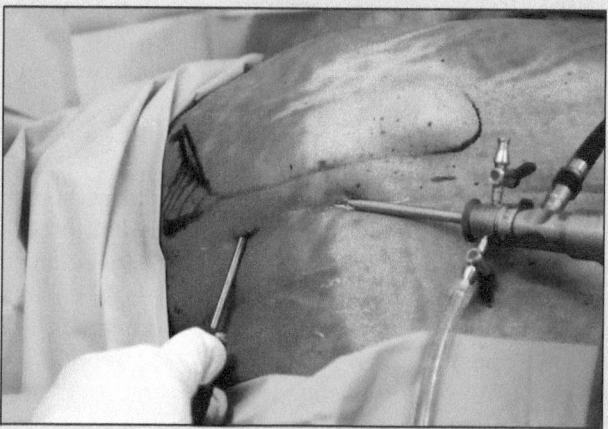

Fig. 53.18 Initial access into the subscapular bursa.

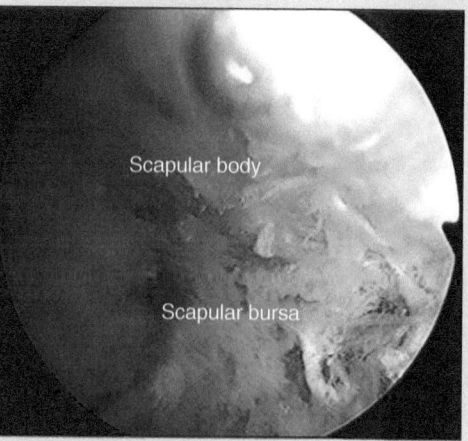

Fig. 53.19 The typical initial visualization upon entering the subscapular bursa. The scapular body is visible superiorly, and the bursa is seen below.

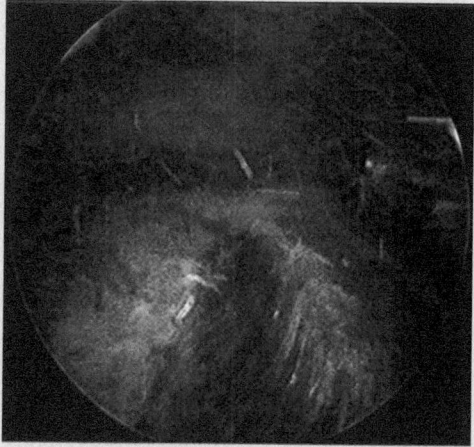

Fig. 53.20 Ribs and intercostal muscles visualized after resection of the serratus anterior (not recommended).

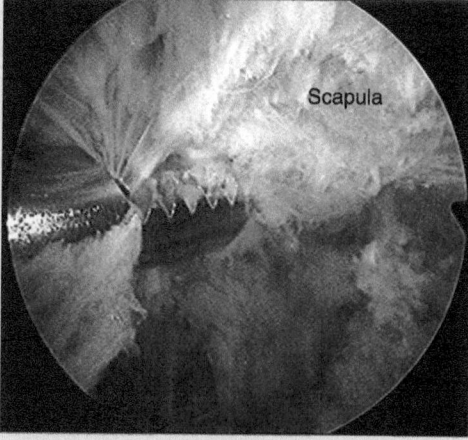

Fig. 53.21 Resection of the subscapular bursa should be carried out from medial to lateral and from inferior to superior.

marking the portal, a spinal needle is inserted into the bursa between the chest wall and serratus anterior, and 30 mL of saline solution is injected to distend the space (Fig. 53.18). Portals should be created by incising the skin only, and a blunt obturator is swept through the bursa, being careful to retain a shallow angle of approach and making frequent contact with the scapular body superiorly. A 4-mm, 30-degree arthroscope is then inserted into this potential space.

The superior portal is then created at the level of, or just below, the scapular spine, offering shaver access to the superior medial angle (Fig. 53.19). Portals placed superior to the scapular spine place the dorsal scapular nerve and artery, spinal accessory nerve, and transverse cervical artery at risk and are generally not recommended. An inferior portal just above the inferior angle can be created to débride the bursa at that location.

A radiofrequency ablation device and motorized burr benefit exposure by elevating muscular insertions and resecting bony prominences, respectively (Fig. 53.20). The camera should be oriented to keep the scapular body superior and look frequently at the position of the instrumentation. Resection should be performed by working from medial to lateral (away from neurovascular structures) and inferior to superior (Fig. 53.21). Muscle fibers, which are easily identified by their appearance, should not be resected to minimize bleeding and to aid in visualization. Pump pressure should be kept at a minimum throughout the procedure (we

🏷 Authors' Preferred Technique

Arthroscopic Bursal Resection—cont'd

use 30 mm Hg), and the scapular spine and medial border should be continuously referenced to avoid neurovascular injury. Occasionally a 70-degree arthroscope is required for visualization and should be available throughout the procedure. The bursal resection should be carried superiorly to expose the superior medial angle of the scapula, and the needle left as a marker should be visualized. For patients with inferior crepitus and tenderness upon palpation, the resection can be carried distally to the inferior angle bursa (Fig. 53.22).

When bursal resection is complete, a radiofrequency device can be used to gently elevate the insertion of the rhomboids, levator scapulae, and supraspinatus from the superomedial angle. A sterile ultrasound probe can be used intraoperatively to identify the superior medial angle if it cannot be readily palpated or the needle has fallen out. A motorized burr is then used to resect the superior medial angle. Resection should be at least 2 cm by 2 cm, using a burr run on reverse or a power rasp to smooth the transition zone. The elevated musculature is allowed to fall back in place and scar down to the scapula (Fig. 53.23). The arm is taken through a ROM to gauge the adequacy of the resection, portals are closed with nylon suture, and a sling is applied for the patient's comfort.

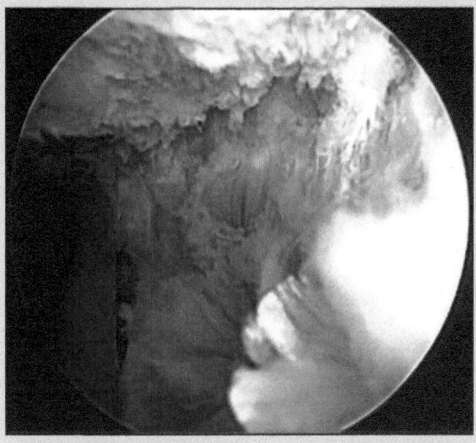

Fig. 53.22 The inferior medial angle is identified and the latissimus insertion is palpated with the radiofrequency device.

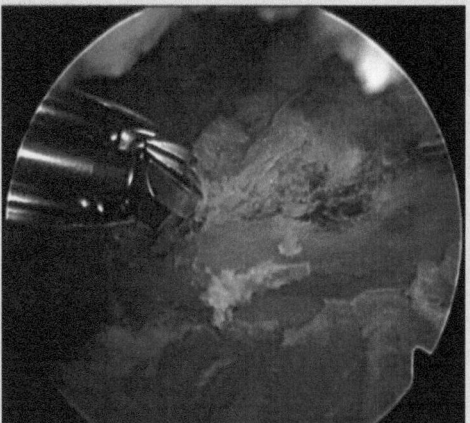

Fig. 53.23 A motorized burr is used to resect the superior medial scapula. A 20-mm by 20-mm area should be resected with the burr, working from lateral to medial. An end-cutting burr is recommended.

Scapular Winging

Scapular winging is most commonly neurologic in origin and in athletes usually results from long thoracic nerve neuropraxia. Treatment is generally nonoperative, focusing on rehabilitation and minimization of deconditioning, with most cases of winging resolving spontaneously. In rare cases when surgery is required, pectoralis major tendon transfers are recommended, with ST fusion reserved for patients for whom a transfer has failed.

Scapular Dyskinesia

Operative treatment is seldom required for persons with SICK scapula syndrome because nearly all patients respond to treatment with physical therapy. Surgery is generally reserved for persons with concomitant pathology or for those that continue to have pain despite extensive and well-directed physical therapy. Provencher et al. have demonstrated good results in these patients with persistent pain and SICK scapula syndrome. They showed that pectoralis minor release improved pain and function while decreasing scapular protraction in 46 patients to levels similar to those patients who responded to nonoperative treatment. No complications were noted, and all patients returned to full activity.[35]

POSTOPERATIVE MANAGEMENT

Our postoperative management begins with a sling and immediate passive range of motion (PROM) exercises.[26,27] At 4 weeks, active and active assisted ROM is begun, and resistance exercises are started at 8 weeks. At 8 weeks post surgery, strengthening of the periscapular musculature is allowed and continued until the strength is equal to the contralateral side.[4]

Return to Play

Patients may safely return to play (RTP) when full, stable, and pain-free ROM with symmetric strength has been achieved. In most cases, RTP generally occurs approximately 3 to 4 months after surgery. For athletes whose sport entails throwing, a return to a throwing program can be initiated at 8 to 12 weeks or once scapular kinematics and strength have been restored. A maintenance program of every-other-day scapular strengthening exercises should begin upon return to play and continue indefinitely. Approximately 10% of patients experience recurrent pain 3 months after discontinuing maintenance exercises.[19]

RESULTS

Pearse et al.[36] published the results of 13 patients who underwent arthroscopic bursectomy and débridement of the superior medial angle of the scapula; 69% of patients reported postoperative improvement, but only 46% returned to their preinjury level of sports. Lehtinen et al.[37] reported improved results with 16 patients who underwent either open or arthroscopic resection, with an 81% satisfaction rate 3 years after surgery. Nicholson and

Duckworth[28] reported on 17 patients, all of whom had satisfactory or better results at 2 years. Of 96 patients treated nonoperatively for SICK scapular syndrome and followed up for 12 months by Burkhart et al.,[19] all successfully returned to their preinjury level of throwing by 4 months.

Complications

Complications from arthroscopic and open bursal resection are extremely rare but have been reported. The most common complication is underresection of the bursa, which can result in persistent pain and crepitus. Other complications include neurovascular injury, postoperative hematoma, heterotopic ossification, and pneumothorax. In a consecutive series of nine patients with open resections, McCluskey and Bigliani[25] reported 89% good or excellent results, with one permanent spinal accessory nerve injury requiring muscle transfers of the medial periscapular musculature (rhomboids, levator scapulae) and trapezius. Care must be taken to maintain proper orientation to prevent resection of a more inferior area of the scapula or inadvertent injury to the surrounding neurovascular structures.

FUTURE CONSIDERATIONS

Scapular disorders remain underrecognized and can be debilitating and frustrating to patients. SICK scapula syndrome is considered to be a precursor to intra-articular pathology and injuries, so timely recognition and treatment are paramount. As future research demonstrates a conclusive link between scapular malposition and labral injuries in athletes who throw, more emphasis will be placed on early recognition and therapy to correct maltracking.

ACKNOWLEDGMENT

We acknowledge the authors of the previous edition on scapulothoracic disorders: Drs. Bryan Hanypsiak, Jeffrey DeLong, and Walter Lowe. We also thank Dr. Gary Mlady and Dr. Jennifer Weaver for assisting in collection of new MRI and radiographic images for this book chapter and video presentation.

For a complete list of references, go to ExpertConsult.com.

SELECTED READINGS

Citation:

Burkhart SS, Morgan CD, Kibler WB. The disabled throwing shoulder: spectrum of pathology. Part III. The SICK scapula, scapular dyskinesis, the kinetic chain, and rehabilitation. *Arthroscopy.* 2003;19(6):641–661.

Level of Evidence:

IV (retrospective case series and current concept series)

Summary:

A spectrum of pathology must be considered when diagnosing and treating a disabled throwing shoulder. Appropriate surgical and nonsurgical treatments, including rehabilitation, can be precisely directed at specific pathophysiologic elements.

Citation:

Kuhn JE, Plancher KP, Hawkins RJ. Scapular winging. *J Am Acad Orthop Surg.* 1995;6:319–325.

Level of Evidence:

Review

Summary:

Scapular winging is caused by a number of pathologic conditions and can be classified as primary, secondary, or voluntary. The evaluation and treatment of these three types are discussed in this article.

Citation:

Kibler WB. The role of the scapula in athletic shoulder function. *Am J Sports Med.* 1998;26(2):325–337.

Level of Evidence:

Current concept review

Summary:

The exact role and the function of the scapula are misunderstood, which often translates into incomplete evaluation and diagnosis of shoulder problems. This review addresses the anatomy of the scapula, the roles the scapula plays in overhead-throwing activities, the normal and abnormal biomechanics of the scapula, and treatment and rehabilitation of scapular problems.

Citation:

Kibler WB, McMullen J. Scapular dyskinesis and its relation to shoulder injury. *J Am Acad Orthop Surg.* 2012;20(6):364–372.

Level of Evidence:

Current concepts review

Summary:

Scapular dyskinesis–altered scapular positioning and motion is found in association with most shoulder injuries. Associated conditions such as shoulder impingement, rotator cuff disease, labral injury, clavicle fracture, acromioclavicular joint injury, and multidirectional instability should be evaluated for scapular dyskinesis and treated accordingly.

Recommended Viewing

Millett PJ. Endoscopic scapulothoracic bursectomy with partial scapulectomy. Available at Vumedi.com.

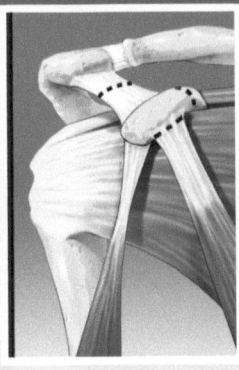

54

Nerve Entrapment

Daniel E. Hess, Kenneth F. Taylor, A. Bobby Chhabra

NERVE ENTRAPMENT IN THE SHOULDER

The incidence of entrapment neuropathies involving the shoulder is largely unknown, but as our understanding of the anatomy and pathology of these conditions grows, earlier and more accurate recognition of these conditions has led to higher rates of treatment. Symptom presentation is most often subtle and insidious in onset, necessitating diagnostic acumen on behalf of the treating physician. Injuries resulting from direct trauma, as with blunt or penetrating mechanisms or from traction across a tethered segment, may present more acutely and be masked by other associated traumatic injuries. A thorough understanding of neurovascular anatomy, common injury mechanisms, and certain at-risk populations should prompt early clinical suspicion. Nerve entrapment is no longer considered simply a diagnosis of exclusion; therefore appropriate advanced imaging and electrodiagnostic examinations are being more readily utilized to confirm the diagnosis. Evidence-based decision-making principles guide operative and nonoperative efforts to return the athlete to competition. This chapter outlines several of the more commonly encountered compressive neuropathies of the shoulder girdle.

SUPRASCAPULAR NERVE PALSY

Anatomy and Biomechanics

The suprascapular nerve arises from the C5 and C6 nerve roots at the upper trunk of the brachial plexus. It passes deep to the trapezius and the omohyoid muscles to enter the supraspinatus fossa through the suprascapular notch beneath the transverse scapular ligament (Fig. 54.1). The suprascapular notch is most commonly U-shaped (48% to 84%) but varies in morphology from flat to enclosed within bone.[1,2] A study of over 200 scapulas described six types of scapular notches and their incidence as follows: (1) absent (8%), (2) shallow V-shape (31%), (3) U-shaped with parallel margins (48%), (4) deep-V shape (3%), (5) type III with partial ossification of the transverse scapular ligament (6%), (6) complete ossification of the ligament.[2] Together, the suprascapular notch and the overlying ligament form the suprascapular fossa. The suprascapular notch has been shown to be approximately 4.5 cm from the posterolateral acromion,[3] a relationship that becomes important in arthroscopic decompression.

The nerve traverses the deep surface of supraspinatus, innervating it with two motor branches. Sensory branches innervate the glenohumeral and acromioclavicular joints, and as recent anatomic studies show additional sensory innervation to the coracohumeral ligament, the coracoclavicular ligament, subacromial bursa, and posterior shoulder capsule.[4] No cutaneous sensory distribution occurs from the suprascapular nerve. Upon reaching the lateral edge of the spine of the scapula, the nerve descends through the spinoglenoid notch, entering the infraspinatus fossa and innervating the infraspinatus.

The spinoglenoid ligament passes from the spine of the scapula to the glenoid neck and posterior shoulder capsule. Its attachment into the posterior capsule results in tightening of the spinoglenoid ligament with cross-body adduction and internal rotation. The ligament is present in 14%[5] to 100%[6] of patients. It may appear as a thin fibrous band, known as type I (60%), or a distinct ligament, known as type II (20%), or it may be absent (20%).[7] The spinoglenoid ligament has been reported to be present more commonly in men (64% to 36%),[8] although in another study it has been reported to be present in equal proportions in men and women.[6] The average distance from the supraglenoid tubercle to the nerve at the suprascapular notch is 3 cm.[9] The distance from the glenoid rim to the spinoglenoid notch is 1.8 to 2.1 cm.[3,9]

The suprascapular nerve is relatively fixed at its origin in the brachial plexus and at its terminal branches into the infraspinatus, putting it at risk for traction injuries and multiple predictable sites of compression.[10] Nerve contact with the suprascapular ligament is accentuated with depression, retraction, or overhead abduction of the shoulder.[2] Extremes of scapular motion also place the nerve under tension.[11–13] Overhead abduction of the shoulder with simultaneous eccentric contraction of the infraspinatus may result in compression of the suprascapular nerve at the spinoglenoid notch.[14] This has been well described in volleyball players.[14–16] Nerve compression against the lateral margin of the spine of the scapula by supraspinatus and infraspinatus tendons at their point of juncture is also thought to result in nerve injury.[14]

"Athletic stress," especially in throwing or serving, produces a backward and forward rotation of the scapula and suprascapular nerve compression at the suprascapular notch.[17] The nerve is often injured in athletes as it passes around the lateral spine of the scapula and enters the spinoglenoid notch, sparing the supraspinatus.[18] Ganglion cysts are a common cause of compressive injury to the suprascapular nerve. These cysts are thought to result from superior labral tears, which are very common in overhead athletes, with the cyst expanding into the posterior

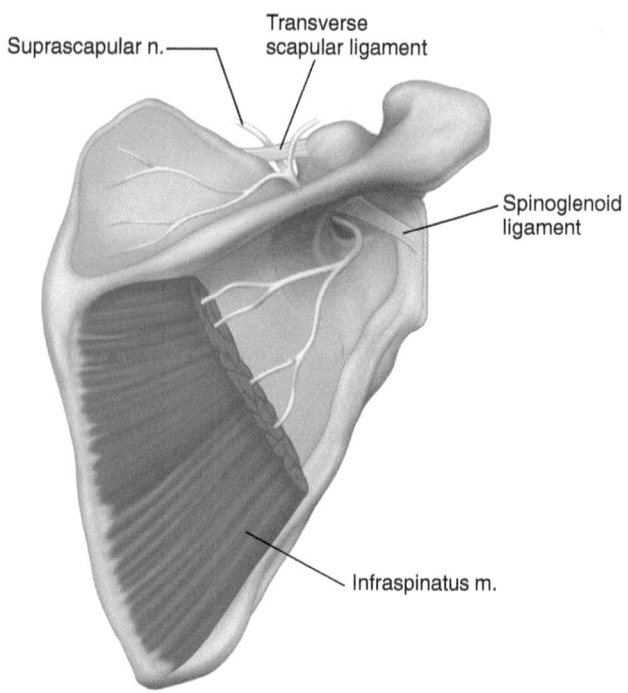

Fig. 54.1 Anatomy of the suprascapular nerve. *n,* Nerve; *m,* muscle. (Modified from Black KP, Lombardo JA. Suprascapular nerve injuries with isolated paralysis of the infraspinatus. *J Sports Med.* 1990;18(3):225–228.)

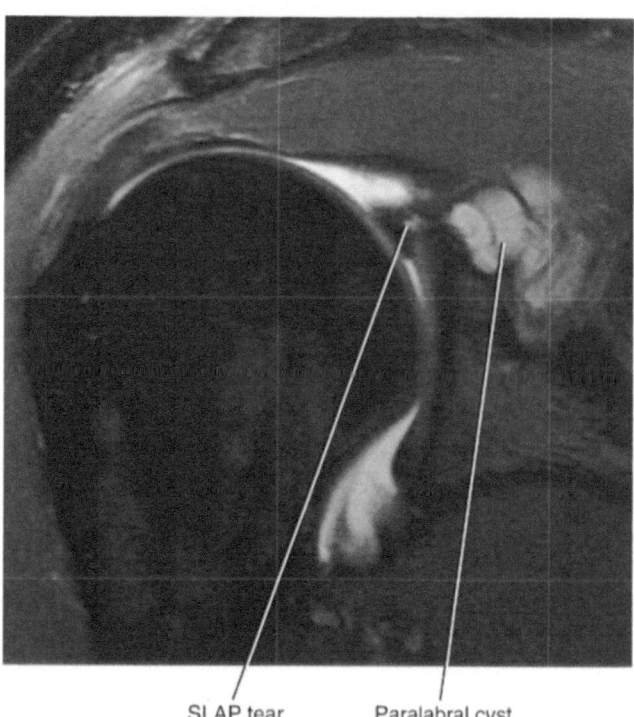

Fig. 54.2 SLAP tear with adjacent paralabral cyst. Coronal T2-weighted image demonstrates a paralabral cyst compressing the suprascapular nerve by mass effect. *SLAP,* superior labrum anterior to posterior.

scapular region, which is devoid of overlying muscle or tendon. Compression of the infraspinatus branch typically occurs as the nerve passes through the spinoglenoid notch (Fig. 54.2),[19] although cysts at the suprascapular notch have been described.[20] Other etiologies of neuropathy are more rare but have also been described. Suprascapular nerve palsy has been reported after distal clavicular fractures and resection of the distal clavicle.[21,22] The nerve is located within 1.5 cm posterior to the clavicle and within 2 to 3 cm of the acromioclavicular joint (Fig. 54.3). Scapular body fractures are also associated with suprascapular nerve palsy.[23] Injury to the axillary or suprascapular artery in overhead athletes can result in microemboli and microvascular infarct of the suprascapular nerve as well.[10] Suprascapular nerve injury has also been reported with acute shoulder dislocation in a cyclist.[24]

Recent attention has been given to the association of suprascapular neuropathy and retracted rotator cuff tears. A cadaveric study showed increased tension on the first motor branch of the suprascapular nerve with medial retraction of the supraspinatus muscle.[25] Clinical studies have suggested that predominant infraspinatus fatty degeneration in the context of a massive rotator cuff tear may be secondary to suprascapular nerve compression at the spinoglenoid notch.[26] Repair of the rotator cuff with appropriate tension, however, has been shown to reverse a significant proportion of suprascapular nerve symptoms in the setting of massive tears.[27]

Clinical Evaluation

Suprascapular nerve injury may present after specific trauma acutely or more commonly chronically. The presentation may be painful range of motion (ROM) or shoulder weakness or

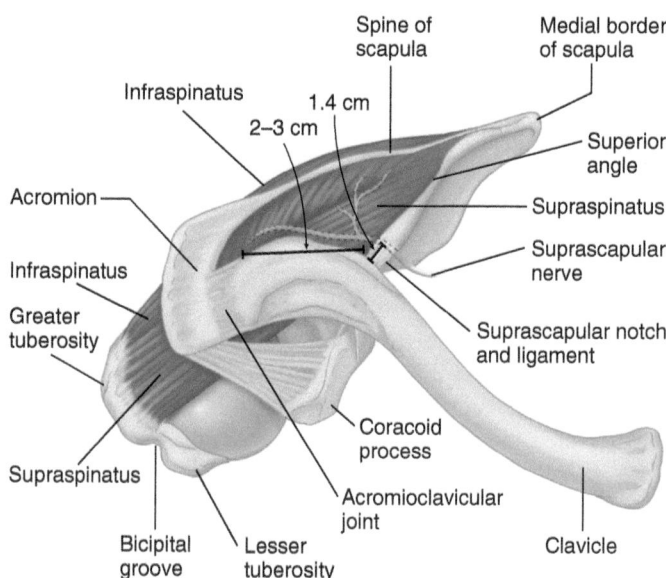

Fig. 54.3 A superior view of the suprascapular nerve showing its proximity to the acromioclavicular joint and posterolateral clavicle. *n,* Nerve.

involve insidious painless muscle atrophy. Athletes who perform repetitive overhead activities—such as baseball players, volleyball players, and swimmers—should be treated with a heightened suspicion for compressive neuropathy.[10,15,28] During the history-taking portion of the exam, all recent upper-extremity and neck injuries, sports-related or not, should be reviewed. A direct blow or forceful scapular protraction may cause traction on

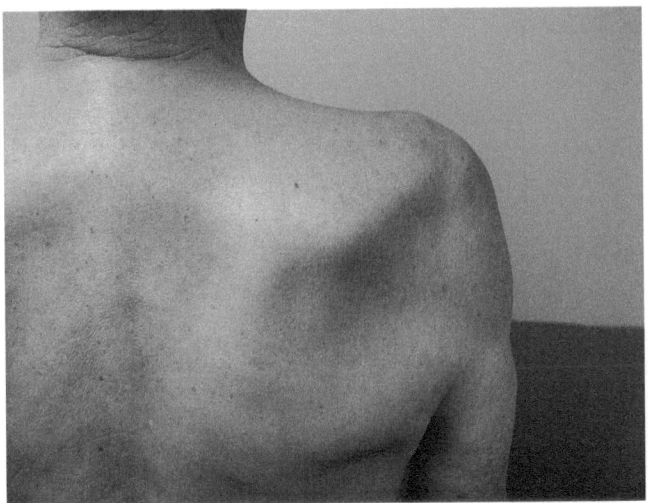

Fig. 54.4 Rotator cuff atrophy.

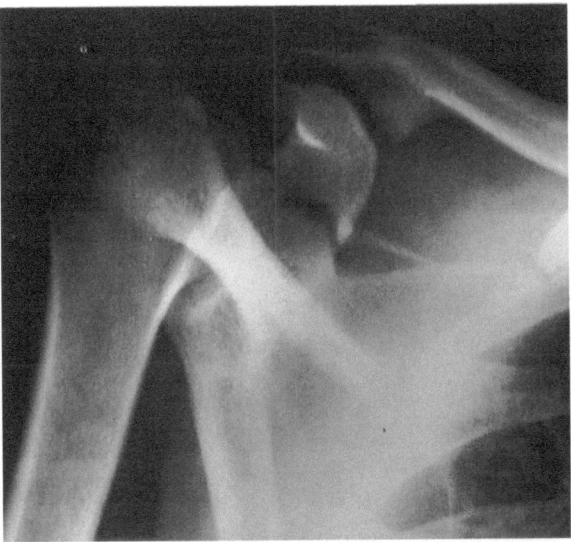

Fig. 54.5 A radiograph of a suprascapular notch fracture with a 30-degree cephalic tilt.

the nerve at the root level or kinking at either the suprascapular or spinoglenoid notch.[29]

The physical exam should begin with general inspection of both shoulders and scapula, concentrating on symmetry of musculature. Scars from trauma or previous surgical incisions should be noted. Active, passive, and resisted ROM is tested, looking for motions that elicit symptoms, the presence of instability, compromised strength, and labral pathology. Tenderness at the suprascapular notch may be elicited with palpation.[30] The inconsistent finding of pain often localizes in the posterior shoulder and radiates to the arm; it may be worse with adduction of the shoulder.[30] An additional physical exam maneuver, the suprascapular nerve stress test, will worsen compression at the suprascapular notch and produce posterior shoulder pain in patients with compressive pathology.[31,32] Bilateral symptoms should raise suspicion for cervical pathology, and the exam should always include a c-spine exam.

When the injury occurs at the suprascapular notch, pain and motor weakness of both the supraspinatus and infraspinatus muscles may result. The complaint is most often a gradual onset of vague posterior shoulder discomfort and weakness. Pain is thought to arise from the articular branches to the acromioclavicular and glenohumeral joints.

Compression of the suprascapular nerve by a ganglion at the spinoglenoid notch is a well-known clinical entity.[33–37] If the lesion is at the spinoglenoid notch, distal to the acromioclavicular and glenohumeral branches, the presentation may be one of painless atrophy of the infraspinatus and external rotation weakness. Posterior shoulder atrophy, especially in the infraspinatus fossa, is an important finding (Fig. 54.4) and should be compared with the contralateral side. Supraspinatus atrophy may be difficult to observe because of the overlying trapezius. Likewise, supraspinatus weakness is not as easily elicited as that of the infraspinatus. Patients with clinical signs suggestive of a labral tear and wasting of the infraspinatus muscle warrant further diagnostic workup, including magnetic resonance imaging (MRI) and electrodiagnostic nerve studies. When the diagnosis is in question, an injection of local anesthetic at the level of the spinoglenoid notch can be helpful to distinguish suprascapular nerve pathology from other causes of shoulder pain.

Diagnostic Studies

Radiographic evaluation should include routine shoulder views and, if clinically indicated, a c-spine series. A 30-degree cephalic tilt radiograph to visualize the suprascapular notch is helpful, especially in patients with fractures (Fig. 54.5).

MRI is useful in the evaluation of patients with suprascapular nerve palsy.[38] Acute entrapment may be differentiated from chronic injury on T2-weighted images based on increased signal in the affected supraspinatus and/or infraspinatus muscles. The high signal intensity of affected muscle returns to normal after recovery, as noted on clinical and electrodiagnostic examination.[39] Chronic compression appears as typical denervation changes, including decreased bulk and fatty infiltration of the muscles.[40] Ganglion cysts in the supraspinatus fossa causing compression of the suprascapular nerve can readily be identified on MRI, as can associated pathology such as superior labrum anterior to posterior (SLAP) and rotator cuff tears. Less common causes of suprascapular nerve palsy such as schwannoma[41] and interneural ganglion[42] have also been identified on MRI.

Ultrasound is also reported to be an effective diagnostic tool for the identification of paralabral cysts and associated rotator cuff tears, although it is very operator-dependent.[43] This modality has the added benefit of facilitating guided aspiration of paralabral cysts, with symptomatic improvement in 86% of patients in one series.[44]

Electrodiagnostic evaluation is the gold standard study for suprascapular nerve pathology. Indications include unexplained persistent shoulder pain, atrophy, and weakness without a concomitant rotator cuff tear or MRI evidence of supraspinatus or infraspinatus atrophy without obvious rotator cuff pathology.[45] A complete test should include both needle electromyography (EMG) of the entire shoulder girdle, including the paraspinal muscles, and nerve conduction velocity (NCV) studies from

Erb's point (2.5 cm superior to the clavicle, representing the convergence of the C5 and C6 nerve roots) to the supraspinatus. Normal conduction latency is 1.7 to 3.7 ms to the supraspinatus and 2.4 to 4.2 ms to the infraspinatus. EMG abnormalities may also be present with brachial neuritis, cervical root compression, and incomplete brachial plexopathies. Conversely, findings of EMG studies may be normal with an obvious clinical supra-scapular nerve deficit,[46,47] confirming the need for the nerve conduction examination. In a study of 79 patients with muscle weakness, EMG and NCV have been shown to have an accuracy of 91% in detecting suprascapular neuropathy.[48] Overall sensitiv-ity and specificity of electrodiagnostic testing is not known and depends on the etiology of the neuropathy. Compression with ganglia may involve only one of the three or four suprascapular nerve branches to the infraspinatus; therefore EMG recordings are performed at more than one location within the muscle.

Decision-Making Principles

Conservative management with activity modification and physical therapy is the treatment of choice for the majority of patients who present with neuropathy secondary to repetitive overhead activities. Depending on the duration of symptoms and the eti-ology, a comprehensive physical therapy regimen will likely decrease pain and improve function. However, muscle bulk may be irreversible once significant atrophy has occurred, even if surgically decompressed.[49] A patient with a chronic condition (i.e., lasting 6 to 12 months) and well-established atrophy that has failed nonoperative measures requires surgical exploration and decompression, as does a patient with suprascapular nerve palsy associated with an acute scapular fracture in the area of the suprascapular notch.[23] Symptomatic patients who have a structural source of compression, such as a ganglion cyst, also benefit from surgical decompression.[20,33–37]

Spinoglenoid Notch Compression

Suprascapular nerve palsy associated with a spinoglenoid ganglion can be treated with arthroscopic techniques to repair or débride associated labral lesions and decompress the labral cyst.[52] The cyst may be decompressed arthroscopically through a preexisting labral tear; however, if no labral tear is present, a capsulotomy is performed with an electrocautery device or a shaver. The cyst is visualized with the arthroscope in the posterior portal. A blunt probe is placed in the labral tear or capsulotomy until the char-acteristic amber-colored cyst fluid is visualized. Decompression is achieved by placing a shaver within the cyst and evacuat-ing the fluid. The cyst wall may be removed with use of the shaver, but care must be taken to avoid iatrogenic injury to the suprascapular nerve. The shaver is pointed at the glenoid neck during removal, and dissection should not extend more than 1 cm medial to the posterior labral attachment to the glenoid.[37] Associated labral pathology is then addressed at the same time as the decompression.

If open decompression of the nerve at the spinoglenoid notch is necessary with excision of ganglia, a surgical approach to the posterior glenoid is performed. This approach is begun with a deltoid split over the glenohumeral joint with limited deltoid detachment laterally from the acromion. The superior edge of

Authors' Preferred Technique
Suprascapular Notch Compression

Traditionally open surgical release methods have been utilized to decompress the suprascapular nerve at the suprascapular notch. This was often difficult to visualize open, as the suprascapular nerve is as small as 2 mm and often required detachment of the trapezius muscle for adequate exposure. As our understanding of the anatomy of the area has improved, along with our arthroscopic techniques, multiple all-arthroscopic surgeries have been described and the all-arthroscopic technique has been reported to be a safe and effective alternative to an open approach; this is now considered the standard of care,[31,50,51] and we prefer to utilize an all-arthroscopic technique at our institution.

The patient is placed in the standard beach-chair position. The all-arthroscopic procedure is as described by Lafosse.[31,51] Standard posterior and lateral sub-acromial portals are utilized for camera visualization. An anterolateral portal and suprascapular nerve portal are used for instrumentation. The suprascapular nerve portal is made under direct visualization approximately 7 cm medial to the lateral border of the acromion between the clavicle and the scapular spine and 2 cm medial to a standard superior-medial portal. Once the glenohumeral joint has been visualized through the posterior portal, we enter the subacromial space. The coracoacromial (CA) ligament is identified, exposed, and traced back to its insertion on the coracoid. The coracoclavicular (CC) ligaments are then identified as the dissection is continued posteriorly and medially from the CA insertion. The transverse scapular ligament's lateral border is just medial to the base of the CC ligaments. The suprascapular portal is then made under direct visualization from the lateral portal. A combination of shavers and radiofrequency ablation devices are used to isolate the ligament. Care is taken to avoid the suprascapular artery, which runs superior to the ligament. Another portal, 1.5 cm lateral to the suprascapular nerve portal, is used with a biter to release the transverse scapular ligament. Gentle manipulation of the nerve with a probe should suffice to determine the adequacy of decompres-sion. A burr can be used to open up the notch if there is residual compression after the ligament is released.

the infraspinatus is identified and, at most, the upper half of that tendon is detached, leaving a humeral side stump for repair.[53] The size of the exposure needed is based on the MRI position of the ganglion and the size of the patient.

Results
Nonoperative

The overall response to conservative management is good, espe-cially in the absence of a rotator cuff tear or space-occupying lesion. For overhead athletes, rest from sports or other inciting causes may be helpful. The timing of return to activity relies on the judgment of the physician and is based on factors in the course of follow-up, including the extent of the initial paralysis, findings of electrical studies, symptoms, and improvements in the muscle examination with therapy. In persons who have pain-less infraspinatus muscle palsy without a cyst, function is usually good with nonoperative care. Asymptomatic ganglia without nerve findings may not require treatment.[14,52,54]

EMG studies have demonstrated that only 30% to 40% of the maximal strength of the infraspinatus is used during overhead throwing; thus in the case of a partial nerve injury, a return to pitching is possible.[18] In a study of asymptomatic volleyball players, it was found that 12 of 96 players had isolated partial infraspinatus paralysis predominantly in the dominant shoulder.

Whereas some players had only electrical abnormalities, others demonstrated muscle atrophy in addition. A 15% to 30% loss of external rotation power was found, although the players retained their ability to play volleyball.[15] The suggested etiology was nerve tension at the spinoglenoid notch when the arm was cocked in maximal external rotation and during follow-through. In a long-term study, subjects with isolated infraspinatus atrophy were reexamined at a mean of 5.5 years. All subjects were still able to play volleyball at a high level with the degree of atrophy unchanged. The incidence of subacromial impingement in this subject population was no higher than that in the general population of volleyball players.[14] Surgical exploration of a well-localized lesion should be performed if 3 to 6 months of conservative management have failed to elicit improvement. Delaying surgery beyond 6 months can lead to irreversible atrophy or incomplete symptom resolution.

Suprascapular Notch Decompression

Most reports show good return of function in selected patients after open surgical decompression.[55–57] A retrospective review of 42 patients at a mean of 18 months demonstrated measurable improvements in motor strength, with supraspinatus strength improving from grades 0 to 2 to grade 4 in 90% of patients. Infraspinatus strength improved from grades 0 to 2 to grade 3 or better in 32% of patients. Pain symptoms improved almost uniformly.[57] In recent years arthroscopic suprascapular notch decompression has gained in popularity and become the preferred method of treatment for many orthopaedic sports surgeons.[31,58] Short- to medium-term follow-up results have been encouraging, restoring patient function and alleviating pain even in the absence of rotator cuff disease.[31,51,59]

Spinoglenoid Notch Decompression

Several authors have reported cyst resolution and return of nerve function after arthroscopic decompression of the cyst.[20,33–37,59] Cyst resolution and return of nerve function after repair or débridement of an associated SLAP lesion without attempts at cyst débridement have been reported.[60] In a large series of patients diagnosed with suprascapular nerve compression, 65 were found to have spinoglenoid notch ganglion cysts associated with glenoid labral tears.[36] Patients with the highest degree of satisfaction (97%) were treated with labral repair and open or arthroscopic decompression of the cyst. Lower satisfaction rates were reported by persons treated with isolated labral repair (67%) or needle aspiration of the cyst (64%) and by those treated nonoperatively (53%).

LONG THORACIC NERVE PALSY

Anatomy and Biomechanics

The long thoracic nerve arises from ventral rami of roots of C5, C6, and C7, which branch shortly after they exit from the intervertebral foramina. Branches of C5 and C6 form the upper trunk of the nerve, which pierces through the middle scalene muscle. It then joins the lower trunk from C7, which passes anterior to the middle scalene to form the long thoracic nerve. This pure motor nerve, with a mean length of 30 cm, courses posterior to

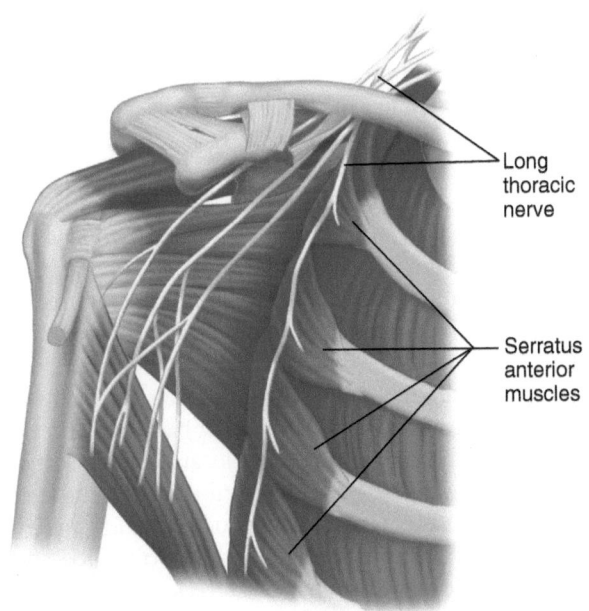

Fig. 54.6 The brachial plexus. (Modified from Haymaker W, Woodhall B. *Peripheral Nerve Injuries*. Philadelphia: WB Saunders; 1956.)

the brachial plexus to perforate the fascia of the proximal serratus anterior (Fig. 54.6).[61] The nerve supplies a single muscle, the serratus anterior, which covers much of the lateral thorax and acts with the trapezius to position the scapula for elevation. It arises from the upper nine ribs and attaches at the deep surface of the scapula along the vertebral border. Innervation of the upper and intermediate portions of the muscle is supplied by the upper division of the long thoracic nerve, which produces shoulder protraction. The lower portion is primarily responsible for scapular stabilization.[62] These portions typically work together to draw the scapula forward and rotate its inferior angle upward. In patients with serratus anterior muscle paralysis, shoulder motion is severely limited because of the lack of scapular rotation. The serratus anterior also acts as an accessory inspiratory muscle, as is seen in runners who fix their scapulas by holding their thighs to catch their breath after a race.

The most common site of compression is where the nerve passes through the middle scalene muscle or angulates over the second rib.[63] A tight fascial band has been identified between the inferior aspect of the brachial plexus and the region of the middle scalene insertion on the first rib.[64] The long thoracic nerve "bowstrings" over this band with shoulder abduction and external rotation. Medial and upward rotation of the scapula further compress the nerve. Asynchronous motion between the arm and scapula has been implicated as a cause of internal traction injury to the nerve.[65]

Clinical Evaluation

Isolated serratus anterior palsy may result from acute injury, chronic irritation, or brachial neuritis. Long thoracic nerve palsy may also occur with prolonged recumbency or intraoperative stretch during thoracic surgery. Sports and repetitive overhead work have been implicated as a cause of isolated serratus anterior palsy, with the proposed mechanism being traction injury (either single or repetitive) to the long thoracic nerve.[24,61,66] In one series the repetitive trauma of tennis and archery was thought to be the cause of the lesion in 5 of 20 patients. Other sports implicated in this type of injury are swimming, basketball, football, golf, gymnastics, ballet, and wrestling.[67,68] Occupational injuries are also certainly possible, with reports from household activities such as hedge clipping or car washing to construction jobs and shoveling.[24,69] Traumatic injuries are typically neuropraxias from sudden depression of the shoulder girdle. Proposed traumatic mechanisms include crushing of the nerve between the clavicle and the second rib, tetanic scalenus medius muscle contraction, and nerve stretch with cervical spine flexion or rotation and lateral tilt with ipsilateral arm elevation or backward arm extension.[61] Because the nerve is in a deep location, a direct blow is unlikely to cause isolated palsy. Serratus anterior rupture has been reported in patients with rheumatoid arthritis,[29] and injury has been reported as a complication of interscalene blocks administered in the course of regional anesthesia.[70] All of a patient's past surgical procedures should be reviewed as iatrogenic causes for injury have been described as well, including lymph node biopsies, clavicular resections, and any other procedure performed at the head/neck/shoulder junction.

The long thoracic nerve is often affected by the poorly understood syndrome of brachial neuritis. Parsonage and Turner[71] coined the term *neuralgic amyotrophy* (brachial neuritis), which they found in 136 military personnel, 30 of whom had isolated serratus anterior paralysis. These investigators also noted a right-sided predominance. Significant pain lasting a variable time, from days to weeks, precedes loss of function in one or more shoulder girdle muscles.[72] Sensory loss does not exclude the syndrome.

A patient with early thoracic nerve palsy may present with subtle changes in the ability to perform his or her sport, along with decreased active ROM of the shoulder and altered scapulohumeral rhythm. The onset may be painful, as in persons with brachial neuritis, or it may be more subtle, involving difficulties with weight lifting or the recognition of pressure from a chair against the "winging" (protruding) scapula while sitting. Scapular winging may not become evident until several weeks after an acute injury, perhaps because a certain amount of time is required for progressive attenuation of the trapezius to occur.[61]

Paralysis of the serratus anterior results in medial winging and poor scapular stabilization, limiting active shoulder elevation to 110 degrees in patients with complete lesions.[61] Scapular winging as a result of long thoracic nerve palsy is characterized by elevation and retraction of the scapula as it moves toward the midline and slightly superior.[65] The deformity is accentuated by resisted active arm elevation or by performing a push-up maneuver while leaning against a wall (Fig. 54.7). A shoulder protraction test can identify long thoracic nerve injuries affecting the upper trunk.[62] In this test, the patient is placed in the supine position and asked to forward flex (protract) the shoulder. Ability to protract the shoulder indicates an intact upper trunk of the nerve. Occasionally a Tinel sign over the trajectory of the long thoracic nerve is present.

The appearance of winging with arm elevation due to serratus anterior palsy differs from that of winging due to trapezius palsy. When the serratus anterior muscle does not function, the inferior

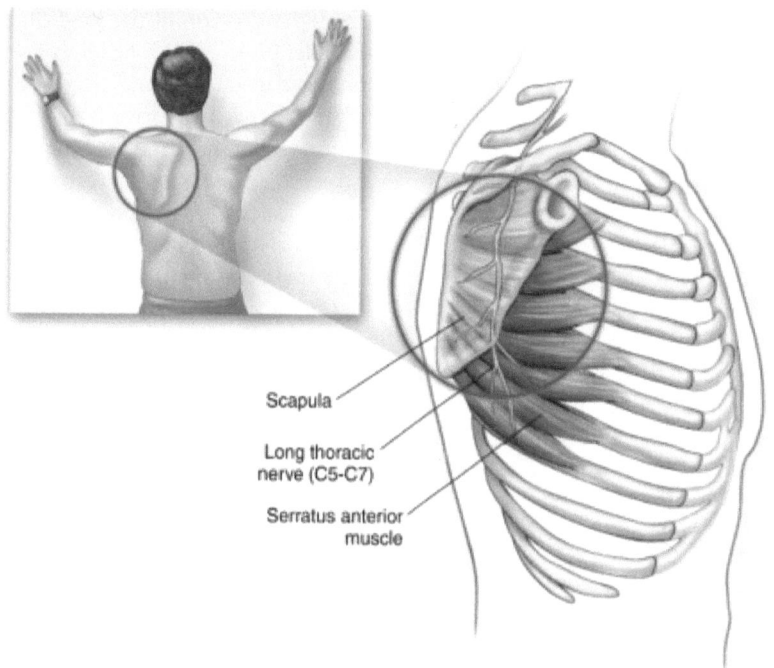

Scapula

Long thoracic nerve (C5-C7)

Serratus anterior muscle

Fig. 54.7 Scapular "winging" is often discovered during weight training as the scapula protrudes with resisted elevation or contacts the flat surface during bench pressing. If weight lifting is thought to be the cause of the problem, participation should cease until nerve function returns. Return to sports by patients with long thoracic nerve palsy depends on the demands placed on the upper extremity by the sport. (From Waldman S. *Atlas of Uncommon Pain Syndromes.* New York: Elsevier; 2014.)

tip of the scapula is pulled medially and posteriorly. With trapezius paralysis, the scapular body is held in position and the medial border merely becomes more prominent, which is a more subtle deformity.

Diagnostic Studies

Plain radiographs of the cervical spine and shoulder may identify contributing arthrosis, fracture malunions, or the presence of accessory ribs and osteochondromas. MRI is generally reserved for patients with shoulder instability or cuff tears,[73] although T2-weighted fast-spin echo with fat saturation may demonstrate increased signal intensity consistent with denervation edema.[74] EMG studies confirm the diagnosis of long thoracic nerve palsy. Conduction studies should be performed from Erb's point to the serratus anterior muscle on the anterolateral chest wall. Repeat nerve studies at 3- to 6-month intervals are helpful to monitor improvement.[73]

Decision-Making Principles

Surgery may be indicated for patients with long thoracic nerve palsy who remain symptomatic and for whom electrodiagnostic studies show no improvement despite 1 to 2 years of nonoperative therapy. Athletes must be counseled that no surgical intervention will provide a reliable return to a competitive sport that requires overhead strength.[75]

Results
Nonoperative

The outcome of acute traction injuries is typically good with conservative management, and spontaneous functional improvement has been well described.[2,73] In a series of 17 patients presenting with various etiologies at a mean of 3 months who were treated with a scapula winger's brace, investigators reported an increase of one motor grade with the brace applied.[83] Six patients demonstrated brace-free recovery to near premorbid function by final follow-up. The investigators hypothesized that the mechanism was proprioceptive feedback preventing muscle overuse or attenuation and transfer of contralateral shoulder mechanics. The prognosis for spontaneous recovery from Parsonage-Turner brachial neuritis is good; 36% of patients diagnosed with this syndrome recover by the end of the first year and 75% recover by the end of the second year.[84] Further improvement may occur beyond 2 years.[24] Recurrent long thoracic nerve palsy is rare.[61]

Pectoralis Major Transfer

No surgical series consisting exclusively of athletes has been reported and functional outcomes and return to work statistics are mixed. A systematic review[82] suggested that interpositional grafts have a higher risk of recurrent medial scapular winging, possibly due to graft attenuation over time. Indirect transfers also had a mean of 12 degrees less postoperative ROM, but functional scores were still equivalent compared with direct pectoralis transfer. Only 46% of patients were able to return to their previous level of work, and although winging may have been resolved, pain because of underlying neuropathy or altered scapulohumeral kinetics often persisted. Forward shoulder flexion was reliably restored in a series of patients who underwent a split tendon transfer at

Long Thoracic Nerve Palsy

Cessation of the activity that is suspected of inciting the injury is important. Shoulder braces cannot begin to normalize rotational balance of the scapula due to the force couple between the serratus anterior and the trapezius. However, in the case of severe serratus winging, braces may prevent progressive attenuation of the trapezius muscle.

Surgical treatment is infrequently indicated. Although pectoralis minor transfer[76,77] to the lateral inferior scapula for dynamic support has been reported, transfer of the pectoralis major sternal head, with or without augmentation, to the inferior border of the scapula is the currently favored reconstruction owed to its similar line of pull, excursion, and cross-sectional area as compared with the serratus anterior.[73,78,79] Indirect transfers with interpositional grafts have been described with equivalent functional results as a direct transfer. The advantage of the interpositional graft is that it avoids overtensioning, which would restrict postoperative ROM[80] and reduce the risk of traction neuropraxia to the medial and lateral pectoral nerves.[81] There is considerable controversy in the literature regarding the most effective surgical technique. A recent study failed to show a consensus among polled shoulder and elbow surgeons regarding the use of the entire tendon or a split tendon technique, direct versus indirect transfers, or regarding graft type.[82]

The patient is placed in the lateral position. A 5-cm incision is made in the inferior deltopectoral groove. The shoulder is abducted to accentuate the interval between the sternal and clavicular heads of the pectoralis major. The sternal head is released sharply from its humeral insertion and bluntly separated from the clavicular head. Care is taken to work medially against the chest wall to avoid the neurovascular structures. Sutures are placed in the tendon to maintain proper orientation during shuttling through the second incision. A second incision is made over the inferior angle of the scapula. The infraspinatus, subscapularis, and serratus anterior are subperiosteally dissected to expose the inferomedial portion of the scapula. A long curved clamp is used to develop a tunnel in the scapulothoracic interval, medial to the coracoid process and conjoined tendon. The transferred pectoral tendon is then secured to the scapula through drill holes with the scapula held in a reduced position.[79] Postoperative immobilization in a sling or scapulothoracic orthosis is emphasized for 6 weeks. Gentle gravity-assisted pendulum exercises and isometrics are allowed during this time. ROM of the shoulder girdle begins 6 weeks after surgery. Return to noncontact athletic activities begins at 12 weeks, but lifting of more than 20 lb is delayed until 6 months after surgery.

a mean of 6 years after their palsy commenced.[79] In a series of 11 consecutive patients who were followed up for a mean of 41 months, one patient demonstrated full recurrence of scapular winging.[85] In a critical analysis of results of 15 patients at a mean of 64 months,[86] all patients demonstrated decreased ROM in the operative shoulder. Seven of 15 had good to excellent results, and 13 returned to their previous employment. Objective scapular winging was measured with the shoulder abducted 90 degrees while holding as much weight as possible. Only one patient had more than mild winging, but no patient lifted more than 25 lb.

SPINAL ACCESSORY NERVE PALSY
Anatomy and Biomechanics

The spinal accessory nerve (cranial nerve XI) exits the jugular foramen at the base of the skull. It penetrates and innervates the upper third of the sternocleidomastoid muscle before crossing the posterior triangle of the neck. It is here that this nerve is superficial and vulnerable to injury. The nerve enters the trapezius and is the predominant motor nerve to that muscle. Root fibers from C3 and C4 also innervate the trapezius and may blend with the accessory nerve, although their contribution may be only proprioceptive.[87] The accessory nerve is a small purely motor nerve, measuring only 1 to 3 mm in diameter.[88]

Scapular stabilization and elevation result from the balance between the trapezius and serratus anterior. The upper trapezius elevates and tilts the scapula, raising the lateral shoulder and assisting in arm elevation, respectively. The lower trapezius works with the rhomboids to retract the scapula and balance the pull of the serratus anterior.

Clinical Evaluation

Spinal accessory nerve injuries are rare in sports. They typically occur as a result of a direct blow, as with a hockey stick or in a traction injury with a cross-face maneuver in wrestling.[89] Stretch injury resulting from distal upper extremity distraction and contralateral head rotation has been reported.[90] Iatrogenic injuries, again, are a common cause of spinal accessory nerve injuries; therefore a patient's surgical history should be reviewed closely.

The patient can present with a sagging shoulder at rest and incomplete arm elevation with loss of strength with shoulder shrug (Fig. 54.8). Trapezius atrophy can also be seen. The symptoms may be quite severe as a result of muscle spasm and brachial plexus traction neuritis or may occur as a more subtle ache, stiffness, and weakness, especially with overhead activity. Examination shows a drooping of the shoulder and a deepening of the supraclavicular fossa after trapezius atrophy has occurred. Winging of the scapula occurs with resisted arm elevation and active external rotation against resistance.[91] The superior angle moves laterally compared with the inferior angle and gives the classic "lateral winging" appearance. The levator scapulae is palpable and is seen as a band of muscle in the neck; rhomboid contraction is also palpable on attempted scapular adduction. The lateral winging is accentuated in abduction but will disappear when

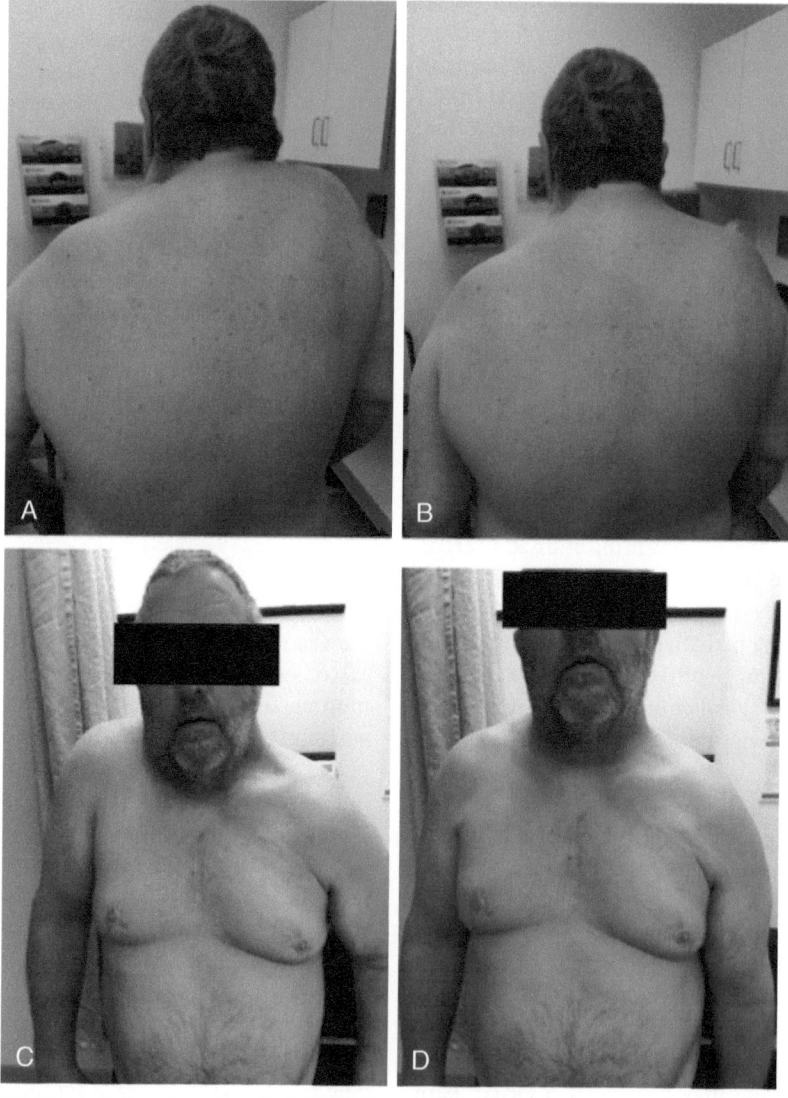

Fig. 54.8 Starting top left and moving clockwise: (A) Posterior view of a patient with a left spinal accessory nerve palsy attempting a shoulder shrug. (B) Note the drooping left shoulder at rest and trapezius atrophy. (C and D) Anterior view of patient attempting shoulder shrug and at rest with a left spinal accessory nerve palsy.

the arm is flexed forward, unlike the medial winging seen with serratus anterior palsy. Lateral winging is typically less obvious and is often less disabling with trapezius palsy than with serratus anterior palsy. However, shoulder function in an athlete with accessory nerve palsy is often inadequate for competition.

Diagnostic Studies

EMG is used to provide the definitive diagnosis, but its role in determining prognosis for recovery has been questioned.[92] Furthermore, low-amplitude compound muscle action potentials and voluntary motor unit potentials may be present in the context of severe spinal accessory nerve injury, warranting surgical exploration.[93]

Decision-Making Principles

Functional results with closed injuries that are treated conservatively are mixed.[65,92,94,95] Spinal accessory nerve palsy does not seem to respond as well to conservative therapy as serratus anterior palsy. Neuropraxic lesions can often be monitored for up to 1 year before considering surgical intervention.[94] If there is complete injury to the nerve, often as it runs in the posterior cervical triangle, and it is diagnosed within 1 year, microsurgical nerve reconstruction should be considered. Symptoms persisting longer than a year typically require the Eden-Lange muscle transfer procedure. Clinical indications for exploration or reconstruction include a symptomatic patient with upper extremity drooping, aching, numbness, and incomplete active arm elevation. Adjacent scapular muscles cannot substitute for a paralyzed trapezius with muscle strengthening alone.

Authors' Preferred Technique
Spinal Accessory Nerve Palsy

The current reconstruction of choice, called the Eden-Lange procedure, involves transferring the levator scapulae, rhomboid minor, and rhomboid major laterally to more functionally advantageous positions to substitute for the upper, middle, and lower trapezius.[95] With the patient in the lateral position, the head of the table is elevated 15 degrees. A longitudinal incision is made midway between the spinous processes and the medial border of the scapula along its entire course. The trapezius is identified and released close to the scapular border, taking care not to injure the underlying rhomboids. The levator scapulae, rhomboid minor, and rhomboid major are separated from each other and then detached from the scapula with a thin strip of insertional bone. These muscles are then elevated with care to avoid injuring the dorsal scapular nerve and transverse cervical artery. Each muscle is tagged individually with a suture, and the infraspinatus is then elevated from its fossa. Six longitudinal drill holes are placed through the scapula 1.5 to 2 cm apart, with the most superior hole 4 to 5 cm lateral to the medial border of the scapula, just inferior to the scapular spine. With a large needle, heavy nylon sutures are passed, taking care not to penetrate the chest wall. The rhomboid minor is secured to the two most superior drill holes, and the rhomboid major is secured to the remaining four drill holes. The infraspinatus muscle is then imbricated over the repair. A second skin incision is made over the scapular spine 3 cm medial to the posterior tip of the acromion, extending medially 4 cm. The trapezius, deltoid, and supraspinatus muscles are then elevated from the scapular spine so that three drill holes can be made through the spine. The levator scapulae is then passed through a tunnel in the trapezius in line with its upper fibers and secured to the scapular spine. After skin closure and application of a dressing, the shoulder is placed in an abduction brace.

Results

In a relatively large series of 27 patients treated for trapezius muscle palsy, 20 underwent neurolysis or repair of the spinal accessory nerve at a mean of 7 months after injury. The remaining 7 patients underwent lateral muscle transfers at a mean of 20 months after the onset of symptoms. Of the 20 patients who underwent nerve surgery, 16 had good or excellent results, with an average follow-up shoulder abduction of approximately 125 degrees. Of 7 patients who underwent muscle transfer, 4 had good or excellent results. Predictors of poor results were patient age greater than 50 years and nerve lesions resulting from radical neck dissection, penetrating injury, or spontaneous spinal accessory nerve palsy.[96] In a series of 7 patients who were followed for a mean of 39 months, 5 had excellent results as demonstrated by full forward flexion, minimal scapular winging and shoulder droop, and improved pain. The remaining 2 patients, who had each undergone a two-stage reconstruction, had residual pain and weakness.[95]

AXILLARY NERVE PALSY
Anatomy and Biomechanics

The axillary nerve arises from the posterior cord of the brachial plexus with contributions from the C5 and C6 nerve roots. The nerve passes close to the coracoid process before coursing posteriorly just inferior to the shoulder joint capsule. It then enters the quadrilateral space, joined by the posterior humeral circumflex artery, and is bound by the humerus laterally, the long head of the triceps medially, the teres minor and infraspinatus superiorly, and the teres major inferiorly (see Fig. 54.8). The axillary nerve divides into anterior and posterior branches, innervating anterior and posterior portions of the deltoid muscle, respectively. A branch from the posterior division also supplies the teres minor muscle and skin overlying the deltoid insertion. Points of relative fixation at the posterior cord, quadrilateral space, and deltoid muscle render it vulnerable to injury.[97] The axillary nerve is vulnerable to traction injury after shoulder dislocation[98] and as a result of direct blunt trauma.[65] Also, considering the close proximity of the axillary nerve to the inferior glenohumeral capsule as it passes from anterior to posterior, it is at risk for compression from an inferior humeral osteophyte from glenohumeral arthritis.[99] Most commonly, quadrilateral (or quadrangular) space syndrome is caused by chronic compression of the posterior humeral circumflex artery and axillary nerve within the quadrilateral space. Fibrotic bands along the inferior edge of teres minor and within the space have been implicated,[100,101] although any space-occupying lesion (e.g., ganglion, aneurysm) or traumatic disruption of the normal anatomy can cause compression.

Clinical Evaluation

Quadrilateral space syndrome is a chronic compressive neuropathy that typically presents in athletes who throw; it is the most common cause of axillary neuropathy.[102] The patient often presents with an insidious onset of abduction weakness, decreased sensation over the deltoid insertion, and eventually deltoid atrophy and glenohumeral subluxation.[65] Symptoms are aggravated by forward flexion and/or abduction with external rotation of the humerus.[100] Resisted shoulder internal rotation in this provocative position also exacerbates symptoms of a dull ache.[103] Discrete point tenderness is noted on palpation posteriorly over the quadrilateral space and a Tinel sign over the quadrilateral space may be elicited.[100] Symptoms are attributed to compression of the axillary nerve, not to arterial occlusion.[101] Although quadrilateral space syndrome is the most common cause of compressive axillary neuropathy, it is certainly not the sole cause of axillary palsy; thus a full history must be taken, focusing on previous injuries and surgeries to the shoulder/neck region, and the duration and quality of symptoms. A full musculoskeletal physical exam should be performed, including aspects of a upper extremity neurologic and vascular exam.

Diagnostic Studies

MRI may demonstrate cysts in the quadrilateral space, inferior labral tears, or fatty atrophy of the teres minor muscle.[104] Muscle edema in the teres minor and/or deltoid may be demonstrated in subacute cases.[105] Electrodiagnostic studies may demonstrate increased latencies on nerve conduction velocities and denervation patterns on EMG of the teres minor muscle.[74,106] Positive subclavian arteriography will demonstrate occlusion of the posterior humeral circumflex artery with the shoulder in abduction and external rotation.[100] An arteriogram may be performed but is not necessary because it suggests associated symptomatic nerve compression only indirectly.[106]

Decision-Making Principles

Conservative measures have been successful in up to 90% of patients.[100] Nonoperative treatment consists of cessation of throwing and management of symptoms. Rehabilitation focuses on shoulder and trunk flexibility, strength, and proper throwing mechanics.[102] In the absence of a space-occupying mass or identifiable lesion, conservative treatment is indicated.[107]

📌 Authors' Preferred Technique

Axillary Nerve Compression in the Quadrilateral Space

Quadrilateral space decompression is performed with the patient in a lateral position. A 3.5-cm longitudinal incision is made over the posterior shoulder at the point of maximal tenderness. The posterior deltoid is elevated superolaterally to expose the fat within the quadrilateral space. Fibrous adhesions are carefully dissected while palpating the axillary nerve and accompanying posterior humeral circumflex artery along the humeral neck. The arm is placed in maximal abduction and external rotation to ensure unrestricted nerve gliding and a palpable arterial pulse as a finger is easily passed through the quadrilateral space and into the axilla.

The shoulder is placed in a sling for postoperative comfort, and the patient is instructed in the immediate use of gravity-assisted pendulum exercises. Active ROM and gentle strengthening exercises are initiated on postoperative day 10. Full abduction with external rotation is avoided until 4 weeks after surgery. A sport-specific therapy program is initiated at 6 weeks.

Results
Nonoperative

Several case reports discuss the nonoperative management of athletes who perform repetitive overhead movements. Two volleyball players demonstrated improved motor strength and resolution of sensory disturbance after abstaining from competitive sports (for 6 months and 1 year, respectively).[16] A competitive baseball pitcher altered his throwing mechanics to a three-quarter overhead motion and successfully returned to competition.[103]

Operative

The surgical solution for axillary nerve palsy depends, as always, on the etiology. A well-described surgical procedure for brachial plexus or axillary nerve injuries in patients with loss of active shoulder abduction is transfer of the triceps branch of the radial nerve to the anterior branch of the axillary nerve. A combined case series showed that the nerve transfer was successful in the majority of patients, increasing shoulder abduction strength and active ROM.[108] In the original series of patients presenting with quadrilateral space syndrome, 18 underwent posterior decompression. Eight experienced complete relief, eight showed improvement, and two did not show any improvement.[100] In a subsequent review of five patients who experienced a traumatic event (two traction injuries and three injuries that occurred as a result of a fall), it was reported that pain symptoms improved and sensory deficits over the lateral arm resolved in all patients. Three patients had persistent limitation of active motion as a result of their associated shoulder joint injuries.[106] In a series confined to athletes who performed repetitive overhead movements, four patients presented with disabling posterior shoulder pain, despite normal findings on electrodiagnostic examination.[109] Upon decompression of the quadrilateral space, three patients were found to have fibrous bands constricting the axillary nerve, and one was found to have constricting venous dilation. All four patients returned to full pain-free activity without restriction by 12 weeks after surgery.

For a complete list of references, go to ExpertConsult.com.

SELECTED READINGS

Citation:

Freehill MT, Shi LL, Tompson JD, et al. Suprascapular neuropathy: diagnosis and management. *Phys Sportsmed.* 2012;40(1):72–83. doi:10.3810/psm.2012.02.1953.

Level of Evidence:

V

Summary:

The authors report a thorough review of the etiology, diagnostic studies of choice, and recent updates in surgical treatment.

Citation:

Lafosse L, Piper K, Lanz U. Arthroscopic suprascapular nerve release: indications and technique. *J Shoulder Elbow Surg.* 2011;20(2 suppl):S9–S13. doi:10.1016/j.jse.2010.12.003.

Level of Evidence:

VII

Summary:

The authors present their own indications and technique for arthroscopic suprascapular nerve release at both the spinoglenoid and suprascapular notch.

Citation:

Chalmers PN, Saltzman BM, Feldheim TF, et al. A comprehensive analysis of pectoralis major transfer for long thoracic nerve palsy. *J Shoulder Elbow Surg.* 2015;24(7):1028–1035. doi:10.1016/j.jse.2014.12.014.

Level of Evidence:

V

Summary:

The authors present the results of a survey of shoulder and elbow surgeons to record a recent snapshot in time their technical preference in pectoralis major transfers for long thoracic nerve palsies. They also provided a systemic review of the outcomes of the differences in technique.

Citation:

Bigliani LU, Perez-Sanz JR, Wolfe IN. Treatment of trapezius paralysis. *J Bone Joint Surg Am.* 1985;67(6):871–877.

Level of Evidence:

IV

Summary:

The authors present a series of patients who sustained an injury to the spinal accessory nerve resulting in paralysis of the trapezius muscle. The rationales for surgical decision-making, surgical technique, and functional outcomes are presented.

Citation:

McAdams TR, Dillingham MF. Surgical decompression of the quadrilateral space in overhead athletes. *Am J Sports Med.* 2008;36(3):528–532. doi:10.1177/0363546507309675.

Level of Evidence:

IV

Summary:

The authors present a series of four athletes who perform repetitive overhead movements and had axillary nerve entrapment within the quadrilateral space, resulting in deltoid muscle paralysis. The authors present a modified surgical technique and report functional outcomes.

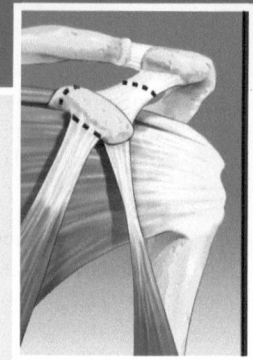

55

Vascular Problems and Thoracic Outlet Syndrome[a]

Matthew A. Posner, Christopher J. Roach, Adam M. Pickett, Brett D. Owens

Vascular problems involving the shoulder are relatively uncommon, but they can result in pain, a profound deleterious effect on an athlete's performance, and, in rare cases, a potentially limb-threatening situation. Acute sports-related vascular injuries are most common in contact sports and can occur as a result of blunt or penetrating trauma. The possibility of penetration of a bone fragment in fractures underscores the need for the rapid assessment of vascular status with a physical examination, plain radiography, and arteriography if necessary. Delayed presentation of vascular injuries can be the result of compression or abnormality within the thoracic outlet. The thoracic outlet, which involves the area of the shoulder girdle in which the subclavian artery and vein exit the chest cavity along with the brachial plexus, is vulnerable to injury because of its crowded confines in combination with the high mobility of the glenohumeral and scapulothoracic articulations.

Thoracic outlet syndrome (TOS) generally defines any compression of brachial plexus elements and/or subclavian vessels as they pass from the intrathoracic area through the ribs into the axilla and proximal arm.[1] However, it is important to identify the particular neurovascular structures involved in attempting to diagnose and treat TOS. Variability in the presenting symptoms of TOS poses a challenge for the clinician and highlights the importance of obtaining a careful history and performing a thorough physical examination. The various names referred to as TOS attest to its confusing nature (Box 55.1).

Historically, the first description of the cervical rib and associated symptoms was presented by the German anatomist Hunald in 1842.[2] After the advent of radiographs, Thomas and Cushing[3] described a brachial plexopathy called the *cervical rib syndrome* and a surgical procedure to correct it in 1903. Neurovascular compression in the thoracic outlet area by structures in addition to the cervical rib were first described by Astley Cooper in 1921.[4] In 1927, Adson and Coffey[5] introduced scalenotomy as a treatment option for cervical rib symptoms. In grouping numerous types of neurovascular compression in the thoracic outlet region, Peet et al.[6] first used the term *thoracic outlet syndrome* in 1956. Surgical management of TOS evolved in 1966, as Roos[7] described the less morbid transaxillary first rib resection. In 1989, Atasoy[8] introduced

a combined approach to TOS consisting of transaxillary first rib resection and transcervical anterior and medial scalenectomy. Today various surgical techniques are used to address any soft tissue or bony structures contributing to compression.

CLASSIFICATION

The current classification of TOS focuses on the particular structures that are injured as opposed to the controversial anatomic factors responsible for the injury. In 1984, Wilbourn[9] developed a classification for the TOS disorders based on the vascular or neural elements injured. This classification includes true neurogenic, arterial, venous, traumatic neurovascular, and nonspecific TOS.[9] Clinical features are quite variable between the neurogenic and vascular subtypes of TOS. Neurogenic TOS accounts for more than 90% of all TOS cases, whereas vascular TOS constitutes 3% to 4% of all cases.[10] Most TOS cases are seen in adults between the ages of 20 and 50 years. Vascular TOS is seen equally in nonathletic men and women, but neurogenic TOS is three to four times more likely to occur in women than in men. Among competitive athletes, venous TOS cases predominantly occur in men in their mid-20s.[11] Other neurovascular pathology in the athlete's shoulder region can be attributed to quadrilateral space syndrome (QSS), scapulothoracic dissociation, shoulder dislocation, and sternoclavicular dislocation.

Patients with neurogenic TOS commonly report a history of neck trauma, such as a motor vehicle accident, a violent collision in a sporting event, or repetitive heavy lifting. Complaints consist of paresthesias or weakness of the hand and arm, as well as pain involving the head, neck, shoulder, and back. Symptoms may also include loss of dexterity, muscle spasm, and a feeling of heaviness of the upper extremity. These clinical findings almost never solely involve pain or weakness in the dermatomes and myotomes associated with C8 or T1 compression. Patients may also report cold intolerance, Raynaud phenomenon, coldness of the hand, and color changes as a result of sympathetic overactivity as opposed to ischemia. Finally, nonspecific complaints such as headaches, tinnitus, and vertigo may also be present.[12] In general, patients with true neurogenic TOS have objective motor and/or sensory deficits, whereas patients with nonspecific neurogenic TOS typically have subjective weakness and/or numbness in the upper extremity. Otherwise, these two entities share the same clinical presentation but may have vastly different treatment protocols.[13]

[a]The views and opinions expressed in this manuscript are those of the authors and do not reflect the official policy of the Department of the Army, the Department of Defense, or the US Government.

BOX 55.1 Synonyms for Thoracic Outlet Syndrome

- Shoulder-hand syndrome
- Paget-Schroetter syndrome
- Cervical rib syndrome
- First thoracic rib syndrome
- Scalenus anterior syndrome
- Brachiocephalic syndrome
- Scalenus minimus syndrome
- Scalenus medius band syndrome
- Costoclavicular syndrome
- Humeral head syndrome
- Hyperabduction syndrome
- Nocturnal paresthetic brachialgia
- Fractured clavicle syndrome
- Pneumatic hammer syndrome
- Cervicobrachial neurovascular compression syndrome
- Effort vein thrombosis
- Rucksack paralysis
- Pectoralis minor syndrome
- Cervicothoracic outlet syndrome
- Subcoracoid syndrome
- Syndrome of the scalenus medius band
- Naffziger syndrome
- Acroparesthesia

Venous TOS, also known as Paget-Schroetter syndrome, has a variety of clinical presentations. This syndrome often occurs in healthy young men who have participated in excessive upper extremity activities; it is caused by a spontaneous thrombosis of the subclavian or axillary vein. Usually no underlying compressive abnormality exists that predisposes the patient to the thrombosis.[14] After the venous occlusion occurs, the limb feels heavy and becomes edematous and possibly even cyanotic. The patient may have neurologic features, such as pain and paresthesias, because of the vascular insult rather than injury to the nerve itself. The three most important factors that lead to venous TOS in athletes are hypertrophy of the pectoral muscle, fibrosis and thickening of the damaged vessel wall from repetitive activity, and damage to the intima of the vein leading to a thrombogenic surface.[15] The term *effort thrombosis* has been used to describe this clinical entity, and this diagnosis has been reported in participants in sports such as swimming, tennis, and weight lifting.[16]

Arterial TOS is the least common form of TOS but may have the most serious potential consequences to life or limb. Flow in the subclavian or axillary artery is obstructed, most likely from compression between the anterior scalene muscle (ASM), or a bony anomaly such as a cervical rib or deformed first thoracic rib. The downstream effects of this arterial compression include vessel damage, turbulent blood flow, aneurysm formation, and thrombus formation.[17] Later consequences can include embolization and ischemia of the digits. Importantly, aneurysm or thrombosis formation may not always be explained by direct arterial vessel compression via nearby structures. Kee et al.[18] reported on ischemia of the throwing hand in professional baseball pitchers because of an embolic occlusion from an axillary artery branch aneurysm. These investigators did not detect any direct inducible compression of the artery but attributed the lesion to repetitive injuries to the artery during the throwing movement.[18] Rohrer et al.[19] showed that the subclavian or axillary artery can undergo considerable compression in arms that were hyperextended into a throwing position. These investigators reported an increase of at least 20 mm Hg in arterial blood pressure in athletes and nonathletes when the arm was placed in that position.[19] This condition may be underdiagnosed because its symptoms can mimic fatigue and musculoskeletal pathology in overhead-throwing athletes.[20] Rarer still, arterial TOS can present in children, in which case making a correct diagnosis often involves a lengthy workup.[21]

QSS in athletes is most commonly diagnosed in baseball pitchers and volleyball players.[22] The quadrilateral space is defined as the area enclosed by the teres minor superiorly, the humeral shaft laterally, the teres major inferiorly, and the long head of the triceps medially. The axillary nerve and posterior humeral circumflex artery traverse this space and are subjected to an often overlooked and position-dependent compressive entrapment. Hypertrophy of any one of the three muscular borders may reduce the space available for the neurovascular bundle, leading to QSS symptoms. Fibrous bands within this space, most commonly between the teres major and long head of the triceps, may contribute to the decreased cross-sectional area of the quadrilateral space.[23] Additionally, the circumflex course of these structures predisposes them to tethering and stretch injuries when the arm is abducted and rotated.[24] Symptoms can be quite vague and overlap with other causes of posterior shoulder pain, such as posterior labral injury, rotator cuff tendinosis, and suprascapular nerve entrapment. Generally no motor or sensory deficits are noted on physical examination. A lidocaine block has been described and is positive if the patient no longer has tenderness to palpation or pain with activity after the injection.[25] The clinician must have a high index of suspicion and should rule out other sources of shoulder pathology before making this diagnosis.

Vascular injuries in the area of the shoulder can be potentially life- or limb-threatening conditions. A high level of awareness should be maintained for athletes who sustain clavicular fractures, proximal humerus fractures, glenohumeral joint dislocations, and other blunt or penetrating shoulder trauma. Most vascular injuries to the shoulder region occur as a result of penetrating bone fragments or a foreign object. However, Carli et al.[26] reported a case of isolated axillary artery dissection due to blunt trauma in an ice hockey player. Vascular injuries after dislocations are also relatively uncommon, with an incidence of 0.97% after shoulder dislocation.[27] Signs and symptoms of axillary artery injury after shoulder dislocation may be subtle, develop slowly, or be absent altogether. Pulses are absent in 93% of cases, but because of an extensive network of collateral vessels, distal pulses may still be present. Pain, swelling, an axillary mass, and a neurologic deficit are other findings to note on physical examination.[28] The clinician must carefully evaluate the potential for injury to the axillary artery or its branches when managing cases of shoulder trauma in an athlete.

ANATOMY

A thorough understanding of the vascular anatomy of the proximal upper extremity is essential in evaluating and treating potential neurovascular injuries in the area of the shoulder (Fig. 55.1). Blood flows from the heart into the subclavian arteries in each upper extremity, with a short traverse through the innominate artery first on the right. The left subclavian artery arises directly from the arch of the aorta. The subclavian artery then enters the thoracic outlet, confined by the upper border of the first rib, the lower border of the clavicle, and the anterior and middle scalene muscles and extends to the lateral border of the first rib. The artery becomes the axillary artery as it exits from the lateral border of the first rib to the inferior border of the latissimus dorsi. The axillary artery is divided into three anatomic sections by the pectoralis minor tendon, with the first section being above the superior border of the pectoralis minor and giving off the superior thoracic artery inferiorly. The second section of the axillary artery lies deep to the pectoralis minor and gives off the lateral thoracic branch and the thoracoacromial artery, which further divides into the clavicular, acromial, deltoid, and pectoral branches. The third and final section of the axillary artery lies distal to the pectoralis minor and contributes the subscapular artery and the anterior and posterior circumflex arteries. The subscapular artery further divides into the scapular circumflex and thoracodorsal arteries. The anterior circumflex artery provides the majority of blood supply to the humeral head near the intertubercular groove through the arcuate artery, which is

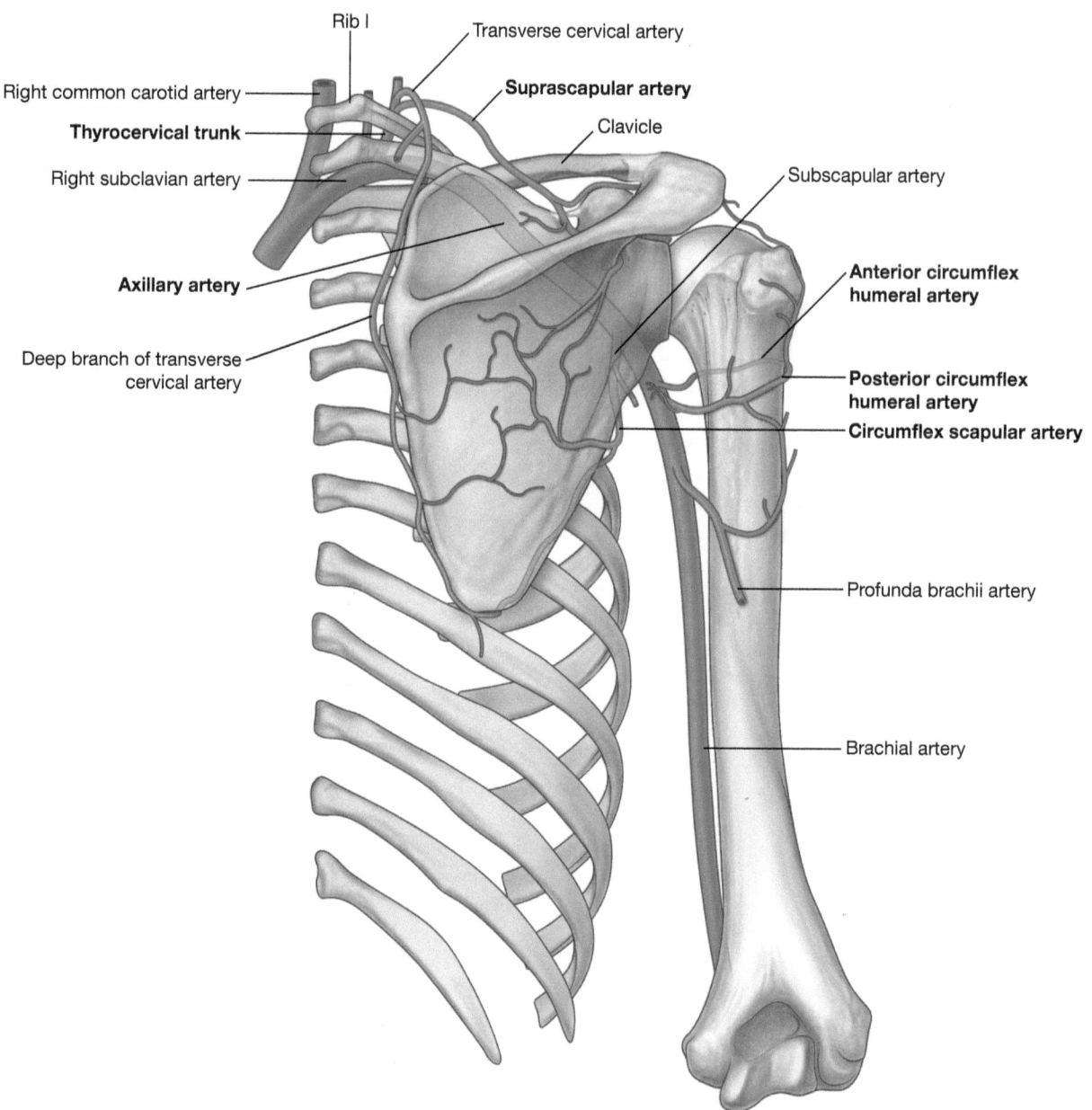

Fig. 55.1 Vascular anatomy of the shoulder. (From Drake RL, Vogl AW, Mitchell AWM. *Gray's Anatomy for Students*, Philadelphia: Elsevier; 2010.)

an anterolateral ascending branch of the anterior circumflex humeral artery.[29]

The basilic vein drains the ulnar portion of the hand and forearm and the medial portion of the arm before becoming the axillary vein at the inferior border of the latissimus dorsi. It then becomes the subclavian vein at the lateral border of the first rib before draining into the brachiocephalic vein medially. The cephalic vein is the more lateral superficial vein in the arm and enters the clavipectoral fascia before emptying into the axillary vein. Together, the axillary and cephalic veins account for the majority of the venous drainage in the shoulder. The shoulder lymphatics end in the thoracic and right lymphatic ducts.[29]

Anatomically, the thoracic outlet spans the general area from the supraclavicular fossa to the axilla and includes the area between the clavicle and the first rib.[17] More specifically, the thoracic outlet comprises three confined spaces in which compression can occur (Fig. 55.2). These compartments include the interscalene triangle, the costoclavicular space, and the retropectoralis minor space.[4,13] The interscalene triangle is bordered anteriorly by the ASM, posteriorly by the middle scalene muscle, and inferiorly by the medial surface of the first rib. The interscalene triangle contains the vast majority of neurovascular compression cases of TOS.[1] The trunks of the brachial plexus and subclavian artery pass through the interscalene triangle, whereas the subclavian vein actually passes anterior to the ASM (Fig. 55.3). The costoclavicular space lies between the clavicle and the first rib posteromedially and the upper border of the scapula posterolaterally. The retropectoralis space lies inferior to the coracoid process beneath the pectoralis minor tendon.

Several bony abnormalities may play a role in compressing structures in the thoracic outlet and causing neurovascular symptoms (Fig. 55.4). Cervical ribs can originate from the seventh cervical vertebra in approximately 1% of the population, with about 10% of those persons having symptoms related to this condition.[30] Various types of cervical ribs can exist, ranging from

short bars of bone, incomplete ribs with fibrous bands, and full ribs articulating with the first rib, manubrium, or sternum.[31] In addition, an elongated C7 transverse process can cause compression. Abnormalities such as exostosis, tumor, callus, or fracture of the first rib or clavicle may also be responsible for compressive symptoms.[32] Complications of clavicular fractures such as malunion, fragmentation, and retrosternal dislocation can also increase the risk of developing TOS.[13,33-35]

Soft tissue abnormalities such as anomalous fibrous bands and anatomic variations of the scalene muscles can create compression in the thoracic outlet. Roos[36] classified 10 types of fibrous bands in the area of the thoracic outlet that may act to compress its neurovascular structures through direct contact or by compromising the space available within the outlet. Scalene muscle variations that may contribute to TOS include anterior scalene

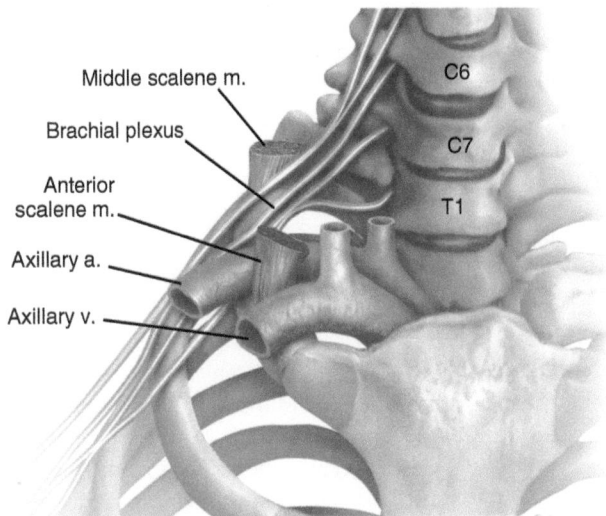

Fig. 55.3 Normal bony anatomy and neurovascular relationships of the thoracic outlet. *a*, Artery; *m*, muscle; *v*, vein.

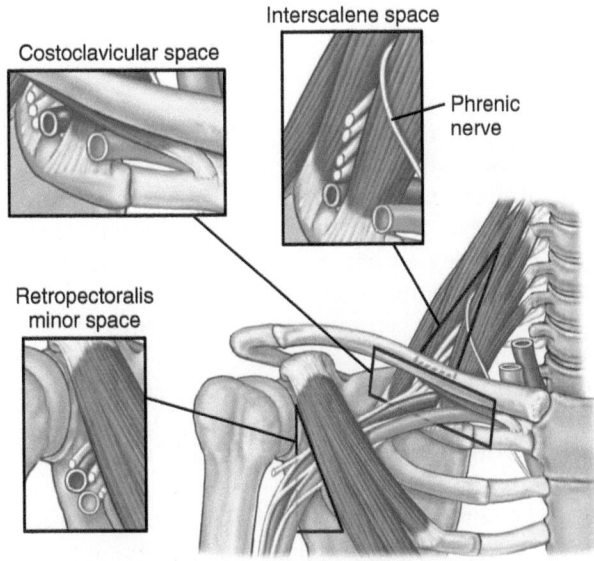

Fig. 55.2 Three spaces in the thoracic outlet that may be responsible for thoracic outlet syndrome.

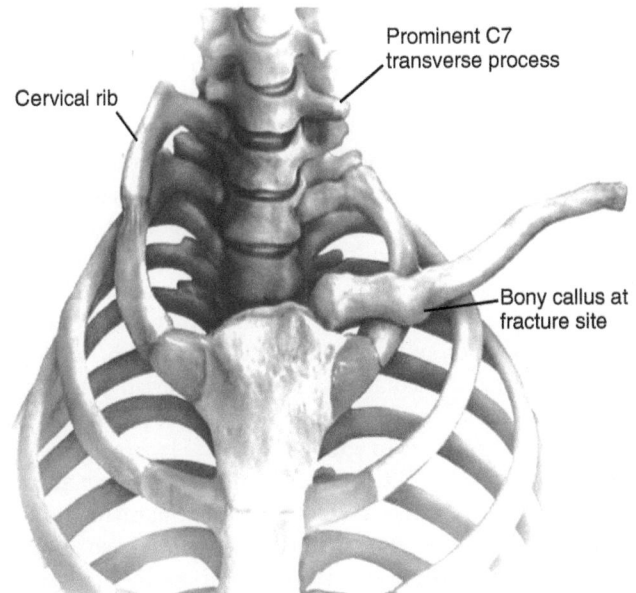

Fig. 55.4 Common bony anomalies in persons with thoracic outlet syndrome.

hypertrophy, passage of the brachial plexus through the substance of the ASM, and a broad, anterior insertion of the middle scalene onto the first rib.[32] Potential loading of the neural tissue may also occur if clavicular motion during upper extremity elevation is compromised, particularly with injuries to the acromioclavicular or sternoclavicular joints.[13] Repetitive trauma to the more vulnerable trunk of the lower brachial plexus and C8–T1 spinal nerve roots can play a role in the pathogenesis of TOS.[1]

HISTORY

The patient's history prior to the onset of symptoms is often the most helpful tool in diagnosing TOS. The history may include a neck injury, clavicular fracture, presence of a cervical rib, unusual postural requirements, or strenuous overhead activities.[37] Patients typically report an aching pain radiating from the back of the shoulder region down into the upper extremity. Pain may be accompanied by numbness, tingling, weakness, swelling, coolness, and discoloration. Occasionally pain spreads up the back and into the side of the neck, with an associated ipsilateral hemicranial headache.[38] These symptoms are often exacerbated by arm elevation and by carrying heavy loads. Furthermore, these symptoms progress despite various conservative treatment modalities, such as physical therapy, medications, injections, biofeedback, and psychotherapy.[39]

The differential diagnoses for TOS include any pathology creating pain or weakness in the neck, arms, or shoulders. The differential can include cervical radiculopathy or arthritis, brachial plexus neuritis, shoulder pathology, peripheral nerve compression, neoplasm, vasculitis or thromboangiitis, rheumatologic conditions, multiple sclerosis, or acute coronary syndrome.[1] In most situations, TOS is a diagnosis of exclusion. For true neurologic TOS, any disorder involving the sensory or motor nerve fibers of the C8 or T1 spinal cord segment must first be investigated and can include anterior horn cell disorders, brachial plexopathies, radiculopathies, or mononeuropathies of the median, ulnar, and radial nerve.[17] Furthermore, traumatic factors such as clavicular fractures, clavicular malunions/nonunions, injuries to the cervical spine, dislocation of the humeral head, and atherosclerosis of the major arteries near the humerus must be considered.[40]

TOS can be seen in athletes who engage in overhead motions, such as pitchers, tennis players, and swimmers. Muscular athletes may be especially susceptible because of hypertrophy of neck, shoulder, and scapular musculature. Athletes in contact sports may sustain traction injuries to the upper arm and chest. Direct trauma that results in rib fractures, transverse process fractures, clavicular fractures, and shoulder injuries may lead to TOS. Effort thrombosis caused by compression of the subclavian vein between the clavicle and first rib is probably the most frequently encountered vascular disorder in young athletes.[11] Hypertrophy of the ASM may be a contributing cause to this compression. Axillary artery lesions are rarely the cause of nontraumatic etiology, although a distinctive lesion can occur in baseball pitchers. Compression and stretching of the axillary artery by the humeral head as it shifts forward during the late cocking phase of pitching may lead to aneurysms and occlusions of the artery itself.[41]

PHYSICAL EXAMINATION

After a thorough history has been obtained that details timing aspects of symptoms and precipitating causes, both upper extremities should be carefully examined for evidence of swelling, discoloration, temperature changes or cold intolerance, ulcerations, muscle atrophy, or nail bed deformities.[22,42] General range of motion (ROM), strength testing (including hand intrinsic muscles), and pulse palpation from the wrist to the shoulder should be documented. A classic finding in true neurogenic TOS is wasting of the abductor pollicis brevis and mild wasting of the interossei and hypothenar muscles, presenting as the Gilliatt-Sumner hand.[43] Blood pressure and an Allen test should be evaluated.[44] The cervical spine, clavicle, and scapula must be thoroughly examined to evaluate for cervical disk pathology, clavicular trauma, scapular winging, or other abnormalities. Sensation should be tested statically and dynamically with two-point discrimination. Muscles and bones should be palpated for areas of tenderness and possible anatomic abnormalities, such as cervical ribs. The extremities also should be examined for evidence of distal nerve compression, especially near common problematic areas such as the carpal tunnel, pronator teres, and cubital and radial tunnels.[42]

Vascular TOS is usually readily identified and differentiated from neurogenic TOS via symptoms, physical examination findings, and diagnostic studies. Arterial TOS commonly involves symptoms and findings distally in the forearm and hand and is less often provoked by scalene palpation, neck rotation, or head tilting. Arterial emboli can produce distal findings of subungual petechiae, digital ischemia, claudication, pallor, coldness, pain, and paresthesias in the hand. Emboli can also lead to obliteration of the radial pulse at rest, and abduction of the arm is unnecessary to detect it. Venous TOS is usually associated with arm swelling, cyanosis, and distended superficial veins not usually seen in arterial or neurogenic TOS (Fig. 55.5).[10]

Neurogenic TOS is classically associated with certain provocative tests, although they display high rates of false positives.[45] All tests are positive if they increase symptoms such as pain, paresthesias, or attenuation of the radial pulse. Tests that more specifically delineate compromise in the interscalene triangle are the Adson test and the supraclavicular pressure test. The costoclavicular or military brace maneuver narrows and emphasizes possible compression in the costoclavicular space. The Wright test compresses and stretches structures in the retropectoral space. The elevated arm test (Roos) evaluates for neural compromise throughout the thoracic outlet. Upper limb tension testing indicates brachial plexus compression; however, it may be in the retropectoral space, interscalene triangle, or cervical spine.

The Adson test is performed with the patient's affected arm extended and slightly abducted, the neck tilted toward the affected side, and the patient inhaling deeply (Fig. 55.6). The physician feels the radial pulse before and during the test and looks for obliteration due to compression of the subclavian artery by the anterior scalene. This test can be positive in a healthy person and can be unreliable for arterial TOS if the pulse is already absent as a result of emboli. Tilting the neck to the opposite side (the reverse Adson test) may be a more reliable test that can produce arm heaviness, fullness, pain, and distal numbness in

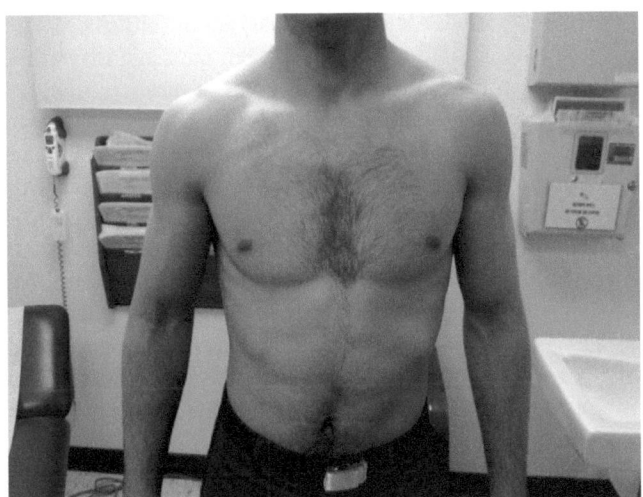

Fig. 55.5 Presentation of a patient with venous thoracic outlet syndrome. Note the engorged superficial veins overlying the right chest.

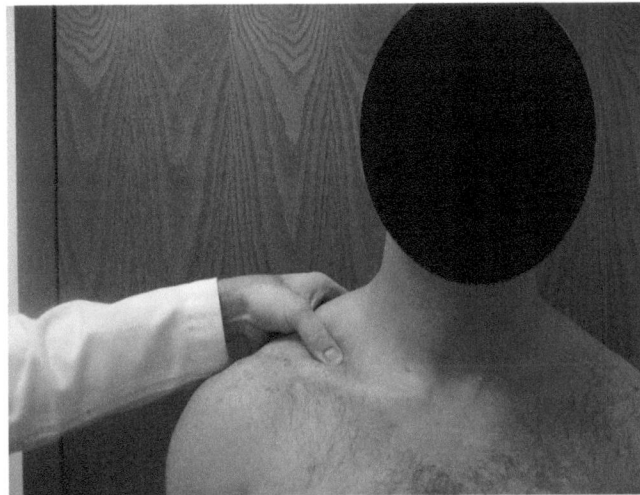

Fig. 55.7 The supraclavicular pressure test is performed by placing compression in the retroclavicular space with the thumb in an attempt to compress the brachial plexus and vascular structures.

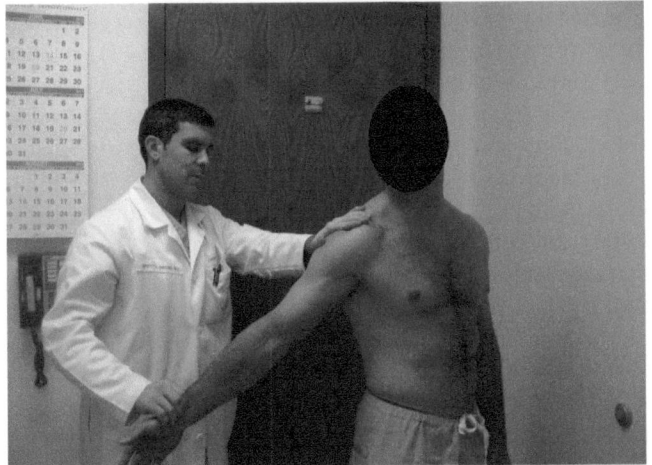

Fig. 55.6 The Adson test is performed with the head tilted to the affected side and the patient's affected arm extended and slightly abducted.

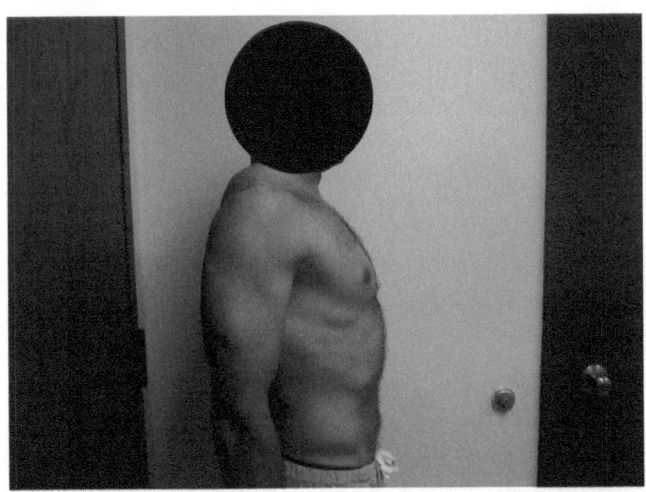

Fig. 55.8 In the costoclavicular maneuver, the patient retracts the shoulders backward and downward to bring the clavicle closer to the first rib in an attempt to elucidate neurogenic or vascular symptoms.

symptomatic patients.[42] The supraclavicular pressure test is performed by placing compression in the retroclavicular space with the thumb in an attempt to compress the brachial plexus and vascular structures (Fig. 55.7). During the costoclavicular maneuver, the patient retracts the shoulders backward and downward to bring the clavicle closer to the first rib in an attempt to elucidate neurogenic or vascular symptoms (Fig. 55.8). The Wright test has the physician hyperabduct and externally rotate the affected extremity of the patient while looking for arm, hand, or pulse changes (Fig. 55.9). The Roos elevated arm test is performed by abducting and externally rotating each of the shoulders 90 degrees while opening and closing the hands rapidly (Fig. 55.10). The test lasts 3 minutes and is positive if the patient feels fatigue, pain, paresthesias, or numbness. Upper limb tension testing is a good screening test for sensitization of neural tissue in the cervical spine, brachial plexus, and upper limb, but it is not specific.[13] The following three positional instructions are performed: (1) abduct both arms to 90 degrees with the elbows straight, (2) dorsiflex both wrists, and (3) tilt the head to one side with the ear to the shoulder and then to the other side.

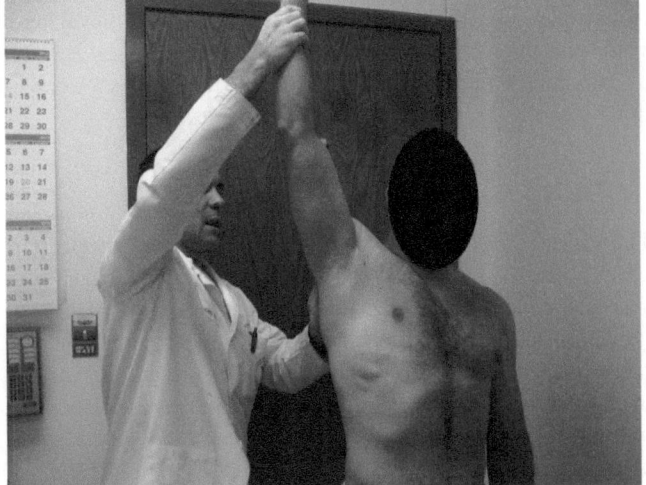

Fig. 55.9 The Wright test has the physician hyperabduct and externally rotate the patient's affected extremity while looking for arm, hand, or pulse changes.

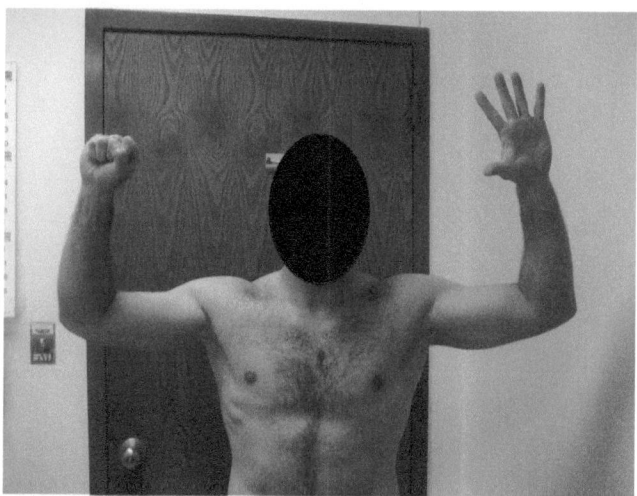

Fig. 55.10 The Roos elevated arm test is performed by abducting and externally rotating each of the shoulders 90 degrees and opening and closing the hands rapidly.

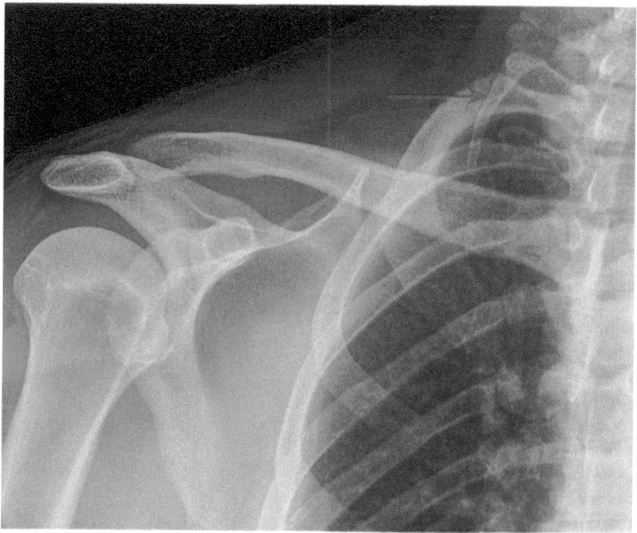

Fig. 55.11 A shoulder radiograph showing a cervical rib *(arrow).*

Ipsilateral symptoms are seen in positions 1 and 2. Contralateral symptoms are seen in position 3. A strong positive test is onset of pain and/or paresthesias in position 1 that increases in positions 2 and 3.[10]

IMAGING

The thoracic outlet consists of three spaces: the interscalene triangle, the costoclavicular space, and the retropectoralis minor space. A leading cause of TOS is the dynamic compression of the neurovascular bundle as it traverses this complex anatomic region. Clinical diagnosis can be difficult; therefore various imaging modalities may be used to show the nature and location of the TOS pathology.[32] Routine radiographs of the cervical spine, chest, and shoulder should be performed at the initial visit to evaluate for degenerative spine disease, cervical ribs (Fig. 55.11), an elongated C7 transverse process, pathologic clavicle fractures, and space-occupying lesions.

Peripheral vascular studies such as pulses, blood pressure measurements, and Doppler studies aid in the diagnosis of thoracic outlet compression and occlusion of the arterial supply in the arm. Nerve conduction studies and electromyography can be helpful assessments in patients with suspected TOS. These studies commonly show the following results: (1) decreased amplitude in ulnar sensory action potentials, (2) decreased amplitude in median compound motor action potentials, (3) normal or slightly decreased ulnar motor potentials, and (4) normal median nerve sensory potentials. Because the lower trunk (C8–T1) is in direct contact with the scalene muscle tendon and first rib, median and ulnar nerve fibers have a predilection to injury as a result of their origin in the brachial plexus.[1] Other nerve compression pathologies—such as cervical radiculopathy, carpal tunnel syndrome, and cubital tunnel syndrome—can be present by themselves or in addition to TOS. Double-crush nerve compression, which was first reported in 1973, can be a real diagnostic challenge.[46] A study by Wood and Bioni[47] in 1990 showed that 44% of patients with TOS had compression of a nerve distally, with the most common site being the carpal tunnel. Therefore providers must be aware of the potential for further distal compression neuropathy in patients with TOS.[47]

Vascular studies such as arteriography and venography can be useful tools to confirm any extrinsic compression of the neurovascular structures transmitted through the thoracic outlet. Because of patient comfort issues and visual acuity of these classic studies, they have been largely replaced by less invasive procedures such as sonography, computed tomography (CT), and magnetic resonance imaging (MRI). The effectiveness of color duplex ultrasonographic examination has been well documented. A study by Demondion et al.[48] showed the utility of analyzing an arterial cross-sectional area at various degrees of arm abduction. These investigators found a significant difference in stenosis between volunteers and affected patients for all degrees of abduction in the costoclavicular space.[48] Another study examined the association of shoulder laxity with upper extremity blood flow in professional male pitchers using duplex ultrasonography of the subclavian and axillary arteries. The authors showed a significant decrease in arterial blood flow in the laxity group compared with the nonlaxity throwers.[49] Duplex ultrasonography has an advantage of providing dynamic studies in a relatively simple fashion.

Arterial compression is well visualized with the use of CT angiography (Fig. 55.12). The bony architecture of the TOS region can be assessed concomitantly with CT imaging for potential sites of compression. Using CT angiography, LeBan et al.[50] demonstrated narrowing of the costoclavicular space in the abduction–external rotation position in more than 50% of patients with a clinical history of TOS.[50] Another study using CT angiography showed a significant difference in the maximum distance between the clavicle and first rib before and after a postural maneuver in 79 patients.[51] Although CT angiography easily shows extrinsic compression of vascular structures, the size of the CT gantry can limit shoulder abduction. Other limitations of CT include limited visualization of the brachial plexus, use of ionizing radiation, and use of an iodinated contrast medium. Newer open MRI has multiple advantages that permit imaging in preferred

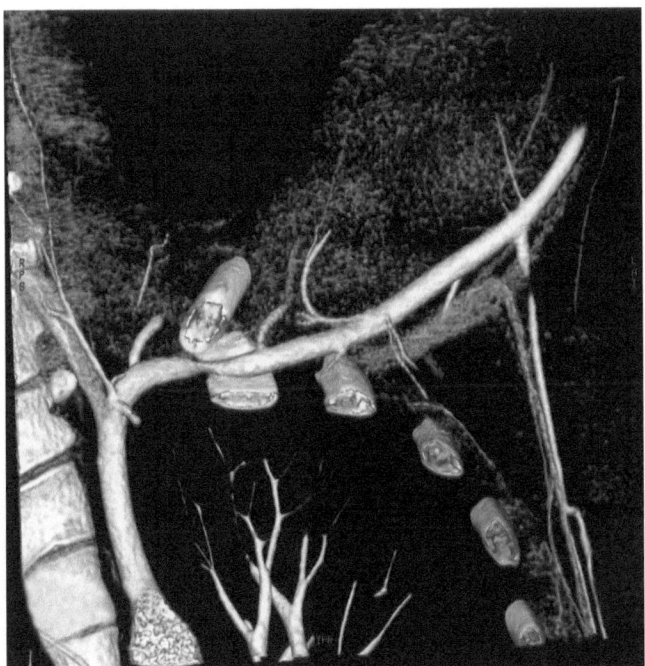

Fig. 55.12 Computed tomographic angiography with the arm in abduction shows subclavian artery compression in this position.

planes at appropriate levels of abduction or other postural maneuvers without the use of contrast material or ionizing radiation. Furthermore, MRI permits good analysis of the brachial plexus and muscle hypertrophy, abnormal muscles, and fibrous bands.[32] Demirbag et al.[52] showed significant differences in MRI findings in patients in neutral versus provocative positions in several anatomic parameters such as costoclavicular distance and retropectoralis minor distance. MRI in the neutral and abducted position has become the preferred screening test for patients suspected of having TOS.

Additionally, expanding techniques in MR neurography (MRN) can isolate the unique water properties of peripheral nerve tissue and locate sites of compression.[53,54] Baumer et al. showed that in a small series of patients with suspected TOS, increased T2W signal within a brachial plexus MRN indicates areas of relative nerve compression.[55] MRN was also helpful in identifying soft tissue anatomic structures that were causing the compression, which correlated with each patient's surgical findings. This emerging technology may assist in diagnosing TOS and developing targeted surgical treatments; however, more research is needed to definitively understand its diagnostic role in patients with TOS.

ASM and pectoralis minor (PMM) muscle injections have been used for diagnostic and therapeutic purposes. Several case series have demonstrated the safety and efficacy of using ultrasound guidance to inject bupivacaine into the muscle belly, even in high-level athletes.[56,57] Furthermore, a good response to injection correlates with a positive outcome after certain surgical treatments for TOS.[57,58] Botulinum toxin has recently been studied as a means of nonsurgical treatment for neurogenic TOS. One study showed that patients experienced substantial pain relief for up to 3 months after a single injection of botulinum toxin into the ASM under CT guidance. This treatment choice may be valuable for nonsurgical patients or may serve as a prognostic tool for surgical intervention.[59]

DECISION-MAKING PRINCIPLES

Acute vascular trauma of the shoulder in the athlete is a rare occurrence and is most often associated with penetrating trauma from foreign objects or bone fragments. Although uncommon and with a majority occurring as a result of motor vehicle accidents in persons who are not athletes, axillary artery injuries from humeral neck and scapular neck fractures have been reported.[60-62] Clavicular fracture can be a common occurrence in athletes participating in contact sports and cycling, and although most do not have significant sequelae, vessel laceration, pseudoaneurysm, or thrombus can occur.[63] Close attention to vascular status and rapid assessment of fracture pattern with plain films is important, moving on to angiography if indicated. Limb ischemia should be minimized by rapid assessment and movement to definitive treatment if acute vascular injury is suspected. Other traumatic events that can lead to vascular injury are scapulothoracic dissociation, glenohumeral dislocation, and posterior sternoclavicular dislocation.

Scapulothoracic dissociation is an uncommon but severe injury of the shoulder girdle and is usually associated with disruption of the subclavian or axillary vessels and brachial plexus components. The injury occurs most often in persons involved in motorcycle and other motor vehicle accidents, but it can also occur after falls from heights.[64] Attention must be directed to the extremities in these patients, who often have multiple traumatic injuries, and a peripheral vascular examination should be performed, although the extensive collateral network in the area of the shoulder may mask a proximal vascular injury.[65] Lateral displacement of the scapula on chest radiographs is pathognomonic for scapulothoracic dissociation.[66] Comparisons may be made between the sternal notch and coracoid or glenoid notch on each side. CT myelography and MRI are the primary studies for determining the anatomic level of injury, and electromyography is helpful in evaluating the severity of the injury. Surgical decisions regarding limb salvage versus amputation are usually guided by the extent of neurologic involvement.[67] Lesser injuries may involve other components of the superior shoulder suspensory complex that require surgical attention.

Shoulder dislocation is a common injury that can occasionally present in association with vascular injury.[27] The axillary artery is vulnerable because of its fixation to the humerus via the circumflex scapular artery and may be damaged by the pectoralis minor tendon, which may act as a fulcrum when the humeral head displaces anteriorly.[68-70] These arterial injuries are not likely to occur in a young, athletic population; however, dislocations in this population are frequent.[71] Luxatio erecta, a glenohumeral dislocation in which the humeral head is displaced inferior to the glenoid with the humeral shaft parallel to the scapular spine, can present with vascular occlusion or injury.[72,73] Suspicious peripheral pulses or swelling should prompt angiography and appropriate revascularization if necessary.

Sternoclavicular injuries account for only approximately 3% of shoulder girdle injuries, with anterior dislocations far more prevalent than posterior dislocations.[74] The proximity of the great vessels, esophagus, and trachea and their possible compression make the posterior sternoclavicular dislocation potentially life threatening. Although motor vehicle accidents are the major cause, up to 21% of these injuries can be sports-related.[75,76] Patients usually have a history of trauma to the sternum or scapulothoracic area and may report dyspnea, dysphagia, dysphonia, pain over the clavicular head, or swelling. Examination should include evaluation of peripheral nerve function and a change in symptoms with arm positioning.[77] CT is ideal for confirming the diagnosis. Closed reduction is usually successful and can be performed with traction in line with the clavicle, with a bolster placed between the scapulae of the supine patient and a thoracic surgeon available if necessary.[75] Spencer and Kuhn[78] have described a figure-eight reconstruction of the sternoclavicular joint with a semitendinosus graft that closely mimics the stability of the intact joint for patients with persistent instability of the medial clavicle.

Vascular TOS does not usually respond to conservative management and requires surgical intervention. Prompt recognition of arterial TOS with appropriate imaging studies is important in an attempt to prevent distal ischemia. Studies with the arm abducted can identify possible compressing structures that may require augmentation surgically along with treatment of the vessel itself.[41] Venous TOS, when diagnosed, is initially treated with anticoagulants and thromboprophylaxis and also usually requires surgical management consisting of thoracic outlet decompression around the axillary and subclavian veins and venous reconstruction if necessary.[11]

Neurogenic TOS can be thought of as either true or nonspecific. True neurogenic TOS warrants surgical management for decompression of the affected brachial plexus structures. True neurogenic TOS tends to be relatively painless and has abnormal neurologic and electrodiagnostic findings. Nonspecific TOS is associated with chronic pain and few definitive neurologic and electrodiagnostic findings.[1] Neurologic findings in persons with true neurogenic TOS involve the lower plexus, with more symptoms in the more tensioned T1 anterior primary rami than the C8 anterior primary rami, which produces a more pronounced effect in the thenar eminence muscles than in any other group.[17] In most cases, nonspecific TOS is treated conservatively, with surgical decompression as the final treatment choice after extensive discussion of the potential risks and possible complications of surgery in the complex thoracic outlet region.[1] A proposed algorithm (Fig. 55.13) may help to guide decisions for treatment.

TREATMENT OPTIONS

Conservative management should be the initial treatment for nonspecific neurogenic TOS. Initial pain relief may be obtained through the judicious use of anti-inflammatory drugs and muscle relaxants. Selective muscular (ASM or PMM) blocks can relieve pain temporarily and can assist in the diagnosis.[57,79] An ASM or PMM injection of botulinum toxin is an additional option for temporary pain relief while physiotherapy is performed.[80] After initial pain relief, conservative management begins with patient education about symptoms and prognosis to help ease anxiety

and increase compliance with home exercise programs. Education also centers on activity modifications such as improving posture while sleeping, working, and driving. Costoclavicular space mobility may be improved by working on the diaphragm and scalene muscles. Mobilization of sternoclavicular, acromioclavicular, and first rib costovertebral joints is also stressed. First rib mobilization and scalene muscle stretching can help widen the posterior scalene triangle. The retropectoral space is mobilized through stretching of the pectoralis major and minor muscles.[13,17] Vanti et al.[81] performed a review of 13 studies of conservative management of TOS and found that 76% to 100% of patients with nonspecific neurogenic TOS had good or very good results at short-term follow-up and 59% to 88% had good or very good results after at least 1 year.[81] Novak et al.[82] found that obesity, worker's compensation, and double crush pathology involving the carpal or cubital tunnels were associated with poor outcomes.[82]

Surgical decompression is warranted in patients with true neurogenic TOS and in those with nonspecific TOS when conservative management has failed. Specific surgical treatment for TOS is controversial because of the complex nature of presenting symptoms, the difficulty of isolating a specific site of neurologic compression, and the pathoanatomy involved. Decompression of offending structures in the thoracic outlet is the goal; this usually involves removal of the first rib, release or removal of portions of the anterior and middle scalene muscles, pectoralis minor tenotomy, supraclavicular decompression, and removal of cervical rib when applicable. Some surgeons prefer to get to the thoracic outlet through the transaxillary approach, first described by Roos in 1966[7] and popularized by Urschel,[83] with the patient in a posterolateral position and the arm elevated above the head.[7,84,85] Advantages include a hidden incision in the axilla and excellent access to the first rib unhindered by the neurovascular structures. The disadvantage is limited access to the neural structures, congenital bands, and cervical ribs that lie behind the vascular structures.[1] The supraclavicular approach is most commonly used for TOS decompression, which allows a wide exposure of the supraclavicular plexus and the middle third of the first rib.[86-89]

Recently endoscopic treatments have been described for TOS. Lafosse et al.[90] described an all-endoscopic technique for infra- and supraclavicular brachial plexus neurolysis and decompression. He has subsequently performed this technique on a series of 21 patients who showed improvement in symptoms and functional scores with no complications reported at 6 months of follow-up.[91] Also, George et al.[92] has described a video-assisted thoracoscopic surgery (VATS) approach to first rib resection for patients with TOS. All 10 patients in his series had resolution of symptoms, with 1 patient experiencing transient mild loss of function and sensation that resolved by 8 months postoperatively. These new techniques require an expert knowledge of the anatomy as well as endoscopic skills.

QSS can be treated in a manner similar to the treatment of nonspecific neurogenic TOS, with conservative management initially. Treatment begins with reassurance, relative rest, observation of and possible changes to athletic biomechanics, and therapy that includes stretching of the posterior capsule and teres minor.[93] Surgical decompression is performed if conservative measures

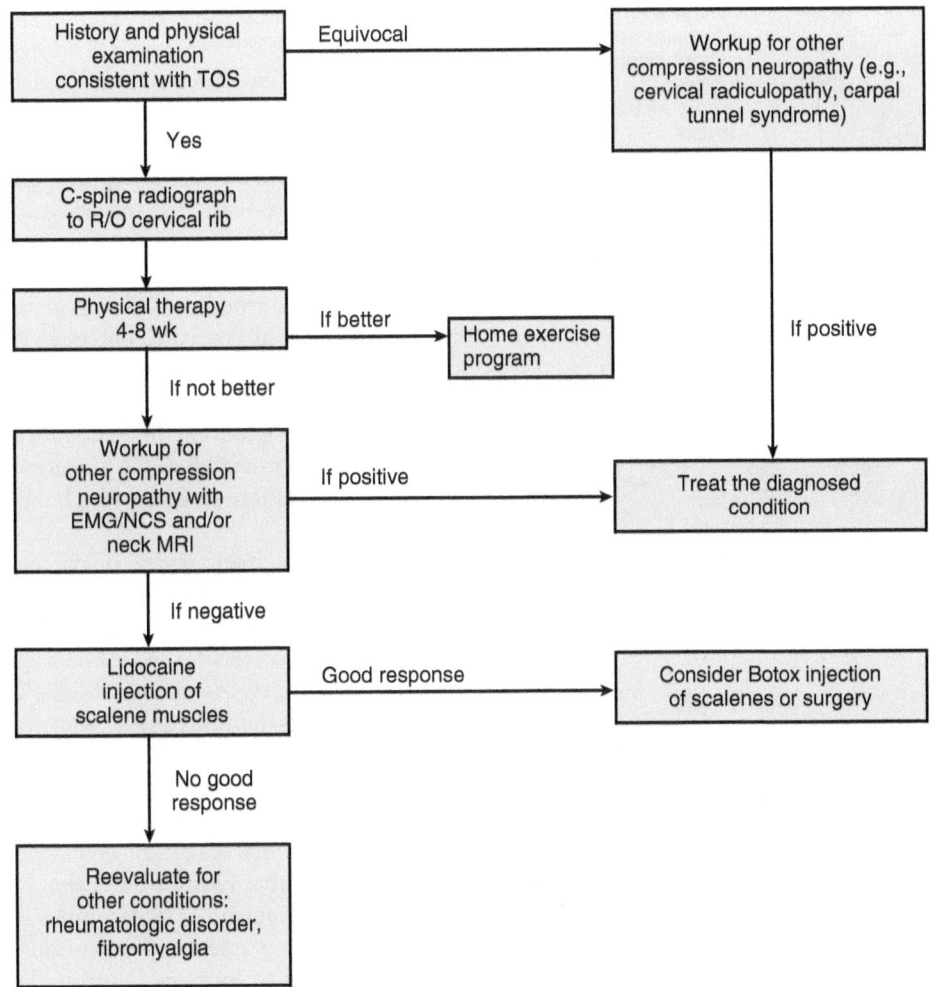

Fig. 55.13 A proposed algorithm for the treatment of thoracic outlet syndrome *(TOS)*. *EMG,* Electromyography; *MRI,* magnetic resonance imaging; *NCS,* nerve conduction study; *R/O,* rule out.

fail, with dynamic testing performed at the time of surgery to ensure complete release of the axillary nerve and maintenance of the radial pulse via the posterior circumflex humeral artery.[25]

Arterial TOS involves surgical treatment of the compression of the vasculature, as well as treatment of the vessel itself. Decompression often involves removal of the cervical and first ribs, scalenectomy, and excision of constricting bands.[41,94] Thrombolytic or balloon angioplasty can be performed for acute ischemia.[95] Arterial degeneration, aneurysm, and intimal damage require bypass grafting or arterial reconstruction.[41,94]

A review of the pathophysiology and treatment of venous TOS is shown in Fig. 55.14. Initial treatment begins with anticoagulation and thrombolysis. The next step in treatment is to decompress the thoracic outlet impingement of the subclavian vein with first rib resection, medial claviculectomy, and scalenectomy as indicated. Venous reconstruction is then performed depending on the status of the vein and symptoms at the time of surgery.[96] Comprehensive surgical management is advocated, with (1) early diagnosis, thrombolysis, and tertiary referral; (2) periclavicular thoracic outlet decompression and frequent use of

venous reconstruction; and (3) temporary postoperative anticoagulation, with an adjunctive arteriovenous fistula if necessary.[11]

RESULTS

Surgical treatment of vascular TOS is generally successful, with outcomes slightly more improved in arterial TOS compared with venous TOS. In the treatment of combined vascular TOS, Davidovic et al.[97] reported complete resolution of symptoms with all cases of arterial TOS but persistent symptoms in patients presenting with axillary-subclavian venous thrombosis when treated with cervical/first rib resection, decompression of all soft tissue elements, and combined vascular procedure.[97] Athletes who engage in overhead movements in their sport have particular success in returning to sport without symptoms after treatment for arterial TOS, including professional baseball players.[20,24] The treatment of venous TOS has evolved from delayed decompression and definitive vascular procedures after a prolonged period of anticoagulation to more rapid decompression after thrombolysis if the condition is diagnosed within 14 days.[96,98] Delayed

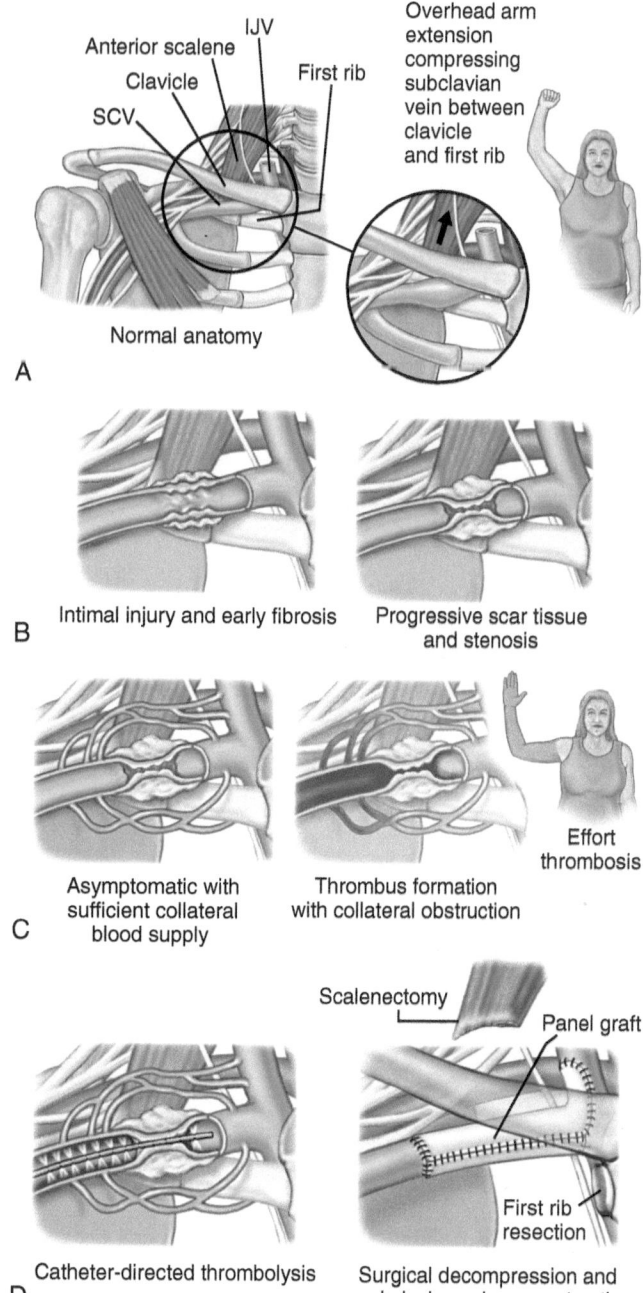

Fig. 55.14 A review of the pathophysiology and treatment of venous thoracic outlet syndrome. *IJV,* Internal jugular vein; *SCV,* subclavian vein.

decompression and definitive vascular procedures yielded only a 40% success rate in 10 patients, with 6 patients requiring additional procedures to achieve venous patency, whereas more rapid decompression after thrombolysis yielded an initial success rate of 83% at 5-year follow-up. A recent report by Melby et al.[11] revealed 100% patency in 32 athletes with effort thrombosis at 10 months, although 7 patients underwent secondary procedures.[11]

Long-term results after the treatment of neurogenic TOS are difficult to elucidate because of differing diagnoses, the complexity of symptoms, and the wide variation of surgical treatments. Mingoli et al.[99] reported a long-term outcome of 81.4% good

to excellent results and a reoperation rate of 15% in a mixed population of patients with TOS treated with a transaxillary extraperitoneal first rib resection and scalene muscle transection.[99] Atasoy[42] also saw improvement in 95 of 102 patients treated with a combined transaxillary first rib resection and transcervical scalenectomy, and 60 patients reported good to excellent results. A retrospective review of patients with mixed TOS treated with a supraclavicular surgical decompression with or without first rib resection at a single institution reported 95% improvement in patients with nonspecific TOS with a minimum 3-year follow-up.[100] Vemuri et al. compared outcomes of patients treated with a pectoralis minor tenotomy versus tenotomy plus supraclavicular decompression, scalenectomy, and first rib resection.[101] They found no significant difference in comparing both groups' outcomes but noted that the tenotomy-plus-decompression group included more patients with a bony anomaly and a history of injury.

A recent systematic review of outcomes following surgical treatment for TOS found more reliable improvement in patients with arterial TOS and venous TOS (90% excellent/good results) as opposed to patients treated for neurogenic TOS.[102] However, 56% to 89% of patients with neurogenic TOS reported improvements in their symptoms and a mean 28.3 point improvement in Disabilities of the Arm, Shoulder, and Hand (DASH) scores.[102] It was difficult to draw conclusions because all studies lacked a standardized method of diagnosing neurogenic TOS, of treating neurogenic TOS, and of obtaining outcome measures. The authors recommended that future studies should focus on these three areas of improvement. QSS decompression seems to be quite successful, with a recent report on four athletes whose sport required overhead motions returning to full activity without symptoms 3 months after undergoing release.[25]

Complications

Surgical complications range from general complications, such as wound healing problems and infection, to those inherent to the delicate anatomy of the thoracic outlet area, including blood vessel damage and possible exsanguination, brachial plexus injuries resulting in severe sensorimotor dysfunction, and nerve injuries and transections (affecting the long thoracic, phrenic, intercostal brachial, supraclavicular, and cutaneous nerves as well as causing Horner syndrome).[17] Apical hematoma, pneumothorax (in up to 33% of patients), hemothorax, chylothorax, and thoracic duct injury have also been encountered.[103] Incomplete resection of the first rib or failure to resect constricting congenital bands can lead to continued symptoms and surgical failure.[103,104] Despite moderately good results in most patients, the risk of devastating complications has prompted some authors to critically evaluate the need for surgery.[105,106] The serious potential for injury emphasizes the need for familiarity with the anatomy of the thoracic outlet.

POSTOPERATIVE MANAGEMENT

The postoperative management of patients with TOS can be simple or complex, depending on the underlying pathophysiology and the surgical procedure used. Surgery ranges from resection of the scalenus anterior to resection of the first thoracic rib. Vascular pathology, such as aneurysm or thromboembolism, must also be addressed at the time of thoracic outlet decompression. After decompression, patients are generally allowed limited ROM of the arm for 3 to 4 weeks for activities of daily living. Active ROM exercises typically begin at 6 weeks after surgery, with return to play (RTP) between 4 and 6 months after surgery.[24] If a patient requires anticoagulation after vascular surgery, early mobilization is not only encouraged for ROM maintenance but may actually reduce the long-term symptoms of postthrombotic syndrome. Athletes may RTP with a gradual increase in intensity and duration after completing their course of anticoagulation.[107] Todd et al.[108] reported on a professional pitcher who returned to the Major League 4 months after saphenous vein interposition grafting of the axillary artery.[108] Bottros et al. also reported on an MLB pitcher who was able to return to pitching in the major leagues one season after surgical treatment of neurogenic TOS.[57] Chang et al.[109] studied the physical and mental component scores on the Short Form–12 scale after surgical decompression of neurogenic TOS and found that the median time to recovery of normal quality of life was 23 months for physical function and 12 months for mental function; however, only 50% of their patients had returned to work at the time of the last follow-up.[109]

SUMMARY

Vascular problems involving the shoulder are relatively uncommon but can result in pain, and may have a profoundly deleterious effect on an athlete's performance; they can also lead to potentially limb-threatening situations. TOS generally comprises any compression of brachial plexus elements and/or subclavian vessels as they pass from the cervical area to the axilla and proximal arm. Although these conditions are rare, the sports medicine surgeon should consider TOS in the differential diagnosis when more common causes of pathology are excluded or the patient's history is suggestive of the condition.

For a complete list of references, go to ExpertConsult.com.

SELECTED READINGS

Citation:
Melby SJ, Vedantham S, Narra VR, et al. Comprehensive surgical management of the competitive athlete with effort thrombosis of the subclavian vein (Paget-Schroetter syndrome). *J Vasc Surg.* 2008;47:809–821.

Level of Evidence:
IV

Summary:
The overall duration of management from symptoms to full athletic activity was significantly correlated with the time interval from venographic diagnosis to surgery and was longer in patients with persistent symptoms or rethrombosis before referral. Optimal outcomes for venous thoracic outlet syndrome depend on early recognition by treating physicians and prompt referral for comprehensive surgical management.

Citation:
Mingoli A, Feldhaus RJ, Farina C, et al. Long-term outcome after transaxillary approach for thoracic outlet syndrome. *Surgery.* 1995;118:840–844.

Level of Evidence:
IV

Summary:
Of 105 patients who were followed up, good to excellent results were obtained in 96 cases (81.4%) and fair to poor results were recorded in 22 cases (18.6%). No major complications were observed. The presence of a long posterior first rib stump, measured from the chest radiograph films, was the strongest determinant of the long-term results among the variables examined. Results suggest that the long-term outcome after surgery for thoracic outlet syndrome was strongly influenced by the extent of the first rib resection.

Citation:
Ciampi P, Scotti C, Gerevini S, et al. Surgical treatment of thoracic outlet syndrome in young adults: single centre experience with minimum three-year follow-up. *Int Orthop.* 2011;35: 1179–1186.

Level of Evidence:
IV

Summary:
The authors' surgical approach consists of performing a supraclavicular decompression without routine first rib resection. This approach allows for the identification and removal of the constricting anatomy in most cases, with satisfactory results in 96.9% of patients and a low complication rate.

Citation:
Peek J, Vos CG, Ünlü Ç, et al. Outcome of surgical treatment for thoracic outlet syndrome: systematic review and meta-analysis. *Ann Vasc Surg.* 2017;40:303–326.

Level of Evidence:
III

Summary:
The authors review the current literature concerning the various surgical treatments of thoracic outlet syndrome and its outcomes. The authors subdivide treatments for arterial TOS, venous TOS and neurogenic TOS. This is a meta-analysis and systematic review of mostly retrospective level III studies. They recommend that further investigations should focus on standardizing diagnostic criteria.

Citation:
Hooper TL, Denton J, McGalliard MK, et al. Thoracic outlet syndrome: a controversial clinical examination. Part 1: Anatomy, and clinical examination/diagnosis. *J Man Manip Ther.* 2010;18(2):74–83.

Level of Evidence:
V

Summary:
The authors provide a simplified method for looking at the controversial entity of thoracic outlet syndrome (TOS). A categorization system for TOS is presented, along with detailed clinical examination techniques.

Citation:

Ferrante MA. The thoracic outlet syndromes. *Muscle Nerve*. 2012;45:780–795.

Level of Evidence:

V

Summary:

An overview of thoracic outlet syndrome (TOS) is presented with a distinction between neurologic and vascular types. Neurogenic TOS is further compared with other upper extremity neuropathies, and distinguishing characteristics are noted.

Citation:

Thompson RW, Driskill M. Neurovascular problems in the athlete's shoulder. *Clin Sports Med*. 2008;27:789–802.

Level of Evidence:

V

Summary:

The authors present an overview of both neurogenic and vascular thoracic outlet syndrome in athletes who engage in overhead motions. Specific attention is given to vascular problems with the axillary artery and subclavian vein and their treatment.

Citation:

Atasoy E. A hand surgeon's further experience with thoracic outlet compression syndrome. *J Hand Surg Am*. 2010;35:1528–1538.

Level of Evidence:

III

Summary:

The author provides an overview of the etiology, symptomatology, examination, and treatment of thoracic outlet syndrome. A retrospective study of surgical outcomes over 20 years is also presented.

Citation:

Hooper TL, Denton J, McGalliard MK, et al. Thoracic outlet syndrome: a controversial clinical condition. Part 2: Non-surgical and surgical management. *J Man Manip Ther*. 2010;18:132–138.

Level of Evidence:

V

Summary:

After reviewing anatomy, examination, and diagnosis of thoracic outlet syndrome (TOS) in part 1 of this article, the authors shift focus to treatment. Concentration is on nonsurgical management for nonspecific neurogenic TOS.

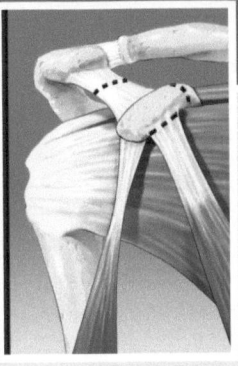

56

Injury to the Acromioclavicular and Sternoclavicular Joints

Connor G. Ziegler, Samuel J. Laurencin, Rachel M. Frank, Matthew T. Provencher, Anthony A. Romeo, Augustus D. Mazzocca

Injuries to the acromioclavicular (AC) joint are common occurrences in the athletic patient population, with approximately 9% of all shoulder injuries involving the AC joint. Injuries to the sternoclavicular (SC) joint are less common, accounting for up to 3% of all shoulder girdle injuries. Damage to either of these joints can lead to significant limitations and pain; therefore it is critical for the orthopedic surgeon to recognize and treat these conditions. Studies have reported that most AC joint injuries occur in young males and that injuries are often incomplete rather than complete.[25,39,64] Although SC injuries are rare, disruptions to this joint can involve the critical airway and vascular structures immediately deep to the sternum, ultimately resulting in life-threatening complications.

Like other major joints, the AC joint is composed of its own joint capsule that contains an intra-articular meniscus-like structure. Eventually, the meniscus-like structure undergoes age-related degeneration and reportedly no function beyond the fourth decade of life.[97,107] Articular cartilage lines both aspects of the articulation; however, the true articular portion of the distal clavicle varies with regard to location and size.[18] In addition to the primary structures of the joint, the AC joint depends on a coordinated function of the AC, coracoclavicular (CC), and coracoacromial (CA) ligaments (Table 56.1). The AC ligament acts as the primary restraint to anterior and posterior displacement of the AC joint.[127] The CC ligament is uniquely composed of the trapezoid and conoid ligaments.[19] The two major functions of the CC ligament include mediating synchronous scapulohumeral motion by attaching the clavicle to the scapula and providing additional strength to the AC articulation. As a result, the CC ligament mainly contributes to vertical stability by preventing superior and inferior translation of the clavicle. Although it is not a primary stabilizer, the CA ligament provides secondary glenohumeral stabilization to prevent anterosuperior displacement of the humeral head in long-standing massive rotator cuff disease. Of note, the normal anatomic CC interspace is approximately 1.1 to 1.3 cm (Figs. 56.1–56.3).[9]

During normal shoulder forward elevation and abduction to 180 degrees, approximately 5 to 8 degrees of motion is detected at the AC joint.[25] The clavicle rotates between 40 and 50 degrees during full overhead elevation. This motion is combined with scapular rotation as opposed to occurring through the AC joint itself. This synchronous motion between the clavicle—which is rotating upward as the scapula rotates downward during abduction—and forward elevation was described by Codman[28] as synchronous scapular-clavicular rotation, which is coordinated by the CC ligaments. The motion of the AC joint is important to understand clinically, because the contribution of different ligaments with regard to resisting translation changes depends on the amount of displacement. For example, with small displacements, the AC ligaments are most important in preventing posterior and superior translation of the clavicle; however, with larger amounts of displacement, the conoid ligament becomes the primary restraint to superior translation. The trapezoid ligament is vital in resisting compression at both small and large amounts of displacement (Fig. 56.4).[41]

The pathologic process of AC joint dislocations involves sequential injury, beginning with the AC ligaments, extending to the CC ligaments, and finally affecting the deltoid and trapezial muscles and fascia. In 1963, Tossy and colleagues[125] originally developed a classification scheme that included types I, II, and III. In 1984, Rockwood[25] expanded the classification, which is purely radiographic, to include types IV, V, and VI (Fig. 56.5). The Rockwood system is generally described as follows: In a type I injury, there is a sprain of the AC ligament with no radiographic abnormality. In type II injuries, the AC ligaments and joint capsule are disrupted, while the CC ligaments are sprained but intact, in addition to a 50% vertical subluxation of the distal clavicle. In type III injuries, the AC ligaments and joint capsule, as well as the CC ligaments, are disrupted with 100% superior displacement of the distal clavicle. In type IV injuries, there is posterior subluxation of the clavicle into the trapezius. A type V injury is an exaggeration of a type III injury with 100% to 300% superior displacement of the clavicle. In the rare type VI injury, there is subacromial or subcoracoid displacement of the clavicle and a reversed CC interspace.

Unlike the AC joint, the SC joint is the only true articulation between the shoulder girdle and the axial skeleton. The bulbous end of the medial clavicle within the SC joint creates a saddle-type joint in the notch of the sternum,[49,50] which nearly functions as a ball-and-socket joint because it can move in almost all planes (up to 35 degrees of upward elevation, 35 degrees of anteroposterior [AP] translation, and 50 degrees of rotation about the

TABLE 56.1	Summary of the Ligamentous Anatomy of the Acromioclavicular Joint			
Ligament	**Origin**	**Attachment**	**Function**	**Notes**
Acromioclavicular: superior, posterior, anterior	Anteromedial edge of the acromion	Lateral aspect of the clavicle	Provides horizontal stability	Flattened tissue that joins the superior surface of the acromioclavicular joint capsule
Trapezoid (coracoclavicular)	Upper coracoid process	Oblique ridge on the inferior clavicle	Provides vertical stability (less than a conoid ligament)	Broad, thin, and quadrilateral; lateral to conoid
Conoid (coracoclavicular)	Base of the coracoid process	Conoid tubercle on the inferior clavicle	Provides vertical stability (more than a trapezoid ligament)	Dense and conical; medial to trapezoid
Coracoacromial	Lateral border of the coracoid	Anterior and inferior surface of the acromion just anterior to the clavicular articular surface	Forms part of the coracoacromial arch, preventing superior migration of the humeral head	Strong, dense, triangular band

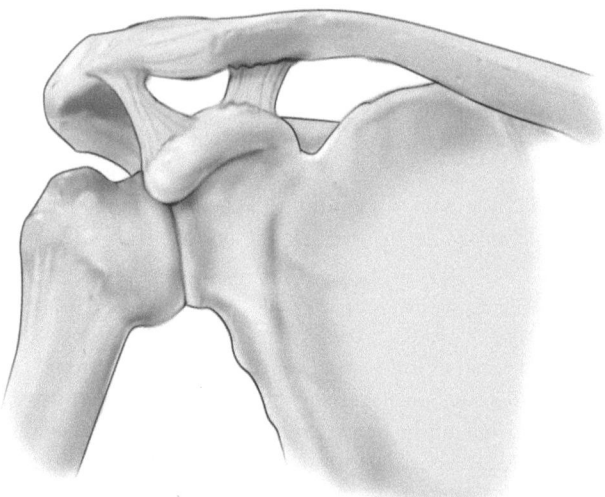

Fig. 56.1 Normal anatomy of the acromioclavicular joint. (From Rockwood CA Jr, Williams GR Jr, Young DC. Disorders of the acromioclavicular joint. In: Rockwood CA Jr, Matsen FA III, Wirth MA, et al, eds. *The Shoulder*. 3rd ed. Philadelphia: Elsevier; 2004.)

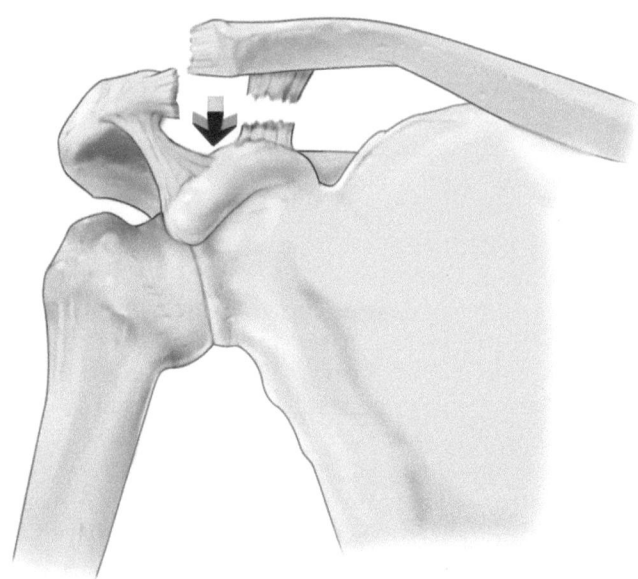

Fig. 56.3 Injury to both coracoclavicular ligaments frequently occurs in the face of acromioclavicular ligament injury and causes an inferior translation of the scapulohumeral complex from the clavicle. In this illustration, it is important to note that the clavicle stays in its normal anatomic position, tethered by the sternoclavicular joint, and the scapulohumeral complex subluxates inferiorly.

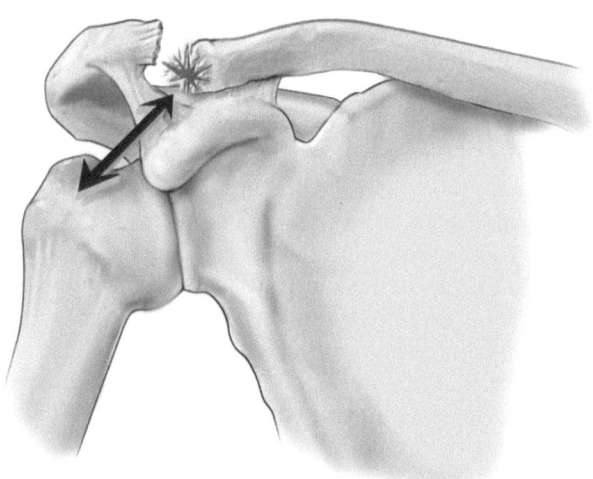

Fig. 56.2 Resection or injury of the acromioclavicular ligaments causes horizontal instability and, if in excess, can cause abutment of the posterior clavicle into the anterior portion of the scapular spine.

longitudinal axis of the clavicle).[59,66,74,104] Typically, the SC joint involves only the articulation between the medial clavicle and the sternum, but approximately 2.5% of patients have an articulation between the medial clavicle and the superior aspect of the first rib.[23]

Nevertheless, the significant ligamentous constraints surrounding the SC joint result in very limited motion at this joint. The stability of the SC joint is reliant solely on soft tissue constraints, including the costoclavicular ligament (rhomboid ligament), SC capsular ligaments, interclavicular ligaments, and intra-articular disk ligament. The intra-articular disk ligament arises from the synchondral junction of the first rib and sternum, which passes through the SC joint with the upper attachment to the superior/posterior aspects of the medial clavicle.[49,50] As a result, the intra-articular disk ligament divides the joint into two spaces, creating a disk that acts to prevent medial displacement of the inner clavicle. The costoclavicular ligament consists of an anterior and posterior fasciculus, which is referred to as

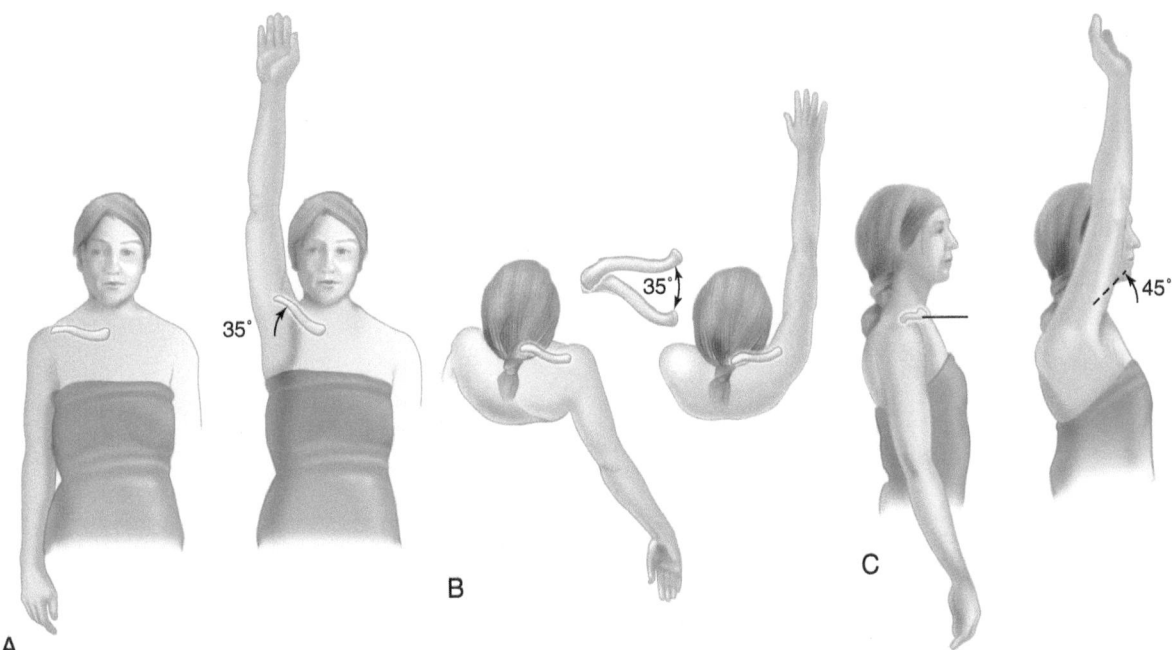

Fig. 56.4 Motions of the clavicle and the sternoclavicular joint. (A) With full overhead elevation, the clavicle is elevated 35 degrees. (B) With adduction and extension, the clavicle displaces anteriorly and posteriorly 35 degrees. (C) The clavicle rotates on its long axis 45 degrees as the arm is elevated to full overhead position. (From Rockwood CA, Green DP, eds. *Fractures in Adults.* 2nd ed. Philadelphia: JB Lippincott; 1984.)

the *rhomboid ligament*.[23,33,50] The anterior fasciculus arises from the anterior medial surface of the first rib and projects superior and laterally, whereas the posterior fasciculus arises lateral to the anterior fibers on the rib and projects superior and medially. The interclavicular ligament spans the top of the sternum, connecting the superomedial aspect of each clavicle, which function to assist the capsular ligaments to hold up the shoulder (also referred to as *shoulder poise*). The capsular ligament covers the anterosuperior and posterior aspects of the joint and represents the thickening of the joint capsule; it is by far the most important structure in preventing upward displacement of the medial clavicle. The importance of the capsular ligament in posterior stability was demonstrated by Spencer et al.[117] in a biomechanical study in which a 50% greater force was required to cause a posterior dislocation versus an anterior dislocation. The capsular ligament is also the strongest ligament of the SC joint and provides a first line of defense against superior displacement of the medial clavicle when a downward force is applied to the lateral aspect of the shoulder.[10]

The spectrum of SC joint dislocations is classified as type I (incomplete tear of the SC and/or CC ligaments), type II (clavicle subluxation with a complete tear of the SC ligament and a possible partial tear of the CC ligament), and type III (a complete tear of both SC and CC ligaments). Historically, SC joint dislocations have been described by either the anatomic direction or the cause of the dislocation. Under the anatomic description, the SC joint dislocation is described based on the direction of the medial clavicle in relation to the sternum. Thus the two types of anatomic dislocations described are anterior and posterior dislocations, with anterior dislocations being the most common. In addition to their anatomic descriptions, SC joint

dislocations have been described based on the cause of the dislocation according to the following categories: sprain or subluxation, acute dislocation, recurrent dislocation, unreduced dislocation, and atraumatic dislocation (see Figs. 56.35–56.38).

Numerous procedures, protocols, and a wealth of biomechanical testing[3,7,11-13,18,29,34,35,37,41,42,62,68,70,74,78-80,87,117,118] have been devised to treat injuries to the AC and SC joints. This multitude of research with its various conflicting outcomes render confusion regarding the appropriate choice of treatment. Moreover, indications for surgical intervention vary based on the evaluation of functional impairment and the assessment of the patient's concern regarding the cosmetic deformity of the injury, particularly in the setting of type III AC joint injuries. In this chapter, we focus on the pertinent patient history, physical examination, clinically relevant anatomy and imaging, decision-making principles, treatment options, and clinical outcomes reported in the literature. Specific attention is given to our preferred operative techniques with video supplementation to this text.

ACROMIOCLAVICULAR JOINT

History

The key element of the history for a patient presenting with a potential AC or SC joint injury is the mechanism of injury, which is usually related to direct trauma. The AC joint is a complex osseous ligamentous structure that is vulnerable to traumatic injury because it lacks additional protection from muscle and adipose tissue because of its subcutaneous position. Direct trauma related to a fall or blow to the acromion with the arm adducted is often described. During such high-energy events, the innate

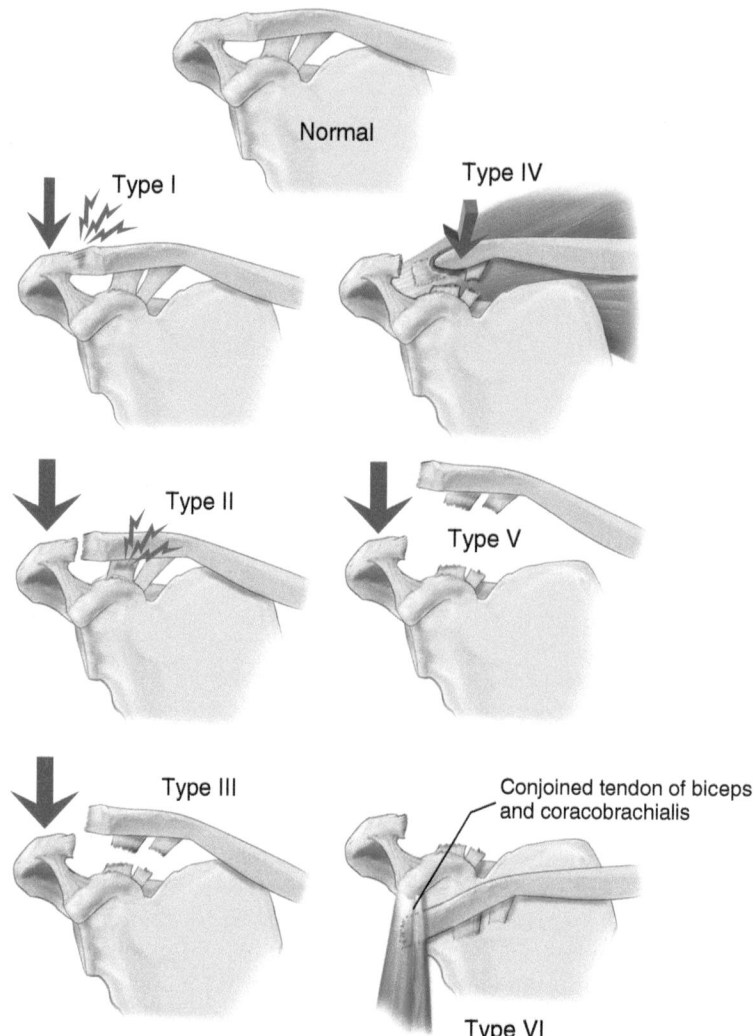

Fig. 56.5 The classification of the ligamentous injuries that can occur to the acromioclavicular (AC) joint. In a type I injury, a mild force applied to the point of the shoulder does not disrupt either the AC or coraco-clavicular (CC) ligament. In a type II injury, a moderate to heavy force applied to the point of the shoulder disrupts the AC ligaments, but the CC ligaments remain intact. In a type III injury, when a severe force is applied to the point of the shoulder, both the AC and the CC ligaments are disrupted. In a type IV injury, not only are the ligaments disrupted, but the distal end of the clavicle is displaced posteriorly into or through the trapezius muscle. In a type V injury, a violent force applied to the point of the shoulder not only ruptures the AC and CC ligaments but also disrupts the muscle attachments and creates a major separation between the clavicle and the acromion. A type VI injury is an inferior dislocation of the distal clavicle in which the clavicle is inferior to the coracoid process and posterior to the biceps and coracobrachialis tendons. The AC and CC ligaments have also been disrupted. (From Rockwood CA Jr, Williams GR Jr, Young DC. Disorders of the acromioclavicular joint. In: Rockwood CA Jr, Matsen FA III, Wirth MA, et al, eds. *The Shoulder*. 3rd ed. Philadelphia: Elsevier; 2004.)

stability of the SC joint results in a transfer of energy to the AC and CC ligaments, resulting in a dislocation of the AC joint. The AC joint also can be subjected to indirect trauma during a fall onto an adducted outstretched hand or elbow, resulting in superior translocation of the humerus, and ultimately resulting in a collision of the humeral head into the acromion. Although rare, nontraumatic injury to the AC joint can result from chronic overuse, referred to as *AC arthrosis,* which often results from a history of weight lifting and repetitive overhead or throwing activities (Fig. 56.6).

Physical Examination

The complete AC joint examination must include inspection, palpation, range of motion (ROM), strength, sensation, and stabilization assessments of both shoulders, after which special tests specific to the AC joint can be performed. An examination for neural, vascular, or additional injuries of the adjoining joints should always be completed. The clinician should be aware of and test for any appropriate cervical spine and/or glenohumeral joint pathologic conditions that, if present, may confuse the clinical picture. Similarly, other disease processes including

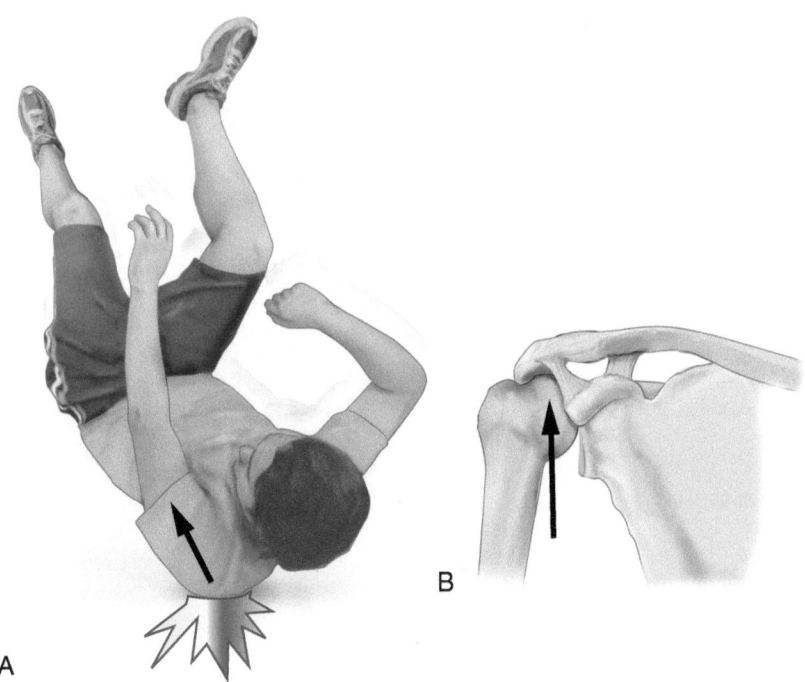

Fig. 56.6 Mechanism of acromioclavicular joint injury. (A) Direct trauma as result of a fall or blow to the acromion with the arm adducted. (B) Indirect injury caused by falling on an adducted outstretched hand or elbow, causing the humerus to translocate superiorly.

gout, pseudogout, and chondromatosis should be considered and ruled out.

The initial physical examination of the patient with a suspected AC joint injury should include observation of the patient either standing or sitting so that the weight of the arm pulling downward stresses the AC joint making any deformity (superior prominence of the distal clavicle) more apparent. When examining a patient for suspected AC joint injuries, the clinician must be sure to examine the entire clavicle and AC joints because of the possibility of biclavicular dislocations.[36,109]

After inspection, the clinician should attempt to isolate the location of the patient's pain via direct palpation. Traumatic pathology of the AC joint is identified by pain, swelling, and point tenderness at the AC joint. In AC joint injuries, the patient most often reports pain originating from the anterosuperior aspect of the shoulder. However, isolating the structure responsible for anterosuperior shoulder pain can be a diagnostic challenge because of the innervation of the AC joint and the superior aspect of the glenohumeral joint. The lateral pectoral nerve provides innervation to the anterior aspect of the AC joint and surrounding structures of the shoulder, whereas the suprascapular nerve provides innervation to the posterior aspect of the AC joint and other posterior structures of the shoulder. Gerber and colleagues[44] evaluated patterns of pain and found that irritation to the AC joint produced pain over the AC joint, in the anterolateral neck, and in the region of the anterolateral deltoid. Irritation of the subacromial space produced pain in the region of the lateral acromion and lateral deltoid muscle but did not produce pain in the neck or the trapezius region. If a patient has more pain than expected for a simple AC joint injury, a coracoid fracture or a type IV injury with displacement of the clavicle through the trapezial fascia should be suspected.

In type III injuries, both the AC and CC ligaments are torn, with no significant disruption of the deltoid or trapezial fascia. The upper extremity is held in an adducted position with the acromion and upper extremity displaced inferior to the horizontal plane of the lateral clavicle. Severe pain persists with motions even 1 to 3 weeks after injury. Patients should be evaluated 3 to 6 weeks after injury to allow for a thorough examination, which is typically not possible in the acute phase due to significant pain. Therefore the patient should be referred to a physiotherapist to improve ROM and re-establish scapular kinematics after initial examination.

Several physical examination techniques are available to help identify and isolate AC joint disease. Diagnostic tests specific to the AC joint: cross-arm adduction test, active compression test, AC resisted extension test, the Paxino test, and the Hawkins-Kennedy sign. Previous studies have reported sensitivities of 77% for the cross-body abduction test, 72% for the AC resistance test, and 41% for the active compression test, respectively; however, the combination of all 3 tests has a reported high specificity of 95%.[26] Of note, several of the AC-specific tests are more specific for AC arthrosis and distal clavicle osteolysis as opposed to unstable AC joint disease. In some cases, the injection of a local anesthetic agent into the AC joint may relieve the pain implicating AC joint etiology. The examination should be performed before and after injection to determine whether changes in symptoms occurred. Likewise, physical examination can help differentiate the different types of AC joint injuries (Table 56.2). For example, type III injuries can often be distinguished from type V injuries by having the patient shrug both shoulders. Type III injuries are reducible with a shoulder shrug because the integrity of the deltotrapezial fascia has not been compromised.[63]

TABLE 56.2   Type of Acromioclavicular Joint Injury and Associated Findings

Type	AC Ligament Injury	CC Ligament Injury	Deltotrapezial Fascia	Clinical Findings	Radiographic Findings
I	Intact	Intact	Intact	AC tenderness	Normal
II	Ruptured	Intact	Intact	Pain with motion; the clavicle is unstable in the horizontal plane	The lateral end of the clavicle is slightly elevated; stress views show <100% separation
IIIA, stable	Ruptured	Ruptured	Mild injury	Clavicle is unstable in both the horizontal and vertical planes and acromion is depressed relative to the clavicle; much improved functionally and with pain after 3–6 weeks nonop management	Radiographs and are abnormal—100% separation; less overriding of clavicle on acromion the IIIB injuries
IIIB, unstable	Ruptured	Ruptured	Mild injury	Continued abnormal scapular movement, pain, weakness, and poor ROM after 3–6 weeks nonop treatment	Cross body stress adduction x-ray showing overriding clavicle on acromion
IV	Ruptured	Ruptured	Injured as the clavicle is posteriorly displaced	Possible skin tenting and posterior fullness	The clavicle is displaced posteriorly on the axillary view
V	Ruptured	Ruptured	Injured and stripped off the clavicle	A more severe type III injury, shoulder with severe droop; if a shoulder shrug does not reduce it, then it is a type V injury	A 100%–300% increase in the clavicle to acromion distance
VI	Ruptured	Ruptured	Possible injury	Rare inferior dislocation of the distal clavicle; accompanied by other severe injuries; transient paresthesias	The clavicle is lodged behind the intact conjoined tendon

AC, Acromioclavicular; *CC,* coracoclavicular; *ROM,* range of motion.

Cross-arm adduction test: This test is performed with the arm elevated to 90 degrees and then adducted across the chest with the elbow bent at approximately 90 degrees. The described motion causes compression across the AC joint, leading to pain. Of note, this motion can also produce pain in the posterior aspect of the shoulder that is associated with a tight posterior capsule or at the lateral aspect of the shoulder, which can be associated with rotator cuff pathology (Fig. 56.7A).

Active compression test (O'Brien test): This test is performed with the arm elevated to 90 degrees and adducted to 10 to 15 degrees with the elbow in extension, followed by maximal pronation of the forearm with obligate internal rotation of the arm as the examiner applies a downward force resisted by the patient. The described positioning of the shoulder causes the greater tuberosity of the humerus to elevate the depressed acromion with the addition of applied resistance resulting in the "lock and load" of the AC joint. Symptoms referred to the top of the shoulder and confirmed by examiner palpation of the AC joint indicate damage to this structure, whereas symptoms referred to the anterior glenohumeral joint suggest labral or biceps disease. Therefore this test can be useful in differentiating AC joint disease from intra-articular disease (see Fig. 56.7B and C).

AC resisted extension test: This test is performed with the arm flexed to 90 degrees and the elbow bent to 90 degrees. The patient is asked to extend the arm against resistance, and the test is positive if pain is reproduced around the AC joint.

Paxino test: To perform this test, the examiner places thumb pressure at the posterior AC joint to cause reproducible pain.

Hawkins-Kennedy sign: This test was originally described regarding the diagnosis of impingement syndrome by causing pain with forced passive internal rotation behind the back and forced adduction with internal rotation. Because impingement syndrome can lead to involvement of the AC joint, the maneuver has been shown to reproduce AC joint-related pain.[53]

Injury to the AC joint not only affects glenohumeral function but also may have a negative effect on scapulothoracic function and scapulohumeral dynamics. The clavicle is the anterior strut supporting the scapula, and proper function of the AC and CC ligaments contributes significantly to the physiologic motion of the scapula.[60,75,110] AC joint instability may position the scapula in a protracted and internally rotated position. Prior studies have reported that scapular dyskinesis may lead to deficits in motion as well as glenohumeral and lateral shoulder pain.[67] Clinical evaluation of the scapula can determine the presence or absence of alterations in scapular position or motion, collectively called "scapular dyskinesis," and can help guide effective treatment for associated functional deficits. A reliable examination can be performed within 10 days after acute injury, when the immediate symptoms have subsided. The clinician should position themselves behind the patient and examine both scapulae to assess resting scapular with both the patient's arms held at their side. It is important to assess for asymmetry of the medial scapular border as prominence indicates excessive scapular internal rotation and/or anterior tilt, which can result in functional deficits in rotator cuff strength and arm motion in flexion and abduction secondary to scapular dyskinesis. This medial scapular border prominence can result when the scapular strut is compromised either from isolated injury to the AC ligaments (type II) or injury to both AC and CC ligaments (type III and higher). Therefore any AC joint separation that results in scapular dyskinesis will potentially create physiologic and biomechanical deficits affecting maximal shoulder function. Patients who demonstrate these

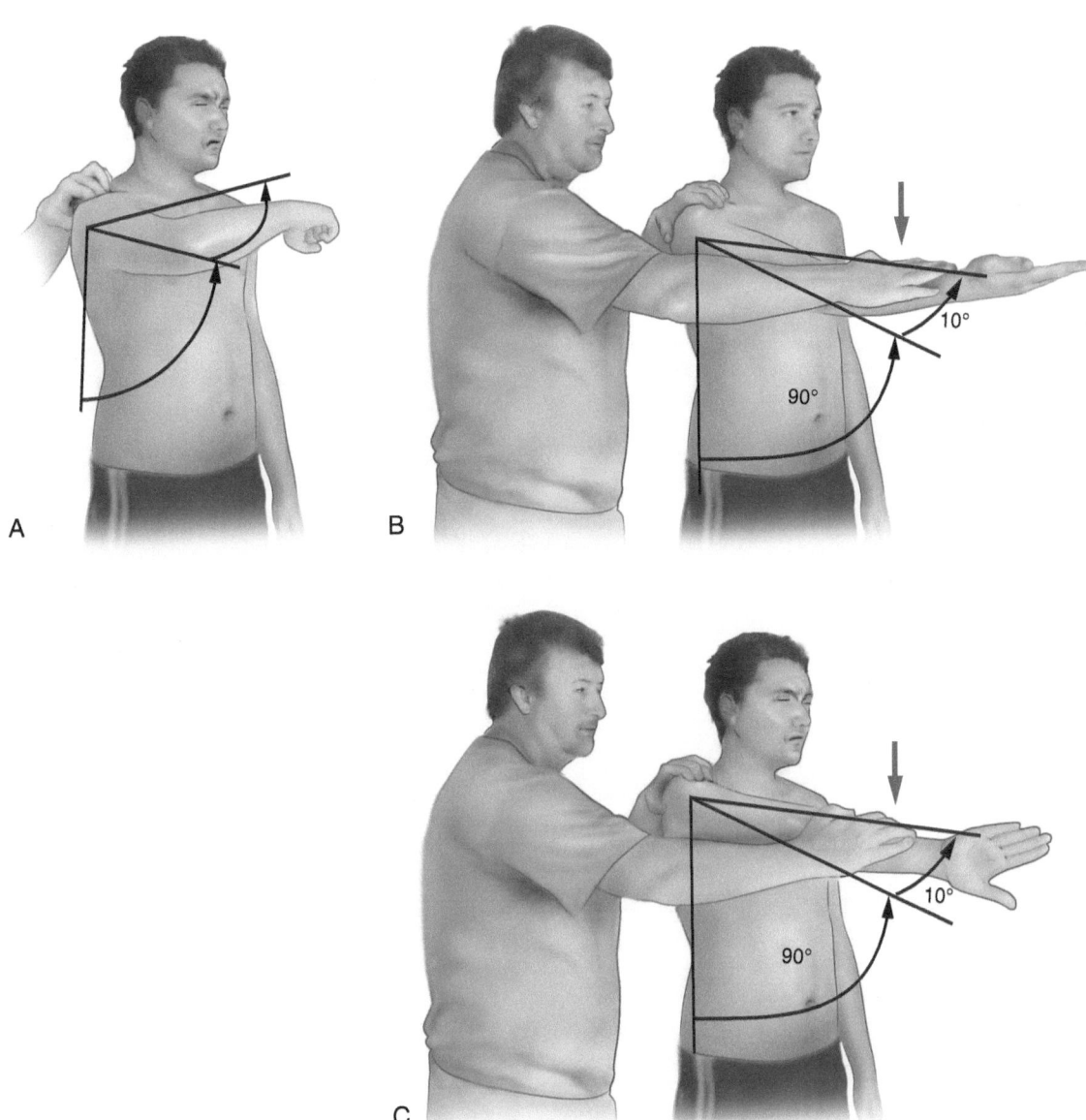

Fig. 56.7 (A) The cross-arm adduction test is performed with the arm flexed to 90 degrees in adduction across the body with a finger placed on the acromioclavicular (AC) joint, indicating pain at that spot only. It is important to understand that this test may produce pain posteriorly if a tight posterior capsule is decreasing internal rotation or in the glenohumeral joint if glenohumeral arthritis is present. This test is positive for AC joint disease only if cross-arm adduction produces pain at the AC joint itself. (B and C) The O'Brien test is performed with the arm flexed to 90 degrees with the elbow in extension and adducted 10 to 15 degrees with maximal supination; it is then performed again in maximal pronation. Symptoms referred to the AC joint with either of these maneuvers or with the arm in supination indicate more of an AC joint disorder, whereas symptoms referred to the anterior glenohumeral joint that are increased in maximal pronation indicate more of a superior labral disorder.

problems on physical exam should be considered for repair or reconstruction of both the AC and CC ligaments.

Overall, the clinical diagnosis of AC joint disease after a traumatic event can be determined via a triad of (1) point tenderness to palpation at the AC joint, (2) pain at the AC joint with cross-arm adduction, and (3) relief of symptoms by injection of a local anesthetic agent. Meanwhile, diagnosis of AC joint pathology resulting from nontraumatic or chronic overuse can often be accomplished via the cross-arm adduction test, the active compression test, and the AC resisted extension test. Chronopoulos et al.[26] reported that the AC resisted extension test combined with the cross-arm adduction test had the greatest sensitivity, whereas the active compression test had the greatest specificity and the highest overall accuracy for diagnosis of these injuries.

Imaging

A complete, standard shoulder radiographic series should be obtained in the setting of an AC joint injury, particularly in high degrees of AC joint dislocation, as associated injuries of the glenohumeral joint are reportedly common.[124] Varying configurations of the AC joint as well as vertical CC translation can be delineated on a standard AP radiograph; however, this shoulder view is not specific to the AC joint. Therefore the radiographic workup AC joint disease should include a bilateral Zanca view, which visualizes the ipsilateral and contralateral AC joints on a single x-ray cassette while maintaining the same orientation of the x-ray beam. The view is obtained by tilting the x-ray beam 10 to 15 degrees cephalad and using only 50% of the standard shoulder AP penetration strength. By visualizing both AC joints on the same cassette, the CC distance can be compared from side to side, also allowing for future comparison of preoperative and postoperative examination findings. The reduced radiographic penetration from that which is standard for the denser glenohumeral joint on an AP shoulder radiograph prevents overpenetration of the AC joint (too dark), which can result in the misinterpretation of subtle pathology. As determined by Zanca,[134] the normal AC joint width is between 1 and 3 mm, although this width diminishes with age (Fig. 56.8). Likewise, the

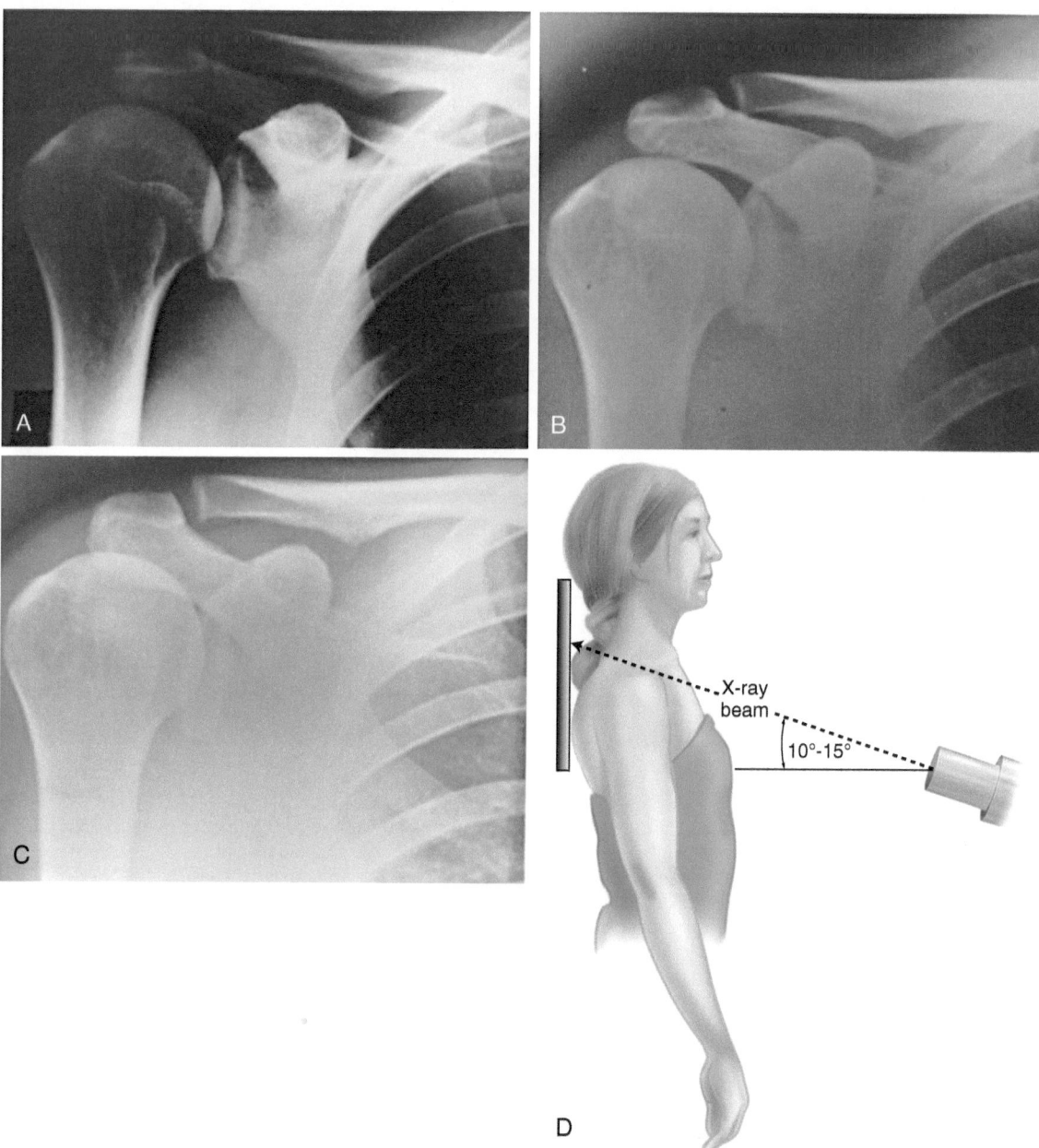

Fig. 56.8 An explanation of why the acromioclavicular (AC) joint is poorly visualized on routine shoulder radiographs. (A) This routine anteroposterior view of the shoulder shows the glenohumeral joint well. However, the AC joint is too dark to be interpreted because that area of the anatomy has been overpenetrated by the x-rays. (B) When the usual exposure for the shoulder films is decreased by two-thirds, the AC joint is well visualized. However, the inferior corner of the AC joint is superimposed on the acromion process. (C) Tilting the tube 15 degrees upward provides a clear view of the AC joint. (D) The position of the patient for the Zanca view: a 10- to 15-degree cephalic tilt of the x-ray tube is required to visualize the AC joint. (From Rockwood CA Jr, Williams GR Jr, Young DC. Disorders of the acromioclavicular joint. In: Rockwood CA Jr, Matsen FA III, Wirth MA, et al, eds. *The Shoulder*. 3rd ed. Philadelphia: Elsevier; 2004.)

normal anatomic CC interspace is approximately 1.1 to 1.3 cm, although this interval does exhibit variability, as demonstrated by Bosworth.[19] Bearden et al.[9] reported a 25% to 50% increase of the CC interval compared with the contralateral shoulder as indicative of complete CC disruption.

An axillary view is useful in visualizing posteriorly displacement of the distal clavicle in relation to the acromion, which occurs in type IV AC joint injury where the scapula displaces anteromedially. However, caution must be taken when diagnosing posterior translation of the distal clavicle based on this view because recent studies have reported difficulties in identifying a posteriorly translated clavicle on an axillary radiograph.[99]

The cross-body adduction radiograph (so-called Basamania view) is reported to differentiate between a stable and unstable AC joint.[8] If the clavicle overrides the acromion on the cross-body adduction view, it indicates instability of the CC ligaments in addition to the AC joint disruption. In this imaging technique, a crossbody adduction AP view of the AC joint with the arm elevated to 90 degrees is used to assess clavicle overlap of the acromion secondary to anteromedial translation of the scapula. In 1949, Alexander described a similar radiographic imaging technique for AC joint instability.[2]

The stress view of the AC joint is obtained by placing 5 lb on each wrist and essentially taking an AP view of both shoulders and is mainly used to differentiate between type II and III dislocations.[58] However, the difference in type II and III injuries is rarely significant, and the classical stress views with distal traction are not typically necessary for diagnosis. Patients who present with a clinically obvious AC injury and deformity suggestive of complete dislocation (types III, IV, V, and VI) often demonstrate maximal CC interspace widening on routine AP view and thus do not require stress views (Fig. 56.9).

The Stryker notch view is useful for determining a coracoid fracture when clinical suspicion is high for AC joint dislocation despite a normal CC interval on the standard AP view of the shoulder (Fig. 56.10). Coracoid process fracture should be suspected when radiographs show AC dislocations with a normal CC distance. This view is taken with the patient supine and his or her palm (affected side) placed on their head while the x-ray beam is tilted 10 degrees cephalad.

Decision-Making Principles

Treatment options for AC joint injuries continue to evolve (Table 56.3). The overall goal, regardless of injury severity or treatment, is to regain full, stable, and pain-free ROM normal strength, and no limitations in activities. The demands on the shoulder will differ among patients, and these demands should be considered during the initial evaluation, as well as ascertaining patient expectations. Initially nonoperative treatment (i.e., use of a sling, ice, analgesics, and immobilization) should be attempted for all patients with incomplete (types I and II) AC joint injuries.[71] Although no current evidence supports the recommendation of surgical intervention for type I or II injuries, some studies have demonstrated persistent symptoms years after nonoperative treatment.[84,88]

For patients with complete AC joint injuries (i.e., types IV, V, and VI), treatment is typically operative because of the significant morbidity associated with persistently dislocated joints and severe soft tissue disruption. In the randomized controlled trial of 12 patients with type V AC joint dislocations, Bannister and colleagues[6] demonstrated superior results with operative treatment with CC screw and AC joint fixation compared with nonoperative treatment.

Treatment of type III injuries remains controversial, with a trend toward initial nonoperative treatment in most cases. Factors involved in the decision-making process include activity level, type of sport/work, timing of injury within the athletic season, and throwing demands on both the injured and the

TABLE 56.3	**Treatment Options**		
Treatment Classification	**Essentials of Repair**	**Clinical and Operative Considerations**	**Level of Evidence**
AC ligament repair	The AC ligament is repaired with reinforcing pin(s), screw, or plate	The implant is usually removed	IV
Dynamic muscle transfer	Transfer of the short head of the biceps with or without coracobrachialis	Partial transfer of structures—may alter shoulder mechanics	IV
CA ligament transfer	Transfer of CA ligament alone or in concert with other procedures	Preserve the length of the CA ligament	IV
CC ligament repair	Traditionally the Bosworth screw technique—wires, suture loops, and grafts have been described	Usually requires a second procedure for hardware removal	IV
Distal clavicle resection with CC reconstruction	Classically, the distal clavicle is excised and the CC is reconstructed using CA ligament	Can also be a salvage procedure for persistent pain after an AC dislocation (especially for type I and II injuries)	IV
Distal clavicle resection without CC reconstruction			IV
Arthroscopic repair and reconstruction	Repair or reconstruction arthroscopically viewed from the subacromial space of CC ligaments	Technical reports have described the efficacy of the procedure	VI
Anatomic reconstruction of the CC ligaments	Reconstruction of CC ligaments using soft tissue grafts to reapproximate the conoid and trapezoid ligaments	Potential advantages of improved horizontal plane stability	IV

AC, Acromioclavicular, *CA,* coracoacromial; *CC,* coracoclavicular.

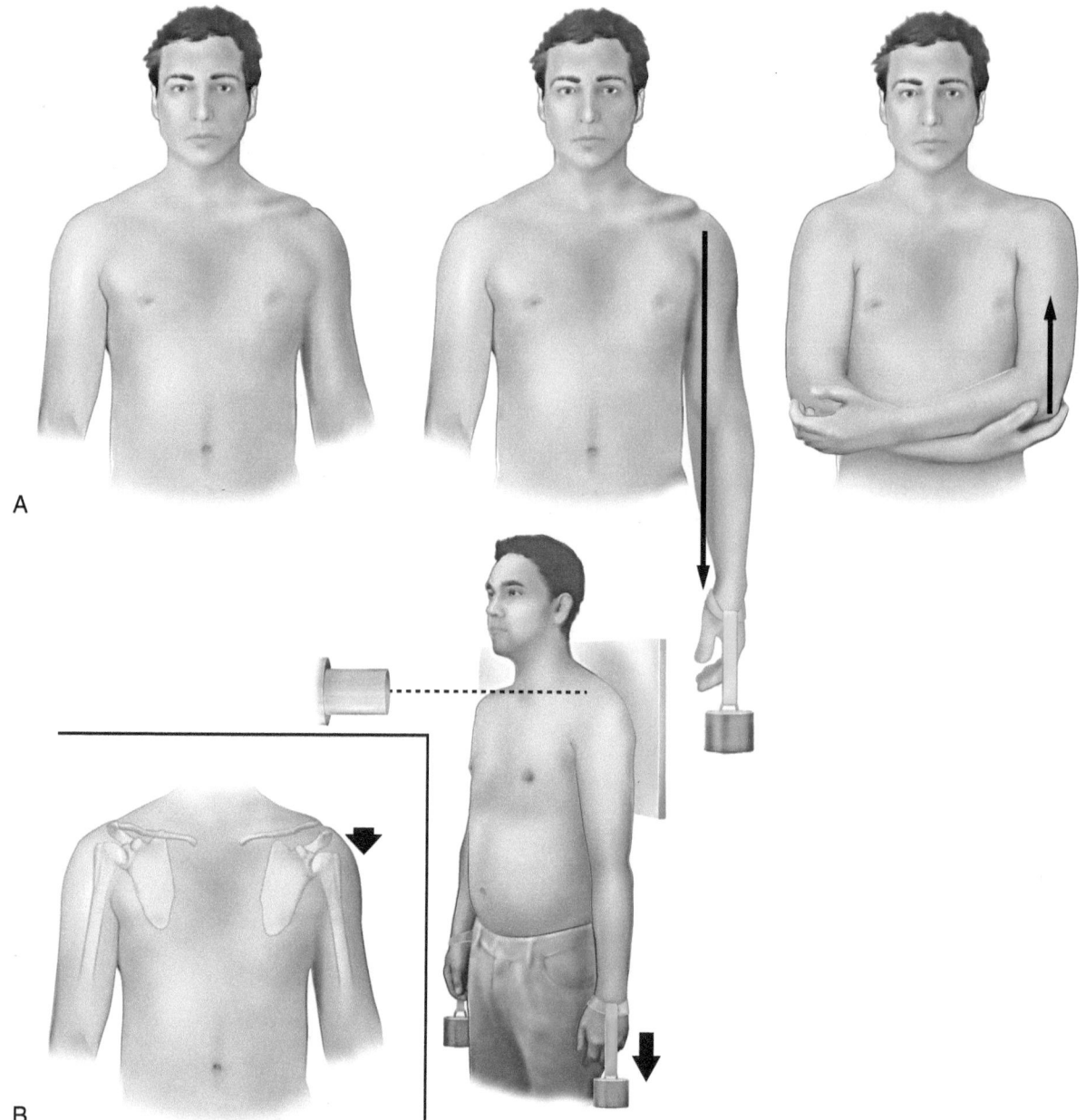

Fig. 56.9 The technique of obtaining stress radiographs of the acromioclavicular (AC) joint. (A) Anteroposterior radiographs are made of both AC joints with 10 to 15 lb of weight hanging from the wrists. (B) The distance between the superior aspect of the coracoid and the undersurface of the clavicle is measured to determine whether the coracoclavicular ligaments have been disrupted. One large horizontally positioned 14- by 17-inch x-ray cassette can be used in small patients to visualize both shoulders on the same film. In large patients, it is better to use two horizontally placed smaller cassettes and take two separate films to obtain the measurement. The arrows indicate the inferior subluxation of the scapulohumeral complex. (From Rockwood CA Jr, Williams GR Jr, Young DC. Disorders of the acromioclavicular joint. In: Rockwood CA Jr, Matsen FA III, Wirth MA, et al, eds. *The Shoulder.* 3rd ed. Philadelphia: Elsevier; 2004.)

contralateral shoulders.[18] The ISAKOS Terminology Project[15] suggested a revision to the Rockwood classification by further subdividing the type III AC joint injuries into type IIIA (stable) and type IIIB (unstable). This subclassification is primarily based upon functional rather than anatomic criteria. Type IIIA injuries are defined as those without overriding of the clavicle on the cross-body abduction radiograph and without significant

scapular dysfunction, while unstable type III injuries demonstrate therapy-resistant scapular dysfunction after 3 to 6 weeks of conservative management and overriding of the clavicle on the cross-body abduction radiograph. Unstable type III lesions (type IIIB) will continue to cause pain (usually on the anterior acromion, rotator cuff, and medial scapular area), weakness during rotator cuff testing, decreased flexion and abduction ROM, and

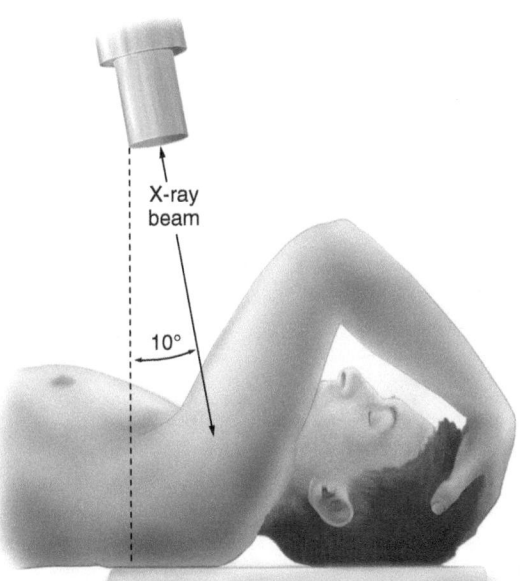

Fig. 56.10 The Stryker notch view.

demonstrable scapular dyskinesis. A basic algorithm has been proposed regarding high-level athletes with type III injuries. If the athlete is currently within his or her playing season, then consideration of an intra-articular injection of lidocaine and return to sport may be considered. If the athlete is not in the midst of his or her playing season, then he or she should undergo functional rehabilitation for up to 3 months followed by either return to full activity (if asymptomatic) or consideration of surgery (if symptomatic).[18] Evidence supporting nonoperative treatment of type III AC dislocations has been reported in a meta-analysis performed by Phillips and colleagues,[137] in which 88% of operatively treated patients and 87% of nonoperatively treated patients (a total of 1172 patients) had satisfactory outcomes. Complications included the need for further surgery (59% operative vs. 6% nonoperative), infection (6% vs. 1%), and deformity (3% vs. 37%). Pain and ROM were not significantly affected regardless of the treatment choice. Overall, based on the available evidence, the authors did not recommend surgery for type III AC joint injuries in young patients. Likewise, a more recent article reported that more than 70% of patients successfully completed nonoperative treatment for type III AC joint injury at a mean follow-up of 3.5 years with excellent outcome scores. Moreover, Petri et al.[98] also reported that patients who failed nonoperative treatment and subsequently underwent AC joint reconstruction had similar outcome scores compared with those who successfully completed nonoperative treatment after a mean follow-up of 3.3 years. These results indicate that a trial of nonoperative treatment is warranted because successful outcomes can be expected even in patients who eventually opt for surgery. However, it should be noted that patients who did not proceed to AC joint reconstruction were less likely to return to their preinjury level of sports participation, suggesting that some amount of shoulder dysfunction may be present despite promising outcome scores.

McFarland and associates[81] published the results of a survey of Major League Baseball team physicians evaluating treatment modalities for a type III injury in pitchers. Of the respondents, 69% reported that they would opt for nonoperative treatment. Of the 32 patients with type III injuries, 20 were treated nonoperatively and 12 were treated operatively. Complete pain relief and normal function was achieved in 80% of the patients treated nonoperatively and in 91% of the patients treated operatively. A recent survey of American Orthopaedic Society for Sports Medicine members indicated that 86% of respondents preferred nonoperative treatment for their patients with type III injuries.[90] In a recent consensus statement published by the International Society of Arthroscopy, Knee Surgery and Orthopaedic Sports Medicine (ISAKOS), a trial of nonoperative treatment was recommended for 3 to 6 weeks in all patients with grade III AC joint injuries. They suggested operative management if, after this period, there was persistent pain and abnormal scapular motion.[15] The decision to pursue operative management should be weighed against the high reported rate of complications (as high as 80%) with current techniques, including coracoid and clavicle fractures, hardware failure, loss of reduction, graft ruptures, and adhesive capsulitis.[85]

Treatment Options

The main goals of treatment, whether surgical or nonsurgical, are to achieve a pain-free shoulder with full ROM, strength, and no limitations in activities. The demands on the shoulder will differ from patient to patient, and these demands should be considered during the initial evaluation. As already discussed, type I and type II AC joint separations are typically treated nonoperatively, and there is merit for nonoperative management of type III injuries with the decision for surgery after an initial 3 to 6 weeks of conservative management. Patients should be evaluated as early as possible by a physiotherapist to regain as much movement and scapular control as possible, which is especially important for those presenting with type III injury. A second evaluation for type III lesions should be performed 3 to 6 weeks after injury and always completed within 3 months. The decision for surgery should be made on a case-by-case basis, considering heavy labor occupation, position/sport requirements (e.g., quarterbacks and pitchers), therapy-resistant scapulothoracic dysfunction, capacity to cooperate with postoperative protocols and risk for reinjury. The new classification of type IIIA and type IIIB lesions helps to differentiate and better identify patients who would benefit from surgical intervention. Some patients will have persistent pain and an inability to return to their sport or job after 3 to 6 weeks of conservative management.[15] Nevertheless, subsequent surgical stabilization will still allow eventual return to sport or work in such cases with reported equivalent outcome scores to those undergoing acute surgical management of type III injuries.[98]

Patients with types IV, V, and VI injuries are generally treated operatively. Some literature supports reduction of the clavicle in type IV, V, and VI injuries, turning them into a type III injury and then treating them conservatively.[92] Numerous surgical procedures for the treatment of injuries greater than type IV exist; however, none has proved to be the gold standard. Likewise,

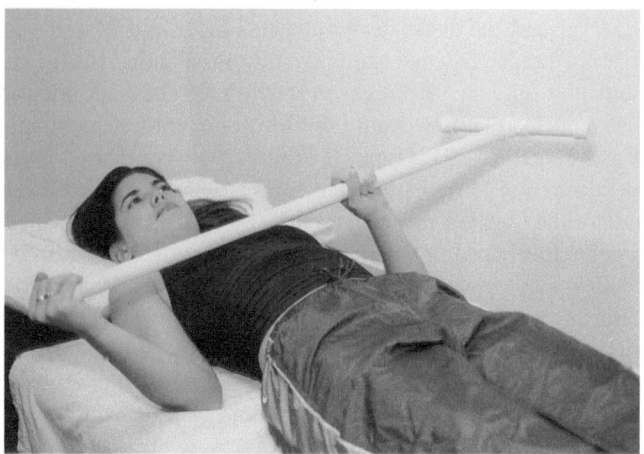

Fig. 56.11 Phase 1: Nonoperative treatment. The goal is to decrease pain, thus allowing early range of motion (ROM). Ice and some short-term immobilization. Active-assisted ROM is begun as early as possible. It is important for the patient to reach the ROM where pain begins but not go beyond this point. Avoid arm elevation in abduction, which stresses the AC joint. Isometric shoulder motions to decrease the atrophy and closed-chain scapular activities that are easily tolerated early in the postinjury period.

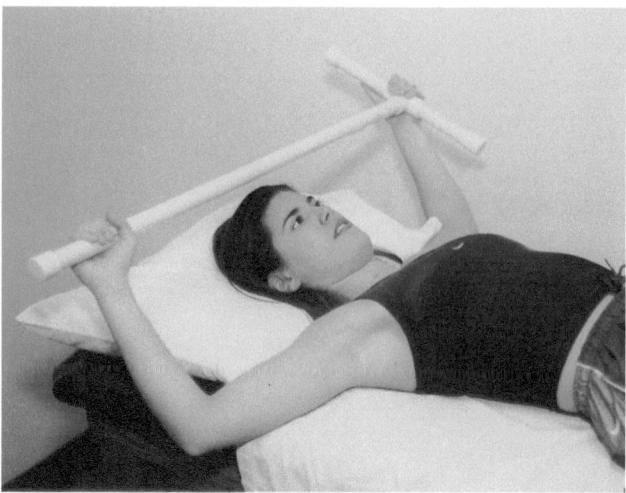

Fig. 56.12 Phase 2: The criteria to advance to phase 2 are (1) 75% of full range of motion (ROM), (2) minimal pain and tenderness on palpation of the AC joint, and (3) a manual muscle test grade of 4 out of 5 for the anterior deltoid, middle deltoid, and upper trapezius. The main goal of phase 2 is to help a patient advance to full painless ROM and increase strength in an isotonic arc through active-assisted motion exercises strengthening.

higher level studies are needed before a gold standard treatment algorithm for type III injuries can be provided.[24,114] Nevertheless, specific criteria should be used when treating AC joint dislocations surgically: (1) Biologic augmentation, namely tendon graft, should be used in the chronic situation (>3 weeks after injury), and (2) anatomic techniques for surgical reconstruction should be favored.[14]

General nonoperative treatment involves the use of a sling with ice and anti-inflammatory agents, as well as a brief period of immobilization typically lasting 3 to 7 days. The use of the sling is recommended until the pain has subsided, which typically takes 1 to 2 weeks for type I injuries and upward of 3 weeks for type II injuries. The patient is encouraged to initiate range-of-motion activities within the first week after injury to attempt reduction of pain and inflammation, and thus decrease associated morbidity.[30] Prior to return to athletic activity, a four-phase rehabilitation protocol has been described by Gladstone and colleagues.[46] Phase 1 includes pain control, sling use, immediate protective ROM, and isometric exercises. We also incorporate closed chain scapular exercises. Phase 2 involves ROM exercises to restore full mobility and a gradual progression of strengthening with the addition of isotonic exercise. Phase 3 involves unrestricted functional participation with the goal of increasing strength, power, endurance, and neuromuscular control. Finally, Phase 4 involves return to activity with sports-specific functional drills (Figs. 56.11–56.14). Full rehabilitation should be achieved within 6 to 12 weeks.

- Phase 1: The first phase of nonoperative treatment (see Fig. 56.11) is to decrease pain, thus allowing early ROM to nourish the cartilage and maintain maximal soft tissue function. Ice and some short-term immobilization can be used in this phase to decrease pain and reduce inflammation. Active-assisted ROM is begun as early as possible for shoulder internal–external rotation and elevation–depression of the arm in the plane

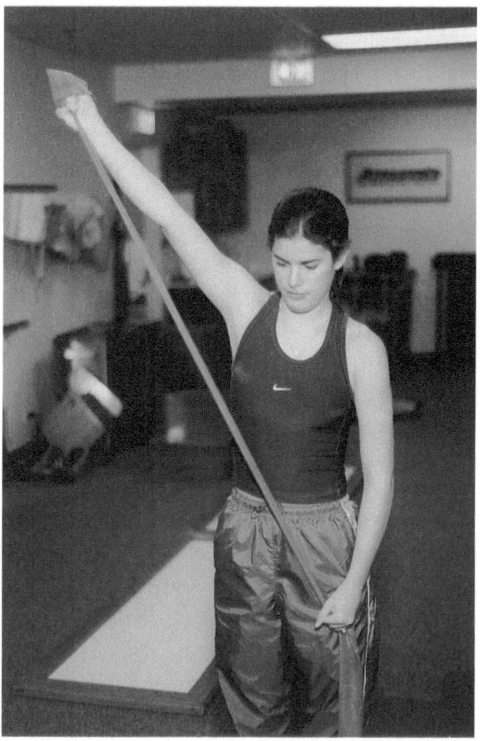

Fig. 56.13 Phase 3: The criteria for advancing from phase 2 to phase 3 are pain-free range of motion, no pain or tenderness on palpation, and strength that is 75% that of the contralateral side.[46] The main goal of phase 3 is to increase strength and endurance of the shoulder and scapula stabilizers. Specific exercises emphasized during this phase are isotonic dumbbell shoulder flexion, abduction, shrugs, and bench press.

of the scapula (30 to 45 degrees of abduction and 30 to 40 degrees of forward flexion). It is important for the patient to reach the ROM where pain begins but not go beyond this point. Arm elevation in abduction allows the clavicle to rotate upward, which stresses the AC ligament and can

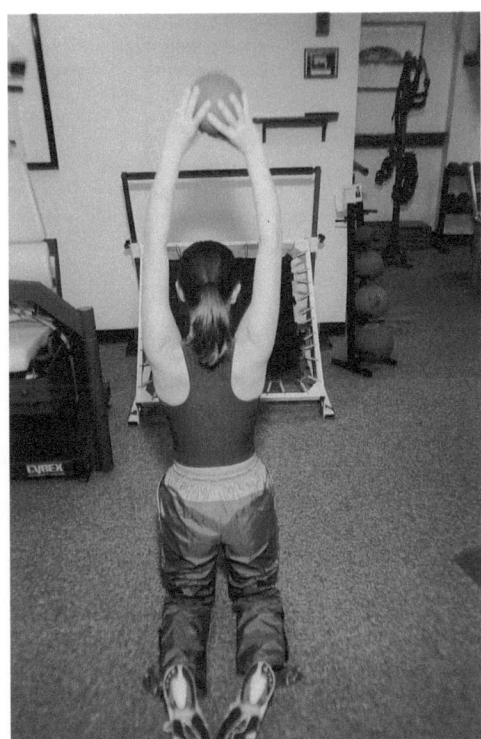

Fig. 56.14 Phase 4: The last rehabilitative stage involves sport-specific exercise and permits throwing after the patient achieves (1) full range of the motion, (2) no pain or tenderness, (3) satisfactory clinical examination, and (4) isokinetic strength approaching 100% and restored range of motion compared with the contralateral uninjured side (if available).

further increase pain and inflammation, and thus the athlete is instructed not to perform this motion. Isometric motions to decrease the atrophy of the surrounding muscular groups in the shoulder are shoulder flexion and internal and external rotation, which do not cause the clavicle to rotate. We prefer to start with closed-chain scapular activities that are easily tolerated early in the postinjury period, allowing the patient to work on scapular strength and motion without provoking undesirable increases in symptoms.[30] The patient or athlete is transitioned to the second phase when the ROM and forward elevation are relatively pain free or with minimal pain up to 140 degrees of flexion and maximal external rotation compared with the contralateral arm. The criteria to advance to phase 2 are (1) 75% of full ROM, (2) minimal pain and tenderness on palpation of the AC joint, and (3) a manual muscle test grade of 4 out of 5 for the anterior deltoid, middle deltoid, and upper trapezius.

- Phase 2: The main goal of phase 2 (see Fig. 56.12) is to help a patient advance to full painless ROM and increase strength in an isotonic arc. Active-assisted motion exercises, allowing up to full forward flexion and internal and external rotation, are performed with 90 degrees of shoulder abduction, as well as with the arm at the patient's side. Strengthening exercises are directed toward the deltoid, trapezius, and rotator cuff. Press maneuvers, such as the bench press or the military shoulder press, are limited because they increase the stress in the AC joint. The criteria for advancing from phase 2 to phase 3 are pain-free ROM, no pain or tenderness on palpation, and strength that is 75% that of the contralateral side.[46]

- Phase 3: The main goal of phase 3 (see Fig. 56.13) is to increase the strength of the entire shoulder complex musculature. Specific exercises emphasized during this phase are isotonic dumbbell shoulder flexion, abduction, shrugs, and bench press (see Fig. 56.14).

- Phase 4: Transition to phase 4, which involves sport-specific exercises, is allowed once the patient achieves (1) full range of the motion, (2) no pain or tenderness, (3) satisfactory clinical examination, and (4) isokinetic strength approaching 100% and restored ROM compared with the contralateral uninjured side (if available). These isokinetic tests are performed at 180 degrees per second and 300 degrees per second (see Fig. 56.14).

Despite the prevalence and success of nonoperative management of AC joint injuries, much of the literature has focused on surgical treatment. Operative treatment of types IV, V, and VI is generally recommended because of morbidity associated with persistent marked displacement of the distal clavicle, although good results with conservative management have been reported.[46] A closed reduction maneuver should be attempted because these types of dislocations can sometimes be reduced into a position that mimics a type III injury, then treated nonoperatively.

The literature is replete with surgical techniques to address complete AC dislocations, with more than 75 different techniques described in various reports. Most techniques are based on several basic types of procedures, including (1) primary AC joint fixation with pins, screws, or rods; (2) coracoacromial ligament transfer (Weaver-Dunn) ± distal clavicle excision; (3) anatomic CC reconstruction; and (4) arthroscopic suture fixation. Nearly all the recently reported "novel" techniques involve combinations of the basic techniques, modifications of these techniques, and/or modifications of the modifications.[18]

In addition to primary repair, these procedures can include reconstruction augmentation with autogenous tissue (coracoacromial ligament), augmentation with absorbable and nonabsorbable suture and prosthetic material, and CC stabilization with metallic screws.[1,7,70,87,113,123,126,128,129] The Weaver–Dunn technique using transfer of the coracoacromial ligament has been the most popular procedure in acute and chronic injuries.[128] Several more recent reports have described good results with modifications of this technique.[69,123,129] However, compromised results have been observed in patients after Weaver-Dunn-based procedures with residual subluxation or dislocation after surgery.[123,129] Ammon and associates[3] performed a biomechanical study comparing the Bosworth screw with a poly-L-lactic acid bioabsorbable screw and found that the Bosworth screw provided superior strength (native ligament, 340 N; poly-L-lactic acid screw, 272 N; and Bosworth screw, 367 N).

From a biomechanical perspective, the importance of the CC ligaments and AC ligaments in controlling superior and horizontal translations has been elucidated.[41,62,68] In fact, failure to surgically reproduce the conoid, trapezoid, and AC ligament function with current techniques may explain the observed incidence of recurrent instability and pain.[62,68] Several authors have advocated using a separate and potentially more robust graft

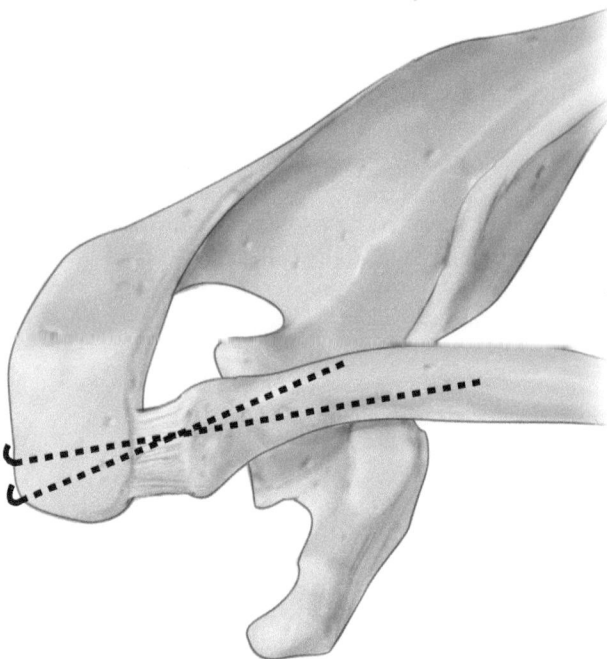

Fig. 56.15 Acromioclavicular ligament repair. The acromioclavicular joint is fixed internally with two unthreaded Kirschner wires. The wires are generally removed about 8 weeks after surgery. (From Justis EJ Jr. Traumatic disorders. In: Canale ST, ed. *Campbell's Operative Orthopedics.* Vol 3. 7th ed. St Louis: Mosby; 1987.)

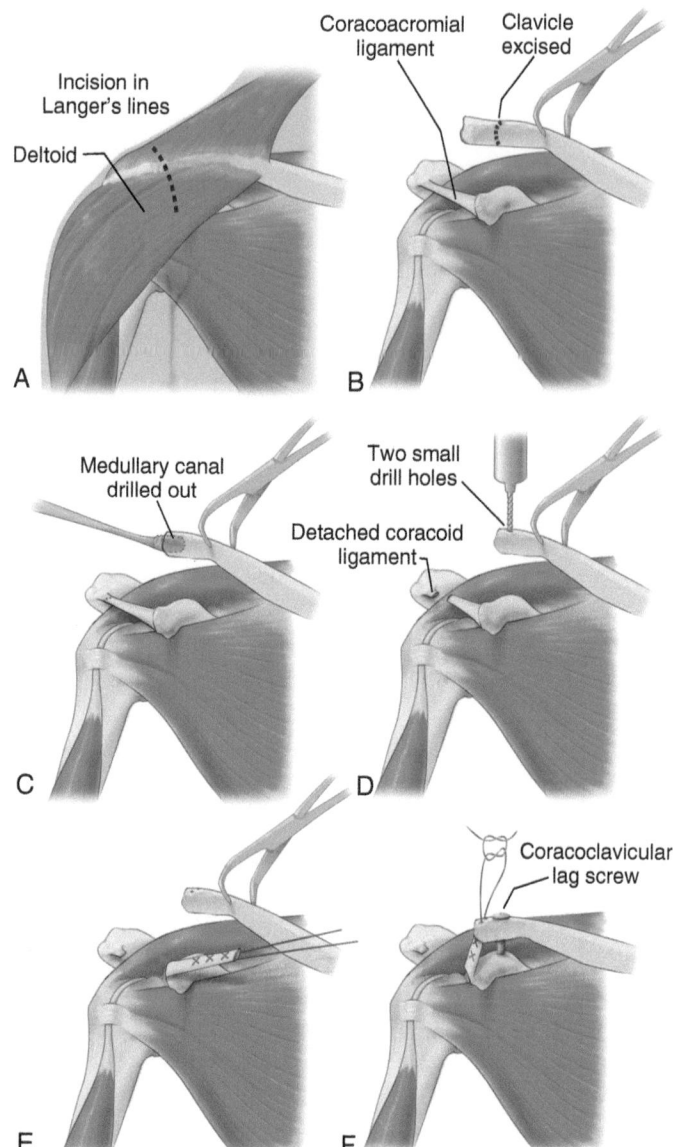

Fig. 56.16 Dr. Charles Rockwood's method of reconstructing a chronic type III, IV, V, or VI acromioclavicular dislocation. (A) The incision is made in Langer's lines. (B) The distal end of the clavicle is excised. (C) The medullary canal is drilled out and curetted to receive the transferred coracoacromial ligament. (D) Two small drill holes are made through the superior cortex of the distal clavicle. The coracoacromial ligament is carefully detached from the acromion process. (E) With the coracoacromial ligament detached from the acromion, a heavy nonabsorbable suture is woven through the ligament. (F) The ends of the suture are passed out through the two small drill holes in the distal end of the clavicle. The coracoclavicular lag screw is inserted, and when the clavicle is reduced to its normal position, the sutures used to pull the ligament snugly up into the canal are tied. (From Rockwood CA Jr, Williams GR Jr, Young DC. Disorders of the acromioclavicular joint. In: Rockwood CA Jr, Matsen FA III, Wirth MA, et al, eds. *The Shoulder.* 3rd ed. Philadelphia: Elsevier; 2004.)

source to improve surgical results.[71] The use of a free autogenous or allograft tendon has been further supported biomechanically.[70] Other reconstruction grafts, such as the lateral half of the conjoined tendon,[113] have also been described. Anatomic reconstruction of the CC ligaments has been shown to be biomechanically superior when compared with previous surgical constructs.[29] Other types of fixation have been biomechanically evaluated, including interference screw fixation, suture cerclage, and suture anchors.[35] Although none of these techniques fully restored native AC joint stability, they were all found to be superior to the Weaver-Dunn procedure.[11,18,29,35,62,78,87] Thus given the biomechanical limitations of CA ligament transfer, newer techniques involve augmentation with CC ligament reconstruction using tendon grafts, suture anchors, screws, or suture loops.

The major surgical options for AC joint reconstruction are included in the following summary:

- Primary AC joint repair involves primary repair of the AC ligament with reinforcement of the superior AC ligament with joint meniscus. The repair is typically augmented with smooth or threaded pins, screws, suture wires, or plates (e.g., an AC joint plate or hook plate). This technique features limited surgical dissection; however, it places the patient at risk for pin migration (Fig. 56.15).
- Coracoacromial ligament transfer (Weaver-Dunn) with or without distal clavicle excision involves transfer of the coracoacromial ligament from the acromion to the clavicle as a substitute for the ruptured CC ligament with or without distal clavicle excision (Fig. 56.16).
- Debate exists regarding distal clavicle excision:

- If the patient's condition is very acute, if AC joint arthrosis is minimal, and/or if stability is of paramount concern, one may consider keeping the distal clavicle, especially because recent biomechanic evidence has suggested increases in horizontal translation with sequential resection.[13]

- If the patient has a chronic injury or preexisting AC joint arthrosis, consideration of excision can be made.
- Modification to the Weaver-Dunn procedure includes transfer of the conjoined tendon to the distal clavicle, augmentation with a suture loop, and augmentation with a semitendinosus autograft or anterior tibialis allograft via a bone tunnel and interference screw fixation.
- Anatomic CC reconstruction involves arthroscopy, distal clavicle excision, and reconstruction with an autograft or allograft. Biomechanically,[78] this technique has been shown to better reapproximate the stiffness of the native CC ligament complex and improve anterior and posterior translation

restriction compared with the Weaver-Dunn procedure, and is described in detail in the Authors' Preferred Technique section.[16,22]
- Arthroscopic suture fixation involves restoration of the CC ligaments arthroscopically using two suture anchors through four drill holes in the clavicle with an associated CC ligament transfer. The suture anchors are thus fixed to the coracoid as the suture is tied over a bone bridge to the clavicle. Similarly, tightrope devices have been used as well, and this technique is also arthroscopic, involving two single tunnels through the clavicle and coracoid through which to feed the tightrope device.

🏃 Authors' Preferred Technique

Anatomic Coracoclavicular Reconstruction (See Video Supplementation)

Exposure
- A curvilinear center incision is placed approximately 3.5 cm from the distal clavicle or AC joint, along Langer's lines toward the coracoid process (Figs. 56.17 and 56.18).
- Control of superficial skin bleeders down to the fascia of the deltoid is accomplished with a needle-tip bovie.
- Once the entire clavicle is palpated, full-thickness flaps are made. Care must be taken to avoid button-holes when creating skin flaps due to poor wound healing potential.
- Care is then taken to remove the deltoid off the clavicle both anteroinferiorly and posterosuperiorly
- Soft-tissue attachments along the medial coracoid are carefully released to allow for later graft passage.
- We do not perform a distal clavicle resection to prevent destabilization of the AC joint.[13]

Graft Preparation
- Selection depends on the surgeon's preference. We prefer peroneus longus allograft fresh-frozen tendon (5 mm) or semitendinosus autograft whip-stitched with no. 2 FiberWire sutures (Arthrex Inc.) in a baseball-type fashion at both

distal tails of the graft (2 to 2.5 cm). An ideal graft models a bullet, where the distal diameter is narrower than the than the proximal diameter. This is accomplished by adding additional stitches to the distal tip of the graft to tabularize (Fig. 56.19).
- The diameter of the graft is measured with a standard tendon-measuring device or using the handle of a repair system (Biotenodesis System, Arthrex Inc.) to determine the graft size (see Fig. 56.19).
- The graft is placed on the table in a moist sponge until the bone tunnels are prepared.

Coracoid Preparation
- The coracoid is carefully dissected making sure to release all soft-tissue attachments laterally and medially all the way to the base.

Clavicle Bone Tunnel Placement
- The AC joint is anatomically repositioned, and bone tunnels are created in the clavicle. It is critical that the bone tunnels are placed anatomically to

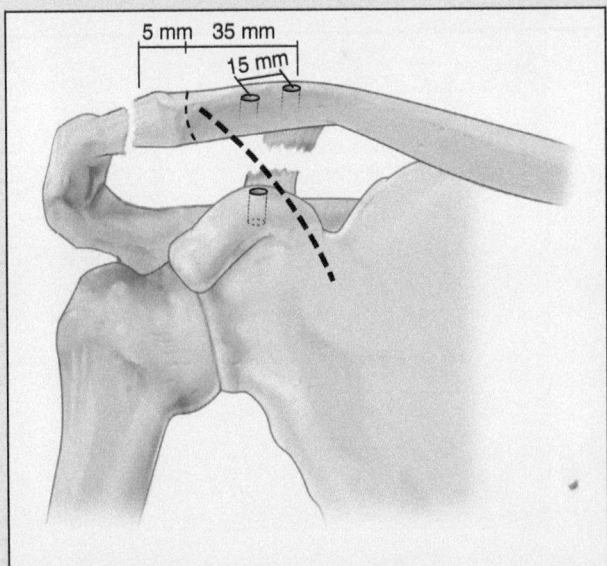

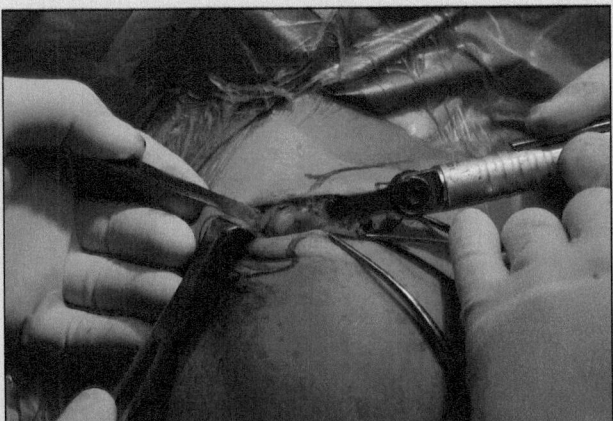

Fig. 56.17 Initial exposure for access to the acromioclavicular joint. The skin incision is made in line with Langer's lines, from anterior to posterior. Once the deltotrapezial fascia is encountered, this layer is incised sharply over the midline to develop full-thickness fascial flaps in a medial to lateral direction. Repair of this layer during closure is an important aspect of the case.

Fig. 56.18 Distances for the distal clavicle excision and bone tunnels are shown. The conoid bone tunnel should start about 45 mm from the acromioclavicular joint, in the posterior one-third of the clavicle. The trapezoid bone tunnel should be positioned 15 mm anteromedial to the conoid bone tunnel.

Continued

Authors' Preferred Technique

Anatomic Coracoclavicular Reconstruction (See Video Supplementation)—cont'd

recreate the CC ligament (Fig. 56.20); these tunnels should be separated by a minimum of 20 mm.

- The first tunnel for the conoid ligament (medial limb). Measuring approximately 45 mm medial from the lateral edge of the distal clavicle and localized to the posterior half of the clavicle, the conoid tunnel is made in a superior-to-inferior direction. The footprint of the conoid ligament is extremely posterior, along the posterior edge of the clavicle, which is why making this bone tunnel as posterior as possible (i.e., in the posterior half of the clavicle) is extremely important.
- The second tunnel is for the trapezoid ligament. This is placed centrally within the clavicle approximately 25 mm from its lateral edge due to the better bone mineral density within the anatomic insertion area of the CC ligaments (between 20 and 50 mm from the lateral end of the clavicle). Low bone mineral density has been shown to correlate with decreased load to failure, so care must be taken not to drill a tunnel too lateral in the clavicle.[43]
- A cannulated reamer guide pin is used for placement of the tunnels. Two guide pins are used before reaming to confirm accurate placement of the tunnels.
- For the conoid ligament tunnel, the guide pin is angled about 45 degrees from the direct perpendicular of the clavicle to re-create the oblique nature of the ligament.

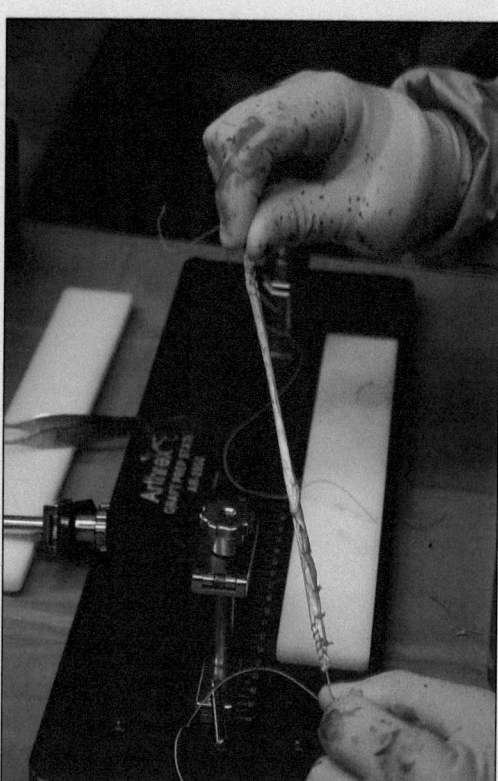

Fig. 56.19 Graft preparation. Here a tibialis anterior allograft is used, and the two ends of the tendon are stitched in Krakow fashion using no. 2 FiberWire (Arthrex Inc.). The graft is then doubled over and measured using graft sizers from the Biotenodesis System (Arthrex Inc.). The doubled-over graft size is usually 6 to 7 mm. If larger, the graft should be trimmed (especially in an allograft situation). The graft is then placed under tension on the back table in preparation for implantation.

- For the trapezoid ligament tunnel, which is a more anterior and lateral structure than the conoid, the guide pin is drilled in the center point of the clavicle, about 25 mm medial to the AC joint.
- A 5-mm reamer is used to create each tunnel with careful attention to confirm that the conoid tunnel is as posterior as possible in the clavicle without "blowing out" the posterior cortical rim (Fig. 56.21). A 5.5-mm tap is then used.
- After tunnel reaming, copious irrigation follows to remove any bone fragments.

Graft Passage Around Coracoid

- The tendon graft is looped around the base of the coracoid process, which can be facilitated with the use of a curved aortic cross-clamp (Satinsky clamp) and a suture-passing device. While the graft is passed, a no. 2 FiberWire or FiberTape (Arthrex Inc.) is also passed around the base of the coracoid, which will serve as a nonbiologic fixation reinforcement and help reduce the clavicle to the scapula (Fig. 56.22).

Interference Screw Fixation of Graft to Clavicle

- The tendon graft limb exiting the conoid tunnel is first fixed using a bioabsorbable or inert (polyetheretherketone [PEEK]) interference screw. We use 5.5 mm diameter screws of 3 different lengths depending on clavicle thickness (5.5 × 8 mm, 5.5 × 10 mm, 5.5 × 12 mm).
- The opposite graft limb exiting the trapezoid tunnel is cyclically tensioned to remove all slack from the system, and a similarly sized screw is subsequently placed into the trapezoid ligament tunnel to fix this end of the graft.
- One limb of the biologic graft is taken and placed through the posterior bone tunnel, recreating the conoid ligament (Fig. 56.23). The other limb is passed through the anterior bone tunnel, recreating the trapezoid ligament.
- While the graft is brought through the tunnel (Fig. 56.24), a no. 2 high-strength suture is also brought through the respective bone tunnels (Fig. 56.25).
- For reduction purposes, superiorly directed displacement of the scapulohumeral complex by the assistant reduces the AC joint. Likewise, large point-of-reduction forceps placed on the coracoid process and the clavicle can further help with reduction while securing the tendon grafts.
- With the AC joint anatomically reduced and with the tendon graft sufficiently taut, a 5.5 mm PEEK interference screw is placed in either the posterior or the midline bone tunnel.
- A no. 2 high-strength suture or FiberTape (Arthrex Inc.) is brought up through this cannulated screw hole, and the second PEEK interference screw is placed in the remaining bone tunnel.
- With both grafts secured using interference screw fixation, the no. 2 suture or FiberTape (Arthrex Inc.) is tied over the top of the clavicle, becoming a nonbiologic fixation for the overreduced AC joint (Figs. 56.26 and 56.27).

Acromioclavicular Ligament Reconstruction (Fig. 56.28)

- The remaining lateral trapezoid graft limb is looped over the top of the AC joint to reinforce the repair and reconstruct the AC joint capsule.
- High-strength nonabsorbable sutures are used to suture the graft limb into the most posterior tissue on the acromial side of the joint.
- The remaining graft is shuttled underneath the AC joint from posterior to anterior and again sutured to the acromial side of the joint and itself.
- Finally, the superior AC capsule is sutured.
- This technique, which involves direct wrapping and suturing of the remaining graft around the AC joint, has been demonstrated to be biomechanically superior to other methods of AC ligament reconstruction and most closely restore native joint biomechanics.[16]
- Alternatively, the remaining graft limbs may be incorporated into the soft-tissue deltoid and trapezial repair to the clavicle.

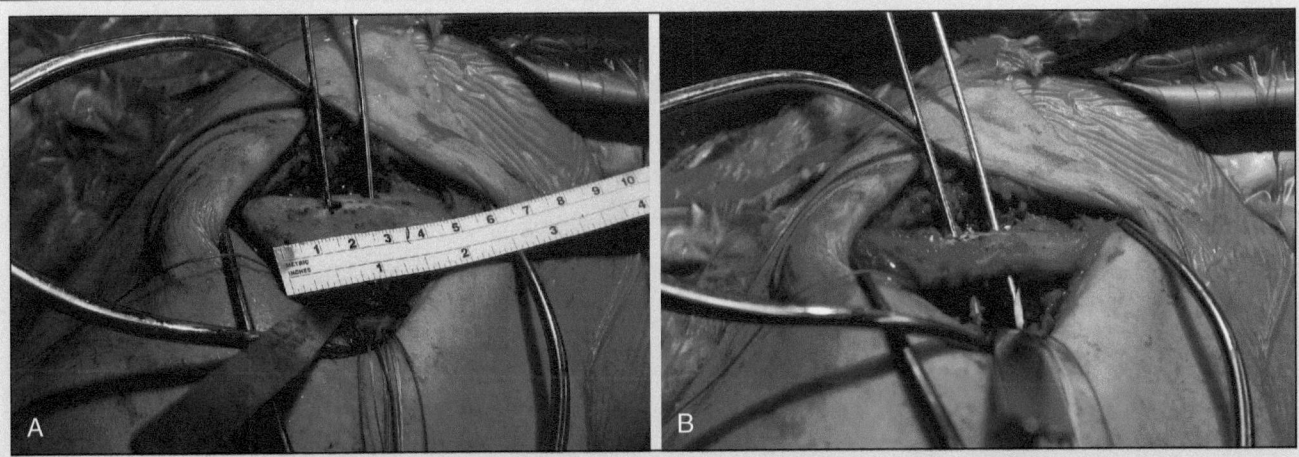

Fig. 56.20 The guide pins are placed into the distal clavicle at points that approximate the attachment sites of the conoid and trapezoid ligaments. The conoid ligament attaches more posteriorly and more medially than the trapezoid ligament. The first tunnel, which is for the conoid process and is extremely posterior, is roughly 45 mm away from the distal end of the clavicle, along the entire posterior edge of the clavicle (A). The guide pin is also angled about 45 degrees from the direct perpendicular of the clavicle to re-create the oblique nature of the ligament. A 6- or 7-mm reamer is used to create the tunnel with careful attention to confirm that the tunnel is as posterior as possible in the clavicle without "blowing out" the posterior cortical rim. Once this position is confirmed, a 15- to 16-mm bone tunnel is created. The same procedure is repeated for the trapezoid ligament, which is a more anterior structure than the conoid and is usually placed in the center point of the clavicle, about 15 mm away from the center portion of the previous tunnel. Two guide pins are used before reaming to confirm accurate placement of the tunnels (B).

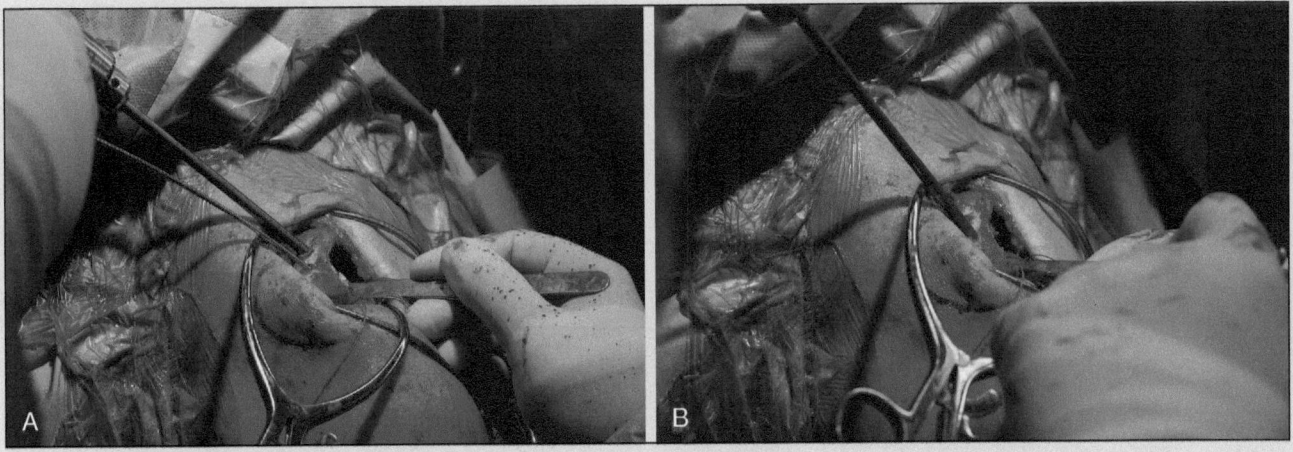

Fig. 56.21 After tunnel reaming of the conoid (A) and trapezoid (B) tunnels, copious irrigation is performed to remove any bone fragments.

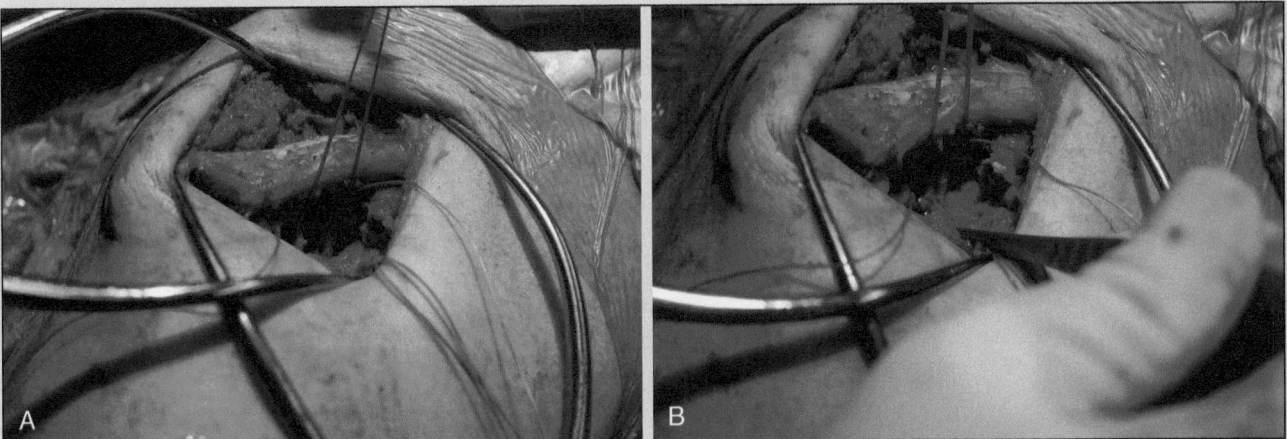

Fig. 56.22 Coracoid graft fixation with soft tissue passed under the coracoid. Suture may be passed around the coracoid (A) and used to shuttle the soft tissue graft under the coracoid. At the same time, a high-strength no. 2 suture (FiberWire or FiberTape, Arthrex Inc.) is used for nonbiologic fixation and left in place once the graft is shuttled underneath the coracoid (B).

Continued

Authors' Preferred Technique

Anatomic Coracoclavicular Reconstruction (See Video Supplementation)—cont'd

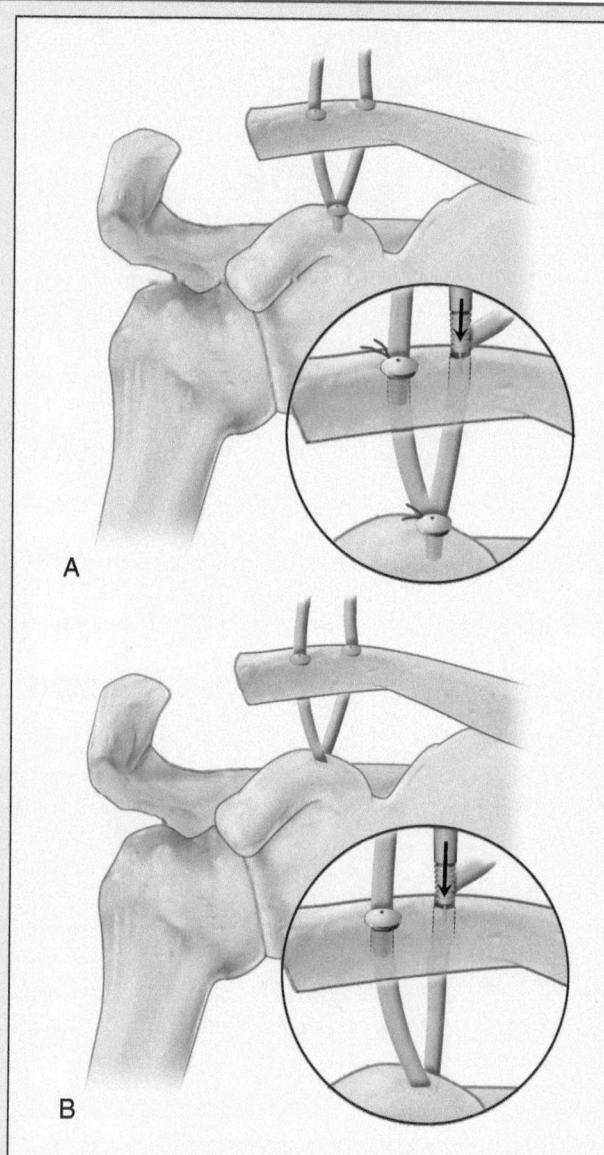

A

B

Fig. 56.23 (A) Fixation of the conoid and trapezoid graft limbs to the reduced clavicle using Biotenodesis screw (Arthrex Inc.) fixation. One limb of the biologic graft is taken and placed through the posterior bone tunnel, re-creating the conoid ligament. The other limb is passed through the anterior bone tunnel, recreating the trapezoid ligament. (B) As an alternative to a screw in the coracoid, we prefer that the graft be placed under the base of the coracoid.

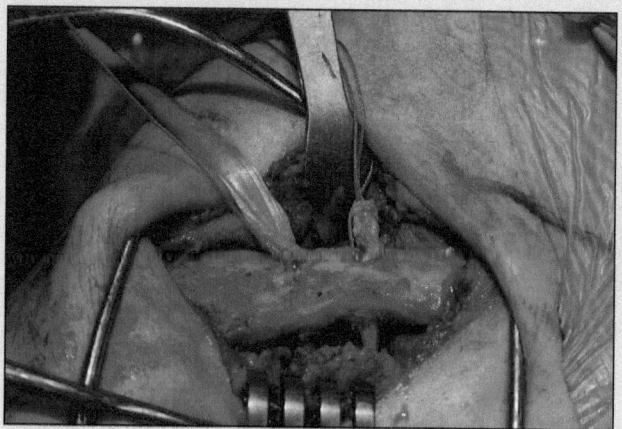

Fig. 56.24 A limb of no. 2 FiberWire (Arthrex Inc.) is also brought out each of the respective bone tunnels with the soft tissue graft. For reduction purposes, superiorly directed displacement of the scapulo-humeral complex by the assistant reduces the acromioclavicular (AC) joint. Likewise, large point-of-reduction forceps placed on the coracoid process and the clavicle can further help with reduction while securing the tendon grafts. With the AC joint anatomically reduced and with the tendon graft sufficiently taut, a 5.5 mm polyetheretherketone (PEEK) interference screw is placed in either the posterior or midline bone tunnel. A no. 2 high-strength suture or FiberTape (Arthrex Inc.) is brought up through this cannulated screw hole, and the second PEEK interference screw is placed in the remaining bone tunnel.

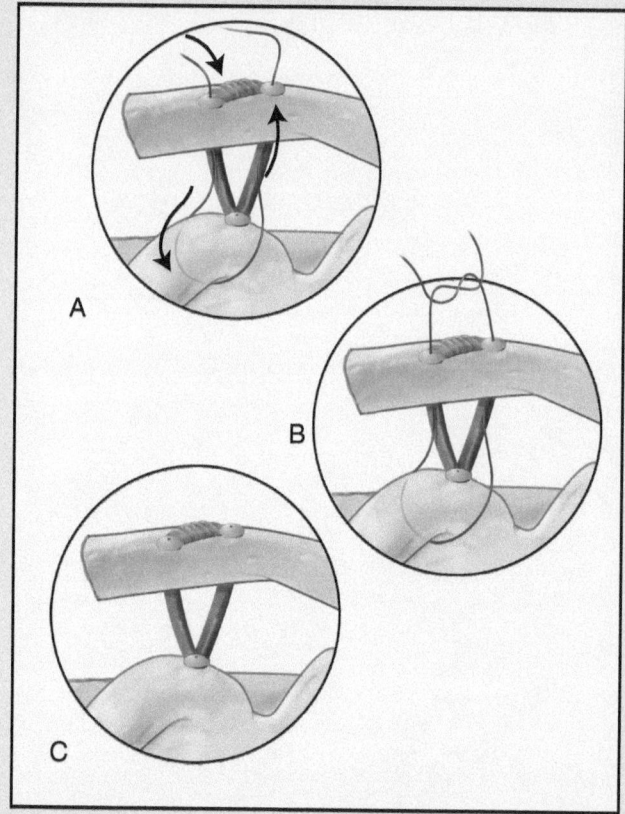

A

B

C

Fig. 56.25 (A and B) With both grafts secured using interference screw fixation, the no. 2 FiberWire (Arthrex Inc.) is tied over the top of the clavicle, becoming a nonbiologic fixation for the overreduced acromioclavicular joint. (C) Alternatively, we prefer that only the graft be used under the coracoid.

🔖 Authors' Preferred Technique

Anatomic Coracoclavicular Reconstruction (See Video Supplementation)—cont'd

Closure

- One of the most important concepts with AC or CC joint reconstruction is closure of the deltotrapezial fascial flaps from the dissection.
- A nonabsorbable suture, in a modified Mason-Allen-type fashion, is placed through the deltoid fascia. Six or seven sutures are used, and the knots are tied on the posterior aspect of the trapezius.
- This closure of the deltotrapezial fascia should completely obscure the grafts, as well as the clavicle.
- If any concern exists regarding the fascial repair, the deltoid can be repaired through small drill holes in the anterior cortex of the clavicle.
- The subdermal skin is closed with 2-0 or 3-0 absorbable sutures, and the skin itself is closed with either a 2-0 running or interrupted nylon suture, everting the skin edges.
- A compression dressing is applied, and the patient is placed in a supportive sling with external rotation to 0 degrees and an upward force on the arm.

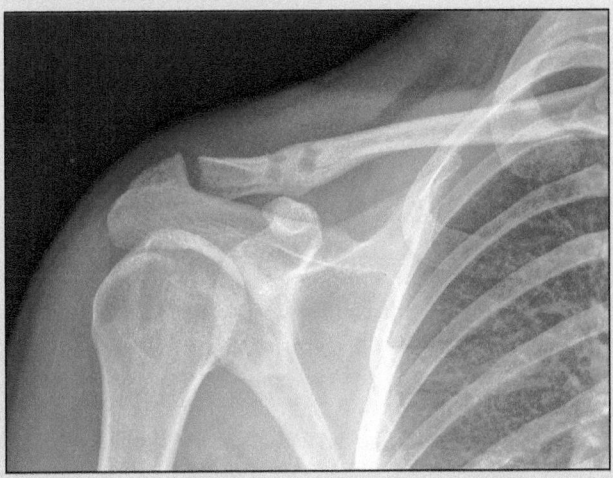

Fig. 56.27 A final anteroposterior radiograph demonstrating reduction of the acromioclavicular joint with the two 5.5-mm clavicular tunnels.

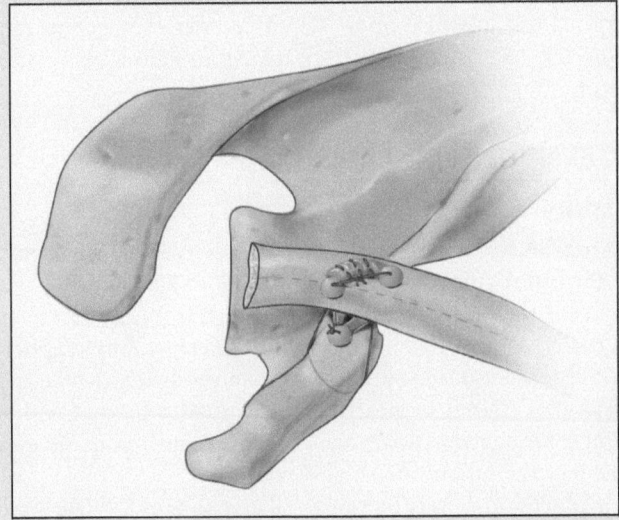

Fig. 56.26 The final view of the anatomic coracoclavicular ligament reconstruction. Note the position of the clavicular bone tunnels in relation to the center line of the clavicle and the interference screw fixation backed up with a nonbiologic no. 2 FiberWire (Arthrex Inc.) suture through the cannulated holes of the interference screws.

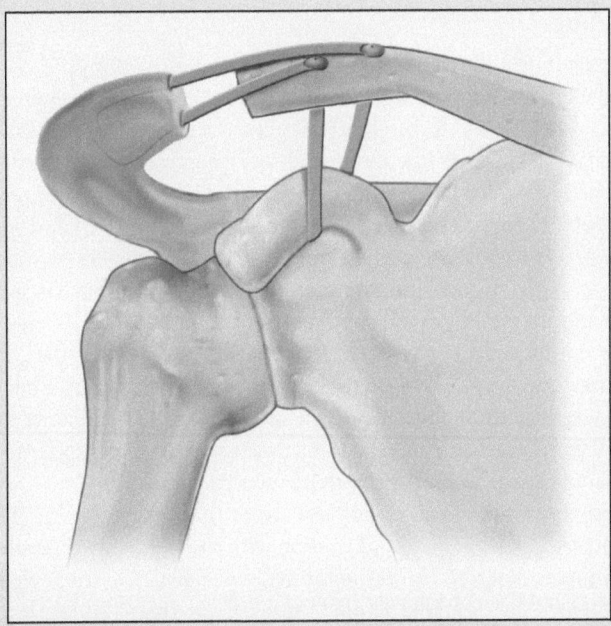

Fig. 56.28 A graft limb (usually the lateral trapezoid limb) may be brought out to the acromion to reconstruct the acromioclavicular joint capsule. This graft limb may be fed into the end of the acromion that articulates with the clavicle and then may exit out the top and return to the clavicle. Significantly less anterior, posterior, and superior translation has been reported with this acromial limb graft technique, which reportedly better reproduces the native joint.[16]

Postoperative Management/Return to Play

Postoperative management after AC joint stabilization depends on the procedure performed. If the procedure includes only a distal clavicle resection, then a short (1- to 3-day) period of immobilization is followed by ROM activities. Strengthening begins at 4 to 6 weeks postoperatively, and return to sports or weight training can begin at 3 months. Of note, power athletes often require 6 to 12 months to return to peak strength.

If the procedure includes CC ligament reconstruction, the operative arm is immediately immobilized in a sling and brace. Gentle ROM activities in the supine position can begin after 7 to 10 days; however, motion exercises with the arm unsupported in an upright position should be delayed until the reconstruction has had time to develop early biologic stability. For an acute repair, this process typically involves 4 to 6 weeks and the brace (e.g., a gunslinger or Lehrman brace) is worn for this duration. For a chronic repair with severe soft tissue involvement; however, achieving stability may take up to 6 to 12 weeks. Patients may begin ROM exercises 6 weeks after surgery. At 12 weeks, strengthening exercises can begin with an emphasis on scapular stabilizers. These muscles decrease the load on the joint by keeping the scapula in a relatively retracted position. After the initiation of strength training, weight training can typically commence at 3 to 4.5 months after surgery. This process is again delayed in chronic cases.

Athletes should be prohibited from returning to contact sports until at least 6 months after undergoing surgery. Before this, the therapist should work with the athlete on sport-specific training exercises and ensure that Cybex upper extremity power testing is within 10% to 15% of the contralateral normal limb. Power athletes and persons whose work entails heavy physical demands take the longest to rehabilitate. Generally, 9 to 12 months are required in these patients to reach peak strength, especially with pressing activities or lifting from the floor (i.e., dead lift).

Results

As previously described, most authors agree on nonoperative management for type I and II injuries and operative management for type IV through VI injuries. Treatment for persons with type III injuries has traditionally been controversial; however, increasing evidence for nonoperative management has gained support. The new classification of type IIIA and type IIIB lesions helps to differentiate and better identify patients who would benefit from surgical intervention. Some patients will have persistent pain and an inability to return to their sport or job after a recommended 3 to 6 weeks of conservative management, thereby warranting surgical intervention.[16] Nevertheless, subsequent delayed surgical stabilization will still allow return to sport or work with reported equivalent outcome scores to those undergoing acute surgical management of type III injuries.[98]

Furthermore, no gold standard currently exists regarding the most appropriate method of fixation with more than 75 different techniques described in the literature. In a 2010 Cochrane review performed by Tamaoki et al.,[120] three trials (two randomized and one quasi-randomized) compared nonoperative and operative treatment of AC dislocation injuries with no significant differences reported regarding functional outcomes or treatment failure eventually requiring surgery. Interpretation of outcomes in the literature can be difficult given the lack of high-level comparative studies.[24,114,120]

A sample of outcomes reported in the literature is included in Table 56.4. It is important to understand that this table contains a subset of the published data and is certainly not comprehensive. Perhaps some of the more important takeaway points from the data include the observation that patients with type III injuries have similar outcomes when comparing operative and nonoperative treatments (depending on the patient population) and that, although anatomic CC reconstruction is biomechanically superior to modified Weaver-Dunn repair techniques, more substantial clinical outcomes data are required before conclusive recommendations can be made.

Complications

Complications after nonoperative treatment of AC joint injuries include the development of late arthrosis, persistent instability, and even distal clavicle osteolysis. Operative complications typically depend on the procedure. Hardware migration and/or failure is a well-described complication that can have devastating consequences, including migration into the lung, spinal canal, and other adjacent core structures. For this reason, the use of smooth pins has essentially been abandoned. Pin migration into the lung, spinal canal, and subclavian artery, as well as posterior to the carotid sheath, has been reported.[73,77,91,111] Another reported complication includes loss of reduction and recurrent instability, which is most often related to noncompliance with immobilization and rehabilitation protocols in younger patients.

Other surgical complications[106] include clavicle fracture either after repeat injury or resulting from stress risers secondary to drilled graft tunnels; infection, aseptic reaction to the reconstruction, calcifications, erosion through the clavicle from nonabsorbable materials used to augment the repair and reconstruction, fracture of the coracoid, osteolysis,[21,101,106] and persistent pain or loss of motion. Reported rates of infection range from 0% to 9% (average, 6%), taking numerous reports into account.[48,54,55,130]

STERNOCLAVICULAR JOINT

History

As previously described for AC joint injuries, the key element of the history for a patient presenting with a potential SC joint injury is the mechanism of injury, which is most often related to direct trauma. Given the significant ligamentous support of the SC joint, it is one of the joints of the body that is least often dislocated. Therefore nearly all patients who present with SC joint injuries report a history of a significant traumatic event. The most common causes of SC injury are motor vehicle collisions followed closely by sports-related injuries.[89,93] During the traumatic event, it is often indirect trauma that ultimately results in the SC joint disruption.[83] Specifically, a force is applied through the SC joint from the anterolateral or posterolateral aspects of the shoulder, resulting in either anterior or posterior displacement of the SC joint. In the event of direct trauma to the SC joint itself, a force is typically applied directly to the anteromedial aspect of the clavicle, causing it to migrate posteriorly behind the sternum. Nearly all SC joint dislocations resulting from direct trauma result in posterior displacement because anatomic constraints prevent an anterior displacement from direct force.[51]

Physical Examination

Several physical examination techniques can be used to help identify and isolate SC joint disease. The complete examination must include inspection, palpation, ROM, strength, sensation, and stabilization assessments of both shoulders. After this, special tests specific to the AC and SC joints can be performed. The clinician should be aware and appropriately assess any suspected cervical spine and/or glenohumeral joint pathologic conditions that, if present, may confuse the clinical picture. Similarly, other

TABLE 56.4   Clinical Outcomes Following Nonsurgical and Surgical Management of Acromioclavicular Joint Injuries

Study	Injury Type	No. of Patients	Average Follow-Up	Treatment	Outcome
Larsen et al.[69]	Type III	41 Surgical 43 Nonsurgical	13 months	Surgical with AC joint fixation	Surgical: 97% good-excellent Nonsurgical: 98% good-excellent
Taft et al.[136]	Type III	63 Surgical 52 Nonsurgical	9.5 years	Surgical with CC screw or AC joint fixation	Surgical: 94% good-excellent Nonsurgical: 91% good-excellent
Bannister et al.[6]	Type III[a]	27 Surgical 33 Nonsurgical	4 years	Surgical with CC screw	Surgical: 78% good-excellent Nonsurgical: 88% good-excellent
Weinstein et al.[129]	Type III	44 (27 acute, 17 chronic [>3 weeks])	4 years	CC fixation with heavy nonabsorbable sutures in all; CA transfer in 15/27 acute repairs; CA transfer in 17/17 chronic repairs	Overall 89% satisfactory results; trend toward better results with earlier repairs; overall 20% loss of reduction
Phillips et al.[137]	Type III	602 Surgical 231 Nonsurgical	Meta-analysis	Multiple methods of surgical fixation	Surgical: 88% satisfactory outcome Nonoperative: 87% satisfactory outcome Complications (surgical vs. nonsurgical): need for further surgery (59% vs. 6%), infection (6% vs. 1%), deformity (3% vs. 37%) Conclusions: The authors did not recommend surgery for type III AC injuries
Mouhsine et al.[88]	Type I/II	17 Type I 16 Type II	6.3 years	Nonoperative	27% required surgery at an average of 26 months after injury; 52% remained asymptomatic
Nicholas et al.[138]	Type V	9	Minimum 1 year (range 1–4)	CC reconstruction using semitendinosus allograft	No strength deficits ASES: 96 SST: 11.6 Overall satisfaction: 89% No loss of reduction radiographically
Mikek[84]	Type I/II	23	10.2 years	Nonoperative	Minor symptoms in 52%; none had major symptoms
Gstettner et al.[139]	Type III	24 Surgical 17 Nonsurgical	34 months	AC joint fixation: HP surgical fixation	Constant score: 80.7 (nonoperative) vs. 90.4 (operative) Mean CC distance: 19.9 mm (nonoperative) vs. 12.1 mm (operative) Failure with HP eroding through the acromion noted at 32 days after surgery
Tomlinson et al.[140]	High grade	10	5 months (minimum, 3)	Arthroscopically assisted subacromial approach passing suture material and tendon graft around the coracoid	100% subjective improvement in pain and function
Murena et al.[141]	Type III–V	16	31 months	Arthroscopic CC double-flip button	Constant score: 97; 25% with radiographic loss of reduction because of distal migration of the flip button
Shin et al.[142]	Type V	29	28 months	CC reconstruction using two 3.5-mm double-loaded suture anchors with two clavicular drill holes with sutures tied over the clavicle, all with CA ligament transfer	Constant score: 97 Return to activities at 3 months 24/29 had anatomic reduction on radiographs
Huang et al.[143]	Complete CC ligament disruption	10	35 months (minimum, 14)	CC interval repair with two no. 5 Ethibond sutures through drill holes in the clavicle and looped around the coracoid	No loss of reduction at final follow-up At 12 months: UCLA, 33.8; WOSI, 93.4

Continued

TABLE 56.4   Clinical Outcomes Following Nonsurgical and Surgical Management of Acromioclavicular Joint Injuries—cont'd

Study	Injury Type	No. of Patients	Average Follow-Up	Treatment	Outcome
Tauber et al.[144]	Type III–V	24 (12 modified WD, 12 ACCR)	35 months	Modified WD (n = 12), autograft semitendinosus graft (n = 12)	ASES: WD, 74 to 86; ACCR, 74 to 96 Constant score: WD, 70 to 81; ACCR, 71 to 93 Mean CC distance: WD, 12.3 mm (14.9 under stress loading); ACCR, 11.4 mm (11.8 under stress loading; $P = 0.27$) Conclusions: ACCR had superior clinical and radiographic results
Yoo et al.[145]	Type IV, V, or chronic III (16 patients) Nonunion distal clavicle fracture with CC separation (5 patients)	21	33 months (minimum, 18)	CC interval repair with three no. 5 Ethibond sutures and semitendinosus autograft through a single tunnel drill hole in the clavicle and looped around the coracoid	48% excellent 42% good Constant score: 84.7 UCLA: 30 81% maintained reduction
Salzman et al.[146]	Type III (3), IV (3), V (17)	23	31 months (minimum, 24)	Arthroscopically assisted anatomic AC reconstruction using two flip-button devices	Constant score: 34 to 94 VAS: 4.5 to 0.25 35% with loss of reduction on radiograph but no difference in clinical outcomes
DeBerardino et al.[147]	Type IV–VI	10	6 months	AC GraftRope system: subacromial arthroscopic approach with subcoracoid button secured by nonabsorbable sutures to clavicle washer, augmentation with a centrally placed soft tissue graft	100% return to preinjury level of activity; no complications; no loss of reduction on radiograph
Carofino and Mazzocca[22]	Type III or V (failed conservative management)	16 (plus 1 failure not included in follow-up statistics)	21 months (minimum, 6)	ACCR with two-bundle semitendinosus allograft and PEEK interference screw fixation in the clavicle via drill holes—2 with distal clavicle excision (1 of whom had SAD)	ASES: 52 to 92 Constant score: 67 to 95 SST: 7 to 12 SANE: 94 3 failures, none from erosion through bone, with 2 revision surgeries
Cohen et al.[148]	Type III or IV	16	12 months	Endoscopically assisted AC reconstruction with synthetic ligament repair	Constant score: 91 (60–100), 2 with revision surgery and 3 with radiographic loss of reduction
Von Heideken et al.[149]	Type V	37 (22 acute with HP, 15 chronic with modified WD augmented with hook plate)	1–8 years	AC joint fixation: Modified WD technique vs. HP technique	Constant score: 91 (HP) vs. 85 (mWD) Less pain at rest and with movement in HP group No difference in AC joint reduction radiographically

[a]Twelve of the 60 patients were found to have severe AC dislocation (type V injury), and these patients fared better with operative compared with nonoperative treatment.

AC, Acromioclavicular; *ACCR,* anatomic coracoclavicular reconstruction; *ASES,* American Shoulder and Elbow Surgeons; *CA,* coracoacromial; *CC,* coracoclavicular; *HP,* hook plate; *mWD,* modified Weaver-Dunn; *PEEK,* polyetheretherketone; *SAD,* subacromial decompression; *SANE,* single assessment numeric evaluation; *SST,* simple shoulder test; *UCLA,* University of California–Los Angeles; *VAS,* visual analogue scale; *WD,* Weaver-Dunn; *WOSI,* Western Ontario Shoulder Instability.

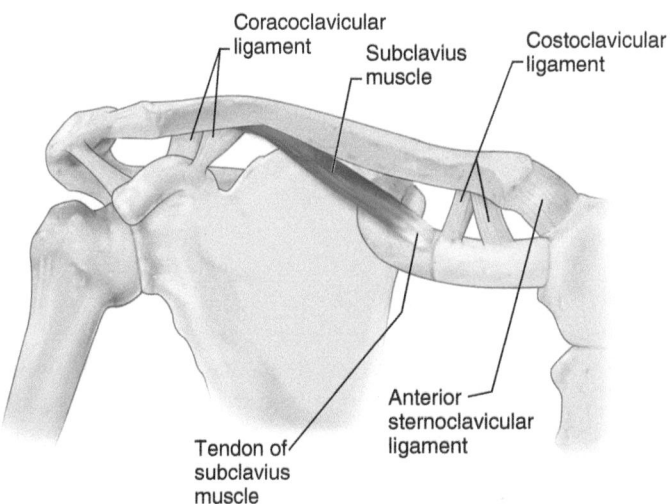

Fig. 56.29 Normal anatomy around the sternoclavicular and acromioclavicular joints. Note that the tendon of the subclavius muscle arises near the costoclavicular ligament from the first rib and has a long tendon structure. (Modified from Rockwood CA, Green DP, eds. *Fractures*. 2nd ed. Philadelphia: JB Lippincott; 1984.)

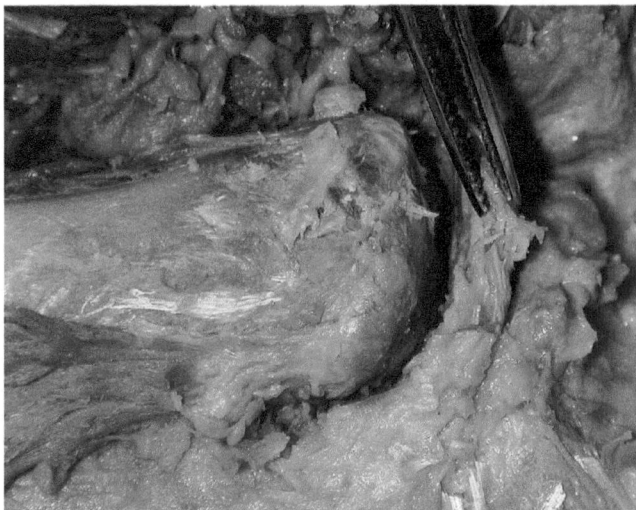

Fig. 56.30 Cadaveric dissection shows how the intra-articular disk ligament (held in forceps) divides the joint into two separate joint spaces.

disease processes including gout, pseudogout, infection, and chondromatosis should be ruled out.

In the event of an SC joint injury, it is often possible to readily observe a gross deformity, especially with an anterior dislocation or subluxation. In these situations, the patient is likely to be seen supporting the affected extremity with his or her head tilted toward the side of injury to decrease stress across the joint. Initial examination of a patient with a suspected SC joint injury should include assessment for secondary injuries to hilar structures. In addition, assessment for brachial plexus and vascular injuries resulting from posterior displacement of the SC joint should be performed.

After inspection, direct palpation of SC joint injuries will elicit maximal tenderness with isolation around the joint, accompanied by restricted ROM due to pain. Furthermore, patients may have a palpable step-off at the SC junction. Careful examination can also help distinguish between the different types of SC joint injuries. In type I (mild sprain) injuries, patients typically have mild pain with movement of the involved arm, and the SC joint itself may be swollen and slightly tender to palpation. In type II injuries, patients have similar findings but may also have a palpable subluxation of the SC joint with manual stress testing, given partial disruption of the ligaments. Finally, in type III injuries, patients often hold the affected extremity in an adducted position with the head tilted toward the injured side. These patients have severe pain with any movement and typically do not tolerate lying supine on the examination table. Understanding SC anatomy is important in better understanding the pathology of these injuries and performing and accurate exam (Figs. 56.29–56.35).

Imaging

Radiographic evaluation of the SC joint can be difficult to interpret despite the development of special projected views. Potential radiographic views of the SC joint include the standard AP view of the chest, the Heinig view, the Hobbs view, and the serendipity

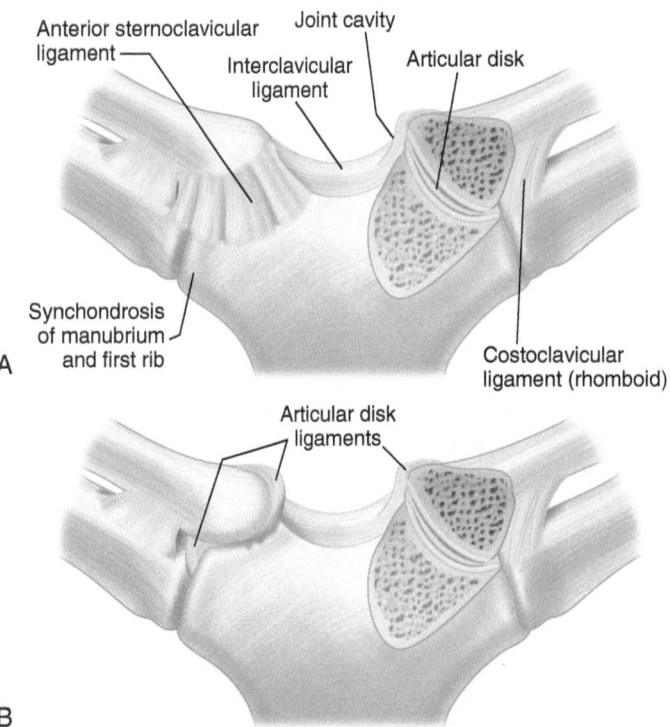

Fig. 56.31 (A) Normal anatomy around the sternoclavicular (SC) joint. Note that the articular disk ligament divides the SC joint cavity into two separate spaces and inserts onto the superior and posterior aspects of the medial clavicle. (B) The articular disk ligament acts as a checkrein for a medial displacement of the proximal clavicle. (Modified from Rockwood CA, Matsen FA, eds. *The Shoulder*. 2nd ed. Philadelphia: WB Saunders; 1998.)

view. Computed tomography (CT) is usually obtained in these cases to assess for subtle side-to-side differences. Although it is not an ideal view for visualization of the SC joint, the AP chest film may help identify asymmetry of the clavicle. This view can also identify a collapsed lung in a patient with suspected posterior SC joint dislocation.

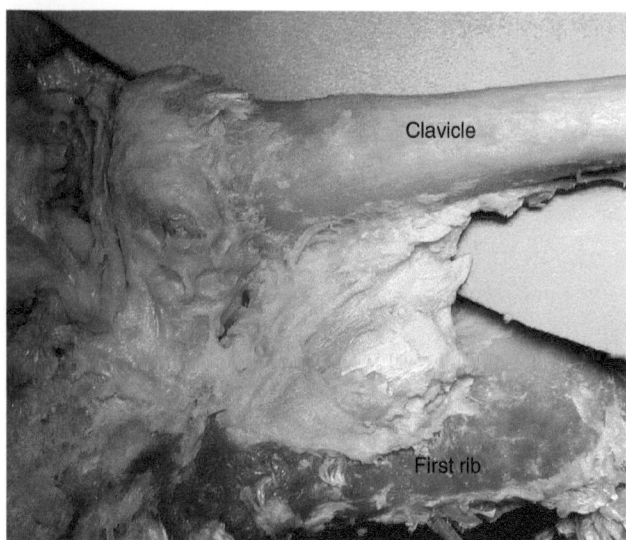

Fig. 56.32 Cadaveric dissection showing the costoclavicular ligament connecting the upper surface of the first rib to the inferior surface of the medial end of the clavicle.

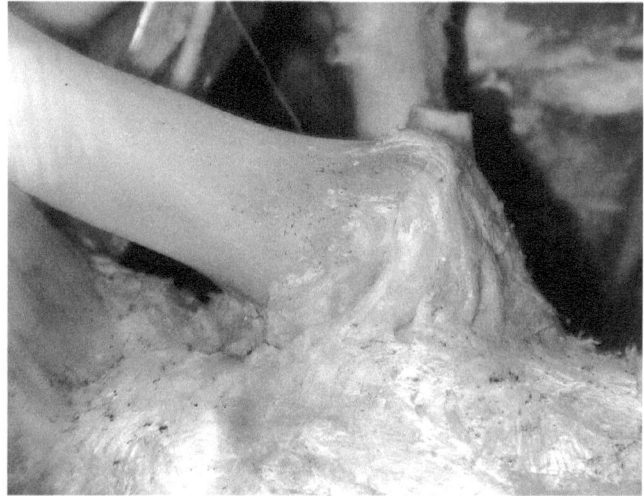

Fig. 56.33 Cadaveric dissection showing the anterior fibers of the capsular ligament of the sternoclavicular joint.

The Heinig and Hobbs views of the SC joint are more beneficial than the standard AP view but nevertheless have limited utility. The Heinig view is obtained when the patient is supine with the x-ray source set up to shoot tangential to the joint and parallel to the opposite clavicle. The Hobbs view is taken with the patient leaning forward over the x-ray cassette and the x-ray source directed over the top of the patient (Figs. 56.36 and 56.37).[56]

Given the anatomic constraints, it is impossible to obtain an ideal view of a true 90-degree cephalic-to-caudal lateral view of the SC joint. Therefore the optimal image developed for identifying SC joint disease has been the serendipity view, which is a 40-degree cephalic tilt view first described by Rockwood.[103] It is performed by tilting the radiograph source 40 degrees off the vertical plane and centering it on the sternum (Fig. 56.38). When interpreting the serendipity view, the key is the relationship of the medial clavicle to the interclavicular line. In the event of an

anterior dislocation, the medial clavicle lies above the interclavicular line, whereas in the posterior dislocation it lies below the interclavicular line (Figs. 56.39 and 56.40).

The shortcomings of plain films can partially be overcome with the use of CT, which is the modality of choice in the evaluation of SC joint injuries. It is capable of distinguishing between fractures and dislocations, as well as only minor subluxations of the joint (Fig. 56.41).

Decision-Making Principles

Treatment options for SC joint injuries are evolving. Although these injuries certainly occur less frequently than AC joint injuries, given the tremendous energy required to disrupt the strong ligamentous constraints of the joint and cause a dislocation, severe pain, deformity, and life-threatening concurrent injuries can occur.

Mild sprains and subluxations (type I and II injuries) are always treated nonoperatively with ice, analgesics, and immobilization with a clavicle strap or a sling and swathe. The immobilization period typically lasts for 6 weeks. If the clavicle is subluxated as in type II injuries, a gentle force directing the shoulders posteromedially can be applied, followed by immobilization with a figure-of-eight brace.

Acute anterior SC joint dislocations (type III) (Fig. 56.42), which are more common than posterior dislocations, require immediate closed reduction that can be accomplished with use of either a local anesthetic with sedation or use of a general anesthetic. After successful reduction, the affected extremity should be immobilized in a figure-of-eight brace for at least 6 weeks.[51] Of note, most anterior SC dislocation injuries are inherently unstable and thus may dislocate again after reduction; however, surgery is rarely indicated.

In the setting of acute posterior SC joint dislocations, the clinician must assess for concomitant injury to local vessels, heart, and/or lung tissue. Although historically the treatment of choice was open reduction,[58,71] currently closed reduction is the initial treatment of choice because the SC joint typically remains stable after reduction.[18,20,38,52,61,82,83,86,96,106,119] Any attempt at closed reduction must be performed in a controlled setting (i.e., an operating room) with the use of a general anesthetic. Furthermore, a cardiothoracic surgeon should be available at the time of reduction in case neurovascular compromise occurs secondary to the dislocation and/or reduction attempt itself.[133] Similar to anterior SC dislocation reduction, after closed reduction the patient should wear a figure-of-eight brace for 4 to 6 weeks to facilitate ligamentous healing. Operative management for posterior SC dislocations is rarely needed given the stability of the joint after closed reduction.

Conservative management is the standard, and surgical stabilization should be avoided when possible because the potential surgical risks outweigh the benefits.[17,51,57] Operative treatment for traumatic SC joint injuries carries substantial risks including infection, recurrence, poor cosmesis, neurovascular injury, and hardware migration; therefore surgery should only be considered if the patient is experiencing chronic symptomatic instability after a period of nonoperative management.[121]

Text continued on p. 673

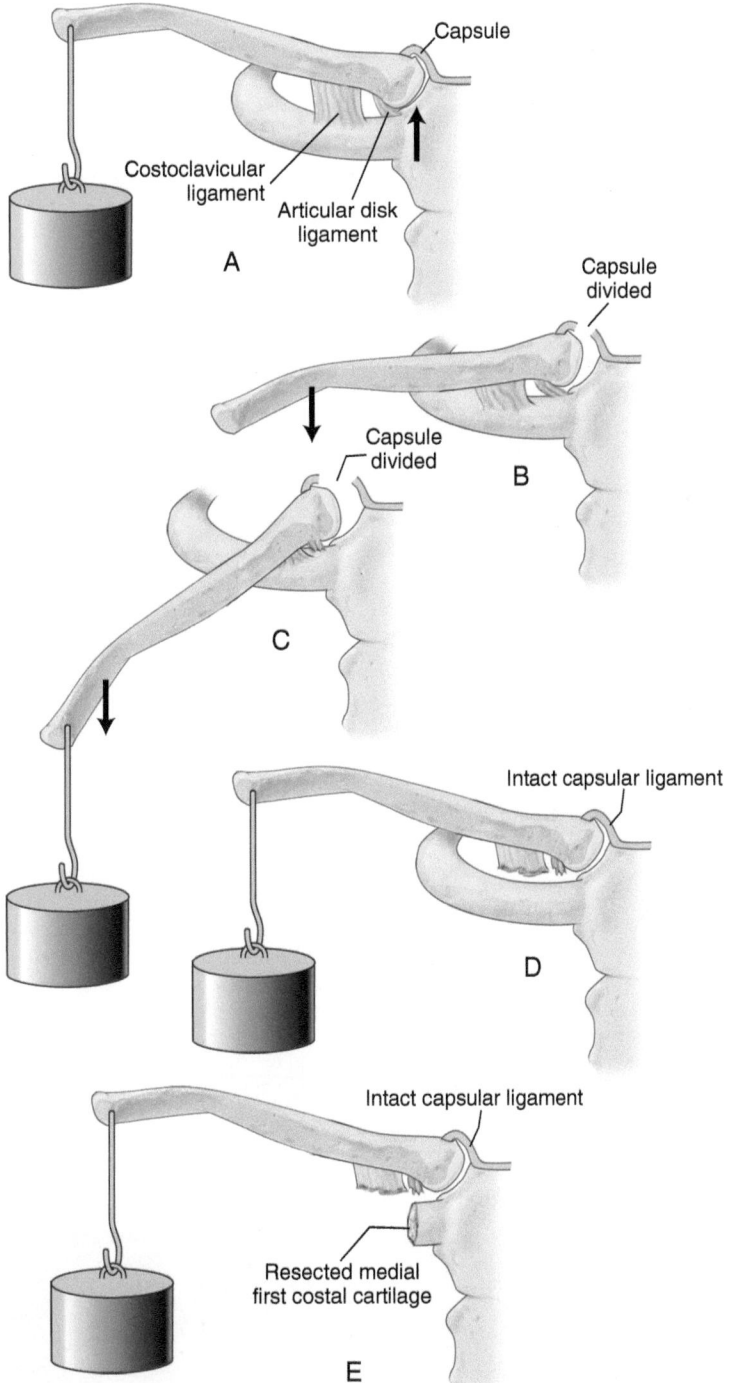

Fig. 56.34 The importance of the various ligaments around the sternoclavicular (SC) joint in maintaining normal shoulder poise. (A) The lateral end of the clavicle is maintained in an elevated position through the SC ligaments. The *arrow* indicates the fulcrum. (B) When the capsule is divided completely, the lateral end of the clavicle descends under its own weight without any loading. The clavicle will appear to be supported by the intra-articular disk ligament. (C) After division of the capsular ligament, it was shown that a weight of less than 5 lb was enough to tear the intra-articular disk ligament from its attachment on the costal cartilage junction of the first rib. The fulcrum was transferred laterally so that the medial end of the clavicle hinged over the first rib near the costoclavicular ligament. (D) After division of the costoclavicular ligament and the intra-articular disk ligament, the lateral end of the clavicle could not be depressed as long as the capsular ligament was intact. (E) After resection of the medial first costal cartilage along with the costoclavicular ligament, no effect was seen on the poise of the lateral end of the clavicle as long as the capsular ligament was intact. (Modified from Beam JG. Direct observation on the function of the capsule of the sternoclavicular joint in clavicular support. *J Anat.* 1967;101:159–170.)

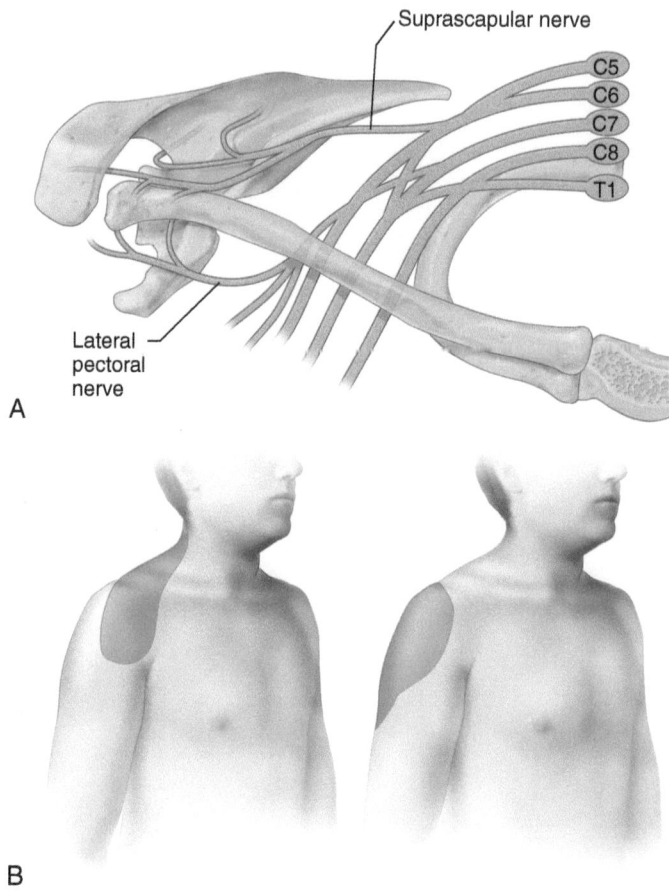

Fig. 56.35 (A) Innervation of the acromioclavicular (AC) joint in the superior aspect of the glenohumeral joint is provided by two nerves. The lateral pectoral nerve provides sensation to the anterior aspect of the shoulder. The suprascapular nerve provides innervation of the posterior aspect of the AC joint and posterior structures. (B) A superficial pain pattern produced by irritation of the AC joint and irritation of the subacromial space. (From Gerber CR, Galantay R, Hersche O. The pattern of pain produced by irritation of the acromioclavicular joint and the subacromial space. *J Shoulder Elbow Surg.* 1998;7[4]:352–355.)

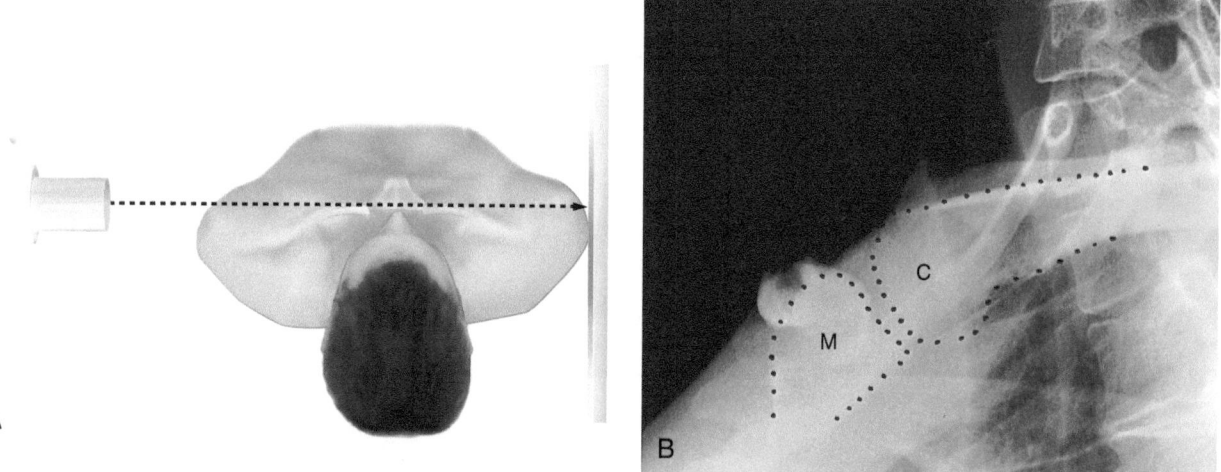

Fig. 56.36 (A) Patient positioning for radiographic evaluation of the sternoclavicular joint, as described by Heinig. (B) The Heinig view demonstrating a normal relationship between the medial end of the clavicle *(C)* and the manubrium *(M)*. (Modified from Rockwood CA, Green DP, Bucholz RW, et al, eds. *Fractures in the Adult.* Philadelphia: JB Lippincott; 1996.)

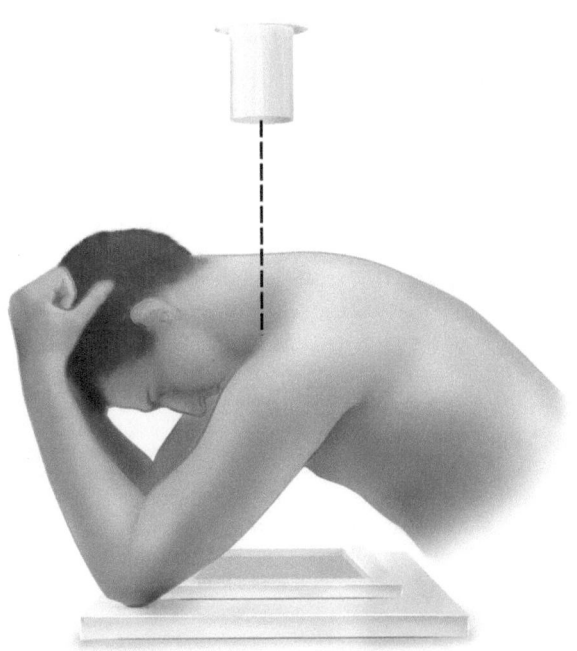

Fig. 56.37 Positioning of the patient for radiographic evaluation of the sternoclavicular joint, as recommended by Hobbs. (Modified from Hobbs DW. The sternoclavicular joint: a new axial radiographic view. *Radiology.* 1968;90:801.)

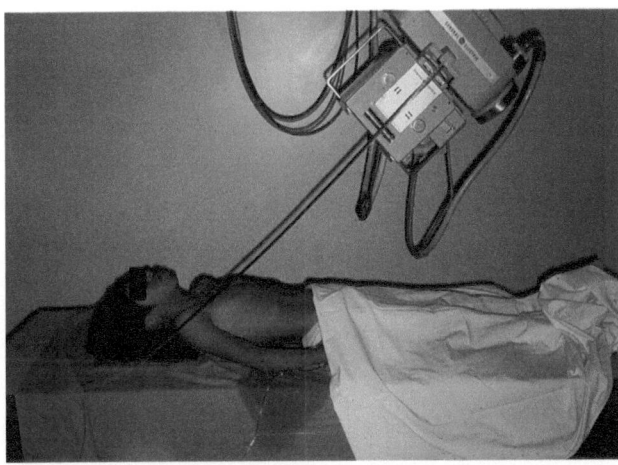

Fig. 56.38 Positioning of the patient to take the serendipity view of the sternoclavicular joints. The x-ray tube is tilted 40 degrees from the vertical position and is aimed directly at the manubrium. The nongrid cassette should be large enough to receive the projected images of the medial halves of both clavicles. In children, the tube distance from the patient should be 45 inches; in adults with thicker chests, the distance should be 60 inches.

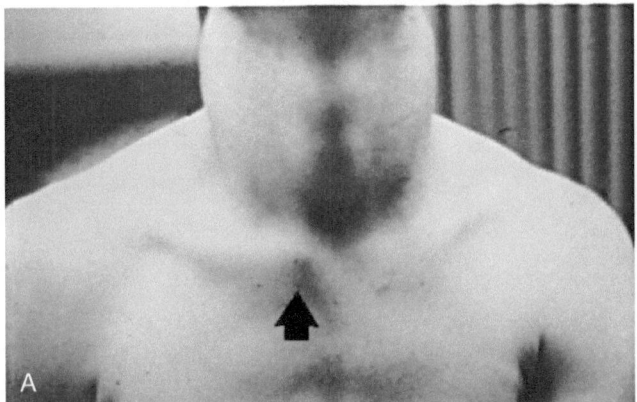

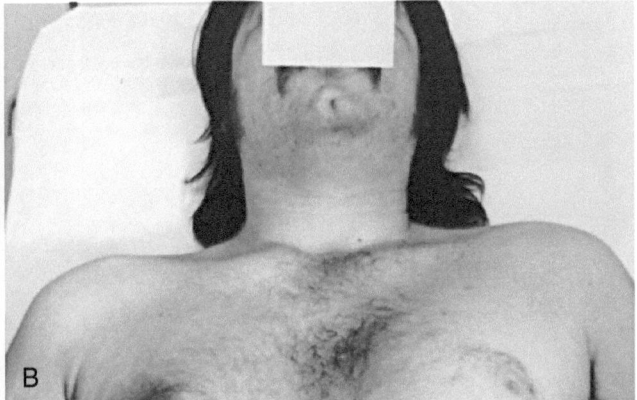

Fig. 56.39 (A) Clinically, an anterior dislocation of the left sternoclavicular joint is evident *(arrow).* (B) When the clavicles are viewed from the patient's feet looking cephalad, it is apparent that the right clavicle is dislocated anteriorly. (From Rockwood CA, Green DP, eds. *Fractures.* 2nd ed. Philadelphia: JB Lippincott; 1984.)

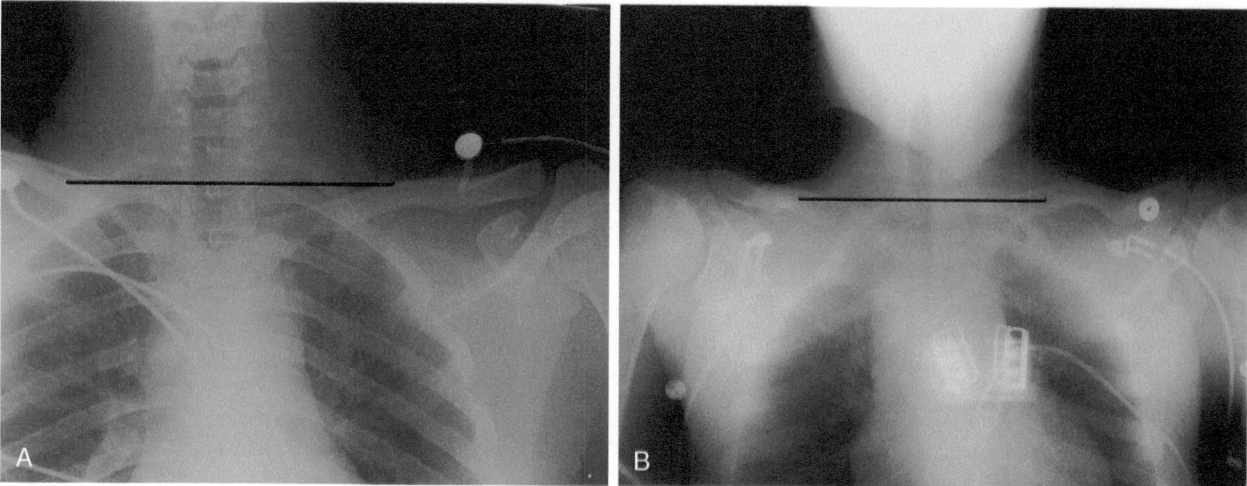

Fig. 56.40 Interpretation of the cephalic tilt radiographs of the sternoclavicular (SC) joints. (A) In a patient with posterior dislocation of the left SC joint, the medial half of the left clavicle is projected below a horizontal line drawn tangential to the superior aspect of the normal left medial clavicle. (B) After manual reduction is performed in the same patient, the medial aspects of both clavicles appear on the same horizontal line.

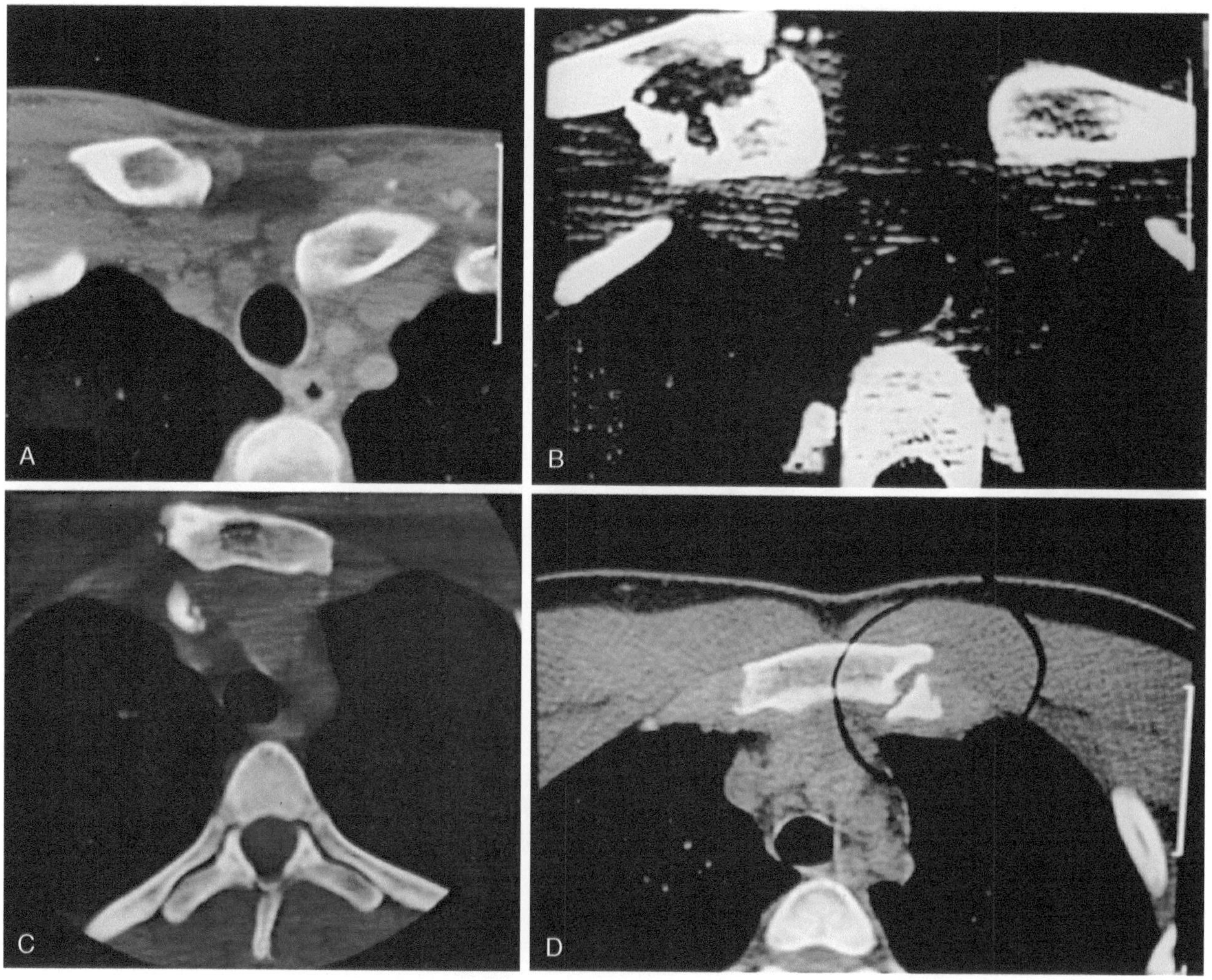

Fig. 56.41 Computed tomographic scans of the sternoclavicular (SC) joint demonstrating various types of injuries. (A) A posterior dislocation of the left clavicle compressing the great vessels and producing swelling of the left arm. (B) A fracture of the medial clavicle that does not involve the articular surface. (C) A fragment of bone displaced posteriorly into the great vessel. (D) A fracture of the medial clavicle into the SC joint.

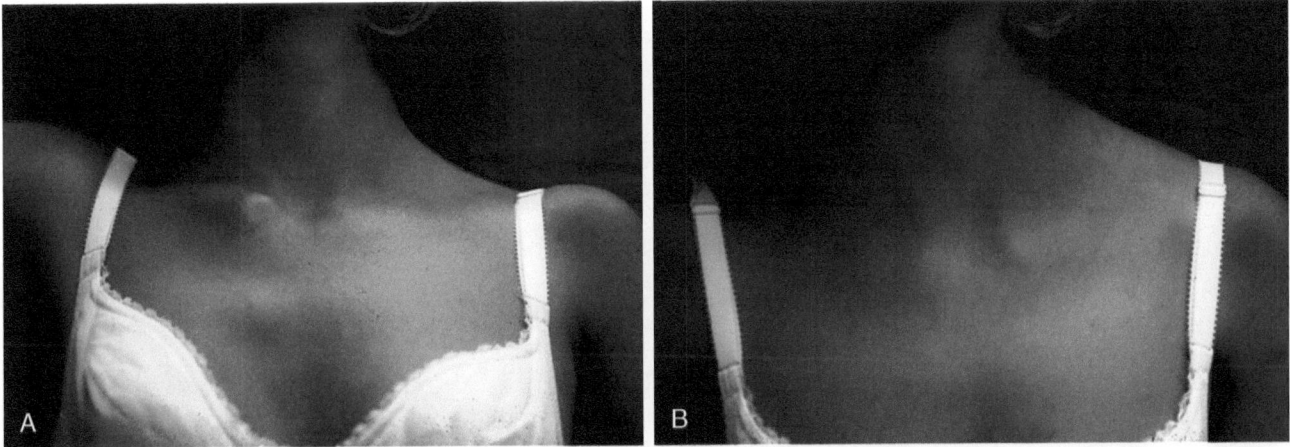

Fig. 56.42 Spontaneous anterior subluxation of the sternoclavicular joint. (A) With the right arm in the overhead position, the medial end of the right clavicle spontaneously subluxes out anteriorly without any trauma. (B) When the arm is brought back down to the side, the medial end of the clavicle spontaneously reduces, which is usually associated with no significant discomfort.

Treatment Options

As mentioned in the preceding section, most traumatic SC joint injuries can be treated effectively with nonoperative management. The following options are the most commonly accepted methods of nonoperative treatment.

Mild and Moderate Sprains (Type I and II Injuries)

- Mild sprains are treated with ice, analgesics, and immobilization in a sling with a gradual return to activities based on the patient's tolerance and comfort level.
- Moderate sprains or subluxations (type II injuries) are treated with ice, analgesics, and immobilization with a clavicle strap, sling, and swathe, or a figure-of-eight bandage for 1 week followed by sling immobilization for an additional 4 to 6 weeks.
- If a subluxation is present, reduction can be attempted in the clinic and/or emergency department setting via application of a gentle force, directing the shoulders posteromedially.

Dislocations (Type III Injuries)

- For an anterior dislocation, closed reduction is performed with the use of either a local anesthetic with sedation or under general anesthesia. With the patient supine, a 3- to 4-inch pad is placed between the shoulders, which allows the scapula to assume a retracted position, pulling the clavicle laterally. A posterior-directed force is then gently applied to the anteromedial clavicle. Postreduction care includes use of a clavicle strap, sling, and swathe or a figure-of-eight bandage for at least 6 weeks with the arm protected for another 2 weeks before undertaking strenuous activity.
- For a posterior dislocation, closed reduction via the abduction–traction technique is performed in the operating room under general anesthesia. With the patient supine, a 3- to 4-inch pad is placed between the shoulders and lateral traction is applied to the abducted arm while it is slowly brought into extension. If the joint does not easily reduce, grasping the

clavicle between the surgeon's fingers and/or using a towel clip can aid with manipulation (Fig. 56.43; also see Fig. 56.44).[33,38,86,102,108] Postreduction care includes the use of a clavicle strap, sling and swathe, or a figure-of-eight bandage for 4 to 6 weeks.
- A cardiothoracic surgeon should be available at the time of reduction in case of neurovascular compromise secondary to the dislocation and/or reduction attempt itself (Fig. 56.45).[132,133] Adjacent structures at risk include the trachea, brachiocephalic vein, brachiocephalic trunk, subclavian artery, and the common carotid artery.[17]

Given the potential risks, surgical intervention should be reserved only in cases of recurrent, symptomatic SC joint instability. Numerous surgical options exist. While posttraumatic arthritis of the SC joint is typically treated with medial clavicle excision or resection arthroplasty,[65] SC joint reconstruction has emerged as the preferred management for the unstable SC joint. Different techniques for SC joint reconstruction have been described including figure-of-eight hamstring tendon[40,98,112,118] or palmaris tendon reconstruction,[31] subclavius tendon reconstruction,[4] suture anchor tendon reconstruction,[5] and plate fixation.[135] Regarding reconstruction options, superior biomechanical properties have been reported after reconstruction with the figure-of-eight tendon reconstruction technique.[118]

Upon moving forward with operative management, proper patient positioning and surgical exposure are crucial. Stabilization of the SC joint via a figure-of-eight hamstring tendon autograft versus allograft reconstruction or medial clavicle excision can then be appropriately performed. Regardless of the technique used, at no point during the surgical stabilization of the SC joint should Kirschner wires or any other type of metallic pin be used to stabilize the joint. Several deaths, near-deaths, or migrations of the Kirschner wire, although rare, have been reported in the literature.[27,45,72,89,95,100,108,115-117,132] A more common complication involves vascular injury resulting from migration of intact or broken wires.

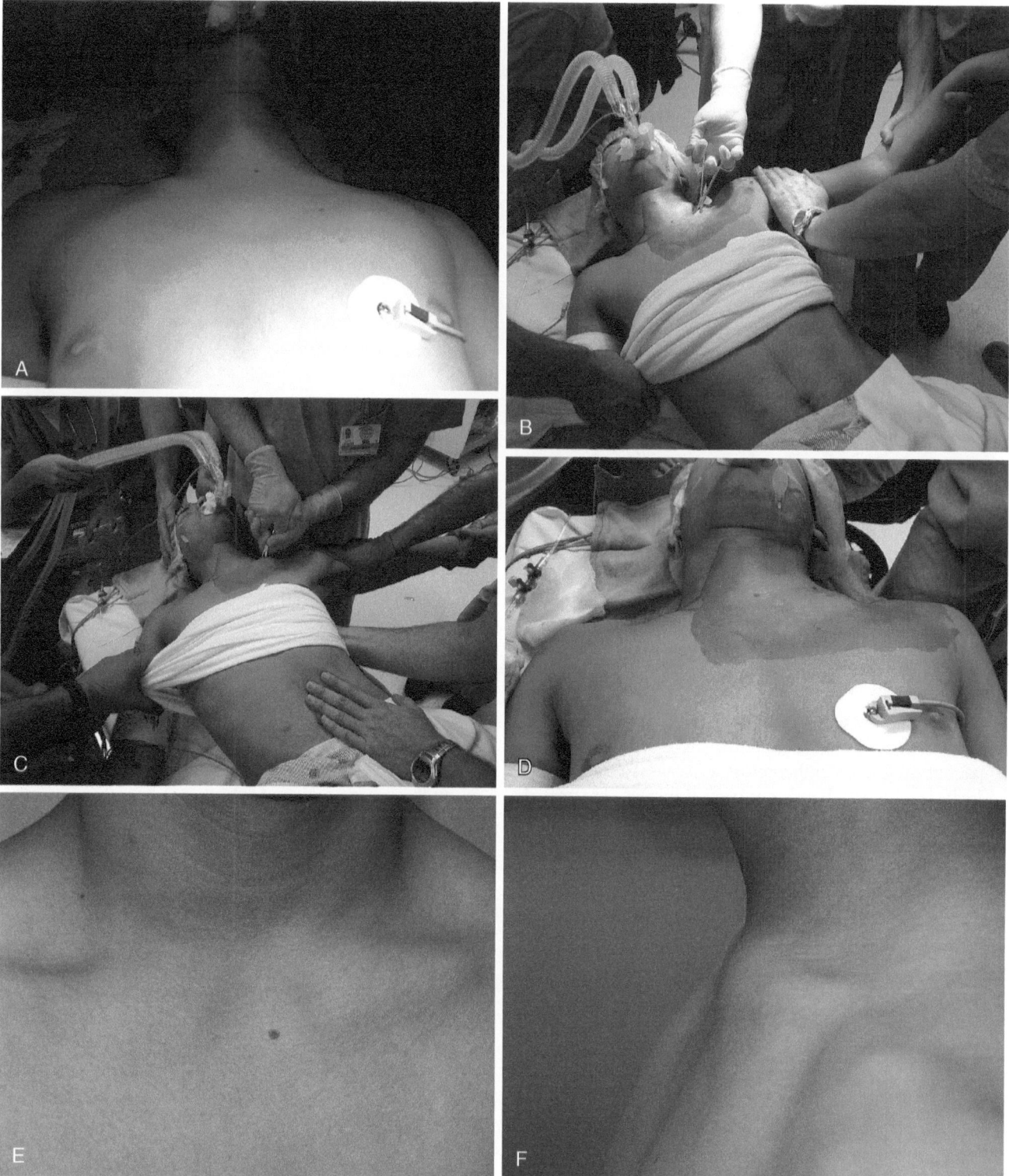

Fig. 56.43 Posterior dislocation of the left sternoclavicular (SC) joint. (A) A 19-year-old male has a 24-hour-old posterior displacement of the left medial clavicle that occurred from direct trauma to the anterior chest wall. He noted the immediate onset of difficulty in swallowing and some hoarseness. Note that the left medial prominence of the clavicle is lost. (B) After a failed attempt at closed reduction after induction of general anesthesia, a sterile towel clip is placed percutaneously around the medial left clavicle after preparing the area with povidone-iodine. (C) While assistants provide countertraction on the torso and traction on the ipsilateral extremity, the surgeon provides a lateral and anterior force on the clavicle with the towel clip. This maneuver results in an audible "pop" as the left SC joint reduces. (D) After reduction, the left medial clavicular prominence can easily be seen. (E and F) Clinical photographs 4 months after reduction demonstrate a stable, healed left SC joint. The patient was asymptomatic with normal range of motion and strength.

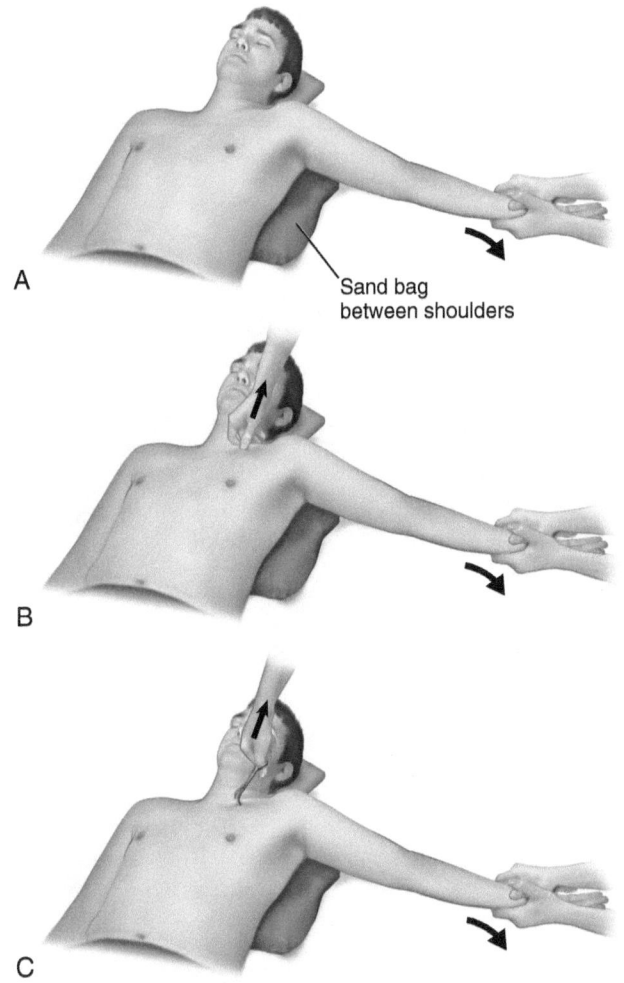

A

B

C

Fig. 56.44 The technique of closed reduction of the sternoclavicular joint. (A) The patient is positioned supine with a sandbag placed between the two shoulders. Traction is then applied to the arm against countertraction in an abducted and slightly extended position. In anterior dislocations, direct pressure over the medial end of the clavicle may reduce the joint. (B) In posterior dislocations, in addition to the traction, it may be necessary to manipulate the medial end of the clavicle with the fingers to dislodge the clavicle from behind the manubrium. (C) In stubborn cases of posterior dislocations, it may be necessary to sterilely prepare the medial end of the clavicle and use a towel clip to grasp around the medial clavicle to lift it back into position. (Modified from Rockwood CA, Green DP, eds. *Fractures*. 2nd ed. Philadelphia: JB Lippincott; 1984.)

Open SC Joint Reduction

- The patient is positioned supine with a bump between the scapulae.
- Draping should keep the involved extremity free to allow for traction.
- Exposure is typically via a 5- to 7-cm incision parallel to the superior border of the medial clavicle, extending over the sternum (Fig. 56.46).
- Care must be taken to preserve as much of the anterior capsule as possible.
- Reduction is performed via traction/countertraction and pulling anteriorly on the clavicle.

Figure-of-Eight Reconstruction

- Hamstring or palmaris tendon harvest via standard technique if using autograft.
- Sternoclavicular joint exposure is created as previously described (see Fig. 56.46).
- Two drill holes are created in the medial clavicle and manubrium.
- The graft is woven through the holes in a figure-of-eight fashion.

Medial Clavicle Excision

- Exposure is created as previously described.
- Subperiosteal exposure of the medial clavicle is achieved.
- Care must be taken to preserve as much of the anterior capsule as possible.
- Resection of the medial clavicle is performed.
- Care must be taken to protect the posterior vascular structures.
- The intra-articular disk and capsular ligaments are transferred into the medullary canal of the clavicle via drill holes and suture passage.
- Sutures are tied to secure the transferred ligament into the clavicle.
- Periosteal sleeve closure is secured, and repair to the costoclavicular ligaments and/or first rib periosteum is performed with multiple sutures.
- The repair is augmented with the previously described reconstruction method if such augmentation is deemed appropriate.

Authors' Preferred Technique

Figure-of-Eight Semitendinosus Allograft Reconstruction

- The patient is positioned supine with a bump between the scapulae.
- Draping should keep the involved extremity free to allow for traction.
- Exposure is via a 5- to 7-cm incision parallel to the superior border of the medial clavicle, extending over the sternum (see Fig. 56.46).
- Care must be taken to preserve as much of the anterior capsule as possible.
- Reduction is performed via traction/countertraction and pulling anteriorly on the clavicle.
- Two 4-mm drill holes are created from anterior to posterior through the medial part of the clavicle and manubrium.
- Free semitendinosus allograft is woven through the holes in a figure-of-eight fashion so that the tendon strands are parallel to each other posterior to the joint, and cross each other anterior to the joint.

- The tendon is tied in a square knot and secured with standard, high strength nonabsorbable suture.
- The deep dermal layer is closed with 2-0 or 3-0 absorbable suture, and the skin itself is closed with either a 2-0 running or interrupted nylon suture, everting the skin edges.
- A compression dressing is applied, along with a supportive sling.

Alternative Approaches

- Delta and other graft configurations are used with small drill holes in the sternum and clavicle.
- Ensure careful protection of the posterior hilar structures at all times.

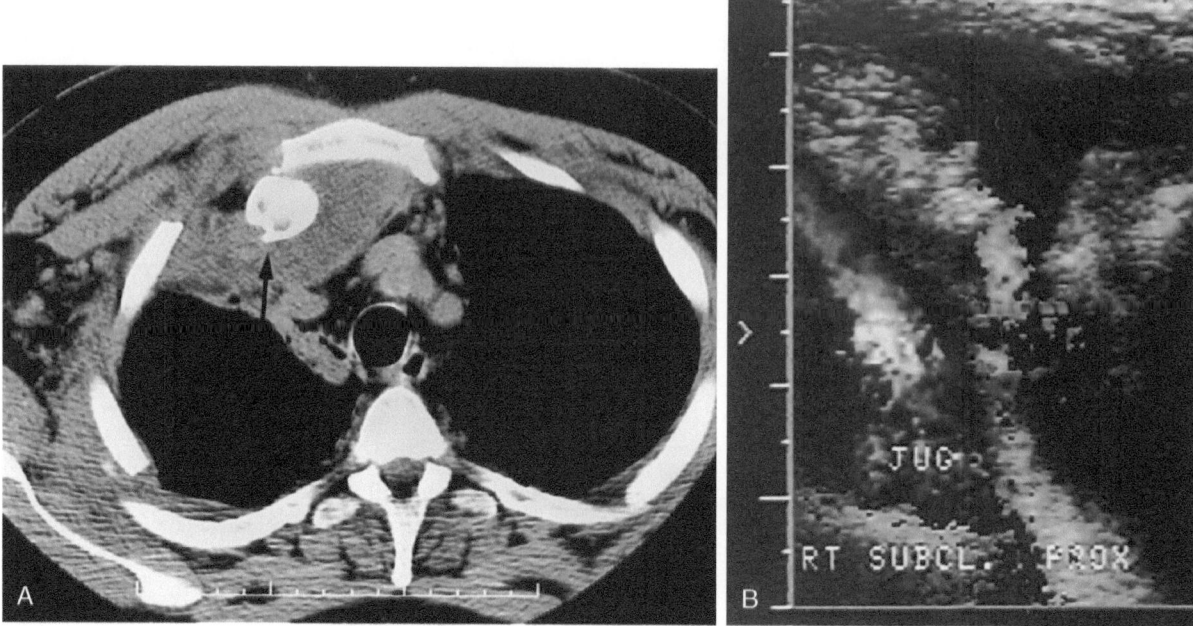

Fig. 56.45 (A) A computed tomographic scan revealing a posterior fracture-dislocation of the sternoclavicular joint *(arrow)* with significant soft tissue swelling and compromise of the hilar structures. (B) A duplex ultrasound study revealing a large pseudoaneurysm of the right subclavian artery. Note the large neck of the pseudoaneurysm, which measured about 1 cm in diameter. (From Rockwood CA, Green DP, Bucholz RW, et al, eds. *Fractures in the Adult.* Philadelphia: JB Lippincott; 1996.)

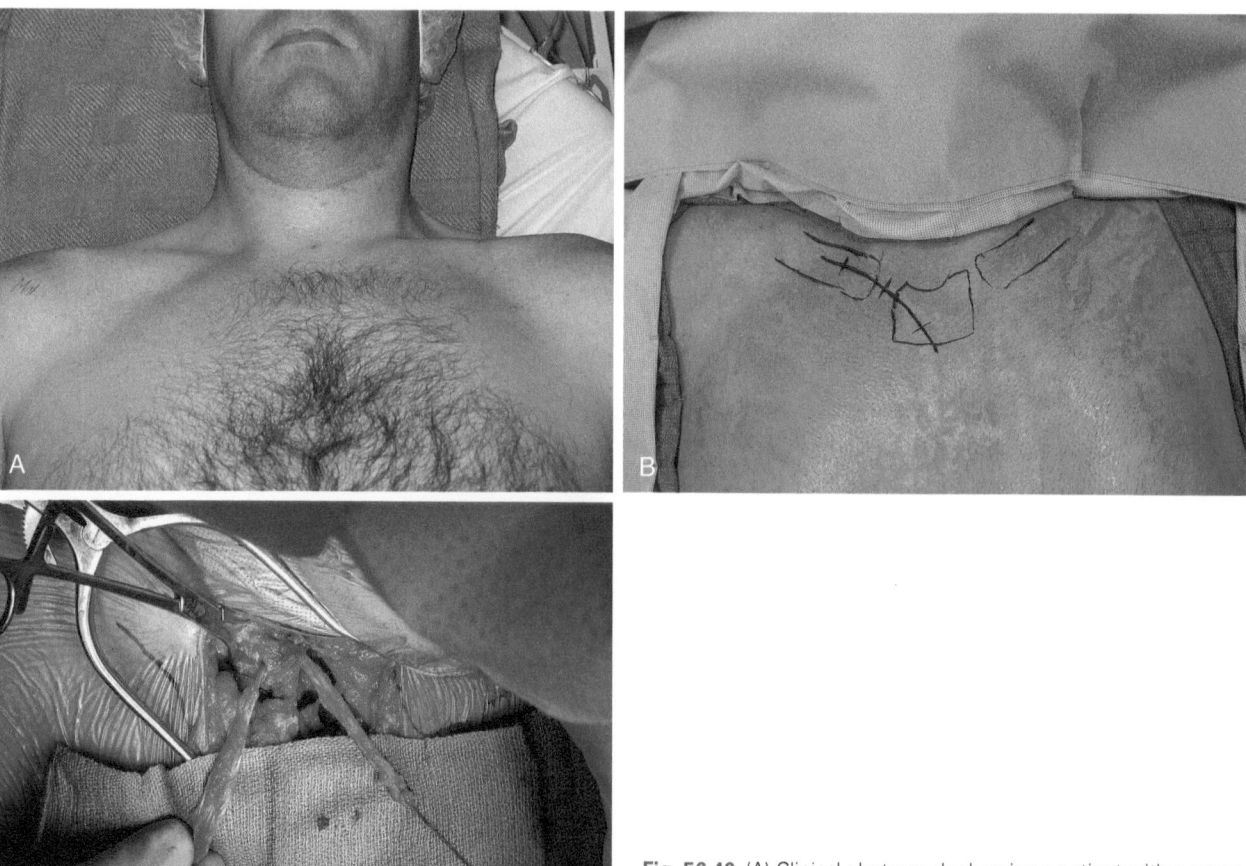

Fig. 56.46 (A) Clinical photograph showing a patient with a symptomatic chronic posterior sternoclavicular dislocation on the right. (B) The proposed skin incision after the patient has been prepared and draped. (C) An intraoperative photograph showing a semitendinosus graft being positioned for a figure-of-eight reconstruction.

Postoperative Management/Return to Play

Postoperative management after SC joint stabilization depends on the surgeon's preferred method of operative fixation. Typically, patients wear a figure-of-eight splint for 4 weeks after surgery and a sling is then used for an additional 6 to 8 weeks. Patients are restricted to minimal use of the involved extremity during this acute phase of rehabilitation (e.g., for hygiene and feeding). Patients can gradually return to strengthening and to contact sports 12 to 14 weeks after surgery to allow adequate time for remodeling and strengthening of the medial clavicle.

Results

Outcomes after both nonoperative and operative treatment for SC joint injuries are more easily interpretable, given the general agreement within the orthopaedic community on nonoperative management for nearly all injuries.[17,32,51,89,104,108,116,131,133] Good to excellent outcomes have been reported with both operative and nonoperative management. In a recent systematic review, Glass and colleagues[47] identified a total of 251 SC dislocations in 24 different studies and found satisfactory results after both nonoperative and operative treatment. Regarding anterior SC dislocations, the authors reported good to excellent results in 69% of patients treated nonoperatively, 85% of patients treated with closed reduction, 80% of patients treated with open reduction after failed closed reduction, and in 75% of patients treated with open reduction. Regarding posterior SC dislocations, the authors reported good to excellent outcomes in 100% of patients treated with closed reduction, 88% of patients treated with open reduction after a failed closed reduction attempt, and in 91% of patients treated with open reduction. Attempts to perform a closed reduction prior to an open reduction did not cause a worse outcome compared with patients who had not undergone an attempt at closed reduction. Of the posterior dislocation cases, 30% (24 of 80) of patients experienced symptoms of mediastinal compression, and 23 of these patients still achieved good to excellent outcomes. Overall, the authors reported better functional outcomes in patients with acute dislocations compared with those who had chronic dislocations.[47] Another recent systematic review reported that chronic SC dislocation is best treated with the tendon tissue woven with the figure-of-eight technique, whereas acute SC dislocation can be managed with repair of the joint capsule alone.[122]

Regarding medical clavicle resection as treatment for SC dislocation, Rockwood and colleagues[105] reviewed a series of patients who had either undergone primary resection arthroplasty of the SC joint in which the costoclavicular ligament was left intact (*n* = 8) or revision resection arthroplasty (after failed resection without maintenance of the costoclavicular ligament) with costoclavicular ligament reconstruction (*n* = 7). At an average of 7.7 years after surgery, all eight patients in the first group had substantially better results, and the authors recommended preservation or reconstruction of the CC ligament in all patients undergoing medial clavicle resection.[105] Nevertheless, current recommendations suggest that resection arthroplasty be reserved for chronic, painful posttraumatic osteoarthritis and degenerative conditions of the SC joint with or without instability, or

following failed SC joint reconstruction[76,94] Moreover, preservation or reconstruction of the costoclavicular ligament and achieving stabilization of the medial clavicular portion to the first rib is essential at the time of resection arthroplasty.

Complications

The most common complication after acute SC joint injury is related to poor cosmesis resulting from a medial prominence at the SC joint after nonoperative management. The most severe complications are related to posterior dislocations, given the proximity of hilar structures. Such complications include acute pneumothorax, laceration or occlusion of the great vessels, esophageal rupture, brachial plexus injury or compression, and injury to the recurrent laryngeal nerve resulting in voice changes. Late complications can also arise and can be devastating, including tracheoesophageal fistula, stridor, and dysphagia. As previously mentioned, operative complications include infection, loss of reduction, posttraumatic arthritis, and neurovascular injury either iatrogenic or resulting from migrating or broken metallic hardware.

FUTURE CONSIDERATIONS

For both AC and SC joint injuries, the goal remains to determine a gold standard treatment through double-blind, randomized, controlled trials. Most of the literature is confined to level IV and V evidence and thus definitive recommendations for the clinician are still needed. This has historically been the case regarding when to operate on persons with type III AC joint injuries or anterior SC joint dislocations, although newer data have helped guide the treatment algorithms for these injuries. Prospective randomized studies using validated outcome measures are needed to identify the best surgical treatment for both AC and SC joint injuries.

For a complete list of references, go to ExpertConsult.com.

SELECTED READINGS

Citation:

Beitzel K, Cote MP, Apostolakos J, et al. Current concepts in the treatment of acromioclavicular joint dislocations. *Arthroscopy*. 2013;29(2):387–397.

Level of Evidence:

V

Summary:

In this excellent recent review article, the authors describe the anatomy, pathophysiology, and management of AC joint injuries. Special attention is given to recent developments and techniques, and outcomes.

Citation:

Martetschläger F, Warth RJ, Millett PJ. Instability and degenerative arthritis of the sternoclavicular joint: a current concepts review. *Am J Sports Med*. 2014;42(4):999–1007.

Level of Evidence:

V

Summary:

In this excellent review article, the authors describe the anatomy, pathophysiology, workup and management of sternoclavicular (SC) joint injuries. They also describe updated surgical techniques and discuss current patient outcomes data available in the literature.

Citation:

Bontempo NA, Mazzocca AD. Biomechanics and treatment of acromioclavicular and sternoclavicular joint injuries. *Br J Sports Med*. 2010;44(5):361–369.

Level of Evidence:

V

Summary:

In this excellent review article, the authors describe the biomechanics and management of AC and SC joint injuries. This article is particularly helpful in understanding the underlying anatomic features of these joints to guide treatment decisions.

Citation:

Beitzel K, Mazzocca AD, Bak K, et al. ISAKOS upper extremity committee consensus statement on the need for diversification of the Rockwood classification for acromioclavicular joint injuries. *Arthroscopy*. 2014;30(2):271–278.

Level of Evidence:

V

Summary:

In this excellent recent review article, the authors describe the radiographic and clinical evaluation or acromioclavicular injuries and discuss an updated classification and treatment algorithm directing the management of these injuries, particularly pertaining to type III AC joint dislocations.

Citation:

Beitzel K, Obopilwe E, Apostolakos J, et al. Rotational and translational stability of different methods for direct acromioclavicular ligament repair in anatomic acromioclavicular joint reconstruction. *Am J Sports Med*. 2014;42(9):2141–2148.

Level of Evidence:

Cadaveric study

Summary:

This cadaveric biomechanics study analyzes different techniques of direct AC ligament reconstruction in addition to anatomic CC reconstructions for horizontal and vertical translation, as well as anterior and posterior rotation. The results indicate that reconstruction of the AC ligament by direct wrapping and suturing of the remaining graft around the AC joint was the most stable method and was the only one to show anterior rotation comparable with the native joint.

Citation:

Spencer EE Jr, Kuhn JE. Biomechanical analysis of reconstructions for sternoclavicular joint instability. *J Bone Joint Surg Am*. 2004;86A(1):98–105.

Level of Evidence:

Cadaveric study

Summary:

In this basic science study, the authors analyze a variety of SC joint repair constructs, including intramedullary ligament reconstruction, subclavius tendon reconstruction, and semitendinosus graft figure-of-eight reconstruction. The results indicate superior biomechanical properties of the semitendinosus graft figure-of-eight reconstruction for sternoclavicular joint instability; however, the need for in vivo correlation is noted.

Elbow, Wrist, and Hand

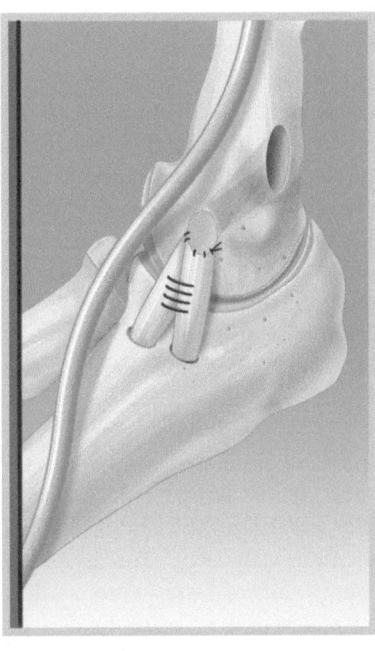

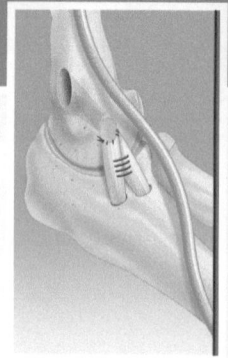

57

Elbow Anatomy and Biomechanics

Marshall A. Kuremsky, E. Lyle Cain Jr., Jeffrey R. Dugas, James R. Andrews, Lucas R. King

Elbow anatomy is complex, but knowledge of its intricate structural makeup is crucial to understanding athletic injuries in this area. Those who provide care for athletes, particularly athletes who participate in overhead-throwing sports, must have the ability to accurately diagnose and treat all forms of elbow injury and pathology. Accurate diagnosis and treatment require a thorough understanding of the interplay between the anatomy and function of the elbow joint.[1]

ANATOMY

Elbow stability is afforded by both static and dynamic constraints.[1,2] The primary static constraints include the ulnohumeral articulation, the anterior bundle of the ulnar collateral ligament (UCL), and the lateral collateral ligament (LCL) complex. Secondary static constraints include the common extensor and flexor pronator tendon origins, the joint capsule, and the radiocapitellar articulation.[2,3] Dynamic stability is conferred by surrounding musculature that crosses the elbow and stabilizes the joint secondarily during active contraction, including the brachialis, biceps, triceps, flexor pronator mass, brachioradialis, extensor carpi radialis brevis, and longus.

Osseous Anatomy

The articular surfaces of the elbow joint consist of the distal humerus, radial head, and proximal ulna. The joint itself has been referred to as a trochleoginglymoid joint and comprises the ulnohumeral joint (hinged or ginglymoid joint) and the radiocapitellar articulation (trochoid).[3,4]

The congruent articulation of the olecranon with the olecranon fossa is pivotal for elbow stability at terminal extension and greater than 120 degrees of flexion.[1,5] In maximal elbow flexion, the coronoid process and radial head are locked into their respective fossae of the distal humerus, thereby imparting maximal stability.[6] The distal humeral shaft has both medial and lateral supracondylar columns, as well as condyles. On the medial side is the spool-like trochlea, whereas on the lateral side is the spherical capitellum.[7] The articular surface of the radial head articulates with the capitellum, whereas the radial head articulates with the sigmoid notch of the proximal ulna.[7] Distally the biceps tendon inserts on the extraarticular radial tuberosity, whereas the triceps tendon inserts on the tip of the olecranon posteriorly.

The normal valgus orientation of the forearm relative to the arm varies as a function of both age and sex. It is smaller in children and averages 3 to 4 degrees more in females.[8,9] The carrying angle represents the orientation of the forearm in reference to the humerus when the elbow is in full extension as viewed from anterior to posterior.[10] It is formed by the valgus tilt of the axis of rotation (humeral articulation) and the valgus orientation of the ulnar shaft in relation to the olecranon.[11–13] The normal angle varies, averaging about 10 degrees in males and 13 degrees in females (Fig. 57.1).

Capsuloligamentous Restraints

The capsule of the elbow joint contains all three bony articulations and incorporates medial and lateral thickenings, which help form the primary ligamentous stabilizers.[7] The distended capsule may hold up to about 30 mL of fluid in the adult.[14] The majority of the stabilizing effects of the capsule are derived from its anterior portion when the elbow is in full extension.[15] In this regard, the anterior capsule resists hyperextension of the elbow, valgus stress, and joint distraction. In contrast, the posterior capsule may resist joint hyperflexion and posterior directed stresses.

The UCL complex, also referred to as the medial collateral ligament, comprises both anterior and posterior bundles and a variable transverse element (Cooper ligament)[16–18] (Fig. 57.2). The anterior bundle of the UCL (aUCL) is the primary ligamentous stabilizer to valgus stress on the elbow. It originates at the anteroinferior aspect of the medial epicondyle and inserts on the sublime tubercle of the medial coronoid process (new[19]). The aUCL is further divided into anterior and posterior bands. These two bands have a cam effect because the origin of the ligament is slightly posterior to the flexion-extension axis.[17] The anterior band of the aUCL is taut in extension and relaxes with further flexion, whereas the posterior band becomes more taut with elbow flexion. The posterior bundle of the UCL represents a capsular thickening and is less well defined.[20] The transverse bundle does not have a large role in joint stability.[17]

The LCL complex is composed of multiple structures, including the radial collateral ligament (RCL), the lateral ulnar collateral ligament (LUCL), the annular ligament, and the accessory lateral collateral ligament (Fig. 57.3). The LCL complex is a key stabilizer for resisting varus stress and posterolateral instability.[21] The RCL and LUCL originate from the isometric point on at the inferior

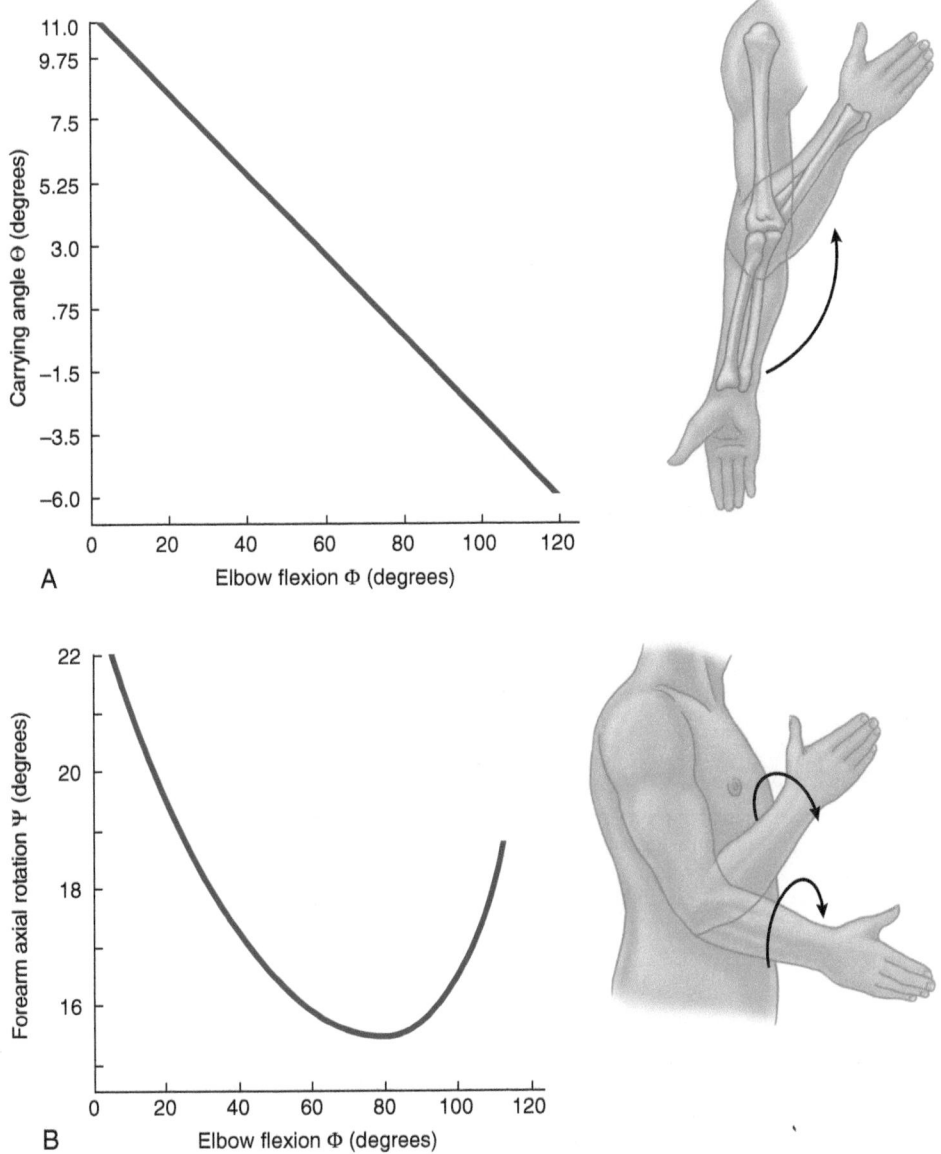

Fig. 57.1 (A) During elbow flexion, the carrying angle changes in a linear fashion from valgus to neutral or varus. (B) The ulna undergoes a slight axial rotation during flexion and extension. (Courtesy the Mayo Foundation.)

aspect of the lateral epicondyle. The RCL inserts into the annular ligament and stabilizes the radial head, whereas the LUCL attaches to the supinator crest of the proximal ulna and resists varus and posterolateral instability. The annular ligament forms a ring of tissue around the radial head, and inserts on the anterior and posterior aspects of the radial notch.

Elbow Musculature

Muscles crossing the elbow joint serve to control motion of the limb and provide dynamic stabilization to help the static structures. The primary groups acting on the joint include the elbow flexors (biceps, brachialis), elbow extensors (triceps), flexor pronator mass (resist valgus forces), and the mobile wad of three (brachioradialis, extensor carpi radialis longus, and extensor carpi radialis brevis—resist varus forces). The anconeus muscle may have a minor role in elbow extension but more importantly

is thought to function as a restraint to varus stress and posterolateral rotatory instability.[6]

ELBOW BIOMECHANICS

Joint Motion

Flexion-Extension

The normal arc of motion during flexion ranges from 0 degrees (full extension) to roughly 140 degrees. The axis of rotation (Fig. 57.4) for elbow flexion passes through the capitellum in line with the bottom of the trochlear sulcus.[7]

Pronation-Supination

Forearm rotation averages nearly 180 degrees through its arc. Pronation typically accounts for 80 to 85 degrees, and supination accounts for 85 to 90 degrees of motion. The axis of forearm

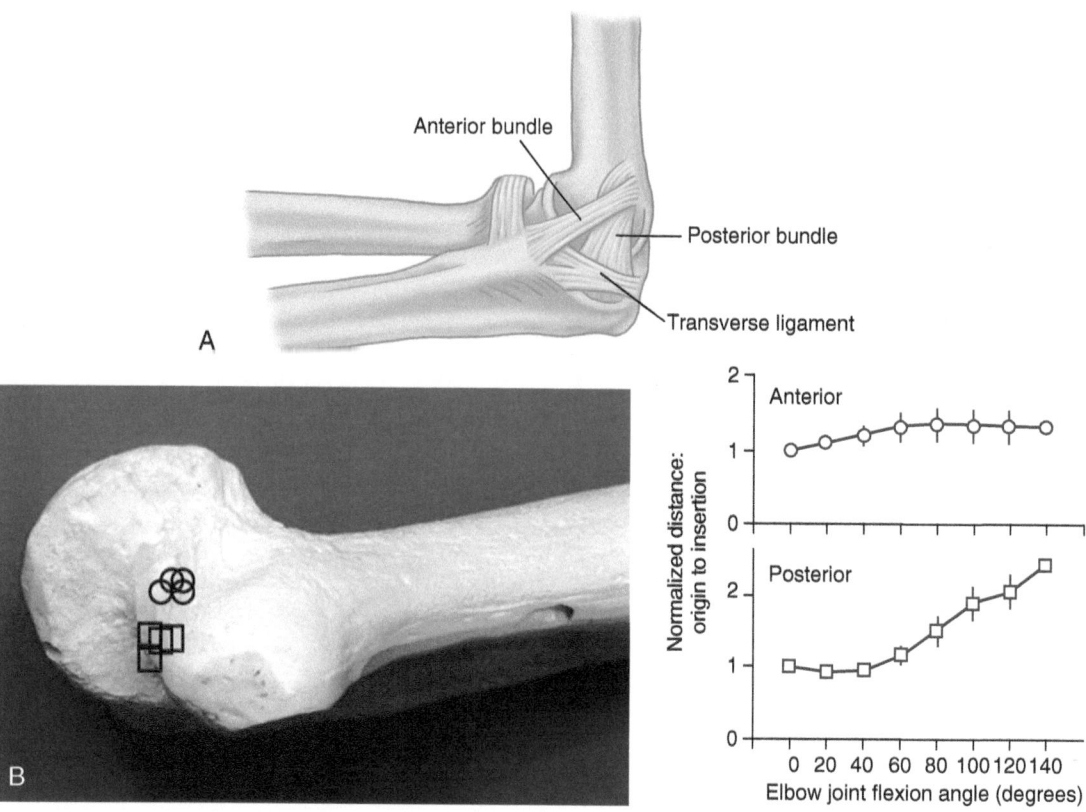

Fig. 57.2 (A) Anatomic distribution of the components of the medial collateral ligament complex. (B) The anterior bundle originates at the locus of the axis of rotation. However, the origin of the posterior bundle does not lie along the axis of rotation, and thus some change in the length of the posterior band is seen with changes in the elbow flexion angle. (Courtesy the Mayo Foundation.)

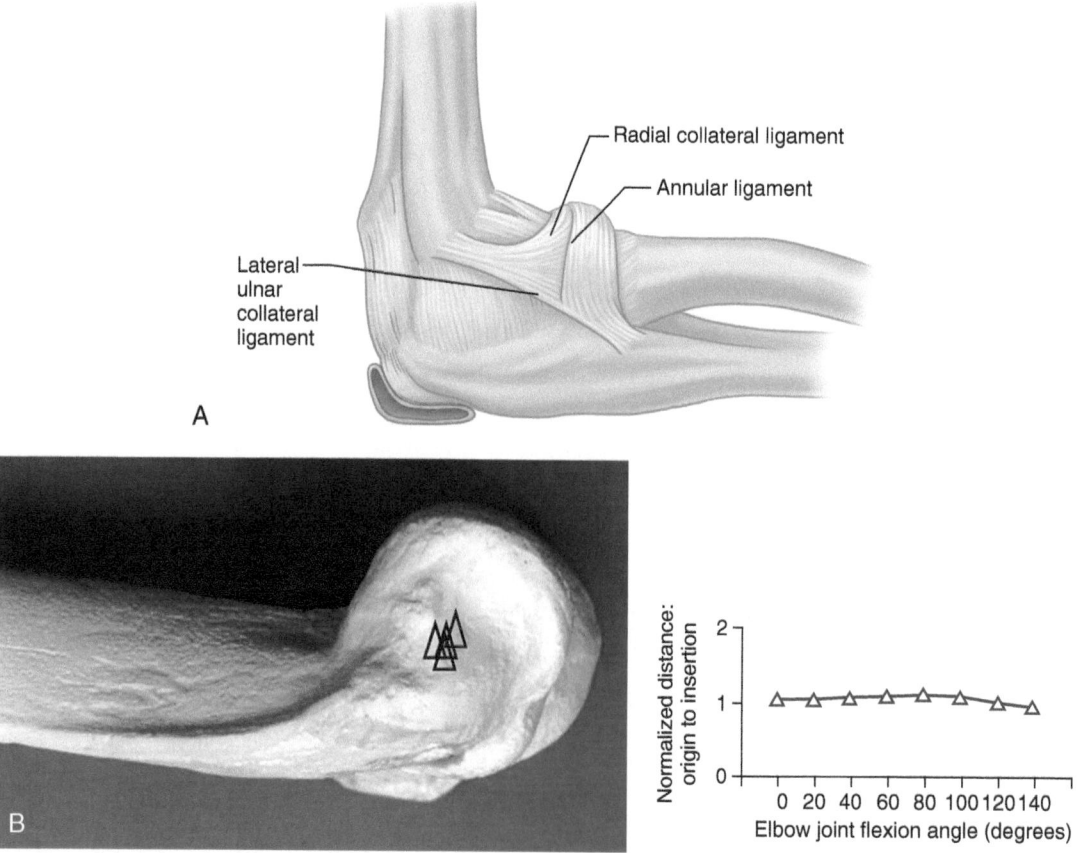

Fig. 57.3 (A) The lateral collateral ligament complex consists not only of the radial collateral ligament but also a lateral ulnar collateral ligament. (B) With flexion, no change occurs in the length of the radial collateral ligament complex, which suggests that the origin is at the axis of rotation. (Courtesy the Mayo Foundation.)

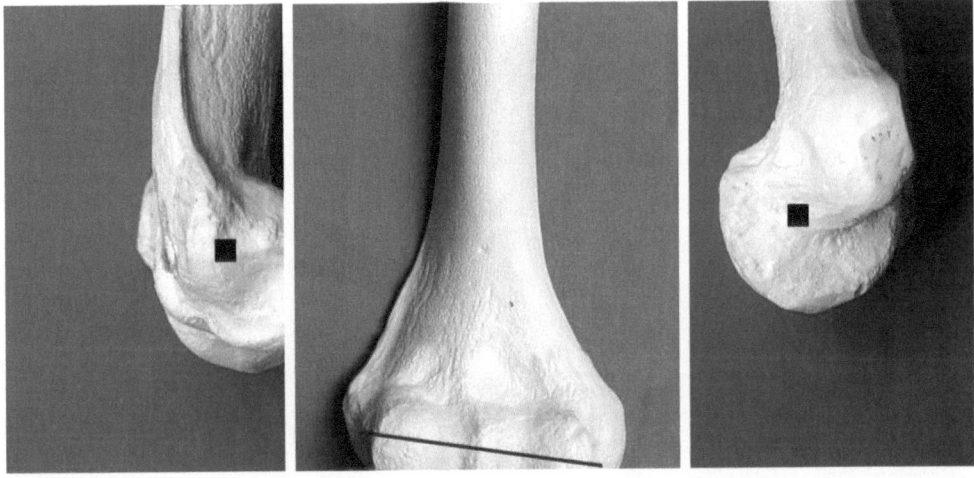

Fig. 57.4 The axis of rotation of the elbow is approximated by a line running through the middle of the lateral epicondyle and the center of the trochlea, emerging on the anterior inferior aspect of the medial epicondyle.

rotation runs from the center of the radial head to the fovea of the ulnar head.[22,23] Ligamentous deficiency is to some degree offset or altered by forearm position; supination may help stabilize the UCL-deficient elbow, whereas pronation can add stability to an elbow with LCL insufficiency.[24,25]

Motion Loss

There are a myriad of causes for elbow stiffness. A loss of flexion may be caused by bony impingement of the radial head or coronoid process against their respective fossae, loose bodies in the anterior capsule, or posterior capsular tightness.[7] Extension may be limited because of posterior osteophyte impingement or anterior capsular tightness, although a mild flexion contracture is an adaptive variation of normal in the dominant throwing arm of many athletes.[26] Numerous studies have examined the question of what constitutes "functional range of motion."[27] Morrey et al.[28] noted that most activities of daily living, such as grooming, feeding, and bathing, could be performed with a total elbow flexion arc of 100 degrees (30 to 130 degrees) and a forearm rotation arc of 100 degrees, with 50 degrees each of both pronation and supination. More recently, Sardelli et al.[29] noted that the use of cell phones requires greater elbow flexion, whereas use of computer keyboards requires more forearm pronation than may have been previously appreciated.

Joint Stability
Osteoarticular Stability

Distal humeral articular anatomy. The distal humerus is composed of two articular surfaces, named the capitellum and the trochlea. The capitellum articulates with radial head in the lateral aspect of the joint. The capitellar shape is hemispherical, accommodating the concave elliptical nature of the radial head. The trochlea is often described as spool-shaped. It angles slightly posteriorly to minimize posterior translation when engaged by the coronoid.[30]

Coronoid process. The coronoid of the proximal ulna is critical to elbow stability.[31] It is composed of anteromedial and anterolateral facets, a body and tip. Given that the tip of the

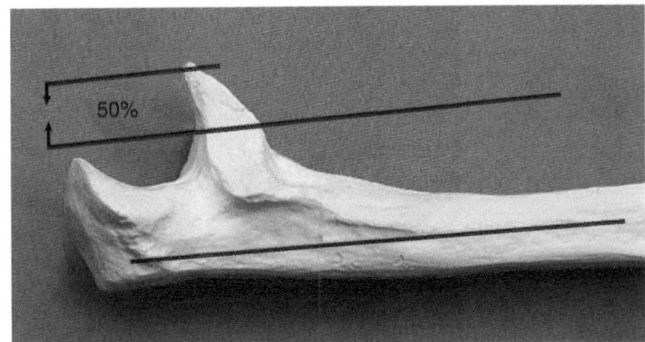

Fig. 57.5 Absence of 50% of the coronoid is estimated by drawing a line from the olecranon tip to the coronoid release. The line is parallel to the shaft at the 50% level.

coronoid is devoid of soft tissue attachments, fractures tend to be secondary to shear and/or axial loading.[3,32] Located on the anteromedial facet is the sublime tubercle to which the aUCL inserts. Studies have shown that fractures involving more than 50% of the coronoid (Fig. 57.5) are associated with increased instability at the elbow in extension.[3,33,34] In addition, in conjunction with the radial head, the coronoid is important for posterolateral stability.[35] Approximately 30% to 40% of the coronoid may be removed without consequent ulnohumeral instability; further resection of the coronoid process, particularly in the setting of concomitant fracture of the radial head, will consistently lead to posterior dislocation.[36] The coronoid is also important for varus stability in conjunction with an intact LCL complex.[37]

Radial head. The radial head is an important secondary static stabilizer of the elbow, particularly under valgus load.[16,38] In this regard, its importance is increased in the setting of UCL insufficiency (Fig. 57.6).[39] Posterolateral rotatory instability may manifest after isolated radial head resection, most likely because of diminished tension on the LCL complex or concurrent injury to the LUCL itself.[40] Furthermore, radial head deficiency in the setting of accompanying interosseous membrane disruption may lead to longitudinal instability, characterized by proximal radial

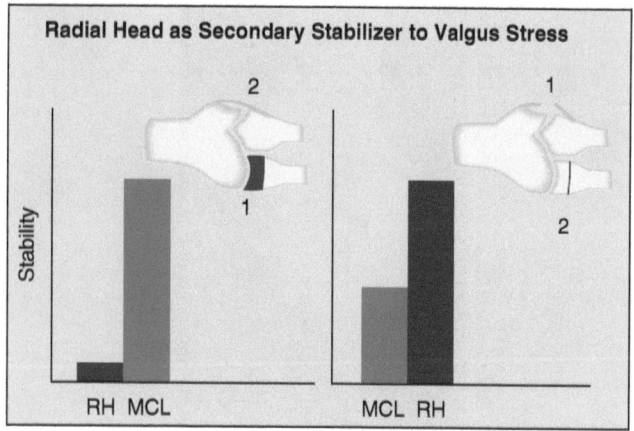

Fig. 57.6 *Left,* Removing the radial head *(RH) (1)* but leaving the medial collateral ligament *(MCL)* intact *(2)* results in no alteration in valgus stability. *Right,* When the MCL is removed first *(1),* the RH is observed to provide some resistance to valgus stress. When both constraints are released *(2),* the elbow is grossly unstable. (Courtesy the Mayo Foundation.)

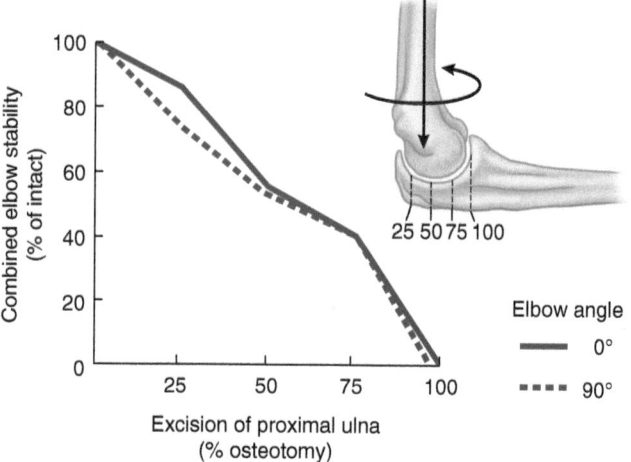

Fig. 57.7 With serial removal of the olecranon, a linear decrease in ulnohumeral stability is observed. Note the 50% loss with 50% resected. (Courtesy the Mayo Foundation.)

head migration, ulnar positive variance, and ulnar-sided wrist pain (Essex-Lopresti injury).

Olecranon process. The olecranon contributes to elbow stability by engaging with the olecranon fossa of the posterior distal humerus as the elbow extends. Not surprisingly, joint contact pressures increase with progressive resection of the olecranon (e.g., as may be performed for a comminuted olecranon fracture).[41] Partial resection of the olecranon may increase coronal plane (varus/valgus) laxity (Fig. 57.7). It has been generically recommended that no more than 50% of the olecranon should be resected, although a recent in vitro study suggested that gross instability does not occur until resection levels greater than 87% are reached.[42] Overhead-throwing athletes may not tolerate larger amounts of olecranon resection over as little as 3 mm because of amplified strain on the UCL with increasing angles of elbow flexion.[43]

Soft Tissue Stability

Ulnar collateral ligament. The aUCL is the primary restraint to valgus force at the elbow.[16,44,45] The anterior band of the aUCL is the primary restraint to valgus loads between 30 and 90 degrees of elbow flexion, and both the posterior and anterior bands function jointly as primary restraints at 120 degrees.[46] The aUCL also has a central band between the anterior and posterior bands that is essentially isometric throughout elbow flexion. With complete release of the aUCL, the elbow is maximally unstable in valgus at 70 degrees of flexion.[3,47] The UCL provides a third of the valgus stability in full extension, compared with half of the stability at 90 degrees of flexion.[30]

As previously mentioned, the UCL has a cam effect during elbow motion. This effect occurs because the ligament complex origin is posterior to the center of rotation, and thus ligament tension has been shown to change throughout the arc of motion, specifically increasing in length when the elbow moves from terminal extension to high angles of flexion.[17]

With an intact MCL, radial head excision does not impart valgus instability to the elbow. If the MCL is additional injured, the joint becomes unstable.

Isolated injury to the posterior bundle of the MCL can lead to posteromedial rotatory instability.

Lateral collateral ligament. Much like its analogous structure at the medial elbow, the LCL complex is the structure primarily responsible for resisting varus stress and external rotation. In contrast to the UCL, the center of rotation passes through the origin of the LCL, ensuring enhanced isometry and the absence of a cam effect.[17] With respect to the annular ligament, the anterior portion is taut during supination, whereas the posterior portion is taut in pronation. O'Driscoll et al.[2] stated that LCL injury is the initial injury in the spectrum of the pathology of elbow dislocations.

The individual anatomic structures of the LCL likely function together as a complex. With an intact annular ligament, both the LUCL and RCL need to be cut to produce gross coronal plane instability or posterolateral rotatory instability.[48] Individual transection of the annular ligament or LUCL produces only minor laxity.[49] In combined injuries with radial head deficiency and LCL complex insufficiency, instability with varus and external rotation forces is more pronounced. Replacement of the radial head restores partial stability, but simultaneous repair or reconstruction of the ligament complex is also necessary in this scenario (Fig. 57.8).[50] In the setting of posterolateral rotatory instability, loads applied across the flexed, supinated elbow can lead to posterior radial head subluxation, lateral elbow pain, and mechanical symptoms.[51]

Experimental in vitro data may be summarized by stating that the articular surfaces provide about 50% of elbow stability and the collateral ligaments provide the remaining 50%. When the elbow is in full extension, the anterior capsule contributes about 15% of the resistance to varus-valgus stress.[10,16]

Muscular contributions and joint reactive forces. Muscles crossing the joint are dynamic stabilizers and are associated with corresponding joint reaction forces.[7] For example, the flexor pronator musculature is consistently active during the throwing

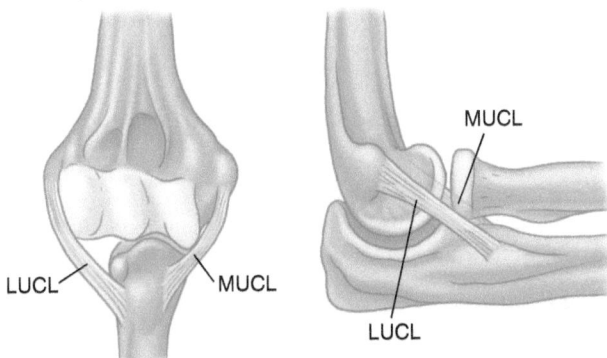

Fig. 57.8 The ulnohumeral joint is stabilized by both medial and lateral constraints, independent of the presence of the radial head. *LUCL,* Lateral ulnar collateral ligament; *MUCL,* medial ulnar collateral ligament. (Courtesy the Mayo Foundation.)

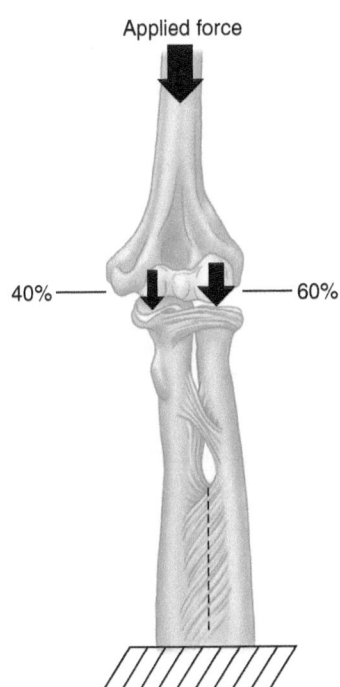

Fig. 57.9 The distributive forces with the elbow in full extension and an axial load placed at the wrist show that about 60% of the force goes across the radiohumeral joint and 40% goes across the ulnohumeral joint; this does not change the section of the interosseous membrane. (Courtesy the Mayo Foundation.)

motion and contributes significantly to the dynamic stability of the elbow, especially if injury to the static restraints has been realized.[1] Evidence of the relative contribution of dynamic muscular stabilization is demonstrated in cadaveric sectioning studies, in which the ultimate tensile failure of the UCL (about 260 N) is less than the tensile forces experienced by the medial elbow during throwing.[44,52] Therefore activation of these muscles provides protection of the static soft tissues. The flexor carpi ulnaris and portions of the flexor digitorum superficialis lie directly over the anterior bundle of the UCL.[53] With the arm relatively extended, approximately 40% of axial load across the elbow joint is experienced at the ulnohumeral joint, with almost 60% of the force transmitted across the radiocapitellar joint (Fig. 57.9).[54] Force transmission across the radial head is greatest in the 0- to 30-degree arc and is also larger with forearm pronation. Absence of the radial head results in higher forces at the ulnotrochlear joint, which is enhanced further in the setting of collateral ligament insufficiency.

The throwing cycle. Knowledge of the throwing cycle aids practitioners who evaluate and treat overhead-throwing athletes with elbow pathology. The overhead-throwing motion can be broken down into six phases: (1) windup, (2) early cocking, (3) late cocking, (4) acceleration, (5) deceleration, and (6) follow-through.[1,55–57] Medial tensile forces and lateral compression forces are generated at the elbow during the late cocking and acceleration phases, whereas deceleration causes high shear stress, especially in the posterior compartment. Biomechanical testing has estimated valgus forces as high as 64 N · m at the elbow during the late cocking and early acceleration phases of throwing, with compressive forces of 500 N at the lateral radiocapitellar articulation as the elbow moves from approximately 110 to 20 degrees of flexion with angular velocities as high as 3000 degrees per second. This combination of large valgus loads and rapid elbow extension produces high tensile stress medially along the soft tissue restraints (UCL, flexor-pronator mass, medial epicondylar apophysis, and ulnar nerve), along with compression stress laterally (radiocapitellar joint) and shear stress in the posterior compartment (posteromedial tip of the olecranon, trochlea, and olecranon fossa). This phenomenon has been termed *valgus extension overload syndrome* and forms the basic pathophysiologic

model explaining the mechanism for the most common elbow injuries in the overhead-throwing athlete.

More recently, the link between shoulder and elbow mechanics—as it relates to the overhead athlete—is becoming clearer. Elbow injuries requiring surgery in throwing athletes have been associated with decreased total shoulder rotation, as well as decreased shoulder forward flexion.[58] Furthermore, Anand et al. found that UCL insufficiency was associated with significant changes in contact area, contact pressure, and valgus laxity—during both relative flexion (such as the late cocking/early acceleration phase) as well as relative extension (deceleration phase) moments during the throwing motion arc.[59]

The anterior bundle of the UCL is the primary restraint to valgus force of the elbow from 20 to 120 degrees of flexion and is subjected to near failure during the acceleration phase of the throwing motion. Repetitive loads near tensile failure result in microtrauma to the anterior band of the UCL and may eventually lead to ligament attenuation or rupture. Continued valgus and extension forces combined with subtle laxity are ingredients for further pathologic deterioration of the thrower's elbow.

For a complete list of references, go to ExpertConsult.com.

SELECTED READINGS

Citation:
Cain EL Jr, Dugas JR. History and examination of the thrower's elbow. *Clin Sports Med.* 2004;23(4):553–566.

Level of Evidence:
V

Summary:

This excellent review article highlights the basic history and examination of the elbow in overhead-throwing athletes.

Citation:

O'Driscoll SW, Jupiter JB, King GJ, et al. The unstable elbow. *Instr Course Lect.* 2001;50:89–102.

Level of Evidence:

V

Summary:

This comprehensive review article covers the diagnosis and treatment of acute injuries to the elbow.

Citation:

Morrey BF. Applied anatomy and biomechanics of the elbow joint. *Instr Course Lect.* 1986;35:59–68.

Level of Evidence:

V

Summary:

This thorough review addresses the biomechanics and anatomy of the elbow.

Citation:

Morrey BF, An KN. Articular and ligamentous contributions to the stability of the elbow joint. *Am J Sports Med.* 1983;11(5):315–319.

Level of Evidence:

V

Summary:

This article describes a basic science study regarding the articular and ligamentous stability of the elbow.

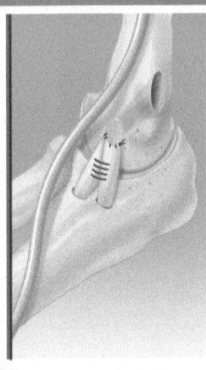

58

Elbow Diagnosis and Decision-Making

Nicholas J. Clark, Bassem T. Elhassan

OVERVIEW OF PATHOLOGIES

The key to diagnosing elbow injuries involves performing a thorough history and physical examination of the elbow. Additionally, to rule out referred pain, the surrounding areas such as the cervical spine, shoulder, wrist, and hand should also be examined. This chapter discusses the elements of a complete elbow history and physical examination, which would include inspection, palpation, range of motion (ROM), strength, neurologic assessment, joint stability testing, and various provocative maneuvers to help identify and characterize different disorders around the athlete's elbow.

Owing to the wide variety of elbow pathologies, a systematic approach is necessary to diagnose the disorders accurately. A helpful strategy is to divide the elbow into four anatomic regions: lateral, medial, anterior, and posterior. This strategy enables the examiner to narrow the range of the differential diagnosis. In addition, knowing the patient's athletic history and any previous history of injury can help focus decision-making regarding treatment.

Pathologic conditions that are present around the lateral aspect of the elbow include lateral epicondylitis, radial nerve compression neuropathies, osteochondritis dissecans (OCD) of the capitellum, posterolateral rotatory instability, and radiocapitellar arthritis. Symptoms arising from the medial aspect of the elbow include medial epicondylitis, cubital tunnel syndrome, flexor-pronator strain, and medial (ulnar) collateral ligament injury. The differential diagnoses for anterior elbow pain include median nerve compression neuropathies, distal biceps tendinopathy, partial or complete distal biceps tendon ruptures, and an anterior capsular strain from a hyperextension injury. Conditions causing symptoms at the posterior elbow include olecranon bursitis; olecranon stress fracture; posteromedial impingement syndrome, such as a valgus extension overload as seen in overhead-throwing athletes; triceps tendinopathy; or a triceps rupture.

HISTORY

Athletes typically present with pain, mechanical symptoms, and a compromised ability to play. The pain may be exacerbated by activity and relieved with rest, or it can be persistent with daily routines. It is therefore helpful to localize the athlete's symptoms into one of the four anatomic regions previously described.

Lateral Elbow

Symptoms involving the lateral elbow are typically related to lateral epicondylitis, radial nerve compression neuropathies, OCD lesion of the capitellum, posterolateral rotatory instability, and/or radiocapitellar arthritis.

Lateral epicondylitis, often known as "tennis elbow," is caused by tendinosis and inflammation at the origin of the extensor carpi radialis brevis (ECRB). Patients often present with a "burning" pain that radiates from the lateral epicondyle distally along the extensor muscles of the forearm. This pain is intensified by a combination of elbow extension, resisted wrist extension, and a tight grip. Eccentric loading during these combined maneuvers, as seen when hitting a backhand late in tennis or catching a golf swing "fat" (i.e., striking the ground before the ball), may trigger the symptoms associated with lateral epicondylitis.

Sharp pain in the lateral aspect of the elbow associated with locking or catching can result from loose bodies in the radiocapitellar joint or an OCD lesion of the capitellum. Patients at risk for OCD lesions include young overhead throwers and gymnasts. Young overhead throwers develop OCD lesions as an overuse injury from increased compression and shear forces during the late cocking phase of throwing across the radiocapitellar articulation. The radiocapitellar joint also experiences 60% of axial load placed across the elbow, which can cause OCD lesions in gymnasts after repetitive loading.[1] These patients often report an insidious onset of symptoms with limitation of elbow motion, particularly elbow extension.[2] Mechanical symptoms involving the elbow are often found in patients with radiocapitellar arthritis, with symptoms most severe at extremes of elbow motion.

Radial nerve compression syndromes include compression neuropathies involving the posterior interosseous nerve (PIN) and radial tunnel syndrome (RTS). PIN syndrome is characterized by a pure motor loss of extension of the thumb and fingers. This syndrome is exceptionally uncommon in athletes in the absence of a mass in the region of the radial neck, prolonged compression as seen in the "Saturday night palsy," or Parsonage-Turner syndrome. RTS is also quite uncommon. It is characterized by pain that is exacerbated with activity and commonly located in the extensor mobile wad and proximal lateral forearm. Throwing athletes may experience this pain at the end of follow through. Symptoms of posterolateral rotatory instability usually follow a history of prior elbow dislocation in an athlete. Complaints include lateral-sided elbow pain, snapping, locking, subjective instability, and recurrent elbow dislocation.

Medial Elbow

Complaints localized to the medial aspect of the elbow may result from cubital tunnel syndrome, medial epicondylitis, and medial (ulnar) collateral ligament injury.

Paresthesias radiating along the medial portion of the forearm to the ring and small finger are typical of cubital tunnel syndrome. Patients often complain of nocturnal symptoms or symptoms exacerbated by prolonged elbow flexion. Popping or snapping along the medial aspect of the elbow may result from a subluxating ulnar nerve or movement of the medial head of the triceps after ulnar nerve transposition.

Medial epicondylitis, also known as "golfer's elbow," is also found in racquet sports and baseball. It is associated with a history of repetitive forceful forearm pronation or wrist flexion. In golfers, it typically involves the dominant arm. A single "fat" shot leading to eccentric loading of the flexor-pronator mass or repetitive loading of the elbow can lead to disruption of the flexor pronator origin, with ischemia and development of angiofibroblastic hyperplasia.[3] Medial epicondylitis has been associated with ulnar nerve symptoms in up to 60% of cases.[4]

Athletes who throw and sustain an isolated acute medial collateral ligament injury will frequently describe a pop, sharp pain, and the inability to continue pitching or throwing. Insidious medial elbow pain with associated loss of velocity and control in throwing athletes are signs of chronic medial collateral ligament injury. Medial elbow discomfort in the setting of acute elbow trauma from higher-energy mechanisms can relate to disruption of the medial collateral ligament. These patients typically have associated injuries, such as radial head fracture, capitellum fracture, or dislocation. Throwing athletes with flexor-pronator strains have a history similar to that of medial collateral ligament injury.

Anterior Elbow

Athletes may present with anterior elbow pain for a number of reasons, including partial or complete distal biceps rupture, distal biceps tendinosis, median nerve compression neuropathies such as pronator or anterior interosseous nerve (AIN) syndrome, and anterior capsular strains.

Distal biceps tendon ruptures are most often reported with a traumatic event involving an unexpected extension force applied to the flexed arm that can occur in weight lifting, rugby, or football. A history of anabolic steroid use is helpful, as this is a significant risk factor for tendon ruptures, most notably in the upper extremity.[5] A distal biceps rupture is usually associated with a pop followed by pain and weakness in the upper extremity. The intense pain recedes quickly, as does the initial weakness of elbow flexion. Patients are usually left with weakness in forearm supination and, rarely, cramping in the arm. Distal biceps tendinosis is associated with anterior elbow pain that is more pronounced with repetitive forearm supination and resisted elbow flexion.

Pronator syndrome is a rare condition that results most commonly from compression of the median nerve as it passes between the two heads of the pronator teres. There are other locations of potential compression; these are described later in the chapter. Patients present with aching pain in the proximal volar forearm and paresthesias radiating into the radial side of the hand, namely the thumb to the radial border of the ring finger. Symptoms may worsen with repetitive forearm rotation as well. AIN syndrome is a pure motor palsy with symptoms found distally in the hand. However, patients may have a vague achy discomfort in the anterior elbow associated with median nerve compression at that level.

Posterior Elbow

Athletes may experience posterior elbow pain due to olecranon bursitis, a stress fracture, posteromedial impingement syndrome (e.g., valgus extension overload syndrome), triceps tendinosis, and triceps tendon rupture. Olecranon bursitis typically occurs after either a single traumatic episode or with repetitive pressure or a shearing force on the apex of the elbow. Olecranon stress fractures are seen most often in gymnasts, athletes who throw, and weight lifters (Fig. 58.1). These athletes present with reports of posterior elbow pain, loss of terminal extension, and in some cases elbow clicking or catching.

Posteromedial impingement syndrome (e.g., valgus extension overload syndrome) is nearly exclusive to throwing athletes who

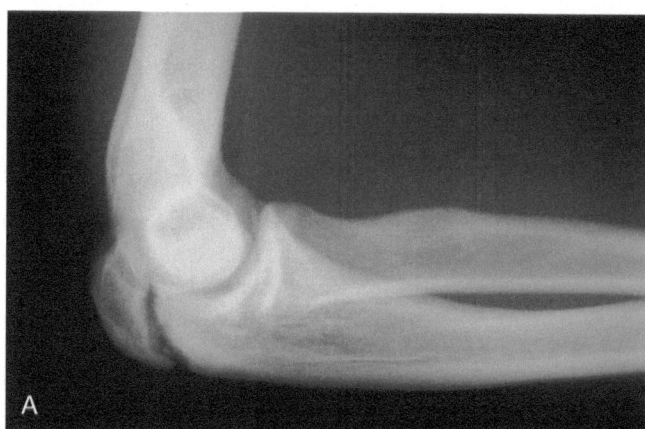
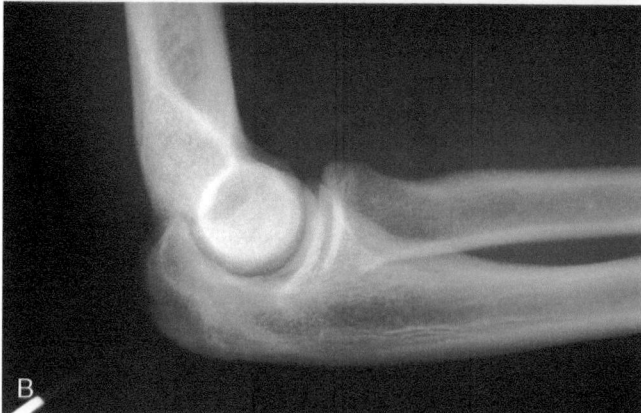

Fig. 58.1 An olecranon stress fracture. Radiographs of a college gymnast who presented with posterior elbow pain are shown. (A) The symptomatic side. (B) The contralateral extremity is shown for comparison.

report pain at the posteromedial aspect of the elbow during the follow-through phase while reaching terminal elbow extension. This is usually secondary to posterior olecranon osteophytes impinging in the fossa at the terminal extension phase.

Patients who have triceps tendinopathy have pain with elbow extension, especially against resistance. An athlete with a distal triceps tendon rupture will often recall a specific traumatic event during resisted elbow extension, followed by intense pain and significant weakness.[6] Rupture may occur with minimal trauma in patients who use anabolic steroids.[5]

Overall, elbow injuries are most commonly found in throwing athletes. The American Academy of Orthopaedic Surgeons (AAOS) reports that 50% to 75% of adolescent baseball players report episodes of elbow pain during play. In taking a history, especially from a throwing athlete, it is important to determine when symptoms occur in the throwing phase. Medial-sided symptoms usually occur during the late acceleration and cocking phase compared with posterior elbow symptoms, which occur during the deceleration and follow-through phase.

PHYSICAL EXAMINATION

For a diagnostic test to be clinically useful, it must be easily performed, reliable, reproducible, and have high sensitivity and specificity. In evaluating elbow injuries, a combination of inspection, palpation, ROM, strength, stability, neurologic assessment, and other provocative maneuvers will assist in the development of a working diagnosis.

Inspection

Inspection is the initial step of the physical examination of the elbow and, if possible, should include a comparison of the injured side with the uninjured side. During inspection, the physician should assess the skin and soft tissue envelope for signs of acute injury such as ecchymosis, swelling, deformity, abnormal muscle contour, and chronic changes such as muscle hypertrophy or atrophy.

During inspection, a measurement of the carrying angle is useful, especially for throwing athletes. The carrying angle of the elbow is the angle between the axis of the humerus and the axis of the forearm measured with the elbow extended and the forearm maximally supinated (the anatomic position) in the coronal plane. Typically, the angle is 7 to 13 degrees of valgus.[7] Paraskevas et al.[8] found that the mean carrying angle of the general population is almost 13 degrees, with men averaging 2 degrees less and women 2 degrees more. The increased angle in women has been attributed to increased joint laxity in women compared with men. Variations in the carrying angle can be due to previous trauma, injury, developmental abnormality, or adaptive changes to repetitive stress.[8,9] In professional throwers, it is common to see carrying angles greater than 15 degrees.[10] Fick submitted the "muscle theory," which accounts for the greater carrying angle in athletes who throw. This theory hypothesizes that the increased strength of the brachioradialis and extensor carpi radialis longus in athletes who throw will cause a greater radial deviation in extension and thus a greater carrying angle. It has also been hypothesized that an increased amount of stress on

the elbow joint in athletes who throw may lead to increased laxity of the joint, which also contributes to a greater carrying angle.

When evaluating patients for atrophy or hypertrophy of muscles of the arm or forearm, girth measurements compared with the contralateral side are useful when appropriate. Hypertrophy of the forearm musculature is often present in the dominant extremity of many types of athletes. Atrophy of the arm and forearm muscle may also indicate disuse because of chronic discomfort or an underlying neurologic disorder.

Palpation

It is important to start with palpation of asymptomatic areas first while progressively moving toward the symptomatic area. Additionally, the physician must understand the qualitative aspect of this portion of the examination and use maneuvers while palpating to understand what exacerbates or relieves symptoms.

Lateral Elbow

Beginning with the lateral elbow, the bony prominences should be palpated, including the lateral epicondyle, radial head, and olecranon process. The radiocapitellar joint line should also be palpated for tenderness. Based on the history, point tenderness of the lateral epicondyle in the setting of trauma can be indicative of lateral collateral ligament disruption.

Tenderness due to lateral epicondylitis may be palpated just anterior and distal to the lateral epicondyle at the ECRB origination and may extend distally from the lateral epicondyle for several centimeters along the common extensor origin. Pain associated with lateral epicondylitis is generally worsened by elbow extension with resisted wrist extension and a clenched fist. Additionally, grip strength decreases in the affected extremity, most notably in elbow extension, and is one of the few objective measures for diagnosing lateral epicondylitis. Dorf described testing grip strength while the elbow was flexed and extended. An 8% difference between flexion and extension grip strength was 83% accurate for diagnosing lateral epicondylitis.[11]

Pain with pressure directly over the radiocapitellar joint, especially when combined with active pronosupination of the forearm with axial loading in midrange elbow flexion (e.g., active radiocapitellar compression test), is indicative of radiocapitellar pathology.[12] In the middle-aged adult patient, point tenderness at the posterolateral elbow points more to radiocapitellar arthritis, although it may be more indicative of an OCD lesion in adolescent patients. These patients often have an effusion over the radiocapitellar joint.

Next, the "soft spot" over the anconeus can be palpated at the center of a triangle drawn between the olecranon, lateral epicondyle, and radial head. An effusion in that area can present with fullness over the soft spot and should raise suspicion for an underlying injury.

Local, vague tenderness in the region of the proximal lateral forearm, especially along the course of the PIN, is more consistent with the diagnosis of RTS versus PIN syndrome and is explained in more detail later in this chapter.

Medial Elbow

Palpation of the medial elbow begins with the medial epicondyle. Tenderness associated with medial epicondylitis is often located on the anteromedial facet of the medial epicondyle where the pronator teres and flexor carpi radialis originate. The involvement of the pronator origin can be isolated by palpating the proximal third of the medial epicondyle while resisting forearm pronation. The flexor carpi ulnaris origin is isolated by palpating the distal third of the medial epicondyle with resisted flexion and ulnar deviation.

The medial (ulnar) collateral ligament is best palpated when the elbow is flexed to 50 to 70 degrees, which anteriorly translates the medial muscles. Tenderness associated with medial collateral ligament tear will be along the course of the ligament either at the origin on the medial epicondyle or at the insertion on the sublime tubercle of the proximal ulna. The ulnar nerve can be palpated directly beneath the medial epicondyle (as described later in this chapter).

Anterior Elbow

Palpation of the anterior elbow begins in the antecubital fossa, where multiple soft tissue structures can be palpated: the distal biceps tendon, brachioradialis, lacertus fibrosus, brachialis, and pronator teres. Distal biceps tendon pathology is the most common source of anterior elbow pain in the athlete, and the tendon is readily palpable in the antecubital fossa with the elbow supinated. The hook test or biceps squeeze test can be performed to assist in the diagnosis of distal biceps tendon rupture; these tests are detailed later in this chapter.[13,14] Tenderness along the distal extent of the tendon with resisted supination in the face of an intact tendon suggests pain from distal biceps tendinosis.

Median nerve compression neuropathies, specifically pronator syndrome, can cause anterior elbow and forearm pain with palpation. Deep palpation or the Tinel test of the median nerve in the antecubital fossa can elicit pain in the proximal forearm and elbow, but median nerve symptoms would also be expected distally in the hand (as discussed later in this chapter).

Posterior Elbow

Palpation of the posterior elbow involves palpating the triceps tendon and the olecranon process. When the elbow is flexed to approximately 30 degrees, the triceps is relaxed, allowing for easier access to the medial and lateral gutters of the posterior compartment. Fullness in these regions is consistent with an intra-articular inflammatory process. Tenderness on the medial or lateral aspect of the trochlea can be seen in association with spurs on the posterior aspect of the distal humerus. Pain with terminal extension can be seen with spurs on the tip of the olecranon process. Boxers can fracture the tip of the olecranon process, particularly in their nondominant elbow, during a jab. Tenderness from this type of fracture may be elicited at the apex of the olecranon process with the elbow slightly flexed.

Pain elicited along the posteromedial aspect of the olecranon in overhead-throwing athletes should immediately warrant a focused exam for posteromedial impingement syndrome. It is also important to carefully evaluate the integrity of the medial collateral ligament because there is an association between medial collateral ligament injury and posteromedial impingement syndrome. The extension impingement and arm bar test are sensitive

physical exam maneuvers that can be used (as discussed later in this chapter).

A palpable defect in the triceps just proximal to the tip of the olecranon is indicative of triceps tendon rupture. Complete ruptures typically involve the posterior superficial portion of the tendon, which is made up of the long and lateral heads of the triceps. This leaves the deep anterior portion of the tendon, which is composed of the medial head of the triceps, intact.

Motion

The normal arc of flexion-extension ranges from 0 to 140 degrees, ±10 degrees.[15] Loss of terminal extension is common in athletes with elbow pathology. Greater variation is found in the pronation-supination arc than in the flexion-extension arc; however, approximately 75 degrees of pronation and 85 degrees of supination are considered to be within normal ranges.[15] The arc of motion required for daily activities ranges from 30 to 130 degrees of flexion-extension and 50 degrees of pronosupination in each direction.[16] Depending on the sport, loss of terminal extension may create a significant impairment. It is important to note at which point in the arc of motion that pain or mechanical symptoms occur because this information may provide clues to the diagnosis.

Neurologic Assessment

The neurologic examination includes an assessment of skin appearance and texture, muscle bulk, strength, sensation, reflexes, and provocative maneuvers for nerve compression. Loss of skin texture and abnormal sweat patterns on the finger pads are signs of significant sensory denervation. Similarly, loss of muscle bulk follows motor denervation or limb disuse.

Elbow flexion strength is best tested with the elbow flexed 90 degrees and the forearm in neutral rotation. The contribution of flexion strength from the brachialis is disproportionate compared with the biceps. The brachialis inserts onto the anterior surface of the coronoid, which causes its line of pull to remain constant regardless of the position of the hand or wrist. This is in contrast to the biceps, which attaches onto the radial tuberosity and then contributes to both flexion and supination. Additionally, the brachialis is positioned closer to the axis of the elbow joint increasing its mechanical advantage compared to the biceps.

Triceps strength is demonstrated by extension of the elbow with and without the aid of gravity and then against increasing resistance. To eliminate the aid of gravity, the patient should be asked to extend the elbow while in the supine position with the arm forward flexed to 90 degrees and the elbow in 90 degrees of flexion (Fig. 58.2). Triceps strength is assessed with resisted elbow extension starting with the elbow in 100 degrees of flexion, which will assess the lateral and middle heads of the triceps. To isolate the medial head of the triceps, the examiner should have the patient place his or her affected hand on the examiner's shoulder with the elbow extended. The examiner then places his or her hands over the patient's antecubital fossa and attempts to flex the patient's elbow while the patient resists the motion. This will isolate the medial head of the triceps.

Pronation and supination are best evaluated with the elbow at 90 degrees of flexion and the forearm starting in neutral

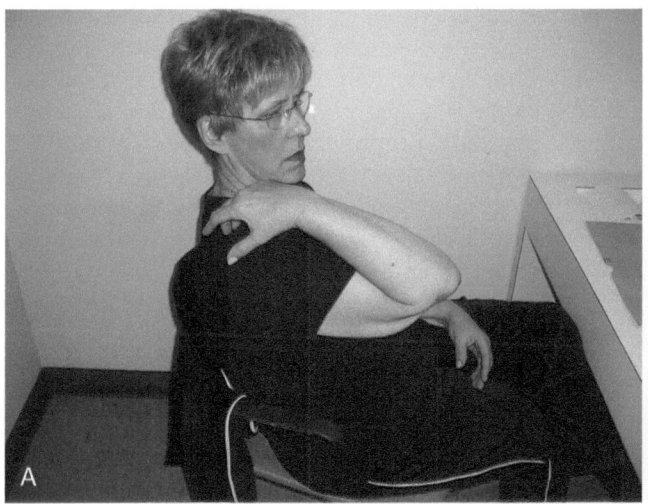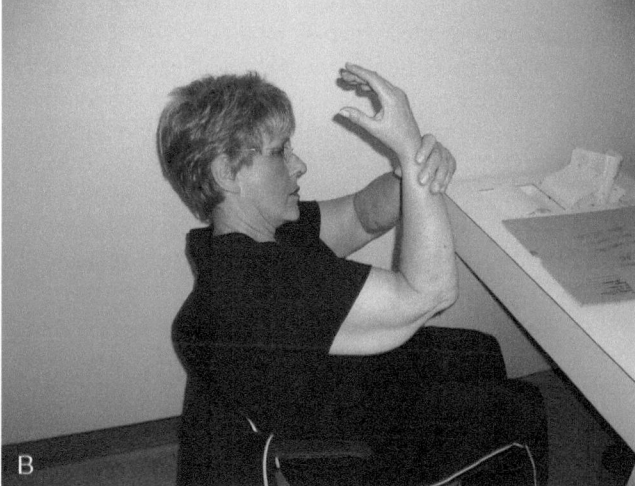

Fig. 58.2 Triceps insufficiency. Triceps function may be first demonstrated by having the patient attempt to extend the elbow against gravity. This maneuver is performed with the patient sitting and the humerus held perpendicular to the torso during elbow extension. The patient was unable to actively extend the elbow (A), although passive extension was possible (B), effectively indicating triceps insufficiency.

rotation. Although not an absolute rule, the dominant extremity has been shown to be approximately 10% stronger than the nondominant extremity.[17,18]

Sensation may be tested by lightly touching the patient in either the dermatomal or peripheral nerve distributions of the hand and forearm. Any decrease in light touch perception or difference from the contralateral side should raise suspicion for neurologic compromise.

COMPRESSION NEUROPATHIES AT THE ELBOW

Tests to detect potential compression neuropathy should also be performed when clinical suspicion is high based on the history and description of symptoms.

Ulnar Nerve Compression (Cubital Tunnel Syndrome)

Cubital tunnel syndrome is one of the most common compression neuropathies of the upper extremity, occurring in 1.8% of the population.[19] Various physical exam maneuvers can be performed to help with diagnostic decision-making. The Tinel test is performed by tapping a nerve (mixed peripheral or cutaneous) over a suspected area of compression or compromise (Fig. 58.3). The test is considered positive if paresthesias are produced in the distribution of the nerve in question.

The ulnar nerve is palpated posterior to the medial epicondyle as it travels through the cubital tunnel and distally into the flexor carpi ulnaris muscle mass. A painful snapping sensation can occur in two situations during elbow flexion: subluxation of the ulnar nerve and subluxation of the medial head of the triceps, with the latter typically occurring after ulnar nerve transposition. However, ulnar nerve hypermobility is present in up to one-third of the general population, with the vast majority of these individuals remaining asymptomatic from this phenomenon.[20]

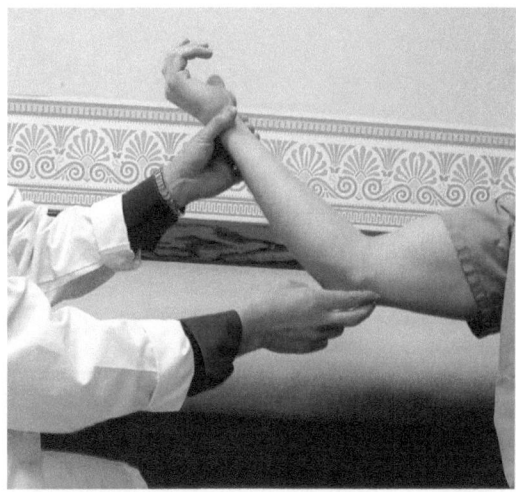

Fig. 58.3 The Tinel test is performed by tapping a nerve over the suspected area of compression or nerve irritation. The test is considered positive if it produces paresthesias in the areas of the nerve's typical distribution.

In addition to the Tinel test, ulnar nerve irritability may be elicited by prolonged maximal elbow flexion, direct pressure at the cubital tunnel, or a combination of the two (elbow flexion-pressure test). Multiple studies have evaluated the sensitivity, specificity, positive predictive value (PPV), and negative predictive value (NPV) for these maneuvers.[21-23] The sensitivity, specificity, PPV, and NPV for a Tinel test at the elbow ranges from 54% to 70%, 53% to 99%, 77% to 97%, and 30% to 98%, respectively.[21-23] The sensitivity, specificity, PPV and NPV for the elbow flexion-pressure maneuver ranges from 46% to 98%, 40% to 99%, 72% to 96%, and 29% to 99%, respectively.[21-23]

The scratch collapse test has also proved to be sensitive and accurate as a provocative maneuver for the diagnosis of cubital tunnel syndrome. In this test, the examiner scratches the patient's skin lightly over the area of nerve compression while the patient performs sustained resisted external rotation of the shoulder bilaterally.[23] Brief loss of muscle resistance will be elicited as a result of nerve-related allodynia. This test does not rely on the patient's report of symptoms but rather provides a more objective evaluation compared with most other examination maneuvers. The scratch collapse test has shown significantly higher sensitivity (69%) than the Tinel test (54%) and the elbow flexion-pressure test (46%) and has an overall accuracy approaching 90% for the diagnosis of cubital tunnel syndrome.[23]

Overall, provocative maneuvers are an essential clinical tool in assisting in the diagnosis of cubital tunnel syndrome. However, the examiner should still be aware that there can be up to a 34% false-positive rate, which was shown in a cohort of asymptomatic individuals with positive elbow flexion and the Tinel sign.[24]

Chronic ulnar nerve compression can result in the development of intrinsic muscle weakness and atrophy (commonly seen in the first dorsal web space). Many characteristic signs of chronic ulnar nerve compression can be found distally in the hand, including the "claw hand," and the Wartenberg, Froment, Masse, and Jeanne signs. The most notable of the chronic signs is clawing of the hand, which is synonymous with the terms *intrinsic minus position* and *the Duchenne sign* (Fig. 58.4). Nevertheless, all these descriptive eponyms describing paralysis of both the lumbrical and interosseous muscles point to an imbalance between the extensors and flexors of the digits. With loss of intrinsic muscle function to the digits, the extensor digitorum communis is unopposed at the metacarpalphalangeal joint, leading to extension at the joint. Additionally, the flexor digitorum superficialis and profundus are no longer opposed by the intrinsics, which causes proximal and distal interphalangeal joint flexion. Clawing is most

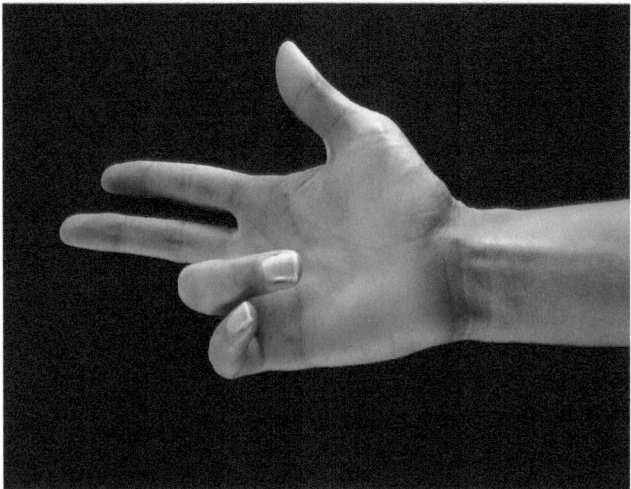

Fig. 58.4 Intrinsic minus or clawing of hand. This condition is caused by compression of the ulnar nerve leading to paralysis of the interossei muscles of the hand and the ulnar two lumbricals. The extensor digitorum comminus (EDC) is then unopposed at the metacarpophalangeal (MCP) joint causing MCP joint extension. The flexor digitorum superficialis (FDS) and flexor digitorum profundus (FDP) are also unopposed leading to flexion at the proximal interphalangeal (PIP) and distal interphalangeal (DIP) joints. Clawing caused by ulnar nerve compression is generally limited to the ring and small fingers as the first and second lumbricals are innervated by the median nerve.

commonly limited to the ring and small fingers and is associated with ulnar nerve lesions that are distal to the innervation of the flexor digitorum profundus to the fourth and fifth digits. Clawing in the index and long fingers is uncommon because of the median nerve's contribution to the lumbrical muscles of those digits. The Masse sign is a flattening of the palmar arch due to hypothenar muscle paralysis and results in a loss of tone across the transverse metacarpal arch. The Wartenberg sign presents as a fixed ulnar deviation and extension of the small finger at rest, with weakness of active adduction. This is secondary to unopposed extensor digiti quinti function, or a weak third palmar interosseous muscle. The Froment sign is a compensatory flexion by the flexor pollicis longus at the interphalangeal joint during key pinch secondary to a weak adductor pollicis brevis. If there is an associated hyperextension of the thumb metacarpophalangeal joint with weakness of thumb adduction, it is called the Jeanne sign.[25]

Radial Nerve Compression Neuropathies

Radial nerve compression neuropathies that occur around the elbow include PIN syndrome and RTS.

Proximal compression of the superficial sensory branch of the radial nerve, also known as Wartenberg syndrome, occurs as the branch courses from a deep to superficial structure along the brachioradialis. Patients usually present with dorsoradial hand and forearm pain with sensory loss except in the elbow.

In assessing PIN compression syndromes, the physician must understand the clinical differences between PIN syndrome and RTS. RTS is a painful condition localized to the proximal lateral forearm, whereas PIN syndrome is a pure motor palsy. Although they are clinically different, both syndromes involve compression of the PIN and other common sites of compression.

Radial Tunnel Syndrome

Roles and Maudsley[26] described maneuvers that elicited pain in a cohort of 36 patients with RTS who were believed to have "resistant" tennis elbow. They most commonly provoked symptoms with resisted supination, wrist extension, and middle finger extension. Traction on the radial nerve can also be maximized by extending the elbow in pronation and flexing the wrist. Palpation of the radial tunnel, located 3 to 5 cm distal to the lateral epicondyle, can elicit pain. This can be performed by using the rule-of-nine test described by Loh,[27] which consists of drawing a square over the anterior portion of the proximal forearm (Fig. 58.5) measured as the width of the elbow crease with the elbow fully extended and fully supinated. This measured width will then serve as the length distally as well. The square is then further subdivided into nine squares, with three columns and three rows. The nine squares are then numbered one to three from proximal to distal in the lateral, middle, and medial columns. The authors found that the nerve was present in the proximal two boxes in the lateral column on all specimens studied. Therefore tenderness over the lateral boxes during palpation indicates irritation consistent with RTS. The other boxes serve as controls, and no tenderness should be noted over these areas.

To help distinguish RTS from lateral epicondylitis, a local anesthetic and/or corticosteroid may be injected along the course

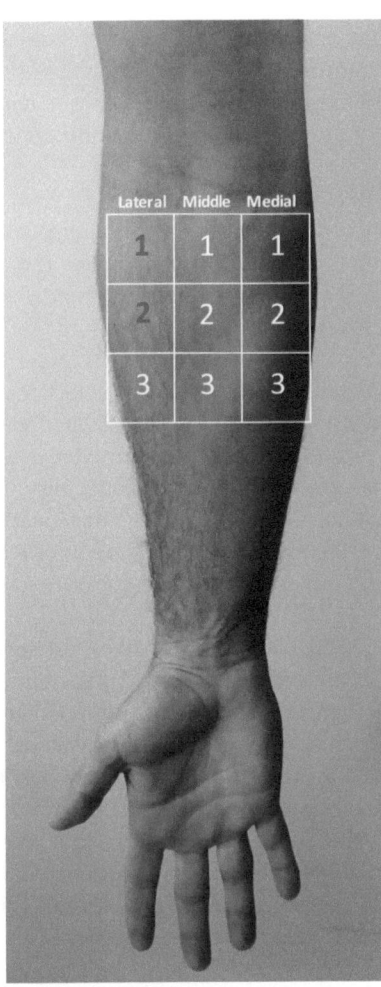

Fig. 58.5 The rule-of-nine test for radial tunnel syndrome. The anterior forearm is subdivided into nine squares. The lateral, middle, and medial columns are divided into three squares numbered proximally to distally. Patients with radial tunnel syndrome will note tenderness over squares one and two in the lateral column where the radial nerve resides in the proximal forearm. The other squares serve as controls.

of the PIN in the proximal forearm approximately 3 to 5 cm distal to the lateral epicondyle. This is more distal than the common source of pain associated with lateral epicondylitis. Despite the justified hesitation of most practitioners, it is recommended that enough lidocaine be administered to provide a temporary PIN motor block to confirm correct placement of the injection.

Sarhadi et al.[28] reported on 25 patients with suspected RTS, 16 of whom showed pain relief at 2 years with an injection of 1% lidocaine (which initially resolved symptoms in all patients) and 40 mg of triamcinolone for long-term pain control. Nonetheless, it is not our practice to inject an anesthetic or steroid in the vicinity of the posterior interosseous nerve for the purpose of diagnosis or treatment. For baseball pitchers, provocative maneuvers that can increase tension on the PIN include elbow extension, forearm pronation, and wrist flexion. This position occurs at the end of ball release; thus reproducing pain in the lateral proximal forearm in this position in the office setting may lend more weight toward a working diagnosis of RTS, especially if there is no motor loss.

Posterior Interosseous Nerve Syndrome

PIN syndrome is distinct from RTS in that patients with PIN syndrome have a significant motor deficit. This includes loss of finger and thumb extension and radial deviation of the wrist during extension because of the consistent PIN innervation of the extensor carpi ulnaris as opposed to the extensor carpi radialis longus (which is usually innervated by the radial nerve proper).[29] This condition may result from atypical (deep) lipomas, inflammatory synovitis, or a local hematoma from trauma. Temporary and even permanent dysfunction of the PIN can follow neurolysis of the PIN during exposure for fracture fixation and surgical decompression for RTS. PIN palsy is also a recognized complication of surgery for a distal biceps tendon rupture, occurring in 2.7% of one-incision approaches and in 0.2% of two-incision approaches.[30]

It is also possible to experience partial or complete PIN dysfunction in association with brachial neuritis, or Parsonage-Turner syndrome. Partial lesions may only involve the medial branch of the PIN, causing weakness of the extensor carpi ulnaris, extensor digiti minimi, and extensor digitorum communis, whereas involvement of the lateral branch can cause weakness of the abductor pollicis longus, extensor pollicis brevis, extensor pollicis longus, and extensor indicis proprius.[31] A thorough and accurate exam is therefore essential to localize lesions that may present with a variable clinical picture.

Median Nerve Compression at the Elbow
Pronator Syndrome

Pronator syndrome is a rare clinical entity that is thought to result from compression of the median nerve as it passes through the two heads of the pronator teres or the proximal aspect of the flexor digitorum superficialis in the proximal forearm. Patients present with volar proximal forearm pain and paresthesias of the first three digits and radial half of the index finger. These symptoms can be exacerbated by repetitive physical activities. Discriminating between pronator syndrome and carpal tunnel syndrome is important and based on the anatomic relationship of the palmar cutaneous branch, which arises 4 to 5 cm proximal to the transverse carpal ligament.[32] A patient with a more proximal compression lesion of the median nerve will have thenar eminence numbness versus a true carpal tunnel compression, which presents with symptoms in the first three digits and radial half of the ring finger and normal sensation of the thenar region. Anterior interosseous nerve syndrome can be differentiated from both carpal tunnel and pronator syndrome because it presents with only motor symptoms, primarily of the flexor pollicis longus and flexor digitorum profundus of the index finger and no loss of sensation.

The provocative maneuvers for pronator syndrome vary. Irritation of the nerve at the level of the pronator teres can be elicited by resisted pronation of the forearm while moving the elbow from flexion to extension.[33,34] Other maneuvers include resisted flexion of the flexor digitorum superficialis to the middle finger and resistance of the forearm in almost full flexion and full supination, which are thought to result from compression at the level of the fibrous arch between the heads of the flexor digitorum superficialis and lacertus fibrosus, respectively.[33-35] Additionally, a positive scratch collapse test and Tinel test may be observed in patients with proximal median neuropathy. The diagnosis of pronator syndrome is sufficiently rare that the accuracy of these provocative maneuvers is based more on expert opinion than on evidence.

Anterior Interosseous Nerve Syndrome

Compression of the AIN is a motor-only palsy associated with vague proximal forearm pain and significant motor deficits of the flexor pollicis longus, flexor digitorum profundus to the index and middle fingers, and pronator quadratus. Having the patient make an "OK" sign while paying specific attention to whether he or she is flexing the thumb interphalangeal joint can quickly assess AIN function. Isolating pronator quadratus function is much more difficult because the pronator teres function overpowers its isolated function. Flexing the elbow maximally can keep the humeral head of the pronator teres from contributing to forearm pronation; however, this still completely isolates pronator quadratus function.

JOINT STABILITY TESTING

Lateral Collateral Ligament

Most patients with recurrent elbow instability secondary to a history of previous trauma (e.g., dislocations or fracture-dislocations of the elbow) or surgical procedures such as tennis elbow surgery can have posterolateral rotatory instability resulting from a deficient lateral collateral ligament complex. Patients will report chronic instability with common daily maneuvers and possibly frank dislocation.

A varus stress test can be used to assess direct stability of the lateral side with the elbow at 30 degrees of flexion. However, the most commonly used test to assess for posterolateral rotary instability is the lateral pivot-shift test. This test was first described by O'Driscoll[36] and is performed with the patient relaxed in the supine position. With the examiner at the patient's head, the forearm is supinated while a valgus stress with an axial load is applied to the elbow. The elbow is then slowly extended from full flexion. The test is considered positive when posterolateral subluxation of the radial head occurs at approximately 40 degrees of extension. Flexion from that point reduces the subluxed radial head. This maneuver produces subluxation 38% of time only in a patient who is awake. Therefore an examination with use of general anesthesia is warranted when the history suggests recurrent posterolateral instability with a positive maneuver elicited in 87.5% to 100% of patients.[37,38]

The combination of elbow extension and forearm supination may elicit a sense of apprehension in an awake patient. In a study of eight patients with posterolateral rotatory instability, the use of a ground or chair push-up test was compared with the lateral pivot-shift test.[37] The push-up test is a maneuver that can be done on the ground or while sitting and involves supination with the elbows flexed to 90 degrees and arms greater than shoulder width apart. A positive test was determined as either guarding or dislocation as the elbows are extended during each maneuver. Although these tests were more sensitive than the lateral pivot-shift test in awake patients, there was no comparison to a negative control group. Performing the push-up test may therefore confound the physician for other potential causes of elbow pain and instability if pain is the only complaint.

Medial (Ulnar) Collateral Ligament

Medial (ulnar) collateral ligament instability is evaluated by numerous tests, including the valgus stress test, the "milking maneuver," and the moving valgus stress test.

The valgus stress test is performed with the shoulder held in abduction and external rotation. The examiner stabilizes the arm and flexes the elbow to 30 degrees to unlock the ulnohumeral joint. A valgus stress is then placed on the elbow. The test is positive if the patient has pain, apprehension, or gross laxity of the medial side. Sensitivity and specificity vary depending on whether the patient has pain with the maneuver versus laxity. Pain elicited by the exam has higher sensitivity (65%) versus laxity (19%) but has lower specificity (50%) versus laxity on exam (100%).[39]

The milking maneuver is performed by extending and externally rotating the humerus to restrict glenohumeral motion. The forearm is then supinated and a valgus stress is applied by pulling on the extended thumb with the elbow flexed at 90 degrees. This can be done by the patient or the examiner. The ligament is palpated during the stress maneuver, and the test is positive if there is pain, apprehension, or gross medial laxity (Fig. 58.6). Attention should be paid to baseball pitchers because they can have increased laxity of the medial collateral ligament of the dominant arm.[40] What is perceived as laxity of the medial collateral ligament can therefore actually be a false-positive result in what is otherwise a normal variant for these athletes.

The moving valgus stress test, developed by O'Driscoll, is a dynamic milking maneuver that addresses concerns regarding the position of the elbow and the sensitivity of a static valgus stress test, arthroscopic valgus stress test, and MRI in the diagnosis of

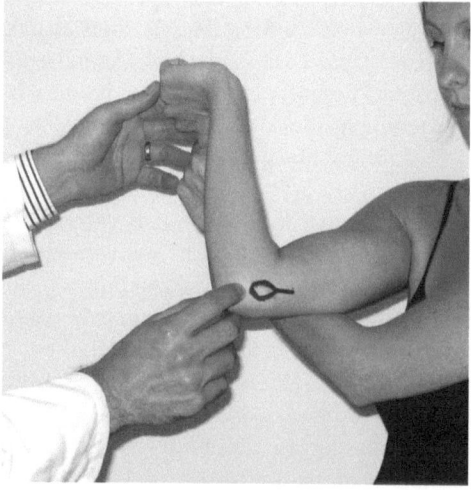

Fig. 58.6 The "milking maneuver" test. This is performed by extending and externally rotating the humerus to restrict glenohumeral motion. The forearm is then supinated and a valgus stress is applied by pulling on the extended thumb with the elbow flexed at 90 degrees. The test is considered positive if it elicits pain.

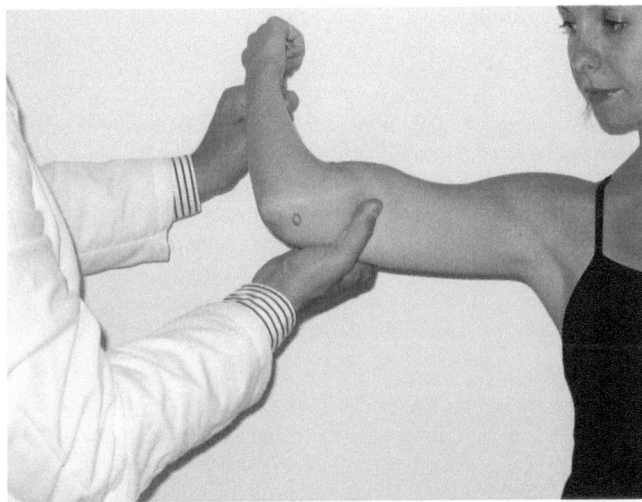

Fig. 58.7 The moving valgus stress test is performed with the shoulder held in abduction and external rotation. The examiner stabilizes the arm and flexes and extends the elbow through an arc of motion. The test is considered positive if the medial elbow pain is reproduced at the ulnar collateral ligament.

medial collateral ligament tears. The patient's arm is placed in the same position as in the milking maneuver but a constant valgus stress is placed at the elbow as it is moved through an arc of flexion and extension (Fig. 58.7). Based on analysis, the moving valgus stress test has a high sensitivity (100%) and specificity (75%) for ulnar collateral ligament injury.[39] The test is considered positive if it reproduces the patient's symptoms between a range of 70 to 120 degrees. The mean angle to reproduce the most pain in patients was 90 degrees.[39]

OTHER PROVOCATIVE MANEUVERS

Distal Biceps Tendon Rupture

For distal biceps tendon ruptures, specific physical exam maneuvers can help to assess the integrity of the tendon at its insertion site. O'Driscoll et al.[13] have described the hook test and Ruland et al.[14] reported on the use of the biceps squeeze test.

The hook test involves the examiner hooking his or her index finger under the intact biceps tendon from the lateral side while the patient fully supinates the forearm and flexes the elbow to 90 degrees. When performing the test, it is beneficial to have the patient make the "thumbs up" sign during supination and hold the arm in almost 90 degrees of abduction. The examiner can also approach the tendon from the medial side underneath the lacertus fibrosus. This is more difficult, however, because the finger cannot be hooked underneath as far. If the examiner can hook his or her finger under the tendon, then it is intact. An abnormal test corresponding to an avulsed tendon would indicate an inability to hook the finger underneath the tendon. In the study by O'Driscoll et al.,[13] the hook test was compared with MRI and intraoperative findings of patients with a distal biceps tendon rupture. The sensitivity and specificity were both 100% with the hook test compared with 92% and 85% for MRI alone.[13]

The biceps squeeze test is similar in concept to the Thompson test for Achilles tendon rupture. The biceps muscle belly is squeezed with one hand while the examiner's other hand squeezes the musculotendinous junction. The patient's arm should be resting at approximately 60 to 80 degrees of flexion. A normal exam would demonstrate forearm supination when squeezing the muscle belly and tendinous junction. A positive test would not demonstrate supination of the forearm. Based on one patient population, this test had a reported sensitivity of 95%, and all patients who had surgery had return of forearm supination when assessed with the biceps squeeze test.[14]

Posteromedial Impingement Syndrome

The extension impingement and arm bar tests are useful for evaluating posterior impingement in athletes secondary to posteromedial impingement syndrome. The extension impingement test is performed by palpating the posteromedial aspect of the olecranon with the patient's arm near full extension at the elbow (20 to 30 degrees) and then quickly extending the elbow fully to terminal extension with a continuous valgus stress. The purpose of this maneuver is to recreate the terminal phase of a valgus extension overload typically seen in overhead-throwing athletes. The valgus stress is necessary to identify whether the pain is primarily from posteromedial impingement and not from instability or other sources of pain. The test can also be performed without valgus or in varus and appropriate comparisons can be made.[41]

The arm bar test is performed with the arm in full internal rotation at 90 degrees of forward flexion with the hand on the examiner's shoulder. The patient's olecranon/distal humerus is pulled down to recreate full extension. A positive test will elicit pain in the patient's posteromedial elbow. This is considered a more sensitive test than the extension impingement test. It therefore may not be unusual to examine a pitcher in the recovery phase who still has a positive arm bar test but a negative extension impingement exam.[42]

CONCLUSION

The elbow is a complicated joint; it can be affected by many associated disorders in the athlete. Therefore a focused history and physical examination of the lateral, medial, anterior, and posterior aspects of the elbow can help the physician to develop a narrow differential diagnosis and guide treatment decisions that will allow the patient's return to play in a timely and safe manner.

ACKNOWLEDGMENT

The authors and editors gratefully acknowledge the contributions of the previous authors,
   Aakash Chauhan, Jeffrey Cunningham, Rishi Bhatnagar, Caroline Baratz, and Mark E. Baratz.
   For a complete list of references, go to ExpertConsult.com.

SELECTED READINGS

Citation:
Cheng C, Mackinnon-Patterson B, Beck JL, et al. Scratch collapse test for evaluation of carpal and cubital tunnel syndrome. *J Hand Surg Am.* 2008;33A:1518–1524.

Level of Evidence:

II

Summary:

This study evaluates the usefulness of a new physical examination test for carpal tunnel syndrome and cubital tunnel syndrome. This test had a higher sensitivity (62%) compared with the Tinel test (32%) and the wrist flexion/compression test (44%) in diagnosing carpal tunnel syndrome. This test also had a higher sensitivity (69%) than the Tinel test (54%) and the elbow flexion/compression test (46%) in diagnosing cubital tunnel syndrome. The overall conclusion is that this physical examination maneuver is highly sensitive and useful in the diagnosis of carpal and cubital tunnel syndrome.

Citation:

Rosenthal EA. Examination of hand and forearm: claw hand deformity & thumb deformity with ulnar palsy. In: Peimer CA, ed. *Surgery of the Hand and Upper Extremity*. New York: McGraw-Hill; 1996:83–87.

Level of Evidence:

V

Summary:

This book chapter details the features of various nerve palsies and how they may manifest in the hand.

Citation:

O'Driscoll SW, Lawton RL, Smith AM. The "moving valgus stress test" for medial collateral ligament tears of the elbow. *Am J Sports Med*. 2005;33:231–239.

Level of Evidence:

II

Summary:

This study evaluates a physical examination maneuver for medial collateral ligament (MCL) injuries of the elbow. The moving valgus stress test was 100% sensitive and 75% specific in assessment of medial elbow pain from MCL injuries compared with other standards of diagnosis. The moving valgus stress test is another highly sensitive physical examination maneuver that can aid clinicians in narrowing the differential diagnosis of medial elbow pain with specific consideration of an MCL injury.

Citation:

O'Driscoll SW, Goncalves LB, Dietz P. The hook test for distal biceps tendon avulsion. *Am J Sports Med*. 2007;35(11):1865–1869.

Level of Evidence:

II

Summary:

This study evaluates the usefulness of the hook test when assessing a potential distal biceps tendon rupture. The hook test was found to have a sensitivity and specificity of 100% for a distal biceps tendon rupture, which is higher than magnetic resonance imaging (92% and 85%, respectively).

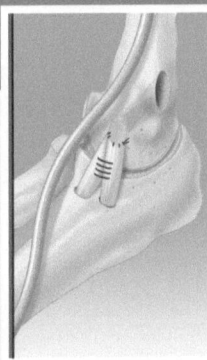

59

Elbow Imaging

Benjamin M. Howe, Michael R. Moynagh

The elbow is a complex joint affected by a variety of pathologic conditions. Advanced imaging of the elbow with computed tomography (CT), magnetic resonance imaging (MRI), MR arthrography, and ultrasound (US) provide powerful tools for diagnosis; however, an understanding of the utility and limitations is required to select the optimal modality to answer each clinical question. Despite the availability of advanced imaging, conventional radiographs remain central to imaging of the elbow. It is important not to overlook conventional radiographs in the evaluation of the elbow; they are recommended in all patients prior to the consideration of advanced imaging techniques. This chapter reviews these imaging modalities and also considers how these modalities can best be utilized in the evaluation and treatment planning of commonly encountered elbow pathology.

IMAGING MODALITIES

Conventional Radiographs

Imaging evaluation of the elbow typically begins with conventional radiographs. Standard radiographic views of the elbow include anteroposterior (AP), lateral, and oblique projections (Fig. 59.1). The AP and oblique views are obtained with the elbow extended and forearm supinated, permitting visualization of the proximal radioulnar and radiocapitellar articulations, medial and lateral epicondyles, and trochlea. The carrying angle of the elbow typically measures 12 to 15 degrees valgus in this anatomic resting position.[1] The lateral view, obtained with the elbow flexed 90 degrees and the forearm in a neutral position, permits evaluation of the radiocapitellar and ulnotrochlear articulations, distal humerus, olecranon, and coronoid processes. An appropriately acquired lateral elbow radiograph clearly shows the ulnotrochlear articulation with minimal overlap of osseous structures. This ulnotrochlear space on the lateral view can be obscured with small amounts of rotation; therefore careful attention should be paid the obtaining well-positioned lateral elbow views. An anatomically positioned radial head is collinear with the capitellum. A dark radiolucent area is normally seen just anterior to the distal humerus, representing the anterior fat pad. Similarly, the posterior fat pad sign is a well-demarcated lucency posterior to the distal humeral metaphysis; its presence tends to indicate a pathologic process.[2] Displacement of these fat pads, produced by an intra-articular effusion or hemarthrosis, resembles the spinnaker on a sailboat and is referred to as the *sail sign*.[3]

Conventional radiographic projections are usually satisfactory for the initial evaluation of the elbow; however, additional projections may be utilized for structures that are difficult to evaluate on standard AP, lateral, and oblique projections. Fractures of the radial head are common and may be challenging to detect when nondisplaced. A specific radial head (radiocapitellar) view may better demonstrate the fracture, characterize the fracture pattern, and aid in classification. With the elbow flexed to 90 degrees, the beam is angled 45 degrees anteriorly from a true lateral.[1] This projection provides an unobstructed view of the radial head without overlap of the proximal ulna. Other common fractures include those involving the epicondyles (especially the medial epicondyle in skeletally immature patients), distal humerus, and olecranon. The "terrible triad" injury includes fractures of the radial head and coronoid process, along with dislocation of the elbow joint. Conventional radiographs are usually sufficient for confirming concentric reduction of the elbow after closed manipulation.

Any patient presenting with non–activity-related pain or a mass at the elbow should first be evaluated with conventional radiographs. Radiographs offer a large amount of information and help guide further imaging workup.

Elbow trauma often involves a combination of osseous and soft tissue injury. When conventional radiographs do not reveal a problem or provide incomplete information, the choice of additional studies is guided by the history and physical examination. These additional studies may include CT, MRI, MR arthrography, fluoroscopy, and bone scan. Some relevant injuries and their imaging findings are highlighted in this chapter to aid the general orthopedic surgeon or sports medicine specialist.

Computed Tomography

Modern CT scanners allow for rapid image acquisition, high spatial resolution, and isovolumetric data sets that can provide multiplanar reformatting of the images. These qualities allow for excellent depiction of bone; they are useful for the detection of subtle fractures, periosteal reaction, and subtle bone lesions that may be difficult to appreciate on conventional radiographs. The high attenuation of cortical bone allows for segmentation and generation of three-dimensional volume-rendered images with minimal manual postprocessing. These images provide important visual information in the planning of complex fracture repairs. CT technology continues to improve, with dose reduction, metal reduction techniques, and quantitative technology.

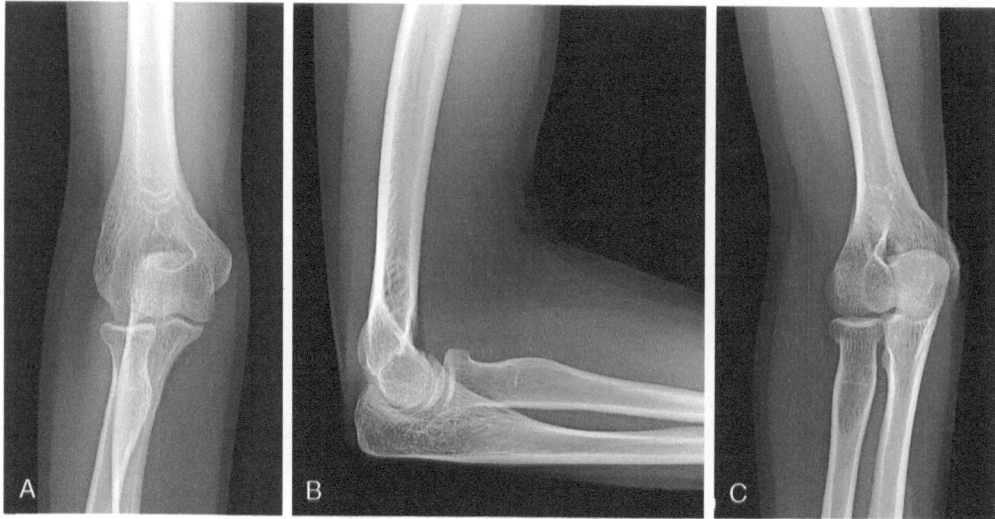

Fig. 59.1 Conventional radiographs of the elbow. (A) Anteroposterior view. (B) Lateral view. (C) Oblique view.

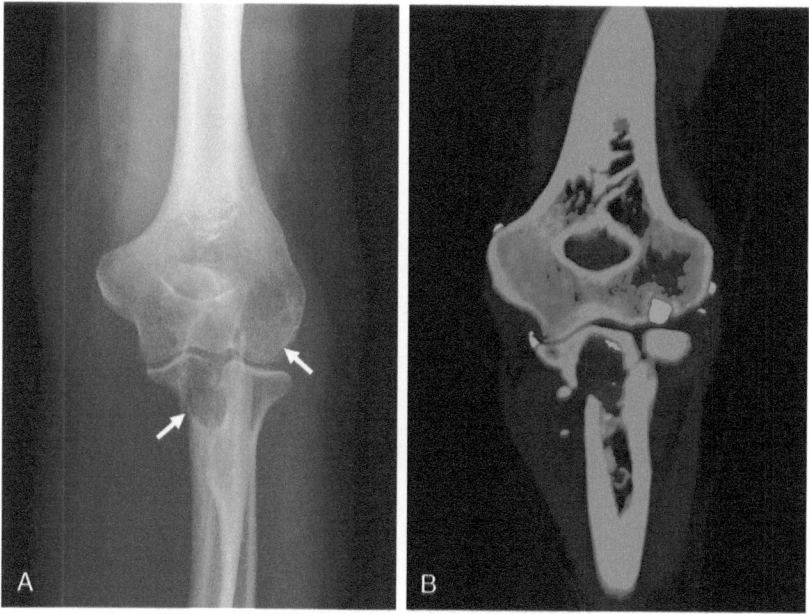

Fig. 59.2 Anteroposterior radiograph of the elbow (A) demonstrates lytic lesions in the proximal ulna and capitellum *(arrows)*. Biopsy of the lytic ulnar lesion was negative for malignancy and demonstrated inflammation. A subsequent dual-energy computed tomography exam (B) confirmed the presence of a large amount of uric acid crystal deposition in the elbow as indicated by the green encoded pixels on the postprocessed coronal image, confirming the diagnosis of gout.

For example, dual-energy CT (DECT) can be used in the musculoskeletal system for the detection of uric acid crystals in gout.[4] The foot and ankle are most commonly imaged with this DECT technique, but it can also be applied to the elbow in challenging diagnostic cases (Fig. 59.2).

Magnetic Resonance Imaging

MRI provides excellent soft tissue contrast and is the modality of choice for evaluating soft tissue masses, ligament injury, tendon injury, nerve-related symptoms, and articular cartilage. It is also the modality of choice in evaluating clinically relevant nonspecific elbow pain not explained by conventional radiographs. There is no single MRI protocol for the elbow, and the MRI technique

should be tailored to the specific clinical question in order to provide the best diagnostic information. T1-weighted, proton density and fluid-sensitive sequences are typically adequate for evaluating the elbow. T1-weighted images better depict osseous pathology and are preferred in the evaluation of a soft tissue mass and of the nerves. Ligaments, tendons, and cartilage are better depicted with proton density sequences. The term *fluid sensitive* refers to an MRI sequence that depicts the protons in fluid/edema as bright while the protons in fat appear dark. Examples of fluid-sensitive sequences include T2-weighted images with chemical fat saturation, intermediate proton density–weighted with chemical fat saturation, short tau inversion recovery (STIR), and Dixon water/fat separation. Intravenous gadolinium contrast is not typically required in elbow MRI but is often used for the evaluation of soft tissue masses, nerve pathology, or synovitis.

Magnetic Resonance Arthrography

MR arthrography may improve the MRI evaluation of locking, limited range of motion (ROM), and ulnar collateral ligament (UCL) injury, but preference between standard MRI and MR arthrogram for these diagnoses varies. The instillation of dilute gadolinium contrast into the elbow may be guided by US or fluoroscopy, depending on availably and the comfort of the proceduralist. The patient is most commonly positioned prone with the elbow above the head, but the injection can also be administered with the patient seated adjacent to the fluoroscopy table and the arm placed on the table. With the elbow flexed at 90 degrees, the elbow is positioned as in a lateral radiograph. A 22-gauge needle is placed in the radiocapitellar joint and a small test of iodinated contrast is used to confirm intra-articular placement. The dilute gadolinium contrast is instilled under intermittent fluoroscopic guidance to ensure intra-articular placement. The MR arthrography sequences differ, as the exam relies heavily on T1-weighted fat-saturated images. This allows for the detection of any gadolinium contrast that may extend into or through a ligament tear, as in the evaluation of an UCL tear.

Ultrasound

US excels at dynamic soft tissue evaluation of the elbow joint and is able to provide an alternative for imaging around surgical hardware. Because of the complex mechanics of hinging and rotation, static imaging may fail to detect dynamic pathology. US has the benefit of high-resolution dynamic image evaluation without ionizing radiation and allows for direct patient communication and "real-time" examination. US is a powerful tool but is user-dependent, requiring a detailed anatomic knowledge and basic understanding of sonographic principles if the operator is to select the correct transducer and be aware of imaging artifacts and pitfalls. Image interpretation can be optimized by using high-frequency linear array transducers (10 to 20 MHz), utilizing standardized imaging acquisition planes and acquiring stored cine clips for subsequent review.

The use of US in the evaluation of the elbow is growing. Currently it is most often used in the evaluation of dynamic pain/snapping, tendon pathology, joint effusion, peripheral nerve evaluation, and for guiding percutaneous procedures about the elbow.

TRAUMA

Fracture

The elbow features complex three-dimensional anatomy and overlapping structures that can make the detection of subtle fractures on conventional radiographs challenging. Interpretation of radiographs of the skeletally immature elbow for trauma requires knowledge of the ossification centers, the time line for development of the ossification centers, and an understanding of the order of growth plate closure. The mnemonic CRITOE can serve as an aid for remembering the order of ossification and closure (C, capitellum; R, radial head; I, internal/medial epicondyle; T, trochlea; O, olecranon; E, external/lateral epicondyle). Avulsion fractures are common injuries of the pediatric elbow, and knowledge of this pattern of growth plate closure helps in their identification.

CT or MRI can help to detect subtle fractures. CT is often preferred, given its availability and lower cost; however, MRI is also excellent for detecting nondisplaced fractures. CT with multiplanar reformatted images is the preferred modality in the presurgical planning of complex elbow fractures.[5] Therefore complex fractures of the distal humerus and medial coronoid facet are commonly evaluated by CT for preoperative planning.

Fracture-Dislocation

Elbow dislocations are evident on conventional radiographs and are characterized by the position of the radius/ulna relative to the humerus. Typically these injuries are not subtle on radiographs, but the associated deformity and difficulty of positioning can limit the detection and characterization of fractures. Traction radiographs may help delineate the fracture pattern but may not be tolerated by all patients owing to the associated pain. CT better depicts complex fracture-dislocations and aids in fracture pattern characterization, degree of fragment displacement, articular surface involvement, and/or the presence of associated intra-articular fracture fragments, which may block concentric reduction and lead to persistent joint subluxation. Failure to identify fractures of stabilizing osseous structures such as the coronoid or radial head may lead to a poor functional outcome.[6] Osseous three-dimensional reconstructions are commonly created from CT data for these complex fractures of the elbow to best demonstrate the relationship of the fracture fragments and for surgical planning. Finally, MRI is the best option for determining the pattern of soft tissue disruption in acutely unstable injuries or those that present with delayed complaints of subjective instability, which may require collateral ligament repair or reconstruction.

Occult Fracture

Persistent tenderness over a suspected injury site despite negative findings of conventional radiographs may be an indication for further evaluation in select cases. The posterior fat pad sign in the setting of trauma corresponds to an occult fracture in more than 75% of patients.[7,8] The radial head is the most frequent site of an occult fracture.[8] Fractures of the coracoid process are best visualized on well-positioned lateral radiographs; however, oblique views may also be helpful in detection and characterization. CT or MRI better detect non-displaced fractures and are indicated with high clinical suspicion of a fracture and negative radiographs. Fluid-sensitive (fat-suppressed T2-weighted or inversion recovery) sequences are the most sensitive for detecting radiographically occult fractures.[7] Fractures show a linear pattern of signal change, with decreased signal on T1-weighted images and increased signal on T2-weighted images (Fig. 59.3A and B). Proton density images are commonly utilized in examining the elbow, but T1 images better demonstrate the linear signal abnormality of a fracture (see Fig. 59.3A). In contrast, osseous contusion produces a nonspecific diffuse increase in signal on T2-weighted images without a discrete fracture line (see Fig. 59.3C).

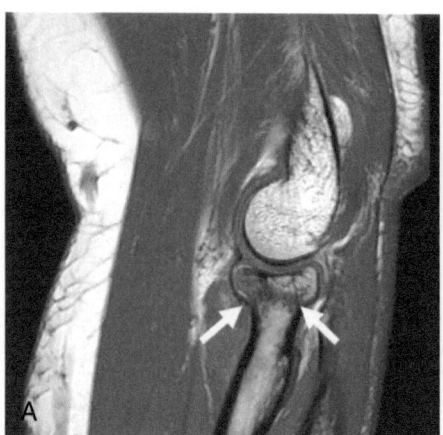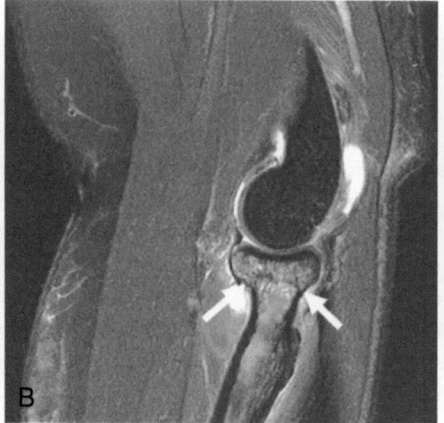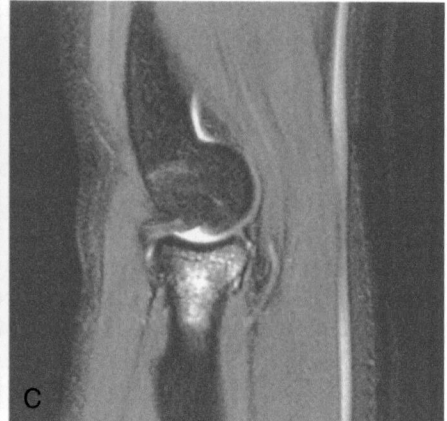

Fig. 59.3 Sagittal T1- (A) and T2-weighted fat-saturated (B) magnetic resonance images of the elbow after trauma demonstrate a radiographically occult acute fracture of the radial head and neck. Note the linear decreased signal abnormality of the fracture on both the T1- and T2-weighted sequences *(arrows)* and the surrounding bone marrow edema. Sagittal T2-weighted fat-saturated image of the radiocapitellar joint (C) in a different patient after trauma demonstrates the appearance of an osseous contusion with amorphous bone marrow edema in the absence of a discrete linear signal abnormality.

Stress Fracture

The olecranon is the most common stress fracture site, and this condition is most often seen in baseball players.[9] When the history and physical examination suggest it, a CT, MRI, or bone scan may be diagnostic.[10] A CT scan typically reveals a subtle fracture line in the olecranon, often with a linear area of sclerosis. Findings on MRI resemble those of occult fractures described previously. A bone scan would reveal abnormal radiotracer uptake at the site of repetitive stress.

DEGENERATIVE ARTHRITIS AND LOOSE BODIES

Pain and limited ROM associated with degenerative arthritis of the elbow can be quite limiting. Prior trauma may accelerate the development of degenerative arthritis, and surgical intervention may be beneficial in restoring function and reducing pain. The goal of imaging is to assist in determining potential pain-generating sites and/or a structural cause limiting ROM. Conventional radiographs may detect intra-articular loose bodies in the coronoid or olecranon fossae and osteophytes that may limit range of flexion or extension. Flexion and extension radiographs may be useful to illustrate how the structural abnormality is affecting the arc of motion. Supplemental oblique or axial projections may be helpful in distinguishing intra-articular and extra-articular calcifications, especially in severe cases of heterotopic ossification. In ambiguous cases, CT is the modality of choice for further information. Singson et al.[11] compared the utility of double-contrast CT arthrography and conventional radiography in patients with pain, locking, and limited elbow motion. They found that double-contrast CT arthrography successfully diagnosed 100% of loose bodies and provided precise information regarding the size, number, and location of the lesions. In contrast, conventional radiographs identified only 50% of the intra-articular loose bodies. Zubler et al.[12] arrived

at the same conclusion, noting greater accuracy of loose body detection with CT than with conventional radiographs, but particularly in the posterior fossae.

On the other hand, not all investigators agree that CT is necessary for loose body detection. Dubberley et al.[13] found that CT and MRI were no more effective than conventional radiography alone for the detection of loose bodies. Quinn et al.[14] recommended MRI for the accurate assessment of elbow intra-articular loose bodies. Current standard CT and MRI techniques are typically adequate for detecting intra-articular bodies without the need for arthrography. An advantage of using MRI is that it enables the detection of cartilaginous or osteocartilaginous fragments[7] associated with osteochondritis dissecans of the capitellum that, in young athletes, may elude characterization by conventional radiography or CT. Furthermore, MRI may distinguish osteophytes and synovial hypertrophy, which often mimic loose body formation.[15]

COLLATERAL LIGAMENT INJURY

Conventional radiographs are usually insufficient for detecting collateral ligament injury of the elbow; however, soft tissue edema or hematoma can be identified. Ligamentous insufficiency may affect elbow alignment on standard radiographs. The normal alignment of the radiocapitellar joint can be altered on conventional radiographs with posterolateral rotatory instability, the most common pattern of elbow instability.[16] Severe posterolateral rotatory instability may alter the radiocapitellar alignment on conventional radiographs with posterolateral subluxation of the radial head. Collateral ligament instabilities of the elbow can be evaluated with stress imaging, including radiographs or US. Elbow instability resulting from collateral ligament injury or varus/valgus stress is applied to visualize asymmetric widening of the joint.[17,18] US has the benefit of dynamic visualization and the ability to compare an image with one of the contralateral elbow (Fig. 59.4). Other examinations—such as CT arthrography, MRI, and MR arthrography—also offer additional information by direct visualization of the ligament.

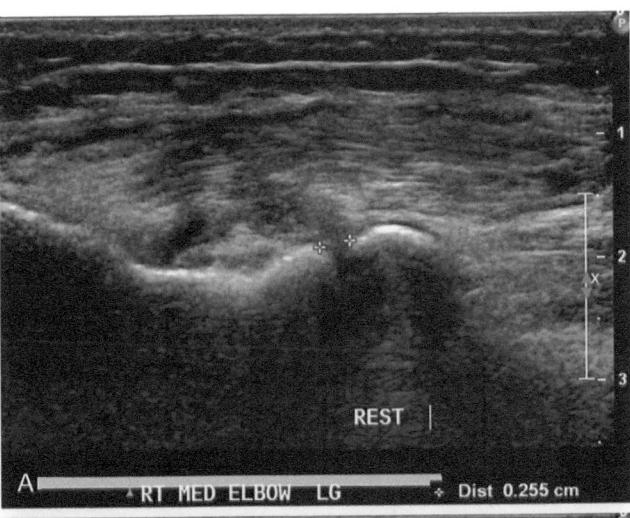

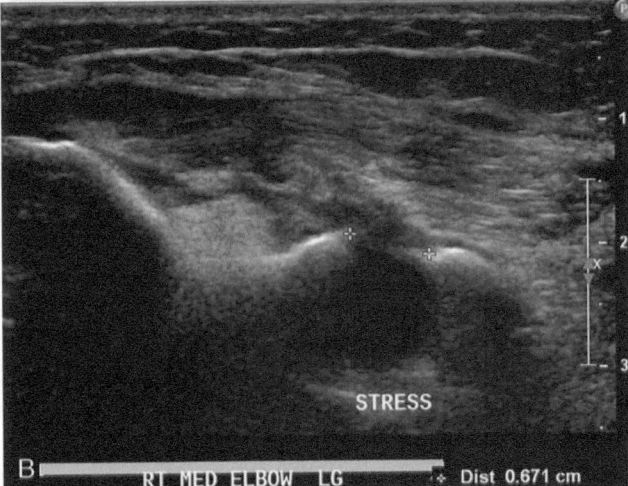

Fig. 59.4 Longitudinal ultrasound images of the medial right elbow were performed at rest (A) and with valgus stress (B). This exam demonstrates 4 mm of medial joint space widening with valgus stress in a patient with a complete ulnar collateral ligament tear.

Ulnar Collateral Ligament Injury

The UCL is an important valgus stabilizer of the elbow and is particularly vulnerable to injury in athletes whose sport involves throwing, such as baseball pitchers and javelin throwers.[19] Interpretation of valgus stress radiography in athletes can be challenging. Several investigators have shown increased valgus laxity in the dominant arm of asymptomatic persons.[17,20,21] When the index of clinical suspicion for a UCL injury is high, MRI provides important additional information. The UCL is a vertically oriented structure coursing between the medial epicondyle and the coronoid process that is uniformly of low signal intensity; it is best depicted on coronal MRI. The UCL is composed of anterior, posterior, and transverse bands. The anterior bundle provides the most valgus elbow stabilization. MRI may detect full-thickness tears of the anterior bundle, with increased signal intensity often found within and adjacent to the discontinuous ligament on fat-suppressed T2-weighted images as a result of edema and/or hemorrhage (Fig. 59.5A).[7,22] MRI is less reliable for the detection of partial-thickness tears. Timmerman et al.[23] found MRI to be 100% sensitive for full-thickness tears but only 14% sensitive for partial-thickness tears. Administration of intra-articular contrast material improves sensitivity[7,22–24] in detecting partial-thickness UCL tears (see Fig. 59.5B). Schwartz et al.[25] reported 86% and 100% sensitivity and specificity, respectively, for the detection of partial-thickness UCL tears with MR arthrography. Variability in the insertion of the anterior bundle, however, complicates MRI interpretation of partial-thickness tears. The distal ulnar attachment of the anterior bundle may insert anywhere between 1 mm of the articular margin of the coronoid process[25] and 3 mm distal to the sublime tubercle of the ulna.[26] This characteristic can create a small recess on MR arthrography along the medial margin of the coronoid process. Partial tears of the distal insertion of the UCL are diagnosed by intra-articular gadolinium extending deep to the insertion, referred to as the

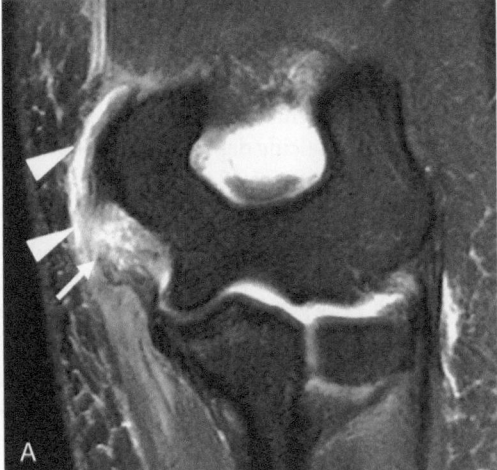

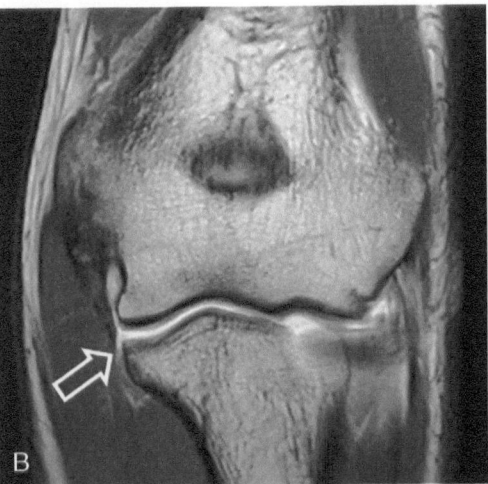

Fig. 59.5 Tears of the ulnar collateral ligament (UCL). (A) Coronal T2-fat-saturated magnetic resonance image demonstrates an acute full-thickness tear of the proximal UCL of the elbow (arrow) and surrounding edema (arrowheads). (B) Coronal T1-weighted elbow arthrogram shows a pitcher with a partial tear of the distal UCL at the undersurface of the insertion at the sublime tubercle (open arrow). This partial undersurface tear of the distal UCL is referred to as the "T-sign," given the appearance of a horizontal T by the intra-articular gadolinium contrast.

"T-sign" (see Fig. 59.5B). Consequently distinguishing between normal anatomy and a pathologic partial undersurface tear at the attachment of the distal ligament can be challenging[27]; therefore clinical correlation is paramount.

US examination of the UCL can aid in the diagnosis of a tear and can evaluate for instability with valgus stress. The UCL is best depicted at 70 degrees of flexion with the transducer placed in a longitudinal manner to the long axis of the ligament (Fig. 59.6).[28] In this position, the anterior band of the UCL should appear taut, with a tear demonstrated as focal hypoechogenicity with fiber disruption.[29] The medial joint margin and UCL can be dynamically evaluated under valgus stress for determining laxity/insufficiency, with greater than 2 mm of widening compared with the contralateral elbow being considered an abnormality of the anterior band of the UCL.[30] The prevalence of UCL thickening, irregularity, and laxity complicates the US evaluation of the UCL in pitchers, and these abnormalities tend to progress over time.[31]

Injury of the Lateral Collateral Ligament

The lateral UCL (LUCL), radial collateral ligament (RCL), and annular ligament form the lateral collateral ligament complex. The LUCL is found posteriorly extending from the lateral humeral

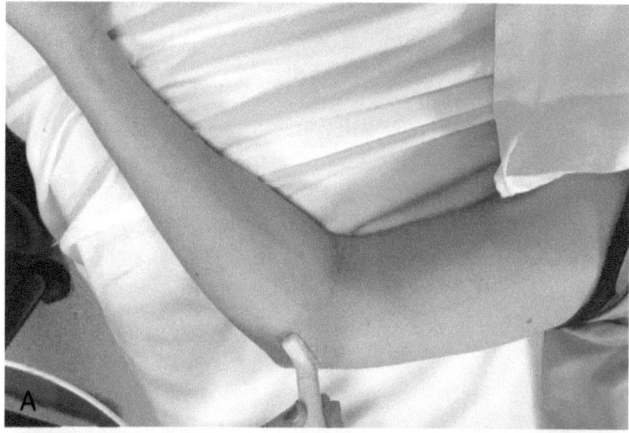

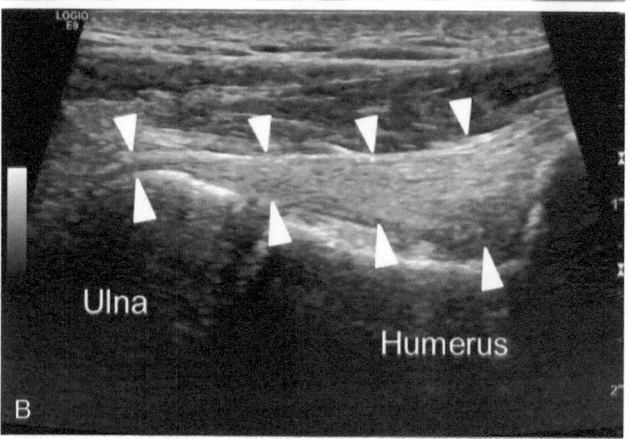

Fig. 59.6 Ultrasound (US) imaging of the ulnar collateral ligament (UCL). A photograph (A) demonstrates the US probe position for evaluating the UCL with the elbow in 70 degrees of flexion. The longitudinal US image (B) was obtained with the Logiq E9 US system (GE Healthcare, Milwaukee, WI) using a wide-band high-frequency probe (8 to 18 MHz). The image demonstrates the normal appearance of the UCL *(arrowheads)*.

condyle to the supinator crest of the ulna. The RCL arises from the lateral humeral epicondyle, deep to the common extensor tendon, and blends into the annular ligament surrounding the radial head. On MRI, the RCL and LUCL are best seen on sequential coronal images with an image slice thickness of 2 mm or less.[32] The annular ligament is optimally seen on axial MRI images.[27] The LUCL is the primary varus elbow stabilizer.

Tears of the lateral collateral ligament complex are common in persons with acute elbow dislocations. MRI findings of acute LUCL and RCL tears include ligament attenuation, redundancy, and discontinuity evident on coronal and/or axial images[22,33]; they are most often seen at the humeral origin of the ligament (Fig. 59.7).[32] Chronic insufficiency of the LUCL, which can lead to posterolateral rotatory instability, is difficult to identify on MRI.[34,35] Terada et al.[36] found that MRI of asymptomatic persons revealed inconsistent signal characteristics within the LUCL or frank inability to identify the structure altogether. In contrast, Potter et al.[37] found that abnormalities in the LUCL could be reliably detected with three-dimensional gradient-recalled and fast spin echo MRI in persons with posterolateral rotatory instability compared with asymptomatic control subjects.[37] The role of MR arthrography in this setting is unclear; it is not currently deemed to be a superior method of characterizing injuries of this ligament complex.

The RLC originates intimately with the origin of the common extensor tendon. The separate RCL structure can be delineated from the common extensor tendon origin with knowledge of the humeral footprint.[38] The LUCL originates with and cannot be readily distinguished from the RCL proximally. The oblique course of the middle and distal LUCL makes US evaluation particularly challenging.[39] Posterolateral ulnohumeral laxity can be quantified by using dynamic US in patients with suspected posterolateral rotatory instability.[40]

LATERAL AND MEDIAL EPICONDYLITIS

Lateral epicondylitis, or "tennis elbow," is the most common overuse disorder of the elbow. Conventional radiographs rarely show any findings in persons with lateral epicondylitis. Pomerance[41] found radiographic abnormalities in only 16% of 294 patients with lateral epicondylitis; the most common manifestation was faint calcific deposits at the origin of the extensor carpi radialis brevis (Fig. 59.8A). MRI has 90% to 100% sensitivity and 83% to 100% specificity for the detection of lateral epicondylitis.[42] However, it is reserved for equivocal or recalcitrant cases in order to exclude concomitant/alternative sources of elbow pain such as degenerative joint disease, osteochondral lesions, radial neuritis, posterolateral rotatory instability, occult fracture, and/or loose bodies.[43] Common MRI findings include high signal intensity on T2-weighted and STIR sequences in a thickened common extensor tendon with or without adjacent soft tissue edema (see Fig. 59.8B and C).[22,33]

Medial epicondylitis, or "golfer's elbow," is the next most common overuse disorder of the elbow. Although conventional radiographs are usually unremarkable in middle-aged patients with degenerative tendinopathies, concomitant medial ulnotrochlear osteophytes may be present in this age group and thus have

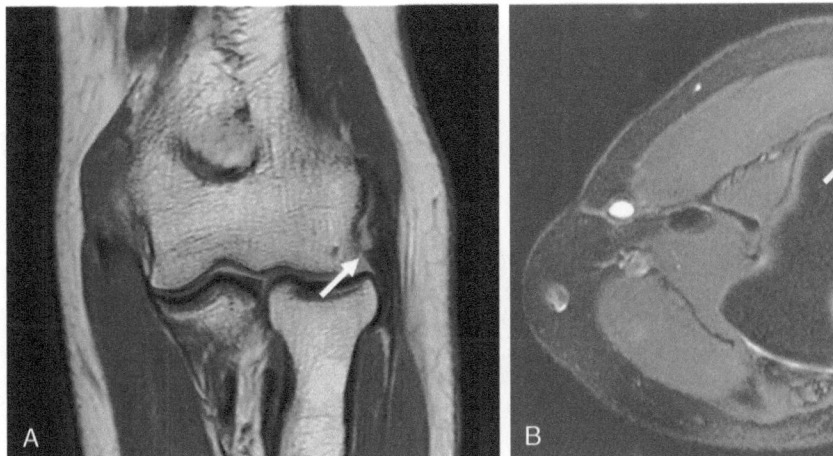

Fig. 59.7 Avulsion of the radial collateral ligament. (A) Coronal proton density weighted magnetic resonance image demonstrates a complete avulsion of the radial collateral ligament *(arrow)*. (B) The axial T2-weighted fat-saturated image confirms complete avulsion of the origin of the radial collateral ligament *(arrow)*. Note that the overlying common extensor tendon remains intact. Exam under anesthesia was positive for posterolateral rotatory instability and followed by surgical confirmation and reconstruction.

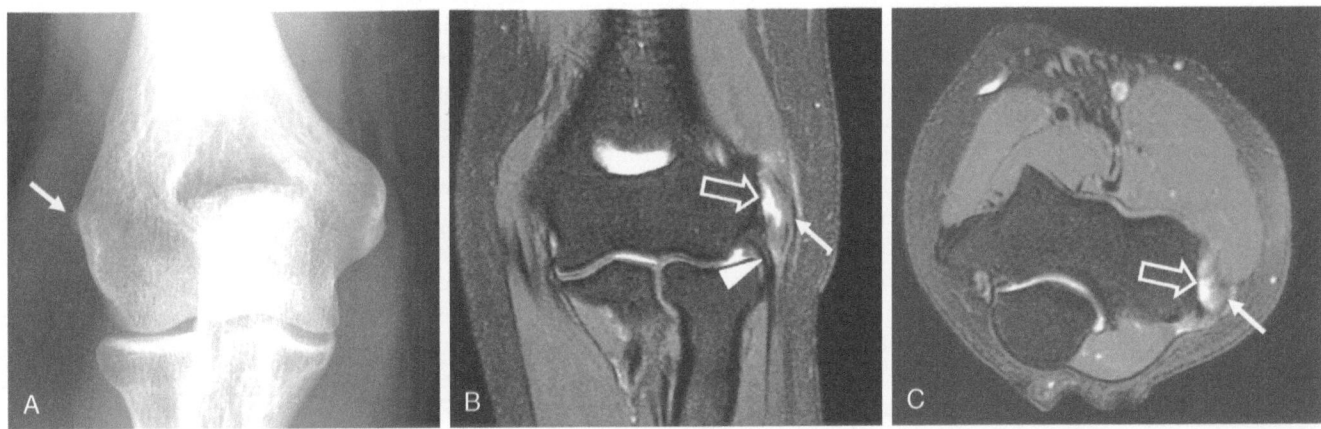

Fig. 59.8 Lateral epicondylitis. (A) Anteroposterior radiographs of the elbow demonstrates faint heterotopic ossification at the origin of the common extensor tendon *(arrow)*. (B) Coronal and (C) axial T2-weighted fat-saturated magnetic resonance imaging (MRI) illustrates the MRI findings in lateral epicondylitis. The common origin of the extensor tendon demonstrates marked thickening and increased intrasubstance signal *(arrows)*. A partial tear at the origin of the common extensor tendon is seen as a cleft of fluid *(open arrows)*. Note the intact underlying radial collateral ligament *(arrowhead)*.

implications for the overall treatment plan. MRI is beneficial only for cases of refractory medial epicondylitis, mostly to exclude other sources of pain such as UCL injury or ulnar neuritis.[27] A thickened common flexor tendon may be seen on T1-weighted sequences, with local soft tissue edema surrounding the medial epicondyle on T2-weighted sequences. Degenerative tendinosis is typically localized to the origins of the flexor carpi radialis and pronator teres.[27]

Abnormal tendon hypoechogenicity, thickening and decreased fibrillary echotexture are the US features of tendinopathy seen in both medial and lateral epicondylitis. A tear appears as a linear anechoic focus with associated fiber disruption.[44]

Distal Biceps Tendon

Diagnosis of distal biceps tendon rupture by conventional radiography is limited because osseous avulsion injuries from the insertion of the radial tuberosity are rare. MRI may distinguish degenerative tendinosis and acute injury and differentiate partial from complete tears of the tendon. Fitzgerald et al.[45] reported a 100% accuracy rate of MRI for the diagnosis of distal ruptures of the biceps tendon. A complete rupture is characterized by an interruption in the low-signal-intensity tendon insertion at the radial tuberosity on axial images combined with an associated large amount of high-signal-intensity fluid and/or hemorrhage in the antecubital fossa seen on T2-weighted images (Fig. 59.9). The degree of tendon retraction is best assessed on sagittal images. Partial tears or nonretracted distal avulsions can be challenging to diagnose and differentiate on standard MRI planes of the elbow. The distal biceps tendon courses to the medial aspect of the radius to insert on the radial tuberosity, which may limit the evaluation of insertional injury. The radial insertion of the biceps is well demonstrated with the elbow flexed 90 degrees,

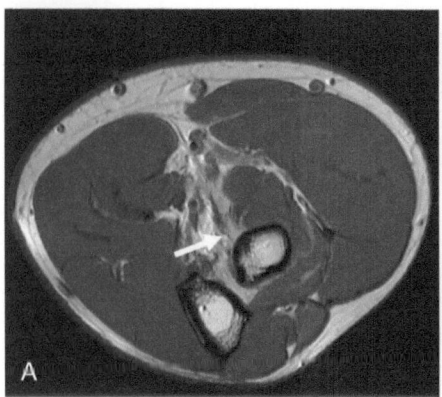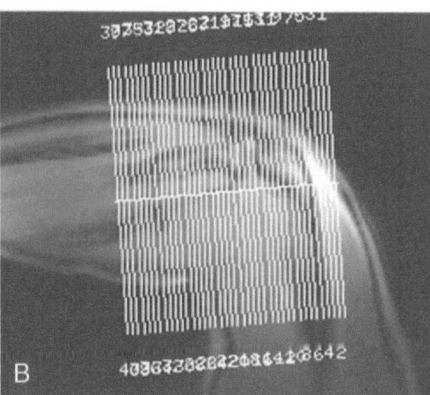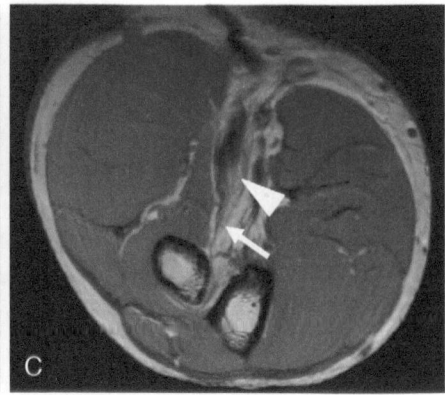

Fig. 59.9 Distal biceps tendon avulsion. (A) Axial proton-density image of the elbow demonstrates a complete avulsion of the distal biceps tendon *(arrow)* at the insertion on the radial tuberosity. To better define the tear and the quality of the distal biceps tendon, the patient was placed in the FABS position (elbow flexion, shoulder abduction, and forearm supination). (B) Scout image in the FABS position shows the plane of acquisition perpendicular to the long axis of the proximal radius. (C) Proton density axial FABS image shows the distal biceps avulsion *(arrow)* and the thickening and increased intrasubstance signal in the biceps tendon stump *(arrowhead)*.

the shoulder abducted, and the forearm supinated. This position is commonly referred to as the FABS position, for Flexed elbow, shoulder ABduction, and Supination of the forearm. Images are acquired perpendicular to the long axis of the proximal radial shaft in the FABS position, allowing for a long segment of the distal biceps tendon to be evaluated on a limited number of slices (see Fig. 59.9B and C).[46] The lacertus fibrosus (bicipital aponeurosis) may prevent proximal tendon retraction after a complete distal rupture.[27] Partial tears of the biceps tendon are usually the result of repetitive microtrauma and tendon degeneration. Thickening of the distal biceps tendon is often seen on T1-weighted and proton density, with increased intratendinous signal intensity representing tendinopathy on T2-weighted sequences. The interval between the individual short- and long-head tendons should not be mistaken for a tear.[47] Partial tears may also produce bone marrow edema at the radial tuberosity or increased fluid in the bicipitoradial bursa on T2-weighted images.[33,48]

US can diagnose both complete and partial tendon tears of the distal biceps. Full-thickness tears are seen as an absence of the distal biceps tendon fibers, often with interposed hematoma and adjacent edema. Partial tears at the radiobicipital origin may be difficult to diagnose on US, given the steep obliquity at the insertion of the bicipital tuberosity; however, sonographic techniques such as using a pronator window approach can improve visualization.[49]

ULNAR NEUROPATHY

Ulnar neuropathy at the cubital tunnel is the most common neuropathy at the elbow. It affects 40% of athletes with valgus elbow instability and 60% of throwers with medial epicondylitis.[50] Possible causes of ulnar neuropathy potentially revealed by conventional radiographs include impinging osteophytes, heterotopic ossification, fracture malunion, and valgus instability.[51] Although the history and physical examination, in conjunction with electrodiagnostic studies, are the mainstays of diagnosis, MRI may be used adjunctively to evaluate recalcitrant cases when nonoperative management or surgical intervention has failed. Vucic et al.[52] have

suggested that MRI may actually be more sensitive than nerve conduction studies in diagnosing ulnar neuropathy at the elbow. Britz et al.[53] compared the efficacy of electrodiagnostic studies and MRI for the diagnosis of ulnar neuropathy. Although the two modalities were comparable for severe cases, these investigators found that when results were stratified by neuropathic severity, sensitivity for the detection of mild cases was 91% and 74% for MRI and electrodiagnostic studies, respectively. MRI findings in compression neuropathy may include constricting anatomy, nerve thickening, nerve edema, or an adjacent space-occupying lesion on T1-weighted sequences (Fig. 59.10A).[7] In the absence of a morphologic case for cubital tunnel syndrome, it may be difficult to confidently diagnose nerve compression. The ulnar nerve commonly demonstrates increased T2-weighted signal as it passes through the cubital tunnel and has been reported in 60% asymptomatic individuals.[54] A reticulated appearance of the adjacent soft tissues or a surrounding fluid collection may represent inflammatory changes on T2-weighted sequences (see Fig. 59.10B). Chronic neuropathy with muscle denervation may produce muscle atrophy and fatty infiltration seen on T1-weighted images or muscle edema seen on T2-weighted images.[55] US is useful to assess for dynamic nerve instability or presence of accessory anconeus epitrochlearis musculature.[56]

CONCLUSION

A thorough understanding of elbow pathology and a familiarity with common imaging findings ensures timely diagnosis, appropriate treatment, and expeditious return to sport for the affected athlete.

ACKNOWLEDGMENT

We would like to extend acknowledgment to the previous authors of this chapter; Ashvin K. Dewan, A. Bobby Chhabra, and Lance M. Brunton.

For a complete list of references, go to ExpertConsult.com.

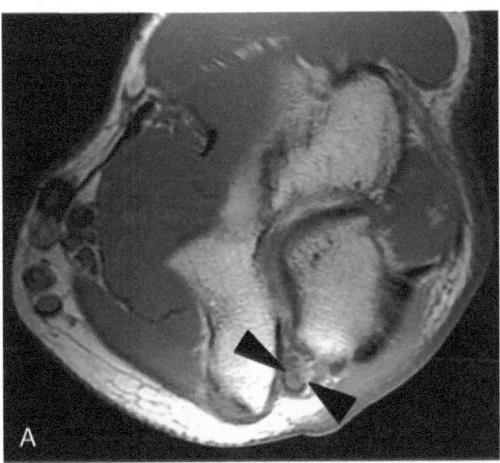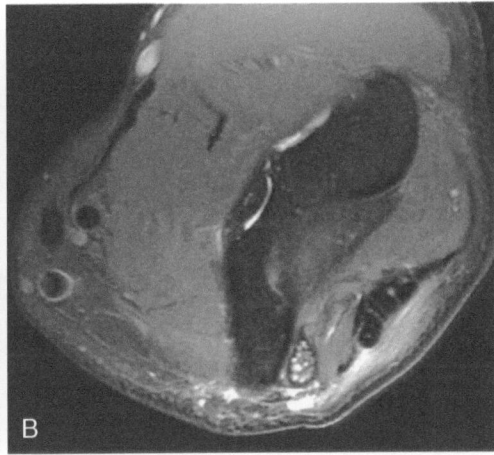

Fig. 59.10 Ulnar neuritis at the cubital tunnel. (A) Axial T1-weighted magnetic resonance imaging at the cubital tunnel demonstrates compression of the ulnar nerve with reduction of the perineural fat *(arrowheads)*. (B) Axial T2-weighted image proximal to the cubital tunnel demonstrates prominent nerve enlargement and hyperintensity of the nerve with fasicular enlargement consistent with nerve edema/inflammation.

SELECTED READINGS

Citation:
Chen AL, Youm T, Ong BC, et al. Imaging of the elbow in the overhead throwing athlete. *Am J Sports Med*. 2003;31(3): 466–473.

Level of Evidence:
III

Summary:
This article provides an excellent overview of elbow pathology and imaging in the overhead-throwing athlete.

Citation:
Norell HG. Roentgenologic visualization of the extracapsular fat; its importance in the diagnosis of traumatic injuries to the elbow. *Acta Radiol*. 1954;42(3):205–210.

Level of Evidence:
III

Summary:
In this retrospective case series, radiographs of 156 elbow fractures were examined. This article includes the original description of the posterior fat pad sign.

Citation:
Ring D, Jupiter JB, Zilberfarb J. Posterior dislocation of the elbow with fractures of the radial head and coronoid. *J Bone Joint Surg Am*. 2002;84(4):547–551.

Level of Evidence:
IV

Summary:
This article describes a clinical series of 11 patients with injuries to the radial head, coronoid, and/or lateral collateral ligament after posterior elbow dislocation. The article emphasizes the importance of recognizing the "terrible triad" and the associated role of advanced imaging.

Citation:
Zubler V, Saupe N, Jost B, et al. Elbow stiffness: effectiveness of conventional radiography and CT to explain osseous causes. *AJR Am J Roentgenol*. 2010;194(6):W515–W520.

Level of Evidence:
III

Summary:
This article describes a retrospective study of computed tomography (CT) and plain radiograph findings in 94 consecutive patients with elbow stiffness. The authors found CT helpful for the diagnosis of loose bodies. The study population was different from that in the study by Dubberley et al. (see the next citation).

Citation:
Dubberley JH, Faber KJ, Patterson SD, et al. The detection of loose bodies in the elbow: The value of MRI and CT arthrography. *J Bone Joint Surg Br*. 2005;87(5):684–686.

Level of Evidence:
III

Summary:
In this retrospective cohort study, magnetic resonance imaging, computed tomography, and conventional radiographic findings were compared with arthroscopic findings for 26 patients with mechanical symptoms of the elbow. The authors found that advanced imaging provided no benefits. Note the differences between this study and the study by Zubler et al. (see the previous citation).

Citation:
Timmerman LA, Schwartz ML, Andrews JR. Preoperative evaluation of the ulnar collateral ligament by magnetic resonance imaging and computed tomography arthrography. Evaluation in 25 baseball players with surgical confirmation. *Am J Sports Med*. 1994;22(1):26–32.

Level of Evidence:
II

Summary:

In this prospective cohort study, use of computed tomography and magnetic resonance imaging for diagnosis of medial-sided elbow pain in baseball players was evaluated. The article describes the "T sign" in partial ulnar collateral ligament tears.

Citation:

O'Driscoll SW, Bell DF, Morrey BF. Posterolateral rotatory instability of the elbow. *J Bone Joint Surg Am*. 1991;73(3):440–446.

Level of Evidence:

IV

Summary:

This article provides the first clinical description of posterolateral rotatory instability of the elbow and the role of the lateral ulnar collateral ligament in maintaining elbow stability.

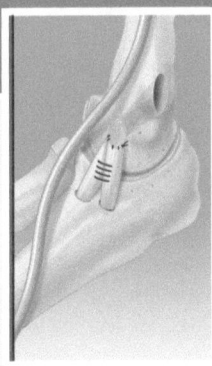

60

Elbow Arthroscopy

Todd A. Rubin, Shawn M. Kutnik, Michael R. Hausman

Arthroscopic and endoscopic techniques were first introduced in the early 1920s and have since revolutionized medical treatments, especially in the field of orthopedic surgery.[1] Widespread application of arthroscopic techniques has been demonstrated in the shoulder and knee; however, its utility in the elbow has been slowly adopted. The elbow joint itself presents unique challenges because of its highly constrained nature and close proximity of neurovascular structures. Advances in instrumentation and the improved understanding of the surgical anatomy have expanded the indications for the use of elbow arthroscopy. Initially, elbow arthroscopy was limited to loose body removal and chondroplasty.[2] The literature now supports the use of elbow arthroscopy for treatment of conditions such as lateral epicondylitis, osteochondritis dissecans (OCD), elbow instability, fracture reduction, excision of heterotopic ossification (HO), contracture release, and septic arthritis. This chapter will discuss the basics of elbow arthroscopy as well as the authors' surgical techniques for loose body removal, OCD, lateral epicondylitis, and instability.

HISTORY

The approach to treatment begins with a detailed history and physical exam. Evaluation of the patient should include the duration of symptoms, mechanism of injury, presence of nighttime symptoms, and neurologic involvement. Of particular concern in the athlete are precipitating activities, the presence of mechanical symptoms, and reduced range of motion (ROM). The type of sport and the patient's related activities should be assessed to elucidate overuse injuries. This is particularly common in young baseball pitchers and gymnasts who engage in repetitive loading of the elbow. They may present with elbow pain and stiffness that improves with rest. They may also present with catching or locking symptoms indicative of loose body formation. Previous treatments should be documented, including use of medication, activity modifications or restrictions, and course of formalized therapy.

PHYSICAL EXAMINATION

A complete physical examination includes a thorough evaluation of the cervical spine, shoulder, elbow, and wrist. The elbow carrying angle and ROM should be compared with the contralateral side. Precise examination may help differentiate pain originating from the capitellum, radial head, common extensor tendon insertion, medial epicondyle, flexor-pronator mass, and posterior medial/lateral ulnohumeral articulations. It is also important to assess coronal plane stability of the elbow and conduct a detailed neurologic assessment. Assessment of ulnar nerve position is essential prior to surgery to avoid iatrogenic injury during portal placement and to prevent aggravation of a mild, preexisting neuropathy.

Specific diagnoses have certain associated findings. For example, loss of terminal extension is often present in patients with OCD, and valgus stress will often recreate pain at the lateral elbow.[3] End-arc limitation of motion with pain is indicative of osteophyte impingement associated with osteoarthritis. Tenderness to palpation at the extensor origin and pain with resisted wrist extension are commonly seen in persons with lateral epicondylitis.[4]

IMAGING

Standard anteroposterior, lateral, and oblique radiographs of the elbow should be obtained for all patients. Contralateral radiographs may be included for comparative purposes. If an OCD lesion of the capitellum is suspected, a 45-degree flexion view can provide improved visualization.[5] Radiographs may be positive for an effusion, loose bodies, and/or subchondral lucency. Ultrasound has also been used to aid in diagnosis (i.e., lateral epicondylitis) though remains largely operator dependent.[6] Computed tomography (CT) is used to assess bony anatomy and may demonstrate loose bodies, fragmentation, and/or collapse of advanced OCD lesions. It may also be helpful for preoperative planning of débridement procedures in patients with elbow arthritis.

If advanced imaging is required, magnetic resonance imaging (MRI) with and without contrast should be obtained. MRI provides detailed images of ligament, chondral, and synovial pathology and is standard in evaluation of OCD. Bowen demonstrated high sensitivity and specificity in identifying these lesions, and specific cartilage-imaging sequences may help with staging.[5,7] Finally, MRI arthrogram may be helpful in detecting inconspicuous loose bodies.

DECISION-MAKING PRINCIPLES AND TREATMENT OPTIONS

The theoretical advantages of arthroscopic treatment of elbow pathology include improved visualization and less tissue disruption compared with open procedures. The surgeon is able to access the entire elbow through small portals, including the neck of the radius, the medial and lateral gutters, and the anterior and posterior compartments. In contrast, obtaining such exposure by open means entails a wider dissection. Nonetheless, one needs to be proficient with elbow arthroscopy, given the risk of injury to adjacent neurovascular structures.

Anesthesia

Elbow arthroscopy may be performed with administration of either a regional or nondepolarizing general anesthetic. The authors prefer to use regional anesthesia with sedation, as it is generally safer than a nondepolarizing general anesthetic and affords improved postoperative pain control. General anesthesia, however, is advantageous for ease of positioning and immediate assessment of postoperative neurologic status. Use of paralytic agents should be avoided, if possible, to improve intraoperative safety.[2,8,9] Paralysis eliminates the possibility of using intraoperative stimulation to identify the location of a nerve and/or observing a response if a nerve is touched and stimulated.

Positioning

Elbow arthroscopy may be performed with the patient in the supine or lateral decubitus position. In our practice, we prefer use of the supine position with a limb-positioning device; in particular, the McConnell arm holder (McConnell Orthopaedic Manufacturing Co., Greenville, TX). The McConnell arm holder allows the extremity to be moved intraoperatively for improved access to the anterior and posterior compartments (Fig. 60.1). The supine position mimics a natural orientation of the joint space, making it conceptually easier to appreciate the surrounding

anatomy by the arthroscopist. Furthermore, the supine position affords the option to convert to an open procedure if necessary.[10]

The prone position, which was originally described by Poehling et al.[11] in 1989, has been largely abandoned because of limited access to the anterior compartment and poor tolerance with the use of regional anesthesia. The lateral decubitus position is frequently used, as it provides complete visualization of the joint and adequate stability of the extremity.[9,11,12] The patient is placed on their side with the operative extremity up and flexed 90 degrees over a padded bolster.

Fluid Management and Instrumentation

Fluid management is critical in elbow arthroscopy. The short distance between the joint capsule and skin causes rapid fluid extravasation with use of conventional, fenestrated cannulae.[9,13] Therefore the use of special cannulae without side vents helps prevent this (Fig. 60.2). Furthermore, increased visualization seen at higher inflow pressures (>35 mm Hg) comes at the expense of significant swelling and markedly decreased working time (maximum 30 to 45 minutes). Maintaining lower pressures of 25 to 30 mm Hg and using strategically placed retractors permit extended working time and improve visualization.[14,15] The use of switching sticks minimizes the number of passes through the tissues once portals are established and decreases the risk of neurovascular injury. A tourniquet should be used to help minimize bleeding. This may ultimately help avoid higher inflow pressures and allow longer working times.

Appropriate instrumentation includes multiple blunt and sharp trocars with paired cannulae, nonfenestrated cannulae to prevent extravasation of fluid, soft tissue shavers (3.5 mm and 4.5 mm), a radiofrequency ablator, and both the 2.7 mm and

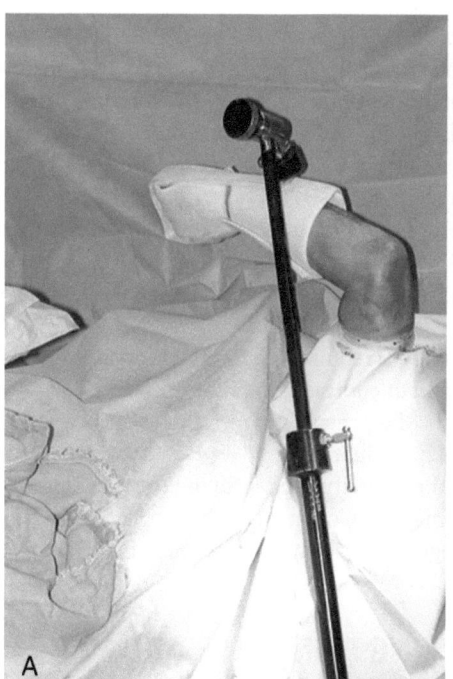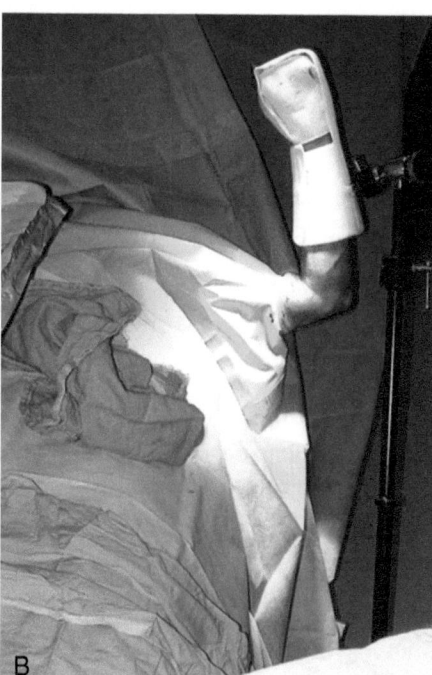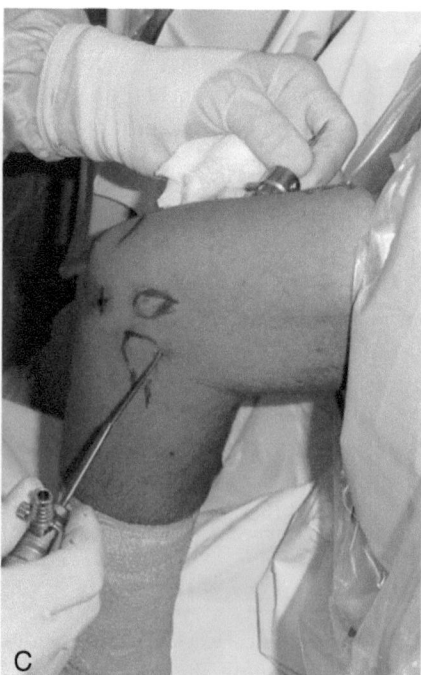

Fig. 60.1 Positioning options for elbow arthroscopy. (A) Supine with use of the McConnell limb positioner (authors preference) for access to the posterior compartment. (B) Positioning for access to the anterior compartment. (C) Alternative lateral decubitus positioning.

4.0 mm arthroscopes. Oftentimes, a 70-degree arthroscope is useful for viewing the coronoid base and the anterior surface of the humerus from the distal posterolateral portal. Adult-sized (3.5 or 4.0 mm) arthroscopes are more commonly used for patients aged 3 and older, while a wrist arthroscope is used for younger children. This may vary according to the individual's anatomy and the type of procedure.

Portal Placement and Precautions

The proximity of critical neurovascular structures has been detailed in multiple anatomic studies (Tables 60.1 and 60.2). Initial insufflation of the elbow joint with approximately 8 to 10 cc saline via the posterior radiocapitellar "soft spot" portal displaces vital structures from offending instruments,[16] although the benefit may be minimal in patients with elbow stiffness.[17] Risk is further minimized by establishing all portals while the elbow is flexed to 90 degrees.[16,18–20] These portals should be made close to the capsular insertion on the supracondylar ridge because

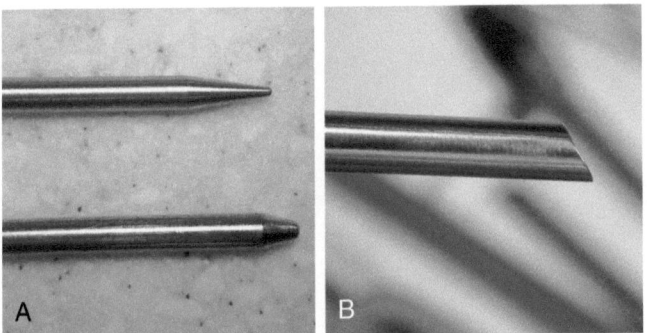

Fig. 60.2 Paired trocars (A) and a nonfenestrated cannulae (B) facilitate joint access and help minimize soft tissue damage.

entrapped tissue between the portal and humerus decreases joint volume and compromises exposure.[17,21]

Standard technique includes making a small incision through skin only using a No. 15 blade, followed by blunt dissection through the subcutaneous tissue and musculature down to the capsular level. In general, blunt-tipped trocars are preferred, although sharp trocars may facilitate capsular penetration in cases with scar or significant contracture.

Standard Anteromedial Portal

The standard anteromedial portal is located 2 cm distal and 2 cm anterior to the medial epicondyle (Fig. 60.3). The arthroscope is aimed toward the center of the joint and passes through the common flexor origin, deep to the median nerve and brachial artery.[2,16,19] The arthroscope provides an excellent view of the anterior compartment of the joint, especially the radiocapitellar joint, mid to lateral coronoid, and trochlea. The proximal radio-ulnar joint articulation may be obstructed by the coronoid process, and the medial ulnohumeral articulation is often difficult to see. Pronation and supination will allow a 260-degree arc of visibility of the radial head.[18]

The structure at greatest risk is the medial antebrachial cutaneous nerve (MABC),[9] which is located on average as little as 1 mm from the trocar, with considerable variability in its branching and location.[18] Blunt subcutaneous tissue dissection is important in this location. The median nerve is located within average 7 to 14 mm.[16,18–20] Considering previous anatomic studies, Verhaar et al.[22] advocated for placement of the anteromedial portal only 1 cm anterior to the medial epicondyle, thereby increasing the safe distance to 18 mm. Either way, the nerve is at increased risk based on its course relative to the portal orientation.[23] In addition, the brachial artery is located lateral to the nerve on average 8 to 17 mm.[16,18–20]

TABLE 60.1	Anterior Portals and Average Proximity to Neurovascular Structures (mm)			
	ANTERIOR PORTALS			
Neurovascular Structure	**Standard Anteromedial**	**Proximal Anteromedial**	**Standard Anterolateral**	**Proximal Anterolateral**
Medial antebrachial cutaneous nerve	1	6	—	—
Median nerve	7	12	—	—
Brachial artery	8	18	—	—
Ulnar nerve	—	12	—	—
Lateral antebrachial cutaneous nerve	—	—	—	6
Posterior antebrachial cutaneous nerve	—	—	13	—
Radial nerve	—	—	1	10

TABLE 60.2	Posterior Portals and Average Proximity to Neurovascular Structures (mm)		
	POSTERIOR PORTALS		
Neurovascular Structure	**Posterior Radiocapitellar**	**Transtriceps**	**Proximal Posterolateral**
Medial antebrachial cutaneous nerve	—	—	25
Ulnar nerve	—	19	25
Lateral antebrachial cutaneous nerve	10	—	—
Posterior antebrachial cutaneous nerve	7	23	25

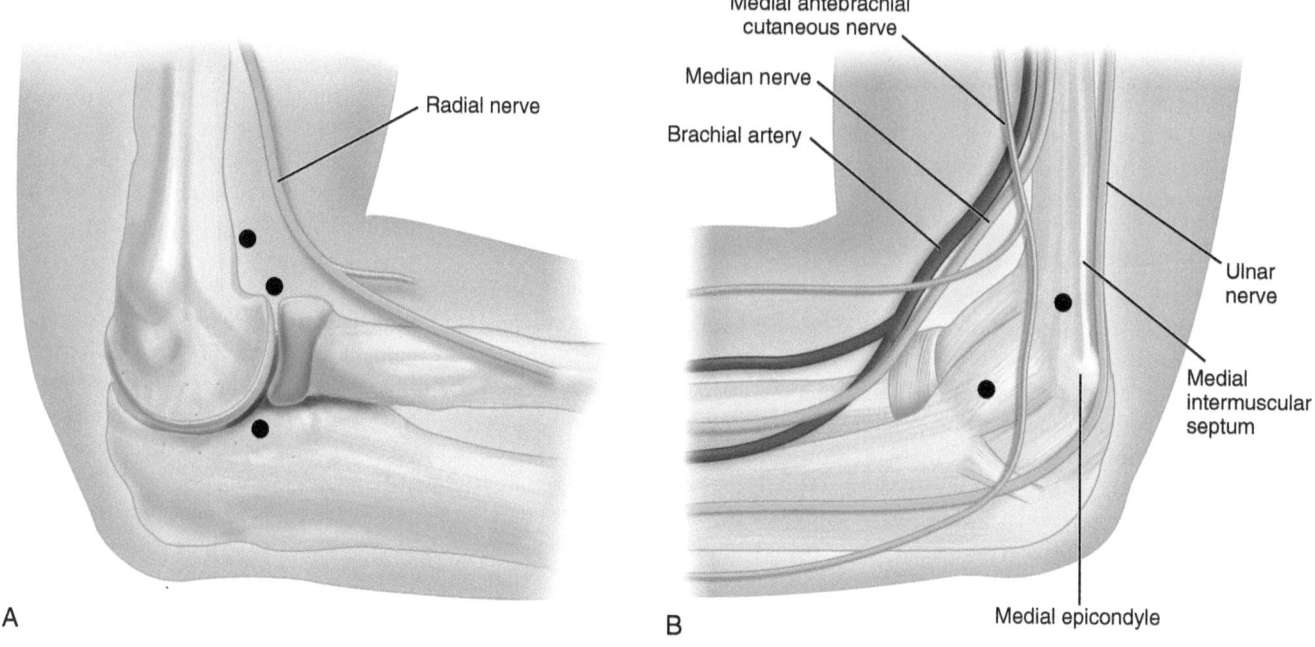

A

B

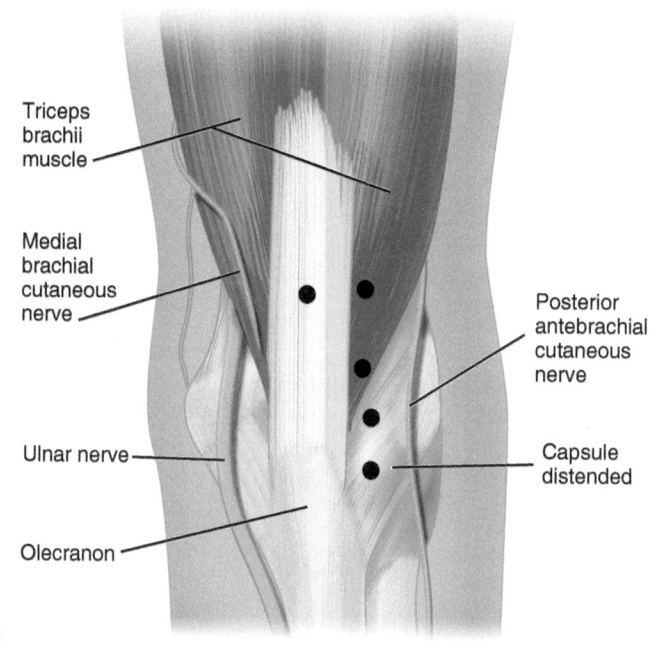

C

Fig. 60.3 Commonly used lateral (A), medial (B), and posterior (C) portals. Refer to the chapter for portal placement and Table 60.1 for proximity to neurovascular structures.

Proximal Anteromedial Portal

Many surgeons advocate for initial placement of the proximal anteromedial portal, as it is safe and provides an excellent view of the anterior compartment.[24] As described by Poehling et al.,[11] this portal is created 2 cm proximal to the medial epicondyle and just anterior to the intermuscular septum to avoid injury to the ulnar nerve (see Fig. 60.3). An additional margin of safety is provided by placing the portal a full 1 cm anterior to the septum,[18,20,22] which, in our experience, improves the mechanical arc of motion of the scope before levering against the supracondylar ridge of the humerus. The blunt trocar should slide along the anterior surface of the humerus while aimed toward the coronoid fossa. If the ulnar nerve tends to subluxate, care must be taken to palpate it and hold it in the normal position posterior to the medial epicondyle while creating the proximal anteromedial portal.

When establishing this portal, the MABC nerve remains at most risk to injury. Anatomic studies have shown that on average it is 6 mm from the cannula, but variations in branching may reduce this distance to within 2 mm.[18–20] If the aforementioned technique is used, the median nerve is relatively safe, at an average distance of 12 to 22 mm.[18–20,23] The brachialis muscle provides an additional layer of protection from penetration of the median nerve.[25] Aiming the trocar more parallel (rather than perpendicular) to the median nerve increases the safety of its introduction.[23]

Further away and at less risk is the brachial artery, at an average distance of 18 mm.[19,20] The ulnar nerve is an average distance of 12 to 25 mm and is considered safe from this portal as long as the trocar is kept anterior to the intermuscular septum.[18–20,23] One case report, however, demonstrated that protection afforded by the septum may be negated if the portal is moved farther proximal than the recommended 2 cm from the medial epicondyle.[26] The surgeon must be aware of the presence of previous ulnar nerve transposition or anterior subluxation before portal placement.

Historically, ulnar nerve transposition was considered a contraindication to the anteromedial portal because of potential nerve injury.[23] More recent studies have maintained that with a thorough preoperative examination and appropriate precautions, safe placement can be performed despite anterior ulnar nerve transposition. A systematic approach to placement of the proximal medial portal was well described in 2010 by Sahajpal et al.[27] In some cases, a mini open procedure was recommended, particularly in those with prior submuscular transposition.

In general, the authors consider a medial portal to be a relative contraindication after a subcutaneous ulnar nerve transposition. Placement of the proximal anteromedial portal is absolutely contraindicated following submuscular ulnar nerve transposition.

Standard Anterolateral Portal

The standard anterolateral portal was originally described by Andrews and Carson[2] as 3 cm distal and 1 cm anterior to the lateral epicondyle (see Fig. 60.3). The value of this portal has been called into question because the proximal anterolateral portal offers the same visualization with less risk.[19,28] The posterior antebrachial cutaneous (PABC) nerve averages 13 mm from the portal. The radial nerve, averaging 1 to 7 mm from this portal, is also at increased risk compared with a more proximal portal (10 to 14 mm).[16,19,20,28]

Proximal Anterolateral Portal

The proximal anterolateral portal is located 2 cm proximal and 1 to 2 cm anterior to the lateral epicondyle (see Fig. 60.3). It allows for a more consistent view of the radiocapitellar joint than the standard anterolateral portal.[19,28] The sheath should be directed toward the center of the joint with the trocar contacting the anterior humerus. The capsule is pierced after traversing the brachioradialis and extensor carpi radialis longus muscles.

The posterior branch of the lateral antebrachial cutaneous (LABC) nerve is located an average of 6 mm from this portal.[19]

The radial nerve is located approximately 10 to 14 mm from the portal with elbow flexion.[19,28] This portal has been advocated as a safe starting point during elbow arthroscopy because it offers similar visualization compared with the standard anterolateral portal though is at a safer distance from the radial nerve.[28]

Posterior Radiocapitellar ("Soft Spot") Portal

The posterior radiocapitellar portal is located within the center of the anatomic triangle bound by the lateral epicondyle, olecranon, and radial head (see Fig. 60.3). This portal allows access to the posterior radiocapitellar and proximal radioulnar joints[8] and is at a relatively safe distance from the LABC nerve (10 mm) and the PABC nerve (7 mm).[8,20] When using this portal, one must ensure that the skin heals appropriately. The lack of subcutaneous tissue overlying the joint capsule in this region makes this portal susceptible to fluid extravasation and sinus tract formation.

Straight Posterior (Transtriceps) Portal

The straight posterior portal is located 3 cm proximal and midline to the olecranon tip centered between the medial and lateral epicondyles (see Fig. 60.3).[29] The trocar passes centrally through the triceps tendon and into the olecranon fossa. This portal allows visualization of the entire posterior compartment, including both the medial and lateral gutters. Compared with other portals, the transtriceps portal is relatively safe within average 19 to 25 mm of the ulnar nerve and 23 to 29 mm of the PABC nerve.[19,20,30]

Proximal Posterolateral Portal

The proximal posterolateral portal is classically placed 4 cm proximal to the olecranon tip and just lateral to the palpable edge of the triceps tendon (see Fig. 60.3).[30] The trocar is again advanced toward the olecranon fossa, passing lateral to the tendon and through the posterolateral capsule. The ulnar and PABC nerves are both approximately 25 mm from the trochar, which minimizes risk during elbow arthroscopy.[8,16,18,20]

Accessory Portals

The distal posterolateral portal is often used in junction with the transtriceps portal for visualization of the posterior compartment, including the lateral gutter, posterior radiocapitellar joint, proximal radioulnar joint, and medial gutter. This portal may be utilized so that a shaver or forceps can be introduced into the transtriceps portal.[15]

Another useful accessory portal is the anterior radiocapitellar portal, just anterior and proximal to the joint. It should only be made under direct visualization from the medial portal because it lies closest to the radial nerve. Extreme caution should be used when inserting the trocar here because anterior deflection along the capsule will place the radial nerve at risk.[15]

A distal ulnar portal described by Van den Ende et al.[31] may augment visualization of the posterior radiocapitellar joint and may offer a better trajectory for instrumentation. This portal is located 3 cm distal to the posterior radiocapitellar joint, lateral to the palpable ulnar edge.

Order of Portal Placement

The authors' preference is to start in the posterior compartment, though this may change depending on the patient's underlying pathology. In regard to the anterior compartment, we prefer to start with a proximal, anteromedial portal because it carries less risk to neurovascular structures, which are anterior to the brachialis muscle. Also, correct placement of the lateral portals is essential, especially if a retractor is needed. By establishing the medial portal first, the lateral portals can be precisely placed under direct vision. Whatever the case, the initial portal should allow ease of entry into the joint in a safe and controlled manner.[24,28]

Authors' Preferred Technique

Diagnostic Arthroscopy and Loose Body Removal

The patient is placed supine on the operating table and the arm is prepped/draped in the standard fashion. A tourniquet is placed high on the arm and the limb is placed overhead using the McConnell limb positioner. Surface landmarks are marked, including the medial and lateral epicondyles, olecranon, proximal ulna, radial head, and radiocapitellar joint. Proposed portals are similarly drawn prior to joint distention (Fig. 60.4). The ulnar nerve is palpated and its position localized. Subluxation of the ulnar nerve should be noted prior to the start of the case.

The limb is then exsanguinated and the tourniquet inflated. The transtriceps portal is established through a stab incision directly down to the bone of the distal humerus, followed by insertion of a 30-degree arthroscope. A fluid pump is used and the pressure is set to 25 to 30 mm Hg to minimize fluid extravasation. The pressure is only increased transiently throughout the case if necessary to identify and control bleeding. The proximal or distal posterolateral portal is established as a working portal in a similar fashion, and a shaver is introduced into the posterior compartment. Fat pad débridement is necessary to establish a viewing space, and dissection is then carried distally to identify the tip of the olecranon and lateral gutter (Fig. 60.5). Intraoperative flexion and extension of the elbow will confirm the location of the joint. The arthroscope is then advanced medially along the tip of the olecranon to visualize the medial gutter and medial column.

The posterior radiocapitellar joint can be visualized by passing the arthroscope along the lateral gutter over the distal humerus until the base of the coronoid and radial head come into view (see Fig. 60.5). A 3.5-mm shaver in the posterior radiocapitellar "soft spot" portal will help débride any localized synovitis. Loose bodies may be removed using a grasper or débrided with the shaver. Larger bodies may be guided with a grasper and then pushed out of the joint via a cannula.

The arm is repositioned by the patient's side with the elbow in approximately 90 degrees of flexion for access to the anterior compartment. The proximal antero-medial portal is first established as a viewing portal. The proximal anterolateral portal is then established under direct visualization and used for instrumentation. The anterior compartment inspection consists of the anterior radiocapitellar joint, proximal radioulnar joint, coronoid, and coronoid fossa (Fig. 60.6). Switching viewing portals allows for complete inspection of the remainder of the joint.

Loose bodies should be removed as encountered to prevent them from "hiding" or "escaping." The loose body may be stabilized against a surface and firmly grasped with an instrument of adequate size. Usually an arthroscopic grasping instrument will suffice, although occasionally a hemostat is needed. The arthroscope can be used to push the loose body as it is pulled. Make the incision large enough that the loose body does not get lost in the subcutaneous tissues.

Once the procedure is completed, portals are tightly closed with interrupted nonabsorbable sutures to prevent drainage and synovial fistulae. Postoperative management depends on the degree of operative intervention and underlying diagnosis.

Results

The results of loose body removal are excellent, with reliable relief of pain and symptoms of catching or locking.[32–35] In patients with synovial chondromatosis, Flury et al.[36] demonstrated good results with both open and arthroscopic loose body removal. There was a trend toward shorter rehabilitation and higher patient satisfaction in the arthroscopic cohort. The results were similar in the arthroscopic treatment of athletic patients with loose bodies and/or impinging osteophytes.[35]

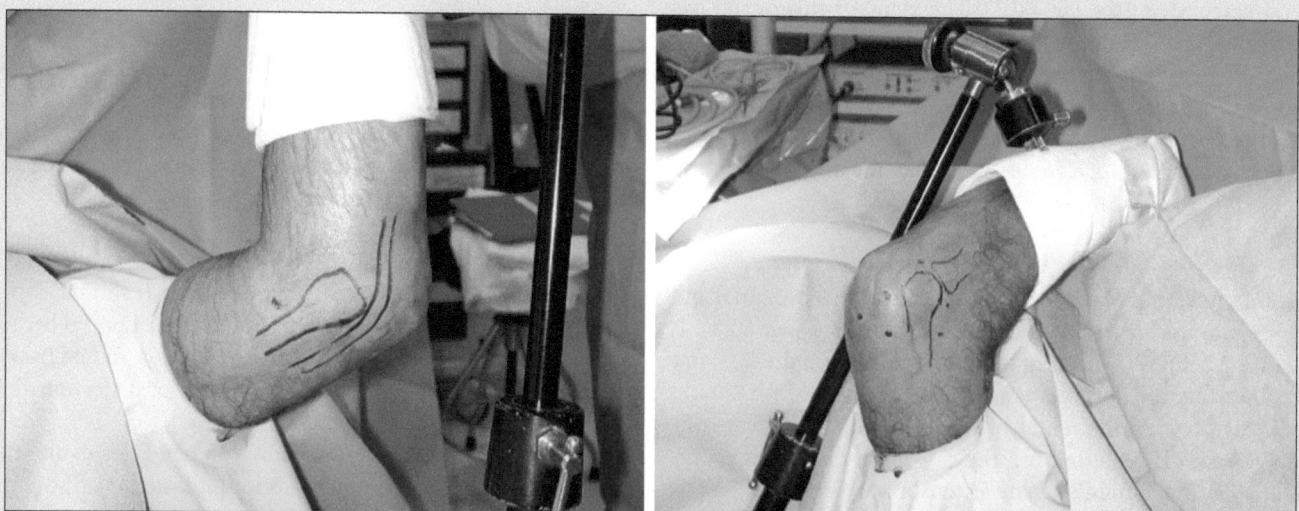

Fig. 60.4 Intraoperative photos depicting bony landmarks, commonly used portals, and location of the ulnar nerve.

📌 **Authors' Preferred Technique**

Diagnostic Arthroscopy and Loose Body Removal—cont'd

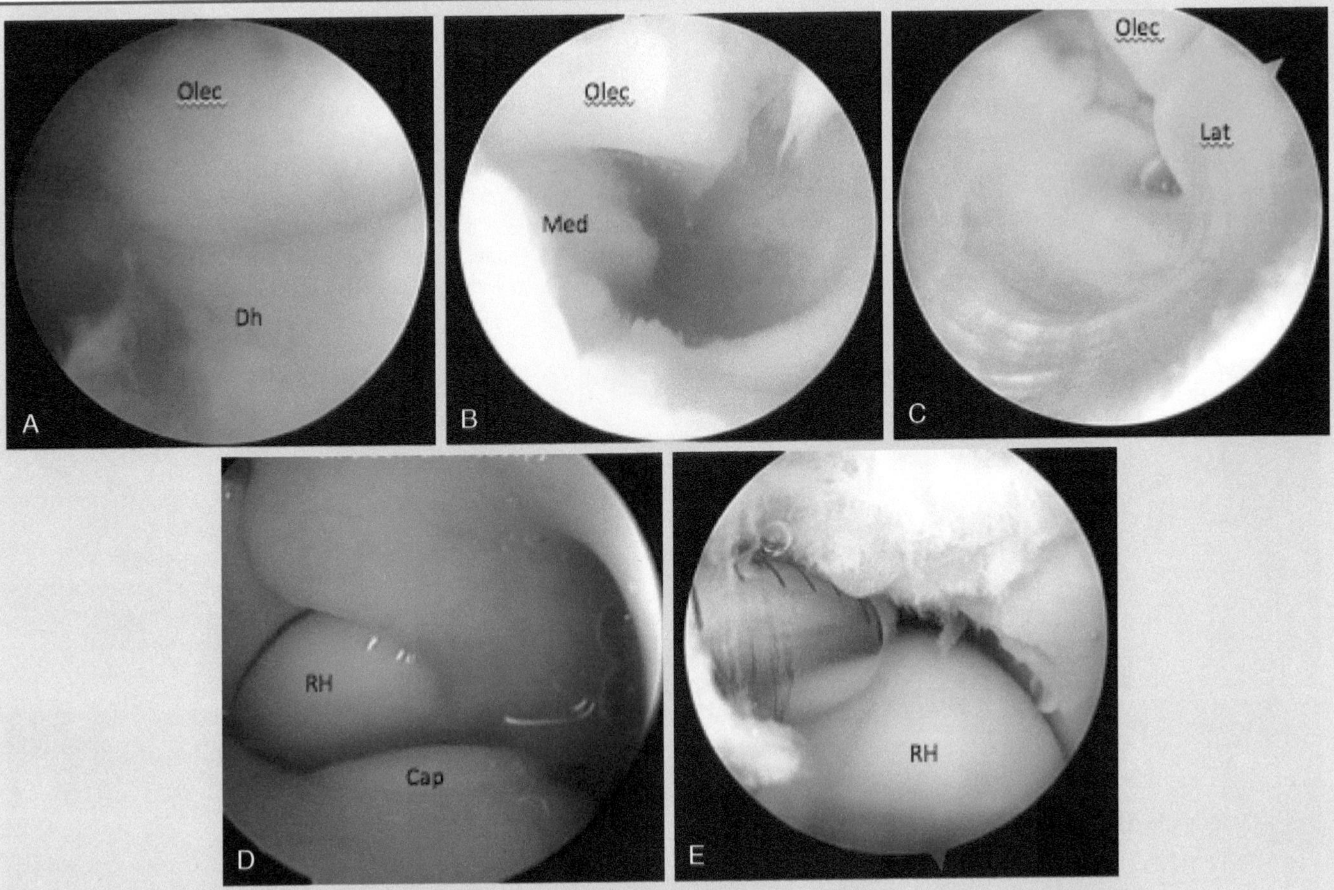

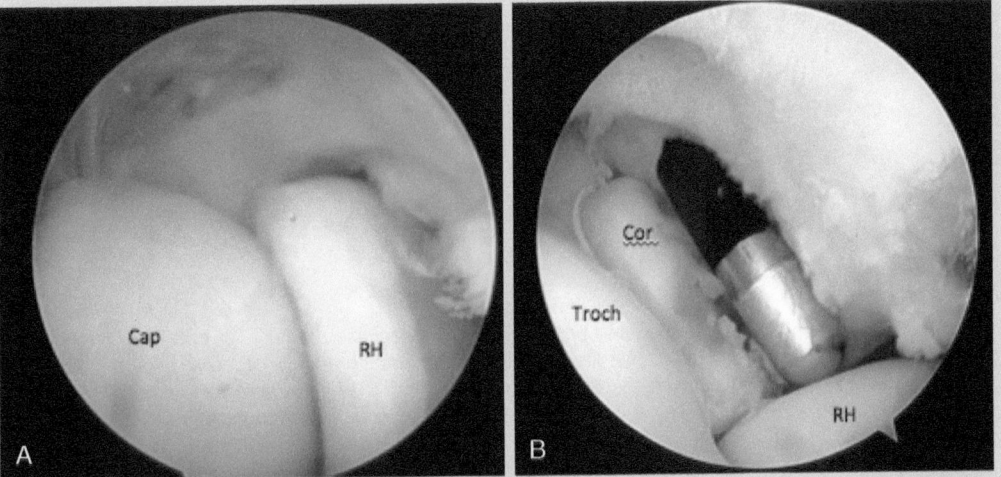

Fig. 60.5 Posterior compartment arthroscopic views. (A) Olecranon and posterior articular surface. (B) Medial gutter. (C) Lateral gutter. (D) View of the posterior radiocapitellar joint with the arthroscope in the transtriceps portal. (E) The radial head with instrumentation in the soft spot portal. *Cap*, Capitellum; *Dh*, distal humerus; *Lat*, lateral trochlear ridge; *Med*, medial trochlear ridge; *Olec*, olecranon; *RH*, radial head.

Fig. 60.6 Anterior compartment arthroscopy. (A) View of the radiocapitellar joint from the proximal antero-medial portal. (B) View of the coronoid and trochlea from the proximal anterolateral portal with instrumentation in the anteromedial portal. *Cap*, Capitellum; *Cor*, coronoid; *RH*, radial head; *Troch*, trochlea.

Authors' Preferred Technique

Osteochondritis Dissecans Débridement

Elbow arthroscopy has increasingly been used in the treatment of OCD. Débridement, microfracture, abrasion arthroplasty, and/or fragment fixation may be performed arthroscopically for patients that have failed nonoperative treatment or for those with unstable lesions. Arthroscopic-assisted osteochondral transplantation using a lateral femoral condyle autograft has also be performed for advanced capitellar lesions.[37]

The primary lesion is often best viewed from the distal posterolateral portal into the posterior radiocapitellar joint, using the "soft spot" portal for instrumentation (Fig. 60.7). A 70-degree arthroscope may improve visualization in specific cases. For drilling, our preference is to "back drill" the lesion from the posterolateral column over a guidewire rather than violating the articular cartilage via a transarticular approach. The guidewire is drilled toward the lesion in a posterior to anterior direction starting from the posterolateral aspect of the humerus. Under direct visualization, the guidewire is advanced toward the lesion, with care not to displace the lesion or penetrate the articular surface. A Freer elevator can be used to prevent dislodgement of the lesion if necessary. Fluoroscopy may also be used to direct the guidewire trajectory appropriately and confirm wire position. The guidewire is ultimately advanced until tenting of the articular surface is visualized arthroscopically. Multiple guidewires or repositioning of a single guidewire may allow for additional drilling locations.

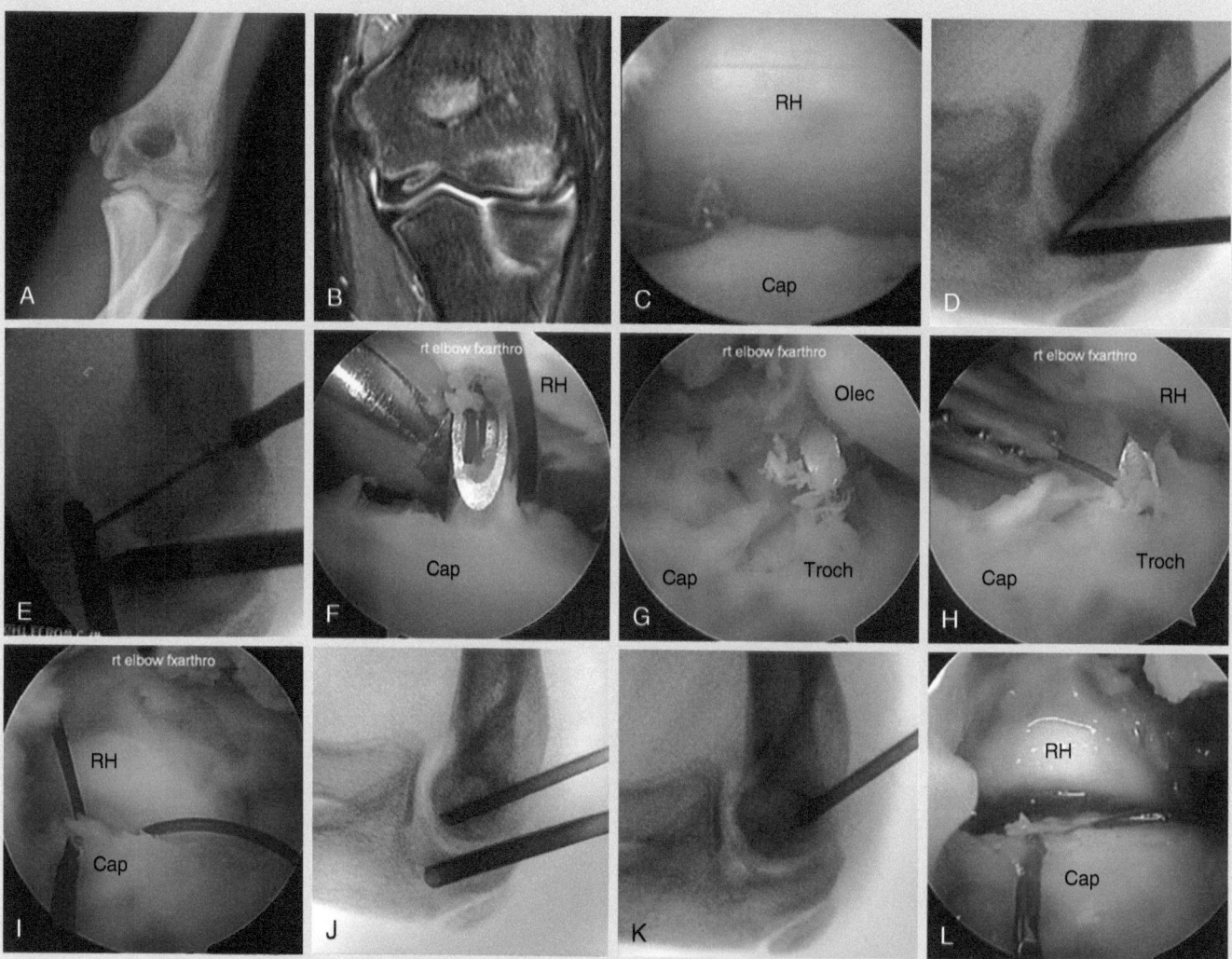

Fig. 60.7 Arthroscopic suture fixation and bone grafting of a capitellar fracture. (A and B) Anteroposterior (AP) radiograph and magnetic resonance imaging (T2) demonstrating a large capitellar osteochondritis dissecans (OCD) fragment. (C) Guidewire placed through the center of the fragment as viewed from the posterior radiocapitellar portal confirmed with fluoroscopy (D). (E) Fluoroscopic image depicting drilling of the OCD lesion from posterior to anterior. An arthroscopic grasper secures the guidewire in place. (F) Spinal needle used to shuttle a 0-polydioxanone suture (PDS) suture with retrieval through an accessory portal. (G) A second point of fixation drilled medial to the defect. (H) A Prolene suture is used to shuttle the PDS fixation suture posteriorly. (I) Multiple fixation points are chosen to adequately secure the fragment. (J) Following OCD fixation, a tunnel is drilled up to the subchondral surface. (K) Drilling allows for insertion of the cannula and placement of the bone graft to support the OCD lesion. Sutures are tied posteriorly and final fixation of the OCD lesion is confirmed (L). *Cap,* Capitellum; *Olec,* olecranon; *RH,* radial head; *Troch,* lateral trochlea.

Authors' Preferred Technique
Osteochondritis Dissecans Débridement—cont'd

Results

The use of accessory portals for arthroscopic treatment of OCD lesions has been previously described. Baumgarten et al.[38] advocated that the soft spot portal was key for lesion visualization. In addition, they reported the use of a second direct lateral portal placed 1 cm distal for cases involving abrasion chondroplasty. Davis et al.[39] found that 78% of the capitellum was accessible through these dual lateral portals. To avoid the close proximity of portals and instrumentation interference, however, Van den Ende et al.[31] described a distal ulnar portal located 3 cm distal to the posterior aspect of the radiocapitellar joint just lateral to the posterior ulnar cortex. The authors reported a more in-line view with easier coordination of movements using this portal. Lastly, Arai et al.[40] demonstrated good results via subchondral drilling through the radial head.

They described a technique whereby the drill is placed through the radial head and advanced into the capitellar OCD lesion. Multiple levels of drilling were achieved via pronation, supination, flexion, and extension of the forearm and elbow. Although this approach is effective in treating capitellar OCD lesions, the long-term consequences of violation of the otherwise normal radial head articular surface remain unknown.

Reports of arthroscopic débridement of OCD lesions are limited to retrospective, short to midterm studies. Furthermore, reported results are difficult to compare for a variety of reasons, including differences in patient population, severity of lesions, and surgical techniques executed.[3] Nevertheless, the literature reflects reproducible pain relief and improvement in elbow ROM. Return to sport is highly variable, as demonstrated by Baumgarten et al.,[38] Brownlow et al.,[41] and Rahusen et al.[42] These authors reported full recovery in the majority of patients treated; however, studies by Byrd and Jones,[43] Ruch et al.,[44] and Jackson et al.[45] reported a low percentage of patients with full return to sport. In general, the size of the OCD lesion has been shown to effect outcome, with a more guarded prognosis in persons with larger lesions.[46]

 ## Authors' Preferred Technique
Osteochondritis Dissecans Suture Fixation and Bone Grafting

A similar approach to the treatment of large, unstable OCD lesions is utilized; however, with the addition of stabilization of the lesion. As previously described, the elbow is flexed to 90 degrees and held over the patient's body to allow access to the posterior compartment. The posterolateral portal is established and the arthroscope is inserted to identify the medial and lateral gutters. The arthroscope is carefully advanced over the distal humerus along the lateral gutter until the posterior radiocapitellar joint is reached. The posterior radiocapitellar or "soft spot" portal is then established and a 3.5-mm shaver is introduced to débride any synovitis. The lesion is inspected and probed to evaluate its integrity and stability. For lesions located more anteriorly, a 70-degree arthroscope may be substituted for improved visualization.

If fixation of the lesion is required, a 3-cm incision is made along the posterior aspect of the lateral column and 2 cm proximal from the viewing portal. The incision is carried down to bone, developing a plane just lateral to the triceps. A guidewire is then drilled through the posterior column and aimed to exit at the center of the capitellar lesion under arthroscopic visualization (see Fig. 60.7). Fluoroscopy can also be used to confirm the correct trajectory and location of the guidewire. An arthroscopic grasper is then used through the posterior radiocapitellar working portal to stabilize the OCD lesion to prevent displacement.

An arthroscopic grasper inserted through the "soft spot" portal can be used to stabilize the guidewire and compress the lesion during drilling. This will also prevent the wire from advancing or being inadvertently withdrawn. A tunnel is drilled through the humerus to just under the subchondral bone using sequentially larger cannulated drills that are 2.5 mm, 3.0 mm, and 3.5 mm in diameter. The wire is removed, and an 18-gauge spinal needle is inserted through the tunnel into the joint. A 0-polydioxanone suture (PDS; Ethicon, Somerville, NJ) is passed through the needle into the joint and retrieved via the "soft spot" portal. This process is repeated as necessary, depending on the number of desired mattress sutures (usually 3).

Another point of fixation is established medial to the defect by drilling a separate guidewire through the posterolateral column to exit out the lateral trochlea under arthroscopic visualization. An 18-gauge spinal needle is inserted through this hole into the joint and is used to pass a 2-0 Prolene suture (Ethicon). This is retrieved through the working portal and secured to one of the 0-PDS sutures that are shuttled out posteriorly. An additional point of fixation can be established along the posterior border of the lesion by passing the 18-gauge spinal needle directly along the posterior border of the distal humerus into the joint deep to the lateral ulnar collateral ligament (LUCL). Again, a 2-0 Prolene suture threaded through an 18-gauge needle is used to shuttle another PDS suture posteriorly. By curving the spinal needle around the lateral border of the distal humerus and shuttling the remaining sutures out posteriorly, a fixation point proximal and lateral to the defect is established. This results in an "umbrella" of fixation, with the mattress sutures securing the unstable fragment.

Once all sutures are passed and collected at the posterolateral incision, morselized, autogenous bone graft is harvested from the iliac crest percutaneously using a trephine. A cannula is placed from the posterolateral incision into the humeral tunnel and advanced to just under the subchondral bone of the defect. This is done under arthroscopic visualization to ensure that the space immediately beneath the defect is firmly and densely packed with bone graft, so that when probed, the lesion feels stable. Patience must be exercised to avoid blocking the tunnel near the posterior entrance. Also, bone graft packing should be done with low or, ideally, no fluid inflow to avoid washing the marrow out of the posterior entrance hole. Unfortunately, some inflow is usually necessary at this step in order for adequate visualization. The cannula is slowly withdrawn as the process continues in order to fill the tunnel as much as possible.

Once bone grafting is completed, the mattress sutures are individually tied along the posterior lateral column using an arthroscopic knot pusher. Lastly, inspection of the joint is performed without inflow to avoid washing out the packed tunnel. The construct is probed to ensure stable fixation of the fragment and appropriate suture placement. The portals are tightly closed with interrupted nylon sutures to prevent drainage and synovial fistula formation. The patient is then placed in a long-arm cast with forearm in neutral position and the elbow flexed to 90 degrees.

Results

Various fixation techniques have been described for OCD lesions, including screws, pullout wires, bone pegs, and absorbable pins. The results of these techniques have been highly successful, with reliable union rates approaching

Continued

Authors' Preferred Technique

Osteochondritis Dissecans Suture Fixation and Bone Grafting—cont'd

100% and return to play (RTP) rates of greater than 90%.[47–51] Nobuta et al.[51] cautioned that lesions greater than 9 mm in thickness had markedly inferior results.

There are few published reports on arthroscopic fixation of OCD lesions in the literature. Hardy et al.[52] published a case report of arthroscopic screw fixation of a type I capitellar fracture with successful healing at 2 months and a residual 15-degree extension deficit at final follow-up. Takeda et al.[47] reported a series of four male athletes with OCD lesions treated with arthroscopic fixation using bioabsorbable pins. Healing was evident on CT scans for three patients, and the other patient showed radiographic improvement. RTP was not reported, but ROM was considerably improved in all patients.

We have previously published our findings of four consecutive patients age 13 to 15 years using arthroscopic suture fixation and bone grafting with greater than 2-year follow-up.[53] The patients were all elite-level athletes competing at the national or international level of play: two gymnasts, one baseball pitcher,

and one lacrosse player. All patients presented complaining of lateral elbow pain, limited ROM, and difficulty with activity and/or throwing motions. Preoperative loss of terminal extension ranged from 10 to 60 degrees, with one patient having loss of terminal flexion of 30 degrees. Union was confirmed on MRI at a mean 3 months post op. At final follow up, mean loss of extension was 2 degrees and flexion was 153 degrees with an average Mayo Elbow score of 88 (SD 7). The mean time to RTP was 4 months, and all patients returned to elite level of competition.

In our practice we have found that the aforementioned technique results in reliable healing of the fragment, improvement in motion, and return to preinjury levels of activity and competition. Despite the postoperative immobilization, none of our patients has required subsequent elbow contracture release, although the possibility should be discussed preoperatively. Notably, the same technique may be applied to treat type II Kocher-Lorenz capitellum fractures, as the osteochondral "shell" fragment cannot typically support screw fixation.

 Authors' Preferred Technique

Lateral Epicondylitis Débridement

Arthroscopic treatment of lateral epicondylitis was first described by Kuklo et al.[54] in 1999 and was developed as a method for releasing the extensor carpi radialis brevis (ECRB) tendon with limited morbidity. Though the exact underlying pathophysiology is unknown, lateral epicondylitis is commonly defined as an overuse injury from repetitive microtrauma and degeneration of the ECRB tendon. The authors additionally believe that the pathophysiology involves a capsular thickening or plica responsible for local abrasion of the radial head and reactive synovitis.[55]

The procedure begins with a standard diagnostic arthroscopic evaluation of the elbow via the posterior transtriceps portal. The radiocapitellar portal is then established to remove degenerative tissue interposed in the posterior radiocapitellar joint using a resector (Fig. 60.8). Next, the anterior compartment is examined via the proximal anteromedial portal, which allows precise placement of the laterally based portal. A high proximal anterolateral portal will allow access to the anterolateral capsule without obstruction by the radial head, and an anterolateral capsulectomy can be performed to "decompress" the radial head. In some cases, this procedure may require resection of the deep ECRB fibers that blend with the annular ligament, but full resection of the common extensor tendon origin is avoided. Great care is taken to protect the LUCL during both the posterior and anterior resections. The LUCL origin on the lateral epicondyle is carefully protected and the resection does not extend posteriorly beyond the equator of the radial head.

Postoperatively, the patient's elbow is immobilized in a sling for 1 to 2 days, and early use of the arm is encouraged. Postoperative pain gradually resolves

over the course of several weeks. Patients are allowed to use the arm as tolerated.

Results

Bunata et al. performed a cadaveric study to evaluate the pathogenesis of lateral epicondylitis.[56] Following the examination of 85 cadaver elbows, the authors concluded that the ECRB tendon is vulnerable to contact and abrasion against the lateral edge of the capitellum during elbow motion.[56] Anatomic variation of the ECRB tendon origin may predispose certain patients. Sasaki et al.[57] further reinforced this concept with retrospective examination of cartilage injury in patients with recalcitrant lateral epicondylitis. Most lesions were located on the lateral aspect of the radial head and capitellum, and cartilaginous injuries were more likely in the absence of ECRB tears.

The increase in tendon thickness seen on ultrasound in patients with lateral epicondylitis moreover suggests that direct impingement may contribute to the pathology.[6]

Many reports have been published on the utility of arthroscopic treatment of lateral epicondylitis. Studies demonstrate good to excellent results in 70% to 85% of patients with regard to symptom relief and return to preinjury activity levels.[55,58–65] In addition, Baker and Baker reported long-term follow-up without deterioration in symptoms.[66] Though arthroscopic approaches may offer similar results compared with open approaches, a percentage of patients in both cohorts may continue to experience pain with overuse and early return to work.[55,62,63]

Authors' Preferred Technique

Lateral Epicondylitis Débridement—cont'd

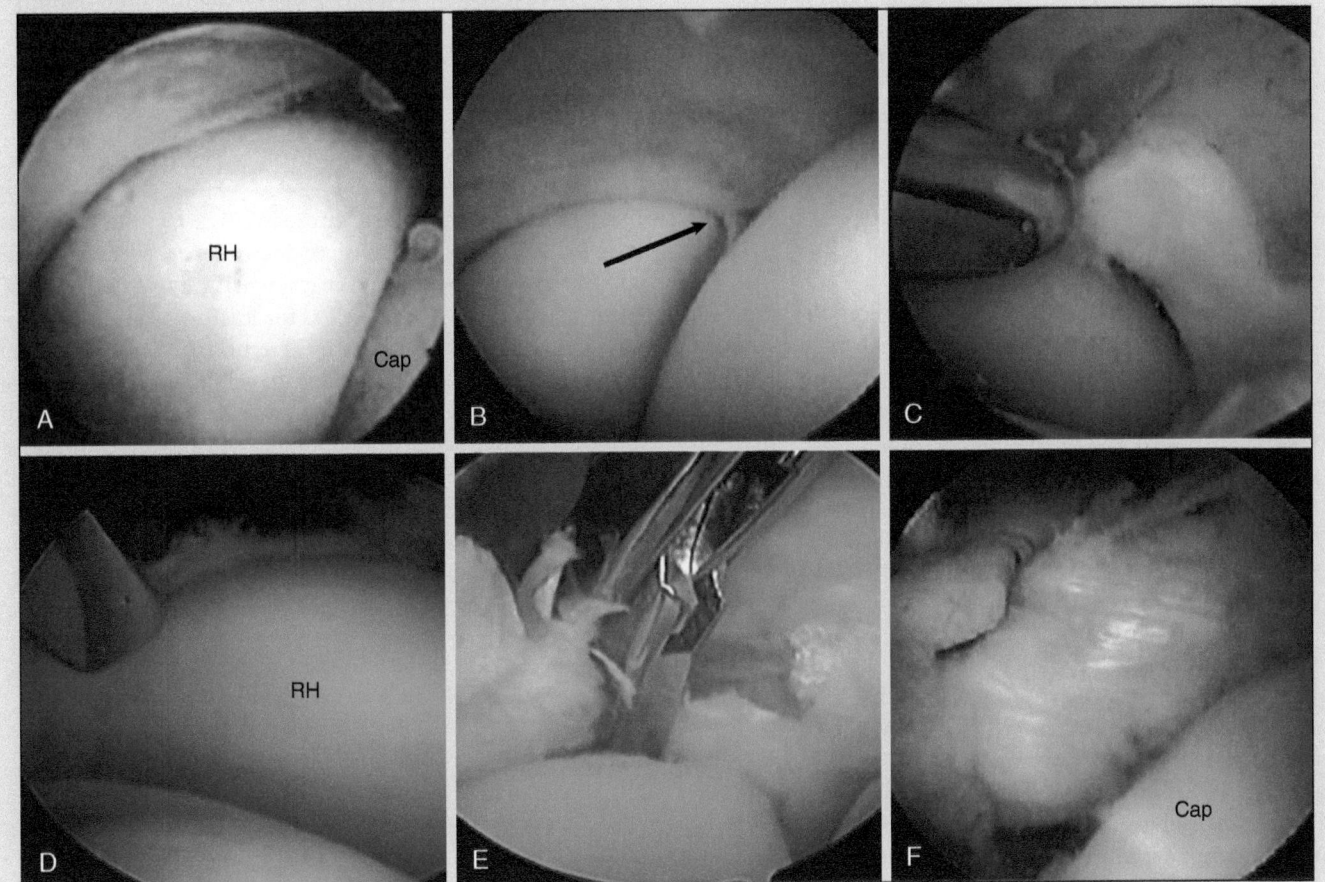

Fig. 60.8 (A) Normal anterolateral capsular morphology of the radiocapitellar joint. (B) Impingement of capsular tissue *(arrow)* and abrasion along the radial head in a patient with lateral epicondylitis. (C and D) Débridement performed using a 3.5-mm shaver via the posterior radiocapitellar portal. (E) Resection of the thickened anterolateral capsule using a resector via the proximal anterolateral portal. (F) Following capsular resection, normal extensor carpi radialis brevis tendon is visualized. *Cap,* Capitellum; *RH,* radial head.

Authors' Preferred Technique

Diagnosis and Treatment of Elbow Instability

Subacute injury to the medial and/or lateral collateral ligament complexes of the elbow following trauma often result in persistent symptoms and may be difficult to diagnose.[67] Timmerman and Andrews[68] proposed an arthroscopic valgus instability stress test to assess for medial collateral ligament (MCL) instability. Through the anterolateral portal, the authors were able to visualize the antero-medial aspect of the ulnohumeral joint and look for gapping along the ulnotrochlear joint. This was used as an indirect measure of MCL injury, given that only a portion of the anterior bundle of the MCL can be visualized during elbow arthros-copy. In a normal elbow with an intact MCL, the elbow is expected to gap less than 1 mm at 70 degrees of elbow flexion along the ulnotrochlear joint. In com-parison, complete sectioning of the anterior bundle of the MCL yielded 3 to 5 mm of gapping along the ulnohumeral joint. The investigators concluded that even though the structural integrity of the MCL cannot be determined directly, an arthroscopic stress test may provide a dependable, reproducible, indirect assess-ment of its competence.[68,69]

The arthroscopic treatment of posterolateral rotatory instability of the elbow was initially described by Smith et al.[70] in 2001 and further expanded upon by Savoie et al.[71] in 2010. In both studies, the authors provided an arthroscopic method for confirming the diagnosis of posterolateral rotatory instability. A pivot shift maneuver was performed during visualization of the anterior compartment via the proximal anteromedial portal. A positive test was described as persistent posterolateral subluxation of the ulna and radial head in the presence of instability. In addition, the presence of a "drive-through" sign (i.e., the ability to drive the arthroscope into the ulnohumeral joint) was present in the unstable elbow but was corrected with appropriate treatment of the instability. The authors additionally described a technique for suture plication of the LUCL in cases of posterolateral rotatory instability. Comparing this procedure with open repair, the arthroscopic technique resulted in similar high rates of success.[71] The authors remarked that in addition to direct visualization of posterolateral subluxation, arthroscopic plication of the attenuated ligament provides an effective alternative approach to joint stabilization.

POSTOPERATIVE MANAGEMENT

Return to Play

Painless, full ROM is the primary goal of all arthroscopic elbow surgery and should serve as a prerequisite to athletic activity. Strength training is gradually increased as tolerated over time and full participation, especially involving contact sports, should be avoided until evidence of complete healing is confirmed clinically and/or radiographically.

COMPLICATIONS

Reports in the adult literature reflect a complication rate of 2% to 15%, including portal sinus tract, major nerve injury, transient neuropraxia, joint infection, compartment syndrome, arthrofibrosis, thromboembolism, and complex regional pain syndrome.[72-75] Persistent portal drainage and fistula formation are the most common problems following elbow arthroscopy; however, with careful, tight portal closure, this can be avoided. If a drain is required, we often place a horizontal mattress suture around the drain left untied so that following drain removal we are able to close the residual hole.

Neurologic Injury

Injury to all three major nerves (median, radial, and ulnar) has been reported following elbow arthroscopy. While the literature reflects an injury rate of 0% to 14%, the exact incidence is unknown and likely underreported.[26,72,75-82] Most injuries are neuropraxias that resolve with time,[73] though complete transections have been described.[80] Nerve injury may result from local injection, compression secondary to severe swelling, crush from arthroscopic instrumentation, direct trauma from trocar insertion, or damage from the use of shavers.

Minimization of such risks requires experience and careful attention to the anatomy. Special consideration should be made for cases involving elbow contractures, rheumatoid arthritis, and HO. Any injury, even to cutaneous nerves, can cause chronic pain and disability.

Infection

Infection following elbow arthroscopy is rare, and superficial injections may be treated with oral antibiotics. Of note, increased rates of septic arthritis have been seen in patients receiving intraarticular steroid injections at the end of the procedure.[73] Thus the routine use of intra-articular steroid injections following elbow arthroscopy should be avoided. We do, however, find steroid injections and/or postoperative steroid protocols beneficial for patients requiring significant bony débridement or contracture release.

Heterotopic Ossification

Although this is a rare complication, HO formation has been reported in the literature following elbow arthroscopy and associated with the extensiveness of the procedure.[83,84] HO has even been reported following arthroscopic removal of a loose body. Thus many surgeons routinely recommend the use of HO prophylaxis with indomethacin or preoperative radiation.[84-86] Currently we do not take any increased precautions for routine arthroscopic procedures other than warning patients of the potential complication. We do utilize indomethacin (25 mg three times per day for 6 weeks) following arthroscopic contracture release. If HO occurs and causes symptoms, treatment involves excision once the lesion is mature.[84,87]

FUTURE CONSIDERATIONS

In experienced hands, the arthroscopic treatment of elbow disorders is safe and effective. As previously described, arthroscopic approaches may be utilized in cases with loose bodies, OCD lesions, instability, HO, as well as for fracture fixation and contracture release. Refinement of these techniques and development of new methods holds tremendous possibility for the treatment of pediatric pathology, instability, and elbow contracture. Additional efforts to understand the biology of wound healing, chondral lesion formation, and scar propagation may further help elucidate treatment options for such patients.

For a complete list of references, go to ExpertConsult.com.

SELECTED READINGS

Citation:

Takahara M, Mura N, Sasaki J, et al. Classification, treatment, and outcome of osteochondritis dissecans of the humeral capitellum: surgical technique. *J Bone Joint Surg Am.* 2008;90A:47–62.

Level of Evidence:

II

Summary:

This article provides a retrospective review of 106 patients treated for osteochondritis dissecans lesions with development of a classification system for stable and unstable lesions as well as a treatment algorithm. The article includes a surgical technique for arthroscopic management of these lesions.

Citation:

O'Driscoll SW, Morrey BF. Arthroscopy of the elbow: diagnostic and therapeutic benefits and hazards. *J Bone Joint Surg Am.* 1992;74A:84–94.

Level of Evidence:

II

Summary:

This retrospective review of 71 elbow arthroscopies outlines the clinical value and functional outcomes of the procedure. The operative technique is discussed in detail.

Citation:

Lynch GJ, Meyer JF, Whipple TL, et al. Neurovascular anatomy and elbow arthroscopy: inherent risks. *Arthroscopy.* 1986;2:190–197.

Level of Evidence:

IV

Summary:

In this cadaveric study, the anatomic relationship of vital neurovascular structures to commonly used arthroscopic portals is investigated. The proper technique of portal entry to minimize risk is emphasized.

Citation:
Sahajpal DT, Blonna D, O'Driscoll SW. Anteromedial elbow
arthroscopy portals in patients with prior ulnar nerve
transposition or subluxation. *Arthroscopy*. 2010;26:1045–1052.

Level of Evidence:
IV

Summary:
This article describes a case series of 59 patients who underwent
elbow arthroscopy with use of the anteromedial portal in patients
with evidence of ulnar nerve subluxation or previous ulnar nerve
transposition. The technique for protection of the nerve in these
circumstances is discussed.

Citation:
Kelly EW, Morrey BF, O'Driscoll SW. Complications of elbow
arthroscopy. *J Bone Joint Surg Am*. 2001;83A:25–34.

Level of Evidence:
III

Summary:
This retrospective review of 473 elbow arthroscopies details the most
common complications associated with the procedure. Most
complications are transient; permanent disabilities are
uncommon following the procedure.

Citation:
Mullett H, Sprague M, Brown G, et al. Arthroscopic treatment of
lateral epicondylitis: clinical and cadaveric studies. *Clin Orthop
Relat Res*. 2005;439:123–128.

Level of Evidence:
IV

Summary:
This article details the underlying etiology of lateral epicondylitis
through a case series and cadaveric study. The authors identify a
redundant capsular complex that results in radiocapitellar
impingement in patients with refractory symptoms. A
classification system is devised based on anatomic variations seen
in cadaver elbows.

Citation:
Bunata RE, Brown DS, Capelo R. Anatomic factors related to the
cause of tennis elbow. *J Bone Joint Surg Am*. 2007;89A:1955–1963.

Level of Evidence:
IV

Summary:
This cadaveric study details anatomic variations of the extensor carpi
radialis brevis origin and its contribution to dynamic abrasion of
the capitellum during motion. Implications for the development
of symptomatic lateral epicondylitis are discussed.

Citation:
Peart RE, Strickler SS, Schweitzer KM Jr. Lateral epicondylitis: a
comparative study of open and arthroscopic lateral release. *Am J
Orthop*. 2004;33:565–567.

Level of Evidence:
II

Summary:
This retrospective review evaluates the outcomes of open versus
arthroscopic release in 75 patients with lateral epicondylitis.

Citation:
Hardy P, Menguy F, Guillot S. Arthroscopic treatment of capitellum
fracture of the humerus. *Arthroscopy*. 2002;18:422–426.

Level of Evidence:
IV

Summary:
This article provides the first published report documenting the
technique for arthroscopic fixation of a capitellar fracture with
review of the associated literature.

Citation:
Takeda J, Takahashi T, Hino K, et al. Arthroscopic technique for
fragment fixation using absorbable pins for osteochondritis
dissecans of the humeral capitellum: a report of 4 cases. *Knee
Surg Sports Traumatol Arthrosc*. 2010;18:831–835.

Level of Evidence:
IV

Summary:
This article provides a description of the arthroscopic technique for
fragment fixation of unstable osteochondritis dissecans lesions
using absorbable pins, with evaluation of the short-term results.

Citation:
Savoie FH 3rd, O'Brien MJ, Field LD, et al. Arthroscopic and open
radial ulnohumeral ligament reconstruction for posterolateral
rotatory instability of the elbow. *Clin Sports Med*.
2010;29:611–618.

Level of Evidence:
IV

Summary:
This article provides a summary of clinical testing for posterolateral
rotatory instability, associated arthroscopic findings, and a
description of a novel technique for arthroscopic repair or
plication of the unstable elbow.

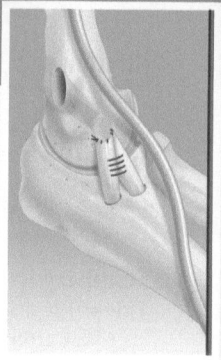

61

Elbow Tendinopathies and Bursitis

Jennifer Moriatis Wolf

Lateral and medial epicondylitis are common elbow tendinopathies involving tendon origins that most commonly present in middle age. These are typically self-limited, with a multitude of conservative and operative options described. In contrast, biceps and triceps tendinitis are insertional tendinopathies. Finally, olecranon bursitis is an inflammation of the dorsal bursa at the elbow. This chapter will evaluate the literature and current evidence about diagnostic maneuvers and treatment options to allow the sports physician to effectively treat patients with these problems.

LATERAL AND MEDIAL EPICONDYLITIS

History

Initially described secondary to lawn tennis,[1] lateral epicondylitis affects approximately 3% of the population during some point in their lives.[2,3] It is far more common than medial epicondylitis, with a 3 to 6:1 ratio.[4] Patients with lateral and medial epicondylitis present with complaints of pain on the respective side of the elbow. Also known as tennis elbow (lateral) or golfer's elbow (medial), these entities present most commonly in persons between 30 and 50 years of age.[5] Men and women are equally affected, with a higher occurrence rate in non-athletes.[6]

Symptoms are typically insidious in onset, although some patients develop complaints after a traumatic incident. The pathophysiology of lateral epicondylitis has been shown to involve the origin of the extensor carpi radialis brevis (ECRB) tendon, with infiltration of vascular buds and fibroblast proliferation termed "angiofibroblastic hyperplasia."[7] Another histologic evaluation noted vascular proliferation and hyaline degeneration, without an inflammatory response.[8] Occasionally, the extensor digitorum communis and extensor carpi radialis longus may also be involved. The most common presenting complaint is pain with lifting. As many activities of daily lifting are performed with the forearm in neutral rotation, lifting in this position requires slight wrist extension, which may cause overuse or microtears of the ECRB tendon origin as the source of pain.[9] Nirschl et al. classified lateral epicondylitis by pathologic and pain phases as a guide to the severity of the problem (Table 61.1).[10]

Medial epicondylitis is less common and is not well understood. Patients complain of an insidious onset of pain at the medial aspect of the elbow. Risk factors for medial epicondylitis are similar to those of lateral epicondylitis and include repetitive overuse and obesity. At surgery, Gabel and Morrey observed a nidus of granulation tissue at the flexor-pronator origin overlying the pronator teres and flexor carpi radialis origin.[11] They noted that this entity often overlaps with symptomatic ulnar nerve compression.

Physical Examination

On examination of the patient with tennis elbow, patients are typically tender at or just distal to the lateral epicondyle with palpation. The most characteristic examination maneuver is the provocation of pain at the lateral elbow with resisted wrist extension of the patient's fist, forearm pronated and the elbow fully extended (Fig. 61.1).[12] The Cozen test is a similar maneuver, except that the examiner grasps the elbow to stabilize it while asking the patient to extend the clenched fist against resistance.[12] To rule out posterolateral rotatory instability due to lateral ulnar collateral ligament injury, the posterolateral rotatory drawer test is performed. This is done with the patient supine, with the arm overhead and held externally rotated; the examiner stabilizes the humerus with one hand and applies a posterolateral rotatory stress by grasping the forearm and attempting to push the radial head posteriorly.[13]

At the medial elbow, patients have tenderness at the flexor-pronator origin at the medial epicondyle. Pain with resisted forearm pronation is felt to be the most sensitive test for medial epicondylitis,[11] while pain with resisted wrist flexion may also be indicative. Because of the overlap of medial epicondylitis and ulnar nerve compression, Tinel's testing over the ulnar nerve posterior to the medial epicondyle should be performed. Gabel and Morrey classified medial epicondylitis by the degree of ulnar nerve involvement, as follows: type IA with no symptoms of ulnar nerve compression; type IB with mild ulnar nerve symptoms; and type II with moderate or severe ulnar nerve compression in association with medial epicondylitis.[11] The medial collateral ligament should be examined to rule out instability with valgus load applied to the elbow at 30 degrees of elbow flexion.

Differential diagnosis of these conditions includes radial tunnel syndrome, characterized by aching pain in the proximal forearm distal to the lateral epicondyle with many similar positive provocative tests,[9] medial triceps tendinitis or snapping,[14] and injury or sprain to the lateral and medial collateral ligaments. In addition, neurologic conditions such as pronator syndrome and cubital tunnel syndrome as well as elbow pathologies such as plica, osteochondral defects, and joint degeneration need to be considered.

TABLE 61.1   Nirschl Classification of Pathology and Pain in Tennis Elbow

Pathology Staging Score	Pain Phase Score
I. Temporary irritation	1. Pain after exercise only, lasting <24 hours before resolution
	2. Pain after exercise, lasting >48 hours, resolves with warming up
II. Permanent tendinosis <50% cross-sectional area	3. Pain with exercise not affecting the activity
III. Permanent tendinosis >50% cross-sectional area	4. Pain with exercise that alters the sports activity
	5. Pain caused with heavy activities of daily living (ADLs)
	6. Intermittent pain at rest, and pain with light ADLs
IV. Partial or complete ECRB tendon rupture	7. Constant pain at rest, pain that wakes patient up from sleep

Modified from Nirschl RP, Ashman ES. Elbow tendinopathy: tennis elbow. *Clin Sports Med.* 2003;22(4):813–836.

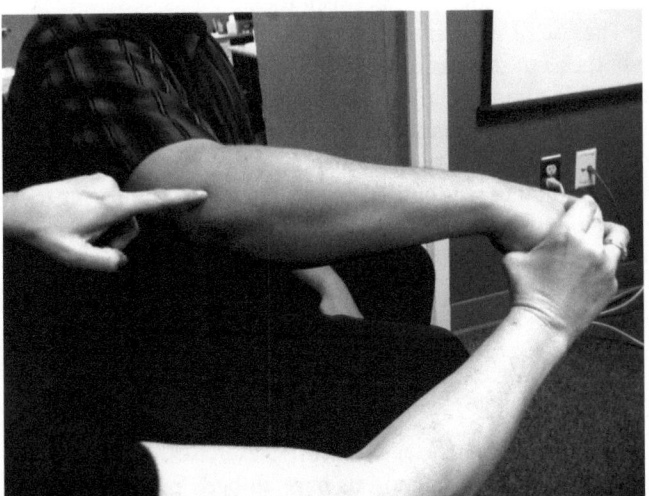

Fig. 61.1 Resisted wrist extension test for lateral epicondylitis.

Imaging

Tennis and golfer's elbow are primarily clinical diagnoses, and the role of imaging is to rule out other conditions about the elbow. Plain radiographs are typically normal, with faint calcifications occasionally seen at the tendon origin (Fig. 61.2). Pomerance evaluated 294 radiographs in patients diagnosed with lateral epicondylitis and noted that 7% had this finding; however, radiographic findings changed management only twice, for patients noted to have osteochondritis dissecans who went on to surgical treatment for this diagnosis.[15]

Ultrasound has been used to evaluate the tendon origin, with findings of decreased echogenicity and peritendinous soft tissue thickening. Abnormalities of the deep fibers of the ECRB may also be visualized.[16] A recent systematic review of 15 diagnostic studies confirmed the utility of gray-scale ultrasound in identification of hypoechogenicity and bone changes at the lateral epicondyle (Fig. 61.3).[17] Heales et al. reported a case-control comparison of ultrasound of patients with lateral epicondylitis, interpreted by blinded radiologists, and noted a sensitivity of 90% and specificity of 47% when greyscale and power Doppler imaging were combined.[18] Magnetic resonance imaging (MRI) may show signal changes at the ECRB origin on T1-weighted images, with fluid or thinning seen at the tendon origin on T2 images, interpreted as enthesopathy or partial tear (Fig. 61.4).[19] van Kollenburg et al. noted that patients with lateral epicondylitis were significantly more likely to have signal changes interpreted

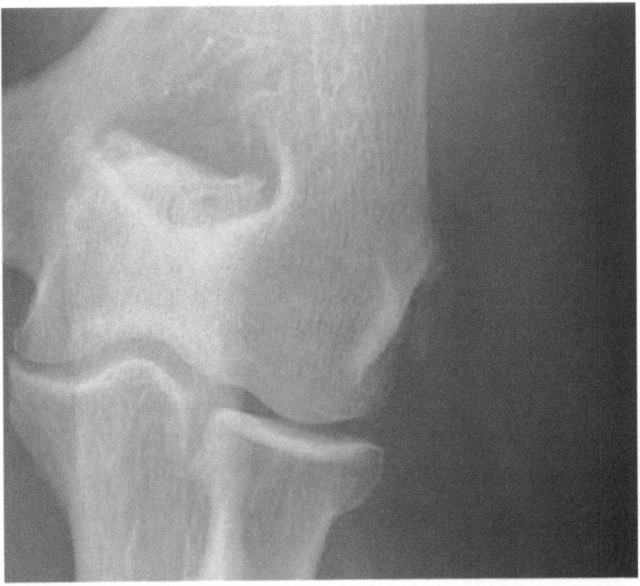

Fig. 61.2 Faint calcifications adjacent to the lateral epicondyle seen on plain radiograph.

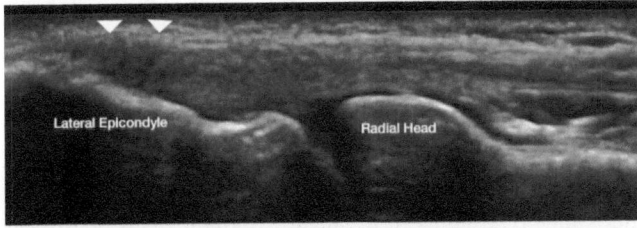

Fig. 61.3 Ultrasound findings in lateral epicondylitis. Arrowheads demonstrate enlargement and hypoechoic areas (black areas) within the proximal common extensor tendon compatible with tendinosis. (Courtesy Leonardo Oliveira, MD.)

as ECRB tendinosis on MRI than controls ($P < .001$), but that both groups had similar proportions of signal changes in the lateral collateral ligament and reading of partial ECRB defect.[19] The same group also evaluated MRI reports of 3374 patients, noting that signal change in the ECRB was common in both symptomatic and asymptomatic elbows, and the incidence of signal change increased over time with increasing age.[20] A recent study suggests that the role of MRI is not for diagnostic or prognostic information but rather to rule out pathology in equivocal or recalcitrant cases of epicondylitis.[21]

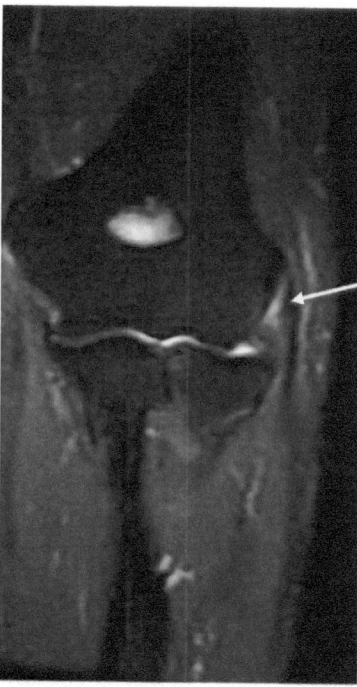

Fig. 61.4 Typical findings on magnetic resonance imaging with signal change in the extensor tendon origin.

Decision-Making Principles

Because the treatment of epicondylitis is primarily nonsurgical, decision-making is based on a discussion with the patient about the evidence regarding various treatment options. It is important for the patient to know that no matter what treatment is chosen, epicondylitis often takes a long time to resolve. Given that no one particular treatment method or algorithm has universal acceptance or been deemed superior to another in these conditions, patients are often initially managed nonoperatively with special considerations given to the individual's vocational and avocational activities. Avoidance of a known aggravating activity is likely where treatment should begin. The remaining methods of treatment are designed to alleviate or reduce symptoms, although their effect may not be immediate or curative. Surgery for epicondylitis is considered as a last resort after other treatments have failed. Although many retrospective studies have reported good outcomes for surgery, more recent meta-analyses have not been able to support a definitive role for surgery for epicondylitis, as the outcomes can be unpredictable.[22]

Treatment Options

There is increasing evidence that lateral and medial epicondylitis are self-limited entities that resolve on their own over time. Smidt et al. performed a randomized controlled trial comparing corticosteroid injection, physiotherapy, or a wait-and-see approach in 185 patients in the Netherlands. At 1 year, success rates were 69% for injections, 91% for therapy, and 83% for wait-and-see, with no significant differences between therapy and observation (see Fig. 61.2).[23] Szabo has recommended reassurance that continued use of the arm will not damage or worsen the tendinosis, and emphasis of the self-limited nature of lateral or medial epicondylitis.[24]

Splinting

The use of a forearm support band or tennis elbow strap has been proposed to reduce stress at the ECRB tendon origin. Meyer et al. noted in a cadaver study that increased band compression caused concomitant force reduction at the ECRB origin.[25] Others noted that wearing a support band increased the rate of fatigue of the wrist extensors, and recommended against their use.[26] A recent randomized trial comparing a forearm band and extensor strengthening exercises showed that both groups improved with time, with no differences between them.[27]

The use of wrist splinting has also been described, with the hypothesis of decreasing the stretch and use of the ECRB. Van de Streek compared a forearm splint to elbow band treatment in 43 patients in a randomized trial and noted no differences in grip or pain after 6 weeks, concluding that both showed some effect.[28] Another randomized trial in 42 patients comparing wrist extension splinting to counterforce strap noted significantly better pain relief with the splint, although there was no difference in measures of function, including the Mayo Elbow Performance score or American Shoulder and Elbow Society (ASES) scores.[29]

Therapy

The use of deep massage, eccentric exercises, strengthening, ultrasound, and iontophoresis have all been proposed as part of therapeutic interventions for epicondylitis; however, there is limited evidence to support one as superior. In Smidt's study comparing therapy, injection, and observation, physiotherapy had the highest success rate at 1 year.[23] The modality of friction massage was described by Cyriax to relieve pain and increase blood flow.[30] A recent randomized trial showed superior results with a supervised exercise program compared to Cyriax physiotherapy for tennis elbow, although both groups improved with respect to pain and function.[31] A meta-analysis evaluating exercise in the treatment of epicondylitis showed that resistance exercises resulted in improvement in tennis elbow symptoms, with eccentric stretching being the most studied.[32] A randomized trial comparing eccentric to concentric exercise showed the largest decrease in pain when eccentric and concentric contractions were combined with isometric exercises.[33]

Ultrasound is thought to provide benefit through deep heating of tissues. Binder et al. noted a significant difference in lateral epicondylitis patients treated with ultrasound compared to placebo treatment;[34] however, later randomized trials have shown no differences between ultrasound and sham-ultrasound treated groups.[35,36] A recent randomized trial comparing exercise and therapeutic ultrasound to corticosteroid injection in 49 subjects demonstrated significant improvement in pain and function in the exercise group at 12 weeks.[37]

Iontophoresis delivers water-soluble medications such as dexamethasone or saline through the skin with the use of electrical current. Stefanou et al. noted short-term benefit of dexamethasone iontophoresis in a randomized study with comparison to injection of dexamethasone.[38] In a double-blind comparison study, however, Runeson and Haker noted no significant differences in 64 patients randomized to iontophoresis or placebo.[39]

Injections

Multiple types of injections have been used for the treatment of epicondylitis. The most common is corticosteroid injection, which has been shown in systematic reviews to have a short-term effect on pain relief for up to 6 weeks (see Fig. 61.3).[40] Given that epicondylitis is a noninflammatory condition, the mechanism of action of steroid injection is uncertain. Randomized trials and a recent meta-analysis of corticosteroid versus placebo injection for tennis elbow showed no differences in outcomes as measured by either Disabilities of the Arm, Shoulder, and Hand (DASH) or pain scores.[41,42]

There has been recent interest in injections of whole blood and platelet-rich plasma (PRP), with the purported mechanism of stimulating reversal of the angiofibroblastic tendinosis by the delivery of humoral mediators and growth factors.[43] Whole or autologous blood contains these factors, and separating blood components by centrifugation to inject plasma concentrates the solution. Edwards and Calandruccio initially described pain relief and functional improvement in two-thirds of a group with chronic lateral epicondylitis treated with one or two autologous blood injections in a retrospective study.[44] Studies of PRP in lateral epicondylitis have shown mixed results, with some randomized trials showing significantly better results compared to corticosteroid,[45,46] while others demonstrated no differences among PRP, corticosteroids, or placebo saline.[47,48] A recent systematic review and network analysis comparing injections of autologous blood to PRP showed comparable outcomes, with both injection types being superior to steroid injections, with a higher risk of complications with autologous blood injection.[49]

Less commonly used injections include botulinum toxin and prolotherapy. Botulinum works by temporary paralysis of the extensor origin, and limited studies have shown effective results in decreasing pain. A randomized multicenter trial showed significantly better results with botulinum injection compared to placebo at 18 weeks, although middle finger extension was weakened by the botulinum temporarily.[50] A different formulation, prolotherapy, consists of either hypertonic glucose or saline injected into the ECRB origin in an effort to sclerose pathologic neovascularization and provide a toxic effect on granulation tissue.[51] While evidence is limited, a recent randomized trial comparing prolotherapy to corticosteroid showed improvement in both groups without significant differences between them.[52]

Surgical Treatment

There are several surgery options for epicondylitis, typically reserved for patients who have failed extensive nonoperative treatment, which include open or arthroscopic débridement, extensor release or repair, extensor repair, and denervation. The classic surgical approach to lateral epicondylitis is termed the "Nirschl procedure" and involves open débridement of all identifiable granulation and/or fibrous tissue at the ECRB origin, (Fig. 61.5) followed by decortication or drilling of the lateral epicondyle prominence to improve blood supply.[7] The overlying

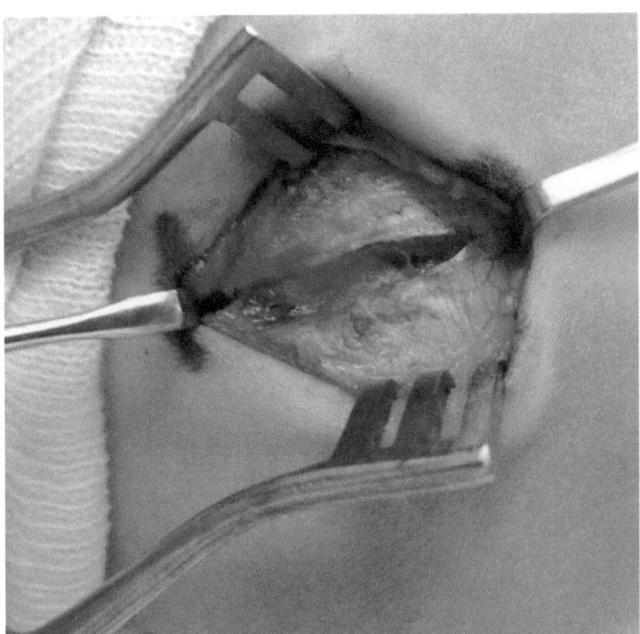

Fig. 61.5 Open surgical débridement for epicondylitis (the Nirschl procedure).

fascial edges of the extensor carpi radialis longus and extensor digitorum communis are closed.

Other authors have described percutaneous[53] or open[54] release of the extensor origin down to the capsule of the elbow, after which the extensors are allowed to retract distally. The extensor muscular origin is attached at multiple points to the surrounding fascial bands and to underlying joint capsule, and thus extensor weakness is not observed after this procedure. A recently described alternative is the use of ultrasound-guided instrumentation to perform microresection and tenotomy at the tendon origin. A retrospectively evaluated cohort of 20 patients showed significant reduction in pain and improved function at 3-year followup.[55]

An alternate procedure involves débridement of devitalized tissue and repair of the ECRB to the lateral epicondyle using suture anchors[56] or bone tunnels.[57] Additionally, denervation of the lateral elbow has been described by Kaplan[58] and others,[59,60] with careful dissection and division of multiple cutaneous radial nerve branches while preserving the posterior interosseous nerve (PIN).

Arthroscopic management of lateral epicondylitis has been demonstrated, with débridement and release of the underside origin of the ECRB. The proposed advantages of arthroscopy are that it is minimally invasive and is able to manage concomitant intra-articular pathology, which has been seen in up to one-third of patients.[61] It is only necessary to access the anterior compartment of the elbow, with use of a modified anterolateral portal established using an inside-out technique, starting 2 to 3 cm proximal and anterior to the lateral epicondyle.[62] Synovitis, identified at the tendon origin and lateral capsule, is débrided using a shaver. The ECRB is then released using monopolar thermal dissection or a shaver, taking care to limit the release to the area anterior to the midline of the radiocapitellar joint in order to preserve the lateral collateral ligament origin. Some surgeons will drill the epicondyle, or débride the exposed underside using an arthroscopic burr.

At the medial epicondyle, it is necessary to first identify and protect the ulnar nerve. The nerve is typically decompressed in situ through a mini-incision, and a limited débridement of the underside of the flexor pronator origin is performed using a shaver. During débridement, the ulnar nerve is retracted medially to protect it.

📌 Author's Preferred Technique

My management of lateral or medial epicondylitis begins with a discussion of the evidence for and against the multiple treatment options. I emphasize the typical self-limited nature of the condition and caution that this tendinosis may remain symptomatic up to 1 to 2 years before resolving, except in a small number of people. I also reassure patients that they are not causing themselves harm or damage by using the arm, and that they are not causing joint instability or tissue damage that will lead to disability. For each patient, I demonstrate eccentric stretching exercises for tendinosis,[32] and discuss that this expectant treatment alone can be sufficient to treat epicondylitis.

I offer referral to therapy and discuss injection options. I always emphasize the limited course of pain relief from steroid injections, approximately 6 weeks in length, but will give one at a patient's request. For patients presenting with greater than 6 months of symptoms and especially with chronic epicondylitis, I will offer an autologous blood injection, as my anecdotal experience has shown that this work bests in that patient group.

For surgical management of lateral epicondylitis, I perform the Nirschl procedure with open débridement of the ECRB origin. This is typically done under Bier block anesthesia, with a longitudinal incision over the lateral epicondyle and ECRB origin. The fascia is incised with retraction of the extensor carpi radialis longus and extensor digitorum communis, exposing the deep ECRB. The origin is débrided of any gray, shiny tissue to leave healthy tendon behind. I typically do not open the elbow joint. I use a rongeur or osteotome to decorticate the prominence of the lateral epicondyle, taking care not to go too inferiorly to protect the origin of the lateral collateral ligament. Sometimes, there may be some degenerative changes on the undersurface of the extensor digitorum communis, which I also débride, as failure to do so may lead to suboptimal results. After irrigation, the fascia of the extensor carpi radialis longus (ECRL) and extensor digitorum communis (EDC) is closed using 2-0 resorbable sutures, and the skin is then closed using a resorbable monocryl subcuticular suture.

For medial epicondylitis, I perform an open débridement of the flexor-pronator origin, focusing on the interval between the pronator teres and the flexor carpi radialis at their attachment to the medial epicondyle. While not typically able to visualize a nidus of abnormal tissue as advocated by Gabel and Morrey, I remove any devitalized tissue at the origin and decorticate the medial epicondyle with a rongeur. Closure and other management are similar to my treatment of lateral epicondylitis.

Postoperative Management

The patient is splinted postoperatively for 2 weeks and then begins therapy for 4 to 6 weeks with a 5-lb lifting limit. Strengthening is begun at 6 weeks, and return to heavy lifting and strenuous sports is not permitted until 3 months.

Return to Play

Resumption of athletic activities is sport-dependent after surgery for lateral or medial epicondylitis. Strenuous or contact sport activity is permitted at 3 months if the patient has tolerated the strengthening phase of rehabilitation. Earlier return, typically at 6 weeks, is allowed for individual sports such as golf, skiing, and swimming, with the elbow taped or supported as necessary.

For nonoperatively treated patients, return to sport is allowed at their tolerance, with the understanding that the elbow may be painful with certain motions or after heavy use.

Results

Open Surgical Management—Lateral Epicondylitis

Dunn et al. reported 10 to 14-year follow-up of the Nirschl open débridement technique in 139 patients in a retrospective review. The authors noted decreased pain scores and improved American Shoulder and Elbow Surgeons' scores, with 84% good to excellent results combining two other functional scales, and 93% of patients who were able to return to sports.[63] A prospective randomized comparative study between percutaneous and open ECRB release showed improvements in both groups, but the percutaneous-release group had significantly better DASH scores, improvement in sports performance, and earlier return to work.[64] Ruch et al. compared open débridement with and without anconeus flap rotation in 57 patients and noted significantly better DASH scores in the group treated with anconeus rotation, but no other differences at 7-month follow-up.[65] A recent Cochrane review of the available evidence for surgical treatment concluded that there was insufficient evidence to support the use of surgical treatment for lateral epicondylitis or the application of one surgical technique as superior.[66]

Arthroscopic Release—Lateral Epicondylitis

Lattermann et al. noted improvement of pain and function scores in a retrospective review of 36 patients treated arthroscopically, although 31% noted mild pain with strenuous activities. Other authors have noted similar positive findings, although heavy laborers and worker's compensation claimants had overall worse outcomes.[67] Szabo et al. compared open, arthroscopic, and percutaneous release of the ECRB in a group of 109 patients with 47.8-month mean follow-up.[68] The authors noted that there was significant improvement in Andrews-Carson scores from pre- to postoperative evaluation, with no differences between groups, and concluded that all three procedures were highly effective in treating lateral epicondylitis. A recent retrospective comparison of arthroscopic to open ECRB débridement showed similar improvement in both groups, but the open procedure cohort had a significantly better pain visual analogue scale (VAS) score during hard or heavy work compared to the arthroscopic group.[69]

Surgical Treatment of Medial Epicondylitis

The majority of reports of treatment for medial epicondylitis involve open débridement of the flexor-pronator origin in patients who have failed lengthy conservative management. Gabel and Morrey noted excellent outcomes in a retrospective review of 26 elbows treated for medial epicondylitis, reporting significantly better results in patients without concomitant ulnar nerve compression neuropathy.[11] A recent retrospective evaluation of 55 patients treated surgically with débridement, medial epicondylectomy, and ulnar nerve release showed significant improvement in pain, grip strength, and DASH and Mayo scores at a minimum

5-year follow-up.[70] Zonno et al. performed a cadaveric study to evaluate the safety of arthroscopic débridement of medial epicondylitis,[71] but this technique has not been reported in clinical studies to date.

Complications

A notable complication of nonoperative treatment is soft tissue atrophy, skin thinning, and hypopigmentation after corticosteroid injections, which is a risk that should be addressed when treating patients with this modality.[72] Subcutaneous injection should be avoided to minimize this complication, and repeated injections increase the risk of atrophy.

Surgical complications include posterolateral rotatory instability if the lateral collateral ligament is damaged in the approach to the common extensors.[73] Kalainov et al. noted this complication after corticosteroid injection in three elbows.[74] The risk of this complication is minimized by taking care not to dissect too far posteriorly on the lateral epicondyle during the surgical approach. Other reported complications are rare, including development of synovial fistulae[75] and transient paresthesias.[76]

Future Considerations

Short-term evidence supports expectant treatment of epicondylitis, with assurance to the patient that this self-limited entity tends to resolve over time. There is a subset of patients, however, who do not resolve their symptoms, eventually leading to surgical treatment. Identification of this group is a focus of continued study. The current evidence for conservative treatment of medial and lateral epicondylitis is strong, with surgery reserved for those who have failed multiple modalities. Potential future considerations include refinement of biologic treatments such as autologous blood and PRP, as well as exploration of the neurologic contributions in patients with chronic epicondylitis.

DISTAL BICEPS AND TRICEPS TENDINITIS

History

Biceps and triceps tendinitis are correctly termed insertional tendinopathies. Similar to epicondylitis and Achilles tendinopathy, they tend to present in middle age with an insidious onset, indicating chronic degenerative changes in aging tendons that do not respond well to overuse.[77] While patients may recall a traumatic event, a careful history will often elicit prodromal aching or pain.

Patients with biceps tendinitis present with anterior elbow pain, which worsens with activities requiring forceful supination (such as application of torque) or elbow flexion.[78] Differential diagnosis includes pronator syndrome, PIN compression, or phlebitis of the brachial vein. Triceps tendinitis is more rarely seen, with patients complaining of posterior elbow soreness, with pain when pushing open doors, or other activities requiring triceps activation without the benefit of gravity.

Physical Examination

In the patient with biceps tendinitis, the most important maneuver is to rule out a complete biceps rupture. This is most effectively done with the biceps hook test, where the examiner has the

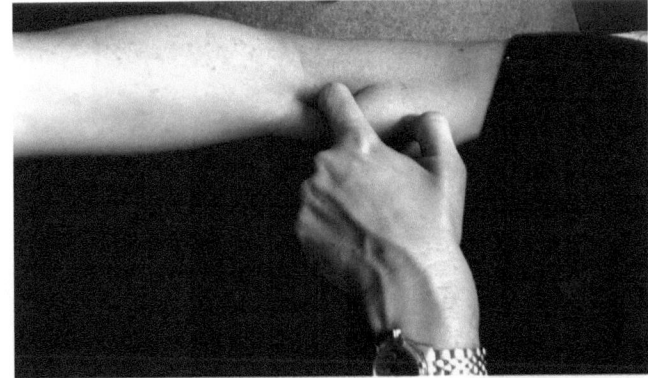

Fig. 61.6 Demonstration of the "hook test" as described by O'Driscoll et al.

shoulder abducted and places the patient's forearm in supination with the elbow flexed at 90 degrees, and then hooks his or her finger around the intact biceps tendon from lateral to medial, lifting it slightly anteriorly (Fig. 61.6). O'Driscoll et al. noted that the hook test was more sensitive and specific for biceps ruptures than MRI in a series of surgically treated individuals.[79]

Once the biceps tendon is determined to be intact, palpation of the tendon may elicit pain in the patient's tendinopathy, and pulling on the tendon during the hook test should reproduce the symptoms. In addition, pain in the antecubital fossa with resisted forearm supination, more than elbow flexion, is indicative of distal biceps tendinitis.

Patients with triceps tendinitis may have tenderness to palpation over the distal triceps, and often have weakness and pain with resisted extension. The literature is limited on this entity and includes partial tendon tears, which also present with a palpable defect of the broad triceps insertion.[80]

Imaging

Plain radiographs are nondiagnostic and should be ordered only if a bony lesion is being ruled out as a cause of symptoms. MRI is most commonly used to evaluate the biceps and triceps tendon integrity.[81] For the best imaging of the biceps tendon, the FABS position (flexed elbow, abducted shoulder, supinated forearm) has been described to produce a true view of the tendon in the longitudinal plane.[82] Tendinosis is characterized by abnormal signal intensity within the tendon on T2-weighted sequences, as well as tendon thickening, abnormal contour, or swelling on any sequence (Fig. 61.7).[77,82] The triceps tendon is best visualized on sagittal MRI, with fluid-filled defects, signal heterogeneity, and other findings similar to biceps tendinosis at the affected insertion.[81]

Ultrasound has also been used for diagnostic purposes in elbow insertional tendinopathies.[83] Biceps tendinitis may be identified with abnormal fluid signal within the distal tendon. The triceps tendon also shows abnormalities on ultrasound and its integrity and thickness may be evaluated for pathologic differences from normal controls.[84]

Decision-Making Principles

Biceps and triceps tendinopathies are challenging entities to treat, because the patients are often quite symptomatic and it is

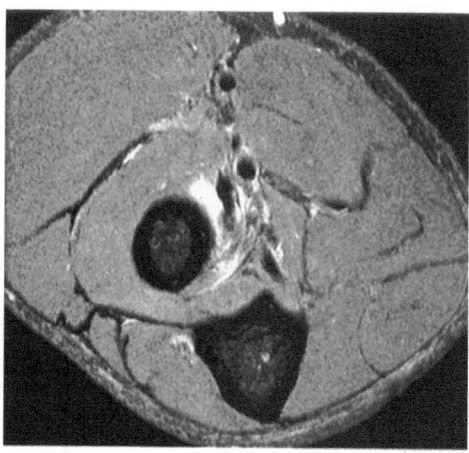

Fig. 61.7 T2-weighted magnetic resonance imaging of biceps tendinosis with fluid in the tendon sheath and high signal surrounding the biceps tendon. (Courtesy George Athwal, MD, FRCSC.)

difficult to modify their elbow use. These insertional tendinopathies are fairly rare, and should be considered typical enthesopathies similar to lateral epicondylitis and Achilles tendinitis when discussing treatment.[77] As such, a trial of nonoperative treatment is always recommended, with assurance of patients that surgery is *not* always necessary. In patients who fail conservative treatment, surgical options have been fairly successful in alleviating symptoms.

Treatment Options and Results

Conservative

Nonoperative treatment of biceps or triceps tendinosis begins with modifying activities that aggravate the patient's symptoms as much as possible. Use of intermittent splinting during heavy loading activities may be considered, with a static elbow splint set between 45 and 90 degrees; however, full-time wear is not recommended due to risks of joint stiffness.[80] Other described conservative measures include nonsteroidal antiinflammatory drugs (NSAIDs) and therapy.[85] More recently, there have been reports of ultrasound-guided PRP for tendinopathy. Sanli reported on 12 patients given a single PRP injection for distal biceps tendinitis using ultrasound, and noted significantly improved pain VAS, biceps strength, and function at 47-month follow-up.[86]

The key in conservative treatment is giving the tendinosis sufficient time, as with epicondylitis, to self-resolve. Mair et al. noted healing of partial triceps ruptures in 6 of 10 professional football players who were treated with time away from competition and protective bracing upon return to play (RTP); one sustained a complete rupture in the splint and the other three had delayed surgery for persistent pain and weakness.[80] Durr et al. reported four patients with partial biceps tendon tears with successful conservative treatment in three-fourths of this group.[87] In general, nonoperative treatment appears to have modest success, possibly associated with the severity of the tendinopathy and demands of the athlete or patient.

Operative

Operative treatment of biceps and triceps tendinosis is indicated when nonoperative treatment has failed. The recommended

length of conservative treatment is controversial and varies between 8 weeks[88] and 1 year.[77] The degenerative biceps tendon is débrided through an anterior incision and then repaired using either the same incision with suture anchors[89] or through bone tunnels using a second posterior incision.[90] Kelly et al. described débridement and reattachment all through a single posterior incision.[88] Rokito et al. débrided and reinserted the biceps tendon and reported good subjective outcomes and recovery of strength in a retrospective report.[78] Vardakas et al. evaluated seven patients who failed a mean of 9.5 months of nonoperative treatment and underwent biceps tendon débridement and reattachment through an anterior incision using suture anchors.[85] All were subjectively satisfied at 6 months, had returned to preinjury activity and sport levels, and strength testing showed greater strength than the unaffected side in all cases. Another study evaluated strength at 32 months after surgical débridement and repair of partial biceps tears, showing greater isometric and dynamic elbow flexion strength than the opposite side, although forearm supination strength was 10% weaker.[91]

Triceps ruptures are repaired through bone tunnels in the olecranon, often with graft augmentation from autogenous palmaris longus[92] or hamstring (Fig. 61.8).[93] van Riet et al. reported the results of 23 triceps repairs and reconstructions at 88-month follow-up, noting that triceps strength was on average 82% of the strength in the unaffected arm.[92]

📌 Author's Preferred Technique

Initially, I treat tendinosis or partial tearing of the biceps or triceps insertion conservatively, and discuss with patients that this is similar to other enthesopathies of middle age, which can often resolve without surgical treatment. I use intermittent splinting, therapy, and modification of aggravating activities. I do not recommend corticosteroid injection, as this poses a higher risk of rupture to a degenerative tendon. The implications of biceps or triceps insertional tendon rupture after steroid injection are more concerning than a similar occurrence from injection at the common extensor or flexor origin for epicondylitis, where functional deficits would be less disabling after iatrogenic rupture. I do not have current experience with PRP injection for these tendinopathies.

When patients have failed 6 to 12 months of conservative therapy, I recommend surgical treatment. For biceps tendinitis, I prefer a two-incision technique, with débridement of the tendon and detachment from the anatomic footprint, after which nonresorbable sutures are placed using a locking Krackow configuration in the tendon. The posterior counter-incision is made after passing a curved clamp ulnarly around the bicipital (radial) tuberosity to the dorsal forearm, using the palpable clamp tip for guidance. Using a burr, a trough for the tendon is created at the tuberosity, with drill holes then placed from dorsal to volar to allow passage of the tendon sutures. The elbow is placed in 90 degrees of flexion and fully pronated, and the tendon sutures are tensioned and tied.

For triceps tendinosis, I have performed arthroscopic débridement in one patient, with partial pain relief reported. This was done in the posterior compartment only, with débridement of an acute area of thickened degenerative-appearing tissue using a 3.5 mm shaver. While I have never had to débride and reattach the triceps for tendinosis, this would be done through a straight posterior incision, with similar nonresorbable sutures placed in a locking Krackow technique in the tendon. Obliquely oriented drill holes in the olecranon and proximal ulna are used to pass the sutures, which are then tied over the dorsal surface of the ulna with the elbow flexed at 45 degrees.

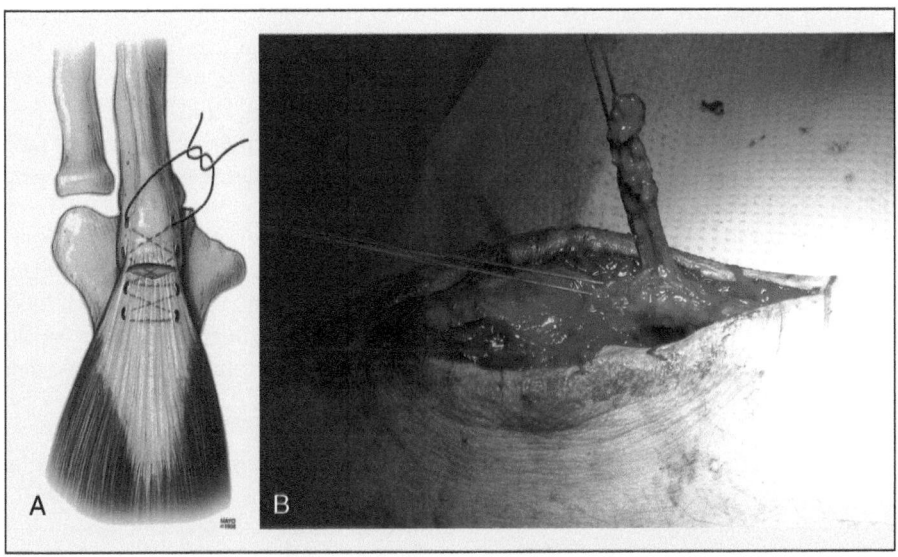

Fig. 61.8 Triceps tendon repair with locking Krackow stitch.

Postoperative Management

After biceps tendon reattachment, the patient is placed in a splint at 90 degrees of elbow flexion with the forearm supinated to decrease tensile forces on the repair. Graded active extension and passive flexion are allowed at 2 to 3 days, and a removable splint in the same position as the immediate postoperative splint is employed and worn between exercises for 4 to 6 weeks. Active elbow flexion and forearm supination are begun at 4 weeks. Strengthening is not begun until 3 months postoperatively.

After triceps tendon surgery, the patient is placed in a splint at 45 degrees of elbow flexion, with graded active flexion and passive extension started within the week. Flexion is slowly increased by 10 to 20 degrees per week. Active extension is begun at 4 to 6 weeks, and similarly to the biceps, strengthening is deferred until 3 months.

In both sets of patients, oral indomethacin is used for one month to prevent heterotopic ossification, unless contraindicated by other co-morbidities. I prefer three times daily dosing, at 25 mg, as opposed to the extended release, as patients seem to tolerate this dosage better.

Return to Play

RTP is allowed as strengthening begins, with protection in a splint initially. Particularly in contact sports, it is critical to defer full participation until the tendon repair is fully healed enough to tolerate heavy use.

Complications

Surgical complications of biceps repair include heterotopic ossification, nerve injuries (median, lateral antebrachial, and PIN), and re-rupture. Heterotopic ossification occurs more frequently with two-incision repairs,[94] but can be seen with both techniques. The worst-case scenario is the development of heterotopic ossification limiting elbow motion or radioulnar synostosis,[95] both of which require secondary surgery. While heterotopic ossification is typically non-bridging, oral indomethacin has been suggested as a prophylactic measure. Anakwenze et al. reported on the outcomes of 34 patients with complete biceps ruptures treated with a two-incision repair and chemoprophylaxis using indomethacin.[96] At a mean of 22 months, the authors noted no heterotopic ossification, reruptures, or synostoses, although they acknowledged the limitation of no comparative control group not treated with indomethacin.

Nerve injuries during biceps repair involve either the lateral antebrachial cutaneous (LABC) nerve or the PIN, both related to excessive retraction in the anterior or single-incision approach. Injury to the LABC is typically neuropraxic, with the patient noting transient numbness on the anterolateral aspect of the forearm. Grewal et al. noted LABC neuropraxia in 19 of 47 patients after a single-incision biceps repair compared to 3 of 43 in the double-incision group, thought due to more extensive retraction time necessary with the single-incision technique.[90] Injury to the PIN, while typically a neuropraxic stretch mechanism as well, is a dreaded complication, causing wrist drop that may take 4 to 5 months to resolve. To decrease the risk of this complication, anterior elbow dissection should be performed with the forearm maximally supinated to move the nerve as far laterally as possible.[97]

Finally, re-rupture may occur, most commonly associated with patient noncompliance, but also potentially due to inadequate fixation methods.[98] This is best prevented by securing the tendon with adequate grasping sutures, using superior tendon-to-bone fixation techniques, and preparing the patient preoperatively for the extent and particular restrictions of postoperative rehabilitation.

Complications of triceps repair include ulnar neuropraxia and rerupture. van Riet noted one case of ulnar neuropraxia, thought likely due to repair of an associated olecranon avulsion with tension-band wiring, and three reruptures after primary repair.[92]

Future Considerations

The natural history of biceps and triceps tendinosis has not been well addressed in the literature, and further prospective studies of these rare entities are needed. Prospective studies could elucidate evidence that supports earlier and more aggressive intervention in these conditions, rather than prolonged and only modestly successful nonoperative management as the standard of care. This is already the prevailing theory for many surgeons, citing that lack of elbow extension and/or forearm supination power may be more debilitating for athletes and manual laborers than the functional deficits engendered by the epicondylitides. Furthermore, protracted conservative care of some individuals may be counterproductive, leading to unnecessary time off work, extended avoidance of competitive sporting activities, and overall frustration on the part of patient and caregiver, when there is little to suggest that these conditions are reliably self-limiting. Detachment and reattachment of the degenerative or partially torn distal biceps tendon, in particular, may reveal more predictable subjective and objective clinical outcomes, especially in high demand patients.

OLECRANON BURSITIS

Olecranon bursitis differs from the other entities described in this chapter in that it is primarily inflammatory in nature. The olecranon bursa is the anatomic "cushion" for the dorsal elbow, which pads the prominent tip of the olecranon (Fig. 61.9). When the subcutaneous bursa becomes inflamed from pressure or trauma, the lining synovial cells produce increased fluid that then distends the bursa. As the bursa is anatomically not connected to the elbow joint, the inflammation is typically limited to the posterior elbow. Olecranon bursitis can be acutely painful, and if contaminated by an open wound due to trauma, may become infected. This section will focus on the evaluation and treatment of nonseptic olecranon bursitis.

History

Olecranon bursitis often presents after an inciting incident, such as a fall directly onto the posterior elbow, other traumatic or overuse mechanism, or repetitive pressure over the dorsal elbow. Patients may complain of pain due to the trauma, but often are

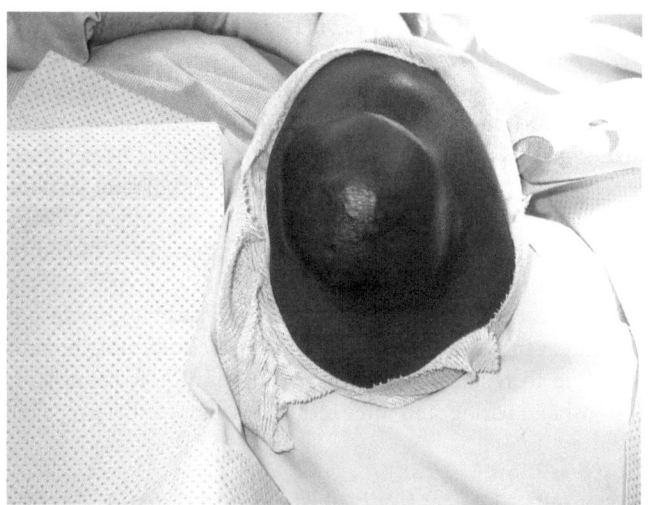

Fig. 61.9 Olecranon bursitis with a large mass over the dorsal elbow.

minimally symptomatic after a short time passes. They note the presence of a large, sometimes boggy sac at the posterior elbow (see Fig. 61.9). These patients may present with either acute or chronic complaints and to variable types of medical settings apart from the orthopaedic or sports medicine specialist (emergency department, urgent care clinic, or primary care physician office).

Other contributing diagnoses include gout, calcium pyrophosphate disease (CPPD), and rheumatoid arthritis. All of these comorbid diseases may present with swelling and inflammation of the olecranon bursa, although they are more likely to have separate and often multiple musculoskeletal complaints.

Physical Examination

On inspection, most patients have fullness over the posterior elbow. Acutely, the examiner may sometimes appreciate a fluid wave. In the chronic presentation, the bursal fullness often feels somewhat solid or thickened, reflecting fibrous organization of inflammatory tissue and synovitis. When a small bursa is present, the examiner should palpate the olecranon tip to evaluate for possible spur formation.

Infectious processes more often demonstrate patchy erythema and exquisite pain over the bursa. Loss of elbow motion is a less reliable predictor of infection, since many patients will have concomitant pathology, such as osteoarthritis, or have variable tolerance to stretching of inflamed or swollen soft tissue. The risk of infection is highest in acute presentations, with associated open wounds over the bursa, and in diabetics. A similar presentation, however, may accompany a crystalline deposition disease, which is often deemed a mimicker of infection regardless of the site of involvement. Aspiration, in these instances, may differentiate the two diagnoses and have obvious implications for the natural course and effective treatment of the offending condition.

Imaging

Plain radiographs of the elbow should be obtained to evaluate for olecranon spurs (enthesophytes), as well as calcifications within the bursa (Fig. 61.10). Saini and Canoso compared the radiographs of the affected and unaffected elbow of 28 patients with traumatic olecranon bursitis, and noted that the presence of olecranon spurs and amorphous calcium deposits were higher in bursitis patients (16 of 28) compared to controls (4 of 28).[99] The presence of an olecranon spur is worth noting, because it should be concurrently addressed if surgical treatment is necessary (see Fig. 61.10).

Decision-Making Principles

In nonseptic olecranon bursitis, both conservative and operative options are available. This author's practice does not include aspiration of the bursa, however, because of the risk of converting a nonseptic situation to a septic olecranon bursitis, mandating antibiotics and often inevitable surgical treatment. This view is in contradistinction to that held by many emergency department and primary care physicians.[100] Other accompanying signs and symptoms may lead to a higher clinical suspicion for infection or crystalline deposition disease, where aspiration may be accordingly

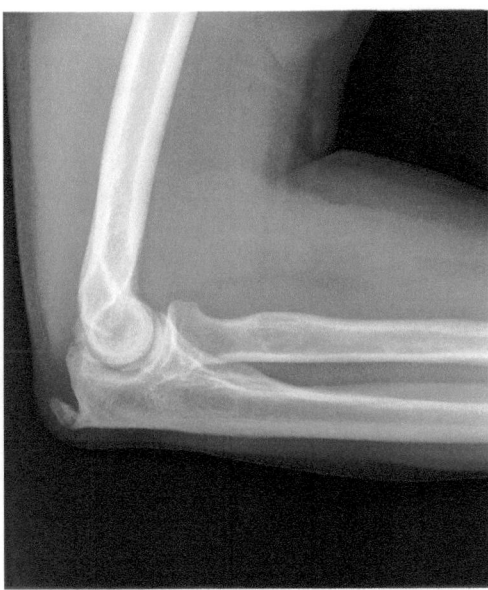

Fig. 61.10 Large olecranon spur and associated soft tissue swelling in the bursa.

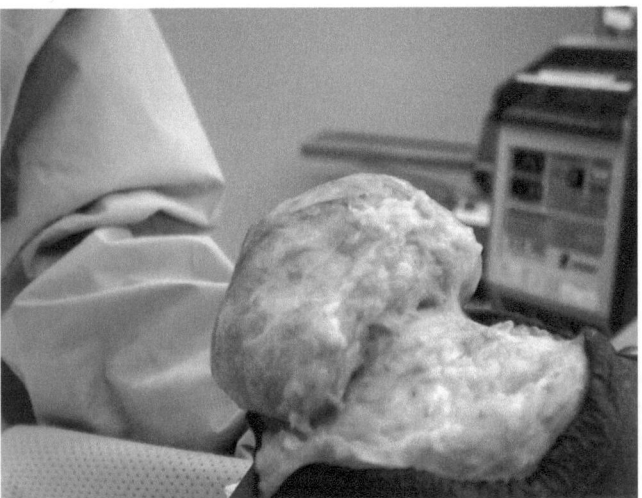

Fig. 61.11 Bursal sac dissected free of skin.

more justified to differentiate between the two diagnoses. In this regard, the results of aspiration have implications for deciding between management with either anti-inflammatory medication and time or aggressive surgical débridement to prevent progression of an infection to involve the elbow joint. In the rare cases where aspiration is indicated, a direct posterior needle track should be avoided. Rather, the needle should be placed from an anterolateral starting point, through the anconeus or extensors, to prevent the development of a sinus tract.

Treatment Options

Initial treatment of olecranon bursitis is supportive, with compressive wrapping and occasionally elbow splinting in 90 degrees of flexion in the acute setting. Even chronic olecranon bursitis can respond to compressive bandaging.[101] The patient should be informed that compressive wrapping often requires 1 to 2 months of consistent compliance before they see evidence of resolution. In addition, judicious use of anti-inflammatory medication may be considered, particularly in patients with a history of gout.[101]

As noted above, the use of aspiration and corticosteroid injection into the bursa has been advocated. Weinstein et al. reported on aspiration alone versus aspiration and corticosteroid injection for nonseptic bursitis in 47 patients, and noted faster resolution of effusion with the addition of corticosteroid.[102] Complications including infection, skin atrophy, and chronic pain, however, developed in 15 of 25 patients treated with corticosteroid. The risks of corticosteroid injection affecting the underlying triceps should also be considered. van Riet et al. noted that one of the triceps rupture patients in their series had been treated with a steroid injection for olecranon bursitis.[92]

Surgical treatment with excision of the bursa is considered after failure of compressive treatment, or if there is an infectious etiology. Open excision involves complete removal of the bursa along with any olecranon spurring, to prevent recurrence, and

the patient is warned about the minimal soft tissue envelope remaining over the olecranon. This surgery is performed under general or regional block, with the patient positioned supine with a bump under the ipsilateral shoulder and the elbow placed across the chest on a pillow. Use of a sterile blanket in addition is helpful.

A posterior incision with a slight curve to avoid the tip of the olecranon is performed and the bursal sac is carefully dissected free of the skin and subcutaneous fat, which is carefully preserved (Fig. 61.11). The bursa is often firmly adherent to the underlying triceps and needs to be peeled up with sharp dissection. When the bursal sac is removed, the skin edges may need to be trimmed to reduce loose skin at closure, depending on the size of the pathologic bursa.

Arthroscopic excision has also been described, with a posterior elbow arthroscopic setup and use of shavers to débride and remove the bursal sac.[103,104] Rhyou et al. recently reported on the use of arthroscopic bursal resection in 30 patients treated for aseptic and septic olecranon bursitis, noting no recurrences and improved pain and quick DASH scores.[105]

Author's Preferred Technique

When a patient presents with nonseptic olecranon bursitis, I discuss nonoperative treatment first, which is principally full-time compressive bandaging, using either an Ace wrap or neoprene sleeve. The patient may add NSAIDs if they wish, but I believe the primary treatment goal is compression to allow the body to naturally resorb the fluid within the bursa. I emphasize that the compressive bandage should be used as much as possible but may take 1 to 2 months to work. As stated above, I do not recommend aspiration of either septic or nonseptic bursitis. If the bursitis is persistent, this is an indication for surgical excision of the bursa, not serial aspirations.

I perform open surgical excision with the positioning as noted in the treatment section, utilizing a straight posterior incision. After bursal excision, the tourniquet is released and careful hemostasis is achieved in order to leave a dry bed prior to closure. I warn patients about the common reaccumulation of fluid. I also trim the skin to allow a smooth closure without skin redundancy. I then place the patient in a compressive dressing and a splint at 90 degrees. Frequently, compressive bandaging is needed for some time postoperatively.

Postoperative Care

Typically, the patient is splinted for 1 to 2 weeks with the forearm neutral at 90 degrees of elbow flexion and the wrist free. Subsequently, compressive wrapping is recommended while the wound heals further, for the next 2 to 4 weeks. Contact sports and heavy lifting may be resumed at 6 to 8 weeks. Therapy is not usually necessary.

Results

There are limited data regarding surgical bursal excision. Stewart et al. reported retrospectively on 16 patients at the Mayo Clinic treated surgically, and noted 15 of 16 with good results and no recurrence.[106] Other authors noted less positive results in a series of 37 patients treated with bursal excision, with recurrence in eight (22%) and wound healing issues in ten (27%).[107] Arthroscopic resection has shown promising results, with reports of full elbow motion and no recurrence in a group of nine patients.[104]

Complications

Noted surgical complications include recurrence, hematoma, and wound healing problems. Recurrence is poorly defined in the few studies existing, and it is possible this refers to re-accumulation of fluid in the soft tissues as well, since excision of the bursal sac should not allow true recurrence. Degreef and De Smet noted a recurrence in 8 of 37 patients (22%) treated with open bursectomy.[107] Stewart noted postoperative hematoma in one patient, which required surgical drainage.[106]

Wound healing problems have been reported. Degreef and De Smet noted fistula formation, persistent draining wounds, and skin loss requiring flap coverage in 10 of 37 patients reviewed retrospectively.[107] Some of these patients were on chronic anticoagulation and the cohort included resections of infected bursae, some of whom had open draining wounds preoperatively. Careful management of the soft tissues is required to decrease the risk of these complications.

Future Considerations

Despite the common presentation of olecranon bursitis, there is minimal literature documenting its treatment and clinical outcomes. Further prospective evaluation would be an addition to our current limited knowledge of this entity.

For a complete list of references, go to ExpertConsult.com.

SELECTED READINGS

Citation:
Nirschl RP, Ashman ES. Elbow tendinopathy: tennis elbow. *Clin Sports Med*. 2003;22:813–836.

Level of Evidence:
V, expert opinion

Summary:
This article provides both historical context and the basis of much of the etiology, as well as conservative and operative treatment options for lateral epicondylitis.

Citation:
Smidt N, van der Windt DA, Assendelft WJ, et al. Corticosteroid injections, physiotherapy, or a wait-and-see policy for lateral epicondylitis: a randomised controlled trial. *Lancet*. 2002; 359:657–662.

Level of Evidence:
II

Summary:
This is the definitive support for expectant treatment of epicondylitis as a self-limited disease, and also shows the short-lived effect of steroids as well as the possible impact of therapy.

Citation:
Pierce TP, Issa K, Gilbert BT, et al. A systematic review of tennis elbow surgery: open versus arthroscopic versus percutaneous release of the common extensor origin. *Arthroscopy*. 2017;S0749-8063 (epub ahead of print).

Level of Evidence:
Systematic review

Summary:
This summarized data from 30 articles, and showed that open and arthroscopic techniques were associated with better Disabilities of the Arm, Shoulder, and Hand scores than percutaneous release, with lower pain scores in arthroscopic and percutaneous techniques. There were no overall differences among the three techniques in satisfaction.

Citation:
Hobbs MC, Koch J, Bamberger HB. Distal biceps tendinosis: evidence-based review. *J Hand Surg Am*. 2009;34:1124–1126.

Level of Evidence:
Review, with some Level V expert opinion

Summary:
This article provides a current review of the limited literature on biceps tendinosis and an objective evaluation of treatment options including nonoperative treatment.

Citation:
Sayegh ET, Strauch RJ. Treatment of olecranon bursitis: a systematic review. *Atch Orthop Trauma Surg*. 2014;124(111):1517–1536.

Level of Evidence:
Systematic review

Summary:
This review included 29 studies using primarily Level IV evidence. This showed that nonsurgical treatment is significantly more effective in resolving olecranon bursitis than surgery, and that aseptic bursitis is more difficult to treat than septic bursitis.

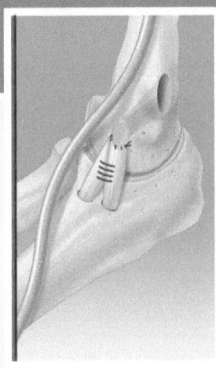

62

Distal Biceps and Triceps Tendon Ruptures

James Bradley, Fotios P. Tjoumakaris, Gregory T. Lichtman, Luke S. Austin

DISTAL BICEPS TENDON RUPTURE

In 1941, Dobbie was the first to report the results of surgical reattachment of the distal biceps tendon. He recommended routine tenodesis of the biceps to the brachialis because of the risks associated with anatomic repair from the surrounding neurovascular structures within the antecubital fossa. Improved surgical techniques and a better understanding of the anatomy and biomechanics of the distal biceps tendon subsequently changed this sentiment. Many orthopedic surgeons now advocate early anatomic surgical repair of the distal biceps tendon in young, active patients.

Controversies continue to exist regarding the optimal treatment of distal biceps tendon ruptures. Many of these controversies focus on patient selection, approach to the radial tuberosity, and tendon fixation techniques. The first half of this chapter reviews the relevant pathoanatomy, workup, and treatment of patients with distal biceps tendon ruptures. The second half of the chapter focuses on triceps tendon rupture and repair.

Epidemiology

The estimated incidence of distal biceps tendon ruptures has risen from 1.2 to 2.55 per 100,000 population per year according to a recent epidemiologic analysis.[1,2] Distal ruptures account for only 3% of biceps brachii tendon injuries.[1,3] The injury is most commonly seen between the fourth and sixth decades of life, with an average age of approximately 50 years (range, 18 to 72 years).[1,3–7] Several patient factors have been associated with distal biceps tendon ruptures, with the most significant factor being male sex. Eighty-six percent of distal biceps tendon ruptures occur in the dominant extremity, and they typically occur in highly active people, often with elevated body mass indices.[1,2,8] Poisson regression analysis of tobacco use yields a 7.5 times increased risk of distal biceps tendon rupture among persons who smoke.[1,4] Middle-aged men who use nicotine and anabolic steroids have a higher incidence of bilateral injuries.[4]

Anatomy

The biceps brachii muscle is contained in the anterior compartment of the arm and is composed of two heads. The long head originates from the supraglenoid tubercle within the shoulder joint, and the short head originates from the coracoid process. The two heads converge at the level of the deltoid tuberosity. The distal tendon gives rise to the lacertus fibrosus (bicipital

aponeurosis) before passing deep through the antecubital fossa and inserting onto the radial tuberosity. Anatomic investigation of the distal tendon reveals two distinct attachment sites, with a mean length of 92 mm and a mean width ranging from 2.9 to 6.1 mm.[9] The tendon of the short head, which is more significant, attaches more distally on the tuberosity, and biomechanically acts as a flexor. The tendon of the long head inserts further from the axis of rotation of the forearm and acts as a strong supinator (Fig. 62.1).[10,11] The lacertus fibrosus spreads out in an ulnar direction and blends into the forearm fascia, ultimately inserting onto the subcutaneous border of the ulna (Fig. 62.2). This aponeurosis may provide stability to the distal tendon.

Innervation of the biceps brachii is via the musculocutaneous nerve, a branch of the lateral cord of the brachial plexus. It penetrates the biceps muscle at an average of 134 mm distal to the acromion[12] and travels between the biceps and the brachialis before it penetrates the deep fascia of the arm and becomes the lateral antebrachial cutaneous nerve, which supplies sensation to the volar-lateral aspect of the forearm.

The biceps brachii is in close proximity to many vital neurovascular structures. The brachial artery, brachial vein, and the median nerve lie just medial to the biceps tendon and directly underneath the lacertus fibrosus. The brachial artery bifurcates into the radial and ulnar arteries at the level of the radial head. The radial recurrent artery arises from the radial artery and crosses laterally through the antecubital fossa, lying within the typical surgical field (Fig. 62.3). Lateral to the biceps tendon, the radial nerve enters the proximal forearm between the brachialis and the brachioradialis. The radial nerve divides into the deep and superficial branch anterior to the lateral humeral condyle.

Biomechanics

Owing to its dual insertion onto the radial tuberosity, the biceps muscle provides power and endurance for forearm supination and assists the brachialis in elbow flexion. The extent to which the biceps brachii contributes to elbow flexion correlates with the position of the forearm, with increasing contribution as the forearm is supinated. Furthermore, the biceps is able to exert maximum supination strength with the elbow at 90 degrees of flexion.

Morrey et al.[13] performed a biomechanical study of 10 patients to evaluate the differences between conservative management and operative reattachment of distal biceps tendon ruptures. Immediate surgical fixation of the tendon to its insertion ultimately restored normal elbow flexion and forearm supination strength. In the group treated conservatively, an average loss of 40% supination strength and 30% flexion strength occurred.[13] Baker and Bierwagen[14] noted an 86% decrease in supination endurance in patients treated conservatively. Surgical management varies highly in the treatment of distal biceps injuries, both in terms of approach and fixation methods. Prud'homme-Foster et al.[15] demonstrated that, when compared with a one-incision approach, a two-incision approach allows for a more anatomic repair. In their cadaveric study, they demonstrated that forearms repaired anatomically via a two-incision approach demonstrated 15% more supination torque at neutral pronosupination and 40% more supination torque at 45 degrees of supination compared with tendons fixed nonanatomically via a one-incision approach.

Classification

Classification of distal biceps tendon ruptures is based on chronicity, degree of tear (partial vs. complete), and extent of retraction. The Ramsey classification uses these three characteristics to help guide treatment by predicting the ability to reattach the distal biceps tendon primarily to the radial tuberosity (Box 62.1).[7]

History

The mechanism of injury is nearly always a forceful, eccentric contraction of the biceps muscle. Examples of this mechanism include a preacher curl performed with excessive weight by a

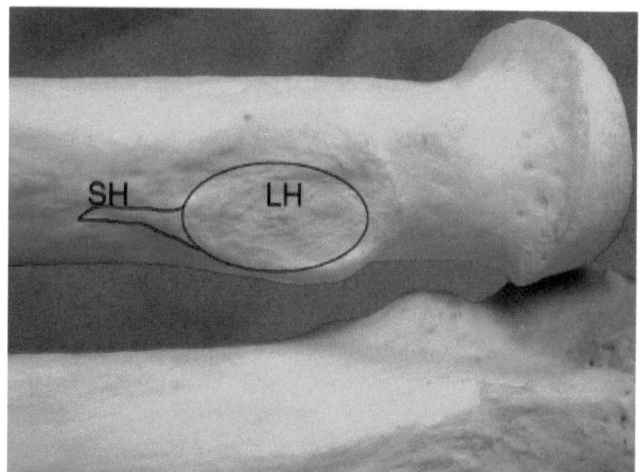

Fig. 62.1 Anatomy of the distal biceps tendon. Note the more distal insertion of the short head *(SH)*, which acts as a strong flexor. The long head *(LH)*, which inserts farther from the axis of rotation, acts as a strong supinator. (From Eames MH, Bain GI, Fogg QA, et al. Distal biceps tendon anatomy: a cadaveric study. *J Bone Joint Surg Am.* 2007;89:1044–1049.)

BOX 62.1   Classification of Distal Biceps Tendon Ruptures

Partial Ruptures
- Insertional
- Intrasubstance (elongation)

Complete Ruptures
- Acute (<4 weeks)
- Chronic (>4 weeks)
- Intact aponeurosis
- Ruptured aponeurosis

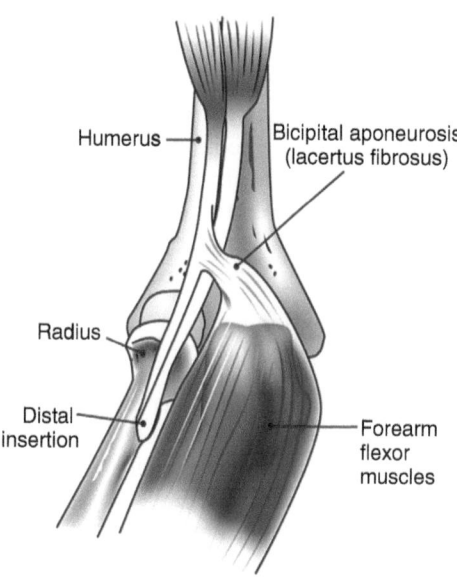

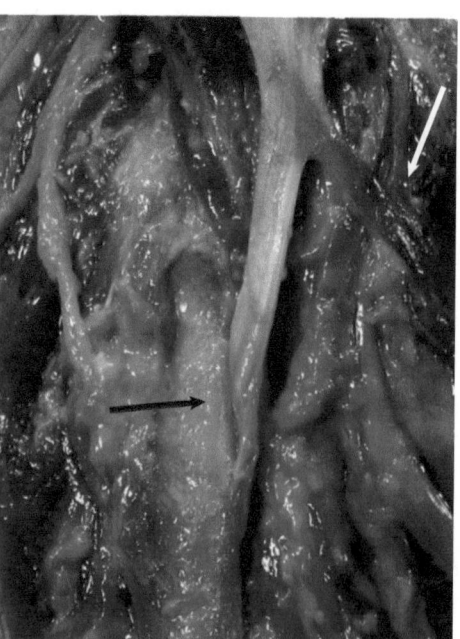

Fig. 62.2 Anatomy of the distal biceps tendon. The *black arrow* indicates the insertion of the distal biceps tendon; the *white arrow* indicates the bicipital aponeurosis. (From Miyamoto RG, Elser F, Millett PJ. Distal biceps tendon injuries. *J Bone Joint Surg Am.* 2010;92[11]:2128–2138.)

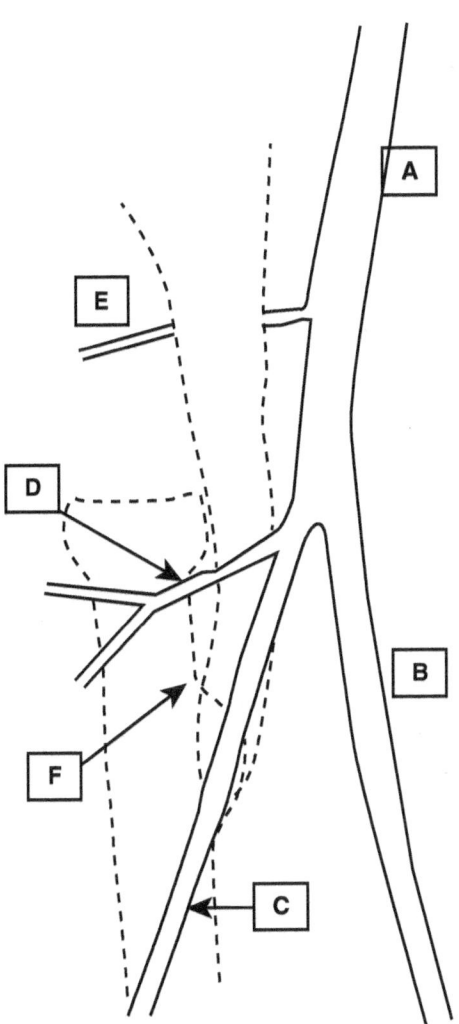

Fig. 62.3 Vascular anatomy surrounding the distal biceps insertion. Proximal radius and biceps tendon are depicted by dotted lines. *A*, Brachial artery; *B*, ulnar artery; *C*, radial artery; *D*, radial recurrent artery; *E*, dorsal radial recurrent artery; *F*, proximal most aspect of radial tuberosity. (From Zeltser DW, Strauch, RJ. Vascular anatomy relevant to distal biceps tendon repair. *J Shoulder Elbow Surg.* 2016;25[2]:238238.)

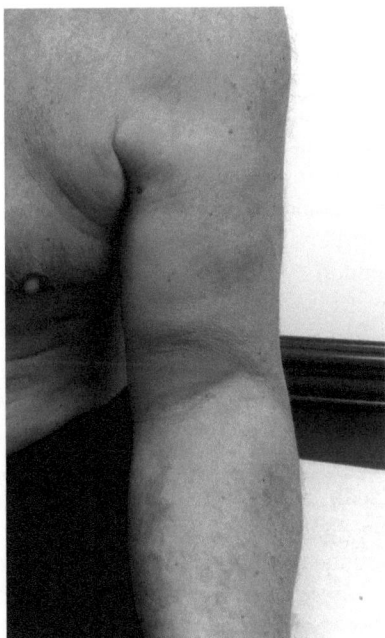

Fig. 62.4 Inspection of an acute distal biceps tendon rupture with proximal muscle retraction and ecchymosis.

weight lifter and forcible extension of the elbow during an attempted tackle by a football player. The most common description and localization of initial pain is an abrupt, intense tearing sensation in the antecubital fossa. A palpable or audible "pop" is frequently recounted. Patients may report sudden and persistent weakness, especially with forearm supination and elbow flexion. As days pass and the swelling diminishes, the patient may notice a cosmetic deformity of the arm as the biceps retracts proximally. Many patients report the slow migration of skin discoloration from the hematoma within the elbow region toward the wrist over time. In patients with a partial biceps tear, the diagnosis is less clear. They may complain of a vague ache like discomfort within the antecubital region, which is exacerbated with forearm supination.

Physical Examination

Inspection of the elbow will often reveal deformity and proximal retraction of the biceps (termed a "Popeye muscle"), swelling,

and ecchymosis within the antecubital fossa and medial aspect of the forearm (Fig. 62.4). Palpation elicits tenderness in the antecubital fossa and a defect of the tendon compared with the contralateral arm. In patients with an intact lacertus fibrosus, the deformity may be less pronounced. Weakness and pain with resisted forearm supination compared with the contralateral side is universally observed in complete ruptures.

Other physical examination tests specific for distal biceps tendon ruptures include the hook test and the biceps squeeze test. The hook test was originally described by O'Driscoll et al.[16] and is performed by first placing the patient's arm at 90 degrees of flexion. Next, the examiner attempts to hook the lateral edge of the biceps tendon with the index finger by pulling from a lateral to medial direction within the antecubital fossa. A positive test elicits an intact cordlike distal biceps tendon. The test is reported to have 100% sensitivity and between 85% and 92% specificity. One needs to be sure that they are feeling for the distal biceps tendon, which occasionally may be tricky as they palpate an intact lacertus fibrosus. The biceps squeeze test[17] is similar to the Thompson test for Achilles tendon ruptures. The examiner squeezes the biceps brachii muscle, and in patients with an intact distal tendon, the forearm should supinate. Pain with palpation over the posterolateral aspect of the radial tuberosity while pronating the forearm is suggestive of distal biceps tendinopathy.

Imaging

A standard elbow radiographic trauma series (i.e., anteroposterior, lateral, and oblique views) should be obtained to evaluate for other causes of anterior elbow pain. Generally there are no signs of acute bony injury, but anterior soft tissue swelling may be appreciated. In rare cases an avulsion fracture of the radial tuberosity may occur and should be visible on radiographs.

Magnetic resonance imaging (MRI) is an excellent modality for assessment of the integrity of the distal biceps tendon, but it is not always necessary to make or confirm the diagnosis.[18] MRI is valuable for differentiating complete from partial tears in equivocal cases, such as in obese patients and persons with an intact lacertus fibrosus. Positioning the arm for an MRI with the elbow flexed, shoulder abducted, and the forearm supination, the so-called "FABS view," allows for complete imaging of the distal biceps tendon, typically on a single image (Fig. 62.5).[19]

Treatment Options

Nonoperative treatment may be considered especially for elderly, low demand individuals and those with partial tendon ruptures wishing to avoid surgery. The typical nonoperative protocol consists of a brief period of immobilization, analgesia, and physical therapy. The goals of physical therapy are the restoration of range of motion (ROM) with gradual elbow flexion and forearm supination strengthening. Patients who elect nonoperative treatment must be counseled on the risk of chronic activity-related pain, fatigue, loss of supination strength between 40% and 60%, and flexion strength of up to 30% and endurance.[13,14,20,21] Patients also must be made aware that outcomes after delayed repair (>4 weeks) may be inferior to those obtained with acute repair and may require tendon grafting or be deemed irreparable.

Once the decision is made to treat a distal biceps tendon rupture surgically, several factors must be carefully taken into consideration prior to proceeding. These include patient factors such as occupation and function, history of anabolic steroids use, how much time has elapsed from the injury, how to expose of the radial tuberosity (one vs. two incisions) and how best fixate the tendon to bone. To date no single surgical plan has demonstrated clear superiority; operative treatment must be tailored to the individual patient and the proficiency of the surgeon.

Injury chronicity is perhaps the most important factor for the surgeon to consider. Early diagnosis may prevent tendon retraction permitting easier reattachment of the biceps tendon to the radial tuberosity regardless of the integrity of the lacertus

fibrosus. In this regard, primary reattachment is generally reliable if performed within 4 weeks of the injury. An intact lacertus fibrosus may minimize tendon retraction and increase the window for reattachment beyond 4 weeks. Concurrent rupture of the lacertus fibrosus will lead to proximal retraction of the tendon and formation of scar tissue with attachment to the adjacent brachialis muscle. Delayed surgery often necessitates extensive scar dissection to liberate the coiled tendon and regain critical length for primary reattachment.

Primary repair may not be possible in persons with chronic injuries, and tendon autograft/allograft reconstruction may be offered to these patients as an alternative to nonoperative care. The most commonly used autografts are semitendinosus and fascia lata, whereas the standard allograft is the Achilles tendon. Delayed reconstruction with use of a tendon graft historically has a less predictable outcome than early anatomic repair of the native tendon. Improvements in strength and endurance are possible, but delayed reconstruction may be reserved for symptomatic patients with significant disability.

Nonanatomic repair or distal biceps tenodesis to the brachialis muscle was first proposed in an effort to decrease complications associated with anatomic reattachment. Several studies have evaluated the efficacy of nonanatomic repair and have found excellent return of flexion strength but, predictably, little or no improvement in forearm supination strength.[22,23] With modern anatomic reattachment techniques, the complication rate has decreased and nonanatomic repair has largely fallen from favor. One exception is a patient with a chronic, irreparable tear who has a chief complaint of activity-related pain and cramping rather than weakness and loss of endurance.

Much debate exists as to whether to perform a one or two incision repair technique. The discussion focuses on the ability to anatomically reattach the biceps tendon to the footprint of the radial tuberosity and the complications associated with each approach. Originally the surgery was performed using a one-incision technique to expose the radial tuberosity through the antecubital fossa. Given the relatively high rate of nerve injury,

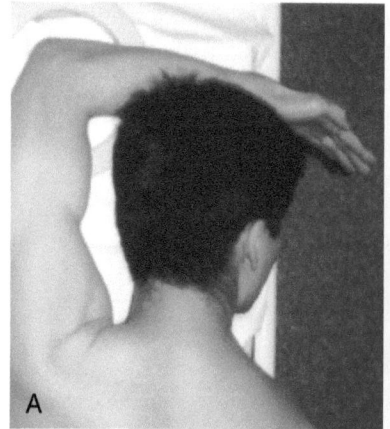 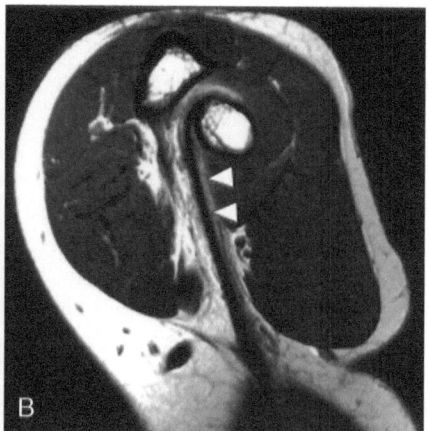

Fig. 62.5 Utilization of the flexed, abducted supinated "FABS view" during magnetic resonance imaging (MRI) for the detection of distal biceps injuries. (A) Patient positioning for the "FABS view": the patient is prone on the MRI table, with the elbow flexed, the shoulder abducted and the hand supinated. (B) Proton density-weighted MR image (TR/TE 3,000/34) in the "FABS" position demonstrating the entire tendon on a single cut. *White arrowheads*, Abnormal signal within the tendon, indicating a partial tear.

Boyd and Anderson[24] developed a two-incision technique to expose the footprint through an additional posterolateral approach. Attachment of the biceps tendon through the posterolateral approach permits a more anatomic reconstruction to the radial tuberosity and requires less extensive anterior exposure, theoretically decreasing the risk of iatrogenic nerve injury. Furthermore, Hasan et al. demonstrated that through a single incision approach, only 9.7% of the repair site was within the original footprint, compared with 73.4% for the double incision approach.[25] Critics of this two-incision approach point to the unique risk of radioulnar synostosis. Failla et al.[26] responded to this drawback by reporting a case series of four patients with radioulnar synostosis who were treated with a modification of the Boyd and Anderson procedure involving a muscle-splitting approach between the common extensor mass and the supinator. This modification allows exposure of the radial tuberosity without violating the ulnar periosteum and decreases the risk of radioulnar synostosis.[26] A subsequent study revealed that the rate of radioulnar synostosis increases if the posterolateral incision is made over the subcutaneous border of the ulna rather than over the common extensors.[27]

Four fixation techniques are presently being used to reattach the distal biceps tendon to the radial tuberosity: transosseous tunnels, suture anchors, interference screws, and cortical fixation buttons (or a combination thereof). Several biomechanical studies have compared fixation strength and stiffness between the different fixation techniques.[28–33] In general, all fixation methods provide adequate fixation strength compared with the intact tendon, with the highest load to failure achieved using a cortical fixation button (Table 62.1).[15,34]

Decision-Making Principles

Acute operative fixation of the distal biceps may be offered to patients who require strength and endurance with elbow flexion and forearm supination. Nonoperative treatment of complete ruptures will yield between 12% and 40% loss of supination strength, up to 86% loss of supination endurance, and consistently decreased Disabilities of the Arm, Shoulder and Hand (DASH) and European Society of Surgery of the Shoulder and Elbow scores. Conversely, early anatomic reconstruction of the distal biceps can restore elbow flexion and supination strength and endurance and demonstrates higher clinical and functional outcomes.[13,14,20,21,35] When considering nonoperative treatment, the practitioner needs to consider the patient's functional status and needs to inform patients of the sequelae should they proceed with this option.

Postoperative Management

Rehabilitation protocols vary depending on the surgical technique and patient compliance. Early in the postoperative course, a period of immobilization or protective splinting is typical. Gentle passive ROM is permissible within the first few weeks. Some surgeons use a hinged brace to block terminal elbow extension initially, which is meant to protect the healing tendon from high tensile forces. After 3 weeks, patients may begin active assisted ROM, and full active motion is usually achieved 6 to 8 weeks after surgery. Resistive exercises are restricted until 8 weeks after surgery, at which time a gradual approach to biceps strengthening exercises is prudent to avoid a repeat tendon rupture. Although many patients prefer a home exercise regimen, it may be wise to refer noncompliant patients to a physical or occupational therapist for guidance and supervision during this phase. Most patients recover ROM and desired strength between 3 and 6 months after surgery.

Cheung et al.[37] evaluated early self-administered passive ROM exercises. After surgery, a hinged elbow brace locked at 90 degrees of flexion was immediately applied. On the first postoperative day, the brace was unlocked to allow passive ROM exercises from 60 degrees to full flexion with full forearm rotation. The elbow extension block was reduced at 2 weeks to 40 degrees, at 4 weeks to 20 degrees, and at 6 weeks to full extension. Strength training was begun at 8 weeks. With this protocol of immediate elbow motion following distal biceps tendon reattachment, no deleterious effects on healing or strength were observed.

Return to sport after distal biceps tendon rupture has not been specifically studied. The general consensus is that patients may return to unrestricted activities at 16 to 20 weeks after surgery. Athletes who participate in contact sports, such as football and rugby players, may need the full 20 weeks to permit tendon maturation and to prevent a repeat rupture.

Results

Several studies have evaluated the outcome of one- and two-incision distal biceps tendon repairs. Both techniques improve DASH scores and elbow flexion and forearm supination strength.[27,38–43]

Karunakar et al.[38] reported on 21 patients after use of the modified Boyd and Anderson technique with bone tunnels. At 44 months all patients reported good to excellent results. Compared with the uninjured arm, endurance was decreased 38% in supination and 33% in flexion. A 15% rate of heterotopic ossification was noted.

TABLE 62.1 Methods for Distal Biceps Tendon Repair: Fixation Strength

Study	LOAD TO FAILURE (N)				
	Intact Tendon	Transosseous Tunnel	Suture Anchor	Interference Screw	Cortical Fixation Button
Berlet et al.[28]		307 (±142)	220 (±54)		
Lemos et al.[31]		203	263		
Idler et al.[32]	204 (±76)	125 (±23)		178 (±54)	
Greenberg et al.[29]		177			584
Mazzocca et al.[33]		310	381	232	440

Authors' Preferred Technique

Distal Biceps Tendon Rupture

Our preferred technique is a single-incision anatomic repair of the distal biceps tendon using a combination of both a fixation button and an interference screw.[36] To perform this technique, a transverse incision is made anterior to the radial tuberosity with the arm in extension, usually 3 to 4 cm distal to the elbow flexion crease. An alternative approach is a longitudinal incision over the radial tuberosity, which is more extensile than a transverse approach. The antecubital veins are ligated or mobilized. The lateral antebrachial cutaneous nerve is identified lateral to the biceps course and carefully protected to avoid traction injury. To access the footprint of the radial tuberosity, the leash of radial recurrent artery is identified and ligated. At this point the ruptured tendon is either found locally (when the lacertus fibrosus is intact) or proximal blunt dissection is carried out if the tendon has retracted (i.e., when the lacertus fibrosus is torn). Along the original course of the tendon, large seromas are frequently discovered and evacuated. As the chronicity of the injury increases, a pseudosheath of fibrous scar tissue may mimic the actual tendon. Often this pseudosheath must be carefully débrided to unveil the native tendon end buried within this "cocoon." Once retrieved, many surgeons will place a clamp (e.g., an Allis clamp) at the terminal tendon and manually release proximal adhesions or even "water ski" with the tendon to achieve maximal excursion. To aid in this, the tourniquet may need to be deflated as this may tether the biceps muscle. Using a heavy nonabsorbable suture (e.g., No. 2 FiberWire, Ticron, or Ethibond), a whipstitch is woven through the distal biceps tendon from proximal to distal, leaving two long limbs exiting the terminus.

The radial tuberosity is exposed with the elbow in full extension and maximal passive supination to protect the posterior interosseous nerve. A retractor may be placed by the radial aspect of the tuberosity, but care must be exercised to avoid excessive lateral retraction to prevent injury to the posterior interosseous

nerve. A 3.2-mm guide pin is then drilled bicortically through the radial tuberosity. An acorn-shaped reamer is passed over the guide pin to create a unicortical tunnel. The suture limbs are passed through a fixation button, and the button is passed bicortically through the radial tuberosity. The tendon is advanced approximately 1 cm into the tunnel and the sutures are tied, securing the biceps tendon within the radial tuberosity (Fig. 62.6). An interference screw is placed into the tunnel, displacing the tendon more distally and ulnar to better recreate the anatomic insertion site.

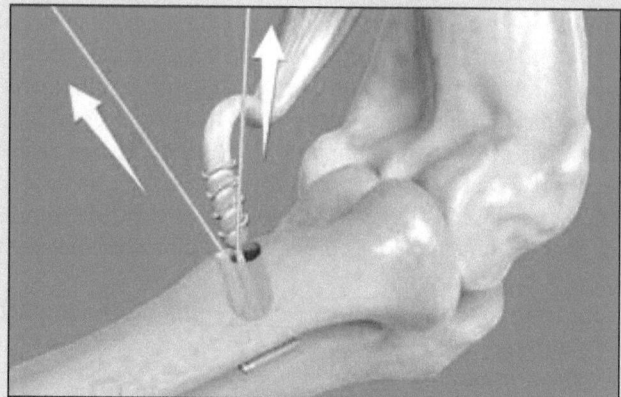

Fig. 62.6 Anatomic repair of a distal biceps tendon. (From Sethi P, Cunningham J, Miller S, et al. Anatomical repair of the distal biceps tendon using the tension-slide technique. *Techniques Shoulder Elbow Surg.* 2008;9[4]:182–187.)

McKee et al.[42] compared one-incision repairs with two suture anchors, using the uninjured arm as a control. At final follow-up, no difference was found in DASH scores. Strength was 96% in flexion and 93% in supination compared with the uninjured side. No differences in ROM were observed.

In a study evaluating outcomes after EndoButton (Smith and Nephew, Andover, MA) fixation, Peeters et al.[44] reported an average Mayo Elbow Performance Score of 94 points. Isokinetic testing showed 80% recovery of flexion strength and 91% recovery for supination. Of 26 patients, 2 experienced asymptomatic heterotopic ossification, and three had asymptomatic disengagement of the EndoButton.

Grewal et al.[45] performed a direct comparison between one-incision repairs using suture anchors and the modified Boyd and Anderson approach using bone tunnels. They found no difference in patient reported outcomes for pain and function at 2 years postoperatively. The one-incision cohort had greater improvement in flexion (142.8 vs. 131.1 degrees) but an overall higher complication rate, with the majority of complications being lateral antebrachial cutaneous nerve palsies. Similarly, Shields et al.[46] found a higher incidence of lateral antebrachial cutaneous neuropraxia following one-incision repairs, but found no difference in strength or ROM and equivalent patient reported outcomes. Schmidt et al.[47] investigated factors that determine strength after distal biceps reattachment and found[47] a two-incision approach to better restore strength than a one-incision

approach with no ultimate differences in forearm motion between groups.

Several fixation techniques may be used to affix the tendon to the radial tuberosity. Fixation techniques and respective load to failure are reviewed in Box 62.2. Techniques that increase the load to failure may allow earlier rehabilitation after surgery.

Chronic tears (i.e., those that occurred >6 weeks earlier) may require tendon grafting. Darlis et al.[48] retrospectively reviewed seven patients with chronic distal biceps tendon ruptures. These investigators sutured Achilles tendon allograft to the distal biceps tendon remnant and secured it to the radial tuberosity with two anchors. Mean elbow flexion was 145 degrees, and mean pronosupination was 170 degrees. Mean supination strength was 87% of the contralateral arm. Wiley et al.[49] compared nonoperative treatment versus operative fixation using a semitendinosus allograft in chronic distal biceps tendon ruptures. At final follow-up, flexion and supination strength returned to normal range in the operative group, and they returned to 20% of normal in the nonoperative group. Endurance in both groups was normal.

Complications

A systematic review of the literature evaluating one- and two-incision distal biceps tendon repairs revealed an 18% complication rate for one-incision repairs and a 16% complication rate for two-incision repairs. The majority of complications were nerve injuries (13%) after one-incision repair and loss of rotation and supination strength after two-incision repairs.[38,41] Heterotopic

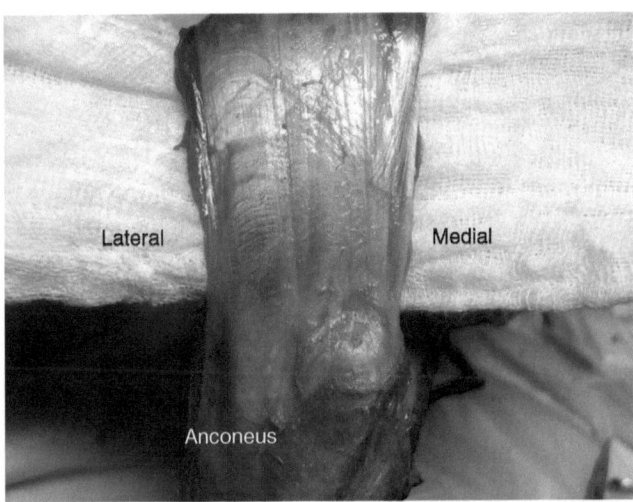

Fig. 62.7 Insertional anatomy of the distal triceps tendon. (From Keener JD, Chafik D, Kim HM, et al: Insertional anatomy of the triceps brachii tendon. *J Shoulder Elbow Surg.* 2010;19[3]:399–405.)

ossification has been reported to be more common following two-incision repairs.[50] More recently, a randomized controlled trial and a meta-analysis demonstrated significantly higher rates of neurapraxia of the lateral antebrachial cutaneous nerve following a single incision approach.[50,51] Although a slight predilection to certain complications appears to exist for each technique, it is important to recognize that no technique completely eliminates the risk of any one complication.

DISTAL TRICEPS TENDON RUPTURE

Elbow flexion is generally regarded as the most essential function of the elbow because gravity can aid in extension. However, the lack of active elbow extension can compromise even the most basic activities of daily living, such as pushing up out of a chair from the seated position. The loss of elbow extension strength is most devastating for athletes of various sports. Therefore prompt recognition and treatment of distal triceps tendon ruptures is warranted.

Epidemiology

Distal triceps tendon ruptures are relatively uncommon injuries. However, their incidence is likely rising because the training of high-performance athletes and the use of performance-enhancing substances has increased over the past two decades.

Distal triceps tendon ruptures occur predominantly in a subset of high-risk people and are exceedingly uncommon in the general population. Strenuous activities, steroid use, and metabolic disease can predispose persons to this condition (see Box 62.2).[52–56] Football players, particularly linemen and powerlifters, are at increased risk because of the nature of their sport and the intensity of their training.[57] Hyperparathyroidism, which is typically a result of chronic renal disease, is also associated with tendon ruptures. Hyperparathyroidism alters the enthesis

of all tendon insertions. The mechanism of insult is not entirely understood but is likely a result of osteoclast overstimulation, leading to the leaching of calcium from the tendon insertion. The enthesis is thus weakened and becomes prone to microfracture and avulsion injuries.

Anatomy and Biomechanics

The triceps brachii is a large muscle encompassing the entire posterior compartment of the arm. Innervation is entirely from the radial nerve (C6-C8). This muscle is composed of three heads: lateral, long, and medial. The medial and lateral heads originate from the posterior humerus and the intermuscular septum and act solely to extend the ulnohumeral joint. The long head originates from the infraglenoid tubercle and may also assist in shoulder adduction and extension.

Keener et al.[58] evaluated the insertional anatomy of the triceps and described a broad footprint on the olecranon measuring 466 mm.[3] The triceps insertion can be divided into the triceps insertion proper and the lateral triceps expansion. Medially, the triceps attaches directly to the olecranon, forming the medial border of the triceps tendon proper. Laterally, the triceps tendon expands beyond the olecranon and becomes continuous with the anconeus and antebrachial fascia and inserts distally on the radial aspect of the proximal ulna (Fig. 62.7).

Classification

In classifying distal triceps tendon ruptures, three characteristics must be evaluated. First, the degree of tendon tear is an important factor in decision-making. Patients with complete tears and high-grade partial tears may be candidates for surgery, whereas low-grade partial tears often respond to conservative treatment. Second, the anatomic location of the tear will influence the choice of surgical technique and strength of fixation, with muscle belly and musculotendinous junction repairs being less stout than their tendinous counterparts. Lastly, the chronicity of the tear is an important factor in determining surgical feasibility and for preoperative planning (i.e., graft augmentation; see Box 62.3).

BOX 62.3   Classification of Distal Triceps Tendon Ruptures

Degree of Tear
- Partial
  - <50%
  - >50%
- Complete
  - Intact lateral expansion
  - Ruptured lateral expansion

Tear Location
- Muscle belly
- Musculotendinous insertion
- Insertional
- Olecranon avulsion fracture

Chronicity of Tear
- Acute (<3 weeks)
- Chronic (>3 weeks)

History

The diagnosis of distal triceps tendon ruptures may not always be straightforward, and thus obtaining a thorough patient history is essential. Because triceps tendon ruptures are rare in the general population, a history of strenuous elbow extension activities, steroid use, and/or metabolic disorder should provide clues to the diagnosis. The most common mechanism of injury is a sudden eccentric triceps contraction that can occur during participation in a sport, weight lifting, and falls onto an outstretched arm.

Pain and swelling over the distal triceps are the most common presenting symptoms. As the pain subsides, patients often report elbow weakness and loss of function. Younger patients may report that they are unable to perform pressing exercises at the gym, whereas older patients may lose the ability to push up from a seated position.

Physical Examination

In the acute injury phase, physical examination reveals swelling, ecchymosis, and tenderness near the triceps insertion. In more chronic injuries, a tendon defect may be palpable along with elbow extension weakness compared with the contralateral arm. Active elbow extension against gravity can help determine the degree of tendon tear, but it is important to recognize that patients with complete tears may have preserved elbow extension as the result of an intact lateral tendon expansion. Furthermore, a thorough examination of the skin, arm, and forearm compartments and determination of distal neurovascular status is important to rule out tendon lacerations, compartment syndrome, and ulnar neuropathy, all of which have been associated with distal triceps brachii tendon ruptures.[59,60]

Imaging

A standard elbow radiographic trauma series (i.e., anteroposterior, lateral, and oblique views) should be ordered to evaluate for bone spurs, bone avulsions, and associated injuries. MRI is an excellent modality for assessment of the integrity of the distal triceps tendon, especially when determining the extent of the tear. MRI may help distinguish between partial and complete tears and determines the extent of retraction in complete tear injuries. Ultrasound has recently demonstrated the ability to accurately identify partial tears of the distal triceps and reliably differentiate them from complete injuries.[61]

Decision-Making Principles

The decision to treat distal triceps tendon ruptures operatively or nonoperatively is based on three factors: (1) the characteristic of the rupture, (2) the patient's medical status, and (3) the patient's functional expectations.

Tear characteristics can be classified using the information in Box 62.3. Partial tears that involve less than 50% of the tendon can often be managed conservatively in patients with adequate active elbow extension. Conservative management of partial tears that involve more than 50% of the tendon and complete tears will typically yield unsatisfactory results, especially in younger, more active patients. In such cases, early primary repair is indicated.[59] Tear location is also an important consideration. Insertional tears allow for more secure surgical fixation than musculotendinous or muscle belly tears. In proximal tear patterns, a more conservative treatment strategy may be appropriate. Tear chronicity should be determined in all patients. In patients for whom surgery is indicated, all attempts should be made to repair the triceps within 3 weeks[59]; however, primary repair has been reported with success up to 8 months after the time of injury.[62] An intact lateral expansion may allow for delayed primary repair by preventing proximal retraction and extensive formation of adhesions.

The patient's general medical condition and functional expectations will also guide treatment decisions. Two distinct patient populations are at risk for distal triceps ruptures: first, young, highly functioning athletes, and second, debilitated patients with metabolic disease. A lower threshold for surgery should be afforded to young athletes. Elderly debilitated patients often respond well to conservative treatment as long as they maintain some active extension and have enough power to rise from a seated position.

Treatment Options
Nonoperative Treatment

Nonsurgical treatment of distal triceps ruptures consists of 4 weeks of splint immobilization at 30 degrees of elbow flexion. At 4 weeks, ROM exercises are started, and strengthening exercises are added after 8 weeks. The outcomes after conservative treatment are not well documented. There is a paucity of evidence to guide nonoperative care, and the results vary widely. Tendon gapping is an important factor to consider when treating patients nonoperatively. Biomechanical studies reveal a 40% loss of extension strength with as little as 2 cm of gapping.[63] Thus in patients in whom significant retraction is observed, nonoperative treatment will likely lead to greater loss of strength and endurance[64–66] and should be considered only in elderly, sedentary patients and persons too ill to undergo surgery. Muscle belly tears are a distinct entity and heal with scar tissue. Although surgical fixation has been reported in high-level athletes, outcomes are not believed to be altered by surgical intervention.[67]

Operative Treatment

The primary goals of surgical treatment are to reduce the gap between the distal triceps and the olecranon, allow healing to occur, and restore normal strength and endurance to the elbow. Primary repair is optimal and can be accomplished in patients who are treated within 3 weeks of the injury.[59] Primary repair may be possible after this time window, but reconstructive options should be available as a backup.

Primary repair should be performed by passing a heavy, non-absorbable suture through the triceps tendon with use of either a Bunnell or Krackow whipstitch. Fixation most commonly is achieved by passing the sutures through drill holes in the olecranon and tying them over a bone bridge (Fig. 62.8). Alternatively, knotless suture anchors may be used to fix the tendon to bone. A recent biomechanical study found less displacement after cyclic loading at the footprint when knotless suture anchors were used in lieu of a traditional transosseous repair with manually tied knots.[68]

Chronic tendon ruptures often require reconstruction, and several options have been described in the literature. An anconeus rotation flap is an excellent option when adequate tissue bulk and quality are available. In one study, however, it was found that this technique was only possible in one of nine cases owing to local tissue quality.[59] The second option is triceps augmentation with either an autograft or allograft. The most commonly used grafts are the palmaris longus and semitendinosus.[59,69] Achilles tendon allografts have also been used. Tissue augmentation is achieved by weaving the graft through the remaining triceps tendon, often in a Bunnell fashion, and then attaching it to the olecranon through drill holes (Fig. 62.9).

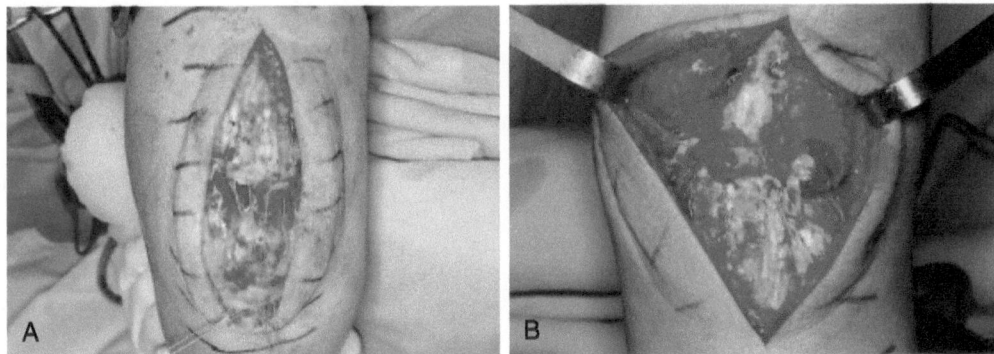

Fig. 62.8 A primary repair using a Krackow suturing technique attached to the olecranon via three drill holes. Sutures are then tied over a bone bridge. (A) Photograph demonstrating suture placement prior to tying. (B) Photographs after suture limbs have been tied over a bone bridge. (From Sierra RJ, Weiss NG, Shrader MW, et al. Acute triceps ruptures: case report and retrospective chart review. *J Shoulder Elbow Surg.* 2006;15[1]:130–134.)

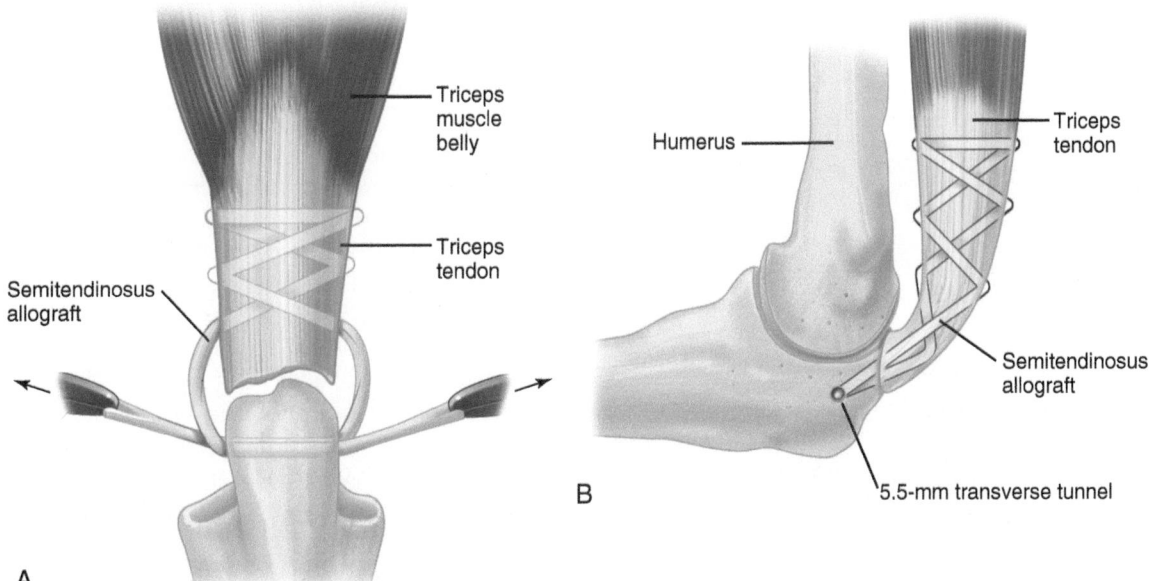

Fig. 62.9 A reconstruction technique using a tendon graft woven through remaining triceps tendon (A) and attached through olecranon drill holes (B). (From Yeh PC, Dodds SD, Smart LR, et al. Distal triceps rupture. *J Am Acad Orthop Surg.* 2010;18[1]:31–40.)

Authors' Preferred Technique

Distal Triceps Tendon Rupture

Recent studies have delineated the anatomy of the distal triceps tendon[58,70] and described an insertional footprint on the olecranon similar to the footprint of the rotator cuff. The footprint measures 466 mm.[3] Information gained from these anatomic studies has led to a new repair technique called the "suture bridge." To perform this technique, a locking Krackow suture is placed through the ruptured triceps tendon, entering and leaving the tendon roughly 2 cm from its distal tip. The olecranon footprint is then identified and excoriated. Two suture anchors are placed at the proximal medial and lateral footprint. Mattress sutures from both anchors are then placed 2 cm from the tendon edge and tied. The sutures from both horizontal mattresses and from the Krackow suture are configured to form a suture bridge and locked into place using two more press-fit suture anchors positioned at the distal end of the footprint (Fig. 62.10).[70] Care is taken to ensure that none of the anchors penetrates the ulnotrochlear joint. The sutures are secured with the arm held in 35 to 40 degrees of flexion.

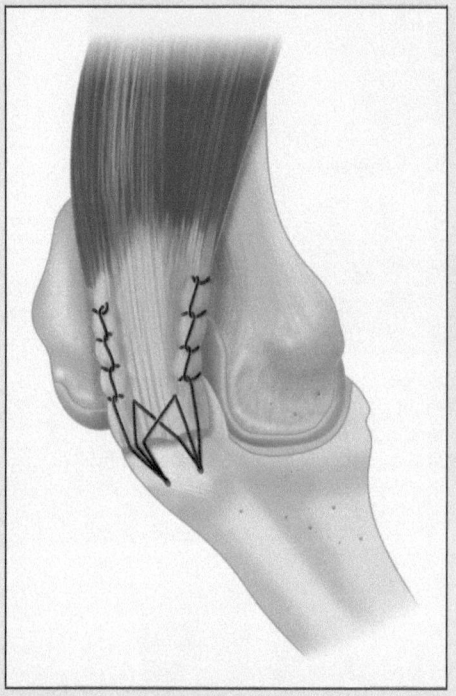

Fig. 62.10 The suture bridge technique. (From Yeh PC, Dodds SD, Smart LR, et al Distal triceps rupture. *J Am Acad Orthop Surg.* 2010;18[1]:31–40.)

Postoperative Management

A standardized postoperative protocol has not been established in the literature. The elbow is often immobilized in a splint at 30 to 40 degrees of flexion for 2 weeks after surgery. At 2 weeks, active-assisted ROM is started if the repair is deemed stable. Some surgeons use a hinged brace to block terminal elbow flexion initially, which is meant to protect the healing tendon from high tensile forces. Light strengthening exercises with a 5-lb weight restriction are started at 6 weeks and progressive resistance exercises, which are best performed under the guidance of a physical therapist, may begin at 8 to 10 weeks. Return to competitive sport or heavy weight lifting is usually prohibited for 4 to 6 months after the repair is performed.

Results

Van Riet et al.[59] evaluated 23 patients, including 13 primary repairs via bone tunnels and 9 reconstructions using a variety of techniques. ROM averaged 8 to 138 degrees of flexion after primary repairs and 13 to 133 degrees after reconstructive procedures. All patients regained 4/5 or 5/5 strength on manual muscle testing. Peak strength averaged 92% of the contralateral extremity in the persons who underwent primary repairs and 66% in the persons who underwent reconstructive procedures. These investigators concluded that early surgical repair (i.e., within 3 weeks) is the optimal treatment for distal triceps tendon ruptures.[59] Yeh et al.[71] performed a biomechanical study evaluating three repair techniques: cruciate repair, suture anchor repair, and anatomic repair (our preferred technique). Load at yield and peak load were similar in all groups; however, the anatomic repair technique most accurately reproduced the anatomic footprint and demonstrated the least amount of displacement after cyclic loading.[71] Recent data have demonstrated excellent results in high demand individuals. Balazs et al.[72] demonstrated a 94% return to active duty in the military population. In active players in the National Football League, Finstein et al.[57] demonstrated a 100% return to play at an average of 165 days.

Complications

In the study of 23 distal triceps brachii repairs by van Riet et al.,[59] complications included one case of ulnar neuropathy, which resolved; one case of prominent hardware that required removal; and repeat tendon rupture in three patients. Balazs et al.[72] demonstrated a retear rate of 12.5% in the military personnel, all of which occurred within the first four months following surgery. Other potential complications include olecranon bursitis and elbow flexion contracture.

Future Considerations

The treatment of distal biceps and triceps tendon ruptures has evolved considerably. As our understanding of insertional anatomy and biomechanics has improved, our surgical techniques have improved as well, allowing for stronger fixation methods, improved outcomes, and fewer complications. Early anatomic repair is indicated in healthy, active patients who do not wish to restrict their activities or lose arm strength. Conservative treatment may be appropriate in select cases and may yield satisfactory outcomes when maximal elbow and forearm strength is not necessary or desired. Because the length of recovery is relatively prolonged after these major tendon injuries, future research will likely focus on preventative strategies and methods to decrease tendon-to-bone healing time when injury does occur. The arena of biologic augmentation for optimal tendon healing continues to grow, and translational research will help elucidate the effects of these substances after injury or surgical treatment.

For a complete list of references, go to ExpertConsult.com.

SELECTED READINGS

Citation:
Morrey BF, Askew LJ, An KN, et al. Rupture of the distal tendon of the biceps brachii: a biomechanical study. *J Bone Joint Surg Am*. 1985;67:418–421.

Level of Evidence:
III

Summary:
This classic article presents the biomechanical results of immediate reattachment versus conservative treatment for distal biceps brachii rupture. At 1-year follow-up, it was found that immediate reattachment restored normal strength to the elbow in all patients. Patients treated conservatively lost a mean of 40% of forearm supination strength and 30% of elbow flexion strength.

Citation:
Baker BE, Bierwagen D. Rupture of the distal tendon of the biceps brachii: operative versus non-operative treatment. *J Bone Joint Surg Am*. 1985;67:414–417.

Level of Evidence:
III

Summary:
Baker and Bierwagen performed a case-control study comparing patients treated with surgery versus patients treated conservatively after a distal biceps tendon rupture. Using a Cybex isokinetic dynamometer, it was determined that the group treated conservatively had a 40% reduction in forearm supination strength, a 79% reduction in supination endurance, and a 30% reduction in elbow flexion strength and endurance compared with the group that underwent surgery.

Citation:
van Riet RP, Morrey BF, Ho E, et al. Surgical treatment of distal triceps ruptures. *J Bone Joint Surg Am*. 2003;85:1961–1967.

Level of Evidence:
IV

Summary:
Primary repair of distal triceps tendon ruptures can always be achieved when surgery is performed within 3 weeks. After repair, isokinetic testing showed peak strength of the involved extremity to be 82% and average endurance to be 99% that of the uninvolved extremity. Results of early repair are favorable compared with results of late reconstruction.

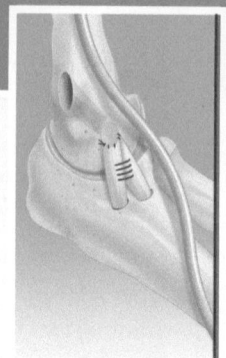

63

Entrapment Neuropathies of the Arm, Elbow, and Forearm

Wajeeh Bakhsh, Warren C. Hammert

ENTRAPMENT NEUROPATHIES

Entrapment neuropathy is a condition wherein compression, or external pressure applied to a nerve, alters function. Multiple potential etiologies exist, including a space-occupying lesion, inflammatory processes, edema, or compression via anatomic structures. Lesions can present as either acute or chronic conditions. If untreated, the sequelae of prolonged compression can result in permanent compromise of function.

The median nerve at the wrist is the most common nerve compression in the upper extremity, but other sites of compression of the median, ulnar, and radial nerves in the arm, elbow, and forearm occur and can be problematic for athletes. Entrapment of a nerve as a result of any pathologic process can progress to neural injury and dysfunction. Initially, nerves experience edema secondary to compression, although this may be clinically silent or intermittent. Sensory fibers are typically affected first due to their lower threshold of injury because they are less invested in protective myelin sheath, with smaller dimensions. Prolonged compression results in an inflammatory response, microvascular changes, and Schwann cell degeneration.[1] A greater degree of severity of compression can progress to include motor dysfunction and may ultimately result in irreversible changes.

The double crush phenomenon is a condition where the axons distal to the injury site are at increased risk of further injury due to affected axonal transport and myelin or Schwann cell injury that propagates distally.[1] Patient recovery and relief of symptoms is dependent on release of all sites of compression along the course of the affected nerve.

History

Patients with entrapment neuropathy may present with motor dysfunction (weakness), sensory dysfunction (numbness), or both, with specific patterns dependent on the nerve and site of compression. Symptoms often follow typical patterns, given the anatomic distribution of the affected nerve, and range from intermittent to constant symptoms that may vary in severity. The duration and severity of symptoms may play a role in projecting outcomes following surgery.

Physical Exam

Examination of an extremity must always begin proximally, especially with nerve-related complaints, to evaluate contributing or confounding factors such as cervical spine pathology or the aforementioned double crush phenomenon. In general, isolated motor neuropathies, such as anterior or posterior interosseous nerve (AIN; PIN) syndrome, will present with weakness or paralysis in the associated motor groups. Sensory findings follow anatomic distributions, presenting as diminished or altered sensation. Altered sensitivity to light touch (determined with Semmes-Weinstein monofilaments) is an early finding, whereas changes in two-point discrimination are a late finding. Entrapment also makes injured nerves susceptible to manual irritation or provocation of sensory symptoms, which can be reliably identified by the presence of a positive Tinel sign or distal paresthesias/sensations, which occur when percussing a nerve in an area of irritation.

Imaging

Radiographic imaging has a limited role in evaluation of entrapment neuropathy. In situations such as heterotopic ossification (HO) or posttraumatic elbow conditions, osseous anatomic anomalies may exist that result in nerve entrapment. Ultrasound is a relatively new modality and appears promising, but at this time there are limited data regarding its role.[2-5] It can be used to help diagnose and classify cubital tunnel syndrome, as the ulnar nerve undergoes changes in cross-sectional area with entrapment at the elbow, and nerve subluxation can be visualized.[6] There is both a diagnostic and therapeutic role in the management of carpal tunnel as well.[7]

Magnetic resonance imaging (MRI) provides information regarding soft tissue anatomy and can occasionally be valuable in entrapment neuropathy. It can be helpful in evaluation of anomalous anatomic structures, space-occupying lesions. Cysts or tumors, such as a lipoma, can cause pressure on the nerve and can be particularly helpful in evaluating radial nerve in the forearm. MRI can also be used for evaluation of nerve integrity following trauma. It can also provide valuable information in the setting of motor dysfunction because degenerative changes in muscles can indicate level of injury or degree of involvement.[8]

Electrophysiologic Testing

Further diagnostic information is available via electrophysiologic evaluation. Nerve compression results in demyelination along the length of the nerve, which progresses distally, impairing conduction velocity. More severe entrapment can progress to asynchronous conduction and even conduction block, with resultant weakness, atrophy, and eventual paralysis.[9]

Electrodiagnostic studies have two components: nerve conduction velocities (NCVs) and electromyogram (EMG). NCV studies can potentially identify sites of slowing, which can help in diagnosing potential double crush injuries. Increased conduction latencies occur due to demyelination. Sensory nerves demonstrate changes earlier in the disease process due to their lower injury threshold and decreased myelin content in comparison to motor nerves. Amplitude of conducted impulses is proportional to the cross-sectional area of functional axons. Increased motor latency and decreasing amplitude indicate more advanced compression. EMG describes the muscles' response to stimulation, including motor recruitment. EMG or motor changes lag behind NCV changes in entrapment neuropathy, indicating more advanced disease. In addition, repeat studies provide useful information in monitoring nerve recovery after intervention, which is most useful in the context of motor function, with nerves such as the AIN and PIN.[10] Early axonal denervation presents with sharp waves and fibrillation potentials, onset 1 to 4 weeks after nerve injury. Chronic injuries demonstrate these patterns but with diminished amplitude. A regenerating/healing nerve will have motor units with polyphasic patterns and nascent, low-amplitude potentials on EMG.[11]

These studies are done with the limb in a resting position. Some athletes only have symptoms with provocation, such as ulnar nerve irritation in throwing athletes. Special circumstances, such as communications or connections with other major nerves, such as the anomalous Martin-Gruber connection, may be present, making it difficult to match the clinical and electrical findings. The Martin-Gruber connection is a motor nerve connection between the median and ulnar nerves and can result in retained distal function in the distribution of the transected nerve.[12] In addition, temperature of the limb undergoing evaluation can influence outcomes, specifically EMG amplitude, due to corresponding variations in fluid distributions within muscle.[13-16] Therefore these results should be interpreted within clinical context.

Decision-Making Principles

With early presentation, a trial of nonoperative treatment is warranted and typically pursued for 3 to 6 months, after which persistence or worsening of symptoms warrants surgical intervention.[17-19] Severe entrapment or symptoms associated with trauma are best treated with early nerve decompression.

Treatment Options

Nonoperative management should include activity modification, with avoidance of the offending position or movement, and use of an orthosis. Antiinflammatory medication can help with mild or moderate symptoms. Corticosteroid injections have a limited role in many entrapment neuropathies of the upper extremity other than carpal tunnel syndrome. Failure of nonoperative management or persistence or worsening of symptoms warrants surgical intervention.

Postoperative Management

Postoperatively, patients should be expected to return to full activity, with timing dependent upon the procedure and sport/position. This is typically a much shorter duration than with osseous or ligamentous injuries, which may be up to 6 months.[20-23] The athletes must demonstrate the ability to safely take the affected limb through the necessary range of motion (ROM) and with the necessary strength and control to return to play (RTP).

Complications

Untreated entrapment neuropathy can eventually progress to chronic degeneration and associated permanent nerve dysfunction and muscle atrophy. Surgical intervention carries risks, including wound complications, iatrogenic nerve injury, inadequate or incomplete surgical decompression, and recurrence of symptoms. A rare but serious complication is the development of complex regional pain syndrome (CRPS), associated with chronic pain, early vasomotor changes, stiffness, and loss of function. It may be associated with chronic nerve entrapment, which can occur with nerve compressions, specific nerve injuries, or trauma in the extremity.[24,25]

Median Nerve

The median nerve is positioned along the anterior aspect of the arm, initially lateral to the brachial artery, although it crosses over to lie medially upon reaching the antecubital fossa. Approximately 1% of the population has an anomalous supracondylar humerus process that can give rise to a fibrous band that inserts at the medial epicondyle, named the ligament of Struthers. The median nerve travels beneath this structure, when present,[26-28] and crosses the antecubital fossa, where it is bordered by the brachial artery (lateral), brachialis (posterior), pronator teres (PT) (medial), and lacertus fibrosus, or bicipital aponeurosis (anterior).[29] The nerve then enters the anterior compartment of the forearm between the heads of the PT.[30] The median nerve travels distally between the flexor digitorum superficialis (FDS) and flexor digitorum profundus (FDP). The AIN branches at a variable location within the proximal forearm. The median nerve becomes more superficial, running between the FDS and flexor pollicis longus (FPL), gives off the palmar cutaneous nerve branch and then enters the carpal tunnel at the wrist. The median nerve innervates the FDS, flexor carpi radialis (FCR), and palmaris longus (PL) muscles in the forearm (Fig. 63.1).

The AIN may divide from the median nerve as proximal as the two heads of the PT, typically in a radial direction. It passes through the FDS arch along with the median nerve and progresses distally volar to the interosseous membrane between the FDP and FPL. The AIN terminates at the pronator quadratus (PQ) muscle after innervating the FPL, variable portions of the radial FDP, and PQ muscles.

Of note, approximately 22% of the population can present with a connection between the AIN or median nerve and the ulnar nerve, known as the Martin-Gruber connection.[31] A potential space-occupying anomaly is the Gantzer muscle, an accessory head of the FPL muscle, which can be present in up to 68% of patients.[32]

Median nerve compression in the arm and forearm is typically associated with high stress, repetitive flexion through the elbow, and repetitive forceful pronation. Sports that rely

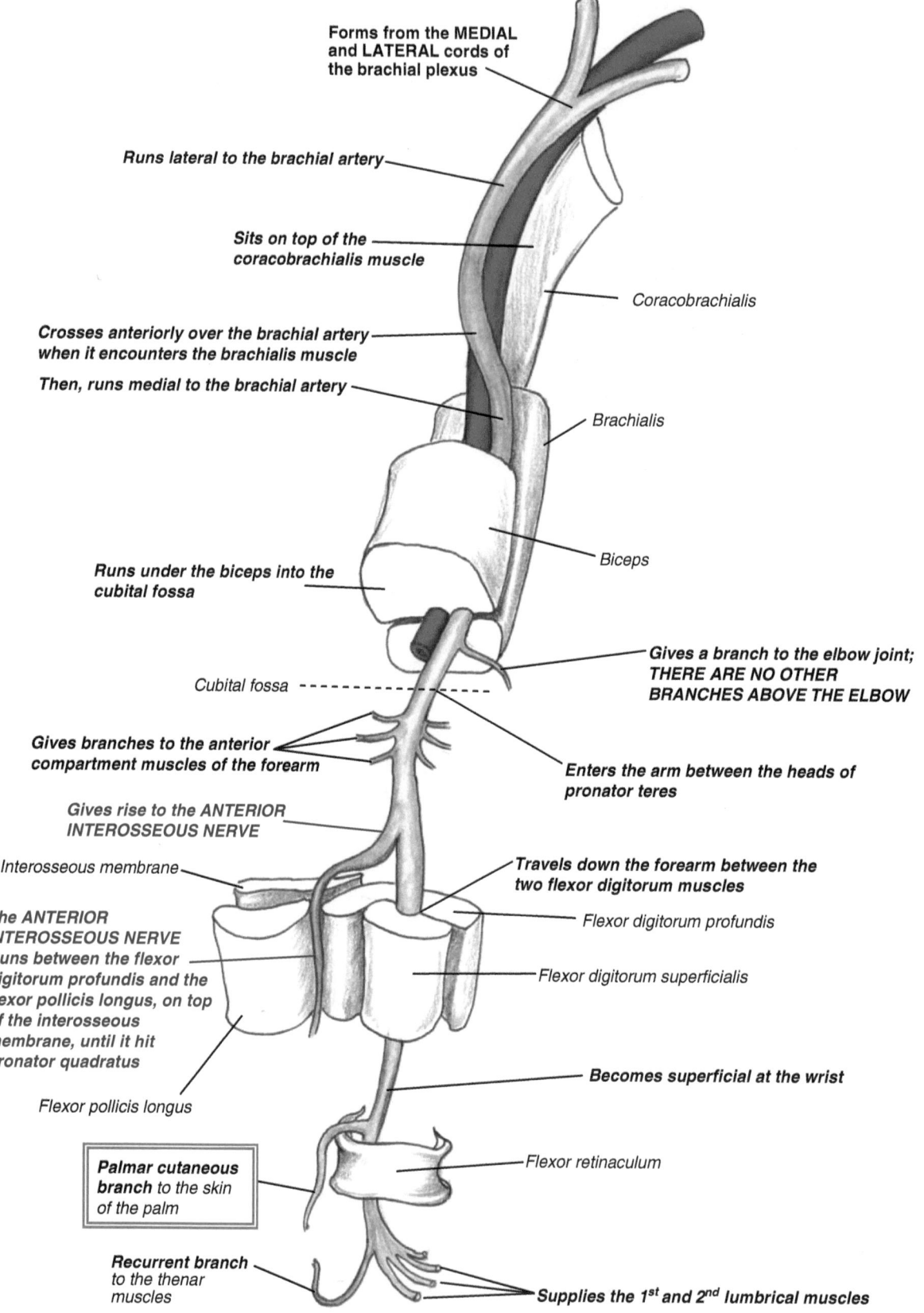

Forms from the MEDIAL and LATERAL cords of the brachial plexus

Runs lateral to the brachial artery

Sits on top of the coracobrachialis muscle

Coracobrachialis

Crosses anteriorly over the brachial artery when it encounters the brachialis muscle

Then, runs medial to the brachial artery

Brachialis

Biceps

Runs under the biceps into the cubital fossa

Gives a branch to the elbow joint; THERE ARE NO OTHER BRANCHES ABOVE THE ELBOW

Cubital fossa

Gives branches to the anterior compartment muscles of the forearm

Enters the arm between the heads of pronator teres

Gives rise to the ANTERIOR INTEROSSEOUS NERVE

Travels down the forearm between the two flexor digitorum muscles

Interosseous membrane

Flexor digitorum profundis

The ANTERIOR INTEROSSEOUS NERVE Runs between the flexor digitorum profundis and the flexor pollicis longus, on top of the interosseous membrane, until it hit pronator quadratus

Flexor digitorum superficialis

Becomes superficial at the wrist

Flexor pollicis longus

Palmar cutaneous branch to the skin of the palm

Flexor retinaculum

Recurrent branch to the thenar muscles

Supplies the 1st and 2nd lumbrical muscles

Fig. 63.1 Diagram depicting the anatomic course of the median nerve.

on these motions include archery, baseball, and automobile racing.[33]

PRONATOR SYNDROME

Pronator syndrome is primarily attributed to median nerve compression between the two heads of the PT in the forearm. Other sites of entrapment include the proximal arch of FDS, the anomalous ligament of Struthers, or the lacertus fibrosus in the antebrachial fossa.[34,35] Sources of potential external compression include tumors and the anomalous Gantzer muscle.[32] Pronator syndrome has also been described with the presence of a persistent median artery.[36,37] The most common sites of median nerve compression are at the deep head of the PT, the FDS arch, and lacertus fibrosus.[38] There are surgeons who feel this is really entrapment at the lacertus fibrosus and isolated decompression at this level will resolve symptoms.[39]

History

Pronator syndrome presents primarily with complaints of pain in the forearm, typically in the proximal, anterior region, with minimal weakness or sensory deficits. A notable differentiating factor from carpal tunnel syndrome is the absence of nocturnal symptoms.[34,35] If sensory deficits are present, they can present as numbness or paresthesia in the thenar eminence, in the distribution of the palmar cutaneous branch of the median nerve, as well as the volar aspect of the thumb, index, middle, and radial aspect of the ring finger, following typical median nerve innervation.[30,40]

Physical Exam

As with other entrapment neuropathies, provocative maneuvers can help determine a site of compression. Reproducible pain with resisted forearm pronation while the elbow is extended suggests compression at the PT. When the site of compression is the fibrous arch of the FDS, resisted contraction of the middle finger proximal interphalangeal (PIP) joint will elicit pain in the volar forearm.[34,35] Pain with resisted elbow flexion while the forearm is held in maximum supination is associated with median nerve compression under the lacertus fibrosus.[41] Compression under the ligament of Struthers is suggested by pain with resisted elbow flexion at 120 to 130 degrees.[30] The patient may also present with weakness of the FPL and FDP of the index finger, similar to findings with AIN neuropathy. The Gainor test involves direct compression of the PT in bilateral upper extremities while at rest. A positive test, which indicates PT compression, is defined as provocative symptoms only in the affected limb.[42] The scratch-collapse test, which is positive with acute ipsilateral weakness in shoulder external rotation upon noxious stimulus to a site of nerve compression, has been previously described with sensitivity and specificity similar to other exam maneuvers. This is performed with the examiner in front of the patient and both arms flexed at the elbow and forearms in neutral rotation. The examiner attempts to bring the hands together while the patient resists. The nerve in question is then scratched, and the examiner again attempts to bring the hands together. A positive result occurs when the patient temporarily

cannot resist the examiner's pressure and the extremity collapses due to the pressure. However, studies find this exam to be operator dependent with variable diagnostic outcomes, and although it may provide an adjunct to EMG or other exam findings, it is not independently diagnostic.[43-45]

Decision-Making Principles

Vague anterior forearm pain is the primary and most reliable reproducible symptom, whereas history and exam maneuvers are not as specific as in other entrapment neuropathies. Electrodiagnostic studies are often normal.[46] Imaging can provide some information because the anomalous supracondylar humerus process associated with the ligament of Struthers can be seen on x-ray.[47] Further imaging, such as MRI or ultrasound, may be warranted with clinical concern for a space-occupying lesion, such as a cyst or tumor, or to evaluate anomalous anatomy.

Initial management should be nonoperative, including activity modification to avoid the offending action, immobilization, and antiinflammatory medications and can result in symptom resolution in 50% to 70% of cases.[40,48]

Treatment Options

Traditional surgical management requires exposure of the antecubital fossa to address all potential sites of compression of the median nerve. The skin incision typically begins 5 cm proximal to the elbow and extends distally to the mid-forearm.[49] Incisions can either follow a lazy-S pattern with or without offset linear incision, or a transverse incision.[50,51] Longitudinal incisions result in more noticeable scarring. Endoscopic assisted decompression has also been described.[49]

The most common approach is via a lazy-S incision that progresses from the mid-arm along the medial aspect of the biceps, curving toward the supracondylar region medially and continuing distally over the flexor-pronator mass to the mid-forearm. Dissection should preserve the cutaneous nerve branches. Supracondylar exposure should be performed, with release of the ligament of Struthers, if indicated clinically or radiographically. The median nerve is identified and traced to identify potential sites of compression. The lacertus fibrosus should be divided and released. The two heads of the PT should be divided and adhesions released. Distally, the FDS arch should be released, with care to protect the AIN, which may have branched proximally. Any space-occupying masses should be excised and sent for pathologic evaluation.

Preferred Technique (Fig. 63.2)

Our preference is a complete decompression of the median nerve from the lacertus fibrosus through the fibrous arch of the FDS, as described previously.

Postoperative Management and Return to Play

Mobilization should take place within 1 week, with therapy directed at nerve gliding, motion, and strengthening. RTP is typically 6 to 8 weeks for most sports and is dependent upon adequate healing, motion, and return of grip strength but may be up to 6 months.[38,49] Endoscopic surgery, or isolated decompression

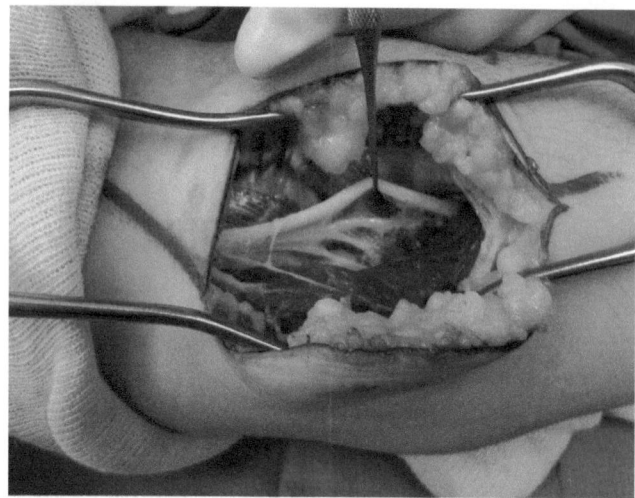

Fig. 63.2 Clinical picture of median nerve decompression. Anterior interosseous nerve and muscular branches are visible following decompression.

at a specific point, will result in a smaller incision and shorter recovery.

Results

Surgical release has been shown to reliably relieve symptoms with good or excellent results in 60% to 80%+ of cases.[38,46,52] This is supported with objective measures such as the Disabilities of the Arm, Shoulder, and Hand (DASH) score and some studies showing 60% of patients with near or complete resolution of symptoms.[49] Outcomes are variable because Olehnik et al. report persistent symptoms in 25% of 39 patients.[53]

Complications

Complications are unusual but include incomplete release, iatrogenic nerve injury, and scarring with recurrence of symptoms. Transient AIN palsy has been documented.[51]

ANTERIOR INTEROSSEOUS NERVE SYNDROME

AIN syndrome is an isolated motor nerve dysfunction, often without associated trauma or injury. There has been no specific pattern of activity or sport that has been associated with this condition. It is often idiopathic, although entrapment is possible.[54] Potential other etiologies include trauma, space-occupying lesions, and anomalous vasculature. If entrapment is the etiology of AIN palsy, the most common site of compression is under the FDS arch.[55] Alternative sites of compression mirror those for pronator syndrome.[56]

History

Clinical presentation often includes a dull ache or pain in the volar forearm.[57] The diagnostic finding is motor dysfunction in the AIN distribution without sensory deficits.[54,58] It is important to rule out Parsonage-Turner syndrome in these patients, or brachial neuritis. Parsonage-Turner syndrome is a prodrome of viral illness–like symptoms, followed by shoulder pain, several days to weeks prior to the onset of muscle weakness suggestive of AIN dysfunction. These patients typically respond to nonoperative management. In addition, sensory deficits may be associated with Parsonage-Turner or carpal tunnel syndrome, which is helpful in diagnosis differentiation.[54,59]

Physical Exam

Motor dysfunction in the AIN distribution is the hallmark of AIN syndrome. Patients often present with loss of flexion of the thumb interphalangeal (IP) joint (secondary to FPL dysfunction) and the index distal interphalangeal (DIP) joint (loss of FDP function). This results in loss of tip pinch between index and thumb (inability to make an "O" when opposing the tip of the thumb to the tip of the index finger). Dysfunction isolated to a single tendon must be evaluated to rule out tendon rupture, especially in patients with inflammatory arthropathies.[60] This can be accomplished through tenodesis, or evaluation of resting passive tension of tendons, which allows for identification of tendon ruptures. When the wrist is flexed, the fingers should extend due to tension on the digital extensors. When the wrist is extended, the fingers should flex, with the ulnar digits flexing slightly more to maintain a normal digital cascade.

Decision-Making Principles

The diagnosis of an AIN syndrome is primarily clinical. However, further workup is required to determine a truly idiopathic AIN pathology from entrapment neuropathy that may possibly benefit from surgical intervention. Electrodiagnostic studies are often normal in idiopathic cases but do provide information regarding the severity of nerve compression in AIN syndrome.[61,62] Advanced imaging such as MRI may be used to rule out space-occupying lesions and also evaluate potential atrophy in AIN-innervated muscle groups. The most reliable MRI finding in AIN syndrome diagnosis is increased signal intensity within the PQ.[8]

Nonoperative management is the primary course of treatment. Rest, immobilization, and analgesia with antiinflammatory medications are the mainstays of early treatment. Avoiding offending actions, especially forceful gripping and repetitive pronation, and use of an orthosis or a sling to maintain rest with the elbow in flexion relieve tension on the AIN. Spontaneous resolution of symptoms often takes up to 9 months.[63] Surgery is indicated for patients with compressive findings on electrodiagnostic testing that have failed nonoperative management, which can be defined as 3 to 6 months without improvement either clinically or via EMG studies.[55,64-66]

Treatment Options

Given that the sites of compression are the similar to pronator syndrome, surgical treatment follows the same approach. Anterior exposure of the distal arm, antecubital fossa, and proximal forearm is required to obtain access to all sites of compression. More extensive dissection at the proximal aspect of the incision helps to expose the origin of the AIN by releasing and reflecting the humeral head of the PT.[67] Division of the lacertus fibrosus and release of the arch of FDS distally are carried out for decompression. The Gantzer muscle, if present, should be released. Innervating branches of the AIN to FPL and FDP must be preserved. Identification of vascular anomalies and mass lesions should be followed by appropriate excision or ligation.

Preferred Technique

Our technique mimics that used for pronator syndrome, because we prefer to release all potential sites of compression unless there is a localized point of compression confirmed on electrodiagnostic studies, in which case we will decompress only that area.

Postoperative Management and Return to Play

AIN syndrome secondary to a compressive etiology often results in progressive return of function postoperatively.[68] RTP depends on return of strength in the affected motor groups, and similar to pronator syndrome, is typically 6 weeks but dependent on sport, position, and level of competition.[49] Studies demonstrate recovery of strength within 6 to 12 months.[55]

Results

Studies have widely variable results, with one study by Werner, et al. that reviewed 69 patients, reporting only 14 confirmed compressive lesions.[69] There are smaller studies that report findings of compression in 60% to 90% of cases.[55]

Postsurgical outcomes demonstrate high rates of function recovery, with a study by Park, et al. demonstrating recovery of motor strength to 4 or greater out of 5 in 10 of 11 surgical cases within 12 months.[55,70] Multiple studies suggest rates of 70% to 90% with good to excellent results.[64,70,71] However, the role of surgical intervention is still unclear, due to the high rates of functional recovery with nonoperative management. A small, but controlled study of 16 patients by Sood and Burke reported no functional difference in outcomes between operative and nonoperative management, although the authors still recommend surgical intervention at 6 months if no improvement in symptoms.[66]

Complications

Due to the potential idiopathic etiology of AIN syndrome symptoms, misdiagnosis of a nerve entrapment is a risk. Similar to pronator syndrome, scar formation and persistent or recurrent symptoms may occur.[51,57] Iatrogenic nerve injury with further or permanent changes to motor function is possible due to the degree of dissection required to achieve decompression.

Ulnar Nerve

The ulnar nerve travels from the anterior compartment to the posterior in the arm, where it pierces the intermuscular septum, descending in front of the medial head of the triceps (Fig. 63.3). Approximately 8 cm proximal to the medial epicondyle, in 80% of individuals, the nerve travels under the arcade of Struthers—an aponeurotic band of tissue from the medial head of the triceps to the intermuscular septum.[72] The nerve travels posterior to the medial epicondyle of the humerus at the elbow, where it passes through the cubital tunnel.

The cubital tunnel extends from the medial epicondyle to the olecranon. The borders include Osborne ligament, or the aponeurosis of both heads of the flexor carpi ulnaris (FCU), which serves as the roof. The floor is formed by the posterior and transverse bands of the medial collateral ligament (MCL)

of the elbow. Walls of the tunnel are formed by the olecranon and medial epicondyle. Distal to the elbow, the nerve sends motor branches to the FCU and ulnar half of FDP. It then traverses between the two heads of the FCU, under the aponeurosis known as arcuate ligament.[73] The nerve travels distal through the forearm under the FCU before entering the Guyon canal at the wrist. Proximal to the wrist and Guyon canal, the dorsal sensory branch separates from the main nerve approximately 5 to 8 cm proximal to the pisiform.[74] Muscles innervated by the ulnar nerve include the FCU, ulnar half of the FDP, intrinsic muscles of the hand, and the hypothenar muscles, as well as the adductor pollicis of the thumb.

Potential anomalous anatomy includes the anconeus epitrochlearis, which is found in approximately 10% of patients. It travels from the medial border of the olecranon to the medial epicondyle and can cause compression of the ulnar nerve.[75] Posttraumatic deformities of the elbow can also cause ulnar neuropathies due to the lack of soft tissue at the elbow and superficial course of the ulnar nerve. This includes lateral condyle trauma with a resultant valgus deformity, which is associated with a tardy ulnar nerve palsy.[76]

Repetitive throwing motions have been well-documented as a cause of ulnar neuropathy at the elbow, due to the position of the ulnar nerve adjacent to the ulnar collateral ligament (UCL).[77] An overhead throwing motion results in significant tensile load on the UCL and can subsequently cause irritation, inflammation, and impingement of the neighboring ulnar nerve.[78] In late cocking of an overhead throw, there is a sixfold increase in the pressure within the cubital tunnel.[79] The acceleration phase of throwing increases pressures on the ulnar nerve to the limits of elasticity and vascular integrity of the ulnar nerve.[80] In vivo anatomic studies demonstrate anterior translation and flattening of the ulnar nerve, worst during stages of throwing with the most elbow flexion.[81] UCL instability is often seen in baseball pitchers due to the chronic valgus extension forces of repetitive throwing.[82] This can result in an acquired valgus deformity and associated strain on the ulnar nerve.[83]

CUBITAL TUNNEL SYNDROME

Cubital tunnel syndrome is caused by entrapment of the ulnar nerve at the elbow, most commonly under the Osborne ligament at the cubital tunnel.[17] Other common sites of entrapment include the arcade of Struthers in the arm, the medial epicondyle, and the arcuate ligament or FCU aponeurosis.[84] Entrapment neuropathy may also be associated with lipomas or other mass lesions, or anomalous anatomy, such as the anconeus epitrochlearis. Specifically for athletes, an additional potential site of compression is under the FCU because muscular hypertrophy can directly increase pressure on the underlying ulnar nerve.[85]

These symptoms of ulnar nerve compression at the elbow are commonly seen in baseball, for reasons of repetitive throwing mechanics as previously described. Similar motions resulting in increased tension on the nerve or compression of the cubital tunnel include activity in the following sports: bicycling, weightlifting, cross-country skiing, wrestling, and martial arts.[33]

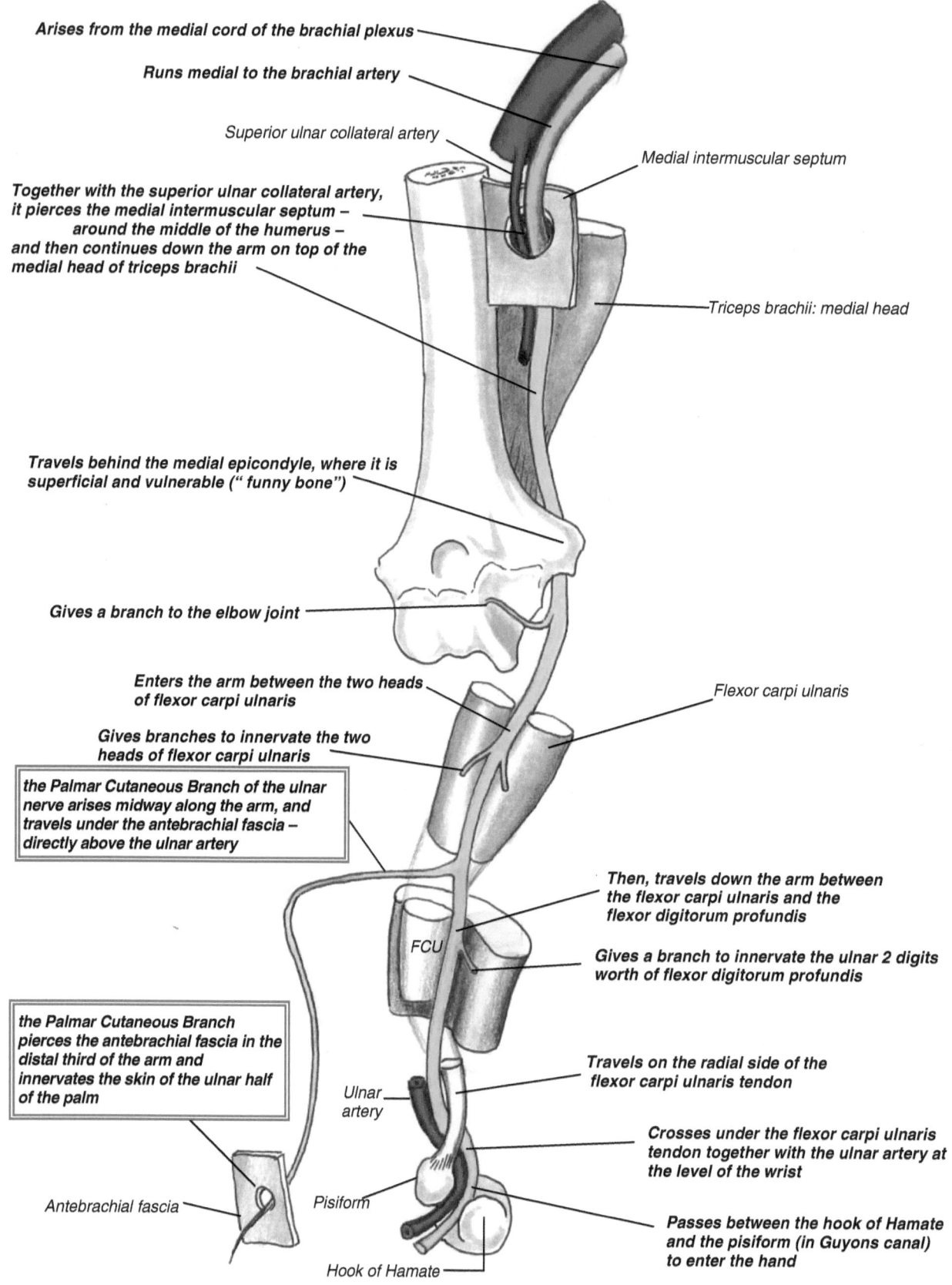

Arises from the medial cord of the brachial plexus

Runs medial to the brachial artery

Superior ulnar collateral artery

Medial intermuscular septum

Together with the superior ulnar collateral artery,
it pierces the medial intermuscular septum –
around the middle of the humerus –
and then continues down the arm on top of the
medial head of triceps brachii

Triceps brachii: medial head

Travels behind the medial epicondyle, where it is
superficial and vulnerable (" funny bone")

Gives a branch to the elbow joint

Enters the arm between the two heads
of flexor carpi ulnaris

Flexor carpi ulnaris

Gives branches to innervate the two
heads of flexor carpi ulnaris

the Palmar Cutaneous Branch of the ulnar
nerve arises midway along the arm, and
travels under the antebrachial fascia –
directly above the ulnar artery

Then, travels down the arm between
the flexor carpi ulnaris and the
flexor digitorum profundis

FCU

Gives a branch to innervate the ulnar 2 digits
worth of flexor digitorum profundis

the Palmar Cutaneous Branch
pierces the antebrachial fascia in the
distal third of the arm and
innervates the skin of the ulnar half
of the palm

Travels on the radial side of the
flexor carpi ulnaris tendon

Ulnar
artery

Crosses under the flexor carpi ulnaris
tendon together with the ulnar artery at
the level of the wrist

Antebrachial fascia

Pisiform

Passes between the hook of Hamate
and the pisiform (in Guyons canal)
to enter the hand

Hook of Hamate

Fig. 63.3 Diagram depicting the anatomic course of the ulnar nerve. *FCU,* Flexor carpi ulnaris.

History

Early clinical presentation is sensory in nature, with paresthesias in the small and ulnar half of the ring fingers. These symptoms are often nocturnal due to elbow flexion while sleeping. Chronic or severe entrapment results in muscle weakness in the innervated groups, although often FCU and FDP are spared due to the topographic distribution of motor innervation of the ulnar nerve.[86,87] In athletes, cubital tunnel may primarily present with medial elbow pain, aggravated by throwing or with elbow flexion. The differential diagnosis includes valgus extension overload syndrome, medial epicondylitis, flexor-pronator muscle strain, and UCL injury.

Physical Exam

Reproducible numbness in the ring and small fingers with elbow flexion through a throwing motion leads to a high index of suspicion for cubital tunnel syndrome. Flexing the elbow and extending the wrist for 1 minute has been demonstrated to be highly accurate for diagnosis of cubital tunnel syndrome.[79] In addition, a positive Tinel sign can often be elicited. Prolonged entrapment progresses to muscle weakness, evidenced with many clinical signs. These include the Wartenberg sign (small finger abduction due to third palmar interosseous muscle weakness), Froment sign (compensatory pinch by use of the FPL due to weakness of adductor pollicis), and late-stage deformity of claw hand due to loss of intrinsic function.[17] Muscle weakness is most noticed by athletes as a decrease in grip strength. Loss of sensation to the dorsum of the small and ring fingers is of specific importance because it denotes compression of the ulnar nerve proximal to take of the dorsal sensory branch. Patients with ulnar neuropathy often present later, when weakness and muscle atrophy are present, but this is the general population and not specific to athletes.[88] Of note, an incompetent Osborne ligament can create a painful snapping or popping sensation involving the ulnar nerve during elbow flexion. Other exam maneuvers should be performed to assess instability of the elbow or medial epicondylitis as indicated.

Decision-Making Principles

Similar to other entrapment neuropathies, diagnosis is largely based on clinical history and exam. Electrodiagnostics are helpful and can delineate the severity of the compression and often the specific site of compression. A review of 50 published series states that 56% of patients with symptomatic cubital tunnel respond to nonoperative management. These improvements may take up to 6 months, which may not be acceptable in high-performing athletes; however, this success rate indicates a trial of nonoperative modalities can be worthwhile.[89] Ultrasound offers some diagnostic information because the nerve can be visualized in a dynamic fashion while the elbow is ranged to evaluate both stability and compression. Van Den Berg and colleagues have demonstrated there is no significant difference in rates of subluxation in patients with ulnar neuropathy than healthy controls, but this may have implications in determining whether to transpose the nerve during surgery.[5] Nonoperative management includes discontinuation of triceps-strengthening

exercises, avoiding application of direct pressure to the medial elbow, blocking elbow flexion at 50 degrees to minimize tension on the ulnar nerve, and using a nighttime orthosis to prevent elbow hyperflexion while sleeping.[17] Nerve-gliding exercises designed to stretch and promote gliding of the nerve can be performed. These include holding the elbow extended, forearm pronated and flexing and extending the wrist, then flexing the elbow while keeping the wrist extended. Extending the elbow and wrist while rotating the forearm through full pronosupination will also allow stretch and gliding of the nerve, but there are inadequate data demonstrating independent efficacy for ulnar compression neuropathies.[17,90]

Sport-specific rehabilitation programs can hasten RTP for athletes.[91] Corticosteroid injections do not demonstrate reliable symptom improvement in ulnar nerve entrapment and are at risk of causing skin hypopigmentation and subcutaneous tissue atrophy.[92]

Earlier operative intervention is indicated for more severe symptoms, including sensory changes or muscle atrophy, because nerve recovery prognosis diminishes over time.[17,93] Surgical intervention also expedites return to activity; studies looking at operative intervention demonstrate RTP of approximately 3 months.[22]

Treatment Options

Many surgical techniques exist for ulnar nerve decompression, with slightly different indications but similar outcomes. Options include open or endoscopic in situ decompression, anterior transposition (subcutaneous, intramuscular, or submuscular), and medial epicondylectomy. Across all options, patients tend to recover well, with improvement of 80% to 90% of symptoms. Gervasio et al. demonstrated no difference between simple decompression and submuscular transposition for severely neuropathic patients, although recent literature suggests there is a higher revision rate following in situ decompression for mild changes on electrical studies.[94,95] Recent evidence indicates no significant difference between open versus endoscopic in situ decompression, between medial epicondylectomy and nerve transposition, and between simple decompression and nerve transposition.[96] Some literature suggests that medial epicondylectomy should not be performed for severe disease, with worse overall outcomes.[97]

In Situ Decompression (Fig. 63.4)

Both open and endoscopic approaches have been described for in situ decompression, with no difference in outcomes.[98] Cochrane Database Review suggests equivalent outcomes to nerve transposition in ulnar neuropathy symptom relief.[96] However, athletes with UCL attenuation or elbow instability may require more than a simple decompression due to the underlying pathology of altered biomechanics creating additional strain on the nerve.

Open decompression is performed via an incision over the course of the ulnar nerve. The length is variable and may be as short as 2 to 3 cm or as long as 14 cm. The nerve should be released along the anterior aspect because this has been demonstrated to decrease the chance of subluxation with elbow flexion. A limited open incision over the medial epicondyle may

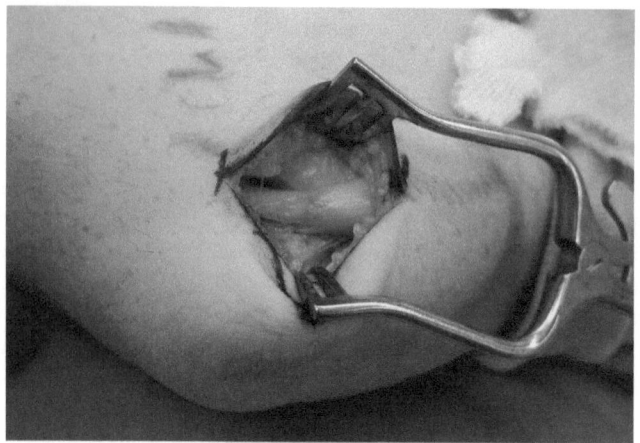

Fig. 63.4 Clinical picture of in situ ulnar nerve decompression. The nerve is perching on the epicondyle but does not subluxate anteriorly.

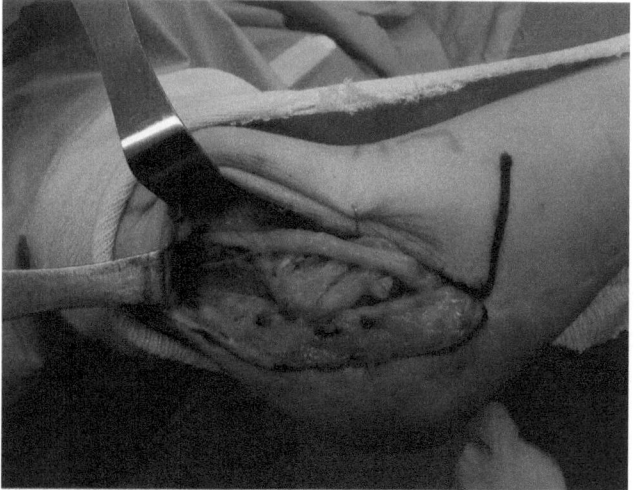

Fig. 63.5 Clinical picture of ulnar nerve following subcutaneous transposition.

be performed, but this typically allows release of only the cubital tunnel itself and decompression at the FCU heads. A more extensile approach involves exposure of the nerve and releasing sites of compression, namely Osborne ligament, but also from the arcade of Struthers proximally to the FCU aponeurosis distally. More thorough release of soft tissues does carry the risk of destabilization of the ulnar nerve, which may increase subluxation. There are currently insufficient data to demonstrate one approach is superior.

Endoscopic decompression uses a 2-cm skin incision with less soft tissue dissection but enables decompression of the nerve up to 10 cm proximal and distal to the medial epicondyle. Outcome studies show similar outcomes to open decompression.[98,99]

Anterior Nerve Transposition: Subcutaneous (Fig. 63.5)

Subcutaneous transposition requires the development of a subcutaneous pocket with release of a portion of the FCU muscle to allow for a straight path for the nerve and does not violate the origin of the flexor-pronator mass. This can be a benefit when treating athletes because protecting the integrity of the

flexor-pronator mass is thought to require less rehabilitation to return to strength and a quicker RTP.[22]

This procedure involves the full incision previously described, with exposure from 8 cm proximal to the medial epicondyle down to 6 cm distal to the medial epicondyle. The incision is centered along the path of the nerve in the cubital tunnel. Care must be taken to protect branches of the medial antebrachial cutaneous nerve (MABCN) because this can be a source of postoperative pain. The ulnar nerve should be identified proximal to the cubital tunnel, with release of the Osborne ligament to decompress the cubital tunnel, and the aponeurosis between the FCU heads. The nerve must be mobilized for transposition, and articular branches to the elbow proximally are sacrificed. Care should be taken to protect motor branches to the FCU.

Proximal dissection involves release of the arcade of Struthers and excision of the intermuscular septum to prevent a new site of compression following transposition.

Release of deep fascia is required prior to transposition. This requires gentle retraction of the nerve, which can be performed with vessel loops. The nerve is then moved anterior to the medial epicondyle, where it lies on top of the flexor-pronator mass. Various techniques can be used to keep the nerve anteriorly, including creation of a fascial sling, closing the cubital tunnel, or suturing the dermis to the epicondyle. The elbow is taken through full flexion and extension to ensure there is no kinking of the nerve at any point. The nerve is protected anteriorly while the skin is closed.

Anterior Nerve Transposition: Intramuscular (Fig. 63.6)

Intramuscular transposition is an established alternative, with a comprehensive description by Kleinman and Bishop in 1989.[100,101] This procedure involves the same incision, decompression, and mobilization of the nerve as described in the subcutaneous transposition. However, when the nerve is laid in a tension-free position on top of the flexor-pronator mass, this position is then developed into a groove in the flexor-pronator musculature. A trough of approximately 5 mm is developed along the predicted course that the nerve will take, and the nerve is seated within it. Removal of the fascial bands, which may be a source of irritation of the nerve, is essential. The flexor-pronator fascia may be left open or closed while the forearm is held in pronation and 90 degrees of flexion to ensure proper positioning. This fascia may be lengthened by creating opposing rectangular flaps to minimize local compression of the transposed nerve.[102]

Benefits of this procedure include a highly vascularized bed of tissue, with soft tissue mass providing protection for the nerve once transposed. However, this requires violation of the flexor-pronator mass, which may delay RTP. In addition, while seated in the muscle bed, the nerve may be subject to tensile stresses and scarring.[103]

Anterior Nerve Transposition: Submuscular (Fig. 63.7)

Submuscular transposition places the nerve beneath the flexor-pronator mass, as described by Learmonth in 1942.[104] The same incision, nerve decompression, and mobilization is performed as previously described. However, prior to nerve transposition, the flexor-pronator muscle mass is elevated from the medial

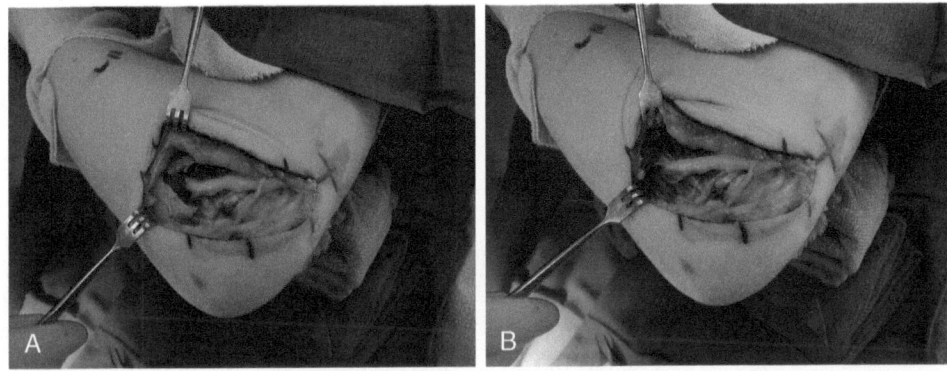

Fig. 63.6 Clinical picture of ulnar nerve transposition in intramuscular plane. The fascia is released and a trough in muscle is created to ensure a straight path for the nerve. (A) Note the kinking of the distally within flexor carpi ulnaris (FCU) muscle. (C) Appearance following resection of a portion of the FCU muscle to allow the nerve to have a straight path.

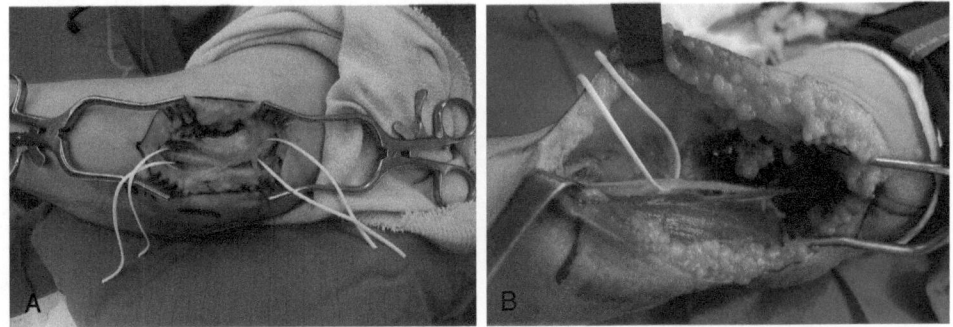

Fig. 63.7 Clinical picture of (A) ulnar nerve following in situ decompression, prior to release of fascia and elevation of flexor pronator muscles (note medial antebrachial cutaneous nerve preserved) and (B) appearance of nerve following anterior transposition prior to fascial and muscular closure over the nerve.

epicondyle. The origin is exposed, and the muscle is divided from the epicondyle, leaving a 1-cm cuff for later repair. The interval between the flexor-pronator mass and FDS is developed with blunt dissection. After reflection of the flexor-pronator mass, the ulnar nerve is transposed so that it lies adjacent and medial to the median nerve. It must lie in a tension-free state, free of all sites of compression. The flexor-pronator mass is then repaired with the forearm flexed to 60 degrees and fully pronated and can be lengthened if necessary.[105]

Del Pizzo et al. argued that submuscular transposition provides better protection for the nerve and may have benefits for athletes.[106] In addition, this procedure seats the nerve in a vascular bed that is likely to remain free of scarring and provides the straightest path for the nerve to follow. Those that oppose submuscular transposition contend that it is a violation of the flexor-pronator mass that can result in prolonged rehabilitation and a longer RTP due to weakness.[22] It also creates iatrogenic injury to the musculature, and due to these concerns, submuscular transposition is not recommended as a primary procedure in throwing athletes.[107]

Medial Epicondylectomy

This procedure is typically indicated for patients with a visibly unstable ulnar nerve. It requires a more limited skin incision, centered just posterior to the medial epicondyle over the cubital tunnel. A portion of the flexor-pronator origin is released medially and the medial condyle is exposed. The original procedure involved excision of the supracondylar ridge, along the medial border to the trochlea, and therefore release of the cubital tunnel. This procedure resulted in potential destabilization of the elbow; studies found only 20% of the anterior aspect of the medial epicondyle can be excised while maintaining the origin of the anterior band of the UCL. More can be excised posteriorly without compromising elbow stability, so a modified oblique technique was developed that has improved postoperative valgus instability.[108,109]

This technique is beneficial due to minimal direct dissection and handling of the nerve. The nerve falls forward and is decompressed by excision of the anatomic restraint. Proponents of this procedure reference that there is no significant difference in outcomes between medial epicondylectomy and nerve transposition.[110] However, this procedure is not recommended in athletes, especially throwers, because the original procedure has potential to interfere with flexor-pronator function, which can limit recovery and RTP.[22] The modified oblique epicondylectomy involves excision of bone closely associated with the UCL, a vital structure in elbow stability that is stressed in a throwing motion. Therefore this is not recommended for concern of iatrogenic instability.

Preferred Technique

For primary ulnar neuropathy at the elbow, our preferred technique is in situ decompression through a small (3 to 4 cm) incision, releasing the cubital tunnel and any proximal or distal sites of compression for 7 to 8 cm from the medial epicondyle. Following release, we flex and extend the elbow. If the nerve perches but does not subluxate anterior to the epicondyle, we leave it in situ. If the triceps is large and appears to be pushing the nerve anteriorly, we will resect a portion of the medial triceps muscle. If the nerve subluxates anterior to the epicondyle, we will transpose it through an extended excision. We perform an intramuscular transposition, so the nerve lies in a straight path and does not kink distally as it enters the FCU. When the patient has had a previous ulnar nerve procedure with persistent or worsening symptoms and we feel revision surgery is warranted, we will transpose and most often, place it in a submuscular location, as described previously.

Postoperative Management and Return to Play

Early mobilization is key and can begin as early as postoperative day 2 in endoscopic procedures.[111] This has been associated with quicker return to work.[112] Mobilization is dependent on incision size and type of procedure, with prolonged postoperative immobilization for more extensive dissection.

Rehabilitation should begin as soon as the patient is comfortable and is earlier for in situ techniques. Gradual strength regimens should accelerate over the first month.[113] It is important to begin sport-specific rehabilitation exercises for rapid return to activity. It is reasonable to expect a RTP within 4 to 12 weeks postoperatively for both throwing and nonthrowing athletes, depending on the procedure (in situ at 4 weeks and submuscular transposition at 12 weeks).[22,114] RTP is again limited by the athlete's demonstration of sufficient strength and control.

Results

The overall success rate is similar across the myriad of described interventions, with rates ranging from 70% to 90%.[115,116] Multiple studies demonstrate 80% or greater improvement in symptoms or return of function with different interventions, and further literature demonstrates no difference in outcomes between the interventions.[96,111,117,118] Prognosis worsens and recovery becomes both unpredictable and incomplete with more severe compression.[119]

Complications

The complications include both general and procedure-specific complications. As with all nerve surgery, iatrogenic damage to the nerve is possible, whether to the ulnar nerve, its motor branches, or the MABCN. The most common reason for failure of cubital tunnel release surgery is incomplete decompression, or kinking of the nerve creating a new iatrogenic compression.[100] Recurrence of symptoms is also possible with chronic postoperative subluxation. Symptom persistence is a risk following in situ decompression.[95] Endoscopic decompression carries a risk of hematoma formation in up to 4% of cases.[111] Scarring and recurrence of symptoms may occur with intramuscular transposition.[103] Submuscular transposition violates the flexor-pronator mass and can lead to weakness, postoperative rupture, and potentially elbow contracture.[107]

Radial Nerve

The radial nerve travels along the posterior compartment of the arm, deep to the lateral head of the triceps. It then courses along the spiral groove of the humerus until 10 cm proximal to the lateral epicondyle, after which it pierces the intermuscular septum. (Fig. 63.8) The nerve then lies between the brachialis and brachioradialis, where it remains as it passes along the anterior elbow.[120,121] The nerve crosses the capsule at the midportion of the capitellum and proceeds distally giving off motor branches to the triceps and mobile wad, and cutaneous branches to the arm.

In the forearm, at the level of the radiohumeral joint line, the radial nerve divides into its terminal branches of the PIN and superficial radial sensory nerve. Together, these travel through the radial tunnel. The borders include the mobile wad musculature laterally and biceps tendon and brachialis medially. The floor is formed by the elbow joint capsule.[122,123] As the PIN travels along this tunnel, it passes beneath the proximal edge of the supinator, known as the arcade of Frohse.[124] It also travels along the fibrous edge of the extensor carpi radialis brevis (ECRB), borders the radial recurrent vessels including the leash of Henry, and encounters the inferior margin of the superficial supinator muscle.[125,126] It then travels down the forearm, beneath the extensor digitorum communis (EDC), and lies on top of the abductor pollicis longus (APL) and extensor pollicis brevis (EPB) muscle bellies. It then dives under the extensor pollicis longus (EPL) tendon and inserts into the wrist joint capsule along the radial aspect of the floor of the fourth extensor compartment. Motor innervation is as follows: the radial nerve is responsible for the triceps, anconeus, brachioradialis, and extensor carpi radialis longus (ECRL). The PIN innervates the ECRB, supinator, and remaining extensors of the forearm.

The superficial radial nerve travels distally along the forearm, directly beneath the brachioradialis, and emerges distally between the tendons of the brachioradialis and ECRL to provide sensation to the radial aspect of the hand.

In the arm, compression of the radial nerve is rare in the absence of prior humeral trauma. Sites of compression include between the heads of the triceps by an overlying fibrous band or at the intermuscular septum.[127,128] These symptoms can improve with nonsurgical management, indicating a trial of 3 months of activity modification and rest before surgical intervention.[129] Nonoperative management should focus on minimizing triceps contracture.

From the elbow to the wrist, compression of the radial nerve and its branches is most exaggerated in positions that involve elbow extension, forearm pronation, and wrist flexion. Sports that involve forceful rotation of the wrist or forearm, including baseball, rowing, track and field, or racquet sports result in positions that cause increased pressure along the radial nerve.[130]

RADIAL TUNNEL SYNDROME

Radial tunnel syndrome is associated with compression most commonly by the arcade of Frohse.[131] Other sites of compression include the fibrous edge of the ECRB or the fibrous band at the distal end of the supinator muscle.[132] Dynamic compression can

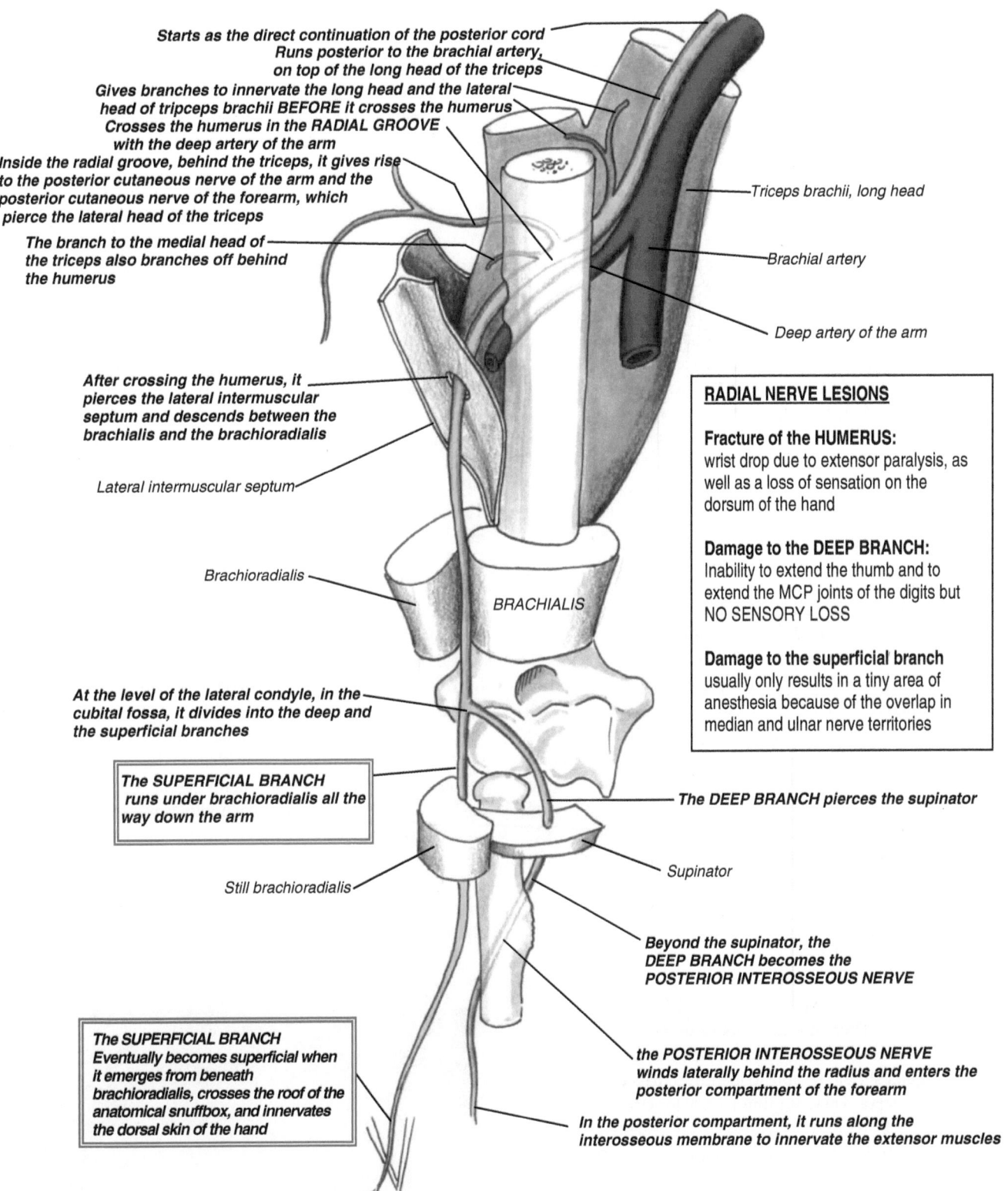

Starts as the direct continuation of the posterior cord
Runs posterior to the brachial artery,
on top of the long head of the triceps
Gives branches to innervate the long head and the lateral
head of tripceps brachii BEFORE it crosses the humerus
Crosses the humerus in the RADIAL GROOVE
with the deep artery of the arm
Inside the radial groove, behind the triceps, it gives rise
to the posterior cutaneous nerve of the arm and the
posterior cutaneous nerve of the forearm, which
pierce the lateral head of the triceps

The branch to the medial head of
the triceps also branches off behind
the humerus

Triceps brachii, long head

Brachial artery

Deep artery of the arm

After crossing the humerus, it
pierces the lateral intermuscular
septum and descends between the
brachialis and the brachioradialis

Lateral intermuscular septum

Brachioradialis

BRACHIALIS

At the level of the lateral condyle, in the
cubital fossa, it divides into the deep and
the superficial branches

The SUPERFICIAL BRANCH
runs under brachioradialis all the
way down the arm

Still brachioradialis

The SUPERFICIAL BRANCH
Eventually becomes superficial when
it emerges from beneath
brachioradialis, crosses the roof of the
anatomical snuffbox, and innervates
the dorsal skin of the hand

RADIAL NERVE LESIONS

Fracture of the HUMERUS:
wrist drop due to extensor paralysis, as
well as a loss of sensation on the
dorsum of the hand

Damage to the DEEP BRANCH:
Inability to extend the thumb and to
extend the MCP joints of the digits but
NO SENSORY LOSS

Damage to the superficial branch
usually only results in a tiny area of
anesthesia because of the overlap in
median and ulnar nerve territories

The DEEP BRANCH pierces the supinator

Supinator

Beyond the supinator, the
DEEP BRANCH becomes the
POSTERIOR INTEROSSEOUS NERVE

the POSTERIOR INTEROSSEOUS NERVE
winds laterally behind the radius and enters the
posterior compartment of the forearm

In the posterior compartment, it runs along the
interosseous membrane to innervate the extensor muscles

Fig. 63.8 Diagram depicting the anatomic course of radial nerve.

be seen in cases of close association with the radial recurrent vessels. Other potential etiologies of radial tunnel entrapment include lipomas or other mass-lesions, and anatomic or vascular anomalies.[133]

History

The chief complaint of patients with radial tunnel syndrome is dorsal forearm pain, despite the PIN being a motor nerve. The pain, which may have a radiating component, is localized along the dorsal aspect of the proximal forearm, several centimeters anterior and distal to the lateral epicondyle, independent from the site of pain typically associated with lateral epicondylitis. Lateral epicondylitis is far more common, with incidence 1% to 3% annually versus 0.003% annually for radial tunnel syndrome.[134] These diagnoses can be concomitant or related, because previous studies have described radial nerve entrapment as an associated finding in cases of resistant lateral epicondylitis.[135] Athletes will often have a high demand of elbow extension or supination, which aggravates pain complaints.[33] Weakness is mild, never the primary complaint, and associated with pain inhibition resulting in early fatigue or weak digit/thumb extension.[136]

Physical Exam

The key diagnostic exam maneuver is localized, focal tenderness to palpation over the PIN. This is accomplished with direct palpation of the dorsal lateral forearm, 3 to 5 cm distal to the lateral epicondyle, which enables differentiation from the presentation of lateral epincondylitis.[137,138] As with other entrapment neuropathies, exacerbation of symptoms with exam maneuvers can be diagnostic. Pain with resisted forearm supination or middle finger extension is a suggestive finding, although middle finger extension is not sensitive.[136,139] Weakness, an uncommon finding, affects the wrist extensors.[140] Concomitant lateral epicondylitis makes diagnosis a challenge, although this will present with tenderness and pain localized to the lateral epicondyle.

Decision-Making Principles

The diagnosis of radial tunnel syndrome is primarily clinical. Routine radiographic evaluation is not indicated. MRI imaging may show edema along the course of the PIN, although these are not specific.[141] There are less data to describe the utility of ultrasound in evaluation of radial tunnel, but an experienced ultrasonographer should be able to identify a mass causing compression of the nerve. There is minimal role for electrodiagnostic studies because EMG and NCV studies are usually normal.[136] Although some studies demonstrate findings with modified NCV exams, it remains a clinical diagnosis.[142,143]

As with other entrapment neuropathies of the forearm, conservative management is indicated primarily. Rest and avoidance of provocative maneuvers are necessary.[139,144] The forearm should be maintained in supination with mild wrist extension. Alternative interventions such as ultrasound have not shown efficacy.[145] Steroid injections may have both a diagnostic and therapeutic role after 6 to 12 weeks of symptoms.[139] Nonoperative management is recommended for a minimum of 3 to 6 months before considering surgical intervention.[136,139]

Treatment Options

Surgical intervention is undertaken with the goal of decompression addressing any lesions or sites of compression along the entire length of the nerve. Different approaches provide varying levels of exposure of the radial tunnel and are therefore indicated by the site of compression.

Posterior Approach

Posteriorly, an incision can be made at the lateral epicondyle, extending 6 to 8 cm distally. Lateral cutaneous nerves to the forearm should be protected. An interval is developed between ECRL and EDC, revealing the supinator muscle deep. Identification of the PIN at the arcade of Frohse is necessary because the supinator fascia is then incised over the extent of the PIN. This addresses only compression localized to the supinator and arcade of Frohse but limits iatrogenic trauma. It also offers an extensile exposure to address concomitant lateral epicondylitis.

Anterolateral Approach (Fig. 63.9)

The anterolateral incision is approximately 5 cm long, curvilinear, extending from just proximal to the lateral epicondyle distally along the interval between the brachioradialis and biceps tendon. Deep dissection requires retraction of the brachioradialis laterally and identification of the radial nerve proximally in the interval between the brachioradialis and biceps. The radial nerve is then traced distally, addressing all sites of compression including the fibrous edge of ECRB. The wrist is then pronated and flexed. Release of the ECRB origin should be performed, if indicated. Next, the leash of Henry or radial recurrent vessels should be ligated and divided. The PIN is identified and followed into the radial tunnel, where the supinator fascia is released along the extent of the PIN. This approach allows release of all potential sites of compression relating to radial tunnel syndrome.

Preferred Technique

In general, we do not treat this condition with surgery. In the absence of objective findings of motor weakness (PIN syndrome)

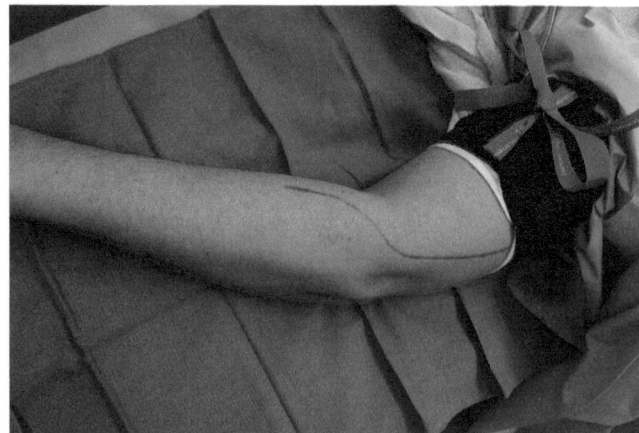

Fig. 63.9 Clinical appearance of an incision outline for radial nerve decompression with anterolateral exposure. Decompression of radial nerve with identification of SBRN and PIN prior to release through supinator.

or NCV/EMG changes, we feel surgery can be unpredictable for pain relief. We reassure the patient that we have not identified a condition with predictable surgical outcomes and recommend nonoperative treatment. In the rare circumstance where we proceed with surgery, we use the posterior approach in the interval between the EDC and ECRL.

Postoperative Management and Return to Play

Postoperatively, splinting with the wrist in neutral is recommended to protect the incision and allow for initial healing. Therapy should focus on stretching of the extensor muscles of the forearm and elbow and forearm motion. This should then progress to sports-specific conditioning with strengthening at week 3 to 4.[136] Release to full activity can take from 6 to 12 weeks, dependent on recovery of sufficient strength and control.[139]

Results

Operative decompression of radial tunnel syndrome has been found effective in 67% to 92% of cases in a systematic review by Huisstede et al.[146] Multiple series report postoperative success and pain relief in 80% to 90% of cases, although this was diminished in patients with concomitant lateral epicondylitis.[138,140,147,148]

Complications

Due to its anatomic course and structure, the superficial radial sensory nerve is at risk with decompression. Paresthesias have been found in up to 31% of cases.[144] Other potential complications include iatrogenic injury to the PIN, symptom persistence, incomplete decompression, scar tissue and related elbow contracture, and injury to the lateral antebrachial cutaneous nerve (LABCN).

POSTERIOR INTEROSSEOUS NERVE SYNDROME

PIN syndrome involves compression of the PIN at the same sites that result in radial tunnel syndrome. Most commonly, the site of compression is at the arcade of Frohse or at the fibrous edge of the ECRB. Trauma involving the radial head or neck, space-occupying lesions (e.g., ganglion cysts), or radiocapitellar joint instability or rheumatoid synovial proliferation can similarly cause compression of the PIN. Muscles innervated by the PIN include the supinator, EDC, extensor carpi ulnaris (ECU), extensor indicis proprius (EIP), extensor digiti minimi (EDM), APL, EPB, and EPL.

History

Clinical presentation is most notable for motor deficits, which differentiate this constellation of symptoms from radial tunnel syndrome. PIN syndrome patients will report weakness as the primary complaint and may present with radial deviation of the wrist due to preservation of ECRB and ECRL innervation. Pain and sensory deficits are uncommon. PIN symptoms can also be associated with brachial neuritis or Parsonage-Turner syndrome, and therefore a thorough history and exam of all major motor nerves of the upper limb are indicated.

Physical Exam

Provocative maneuvers have a limited role. Evaluation of PIN syndrome is centered on testing the strength of the muscles innervated by PIN. Specific maneuvers to evaluate include digit extension, thumb extension, and wrist extension. Resting wrist position and tracking with active extension should be examined. The physical exam is vital to differentiating an isolated tendon rupture.

Decision-Making Principles

Diagnosis of PIN syndrome is largely clinical, with weakness of finger, thumb, or wrist extension. Radiographs should be obtained to ensure there is not an underlying osseous abnormality. Electrodiagnostic studies can be used to diagnose and objectively evaluate the degree of denervation of affected muscles.[149] MRI is routinely obtained to evaluate for a potentially compressive soft tissue mass, although ultrasound could be used for preliminary evaluation in the setting of superficial lesions.

Nonoperative management is indicated for entrapment neuropathy without a space-occupying lesion. Rest and avoiding aggravating activities, with or without immobilization in a wrist cock-up position, should be followed by passive ROM to prevent contractures. Progression to a targeted strengthening regimen should occur as tolerated. Surgical intervention is indicated with persistence of symptoms for greater than 3 months, because spontaneous recovery is unlikely, or when there is severe weakness/loss of extension.[139] Studies have noted excellent results with early neurolysis.[150] Muscle fibrosis can occur at 18 months, which may necessitate tendon transfers.[151]

Treatment Options

Surgical approaches to obtain the necessary exposure for dissection and release of the nerve are the same as detailed above in management of radial tunnel syndrome. The keys to surgical intervention remain thorough decompression of the nerve at all sites, excision of any space-occupying lesions, and careful soft tissue dissection to prevent iatrogenic injury.

Preferred Technique

Our preference is to decompress the radial nerve from above the elbow through the supinator muscle, unless there is a clear site of compression, as with a mass identifiable on MRI. In this scenario, we use the anterior approach from the distal humerus through the supinator.

Postoperative Management and Return to Play

Initial immobilization with the wrist in extension is followed with stretching exercises. Sport-specific conditioning and strengthening should begin at week 2 to 3, with myofascial release and soft tissue mobilization techniques. Full RTP can be expected in 5 to 6 weeks.[152]

Results

With early diagnosis and intervention, patients experience a greater resolution of symptoms and recovery of function.[139] Surgical decompression of a space-occupying lesion is a reliable

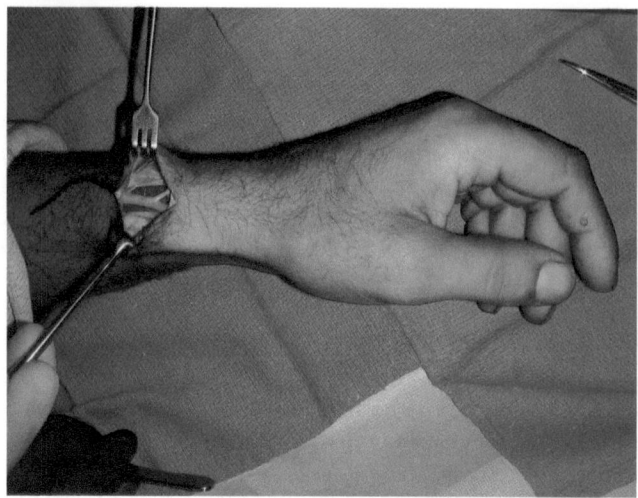

Fig. 63.10 Appearance of the sensory branch of the radial nerve following decompression. Neurolysis has been performed, and due to localized scarring, the brachioradialis tendon was not partially resected.

means of symptom relief. A large, single-center retrospective review across 20 years found excellent results with full return of function in 9 of 15 cases.[150]

Complications

Potential complications include iatrogenic injury to the PIN, superficial radial nerve, or LABCN, and similarly to radial tunnel syndrome surgery, scar formation, persistence of symptoms with incomplete decompression, and possible elbow contracture.

RADIAL SENSORY NERVE COMPRESSION

Compression of the radial sensory nerve (RSN) (Wartenberg syndrome) is not common in the general population, and there is no specific association with sports or athletes. The RSN travels deep to the brachioradialis and becomes subcutaneous between the brachioradialis and ECRL in the mid-forearm. Compression of the RSN can occur between the brachioradialis and ECRL with repetitive pronation and ulnar deviation, making it more likely in sports such as tennis.

De Quervain tenosynovitis is much more common but can coexist with Wartenberg syndrome. Electrodiagnostic studies are rarely helpful, but a Tinel sign is often noted over the RSN. Finkelstein test, performed by the patient's maintaining thumb flexion while ulnarly deviating the wrist, is up to 80% sensitive in diagnosis of de Quervain tenosynovitis and also provokes radial nerve symptoms in Wartenberg syndrome via traction on the nerve.[153] Initial treatment is activity modification, with avoidance of repetitive forearm rotation. In the rare event surgical treatment is deemed necessary, the nerve is exposed through a longitudinal or curvilinear incision along the radial aspect of the forearm. (Fig. 63.10) A portion of the brachioradialis tendon

can be resected and the nerve decompressed proximally and distally. The forearm is rotated and the nerve visualized ensuring complete decompression of the nerve with motion. Return to sports and activities progress as the wound heals and formal therapy is rarely necessary.

For a complete list of references, go to ExpertConsult.com.

SELECTED READINGS

Citation:
Boone S, Gelberman RH, Calfee RP. The management of cubital tunnel syndrome. *J Hand Surg Am.* 2015;40(9):1897–1904.

Level of Evidence:
IV

Summary:
This comprehensive review of the etiology, presentation, and management of cubital tunnel syndrome offers a thorough analysis in a concise format.

Citation:
Caliandro P, La Torre G, Padua R, et al. Treatment for ulnar neuropathy at the elbow. *Cochrane Database Syst Rev.* 2016;(11):CD006839.

Level of Evidence:
I

Summary:
This review paper further explores the multitude of surgical options available to manage ulnar neuropathies about the elbow, a common issue for athletes. It provides comparisons among surgical indications and outcomes.

Citation:
Naam NH, Nemani S. Radial tunnel syndrome. *Orthop Clin North Am.* 2012;43(4):529–536.

Level of Evidence:
Review article

Summary:
In offering a discussion of radial nerve pathologies in the upper extremity, this study is an invaluable as a resource for anatomy, pathology, and management options available to address radial nerve entrapment.

Citation:
Krogue JD, Aleem AW, Osei DA, et al. Predictors of surgical revision after in situ decompression of the ulnar nerve. *J Shoulder Elbow Surg.* 2015;24(4):634–639.

Level of Evidence:
III

Summary:
This case-control study analyzes factors that contribute to surgical revision after in situ decompression of the ulnar nerve. It also presents a thorough discussion of indications, surgical interventions, and potential complications.

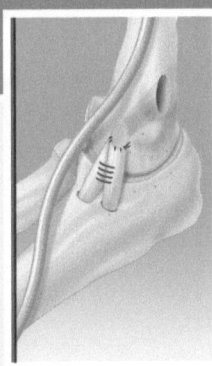

64

Elbow Throwing Injuries

Marshall A. Kuremsky, E. Lyle Cain Jr., Jeffrey R. Dugas, James R. Andrews, Christopher A. Looze

Elbow injuries in the throwing athlete are often the result of high valgus and extension forces that act on the elbow during the throwing motion. These forces place tensile stress on medial structures, compression stress on lateral structures, and shear stress posteromedially. Identification of the disorder and provision of appropriate treatment requires an accurate history, a thorough physical examination, and adequate ancillary testing. Common diagnoses in the throwing athlete with medial elbow pain include ulnar neuritis, ulnar collateral ligament (UCL) insufficiency or tear (valgus instability), flexor pronator strain or tendinopathy, and medial epicondylar apophysitis or avulsion (particularly in athletes whose skeletons are immature). Lateral elbow pain may result from osteochondritis dissecans of the capitellum, loose bodies, lateral epicondylitis, or radial nerve entrapment. Finally, posterior pain may indicate valgus extension overload (VEO) syndrome with posteromedial ulnohumeral osteophytes, trochlear chondromalacia, olecranon stress fracture, or distal triceps tendinopathy.

A thorough understanding of the complex anatomy and function of the elbow joint as well as of throwing biomechanics, is essential for physicians who treat overhead-throwing athletes. This chapter reviews elbow injuries in such athletes, focusing primarily on young skeletally mature adults, with an emphasis on pertinent anatomy and biomechanics where appropriate.[1]

HISTORY

A careful history is the cornerstone of the systematic approach to all elbow pathology. Frequently the diagnosis and foundation of treatment are quickly elicited from a clear description of the thrower's injury or development of symptoms. Important features include symptom duration, location, timing within the throwing motion, previous injuries and treatments, and associated symptoms.[1-4]

The timing of symptoms, whether acute or insidious in onset, should be noted first. Subtle clues tied to symptom onset are often revealing, such as a change in workout regimen or intensity; position changes; or advancement to a new league, level, or team. Changes in stamina, arm strength, velocity, or ball control are additional pieces of valuable information. A prior history of shoulder injury or pain may alert the clinician to a variation in throwing mechanics or muscle strength as the source of newfound elbow pain. It is therefore common for throwers to report elbow symptoms after undergoing treatment for a shoulder problem, and vice versa.

Elbow pain in the thrower often presents as an acute event superimposed on a chronic or subacute overuse injury. About half of patients with a UCL injury will present after an acute episode. The examiner should discern the competence of the UCL and the possibility of valgus instability as the primary pathology; often these athletes will report a history or treatment history of tendinopathy or ulnar neuritis for medial-sided pain or persistent posterior pain that was not relieved after arthroscopy for isolated posterior decompression.[3,5,6] The location of symptoms is also critically important and is closely linked to the physical examination.

Knowledge of the six phases of the throwing motion is mandatory for the clinician because certain pathologies demonstrate symptoms at specific phases that can be reproduced by the athlete (Fig. 64.1).[4,7,8] Of athletes with medial elbow instability (UCL insufficiency), nearly 85% will experience pain during the acceleration phase of throwing whereas fewer than 25% will experience pain during the deceleration phase.[9] Pain during late acceleration and cocking is often due to medial tensile stress (e.g., UCL insufficiency, medial epicondylitis, flexor-pronator strain, or ulnar neuritis), whereas pain with deceleration and follow-through often signifies posterior pathology (e.g., VEO, ulnohumeral osteophyte formation, loose bodies, or triceps tendinopathy).[1-3,10-12]

Other less common symptoms of a neurovascular etiology may occur in overhead-throwing athletes such as the development of cold intolerance, paresthesias in the hand or fingertips, or deterioration of fine motor skills and coordination. Although the ulnar nerve is most at risk in this population, compressive neuropathies of the radial or median nerves should be kept in mind.[7]

Pitch intensity may also influence symptoms. Throwers with UCL insufficiency often remain asymptomatic at low levels of throwing intensity but have pain with throwing attempts at greater than 75% effort. Other throwers can long toss to 120 feet with high velocity but are unable to throw from a mound without significant pain.[1]

Most acute UCL injuries occur at some point during regular-season competition, whereas injuries due to improper mechanics

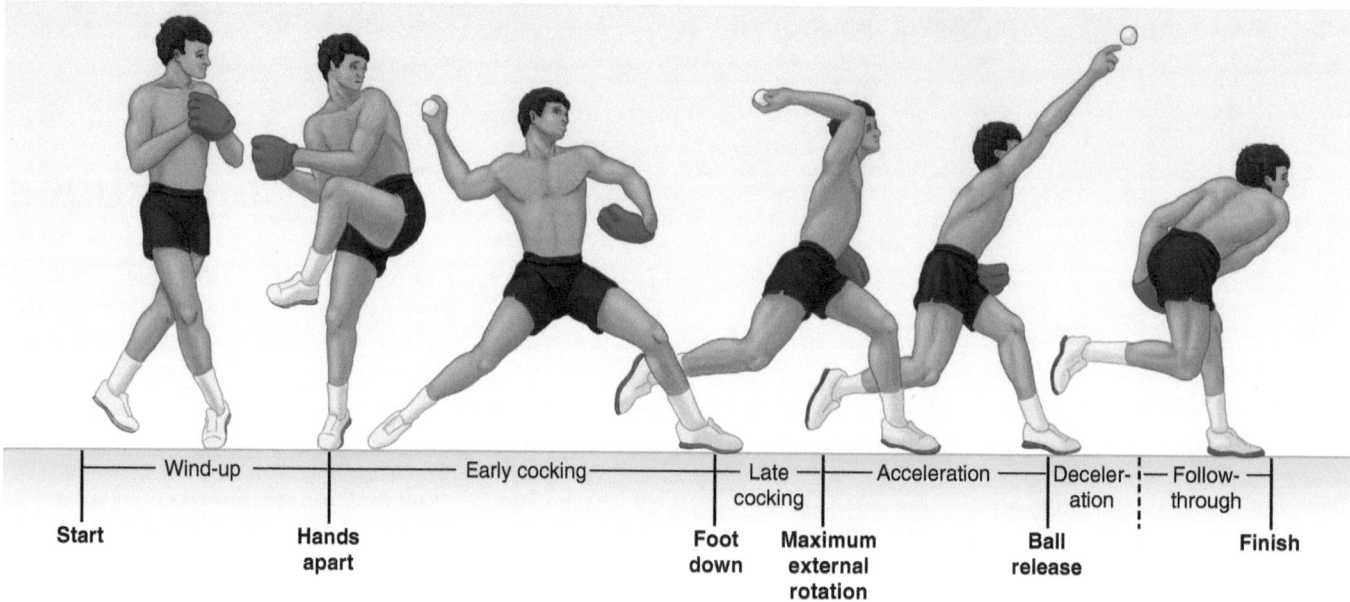

Fig. 64.1 The six phases of the overhead-throwing cycle. (From Meister K. Injuries to the shoulder in the throwing athlete. *Am J Sports Med.* 2000;28[2]:265–275.)

or training, such as flexor pronator tendinopathy or muscle strain, often present during early preparation or spring training.[6] The clinician should specifically ask about warm-up, preseason preparation, "getting the arm in throwing shape," and excessive pitch counts, because all these factors have been implicated in elbow injuries.[4,13,14] Acute injuries are also seen when a position player attempts to begin pitching during a contest without adequate warm-up or preparation to condition the soft tissues. Overthrowing, or trying to exceed maximal velocity, is seen during tryouts or "showcases" and may herald injury. Year-'round throwing without adequate rest and recovery has been implicated in the increased incidence of elbow injuries (especially involving the UCL) in young throwers.[3] Many authors have commented on strategies aimed at preventing or minimizing elbow UCL injuries, particularly in the adolescent and teenage population of overhead athletes.[15] Some strategies include utilizing pitch counts and limits, avoidance of year-round throwing or participation in throwing sports, and a focus on proper throwing technique and mechanics.[15]

PHYSICAL EXAMINATION

Examination of the elbow includes inspection, palpation, range of motion (ROM), and special tests to elucidate specific pathology.

The resting position of the elbow is first inspected for the carrying angle, which is formed by the long axis of the humerus and forearm at their articulation, with the elbow maximally extended. Normal values for the carrying angle are 11 to 13 degrees of valgus.[16] In the elbows of overhead throwing athletes, however, the carrying angle may be increased as a result of the adaptive changes of repetitive stress.

The lateral "soft spot" between the capitellum, radial head, and olecranon should be assessed for soft tissue fullness and swelling, which could indicate the presence of a joint effusion.

In this case, the patient will often maintain the elbow in 70 to 80 degrees of flexion, the position that maximizes the capsular volume.

Normal ROM of the elbow is from full extension—which may include slight hyperextension—to flexion at or slightly beyond 140 degrees. Motion should be symmetric to the contralateral side. In the overhead throwing athlete, loss of elbow extension may be either developmental or pathologic, and a flexion contracture of up to 15 or 20 degrees is not uncommon.

Both active and passive motion should be evaluated. A solid end point in flexion may be due to an impinging osteophyte within the coronoid fossa, whereas a firm block during terminal extension may be due to a posterior osteophyte on the tip of the olecranon or within the olecranon fossa. In either case, the end point will be firm, and attempts at further passive motion will often be painful. Softer end points may be a result of soft tissue swelling, capsular contracture, or a joint effusion.

Palpation of individual anatomic structures should be carried out sequentially to determine the most common potential sites of pathology. A key stabilizing structure in the elbow of the overhead throwing athlete is the UCL (Fig. 64.2). Palpation of this structure is performed with the elbow between 50 and 70 degrees of flexion, which will move the flexor pronator mass anterior to the UCL.

Tenderness along the course of the ligament, which runs from the inferior medial epicondyle to the sublime tubercle of the proximal ulna, may indicate injury. UCL injury may be differentiated from epicondylitis by performing the valgus stress test with the wrist in passive flexion and the forearm in pronation to eliminate tension on the flexor pronator mass. Heightening of medial-sided elbow pain with this modification likely indicates UCL injury rather than medial epicondylitis or muscle strain.[17]

Lateral-sided structures of interest include the radial head, capitellum, lateral epicondyle, and extensor muscle mass. Crepitus

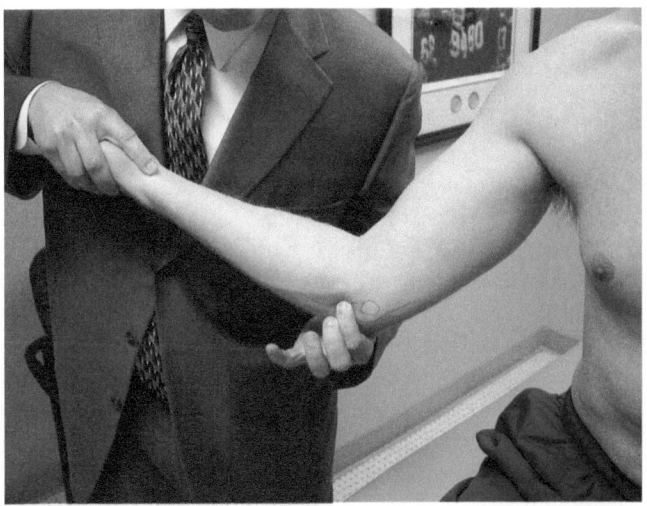

Fig. 64.2 Identification and palpation of the ulnar collateral ligament.

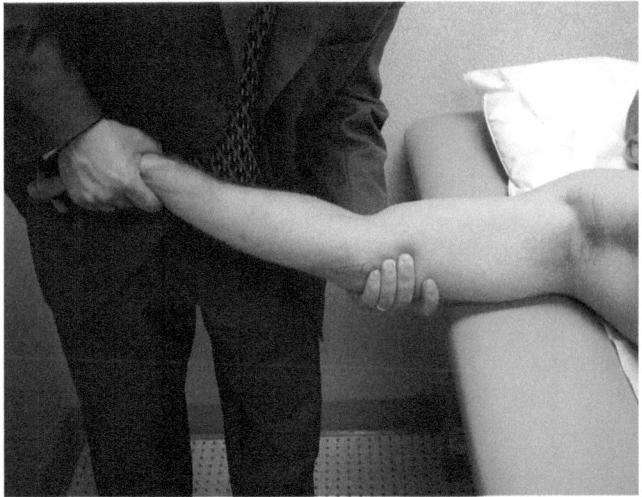

Fig. 64.3 The supine valgus stress test, which is used to evaluate medial elbow stability.

over the radiocapitellar joint may indicate chondral injury or loose bodies. The radiocapitellar compression test can be used to diagnose radiocapitellar chondral degeneration and is performed by applying an axial load to the lateral elbow with neutral wrist position and repeated pronation and supination to elicit symptoms.[18] In those with lateral epicondylitis, pain will be experienced with resisted wrist or long finger extension. In persons with radial tunnel syndrome, deep, aching pain is often experienced with palpation of the middle and distal forearm.[1]

Anteriorly, the distal biceps tendon, brachialis muscle, and anterior capsule are evaluated. Posteriorly, the olecranon and distal triceps tendon are palpable and easily assessed. Tenderness over the posteromedial olecranon usually indicates VEO with osteophyte formation, whereas posterolateral tenderness may be associated with an olecranon stress fracture.

The ulnar nerve may be palpated proximal to the medial epicondyle, then through the cubital tunnel, and distally as far as possible into the flexor carpi ulnaris muscle mass. Gentle percussion of the nerve should not cause pain or discomfort in an otherwise healthy elbow. The Tinel sign may be elicited with radiating symptoms coursing distally into the ring and small fingers. If the nerve is unstable, it may subluxate or dislocate anterior to the medial epicondyle when the elbow is brought into maximal flexion.[19,20] Anomalous bands of the distal triceps insertion have been described as a cause of ulnar nerve impingement and may cause a "snapping" sensation as they move across the medial epicondyle.

Certain special tests can be performed in the thrower's elbow to evaluate common throwing injuries.[2,3,10] The most important structure to evaluate is, again, the UCL. Valgus stress testing is performed to evaluate injury to the anterior bundle of the UCL. Although cadaveric cutting studies have suggested 70 to 90 degrees of elbow flexion as the optimal position to isolate the contribution of the UCL to valgus stability, it is difficult to control humeral rotation and apply valgus stress at that angle; therefore testing is best performed at 20 to 30 degrees elbow flexion with the forearm pronated. Valgus stress testing may be performed with the patient seated upright, supine, and/or prone. Norwood and

colleagues[21] have described valgus stress testing with the forearm supinated and the elbow at 15 to 20 degrees of flexion to unlock the olecranon from the olecranon fossa. It is now recognized that forearm pronation prevents subtle posterolateral instability from mimicking medial laxity and is the preferred forearm position for valgus stress testing.[22]

To perform the valgus instability test on the right elbow in the seated or supine position, the examiner stabilizes the humerus with the left hand just above the humeral condyles and applies a valgus moment with the right hand while grasping the patient's pronated forearm (Fig. 64.3). In the prone position, the examiner stabilizes the humerus in 90 degrees of shoulder abduction with the right hand above the humeral condyles, flexes the elbow 20 to 30 degrees, and applies valgus stress with the left hand on the patient's pronated forearm. Comparison is made to the opposite elbow for both medial-sided joint opening and reproduction of pain. Detection of instability is often very subtle in the overhead throwing athlete because of the relatively small degree of medial opening that corresponds to a significant ligament injury. Field and colleagues[23,24] have demonstrated that complete sectioning of the anterior bundle of the UCL increases medial opening by only 1 to 2 mm.

The "milking maneuver" has been described as a way to evaluate valgus stability.[2,3,10] With the patient seated, the examiner grasps the thrower's thumb with the arm in the cocked position (90 degrees of shoulder abduction and 90 degrees of elbow flexion) and applies valgus stress by pulling down on the thumb (Fig. 64.4). A variation of this test is performed with the examiner beginning in the position of the milking maneuver and slowly extending the elbow from 90 degrees of flexion to 20 degrees of flexion while applying valgus stress (i.e., pulling the thumb toward the floor).

The VEO test may be performed to identify the presence of a posteromedial olecranon osteophyte or overgrowth in the olecranon fossa (Fig. 64.5). With the humerus stabilized with one hand, the examiner's opposite hand pronates the forearm and applies a valgus force while quickly and maximally extending the elbow. A positive VEO test will cause pain

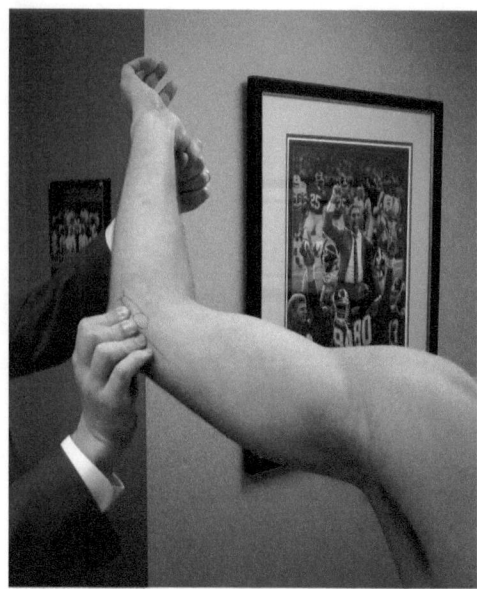

Fig. 64.4 The milking maneuver, which is used to test the integrity of the ulnar collateral ligament.

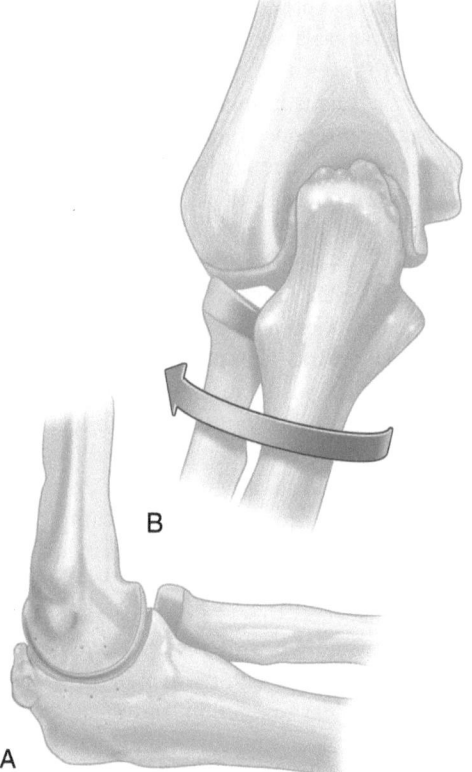

Fig. 64.5 Valgus extension overload (A) and an illustration of force (B), showing pathomechanics.

posteromedially as the olecranon osteophyte engages the olecranon fossa.[2,3,10]

IMAGING

Our standard radiographic series of the thrower's elbow includes anteroposterior (AP), lateral, and axial views and two oblique views of the affected side. An oblique axial view taken with the elbow in 110 degrees of flexion may be helpful to demonstrate posteromedial olecranon osteophytes.[2,12] If medial instability is suspected, stress AP radiographs may be performed with use of a valgus stress radiography machine (Telos, Weiterstadt, Germany). We typically obtain AP views with 0, 5, 10, and 15 N of valgus stress applied to each elbow at 25 degrees of flexion. An increase in the medial-sided joint opening with increasing stress, compared with the uninjured side, is indicative of UCL injury, although reference values for normal, healthy elbows have not been clearly established (Fig. 64.6).[25] Radiographs are evaluated for the presence of olecranon osteophytes, calcification within the UCL (possibly indicating previous injury), osteochondral damage to the capitellum, or osseous loose bodies.[2] A bone scan and/or computed tomography (CT) may be useful for detecting olecranon stress fractures.

Magnetic resonance arthrography (MRA) with the use of intra-articular contrast or saline enhancement has emerged as our imaging modality of choice to assess intra-articular pathology in the thrower's elbow. Schwartz et al.[26,27] reported 92% sensitivity and 100% specificity with saline-enhanced MRA in the diagnosis of UCL tears, with sensitivity for accurate diagnosis of complete tears greater than that for partial tears (Fig. 64.7). The lateral soft spot is the entry point for injection of saline solution, and extravasation through the UCL is diagnostic for full-thickness injury. Other advantages of MRA include assessment of possible osteocartilaginous loose bodies, osteochondral fragments, and bone marrow edema that may suggest a stress reaction or fracture.[2,26]

Other authors have advocated the use of musculoskeletal ultrasound for assessing normal and abnormal anatomy of the UCL. This has the advantage of being able to study the ligament and surrounding anatomy in static or dynamic fashion, is non-invasive, and can also have the benefit of comparing the contralateral side via examination in the same setting.[28,29]

DECISION-MAKING PRINCIPLES

The cornerstone for successful management of the overhead throwing athlete with elbow pain is accurate diagnosis of the problem. To this end, the history and physical examination form the framework for identifying potential pathologic conditions. Ancillary imaging modalities or other tests are then used to confirm the diagnosis and extent of pathology.

Once an accurate diagnosis has been established, a few core principles may be followed to help guide the clinician in management issues. First, full-thickness and many high-grade partial-thickness tears of the UCL may be tolerated in nonthrowers during routine activities of daily living, but they are frequently poorly tolerated in overhead throwing athletes because of the high tensile stresses and valgus force across the medial elbow during these activities. This subgroup of patients often requires surgery to diminish symptoms and pain if they wish to continue overhead throwing. Second, a majority of other injuries, and certainly many partial UCL tears or strains, can be successfully treated nonsurgically; therefore a formal rehabilitative program specific to overhead throwing athletes is critical to management

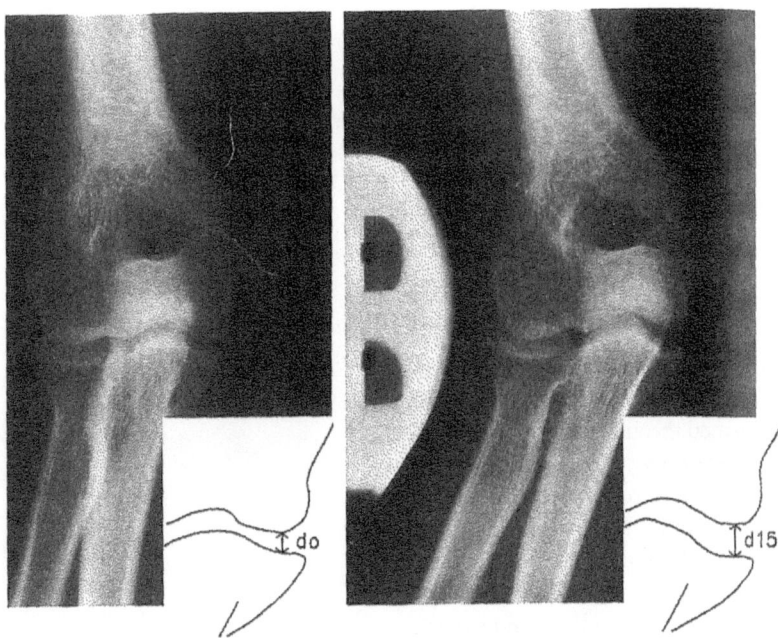

Fig. 64.6 Plain radiograph and schematic *(left)* of the elbow compared with a stress radiograph *(right)*; note the widening of the medial joint space showing laxity/incompetence of the ulnar collateral ligament. (From Ellenbecker TS, Mattalino AJ, Elam EA, et al. Medial elbow joint laxity in professional baseball pitchers: a bilateral comparison using stress radiography. *Am J Sports Med.* 1998;26:420–424.)

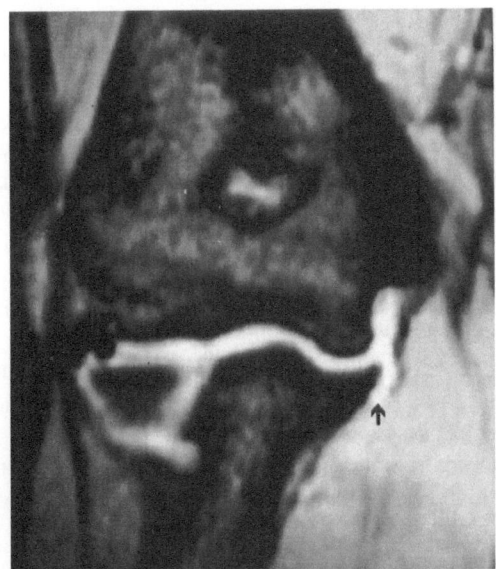

Fig. 64.7 Magnetic resonance arthrogram of an elbow showing a complete distal tear of the ulnar collateral ligament. (From Timmerman LA, Schwartz ML, Andrews JR. Preoperative evaluation of the ulnar collateral ligament by magnetic resonance imaging and computed tomography arthrography. Evaluation in 25 baseball players with surgical confirmation. *Am J Sports Med.* 1994;22(1):26–31.)

and outcome. The return-to-play (RTP) throwing program that we implement for the overwhelming majority of our patients is detailed later in this chapter.

The final issue in decision-making relates to the patient's level of competitive play and the time point within the season (or off season). Most UCL injuries occur during regular season competition, whereas injuries relating to improper mechanics or training (e.g., flexor pronator strain or tendinopathy) often present during early preparation or spring training.[3,6] Given the lengthy time until RTP after UCL reconstruction, professional pitchers must consider contractual issues, and the clinician may be wise to include input from family members, coaches, trainers, agents, and other support staff during the evaluation and treatment process.

TREATMENT OPTIONS

Tendinopathy

Tendon injuries around the elbow range from minor degeneration to complete rupture of the flexor pronator musculature.[21,30,31] Flexor pronator tendinosis is common in throwers because of the muscles' dynamic contribution to elbow stability during the valgus torque produced during cocking and arm acceleration.[21,32] The flexor carpi ulnaris is the primary dynamic stabilizer against valgus stress. In such cases of tendinopathy, patients have tenderness to palpation immediately distal to the common tendon origin at the medial epicondyle and increased pain with valgus stress. Careful attention to the location of pain will likely distinguish tendinopathy from UCL injury, which usually elicits tenderness more distally and posteriorly. Resisted forearm pronation and wrist flexion is more likely to cause pain in cases of tendinopathy compared with UCL injury. Distal triceps tendinopathy is also seen in throwers as a result of the rapid elbow extension required during the acceleration phase. In these cases, the pain is easily traced to the distal triceps tendon insertion at the olecranon tip. In addition, resisted elbow extension may exacerbate symptoms.

As with other locations of tendinopathy, the treatment begins with rest from aggravating activities and use of anti-inflammatory medication, followed by a stretching and strengthening program. Therapeutic modalities and occasional corticosteroid injection have also demonstrated some beneficial effect. In general corticosteroid injection is reserved for recurrent or recalcitrant cases of tendinopathy. With progressive stretching and strengthening of the injured tendon structure of interest (typically the origin or insertion of the tendon), many players can return to competition after 1 to 3 weeks of treatment. In more chronic or recurrent cases, the required period of rest and treatment may be prolonged. In the few cases in which conservative measures fail to result in improvement, operative débridement of the flexor pronator origin or triceps insertion may be performed through an open approach. Similarly, in cases of chronic degenerative tendinosis, we prefer open débridement and repair of the flexor pronator mass. In these cases we reattach the healthy tendon origin to the medial epicondyle using a suture anchor. Although the results of operative treatment are excellent, most cases do not require this type of management. In fact, if nonoperative methods fail and surgery is considered necessary, a concomitant injury such as UCL insufficiency must be considered.

Ulnar Collateral Ligament Injuries

Treatment options for UCL injury include nonoperative rehabilitation, direct repair of the ligament, or reconstruction using a free tendon graft.

Nonoperative treatment of UCL injuries is generally indicated in nonthrowing athletes or for injuries to the nondominant elbow; it has acceptable results in this lower-demand population.[11,33] UCL-deficient athletes in sports that involve throwing and that place a high demand on the elbow do not respond well to nonoperative management on a consistent basis.[6,34]

Rehabilitation for a patient with an injured UCL should begin with a period of active rest. During the initial 2 to 6 weeks after the injury, throwing should cease while the patient focuses on cryotherapy, motion recovery, and strengthening of wrist flexors and the flexor-pronator mass at the elbow. Weakness of the throwing shoulder may increase the stresses on the elbow during the throwing motion, and thus rehabilitation of any elbow injury must include strengthening of the shoulder girdle, rotator cuff, and scapular stabilizers. Significant internal rotation deficits of the glenohumeral joint should be addressed with posterior capsular stretching. As soreness dissipates, strengthening of the flexor pronator muscles of the forearm should begin.[2,3,10]

Once the inflammatory phase has subsided, a detailed program of elbow rehabilitation begins—including functional exercises, plyometrics, and sport-specific exercises—concluding with an interval throwing program.[6,12] RTP may be considered after completion of the entire program and if the athlete remains free of pain. There is growing utilization and research conducted on use of treatments such as platelet-rich plasma (PRP) for partial UCL injuries or in very young, skeletally immature athletes; these have met with reasonable success[35] and represent an area of ongoing research.

Operative treatment of the UCL is indicated in the symptomatic overhead throwing athlete with a complete tear of the anterior bundle of the UCL as determined by history, physical examination,

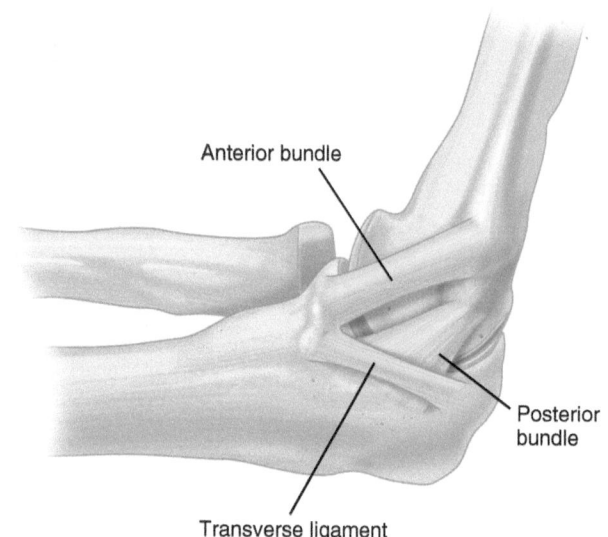

Fig. 64.8 Ulnar collateral ligament anatomy.

and imaging studies (Fig. 64.8). In general surgery is necessary if the athlete wishes to return to competitive throwing. Surgery is also considered in athletes with a partial UCL injury who fail to return to their prior level of competition after undergoing a comprehensive rehabilitation program. Certainly a thrower who places high demands on the elbow—such as a baseball pitcher, quarterback, or javelin thrower—is much more likely to require UCL reconstruction even with a more minor partial injury. These athletes may not respond favorably to nonoperative management.[2,34]

Direct primary UCL repair in the overhead throwing athlete has been reported in several series, but in general results have been inferior compared with results of reconstructive procedures.[21] Conway et al.[9] have described treatment of UCL deficiency in overhead throwing athletes with either repair or reconstruction. At follow-up examination, 50% (7 of 14) of the group that underwent repair had returned to the same level of sport, compared with 68% (38 of 56) of the reconstruction group. Overall, 80% of the reconstruction group had good or excellent results, compared with 71% of the primary repair group, indicating improved results with reconstruction versus repair.

Timmerman and colleagues[36,37] also documented better outcomes with reconstruction rather than repair in a subset of professional baseball players. In this group, neither of the two patients who underwent direct UCL repair was able to RTP, compared with 12 of 14 patients (86%) who underwent reconstruction.

Azar and colleagues[6] reported on the treatment of UCL deficiency in athletes with either reconstruction or repair. Of the eight patients who underwent primary repair, five (63%) were able to RTP at the same or a higher level of competition versus 81% (48 of 59) in the reconstruction group. The authors concluded that UCL reconstruction is superior to repair in overhead throwing athletes. For these reasons isolated direct primary repair of UCL injury is not performed at our institution.

Jobe and colleagues[38] first described the technique for UCL reconstruction using a free tendon graft in a figure-eight fashion through bone tunnels, suturing the graft to itself. The flexor pronator mass was detached from the medial epicondyle and submuscular ulnar nerve transposition was performed. Since that time several modifications have been made to Jobe's original method.[9] Andrews modified the procedure by elevating the flexor-pronator mass without detaching it from the medial epicondyle and performing a subcutaneous ulnar nerve transposition.[6] Others split the muscle and leave the nerve in situ. Rohrbough and coauthors[39] secured the tendon graft through a single humeral tunnel, calling it the *docking procedure*. This involves passing the graft through the ulna (described further on under Authors' Preferred Technique: UCL Reconstruction); however, the medial epicondyle is opened using a 3-mm round burr without exiting the proximal aspect of the medial epicondyle. A small dental drill is then used to make two smaller converging tunnels in the epicondyle connecting to the larger burr hole. The two tails of the graft are passed from distal to proximal in a divergent manner through the two tunnels and tied to one another atop the epicondyle.[40-42] This technique does not typically include ulnar nerve transposition and has been noted to involve less soft tissue dissection than the standard technique first described by Jobe and colleagues (Figs. 64.9 and 64.10). Another technique[43] involves a single tunnel at both the medial epicondyle and sublime tubercle, with graft fixation achieved by using soft tissue bioabsorbable interference screws.

Valgus Extension Overload and Loose Bodies

UCL injury is not the only cause of medial elbow pain in the overhead throwing athlete. VEO is a condition precipitated by the forces of the throwing motion acting at the elbow joint in which impingement of the posteromedial olecranon tip against

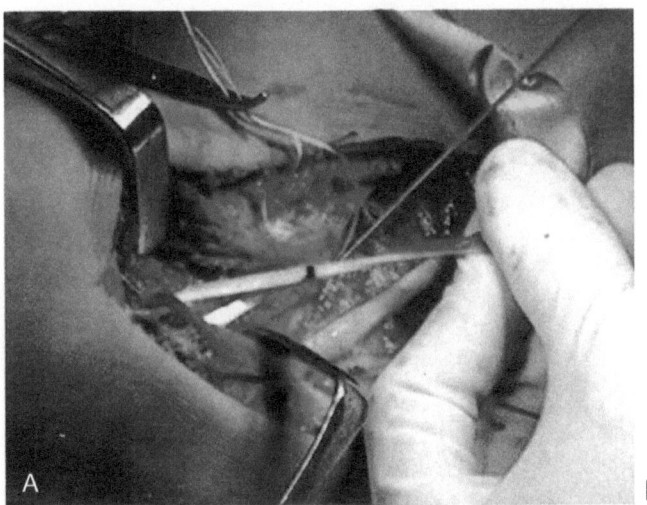
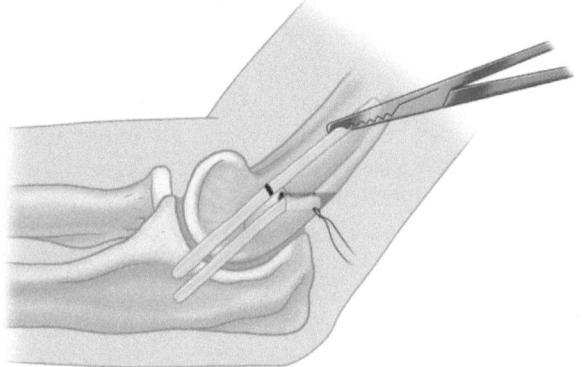

Fig. 64.9 Ulnar collateral ligament reconstruction using the docking technique—assessment of graft length and tensioning. Clinical photograph (A) and drawing (B) showing assessment of tensioning prior to securing the graft. An ink pen marks the point on the tendon graft that should be docked into the bone tunnel; this line is drawn at the edge of the bone tunnel where the tendon would insert. (From Dodson CC, Thomas A, Dines JS, et al. Medial ulnar collateral ligament reconstruction of the elbow in throwing athletes. *Am J Sports Med.* 2006;34(12):1926–1932.)

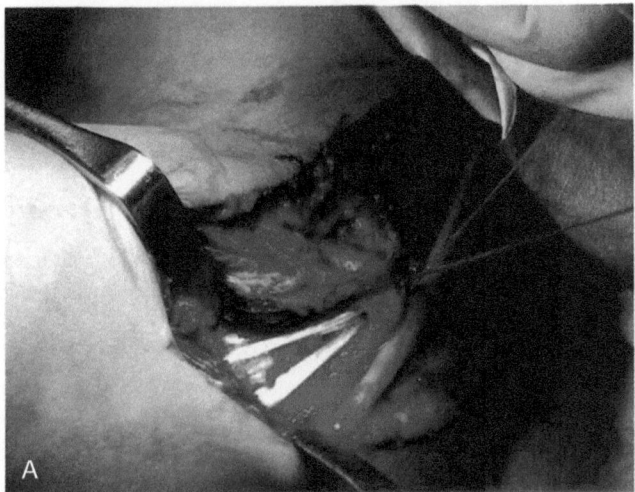
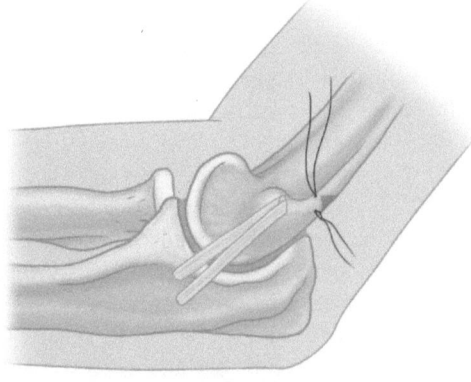

Fig. 64.10 Final tensioning of the graft and suture tying using docking technique. Clinical photograph (A) and drawing (B) showing the proper tensioning of the tendon graft and suture passage. Note that the ink line drawn on the tendon in Fig. 64.9 is now just inside the bone tunnel, indicating that the surgeon has set the desired tension. The graft is now securely sutured to itself on the far side of the bone tunnel. (From Dodson CC, Thomas A, Dines JS, et al. Medial ulnar collateral ligament reconstruction of the elbow in throwing athletes. *Am J Sports Med.* 2006;34(12):1926–1932.)

the medial wall of the olecranon fossa occurs. With repeated impingement, osteophytes may emerge at the ulnohumeral point of contact, typically posteriorly or posteromedially. Olecranon osteophytes may fracture and produce loose bodies capable of migrating into any intra-articular compartment. Bony overgrowth within the olecranon fossa of the distal humerus is also common. Additional symptoms of pain and swelling may be due to localized synovial hypertrophy in the same region. Throwers typically report posteromedial elbow pain at the initiation of the acceleration phase, although symptoms may also be elicited during the deceleration and follow-through phases.[12] The distinction between this condition and UCL injury is difficult but can usually be made by carefully determining the exact location of the pain that the patient experiences. With VEO, the pain of greatest magnitude is typically more proximal with direct palpation of the posteromedial tip of the olecranon. The provocative test for VEO is the VEO test, which is an important aspect of this diagnosis. In the case of UCL injury, the VEO test may also elicit pain, which is generally located more distal in the area of the ligament's insertion.

Once VEO is diagnosed, a conservative treatment protocol similar to those described earlier should be instituted, including active rest and rehabilitation that entails both shoulder and elbow exercises with avoidance of throwing. A return to graduated interval throwing can be permitted once symptoms diminish.

When conservative measures fail to resolve the problem, open or arthroscopic débridement of impinging osteophytes and removal of associated loose bodies is undertaken, followed by an appropriate rehabilitative program. Park et al. reported on a small group of adolescent baseball players who underwent arthroscopic excision of the olecranon tip with favorable outcomes at a minimum 2-year follow-up.[44]

Olecranon Stress Fracture

Although traumatic elbow fractures are possible in the pediatric population, olecranon stress fractures are more common in adult throwers. The olecranon process is the most common stress fracture site among baseball players.[45] These overuse injuries typically present with pain during the acceleration phase of throwing, which is localized to the posterior and sometimes the lateral border of the ulna at the level of the olecranon articular surface. Physical examination in these cases is unlikely to yield pain with valgus stress. Rather, these throwers will have point tenderness to palpation over the affected site. In the more chronic cases, these stress fractures are apparent on plain radiographs (Fig. 64.11), indicated by a focal sclerotic reaction. CT, bone scan, or MRI are viable imaging modalities when plain films are negative, but a high clinical suspicion exists (Fig. 64.12). Early lesions diagnosed by advanced imaging may be managed nonoperatively. Injuries that present later with sclerotic changes are more resistant to nonoperative treatment and may therefore benefit from operative treatment.[1]

There have been no large clinical series to guide treatment of this overuse condition. Several anecdotal reports have demonstrated some success with both conservative and operative management.[46-48] In our clinic, treatment of stress fractures of the olecranon begins with rest from throwing along with strictly enforced lifting restrictions. Rotator cuff exercises, along with

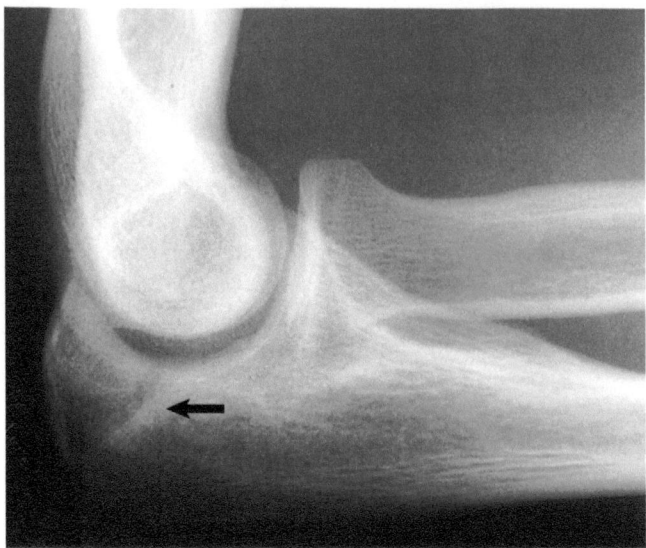

Fig. 64.11 A plain lateral radiograph of the elbow in an overhead throwing athlete with posterior elbow pain. The *arrow* indicates lucency through the proximal olecranon, consistent with a stress fracture. Typically these types of injury cause pain with rapid extension of the elbow, as seen in throwers. Also, pain on palpation of the stress fracture site is typically present.

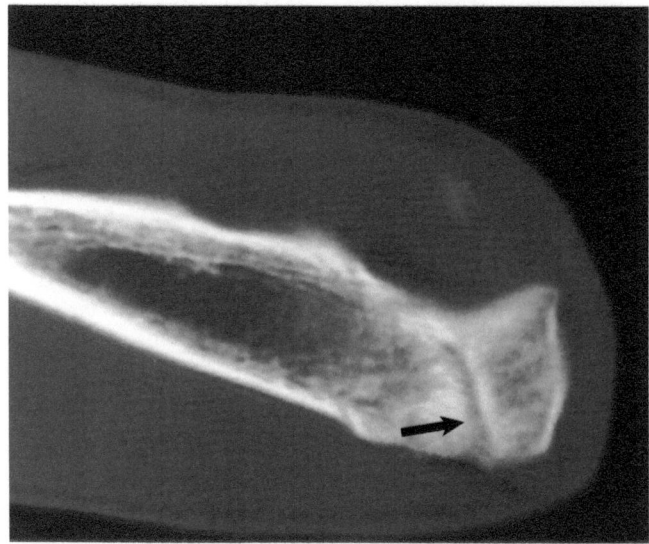

Fig. 64.12 A computed tomography scan of the same elbow depicted in Fig. 64.11. This scan demonstrates the olecranon stress fracture in this thrower *(arrow)*.

plyometrics and light triceps and biceps strengthening, may be initiated once the point tenderness ceases. A bone growth stimulator may be used to expedite union. Once clinical symptoms dissipate and radiographic union is confirmed, rehabilitation may progress to an interval throwing program. If symptoms persist despite this algorithm, surgical intervention is considered. A single longitudinally oriented 6.5- or 7.3-mm cannulated partially threaded screw inserted through the distal triceps tendon is our treatment of choice in these cases (Fig. 64.13). Early ROM exercises are instituted, followed by strengthening and return to throwing when healing is apparent, which typically is around 6 weeks after surgery. Screw removal is entertained only if the

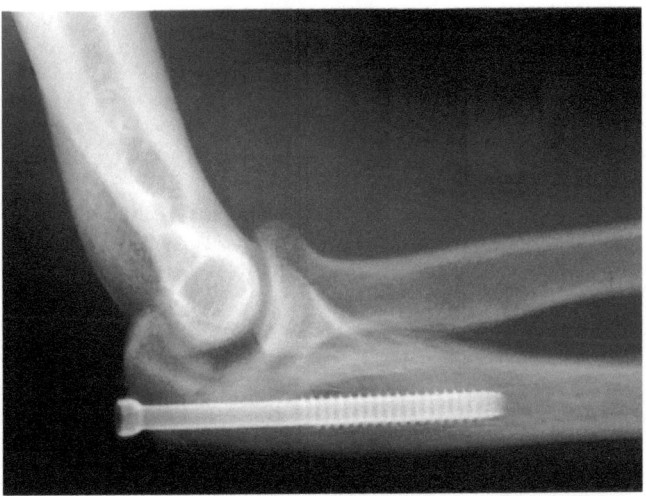

Fig. 64.13 After failure of conservative management, a percutaneous cannulated screw was placed.

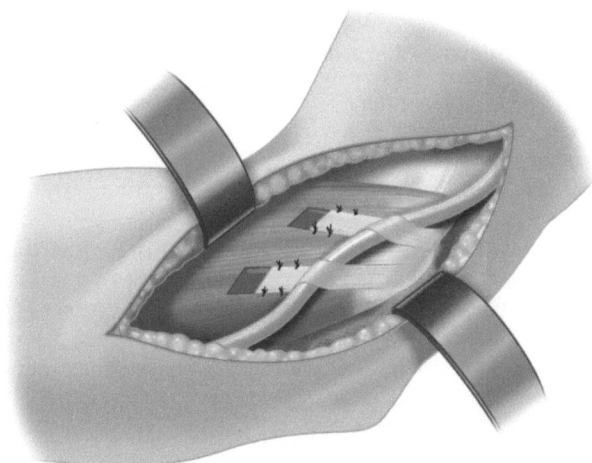

Fig. 64.14 Anterior subcutaneous transposition of the ulnar nerve.

patient has obvious symptoms and union has been confirmed. Not all throwers will require removal of the screw.[1,2]

Ulnar Neuritis

Irritation or compromise of the ulnar nerve related to repeated valgus stress at the elbow has been seen in overhead throwing athletes with medial elbow instability.[9] A significant amount of stress is exerted on the ulnar nerve during the throwing motion. A study by Aoki and colleagues[49] found that the maximal strain on the ulnar nerve during the acceleration phase was close to the elastic and circulatory limits of the nerve.[49] Besides the propagated tensile stresses, other factors thought to affect the nerve included friction, compression from local adhesions, regional osteophytes or muscle hypertrophy, or the presence of an anconeus epitrochlearis muscle over the cubital tunnel.[19,20] Symptomatic throwers may report intermittent paresthesias in the medial forearm radiating to the ring and small finger as well as aching discomfort in the medial elbow or forearm. Patients may demonstrate a Tinel sign or symptoms with compression over the affected portion of the nerve.[50-52] The situation may be worsened by ulnar nerve instability, although evident subluxation may be symmetric with the nonthrowing arm or may itself be asymptomatic.[53,54] Nonoperative measures to consider include periodic splinting of the elbow in extension or the use of an elbow pad to minimize external pressure on an inflamed, irritated nerve.[2] If symptoms fail to improve after short-term rest, use of anti-inflammatory medication, and physical therapy, ulnar nerve decompression and transposition may be recommended.[2]

Our current preferred method of surgical treatment for recalcitrant ulnar neuritis or neuropathy is anterior subcutaneous transposition (Fig. 64.14). A 4- to 5-cm medial incision is centered over the medial epicondyle. Traversing posterior branches of the medial antebrachial cutaneous nerve are identified and protected and the ulnar nerve is carefully dissected from the cubital tunnel. Complete release is performed beginning at the arcade of Struthers proximally and extending 2 to 3 cm into the flexor carpi ulnaris muscle. A slip of the medial intermuscular septum is developed to use later for the transposition, and the flexor pronator fascia is closed. The ulnar nerve is transposed subcutaneously, anterior to the medial epicondyle, and held loosely in place by suturing the distally based slip of medial intermuscular septum to the flexor fascia. Care must be taken to make sure that the fascia does not act as a point of nerve impingement. The posterior triceps fascia is then sutured to the medial epicondyle to close the cubital tunnel, and the flexor carpi ulnaris fascial split is reapproximated loosely. A drain is placed and the wound is closed in two layers with a subcuticular closure. The elbow is splinted in 90 degrees of elbow flexion for the first week postoperatively to allow soft tissue healing, followed by progressive motion and rehabilitation.[2]

✎ Authors' Preferred Technique

Ulnar Collateral Ligament Reconstruction With Ipsilateral Palmaris Longus Autograft

Our preferred method for UCL reconstruction is a modification of the original technique described by Jobe et al.[38] These modifications include elevation rather than detachment of the flexor-pronator muscle mass and subcutaneous rather than submuscular ulnar nerve transposition.[2,6]

The procedure requires the patient to be positioned supine with the arm on a hand table. After induction of general anesthesia, a nonsterile tourniquet is inflated to 250 mm Hg. The incision is made, extending from 4 cm above the medial epicondyle to 6 cm distal to it. Cutaneous nerve branches are protected.

The ulnar nerve is isolated above and below the medial epicondyle, and both regions of the nerve are tagged with vessel loops. Ulnar nerve release must continue proximally to the arcade of Struthers and distally into the flexor carpi ulnaris muscle mass. The medial intermuscular septum is excised to prevent tethering of the nerve when it is transposed. Next, the flexor-pronator mass is elevated off the underlying joint capsule until the UCL complex is completely visualized. The origin of the flexor-pronator tendon is left attached to the medial epicondyle. The anterior band of the UCL is identified at its distal attachment at

Continued

📌 Authors' Preferred Technique

Ulnar Collateral Ligament Reconstruction With Ipsilateral Palmaris Longus Autograft—cont'd

the sublime tubercle. The native ligament is split longitudinally in line with its fibers to expose the underlying ulnohumeral joint as well as to visualize potential pathology within the deep portion of the ligament. The torn or degenerative ligament tissue may be débrided at this stage of the operation, although débridement is not mandatory (Fig. 64.15).

If concomitant valgus extension overload is suspected, then a vertically oriented posterior capsulotomy is performed proximal to the fibers of the posterior band of the UCL to visualize any osteophytes that may be present at the tip of the olecranon. If osteophytes are present, a small osteotome and/or a high-speed burr can be used to remove them. At this time the posterior compartment should also be inspected for loose bodies or damage to the articulating chondral surfaces, representing a potential "kissing lesion" of the trochlea. The capsulotomy should then be closed with absorbable suture.[18]

Next, the graft is harvested. The ipsilateral palmaris longus tendon is our current graft of choice, followed by the contralateral palmaris longus, gracilis, plantaris, or toe extensor tendon. The palmaris longus tendon is harvested with three small incisions on the volar forearm beginning at the proximal wrist crease. Care must be taken to ensure harvest of the palmaris longus tendon rather than the similar-appearing flexor carpi radialis tendon. The median nerve lies deep to the palmaris longus tendon and should be protected during harvest by avoiding deep dissection below the forearm fascia. The minimum graft length necessary for UCL reconstruction is 12 cm.

A 9/64 drill bit is then used to create two connecting holes in the sublime tubercle of the proximal ulna, one from medial to lateral and one from anterior to posterior, leaving an adequate bone bridge (Fig. 64.16). Curved curets can be used to connect the two holes if necessary. The same-sized drill bit is used to make two converging holes in the medial epicondyle, one from proximal to distal and one from medial to distal. These two holes should converge to exit the epicondyle at the origin of the UCL. Straight curets may be used to connect these holes if necessary. Suture passers are then used to pull suture loops through these tunnels. The distal end of the native ligament is repaired side to side using nonabsorbable suture for supplemental stability, leaving the most proximal ligament unrepaired. By closing the native ligament, the joint surfaces are also covered, which protects the graft from abrasion. The proximal ligament is not repaired at this time so that the entrance to the epicondylar tunnels can be

visualized. If the native ligament was torn away from either insertion, sutures may be placed in the leading edges of the ligament for the purpose of repair through the tunnels for the graft. Nonabsorbable braided sutures are placed at each end of the graft tissue in Bunnell or Krackow fashion. The graft is then passed through the tunnels using suture passers and sewn to itself with the elbow positioned at 30 degrees of flexion and the joint reduced with varus stress (Fig. 64.17). The graft is secured side to side with multiple nonabsorbable sutures. We routinely perform subcutaneous transposition of the ulnar nerve at the time of UCL reconstruction. The nerve is held in place with a single fascial sling from either the flexor-pronator muscle fascia or the released intermuscular septum, which is left attached to the medial epicondyle. The sling is created with loose tension to prevent any excessive compression of the ulnar nerve with elbow motion. The skin is closed with subcuticular suture, and the elbow is splinted at 90 degrees of flexion for the first week after surgery to allow soft tissue healing. A supervised four-phase postoperative rehabilitation program follows (see later).[2,6]

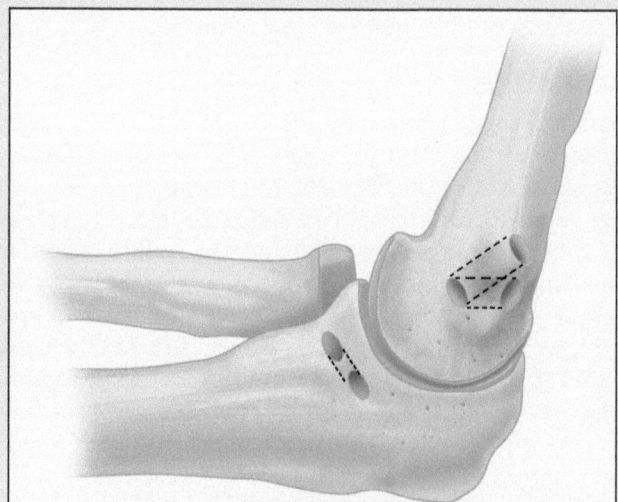

Fig. 64.16 Bone tunnels for ulnar collateral ligament reconstruction.

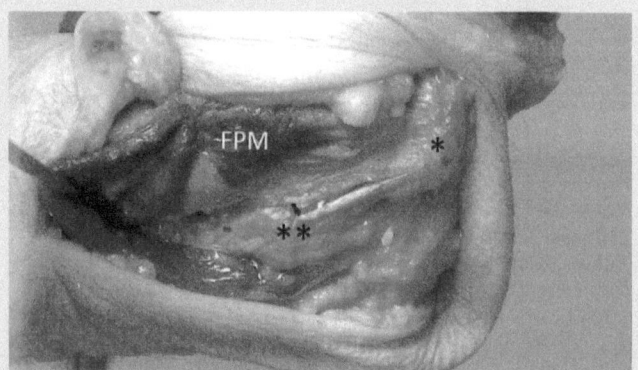

Fig. 64.15 Longitudinal split in the native ulnar collateral ligament to inspect the joint and the pathologic ligament tissue. *FPM,* Flexor pronator mass; *,* ulnar collateral ligament origin; **,** ulnar collateral ligament insertion. (From Dugas JR, Walters BL, Beason DP, et al. Biomechanical comparison of ulnar collateral ligament repair with internal bracing versus modified Jobe reconstruction. *Am J Sports Med.* 2016;44(3):735–741.)

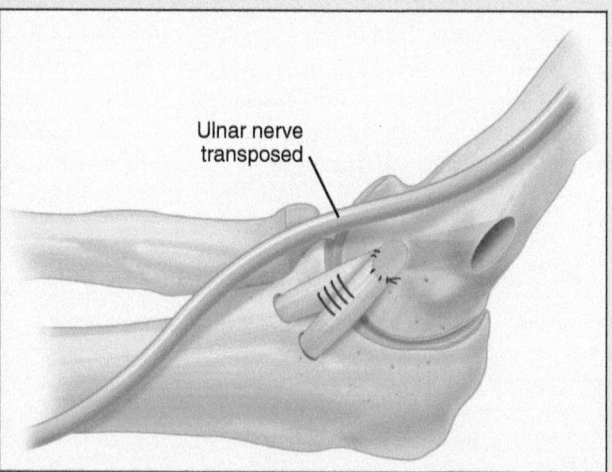

Fig. 64.17 A graft passed through tunnels and sutured in place.

Ulnar nerve transposed

Authors' Preferred Technique
Elbow Arthroscopy With or Without Posterior Decompression

Arthroscopic elbow débridement may be performed with the patient in the supine, prone, or lateral decubitus position. We prefer the supine position with the arm in 90 degrees of abduction and the elbow in 90 degrees of flexion, suspended by an overhead traction device. A tourniquet set at 250 mm Hg is routinely used, and use of a pressure-sensitive arthroscopic pump is helpful to allow adequate visualization and prevent over distention of the joint. Initially all bony landmarks and portal locations are marked with a methylene blue pen, as described by Andrews and Carson,[55] and the elbow is injected with 30 mL of saline solution through the lateral soft spot[2,56] (Fig. 64.18). A detailed knowledge of elbow anatomy is critical for proper portal placement. The anterolateral portal is established; diagnostic arthroscopy of the anterior compartment is performed through this portal. An anteromedial portal is established, with use of a spinal needle to assist with proper placement; however, in overhead throwing athletes, the anteromedial portal may not be created if no overt pathology is seen from the anterolateral portal. The anterior compartment is thoroughly evaluated for (1) loose bodies; (2) evidence of chondral damage to the coronoid process, capitellum, or radial head; or (3) osteophyte formation in the coronoid fossa. Because loose bodies from the posterior or lateral compartments often migrate to the anterior compartment or vice versa, all compartments must be thoroughly visualized.

An arthroscopic valgus stress test is performed at 70 degrees of elbow flexion to evaluate the stability of the ulnar collateral ligament, with a medial opening of greater than 1 to 2 mm suggesting UCL insufficiency.[24] A lateral soft spot portal is then established for the 2.7-mm arthroscope at the site of initial elbow injection. A second lateral portal may be placed approximately 1 cm distal to the first lateral portal for instrumentation of the lateral compartment or removal of loose bodies.

A posterolateral portal is established for placement of the 4.0-mm arthroscope, and an accessory straight posterior portal is then established through the triceps tendon, with care taken to avoid the ulnar nerve within the cubital tunnel. With the arthroscope in the posterolateral portal, a shaver is introduced through the accessory (straight) posterior portal to débride synovitis and soft tissue from the olecranon tip and olecranon fossa so that the entire bony margin of the olecranon tip can be visualized and associated loose bodies identified. The kissing lesion at the medial ulnotrochlear articulation is also débrided. The olecranon osteophyte is then excised with a sharp osteotome and burr. The amount of olecranon osteophyte that can safely be excised is unknown (Fig. 64.19). We remove only enough bone to allow full elbow extension without bony impingement—approximately 3 to 5 mm.[57] A lateral radiograph is then obtained intraoperatively to ensure that adequate bone has been removed and that no bone debris remains in the extra-articular soft tissues around the elbow. A compressive dressing is applied, and the arm is iced and elevated postoperatively. Early rehabilitation, with an emphasis on early recovery of motion, is initiated after surgery.

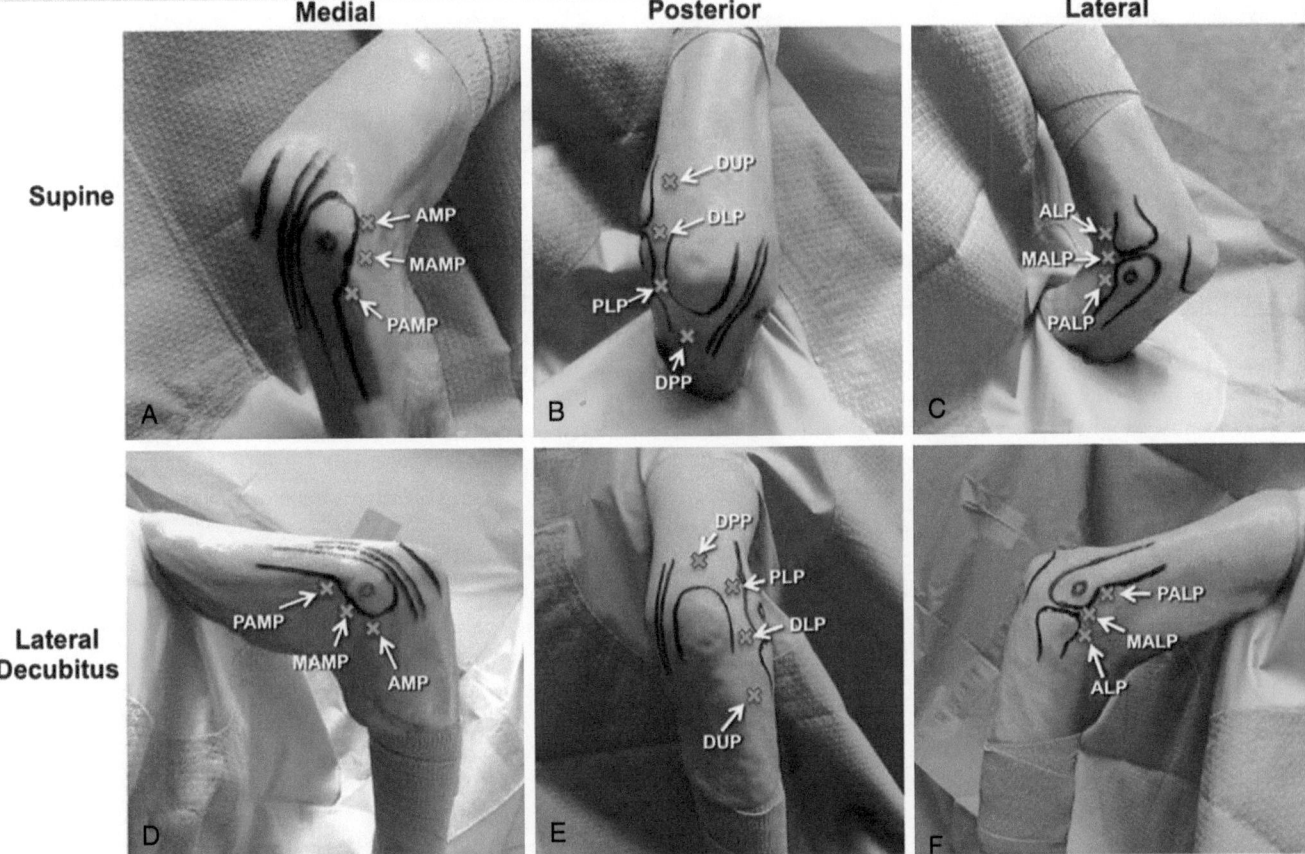

Fig. 64.18 Overview of portal locations for elbow arthroscopy portal locations for both supine and lateral decubitus positioning. *ALP,* anterolateral portal; *AMP,* anteromedial portal; *DLP,* direct lateral portal; *DPP,* direct posterior portal; *DUP,* distal ulnar portals; *MALP,* mid-anterolateral portal; *MAMP,* mid-anteromedial portal; *PALP,* proximal anterolateral portal; *PAMP,* proximal anteromedial portal; *PLP,* posterolateral portal. (From Camp CL, Degen RM, Sanchez-Sotelo J, et al. Basics of elbow arthroscopy part 1: surface anatomy, portals, and structures at risk. *Arthrosc Tech.* 2016;5(6):e1339–e1343.)

Continued

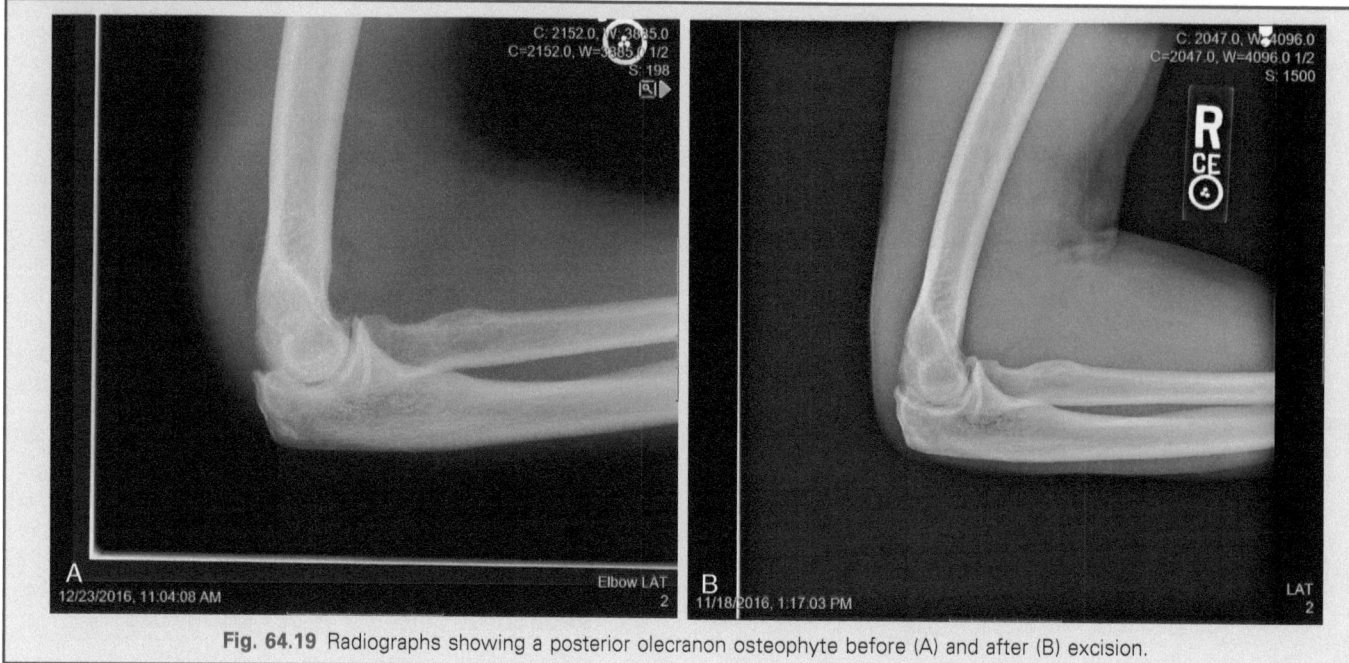

Fig. 64.19 Radiographs showing a posterior olecranon osteophyte before (A) and after (B) excision.

POSTOPERATIVE MANAGEMENT AND RETURN TO PLAY

UCL reconstruction requires the longest as well as most dedicated postoperative rehabilitative course. A standardized postoperative four-phase rehabilitation program as described by Wilk and colleagues[58-61] is implemented. The first phase begins immediately after surgery and continues for 3 weeks. At surgery a compression dressing is applied to the patient's elbow and a posterior splint is used to immobilize the elbow in 90 degrees of elbow flexion for 1 week to allow initial healing. During the first week, the patient performs wrist and digit ROM and hand-grasping exercises. Eight days after surgery, a hinged elbow ROM brace is applied and adjusted to allow motion from 30 to 100 degrees of flexion. During the third week after surgery, the brace is adjusted to permit 15 degrees to 110 degrees of motion; every week thereafter, motion is increased by 5 degrees to 10 degrees of extension and 10 degrees of flexion. Forearm pronosupination is permitted while the brace is worn. The goal is to restore full motion by the end of the fifth to sixth week after surgery. Use of the elbow ROM brace is discontinued at the end of the eighth week. During phase I (week 2), submaximal isometric strengthening is performed for the shoulder, scapular, and arm musculature. During week 3, active ROM exercises of the shoulder and arm are permitted. During phase II (weeks 4 to 10), full ROM is restored and a progressive isotonic strengthening program is initiated along with the Thrower's Ten Program for overhead throwing athletes.[62-64] During the advanced strengthening phase (phase III) from weeks 10 to 16, a sport-specific exercise and rehabilitation program is initiated. Phase IV, the return-to-activity phase (week 16 and beyond), is characterized by the initiation of an interval throwing program. Currently most of the rehabilitation protocols are designed around baseball, but these protocols can be extrapolated to meet the demands and needs of athletes in other sports.[58,65-67] In general return to throwing after UCL reconstruction takes an estimated 9 to 12 months, and the athlete and his or her family, coaches, and trainers should be aware of this lengthy time course.

After elbow arthroscopy, ulnar nerve transposition, and other procedures, a general framework for postoperative rehabilitation can be followed. This framework includes early shoulder ROM and strengthening, including scapular stabilization and parascapular muscle activation. Once surgical wounds have healed, gentle early elbow ROM should be initiated. Gradual forearm and elbow muscle strengthening should commence, followed by plyometric and sport-specific activities. Last, the interval throwing program is a common final pathway for most overhead throwing athletes.

It is reasonable to expect that the athlete may RTP when he or she has pain-free motion and function and has completed a dedicated rehabilitation protocol and, if necessary, an interval throwing program as well. The time course for this process varies greatly depending not only on the individual but also on the specific surgical procedure performed and the underlying pathology that was addressed.

RESULTS

Ulnar Collateral Ligament Injury

Dugas et al. have reported encouraging results with direct repair of the UCL. Here, an "internal brace" using a strong collagen-coated tape (FiberTape, Arthrex, Naples, Florida) attached at the anatomic insertions of the ligament using nonabsorbable anchors allows for direct repair of partial-thickness or avulsion-type injuries with good healthy ligament tissue while spanning the entire native ligament. A cadaveric biomechanical comparison with the modified Jobe reconstruction (authors' preferred technique) showed the two techniques to have similar time-zero strength and ultimate failure load.[68,69]

The largest series to date on outcomes of UCL reconstruction was published by Cain et al.[58] In this series, 1266 athletes underwent UCL reconstruction and subcutaneous ulnar nerve transposition. At a minimum 2-year follow-up, 83% of respondents ($n = 743$ patients) returned to play at the same or higher level when compared with their level before surgery. The average time to return to a throwing program was 4.4 months, and the mean time to return to full competition was 11.6 months. These study results have been updated by the same study group in a more recent study on the same patient population but with a minimum of 10-year follow-up from UCL reconstruction via the modified Jobe technique.[70] Most baseball players were satisfied after the operation; they were able to return to the same or higher level of play in less than 1 year with acceptable career longevity.

In the original report by Jobe and colleagues,[38] 10 of 16 overhead throwing athletes (63%) were able to return to their previous level of competition. In Conway's group of 70 patients, only 50% of the athletes who underwent repair of the ligament returned to competition, compared with 68% (45 of 56) of those who underwent UCL reconstruction.[9] Later, Andrews and Timmerman[5] reported on 72 professional baseball players with elbow disorders, 14 of whom underwent UCL reconstruction, with 12 of those players (86%) returning to their previous level of competition. Azar and colleagues then reported on 67 patients, with 81% (48 of 59) of those who underwent UCL reconstruction returning to the same or higher level of play; return to competition took approximately 1 year.[6] Thompson and colleagues[71] reported that 93% of 33 patients had an excellent result with UCL reconstruction. In a study by Paletta and Wright,[72] 92% of 25 professional and collegiate baseball players were able to return to their preinjury level of competition. Ninety percent of 100 patients evaluated by Dodson and coworkers[73] were able to compete at the same or a higher level.

Several recent studies have compared versions of these modified techniques for UCL reconstruction.[74-78] Armstrong and associates[77] reported that the docking technique and an Endo button technique were stronger than the interference screw or figure-eight technique, with all four techniques demonstrating inferior peak load to failure compared with an intact ligament. A comprehensive literature review by Langer and colleagues[78] revealed that decreased dissection of the flexor-pronator mass and decreased handling of the ulnar nerve led to improved outcomes. Paletta and coworkers[76] found that neither the docking nor the figure-eight technique reproduced the biomechanical profile of the native UCL, but they did suggest that the docking construct may offer an initial biomechanical advantage over the figure-eight construct. A study by McAdams and associates[75] that compared the effects of cyclic valgus loading on the docking and interference screw procedures demonstrated increased valgus angle widening with the docking technique after 10 and 100 cycles but no difference between the two techniques at 1000 cycles. Finally, Large and colleagues[74] biomechanically compared

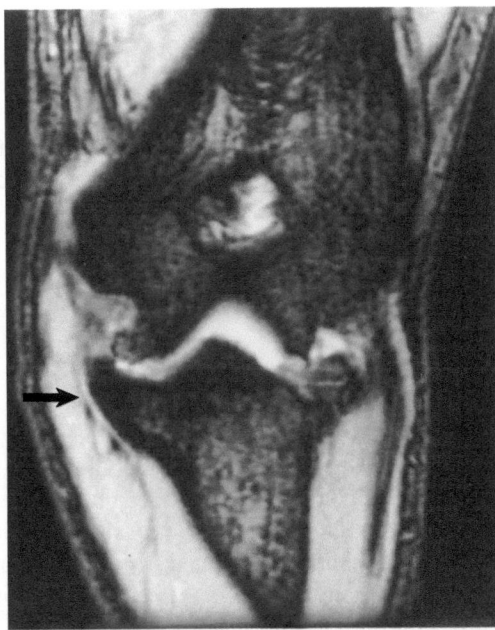

Fig. 64.20 A magnetic resonance image of the elbow with use of contrast material demonstrates a bony osteophyte of the medial proximal ulna. In such cases the ulnar collateral ligament attaches to the tip of the osteophyte. The bone is acting in a tension mode, which places it at risk for failure. If the ulnar collateral ligament is reconstructed in a person with osteophytes, as pictured here (arrow), it is important to obtain a graft that can replace the native ligament because the distal ligament is deficient after removal of the bony prominence.

the transosseous figure-eight and interference screw reconstructions. Their study showed that failure strength, as well as initial and overall stiffness of the transosseous figure-eight technique, was superior to the interference screw procedure.

The UCL originates on the distal aspect of the medial epicondyle and inserts onto the sublime tubercle of the medial proximal ulna. Many adult throwers have either a bony extension from the sublime tubercle directed proximally along the course of the ligament or one or more small ossicles of bone within the ligament (Fig. 64.20). In most cases, the bony ossicles represent old avulsion fractures that likely occurred during the patient's childhood or adolescent years. The same may be true of the development of a bony excrescence from the sublime tubercle, although the exact cause of this finding is uncertain. These bony findings are critical in the treatment of elbow instability in throwers. Because bone is stronger in compression than in tension, these aberrancies potentially create a weak link in the medial stabilizing tissues. Both the ossicles and the bony excrescence are actually within the substance of the UCL. In the case of the bony projection from the ulna, the terminal distal fibers of the UCL actually insert onto the prominence. The presence of these bony proliferations may make the decision to proceed with UCL reconstruction somewhat less difficult. If the decision is made to perform UCL reconstruction in these patients, a larger graft should be used, if possible, because of the soft tissue deficiency that will result from bone débridement from within the native ligament substance. In the absence of such findings, the native ligament can be left in place or reattached at the site of rupture along with palmaris longus reconstruction, creating significant tissue augmentation. In fact, the native ligament is usually placed beneath the tendon graft to protect the ligament reconstruction from abrasion by the joint surfaces. If the native ligament either cannot be retained or if it is insufficient, a graft with a greater thickness should be used to make up for the deficiency. We prefer to use the gracilis tendon in such cases.[79]

Other authors have reported on UCL reconstruction in athletes engaged in sports other than baseball, such as javelin throwers,[80] and numerous other basic science and clinical studies pertaining to ulnar collateral ligament reconstruction have been performed.[58,80-85]

Valgus Extension Overload

When the throwing program is completed, the athlete may return to competition, with the entire process typically taking 3 to 4 months. Andrews and Timmerman[5] reported on 56 professional baseball players who underwent excision of the posteromedial olecranon osteophyte either as an isolated arthroscopic procedure or as a part of UCL reconstruction. In their report, 68% returned to play for at least one season; however, 41% required a repeat operation. The authors concluded that arthroscopic débridement was superior to open techniques but warned against overresection, which can eventually lead to medial instability. Finally, Reddy and colleagues[86] reported on 187 elbow arthroscopies, noting that posterior olecranon impingement was the most common diagnosis (51%). In their series, 47 of 55 professional athletes (85%) returned to their previous level of competition. These investigators also noted that players with either loose bodies or VEO tended to have better results than did players with degenerative disease in the elbow.

Ulnar Neuritis

Results of ulnar nerve transposition in overhead throwing athletes are generally good.[2] Rettig and Ebben[87] reported excellent results with anterior subcutaneous transposition of the ulnar nerve in 20 athletes for whom nonoperative management had failed. At an average follow-up of 19 months, 95% were asymptomatic, without any symptoms interfering with sporting activity. Average RTP was 12.6 weeks.[87]

Andrews and Timmerman[5] reported on eight professional baseball players after anterior subcutaneous ulnar nerve transposition, including six patients who also had posteromedial olecranon osteophyte excision. Of the eight athletes, seven (88%) returned to play for at least one season at the professional level.[5]

In the setting of concomitant ulnar collateral ligament insufficiency, it is widely recognized that isolated treatment of the neuritic ulnar nerve will fail unless the ligament insufficiency is addressed concomitantly.[88] However, the technique of ulnar collateral ligament reconstruction itself may also place the ulnar nerve at risk of injury. Originally Jobe et al.[38] and Conway et al.[9] reported 31% and 21% incidences, respectively, of postoperative ulnar nerve dysfunction after ulnar collateral ligament reconstruction despite submuscular transposition of the ulnar nerve in all but one case. On the basis of this experience, Jobe and other investigators have recommended performing nerve transposition only in the setting of preoperative symptoms or the need for exploration of the posterior compartment.[89-92]

Azar et al.[6] reported resolution of preoperative ulnar nerve symptoms in 9 of 10 patients when subcutaneous ulnar nerve transposition was performed in conjunction with ulnar collateral ligament reconstruction. On the basis of these and other results, subcutaneous transposition may offer less morbidity compared with submuscular transposition in the setting of ulnar collateral ligament reconstruction. At our institution we currently favor anterior subcutaneous transposition.

Recurrent ulnar nerve subluxation, which is reported to occur with an incidence of 16% in the general population, may cause ulnar neuritis in the overhead throwing athlete.[92] In a study by Rettig and Ebben,[87] 16 of 20 patients were successfully treated with anterior subcutaneous transposition. Preoperatively all had been noted to have ulnar nerve subluxation.

COMPLICATIONS

In the setting of nonoperative management of elbow injuries, the primary drawback is time lost from competition if this initial management path proves unsuccessful. In certain circumstances, time away from competition can have a significant impact on the athlete's career, particularly at the professional level. In contrast, the list of potential complications from surgical intervention is lengthy. This list includes risk of iatrogenic nerve or vessel injury, recurrent UCL ligament tear, recurrent ulnar neuritis, wound complications, and persistent drainage from arthroscopic portals. Revision UCL reconstruction does not carry the same level of success for return to sport as does primary reconstruction.[93] Persistent portal drainage is likely the most common complication, but nerve injury or dysfunction is the most severe and dreaded complication arising from elbow arthroscopy. Revision surgery for failed UCL reconstruction carries a higher complication rate as well as a lower return to previous level of competition as compared with primary UCL reconstruction.[58] The incidence of ulnar neuritis from UCL reconstruction appears to have decreased in recent years, perhaps because of subcutaneous (as opposed to submuscular) transposition as well as use of a slip from the medial intermuscular septum, which may allow for less constraint and compression on the transposed nerve.[58]

FUTURE CONSIDERATIONS

Future investigations will likely enhance our understanding of elbow injury prevention, particularly in adolescent overhead throwing athletes. Attention to proper pitching mechanics and adherence to guidelines regarding pitch counts and pitch types depending on age may help decrease the incidence of injury over time. Surgical fixation methods for ulnar collateral ligament reconstruction will continue to evolve and improve. A final focus is optimizing the rehabilitation of persons with ulnar collateral ligament injuries. Currently RTP after surgical reconstruction averages close to 12 months. Decreasing recovery time either through improved surgical techniques or postoperative protocols will likely prove challenging but potentially beneficial for the athlete, team, school, or organization.

For a complete list of references, go to ExpertConsult.com.

SELECTED READINGS

Citation:
McCall BR, Cain EL Jr. Diagnosis, treatment, and rehabilitation of the thrower's elbow. *Curr Sports Med Rep.* 2005;4(5):249–254.

Level of Evidence:
Review

Summary:
This article provides a summary of the diagnosis, treatment, and rehabilitation of throwing elbow injuries. It also summarizes common clinical conditions and pearls from the history and physical examination.

Citation:
Cain EL Jr, Dugas JR, Wolf RS, et al. Elbow injuries in throwing athletes: a current concepts review. *Am J Sports Med.* 2003;31(4):621–635.

Level of Evidence:
Review

Summary:
This article provides a comprehensive review of the surgical techniques, history, physical examination, and diagnoses of elbow injuries in athletes, including arthroscopic and reconstructive surgery.

Citation:
Cain EL Jr, Dugas JR. History and examination of the thrower's elbow. *Clin Sports Med.* 2004;23(4):553–566.

Level of Evidence:
Review

Summary:
This articles provides an overview of the pitching cycle, history, and examination of acute and chronic injuries to the overhead throwing athlete's elbow.

Citation:
Azar FM, Andrews JR, Wilk KE, et al. Operative treatment of ulnar collateral ligament injuries of the elbow in athletes. *Am J Sports Med.* 2000;28(1):16–23.

Level of Evidence:
III, therapeutic study

Summary:
This study includes 3-year follow-up data for more than 90 patients who underwent UCL reconstructions and ulnar nerve transpositions and shows that the average time to return to competitive throwing was 10 months. Approximately 80% of patients returned to their prior level of competition.

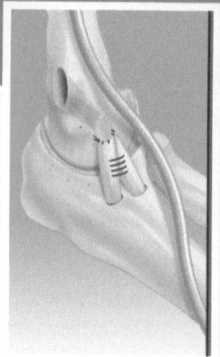

65

Loss of Elbow Motion

Timothy J. Luchetti, Debdut Biswas, Robert W. Wysocki

Acute and chronic disorders of the elbow are frequently observed in both recreational and professional athletes, particularly athletes who participate in sports that involve throwing. Although clinicians most frequently evaluate athletes in throwing-related sports who have elbow pathology related to overuse injuries, including ulnar collateral ligament insufficiency, valgus extension overload syndrome, and epicondylitis, acute elbow trauma may affect athletes in all sports. These acute injuries most commonly include elbow fractures/dislocations after falls onto an outstretched hand. The injuries may occur in sports such as wrestling, as a result of the combination of compression and torque applied to the arm when competitors are driven into the mat, or weightlifting, as a result of spontaneous dislocation from massive exertion. Elbow osteoarthritis is almost uniquely seen in middle-aged muscular men who may have been involved in repetitive, strenuous athletic endeavors, especially boxing and weightlifting.

Loss of mobility is the most common complication after elbow injury. The predisposition of the elbow to the development of posttraumatic contracture has been attributed to several factors, including the intrinsic congruity of the ulnohumeral articulation, the presence of three articulations within a synovium-lined cavity, and the intimate relationship of the joints to the intracapsular ligaments and extracapsular muscles.[1-3] Several authors have studied the degree of elbow motion necessary to complete daily activities. Their conclusions have yielded a functional arc of 100 degrees (range, 30 to 130 degrees) of flexion and extension of the elbow and 100 degrees of rotation of the forearm (50 degrees each for pronation and supination).[4] The inability of the elbow to achieve this degree of flexibility after trauma may lead to substantial impairment of upper extremity function. For patients whose elbow contracture is refractory to conservative management, surgical débridement and release of the elbow is offered to restore functional motion of the joint. Although open approaches have classically been described for the surgical treatment of the posttraumatic elbow contracture, arthroscopic techniques have recently emerged as a less invasive alternative with similar efficacy for the treatment of elbow stiffness, especially when secondary to intrinsic contracture.

Although several authors have attempted to formulate classification schemes to grade the severity of elbow stiffness, the system devised by Morrey[5] most accurately accounts for both osseous and soft tissue pathology contributing to loss of motion. Morrey divides the etiologies of elbow stiffness into either intrinsic or extrinsic factors. Intrinsic factors include intra-articular adhesions and loose bodies, articular malalignment, and loss of articular cartilage, whereas extrinsic factors include capsular and ligamentous contracture, heterotopic ossification (HO), extra-articular malunion, ulnar neuropathy, and postburn contracture of the superficial soft tissues. All of these potential sources of motion loss should be considered and separately addressed in patients who present with a stiff elbow.

HISTORY

Assessing Impairment

It is imperative for the practitioner to determine the extent to which the loss of elbow motion compromises a patient's functional capabilities. The magnitude of functional impairment, rather than absolute loss of motion, ultimately directs management decisions when treating the patient with posttraumatic contracture of the elbow. In this regard, the chief complaint is often related to functional loss rather than pain, swelling, deformity, or another manifestation of previous trauma. From the standpoint of activities of daily living, loss of flexion can restrict the ability to bring the hand to the face and head, which makes it challenging to button clothing, eat, and wash the face and hair. A loss of extension is less functionally significant with regard to activities of daily living because most patients can make accommodations for this deficit by moving closer to an object, but it can cause problems with overhead reaching. In modern society, loss of pronation is often reported because it causes difficulties with writing and typing; however, further abducting the shoulder as necessary can help to compensate for this deficit. Loss of supination is less commonly a problem, although it may present difficulties with activities such as carrying an item with two hands, holding a bowl/plate, or using a drive-through window, especially because no effective compensatory motions exist for a lack of supination.

When participating in a sport, lack of extension even to a mild degree often has greater consequences than interfering with activities of daily living alone. Two-handed weight training for which symmetry is important (e.g., bench press and military press) are affected for all athletes, and basketball players and throwing athletes especially struggle as they lose follow-through. Gymnasts' mechanics and ability to propel themselves are affected by loss of extension as well. With the possible exception of quarterbacks, football, hockey, and lacrosse players tend to accommodate very well to mild or even moderate elbow flexion contractures.

Intrinsic Causes

Several elements of the history can help the practitioner to determine if elbow stiffness is related to intrinsic pathology. When the patient has a history of an intra-articular fracture, radiographs and preferentially a computed tomography (CT) scan should be closely reviewed for evidence of intra-articular malunion or resultant osteoarthritis, especially when the trauma is remote. An inability to achieve full range of motion (ROM) in the setting of malunion may suggest a true bony impingement, whereas a gradual decline over several years is more suggestive of post-traumatic arthritis as the cause of stiffness. The history should determine if the patient has mechanical symptoms such as locking or catching that would be suggestive of intra-articular loose bodies, which can be confirmed by a CT scan, magnetic resonance imaging, or preferably CT combined with an arthrogram.

Stiffness from elbow osteoarthritis presents with months to years of gradually progressive loss of motion and pain at terminal flexion and extension, usually with less pain within the mid arc of motion until the process is very advanced. These patients usually identify pain with triceps- and biceps-strengthening exercises from the forced terminal motion, and fluctuations of pain and swelling often occur that increase in severity the more the elbow is used.

Extrinsic Causes

When evaluating a patient for extrinsic causes of elbow stiffness, it is important to elicit the length of the immobilization period after an acute injury, because immobilization for longer than 7 to 14 days after elbow trauma predisposes the joint to capsular contracture. Except in rare circumstances of persistent instability despite surgical intervention, acute elbow fractures and dislocations should either be inherently stable enough to allow ROM to begin within 7 to 14 days, or the elbow should be surgically stabilized from a bony and/or soft tissue standpoint to allow ROM within that time frame. HO, if it occurs, typically starts to appear within a few weeks of injury and can continue to progress and mature for months. Patients with symptomatic HO initially demonstrate appropriate progress with ROM and then their condition deteriorates as the HO progresses. Surgical intervention for posttraumatic HO should be delayed until it appears to be mature radiographically, typically 3 to 6 months later.

The practitioner should specifically inquire about any associated symptoms of ulnar neuropathy because, in addition to accompanying a loss of flexion, ulnar neuropathy may also cause a loss of flexion after a relatively innocuous elbow trauma. A history of a burn, a degloving injury, or infection of the skin and soft tissues should raise suspicion that the soft tissues are contributing to the contracture, although this situation is uncommon.

Forearm Contracture

Stiffness specific to loss of forearm rotation has several causes. Although one must consider causes intrinsic to the elbow, such as radial head fracture malunion and HO affecting the ulnohumeral and proximal radioulnar joints, other injuries such as a Monteggia fracture, a Galeazzi fracture, and fractures of both bones of the forearm are more common scenarios for isolated forearm contracture. Even with appropriate treatment, a loss of 10 to 20 degrees of forearm rotation is not uncommon after these injuries. Performing a corrective osteotomy in this setting is technically challenging with somewhat poorly reproducible results, and thus the corrective osteotomy is reserved for persons with more severe contractures.

A unique complication of distal biceps tendon reattachment, especially two-incision techniques, is HO at the level of the radial tuberosity that limits forearm rotation. This condition can be treated very successfully through resection of the HO, with excellent return of ROM and biceps strength[6] and improved outcomes compared with HO resection associated with other forearm trauma.[7]

Prior Treatment

If prior operative treatment was performed, it is especially important to obtain and review any operative documentation and arthroscopic images where applicable, especially when further surgical treatment is being considered. Complications related to initial treatments, including infection or neurologic deficits, can potentially account for posttraumatic stiffness and should be investigated. The physician should also ascertain the duration of physical therapy that has already been undertaken, the types of splinting that have been used (e.g., static progressive or dynamic), and to what degree progress has plateaued.

PHYSICAL EXAMINATION

Physical examination begins with inspection of the entire upper extremity, specifically evaluating for soft tissue contracture, deformity, swelling, and muscle atrophy, while noting the location of any previous arthroscopic portal sites or surgical incisions that would influence further surgical planning.

ROM evaluation should include the hand, wrist, forearm, and elbow and be compared with the contralateral, unaffected extremity. Crepitus, locking, and mechanical symptoms may occur as a result of loose bodies or osteochondral injuries. Pain at the extremes of motion with mechanical blocks may be the result of osteophyte formation and impingement in the coronoid fossa at terminal flexion or within the olecranon fossa at terminal extension. Pain during the mid arc of motion in a young athlete is frequently due to osteochondral lesions. The examiner should test both active and passive motion and characterize the type of end point at the extremes of motion. A gradual passive stretch obtained after the initial limitation in active ROM is suggestive of a residual myostatic contracture that usually would be expected to resolve with time. Varus and valgus stress testing, especially posterolateral drawer testing, is imperative, particularly in the setting of previous trauma, because posttraumatic posterolateral rotatory instability can often present with stiffness as the chief complaint rather than subtle instability.

Performing a careful neurologic examination is essential. As it traverses the cubital tunnel adjacent to the medial joint capsule, the ulnar nerve may become entrapped in scar tissue along the medial elbow after trauma, resulting in posttraumatic ulnar

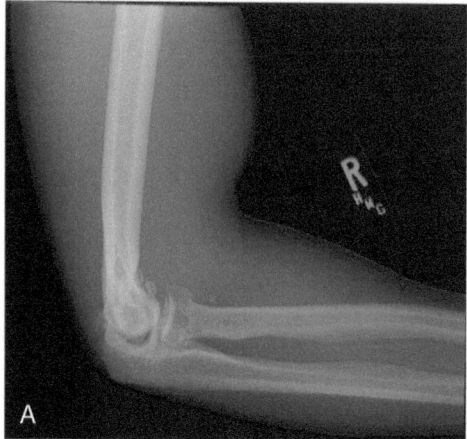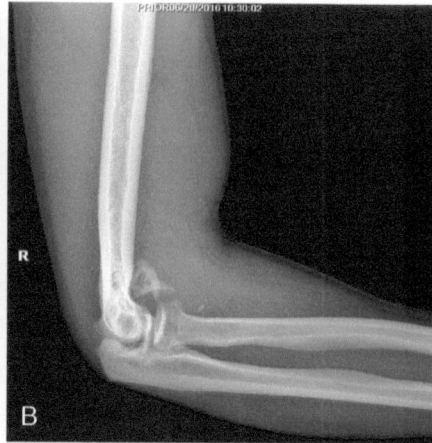

Fig. 65.1 (A) Heterotopic ossification is readily identifiable on radiographs and gradually progresses from a more poorly defined "fluffy" appearance when immature to (B) a well-defined morphology with clearly visible borders when mature.

neuropathy. Traction ulnar neuritis of the elbow may manifest as medial elbow tenderness and subjective paresthesias in an ulnar nerve distribution (medial forearm into the small finger and ulnar border of the ring finger), particularly with elbow flexion. Patients with posttraumatic ulnar neuropathy may present simply with loss of flexion and medial elbow pain in the absence of overt symptoms of ulnar neuropathy. Two-point discrimination, grip-and-pinch strength, and intrinsic muscle function should be documented.

IMAGING

Standard plain radiographs of the elbow are obtained and include anteroposterior, lateral, and oblique projections. Radiographs may demonstrate evidence of malunion of distal humerus, radial head/neck, or proximal ulna fractures, as well as bony loose bodies and degenerative changes in the ulnohumeral or radiocapitellar joints. HO is readily identifiable on radiographs and gradually progresses from a more poorly defined "fluffy" appearance when immature to a well-defined morphology with clearly visible borders when mature (Fig. 65.1).

A CT scan can help to localize HO, intra-articular loose bodies, and degenerative joint disease within the elbow when surgical intervention is being considered (Fig. 65.2). Although plain radiographs are typically sufficient for establishing a diagnosis for these conditions, they often underestimate the pathology. Accordingly, two- and three-dimensional CT reconstructions are helpful in further delineating bony and articular anatomy. CT arthrography demonstrates filling defects around osseous and nonosseous loose bodies, as well as areas of osseous impingement resulting from overgrowth in the olecranon or coronoid fossae and at the tips of the coronoid and olecranon processes.

For posttraumatic HO, we favor standard CT imaging without arthrography because loose bodies are less often present and the HO is better appreciated without intra-articular contrast obscuring its borders. The use of CT is less common but also beneficial when evaluating intra-articular malunion if corrective osteotomy

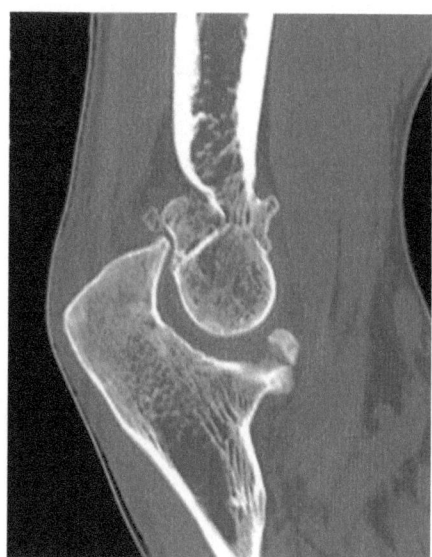

Fig. 65.2 A sagittal computed tomography image demonstrating complex osteophytes in the olecranon and coronoid fossae.

is being considered. We have found that magnetic resonance imaging has a limited role for the evaluation of stiff elbows.

DECISION-MAKING PRINCIPLES AND TREATMENT OPTIONS

Nonoperative management remains the initial means of treatment and prevention of elbow contracture after acute injuries and typically includes early ROM and supervised therapy as long as the elbow joint and any internal fixation are deemed stable enough to withstand it. Motion is typically initiated no later than 2 to 3 weeks after elbow trauma as long as the injury is stabilized by operative or nonoperative means. In most cases, active or active assisted motion commences prior to passive motion. When posttraumatic HO is identified, patients usually continue to undergo supervised therapy until their ROM plateaus and the HO is mature radiographically.

For cases of elbow stiffness due to osteoarthritis and loose bodies, physical therapy typically does not have a role given the mechanical nature of the disease process, although cortisone injection can be safe and effective in the short term for athletes trying to complete their season.

Static progressive or dynamic splinting for passive stretch of the soft tissues is an effective adjunct to physical therapy once sufficient bony and/or ligamentous healing is present at 6 to 8 weeks after an acute injury. These types of splints should also be used for patients who present with an established contracture after prolonged immobilization and can be used for contractures in either forearm rotation or elbow flexion/extension. Static progressive splints are adjusted by the patient and apply a constant tension to the soft tissues; these splints are generally locked in a given position and do not allow motion of the elbow while the splint is applied. Dynamic splints work by applying a constant tension through an elastic-based mechanism but do permit motion; they usually require a longer continuous period of use, typically 4 to 6 hours. We tend to favor static splints in our practice because patient compliance has been better than with dynamic splints because static splints are generally worn for only approximately 30 minutes per day (Fig. 65.3).

Splinting, either flexion or extension depending on the primary deficit, is most useful during the first 3 to 6 months after an injury, particularly for patients whose stiffness is due to extrinsic soft tissue contracture and who do not show radiographic evidence of bony deformity, arthrosis, or osteophyte impingement. Recent level I evidence has demonstrated that static progressive and dynamic splinting have equivalent results with benefits still observed as long as 12 months after injury.[8,9] These results have been demonstrated regardless of the cause of the contracture.[9] We typically reexamine patients at monthly intervals to document continued improvements with their splinting regimen and discontinue use of the splints when no improvement is demonstrated at successive visits, especially given their cost and time investment.

Surgical management is indicated for patients who continue to experience significant loss of mobility with resultant impairment of upper extremity function and limitation with daily activities or sport. Although a flexion contracture of at least 25 to 30 degrees and/or less than 110 to 115 degrees of active flexion was historically reported as an indication for elbow contracture release, operative management may also be offered to persons with greater motion requirements for specific lifestyle, occupational, or athletic demands. Most importantly, patients must be willing to comply with extensive postoperative therapy, because operative outcomes depend on diligent participation in a structured rehabilitation program. Compliance with extensive postoperative therapy is especially important for adolescents, who may be less dedicated to improving their elbow motion than other patients whose livelihood depends on maximal functional recovery.

In the setting of acute stiffness after elbow trauma, 4 to 6 months are typically required for swelling and inflammation to decrease sufficiently for "tissue equilibrium" to be achieved, after which surgery is advisable for patients who fail to progress with use of the aforementioned nonoperative methods.

Although patients with degenerative disease that results from anterior or posterior impinging osteophytes are good candidates for débridement, persons with diffuse joint space narrowing and pain throughout the arc of motion are better candidates for salvage-type procedures such as interposition arthroplasty or total elbow arthroplasty.[10]

The timing of operative débridement for osteoarthritis is flexible, and many athletes elect to manage the condition with intra-articular steroid injections during the playing season and then have surgery during the off-season, with an expectation that 4 to 6 months will pass before they are capable of returning to their sport.

Treatment of a stiff yet unstable elbow is particularly challenging. Subtle elbow instability may exist concurrently with loss of motion after elbow fracture-dislocation. Accordingly, special attention should be devoted to evaluating elbow stability either with stability testing or stress radiographs. If instability is present, ligament reconstruction may be combined with capsular release in certain patients,[11,12] although most cases should be treated with a staged procedure. The priority should be to

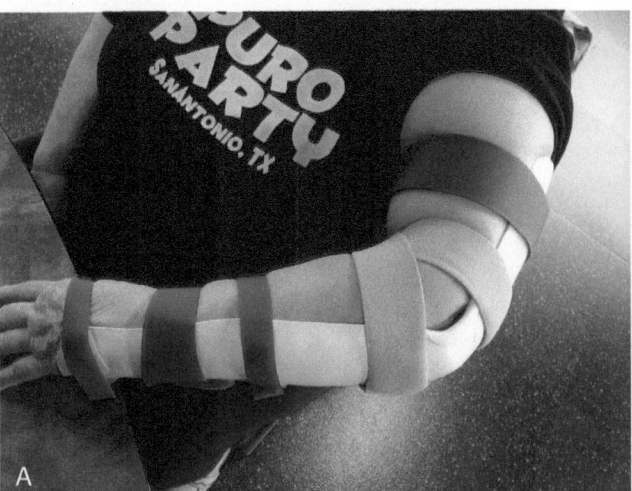
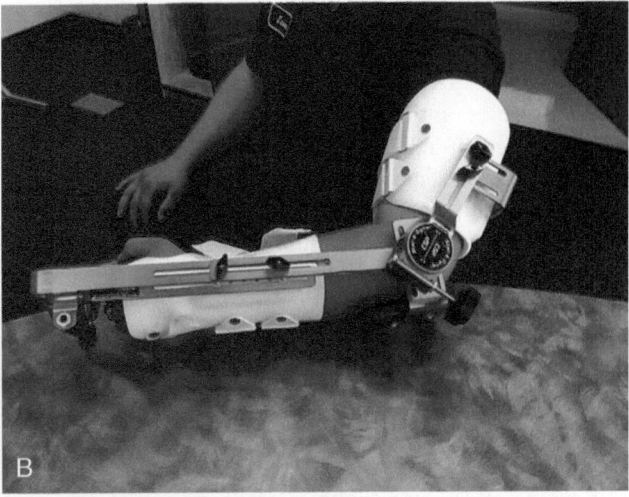

Fig. 65.3 (A) We tend to favor static splints in our practice because patient compliance has been better than with (B) dynamic splints, as static splints are generally worn for only approximately 30 minutes per day.

achieve stability first and restore motion later with an elbow release procedure if necessary.

SURGICAL TECHNIQUES

Open and arthroscopic techniques are well described for the treatment of elbow contracture. Although success has been reported with use of open release via posterior, lateral, medial, and combined approaches, isolated releases from the medial or lateral side are now most commonly used. The choice of approach may be contingent on previous surgery, the location of the primary offending pathology, or simply the surgeon's preference based on his or her comfort level and experience with the approach. The anterior and posterior ulnohumeral joint articular surfaces and capsular tissues can be adequately exposed for débridement from either the medial or lateral side. However, significant involvement of the radiocapitellar joint requires a lateral exposure, whereas posteromedial osteophytes and associated ulnar neuropathy require a medial approach. Although a combined approach can be performed through a universal posterior incision, evidence suggests that ROM gains are less impressive with this technique.[13] For this reason, we recommend the use of separate medial and/or lateral incisions.

Arthroscopy has emerged as a less invasive method of restoring motion, particularly for intrinsic contractures. Although this technique is technically demanding, advances in instrumentation and arthroscopic equipment have resulted in expanding indications for arthroscopic elbow release. Although arthroscopic release has the theoretical benefit of less morbidity and a more rapid return to function, these benefits have yet to be convincingly demonstrated in the literature.

In a systematic review of the literature in 2013, a total of three comparative series of different treatment options for elbow stiffness were included. Also included were 27 retrospective case series. The authors observed that arthroscopic release is associated with the lowest overall complications rates, at an aggregate of 5% from the included studies.[14] In general, they recommended performing the most minimally invasive approach possible to minimize complication rates. Cohen et al. reported on a prospective, nonrandomized study comparing outcomes after the Outerbridge-Kashiwagi (O-K) procedure with an arthroscopic débridement of the olecranon fossa for mild osteoarthritis of the elbow. The authors found that the O-K procedure resulted in significantly better motion, whereas the arthroscopic procedure provided suitable pain relief.[15]

Relative contraindications to arthroscopic elbow release include the most severe elbow contractures, prior ulnar nerve transposition surgery, the presence of significant HO, and previous surgery involving the radial head, which may render the radial nerve susceptible to iatrogenic injury. Patients with these conditions are more reliably treated with open release with direct visualization and protection of neurovascular structures. Surgeons considering arthroscopic elbow release should inquire about previous ulnar nerve transposition and acquire records to confirm the exact nerve location.

Until comparative studies with matched treatment groups have been performed, no definitive conclusions can be made about the superiority of open or arthroscopic elbow release. Given the risks of nerve injury with complex elbow arthroscopy, the surgeon must still choose the procedure that is safest and most effective in his or her hands. Although some surgeons can perform arthroscopic release in nearly all cases, the most reproducible arthroscopic releases to perform are those in cases of stiffness secondary to mild or moderate elbow osteoarthritis where the borders of osteophytes and normal bony contours can be easily appreciated. Posttraumatic contractures without a history of previous surgery and with mild HO are also typically less challenging releases. Cases become increasingly complex in the face of previous surgery and more widespread HO that either approaches neurovascular structures or obliterates the normal bony anatomy.

Arthroscopic Release

Arthroscopic elbow release is a demanding procedure that requires intimate knowledge of intra-articular elbow anatomy and advanced skills in elbow arthroscopy. Multiple portals are required and diligent fluid management is essential, especially because capsulectomy consequently creates unreliable joint distention. The use of joint retractors improves visualization and facilitates appropriate surgical débridement of contracted or impinging structures.[16-20]

From a mechanical standpoint, posterior débridement improves elbow extension and anterior débridement improves elbow flexion. However, optimal results are possible when the entire joint is considered regardless of the major motion deficiency and primary pathology. To increase extension, any cause of posterior impingement must be removed between the olecranon tip and the olecranon fossa. The fossa may require deepening to achieve terminal elbow extension. The anterior joint capsule and adhesions between the brachialis muscle and distal humerus must also be released. To increase flexion, any cause of anterior impingement must be eliminated in the region of the coronoid and radial fossae. For full flexion to occur, deep concavities must be restored at the fossae to accept the coronoid process centrally and the radial head laterally (Fig. 65.4). The posterior and posteromedial joint capsules and adhesions between the triceps muscle and distal humerus must be released.

Anesthesia and Positioning

We favor use of a regional block rather than general anesthesia when feasible. We position the patient in the lateral decubitus position with the affected extremity over a cradle and all bony prominences well padded. It is helpful to position the patient slightly overrotated toward the surgeon to prevent the arm from "sliding away" during the procedure. The shoulder is positioned at 90 degrees of abduction and adequate extension to keep the elbow elevated higher and allow enough clearance for maximal freedom of passive motion (Fig. 65.5A). After the extremity is sterilely prepared and draped up to the axilla, the hand and forearm are wrapped with an elastic bandage to limit fluid extravasation and a sterile pneumatic tourniquet is placed as proximally as possible around the arm.

The major external landmarks and portal sites are then marked, including the olecranon tip, the medial and lateral epicondyles,

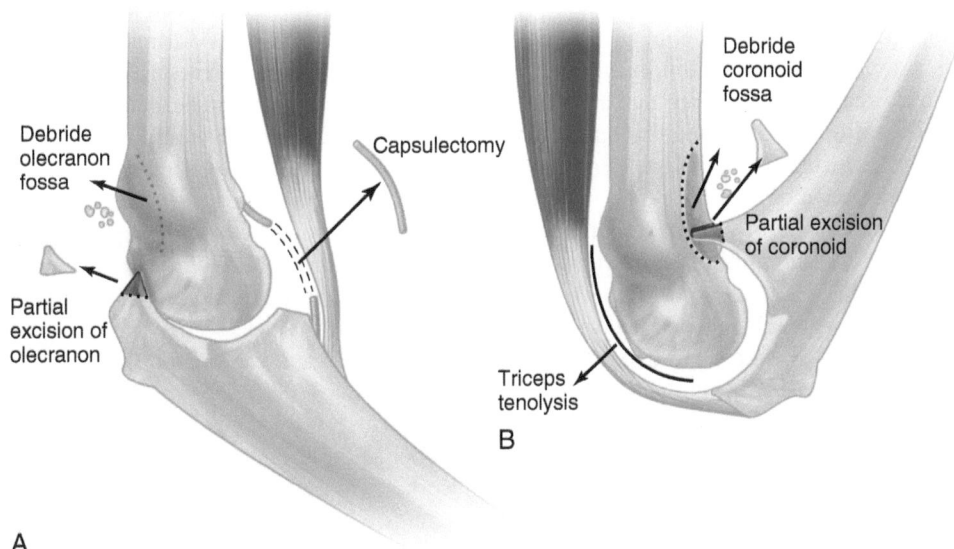

Fig. 65.4 (A) Improvement of elbow extension requires removal of posterior bony impingement and release of the anterior joint capsule. (B) Improvement of flexion requires posterior soft tissue release and removal of any soft tissue or bony impingement anteriorly. (Courtesy Hill Hastings, MD, Indiana Hand Center, Indianapolis, IN.)

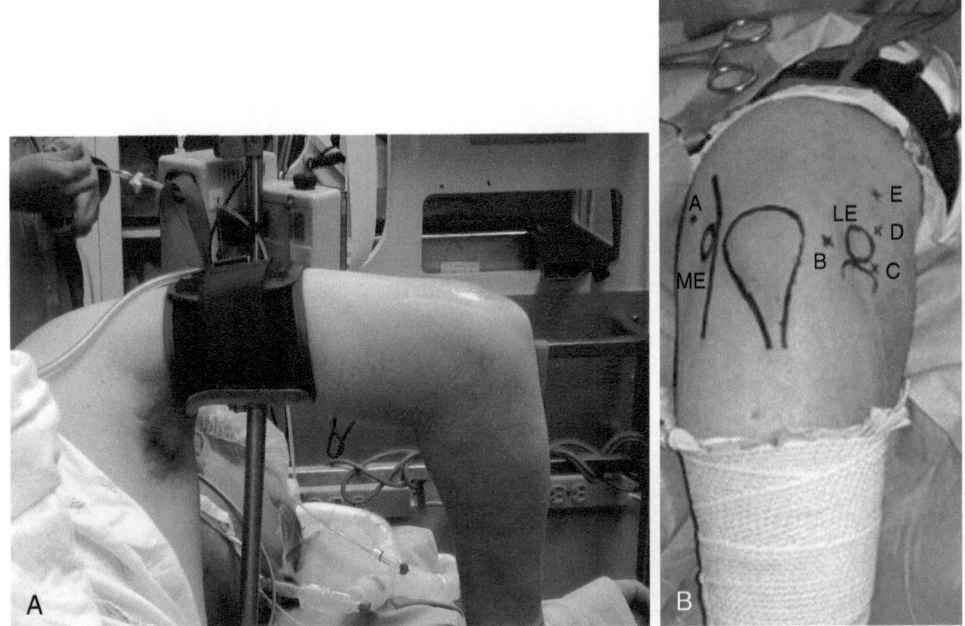

Fig. 65.5 (A) The arm is positioned over a cradle, allowing sufficient space for full flexion. (B) Anatomic landmarks are marked: lateral epicondyle *(LE)*, medial epicondyle *(ME)*, proximal anteromedial portal *(A)*, soft-spot portal *(B)*, standard anterolateral portal *(C)*, modified anterolateral portal *(D)*, and proximal anterolateral portal *(E)*. The expected path of the ulnar nerve is also depicted.

and the course of the ulnar nerve (see Fig. 65.5B). The extremity is exsanguinated with a compressive elastic bandage, and the tourniquet is inflated.

Surgical Landmarks, Incisions, and Portals

The elbow joint is first insufflated with 30 mL of normal sterile saline solution through the soft spot outlined by the lateral

epicondyle, radial head, and olecranon tip to facilitate joint entry with the arthroscope (Fig. 65.6).

Anteromedial portal. The proximal anteromedial portal is created through a stab skin-only incision, 2 cm proximal and 2 cm anterior to the medial epicondyle, just anterior to the medial intermuscular septum. Subcutaneous tissue is spread with a hemostat clamp (Fig. 65.7A), and the blunt trocar for the arthroscope is inserted, aiming straight medial to lateral. The surgeon should be able to sense the trocar flipping back and forth from posterior to anterior along the septum, ensuring that the trajectory is anterior to the septum to protect an anatomically positioned ulnar nerve. It should be noted that entry into the joint might be difficult, particularly in cases involving post-traumatic stiffness with a contracted capsule. Care must be taken to pass directly along the anterior humeral cortex because the capsule may be quite adherent, pushing the instrument into an extraarticular plane.

The anterior joint compartment is then penetrated with the tip of the trocar directed laterally toward the radial head (see Fig. 65.7B). The trocar is then advanced gently through the capsule and exchanged for a long standard 4.0-mm 30-degree arthroscope (or occasionally a 2.7-mm 30-degree arthroscope for small elbows). Gravity inflow of sterile saline solution is established to allow for distention of the elbow capsule. Specialized cannulas that do not have any holes near the tip (Fig. 65.8) may be helpful

because standard cannulas can lead to the inadvertent entry of fluid into the soft tissues during visualization of the joint.

This medial portal allows excellent inspection of the lateral joint including the radial head, capitellum, and lateral capsule. An examination of the anterior elbow joint compartment is performed to evaluate for loose bodies, synovitis, and cartilage injury. The arthroscope is then directed laterally, and the camera is rotated to visualize the radiocapitellar joint in the horizontal plane. If visualization is difficult, a retractor or freer elevator can be introduced through a proximal anterolateral portal (described in the next section). Improved visualization of the lateral capsule and soft tissues is achieved by providing tension to the capsule anteriorly.

Anterolateral portal. After diagnostic arthroscopy of the anterior elbow through the medial portal, a modified anterolateral "working" portal is created with use of either an inside-out

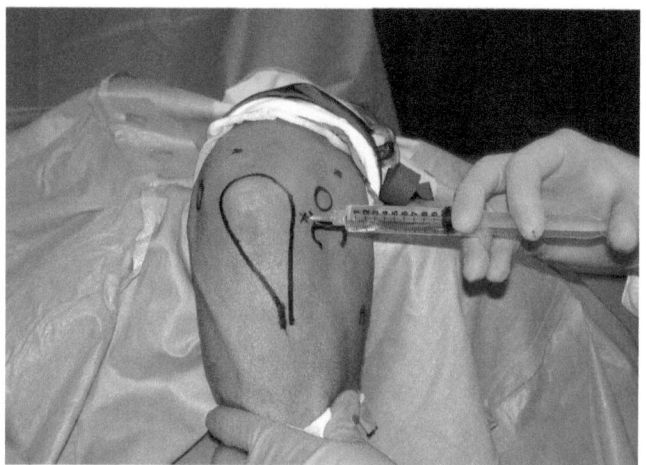

Fig. 65.6 The elbow joint is insufflated with sterile saline solution through the lateral soft spot.

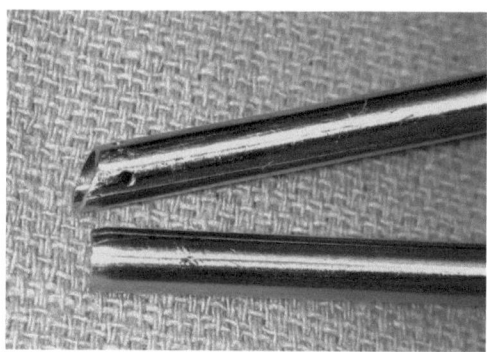

Fig. 65.8 A close-up view of the arthroscopic cannulas used for the elbow. Traditional cannulas *(top)* for larger joints commonly have an oblique end with holes near the tip to facilitate flow. Specialized cannulas *(bottom)* for the elbow do not have outflow holes. This distinction is important because the distance between the cannula tip and the joint capsule can be quite small in the elbow, allowing fluid to extravasate inadvertently into the soft tissues. Fluid management is important when performing an elbow release arthroscopically.

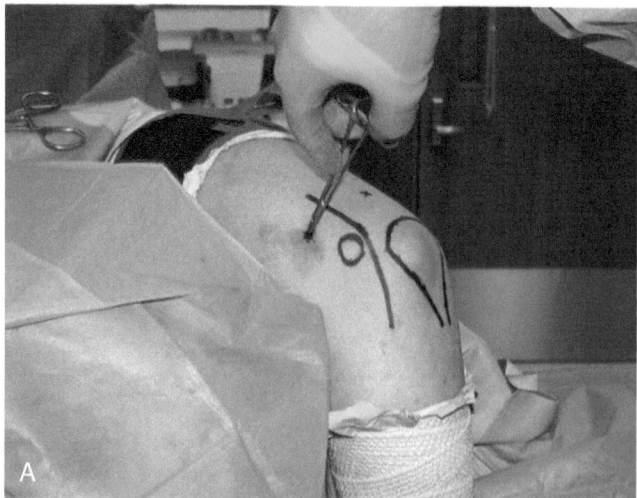

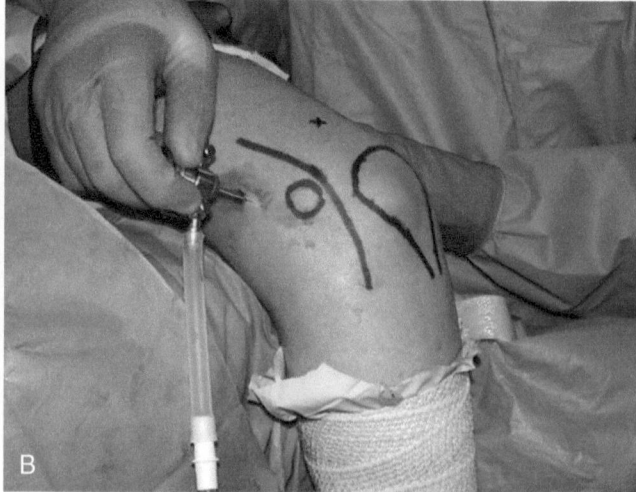

Fig. 65.7 (A) Subcutaneous tissue is first spread with a hemostat clamp when placing the anteromedial portal. (B) The trocar is then introduced and directed inferolaterally toward the radial head and through the anterior elbow capsule.

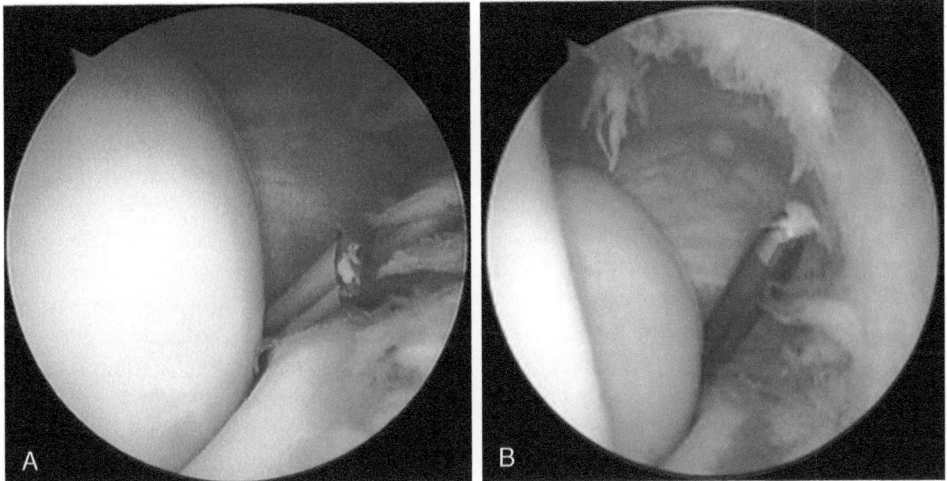

Fig. 65.9 An arthroscopic view of the elbow joint as viewed from a medial portal with localization of an anterolateral portal with an 18-gauge spinal needle (A) followed by placement of a blunt trocar through the joint (B).

technique with a switching stick or direct needle localization while viewing the field from the medial side.

The portal is typically 1 cm proximal and 1 cm anterior to the superior aspect of the capitellum. Any lateral synovitis may be débrided through this portal (Fig. 65.9) with a resector. It is of utmost importance to understand the position of the posterior interosseous nerve just anterior to the midline of the radiocapitellar joint to avoid iatrogenic injury when advancing cutting or thermal instruments in the working portals.

Anterior release. After placement of anteromedial and anterolateral portals, the anterior joint is cleared of any synovitis or adhesions that are present. Typically the arthroscope is introduced through the anteromedial portal, whereas instruments to be used for débridement are initially placed through the anterolateral portal. Mechanical instruments (e.g., a shaver) are commonly used for débridement, although thermal devices may more easily facilitate the removal of soft tissue. If a surgeon elects to use thermal instruments, inflow should be gradually increased to avoid heat generation within the joint. The coronoid and radial fossae are débrided of any fibrous tissue down to the bony floor to allow visualization of the articulation of the coronoid and radial head, respectively, with the distal humerus during elbow flexion. Once the locations of bony impingement are clearly identified, they are resected with a high-speed burr until concavities are created within the fossae to permit further flexion of the coronoid process and radial head without impedance (Figs. 65.10 and 65.11). The arthroscope and the working instruments must be alternated efficiently and effectively from medial to lateral positions during débridement.

After débridement of the coronoid and radial fossae, attention is next turned toward the anterior capsule. Special care is devoted to the radial nerve, which lies directly anterior to the capsule near the midline of the radiocapitellar joint. Accordingly, débridement of the anterior capsule directly off of the humerus proximal to the trochlea is much safer than at its distal origin. The capsulotomy is usually initiated with a wide-mouthed duckling punch in a medial to lateral direction with viewing through the

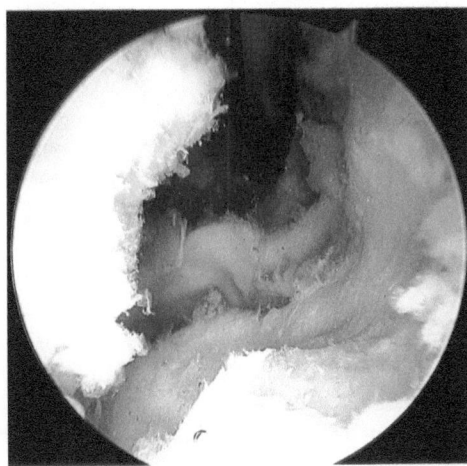

Fig. 65.10 The coronoid and radial fossa have been débrided of any tissue that would cause impingement in flexion; a concavity is produced above the articular surface.

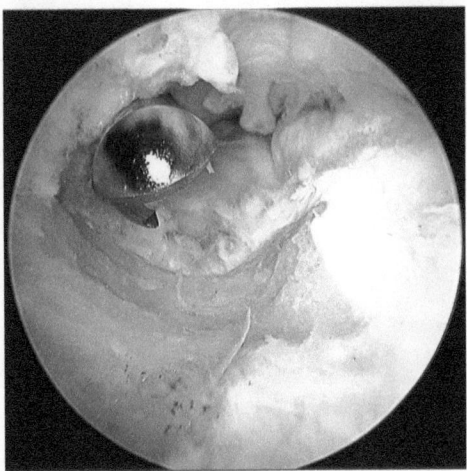

Fig. 65.11 The concavity proximal to the trochlea is viewed from the lateral portal.

anterolateral portal; dissection in this direction is technically easier because the interval between the capsule and the brachialis muscle is more defined on the medial side. The portals are then reversed so that a medial view is achieved and working instruments are passed from the lateral portal, while continuing to strip the anterior capsule off its humeral origin. Use of a knife to extend the capsulotomy down to the level of the collateral ligaments on each side completes the capsulotomy. The capsular attachments should be resected off the distal humerus as far as the supracondylar ridges both medially and laterally.

A capsulectomy is then performed. Débridement performed more distally near the level of the joint must be conducted with extreme diligence to avoid iatrogenic injury to the radial nerve. The capsulectomy should be performed on the medial side extending from a proximal to distal direction. The lateral capsule should then be excised proximally and distally. This excision is the most dangerous aspect of the anterior release because the radial nerve is vulnerable immediately behind the capsule, just anterior to the radial head, between the brachialis muscle and extensor carpi radialis brevis tendon origin. If significant doubt exists regarding the tissue planes intraoperatively and working toward a complete capsulectomy is placing the radial nerve at risk, a simple capsulotomy off the humerus often suffices for motion restoration (Fig. 65.12).

The use of retractors during anterior capsulectomy is strongly advocated because they greatly aid in visualization, can obviate the need for increased fluid pressure, and can aid in fluid management, which is especially true after the capsulectomy has begun, because fluid distention is less effective and extravasation into the periarticular soft tissues occurs more rapidly. Bony work should be limited after a capsulectomy because it is much more difficult to work within the elbow after a significant amount of fluid has extravasated. Retractor portals, both medially and laterally, are typically placed 2 cm proximal to the already described medial and lateral portals.

Posterior release. After anterior release, we recommend maintaining a cannula in the anterior joint during the posterior release to establish outflow for the remainder of the procedure. The posterior portals may then be placed. The posterolateral portal is started approximately 1 cm proximal to the midpoint between a line drawn from the olecranon tip to the lateral epicondyle. The posterior portal is established 3 to 4 cm above the olecranon tip in the midline. With the elbow extended to protect the posterior trochlea, a blunt elevator is used to blindly strip and clear the olecranon fossa and elevate the posterior joint capsule using tactile feedback.

With the arthroscope in the posterolateral portal and the shaver in the posterior portal, a view is first established by débriding the olecranon fossa (Fig. 65.13). Visualization may be difficult initially, and all débridement should begin lateral of midline to avoid inadvertent injury to the ulnar nerve. Once a view is established, the shaver or a radiofrequency ablation device can be used to débride dense scar tissue and synovium, taking care to preserve the capsule to more easily perform the capsulotomy later. If necessary, the posterior capsule is partially freed from the humerus proximally with a shaver or periosteal elevator and can be partially resected to improve visualization. Typically, this capsule is less hypertrophic than the anterior capsule. Placing a retractor in a proximal posterolateral portal 1 to 2 cm proximal to the posterolateral portal is useful to maintain that space.

Bony resection is then carried out with a high-speed burr, particularly near the tip of the olecranon, within the olecranon fossa, and at the medial and lateral corners (Fig. 65.14). Special care must be taken medially to either fully delineate the medial gutter and protect the ulnar nerve or perform débridement through a small, open medial approach to directly visualize the nerve, particularly when significant posteromedial bone is encountered and extensive débridement is anticipated. After bony and synovial débridement, the posterior capsule is then resected, which is most easily performed with a shaver or radiofrequency ablation device through the posterolateral portal. The posterolateral capsule is initially resected, and the posteromedial capsule is released in cases in which there is a significant loss of flexion (i.e., flexion limited to less than 90 to 110 degrees).

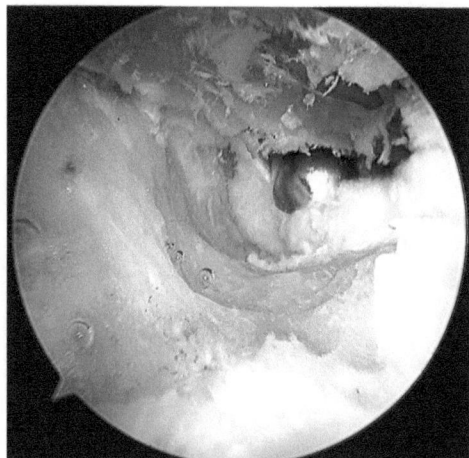

Fig. 65.12 A capsulectomy has been performed anteriorly, revealing the undersurface of the brachialis. The capsular resection is performed proximal to the joint line; capsular débridement distal to the radiocapitellar joint would place the radial nerve, which lies directly anterior to the capsule at the joint line, at risk.

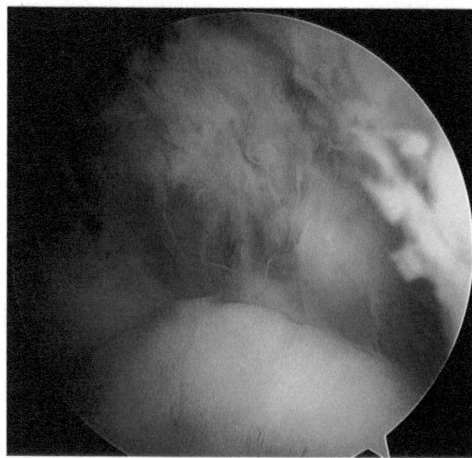

Fig. 65.13 An arthroscopic view of the posterior joint, including fibrous tissue within the olecranon fossa.

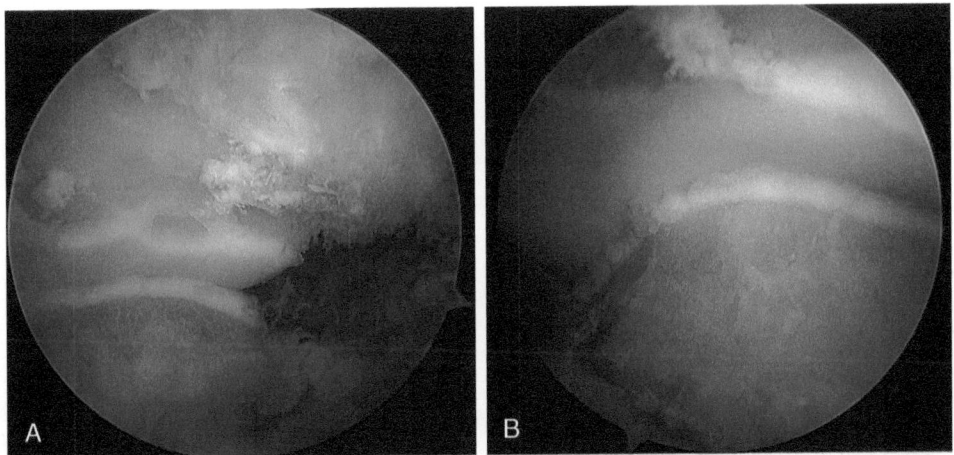

Fig. 65.14 Lateral (A) and medial (B) views of the olecranon, demonstrating that the olecranon fossa and olecranon tip have been débrided of scar and osteophytes, thus removing any structures causing impingement and preventing extension.

Posteromedial capsulectomy and ulnar nerve decompression. The ulnar nerve lies along the medial joint capsule in the cubital tunnel and may become enveloped in scar tissue and develop adhesions to the soft tissues after trauma. We recommend that the ulnar nerve be decompressed and/or transposed in all cases when preoperative symptoms exist either at rest or with provocative positioning or testing (i.e., a positive Tinel sign or a positive elbow flexion test). This procedure is also recommended when significant preoperative loss of flexion exists, for which postoperative restoration in joint flexion may precipitate ulnar nerve symptoms. It has generally been recommended that ulnar nerve decompression be considered when preoperative elbow flexion is limited (less than 90 to 110 degrees).[21]

In cases in which a posteromedial capsulectomy is considered, any mechanical or thermal instruments used along the medial ulnohumeral joint and medial gutter render the ulnar nerve susceptible to injury. The concomitant use of suction makes the use of mechanical burrs and shavers even more dangerous. Although the posteromedial capsulectomy may be performed arthroscopically, our preference is to first identify and decompress the ulnar nerve through a limited open approach prior to arthroscopic elbow release, particularly in cases in which a posteromedial release is anticipated. If a limited open approach is chosen for the nerve, it is much easier to perform before the arthroscopic joint release because fluid extravasation and resultant swelling of the soft tissues can obscure tissue planes and local anatomy, rendering nerve dissection more difficult.

After ulnar nerve decompression, the posteromedial capsulectomy may be more safely performed. During the posteromedial release, it is important to understand that the ulnar nerve is closer to the epicondyle than the tip of the olecranon, and thus release of the capsule is safer along the olecranon. A retractor placed in the proximal posterolateral portal, or even in a proximal posterior portal (sometimes using two retractors), is invaluable at this stage.

After anterior and posterior release, intraoperative passive elbow ROM is documented with an expectation for near full terminal flexion and extension regardless of soft tissue swelling.

If the ulnar nerve was decompressed, it may be left in the cubital tunnel (i.e., in situ decompression) or formally transposed anteriorly, depending on the surgeon's preference.

Closure. We prefer to place a drain posteriorly through a separate exit wound rather than through a portal to help prevent formation of a synovial fistula. Portal sites and the ulnar nerve incision, if used, are closed. The elbow is wrapped in a soft compressive dressing; in our practice, we prefer to cut out some of the dressing anteriorly (in the antecubital fossa) to allow more flexion postoperatively because we start continuous passive motion (CPM) immediately.

Open Release

Open débridement should be considered in cases featuring severe elbow contractures with minimal joint motion, prior ulnar nerve transposition surgery, or the presence of significant HO that obliterates normal bony anatomy. For many surgeons these patients are more reliably treated with extensive open débridement rather than arthroscopic débridement to restore motion effectively and safely.

The exposure may include either a medial or lateral approach, although we prefer to use a lateral approach for simple contractures because of its simplicity and access to the radiocapitellar, ulnohumeral, and proximal radioulnar joints. The lateral approach posteriorly uses the internervous Kocher interval between the anconeus and the extensor carpi ulnaris, reflecting the anconeus posteriorly while reflecting the triceps posteriorly from the supracondylar ridge of the humerus. A triceps tenolysis may be performed at this stage. Excising the elbow capsule proximal to the lateral collateral ligament and annular ligamentous complex carries out the deeper exposure of the joint. The radiocapitellar joint may be visualized along with the posterior ulnohumeral joint, where osteophytes may be resected and the radial and olecranon fossae can be débrided of any offending tissue that may cause impingement. The anterior aspect of the joint and anterior capsule is exposed by dissecting the brachialis from the supracondylar ridge proximally and developing the interval between the extensor carpi radialis longus and extensor carpi brevis distally. A tenolysis of the brachialis may be performed; the capsule is then excised from the humerus and the radial and coronoid fossa are cleared of any fibrous or bony tissue responsible for anterior impingement. The posterior and anterior capsules are resected through the posterior and anterior exposures, respectively.

An analogous medial approach may be considered in cases in which significant contracture is present despite joint release from a lateral approach or if the ulnar nerve requires formal exposure and decompression. The subcutaneous tissues are carefully divided, preserving all branches of the medial antebrachial cutaneous nerve. The ulnar nerve is exposed proximal and distal to the joint and is reflected anteriorly. The triceps is then reflected posteriorly from the intermuscular septum, and the posterior ulnohumeral joint is débrided with use of the same technique as described for the lateral approach. The anterior aspect of the joint is exposed by reflecting the brachialis from the supracondylar ridge and dividing the flexor-pronator muscle origin through the juncture of the middle and posterior thirds of the muscle mass. The anterior joint capsule is exposed and débridement can then be carried out as described for the lateral approach. We prefer to transpose the ulnar nerve in a subcutaneous position after joint débridement.

POSTOPERATIVE MANAGEMENT

Follow-up

It is imperative for the surgeon to diligently follow up on these patients in the postoperative period. Patients are typically seen in the office between 10 and 14 days after surgery for suture removal. Although the majority of elbow motion is recovered during the first 6 to 8 weeks, patients can continue to make gains in terminal flexion and extension for several months postoperatively. This phenomenon may occur to a larger degree in patients who had the most severe contractures preoperatively.[13] On the other hand, patients with minor contractures (i.e., total arc >90 degrees preoperatively) may actually lose motion after the release.[13] Patient selection is clearly important, and patients with minor preoperative contractures should be monitored closely.

Rehabilitation

We typically prefer that CPM begin immediately in the recovery room and continue overnight until discharge the following day. Formal therapy is commonly begun on postoperative day 1, at which time the dressing is removed and edema-control modalities (e.g., an edema sleeve or an athletic wrap) are used to limit swelling. Weighted stretches and unrestricted active and passive elbow motion are immediately initiated, and patients use CPM and receive static progressive elbow bracing 2 to 3 times per day after discharge. Flexion and extension are alternated based on the preoperative deficit and the early progress of the elbow. CPM should be continued at home for 3 to 4 weeks along with a formal supervised rehabilitation program.

A nonsteroidal antiinflammatory agent (NSAID) (e.g., indomethacin) is commonly prescribed as prophylaxis against HO for several weeks after surgery. Use of such an agent also helps to limit inflammation of the periarticular soft tissues during rehabilitation. A single dose of radiation therapy (XRT) within 48 hours of surgery, typically 5 to 7 Gy, is considered in select cases with abundant HO, typically in cases that required open capsular release and significant bony resection. XRT has been shown to be effective in preventing the recurrence of HO after elbow release, even for patients at high risk for HO. However, patients are at risk for wound complications with XRT.[22] Therefore we recommend using NSAIDs whenever possible.

Return to Sport

Patients are extensively counseled that strengthening will not commence until the soft tissues have reached equilibrium and postoperative ROM has maximally improved, typically at 2.5 to 3 months after surgery. Return to sport is typically considered at 4 to 6 months after surgery, depending on the needs and demands specific to a given sport. However, the duration between surgery and return to sport is quite variable, and is based on the exact pathology present and the surgical procedure undertaken. A patient with mild stiffness from a loose body that resolves after loose body excision may typically return to sport within several weeks, whereas a patient who has severe stiffness from HO and must undergo open release may require more than 6 months before returning to athletic competition after surgery.

RESULTS

With proper patient selection and surgical indications, excellent outcomes may be achieved with predictable recovery of a functional arc of elbow motion and substantial pain relief. Several studies have reported the efficacy of both arthroscopic and open elbow contracture release procedures (Table 65.1).[18,23-25] It is widely reported that patients regain approximately 50% of lost motion after either treatment. A meta-analysis of the literature suggests that 90% to 95% of patients regain lost motion (defined by at least a 10-degree increase in the arc of motion) and approximately 80% obtain a functional arc of motion (defined as ranging from 30 to 130 degrees); another 5% to 10% get to within 5 to 10 degrees at each end of this functional range.

The use of CPM remains controversial. Early studies demonstrated improved postoperative ROM with CPM, and the use of postoperative CPM was found to improve the total arc of motion after anterior capsulectomy for posttraumatic flexion contracture.[26] However, a more recent retrospective series documented no clinical benefit of CPM after open contracture release.[27]

Complications

Pathologic HO after contracture release has become rare, especially with the development of structured, supervised rehabilitation protocols in the immediate postoperative period. The use of pharmacologic prophylaxis has also limited the development of HO. Although reports are limited regarding the efficacy of postoperative XRT or nonsteroidal antiinflammatory medications as postoperative prophylaxis for HO, the use of these modalities has been demonstrated to be effective

TABLE 65.1   Outcomes After Arthroscopic Release of Elbow Contracture

Author	Methodology	Results
Savoie et al.[19]	24 patients; arthroscopic débridement of coronoid/olecranon processes; olecranon fossa 18 patients underwent radial head resection	Average arc of motion 131 degrees, improvement of 81 degrees; significant decrease in VAS pain score (preoperative 8.2; postoperative 2.2)
Ball et al.[14]	14 patients, arthroscopic contracture release	Average VAS satisfaction 8.4/10, VAS pain score 4.6/10; mean flexion increased from 117.5 to 133 degrees, and extension improved from 35.4 to 9.3 degrees; mean self-reported functional ability score was 28.3/30
Nguyen et al.[30]	22 patients, arthroscopic contracture release	Mean flexion improved from 122 to 141 degrees ($P < .001$); extension improved from 38 to 19 degrees ($P < .001$); mean arc improvement was 38 degrees ($P < .001$); the mean ASES-e score was 31/36
Kelly et al.[16]	25 elbows, arthroscopic débridement	24 were "better" or "much better" postoperatively, with 21 patients reporting minimal or no pain; the average flexion-extension arc improved by 21 degrees

ASES-e, American Shoulder and Elbow Surgeons–Elbow; *VAS,* visual analog scale.

in the prevention of HO formation after surgical procedures of the hip.[28] Our institution recently published a retrospective review demonstrating the efficacy of combined XRT and the use of indomethacin after surgical resection of HO around the elbow, as well as after surgical procedures that carry a high risk of the development of HO. We typically prescribe 75 mg of oral indomethacin to be taken twice daily for 2 weeks after surgery.[29] However, diligent radiographic follow-up is the best way to monitor these patients for the development of this complication.

In a retrospective review of elbow arthroscopies performed for various orthopedic conditions, Kelly et al.[18,19] reported four cases of deep infection, 33 cases of prolonged drainage or superficial infection at a portal site, and 12 transient nerve palsies (affecting five ulnar nerves, four superficial radial nerves, one posterior interosseous nerve, one medial antebrachial cutaneous nerve, and one anterior interosseous nerve). Several other cadaveric studies have carefully described the relationship between neurovascular structures to portal sites and cannula positions; the work of these authors has improved the understanding of anatomy in the area of the elbow and emphasized the importance of judicious portal placement.[30,31]

Several authors have suggested that the risk of nerve injury may be higher with arthroscopic versus open contracture release, which may be attributed to several factors, including the surgeon's experience and the complexity of the surgery. The majority of iatrogenic nerve injuries occurred early during the initial reports of arthroscopic contracture release.[15,16,32,33] Based on our experience, we believe that the majority of intraoperative nerve injuries can be avoided through the diligent use of retractors, the avoidance of suction near a nerve, the use of a shaver instead of a burr near a nerve to avoid the "power-takeoff" effect in which the burr wraps tissue and pulls the nerve into it, and a thorough knowledge and understanding of where the nerves are and/or actually visualizing and retracting them. Most importantly, however, the surgeon may avoid a majority of these complications by recognizing the limits of arthroscopic technique and switching to an open approach in situations in which contracture release is difficult or cannot be safely performed.

For a complete list of references, go to ExpertConsult.com.

SELECTED READINGS

Citation:
Morrey BF. The posttraumatic stiff elbow. *Clin Orthop Relat Res.* 2005;431:26–35.

Level of Evidence:
IV

Summary:
This review article summarizes the surgical treatments for posttraumatic contractures of the elbow, including open débridement and arthroscopic release. Salvage procedures such as interposition arthroplasty and total elbow arthroplasty are also discussed.

Citation:
Jupiter JB, O'Driscoll SW, Cohen MS. The assessment and management of the stiff elbow. *Instr Course Lect.* 2003;52:93–111.

Level of Evidence:
IV

Summary:
The instruction course lecture describes the evaluation of the patient with posttraumatic contracture of the elbow and discusses both nonoperative and operative treatments for restoring elbow motion.

Citation:
Cohen AP, Redden JF, Stanley D. Treatment of osteoarthritis of the elbow: a comparison of open and arthroscopic debridement. *Arthroscopy.* 2000;16(7):701–706.

Level of Evidence:
II

Summary:
This prospective, nonrandomized series compared outcomes after the Outerbridge-Kashiwagi (O-K) procedure with an arthroscopic débridement of the olecranon fossa for mild osteoarthritis of the elbow. The authors found that the O-K procedure resulted in significantly better motion, whereas the arthroscopic procedure provided suitable pain relief.

Citation:
Savoie FH 3rd, Nunley PD, Field LD. Arthroscopic management of the arthritic elbow: indications, technique, and results. *J Shoulder Elbow Surg.* 1999;8(3):214–219.

Level of Evidence:
II

Summary:
The authors report the outcomes of 24 patients who underwent an arthroscopic modification of the Outerbridge-Kashiwagi procedure for elbow stiffness as a result of arthrosis of the joint. The average arc of motion was 131 degrees, representing an 81-degree improvement from preoperative motion.

Citation:
Marshall PD, Fairclough JA, Johnson SR, et al. Avoiding nerve damage during elbow arthroscopy. *J Bone Joint Surg Br.* 1993;75B(1):129–131.

Level of Evidence:
III

Summary:
The authors conducted a cadaveric study investigating the position of portals in arthroscopy relative to the position of motor and sensory nerves within the elbow. Dissection of 20 specimens was undertaken, and the relative positions of the radial, median, and ulnar nerves are reported.

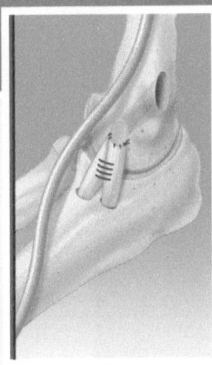

66

Anatomy and Biomechanics of the Hand and Wrist

Raj M. Amin, John V. Ingari

HAND

The human hand is the athlete's tactile connection to his or her sport. Our hands are virtually linked to every sport via a handle, a stick, a glove, or even the bare fingers. Athletes may be said to have good hand-eye coordination, good ball-handling skills, or even quick hands, but in each case the relationship between the sport and the athlete's hands is obvious. Hand anatomy and biomechanics form the framework for understanding the human ability to grip, let go, cup, spread, flex, extend, and even strike, using the most complex anatomic tool of our bodies. The wrist, forming the linkage between the forearm and the hand, is discussed later in this chapter because it allows the hands to be placed in a multitude of positions and is integral to the interactions that lead to throwing, catching, twisting, or any of the innumerable actions that the hands can perform.

Skin

The skin of the hand is specialized to allow the many activities we take for granted. Complex dermatoglyphics, or "fingerprints," are both unique to each individual and allow the fingers to grip of smooth objects. This is similar to the function of a ribbed sole on a running shoe, which allows grip to the smooth surface of a basketball court.[1] Even the moisture on our fingertips is modulated for optimal grip.[1]

The skin on the palmar surface of the hand is tethered to the underlying deeper tissue and ligamentous structures by specialized structures known as the septa of Legueu and Juvara. This arrangement minimizes the natural tendency of the skin to slide over underlying fat and fascia, thereby optimizing grip and creating a sturdy surface for tight grasping.[2] This is in stark contrast to the skin of the dorsal hand (Fig. 66.1A), which is easily pulled and stretched (see Fig. 66.1B). Several reproducible lines on the palms of our hands allow not only flexion of the fingers but also controlled "collapse" of the skin on the palms as well. The thenar, proximal palmar, and distal palmar creases are the visible lines that are evident on uninjured hands (Fig. 66.2A). The creases on the palmar side of the fingers—namely the palmar digital crease, proximal interphalangeal (PIP) flexion crease, and distal interphalangeal (DIP) flexion crease—also accommodate the specialized tethered skin on the palms and fingers while allowing full flexion and extension (see Fig. 66.2B). The creases of the palm and digits also allow communication of anatomic locations on the hand. For example, "a 1-cm transverse laceration at the level of the proximal palmar crease in line with the middle finger ray" communicates the exact location of a hand laceration within the palm. Additionally, these creases often provide frames of reference for underlying structures, which aids in planning surgical incisions.

Nerves

Sensory nerves in the hand are the terminal branches of the radial, ulnar, and median nerves. The nerves of the fingertip pads that allow fine sensation are the terminal branches of the median and ulnar nerves. Although anatomic variability exists, the median nerve innervates the volar thumb and the index, middle, and radial half of the ring finger, whereas the ulnar half of the ring finger and the small finger are innervated by terminal branches of the ulnar nerve. The main nerve branches within the fingers are termed *proper digital nerves* and are further designated as radial or ulnar based on which half of the finger is being described (Fig. 66.3). The radial nerve provides sensation to the dorsum of the hand and digits, but its terminal branches do not technically reach the tip of any digit. Dermatomal diagrams delineate the actual areas innervated by individual nerve roots (primarily C6-C8 in the hand), although some individual variation exists. It is the fine tactile sensation in the hand that allows us to "feel" surfaces, easily sensing the difference between the edge of a quarter and the edge of a nickel, for example. Normal two-point discrimination, our ability to sense two separate points of contact on our fingertips, is generally accepted as 5 mm (Fig. 66.4A and B).

Muscles and Tendons

The muscles and tendons of the hand are the "motors" and linkages that work the joints, allowing the flexion, extension, abduction, adduction and opposition that occur fluidly and seemingly effortlessly in our hands with nearly every task of daily life. The muscles are divided into those that are intrinsic to the hand, meaning that they originate and terminate within the hand, and the extrinsic muscles, which originate more proximally in the forearm but terminate in the hand. The intrinsic muscles are the lumbrical, dorsal, and palmar interossei and the thenar and hypothenar muscles. The thenar muscles are specifically named abductor pollicis brevis, flexor pollicis brevis, and opponens pollicis. The hypothenar muscles, similarly, are named abductor digiti minimi, flexor digiti minimi, and opponens digiti minimi. Four dorsal interosseous muscles serve to abduct

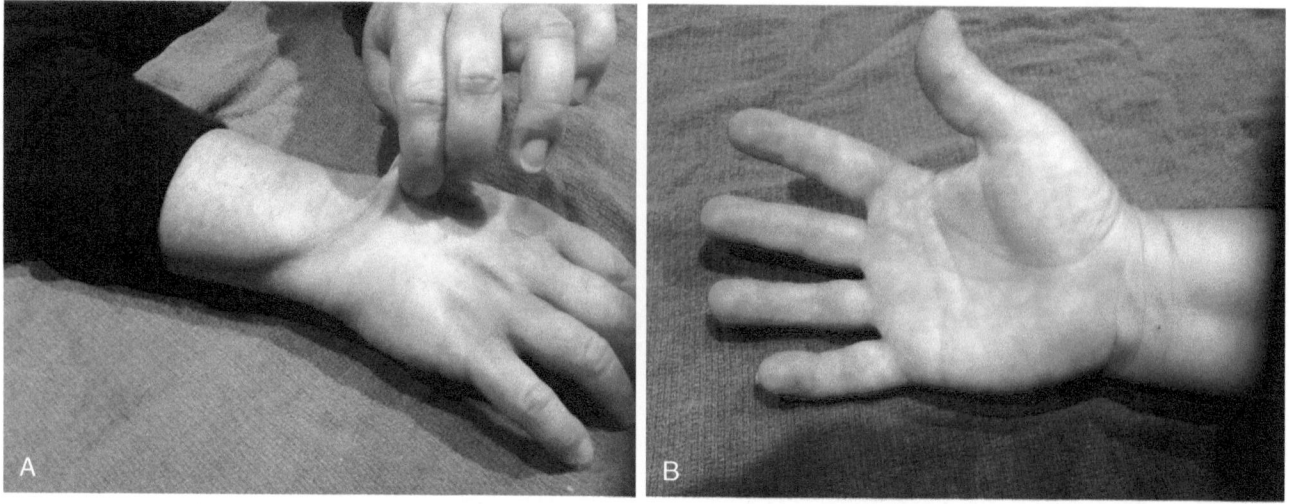

Fig. 66.1 (A) The skin on the dorsum of the hand is relatively smooth and elastic, allowing the skin to be easily slid or stretched, as seen here. (B) The palmar skin is creased, fingerprinted, and tethered to the underlying tissues to allow optimal grip and tactile sensation of objects held in the hand.

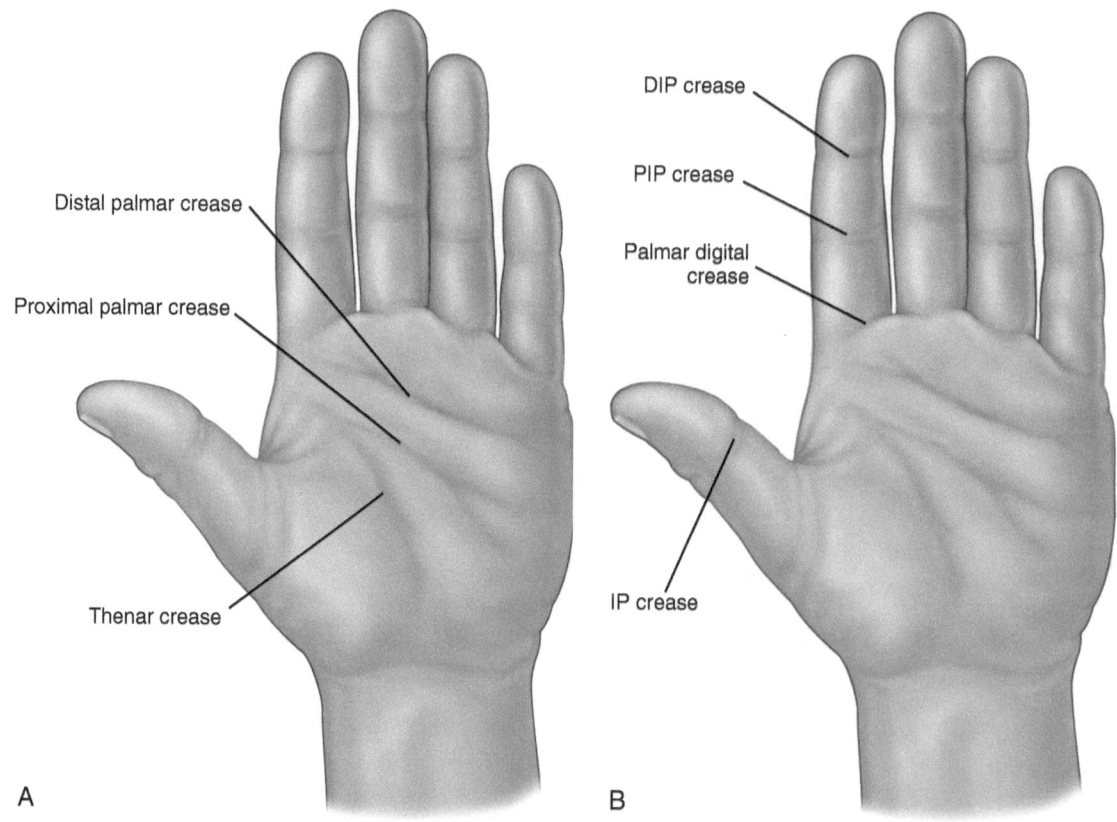

Fig. 66.2 (A) The proximal palmar crease, distal palmar crease, and thenar crease are normal creases found in most hands. Occasional variations occur. (B) The creases of the thumb and digits are shown, including the palmar digital crease, the proximal interphalangeal *(PIP)* crease, and the distal interphalangeal *(DIP)* crease. The thumb has only an interphalangeal *(IP)* crease, as shown.

the digits, whereas the three palmar interosseous muscles cause adduction of the fingers. All of the interossei are innervated by the ulnar nerve. The lumbrical muscles have been given the moniker "workhorse of the extensor mechanism."[3] The lumbrical muscles course on the radial side of each metacarpal and then travel via the radial lateral bands to join in confluence with the

extensor mechanism. The lumbrical muscles and their tendinous extension run palmar to the axis of rotation at the metacarpopha-langeal (MCP) joint but dorsal to the axis of rotation at the PIP and DIP joints. Therefore when the lumbrical muscles contract, flexion occurs at the MCP joint and extension occurs at the PIP and DIP joints (Fig. 66.5 A and B). The lumbrical muscles originate on the flexor digitorum profundus (FDP) tendon just distal to the carpal tunnel and then insert via the radial lateral bands into the extensor mechanism. The actions of the FDP and lumbrical muscles are antagonistic; thus this unique arrangement allows the contraction of one muscle to maximally relax the other.

The extrinsic flexors in the hand are the flexor pollicis longus, which causes flexion of the interphalangeal joint of the thumb, and the flexor digitorum superficialis and FDP, which flex the proximal and DIP joints in the fingers, respectively (Fig. 66.6A and B). Both the flexor digitorum superficialis and FDP tendons run through the carpal tunnel, across the hand, and into the fingers. The extrinsic extensor muscles of the hand are discussed in the wrist section because all of these muscles cross the wrist joints but may act at the wrist, digits, or thumb.

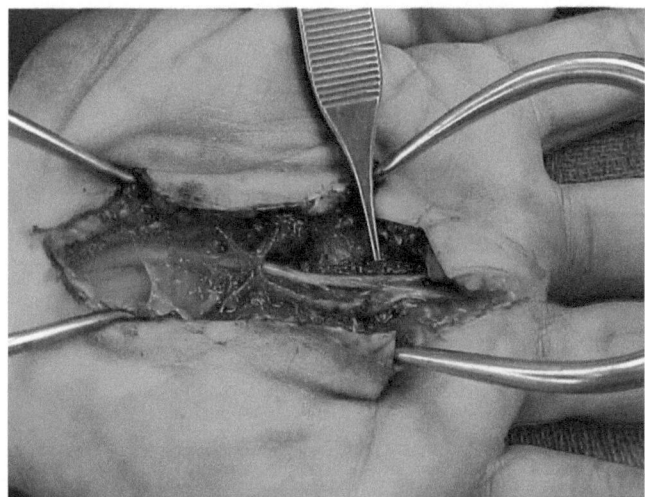

Fig. 66.3 The common digital nerve to the middle and ring fingers in the palm can be seen to bifurcate and give off the radial digital nerve to the ring finger and the ulnar digital nerve to the middle finger.

Joints

The joints in the hand are primarily hinge, or ginglymus, joints, but they also allow some translational and rotational moments. This mechanism is especially true at the MCP joints; it enables the ability to spread the fingers, slightly rotate them, and fine-tune their grip on both large and small objects.

Metacarpophalangeal Joint of the Fingers

The bony architecture of the MCP joint allows for significant motion, including hyperextension and flexion in the sagittal plane, adduction/abduction in the frontal plane, and rotatory motion of the base of the proximal phalanx (P-1) on the metacarpal head. The cartilaginous surface of the metacarpal head has a trapezoidal shape, being broader on the palmar surface. MCP joint stability is dependent on surrounding collateral and accessory collateral ligaments, volar plate, capsule, and extrinsic flexor and extensor tendons.[4] The collateral and accessory collateral ligaments provide lateral static stability. The collateral ligaments originate dorsal to the metacarpal head's axis of motion and insert into tubercles on the sides of the P-1. Accessory collateral ligaments have their origin palmar to the proper collateral ligaments and insert into the palmar base of P-1 and the volar plate.[2] Because of the dorsal metacarpal origin of the collateral ligaments and the cam shape of the metacarpal head in the sagittal plane, the ligaments have laxity in extension but are taut in flexion.[2] This characteristic is the basis for the recommendation that most hand injuries be splinted with the MCP joints in full flexion, or the so-called "safe position."[5] The safe position for the interphalangeal joints is in extension because of disparate anatomy at the PIP and DIP joints.[6] Accessory collateral ligaments, along with interosseous and lumbrical tendons, provide additional lateral (adduction/abduction) stability. The volar plate provides a block to hyperextension and constitutes the third side of the anatomic box, which provides static MCP stability. The volar plate has a broad, firm distal attachment to P-1 and a membranous loose

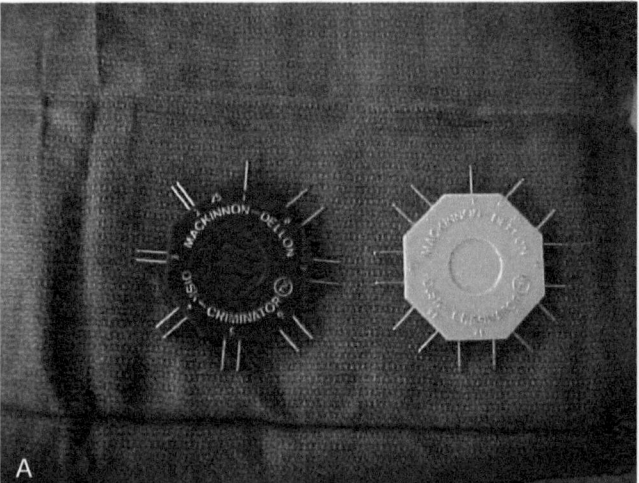

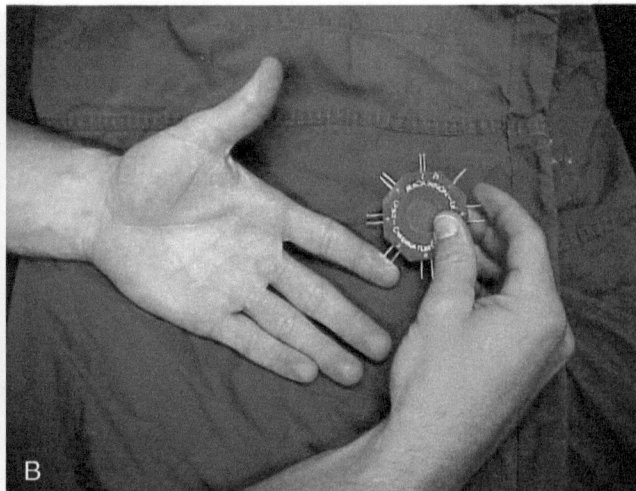

Fig. 66.4 (A) Two-point discriminators, such as the pictured, are necessary tools to evaluate the sensory examination of the fingertips. (B) Normal two-point discrimination is 5 mm or less. The patient should be able to feel the two metal prongs as two separate stimuli when they are 5 mm apart. If the patient is unable to feel two points at a spread of 15 mm, the area is completely insensate.

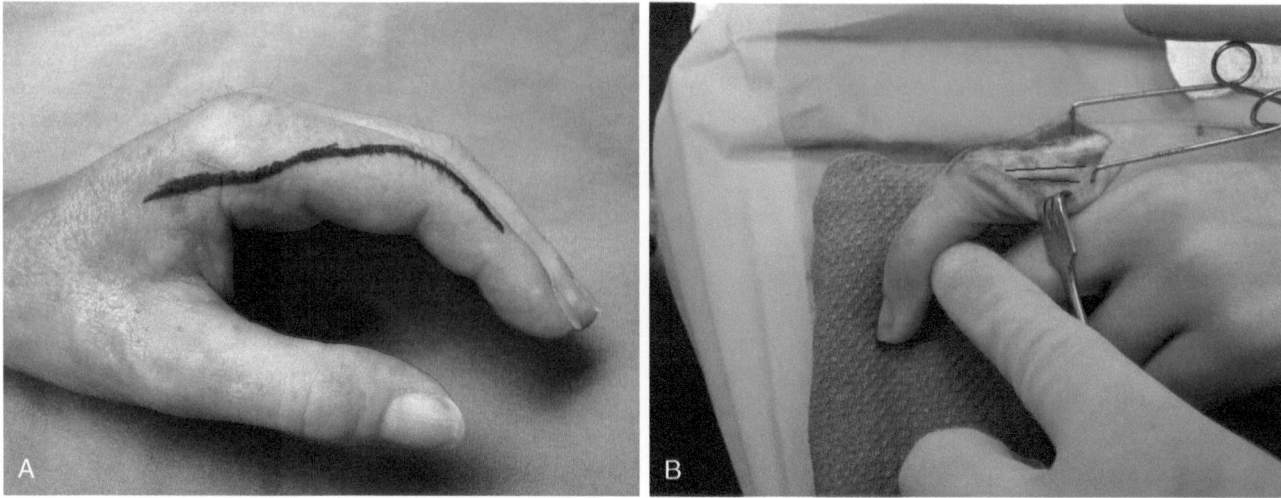

Fig. 66.5 (A) The lumbrical musculotendinous unit runs palmar to the axis of rotation at the metacarpophalangeal (MCP) joint, then courses dorsal to the axis of rotation at the proximal interphalangeal and distal interphalangeal joints. (B) The lateral band of the extensor mechanism is outlined in this surgical case. Notice that it is palmar to the axis of rotation at the MCP joint and then becomes dorsal as it travels distally.

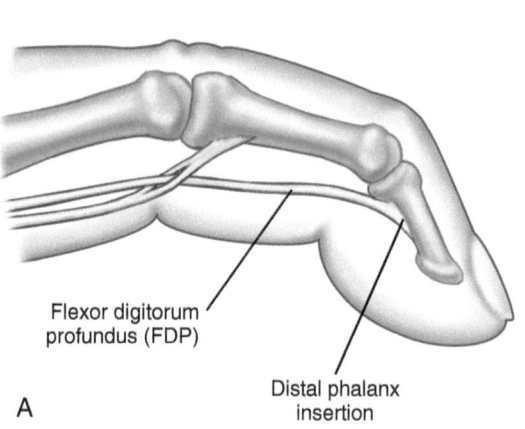

Flexor digitorum
profundus (FDP)

Distal phalanx
insertion

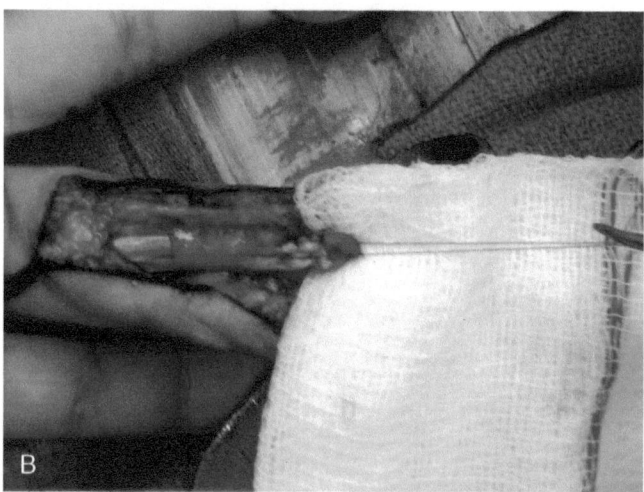

Fig. 66.6 (A) The flexor digitorum profundus *(FDP)* tendon, schematically shown here, inserts into the palmar aspect of the distal phalanx, causing flexion of the distal interphalangeal (DIP) joint when the muscle belly contracts. (B) This surgical image depicts the actual FDP tendon just prior to being reattached after rupture. Reattaching the tendon surgically restores the ability to flex the DIP joint.

origin from the metacarpal neck. The laxity of the collateral ligaments in extension places the volar plate at risk of rupture (usually proximally) with excessive or forceful MCP hyperextension. The dorsal capsule is relatively loose, and the extrinsic extensor tendons extend the MCP joint through the sagittal bands' attachment to the base of P-1 and the volar plate.[3]

Proximal Interphalangeal Joint

The PIP joint is a highly congruous hinge joint, with stability provided by the matching articular surfaces of the phalanges and the combination of a thick volar plate and stout collateral ligaments. The tight fit of the opposing articular contours increases stability, especially when the PIP is under axial load.[3] The collateral ligaments are thick and composed of proper and accessory components. The proper ligaments insert into the base of the middle phalanx (P-2) and the volar plate, whereas the accessory collateral ligaments insert only into the volar plate. The volar plate is very thick distally where it inserts into the volar lip of P-2, whereas proximally it thins out and has two proximal projections that attach to P-1, called the *check rein ligaments*. This arrangement allows the PIP joint to flex more than 110 degrees. The condyles of the head of P-1 are not cam-shaped; therefore the PIP joint does not become as stiff as other joints in the hand, relatively speaking, when immobilized in full extension for a short period as the collateral ligaments stay stretched. On the contrary, the PIP joint has a propensity to develop flexion contracture, with shortening of the volar plate, when immobilized or held in a flexed position as the result of an injury. PIP flexion contractures are most pronounced after trauma to the ring and small digits. Eaton described the soft tissue constraints of the PIP joint as three sides of a box; instability occurs when at least two sides of this box are disrupted.[4] The central slip of the extensor apparatus attaches at the dorsal epiphysis of P-2 and is frequently avulsed in volar PIP dislocations from a hyperflexion mechanism of injury. The PIP joint is notorious for the challenges posed by intraarticular injury and the consequences of poor management, often leading to recalcitrant stiffness.

Distal Interphalangeal Joint

Like the PIP joint, the DIP joint acts as a hinge. It allows flexion and extension, but its bony and ligamentous anatomy effectively eliminates lateral motion and minimizes rotation. Digital DIP flexion is provided through contraction of the FDP, and DIP extension occurs via the contraction of the lateral bands, which coalesce into a terminal extensor tendon insertion at the distal phalanx dorsal epiphysis.[3] Common sports-related injuries involving the DIP joint are "mallet finger," which refers to an avulsion of the terminal extensor mechanism, and "jersey finger," which refers to a disruption to the FDP tendon at its insertion (Fig. 66.7A and B).

Thumb

The human thumb is unique in its ability to provide circumduction and opposition to the other digits, giving the human hand its superb functional capacity to grasp, pinch, and oppose. Athletes and physicians alike are familiar with the thumb's crucially important role in hand function through sporting activity. Whether an athlete handles a ball, a pole, or a stick or checks reins, the opposable thumb's function is indispensable in the interaction of the athlete with his or her competitive environment. Essential functions of large-object (cylindrical) grasp, key (power) pinch, and tip (precision) pinch are dependent on normal thumb stability, mobility, sensibility, and length. The thumb is frequently injured owing it its "at risk" position out of the plane of the palm and its involvement in the most demanding of tasks.

Because of the thumb's specific osseous makeup, with a specialized basilar joint, along with its at-risk position, injury patterns in the thumb are unique. For example, the MCP joint is more exposed than the corresponding joint in the digits, leading to a higher incidence of collateral ligament tears in the thumb. Injuries to the thumb require special attention because the thumb's functions are unique and highly dependent on ligamentous, bony, and tendinous integrity.

WRIST

The hand and wrist are intimately linked; therefore any study of the anatomy and biomechanics of the hand and wrist as a single functional unit is both appropriate and essential. Although the biomechanics of each individual articulation in the wrist are unique and separate from the biomechanics in each of the digits, the conglomerate actions of both hand and wrist are necessary in essentially all sports. Throwing a baseball, for example, involves complex interactions of finger flexion, grip, and extension coupled with motions of wrist extension and radial deviation; these are followed by wrist flexion and ulnar deviation to achieve the goal of directed accurate ball release.[7] Virtually all sports—from baseball, basketball, football, swimming, and even ping-pong—depend on the complex interactions of the hand and wrist for successful performance.[8] This section focuses on the integral linkage of the hand to the forearm.

The wrist in the adult athlete is amazingly complex. An understanding of wrist anatomy and kinematics helps to explain why this complex arrangement of bones, ligaments, tendons, and neurovascular structures is susceptible to athletic injury. In the following paragraphs the anatomy, kinematics, and some pertinent physical examination findings in the wrist are outlined. Discussion of the various specific injuries, their diagnosis, treatment options, and authors' preferred methods are presented in other chapters, with emphasis on the athlete as the patient and return to sports as the goal.

Wrist Anatomy and Biomechanics

The bony anatomy of the wrist, or carpus, comprises eight carpal bones and their articulations with one another as well as with the radius, ulna, and metacarpals (Fig. 66.8). The scaphoid, lunate, triquetrum, hamate, capitate, trapezoid, trapezium, and pisiform create a uniquely mobile, interconnected bony network that allows motion in a limitless number of planes. For example, the motion involved in throwing a dart exemplifies the combination of the wrist moving from relative extension and radial deviation to a position of flexion and ulnar deviation in a fluid, almost effortless action.[8–10] The simple motion of the dart throw belies the complexity of the muscle action, tendon excursions, and carpal bone movements occurring in the wrist simultaneously with grip and release in the hand. Most of this natural motion occurs not through the radiocarpal joint but rather through the

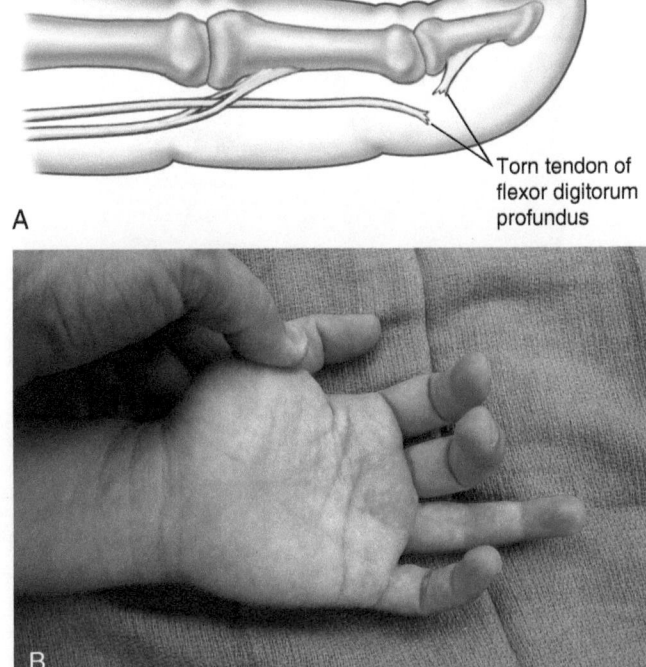

Torn tendon of flexor digitorum profundus

Fig. 66.7 A jersey finger occurs when the flexor digitorum profundus tendon is disrupted or torn from its attachment to the distal phalanx (A). There is resultant loss of the normal flexion cascade of the digits, and the involved finger remains extended at rest (B).

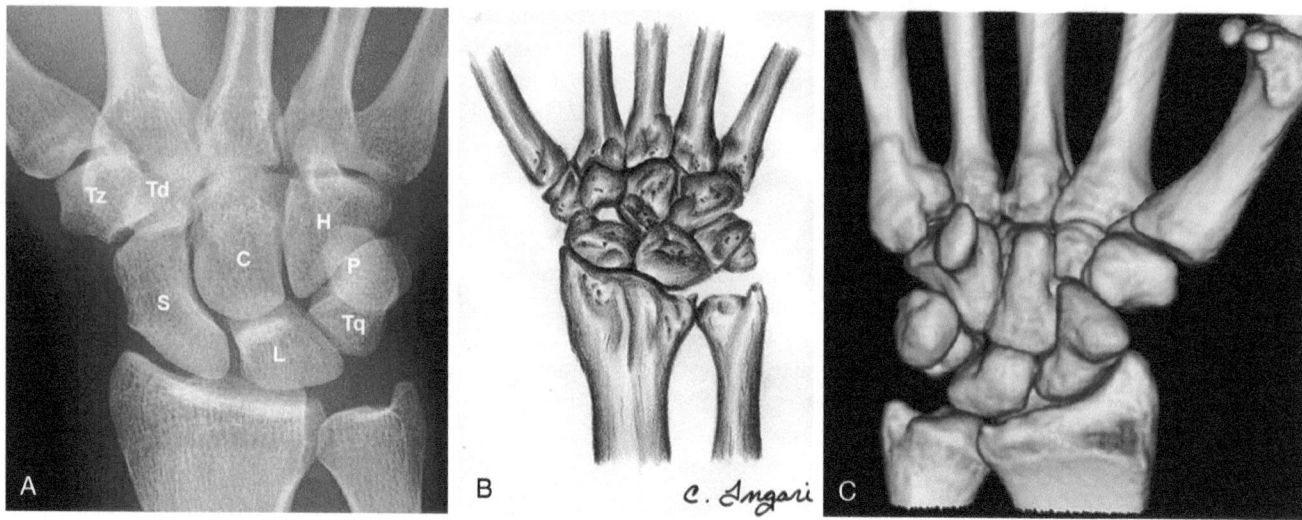

Fig. 66.8 (A) A posteroanterior radiograph of the carpus, with each of the carpal bones identified. (B) Artist's rendering of the dorsal view of the carpus. (C) A three-dimensional computed tomography scan depicting a volar view of the carpus. Notice how the hook of the hamate projects palmarly. *C,* Capitate; *H,* hamate; *L,* lunate; *P,* pisiform; *S,* scaphoid; *Td,* trapezoid; *Tq,* triquetrum; *Tz,* trapezium.

midcarpal joint, which obviously has implications not only for the initial understanding of injury but also for methods of rehabilitation after the nonoperative and operative treatment of various injuries.

The basic carpal anatomy and kinematics have been likened to an oval ring,[6,11] a proximal and distal row,[12–14] and three columns[15] as well as combinations of these. Each of the carpal bones except the capitolunate joint has a ligamentous attachment to the adjacent bone within its row. These attachments are the intrinsic intercarpal ligaments, such as the scapholunate ligament and lunotriquetral ligament joining the adjacent bones in the proximal row. The scapholunate ligament is stouter on the dorsal aspect, whereas the lunotriquetral ligament is stouter on the palmar aspect. The extrinsic ligaments, conversely, provide connection between the carpals and the radius and ulna proximally as well as to the metacarpals distally. Extrinsic ligaments include the radiocarpal ligaments and the carpometacarpal ligaments. The radiocarpal ligaments are more stout on the palmar aspect than on the dorsal aspect and are usually best seen during wrist arthroscopy from within the joint.[16] Viewed arthroscopically, the most radial volar extrinsic ligament is the radioscaphocapitate ligament. Progressing in the ulnar direction, next is the long radiolunate ligament, followed by the radioscapholunate (RSL) ligament. The RSL ligament is directly in line with the articulation between the scaphoid and the lunate when viewed arthroscopically and is otherwise known as the ligament of Testut. It is primarily a vascular structure, contributing little structural support. Immediately ulnar to the RSL ligament is the short radiolunate ligament. Continuing ulnarly is the ulnolunate ligament, followed by the ulnotriquetral ligament. The two primary dorsal extrinsic radiocarpal ligaments are the dorsal radiotriquetral (radiocarpal) ligament and the dorsal intercarpal ligament. All extrinsic wrist ligaments are thickenings of the joint capsule, which underscores the complexity of providing stability while allowing free, unhindered movement of the wrist. Pathology involving any of these ligaments, whether intrinsic or extrinsic,

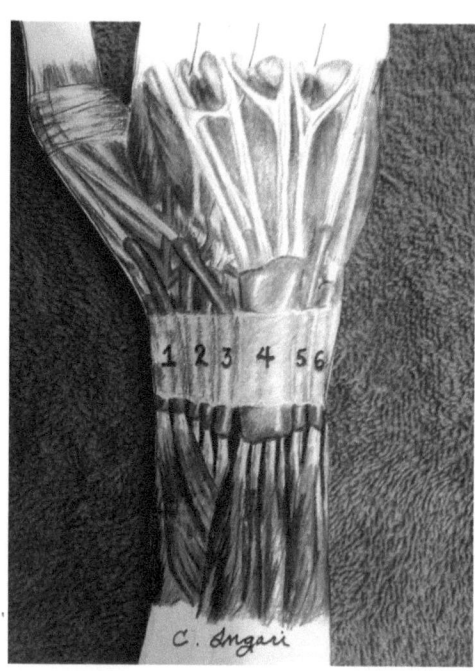

Fig. 66.9 The extensor compartments of the wrist are depicted here in an artist's rendering. The compartments from radial to ulnar are as follows: *1,* abductor pollicis longus and extensor pollicis brevis; *2,* extensor carpi radialis longus and extensor carpi radialis brevis; *3,* extensor pollicis longus; *4,* extensor digitorum communis and extensor indicis proprius; *5,* extensor digiti minimi; and *6,* extensor carpi ulnaris.

may lead to pain, limitation of motion, and eventually carpal arthritis and collapse.[15]

Extensor Tendons of the Wrist and Hand

Any thorough discussion of wrist anatomy must include the extensor tendons as they cross the wrist. The six dorsal compartments of the wrist are arranged in numeric order from radial to ulnar, and each compartment houses one or more wrist, hand, or digital extensors (Fig. 66.9). Beginning radially, the first dorsal

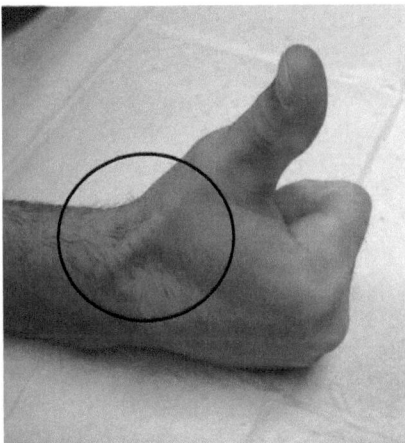

Fig. 66.10 The extensor pollicis longus tendon, seen coursing obliquely across the dorsal wrist and hand, extends the interphalangeal joint of the thumb.

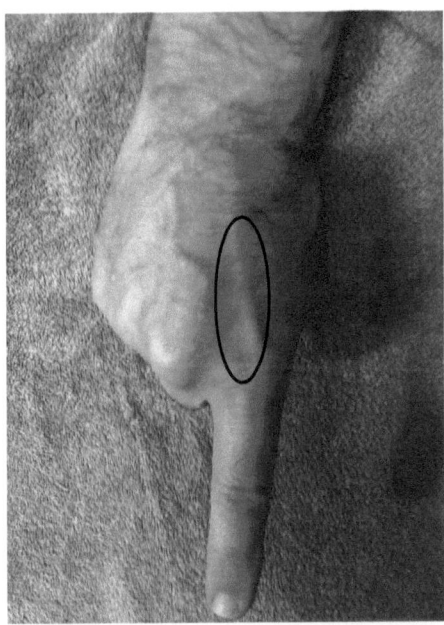

Fig. 66.11 The extensor indicis proprius allows independent extension of the index finger even when the other digits are maximally flexed.

compartment contains the tendons of the abductor pollicis longus (APL) and the extensor pollicis brevis. The APL inserts on the base of the thumb metacarpal and abducts the thumb ray. The extensor pollicis brevis, a more diminutive tendon that lies dorsal to the APL, is attached to the base of the proximal phalanx of the thumb, and its action is extension of the thumb MCP joint. These tendons may lie within or in different subsheaths within the first dorsal compartment. The second dorsal compartment comprises two tendons, the extensor carpi radialis longus and the extensor carpi radialis brevis. These wrist extensors insert dorsally at the bases of the index and middle finger metacarpals, respectively. The third dorsal compartment has only a single tendon, the extensor pollicis longus. The tendon turns 40 degrees radially as it courses around the ulnar aspect of Lister's tubercle and then runs obliquely across the carpus, inserting into the dorsum of the base of the distal phalanx of the thumb. Its primary action is to extend the interphalangeal joint of the thumb but also to act as an adductor of the thumb (Fig. 66.10). The fourth dorsal compartment houses the tendons of the extensor digitorum communis and extensor indicis proprius. These tendons, via the central slips of the extensor mechanism, insert onto the dorsal aspect of the base of the middle phalanx of the index through small fingers. Although the primary function of these tendons is MCP extension through the sagittal bands, they also participate via a complex mechanism in the extension of the interphalangeal joints along with the lumbrical and interosseous muscles. The extensor indicis proprius allows independent extension of the index finger even when the remaining digits are held in flexion (Fig. 66.11). The fifth dorsal compartment, which overlies the distal radioulnar joint, contains the tendon of the extensor digiti minimi. This tendon allows independent extension of the small finger via its insertion onto the dorsal aspect of the middle phalanx of small finger. The sixth dorsal compartment, coursing intimately upon the dorsal ulnar aspect of the ulnar head, comprises the tendon of the extensor carpi ulnaris. This tendon, via its insertion at the base of the small finger metacarpal, allows wrist extension and ulnar deviation simultaneously.

Wrist Flexors

Three primary wrist flexors cross the wrist, with their respective muscle bellies lying further proximal in the forearm. They are the flexor carpi radialis (FCR), flexor carpi ulnaris (FCU), and palmaris longus (PL). The FCR courses adjacent to the scaphotrapezial articulation and inserts at the base of the second metacarpal. The FCU blends into the sesamoid pisiform at the volar ulnar wrist. Interestingly, 13% to 15% of normal adults do not have a PL, although the actual number varies depending on the population studied.[7] The PL is often used as a tendon autograft in upper extremity reconstructive procedures to replace tendinous deficits or augment ligamentous stability.

Vascular Anatomy

The vascular supply to the wrist and hand is from a rich network of anastomosing vessels that originate primarily from the radial artery, ulnar artery, and interosseous arteries (Fig. 66.12). Gelberman's classic cadaveric studies[17,18] delineated three dorsal arches and three palmar arches that are longitudinally fed by the radial artery laterally and the ulnar artery medially.[17] These arches, along with several recurrent branches, form a rich network of vessels supplying the carpus and hand. On the palmar side, the most distal arch is the superficial palmar arch, formed by the main continuation of the ulnar artery with an anastomosis to the radial artery in most hands. The deep palmar arch is located more proximally and is formed by the anastomosis of the radial artery and the deep branch of the ulnar artery. The superficial palmar arch courses immediately distal to the distal edge of the transverse carpal ligament. Gelberman et al.[17,18] also described the arterial anatomy of the carpal bones themselves and specifically noted that single vessels supply the scaphoid, capitate, and 87% of lunates examined, which explains why those three bones are at risk for vascular compromise with fractures or other trauma.

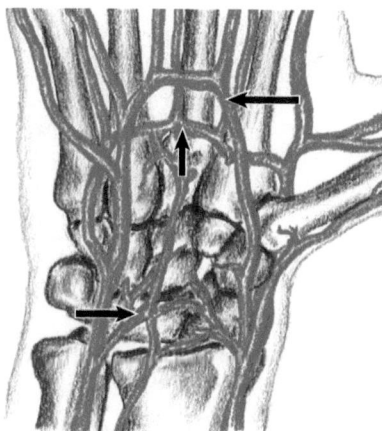

C. Ingari

Fig. 66.12 Vascular anatomy of the carpus. The proximal and distal palmar arches are part of a rich anastomotic blood supply of the wrist. *Bottom arrow*, radiocarpal arch; *middle arrow*, deep palmar arch; *top arrow*, superficial palmar arch.

The vascular anatomy of the wrist and the carpal bones most at risk for osteonecrosis have been reexamined by Botte et al.,[19] confirming Gelberman's original work.

SUMMARY

The hand and wrist comprise a complex array of tendons, muscles, nerves, arteries, and bones that all come together not just anatomically but functionally to allow the athlete to effortlessly throw a baseball or a dart, swing a tennis racket or a baseball bat, and virtually move in any and all directions during sporting activity. The actions of the hand and wrist are intimately coordinated, as ball release—mainly a finger function—follows closely after the wrist is snapped from a dorsal and radial "cocked" position into a palmar and ulnar "follow through" position. Any injury to the hand or wrist may lead to a loss of function as well as pain, impairing participation in virtually all athletic endeavors. This chapter, in outlining the anatomy and biomechanics of the wrist and hand, provides the reader with a basic understanding of the underpinnings of their structure and function as well as some general history, physical description, and radiologic evaluation tools that are such a vital part of what we do daily as physicians.

For a complete list of references, go to ExpertConsult.com.

SELECTED READINGS

Citation:

Garcia-Elias M. Carpal instabilities and dislocations. In: Green DP, Hotchkiss RN, Pederson WC, eds. *Green's Operative Hand Surgery.* Vol 1. 5th ed. New York: Elsevier; 2005.

Level of Evidence:

I

Summary:

This comprehensive textbook chapter delineates the anatomy and biomechanics of the carpus along with pathologic injury to the wrist and is the single most important current compilation of existing works regarding wrist biomechanics and associated pathology.

Citation:

Wolfe SW, Crisco JJ, Orr CM, et al. The dart-throwing motion of the wrist: is it unique to humans? *J Hand Surg Am.* 2006;31:1429–1437.

Level of Evidence:

V

Summary:

The standard motion from dorsoradial to palmar-ulnar in the "dart-throw" motion is examined in this thoughtful summary. The evolution of the dart-throw motion is discussed.

Citation:

Pappas AM, Morgan WJ, Schulz LA, et al. Wrist kinematics during pitching. A preliminary report. *Am J Sports Med.* 1995;23:312–315.

Level of Evidence:

V

Summary:

An in-depth evaluation of the biomechanics of wrist motion during baseball pitching is described. Unique baseball throwing motions and carpal biomechanics are discussed.

Citation:

Smith RJ. Intrinsic muscles of the fingers: function, dysfunction and surgical reconstruction. *AAOS Instr Course Lect.* 1975;200–220.

Level of Evidence:

I

Summary:

This instructional course lecture by Richard Smith is considered a classic work on the anatomy and biomechanics of the hand. No anatomic study of the hand or wrist is complete without referencing Smith's brilliant evaluations of the intrinsic muscles of the hand.

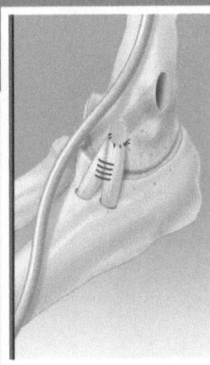

67

Hand and Wrist Diagnosis and Decision-Making

Patrick G. Marinello, R. Glenn Gaston, Eliott P. Robinson, Gary M. Lourie

OVERVIEW

Athletic participation frequently places the hand and wrist at risk of injury, which may lead to sprains, fractures, and dislocations. Reports in the literature suggest that 3% to 25% of all athletic injuries involve the hand and wrist.[1-4] Additionally, overuse in competition and training may lead to tendinopathy and tendon rupture. Certain injuries are more common in particular sports and various playing positions. For instance, baseball players are subject to repeated blunt trauma to the palm from catching and batting; consequently fractures to the hook of the hamate are high on the differential diagnosis. For cyclists, gripping of the handlebar may cause compression of the ulnar nerve at the wrist.[5] Certain sports place exceedingly high demands on the hand and wrist. For instance, gymnasts are reported to have a 49% to 87% incidence of wrist injury over the course of their participation.[6,7]

Consultants must therefore be familiar with the spectrum of pathology affecting the athlete's hand and wrist and then use a thorough and methodical history and physical examination to narrow the differential diagnosis. With the numerous pathologic conditions that may affect the wrist, we suggest a four-quadrant approach for describing the hand and wrist anatomically. These quadrants are as follows: the *radial quadrant*, defined by the area from the flexor carpi radialis (FCR) to the extensor carpi radialis longus (ECRL); the *dorsal quadrant*, defined by the area between the ECRL and the extensor carpi ulnaris (ECU); the *ulnar quadrant*, defined by the area from the ECU to the flexor carpi ulnaris (FCU); and the *volar quadrant*, from the FCU to the FCR. This chapter discusses specific conditions encountered within each of these quadrants in an effort to compartmentalize the possible differential diagnosis of an injured athlete (Table 67.1). Such a differential diagnosis is critical to have in mind in examining the athlete's hand and wrist.

HISTORY AND PHYSICAL EXAM

As with any patient encounter, general information should initially be gathered on all patients, including the individual's age, sport, position, hand dominance, any preexisting pain or injury to the involved hand/wrist, worsening or alleviating factors, and associated medical conditions.[8] In obtaining a history, the patient should be asked about the chronicity, mechanism of injury, initial management, subjective weakness, and any associated loss of

consciousness. For athletes, it is important to know the player's sport and position as well as the time of season to accurately understand the specific stresses placed on the hand and wrist. This is important not only for diagnosis of the injury but also to guide appropriate return to play (RTP). The identical injury in the throwing hand of a quarterback will likely be managed very differently than the same injury in a defensive lineman.

In examining a patient's wrist and forearm, the examiner should be seated across from the patient with the patient's elbow resting on the examination table, the hand toward the ceiling, and the forearm in neutral rotation (Fig. 67.1). General inspection should include any focal areas of swelling, ecchymosis, effusion, open wound or laceration, and any finger or joint misalignment. The patient should be asked to point to the area of maximal tenderness, which should be evaluated last. This is important not only to effectively rule out associated pathology but also to make the patient as comfortable as possible and gain his or her trust.

Next, active and passive range of motion (ROM) should be evaluated with the use of a goniometer. This should be determined for all relevant joints of the digits, thumb, and wrist. Specifically, active and passive motion of the wrist includes flexion and extension, radial and ulnar deviation, as well as pronation and supination. During active or passive motion, any pain or mechanical symptoms of locking or popping should be documented. It is quite common for true carpal pathology to involve some loss of wrist flexion. Normal wrist active ROM is approximately 80 degrees flexion, 70 degrees extension, 30 degrees ulnar deviation, 20 degrees radial deviation, and 90 degrees of both pronation and supination. ROM is always compared with the opposite side.

Next, grip strength should be obtained with the use of a dynamometer and compared with the contralateral, unaffected side. Weakness of grip strength is a very sensitive global assessment tool for wrist and hand pain and can be used to track improvement in subsequent visits and also aid in RTP decisions (many physicians use 85% grip strength as a relative guideline in the RTP algorithm).

The most useful tool in ascertaining the correct diagnosis for hand and wrist pathologies is knowledge of the surface anatomy. The majority of hand and wrist structures are directly palpable once the examiner learns their exact locations. The point of maximal tenderness is the most critical physical examination maneuver in obtaining the correct diagnosis in the hand and wrist.

TABLE 67.1 Differential Diagnosis Based on Quadrant Location in the Wrist

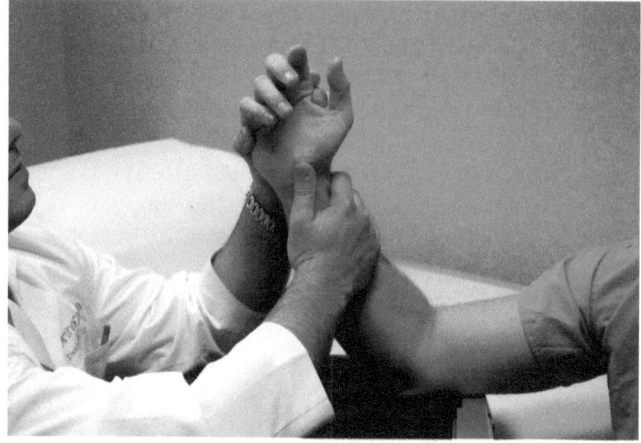

Radial Quadrant	Dorsal Quadrant	Ulnar Quadrant	Volar Quadrant

• De Quervain tenosynovitis
• Intersection syndrome
• FCR tendinopathy
• Scaphoid fracture
• CMC fracture/dislocation
• Trapezial ridge fracture
• CMC synovitis
• Volar wrist ganglion
• Superficial radial nerve entrapment
• CMC or STT arthritis
	• Carpal instability (SL ligament tears, midcarpal instability)
	• Perilunate injuries
	• Extensor tendinopathy
	• Carpal boss
	• Distal radius fractures
	• Capitate and lunate fractures
	• Kienbock disease
	• Dorsal ganglion cysts
		• ECU tendinopathy
		• TFCC tear
		• DRUJ arthritis
		• FCU tendonitis
		• Ulnar impaction
		• LT ligament tear
			• Pisiform
			  • Arthritis
			  • Fracture
			  • FCU insertional tendonitis
			• Hamate hook fracture
			• Ulnar nerve and artery injuries/compression
			• Median nerve injuries/compression

CMC, Carpometacarpal; *ECU,* extensor carpi ulnaris; *FCR,* flexor carpi radialis; *FCU,* flexor carpi ulnaris; *LT,* lunotriquetral; *SL,* scapholunate; *STT,* scaphotrapezotrapezoidal.

Fig. 67.1 Proper position for wrist examination.

Lastly no physical examination is complete without a detailed neurovascular examination. Radial and ulnar pulses as well as capillary refill to all fingertips should be documented in all patients. If there is any concern for vascular compromise, an Allen test should be performed. This is described in detail in the physical examination portion of this chapter. Median, ulnar, and radial sensory examination should be carried out preferably with a two-point discriminator, with normal being less than 5 mm. Intrinsic and extrinsic muscle strength should be documented, along with any associated muscle atrophy. Sport-specific neurovascular pathologies exist, such as ulnar nerve entrapment in Guyon's canal in cyclists,[9,10] ulnar digital nerve injuries in bowlers, and hypothenar hammer syndrome in baseball catchers[11]; these can help the examiner to focus the exam.

Although discussed in a different chapter, the elbow should always be evaluated as well, since concomitant injuries can occur and be overlooked in the presence of a hand or wrist injury. Finally, the physical examination of the wrist should proceed in a systematic fashion. Each examiner will develop a personal approach, but in general a quadrant-based approach culminating with the region of maximal tenderness is recommended. The remainder of this chapter is devoted to exploring the physical exam of the hand and wrist and a discussion of associated pathology.

RADIAL QUADRANT

The radial quadrant is defined as the area extending from the FCR to the ECRL (Fig. 67.2). Common pathologies affecting the radial quadrant include FCR tendinopathy, scaphoid or trapezial ridge fractures, De Quervain tenosynovitis, intersection syndrome, thumb carpometacarpal (CMC) synovitis, fracture or dislocation, volar wrist ganglion, superficial radial nerve entrapment, and scaphotrapezotrapezoidal (STT) or thumb CMC arthritis.

On examination, the FCR tendon is subcutaneous and can be palpated in its entirety from the musculotendinous junction until it enters the fibro-osseous FCR tunnel at the STT joint on its way to insert on the second metacarpal base. The FCR can be more easily visualized by placing the wrist in flexion and slight radial deviation and having the patient resist wrist flexion. Tenderness along the FCR tendon distally is seen in FCR tendinopathy or FCR tunnel syndrome and may be exacerbated with resisted wrist flexion. Just distal to the wrist flexion crease and in line with the course of the FCR is the bony protuberance of the distal pole of the scaphoid (volar tubercle or scaphoid

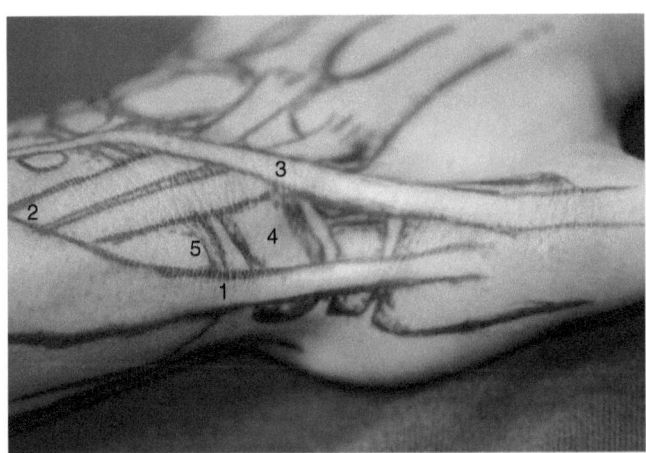

Fig. 67.2 Illustrated surface anatomy of the radial compartment. *1*, First dorsal compartment (APL and EPB) and location of pain in De Quervain tenosynovitis. *2*, ECRL next to ECRB as they cross below APL and EPB and location of pain in intersection syndrome. *3*, EPL. *4*, Scaphoid waist in the anatomic snuffbox. *5*, Radial styloid.

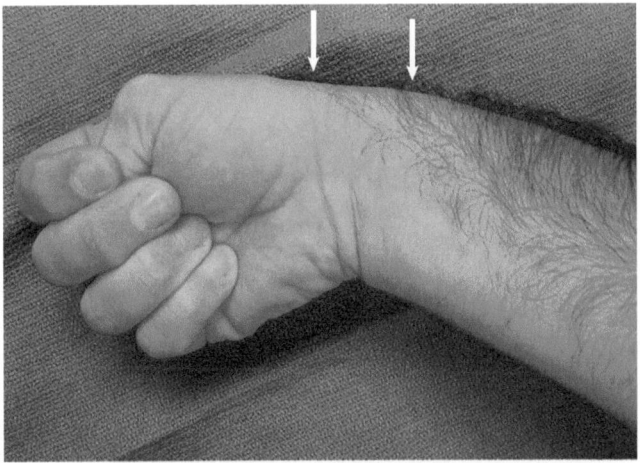

Fig. 67.3 The Finkelstein test demonstrated with thumb grasped in the palm with ulnar deviation of the wrist. The elbow should be in extension.

tuberosity). This is a critical structure to be able to palpate reliably. It will become more prominent with wrist radial deviation and flexion and less palpable with ulnar deviation and extension. This anatomic landmark is critical for wrist examination and for performing a Watson scaphoid shift test, which is described later in this chapter. Distal pole scaphoid fractures and even scaphoid waist fractures and scapholunate (SL) ligament tears will have pain reproduced with a dorsally applied pressure to the volar tubercle.

Trapezial ridge fractures will present with pain in the thenar region after a fall. The trapezial ridge serves as the radial attachment of the transverse carpal ligament and can be avulsed with a sizable bony fragment. A carpal tunnel radiographic view or computed tomography (CT) scan aids in the diagnosis of this easily overlooked fracture.

Moving slightly radial to the FCR, the radial artery is easily palpable. A pulse exam and an Allen test should be documented. The superficial branch of the radial artery can be palpated as it courses obliquely across the volar-radial aspect of the wrist just proximal to the scaphoid tuberosity. The deep branch of the radial artery dives beneath the first dorsal compartment into the proximal aspect of the anatomic snuffbox.

Moving dorsal and radial, the next palpable structure is the radial styloid and first dorsal compartment (abductor pollicis longus [APL] and extensor pollicis brevis [EPB]). The very tip of the radial styloid is easily palpable and represents the distal edge of the first dorsal compartment's tendon sheath. Tenderness at this location may represent radial styloid fracture or radiocarpal ligament sprain in the acute injury setting or, more often, De Quervain tenosynovitis in the subacute or insidious presentation. In the athletic population, De Quervain tendonitis is the most common wrist tendonitis, particularly in racquet sport and rowing athletes.[12–14] A Finkelstein test has been shown to be reliable and very sensitive (though not always specific) for De Quervain tenosynovitis. The Finkelstein test is performed by the examiner passively flexing the patient's thumb and assessing for pain,[15] whereas the Eichoff test is performed by having the patient

place the thumb within a closed fist and ulnarly deviate the wrist (Fig. 67.3). Pain may also be elicited with resisted thumb abduction and extension. Similar pain located about 4 to 5 cm proximal to the radial styloid and slightly more ulnar is typically due to intersection syndrome. Intersection syndrome is caused by inflammation between the first and second extensor compartments, which contain the APL and EPB and the ECRL and extensor carpi radialis brevis (ECRB), respectively. Often, intersection syndrome is accompanied by audible or palpable crepitation at this precise location and may also manifest a positive Finkelstein test.[13] This is frequently seen in rowers, weight lifters, football linemen, and powder skiers due to the repetitive wrist extension and radial deviation that these activities require.[16–19]

Dorsal to the first extensor compartment is the anatomic snuffbox (bordered by the first extensor compartment volarly, the extensor pollicis longus [EPL] dorsally, and the radial styloid proximally). The location of the scaphoid waist correlates with the anatomic snuffbox. Normally, it has a concave appearance, and fullness with tenderness in this region should always raise suspicion for a scaphoid fracture.

Fractures are common after a collision or fall in sports. These present with immediate pain, swelling, and tenderness. The scaphoid is the most commonly fractured carpal bone, representing roughly two-thirds of all carpal fractures; therefore so a high index of suspicion should always be maintained. The typical mechanism of injury is a fall onto an outstretched hand. These injuries are very common in sports such as, basketball, skiing, snowboarding, and skateboarding.[20–24] It has been recommended that all athletes with radial-sided wrist pain should carry the diagnosis of scaphoid fracture until proven otherwise and all patients with snuffbox tenderness should have dedicated radiographs to rule out a possible scaphoid fracture.[25,26] Less common and at times easily missed are fractures of the trapezial ridge. The mechanism of injury is often the same as for a scaphoid fracture but the pain is located in the thenar eminence. If missed, a malunited trapezial ridge fracture has been reported to lead to FCR tendonitis in a professional baseball player. We have seen one case of FCR rupture in a professional football player after this injury (Fig. 67.4).[27]

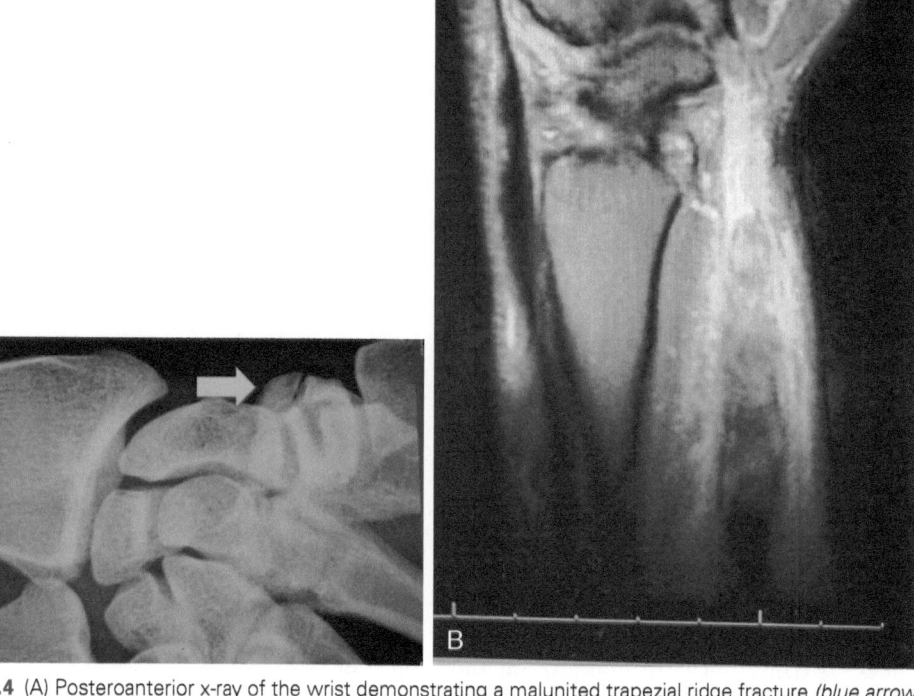

Fig. 67.4 (A) Posteroanterior x-ray of the wrist demonstrating a malunited trapezial ridge fracture *(blue arrow)*. (B) Magnetic resonance imaging demonstrating a flexor carpi radialis rupture from a malunited trapezial ridge fracture.

Degenerative processes such as STT and CMC arthritis are common in aging athletes and most often present insidiously; however, often an acute event will exacerbate an only mild pre-existing pain. Traditionally CMC arthritis is assessed with a CMC axial grind test,[28] but more recently Gelberman and colleagues described thumb adduction and extension provocative testing, which was shown to be more sensitive than the grind test.[29] This is performed by stabilizing the patient's trapezium in one hand (located at the distal edge of the anatomic snuffbox) and loading the thumb axially, all while passively circumducting the thumb ray with the other hand. Pain and crepitation are hallmarks of CMC arthritis with this maneuver. Tenderness over the thumb CMC joint in the setting of trauma should heighten concern for a thumb metacarpal base fracture, including extra-articular metaphyseal base fractures, Bennett, and Rolando fractures. The thumb CMC joint is most easily palpable along the radial side of the thumb metacarpal at the distal edge of the snuffbox, whereas the STT joint is more easily palpable volarly, just distal to the scaphoid distal pole.

Wartenberg syndrome can be a source of radial quadrant pain. This superficial radial nerve entrapment underneath the brachioradialis produces pain, paresthesia, dysesthesia, and/or a positive Tinel sign typically 1 to 2 cm proximal to the radial styloid. This too can produce a falsely positive Finkelstein maneuver.

The radial quadrant is the second most common location for a ganglion cyst (dorsal adjacent to the SL ligament being the most common).[30] Volar wrist ganglions are typically intimately associated with the radial artery adjacent to the FCR tendon and represent the most commonly encountered mass in the radial quadrant. They typically arise from either the FCR tendon sheath

or radioscaphoid joint and can be a source of radial quadrant pain. A differential diagnosis of a ganglion cyst in this location is an adventitial cyst, which is a cyst emanating off a branch of the radial artery.

DORSAL QUADRANT

Wrist pathology affecting the dorsal quadrant includes carpal instability (SL ligament tears, midcarpal instability, perilunate injuries); extensor tendinopathy and carpal boss; distal radius, capitate and lunate fractures, Kienbock disease; and dorsal ganglion cysts. Lister's tubercle is the key landmark for identifying dorsal quadrant pathology (Fig. 67.5). This raised dorsal bony prominence of the distal radius separates the second compartment (ECRL and ECRB) from the third compartment (EPL). With wrist ROM, this prominence will remain stationary.

As in the radial quadrant, pain from tendinopathy is most often seen from overuse and repetitive sports injuries. Extensor tendonitis can at times present with rather impressive swelling and pain over the wrist or digital extensor tendons residing just radial and ulnar, respectively, to Lister's tubercle. A bony prominence known as a carpal boss can exist at the insertion of the radial wrist extensors. Although often clinically silent, they can become symptomatic with overuse or after a direct blow to this area is sustained. Grasping the second and third metacarpal heads and shucking one palmar and one dorsal may reproduce pain from a carpal boss.[30] Moving from Lister's tubercle distally about 1 cm toward the long finger, the examiner's finger falls into the concavity of the radiocarpal joint. This point is directly over the dorsal SL ligament and is known as the SL interval. With

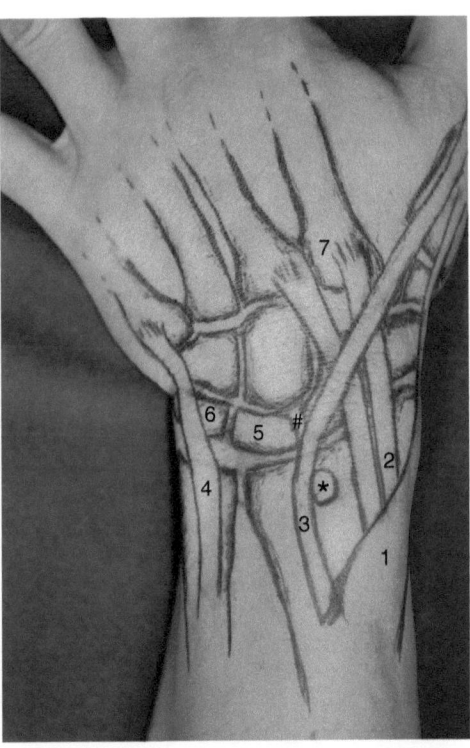

Fig. 67.5 Illustrated surface anatomy of the dorsal quadrant. *, Lister's tubercle. #, Scapholunate interval. *1*, First dorsal compartment (APL and EPB). *2*, Second dorsal compartment (ECRL and ECRB) and location of intersection syndrome. *3*, Third dorsal compartment (EPL); the fourth and fifth compartments have been omitted for clarity. *4*, Sixth dorsal compartment (ECU). *5*, Lunate. *6*, Triquetrum. *7*, Insertion of ECRL and ECRB and location of carpal boss.

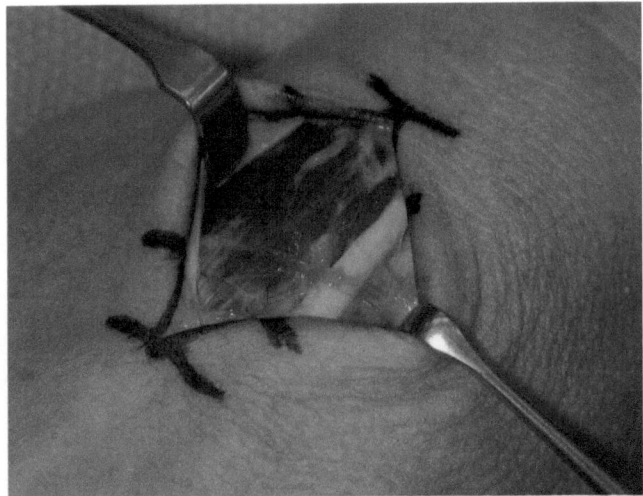

Fig. 67.6 Dorsal surgical exposure to the hand demonstrating the anomalous muscle, extensor digitorum brevis manus. Radially, the extensor digitorum communis tendon to the long finger is present.

wrist flexion, the proximal pole of the scaphoid can be palpated just radial to this point and the lunate just ulnar to this point. Tenderness over the proximal pole of the scaphoid may indicate either fracture or scaphoid impaction. Scaphoid impaction, often seen in gymnasts and weight lifters, occurs with repetitive wrist hyperextension resulting in the scaphoid impinging on the dorsal edge of the radius; it presents with pain upon wrist extension with the potential for osteophyte formation.[31]

The SL interval is the most typical location for a dorsal ganglion cyst. In addition to an injury to the SL ligament, an occult dorsal ganglion can produce pain to palpation over this location. Less commonly, anomalous muscles such as the extensor digitorum brevis manus can be located in this area and produce a soft tissue mass and accompanying pain mimicking a ganglion (Fig. 67.6).[32] If uncertainty exists as to whether a mass is a ganglion, simple transillumination or aspiration can easily distinguish a ganglion from anomalous muscles or solid tumors. Along the ulnar edge of the SL interval, the lunate is palpable, particularly with wrist flexion. Tenderness here may represent an SL ligament tear, lunate fracture, lunotriquetral (LT) tear, or Kienbock disease.

Testing the stability of the SL ligament is a critical examination skill for anyone caring for wrist injuries. Carpal instability encompasses a broad spectrum of ligamentous deficiency, including acute and chronic conditions from traumatic and atraumatic causes. In athletes, the most common of these, particularly following an acute traumatic event, is injury of the SL ligament. These are very common injuries in contact sports and

the examiner should always have a high index of suspicion, since missed injuries can lead to a chronic debilitating wrist arthritis known as scapholunate advanced collapse (SLAC).

The classic scaphoid shift test was described by Watson and is the most important provocative maneuver in testing SL stability.[33,34] The maneuver is performed beginning with the patient's wrist in extension and ulnar deviation. The examiner places his or her hand with the thumb over the distal pole of the scaphoid and fingers wrapped around the ulnar side of the patient's hand for stability. The patient's hand is then passively brought into flexion and radial deviation while dorsal pressure is applied to the scaphoid distal pole, resisting its tendency for volar translation (Fig. 67.7). In the setting of a significant SL ligament disruption, the proximal pole of the scaphoid will be temporarily forced onto the dorsal rim of the radius and then clunk back into the scaphoid fossa when pressure is released. The results of the test should always be compared with the opposite side for both stability and pain elicited by the maneuver. It is very common for patients without a history of wrist trauma, especially those with generalized ligamentous laxity, to have painless or minimally painful clunks with a scaphoid shift test.[35,36] Easterling found that 32% of asymptomatic patients without a history of trauma had bilateral painless "clunking" and another 14% with unilateral painless findings. Asymmetric pain and instability combined with a feasible mechanism of injury are most consistent with an SL ligament tear. When the scaphoid shift test produces only pain, the differential diagnosis includes occult dorsal carpal ganglion, scaphoid impaction, and radioscaphoid or STT chondromalacia.[34] Additional maneuvers to test for SL stability include the scaphoid lift test and scaphoid thrust test, but these are much less comprehensively described and practiced.[37,38] Both tests seek to understand abnormal carpal motion during dynamic stress testing. Chronic cases of SL instability may lead to pain attributed to a predictable pattern of degenerative changes known as SLAC wrist.

Midcarpal instability may be reproduced with a catch-up clunk test.[39] This maneuver involves the patient beginning with the forearm pronated and the wrist radially deviated. The patient is then asked to move the wrist from radial deviation (during

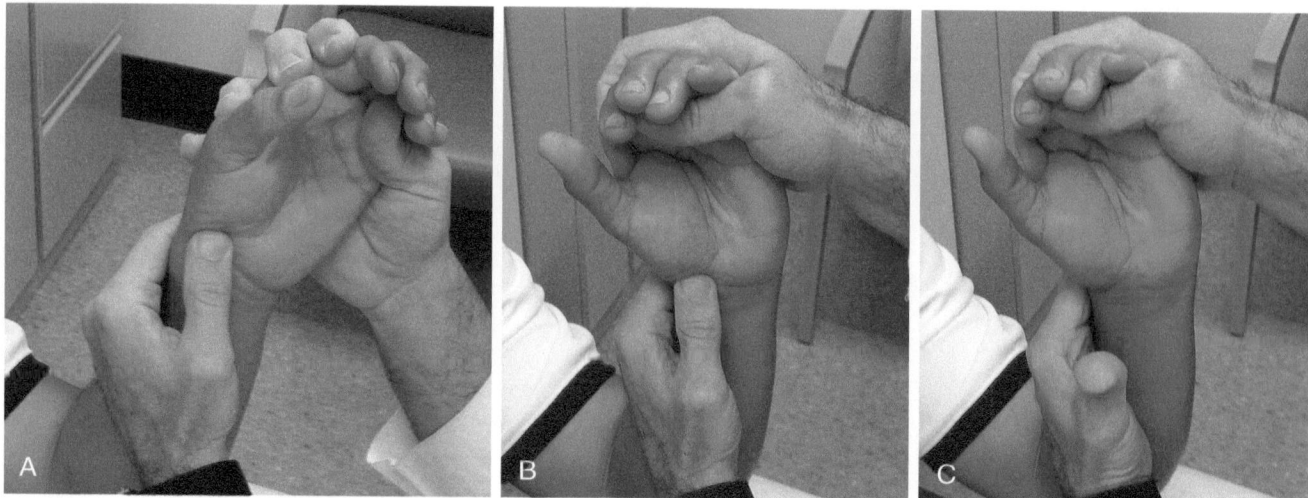

Fig. 67.7 The Watson scaphoid shift test. (A) The examiner places his or her hand with the thumb over the distal pole of the scaphoid and fingers wrapped around the ulnar side of the patient's hand for stability. (B) The patient's hand is then passively brought into flexion and radial deviation while dorsal pressure is applied to the scaphoid distal pole, resisting its tendency for volar translation. (C) In a positive test, once the scaphoid is released, it will clunk back into the scaphoid fossa.

which time the proximal row is flexed and the distal row relatively volar) into ulnar deviation (which extends the proximal row and translates the distal row dorsally). Midway into this maneuver, a visible and audible clunk will occur in the setting of midcarpal instability as the distal row suddenly shifts dorsal and the proximal row shifts into extension. Since an identical clunk can occur in the setting of radiocarpal instability as the proximal row shifts dorsally (rather than into extension as seen in midcarpal instability), this test lacks specificity.[39,40] An additional test for midcarpal instability reported by Lichtman et al.[39] is the midcarpal shift test. In this test the patient's forearm is placed in pronation with the wrist secured in neutral while a volarly directed pressure is applied to the dorsum of the capitates. The amount of midcarpal translation is noted and compared with the opposite wrist. Next, an axial load is applied, and the wrist is passively deviated ulnarly. The presence of a clunk or report of pain is noted. A grading system of 1 to 4 has been developed and correlated with measured amounts of translation.[41]

Isolated injuries to the capitate are rare; these more commonly represent a spectrum of greater arc injuries including scaphoid waist and capitate neck fractures, termed "scaphocapitate syndrome."[42–44] Capitate stress fractures can also be seen in athletes involved in racquet sports. The head of the capitate is palpable just distal to the SL ligament, especially with slight wrist flexion.

Finally, Kienbock disease must be considered in patients with unexplained dorsal wrist pain. Mild insidious complaints of generalized pain, stiffness, or weakness without a history of substantial trauma should prompt further workup for Kienbock. Examination may be largely nonspecific, with lunate tenderness, minor deficits of motion, and reduced grip strength as compared with the contralateral wrist.

ULNAR QUADRANT

Historically the ulnar quadrant has been the least well understood quadrant of wrist pathology and has been termed "the black

box" by Kleinman and others. Ulnar-sided wrist pain is arguably the most common athletic wrist complaint and often imparts a diagnostic challenge to even the most experienced specialists.[45,46] Recent advancements in our understanding of ulnar-sided wrist pain have led to much improved diagnostic and therapeutic care for these injuries. It is useful to distinguish between pathology arising from the radio ulnar, ulnocarpal, and intercarpal articulations and pathology that is extra-articular. This is due to the numerous intimately positioned structures that are prone to traumatic, inflammatory, or degenerative injury. The pathologies include ECU tendinopathy, triangular fibrocartilage complex (TFCC) injuries, distal radioulnar joint (DRUJ) instability, and FCU tendonitis, ulnar impaction, and LT ligament tears.

Most dorsal in the ulnar quadrant of the wrist is the ECU tendon, residing within the sixth dorsal extensor compartment (Fig. 67.8). Physical examination will often show tenderness and sometimes swelling over the course of the ECU tendon (Fig. 67.9). Pain will typically be recreated with resisted wrist extension and ulnar deviation.[47] Tendinopathy of the ECU is extremely common in the athlete, second only to the incidence of De Quervain.[48–50] There is a predilection for baseball, hockey, golf, and racquet sports, typically with pain generated by backhand volley.[51] When the forearm is pronated and the wrist is in neutral, the tendon has a direct course through its sheath toward its insertion on the base of the fifth metacarpal. This angle increases, however, when the wrist is positioned in supination, ulnar deviation and wrist extension. Excessive extension, as well as rapid flexion, ulnar deviation, and supination can cause tendinopathy or lead to attritional or traumatic ruptures of the ECU subsheath, resulting in painful subluxation or dislocation of the tendon, often associated with a snapping sensation.[51]

Unfortunately tenderness to palpation over the sixth compartment is not specific, as it loads nearby potential sources of pain. To reduce ambiguity, Ruland et al. described the "ECU synergy test": With the elbow at 90 degrees of flexion and the forearm fully supinated, the examiner grasps the thumb and

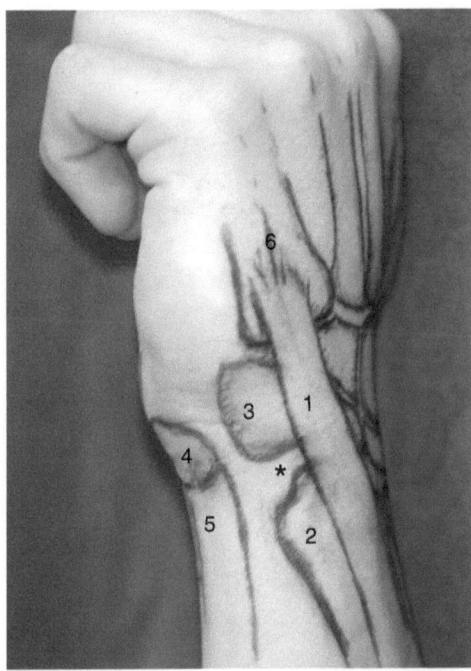

Fig. 67.8 Illustrated surface anatomy of the ulnar quadrant. *, Fovea. *1*, ECU tendon. *2*, Distal ulna and styloid. *3*, Triquetrum. *4*, Pisiform. *5*, FCU tendon. *6*, Base of the fifth metacarpal.

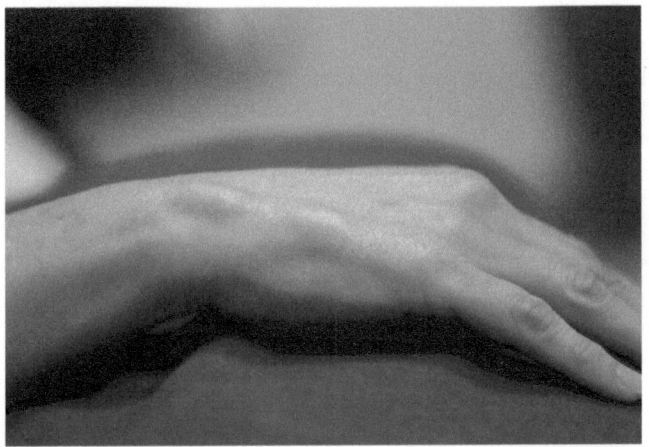

Fig. 67.9 Photograph showing significant tendonitis of the extensor carpi ulnaris. Note the swelling along the entire course of the sixth compartment.

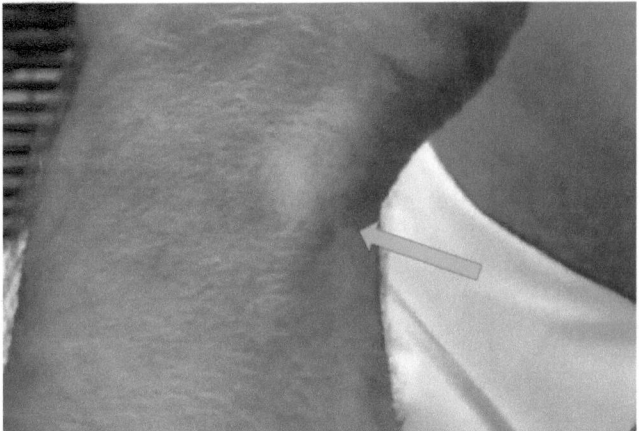

Fig. 67.10 Demonstrates instability of the extensor carpi ulnaris tendon during flexion, ulnar deviation, and supination maneuvers. The *blue arrow* points to the subluxed extensor carpi ulnaris tendon.

long finger. When the patient then radially deviates the thumb against resistance, the ECU contracts isometrically and recreates the patient's pain.[52] Instability of the ECU tendon may be elicited with the "FUSS maneuver"—flexion, ulnar deviation, and supination leading to subluxation. This "ice cream scoop" motion[53] will recreate pain with visible or palpable subluxation of the tendon (Fig. 67.10).

Athletic endeavors that involve high-energy or repetitive axial or torsional forces may lead to ulnar impaction syndrome, tearing of the TFCC, and DRUJ instability. Individuals with ulnar positive variance are known to be at higher risk for developing ulnar impaction. Although the incidence of ulnar positive wrists in athletes is not known, it has been noted that football lineman and gymnasts may be at higher risk for developing ulnar positive

variance due to chronic distal radial physeal loading and premature arrest.[54,55]

The TFCC is encountered in the "soft spot" between the ECU and FCU known as the fovea. Foveal tenderness has high sensitivity and specificity (95% and 87%) for TFCC tear.[56] The Nakamura ulnar impaction test loads the TFCC and will cause pain with abutment or tear.[57] While stabilizing the forearm, the examiner takes the patient's ulnarly deviated hand though supination and pronation, all while applying a proximally directed axial load.[57] Ulnar styloid–triquetral impaction (USTI) occurs in supination, as this is the position in which the ulnar styloid is closest to the carpus. A typical history would include pain in the supinated wrist while holding a hockey stick.[58] The USTI test is positive when pain is elicited as the dorsiflexed wrist is taken from pronation to supination.[59] The "press test," in which the seated patient pushes out of a chair, places the wrist in the same position. This simple test was reported to have 100% sensitivity for TFCC tearing.[60] It should be kept in mind that while they are sensitive, these ulnocarpal loading maneuvers are not specific to TFCC pathology, as they also load the nearby intercarpal joints as well.[61]

Assessment of DRUJ stability completes the evaluation of the TFCC. Injuries that affect the stability of this joint may be isolated or associated with other injuries ranging from frank traumatic dislocation with rotatory mechanical block to more indolent chronic pain and dysfunction with pronosupination activities. On physical examination, the DRUJ is loaded when the ulna is compressed against the radius. Subsequent pain with forearm rotation indicates DRUJ pathology.[62] Increased anterior-to-posterior translation of the radius relative to the ulna indicates instability.[63] Several variations of this test have been described. In the radioulnar ballottement test, the examiner applies palmar and then dorsal pressure to the ulnar head and notes translation relative to the radius in neutral, pronated, and supinated positions.[47] A cadaveric study showed statistically significant examiner accuracy in detecting DRUJ instability with the ballottement test after complete TFCC section,[64] but the performance of these tests in incomplete tears or in the clinical setting is unknown.

Moving distally on the dorsal-ulnar wrist, the intercarpal and CMC articulations are examined. Injury to the LT ligament may occur with a fall, particularly with hyperextension and twisting, although the exact mechanism is controversial.[33] Several maneuvers have been described to specifically elicit instability and pain originating from this joint. First, pain may be elicited with direct palpation of the ligament on the dorsum of the wrist, about a fingerbreadth distal to the DRUJ. Compression of the triquetrum against the lunate with ulnar-to-radial pressure by the examiner may recreate symptoms and has been recommended by some as having the highest sensitivity and specificity.[61] This is similar to the TFCC foveal test, but the anatomic location is immediately dorsal to the pisiform instead of immediately distal to the ulnar styloid. Other tests include the LT "ballottement" as described by Regan[33,65] or the LT "shear" test as described by Kleinman.[66] Both involve stabilizing the lunate with one hand and the pisotriquetral unit in the other while applying forces in opposite directions across the joint.

CMC fractures at the base of the fifth metacarpal are common following blunt-force injury or after striking with the ulnar side of the hand. Dorsal triquetral fractures are also common after a fall during sports and should be kept in mind when there is focal pain over the dorsal aspect of the triquetrum. A pronated oblique radiograph is sometimes necessary to find this small avulsion fracture. Anatomically, this represents more of an extrinsic ligamentous avulsion than a true carpal fracture.

Due to the proximity of pathology affecting the wrist in the ulnar quadrant, differentiating between one or more diagnoses can be challenging. For example, ECU tendinopathy and TFCC injuries commonly overlap. It can be advantageous to perform a differential lidocaine injection test, which we frequently supplement with corticosteroid once the main area of involvement is discerned. The first location is chosen and a small amount of anesthetic (typically 0.05 mL) is administered. After a few minutes, the amount of pain improvement is noted. It is important to have the patient try to reproduce the previous pain with aggravating wrist positions or offending loading maneuvers. Another selective injection is given at a second (or even third) area and this response of pain improvement is compared to the first response.[40] If performed properly and patiently, this exercise is a powerful diagnostic adjunct with the potential for more accurate therapeutic intervention.

VOLAR QUADRANT

The volar quadrant houses the most critical neurovascular structures of the hand and wrist (Fig. 67.11). The ulnar artery and nerve course deep and radial to the FCU tendon and enter the wrist at Guyon's canal. In this location the ulnar artery is relatively superficial and may be compressed against the underlying hamate. Repetitive blunt trauma may therefore cause local arterial occlusion or aneurysmal dilation. This may further lead to distal embolization[67] or compression of the nearby ulnar nerve. These clinical findings are referred to as the *hypothenar hammer syndrome*, which is well described in baseball catchers as well as some tennis players and golfers.[68] It usually presents as dysaesthesia or cold intolerance of the ring and small fingers.[69]

The ulnar nerve is more commonly compressed at the elbow, particularly in throwing athletes. Compression or irritation at

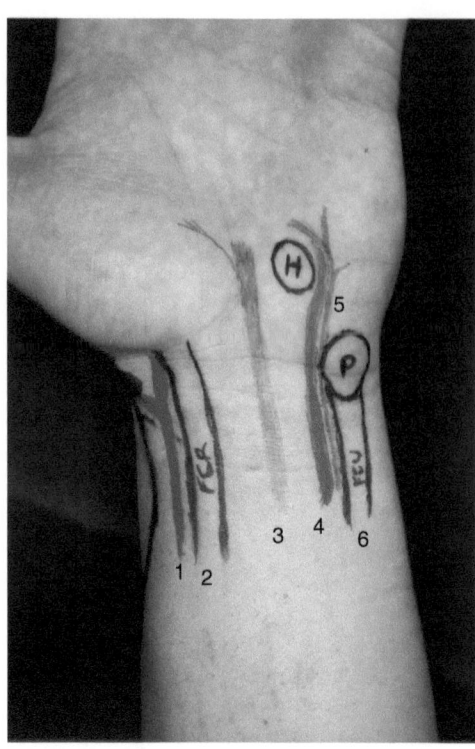

Fig. 67.11 Illustrated surface anatomy of the volar quadrant. *1*, Radial artery. *2*, Flexor carpi radialis tendon. *3*, Median nerve. *4*, Ulnar artery. *5*, Ulnar nerve. *6*, Flexor carpi ulnaris tendon. *H*, Hamate. *P*, pisiform.

the wrist, however, may also occur at the Guyon canal. This may be due to an extrinsic mass effect such as ganglion, lipoma, or aneurysmal dilation of the ulnar artery as well as focal prolonged external compression. This last entity is well described in cyclists.[9]

The median nerve, along with the digital flexor tendons, crosses the wrist in a fibro-osseous sheath known as the carpal tunnel. Compression of the median nerve within this sheath is the most common peripheral compression neuropathy but is not considered particularly common in the athletic population. Nevertheless, it has been described in sports that require forceful or prolonged gripping such as cycling[9] and rock climbing[70] or repeated direct volar pressure on the extended wrist as in wheelchair rim propulsion.[71] Additionally, exposure to vibration has been associated with a risk of carpal tunnel syndrome, with implications for motor racing athletes.[72,73]

From an osseous standpoint, the pisiform and hook of the hamate are important to consider, given their higher predilection for injury during sport. The pisiform is a mobile sesamoid within the FCU tendon, which may then continue to insert on portions of the hamate and base of the fifth metacarpal. The hamate hook protrudes from the hamate body and is a site of muscular and ligamentous attachment. Injuries to these ulnar-sided carpal bones are relatively rare but should be considered in athletes who use bats, racquets, clubs, or sticks, as errant impact is transmitted directly to the hypothenar region of the nondominant palm. A history of a "check swing" in baseball or a "fat" shot in golf should further raise suspicion. A fall onto the outstretched hand may also be responsible for fractures of these structures. Increased participation in sports has led to a recent increase in the prevalence of acute ulnar carpal fractures and chronic stress fractures.[74,75] Additionally, arthritis may develop between the pisiform and the triquetrum with which it articulates.

Inserting onto the pisiform, the FCU can be a source of volar-ulnar wrist pain. Tendinosis[76] may develop with repetitive microtrauma such as occurs in racquet sports. Occasionally acute calcific tendinitis may develop, which may be mistaken for infection or gout due to the sometimes dramatic erythema and intense pain associated with this condition.[77,78]

In the volar quadrant, physical examination begins with searching for bony tenderness at prominences of the pisiform and then the hook of the hamate. The pisiform is subcutaneous and easy to locate at the level of the wrist flexion crease, but the hamate hook is deep to the hypothenar musculature. It can be located by placing the examiner's thumb IP flexion crease on the pisiform and aiming the tip of the examiner's thumb radially and distally toward the patient's long finger, but this requires deep palpation. In addition to direct tenderness, a hamate hook fracture will often produce pain with resisted small- and ring-finger flexion, as the hamulus serves as a pulley for these tendons traversing the carpal canal. Delayed flexor tendon injuries may be associated with fractures of the hook of the hamate in up to 17% of cases.[79] It should be kept in mind that fractures of the hook of the hamate may be associated with median or ulnar neuropathy[80] due to the hook's location between the carpal tunnel and Guyon's canal, so concurrent neurologic and vascular assessment is paramount. The pisotriquetral grind test indicates arthritis in this joint and is performed by compressing the pisiform to the triquetrum while flexing and extending the wrist or moving the pisiform medially and laterally. Lastly, radiographic identification of injury to these carpal bones may be difficult because of their three-dimensional shape and overlap with the rest of the carpus. A supinated oblique radiograph of the wrist shows the pisiform in profile well. A carpal tunnel view may identify a fracture of the hook of the hamate, although a CT scan is sometimes necessary for diagnosis in equivocal cases.

More proximally, the FCU tendon is inspected. Physical examination typically reveals tenderness along the tendon proximal to the pisiform as well as pain with wrist flexion and pronation.[76]

Examination of the volar ulnar side of the wrist is not complete without assessing the status of its neurologic and vascular structures. Vascular examination includes examining distal perfusion to the digits and thumb. Altered color, decreased temperature, loss of tissue turgor, sluggish capillary refill, and even ulcerated or gangrenous tips all indicate critical ischemia. Next, the presence of an ulnar artery pulse should be established. Examination with a handheld Doppler is a reliable method for evaluating areas of occlusion, pathways of perfusion, and even the quality of blood flow. The Allen test establishes the patency of the radial and ulnar arteries and the state of the superficial palmar arch connecting them. This test is performed by manually compressing the radial and ulnar arteries and then having the patient open and close his or her fist several times to exsanguinate the hand. Pressure is then released from one of the arteries, which in a normal state (complete superficial palmar arch) should reperfuse the entire hand in less than 3 seconds. The test is then repeated with release of the other artery, and resulting flow is documented (Fig. 67.12).

The function of the ulnar nerve should be assessed by testing two-point sensibility along the small finger. Intrinsic muscle bulk, tone, and function should likewise be examined. The Froment sign assesses key grip and the function of the adductor pollicis, which is innervated by the terminal deep motor branch of the ulnar nerve. The patient is asked to forcefully key pinch a piece of paper, which the examiner attempts to pull away. If the adductor is weak, the flexor pollicis longus (FPL) is recruited as a compensatory mechanism and the IP joint assumes a flexed posture (Fig. 67.13).

Concluding the examination of the volar surface of the wrist is an assessment of the median nerve. History will include numbness in the radial digits during offending activities. Physical examination of the carpal tunnel is well described. Durkan's compression test, which is performed by applying pressure over the carpal tunnel for 30 seconds, is reported to be the provocative test with the highest sensitivity and specificity.[81] Two-point discrimination should be tested for in the volar thumb and index. The thenar musculature should be inspected for atrophy. Asking the patient to keep their thumb out of their palm against resistance tests the motor function of the abductor pollicis brevis.

HAND AND DIGITS

The hand and digits are especially vulnerable to injury during athletic participation and in fact are the most commonly fractured body sites, making up 32% of all high school sports–related fractures.[82] Both phalangeal and metacarpal fractures are extremely common in sports, with phalangeal fractures representing over half of all sports-related hand fractures.[83] Additionally, injuries to certain ligaments and tendons occur with such frequency that they carry the name of the offending sport, such as skier's thumb or boxer's knuckle.

History should center on the activity and mechanism of injury and acuity or chronicity of the complaint. A relatively violent mechanism with sudden onset of pain—along with swelling, ecchymosis, and crepitus—typically creates a high level of suspicion for fracture. Following any hand injury, radiographs must be obtained to rule out fracture or joint incongruity. Angulation and rotational deformity are noted. Evaluation of neurologic and vascular status as well as that of the overlying skin is emphasized.

DISTAL INTERPHALANGEAL JOINT

Fingertip crush injuries are extremely common in sport and may result in distal phalangeal fractures and nail bed injuries. Distal phalangeal fractures are the most common of all hand fractures. In the skeletally immature athlete, a unique dorsally displaced transphyseal distal phalanx fracture known as a Seymour fracture can present with associated nail bed incarceration in the fracture site (Fig. 67.14). Axial loads to the end of the finger can rupture the terminal tendon producing the inability to extend the distal interphalangeal joint (DIP) joint, which is termed "mallet finger" or "baseball finger."[84] This injury is particularly common in baseball, football, and basketball and is the most common closed tendon injury in athletes.[85] On the opposite side of the digit, an avulsion of the flexor digitorum profundus

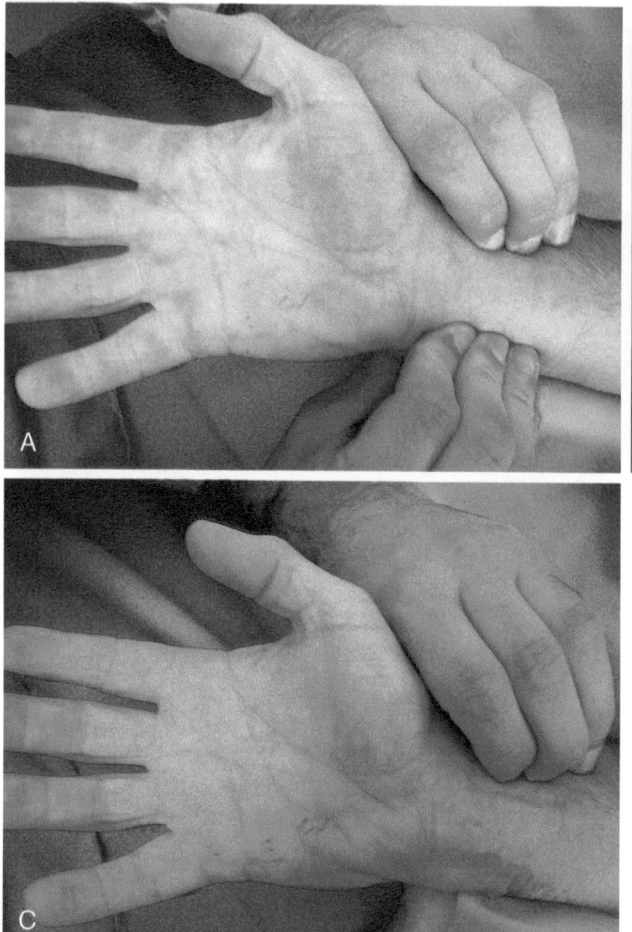
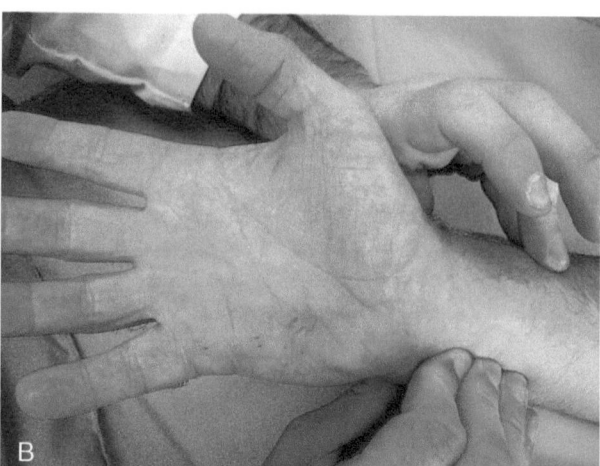

Fig. 67.12 The Allen test to assess the vascular supply of the hand. (A) This test is performed by manually compressing the radial and ulnar arteries, then having the patient open and close his or her fist several times to exsanguinate the hand. (B) Pressure is then released from one of the arteries, which in a normal state (complete superficial palmar arch), should reperfuse the entire hand in less than 3 seconds. (C) The test is then repeated with the release of the other artery, and the resulting flow is documented.

(FDP) from its insertion may occur with swift pulling away of a forcefully flexed finger. This frequently occurs while grabbing the jersey of an opponent in football or rugby and therefore is commonly called "jersey finger." The ring finger is involved in over 75% of cases, although this injury has been reported in all digits.[85] It is well established that timely repair of the flexor tendon, especially when it is retracted into the palm, improves results.[86,87]

Physical examination starts with noting the resting posture of the affected digit during a passive wrist tenodesis test. The DIP joint will be abnormally extended in the setting of FDP avulsion, particularly when the wrist is passively extended. In this setting, the patient will be unable to flex the DIP joint but should be able to independently flex the proximal interphalangeal joint (PIP) joint, since the FDS is typically not involved simultaneously. Active DIP joint flexion should be tested while blocking PIP and MCP joint motion, as should the adjacent digits. PIP joint flexion may be diminished, however, due to the avulsed FDP tendon stump lodged in the flexor sheath, which impedes the gliding of the FDS tendon of the involved digit.

Impact to the extended finger may rupture the terminal tendon, which is the insertion of the extensor mechanism on the dorsal epiphyseal portion of the distal phalanx. Examination of these "mallet fingers" reveals a flexed DIP joint posture and inability to fully extend it actively. Typically full passive extension is possible, and tenderness is present dorsally at the DIP joint. There may be an associated hyperextension posture of the PIP joint or a swan-neck deformity, particularly in a chronic mallet finger or individual with PIP volar plate laxity. Radiographic evaluation differentiates between bony or purely tendinous injury and assesses congruity of the joint.

PROXIMAL INTERPHALANGEAL JOINT

The PIP joint is next considered. According to Rettig, the PIP joint is the most commonly injured structure of the hand in athletes.[88] Disruption of the extensor mechanism, collateral ligaments, and/or volar plate may occur in this highly constrained hinge joint. These are usually partial injuries, often referred to as the "jammed finger," but they can range from minor sprains to open fracture/dislocations. A 10-year review of the National Football League database found dorsal PIP dislocations to be the most common hand injury.[89] Dislocations present with gross malalignment and are often reduced "on the field" by the player or trainer with manual traction. Following closed reduction, the joint should be assessed clinically by applying gentle angular force and ensuring that a stable, concentric ROM is present. It should also be evaluated radiographically to rule out associated

Fig. 67.13 Froment sign. The Froment sign assesses key grip and the function of the adductor pollicis, which is innervated by the terminal deep motor branch of the ulnar nerve. The patient is asked to forcefully key pinch a piece of paper, which the examiner attempts to pull away. If the adductor is weak, the FPL is recruited as a compensatory mechanism and the IP joint assumes a flexed posture.

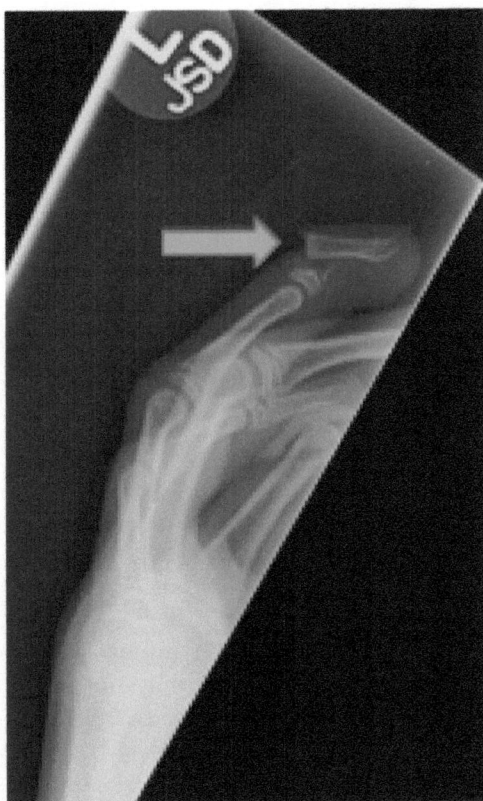

Fig. 67.14 X-ray evaluation demonstrating a displaced transphyseal distal phalanx fracture (*blue arrow*), known as a Seymour fracture, which can present with associated nail bed incarceration in the fracture site.

fracture and confirm congruent reduction is present. Radiographic stress views may be helpful in detecting subtle instability.

At the level of the PIP joint, the insertion of the extensor mechanism dorsally is known as the *central slip*. Disruption of the central slip can lead to a boutonnière deformity, and prompt recognition of this injury is paramount.

The extensor mechanism at this joint may be injured in a manner similar to mallet finger but with force concentrated at the middle phalanx instead of the distal phalanx. This may lead to rupture of the central slip, which is the insertion of the extensor mechanism on the dorsal middle phalanx base. The patient may be able to extend the PIP joint in the acute setting, but over time an extension lag and boutonnière deformity may develop.[88] This refers to a posture of flexion at the PIP joint and hyperextension at the DIP joint as well as inability to initiate PIP joint flexion due to volar subluxation of the lateral bands. In the acute setting, an Elson test can aid in the diagnosis of a central slip injury before a boutonnière deformity develops. This test is performed by having the patient flex the involved PIP joint 90 degrees over the end of a table. The examiner then blocks active PIP joint extension with counterpressure over the dorsum of the middle phalanx. In a normal state, there is supple passive flexion of the DIP joint by the examiner, but in the setting of an acute central slip injury, force transmission to the terminal tendon places the DIP joint in rigid extension (Fig. 67.15).

A pseudoboutonnière deformity refers to an isolated flexion contracture at the PIP joint without concurrent DIP joint hyperextension. This deformity is secondary to scar contraction of the volar plate after sprain or rupture. It often develops when a small bony avulsion of the volar plate insertion at the middle phalanx base is present and the joint is mistakenly immobilized for a prolonged period. The examiner must distinguish greater tenderness at the volar plate than at the dorsal central slip and also confirm a negative Elson test.[90]

METACARPOPHALANGEAL JOINT

At the MCP joint, dorsal pain is common following athletic injuries. Causes may include collateral ligamentous injuries, sagittal band ruptures, dorsal capsule ruptures, and fracture. Often associated with striking, injuries in this area carry eponyms such as "boxer's fracture" (fifth metacarpal neck fracture) and "boxer's knuckle." Boxer's knuckle classically refers to disruption of the dorsal MP capsule but has been applied to closed sagittal band ruptures as well by some authors.[73] On the volar side of this joint pain may result from volar plate injury, sesamoid fracture, or the common trigger finger.

The common extensor tendon glides over the dorsal MCP joint capsule. It is held in this position by the balanced tension of the adjacent investing sagittal bands. This capsuloligamentous apparatus is termed *the dorsal hood*. Injury to this complex may occur with repetitive blunt trauma to the area and is sometimes referred to as boxer's knuckle. Rupture of the dorsal MCP capsule or partial injury to the extensor mechanism investments may present only with swelling and pain, but complete rupture of a sagittal band may also lead to coronal plane subluxation of the common extensor tendon over the metacarpal head.[91] In the

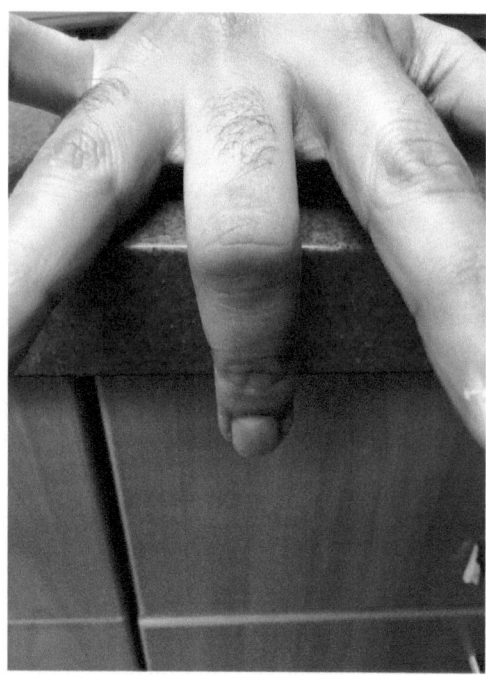

Fig. 67.15 Elson test. This test is performed by having the patient flex the involved proximal interphalangeal (PIP) joint 90 degrees over the end of a table. The examiner then blocks active PIP joint extension with counterpressure over the dorsum of the middle phalanx. In a normal state, there is supple passive flexion of the distal interphalangeal (DIP) joint by the examiner, but in the setting of an acute central slip injury, force transmission to the terminal tendon places the DIP joint in rigid extension.

latter scenario, the athlete may demonstrate inability to fully extend the MCP joint starting from a flexed position, but once the digit is placed in full extension passively by the examiner, the extensor mechanism is once again centralized and active extension can be maintained. Sagittal band injuries have also been termed the "flea-flicker" injury, describing one of the possible mechanisms for their occurrence when the flexed MCP joint is suddenly extended against resistance.

THUMB ULNAR COLLATERAL

Although all digits are subject to collateral ligament injuries from sports-related trauma, the thumb collateral ligaments warrant additional discussion owing to their critical role in stable pinch-and-grip in athletes. Although the acute injury derives its name from downhill skiing ("skier's thumb"), ulnar collateral ligament (UCL) injuries are very common in many athletic pursuits including racquet, ball, and stick sports. Patients with acute thumb UCL injuries will present with pain, swelling, and bruising at the thumb MCP joint and may recall a valgus load to the vulnerable thumb. Point tenderness over the UCL is present and may be accompanied by a palpable lump corresponding to a Stener lesion, which represents the torn UCL residing superficial to the adductor aponeurosis after a distal avulsion and necessitates surgical reattachment (Fig. 67.16). Prior to stressing the joint, radiographs should be obtained to rule out fracture of either the proximal phalanx or metacarpal. If radiographs are negative, the

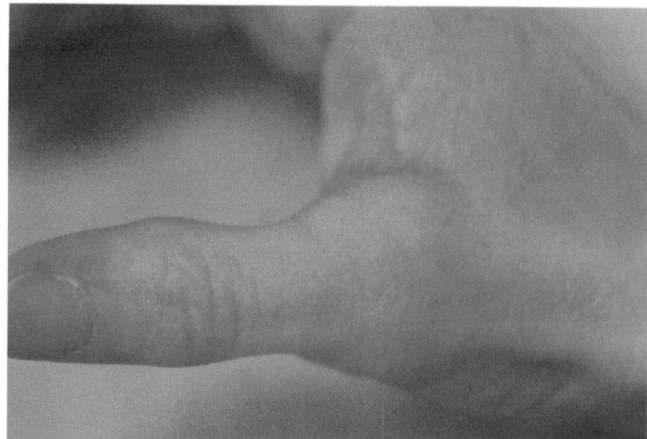

Fig. 67.16 Stener lesion. This lesion represents the torn ulnar collateral ligament residing superficial to the adductor aponeurosis after a distal avulsion and necessitates surgical reattachment.

MCP joint should be stressed both in extension and 30 degrees of flexion (the position that assesses the accessory and proper collateral ligaments, respectively). Greater than 30 degrees of angulation or more than 15 degrees of opening compared with the contralateral side are suggestive of a ligament tear. If a reliable examination is precluded by pain inhibition, a local anesthetic digital block will allow for patient comfort during stress testing. Although less commonly encountered than a UCL injury, trauma to the radial collateral ligament is evaluated similarly; when this is accompanied by dorsal MCP capsular involvement, there may be evidence of volar subluxation of the proximal phalanx relative to the metacarpal head.

Flexor Pulley Injury

One last uncommon but important athletic hand injury to mention is flexor pulley ruptures.[92] The digital flexor tendons are stabilized by a system of annular and cruciate pulleys, with the A2 and A4 pulleys overlying the proximal and middle phalanges, respectively. These two pulleys are the most critical to prevent bowstringing of the flexor tendons. Sustained resistive flexion forces on the fingers may result in acute pulley ruptures. This is most commonly seen in rock climbers engaging in a crimp position hold. Isolated A4 ruptures have also been reported in professional baseball pitchers.[93] We have seen cases of this as well in everyday athletes doing fingertip pull-ups. Tenderness directly over the involved pulley, especially when combined with palpable flexor tendon bowstringing and consequent motion loss, should heighten awareness of this rare diagnosis.

▌ SUMMARY

Injuries to the hand and wrist are extremely common in athletes. It is paramount to have a comfortable understanding of the anatomy of the hand and wrist as well as the physical exam of such structures. Working through the exam in a systematic way, using the anatomic quadrants as a guide, will help the clinician effectively perform the exam and account for the many possible conditions that can affect the athlete's hand and wrist.

For a complete list of references, go to ExpertConsult.com.

SELECTED READINGS

Citation:
Hand Clin. 2017 Feb;33(1):1–228.

Level of Evidence:
V

Summary:
The February 2017 issue of *Hand Clinic* is devoted to optimizing the treatment of upper extremity injuries in athletes. This issue focuses on the entire upper extremity with an emphasis on care and return to play of the athlete's hand and wrist.

Citation:
Goldfarb CA, Puri SK, Carlson MG. Diagnosis, treatment and return to play for four common sports injuries of the hand and wrist. *J Am Acad Orthop Surg.* 2016;24:853–862.

Level of Evidence:
V

Summary:
A well-written review article on the diagnosis and treatment of flexor digitorum profundus avulsion, flexor pulley rupture, extensor carpi ulnaris dislocation and injury to the thumb ulnar collateral ligament.

Citation:
Sports Med Arthrosc Rev. 2014 Mar;22(1):1–70.

Level of Evidence:
V

Summary:
The March 2014 issue of *Sports Medicine and Arthroscopy Review* is devoted to the diagnosis and treatment of hand and wrist injuries in sports medicine. Several review articles describe treat of many common conditions encountered in caring for athletes.

Citation:
Hand Clin. 2012 Aug;28(3):253–452.

Level of Evidence:
V

Summary:
The August 2012 issue of *Hand Clinic* is devoted solely to hand and wrist injuries in the elite athlete. It focuses on the treatment on a wide range of sport-specific hand and wrist injuries in athletes. The issue was written by a selected group of hand surgeons who are all consultants for professional sports teams.

Citation:
Kleinman WB. Stability of the distal radioulna joint: biomechanics, pathophysiology, physical diagnosis, and restoration of function what we have learned in 25 years. *J Hand Surg.* 2007;32(7):1086–1106.

Level of Evidence:
V

Summary:
Dr. Kleinman discusses the anatomy, pathophysiology, and treatment of disruption of the DRUJ. This is perhaps the best-written and illustrated article on this complex topic.

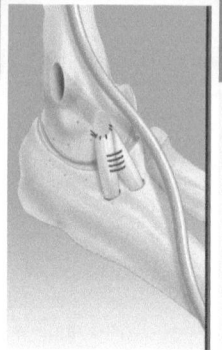

68

Imaging of the Wrist and Hand

Kimberly K. Amrami

Imaging evaluation of hand and wrist injuries in the athlete should always begin with conventional radiographs. Radiographs are excellent for detecting osseous injuries or malalignment in osseous structures as a result of ligament disruption. A standard wrist series includes posteroanterior (PA), lateral, and oblique views (Fig. 68.1).

A standard PA view is obtained with the shoulder abducted, the elbow flexed 90 degrees, and the forearm in a neutral position (see Fig. 68.1A). Evaluation begins with examination of the distal radius and ulna. Any cortical disruption in a skeletally mature patient may be indicative of fracture. Standard parameters to be checked include radial inclination, radial height, and ulnar variance. Radial inclination describes the angulation of the distal radius articular surface relative to the long axis of the radius, typically 23 degrees (range, 16 to 30 degrees).[1] Radial height is the distance measured between two parallel lines perpendicular to the radial shaft, one drawn across the tip of the radial styloid and the second across the distal ulna surface. The radial height averages 11 mm (range, 10 to 13 mm).[1] Deviations of these indices suggest an underlying abnormality.

Ulnar variance is the relative difference in height at the distal ulna and radius articular surfaces. When the wrist is at ulnar neutral variance, the distal ulna and distal radius articulations form a contiguous line where they meet. Deviation of the distal ulna head distal to the adjacent distal radius articulation is considered positive ulnar variance, and conversely, proximal migration of the distal ulna head relative to the distal radius articulation is considered negative ulnar variance. Pronation or supination of the forearm will alter ulnar variance, and therefore the image must be obtained with the forearm in the neutral position for accuracy and compared with the contralateral wrist. It is important to note the relationship of the distal radioulnar joint (DRUJ). Diastasis between the radius and ulna at the DRUJ can be pathologic. The carpal bones form three contiguous, smooth, parallel arcs along the proximal articular margins of the proximal carpal row, the distal articular margins of the proximal carpal row, and the proximal articular margins of the distal carpal row. Any disruption of these "arcs of Gilula" suggests disruption of carpal alignment.[2] Finally, each intercarpal and carpometacarpal joint space should be scrutinized individually for congruency.

On a true lateral radiograph of the wrist (see Fig. 68.1B) in neutral rotation, the axis of the radius, lunate, capitate, and third metacarpal should be collinear. On an appropriately obtained lateral wrist image, the volar edge of the pisiform lies between the distal pole of the scaphoid and the palmar aspect of the capitate head with the pisiform ideally bisected by the palmar cortex of the capitate. The scapholunate angle is subtended by a line parallel to the long axis of the lunate and a line parallel to the long axis of the scaphoid. Normally it measures 45 degrees (range, 30 to 60 degrees).[3] Palmer tilt, which measures the slope of the distal radius articular surface relative to a line perpendicular to the long axis of the radius, is usually 0 to 20 degrees, with a mean of 12 degrees.[1] Any degree of dorsal tilt is considered abnormal.

A standard series of radiographs for evaluation of the hand also includes PA, lateral, and oblique views. If an injury or problem is truly isolated to the thumb or a digit, individual radiographs of these digits are best. An appropriate lateral hand view is obtained with the fingers spread in a cascade to profile the phalanges and interphalangeal joints. Hand injuries are often subtle, and additional rotated views are often necessary to evaluate the metacarpophalangeal (MCP) and carpometacarpal joints in particular.

Any patient presenting with pain at rest or a "mass" at the wrist or hand is first evaluated with conventional radiographs. Occasionally radiographs are pathognomonic for entities such as Kienböck disease or Madelung deformity. Atypical imaging findings, such as a calcified soft tissue mass or lytic osseous lesion, may prompt further evaluation by an upper extremity or oncologic orthopedic specialist.

Many injuries of the wrist and hand involve a combination of osseous and soft tissue structures. When conventional radiographs are unrevealing or provide incomplete information, the choice of additional studies is guided by the history and physical examination. These additional studies may include computed tomography (CT), magnetic resonance imaging (MRI), magnetic resonance arthrography, real-time fluoroscopy, or bone scan.[4] Newer combined modalities such as positron emission tomography (PET) combined with CT or MRI may in rare instances be indicated. Some relevant injuries and their classic imaging findings are highlighted in this chapter to aid the general orthopedic surgeon or sports medicine specialist.

WRIST INJURIES

Distal Radius Fractures

Standard views of the wrist are mandatory and typically adequate to discern extra-articular and simple intra-articular fracture patterns. Obtaining the same views with traction takes advantage

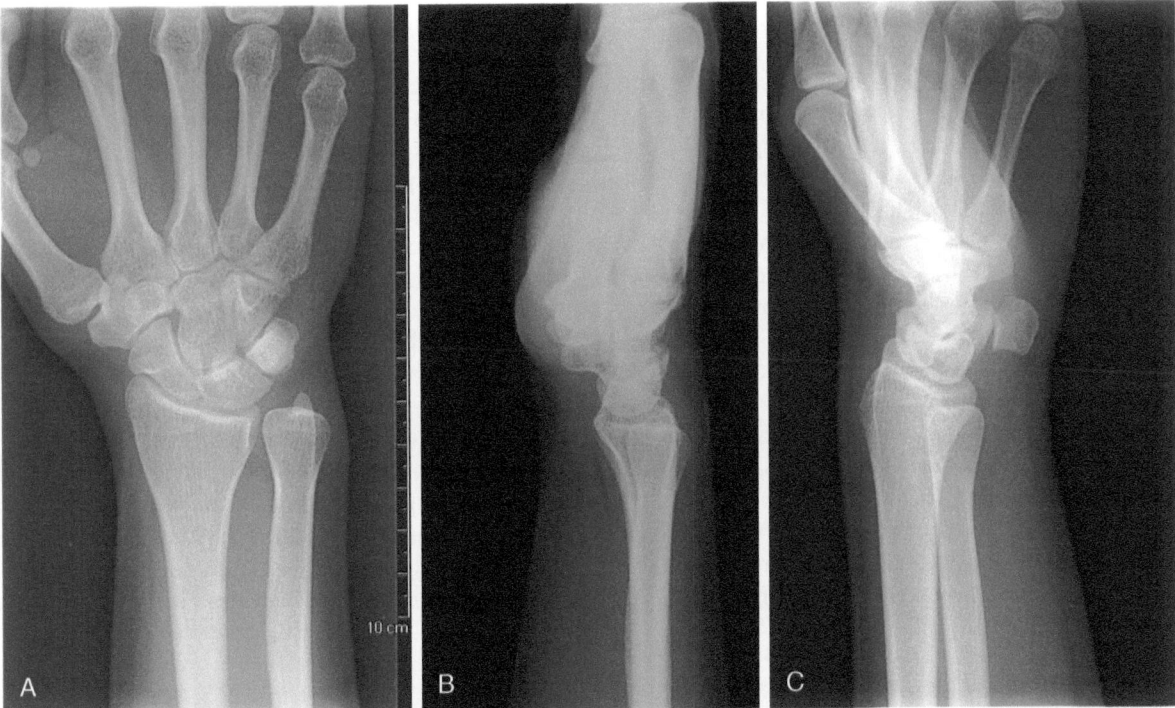

Fig. 68.1 Conventional radiographs of the wrist. (A) Posteroanterior view. (B) Lateral view. (C) Oblique view.

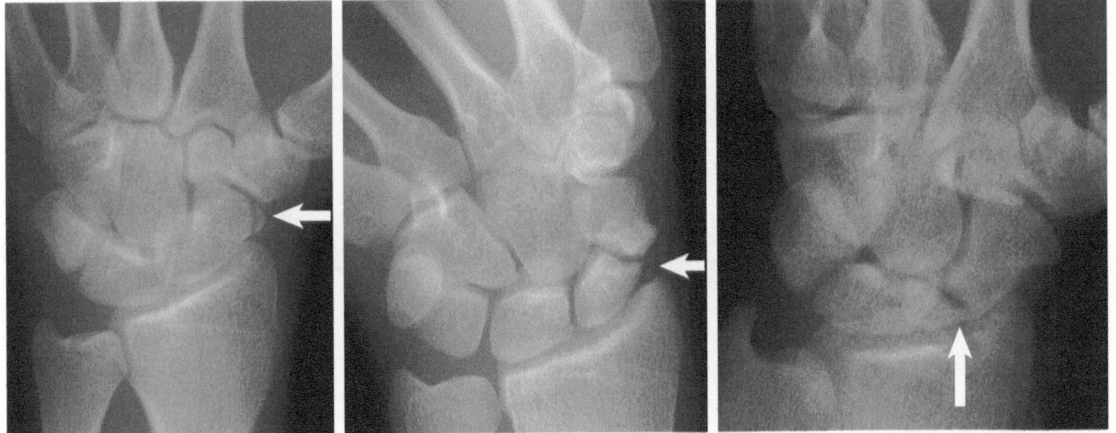

Fig. 68.2 Scaphoid fractures *(arrows)*. From left to right, radiographs show a distal scaphoid tuberosity fracture, a scaphoid waist fracture, and a proximal pole fracture. The fracture location has implications for healing and treatment options.

of ligamentotaxis that can better align fracture fragments and decompress areas of impaction and/or comminution. Although some debate has ensued about "normal" radiographic parameters after reduction of a distal radius fracture depending on the characteristics of the given patient, the American Association of Orthopaedic Surgeons has provided recommendations in published clinical practice guidelines. Operative fixation is suggested for fractures with more than 3 mm of radial shortening, 10 degrees of dorsal tilt, and 2 mm of intra-articular incongruity.[5] CT scans are sometimes used to better characterize complex intra-articular fracture patterns, especially when surgery is planned and the best approach for internal fixation is equivocal. Katz et al.[6] established that CT increased interobserver reliability in the management of complex distal radius fractures. MRI is rarely

necessary for distal radius fracture management, although it may be helpful in assessing ligamentous injuries often associated with distal radius fracture or in cases where fracture impaction results in symptoms of ulnar impaction.

Carpal Fractures
Scaphoid Fracture
In addition to the standard wrist series, special views may be necessary to identify scaphoid fractures. The scaphoid or "navicular" view, obtained with the wrist partially extended and in maximal ulnar deviation, and the 45-degree semipronated radiographic views are best for scrutinizing the scaphoid in profile (Fig. 68.2). When these initial radiographs are unrevealing and a high clinical suspicion for occult fracture exists, MRI is considered the

gold standard for identifying radiographically "occult" scaphoid fractures[7,8] with nearly 100% sensitivity and specificity. Additional or delayed radiographic views are rarely informative, primarily due to poor interobserver reliability and low predictive value even among experienced clinicians and radiologists.[9] CT can be useful but has lower sensitivity and specificity than MRI with a recent meta-analysis of 30 studies by Yin et al. showing decreased sensitivity of CT compared with other modalities, including radiography.[8] Early detection is critical in athletes because treatment decisions are often dictated by how quickly they can return to sport and also results in cost savings related to unnecessary or delayed treatments, particularly when non-hospital costs are considered.[7,10] Multiple studies have shown that MRI is the best modality for the early detection of a occult scaphoid fracture, and the American College of Radiology recommends MRI as the first choice, second line investigation.[4,7,8,11,12] When the x-ray is negative (Fig. 68.3A and B) and a fracture is present, T1-weighted images show the fracture as a distinct low-signal-intensity line surrounded by high-signal marrow fat (see Fig. 68.3C). Fat-suppressed T2-weighted images show high-signal marrow edema surrounding the fracture line (see Fig. 68.3D). MRI is also helpful in separating true fractures from incomplete fractures or contusions that may show edema but lack the discrete low signal line indicating a fracture. Consistent application of this standard will help distinguish a true fracture from contusions or microtrabecular fracture that might heal on its own with immobilization. A scaphoid fracture that is visible on initial radiographs should be further evaluated with CT to determine the degree of comminution and displacement, which may be difficult to determine on plain radiographs.

Trapezium Fracture

Displaced fractures of the trapezium body are readily seen on conventional radiographs of the wrist; however, more subtle fractures of the trapezial ridge can be missed.[13] Specific radiographs of the thumb, including dedicated PA, lateral, and Roberts views, are better for detecting these injuries and determining displacement.[14] The Roberts view is essentially a true anteroposterior

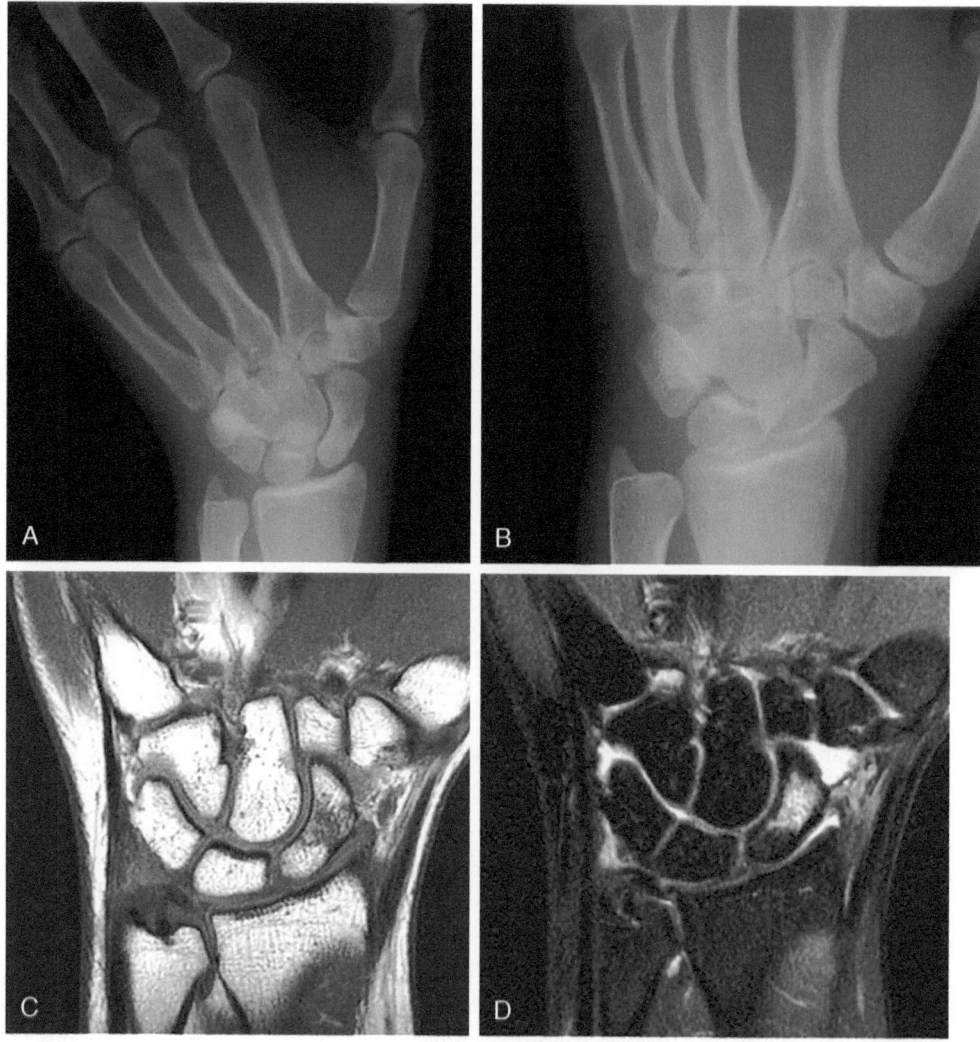

Fig. 68.3 An occult scaphoid fracture. The posteroanterior (A) and ulnar deviated (B) radiographs were read as normal. No obvious fracture line is visible. (B) Because of clinical suspicion, a magnetic resonance imaging scan was obtained, which showed a scaphoid waist fracture. Note low signal line on the T1 (C) and bone marrow edema and fluid in the fracture line on T2 with fat saturation (D).

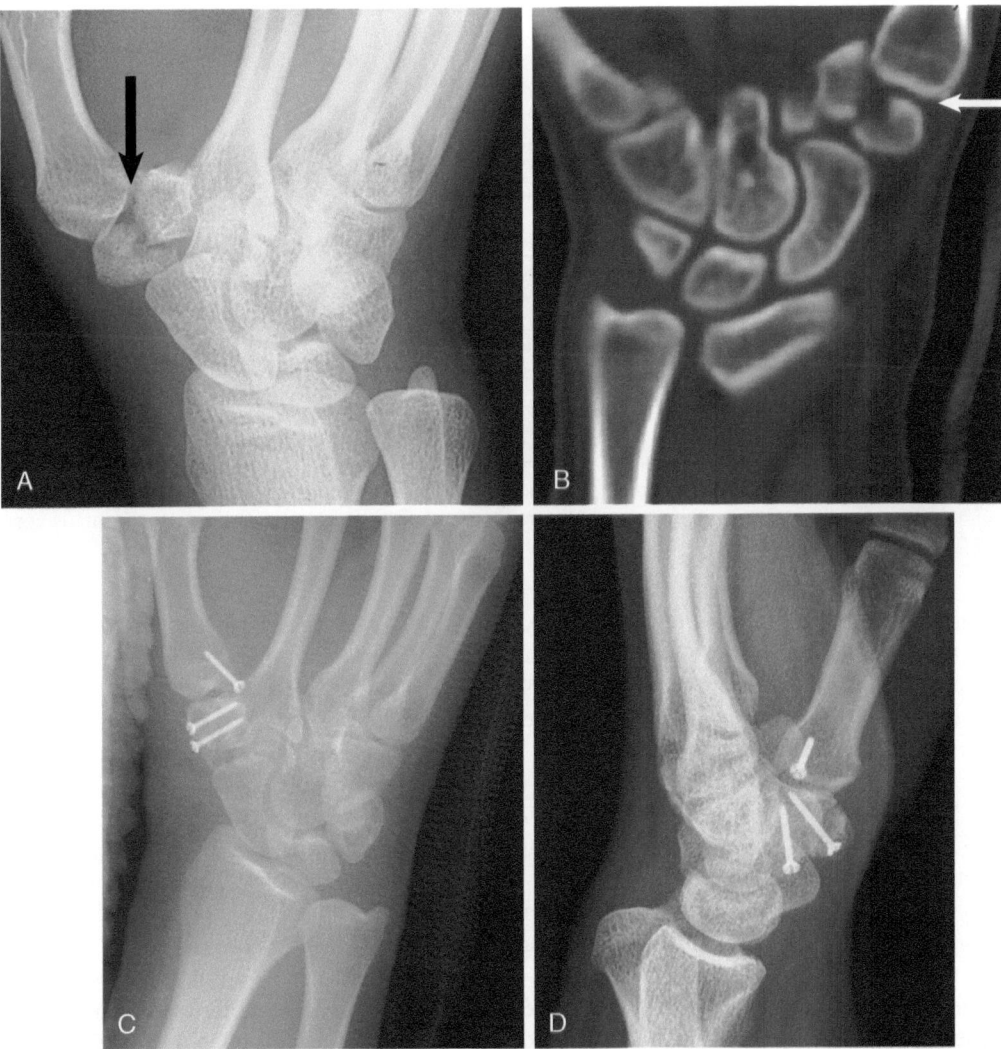

Fig. 68.4 A trapezium fracture. (A) A vertical fracture of the trapezium with intra-articular involvement both proximally and distally. (B) Computed tomography can help identify main fracture fragments for surgical plans. Oblique (C) and lateral (D) radiographic views of the wrist after open reduction and internal fixation of the fracture to restore articular congruity. An additional thumb metacarpal base fracture was also stabilized.

view of the first MCP joint taken with the hand in hyperpronation, with the dorsum of the thumb resting on the radiograph cassette. A carpal tunnel view may also help identify fractures of the trapezial ridge.[15] For additional osseous detail or surgical planning, a CT scan is preferred (Fig. 68.4).

Capitate Fracture

A displaced fracture of the capitate typically results in inversion of the proximal capitate fragment that is easy to detect on conventional radiographs of the wrist. Additional views that are helpful in visualizing the fracture include the semipronated 45-degree oblique view and a clenched-fist PA view. A nondisplaced capitate fracture may be difficult to detect with conventional radiographs. Other modalities such as CT and MRI are indicated if conventional radiographs are negative and there is clinical suspicion of an injury at this location.[16,17] These injuries occur more frequently as part of a greater arc perilunate dislocation than in isolation. MRI is preferred if avascular necrosis (AVN) is suspected based on radiographs or CT.

Hamate Fracture

Routine radiographic examination is typically inadequate for hamate fracture detection.[18] A carpal tunnel view or a semisupinated oblique view makes it easier to visualize the hamate profile and its volarly projecting hook.[19,20] In cases where the initial radiograph is negative and the clinician has a high index of suspicion for a hamate injury, CT is the test of choice.[19–21] In cases of chronic hamate hook nonunion, MRI may reveal flexor tendon injury within the carpal canal or extrinsic compression on the ulnar nerve as it travels through the Guyon canal.

Perilunate Dislocation

For the astute observer, standard wrist views are adequate for recognizing perilunate dislocations. The PA view alone, however, may look deceptively normal, and up to 25% of these injuries are missed at initial presentation.[22] On the lateral view, the capitate is dislocated dorsal to the lunate, which may either remain in its fossa at the distal radius (Mayfield stage III) or dislocate

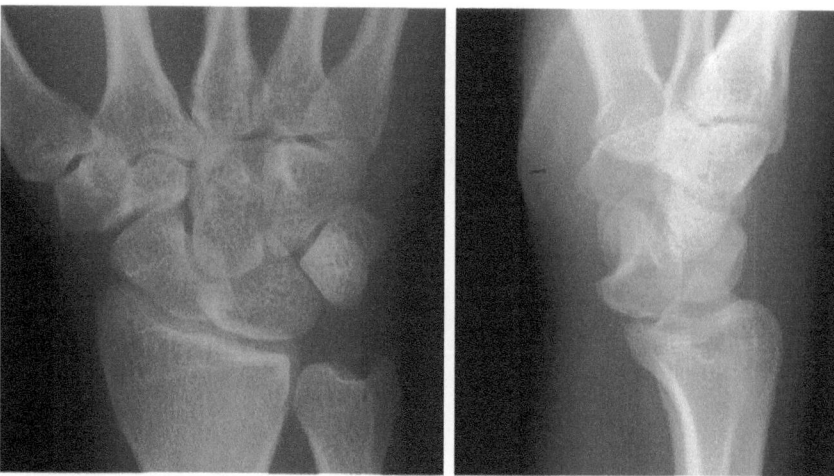

Fig. 68.5 Posteroanterior *(left)* and lateral *(right)* radiographs of a perilunate dislocation. Notice the difficulty of assessing the dislocation on the posteroanterior view alone. On the lateral radiograph, the lunate is seen to be completely dislocated.

volarly (Mayfield stage IV; Fig. 68.5).[22] Because of the difficulty in achieving a stable closed reduction and the high incidence of acute carpal tunnel syndrome, clinical urgency typically precludes additional imaging studies.[23] These injuries require definitive surgical treatment without exception.

Ulnar Impaction Syndrome

Ulnar impaction syndrome describes chronic abutment of the lunate and/or triquetrum with a prominent distal ulna articulation. Ulnar positive variance is a common finding, along with subchondral sclerosis and/or cyst formation at the distal ulna and proximal carpal row.[24] Upon MRI evaluation, ulnar impaction syndrome is characterized by a combination of degenerative central triangular fibrocartilage complex (TFCC) perforation, articular cartilage thinning, possible lunotriquetral ligament tear, and focal signal alteration at the impacted areas of the carpus and distal ulna.[25] Subchondral cysts at the point of impaction on the ulna and carpus are common. The increased signal intensity within the lunate on T2-weighted images is focal rather than diffuse, which helps distinguish this process from Kienböck disease.

Kienböck Disease

Kienböck disease is idiopathic osteonecrosis of the lunate. It is often associated with negative ulnar variance. Progression of the disease is characterized by imaging findings and progressive pain and disability. In the earliest stage of the disease, conventional radiographs are normal, but T1-weighted MRI sequences reveal diffuse low-signal intensity throughout the lunate. T2-weighted MRI sequences correlate with prognosis, with increased signal intensity directly proportional to lunate vascularization. In the second stage, sclerosis becomes apparent on conventional radiographs but is sometimes confused with increased density in the bone related to reactive edema rather than true necrosis, making MRI generally a better test at this stage.[26] By the third stage, the lunate breaks into fragments and collapses, and carpal malalignment follows. In the fourth stage, pancarpal arthritis is evident.[27] Early diagnosis by MRI is critical because early

surgical intervention such as vascularized bone grafting may slow the progression of disease and prevent lunate collapse with subsequent arthritis. Although more commonly applied to the scaphoid, some centers use dynamic contrast enhanced MRI to show whether or not vascularity of the lunate is preserved, but results have been inconsistent, possibly related to inconsistent techniques and analysis.[28-30] A recent prospective study of patients with suspected early Kienböck disease showed that conventional MRI and thin section CT with clinical information provided the best diagnostic accuracy without additional value from either 3T MRI or contrast enhancement.[30] The role of trauma in the evolution of lunate AVN is controversial. Vertical fractures of the lunate are commonly present in more advanced cases at presentation, but it is often unclear whether this is a sequela or the inciting event in the development of lunate osteonecrosis.

Intrinsic Carpal Ligament Injury

The scapholunate and lunotriquetral ligaments are the most important intrinsic ligaments of the wrist and the most susceptible to traumatic injury. For scapholunate dissociation, notable findings on the standard PA view include foreshortening of the scaphoid, widening of the scapholunate interval (normally 2 to 3 mm),[31] and a triangular appearance of the lunate because of its extended posture. The PA view may reveal a "cortical ring sign," where the abnormally flexed scaphoid creates superimposition of its distal pole and waist.[3] Lunotriquetral ligament disruption may produce an offset of the Gilula arc at the proximal articulation of the lunate or triquetrum or a widened lunotriquetral interval on a PA view, although this finding is more infrequent than with the corresponding pathology at the scapholunate interval. On a lateral wrist radiograph, a scapholunate angle of more than 60 degrees indicates dorsal intercalated segmental instability and scapholunate dissociation (Fig. 68.6).[3] Conversely, a scapholunate angle of less than 30 degrees suggests volar intercalated segmental instability and possible lunotriquetral ligament disruption.[3] The relative position of the lunate in the sagittal plane, with the wrist at neutral, predicts the instability pattern (Fig. 68.7). Additional specialized radiographic views

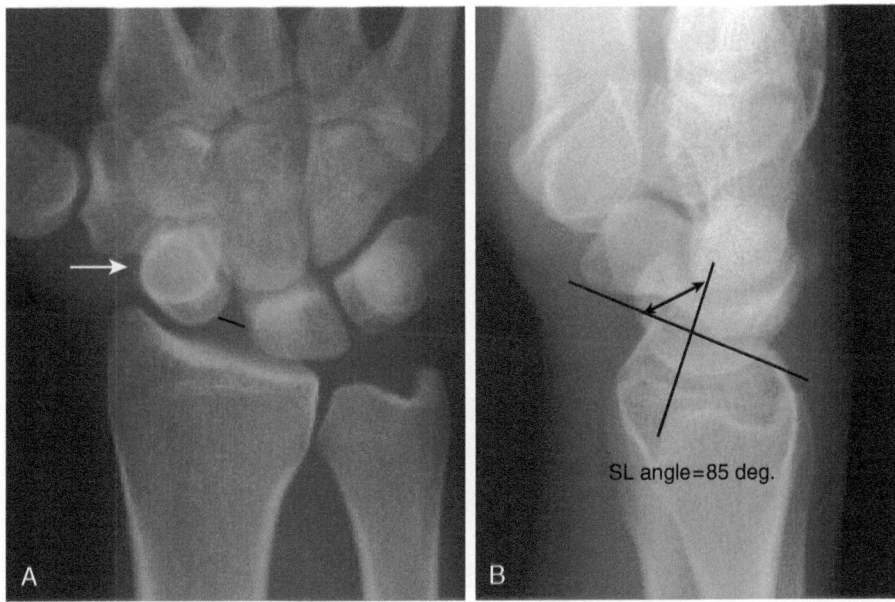

Fig. 68.6 A scapholunate *(SL)* ligament injury. (A) An anteroposterior radiograph depicting an SL ligament injury. Notice the foreshortened scaphoid, with a cortical ring sign *(arrow)*, as well as the widened SL interval *(black line)*. (B) A lateral radiograph of the wrist showing an SL ligament disruption. Notice the dorsiflexed posture of the lunate and the increased SL angle.

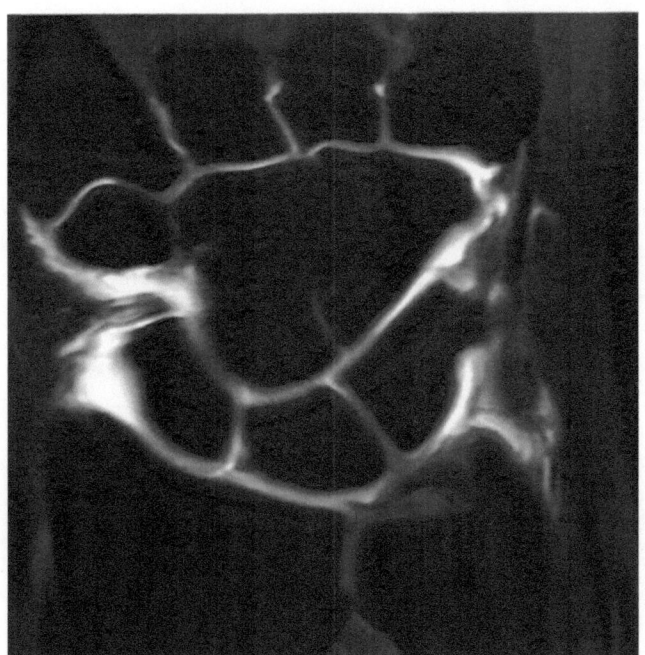

Fig. 68.7 Coronal T1-weighted image with fat suppression from a magnetic resonance arthrogram shows bright contrast communicating to the midcarpal joint through a complete tear of the scapholunate ligament after a radiocarpal joint injection.

for suspected scapholunate dissociation include the semipronated 45-degree oblique view, a clenched-fist anteroposterior view, and a PA view in ulnar deviation with the beam centered on the scaphoid. Ulnar deviation also stresses the scapholunate ligament and accentuates scapholunate widening. These studies are often performed of both wrists, as ligamentous laxity is common and comparison to the asymptomatic side and clinical findings is

critical. Abnormal carpal kinematics maybe elicited only under physiologic loading conditions, and pathology may be missed on static radiographs. Dynamic fluoroscopy is an adjunctive test that can show asynchronous carpal motion during certain wrist positions or when stress is applied. Compared with wrist arthroscopy, cineradiography has a specificity and sensitivity of 95% and 86%, respectively, for detecting scapholunate ligament tears.[32]

MRI is typically preferred to stress radiography and wrist arthrography for the diagnosis of intrinsic carpal ligament disruptions.[33] Hobby et al. performed a meta-analysis of studies examining the use of 0.5- to 1.5-tesla MRI for the detection of intrinsic ligament tears.[34] Six studies on scapholunate ligament tear detection with 159 pooled patients showed sensitivity, specificity, and accuracy of 70%, 90%, and 85%, respectively, for MRI compared with arthroscopy.[34] Similarly, six studies on lunotriquetral ligament tear detection with 142 pooled patients showed a sensitivity, specificity, and accuracy of 56%, 91%, and 82%, respectively, for MRI compared with arthroscopy.[34] The increasing availability of 3.0 Tesla MRI has improved its sensitivity for the detection of scapholunate and lunotriquetral tears to at least 89% and 82%, respectively.[35] Anderson et al.[36] showed a trend of improved sensitivity for scapholunate ligament tears with 3T compared with 1.5T, but the differences did not reach statistical significance.

In addition to detecting complete tears, MRI has the ability to detect partial tears involving either the volar or dorsal components of the scapholunate ligament and will often show tiny associated ganglion cysts that contribute to diagnostic confidence. If the diagnosis remains unclear, magnetic resonance arthrography has been proposed to improve sensitivity and specificity.[37,38] Single compartment direct gadolinium arthrography is commonly performed, but the communication between compartments is better seen with conventional arthrography at the time of the injection that can show subtle communications,[37] improving sensitivity and specificity compared with unenhanced MRI. It is important to recognize with all wrist arthrography, however, that communication between the radiocarpal compartment and other compartments during arthrography is encountered in 13% to 47% of asymptomatic patients.[35]

Tendon Injuries

With the exception of calcific tendinitis, conventional radiographs are generally unremarkable when tendon pathology is present. Overuse tendinopathies are common in athletes. Repetitive tendon irritation may produce a nonseptic tenosynovitis of any of the flexor or extensor tendons of the hand and wrist, producing tendon sheaths distended with fluid of high intensity signal on T2-weighted MRI.[25] For example, De Quervain's stenosing tenosynovitis is an overuse tendinopathy of the first dorsal extensor compartment that commonly affects golfers and racquet sport players (Fig. 68.8).[39] In addition to the tendon sheath distention previously described, Jackson et al. noted a 70% incidence of a septum separating the first extensor compartment tendons (abductor pollicis longus and extensor pollicis brevis) on axial MRI studies of the wrist in cases requiring surgical release.[26] Intersection syndrome describes tendinopathy of the second extensor compartment tendons at the site where the first extensor compartment tendons cross over them in the distal forearm.[40] The intersection, approximately 4 to 8 cm proximal to the radiocarpal joint, is often more proximal than the field of a typical wrist MRI. Therefore to acquire adequate MRI studies, it is important to communicate this clinical consideration. MRI is not necessary for the diagnosis of De Quervain tenosynovitis or intersection syndrome. Tendinosis describes a chronic degenerative process that lacks the inflammatory component of tenosynovitis. Tendinosis causes fusiform focal areas of tendon

thickening apparent on MRI.[40] Increased intrasubstance signal can be present on T1-weighted images, but T2 hyperintensity is typical of later-stage degeneration and/or partial tearing.[40]

Chronic, repetitive stress injury to the extensor carpi ulnaris (ECU) tendon is commonly seen in tennis and other types of racquet sports. This can range from chronic tendinopathy and partial tearing to subluxation and even dislocation from the ulnar groove with associated tearing of the ECU subsheath attachments at the ulnar TFCC. MRI can show the status of the tendon, but dynamic imaging of the ECU in pronation and supination can be performed with ultrasound (US) and correlated with symptoms in real time.[41]

Traumatic tendon rupture is visualized on MRI as an interruption in tendon continuity with separation of the tendon ends and fluid tracking between the torn margins (Fig. 68.9). Gap distance may guide the decision between primary repair and graft reconstruction. Flexor tendon injuries are usually classified by the anatomic zone of injury. "Jersey finger" describes a zone 1 distal avulsion of the flexor digitorum profundus tendon from its distal phalanx insertion.[42] Unless the rupture involves a small bony avulsion injury, conventional radiographs are not helpful in determining the level of retraction. MRI can be used for assessment of tendon ruptures and retraction, but care must be taken to extend imaging proximally to the point where the torn and retracted tendon can be seen, often within the palm in the case of flexor tendon injuries. US is increasingly used with tendon injuries in the hand and wrist on its own or as a complement to MRI. Increasing expertise in musculoskeletal US has become more widely available, which has improved reliability and consistency, but the modality remains challenging due to its dependence on operator experience.

Supplemental imaging is rarely necessary to diagnose distal extensor tendon injuries such as mallet or boutonnière finger.

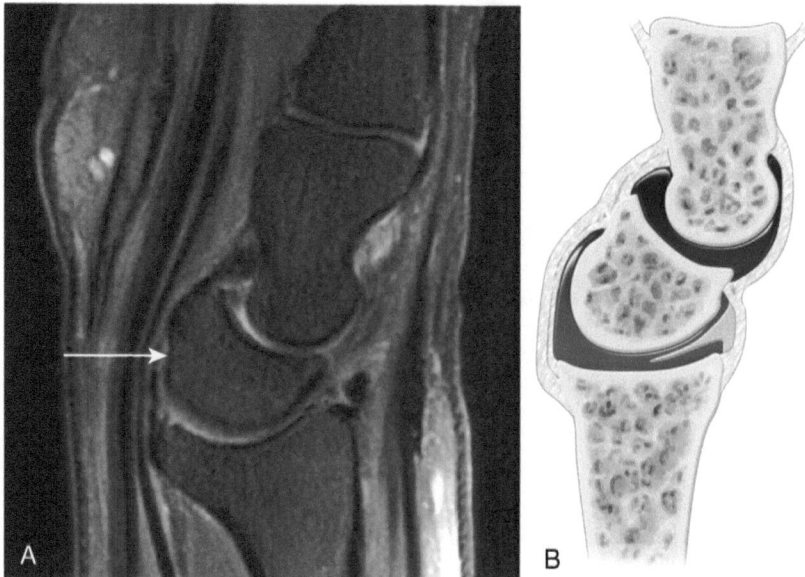

Fig. 68.8 Dorsal intercalary segmental instability. (A) The dorsal intercalary segmental instability (DISI) posture of the lunate as seen on a sagittal plane magnetic resonance image in a patient with scapholunate dissociation. The *arrow* is pointing to the intercalary segment, the lunate, which is seen to tip dorsally. (B) An artist's rendition of the DISI pattern.

However, MRI may serve a role in elucidating some extensor and collateral ligament injuries at the MCP joint. Collateral ligament injury can sometimes be best evaluated on MRI with the fist clenched as an adjunct to conventional imaging. Traumatic injury to the sagittal band and/or dorsal capsule overlying the MCP joint, also known as "boxer's knuckle," can produce painful swelling, subluxation of the extensor tendon, and occasional joint instability.[25] On axial MRI studies, sagittal band injury appears as an interruption in the fine, low-signal-intensity, linear structure distributed circumferentially from the central tendon to the volar plate.[43] Deeper disruption to the joint capsule with accompanying synovial fluid extravasation also may be evident. US can also be useful for imaging injuries to the collateral ligaments,

sagittal bands, and extensor hood. When evaluating tendons, an appreciation of the "magic angle" phenomenon is important. This phenomenon affects all structures with high collagen content, such as tendons and ligaments. Asymptomatic, spuriously increased intrasubstance signal alteration may be seen in wrist flexor and extensor tendons as a result of the magnetic field orientation during image acquisition. At approximately 55 degrees relative to the static magnetic field, imaging sequences may show artificially increased intratendinous signal intensity that disappears on more heavily T2-weighted sequences.[27] The tendons most often affected are the ECU, extensor carpi radialis longus, extensor pollicis longus, flexor carpi radialis, and flexor carpi ulnaris.

Adjustments in technique, particularly increasing the echo time (TE), can be made if there is persistent uncertainty regarding intratendinous increased signal on MRI.

Triangular Fibrocartilage Complex Injury

Conventional radiographs are usually unrevealing in the setting of TFCC injury, although TFCC injuries can be associated with radius fractures and DRUJ instability.[44] MRI may be used to evaluate the major TFCC components—the fibrocartilaginous articular disc, dorsal and volar radioulnar ligaments, ulnolunate ligament, ulnotriquetral ligament, and ECU tendon subsheath.[24,27,33] MRI has been shown to have high sensitivity and specificity for imaging the components of the TFCC.[35,36,45] TFCC abnormalities have traditionally been classified as degenerative or traumatic, but it is rare to diagnose acute injuries to the TFCC (Fig. 68.10). A more relevant approach will assess radial or central tears versus injury to the ulnar attachments, which are more commonly associated with joint instability. Ulnar wrist pain is a challenging clinical problem, and MR imaging the ulnar attachments of the TFCC, specifically including the ulnotriquetral and ulnar foveal attachments, requires close attention to detail. Techniques are

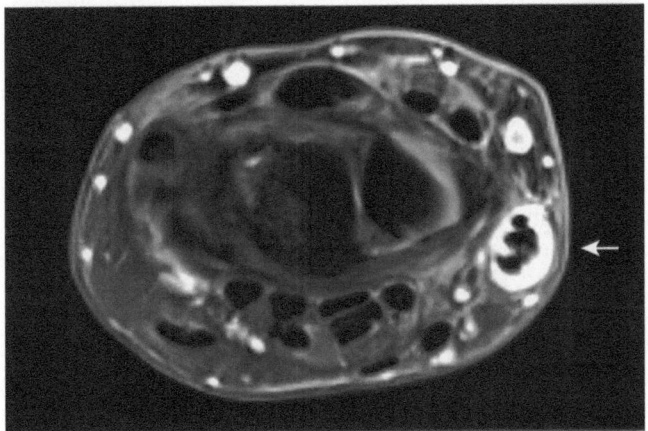

Fig. 68.9 An axial fat-suppressed T2-weighted magnetic resonance image reveals high-signal intensity fluid distending the sheath of the first extensor compartment, with thickening of the abductor pollicis longus and extensor pollicis brevis tendons *(arrow)* compatible with De Quervain tenosynovitis.

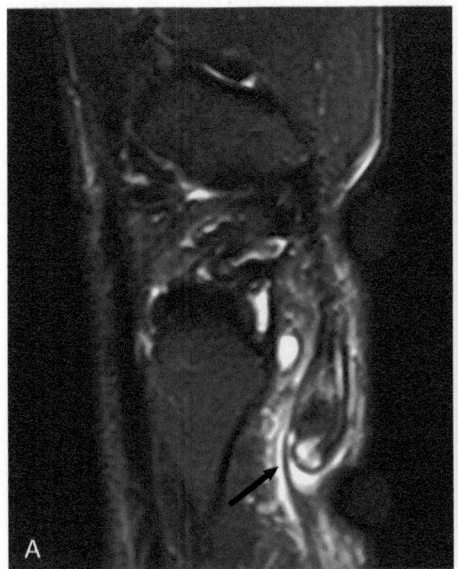
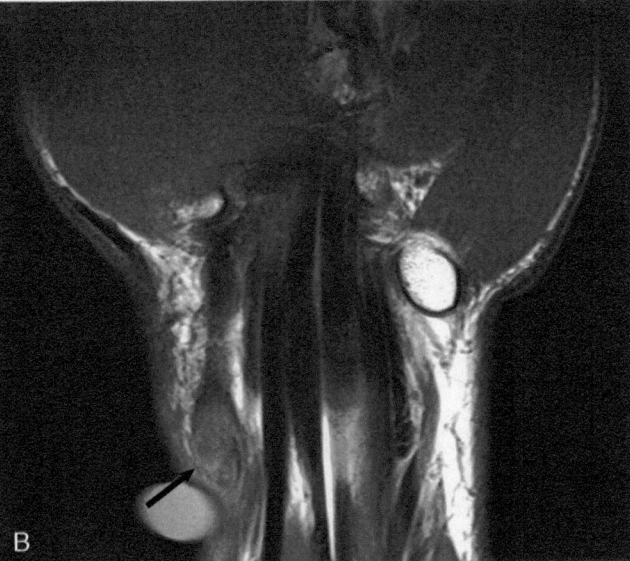

Fig. 68.10 (A) A sagittal T2-weighted magnetic resonance image of the wrist showing complete rupture of the flexor carpi radialis tendon with thickening and a diffusely abnormal signal at its torn margin *(arrow)*. The proximal portion of the tendon was retracted and outside of the field of view. (B) A coronal T1-weighted magnetic resonance image of the wrist for the same patient showing complete rupture of the flexor carpi radialis tendon with thickening and diffusely abnormal signal at its torn margin *(arrow)*.

challenging to assess and optimized imaging in three planes with dedicated wrist coils and high field technique is required. Some studies have shown improvement in sensitivity with imaging at 3T compared with 1.5T,[35,36] and in general if 3T is available, it is preferred for wrist imaging compared with lower field imaging. Dorsal displacement of the DRUJ on pronated axial MR images and correlation with clinical findings such as the "foveal sign" may improve the detection of ulnotriquetral and foveal tears with instability.[46,47] CT can also be performed with progressive pronation against resistance to evoke instability at the DRUJ.[48] Radial-sided tears and central perforations of the articular disk are common and generally well seen on conventional MRI (Figs. 68.11A and B).

Of the available diagnostic tools, wrist arthroscopy remains the gold standard, and imaging modalities are compared for accuracy against this standard.[27,33] A meta-analysis of the 0.5- to 1.5-tesla MRI examinations of 410 patients performed for the detection of TFCC tears revealed a sensitivity, specificity, and accuracy of 83%, 80%, and 81%, respectively, when compared with arthroscopy.[34] Newer, more powerful, 3.0-tesla magnets have improved the detection of TFCC tears, with a sensitivity and specificity approaching 86% and 100%, respectively.[35] Magnetic resonance three-compartment arthrography of the wrist is typically not used for TFCC tears due to the large number of false-positive findings because of microperforations that are present in 7% to 35% of the population.[35]

HAND INJURIES

Pulley Injuries

Pulley injuries commonly occur in rock climbers. Normal digital flexion power requires integrity of the pulley system.[40] Direct visualization of the disrupted pulley in the transverse plane or the absence of a pulley in the sagittal plane is diagnostic on MRI.[40] A pulley rupture results in an increased distance between the phalanx and flexor tendon, known as "bowstringing." US

can be used to directly visualize the pulley structures but does not display the bone relative to the tendon in the same as MRI and CT. Any distance of the flexor tendon of more than 1 mm from the bone is considered pathologic. Widening of 1 to 4 mm from the bone is associated with complete A2 pulley ruptures. A combination of A2 and A3 pulley ruptures may increase the distance up to 7 mm. In the setting of a high clinical suspicion, acquiring images with the affected digit in maximal flexion enhances these findings.[40]

Thumb Ulnar Collateral Ligament Injury

The thumb ulnar collateral ligament (UCL), the primary restraint to hyperabduction at the MCP joint, is commonly injured by skiers. The diagnosis of acute thumb UCL injury is based primarily on history and physical examination.[49] When UCL injury is suspected, conventional radiographs should precede stress testing to prevent potential displacement of an associated avulsion fracture.[37] Once a fracture is ruled out, a thumb abduction stress PA radiograph may help in the comparison of side-to-side differences in joint stability and aid in surgical decision-making.[50] When stress testing is equivocal, MRI can often differentiate partial from complete ligament injuries, especially in cases that do not respond to initial nonoperative management (Fig. 68.12A–C).[51] The displacement of a distally torn UCL to a position superficial to the aponeurosis of the adductor pollicis muscle is called a Stener lesion.[27] MRI may detect a Stener lesion in the coronal plane, parallel to the plane of the collateral ligaments, but US also has utility, especially with acute injuries or instances where dynamic movement and stress imaging can display free edge of the torn tendon. It is important to detect Stener lesions, because most athletes with these complete UCL tears require surgical treatment.[33]

Metacarpal Fracture

Metacarpal fractures are easily seen on conventional radiographs. If on routine radiographs a subtle interruption of the cortices

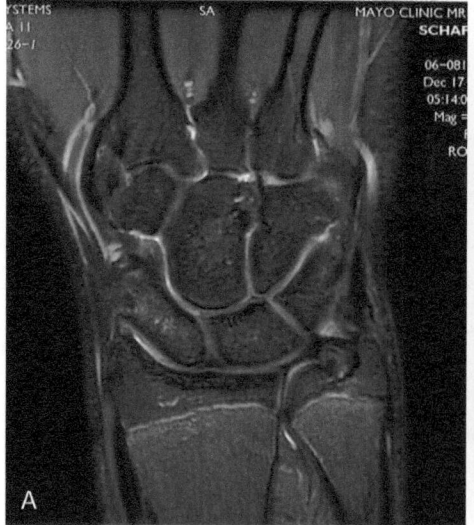
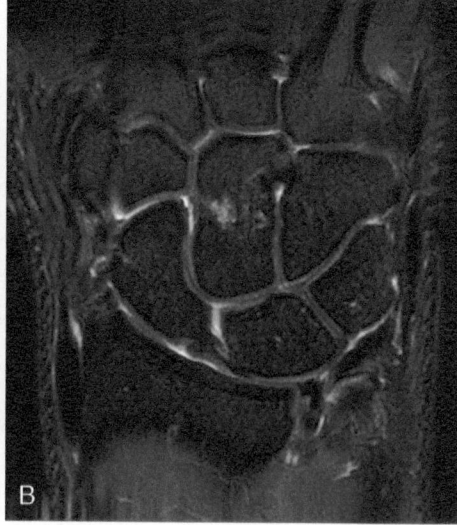

Fig. 68.11 T2-weighted coronal images of the wrist with fat suppression from two different patients showing a normal (A) triangular fibrocartilage complex and a distracted tear (B) of the central disk and radial attachment.

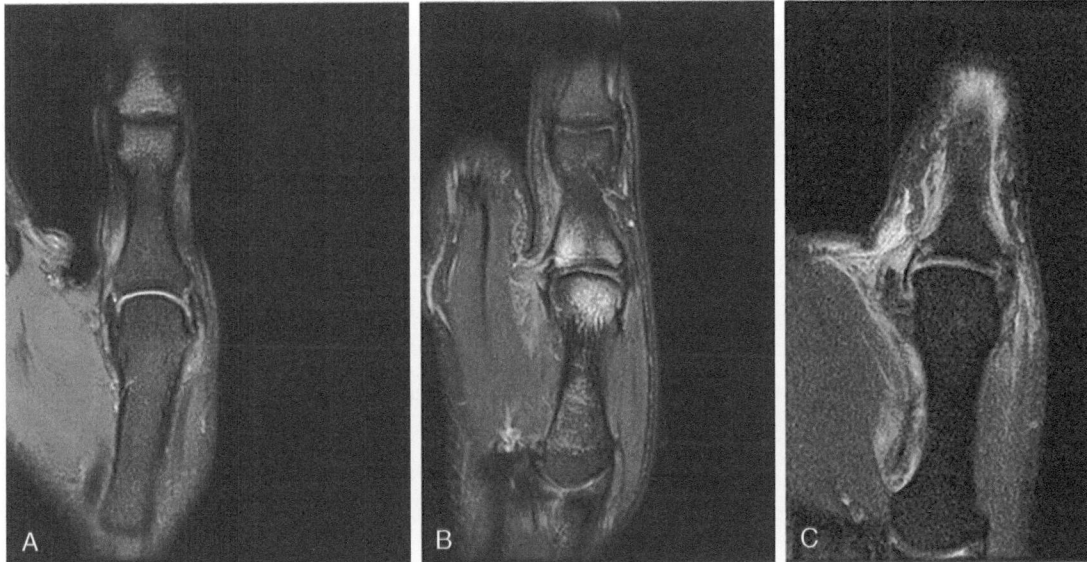

Fig. 68.12 Coronal T2-weighted 3T magnetic resonance images of the thumb with fat suppression from three different patients showing (A) a partial tear of the ulnar collateral ligament; (B) a complete tear of the ulnar collateral ligament with the torn end of the adductor pollicis tendon just at the aponeurosis; and (C) a complete tear of the ulnar collateral ligament with the tendon completely superficial to the aponeurosis representing a Stener lesion.

is noted, a 30-degree pronated lateral or a 30-degree supinated lateral view for visualizing the index and long or ring and small metacarpals, respectively, can be obtained. If metacarpal head disruption is suspected, a Brewerton view with the supinated hand resting on the cassette and the MCP joints flexed 40 degrees can help.[52] CT may be necessary to rule out occult intra-articular injuries. Fracture of neighboring metacarpals is not an uncommon finding because of the strong interosseous ligaments between adjacent metacarpals.

Fractures at the carpometacarpal joint of the thumb deserve special attention. The thumb's opposable orientation relative to the other digits warrants specialized imaging for better visualization. A Robert's view provides a true anteroposterior projection of the thumb. A true lateral view of the carpometacarpal joint is obtained with the forearm flat on the table, the hand pronated 20 degrees, the thumb flat on a cassette, and the gantry angled 10 degrees from vertical in the distal to proximal projection. These views permit evaluation of metacarpal displacement and assessment of the number, size, and position of the intra-articular fracture fragments. Intra-articular metacarpal base fractures of the thumb may be partial[53] or complete[54] types. A Bennett fracture produces an intra-articular oblique volar lip avulsion fragment at the ulnar base of the thumb metacarpal (Fig. 68.13).[53] In contrast, a Rolando fracture has more complex intra-articular involvement and potential comminution.[54] Distinguishing the fracture types is important for treatment and prognosis.

CONCLUSION

A thorough understanding of hand and wrist pathology and a familiarity with common imaging findings ensures timely diagnosis, appropriate treatment, and expeditious return to sport for the affected athlete.

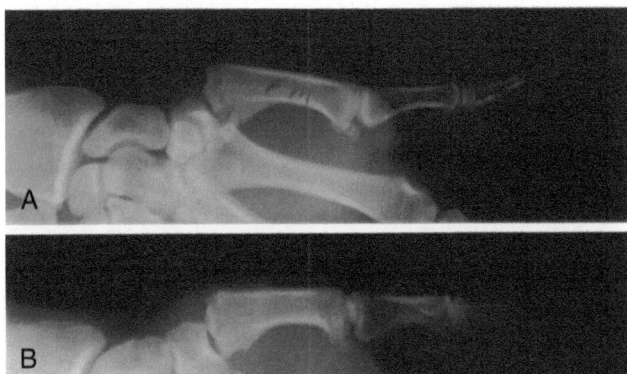

Fig. 68.13 True lateral radiographs of the thumb base showing a Bennett fracture subluxation of the thumb carpometacarpal joint before (A) and after (B) reduction.

ACKNOWLEDGMENT

The author wishes to thank Drs. Ashvin K. Dewan, Avneesh Chhabra, and Lance M. Brunton for their excellent chapter on this topic in the fourth edition.

For a complete list of references, go to ExpertConsult.com.

SELECTED READINGS

Citation:

Potter HG, Asnis-Ernberg L, Weiland AJ, et al. The utility of high-resolution magnetic resonance imaging in the evaluation of the triangular fibrocartilage complex of the wrist. *J Bone Joint Surg Am.* 1997;79(11):1675–1684.

Level of Evidence:

II

Summary:
This article details a prospective evaluation of high-resolution magnetic resonance imaging of the wrist in 77 patients who subsequently underwent arthroscopy for wrist pain. Sensitivity, specificity, and accuracy were compared against arthroscopy as a goal standard.

Citation:
Pliefke J, Stengel D, Rademacher G, et al. Diagnostic accuracy of plain radiographs and cineradiography in diagnosing traumatic scapholunate dissociation. *Skeletal Radiol.* 2008;37(2):139–145.

Level of Evidence:
III

Summary:
In this retrospective study of 102 patients with a hyperextension injury of the wrist, diagnostic accuracy of scapholunate ligament tears using magnetic resonance imaging and diagnostic arthroscopy is evaluated.

Citation:
Karl JW, Swart E, Strauch RJ. Diagnosis of occult scaphoid fractures: a cost-effectiveness analysis. *J Bone Joint Surg Am.* 2015;97(22):1860–1868.

Level of Evidence:
IV

Summary:
This is an exceptionally high-quality study that uses formal cost-effectiveness measures to model to evaluate a scenario where a patient presents with clinical suspicion of scaphoid fracture and negative radiographs. The most important determining factor of cost (including the total episode of care and impact on Quality Adjusted Life Years) was the use of advanced imaging in the emergency setting. Magnetic resonance imaging was slightly more cost effective than computed tomography, but the authors conclude that either is acceptable, depending on local institutional factors such as access.

Citation:
Yin ZG, Zhang JB, Kan SL, et al. Diagnostic accuracy of imaging modalities for suspected scaphoid fractures: meta-analysis combined with latent class analysis. *J Bone Joint Surg Br.* 2012;94(8):1077–1085.

Level of Evidence:
IV

Summary:
This is a comprehensive, meta-analysis of 30 studies comparing the sensitivity and specificity of radiographs, magnetic resonance imaging (MRI), computed tomography, and bone scan in the diagnosis of suspected scaphoid fractures. The conclusion supports the use of MRI as a first choice, second line tool.

Citation:
Bennett EH. Fractures of the metacarpal bones. *Dublin J Med Sci.* 1882;73:72–75.

Level of Evidence:
IV

Summary:
This article features the original description of the Bennett fracture.

Citation:
Rolando S. Fracture of the base of the first metacarpal and a variation that has not yet been described: 1910 (translated by Roy Meals). *Clin Orthop Relat Res.* 2006;445:15–18.

Level of Evidence:
IV

Summary:
This article features the original description of the Rolando fracture.

Citation:
Lichtman DM, Bindra RR, Boyer MI, et al. American Academy of Orthopaedic Surgeons clinical practice guideline on the treatment of distal radius fractures. *J Bone Joint Surg Am.* 2011;93(8):775–778.

Level of Evidence:
V

Summary:
This article provides evidence-based guidelines and consensus recommendations regarding treatment of distal radius fractures from the American Academy of Orthopaedic Surgeons.

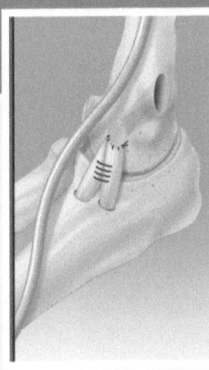

69

Wrist Arthroscopy

William B. Geissler, David A. Rush, Christopher A. Keen

Arthroscopy has revolutionized the practice of orthopedics by providing the technical capacity to examine and treat intraarticular abnormalities under magnified and brightened conditions. The development of wrist arthroscopy was a natural progression in the successful application of arthroscopy to other larger joints. The wrist itself is a labyrinth of eight carpal bones, multiple articular surfaces, intrinsic and extrinsic ligaments, and a triangular fibrocartilage complex (TFCC), all within a 5 cm interval. Wrist arthroscopy has continued to undergo considerable development since Whipple and colleagues[1] originally reported the techniques they developed. This complex joint continues to challenge clinicians with an array of potential diagnoses, pathology, and treatment options.

Indications for wrist arthroscopy continue to expand, as new techniques and instrumentation are constantly being developed and improved. Diagnostic indications include assessment of the interosseous ligaments, which show a spectrum of injury, as well as evaluation of the array of pathology that may occur on the ulnar side of the wrist—particularly the TFCC.[2-4] The use of wrist arthroscopy in managing fractures continues to grow, with management of both distal radius and scaphoid fractures now possible.[5,6] Wrist arthroscopy is extremely sensitive in detecting chondral defects of both the radiocarpal and midcarpal joints, which are frequently difficult to evaluate with imaging studies alone. These defects may be a source of chronic wrist pain of unknown etiology.[7]

The purpose of this chapter is to present a variety of wrist arthroscopy techniques and describe how they may be applied to an array of pathologic conditions of the wrist.

GENERAL SET-UP FOR WRIST ARTHROSCOPY

Instrumentation

The use of instruments tailored for small joints is absolutely essential in wrist arthroscopy.[8] The use of instruments developed for arthroscopy of large joints is not appropriate for the small joint of the wrist. In general, a small joint arthroscope that measures 2.7 mm or smaller is used with either a 30- or 70-degree visualization angle. Small joint punches and graspers are used, particularly for management of tears to the articular disk of the TFCC. A small joint shaver that measures 3.5 mm or smaller with varied tips should be available for joint débridement.

The use of traction is essential for visualization.[9] A commercial traction tower may be used, which involves stabilization of the forearm and application of longitudinal force to finger traps that are placed on two or more of the digits. The amount of traction may be adjusted by means of a gear mechanism. Traction towers are now being made with the traction bar at the side of the forearm rather than in the middle, which facilitates the use of fluoroscopy and expands the indication of wrist arthroscopy for the management of carpal instability and fractures. An advantage of using the traction tower is that it applies constant traction to the wrist while it is slightly flexed. The slightly flexed position of the wrist makes it easier to insert the wrist arthroscope and other instruments. The improved visualization and increased ability to use instruments in the wrist with newer traction towers continue to expand the indications for treating various wrist pathologies (Fig. 69.1).

If a traction tower is not available, a shoulder holder may be used overhead to support the wrist. A countertraction band is placed around the arm. The wrist may be aligned in a horizontal manner on a hand table, which allows it to be stabilized by a pulley attached to the hand table with weights hanging over the end of the table (Fig. 69.2). Some surgeons prefer the horizontal position for wrist arthroscopy. In general, approximately 10 lb. (4.5 kg) of traction is applied.

Portal Placement

Accurate portal placement is vital in wrist arthroscopy because of the small space available in the wrist joint.[10,11] Appropriate portal placement begins with palpation of anatomic landmarks, first marking the base of the index, long, and ring metacarpals. Next, the radial and ulnar borders of the extensor carpi ulnaris (ECU) tendon are identified and marked. The radiocarpal joint space may be palpated and marked by rolling the surgeon's thumb over the dorsal rim of the distal radius and making an impression with the fingernail. The tendons of the extensor pollicis longus and extensor digitorum communis are palpated and marked unless they are obscured by swelling from an acute injury.

After traction is applied, all portals should be drawn on the skin before any incisions are made (Fig. 69.3). The portals are named by their position relative to the dorsal (extensor) tendon compartments. The 3-4 portal is the most common viewing portal and passes between the third and fourth dorsal compartments. It is located by palpating the Lister tubercle and then moving the finger about 1 cm distal until a soft spot is felt between the coursing tendons. In addition, the 3-4 portal is in line with the radial border of the long finger. The 4-5 portal, which is

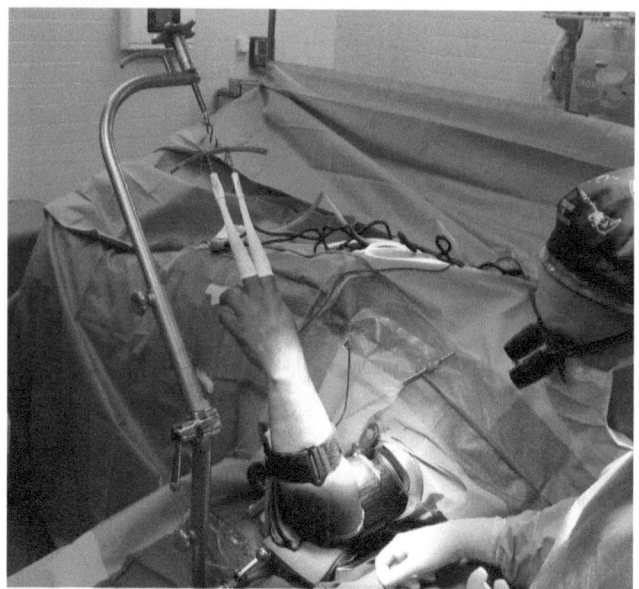

Fig. 69.1 The general setup for wrist arthroscopy. The upper area is stabilized to the traction tower with Velcro straps. The forearm is stabilized via a volar brace, allowing various degrees of wrist flexion. All points of contact with the traction tower are padded. Approximately 10 lb of traction is applied to the index and middle finger via finger traps.

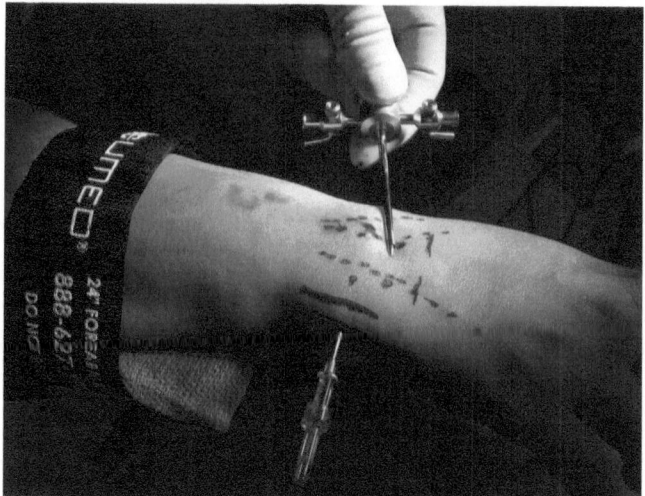

Fig. 69.3 Portal sites are drawn on the skin after application of traction to the wrist. The inflow needle may be seen entering the 6-U portal. A horizontal line represents the base of the middle and ring metacarpals. The extensor carpi ulnaris (ECU) tendon is outlined by the solid lines next to the inflow needle. The 6-R portal is marked by the proximal dot on the radial side of the ECU tendon. The two midcarpal portals are seen approximately 1 cm distal to the 3-4 portal and the 4-5 portal.

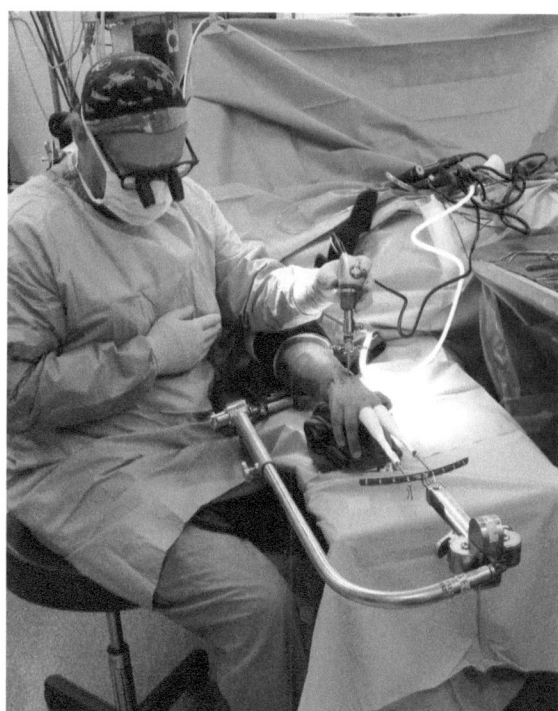

Fig. 69.2 Horizontal positioning of the traction tower. Traction also may be accomplished with a countertraction band around the arm and a pulley attached to the end of the hand table.

located between the fourth and fifth dorsal compartments, is the primary working portal. This portal is located by palpating the ulnar aspect of the fourth compartment and identifying the soft spot opposite the 3-4 portal. As a general rule, the 4-5 portal lies slightly more proximal than the 3-4 portal because of the normal radial inclination of the distal radius and is in line with

the mid axis of the ring finger. The 1-2 portal is located between the first and second extensor compartments just distal to the radial styloid. It is important to be mindful of the adjacent neurovascular structures when utilizing this portal. One study showed that the radial artery was located 3 mm radial to the portal, and the branches of the dorsal sensory branch of the radial nerve were within 3 mm radial and 5 mm ulnar to the portal.[12] The 6-R and 6-U portals are named according to their position relative to the ECU tendon, with the 6-R portal being radial and the 6-U portal being ulnar to the tendon. The 6-R portal is generally a working portal, whereas the 6-U portal is frequently used for inflow. Normally 3 to 5 mL of irrigation fluid is injected into the radiocarpal space through an inflow cannula established at the 6-U portal. As the wrist joint is inflated with irrigation fluid, the dorsal aspect of the 3-4 portal bulges, which further helps localize the proper position of the 3-4 portal. A pressurized pump may include a feedback mechanism to provide uniform pressure flow of irrigation into the joint. When a pump is not available, gravity flow of irrigation fluid is usually sufficient for wrist arthroscopy. Outflow is provided through the arthroscope cannula.

The wrist is suspended in the traction tower with slight flexion. This position facilitates insertion of the arthroscope and other instruments. Before committing to a portal, a 22-gauge needle should be placed in the proposed portal location to ensure that it passes easily into the joint without affecting the distal radius, ulna, or carpus. Portal incisions may be longitudinal or transverse. Transverse portals may be more cosmetic but pose a slightly higher risk of injury to the underlying dorsal radial or dorsal ulnar sensory nerve branches. To avoid injury to these cutaneous nerves, the surgeon uses his or her thumb to pull the skin against the tip of a number 11 scalpel blade along the length of incision (Fig. 69.4). Blunt dissection is carried out with a hemostat to

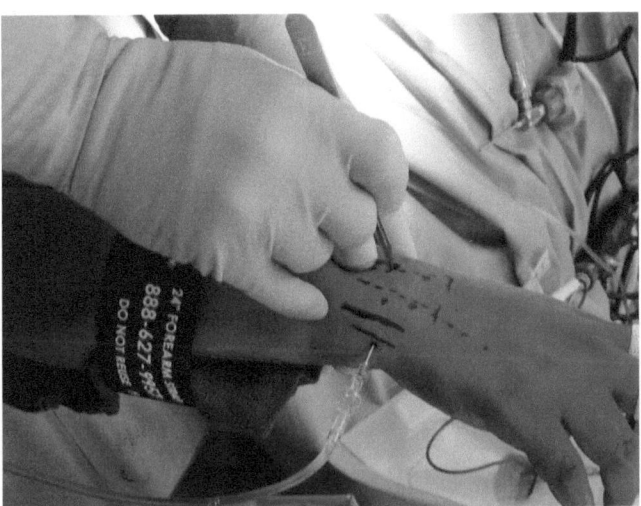

Fig. 69.4 Vertical skin incisions are used to decrease the risk of injury to superficial sensory nerves. The skin is placed under tension with the left thumb, and a No. 11 blade is used to incise the skin only. A hemostat is then used to bluntly dissect the soft tissue.

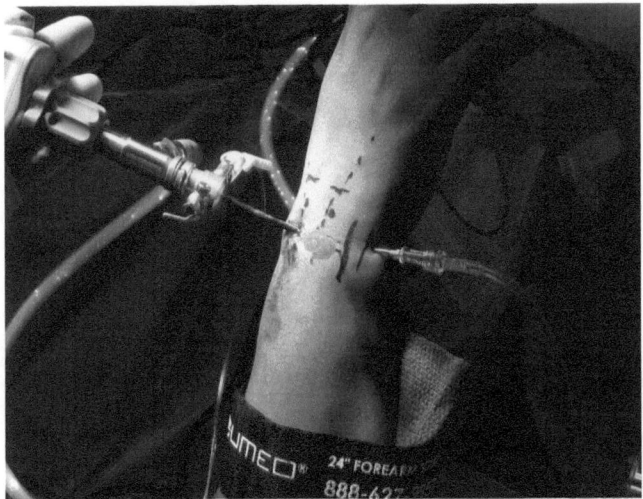

Fig. 69.5 The 2.7 mm arthroscope view through the 3-4 portal. Note the 10-degree inclination of the arthroscope to accommodate the normal volar tilt of the distal radius. An 18-gauge needle is first used to localize the 6-R portal under arthroscopic visualization.

the level of the joint capsule. The arthroscopic cannula with a blunt trocar is placed at an approximate 10-degree angle relative to the long axis of the forearm, to enter the radiocarpal joint in line with the normal volar slope of the distal radius (Fig. 69.5).

The radial and ulnar midcarpal portals are made approximately 1 cm distal to the 3-4 and 4-5 portals, respectively.[13] The midcarpal space is somewhat tighter than the radiocarpal space, and care should be taken when entering it with a blunt trocar. A needle is always used first to identify the precise position of the midcarpal portals before incising the skin. The radial midcarpal portal has slightly less room compared with the ulnar midcarpal portal. If the surgeon has difficulty entering the radial midcarpal portal, the arthroscope can be placed in the ulnar midcarpal space first, where more room is available to enter the joint. This may be seen, for example, if the patient has a scapholunate ligament

injury with carpal malreduction. Inflow is provided through the arthroscopic cannula, and a needle is used to provide outflow in the intercarpal space to improve visualization.

The volar radiocarpal (VR) portal is made between the interval of the radioscaphocapitate ligament and the long radiolunate ligament. This portal is most easily established by placing the arthroscope directly at that interval while viewing the volar extrinsic ligaments from the 3-4 portal. A blunt trocar is then inserted into the cannula and gently passed through the volar capsule, tinting the skin on the volar aspect of the wrist. An incision is made and a second slightly larger cannula may be placed over the arthroscopic cannula or a guidewire passed through the arthroscopic cannula. The trocar then enters the volar aspect of the wrist with this inside-out technique, with care taken to protect the adjacent structures—namely the radial artery (which lies radial to the portal) and the ulnarly based flexor carpi radialis tendon and the median nerve. The volar ulnar (VU) portal, described by Slutsky,[14] is established by making a 2 cm longitudinal or zigzag incision just proximal to the wrist crease along the ulnar edge of the finger flexor tendons. The flexor carpi ulnaris (FCU) and ulnar neurovascular bundle are retracted ulnarly, while the common flexor tendons are retracted radially. The radiocarpal joint space is localized with a 22-gauge needle just distal to the pronator quadratus, and the capsule is opened bluntly, followed by insertion of the trocar/cannula. The VU portal can also be made using an inside-out technique. While the arthroscope is in the 3-4 portal, a blunt trocar is placed in the 6-U portal and pushed volarly through the ulnar carpal joint complex between the ulnolunate and triquetrum ligaments, exiting the floor of the flexor tendons. It is important to remember that the ulnar neurovascular bundle is generally found approximately 5 mm ulnar to the trocar; the median nerve is protected by the flexor tendons.

DRY ARTHROSCOPY

Dry arthroscopy is an alternative technique, where traction through the fingers alone maintains a suitable joint space for viewing.[15] It is very useful in situations where larger portals or mini-open incisions are needed, while avoiding the normal tissue plane disruption seen in wet arthroscopy and the potential risk of compartment syndrome.[2,15] It is important to keep the side valve on the cannula open to air so that suction does not collapse the joint capsule. Suction should be used sparingly. In the setting of fracture, initial washing of the joint with 10 to 20 mL of fluid through a syringe attached to the side valve of the arthroscope sheath may be useful for evacuating hematoma or debris. The wrist arthroscope can be dried with small surgical padding inserted through a separate portal. *Tip:* To improve visualization, immerse the tip of the arthroscope in warm water to prevent condensation. Dry arthroscopy is contraindicated in the setting where heat generators such as cautery or lasers are used.

ARTHROSCOPIC ANATOMY

Arthroscopic evaluation of the radiocarpal space begins with the arthroscope in the 3-4 portal and progresses systematically from a radial to ulnar direction. The radial styloid process and distal radius scaphoid facet articulate with the proximal aspect of the scaphoid, and this region is examined for any signs of chondromalacia or synovitis, which may be seen in persons with degenerative arthritis. The volar extrinsic ligaments are then evaluated. The radioscaphocapitate ligament is the most radial extrinsic ligament.[16] The long radiolunate ligament is just ulnar to the radioscaphocapitate ligament and may be two to three times wider (Fig. 69.6).[13,17] Ulnar to the long radiolunate ligament is the short radiolunate ligament, and the variable radioscapholunate ligament (the ligament of Testut) is actually a neurovascular structure passing at the scapholunate interval.

The normal concave appearance of the scapholunate interosseous ligament is found between the scaphoid and the lunate (Fig. 69.7). The lunate facet of the distal radius and the articular surfaces of the proximal carpal row are inspected for areas of chondromalacia. The articular disk of the TFCC inserts adjacent to the central ulnar rim of the distal radius. The normal thickening of the volar and dorsal radioulnar ligaments is typically well visualized.

A metal probe may be inserted in either the 4-5 or 6-R portal to palpate the TFCC articular disk. This region may be palpated and confirmed to be uniformly taut, similar to the effect on a trampoline. In addition, Greene and Kakar described the suction test that can be used to determine the tension within the TFCC articular disk.[18] A 2.5 or 3.5 mm shaver is placed in the 4-5 or 6R portal, and suction through the shaver will help delineate the TFCC's stability. The prestyloid recess is located dorsal to the ulnocarpal ligaments (Fig. 69.8). The prestyloid recess is a normal anatomic finding that is not to be confused with a peripheral tear of the TFCC. The 6-U inflow cannula is traditionally placed through this recess. The extrinsic volar ulnocarpal ligaments and lunotriquetral interosseous ligament are best visualized with the arthroscope in either the 4-5 or 6-R portal. The ulnolunate and ulnotriquetral ligaments are capsular thickenings that are considered part of the TFCC. The lunotriquetral interosseous ligament should have a normal concave appearance between the lunate and triquetrum, very similar to that of the scapholunate interosseous ligament.

The midcarpal space is evaluated next.[19] The arthroscope is usually placed in the radial midcarpal space initially, although in smaller wrists, it may be easier to start the examination with the arthroscope in the ulnar midcarpal portal. Once the arthroscope is established in the radial midcarpal portal, the head of the capitate and scapholunate interval are initially identified (Fig. 69.9). The proximal hamate and lunotriquetral interval are viewed as the arthroscope is translated ulnarly (Fig. 69.10). The arthroscope may then be translated radially and distally between the scaphoid and the capitate to visualize the scaphotrapezial-trapezoid joint. Accordingly, the trapezoid is found in the foreground and the trapezium is found in the background.

DISTAL RADIOULNAR JOINT ARTHROSCOPY

Distal radioulnar joint arthroscopy is useful for evaluating the articular cartilage of the ulnar head and sigmoid notch, as well as assessment of soft tissue disorders that cannot be seen from

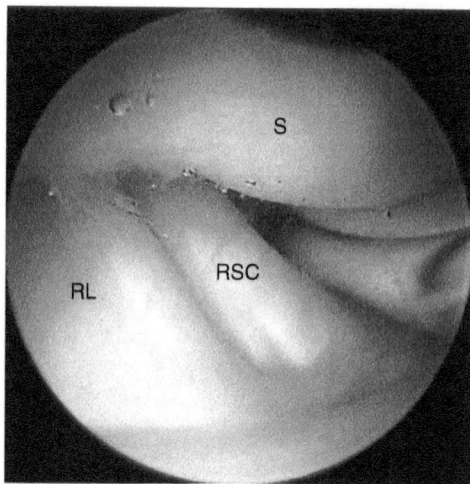

Fig. 69.6 An arthroscopic image of the long radiolunate *(RL)* ligament and the radioscaphocapitate *(RSC)* ligament. Note that the RL ligament is two to three times the width of the RSC ligament. The scaphoid *(S)* is seen superiorly.

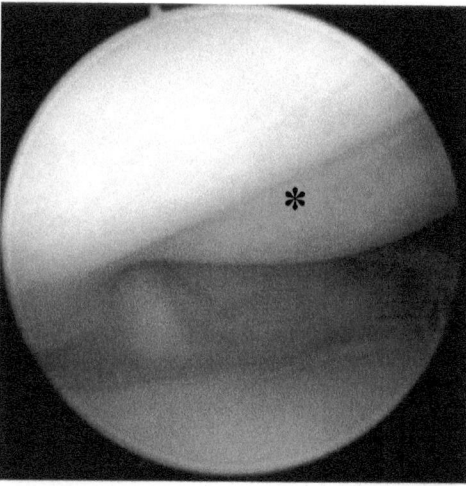

Fig. 69.7 An arthroscopic image of the scapholunate interosseous ligament *(asterisk)* as seen from the 4-5 portal. The short radiolunate, long radiolunate, and radioscaphocapitate ligaments are seen in the background.

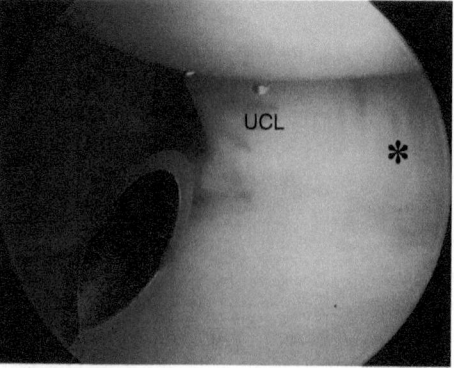

Fig. 69.8 An arthroscopic image as viewed from the 4-5 portal showing the inflow needle entering through the prestyloid recess. The ulnar collateral ligament *(UCL)* and dorsal ulnocarpal ligaments *(asterisk)* can be seen to the right of the inflow needle.

the radiocarpal space.[20] Indications include débridement of undersurface flap tears of the articular disk, removal of loose bodies, examination of the foveal insertion of the TFCC, diagnosis and evaluation of sigmoid notch arthritis, capsulorrhaphy for arthrofibrosis, and débridement/resection of the ulnar head for class II degenerative lesions of the TFCC. Four portals have been described: two dorsal, one volar, and one foveal. It is generally recommended to use a smaller 1.9-mm arthroscope and

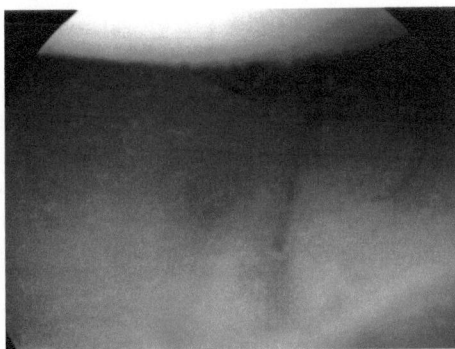

Fig. 69.9 An arthroscopic image of the midcarpal space. The scapholunate interval is seen without gapping or separation of the interval. The capitate head is situated at the top of the image.

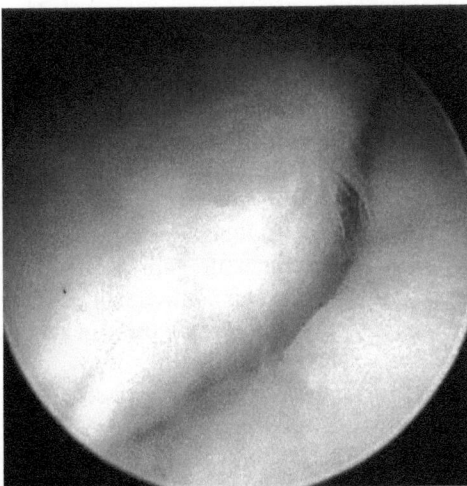

Fig. 69.10 An arthroscopic image of the lunotriquetral interval as seen from the midcarpal space. Note the 1-mm separation, which is normal for the lunotriquetral interval as opposed to the scapholunate interval, where no separation should be seen.

decrease traction to help reduce tension on the capsule so as to improve visualization.

CARPAL INSTABILITY

Both the radiocarpal and midcarpal space should be evaluated arthroscopically when carpal instability is suspected. The key to arthroscopic management of carpal instability is the recognition of what is normal and what is pathologic when viewing the integrity of the interosseous ligaments and the overall alignment of the carpal bones. The interosseous ligaments may stretch and deform significantly before they eventually tear. Consequently, bulging of the interosseous ligament and rotation of the carpal bones are possible prior to true intercarpal dissociation. Extrinsic ligaments also contribute to wrist stability. A combination of both intrinsic and extrinsic pathology may lead to carpal malalignment and clinical instability. The scapholunate and lunotriquetral interosseous ligaments should have a normal concave appearance, as seen from the radiocarpal space. The scapholunate interosseous ligament is best seen with the arthroscope in the 3-4 portal, and the lunotriquetral interosseous ligament is best seen with the arthroscope in either the 4-5 or 6-R portal. As viewed from the midcarpal space, the scapholunate interval should be highly congruent without any notable step-off between carpal bones. The lunotriquetral interval should also be congruent, but a 1-mm distal step-off between carpal bones is normally seen. A small amount of motion is possible at the lunotriquetral interval and should not be mistaken for instability.

A limited type of intraoperative arthrogram (poor man's arthrogram) may be performed for evaluation of carpal instability. To perform this procedure, a needle is placed in either the radial or ulnar midcarpal portal, and a tear of the interosseous ligament is strongly suspected when a free flow of irrigation fluid occurs from the radiocarpal space and exits the needle.

A spectrum of interosseous ligament injury is possible. The ligament progresses from attenuation to frank tearing in a volar to dorsal direction. Geissler et al.[21] devised an arthroscopic classification of carpal instability based on observations of injury to the scapholunate and lunotriquetral interosseous ligaments when associated with fractures of the distal radius (Table 69.1).

In grade I injuries, the normal concave appearance between the carpal bones is lost. The interosseous ligament bulges with a convex appearance, as seen with the arthroscope in the radiocarpal space. Evaluation of the midcarpal space shows the carpal

TABLE 69.1	Carpal Instability Chart	
Grade	Description	Management
I	Attenuation or hemorrhage of interosseous ligament as seen from the radiocarpal space. No incongruence of carpal alignment in mid carpal space.	Cast immobilization
II	Attenuation or hemorrhage of interosseous ligament as seen from radiocarpal space. Incongruence or step-off seen in mid carpal space. There may be a slight gap (less than width of probe) between carpal bones.	Arthroscopic pinning
III	Incongruence or step-off of carpal alignment as seen from both radiocarpal and mid carpal space. Probe may be passed through gap between carpal bones	Arthroscopic pinning/ open repair
IV	Incongruence or step-off of carpal alignments as seen from both radiocarpal and mid carpal space. There is gross instability with manipulation. A 2.7 mm arthroscope may be passed through gap between carpal bones.	Open repair

bones to be highly congruent without step-off. In grade II injuries, the interosseous ligament is again convex, as seen with the arthroscope in the radiocarpal space. From the midcarpal space, the carpal bones are no longer congruent (Fig. 69.11). With early scapholunate instability, the scaphoid is observed to flex, as the dorsal edge is distal to the lunate; however, the gap is minimal. Slight motion at the lunotriquetral articulation is not pathologic in most instances and should be correlated with ligament integrity and degree of interval dissociation. In grade III injuries, the interosseous ligament begins to tear and a larger gap is seen between the carpal bones from both the radiocarpal and midcarpal spaces (Fig. 69.12). In grade IV injuries, the interosseous ligament is completely detached, and the arthroscope may be passed freely from the radiocarpal to the midcarpal space through the affected interval, which is designated as the "drive-through sign." This sign often corresponds with an excessively widened scapholunate (or lunotriquetral) gap on a posteroanterior radiograph of the wrist, indicative of intercarpal dissociation.

Another arthroscopic classification for scapholunate instability is the European Wrist Arthroscopy Society (EWAS) classification, described by Messina et al.[22] It characterizes the specific location of a scapholunate interosseous ligament tear, indicates whether the tear is complete or partial, and describes whether or not

there is extrinsic ligament involvement. An increase in the arthroscopic stage indicates a more severe injury.

Geissler grade I injuries are considered mild wrist sprains that typically resolve with conservative management. If detected intraoperatively at the time of concurrent evaluation and treatment of other wrist injuries, arthroscopic débridement of the partially injured interosseous ligament may be performed. Acute Geissler grade II (and some grade III) tears of the scapholunate or lunotriquetral interosseous ligaments that result in incongruence from the midcarpal space, however, may be arthroscopically reduced and temporarily pinned to provide stabilization. Two or three 0.045 Kirschner wires (K-wires) are placed just distal to the radial styloid into the scaphoid under fluoroscopic guidance. It is important to place the guidewires either through a protective cannula or in oscillation mode to avoid injury to traversing cutaneous nerve branches. The wrist is then suspended in the traction tower, and the arthroscope is placed in the ulnar midcarpal portal. A joystick K-wire may be placed into the lunate to help control rotation. The scapholunate interval is anatomically reduced, as viewed from the midcarpal space, and the K-wires are advanced across the scapholunate interval. Frequently droplets of fat are seen exiting the scapholunate interval. These wires are left in position for approximately 8 weeks. The wrist is immobilized in a below-elbow cast. The decision about whether to leave the K-wires protruding from the skin is made by the surgeon. Digital range of motion (ROM) is encouraged. The wires are removed at 8 weeks and the wrist is immobilized for an additional 4 weeks. Outpatient therapy for ROM and strengthening is initiated after a 3-month interval.

Management of Geissler grade II or III acute tears of the lunotriquetral interosseous ligament is essentially the same, except that the arthroscope is placed in the radial midcarpal space as the pins are driven across the lunotriquetral interval from ulnar to radial. Again, protective measures are undertaken to prevent iatrogenic cutaneous nerve injury. Anecdotally, reduction of the lunotriquetral interval is usually less difficult compared with reduction of the scapholunate interval.

In persons with Geissler grade IV interosseous ligament dissociation, arthroscopic management alone may be inadequate to restore alignment and stability, and an open approach is recommended. Kirschner wires are effective for stabilization, but they can only be left in for a short period of time (6 to 8 weeks) because of problems with pin irritation and potential pin tract infection. They can also limit rehabilitation. The concern is that the interosseous ligaments may take a longer time to heal than the wires can safely be left in place.

The scapholunate-intercarpal-carpal (SLIC) screw (Acumed, Hillsboro, OR) was specifically designed for acute carpal instability (Fig. 69.13). A SLIC screw rotates in its midsection and has approximately 20 degrees of toggle. It can be left in for a prolonged period of time (6 to 9 months), allowing rotation of the scaphoid and lunate in the sagittal plane while the ligament heals. The cannulated screw can be removed in the future.

Whipple[23] reviewed the results of arthroscopic treatment of scapholunate instability in patients who were followed up for a duration of 1 to 3 years. Patients were classified in two distinct groups of 40 patients, each according to the duration of symptoms

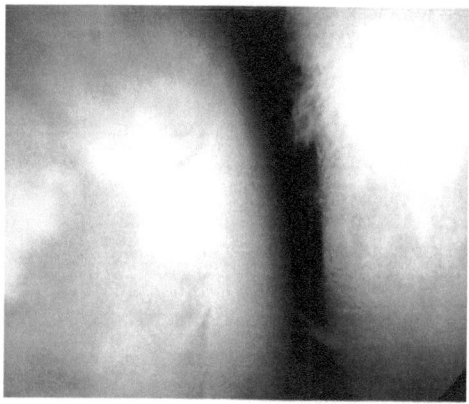

Fig. 69.11 An arthroscopic image of the scapholunate interval as viewed from the midcarpal space. Abnormal gapping of the interval denotes a grade II injury to the scapholunate interosseous ligament.

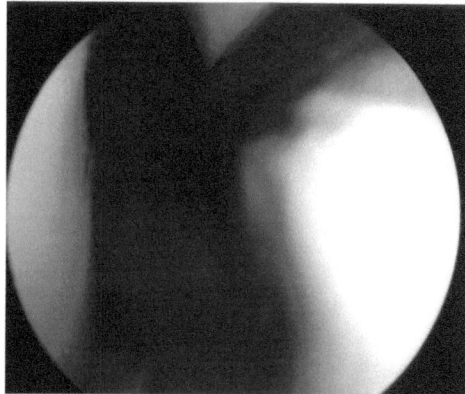

Fig. 69.12 An arthroscopic image of a grade III injury to the scapholunate interosseous ligament with significant gapping of the interval as seen from the midcarpal space.

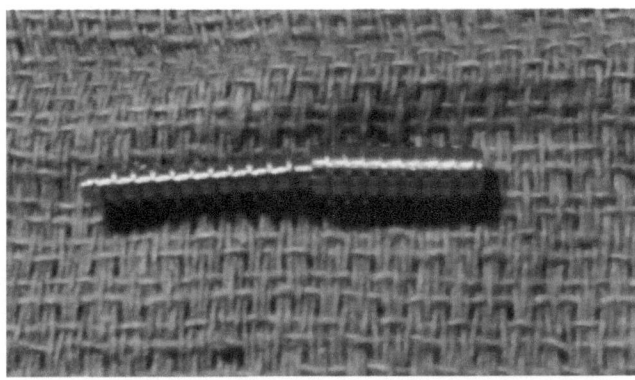

Fig. 69.13 Radial styloid fractures are highly associated with scapholunate interosseous ligament *(SLIL)* injuries. Arthroscopic evaluation confirmed a complete tear of the SLIL, which was stabilized with a SLIC screw (Acumed, Hillsboro, OR).

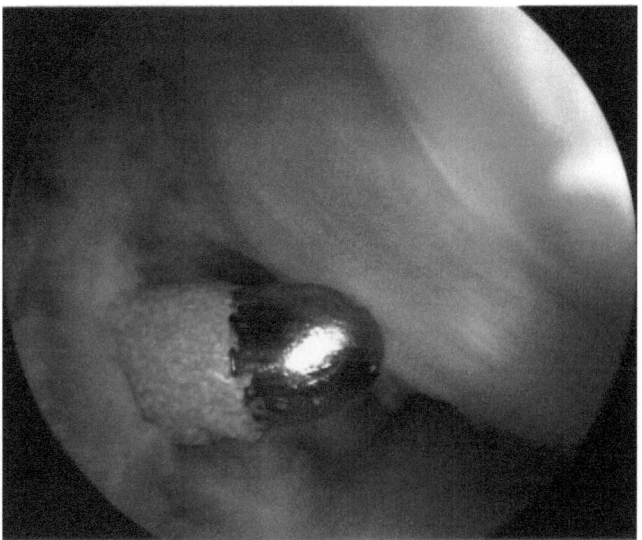

Fig. 69.14 An arthroscopic image of a grade II scapholunate injury after electrothermal shrinkage. The ligament has now returned to its concave appearance, and areas of spot welds are present on the membranous portion of the scapholunate ligament.

and the side-to-side scapholunate gap. Eighty-three percent of patients who had scapholunate instability of 3 months or less and a gap of 3 mm or less experienced relief of their symptoms, compared with only 21 patients (63%) who had symptoms longer than 3 months and more than a 3-mm side-to-side difference. The conclusion from the study was that arthroscopic pinning should be reserved for patients with an acute injury rather than a chronic, complete tear.

Osterman and Seidman[24] reviewed their results of arthroscopic treatment of acute lunotriquetral instability in 20 patients who did not have volar intercalated segment instability. Follow-up was an average of 32 months, and 16 patients had good to excellent relief of pain. Grip strength improved in 18 patients.

Weiss and colleagues reviewed their results of arthroscopic débridement alone of interosseous ligament tears with an average of 27 months of follow-up after the procedure.[25] In this study, 31 of 36 patients who had a partial tear of the scapholunate interosseous ligament had complete resolution or a decrease in their symptoms, compared with 19 of 21 patients who had a complete tear of the scapholunate interosseous ligament. All 42 patients who had a partial tear of the lunotriquetral interosseous ligament and 26 of 33 patients who had a complete tear of the lunotriquetral interosseous ligament experienced complete resolution or a decrease in their symptoms. Grip strength improved an average of 23% in this study. The investigators concluded that débridement of lunotriquetral interosseous ligament tears had a better result compared with injury to the scapholunate interosseous ligament. In addition, débridement of partial tears provided better results compared with complete tears.

Although electrothermal shrinkage of ligaments has failed to show consistent effectiveness elsewhere, this technique may play a role in the management of chronic partial tears of the interosseous wrist ligaments. Electrothermal shrinkage is based on heating and denaturing of collagen, resulting in fiber contraction, and likely is best for a grade I or II partial interosseous ligament injury. After débridement of the torn ligament edges, an electrothermal probe is used to shrink the uninjured portion of the ligament. A monopolar or bipolar probe may be used. The monopolar probe has been shown to have deeper penetration of heat than the bipolar probe. On the other hand, bipolar probes

yield higher surface temperatures, which may have the undesirable effect of increasing the temperature of the irrigation fluid medium. It is important not to paint the entire tissue but rather to spot weld and leave viable tissue in between the contracted areas (Fig. 69.14). The probe is primarily directed at the membranous portion of the interosseous ligament, but the dorsal and volar wrist capsule may be included in the procedure. It is extremely important to increase the flow of irrigation fluid into the wrist joint to maximally dissipate heat emanating from the probe. In this regard, separate inflow is established through the 6-U portal. The temperature of the irrigation fluid exiting the wrist should be monitored to prevent skin burns.

Few protocols have been developed to guide postoperative management after use of thermal shrinkage procedures. The use of concurrent K-wire stabilization is controversial. The wrist is generally immobilized for approximately 8 weeks, followed by an additional 4 weeks in a removable brace as therapeutic exercises are initiated. Theoretically, prolonged postoperative immobilization of the wrist may allow the contracted collagen to mature.

Geissler and Savoie[5] reviewed the results of chronic isolated interosseous ligament tears managed by thermal shrinkage in 19 patients. A chronic injury was defined as the presence of symptoms for more than 6 months. The authors noted that grade II tears of the scapholunate and lunotriquetral interosseous ligaments had significantly better results compared with grade III tears. No real difference is seen between scapholunate and lunotriquetral interosseous ligament tears in the study.

Wrist arthroscopy may also serve as a valuable adjunct in the management of chronic injuries to the interosseous ligaments beyond thermal shrinkage. Wrist arthroscopy may be used to evaluate the degree and extent of articular cartilage degeneration in patients with posttraumatic scapholunate advanced collapsed osteoarthrosis. In particular, arthroscopic evaluation of the capitate head helps determine the most appropriate salvage procedure between proximal row carpectomy (healthy capitate) and scaphoid excision four-corner fusion (unhealthy capitate). In select patients with early scapholunate advanced collapsed changes limited to the radioscaphoid joint, arthroscopic radial styloidectomy is a viable option. In this procedure, the arthroscope is placed in the 3-4 portal and a high-speed burr is carefully placed in the 1-2 portal. Approximately 4 mm of the tip of the radial styloid may be excised while preserving the origin of the radioscaphocapitate ligament to avoid consequent ulnar translation of the wrist. The degree of chondromalacia at the tip of the radial styloid determines the extent of ulnar resection during the procedure. Generalized débridement and/or local synovectomy may also be considered for temporary symptom relief in patients with any form of arthropathy.

Wrist arthroscopy is valuable in the management of chondral defects in the midcarpal space. For example, chondral defects involving the hamate are being increasingly recognized as a source of ulnar-sided wrist pain.[26] A partial resection of the proximal aspect of the hamate, in the so called Hamate Arthrosis Lunotriquetral Joint instability (HALT), is performed arthroscopically with the arthroscope placed in the radial midcarpal portal and the high-speed burr placed in the ulnar midcarpal portal.

FRACTURE MANAGEMENT

Scaphoid Fractures

The scaphoid is the most commonly fractured carpal bone, accounting for 60% to 70% of all carpal fractures. The majority of scaphoid fractures are low-energy injuries arising from either a sporting event or a fall onto an outstretched, extended, and radially deviated wrist. It is well known that the majority of scaphoid fractures occur in young adult males. The carpal bones are aligned in two rows of matching concave and convex gliding surfaces, and the scaphoid links these rows. Approximately 80% of the scaphoid surface area is covered by articular cartilage, and its retrograde blood supply makes it susceptible to relatively high rates of nonunion and osteonecrosis when injuries are poorly managed.

Many nondisplaced scaphoid fractures may be effectively treated by cast immobilization with an expected healing rate of 85% to 95%. However, risks of prolonged casting include wrist stiffness, muscle atrophy, disuse osteopenia, and longer return to play in the young, athletic population. Early internal fixation has proved to be cost-effective and is associated with shorter union times and minimal morbidity.[27] Several operative techniques are available, including percutaneous, mini open, and arthroscopic fixation methods. Only the arthroscopic technique is discussed here, because a separate chapter is devoted to scaphoid and other carpal bone injuries.

Arthroscopic Reduction of Selected Scaphoid Nonunions

Geissler and Slade[29] developed a classification of scaphoid nonunions (Table 69.2). In 15 patients with type I-III scaphoid nonunions, Geissler[30] described using Slade's dorsal percutaneous fixation technique[31] with excellent results. Patients were treated with a headless cannulated screw without bone grafting. All healed in an average of 3 months.

In patients with a type IV cystic scaphoid nonunion, Geissler and Slade[29] described a technique for arthroscopic fixation with percutaneous demineralized bone matrix (DBM) putty insertion at the nonunion site. When using this technique, the guidewire is placed arthroscopically as previously described. The scaphoid is then reamed with a cannulated reamer. A bone biopsy needle

---

⚑ Authors' Preferred Technique

Arthroscopic Reduction

The arthroscopic fixation technique may be used for both acute fractures and selected scaphoid nonunions.[28] Inserting the guidewire at the optimal starting point, reducing the fracture, and burying the headless compression screw beneath articular cartilage may be ensured by direct visualization. In experienced hands, this method may prove simpler than percutaneous approaches that rely solely on fluoroscopic guidance for correct placement of the implant. The wrist is initially placed in the traction tower and the arthroscope is placed in the 3-4 portal to evaluate any associated soft tissue injuries. The arthroscope is then transferred into the 6-R portal and the wrist is partially flexed approximately 30 degrees. A 14-gauge needle is inserted through the 3-4 portal and used to confirm the ideal dorsal starting point near the scapholunate ligament origin at the central one third of the proximal pole. The needle is then advanced and impaled into the proximal pole of the scaphoid (Fig. 69.15). If the starting point appears accurate throughout a series of fluoroscopic images, it may be further advanced and ultimately replaced with a guidewire. The optimal position is within the central one third of the entire scaphoid, ending at the subchondral bone of the distal pole. A second guidewire is then placed against the proximal pole of the scaphoid, and the length of the screw is determined by the difference of the two guidewires. A headless compression screw that is 4 mm shorter than measured between the two guidewires is recommended for most fractures.

The arthroscope is then placed in the midcarpal space to evaluate the fracture reduction (Fig. 69.16). Fractures of the proximal pole are best seen with the

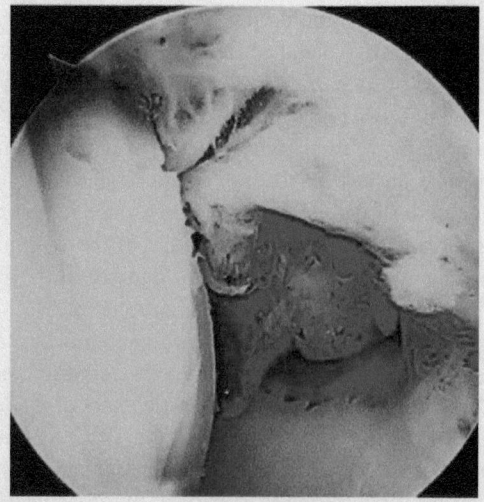

Fig. 69.15 The starting point for arthroscopic screw fixation of a scaphoid fracture is viewed from either the 6-R or 4-5 portal. A 14-gauge needle is inserted through the 3-4 portal and placed 1 to 2 mm from the radial border of the scapholunate ligament.

Authors' Preferred Technique

Arthroscopic Reduction—cont'd

arthroscope in the ulnar midcarpal portal, and fractures of the waist are best visualized with the arthroscope in the radial midcarpal portal. If the fracture reduction is anatomic, the guidewire is then advanced to exit the volar aspect of the wrist. If the reduction is unsatisfactory, the guidewire is withdrawn into one fracture fragment alone so a joystick can be used to manipulate the reduction; this technique may require additional manual manipulation of the wrist in several planes to achieve reduction. After arthroscopic confirmation of a satisfactory reduction, the guidewire may then be advanced across the fracture plane for security. At this point, the guidewire should be exiting from the volar and dorsal aspects of the wrist. If the guidewire breaks, it is easily retrievable. The scaphoid is then reamed through a trocar to protect the extensor tendons and cutaneous nerves. A cannulated headless screw is then placed over the guidewire. The position of the screw is evaluated under fluoroscopic guidance in multiple planes. The wrist is then evaluated arthroscopically both from the midcarpal and radiocarpal spaces. From the midcarpal space, the reduction and compression of the scaphoid fracture are evaluated. In the radiocarpal space, it is imperative to verify that the headless cannulated screw has been buried deep to the articular cartilage surface (Fig. 69.17), which offers an advantage over percutaneous techniques that depend on fluoroscopy to determine whether the screw is prominent.

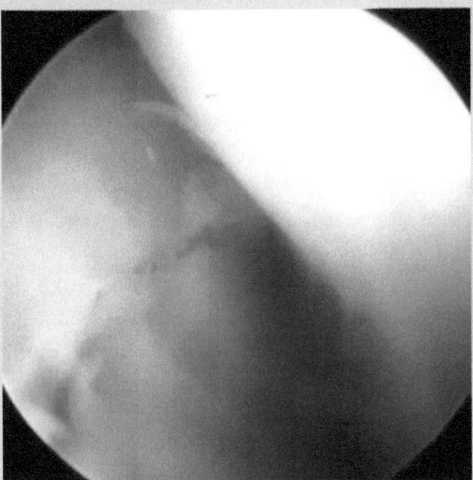

Fig. 69.16 After a guidewire is placed, the reduction of the scaphoid may be visualized best from the radial midcarpal portal, as seen above.

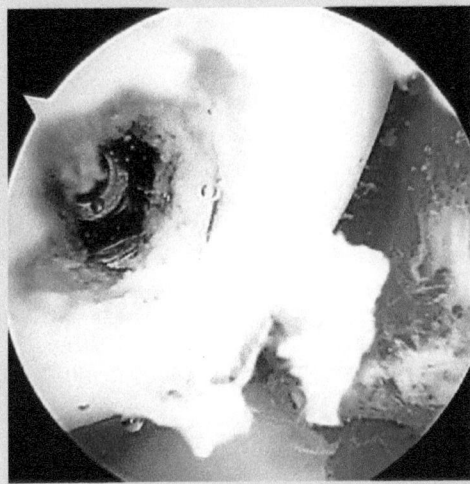

Fig. 69.17 After insertion of a cannulated screw, the subchondral placement is confirmed arthroscopically. Because fluoroscopic images may be deceiving, it is imperative to confirm the depth of screw insertion arthroscopically to avoid prominence of the screw head.

TABLE 69.2   Scaphoid Nonunion Classification

Slade and Geissler
- Type I
  Delayed presentation 4–12 weeks
- Type II
  Fibrous union, minimal fracture line
- Type III
  Minimal sclerosis <1 mm
- Type IV
  Cystic formation, between 1 and 5 mm
- Type V
  Humpback deformity, >5 mm cystic change
- Type VI
  Wrist arthrosis

From Geissler WB. *Wrist Arthroscopy*. New York: Springer-Verlag; 2004.

is filled with DBM putty and placed directly over the guidewire into the cystic nonunion site of the scaphoid. The guidewire is then retracted distally but still remains in the distal pole of the scaphoid. The DBM putty is then injected through the bone biopsy needle directly into the central aspect of the scaphoid at the nonunion site that has been previously reamed. The guidewire is then advanced back through the bone biopsy needle from a volar to dorsal direction out the dorsum of the wrist after the putty has been injected. In this manner, the guidewire passes through the original path of the proximal pole of the scaphoid and out the soft tissues. A headless cannulated screw is inserted over the guidewire across the scaphoid nonunion site. As before, both the radiocarpal and midcarpal spaces are reevaluated arthroscopically to confirm the position of the screw and reduction of the scaphoid nonunion.

Geissler and Slade[29] reported their technique in 15 patients with cystic scaphoid nonunions without a humpback deformity (type IV). Fourteen of the 15 patients healed successfully, and all had good to excellent results according to the Modified Mayo Wrist Score.

Transscaphoid Perilunate Fracture-Dislocations

Transscaphoid perilunate fracture dislocations are uncommon high-energy injuries that have traditionally been managed with an open approach. The senior author has described an all-arthroscopic technique for management of these injuries (Fig. 69.18).[32] With this technique, the wrist is initially arthroscopically evaluated to confirm a tear to the lunotriquetral interosseous ligament. Once confirmed, K wires or a SLIC screw (Acumed, Hillsboro, OR), percutaneously inserted over a guidewire, is used

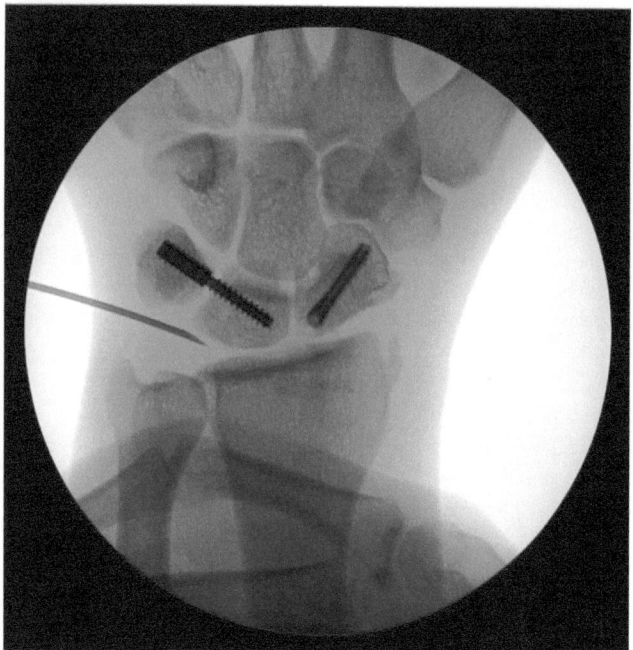

Fig. 69.18 A fluoroscopic view demonstrating an anatomically reduced and stabilized transscaphoid perilunate dislocation. A percutaneous scapholunate-intercarpal-carpal screw (Acumed, Hillsboro, OR) is placed in the lunotriquetral interval, and a headless compression screw is placed across the scaphoid fracture.

to stabilize the lunotriquetral interval. The wrist is then suspended in a traction tower, and the scaphoid is arthroscopically stabilized as previously described (Fig. 69.19).[28] In seven patients treated with this technique, all fractures healed at 3 months and the wrist flexion–extension arc ranged from 70 to 120 degrees. Five of the seven patients had no pain. Stabilization without Kirschner wires allowed patients to participate in physical therapy at an earlier stage and resulted in a very functional ROM at 3 months postoperatively.[32]

Fractures of the Distal Radius

Intra-articular fractures of the distal radius are usually the result of a high-energy injury and are less amenable to the traditional methods of closed manipulation and casting. The prognosis for these injuries depends on restoration of original length, articular inclination, and articular congruity at the radiocarpal and distal radioulnar joints.[33–36] The prevailing recommendation to accept 2 mm or less displacement is a well-established clinical threshold for intra-articular congruity of the distal radius.[19] Other investigations have indicated that the tolerance may be as low as 1 mm before an unacceptably high rate of posttraumatic osteoarthrosis occurs.[37–41]

Arthroscopic-assisted fixation of intra-articular distal radius fractures permits reduction of the joint surface under bright light and magnified conditions. This technique permits lavage

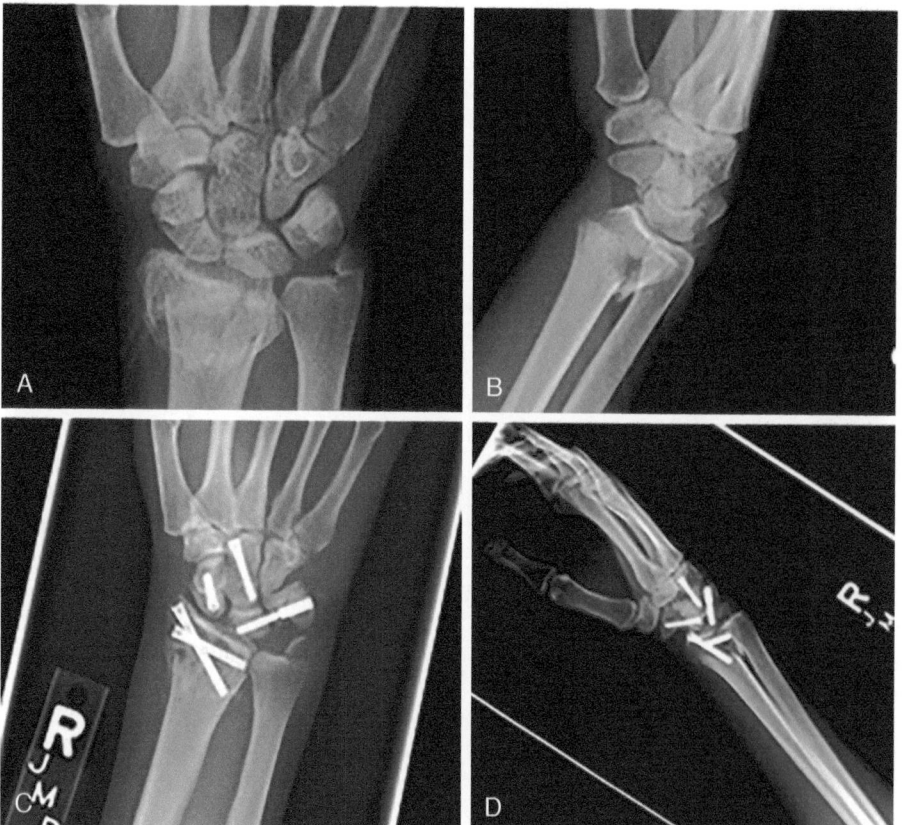

Fig. 69.19 (A and B) Preoperative and (C and D) postoperative views of a greater arc perilunate dislocation entirely by arthroscopic and percutaneous techniques.

of a hematoma and multiple joint debris, along with management of concurrent soft tissue injuries associated with these fracture patterns.

Arthroscopic-assisted fixation may be used for simple intra-articular fractures that have large, well-defined fragments, such as radial styloid, die-punch, and Barton-type fractures. Wrist arthroscopy may serve an adjunctive role in the management of three-part and four-part intra-articular fractures with metaphyseal comminution. Both intra- and extra-articular fractures of the distal radius have a high prevalence of associated ligamentous injuries. In this setting, TFCC injuries are most frequently encountered[42] and may lead to persistent ulnar-sided wrist pain after fracture healing if these injuries are underappreciated. A recent study shows a higher than expected incidence of concurrent scapholunate ligament tears accompanying distal radius fractures.[43,44]

Operative Technique

Patients with displaced, unstable intra-articular fractures of the distal radius are taken to the operating room within approximately 10 days of the date of the injury. A delay of at least 48 hours helps minimize bleeding from the fracture and poor visualization during arthroscopy.[43] Fractures that are more than 10 days old may be difficult to reduce with minimally invasive methods. The operating room is set up so that both fluoroscopy and arthroscopy may be used simultaneously. The wrist is suspended with 10 lb. of traction in a standard traction tower. The standard 3-4, 6-R, and 6-U portals are created. It is helpful to lavage the joint to remove fracture debris and blood from a hematoma before introduction of the arthroscope. Lavage is performed by placing the inflow through the 6-U portal and the arthroscopic cannula in the 3-4 portal. After lavage is completed, the arthroscope is placed in the 3-4 portal and a shaver is brought in through the 6-R portal to remove any further fracture debris. A traditional diagnostic wrist arthroscopy procedure is then performed.

Fractures of the radial styloid are ideally suited for arthroscopic management. Rotation is best judged by looking across the wrist. Under fluoroscopy, one or two guidewires are placed in oscillation mode at the tip of the displaced radial styloid fragment without crossing the fracture site. The arthroscope is placed in the 6-R portal to best visualize the radial styloid fracture line. With the guidewire in the radial styloid fragment and the trocar placed in the 3-4 portal, the radial styloid fragment may be manipulated and anatomically reduced (Fig. 69.20). The guidewire is then advanced across the fracture site for provisional stabilization. Fluoroscopy confirms reduction, and additional guidewires control fragment rotation. One or two headless cannulated screws are placed over the guidewires, allowing for fracture compression and early wrist mobilization. If using wet arthroscopy, care must be given during the procedures to guard against fluid extravasation within the forearm, which may cause compartment syndrome.

In three-part intra-articular fractures of the distal radius without metaphyseal comminution, the radial styloid fragment may be manually reduced and provisionally pinned with K-wires under fluoroscopy, which will serve as a stable foundation to

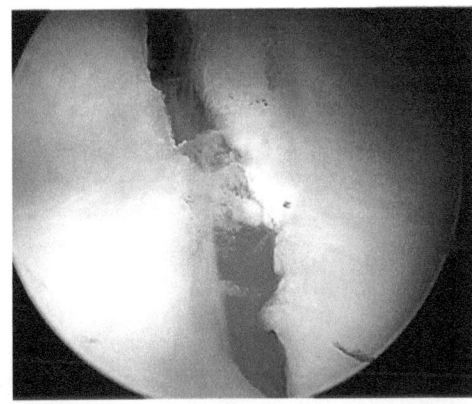

Fig. 69.20 An arthroscopic image of a radial styloid fracture showing 1 to 2 mm of articular incongruity. Kirschner wires can be placed in the radial styloid fragment and used as joysticks for fracture reduction into anatomic alignment. Following anatomic intra-articular reduction, a cannulated screw, fragment-specific plate, or small locking plate may be placed to stabilize the distal fragment.

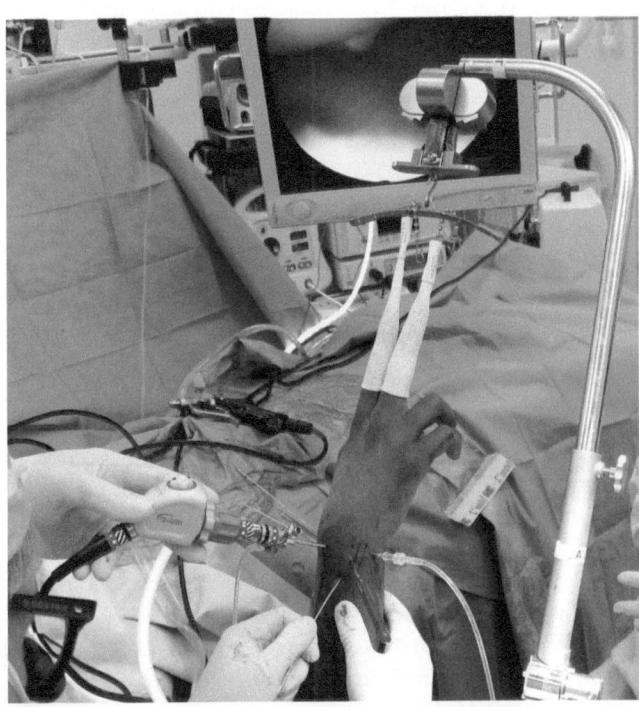

Fig. 69.21 After the lunate facet die-punch fragment is visualized arthroscopically, a Steinmann pin is used to lever the die-punch fragment into appropriate reduction with the radial styloid fragment.

elevate the lunate facet into anatomic position. The wrist is then suspended in a traction tower and the articular surface is evaluated directly. A headless cannulated screw may be placed in the radial styloid fragment as previously described. The lunate facet fragment is identified with the arthroscope in the 3-4 portal, and a needle is placed over the fragment percutaneously. This landmark permits accurate Steinman pin placement 2 cm proximally to elevate the depressed facet fragment (Fig. 69.21). Once the fragment is elevated and judged to be anatomic, a guidewire is placed transversely beneath the articular surface to stabilize the fragment. It is important to pronate and supinate the wrist to ensure the guide pin does not violate the distal radioulnar joint. An additional headless cannulated screw is then placed transversely over the guidewire to support the lunate facet fragment.

Volar wrist approaches for open reduction and internal fixation of distal radius fractures are presently commonplace, but joint reduction must be estimated fluoroscopically because the approach does not allow for direct inspection of the articular surface. Dry or conventional wrist arthroscopy may be used to confirm adequate articular reduction in persons with more complicated intra-articular fracture patterns that have been stabilized with volar plating. Furthermore, intra-articular penetration of distal locking screws may be grossly underestimated with the use of fluoroscopy alone.[45] Concurrent soft tissue injuries may be diagnosed and treated accordingly.

TRIANGULAR FIBROCARTILAGE COMPLEX

Surgical Anatomy

The TFCC comprises an intricate soft tissue support at the ulnar aspect of the wrist. It acts as an extension of the articular surface of the distal radius to support the proximal carpal row and stabilizes the distal radial ulnar joint. Palmer[46] classically described the components as the fibrocartilage articular disk, the dorsal and volar radioulnar ligaments, the ulnolunate and ulnotriquetral ligaments, the meniscus homologue, and the subsheath of the ECU.

The volar aspect of the articular disk has two bundles; one bundle is directed superficially toward the ulnar styloid, and the second bundle is directed deep toward the fovea of the distal ulna. The proximal limbs of the volar and dorsal radioulnar ligaments are conjoined at the fovea just radial to the base of the ulnar styloid. This structure has been referred to as the *ligamentum subcruentum*. This deep layer represents the more robust stabilizing component of the TFCC, but it cannot be directly seen arthroscopically from the radiocarpal joint. Conversely, the distal superficial portions of the volar and dorsal radioulnar ligaments are more easily visualized at their ulnar styloid insertion. The superficial and deep limbs of the TFCC likely behave independently of each other, although the question of which is under more tension in different positions of wrist pronosupination is controversial. Dorsally the TFCC blends with the ECU subsheath and is a frequent area of peripheral detachment of the articular disk. The subsheath is a thick fibrous investment that is ideally suited for fixation of sutures with an outside-in arthroscopic technique. Studies suggest that the richest blood supply through the TFCC resides at the periphery, implying that tears in this region are the most amenable to fixation and reliable healing.[47,48]

Clinical Features

Injuries to the TFCC typically occur from a fall on an outstretched hand or a forceful twisting mechanism. TFCC injuries are common in athletes who participate in racquet and stick sports. Patients report deep, diffuse pain across the ulnar side of the wrist, particularly with lifting or turning activities. Frequently they report weakness when gripping, as well as a palpable or

audible clicking sensation with rotation of the forearm. Tenderness may be elicited at the dorsal distal radioulnar joint or at the fovea, located just volar to the styloid process, and is accentuated with the extremes of forearm rotation. Massive disruptions of the TFCC may result in gross distal radioulnar instability with stress testing compared with the contralateral wrist. The chronicity of complaints has implications for treatment, and plain radiographs should determine ulnar variance in all patients with suspected TFCC pathology.

Palmer[46] proposed a classification for tears of the TFCC that divided injuries into class I (traumatic injuries) and class II (degenerative injuries; Table 69.3). In class I injuries, tears are further divided regarding the anatomic location of the tear, which may consequently determine the ease or difficulty of potential arthroscopic management. Class II degenerative lesions result from ulnar impaction syndrome and are usually treated with arthroscopic débridement followed by an ulnar shortening osteotomy.

TABLE 69.3 Traumatic Triangular Fibrocartilage Complex Injuries

Subclassification	Description
Traumatic Injuries—Class I	
Class IA	Tears or perforations of the horizontal portion of the TFCC
	Usually 1–2 mm wide
	Dorsal palmar slit located 2–3 mm medial to the radial attachment of the sigmoid notch
Class IB	Traumatic avulsion of TFCC from insertion into the distal ulna
	May be accompanied by a fracture of the ulnar styloid at its base
	Usually associated with distal radiocarpal joint instability
Class IC	Tears of the TFCC, which result in ulnocarpal instability such as avulsion of the TFCC from the distal attachment of the lunate or triquetrum
Class ID	Traumatic avulsions of the TFCC from the attachment at the distal sigmoid notch
Degenerative Lesions—Class II	
Class IIA	Wear of the horizontal portion of the TFCC distally, proximally, or both, with no perforation
	Possible ulnar plus syndrome
Class IIB	Wear of the horizontal portion of the TFCC and chondromalacia of lunate and/or ulna
Class IIC	TFCC perforation and chondromalacia of the lunate and/or ulna
Class IID	TFCC perforation and chondromalacia of the lunate and/or ulna
	Perforation of the lunotriquetral ligament
Class IIE	TFCC perforation and chondromalacia of the lunate and/or ulna
	Perforation of the lunotriquetral ligament
	Ulnocarpal arthritis

TFCC, Triangular fibrocartilage complex.

ARTHROSCOPIC MANAGEMENT OF TRAUMATIC CLASS I INJURIES

Class IA tears are perforations of the articular disk that are usually 1 to 2 mm wide and located approximately 2 to 3 mm ulnar to the distal radius rim (Fig. 69.22). Arthroscopic débridement is recommended. The arthroscope is placed in the 3-4 portal, and a small banana blade is inserted through the 6-R portal. Unstable flaps are outlined with a banana blade, and a grasper is used to remove loose disk fragments. The arthroscope is then transferred to the 6-R portal, and a small punch is inserted through the 3-4 portal to further débride the most ulnar aspect of the tear. A small joint shaver is then used to smooth the remaining portion of the articular disk and address any associated local synovitis. Approximately two-thirds of the articular disk may be excised without causing distal radioulnar joint instability (Fig. 69.23). In this regard, leaving an approximate 2-mm peripheral rim is

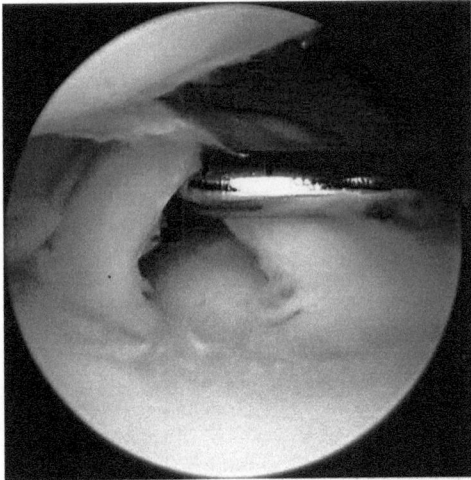

Fig. 69.22 An arthroscopic image of a central IA tear of the triangular fibrocartilage complex. The probe is shown elevating the tear, and the ulnar head is seen inferiorly.

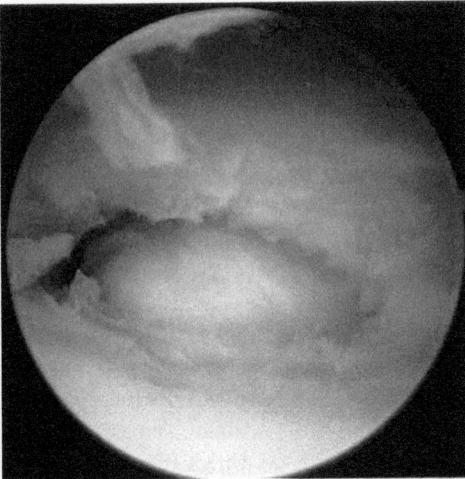

Fig. 69.23 After débridement of a central triangular fibrocartilage complex tear, at least a 2-mm rim should be left to prevent destabilization of the distal radioulnar joint.

usually sufficient. Care should be taken to avoid iatrogenic injury to the dorsal and volar radioulnar ligaments.

Class IB injuries are traumatic avulsions of the TFCC from its ulnar insertion. Several techniques for repair have been described in the literature. Whipple[49] described an outside-in technique in which sutures are placed longitudinally to reattach the articular disk to the floor of the ECU tendon sheath. With this method, the arthroscope is placed in the 3-4 portal and the peripheral tear is débrided with a small motorized shaver to help further identify the site of detachment. The 6-R portal is then elongated for approximately 1.5 cm, and the retinaculum of the ECU tendon sheath is opened. Care is taken to identify and protect the branches of the dorsal sensory branch of the ulnar nerve. The tendon is retracted ulnarly to expose the ECU subsheath. An 18-gauge needle is then placed as vertically as possible through the subsheath and into the articular disk. A 2-0 polydioxanone suture (PDS) is advanced through the needle into the joint space. A suture retriever is directed in a manner that allows for mattress repair of the peripheral tear, with all suture limbs exiting the subsheath superficially. This procedure may be repeated several times, depending on the size of the detachment and the quality of repair necessary. Traction is removed and the wrist is placed in slight supination when the sutures are tied externally. A sliding knot facilitates proper tensioning of the disk to its insertion through such a small window. The retinaculum is closed separately (Fig. 69.24).

Ekman and Poehling[9] described a Tuohy needle technique for repair of peripheral ulnar-sided tears of the articular disk. With the arthroscope in the 4-5 portal, a 20-gauge anesthetic Tuohy needle is placed into the radiocarpal space through either the 1-2 or 3-4 portal. The needle is passed across the wrist to the torn edge of the articular disk above the ulnar styloid process and advanced out the skin. A grasper may be helpful in directing the needle across the wrist and in perforating the articular disk. A 2-0 absorbable suture is threaded through the entire needle and exits the skin. A hemostat is placed on the suture exiting the skin. The needle is retrieved into the radiocarpal space and passed again through the edge of the articular disk and advanced out the skin so that a mattress suture is placed. The loop of suture that is exiting the needle is then pulled out the ulnar side of the wrist. This process may be repeated two or three times to form a horizontal mattress suture. Blunt dissection is carried out and the sutures are tied over the joint capsule. It is very important to ensure that branches of the dorsal sensory branch of the ulnar nerve are not trapped underneath the sutures as they are tied down to the capsule.

Most recently, Geissler[6] described an all-arthroscopic knotless technique for repair of peripheral ulnar-sided tears. In this technique, the standard 3-4 and 6-R portals are made. An accessory 6-R portal is made approximately 1.5 cm distal to the standard 6-R portal. It is helpful if the wrist is flexed 20 to 30 degrees for easier access to the distal ulna. A suture lasso is then inserted through the accessory 6-R portal into the joint space. The curved suture lasso is then passed with a gentle twisting motion through the articular disk in a proximal to distal direction. A Nitrol suture passer is inserted through the suture lasso and is retrieved through the 6-R portal with a suture grasper. A 2-0 FiberWire suture is

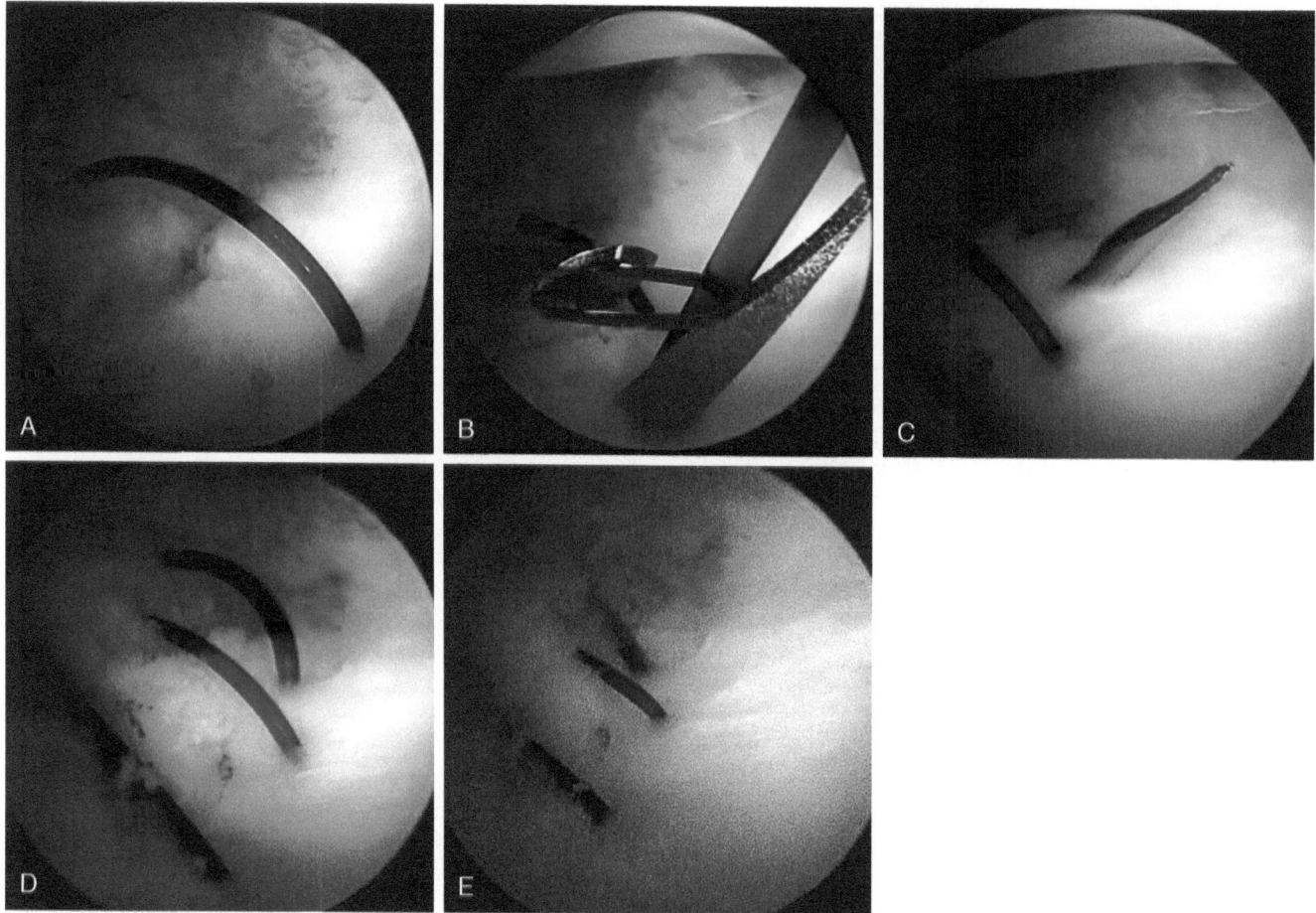

Fig. 69.24 (A) A single loop of 2-0 polydioxanone suture placed across a peripheral triangular fibrocartilage complex tear. (B) A second suture being passed across the peripheral tear. An 18-gauge needle is used to pierce the articular disk, and a suture is fed through the needle and retrieved with a suture lasso. (C) A third suture being placed. (D) All sutures have been placed without being tied at this point. (E) The sutures are tensioned to show closure of the tear. The arthroscope is removed and the wrist is taken out of traction before tying the sutures over the floor of the extensor carpi ulnaris tendon.

then passed through the wire retriever and pulled out the suture lasso distally through the handle. The suture lasso is then backed out of the articular disk and reinserted either anterior or posterior to the original perforation so that a horizontal mattress suture is placed. As the suture lasso passes through the articular disk for the second time, a loop of suture is formed that will be retrieved through the 6-R portal with a suture retriever. At this stage, both suture limbs are not exiting the 6-R portal.

A cannula is then inserted through the accessory 6-R portal into the joint space. The crochet hook is then used to retrieve both sutures distally through the cannula in the accessory 6-R portal. The cannula is then advanced directly onto the bone and held in position, and the two suture limbs are pulled out of the slot in the cannula so that they will not be twisted as the ulna is drilled. The drill is inserted through the cannula, and the base of the ulna is drilled as the cannula is held firmly against the insertion site. The two suture limbs are advanced into a push lock anchor, and the anchor is inserted through the cannula and into the predrilled hole. Tension is applied to the sutures as the anchor is advanced into the ulnar head. After the anchor has been seated, moderate tension is applied to the handle to ensure

that the anchor and sutures cannot be pulled out. If resistance is noted, the anchor has been inserted correctly. The anchor has a tendency to slide off the volar aspect of the ulna. If this event occurs, the anchor will easily pull out with minimal tension on the handle. Upon secure fixation, the sutures are cut with a small upbiter (Fig. 69.25).

Postoperatively, the patient's wrist is protected in an above-elbow splint. Gentle wrist flexion and extension may be started immediately in select patients, but pronosupination is restricted for at least 4 weeks after repair. At 7 weeks after surgery, a therapy program is begun for grip strengthening and ROM.

Class IC tears are rare injuries involving the distal attachment of the articular disk to the volar extrinsic ulnocarpal ligaments. Such a tear may result in ulnocarpal instability or ulnar translocation of the carpus. Trumble and colleagues[50] have advocated arthroscopic suture repair of these injuries with good results. Other management options include arthroscopic débridement and electrothermal shrinkage, which may restore tension back to the ulnar carpal ligaments. Class ID lesions of the TFCC involve a traumatic avulsion of the articular disk from the attachment at the sigmoid notch of the distal radius and often include

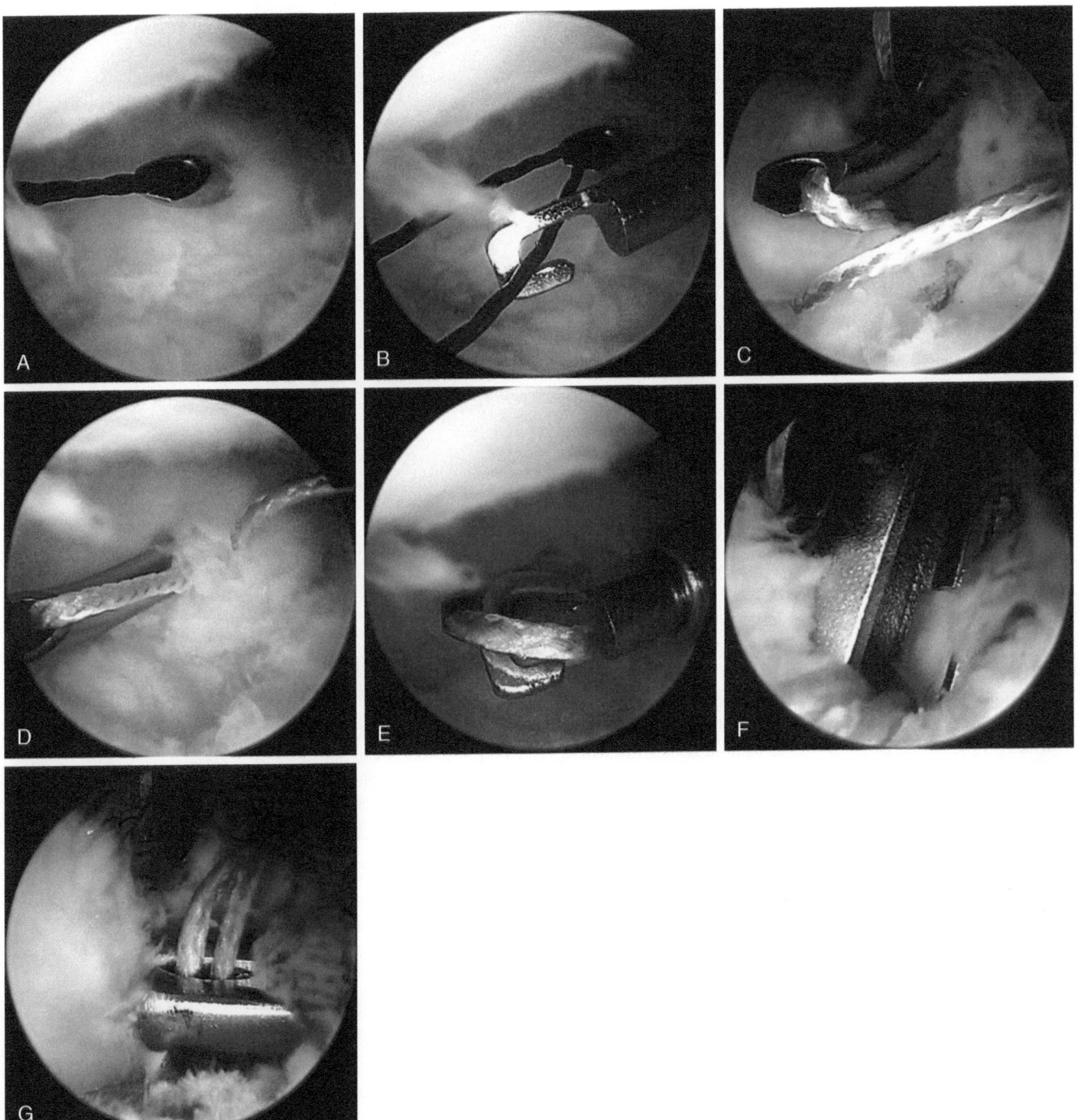

Fig. 69.25 (A) A suture lasso enters from the accessory 6-R portal and pierces the articular disk of the triangular fibrocartilage complex. (B) The suture wire retrieved by the crochet hook and pulled out of the 6-R portal. A 2-0 FiberWire suture is loaded into the loop of the suture wire and pulled through the articular disk and out the suture lasso. (C) The suture lasso is then pulled out from the articular disk and a loop is created with the FiberWire. (D) The suture lasso is then passed back through the articular disk. (E) The FiberWire loop is retrieved with the crochet hook from the 6-R portal. (F) The suture limbs are then both retrieved through the cannula in the accessory 6-R portal, the anchor site is drilled, and a PushLock anchor is inserted in the ulna to secure the repair. (G) A small punch is used to cut the sutures.

the volar and/or dorsal radioulnar ligaments. These lesions may be associated with a fracture of the distal radius involving the sigmoid notch. Sagerman and Short[51] described arthroscopic treatment of radial-sided TFCC tears. In this technique, a cannula is placed in the 6-U portal with the arthroscope in the 3-4 portal.

A 0.062-inch K-wire is used through the cannula to create three drill holes starting at the sigmoid notch insertion, traversing the distal radius, and exiting the skin radially. Long meniscus repair needles are then inserted through the 6-U portal through the articular disk and into the drill holes sequentially. A grasper is helpful at the 6-R portal to invert the disk and promote passage of the meniscus repair needle. Then 2-0 nonabsorbable sutures are placed in horizontal mattress fashion and tied over bone through a small radial-sided wrist approach that reduces iatrogenic cutaneous nerve injury.

ARTHROSCOPIC MANAGEMENT OF CLASS II DEGENERATIVE INJURIES

Degenerative tears of the TFCC are characterized by either thinning or central perforations of the articular disk that may vary in magnitude and ultimately lead to chondromalacia of the proximal carpal row if untreated. The underlying problem is ulnar positive variance, which may result from multiple etiologies and must be simultaneously addressed to predictably resolve symptoms of ulnar-sided wrist pain in these patients. Class IIA and IIB lesions without perforation are often treated with arthroscopic débridement and an ulnar shortening osteotomy.[52,53] For class IIC lesions with a central TFCC perforation, the prominent distal ulnar head may be partially resected arthroscopically in lieu of open ulnar shortening. Normally, 3 to 4 mm of bone is resected with a high-speed burr. Fluoroscopy is strongly encouraged to monitor the amount of resection because arthroscopic magnification makes the amount of resection difficult to judge. The articulation of the ulnar head with the sigmoid notch should not be violated. Wnorowski et al. demonstrated that shortening the ulnar head by 3 mm decreased the force across the ulna by 50%.[54] Class IID and IIE lesions involve other components of soft tissue and articular cartilage degeneration, and arthroscopic management alone is inadequate to fully address the degree of pathology.

ARTHROSCOPIC GANGLIONECTOMY

Arthroscopic resection of dorsal ganglions was popularized by Osterman and Rafael,[26] who reported initial excellent results. Open excision of dorsal ganglions is not a benign procedure, and patients occasionally report wrist stiffness in flexion. The arthroscopic procedure may be performed with much less scarring, improved cosmesis, and faster motion recovery. The recurrence rate appears to be extremely low and comparable with that of open procedures.[53] The arthroscope is initially placed in the 4-5 and 6-R portals, with inflow provided through the 6-U portal. A needle is then placed through the sac of the ganglion and into the radiocarpal space. The sac of the ganglion is usually located more distal than the 3-4 portal, requiring an oblique advancement of the needle into the joint. The needle typically enters the joint over the dorsal capsule at the level of the scapholunate interosseous ligament. A portal is established adjacent to the needle path, and a small joint shaver is inserted. The shaver creates an approximate 1-cm full-thickness dorsal capsular defect near its confluence with the scapholunate ligament. The residual ganglion stalk is identified and débrided. Visualizing a dorsal extensor tendon ensures adequate ganglion decompression (Fig. 69.26). Simultaneous external palpation of the ganglion cyst as the capsule is being resected usually demonstrates a sudden blush because the cyst and stalk have been débrided.

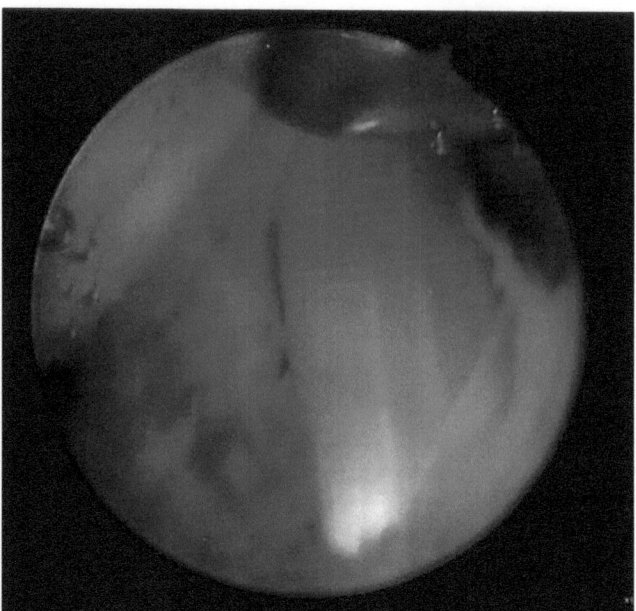

Fig. 69.26 An arthroscopic image after débridement of a dorsal ganglion viewed from the 6-R portal. Note the full thickness débridement of capsule with exposure of underlying extensor tendon.

TABLE 69.4   Bain and Begg Arthroscopic Classification

Grade	Description
0	All functional surfaces are working
I	One nonfunctional articular surface—usually the proximal articular surface of the lunate
II	Two nonfunctional articular surfaces divided into types A and B
IIA	Proximal lunate facet of the radius
IIB	Proximal surface of the lunate and distal articular surface of the lunate
III	Three nonfunctional articular surfaces—lunate facet of the radius, proximal, and distal articular surfaces of the lunate with a preserved head of the capitate
IV	All functional surfaces are nonfunctional

Occasionally a small joint punch may facilitate capsulectomy. It is uncommon, but not impossible, to injure the overlying extensor tendons because the small joint shavers and punches are minimally aggressive. The patient is encouraged to begin ROM exercises the day after surgery; initiation of formal therapy is usually unnecessary. Patients regain ROM earlier compared with open excision.

Kienböck Disease

Wrist arthroscopy has become a reliable method to judge the extent of Kienböck disease by directly visualizing the involved articular surfaces in the radiocarpal and midcarpal joints. Bain and Begg described their arthroscopic classification in 2006 (Table 69.4).[55] The classification system is based on the number of nonfunctional articular surfaces. A normal articular surface was defined as having a glistening appearance or minor fibrillation

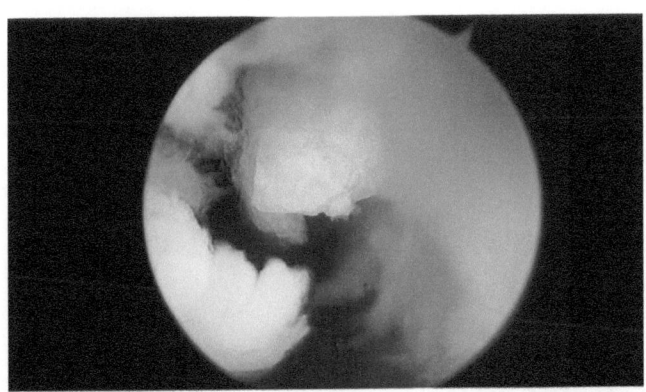

Fig. 69.27 An arthroscopic image of a necrotic lunate in Kienböck disease.

with normal hard subchondral bone with probing. A nonfunctional articular surface was defined as having extensive fibrillation, fissuring, localized or extensive articular loss, floating articular surface, or fracture (Fig. 69.27). The scale is from grade 0 to grade 4, with grade 2 subdivided into types A and B. The number of nonfunctional articular surfaces determines the grade. In the Bain and Begg study series, they found a consistent pattern of changes within the lunate, and changes always occurred initially on the proximal articular surface of the lunate.

Bain and Durrant developed a treatment algorithm based on their arthroscopic grading.[56] The basis of treatment was to remove only the nonfunctional surfaces while maintaining ROM. In grade 0, all the articular surfaces are functional. Arthroscopic synovectomy is performed and further treatment may include an unloading procedure, revascularization, arthroscopic or open core decompression, or bone grafting. Arthroscopic core decompression is recommended only for patients with a neutral or positive ulnar variance.[56]

Grade I Kienböck disease is defined by a nonfunctioning proximal lunate articular surface. Treatment options include proximal row carpectomy or radioscapholunate fusion. In grade IIA, both the proximal articular surface of the lunate and the lunate fossa are nonfunctional. Radioscapholunate fusion is recommended in this case and maintains normal midcarpal kinematics. In grade IIB, the proximal and distal articular surfaces of the lunate are nonfunctional. Bain and Begg feel a proximal row carpectomy is the treatment of choice, provided the lunate articular facet of the radius is intact.

In grade III Kienböck, three articular surfaces are nonfunctional, while the capitate articular surface usually is preserved. In this instance, Bain and Begg recommend a salvage procedure such as a total wrist fusion or arthroplasty. A third option is a resurfacing hemiarthroplasty of the distal radius that articulates with the head of the capitate. In grade IV Kienböck, all four articular surfaces are nonfunctional, and a total wrist fusion or arthroplasty is recommended.

Tatebe et al. performed arthroscopy on 57 patients with Kienböck disease and classified the extent of involvement using the Bain and Begg classification.[57] They found that the number of articular surfaces involved did not correlate with the Lichtman radiographic stage or the duration from onset to surgery. Furthermore, they found that all but two patients had cartilage lesions in the proximal articular surface of the lunate, and loss of additional articular surfaces correlated with patient age.

COMPLICATIONS

Complications of wrist arthroscopy are relatively rare and usually preventable.[49] A needle should be used to determine precise portal placement, because a few millimeters of altered positioning may inadvertently increase the technical difficulty of the procedure. The needle should pass easily into the joint without impaling osseous structures. Blunt trocars prevent iatrogenic cartilage damage as the cannula is introduced. Repeated futile attempts to enter a joint space should be minimized. Separate inflow and outflow portals limit soft tissue fluid extravasation. The risk of compartment syndrome is diminished through the use of physiologic solutions (e.g., lactated Ringer solution), which readily reabsorb, and by adhering to the tenets of careful dressing placement and postoperative elevation. When performing fracture or carpal instability work, K-wires should be inserted with the use of a soft tissue protector or oscillating drill to limit any potential damage to the sensory nerve branches surrounding the wrist.

FUTURE CONSIDERATIONS

In conclusion, wrist arthroscopy continues to grow in popularity as a valuable adjunct in both the diagnosis and management of complex disorders of the wrist. It permits intra-articular structures to be evaluated under bright light and magnified conditions with minimal morbidity. Expanded indications will likely emerge as more surgeons are exposed to the techniques of wrist arthroscopy and better instrumentation is developed.

For a complete list of references, go to ExpertConsult.com.

SELECTED READINGS

Citation:
Whipple TL. The role of arthroscopy in the treatment of scapholunate instability. *Hand Clin.* 1995;11:37–40.

Level of Evidence:
IV

Summary:
In this classic article, Dr. Whipple defined the role of arthroscopy in the management of carpal instability. He noted that results of arthroscopic management of acute carpal instability were better than results for chronic carpal instability.

Citation:
Viegas SF. Midcarpal arthroscopy: anatomy and portals. *Hand Clin.* 1994;10:577–587.

Level of Evidence:
IV

Summary:
This classic article describes the role of midcarpal arthroscopy, particularly focusing on the variations of anatomy that occur in the midcarpal space and the portals used to assess it.

Citation:

Geissler WB, Hammit MD. Arthroscopic aided fixation of scaphoid fractures. *Hand Clin.* 2001;17:575–588.

Level of Evidence:

IV

Summary:

This article is one of the first to define arthroscopic fixation of scaphoid fractures. It defined the advantage of arthroscopy for the management of scaphoid fractures compared with percutaneous reduction.

Citation:

Geissler WB. Arthroscopic knotless peripheral ulnar-sided TFCC repair. *Hand Clin.* 2011;27:273–279.

Level of Evidence:

IV

Summary:

This article describes a new technique for arthroscopic knotless repair of peripheral ulnar-sided tears of the triangular fibrocartilage complex. It defines the advantages of direct repair of the articular disk back down to bone compared with previous techniques, which potentially left knots that could cause symptoms.

Citation:

Slade JF, Geissler WB, Gutow AP, et al. Percutaneous internal fixation of selected scaphoid nonunions with an arthroscopically assisted dorsal approach. *J Bone Joint Surg Am.* 2003;85A:20-32.

Level of Evidence:

IV

Summary:

In this classic article, it is noted that percutaneous fixation of selected fibrous nonunions of the scaphoid can be successfully managed without bone grafting. The article showed superior results for range of motion with percutaneous techniques and showed that bone grafting was not required for every scaphoid nonunion.

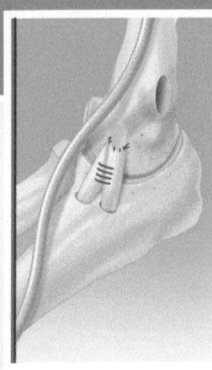

70

Carpal Injuries

Gabrielle M. Paci, Jeffrey Yao

Carpal injuries represent 3% to 9% of all sports-related ailments, with carpal fractures comprising 8% to 19% of hand injuries.[1] Carpal fractures, ligament injury, and instability can occur as a result of acute injury or overuse.[2] Contact sports, such as football, have the highest incidence of carpal injury. These injuries are also frequently seen in gymnasts, mixed martial artists, and boxers, although any participant in sport will be at risk.[2,3] These injuries may be career-threatening for the high-level athlete; therefore timely diagnosis is critical. One major challenge in management is to balance the desire to allow early return to play (RTP) where appropriate, while minimizing the risk of re-injury, future pain, and disability that may result when injuries are treated too aggressively. Treatment is tailored to the individual, accounting for injury severity, concomitant injury, demands of the sport, and career goals. Open communication among the athlete, family, coaches, trainers, and the physician is paramount. This chapter reviews carpal anatomy and kinematics, patterns of injury, and management options with the specific needs of the athlete in mind.

ANATOMY AND KINEMATICS

The wrist is a diarthrodial joint composed of eight carpal bones arranged in two rows. The geometry of the carpal bones and their attachments allows motion in two primary planes: flexion-extension and radial-ulnar deviation. The flexion-extension arc is derived from roughly equal motion through both the radio-carpal and the midcarpal articulations. Radial-ulnar deviation is similarly distributed, with the radiocarpal joint contributing 40% and the midcarpal joint contributing 60%.[4] Meanwhile, axial load bearing at the wrist occurs 80% through the radiocarpal joint and 20% through the ulnocarpal articulation.[5]

Several theories have been proposed to explain carpal kinematics and function. Navarro[6] proposed that the carpus was arranged in three rigid, vertical columns. In 1984, Weber[7] introduced the longitudinal column theory. The column theories provided a model to account for axial load transmission from hand to forearm but did not account for the coupled motion between the proximal and distal rows and the small but significant independent motion present between the carpal bones.[8]

The row theory was introduced in the 1980s and suggested that the proximal and distal rows behave as separate functional units.[4,8,9] The interosseous ligaments and the articular geometry allow the carpal bones to move in unison during wrist motion. Linscheid and Dobyns[10] noted that as the wrist deviates radially,

the scaphoid and proximal row flex. They believed that scaphoid flexion occurs in response to the pressure exerted by the trapezium and trapezoid. Weber[7] postulated that it is the helicoid geometry of the triquetrohamate articulation that forces the distal row to translate palmarly during radial deviation, creating a flexion moment on the proximal row. Conversely, during ulnar deviation, the distal row is forced to translate dorsally, creating an extension moment on the proximal row.

Different theories on kinematics have provided a greater understanding of the coordinated motion between rows and the tendencies for abnormal motion when the system breaks down. Given that no one concept adequately describes the complexity of carpal motion, most investigators agree that carpal kinematics can best be explained by a combination of these theories. It is evident that in the intact wrist, a complex synchrony exists between the carpal bones and between the carpal rows.

Intrinsic and extrinsic ligaments of the wrist link and stabilize the carpal bones. Intrinsic ligaments, also known as interosseous ligaments, connect carpal bones to one another. Extrinsic ligaments connect the carpal bones to the radius and ulna and tend to be stronger than their intrinsic counterparts. With the exception of the pisiform, tendons do not directly insert on the carpal bones but help to stabilize their motion when actively contracting. Wrist motion is initiated by the distal carpal row and metacarpals, which move as a unit. Radioulnar motion occurs primarily through the midcarpal joint. Radial deviation of the wrist causes the distal row to incline radially, extend, and supinate while the proximal row remains flexed with minimal translation. Conversely, during ulnar deviation, the distal row inclines ulnarly, flexes, and pronates while the proximal row extends with minimal translation.[11]

CARPAL FRACTURES

Scaphoid

History

The scaphoid is the most commonly injured carpal bone, accounting for nearly 70% of carpal bone fractures.[12] A scaphoid fracture is typically seen after a fall onto an outstretched, pronated, and ulnar-deviated hand but can also be seen after a direct blow or as an occult injury.[13] Patterns of injury include waist (the most common), distal pole, or proximal pole fractures. Any athlete presenting with radial-sided wrist pain should be considered to have a scaphoid fracture until proven otherwise.[14]

Physical Exam

Scaphoid fractures classically present with anatomic snuffbox swelling and tenderness. Palpation over the volar scaphoid tubercle and scaphoid compression with axial load of the thumb metacarpal may also elicit pain.[13,15] Duckworth et al.[16] found that the combination of snuffbox tenderness and pain with ulnar wrist deviation was 91% specific for scaphoid fracture in males with sports-related injuries.

Imaging

Radiographs, including posteroanterior (PA), lateral and oblique views, should be obtained. Additionally, a scaphoid-specific view taken as a PA at 45 degrees of pronation and ulnar deviation should be taken. False-negative results on initial plain radiographs have been estimated to be as high as 25%.[17] Additional studies early in an acutely injured athlete can help define the injury and can be cost-effective. Magnetic resonance imaging (MRI) is the gold standard for diagnosing occult scaphoid fractures.[18,19] Computed tomography (CT) scans can be helpful in providing detail of the fracture and, when obtained, should be done in 1-mm cuts in the longitudinal axis of the scaphoid.

Decision-Making Principles

Fractures of the distal pole and nondisplaced fractures of the waist are considered stable and demonstrate a high rate of healing with nonoperative treatment. Non-skill position players (e.g., a football player who does not have to handle the ball) can be treated with a padded short arm thumb spica cast for most nondisplaced fractures, with the caveat that this may increase the risk of nonunion.[20,21] Athletes who require wrist motion to perform (e.g., a quarterback, running back, or wide receiver in football) may be able to RTP earlier with early internal fixation.[22-25]

Proximal pole fractures require a longer time to union and have higher rates of nonunion due to interruption of the integrity of the dorsal vascular supply and retrograde intraosseous blood supply. Therefore early fixation may be recommended for nondisplaced proximal pole fractures.[26] Ultimately the weakness and stiffness that result from extended immobilization are significant setbacks for the athlete; therefore early surgical intervention for scaphoid fractures in the athlete should be considered.

Treatment Options

Nonoperative treatment is carried out with cast immobilization for 6 to 12 weeks.[13,27,28] Whether to use a long arm, short arm, or thumb spica cast has been debated.[28-30] However, it is reasonable to consider a long arm cast in any patient with concern for noncompliance. Surgical techniques include percutaneous, open, or arthroscopic-assisted approaches to fixation with a headless compression screw.

Postoperative Management

Patients are placed in a thumb spica splint following surgery and transitioned to a short arm cast at their 2-week clinic follow up. A playing cast can be considered for noncontact athletes at this juncture.[2] For contact athletes, the cast is removed at 6 weeks

postoperatively if union is achieved. For proximal pole fractures or where there is a concern for incomplete union, the cast may be continued for up to 12 weeks postoperatively. If early RTP is critical, CT scans should be obtained at 6-week intervals to assess for union. Once the fracture has achieved at least 50% bony bridging and the patient is free of pain with at least 80% of preoperative grip strength and good motion, RTP is considered.[15] These recommendations are strictly guidelines and the most appropriate postoperative plan should be individualized to the athlete.

Results

Surgical fixation of scaphoid fractures achieves excellent rates of union with a shorter period of immobilization and faster gains in strength and motion compared with nonoperative treatment in a cast. Whether percutaneous techniques in particular allow for shorter time to union compared with nonoperative treatment remains an area of debate.[31-34] However, it is clear that surgical treatment is associated with an increased risk of complications.[35]

Complications

Complications of scaphoid fractures include avascular necrosis (up to 40%), malunion (up to 50% of displaced fractures), nonunion (up to 5% of nondisplaced and 55% of displaced fractures), carpal instability and posttraumatic arthritis or development of scaphoid nonunion with advanced collapse.[13] Complications of surgical treatment include displacement of nondisplaced fractures, injury to the radial artery, and over- or underdrilling, which can lead to poor screw purchase or distraction across the fracture site, respectively.[36]

Triquetrum

History

The triquetrum is the second most commonly injured carpal bone, representing up to 18% of all carpal fractures.[37-39] Fracture patterns include dorsal cortical avulsion fractures, fractures through the body, and volar cortical fractures. Dorsal cortical avulsion fractures are most prevalent, accounting for 93% of all triquetral fractures.[38] The mechanism of injury for dorsal cortical fractures primarily involves either palmar flexion and radial deviation[39,40] or dorsiflexion and ulnar deviation of the wrist.[41-43] During wrist hyperflexion, the dorsal extrinsic ligaments (which attach to the triquetrum) are placed under stress and lead to an avulsion of the dorsal triquetrum. During wrist dorsiflexion and ulnar deviation, it is surmised that the ulnar styloid drives into the triquetrum, leading to a "dorsal chip." Triquetral body fractures occur with the wrist in extension and ulnar deviation. Body fractures typically follow high-energy mechanisms, and the clinician should suspect related injuries. Perilunate dislocations are present in 12% to 25% of body fractures.[44] Finally, volar cortical injuries are rare and can represent a lunotriquetral ligament avulsion.

Physical Exam

Triquetral fractures present with ulnar-sided wrist pain. Associated soft tissue swelling may represent ligamentous injury.

Authors' Preferred Technique

For nondisplaced scaphoid fractures, we prefer a minimally invasive approach with a cannulated, headless compression screw. This approach has the advantage of minimizing soft tissue disruption and damage to the blood supply, which may optimize conditions for achieving union and maximizing range of motion (ROM). For displaced fractures, however, anatomic reduction requires direct visualization through an open approach. For proximal pole fractures, this is achieved through a dorsal approach. (Fig. 70.1). Distal pole fractures and any humpback deformities are addressed through a volar approach, which affords superior visualization. Waist fractures may be addressed from either approach.

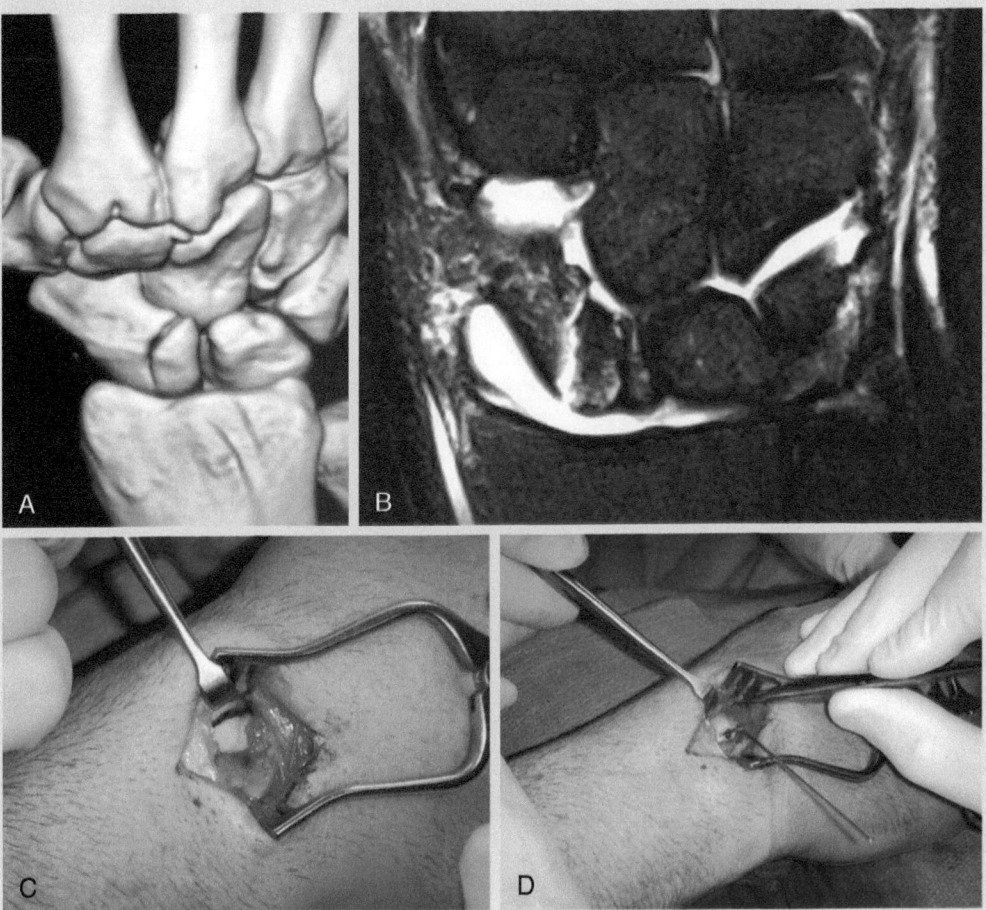

Fig. 70.1 A displaced fracture of the proximal third of the scaphoid in a Major League Baseball player. (AB) Magnetic resonance imaging and three-dimensional computed tomography reconstruction can aid in identifying the fracture pattern. (C) A mini-open approach was used through a 1- to 2-cm dorsal incision. (D) The fracture was reduced using K-wires as joysticks and fixed with a cannulated screw down the central axis of the scaphoid.

Considering the likelihood of concomitant injuries and the close proximity to other ulnar structures such as the triangular fibrocartilage complex, eliciting point tenderness over the triquetrum may be challenging. Direct tenderness and pain with wrist motion are often present with dorsal avulsion injuries.

Imaging

Radiographs—including PA, lateral, and oblique views—are typically sufficient for the diagnosis of a triquetral fracture. A CT scan can provide additional detail of the fracture pattern. An MRI can be ordered in instances in which there is significant soft tissue swelling or recovery does not progress and a concurrent scapholunate or lunotriquetral tear is suspected.

Decision-Making Principles

Fractures of the dorsal cortex and nondisplaced triquetral body fractures are generally considered stable and amenable to nonoperative treatment. Significant soft tissue swelling should raise suspicion for ligamentous injury and requires a longer period of immobilization.[37] Athletes should be counseled regarding fracture fibrous nonunion, a common result with little potential consequence. Surgical treatment is reserved for symptomatic nonunion. Though rare, displaced fractures of the body, as well as body or volar cortical fractures with associated ligamentous injury, are inherently unstable and should be treated surgically.

Treatment Options

Triquetral fractures of the dorsal cortex and nondisplaced body fractures can be treated with a brace or a short arm cast for 3 to 6 weeks or longer depending on the condition of the soft tissues (Fig. 70.2).[45,46] In the event of fibrous nonunion that is symptomatic, surgical excision of the fragment with reattachment of the extrinsic ligaments to the remaining triquetrum may be performed.

Displaced body fractures may be treated with open reduction and surgical fixation. This can be done using a headless compression screw through a dorsal approach along the extensor carpi ulnaris (ECU) tendon. Treatment of body or volar cortical fractures with associated ligamentous injury focuses on surgical stabilization of the surrounding intercarpal articulations. In cases of symptomatic malunion, nonunion, or pisotriquetral arthritis, excision of the pisiform may provide adequate symptom relief.[47–49]

📌 Authors' Preferred Technique

For acute fractures of the dorsal cortex with mild to moderate swelling, a cast or splint is applied for 2 to 4 weeks and the athlete is reexamined at weekly intervals until he or she is asymptomatic and ready for unrestricted play. When a triquetral body fracture is associated with a perilunate dislocation, it is our practice to pin the lunotriquetral joint along with the scapholunate joint and midcarpal joints and bypassing fixation of the triquetral fracture.

Postoperative Management

Postoperatively, triquetral injuries should be immobilized and any Kirschner wires (K-wires) should be left in place for a minimum of 4 weeks.

Results

Most fractures of the triquetral dorsal cortex go on to fibrous nonunion that is asymptomatic. Unstable patterns have more variable outcomes and do best when identified and treated promptly.[50]

Complications

The most common complication following fracture of the triquetrum is a delay in diagnosis, which can result in chronic instability due to an untreated associated triangular fibrocartilage complex, perilunate or lunotriquetral ligament injury with associated pain, stiffness, and pisotriquetral arthritis.[37]

Trapezium
History

Four to 5% of carpal fractures involve the trapezium.[51–53] Fractures can involve the body or the volar ridge at the attachment of the transverse carpal ligament. Body fractures are most common and are divided into sagittal split, horizontal split, transarticular, dorsoradial tuberosity, and comminuted subtypes. Volar trapezial ridge fractures are subdivided into base (type I) and tip avulsion (type II) fractures.

The mechanism of injury involves an axial load on a dorsiflexed wrist, whereby the thumb metacarpal is driven into the trapezium. Other described mechanisms include a load onto the radially deviated wrist with the thumb abducted and hyperextended, whereby the radial styloid is driven into the trapezium. Most injuries occur as a result of high-energy motor vehicle collisions or falls onto an outstretched hand.[46,54]

Physical Exam

Physical examination reveals point tenderness distal to the scaphoid tubercle at the volar base of the thumb. Pain or weakness can occur with pinch-related activities and may worsen with wrist flexion because of the proximity of the flexor carpi radialis (FCR) tendon to the trapezial ridge (Fig. 70.3). The clinician must evaluate for commonly associated injuries to the distal radius, scaphoid, hamate, and first metacarpal.[7,54,55]

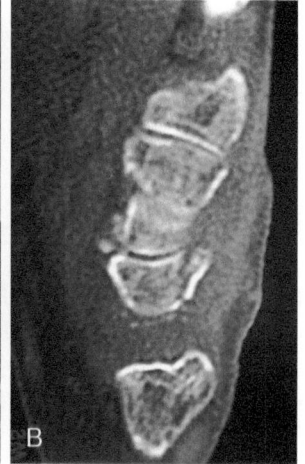

Fig. 70.2 (A) A patient was noted to have tenderness over the triquetrum. (B) A computed tomography scan was obtained, which revealed a dorsal triquetral fracture. The patient was treated nonoperatively in a short arm cast for 6 weeks. Patients should be counseled that a fracture may proceed to an asymptomatic fibrous union.

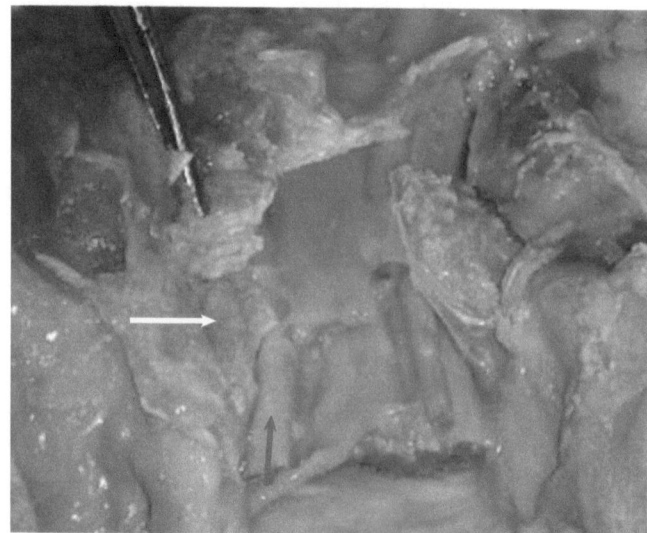

Fig. 70.3 Anatomic dissection revealing the proximity of the trapezial ridge *(white arrow)* to the flexor carpi radialis tendon *(green arrow)*.

Imaging

Radiographs—including PA, lateral and oblique views—should be obtained and will typically demonstrate a trapezium fracture when present (Fig. 70.4). Bett's view is an anteroposterior view of the wrist in pronation that allows for better visualization of the trapeziometacarpal articulation. The carpal canal views better depict the volar trapezial ridge. CT is also useful to delineate fracture details and identify concurrent fractures of the neighboring bones.

Decision-Making Principles

Nonoperative treatment is reserved for nondisplaced trapezial fractures. Displaced fractures of the volar trapezial ridge are at risk of nonunion due to the pull of the transverse carpal ligament. Trapezial body fractures with displacement greater than 2 mm or carpometacarpal (CMC) subluxation require reduction and surgical fixation.[54]

Treatment Options

Nonoperative treatment consists of immobilization in a thumb spica cast for 4 to 6 weeks. Trapezial ridge fractures resulting in symptomatic nonunion can be treated with excision of the fracture fragment (Fig. 70.5). For displaced fractures of the body, open reduction and internal fixation with K-wires or screws may be performed (Fig. 70.6). Comminuted fractures may be amenable to external fixation or oblique dynamic traction splinting for early motion.[17,54]

Postoperative Management

Postoperatively, trapezial fractures should be immobilized and any K-wires should be left in place for a minimum of 4 weeks.

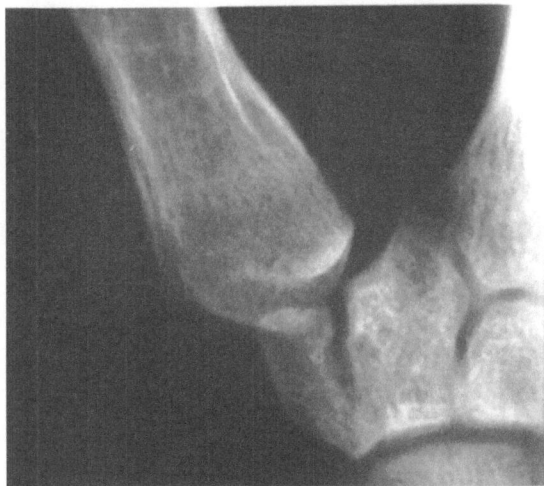

Fig. 70.4 The oblique view (pronated) of the wrist reveals a longitudinal fracture of the body of the trapezium. (Courtesy Michael Hayton, MD, Manchester, UK.)

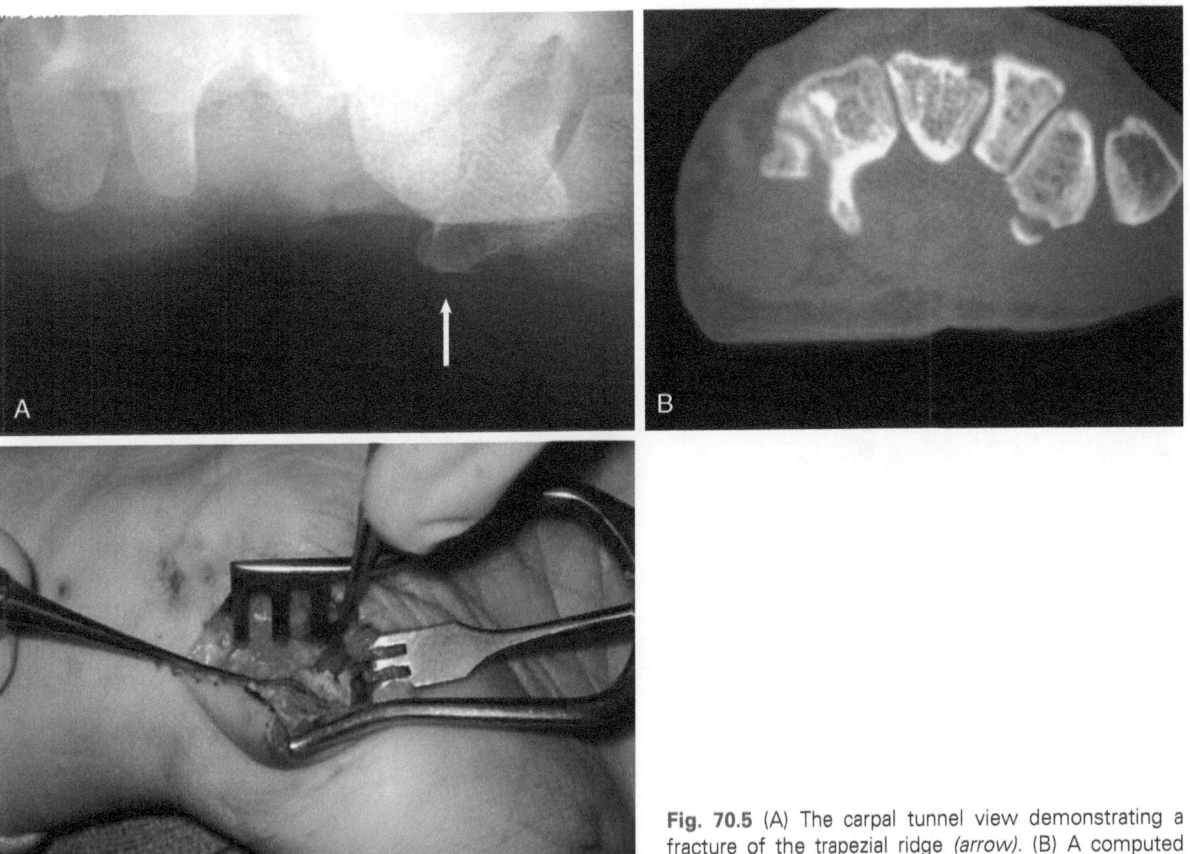

Fig. 70.5 (A) The carpal tunnel view demonstrating a fracture of the trapezial ridge (arrow). (B) A computed tomography scan demonstrating fracture of the trapezial ridge. (C) The incision near the base of the thenar eminence with resection of the fractured trapezial ridge.

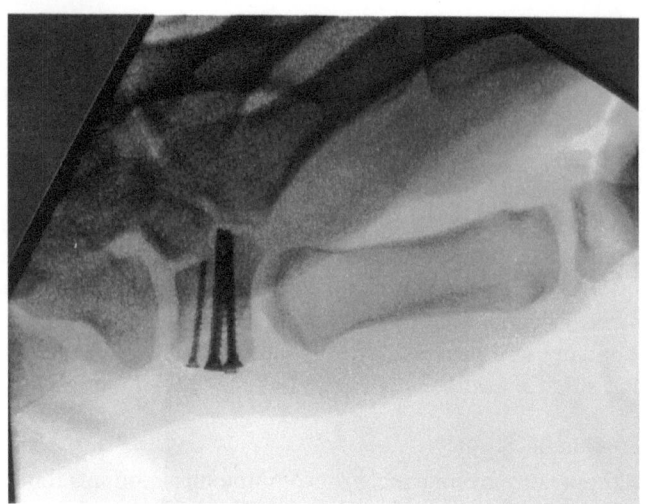

Fig. 70.6 Open reduction and internal fixation of a displaced trapezial body fracture with screws.

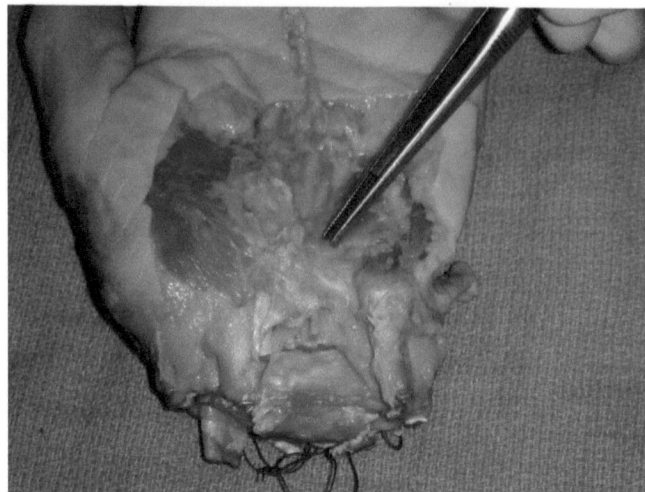

Fig. 70.8 The transverse carpal ligament forms the roof of the carpal canal and attaches to the hook of the hamate. Pull of the thenar muscles through the transverse carpal ligament can displace the hook of the hamate fracture. Injuries can lead to paresthesias in the ulnar and median nerve distribution.

Authors' Preferred Technique

When operative treatment is chosen, we prefer the volar Wagner approach to the trapezium. The skin incision follows the thenar eminence at the junction of the glabrous skin of the palm and the dorsal skin of the wrist and curves in a volar direction. Dissection follows beneath the thenar musculature. Careful attention should be directed to protecting the branches of the radial sensory nerve and the radial artery (Fig. 70.7). Reduction under direct visualization is achieved and fixation established with the use of K-wires or minifragment screws.

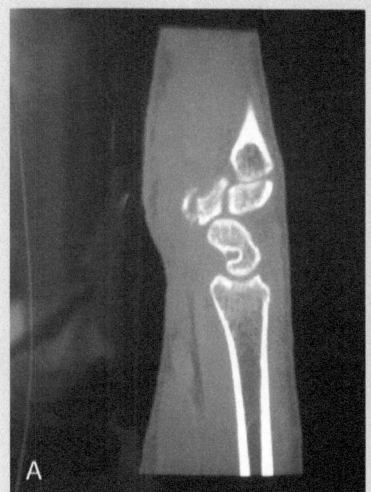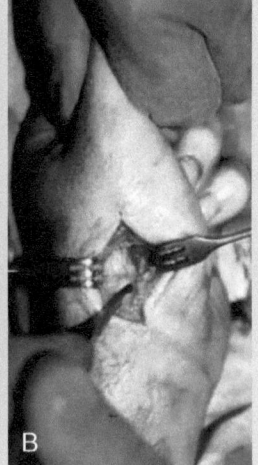

Fig. 70.7 (A) A sagittal computed tomography image illustrating a coronal fracture through the body of the trapezium. (B) The skin incision for the Wagner approach to the trapezium body fractures is along the glabrous skin of the palm and the dorsal skin of the wrist. This approach places the branches of the radial artery and nerve at risk.

Results

Outcomes studies in the literature are limited to small series of patients. Overall, cast immobilization alone has demonstrated poor outcomes for displaced or comminuted fractures due to the resultant incongruence of the CMC articulation. Surgical

treatment with restoration of the articular surface yields good functional outcomes.[54]

Complications

Complications of trapezial fractures include nonunion, FCR tendonitis or rupture, carpal tunnel syndrome, stiffness of the CMC joint, posttraumatic arthritis, and loss of pinch strength.[37,49,56]

Hamate
History

Hamate fractures represent close to 2% of all carpal fractures.[12] The hamate lies in close proximity to surrounding neurovascular structures. It forms the radial border of Guyon canal and serves as an attachment site for the transverse carpal ligament at the ulnar border of the carpal tunnel. As a result, hamate injuries may lead to paresthesias and/or motor dysfunction in the ulnar or median nerve distribution (Fig. 70.8).

Mechanisms of injury for fractures of the hook of the hamate involve direct compression or shear forces from adjacent tendons during forceful twisting of the wrist.[57] The superficial position of the hook predisposes it to injury from compressive trauma to the palm. The most common activities relating to this injury include baseball and golf, where they affect the nondominant hand, and various racquet-related sports, where the dominant hand is affected. Body fractures of the hamate are rare but may occur as a result of high-energy axial load through the fourth and fifth metacarpals. These fractures are classified as either coronal or transverse.[58] Small finger CMC dislocations may accompany these injuries (Fig. 70.9).[45,59] Clinical diagnosis can be difficult and these fractures are frequently missed, so a high index of suspicion is needed.[60,61]

Physical Exam

Hamate fractures present as ulnar-sided palm or wrist pain that may be worsened with grasping.[62] Tenderness can often

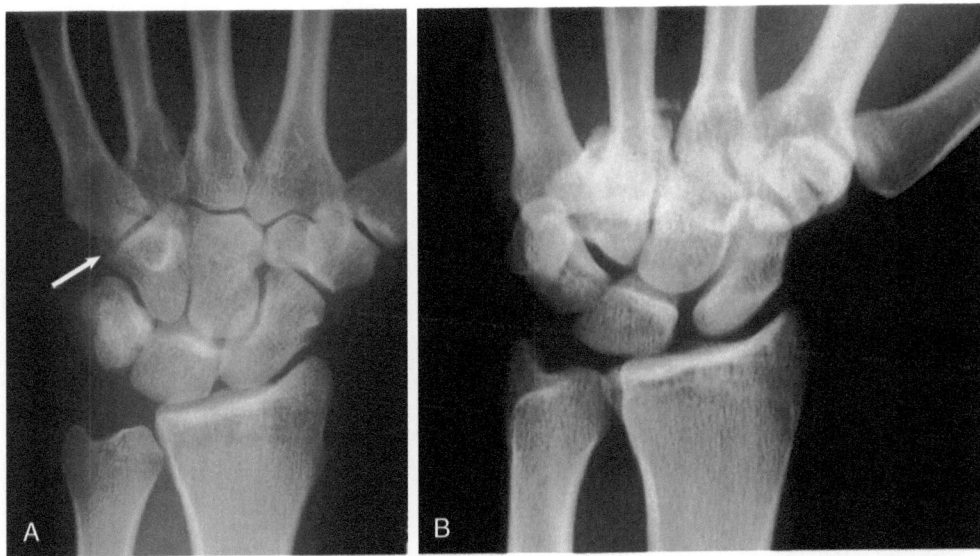

Fig. 70.9 (A) Posteroanterior plain radiographs of the wrist allow visibility of the joint space between the base of the fifth metacarpal and the hamate *(arrow)*. (B) Obliteration of the joint space in a patient with a III to V carpometacarpal fracture dislocation.

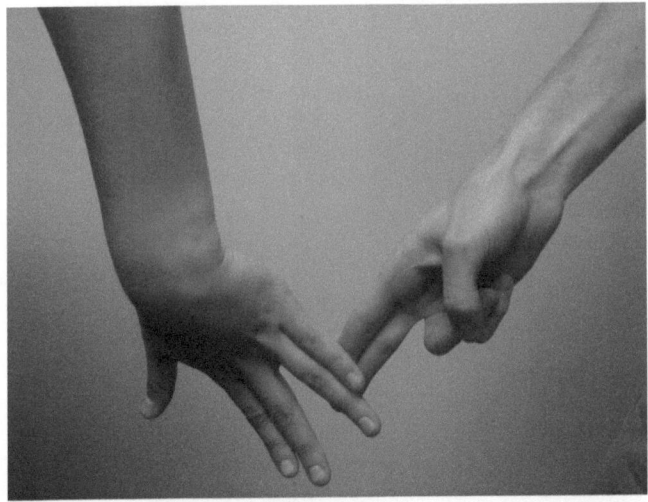

Fig. 70.10 Resisted wrist flexion and ulnar deviation elicits pain; a provocative test evaluates injury to the hook of the hamate.

be elicited over the hook. The hook of hamate pull test is performed with resisted flexion of the ring and small fingers and is positive when resultant hamate fracture displacement causes pain. (Fig. 70.10).[57,63] A thorough motor and sensory examination is important. Irritation of the adjacent ulnar and median nerves may lead to paresthesias. Abrasion of the adjacent flexor tendons against the fractured hook may lead to tendinosis or flexor tendon rupture (Fig. 70.11). Body fractures are often seen with significant swelling and associated CMC joint dislocation.

Imaging

Standard radiographs are often insufficient for detecting hamate fractures. The oblique joint space of the CMC articulation is obliterated in the setting of dislocation. A cortical circular ring, representing the end-on view of the hook of the hamate on PA views, may be missing on injury radiographs. When images demonstrate increased

sclerosis around the circular ring, a nondisplaced nonunion should be considered.[64] A CT scan is used to confirm diagnosis, delineate fracture pattern, and distinguish between occult fracture versus an anatomic variant, the os hamuli (Fig. 70.12).[65,66] Specialized radiographic views can assist with diagnosis and include (1) the carpal tunnel view (Fig. 70.13),[67] (2) the supinated oblique view with the wrist in dorsiflexion,[68,69] and (3) the lateral view through the first web with the thumb abducted.[70]

Decision-Making Principles

Nondisplaced hamate fractures are considered stable, with good healing potential if treated within 1 week of injury.[71] They do, however, require prolonged immobilization (up to 11 weeks). In the athlete, this lengthy period of immobilization and the risk of associated flexor tendon rupture make nonoperative treatment less practical. Furthermore, the tenuous blood supply to the hook of the hamate leads to a high risk of nonunion or avascular necrosis following distal hook fractures. In general, early surgical treatment of all hamate fractures may allow for faster RTP and should be strongly considered.

Treatment Options

Nonoperative treatment consists of early cast immobilization with the wrist in slight flexion and the fourth and fifth metacarpophalangeal joints in maximum flexion to minimize shear forces on the hook from the flexor tendons. Thumb immobilization may help to minimize displacing forces from the pull of the transverse carpal ligament.[50] Surgical treatment is most commonly carried out with excision of the fracture fragment via a volar or lateral approach. However, open reduction and internal fixation with either K-wires or screws has also been described.[62,72,73]

Postoperative Management

Postoperatively the wrist should be splinted for 3 to 5 days. The wound is checked, and if it has sealed, a soft dressing is applied

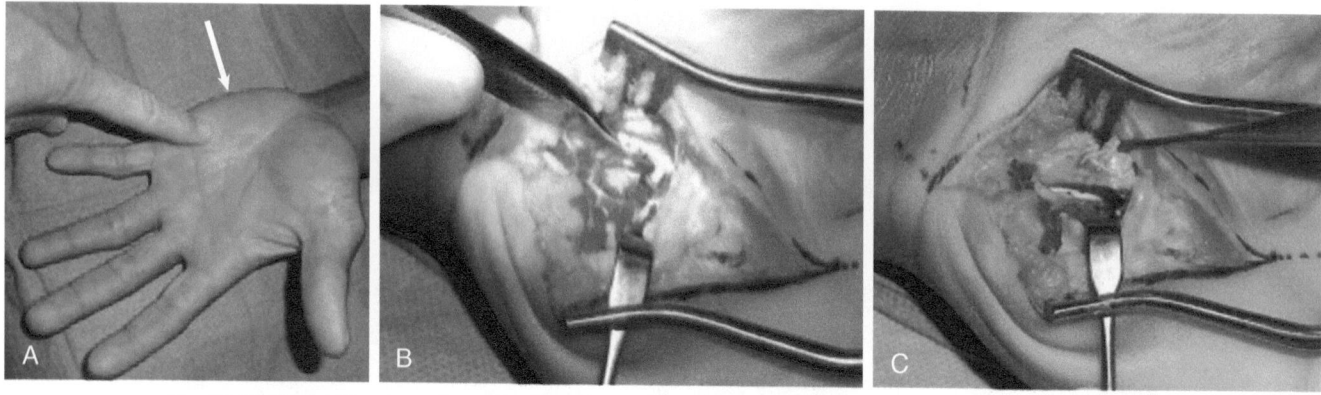

Fig. 70.11 (A) A callus *(arrow)* over the hypothenar eminence in a baseball player with flexor tendonitis and ulnar-sided palm pain. (B) A fracture was found over the distal margin of the hamate at the carpometacarpal joint. The hamate hook was not fractured. (C) A partial flexor tendon laceration was encountered from abrasion against the fractured hamate.

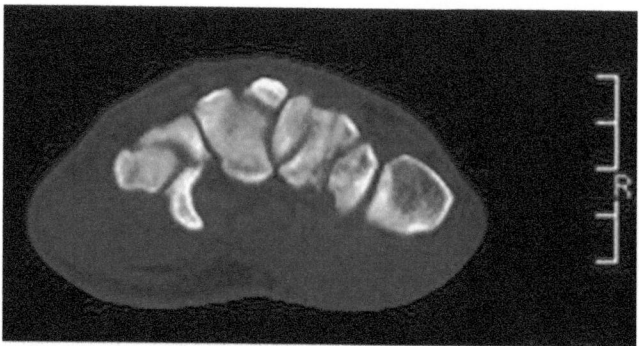

Fig. 70.12 A computed tomography image of the carpal canal demonstrating a hook of the hamate fracture.

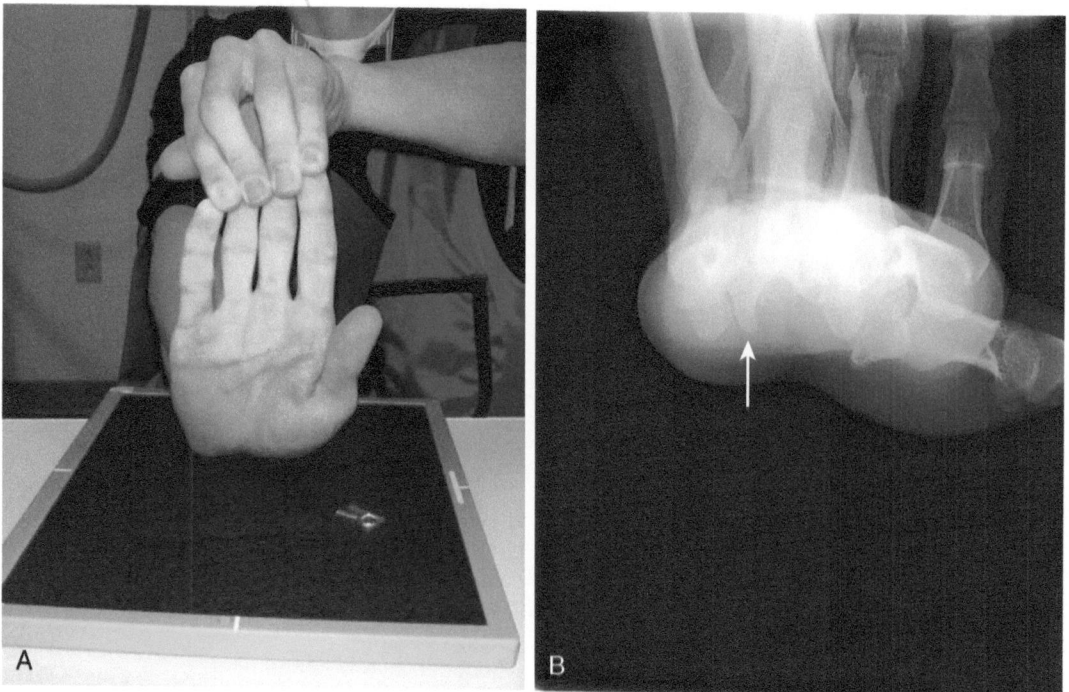

Fig. 70.13 (A) A hand held in maximum extension to obtain the carpal tunnel view. (B) The carpal tunnel view demonstrates the hamate hook *(arrow)*.

✎ Authors' Preferred Technique

We prefer hook of hamate excision for both acute fractures and nonunion. When approaching the hook of the hamate, particular attention should be directed to the proximity of the deep motor branch of the ulnar nerve. An S-shaped incision is centered over the hook. We avoid crossing the wrist flexion creases to minimize scar sensitivity and facilitate RTP. The ulnar nerve and artery are dissected proximal to distal toward the hook. The ulnar motor branch, which exits dorsal and ulnar to the ulnar nerve proper, dives deep as it travels in a radial direction toward and around the ulnar border of the hamate hook.[74] Once mobilized and retracted, the hook can be exposed; the periosteum is elevated, and the hook is uncovered (Fig. 70.14). Removal of the entire hook is preferred to avoid irritating the adjacent flexor tendons with residual exposed bone.

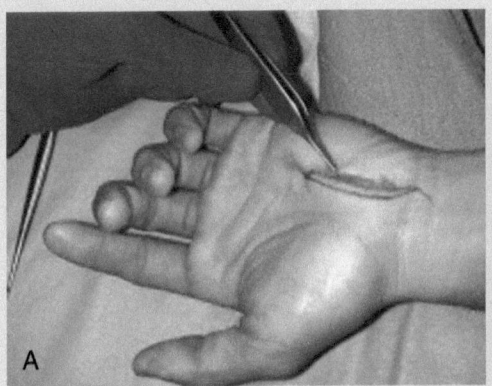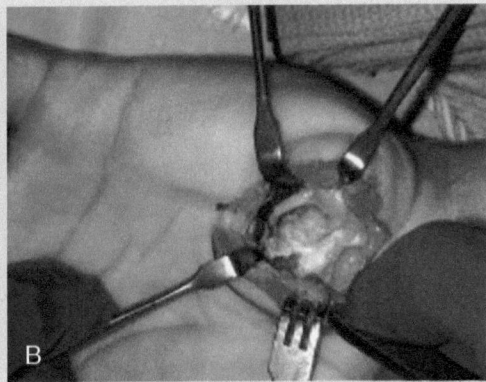

Fig. 70.14 (A) Exposure of the hamate hook through a curvilinear incision in the palm. (B) Exposed hamate hook.

and the athlete is allowed to perform wrist motion and aerobic workouts. Return to competition is sport-specific. At 2 to 3 weeks, baseball, tennis, and squash players are permitted "dry swings" with a padded glove; golfers are allowed to putt and chip. Contact off a tee in baseball, light volleying in racquet sports, and half swings off a mat in golf may be initiated at 3 weeks, with gradual progression to normal play at 4 to 6 weeks. Athletes can expect scar sensitivity that will improve over time but should be counseled that complete relief may not occur for up to 4 to 6 months after surgery.

Results

Although cadaver studies have demonstrated a loss of grip strength following hamate excision, clinical studies have shown no impact on functional performance in high-level athletes.[73,75–77] The literature on outcomes following open reduction with internal fixation is limited to small series and suggests that there may be high rates of nonunion.[60]

Complications

Complications of hamate fractures include rupture of either the small or ring finger flexor tendons, which can occur in up to 14% of injuries. Osteonecrosis and nonunion of the hamate body or hook have also been reported.[78–81] After surgery, the patient should be aware that there is a 3% risk of complication, with nerve injury being the most common untoward event.[82]

Capitate
History
Capitate fractures represent 1% to 2% of carpal fractures.[12] They are divided into four types, including transverse pole, transverse body, coronal, and parasagittal. Transverse body fractures are most common.

The capitate can fracture with axial loads directed on the third metacarpal with the wrist in flexion.[83] Other proposed mechanisms include hyperextension with the wrist in ulnar deviation, resulting in dorsal impaction of the distal radius onto the capitate waist. Isolated injuries are rare and more commonly occur in association with greater arc injuries where the force is transmitted through a combination of ligament and bone, including the scaphoid. Wrist hyperextension and radial deviation can lead to transscaphoid, transcapitate, and perilunate fracture dislocations. Scaphocapitate fracture syndrome is a high-energy perilunate injury with dissipation of energy through the scaphoid waist and neck of the capitate, resulting in the 180-degree rotation of the proximal fragment.

Physical Exam
As with other carpal injuries, patients frequently present with a swollen hand and a painful wrist. If the hand is particularly swollen and the carpus is palpable dorsally, a perilunate injury is likely to have occurred. Tenderness over the dorsal surface of the capitate is a relatively common examination finding for the less common isolated capitate fracture.[37]

Imaging
Although displaced capitate fractures may be apparent on plain radiographs, these can be subtle and difficult to visualize. Advanced imaging with CT or MRI can help to identify fractures and fracture displacement, particularly those that occur in the coronal plane. MRI has the added benefit of detailing any associated ligamentous injuries as well as the blood supply to the proximal fragment.[37]

Decision-Making Principles

Because of a retrograde blood supply, capitate fractures are at risk of avascular necrosis and nonunion. Nondisplaced fractures are amenable to nonoperative treatment with casting and close surveillance. When healing is in question, a CT scan can identify crossing trabeculae at the site of union. Displaced fractures should be treated surgically in order to minimize the risk of nonunion and allow for early RTP. In the athlete, consideration should be given to early surgical treatment of all capitate fractures in order to decrease the setbacks associated with prolonged immobilization and to expedite RTP.

Treatment Options

Nonoperative treatment is carried out with short arm casting for 4 to 8 weeks. Surgical treatment can be achieved with open reduction and internal fixation using K-wires or headless compression screws.

Postoperative Management

Depending on the extent of concomitant injury, athletes can begin ROM exercises as early as 2 weeks postoperatively following screw fixation. For associated scaphoid or perilunate pathology, a minimum of 6 weeks of immobilization should be undertaken, after which K-wires are removed.

📌 Authors' Preferred Technique

We favor surgical fixation of capitate fractures with headless compression screws. This procedure is accomplished via a dorsal approach through the third and fourth extensor compartments along the radial border of the long finger. The approach allows for fixation of the capitate, scaphoid, and associated ligamentous injuries in those with scaphocapitate syndrome (Fig. 70.15).

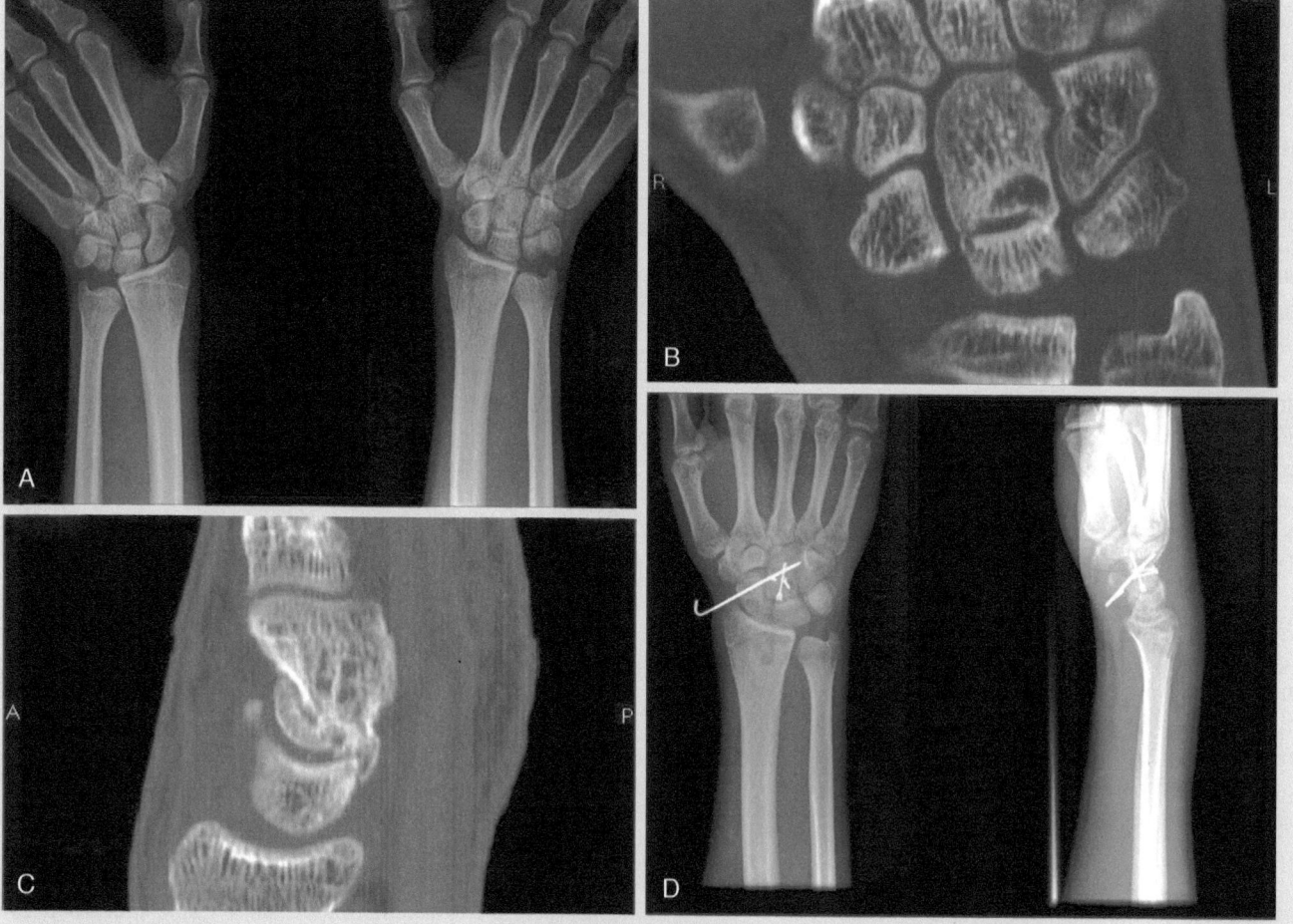

Fig. 70.15 A 17-year-old male presented 7 weeks after punching a tree. He sustained an isolated fracture of the capitate as seen on plain radiographs (A) and coronal (B) and sagittal (C) computed tomography images. (D) Postoperative radiographs after open reduction and internal fixation with a headless compression screw.

Results

Prognosis is guarded depending on the severity of injury to bone and soft tissue. Athletes should understand that this injury can end their season or even their career.

Complications

The most common complication after capitate fracture is non-union, which may occur in up to 50% of isolated injuries.[44] Other complications include avascular necrosis and midcarpal instability. In the setting of perilunate dislocation, stiffness and midcarpal arthritis are common sequelae.

Trapezoid
History

Trapezoid fractures make up less than 1% of carpal fractures.[60] The trapezoid is a keystone-shaped bone with a dorsal length that is two times the distance of the volar length. Trapezoid fractures may occur at the dorsal rim or the body and are most commonly seen with associated fractures of neighboring bones. The trapezoid is protected by surrounding metacarpals, carpals, and strong volar ligamentous attachments. Because of these attachments, dorsal fracture displacement or dislocation is more likely, but volar dislocations have been described.[37,84,85] Fracture and/or dislocation usually occurs when high-energy axial load is transmitted through the second metacarpal.

Physical Exam

Examination reveals tenderness at the base of the index metacarpal. Gentle motion of the metacarpal can elicit pain. If deformity is present, the trapezoid may be dorsally displaced or dislocated.

Imaging

Trapezoid fractures are the most commonly missed fractures on radiographic analysis owing to the adjacent overlying structures. Nevertheless, standard radiographs including PA, lateral, and oblique views may be adequate for diagnosing fractures of the trapezoid. PA images demonstrate not only fracture but may also reveal proximal migration of the second metacarpal, suggesting trapezoidal dislocation.[84] CT or MRI is useful in identifying occult fracture and should be ordered for patients who have normal radiographs but report localized, persistent pain after trauma in this region.[86]

Decision-Making Principles

Nondisplaced trapezoid fractures are amenable to nonoperative treatment. Seventy percent of the trapezoid's blood supply arrives dorsally, making displaced fractures prone to avascular necrosis.[37] Therefore displaced fractures should be treated surgically, as should those with an incongruent CMC joint.

Dislocations should be managed with initial closed reduction. The closed reduction maneuver involves gentle traction of the second metacarpal followed by wrist flexion while simultaneously placing direct pressure over the dorsal side of the trapezoid.[84,87] If the trapezoid is unstable and continues to subluxate dorsally, surgical treatment is warranted.

Treatment Options

Nonoperative treatment is carried out with immobilization in a short arm cast for 4 to 6 weeks. Open reduction and internal fixation for displaced fractures can be performed with K-wires or compression screws.[88] In cases of isolated trapezoid dislocation, percutaneous pin fixation alone may be sufficient following a successful closed reduction. Highly comminuted fractures or those that result in symptomatic malunion or nonunion can be treated with fusion of the CMC joint.[37,44]

> ### 📌 Authors' Preferred Technique
>
> We approach the trapezoid via a dorsal curvilinear transverse incision just distal to the radial styloid. Superficial branches of the radial nerve and the dorsal radial artery are identified and protected. The distal aspect of the extensor retinaculum is then incised along the extensor pollicis longus tendon and a transverse incision is made in the capsule between extensor carpi radialis longus and brevis tendons. With the trapezoid exposed, surgical fixation is achieved with a headless compression screw. Concomitant ligamentous or bony injuries should be addressed with K-wire fixation as appropriate.

Postoperative Management

Depending on the extent of concomitant injury, athletes can begin ROM as early as 2 weeks postoperatively following screw fixation. If K-wires are used to stabilize associated ligamentous injury, these are left in position for 6 to 8 weeks, which precludes this early ROM protocol. Full RTP is resumed at 12 weeks postoperatively.

Results

The literature is scarce regarding outcomes following these rare injuries. Small series have reported excellent union rates and functional outcomes following both closed treatment of nondisplaced trapezoid fractures and surgical treatment of those that are displaced.[89]

Complications

Complications after trapezoid fracture include avascular necrosis, nonunion, and posttraumatic arthritis.

Lunate
History

Lunate fractures account for fewer than 1% of all carpal fractures.[90] Five fracture types have been observed: volar pole, dorsal pole, transverse body, sagittal body, and osteochondral/chip fractures. The volar pole fracture is the most common. The mechanism of injury usually involves wrist hyperextension and ulnar deviation. Falls on an outstretched hand and direct blow injuries in line with the forearm have been described.[91] These fractures are most commonly seen in upper extremity weight-bearing sports such as gymnastics and weight-lifting.[2]

Physical Exam

Physical examination reveals tenderness over the dorsal lunate, and pain may worsen with wrist motion.

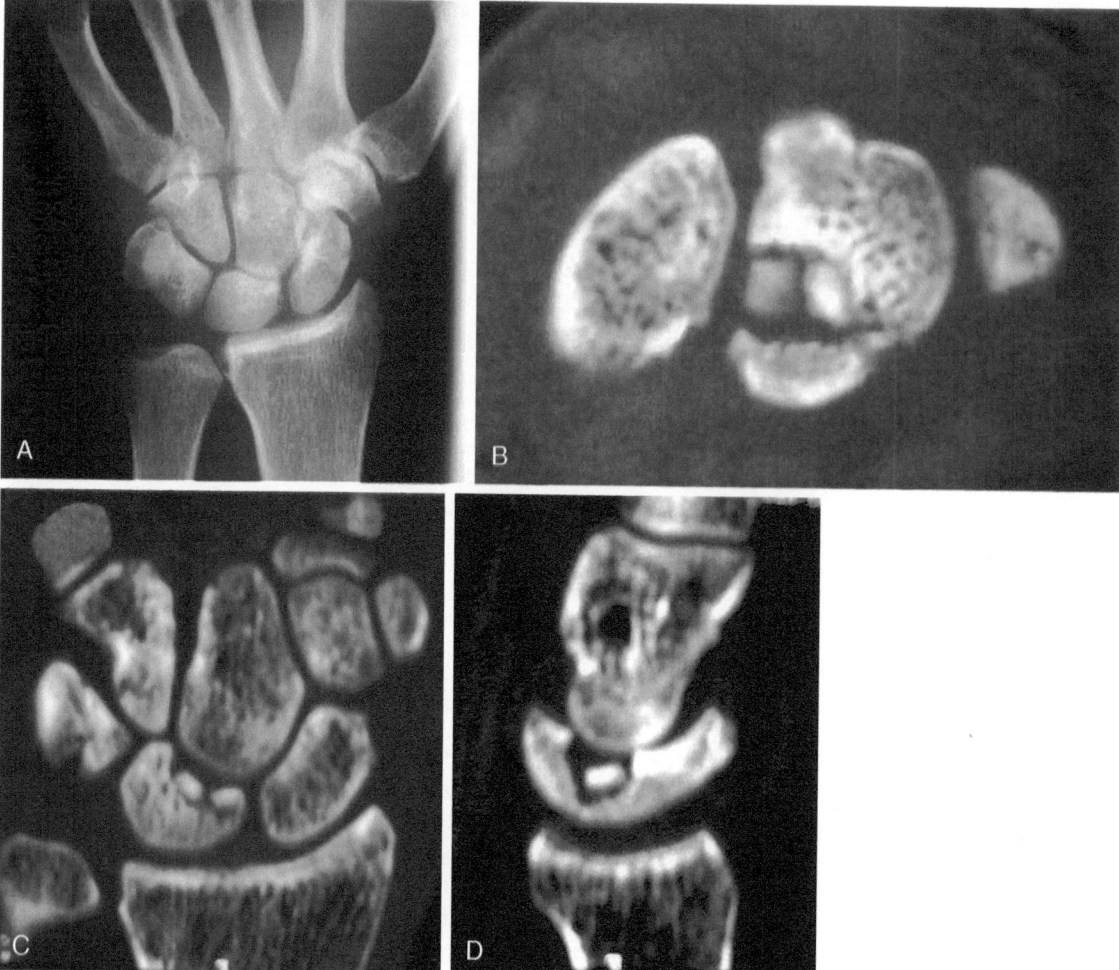

Fig. 70.16 The curvature of the lunate surfaces and position of the bone in the proximal row can obscure lunate body fractures on standard radiographs (A). Computed tomography clearly illustrates a lunate body fracture on axial (B), coronal (C), and sagittal (D) views.

Imaging

Radiographs—including PA, lateral, and oblique views—are typically sufficient for the diagnosis of a lunate fracture. A CT scan may be ordered to confirm or provide detail of the injury (Fig. 70.16). MRI may be helpful to distinguish old dorsal chip fractures from acute interosseous ligament avulsions and to identify preexisting avascular necrosis, as in Kienbock disease.

Decision-Making Principles

The lunate is devoid of soft tissue attachments and 20% of the population have only a single volar nutrient blood supply. It is therefore susceptible to avascular necrosis following volar pole fracture. Isolated nondisplaced dorsal chip fractures are amenable to nonoperative treatment. Imaging should be closely reviewed for evidence of ligamentous injury with associated volar or dorsal intercalated segmental instability (DISI). Volar chip fractures and displaced body fractures of the lunate should be treated surgically to minimize the risk of avascular necrosis and address associated ligamentous instability. Dorsal pole fractures with associated ligamentous injury also require surgical treatment.[37]

Treatment Options

Nonoperative treatment is carried out with a brace or a short arm cast for 4 to 6 weeks or longer depending on any associated ligamentous injuries. Surgical treatment utilizes a volar or dorsal approach depending on the pattern of injury, and fixation is achieved with K-wires or compression screws. Chronic injuries that have progressed to posttraumatic arthritis or severely comminuted fractures can be treated with salvage procedures such as limited arthrodesis or proximal row carpectomy.[44]

Postoperative Management

Postoperatively, lunate injuries should be immobilized and any K-wires should be left in place for a minimum of 6 weeks.

Results

Early diagnosis and treatment give the best chance of a good clinical outcome. The causal relationship between lunate fractures and development of Kienbock disease is not well understood. Some long-term data have failed to show development of avascular necrosis following acute fracture of the lunate.[91] Nonetheless,

Authors' Preferred Technique

For nondisplaced dorsal chip fractures, a cast or splint is applied for 1 week and weekly reexaminations are performed to avoid missed concomitant injury and to monitor steady improvement. For volar fractures requiring surgical fixation, we favor an extended carpal tunnel approach through a zigzag incision with a headless compression screw for fixation. In the case of a small bony avulsion with ligamentous injury, a suture anchor may be used instead. K-wire stabilization of the scapholunate and lunotriquetral ligaments may be needed. A K-wire stabilizing the capitate to the scaphoid avoids proximal migration of the capitate and compression on the lunate. Dorsal fractures and fractures that propagate into the body of the lunate with intra-articular extension are exposed through a dorsal approach between the third and fourth extensor compartments. Modular hand screws or cancellous bone graft may be used for fractures with comminution.[92]

athletes should understand that complications associated with lunate fracture can be career-ending.

Complications

Complications include avascular necrosis, nonunion, chronic instability, and posttraumatic arthritis.

Pisiform

History

Pisiform fractures account for 1% to 2% of carpal fractures.[60] The pisiform articulates with the trapezium on its dorsal surface and serves as an attachment site for the flexor carpi ulnaris, pisohamate, and pisotriquetral ligaments, the abductor digiti minimi, and the transverse carpal ligament. It forms the ulnar border of Guyon canal, placing the ulnar artery and nerve at risk at the time of fracture. Types of pisiform fractures include transverse, parasagittal, comminuted, and impaction varieties.[93] Fifty percent of pisiform fractures occur with other carpal injuries.[44]

The mechanism of injury commonly involves a direct blow, as from a fall, a racquet sport,[94] or the firing of a handgun.[46] Forceful contraction of the flexor carpi ulnaris tendon during resisted hyperextension can result in transverse bony avulsion. When there is a displaced fracture of the pisiform, a concomitant flexor carpi ulnaris tendon rupture may be present.[95] Dislocations also can occur with direct blows or falls on an outstretched hand.[96,97]

Physical Exam

Patients with pisiform fractures report palmar and ulnar-sided wrist pain. The apex of the pisiform is tender, and pain can be elicited with resisted wrist flexion due to the pull of the flexor carpi ulnaris.[50] Ulnar nerve function should be assessed and documented.

Imaging

Radiographs, including PA and lateral views, may be insufficient for the diagnosis of a pisiform fracture. Reverse oblique views, performed with the wrist in 45 degrees of supination and extension, show the pisiform in profile and should be obtained (Fig. 70.17). A pisotriquetral joint injury should be considered if bone surfaces are more than 20 degrees from parallel or if the distance between bones is greater than 3 mm.[98] Joint space widening greater than 4 mm should raise suspicion for dislocation.[95] A CT scan can be useful in confirming the diagnosis.

Decision-Making Principles

Nondisplaced pisiform fractures are amenable to nonoperative treatment and commonly result in asymptomatic fibrous nonunion. Displaced fractures or those associated with flexor carpi ulnaris dysfunction, severe comminution, or persistent ulnar nerve palsy require surgical treatment. Given the setbacks associated with immobilization, clinicians should have a low threshold to consider surgical treatment of pisiform fractures, with speedy RTP in mind.

Treatment Options

Nonoperative treatment is undertaken with short arm cast immobilization for 4 to 6 weeks. Operative intervention for displaced fractures or symptomatic nonunion is pisiform excision carried out through a volar or a lateral approach.[1,37]

Postoperative Management

RTP after pisiform excision is nearly identical to that following hamate hook excision. We splint the wrist for 3 to 5 days. The

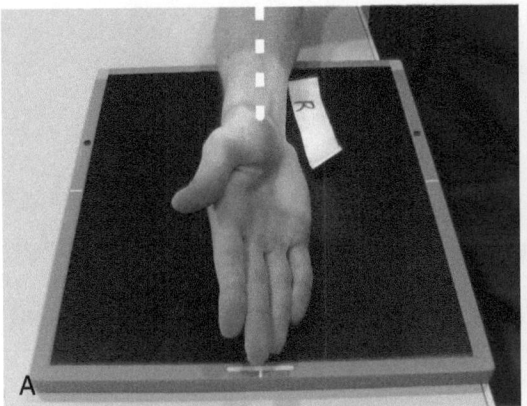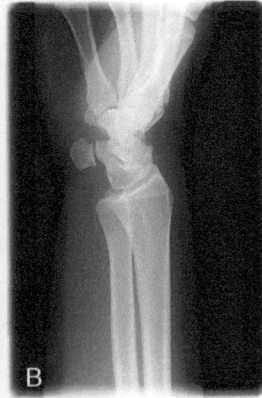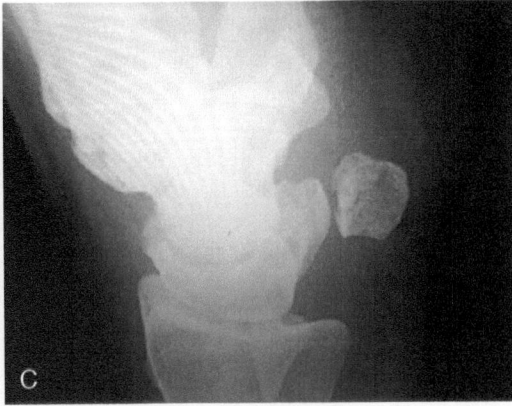

Fig. 70.17 The reverse oblique carpal view with the hand in a semisupinated position (A), with 30-degree supination on the cassette is useful to demonstrate the pisotriquetral joint (B) and evaluate pisiform fractures (C).

> ### Authors' Preferred Technique
>
> We prefer early pisiform excision via a volar approach. This approach avoids blind release of the radial attachments of the pisiform, which lie in close proximity to the ulnar nerve. During the volar approach, the ulnar nerve is identified proximally and retracted radially. A penetrating towel clip is a useful instrument to provide traction on the pisiform during excision. The pisiform resembles the shape of a top hat, and dissection should proceed from the top of the hat, the apex, and move around the brim while protecting the ulnar nerve.

wound is checked, and if it has sealed, a soft dressing is applied and the athlete is allowed to perform wrist motion and aerobic workouts. Return to competition is sport-specific. At 2 to 3 weeks, athletes begin light contact with a padded glove and progress to normal play at 4 to 6 weeks.

Results

Numerous studies have reported resolution of pain and complete return of wrist function following pisiform excision.[99–101]

Complications

A common complication after a pisiform injury is ulnar neurapraxia.[102] Most neurapraxias resolve with simple observation. If ulnar nerve dysfunction continues past 12 weeks, nerve exploration is performed in combination with pisiform excision. The ulnar nerve may be stretched during the surgical dissection as well. In this scenario, if the nerve was well visualized during the procedure, the deficit can be observed and most will resolve. If the nerve was not well visualized at the time of surgery and either 2-point discrimination is greater than 15 mm or obvious intrinsic weakness is present, it is appropriate to perform further nerve exploration and treatment as indicated.

CARPAL LIGAMENT INJURY AND INSTABILITY

History

The most commonly injured carpal ligaments are the scapholunate interosseous ligament (SLIL) and the lunotriquetral interosseous ligament (LTIL). SLIL injury is about six times more common than LTIL injury.[2] The thickest region of the SLIL is dorsal, whereas the LTIL is strongest volarly. Injury to these structures and adjacent extrinsic ligaments leads to altered carpal mechanics, called *carpal instability dissociative*, whereas disruption that alters motion between the proximal and distal carpal rows or between the distal radius and proximal carpal row has been termed *carpal instability nondissociative*. A multiligamentous disruption occurring both within a row and between rows has been designated *carpal instability complex*.[103]

Carpal ligament injuries are most often associated with a fall into forced hyperextension of the wrist.[104] These patients often present with dorsal wrist pain and swelling along with reduced wrist motion and grip strength.

Physical Exam

Examination may reveal tenderness over the carpus, a prominent proximal pole of the scaphoid, boggy synovitis over the radioscaphoid joint, and tenderness over the scapholunate ligament, which lies just distal to Lister tubercle with the wrist in a degree of flexion. Scapholunate instability can be evaluated with the Watson test, whereby the examiner's thumb is placed over the scaphoid tubercle while the wrist is ranged from ulnar to radial deviation. The test is positive when a palpable clunk is felt as the scaphoid subluxates dorsally with radial deviation and then reduces into its fossa with ulnar deviation.[105] Lunotriquetral instability can be tested using either Reagan ballottement test or Kleinman shear test, whereby the triquetrum is translated dorsal and palmarly while the lunate is stabilized. Pain, crepitus, or an appreciable clunk indicate a lunotriquetral injury.[106,107]

Imaging

Standard radiographs—including PA, lateral, and oblique views—should be obtained with contralateral views if there is concern for subtle changes. Radiographs should be scrutinized for congruity of Gilula lines (Fig. 70.18), intercarpal distance, and angular associations between carpal bones. Normal balance is assessed by the collinear alignment of the radius, lunate, capitate, and third metacarpal (Fig. 70.19). Deviated values for the scapholunate angle (30 to 60 degrees), radiolunate angle (<15 degrees), and carpal height ratio (>0.5) provide objective evidence of injury. Standard PA and lateral views can demonstrate static instability patterns. Static instability is defined as carpal instability that can be detected with standard radiographs. The appearance of a cortical ring sign on PA view is consistent with a palmar flexed scaphoid in which the distal pole cortex is seen on end. This finding should direct the clinician to consider a SLIL injury. Scapholunate dissociation will demonstrate scapholunate widening of greater than 3 mm on the PA film and may lead to instability of the dorsal intercalated segment with a scapholunate angle of greater than 70 degrees on the lateral view. Lunotriquetral ligament injury may be seen on radiographs as a decreased scapholunate angle (<30 degrees), increased capitolunate angle (>15 degrees), or proximal migration of the triquetrum. Sometimes there may be a subtle break of Gilula lines. Once the

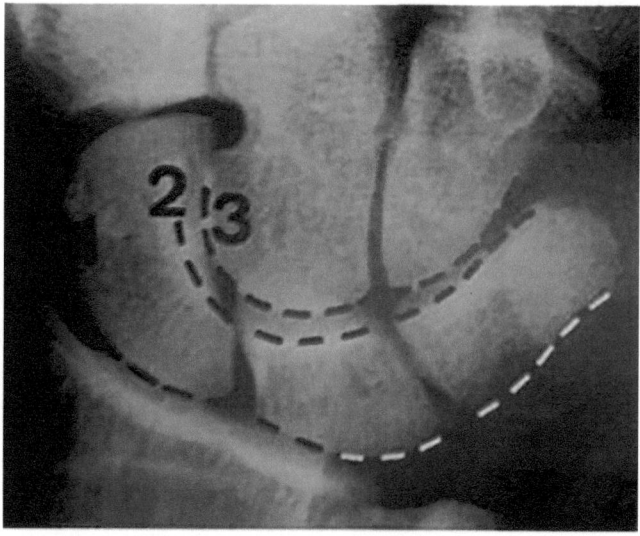

Fig. 70.18 Posteroanterior plain radiograph of intact Gilula lines.

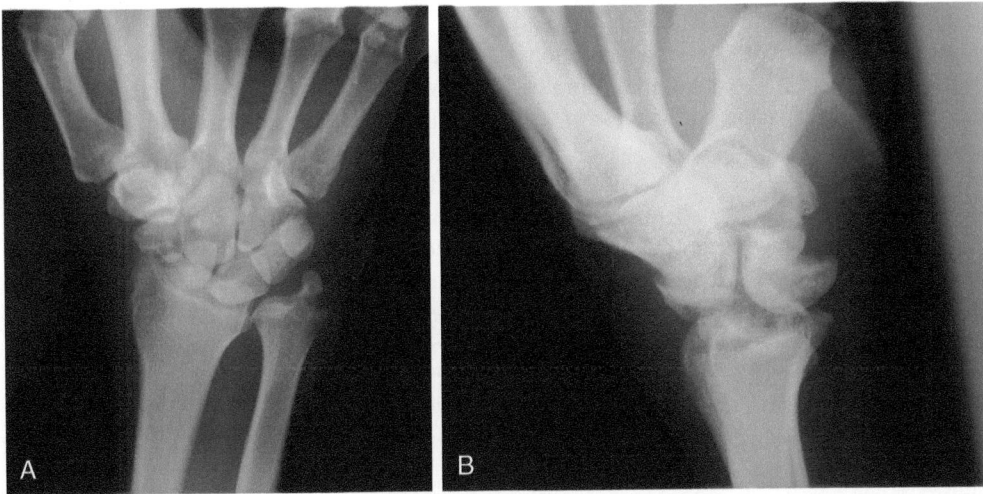

Fig. 70.19 Posteroanterior (PA) and lateral plain radiographs of a transscaphoid perilunate dislocation. (A) The PA view demonstrates a loss of carpal arcs, and the lunate appears triangular. (B) The lateral image demonstrates alteration of the collinear alignment of the radius, lunate, and capitate.

secondary extrinsic ligament stabilizers (dorsal radiocarpal, dorsal intercarpal, and palmar ulnocarpal ligaments) are injured, the lunate may become palmar flexed and appear triangular on the PA image. Instability of the volar intercalated segment may appear as a scapholunate angle less than 30 degrees on the lateral view.

Dynamic instability patterns require special views (i.e., axial loading view, ulnar deviation view, clenched fist view, and distraction view) to illuminate carpal malalignment. Radiographs should also be examined to decipher the chronicity of injury. Arthritis of the radial styloid, radioscaphoid, and midcarpal joints or carpal collapse indicate that the injury did not occur in the acute or subacute time frame. Fluoroscopy, CT scan, and MRI may all be useful adjuncts to plain images.

Decision-Making Principles

SLIL tears primarily affect proximal row mechanics. An associated injury to a secondary soft tissue restraint, such as the radiocarpal extrinsic ligaments, will allow the scaphoid to flex independently, while the lunate follows the triquetrum in relative extension. This pattern is aptly termed *scapholunate dissociation*.[108,109] Depending on the severity of energy, the spectrum of SLIL injuries can vary from dynamic instability to static dissociation with DISI. Observational studies have shown that when these injuries are left untreated, a predictable pattern of carpal deterioration occurs, starting at the radioscaphoid joint and proceeding to the capitolunate joint, which is known as the arthritic progression of scapholunate advance collapse (SLAC).[110,111] LTIL tears usually have an associated dorsal radiocarpal ligament tear[112] as well as an ulnocapitate ligament injury.[113] LTIL injuries also disrupt the synchrony of the proximal row, allowing the lunate to follow the scaphoid into flexion while the triquetrum remains in extension. This pattern is also known as volar intercalated segmental instability (VISI).

Treatment of partial tears of the SLIL or LTIL typically begins with nonoperative measures such as splinting and dedicated therapy (for SLIL injuries, strengthening of the FCR and extensor carpi radialis brevis [ECRB] and for the LTIL would be ECU-strengthening). Acute (<3 weeks from injury) and chronic complete tears may be treated surgically. Various surgical procedures have been developed to address complete injuries to improve pain and function while preventing the potential for delayed carpal arthritis. The existing literature suggests that operative treatment may help but the outcomes can be unpredictable.[114,115] This type of injury places the elite athlete in a difficult situation. Treatment means loss of the season, and full recovery of strength and motion is rare. Athletes often present weeks to months after sustaining what was thought to be a "sprained" wrist. Delayed treatment results in a worse ultimate outcome, and even with treatment, it cannot be guaranteed that posttraumatic arthritis will be avoided.

The scenario that leads to the most difficulty in making a treatment decision is when an athlete presents 3 months after injury with nearly full motion and minimal discomfort. A frank discussion should include the option of providing no treatment with the possibility of performing reconstructive surgery in the future. Ultimately the treatment plan for any carpal ligament injury in the athlete will be personal, involving a discussion between the athlete, training staff, and agent with consideration of their sport-specific demands, timing in the season, and career goals.

Treatment Options

Nonoperative treatment of carpal ligament injury consists of short arm cast immobilization for 4 weeks, after which time a gradual return to full play is allowed if symptoms have resolved. Arthroscopic débridement, with or without thermal ligament shrinkage, has been shown to be a satisfactory option for partial injuries that do not respond to a trial of immobilization.[116–118]

For acute injuries, a combination of primary ligament repair and K-wire fixation has been used with or without capsulodesis to maintain carpal alignment.[119–121] K-wires are inserted into the carpal bones as joysticks to assist in reduction of the scapholunate or lunotriquetral articulations. Once reduction has been achieved, the SLIL is repaired with suture anchors. The carpus is then stabilized with 0.045-inch K-wires. A biomechanical study evaluating the loads to failure after five different K-wire configurations for scapholunate dissociation found that scapholunate pinning coupled with scaphocapitate fixation achieved the greatest stabilization of both carpal rows.[122]

An alternative technique was recently described using a scapholunate intercarpal screw in conjunction with primary SLIL repair. The screw allows free rotation and toggle at its midsection to simulate anatomic motion across the scapholunate interval. The authors allow their patients to RTP at 1 to 2 weeks postoperatively with a removable wrist splint. Outcomes have not yet been reported for this technique.[104]

Dorsal capsulodesis can be used to augment the primary ligament repair. For SLIL injury, this can be performed using a Blatt, modified Berger, or Szabo technique, which involve radially based or triquetral-based dorsal capsular flaps fixed to the scaphoid or lunate.[123–125] For LTIL injury, a dorsal radiocarpal ligament flap is anchored to the lunate.[126]

In the setting of chronic (more than 6 months from injury) complete carpal ligament injury with reducible proximal row subluxation and absence of arthritis, options shift to a number of ligament reconstruction techniques. A bone-retinaculum-bone graft taken from the third dorsal compartment and inserted into the scaphoid and lunate was one of the first techniques described for ligament reconstruction.[127] The modified Brunelli reconstruction, or three-ligament tenodesis, uses the FCR tendon, with its insertion on the second metacarpal intact, tunneled through the scaphoid and attached to the dorsal lunate to reconstruct the SLIL.[128,129] The reduction and association of the scaphoid and lunate (RASL) procedure, utilizing screw fixation across the scapholunate joint, has been described as an open[130] or arthroscopic technique.[131] Reconstruction of the LTIL is performed by tunneling

the ECU tendon through the triquetrum and lunate and then securing it onto itself.[132]

When the scapholunate joint or lunotriquetral joint is not reducible or when posttraumatic arthritis is present, options are limited to salvage procedures. These include proximal row carpectomy or scaphoid excision with capitolunate fusion with or without incorporation of the hamate and triquetrum in the fusion mass as in a four-corner arthrodesis.

Authors' Preferred Technique

For nonskill athletes, we recommend a trial of nonoperative treatment for partial ligament injuries in a padded short-arm cast for 4 weeks. If this fails or the athlete is unable to tolerate casting and for all athletes who require wrist motion to perform, we favor early surgical treatment with arthroscopy, débridement, and possible thermal shrinkage or pinning for instability.

For ligament reconstruction of the SLIL, we prefer the scapholunate axis method (SLAM). (Fig. 70.20) In this technique, a tunnel is made through an incision over the anatomic snuffbox and across the central axis of the scaphoid and lunate for a tendon graft (palmaris or FCR) to be passed. This graft is anchored to the proximal-ulnar corner of the lunate and tensioned with an interference screw into the scaphoid.[133] The multiplanar tether of the tendon graft allows for restoration of scaphoid extension, scaphoid pronation, and the scapholunate interval. More importantly, the central axis reconstruction stabilizes the scapholunate interval uniformly rather than preferentially reconstructing the dorsal ligament alone as described by earlier techniques. A similar technique of central axis reconstruction has been described in a small series incorporating the scaphoid, lunate, and triquetrum for LTIL reconstruction.[134]

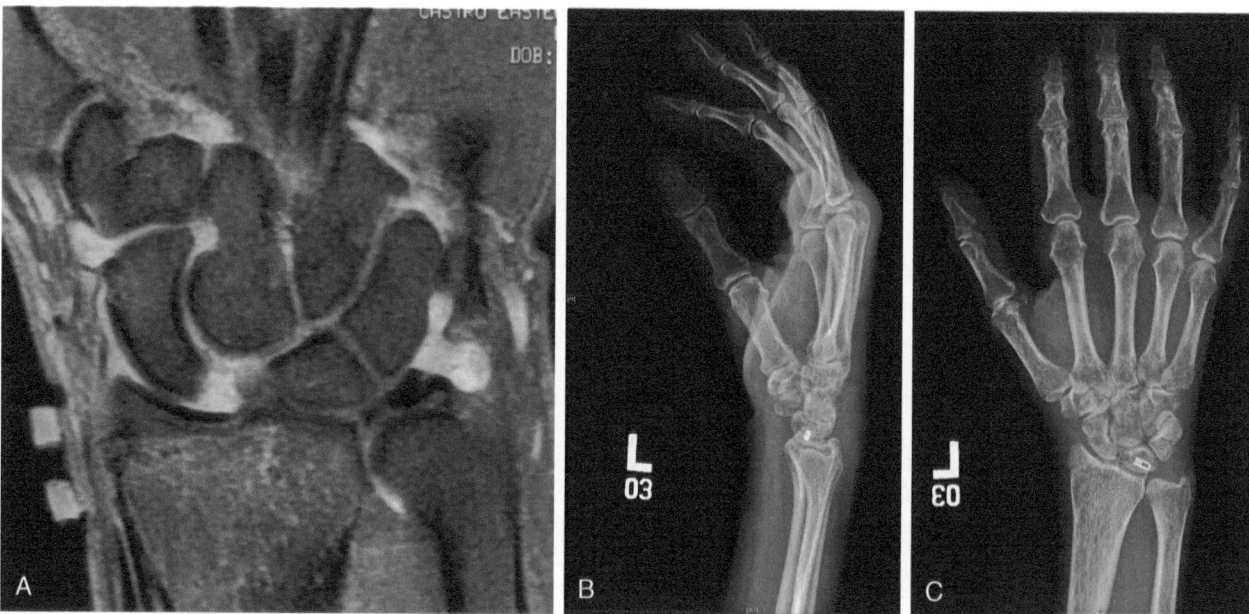

Fig. 70.20 (A) Magnetic resonance imaging demonstrating scapholunate ligament injury. Posteroanterior (B) and lateral (C) plain radiographs at 4-year postoperative follow-up after treatment with the scapholunate axis method technique.

Finally, in athletes with disabling arthritic pain who place a high demand on their wrists, we would offer a scaphoid excision and capito-lunate-triquetrum-hamate fusion. This may be done between seasons or at the end of the athlete's career.

Postoperative Management

Following primary ligament repair or reconstruction, patients are placed in a short arm cast for 6 to 8 weeks. At this time the cast and K-wires are removed. Transition is made to a removable splint for an additional 4 weeks while gentle ROM exercises are begun. RTP is at 4 to 6 months postoperatively.

Results

In one recent study, injuries treated with primary repair more than 6 weeks after carpal ligament injury had an increased failure rate and worse radiographic outcomes, emphasizing the importance of timing in patient selection.[135] Although short-term results in professional basketball players have been promising following primary ligament repair with capsulodesis for acute SLIL injury, some have suggested that outcomes may deteriorate over time in high-demand patients.[136,137] Ligament reconstruction techniques have demonstrated variable short-term outcomes with most achieving some pain relief, but at the expense of ROM.[136,138] A recent study of professional athletes reported 79% RTP 4 months after modified Brunelli SLIL reconstruction, but only 64% were able to return to their preinjury level of competition.[139]

Complications

Complications include pin-site infections, injury to superficial radial sensory nerve branches, persistent instability, and development of posttraumatic arthritis.

PERILUNATE INSTABILITY

History

Perilunate instability describes a predictable disruption of the carpal anatomy and comprises 7% of all injuries involving the carpus. The defining feature of perilunate injury is dissociation of the capitate from the lunate. The vast majority (~97%) are dorsal perilunate dislocations (i.e., dorsal displacement of the capitate with respect to the longitudinal axis).

Mayfield and colleagues described the characteristic sequence of carpal disruption around the lunate that occurs under axial loading in wrist extension, ulnar deviation, and supination.[140] This sequential disruption occurs in four stages. In stage I, the scapholunate ligament is disrupted and the radioscapholunate ligament is torn. The force is then transmitted to the lunocapitate articulation, resulting in stage II. This results in capitate dislocation and is accompanied by injury to the radioscaphocapitate ligament, dorsal intercarpal ligament, and radial collateral ligament. In stage III, energy propagates into the lunotriquetral joint, tearing the lunotriquetral ligament. A triquetral dissociation results, but the lunate remains aligned with the radius. Finally, in stage IV, the lunate dislocates as a result of ulnotriquetral and dorsal radiocarpal tears. The lunate no longer remains within the lunate fossa of the radius and displaces volarly. The volar

extrinsic ligaments, which usually remain intact, cause the lunate to rotate into the carpal tunnel.

Perilunate instability can occur via ligament injury alone or in combination with fracture. Johnson[141] described the isolated perilunate dislocations as lesser arc injuries, while the perilunate fracture dislocations are referred to as greater arc injuries. Bain and colleagues[142] modified Johnson's classification to describe a third pattern of injury termed *translunate arc,* which occurs through the lunate (Fig. 70.21). Common perilunate injuries include transscaphoid or transstyloid patterns. Less common variants include transtriquetral and transcapitate injuries. The mechanism of injury is typically high-energy.

Physical Exam

Physical examination often reveals a prominent, palpable dorsal capitate. In acute injuries, soft tissue swelling may obscure bone landmarks. If the lunate is dislocated, it can encroach on the carpal tunnel and cause symptoms consistent with median nerve compression. The incidence of acute carpal tunnel syndrome with perilunate injuries ranges from 16% to 46%.[143]

Imaging

Standard radiographs—including PA, lateral, and oblique views—will reveal abnormalities on careful inspection. However, as many as 25% of perilunate injuries are missed at initial presentation, emphasizing the importance of a heightened awareness and high index of suspicion following high-energy mechanism.[144] The PA

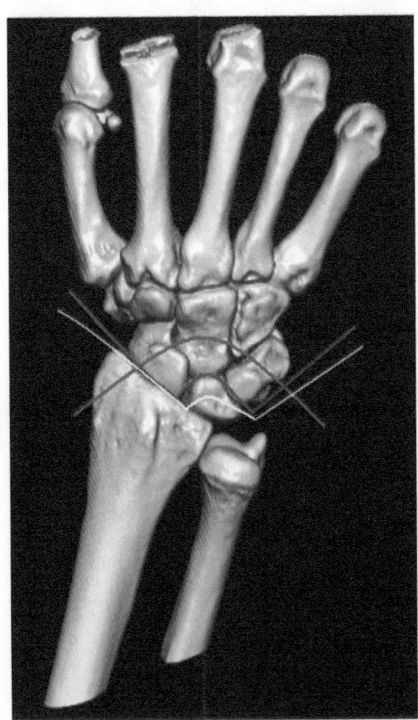

Fig. 70.21 A computed tomography image of the wrist demonstrating Bain's modification of Johnson's original classification of perilunate injury. The *red line* depicts a greater arc injury with fracture to the bones surrounding the lunate, which can include the radial styloid, scaphoid, capitate, hamate, and triquetrum. The *blue line* depicts a lesser arc injury, representing disruption to the ligaments around the lunate. The *yellow line* describes a third pattern of injury that occurs through the lunate.

view will demonstrate a loss of Gilula carpal arcs.[145] Radiographic findings may be similar to those seen with SLIL or LTIL injury. The lunate may appear triangular and will be displaced relative to the extent of energy imparted. (Fig. 70.22) Loss of articular alignment, overlap of carpal bones, and fractures may also be present. The lateral image will demonstrate alteration of the collinear alignment of the radius, lunate, and capitate. The capitate is commonly displaced in a dorsal direction while the lunate is displaced volarly. The lunate may be rotated 90 or 180 degrees,

resembling a spilled teacup.[146] A CT scan can delineate subtle fracture lines that may be present.

Decision-Making Principles

Initial closed reduction relieves pressure on the median nerve and should be performed promptly on presentation. Persistent and evolving carpal tunnel symptoms following closed reduction necessitates emergent surgical intervention to release the transverse carpal ligament. Open injury or the inability to achieve closed reduction are also indications for expedient open treatment. If reduction is acceptable and median nerve symptoms are mild or nonprogressive, surgical treatment can be performed on a nonurgent basis. Perilunate injuries as a whole are unstable patterns of injury, with significant osteochondral and ligamentous disruption, and have been shown to have better results with early surgical treatment.[147,148]

Treatment Options

Treatment for perilunate injury has evolved over the years. Although an early approach to treatment involved closed reduction and percutaneous fixation,[149,150] more anatomic surgical treatments have emerged and include external fixation with or without internal fixation,[151] open reduction and surgical fixation,[144,152–155] lunate excision,[156] proximal row carpectomy,[157] and four-corner fusion.[151] The technique for fixation varies but can include K-wires, headless compression screws, and lag screws (Fig. 70.23).

A dorsal midline,[155] volar,[153] or combined approach may be necessary and is often chosen on the basis of the surgeon's preference.[120] Arthroscopy may be used as an adjunct. The dorsal approach provides excellent visualization for carpal reduction, interosseous ligament repair, and fracture fixation. The volar approach allows decompression of the carpal tunnel and volar capsule repair. After open reduction and internal fixation of the scaphoid in transscaphoid perilunate dislocations, it is important

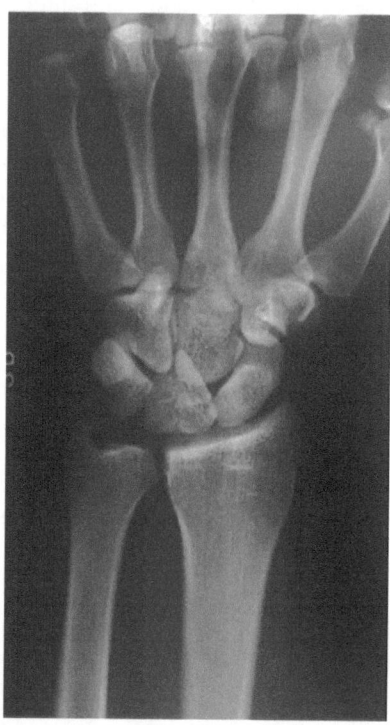

Fig. 70.22 Posteroanterior plain radiograph of perilunate injury demonstrating the triangular appearance of the lunate.

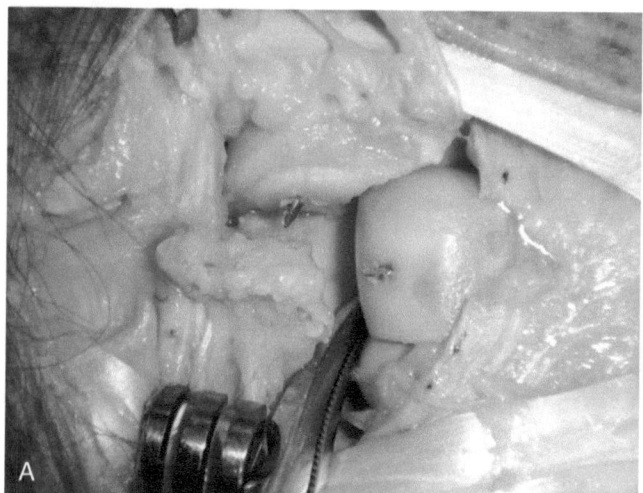
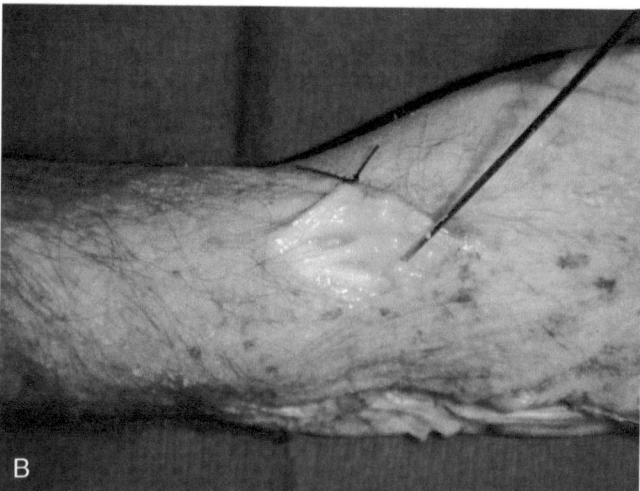

Fig. 70.23 Demonstration of the technique for fixation of perilunate injuries. K-wires are placed in a retrograde fashion through the scaphoid starting at its articulation with the lunate (A). Another wire is placed into the head of the capitate and advanced so it exits the zone between the radial wrist extensors and finger extensors. A counterincision is made over the radial aspect of the wrist to visualize and protect the radial sensory nerve (B).

to evaluate the integrity of the SLIL and LTIL. Garcia-Elias and colleagues[158] found that transscaphoid patterns have a 3.8% incidence of associated complete SLIL disruption. K-wires can be useful as joysticks to obtain adequate reduction of the scapholunate and lunotriquetral articulations. The SLIL often tears from the scaphoid and can be repaired with braided polyester suture or suture anchors (Fig. 70.24). Although the strongest fibers of the LTIL are located volarly, some have advocated pinning of the lunotriquetral joint through a dorsal approach without ligament repair.[159,160] Following ligament repair, intercarpal K-wires or screws should remain in place for stabilization of the reduction (Fig. 70.25).

The extent of chondral injury should be documented during the procedure. Transscaphoid patterns should undergo fixation of the scaphoid with a headless compression screw or K-wires and concomitant SLIL or LTIL injury should be repaired if present (Fig. 70.26). In the translunate arc injury, the lunate can be stabilized with screws or K-wires (Fig. 70.27).[92,142]

Postoperative Management

Neurovascular checks should be performed as part of the postoperative protocol. A cast is typically used for 6 to 8 weeks,

> ### 🗡 Authors' Preferred Technique
>
> Perilunate injuries are complex, and we prefer an individualized approach to treatment. The most important principle with regard to technique is to optimize the chances of obtaining an anatomic reduction and a stable carpus. We typically prefer the dorsal-only approach but have a low threshold to use a combined approach when it is needed to release the carpal tunnel, repair the volar capsule, provide adequate visualization, and ensure anatomic stabilization.

followed by a removable splint for an additional 4 weeks. If K-wires are used for fixation, they are typically removed at 12 weeks postoperatively.

Results

Results following perilunate injury depend on the severity of the initial injury, accurate and timely diagnosis, and the quality of the reduction. Patients should be counseled that loss of motion and diminished grip strength are common consequences even in the face of appropriate treatment. The development of posttraumatic arthritis may occur radiographically in as many as 70% of patients. Although these radiographic results have not

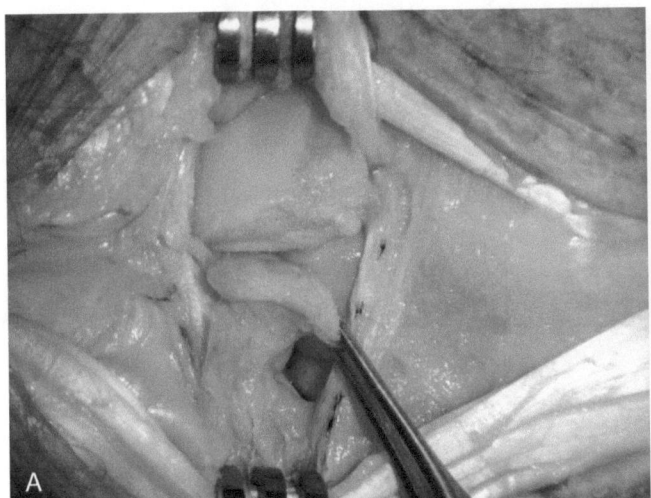
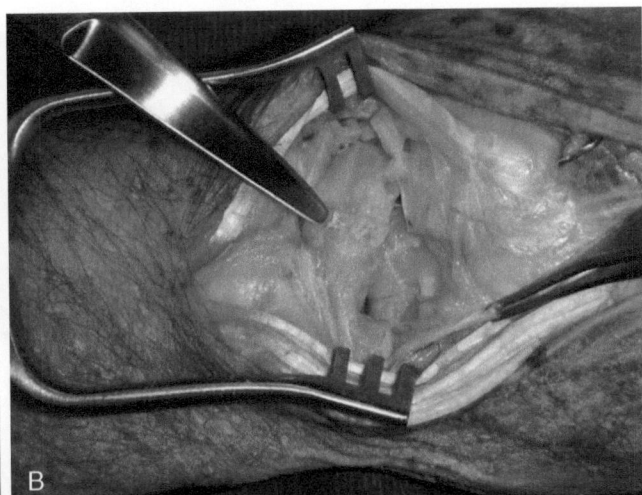

Fig. 70.24 (A and B) The dorsal fibers of the scapholunate interosseous ligament often tear off its scaphoid attachment. The repair can be made primarily to bone using braided polyester sutures or suture anchors.

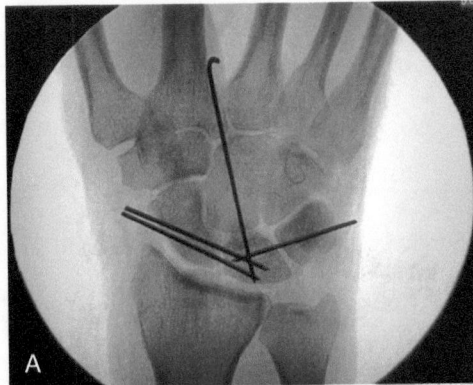
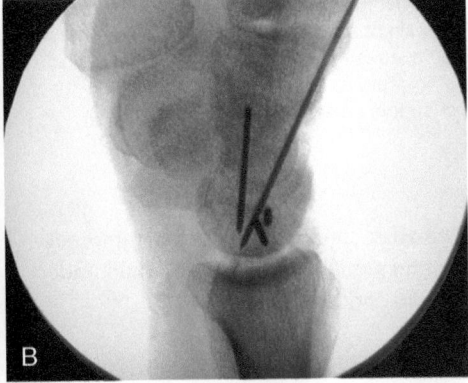

Fig. 70.25 (A and B) Posteroanterior and lateral plain radiographs demonstrating the appropriate position of intercarpal pins after reduction and ligamentous stabilization of a perilunate dislocation.

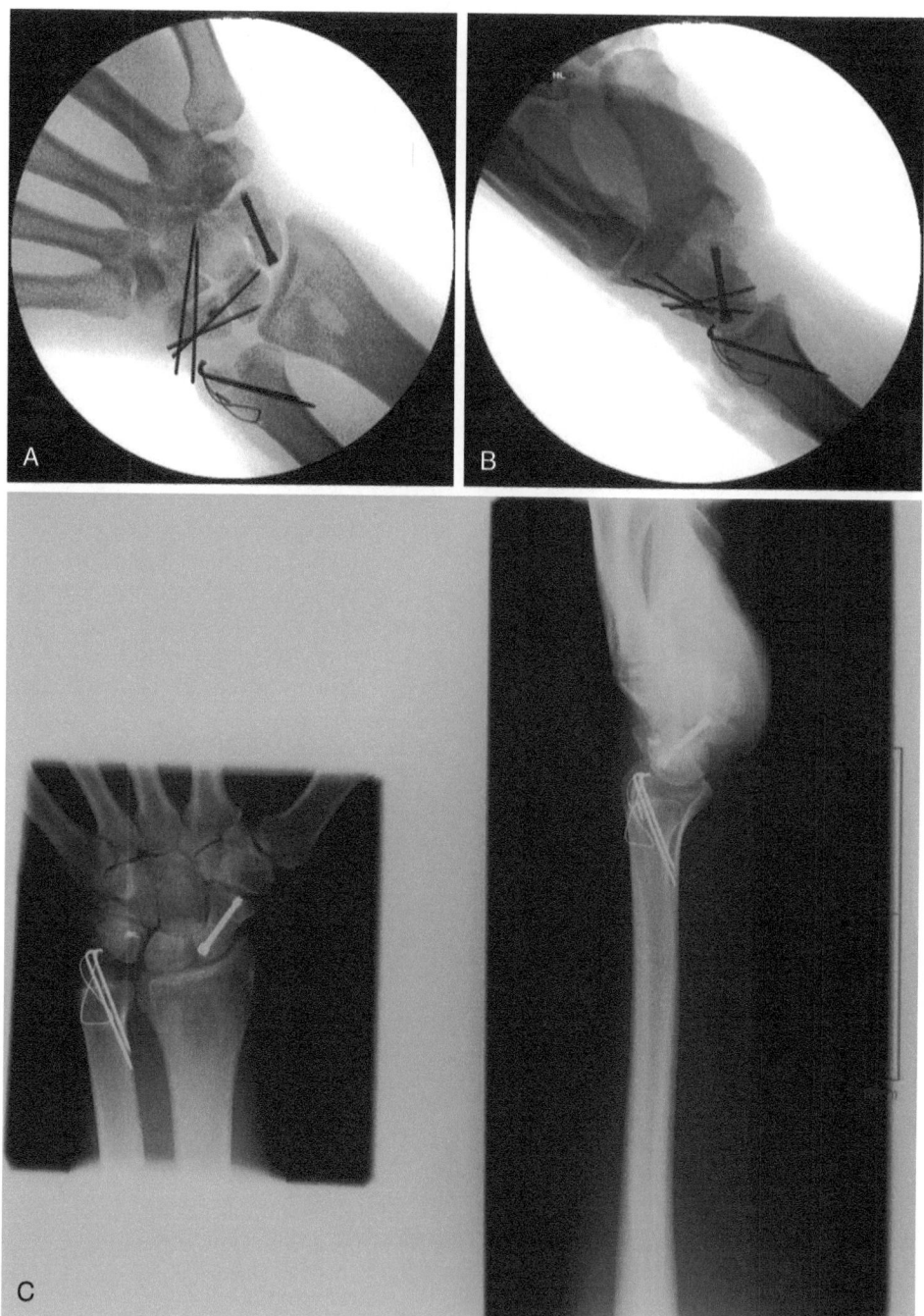

Fig. 70.26 (A and B) Posteroanterior and lateral plain radiographs of a perilunate dislocation after repair. The scaphoid fracture was treated with cannulated screw fixation, and the lunotriquetral ligament was repaired with the aid of a suture anchor. The lunotriquetrum and pisohamate were pinned with 0.045-inch K-wires to hold an adequate reduction, and the ulnar styloid was fixed using the tension band technique. Ten months after the repair was made, the patient had functional range of motion. Two-year radiographic follow-up demonstrates preserved carpal alignment (C).

been found to correlate with clinical outcomes, symptomatic arthritis remains a common sequela, and athletes should understand that this injury could end their career.[161]

Complications

Complications following perilunate injury include delayed diagnosis, stiffness, persistent instability, and posttraumatic arthritis.

Surgical complications can include acute carpal tunnel syndrome as well as pin-site infection.

FUTURE CONSIDERATIONS

Many options are available to treat carpal instability. The lack of consensus reveals that optimal management is unclear. Our

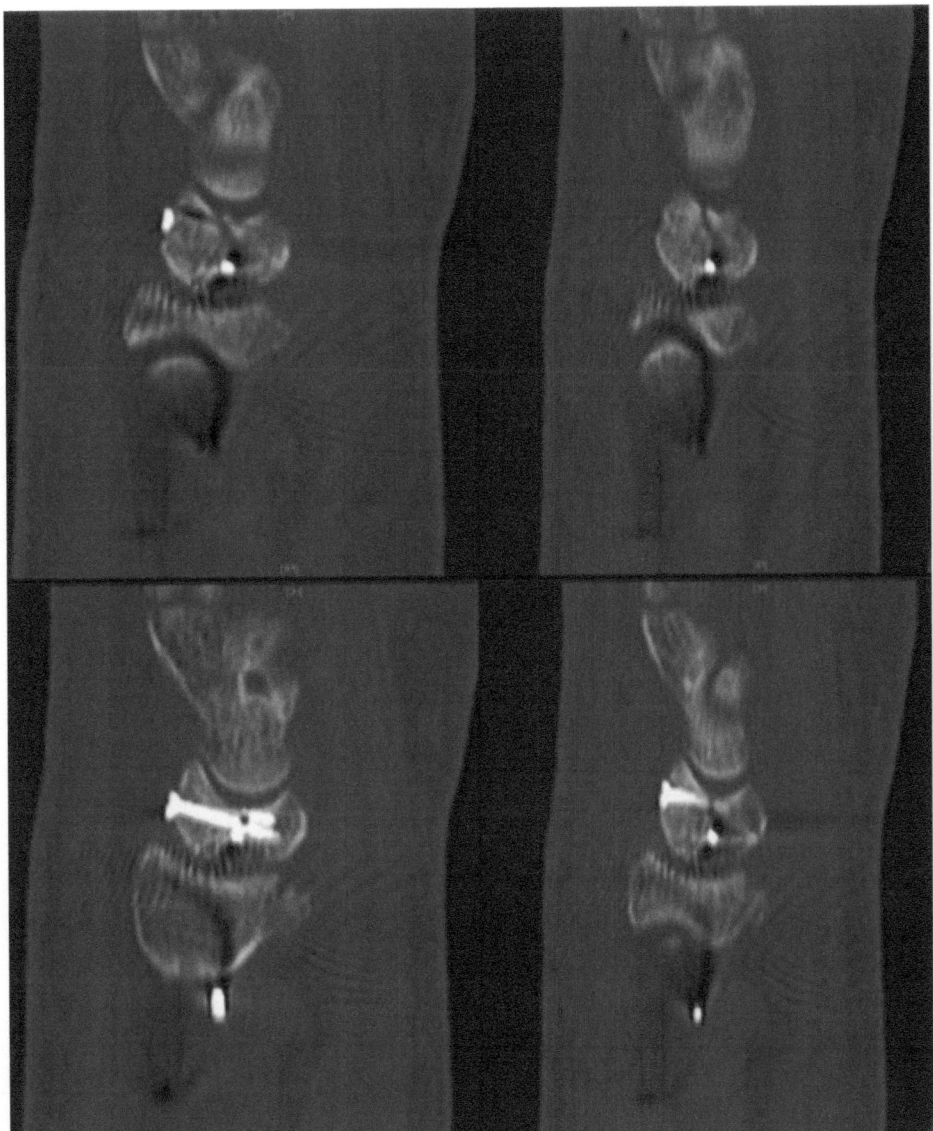

Fig. 70.27 A sagittal computed tomography image obtained postoperatively following open reduction and internal fixation of a coronal fracture through the lunate.

greatest challenge is to develop a reliable technique to manage scapholunate dissociation, particularly for patients who present in a delayed fashion following injury.

Posttraumatic arthritis is a major cause of morbidity after carpal fractures and perilunate injuries. At present the surgeon can do little to prevent it; future studies should attempt to provide a solution to this unavoidable issue. Long-term large-scale prospective studies may serve to identify predictors of posttraumatic arthritis. If a particular pattern of injury, whether involving bone or purely ligamentous, could be shown to predispose to degenerative disease, this information would provide assistance in making treatment decisions and developing new management protocols in elite athletes.

ACKNOWLEDGMENT

The authors would like to thank Prasad J. Sawardeker, MD, and Mark E. Baratz, MD, for their contribution to this chapter.

For a complete list of references, go to ExpertConsult.com.

SELECTED READINGS

Citation:

Kuo CE, Wolfe SW. Scapholunate instability: current concepts in diagnosis and management. *J Hand Surg Am.* 2008;33(6):998–1013.

Level of Evidence:

Review

Summary:

This review article discusses anatomy, kinematics, and biomechanical properties of the scapholunate articulation and proposes an algorithm for management based on the severity of the injury, ligamentous damage, and the presence of arthritic disease. The authors devise a classification scheme with treatment implications, dividing the disorder into stages: static versus dynamic instability, repairable versus irreparable ligament, reducible versus irreducible deformity, and combined coronal and sagittal plane pathology.

Citation:

Kremer T, Wendt M, Riedel K, et al. Open reduction for perilunate injuries—clinical outcome and patient satisfaction. *J Hand Surg Am*. 2010;35(10):1599–1606.

Level of Evidence:

IV

Summary:

This article provides a retrospective analysis of the postoperative radiographic results, range of motion, pain, sensitivity, grip strength, Mayo and Krimmer wrist scores, and patient disability scores in 39 patients with perilunate dislocations (Mayfield stage 3/4) who were followed up for an average of 65.5 months. The authors discovered that despite adequate treatment of perilunate injuries, common findings include loss of reduction, loss of grip strength, loss of motion, and posttraumatic arthrosis; radiographic results do not, however, correlate with functional outcomes.

Citation:

Herzberg G, Comtet JJ, Linscheid RL, et al. Perilunate dislocations and fracture-dislocations: a multicenter study. *J Hand Surg Am*. 1993;18:768–779.

Level of Evidence:

III

Summary:

The authors of this article provide a retrospective review of 166 perilunate dislocations from seven specialized institutions and evaluate patient demographics, mechanism, associated injuries, patterns, and treatment outcomes. The diagnosis was missed initially in 25% of injuries. Despite early treatment, a 56% incidence of posttraumatic arthritis was noted. Open injury and delay of treatment had an adverse effect on outcome.

Citation:

Geissler W, Slade JF. Fractures of the carpal bones. In: Wolfe SW, Hotchkiss RN, Pederson WC, et al, eds. *Green's Operative Hand Surgery*. 6th ed. Philadelphia: Churchill Livingstone; 2010:639–707.

Level of Evidence:

Review

Summary:

This chapter provides a well-written, comprehensive review of carpal fractures, functional anatomy, and related injuries.

Citation:

Garcia RM, Ruch DS. Management of scaphoid fractures in the athlete: open and percutaneous fixation. *Sports Med Arthrosc Rev*. 2014;22(1):22–28.

Level of Evidence:

Review

Summary:

This article reviews the diagnosis and treatment of scaphoid fractures. It includes a discussion of nonoperative and operative treatment strategies, including casting, percutaneous, open and arthroscopic-assisted options.

Citation:

Ibrahim T, Qureshi A, Sutton AJ, et al. Surgical versus nonsurgical treatment of acute minimally displaced and undisplaced scaphoid waist fractures: pairwise and network meta-analyses of randomized controlled trials. *J Hand Surg Am*. 2011;36(11):1759–1768.e1.

Level of Evidence:

I

Summary:

This article describes a pairwise meta-analysis of randomized controlled trials to evaluate the effectiveness of surgical intervention compared with nonsurgical intervention for minimally displaced scaphoid waist fractures. Six studies were eligible for inclusion, and outcomes for 363 patients with minimally displaced scaphoid waist fractures were compared. The authors found that although surgical treatment was favored in terms of fracture union, this did not reach statistical significance; rather, surgery was associated with an increased risk of complications.

Citation:

Walsh JJ, Bishop AT. Diagnosis and management of hamate hook fractures. *Hand Clin*. 2000;16(3):397–403.

Level of Evidence:

Review

Summary:

This article provides an excellent review of hook of hamate fractures. The authors describe how a careful understanding of the functional anatomy, presentation, and appropriate imaging can be used to help establish a diagnosis and guide treatment.

Citation:

Urch EY, Lee SK. Carpal fractures other than scaphoid. *Clin Sports Med*. 2015;34:51–67.

Level of Evidence:

Review

Summary:

This article reviews the diagnosis and treatment of carpal fractures excluding the scaphoid. It includes an up-to-date discussion of the pertinent anatomy, imaging, and treatment options following these injuries.

Citation:

Slade JF, Milewski MD. Management of carpal instability in athletes. *Hand Clin*. 2009;25:395–408.

Level of Evidence:

Review

Summary:

This article includes a succinct review of carpal fractures as well as ligamentous and perilunate injuries in the athlete. It poses guidelines for return to play, including a sport-specific chart outlining the timing of return to play following scaphoid fracture fixation.

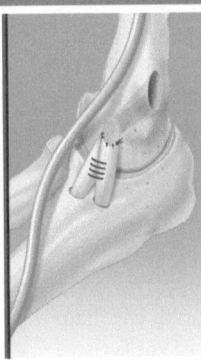

71

Wrist Tendinopathies

Raj M. Amin, John V. Ingari

Tendinopathies are extremely common in athletes. Any sport that requires a repetitive motion, such as a tennis serve or volley, a basketball free throw, or "turning the wrists over," as in the completion of a golf or baseball swing, puts an athlete at risk for tendon inflammation, instability, degeneration, or even rupture.[1,2] Even recreational rock climbing, which is well known for its association with flexor pulley rupture, has been implicated in tendinopathy of the wrist.[3,4] Swimming, bowling, gymnastics, weightlifting, cycling, and skiing are among the many other sports associated with repetitive use tendinopathy.[5]

Montalvan et al.[6] categorized extensor carpi ulnaris (ECU) tendinopathy in 28 elite tennis players. The authors divided ECU tendon injuries into three categories: tendinopathy, instability, or rupture. Allende and Le Viet[7] reported on 28 patients who underwent surgical treatment for ECU tendinopathy between 1990 and 2002. Seventeen of the 28 patients reported onset of symptoms after sports activity. Of the 28 patients, 15 had tenosynovitis or tendinosis, 5 had dislocation of the tendon, 4 had subluxation, and 4 had a tendon rupture.[7] Twenty-two of the 28 patients were able to return to their previous level of activity at a mean of 23 months after surgery.

The first dorsal compartment, which contains the abductor pollicis longus (APL) and extensor pollicis brevis (EPB) tendons, is also subject to wrist tendinopathy, specifically de Quervain tenosynovitis, especially in persons who participate in sports involving a racquet.[8]

Soejima et al.[9] reported a case of flexor carpi radialis (FCR) tendinopathy in a professional baseball player that was associated with a malunited trapezial ridge fracture.[9] The patient was successfully treated with excision of the trapezial ridge. Buterbaugh and colleagues,[10] in evaluating ulnar-sided wrist pain in seven hockey or baseball professional athletes, reported acute calcific flexor carpi ulnaris (FCU) tendinitis as one of the contributing sources. Some sports that require repetitive wrist extension and radial deviation, such as rowing and powder skiing, have been found to be associated with intersection syndrome.[5,8,11]

Even the extensor retinaculum, the soft tissue layer that provides a sheath-like investing roof for the extensor tendons over the dorsal aspect of the distal radius and carpus, has been implicated in athletes as a source of pain. Thickening and diffuse proliferation of this tissue may result from hyperextension activities required in certain athletic pursuits. This particular scenario has been termed *extensor retinaculum impingement*.[12]

For all of the tendinopathies described in sports, early diagnosis and nonoperative treatment with activity modification, use of a splint or brace, and use of nonsteroidal antiinflammatory drugs (NSAIDs) has been the cornerstone of management. This chapter presents a discussion of the history and physical examination and the common tendinopathies associated with sports, as well as treatment options, with return to sports as the ultimate goal.

HISTORY

The history is a critical component in making a correct diagnosis. Tendons are the structures that connect muscle bellies to bones and allow for confluent joint and extremity motion. Therefore any repetitive wrist or hand motions that elicit pain are an important focus in a person with a suspected tendinopathy. If active wrist flexion causes pain, then the flexor tendons may be inflamed. Similarly, if active extension is painful, then extensor tendons may be implicated in the pathology. Conversely, passive stretching of an irritated tendon also causes pain and can be a clue as to which tendon, or tendons, are involved.

The location of the pain is very important. Often when tendinopathy is present, an athlete runs his or her hand longitudinally along the tendon(s) involved, offering a key diagnostic clue. A fracture is often painful at a specific place, whereas tendons tend to "hurt" along the longitudinal course of the tendon. At this point, it is important to note that "pain" is a historic, or subjective, complaint, whereas "tenderness" is a component of the physical examination in which the examiner elicits pain through palpation or pressure.

Next, the timing of the injury is important. Is the pathology the result of repetitive activity, or did it occur after one specific incident? For example, a tendon rupture typically occurs suddenly, after a single event, whereas tendinosis tends to be the result of repetitive movements of the hand or wrist, such as is seen in ping pong, tennis, or sports that involve throwing. Often with tendinosis, the pain recurs with the specific exacerbating motion, such as flexion, extension, radial or ulnar deviation, and, in some cases, pronation and supination of the wrist. All of these questions should be included in the history to help elucidate the correct diagnosis. Any exacerbating or alleviating events should also be ascertained. It is important to know if placing the wrist in a certain position or if performing certain motions or maneuvers worsen (or lessen) the pain; these facts also may provide a clue to the diagnosis. Any prior treatments, no matter how menial, are important historic data. If therapy has been initiated, which is often the case in high-level athletics, it is important to distinguish between exercises or modalities that have proven beneficial or detrimental to recovery. For example, stretching programs may exacerbate the symptoms of tendinopathy when they are implemented before tendon healing, which helps lead the interviewer to the correct diagnosis.

PHYSICAL EXAMINATION

Direct evaluation of the wrist should always begin with inspection. Any visible swelling or asymmetry when compared with the other wrist is a very important clue in diagnosing wrist tendon pathology. In the case of de Quervain tenosynovitis, which involves the tendons of the first dorsal compartment, it is quite common for swelling to occur over the radial aspect of the wrist at the level of the radial styloid. When the wrists are placed side by side, the asymmetric swelling often becomes evident.

The hallmark of physical examination in persons with acute calcific tendinitis is severe tenderness to palpation along the course of the tendon. Whereas tenderness in a fracture occurs at the point of fracture, tenderness associated with tendinosis is often more diffusely felt along the course of the involved tendon. The exception may be insertional tendinopathy, in which case the maximal tenderness is elicited at the insertion point of the involved tendon onto bone. The pain is exacerbated by passive stretch of the involved tendon, further aiding diagnosis. Arthritis pain, conversely, tends to increase with compression across a joint, whereas passive stretching may actually alleviate the pain associated with arthritis or joint pathology.

Certain tests have been determined to be associated with specific tendon pathology. The Finkelstein test, in which the examiner grasps the patient's thumb and ulnarly deviates the wrist to passively stretch the APL and EPB tendons—that is, the tendons of the first dorsal compartment—aids in diagnosing de Quervain tenosynovitis. This maneuver will reproduce pain in most patients with this condition.

Other palpation techniques include the detection of tendon snapping or popping during wrist motion. For example, the ECU tendon may snap over the ulnar styloid when the extended wrist is brought actively from a pronated to a fully supinated position. The patient often feels the tendon snap with the supination maneuver, and the examiner's index finger, when lightly placed over the ulnar styloid, may confirm the abnormal tendon subluxation or frank dislocation.

Range of motion (ROM) may be diminished in tendinopathies such as wrist extension in the case of flexor tendon irritation. To comprehensively assess motion, the patient should be asked to flex and extend, radially and ulnarly deviate, and pronate and supinate the wrist in sequence. Repeating these motions against resistance may reveal subtle tendon pathology. Because variations of normal exist, comparing the ROM with the contralateral wrist is necessary to detect loss of motion in any direction.

In addition to the tendinitis, deciding whether bone, joint, ligament, nerve, or even a vascular structure is concurrently injured depends on the examiner's ability to synthesize appropriate history

clues with key physical examination findings. This approach will help the practitioner avoid compartmentalizing every athletic wrist complaint as a tendon-related pathology and steer him or her toward appropriate adjunctive imaging studies.

IMAGING

Tendinopathy of the wrist is not a bony pathology, but plain radiographs and advanced imaging, when indicated, can help determine and finely hone diagnostic evaluations of the wrist.[13] Imaging can either eliminate or support the diagnosis of fracture, carpal instability, and Kienböck disease, for example, which are in the differential diagnosis of the athlete with wrist pain (Fig. 71.1).

At the minimum, imaging should include two orthogonal views; a posteroanterior (PA) view and a lateral view of the wrist should be obtained. A 45-degree semipronated oblique view and a PA view in ulnar deviation to maximally delineate the scaphoid are also valuable in examining for scaphoid pathology.[14] A clenched-fist anteroposterior view is a form of stress view that may suggest a scapholunate ligament injury and potential carpal instability. Whenever doubt exists, a radiograph of the contralateral wrist is warranted, because widening of the scapholunate interval, for example, may be a bilateral finding and not indicative of a specific injury. In addition, in-office imaging with ultrasound may be of benefit. Ultrasound has the advantage over radiographs in its ability to dynamically assess for tendon pathology including ECU instability, but is highly operator dependent.[15,16]

Additional studies should be directed by history and physical examination findings and should be used to confirm or deny the presence of a suspected injury rather than as a "shotgun" element of the workup. A MRI study, with or without intra-articular administration of gadolinium, may be performed to assess the presence of intrinsic ligamentous or triangular fibrocartilage complex (TFCC) injury.[17] Gadolinium injected into the radiocarpal joint may be seen to leak into either the midcarpal joint or into the distal radioulnar joint if a significant ligament injury is present. This magnetic resonance arthrogram (MRA) is an extremely useful tool when correlated with history, physical examination, and plain radiographic findings that suggest a specific injury. However as with any imaging modality, MRA is not 100% sensitive, and may be negative in the setting of true pathology.[18] Thus imaging must be taken into account with physical exam when determining clinical significance.

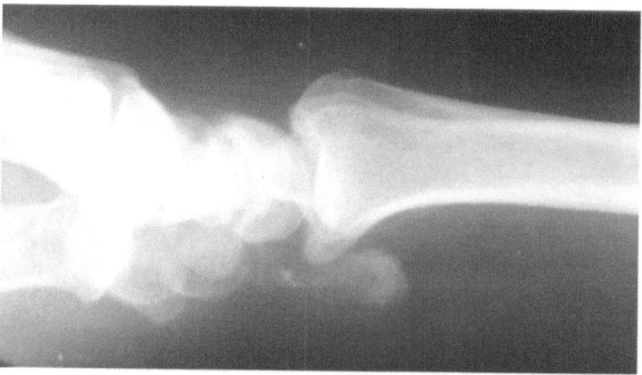

Fig. 71.1 Plain radiograph demonstrating acute calcific tendinitis.

Nuclear medicine studies such as bone scintigraphy (a bone scan) can be helpful as a sensitive indicator of acute injury, such as occult scaphoid fracture, but may lack the specificity to define an exact injury.[19] Bone scans should be ordered no less than 24 to 48 hours after injury to eliminate the possibility of false-negative results. Practically speaking, given the widespread availability of MRI, bone scans have fallen out of favor as a preferred imaging modality for wrist pathology.

COMMON WRIST TENDINOPATHIES

De Quervain Tenosynovitis

Tendinopathy of the first dorsal compartment involves the APL and EPB tendons. It is more common in women than in men, as has been associated with pregnancy and the postpartum period, but has also been noted with certain sports, especially rowing and racquet sports.[20–24] De Quervain tenosynovitis has also been described in volleyball players and should be suspected in any athlete who uses repetitive forceful wrist motions.[25] The area deep to the extensor retinaculum, which overlies the radial styloid, may be swollen and markedly tender. When performing Finkelstein's test, the examiner holds the patient's thumb inside a closed fist and the examiner then passively, ulnarly deviates the wrist. This maneuver reproduces pain in persons with de Quervain tenosynovitis. In the Eichhoff test, the patient is asked to clasp his or her thumb inside the flexed fingers of the hand and then ulnarly deviate the wrist (Fig. 71.2). Specific tenderness is elicited when digital pressure is placed over the radial styloid area.

Imaging can be helpful in the diagnosis of de Quervain tenosynovitis. Plain radiographs can reveal the presence of a bony spur in the floor of the first dorsal compartment. MRI can demonstrate both intrinsic tendon changes and extrinsic inflammation (Fig. 71.3). Ultrasound may demonstrate thickening involving the tendons and their sheaths as well as any instability.[16]

Treatment Options

The treatment of de Quervain tenosynovitis begins with immobilization in a thumb spica splint or cast. NSAIDs are also useful. Injection of a corticosteroid into the first dorsal compartment is another option although patients should be cautioned over

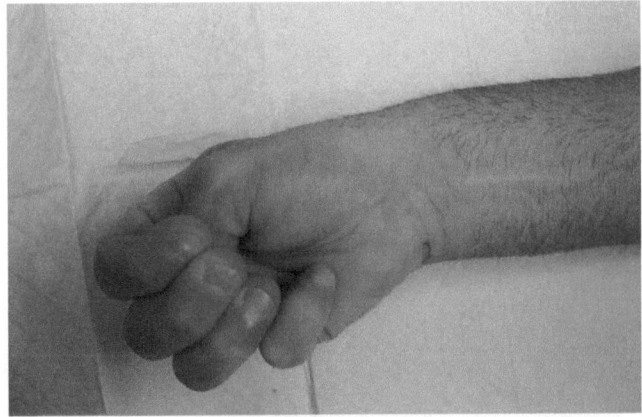

Fig. 71.2 Eichhoff test. With the thumb clasped into the palm, ulnar deviation of the wrist produces pain, or a positive test.

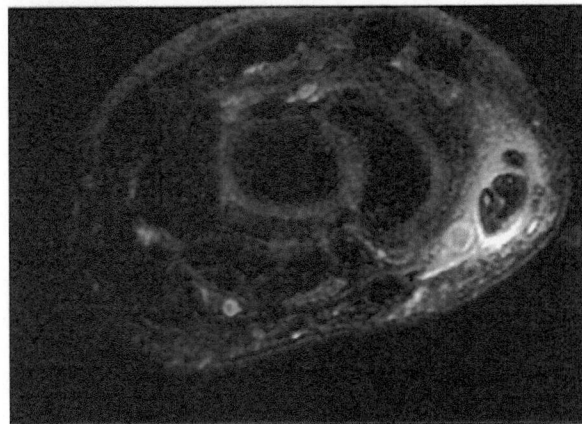

Fig. 71.3 A magnetic resonance imaging T2-weighted scan shows increased signal intensity around the tendons of the first dorsal compartment, indicating de Quervain tendinitis.

the risk of skin hypopigmentation and atrophy if placed too superficial. Avci and colleagues[21] compared the efficacy of cortisone injection with that of splinting in pregnant or lactating women and found that cortisone injection was superior in alleviating symptoms. Lastly, when these treatments are not effective, surgical release of the first dorsal compartment may be indicated. During this procedure, care must be taken to identify both the APL and EPB based on tendon actions.

 ## Authors' Preferred Technique

De Quervain Tenosynovitis

We prefer a stepwise treatment plan for persons with de Quervain tenosynovitis. The diagnosis is largely clinched by history and physical examination findings, as previously noted. Radiographs may help distinguish de Quervain tenosynovitis from problems related to the thumb carpometacarpal, scaphotrapeziotrapezoidal, or radiocarpal joints. Our initial treatment is oral administration of an NSAID, coupled with use of a thumb spica splint or cast and activity modification. We provide a corticosteroid injection if a patient continues to have symptoms after 4–6 weeks of wearing a splint. We use 1 mL of dexamethasone (10 mg/mL) mixed with 1 mL of 1% lidocaine without epinephrine. Patients who have persistent pain despite 3 months of nonoperative management are offered elective release of the first dorsal compartment (Fig. 71.4). We prefer making a 2-cm transverse incision centered approximately 1 cm proximal to the radial styloid. Care is taken to identify and protect branches of either the superficial branch of the radial nerve or the lateral antebrachial cutaneous nerve, which are inevitably encountered during the subcutaneous dissection. The investing extensor retinaculum overlying the first compartment is incised from distal to proximal under direct visualization, cheating dorsally (i.e., staying more dorsal to the midaxial line with the retinacular incision) thereby preventing volar subluxation of the tendons with wrist flexion. We ensure that the tendons are fully released by using a small retractor to pull on the tendons, ascertaining that both the APL and EPB tendons have been released independently. Based on passive extension of the thumb metacarpal and proximal phalanx when the appropriate tendon is pulled, full release of both tendons is thus verified. We believe this step is important because the APL may have multiple tendon slips, and a vertical septum may separate the smaller EPB tendon into a separate "chamber" within the first dorsal compartment. These anatomic aberrancies have been historically cited as predisposing persons to this condition.

Continued

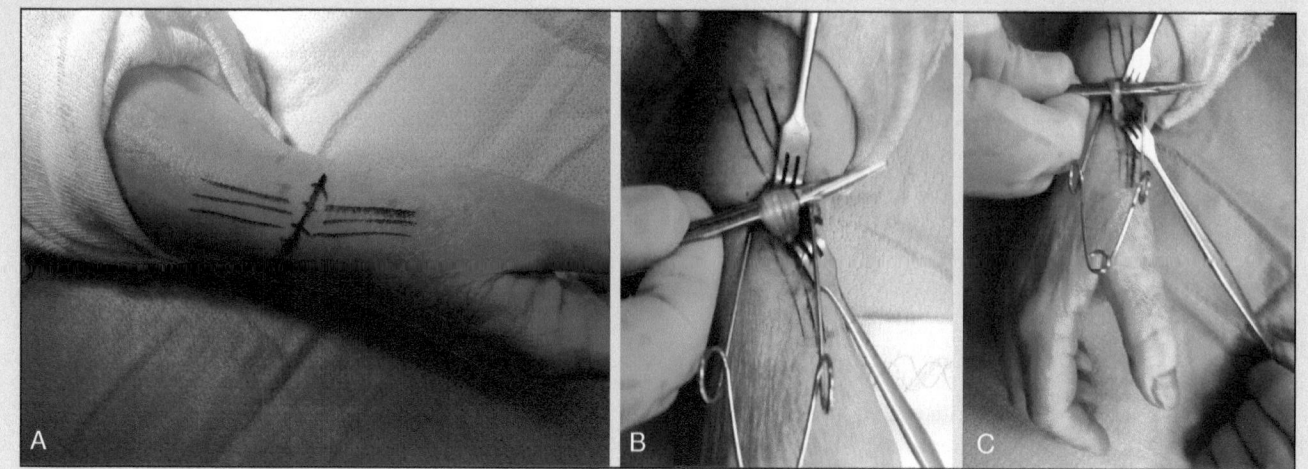

Fig. 71.4 (A) Planned incision for surgical release of the first dorsal compartment for de Quervain tenosynovitis. (B) The abductor pollicis longus (APL) tendon is visible in the incision once the overlying retinaculum is incised. Notice that three separate tendon slips are visible in this case. (C) The extensor pollicis brevis tendon is smaller than the APL but must be released as well. Pulling on the tendon should cause extension of the proximal phalanx of the thumb.

Postoperative Management and Return to Sports

A plaster thumb spica splint is placed immediately after surgical treatment for de Quervain tenosynovitis, and the patient is seen 10 to 14 days after surgery for suture removal and placement of a removable thumb spica splint. Athletes who require surgical release for refractory de Quervain tenosynovitis typically require 6 weeks of postoperative splinting to allow symptoms to resolve. Return to sports is allowed once ROM of the thumb and strength return. For athletes who do not require surgery, return to sports is permissible with use of a functional brace or cast when practical. Use of a functional brace or cast may be virtually impossible in sports such as basketball or gymnastics that require freedom at the wrist. Otherwise, athletes are allowed to return to sports when symptoms resolve and return of motion and strength are demonstrated.

Intersection Syndrome

Intersection syndrome has been associated with sports that involve repetitive extension and radial deviation of the wrist, such as skiing, weightlifting, rowing, and racquet sports.[5,8,11,22] Radial-sided dorsal wrist pain is the hallmark symptom, but it is typically perceived as more proximal than the pain associated with de Quervain tenosynovitis (Fig. 71.5).[26] Athletes may refer to intersection syndrome as "crossover tendinitis" because it occurs in the region of the distal forearm where the tendons of the first dorsal compartment intersect, or cross over, the tendons of the second dorsal compartment (extensor carpi radialis longus and brevis).[5] The inflammatory component is located within the second dorsal compartment. Clinical findings include localized tenderness and, in more severe cases, crepitus with wrist extension at this intersection, approximately 4 cm proximal to the wrist joint. There may be a "wet leather sign" with wrist extension versus resistance, where a sound often described as the one made

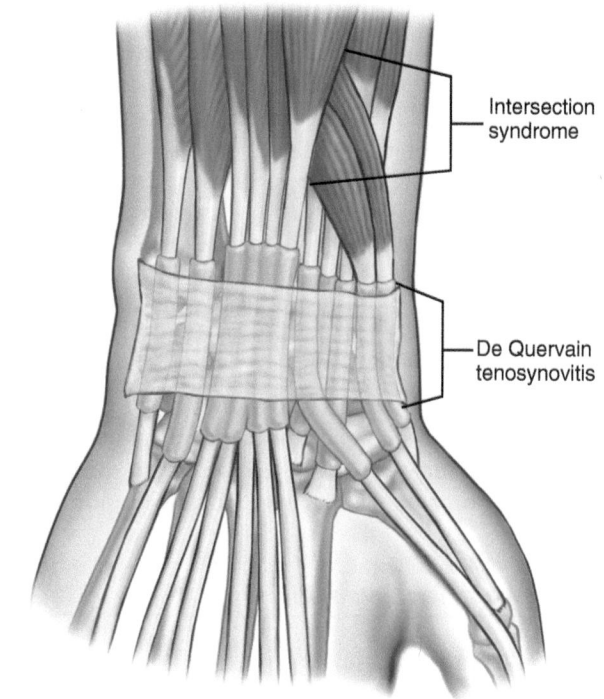

Intersection syndrome

De Quervain tenosynovitis

Fig. 71.5 The specific area of tenderness elicited in persons with intersection syndrome is typically more proximal than that of de Quervain tenosynovitis, as shown in this anatomic drawing.

when rubbing wet leather is heard. MRI is a useful adjunct in making the diagnosis, with increased peritendinous signal evident on T2-weighted images at the offending location.[27]

Treatment Options

Treatment is directed at resting the involved tendons in a thumb spica cast or brace, with oral administration of NSAIDs and cessation of the exacerbating activity. Grundberg and Reagan[28] demonstrated that the pathologic anatomy is a stenosing tenosynovitis of the investing sheath of the extensor carpi radialis longus and extensor carpi radialis brevis tendons. Refractory cases may require release of the stenotic sheath of the second dorsal compartment and débridement of associated tendinosis and hypertrophic tenosynovium.[28]

Authors' Preferred Technique

Intersection Syndrome

Rest, ice, and a forearm-based thumb spica splint are the cornerstones of management. NSAIDs are also prescribed. Corticosteroid injections are infrequently necessary. Use of nonoperative management without the need for surgery has been the experience of most wrist specialists treating this condition. Though we have never had to surgically treat intersection syndrome, we agree with *Green's Operative Hand Surgery*[20] adaptation of the Grundberg and Reagan approach to surgical treatment of intersection syndrome. In this method, a longitudinal incision is made from the area of swelling distally to the radial wrist extensors. The deep fascia overlying the second dorsal compartment is then released and the tendons débrided of any tenosynovitis.

Return to Sports

Athletes are allowed to return to sports once the symptoms have dissipated, or alternatively while still wearing a thumb spica cast or splint if practical for the sport in question.

Extensor Carpi Ulnaris Tendinopathy

Situated in the sixth dorsal compartment at the ulnar aspect of the wrist, the ECU tendon is commonly compromised by sporting activities. Golfers, tennis players, and other participants in racquet sports are at particular risk for injuries to the ECU.[6,7,29,30] ECU tendon problems may manifest as inflammatory tendinitis, degenerative tendinosis, instability (subluxation or dislocation), or rupture.[7] One specific form of tendinopathy, acute calcific tendinitis, presents with intense pain in the area of the involved tendon, and the etiology that differentiates it from degenerative tendinosis is poorly understood.[20]

Anatomically the ECU is adjacent to the ulnar styloid, and dorsal-to-palmar dislocation or subluxation of the tendon can lead to a painful snapping sensation when the wrist undergoes simultaneous extension and rotation.[1,21] Because the floor of the ECU sheath is inherently considered a part of the TFCC, tendinopathy can and does coexist with TFCC injury in some cases.[29] Given the aforementioned complex, and potentially multifaceted, etiology of ulnar-sided wrist pain, Kakar et al. recently described a "four-leaf clover" diagnostic algorithm to guide treatment. The algorithm consists of four questions including whether the ECU is unstable, if there is a concomitant TFCC injury, and if any chondral defect or bony deformity exists. This algorithm allows surgeons to ensure all components of ulnar-sided wrist pain are addressed. In the case of multiple positive answers to the above questions, treatment consists of addressing each of these injuries.[31]

Classification

Differentiating between three types of tendon pathology for the ECU is useful in directing treatment. As previously stated,

Montalvan et al.[6] classified ECU tendon pathology into three categories: acute instability, intrinsic tendinopathy, and rupture. The authors indicate that treatment differs for each of the tendon pathology subtypes, making the classification relevant and important. For any athlete who presents with acute onset of ulnar-sided wrist pain, ECU tendinopathy is high on the list of differential diagnoses. Because it may exist in the presence of other pathology, such as TFCC injury, the exact etiology may be elucidated using the aforementioned "four-leaf clover" diagnostic algorithm.

Occasionally, swelling over the ECU tendon sheath is present, and active extension with ulnar deviation of the wrist elicits pain. The practitioner should inquire about a history of snapping, especially when it is associated with twisting movements of the wrist. Any sudden loss of motion, especially extension combined with ulnar deviation, may provide evidence that rupture is possible.

Special Tests

Tenderness in the area of the ulnar head with circumduction of the wrist, and pronation and supination with the wrist extended, suggests a component of ECU tendinopathy. Tenderness along the ECU tendon should be expected. Any instability of the tendon, as mentioned in the physical examination section, should also be tested. In order to do this, the examiner may feel the ECU become unstable during resisted flexion, ulnar deviation and supination of the wrist. A painful snap indicates ECU instability. Additionally pain with resisted adduction of the thumb and long finger with the forearm in full supination and the wrist in neutral extension, otherwise known as the ECU Synergy Test, is a highly sensitive and specific method of diagnosing ECU tendonitis, and helps differentiate other etiologies of pain including TFCC tears.[32] Lastly, an inability to extend and ulnarly deviate the wrist may be an indication of rupture.

Treatment Options

For cases of acute tendonitis or degenerative tendinosis without instability, immobilization in a short-arm cast, splint, or brace is warranted, along with the administration of oral NSAIDs. Selective use of corticosteroid injection for symptoms unresponsive to splinting and oral medications can be attempted, but patients need to be warned about the theoretical risk of tendon rupture.[7]

Early immobilization for instability involves the use of a long-arm splint or cast with the wrist in pronation, extension, and slight radial deviation, because the supinated wrist, when brought from extension into ulnar deviation and flexion, may elicit the painful snap.[20] If splinting fails to alleviate subjective and objective instability, surgical reconstruction of the ECU tendon sheath to reroute and stabilize the tendon radial and dorsal to the ulnar head is justified.[33] For tendon rupture, primary repair may be needed to rebalance wrist extension and maximize function in the competitive athlete.

Criteria for Return to Sports

After nonoperative management, the timing for return to sport is based on symptom resolution, which may vary from 1 or 2 weeks to 3 months in some cases. For surgical release, a simple Z cut is made in the ECU tendon sheath to release investing compartment. This is followed by loose approximation of the sheath to prevent instability. Postoperatively the patient is splinted for 2 weeks followed by early therapy directed at restoring motion and strength. When the patient demonstrates full painless motion and adequate strength similar to that of the contralateral side, return to sport is allowed, typically 6 weeks after surgery.

In the case of ECU tendon sheath reconstruction, a long-arm splint is used for 6 weeks after surgery, followed by an additional 6 weeks of therapy (ROM, strengthening, and proprioception training) before the athlete is allowed to return to his or her sport. Resolution of pain and instability, coupled with near-normal strength (>80% compared to the contralateral side) and motion, are the benchmarks for permitting a safe return to sports. Recovery time varies per individual. The pain-free swing of a baseball bat is likely to take far longer to recover compared to that of a ping-pong–paddle swing, and as such recovery time can be as short as 6 weeks, and up to 3 months. If it is practical for the given sport, intermittent use of a protective short-arm wrist brace is encouraged until confidence in the strength of the wrist is restored.

Flexor Carpi Radialis Tendinopathy

Tendinopathy of the FCR is distinguished by its involvement at the volar radial aspect of the wrist, with exacerbation by flexion and radial deviation of the wrist against resistance.[34] The FCR tendon is closely associated with the trapezium, scaphoid, and trapezoid; it courses in a fibro-osseous tunnel through the carpus and is especially vulnerable to degenerative changes as it courses adjacent to the ridge of the trapezium on its way to insertion on the volar aspect of the bases of the index and sometimes middle metacarpals.[35,36] Arthritic conditions of the scaphoid, trapezium, or trapezoid can lead to FCR tendinosis and even rupture.[37] Soejima et al.[9] described FCR tendinopathy that was associated with a malunited trapezial ridge fracture in a professional baseball player. Resolution of the condition required excision of the malunited trapezial ridge. Most commonly, repetitive wrist motion, especially flexion with radial deviation, can lead to a tendinopathy of the FCR.[34] Treatment varies according to the exact etiology, but initial splint treatment with use of oral NSAIDs is usually indicated. Conservative treatment with activity modification, splints, and nonsteroidal agents is highly successful in the treatment of primary FCR tendinopathy. Corticosteroid injections are usually unnecessary in this patient population. The use of a thumb spica splint for FCR tendinopathy is not necessary. In the unusual case that it is unresponsive to conservative care, carefully planned surgical release of the FCR tunnel, along with any other offending pathology, such as trapezial ridge malunion, can be extremely beneficial.[34]

Flexor Carpi Ulnaris Tendinopathy

In an athlete presenting with ulnar-sided wrist pain, tendinopathy of the FCU should be considered in the differential diagnosis. The clinical presentation of volar ulnar wrist pain, exacerbated with active flexion and ulnar deviation, is classic. The possibility of other etiologies, such as TFCC tears, fractures of the hook of the hamate or pisiform, lunotriquetral ligament injury, and even

---

📌 Authors' Preferred Technique

Extensor Carpi Ulnaris Tendinopathy

In all cases of ECU tendinopathy without instability, we prefer to immobilize the tendon in a short-arm brace or cast for a period of 4 weeks, along with prescription of an oral NSAID. This approach is typically effective for cases of early degenerative tendinosis or acute calcific tendonitis. If splinting and medication are ineffective, we offer a corticosteroid injection, followed by an additional period of protective splinting. We prefer to use 1 mL of 10 mg/mL dexamethasone mixed with 1 mL of 1% lidocaine without epinephrine. Patients are counseled about the possibility of tendon rupture after a steroid injection and are free to decline this treatment. Surgery is warranted only in recalcitrant cases unless persistent instability is present. Surgical release of stenosing tenosynovitis typically brings a good degree of relief.[7] We use an incision that overlies the course of the dorsal sensory branch of the ulnar nerve so it can be identified and protected. The extensor retinaculum is incised over the ECU tendon from proximal to distal. No cases of late instability have been reported after surgical release of the ECU tendon from its sheath.[20]

In cases of acute instability, on the other hand, a 6-week period of immobilization in a pronated long-arm splint is tried first. In cases refractory to initial splinting or for recurrent episodes of symptomatic dislocation, surgical reconstruction of the ECU tendon sheath with the extensor retinaculum is preferred (Fig. 71.6). The tendon is immobilized in a long-arm splint in pronation for 6 weeks after surgery, followed by a period of motion recovery and progressive strengthening exercises.

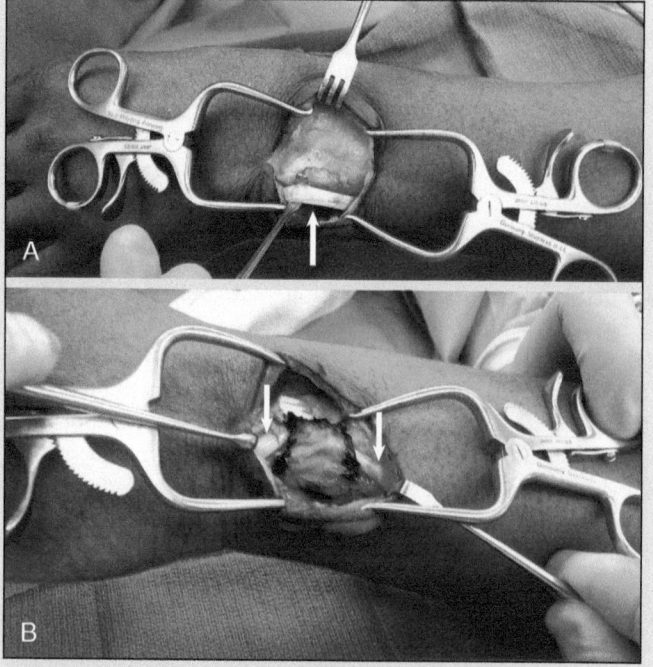

Fig. 71.6 (A) An unstable extensor carpi ulnaris (ECU) tendon is visible outside the normal tendon sheath *(arrow)*. (B) ECU tendon sheath reconstruction using available extensor retinaculum. Notice that the tendon is placed radial to the ulnar head *(arrows)*.

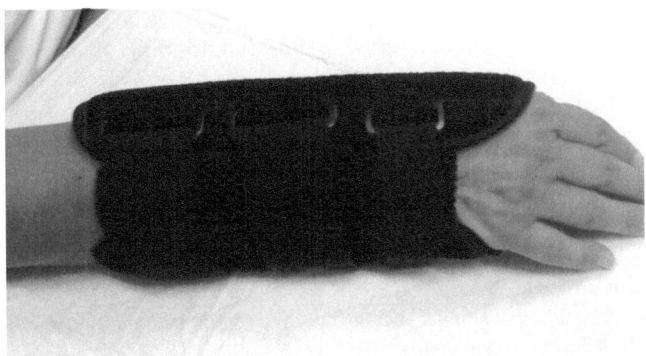

Fig. 71.7 A standard commercially available wrist brace that is useful for many types of wrist tendinopathies. Such a wrist brace is a mainstay of nonoperative care.

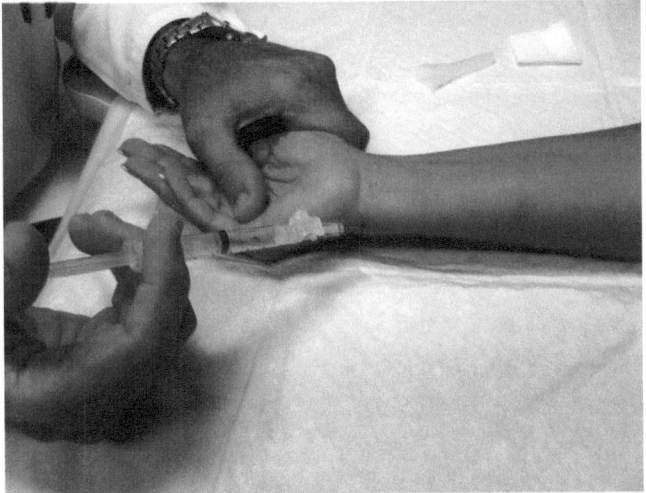

Fig. 71.8 An injection of a corticosteroid as adjunctive treatment for flexor carpi ulnaris tendinosis. Care must be taken to avoid inadvertently injecting the ulnar neurovascular bundle.

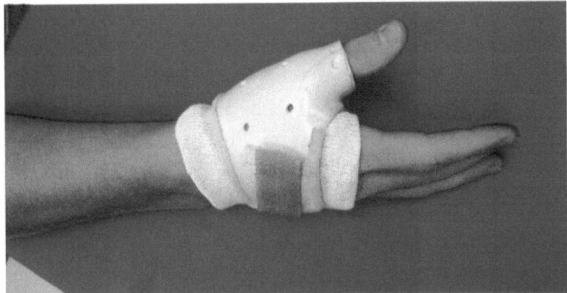

Fig. 71.9 Custom-molded splints may expedite return to play during tendon healing. These splints are made specifically to protect involved tendons while allowing participation in sports.

ECU tendinitis should also be considered. MRI may be helpful but its findings must be correlated with history and physical examination because incidental abnormalities are commonly reported.[38] A diagnosis of FCU tendinopathy is probable with a history of repetitive or forceful combined wrist flexion and ulnar deviation, along with clinical examination findings of tenderness over the FCU tendon, exacerbation of pain against resistance, and irritation with passive wrist extension. A trial of NSAIDs and use of a splint or brace, coupled with activity modification, are warranted (Fig. 71.7). Corticosteroid injection may be attempted for more severe cases (Fig. 71.8). If simple conservative measures are not helpful, then adjunctive studies, including MRI, may be warranted to help differentiate FCU tendinopathy from other sources of ulnar-sided wrist pain.[10] This entity rarely requires surgical intervention for alleviation of symptoms.

RESULTS

Treatment results for tendinopathy are usually quite good; full resolution of symptoms is expected by approximately 3 months

with nonoperative treatment. Certain athletes may be allowed to play with protective splints or casts during the healing process, with the understanding that doing so poses the risk of further injury or even tendon rupture (Fig. 71.9). If surgery is required, both the surgeon and the athlete must recognize that adequate healing time, as well as postoperative rehabilitation, are important and necessary factors for a safe return to play. Reinjury can occur, especially if return to sports is premature, which then requires "restarting the clock" on healing time.

COMPLICATIONS

Common complications faced during the management of wrist tendinopathies include persistent pain despite treatment and prolonged healing times. Many surgeons consider these conditions very stubborn, and they often fail to respond to typical treatment methods because athletes often have difficulty avoiding activities that aggravate the injury. The complication that causes the most concern, however, is the possibility of a tendon rupture. Overuse of steroid injections has been associated with potential tendon rupture, and the athlete should be counseled about the possibility of rupture whenever injections are used.[39] Bilateral extensor pollicis longus tendon ruptures have been described in a hockey goalie after steroid injection.[40] Steroid injections themselves have their own possible adverse effects, which include subcutaneous fat atrophy and skin hypopigmentation in the vicinity of the steroid administration.

Failure of conservative treatment may simply manifest as persistent pain or may involve tendon thickening or tenosynovitis, which may require surgical débridement for optimal resolution of symptoms. Rupture of affected tendons has been described after tenolysis procedures as well and should be part of the informed consent prior to any tendon surgery.[41]

FUTURE CONSIDERATIONS

The future of tendon treatment, especially in the athletic population, is already unfolding, with platelet-rich plasma (PRP) injections playing a controversial but definite role in the attempt to speed recovery of injured tendons. The literature remains mixed, with some studies showing a benefit and other studies showing no difference in tendon healing times with PRP versus placebo.[42–44] Athletes may actively seek PRP injection, because it has become a popular sports medicine treatment in recent years, but this treatment has yet to be proven superior to other methods. Injection of other growth factors has been considered to speed healing, but to date, well-designed controlled studies are needed before any definitive recommendations can be made.[45]

For a complete list of references, go to ExpertConsult.com.

SELECTED READINGS

Citation:

Wolfe SW. Tendinopathy. In: Wolfe SW, Hotchkiss RN, Pederson WC, et al, eds. *Green's Operative Hand Surgery*. 2nd vol. 6th ed. Philadelphia: Churchill Livingstone; 2010:2067–2088.

Level of Evidence:

V

Summary:

This expert author's chapter on tendinopathy in a comprehensive hand surgery textbook covers anatomy, pathophysiology, and the author's preferred treatment options. The chapter includes reviews of multiple level I studies currently available in the literature.

Citation:

VanHeest AE, Luger NM, House JH, et al. Extensor retinaculum impingement in the athlete: a new diagnosis. *Am J Sports Med*. 2007;35:2126–2130.

Level of Evidence:

V

Summary:

In this article, expert authors discuss a newly diagnosed form of wrist impingement involving the extensor retinaculum with wrist extension. Although not a true tendinopathy, impingement of the extensor retinaculum is a valid consideration in the athlete with dorsal wrist pain.

Citation:

Banks KP, Ly JQ, Beall DP, et al. Overuse injuries of the upper extremity in the competitive athlete: magnetic resonance imaging findings associated with repetitive trauma. *Curr Probl Diagn Radiol*. 2005;34:127–142.

Level of Evidence:

V

Summary:

This article includes an anatomic discussion of findings on magnetic resonance imaging in persons with repetitive trauma injuries, including tendinopathy.

Citation:

Allende C, Le Viet D. Extensor carpi ulnaris problems at the wrist—classification, surgical treatment and results. *J Hand Surg [Br]*. 2005;30B:265–272.

Level of Evidence:

V

Summary:

This article provides expert author opinions, classifications, and surgical treatment for extensor carpi ulnaris tendonitis. It provides an excellent overview of extensor carpi ulnaris tendinitis, including subluxation and dislocations.

Citation:

Rossi C, Cellocco P, Margaritondo E, et al. De Quervain disease in volleyball players. *Am J Sports Med*. 2005;33:424–427.

Level of Evidence:

III, retrospective cohort study

Summary:

This article describes the occurrence of de Quervain tendinitis in volleyball players, with specific reference to hand and wrist positioning in the sport leading to tendon inflammation of the abductor pollicis longus and extensor pollicis brevis.

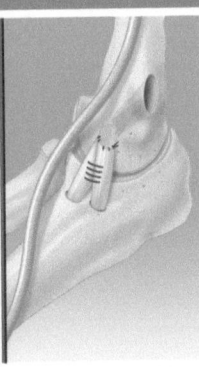

72

Disorders of the Distal Radioulnar Joint

Julie E. Adams

Disorders of the distal radioulnar joint (DRUJ) include those associated with pain or instability or both. In addition, one should consider pathology of degenerative or traumatic etiology. Injury to the triangular fibrocartilage complex can result in pain or instability or both, and may be traumatic or degenerative. Athletes, particularly those engaged in activities with repetitive axial loading, radial or ulnar deviation, and forearm rotation may especially be vulnerable, such as golfers, or those engaged in stick or racquet sports.[1–7] Other pathology of DRUJ can include arthritis, which is beyond the scope of this chapter.

The triangular fibrocartilage complex (TFCC) is a ligamentous complex that has load-bearing and load-sharing functions, stabilizes the DRUJ, and acts as a suspensory structure for the ulnar carpus. In the setting of an injury, it can represent a source of pain and dysfunction.

Patients with TFCC pathology may present with ulnar-sided wrist pain with or without DRUJ instability. Other pathology that should be excluded in evaluation of the patient with a suspected TFCC injury include lunotriquetral ligament tears, pisiform pathology (instability, arthritis, fractures), triquetral fracture, hamate fracture, HALT (hamate arthritis lunotriquetral tear) syndrome, ECU pathology, DRUJ instability or arthritis, systemic arthritides, Kienböck disease, vasoocclusive disorders, compression of the ulnar nerve at Guyon canal, and others.

ANATOMY

The DRUJ functions to allow rotation of the forearm. The ulna is the fixed unit of the forearm and the radius rotates around it at the sigmoid notch.[8] Given that the radius of curvature of the sigmoid notch and the ulnar head differ, motion at this joint consists not only of rotation but also dorsal and volar translation. In addition, the lack of bony congruity also means that the DRUJ relies heavily on soft tissue constraints for stability. The TFCC consists of the central articular disk, dorsal and volar radioulnar ligaments, ulnolunate ligament, ulnotriquetral ligament, meniscal homologue, and the subsheath of the ECU tendon (Fig. 72.1). These structures function as load sharing and load bearing, and also provide soft tissue stabilization. The radii of curvature of the sigmoid notch of the radius and the distal ulna are markedly different; thus the osseous structure of the DRUJ provides very little stability and stability relies heavily on soft tissue contributors, which include the dynamic stabilizers of the muscles, and the distal interosseous membrane, as well as the ligamentous structures of the TFCC complex.[8,9]

The main static soft tissue stabilizers of the DRUJ are the dorsal and volar radioulnar ligaments. These ligaments form the dorsal and volar margins of the TFCC and insert into the ulnar; the superficial fibers insert into the ulnar styloid tip whereas the deeper fibers, classically known as the ligamentum subcruentum, insert into the base or fovea of the distal ulna (Fig. 72.2). The dorsal and volar radioulnar ligaments originate from the dorsal and volar ulnar corners of the distal radius. When viewed from distal to proximal, the arrangement of these ligaments with the sigmoid notch of the radius is triangular, hence the nomenclature of the TFCC. The deep and superficial fibers of the dorsal and volar radioulnar ligaments act differentially to provide stability, analogous to the reins of a "four in hand" team of horses. It is now known that the dorsal superficial and the palmar deep fibers of the ligamentum subcruentum tighten in pronation to stabilize the DRUJ, while the palmar superficial and the dorsal deep fibers are tight in supination, stabilizing the DRUJ.[8–13]

The central articular disk, which mainly consists of fibrocartilage, is bounded by the dorsal and volar radioulnar ligaments and the most ulnar aspect of the distal radius. It serves in load transmission from the ulnocarpal joint but does not itself confer considerable stability to the DRUJ. Consequently, many central disk tears may be simply débrided or left untreated without resulting clinical DRUJ instability.

The ulnolunate and ulnotriquetral ligaments are extrinsic structures that represent thickenings of the volar capsule. Although the name implies that the ligaments arise from the ulna and attach to the lunate and triquetrum, respectively, histologic studies have shown otherwise. These ligaments emanate from the volar portion of the volar radioulnar ligament and the central articular disk, not directly from the ulna.[14] They add to the dorsal stability of the DRUJ and prevent excessive dorsal translation of the distal ulna relative to the carpus.

The meniscal homologue refers to a broad expansion of tissue traversing in a radioulnar direction from the central articular disk to the ulnar styloid and the surrounding joint capsule. It is composed of loose connective tissue and is itself not a major contributor to structural integrity of the TFCC.[14] A nearby ulnar opening in the meniscal homologue is known as the prestyloid recess, which may be confused as a peripheral tear. It is not uncommon to see synovitis in the region of the prestyloid recess, which makes this distinction difficult at times.

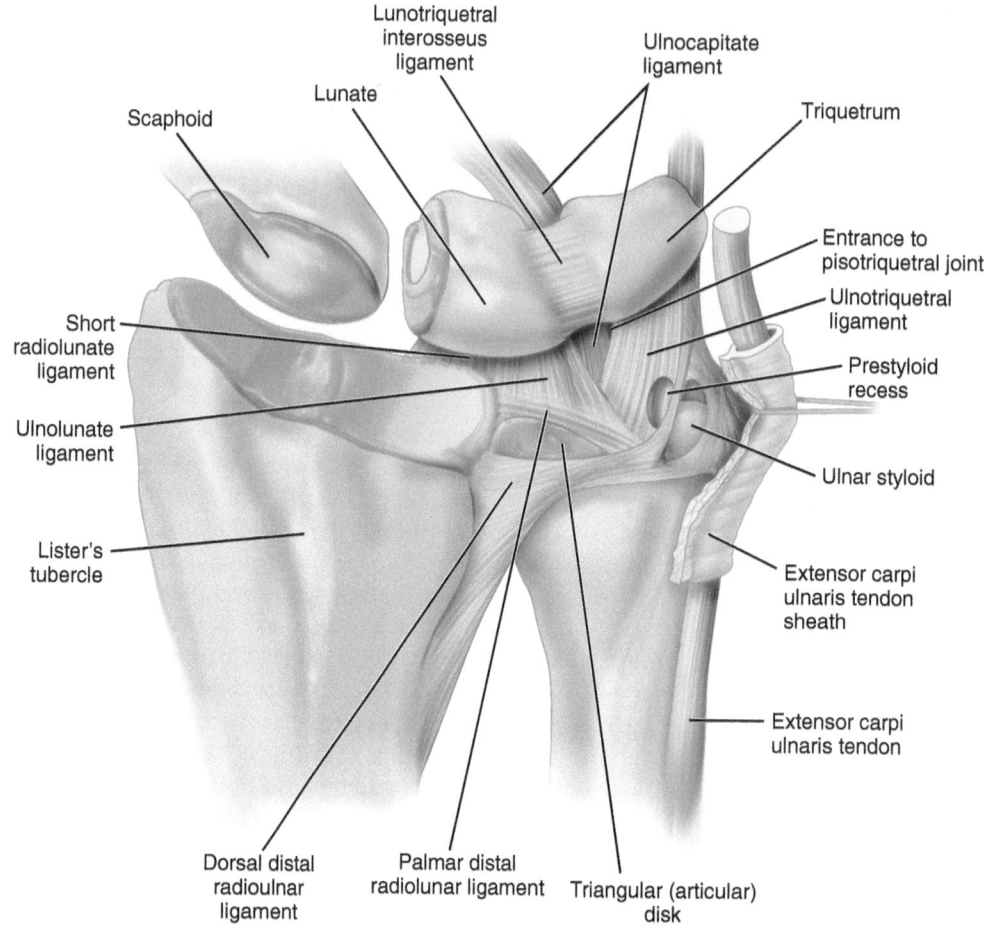

Fig. 72.1 Anatomy of the triangular fibrocartilage complex and associated structures. (From Kovachevich R, Elhassan BT. Arthroscopic and open repair of the TFCC. *Hand Clin.* 2010;26[4]:485–494.)

The floor of the sixth dorsal extensor compartment is the ECU subsheath, which is continuous with the dorsal radioulnar ligament and meniscal homologue.[14]

Blood Supply

The blood supply to the TFCC originates from the terminal branches of the anterior and posterior interosseous arteries. Similar to the knee meniscus, the peripheral TFCC is well perfused via blood supply from the capsular attachments; however, the more central and radial aspects are poorly vascularized; thus only the peripheral 10% to 30% of the TFCC has a vascular supply, which results in the improved healing potential of peripheral compared to more central tears.[15,16]

TRIANGULAR FIBROCARTILAGE COMPLEX TEARS

TFCC tears can result in ulnar-sided wrist pain as well as potentially DRUJ instability. TFCC tears are more common in those with ulnar positive or neutral variance than those with ulnar negative variance, who also have thicker articular disks.

The Palmar classification[17] divides TFCC tears into traumatic versus degenerative (I vs. II) and secondarily into location (IA-D) versus progression (IIA-D) (Table 72.1).

Class I Tears (Traumatic)

The mechanism of injury with traumatic tears is believed to be an extension and pronation moment applied to an axially loaded wrist, although tears may also occur with hypersupination. Traumatic tears commonly occur in association with displaced distal radius fractures.[18]

Class 1 tears are further subdivided based upon location (A, B, C, D). Class 1A represent a central perforation of the TFCC central articular disk and do not result in DRUJ instability. Class 1B tears represent an ulnar avulsion of the TFCC from the fovea and may be accompanied by an ulnar styloid fracture. Depending upon the extent of involvement of the distal radioulnar ligaments, patients may also have DRUJ instability. Class 1C tears involve the ulnolunate or ulnotriquetral ligaments, while the very rare 1D tear represents a radial-sided avulsion of the TFCC.

Class II Tears (Degenerative)

Class 2 tears represent the sequelae of ulnar impaction and are subdivided further by progression (A-E). Class 2A TFCC lesions represent wear or thinning of the TFCC, 2B lesions are those that demonstrate the findings seen in 2A plus ulnocarpal impaction with lunate or ulnar chondromalacia, 2C are those with the findings in 2B plus perforation of the TFCC, while 2D lesions

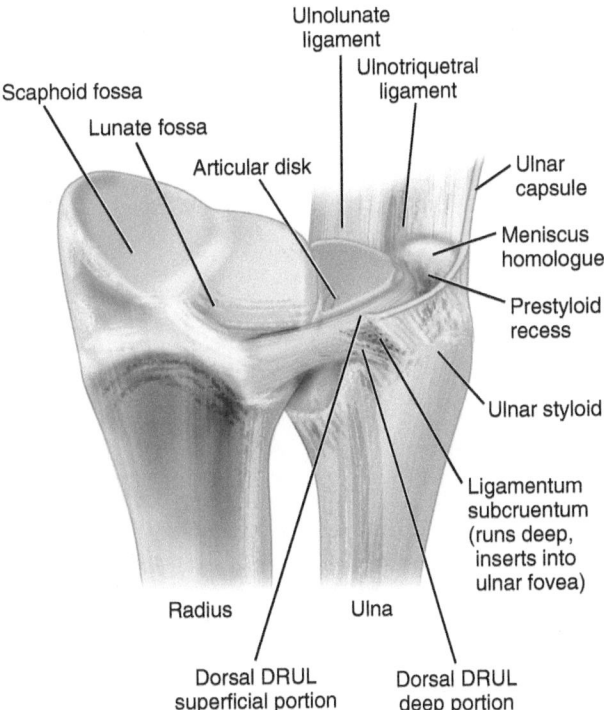

Fig. 72.2 Anatomy of the foveal attachment of the triangular fibrocartilage complex and the ligamentum subcruentum. *DRUL,* Distal radioulnar ligament. (From Ko JH, Wiedrich TA. Triangular fibrocartilage complex injuries in the elite athlete. *Hand Clin.* 2012;28[3]:307–321.)

TABLE 72.1 Palmer Classification for Triangular Fibrocartilage Complex Injury

Type	Description
I	Traumatic
IA	Central perforation of articular disk
IB	Foveal insertional tear, with or without ulnar styloid fracture
IC	Tear of ulnocarpal ligaments (ulnolunate and ulnotriquetral)
ID	Radial-sided insertional tear
II	Degenerative
IIA	Central wear of TFCC
IIB	Wear with chondromalacia of the lunate or ulnar head
IIC	TFCC perforation with chondromalacia
IID	TFCC perforation with chondromalacia and wear or tear of the LT ligament
IIE	TFCC perforation with chondromalacia and wear or tear of the LT ligament, with ulnocarpal arthritis

LT, Lunotriquetral; *TFCC,* triangular fibrocartilage complex.
From Kovachevich R, Elhassan BT. Arthroscopic and open repair of the TFCC. *Hand Clin.* 2010;26(4):485–494.

demonstrate lunotriquetral ligament changes in addition to the findings of 2C. Lastly, 2E represents ulnocarpal arthritis.

HISTORY

Patients with TFCC injuries most commonly present with ulnar-sided wrist pain. However, the differential diagnosis of ulnar-sided wrist pain includes many different pathologies that must be excluded (Table 72.2).

Patients may describe a history of a known acute injury or alternatively may relate a more insidious onset of ulnar-sided wrist discomfort. Although Class 2 tears are degenerative in nature, patients may have findings of ulnar impaction but may be asymptomatic or minimally symptomatic until after a traumatic episode that exacerbates their discomfort and brings symptoms to a level at which they complain. Pain is typically worsened with activities that involve pronosupination, twisting, gripping, or any element of ulnar deviation. Patients may describe instability or clicking or clunking with forearm rotation if DRUJ instability is a component. Specific inquiry into the location, onset of pain, relieving and exacerbating activities, and the results of any prior treatment is included in the history.

Patients with DRUJ instability often describe a single traumatic injury, although this may present insidiously over time. Patients often describe a clunk and pain with forearm rotation as the joint subluxates. They may note pain and worsening instability with axial loading (such as getting up from a chair) or complain of limited forearm rotation.

PHYSICAL EXAMINATION

The physical examination begins with inspection of the skin for any lesions, trophic changes, scars, or deformities. Sensibility is assessed. Range of motion (ROM) in the flexion-extension, radial-ulnar deviation, and pronosupination planes is documented and compared to the contralateral side. Typically grip strength is measured on both sides and side-to-side comparisons are made, using a dynamometer at settings 1, 3, and 5. One can anticipate a normal bell-shaped curve over the three settings with appropriate effort, and typically the nondominant side (in a normal patient) will be 80% of the dominant side's strength. Grip strength is useful to evaluate success of treatment as well as to determine effort and compliance with the examination.

The wrist is palpated to determine areas of tenderness. In the setting of TFCC pathology, patients will usually have tenderness at the ulnar snuffbox (fovea).[19] Alternatively or concomitantly

TABLE 72.2 Differential Diagnoses of Ulnar-Sided Wrist Pain

Ulnar Impaction	Pisiform Pathology (Instability, Arthritis, Fractures)	ECU Instability	Vasoocclusive Disorders
TFCC tear	Triquetral fracture	DRUJ instability	DRUJ arthritis
Lunotriquetral tear	Hamate fracture	Ulnar tunnel syndrome	Systemic or crystalline arthropathy
Inflammatory arthritis	ECU tendinosis	HALT (hamate arthritis lunotriquetral tear) syndrome	Kienböck disease

DRUJ, Disorders of the distal radioulnar joint; *ECU,* extensor carpi ulnaris; *TFCC,* triangular fibrocartilage complex.

with TFCC pathology, patients may have tenderness over the lunotriquetral (LT) interval, the extensor carpi ulnaris (ECU) tendon, and the DRUJ. It is important to distinguish between other causes of ulnar-sided wrist pain including hook of hamate fracture (tenderness over the hook of the hamate); pisotriquetral instability or arthritis (pisotriquetral grind testing) with or without secondary flexor carpi ulnaris (FCU) pathology (tenderness over the FCU tendon and pain over the FCU with resisted wrist flexion); ECU tendonitis (ECU synergy test[20]) or ECU subluxation (instability of the ECU particularly with pronosupination); DRUJ instability (piano key testing, subluxation or instability with pronosupination); or DRUJ arthritis (crepitus and pain with forearm rotation, pain with compression of the DRUJ). The TFCC stress test,[21] performed by axially loading the wrist in ulnar deviation with pronosupination, may be positive (cause pain) in the setting of a TFCC tear, but is relatively nonspecific as it can also be painful in the setting of LT tears. Patients may be asked to "push up" from a chair (with the forearm pronated and axially loaded); pain can indicate TFCC pathology.

It is often quite helpful to consider diagnostic as well as potentially therapeutic differential injections with local anesthesia and/or corticosteroid to further clarify the site of pathology and to assess the patient's potential response to intervention at that site.

IMAGING

Radiographs

Typical plain radiographs obtained in the setting of ulnar-sided wrist pain include posteroanterior, lateral, and oblique films. If pisotriquetral arthritis or a hook of hamate fracture is suspected, semi-supinated oblique views and or a carpal tunnel view may be obtained. If a TFCC tear is suspected, PA grip views of the affected and unaffected (for comparison) wrists on separate cassettes may be taken to evaluate for dynamic ulnar variance. PA grip views on the same cassette may be rotated and make evaluation of ulnar variance difficult. In any case, the appropriate positioning of the patient to evaluate ulnar variance involves the shoulder abducted, the elbow flexed, and the forearm in neutral position (Fig. 72.3). Lateral x-rays are specifically examined to assess congruity of the distal radioulnar joint.

Computed Tomography

Computed tomography (CT) scans are particularly useful to evaluate for DRUJ congruity and changes in forearm rotation especially on the axial cuts obtained in pronation, supination, and neutral. In addition, in selected cases, it is often useful to image the contralateral wrist in similar positions of forearm rotation.[22] When DRUJ instability occurs following, for example, after a distal radius fracture, it can be useful to examine the CT scan to determine if a malunited distal radius fracture or changes in the DRUJ are the primary cause of the instability as opposed to soft tissue problems such as a TFCC tear or disruption of the distal radioulnar ligaments. CT arthrography is mentioned for completeness, of mostly historical significance, and has largely been supplanted by magnetic resonance imaging (MRI) and MR arthrography. It is still occasionally used in patients who are unable to have a MRI.

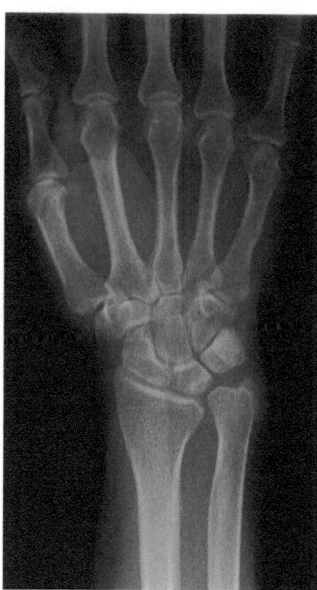

Fig. 72.3 A posteroanterior wrist view showing significant ulnar positive variance. The distal surface of the ulna can be seen distal to the lunate fossa of the distal radius. (From Sammer DM, Rizzo M. Ulnar impaction. *Hand Clin.* 2010;26[4]:549–557.)

Magnetic Resonance Imaging

Aside from inspection during arthroscopy, MRI is the most sensitive and specific imaging modality for evaluation of TFCC pathology (Fig. 72.4). The preferred imaging is done with a dedicated wrist coil in a 3.0 T scanner or better, although satisfactory images may be obtained with a 1.5 T machine if needed. Anderson and colleagues[23] demonstrated improved sensitivity of 94% with a 3.0 T scanner versus 85% sensitivity with a 1.5 T scanner. However, it is important to recall that although sensitivity and specificity to detect a tear is high, there is a high rate of communicating defects in the TFCC that have little clinical significance, and with increasing age, there is an increasing incidence of mostly asymptomatic TFCC pathology.[24] As such, all imaging must be interpreted in the setting of clinical examination and history.[25–27]

Use of MR arthrogram is a subject of controversy, with some centers noting that a high-resolution machine with a dedicated wrist coil is sufficient to detect most pathology without the risk of injection for arthrogram.[28]

Treatment

In the setting of acute DRUJ instability, nonoperative treatment may have a role. In cases of acute DRUJ dislocation, the DRUJ is reduced and the forearm splinted for 6 weeks in supination for dorsal dislocations or pronation for rare palmar dislocations. Chronic injury consisting of TFCC tears with DRUJ instability represent an indication for surgery, with either open or arthroscopic repair of TFCC to the fovea if the TFCC is reparable, or a DRUJ stabilization procedure if the TFCC is not reparable.

In the absence of DRUJ instability, the appropriate initial treatment of TFCC tears is nonoperative. In such cases, patients may benefit from reassurance about their condition, particularly in the setting of known or suspected TFCC pathology in association

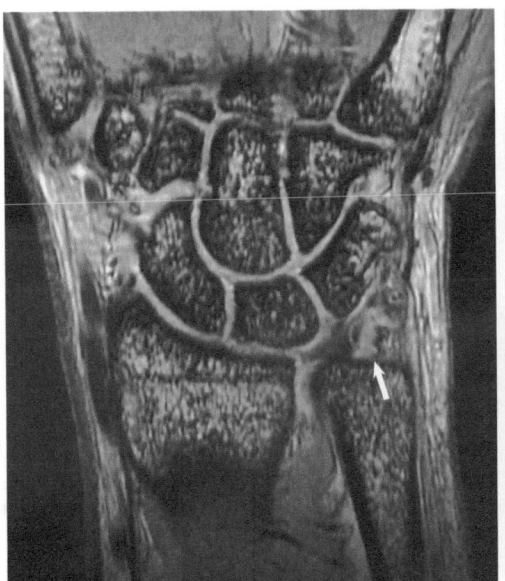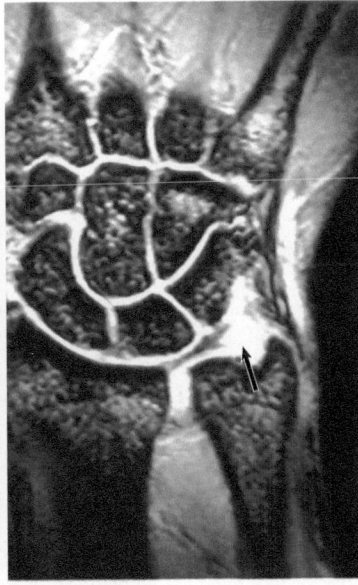

Fig. 72.4 Magnetic resonance imaging cuts showing a class IB triangular fibrocartilage complex (TFCC) tear. Note the loss of the low signal of the TFCC at the foveal attachment *(white arrow)* in the image on the left, with the concomitant high signal intensity at the region of the fovea *(black arrow).* (From Nakamura T, Sato K, Okazaki M, et al. Repair of foveal detachment of the triangular fibrocartilage complex: open and arthroscopic transosseous techniques. *Hand Clin.* 2011;27[3]:281–290.)

with distal radius fractures, in which TFCC pathology may resolve on its own within 6 to 12 months. Alternatively, patients may consider splinting for comfort, activity modification, and symptomatic care (nonsteroidal antiinflammatory drugs [NSAIDs], ice, therapy modalities), or injection of corticosteroid. Although immobilization is commonly used, there is no consensus regarding the benefits of full-time casting versus intermittent splinting, long arm versus short arm, or duration of splinting.[29]

Patients who fail nonoperative treatment may be considered for surgery. Surgical options include open versus arthroscopic management. My preference is for open surgery for TFCC tears associated with DRUJ instability.

Arthroscopy begins with examination of the radiocarpal joint through the 3,4 and 6R portal. The TFCC is visualized and inspected and a probe placed on the TFCC to assess for any laxity with the "trampoline test." I prefer to leave the tourniquet uninflated to better visualize any synovitis. Visualization from the 3,4 and 6R portal allows for assessment of the TFCC, as well as the lunotriquetral ligament and joint, in order to evaluate for ulnar impaction. Radial and ulnar midcarpal portals are placed to visualize in particular the lunotriquetral interval and the capitohamate interval, again, assessing for ulnar impaction or alternative pathologies. Once the diagnostic arthroscopy is completed, the TFCC and any synovitis can be débrided (Palmar 1A, 1D, and 2 lesions) or repaired (Palmar 1B), as described in Chapter 69 on wrist arthroscopy. Briefly, arthroscopic techniques for 1B tears involve either use of a suture anchor or passage of sutures via hollow-bore needles aimed from outside to in. Sutures are passed through the TFCC and repair is effectively to the capsule. In general, use of a 2-0 PDS suture is made and a small incision is made ulnarly to tie the sutures over the capsule and to avoid branches of the dorsal ulnar sensory nerve. Alternatively, a suture anchor may be placed into the fovea for a more anatomic

repair. A high rate of good to excellent results may be anticipated with arthroscopic TFCC repair techniques.[23,30–33]

In the setting of DRUJ instability, my preference is for open repair of the TFCC. In such cases, arthroscopy may be done as a diagnostic or confirmatory tool, but then an open incision is made (Fig. 72.5). A longitudinal incision is made over the fifth extensor compartment that is opened and released. A horizontal capsulotomy is made parallel to the dorsal radioulnar ligament. I use a braided slowly absorbable suture or Prolene or PDS passed through the TFCC, then through holes drilled up into the foveal region and tied over the ulnar metaphyseal region. Use of Keith needles loaded on a mini-driver to pass through the bone facilitates passage of the sutures. An alternative is the use of a suture anchor either open or arthroscopically. In general, I do not repair 1D tears as the results following simple arthroscopic débridement are equally favorable with fewer complications.

For Class 2 TFCC lesions, treatment options may include TFCC débridement alone or can include a joint leveling procedure, such as an arthroscopic or open-wafer procedure or an ulnar shortening osteotomy. Joint leveling procedures, such as an ulnar-shortening osteotomy, may result in more postoperative pain in the initial healing period, a requirement for cast or splint immobilization, and risk of failure to heal. If patients want definitive treatment in the setting of ulnar impaction, they may be offered TFCC débridement with joint leveling procedure at the same setting, accepting the increased risk and investment in time and recovery. Alternatively, if they wish to undergo the TFCC débridement alone they may be counseled that there is a higher risk of residual or recurrent discomfort, although it is possible these patients may respond to the lesser procedure.

Chronic DRUJ instability in the setting of an irreparable TFCC tear without DRUJ arthritis represents an indication for DRUJ stabilization and reconstruction procedure. There are

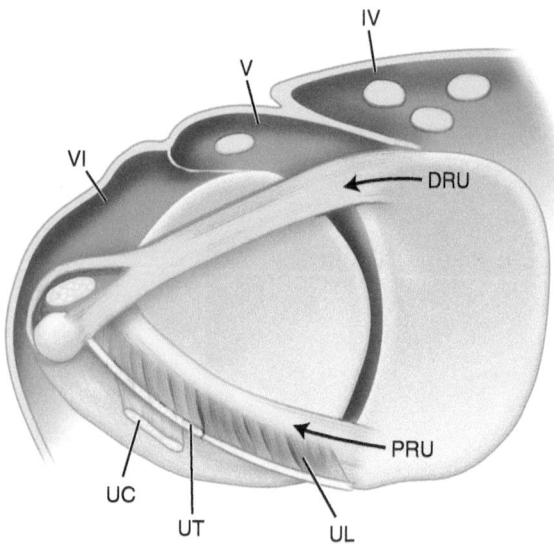

Fig. 72.5 A cross-sectional diagram of the ulnar side of the wrist. Surgical approaches for open repair of the triangular fibrocartilage complex may be performed through the septum of the fourth *(IV)* and fifth *(V)* compartments, the fifth and sixth *(VI)* compartments, or through the sixth compartment and subsequently the extensor carpi ulnaris subsheath as well. *DRU,* Dorsal radioulnar ligament; *PRU,* palmar (volar) radioulnar ligament; *UC,* ulnocapitate ligament; *UL,* ulnolunate ligament; *UT,* ulnotriquetral ligament. (From Tay SC, Berger RA, Parker WL. Longitudinal split tears of the ulnotriquetral ligament. *Hand Clin.* 2010;26[4]:495–501.)

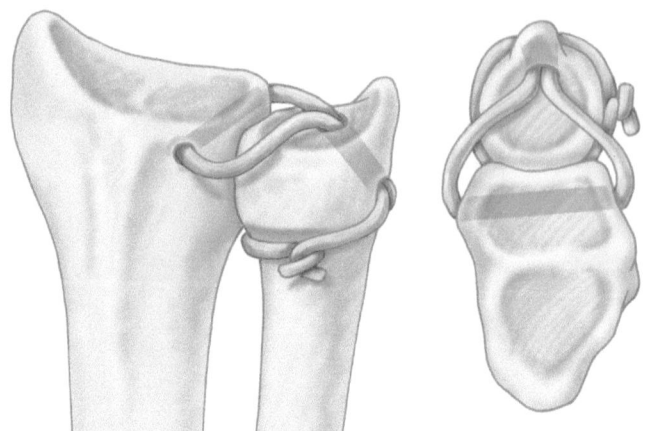

Fig. 72.6 Tendon graft reconstruction to stabilize the distal radioulnar joint. (From Lawler E, Adams BD. Reconstruction for DRUJ Instability. *HAND.* 2007;2:123–126. Copyright American Association for Hand Surgery 2007.)

a number of techniques that can be used including a distally based strip of the ECU tendon through the TFCC.[34] More commonly, the use of a palmaris longus (PL) graft (or a strip of the flexor carpi ulnaris [FCU] if the PL is absent) is performed to reconstruct the distal radioulnar ligaments.[35] A longitudinal incision is made over the fifth extensor compartment, the fifth compartment is opened, and the extensor digiti minimi (EDM) retracted. An "L"-shaped capsulotomy is made, with one limb proximal and parallel to the dorsal radioulnar ligament and the second limb along the sigmoid notch. The fovea is débrided of any scar tissue, retaining any functional remnants of the TFCC. The bone under the fourth extensor compartment is exposed along the dorsal margin of the sigmoid notch such that an area 5 mm proximal to the radiolunate joint and 5 mm radial to the sigmoid notch is revealed. This will be the site of a drill hole for passage of the tendon graft. A K wire is placed at this site from dorsal to volar and overdrilled with a 3.5-mm cannulated drill bit. A longitudinal volar-based incision just radial to the ulnar neurovascular bundle is made for exposure of the volar drill hole. The deep dissection goes between the digital flexors and the ulnar neurovascular bundle. A second tunnel site is identified from the fovea at the base of the ulnar styloid to the metaphyseal ulnar neck region. This may be created by flexing the wrist and placing a K wire from the fovea out ulnarly and proximally or alternatively from proximal ulnar to distal radially. A cannulated 3.5- to 4.0-mm drill bit is used to overdrill this site. Care is taken to avoid an iatrogenic fracture. The tendon graft is passed from volar to dorsal and retrieved (Fig. 72.6). A hemostat is passed from dorsal to volar over the ulnar head and proximal to the remnants of the TFCC, exiting through the volar DRUJ

capsule to grasp and retrieve the tendon graft, which is pulled into the dorsal wound. The two limbs of the tendon graft are then passed through the ulnar tunnel to exit at the ulnar border of the forearm. The two limbs are crossed then passed in opposite directions around the ulnar neck with the more dorsal one placed under the ECU, and after compression of the DRUJ and tensioning in neutral rotation, they are tied to each other, sutured in place, and cut. The DRUJ capsule is closed with nonabsorbable braided sutures and the EDM is left out of its retinacular sheath.[36–39]

POSTOPERATIVE MANAGEMENT

Following TFCC repair, most surgeons immobilize the patient for approximately 6 weeks, although there is no consensus regarding use of a long- versus short-arm cast of splint (Fig. 72.7). I typically immobilize patients in a sugar-tong splint or a muenster cast for a total of 6 weeks following TFCC repair by any technique. Following this time period, the patient begins a progressive ROM and strengthening program with anticipated return to unrestricted and full activity by 3 months postop. Return to sport is generally allowed at this point, but may be dictated by return of motion and grip strength as well as the functional demands of the specific sport. For DRUJ reconstruction with a tendon graft, the patient is immobilized again for approximately 6 weeks, typically in a sugar-tong or muenster cast or splint for the first 3 to 4 weeks and either a muenster cast or a short arm cast for the remaining time.

COMPLICATIONS

Complications of surgical treatment of TFCC tears or DRUJ instability include persistent wrist pain (particularly in the setting of TFCC débridement alone for ulnar impaction). In patients with known or suspected ulnar impaction who elect for TFCC débridement surgery, I counsel them prior to surgery and offer them one of two options: a TFCC débridement and if indicated,

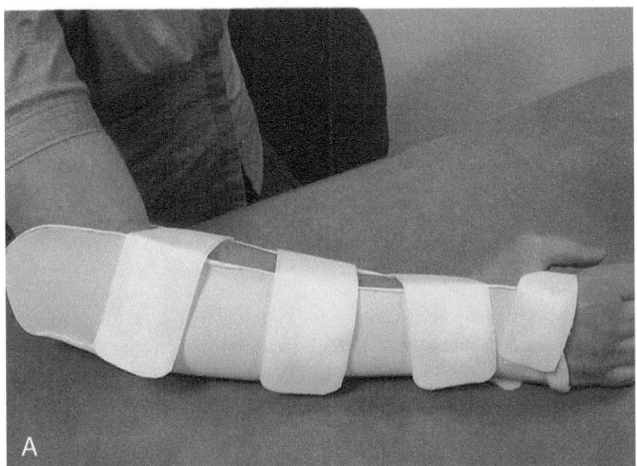

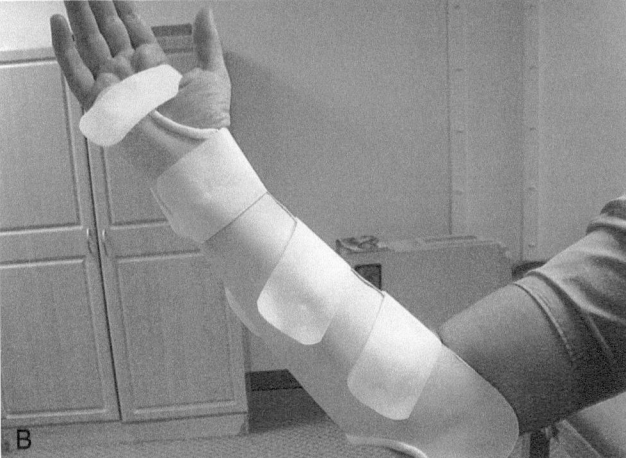

Fig. 72.7 A custom Muenster brace. (From Kaiser GL. Functional outcomes after arthroplasty of the distal radioulnar joint and hand therapy: a case series. *J Hand Ther.* 2008;21[4]:398–409.)

proceeding to simultaneous ulnar shortening osteotomy at the same surgical time versus simply proceeding with a TFCC débridement alone. TFCC débridement alone has a quicker recovery time and no risk of nonunion, but a heightened risk of recurrent or residual pain, but if it works for the patient, he or she may avoid the bigger procedure. Alternatively, if they elect for this option, patients should understand the risk of returning with residual or recurrent pain and desiring a future surgical procedure. Other risks associated with surgery include those inherent to surgery or wrist arthroscopy, as well as risk of dorsal ulnar sensory nerve neuritis, particularly with soft tissue or capsular repairs. Risks of DRUJ reconstruction include persistent or recurrent instability, worsening of any under-appreciated or unrecognized arthritis, and stiffness. If the tunnels are placed incorrectly, fracture of bony tunnels or entry into the joint can be problematic.

ACKNOWLEDGMENT

The author wishes to acknowledge the work of Drs. Corey A Pacek and Glenn Buterbaugh who were the authors of a chapter focused on injuries of the TFCC in the prior edition.

For a complete list of references, go to ExpertConsult.com.

SELECTED READINGS

Citation:
Elite athlete's hand and wrist injury. *Hand Clin.* 2012;28(3).

Level of Evidence:
Multiple articles at levels IV and V

Summary:
This issue of *Hand Clinics* focuses on multiple hand and wrist issues specific to the elite athlete. Several articles focus on triangular fibrocartilage complex (TFCC) injuries specifically. Some articles provide expert opinion on treatment of specific TFCC injuries, whereas others serve as good review articles on TFCC injury in general, with further discussion on anatomy, diagnosis, treatment, and subsequent outcomes.

Citation:
Sachar K. Ulnar-sided wrist pain: evaluation and treatment of triangular fibrocartilage complex tears, ulnocarpal impaction syndrome, and lunotriquetral ligament tears. *J Hand Surg Am.* 2012;37A:1489–1500.

Level of Evidence:
IV and V, (review article)

Summary:
This review article provides an excellent overview of the basic anatomy, physical examination, workup, treatment, and outcomes relating to triangular fibrocartilage complex. Many articles cited for further reading consist of a variety of levels of evidence, mostly levels IV and V, and focus on small case series, expert opinion, and techniques.

Citation:
Kovachevich R, Elhassan BT. Arthroscopic and open repair of the TFCC. *Hand Clin.* 2010;26(4):485–494.

Level of Evidence:
IV

Summary:
This review article compares the literature on arthroscopic and open repair. Multiple repair techniques are described, along with the outcome articles to accompany the techniques. Most articles are level IV, with some level III evidence. No clear benefit is seen with either arthroscopic or open repair.

Citation:
Geissler WB. Arthroscopic knotless peripheral ulnar-sided TFCC repair. *Hand Clin.* 2011;27(3):273–279.

Level of Evidence:
V

Summary:
This technique article reviews an arthroscopic, knotless repair of peripheral triangular fibrocartilage complex tears. Great detail is taken to thoroughly describe the technique, and excellent pictures and figures are provided.

Citation:
McAdams TR, Swan J, Yao J. Arthroscopic treatment of triangular fibrocartilage wrist injuries in the athlete. *Am J Sports Med.* 2009;37(2):291–297.

Level of Evidence:
IV

Summary:
This case series examines 16 elite athletes with triangular fibrocartilage complex injuries. All the athletes were treated arthroscopically with either débridement (in five athletes who had stable tears) or repair (in 11 athletes who had unstable tears). Average return to play was 3.3 months (range, 3 to 7 months). Only two patients did not return to play at 3 months, both of whom had associated conditions (ulnar impaction syndrome and extensor carpi ulnaris pathology). The authors concluded that an arthroscopic approach could reliably facilitate return to play in competitive athletes and that return to play is often slowed when associated injuries are present.

Citation:
Anderson ML, et al. Clinical comparison of arthroscopic versus open repair of triangular fibrocartilage complex tears. *J Hand Surg Am.* 2008;33A(5):675–682.

Level of Evidence:
III

Summary:
This retrospective study compared all triangular fibrocartilage complex repairs over a 10-year period at a single institution (75 total; 36 arthroscopic and 39 open) and evaluated range of motion; grip strength; preoperative and postoperative Mayo Modified Wrist Scores; Disabilities of the Arm, Shoulder and Hand scores; and visual analog scores. Average follow-up was 43 ± 11 months, with one patient lost to follow-up. No statistically significant difference was found between arthroscopic and open repair. A trend toward more superficial ulnar nerve pain was found in the open repair group, but this finding did not reach statistical significance. A statistically significant reoperation rate was found to be associated with female gender but did not depend on the type of repair.

Citation:
Iordache SD, et al. Prevalence of triangular fibrocartilage complex abnormalities on MRI scans of asymptomatic wrists. *J Hand Surg Am.* 2012;37A(1):98–103.

Level of Evidence:
III

Summary:
In this study, a magnetic resonance imaging scan of the wrists was performed for 103 healthy, asymptomatic volunteers. All studies were evaluated independently by three observers (two musculoskeletal radiologists and one orthopedic surgeon). Thirty-nine abnormal scans were seen, with a statistically significant correlation between increasing age and abnormality of the triangular fibrocartilage complex. The authors concluded that given the high incidence of asymptomatic abnormality, especially in patients older than 50 years, abnormal results should be carefully tempered with findings of the history and physical examination.

Citation:
Smith TO, et al. Diagnostic accuracy of magnetic resonance imaging and magnetic resonance arthrography for triangular fibrocartilaginous complex injury: a systematic review and meta-analysis. *J Bone Joint Surg Am.* 2012;94A(9):824–832.

Level of Evidence:
III

Summary:
This meta-analysis was performed to evaluate the sensitivity and specificity of magnetic resonance imaging (MRI) versus magnetic resonance arthrography (MRA) for triangular fibrocartilage complex injuries. A total of 982 pooled wrist studies showed a combined sensitivity and specificity for MRI of 0.75 and 0.81, respectively. The combined sensitivity and specificity for MRA was found to be 0.84 and 0.95, respectively. The authors recommend that this information be used when choosing the appropriate test for further diagnostic evaluation of patients with ulnar-sided wrist pain.

Citation:
Kleinman WB. Stability of the distal radioulna joint biomechanics, pathophysiology, physical diagnosis, and restoration of function what we have learned in 25 years. *J Hand Surg.* 2007;32(7):1086–1106.

Level of Evidence:
V

Summary:
This comprehensive and classic article expounds upon what is known about the DRUJ and TFCC. Well-done figures and prose make clear some of the complexities of this part of the wrist.

Citation:
Adams B, Lawler E. Surgical techniques: chronic instability of the DRUJ. *JAAOS.* 2007;14:571–575.

Level of Evidence:
V

Summary:
This review describes evaluation and treatment of patients with chronic DRUJ instability by distal radioulnar ligament reconstruction or osteoplasty of the sigmoid notch.

Citation:
Pang EQ, Yao J. Ulnar sided wrist pain in the athlete. *Curr Rev Musculoskelet Med.* 2017;10(1):53–61.

Level of Evidence:
V

Summary:
This review of causes of ulnar-sided wrist pain in the athlete explores the various presentations, evaluation, and treatment of wrist pathology.

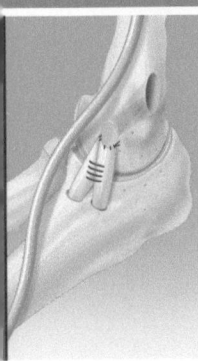

73

Tendon Injuries in the Hand

Robin N. Kamal, Jacob D. Gire

Although not every team physician needs to be a "hand surgeon," the frequency of hand and wrist injuries caused by sporting activity requires expertise in the diagnosis and evaluation of these injuries. Regardless of the sport, an athlete with a hand injury intuitively appreciates the effect that a hand injury has on function and competitive ability. The injuries often sustained in each individual sport generally have distinguishing characteristics, because most sports place specific demands on an athlete's hands in a consistently reproducible manner. Accordingly, certain types of athletes are more prone to certain injuries.[1–4]

Caring for athletes requires an understanding of their preferences for the tradeoffs that exist for various treatments. As treating physicians, surgeons need to appreciate the nuances of patient wishes, risk tolerance, and expectations to guide a shared decision on treatment. Restoring the athlete's unique skill set after these injuries provides professional challenges that often require consultation with a hand and upper extremity specialist.

Four mechanisms responsible for athletic hand injuries have been proposed by Mirabello and colleagues[5]: throwing, weight bearing, twisting, and impact. Usually the injury is a combination of factors. Werner and Plancher[6] categorized the potential for injury based on the type of sport. Mechanisms included were impact with a ball or competitor; contact with a racquet, stick, or club; and external contact, as is seen in gymnastics, rock climbing, and weight lifting. Although almost any injury can be seen in any athlete, certain sport-specific patterns of injury have been recognized. For example, interphalangeal (IP) fracture/dislocations are frequent in ball sports such as volleyball and basketball. Hamate fractures are often diagnosed in golfers, baseball hitters, and tennis players. Some injuries are notoriously easy to miss, such as a flexor digitorum profundus (FDP) tendon avulsion in a football or rugby player. Because of the small margin for diagnostic error and the temporal nature of most recommended interventions, neglect and/or misguided treatment algorithms are certain to lead to a poor outcome. Maintaining a high index of suspicion for the worst-case scenario may be the first step in evaluating the injured hand of an athlete.

In general, providing care for an athlete can be challenging for certain populations, such as elite athletes, as expectations and time from play have greater significance. Coaches, managers, agents, and parents may all have various levels of understanding about injuries and disparate expectations for return to play (RTP). At times, these misaligned goals can be counterproductive. Our initial goals are to make an accurate diagnosis, present options

comprehensively, communicate effectively, and create an environment for shared decision-making. The patient management questions set forth by Green and Strickland[7] create a solid framework for treatment algorithms:

1. Is the method of treatment expected to provide the best long-term result?
2. Would we manage this injury in a similar manner in a nonathlete?
3. Are the potential complications of my treatment significantly greater than might be expected from a more conservative approach?
4. Will the treatment allow the athlete to return to competition with little risk for reinjury?
5. Would reinjury unfavorably influence the prognosis for a satisfactory recovery?

These guidelines apply across the entire scope of sports medicine. Confidentiality, attentive communication, and a patient-centered attitude are all essential to gain the athlete's trust and maximize outcome.

This chapter focuses on the tendon injuries most commonly encountered by the general orthopaedic surgeon or sports medicine specialist who is acting as first responder. Consequently, only the most pertinent elements of the history and physical examination, followed by key imaging findings and treatment options, are presented here. Clinical pearls, decision-making principles, and our preferred surgical techniques are interspersed within the text. Given that most sports involve intensive use of the hands, both open and closed injuries to the flexor and extensor tendons happen routinely. For open injuries, examination, exploration, and repair of damaged structures are performed expediently. Closed tendon injuries in the hand may be subtle and overlooked, but they can cause sufficient morbidity that they deserve special attention. Extensor mechanism injuries are possible at the distal interphalangeal (DIP), proximal interphalangeal (PIP), and metacarpophalangeal (MCP) joint levels, with each producing consistent findings that must be diagnosed by the treating physician. On the flexor side, a FDP avulsion, or "jersey finger," is a serious and often neglected injury that will compromise composite digital flexion if it is not treated (Fig. 73.1).

MALLET FINGER

The anatomy of the dorsal apparatus of the finger is a complex and intricate structure.[8–10] Disruption of the attachment of the

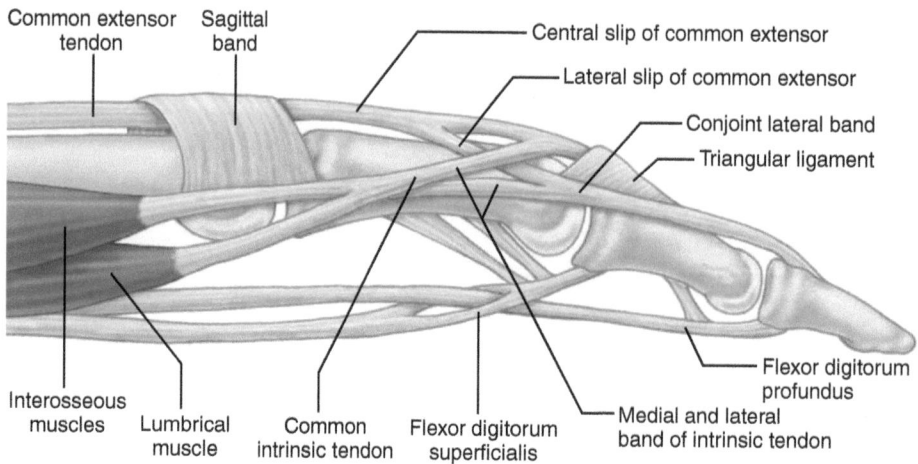

Common extensor tendon
Sagittal band
Central slip of common extensor
Lateral slip of common extensor
Conjoint lateral band
Triangular ligament
Flexor digitorum profundus
Medial and lateral band of intrinsic tendon
Flexor digitorum superficialis
Common intrinsic tendon
Lumbrical muscle
Interosseous muscles

Fig. 73.1 Anatomy of the flexor and extensor apparatus.

terminal extensor tendon into the dorsal base of the distal phalanx has been termed *mallet finger*. Synonyms for this injury are *baseball finger* and *drop finger*, and "jamming" or "stoving" injuries in ball sports. Axial load and forced flexion of the DIP joint can stretch the terminal tendon, avulse the tendon attachment, or cause an avulsion of bone from the dorsal epiphyseal ridge of the distal phalanx. Warren and associates[11] described an area of terminal tendon hypovascularity as the site of vulnerability. The physical examination demonstrates the drooped posture of the DIP joint and the inability to completely extend the joint actively. The degree of dorsal swelling and tenderness is variable. Players may also present with an inability to extend the DIP joint after this injury with PIP joint volar plate laxity with obvious hyperextension and a resulting swan neck deformity. Radiographs are obtained to define any bony injuries, with close attention paid to large avulsion fractures associated with volar subluxation of the DIP joint. It is more common to see a smaller avulsion fracture with variable displacement but without significant joint malalignment.

Extension splinting is the treatment of choice for virtually all mallet finger injuries.[12–16] A comfortable DIP joint extension splint is placed; hyperextension is avoided because it may lead to dorsal skin necrosis, and the PIP joint is left free to avoid unnecessary proximal joint stiffness. Use of a dorsal, volar, or custom thermoplastic splint produce equivalent results.[17] Splints are worn full time for 6 weeks, with care taken to avoid skin breakdown. Traditionally this has been followed by nighttime splinting; however, a recent randomized controlled trial found that this is unnecessary.[18] Interestingly, as long as the joint is passively supple to full extension, nonoperative treatment may be commenced up to 3 months after the injury was sustained with comparable outcomes.

A rare unstable fracture/dislocation of the DIP joint may warrant surgical treatment (Fig. 73.2). Some have advocated for operative intervention when there is more than one-third of the articular surface involved;[19,20] however, in the absence of high grade joint subluxation, extension block pinning was not superior to splint immobilization. Instead, the authors reserved operative fixation for those with high grade subluxation, defined as volar displacement of the dorsal cortex of the distal phalanx beyond

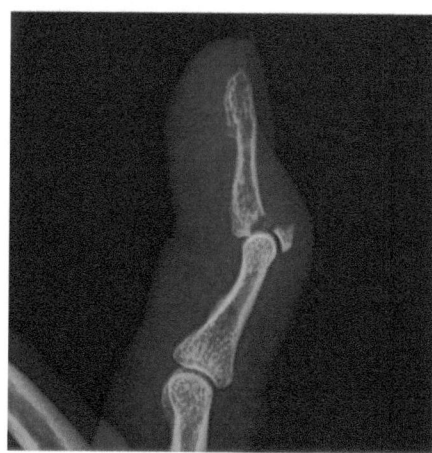

Fig. 73.2 Fracture dislocation of the distal interphalangeal joint with joint subluxation.

the central point of the middle phalangeal head on the lateral view.[21] Complications with surgical treatment have previously been observed in up to 41% of operatively treated injuries.[22] The most commonly observed complication was marginal skin necrosis of the distal phalanx, but recurrent flexion deformity, permanent nail deformities, transient infections of the pin tracts, pullout wires or suture, dorsal prominence, and osteomyelitis were also observed.

We collectively treat all but a few select mallet finger injuries nonoperatively. The use of a comfortable volar-based thermoplastic DIP extension splint is preferred. The splint may be further secured with use of 0.5-inch adhesive tape or Coban wrap. A second splint might be provided for wear during showering and should be exchanged on a hard surface that supports the joint in full extension. Splinting is continued for 6 weeks. Athletes who either remove the splint prematurely or inadvertently dislodge and flex the DIP joint must essentially "start the clock over." As such, agreement on the part of the athlete to partake in the entire length of treatment is necessary prior to initiating treatment. Simultaneous volar and dorsal splinting or digit extension casting can be provided to athletes in contact sports who want to play during the period of immobilization, with the added risk of maceration, loss of immobilization, and injury to other joints. Inclusion of the entire digit with buddy taping to the adjacent finger should be considered during sport to provide additional stability and protect the adjacent joints.[23]

For those that wish to undergo treatment but external splinting is not tolerated, transarticular fixation of the DIP joint in extension with an oblique k-wire buried underneath the skin has been previously utilized[24]; however, this does place the athlete at risk for pin migration or pin breakage with play.[23,25] For those that cannot play their sport effectively with the DIP joint in full extension, such as in ball throwing sports, options include immediate splinting with return to sport after 6 weeks, delayed splinting after the season has completed, and no treatment. For many athletes, delayed or no treatment may be preferred and is generally well tolerated and allows immediate return to sport with pain treated symptomatically.[25] If electing to delay or forego treatment, the athlete should be made aware of the risk of developing swan neck deformity or functional/cosmetic impairment.

In neglected cases or in those undergoing delayed treatment, splinting is prescribed for a longer period until satisfactory clinical results are achieved. Results are generally acceptable to the patient; however, even with proper treatment, a residual extensor deficit of 20 degrees or more is present in about a third of patients, with greater extensor lag at presentation predictive of worse final function. Fortunately this does not correlate with patient satisfaction with treatment or disability.[18] Persons with PIP volar laxity are fitted with a figure-of-eight–type splint to block PIP hyperextension. Chronic mallet injuries may lead to swan neck deformity, and chronic rigid deformities or those with symptomatic DIP instability are referred to hand specialists for consideration of tenodermodesis or DIP fusion.

Less common than digit mallet finger injury is the mallet thumb, which is a tear of the extensor pollicis longus (EPL) insertion at the distal phalanx base. The distal phalanx of the thumb is longer, thicker, and wider than the distal phalanges of the digits. In addition, the terminal insertion of the EPL tendon into the dorsal epiphysis of the thumb's distal phalanx is wider and thicker than the terminal tendon insertion in the fingers. The IP joint of the thumb has variability in its arc of motion. Full extension may range from 0 to 60 degrees of hyperextension.

If the presentation is delayed, it is important to obtain the actual injury date from the athlete. As with mallet finger injuries, active extension of the thumb IP joint is markedly less than on the uninjured side. Tenderness at the dorsal prominence of the distal phalanx base is usually present in isolated mallet injuries and helps rule out a proximal EPL tendon lesion. In axial load or contact mechanisms of injury, concomitant fractures, IP joint collateral ligament injuries, and proximal thumb injuries are possible and should be carefully examined. Radiographs should be obtained, and the relationship between the phalanges is noted at the thumb IP joint on the lateral view.

Most published reports of treatment of this injury are limited to small case series. Operative treatment has been recommended by some investigators[26–28]; however, equivalent results have been documented with closed treatment.[29–33] Some athletes may elect for operative repair to decrease the amount of full-time immobilization. The fixation of a terminal phalanx avulsion fracture has similar complications as operative treatment of bony mallet fingers, and caution should be observed.

The athlete may be best served by not playing for at least 6 weeks regardless of the treatment regimen, especially in contact sports. It is virtually impossible to protect the thumb's IP joint while having a functioning thumb ray that can meet the demands of competition. For this reason, some athletes choose to delay definitive management of these injuries until the off-season.

CLOSED BOUTONNIÈRE (CENTRAL SLIP RUPTURE)

The extensor digitorum communis tendon divides into three parts over the PIP joint of the digit. The central slip inserts into the dorsal base of the middle phalanx at the epiphysis. Two lateral slips of the extrinsic extensor tendon separate from the central slip just proximal to the PIP joint and accept a tendinous contribution from the intrinsic musculature to become the conjoined lateral bands at the level of the middle phalanx. These conjoined lateral bands are joined by the oblique retinacular ligament, which facilitates conjugate extension of the PIP and DIP joints. In a closed injury, with forced flexion of the PIP joint, the central slip can rupture from its insertion. Concurrent injury to the tenuous triangular ligament allows volar subluxation of the lateral bands relative to the PIP joint axis of rotation. The boutonnière posture is defined by the resulting flexion moment at the PIP joint and hyperextension moment on the DIP joint from the malpositioned lateral bands (Fig. 73.3). Avulsion fractures at the central slip attachment site can also cause this deformity.[34] Boutonnière deformities may be classified as either acute or chronic and as either supple or rigid.

The Elson test has been shown to diagnose central slip ruptures most accurately (Fig. 73.4).[35,36] The affected digit is flexed 90 degrees over the edge of a table, and the patient is asked to actively extend the PIP joint against resistance. If the central slip is intact, the DIP joint remains supple. If the central slip is ruptured, the DIP joint remains rigid. This test will not diagnose a partial injury to the central tendon and may be inhibited by pain or lack of patient cooperation. As a confirmatory test, the PIP joint is held passively extended and the athlete is asked to flex the DIP joint. The inability to flex the DIP joint indicates a tear of the central slip.

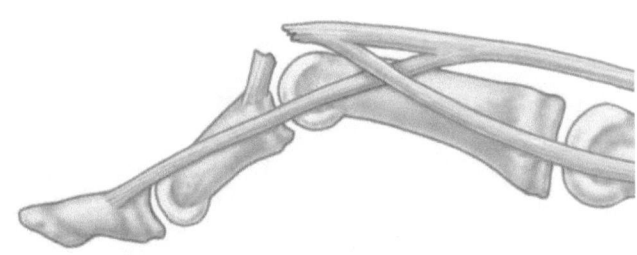

Fig. 73.3 Boutonnière deformity resulting from a central slip rupture with distal interphalangeal joint hyperextension.

Acute open lacerations of the central slip may be repaired with the PIP joint protected with a dynamic extension splint for 6 weeks. Although operative repair of a closed boutonnière deformity has been reported, preferred treatment for most of these deformities is with PIP extension splinting, leaving the DIP joint free (Fig. 73.5).[37,38] DIP flexion is encouraged because it draws the lateral bands dorsally and thereby promotes an extension force to the PIP joint.[39–41] Extension splinting with the aid of a hand therapist requires strict attention and must be uninterrupted. If compliance is an issue, percutaneous pinning of the PIP joint is an option, with pin removal at no later than 3 weeks and protected mobilization with an extension splint for an additional 2 to 4 weeks. Return to sports in the nonprofessional athlete at 6 weeks is possible with buddy taping of the finger. In the elite athlete, many factors need to be weighed to arrive at the best treatment for the individual. Some players in certain sports will opt to accept the cosmetic deformity and return to active play without splinting once the pain subsides,

given the stiffness that may develop with nonoperative or operative treatment of the digit.[42]

For the athlete who presents with severe DIP hyperextension (indicating significant retraction of the central slip), operative repair of the central slip with a suture anchor (Fig. 73.6) and joint pinning for 2 to 3 weeks may be an option. With a neglected or chronic boutonnière deformity, the PIP contracture can be supple or fixed. If passive PIP extension is full, splinting can be tried, unless the athlete is unable to devote the 6 to 8 weeks necessary for successful closed treatment. If the PIP contracture is fixed, active splinting or serial casting is performed to effect full PIP extension. Once full passive extension is attained, static PIP splinting is maintained for 6 weeks. Rarely, release is performed by cutting the check rein ligaments located proximal to the volar plate, which is sometimes combined with open reconstruction of the central slip and mobilization of the lateral bands, or staged reconstruction.[43]

It should be reinforced that a "pseudoboutonnière" follows a ligamentous injury as a result of a hyperextension mechanism, with resultant scarring and contracture of the volar plate. This mechanism postures the PIP joint in flexion, mimicking a

Fig. 73.4 Elson test to evaluate for central slip ruptures.

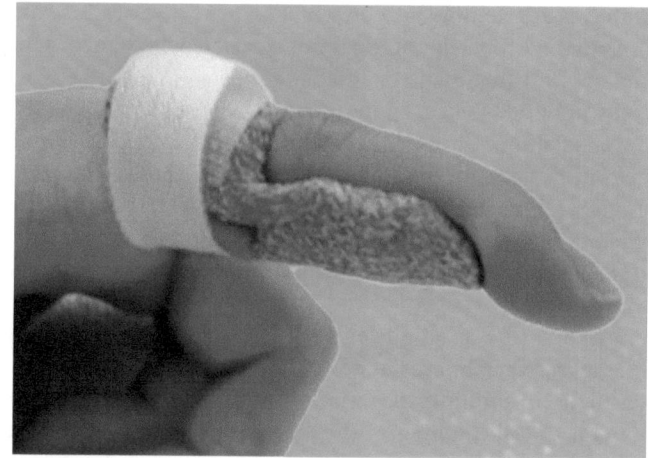

Fig. 73.5 A proximal interphalangeal extension splint allowing distal interphalangeal flexion for treatment of a boutonnière deformity.

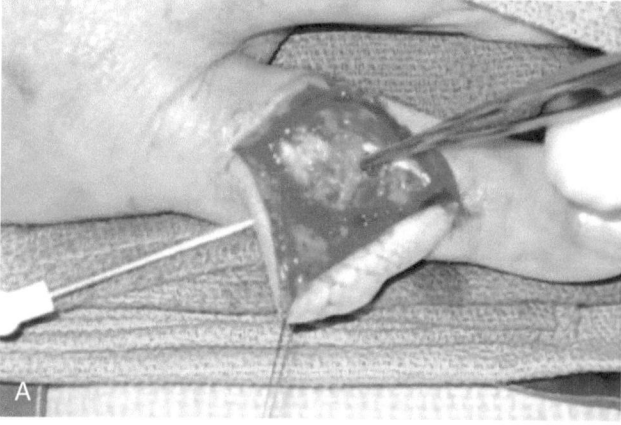

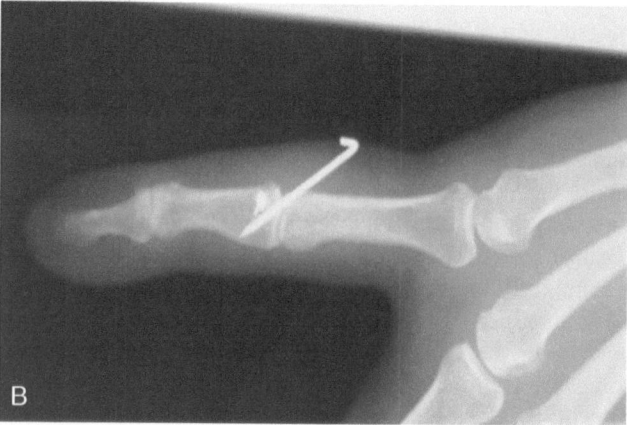

Fig. 73.6 (A) The dorsal approach for repair of a central slip rupture with pinning of the proximal interphalangeal (PIP) joint. (B) Central slip repair with a suture anchor and PIP joint pinning.

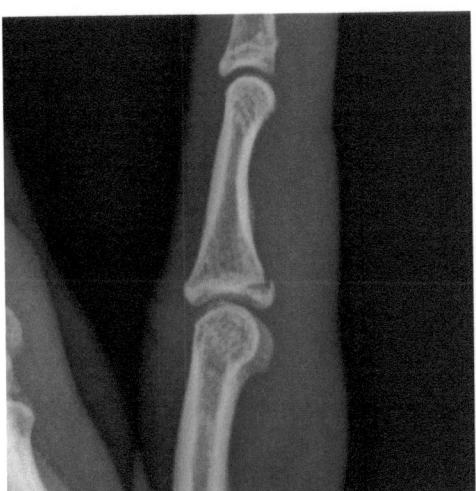

Fig. 73.7 Volar plate avulsion from the middle phalanx after hyperextension injury of the proximal interphalangeal joint.

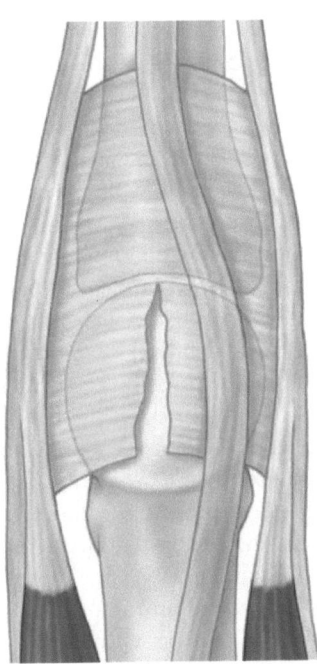

Fig. 73.8 Radial sagittal band tear resulting in ulnar subluxation of the extensor tendon.

boutonnière position.[44,45] However, the hyperextension mechanism of injury and subsequent examination can readily distinguish a true boutonnière from a pseudoboutonnière. In the latter, a chip avulsion fracture fragment is often seen near the volar lip of the middle phalanx where the injury occurred (Fig. 73.7).[46] In addition, with a pseudoboutonnière, the tenderness is almost exclusively at the volar side of the PIP joint, and the DIP motion is essentially normal. Treatment of pseudoboutonnière is directed at progressive stretching of the PIP volar plate, with the introduction of dynamic splinting if necessary.

SAGITTAL BAND RUPTURE

The extensor digitorum communis tendons are maintained over the dorsal apex of the MCP joints by a dorsal sling of adjacent transverse fibers, termed the *sagittal bands* (Fig. 73.8). The sagittal bands act as a tether to prevent either radial or ulnar subluxation of the communis tendon at the level of the MCP joint. The sagittal band invests the extensor mechanism, crossing both volar and dorsal to it, ultimately blending into the volar plate.[47] Radial sagittal band rupture can occur from forceful finger extension (a "flea-flicker" injury), a direct blow such as in a boxer, or an ulnarly directed force.[48] The radial sagittal band of the long finger ruptures most commonly, although ulnar sagittal band ruptures have been reported.[49] Pain and snapping may occur, and a careful examination will document the tendon subluxation or dislocation. Clinically passive extension of the MCP joint is possible and the patient can then usually maintain the finger in an extended position with the extensor tendon centralized; however, the patient may not be able to obtain MCP extension from full flexion. Tendon subluxation is promptly reproduced upon active MCP flexion.

Acute sagittal band ruptures can be treated with a static MCP extension splint, relative motion extension splint, or sagittal band bridge.[50–52] Preference is a hand based volar MCP extension splint or a relative motion extension splint, continued for approximately 4 to 6 weeks or until central

extensor tendon tracking over the MCP joint returns when actively making a fist. Treatment of this condition represents a rare instance in which the MCP is immobilized in extension, counter to the "safe" position of the hand where the MCP joints are maximally flexed to prevent collateral ligament scarring in a lengthened position. For chronic cases, a trial of nonoperative treatment is attempted; however, in those with symptomatic persistent dislocation of the extensor tendon, repair may be indicated. One option includes primary repair of the torn sagittal band with realignment of the extensor tendon by releasing the opposing sagittal band.[53–56] Alternatively, various reconstructive techniques have been described that utilize adjacent structures to restrain the extensor tendon. These techniques include use of adjacent juncturae, anomalous tendons (e.g., extensor medius proprius or extensor indicis et medii communis), palmaris autograft, or distally based slips of the injured extensor tendon to create a restraint to tendon subluxation.[57–62]

The sagittal bands are approached via a curvilinear dorsal incision and torn fibers are primarily repaired. If there is redundant tissue, such as in chronic scenarios, this is imbricated and the opposing sagittal band and/or junctura may necessitate release to allow for centralization of the tendon. The ulnar junctura tendinum can be flipped over and sutured to the palmar radial sagittal band remnant of the deep intermetacarpal ligament to provide additional restraint against ulnar subluxation.[59] Alternatively, the ulnar slip of EDC can be cut proximally, maintaining its distal insertion and routed around the extensor tendon and radial collateral ligament and sutured to itself. Post repair, a relative motion splint may be utilized to facilitate early ROM.[63,64] RTP is delayed for 8 to 12 weeks post-op to allow adequate soft tissue healing.

Few athletes will be comfortable enough to continue competitive play in the acute phase. This situation, coupled with the possibility of further damage to the extensor hood or underlying dorsal capsule from repetitive trauma, leads to the decision to provide treatment in-season in the majority of cases. Mild injuries without subluxation may require only a short period of missed play, with buddy taping utilized upon return, whereas more severe injuries may prevent athletes from competing for several months. We are not aware of ways to manage this pathology safely and effectively while allowing athletes (such as baseball or basketball players) to compete at a high level for the remainder of a season as they await out-of-season surgery. The orthosis limits functional RTP and places the hand at risk for further injury.

Although the hands of any boxer can be subjected to a multitude of injuries, *boxer's knuckle* specifically refers to chronic attritional disruption of the dorsal anatomy at the MCP joint. This disruption may include the central extensor tendon, sagittal band, and/or dorsal capsule.[53,65] A large capsular rent may allow for metacarpal head protrusion and persistent flow of synovial fluid from the joint cavity to the subcutaneous space. Metacarpal head osteochondral defects may be present. Athletes who engage in punching and have early symptoms may possibly continue if proper protection is used and supervision is provided. Operative treatment is comparable to sagittal band repair with repair, reconstruction, or débridement of the dorsal capsule also performed.[53,58,65] As dorsal capsular repairs may lead to a loss of MCP flexion, excisional débridement of the dorsal capsule when a rent is encountered leaving the capsule open is preferred.[66] Post operatively, immobilization is brief (2 to 3 weeks), with the MCP joint flexed 60 degrees to minimize loss of joint flexion. Wrapping and gloving strategies with shock-absorbing padding may decrease further injury, but competition rules may restrict the use of some of the more effective types of equipment for these athletes.

JERSEY FINGER

"Jersey finger" is an avulsion of the FDP from its insertion on the distal phalanx (Fig. 73.9). This injury classically occurs when an athlete, such as a football or rugby player, forcefully grabs an opponent's jersey with flexed fingers as the opponent duly escapes the grasp. Various theories have been proposed to explain why the ring finger, as opposed to the long finger, is most commonly affected.[67] The strength of the FDP insertion of the ring finger is significantly less than that of the adjacent digits.[68] As one grips, the distal segment of the ring finger projects farther and becomes more prominent because of the increased mobility at the ring finger carpometacarpal (CMC) joint.[69]

Leddy and Packer[70] described three types of injury, based on the following factors: (1) the presence or absence of a bony fragment radiographically, (2) the level to which the tendon retracted, and (3) the status of the blood supply of the avulsed tendon. The tendon can avulse with or without a bony fragment. The level of the bony fragment as shown on a lateral radiograph does not reliably predict the level of tendon retraction because the tendon end and bone fragment may separate.[71] In a type I injury, the tendon has retracted into the palm, without the

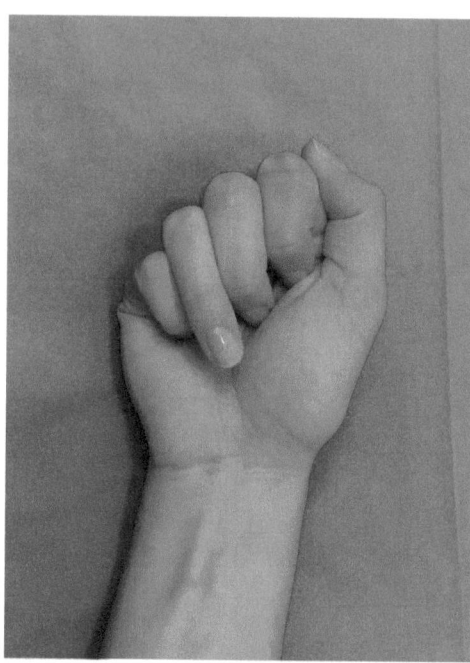

Fig. 73.9 Jersey finger injury results in loss of distal interphalangeal flexion.

presence of a bony fragment. Repair within a week is required for this injury because retraction of the tendon into the palm and loss of blood supply lead to contraction. Type II avulsions often are accompanied by a small bone fragment and retract only to the level of the PIP joint, and the vinculum longum may still be intact. This injury can be successfully repaired up to 6 weeks after the injury occurs because the tendon length has been maintained. Type III injuries are accompanied by a large bony fragment and are restrained distally by the A-4 pulley (Fig. 73.10). These injuries also can be successfully repaired weeks after the injury is sustained. After the original three-part description by Leddy and Packer in 1977, a fourth type was added to the classification scheme. This fourth type involves an intra-articular fracture of the distal phalanx and separation of the tendon from the fracture fragment (see Fig. 73.10).[72]

Loss of isolated DIP joint flexion is the *sine qua non* of this injury and is tested by blocking the PIP joint in an extended position while profundus function is checked (Fig. 73.11A). The middle, ring, and small finger profundus tendons are connected to a shared muscle belly in the forearm, whereas the index profundus typically has its own separate muscle belly. Examination may reveal a prominence where the proximal ruptured tendon end is located. For instance, fullness and tenderness at the A-1 pulley area may indicate a type I injury with retraction to the palm level. Radiographs are important and help determine whether there is an associated fracture or avulsion. Ultrasonography and magnetic resonance imaging (MRI) may be useful adjuncts in equivocal cases, in which the timing of surgery may be dictated by the classification of injury (Fig. 73.12).

Surgical repair is best carried out within a week of the injury, especially for type I injuries where the FDP is retracted into the palm and any further delay may limit the ability to restore the FDP back to its insertion on the distal phalanx. Because it is not possible to know the exact position of the avulsed tendon end by examination alone, proceeding with acute repair of all jersey fingers in athletes is justified.[73] The distal FDP insertion site is exposed with either a Bruner incision or use of the midaxial approach. If the tendon has migrated proximally into the palm, the pulley system and fibro-osseous canal must be maximally

preserved. The tendon can be passed distally with a pediatric feeding tube as a leader or by "milking" the tendon distally with smooth forceps from the palm just proximal to the level of the A-1 pulley. Distal insertional repair was historically performed with a pullout suture, although suture anchor fixation has gained popularity.[74] More recently, an all inside technique has been

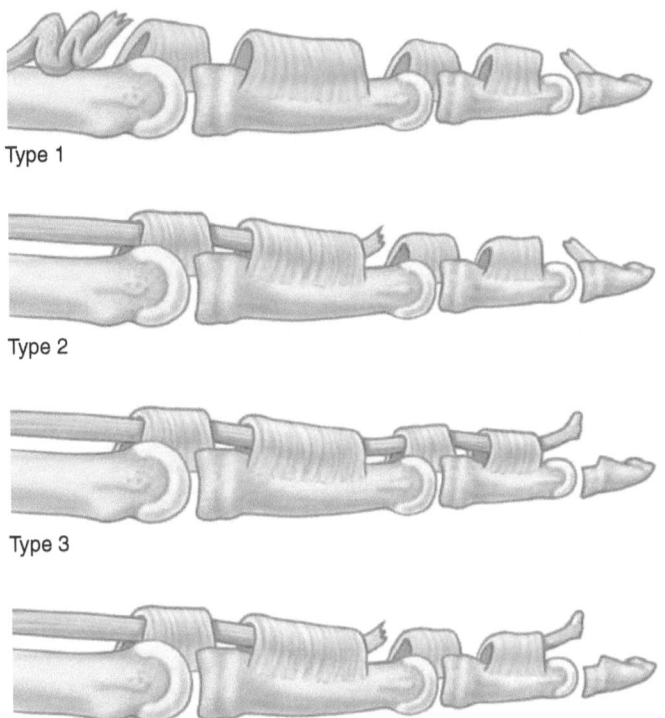

Type 1

Type 2

Type 3

Type 4

Fig. 73.10 Classification of zone 1 flexor digitorum profundus injury.

Fig. 73.12 T2-weighted sagittal image of the long finger after injury demonstrating flexor digitorum profundus rupture with retraction to the A2 pulley.

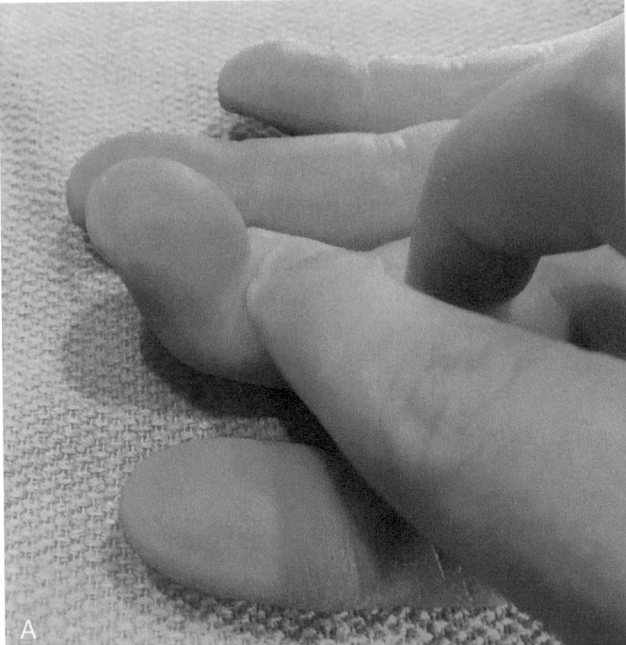

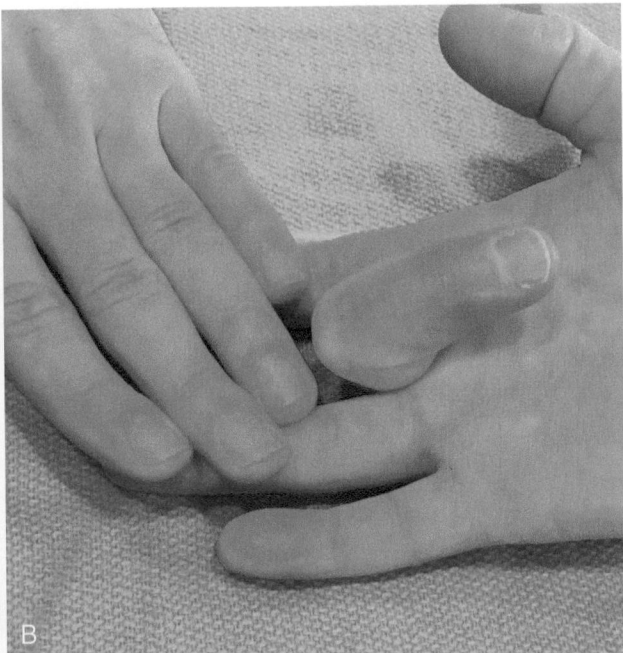

Fig. 73.11 Examination of the (A) flexor digitorum profundus and (B) flexor digitorum superficialis tendons.

described, with the FDP tendon attached to bone with two 3-0 nonabsorbable sutures passed through the phalanx and tied over the dorsal aspect of distal phalanx.[75] There is wide variation in described techniques, none of which have emerged superior.[76] If additional fracture fragments are present, they are fixed with mini screws (Fig. 73.13B) before tendon repair. Utilization of the wide awake local anesthesia—no tourniquet technique allows for intraoperative evaluation of repair and may lead toward increased use of earlier active ROM protocols.[77] After repair, protective dorsal block splinting is provided and a passive Duran flexor tendon protocol is initiated under the supervision of an occupational therapist for the first 4 to 6 weeks. Graduated active flexion is encouraged beginning with place and holds at 2 to 3 weeks. Resistive grasp and return to sports are delayed until 10 to 12 weeks after the repair is made.

Players may not seek immediate treatment for an FDP avulsion injury for a number of reasons. They may believe it is a minor injury that can be treated after the season is over, or they may not want to miss playing for a large part of their season. Informing the player of the long-term consequences of neglecting this injury is imperative, and the need for detailed documentation of conversations with the player cannot be overemphasized. Treating a neglected FDP avulsion is never as satisfying as performing a primary repair, and the clinical results are not nearly as functional. The following treatment options can be considered for a neglected FDP avulsion:

1. Late reinsertion: Late reinsertion is unlikely to be possible if the tendon has retracted a significant amount and the time from injury is beyond 6 weeks.
2. Acute single-stage reconstruction with a tendon graft: This option is fraught with potential complications, including loss of additional ROM (in the PIP joint), scarring, and worsening of FDP function.
3. Two-stage flexor tendon reconstruction: This approach requires a large amount of effort by the patient, surgeon, and therapist and will probably be considered too aggressive a course to regain a small amount of DIP joint flexion. The first stage includes placement of a silicone rod to reconstitute the flexor tendon sheath, followed by exchange for a tendon graft at least 3 months later. A third flexor tenolysis surgery is probable in this treatment course as well.
4. Stabilization of the DIP joint by fusion or capsulodesis: Stabilization is often the most acceptable choice for the patient when risks and benefits are carefully considered.
5. Excision: If a retracted tendon is a tender mass in the palm, simple excision of the scarred proximal tendon end may relieve discomfort with grasping activities.
6. Nonsurgical treatment: Some players choose to do nothing after weighing the pros and cons of the aforementioned possibilities, and the desire to avoid a possible threat to PIP function is not entirely inappropriate.

PULLEY INJURY

The fibro-osseous canal and system of pulleys within the digits were elegantly described by Doyle and Blythe[78] in 1977 (Fig. 73.14). Biomechanically the A-2 and A-4 pulleys are critical for normal flexor tendon function and the prevention of "bowstringing."[79,80] The A-2 pulley overlies the proximal aspect of the proximal phalanx, whereas the A-4 pulley is at the level of the middle phalanx. Attenuation or frank rupture of a digital pulley occurs most often in rock climbers and baseball pitchers[81–83] as a result of acute or chronic exposure to forceful contraction of the FDP tendon against a greater than physiologic load. In "free" rock climbers, the flexed DIP joint incredibly supports body weight repetitively and for prolonged intervals of the activity. The rock climbing hand posture of "crimping" specifically places significant strain on the distal part of the A-2 pulley and may understandably

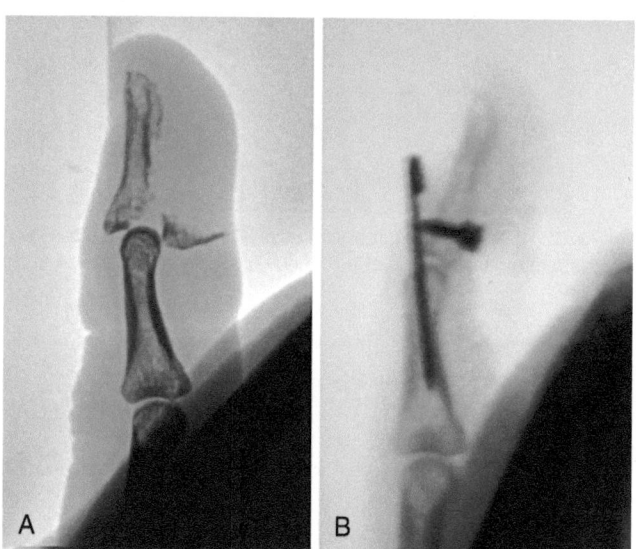

Fig. 73.13 (A) A flexor digitorum profundus avulsion with fracture of the distal phalanx. (B) Fracture fixation and pinning of distal interphalangeal joint subluxation.

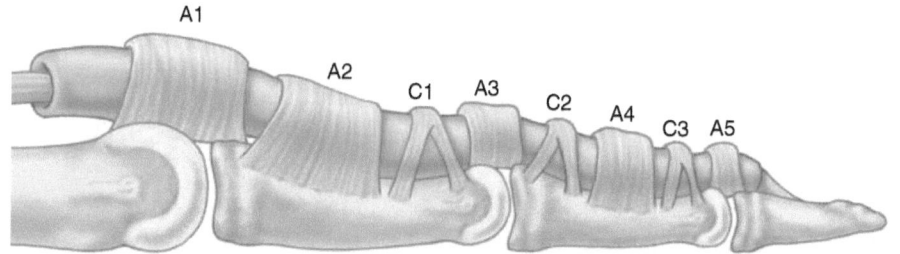

Fig. 73.14 Anatomy of the normal flexor pulley system with associated annular (A) and cruciate (C) pulleys labeled.

result in pulley rupture.[84] Injury to the thumb pulley system is exceedingly rare. The thumb anatomy differs from the digits, with four components consisting of three annular pulleys, the proximal A-1 at the MCP joint, and distal A-2, which attaches to the IP volar plate and the variable annular pulley. Between the variable and distal annular pulleys, the oblique pulley overlies the proximal phalanx.[85] Bowstringing can occur if both the A-1 and oblique pulleys are ruptured.[86]

An athlete may complain of an audible pop or tearing sensation when pulley rupture occurs. On clinical examination, the patient reports pain over the flexor sheath. Swelling over the pulley may be present, and loss of terminal DIP flexion may be noted. Discomfort often occurs with active digit flexion. The athlete may perceive weakness, and pitchers will lose fastball velocity. The spectrum of injury ranges from partial injury of a pulley to complete rupture of multiple pulleys with overt bowstringing of the flexor tendons. Rarely both the A-2 and A-4 pulleys fail simultaneously. MRI can aid in confirming the diagnosis and may show edema within the flexor tendon sheath and tendon bowstringing when the images are obtained with applied digital resistance (Fig. 73.15).[87] Ultrasound may also be utilized to evaluate for pulley rupture, which also allows for dynamic evaluation of the flexor tendon system.[88]

Grading systems for pulley injury have been developed and may help guide treatment.[89] Grade 1 injuries are pulley sprains, and do not require immobilization. Return to sport may be allowed after 4 weeks, with symptoms initially managed with ice and antiinflammatory medications. Complete rupture of the A4 or partial injury of A2 or A3 represent grade 2 injuries and are treated with brief immobilization, symptom management

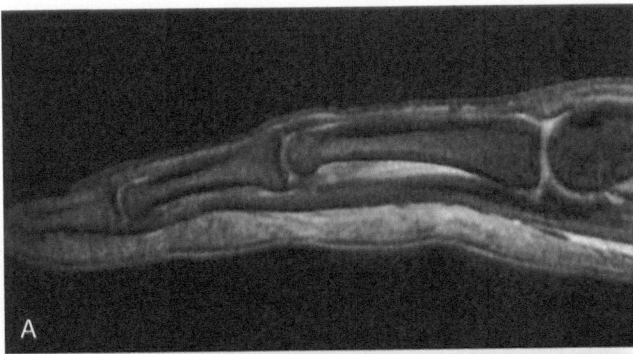

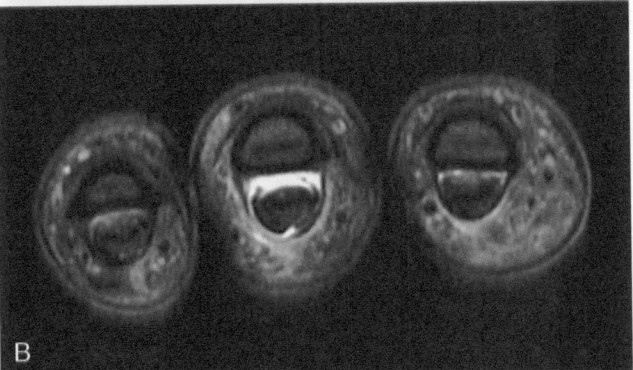

Fig. 73.15 (A) Sagittal proton density fat suppressed and (B) axial T2-weighted magnetic resonance images demonstrating rupture of the A2 pulley with increased bone to tendon distance.

as with grade 1 injuries, pulley support taping, and gentle ROM as edema decreases. Corticosteroid injection is avoided, as it may precipitate pulley rupture and delay healing. Initiation of easy sport specific activities is allowed after 4 weeks.[90] For grade 3 injury with complete rupture of the A-2 and A-3 pulley, an occupational therapist may fashion an external pulley ring for use in addition to support tape to relieve stress on the pulley system. Return to sport is allowed after 6 weeks, with utilization of digit taping in addition to the pulley ring to prevent skin maceration and reduce ring translation.[23,42] Return of complete ROM is frequently delayed. PIP flexion contractures can complicate the postinjury course.

With grade 4 injuries where rupture of the entire pulley system has occurred, loss of motion and bowstringing are evident. This may require surgical reconstruction of the A-2 and/or A-4 pulleys if symptomatic. The principles of reconstruction are to maintain the flexor tendons near the PIP and DIP centers of rotation. Reconstructed pulleys must be sufficiently strong to allow for early mobilization. A tendon autograft (e.g., the palmaris longus, plantaris, or partial flexor digitorum superficialis) or dorsal wrist retinaculum is used to reconstruct the pulleys.[91,92] These may be encircling or nonencircling reconstructions, with looped encircling reconstructions shown to be mechanically superior.[93] We utilize a looped reconstruction with palmaris autograft for most cases. All scar posterior to the tendon is excised. At the A-2 pulley level, the graft is placed beneath the extensor mechanism and then three separate loops envelop the flexor tendons.[94] At the A-4 level, however, the graft is placed over the extensor apparatus with two separate loops. Careful intraoperative tensioning is important, as over tensioning can result in loss of flexion and stiffness, whereas under tensioning can result in failure to improve function. Utilization of wide awake local anesthesia techniques, without tourniquet,[95] can facilitate appropriate tensioning and tendon tracking can be observed intraoperatively with active movement. Postoperatively, passive tendon gliding protocols with place and holds are used, and ring splints help minimize stress to the newly reconstructed pulleys. Full return to sport after reconstruction is delayed for 3 to 6 months, and pulley ring or pulley taping may be necessary for up to 6 months.[92] Reoperation after pulley reconstruction has been reported at 6%, most commonly for tenolysis.[96] Other reported complications include stiffness, flexion contracture, synovitis, ischemia of the phalanx resulting in fracture after encircling techniques, and pulley rerupture.[97,98]

TENDON INJURY COMPLICATIONS

Generally speaking, complications after hand surgery are minimized by careful attention to treatment principles, meticulous surgical technique, and appropriate postoperative rehabilitation. Because small joint stiffness is a pervasive problem throughout the spectrum of hand injury,[99] prolonged immobilization beyond a couple of weeks is usually not recommended. Techniques or strategies to initiate early motion recovery are advocated after most injuries except for specific closed disruptions of the extensor mechanism. Tendon repair can be complicated by adhesion formation, tendon rerupture, joint contracture, and quadriga.

Some of these complications may decrease as wide-awake flexor tendon surgery is popularized and direct dynamic assessment of tension after repair is performed.[77]

Missed injuries have variable consequences. For example, a chronic nonunion of the hamate hook may require nothing more than simple excision once it is detected, with relief of pain and RTP that is typically fast and predictable. On the other hand, mechanical abrasion of the adjacent ulnar-sided digital flexor tendons by the fragment could lead to rupture and the need for surgical reconstruction, which has huge implications with regard to early restrictions, rehabilitation time, and overall recovery of grasping strength. Missing a jersey finger injury has fewer consequences when the proximal tendon end is discovered close to its insertion rather than retracted into the palm.

Postoperative infection after ambulatory hand surgery is rare. In a retrospective review of almost 9000 outpatient hand surgery cases, the overall surgical site infection rate was 0.35%.[100] Prophylactic preincision antibiotics are typically administered only in prolonged cases or when an implant is used. Risk factors for poor wound healing, such as the presence of diabetes mellitus or heavy tobacco use, may also warrant administration of antibiotics.

Masterful knowledge of both normal and aberrant anatomy, as well as careful surgical dissection, is necessary to avoid iatrogenic injury to cutaneous nerve branches found in the hand, which may lead to dysesthesia, formation of a neuroma, failure to progress with rehabilitation, and a potential second surgery in recalcitrant cases. For example, meticulous dorsal dissection during extensor tendon repair is required to prevent injury to the traversing cutaneous nerves. In our experience, this type of close attention to detail may provide the difference between a stiff, painful hand leading to secondary neuroma excision and tenolysis, and a hand that regains nearly immediate full ROM without pain and a prompt return to sport after fracture healing.

FUTURE CONSIDERATIONS

The future of hand surgery as it pertains to the athlete will likely continue to optimize the art of diagnosis, treatment, and rehabilitation to expedite the quickest and safest return to sport. The in-office use of ultrasound techniques by the practicing surgeon has the potential to facilitate the diagnosis of closed tendon injuries, thus avoiding use of expensive MRI scans and possibly altering treatment plans in some circumstances. Emerging technologies will continue to advance surgical fixation methods, some of which may offer a level of strength that allows for early mobilization and swifter RTP. Increased use of wide awake surgery will allow for intraoperative dynamic evaluation of tendon repairs, with immediate correction of any observed gaping. Better treatment methods will only be as good as the rehabilitative protocols that follow, challenging our surgeons and therapists to create strategies that safely accelerate the RTP process.

ACKNOWLEDGMENT

The authors and editors gratefully acknowledge the contributions of the previous authors, Lance M. Brunton, Thomas J. Graham, and Robert E. Atkinson.

For a complete list of references, go to ExpertConsult.com.

SELECTED READINGS

The following collection of articles represents some of the most comprehensive and well-written expert reviews regarding tendon injuries in athletes.

Citation:
Netscher DT, Pham DT, Staines KG. Finger injuries in ball sports. *Hand Clin.* 2017;33:119–139.

Level of Evidence:
V

Citation:
Freilich AM. Evaluation and treatment of jersey finger and pulley injuries in athletes. *Clin Sports Med.* 2015;34:151–166.

Level of Evidence:
V

Citation:
Marino JT, Lourie GM. Boutonnière and pulley rupture in elite athletes. *Hand Clin.* 2012;28:437–445.

Level of Evidence:
V

Citation:
McMurtry JT, Isaacs J. Extensor tendons injuries. *Clin Sports Med.* 2015;34:167–180.

Level of Evidence:
V

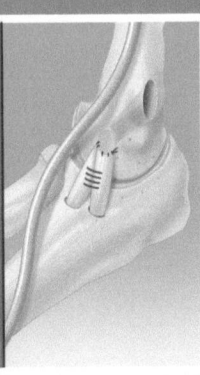

74

Digit Fractures and Dislocations

Christopher L. Stockburger, Ryan P. Calfee

Finger fractures and dislocations can range from minor, self-treated simple proximal interphalangeal joint (PIP) dislocations to some of the most complex and difficult problems in orthopedics. They are some of the most common injuries in various sports, from football to cycling.[1,2] Athletes' significant reliance on their hands for diverse purposes leads to unique challenges in the treatment and rehabilitation of these injuries. Fundamentally, digit fractures and dislocations create a challenge in balancing healing and motion. Both stability and range of motion (ROM) are important for optimal hand function, and balancing surgical intervention and early return to play (RTP) can at times put both at risk.

This chapter focuses on the osseous and soft tissue injuries most commonly encountered by the athletic trainer, general orthopedic surgeon, or sports medicine specialist who is acting as a first responder. Consequently, the most pertinent elements of the history and physical examination, followed by key imaging findings and treatment options, are presented here. Clinical pearls, decision-making principles, and our preferred surgical techniques are interspersed in keeping with the format of this textbook.

LIGAMENTOUS INJURIES AND DISLOCATIONS

A dislocation of the carpometacarpal (CMC), metacarpophalangeal (MCP), or interphalangeal (IP) joint is a frequently encountered sports injury. The hand is the second most common site of dislocation injury, second only to the shoulder.[3] Awkward falls, contact with other competitors, or entanglement with equipment explain many of these incidents. Dislocations may occur from either hyperextension or hyperflexion forces, often combined with torsional and/or axial stress, the result of which dictates the direction of maximal displacement. IP joint dislocations are most often amenable to closed reduction (with the exception of rotatory dislocation of the proximal IP joint), whereas MCP and CMC dislocations are more frequently irreducible and require surgical treatment.

Metacarpophalangeal Joint

Collateral ligament injuries of the digit are much less common than those that occur at the thumb MCP joint (see the section on thumb injuries later in this chapter). Hyperabduction injuries usually occur in an ulnar direction when the finger is flexed and the ligament is taut, and hence the radial collateral ligaments (RCL) of the three ulnar-most digits are most at risk.[3] Most

hyperabduction injuries are partial injuries (grade I or II sprains) that may be treated with early active ROM and "buddy taping" to the adjacent finger for comfort. A radiograph should be obtained for all suspected collateral ligament injuries to assess for avulsion fractures. In a complete (grade III) tear, avulsion fractures may be evident, and the joint is often unstable in the coronal plane. Testing of the affected collateral ligament is performed with the MCP in flexion as that position places the collateral ligaments on maximal tension. If the joint is mechanically unstable or if an avulsion fragment displaces a substantial amount of the articular surface, an open repair is preferred. In pure ligamentous injuries or in those avulsion fractures with extremely small pieces of bone, a suture anchor works well for fixation. If the fracture fragment is large enough, we prefer to use Kirschner wires or mini fragment screw fixation (Fig. 74.1A and B). The avulsed fragment is on the volar half of the proximal phalanx, but we prefer a dorsal approach, as it provides excellent visualization of the entire articular surface. Immobilization of the joint in flexion (intrinsic plus or "safe" position) prevents the development of an extension contracture. For chronic tears presenting in a delayed fashion with pain and instability, temporary pinning of the MCP joint in flexion may be indicated for 2 to 3 weeks, with active motion begun thereafter. Proper diagnosis and treatment at the time of injury in important, because there is evidence that surgical repair of chronic grade III tears have inferior outcomes.[4]

Although MCP dislocations may occur in any digit, the index and small fingers are most vulnerable as border digits. Volar MCP dislocations are relatively rare.[5] Dorsal MCP dislocations are classified as simple (easily reduced) or complex (irreducible by closed reduction). Simple dislocations present with the MCP hyperextended between 70 and 90 degrees (Fig. 74.2). The reduction maneuver combines gentle flexion, slight traction, and a volarly directed pressure at the base of the proximal phalanx (Fig. 74.3). Complex dislocations are often characterized by interposition of the volar plate between the articular surfaces, rendering them irreducible by closed means (Fig. 74.4). The lumbrical muscle is tethered around the radial side of the metacarpal head, and the flexor tendons loop around its ulnar side. Simple traction will only tighten this interval and prevent reduction. Dimpling of the palmar skin around the metacarpal head is one sign of an irreducible dislocation. Sesamoid bones may also be interposed in the index or small finger MCPs.[6] Postero-anterior radiographs may show joint space narrowing or even bayonet apposition. A Brewerton view, taken with the forearm

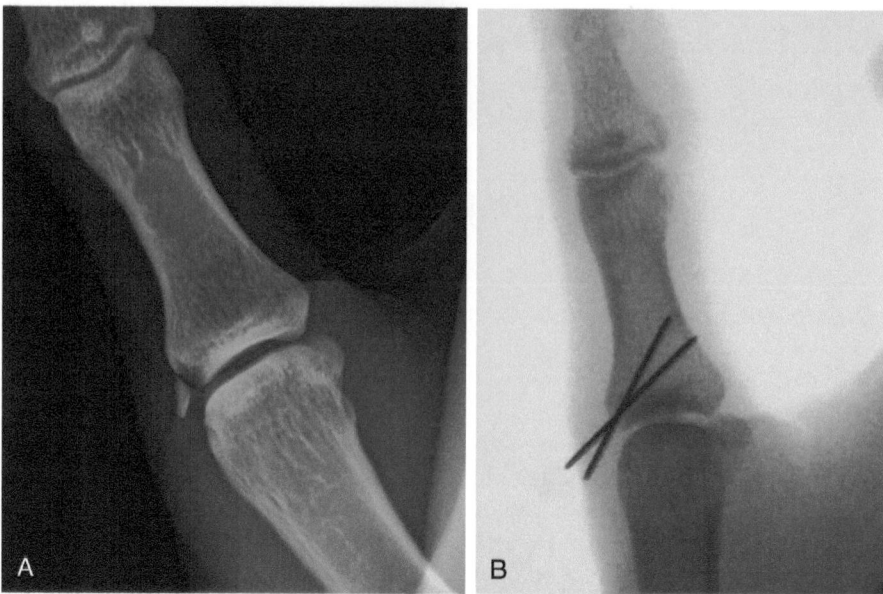

Fig. 74.1 Anteroposterior x-ray of thumb from a 31-year-old patient who fell on the radial thumb. Avulsion fracture with malrotation (A). This fracture fragment was reduced with an open approach and fixed with diverging Kirschner wires (B).

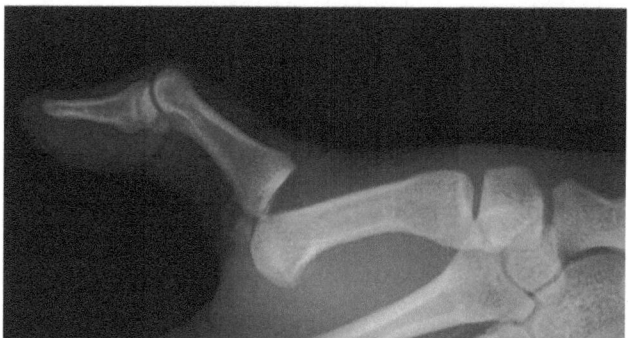

Fig. 74.2 Sesamoids and the attached volar plate perched at the dorsal metacarpal head.

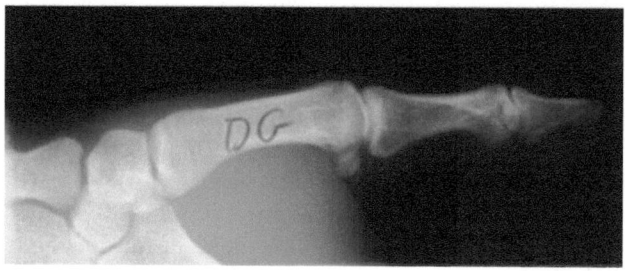

Fig. 74.3 Reduction of the metacarpophalangeal joint with the volar plate in its normal position.

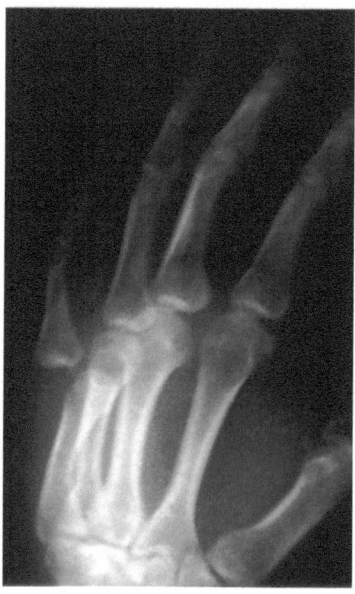

Fig. 74.4 Parallel alignment of the metacarpal and proximal phalanx (a complex metacarpophalangeal dislocation).

supinated and the MCP joints against the x-ray plate, may show an associated metacarpal head fracture.[7]

Every athlete deserves an attempt at closed reduction for a dislocated MCP joint. Although performing immediate reduction "on the field" is tempting, this procedure is best performed with adequate anesthesia and patient comfort. Attempts at longitudinal distraction or exaggeration of the hyperextension deformity risk converting a reducible subluxation into an irreducible dislocation

by permitting the volar plate to fall dorsally between the metacarpal head and the base of the proximal phalanx. If the joint is successfully reduced with digit flexion and volarly directed pressure at the base of the proximal phalanx, a dorsal blocking splint may be applied, preventing hyperextension beyond neutral. Early active motion is started under the supervision of a therapist within 1 week.

When an attempt to perform a closed reduction is unsuccessful, we prefer to use a dorsal approach to perform an open reduction.[8] In this approach, the dorsal capsule is opened, and the interposed volar plate is longitudinally split down its midline to achieve reduction. The dorsal approach also provides excellent access for fixation of the occasional osteochondral shear fracture of the metacarpal head. Volar approaches are also reasonable but require vigilance when dissecting around malpositioned digital nerves. In particular, the radial digital nerve is displaced centrally and superficially by index MCP dislocations, and the ulnar digital nerve is displaced by small MCP dislocations. Care must be taken immediately after skin incision if this approach is chosen. Alternatively, a percutaneous approach to reducing complex dislocations has been reported.[9] Return to sports is guided by return of ROM and comfort level, because chronic instability of this joint is unlikely. Long-term follow-up of complex MCP dislocations has shown good outcomes if the injury is treated appropriately.[10] An early return to sports (within 1 to 2 weeks) is possible with buddy taping and the use of a protective customized orthosis for athletes who participate in contact sports.

Proximal Interphalangeal Joint

Many athletes are subject to injuries of the soft tissue stabilizers of the proximal interphalangeal (PIP) joint over the course of their careers. Pure hyperextension forces produce volar plate injuries, whereas hyperflexion forces may disrupt the central slip of the extensor tendon. The collateral ligaments are susceptible to torsional and angular stresses (Fig. 74.5).[11] Frequently the athlete relates a history of "jamming" the finger. When additional energy is imparted to the digit(s), simple sprains may escalate to disabling complex fractures/dislocations.

The athlete's account of the injury may provide verbal or even visual clues as to "which way the finger went." If stated definitively, the pathoanatomy is almost instantly determined. When the patient cannot recall the sequence of events leading to the injury, the physical examination is paramount. After radiographic evaluation, the examiner must try to discern the area of maximal tenderness—dorsal, volar, radial, or ulnar—which is easiest for injuries of the mildest form. As the severity increases, it becomes more difficult to characterize the injury, especially in the acute phase when swelling and sensitivity to manipulation are heightened. Any deformity in the resting position is noted. Reproduction of the mechanism of injury will be uncomfortable. ROM is often limited by pain at first presentation and is not predictive of a certain pathology.

A central slip injury or avulsion should be suspected in all PIP injuries for which the athlete has predominantly dorsal tenderness. Three tests can be performed to ensure that the central slip is still attached to the dorsal base of the middle phalanx. First, "tenodesis extension" of the PIP joint is checked with the MCP joint in full flexion. The PIP joint should passively extend to within 15 degrees of full extension. Next, passively extend the PIP joint and ask the patient to flex the distal interphalangeal (DIP) joint. Inability to flex this joint implies retraction of a ruptured central slip, with extension forces concentrated at the DIP joint through the lateral bands. Finally, perform the Elson test by flexing the PIP joint to 90 degrees. If the DIP joint becomes rigid to passive flexion as the digit is actively extended, then the central slip is ruptured and extension is occurring through the lateral bands.[12,13] Although difficult to perform very early after injury in the setting of substantial pain, we prefer the Elson test to diagnose these extensor tendon avulsions.

Mild PIP joint hyperextension injuries produce partial injury to the volar plate and on examination are stable with both active and passive extension. Treatment involves buddy taping for 3 to 4 weeks, with Coban elastic wrap used carefully at night to decrease edema. Patients must be instructed on how to safely apply Coban to prevent compromising blood flow secondary to excessively tight compression. Isolated collateral ligament sprains are treated similarly. Flexion contractures notoriously develop after mild hyperextension injuries and small volar plate bony avulsions from the base of the middle phalanx, which are seen best on perfect lateral radiographs of the digit (Fig. 74.6). These contractures are correctly termed "pseudoboutonnière" deformity, where the presenting flexion deformity at the PIP joint could be mistaken for the resultant posture after a central slip injury.[14] However, careful inspection fails to reveal obligate DIP hyperextension (restricting passive DIP flexion) that accompanies disruption of the central slip, and the Elson test is negative.

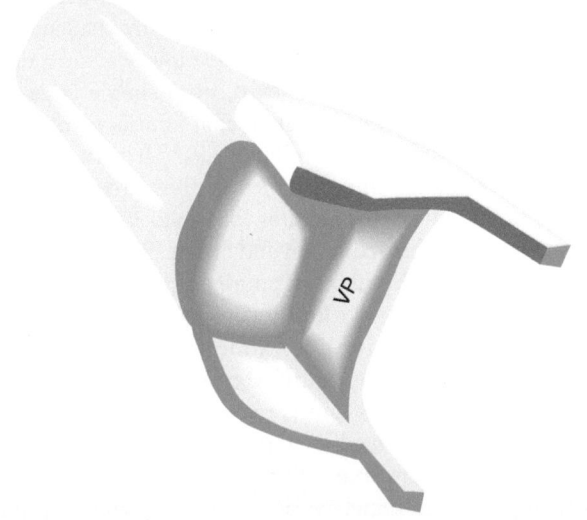

Fig. 74.5 Eaton's three-sided box depiction of the proximal interphalangeal joint. *VP,* Volar plate.

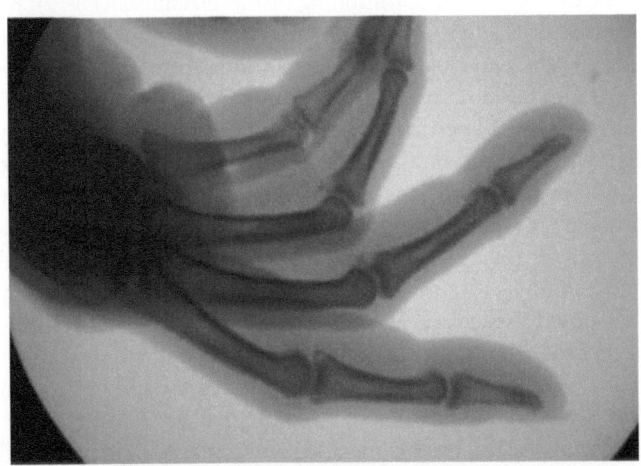

Fig. 74.6 Lateral x-ray demonstrating volar plate avulsion fractures from the index, long, and ring fingers in a 41-year-old female after falling from standing.

Therefore aggressive early motion recovery is the mainstay of treatment of volar plate sprains at the PIP joint. Static progressive or dynamic extension splinting may be necessary in recalcitrant cases of PIP flexion contracture. Patients should be counseled on the persistent discomfort and swelling that can last for upwards of 9 months with these seemingly innocuous injuries. At least to some degree, residual loss of motion is common.

PIP dislocations are often self-diagnosed and self-treated. Delayed presentation is frequent when self-relocation is successful, because many athletes do not question the persistent pain and swelling of the joint until sometimes weeks or even months after the incident. Most PIP dislocations are closed injuries, but open dislocations are *not* uncommon and require appropriate irrigation and débridement. Open PIP dislocations have occurred in soccer goalkeepers, softball players, and martial arts experts.[15]

When a dorsal PIP dislocation occurs, the volar plate and collaterals are injured, but the articular surfaces of the joint are still in congruent contact upon reduction. Stable reductions are treated with buddy taping and early ROM. When the joint has a tendency to hyperextend, possibly as a result of baseline PIP volar plate laxity, a splint is fashioned to sit dorsally and keep the joint partially flexed (i.e., a dorsal block splint). In the setting of any instability, we recommend determining the flexion necessary to keep the joint concentrically reduced before fashioning an orthosis to maintain the joint in 10 to 20 degrees of flexion greater than the degree at which the joint subluxates (Fig. 74.7). Even simple dislocations are quite painful, and the athlete will need to work continuously with his or her trainer or occupational therapist to regain full flexion within the first 3 weeks after injury. At 3 weeks, active extension is emphasized to combat the development of flexion contractures, with use of a resting/nighttime splint in full PIP extension. If a flexion contracture remains 5 weeks after injury, dynamic PIP extension splinting should be prescribed. An accelerated return to certain sports is possible within 7 to 14 days, depending on the degree of pain, swelling, and improvement in digital motion combined with the anticipated demands of the particular sport.

Complex PIP dislocations may present with displaced articular surfaces and bayonet positioning of the phalanges (Fig. 74.8). Rupture of the volar skin can occur from an inside-to-outside mechanism, and residual stiffness is more common after treatment.[16] In the absence of a large accompanying fracture, a closed reduction with anesthesia from a digital block is attempted by gently pushing the middle phalanx (P-2) over the articular surface of the proximal phalanx (P-1). Soft tissues occasionally may become entrapped, necessitating an open reduction through a dorsal approach. The dorsal surgical approach splits the interval between the central slip and the lateral band on one side. Any interposed tissue is extracted and the joint is reduced. Stability is checked after the reduction is performed, and a dorsal splint that blocks terminal extension is fabricated for use in the first 2 to 3 weeks, with the PIP joint in approximately 20 to 30 degrees of flexion. Again, residual flexion contracture is a concern, and active extension is emphasized by 3 weeks. Return to sports, especially if contact is anticipated, is delayed for 3 to 4 weeks with these more severe injuries. Buddy taping or a protective

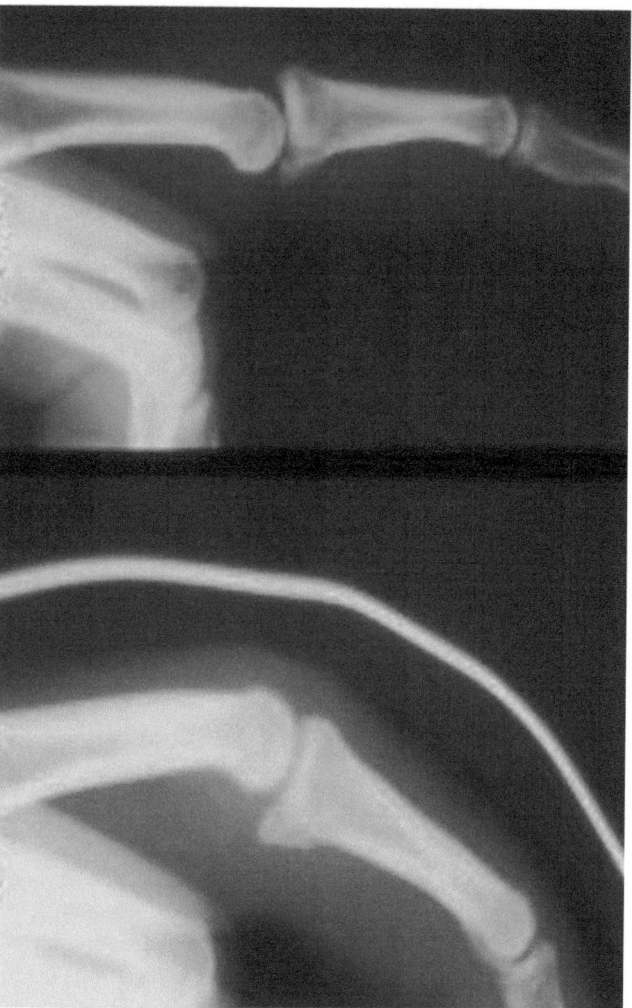

Fig. 74.7 Lateral x-rays demonstrating dorsal subluxation after reduction of dislocation *(upper image)* and restoration of a congruent proximal interphalangeal joint after increased flexion *(lower image)*.

orthosis is recommended during the respective sporting activity until 6 weeks after injury or until nearly full motion is achieved.

Dislocations associated with significant volar fracture fragments at the base of P-2 are almost uniformly challenging to treat. Various authors have classified these injuries, and a variety of fracture configurations may exist, from simple large volar fragments to complex comminuted pilon injuries involving the entire articular surface of P-2 (Fig. 74.9).[17] It may be helpful initially to categorize these injuries by the percentage of the articular surface involved. Fractures with up to 30% involvement are usually stable after reduction and can be treated with dorsal block splinting or a dorsal block pinning with a K wire inserted into the head of P-1, under fluoroscopic guidance, to block the last 30 degrees of extension. Ideally the K wire is placed slightly eccentrically between the central slip and lateral band of the extensor mechanism. The pin is removed at 3 to 6 weeks, but active flexion is encouraged starting immediately after surgery.[18] In our experience, the amount of motion performed with the K wire in place is extremely variable between patients. Injuries involving the "gray zone" of 30% to 50% of the joint surface are potentially unstable, and care is dictated by the degree of

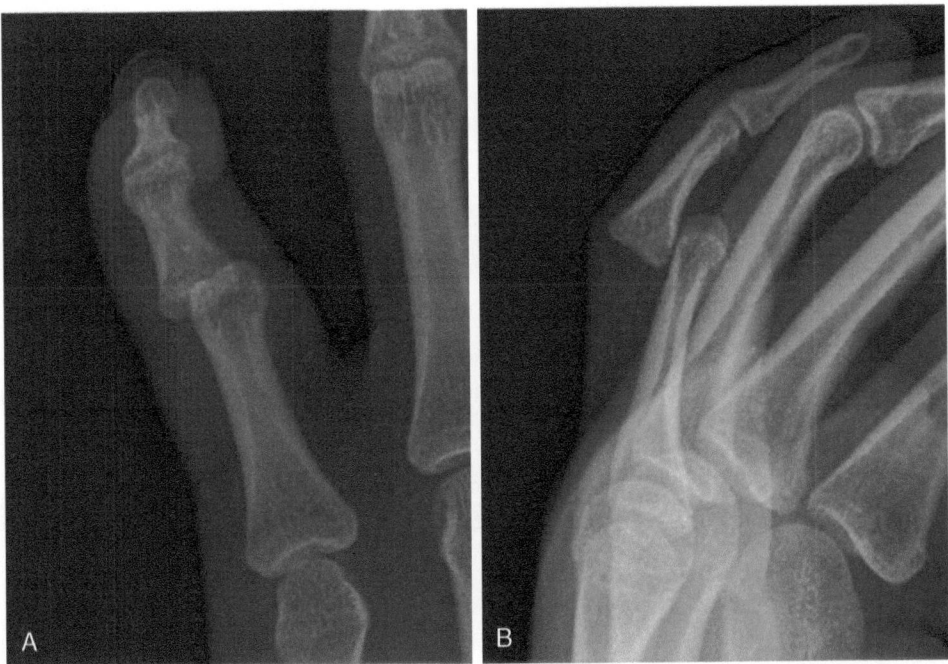

Fig. 74.8 The phalanges shown in the bayonet position on anteroposterior x-ray (A) and on lateral x-ray (B).

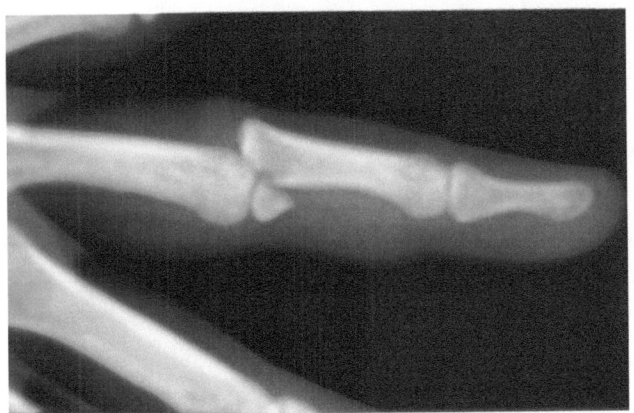

Fig. 74.9 Dorsal subluxation of the proximal interphalangeal joint with an impacted fracture at the base of the middle phalanx (P-2).

instability. Fractures with involvement of more than 50% of the joint surface are consistently unstable and require surgical intervention. These joints will not remain reduced in a splint, as there is no volar bony buttress for the joint and all collateral ligament insertion is on the fracture fragment(s). Generally speaking, if a stable closed reduction cannot be obtained with 45 degrees of flexion, operative fixation is indicated.

If the volar fragments are large, direct fixation may be attempted with mini screws (Fig. 74.10) or K wires (Fig. 74.11) through a formal volar approach.[19] For the open approach, a Bruner or curvilinear incision is made and the flexor tendon sheath is opened between the A-2 and A-4 pulleys to retract the tendons for exposure to the joint. The volar fragments are reduced and held with 1.3- or 1.5-mm screws (Fig. 74.12). This procedure is technically demanding, and most patients will have some degree of permanent PIP stiffness. A percutaneous technique has been

described recently in a small case series.[20] If the volar fragments are comminuted, open reduction may be bypassed for external fixation, either statically or with dynamic traction.[21] Badia and associates[22] described a modification of a traction technique that was originally reported by Gaul and Rosenberg (Fig. 74.13).[23] Once the fixator is applied, a limited open reduction can be effected through a midaxial approach to elevate any articular fragments not reduced by the traction device.

It is surprising how many athletes ignore an injured, stiff PIP joint. When a PIP fracture/subluxation or fracture/dislocation is chronic (i.e., older than 4 weeks), a reconstructive procedure may be the only remaining option to improve PIP function. Although a detailed description is beyond the scope of this chapter, both volar plate arthroplasty[24,25] and hemihamate arthroplasty for reconstruction of the base of P-2 are effective options.[26] The hemihamate reconstruction is preferred in young active patients with a neglected PIP fracture/dislocation because it comes closest to restoring normal anatomy (Fig. 74.14). Volar plate arthroplasty is where the volar plate is advanced into the articular defect at the base of the middle phalanx and is effectively used as a checkrein to avoid dorsal PIP joint instability. It may lead to increased risk of flexion contracture and is not our preferred procedure.[27]

Volar dislocations of the PIP joint are rare but must not be missed,[28,29] because treating them after a delayed presentation results in suboptimal function. An avulsion of the central slip occurs with volar dislocations. Closed reduction of most acute volar dislocations is successful, and the central slip avulsion is allowed to heal with the PIP joint splinted in full extension for approximately 6 weeks. The DIP joint is kept free for maintenance of active flexion during this phase. Encouraging DIP flexion maximizes DIP motion but more importantly pulls the central slip distally and keeps the lateral bands more dorsal while the PIP is immobilized. After 6 weeks, active PIP flexion is initiated

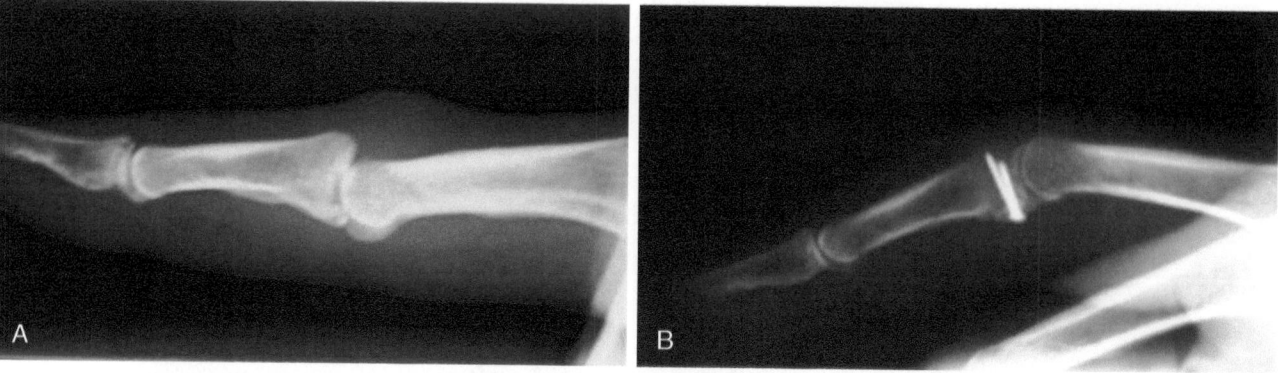

Fig. 74.10 (A) An impacted proximal interphalangeal (PIP) articular surface with joint subluxation. (B) Reduction of PIP joint alignment and fixation of volar articular fragments with 1-mm screws.

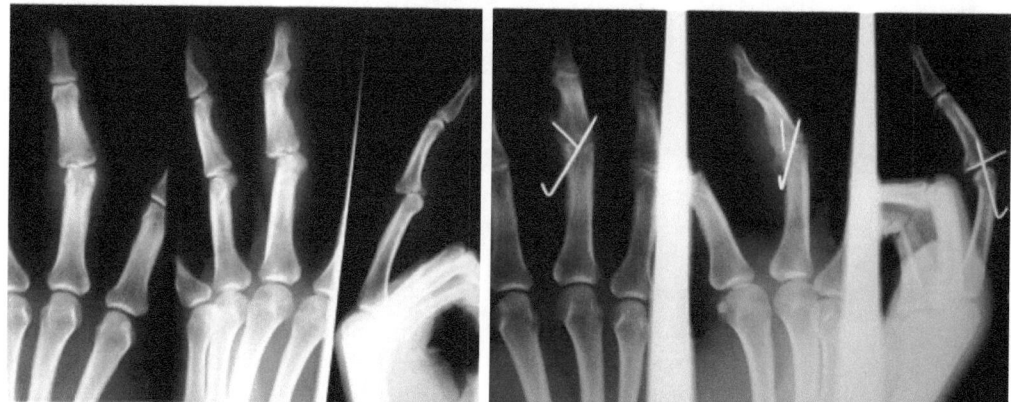

Fig. 74.11 Proximal interphalangeal joint fracture/subluxation *(left)* treated with static pinning, with restoration of the joint surface *(right)*.

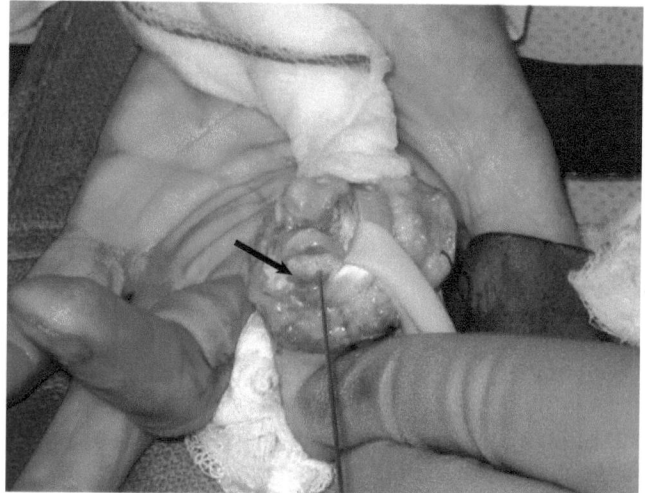

Fig. 74.12 The volar approach for fixation of a middle phalanx (P-2) volar lip and pilon fracture. The *arrow* points to the volar fragment.

and a nighttime static PIP extension splint and/or daytime dynamic extension splint is used for an additional 6 weeks.

An open dorsal approach is used for repair of volar PIP dislocations with avulsion fractures of the central slip attachment or central slip avulsion. A tension band technique is used with 26-gauge wire, a mini fragment (1.0- or 1.3-mm) screw, or a

suture anchor (Fig. 74.15). We would typically supplement any central slip repair with transarticular pinning for 6 weeks. Rehabilitation entails protecting the dorsal central slip insertion for at least 6 weeks. Return to sports is variable after this injury. If the sport involves minimal finger force or motion, then early return in an orthosis is possible. If finger flexion is necessary, then return to sport is not considered in the first 6 weeks and likely will be difficult for up to 3 months as the athlete works to restore motion.

Distal Interphalangeal Joint or Thumb Interphalangeal Joint

Dislocations of the DIP joints of the fingers and the IP joint of the thumb are less common than PIP joint dislocations. This phenomenon is explained by the short lever arm of the distal bony segment, highly congruous articular surfaces, and tight-fitting collaterals inserting at the lateral tubercles of the distal phalanx base (P-3 of the digit and technically P-2 of the thumb). Dislocations of the terminal phalanx occur dorsally or laterally and are often associated with open wounds. Concomitant fractures and injuries to the flexor and extensor tendon insertions must be considered.

Once radiographs are performed to assess for an accompanying fracture, a closed dislocation is readily reduced with use of digital block anesthesia. The reduction is performed with traction

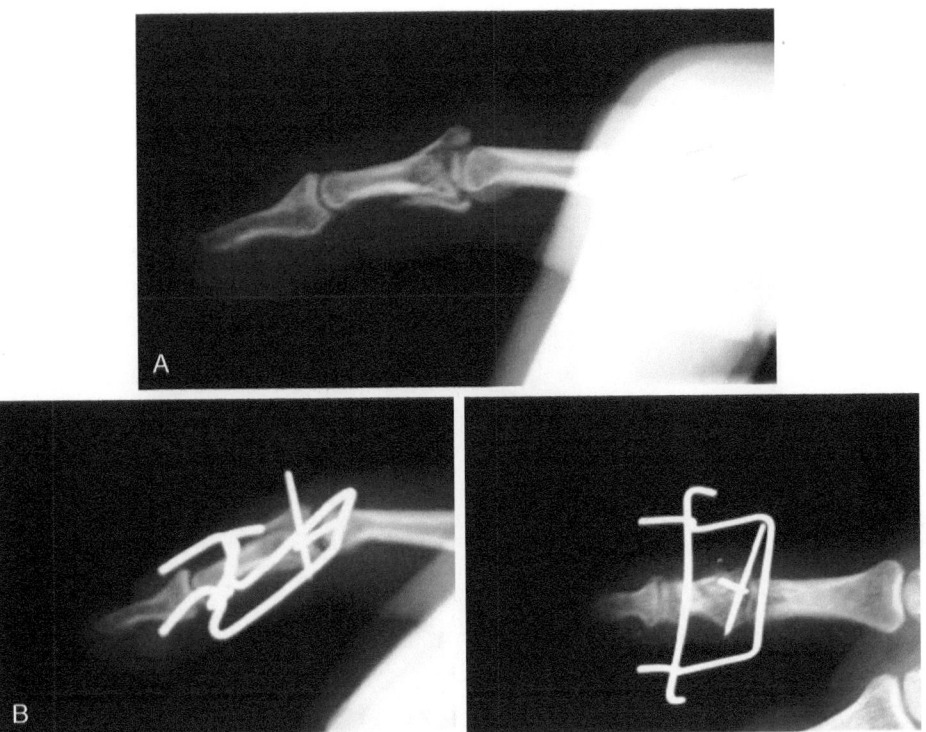

Fig. 74.13 (A) A proximal interphalangeal joint pilon fracture with comminution. (B) Reduction of the joint surface with K wires and a traction device (the Rosenburg technique).

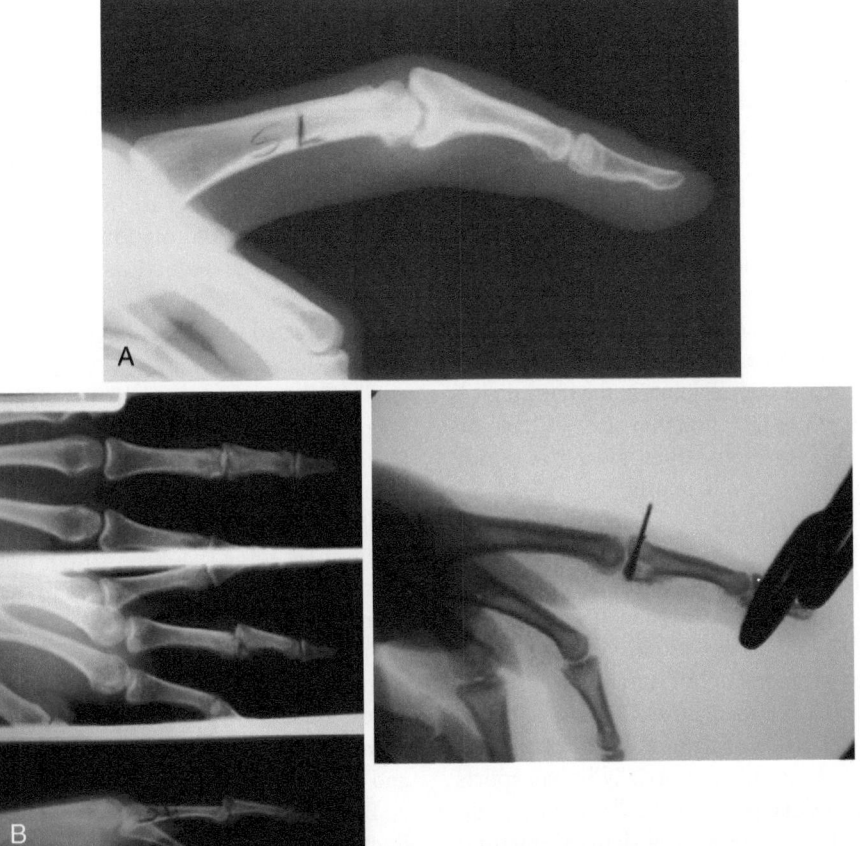

Fig. 74.14 (A) A neglected proximal interphalangeal joint fracture/subluxation with resulting degenerative changes. (B) A chronic dorsal fracture/subluxation may be treated with hemihamate arthroplasty.

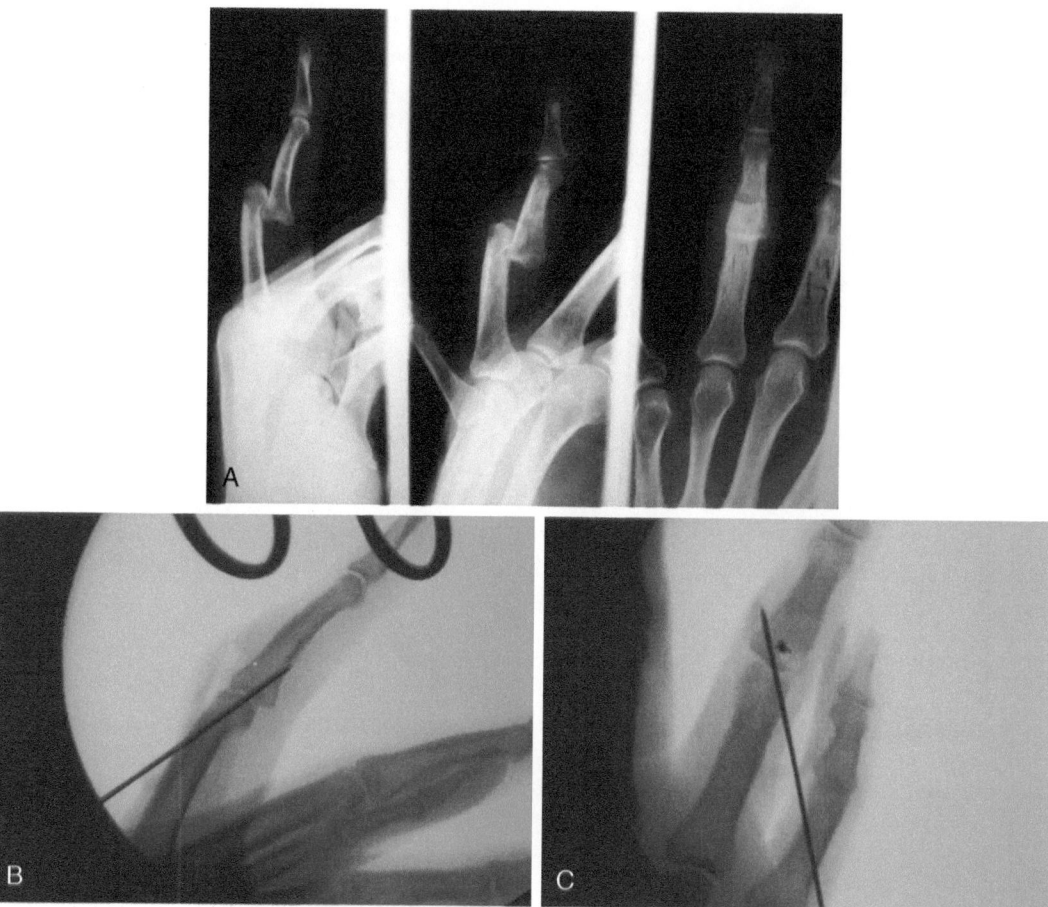

Fig. 74.15 (A) A rare volar proximal interphalangeal (PIP) joint dislocation. (B) A reduced volar PIP dislocation. (C) A central slip avulsion fixed with a suture anchor.

and a dorsal to volar pressure is applied to the dorsal aspect of P-3 (or P-2 of the thumb). Stability is checked after the reduction is performed, and the digit initially is splinted in slight flexion. Active motion can begin after 5 to 7 days, with a block to terminal extension at about 20 degrees.[28] Dorsal block splinting can be removed altogether by 3 weeks. Open injuries require irrigation and débridement in a sterile setting. Irreducible dislocations have been reported but are rare.[30,31] Also seldom reported are simultaneous dislocations of both IP joints in the same digit.[32] Checking flexor and extensor tendon function after a successful closed reduction is critical. Low-profile splinting and/or buddy taping may allow for an early return to sports.

Phalangeal Fractures

Open fractures at the phalanges are much more common than open injuries at the metacarpal level. Associated injuries to neurovascular bundles and tendons, as well as the condition of the soft tissue envelope, have a great deal of influence on the patient's ultimate recovery after phalangeal fractures.[33] While at times early RTP can be safe and effective, phalangeal fractures can lead to prolonged time out of competition, especially in ball sports requiring both hands for optimal performance.[34,35] In one study, the worst functional results were seen in phalangeal fractures associated with tendon injuries.[36] This information can help the treating physician counsel the athlete with an open phalangeal

fracture or a fracture associated with a tendon disruption. As a general rule of thumb, the more tissue types (e.g., bone, tendon, nerve, artery, skin) that are injured, the worse the outcome after that digit injury. Malrotation of P-1 fractures is common and necessitates open reduction and internal fixation (ORIF) to ameliorate finger "scissoring" or "splaying." Comminuted fractures are best treated with percutaneous pinning (Fig. 74.16) or even, rarely, external fixation.

The extensor apparatus is closely applied to the dorsal and lateral surfaces of P-1 and P-2. Either interference with this gliding structure or shortening of the dorsal apparatus can cause loss of motion at the IP joints. Shortening of proximal phalangeal fractures relatively lengthens the dorsal apparatus and causes an extensor lag at the IP joints without restriction in passive extension.[37] The PIP joint is spherical in the sagittal plane, and collateral ligaments on each side of the PIP joint do not shorten with PIP motion. As opposed to the MCP joints, the safe position of immobilization for the PIP joint is in full extension. The volar plate is also sensitive to injury, immobilization, and posttraumatic edema. Contracture of the volar plate leads to PIP joint stiffness and a flexion contracture.

Because soft tissue injuries frequently accompany phalangeal fractures, an accurate assessment on physical examination is important. Injured structures are repaired at the time of fracture fixation, and the postoperative regimen is adjusted accordingly.

Proper digit rotation is indicated by parallel nail plates in extension and flexion, although malrotation is generally more readily appreciated in flexion toward a composite fist. Among numerous possible phalangeal fracture patterns, we discuss the specific treatment of spiral oblique shaft fractures and unstable transverse metaphyseal fractures in this chapter.

Torsional injuries are common in all sports and often result in oblique fractures of P-1 (Fig. 74.17A). Displaced, shortened, and malrotated oblique fractures are all indications for operative fixation. Techniques that are minimally invasive yet afford maximal strength are ideally suited for earlier RTP in high-demand athletes who sustain fractures that require operative reduction.[38] ORIF with lag screws is recommended when the fracture length is at least twice as long as the bone diameter. Minimal operative disruption of the extensor apparatus is critical to accelerate postoperative recovery. Sometimes one "wing" of the lateral bands needs to be resected to allow reduction and fixation. Lag screws of 1.3-, 1.5-, or 2.0-mm diameter are used, based on fracture length and bone morphology (see Fig. 74.17B). If bone loss or comminution is present, a plate and screw constructs are considered.[39,40] Operative fluoroscopy is necessary to document reduction and appropriate screw lengths. When used properly with the injured hand positioned against the image intensifier, a mini fluoroscopy unit offers the advantage of limited radiation exposure and is preferred by most hand specialists.

Transverse metaphyseal fractures of the proximal phalanx are notoriously unstable, especially if significant displacement was evident on injury films (Fig. 74.18A). Comminution and complex injuries may require either mini plate fixation (see Fig. 74.18B) or external fixation. Preferential positioning of the plate (1.5 or 2.0 mm) laterally potentially reduces extensor tendon adhesions and may maximize recovery of ROM.[41,42] We have also preferred to close periosteum over hardware when possible. Simple angulated fractures (Fig. 74.19A and B) may be treated with closed reduction and percutaneous fixation by crossing two pins (0.045 inch) across the fracture site starting from each lateral tubercle of the proximal phalanx base.[43] Neither the MCP nor PIP joints are violated by this fixation strategy (see Fig. 74.19C). Pins are removed at 3 weeks, but some MCP and PIP motion can begin before pin removal depending on patient comfort, compliance, and soft tissue envelope. More recently some practitioners have had success with minimally invasive cannulated headless compression screws for transverse fractures of phalanges.[44]

In general, many athletes can RTP immediately or within a month of a stable, nonoperative metacarpal or phalangeal fracture. Morse et al. documented the RTP in National Basketball

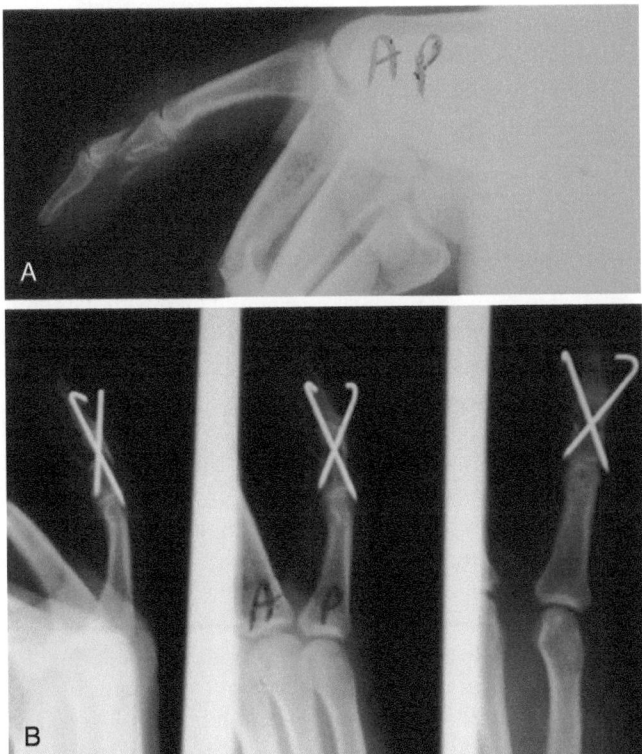

Fig. 74.16 (A) A comminuted middle phalanx (P-2) fracture. (B) Crossed pinning of a P-2 fracture with the proximal interphalangeal joint free.

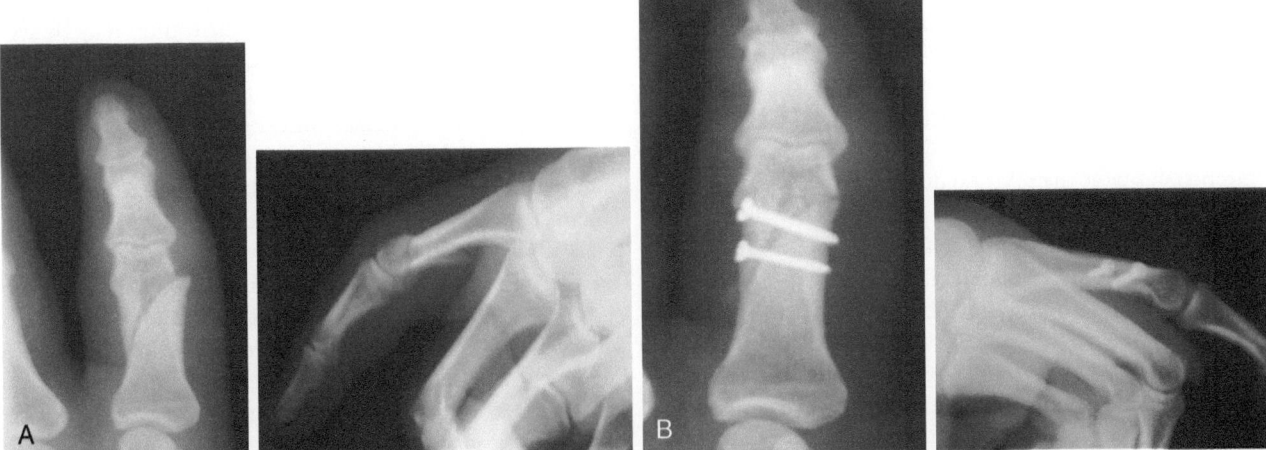

Fig. 74.17 (A) An oblique proximal phalanx (P-1) fracture. (B) Open reduction and internal fixation of a P-1 fracture with lag screws.

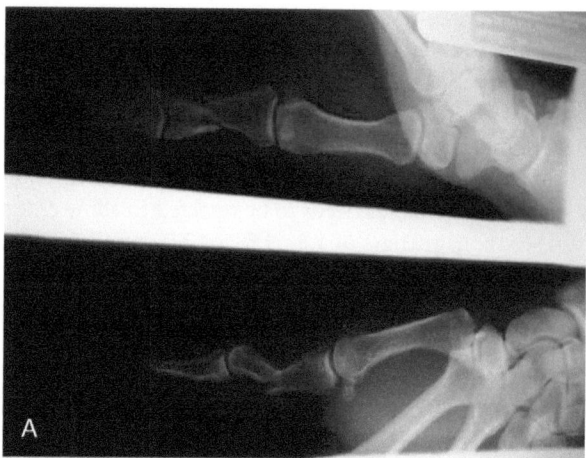
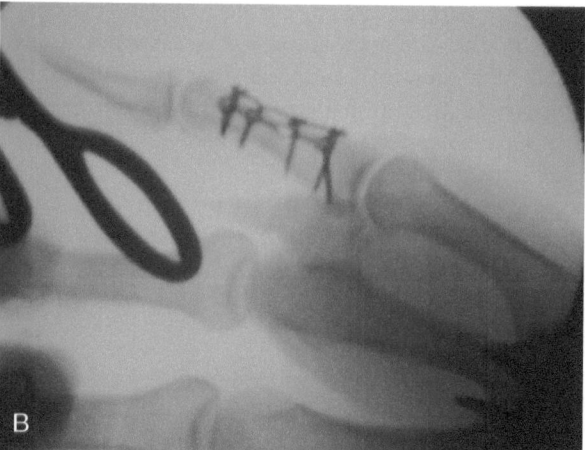

Fig. 74.18 (A) An angulated thumb proximal phalanx (P-1) fracture. (B) Open reduction and internal fixation of a P-1 fracture with a 1.5-mm ladder plate.

Association (NBA) basketball players with hand injuries and showed that nonoperative phalangeal fractures were out an average of 33 days, while operative metacarpal fractures were out the longest for hand fractures with an average of 57 days.[35] In sports where dexterity is less crucial than basketball, bracing and buddy taping can allow for earlier RTP. Experienced hand therapists can design custom-molded orthoses that adequately protect hand injuries yet allow for speedier return to participation in the athlete's specific activity. Clearly certain activities such as weight lifting or extreme contact sports may require a longer period of protection to prevent reinjury.

OSSEOUS AND SOFT TISSUE INJURIES OF THE THUMB

Athletes and physicians alike are familiar with the thumb's crucially important role in hand function and sports activities. Whether the athlete is handling a ball, pole vaulting, handling a stick, or checking the reins, the function of the opposable thumb is indispensable for the interaction of the athlete with his or her competitive environment. Essential functions of large-object (cylindrical) grasp, key, and tip pinch are dependent on normal thumb stability, mobility, sensibility, and length. The thumb is frequently injured because of its location out of the plane of the palm and its involvement in the most demanding of tasks. Thumb injuries are particularly prevalent in men's lacrosse compared with other sports involving a stick and glove.[45]

Thumb stability at the CMC and MCP joints is crucial for opposing the thumb in pinching and grasping. Stout dorsal and palmar ligaments at the CMC level and collateral ligaments at the MCP level maintain normal stability.[46] The thumb's unique osseous structure, with a specialized basilar joint, along with its at-risk position, lead to unique injury patterns. The MCP joint is particularly susceptible, and collateral ligaments are frequently compromised. Torn or chronically incompetent ligaments at either level lead to weakness, degenerative joint disease, and painful dysfunction. In this section, we review injuries of the thumb.

Metacarpophalangeal Dislocation

The MCP joint of the thumb is an ellipsoid joint with the elliptical articular surface of the proximal phalanx moving over a convex metacarpal head. The morphology of the thumb metacarpal head is disparate from its shape at the digits; it is wider dorsally and flatter in the frontal plane. ROM in the thumb MCP joint varies widely, which is attributed to differences in the curvature of the metacarpal head among individuals. Spherical metacarpal heads are associated with more motion (greater flexion). Accordingly, ROM may vary from 10 to 90 degrees of flexion. The metacarpal head is surrounded on three sides by strong stabilizers. The ulnar and RCLs provide lateral support, and the volar plate prevents hyperextension. The most common thumb MCP dislocation occurs dorsally. A hyperextension force produces disruption of the volar plate, while the collateral ligaments may fail secondary to torsional forces. In our experience, thumb MCP dislocations rarely demonstrate complete collateral ligament disruptions. These dislocations may be simple (reducible by closed means) or complex (irreducible). In a simple dislocation, some contact of the base of P-1 with the metacarpal head still occurs. Similar to simple MCP dislocation of the other digits, a hyperextension posture of the thumb may be seen on the lateral radiograph. Irreducible dislocations of the MCP joint are often the result of volar plate and/or sesamoid entrapment, interposed between the base of P-1 and the metacarpal head.[47,48] The proximal phalanx is usually parallel to the metacarpal in complex dislocations. Rupture of the volar plate occurs in MCP dislocations, and it usually occurs proximally at the metacarpal neck area.

Closed reduction of a simple dislocation is performed with use of a wrist block, augmented with a local hematoma block at the MCP joint area. The key to the reduction maneuver is to *avoid traction* and instead gently push P-1 over the metacarpal head. Axial traction, while tempting, can convert a simple MCP dislocation into a complex dislocation by interposing the volar plate. An adequate block, relaxed patient and even conscious sedation can help in an attempt to gently slide P-1

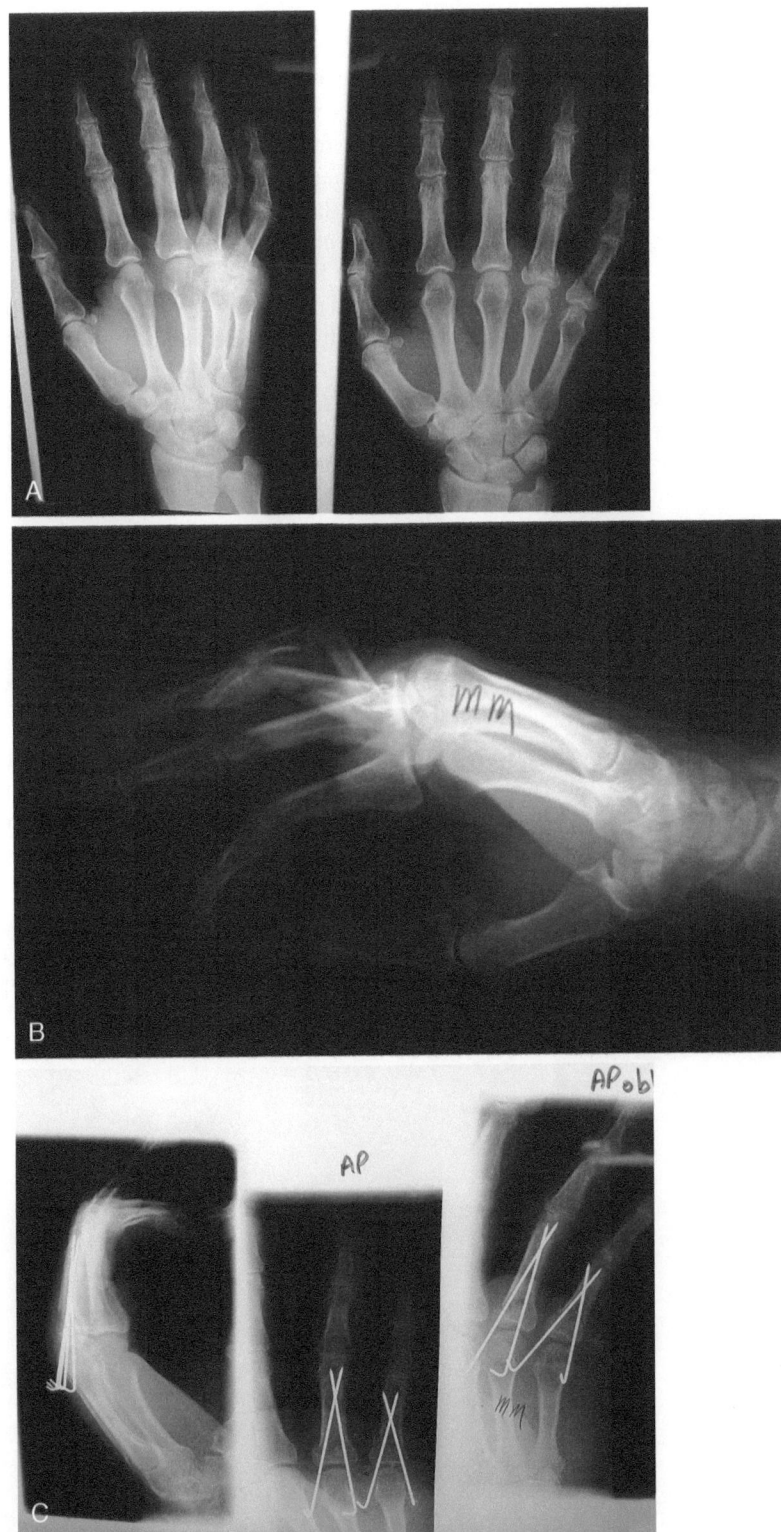

Fig. 74.19 (A) Angulated P-1 metaphyseal fractures of the ring and small fingers. (B) Apex volar angular deformities. (C) Reduction and percutaneous pinning.

over the metacarpal head. Counterpressure at the metacarpal neck may aid in the reduction. If the P-1 will not slide, aggressive attempts at reduction should be avoided, as there likely is interposed tissue. Simple MCP dislocations are usually stable on reduction. After reduction, the thumb may be immobilized

for 2 to 3 weeks positioned with approximately 20 degrees of flexion at the MCP joint.

Complex dislocations require open reduction through either a dorsal or volar approach.[49] We prefer to use the dorsal approach, which has proved to be consistently safe and effective.[50] A volar approach risks injury to traversing digital nerves that may be draped over the prominent metacarpal head. A freer elevator or other instrument may be used to extricate the offending structures from a dorsal vantage point, or a longitudinal incision may be made in the volar plate to loosen its stranglehold. The proximal phalanx is levered into a reduced position, and no soft tissue repairs are required. After open reduction of a complex dislocation, the MCP joint is immobilized for 2 to 3 weeks in gentle flexion and active ROM is then begun, with provision of a resting hand-based orthosis.

Rarely a volar MCP dislocation of the thumb occurs that is usually the result of direct dorsal trauma. This dislocation results in a torn dorsal capsule and, frequently, tearing of one or both collateral ligaments. In addition, the extensor pollicis brevis insertion may be torn from the base of the proximal phalanx. These injuries frequently require open reduction and stress testing of collateral ligaments, with collateral ligament repair as needed.[51] Because the development of osteoarthrosis is highly likely and the arc of motion after reduction of a chronic dislocation is typically minimal, MCP fusion for neglected dislocations has been advocated.

Timing of return to sports for athletes with these injuries depends on treatment (closed versus open) and return of ROM and strength. Taping and static orthoses are recommended on return to contact sports or sports that require intense use of the hands. Elite and professional athletes may return to sports earlier, especially after a closed reduction.

Collateral Ligament Injuries of the Metacarpophalangeal Joint

The thumb functions out of the plane of the palm and is called on frequently to participate in cylindrical grasping. Radial and ulnar deviation stresses on the MCP joint are resisted primarily by the collateral ligaments and volar plate. Ulnar collateral ligament (UCL) injuries are more common than those involving the RCL. The importance of UCL integrity for tip (precision) and power (key) pinch is indisputable.[52] Although a Stener lesion with interposed adductor between the ruptured UCL and its insertion is the only absolute surgical indication, most complete tears of the UCL are repaired or reattached in athletes who place a high demand on their hands (Fig. 74.20A and B). A complete tear of the RCL, although less common, may lead to volar-ulnar subluxation at the MCP joint with resultant pain, instability, and weakness. This scenario is especially true when the dorsal capsule is simultaneously torn or stretched. Complete tears of the RCL, although somewhat more controversial, are also typically treated surgically.[53,54]

The proper UCL has a predictable angular orientation from dorsal at the metacarpal head to volar at the proximal phalanx (P-1) base as it courses distally.[55] The fibers of the accessory collateral ligament blend between the proper UCL and the volar plate. The vast majority (>80%) of complete UCL tears occur at the distal insertion. The adductor aponeurosis, a thin sheet of fascial tissue, lies superficial to the UCL. This thin expansion

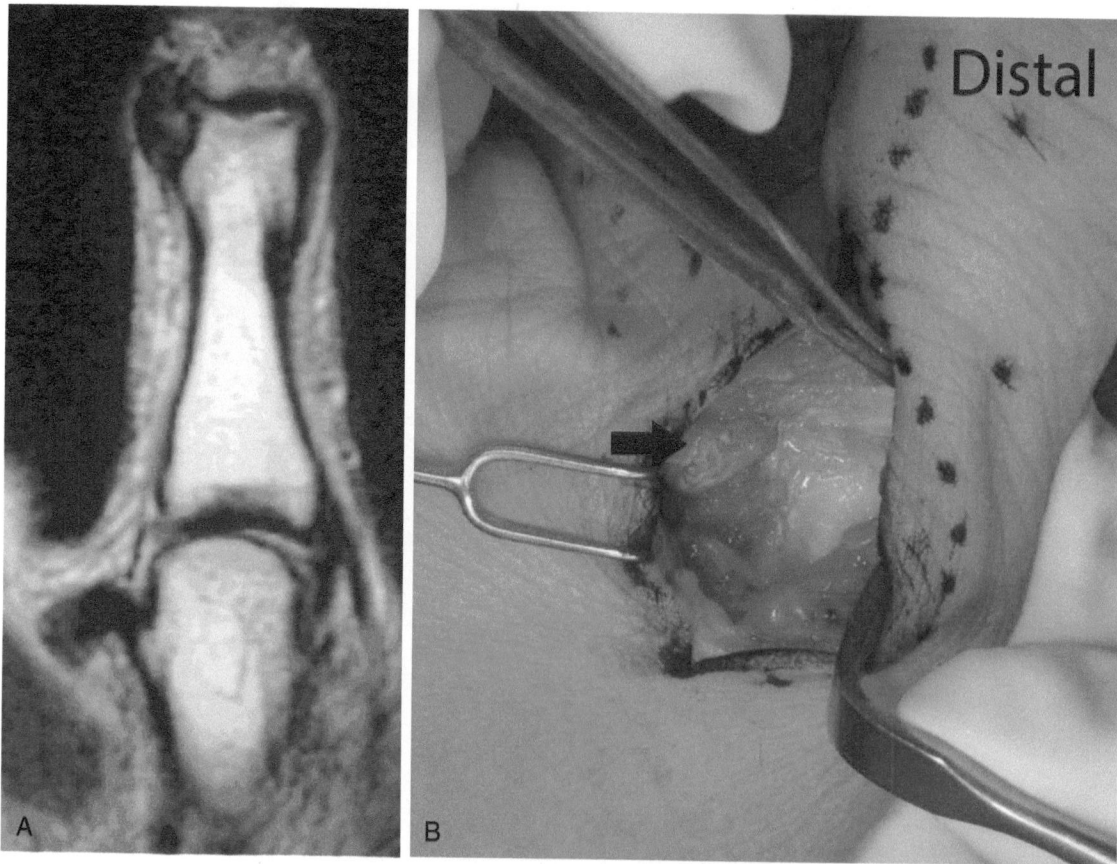

Fig. 74.20 MRI (A) and intraoperative photograph (B—Ulnar collateral ligament [UCL] marked with *arrow*) of a Stener lesion with UCL avulsed from proximal phalanx and displaced superficial to adductor insertion.

inserts onto the extensor pollicis longus (EPL) tendon. Stener[56] described the interposition of this adductor expansion between the torn distal end of the UCL and its attachment at the base of P-1. This interposition precludes adequate healing of the torn ligament edge to its anatomic distal insertion and is an absolute indication for surgical treatment when it is suspected clinically. On careful examination, the Stener lesion is appreciated as a thickening in the soft tissues just proximal and dorsal to the joint line over the ulnar border of the metacarpal head.

"UCL rupture," "skier's thumb," and "gamekeeper's thumb" all imply loss of continuity of the UCL at the MCP joint, although "gamekeeper's thumb" implies a chronic stretch toward incompetence of the ligament. The mechanism of injury is radial deviation of P-1 on the metacarpal head due to the combined forces of hyperabduction and hyperextension of the thumb. Palpable fullness at the ulnar MCP joint after this initiation of this mechanism implies a Stener lesion and has been found to be the most reliable sign of complete UCL rupture.[57] Surgical intervention is recommended for ruptures with Stener lesions. Although we are unaware of any cases of physical examination displacing UCL avulsion fractures, it is generally recommended that a stress examination be performed after radiographs rule out a nondisplaced avulsion injury at the base of the proximal phalanx that may otherwise be treated nonoperatively. A displaced avulsion fracture is treated with surgery. In cases without a fracture, radial deviation stress should be applied with the MCP joint flexed approximately 30 degrees to reduce the contribution of the volar plate and accessory collateral to MCP stability. The lack of a firm end point indicates a substantial tear (Fig. 74.21). If less than a 10-degree side-to-side difference in joint opening is noted, a partial tear may be present, and closed treatment of these lesions may yield satisfactory results. A stress radiograph (Fig. 74.22) may help measure the side-to-side difference and aid in decision-making regarding surgery. Greater than 15 to 30 degrees of joint opening compared with the contralateral side has long been considered the threshold for operative repair. Cadaver studies have demonstrated that stress radiographs demonstrate hinging with incomplete tears of the UCL, compared with true translation of the proximal phalanx when there is a complete tear.[58] When stress testing is equivocal, MRI or ultrasound may better characterize the degree of injury.[59,60] Alternatively, a stress examination may be performed after anesthesia with a local digital block to eliminate pain inhibition.

Partial injuries of the thumb UCL are treated with immobilization in a cast, splint, or brace to block thumb abduction, and the injury is reassessed after 4 to 6 weeks. In one comparative study of splinting versus casting, it was found that the type of immobilization resulted in no difference in functional outcomes or pinch strength.[61] Although a cast must be applied when patients are not compliant with treatment, most athletes will comply with the use of custom-molded splinting that allows for both gentle ROM of unaffected joints and hygiene. A quick return to sport after these injuries is challenging for most athletes. Some suggested criteria for return to sport are a painless thumb that demonstrates a firm end point with radial deviation stress and a recovery of at least 80% ROM and pinch strength. A prolonged recovery of 8 to 12 weeks before unrestricted return to sport is not unusual, especially for athletes involved in sports that involve use of a stick or heavy contact. Werner and colleagues showed that in college football players, skilled players had longer RTP time (mean 7 weeks) than nonskilled players (4 weeks), but both had reliable return to sport and excellent long term outcome after UCL suture anchor repair.[62]

Complete ligament avulsions of the UCL, along with displaced avulsion fractures, are treated surgically.[63,64] Functional results are generally good, with some loss of MCP ROM after operative repair. This stiffness, however, is generally well tolerated. Pinch strength may nearly reach that of the uninjured side after adequate rehabilitation. The operative approach itself causes minimal postoperative morbidity as long as the dorsal ulnar sensory nerve branch is identified and protected. Fixation techniques have evolved, although the use of small suture anchors currently predominates.[65]

For acute complete tears ("skier's thumb"), we prefer to use an appropriately sized suture anchor rather than a pullout suture via a bone tunnel. A curvilinear incision is made at the ulnar aspect of the thumb MCP joint, with the distal limb slightly volar to the midaxis of P-1 to parallel the course of the UCL.

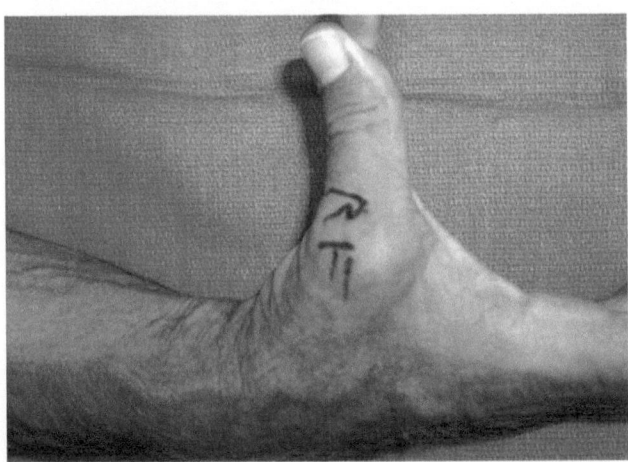

Fig. 74.21 A positive ulnar collateral ligament stress test.

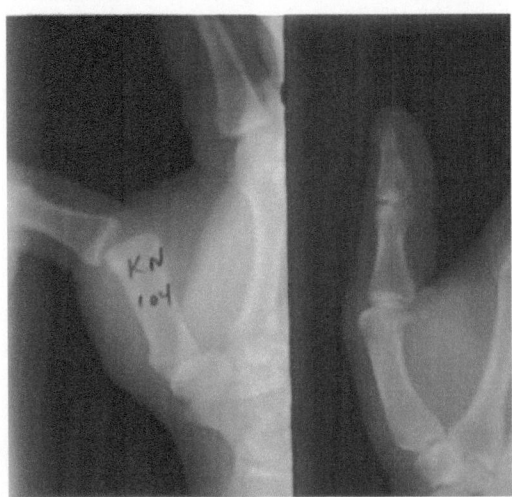

Fig. 74.22 An ulnar collateral ligament rupture with a positive stress radiograph.

Dorsal sensory nerves are protected, and the adductor aponeurosis is incised parallel to the EPL tendon and reflected volarly. Although the vast majority of these injuries are disrupted at the distal insertion, proximally based injuries and midsubstance ruptures are also possible. The torn collateral ligament is teased out, and the insertion site is roughened with a curette. The joint is inspected for rare cartilage defects and subsequently irrigated. The suture anchor is drilled and placed just distal to the ligament's insertion site, aiming away from the articular surface of P-1. This insertion is in the volar half of the proximal phalanx. The anchor should contain either 2-0 or 3-0 nonabsorbable suture in most instances. Temporary pinning of the reduced MCP joint with a 0.045-inch K wire is performed at the discretion of the surgeon. We often transfix the joint with a K wire to simplify ligament repair and ensure proper tensioning, although we determine whether or not to maintain the K wire for the first 2 to 4 weeks of healing based on a case-by-case basis. The torn ligament edge is captured and tied down to its insertion. The adductor aponeurosis is separately repaired to form a layer over the underlying suture knot. Finally, the incision is closed and a splint is placed.

Postoperative full-time immobilization ranges from 2 to 4 weeks, followed by progressive ROM exercises and protective splinting, as mentioned previously. Reliable, motivated athletes may begin earlier protected ROM, but pinching activities should be avoided for 4 to 6 weeks to avoid placing stress on the repaired ligament.[66] Unrestricted return to some high-demand sports may take anywhere from 3 to 6 months, depending on the specific activities involved, the position played by the athlete, and clinical examination findings. Participation is often contingent on the ability to protect the thumb in the early days after RTP.

If a sizable avulsion fracture is present, it may be reduced and pinned; for even larger fractures, a mini fragment screw is used for maximal stabilization. These fractures most commonly require operative treatment for malrotation of the articular surface. When opened, they typically involve more of the articular surface than anticipated but are still small enough to require K wires for fixation. K wires are removed at 6 weeks or when a radiograph suggests that healing has occurred. Bony injuries theoretically heal more quickly and reliably than their soft tissue counterparts, with obvious implications for rehabilitation and return to sport considerations. Tiny avulsion fragments may be excised, and the torn ligament is reinserted with an anchor as previously described.

Chronic UCL laxity ("gamekeeper's thumb") is easily recognized, and operative treatment with ligament reconstruction is largely effective.[67] Glickel[68] and others have described the technique for UCL reconstruction, with the use of an ipsilateral palmaris longus tendon autograft when available. The tendon graft is placed through a bony tunnel in the proximal phalanx (Fig. 74.23). An apex proximal triangular configuration has been found to be the strongest biomechanically.[69] The tendon graft is sutured to the collateral ligament stump proximally, or an anchor in the metacarpal head may aid in fixation of the graft. Because a good reconstructive option exists for chronic UCL laxity, MCP fusion is reserved for cases in which degenerative

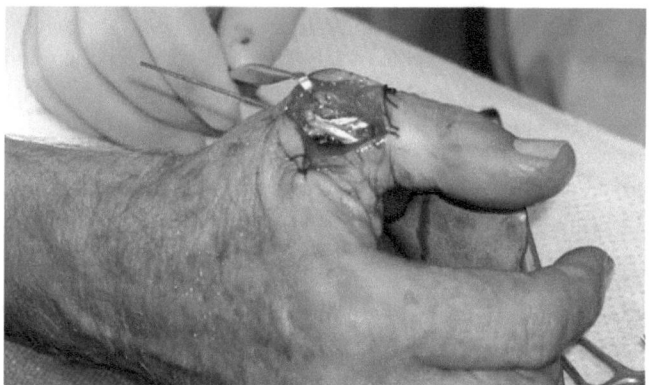

Fig. 74.23 Reconstruction of the collateral ligament with a palmaris longus tendon graft.

joint changes are present. However, we do favor MCP arthrodesis for the patient with minimal flexion-extension arc in the contralateral thumb MCP since it provides the most rapid and reliable stable, pain-free thumb MCP joint.

RCL tears are encountered less frequently, and thus a high index of clinical suspicion is necessary in the athlete with disproportionate radial-sided thumb pain after an MCP joint injury. The history may include a fall on or contact with a flexed or hyperadducted thumb. The adductor expansion overlying the UCL has no radial counterpart. The diagnostic examination and criteria for instability are similar to those used for UCL tears. Most injuries are incomplete but may include portions of the dorsal capsule that blends with the RCL. Partial injuries are uniformly treated with a cast or a functional splint until healing occurs. Symptom resolution often takes longer than expected with nonoperative management. Radiographs are mandatory in every case, and special attention is given to overall alignment of the MCP joint in both planes. Comparison to the contralateral side is recommended, because some volar positioning of the proximal phalanx relative to the metacarpal is possible in the uninjured, asymptomatic thumb. Volar or ulnar joint subluxation that is evident only on the injured side may indicate a complete (type III) rupture of the dorsal-radial restraints, and surgical repair with ligament reconstruction with or without joint pinning is indicated in this situation. Some surgeons have reported acceptable results with RCL soft tissue sleeve advancement only in cases of chronic RCL instability, but we do not have any personal experience with that technique.[70] Other surgeons prefer to use a reconstructive procedure with a tendon autograft for chronically unstable RCL injuries.[71] A neglected injury with joint subluxation will theoretically lead to posttraumatic osteoarthrosis of the MCP joint, which necessitates arthrodesis when it is symptomatic and disabling.

For a complete list of references, go to ExpertConsult.com.

SELECTED READINGS

Citation:
Kodama N, Takemura Y, Ueba H, et al. Operative treatment of metacarpal and phalangeal fractures in athletes: early return to play. *J Orthop Sci.* 2014;19:729–736.

Level of Evidence:

V

Summary:

This article reviews 105 athletes with metacarpal or phalangeal fractures and demonstrates that good outcomes can be achieved with early return to play in certain clinical situations.

Citation:

Kozin SH, Thoder JJ, Lieberman G. Operative treatment of metacarpal and phalangeal shaft fractures. *J Am Acad Orthop Surg*. 2000;8:111–121.

Level of Evidence:

V

Summary:

This article is a straightforward review of operative indications for metacarpal and phalangeal shaft fractures.

Citation:

Lee AT, Carlson MG. Thumb metacarpophalangeal joint collateral ligament injury management. *Hand Clin*. 2012;28:361–370.

Level of Evidence:

V

Summary:

This article is a useful review of UCL and RCL injuries, with focused review of relevant anatomy, operative evaluation, and surgical techniques.

Citation:

Singletary S, Geissler WB. Bracing and rehabilitation for wrist and hand injuries in collegiate athletes. *Hand Clin*. 2009;25:443–448.

Level of Evidence:

This article is a cowritten with therapist, and is an excellent review of rehabilitation and protective splinting for athletes after injury to the hand and digit.

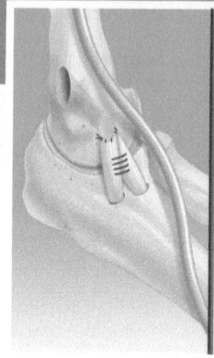

75

Neuropathies of the Wrist and Hand

Gwendolyn Hoben, Amy M. Moore

Although athletes at all levels of participation may experience the same entrapment neuropathies as the general population, some sport-specific peripheral nerve factors must be considered with regard to the wrist and hand. Neuropathies may occur as a result of chronic repetitive motion or acute isolated trauma experienced during athletic activities. Just as with other pathologies that may have an effect on, or be affected by, sports participation, the type and timing of treatment will vary depending on severity and "sport season" considerations. Although "playing with pain" may be an acceptable choice in the presence of some repetitive traumatic injuries, hand and wrist neuropathies often necessitate careful and timely treatment to prevent irreversible damage. Although a multitude of potential upper extremity neuropathies exist, this chapter focuses on the ones that are most typical and/or cause the most concern involving the wrist and hand.

Wrist and hand neuropathies are more common with certain athletic activities. Median neuropathy at the wrist may result from activities that (1) apply prolonged direct compression, such as bicycling or wheelchair events, (2) elicit vibratory stimuli, such as motocross racing, or (3) require repetitive power gripping, such as in weightlifting and ice hockey.[1-4] In addition to similar mechanisms of injury for the ulnar nerve at the wrist, secondary extrinsic causes of compression dominate, including a high prevalence of hook of hamate fractures as a result of using a stick in certain sports and ulnar artery aneurysm/thrombosis (hypothenar hammer syndrome) that occurs as a result of the repetitive blunt palmar trauma commonly experienced by baseball catchers and martial arts practitioners.[5-7] The superficial sensory radial nerve is susceptible to either direct blunt trauma, which is most commonly associated with football, lacrosse, and ice hockey, or repetitive traction forces, which are often experienced by competitive rock climbers and powerlifters.[8] Furthermore, the perpetual use of compressive wrist bands or athletic tape, which is frequently seen in athletes whose sport entails use of a racquet, may cause local irritation of the radial nerve at the wrist.[9] The ulnar digital nerve of the thumb is vulnerable in bowlers, and the radial digital nerve of the index finger may be affected in tennis, racquetball, or squash players.[10,11]

HISTORY

The symptoms of sports-related wrist and hand neuropathies may include subjective paresthesias and weakness in the affected nerve's distribution, loss of coordination, and a variable level of pain. Depending on the reported distribution of symptoms, further questioning should focus on potential areas of nerve compression or repetitive trauma precipitated by the athlete's activity requirements. Direct questioning of the athlete will also reveal if the symptoms worsen or improve in certain positions or occur while the athlete is sleeping. Determining the onset, frequency, and intensity of nerve symptoms may be helpful in deciding what type of an approach to take with further workup and treatment. The benefit or futility of prior treatment should be elicited. The practitioner should also remember that although symptoms and signs may be present in the wrist and hand, the true site of pathology may be more proximal, and therefore an inventory of proximally generated symptoms should be conducted.

As with most pathologies, the patient's history typically directs one to the diagnosis. It is important to avoid asking patients leading questions. Instead, allowing athletes to describe their own symptoms, exacerbating and remitting factors, and prior treatments often leads to the correct diagnosis and determines the course of further management.

PHYSICAL EXAMINATION

The athlete's subjective complaints direct the focus of the physical examination. However, having a systematic approach to the upper extremity nerve exam is helpful. This includes visual inspection, a thorough sensory and a functional motor exam. Performing these tests on every patient allows the practitioner to pick up subtle clues on causation of the patient's symptoms.

When entering the examination room, it is important to visually assess the patient. During your history taking, is the patient demonstrating a posture of pain, such as slouching to one side and/or holding the extremity in a position of protection? Are there obvious differences in shoulder height or discrepancy in muscle bulk of the shoulders, arms, forearms, and hands? Unilateral atrophy is an important sign that a more proximal injury or lesion is present or there has been compensation because of a nerve compression/neuropathy that is distal. For example, if the patient lacks dexterity and has trouble gripping due to an ulnar neuropathy at the wrist, then there may be disuse atrophy of the forearm, which can be a late sign but visible on exam.

A complete sensory exam is important when evaluating for hand or wrist neuropathies. Rating light touch sensation in the distribution of the symptomatic nerve relative to the asymptomatic wrist and hand is fast, easy, and helpful. This determination of

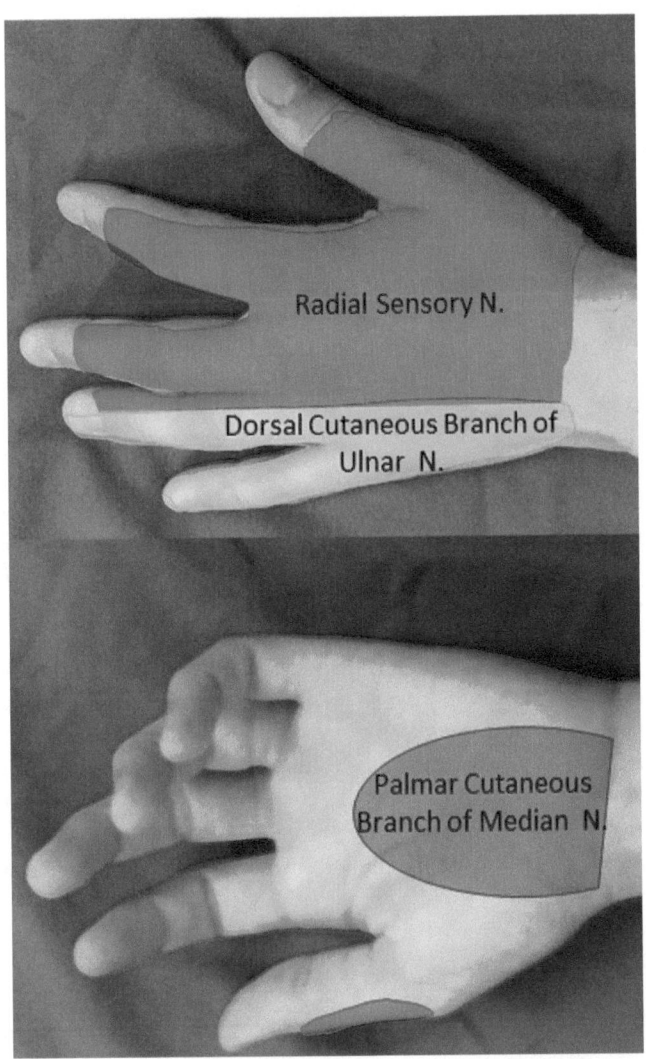

Fig. 75.1 Critical sensory nerve distributions of the arm: Numbness in the palmar cutaneous distribution of the median nerve suggests pathology proximal to the carpal tunnel. Likewise, sensory paresthesias of the dorsal cutaneous branch of the ulnar nerve indicate pathology proximal to Guyon canal. Pain or numbness in the distribution of the radial sensory nerve in absence of motor symptoms can indicate compression where the nerve becomes superficial between the extensor carpi radialis longus and brachioradialis.

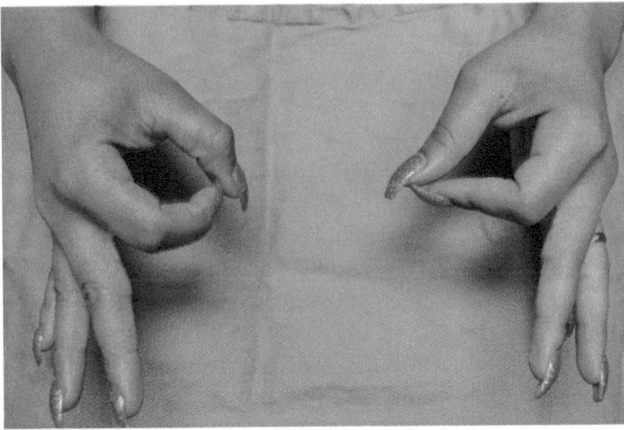

Fig. 75.2 Anterior interosseous nerve neuropathy can be testing by having the patient make an "OK" sign with their hand. When the flexor pollicis longus and flexor digitorum profundus to the index finger are not working, rather than an O, the sign appears more like an oval, as seen here in the patient's left hand.

light touch sensation should include the dorsal sensory branch of the ulnar nerve, the palmar cutaneous branch of the median nerve, and the dorsal sensory branch of the radial nerve (Fig. 75.1). Involvement of these terminal cutaneous nerve components is helpful in confirming the site of peripheral nerve compression or disease. For example, normal findings of a sensory examination over the dorsal ulnar hand in the setting of other ulnar nerve symptoms typically indicate ulnar nerve pathology in the wrist or hand rather than at the elbow. Altered sensation in the central palmar aspect of the hand indicates median nerve pathology proximal to the level of the carpal tunnel due to involvement of the palmar cutaneous branch of the median nerve. For digital neuropathies, such as bowler's thumb, altered sensation in the digital nerve is expected, and a palpable mass may be present.

Another fast and easily communicated way of assessing light touch sensation is the Strauch 10-10 test.[12,13] The patient rates the level of light touch sensation in an injured area on a scale of 0 to 10, with 0 = no sensation, 10 = normal sensation, generally as compared with the unaffected contralateral hand (note: the original scale was 1 to 10, but we find patients better understand 0 = no sensation). More advanced sensory examinations, such as static and moving two-point discrimination, vibratory sense, and Semmes-Weinstein monofilament testing, provide good objective and standardized data points that are monitored for the progression or resolution of neuropathy.

A thorough motor exam is important to perform in all patients with suspected neuropathy. A quick assessment of peripheral nerve motor function can be performed by having the athlete make the "OK" sign (median nerve), cross the index and long fingers (ulnar nerve), and extend the index finger and thumb (radial nerve). When making the OK sign, it is important for the patient to make a rounded circle with the thumb and index finger; flattening of the circle into a more oval shape is an abnormal result that indicates proximal involvement of the anterior interosseous nerve (Fig. 75.2). Other nerve-specific maneuvers include having the athlete oppose the thumb to the base of the small finger (distal median and ulnar innervated thenar muscles), pinch a piece of paper between the thumb and clenched index finger (Froment sign: denervation or atrophy of ulnar innervated adductor pollicis requires the thumb to flex to pinch the paper) (Fig. 75.3), and abduct the small finger against resistance (ulnar innervated abductor digiti minimi). Clawing of the ring and small fingers indicates significant ulnar neuropathy distal to the digital flexor muscles in the forearm. Formal tip-pinch, key-pinch, and grip strength measurements with dynamometers should be performed and provide objective results that are tracked over time.

Tinel testing along the course of the symptomatic peripheral nerve may help determine a specific site of chronic trauma or compressive neuropathy. It is usually helpful to initially tap lightly for this test to get a sense of the hypersensitivity/reactivity of the symptomatic nerve. The Finkelstein test (i.e., ulnar deviation of the athlete's wrist with the thumb in palm by the examiner) may cause dorsal radial sensory nerve symptoms. These symptoms should be differentiated from symptoms caused by de Quervain first extensor compartment tenosynovitis (i.e., pain at the radial styloid) by checking for the presence of nerve symptoms and a positive Tinel sign proximal to the radial styloid at the level where the brachioradialis (BR) and extensor carpi radialis longus (ECRL) meet and the dorsal radial sensory nerve exits.

A limitation of Tinel testing is that it depends on the patient reporting whether symptoms are elicited. The scratch collapse test is a maneuver thought to be based upon an inhibitory spinal reflex such that when the site of compression is stimulated (i.e., *scratched*), the patient is no longer able to sustain resisted shoulder external rotation.[14] In brief, the patient sits with shoulders externally rotated, elbows bent to 90 degrees, hands outstretched with wrists neutral. The examiner applies bilateral adduction and internal rotation pressure to the patient's forearms. Next, the examiner scratches the compression point while the patient holds his or her arms steady. The examiner then applies pressure as before, and if the patient is unable to resist the force and collapses, it is considered a positive test indicative of nerve compression at that site. A *hierarchical* scratch collapse test can be done by "freezing out" compression points with ethyl chloride to unmask secondary compression points.[15] Multiple prospective studies have examined this test for reliability in carpal tunnel syndrome and have demonstrated a relatively low sensitivity, 24% to 33%, and specificity ranged 60% to 61%.[16–18] In contrast,

Cheng et al. reported a significantly greater sensitivity of 64% and specificity of 99%.[14] We generally find there is a significant learning curve with the test before it can be considered reliable by the practitioner and can be considered as a helpful component of a full and comprehensive evaluation.

Direct compression and/or flexion/extension tests along the course of the symptomatic nerve may also be helpful in localizing the site of compression. These tests are typically performed for 30 to 60 seconds or until symptoms occur, whichever comes first. The Phalen test for carpal tunnel/median nerve compression requires placing the wrist in full flexion and holding this for 60 seconds. For ulnar nerve symptoms at the wrist and hand, the practitioner should also consider a vascular examination because of possible associated ulnar artery aneurysm and/or thrombosis. This examination includes examining the athlete's nails for streaking (splinter hemorrhages) that could indicate thrombotic/embolic events and checking for ulcerations or skin breakdown due to ischemia, especially in the palmar fingertips. An Allen test can also be performed to determine to determine if there is a complete palmar arch.

As mentioned earlier, consideration of more proximal nerve disorders that could manifest symptoms distally in the hand and wrist is important. Symptoms and signs dictate whether the cervical spine, brachial plexus, thoracic outlet, arm, or proximal forearm should be scrutinized for the source of the problem. Cervical radiculopathy, thoracic outlet syndrome, and brachial plexopathy are not uncommon conditions in athletes who participate in contact sports.

IMAGING

In general, radiographic and advanced imaging is not necessary for evaluation of hand and wrist neuropathies, although special circumstances may spur the examiner to pursue imaging. For example, ulnar nerve symptoms in an athlete with chronic trauma to the ulnar-palmar aspect of the hand may be a sign of a hamate fracture or vascular injury such as with hypothenar hammer syndrome (Fig. 75.4). Plain radiographs are a recommended first step. Although the carpal tunnel view is an often-cited special view for assessing the hamate hook, an alternative view is much easier to perform reproducibly, especially with use of fluoroscopy. To achieve this view, start with the wrist in radial deviation and the thumb abducted, as if the patient were holding a cup. The wrist is then slightly supinated from a

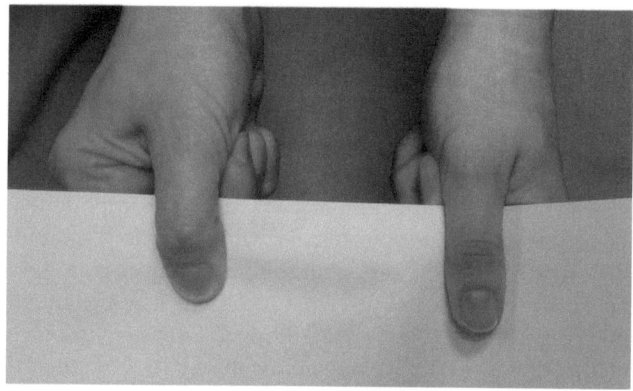

Fig. 75.3 A positive Froment sign shows flexor pollicis longus flexion in order to pinch and hold the paper between the thumb and clenched fist secondary to denervation of the ulnar innervated adductor pollicis. The right hand has a proximal ulnar nerve compression.

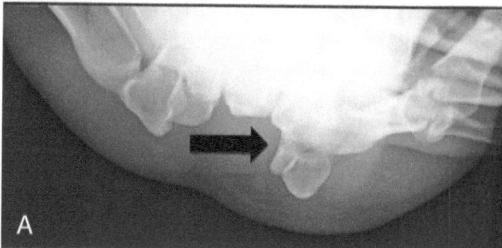
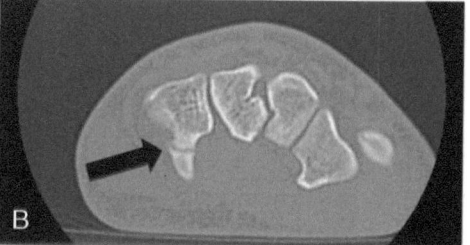

Fig. 75.4 Hook of hamate fractures may be difficult to visualize on x-ray without a special view, such as the carpal tunnel view shown here (A). Although computed tomography is still considered by most to be the "gold standard" for evaluating the hook of the hamate, when such a fracture is clinically suspected, magnetic resonance imaging can provide excellent visualization as well (B). (Photos courtesy of Dr. Mark Vitale MD.)

TABLE 75.1   Interpretation and Application of Electrodiagnostic Studies to Patient Treatment and Recovery

Nerve Changes	Signs and Symptoms	Electrodiagnostics	Treatment Options	Recovery
Dynamic ischemic changes	Intermittent pain and paresthesias	NCVs: normal EMG: normal	Night splinting, corticosteroid injection	Can expect full recovery
Demyelination injury	Pain and paresthesias, may be intermittent or constant; reduced nerve conduction velocities	NCVs: reduced velocities EMG: normal	Operative decompression	Can expect full recovery in 3–4 months
Axonal injury	Constant pain and paresthesias, weakness and clumsiness with fine hand movements, appearance of muscle wasting	NCVs: reduced velocities EMG: fibrillations, chronic and severe may have loss of MUPS	Operative decompression	Full or partial recovery at a rate of 1 in/month

EMG, Electromyography; *MUPS*, motor unit potentials; *NCVs*, nerve conduction velocities.

lateral x-ray view position to generate a slightly oblique view. In this position, the x-ray beam is directed between the thumb and finger metacarpals and the hamate hook is seen projecting palmarly. For athletes with symptoms and signs of proximal median nerve compression, elbow or humerus radiographs may reveal a supracondylar process. In the absence of a supracondylar process, magnetic resonance imaging (MRI) may be justified to evaluate for an occult forearm mass causing extrinsic compression on the median nerve.

Ultrasound (US) can also be used as an imaging modality to evaluate nerve compression, nerve ganglions, or masses causing compression of the nerve. It is inexpensive and is gaining acceptance as a diagnostic tool. Furthermore, US can also assess vascular abnormalities, such as aneurysms, pseudoaneurysms, and arteriovenous fistulas, thus providing significant information in a patient with the vague presentation of numbness or pain.[19]

MRI is not commonly used in the evaluation of compression neuropathies but can have utility for evaluating mass lesions resulting in compression, when there may be a superimposed proximal or systemic neuropathy on a focal compression point, and in patients who cannot tolerate electrodiagnostic studies. Although a less common cause of compression neuropathy, schwannomas and other more rare tumors may present with compression symptoms, and any palpable masses should be evaluated with MRI for diagnosis and surgical planning.[20] In cases such as bowler's thumb, MRI is the only modality that can preoperatively determine nodular neuroma formation versus perineurial fibrosis, which may present in a similar fashion.[21,22]

DECISION-MAKING PRINCIPLES

As with any other athletic injury, decision-making is based on the nature and extent of the pathology and sport-specific considerations for the athlete. The patient's history of symptoms, presence of atrophy, and electrodiagnostic tests help to delineate the degree of nerve damage and the likelihood of success with different interventions. Although the diagnosis of carpal or cubital tunnel syndrome is considered "clinical," we generally obtain neurodiagnostic tests including nerve conduction velocities (NCVs) and electromyography (EMG). NCV values show the integrity of the nerve: the speed of conduction reflects myelin integrity and nerve compression, whereas the amplitude reflects the number of conducting axons within the nerve. EMG directly samples muscle fibers, and the presence of motor unit potentials (MUPs) shows the connectivity of the spinal cord to the muscle in the form of MUPs. These tests confirm the diagnosis and severity and allow for accurate prediction of recovery because they can often differentiate ischemic versus myelin versus axonal injury (Table 75.1). Ischemic changes are often dynamic and dependent on positioning; there is no break in the link between the spinal cord and muscle. Thus the EMG is normal, and similarly, NCV values are normal because the myelin is intact. With progressive compression, there is loss of myelin and a conduction block develops, reducing the NCV values, but the EMG remains normal. With axonal loss there is reduced amplitude in the NCV and loss of MUPs on EMG.

In the presence of recent symptoms or clear inciting actions and no slowing of nerve conduction, conservative and nonoperative treatment strategies are reasonable. When the symptoms have been present for longer and there are changes on nerve conduction studies and/or EMG, surgical intervention is most reasonable to prevent permanent sequelae. In cases of overt clawing or intrinsic wasting, a comprehensive work-up and surgical intervention, without delay, are paramount because there are already irreversible changes. However, in the context of the athlete, it is often helpful to present treatment options as they relate to the athlete's season, career, and remainder of his or her life, which helps the athlete to put the different choices into perspective.

TREATMENT OPTIONS

Treatment options for the various peripheral nerve pathologies depend on the particular nerve involved, the severity of the involvement, and the type and timing of the patient's athletic activities. In general, wrist-neutral nighttime bracing is started and daytime and/or athletic-activity wrist-neutral bracing is attempted as much as possible. Note that most commercially available wrist braces are in mild wrist extension and must be flattened to neutral to be most helpful, because both wrist flexion and extension increase pressure in the carpal tunnel and can contribute to persistent symptoms.[23] Although the use of oral antiinflammatory drugs along with bracing may be beneficial, using these drugs in isolation has not been shown to be effective. Modification of activities that worsen symptoms is helpful and may be facilitated by therapists and athletic trainers. There is also growing evidence that sleep position may predispose to carpal tunnel syndrome and that sleeping supine with wrists and elbows are extended may also reduce compressive symptoms.[24,25] A 6- to 8-week trial of splinting and activity modification is reasonable before reassessing symptoms.

If there is no improvement after splinting or the presenting signs and symptoms are severe, surgical decompression is offered. Proceeding with surgery is often based on the patient's immediate, short-term, and long-term athletic schedule. For example, if it is off-season, the athlete may elect to proceed with surgical release as the most definitive treatment so he or she will not have persistent or worsening issues during the season. However, if the athlete is in the middle of a playoff run or a similar competitive scenario and taking time off for surgery is impossible, a corticosteroid injection, in addition to night splinting, is potentially helpful to improve symptoms over the course of several weeks to months.[26]

For ulnar neuropathies of the wrist and hand, activity modification and intermittent bracing may be helpful. One difference in the treatment of ulnar neuropathy at the wrist involves the presence of motor involvement. Intrinsic muscle weakness or atrophy resulting from identifiable secondary pathology, such as a hamate hook fracture, ulnar artery thrombosis, or other mass, should prompt the surgeon to address the offending source of compression sooner rather than later. A 6- to 8-week period of observation and activity modification is reasonable if secondary pathology is absent. Situations typically occur in which a single acute trauma (e.g., a direct blow) or a few episodes of direct compression (e.g., from cycling) cause the ulnar nerve palsy. Steady clinical improvement warrants further observation without repeat neurodiagnostic tests, and many palsies resolve completely within this time frame with activity modification alone. Neurodiagnostic tests precede surgical intervention for cases that fail to resolve after the observation period. It is important to assess for any signs of ulnar deep motor branch compression in a patient with carpal tunnel syndrome because returning to the operating room to decompress the Guyon canal in an already operated field increases the difficulty of safe decompression due to scar tissue.

Although proximal radial neuropathy may cause both motor and sensory loss, involvement at the level of the wrist and hand is purely sensory in nature. Idiopathic neuropathy originating between the BR and ECRL is called *Wartenberg syndrome*, or cheiralgia paresthetica. The main goals of treatment for this condition are to improve symptoms and prevent worsening, which may lead to complex regional pain syndrome type II, also known as *causalgia*. The most common nonoperative treatment for radial neuropathy at the wrist is removal of any constrictive external devices, wraps, or bands. Avoiding power pronosupination and splinting may have a limited benefit; 37% of patients with radial sensory nerve compression can be managed successfully nonoperatively.[27] For recalcitrant cases of radial sensory nerve disturbance at the wrist, an injection of a local anesthetic may

be attempted, more for diagnostic than therapeutic purposes. If symptoms persist despite several (usually at least 6) months of conservative management or in the case of relief with diagnostic injection of a local anesthetic, surgical treatment can be offered. Surgical decompression of the radial sensory nerve is performed through a dorsoradial incision centered approximately 9 cm from the radial styloid. The radial sensory nerve is identified between the ECRL and BR, the tight fascia joining the BR and ECRL is released and full BR tenotomy is performed, if needed. Alternatively, the constricting portion of the BR and ECRL may be excised to ensure full nerve decompression.[27,28]

Digital neuropathies that result from bowling, baseball, or racquet sports typically respond to nonoperative measures such as grip modification, padding, or other equipment changes. Several months of nonoperative treatment is warranted before considering surgery. Bowler's thumb is most notable and is due to repeat trauma to the ulnar aspect of the thumb and resultant subcutaneous and perineurial fibrosis. In severe cases this can develop into a true digital nerve neuroma. Rest and a plastic thumb guard are sufficient for most cases. Although it is uncommon to treat digital neuropathy surgically, procedures such as neurolysis and fibrotic synovectomy or nerve transposition have been described in cases of chronic compression and pain that have failed nonoperative management.[29–31] For example, the ulnar digital nerve can be transposed dorsal to the adductor pollicis to prevent continued local mechanical trauma.[11,30,31]

There are few medications that may reduce the severity of neurogenic pain and paresthesias. If neurogenic pain is severe, then a multidisciplinary approach must be taken. This includes the primary care physicians, pain management specialists, and the occupational therapists. Medications to treat nerve pain act centrally and have common adverse effects; thus it is rare that they are used to treat compression syndromes in the athlete.

POSTOPERATIVE MANAGEMENT AND RETURN TO PLAY

After carpal tunnel release, finger motion is encouraged immediately but patients are instructed to not lift anything heavier than a pen or piece of paper for 2 weeks. The dressing is removed in 5 days, and the patients are allowed to shower. The skin is usually healed by 2 weeks after surgery, and if range of motion is full or nearly full, the athlete can start gradually increasing their activities as permitted by their level of pain and the condition of their soft tissues. Strengthening exercises and full-weight bearing is usually initiated by 4 weeks. Pain, swelling, and other postoperative symptoms usually wax and wane depending on activities performed and dictate how rapidly and aggressively the athlete can progress. Once the skin is healed, athletes may return to play (RTP) if time is of the essence and if it seems physically possible for them to compete at a high level. This decision typically depends on their pain tolerance, strength, and overall coordination. Otherwise, if early RTP is less critical, a more measured approach may involve a gradual return to athletic participation once strength is 50% to 75% of the unaffected contralateral side, which is a good postoperative rule of thumb for other nerve-related procedures involving the wrist and hand

🔖 Authors' Preferred Technique
Carpal Tunnel Release and Guyon Canal Release

Endoscopic carpal tunnel release has proven to be safe and effective, although not superior to the traditional open method. An earlier RTP is theoretically possible for most athletes and sports and is often cited as an early short-term advantage of this technique (extrapolating from return-to-work data).[32,33] In terms of safety, median nerve injury is very rare with either technique, although the risk of nerve injury has been shown to be higher with endoscopic releases in one study.[33] In the end, we recommend that the surgeon should do the technique with which they are most comfortable: that technique will be the most safe. At our institution we prefer the open technique. If there is any concern for ulnar nerve entrapment at the wrist, we also perform Guyon canal release.

Induction of anesthesia according to the surgeon's preference and sterile skin preparation and draping of the patient's upper extremity are performed. A tourniquet can be placed on the proximal forearm if desired. A 3-cm linear incision is marked slightly ulnar and parallel to the thenar skin crease extending from the wrist crease distally (Fig. 75.5A). The incision is made ulnar to the thenar crease to protect the course of the palmar cutaneous branch of the median nerve and to avoid a possible transligamentous thenar branch. A Bruner-style incision is marked across the distal wrist crease to be used if necessary to fully release the antebrachial fascia (see Fig. 75.5B). The palmar fascia is opened longitudinally in line with the skin incision. Dissection proceeds to expose the transverse carpal ligament and the distal border of the release is visualized, which forms a "V" from confluence of the thenar and hypothenar musculature. The transverse carpal ligament is completely released from the distal volar wrist crease to the "V." The fat pad protecting the superficial palmar arch and common digital nerve

branches is visualized and protected. To ensure complete release the antebrachial fascia, it is helpful for the surgeon to move to the end of the hand table. Under direct visualization, the fascia can be released in a controlled manner. This fascia can be surprisingly tight in muscular forearms of athletes and may extend well proximal to the volar wrist crease. Do not hesitate to extend the incision proximal across the wrist crease if needed to avoid an incomplete release.

If a Guyon canal release is also indicated in the patient, then this release is approached prior to the carpal tunnel release. The palmaris brevis and palmar aponeurosis are divided, and ulnar sensory branches (one large branch is commonly encountered 2.5 cm distal to the wrist crease and 1 cm ulnar to the thenar crease) are carefully avoided. The neurovascular bundle is identified and swept ulnarly with a blunt retractor. The hook of hamate is palpated and the leading edge of the hypothenar musculature is identified. The motor branch of the ulnar nerve is not visualized until the fascia of the hypothenar muscle is released. Decompression of the motor branch can be achieved with release of the fascia of the hypothenar musculature. Once released, the dissection of the soft tissue is carried radially and the transverse carpal ligament is identified and released as described previously.

Once a complete release has been confirmed with direct visualization, the tourniquet (if used) is released and hemostasis is achieved. The choice regarding the type of suture and technique to be used for skin closure is made by the surgeon, but horizontal mattress eversion of the skin edges with 4-0 nylon is standard. A bulky dressing is applied, and the patient is encouraged to move their fingers often.

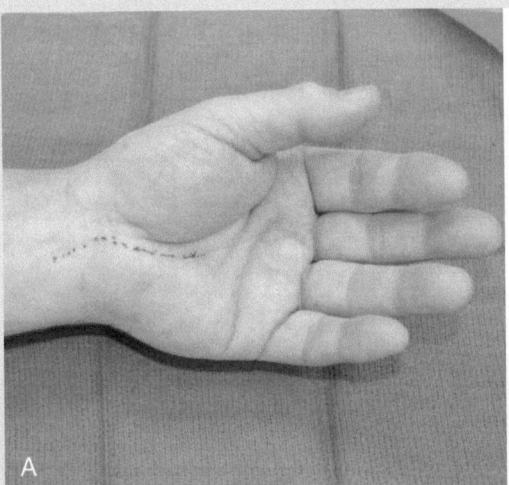
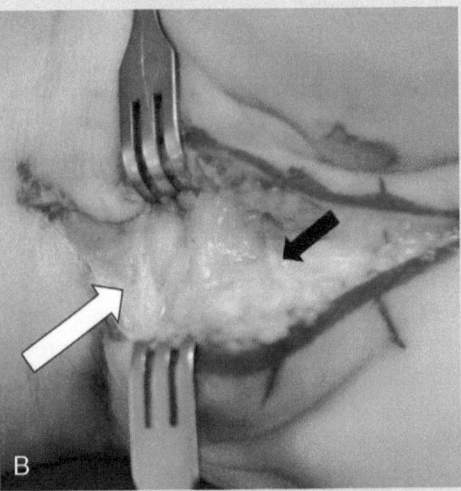

Fig. 75.5 Carpal tunnel and Guyon release: (A) The typical incision planned for carpal tunnel and Guyon canal release, just ulnar to the thenar crease. (B) The *black arrow* indicates an ulnar sensory branch that should be protected in the dissection. Thickened and compressive antebrachial fascia is indicated by the *white arrow*.

as well. Formal therapy is recommended for athletes because they may benefit from work with a therapist and/or an athletic trainer to facilitate an earlier RTP.

RESULTS

If the diagnosis of carpal tunnel syndrome is correct and the surgical release is performed, postoperative results should be consistently satisfactory. Most authors report improvement for

more than 90% of patients.[34] However, the degree to which patients improve is harder to predict. If the athlete experienced nocturnal symptoms or positional aggravation, these symptoms often improve first and potentially immediately. Daytime pain and paresthesias improve on a less predictable timetable and may never fully resolve.[35] The patient's strength is usually the last thing to improve, and full recovery of strength is usually incomplete.[36] Any preoperative thenar atrophy will likely remain visible. Results for ulnar, radial, and digital nerve procedures at the wrist and hand for athletes are less predictable unless a secondary extrinsic inciting cause is eliminated by the surgery.[37] One of the main reasons for this current unpredictability is the relative paucity of outcomes published for these non–carpal tunnel syndrome neuropathies, especially when they are idiopathic. Most publications concerning these nerve syndromes are small case series or case reports for particular causes of the peripheral nerve condition.

Complications

Fortunately, major complications after carpal tunnel release are relatively uncommon. However, iatrogenic injuries to the median and ulnar nerves, ulnar artery/superficial arch, and digital flexor tendons have been reported for all techniques described in the literature.[38] The surgeon should use the utmost caution during the procedure, to avoid these devastating complications. A more common complication is persistent or recurrent carpal tunnel syndrome. Persistent carpal tunnel syndrome is defined as having unchanged or worse symptoms after surgery, in contrast to patients who have steady improvement as part of the natural history of the postoperative course. True recurrence is defined as having had a significant interval of symptom relief after surgery followed by a return of symptoms. Recurrence, when it does happen, usually does not occur until the late postoperative period (often years after surgery). Recurrence or persistence rates vary between 1% and 10% over the lifetime of the patient after carpal tunnel release.[39–41]

Severe and acute worsening of median nerve symptoms after carpal tunnel release may be due to direct median nerve injury, hematoma, or infection. If these early causes of median nerve compromise are evident, an urgent return to the operating room is strongly recommended.

Infection after carpal tunnel release is rare, and routine administration of preoperative antibiotics is unnecessary.[42] Administration of preoperative antibiotics for clean hand procedures generally also can be considered for patients who smoke or have diabetes and for procedures that may last longer than 2 hours. However, even for these potential indications for use of preoperative antibiotics in higher risk patients, it is currently unknown if antibiotic use actually helps to prevent infection.[43,44] Postoperative infections are treated with oral antibiotics and local wound care if they are superficial and with operative débridement if they are deep or nonresponsive to nonoperative care. Wound dehiscence occurs more frequently than true wound infection and heals reliably with moist to dry dressing changes and time. Patients often experience "pillar pain" along the radial and ulnar borders of the carpal canal for several weeks to months after surgery, which is usually considered a consequence, as opposed to a complication, of the procedure.

FUTURE CONSIDERATIONS

Nerve compression in the hand and wrist is not a novel concept in the athlete, but there are a few newer diagnostic and therapeutic tools to consider. With regards to diagnosis, nerve US is gaining ground. Multiple studies have compared cross-sectional area of the median nerve with nerve conduction studies to accurately diagnose carpal tunnel syndrome.[45–47] The use of US may emerge as a more valuable diagnostic tool in this arena and perhaps even replacing electrodiagnostic testing. Magnetic resonance neurography may also become more clinically available as an adjuvant study in the work-up of nerve-related pathology.[48,49]

With regards to therapeutic advances, surgical techniques and intraoperative adjunctive therapies continue to be developed and evaluated. As previously stated, comparison of endoscopic and open techniques has validated the efficacy and safety of both procedures, future studies will need to determine cost efficacy. Recent work has shown that endoscopic procedures are slightly more expensive in total cost, but full analysis of the sources of extra cost is forthcoming.[50,51] As an adjunct to the standard techniques, electrical stimulation is showing promise.[52] In a preliminary randomized controlled clinical study, 1 hour of electrical stimulation following carpal tunnel release surgery resulted in accelerated motor and sensory conduction speed and improved thenar musculature reinnervation versus carpal tunnel release surgery only controls. However, these improvements did not correlate to improved clinical functional outcome measures, including Semmes-Weinstein monofilament testing, Purdue Pegboard Test, and Levine Carpal Tunnel Syndrome Questionnaire.[53]

Early recognition and response to symptomatology will likely remain the best safeguard to prevent permanent and often debilitating neurologic deterioration regardless of the cause. Future studies should also help to delineate the most cost-effective and time-effective evaluation and management options for compressive neuropathies in the general population and among athletes or other patients who require or seek the most rapid recuperation with the highest function possible.

For a complete list of references, go to ExpertConsult.com.

SELECTED READINGS

Citation:
Ashworth NL. Carpal tunnel syndrome. *Clin Evid.* 2011;1114.

Level of Evidence:
II

Summary:
This listing indicates the current best evidence for the safety and effectiveness of several nonoperative and operative interventions for carpal tunnel syndrome, including acupuncture, corticosteroids and other medications, therapy modalities, and open versus endoscopic surgical release.

Citation:
Ono S, Clapham PJ, Chung KC. Optimal management of carpal tunnel syndrome. *Int J Gen Med.* 2010;3:255–261.

Level of Evidence:
I

Summary:
This article serves as an update to the original 2009–2010 American Academy of Orthopaedic Surgeons publication of clinical guidelines regarding evaluation and management of carpal tunnel syndrome. Significant changes include a current trend for earlier recommendations for surgical intervention even without evidence of median nerve denervation, although definitive

recommendations have not yet been made. The four accepted treatment methods for carpal tunnel syndrome based on current best evidence are splinting, corticosteroids, ultrasound, and surgical release, with ultrasound having the lowest level of evidence to support its use.

Citation:

Keith MW, Masear V, Chung KC, et al. American Academy of Orthopaedic Surgeons Clinical Practice Guideline on diagnosis of carpal tunnel syndrome. *J Bone Joint Surg Am.* 2009;91A(10):2478–2479.

Levels of Evidence:

I-V

Summary:

This document is intended to be an initial practice guideline for the diagnosis of carpal tunnel syndrome based on current best evidence. Important points include the relatively limited amount of high-level evidence available regarding the diagnosis of carpal tunnel syndrome, as well as the recommended use of electrodiagnostic testing preoperatively.

Citation:

Keith MW, Masear V, Chung KC, et al. American Academy of Orthopaedic Surgeons clinical practice guideline on the treatment of carpal tunnel syndrome. *J Bone Joint Surg Am.* 2010;92A(1):218–219.

Levels of Evidence:

I-V

Summary:

Recommendations with a high level of evidence include performing a trial of nonoperative treatments for carpal tunnel syndrome before considering surgery, complete division of the flexor retinaculum if surgical release is performed, and avoidance of additional surgical procedures during carpal tunnel release such as an epineurotomy or skin nerve preservation. The authors also recommend avoiding immobilization after carpal tunnel release.

Citation:

Tang D, Barbour J, Davidge K, et al. Nerve entrapment: update. *Plast Reconstr Surg.* 2015;135:199e.

Levels of Evidence:

I–V

Summary:

Review of upper extremity compression neuropathies including comprehensive patient examination, neurodiagnostic testing, and operative decision-making. Special focus is placed on the scratch-collapse test, thoracic outlet compression, and nerve transfers for ulnar intrinsic atrophy.

Citation:

Scholten RJ, Mink van der Molen A, Uitdehaag BM, et al. Surgical treatment options for carpal tunnel syndrome (review). *Cochrane Database Syst Rev.* 2007;(4):CD003905.

Level of Evidence:

I

Summary:

Comprehensive comparison of 33 studies comparing endoscopic and open carpal tunnel release. Symptom relief, time to return to week, and complications are reviewed. The authors conclude long- and short-term results are similar between the methods and that major complications are also not different, with the caveat that "problem" carpal tunnels are often excluded from endoscopic treatment. The return to work was an average of 6 days fewer with endoscopic treatment.

INDEX

Page numbers followed by "*f*" indicate figures, "*t*" indicate tables, and "*b*" indicate boxes.

A

Abductor testing, 933
Abductors, of hip, 917
Abrasions, 253–254
  synovial, 1148
Abscess, skin, 203–204, 203*f*
Acceleration, 17–19, 17*t*, 18*f*
Accessory navicular, 1727–1728, 1728*f*
Accessory obturator nerve, of hip, 916
Accessory portal, 711, 951, 951*f*
Acetabulum
  cup depth, 938
  depth of, 908
  development, 907, 908*f*
  inclination, 938
  labrum, 313, 911, 911*f*–912*f*
  version, 907–908, 938
  volume of, 908
Acetaminophen, perioperative pharmacology, 338
Achilles tendon
  imaging, 1381–1383, 1382*f*–1383*f*
  injuries, 1476–1482
    complications, 1482
    decision-making principles, 1478–1479
    future considerations, 1482
    history, 1476
    imaging, 1477–1478, 1478*f*
    physical examination, 1477, 1477*f*
    postoperative management, 1480–1481
    results, 1481–1482
    treatment options, 1479–1480, 1479*t*,
      1480*b*–1481*b*, 1480*f*
  repair, platelet-rich plasma for, 54
ACL. *See* Anterior cruciate ligament
ACL-Return to Sport After Injury (ACL-RSI)
  scale, 387–389
Acne mechanica, 254–255, 255*f*
Acoustic shadowing, in ultrasonography, 79–80,
  80*f*
Acquired disease, hip, 1693–1694
Acromioclavicular (AC) joint, 397
  injuries, 645–678
    anatomy, 646*f*–647*f*, 646*t*
    classification, 645, 648*f*
    complications, 664
    decision-making principles, 653–655, 653*t*
    future considerations, 677
    history, 647–648, 649*f*
    imaging, 651–653, 652*f*, 654*f*–655*f*
    physical examination, 648–651, 650*t*, 651*f*
    postoperative management, 663–664
    results, 664, 665*t*–666*t*
    return-to-play guidelines, 663–664
    treatment, 655–659, 656*f*–658*f*
      anatomic coracoclavicular reconstruction,
        659*b*–663*b*, 659*f*–663*f*
  pathologies, 406
Acromion, imaging, 414–415, 414*f*–415*f*
  magnetic resonance imaging, 415–417, 416*f*,
    418*f*
Actifit implant, 42
Action plan, emergency, 150, 151*b*
Action-reaction, 19, 19*f*–20*f*
Acute bronchitis, 209
Acute compartment syndrome (ACS), 154
Acute kidney injury, 229

Acute mountain sickness (AMS), 242–243, 243*b*
Acute otitis externa, 213–214
Acute pneumonia, 209–210
Acute rotator cuff trauma, 548
Adaptive sports equipment
  amputee athlete, 317
  cerebral palsy, 321
  intellectually disabled athletes, 323
  visually impaired athletes, 323
  wheelchair athlete, 320
Adductor
  anatomy, 1007–1008, 1008*f*
  hip, 920
  pathology, 1007–1017
  strains, 1011–1012, 1050–1051
    complications, 1051
    decision-making principles, 1051
    future considerations, 1051
    history, 1050
    imaging, 1050, 1050*f*
    nonoperative management, 1011
    operative management, 1011–1012
    physical examination, 1050
    results, 1051
    return to play, 1051
    treatment options, 1013*b*, 1013*f*, 1050–1051,
      1051*b*
  tenotomy, 1016
Adductor canal nerve block, 333, 333*f*
Adenovirus, waterborne diseases, 212–213
Adhesive capsulitis, 407, 424, 425*b*, 426*f*
  in female athlete, 310–312, 311*t*
  idiopathic, 581–582
Adipose-derived stem cells (ADSCs), 57–58, 58*f*
Adolescent bunion, 1727
Adrenal hormones, 69*t*, 70
Adson test, 636–638, 637*f*
Adult involvement, in pediatric sports, 1610
Age/aging
  anterior cruciate ligament injuries, 1188–1189
  anterior shoulder instability, 452
  articular cartilage lesions, 1164
  articular cartilage repair, 12
  skeletal muscle and, 68
Alcohol, 290–291
Allergic contact dermatitis, 258
Allergies
  anesthesia, 339
  preparticipation physical evaluation, 149
Allograft, 31–32
  augmentation of, 32
  autograft *vs.*, healing of, 32–33
  meniscal, transplantation, 1142
  osteochondral, 1166, 1173*f*–1174*f*, 1176
  particulated juvenile cartilage, 1165–1166,
    1172*f*, 1176
Alpha angle, 938
Altitude sickness. *See* Acute mountain sickness
American football injuries. *See* Football injuries
Amputation, traumatic, 154
Amputee athletes, 316–317
  adaptive sports equipment, 317
  exercise, 316, 316*t*
  medical considerations, 316–317
    bone spurs, 317
    dermatologic conditions, 316–317

Amputee athletes (*Continued*)
  heterotopic ossification, 317
  musculoskeletal injuries, 316
  neuroma, 317
AMS. *See* Acute mountain sickness
Amylin analog therapy, 221
Anabolic-androgenic steroids, 284–287, 1611
  adverse effects, 285–287
    cardiovascular, 286
    hepatic, 286
    musculoskeletal, 286
    psychiatric, 286–287
  athletic performance considerations, 285
  physiologic considerations, 284–285
Analgesic medications, for knee arthritis, 1279
Anaphylaxis, 153
Anatomic coordinate system, 16
Anatomic coracoclavicular reconstruction,
  659*b*–663*b*, 659*f*–663*f*
Anatomic reconstructions, for lateral and
  posterolateral corner injuries of knee,
  1255–1256
Androstenedione, 287
Anemia, 196. *See also* Red blood cells, disorders of
Anesthesia
  arthroscopy
    elbow, 708
    principles, 110, 110*f*
    synovectomy, 1129
  intraoperative care, 327–329. *See also* Regional
    anesthesia
    positioning, 329
    tourniquets, 328–329
  neuraxial, 329
  perioperative complications, 339–340
    allergic reactions, 339
    Parsonage-Turner syndrome, 339–340
  perioperative medicine and, 325–340
    cardiac considerations, 326–327
    diabetes mellitus, 327
    respiratory considerations, 325–326, 326*f*
  perioperative pharmacology, 335–339
    acetaminophen, 338
    buprenorphine, 337–338
    dexmedetomidine, 338–339
    ketamine, 338
    methadone, 337
    nonsteroidal antiinflammatory drugs, 338
    opioids, 337
    propofol, 338
  regional, 328
    arm, 330
    benefits, 328
    complications, 328
    contraindications, 328
    elbow, 330–332
    femur, 332–333
    forearm, 330–332
    hand, 330–332
    hip, 332–333
    intravenous, 334
    knee, 332–333
    neuraxial anesthesia, 329
    orthopaedic surgeries and, 327
    patient characteristics, 327
    peripheral nerve block, 329–330

Anesthesia (Continued)
    shoulder, 330
    techniques, 329–335
    thigh, 332–333
Angiography, of popliteal artery entrapment
        syndrome, 1353–1354, 1354f
Angular kinematics, 22
Ankle
    arthrodesis, 1427b, 1427f
    arthroscopy, 1421–1435, 1422f
        calcaneoplasty, 1433–1435
        endoscopic Haglund resection, 1433–1435
        soft tissue conditions, 1421–1428, 1422f
        subtalar arthroscopy, 1428–1433
    biomechanics, 1359–1369
    decision-making, 1370–1379
    diagnosis, 1370–1379
    forefoot, 1515–1526
        hallux rigidus, 1523–1526
        metatarsalgia, 1519–1522
        sesamoid dysfunction, 1516–1519,
            1517b–1518b
        turf toe, 1515–1516, 1516b
    history, 1372–1379, 1373f–1378f
    imaging, 1380–1392
        computed tomography, 1380
        ligaments, 1387–1388, 1388f
        magnetic resonance imaging, 1380–1381
        nerve entrapment, 1389–1391
        osteochondral lesions, 1388–1389, 1389f
        plantar fasciitis, 1391, 1391f
        radiographs, 1380, 1381f
        tendons, 1381–1386, 1381f
        ultrasound, 1380
    injuries
        in adolescent athlete, 1725–1740
            fractures, 1729–1733, 1729f, 1732f–1734f,
                1732t
            orthotics, 1739
            shoes, 1739
            soft tissue, 1728–1729, 1728f
            systemic illness, 1739
            variations of normal anatomy, 1725–1728
        articular cartilage, 1484–1503
        in female athlete, 305–306
        figure skating, 117–118
        lacrosse, 122
        ligamentous, 1444–1461
        tendons, 1462–1483
        volleyball, 127
    joint, biomechanics, 1360–1363, 1361f–1362f
    lateral ligament, reconstruction, 1426b
    pathologies, 1370–1371
    pediatric, 1633–1635
        acute injuries, 1633, 1634f
        overuse injuries, 1633–1635, 1634f
    peripheral nerve entrapment around,
            1402–1420
        deep peroneal nerve, 1415–1416, 1415f
        interdigital neuralgia (Morton neuroma),
            1416–1419
        lateral plantar nerve, 1411–1412
        medial plantar nerve, 1412–1413
        saphenous nerve, 1405–1407, 1405f–1406f
        superficial peroneal nerve, 1413–1415, 1413f
        sural nerve, 1402–1405, 1403f
        tarsal tunnel syndrome, 1407–1411, 1407f
    physical examination, 1371–1372
    plantar fasciitis, 1509–1513
        complications, 1513
        decision-making principles, 1510
        future considerations, 1513
        history, 1509
        imaging, 1509, 1509f
        physical examination, 1509
        postoperative management, 1511

Ankle (Continued)
        results, 1511–1513
        treatment options, 1510–1511, 1510f, 1511b,
            1512f
    posterior heel pain, 1504–1508, 1505f
        complications, 1508
        decision-making principles, 1505–1506
        future considerations, 1508
        history, 1504
        imaging, 1504–1505, 1505f–1506f
        physical examination, 1504, 1505f
        postoperative management, 1508
        results, 1508
        treatment options, 1506–1507
    sprains, 115, 371, 380–381
        balance, 381, 382f–383f
        bracing, 380–381
        coordination, 381
        dorsiflexion range of motion, 381
        education of risk, 381
        hypomobility issues, 381
        lateral, 1444–1450, 1445f
        medial, 1450–1453
        strength training, 381
        taping, 369, 369f–370f, 380–381
Ankle block, 333–334
Ankle-brachial index (ABI) testing, 1395
Anomalous coronary artery, 168
Anterior arthroscopic débridement, 1425b
Anterior center edge angles, 937–938
Anterior compartment
    arthroscopic synovectomy, of knee, 1129, 1130t
    release, 1399
Anterior cruciate ligament (ACL)
    anatomy, 1069, 1070f, 1185–1186, 1186f
    basic science, 1186–1187
    biology, 1187
    biomechanics, 1185–1186, 1186f
    chronic insufficiency, 1284, 1284f
    injuries, 1185–1198
        biofeedback, 1196
        clinical history, 1187
        complications, 1197–1198
        decision-making principles, 1188–1190
        electrical stimulation, 1196
        epidemiology, 1187, 1199
        in female athlete, 307, 308t–309t, 309f
        functional training, 1196–1197
        future considerations, 1198
        graft type, 1197
        history, 1185
        imaging, 1188, 1188f
        muscle training, 1195–1196, 1196f
        pediatrics, 1697–1703
            complications, 1702
            decision-making principles, 1698
            future direction, 1703
            history, 1697
            imaging, 1697–1698
            partial tears, 1698
            physical examination, 1697
            postoperative management, 1701–1702
            reconstruction, 1700–1701, 1700f–1702f,
                1701b
            rehabilitation, 1701–1702
            treatment, 1698–1700, 1699f
        physical examination, 1187–1188
        postoperative management, 1192–1197
        proprioception, 1196
        reconstruction, 1193b–1195b, 1193f–1195f
            causes of failure, 1202–1203
            in female athlete, 310
            primary graft choice, 1203
            results, 1197–1198
            two-stage, 1207
        rehabilitation, 1192–1195, 1197

Anterior cruciate ligament (ACL) (Continued)
        return to play, 389t, 1197
        revision, 1189–1190, 1192, 1199–1210, 1208b
            advanced imaging, 1202, 1202f
            complications in, 1209
            decision-making principles, 1202–1204
            future considerations, 1209
            history, 1199–1200
            imaging, 1200–1202, 1200f
            multiple, 1209
            physical exam, 1200
            postoperative management, 1207–1209
            results, 1209
            treatment options, 1204–1207
        single vs. double bundle, 1197
        surgery, platelet-rich plasma for, 54–55
        tear, 377–380, 378f–379f
        treatment options, 1190–1192
    microanatomy, 1186
    MRI, 1110–1111, 1111f–1112f
    multiligament knee injuries and, 1267–1268
    partial tear, 1189
Anterior drawer test, 1377–1379, 1444, 1446f
Anterior interosseous nerve neuropathy, 899f
Anterior interosseous syndrome (AIN), 694,
        746–747
    complications, 747
    decision-making principles, 746
    history, 746
    physical examination, 746
    postoperative management, 747
    results, 747
    return-to-play guidelines, 747
    treatment, 746
Anterior intramuscular transposition, 750, 751f
Anterior shoulder instability, 440–462
    anatomy, 440–441, 441f–442f
    decision-making principles, 450–454
        age, 452
        associated injuries, 453–454
        contact sports, 453
        first-time vs. recurrent instability, 452–453
        in-season management, 453
        synthesis, 454, 454t
    future considerations, 461–462
    history, 447
    imaging, 448–450, 450f–452f
    pathoanatomy, 441–447, 443f–444f, 443t, 446f
    physical examination, 447–448, 448f–449f
    treatment options, 454–461
        complications, 461
        emergency department, 455
        nonoperative sling immobilization, 455
        on-field management, 454–455
        rehabilitation, 455
        results, 461
        surgical management, 455–461, 456b
Anterior subcutaneous transposition, 750, 750f
Anterior submuscular transposition, 750–751, 751f
Anterior tibial tendons, 1386, 1387f
    injuries, 1462–1464
        complications, 1464
        decision-making principles, 1462
        history, 1462
        imaging, 1462
        physical examination, 1462, 1463f
        postoperative management, 1463
        results, 1463–1464
        treatment options, 1462–1463, 1463b–1464b,
            1464f
    translation of, 1247–1248
Anteroinferior iliac spine, 908
Anterolateral ligament, of knee, 1070–1071, 1071f
Anterolateral portal, 778–779, 950–951, 950f
Anteromedial portal, 777–778
Anteroposterior view, 408, 409f

Antiepileptic drug (AED), 231
Apophyseal ring fractures, 1753, 1756*f*
Appositional ossification, 14
"Apprehension test", 404
Arachnoid mater, 1528
Arch taping, 368–369
Arcuate ligament complex, 1246
Arm. *See also* Entrapment neuropathies
   radial nerve, 752
   regional anesthesia, 330
Arrhythmias, 172–173
   atrial fibrillation, 172
   catecholamine polymorphic ventricular
      tachycardia (CPVT), 172–173, 173*f*
   channelopathies, 172–173
   Wolff-Parkinson-White syndrome, 172
Arrhythmogenic right ventricular cardiomyopathy
   (ARVC), 168
Arthritis
   glenohumeral, 592–608
     classification, 592–595
     complications, 606, 607*t*
     decision-making principles, 603–604
     epidemiology, 592
     future considerations, 607
     history, 595
     physical examination, 595–596
     postoperative management, 605–606, 606*t*
     presentation, 595
     prior operative notes, 596
     return-to-play guidelines, 606
     treatment, 596–603, 604*b*, 604*f*–605*f*
   hip, 1053–1060
     complications, 1060
     decision-making principles, 1057
     future direction, 1060
     history, 1053
     imaging, 1055–1057, 1055*f*–1056*f*, 1055*t*
     physical examination, 1053–1055
     postoperative management in, 1059
     results, 1059–1060
     surgical treatment, 1058–1059
     treatment options, 1057, 1060*b*
   knee, 1277–1292
     decision-making principles, 1283–1284
     history, 1277, 1278*t*
     imaging, 1277–1279, 1278*f*–1279*f*
     postoperative management, 1289, 1289*t*
     results, 1289, 1290*t*
     treatment options, 1279–1283, 1280*f*, 1284*f*
       nonoperative, 1279–1280
       not recommended, 1280
       operative, 1280–1283
   rheumatoid, 594–595, 594*f*
Arthrodesis
   ankle, 1427*b*, 1427*f*
   arthroscopic ankle, 1427*b*, 1427*f*
   metatarsophalangeal, 1525, 1525*f*
Arthrography, 76–77, 76*f*–77*f*
   computed tomography, 87, 87*f*
   magnetic resonance imaging, 415–417, 416*f*
   rotator cuff, 417–422
   shoulder, 410–411, 410*f*
Arthropathy
   capsulorrhaphy, 593, 593*f*
   dislocation, 593
   instability, 592–595
     chondrolysis, 593–594
     osteonecrosis, 595, 595*f*, 595*t*
     rheumatoid arthritis, 594–595, 594*f*
Arthroplasty, 605–606
   for knee arthritis, 1283
   return to sport after, 1283
   total hip, 1059

Arthroscope, 105–107, 106*f*
Arthroscopic ankle arthrodesis, 1427*b*, 1427*f*
Arthroscopic biceps tenodesis, 532
Arthroscopic bursal resection, 617*b*–619*b*,
   617*f*–619*f*
Arthroscopic capsular release, 585–586
Arthroscopic plication, 481
Arthroscopic portals, 110, 817–819, 818*f*–819*f*
   accessory, 711
   hip, 950–952
     anterolateral, 950–951, 950*f*
     distal anterolateral accessory, 951, 951*f*
     modified mid-anterior, 951, 951*f*
     posterolateral, 951–952
   posterolateral, 951–952
Arthroscopic posterior shoulder stabilization,
   470*b*–472*b*, 470*f*–472*f*
Arthroscopic probe, 107
Arthroscopic subtalar arthrodesis, 1430*b*–1431*b*
Arthroscopic subtalar débridement, 1429*b*–1430*b*,
   1429*f*–1430*f*
Arthroscopic suprapectoral biceps tenodesis,
   533*b*, 533*f*–534*f*
Arthroscopic synovectomy, of knee, 1127–1131
   anesthesia, 1129
   complications, 1130
   decision-making principles, 1128–1130,
     1128*f*–1129*f*
   future direction, 1130–1131
   history, 1127
   imaging, 1127–1128
   physical examination, 1127
   positioning, 1129
   postoperative management, 1130
   results, 1130
   surgical steps, 1129–1130
     anterior compartments, 1129, 1130*t*
     posterior compartments, 1129–1130
   treatment options, 1128–1129, 1129*b*
Arthroscopy, 105–113
   anesthesia, 110, 110*f*
   ankle, 1421–1435, 1422*f*
     calcaneoplasty, 1433–1435
     endoscopic Haglund resection, 1433–1435
     soft tissue conditions, 1421–1428, 1422*f*
   applications of, 105
   for calcaneal fractures, 1431*b*
   complications, 110–112
   diagnostic, 110
   elbow, 707–719, 767*b*, 767*f*–768*f*
     complications, 718
     decision-making principles, 707–712
     fluid management, 708–709
     future considerations, 718
     history, 707
     imaging, 707
     instrumentation, 708–709, 709*f*
     physical examination, 707
     portal placement, 709–711, 709*t*
     postoperative management, 718
     return-to-play guidelines, 718
     treatment, 707–712, 717*b*
   equipment in, 105–109, 106*f*
     arthroscope, 105–107, 106*f*
     arthroscopic probe in, 107
     basket forceps in, 107–108, 108*f*
     cannulas in, 108
     electrocautery in, 108–109
     fluid pump, 107
     grasping forceps in, 108
     instruments and, 107
     knives in, 108
     motorized shavers in, 107–108
     radiofrequency instruments and, 108–109

Arthroscopy (*Continued*)
   scissors in, 108
   switching sticks in, 108
   hip, 947–956, 1058–1059, 1058*f*
     contraindications, 947
     femoroacetabular impingement, 965–967,
       966*f*, 966*t*
     indications, 947–948
     learning curve for, 948
     operating room set-up, 948–950
     positioning for, 948–950
     procedure for, 950–955
   knee, 1121–1126, 1280–1281
     complications, 1125–1126
     diagnostic, 1123–1125, 1125*f*
     indications, 1121
     instrumentation, 1125
     lateral and posterolateral corner injuries,
       1254, 1254*f*
     portal placement, 1121–1123, 1122*f*–1124*f*
     positioning, 1121, 1122*f*
     postoperative care, 1125
     preoperative evaluation, 1121
   lateral epicondylitis, 724
   for meniscal injuries, 1140
   motion, loss, in elbow, 776–781, 777*f*–781*f*
     anterolateral portal, 778–779
     anteromedial portal, 777–778
   pediatric, 1612–1614, 1612*f*–1615*f*
   posterior hindfoot, 1470*b*, 1471*f*
   principles, 109–110
     anesthesia, 110, 110*f*
     arthroscopic portals in, 110
     diagnostic arthroscopy, 110
     patient positioning, 109–110, 109*f*–110*f*
     preoperative, 109
     preparation, 109–110, 109*f*–110*f*
     surgical technique, 109
   reduction, 824*b*–825*b*, 824*f*–825*f*
   scaphoid nonunions, reduction of, 824–825,
     825*t*
   shoulder, 433–439
     anatomy, 435–436
     background, 433
     complications, 438–439
     contraindications, 433
     diagnostic examination, 436–438,
       437*f*–438*f*
     indications, 433
     open procedures *vs.*, 433
     portal placement, 435–436, 436*f*
     positioning, 434–435, 434*f*
     preoperative imaging, 433–434
     setup, 435
     visualization, 435
   subtalar, 1428–1433
     complications, 1432–1433
     decision-making principles, 1429
     history, 1429
     imaging, 1429
     physical examination, 1429
     postoperative management, 1431
     results, 1431–1432
   triangular fibrocartilage complex, 828, 828*t*
   wrist, 817–834
     anatomy, 819–820, 820*f*–821*f*
     carpal instability, 821–824, 821*t*, 822*f*–823*f*
     class I traumatic injuries, 829–832,
       829*f*–831*f*
     class II degenerative injuries, 832
     complications, 833
     fracture, 824–828
     future considerations, 833
     ganglionectomy, 832–833, 832*f*

Arthroscopy *(Continued)*
  management, 829–832, 829*f*–831*f*
  set-up, 817–819, 818*f*–819*f*
  triangular fibrocartilage complex, 828, 828*t*
Articular cartilage, 9–12
  cell-matrix interactions, 11
  clinical relevance and further developments in, 12
  defects, 1179*f*
    depth, 12
    size, 12
    surgical management, 1178–1184
      palliative, 1179
      reparative, 1179–1181, 1180*f*–1181*f*
      restorative, 1181–1184, 1182*f*
    treatment, 1178–1184
  extracellular matrix, 11
  hip, 913–914
  injuries, 1484–1503. *See also* Osteochondral lesions
    revision anterior cruciate ligament injuries and, 1203–1204
  lesions (ACL), 1161–1177
    anatomy, 1161–1162
    biomechanics, 1161–1162
    classification, 1162, 1162*t*
    complications, 1176
    decision-making principles, 1163–1164
    future considerations, 1176–1177
    history, 1162–1163
    imaging, 1163
    physical examination, 1163
    postoperative management, 1166–1167
    results, 1174–1176
    return to play, 1167
    treatment options, 1164–1166, 1167*b*–1173*b*, 1168*f*
  repair, 11–12
  structure and composition, 10–11, 10*f*
  zones of, 10–11, 10*f*
Articular hyaline cartilage, restoration of, 1488
Articular surfaces, 431–432, 431*f*–432*f*
Articulation, scapulothoracic, 398
Artifacts, magnetic resonance, 98–99
ARVC. *See* Arrhythmogenic right ventricular cardiomyopathy
Aseptic meningitis, 214
  waterborne diseases, 212–213
Aspirin, 191–192
Asthma, 190, 325
Athlete. *See also* Elite athlete
  amputee, 316–317
    adaptive sports equipment, 317
    exercise physiology, 316
    medical considerations, 316–317, 316*t*
  with cerebral palsy, 320–321
    adaptive equipment, 321
    exercise, 320–321, 320*b*
    medical considerations, 321
  collegiate, 155
  in contact sports, 453
  with diabetes, 218–226. *See also* Diabetes
    diagnosis, 218–219
    epidemiology, 218
    exercise, physiologic changes of, 221–223, 221*f*, 222*t*
    management, 223–225, 223*f*
    treatment, 219–221
  exercise-induced bronchoconstriction, risk for, 175
  female. *See* Female athlete
  gastrointestinal medicine in, 189–195
  genitourinary trauma in, 227–229
  hematologic medicine, in, 196–200
  high school, 155
  infectious diseases in, 201–217

Athlete *(Continued)*
  injured, approach to, 1554–1556, 1554*f*
  intellectually disabled, 321–323
    adaptive equipment, 323
    exercise physiology, 322
    medical considerations, 322–323
  posterior cruciate ligament injuries, 1211–1212, 1212*f*
  professional, 155
  with special needs, 150
  visually impaired, 323
  wheelchair, 317–320
    adaptive, 320
    exercise, 317–318
    medical considerations, 318–320
"Athlete's foot" (tinea pedis), 249, 250*f*
Athlete's nodules (collagenomas), 255, 255*f*
Athletic heart syndrome, 326
Athletic pubalgia, 1007–1017
  anatomy, 1007–1008, 1008*f*
  complications, 1016
  decision-making principles, 1011
  future considerations, 1016
  historical background, 1008
  history, 1009
  imaging, 1010–1011
    dynamic ultrasonography, 1010–1011
    magnetic resonance imaging, 1010, 1010*f*–1011*f*
    radiographic analysis, 1010, 1010*f*
  pediatrics, 1692
  physical examination, 1009, 1009*f*
    diagnostic injections, 1009
  treatment options, 1011–1016, 1014*b*
    adductor strain, 1011–1012, 1013*b*, 1013*f*
    osteitis pubis, 1014–1016, 1016*b*
    sports hernia, 1012–1014, 1014*b*, 1014*f*
Athletic trainer, 342–346
  education, 342–343, 343*b*, 343*t*
  regulation, 343, 344*t*
  scope of practice, 344–346
    clinical diagnosis, 344, 345*f*
    emergent care, 344–345
    health care administration, 346
    health promotion, 344
    immediate care, 344
    injury prevention, 344
    psychosocial strategies, 345–346
    referral, 345–346
    therapeutic interventions, 345, 345*f*
    working relationship, 344
Athletic training, 342, 343*b*. *See also* Training
Atlantoaxial instability, 1758
  in Down syndrome, 1758–1759
    decision-making principles, 1758, 1759*f*
    history, 1758
    imaging, 1758
    physical examination, 1758
    results, 1759
    treatment, 1759, 1760*f*
Atlas, spine, 1533
Atraumatic hip microinstability, 977–978
Atraumatic instability, 1654–1655
  history, 1654
  imaging, 1655, 1655*f*
  physical examination, 1654–1655, 1654*f*
  treatment options, 1655, 1655*f*
Atria, 160–161
Atrial fibrillation, 172
Augmentation
  allograft, 32
  autograft, 30–31
  ligament, 5–7
  meniscal repair, 9
  tendon, 5–7

Auto racing injuries, 117
Autogenous cancellous bone grafting, 1491
Autograft, 30
  allograft *vs.*, 32–33
  augmented, 30–31
  bone-tendon-bone, 30
  osteochondral, 1165, 1167*b*–1173*b*, 1169*f*–1171*f*, 1175
  semitendinosus, 31
  soft tissue, 31
Autologous chondrocyte implantation, 42–43, 1165, 1167*b*–1173*b*, 1171*f*, 1175–1176, 1489
Autologous matric induced chondrogenesis (AMIC), 1489
Autonomic dysreflexia, 319–320
AVPU scale, for injured athlete, 1554–1555
Avulsion fractures, 928, 1052, 1688, 1689*f*
Axial neck pain, 1593–1594
Axillary brachial plexus block, 332
Axillary lateral view, 408, 409*f*
Axillary nerve compression, 630*b*
Axillary nerve palsy, 629–630
  anatomy, 629
  biomechanics, 629
  clinical evaluation, 629–630
  decision-making principles, 630
  diagnostic studies, 630
  results, 630

B

Back. *See also* Spine
  injuries, 118–121, 126
  pain, 128, 1598
Bacterial infections, 246–249
  cellulitis/erysipelas, 247–248, 248*f*
  erythrasma, 248–249, 249*f*
  folliculocentric infections, 246, 247*f*
  impetigo, 246–247, 247*f*
  pitted keratolysis, 248, 248*f*
  pseudomonal folliculitis (hot tub folliculitis), 249, 249*f*
  skin, 203–205
    definition, 203
    diagnosis, 203–204, 203*f*–204*f*
    epidemiology, 203
    pathobiology, 203
    prevention, 204
    return-to-play guidelines, 204–205
    treatment, 204
Balance, 381, 382*f*–383*f*
Balance Error Scoring System (BESS), 1744, 1744*b*
Bankart repair, arthroscopic, 457*b*–459*b*, 458*f*, 461
Baseball injuries, 114–115
  elbow, 115
  lower extremity, 115
  pediatric, 115
  shoulder, 114–115
  sliding, 115
Basketball injuries, 115–116
  ankle sprains, 115
  concussion, 116
  dental, 116
  facial, 116
  finger, 116
  hand, 116
  knee, 115–116
  sudden death, 116
  tendinitis, 116
Basket forceps, 107–108, 108*f*
"Baxter's nerve", 1411
Beach chair position, 329
Bear-hug test, 404, 559
Beighton scoring method, 1446*t*
Belly-press test, 404, 559

Biceps
distal
tendinitis, 725–728
complications, 727
decision-making principles, 725–726
future considerations, 727–728
history, 725
imaging, 725, 726f
physical examination, 725, 725f
postoperative management, 727
results, 726
return-to-play guidelines, 727
treatment, 726, 726b
tendon rupture, 731–741
anatomy, 731, 732f–733f
biomechanics, 731–732
classification, 732, 732b
complications, 736–737
decision-making principles, 735
epidemiology, 731
history, 732–733
imaging, 733–734, 734f
physical examination, 733, 733f
postoperative management, 735
results, 735–736
treatment, 734–735, 735t, 736b, 736f
imaging, 422–424, 425f
tendon, long head of, 424–427, 427f
tenodesis, 524, 532, 1254–1255
tenosynovitis, 548
tenotomy, 531–532
Biceps femoris muscle, 1245–1246
long head of, 1245–1246
short head of, 1246
Biceps pulley, 422–424, 425f
Bicuspid aortic valve, 168–169, 170f–171f
Bier block, 334
Bifurcate ligament sprain, 1456–1457
complications, 1458
decision-making principles, 1457
history, 1457
imaging, 1457
physical examination, 1457
postoperative management, 1457
results, 1457–1458
treatment, 1457, 1457b
Bioabsorbable implants, 1204
BioCart II, 44
Biofeedback, 1196
Biologic augmentation, repair with, 571
Biologic stimulation, 1147–1150
Biomechanics, 16–29
ankle, 1359–1369
joints, 1360–1363, 1361f–1362f
anterior cruciate ligament, 1185–1186, 1186f
articular cartilage lesions, 1161–1162
axillary nerve palsy, 629
basic concepts, 16–19
coordinate systems, 16
degrees of freedom, 16–17, 18f
Newton's laws, 17–19, 17t
scalars, 16
units of measure, 16, 17t
vectors, 16, 18f
distal biceps tendon rupture, 731–732
distal triceps tendon rupture, 737
dynamics, 22–23
joint motions in, 22–23, 23f
kinematics, 22
kinetics, 23
relative motion, 22
elbow, 681–685
extensor mechanism injuries, 1319, 1320f

Biomechanics (Continued)
factors affecting properties, 27
foot, 1359–1369
head, 1535, 1535f
injuries, 1538, 1539f
hip, 907–924
gait cycle in, 921–922
joint, forces around, 922–923
motions in, 921
spine and, relationship of, 923–924, 923f
stability in, 921
knee, 1072–1073, 1073f
joint, 1077–1080
lateral and posterolateral corner injuries, 1246, 1247f
ligament, 1075–1077, 1076f
meniscal, 1080–1082
patellofemoral joint, 1082–1087
techniques, 1073–1074, 1074f
tibiofemoral joint, 1074–1080
lateral corner injuries, 1246, 1247f
long thoracic nerve palsy, 625, 625f
mechanics, classes of, 23–24
fluid mechanics, 23–24
rigid body mechanics, 23
viscoelasticity and, 24, 24f–25f
meniscus, 1134–1135
methods, 24–29
functional tissue engineering, 28–29
improving performance, 28
injury prevention, 28
mechanical properties, 25–27, 26f–27f
practical application, 27–29
stiffness vs. flexibility testing, 27
structural properties, 24–25, 25f–26f
surgical reconstruction, 28
patellofemoral joint, 1082–1087
pediatrics
concussion, 1741, 1742f
throwing, 1663–1665
rotator cuff and impingement lesions, 542–543
biceps function, 542, 543f
function, 542, 542f
scapular function, 543
static stabilizers, 542–543
spinal accessory nerve palsy, 627–628
spine, 1535, 1535f
statics in, 19–22
force vectors, 21
free-body diagrams, 20f, 21
ligament and joint contact forces in, 21–22
moment/torque vectors, 21
subtalar joint, 1363–1365, 1363t, 1364f–1366f
suprascapular nerve palsy, 621–622, 622f
throwing, 1663–1665
transverse tarsal joints, 1365, 1367f
wrist, 789–790, 790f, 835
BioSeed-C, 44
Birth control, in female athlete, 301, 301t
Bladder
injuries, 227
neurogenic, 319
Blisters, friction, 254
Blood-borne infections, 210
BMAC. See Bone marrow aspirate concentrate (BMAC)
Bone, 12–15
appositional ossification, 14
cellular biology, 13
circulation, 13
formation, 14
fracture healing in, biology, 14–15, 14t–15t
injuries, hip, 925–926

Bone (Continued)
matrix, 13
pediatrics, 1688–1691
realignment of, procedures for, 1300–1301
remodeling, 13
tissue surrounding, 13–14
types, 12–13, 12f
Bone grafting, 715b–716b, 1204
Bone marrow aspirate (BMA), 1489
Bone marrow aspirate concentrate (BMAC), 57, 57f
Bone scans, 88–89, 89f
meniscal transplantation, 1155
posterior cruciate ligament injuries, 1214
Bone-tendon-bone autograft, 30
Bony anatomy
hip, 907–911
pertinent, patellar instability, 1294, 1294f
Borderline dysplasia, 977
Bowel, neurogenic, 319
Boxing
injuries, 116–117
facial, 116–117
neurologic, 117
upper extremity, 117
professional vs. amateur, 116
Braces
ankle sprains, 380–381
knee arthritis, 1279–1280
Brachial plexus, 330, 331f
Brain, 1528–1529
injury, 1562–1569
background, 1562–1564
clinical presentation, 1563–1564
definition, 1562–1563
epidemiology, 1563
imaging, 1566
interventions, 1567–1568
management, 1566–1567
pathophysiology, 1563
physical examination, 1564–1566
retiring athlete, 1567
return-to-play, 1567, 1567t
Brainstem, 1528–1529
Bronchitis, acute, 209
Bronchodilators, for exercise-induced bronchoconstriction, 177
BST-CarGel, 44
Bunion, adolescent, 1727
Buprenorphine, perioperative pharmacology, 337–338
Burners, 406, 1579
Burning hands syndrome, 1579
Bursae
around hip joint, 920–921
iliopsoas, 921
knee, 1068–1069
trochanteric, 920–921
Bursitis
iliopsoas, 980
olecranon, 728–730, 728f
complications, 730
decision-making principles, 728–729
future considerations, 730
history, 728, 728f
imaging, 728, 729f
physical examination, 728
postoperative care, 730
results, 730
treatment, 729, 729b, 729f
pediatrics, 1692
trochanteric, 1001–1002, 1002b
Burst fractures, of thoracolumbar spine, 1584, 1585f

C

C sign, 929–930, 930f
Caffeine, 290
  historical perspectives, 290
  mechanism of action, 290
  side effects, 290
Calcaneoplasty, 1433–1435
  complications, 1435
  decision-making principles, 1433
  history, 1433
  imaging, 1433
  physical examination, 1433
  postoperative management, 1434
  results, 1434
Calcaneum fracture, 1456–1457
  arthroscopically assisted treatment, 1431b
Calcified cartilage zone, 11
Calcium, 279
Calluses, 254
Cam impingement, 927–928, 957, 958f
Cancellous bone, 12f, 13
Cannulas, in arthroscopy, 108
Capacity, to exercise, 71–73, 71f
Capitate carpal injuries, 843–845, 844b, 844f
Capitate fracture, 809
Capsule
  innervation, 914–916
    accessory obturator nerve, 916
    femoral nerve, 916
    inferior gluteal nerve, 916
    obturator nerve, 916
    quadratus femoris, nerve to, 916
    sciatic nerve, 916
    superior gluteal nerve, 916
  joint
    capsular ligaments, 914
    safe zone, 916, 916f
    zona orbicularis in, 914
  structure, 427–431
    anatomy, 427–428
    anterior, 428–429, 429f–430f
    instability, 426f, 428
    multidirectional, 430, 430f
    posterior, 429, 430b, 430f
  vascularization, 916, 917f
Capsuloligamentous restraints, 680–681, 682f
Capsulorrhaphy arthropathy, 593, 593f
Carbohydrates, 277–278, 278t
Carbuncles, 246, 247f
Cardiac arrest, 153
Cardiorespiratory response, to exercise, 72, 72f, 72t
Cardiovascular system
  abnormalities, in intellectually disabled
    athletes, 322–323
  elite athlete
    electrocardiogram and electrophysiologic
      adaptations, 161, 161f
    rigorous athletic training and, 160–161
    screening, 162–166, 163b
    structural adaptations, 160–161
  preoperative care, 326–327
    athletic heart syndrome, 326
    hypertrophic cardiomyopathy, 326–327
  preparticipation physical evaluation, 145–147,
    145b–146b
Carpal tunnel release, 903b, 903f
Carpals
  fractures, 807–809
    capitate, 809
    hamate, 809
    imaging, 807–809
    scaphoid, 807–808, 807f–808f
    trapezium, 808–809, 809f
  injuries, 835–856
    anatomy, 835
    biomechanics, 835

Carpals (Continued)
    capitate, 843–845, 844b, 844f
    future considerations, 854–855
    hamate, 840–843, 840f–843f, 843b
    instability, 848–851, 848f–850f, 850b
    Kienböck disease, 846–847
    ligament, anatomy and mechanics, 848–851,
      848f–850f, 850b
    lunate, 845–847, 846f, 847b
    lunotriquetral injuries, 848
    perilunate instability, 851–854, 851f–855f,
      853b
    pisiform, 847–848, 847f, 848b
    scaphoid, 835–836, 837b, 837f
    scapholunate injuries, 848
    trapezium, 838–840, 838f–840f, 840b
    trapezoid, 845, 845b
    triquetrum, 836–838, 838b, 838f
  instability, 821–824, 821t, 822f–823f
Cartiform, 1183–1184
Cartilage
  articular, 9–12, 913–914
    cell-matrix interactions, 11
    clinical relevance and further developments
      in, 12
    defect
      depth, 12
      size, 12
    extracellular matrix, 11
    repair, 11–12
    structure and composition, 10–11, 10f
    zones of, 10–11, 10f
  knee, 1116–1118, 1118f–1119f
  repair, 42–45, 59–60
  restoration
    indications, 1163
    platelet-rich plasma, 55
Cartilage Autograft Implantation System (CAIS),
  44
Cartilage Regeneration System (CaReS), 43
CartiONE, 1182
Cartistem, 1181–1182
Cartiva, 44
Catecholamine polymorphic ventricular
  tachycardia (CPVT), 172–173, 173f
Causalgia, 902
Cavus foot, 1728
Celiac disease, 194–195
Cell-matrix interactions, 11
Cellulitis, 203–204, 203f, 247–248, 248f
Central compartment
  femoroacetabular impingement, 967
  hip arthroscopy, 952–954, 952f–953f
Cerebellum, 1528–1529
Cerebral edema, high-altitude, 242–243
Cerebral palsy, 320–321
  adaptive equipment, 321
  exercise, 320–321, 320b
  medical considerations, 321
    epilepsy/seizures, 321
    medications, 321
    musculoskeletal injuries, 321
    spasticity, 321
Cerebrum, 1528–1529
Cervical disc herniation, 405–406
Cervical motion segment, 1593
Cervical spine, 1533
  congenital anomalies of, 1762–1763
  degenerative, 1593–1604
    axial neck pain, 1593–1594
    cervical spondylosis, 1594–1596,
      1594f–1596f
    ossified posterior longitudinal ligament,
      1597, 1597f
    rheumatoid cervical spondylitis, 1596–1597,
      1596f

Cervical spine (Continued)
    uncovertebral joints, 1594
  injuries, 1578–1581
    decision-making principles, 1579–1580
    diagnosis, 1579–1580
    history, 1578
    imaging, 1578–1579
    on-field emergencies, 152–153
    on-field evaluation, 1578
    physical examination, 1578
    return to play, 1580–1581, 1580f–1581f
    sprain, 1579
    strain, 1579
    treatment, 1579–1580
  unstable fractures and dislocations
    decision-making principles, 1542
  unstable fractures and dislocations of,
    1541–1543
    complications, 1543
    future considerations, 1543
    history, 1541
    imaging, 1541–1542, 1542f
    physical examination, 1541
    postoperative management, 1543
    results, 1543
    treatment options, 1542–1543, 1542b
Cervical spondylosis, 405
Cervical stenosis, 405
Cervical strain, 405
Chance fractures, 1584, 1586f, 1753–1755
Channelopathies, 172–173
Cheilectomy, 1524, 1524f
Cheiralgia paresthetica, 902
Chilblains (perniosis), 257, 258f
Children. See Pediatrics
Chondral injuries, 942, 943f, 967
Chondrocytes, 11
Chondrofix, 1183
Chondrolysis, 593–594
ChondroMimetic, 43
Chronic anterior cruciate ligamentous
  insufficiency, 1284, 1284f
Chronic pain, in stiff shoulder, 580, 580b
Chronic peroneal tendon dislocation, 1474f,
  1475f
Chronic proximal hamstring tendinopathy, 1041
Chronic rotator cuff disease, 548
Chronic traumatic encephalopathy (CTE), 1747
Circulation, bone, 13
Class II degenerative injuries, 832
Class I traumatic injuries, 829–832, 829f–831f
Clavicle
  anatomy, 1637, 1638f
  fractures, 139, 139f
  medial, excision, 675
  midshaft fractures, 1637–1640, 1639f–1640f
  physeal fractures, 1637–1644
    lateral, 1640–1642, 1641f–1642f
    medial, 1642–1644, 1642f–1644f
Clinical Decision Rules for Cervical Spine
  Imaging, 1559f
Clinical diagnosis, 344, 345f. See also Physical
  examination
Closed boutonnière (central slip rupture),
  875–877, 875f–877f
Closed kinetic chain, 1195–1196, 1196f
Coaches, disagreements with, 157
Cocaine, 292
Coils, in magnetic resonance imaging, 99–100,
  100f
Cold injury, 240–242
  frostbite, 241–242
  hypothermia, 240–241
Cold water immersion, 358
Collagen meniscus implant (CMI), 41–42
Collagenomas, 255, 255f

Collapsed athlete, 151–152, 151t
Collateral ligament
  assessment, posterior cruciate ligament injuries, 1213–1214
  injury, 700–702
    imaging, 700–702, 701f
    lateral, 702, 703f
    ulnar, 701–702, 701f–702f
  knee, 1069–1071
  multiligament knee injuries, 1267
Collegiate athletics, ethical/legal issues with, 155
Colonic ischemia, 194
Combined impingement, 927–928
Common warts, 251–252, 252f
Commotio cordis, 173
Compact bone, 12–13, 12f
Compartment testing, 1397–1398, 1397t
Competition, diabetic athlete, 223
Complex lacerations, 262–263, 264f
Complex regional pain syndrome, 1316
Compression, 624
  intermittent, 362, 362f
  radial sensory nerve, 756, 756f
Compression fractures, of thoracolumbar spine, 1583–1584, 1584f
Compression neuropathies, elbow, 691–694
  median nerve, 693–694
  radial nerve, 692–693
  ulnar nerve, 691–692, 691f–692f
Computed tomographic angiography (CTA), 1353, 1353f
Computed tomography (CT), 85–88
  advantages, 87, 87f–88f
  ankle, 1380
  arthrography, 87, 87f
  disadvantages, 87–88, 88f
  elbow, 697–698
  femoroacetabular impingement, 964, 965f
  foot, 1380
  glenohumeral joint, 411, 411f
  hip, 938–939
  knee, 1105f
  medial clavicle physeal fractures, 1643, 1643f
  patellar instability, 1298, 1299f
  popliteal artery entrapment syndrome, 1353, 1353f
  positron emission tomography, 90, 93f
  scapulothoracic disorders, 614
  single photon emission, 88, 89f
  spine, 1546, 1546f
  technical considerations, 85–87, 86f–87f
Concomitant injury, 1249
Concomitant intra-articular pathology, revision anterior cruciate ligament injuries and, 1203
Concussion, 1530–1531, 1562–1569
  background, 1562–1564
  basketball, 116
  clinical presentation, 1563–1564
  definition, 1562–1563
  epidemiology, 1563
  in female athlete, 303–304, 304t
  imaging, 1566
  interventions, 1567–1568
  lacrosse, 122
  management, 1566–1567
  pathophysiology, 1563
  physical examination, 1564–1566
    baseline (preseason) assessment, 1564–1565
    comprehensive assessment, 1566
    sideline assessment, 1565–1566
  retiring athlete, 1567
  return-to-play, 1567, 1567t

Concussion (Continued)
  in skeletally immature athletes, 1741–1747
    biomechanics, 1741, 1742f
    complications, 1746–1747, 1747t
    decision-making principles, 1745
    epidemiology, 1741–1743
    future considerations, 1747
    history, 1743, 1743t
    imaging, 1744–1745, 1745b
    pathophysiology, 1741, 1742f
    physical examination, 1743–1744
    return to play, 1746, 1746t
    treatment options, 1745–1746
  soccer, 125–126
  volleyball, 128
Conditioning, in female athlete, 294–296, 296t
Confidentiality, 155
Congenital disease, in elite athlete, 166–169
Contact sports, athletes in, 453
Continuous catheter techniques, 334
Contra coup contusion, 1112
Contractions, of skeletal muscle
  physiology, 62–64, 64f
  types, 65
Contrast agents, 99, 99f
Contrast tissue, 95, 95f–96f, 96t
Contusions, 1043–1052
  groin, 1047, 1047f
  iliac crest, 1043–1044, 1044f
    complications, 1044
    history, 1043
    imaging, 1043, 1044f
    physical examination, 1043
    results, 1044
    return to play, 1044
    treatment options, 1043, 1043b
  quadriceps, 1044–1047, 1044t
    complications, 1047
    decision-making principles, 1046
    future considerations, 1047
    history, 1044–1045
    imaging, 1045, 1045f
    physical examination, 1045
    results, 1046
    return to play, 1046
    treatment options, 1045–1046, 1046b
  thoracolumbar spine, 1585–1588
Conventional radiography, 74–78
  advantages, 77
  arthrography, 76–77, 76f–77f
  disadvantages, 77–78, 78f
  fluoroscopy, 75–76, 75f–76f
  technical considerations, 74–75, 75f
Coordinate systems, 16
Coordination training, 381
Coracoclavicular reconstruction, anatomic, 659b–663b, 659f–663f
Core muscle injury, 1007–1017
Core strength, 69
Corneal abrasion, 269
Corns, 254
Coronary artery disease (CAD), 169
Coronoid process, 683, 683f
Cortical bone, 12–13, 12f
Corticosteroids
  exercise-induced bronchoconstriction, 177
  knee arthritis, 1280
  platelet-rich plasma vs., 53
Costoclavicular maneuver, 636–638, 637f
Countercoup injury, 1538, 1539f
Coup injury, 1538, 1539f
Coxa saltans, 925, 996–1001, 1692–1693
  external, 999–1001
  internal, 996–997

CPVT. See Catecholamine polymorphic ventricular tachycardia
Cranial meninges, 1528
Cranial nerve (CN), 1529
Cranium, 1528, 1529f
Creatine, 288–289
  adverse effects, 289
  historical perspectives, 288
  physiology, 288–289
Crepitus, 581, 609, 611b, 611f, 611t, 614–615, 616f–617f
Criteria for Spinal Motion Restriction (SMR), 1557f
Critical limb ischemia (CLI), 1351
Cross-table lateral view, 935, 936f
Cruciate ligaments
  anterior, 1069, 1070f
  in joint biomechanics, 1077–1079
  knee, 1069
  posterior, 1069, 1070f
  reconstruction, for multiligament knee injuries, 1267
Cryotherapy, for pain, 358–359
Cryptosporidiosis, 211–212
CT. See Computed tomography
CTA. See Computed tomographic angiography
Cubital tunnel syndrome, 691–692, 691f–692f, 747–752, 748f
  complications, 752
  decision-making principles, 749
  history, 749
  physical examination, 749
  postoperative management, 752
  results, 752
  return-to-play guidelines, 752
  treatment, 749–751
    anterior intramuscular transposition, 750, 751f
    anterior subcutaneous transposition, 750, 750f
    anterior submuscular transposition, 750–751, 751f
    medial epicondylectomy, 751
    in situ decompression, 749–750, 750f
    technique, 751–752
Curettage, 1487–1488
Cutaneous infections, 246–253
  bacterial infections, 246–249
  fungal infections, 249–250
  mycobacterial infections, 252
  parasitic infections, 252–253
  viral infections, 250–252
Cutaneous larva migrans, 253, 253f
Cytokine, in meniscal injuries, 1149

D

Dashboard injury, posterior cruciate ligament injuries and, 1211
Débridement
  Achilles tendon rupture, 1480b–1481b, 1480f
  anterior arthroscopic, 1425b
  arthroscopic subtalar, 1429b–1430b, 1429f–1430f
  lateral epicondylitis, 716b, 717f
  osteochondral lesions, 1487–1488
  osteochondritis dissecans, 714–715b, 714f
  posterior tibial tendon injury, 1467b–1468b, 1467f
  revision rotator cuff repair, 569
  SLAP tear, 524
Decision-making principles
  acromioclavicular joint, 653–655, 653t
  adductor strains, 1051

Decision-making principles (*Continued*)
  AIN syndrome, 746
  ankle, 1370–1379
  anterior cruciate ligament injuries, 1188–1190
    age, 1188–1189
    associated injuries, 1189
    gender, 1189
    operative *vs.* nonoperative treatment, 1188
    partial tear, 1189
    revision, 1189–1190
  anterior shoulder instability, 450–454
    age, 452
    associated injuries, 453–454
    contact sports, 453
    first-time *vs.* recurrent instability, 452–453
    in-season management, 453
    synthesis, 454, 454*t*
  articular cartilage lesions, 1163–1164
    age, 1164
    cartilage restoration, 1163
    contraindications, 1163
    defect chronicity, 1164
    osteochondritis dissecans lesions, 1164
    treatment algorithm, 1164
  athletic pubalgia, 1011
  atlantoaxial instability, 1758, 1759*f*
  atraumatic hip microinstability, 977–978
  axillary nerve palsy, 630
  borderline dysplasia, 977
  calcaneoplasty, 1433
  cervical spine
    dislocations, 1542
    injuries, 1579–1580
    unstable fractures and dislocations, 1542
  cubital tunnel syndrome, 749
  distal biceps tendinitis, 725–726
  distal biceps tendon rupture, 735
  distal triceps tendon rupture, 738, 738*b*
  elbow, 687–696
    history, 687–689, 688*f*
    motion, loss, 774–776, 775*f*
    pathologies, 687
    physical examination, 689–691
    throwing injuries, 760–761
  entrapment neuropathies, 743
  exertional compartment syndromes, 1396–1397, 1396*t*–1397*t*
  extensor mechanism injuries, 1327
  external coxa saltans, 999, 1000*b*
  flexor hallucis longus injuries, 1470
  foot, 1370–1379
  glenohumeral arthritis, 603–604, 604*b*, 604*f*–605*f*
  gluteus medius and minimus tears, 990, 991*b*
  Haglund resection, 1433
  hallux rigidus, 1523–1524
  hamstring injuries, 1037
  hand, 793–805
  head injuries, 1540
  hip, 925–934
    arthritis, 1057
    dysplasia, 975–978, 975*f*–976*f*
  interdigital neuralgia, 1418
  internal coxa saltans, 997, 997*b*
  ischiofemoral impingement, 1004, 1005*b*, 1005*f*
  knee, 1089–1103, 1101*f*–1102*f*
    arthritis, 1283–1284
    arthroscopic synovectomy, 1128–1130, 1128*f*–1129*f*
    lateral and posterolateral corner injuries, 1253
    motion, loss of, 1337–1338, 1337*t*, 1338*f*
  lateral epicondylitis, 722
  lateral plantar nerve entrapment, 1411
  leg, 1370–1379
    pain, 1396–1397, 1396*t*–1397*t*

Decision-making principles (*Continued*)
  long thoracic nerve palsy, 627
  medial collateral ligament and posterior medial corner injuries, 1234–1235
  medial epicondylitis, 722
  medial plantar nerve entrapment, 1413
  meniscal injuries, 1142–1147
  metatarsalgia, 1520
  Morton neuroma, 1418
  multidirectional instability, 479–480
  multiligament knee injuries, 1266–1267
  olecranon bursitis, 728–729
  olecranon osteochondrosis, 1674
  osteochondral lesions, 1486, 1486*f*–1487*f*
  osteochondritis dissecans, 1669, 1669*t*
  patellar instability, 1299–1301
  pediatrics
    anterior cruciate ligament (ACL) injuries, 1698
    concussion, 1745
    discoid meniscus, 1706
    distal radial physeal stress reaction, 1684
    finger fractures, 1678
    jammed finger, 1682
    lateral epicondylitis, 1675
    Little League elbow, 1667
    medial collateral ligament injury, 1672
    medial epicondyle avulsion fractures, 1671
    medial epicondylitis, 1675
    meniscal injuries, 1703
    osteochondritis dissecans, 1669, 1669*t*, 1714–1715
    Panner disease, 1669, 1669*t*
    patellar instability, 1709
    physeal fractures, 1719–1720
    posterior elbow pathologic conditions, 1674
    scaphoid fracture, 1685
  PIN syndrome, 755
  piriformis syndrome, 1003, 1003*b*
  plantar fasciitis, 1510
  posterior heel pain, 1505–1506
  posterior medial corner injuries, 1234–1235, 1235*f*
  posterior shoulder instability, 468
  posterolateral corner injuries, 1253
  posteromedial impingement, 1674
  pronator syndrome, 745
  quadriceps contusion, 1046
  quadriceps strains, 1049
  radial tunnel syndrome, 752–755
  revision anterior cruciate ligament injuries, 1202–1204
  revision rotator cuff repair, 568–569, 569*t*, 570*f*
  revision shoulder instability, 493–494
  rotator cuff and impingement lesions, 547–548
    acute rotator cuff trauma, 548
    chronic rotator cuff disease, 548
    subacromial impingement and biceps tenosynovitis, 548
  scapulothoracic disorders, 614–615
    crepitus, 614–615
    injection, 615, 615*f*
    pain, 614–615
    pathologies, 615
    treatment, 615
  sesamoid dysfunction, 1517
  soft tissue conditions, ankle arthroscopy, 1424
  spinal accessory nerve palsy, 629
  sternoclavicular joint, 668, 673*f*
  stiff shoulder, 585
  subscapularis injury, 559–560
  subtalar arthroscopy, 1429
  superficial peroneal nerve entrapment, 1414
  superior labrum anterior to posterior (SLAP) tears, 505–506, 506*f*

Decision-making principles (*Continued*)
  suprascapular nerve palsy, 624
  tarsal tunnel syndrome, 1408
  thoracic outlet syndrome, 639–640
  thoracolumbar spine injuries, 1583–1591
  triceps tendinitis, 725–726
  trochanteric bursitis, 1002, 1002*b*
  turf toe, 1515–1516
  wrist, 793–805
Decompression
  endoscopic, for posterior hip pain, 1027–1030, 1028*t*–1029*t*, 1029*f*–1030*f*
  in situ, 749–750, 750*f*
  spinoglenoid notch, 625
  suprascapular notch, 625
Deep bursae, 920
Deep gluteal syndrome, 1020–1024
  anatomy, 1020–1021, 1021*f*
  etiology, 1021–1024, 1021*f*–1023*f*
  operative treatment, 1027–1030
  physical examination, 1024–1026, 1024*f*–1026*f*
  preoperative and postoperative rehabilitation, 1027–1030, 1027*f*–1028*f*
Deep peroneal nerve entrapment, 1415–1416, 1415*f*
  history, 1415
  imaging, 1416
  physical examination, 1415–1416
  postoperative management, 1416
  results, 1416
  treatment options, 1416, 1416*b*
Deep venous thrombosis (DVT), 180–188
  clinical manifestations, 182–184
  diagnosis, 182–184
  imaging, 182–184, 185*f*–186*f*
  laboratory findings, 182–184
  normal physiology, 180, 181*f*
  return to play, 185–186
  risk factors, preoperative, 180–181
  sports issues in, 185–186
  thromboembolic prophylaxis, 182, 183*t*–185*t*
  travel and, 185–186
  treatment, 184–185, 187*t*
Deep zone, of articular cartilage, 11
Degenerative arthritis, in female athlete, 303
Degenerative cervical spine, 1593–1604
  axial neck pain, 1593–1594
  cervical spondylosis, 1594–1596, 1594*f*–1596*f*
  imaging, 1550–1551
  ossified posterior longitudinal ligament, 1597, 1597*f*
  rheumatoid cervical spondylitis, 1596–1597, 1596*f*
  uncovertebral joints, 1594
Degenerative joint disease, of hip, 926, 927*f*
Degenerative thoracolumbar spine, 1597–1604
  discogenic low back pain, 1598–1599
  low back pain, 1598
  lumbar disc herniation, 1599–1601, 1601*f*
  lumbar spinal stenosis, 1602–1603, 1602*f*
  lumbar spine, 1598–1604
  radiculopathy, 1599–1601, 1600*f*
  spondylolisthesis, 1603–1604, 1603*f*–1604*f*
  synovial facet cysts, 1601–1602
  thoracic spine, 1597–1598
Degrees of freedom, 16–17, 18*f*
Dehydroepiandrosterone (DHEA), 287
Delayed gadolinium, for magnetic resonance imaging, 101
Delayed-onset muscle soreness, 68
Deltoid ligament injury. *See* Medial ankle sprains
DeNovo Natural Tissue, 1182
Dental injuries, 269–270. *See also* Teeth
  basketball, 116
  fractured teeth, 270

Dental injuries (Continued)
 handball, 122
 periodontal/displacement injuries (loose teeth),
  270
 primary vs. permanent teeth, 269, 270f
Dephasing, in magnetic resonance imaging, 95
De Quervain tenosynovitis, 859–860, 859f
 postoperative management and return to
  sports, 860
 treatment options, 859, 859b, 860f
Dermatology, 149
 amputee athletes and, 316–317
Dermatophytoses, 249–250, 250f
Dermatoses, 246–259
 cutaneous infections, 246–253
  bacterial infections, 246–249
  fungal infections, 249–250
  mycobacterial infections, 252
  parasitic infections, 252–253
  viral infections, 250–252
 environmental dermatoses, 256–257
  aquatic dermatoses, 256
  irritant contact dermatitis, 256–257
  photodermatoses, 256
  thermal damage, 257, 257f
 mechanical dermatoses, 253–256
  abrasions/lacerations, 253–254
  acne mechanica, 254–255, 255f
  athlete's nodules (collagenomas), 255, 255f
  calluses and corns, 254
  friction blisters, 254
  hemorrhage, 254, 254f–255f
  hidradenitis suppurativa, 255–256, 256f
  striae, 254, 255f
 urticaria, anaphylaxis, and immunologic
  disorders, 257–258
Dexmedetomidine, perioperative pharmacology,
 338–339
dGEMRIC MRI, 101
DHEA. See Dehydroepiandrosterone
Diabetes
 athlete with, 218–226
  definition, 218
  diagnosis, 218–219
   morning after, 219
  epidemiology, 218
  exercise, physiologic changes of, 221–223,
   221f, 222t
  management, 223–225, 223f
  treatment, 219–221
   amylin analog therapy, 221
   incretin, 221
   insulin, 220, 221t
   insulin analogs, 220
   medical nutrition therapy, 219–220
   oral hypoglycemic agents, 220
 gestational, 218
 overt, 218
 prediabetes, 218
 type 1, 218, 221, 221f
  management, 224–225
 type 2, 218
  management, 225
Diabetes mellitus, 218, 327
 pathophysiologic responses to exercise,
  222–223
Diagnosis, 344, 345f
Diagnostic arthroscopy, 110, 1123–1125,
 1125f
 lateral and posterolateral corner injuries of
  knee, 1254, 1254f
 meniscal insufficiency, 1157
 proximal biceps tendon pathology, 531–532
Dial test, 932, 1213, 1250, 1250f

Diarrhea, 192–194, 212
Dietary Supplement Health and Education Act in
 1994, 1611
Diffusion weighted imaging, 100, 100f
Digits, 801. See also Fingers
 distal interphalangeal joint, 801–802, 803f
 flexor pulley injury, 804
 fractures and dislocations, 883–897
  ligamentous injuries and dislocations,
   883–892
  osseous and soft tissue injuries of thumb,
   892–896
 metacarpophalangeal joint, 803–804
 proximal interphalangeal joint, 802–803, 804f
 ulnar collateral ligament, 804, 804f
DIP joint. See Distal interphalangeal (DIP) joint
Disagreements, with coaches, 157
Disc degeneration, 1543
Disc herniation
 cervical, 405–406, 1595
 lumbar, 1599–1601, 1601f
 thoracolumbar spine, 1588, 1588f
Discogenic pain
 cervical spondylosis, 1594–1595
 low back, 1598–1599
Discoid meniscus, 1140–1142, 1141f–1142f,
 1705–1708
 classification, 1705–1706, 1706f
 complications, 1707
 decision-making principles, 1706
 future considerations, 1707–1708
 history, 1706
 imaging, 1706
 physical examination, 1706
 postoperative management, 1707
 results, 1707
 treatment options, 1706–1707
Dislocation
 arthropathy, 593
 cervical spine, 1541–1543
  complications, 1543
  decision-making principles, 1542
  future considerations, 1543
  history, 1541
  imaging, 1541–1542, 1542f
  physical examination, 1541
  postoperative management, 1543
  results, 1543
  treatment options, 1542–1543, 1542b
 chronic peroneal tendon, 1474f, 1475b
 distal interphalangeal joint, 888–890
 elbow, 699
 hip, 942, 944f–945f, 1690–1691, 1691f
 knee, 154, 1345–1349, 1346f
  anterior, 1345
  clinical presentation, 1346–1347, 1346t,
   1347f
  complications, 1349
  imaging, 1348
  physical examination and testing of,
   1347–1348, 1347f
  popliteal artery repair, 1349b
  posterior, 1345–1346
  postoperative management, 1349
  treatment options, 1348–1349
  vascular injury, 1346
 metacarpophalangeal, 892–894
 patellar, 1293
 perilunate, 809–810, 810f
 proximal interphalangeal joint, 885–888,
  885f–890f
 sternoclavicular joint, 673, 674f–676f
 transscaphoid perilunate fracture, 825–826,
  826f

Displacement injuries (loose teeth), 270
Distal anterolateral accessory portal (DALA), in
 hip arthroscopy, 951, 951f
Distal biceps tendon
 rupture, 695, 703–704, 704f, 731–741
  anatomy, 731, 732f–733f
  biomechanics, 731–732
  classification, 732, 732b
  complications, 736–737
  decision-making principles, 735
  epidemiology, 731
  history, 732–733
  imaging, 733–734, 734f
  physical examination, 733, 733f
  postoperative management, 735
  results, 735–736
  treatment, 734–735, 735t, 736b, 736f
 tendinitis, 725–728
  complications, 727
  conservative, 726
  decision-making principles, 725–726
  future considerations, 727–728
  history, 725
  imaging, 725, 726f
  operative, 726, 727f
  physical examination, 725, 725f
  postoperative management, 727
  results, 726
  return-to-play guidelines, 727
  treatment, 726, 726b
Distal femoral osteotomy, 1282
Distal humerus, anatomy, 683
Distal interphalangeal (DIP) joint, 789, 801–802,
 803f
 dislocations, 888–890
Distal radial physeal stress reaction, pediatrics,
 1683–1684
 complications in, 1684
 decision-making principles, 1684
 future consideration in, 1684
 history, 1683
 imaging, 1683–1684, 1683f
 physical examination, 1683
 postoperative management, 1684
 results, 1684
 treatment options, 1684, 1684b
Distal radioulnar joint, disorders of, 865–872
 anatomy, 865–866, 866f–867f
  blood supply, 866
 complications, 870–871
 history, 867, 867t
 imaging, 868–870
  computed tomography, 868
  magnetic resonance imaging, 868, 869f
  radiographs, 868, 868f
  treatment, 868–870, 870f
 physical examination, 867–868
 postoperative management, 870, 871f
 triangular fibrocartilage complex tears,
  866–867
  class 1 tears (traumatic), 866
  class 2 tears (degenerative), 866–867
  Palmer Classification, 867t
Distal radius fractures, 806–807, 826–827
Distal tibial plafond, osteochondral lesions of,
 1500–1501, 1500f–1501f
Distal triceps tendon rupture, 737–740
 anatomy, 737, 737f
 biomechanics, 737
 classification, 737
 complications, 740
 decision-making principles, 738, 738b
 epidemiology, 737, 737b
 future considerations, 740

Distal triceps tendon rupture (Continued)
    history, 738
    imaging, 738
    physical examination, 738
    postoperative management, 740
    results, 740
    treatment, 738–739
        nonoperative, 738
        operative, 739, 739f
        technique, 740b, 740f
Dominant deep bursa, 920
DOMS. See Delayed-onset muscle soreness
Doping, 283–293
    erythropoietin, 287–288
    historical perspectives, 287
    mechanism of action, 288
    side effects, 288
    testing, 288
Dorsal quadrant, 794t, 796–798, 797f–798f
Dorsiflexion range of motion, 381
Double-bundle reconstruction
    posterior cruciate ligament injuries, 1218–1219,
        1218f, 1225–1229
    in revision setting, 1206–1207
Down syndrome, atlantoaxial instability in,
    1758–1759
    decision-making principles, 1758, 1759f
    history, 1758
    imaging, 1758
    physical examination, 1758
    results, 1759
    treatment, 1759, 1760f
Draping, hip arthroscopy, 949–950, 950f
Drilling, 1487–1488
Drugs. See also Medications; Medicine
    ergogenic, 283–290
        anabolic-androgenic steroids, 284–287
        caffeine, 290
        creatine, 288–289
        doping, 287–288
        growth hormone, 289–290
        steroid supplements, 287
        testosterone, historical perspectives, 283–284
    recreational, 290–293
        alcohol, 290–291
        cocaine, 292
        inhalants, 293
        marijuana, 291–292
        tobacco, 292
    using, 156
Dunn view, 935, 937f
Duplex ultrasonography, of popliteal artery
    entrapment syndrome, 1352, 1352f
Dura mater, 1528
DVT. See Deep venous thrombosis
Dynamic contrast enhancement, in MRI,
    101–103
Dynamic imaging, in forces, of hip joint, 923
Dynamics, in biomechanics, 22–23
    joint motions in, 22–23, 23f
    kinematics, 22
    kinetics, 23
    relative motion, 22
Dynamometer, 386, 386f
Dyspepsia, 191–192
Dysphagia, 192
Dysplasia, hip, 971–978
    decision-making, 975–978
        atraumatic hip microinstability, 977–978
        borderline dysplasia, 977
        dysplasia, 975–978, 975f–976f
    history, 973
    imaging, 974–975, 975f
    pathologies, 971–973
        dysplasia and, 971–973, 972f–973f
    physical examination, 973–974

E
EAMC. See Exercise-associated muscle cramps
Ears, preparticipation physical evaluation, 145
Echo
    gradient, 96–97, 97f
    sequence, ultrashort time to, 100–101
    spin, 96, 97f
    time, 95
    train, 96
Education, for athletic trainer, 342–343, 343b,
    343t
EHS. See Exertional heat stroke
EIB. See Exercise-induced bronchoconstriction
Elastin, 3
Elastography, ultrasound, 83–84, 83f
Elbow, 680–686, 720–730. See also Entrapment
    neuropathies
    anatomy, 680–681
        capsuloligamentous restraints, 680–681, 682f
        elbow musculature, 681
        osseous, 680, 681f
    anterior
        history, 688
        palpation, 690
    arthroscopy, 707–719
        complications, 718
        decision-making principles, 707–712
        fluid management, 708–709
        future considerations, 718
        history, 707
        imaging, 707
        instrumentation, 708–709, 709f
        physical examination, 707
        portal placement, 709–711, 709t
        postoperative management, 718
        return-to-play guidelines, 718
        treatment, 707–712, 717b
    biomechanics, 681–685
    compression neuropathies, 691–694
    decision-making principles, 687–696
    diagnosis, 687–696
    distal biceps tendinitis, 725–728
        decision-making principles, 725–726
        history, 725
        imaging, 725, 726f
        physical examination, 725, 725f
        postoperative management, 727
        results, 726
        treatment, 726, 726b
    history, 687–689, 688f
    imaging, 697–706, 698f
        collateral ligament injury, 700–702, 701f
        computed tomography, 697–698
        conventional radiographs, 697
        lateral epicondylitis, 702–704, 703f
        loose bodies, 700
        magnetic resonance arthrography, 699
        magnetic resonance imaging, 698–699
        medial epicondylitis, 702–704
        tendon ruptures, 703–704, 704f
        trauma, 699–700
        ulnar neuropathy, 704, 705f
        ultrasound, 699
    injuries
        baseball, 115
        golf, 119–120
        throwing, 757–771
    inspection, 689
    joints, stability, 694–695
    lateral
        history, 687–688
        palpation, 689
    lateral epicondylitis, 720–725
        decision-making principles, 722
        history, 720, 721t
        imaging, 721, 721f–722f

Elbow (Continued)
        physical examination, 720, 721f
        postoperative management, 724
        treatment, 721f, 722–724
    Little League, 1612, 1612f
    medial
        history, 688
        palpation, 689–690
    medial epicondylitis, 720–725
        decision-making principles, 722
        history, 720, 721t
        imaging, 721, 721f–722f
        physical examination, 720, 721f
        postoperative management, 724
        treatment, 721f, 722–724
    motion, 681–683, 772–784
        complications, 782–783
        decision-making principles, 774–776, 775f
        follow-up, 782
        history, 772–773
        imaging, 774, 774f
        physical examination, 773–774
        postoperative management, 782
        rehabilitation, 782
        results, 782–783, 783t
        return-to-play guidelines, 782
        surgery, 776–782, 777f
        treatment, 774–776, 775f
    musculature, 681
    olecranon bursitis, 728–730, 728f
        complications, 730
        decision-making principles, 728–729
        future considerations, 730
        history, 728, 728f
        imaging, 728, 729f
        physical examination, 728
        postoperative care, 730
        results, 730
        treatment, 729, 729b, 729f
    palpation, 689–690
    pathologies, 687
    pediatrics, 1619–1623
        acute injuries, 1619, 1621f
        development, 1619
        injuries, 1661–1676
        Little League, 1621–1623, 1622f–1623f,
            1665–1668
        overuse injuries, 1619–1623
    physical examination, 689–691
    posterior
        history, 688–689
        palpation, 690
        pediatrics, 1673–1674, 1673f
    regional anesthesia, 330–332
    stability, 683–685
    trauma, 699–700
        fracture, 699
        occult, 699, 700f
        stress, 700
    triceps tendinitis, 725–728
        decision-making principles, 725–726
        history, 725
        imaging, 725, 726f
        physical examination, 725, 725f
        postoperative management, 727
        results, 726
        treatment, 726, 726b
Electrical stimulation, 359, 1196
Electrocardiogram, 161, 161f, 163–164, 164f
Electrocautery, 108–109
Electromyography, 614
Electrophysiology, 161, 161f, 742–743
Elite athlete, 158–174
    acquired cardiovascular conditions, 169–173
        arrhythmias, 172–173
        atrial fibrillation, 172

Elite athlete (Continued)
  catecholamine polymorphic ventricular
    tachycardia (CPVT), 172–173, 173f
  channelopathies, 172–173
  commotio cordis, 173
  coronary artery disease (CAD), 169
  hyperlipidemia, 172
  hypertension, 169–172
  myocarditis, 169, 171f
  postural orthostatic tachycardia syndrome
    (POTS), 173
  syncope, 173
  Wolff-Parkinson-White syndrome, 172
  cardiovascular care
    electrocardiogram and electrophysiologic
      adaptations, 161, 161f
    rigorous athletic training and, 160–161
    screening, 162–166, 163b
    structural adaptations, 160–161
  future, 173–174
  gender, 161–162, 162f
  genetics, 161–162, 162f
  historical perspective, 158–159
  medical home of, 159–160
  race, 161–162, 162f
  structural/congenital disease, 166–169
    arrhythmogenic right ventricular
      cardiomyopathy, 168
    bicuspid aortic valve, 168–169, 170f–171f
    congenital anomalous coronary artery, 168
    hypertrophic cardiomyopathy, 167
    Marfan syndrome, 169, 171f
Elson test, 875, 876f
Emergencies
  action plan, 150, 151b, 1553
  on-field, 150–155
    anaphylaxis, 153
    cardiac arrest, 153
    cervical spine injury, 152–153
    collapsed athlete, 151–152, 151t
    emergency action plan, 150, 151b
    environmental factors, 154
    head injury, 152
    limb-threatening injuries, 154
    tension pneumothorax, 153
  spine injuries, 1553–1561, 1559f
    common acute, 1559–1560, 1560f
    emergency management, 1553–1561, 1559f
    field-side management, 1553–1561,
      1554f–1558f
Emergency department, 455
Emergency medical services (EMS), 1553
Emergent care, 344–345
Encephalitis, 214–215
Endochondral bone formation, 14
Endocrine system, preparticipation physical
  evaluation, 149
Endoscopic Haglund resection, 1433–1435
  complications, 1435
  decision-making principles, 1433
  history, 1433
  imaging, 1433
  physical examination, 1433
  postoperative management, 1434
  results, 1434
  treatment, 1433b–1434b, 1434f
Endoscopy, for hamstring injuries, 1037–1039,
  1038f
Endotenon, 2, 3f
Endothelial damage, 180
Endurance training, 1607–1608
Energy metabolism, of skeletal muscle, 65–66,
  65f
Enthesis, fibrocartilaginous, 2–3

Entrapment neuropathies, 742–756
  complications, 743
  decision-making principles, 743
  history, 742
  imaging, 742
  median nerve, 743–745, 744f
  physical examination, 742
  postoperative management, 743
  radial nerve, 752, 753f
  testing, 742–743
  treatment, 743
  ulnar nerve, 747, 748f. See also Cubital tunnel
    syndrome
Environmental dermatoses, 256–257
  aquatic dermatoses, 256
    hair discoloration, 256
    swimmer's itch and seabather's eruption,
      256, 257f
  irritant contact dermatitis, 256–257
  photodermatoses, 256
    skin cancer, 256
    sunburn, 256
  thermal damage, 257, 257f
Environmental factors, during on-field
  emergencies, 154
Environmental illness, 235–245
  cold injury, 240–242
    frostbite, 241–242
    hypothermia, 240–241
  exertional heat illness
    definition, 235
    epidemiology, 235
    exercise-associated collapse, 237
    exercise-associated hyponatremia, 239–240
    exercise-associated muscle cramps, 236–237
    exertional heat exhaustion, 235–236
    exertional heat stroke, 236
    exertional rhabdomyolysis, 237–238
    exertional sickling collapse, 238–239
    heat syncope, 237
  high-altitude illness, 242, 244t
    acute mountain sickness, 242–243
    high-altitude cerebral edema, 242–243
    high-altitude headache, 242–243
    high-altitude pulmonary edema, 243–245
EOS 2D/3D x-ray imaging system, of spine,
  1545–1546, 1545f
Epicondylectomy, medial, 751
Epicondylitis
  lateral, 687, 702–704, 703f, 720–725
    complications, 725
    decision-making principles, 722
    future considerations, 725
    history, 720, 721t
    imaging, 721, 721f–722f
    physical examination, 720, 721f
    postoperative management, 724
    results, 724–725
    return-to-play guidelines, 724
    splinting, 722
    treatment, 721f, 722–724
  medial, 688, 702–704, 720–725
    complications, 725
    decision-making principles, 722
    future considerations, 725
    history, 720, 721t
    imaging, 721, 721f–722f
    physical examination, 720, 721f
    postoperative management, 724
    results, 724–725
    return-to-play guidelines, 724
    splinting, 722
    treatment, 721f, 722–724
  surgical management, 724

Epidural hematoma, 1745
Epilepsy, 230–234. See also Seizure
  cerebral palsy, 321
  classification, 230
  diagnosis, 230–231
  evaluation, 230–231
  intellectually disabled athletes, 322
  safety considerations of, 232–234, 233b
  terminology of, 230
  treatment, 231
Epilepsy syndrome, 230
Epimysium, 62, 63f
Epitenon, 2, 3f
EPO. See Erythropoietin
Equipment. See also Instruments
  adaptive sports
    amputee athlete, 317
    cerebral palsy, 321
    intellectually disabled athletes, 323
    visually impaired athletes, 323
    wheelchair athlete, 320
  arthroscopic, 105–109, 106f
    arthroscope, 105–107, 106f
    arthroscopic probe in, 107
    basket forceps in, 107–108, 108f
    cannulas in, 108
    electrocautery in, 108–109
    fluid pump, 107
    grasping forceps in, 108
    instruments and, 107
    knives in, 108
    motorized shavers in, 107–108
    radiofrequency instruments and, 108–109
    scissors in, 108
    switching sticks in, 108
Ergogenic drugs, 283–290
  anabolic-androgenic steroids, 284–287
  caffeine, 290
  creatine, 288–289
  doping, 287–288
  growth hormone, 289–290
  steroid supplements, 287
  testosterone, historical perspectives, 283–284
Erysipelas, 247–248, 248f
Erythrasma, 248–249, 249f
Erythropoietin (EPO), 197, 287–288
Ethical/legal issues, in sports medicine, 155–157
  collegiate athletics, 155
  confidentiality, 155
  disagreements with coaches, 157
  drug use, 156
  high school athletics, 155
  informed consent, 156, 156t
  professional athletics, 155
Eucapnic voluntary hyperventilation (EVH),
  176–177
Exacerbating factors, for stiff shoulder, 580–581
Excision, 1487–1488
Exercise
  amputee athletes and, 316, 316t
  capacity, 71–73, 71f
  cardiorespiratory response to, 72, 72f, 72t
  cerebral palsy, 320–321, 320b
  core strength, 69
  diabetic athlete, physiologic changes of,
    221–223, 221f, 222t
  hormonal adaptation to, 69–71, 69t
    adrenal hormones, 69t, 70
    gonadal hormones, 69t, 70–71
    pancreatic hormones, 69t, 71
    pituitary, 69–70, 69t
  immune system, 201–202, 202f
  intellectually disabled athletes, 322
  low-impact, for knee arthritis, 1279

Exercise *(Continued)*
  muscle during
    delayed-onset soreness of, 68
    fatigue, 67
  neuromuscular adaptation to, 67–68
  pediatrics, 1607–1609
    endurance training, 1607–1608
    heat-related injuries, 1609
    strength training, 1608–1609
    thermoregulation, 1609
  physiology, 62–73
  respiratory response to, 72–73
  seizure and, 231–232
  visually impaired athletes, 323
  wheelchair athletes, 317–320
Exercise-associated collapse (EAC), 237
Exercise-associated hyponatremia (EAH), 239–240
Exercise-associated muscle cramps (EAMC), 236–237
Exercise-induced anaphylaxis, 257–258
"Exercise-induced arterial hypoxemia", 73
Exercise-induced bronchoconstriction (EIB), 175–179
  athletic populations at risk, 175
  clinical presentation, 175–176, 176b
  complications, 178–179
  definition, 175
  diagnosis, 176–177
    differential, 176, 176b
    history, 176
    objective testing, 176–177
  prevalence of, 175, 176t
  return to play, 179, 179f
  sideline management, 178, 178b, 179f
  treatment options, 177
    nonpharmacologic therapy, 177
    pharmacologic therapy, 177, 177t
    technique, 178b, 178f
Exertional compartment syndromes, 1393–1401, 1394t
  anatomy, 1393–1394, 1394f, 1394t
  classification, 1394–1395
  compartment testing, 1397–1398, 1397t
  complications, 1400
  decision-making principles, 1396–1397, 1396t–1397t
  diagnostics/imaging, 1395–1396, 1396f
  epidemiology, 1393
  history, 1395
  pathophysiology, 1394
  physical examination, 1395
  postoperative care, 1398
  results, 1400
  return to play, 1400
  treatment options, 1398
Exertional heat exhaustion (EHE), 235–236
  diagnosis, 235
  prevention, 236
  return to play, 235–236, 236b
  treatment, 235
Exertional heat illness (EHI)
  definition, 235
  epidemiology, 235
  exercise-associated collapse, 237
  exercise-associated hyponatremia, 239–240
  exercise-associated muscle cramps, 236–237
  exertional heat exhaustion, 235–236
  exertional heat stroke, 236
  exertional rhabdomyolysis, 237–238
  exertional sickling collapse, 238–239
  heat syncope, 237
Exertional heat stroke (EHS), 236, 236b
Exertional rhabdomyolysis (ER), 237–238, 238b
Exertional sickling collapse, 238–239, 238t

Extension/extension-distraction injuries, of thoracolumbar spine, 1584–1585
Extensor carpi ulnaris tendinopathy, 861–862
Extensor mechanism, 1113–1116, 1115f–1117f
  injuries, 1318–1334, 1330b
    anatomy, 1318–1319, 1319f
    biomechanics, 1319, 1320f
    clinical outcomes, 1331–1333
    complications, 1333
    decision-making principles, 1327
    future considerations, 1333
    history, 1322–1323
    imaging, 1324–1326
    patella, 1318–1319
    patellar and quadriceps tendon structure in, 1320, 1320f–1321f
    patient evaluation, 1322–1326
    physical examination, 1323–1324
    postoperative management, 1330–1331
    quadriceps tendon, 1318
    treatment options, 1327–1330
Extensor tendons, 790–791, 790f–791f
Extensors, of hip, 919–920
External coxa saltans, 999–1001
  complications, 1000
  decision-making principles, 999, 1000b
  future considerations, 1000–1001
  history, 999
  imaging, 999
  physical examination, 999, 999f
  postoperative management, 1000
  results, 1000, 1001t
  techniques, 1000b, 1000f–1001f
  treatment options, 999–1000
External rotation, 1247
  recurvatum test, 1250, 1250f
External rotators, of hip, 920
Extra-articular augmentation, 1192
Extracellular matrix
  articular cartilage, 11
  bone, 13
  cell-matrix interactions, 11
  ligaments, 3
  meniscus, 8
  tendons, 3
Eyes
  injuries, 269
    corneal abrasion, 269
    hyphema, 269
    iridodialysis, 269
    retinal detachment, 269
    ruptured globe, 269
  preparticipation physical evaluation, 145

F
Fabellofibular ligament, 1246
Face
  fractures, 264–268
    evaluation, 264–266, 266b
    frontal sinus fractures, 268
    mandible fractures, 267, 267f
    midface fractures, 267–268
    nasal fractures, 266–267, 266f–267f
    orbital fractures, 268, 268f
  injuries
    basketball, 116
    boxing, 116–117
    handball, 122
  soft tissue injuries to, 260–263, 262f
    general considerations, 260–262
      anesthesia, 260
      antibiotics, 261
      choice of closure, 261
      cleaning, 260–261

Face *(Continued)*
      postclosure wound care, 261–262
      timing of repair, 260
    management, 262–263
      complex lacerations, 262–263, 264f
      intraoral/tongue lacerations, 263
      lateral face lacerations, 263, 265f
      lip lacerations, 263, 264f
      periorbital lacerations, 263
      simple lacerations, 262, 262f–263f
      soft tissue ear injuries, 263
Facemask removal, in athlete, 1555, 1556f
Facets, 1593–1594
False-profile view, 936, 937f
Fasciotomy, 1398
Fast spin-echo, 96, 97f
Fat, 277–278, 278t
  suppression, 98, 99f
Fatigue, muscle, 67
Fatty infiltration, 422, 423f
Fecally derived recreational water-related illness, 211
  non-, 213–214
    acute otitis externa, 213–214
    hot tub folliculitis, 213
    Pseudomonas infections, 213
  other, 212–213
Female athlete, 294–314
  anterior cruciate ligament tears, 377–380, 378f–379f
  general considerations, 294–304
    birth control, 301, 301t
    concussion, 303–304, 304t
    conditioning, 294–296, 296t
    degenerative arthritis, 303
    female athlete triad, 298–299, 298f, 299t
    hydration, 296–298
    nutrition, 296–298, 297t–298t
    osteopenia, 299–301, 300f, 300t
    osteoporosis, 299–301, 300f, 300t
    pregnancy, 301–302, 302t
    psychological issues, 302–303
  importance and recognition of, 294, 295t
  orthopaedic injuries, 304–314
    acetabular labral injuries, 313
    ankle, 305–306
    anterior cruciate ligament injuries, 307, 308t–309t, 309f
    anterior cruciate ligament reconstruction, 310
    epidemiology, 304–305
    femoroacetabular impingement, 313
    foot, 305–306, 305t, 306f
    frozen shoulder/adhesive capsulitis, 310–312, 311t
    idiopathic scoliosis, 313–314
    noncontact anterior cruciate ligament injury, 307–309, 308f, 310f
    patellofemoral pain syndrome, 306–307, 306t
    shoulder instability, 312–313, 312f
    stress fractures, 314
  triad, 298–299, 298f, 299t
Femoral neck stress fractures, 132–133, 132f–133f
Femoral nerve, of hip, 916
Femoral nerve block, 332–333, 333f
Femoral nerve stretch test, 933
Femoral osteotomy, 1301
Femoral tunnel, for revision anterior cruciate ligament injuries, 1205–1206, 1206f
Femoroacetabular impingement (FAI), 313, 957–970, 958f
  complications, 969
  diagnosis, 960–965
    computed tomography, 964, 965f
    magnetic resonance arthrography, 964

Femoroacetabular impingement (FAI)
(Continued)
   magnetic resonance imaging, 963–964,
     963f–964f
   plain radiographs, 960–963, 961f–963f
   ultrasonography, 964–965
  history, 958–959, 959f
  imaging, 942, 944f
  intra-articular injection, 965–969
  management, 965–969
   hip arthroscopy, 965–967, 966f, 966t
   nonoperative, 965
   open surgical dislocation, 965
   operative, 965
   outcomes, 969
   rehabilitation, 967–969
  pediatrics, 1693
  physical examination, 959–960, 959t, 960f
Femur
  anatomy, 1064–1065, 1065f
  head-neck junction of, 909–910
  neck
   internal bony architecture of, 910, 910f
   version, 909
  proximal, development, 908–909
  regional anesthesia, 332–333
Fibrin clot augmentation, 1148
Fibroblasts, tendon-specialized. See Tenocytes
Fibrocartilaginous enthesis, 2–3
Fibula-based reconstruction, 1256
Fibular collateral ligament, 1070, 1071f, 1113,
  1244–1245
Field-side management, of spine injuries,
  1553–1561, 1554f–1558f
Figure-of-eight reconstruction, 675, 675b, 676f
Figure skating injuries, 117–118
Fingers. See also Digits
  fractures, pediatrics, 1677–1681
   complications, 1680–1681
   decision-making principles, 1678
   future considerations, 1681
   history, 1677
   imaging, 1678, 1678f–1679f
   physical examination, 1677–1678, 1678f
   postoperative management, 1680
   results, 1680
   treatment options, 1678–1680, 1680f, 1681b
  injuries
   basketball, 116
   volleyball, 127–128
  jammed, 1681–1683
   complications, 1683
   decision-making principles, 1682
   history, 1681
   imaging, 1682, 1682f
   physical examination, 1681–1682
   postoperative management, 1683
   results, 1683
   treatment options, 1682, 1682b
  jersey, 878–880, 878f–880f
  mallet, 873–875, 874f
  metacarpophalangeal joints, 787–788
Fixation
  for posterior cruciate ligament injuries, 1219
  for revision anterior cruciate ligament injuries,
   1204, 1204f
Flexibility testing, stiffness testing vs., 27
Flexion, abduction, and external rotation
  (FABER) test, 932
Flexion-extension, elbow, 681, 683f
Flexors
  hip, 917–919
  pulley injury, 804
  wrist, 791

Flexor carpi radialis tendinopathy, 862
Flexor carpi ulnaris tendinopathy, 862–863, 862b,
  862f–863f
Flexor digitorum longus tendon transfer
  for Achilles tendon rupture, 1480b–1481b
  for posterior tibial tendon injury, 1467b–1468b
Flexor hallucis longus, 1384–1385, 1385f
  injuries, 1469–1472
   complications, 1471–1472
   decision-making principles, 1470
   future considerations, 1472
   history, 1469
   imaging, 1469, 1470f
   physical examination, 1469
   postoperative management, 1471
   results, 1471
   treatment options, 1470, 1470b, 1471f
Flexor retinaculum reconstruction, for posterior
  tibial tendon injury, 1467b–1468b
Flight dysrhythmia, 323
Flip angle, in magnetic resonance imaging, 94
Fluid mechanics, 23–24
Fluid pump, 107
Fluoroscopy, 75–76, 75f–76f
Focal seizures, 230
Foot
  biomechanics, 1359–1369
  decision-making, 1370–1379
  diagnosis, 1370–1379
  forefoot, 1515–1526
   hallux rigidus, 1523–1526
   metatarsalgia, 1519–1522
   sesamoid dysfunction, 1516–1519,
    1517b–1518b
   turf toe, 1515–1516, 1516b
  imaging, 1380–1392
   computed tomography, 1380
   ligaments, 1387–1388, 1388f
   magnetic resonance imaging, 1380–1381
   nerve entrapment, 1389–1391
   osteochondral lesions, 1388–1389, 1389f
   plantar fasciitis, 1391, 1391f
   radiographs, 1380, 1381f
   of tendons, 1381–1386, 1381f
   ultrasound, 1380
  injuries, 117
   in adolescent athlete, 1725–1740
    fractures, 1733–1739, 1735f–1737f
    orthotics and, 1739
    shoes and, 1739
    soft tissue injuries of, 1728–1729, 1728f
    systemic illness and, 1739
   articular cartilage, 1484–1503
   in female athlete, 305–306, 305t, 306f
   ligamentous, 1444–1461
   tendons, 1462–1483
  metatarsal break in, 1365–1367, 1367f–1368f
  orthoses, 1436–1439
   clinical application, 1437–1439, 1438t–1439t,
    1440f
   research in, 1436–1437, 1437f
  orthotics, 372–374
  osteochondroses in, 1737–1739, 1738f–1739f
  pathologies, 1370–1371
  pediatric, 1633–1635
   acute injuries, 1633, 1634f
   cavus, 1728
   overuse injuries, 1633–1635, 1634f
  peripheral nerve entrapment around,
   1402–1420
   deep peroneal nerve, 1415–1416, 1415f
   interdigital neuralgia (Morton neuroma),
    1416–1419
   lateral plantar nerve, 1411–1412

Foot (Continued)
   medial plantar nerve, 1412–1413
   saphenous nerve, 1405–1407, 1405f–1406f
   superficial peroneal nerve, 1413–1415,
    1413f
   sural nerve, 1402–1405, 1403f
   tarsal tunnel syndrome, 1407–1411, 1407f
  physical examination, 1372–1379, 1373f–1378f
  plantar fasciitis, 1509–1513
   complications, 1513
   decision-making principles, 1510
   future considerations, 1513
   history, 1509
   imaging, 1509, 1509f
   physical examination, 1509
   postoperative management, 1511
   results, 1511–1513
   treatment options, 1510–1511, 1510f, 1511b,
    1512f
  posterior heel pain, 1504–1508, 1505f
   complications, 1508
   decision-making principles, 1505–1506
   future considerations, 1508
   history, 1504
   imaging, 1504–1505, 1505f–1506f
   physical examination, 1504, 1505f
   postoperative management, 1508
   results, 1508
   treatment options, 1506–1507
  shoes, 1439–1442
   anatomy, 1440, 1441f
   insole, 1441
   midsole, 1440–1441
   outsole, 1440
   selection and fitting of, 1442, 1442t
   upper, 1441–1442
  taping, 368–372, 369f
  variations of normal anatomy, 1725–1728
  windlass mechanism, 1365–1367, 1367f–1368f
Foot-strike hemoglobinuria, 196
Football injuries, 118–119
  head, 118
  lower extremity, 118–119
  neck, 118
  upper extremity, 118
Foraminal stenosis, cervical, 1595
Force
  around hip joint, 922–923
  ground reaction, 19
  joint contact, 21–22
  joint reaction, 19, 19f–20f
  production of skeletal muscle, 64–65
  vectors, 21
Forced flexion, adduction, and internal rotation
  of hip (FADIR), 932
Forearm. See also Entrapment neuropathies
  contracture, 773
  regional anesthesia, 330–332
Forefoot, 1515–1526
  hallux rigidus, 1523–1526
   complications, 1526
   decision-making principles, 1523–1524
   examination of, 1523, 1523f
   history, 1523
   imaging, 1523
   results, 1525
   treatment options, 1524–1525
  metatarsalgia, 1519–1522
   complications, 1522
   decision-making principles, 1520
   future considerations of, 1522
   history, 1519
   imaging, 1520
   physical examination, 1519–1520

Forefoot *(Continued)*
  postoperative management, 1521–1522
  results, 1522
  treatment options, 1520–1521, 1521*f*–1522*f*,
    1522*b*
  sesamoid dysfunction, 1516–1519, 1516*b*
    complications, 1519
    decision-making principles, 1517
    history, 1517
    imaging, 1517, 1518*f*
    physical examination, 1517
    postoperative management, 1518–1519
    results, 1519
    treatment options, 1517–1518, 1518*b*,
      1519*f*
  turf toe, 1515–1516
    anatomic classification, 1518*t*
    complications, 1516
    decision-making principles, 1515–1516
    history, 1515
    imaging, 1515, 1516*b*
    physical examination, 1515
    postoperative management, 1516
    results, 1516
    treatment options, 1516, 1517*b*, 1517*f*
45-degree Dunn view, 935, 937*f*
Fracture-dislocations, of thoracolumbar spine,
  1584, 1586*f*–1587*f*
Fractures, 131–142, 1690
  ankle, 1729–1733, 1729*f*, 1732*f*–1734*f*, 1732*t*
  calcaneum, 1456–1457
  capitate, 809
  carpal, 807–809
  cervical spine injuries, 1579
  clavicle, 139, 139*f*
  distal radius, 826–827
  elbow, 699
    occult, 699, 700*f*
    stress, 700
  in foot, 1733–1739, 1735*f*–1737*f*
  hamate, 809
  imaging, 807–809
  metacarpals, 814–815, 815*f*
  patellar, 1322, 1322*b*
    clinical outcomes, 1332–1333
    complications, 1333
    decision-making principles, 1327
    history, 1323
    imaging, 1326, 1326*f*
    nonoperative treatment, 1327–1328,
      1328*f*
    operative treatment, 1329–1330
    physical examination, 1324
    postoperative management, 1331
  pediatrics
    apophyseal ring, 1753, 1756*f*
    avulsion, 1688, 1689*f*
    Chance, 1753–1755
    clavicle physeal, 1637–1644
    finger, 1677–1681
    hip, 1690
    lesser tuberosity, 1647
    medial epicondyle avulsion, 1670–1672
    physeal, 1718–1721
    proximal humerus, 1644–1647
    sacral facet, 1755, 1756*f*
    scaphoid, 1684–1686
    stress, 1688–1690, 1690*f*
  repair, 14–15
  return to sport, 139–142, 140*f*–141*f*
  rib, 137–139
  Salter-Harris
    type I, 1729*f*, 1730
    type II, 1729*f*, 1730, 1733*f*
    type III, 1729*f*, 1730
    type IV, 1729*f*–1731*f*, 1730–1731

Fractures *(Continued)*
  scaphoid, 807–808, 807*f*–808*f*, 824
  stress, 131–139
    biomechanical factors of, 131–132
    classification, 132*t*
    elbow, 700
    fatigue and training errors causing, 132
    in female athlete triad, 131
    femoral neck, 132–133, 132*f*–133*f*
    genetic factors, 132
    metatarsal, 135–136
    navicular, 136, 137*f*
    nutrition and, 132
    olecranon, 764–765, 764*f*–765*f*
    pars, 136–137, 138*f*
    proximal fifth metatarsal, 134–135,
      135*f*–136*f*
    tibial, 133–134, 134*f*–135*f*
  teeth, 270
  thoracolumbar, 1583
    burst, 1584, 1585*f*
    Chance, 1584, 1586*f*
    compression, 1583–1584, 1584*f*
    stress, 1584–1585
    vertebral body apophyseal avulsion, 1585
  transscaphoid perilunate, 825–826, 826*f*
  trapezium, 808–809, 809*f*
  wrist arthroscopy, 824–828
    arthroscopic reduction, 824*b*–825*b*,
      824*f*–825*f*
    scaphoid nonunions, 824–825, 825*t*
    technique, 827–828, 827*f*
Free-body diagrams, 20*f*, 21
Freiberg disease, 1738, 1738*f*
Frequency selective fat saturation, 98
Fresh-frozen allografting, 1488–1489
Friction blisters, 254
Frog-leg lateral view, 935, 937*f*
Froment sign, 900*f*
Frontal sinus fractures, 268
Frostbite, 241–242
  diagnosis, 241
  laboratory, 241
  pathophysiology, 241
  prevention, 242
  treatment, 241–242
Frozen shoulder, 310–312, 311*t*, 581
FTE. *See* Functional tissue engineering
Functional heartburn, 191
Functional leg lengths, 936
Functional metabolic imaging, of spine, 1549
Functional tissue engineering, 28–29
Functional training, 1196–1197
Fungal infections, 249–250
  dermatophytoses, 249–250, 250*f*
  Malassezia, 250, 251*f*
  skin, 205–206
Furuncles, 246, 247*f*

G

Gadolinium, delayed, 101
Gait
  alignment of, posterior cruciate ligament and,
    1214
  cycle, 921–922, 1359, 1360*f*
  examination of
    lateral and posterolateral corner injuries of
      knee, 1251
    medial collateral ligament and posterior
      medial corner injuries, 1231
    multiligament knee injuries, 1265
    patellar instability, 1296
  kinetics, 1359–1360, 1360*f*
Gallium scans, 90, 92*f*–93*f*
Ganglionectomy, 832–833, 832*f*

Gastrocnemius tendon, lateral, 1246
Gastroesophageal reflux disease (GERD),
  190–191
Gastrointestinal system
  medicine
    in athlete, 189–195
      lower gastrointestinal tract conditions,
        192–195, 193*t*
      pathophysiology, 189
      upper gastrointestinal tract conditions,
        189–192
    preparticipation physical evaluation, 148
Gastrointestinal tract ischemia, 189
Geissler technique, 824–825
Gender
  anterior cruciate ligament injuries, 1189
  of elite athlete, 161–162, 162*f*
Generalized seizures, 230
Genetics, of elite athlete, 161–162, 162*f*
Genitourinary system
  preparticipation physical evaluation, 148
  trauma, 227–229
    classification, 227, 228*t*
    definition, 227, 228*t*
    diagnosis, 227–228
    epidemiology, 227
    pathobiology, 227
    pathophysiology, 227
    return-to-play guidelines, 229
    treatment, 228–229
GERD. *See* Gastroesophageal reflux disease
Gestational diabetes, 218
GIRD. *See* Glenohumeral internal rotation deficit
Glasgow Coma Scale, to injured athlete,
  1554–1555, 1555*f*
Glenohumeral arthritis, 407
Glenohumeral internal rotation deficit (GIRD),
  431
  pathophysiology, 514
  treatment options, 518
Glenohumeral joint, 395–396, 395*f*–396*f*
  arthritis, 592–608
    classification, 592–595
    complications, 606, 607*t*
    decision-making principles, 603–604
    epidemiology, 592
    future considerations, 607
    history, 595
    physical examination, 595–596
      arthroscopic images, 596
      imaging, 596, 597*f*–598*f*
    presentation, 595
    prior operative notes, 596
    return-to-play guidelines, 606
    treatment, 596–603, 604*b*, 604*f*–605*f*
  capsule, 396–397
  imaging, 408–432
    abnormalities, 414–432
    arthrography, 410–411, 410*f*
    computed tomography, 411, 411*f*
    conventional radiography, 408–410, 409*b*
    magnetic resonance imaging, 412–414, 413*f*,
      413*t*
    ultrasonography, 411–412, 412*f*, 412*t*
  instability, 1647–1648
Glucose, 221, 221*f*, 222*t*
Gluteal nerves, superior and inferior, 1032–1033,
  1032*f*, 1032*t*
Gluteus maximus, 920
Gluteus medius, 917
  tears, 990–996
    complications, 996
    decision-making principles, 990, 991*b*
    future considerations, 996
    history, 990
    imaging, 990, 991*f*

Gluteus medius *(Continued)*
    physical examination, 990
    postoperative management, 995
    results, 995, 996*t*
    techniques, 991*b*–992*b*, 992*f*–995*f*
    treatment options, 990
Gluteus minimus, 917
    tears, 990–996
        complications, 996
        decision-making principles, 990, 991*b*
        future considerations, 996
        history, 990
        imaging, 990, 991*f*
        physical examination, 990
        postoperative management, 995
        results, 995, 996*t*
        techniques, 991*b*–992*b*, 992*f*–995*f*
        treatment options, 990
Glycolytic energy system, 65–66
Godfrey test, for posterior cruciate ligament
    injuries, 1212–1213, 1213*f*
Golf injuries, 119–120
    elbow, 119–120
    forearm, 119–120
    hand, 120
    lower back, 119
    shoulder, 120
    wrist, 120
Gonadal hormones, 69*t*, 70–71
Gore-Tex implant, 39
Gradient echo, 96–97, 97*f*
Graft/grafting
    bone, 715*b*–716*b*
    harvest, 1191
    healing, 1192
    for multiligament knee injuries, 1267
    for posterior cruciate ligament injuries, 1219
    for revision anterior cruciate ligament injuries,
        1207
    selection, 1190–1191
    tension and fixation, 1191–1192
    timing, 1190–1192
    tissue, 30–34
        allograft, 31–32
        autograft, 30
        future direction, 33
    type, 1197
Granuloma, swimming pool/fish tank, 252, 252*f*
Grasping forceps, 108
Great arteries, 161
Great veins, 161
Greater trochanter, 910, 910*f*
Greater trochanteric pain syndrome (GTPS), 925
Groin contusions, 1047
Ground reaction force, 19
Growth factor modulation, in meniscal injuries,
    1149
Growth hormone, 289–290
    adverse effects, 289–290
    historical perspectives, 289
    mechanism of action, 289
GTPS. *See* Greater trochanteric pain syndrome
Guyon canal release, 903*b*, 903*f*
Gymnastics injuries, 120–121

H

HACE. *See* High-altitude cerebral edema
Haglund deformity, 1477
Haglund resection, endoscopic, 1433–1435
    complications, 1435
    decision-making principles, 1433
    history, 1433
    imaging, 1433

Haglund resection, endoscopic *(Continued)*
    physical examination, 1433
    postoperative management, 1434
    results, 1434
    treatment, 1433*b*–1434*b*, 1434*f*
Hair discoloration, 256
Hallux rigidus, 1523–1526
    complications, 1526
    decision-making principles, 1523–1524
    examination of, 1523, 1523*f*
    history, 1523
    imaging, 1523
    results, 1525
    treatment options, 1524–1525
        nonoperative, 1524
        operative, 1524–1525, 1524*f*–1525*f*
        technique, 1526*b*
Hamate carpal injuries, 840–843, 840*f*–843*f*, 843*b*
Hamate fracture, 809
Hamstring injuries
    open surgery, 1037, 1038*f*
Hamstrings, 919–920, 919*f*
    injuries, 1034–1042, 1035*f*
        complications, 1041–1042
        decision-making principles, 1037
        future considerations, 1042
        history, 1034–1035
        imaging, 1036–1037, 1036*f*–1037*f*
        physical examination, 1035–1036
        postoperative management, 1039–1040
            rehabilitation in, 1039–1040
        results, 1040–1041
        treatment options, 1037–1039
            nonoperative, 1037
            surgical, 1037–1039
            techniques, 1039*b*, 1039*f*–1040*f*
    strains, 376
        causes, 376
        preventing, 377, 377*f*, 377*t*
        risk factors, 376–377
Hand, 785–792
    decision-making principles, 793–805
    diagnosis, 793–805
    extensor tendons of, 790–791, 790*f*–791*f*
    history, 793–794
    imaging, 806–816
        metacarpal fracture, 814–815, 815*f*
        pulley injuries, 814
        thumb ulnar collateral ligament injury, 814,
            815*f*
    injuries. *See also* Wrist/hand injuries
        basketball, 116
        golf, 120
    joints, 787–789
        distal interphalangeal, 789, 789*f*
        metacarpophalangeal, of fingers, 787–788
        proximal interphalangeal, 788–789
        thumb, 789
    muscles, 785–787, 788*f*
    nerves, 785, 787*f*
    neuropathies, 898–905
        decision-making principles, 901
        future considerations, 904
        history, 898
        imaging, 900–901, 900*f*, 901*t*
        physical examination, 898–900, 899*f*–900*f*
        postoperative management and return to
            play, 902–903, 903*b*, 903*f*
        results, 903–904
        treatment options, 901–902
    physical examination, 793–794, 794*f*
    quadrants
        dorsal, 794*t*, 796–798, 797*f*–798*f*
        radial, 794–796, 794*t*, 795*f*–796*f*

Hand *(Continued)*
        ulnar, 794*t*, 798–800, 799*f*
        volar, 794*t*, 800–801, 800*f*, 802*f*–803*f*
    regional anesthesia, 330–332
    skin, 785, 786*f*
    tendons, 785–787, 788*f*
Handball injuries, 121–122
Hardware complications, of subscapularis injury,
    565
Hawkins test, 404, 545*f*
HBV. *See* Hepatitis B virus
HCM. *See* Hypertrophic cardiomyopathy
HCV. *See* Hepatitis C virus
Head
    anatomy, 1528, 1529*f*
        brain, 1528–1529
        intervertebral disk, 1534
        ligaments, 1534
        muscles, 1534
        neurologic tissues, 1534–1535, 1534*f*
        skull (cranium), 1528, 1529*f*
        spine, 1531–1533, 1532*f*–1533*f*
    biomechanics, 1535, 1535*f*
    brain injury, 1562–1569
        background, 1562–1564
        clinical presentation, 1563–1564
        definition, 1562–1563
        epidemiology, 1563
        imaging, 1566
        interventions, 1567–1568
        management, 1566–1567
        pathophysiology, 1563
        physical examination, 1564–1566
        retiring athlete, 1567
        return-to-play, 1567, 1567*t*
    concussion, 1530–1531, 1562–1569
        background, 1562–1564
        clinical presentation, 1563–1564
        definition, 1562–1563
        epidemiology, 1563
        imaging, 1566
        interventions, 1567–1568
        management, 1566–1567
        pathophysiology, 1563
        physical examination, 1564–1566
        retiring athlete, 1567
        return-to-play, 1567, 1567*t*
    injuries, 1529–1530, 1530*f*–1531*f*, 1538–1541
        anatomy, 1538
        biomechanics, 1538, 1539*f*
        complications, 1540–1541
        decision-making principles, 1540
        football, 118
        future considerations, 1541
        history, 1539
        ice hockey, 121
        imaging, 1539–1540
        on-field emergencies, 152
        pathophysiology, 1538–1539
        physical exam, 1539
        results, 1540
        in skeletally immature athletes, 1741–1748.
            See also Concussion
        treatment options, 1540, 1540*b*
    preparticipation physical evaluation, 145
    stingers, 1570–1577
        classification, 1573–1574, 1574*t*
        decision-making principles, 1573–1574
        future considerations, 1576, 1576*f*
        history, 1570
        imaging, 1571–1573, 1573*f*
        mechanism of, 1573, 1574*f*
        physical examination, 1570–1571, 1571*f*–
            1572*f*, 1572*t*

Head *(Continued)*
 return to play criteria, 1576
 sequela, 1576
 treatment options, 1574–1575, 1575b, 1575f
Head-neck offset, 938
Head sphericity, 938
Headache, high-altitude, 242–243
Healing. *See also* Repair
 autograft *vs.* allograft, 32–33
 bone, biology, 14–15, 14t–15t
 graft, 1192
 tendon and ligament
  factors affecting, 5, 6t
  methods for augmentation of, 5–7
Health promotion, 344
Heartburn, functional, 191
Heat
 balance, 240
 exertional illness
  definition, 235
  epidemiology, 235
  exercise-associated collapse, 237
  exercise-associated hyponatremia, 239–240
  exercise-associated muscle cramps, 236–237
  exertional heat exhaustion, 235–236
  exertional heat stroke, 236
  exertional rhabdomyolysis, 237–238
  exertional sickling collapse, 238–239
  heat syncope, 237
 illness, 149–150
 loss, 240
 production, 240
 related injuries, 1609
 stroke, exertional, 236, 236b
Heat syncope (HS), 237
Heel pain, posterior, 1504–1508, 1505f
 complications, 1508
 decision-making principles, 1505–1506
 future considerations, 1508
 history, 1504
 imaging, 1504–1505, 1505f–1506f
 physical examination, 1504, 1505f
 postoperative management, 1508
 results, 1508
 treatment options, 1506–1507
  nonoperative therapy, 1506–1507
  operative therapy, 1507
  technique, 1507b, 1507f
Heel strike, 932
Hematologic disease, preparticipation physical evaluation, 148–149
Hematologic medicine, in athlete, 196–200
 hemostasis disorders, 198–200
 red blood cells disorders, 196–198
Hematuria, exercise-induced, 228
Hemispheres, brain, 1528–1529
Hemoglobin S, 197
Hemoglobinopathies, 196
Hemophilia, 199
Hemorrhage, 254, 254f–255f
Hemostasis, disorders of, 198–200
 definition, 198–199, 199f
 diagnosis, 199–200
 epidemiology, 199
 pathophysiology, 199
 return-to-play guidelines, 200
 treatment, 200
Hepatitis A, waterborne diseases, 212
Hepatitis B virus (HBV), 210
Hepatitis C virus (HCV), 210
Hepcidin, 197
Hernia, sports, 1007, 1012–1014, 1014b, 1014f
Herniation, disk, 1579
Herpes gladiatorum, 251f
Herpes simplex, 250–251, 251f

Herpes simplex virus (HSV), 205
 definition, 205
 diagnosis, 205
 epidemiology, 205
 pathobiology, 205
 return-to-play guidelines, 205, 205t
 treatment, 205
Heterotopic ossification (HO), 317, 319, 718
Hidradenitis suppurativa, 255–256, 256f
High-altitude cerebral edema (HACE), 242–243
High-altitude headache (HAH), 242–243
High-altitude illness (HAI), 242, 244t
 acute mountain sickness, 242–243
 high-altitude cerebral edema, 242–243
 high-altitude headache, 242–243
 high-altitude pulmonary edema, 243–245
High-altitude pulmonary edema (HAPE), 243–245
High school athletics, ethical/legal issues with, 155
High tibial osteotomy, for chronic PCL injuries, 1219–1220
Hilton's law, 929
Hindfoot conditions, 1504–1514
 plantar fasciitis, 1509–1513
 posterior heel pain, 1504–1508, 1505f
Hip
 anatomy, 907–924
  bony, 907–911
 arthritis, 1053–1060
  arthroscopy, 1058–1059, 1058f
  complications, 1060
  decision-making principles, 1057
  future direction, 1060
  history, 1053
  imaging, 1055–1057, 1055f–1056f, 1055t
  physical examination, 1053–1055
  postoperative management in, 1059
  results, 1059–1060
  resurfacing for, 1058
  surgical treatment, 1058–1059
  techniques, 1060b
  treatment options, 1057
 arthroscopy, 947–956
  contraindications, 947
  femoroacetabular impingement, 965–967, 966f, 966t
  indications, 947–948
  learning curve for, 948
  operating room set-up, 948–950
  positioning for, 948–950
  procedure for, 950–955
 biomechanics, 907–924
  gait cycle in, 921–922
  joint, forces around, 922–923
  motions in, 921
  spine and, relationship of, 923–924, 923f
  stability in, 921
 bone injuries, 925–926
 center position, 938
 contusions, 1043–1052
  groin, 1047, 1047f
  iliac crest, 1043–1044, 1044f
  quadriceps, 1044–1047, 1044t
 decision-making, 925–934
 degenerative joint disease in, 926, 927f
 diagnosis, 925–934
 dysplasia and instability
  decision-making, 975–978, 975f–976f
   atraumatic hip microinstability, 977–978
   borderline dysplasia, 977
 dysplasia and instability of, 971–978
  history, 973
  imaging, 974–975, 975f
  pathologies, 971–973, 972f–973f
  physical examination, 973–974

Hip *(Continued)*
 history, 928–929, 928f, 929b
 imaging, 935–946
  computed tomography, 938–939
  magnetic resonance evaluation, 939–946
  plain radiographic images, interpretation, 936–938
  radiographic techniques, 935–936
  ultrasound, 946
 infection, 928
 injuries, 118
 inspection, 929
 instability, 926, 971–978
  decision-making, 975–978, 975f–976f
   atraumatic hip microinstability, 977–978
   borderline dysplasia, 977
  history, 973
  imaging, 974–975, 975f
  pathologies, 971–973, 972f–973f
  physical examination, 973–974
 intra-articular, 911–914
  acetabular labrum, 911, 911f–912f
  articular cartilage, 913–914
  ligamentum teres, 912, 913f
  pathology, 927–928
 joint
  bursae around, 920–921
  capsule, 914–916
  muscles around, 916–920, 918t
  prenatal, development, 907
 kinematics of, 921–924
  gait cycle in, 921–922
  joint, forces around, 922–923
  motions in, 921
  spine and, relationship of, 923–924, 923f
  stability in, 921
 ligamentous laxity, evaluation, 932
 measurements of, 930–931
 nerve entrapment injuries, 927
 pain, posterior, 1018–1033
 pathologies, 925–928, 926b
 pediatrics, 928, 1625–1628, 1688–1696
  acute injuries, 1625–1626, 1626f
  overuse injuries, 1626–1628, 1627f–1628f
 physical examination, 929–933
 range of motion of, 930–931, 931t
 regional anesthesia, 332–333
 soft tissue injuries, 925
 special maneuvers, 932–933
 sprain and dislocation, 942, 944f–945f
 strains, 1043–1052
  adductor, 1050–1051
  classification, 1047, 1047t
  quadriceps, 1047–1050
 symptom localization, 929–930, 930f–931f
History of patient
 Achilles tendon injuries, 1476
 acromioclavicular joint injuries, 647–648, 649f
 adductor strains, 1050
 AIN syndrome, 746–747
 anterior cruciate ligament injuries, 1185
 anterior shoulder instability, 447
 arthroscopic synovectomy, of knee, 1127
 articular cartilage lesions, 1162–1163
 athletic pubalgia, 1009
 calcaneoplasty, 1433
 cervical spine
  injuries, 1578
  unstable fractures and dislocations of, 1541
 cubital tunnel syndrome, 749
 deep peroneal nerve entrapment, 1415
 distal biceps tendinitis, 725
 distal biceps tendon rupture, 732–733
 distal triceps tendon rupture, 738

History of patient *(Continued)*
elbow, 687–689, 688f, 757–758, 758f, 772–773
endoscopic Haglund resection, 1433
entrapment neuropathies, 742
exercise-induced bronchoconstriction, 176
exertional compartment syndromes, 1395
extensor mechanism injuries, 1322–1326
external coxa saltans, 999
femoroacetabular impingement, 958–959, 959f
flexor hallucis longus injuries, 1469
glenohumeral arthritis, 595
gluteus medius and minimus tears, 990
hallux rigidus, 1523
hamstring injuries, 1034–1035
hand, 793–794
head injuries, 1539
hip, 928–929, 928f, 929b
    arthritis, 1053
    arthroscopy, 947
    dysplasia and instability, 973
iliac crest contusion, 1043
iliopsoas pathology, 982
interdigital neuralgia, 1417
internal coxa saltans, 996
ischiofemoral impingement, 1003–1004, 1004f
knee, 1089–1091, 1090t
    arthritis, 1277, 1278t
    lateral and posterolateral corner injuries,
        1248–1249
    motion loss, 1335–1336
lateral epicondylitis, 720, 721t
lateral plantar nerve entrapment, 1411
leg pain, 1395
medial epicondylitis, 720, 721t
medial plantar nerve entrapment, 1412
meniscus, 1132, 1137
metatarsalgia, 1519
Morton neuroma, 1417
multidirectional instability, 477
multiligament knee injury, 1264
olecranon bursitis, 728, 728f
osteochondral lesions, 1484
patellar instability, 1293, 1294f
patellofemoral pain, 1309–1310
pediatrics, 1052
    anterior cruciate ligament (ACL) injuries,
        1697
    apophyseal ring fractures, 1753
    atraumatic instability, 1654
    cervical spine, 1762
    concussion, 1743, 1743t
    discoid meniscus, 1706
    distal radial physeal stress reaction, 1683
    Down syndrome, atlantoaxial instability in,
        1758
    finger fractures, 1677
    jammed finger, 1681
    lateral clavicle physeal fractures, 1640
    lateral epicondylitis, 1675
    lesser tuberosity fractures, 1647
    Little League elbow, 1665–1666, 1665f
    medial clavicle physeal fractures, 1643
    medial collateral ligament injury, 1672
    medial epicondyle avulsion fractures,
        1670–1671
    medial epicondylitis, 1675
    meniscal injuries, 1703
    odontoid fractures, 1761
    osteochondritis dissecans, 1668, 1712, 1713f
    osteochondrosis, 1668
    Panner disease, 1668
    patellar instability, 1708–1709
    physeal fractures, 1719
    posterior elbow pathologic conditions, 1674

History of patient *(Continued)*
    proximal humerus epiphysiolysis, 1656
    proximal humerus fracture, 1644
    rotatory atlantoaxial subluxation, 1759
    scaphoid fracture, 1684
    scoliosis, 1755–1757
    spinal cord injury without radiographic
        abnormality, 1763
    spinal injuries, 1749–1750, 1750b
    spondylolisthesis, 1751–1752
    spondylolysis, 1751–1752
    traumatic anterior instability, 1648, 1648f
    traumatic posterior instability, 1651–1652
peroneal tendon injuries, 1472–1476
PIN syndrome, 755
piriformis syndrome, 1002
plantar fasciitis, 1509
popliteal artery entrapment syndrome, 1350
posterior heel pain, 1504
posterior shoulder instability, 465
preparticipation physical examination,
    145–150
pronator syndrome, 745
quadriceps contusion, 1044–1045
quadriceps strains, 1048
radial tunnel syndrome, 754
revision shoulder instability, 489
saphenous nerve entrapment, 1405
scapulothoracic disorders, 609–611
sesamoid dysfunction, 1517
soft tissue, ankle arthroscopy, 1423
sprains
    ankle, 1444–1446, 1450–1451
    bifurcate ligament, 1457
    Lisfranc, 1458
    syndesmosis, 1453–1454
sternoclavicular joint injuries, 664
stiff shoulder, 579–583
    crepitus, 581
    exacerbating factors, 580–581
    pain, 579–581, 580b
    relieving factors, 580–581
    stiffness, 581
    weakness, 581
stingers, 1570
subscapularis injury, 558–559, 558f
subtalar arthroscopy, 1429
superficial peroneal nerve entrapment, 1413
superior labrum anterior to posterior (SLAP)
    tears, 502
sural nerve entrapment, 1402
tarsal tunnel syndrome, 1408
thoracic outlet syndrome, 636
thoracolumbar spine injuries, 1582
triceps tendinitis, 725
trochanteric bursitis, 1001–1002
turf toe, 1515
wrist, 793–794, 857–858
HIV. *See* Human immunodeficiency virus
Hook of hamate fractures, 900f
Hop tests, 388f
Hormones
    adaptation to exercise of, 69–71, 69t
    adrenal, 69t, 70
    gonadal, 69t, 70–71
    pancreatic, 69t, 71
    pituitary, 69–70, 69t
Hot tub folliculitis, 213
HSV. *See* Herpes simplex virus
Hueter-Volkmann law, in bone remodeling, 13
Human immunodeficiency virus (HIV), 210
Humerus, proximal, 1637, 1638f
Hyalofast, 1181
Hyalograft C, 43–44

Hydration, 278–279, 279t
    considerations, 278
    gastrointestinal tract conditions, 189
    monitoring, 278–279
Hydrodilatation, 585
Hygiene, for preventing infectious disease, 202
Hypercoagulability, 180
Hyperlipidemia, 172
Hypertension, 169–172
Hypertrophic cardiomyopathy (HCM), 167,
    326–327
Hyphema, 269
Hypomobility issues, 381
Hyponatremia, 229
    exercise-associated, 239–240
Hypothalamic-pituitary-testicular (HPT) axis, 70
Hypothermia, 240–241
    diagnosis, 240–241
    heat balance, 240
    pathophysiology, 240
    prevention, 241
    thermal balance, 240
    treatment, 241

I

IBS. *See* Irritable bowel syndrome
Ice hockey injuries, 121
Idiopathic adhesive capsulitis, 581–582
Idiopathic anterior knee pain, 1314–1315
Idiopathic scoliosis, 313–314
Idiopathic thrombocytopenic purpura (ITP), 199
IFI. *See* Ischiofemoral impingement
ILFL. *See* Iliofemoral ligament
Iliac crest contusion, 1043–1044, 1044f
    complications, 1044
    history, 1043
    imaging, 1043, 1044f
    physical examination, 1043
    results, 1044
    return to play, 1044
    techniques, 1043b
    treatment options, 1043
Iliocapsularis muscle, 919
Iliofemoral ligament (ILFL), 914, 915f
Iliopsoas, 917–919
    anatomy, 979–980, 980f–981f
    bursa, 921
    bursitis, 980
    complications, 987–988
    function of, 979–980, 980f–981f
    history, 982
    imaging, 983–984
    impingement, 980–983, 982f, 986–987
    pathology, 979–989
    physical exam, 982–983
    postoperative management, 984
    results, 984–987
    snapping, 980, 981f, 982, 983f, 984–986
    techniques, 986b–987b, 987f
    tendonitis, 980
    treatment options, 984, 984f–986f
Iliotibial band, 1244
Imaging, 74–104. *See also specific imaging
    modalities*
    acromioclavicular joint injuries, 651–653, 652f,
        654f–655f
    adductor strains, 1050, 1050f
    ankle, 1380–1392
        computed tomography, 1380
        ligaments, 1387–1388, 1388f
        magnetic resonance imaging, 1380–1381
        nerve entrapment, 1389–1391
        osteochondral lesions, 1388–1389, 1389f

Imaging (*Continued*)
    plantar fasciitis, 1391
    radiographs, 1380, 1381*f*
    tendons, 1381–1386, 1381*f*
    ultrasound, 1380
  anterior cruciate ligament injuries, revision,
    1200–1202, 1200*f*
  anterior shoulder instability, 448–450,
    450*f*–452*f*
  apophyseal ring fractures, 1753, 1756*f*
  arthroscopic synovectomy, of knee, 1127–1128
  articular cartilage lesions, 1163
  athletic pubalgia, 1010–1011
    dynamic ultrasonography, 1010–1011
    magnetic resonance imaging, 1010,
      1010*f*–1011*f*
    radiographic analysis, 1010, 1010*f*
  brain injury, 1566
  calcaneoplasty, 1433
  cervical spine
    congenital anomalies of, 1762
    injuries, 1578–1579
    unstable fractures and dislocations of,
      1541–1542, 1542*f*
  collateral ligament injury, 700–702, 701*f*
  computed tomography, 85–88
    advantages, 87, 87*f*–88*f*
    disadvantages, 87–88, 88*f*
    technical considerations, 85–87, 86*f*–87*f*
  concussion, 1566
  conventional radiography, 74–78, 1104, 1105*f*
    advantages, 77
    arthrography, 76–77, 76*f*–77*f*
    disadvantages, 77–78, 78*f*
    fluoroscopy, 75–76, 75*f*–76*f*
    technical considerations, 74–75, 75*f*
  deep venous thrombosis, 182–184, 185*f*–186*f*
  diffusion weighted, 100, 100*f*
  distal biceps tendon rupture, 733–734, 734*f*
  distal triceps tendon rupture, 738
  Down syndrome, atlantoaxial instability in,
    1758
  elbow, 697–706, 698*f*
    collateral ligament injury, 700–702, 701*f*
    computed tomography, 697–698
    conventional radiographs, 697
    distal biceps, 725, 726*f*
    lateral epicondylitis, 702–704, 703*f*, 721,
      721*f*–722*f*
    loose bodies, 700
    magnetic resonance arthrography, 699
    magnetic resonance imaging, 698–699
    medial epicondylitis, 702–704, 721,
      721*f*–722*f*
    motion, loss, 774, 774*f*
    olecranon bursitis, 728, 729*f*
    tendon ruptures, 703–704, 704*f*
    throwing injuries, 760, 761*f*
    trauma, 699–700
    triceps tendinitis, 725, 726*f*
    ulnar neuropathy, 704, 705*f*
    ultrasound, 699
  endoscopic Haglund resection, 1433
  exertional compartment syndromes, 1395–
    1396, 1396*f*
  extensor mechanism, 1113–1116,
    1115*f*–1117*f*
    injuries, 1324–1326
  external coxa saltans, 999
  femoroacetabular impingement
    computed tomography, 964, 965*f*
    magnetic resonance arthrography, 964
    magnetic resonance imaging, 963–964,
      963*f*–964*f*
    plain radiographs, 960–963, 961*f*–963*f*
    ultrasonography, 964–965

Imaging (*Continued*)
  foot, 1380–1392
    computed tomography, 1380
    ligaments, 1387–1388, 1388*f*
    magnetic resonance imaging, 1380–1381
    nerve entrapment, 1389–1391
    osteochondral lesions, 1388–1389, 1389*f*
    plantar fasciitis, 1391
    radiographs, 1380, 1381*f*
    tendons, 1381–1386, 1381*f*
    ultrasound, 1380
  genitourinary trauma, 228
  glenohumeral arthritis, 596, 597*f*–598*f*
  gluteus medius and minimus tears, 990,
    991*f*
  hallux rigidus, 1523
  hamstring injuries, 1036–1037, 1036*f*–1037*f*
  hand, 806–816
    metacarpal fracture, 814–815, 815*f*
    pulley injuries, 814
    thumb ulnar collateral ligament injury, 814,
      815*f*
  head injuries, 1539–1540
  hip, 935–946
    arthritis, 1055–1057, 1055*f*–1056*f*, 1055*t*
    computed tomography, 938–939
    dysplasia and instability, 974–975, 975*f*
    magnetic resonance evaluation, 939–946
    plain radiographic images, interpretation,
      936–938
    radiographic techniques, 935–936
    ultrasound, 946
  iliac crest contusion, 1043, 1044*f*
  iliopsoas, 983–984
  interdigital neuralgia, 1417–1418
  internal coxa saltans, 996–997
  ischiofemoral impingement, 1004
  key points, 104
  knee, 1104–1120
    arthritis, 1277–1279, 1278*f*–1279*f*
    background, 1104
    cartilage, 1116–1118, 1118*f*–1119*f*
    computed tomography, 1105*f*
    dislocation in, 1348
    ligaments, 1110–1113, 1111*f*–1115*f*
    magnetic resonance imaging, 1105–1106
    motion, loss, 1336–1337, 1337*f*
    musculotendinous structures, 1110, 1111*f*
    osseous structures, 1116–1118, 1118*f*–1119*f*
    pitfalls, 1109–1110, 1110*f*
  lateral and posterolateral corner injuries of
    knee, 1251–1253
    magnetic resonance imaging, 1251–1253,
      1252*f*
    radiographs, 1251, 1251*f*
    ultrasound, 1253
  latissimus dorsi injuries, 576, 577*f*
  leg pain, 1395–1396, 1396*f*
  magnetic resonance, 92–100
    advantages, 102
    contraindications, 102–103
    delayed gadolinium for, 101
    Dgemric, 101
    diffusion weighted imaging, 100, 100*f*
    disadvantages, 102, 102*f*
    dynamic contrast enhancement in, 101–103
    image formation of, 94–95
    image quality in, 100
    protocols for, 93, 94*f*
    proton density in, 95, 96*f*, 96*t*
    pulse sequences, 95–98
    T1, 95, 95*f*, 96*t*
    T2, 95, 96*t*
    technical considerations of, 93–100
    ultrashort time to echo sequence for,
      100–101

Imaging (*Continued*)
  medial collateral ligament and posterior medial
    corner injuries, 1232–1234, 1233*f*–1235*f*
  meniscus, 1106–1109, 1106*f*–1109*f*
    injuries, 1138–1139, 1138*f*
  metatarsalgia, 1520
  Morton neuroma, 1416–1419
  multiligament knee injuries, 1265–1266,
    1265*f*–1266*f*
  nerve entrapment
    deep peroneal nerve, 1416
    lateral plantar nerve, 1411
    medial plantar nerve, 1413
    saphenous nerve, 1406
    superficial peroneal nerve, 1414
    sural nerve, 1403–1404
  nuclear medicine, 88–92
    advantages, 90, 93*f*
    bone scans in, 88–89, 89*f*
    disadvantages, 90–92, 94*f*
    gallium scans in, 90, 92*f*–93*f*
    labeled white blood cell scans in, 89–90, 91*f*
    PET/CT scans, 90, 93*f*
    planar imaging, 88, 89*f*
    SPECT/CT imaging, 88, 89*f*
    technical considerations, 88
  odontoid fractures, 1761–1762, 1761*f*
  patella
    fractures, 1326, 1326*f*
    instability, 1297–1299, 1298*f*–1299*f*
    tendinopathy, 1324–1325, 1324*f*–1325*f*
    tendon ruptures, 1325–1326, 1325*f*–1326*f*
  pectoralis major muscle injuries, 575
  pediatrics, 1052
    anterior cruciate ligament (ACL) injuries,
      1697–1698
    atraumatic instability, 1655, 1655*f*
    concussion, 1744–1745, 1745*b*
    discoid meniscus, 1706
    distal radial physeal stress reaction,
      1683–1684, 1683*f*
    finger fractures, 1678, 1678*f*–1679*f*
    jammed finger, 1682, 1682*f*
    lateral clavicle physeal fractures, 1641
    lateral epicondylitis, 1675
    lesser tuberosity fractures, 1647
    Little League elbow, 1667
    medial clavicle physeal fractures, 1643,
      1643*f*
    medial collateral ligament injury, 1672
    medial epicondyle avulsion fractures, 1671
    medial epicondylitis, 1675
    meniscal injuries, 1703–1704
    osteochondritis dissecans, 1668–1669, 1669*f*
    osteochondrosis, 1668–1669, 1669*f*
    Panner disease, 1668–1669, 1669*f*
    patellar instability, 1709, 1709*f*
    physeal fractures, 1719, 1720*f*–1721*f*
    posterior elbow pathologic conditions,
      1674
    proximal humerus epiphysiolysis, 1656,
      1656*f*
    proximal humerus fractures, 1644–1645,
      1645*f*–1646*f*
    scaphoid fracture, 1684–1685
    traumatic anterior instability, 1648–1649,
      1649*f*–1650*f*
    traumatic posterior instability, 1652, 1653*f*
  piriformis syndrome, 1003
  plantar fasciitis, 1509, 1509*f*
  popliteal artery entrapment syndrome,
    1352–1354
    angiography, 1353–1354, 1354*f*
    computed tomography and computed
      tomographic angiography, 1353, 1353*f*
    duplex ultrasonography, 1352, 1352*f*

Imaging (Continued)
  magnetic resonance angiography, 1352–1353, 1353f
  magnetic resonance imaging, 1352–1353, 1353f
  posterior heel pain, 1504–1505, 1505f–1506f
  posterior shoulder instability, 467–468, 467f–468f, 468t
  postoperative, 1118–1120, 1119f–1120f
  preoperative, 433–434
  quadriceps contusion, 1045, 1045f
  quadriceps strains, 1048, 1048f
  radiation exposure in, 103–104, 103t
  revision rotator cuff repair, 568
  revision shoulder instability, 490–493, 491f–492f
  rotator cuff and impingement lesions, 547
    magnetic resonance imaging, 547, 547f
    plain radiographs, 547
    ultrasonography, 547
  rotatory atlantoaxial subluxation, 1760, 1761f
  scapulothoracic disorders, 614
    computed tomography, 614
    electromyography, 614
    magnetic resonance imaging, 614
    radiographs, 614
    ultrasound, 614, 614f–615f
  scoliosis, 1757
  sesamoid dysfunction, 1517, 1518f
  soft tissue, ankle arthroscopy, 1423–1424
  spinal cord injury without radiographic abnormality, 1763
  spine, 1544–1552
    computed tomography, 1546, 1546f
    degenerative, 1550–1551
    EOS 2D/3D x-ray imaging system, 1545–1546, 1545f
    functional metabolic imaging, 1549
    future considerations, 1551
    interventional radiology, 1550
    magnetic resonance imaging, 1547, 1547f
    myelography, 1548
    nuclear scintigraphy, 1548–1549, 1549f
    radiographs, 1544, 1545f
    single photon emission computed tomography, 1549–1550
    study interpretation, 1551
  spondylolisthesis, 1752, 1752f
  spondylolysis, 1752, 1752f
  sternoclavicular joint injuries, 667–668, 670f–672f
  stiff shoulder, 584–585
  stingers, 1571–1573, 1573f
  subscapularis injury, 559, 559f
  subtalar arthroscopy, 1429
  superior labrum anterior to posterior (SLAP) tears, 503–504, 505f
  tarsal tunnel syndrome, 1408
  techniques, 74–103
  tendons, ruptures, 703–704, 704f
  thoracic outlet syndrome, 638–639, 638f–639f
  thoracolumbar spine injuries, 1583
  3D acquisitions in, 98, 98f
  thrower's shoulder, 515–516, 516f
  trochanteric bursitis, 1002
  turf toe, 1515, 1516b
  2D acquisitions in, 98, 98f
  ulnar neuropathy, 704, 705f
  ultrasonography, 78–85, 1104–1105, 1106f
    advantages, 84
    disadvantages, 84–85, 85f
    dynamic, 84, 84f
    elastography, 83–84, 83f
    musculoskeletal, 79–83, 80f–83f
    technical considerations, 78–79, 79f

Imaging (Continued)
  wrist, 806–816, 807f
    carpal fractures, 807–809
    distal radius fractures, 806–807
    intrinsic carpal ligament injury, 810–812, 811f
    Kienböck disease, 810
    perilunate dislocation, 809–810, 810f
    tendinopathies, 858–859, 858f
    tendon injuries, 812–813, 812f–813f
    triangular fibrocartilage complex injury, 813–814, 813f–814f
    ulnar impaction syndrome, 810
Immature bone, 12, 12f
Immediate care, 344
Immune system, exercise and, 201–202, 202f
Immunizations, 149, 202
Impairment-based rehabilitation programs, 355–357, 356f
Impetigo, 246–247, 247f
Impingement. See also Rotator cuff and impingement lesions
  cam, 957, 958f
  femoroacetabular, 942, 944f, 957–970, 958f, 1693
    complications, 969
    diagnosis, 960–965
    history, 958–959, 959f
    intra-articular injection, 965–969
    management, 965–969
    physical examination, 959–960, 959t, 960f
  iliopsoas, 980–983, 982f, 986–987
  ischiofemoral, 1003–1006
    complications for, 1006
    decision-making principles, 1004, 1005b, 1005f
    future considerations, 1006
    history, 1003–1004, 1004f
    imaging, 1004
    physical examination, 1004
    results, 1006
    treatment options, 1004–1006
  pincer, 958f, 967
  posterior, 1426b, 1426f
  posteromedial, 1673–1674, 1673f
    complications, 1674
    decision-making principles, 1674
    history, 1674
    imaging, 1674
    physical examination, 1674
    results, 1674
    treatment, 1674
  syndrome, 406
  test, 614, 614f, 933
Implants, 35–49
  cartilage repair, 42–45
  ligament reconstruction, 38–41
  meniscus repair, 41–42
  osteochondral repair, 42–45
  suture anchors for, 46–47
  sutures for, 45–46
  tendon repair, 35–38
In-season management, of anterior shoulder instability, 453
In silico studies, in forces, of hip joint, 922, 923f
In situ decompression, 749–750, 750f
Incretin, 221
Inertia, 17, 17t, 18f
Infections
  bacterial skin, 203–205
  blood-borne, 210
  elbow arthroscopy, 718
  fungal skin, 205–206

Infections (Continued)
  hip, 928
  lower respiratory tract, 209–210
  neurologic, 214–215
  Pseudomonas, 213
  skin and soft tissue, 203–206
  unusual, 215–216
  upper respiratory tract, 206–209
Infectious diarrhea, 212
Infectious diseases, 201–217
  blood-borne infections, 210
    hepatitis B virus, 210
    hepatitis C virus, 210
    human immunodeficiency virus, 210
  epidemiology, 201
  exercise and immune system, 201–202, 202f
  lower respiratory tract infections, 209–210
    acute bronchitis, 209
    acute pneumonia, 209–210
  neurologic infections, 214–215
    encephalitis, 214–215
    meningitis, 214–215
  preparticipation physical evaluation, 148–149
  prevention, 202–203
  skin and soft tissue infections, 203–206
    bacterial skin infections, 203–205
    fungal skin infections, 205–206
    herpes simplex virus, 205
  unusual infections, 215–216
    leptospirosis, 215
    Naegleria fowleri, 215–216
    schistosomiasis, 216
  upper respiratory tract infections, 206–209
    infectious mononucleosis, 207–208
    measles, 208–209
  waterborne diseases and recreational water-related illness, 210–213
    cryptosporidiosis, 211–212
    fecally derived, 211
    infectious diarrhea, 212
    nonfecally derived, 213–214
Infectious mononucleosis (IM), 207–208
Inferior gluteal nerve, 916, 1032–1033, 1032f, 1032t
Inflammatory phase, of tendon and ligament repair, 4
Informed consent, 156, 156t
Infraclavicular block, 332
Inhalants, 293
Injections
  diagnostic, for athletic pubalgia, 1009
  knee arthritis, 1280
  lateral epicondylitis, 721f, 723
  medial epicondylitis, 721f, 723
  scapulothoracic disorders, 615, 615f
Injuries, 114–130
  acetabular labral, 313
  Achilles tendon, 1476–1482
    complications, 1482
    decision-making principles, 1478–1479
    future considerations, 1482
    history, 1476
    imaging, 1477–1478, 1478f
    physical examination, 1477, 1477f
    postoperative management, 1480–1481
    results, 1481–1482
    treatment options, 1479–1480, 1479t, 1480b–1481b, 1480f
  acromioclavicular joint, 645–678
    anatomy, 646f–647f, 646t
    classification, 645, 648f
    complications, 664

Injuries (Continued)
decision-making principles, 653–655, 653t
future considerations, 677
history, 647–648, 649f
imaging, 651–653, 652f, 654f–655f
physical examination, 648–651, 650t, 651f
postoperative management, 663–664
results, 664, 665t–666t
return-to-play guidelines, 663–664
treatment, 655–659, 656f–658f
ankle, in adolescent athlete, 1725–1740
anterior cruciate ligament
in female athlete, 307, 308t–309t, 309f
knee, 1185–1198
anterior tibial tendon, 1462–1464
complications, 1464
decision-making principles, 1462
history, 1462
imaging, 1462
physical examination, 1462, 1463f
postoperative management, 1463
results, 1463–1464
treatment options, 1462–1463, 1463b–1464b, 1464f
articular cartilage, 1484–1503
back, 118–121, 126
bone, 925–926
brain, 1562–1569
background, 1562–1564
clinical presentation, 1563–1564
definition, 1562–1563
epidemiology, 1563
imaging, 1566
interventions, 1567–1568
management, 1566–1567
pathophysiology, 1563
physical examination, 1564–1566
retiring athlete, 1567
return-to-play, 1567, 1567t
carpal, 835–856
anatomy, 835
biomechanics, 835
capitate, 843–845, 844b, 844f
carpal instability, 848–851, 848f–850f, 850b
future considerations, 854–855
hamate, 840–843, 840f–843f, 843b
Kienböck disease, 846–847
ligament, anatomy and mechanics, 848–851, 848f–850f, 850b
lunate, 845–847, 846f, 847b
lunotriquetral injuries, 848
perilunate instability, 851–854, 851f–855f, 853b
pisiform, 847–848, 847f, 848b
scaphoid, 835–836, 837b, 837f
scapholunate injuries, 848
trapezium, 838–840, 838f–840f, 840b
trapezoid, 845, 845b
triquetrum, 836–838, 838b, 838f
cervical spine, 1578–1581
chest, 123
cold, 240–242
frostbite, 241–242
hypothermia, 240–241
collateral ligament, 700–702
imaging, 700–702, 701f
lateral, 702, 703f
ulnar, 701–702, 701f–702f
concomitant, 1249
dental, 269–270
basketball, 116
fractured teeth, 270
handball, 122
periodontal/displacement injuries (loose teeth), 270
primary vs. permanent teeth, 269, 270f

Injuries (Continued)
elbow
baseball, 115
golf, 119–120
throwing, 757–771
extensor mechanism, 1318–1334, 1330b
anatomy, 1318–1319, 1319f
biomechanics, 1319, 1320f
clinical outcomes, 1331–1333
complications, 1333
decision-making principles, 1327
future considerations, 1333
history, 1322–1323
imaging, 1324–1326
patella, 1318–1319
patellar and quadriceps tendon structure in, 1320, 1320f–1321f
patient evaluation, 1322–1326
physical examination, 1323–1324
postoperative management, 1330–1331
quadriceps tendon, 1318
treatment options, 1327–1330
eyes, 269
corneal abrasion, 269
hyphema, 269
iridodialysis, 269
retinal detachment, 269
ruptured globe, 269
facial
basketball, 116
boxing, 116–117
handball, 122
finger
basketball, 116
volleyball, 127–128
flexor hallucis longus, 1469–1472
complications, 1471–1472
decision-making principles, 1470
future considerations, 1472
history, 1469
imaging, 1469, 1470f
physical examination, 1469
postoperative management, 1471
results, 1471
treatment options, 1470, 1470b, 1471f
flexor pulley, 804
foot, 1725–1740
hamstrings, 1034–1042, 1035f
complications, 1041–1042
decision-making principles, 1037
future considerations, 1042
history, 1034–1035
imaging, 1036–1037, 1036f–1037f
physical examination, 1035–1036
postoperative management, 1039–1040
rehabilitation in, 1039–1040
results, 1040–1041
treatment options, 1037–1039
nonoperative, 1037
surgical, 1037–1039
techniques, 1039b, 1039f–1040f
hand
basketball, 116
golf, 120
head
football, 118
ice hockey, 121
on-field emergencies, 152
in skeletally immature athletes, 1741–1748
heat-related, 1609
intrinsic carpal ligament, 810–812, 811f
knee
basketball, 115–116
figure skating, 118
lacrosse, 122
rowing, 123

Injuries (Continued)
skiing, 124
swimming, 126
volleyball, 127
lateral corner, 1244–1263
latissimus dorsi muscle, 576–578
anatomy, 576
classification, 576
imaging, 576, 577f
mechanisms of, 576
physical examination, 576, 577f
teres major, 578
treatment, 576–578, 578f
ligaments, 3–4
collateral ligament injuries of metacarpophalangeal joint, 894–896, 894f–896f
distal interphalangeal joint, 888–890
metacarpophalangeal joint, 883–885, 884f
phalangeal fractures, 890–892, 891f–893f
platelet-rich plasma for, 53–54
proximal interphalangeal joint, 885–888, 885f–890f
limb-threatening, 154
acute compartment syndrome, 154
knee dislocation, 154
traumatic amputation, 154
lower back, 119
lower extremity
basketball, 115
football, 118–119
gymnastics, 120
ice hockey, 121
snowboarding, 125
soccer, 125
tennis, 126–127
lumbar spine, 123
lunotriquetral, 848
medial collateral ligament, 1231–1243, 1672–1673
meniscal, 1703–1705
anatomy, 1703
complications, 1705
decision-making principles, 1704
development, 1703, 1703f
future considerations, 1705
history, 1703
imaging, 1703–1704
physical examination, 1703
postoperative management, 1704–1705
results, 1705
treatment options, 1704
muscle, 574–578
latissimus dorsi, 576–578
other, 574–578
pectoralis major, 574–576
platelet-rich plasma for, 56
musculoskeletal, 128–129
amputee athletes, 316
cerebral palsy, 321
intellectually disabled athletes, 322
visually impaired athletes, 323
neck, 118
neurologic, 117, 718
pectoralis major, 574–576
anatomy, 574
classification, 574–575
imaging, 575
mechanisms of, 574
physical examination, 575
treatment, 575–576, 576f
pediatric. See Pediatrics
peroneal tendon, 1472–1476
complications, 1476
decision-making principles, 1473–1474
future considerations, 1476

Injuries (Continued)
history, 1472
imaging, 1473, 1473f
physical examination, 1472–1473, 1472f
postoperative management, 1475
results, 1475–1476
treatment options, 1474–1475, 1474f–1475f, 1475b
posterior cruciate ligament, 1211–1230, 1220b–1222b, 1221f–1223f
posterior medial corner, 1231–1243
complications in, 1242
decision-making principles, 1234–1235, 1235f
future considerations, 1243
history, 1231
imaging, 1232–1234, 1233f–1235f
physical exam, 1231–1232
postoperative management, 1239–1240
results, 1240–1242
return-to-play guidelines, 1240b
treatment options, 1235–1236
posterolateral corner, 1244–1263
prevention, 344, 376–384
ankle sprains, 380–381
anterior cruciate ligament tears, 377–380, 378f–379f
biomechanics, 28
hamstring muscle strains, 376
taping for, 371
ankle sprains, 371
patellofemoral pain, 371
plantar fasciitis, 371
plantar fasciosis, 371
psychological adjustment to, 272–276
complications, 275
decision-making principles, 273
future considerations, 275
historical perspective and evolution, 272–273
postinjury management and outcome, 275
preparticipation screening, 273
treatment options, 274b
pulley, 814
return to activity and sport after, 385–391
scapholunate, 848
shoulder
anterior instability, 453–454
baseball, 114–115
golf, 120
handball, 122
skiing, 124
swimming, 126
volleyball, 128
soft tissue
foot and ankle, 1728–1729, 1728f
hip, 1691–1693
wrestling, 129
spine
common acute, 1559–1560, 1560f
emergency management, 1553–1561, 1559f
epidemiology, 1553
field-side management, 1553–1561, 1554f–1558f
sport-specific, 114–130. See also specific sports
auto racing, 117
baseball, 114–115
basketball, 115–116
boxing, 116–117
figure skating, 117–118
football, 118–119
golf, 119–120
gymnastics, 120–121
handball, 121–122
ice hockey, 121

Injuries (Continued)
lacrosse, 122
rowing, 123
rugby, 123–124
running, 124
skiing, 124–125
snowboarding, 124–125
soccer, 125–126
swimming, 126
tennis, 126–127
volleyball, 127–128
wrestling, 128–129
sternoclavicular joint, 664–677
anatomy, 667, 667f–670f
complications, 677
decision-making principles, 668, 673f
future considerations, 677
history, 664
imaging, 667–668, 670f–672f
physical examination, 664–665
postoperative management, 677
results, 677
return-to-play guidelines, 677
treatment, 673
stress, 942–944, 945f
subscapularis, 556–566, 557f
anatomy, 556–557
classification, 558
decision-making principles, 559–560
function of, 557
future considerations of, 565–566
history, 558–559
imaging, 559, 559f
mechanism of, 557–558
physical examination, 558–559, 558f
treatment options, 560–565, 561f–562f
tendon, 3–4, 873–882, 874f
closed boutonnière (central slip rupture), 875–877, 875f–877f
complications, 881–882
future considerations, 882
Jersey finger, 878–880, 878f–880f
mallet finger, 873–875, 874f
platelet-rich plasma for, 53–54
pulley injury, 880–881, 880f–881f
sagittal band rupture, 877–878, 877f
throwing, 757–771
complications, 770
decision-making principles, 760–761
future considerations, 770
history, 757–758, 758f
imaging, 760, 761f
physical examination, 758–760, 759f–760f
postoperative management, 768
results, 768–770
return to play, 768
treatment, 761–765
thumb, 124
triangular fibrocartilage complex, 813–814, 813f–814f
ulnar collateral ligament, 700–702
upper extremity
figure skating, 118
football, 118
gymnastics, 120
ice hockey, 121
rowing, 123
snowboarding, 124–125
soccer, 125
tennis, 127
weight-loss-related, 129
wrist
class I traumatic, 829–832, 829f–831f
class II degenerative, 832

Injuries (Continued)
golf, 120
tendons, 812–813, 812f–813f
volleyball, 127–128
Innervation, of knee, 1072
Insole, 1441
Inspection
elbow, 689
hip, 929
knee, 1091–1092, 1091b, 1091f–1092f
patellofemoral pain, 1310–1311, 1311f–1312f
scapulothoracic disorders, 611–612
Instability arthropathy, 592–595
capsulorrhaphy arthropathy, 593, 593f
chondrolysis, 593–594
dislocation arthropathy, 593
osteonecrosis, 595, 595f, 595t
rheumatoid arthritis, 594–595, 594f
Instruments. See also Equipment
arthroscopic, 107
hip arthroscopy, 948, 948f–949f
knee arthroscopy, 1125
radiofrequency, 108–109
wrist arthroscopy, 817, 818f
Insulin, 220, 221t
Insulin analogs, 220
Intellectually disabled athletes, 321–323
adaptive equipment, 323
exercise, 322
medical considerations, 322–323
cardiac abnormalities, 322–323
epilepsy/seizures, 322
musculoskeletal injuries, 322
visual impairment, 322
Interdigital nerve, magnetic resonance imaging, 1389–1390, 1390f
Interdigital neuralgia, 1416–1419
complications, 1418–1419
decision-making principles, 1418
etiologies of, 1417
history, 1417
imaging, 1417–1418
pathomechanism of, 1417
physical examination, 1417
postoperative management, 1418
results, 1418
treatment options, 1418, 1419b, 1419f
Intermittent compression, 362, 362f
Internal coxa saltans, 996–997
author's preferred techniques, 998b, 998f
complications, 997
decision-making principles, 997, 997b
history, 996
imaging, 996–997
physical examination, 996, 997f
postoperative management, 997
results, 997, 998t
treatment options, 997
Internal fixation, 1488, 1488f
Internal impingement
pathophysiology, 513, 513f
treatment options, 517
Internal rotators, of hip, 917
Interscalene block, 330, 332f
Intersection syndrome, 860–861, 860f
return to sports, 861
treatment options, 860–861, 861b
Interventional radiology (IR), of spine, 1550
Intervertebral disks, 1534, 1593
Intra-articular pathology, of hip, 927–928
Intracerebral hematoma, 1745
Intramembranous bone formation, 14

Intraoperative care, during anesthesia, 327–329.
   See also Regional anesthesia
   positioning, 329
   tourniquets, 328–329
Intraoral/tongue lacerations, 263
Intraosseous hypertension, of patella, 1316
Intravascular hemolysis, 196
Intrinsic carpal ligament injury, 810–812, 811*f*
Inversion recovery, 97–98, 97*f*
Iontophoresis, 360–361
Iridodialysis, 269
Iron, 279
Irritable bowel syndrome (IBS), 194
Ischemic conditions, of lower gastrointestinal
   tract, 194
Ischiofemoral distance (IFD), 911
Ischiofemoral impingement (IFI), 1003–1006
   complications for, 1006
   decision-making principles, 1004, 1005*b*, 1005*f*
   future considerations, 1006
   history, 1003–1004, 1004*f*
   imaging, 1004
   physical examination, 1004
   results, 1006
   treatment options, 1004–1006
Ischiofemoral ligament (ISFL), 914
Isokinetic strength testing, 386, 387*f*
Isolated structure reconstruction, 1255–1256
ITP. *See* Idiopathic thrombocytopenic purpura

J

Jammed finger, 1681–1683
   complications, 1683
   decision-making principles, 1682
   history, 1681
   imaging, 1682, 1682*f*
   physical examination, 1681–1682
   postoperative management, 1683
   results, 1683
   treatment options, 1682, 1682*b*
Jersey finger, 878–880, 878*f*–880*f*
Jobe's test, 546*f*
"Jock itch" (tinea cruris), 249, 250*f*
Jogger's foot, 1412
Joints
   biomechanics
     ankle, 1360–1363, 1361*f*–1362*f*
     cruciate ligaments, 1077–1079
     medial and lateral collateral ligaments,
       1079–1080
     patellofemoral, 1082–1087
     tibiofemoral, 1074–1080
   capsule
     hip, 914–916
     knee, 1071–1072, 1072*f*
   contact forces, ligament and, 21–22
   distal interphalangeal, 801–802, 803*f*
   elbow
     motion, 681–683
     stability, 683–685
   glenohumeral, 395–396, 395*f*–396*f*, 408–432
   hand, 787–789
     distal interphalangeal, 789, 789*f*
     metacarpophalangeal, of fingers, 787–788
     proximal interphalangeal, 788–789
     thumb, 789
   hip
     bursae around, 920–921
     muscles around, 916–920, 918*t*
     prenatal, development, 907
   metacarpophalangeal, 803–804
   metatarsophalangeal, 1365–1367, 1367*f*–1368*f*
   motions, 22–23, 23*f*
   proximal interphalangeal, 788–789, 802–803,
     804*f*

Joints (*Continued*)
   reaction force, 19, 19*f*–20*f*
   resurfacing techniques, 599–603, 600*f*–601*f*
   shoulder, 395–398
     acromioclavicular joint, 397
     glenohumeral, 395–396, 395*f*–396*f*
     glenohumeral joint capsule, 396–397
     scapulothoracic articulation, 398
     sternoclavicular joint, 397, 397*f*
   stability, 694–695, 1081–1082
   sternoclavicular, 664–677
     anatomy, 667, 667*f*–670*f*
     complications, 677
     decision-making principles, 668, 673*f*
     future considerations, 677
     history, 664
     imaging, 667–668, 670*f*–672*f*
     physical examination, 664–667
     postoperative management, 677
     results, 677
     return-to-play guidelines, 677
     treatment, 673
   subtalar, biomechanics, 1363–1365, 1363*t*,
     1364*f*–1366*f*
   transverse tarsal, 1365
Joint cryotherapy, 366
Joint loading, in articular cartilage repair, 11–12
Joint mobility, 350
Joint reactive forces, muscular contributions and,
   684–685, 685*f*
Joint space width, 938
Joint-sparing techniques, 598–599, 599*f*
J sign, dynamic change in, patellar instability and,
   1296, 1296*f*

K

Ketamine, perioperative pharmacology, 338
Kienböck disease, 810, 832–833, 832*t*, 833*f*,
   846–847
Kinematics, 22
   ankle joint, 1360–1363
   hip, 921–924
     gait cycle in, 921–922
     joint, forces around, 922–923
     motions in, 921
     spine and, relationship of, 923–924, 923*f*
     stability in, 921
   subtalar joint, 1363–1365, 1363*t*, 1364*f*–1366*f*
   transverse tarsal joints, 1365, 1367*f*
Kinetic chain, 1195–1196, 1196*f*
Kinetics, 23, 1359–1360, 1360*f*
Klippel-Feil syndrome, 1762
Knee
   anatomy, 1062–1063
     bursae, 1068–1069
     joint capsule, 1071–1072, 1072*f*
     ligaments, 1069–1071
     muscular, 1065–1068, 1066*f*
     neurovascular, 1072
     osseous, 1063–1065, 1064*f*
     superficial, 1062–1063, 1063*f*
     synovial membrane, 1071–1072, 1072*f*
   arthritis, 1277–1292
     decision-making principles, 1283–1284
     history, 1277, 1278*t*
     imaging, 1277–1279, 1278*f*–1279*f*
     nonoperative treatment, 1279–1280
     operative options for, 1280–1283
     postoperative management, 1289, 1289*t*
     results, 1289, 1290*t*
     treatment not recommended, 1280
     treatment options, 1279–1283, 1280*f*, 1284*f*
   arthroscopic synovectomy of, 1127–1131
     anesthesia, 1129
     complications, 1130

Knee (*Continued*)
     decision-making principles, 1128–1130,
       1128*f*–1129*f*
     future direction, 1130–1131
     history, 1127
     imaging, 1127–1128
     physical examination, 1127
     positioning, 1129
     postoperative management, 1130
     results, 1130
     surgical steps, 1129–1130
     technique, 1129*b*
     treatment options, 1128–1129
   arthroscopy, 1121–1126
     complications, 1125–1126
     diagnostic, 1123–1125, 1125*f*
     indications, 1121
     instrumentation, 1125
     portal placement, 1121–1123, 1122*f*–1124*f*
     positioning, 1121, 1122*f*
     postoperative care, 1125
     preoperative evaluation, 1121
   articular cartilage lesions, 1161–1177
     anatomy, 1161–1162
     biomechanics, 1161–1162
     classification, 1162, 1162*t*
     complications, 1176
     decision-making principles, 1163–1164
     future considerations, 1176–1177
     history, 1162–1163
     imaging, 1163
     physical examination, 1163
     postoperative management, 1166–1167
     results, 1174–1176
     return to play, 1167
     treatment options, 1164–1166, 1167*b*–1173*b*,
       1168*f*
   biomechanics, 1072–1073, 1073*f*
     joint, 1077–1080
     ligament, 1075–1077, 1076*f*
     meniscal, 1080–1082
     patellofemoral joint, 1082–1087
     techniques, 1073–1074, 1074*f*
     tibiofemoral joint, 1074–1080
   decision-making, 1089–1103, 1101*f*–1102*f*
   diagnosis, 1089–1103
   dislocation, 154, 1345–1349, 1346*f*
     anterior, 1345
     clinical presentation, 1346–1347, 1346*t*,
       1347*f*
     complications, 1349
     imaging, 1348
     physical examination and testing of,
       1347–1348, 1347*f*
     popliteal artery repair, 1349*b*
     posterior, 1345–1346
     postoperative management, 1349
     treatment options, 1348–1349
     vascular injury, 1346
   history, 1089–1091, 1090*t*
   imaging, 1104–1120
     background, 1104
     cartilage, 1116–1118, 1118*f*–1119*f*
     computed tomography, 1105*f*
     extensor mechanism, 1113–1116,
       1115*f*–1117*f*
     ligaments, 1110–1113, 1111*f*–1115*f*
     magnetic resonance imaging, 1105–1106
     menisci in, 1106–1109, 1106*f*–1109*f*
     musculotendinous structures, 1110, 1111*f*
     osseous structures, 1116–1118,
       1118*f*–1119*f*
     pitfalls, 1109–1110, 1110*f*
     postoperative, 1118–1120, 1119*f*–1120*f*
     radiographs, 1104, 1105*f*
     ultrasound, 1104–1105, 1106*f*

Knee (Continued)
  injuries
    basketball, 115–116
    figure skating, 118
    lacrosse, 122
    rowing, 123
    skiing, 124
    swimming, 126
    volleyball, 127
  inspection, 1091–1092, 1091b, 1091f–1092f
  instability, 1282
  lateral and posterolateral corner injuries,
        1244–1263
    anatomy, 1244–1248
    classification, 1248, 1248t
    complications in, 1260–1261, 1262f
    decision-making principles, 1253
    future considerations, 1262
    history, 1248–1249
    imaging, 1251–1253, 1251f–1252f
    layers of lateral side of, 1244
    nonoperative management, 1253
    pediatric, 1262
    physical examination, 1249–1251,
        1249f–1250f
    postoperative management, 1256–1260,
        1259t
    repair vs. reconstruction, 1253
    results, 1260, 1260t–1261t
    return to play, 1260
    structures, 1244–1246, 1245f
    surgical considerations, 1254–1256
    techniques, 1257b, 1257f–1258f
    timing of diagnosis, 1253
    treatment options, 1253–1256
  ligamentous stability in, 1097–1101,
        1098f–1101f
  meniscus, 1096–1097, 1097f
    injuries, 1132–1153
      arthroscopy, 1140
      biologic stimulation, 1147–1150
      classification, 1136–1137, 1136f–1137f
      complications, 1151–1152
      critical points in, 1152
      decision-making principles, 1142–1147
      future considerations, 1152
      history, 1137
      imaging, 1138–1139, 1138f
      physical examination, 1137–1138
      postoperative management, 1150–1151
      results, 1151
      return to play, 1151
      surgery for, 1139–1140, 1143–1147
      treatment options, 1139–1142
  motion, loss of, 1335–1344
    complications, 1342
    decision-making principles, 1337–1338,
        1337t, 1338f
    future considerations, 1343
    history, 1335–1336
    imaging, 1336–1337, 1337f
    physical examination, 1336, 1336f
    postoperative management, 1340–1342,
        1340f–1341f
    results, 1342
    return to sports and, 1342
    treatment options, 1338–1339, 1339b–1340b,
        1339f–1340f
  multiligament injuries, 1264–1276, 1269b–
        1273b, 1269f–1273f
    acute management, 1267
    complications, 1274
    decision-making principles, 1266–1267
    future considerations, 1274–1276

Knee (Continued)
    history, 1264
    imaging, 1265–1266, 1265f–1266f
    nonoperative treatment, 1266
    operative treatment, 1266
    physical examination, 1264–1265
    postoperative management, 1273–1274
    results, 1274, 1275t
    special considerations, 1267
    surgical timing of, 1266
    treatment options, 1267–1269
  palpation, 1092–1094, 1093f
  patella, 1095–1096, 1095f–1096f
  patellofemoral pain, 371, 1308–1317
  pediatrics, 1628–1633
    acute injuries, 1628–1630, 1629f–1630f
    injuries, 1697–1724
    osteochondroses, 1717–1718
    overuse injuries, 1630–1633, 1631f–1633f
  physical examination, 1091
  popliteal artery entrapment syndrome in,
        1349–1356
    classification, 1350–1351, 1350f
    clinical presentation, 1351
    complications, 1356
    criteria for return to play, 1356
    history, 1350
    imaging, 1352–1354, 1352f–1353f
    physical examination and testing of,
        1351–1352
    postoperative management, 1356
    treatment options, 1354–1356, 1355f,
        1356b
  range of motion of, 1094–1095, 1094f–1095f
  regional anesthesia, 332–333
  stability, 369–370, 370f
  strength testing, 1094–1095, 1094f–1095f
  synthesis in, 1101–1102, 1101f–1102f
  taping, 369–370
  vascular problems, 1345–1357
    dislocations of, 1345–1349, 1346f
    vascular problems of, 1345–1357
Knives, in arthroscopy, 108
Kohler syndrome, 1738, 1738f
Kyphotic thoracic spine, 1533

L
Labeled white blood cell scans, 89–90, 91f
Labrum, 427–431
  conditions, 939
  injuries, 967, 967f
  superior labrum, anterior, and posterior
        (SLAP) tears, 430–431, 430f, 431t
  tears, 941–942, 942f
    hip, 1614, 1614f
    pediatrics, 1693, 1693f
  variant, 939, 939f–941f
Lacerations
  face
    complex, 262–263, 264f
    lateral, 263, 265f
    intraoral/tongue, 263
    lip, 263, 264f
  mechanical dermatoses, 253–254
  periorbital, 263
Lacrosse injuries, 122
Lactate, 66
Lag signs, 404
Laryngopharyngeal reflux disease (LPRD), 190
Laser, 361–362
Latarjet-Patte coracoid transfer, 459b–461b, 460f,
        461
Lateral ankle ligament reconstruction, 1426b

Lateral ankle sprain, 1444–1450, 1445f
  classification, 1447t
  complications, 1450
  decision-making principles, 1447
  history, 1444–1446
  imaging, 1446–1447, 1447f
  physical examination, 1444–1446, 1446f, 1446t
  postoperative management, 1450
  results, 1450
  treatment, 1447–1449
    conservative, 1447–1448
    surgical, 1448–1449, 1448f
    technique, 1449b, 1449f
Lateral capsular ligament, mid-third, 1246
Lateral center edge angles, 937
Lateral clavicle physeal fractures, 1640–1642,
        1641f
  complications, 1642
  history, 1640
  imaging, 1641
  physical examination, 1640–1641
  results, 1642
  treatment options, 1641–1642, 1642f
Lateral closing wedge high tibial osteotomy, 1281,
        1282t
Lateral collateral ligaments, 684, 685f, 694,
        1079–1080
Lateral compartment osteoarthritis, 1284, 1284f
  osteotomy for, 1282
Lateral compartment release, 1399
Lateral corner injuries, 1244–1263
  anatomy, 1244–1248
  biomechanics, 1246, 1247f
  classification, 1248, 1248t
  complications in, 1260–1261, 1262f
  decision-making principles, 1253
  future considerations, 1262
  history, 1248–1249
  imaging, 1251–1253, 1251f–1252f
    magnetic resonance imaging, 1251–1253,
        1252f
    radiographs, 1251, 1251f
    ultrasound, 1253
  layers of lateral side of, 1244
  neurovascular structures, 1246
  nonoperative management, 1253
    grade I injuries, 1253
    grade II injuries, 1253
    grade III injuries, 1253
  pediatric, 1262
  physical examination, 1249–1251, 1249f–1250f
  postoperative management, 1256–1260,
        1259t
  repair vs. reconstruction, 1253
  results, 1260, 1260t–1261t
  return to play, 1260
  structures, 1244–1246, 1245f
    arcuate ligament complex, 1246
    biceps femoris muscle, 1245–1246
    biomechanics, 1246, 1247f
    fabellofibular ligament, 1246
    fibular collateral ligament, 1244–1245
    iliotibial band, 1244
    lateral gastrocnemius tendon, 1246
    mid-third lateral capsular ligament, 1246
    neurovascular, 1246
    popliteus tendon complex, 1245
  surgical considerations, 1254–1256
    diagnostic arthroscopy, 1254, 1254f
    primary repair, 1254, 1254f
    reconstruction techniques, 1254–1255
  techniques, 1257b, 1257f–1258f
  timing of diagnosis, 1253
  treatment options, 1253–1256

Lateral epicondylitis, 687, 702–704, 703f, 720–725, 1674–1676
  arthroscopy, 724
  complications, 725, 1676
  decision-making principles, 722, 1675
  future considerations, 725
  history, 720, 721t, 1675
  imaging, 721, 721f–722f, 1675
  physical examination, 720, 721f, 1675
  postoperative management, 724
  results, 724–725, 1675–1676
  return-to-play guidelines, 724
  splinting, 722
  treatment, 721f, 722–724, 1675
    injections, 721f, 723
    management, 724b
    splinting, 722
    surgery, 723–724, 723f
    therapy, 722–723
Lateral face lacerations, 263, 265f
Lateral gastrocnemius tendon, 1246
Lateral impingement test, 932
Lateral meniscus, 1069, 1069f
Lateral patella compression syndrome, 1316
Lateral plantar nerve entrapment, 1411–1412
  complications, 1412
  decision-making principles, 1411
  history, 1411
  imaging, 1411
  physical examination, 1411
  postoperative management, 1412
  results, 1412
  treatment options, 1411–1412, 1412b, 1412f
Lateral position, 933
Latissimus dorsi muscle, injuries to, 576–578
  anatomy, 576
  classification, 576
  imaging, 576, 577f
  mechanisms of, 576
  physical examination, 576, 577f
  teres major, 578
  treatment, 576–578, 578f
Lavage, 1487–1488
LCPD. See Legg-Calvé-Perthes disease
Left ventricle, 160
Leg
  decision-making, 1370–1379
  diagnosis, 1370–1379
  exertional compartment syndromes, 1393–1401, 1394t
    anatomy, 1393–1394, 1394f, 1394t
    classification, 1394–1395
    compartment testing, 1397–1398, 1397t
    complications, 1400
    decision-making principles, 1396–1397, 1396t–1397t
    diagnostics/imaging, 1395–1396, 1396f
    epidemiology, 1393
    history, 1395
    pathophysiology, 1394
    physical examination, 1395
    postoperative care, 1398
    results, 1400
    return to play, 1400
    treatment options, 1398
  history, 1372–1379, 1373f–1378f
  pain, 1393–1401, 1394t
    anatomy, 1393–1394, 1394f, 1394t
    classification, 1394–1395
    compartment testing, 1397–1398, 1397t
    complications, 1400
    decision-making principles, 1396–1397, 1396t–1397t
    diagnostics/imaging, 1395–1396, 1396f
    epidemiology, 1393
    history, 1395

Leg (Continued)
    pathophysiology, 1394
    physical examination, 1395
    postoperative care, 1398
    results, 1400
    return to play, 1400
    treatment options, 1398
  pathologies, 1370–1371
  physical examination, 1371–1372
Legg-Calvé-Perthes disease (LCPD), 928, 1693–1694, 1694f
Leptospirosis, 215
Les Autres group, 323
Lesions. See also specific lesions
  articular cartilage, 1161–1177
  osteochondral, 1388–1389, 1389f. See also Talus, osteochondral lesions of
  pathologic, 1691
Lesser trochanter, 911
Lesser tuberosity fractures, 1647
  complications, 1647
  history, 1647
  imaging, 1647
  physical examination, 1647
  treatment options, 1647, 1647f
Leukotriene modifiers, for exercise-induced bronchoconstriction, 177
Lift-off test, 404, 546f, 558–559
Ligaments, 2–7
  ankle, 1387–1388, 1388f
  anterior cruciate
    MRI, 1110–1111, 1111f–1112f
    partial tear, 1189
    revision, 1189–1190, 1192
  arcuate, 1246
  bifurcate, sprain, 1456–1457
    complications, 1458
    decision-making principles, 1457
    history, 1457
    imaging, 1457
    physical examination, 1457
    postoperative management, 1457
    results, 1457–1458
    treatment, 1457, 1457b
  biomechanics, 1075–1077, 1076f
  capsular, 914
  carpal injuries, 848–851, 848f–850f, 850b
  collateral, 1069–1071, 1079–1080
  cruciate, 1069, 1077–1079
    anterior, 1069, 1070f
    in joint biomechanics, 1077–1079
    posterior, 1069, 1070f
  fabellofibular, 1246
  fibular collateral, 1113, 1244–1245
  foot, 1387–1388, 1388f
  force measurement of, 1074–1075
  head, 1534
  healing
    factors affecting, 5, 6t
    methods for augmentation of, 5–7
  iliofemoral, 914, 915f
  imaging, 1110–1113, 1111f, 1115f
  injuries, 3–4
    ankle, 1444–1461
    collateral ligament injuries of metacarpophalangeal joint, 894–896, 894f–896f
    distal interphalangeal joint, 888–890
    foot, 1444–1461
    metacarpophalangeal joint, 883–885, 884f
    phalangeal fractures, 890–892, 891f–893f
    platelet-rich plasma for, 53–54
    proximal interphalangeal joint, 885–888, 885f–890f
  intrinsic carpal, 810–812, 811f
  ischiofemoral, 914, 915f

Ligaments (Continued)
  joint contact forces and, 21–22
  knee, 1069–1071
  lateral ankle, reconstruction, 1426b
  laxity, 1187–1188
    evaluation, 932
    untreated, revision anterior cruciate ligament injuries and, 1203
  medial collateral, MRI in, 1113, 1114f
  mid-third lateral capsular, 1246
  pediatrics, 1661–1662, 1662f–1663f, 1697–1703
  posterior cruciate, 1112
  pubofemoral, 914, 915f
  reconstruction, implants for, 38–41
  repair, 4–5
    platelet-rich plasma for, 53–55
  spine, 1534
  stability, in knee, 1097–1101, 1098f–1101f
  strain measurement of, 1075
  structure of, 2–3
  ulnar collateral, 701–702, 701f–702f, 804, 804f
    injuries, 814, 815f
Ligamentum teres, 912, 913f, 932–933
Lightning, 154
Limb-threatening injuries, 154
  acute compartment syndrome, 154
  knee dislocation, 154
  traumatic amputation, 154
Linear kinematics, 22
Lip lacerations, 263, 264f
Lisfranc sprains, 1458–1460
  complications, 1460
  decision-making principles, 1459
  history, 1458
  imaging, 1458–1459, 1459f
  physical examination, 1458
  postoperative management, 1459–1460
  results, 1460
  treatment, 1459, 1460b, 1460f
Little League elbow, 1612, 1612f, 1621–1623, 1622f–1623f, 1665–1668
  complications, 1668
  decision-making principles, 1667
  history, 1665–1666, 1665f
  imaging, 1667
  physical examination, 1666–1667
  results, 1668
  treatment options, 1667–1668
Little League shoulder, 1612, 1612f, 1655–1656
  complications, 1656
  history, 1656
  imaging, 1656, 1656f
  physical examination, 1656
  treatment, 1656
"Load and shift test", 405
Load transmission, 1080–1081
Local anesthetic agents, 334–335
  systemic toxicity, 334–335, 335t
Localization pain, 580, 580b
Log roll test, 932
Long thoracic nerve palsy, 625–627
  anatomy, 625, 625f
  biomechanics, 625, 625f
  clinical evaluation, 625–627, 626f
  decision-making principles, 627
  diagnostic studies, 627
  results, 627
  technique, 627b
Loose bodies, 700, 763–764
  removal, 712b, 712f–713f
Low-impact exercise, for knee arthritis, 1279
Lower back injuries, 119
Lower extremity
  injuries
    basketball, 115
    football, 118–119

Lower extremity (Continued)
  gymnastics, 120
  ice hockey, 121
  snowboarding, 125
  soccer, 125
  tennis, 126–127
innervation, 332
strength, restoration of, 386, 386f–387f
Lower gastrointestinal tract conditions, 192–195, 193t
  celiac disease, 194–195
  diarrhea, 192–194
  irritable bowel syndrome, 194
  ischemic conditions, 194
  lower gastrointestinal bleeding, 194
Lower respiratory tract infections, 209–210
  acute bronchitis, 209
  acute pneumonia, 209–210
Lumbar disc herniation, 1599–1601, 1601f
Lumbar spine
  anatomy, 1598
  degenerative, 1598–1604
  injuries, 123
  stenosis, 1602–1603, 1602f
Lunate carpal injuries, 845–847, 846f, 847b
Lunotriquetral injuries, 848

M

Maddocks questions, 1744
Magnetic field strength, 99
Magnetic resonance angiography (MRA)
  elbow, 699
  popliteal artery entrapment syndrome, 1352–1353, 1353f
Magnetic resonance arthrography, 99, 99f
  femoroacetabular impingement, 964
  hip dysplasia and instability, 974
  revision rotator cuff repair, 568
Magnetic resonance imaging (MRI), 92–100
  advantages, 102
  ankle, 1380–1381
    ligaments, 1387–1388, 1388f
  anterior tibial tendons, 1386, 1387f
  athletic pubalgia, 1010, 1010f–1011f
  contraindications, 102–103
  delayed gadolinium for, 101
  Dgemric, 101
  diffusion weighted imaging, 100, 100f
  disadvantages, 102, 102f
  dynamic contrast enhancement in, 101–103
  elbow, 698–699
  entrapment neuropathies, 742
  femoroacetabular impingement, 963–964, 963f–964f
  flexor hallucis longus, 1384–1385, 1385f
  foot, 1380–1381
    ligaments, 1387–1388, 1388f
  glenohumeral joint, 412–414, 413f, 413t
    acromion, 415–417, 416f–418f, 417b
    osseous outlet, 415–417, 416f–418f, 417b
    rotator cuff, 419–422, 420f–424f, 423b
  hip, 939–946
    chondral injury, 942, 943f
    dysplasia and instability, 974
    femoroacetabular impingement, 942, 944f
    hip sprain and dislocation, 942, 944f–945f
    labral conditions, 939
    labral variant, 939, 939f–941f
    labrum tear, 941–942, 942f
    stress injuries, 942–944, 945f
  iliopsoas, 979, 983–984
  interdigital nerve, 1389–1390, 1390f

Magnetic resonance imaging (MRI) (Continued)
  knee, 1105–1106
    arthritis, 1278–1279
    lateral and posterolateral corner injuries of knee, 1251–1253, 1252f
    medial collateral ligament and posterior medial corner injuries, 1232–1234, 1234f
    meniscal transplantation, 1155, 1155f
    multiligament knee injuries, 1265, 1266f
    osteochondral lesions, 1388–1389, 1389f
    patellar instability, 1298–1299, 1299f
    patellofemoral pain, 1313–1314, 1315f
    pediatrics
      of traumatic anterior instability, 1648–1649, 1650f
      of traumatic posterior instability, 1652, 1653f
    peroneal tendon, 1385–1386, 1385f–1386f
    popliteal artery entrapment syndrome, 1352–1353, 1353f
    posterior cruciate ligament injuries, 1214
    posterior tibial tendon, 1383–1384
    revision rotator cuff repair, 568
    scapulothoracic disorders, 614
    spine, 1547, 1547f
    technical considerations, 93–100
      artifacts, 98–99
      coils, 99–100, 100f
      contrast agents, 99, 99f
      fat suppression, 98, 99f
      image formation, 94–95
      image quality, 100
      imaging protocols, 93, 94f
      magnetic field strength, 99
      proton density, 95, 96f, 96t
      pulse sequences, 95–98
      T1, 95, 95f, 96t
      T2, 95, 96t
      tissue contrast, 95, 95f–96f, 96t
    ultrashort time to echo sequence for, 100–101
Malassezia, 250, 251f
Mallet finger, 873–875, 874f
Mandible fractures, 267, 267f
Manipulation, 363
  under anesthesia (MUA), 585–586
Manual therapy, 354–355, 355f, 356t
  for pain, 357, 358t
March hemoglobinuria, 196
Marfan syndrome, 169, 171f
Marijuana, 291–292
Marrow stimulation, 1164–1165, 1167b–1173b, 1169f, 1174–1175
Mast cell stabilizers, for exercise-induced bronchoconstriction, 177
Matrix
  bone, 13
  extracellular, 11
    cell-matrix interactions, 11
    meniscus, 8
    tendons and ligaments, 3
Matrix-assisted chondrocyte implantation (MACI), 43
Maximum oxygen uptake (Vo₂ max)
  adrenal hormones and, 70
  in exercise capacity, 71
McCarthy test, 932
MCP joint. See Metacarpophalangeal (MCP) joints
MDI. See Multidirectional instability
Measles, 208–209
Measure, units of, 16, 17t
Mechanical dermatoses, 253–256
  abrasions/lacerations, 253–254
  acne mechanica, 254–255, 255f
  athlete's nodules (collagenomas), 255, 255f

Mechanical dermatoses (Continued)
  calluses and corns, 254
  friction blisters, 254
  hemorrhage, 254, 254f–255f
  hidradenitis suppurativa, 255–256, 256f
  striae, 254, 255f
Mechanics
  classes, 23–24
  fluid, 23–24
  rigid body, 23
  viscoelasticity and, 24, 24f–25f
Medial ankle sprains, 1450–1453
  complications, 1452–1453, 1453f
  decision-making principles, 1451
  history, 1450–1451
  imaging, 1451, 1451f
  physical examination, 1450–1451
  results, 1452
  treatment, 1452, 1452b
Medial clavicle
  excision, 675
  physeal fractures, 1642–1644, 1642f
    complications, 1644
    history, 1643
    imaging, 1643, 1643f
    physical examination, 1643
    treatment options, 1643–1644, 1644f
Medial collateral ligament (MCL), 694–695, 694f–695f
  injuries, 1231–1243, 1672–1673
    complications, 1242, 1673
    decision-making principles, 1234–1235, 1235f, 1672
    future considerations, 1243
    history, 1231, 1672
    imaging, 1232–1234, 1233f–1235f, 1672
    physical exam, 1231–1232, 1233f, 1233t
    physical examination, 1672
    postoperative management, 1239–1240, 1239t
    results, 1240–1242, 1673
    return-to-play guidelines, 1240b
    treatment options, 1235–1236, 1236b–1238b, 1236f–1238f, 1672–1673, 1673f
  joint biomechanics, 1079–1080
  knee, 1069–1070, 1070f
  MRI, 1113, 1114f
Medial collateral osteoarthritis, 1284b
Medial compartment osteoarthritis, 1283, 1283t
  arthroplasty for, 1283
  osteotomy for, 1281, 1281f
Medial displacement calcaneal osteotomy, for posterior tibial tendon injury, 1467b–1468b
Medial epicondyle avulsion fractures, 1670–1672
  complications, 1672
  decision-making principles, 1671
  history, 1670–1671
  imaging, 1671
  physical examination, 1671, 1671f
  results, 1671–1672
  treatment, 1671
Medial epicondylitis, 688, 720–725, 751, 1674–1676
  complications, 725, 1676
  decision-making principles, 722, 1675
  future considerations, 725
  history, 720, 721t, 1675
  imaging, 721, 721f–722f, 1675
  physical examination, 720, 721f, 1675
  postoperative management, 724
  results, 724–725, 1675–1676
  return-to-play guidelines, 724
  splinting, 722

Medial epicondylitis (Continued)
  treatment, 721f, 722–724, 1675
    injections, 721f, 723
    management, 724b
    splinting, 722
    surgery, 722–724, 723f
Medial meniscus, 1068
Medial opening wedge high tibial osteotomy, 1281, 1282t, 1285b–1288b, 1285f–1288f
Medial patellofemoral reconstruction, 1301b–1302b, 1302f–1303f
Medial plantar nerve entrapment, 1412–1413
  decision-making principles, 1413
  history, 1412
  imaging, 1413
  physical examination, 1412
  postoperative management, 1413
  treatment options, 1413
Medial tibial stress syndrome (MTSS), 1393
Median nerve, 743–745, 744f
  AIN syndrome, 746–747
    complications, 747
    decision-making principles, 746
    history, 746
    physical examination, 746
    postoperative management, 747
    results, 747
    return-to-play guidelines, 747
    treatment, 746
  pronator syndrome, 745–746
    complications, 746
    decision-making principles, 745
    history, 745
    physical examination, 745
    postoperative management, 745–746
    results, 746
    return-to-play guidelines, 745–746
    technique, 746f
    treatment, 745
Median nerve compression, elbow, 693–694
Medical home, of elite athlete, 159–160
Medical nutrition therapy, 219–220
Medications. See also Drugs
  cerebral palsy, 321
  preparticipation physical evaluation, 149
Medicine. See also Medications; Nuclear medicine
  gastrointestinal, 189–195
    lower gastrointestinal tract conditions, 192–195, 193t
    pathophysiology, 189
    upper gastrointestinal tract conditions, 189–192
  hematologic, 196–200
    hemostasis disorders, 198–200
    red blood cells disorders, 196–198
Meningitis, 214–215
  aseptic, waterborne diseases, 212–213
  classification, 214
  definition, 214
  diagnosis, 214–215
  epidemiology, 214
  pathobiology, 214
  prevention, 215
  return-to-play guidelines, 215
  treatment, 215
Meningoencephalitis, 214
Meniscal insufficiency
  history, 1154
  physical examination, 1154–1155, 1155f
  treatment options, 1156–1158, 1157b
    bone plug and trough, 1158
    diagnostic arthroscopy, 1157
    nonoperative management, 1156
    operative management, 1156
    positioning, 1157
Meniscal regeneration, 9

Meniscal transplantation, 1154–1160
  complications, 1159–1160
  contraindications, 1156
  contributing factors, 1156, 1156f
  decision-making principles, 1155–1156
  future considerations, 1160
  imaging, 1155
  indications, 1155–1156
  lateral, 1157, 1157f
  medial, 1157–1158, 1158f
  pathophysiology, 1155–1156
  postoperative management, 1159
  results, 1159
Meniscectomy, 1143–1144, 1144f
Meniscus, 7–9, 1068–1069, 1068f
  allograft transplantation, 1142
  anatomy, 1132–1134, 1133f–1134f
  biomechanics, 1080–1082, 1134–1135, 1135f
  cysts, 1140
  discoid, 1140–1142, 1141f–1142f
  epidemiology, 1135–1136
  extracellular matrix, 8
  function of, 1134–1135, 1135f
  history, 1132
  injuries, 8–9, 1132–1153, 1703–1705
    anatomy, 1703
    arthroscopy, 1140
    biologic stimulation, 1147–1150
    classification, 1136–1137, 1136f–1137f
    complications, 1151–1152, 1705
    critical points in, 1152
    decision-making principles, 1142–1147, 1704
    development, 1703, 1703f
    future considerations, 1152, 1705
    history, 1137, 1703
    imaging, 1138–1139, 1138f, 1703–1704
    physical examination, 1137–1138, 1703
    postoperative management, 1150–1151, 1704–1705
    results, 1151, 1705
    return to play, 1151
    revision anterior cruciate ligament injuries, 1203
    surgery for, 1139–1140, 1143–1147
    treatment options, 1139–1142, 1704
  in joint stability, 1081–1082
  knee, 1096–1097, 1097f, 1106–1109, 1106f–1109f
  lateral, 1069, 1069f
    fascicular tears, 1140
  load transmission, 1080–1081
  medial, 1068
  pediatrics
    anatomy, 1703
    discoid, 1705–1708
    injuries, 1703–1705
  repair, 9
    all-inside, 1147, 1148f
    augmentation in, 9
    in avascular portions, 9
    basics of, 1144
    cell-based approaches, 1149
    factors affecting, 9
    implants for, 41–42
    inside-out, 1144–1146, 1145f–1146f
    outside-in, 1146–1147, 1147f
    platelet-rich plasma, 55–56
    scaffolds for, 9, 1149–1150
    stem cell-based therapy, 60
    techniques, 1143b, 1143f
    in vascular regions, 9
  root tears, 1140
  structure of, 7–8, 7f, 1132–1134, 1133f–1134f
  variants, 1140–1142, 1141f–1142f
Meralgia paresthetica, 927

Mesenchymal stem cells (MSCs)
  in allograft, 32
  silk-based scaffold and, 39
  three-dimensional matrices, 1181–1182
Metabolism, energy, 65–66, 65f
Metacarpal fracture, 814–815, 815f
Metacarpophalangeal (MCP) joints, 803–804
  collateral ligament injuries of, 894–896, 894f–896f
  fingers, 787–788
  ligamentous injuries and dislocations, 883–885, 884f
Metatarsal
  break, 1365–1367, 1367f–1368f
  first, osteochondral lesions of, 1501, 1502f
  stress fractures, 135–136
Metatarsalgia, 1519–1522
  complications, 1522
  decision-making principles, 1520
  future considerations of, 1522
  history, 1519
  imaging, 1520
  physical examination, 1519–1520
  postoperative management, 1521–1522
  results, 1522
  treatment options, 1520–1521
    nonoperative, 1520–1521
    operative, 1521, 1521f
    technique, 1522b, 1522f
Metatarsophalangeal arthrodesis, 1525, 1525f
Metatarsophalangeal joint, 1365–1367, 1367f–1368f
Methadone, perioperative pharmacology, 337
Methicillin-resistant Staphylococcus aureus (MRSA), skin infections, 203–204, 204f
Microfracture, 1164–1165, 1487–1488
Microinstability, atraumatic hip, 977–978
Mid-anterior portal, modified, in hip arthroscopy, 951, 951f
Midface fractures, 267–268
Midsole, 1440–1441
Minced cartilage techniques, 1182, 1183f
Mineralization, endochondral bone formation and, 14
Mitochondrial respiration, 66
Mobilization, 363, 364f–365f
  with movement, 363–365, 365f
Modalities. See Imaging
Modified mid-anterior portal, in hip arthroscopy, 951, 951f
Modified Thomas test, 933
Molluscum contagiosum, 252, 252f
Moment/torque vectors, 21
Montelukast, for exercise-induced bronchoconstriction, 177
Morton neuroma, 1416–1419
  complications, 1418–1419
  decision-making principles, 1418
  etiologies of, 1417
  history, 1417
  imaging, 1417–1418
  pathomechanism of, 1417
  physical examination, 1417
  postoperative management, 1418
  results, 1418
  treatment options, 1418, 1419b, 1419f
Mosaicplasty, 1488
Motion. See also Range of motion
  dorsiflexion range of, 381
  elbow, 681–683, 690, 772–784
    arthroscopy, 776–781, 777f–781f
    complications, 782–783
    decision-making principles, 774–776, 775f
    follow-up, 782
    history, 772–773
    imaging, 774, 774f

Motion (Continued)
  physical examination, 773–774
  postoperative management, 782
  rehabilitation, 782
  results, 782–783, 783t
  return-to-play guidelines, 782
  surgery, 776–782, 777f
  treatment, 774–776, 775f
hip, 921
joint, 22–23, 23f
  mobility, 350
loss, knee, 1335–1344
  complications, 1342
  decision-making principles, 1337–1338,
    1337t, 1338f
  future considerations, 1343
  history, 1335–1336
  imaging, 1336–1337, 1337f
  physical examination, 1336, 1336f
  postoperative management, 1340–1342,
    1340f–1341f
  results, 1342
  return to sports and, 1342
  treatment options, 1338–1339, 1339b–1340b,
    1339f–1340f
maintenance of, 349–350
relative, 22
restoration of, 349–350
rolling, 22–23, 23f
sliding, 22–23, 23f
spinning, 22–23, 23f
throwing, 1663–1665, 1663f–1664f
varus, 1246–1247
Motion-sparing procedures, in advanced
  degeneration, 1525
Motor testing, for ankle, foot, and leg,
  1374–1375
Motor unit, 62
Motorized shavers, 107–108
MRA. See Magnetic resonance angiography
MRI. See Magnetic resonance imaging
MSCs. See Mesenchymal stem cells (MSCs)
Multibody dynamics, 922, 922f
Multidirectional instability (MDI), 476–488, 482b,
  482f, 1654–1655
  decision-making principles, 479–480
  future considerations, 480–481
  history, 477, 1654
  imaging, 479, 479f, 1655, 1655f
  physical examination, 477–479, 477t–478t, 478f,
    1654–1655, 1654f
  postoperative management, 481–483, 483f
  results, 483–487, 484t–485t
    complications, 486–487
    return to sport, 485–486, 486t
  treatment options, 480–481, 1655, 1655f
    arthroscopic plication, 481
    open inferior capsular shift, 480–481, 480f
Multiligament knee injuries, 1264–1276,
  1269b–1273b, 1269f–1273f
  acute management, 1267
  complications, 1274
  decision-making principles, 1266–1267
  future considerations, 1274–1276
  history, 1264
  imaging, 1265–1266, 1265f–1266f
  nonoperative treatment, 1266
  operative treatment, 1266
  physical examination, 1264–1265
  postoperative management, 1273–1274
  results, 1274, 1275t
  special considerations, 1267
  surgical timing of, 1266
  treatment options, 1267–1269

Muscles
  balance of, patellar instability and, 1296–1297,
    1297f
  biceps femoris, 1245–1246
    long head of, 1245–1246
    short head of, 1246
  cramps, exercise-associated, 236–237
  delayed-onset soreness of, 68
  elbow, 681
  energy technique, 366–367
  fatigue, 67
  fibers, classification, 62, 63t
  hand, 785–787, 788f
  head, 1534
  hip joint, 916–920, 918t
    abductors, 917
    adductors, 920
    extensors, 919–920
    external rotators, 920
    flexors, 917–919
    internal rotators, 917
  injuries
    latissimus dorsi, 576–578
    other, 574–578
    pectoralis major, 574–576
  knee, 1065–1068, 1066f
    anterior, 1066
    lateral, 1068
    medial, 1067–1068, 1067f
    posterior, 1066–1067, 1067f
  pediatrics, 1691
  performance
    restoration of, 350–351
      hypertrophy vs. motor learning, 350–351
      inhibition/activation, 350
  shoulder
    rotator cuff, 398–399, 398f
    scapular muscles, 399
  spine, 1534
  training, 66–67, 1195–1196, 1196f
Musculoskeletal system
  injuries, 128–129
    amputee athletes, 316
    cerebral palsy, 321
    intellectually disabled athletes, 322
    visually impaired athletes, 323
    wheelchair athletes, 318
  preparticipation physical evaluation, 148, 148b
  tissues
    articular cartilage, 9–12
    bone, 12–15
    meniscus, 7–9
    physiology pathophysiology, 2–15
    tendon and ligament in, 2–7
  ultrasound, 79–83, 80f–83f
Mycobacterial infections, 252
Mycobacterium marinum (swimming pool or fish
  tank granuloma), 252, 252f
Myelography, of spine, 1548
Myelopathy, cervical, 1595–1596
Myocarditis, 169, 171f
myofascial release, 367
Myositis ossificans, 1046–1047, 1046f

N

Naegleria fowleri, 215–216
Nanofiber scaffolds, 37–38
Nasal fractures, 266–267, 266f–267f
Natural supplements, 1611
Nausea, 192
Navicular stress fractures, 136, 137f
Neck shaft angle, 909, 936–937
Neer test, 404, 545f

Nerve entrapment, 621–631
  ankle, 1389–1391, 1390f–1391f
  axillary nerve palsy, 629–630
    anatomy, 629
    biomechanics, 629
    clinical evaluation, 629–630
    decision-making principles, 630
    diagnostic studies, 630
    results, 630
  deep peroneal nerve, 1415–1416, 1415f
    history, 1415
    imaging, 1416
    physical examination, 1415–1416
    postoperative management, 1416
    results, 1416
    treatment options, 1416, 1416b
  foot, 1389–1391, 1390f–1391f
  hip, 927
  interdigital neuralgia (Morton neuroma),
    1416–1419
    complications, 1418–1419
    decision-making principles, 1418
    etiologies of, 1417
    history, 1417
    imaging, 1417–1418
    pathomechanism of, 1417
    physical examination, 1417
    postoperative management, 1418
    results, 1418
    treatment options, 1418, 1419b, 1419f
  lateral plantar nerve, 1411–1412
    complications, 1412
    decision-making principles, 1411
    history, 1411
    imaging, 1411
    physical examination, 1411
    postoperative management, 1412
    results, 1412
    treatment options, 1411–1412, 1412b,
      1412f
  long thoracic nerve palsy, 625–627
    anatomy, 625, 625f
    biomechanics, 625, 625f
    clinical evaluation, 625–627, 626f
    decision-making principles, 627
    diagnostic studies, 627
    results, 627
    technique, 627b
  medial plantar nerve, 1412–1413
    decision-making principles, 1413
    history, 1412
    imaging, 1413
    physical examination, 1412
    postoperative management, 1413
    treatment options, 1413
  peripheral, 1402–1419
  saphenous nerve, 1405–1407, 1405f–1406f
    history, 1405
    imaging, 1406
    physical examination, 1405–1406
    results, 1406–1407
    treatment options, 1406
  shoulder, 621
  spinal accessory nerve palsy, 627–629
    anatomy, 627–628
    biomechanics, 627–628
    clinical evaluation, 628–629, 628f
    decision-making principles, 629
    diagnostic studies, 629
    results, 629
    technique, 629b
  superficial peroneal nerve, 1413–1415, 1413f
    decision-making principles, 1414
    history, 1413

Nerve entrapment *(Continued)*
  imaging, 1414
  physical examination, 1413–1414
  postoperative management, 1415
  results, 1415
  treatment options, 1414–1415, 1414b, 1414f
  suprascapular nerve palsy, 621–625
    anatomy, 621–622, 622f
    biomechanics, 621–622, 622f
    clinical evaluation, 622–623, 623f
    decision-making principles, 624
    diagnostic studies, 623–624, 623f
    results, 624–625
  sural nerve, 1402–1405, 1403f
    history, 1402
    imaging, 1403–1404
    physical examination, 1402–1403
    postoperative management, 1405
    results, 1405
    treatment options, 1404, 1404b, 1404f
Nerves. *See also* Neuropathies
  accessory obturator, 916
  capsular innervation, 914–916
    accessory obturator nerve, 916
    femoral nerve, 916
    inferior gluteal nerve, 916
    obturator nerve, 916
    quadratus femoris, nerve to, 916
    sciatic nerve, 916
    superior gluteal nerve, 916
  femoral, 916
  hand, 785, 787f
  inferior gluteal, 1032–1033, 1032f, 1032t
  median, 743–745, 744f
    AIN syndrome, 746–747
    pronator syndrome, 745–746
  obturator, 916
  quadratus femoris, 916
  radial, 752
    PIN syndrome, 755–756
    radial tunnel syndrome, 752–755, 753f
  sciatic, 1018–1020, 1019f–1020f
  superior gluteal, 1032–1033, 1032f, 1032t
  ulnar, 747, 748f. *See also* Cubital tunnel syndrome
Neuraxial anesthesia, 329
Neurologic infections, 214–215
  encephalitis, 214–215
  meningitis, 214–215
Neurologic system
  assessment, 690–691, 691f
  injuries, 117, 718
  preparticipation physical evaluation, 148
  tissues, 1534–1535, 1534f
Neuroma, 317
  Morton, 1416–1419
    complications, 1418–1419
    decision-making principles, 1418
    etiologies of, 1417
    history, 1417
    imaging, 1417–1418
    pathomechanism of, 1417
    physical examination, 1417
    postoperative management, 1418
    results, 1418
    treatment options, 1418, 1419b, 1419f
Neuromuscular electrical stimulation, 366
Neuromuscular training, 69
Neuropathies
  entrapment, 742–756
    complications, 743
    decision-making principles, 743
    history, 742
    imaging, 742
    median nerve, 743–745, 744f
    physical examination, 742

Neuropathies *(Continued)*
    postoperative management, 743
    radial nerve, 752, 753f
    testing, 742–743
    treatment, 743
    ulnar nerve, 747, 748f. *See also* Cubital tunnel syndrome
  wrist and hand, 898–905
    decision-making principles, 901
    future considerations, 904
    history, 898
    imaging, 900–901, 900f, 901t
    physical examination, 898–900, 899f–900f
    postoperative management and return to play, 902–903, 903b, 903f
    results, 903–904
      complications, 904
    treatment options, 901–902
Neurovascular anatomy, of knee, 1072
Neutral Ober test, 933
Newton's laws, 17–19, 17t
  first law (inertia), 17, 17t, 18f
  second law (acceleration), 17–19, 17t, 18f
  third law (action-reaction), 19, 19f–20f
Night pain, in stiff shoulder, 580, 580b
90-degree Dunn view, 935, 937f
Noncontact anterior cruciate ligament injury, in female athlete, 307–309, 308f, 310f
Nonfecally derived waterborne diseases, 213–214
  acute otitis externa, 213–214
  hot tub folliculitis, 213
  Pseudomonas infections, 213
Nonoperative sling immobilization, 455
Nonsteroidal antiinflammatory drugs (NSAIDs)
  dyspepsia, 191–192
  knee arthritis, 1279
  perioperative pharmacology, 338
Nonthermal ultrasound treatments, 360–363
  compression, 362, 362f
  iontophoresis, 360–361
  laser, 361–362
  phonophoresis, 360
  range of motion, 362
  stress fracture healing, 360, 361f
  superficial heat, 362–363
Nose, preparticipation physical evaluation, 145
NSAIDs. *See* Nonsteroidal antiinflammatory drugs
Nuclear medicine, 88–92
  advantages, 90, 93f
  bone scans in, 88–89, 89f
  disadvantages, 90–92, 94f
  gallium scans in, 90, 92f–93f
  labeled white blood cell scans in, 89–90, 91f
  PECT/CT scans, 90, 93f
  planar imaging, 88, 89f
  SPECT/CT imaging, 88, 89f
  technical considerations, 88
Nuclear scintigraphy, of spine, 1548–1549, 1549f
Nutrition
  carbohydrates, 277–278, 278t
  fat, 277–278, 278t
  gastrointestinal tract conditions, 189
  hydration, 278–279, 279t
    considerations, 278
    in female athlete, 296–298, 297t–298t
    gastrointestinal tract conditions, 189
    monitoring, 278–279
  pediatrics, 1610–1611

O

Ober testing, 933
Obstructive sleep apnea (OSA), 325–326, 326f
Obturator nerve, of hip, 916
Occult fracture, 699, 700f

OCD. *See* Osteochondritis dissecans (OCD)
OCLs. *See* Osteochondral lesions
Odontoid fractures, 1761–1762
  classification, 1761
  history, 1761
  imaging, 1761–1762, 1761f
  physical examination, 1761
  treatment, 1762
Off-the-shelf surface allograft transplantation, 1182–1184, 1183f
OHAs. *See* Oral hypoglycemic agents
Olecranon bursitis, 728–730, 728f
  complications, 730
  decision-making principles, 728–729
  future considerations, 730
  history, 728, 728f
  imaging, 728, 729f
  physical examination, 728
  postoperative care, 730
  results, 730
  treatment, 729, 729b, 729f
Olecranon osteochondrosis, 1673–1674, 1673f
  complications, 1674
  decision-making principles, 1674
  history, 1674
  imaging, 1674
  physical examination, 1674
  results, 1674
  treatment, 1674
Olecranon process, 684, 684f
Olecranon stress fracture, 764–765, 764f–765f
On-field emergencies, 150–155
  anaphylaxis, 153
  anterior shoulder instability, 454–455
  cardiac arrest, 153
  cervical spine injuries, 152–153, 1578
  for collapsed athlete, 151–152, 151t
  emergency action plan, 150, 151b
  environmental factors, 154
  head injury, 152
  limb-threatening injuries, 154
    acute compartment syndrome, 154
    knee dislocation, 154
    traumatic amputation, 154
  tension pneumothorax, 153
Open biceps tenodesis, 532
Open inferior capsular shift, 480–481, 480f
Open kinetic chain, 1195–1196, 1196f
Operating room set-up, in hip arthroscopy, 948–950
Opioids, perioperative pharmacology, 337
Oral hypoglycemic agents (OHAs), 220
Orbital fractures, 268, 268f
Orthobiologics, 50–61
  platelet-rich plasma
    in cartilage restoration, 55
    composition, 50–53, 52f, 52t
    definitions, 50
    growth factors, 51, 53t
    ligament-related disorders/repair, 53–55
    in meniscal repair, 55–56
    for muscle injuries, 56
    preparation, 50–53, 52f, 52t
    properties of, 50
    sports medicine and, 50–53, 51f
    tendon-related disorders/repair, 53–55
  stem cell-based therapy
    application, 58
    in cartilage repair, 59–60
    definitions, 56–58, 57f–58f
    in meniscal repair, 60
    preparations, 56–58, 57f–58f
    in sports medicine, 56–58, 57f
Orthopaedic injuries, in female athlete, 304–314
  acetabular labral injuries, 313
  ankle, 305–306

Orthopaedic injuries, in female athlete (Continued)
  anterior cruciate ligament
    injuries, 307, 308t–309t, 309f
    reconstruction, 310
  epidemiology, 304–305
  femoroacetabular impingement, 313
  foot, 305–306, 305t, 306f
  frozen shoulder/adhesive capsulitis, 310–312, 311t
  idiopathic scoliosis, 313–314
  noncontact anterior cruciate ligament injury, 307–309, 308f, 310f
  patellofemoral pain syndrome, 306–307, 306t
  shoulder instability, 312–313, 312f
  stress fractures, 314
Orthopaedic surgeries, 327
Orthoses, foot, 1436–1439
  clinical application, 1437–1439, 1438t–1439t, 1440f
  research in, 1436–1437, 1437f
Orthotics, 372–374, 1739
  foot evaluation, 372
  materials, 373, 373f
  overuse issues, 373–374
  types, 373, 373f
OSA. See Obstructive sleep apnea
Osgood-Schlatter disease, 1717–1718, 1717f
Osseous, 680, 681f
  knee, 1063–1065, 1064f, 1116–1118, 1118f–1119f
    femur, 1064–1065, 1065f
    patella, 1065, 1065f–1066f
    tibia, 1065
  outlet, 415–417, 416f–418f, 417b
    imaging, 414–415, 414f
Ossification
  appositional, 14
  heterotopic, 317, 319, 718
Ossified posterior longitudinal ligament (OPLL), 1597, 1597f
Osteitis pubis, 1007, 1014–1016
  complications, 1016
  nonoperative management, 1014–1015
  operative management, 1015–1016
  treatment, 1016b
Osteoarthritis
  lateral compartment, 1284, 1284f
  medial collateral, 1284b
  medial compartment, 1283, 1283t
    arthroplasty for, 1283
    osteotomy for, 1281, 1281f
  primary, 592
  tricompartmental, arthroplasty for, 1283
Osteoarticular stability, elbow, 683–684, 683f–684f
Osteoblasts, 13
Osteochondral allografts, 1488–1489
  transplantation, 1166, 1173f–1174f, 1176
Osteochondral autografts, 1488–1489
  transfer, 1165, 1167b–1173b, 1169f–1171f, 1175
Osteochondral lesions (OCLs)
  distal tibial plafond, 1500–1501, 1500f–1501f
  first metatarsal, 1501, 1502f
  imaging, 1388–1389, 1389f
  talus, 1484–1500, 1734–1737
    decision-making principles, 1486, 1486f–1487f
    diagnosis, 1484–1486
    history, 1484
    imaging, 1484–1486, 1485f
    physical examination, 1484
    postoperative management, 1500
    results, 1490–1493, 1490b

Osteochondral lesions (OCLs) (Continued)
    return to play, 1500
    treatment options, 1486–1490
Osteochondral repair, implants for, 42–45
Osteochondritis dissecans (OCD), 1668–1670
  complications, 1670
  débridement, 714b–715b, 714f
  decision-making principles, 1669, 1669t
  history, 1668
  imaging, 1668–1669, 1669f
  knee, 1614f–1615f
  lesions, 1164
  pediatrics, 1712–1717
    complications, 1716–1717
    decision-making principles, 1714–1715
    etiology, 1712
    future considerations, 1717
    history, 1712, 1713f
    physical examination, 1712, 1713f
    radiographs, 1713–1714, 1713f–1714f
    results, 1715–1716
    treatment options, 1715, 1716b, 1716f
  physical examination, 1668
  results, 1670
  suture fixation, 715b–716b
  treatment, 1669–1670
Osteochondrosis, 1668–1670
  complications, 1670
  decision-making principles, 1669, 1669t
  in foot, 1737–1739, 1738f–1739f
  history, 1668
  imaging, 1668–1669, 1669f
  knee, 1717–1718, 1717f–1718f
  olecranon, 1673–1674, 1673f
    complications, 1674
    decision-making principles, 1674
    history, 1674
    imaging, 1674
    physical examination, 1674
    results, 1674
    treatment, 1674
  physical examination, 1668
  results, 1670
  superior pole, 1718
  treatment, 1669–1670
Osteoclasts, 13
Osteocytes, 13
Osteology, 1661, 1662f
Osteonecrosis, 595, 595f, 595t
Osteopenia, 299–301, 300f, 300t
Osteoperiosteal bone graft, 1489
Osteoporosis, 299–301, 300f, 300t
Osteotomy, 1524–1525
  distal femoral, 1282
  femoral, 1301
  high tibial
    for chronic PCL injuries, 1219–1220
    lateral closing wedge, 1281, 1282t
    medial opening wedge, 1281, 1282t, 1285b–1288b, 1285f–1288f
    patient satisfaction after, 1283
  hip arthritis, 1058
  knee arthritis, 1281–1283, 1281b
  lateral compartment osteoarthritis, 1282
  medial displacement calcaneal, for posterior tibial tendon injury, 1467b–1468b
  proximal tibial, 1255, 1255f, 1259b, 1259f, 1282
  return to sport after, 1283
  tibial tuberosity, 1300–1301, 1305b
Outsole, 1440
Overt diabetes, 218
Overuse injuries, pediatrics, 1655–1659
Oxidative system, 66

P
PAES. See Popliteal artery entrapment syndrome
Paget-Schroetter syndrome, 633
Pain
  back, 128, 1598
  chronic, 580, 580b
  combined with instability
    arthroplasty for, 1283
    osteotomy for, 1282–1283
  leg, 1393–1401, 1394t
    anatomy, 1393–1394, 1394f, 1394t
    classification, 1394–1395
    compartment testing, 1397–1398, 1397t
    complications, 1400
    decision-making principles, 1396–1397, 1396t–1397t
    diagnostics/imaging, 1395–1396, 1396f
    epidemiology, 1393
    history, 1395
    pathophysiology, 1394
    physical examination, 1395
    postoperative care, 1398
    results, 1400
    return to play, 1400
    treatment options, 1398
  localization, 580, 580b
  modulation, 357, 357t
  night, 580, 580b
  patellofemoral, 371, 1308–1317
    anatomy, 1308–1309, 1309f
    diagnostic studies, 1313–1314, 1314f–1315f
    differential diagnosis, 1310t
    history, 1309–1310
    inspection, 1310–1311, 1311f–1312f
    palpation, 1311
    patient evaluation, 1309–1314
    physical examination, 1310–1311
    provocative tests, 1312–1313, 1312f–1313f
    range of motion and strength in, 1311–1312
    specific conditions, 1314–1316
      complex regional pain syndrome, 1316
      idiopathic anterior knee pain/ patellofemoral pain syndrome, 1314–1315
      intraosseous hypertension of patella, 1316
      lateral patella compression syndrome and, 1316
      synovial impingement syndromes, 1315–1316, 1316f
  posterior heel, 1504–1508, 1505f
    complications, 1508
    decision-making principles, 1505–1506
    future considerations, 1508
    history, 1504
    imaging, 1504–1505, 1505f–1506f
    physical examination, 1504, 1505f
    postoperative management, 1508
    results, 1508
    treatment options, 1506–1507
  posterior hip, 1018–1033
    deep gluteal syndrome in, 1020–1024
    operative treatment, 1027–1030
    physical examination, 1024–1026, 1024f–1026f
    preoperative and postoperative rehabilitation, 1027–1030, 1027f–1028f
    pudendal nerve entrapment in, 1030–1032, 1031f–1032f, 1031t
    sciatic nerve
      characteristics, 1018–1020, 1019f–1020f
      entrapment, 1020–1024
    superior and inferior gluteal nerves in, 1032–1033, 1032f, 1032t
  scapulothoracic disorders, 614–615
  stiff shoulder, 579–581, 580b

Pain (Continued)
  treatments, 357–360
    cryotherapy, 358–359
    edema/inflammation, 359
    electrical stimulation, 359
    manual therapy, 357, 358t
    transcutaneous electrical nerve stimulation, 359
    ultrasound, 359–360
Palpation
  elbow, 689–690
  knee, 1092–1094, 1093f
  patellofemoral pain, 1311
  scapulothoracic disorders, 612–613
  stiff shoulder, 583–584
Palsy. See also Cerebral palsy
  axillary nerve, 629–630
    anatomy, 629
    biomechanics, 629
    clinical evaluation, 629–630
    decision-making principles, 630
    diagnostic studies, 630
    results, 630
  long thoracic nerve, 625–627
    anatomy, 625, 625f
    biomechanics, 625, 625f
    clinical evaluation, 625–627, 626f
    decision-making principles, 627
    diagnostic studies, 627
    results, 627
    technique, 627b
  spinal accessory nerve, 627–629
    anatomy, 627–628
    biomechanics, 627–628
    clinical evaluation, 628–629, 628f
    decision-making principles, 629
    diagnostic studies, 629
    results, 629
    technique, 629b
  suprascapular nerve, 621–625
    anatomy, 621–622, 622f
    biomechanics, 621–622, 622f
    clinical evaluation, 622–623, 623f
    decision-making principles, 624
    diagnostic studies, 623–624, 623f
    results, 624–625
Pancreatic hormones, 69t, 71
Panner disease, 1668–1670
  complications, 1670
  decision-making principles, 1669, 1669t
  history, 1668
  imaging, 1668–1669, 1669f
  physical examination, 1668
  results, 1670
  treatment, 1669–1670
Para-athlete, 315–324
  amputee athlete, 316–317
    adaptive sports equipment, 317
    exercise physiology, 316
    medical considerations, 316–317, 316t
  cerebral palsy, 320–321
    adaptive equipment, 321
    exercise, 320–321, 320b
    medical considerations, 321
  classification, 315
  intellectually disabled athlete, 321–323
    adaptive equipment, 323
    exercise physiology, 322
    medical considerations, 322–323
  Les Autres group, 323
  visually impaired athletes, 323
  wheelchair athlete, 317–320
    adaptive equipment, 320
    exercise, 317–318
    medical considerations, 318–320

Parasitic infections, 252–253
  cutaneous larva migrans, 253, 253f
  pediculosis capitis, 252–253
  scabies, 253, 253f
Paratenon, 2, 3f
Paratenonitis, 1320–1321
Paresthesias, 688
Pars stress fractures, 136–137, 138f
Parsonage-Turner syndrome, 339–340
Partial anterior cruciate ligament tears, 1189
Particulated juvenile cartilage allograft, 1165–1166, 1172f, 1176, 1489, 1490f
Patella, 1095–1096, 1095f–1096f, 1318–1319
  anatomy, 1065, 1065f–1066f
  fractures
    decision-making principles, 1327
  fractures of, 1322, 1322b
    clinical outcomes, 1332–1333
    complications, 1333
    history, 1323
    imaging, 1326, 1326f
    nonoperative treatment, 1327–1328, 1328f
    operative treatment, 1329–1330
    physical examination, 1324
    postoperative management, 1331
  instability, 1293–1307, 1708–1712
    complications, 1304–1306, 1304b, 1304f
    decision-making principles, 1299–1301, 1709
    embryology, 1708, 1708f
    episode of
      acute, 1295–1296, 1299–1300
      subacute, first-time, 1300–1301
      subacute, recurrent, 1300–1301
    examination overview for, 1295–1297
    future considerations, 1306, 1712
    history, 1293, 1294f, 1708–1709
    imaging, 1297–1299, 1298f–1299f, 1709, 1709f
    pathoanatomy, 1708
    physical examination, 1294–1295, 1708–1709
    postoperative management, 1304–1306, 1711
    prone examination of, 1297
    results, 1304, 1306, 1711–1712
    risk factors for, 1708
    sitting examination, 1296, 1296f
    static standing and gait examination of, 1296
    supine examination of, 1296–1297, 1297f
    treatment options, 1299–1301, 1709–1711, 1710f
  intraosseous hypertension of, 1316
  rupture, 1321–1322
    clinical outcomes, 1332
    complications, 1333
    decision-making principles, 1327
    history, 1323
    imaging, 1325–1326, 1325f–1326f
    nonoperative treatment, 1327
    operative treatment, 1328–1329, 1329f
    physical examination, 1324, 1324f
    postoperative management, 1330–1331
  structure of, 1320, 1320f–1321f
  tendinopathy, 1320–1321
    clinical outcomes, 1331–1332, 1332f
    complications, 1333
    history, 1322–1323
    imaging, 1324–1325, 1324f–1325f
    physical examination, 1323–1324, 1323t
    postoperative management, 1330
Patellar apprehension test, 1297
Patellar ballottement test, 1277
Patellar glide test, 1296–1297, 1297f
Patellar tilt test, 1296, 1297f
Patellofemoral joint
  biomechanics, 1082–1087
  contact area, 1082–1084, 1083f
  force transmission, 1084–1087, 1084f–1086f

Patellofemoral pain, 370–371, 1308–1317
  anatomy, 1308–1309, 1309f
  diagnostic studies, 1313–1314, 1314f–1315f
  differential diagnosis, 1310t
  history, 1309–1310
  inspection, 1310–1311, 1311f–1312f
  palpation, 1311
  patient evaluation, 1309–1314
  physical examination, 1310–1311
  provocative tests, 1312–1313, 1312f–1313f
  range of motion and strength in, 1311–1312
  specific conditions, 1314–1316
    complex regional pain syndrome, 1316
    idiopathic anterior knee pain/patellofemoral pain syndrome, 1314–1315
    intraosseous hypertension of patella, 1316
    lateral patella compression syndrome and, 1316
    synovial impingement syndromes, 1315–1316, 1316f
  taping, 370, 370f
Patellofemoral pain syndrome (PFPS), 306–307, 306t, 1314–1315
Pathologic bone, 12, 12f
Pathologic lesions, 1691
Pathologies
  adductor, 1007–1017
  ankle, 1370–1379
  elbow, 687
  foot, 1370–1379
  hip dysplasia and instability, 971–973, 972f–973f
  iliopsoas, 979–989
  leg, 1370–1379
  proximal biceps tendon, 526–539
  scapulothoracic disorders, 615
Patient, satisfaction of, after high tibial osteotomy, 1283
Patient history. See History of patient
Patrick test, 932
Patterned electrical nerve stimulation, 366, 366f
Pectineus, 919
Pectoralis major muscle, injuries to, 574–576
  anatomy, 574
  classification, 574–575
  imaging, 575
  mechanisms of, 574
  physical examination, 575
  treatment, 575–576, 576f
Pediatrics, 1606–1614
  ankle injuries, 1633–1635, 1725–1740
    acute, 1633, 1634f
    fractures, 1729–1733, 1729f, 1732f–1734f, 1732t
    normal anatomy, 1725–1728
    orthotics and, 1739
    overuse, 1633–1635, 1634f
    shoes and, 1739
    soft tissue injuries of, 1728–1729, 1728f
    systemic illness and, 1739
  arthroscopy, 1612–1614, 1612f–1615f
  baseball injuries, 115
  concussion, 1741–1747
    biomechanics, 1741, 1742f
    complications, 1746–1747, 1747t
    decision-making principles, 1745
    epidemiology, 1741–1743
    future considerations, 1747
    history, 1743, 1743t
    imaging, 1744–1745, 1745b
    pathophysiology, 1741, 1742f
    physical examination, 1743–1744
    return to play, 1746, 1746t
    treatment options, 1745–1746
  elbow injuries, 1619–1623, 1661–1676
    acute, 1619, 1621f
    anatomy, 1661–1665

Pediatrics (Continued)
  biomechanics, 1661–1665
  development, 1619
  lateral epicondylitis, 1674–1676
  ligaments, 1661–1662, 1662f–1663f
  Little League, 1621–1623, 1622f–1623f,
    1665–1668
  medial collateral ligament injury, 1672–1673
  medial epicondyle avulsion fractures,
    1670–1672
  medial epicondylitis, 1674–1676
  osteochondritis dissecans, 1668–1670
  osteology, 1661, 1662f
  overuse, 1619–1623
  Panner disease, 1668–1670
  pathologies, 1665–1676
  soft-tissue, 1661–1662, 1662f–1663f
  epidemiology, 1606–1607
  exercise, 1607–1609
  foot injuries, 1633–1635, 1725–1740
    acute, 1633, 1634f
    fractures, 1733–1739, 1735f–1737f
    orthotics and, 1739
    overuse, 1633–1635, 1634f
    shoes and, 1739
    soft tissue injuries of, 1728–1729, 1728f
    systemic illness and, 1739
  fractures
    avulsion, 1688, 1689f
    hip, 1690
    lesser tuberosity, 1647
    proximal humerus, 1644–1647
    stress, 1688–1690, 1690f
  head injuries, 1741–1748
  hip, 1625–1628
    conditions, 928
    injuries, 1688–1696
      acute, 1625–1626, 1626f
      overuse, 1626–1628, 1627f–1628f
  injury, 1606–1607
  knee injuries, 1628–1633, 1697–1724
    acute, 1628–1630, 1629f–1630f
    anterior cruciate ligament (ACL) injuries,
      1697–1703
    discoid meniscus, 1705–1708
    meniscal injuries, 1703–1705
    osteochondritis dissecans, 1712–1717
    osteochondroses, 1717–1718
    overuse, 1630–1633, 1631f–1633f
    patellar instability, 1708–1712
    physeal fractures, 1718–1721
  lower leg, 1633–1635
    acute injuries, 1633, 1634f
    overuse injuries, 1633–1635, 1634f
  nutrition, 1610–1611
  pathophysiology, 1616
  performance-enhancing substances, 1611
  shoulder, 1616–1618, 1637–1660
    acute injuries, 1617–1618, 1618f–1619f
    development, 1616–1617, 1617f
    overuse injuries, 1618, 1620f–1621f
  soccer injuries, 126
  spine issues in, 1635–1636, 1635f, 1749–1764
    apophyseal ring fractures, 1753
    atlantoaxial instability, 1758
    Down syndrome, atlantoaxial instability in,
      1758–1759
    rotatory atlantoaxial subluxation, 1759–1761
    sacral facet fractures, 1755
    scoliosis, 1755–1758
    spinal cord injury without radiographic
      abnormality (SCIWORA), 1763
    spondylolisthesis, 1750–1753
    spondylolysis, 1750–1753

Pediatrics (Continued)
  sports participation, 1606
  strength training in, 68
  wrist and hand injuries, 1623–1625, 1677–1687
    acute, 1623–1624, 1623f
    distal radial physeal stress reaction,
      1683–1684
    finger fractures, 1677–1681
      complications, 1680–1681
      decision-making principles, 1678
      future considerations, 1681
      history, 1677
      imaging, 1678, 1678f–1679f
      physical examination, 1677–1678, 1678f
      postoperative management, 1680
      results, 1680
      treatment options, 1678–1680, 1680f,
        1681b
    jammed finger, 1681–1683
      complications, 1683
      decision-making principles, 1682
      history, 1681
      imaging, 1682, 1682f
      physical examination, 1681–1682
      postoperative management, 1683
      results, 1683
      treatment options, 1682, 1682b
    overuse, 1624–1625, 1624f–1626f
    scaphoid fracture, 1684–1686
      complications, 1685
      decision-making principles, 1685
      future considerations, 1686
      history, 1684
      imaging, 1684–1685
      physical examination, 1684
      postoperative management, 1685
      results, 1685
      treatment options, 1685, 1685b, 1686f
Pediculosis capitis, 252–253
Pedowitz criteria, for chronic exertional
    compartment syndrome, 1396, 1396t–1397t
Pelvis injuries
  figure skating, 118
  gymnastics, 120–121
Performance, biomechanics for improving, 28
Performance-enhancing substances, 1611
Performance enhancing supplements (PES), 280,
    281t
Periacetabular osteotomy (PAO), 971
Perilunate dislocation, 809–810, 810f
Perilunate instability, 851–854, 851f–855f, 853b
Perimysium, 62, 63f
Periodontal/displacement injuries (loose teeth),
    270
Perioperative complications, with anesthesia,
    339–340
  allergic reactions, 339
  Parsonage-Turner syndrome, 339–340
Perioperative pain management, 335
Perioperative pharmacology, 335–339
  acetaminophen, 338
  buprenorphine, 337–338
  dexmedetomidine, 338–339
  ketamine, 338
  methadone, 337
  nonsteroidal antiinflammatory drugs, 338
  opioids, 337
  perioperative pain management, 335, 336t–337t
  propofol, 338
Periorbital lacerations, 263
Periosteum, 13–14
Peripheral compartment
  femoroacetabular impingement, 967, 968f
  hip arthroscopy, 954–955, 954f–955f

Peripheral nerve entrapment, 319, 1402–1420
  deep peroneal nerve, 1415–1416, 1415f
    history, 1415
    imaging, 1416
    physical examination, 1415–1416
    postoperative management, 1416
    results, 1416
    treatment options, 1416, 1416b
  interdigital neuralgia (Morton neuroma),
      1416–1419
    complications, 1418–1419
    decision-making principles, 1418
    etiologies of, 1417
    history, 1417
    imaging, 1417–1418
    pathomechanism of, 1417
    physical examination, 1417
    postoperative management, 1418
    results, 1418
    treatment options, 1418, 1419b, 1419f
  lateral plantar nerve, 1411–1412
    complications, 1412
    decision-making principles, 1411
    history, 1411
    imaging, 1411
    physical examination, 1411
    postoperative management, 1412
    results, 1412
    treatment options, 1411–1412, 1412b,
      1412f
  medial plantar nerve, 1412–1413
    decision-making principles, 1413
    history, 1412
    imaging, 1413
    physical examination, 1412
    postoperative management, 1413
    treatment options, 1413
  saphenous nerve, 1405–1407, 1405f–1406f
    history, 1405
    imaging, 1406
    physical examination, 1405–1406
    results, 1406–1407
    treatment options, 1406
  superficial peroneal nerve, 1413–1415, 1413f
    decision-making principles, 1414
    history, 1413
    imaging, 1414
    physical examination, 1413–1414
    postoperative management, 1415
    results, 1415
    treatment options, 1414–1415, 1414b, 1414f
  sural nerve, 1402–1405, 1403f
    history, 1402
    imaging, 1403–1404
    physical examination, 1402–1403
    postoperative management, 1405
    results, 1405
    treatment options, 1404, 1404b, 1404f
  tarsal tunnel syndrome, 1407–1411, 1407f
    decision-making principles, 1408
    electrodiagnostic studies, 1408
    etiologies of, 1407–1408, 1407t
    history, 1408
    imaging, 1408
    physical examination, 1408
    postoperative management, 1410
    results, 1410–1411
    treatment options, 1408–1409, 1409b–1410b,
      1409f–1410f
Peritenon, 2
Peritrochanteric disorders, 990–1006
  coxa saltans, 996–1001
  gluteus medius and minimus tears, 990–996
  ischiofemoral impingement, 1003–1006

Peritrochanteric disorders (Continued)
  piriformis syndrome, 1002–1003
  trochanteric bursitis, 1001–1002
Peroneal nerve entrapment
  deep, 1415–1416, 1415f
    history, 1415
    imaging, 1416
    physical examination, 1415–1416
    postoperative management, 1416
    results, 1416
    treatment options, 1416, 1416b
  superficial, 1413–1415, 1413f
    decision-making principles, 1414
    history, 1413
    imaging, 1414
    physical examination, 1413–1414
    postoperative management, 1415
    results, 1415
    treatment options, 1414–1415, 1414b, 1414f
Peroneal tendons, 1385–1386, 1385f–1386f
  injuries, 1472–1476
    complications, 1476
    decision-making principles, 1473–1474
    future considerations, 1476
    history, 1472
    imaging, 1473, 1473f
    physical examination, 1472–1473, 1472f
    postoperative management, 1475
    results, 1475–1476
    treatment options, 1474–1475, 1474f–1475f, 1475b
Pertinent bony shoulder, 393–395, 394f
PET/CT scans. See Positron emission tomography/computed tomography scans
PFPS. See Patellofemoral pain syndrome
Phalangeal fractures, 890–892, 891f–893f
Phonophoresis, 360
Phosphagen energy system, 65
Physeal fractures, 1718–1721
  complications, 1720–1721
  decision-making principles, 1719–1720
  history, 1719
  imaging, 1719, 1720f–1721f
  lesser tuberosity fractures, 1647
    complications, 1647
    history, 1647
    imaging, 1647
    physical examination, 1647
    treatment options, 1647, 1647f
  physical examination, 1719
  proximal humerus fractures, 1644–1647, 1644f–1645f
    complications, 1647
    history, 1644
    imaging, 1644–1645, 1645f–1646f
    physical examination, 1644
    treatment, 1645–1646, 1646f
  treatment options, 1719–1720, 1722f–1723f
Physical examination
  Achilles tendon injuries, 1477, 1477f
  acromioclavicular joint, 648–651, 650t, 651f
  for adductor strains, 1050
  AIN syndrome, 746
  ankle, 1372–1379, 1373f–1378f
  anterior cruciate ligament injuries, 1187–1188
  anterior shoulder instability, 447–448, 448f–449f
  articular cartilage lesions, 1163
  athletic pubalgia, 1009, 1009f
  brain injury, 1564–1566
  calcaneoplasty, 1433
  cervical spine
    injuries, 1578
    unstable fractures and dislocations of, 1541
  concussion, 1564–1566
  cubital tunnel syndrome, 749

Physical examination (Continued)
  digits, 801
  distal biceps, 725, 725f, 733, 733f
  distal triceps, 738
  elbow, 689–691
    inspection, 689
    joint stability, 694–695
    maneuvers, 695
    motion, loss, 773–774
    neurologic assessment, 690–691, 691f
    palpation, 689–690
    throwing injuries, 758–760, 759f–760f
  endoscopic Haglund resection, 1433
  exertional compartment syndromes, 1395
  extensor mechanism injuries, 1323–1324
  external coxa saltans, 999, 999f
  femoroacetabular impingement, 959–960, 959t, 960f
  flexor hallucis longus injuries, 1469
  foot, 1372–1379, 1373f–1378f
  glenohumeral arthritis, 595–596
    arthroscopic images, 596
    history, 595
    imaging, 596, 597f–598f
    presentation, 595
    prior operative notes, 596
  gluteus medius and minimus tears, 990
  of hallux rigidus, 1523, 1523f
  hamstring injuries, 1035–1036
  hand, 793–794, 794f
  head injuries, 1539
  hip, 929–933
    arthritis, 1053–1055
    dysplasia and instability, 973–974
    inspection, 929
    ligamentous laxity, evaluation, 932
    measurements in, 930–931
    range of motion, 930–931, 931t
    special maneuvers, 932–933
    symptom localization, 929–930, 930f–931f
  iliac crest contusion, 1043
  iliopsoas, 982–983
  interdigital neuralgia, 1417
  internal coxa saltans, 996, 997f
  ischiofemoral impingement, 1004
  knee, 1091
    arthroscopic synovectomy of, 1127
    dislocation, 1347–1348, 1347f
    lateral and posterolateral corner injuries, 1249–1251, 1249f–1250f
    loss of motion, 1336, 1336f
    popliteal artery entrapment syndrome in, 1351–1352
  lateral epicondylitis, 720–725
  latissimus dorsi muscle, 576, 577f
  leg, 1372–1379, 1373f–1378f
    pain, 1395
  medial collateral ligament and posterior medial corner injuries, 1231–1232, 1233f, 1233t
  medial epicondylitis, 720
  meniscal injuries, 1137–1138
  metatarsalgia, 1519–1520
  Morton neuroma, 1417
  multidirectional instability, 477–479, 477t–478t, 478f
  multiligament knee injuries, 1264–1265
  nerve entrapment
    deep peroneal, 1415–1416
    lateral plantar, 1411
    medial plantar, 1412
    of saphenous, 1405–1406
    superficial peroneal, 1413–1414
    sural, 1402–1403
  olecranon bursitis, 728
  osteochondral lesions, 1484

Physical examination (Continued)
  patella
    instability, 1294–1295
      pertinent bony anatomy, 1294, 1294f
      pertinent soft tissue anatomy, 1294–1295, 1295f
    tendinopathy, 1323–1324, 1323t
    tendon ruptures, 1324, 1324f
  patellofemoral pain, 1310–1311
  pectoralis major muscle, 575
  pediatrics, 1052
    anterior cruciate ligament (ACL) injuries, 1697
    apophyseal ring fractures, 1753
    atraumatic instability, 1654–1655, 1654f
    cervical spine, congenital anomalies of, 1762
    concussion, 1743–1744
    discoid meniscus, 1706
    distal radial physeal stress reaction, 1683
    Down syndrome, atlantoaxial instability in, 1758
    finger fractures, 1677–1678, 1678f
    jammed finger, 1681–1682
    lateral clavicle physeal fractures, 1640–1641
    lateral epicondylitis, 1675
    lesser tuberosity fractures, 1647
    Little League elbow, 1666–1667
    medial clavicle physeal fractures, 1643
    medial collateral ligament injury, 1672
    medial epicondyle avulsion fractures, 1671, 1671f
    medial epicondylitis, 1675
    meniscal injuries, 1703
    odontoid fractures, 1761
    osteochondritis dissecans, 1668, 1712, 1713f
    osteochondrosis, 1668
    Panner disease, 1668
    patellar instability, 1708–1709
    physeal fractures, 1719
    posterior elbow pathologic conditions, 1674
    proximal humerus epiphysiolysis, 1656
    proximal humerus fractures, 1644
    rotatory atlantoaxial subluxation, 1759
    scaphoid fracture, 1684
    scoliosis, 1755–1757
    spinal cord injury without radiographic abnormality, 1763
    spine, 1749–1750, 1751b
    spondylolisthesis, 1751–1752
    spondylolysis, 1751–1752
    traumatic anterior instability, 1648, 1649f
    traumatic posterior instability, 1652, 1652f
  peroneal tendon injuries, 1472–1473, 1472f
  PIN syndrome, 755
  piriformis syndrome, 1002–1003
  plantar fasciitis, 1509
  posterior cruciate ligament injuries, 1212–1214
    collateral ligament assessment, 1213–1214
    external rotation of tibia (Dial test) in, 1213
    gait and limb alignment in, 1214
    posterior drawer test, 1212, 1213f
    posterior sag test (Godfrey test) in, 1212–1213, 1213f
    quadriceps active test, 1212–1213
    reverse pivot-shift test, 1213
  posterior heel pain, 1504, 1505f
  posterior hip pain, 1024–1026, 1024f–1026f
  posterior shoulder instability, 465–467, 466f, 466t
  preparticipation, 144–150
    allergies, 149
    athletes with special needs, 150
    cardiovascular system, 145–147, 145b–146b
    dermatology, 149
    ears, 145
    endocrine system, 149

Physical examination (Continued)
eyes, 145
gastrointestinal system, 148
genitourinary system, 148
goals, 144
head, 145
heat illness, 149–150
hematologic disease, 148–149
history, 145–150
immunizations, 149
infectious disease, 148–149
medications, 149
musculoskeletal system, 148, 148b
neurologic system, 148
nose, 145
objectives, 144
organization, 144–145
physical examination, 145–150
pulmonary system, 147–148
setting, 144–145, 145t
throat, 145
timing, 144–145
pronator syndrome, 745
quadriceps contusion, 1045
quadriceps strains, 1048
radial tunnel syndrome, 754
revision anterior cruciate ligament injuries, 1200
revision rotator cuff repair, 568
revision shoulder instability, 489–490, 490f
rotator cuff and impingement lesions, 543–547, 544f–546f
scapulothoracic disorders, 611–614
inspection, 611–612
palpation, 612–613
range of motion, 613
strength, 613
testing, 613–614
sesamoid dysfunction, 1517
soft tissue, ankle arthroscopy, 1423
sprains
ankle, 1444–1446, 1446f, 1446t, 1450–1451
bifurcate ligament, 1457
Lisfranc, 1458
syndesmosis, 1453–1454
sternoclavicular joint, 664–677
stingers, 1570–1571, 1571f–1572f, 1572t
subscapularis injury, 558–559, 558f
subtalar arthroscopy, 1429
superior labrum anterior to posterior (SLAP) tears, 502–503, 504t
tarsal tunnel syndrome, 1408
thoracic outlet syndrome, 636–638, 637f–638f
thoracolumbar spine injuries, 1582–1583
thrower's shoulder, 514–515
triceps tendinitis, 725, 725f
trochanteric bursitis, 1002
turf toe, 1515
wrist, 793–794, 794f
tendinopathies, 858
Physical therapy, for knee arthritis, 1280
Pia mater, 1528
Pill esophagitis, 192
PIN syndrome. See Posterior interosseous nerve (PIN) syndrome
Pincer impingement, 927–928, 957–958, 958f, 967
Piriformis syndrome, 1002–1003, 1003b
Pisiform carpal injuries, 847–848, 847f, 848b
Pitted keratolysis, 248, 248f
Pituitary hormones, 69–70, 69t
Pityrosporum folliculitis, 251f
Plain radiography
femoroacetabular impingement, 960–963, 961f–963f

Plain radiography (Continued)
interpretation, 936–938
acetabular cup depth, 938
acetabular inclination, 938
acetabular version, 938
alpha angle, 938
anterior center edge angles, 937–938
functional leg lengths, 936
head-neck offset, 938
head sphericity, 938
hip center position, 938
joint space width, 938
lateral center edge angles, 937
neck shaft angle, 936–937
trabecular pattern, 937
rotator cuff and impingement lesions, 547
Planar imaging, 88, 89f
Plantar fascia, 368–369
Plantar fasciitis, 371, 1391, 1391f, 1509–1513
complications, 1513
decision-making principles, 1510
future considerations, 1513
history, 1509
imaging, 1509, 1509f
physical examination, 1509
postoperative management, 1511
results, 1511–1513
treatment options, 1510–1511, 1510f, 1511b, 1512f
Plantar fasciosis, 371
Plantar midfoot ecchymosis, 1373, 1373f
Plantar nerve entrapment
lateral, 1411–1412
complications, 1412
decision-making principles, 1411
history, 1411
imaging, 1411
physical examination, 1411
postoperative management, 1412
results, 1412
treatment options, 1411–1412, 1412b, 1412f
medial, 1412–1413
decision-making principles, 1413
history, 1412
imaging, 1413
physical examination, 1412
postoperative management, 1413
treatment options, 1413
Platelet-rich plasma, 1148–1149
in cartilage restoration, 55
composition, 50–53, 52f, 52t
definitions, 50
growth factors, 51, 53t
for knee arthritis, 1280
ligament-related disorders/repair, 53–55
in meniscal repair, 55–56
for muscle injuries, 56
preparation, 50–53, 52f, 52t
properties of, 50
sports medicine and, 50–53, 51f
tendon and ligament-related disorders/repair, 53–55
Achilles tendon repair, 54
anterior cruciate ligament surgery and, 54–55
ligament injuries, 53–54
rotator cuff repair, 54
tendon injuries, 53–54
Pneumonia, acute, 209–210
Pneumothorax, tension, 153
Polyetheretherketone (PEEK), as suture anchors, 47
Polymethylmethacrylate (PMMA), for bone fixation, 39

Polytetrafluoroethylene (PTFE), for ACL reconstruction, 39
Popliteal artery entrapment syndrome (PAES), 1349–1356
classification, 1350–1351, 1350f
clinical presentation, 1351
complications, 1356
criteria for return to play, 1356
history, 1350
imaging, 1352–1354, 1352f–1353f
angiography, 1353–1354, 1354f
computed tomography and computed tomographic angiography, 1353, 1353f
duplex ultrasonography, 1352, 1352f
magnetic resonance angiography, 1352–1353, 1353f
magnetic resonance imaging, 1352–1353, 1353f
physical examination and testing of, 1351–1352
postoperative management, 1356
treatment options, 1354–1356, 1355f, 1356b
Popliteal artery repair, in knee dislocation, 1349b
Popliteus tendon complex, 1245
Portal placement
arthroscopic, 110
elbow arthroscopy, 709–711, 709t
accessory portal, 711
order of, 712
posterior radiocapitellar portal, 711
proximal anterolateral portal, 711
proximal anteromedial portal, 710–711
proximal posterolateral portal, 711
standard anterolateral portal, 711
standard anteromedial portal, 709, 710f
straight posterior portal, 711
hip arthroscopy, 950–952
anterolateral, 950–951, 950f
distal anterolateral accessory, 951, 951f
modified mid-anterior, 951, 951f
posterolateral, 951–952
knee arthroscopy, 1121–1123, 1122f–1124f
shoulder arthroscopy, 435–436, 436f
wrist arthroscopy, 817–819, 818f–819f
Position/positioning
arthroscopic synovectomy, of knee, 1129
during arthroscopy, 109–110, 109f–110f
beach chair, 329
elbow arthroscopy, 708, 708f
hip arthroscopy, 948–950
hip center, 938
knee arthroscopy, 1121, 1122f
shoulder arthroscopy, 434–435, 434f
Positron emission tomography/computed tomography scans, 90, 93f
Postclosure wound care, for face facial injuries, 261–262
Postconcussion syndrome (PCS), 1540–1541, 1746, 1747t
Posterior apprehension test, 404–405, 932
Posterior compartment release, 1399, 1399f
Posterior compartments, in arthroscopic synovectomy, of knee, 1129–1130
Posterior cruciate ligament
injuries, 1211–1230, 1220b–1222b, 1221f–1223f
complications in, 1229
decision-making, 1214–1216
future considerations, 1229
history, 1211–1212
imaging, 1214
bone scan and, 1214
magnetic resonance imaging, 1214
radiography, 1214
isolated, 1224–1225, 1227t

Posterior cruciate ligament *(Continued)*
nonoperative treatment, 1216
decision-making, 1215–1216
operative treatment, 1216–1217
results, 1224–1229
physical examination, 1212–1214
collateral ligament assessment, 1213–1214
external rotation of tibia (Dial test) in, 1213
gait and limb alignment in, 1214
posterior drawer test, 1212, 1213*f*
posterior sag test (Godfrey test) in, 1212–1213, 1213*f*
quadriceps active test, 1212–1213
reverse pivot-shift test, 1213
postoperative management, 1224, 1224*b*
treatment options, 1216–1220, 1216*f*–1217*f*
graft choice and fixation, 1219
high tibial osteotomy in, 1219–1220
single-bundle *vs.* double-bundle reconstruction, 1218–1219, 1218*f*, 1225–1229
transtibial tunnel *vs.* tibial inlay techniques, 1217–1218, 1225, 1228*t*
knee, 1069, 1070*f*
MRI, 1112
multiligament knee injuries, 1268
Posterior drawer test, for posterior cruciate ligament injuries, 1212, 1213*f*
Posterior elbow pathologic conditions, 1673–1674, 1673*f*
complications, 1674
decision-making principles, 1674
history, 1674
imaging, 1674
physical examination, 1674
results, 1674
treatment, 1674
Posterior heel pain, 1504–1508, 1505*f*
complications, 1508
decision-making principles, 1505–1506
future considerations, 1508
history, 1504
imaging, 1504–1505, 1505*f*–1506*f*
physical examination, 1504, 1505*f*
postoperative management, 1508
results, 1508
treatment options, 1506–1507
nonoperative therapy, 1506–1507
operative therapy, 1507
technique, 1507*b*, 1507*f*
Posterior hindfoot arthroscopy, 1470*b*, 1471*f*
Posterior hip pain, 1018–1033
deep gluteal syndrome in, 1020–1024
operative treatment, 1027–1030
endoscopic decompression in, 1027–1030, 1028*t*–1029*t*, 1029*f*–1030*f*
physical examination, 1024–1026, 1024*f*–1026*f*
preoperative and postoperative rehabilitation, 1027–1030, 1027*f*–1028*f*
pudendal nerve entrapment in, 1030–1032, 1031*f*–1032*f*, 1031*t*
sciatic nerve
characteristics, 1018–1020, 1019*f*–1020*f*
entrapment, 1020–1024
superior and inferior gluteal nerves in, 1032–1033, 1032*f*, 1032*t*
Posterior impingement, 431, 1426*b*, 1426*f*
Posterior interosseous nerve (PIN) syndrome, 687–688, 693, 755–756
complications, 756
decision-making principles, 755
history, 755
postoperative management, 755
results, 755–756
return-to-play guidelines, 755

Posterior interosseous nerve (PIN) syndrome *(Continued)*
technique, 755
treatment, 755
Posterior medial corner injuries, 1231–1243
complications in, 1242
decision-making principles, 1234–1235, 1235*f*
future considerations, 1243
history, 1231
imaging, 1232–1234, 1233*f*–1235*f*
physical exam, 1231–1232
postoperative management, 1239–1240
results, 1240–1242
return-to-play guidelines, 1240*b*
treatment options, 1235–1236
Posterior radiocapitellar portal, 711
Posterior sag test (Godfrey test), for posterior cruciate ligament injuries, 1212–1213, 1213*f*
Posterior shoulder instability, 463–475
arthroscopic posterior shoulder stabilization for, 470*b*–472*b*, 470*f*–472*f*
background, 463
complications, 474–475
decision-making principles and, 468
future considerations, 475
history, 465
imaging, 467–468, 467*f*–468*f*, 468*t*
pathogenesis of, 463–465, 464*f*–465*f*
physical examination, 465–467, 466*f*, 466*t*
postoperative management, 469–473
results, 473–474
treatment options, 468–469
contraindications, 469
indications, 469
Posterior tibia
tendon, 1383–1384, 1383*f*–1384*f*
tendon, injuries, 1464–1469
complications, 1469
decision-making principles, 1466
future considerations, 1469
history, 1465
imaging, 1465–1466, 1465*f*
physical examination, 1465, 1465*f*
postoperative management, 1468
results, 1468–1469
treatment options, 1466–1467, 1466*f*–1467*f*, 1467*b*–1468*b*
translation of, 1247–1248
Posterolateral corner injuries, 1244–1263
anatomy, 1244–1248
classification, 1248, 1248*t*
complications in, 1260–1261, 1262*f*
decision-making principles, 1253
future considerations, 1262
history, 1248–1249
imaging, 1251–1253
magnetic resonance imaging, 1251–1253, 1252*f*
radiographs, 1251, 1251*f*
ultrasound, 1253
layers of lateral side of, 1244
nonoperative management, 1253
grade I injuries, 1253
grade II injuries, 1253
grade III injuries, 1253
pediatric, 1262
physical examination, 1249–1251, 1249*f*–1250*f*
postoperative management, 1256–1260, 1259*t*
repair *vs.* reconstruction, 1253
results, 1260, 1260*t*–1261*t*
return to play, 1260
structures, 1244–1246, 1245*f*
anterior/posterior tibial translation, 1247–1248
arcuate ligament complex, 1246
biceps femoris muscle, 1245–1246

Posterolateral corner injuries *(Continued)*
biomechanics, 1246, 1247*f*
external rotation, 1247
fabellofibular ligament, 1246
fibular collateral ligament, 1244–1245
iliotibial band, 1244
lateral gastrocnemius tendon, 1246
mid-third lateral capsular ligament, 1246
neurovascular, 1246
popliteus tendon complex, 1245
varus motion, 1246–1247
surgical considerations, 1254–1256
diagnostic arthroscopy, 1254, 1254*f*
primary repair, 1254, 1254*f*
reconstruction techniques, 1254–1255
techniques, 1257*b*, 1257*f*–1258*f*
timing of diagnosis, 1253
treatment options, 1253–1256
Posterolateral corner sling procedure, 1255
Posterolateral drawer test, 1249, 1249*f*–1250*f*
Posterolateral portal, in hip arthroscopy, 951–952
Posteromedial impingement, 1673–1674, 1673*f*
complications, 1674
decision-making principles, 1674
history, 1674
imaging, 1674
physical examination, 1674
results, 1674
treatment, 1674
Postoperative rehabilitation, for posterior hip pain, 1027–1030, 1027*f*–1028*f*
Postural orthostatic tachycardia syndrome (POTS), 173
Power stroke, 63
Pre-event planning, in spine injuries, 1553–1554
Prediabetes, 218
Pregnancy, in female athlete, 301–302, 302*t*
Preoperative arthroscopy, 109
Preoperative imaging, 433–434
Preoperative rehabilitation, for posterior hip pain, 1027–1030, 1027*f*–1028*f*
Preparticipation physical evaluation, 144–150
allergies, 149
athletes with special needs, 150
cardiovascular system, 145–147, 145*b*–146*b*
dermatology, 149
ears, 145
endocrine system, 149
eyes, 145
gastrointestinal system, 148
genitourinary system, 148
goals, 144
head, 145
heat illness, 149–150
hematologic disease, 148–149
history, 145–150
immunizations, 149
infectious disease, 148–149
medical home, 159–160
medications, 149
musculoskeletal system, 148, 148*b*
neurologic system, 148
nose, 145
objectives, 144
organization, 144–145
physical examination, 145–150
pulmonary system, 147–148
setting, 144–145, 145*t*
throat, 145
timing, 144–145
Pressure sores, 319
Primary anterior cruciate ligament reconstruction, 1193*b*–1195*b*, 1193*f*–1195*f*
Primary osteoarthritis, 592
Primary *vs.* permanent teeth, 269, 270*f*
Probe, arthroscopic, 107

Physical examination (Continued)
  eyes, 145
  gastrointestinal system, 148
  genitourinary system, 148
  goals, 144
  head, 145
  heat illness, 149–150
  hematologic disease, 148–149
  history, 145–150
  immunizations, 149
  infectious disease, 148–149
  medications, 149
  musculoskeletal system, 148, 148b
  neurologic system, 148
  nose, 145
  objectives, 144
  organization, 144–145
  physical examination, 145–150
  pulmonary system, 147–148
  setting, 144–145, 145t
  throat, 145
  timing, 144–145
pronator syndrome, 745
quadriceps contusion, 1045
quadriceps strains, 1048
radial tunnel syndrome, 754
revision anterior cruciate ligament injuries, 1200
revision rotator cuff repair, 568
revision shoulder instability, 489–490, 490f
rotator cuff and impingement lesions, 543–547, 544f–546f
scapulothoracic disorders, 611–614
  inspection, 611–612
  palpation, 612–613
  range of motion, 613
  strength, 613
  testing, 613–614
sesamoid dysfunction, 1517
soft tissue, ankle arthroscopy, 1423
sprains
  ankle, 1444–1446, 1446f, 1446t, 1450–1451
  bifurcate ligament, 1457
  Lisfranc, 1458
  syndesmosis, 1453–1454
sternoclavicular joint, 664–677
stingers, 1570–1571, 1571f–1572f, 1572t
subscapularis injury, 558–559, 558f
subtalar arthroscopy, 1429
superior labrum anterior to posterior (SLAP) tears, 502–503, 504t
tarsal tunnel syndrome, 1408
thoracic outlet syndrome, 636–638, 637f–638f
thoracolumbar spine injuries, 1582–1583
thrower's shoulder, 514–515
triceps tendinitis, 725, 725f
trochanteric bursitis, 1002
turf toe, 1515
wrist, 793–794, 794f
  tendinopathies, 858
Physical therapy, for knee arthritis, 1280
Pia mater, 1528
Pill esophagitis, 192
PIN syndrome. See Posterior interosseous nerve (PIN) syndrome
Pincer impingement, 927–928, 957–958, 958f, 967
Piriformis syndrome, 1002–1003, 1003b
Pisiform carpal injuries, 847–848, 847f, 848b
Pitted keratolysis, 248, 248f
Pituitary hormones, 69–70, 69t
Pityrosporum folliculitis, 251f
Plain radiography
  femoroacetabular impingement, 960–963, 961f–963f

Plain radiography (Continued)
  interpretation, 936–938
    acetabular cup depth, 938
    acetabular inclination, 938
    acetabular version, 938
    alpha angle, 938
    anterior center edge angles, 937–938
    functional leg lengths, 936
    head-neck offset, 938
    head sphericity, 938
    hip center position, 938
    joint space width, 938
    lateral center edge angles, 937
    neck shaft angle, 936–937
    trabecular pattern, 937
  rotator cuff and impingement lesions, 547
Planar imaging, 88, 89f
Plantar fascia, 368–369
Plantar fasciitis, 371, 1391, 1391f, 1509–1513
  complications, 1513
  decision-making principles, 1510
  future considerations, 1513
  history, 1509
  imaging, 1509, 1509f
  physical examination, 1509
  postoperative management, 1511
  results, 1511–1513
  treatment options, 1510–1511, 1510f, 1511b, 1512f
Plantar fasciosis, 371
Plantar midfoot ecchymosis, 1373, 1373f
Plantar nerve entrapment
  lateral, 1411–1412
    complications, 1412
    decision-making principles, 1411
    history, 1411
    imaging, 1411
    physical examination, 1411
    postoperative management, 1412
    results, 1412
    treatment options, 1411–1412, 1412b, 1412f
  medial, 1412–1413
    decision-making principles, 1413
    history, 1412
    imaging, 1413
    physical examination, 1412
    postoperative management, 1413
    treatment options, 1413
Platelet-rich plasma, 1148–1149
  in cartilage restoration, 55
  composition, 50–53, 52f, 52t
  definitions, 50
  growth factors, 51, 53t
  for knee arthritis, 1280
  ligament-related disorders/repair, 53–55
  in meniscal repair, 55–56
  for muscle injuries, 56
  preparation, 50–53, 52f, 52t
  properties of, 50
  sports medicine and, 50–53, 51f
  tendon and ligament-related disorders/repair, 53–55
    Achilles tendon repair, 54
    anterior cruciate ligament surgery and, 54–55
    ligament injuries, 53–54
    rotator cuff repair, 54
    tendon injuries, 53–54
Pneumonia, acute, 209–210
Pneumothorax, tension, 153
Polyetheretherketone (PEEK), as suture anchors, 47
Polymethylmethacrylate (PMMA), for bone fixation, 39

Polytetrafluoroethylene (PTFE), for ACL reconstruction, 39
Popliteal artery entrapment syndrome (PAES), 1349–1356
  classification, 1350–1351, 1350f
  clinical presentation, 1351
  complications, 1356
  criteria for return to play, 1356
  history, 1350
  imaging, 1352–1354, 1352f–1353f
    angiography, 1353–1354, 1354f
    computed tomography and computed tomographic angiography, 1353, 1353f
    duplex ultrasonography, 1352, 1352f
    magnetic resonance angiography, 1352–1353, 1353f
    magnetic resonance imaging, 1352–1353, 1353f
  physical examination and testing of, 1351–1352
  postoperative management, 1356
  treatment options, 1354–1356, 1355f, 1356b
Popliteal artery repair, in knee dislocation, 1349b
Popliteus tendon complex, 1245
Portal placement
  arthroscopic, 110
  elbow arthroscopy, 709–711, 709t
    accessory portal, 711
    order of, 712
    posterior radiocapitellar portal, 711
    proximal anterolateral portal, 711
    proximal anteromedial portal, 710–711
    proximal posterolateral portal, 711
    standard anterolateral portal, 711
    standard anteromedial portal, 709, 710f
    straight posterior portal, 711
  hip arthroscopy, 950–952
    anterolateral, 950–951, 950f
    distal anterolateral accessory, 951, 951f
    modified mid-anterior, 951, 951f
    posterolateral, 951–952
  knee arthroscopy, 1121–1123, 1122f–1124f
  shoulder arthroscopy, 435–436, 436f
  wrist arthroscopy, 817–819, 818f–819f
Position/positioning
  arthroscopic synovectomy, of knee, 1129
  during arthroscopy, 109–110, 109f–110f
  beach chair, 329
  elbow arthroscopy, 708, 708f
  hip arthroscopy, 948–950
  hip center, 938
  knee arthroscopy, 1121, 1122f
  shoulder arthroscopy, 434–435, 434f
Positron emission tomography/computed tomography scans, 90, 93f
Postclosure wound care, for face facial injuries, 261–262
Postconcussion syndrome (PCS), 1540–1541, 1746, 1747t
Posterior apprehension test, 404–405, 932
Posterior compartment release, 1399, 1399f
Posterior compartments, in arthroscopic synovectomy, of knee, 1129–1130
Posterior cruciate ligament
  injuries, 1211–1230, 1220b–1222b, 1221f–1223f
    complications in, 1229
    decision-making, 1214–1216
    future considerations, 1229
    history, 1211–1212
    imaging, 1214
      bone scan and, 1214
      magnetic resonance imaging, 1214
      radiography, 1214
    isolated, 1224–1225, 1227t

Posterior cruciate ligament (Continued)
  nonoperative treatment, 1216
    decision-making, 1215–1216
  operative treatment, 1216–1217
    results, 1224–1229
  physical examination, 1212–1214
    collateral ligament assessment, 1213–1214
    external rotation of tibia (Dial test) in, 1213
    gait and limb alignment in, 1214
    posterior drawer test, 1212, 1213f
    posterior sag test (Godfrey test) in, 1212–1213, 1213f
    quadriceps active test, 1212–1213
    reverse pivot-shift test, 1213
  postoperative management, 1224, 1224b
  treatment options, 1216–1220, 1216f–1217f
    graft choice and fixation, 1219
    high tibial osteotomy in, 1219–1220
    single-bundle vs. double-bundle reconstruction, 1218–1219, 1218f, 1225–1229
    transtibial tunnel vs. tibial inlay techniques, 1217–1218, 1225, 1228t
  knee, 1069, 1070f
  MRI, 1112
  multiligament knee injuries, 1268
Posterior drawer test, for posterior cruciate ligament injuries, 1212, 1213f
Posterior elbow pathologic conditions, 1673–1674, 1673f
  complications, 1674
  decision-making principles, 1674
  history, 1674
  imaging, 1674
  physical examination, 1674
  results, 1674
  treatment, 1674
Posterior heel pain, 1504–1508, 1505f
  complications, 1508
  decision-making principles, 1505–1506
  future considerations, 1508
  history, 1504
  imaging, 1504–1505, 1505f–1506f
  physical examination, 1504, 1505f
  postoperative management, 1508
  results, 1508
  treatment options, 1506–1507
    nonoperative therapy, 1506–1507
    operative therapy, 1507
    technique, 1507b, 1507f
Posterior hindfoot arthroscopy, 1470b, 1471f
Posterior hip pain, 1018–1033
  deep gluteal syndrome in, 1020–1024
  operative treatment, 1027–1030
    endoscopic decompression in, 1027–1030, 1028t–1029t, 1029f–1030f
  physical examination, 1024–1026, 1024f–1026f
  preoperative and postoperative rehabilitation, 1027–1030, 1027f–1028f
  pudendal nerve entrapment in, 1030–1032, 1031f–1032f, 1031t
  sciatic nerve
    characteristics, 1018–1020, 1019f–1020f
    entrapment, 1020–1024
  superior and inferior gluteal nerves in, 1032–1033, 1032f, 1032t
Posterior impingement, 431, 1426b, 1426f
Posterior interosseous nerve (PIN) syndrome, 687–688, 693, 755–756
  complications, 756
  decision-making principles, 755
  history, 755
  postoperative management, 755
  results, 755–756
  return-to-play guidelines, 755

Posterior interosseous nerve (PIN) syndrome (Continued)
  technique, 755
  treatment, 755
Posterior medial corner injuries, 1231–1243
  complications in, 1242
  decision-making principles, 1234–1235, 1235f
  future considerations, 1243
  history, 1231
  imaging, 1232–1234, 1233f–1235f
  physical exam, 1231–1232
  postoperative management, 1239–1240
  results, 1240–1242
  return-to-play guidelines, 1240b
  treatment options, 1235–1236
Posterior radiocapitellar portal, 711
Posterior sag test (Godfrey test), for posterior cruciate ligament injuries, 1212–1213, 1213f
Posterior shoulder instability, 463–475
  arthroscopic posterior shoulder stabilization for, 470b–472b, 470f–472f
  background, 463
  complications, 474–475
  decision-making principles and, 468
  future considerations, 475
  history, 465
  imaging, 467–468, 467f–468f, 468t
  pathogenesis of, 463–465, 464f–465f
  physical examination, 465–467, 466f, 466t
  postoperative management, 469–473
  results, 473–474
  treatment options, 468–469
    contraindications, 469
    indications, 469
Posterior tibia
  tendon, 1383–1384, 1383f–1384f
  tendon, injuries, 1464–1469
    complications, 1469
    decision-making principles, 1466
    future considerations, 1469
    history, 1465
    imaging, 1465–1466, 1465f
    physical examination, 1465, 1465f
    postoperative management, 1468
    results, 1468–1469
    treatment options, 1466–1467, 1466f–1467f, 1467b–1468b
  translation of, 1247–1248
Posterolateral corner injuries, 1244–1263
  anatomy, 1244–1248
  classification, 1248, 1248t
  complications in, 1260–1261, 1262f
  decision-making principles, 1253
  future considerations, 1262
  history, 1248–1249
  imaging, 1251–1253
    magnetic resonance imaging, 1251–1253, 1252f
    radiographs, 1251, 1251f
    ultrasound, 1253
  layers of lateral side of, 1244
  nonoperative management, 1253
    grade I injuries, 1253
    grade II injuries, 1253
    grade III injuries, 1253
  pediatric, 1262
  physical examination, 1249–1251, 1249f–1250f
  postoperative management, 1256–1260, 1259t
  repair vs. reconstruction, 1253
  results, 1260, 1260t–1261t
  return to play, 1260
  structures, 1244–1246, 1245f
    anterior/posterior tibial translation, 1247–1248
    arcuate ligament complex, 1246
    biceps femoris muscle, 1245–1246

Posterolateral corner injuries (Continued)
    biomechanics, 1246, 1247f
    external rotation, 1247
    fabellofibular ligament, 1246
    fibular collateral ligament, 1244–1245
    iliotibial band, 1244
    lateral gastrocnemius tendon, 1246
    mid-third lateral capsular ligament, 1246
    neurovascular, 1246
    popliteus tendon complex, 1245
    varus motion, 1246–1247
  surgical considerations, 1254–1256
    diagnostic arthroscopy, 1254, 1254f
    primary repair, 1254, 1254f
    reconstruction techniques, 1254–1255
  techniques, 1257b, 1257f–1258f
  timing of diagnosis, 1253
  treatment options, 1253–1256
Posterolateral corner sling procedure, 1255
Posterolateral drawer test, 1249, 1249f–1250f
Posterolateral portal, in hip arthroscopy, 951–952
Posteromedial impingement, 1673–1674, 1673f
  complications, 1674
  decision-making principles, 1674
  history, 1674
  imaging, 1674
  physical examination, 1674
  results, 1674
  treatment, 1674
Postoperative rehabilitation, for posterior hip pain, 1027–1030, 1027f–1028f
Postural orthostatic tachycardia syndrome (POTS), 173
Power stroke, 63
Pre-event planning, in spine injuries, 1553–1554
Prediabetes, 218
Pregnancy, in female athlete, 301–302, 302t
Preoperative arthroscopy, 109
Preoperative imaging, 433–434
Preoperative rehabilitation, for posterior hip pain, 1027–1030, 1027f–1028f
Preparticipation physical evaluation, 144–150
  allergies, 149
  athletes with special needs, 150
  cardiovascular system, 145–147, 145b–146b
  dermatology, 149
  ears, 145
  endocrine system, 149
  eyes, 145
  gastrointestinal system, 148
  genitourinary system, 148
  goals, 144
  head, 145
  heat illness, 149–150
  hematologic disease, 148–149
  history, 145–150
  immunizations, 149
  infectious disease, 148–149
  medical home, 159–160
  medications, 149
  musculoskeletal system, 148, 148b
  neurologic system, 148
  nose, 145
  objectives, 144
  organization, 144–145
  physical examination, 145–150
  pulmonary system, 147–148
  setting, 144–145, 145t
  throat, 145
  timing, 144–145
Pressure sores, 319
Primary anterior cruciate ligament reconstruction, 1193b–1195b, 1193f–1195f
Primary osteoarthritis, 592
Primary vs. permanent teeth, 269, 270f
Probe, arthroscopic, 107

ProChondrix, 1183
Professional athletics, ethical/legal issues with, 155
Progression, criterion-based, principles, 351–352
  key criteria for rehabilitation protocols and
      progression
    balance, 352, 352f
    movement quality, 352
    muscle performance, 351–352
    outcome measures, 351
    pain, 351
    range of motion, 351
  return-to-sport considerations, 352
Progressive loading, 389, 390f–391f
Pronation-supination, elbow, 681–683
Pronator syndrome, 688, 693–694, 745–746
  complications, 746
  decision-making principles, 745
  history, 745
  physical examination, 745
  postoperative management, 745–746
  results, 746
  return-to-play guidelines, 745–746
  technique, 746f
  treatment, 745
Prone examination
  hip, 933
  patellar instability, 1297
Prophylaxis, thromboembolic, 182, 183t–185t
Propofol, perioperative pharmacology, 338
Proprioception, anterior cruciate ligament
    injuries, 1196
Protective equipment, removal of, in injured
    athlete, 1558f
Protein, 277–278, 278t
Protocols
  in magnetic resonance imaging, 93, 94f
  in rehabilitation, 1208–1209
Proton density, 95, 96f, 96t
Provocative tests, for patellofemoral pain,
    1312–1313, 1312f–1313f
Proximal anteromedial portal, 710–711
Proximal biceps tendon pathology, 526–539
  complications, 538
  decision-making principles, 529–530, 530f
  future considerations, 538
  history, 526
  imaging, 528–529, 529f
  introduction, 526
  physical examination, 526–528, 527t, 528f
  postoperative management, 534–538
    biceps tenodesis rehabilitation protocol,
        534–535
    biceps tenotomy rehabilitation protocol, 534
    phase I: protective phase (day 1 to week 6),
        535
    phase II: moderate protection phase (weeks
        7 to 12), 535–538
    phase III: minimum protection phase (weeks
        13 to 20), 538
    phase IV: advanced strengthening phase
        (weeks 21 to 26), 538
  results, 537t, 538
  treatment options, 530–534
    nonoperative management, 530
    open subpectoral biceps tenodesis, 534, 535f
    surgical management, 530–532, 531f
Proximal femur, development, 908–909
Proximal fifth metatarsal stress fractures,
    134–135, 135f–136f
Proximal hamstring tendinopathy, chronic, 1041
Proximal humerus, 1637, 1638f
  epiphysiolysis, 1655–1656
    complications, 1656
    history, 1656

Proximal humerus (Continued)
    imaging, 1656, 1656f
    physical examination, 1656
    treatment, 1656
  fractures, 1644–1647, 1644f–1645f
    complications, 1647
    history, 1644
    imaging, 1644–1645, 1645f–1646f
    physical examination, 1644
    treatment, 1645–1646, 1646f
Proximal interphalangeal joint, 788–789, 802–803,
    804f
  ligamentous injuries and dislocations, 885–888,
      885f–890f
Proximal posterolateral portal, 711
Proximal tibial osteotomy, 1255, 1255f, 1259b,
    1259f, 1282
Proximal tibiofibular joint instability, 1259b, 1259f
Pseudoanemia, 196
Pseudomonal folliculitis (hot tub folliculitis), 249,
    249f
Pseudomonas infections, 213
Psoas minor, 979
Psychological adjustment, to athletic injury,
    272–276
  complications, 275
  decision-making principles, 273
  future considerations, 275
  historical perspective and evolution, 272–273
  postinjury management and outcome, 275
  preparticipation screening, 273
  treatment options, 274b
Psychological issues, in female athlete, 302–303
Psychosocial strategies, 345–346
Pubofemoral ligament (PFL), 914
Pudendal nerve entrapment, 1030–1032,
    1031f–1032f, 1031t
Pulley injuries, 814, 880–881, 880f–881f
Pulmonary edema, high-altitude, 243–245
Pulmonary embolism, 180–188
  clinical manifestations, 182–184
  diagnosis, 182–184
  imaging, 182–184, 185f–186f
  laboratory findings, 182–184
  normal physiology, 180, 181f
  return to play, 185–186
  risk factors, preoperative, 180–181
  sports issues in, 185–186
  thromboembolic prophylaxis, 182, 183t–185t
  travel and, 185–186
  treatment, 184–185, 187t
Pulmonary system, preparticipation physical
    evaluation, 147–148
Pulse check, in unconscious athlete, 1555
Pulse sequences, in magnetic resonance imaging,
    95–98
  2D acquisitions, 98, 98f
  3D acquisitions, 98, 98f
  gradient echo, 96–97, 97f
  inversion recovery, 97–98, 97f
  spin echo, 96, 97f

Q
Quadrants, of hand/wrist
  dorsal, 794t, 796–798, 797f–798f
  radial, 794–796, 794t, 795f–796f
  ulnar, 794t, 798–800, 799f
  volar, 794t, 800–801, 800f, 802f–803f
Quadratus femoris, nerve to, 916
Quadriceps
  contusion, 1044–1047, 1044t
    complications, 1047
    decision-making principles, 1046

Quadriceps (Continued)
    future considerations, 1047
    history, 1044–1045
    imaging, 1045, 1045f
    physical examination, 1045
    results, 1046
    return to play, 1046
    techniques, 1046b
    treatment options, 1045–1046
  strains, 1047–1050
    complications, 1049
    decision-making principles, 1049
    future considerations, 1050
    history, 1048
    imaging, 1048, 1048f
    physical examination, 1048
    results, 1049, 1049f
    return to play, 1049
    techniques, 1049b
    treatment options, 1048–1049, 1048t,
        1049f
  tendinopathy
    decision-making principles, 1327
  tendinopathy of, 1320–1321
    clinical outcomes, 1331–1332, 1332f
    history, 1322–1323
    imaging, 1324–1325, 1324f–1325f
    physical examination, 1323–1324, 1323t
  tendon rupture, 1321–1322
    clinical outcomes, 1332
    complications, 1333
    history, 1323
    imaging, 1325–1326, 1325f–1326f
    nonoperative treatment, 1327
    operative treatment, 1328–1329, 1329f
    physical examination, 1324, 1324f
    postoperative management, 1330–1331
  tendon structure of, 1320, 1320f–1321f
Quadriceps active test, for posterior cruciate
    ligament injuries, 1212–1213
Quadriceps angle
  patellar instability and, 1296, 1296f
  patellofemoral pain and, 1310–1311
Quadrilateral space syndrome (QSS), 629–630
Quadriplegia, transient, 1579

R
Race, of elite athlete, 161–162, 162f
Radial head, elbow, 683–684, 684f
Radial nerve, 752
  compression neuropathies, 692–693
  PIN syndrome, 755–756
    complications, 756
    decision-making principles, 755
    history, 755
    postoperative management, 755
    results, 755–756
    return-to-play guidelines, 755
    technique, 755
    treatment, 755
  radial tunnel syndrome, 752–755, 753f
    complications, 755
    decision-making principles, 754
    history, 754
    physical examination, 754
    postoperative management, 755
    results, 755
    return-to-play guidelines, 755
    technique, 754–755
    treatment, 754
Radial quadrant, 794–796, 794t, 795f–796f
Radial sensory nerve compression, 756,
    756f

Radial tunnel syndrome (RTS), 687–688, 692–693, 693f, 752–755, 753f
  complications, 755
  decision-making principles, 754
  history, 754
  physical examination, 754
  postoperative management, 755
  results, 755
  return-to-play guidelines, 755
  technique, 754–755
  treatment, 754
    anterolateral approach, 754, 754f
    posterior approach, 754
Radiation exposure, in imaging, 103–104, 103t
Radiculopathy
  cervical, 1595
  lumbar, 1599–1601, 1600f
Radiofrequency excitation pulse, in magnetic resonance imaging, 94
Radiofrequency instruments, for arthroscopy, 108–109
Radiographic densities, 75, 75f
Radiographic tunnel positioning, for revision anterior cruciate ligament injuries, 1200–1202, 1201f
Radiography. See also Plain radiography
  ankle, 1380, 1381f
  athletic pubalgia, 1010, 1010f
  conventional, 74–78
    advantages, 77
    arthrography, 76–77, 76f–77f
    disadvantages, 77–78, 78f
    fluoroscopy, 75–76, 75f–76f
    technical considerations, 74–75, 75f
  elbow, 697
  foot, 1380, 1381f
  glenohumeral joint, 408–410, 409b
    acromioclavicular articulation views, 410
    anteroposterior view, 408, 409f
    axillary lateral view, 408, 409f
    Grashey view, 408
    scapular Y view, 408–409, 409f
    Stryker notch view, 409–410
  hip, 935–936
    cross-table lateral view, 935, 936f
    dysplasia and instability, 974
    false-profile view, 936, 937f
    45-degree Dunn view, 935, 937f
    frog-leg lateral view, 935, 937f
    90-degree Dunn view, 935, 937f
    standing anteroposterior pelvic view, 935, 936f
  iliopsoas, 983–984
  knee, 1104, 1105f
    arthritis, 1277–1278, 1278f–1279f
    lateral and posterolateral corner injuries, 1251, 1251f
    medial collateral ligament and posterior medial corner injuries, 1232, 1233f
    meniscal transplantation, 1155
    multiligament knee injuries, 1265, 1265f
    patellar instability, 1297–1298, 1297t, 1298f
    patellofemoral pain, 1313, 1313f–1314f
  pediatrics
    of medial clavicle physeal fractures, 1643
    of osteochondritis dissecans, 1713–1714, 1713f–1714f
    of traumatic anterior instability, 1648–1649
    of traumatic posterior instability, 1652
  posterior cruciate ligament, 1214
  scapulothoracic disorders, 614
  spine, 1544, 1545f
Range of motion (ROM), 349–350, 362
  active, 350
  ankle, 1375

Range of motion (ROM) (Continued)
  elbow, 683, 690
  hip, 930–931, 931t
  immobilization and, 350
  knee, 1094–1095, 1094f–1095f
  passive, 350
  patellofemoral pain, 1311–1312
  restoration, 385–386, 386f
  scapulothoracic disorders, 613
  stiff shoulder, 583, 584b
Readiness for sport, 1609–1610
Reconstruction
  anatomic coracoclavicular, 659b–663b, 659f–663f
  anterior cruciate ligament, 1193b–1195b, 1193f–1195f, 1700–1701, 1700f–1702f, 1701b
    causes of failure, 1202–1203
    primary graft choice, 1203
    treatment options, 1204–1207
    two-stage, 1207
  figure-of-eight, 675, 675b, 676f
  flexor retinaculum, for posterior tibial tendon injury, 1467b–1468b
  for lateral and posterolateral corner injuries of knee, 1254–1255
    anatomic, 1255–1256
    biceps tenodesis, 1254–1255
    fibula-based, 1256
    posterolateral corner sling procedure in, 1255
    proximal tibial osteotomy, 1255, 1255f, 1259b, 1259f
    split biceps tendon transfer, 1255
  lateral ankle ligament, 1426b
  ligament, implants for, 38–41
  surgical, 28
Recreational drug use, 290–293
  alcohol, 290–291
  cocaine, 292
  inhalants, 293
  marijuana, 291–292
  tobacco, 292
Recreational water-related illness, 210–213
  cryptosporidiosis, 211–212
  fecally derived, 211
  non, 213–214
  other, 212–213
  infectious diarrhea, 212
Rectus femoris, 919
Recurrent instability
  anterior cruciate ligament injuries, 1199
  anterior shoulder instability, 452–453
Red blood cells, disorders of, 196–198
  definition, 196
  diagnosis, 197–198, 197f
  epidemiology, 196
  pathophysiology, 196–197, 197t
  return-to-play guidelines, 198
  treatment, 198
Referral, 345–346
Referred pain
  intrathoracic source, 406
  the neck, 405–406
Regional anesthesia, 328
  arm, 330
  benefits, 328
  complications, 328
  contraindications, 328
  elbow, 330–332
  femur, 332–333
  forearm, 330–332
  hand, 330–332
  hip, 332–333
  intravenous, 334
  knee, 332–333

Regional anesthesia (Continued)
  neuraxial anesthesia, 329
  orthopaedic surgeries and, 327
  patient characteristics, 327
  peripheral nerve block, 329–330
  shoulder, 330
  techniques, 329–335
  thigh, 332–333
Regional pain syndrome, complex, 1316
Regulation, of athletic trainer, 343, 344t
Rehabilitation, 345–346
  anterior cruciate ligament injuries, 1192–1195, 1197
  anterior shoulder instability, 455
  femoroacetabular impingement, 967–969
  glenohumeral arthritis, 605–606
  hamstring injuries, 1039–1040
  motion, loss in elbow, 782
  posterior hip pain, 1027–1030, 1027f–1028f
  principles, 347–353, 1207–1208
    chronic workload ratio, 347–348, 348f
    envelope of function and, 347, 348f
    matched dosing of internal and external load, 348, 348f
    patient modifiers, 349
    tissue healing considerations, 348–349
    tissue-specific considerations, 349
      articular cartilage, 349
      bone, 349
      labral/meniscal, 349
      ligament, 349
      tendon, 349
  protocol for, 1208–1209
Relative motion, 22
Relieving factors, for stiff shoulder, 580–581
"Relocation test", 404
Remodeling phase
  of fracture repair, 14
  of tendon and ligament repair, 5
Renal medicine, 227–229
Renal sports medicine, metabolic problems in, 229
Repair. See also Healing
  Achilles tendon, platelet-rich plasma for, 54
  articular cartilage, 11–12
  cartilage, 42–45
    stem cell-based therapy, 59–60
  fracture, 14–15
  for lateral and posterolateral corner injury of knee, 1254, 1254f
  ligament, 4–5
    platelet-rich plasma for, 53–55
  meniscal, 9, 41–42
    all-inside, 1147, 1148f
    augmentation in, 9
    in avascular portions, 9
    basics of, 1144
    factors affecting, 9
    inside-out, 1144–1146, 1145f–1146f
    outside-in, 1146–1147, 1147f
    platelet-rich plasma, 55–56
    scaffolds for, 9
    stem cell-based therapy, 60
    techniques, 1143b, 1143f
    in vascular regions, 9
  osteochondral, 42–45
  rotator cuff, platelet-rich plasma for, 54
  tendon, 35–38
    platelet-rich plasma for, 53–55
Reparative phase, of tendon and ligament repair, 5
Repetition time, in magnetic resonance imaging, 95
Resistance exercises, for subscapularis injury, 564

Resisted internal rotation test, 933
Resonant frequency, in magnetic resonance imaging, 94
Respiration, mitochondrial, 66
Respiratory considerations, preoperative care, 325–326
  asthma, 325
  obstructive sleep apnea, 325–326, 326f
Respiratory response, to exercise, 72–73
Respiratory tract infections
  lower, 209–210
    acute bronchitis, 209
    acute pneumonia, 209–210
  upper, 206–209
    diagnosis, 207
    epidemiology, 206
    infectious mononucleosis, 207–208
    measles, 208–209
    pathobiology, 206–207
    prevention, 207
    return-to-play guidelines, 207
    treatment, 207
Retinal detachment, 269
Retiring, 1567
Return to play
  acromioclavicular joint, 663–664
  acute bronchitis, 209
  acute otitis externa, 214
  acute pneumonia, 210
  adductor strains, 1051
  after arthroplasty, 1283
  after osteotomy, 1283
  AIN syndrome, 747
  anterior cruciate ligament injuries, 1197
  articular cartilage lesions, 1167
  bacterial skin infections, 204–205
  brain injury, 1567, 1567t
  concussion, 1567, 1567t, 1746, 1746t
  cryptosporidiosis, 212
  cubital tunnel syndrome, 752
  deep venous thrombosis, 185–186
  distal biceps, 727
  elbow, 718, 768
  encephalitis, 215
  exercise-associated collapse, 237
  exercise-associated hyponatremia, 239
  exercise-associated muscle cramps, 237
  exercise-induced bronchoconstriction, 179, 179f
  exertional heat exhaustion, 235–236, 236b
  exertional heat stroke, 236, 236b
  exertional rhabdomyolysis, 238b
  fractures, 139–142, 140f–141f
  fungal skin infections, 206
  genitourinary trauma, 229
  glenohumeral arthritis, 606
  heat syncope, 237
  hemostasis disorders, 200
  herpes simplex virus, 205, 205t
  iliac crest contusion, 1044
  infectious diarrhea, 212
  infectious disease prevention, 202–203
  infectious mononucleosis, 208
  lateral epicondylitis, 724
  loss of knee motion, 1342
  measles, 209
  medial collateral ligament and posterior medial corner injuries, 1240b
  medial epicondylitis, 724
  meningitis, 215
  meniscal injuries, 1151
  motion, loss in elbow, 782
  osteochondral lesions, 1500
  PIN syndrome, 755

Return to play (Continued)
  popliteal artery entrapment syndrome, 1356
  pronator syndrome, 745–746
  quadriceps contusion, 1046
  quadriceps strains, 1049
  radial tunnel syndrome, 755
  red blood cells disorders, 198
  scapulothoracic disorders, 619
  seizure, 232–234
  sternoclavicular joint, 677
  stingers, 1576
  thoracolumbar spine injuries, 1592
  triceps tendinitis, 727
  upper respiratory tract infections, 207
Reverse pivot-shift test, 1213, 1251
Revision anterior cruciate ligament, 1189–1190, 1192
  injuries, 1199–1210, 1208b
    advanced imaging, 1202, 1202f
    complications in, 1209
    decision-making principles, 1202–1204
    future considerations, 1209
    history, 1199–1200
    imaging, 1200–1202, 1200f
    multiple, 1209
    physical exam, 1200
    postoperative management, 1207–1209
    results, 1209
Revision rotator cuff repair, 567–573
  complications, 571–573, 572t–573t
  decision-making principles, 568–569, 569t, 570f
  future considerations of, 573
  history patient with, 567–568
  imaging, 568
  noncuff tear etiologies of, 568t
  physical examination, 568
  postoperative management, 571
  results, 571–573, 572t–573t
  treatment options, 569–571
    with biologic augmentation, 571
    débridement alone, 569
    nonoperative, 569
    revision repair, 569–571
    technique, 571b, 572f
Revision shoulder instability, 489–501
  complications, 499–500
  decision-making principles, 493–494
  future considerations, 500, 500f
  history, 489
  imaging, 490–493, 491f–492f
  physical exam, 489–490, 490f
  postoperative management, 498–499
  preferred surgical technique, 495–498, 496f–499f
  results, 499
  treatment options, 494–495, 494f
Rhabdomyolysis, 229
  exertional, 237–238, 238b
Rheumatoid arthritis, 594–595, 594f
Rheumatoid cervical spondylitis, 1596–1597, 1596f
Rib, fractures, 137–139
Right ventricle, 160
Rigid body mechanics, 23
Rigorous athletic training, cardiovascular adaptations and, 160–161
"Ringworm" (tinea corporis), 249
"Roller-wringer effect", 557
Rolling motion, 22–23, 23f
ROM. See Range of motion
Roos elevated arm test, 636–638, 638f
Rosenberg view, knee arthritis and, 1278, 1278f–1279f

Rotator cuff, 35–36, 398–399, 398f, 417–422
  débridement, 522–523
  magnetic resonance imaging, 419–422, 419f–424f, 419t, 423b
  pathology, 406–407
  repair, 523–524
    platelet-rich plasma for, 54
  revision, 567–573
    complications, 571–573, 572t–573t
    decision-making principles, 568–569, 569t, 570f
    future considerations of, 573
    history patient with, 567–568
    imaging, 568
    noncuff tear etiologies of, 568t
    physical examination, 568
    postoperative management, 571
    results, 571–573, 572t–573t
    treatment options, 569–571
      with biologic augmentation, 571
      débridement alone, 569
      nonoperative, 569
      revision repair, 569–571
      technique, 571b, 572f
  tears, 406, 1656–1658, 1657f–1658f
Rotator cuff and impingement lesions, 540–555
  anatomy, 540–542, 541f
  biomechanics, 542–543
    biceps function, 542, 543f
    function, 542, 542f
    scapular function, 543
    static stabilizers, 542–543
  decision-making principles, 547–548
    acute rotator cuff trauma, 548
    chronic rotator cuff disease, 548
    subacromial impingement and biceps tenosynovitis, 548
  future considerations, 554
  historical perspective, 540
  history, 543
  imaging, 547
    magnetic resonance imaging, 547, 547f
    plain radiographs, 547
    ultrasonography, 547
  physical examination, 543–547, 544f–546f
    impingement test, 546–547
  treatment options, 548–554
    complications, 554
    nonoperative, 549–550
    operative, 550–554, 550b–553b, 551f–552f
    preventive, 548–549, 549f
Rotator interval, 422–424, 425f
Rotatory atlantoaxial subluxation, 1759–1761
  history, 1759
  imaging, 1760, 1761f
  physical examination, 1759
  treatment, 1760–1761
Rowing injuries, 123
  chest, 123
  knee, 123
  lumbar spine, 123
  upper extremity, 123
Rugby injuries, 123–124
Runner's diarrhea, 193
"Runner's trots", 193
Running injuries, 124
Ruptured globe, 269

S

Sacral facet fractures, 1755, 1756f
Sacral stress fracture, 926
Sacroiliac joint, injuries of, thoracolumbar spine and, 1591

Sagittal band rupture, 877–878, 877*f*
Salter-Harris fracture
    type I, 1729*f*, 1730
    type II, 1729*f*, 1730, 1733*f*
    type III, 1729*f*, 1730
    type IV, 1729*f*–1731*f*, 1730–1731
Saphenous nerve block, 333
Saphenous nerve entrapment, 1405–1407,
    1405*f*–1406*f*
    history, 1405
    imaging, 1406
    physical examination, 1405–1406
    results, 1406–1407
    treatment options, 1406
Sarcomeres, 62, 63*f*
Sarcopenia, 68
Sartorius, 919
Scabies, 253, 253*f*
Scaffolds
    meniscal, 1149–1150
    for meniscal repair, 9
Scalars, 16
Scaphoid
    carpal injuries, 835–836, 837*b*, 837*f*
    fractures, 807–808, 807*f*–808*f*, 824, 1684–1686
        complications, 1685
        decision-making principles, 1685
        future considerations, 1686
        history, 1684
        imaging, 1684–1685
        physical examination, 1684
        postoperative management, 1685
        results, 1685
        treatment options, 1685, 1685*b*, 1686*f*
    nonunions, 824–825, 825*t*
Scapholunate injuries, 848
Scapula, 1637, 1638*f*
Scapular bursitis, 609, 611*b*, 611*f*, 611*t*, 616–617,
    616*f*–617*f*
Scapular dyskinesia, 619
    pediatrics, 1659, 1659*f*
Scapular dyskinesis, 609, 612*f*–613*f*, 616*t*
Scapular lag, 543
Scapular muscles, 399
Scapular retraction test, 614
Scapular winging, 609, 612*f*–613*f*, 612*t*, 619
Scapular Y view, 408–409, 409*f*
Scapulothoracic articulation, 398
Scapulothoracic disorders, 609–620, 610*f*, 610*t*
    complications, 620
    crepitus, 609, 611*b*, 611*f*, 611*t*
    decision-making principles, 614–615
        crepitus, 614–615
        injection, 615, 615*f*
        pain, 614–615
        pathologies, 615
        treatment, 615
    future considerations, 620
    history, 609–611
    imaging, 614
        computed tomography, 614
        electromyography, 614
        magnetic resonance imaging, 614
        radiographs, 614
        ultrasound, 614, 614*f*–615*f*
    physical examination, 611–614
        inspection, 611–612
        palpation, 612–613
        range of motion, 613
        strength, 613
        testing, 613–614
    postoperative management, 619
    results, 619–620
    return-to-play guidelines, 619
    scapular bursitis, 609, 611*b*, 611*f*, 611*t*
    scapular dyskinesis, 609, 612*f*–613*f*, 616*t*

Scapulothoracic disorders (*Continued*)
    scapular winging, 609, 612*f*–613*f*, 612*t*
    treatment, 615–619
        arthroscopic bursal resection, 617*b*–619*b*,
            617*f*–619*f*
        nonoperative, 615–616
        operative, 616–619
Schistosomiasis, 216
Sciatic nerve
    characteristics, 1018–1020, 1019*f*–1020*f*
    of hip, 916
Sciatic nerve block, 333
Sciatic nerve entrapment, 1020–1024
    anatomy, 1020–1021, 1021*f*
    etiology, 1021–1024, 1021*f*–1023*f*
    operative treatment, 1027–1030
    physical examination, 1024–1026, 1024*f*–1026*f*
    preoperative and postoperative rehabilitation,
        1027–1030, 1027*f*–1028*f*
Scintigraphy, nuclear, 1548–1549, 1549*f*
Scissors, in arthroscopy, 108
Scoliosis, 1755–1758
    history, 1755–1757
    idiopathic, 313–314
    imaging, 1757
    physical examination, 1755–1757
    sports participation, 1757–1758
    treatment, 1757
Scour test, 932
Scratch collapse test, 691–692
Screening, for cardiovascular system, 162–166,
    163*b*
    electrocardiogram, 163–164, 164*f*
    transthoracic echocardiography, 164–166,
        165*f*–167*f*
SCT. *See* Sickle cell trait
Seabather's eruption, 256, 257*f*
Second-impact syndrome, 1746–1747
Secondary deep bursa, 920
Sedation, in orthopedic patient, 339, 339*t*
Seizure, 230. *See also* Epilepsy
    acute management, 232
    exercise and, 231–232
    return-to-activity guidelines of, 232–234
Semitendinosus autograft, 31
Septic arthritis, of hip, 928
Septic meningitis, 214
Sesamoid dysfunction, 1516–1519, 1516*b*
    complications, 1519
    decision-making principles, 1517
    history, 1517
    imaging, 1517, 1518*f*
    physical examination, 1517
    postoperative management, 1518–1519
    results, 1519
    treatment options, 1517–1518
        nonoperative, 1517
        operative, 1518, 1519*f*
        technique, 1518*b*
Sever disease, 1738–1739, 1739*f*
Shavers, motorized, 107
Shoes, 1739
    sports, 1439–1442
        anatomy, 1440, 1441*f*
        insole, 1441
        midsole, 1440–1441
        outsole, 1440
        selection and fitting of, 1442, 1442*t*
        upper, 1441–1442
Short external rotators, 920
Short tau inversion recovery (STIR), 97–98
Shoulder, 393–401
    anatomy, 393–395, 394*f*
    anterior instability, 440–462
        anatomy, 440–441, 441*f*–442*f*
        decision-making principles, 450–454

Shoulder (*Continued*)
    future considerations, 461–462
    history, 447
    imaging, 448–450, 450*f*–452*f*
    pathoanatomy, 441–447, 443*f*–444*f*, 443*t*,
        446*f*
    physical examination, 447–448, 448*f*–449*f*
    treatment options, 454–461
        complications, 461
        emergency department, 455
        nonoperative sling immobilization, 455
        on-field management, 454–455
        rehabilitation, 455
        results, 461
        surgical management, 455–461, 456*b*
    arthrography, 410–411, 410*f*
    arthroscopy, 433–439
        anatomy, 435–436
        background, 433
        complications, 438–439
        contraindications, 433
        diagnostic examination, 436–438, 437*f*–438*f*
        indications, 433
        open procedures *vs.*, 433
        portal placement, 435–436, 436*f*
        positioning, 434–435, 434*f*
        preoperative imaging, 433–434
        setup, 435
        visualization, 435
    biomechanics, 400
    complex, 399–400
    decision-making, 402–407
    diagnosis, 402–407
    examination of, 568
    history, 402–403
    imaging
        abnormalities, 402
        glenohumeral joint, 408–432
    injuries
        baseball, 114–115
        golf, 120
        handball, 122
        pediatrics, 1637–1660
        skiing, 124
        snowboarding, 124–125
        swimming, 126
        volleyball, 128
    instability, 406–407
    joints, 395–398
        acromioclavicular joint, 397
        glenohumeral, 395–396, 395*f*–396*f*
        glenohumeral joint capsule, 396–397
        scapulothoracic articulation, 398
        sternoclavicular joint, 397, 397*f*
    kinetics, 400
    little league, 1612, 1612*f*
    multidirectional instability, 476–488, 482*b*, 482*f*
        decision-making principles, 479–480
        future considerations, 480–481
        history, 477
        imaging, 479, 479*f*
        physical examination, 477–479, 477*t*–478*t*, 478*f*
        postoperative management, 481–483, 483*f*
        results, 483–487, 484*t*–485*t*
            complications, 486–487
            return to sport, 485–486, 486*t*
        treatment options, 480–481
            arthroscopic plication, 481
            open inferior capsular shift, 480–481, 480*f*
    muscles, 398–400
        rotator cuff, 398–399, 398*f*
        scapular muscles, 399
    nerve entrapment, 621
    pathologies, 406–407
        acromioclavicular joint, 406
        rotator cuff, 406–407

Shoulder *(Continued)*
  pediatric, 1616–1618
    acute injuries, 1617–1618, 1618f–1619f
    development, 1616–1617, 1617f
    overuse injuries, 1618, 1620f–1621f
  pertinent bony, 393–395, 394f
  physical examination, 403–405
  posterior instability, 463–475
    arthroscopic posterior shoulder stabilization, 470b–472b, 470f–472f
    background, 463
    complications, 474–475
    decision-making principles, 468
    future considerations, 475
    history, 465
    imaging, 467–468, 467f–468f, 468t
    pathogenesis, 463–465, 464f–465f
    physical examination, 465–467, 466f, 466t
    postoperative management, 469–473
    results, 473–474
    treatment options, 468–469
      contraindications, 469
      indications, 469
  regional anesthesia, 330
  stiff, 579–591
    acquired causes, 582–583
    anatomy, 579
    complications, 589–590
    decision-making principles, 585
    future considerations, 590
    history, 579–583
    idiopathic adhesive capsulitis, 581–582
    imaging, 584–585
    pain, 579–581, 580b
    pathologies causing, 581b
    physical examination, 583–584
    postoperative management, 586–589
    primary causes, 581–582
    results, 589, 589t
    secondary causes, 582–583
    treatment options, 585–586, 586b
Shoulder instability, 1612, 1612f
  in female athlete, 312–313, 312f
  revision, 489–501
    complications, 499–500
    decision-making principles, 493–494
    future considerations, 500, 500f
    history, 489
    imaging, 490–493, 491f–492f
    physical exam, 489–490, 490f
    postoperative management, 498–499
    preferred surgical technique, 495–498, 496f–499f
    results, 499
    treatment options, 494–495, 494f
Sickle cell trait (SCT), 196, 238
Silk-based scaffold, 39
Simple lacerations, 262, 262f–263f
Sinding-Larsen-Johansson disease, 1718, 1718f
Single-bundle reconstruction, for posterior cruciate ligament injuries, 1218–1219, 1218f, 1225–1229
Single photon emission computed tomography, 88, 89f
  of spine, 1549–1550
Single photon emission computed tomography/ computed tomography imaging, 88, 89f
Sitting examination, of patellar instability, 1296, 1296f
Skeletal muscle
  aging effects on, 68
  contractions
    physiology, 62–64, 64f
    types, 65

Skeletal muscle *(Continued)*
  energy metabolism, 65–66, 65f
  force production, 64–65
  physiology, 62–66, 63t
  structure, 62, 63f
Skeletally immature athletes, 1616–1636
Skiing injuries, 124–125
Skin
  cancer, 256
  of hand, 785, 786f
  in medial collateral ligament and posterior medial corner injuries, 1231–1232
  soft tissue infections, 203–206
    bacterial skin infections, 203–205
    fungal skin infections, 205–206
    herpes simplex virus, 205
Skull, 1528, 1529f
SLAP tears. *See* Superior labrum anterior to posterior (SLAP) tears
"Sliding filament theory", 62–63
Sliding injuries, 115
Sliding motion, 22–23, 23f
Slipped capital femoral epiphysis, 928, 1694, 1695f
Snapping, iliopsoas, 980, 981f, 982, 983f, 984–986
Snapping hip syndrome, 925
  pediatrics, 1692–1693
Snapping scapula, pediatrics, 1658–1659, 1658f
Snowboarding injuries, 124–125
Soccer injuries, 125–126
"Soft spot" portal, 711
Soft tissue
  anatomy, patellar instability, 1294–1295, 1295f
  ankle arthroscopy, conditions amenable to, 1421–1428, 1422f
    complications, 1428
    decision-making principles, 1424
    future considerations, 1428
    history, 1423
    imaging, 1423–1424
    nonoperative management, 1424
    physical examination, 1423
    postoperative management, 1427
    results, 1427–1428
    surgical technique, 1424–1426, 1425f
  autograft, 31
  elbow, stability of, 684–685, 685f
  injuries
    ear, 263
    foot and ankle, 1728–1729, 1728f
    hip, 925, 1691–1693
    pediatrics, 1661–1662, 1662f–1663f
Soreness, delayed-onset muscle, 68
Spasticity, 319, 321
Special needs, athletes with, 150
Special tests, patellar instability and, 1296–1297, 1297f
SPECT. *See* Single photon emission computed tomography
SPECT/CT imaging. *See* Single photon emission computed tomography/computed tomography imaging
Speed test, 405
Spin echo, 96, 97f
Spin lattice relaxation, 95
Spin-spin relaxation, 95
Spinal accessory nerve palsy, 627–629
  anatomy, 627–628
  biomechanics, 627–628
  clinical evaluation, 628–629, 628f
  decision-making principles, 629
  diagnostic studies, 629
  results, 629
  technique, 629b
Spinal cord injury, 1559

Spinal cord injury without radiographic abnormality (SCIWORA), 1763
Spinal stability, in thoracolumbar spine injuries, 1583
Spinal stenosis, cervical, 1595–1596, 1595f–1596f
Spine, 1531–1533, 1532f–1533f. *See also* Back
  anatomy, 1528, 1529f
    brain, 1528–1529
    intervertebral disk, 1534
    ligaments, 1534
    muscles, 1534
    neurologic tissues, 1534–1535, 1534f
    skull (cranium), 1528, 1529f
  biomechanics, 1535, 1535f
  cervical
    congenital anomalies of, 1762–1763
    injuries, 152–153, 1578–1581
  hip and, 923–924, 923f
  imaging, 1544–1552
    computed tomography, 1546, 1546f
    degenerative, 1550–1551
    EOS 2D/3D x-ray imaging system, 1545–1546, 1545f
    functional metabolic imaging, 1549
    future considerations, 1551
    interventional radiology, 1550
    magnetic resonance imaging, 1547, 1547f
    myelography, 1548
    nuclear scintigraphy, 1548–1549, 1549f
    radiographs, 1544, 1545f
    single photon emission computed tomography, 1549–1550
    study interpretation, 1551
  injuries, 1541
    common acute, 1559–1560, 1560f
    emergency management, 1553–1561, 1559f
    epidemiology, 1553
    field-side management, 1553–1561, 1554f–1558f
  issues, in skeletally immature athletes, 1749–1764
    anatomy, 1749, 1750f–1751f
    history, 1749–1750, 1750b
    physical examination, 1749–1750, 1751b
  pediatric, 1635–1636, 1635f
Spinning motion, 22–23, 23f
Spinoglenoid notch compression, 624
Spinoglenoid notch decompression, 625
Splinting, 722
Split biceps tendon transfer, 1255
Spondylolisthesis, 1750–1753
  classification, 1751, 1751f
  degenerative, 1603–1604, 1603f–1604f
  history, 1751–1752
  imaging, 1752, 1752f
  physical examination, 1751–1752
  results, 1753, 1755f
  thoracolumbar spine, 1588–1591, 1590f
  treatment, 1752–1753, 1752f, 1754f
Spondylolysis, 1750–1753
  classification, 1751, 1751f
  history, 1751–1752
  imaging, 1752, 1752f
  physical examination, 1751–1752
  results, 1753, 1755f
  thoracolumbar spine, 1588, 1589f–1590f, 1591
  treatment, 1752–1753, 1752f, 1754f
Spondylosis, cervical, 405, 1594–1596
  disc herniation, 1595
  discogenic pain, 1594–1595
  epidemiology, 1594, 1594f
  foraminal stenosis, 1595
  myelopathy, 1595–1596
  pathoanatomy, 1594

Spondylosis, cervical *(Continued)*
  radiculopathy, 1595
  rheumatoid, 1596–1597, 1596*f*
  spinal stenosis, 1595–1596, 1595*f*–1596*f*
Spontaneous osteonecrosis, 1117
Sport Concussion Assessment Tool version 5
    (SCAT5), 1744
Sport-specific injuries, 114–130. *See also* specific
    sports
  auto racing, 117
  baseball, 114–115
  basketball, 115–116
  boxing, 116–117
  figure skating, 117–118
  football, 118–119
  golf, 119–120
  gymnastics, 120–121
  handball, 121–122
  ice hockey, 121
  lacrosse, 122
  rowing, 123
  rugby, 123–124
  running, 124
  skiing, 124–125
  snowboarding, 124–125
  soccer, 125–126
  swimming, 126
  tennis, 126–127
  volleyball, 127–128
  wrestling, 128–129
Sports
  epilepsy and, 230–234
  forefoot problems in, 1515–1526
  shoes and orthoses, 1436–1443
Sports equipment. *See Equipment*
Sports hernia, 1007, 1012–1014, 1014*b*, 1014*f*
Sports medicine rehabilitation, 354–367
  impairment-based rehabilitation programs,
      355–357
  joint cryotherapy, 366
  manipulation, 363
  manual therapy, 354–355, 356*t*
  mobilization, 363, 364*f*–365*f*
    with movement, 363–365, 365*f*
  modalities, 354, 355*f*
  muscle dysfunction, 365–366
  muscle energy technique, 366–367
  myofascial release, 367
  neuromuscular electrical stimulation, 366
  nonthermal ultrasound treatments, 360–363
    compression, 362, 362*f*
    iontophoresis, 360–361
    laser, 361–362
    phonophoresis, 360
    range of motion, 362
    stress fracture healing, 360, 361*f*
    superficial heat, 362–363
  pain modulation, 357
  patterned electrical nerve stimulation, 366, 366*f*
  thermal effects of ultrasound, 363
  treatments for pain, 357–360
    cryotherapy, 358–359
    edema/inflammation, 359
    electrical stimulation, 359
    manual therapy, 357, 358*t*
    transcutaneous electrical nerve stimulation,
        359
    ultrasound, 359–360
  trigger point therapy, 367, 367*f*
Sports nutrition, 277–282
  carbohydrate, 277–278, 278*t*
  energy balance, 277
  fat, 277–278, 278*t*
  hydration, 278–279, 279*t*
    considerations, 278
    monitoring, 278–279

Sports nutrition *(Continued)*
  minerals, 279–280
  nutrient timing, 280, 280*t*
  protein, 277–278, 278*t*
  sports supplementation, 280, 281*t*
  vitamins, 279–280
Sports participation, in pediatrics, 1606
  adult involvement, 1610
  psychosocial development, 1609
  readiness for sport, 1609–1610
Sports pharmacology
  ergogenic drugs, 283–290
    anabolic-androgenic steroids, 284–287
    caffeine, 290
    creatine, 288–289
    doping, 287–288
    growth hormone, 289–290
    steroid supplements, 287
    testosterone, historical perspectives, 283–284
  recreational drug use, 290–293
    alcohol, 290–291
    cocaine, 292
    inhalants, 293
    marijuana, 291–292
    tobacco, 292
Sprains
  ankle, 115, 371, 380–381
    balance, 381, 382*f*–383*f*
    bracing, 380–381
    coordination, 381
    dorsiflexion range of motion, 381
    education of risk, 381
    hypomobility issues, 381
    lateral, 1444–1450, 1445*f*
    medial, 1450–1453
    strength training, 381
    taping, 380–381
  bifurcate ligament, 1456–1457
    complications, 1458
    decision-making principles, 1457
    history, 1457
    imaging, 1457
    physical examination, 1457
    postoperative management, 1457
    results, 1457–1458
    treatment, 1457, 1457*b*
  cervical spine injuries, 1579
  hip, 942, 944*f*–945*f*
  Lisfranc, 1458–1460
    complications, 1460
    decision-making principles, 1459
    history, 1458
    imaging, 1458–1459, 1459*f*
    physical examination, 1458
    postoperative management, 1459–1460
    results, 1460
    treatment, 1459, 1460*b*, 1460*f*
  sternoclavicular joint, 673
  syndesmosis, 1453–1456
    complications, 1456
    decision-making principles, 1454
    history, 1453–1454
    imaging, 1454, 1455*f*
    physical examination, 1453–1454
    postoperative management, 1456
    results, 1456
    treatment, 1454–1456, 1456*b*
  of thoracolumbar spine, 1585–1588
Standard anterolateral portal, 711
Standard anteromedial portal, 709, 710*f*
Standing anteroposterior pelvic view, 935,
    936*f*
Standing apprehension test, 1250–1251, 1250*f*
Stasis, 180
Static standing, examination of, for patellar
    instability, 1296

Statics, 19–22
  force vectors, 21
  free-body diagrams, 20*f*, 21
  ligament and joint contact forces,
      21–22
  moment/torque vectors, 21
Stem cell-based therapy
  application, 58
  cartilage repair, 59–60
  definitions, 56–58, 57*f*–58*f*
  meniscal repair, 60
  preparations, 56–58, 57*f*–58*f*
  sports medicine, 56–58, 57*f*
Stem cells, for knee arthritis, 1280
Stenosis, cervical, 405
Sternoclavicular joint, 397, 397*f*
  injuries, 664–677
    anatomy, 667, 667*f*–670*f*
    complications, 677
    decision-making principles, 668, 673*f*
    future considerations, 677
    history, 664
    imaging, 667–668, 670*f*–672*f*
    physical examination, 664–667
    postoperative management, 677
    results, 677
    return-to-play guidelines, 677
    treatment, 673
Steroids, anabolic-androgenic, 1611
Stiff shoulder, 579–591
  acquired causes, 582–583
  anatomy, 579
  complications, 589–590
  decision-making principles, 585
  future considerations, 590
  history, 579–583
    crepitus, 581
    exacerbating factors, 580–581
    pain, 579–581, 580*b*
    relieving factors, 580–581
    stiffness, 581
    weakness, 581
  idiopathic adhesive capsulitis,
      581–582
  imaging, 584–585
  pathologies causing, 581*b*
  physical examination, 583–584
    inspection, 583, 583*f*
    motion, 584, 584*b*
    special testing, 584, 584*b*
    strength, 584, 584*b*
  postoperative management, 586–589
  primary causes, 581–582
  results, 589, 589*t*
  secondary causes, 582–583
  treatment options, 585–586, 586*b*
  technique, 586*b*–588*b*, 586*f*–588*f*
Stiffness, flexibility testing *vs.*, 27
Stimulation, electrical, for pain, 359
Stinchfield test, 932
Stingers, 406, 1570–1577, 1579
  classification, 1573–1574, 1574*t*
  decision-making principles, 1573–1574
  future considerations, 1576, 1576*f*
  history, 1570
  imaging, 1571–1573, 1573*f*
  mechanism of, 1573, 1574*f*
  physical examination, 1570–1571, 1571*f*–1572*f*,
      1572*t*
  return to play criteria, 1576
  sequela, 1576
  treatment options, 1574–1575, 1575*b*,
      1575*f*
Straight-leg raise (SLR) test, 932
Straight posterior portal, 711
Strain energy density, 26

Strains, 25–26, 26f, 1043–1052
  adductor, 1011–1012, 1050–1051
    complications, 1051
    decision-making principles, 1051
    future considerations, 1051
    history, 1050
    imaging, 1050, 1050f
    physical examination, 1050
    results, 1051
    return to play, 1051
    technique, 1051b
    treatment options, 1050–1051
  cervical, 405
    spine injuries, 1579
  hamstring, 376
    causes, 376
    preventing, 377, 377f, 377t
    risk factors, 376–377
  quadriceps, 1047–1050
    complications, 1049
    decision-making principles, 1049
    future considerations, 1050
    history, 1048
    imaging, 1048, 1048f
    physical examination, 1048
    results, 1049, 1049f
    return to play, 1049
    technique, 1049b
    treatment options, 1048–1049, 1048t, 1049f
  of thoracolumbar spine, 1585–1588
Strength testing
  in knee, 1094–1095, 1094f–1095f
  shoulder, 404
Strength training, 381
  muscular response to, 66–67
  pediatrics, 1608–1609
  in young athletes, 68
Stress, 25–26, 26f
Stress fractures, 131–139
  biomechanical factors, 131–132
  classification system, 132t
  elbow, 700
  fatigue and training errors causing, 132
  in female athlete, 131, 314
  femoral neck, 132–133, 132f–133f
  genetic factors, 132
  healing, 360, 361f
  metatarsal, 135–136
  navicular, 136, 137f
  nutrition and, 132
  olecranon, 764–765, 764f–765f
  pars, 136–137, 138f
  pediatrics, 1688–1690, 1690f
  proximal fifth metatarsal, 134–135, 135f–136f
  in thoracolumbar spine, 1584–1585
  tibial, 133–134, 134f–135f
Stress injuries, 942–944, 945f
Striae, 254, 255f
Structural disease, in elite athlete, 166–169
Stryker Intra-Compartmental Pressure Monitor,
  for compartment pressure measurement,
  1397
Subacromial decompression and rotator cuff
  repair, 550
Subacromial impingement, 548
Subarachnoid hemorrhage, 1745
Subdural hematoma, 1745
Subscapularis injury, 556–566, 557f
  anatomy, 556–557
  classification, 558
  decision-making principles, 559–560
  function, 557
  future considerations, 565–566
  history, 558–559, 558f

Subscapularis injury (Continued)
  imaging, 559, 559f
  mechanism, 557–558
  physical examination, 558–559, 558f
  treatment options, 560–565, 561f–562f
    complications, 565
    postoperative rehab, 562–564
    results, 564–565
    technique, 563b–564b, 563f–564f
Substances, performance-enhancing, 1611
Subtalar arthroscopy, 1428–1433
  complications, 1432–1433
  decision-making principles, 1429
  history, 1429
  imaging, 1429
  physical examination, 1429
  postoperative management, 1431
  results, 1431–1432
Subtalar joint, biomechanics, 1363–1365, 1363t,
  1364f–1366f
Sudden death, 116
"Sulcus sign", 405
Sunburn, 256
Superficial anatomy, of knee, 1062–1063, 1063f
Superficial bursa, 920
Superficial heat, 362–363
Superficial peroneal nerve entrapment, 1413–
  1415, 1413f
  decision-making principles, 1414
  history, 1413
  imaging, 1414
  physical examination, 1413–1414
  postoperative management, 1415
  results, 1415
  treatment options, 1414–1415, 1414b, 1414f
Superficial zone, of articular cartilage, 10, 10f
Superior gluteal nerve, 1032–1033, 1032f, 1032t
  of hip, 916
Superior labrum anterior to posterior (SLAP)
  tears, 407, 502–510, 503f–504f, 507b–508b,
  507f–508f
  débridement, 524
  decision-making principles, 505–506, 506f
  future considerations, 509
  history, 502
  imaging, 503–504, 505f
  physical examination, 502–503, 504t
  repair, 524
  treatment options, 506–509, 507f
    complications, 509
    postoperative management, 508
    results, 508–509
Superior pole osteochondrosis, 1718
Supine position, 932–933
  hip arthroscopy, 948
Supraclavicular block, 330–332, 332f
Supraclavicular pressure test, 636–638, 637f
Suprascapular block, 330
Suprascapular nerve palsy, 621–625
  anatomy, 621–622, 622f
  biomechanics, 621–622, 622f
  clinical evaluation, 622–623, 623f
  decision-making principles, 624
  diagnostic studies, 623–624, 623f
  results, 624–625
Suprascapular notch compression, 624b
Suprascapular notch decompression, 625
Sural nerve entrapment, 1402–1405, 1403f
  history, 1402
  imaging, 1403–1404
  physical examination, 1402–1403
  postoperative management, 1405
  results, 1405
  treatment options, 1404, 1404b, 1404f

Surface landmarks, in hip arthroscopy, 950
Surgery
  arthroscopic synovectomy, of knee, 1129–1130
    anterior compartments, 1129, 1130t
    posterior compartments, 1129–1130
  hamstring injuries, 1037–1039
  hip arthritis, 1058–1059
  lateral epicondylitis, 722–723, 723f
  medial epicondylitis, 722–723, 723f
  meniscal injuries
    indications, 1139–1140
    techniques, 1143–1147, 1144f
  meniscectomy, 1143–1144, 1144f
  motion, loss in elbow, 776–782, 777f
    arthroscopy, 776–781, 777f–781f
    open release, 781–782
  multiligament knee injuries, timing of, 1266
  orthopaedic, 327
  shoulder, 455–461, 456b
Surgical considerations, for lateral and
  posterolateral corner injuries of knee,
  1254–1256
  diagnostic arthroscopy, 1254, 1254f
  primary repair, 1254, 1254f
  reconstruction techniques, 1254–1255
Suture anchors, 46–47
Sutures
  anchors, 46–47
  for implants, 45–46
Sweat rate measurement, 240b
Swimmer's itch, 256
Swimming injuries, 126
  back, 126
  knee, 126
  shoulder, 126
Swipe test, 1277
Switching sticks, in arthroscopy, 108
Symptom localization, of hip, 929–930, 930f–931f
Syncope, 173
Syndesmosis sprain, 1453–1456
  complications, 1456
  decision-making principles, 1454
  history, 1453–1454
  imaging, 1454, 1455f
  physical examination, 1453–1454
  postoperative management, 1456
  results, 1456
  treatment, 1454–1456, 1456b
Synovial abrasion, 1148
Synovial facet cysts, 1601–1602
Synovial impingement syndrome, 1315–1316,
  1316f
Synovial joints, 9. See also Articular cartilage
Synovial membrane, of knee, 1071–1072, 1072f
Synthesis, in knee, 1101–1102, 1101f–1102f
Systemic illness, foot pain and, 1739

T

T1 magnetic resonance imaging, 95, 95f, 96t
T2 magnetic resonance imaging, 95, 96t
Talar tilt test, for lateral ankle sprain, 1445–1446,
  1446f
Talon noir, 254, 254f
Talus, osteochondral lesions of, 1484–1500
  complications, 1501–1502
  decision-making principles, 1486, 1486f–1487f
  diagnosis, 1484–1486
  history, 1484
  imaging, 1484–1486, 1485f
  physical examination, 1484
  postoperative management, 1500
  results, 1490–1493, 1490b
  return to play, 1500

Talus, osteochondral lesions of (Continued)
    treatment options, 1486–1490
        nonoperative, 1486–1487
        operative, 1487–1490, 1487b, 1488f
        technique, 1493b–1498b, 1494f–1498f, 1499t
Taping, 368
    ankle sprains, 380–381
    arch, 368–369
    cost effectiveness, 372
    effectiveness, 370–371
    injury prevention, 371
        ankle sprains, 371
        patellofemoral pain, 371
        plantar fasciitis, 371
        plantar fasciosis, 371
    length of effectiveness, 372
    summary, 372
    techniques
        ankle, 369, 369f–370f
        criticisms of, 371–372
        foot, 368–372, 369f
        knee, 369–370
        toe, 369
Tarsal coalition, 1725–1727, 1726f
Tarsal tunnel, magnetic resonance imaging,
    1390–1391, 1390f–1391f
Tarsal tunnel syndrome, 1407–1411, 1407f
    decision-making principles, 1408
    electrodiagnostic studies, 1408
    etiologies, 1407–1408, 1407t
    etiologies of, 1407–1408, 1407t
    history, 1408
    imaging, 1408
    physical examination, 1408
    postoperative management, 1410
    results, 1410–1411
    treatment options, 1408–1409, 1409b–1410b,
        1409f–1410f
Team medical coverage, 144–157
    ethical/legal issues in sports medicine, 155–157
        collegiate athletics, 155
        confidentiality, 155
        disagreements with coaches, 157
        drug use, 156
        high school athletics, 155
        informed consent, 156, 156t
        professional athletics, 155
    on-field emergencies, 150–155
        anaphylaxis, 153
        cardiac arrest, 153
        cervical spine injury, 152–153
        for collapsed athlete, 151–152, 151t
        emergency action plan, 150, 151b
        environmental factors, 154
        head injury, 152
        limb-threatening injuries, 154
        tension pneumothorax, 153
    preparticipation physical evaluation, 144–150
        allergies, 149
        athletes with special needs, 150
        cardiovascular system, 145–147, 145b–146b
        dermatology, 149
        ears, 145
        endocrine system, 149
        eyes, 145
        gastrointestinal system, 148
        genitourinary system, 148
        goals, 144
        head, 145
        heat illness, 149–150
        hematologic disease, 148–149
        history, 145–150
        immunizations, 149
        infectious disease, 148–149
        medications, 149
        musculoskeletal system, 148, 148b

Team medical coverage (Continued)
        neurologic system, 148
        nose, 145
        objectives, 144
        organization, 144–145
        physical examination, 145–150
        pulmonary system, 147–148
        setting, 144–145, 145t
        throat, 145
        timing, 144–145
Teeth
    fractures, 270
    primary vs. permanent, 269, 270f
Tendinitis, 4, 1320–1321
    triceps, 725–728
        complications, 727
        decision-making principles, 725–726
        future considerations, 727–728
        imaging, 725, 726f
        physical examination, 725, 725f
        postoperative management, 727
        results, 726
        return-to-play guidelines, 727
        treatment, 726, 726b
Tendinopathies, 4, 761–762
    chronic proximal hamstring, 1041
    elbow, 720–730
    patellar and quadriceps, 1320–1321
        clinical outcomes, 1331–1332, 1332f
        complications, 1333
        decision-making principles, 1327
        history, 1322–1323
        nonoperative treatment, 1327
        operative treatment, 1328
        physical examination, 1323–1324, 1323t
        postoperative management, 1330
Tendon mobilization, of subscapularis injury,
    560
Tendon repair, implants for, 35–38
Tendonitis, iliopsoas, 980
Tendons, 2–7. See also Ligaments
    Achilles, 1381–1383, 1382f–1383f
    ankle, 1381–1386
    anterior tibial, 1386, 1387f
    distal biceps rupture, 731–741
        anatomy, 731, 732f–733f
        biomechanics, 731–732
        classification, 732, 732b
        complications, 736–737
        decision-making principles, 735
        epidemiology, 731
        history, 732–733
        imaging, 733–734, 734f
        physical examination, 733, 733f
        postoperative management, 735
        results, 735–736
        treatment, 734–735, 735t, 736b, 736f
    distal triceps rupture, 737–740
        anatomy, 737, 737f
        biomechanics, 737
        classification, 737
        complications, 740
        decision-making principles, 738, 738b
        epidemiology, 737, 737b
        future considerations, 740
        history, 738
        imaging, 738
        physical examination, 738
        postoperative management, 740
        results, 740
        treatment, 738–739
    extensor
        hand, 790–791, 790f–791f
        wrist, 790–791, 790f–791f
    extracellular matrix, 3
    foot, 1381–1386

Tendons (Continued)
    gastrocnemius, 1246
    hand, 785–787, 788f
    healing
        factors affecting, 5, 6t
        methods for augmentation of, 5–7
    injuries, 3–4
        imaging, 812–813, 812f–813f
        platelet-rich plasma for, 53–54
        wrist, 812–813, 812f–813f
    long head of biceps, 424–427, 427f–428f
    peroneal, 1385–1386, 1385f–1386f
    popliteus, 1245
    posterior tibial, 1383–1384, 1383f–1384f
    quadriceps, 1318
        rupture, 1321–1322
        structure, 1320, 1320f–1321f
        tendinopathy, 1320–1321
    repair, 4–5
        platelet-rich plasma for, 53–55
    ruptures, 703–704, 704f
        distal biceps tendon, 703–704, 704f
    structure of, 2–3, 3f
    tibia
        anterior, 1386, 1387f
        injuries, 1462–1464
        posterior, 1383–1384, 1383f–1384f
Tendoscopy, for posterior tibial tendon injury,
    1467b–1468b, 1467f
Tennis injuries, 126–127
Tenocytes, 3
Tenosynovectomy, for posterior tibial tendon
    injury, 1467b–1468b
Tenosynovium, 2
Tenovagina, 2
Tension pneumothorax, 153
Tensor fascia lata, 917
Testes, injuries, 227
Testing rate, 27
Thalassemia, 196
Therapeutic interventions, 345, 345f
Thermal balance, 240
Thermogenesis, 240
Thermoregulation, 319, 1609
Thigh
    contusions, 1043–1052
        groin, 1047, 1047f
        iliac crest, 1043–1044, 1044f
        quadriceps, 1044–1047, 1044t
    regional anesthesia, 332–333
    strains, 1043–1052
        adductor, 1050–1051
        classification, 1047, 1047t
        quadriceps, 1047–1050
Thomas test, 932
Thompson test, for Achilles tendon injuries, 1477,
    1477f
Thoracic outlet syndrome (TOS), 633b
    anatomy, 634–636, 634f–635f
    classification, 632–633
    complications, 642
    decision-making principles, 639–640
    history, 636
    imaging, 638–639, 638f–639f
    physical examination, 636–638, 637f–638f
    postoperative management, 642–643
    results, 641–642
    treatment, 640–641, 641f–642f
    vascular problems and, 632–644
Thoracic spine, degenerative, 1597–1598
Thoracolumbar spine
    degenerative, 1597–1604
        discogenic low back pain, 1598–1599
        low back pain, 1598
        lumbar disc herniation, 1599–1601, 1601f
        lumbar spinal stenosis, 1602–1603, 1602f

Thoracolumbar spine *(Continued)*
    lumbar spine, 1598–1604
    radiculopathy, 1599–1601, 1600*f*
    spondylolisthesis, 1603–1604, 1603*f*–1604*f*
    synovial facet cysts, 1601–1602
    thoracic spine, 1597–1598
   injuries, 1582–1592
    burst fractures, 1584, 1585*f*
    Chance fractures, 1584, 1586*f*
    classification and severity, 1584*t*
    compression fractures, 1583–1584, 1584*f*
    contusions, 1585–1588
    decision-making principles, 1583–1591
    disc herniation, 1588, 1588*f*
    extension/extension-distraction,
      1584–1585
    fracture-dislocations, 1584, 1586*f*–1587*f*
    history, 1582
    imaging, 1583
    physical examination, 1582–1583
    postoperative management, 1592
    return to play, 1592
    risk factors, 1582, 1583*t*
    sacroiliac joint, 1591
    spinal stability, 1583
    spondylolisthesis, 1588–1591, 1590*f*
    spondylolysis, 1588, 1589*f*–1590*f*, 1591
    sprains, 1585–1588
    strains, 1585–1588
    stress fractures, 1584–1585
    thoracolumbar fractures, 1583
    treatment options, 1591
    vertebral body apophyseal avulsion fracture,
      1585
3D acquisitions, in magnetic resonance imaging,
   98, 98*f*
Throat, preparticipation physical evaluation, 145
Thromboembolic prophylaxis, 182, 183*t*–185*t*
Thromboembolism, 180
Thrombophilia, 180
Thrombosis, 180
Thrower's shoulder, 511–525
   adaptations to, 511–512
   biomechanics throwing, 512–513, 512*f*
   complications, 524
   decision-making principles, 516–517, 516*f*
   future considerations, 524–525
   history, 514
   imaging, 515–516, 516*f*
   pathophysiology, 513–514
    dynamic shoulder and scapular stability,
      513–514
    glenohumeral internal rotation deficit,
      514
    internal impingement, 513, 513*f*
   physical examination, 514–515
   results, 521–524
   treatment options, 517–518, 518*b*–521*b*,
    518*f*–520*f*
    biceps tenodesis, 518
    glenohumeral internal rotation deficit,
      518
    internal impingement, 517
    interval throwing program, 522*t*
    partial-thickness rotator cuff tears, 517
    pitching program, 523*t*
    posterior capsular contracture, 518
    SLAP tear, 517–518
Throwing
   biomechanics, 1663–1665
   injuries, 757–771
    complications, 770
    decision-making principles, 760–761
    future considerations, 770

Throwing *(Continued)*
    history, 757–758, 758*f*
    imaging, 760, 761*f*
    physical examination, 758–760, 759*f*–760*f*
    postoperative management, 768
    results, 768–770
    return to play guidelines, 768
    treatment, 761–765
   motion, 1663–1665, 1663*f*–1664*f*
Throwing cycle, 685
Thumb
   distal interphalangeal joints, 789
   injuries, 124
   ulnar collateral ligament injury, 804, 804*f*, 814,
    815*f*
Tibia
   anatomy, 1065
   proximal osteotomy, 1255, 1255*f*, 1259*b*,
    1259*f*
   stress fractures, 133–134, 134*f*–135*f*
   tendons
    anterior, 1386, 1387*f*
    injuries, 1462–1464
    posterior, 1383–1384, 1383*f*–1384*f*
   translation of, anterior/posterior, 1247–1248
Tibial inlay techniques, for posterior cruciate
   ligament injuries, 1217–1218, 1225, 1228*t*
Tibial slope, role of, 1192
Tibial spine fracture, 1615*f*
Tibial tendons
   anterior, 1386, 1387*f*
   posterior, 1383–1384, 1383*f*–1384*f*
Tibial tuberosity osteotomy (TTO), 1300–1301,
   1305*b*
Tibial tunnel, for revision anterior cruciate
   ligament injuries, 1206
Tibiofemoral joint
   biomechanics, 1074–1080
   ligaments
    biomechanics, 1075–1077, 1076*f*
    cruciate, 1077–1079
    force measurement of, 1074–1075
    lateral collateral, 1079–1080
    medial collateral, 1079–1080
    strain measurement of, 1075
Tillaux fractures, juvenile, 1730, 1730*f*
Tinea versicolor, 250*f*
Tinel test, 691, 691*f*
Tissue contrast, in MRI, 95, 95*f*–96*f*, 96*t*
Tissue engineering
   polymer fibers in, 38
   scaffolds in, 35
TissueMend implant, for tendon repair, 36
Tissues
   engineering, functional, 28–29
   graft, 30–34
    allograft, 31–32
    autograft, 30
    future direction, 33
   musculoskeletal
    articular cartilage, 9–12
    bone, 12–15
    meniscus, 7–9
    physiology pathophysiology, 2–15
    tendon and ligament in, 2–7
   neurologic, 1534–1535, 1534*f*
   storage, 27
Titin, 64
Tobacco, 292
Toe
   taping, 369
   turf, 1515–1516
    anatomic classification, 1518*t*
    complications, 1516

Toe *(Continued)*
    decision-making principles, 1515–1516
    history, 1515
    imaging, 1515, 1516*b*
    physical examination, 1515
    postoperative management, 1516
    results, 1516
    treatment options, 1516, 1517*b*, 1517*f*
Tonnis angle, 938
Torque vectors, 21
Total hip arthroplasty, hip arthritis, 1059
Tourniquets, 328–329
Trabecular pattern, 937
Traction, hip arthroscopy, 948–949
Training
   athletic, 342, 343*b*
   coordination, 381, 382*f*–383*f*
   diabetic athlete, 223
   endurance, 1607–1608
   functional, 1196–1197
   muscle, 1195–1196, 1196*f*
   muscular response to, 66–67
   neuromuscular, 69
   strength, 381, 1608–1609
   strength, in young athletes, 68
Transient quadriplegia, 1579
Transitional zone, of articular cartilage, 10, 10*f*
Transplantation, meniscal allograft, 1142
Transport, of injured athlete, 1556–1558,
   1557*f*
Transposition
   anterior intramuscular, 750, 751*f*
   anterior subcutaneous, 750, 750*f*
   anterior submuscular, 750–751, 751*f*
Transthoracic echocardiography (TTE), 164–166,
   165*f*–167*f*
Transtibial tunnel, for posterior cruciate ligament
   injuries, 1217–1218, 1225, 1228*t*
Transtriceps portal, 711
Transverse tarsal joints, kinematics and
   biomechanics, 1365, 1367*f*
Trapezium carpal injuries, 838–840, 838*f*–840*f*,
   840*b*
Trapezium fracture, 808–809, 809*f*
Trapezoid carpal injuries, 845, 845*b*
Trauma
   elbow, 699–700
   genitourinary, in athlete, 227–229
    classification, 227, 228*t*
    definition, 227, 228*t*
    diagnosis, 227–228
    epidemiology, 227
    pathobiology, 227
    pathophysiology, 227
    return-to-play guidelines, 229
    treatment, 228–229
   imaging, 699–700
Traumatic anterior instability, 1648–1651
   complications, 1651
   history, 1648, 1648*f*
   imaging, 1648–1649, 1649*f*–1650*f*
   physical examination, 1648, 1649*f*
   treatment options, 1649–1651, 1650*f*, 1651*b*,
    1652*f*
Traumatic posterior instability, 1651–1653
   history, 1651–1652
   imaging, 1652, 1653*f*
   physical examination, 1652, 1652*f*
   treatment options, 1653, 1653*f*–1654*f*
Trendelenburg gait, 929
Trephination, 1147–1148
Triangular fibrocartilage complex (TFCC)
   injuries, 813–814, 813*f*–814*f*
   arthroscopy, 828, 828*t*

Triangular fibrocartilage complex tears, 866–867
  class 1 tears (traumatic), 866
  class 2 tears (degenerative), 866–867
  Palmer classification, 867t
Triceps
  distal rupture, 737–740
    anatomy, 737, 737f
    biomechanics, 737
    classification, 737
    complications, 740
    decision-making principles, 738, 738b
    epidemiology, 737, 737b
    future considerations, 740
    history, 738
    imaging, 738
    physical examination, 738
    postoperative management, 740
    results, 740
    treatment, 738–739
  strength test, 690, 691f
  tendinitis, 725–728
    complications, 727
    decision-making principles, 725–726
    future considerations, 727–728
    history, 725
    imaging, 725, 726f
    physical examination, 725, 725f
    postoperative management, 727
    results, 726
    return-to-play guidelines, 727
    treatment, 726, 726b
      conservative, 726
      operative, 726, 727f
Tricompartmental osteoarthritis, arthroplasty for, 1283
Trigger point therapy, 367, 367f
Triquetrum carpal injuries, 836–838, 838b, 838f
Trochanteric bursae, 920–921
Trochanteric bursitis, 1001–1002, 1002b
Trochleoplasty, 1301
TruFit CB plug, 44
Tunnel grafting, 1204–1205, 1205f
Tunnel malpositioning, 1203
  correction of, 1204, 1204f
Turf toe, 1515–1516
  anatomic classification, 1518t
  complications, 1516
  decision-making principles, 1515–1516
  history, 1515
  imaging, 1515, 1516b
  injuries, 1367
  physical examination, 1515
  postoperative management, 1516
  results, 1516
  treatment options, 1516
    nonoperative, 1516
    operative, 1516
    technique, 1517b, 1517f
2D acquisitions, in magnetic resonance imaging, 98, 98f
Type 1 diabetes, 218, 221, 221f
  management, 224–225
Type 2 diabetes, 218
  management, 225

U
Ulnar collateral ligament, 684
Ulnar collateral ligament (UCL) injuries, 701–702, 701f–702f, 762–763, 762f–763f, 765b–766b, 766f, 768–770, 769f
  reconstruction, 763f
  thumb, 804, 804f, 814, 815f
Ulnar impaction syndrome, 810
Ulnar nerve, 747, 748f

Ulnar nerve compression, 691–692, 691f–692f
Ulnar neuritis, 765, 765f, 770
Ulnar neuropathy, 704, 705f. See also Cubital tunnel syndrome
Ulnar quadrant, 794t, 798–800, 799f
Ulnar styloid fracture, 1613f
Ultimate load, in biomechanics, 24–25
Ultrashort time to echo sequence, 100–101
Ultrasonography, 78–85, 946
  advantages, 84
  ankle, 1380
  disadvantages, 84–85, 85f
  dynamic, 84, 84f
    in athletic pubalgia, 1010–1011
  elastography, 83–84, 83f
  femoroacetabular impingement, 964–965
  foot, 1380
  glenohumeral joint, 411–412, 412f, 412t
  iliopsoas, 979, 983–984
  knee, 1104–1105, 1106f
  lateral and posterolateral corner injuries of knee, 1253
  musculoskeletal, 79–83, 80f–83f
  revision rotator cuff repair, 568
  scapulothoracic disorders, 614, 614f–615f
  technical considerations, 78–79, 79f
  thermal effects, 363
Uncovertebral joints, 1594
Units of measure, 16, 17t
Unstable fractures, of cervical spine, 1541–1543
  complications, 1543
  decision-making principles, 1542
  future considerations, 1543
  history, 1541
  imaging, 1541–1542, 1542f
  physical examination, 1541
  postoperative management, 1543
  results, 1543
  treatment options, 1542–1543, 1542b
Upper extremity
  injuries
    figure skating, 118
    football, 118
    gymnastics, 120
    ice hockey, 121
    rowing, 123
    snowboarding, 124–125
    soccer, 125
    tennis, 127
  innervation, 330
Upper gastrointestinal tract conditions, 189–192
  dyspepsia, 191–192
  dysphagia, 192
  functional heartburn, 191
  gastroesophageal reflux disease, 190–191
  nausea, 192
  vomiting, 192
Upper respiratory tract infections (URTIs), 206–209
  diagnosis, 207
  epidemiology, 206
  infectious mononucleosis, 207–208
  measles, 208–209
  pathobiology, 206–207
  prevention, 207
  return-to-play guidelines, 207
  treatment, 207
Urticaria, 257, 258f
URTIs. See Upper respiratory tract infections

V
Vail Sport Test, 387
Valgus extension overload (VEO), 763–764, 770
Valgus stress testing, in medial collateral ligament and posterior medial corner injuries, 1232

Varus motion, 1246–1247
Varus talar tilt test, 1377–1379
Vascular system, thoracic outlet syndrome, 632–644
Vascular tendons, 2
Vascularization
  capsule, 916, 917f
  knee, 1072
Vectors, 16, 18f
  force, 19f–20f, 21
  moment/torque, 21
Velocity, 22
Venous thromboembolism (VTE), 180–181
Ventilator anaerobic threshold, 71–72
VEO. See Valgus extension overload
Verruca vulgaris (common warts), 251–252, 252f
Vertebral body apophyseal avulsion fracture, 1585
Vincula, 2
Viral infections, 250–252
  herpes simplex, 250–251, 251f
  molluscum contagiosum, 252, 252f
  verruca vulgaris (common warts), 251–252, 252f
Virchow triad, 180
Viscoelasticity, 24, 24f–25f
Viscosupplementation, for knee arthritis, 1280
Visually impaired athletes, 323
  adaptive equipment, 323
  exercise, 323
  medical considerations, 323
    flight dysrhythmia, 323
    musculoskeletal injuries, 323
Vitamin D, 279–280
Vitamins, 279–280
Volar quadrant, 794t, 800–801, 800f, 802f–803f
Volleyball injuries, 127–128
  ankle, 127
  back pain, 128
  concussion, 128
  finger, 127–128
  knee, 127
  shoulder, 128
  wrist, 127–128
Vomiting, 192
von Willebrand disease (vWD), 199
VTE. See Venous thromboembolism

W
Wall push-up, 613
Wartenberg syndrome, 902
Warts, common, 251–252, 252f
Waterborne diseases, 210–213
  cryptosporidiosis, 211–212
  fecally derived, 211
    non, 213–214
    other, 212–213
  infectious diarrhea, 212
Weight loss, knee arthritis and, 1279
Weight-loss-related injuries, 129
Wheelchair athletes, 317–320
  adaptive equipment, 320
  exercise physiology, 317–318
  medical considerations, 318–320
    autonomic dysreflexia, 319–320
    heterotopic ossification, 319
    musculoskeletal injuries, 318
    neurogenic bladder and bowel, 319
    peripheral nerve entrapment, 319
    pressure sores/ulcers, 319
    spasticity, 319
    thermoregulation, 319
Whiplash injury, 405
White blood cell scans, labeled, 89–90, 91f
Windlass mechanism, 1365–1367, 1367f–1368f
Wolff-Parkinson-White (WPW) syndrome, 172

Women. *See Female athlete*
WPW. *See* Wolff-Parkinson-White (WPW)
    syndrome
Wrestling injuries, 128–129
    musculoskeletal, 128–129
    skin infections, 129
    soft tissue, 129
    weight-loss-related issues, 129
Wright test, 636–638, 637f
Wrist, 785–792
    anatomy, 789–790, 790f, 792f
    arthroscopy, 817–834
        anatomy, 819–820, 820f–821f
        carpal instability, 821–824, 821t, 822f–823f
        class I traumatic injuries, 829–832, 829f–831f
        class II degenerative injuries, 832
        complications, 833
        fracture, 824–828
        future considerations, 833
        ganglionectomy, 832–833, 832f
        management, 829–832, 829f–831f
        set-up, 817–819, 818f–819f
        triangular fibrocartilage complex, 828, 828t
    biomechanics, 789–790, 790f, 835
    carpal injuries, 835–848
    decision-making principles, 793–805
    diagnosis, 793–805
    extensor tendons, 790–791, 790f–791f
    flexors, 791
    history, 793–794
    imaging, 806–816, 807f
        carpal fractures, 807–809
        distal radius fractures, 806–807
        intrinsic carpal ligament injury, 810–812,
            811f
        Kienböck disease, 810
        perilunate dislocation, 809–810, 810f

Wrist *(Continued)*
        tendon injuries, 812–813, 812f–813f
        triangular fibrocartilage complex injury,
            813–814, 813f–814f
        ulnar impaction syndrome, 810
    injuries
        golf, 120
        rowing, 123
        tendons, 812–813, 812f–813f
        volleyball, 127–128
    neuropathies, 898–905
        decision-making principles, 901
        future considerations, 904
        history, 898
        imaging, 900–901, 900f, 901t
        physical examination, 898–900, 899f–900f
        postoperative management and return to
            play, 902–903, 903b, 903f
        results, 903–904
        treatment options, 901–902
    pediatric, 1623–1625
        acute injuries, 1623–1624, 1623f
        overuse injuries, 1624–1625, 1624f–1626f
    physical examination, 793–794, 794f
    quadrants
        dorsal, 794t, 796–798, 797f–798f
        radial, 794–796, 794t, 795f–796f
        ulnar, 794t, 798–800, 799f
        volar, 794t, 800–801, 800f, 802f–803f
Wrist/hand injuries
    pediatrics, 1677–1687
        distal radial physeal stress reaction,
            1683–1684
        finger fractures, 1677–1681
        future considerations, 1684
        jammed finger, 1681–1683
        scaphoid fracture, 1684–1686

Wrist tendinopathies, 857–864
    complications, 863
    De Quervain tenosynovitis, 859–860, 859f
        postoperative management and return to
            sports, 860
        treatment options, 859, 859b, 860f
    extensor carpi ulnaris tendinopathy, 861–862
        classification, 861
        criteria for return to sports, 861–862
        special tests, 861
        treatment options, 861
    flexor carpi radialis tendinopathy, 862
    flexor carpi ulnaris tendinopathy, 862–863,
        862b, 862f–863f
    future considerations, 863–864
    history, 857–858
    imaging, 858–859, 858f
    intersection syndrome, 860–861, 860f
        return to sports, 861
        treatment options, 860–861, 861b
    physical examination, 858
    results, 863, 863f

Y

Y-balance test, 387, 388f
Yergason test, 405
Young athlete, 1606–1614. *See also* Pediatrics

Z

Zimmer Collagen Repair Patch, 36–37
Zona orbicularis, 914

FIFTH EDITION

DeLee, Drez, & Miller's
Orthopaedic Sports Medicine

Principles and Practice

Mark D. Miller, MD
S. Ward Casscells Professor of Orthopaedic Surgery
Head, Division of Sports Medicine
University of Virginia
Charlottesville, Virginia
Adjunctive Clinical Professor and Team Physician
James Madison University
Harrisonburg, Virginia

Stephen R. Thompson, MD, MEd, FRCSC
Associate Professor of Sports Medicine
Eastern Maine Medical Center
University of Maine
Bangor, Maine

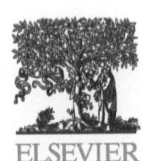

ELSEVIER

DELEE, DREZ, & MILLER'S ORTHOPAEDIC SPORTS MEDICINE,
FIFTH EDITION

ISBN: 978-0-323-54473-3

Notices

Knowledge and best practice in this field are constantly changing. As new research and experience
broaden our understanding, changes in research methods, professional practices, or medical treatment
may become necessary.

Practitioners and researchers must always rely on their own experience and knowledge in evaluating
and using any information, methods, compounds, or experiments described herein. In using such
information or methods they should be mindful of their own safety and the safety of others, including
parties for whom they have a professional responsibility.

With respect to any drug or pharmaceutical products identified, readers are advised to check the most
current information provided (i) on procedures featured or (ii) by the manufacturer of each product to
be administered, to verify the recommended dose or formula, the method and duration of
administration, and contraindications. It is the responsibility of practitioners, relying on their own
experience and knowledge of their patients, to make diagnoses, to determine dosages and the best
treatment for each individual patient, and to take all appropriate safety precautions.

To the fullest extent of the law, neither the Publisher nor the authors, contributors, or editors, assume
any liability for any injury and/or damage to persons or property as a matter of products liability,
negligence or otherwise, or from any use or operation of any methods, products, instructions, or ideas
contained in the material herein.

Previous editions copyrighted 2015, 2010, 2003, 1994.

International Standard Book Number: 978-0-323-54473-3

Senior Content Strategist: Kristine Jones
Senior Content Development Specialist: Joan Ryan
Publishing Services Manager: Catherine Jackson
Senior Project Manager: Amanda Mincher
Design Direction: Ryan Cook

Printed in the United States of America

Last digit is the print number: 9 8 7 6 5 4

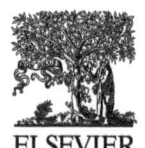

1600 John F. Kennedy Blvd.
Ste 1600
Philadelphia, PA 19103-2899

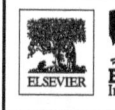

Working together
to grow libraries in
developing countries

www.elsevier.com • www.bookaid.org

Amiethab A. Aiyer, MD
Assistant Professor, Chief Foot and Ankle Service
Department of Orthopaedics
University of Miami, Miller School of Medicine
Miami, Florida
Leg, Ankle, and Foot

Asheesh Bedi, MD
Chief, Sports Medicine and Shoulder Surgery
Professor of Orthopaedics
Head Orthopaedic Team Physician
University of Michigan
Ann Arbor, Michigan
Basic Principles

Stephen F. Brockmeier, MD
Associate Professor
Department of Orthopaedic Surgery
Fellowship Director, University of Virginia Sports Medicine
Fellowship
University of Virginia School of Medicine
Charlottesville, Virginia
Shoulder

Rajwinder Deu, MD
Assistant Professor
Department of Orthopaedics
Johns Hopkins University
Baltimore, Maryland
Medical

F. Winston Gwathmey, Jr., MD
Associate Professor of Orthopaedic Surgery
University of Virginia School of Medicine
Charlottesville, Virginia
Pelvis, Hip, and Thigh

Joe M. Hart, PhD, ATC
Associate Professor
Department of Kinesiology
University of Virginia
Charlottesville, Virginia
Rehabilitation and Injury Prevention

Anish R. Kadakia, MD
Associate Professor of Orthopaedic Surgery
Northwestern Memorial Hospital
Northwestern University Feinberg School of Medicine
Chicago, Illinois
Leg, Ankle, and Foot

Sanjeev Kakar, MD, FAOA
Professor of Orthopaedic Surgery
Mayo Clinic
Rochester, Minnesota
Elbow, Wrist, and Hand

Morteza Khodaee, MD, MPH, FACSM, FAAFP
Associate Professor
University of Colorado School of Medicine
Department of Family Medicine and Orthopaedics
Denver, Colorado
Medical

Bryson Lesniak, MD
Associate Professor
University of Pittsburgh Medical Center
Rooney Sports Complex
Pittsburgh, Pennsylvania
Basic Principles

Eric C. McCarty, MD
Chief, Sports Medicine and Shoulder Surgery
Associate Professor
Department of Orthopaedics
University of Colorado School of Medicine
Director Sports Medicine, Head Team Physician
University of Colorado Department of Athletics
Associate Professor, Adjunct
Department of Integrative Physiology
University of Colorado
Boulder, Colorado
Knee

Matthew D. Milewski, MD
Assistant Professor
Division of Sports Medicine
Department of Orthopaedic Surgery
Boston Children's Hospital
Boston, Massachusetts
Pediatric Sports Medicine

Francis H. Shen, MD
Warren G. Stamp Endowed Professor
Division Head, Spine Division
Co-Director, Spine Center
Department of Orthopaedic Surgery
University of Virginia
Charlottesville, Virginia
Spine and Head

What's in a name? In developing and editing the fifth edition of DeLee, Drez, & Miller's Orthopaedic Sports Medicine: Principles and Practices, we considered removing "orthopaedic" from the title. In an effort to keep pace with the rapidly growing specialty of sports medicine that includes internal medicine, pediatrics, rehabilitation medicine, athletic training, as well as orthopedics and many other disciplines, it is essential to expand the book's focus beyond orthopedics and address a more all-inclusive vision of sports medicine. Regardless of how sports medicine touches your individual practice, this updated version of this classic textbook remains the most comprehensive in the field.

As sports medicine continues to evolve, the need to include additional topics is essential. For this fifth edition, one focus is addressing problems of revision surgery. Important new chapters have been added on revision shoulder instability, revision rotator cuff, and revision anterior cruciate ligament surgery. Additionally, we have fine-tuned the organization of chapters under the dutiful watch of section editors. The hand section has been revised to include more comprehensive chapters on sports-related injuries. The hip section has been updated to reflect the current thinking on the hottest new topics in sports medicine, including new chapters on posterior hip pain and peritrochanteric lesions.

And the non-operative sections have been extensively edited and expanded, to include new information on sports nutrition, psychological adjustment to athletic injury and genitourinary trauma in the athlete.

Incredibly, there are over 300 contributors to this new edition, many of whom are widely regarded as the foremost experts in their fields. To each of them, we extend heartfelt gratitude for their willingness to participate and share their knowledge. Similarly, we would be remiss if we did not thank our outstanding section editors: Drs. Bedi, Lesniak, Khodaee, Deu, Hart, Brockmeier, Kakar, Gwathmey, McCarty, Kadakia, Aiyer, Shen, and Milewski. They did the heavy lifting in the publishing process and we are deeply appreciative of their efforts.

It remains a distinct honor and pleasure to continue the tradition of Drs. Jesse DeLee and David Drez, who first produced this text in 1994. We hope it enables practitioners to remain on the cutting edge of sports medicine to the benefit of the widest possible spectrum of athletes and patients under our collective care.

Mark D. Miller
Stephen R. Thompson

CONTRIBUTORS

Kathleen C. Abalos, MD
Department of Medicine
Beth Israel Deaconess Medical Center
Boston, Massachusetts

Jeffrey S. Abrams, MD
Clinical Professor
School of Graduate Medicine
Seton Hall University
South Orange, New Jersey
Clinical Associate Professor
Penn Medicine Princeton Medical Center
Princeton, New Jersey

Julie E. Adams, MD
Professor of Orthopedic Surgery
Mayo Clinic Health System
Austin, Minnesota and Rochester, Minnesota

Bayan Aghdasi, MD
Orthopaedic Surgery
University of Virginia
Charlottesville, Virginia

Amiethab A. Aiyer, MD
Assistant Professor, Chief Foot and Ankle
    Service
Department of Orthopaedics
University of Miami, Miller School of
    Medicine
Miami, Florida

Nourbakhsh Ali, MD
Spine Surgeon
Wellstar Atlanta Medical Center
Atlanta, Georgia

David W. Altchek, MD
Co-Chief Emeritus
Sports Medicine and Shoulder Service
Hospital for Special Surgery
New York, New York

Raj M. Amin, MD
Resident Physician
Department of Orthopaedic Surgery
The Johns Hopkins Hospital
Baltimore, Maryland

Kimberly K. Amrami, MD
Professor of Radiology
Chair, Division of Musculoskeletal Radiology
Mayo Clinic
Rochester, Minnesota

Christian N. Anderson, MD
Orthopaedic Surgeon
Tennessee Orthopaedic Alliance/The
    Lipscomb Clinic
Nashville, Tennessee

Lindsay M. Andras, MD
Assistant Professor of Orthopaedic Surgery
Children's Orthopedic Center
Children's Hospital Los Angeles
Los Angeles, California

James R. Andrews, MD
Medical Director
The Andrews Institute
Gulf Breeze, Florida
Medical Director
The American Sports Medicine Institute
Birmingham, Alabama

**Michael Antonis, DO, RDMS, FACEP,
CAQSM**
Emergency Medicine & Sports Medicine
Georgetown University
Washington, District of Columbia

Chad A. Asplund, MD, MPH
Director, Athletic Medicine
Associate Professor, Health and Kinesiology
Georgia Southern University
Statesboro, Georgia

Rachid Assina, MD, RPH
Assistant Professor
Department of Neurological Surgery
Rutgers–New Jersey Medical School
Newark, New Jersey

Ashley V. Austin, MD
Resident
Family Medicine and Physical Medicine and
    Rehabilitation
University of Virginia
Charlottesville, Virginia

Luke S. Austin, MD
Associate Professor of Orthopaedics
Rothman Institute
Egg Harbor Township, New Jersey

John T. Awowale, MD
Orthopedic Surgery
University of Wisconsin Hospitals and
    Clinics
University of Wisconsin
Madison, Wisconsin

Derek P. Axibal, MD
Department of Orthopedics
University of Colorado School of Medicine
Aurora, Colorado

Bernard R. Bach Jr., MD
The Claude Lambert-Helen Thompson
    Professor of Orthopedic Surgery
Rush University Medical Center
Chicago, Illinois

Aaron L. Baggish, MD
Director, Cardiovascular Performance
    Program
Massachusetts General Hospital
Boston, Massachusetts

Wajeeh Bakhsh, MD
Surgical Resident, Department of
    Orthopaedics
University of Rochester Medical Center
Rochester, New York

Christopher P. Bankhead, MD
Resident, Orthopaedic Surgery
University of New Mexico
Albuquerque, New Mexico

Michael G. Baraga, MD
Assistant Professor of Orthopaedics
UHealth Sports Medicine Institute
University of Miami, Miller School of
    Medicine
Miami, Florida

Jonathan Barlow, MD, MS
Mayo Clinic
Rochester, Minnesota

Robert W. Battle, MD
Team Cardiologist
Associate Professor of Medicine and
    Pediatrics
Department of Cardiology
University of Virginia Medical Center
Charlottesville, Virginia

Matthew Bessette, MD
Sports Medicine Fellow
The Cleveland Clinic Foundation
Cleveland, Ohio

Thomas M. Best, MD, PhD
Professor of Orthopaedics
Research Director of Sports Performance
    and Wellness Institute
University of Miami Sports Medicine Institute
Miami, Florida

Bruce Beynnon, PhD
McClure Professor of Musculoskeletal
    Research
Director of Research
Department of Orthopaedics and
    Rehabilitation
University of Vermont College of Medicine
McClure Musculoskeletal Research Center
Burlington, Vermont

Kieran Bhattacharya, BS
Research Assistant
Department of Orthopaedic Surgery
University of Virginia
Charlottesville, Virginia

Debdut Biswas, MD
Hinsdale Orthopaedics
Chicago, Illinois

Matthew H. Blake, MD
Assistant Director, Sports Medicine
Orthopaedic Sports Medicine
Avera McKennan Hospital and University
    Health Center
Sioux Falls, South Dakota

Liljiana Bogunovic
Assistant Professor
Department of Orthopaedic Surgery
Washington University School of Medicine
St. Louis, Missouri

Margaret Boushell, PhD
Department of Biomedical Engineering
Biomaterials and Interface Tissue
    Engineering Laboratory
Columbia University Medical Center
New York Presbyterian Hospital
New York, New York

James P. Bradley, MD
Clinical Professor
Orthopaedic Surgery
University of Pittsburgh Medical Center
Pittsburgh, Pennsylvania

William Brady, MD, FAAEM, FACEP
Professor of Medicine and Emergency
    Medicine
University of Virginia
Charlottesville, Virginia

Jonathan T. Bravman, MD
Assistant Professor
Director of Sports Medicine Research
CU Sports Medicine
Division of Sports Medicine and Shoulder
    Surgery
University of Colorado
Denver, Colorado

Stephen F. Brockmeier, MD
Associate Professor
Department of Orthopaedic Surgery
Fellowship Director, University of Virginia
    Sports Medicine Fellowship
University of Virginia School of Medicine
Charlottesville, Virginia

Jeffrey Brunelli, MD
Assistant Professor of Orthopaedic Surgery
    and Rehabilitation
Chief, Sports Medicine and Shoulder
    Surgery
University of Florida-Jacksonville College of
    Medicine
Jacksonville, Florida

Jackie Buell, PhD, RD, CSSD, LD, ATC
Assistant Professor, Clinical Health Sciences
    and Medical Dietetics
The Ohio State University
Columbus, Ohio

Alissa J. Burge, MD
Assistant Professor of Radiology
Weill Cornell Medicine
New York, New York

**Jessica L. Buschmann, MS, RD, CSSD,
LD**
Clinical Dietician—Board Certified
    Specialist in Sports Dietetics Sports
    Medicine
Nationwide Children's Hospital
Columbus, Ohio

Brian Busconi, MD
Associate Professor of Orthopaedic Surgery
Sports Medicine
University of Massachusetts
Worcester, Massachusetts

Charles A. Bush-Joseph, MD
Professor of Orthopaedic Surgery
Division of Sports Medicine
Rush University Medical Center
Chicago, Illinois

Kadir Buyukdogan, MD
Department of Orthopaedic Surgery
University of Virginia
Charlottesville, Virginia

E. Lyle Cain Jr., MD
Founding Partner
Andrews Sports Medicine and Orthopaedic
    Center
Fellowship Director
American Sports Medicine Institute
Birmingham, Alabama

Jon-Michael E. Caldwell, MD
Resident, Department of Orthopedic
    Surgery
Columbia University Medical Center
New York Presbyterian Hospital
New York, New York

Mary E. Caldwell, DO
Assistant Professor of Physical Medicine and
    Rehabilitation and Sports Medicine
Medical College of Virginia
Virginia Commonwealth University
Richmond, Virginia

Ryan P. Calfee, MD, MSc
Associate Professor of Orthopedics
Washington University School of Medicine
St. Louis, Missouri

Christopher L. Camp, MD
Assistant Professor of Orthopedics
Mayo Clinic
Rochester, Minnesota

John T. Campbell, MD
Attending Orthopaedic Surgeon
Institute for Foot and Ankle Reconstruction
Mercy Medical Center
Baltimore, Maryland

Kevin Caperton, MD
Department of Orthopedics and Sports
    Medicine
Georgetown Orthopedics
Georgetown, Texas

Robert M. Carlisle, MD
Resident, Orthopaedic Surgery
Greenville Health System
Greenville, South Carolina

Rebecca A. Cerrato, MD
Attending Orthopaedic Surgeon
Institute for Foot and Ankle Reconstruction
Baltimore, Maryland

Courtney Chaaban, PT, DPT, SCS
Doctoral Student
Sports Medicine Research Laboratory
Department of Exercise and Sport Science
University of North Carolina at Chapel Hill
Chapel Hill, North Carolina

Jorge Chahla, MD
Regenerative Sports Medicine Fellow
Center for Regenerative Sports Medicine
Steadman Philippon Research Institute
Vail, Colorado

Peter N. Chalmers, MD
Assistant Professor
University of Utah Department of
    Orthopaedic Surgery
Salt Lake City, Utah

Angela K. Chang, MD
Center for Outcomes-Based Orthopaedic
    Research
Steadman Philippon Research Institute
Vail, Colorado

Sonia Chaudhry, MD
Assistant Professor of Orthopaedic Surgery
University of Connecticut School of
    Medicine
Pediatric Orthopaedic, Hand, and
    Microvascular Surgery
Connecticut Children's Medical Center
Hartford, Connecticut

Austin W. Chen, MD
Hip Preservation and Sports Medicine
BoulderCentre for Orthopedics
Boulder, Colorado
Academic Faculty
American Hip Institute
Chicago, Illinois

Edward C. Cheung, MD
Resident Physician
Orthopaedic Surgery
University of California, Los Angeles
    Medical Center
Los Angeles, California

A. Bobby Chhabra, MD
Lillian T. Pratt Distinguished Professor and
    Chair
Orthopaedic Surgery
University of Virginia Health System
Charlottesville, Virginia

Woojin Cho, MD, PhD
Assistant Professor, Orthopaedic Surgery
Albert Einstein College of Medicine
Chief of Spine Surgery
Orthopaedic Surgery
Research Director
Multidisciplinary Spine Center
Montefiore Medical Center
New York, New York

Joseph N. Chorley, MD
Associate Professor of Pediatrics
Baylor College of Medicine
Houston, Texas

John Jared Christophel, MD, MPH
Assistant Professor of Otolaryngology—
    Head and Neck Surgery
University of Virginia
Charlottesville, Virginia

Philip Chuang, PhD
Department of Biomedical Engineering
Biomaterials and Interface Tissue
    Engineering Laboratory
Columbia University Medical Center
New York Presbyterian Hospital
New York, New York

Nicholas J. Clark, MD
Orthopedic Surgeon
Mayo Clinic
Rochester, Minnesota

John C. Clohisy, MD
Professor of Orthopaedic Surgery
Washington University School of Medicine
St. Louis, Missouri

Christopher Coleman, MD
Department of Radiology
University of Colorado
Aurora, Colorado

Francisco Contreras, MD
Department of Radiology
Jackson Memorial Hospital
University of Miami Hospital
Miami, Florida

Joseph D. Cooper, MD
Resident, Orthopaedic Surgery
University of Southern California
Los Angeles, California

Chris A. Cornett, MD, MPT
Associate Professor of Orthopaedic Surgery
University of Nebraska Medical Center
Department of Orthopaedic Surgery and
    Rehabilitation
Medical Director Physical/Occupational
    Therapy
Co-Medical Director, Spine Program
Nebraska Medicine
Omaha, Nebraska

Paul S. Corotto, MD
Chief Fellow
Department of Cardiology
University of Virginia Medical Center
Charlottesville, Virginia

Ryan P. Coughlin, MD, FRCSC
Department of Orthopaedic Surgery
Duke University
Durham, North Carolina

Jared A. Crasto, MD
Resident, Department of Orthopaedic
    Surgery
University of Pittsburgh Medical Center
Pittsburgh, Pennsylvania

Shannon David, PhD, ATC
Assistant Professor
Coordinator of Clinical Education
North Dakota State University
Fargo, North Dakota

Thomas M. DeBerardino, MD
Orthopaedic Surgeon
The Orthopaedic Institute
Medical Director
Burkhart Research Institute for
    Orthopaedics
The San Antonio Orthopaedic Group
Co-Director, Combined Baylor College of
    Medicine and The San Antonio
    Orthopaedic Group, Texas Sports
    Medicine Fellowship
Professor of Orthopaedic Surgery
Baylor College of Medicine
San Antonio, Texas

Richard E. Debski, PhD
Professor
Departments of Bioengineering and
    Orthopaedic Surgery
University of Pittsburgh
Pittsburgh, Pennsylvania

Marc M. DeHart, MD
Associate Professor of Orthopaedic Surgery
Chief of Adult Reconstruction
UT Health San Antonio
San Antonio, Texas

Arthur Jason De Luigi, DO, MHSA
Professor of Rehabilitation Medicine and
    Sports Medicine
Georgetown University School of Medicine
Washington, District of Columbia

Elizabeth R. Dennis, MD, MS
Resident, Department of Orthopedic
    Surgery
Columbia University Medical Center
New York Presbyterian Hospital
New York, New York

John J. Densmore, MD, PhD
Associate Professor of Clinical Medicine
Division of Hematology/Oncology
University of Virginia
Charlottesville, Virginia

Joshua S. Dines, MD
Sports Medicine and Shoulder Service
Hospital for Special Surgery
New York, New York

Benjamin G. Domb, MD
Founder
American Hip Institute
Chicago, Illinois

Jason Dragoo, MD
Associate Professor of Orthopaedic Surgery
Stanford University
Stanford, California

Jeffrey R. Dugas, MD
Surgeon
Andrews Sports Medicine and Orthopaedic
    Center
American Sports Medicine Institute
Birmingham, Alabama

Guillaume D. Dumont, MD
Assistant Professor of Orthopaedic Surgery
University of South Carolina School of
    Medicine
Columbia, South Carolina

Eric W. Edmonds, MD
Associate Professor of Clinical Orthopedic
    Surgery
University of California, San Diego
Director of Orthopedic Research and Sports
    Medicine
Division of Orthopedic Surgery
Rady Children's Hospital San Diego
San Diego, California

Karen P. Egan, PhD
Associate Sport Psychologist
Department of Athletics
University of Virginia
Charlottesville, Virginia

Bassem T. Elhassan, MD
Orthopedic Surgeon
Mayo Clinic
Rochester, Minnesota

Claire D. Eliasberg, MD
Resident, Orthopaedic Surgery
Hospital for Special Surgery
New York, New York

Fatih Ertem, MSc
Department of Biomechanics
Dokuz Eylul University Health Science
    Institute
Inciralti, Izmir, Turkey
Visiting Graduate Researcher
Department of Orthopaedics and
    Rehabilitation
McClure Musculoskeletal Research Center
Burlington, Vermont

Norman Espinosa Jr., MD
Head of Foot and Ankle Surgery
Institute for Foot and Ankle Reconstruction
FussInsitut Zurich
Zurich, Switzerland

Anthony Essilfie, MD
Resident Physician
Orthopaedic Surgery
University of Southern California
Los Angeles, California

Jack Farr, MD
Professor of Orthopedics
Indiana University School of Medicine
OrthoIndy Knee Preservation and Cartilage
    Restoration Center
Indianapolis, Indiana

Derek M. Fine, MD
Associate Professor of Medicine
Fellowship Director
Division of Nephrology
The Johns Hopkins University School of
    Medicine
Baltimore, Maryland

Jake A. Fox, BS
Research Assistant
Center for Outcomes-Based Orthopaedic
    Research
Steadman Philippon Research Institute
Vail, Colorado

Salvatore Frangiamore, MD, MS
Summa Health Orthopaedic and Sports
    Medicine
Akron, Ohio

Rachel M. Frank, MD
Department of Orthopaedic Surgery
Rush University
Chicago, Illinois

Heather Freeman, PT, DHS
Physical Therapist
Assistant Research Coordinator
University of Indianapolis, Krannert School
    of Physical Therapy
Indianapolis, Indiana

Jason Freeman, PhD
Sport Psychologist
Department of Athletics
University of Virginia
Charlottesville, Virginia

Nikhita Gadi, MD, MScBR
Internal Medicine Resident, PGY-1
Hackensack University Medical Center
Hackensack, New Jersey

Seth C. Gamradt, MD
Associate Clinical Professor
Director of Orthopaedic Athletic Medicine
Orthopaedic Surgery
University of Southern California
Los Angeles, California

J. Craig Garrison, PhD, PT, ATC, SCS
Director, Sports Medicine Research
Texas Health Sports Medicine
Texas Health
Fort Worth, Texas

R. Glenn Gaston, MD
Hand and Upper Extremity Surgeon
OrthoCarolina
Chief of Hand Surgery
Division of Orthopedics
Carolinas Medical Center
Charlotte, North Carolina

William B. Geissler, MD
Alan E. Freeland Chair of Hand Surgery
Professor and Chief
Division of Hand and Upper Extremity
    Surgery
Chief, Arthroscopic Surgery and Sports
    Medicine
Department of Orthopaedic Surgery and
    Rehabilitation
University of Mississippi Health Care
Jackson, Mississippi

Brandee Gentile, MS, ATC
Athletic Trainer
Department of Neurosurgery
Rutgers–New Jersey Medical School
Newark, New Jersey

J. Robert Giffin, MD, FRCSC, MBA
Professor of Orthopedic Surgery
Western University
London, Ontario, Canada

Todd M. Gilbert, MD
Department of Orthopaedic Surgery and
    Rehabilitation
University of Nebraska Medical Center
Omaha, Nebraska

G. Keith Gill, MD
Department of Orthopaedics
University of New Mexico Health Sciences
    Center
Albuquerque, New Mexico

Thomas J. Gill, MD
Professor of Orthopedic Surgery
Tufts Medical School
Chairman, Department of Orthopedic
    Surgery
St. Elizabeth's Medical Center/Steward
    Healthcare Network
Boston, Massachusetts

Jacob D. Gire, MD
Department of Orthopaedic Surgery
Stanford University
Palo Alto, California

Pau Golanó, MD
Professor of Human Anatomy
Laboratory of Arthroscopic and Surgical
    Anatomy
Human Anatomy and Embryology Unit
Department of Pathology and Experimental
    Therapeutics
University of Barcelona–Spain
Department of Orthopaedic Surgery
University of Pittsburgh School of Medicine
Pittsburgh, Pennsylvania

Jorge E. Gómez, MD, MS
Associate Professor of Adolescent Medicine
    and Sports Medicine
Baylor College of Medicine
Houston, Texas

Juan Gomez-Hoyos, MD
Baylor University Medical Center at Dallas
Hip Preservation Center
Dallas, Texas

Howard P. Goodkin, MD, PhD
The Shure Professor of Pediatric Neurology
Director
Division of Pediatric Neurology
Departments of Neurology and Pediatrics
University of Virginia
Charlottesville, Virginia

Gregory Grabowski, MD, FAOA
Associate Professor
University of South Carolina School of
    Medicine
Department of Orthopedic Surgery
Co-Medical Director
Palmetto Health USC Spine Center
Residency Program Director
Palmetto Health USC Orthopedic Center
Columbia, South Carolina

Tinker Gray, MA
The Shelbourne Knee Center at Community
    East Hospital
Indianapolis, Indiana

James R. Gregory, MD
Assistant Professor of Pediatric Orthopedic
    Surgery
Department of Orthopedic Surgery
University of Oklahoma College of
    Medicine
Oklahoma City, Oklahoma

Phillip Gribble, PhD
Professor of Rehabilitation Sciences
University of Kentucky
Lexington, Kentucky

Letha Y. Griffin, MD, PhD
Team Physician
Georgia State University
Atlanta, Georgia
Staff
Peachtree Orthopedics
Atlanta, Georgia

Warren C. Hammert, MD
Professor of Orthopaedic Surgery and
    Plastic Surgery
Chief, Hand Surgery
Department of Orthopaedics and
    Rehabilitation
University of Rochester Medical Center
Rochester, New York

Kyle E. Hammond, MD
Assistant Professor, Department of
    Orthopaedic Surgery
Emory Sports Medicine Center
Atlanta, Georgia

**Joseph Hannon, PhD, PT, DPT, SCS,
CSCS**
Research Physical Therapist
Texas Health Sports Medicine
Texas Health
Fort Worth, Texas

Colin B. Harris, MD
Assistant Professor
Department of Orthopaedics
Rutgers–New Jersey Medical School
Newark, New Jersey

Joshua D. Harris, MD
Orthopedic Surgeon
Associate Professor, Institute for Academic
    Medicine
Houston Methodist Orthopedics and Sports
    Medicine
Houston, Texas
Assistant Professor of Clinical Orthopedic
    Surgery
Weill Cornell Medical College
New York, New York

Andrew Haskell, MD
Chair, Department of Orthopedics
Geographic Medical Director for Surgical
    Services
Palo Alto Medical Foundation
Palo Alto, California
Associate Clinical Professor
Department of Orthopaedic Surgery
University of California, San Francisco
San Francisco, California

Hamid Hassanzadeh, MD
Assistant Professor
Department of Orthopaedic Surgery
University of Virginia
Charlottesville, Virginia

Michael R. Hausman, MD
Professor of Orthopaedic Surgery
Mount Sinai Medical Center
New York, New York

Stefan Hemmings, MBBS
Post-Doctorate Fellow
Division of Nephrology
The Johns Hopkins University School of
    Medicine
Baltimore, Maryland

R. Frank Henn III, MD
Associate Professor of Orthopaedics
University of Maryland School of Medicine
Baltimore, Maryland

Daniel Herman, MD, PhD
Assistant Professor
Department of Orthopedics and Rehabilitation
Divisions of Physical Medicine and
    Rehabilitation, Sports Medicine, and
    Research
University of Florida
Gainesville, Florida

Jay Hertel, PhD, ATC, FNATA
Joe H. Gieck Professor of Sports Medicine
Departments of Kinesiology and
    Orthopaedic Surgery
University of Virginia
Charlottesville, Virginia

Daniel E. Hess, MD
Department of Orthopaedic Surgery
University of Virginia
Charlottesville, Virginia

Carolyn M. Hettrich, MD
University of Iowa
Iowa City, Iowa

Benton E. Heyworth, MD
Assistant Professor of Orthopedic Surgery
Harvard Medical School
Attending Orthopedic Surgeon
Department of Orthopedic Surgery
Division of Sports Medicine
Boston Children's Hospital
Boston, Massachusetts

Ben Hickey, BM, MRCS, MSc, FRCS (Tr & Orth), MD
Consultant Orthopaedic Foot and Ankle Surgeon
Wrexham Maelor Hospital
Wrexham, Wales, United Kingdom

Michael Higgins, PhD, ATC, PT, CSCS
Professor, Kinesiology
University of Virginia
Charlottesville, Virginia

Betina B. Hinckel, MD, PhD
Department of Orthopaedic Surgery
Brigham and Women's Hospital
Harvard Medical School
Boston, Massachusetts

Gwendolyn Hoben, MD, PhD
Instructor
Plastic and Reconstructive Surgery
Medical College of Wisconsin
Milwaukee, Wisconsin

Christopher Hogrefe, MD, FACEP
Assistant Professor
Departments of Emergency Medicine,
    Medicine—Sports Medicine, and
    Orthopaedic Surgery—Sports Medicine
Northwestern Medicine
Northwestern University Feinberg School of
    Medicine
Chicago, Illinois

Jason A. Horowitz, BA
Research Fellow
Department of Orthopaedic Surgery
University of Virginia
Charlottesville, Virginia

Benjamin M. Howe, MD
Associate Professor of Radiology
Mayo Clinic
Rochester, Minnesota

Korin Hudson, MD, FACEP, CAQSM
Associate Professor of Emergency Medicine
Team Physician, Department of Athletics
Georgetown University
Washington, District of Columbia

Catherine Hui, MD, FRCSC
Associate Clinical Professor
Division of Orthopaedic Surgery
University of Alberta
Edmonton, Alberta, Canada

R. Tyler Huish, DO
First Choice Physician Partners
La Quinta, California

John V. Ingari, MD
Division Chair, Hand Surgery
Department of Orthopaedic Surgery
The Johns Hopkins Hospital
Baltimore, Maryland

Mary Lloyd Ireland, MD
Professor
Department of Orthopaedics
University of Kentucky
Lexington, Kentucky

Todd A. Irwin, MD
Director of Research
OrthoCarolina Foot and Ankle Institute
Associate Professor
Carolinas Medical Center
Charlotte, North Carolina

Nona M. Jiang, MD
Department of Medicine
University of Virginia
Charlottesville, Virginia

Darren L. Johnson, MD
Director of Sports Medicine
University of Kentucky
Lexington, Kentucky

Jared S. Johnson, MD
St. Luke's Clinic–Sports Medicine: Boise
Boise, Idaho

Grant L. Jones, MD
Associate Professor of Orthopaedic Surgery
The Ohio State University
Columbus, Ohio

Jean Jose, DO, MS
Associate Chief of Musculoskeletal
    Radiology
Associate Professor of Clinical Radiology
Division of Diagnostic Radiology
University of Miami Hospital
Miami, Florida

Scott G. Kaar, MD
Associate Professor of Orthopaedic Surgery
Saint Louis University
St. Louis, Missouri

Anish R. Kadakia, MD
Associate Professor of Orthopaedic Surgery
Northwestern Memorial Hospital
Northwestern University Feinberg School of
    Medicine
Chicago, Illinois

Samantha L. Kallenbach, BS
Steadman Philippon Research Institute
The Steadman Clinic
Vail, Colorado

Robin N. Kamal, MD
Assistant Professor of Orthopaedic Surgery
Chase Hand and Upper Limb Center
Stanford University
Palo Alto, California

Thomas Kaminski, PhD, ATC, FNATA
Professor of Kinesiology and Applied
    Physiology
University of Delaware
Newark, Delaware

Abdurrahman Kandil, MD
Stanford University
Stanford, California

Jonathan R. Kaplan, MD
Attending Orthopaedic Surgeon
Orthopaedic Specialty Institute
Orange, California

Christopher A. Keen, MD
Citrus Orthopedic and Joint Institute
Lecanto, Florida

Mick P. Kelly, MD
Resident, Department of Orthopaedic
    Surgery
Rush University Medical Center
Chicago, Illinois

A. Jay Khanna, MD, MBA
Professor and Vice Chair of Orthopaedic
    Surgery
Department of Orthopaedic Surgery
The Johns Hopkins University School of
    Medicine
Baltimore, Maryland

Anthony Nicholas Khoury
Baylor University Medical Center at Dallas
Hip Preservation Center
University of Texas at Arlington
Bioengineering Department
Dallas, Texas

Christopher Kim, MD
Instructor of Orthopaedic Surgery
Saint Louis University
St. Louis, Missouri

Lucas R. King, MD, BS
Sports Orthopedic Surgeon
Department of Orthopedic Surgery
Parkview Medical Center
Pueblo, Colorado

Susan E. Kirk, MD
Associate Professor of Internal Medicine
and Obstetrics and Gynecology
Division of Endocrinology and Metabolism,
Maternal–Fetal Medicine
Associate Dean, Graduate Medical
Education
University of Virginia Health System
Charlottesville, Virginia

Georg Klammer, MD
Consultant
Institute for Foot and Ankle Reconstruction
FussInsitut Zurich
Zurich, Switzerland

Derrick M. Knapik, MD
Orthopaedic Surgery
University Hospitals
Cleveland Medical Center
Cleveland, Ohio

Lee M. Kneer, MD, CAQSM
Assistant Professor, Department of
Orthopaedic Surgery
Assistant Professor, Department of Physical
Medicine and Rehabilitation
Emory Sports Medicine Center
Atlanta, Georgia

Mininder S. Kocher, MD, MPH
Professor of Orthopaedic Surgery
Harvard Medical School
Associate Director
Division of Sports Medicine
Department of Orthopaedic Surgery
Boston Children's Hospital
Boston, Massachusetts

Gabrielle P. Konin, MD
Assistant Professor of Radiology
Weill Cornell Medicine
New York, New York

Matthew J. Kraeutler, MD
Department of Orthopaedic Surgery
Seton Hall-Hackensack Meridian School of
Medicine
South Orange, New Jersey

Alexander B. Kreines, DO
Resident, Orthopaedic Surgery
Rowan University
Stratford, New Jersey

Vignesh Prasad Krishnamoorthy, MD
Section of Young Adult Hip Surgery
Division of Sports Medicine
Department of Orthopedic Surgery
Rush Medical College
Rush University Medical Center
Chicago, Illinois

Marshall A. Kuremsky, MD
Orthopaedic Surgeon
Hand and Upper Extremity Surgeon
Sports Medicine and Arthroscopic Surgeon
EmergeOrtho
Raleigh, North Carolina

Shawn M. Kutnik, MD
Orthopedic Surgeon
Archway Orthopedics and Hand Surgery
St. Louis, Missouri

Michael S. Laidlaw, MD
Department of Orthopaedic Surgery
University of Virginia
Charlottesville, Virginia

Joseph D. Lamplot
Chief Resident
Department of Orthopaedic Surgery
Washington University School of Medicine
St. Louis, Missouri

Drew Lansdown, MD
Section of Young Adult Hip Surgery
Division of Sports Medicine
Department of Orthopedic Surgery
Rush Medical College
Rush University Medical Center
Chicago, Illinois

Matthew D. LaPrade, BS
Steadman Philippon Research Institute
The Steadman Clinic
Vail, Colorado

Robert F. LaPrade, MD, PhD
Chief Medical Research Officer
Steadman Philippon Research Institute
The Steadman Clinic
Vail, Colorado

Christopher M. Larson, MD
Minnesota Orthopedic Sports Medicine
Institute
Twin Cities Orthopedics
Edina, Minnesota

Evan P. Larson, MD
University of Nebraska Medical Center
Department of Orthopaedic Surgery and
Rehabilitation
Omaha, Nebraska

Samuel J. Laurencin, MD, PhD
Department of Orthopaedic Surgery
University of Connecticut School of
Medicine
Farmington, Connecticut

Peter Lawrence, MD
Wiley Barker Professor of Surgery
Chief, Division of Vascular and
Endovascular Surgery
University of California, Los Angeles
Los Angeles, California

Adrian D.K. Le, MD
Department of Orthopedic Surgery
Stanford University
Stanford, California

Nicholas LeCursi, CO
Certified Orthotist
Vice President, Services
Chief Technology Officer
Becker Orthopedic
Troy, Michigan

Sonya B. Levine, BA
Department of Orthopedic Surgery
Columbia University Medical Center
New York Presbyterian Hospital
New York, New York

William N. Levine, MD, FAOA
Frank E. Stinchfield Professor and
Chairman of Orthopedic Surgery
Columbia University Medical Center
New York Presbyterian Hospital
New York, New York

Xudong Joshua Li, MD, PhD
Associate Professor of Orthopaedic Surgery
and Biomedical Engineering
University of Virginia
Charlottesville, Virginia

Gregory T. Lichtman, DO
Department of Orthopedic Surgery
Rowan University School of Osteopathic
Medicine
Stratford, New Jersey

Christopher A. Looze, MD
Orthopaedic Surgeon
MedStar Franklin Square
Baltimore, Maryland

Gary M. Lourie, MD
Hand Surgeon
The Hand and Upper Extremity Center of
Georgia
Atlanta, Georgia

Helen H. Lu, PhD
Professor of Biomedical Engineering
Vice Chair, Department of Biomedical
Engineering
Columbia University Medical Center
New York Presbyterian Hospital
New York, New York

Timothy J. Luchetti, MD
Resident, Orthopedic Surgery
Rush University Medical Center
Chicago, Illinois

Jessica A. Lundgren, MD
Lecturer
Department of Internal Medicine
Division of Endocrinology and Metabolism
University of Virginia Health System
Charlottesville, Virginia

Travis G. Maak, MD
Associate Professor of Orthopaedic Surgery
University of Utah
Salt Lake City, Utah

John M. MacKnight, MD
Professor of Internal Medicine and
    Orthopaedic Surgery
Team Physician and Medical Director
UVA Sports Medicine
University of Virginia Health System
Charlottesville, Virginia

Nancy Major, MD
Department of Radiology
University of Colorado School of Medicine
Aurora, Colorado

Francesc Malagelada, MD
Foot and Ankle Unit
Department of Trauma and Orthopaedic
    Surgery
Royal London Hospital
Barts Health National Health Service Trust
London, England, United Kingdom

Michael A. Marchetti, MD
Assistant Attending, Dermatology Service
Department of Medicine
Memorial Sloan Kettering Cancer Center
New York, New York

Patrick G. Marinello, MD
Hand and Upper Extremity Surgeon
Capital Region Orthopaedic Group
Bone and Joint Center
Albany, New York

Hal David Martin, DO
Medical Director
Baylor University Medical Center at Dallas
Hip Preservation Center
Dallas, Texas

Scott D. Martin, MD
Director, MGH Joint Preservation Service
Director, Harvard/MGH Sports Medicine
    Fellowship Program
Associate Professor of Orthopaedic Surgery
Harvard Medical School
Department of Orthopaedic Surgery
Massachusetts General Hospital
Boston, Massachusetts

Rebecca Martinie, MD
Assistant Professor of Pediatrics
Baylor College of Medicine
Houston, Texas

**Lyndon Mason, MB BCh, MRCS (Eng),
FRCS (Tr & Orth)**
Trauma and Orthopaedic Consultant
Aintree University Hospital
Liverpool, England, United Kingdom

Augustus D. Mazzocca, MD
Department of Orthopaedic Surgery
University of Connecticut School of
    Medicine
Farmington, Connecticut

David R. McAllister, MD
Chief, Sports Medicine Service
Professor and Vice Chair
Department of Orthopaedic Surgery
David Geffen School of Medicine
University of California, Los Angeles
Los Angeles, California

Meagan McCarthy, MD
Fellowship Trained Orthopaedic Sports
    Medicine Surgeon
Reno Orthopaedic Clinic
Reno, Nevada

Eric C. McCarty, MD
Chief, Sports Medicine and Shoulder
    Surgery
Associate Professor
Department of Orthopaedics
University of Colorado School of Medicine
Director Sports Medicine, Head Team
    Physician
University of Colorado Department of
    Athletics
Associate Professor, Adjunct
Department of Integrative Physiology
University of Colorado
Boulder, Colorado

Sean McMillan, DO
Chief of Orthopedics
Director of Orthopedic Sports Medicine
    and Arthroscopy
Lourdes Medical Associates
Lourdes Medical Center at Burlington
Burlington, New Jersey

Heather Menzer, MD
Fellow, Orthopaedic Surgery
University of Virginia
Charlottesville, Virginia

Sean J. Meredith, MD
Resident Physician
Department of Orthopaedics
University of Maryland School of Medicine
Baltimore, Maryland

Dayne T. Mickelson, MD
Department of Orthopaedic Surgery
Duke University
Durham, North Carolina

Michael R. Mijares, MD
Department of Orthopaedics
Jackson Memorial Hospital
Jackson Health System
Miami, Florida

Matthew D. Milewski, MD
Assistant Professor
Division of Sports Medicine
Department of Orthopaedic Surgery
Boston Children's Hospital
Boston, Massachusetts

Mark D. Miller, MD
S. Ward Casscells Professor of Orthopaedic
    Surgery
Head, Division of Sports Medicine
University of Virginia
Charlottesville, Virginia
Adjunctive Clinical Professor and Team
    Physician
James Madison University
Harrisonburg, Virginia

Dilaawar J. Mistry, MD
Team Physician
Primary Care Sports Medicine
Western Orthopedics and Sports Medicine
Grand Junction, Colorado

Erik Mitchell, DO
Valley Health Orthopaedics Front Royal
Front Royal, Virginia

Andrew Molloy, MBChB, MRCS
Consultant Orthopaedic Surgeon
Trauma and Orthopaedics
University Hospital Aintree
Honorary Clinical Senior Lecturer
Department of Musculoskeletal Biology
University of Liverpool
Consultant Orthopaedic Surgeon
Spire Liverpool
Liverpool, England, United Kingdom

Timothy S. Mologne, MD
Sports Medicine Center
Appleton, Wisconsin

Scott R. Montgomery, MD
Franciscan Orthopedic Associates at St. Joseph
Tacoma, Washington

Amy M. Moore, MD, FACS
Associate Professor of Surgery
Plastic and Reconstructive Surgery
Washington University School of Medicine
St. Louis, Missouri

Claude T. Moorman III, MD
Professor of Orthopaedic Surgery
Duke Center for Integrated Medicine
Durham, North Carolina

Gina M. Mosich, MD
Resident Physician
Orthopaedic Surgery
University of California, Los Angeles
Los Angeles, California

Michael R. Moynagh, MBBCh
Assistant Professor of Radiology
Mayo Clinic
Rochester, Minnesota

Andrew C. Mundy, MD
Department of Orthopaedic Surgery
The Ohio State University
Columbus, Ohio

Colin P. Murphy, BA
Research Assistant
Center for Outcomes-Based Orthopaedic
    Research
Steadman Philippon Research Institute
Vail, Colorado

Volker Musahl, MD
Assistant Professor
Department of Orthopaedic Surgery
University of Pittsburgh Medical Center
Pittsburgh, Pennsylvania

Jeffrey J. Nepple, MD
Assistant Professor of Orthopaedic Surgery
Director
Young Athlete Center
Washington University School of Medicine
St. Louis, Missouri

Shane J. Nho, MD, MS
Assistant Professor
Head, Section of Young Adult Hip Surgery
Division of Sports Medicine
Department of Orthopedic Surgery
Rush Medical College
Rush University Medical Center
Chicago, Illinois

Carl W. Nissen, MD
Professor
Department of Orthopaedics
University of Connecticut
Elite Sports Medicine
Connecticut Children's Medical Center
Farmington, Connecticut

Blake R. Obrock, DO
Sports Medicine Fellow
Department of Orthopaedics
University of New Mexico
Albuquerque, New Mexico

James Onate, PhD, ATC, FNATA
Associate Professor
School of Health and Rehabilitation
    Sciences
The Ohio State University
Columbus, Ohio

Scott I. Otallah, MD
Carilion Children's Pediatric Neurology
Roanoke, Virginia

Brett D. Owens, MD
Professor of Orthopedics
Brown Alpert Medical School
Providence, Rhode Island

Gabrielle M. Paci, MD
Physician
Orthopaedic Surgery
Stanford University
Palo Alto, California

Richard D. Parker, MD
Department of Orthopaedic Surgery
The Cleveland Clinic Foundation
Cleveland, Ohio

Jonathan P. Parsons, MD
Professor of Internal Medicine
Department of Pulmonary, Critical Care,
    and Sleep Medicine
Wexner Medical Center
The Ohio State University
Columbus, Ohio

Neel K. Patel, MD
Department of Orthopaedic Surgery
University of Pittsburgh Medical Center
Pittsburgh, Pennsylvania

Thierry Pauyo, MD
Fellow
Department of Orthopaedic Surgery
University of Pittsburgh Medical Center
Pittsburgh, Pennsylvania

Evan Peck, MD
Section of Sports Health
Department of Orthopaedic Surgery
Cleveland Clinic Florida
Weston, Florida
Affiliate Assistant Professor of Clinical
    Biomedical Science
Charles E. Schmidt College of Medicine
Florida Atlantic University
Boca Raton, Florida

Liam Peebles, BA
Research Assistant
Center for Outcomes-Based Orthopaedic
    Research
Steadman Philippon Research Institute
Vail, Colorado

Andrew T. Pennock, MD
Associate Clinical Professor
Orthopedic Surgery
University of California, San Diego
San Diego, California

**Anthony Perera, MBChB, MRCS,
MFSEM, PGDip Med Law, FRCS (Tr &
Orth)**
Consultant, Orthopaedic Foot and Ankle
    Surgeon
University Hospital of Wales
Cardiff, Wales, United Kingdom

Jose Perez, BS
Research Fellow
Department of Orthopedics
Sports Medicine
Miami, Florida

William A. Petri Jr., MD, PhD
Chief, Division of Infectious Disease and
    International Health
Wade Hampton Frost Professor of
    Epidemiology
University of Virginia
Charlottesville, Virginia

Frank A. Petrigliano, MD
Assistant Professor of Orthopaedic Surgery
David Geffen School of Medicine
University of California, Los Angeles
Los Angeles, California

Adam M. Pickett, MD
Faculty, West Point Sports Medicine
    Fellowship
Department of Orthopaedic Surgery
United States Military Academy
West Point, New York

Matthew A. Posner, MD
Director, West Point Sports Medicine
  Fellowship
Department of Orthopaedic Surgery
United States Military Academy
West Point, New York

Tricia R. Prokop, PT, EdD, MS, CSCS
Assistant Professor of Physical Therapy
Department of Rehabilitation Sciences
University of Hartford
West Hartford, Connecticut

Matthew T. Provencher, MD, CAPT, MC, USNR
Professor of Surgery and Orthopaedics
Uniformed Services University of the Health
  Services
Complex Shoulder, Knee, and Sports
  Surgeon
The Steadman Clinic
Vail, Colorado

Rabia Qureshi, MD
Research Fellow
Department of Orthopedic Surgery
University of Virginia
Charlottesville, Virginia

Fred Reifsteck, MD
Head Team Physician
University Health Center
University of Georgia
Athens, Georgia

David R. Richardson, MD
Associate Professor of Orthopaedic Surgery
University of Tennessee–Campbell Clinic
Memphis, Tennessee

Dustin Richter, MD
Assistant Professor, Sports Medicine
Sports Medicine Fellowship Assistant
  Director
Director of Orthopaedics Sports Medicine
  Research
University of New Mexico
Albuquerque, New Mexico

Andrew J. Riff, MD
Assistant Professor of Clinical Orthopaedic
  Surgery
Indiana University Health Orthopedics and
  Sports Medicine
Indianapolis, Indiana

Christopher J. Roach, MD
Chairman, Orthopaedic Surgery
San Antonio Military Medical Center
San Antonio, Texas

Eliott P. Robinson, MD
Orthopedic Surgeon
OrthoGeorgia Orthopaedic Specialists
Macon, Georgia

Scott A. Rodeo, MD
Professor of Orthopaedic Surgery
Weill Cornell Medical College
Co-Chief Emeritus, Sports Medicine and
  Shoulder Service
Attending Orthopaedic Surgeon
Hospital for Special Surgery
New York, New York

Anthony A. Romeo, MD
Department of Orthopaedic Surgery
Rush University
Chicago, Illinois

Kyle Rosen, MD
Dartmouth College
Hanover, New Hampshire

William H. Rossy, MD
Clinical Associate Professor
Penn Medicine Princeton Medical Center
Princeton, New Jersey

Paul Rothenberg, MD
Resident Physician
Department of Orthopaedics
University of Miami
Miami, Florida

Todd A. Rubin, MD
Orthopaedic Surgeon
Hughston Clinic Orthopaedics
Nashville, Tennessee

Robert D. Russell, MD
Orthopaedic Surgeon
OrthoTexas
Frisco, Texas

David A. Rush, MD
Department of Orthopaedic Surgery and
  Rehabilitation
University of Mississippi Medical Center
Jackson, Mississippi

Joseph J. Ruzbarsky, MD
Resident, Orthopedic Surgery
Department of Orthopaedics
Hospital for Special Surgery
New York, New York

Marc Safran, MD
Professor of Orthopedic Surgery
Associate Director
Department of Sports Medicine
Stanford University
Redwood City, California

Susan Saliba, PhD, ATC, MPT
Professor, Kinesiology
University of Virginia
Charlottesville, Virginia

Adil Samad, MD
Florida Orthopaedic Institute
Tampa, Florida

Anthony Sanchez, BS
Medical Doctor Candidate
Oregon Health and Science University
Portland, Oregon

Laura W. Scordino, MD
Orthopaedic Surgeon
OrthoNY
Albany, New York

Virgil P. Secasanu, MD
Clinical Instructor, Housestaff
Department of Pulmonary, Critical Care,
  and Sleep Medicine
Wexner Medical Center
The Ohio State University
Columbus, Ohio

Terrance Sgroi, PT
Sports Medicine and Shoulder Service
Hospital for Special Surgery
New York, New York

Jason T. Shearn, MD
Associate Professor
Department of Biomedical Engineering
University of Cincinnati
Cincinnati, Ohio

K. Donald Shelbourne, MD
The Shelbourne Knee Center at Community
  East Hospital
Indianapolis, Indiana

Seth L. Sherman, MD
Department of Orthopaedic Surgery
University of Missouri, Columbia
Columbia, Missouri

Ashley Matthews Shilling, MD
Associate Professor of Anesthesiology
University of Virginia Medical Center
Charlottesville, Virginia

Adam L. Shimer, MD
Assistant Professor of Orthopaedic Surgery
University of Virginia
Charlottesville, Virginia

Anuj Singla, MD
Instructor, Orthopaedics
University of Virginia
Charlottesville, Virginia

David L. Skaggs, MD, MMM
Professor of Orthopaedic Surgery
Keck School of Medicine of USC
University of Southern California
Chief, Orthopaedic Surgery
Children's Hospital Los Angeles
Los Angeles, California

Mia Smucny, MD
University of Washington
Seattle, Washington

Niall A. Smyth, MD
Resident, Orthopaedic Surgery
University of Miami, Miller School of
    Medicine
Miami, Florida

Frederick S. Song, MD
Clinical Associate Professor
Penn Medicine Princeton Medical Center
Princeton, New Jersey

Kurt Spindler, MD
Cleveland Clinic Foundation
Cleveland, Ohio

Chad Starkey, PhD, AT, FNATA
Professor
Division of Athletic Training
Ohio University
Athens, Ohio

Siobhan M. Statuta, MD
Associate Professor of Family Medicine and
    Physical Medicine and Rehabilitation
University of Virginia
Charlottesville, Virginia

Samuel R. H. Steiner, MD
Orthopedic Surgery
Orthopaedic Associates of Wisconsin
Pewaukee, Wisconsin

John W. Stelzer, MD, MS
Research Fellow
Department of Orthopaedic Surgery
Harvard Medical School
Massachusetts General Hospital
Boston, Massachusetts

Christopher L. Stockburger, MD
Department of Orthopedic Surgery
Washington University School of Medicine
St. Louis, Missouri

J. Andy Sullivan, MD
Clinical Professor of Pediatric Orthopedic
    Surgery
Department of Orthopedic Surgery
University of Oklahoma College of
    Medicine
Oklahoma City, Oklahoma

Eric Swanton, MBChB, FRACS (Orth)
Orthopaedic Consultant
Department of Orthopaedics
North Shore Hospital, Waitemata District
    Health Board
Auckland, New Zealand

Matthew A. Tao, MD
Assistant Professor
Orthopaedic Surgery
University of Nebraska Medical Center
Omaha, Nebraska

Sandip P. Tarpada, BS
Department of Orthopaedic Surgery
Montefiore Medical Center
Albert Einstein College of Medicine
New York, New York

Kenneth F. Taylor, MD
Department of Orthopaedics and
    Rehabilitation
The Pennsylvania State University
Milton S. Hershey Medical Center
Hershey, Pennsylvania

Michael Terry, MD
Professor
Department of Orthopaedic Surgery
Northwestern Medicine
Northwestern University Feinberg School of
    Medicine
Chicago, Illinois

Charles A. Thigpen, PhD, PT, ATC
Senior Director of Practice Innovation and
    Analytics
ATI Physical Therapy
Director, Program in Observational Clinical
    Research in Orthopedics
Center for Effectiveness in Orthopedic
    Research
Arnold School of Public Health
University of South Carolina
Greenville, South Carolina

Stavros Thomopoulos, PhD
Director, Carroll Laboratories for
    Orthopedic Surgery
Vice Chair, Basic Research in Orthopedic
    Surgery
Robert E. Carroll and Jane Chace Carroll
    Professor of Biomechanics (in
    Orthopedic Surgery and Biomedical
    Engineering)
Columbia University Medical Center
New York Presbyterian Hospital
New York, New York

Jason Thompson, MD
Orthopedic Surgery Resident, UT Health
    San Antonio
Adult Reconstructive Surgery Fellow
University of Western Ontario
London Health Sciences Centre
London, Ontario, Canada

**Stephen R. Thompson, MD, MEd,
FRCSC**
Associate Professor of Sports Medicine
Eastern Maine Medical Center
University of Maine
Bangor, Maine

Fotios P. Tjoumakaris, MD
Associate Professor
Department of Orthopedic Surgery
Sidney Kimmel College of Medicine
Thomas Jefferson University
Philadelphia, Pennsylvania

Drew Toftoy, MD
Sports Medicine Fellow
University of Colorado
Aurora, Colorado

John M. Tokish, MD, USAF MC
Orthopedic Surgery Residency Program
    Director
Tripler Army Medical Center
Honolulu, Hawaii

Gehron Treme, MD
Associate Professor, Orthopaedics
University of New Mexico
Albuquerque, New Mexico

Rachel Triche, MD
Attending Orthopaedic Surgeon
Santa Monica Orthopaedic and Sports
    Medicine Group
Santa Monica, California

David P. Trofa, MD
Resident, Department of Orthopaedic
    Surgery
Columbia University Medical Center
New York, New York

Gift Ukwuani, MD
Section of Young Adult Hip Surgery
Division of Sports Medicine
Department of Orthopedic Surgery
Rush Medical College
Rush University Medical Center
Chicago, Illinois

M. Farooq Usmani, MSc
Department of Orthopaedic Surgery
The Johns Hopkins University School of
    Medicine
Baltimore, Maryland

Ravi S. Vaswani, MD
Resident, Department of Orthopaedic
  Surgery
University of Pittsburgh Medical Center
Pittsburgh, Pennsylvania

Aaron J. Vaughan, MD
Family Physician
Sports Medicine Director
Mountain Area Health Education Center
Asheville, North Carolina

Jordi Vega, MD
Orthopaedic Surgeon
Etzelclinic
Pfäffikon, Schwyz, Switzerland

Evan E. Vellios, MD
Resident Physician
Department of Orthopedic Surgery
David Geffen School of Medicine
University of California, Los Angeles
Los Angeles, California

Armando F. Vidal, MD
Associate Professor
Department of Orthopedics
University of Colorado School of Medicine
Aurora, Colorado

Michael J. Vives, MD
Professor and Chief of Spine Surgery
Department of Orthopedics
Rutgers–New Jersey Medical School
Newark, New Jersey

James E. Voos, MD
Associate Professor of Orthopaedic Surgery
Division Chief, Sports Medicine
Medical Director, Sports Medicine Institute
University Hospitals
Cleveland Medical Center
Cleveland, Ohio

Dean Wang, MD
Fellow in Sports Medicine and Shoulder
  Surgery
Hospital for Special Surgery
New York, New York

Robert Westermann, MD
University of Iowa
Iowa City, Iowa

Barbara B. Wilson, MD
Associate Professor of Dermatology
University of Virginia
Charlottesville, Virginia

Benjamin R. Wilson, MD
Resident Physician
Orthopaedic Surgery and Sports Medicine
University of Kentucky
Lexington, Kentucky

Brian F. Wilson, MD
Director of Orthopaedic Surgery Stormont
  Vail Health
Washburn University Orthopaedic Sports
  Medicine
Topeka, Kansas

Jennifer Moriatis Wolf, MD
Professor
Department of Orthopaedic Surgery and
  Rehabilitation
University of Chicago Hospitals
Chicago, Illinois

Rick W. Wright, MD
Jerome J. Gilden Distinguished Professor
Executive Vice Chairman
Department of Orthopaedic Surgery
Washington University School of Medicine
St. Louis, Missouri

Frank B. Wydra, MD
Department of Orthopedics
University of Colorado School of Medicine
Aurora, Colorado

James Wylie, MD, MHS
Director of Orthopedic Research
Intermountain Healthcare
The Orthopedic Specialty Hospital
Murray, Utah

Robert W. Wysocki, MD
Rush University Medical Center
Chicago, Illinois

Haoming Xu, MD
Dermatology Service
Department of Medicine
Memorial Sloan Kettering Cancer Center
New York, New York

Kent T. Yamaguchi, MD
Resident Physician
Orthopaedic Surgery
University of California, Los Angeles
Los Angeles, California

Jeffrey Yao, MD
Associate Professor of Orthopedic Surgery
Stanford University Medical Center
Palo Alto, California

Yi-Meng Yen, MD, PhD
Assistant Professor, Harvard Medical School
Boston Children's Hospital
Department of Orthopaedic Surgery
Division of Sports Medicine
Boston, Massachusetts

Jane C. Yeoh, MD, FRCSC
Vancouver, British Columbia, Canada

M. Christopher Yonz, MD
Summit Orthopaedics
Southeast Georgia Health System
St. Marys, Georgia

Tracy Zaslow, MD, FAAP, CAQSM
Assistant Professor
University of Southern California, Los
  Angeles
Children's Orthopaedic Center (COC) at
  Children's Hospital–Los
Angeles
Medical Director
COC Sports Medicine and Concussion
  Program
Team Physician, LA Galaxy
Los Angeles, California

Andrew M. Zbojniewicz, MD
Department of Radiology
Michigan State University
College of Human Medicine
Advanced Radiology Services
Grand Rapids, Michigan
Division of Pediatric Radiology
Cincinnati Children's Hospital Medical
  Center
Cincinnati, Ohio

Connor G. Ziegler, MD
New England Orthopedic Surgeons
Springfield, Massachusetts

Mary L. Zupanc, MD
Professor and Division Chief
Neurology and Pediatrics
University of California, Irvine
Children's Hospital of Orange County
Orange, California

CONTENTS

Volume I

SECTION 1 Basic Principles
Asheesh Bedi, Bryson Lesniak

1. **Physiology and Pathophysiology of Musculoskeletal Tissues,** 2
   Dean Wang, Claire D. Eliasberg, Scott A. Rodeo
2. **Basic Concepts in Biomechanics,** 16
   Richard E. Debski, Neel K. Patel, Jason T. Shearn
3. **Basic Science of Graft Tissue in Sports Medicine,** 30
   Mia Smucny, Carolyn M. Hettrich, Robert Westermann, Kurt Spindler
4. **Basic Science of Implants in Sports Medicine,** 35
   Elizabeth R. Dennis, Jon-Michael E. Caldwell, Sonya B. Levine, Philip Chuang, Margaret Boushell, Stavros Thomopoulos, Helen H. Lu, William N. Levine
5. **Orthobiologics: Clinical Application of Platelet-Rich Plasma and Stem Cell Therapy,** 50
   Adrian D.K. Le, Jason Dragoo
6. **Exercise Physiology,** 62
   Thomas M. Best, Chad A. Asplund
7. **Imaging Overview,** 74
   Francisco Contreras, Jose Perez, Jean Jose
8. **Basic Arthroscopic Principles,** 105
   Michael R. Mijares, Michael G. Baraga
9. **Overview of Sport-Specific Injuries,** 114
   Jared A. Crasto, Ravi S. Vaswani, Thierry Pauyo, Volker Musahl
10. **Commonly Encountered Fractures in Sports Medicine,** 131
    Christopher Kim, Scott G. Kaar

SECTION 2 Medical
Rajwinder Deu, Morteza Khodaee

11. **Team Medical Coverage,** 144
    Daniel Herman, Nikhita Gadi, Evan Peck
12. **Comprehensive Cardiovascular Care and Evaluation of the Elite Athlete,** 158
    Paul S. Corotto, Aaron L. Baggish, Dilaawar J. Mistry, Robert W. Battle
13. **Exercise-Induced Bronchoconstriction,** 175
    Virgil P. Secasanu, Jonathan P. Parsons
14. **Deep Venous Thrombosis and Pulmonary Embolism,** 180
    Jason Thompson, Marc M. DeHart
15. **Gastrointestinal Medicine in the Athlete,** 189
    John M. MacKnight
16. **Hematologic Medicine in the Athlete,** 196
    John J. Densmore
17. **Infectious Diseases in the Athlete,** 201
    Nona M. Jiang, Kathleen C. Abalos, William A. Petri Jr.

18. **The Athlete With Diabetes,** 218
    Jessica A. Lundgren, Susan E. Kirk
19. **Renal Medicine and Genitourinary Trauma in the Athlete,** 227
    Stefan Hemmings, Derek M. Fine
20. **Sports and Epilepsy,** 230
    Mary L. Zupanc, Scott I. Otallah, Howard P. Goodkin
21. **Environmental Illness,** 235
    Jorge E. Gómez, Joseph N. Chorley, Rebecca Martinie
22. **Dermatologic Conditions,** 246
    Haoming Xu, Barbara B. Wilson, Michael A. Marchetti
23. **Facial, Eye, Nasal, and Dental Injuries,** 260
    John Jared Christophel
24. **Psychological Adjustment to Athletic Injury,** 272
    Karen P. Egan, Jason Freeman
25. **Sports Nutrition,** 277
    Jessica L. Buschmann, Jackie Buell
26. **Doping and Ergogenic Aids,** 283
    Siobhan M. Statuta, Aaron J. Vaughan, Ashley V. Austin
27. **The Female Athlete,** 294
    Letha Y. Griffin, Mary Lloyd Ireland, Fred Reifsteck, Matthew H. Blake, Benjamin R. Wilson
28. **The Para-Athlete,** 315
    Daniel Herman, Mary E. Caldwell, Arthur Jason De Luigi
29. **Anesthesia and Perioperative Medicine,** 325
    Ashley Matthews Shilling

SECTION 3 Rehabilitation and Injury Prevention
Joe M. Hart

30. **The Athletic Trainer,** 342
    Chad Starkey, Shannon David
31. **Principles of Orthopaedic Rehabilitation,** 347
    Courtney Chaaban, Charles A. Thigpen
32. **Modalities and Manual Techniques in Sports Medicine Rehabilitation,** 354
    Susan Saliba, Michael Higgins
33. **Basics of Taping and Orthotics,** 368
    Phillip Gribble
34. **Injury Prevention,** 376
    Jay Hertel, James Onate, Thomas Kaminski
35. **Return to Activity and Sport After Injury,** 385
    J. Craig Garrison, Joseph Hannon

SECTION 4 Shoulder
Stephen F. Brockmeier

36. **Shoulder Anatomy and Biomechanics,** 393
    Timothy S. Mologne
37. **Shoulder Diagnosis and Decision-Making,** 402
    Thomas J. Gill

38. **Glenohumeral Joint Imaging**, 408
   Alissa J. Burge, Gabrielle P. Konin
39. **Shoulder Arthroscopy**, 433
   Thomas M. DeBerardino, Laura W. Scordino
40. **Anterior Shoulder Instability**, 440
   Stephen R. Thompson, Heather Menzer, Stephen F. Brockmeier
41. **Posterior Shoulder Instability**, 463
   James Bradley, Fotios P. Tjoumakaris
42. **Multidirectional Instability of the Shoulder**, 476
   Robert M. Carlisle, John M. Tokish
43. **Revision Shoulder Instability**, 489
   Salvatore Frangiamore, Angela K. Chang, Jake A. Fox, Colin P. Murphy, Anthony Sanchez, Liam Peebles, Matthew T. Provencher
44. **Superior Labrum Anterior to Posterior Tears**, 502
   Sean J. Meredith, R. Frank Henn III
45. **The Thrower's Shoulder**, 511
   Matthew A. Tao, Christopher L. Camp, Terrance Sgroi, Joshua S. Dines, David W. Altchek
46. **Proximal Biceps Tendon Pathology**, 526
   Samuel R.H. Steiner, John T. Awowale, Stephen F. Brockmeier
47. **Rotator Cuff and Impingement Lesions**, 540
   Gina M. Mosich, Kent T. Yamaguchi, Frank A. Petrigliano
48. **Subscapularis Injury**, 556
   William H. Rossy, Frederick S. Song, Jeffrey S. Abrams
49. **Revision Rotator Cuff Repair**, 567
   Joseph D. Cooper, Anthony Essilfie, Seth C. Gamradt
50. **Other Muscle Injuries**, 574
   James E. Voos, Derrick M. Knapik
51. **Stiff Shoulder**, 579
   Jonathan Barlow, Andrew C. Mundy, Grant L. Jones
52. **Glenohumeral Arthritis in the Athlete**, 592
   Jeffrey Brunelli, Jonathan T. Bravman, Kevin Caperton, Eric C. McCarty
53. **Scapulothoracic Disorders**, 609
   G. Keith Gill, Gehron Treme, Dustin Richter
54. **Nerve Entrapment**, 621
   Daniel E. Hess, Kenneth F. Taylor, A. Bobby Chhabra
55. **Vascular Problems and Thoracic Outlet Syndrome**, 632
   Matthew A. Posner, Christopher J. Roach, Adam M. Pickett, Brett D. Owens
56. **Injury to the Acromioclavicular and Sternoclavicular Joints**, 645
   Connor G. Ziegler, Samuel J. Laurencin, Rachel M. Frank, Matthew T. Provencher, Anthony A. Romeo, Augustus D. Mazzocca

SECTION 5 Elbow, Wrist, and Hand
Sanjeev Kakar

57. **Elbow Anatomy and Biomechanics**, 680
   Marshall A. Kuremsky, E. Lyle Cain Jr., Jeffrey R. Dugas, James R. Andrews, Lucas R. King
58. **Elbow Diagnosis and Decision-Making**, 687
   Nicholas J. Clark, Bassem T. Elhassan
59. **Elbow Imaging**, 697
   Benjamin M. Howe, Michael R. Moynagh

60. **Elbow Arthroscopy**, 707
   Todd A. Rubin, Shawn M. Kutnik, Michael R. Hausman
61. **Elbow Tendinopathies and Bursitis**, 720
   Jennifer Moriatis Wolf
62. **Distal Biceps and Triceps Tendon Ruptures**, 731
   James Bradley, Fotios P. Tjoumakaris, Gregory T. Lichtman, Luke S. Austin
63. **Entrapment Neuropathies of the Arm, Elbow, and Forearm**, 742
   Wajeeh Bakhsh, Warren C. Hammert
64. **Elbow Throwing Injuries**, 757
   Marshall A. Kuremsky, E. Lyle Cain Jr., Jeffrey R. Dugas, James R. Andrews, Christopher A. Looze
65. **Loss of Elbow Motion**, 772
   Timothy J. Luchetti, Debdut Biswas, Robert W. Wysocki
66. **Anatomy and Biomechanics of the Hand and Wrist**, 785
   Raj M. Amin, John V. Ingari
67. **Hand and Wrist Diagnosis and Decision-Making**, 793
   Patrick G. Marinello, R. Glenn Gaston, Eliott P. Robinson, Gary M. Lourie
68. **Imaging of the Wrist and Hand**, 806
   Kimberly K. Amrami
69. **Wrist Arthroscopy**, 817
   William B. Geissler, David A. Rush, Christopher A. Keen
70. **Carpal Injuries**, 835
   Gabrielle M. Paci, Jeffrey Yao
71. **Wrist Tendinopathies**, 857
   Raj M. Amin, John V. Ingari
72. **Disorders of the Distal Radioulnar Joint**, 865
   Julie E. Adams
73. **Tendon Injuries in the Hand**, 873
   Robin N. Kamal, Jacob D. Gire
74. **Digit Fractures and Dislocations**, 883
   Christopher L. Stockburger, Ryan P. Calfee
75. **Neuropathies of the Wrist and Hand**, 898
   Gwendolyn Hoben, Amy M. Moore

Volume II

SECTION 6 Pelvis, Hip, and Thigh
F. Winston Gwathmey, Jr.

76. **Hip Anatomy and Biomechanics**, 907
   Marc Safran, Abdurrahman Kandil
77. **Hip Diagnosis and Decision-Making**, 925
   Austin W. Chen, Benjamin G. Domb
78. **Hip Imaging**, 935
   Brian Busconi, R. Tyler Huish, Erik Mitchell, Sean McMillan
79. **Hip Arthroscopy**, 947
   Joshua D. Harris
80. **Femoroacetabular Impingement in Athletes**, 957
   Shane J. Nho, Vignesh Prasad Krishnamoorthy, Drew Lansdown, Gift Ukwuani
81. **Hip Dysplasia and Instability**, 971
   Jeffrey J. Nepple, John C. Clohisy

82. **Iliopsoas Pathology,** 979
   Christian N. Anderson
83. **Peritrochanteric Disorders,** 990
   John W. Stelzer, Scott D. Martin
84. **Athletic Pubalgia/Core Muscle Injury and Adductor Pathology,** 1007
   Christopher M. Larson, Jeffrey J. Nepple
85. **Posterior Hip Pain,** 1018
   Hal David Martin, Anthony Nicholas Khoury, Juan Gomez-Hoyos
86. **Hamstring Injuries,** 1034
   Kyle E. Hammond, Lee M. Kneer
87. **Hip and Thigh Contusions and Strains,** 1043
   Blake R. Obrock, Christopher P. Bankhead, Dustin Richter
88. **Hip Arthritis in the Athlete,** 1053
   Guillaume D. Dumont, Robert D. Russell

SECTION 7 Knee
   Eric C. McCarty

89. **Knee Anatomy and Biomechanics of the Knee,** 1062
   Matthew J. Kraeutler, Jorge Chahla, Francesc Malagelada, Jordi Vega, Pau Golanó, Bruce Beynnon, Fatih Ertem, Eric C. McCarty
90. **Knee Diagnosis and Decision-Making,** 1089
   Andrew J. Riff, Peter N. Chalmers, Bernard R. Bach Jr.
91. **Imaging of the Knee,** 1104
   Nancy Major, Christopher Coleman
92. **Basics of Knee Arthroscopy,** 1121
   Stephen R. Thompson, Mark D. Miller
93. **Arthroscopic Synovectomy of the Knee,** 1127
   Mick P. Kelly, Charles A. Bush-Joseph
94. **Meniscal Injuries,** 1132
   Joseph J. Ruzbarsky, Travis G. Maak, Scott A. Rodeo
95. **Meniscal Transplantation,** 1154
   Frank B. Wydra, Derek P. Axibal, Armando F. Vidal
96. **Articular Cartilage Lesions,** 1161
   Michael S. Laidlaw, Kadir Buyukdogan, Mark D. Miller
97. **Frontiers in Articular Cartilage Treatment,** 1178
   Rachel M. Frank, Armando F. Vidal, Eric C. McCarty
98. **Anterior Cruciate Ligament Injuries,** 1185
   Edward C. Cheung, David R. McAllister, Frank A. Petrigliano
99. **Revision Anterior Cruciate Ligament Injuries,** 1199
   Joseph D. Lamplot, Liljiana Bogunovic, Rick W. Wright
100. **Posterior Cruciate Ligament Injuries,** 1211
   Frank A. Petrigliano, Evan E. Vellios, Scott R. Montgomery, Jared S. Johnson, David R. McAllister
101. **Medial Collateral Ligament and Posterior Medial Corner Injuries,** 1231
   M. Christopher Yonz, Brian F. Wilson, Matthew H. Blake, Darren L. Johnson
102. **Lateral and Posterolateral Corner Injuries of the Knee,** 1244
   Ryan P. Coughlin, Dayne T. Mickelson, Claude T. Moorman III
103. **Multiligament Knee Injuries,** 1264
   Samantha L. Kallenbach, Matthew D. LaPrade, Robert F. LaPrade
104. **Knee Arthritis,** 1277
   Catherine Hui, Stephen R. Thompson, J. Robert Giffin

105. **Patellar Instability,** 1293
   Seth L. Sherman, Betina B. Hinckel, Jack Farr
106. **Patellofemoral Pain,** 1308
   Meagan McCarthy, Eric C. McCarty, Rachel M. Frank
107. **Extensor Mechanism Injuries,** 1318
   Matthew Bessette, Drew Toftoy, Richard D. Parker, Rachel M. Frank
108. **Loss of Knee Motion,** 1335
   K. Donald Shelbourne, Heather Freeman, Tinker Gray
109. **Vascular Problems of the Knee,** 1345
   Peter Lawrence, Kyle Rosen

SECTION 8 Leg, Ankle, and Foot
   Amiethab A. Aiyer, Anish R. Kadakia

110. **Foot and Ankle Biomechanics,** 1359
   Andrew Haskell
111. **Leg, Ankle, and Foot Diagnosis and Decision-Making,** 1370
   Anish R. Kadakia, Amiethab A. Aiyer
112. **Imaging of the Foot and Ankle,** 1380
   Anish R. Kadakia, Amiethab A. Aiyer
113. **Leg Pain and Exertional Compartment Syndromes,** 1393
   Christopher Hogrefe, Michael Terry
114. **Peripheral Nerve Entrapment Around the Foot and Ankle,** 1402
   Norman Espinosa Jr., Georg Klammer
115. **Ankle Arthroscopy,** 1421
   Niall A. Smyth, Jonathan R. Kaplan, Amiethab A. Aiyer, John T. Campbell, Rachel Triche, Rebecca A. Cerrato
116. **Sports Shoes and Orthoses,** 1436
   Nicholas LeCursi
117. **Ligamentous Injuries of the Foot and Ankle,** 1444
   Paul Rothenberg, Eric Swanton, Andrew Molloy, Amiethab A. Aiyer, Jonathan R. Kaplan
118. **Tendon Injuries of the Foot and Ankle,** 1462
   Todd A. Irwin
119. **Articular Cartilage Injuries and Defects,** 1484
   David R. Richardson, Jane C. Yeoh
120. **Heel Pain and Plantar Fasciitis: Hindfoot Conditions,** 1504
   Anish R. Kadakia, Amiethab A. Aiyer
121. **Forefoot Problems in Sport,** 1515
   Ben Hickey, Lyndon Mason, Anthony Perera

SECTION 9 Spine and Head
   Francis H. Shen

122. **Head and Spine Anatomy and Biomechanics,** 1528
   Colin B. Harris, Rachid Assina, Brandee Gentile, Michael J. Vives
123. **Head and Spine Diagnosis and Decision-Making,** 1538
   Rabia Qureshi, Jason A. Horowitz, Kieran Bhattacharya, Hamid Hassanzadeh
124. **Imaging of the Spine,** 1544
   Adil Samad, M. Farooq Usmani, A. Jay Khanna

125. **Emergency and Field-Side Management of the Spine-Injured Athlete,** 1553
Korin Hudson, Michael Antonis, William Brady

126. **Concussion and Brain Injury,** 1562
David P. Trofa, Jon-Michael E. Caldwell, Xudong Joshua Li

127. **Stingers,** 1570
Sandip P. Tarpada, Woojin Cho

128. **Traumatic Injuries of the Cervical Spine in the Athlete,** 1578
Adam L. Shimer, Bayan Aghdasi

129. **Traumatic Injuries of the Thoracolumbar Spine in the Athlete,** 1582
Nourbakhsh Ali, Anuj Singla

130. **Degenerative Conditions of the Cervical and Thoracolumbar Spine,** 1593
Gregory Grabowski, Todd M. Gilbert, Evan P. Larson, Chris A. Cornett

SECTION 10 Pediatric Sports Medicine
Matthew D. Milewski

131. **The Young Athlete,** 1606
Benton E. Heyworth, Mininder S. Kocher

132. **Imaging Considerations in Skeletally Immature Athletes,** 1616
Andrew M. Zbojniewicz

133. **Shoulder Injuries in the Young Athlete,** 1637
Andrew T. Pennock, Eric W. Edmonds

134. **Elbow Injuries in Pediatric and Adolescent Athletes,** 1661
James P. Bradley, Luke S. Austin, Alexander B. Kreines, Fotios P. Tjoumakaris

135. **Wrist and Hand Injuries in the Adolescent Athlete,** 1677
Sonia Chaudhry

136. **Pediatric and Adolescent Hip Injuries,** 1688
Yi-Meng Yen, Mininder S. Kocher

137. **Knee Injuries in Skeletally Immature Athletes,** 1697
Matthew D. Milewski, James Wylie, Carl W. Nissen, Tricia R. Prokop

138. **Foot and Ankle Injuries in the Adolescent Athlete,** 1725
J. Andy Sullivan, James R. Gregory

139. **Head Injuries in Skeletally Immature Athletes,** 1741
Tracy Zaslow

140. **Spine Issues in Skeletally Immature Athletes,** 1749
Lindsay M. Andras, David L. Skaggs

Index, I1

VIDEO TABLE OF CONTENTS

Chapter 1
Video 1.1   Physiology and Pathophysiology of Musculoskeletal Tissues—Dean Wang, Claire D. Eliasberg, and Scott A. Rodeo

Chapter 2
Video 2.1   Basic Concepts in Biomechanics—Richard E. Debski, Neel K. Patel, and Jason T. Shearn

Chapter 4
Video 4.1   Basic Science of Implants in Sports Medicine—Elizabeth R. Dennis, Jon-Michael Caldwell, Sonya B. Levine, Philip Chuang, Margaret Boushell, Stavros Thomopoulos, Helen H. Lu, and William N. Levine

Chapter 5
Video 5.1   Orthobiologics: Clinical Application of Platelet-Rich Plasma and Stem Cell Therapy—Adrian D.K. Le and Jason Dragoo

Chapter 7
Video 7.1   Imaging Overview—Francisco Contreras, Jose Perez, and Jean Jose

Chapter 8
Video 8.1   Basic Arthroscopic Principles—Michael R. Mijares and Michael G. Baraga

Chapter 9
Video 9.1   Overview of Sport-Specific Injuries—Jared A. Crasto, Ravi S. Vaswani, Thierry Pauyo, and Volker Musahl

Chapter 10
Video 10.1   Commonly Encountered Fractures in Sports Medicine—Christopher Kim and Scott G. Kaar

Chapter 11
Video 11.1   Team Medical Coverage—Daniel Herman, Nikhita Gadi, and Evan Peck

Chapter 12
Video 12.1   Comprehensive Cardiovascular Care and Evaluation of the Elite Athlete—Paul S. Corotto, Robert W. Battle, Dilaawar J. Mistry, and Aaron L. Baggish

Chapter 13
Video 13.1   Exercise-Induced Bronchoconstriction—Virgil P. Secasanu and Jonathan P. Parsons

Chapter 14
Video 14.1   Deep Venous Thrombosis and Pulmonary Embolism—Marc M. DeHart and Jason Thompson

Chapter 15
Video 15.1   Gastrointestinal Medicine in the Athlete—John M. MacKnight

Chapter 16
Video 16.1   Hematologic Medicine in the Athlete—John J. Densmore

Chapter 17
Video 17.1   Infectious Diseases in the Athlete—Nona M. Jiang, Kathleen C. Abalos, and William A. Petri Jr.

Chapter 18
Video 18.1   The Athlete with Diabetes—Jessica A. Lundgren and Susan E. Kirk

Chapter 19
Video 19.1   Renal Medicine and Genitourinary Trauma in the Athlete—Stefan Hemmings and Derek M. Fine

Chapter 22
Video 22.1   Dermatologic Conditions—Haoming Xu, Barbara B. Wilson, and Michael A. Marchetti

Chapter 23
Video 23.1   Facial, Eye, Nasal, and Dental Injuries—John Jared Christophel

Chapter 25
Video 25.1   Sports Nutrition—Jessica L. Buschmann and Jackie Buell

Chapter 26
Video 26.1   Doping and Ergogenic Aids—Siobhan M. Statuta, Aaron J. Vaughan, and Ashley V. Austin

Chapter 27
Video 27.1   The Female Athlete—Letha Y. Griffin, Mary Lloyd Ireland, Fred Reifsteck, Matthew H. Blake, and Benjamin R. Wilson
Video 27.2   The Female Athlete—Letha Y. Griffin, Mary Lloyd Ireland, Fred Reifsteck, Matthew H. Blake, and Benjamin R. Wilson

Chapter 28
Video 28.1   The Para-Athlete—Daniel Herman, Mary E. Caldwell, and Arthur Jason De Luigi

Chapter 30
Video 30.1   The Athletic Trainer—Chad Starkey and Shannon David

Chapter 31
Video 31.1 Principles of Orthopaedic Rehabilitation—Courtney Chaaban and Charles A. Thigpen

Chapter 32
Video 32.1 Modalities and Manual Techniques in Sports Medicine Rehabilitation—Susan Saliba and Michael Higgins

Chapter 38
Video 38.1 Glenohumeral Joint Imaging—Alissa J. Burge and Gabrielle P. Konin

Chapter 41
Video 41.1 Posterior Shoulder Instability—James Bradley and Fotios P. Tjoumakaris

Chapter 42
Video 42.1 Multidirectional Instability of the Shoulder—Robert M. Carlisle and John M. Tokish

Chapter 44
Video 44.1 SLAP Tears—Sean Meredith and R. Frank Henn III

Chapter 45
Video 45.1 The Thrower's Shoulder—Matthew A. Tao, Christopher L. Camp, Terrance Sgroi, Joshua S. Dines, and David W. Altchek

Chapter 46
Video 46.1 Proximal Biceps Tendon Pathology—Samuel R.H. Steiner, John T. Awowale, and Stephen F. Brockmeier

Chapter 47
Video 47.1 Rotator Cuff and Impingement Lesions—Gina M. Mosich, Kent T. Yamaguchi, and Frank A. Petrigliano

Chapter 48
Video 48.1 Subscapularis Injury—William H. Rossy, Frederick S. Song, and Jeffrey S. Abrams

Chapter 49
Video 49.1 Revision Rotator Cuff Repair—Joseph D. Cooper, Anthony Essilfie, and Seth C. Gamradt

Chapter 52
Video 52.1 Glenohumeral Arthritis in the Athlete—Jeffrey Brunelli, Jonathan T. Bravman, Kevin Caperton, and Eric C. McCarty

Chapter 53
Video 53.1 Scapulothoracic Disorders—G. Keith Gill, Gehron Treme, and Dustin Richter

Chapter 54
Video 54.1 Nerve Entrapment—Daniel E. Hess, Kenneth F. Taylor, and A. Bobby Chhabra

Chapter 55
Video 55.1 Vascular Problems and Thoracic Outlet Syndrome—Matthew A. Posner, Christopher J. Roach, Adam M. Pickett, and Brett D. Owens

Chapter 56
Video 56.1 Injury to the Acromioclavicular and Sternoclavicular Joints—Connor G. Ziegler, Samuel J. Laurencin, Rachel M. Frank, Matthew T. Provencher, Anthony A. Romeo, and Augustus D. Mazzocca

Chapter 57
Video 57.1 Elbow Anatomy and Biomechanics—Marshall A. Kuremsky, E. Lyle Cain Jr., Jeffrey R. Dugas, James R. Andrews, and Lucas R. King

Chapter 58
Video 58.1 Elbow Diagnosis and Decision-Making—Nicholas J. Clark and Bassem Elhassan

Chapter 59
Video 59.1 Elbow Imaging—Benjamin M. Howe and Michael R. Moynagh

Chapter 61
Video 61.1 Elbow Tendinopathies and Bursitis—Jennifer Moriatis Wolf

Chapter 62
Video 62.1 Distal Biceps and Triceps Tendon Ruptures—James Bradley, Fotios P. Tjoumakaris, Gregory T. Lichtman, and Luke S. Austin

Chapter 63
Video 63.1 Entrapment Neuropathies of the Arm, Elbow, and Forearm—Wajeeh Bakhsh and Warren C. Hammert

Chapter 64
Video 64.1 Elbow Throwing Injuries—Marshall A. Kuremsky, E. Lyle Cain Jr, Jeffrey R. Dugas, James R. Andrews, and Christopher A. Looze

Chapter 65
Video 65.1 Loss of Elbow Motion—Timothy J. Luchetti, Debdut Biswas, and Robert W. Wysocki

Chapter 66
Video 66.1 Anatomy and Biomechanics of the Hand and Wrist—Raj M. Amin and John V. Ingari

Chapter 67
Video 67.1 Hand and Wrist Diagnosis and Decision-Making—Patrick G. Marinello, R. Glenn Gaston, Eliott P. Robinson, and Gary M. Lourie

Chapter 68
Video 68.1 Imaging of the Wrist and Hand—Kimberly K. Amrami

Chapter 69
Video 69.1 Wrist Arthroscopy—William B. Geissler, David A. Rush, and Christopher A. Keen

Chapter 71
Video 71.1 Wrist Tendinopathies—Raj M. Amin and John V. Ingari

Chapter 72
Video 72.1 Disorders of the Distal Radioulnar Joint—Julie E. Adams

Chapter 73
Video 73.1 Tendon Injuries in the Hand—Robin N. Kamal and Jacob D. Gire

Chapter 74
Video 74.1 Digit Fractures and Dislocations—Christopher L. Stockburger amd Ryan P. Calfee

Chapter 75
Video 75.1 Neuropathies of the Wrist and Hand—Gwendolyn Hoben and Amy M. Moore

Chapter 76
Video 76.1 Hip Anatomy and Biomechanics—Marc Safran and Abdurrahman Kandil

Chapter 77
Video 77.1 Hip Diagnosis and Decision-Making—Benjamin G. Domb and Austin W. Chen

Chapter 78
Video 78.1 Hip Imaging—Brian Busconi, R. Tyler Huish, Erik Mitchell, and Sean McMillan

Chapter 79
Video 79.1 Hip Arthroscopy—Joshua D. Harris

Chapter 80
Video 80.1 Femoroacetabular Impingement in Athletes—Shane J. Nho, Vignesh Prasad Krishnamoorthy, Drew Lansdown, Gift Ukwuani

Chapter 82
Video 82.1 Iliopsoas Pathology—Christian N. Anderson

Chapter 83
Video 83.1 Peritrochanteric Disorders—John W. Stelzer and Scott D. Martin
Video 83.2 Peritrochanteric Disorders—John W. Stelzer and Scott D. Martin
Video 83.3 Peritrochanteric Disorders—John W. Stelzer and Scott D. Martin

Chapter 85
Video 85.1 Posterior Hip Pain—Hal David Martin, Anthony Nicholas Khoury, and Juan Gomez-Hoyos

Chapter 87
Video 87.1 Hip and Thigh Contusions and Strains—Blake R. Obrock, Christopher P. Bankhead, and Dustin Richter

Chapter 89
Video 89.1 Knee Anatomy and Biomechanics of the Knee—Matthew J. Kraeutler, Jorge Chahla, Francesc Malagelada, Jordi Vega, Pau Golanó, Bruce Beynnon, Fatih Ertem, and Eric C. McCarty

Chapter 90
Video 90.1 Knee Diagnosis and Decision-Making—Andrew J. Riff, Peter N. Chalmers, and Bernard R. Bach Jr.

Chapter 92
Video 92.1 Basics of Knee Arthroscopy—Stephen R. Thompson and Mark D. Miller

Chapter 94
Video 94.1 Meniscal Injuries—Joseph J. Ruzbarsky, Travis G. Maak, and Scott A. Rodeo

Chapter 96
Video 96.1 Articular Cartilage Lesions—Michael S. Laidlaw, Kadir Buyukdogan, and Mark D. Miller

Chapter 98
Video 98.1 Anterior Cruciate Ligament Injuries—Edward C. Cheung, David R. McAllister, and Frank A. Petrigliano

Chapter 99
Video 99.1 Revision Anterior Cruciate Ligament Injuries—Joseph D. Lamplot, Liljiana Bogunovic, and Rick W. Wright

Chapter 100
Video 100.1 Posterior Cruciate Ligament Injuries—Frank A. Petrigliano, Evan E. Vellios, Scott R. Montgomery, Jared S. Johnson, and David R. McAllister

Chapter 101
Video 101.1 Medial Collateral Ligament and Posterior Medial Corner Injuries—M. Christopher Yonz, Brian F. Wilson, Matthew H. Blake, and Darren L. Johnson

Chapter 102
Video 102.1 Lateral and Posterolateral Corner Injuries of the Knee—Ryan P. Coughlin, Dayne T. Mickelson, and Claude T. Moorman III

Chapter 103
Video 103.1 Multiligament Knee Injuries—Samantha L. Kallenbach, Matthew D. LaPrade, and Robert F. LaPrade

Chapter 108
Video 108.1 Loss of Knee Motion—K. Donald Shelbourne, Heather Freeman, and Tinker Gray

Chapter 110
Video 110.1 Foot and Ankle Biomechanics—Andrew Haskell

Chapter 115
Video 115.1 Ankle Arthroscopy—Niall A. Smyth, Jonathan R. Kaplan, Amiethab A. Aiyer, John T. Campbell, Rachel Triche, and Rebecca A. Cerrato

Chapter 117
Video 117.1 Ligamentous Injuries of the Foot and Ankle—Paul Rothenberg, Eric Swanton, Andrew Molloy, Amiethab A. Aiyer, and Jonathan R. Kaplan

Chapter 118
Video 118.1 Tendon Injuries of the Foot and Ankle—Todd A. Irwin

Chapter 119
Video 119.1 Articular Cartilage Injuries and Defects—David R. Richardson and Jane C. Yeoh

Chapter 121
Video 121.1 Forefoot Problems in Sport—Ben Hickey, Lyndon Mason, and Anthony Perera

Chapter 122
Video 122.1 Head and Spine Anatomy and Biomechanics—Colin B. Harris, Rachid Assina, Brandee Gentile, and Michael J. Vives

Chapter 123
Video 123.1 Head and Spine Diagnosis and Decision-Making—Rabia Qureshi, Jason A. Horowtiz, Kieran Bhattacharya, and Hamid Hassanzadeh

Chapter 124
Video 124.1 Imaging of the Spine—Adil Samad, M. Farooq Usmani, and A. Jay Khanna

Chapter 125
Video 125.1 Emergency and Field-Side Management of the Spine-Injured Athlete—Korin Hudson, Michael Antonis, and William Brady

Chapter 132
Video 132.1 Imaging Considerations in Skeletally Immature Athletes—Andrew M. Zbojniewicz

Chapter 133
Video 133.1 Shoulder Injuries in the Young Athlete—Andrew T. Pennock and Eric W. Edmonds

Chapter 134
Video 134.1 Elbow Injuries in Pediatric and Adolescent Athletes—James P. Bradley, Luke S. Austin, Alexander B. Kreines, and Fotios P. Tjoumakaris

Chapter 137
Video 137.1 Knee Injuries in Skeletally Immature Athletes—Matthew D. Milewski, James Wylie, Carl W. Nissen, and Tricia R. Prokop

Chapter 138
Video 138.1 Foot and Ankle Injuries in the Adolescent Athlete—J. Andy Sullivan and James R. Gregory

Chapter 139
Video 139.1 Head Injuries in Skeletally Immature Athletes—Tracy Zaslow

Pelvis, Hip, and Thigh

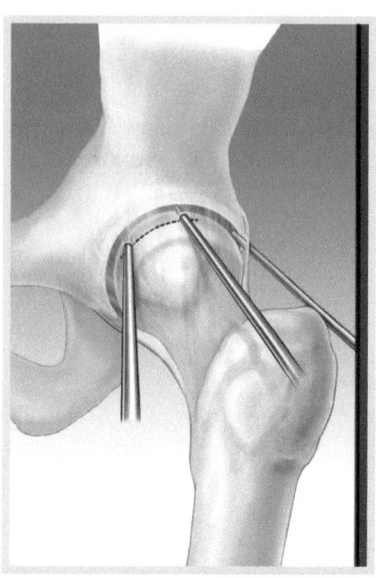

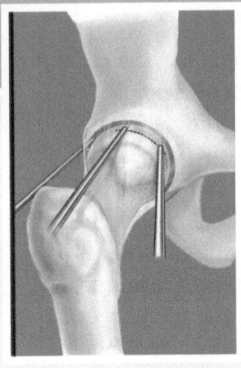

76

Hip Anatomy and Biomechanics

Marc Safran, Abdurrahman Kandil

The hip joint (*coxa* in Latin) is the articulation connecting the pelvis and the femur. It is an encapsulated synovial joint with a ball-and-socket architecture in which the femoral head is the ball and the acetabulum is the socket. Although its structure may seem simple, it is actually very complex, with more than 20 muscles spanning the joint and a three-dimensional (3D) bony morphology that may vary widely among subjects. The acetabulum may be described as retroverted or anteverted, shallow or deep, and with high or low inclination of the weight-bearing surface. The femoral head may be overcovered by the acetabulum or undercovered, and the offset of the femoral head-neck junction may be reduced or normal. The proximal femur may have a short or long neck, a high or low femoral neck-shaft angle, and be retroverted or anteverted. To further complicate matters, the head is not a completely round sphere, the socket is horseshoe shaped, and the center of the femoral head moves relative to the socket; therefore this is not a true ball-and-socket joint. Giorgi et al. showed that a full range of symmetric prenatal movements helps to maintain acetabular depth and femoral head sphericity, whereas reduced or absent movements can lead to decreased sphericity and acetabular coverage of the femoral head.[1]

The main function of the hip is to support the weight of the body in both static (e.g., standing) and dynamic (e.g., walking or running) situations. To address the biomechanical principles involved in the function of the human hip, it is essential to understand the anatomy of the proximal femur and pelvis as well as the muscles, ligaments, and bony structures, which all contribute to the equilibrium of forces needed to control hip joint motion.

PRENATAL HIP JOINT DEVELOPMENT

Knowledge regarding hip joint development is beneficial to the understanding of hip joint anatomy and biomechanics. Limb formation begins by the fourth week of embryonic life. By the sixth week, primitive chondroblasts accumulate at the proximal, central, and distal ends of the cellular femoral template, forming chondrification centers, and a club-shaped cartilage model of the future femur arises from those centers. At the same time a shallow acetabulum begins to form proximal to the femoral head by future ilium, ischium, and pubis precursor cells. Later, the chondrification process of these bones continues until fusion occurs. By the seventh week of development, the cartilage models of both the femur and the acetabulum are complete. By the eight

week, the capsule, acetabular labrum, ligamentum teres, and transverse ligament can be identified microscopically, and 3 weeks later they can be identified macroscopically.[2] At 16 weeks, ossification of the femur is complete up to the lesser trochanter, and primary ossification centers will have appeared in the three pelvic bones. The ossification centers of the acetabulum do not appear until adolescence. Through the 20th week of gestation, differentiation of the hip joint ends and the process shifts to growth and maturation.[3]

BONY ANATOMY

Acetabular Development

The acetabulum has two components: the triradiate cartilage in the center (Fig. 76.1) and the acetabular cartilage complex, which is formed by fusion of the ilium, ischium, and pubis.[2,3] The triradiate cartilage forms the nonarticular medial wall of the acetabulum and its growth is crucial for acetabular height and depth. The acetabular cartilage complex, which is composed mainly of hyaline cartilage, forms the cup-shaped articular portion of the acetabulum.[3] Around the age of 8 to 9 years, secondary ossification centers appear at the acetabular rim (os acetabuli). In 1922, Perna identified three distinct os acetabuli—anterior, posterior, and superior.[4-6] Those ossification centers have an important role in the development of the acetabular rim and its depth.[7] In most cases, the superior os acetabulum fuses by adulthood; however, occasionally its fusion is delayed, and radiographically this may mimic a fracture of the acetabular rim. Normal acetabular development depends heavily on the interaction with the spherical femoral head as a template about which it forms.[3] Complete absence of the proximal femur yields an absent acetabulum.[8]

Acetabular Version

The normal acetabulum is angled 15 to 20 degrees anteriorly, or anteverted.[9] The acetabular version can be estimated by the appearance of the anterior and posterior acetabular walls on a straight (not tilted) anteroposterior (AP) pelvic radiograph, whereas computed tomography (CT) can be used to measure the acetabular version.[9,10] The anteverted acetabulum allows for hip flexion that is greater than hip extension. A retroverted acetabulum occurs when the acetabulum is angled less than 15 degrees anteriorly. The acetabulum may have a relative retroversion (still anteverted, but <15 degrees) or be truly retroverted,

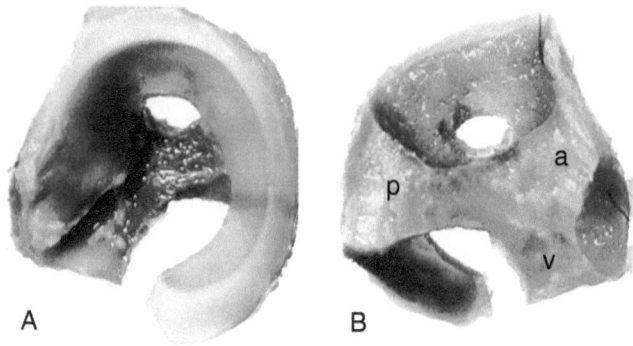

Fig. 76.1 Triradiate cartilage. Lateral view (A) and medial view (B) of the normal acetabular cartilage complex of a 1-day-old infant. The ilium, ischium, and pubis have been removed with a curette. The lateral view shows the cup-shaped acetabulum, and the medial view shows the three flanges of the triradiate cartilage. The anterior flange *(a)* is located between the ilium and pubis and is slanted superiorly; the posterior flange *(p)* is horizontal and located between the ilium and ischium; and the vertical flange *(v)* is located between the pubis and ischium. (Modified from Ponseti IV. Growth and development of the acetabulum in the normal child: anatomical, histological, and roentgenographic studies. *J Bone Joint Surg Am.* 1978;60[5]:576.)

angled posteriorly. Additionally, cranial retroversion may be present, in which the anterior acetabular wall projects more laterally than the posterior wall only superiorly, demonstrating a positive "crossover sign" on radiographs.

Acetabular Depth and Volume

In a cadaveric study of 154 hips, the mean values for the acetabular depth and diameter were 29.49 ± 4.2 and 54.29 ± 3.8 mm, respectively. The maximum and minimum measurements of acetabular diameter were 65.5 and 44.8 mm, respectively, and acetabular depth ranged from 38.6 to 22.6 mm, respectively.[11]

Recently Liu et al. studied a random sample of 545 cadaveric skeletons and found that female cadavers had smaller femoral heads and acetabular volumes than male cadaveric hips, although the femoral head volume/acetabular volume ratio was unchanged.[12]

Another reported measure of acetabular depth can be determined from axial magnetic resonance or CT views of the hip joint as the distance between the center of the femoral head and the line connecting the anterior acetabular rim to the posterior acetabular rim. The value is positive if the center of the femoral neck is lateral to the line connecting the acetabular rim and negative if medial to it. A positive value indicates a shallower acetabulum, whereas a negative value suggests a deeper acetabulum.[13] Murtha et al. studied the acetabular anatomy using 3D surface models of the normal hemipelvis derived from volumetric CT data on 42 patients. For the 22 female subjects, the mean acetabular depth was 0.79 mm (0.56 to 1.04), and for the 20 male subjects it was 0.85 mm (0.65 to 0.99).[14]

Zeng et al. studied acetabular morphologic differences between genders in a Chinese population; they measured the acetabular width as the inferior distance between the superolateral and lowermost points of the acetabulum and the acetabular depth as the perpendicular distance between the top and bottom of the acetabulum on an AP tomogram. Both width and depth

were significantly smaller in women than in men, but the difference was not significant when adjusted for body height.[15]

The acetabular depth can also be quantified radiographically on an AP pelvic view by the center edge angle (of Wiberg). This angle is formed by a line drawn from the center of the femoral head to the outer edge of the acetabular roof and a vertical line drawn from the center of the femoral head directly superior.[6,16] Although currently somewhat a matter of controversy, the normal values of the center edge angle are between 25 and 35 degrees. A center edge angle of 20 to 25 degrees is often considered "borderline dysplasia," whereas the upper limits of the center edge angle may be reported as up to 40 degrees. The anterior center edge angle of Lequesne is composed of a vertical line through the center of the femoral head and a second line through the center of the hip and the foremost aspect of the acetabulum as seen on a false-profile radiograph. This angle quantifies the anterior cover of the femoral head, and angles of less than 20 degrees are considered abnormal.[17]

A deep acetabulum (profunda or protrusio) may result in pincer-type impingement, whereas on the other end of the spectrum the acetabulum may not be deep enough. Failure of the secondary ossification centers to develop the acetabular rim and adequate depth results in a shallow socket, also known as hip dysplasia.[7,18-20]

Anteroinferior Iliac Spine

The anteroinferior iliac spine (AIIS) is a bony prominence above the acetabulum that serves as the attachment of the origin of the direct head of the rectus femoris and the iliocapsularis muscle. It is a structure of increasing interest to those concerned about nonarthritic hip pain. "Subspinal impingement" is defined as abutment of the femoral head or neck on the AIIS and is becoming more recognized as a diagnosis, with treatment often involving recession of the bony prominence performed either arthroscopically or, less commonly, through an open procedure. Amar et al. studied the anatomy of the AIIS using CT and found that there was no significant difference between male and female patients' AIIS anatomy or their left and right sides except for AIIS width, which differed in males versus females.[21]

Philippon et al. largely corroborated the results of Amar and colleagues and found, using CT, that the average horizontal distance from the anteriormost point of the AIIS to the acetabular rim was 21.8 mm, and the direct distance of the inner rim of the acetabulum to the inferolateral corner of the direct head of the rectus femoris footprint was 19.2 mm.[22]

Proximal Femoral Development

At birth, ossification of the femoral shaft reaches the greater trochanter and the femoral neck. A few months later, two ossification centers appear, one in the center of the femoral head and one in the greater trochanter. Three growth plates are defined: longitudinal (between the femoral head and the neck), trochanteric (between the femoral neck and the greater trochanter), and the femoral neck isthmus.[3] These growth plates are essential for the growth and shape of the proximal femur.

The pressure exerted on the femoral head by the acetabulum is necessary to result in a spherical femoral head. Overall, the development of both the proximal femur and the acetabulum are related to correct development and each other's positioning.

Blood Supply

The main artery of the lower limb is the femoral artery, which is a continuation of the external iliac artery distal to the ilioinguinal ligament. The profunda femoris is a large lateral branch of the femoral artery that appears about 3.5 cm below the inguinal ligament. Branches from the profunda include the lateral circumflex, the medial circumflex, perforating arteries to the femur, muscular branches, and the descending genicular artery.[23]

The proximal femur is supplied by three main blood sources: (1) the nutrient artery of the shaft that arises from the perforating arteries, (2) the retinacular vessels of the capsule that arise from the circumflex arteries, and (3) the foveal artery of the ligamentum teres.

The nutrient artery enters the midshaft of the femur and may be single or double; its superior branch runs in the medullary cavity and anastomoses with the retinacular vessels in the metaphysis. In adults over 13 years of age, the nutrient artery has been found to cross the epiphyseal plate from the metaphysis to the epiphysis.[24]

The retinacular vessels penetrate the capsule near its distal attachment and are the main blood supply to the femoral epiphysis and femoral head at all ages.[25,26] The three main groups of retinacular vessels—superior, inferior, and anterior—are all intracapsular and covered with a synovial membrane, sometimes in a mesenteric-like fold. The anterior retinacular vessels are the smallest of the three, branching from the lateral femoral circumflex artery, and are less consistent. Overall, the lateral femoral circumflex artery contributes little to the vascularity of the femoral head.[25] The superior and inferior retinacular vessels arise from the deep branch medial femoral circumflex artery and run along the upper and lower borders of the femoral neck. The medial circumflex femoral artery supplies blood to the neck of the femur and femoral head. It arises from the medial and posterior aspects of the profunda femoris artery and winds around the medial side of the femur, passing first between the iliopsoas and pectineus muscles and then between the obturator externus and adductor brevis. These two groups are fairly large and consistent between specimens. The superior group, which runs in the lateral retinacular fold, is larger, supplies the weight-bearing part of the femoral head, and may be the sole blood supply to the epiphysis.[24] Anastomoses of the deep branch of the medial femoral circumflex artery with other arteries have been described; a significant and consistent anastomosis with a branch of the inferior gluteal artery is found along the piriformis; in some cases the inferior gluteal artery has been found to be the main blood supply of the hip.[25,26]

The foveal artery, running within the ligamentum teres, is formed by the acetabular branches of the obturator or the medial circumflex or from both; often its contribution to the femoral head blood supply is minute.[23,24] In some cases it is found to be anastomosing with the epiphyseal arteries, whereas in other cases it is found to supply only the area of insertion of the ligamentum teres to the fovea.[24] A recent study found no significant vascular contribution by the foveal artery.[26]

Recently Zhao et al. reconstructed the 3D structures of the intraosseous blood supply of 30 uninjured normal human femoral heads using angiographic methods and micro-CT scans. They found that the epiphyseal arterial network is the most widely distributed and the primary network structure in the femoral head. They also found that the main stems of the epiphyseal arteries have fewer anastomoses than the network located in the central region and that the inferior retinacular artery has a relatively large caliber as compared with the round ligament artery and anterior retinacular artery.[27]

Femoral Neck Version

The femoral neck version is the angle between the femoral neck and the axis that crosses the distal femoral condyles; this angle can be measured through CT or magnetic resonance imaging (MRI) that includes both the knee and the hip.[28] Normally the proximal femur is anteverted. Femoral anteversion is greatest at birth and decreases with growth. Normal average anteversion ranges between 35 and 45 degrees at the time of birth, is 31 degrees at the age of 1 year, and decreases to 15.4 degrees by skeletal maturity (16 years of age).[29] Clinically, increased femoral anteversion can be seen as an "in toed" appearance of the lower limb in a standing person, or squinting patellae, where the patellae point toward the midline.[9]

Neck Shaft Angle

The neck shaft angle is the angle measured between the axis of the femoral neck and the femoral shaft. This angle can be measured on plain AP pelvic radiographs, but internal or external rotation of the hip may increase the measured angle. Similar to the version angle, the neck shaft angle is highest at birth and declines with growth. The normal neck shaft angle is approximately 136 degrees at 1 year of age and decreases to 127 degrees by age 18 years.[3]

Femoral Head-Neck Junction

Normally the femoral head-neck junction is waist shaped, with the femoral neck narrower than its head. The head-neck junction morphology can be quantified by the anterior offset or the alpha angle.[30-34] The offset is the difference between the anterior contour of the head and femoral neck on axial MRI or CT scans. On axial radiographs (cross-table or Dunn view), it is defined as the distance between the widest diameter of the femoral head and the most prominent part of the femoral neck.[35] The offset can be measured as the ratio between the femoral head and neck radii or as an absolute distance, which is normally measured as around 10 mm.[35]

The alpha angle was described by Notzli et al. in 2002 as a measurement on angled axial MRI cuts parallel to the axis of the femoral neck.[34] The alpha angle is a simple method to quantify the concavity at femoral head-neck junction, and it was shown to correlate with anterior hip impingement. The alpha angle is composed of a line that connects the center of the femoral neck at its narrowest diameter to the center of the femoral head. The second line that composes the alpha angle is from the center of the femoral head to a point where the femoral head loses its sphericity, and thus where femoral head exceeds the normal radius of the femoral head. The alpha angle can also be measured on plain radiographs and was found to correlate well with the MRI values.[36-38] In general, normal alpha angle perimeters have fluctuated since the original report, being less than 50 or 55 degrees.

Internal Bony Architecture of the Femoral Neck

The first description of the bony trabecular orientation in the femoral neck is attributed to Ward in *Human Anatomy,* which was published in London in 1838; in 1961 it was cited by Garden, who likened the trabecular structure within the femoral neck to that of a lamp bracket.[39] Many other analogies of the trabecular pattern to other 3D weight-bearing subjects, such as cranes, are common as well.[40] Because the proximal femur is exposed to tensile and compressive forces during weight bearing, those forces lead to functional internal bony architecture of the femoral neck trabeculae lines, as stated by Wolff's law of bone remodeling.[41] These trabeculae consist of a primary compressive group, which arises from the medial subtrochanteric cortex and ascends superiorly into the weight-bearing femoral head, and a primary tensile group, which spans from the foveal area of the femoral head, through the superior femoral neck, and into the lateral subtrochanteric cortex (Fig. 76.2).[42] Secondary compressive, secondary tensile, and a greater trochanteric group complete the pattern of trabecular orientation. The calcar femorale was precisely defined anatomically by Merkle in 1874 as a dense plate of bone extending laterally from the posteromedial femoral cortex to the posterior aspect of the greater trochanter.[43] This bone spur is thickest medially and gradually thins as it extends laterally. However, although defined anatomically as a cancellous bone spur, the term "calcar" is frequently (and some say mistakenly)

used to describe the medial cortical bone of the femoral neck, which is the thickest cortex of the femur and the strongest bone in the hip. The medial cortex is also known as Adam's arch.[44]

Greater Trochanter

The greater trochanter can be divided into four facets—anterior, lateral, posterior, and superoposterior.[45] Those facets are the insertions of the abductor complex; the gluteus medius muscle attaches to the superoposterior and lateral facets, and the gluteus minimus muscle attaches to the anterior facet. A bald spot was described on the lateral facet of the greater trochanter, devoid of tendon insertion and bordered anteriorly and distally by the gluteus minimus, posteriorly by the gluteus medius, and proximally by the piriformis tendon (Fig. 76.3).[46] Blood supply to the greater trochanteric area arises from the trochanteric branch of the medial femoral circumflex artery.[25]

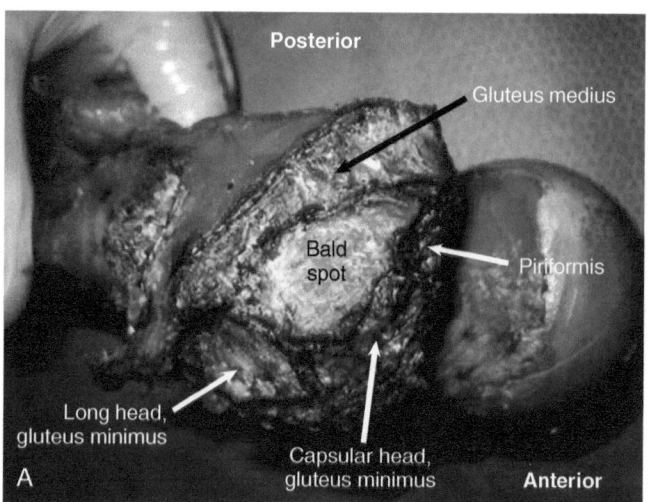

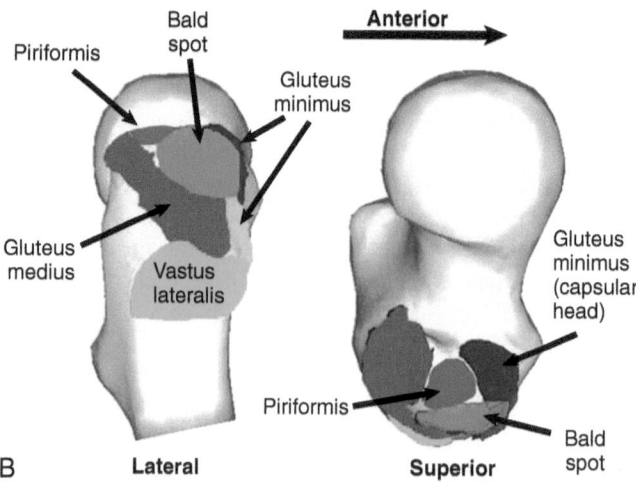

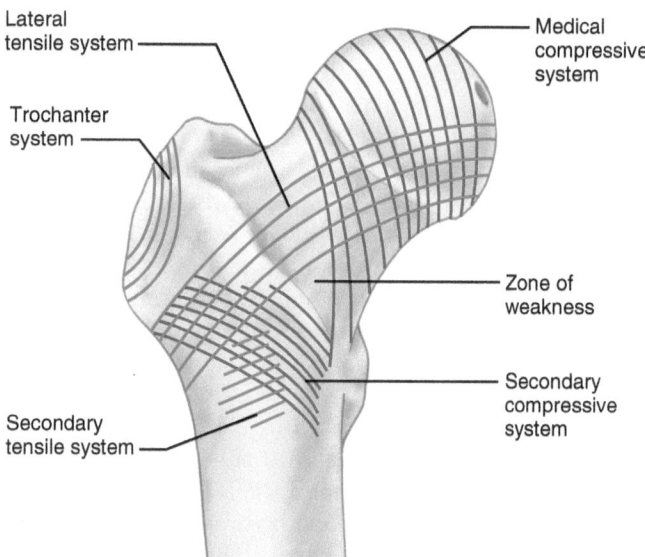

Fig. 76.2 Trabecular pattern. An anteroposterior radiograph of the hip illustrating the primary and secondary compressive and tensile trabecular bone groups. A greater trochanteric group completes the pattern of trabecular orientation. (From Hughes PE, Hsu JC, Matava MJ. Hip anatomy and biomechanics in the athlete. *Sports Med Arthrosc Rev.* 2002;10[2]:103–114.)

Fig. 76.3 The bald spot is bordered posteriorly by the gluteus medius, anteriorly by the two heads of the gluteus minimus, and superiorly and medially by the piriformis. Examples of (A) a gross specimen and (B) the bone morphing model after navigated determination of tendon footprints are shown. (From Gardner MJ, Robertson WJ, Boraiah S, et al. Anatomy of the greater trochanteric "bald spot": a potential portal for abductor sparing femoral nailing? *Clin Orthop Relat Res.* 2008;466[9]:2196–2200.)

Lesser Trochanter

The lesser trochanter is a pyramidal process that projects from the lower and posterior part of the base femoral neck. Medially it is in continuation with the lower border of the femoral neck, laterally with the intertrochanteric crest, and inferiorly with the linea aspera. The lesser trochanter is the insertion point of the iliopsoas muscle. The lesser trochanter varies in size in different subjects: its height is approximately 1.2 cm, and its width can range between 2 and 4.5 cm.[47]

Ischiofemoral distance (IFD) is the smallest distance between the lateral cortex of the ischial tuberosity and the posteromedial cortex of the lesser trochanter. Ischiofemoral impingement (IFI) may result if there is a reduction in IFD. A recent study found that the IFD increased by 1.06 mm for each 1 mm of offset and dropped by 0.09 mm with each year of age. However, the neck-shaft angle did not show any significant correlation with the IFD.[48] In seeking to define the pathomechanics associated with IFI and validate clinical tests to diagnose IFI, Kivlan et al. found that the lesser trochanter is closest to the ischium in lateral hip rotation and furthest away in medial hip rotation when the hip is in neutral flexion-extension/abduction-adduction.[49]

INTRA-ARTICULAR STRUCTURES

Acetabular Labrum

The acetabular labrum is a horseshoe-shaped structure attached to the acetabular rim. Inferiorly the labrum joins the transverse ligament to bridge the acetabular notch, forming a complete circle.[50] It is triangular in its cross-sectional shape, with its base attached to the acetabulum and its apex forming a free edge (Fig. 76.4).[51] Petersen et al. looked at the labrum under light microscopy and found that the majority of the collagen fibers have a circumferential orientation.[52] The capsular side of the labrum is composed of dense connective tissue mainly consisting

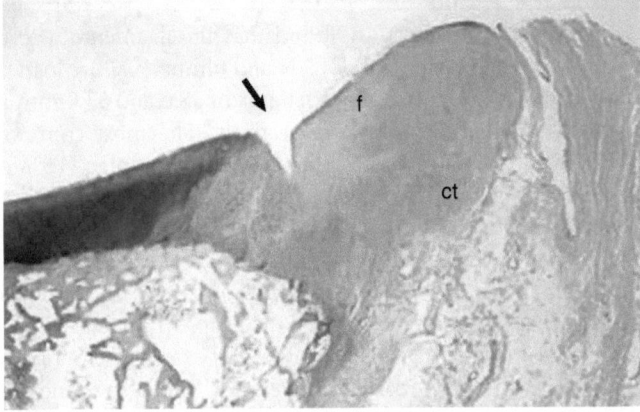

Fig. 76.4 Histology of the labrum. Cross-sectional histology of the labrum: The labrum is separated from the articular cartilage by a physiologic cleft *(arrow)* and is composed of two different tissues, fibrocartilage *(f)* on the articular side and connective tissue *(ct)* on the capsular side. This physiologic cleft is seen more often in the posterior labrum. (From Petersen W, Petersen F, Tillmann B. Structure and vascularization of the acetabular labrum with regard to the pathogenesis and healing of labral lesions. *Arch Orthop Trauma Surg.* 2003, 123[6]:283–288.)

of collagen types I and III, whereas the articular side is composed of fibrocartilage. At the articular side, the labrum is often separated from the articular cartilage by a physiologic cleft that is seen more frequently posteriorly, whereas anteriorly this cleft is usually absent and the transition between the labrum and articular cartilage is smooth.

Seldes et al. also studied the labrum histologically and found it to be widest in its inferior half and thickest at its superior half.[51] On average, the acetabular labral size ranges from 4 to 8 mm. The average labral width as reported by Seldes et al. ranged from 3.8 mm posterosuperiorly to 6.4 mm posteroinferiorly. However, the labral width may vary according to the forces that act on it. It appears that the labral size may be inversely proportional to the depth of the bony acetabular socket contribution to femoral head coverage. Thus the labrum may be small, with a width of less than 3 mm in coxa profunda, or it may be large/hypertrophic, with a width of up to 14 mm in a dysplastic hip.

Inferiorly, the labrum appears to be continuous with the transverse acetabular ligament over the cotyloid notch; however, a distinction is seen between the labrum and the transverse ligament. A bony acetabular tongue exists within the labrum with the labrum firmly attached to it with a well-defined tidemark. Histologically the acetabular labrum merges with the articular hyaline cartilage of the joint surface of the acetabulum through a transition zone of 1 to 2 mm, particularly anteriorly.

The labrum is continuous with the articular cartilage of the acetabulum; however, differences exist in the transition between the anterior and posterior transition zones. The anterior labral-chondral transition is sharp and abrupt, with minimal interdigitation of fibers, whereas the posterior labral-chondral transition is smooth and gradual. This appearance is due to differences in the orientation of collagen fibers of the labrum; the anterior fibers are parallel to the labral-chondral junction, whereas posterior fibers are oriented perpendicularly.[53]

Historically the clock face has been employed to define the position of labral pathology in relation to identifiable arthroscopically relevant acetabular landmarks. Recently Philippon et al. proposed the superior margin of the anterior labral sulcus (psoas-u) as a new standard reference point that is located in close proximity to the usual location of labral pathology as an alternative to the historic landmark, which is the midpoint of the transverse acetabular ligament.[54]

Blood Supply

The main vascular supply of the labrum arises from radial vessels on its capsular side embedded in a loose connective tissue between the labrum and the capsule (Fig. 76.5).[52,55,56] These vessels seem to supply only the outer third of the labrum. Kalhor et al. used a silicon injection technique to show a periacetabular vascular ring supplying the labrum, originating from the superior and inferior gluteal vessels, the medial and lateral femoral circumflex arteries, and the intrapelvic vascular system.[55]

The acetabular bony rim that is embedded in the base of the labrum is another source of blood supply to the labrum. McCarthy et al., in an immunohistochemical study, showed abundant vessels within the bony acetabulum that reach the junction with the labrum.[57] Seldes et al. identified a group of three to four vessels

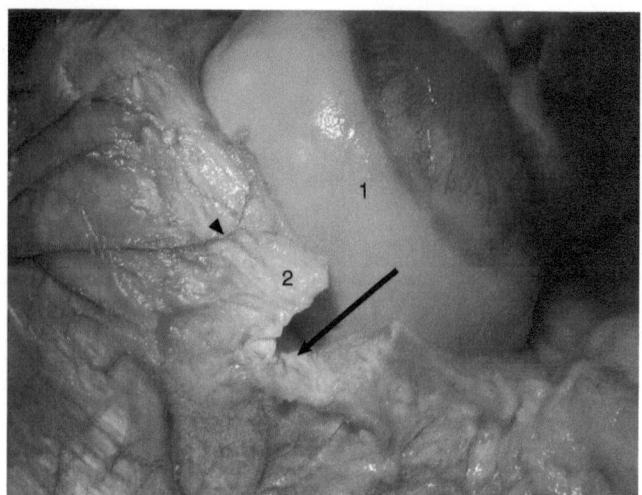

Fig. 76.5 Vascular supply of the labrum. The posterior aspect of a right hip after resection of a segment of the labrum. The *arrow* points to the osseolabral junction and shows the absence of visible vessels traversing this boundary. The radial vessels on the labrum can be seen embedded in a layer of loose connective tissue. *1,* Femoral head; *2,* labrum. The *arrowhead* points to a radial vessel on the labrum that can be seen embedded in a layer of loose connective tissue.[58] (From Kalhor M, Horowitz K, Beck M, et al. Vascular supply to the acetabular labrum. *J Bone Joint Surg Am.* 2010;92[15]:2570–2575.)

located in the substance of the labrum that travels circumferentially around the labrum at its attachment site on the outer surface of the bony acetabular extension.[51]

Innervation

The labrum has been shown to be richly populated by many neurologic structures. Kim and Azuma found sensory nerves and organs such as Vater-Pacini, Golgi-Mazzoni, Ruffini, and Krause corpuscles within the acetabular labrum.[58] Most of these sensory nerve end organs (86%) are in the articular side of the labrum. The corpuscles observed are receptors of pressure, deep sensation, and temperature sense. In addition, no differences in number or type of nerves and organs were found based on the age of the specimens, but more unmyelinated nerve endings, which function to sense pain, were identified in the superior and anterior quarters of the labrum. Additionally, Gerhardt et al. found that the anterior zone of the labrum contained the highest concentration of mechanoreceptors and sensory fibers, specifically Ruffini corpuscles.[59] Thus the labrum may function to provide proprioceptive input, and a damaged labrum may be a source of hip pain.

Biomechanical Properties

The labrum deepens the acetabulum and acts as a suction seal, adding stability to the joint and protecting the articular cartilage. Seldes et al. have shown that the labrum increases the acetabular surface area and volume by 22% and 33%, respectively.[51,60] Furthermore, the labrum creates a seal that opposes the flow of synovial fluid in and out of the central compartment. Safran et al. have shown that the labrum has strain at rest, which increases and decreases in different locations of the labrum as the hip

is taken through range of motion (ROM).[61] According to biomechanical studies, with an intact labrum, the acetabular and femoral cartilage surfaces do not come into direct contact with each other because of a film of fluid contained by the labrum. Ferguson et al. have found that hydrostatic fluid pressure within the intra-articular space was greater within the labrum than without, which may enhance joint lubrication, whereas labrum resection resulted in faster cartilage consolidation.[62] Haemer et al. found that an intact hip labrum is important for limiting fluid exudation from articular cartilage in the hip.[63] Song et al. also found that the acetabular labrum plays a role in maintaining a low-friction environment, possibly by sealing the joint from fluid exudation, because both complete and focal labral débridement resulted in increased joint friction, a condition that is thought to be detrimental to articular cartilage and leads to osteoarthritis.[64] The sealing function of the labrum also helps maintain the negative intra-articular pressure that occurs in all joints. This negative intra-articular pressure helps resist distraction of the femoral head from the socket; this function is called the "suction effect" and is thought to improve the stability of the joint.[65]

Ligamentum Teres

The ligamentum teres, otherwise known as the round ligament of the femur, is a triangular double-band ligament with a length of 30 to 35 mm that attaches the femoral head to the acetabulum.[66-68] Medially it is attached to either side of the acetabular notch by two bands that originate from the acetabular transverse ligament and the pubic and ischial margins. Laterally its apex extends to the anterosuperior portion of the femoral head, merging with the fovea capitis femoris.

The ligament is composed of thick, well-organized, parallel and slightly undulating or wavy fibers of collagen bundles that are composed of collagen types I, III, and V. Embryonically the ligamentum teres is defined at around 8 weeks of intrauterine life as the joint space expands and is seen to attach to the medial border of the acetabular fossa, separating from the transverse acetabular ligament.

A recent anatomic study found that the ligamentum teres achieved a mean yield load of 75 N and ultimate failure load of 204 N. The ligament had mean lengths of 38.0 and 53.0 mm at its yield and failure points, respectively. The most common mechanism of failure was tearing at the fovea capitis (75% of specimens). The mean initial length and cross-sectional area were 32 mm and 59 mm², respectively. The authors suggest that the ligamentum teres may be more important as a static stabilizer of the hip than previously recognized.[69] Martin et al. conducted a biomechanical model that found the ligamentum teres to have the greatest excursion when the hip was externally rotated in flexion and internally rotated in extension. They also found that patients with complete ruptures of the ligamentum teres had had laxity during dynamic impingement testing when their hip was in a position of external rotation and flexion.[70]

Blood Supply

An anterior branch of the posterior division of the obturator artery provides the blood supply to the ligamentum teres

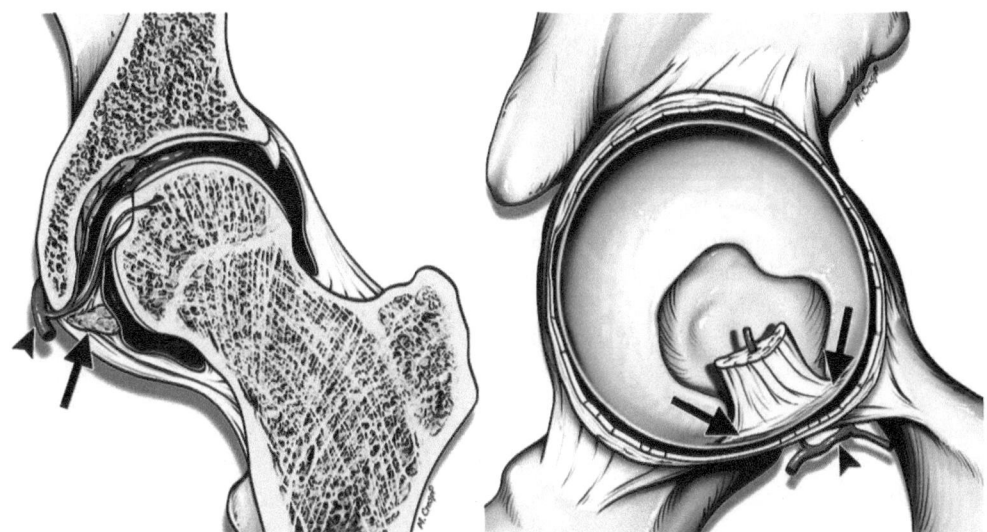

Fig. 76.6 Ligamentum teres. These diagrams show the normal anatomy of the ligamentum teres. It has a broad origin that blends with the entire transverse ligament of the acetabulum *(arrows)* and is attached to the ischial and pubic sides of the acetabular notch by two bands. It inserts into the fovea capitis femoris, and its arterial supply is provided by the anterior branch of the posterior division of the obturator artery *(arrowhead)*. Vascular canals extend a short distance from the fovea capitis into the femoral head. (From Cerezal L, Kassarjian A, Canga A, et al. Anatomy, biomechanics, imaging, and management of ligamentum teres injuries. *Radiographics.* 2010;30[6]:1637–1651.)

(Fig. 76.6). Vascular canals extend from the fovea capitis of the femoral head to supply the epiphysis of the femoral head; however, these arteries are not patent in a third of the population. These vessels do not anastomose with the distal arterial terminals in the femoral head until around age 15 years, when ossification of the head is nearly complete.[71]

Biomechanical Properties

The biomechanical role of the ligamentum teres has been debated in the medical literature since the 19th century, with proposed functions including that of a stabilizer, a fluid and force distributor in the acetabulum, and an embryonic remnant with no specific role in adults.[72-74] The ligamentum teres has also been previously described as a possible transmitter of somatosensory signals that act to help the hip avoid painful and excessive ranges of motion.[75] More recently, the ligamentum teres in the hip has been thought to provide functions comparable with the anterior cruciate ligament in the knee; with similar tensile strength, it has been proposed to provide some degree of stability in the hip, resisting dislocation and microinstability.[76] However, many other studies report that the ligamentum teres plays little role in the stability of the hip joint and suggest that it is possibly a mere embryonic remnant.[77]

The ligamentum teres has been found to be taut in flexion, adduction, and external rotation; thus it may play a role in stability of the hip joint in those positions.[66,67,76] In a recent study, Domb et al. have found that the arthroscopic presence of ligamentum teres tears was associated with acetabular bony morphology and age.[78] Ligamentum teres tears were less frequent in hips with a high lateral coverage index (center edge angle minus acetabular inclination) and also less frequent in patients younger than 30 years.

Innervation

Two histologic studies have found type IVa free nerve endings in the ligamentum teres, which are nociceptors and mechanoreceptors.[75,79] Leunig et al. suggested that in addition to its mechanical and structural functions, the ligamentum teres may be involved in transmitting specific somatosensory afferent signals to the spinal and cerebral regulatory systems.[75] Hence the ligamentum teres may be part of an integral reflex system involved in joint protection, acting as a rein to avoid excessive motion that may be potentially harmful to the joint. Alternatively, Gerhardt et al. identified a paucity of neural fibers in the ligamentum and did not find any sensory nerve fibers within it.[59] Although the function of the ligamentum teres has yet to be determined, its role as a source of hip pain after a full or a partial tear has been more clearly elucidated.[80-87]

Articular Cartilage

The articular cartilage of the hip, both on the acetabular side and the femoral side, has been shown to be highly inhomogeneous in thickness distribution. Von Eisenhart et al. studied the cartilage thickness and pressure on eight fresh cadaveric hip specimens during the phases of gait cycle.[88] Maximum cartilage thickness was found ventrosuperiorly in the acetabulum and in the femoral head. The location of maximum thickness corresponded with the ventrosuperior location of maximum pressure recorded during the walking cycle; the maximal thickness ranged from 2.6 to 4.3 mm in the acetabulum (average, 3.3 mm) and from 2.4 to 5.3 mm in the femoral head (average, 3.5 mm). In general, cartilage thickness decreased with age. No statistical difference was found between the values for maximum thickness on both surfaces, although the mean thickness of the femoral cartilage (1.5 to 2.0 mm, with an average of 1.7 mm) was higher ($P < .01$) than that of the acetabulum (1.1 to 1.7 mm, with an average of 1.4 mm).

HIP JOINT CAPSULE

The hip capsule is made up of internal fibers (within the joint) and external fibers (outside or away from the joint). The external fibers run longitudinally and comprise the iliofemoral ligament, ischiofemoral ligament (ISFL), and pubofemoral ligament (PFL). The inner fibers comprise the zona orbicularis, which forms a collar around the femoral neck.[89,90] The capsule inserts on the bony acetabulum proximal to and distinct from the labrum, forming a recess between the two that ranges between 6.6 and 7.9 mm from the anteroinferior and posteroinferior quadrants, respectively.[51] From its acetabular attachment, the capsule extends to surround the femoral head and neck in a spiral fashion and is attached anteriorly to the intertrochanteric line, superiorly to the base of the femoral neck, superomedially to the intertrochanteric crest, and inferiorly to the femoral neck near the lesser trochanter.[89,91]

One theory regarding the spiral architecture of the capsule is that it originated as humans began to walk upright. As humans transitioned from quadruped to biped, the hips were brought into relative extension, thus causing the capsular fibers to twist into a spiral pattern.[92-94] In normal stance, if the upper body is leaned slightly posteriorly, stability is provided primarily by the static restraints of the anterior capsule (mainly the iliofemoral ligament). If the anterior capsule is damaged or lax, maintaining the upright position may be difficult because the anterior muscle strength is not as powerful as the posterior muscle strength.

Hip capsular thickness has recently been studied by Philippon et al. These authors dissected 13 nonpaired fresh-frozen cadaveric hemipelves using a coordinate measuring device. They found that the hip capsule was thickest between the 1 and 2 o'clock positions for all measured distances from the acetabular labrum and that it reached its maximum thickness at 2 o'clock, which corresponds to the location of the iliofemoral ligament.[95]

Capsular Ligaments
Iliofemoral Ligament

The iliofemoral ligament (ILFL), also known as the *Y ligament of Bigelow,* is shaped like an inverted "Y" and distally splits into two distinct arms, medial and lateral (Fig. 76.7). The single proximal insertion abuts the AIIS, wrapping around the base like a crescent, and extends within a few millimeters of the acetabular rim along the anterior and anterolateral acetabulum. Distally, the ILFL lateral arm crosses the joint obliquely and inserts on the anterior prominence of the greater trochanteric crest, just superior to the origin of the intertrochanteric line, with an elongated oval-shaped footprint. The medial arm passes almost vertically inferior and inserts on a subtle angulated prominence of the anteroinferior femur at the level of the lesser trochanter, with a circular-shaped footprint. The individual arms of the ILFL diverge 57 mm (range, 50 to 64 mm) distal to the most superior aspect of the proximal attachment footprint; the medial and lateral insertional footprints are a few millimeters apart

on intertrochanteric line.[91] The ILFL restricts external rotation in both flexion and extension and internal rotation in flexion.[96]

Recently van Arkel et al. performed a cadaveric study showing that the ILFL and ischiofemoral ligaments were the primary stabilizers preventing dislocation of the native hip joint, with the labrum playing the role of a secondary stabilizer in positions of low flexion/extension.[97]

Pubofemoral Ligament

The PFL originates on the iliopectineal eminence of the superior pubic ramus with a triangle-shaped insertional footprint (see Fig. 76.7). The most inferomedial aspect of the insertional footprint extends to within a few millimeters of the acetabular rim. The PFL crosses inferoposteriorly under the medial arm of the ILFL and wraps around the femoral head like a sling or hammock, proximal to the zona orbicularis. The PFL terminates abruptly by blending with the proximal ISFL, near the acetabular rim, beneath the inferior aspect of the femoral neck (see Fig. 76.7B); the PFL lacks a bony femoral attachment.[91] The PFL blends anteriorly with the medial ILFL. The PFL controls external rotation in extension.[96]

Ischiofemoral Ligament

The ISFL resembles a large asymmetric triangle with a long tapered apex and consists of a single band (see Fig. 76.7). The proximal insertional footprint on the ischial acetabular margin is shaped like a broad triangle, beginning near the root of the ischial ramus and extending to within a few millimeters of the acetabular rim. The ISFL spirals superolaterally to insert at the base of the greater trochanter at the femoral neck-trochanteric junction, slightly anterior to the femoral neck axis; the distal ISFL footprint does not have a consistent shape.[91] The ISFL was noted to be the most significant restrictor of internal rotation both in internal and external rotation.[96]

Zona Orbicularis

The zona orbicularis is a thickening of the capsule, just distal to the femoral head-neck junction, that runs around the femoral neck perpendicular to the axis of the femoral neck. The zona orbicularis has leash-like fibers organized in a spiral configuration; together with the anterior capsular ligaments, they tighten in a "screw home" mechanism during terminal extension and external rotation, further stabilizing the joint.[98] Additionally, the zona orbicularis may limit distraction of the femoral head from the acetabulum.[90]

Capsular Innervation

Sensory innervation of the hip capsule for proprioception and nociception has been studied extensively in the modern literature.[99-105] The capsule is generally thought to receive its innervation from branches of the obturator, femoral, sciatic, and superior gluteal nerves, the nerve to quadratus femoris, and possibly from the accessory obturator nerve. The complexity of the hip joint innervation results in a nonhomogenic pattern of pain referred from the hip joint, with hip pathology causing pain in the groin, all around the thigh, in the buttock, below the knee, and even in the foot.[106]

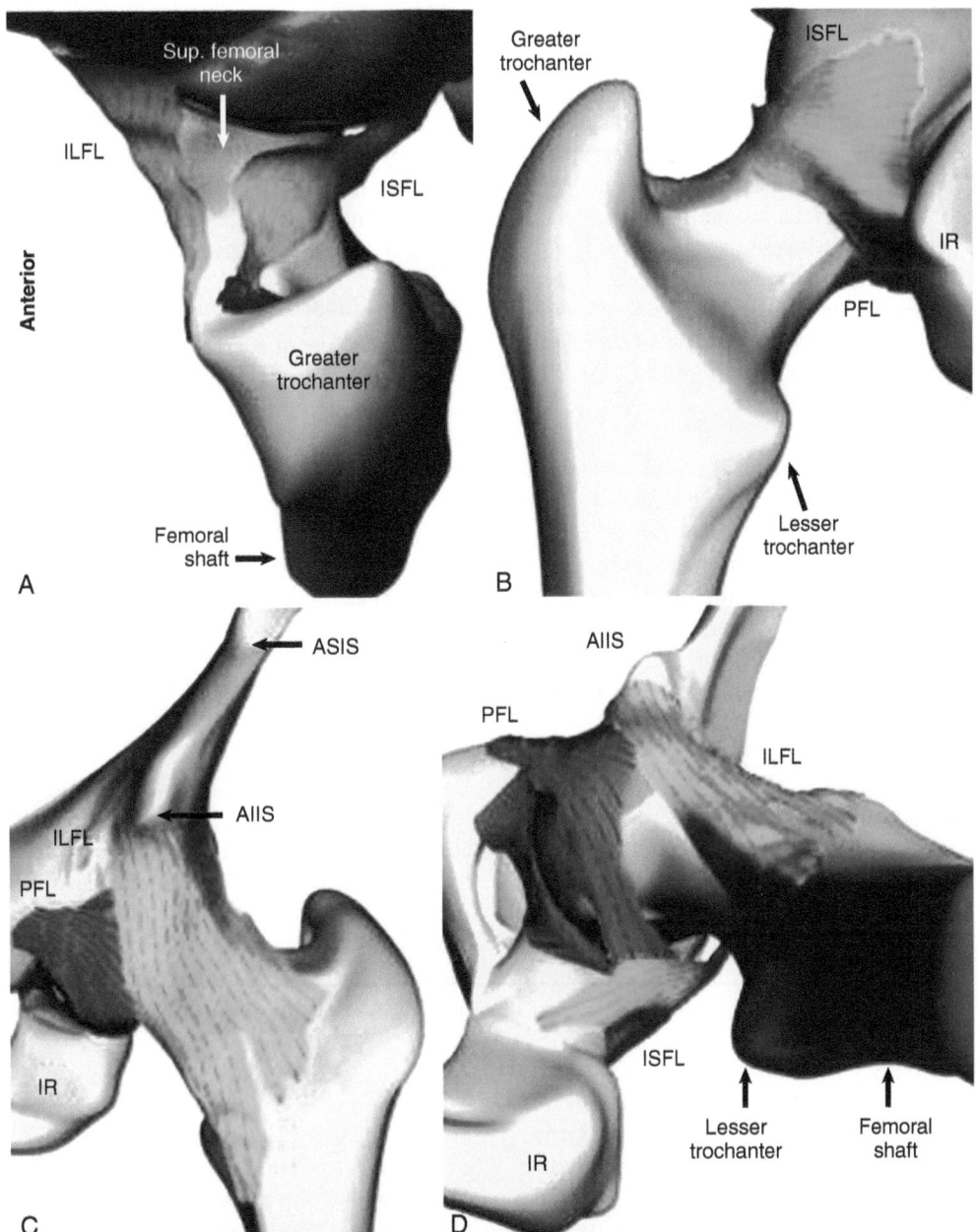

Fig. 76.7 Ligamentous relationships of the hip capsule. (A) A computer model demonstrating the relationship of the distal lateral iliofemoral ligament *(ILFL)* and the distal ischiofemoral ligament *(ISFL)*, viewed from a superior position looking down the femoral shaft. (B) A computer model showing the posterior blend of the pubofemoral ligament *(PFL)* and the ISFL. (C) A computer model showing the anterior blend of the PFL and the ILFL. (D) The relationships of all three ligaments as viewed from an inferior position looking upward at the inferior aspect of the femoral head. *AIIS*, Anterior inferior ischial spine; *ASIS*, anterior superior ischial spine; *IR*, ischial ramus.

Birnbaum et al. examined 11 formalin-mounted human hips and described a separation between the anterior innervation of the capsule (obturator and femoral nerve) and its posterior innervation (sciatic nerve, superior gluteal nerve, and the nerve to the quadratus femoris).[99] Recently Kampa et al. dissected 20 formalin-fixed human hips to further explore the innervation of the capsule and to define its pattern more accurately.[102] They chose to illustrate the capsular innervation arrangement by depicting the capsule as the face of a clock. The reference point from which measurements were taken was the inferior acetabular notch to depict the 6 o'clock position. Therefore the position between 12 and 6 o'clock represented the anterior aspect of the capsule and the position between 6 and 12 o'clock represented the posterior position. Their findings, discussed later in this chapter, were consistent with previous reports and demonstrate a richly innervated structure, innervated by five to seven nerves and a variable number of their branches (direct or muscular).[99]

Femoral Nerve

The femoral nerve is formed by the L2 to 4 nerve roots in the lumbar plexus. It courses along the iliacus muscle and alongside the psoas, descends under the inguinal ligament, innervates the anterior thigh musculature, and provides cutaneous innervation to the lower leg through its terminal branch of the saphenous nerve. The femoral nerve travels with (and lateral to) the femoral artery and vein. The capsular branches of the femoral nerve, which travel along the anterior margin of the capsule, pierce the capsule either medially or laterally over an arc of 75 degrees between the half-past 2 and 5 o'clock positions.[102]

Obturator Nerve

The obturator nerve roots from L2 to L4 descend through the fibers of the psoas major and emerge from the medial border and later enter the thigh through the obturator canal. The capsular branches of the obturator nerve travel along the antero-inferior margin of the capsule, entering the capsule primarily medially over an arc of 105 degrees between 3 o'clock and half past 6 o'clock, with an equal contribution from both the anterior and posterior branches.[73] The obturator nerve also provides innervation to the knee joint.

Accessory Obturator Nerve

In the past the accessory obturator nerve has been described as being present in between 10% and 30% of people.[100,101,103,105] However, Birnbaum et al. did not find it at all in 11 specimens, and Kampa et al. found it in only 1 of 20 hips (5%), where it crossed the anteroinferior margin of the capsule and it entered medially over an arc of 15 degrees between half past 5 and 6 o'clock.[99,102]

Superior Gluteal Nerve

Originating at the sacral plexus from the L4 to S1 sacral nerves, the superior gluteal nerve leaves the pelvis through the greater sciatic foramen above the piriformis, accompanied by the superior gluteal artery and the superior gluteal vein. Kampa et al. found that the superior gluteal nerve branches to the capsule are small and have a leash of vessels; they cross the superior and postero-lateral aspects of the capsule and enter it medially or more commonly laterally over an arc of 75 degrees between half past 10 and 1 o'clock.[102]

Inferior Gluteal Nerve

The inferior gluteal nerve, a branch of the sacral plexus, leaves the pelvis through the lower part of the greater sciatic foramen, below the piriformis, and terminates by innervating the gluteus maximus. Kampa et al. have found a contribution to capsular innervation from the inferior gluteal nerve in only two specimens (10%) and noted that the nerve entered the capsule laterally at 8 o'clock.[102]

Sciatic Nerve

The sciatic nerve is formed by the joining of the L4 to S3 roots. The nerve courses laterally through the pelvis, exits at the greater sciatic foramen, and travels distally deep to the piriformis and superficially to the short external rotators. The nerve divides along the course of the posterior thigh into the common peroneal trunk and the tibial trunk. The common peroneal trunk lies more laterally. The area of the capsule supplied by the sciatic nerve overlaps with that of the superior gluteal nerve, with its branches traveling along the posterior margin of the capsule and entering the capsule mainly medially but also laterally over an arc of 90 degrees between 9 and 12 o'clock.[102]

Nerve to Quadratus Femoris

The nerve to the quadratus femoris is a sacral plexus nerve that arises from L4 to S1 and leaves the pelvis through the greater sciatic foramen. Its branches to the capsule supply the quadratus femoris posteroinferiorly and enter it predominantly medially and occasionally laterally over an arc of 105 degrees between half past 6 and 10 o'clock.[102]

Safe Zone of the Capsule

Kampa et al. found that anterosuperiorly, between 1 o'clock and half past 2 o'clock, no nerves enter the capsule. This internervous plane, which is poorly innervated, was named the "safe zone" of the capsule (Fig. 76.8).[102]

Capsule Vascularization

Kalhor et al. have studied the vascularization of the hip capsule using intra-arterial injection of colored silicon in 20 hips.[107] In all specimens, contributions to the hip capsule;s vasculature arose from the medial femoral circumflex artery, lateral femoral circumflex artery, superior gluteal artery, and inferior gluteal artery. The circumflex arteries supplied the anterior capsule, whereas the posterior capsule was supplied by the gluteal arteries, augmented by contributions from the circumflex arteries (Fig. 76.9).

MUSCLES AROUND THE HIP JOINT

More than 20 muscles cross the hip joint (Table 76.1). They can be grouped according to their main function and innervation. The hip abductors and internal rotators (gluteus medius, gluteus minimus, and tensor fascia lata) are innervated by the superior gluteal nerve; the hip flexors (iliopsoas, rectus femoris, sartorius,

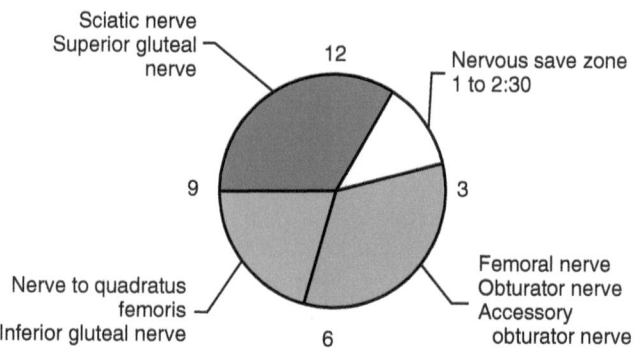

Fig. 76.8 The capsule as the face of a clock. The pie chart demonstrates the different zones of innervation of the capsular and the internervous safe zone anterosuperiorly. (From Kampa RJ, Prasthofer A, Lawrence-Watt DJ, et al. The internervous safe zone for incision of the capsule of the hip: a cadaver study. *J Bone Joint Surg Br.* 2007;89-B[7]:971–976.)

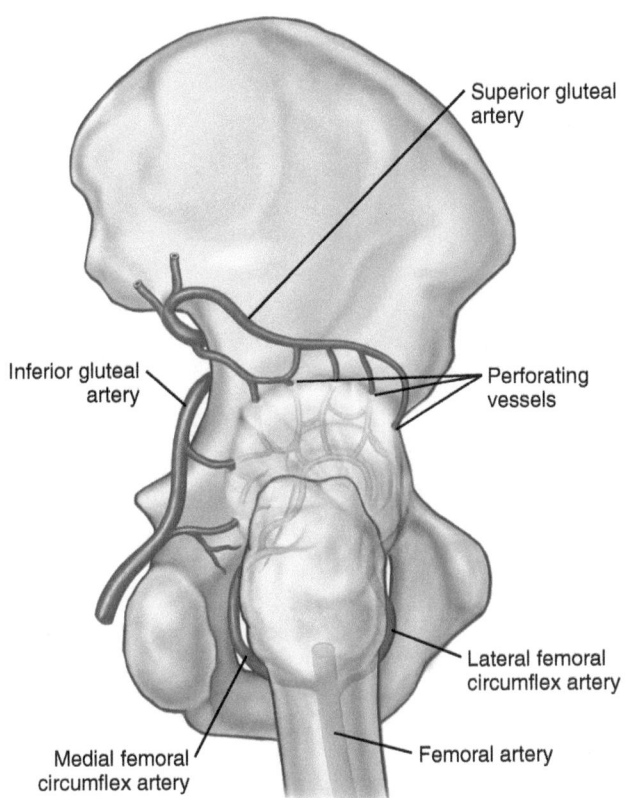

Fig. 76.9 The hip from the posterior view, demonstrating the periacetabular vascular ring and anastomoses between distal and proximal vessels. *1*, Superior gluteal artery; *2*, inferior gluteal artery; *3*, medial femoral circumflex artery; *4*, lateral femoral circumflex artery; *5*, perforating vessels (cut surface). (From Kalhor M, Beck M, Huff TW, et al. Capsular and pericapsular contributions to acetabular and femoral head perfusion. *J Bone Joint Surg Am.* 2009;91[2]:409–418.)

and pectineus) are innervated by the femoral nerve; the hip adductors (adductor magnus, adductor longus, adductor brevis, and gracilis) are innervated by the obturator nerve; and the muscles of the hip extensors have mostly unique nerves that are named after the muscle they innervate.

Abductors and Internal Rotators

The gluteus medius, gluteus minimus, and tensor fascia lata are abductors and internal rotators of the hip joint; all are innervated by the superior gluteal nerve, which originates from the sacral plexus (see Table 76.1).

Gluteus Medius

The proximal attachment of the gluteus medius is at the anterosuperior iliac spine, along the outer edge of the iliac crest to the posterosuperior iliac spine.[108-110] The line of attachment is approximately 1 cm broad and limited to the iliac crest. Robertson et al. found that the gluteus medius tendon inserts into the greater trochanter by way of two distinct attachment sites, the superoposterior facet and the lateral facet.[110] However, Gottschalk et al. define the tendon attachment to be at the anterosuperior portion of the greater trochanter and not at its lateral aspect.[109]

The muscle belly of the gluteus medius is composed of three distinct parts—anterior, middle, and posterior—and all three create a curved and fan-shaped muscle that tapers down to a flat tendon.[109-111] The muscle fibers of the posterior part are parallel to the femoral neck, whereas the fibers of the anterior part are nearly vertical. Each one of the three parts of the gluteus medius is innervated by a separate branch of the superior gluteal nerve and has a different biomechanical function. The posterior part together with the gluteus minimus is thought to stabilize the femoral head in the acetabulum. The middle is thought to initiate hip abduction. The anterior portion has two functions: its vertical fibers aid in abduction and its anterior fibers internally rotate the hip to allow pelvic rotation and swing-through of the contralateral lower limb.[109,110]

Gluteus Minimus

The gluteus minimus is a hip abductor along with the gluteus medius. The gluteus minimus muscle attaches proximally on the iliac wing from the AIIS to the posteroinferior iliac spine, along the middle gluteal line. Its distal attachment is on the anterior facet of the greater trochanter.[109,110] The fibers of this muscle tend to be horizontally oriented and run parallel to the neck of the femur. The gluteus minimus is also innervated by the superior gluteal nerve. Both the gluteus medius and minimus have additional bursae deep to their respective tendons in the peritrochanteric area.

Tensor Fascia Lata

The tensor fasciae lata works with the gluteus medius and minimus muscles to abduct and medially rotate the femur. The tensor fascia lata arises from the anterosuperior iliac spine and the outer lip of the anterior iliac crest; it inserts distally between the two layers of the iliotibial band of the fascia lata and is innervated by the superior gluteal nerve.

Flexors
Iliopsoas

The iliopsoas muscle is the main flexor of the hip joint; in addition, it acts as an external rotator. It is formed by two muscles, the iliacus and the psoas major, and is innervated by the femoral nerve. The iliacus muscle originates from the medial side of the iliac wing, whereas the psoas major arises from the transverse processes of the lumbar vertebrae, the intervertebral disks, adjacent vertebral margins of T12 to L5, and the tendinous arches.[112] Distally the iliopsoas attaches to the lesser trochanter in a unique muscle-tendon attachment, where there is a direct muscular attachment in addition to the tendinous attachment. At the level of the joint, the muscle/tendon ratio is around 50%.[113,114] As the iliopsoas travels distally, a greater percentage of the structure's area is tendon. The tendon passes anterior to the iliopectineal eminence and the anterior capsuloligamentous structures of the hip joint, with the iliopsoas bursa lying in between. The iliopsoas is also one of the dynamic stabilizers of the hip joint; its role as a stabilizer is more prominent in cases of inherent hip instability.[115]

A recent anatomic cadaver study found significant variance between iliopsoas specimens. The investigators found that the prevalence of a single-, double-, and triple-banded iliopsoas

TABLE 76.1   Muscles Around the Hip Joint Sorted by Function

Muscle	Origin	Insertion	Innervation	Spinal Level	Additional Function	Notes
Hip Abductors and Internal Rotators						
Gluteus medius	Ilium (between posterior-anterior gluteal lines)	Greater trochanter	Superior gluteal	L4–S1		
Gluteus minimus	Ilium (between anterior/inferior gluteal lines)	Greater trochanter	Superior gluteal	L4–S1		
Tensor fasciae latae	Anterior iliac crest	Iliotibial band (the Gerdy tubercle)	Superior gluteal	L4–S1		
Hip Flexors						
Iliopsoas	Iliac fossa (iliacus) transverse process L1–L5 (psoas)	Lesser trochanter	Femoral	L2–4	External rotation	Strongest hip flexor
Pectineus	Pectineal line of pubis bone	Pectineal line of femur	Femoral	L2–4	Adduction	
Rectus femoris	AIIS (straight head) anterior acetabular rim (reflected head)	Patella	Femoral	L2–4		Biarthrodial muscle
Sartorius	ASIS	Proximal medial tibia	Femoral	L2–4	External rotation	Biarthrodial muscle
Hip External Rotators						
Gluteus maximus	Ilium along crest posterior to posterior gluteal line	Iliotibial band/posterior femur	Inferior gluteal	L5–S2	Extension	
Piriformis	Anterior sacrum, through sciatic notch	Proximal greater trochanter (piriformis fossa)	Piriformis	S1–S2		
Obturator externus	Ischiopubic rami and external surface of the obturator membrane	Medial greater trochanter	Obturator (posterior branch)	L2–4	Adduction	
Obturator internus	Ischiopubic rami/obturator membrane	Medial greater trochanter	Obturator internus	L5–S2		
Superior gemellus	Ischial spine	Medial greater trochanter	Obturator internus	L5–S2		
Inferior gemellus	Ischial tuberosity	Medial greater trochanter	Quadratus femoris	L4–S1		
Quadratus femoris	Ischial tuberosity	Quadrate line of femur	Quadratus femoris	L4–S1		
Hip Extensors						
Gluteus maximus	Ilium along crest posterior to posterior gluteal line	Iliotibial band/posterior femur	Inferior gluteal	L5–S2	External rotation	
Long head of biceps femoris	Medial ischial tuberosity	Fibular head/lateral tibia	Tibial	L5–S2		Biarthrodial muscle, also flex the knee
Semitendinosus	Distal medial ischial tuberosity	Anterior tibial crest	Tibial	L5–S2		Biarthrodial muscle, also flex the knee
Semimembranosus	Proximal lateral ischial tuberosity	Posterior/medial tibia, posterior capsule, medial meniscus, popliteus, popliteal ligament	Tibial	L5–S2		Biarthrodial muscle, also flex the knee
Hip Adductors						
Adductor magnus	Inferior pubic ramus/ischial tuberosity	Linea aspera/adductor tubercle	Obturator (posterior branch) sciatic (tibial)	L2–4	Flexion, external rotation, extension	
Adductor brevis	Inferior pubic ramus	Linea aspera/pectineal line	Obturator (posterior branch)	L2–4	Flexion, external rotation	
Adductor longus	Anterior pubic ramus	Linea aspera	Obturator (anterior branch)	L2–4	Flexion, internal rotation	
Gracilis	Inferior symphysis/pubic arch	Proximal medial tibia	Obturator (anterior branch)	L2–4	Flexion, internal rotation	Biarthrodial muscle, also flex the knee

AIIS, Anterior inferior ischial spine; *ASIS,* anterior superior ischial spine.

tendon was 28.3%, 64.2%, and 7.5%, respectively. The psoas major tendon was consistently the most medial tendinous structure, and the primary iliacus tendon was found immediately lateral to the psoas major tendon within the belly of the iliacus muscle. When present, an accessory iliacus tendon was located adjacent to the primary iliacus tendon, lateral to the primary iliacus tendon. These findings have implications when it comes to arthroscopic release of the iliopsoas tendon.[116]

Pectineus

The pectineus is a flat quadrangular muscle originating from the pectineal line on the superior ramus pubis and inserting to the femur distal to the lesser trochanter into the pectineal line of the femur. Its main functions are flexion and adduction of the hip. It is innervated mainly by the femoral nerve and sometimes has additional innervation from the obturator nerve.

Rectus Femoris

The rectus femoris is the only one of the four quadriceps muscles that crosses the hip joint. It is innervated by the femoral nerve and originates by two tendons: the anterior or straight head, from the AIIS, and the posterior or reflected head, from a groove above the rim of the acetabulum. It is a biarthrodial muscle and inserts distally to the tibial tubercle with the patella within the combined quadriceps tendon. Its function is to flex the hip and extend the knee.

Sartorius

The sartorius is the longest muscle in the body. It originates from the anterosuperior iliac spine and inserts to the anteromedial surface of the upper tibia in the pes anserinus. The sartorius is innervated by the femoral nerve; it is a biarthrodial muscle that functions as a hip flexor and external rotator and also as a knee extensor.

Iliocapsularis

The iliocapsularis muscle is a little-known muscle that once was thought to be part of the iliopsoas muscle. It lies in the anterior aspect of the hip joint, originating from the inferior part of the anteroinferior iliac spine and the anterior capsule, spanning directly on the anterior capsule, and inserting distal to the lesser trochanter.[117] It is believed to play an important role in stabilizing dysplastic hips and was shown to be hypertrophic in that condition.[118]

Extensors

Hip extension is achieved by a synchronous activation of the gluteus maximus and hamstring muscle complex.

Hamstrings

The hamstrings are a two-joint muscle complex crossing both the hip and the knee. Their function is to extend the hip and flex the knee. The proximal hamstring complex is composed of the semimembranosus (SM), the semitendinosus, and the long heads of the biceps femoris; they cross over the posterior hip joint and are innervated by the tibial nerve. The semitendinosus and the long head of the biceps have a common

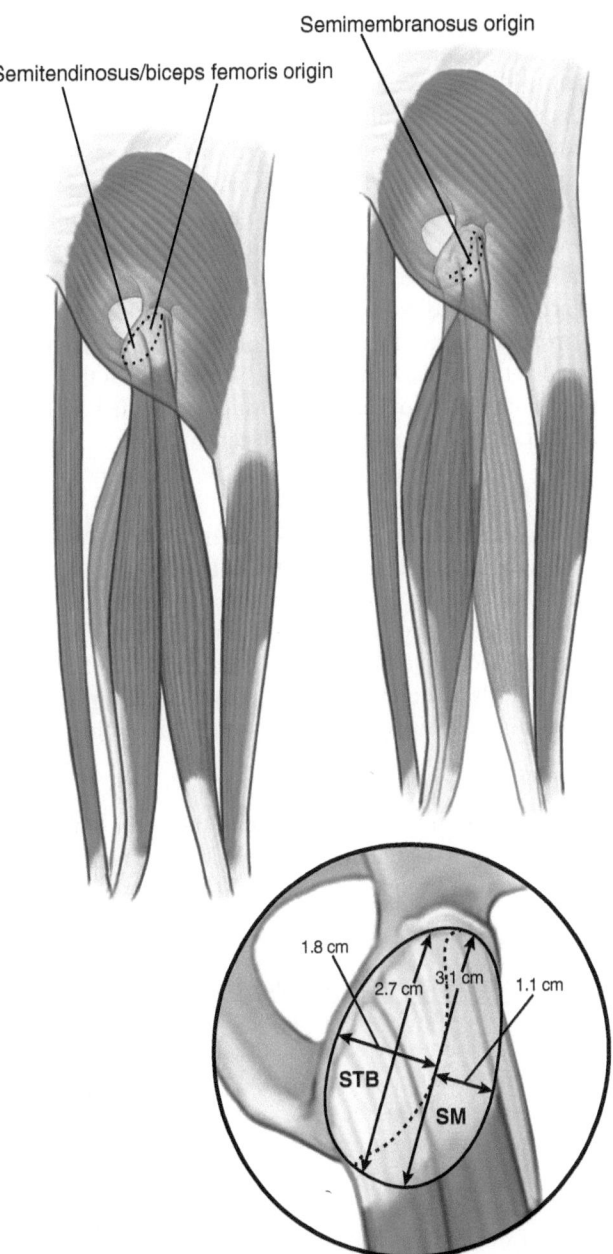

Fig. 76.10 Posterior, right-sided views showing that the origin of the common tendon of the semitendinosus/biceps femoris *(STB)* is oval and measures 2.7 ± 0.5 cm from proximal to distal and 1.8 ± 0.2 cm from medial to lateral and that the semimembranosus *(SM)* origin is crescent shaped and measures 3.1 ± 0.3 cm from proximal to distal and 1.1 ± 0.5 cm from medial to lateral. The semimembranosus originates lateral to the common tendon of the semitendinosus/biceps femoris. (From Miller SL, Gill J, Webb GR. The proximal origin of the hamstrings and surrounding anatomy encountered during repair: a cadaveric study. *J Bone Joint Surg Am.* 2007;89[1]:44–48.)

tendon attaching on the medial side of the ischial tuberosity, whereas the SM attaches laterally via a smaller footprint (Fig. 76.10).[119]

The short head of the biceps femoris is also part of the hamstring complex; however, it does not cross the hip joint. It attaches to the posterior aspect of the femur—the linea aspera—and is innervated by the common peroneal nerve; thus it does not affect hip joint motions directly.

Recently Philippon et al. performed a quantitative and qualitative anatomic analysis of the proximal hamstrings and found that the semitendinosus and long head of the biceps femoris shared a proximal origin (conjoined tendon), having an oval footprint with an average area of 567.0 mm². The SM footprint was crescent shaped and located anterolateral to the conjoined tendon, with an average area of 412.4 mm². The SM footprint had an accessory tendinous extension that extended anteromedially forming a distinct footprint. A consistent bony landmark was found at the medial ischial margin, 14.6 mm from the center of the conjoined tendon footprint, which coincided with the distal insertion of the sacrotuberous ligament.[120]

Gluteus Maximus

The gluteus maximus is the largest of the three gluteal muscles. It is a wide, flat muscle that is responsible for hip extension and external rotation and is innervated by the inferior gluteal nerve. It has a wide origin proximally on the outer side of the ilium, lumbar fascia, sacrum, and sacrotuberous ligament. Its fibers are directed obliquely in the lateral-inferior direction; distally it inserts to the gluteal tuberosity on the femur and the iliotibial band.

External Rotators

External rotation of the hip is performed by the gluteus maximus and the short external rotators, all of which originate from the posterior side of the pelvic ring.

Short External Rotators

The short external rotators muscles include the piriformis, obturator externus, obturator internus, superior gemellus, inferior gemellus, and quadratus femoris. All the short external rotators are innervated by unique nerves named after the muscles they innervate. The piriformis is the superior muscle of the short rotators, originating from the anterior side of the sacrum, going posteriorly through the sciatic notch, and inserting to the piriformis fossa on the proximal greater trochanter. The obturator internus, originating from the internal side of the obturator membrane and the posterior bony margins of obturator foramen, goes in between the superior and inferior gemelli, with all three of them joining together to form the conjoined tendon that inserts into the medial side of the greater trochanter. The obturator externus originates from the ischiopubic rami and external surface of the obturator membrane and inserts to the posteromedial surface of the greater trochanter. The quadratus femoris is the inferior muscle of the short rotators; it originates from the ischial tuberosity and inserts to the quadrate line of the femur.

Adductors

Adduction of the hip is performed by the adductor magnus, adductor brevis, adductor longus, and gracilis, all of which are innervated by the obturator nerve. The pectineus muscles also aid in adduction, and they are innervated by the femoral nerve. All the adductors originate in and around the pubic bone: the pectineus at the superior ramus pubis; the adductor longus at the anterior surface of the body of pubis, just lateral to the pubic symphysis; the adductor brevis at the anterior surface of inferior pubic ramus, inferior to origin of adductor longus; and the gracilis at the inferior margin of pubic symphysis. All adductors but the gracilis insert at the medioposterior side of the femur and the linea aspera, whereas the gracilis inserts at the medial surface of the proximal tibial shaft, just posterior to the sartorius and proximal to the semitendinosis (see Table 76.1).

The adductor magnus is composed of two parts: adductor and hamstring. The adductor part originates from the inferior pubic ramus and has relatively short horizontal fibers that insert onto the rough line leading from the greater trochanter to the linea aspera, medial to the gluteus maximus. This part is innervated by the posterior branch of the obturator nerve. The hamstring component originates from the ischial tuberosity and inserts at the adductor tubercle on the medial condyle of the distal femur. This hamstring part of the adductor magnus is innervated by the tibial nerve. In addition to adducting the hip, the adductor muscles are also important flexors or extensors of the hip. Regardless of hip position, the adductor magnus (especially the hamstring part) is an effective extensor of the hip, similar to the hamstring muscles. Most other adductor muscles, however, are considered flexors from the anatomic (extended) position.[121]

BURSAE AROUND THE HIP JOINT

Trochanteric Bursae

The bursae in the greater trochanteric region, often referred as the *trochanteric bursae,* are a complex of several bursae that are intimately associated with the greater trochanter and the gluteal tendons. The three major bursae are the subgluteus maximus, the subgluteus medius, and the gluteofemoral bursae. The gluteus minimus bursa is a minor bursa located cephalad and ventral to the greater trochanter.[122] Dunn et al. found a subgluteus-maximus bursa in 13 of 14 patients undergoing primary hip surgery.[123] This bursa exists directly superficial to the common attachment of the gluteus medius, minimus, and vastus lateralis muscles onto the greater trochanter. It was termed the *deep bursa* or *dominant deep bursa* and *secondary deep bursa* if more than one was present. In five specimens, two bursae were present and could be separated easily through a fascial plane. The size of the deep bursae ranged from 1.5 to 4.7 cm long and 1.7 to 5.1 cm wide. In about half of the specimens, a smaller bursa was located on the deep surface of the gluteus maximus muscle and was termed the *superficial bursa.* In all specimens an additional deep bursa was located more distally, the gluteofemoral bursa, which was seen between the gluteus maximus and vastus lateralis muscles where the gluteus maximus muscle fibers insert onto the femur. In two specimens, branches of the inferior gluteal nerve (L5 to S2) were seen entering subgluteus-maximus bursae and the surrounding tissues.

Woodley et al. also studied the bursae around the greater trochanter region in 18 embalmed human hips with use of macrodissection and histologic techniques. They demonstrated that multiple bursae are associated with the greater trochanter and are arranged in three distinct layers as determined by the planes of the gluteal tendons.[124] Bursae in each layer differ with respect to morphology and location, although the centers of all bursae are positioned inferior to the apex of the greater trochanter. The mean number of bursae per hip was six, with a minimum of four and a maximum of nine being found in any one specimen.

Iliopsoas Bursa

The iliopsoas bursa lies between the anterior capsule of the hip joint and the iliopsoas tendon. It has been described as the largest bursa in the body, measuring up to 7 cm long and 4 cm wide.[125,126] The portion of the anterior hip capsule between the iliofemoral and PFLs adjacent to the iliopsoas bursa is thin, with a communication between the hip joint and the bursa present in 14% to 25% of cadavers.[127-129]

GENERAL HIP KINEMATICS/BIOMECHANICS

The hip joint is a ball-and-socket joint, with the acetabulum being the socket and the femoral head the ball. As with all ball-and-socket joints, it has six degrees of freedom: three planes of motion (flexion-extension, abduction-adduction, and internal-external rotation), and three planes of translations (AP, mediolateral, and proximodistal). Recent research has shown that the center of the femoral head moves relative to the acetabulum.[130,131] The joint motions are limited both by the bony anatomy and the soft tissues that surround the joint, mainly the hip capsule and ligaments.

Hip Motions

Hip ROM may be affected by the bony morphology or ligamentous and muscle laxity. In general, a dysplastic acetabulum allows greater ROM than a profunda acetabulum. However, hypermobility of a well-covered femoral head may be achieved by ligamentous and muscle laxity. In the standard hip, the ROM is greatest in the sagittal plane; however, because many biarthrodial muscles (see Table 76.1) cross both the hip and the knee, the hip motion is also affected by the knee position. Hip flexion is around 120 to 140 degrees with the knee flexed actively and passively, and 90 degrees with the knee fully extended. Active hip extension is 10 to 20 degrees, and passive extension is as much as 30 degrees. Normal hip abduction is at least 50 degrees and adduction is 30 degrees (limited by the opposite extremity and the tensor fascia lata). Internal and external rotation of the flexed hip may range up to 70 and 90 degrees, respectively. Internal rotation is limited by the short external rotator muscles (obturator internus and externus, superior and inferior gemelli, quadratus femoris, and piriformis) and the ISFL. External rotation is limited by the lateral band of the ILFL, the PFL, the internal rotator muscles, and the degree of femoral neck anteversion.[42] Kivlan et al. performed a cadaveric study and found that multiplanar movement of flexion and abduction moved the ligamentum teres into an anteroinferior position relative to the femoral head and prevented the femoral head from anterior/inferior subluxation. The ligamentum teres endpoint was obtained at a combined average position of 100.6 and 20.0 degree flexion and abduction angle.[132] Martin et al. performed a cadaveric study and found that the major function of the ligamentum teres is controlling hip rotation, because it functions as an end-range

stabilizer to hip rotation dominantly at 90 degrees or greater of hip flexion.[133]

Hip Stability

Overall, the hip is considered a stable joint because of its bony architecture.[134-136] However, soft tissue has been shown to play a major role in the stability of the joint throughout a physiologic and supraphysiologic ROM. Biomechanical studies have suggested that the hip capsule works together with other static soft tissue stabilizers such as the acetabular labrum and transverse acetabular ligament.[135-137] In addition, dynamic stabilizers such as the iliopsoas, iliocapsularis, rectus femoris, and abductor complex also contribute to the overall maintenance of proper joint kinematics and force-coupled compression that enhance hip joint stability.[92,98] Nonetheless, the femoral head has been shown to move up to 3 mm relative to the acetabulum in intact cadaveric studies in which the hip is taken through the extremes of motion; average translation was 3.3 ± 2.8 mm mediolateral, 1.4 ± 1.8 mm AP, and 0.3 ± 1.5 mm proximodistal; except for mediolateral displacement, these translations increased as more soft tissue was removed.[115] In another study, ballet dancers with normal bony morphology were shown to have 1 to 6 mm of femoral head translation relative to the acetabulum when routine dancing motions were analyzed using optical tracker and 3D MRI.[130]

According to a recent study, tensile properties of the hip joint ligaments are largely variable and age-dependent. The ischiofemoral ligament and PFLs were found to change age-dependently based on data obtained from a cadaveric study. Though the hip ligaments contribute to hip stability, the ischiofemoral and cranial iliofemoral may not prevent dislocation owing to their elasticity.[138]

Gait Cycle

The gait cycle consists of two main phases: stance, while the foot is touching the ground, and swing, while the foot is in the air. In walking, the stance phase is longer and consists of about 60% of the gait cycle; thus there is a double-support phase in which both feet are on the ground for approximately 20% of the total gait cycle. The double-support phase defines walking and occurs at the beginning and end of each stance phase. When running, the stance phase is shorter than 50% of the gait cycle; thus a float phase occurs in which both legs are in the air, and at no time are both feet on the ground simultaneously.[139-141] As the velocity of running increases, the stance phase shortens, and it has been reported to be 22% of the cycle in sprinting.

The main motion of the hip during walking and running is in the sagittal plane—flexion and extension. During the stance phase, the hip extends, adducts, and rotates internally, whereas during the swing phase, the hip flexes, abducts, and rotates externally.[42,140-142] During normal walking the hip flexes to about 30 degrees and extends to around 10 degrees. Flexion increases with running by approximately 20 degrees and another 10 to 15 degrees with sprinting. Extension of the hip was found to differ slightly with running and was even reported to decrease with sprinting.[139,143] Anterior pelvic tilt is also a normal motion during both walking and running, and peak anterior pelvic tilt was found to have a significant positive correlation with peak hip extension.

Another difference between running and walking is that during walking, a wider base is found between the feet. In running, the base narrows so that foot strike is more on the center line of progression. Hip adduction is 5 to 10 degrees in walking and 15 to 20 degrees during running.[142]

In general the muscles around the hip joint work in conjunction with each other. Using electromyography, different activation patterns during walking and running beside the amplitude have been shown.[144] Hip flexors are active mainly during the swing phase and extensors are active during the stance phase. The gluteus maximus and hamstrings also function at the same time to help decelerate the swinging thigh.[139,144] Hip adductor muscles are active throughout the running cycle, whereas in walking they are active only from the swing phase to the middle of the stance phase.[140] The gluteus medius and tensor fascia lata help stabilize the pelvis; during running they are active during the swing and early stance phases, whereas in walking they are active mainly during the stance phase.[144]

Forces Around the Hip Joint

The hip joint is complicated biomechanically and is difficult to study, because measuring the forces directly in a live person would require surgical intervention and implantation of transducers. Nonetheless many methods have been used to investigate the forces throughout the hip joint: (1) simplification of the macro forces around the hip joint, also known as multibody dynamics; (2) measurement of forces in vivo in an implanted hip prosthesis; (3) in silico (computational simulation) micromechanics, also known as finite element analysis; (4) cadaveric studies; and (5) dynamic imaging studies with live volunteers.

Multibody Dynamics

A simple diagram of the forces around the hip joint during single leg stance is the most common use of multibody dynamics (Fig. 76.11).[142] The parameters in the equation are body weight (W) minus one leg weight (W – 1/6W), the abductor muscle's force (A), the joint reaction force according to Newton's first law of motion (F), the moment arm from the center of gravity to the center of the hip joint (d), and the abductor muscle's moment arm (l). The calculation takes into account that when standing on one leg the pelvis is in equilibrium; thus the abductor muscle's force (A) multiplied by the abductor muscle's moment arm (l) is equal to the body weight (W) minus one leg (1/6W) multiplied by moment arm from the center of gravity to the center of the hip joint (d) or $A \times l = (W - 1/6W) \times d$. The joint reaction force (F) according to Newton's first law of motion is the force resulting in response to the weight and the abductor muscle's contraction. In general when a person is standing on one leg the center of gravity shifts away from the stance leg, forcing the abductors to work harder and, as a result, increasing the joint force to 2.7 times the body weight with walking (see Fig. 76.11).

In Vivo Studies

Bergmann et al. studied hip contact forces based on gait patterns during daily activities using instrumented implants—that

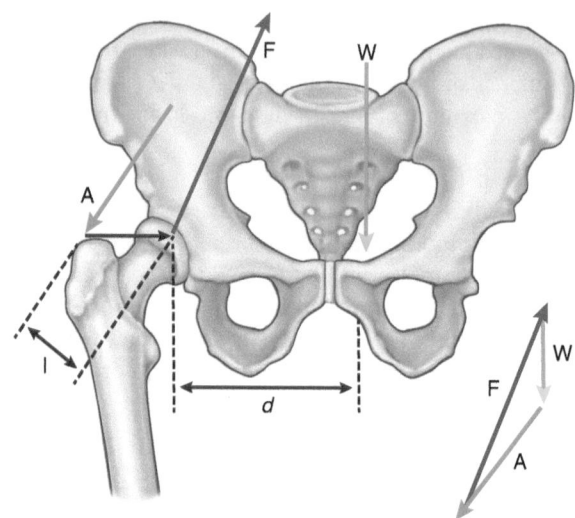

Fig. 76.11 Forces acting on the hip joint during single-leg stance under conditions of equilibrium. Gravitational force (W), abductor muscle force (A), hip joint reaction force (F), abductor muscle moment arm (l), and force of gravity moment arm (d).

is, implant pressure transducers into total hip prosthesis components.[145,146] This method allows direct measurement of all the forces acting on the prosthetic hip joint. The measured forces were found to change with different gait activities: approximately 80% to 100% of body weight during two-legged stance, 250% during one-legged stance, 300% during slow walking, 350% to 400% with quick walking, up to 500% during jogging, to a maximum of more than 800% during stumbling.[146] The fact that the force during two-legged stance was not half of the body weight is attributed to the persistent muscle forces acting on the hips.[142]

In Silico Studies

Finite element analysis methodology can simulate complex geometries and complex loads when all of the elements are reassembled during the solution process. This solution enables a simulation of static and dynamic situations. Typically finite element analysis mesh geometries of musculoskeletal tissues are generated from CT and MRI data, whereas material properties are usually extrapolated from in vitro measurements.[147] This methodology has been used to calculate the forces throughout the femoral neck in stress fractures or pressure distribution within the hip joint. Russell et al. used finite element analysis to calculate the contact force distribution throughout the acetabulum during the gait cycle phases from the resultant contact force applied during gait stance phase kinematics.[148] Maximal load of twice the body weight was calculated within the joint during the midstance phase (Fig. 76.12).

In Vitro Studies

Cadaveric biomechanics studies have been used for many years to measure forces and motion in and around the hip joint. The main limitation of this method is the lack of muscle force and body weight, which must be created artificially. Day et al. have shown an increase of up to five times normal pressure in areas with thin fibrocartilage, mainly at the zenith of the acetabulum.[149] Konrath et al. measured the distribution of contact area and

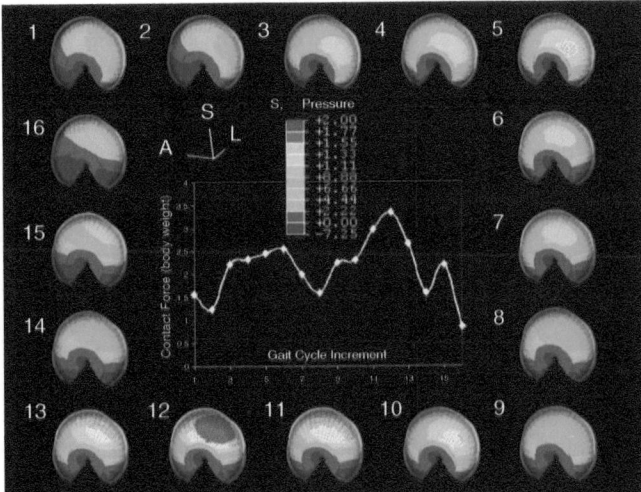

Fig. 76.12 Acetabular loads. Applied loads and normal hip contact contours. Finite element control hip contact pressure contours at each gait cycle increment developed from the resultant contact force *(inset)* applied during gait stance phase kinematics. Maximal load of twice the body weight within the joint was found during the midstance phase. (From Russell ME, Shivanna KH, Grosland NM, et al. Cartilage contact pressure elevations in dysplastic hips: a chronic overload model. *J Orthop Surg Res.* 2006;1:6.)

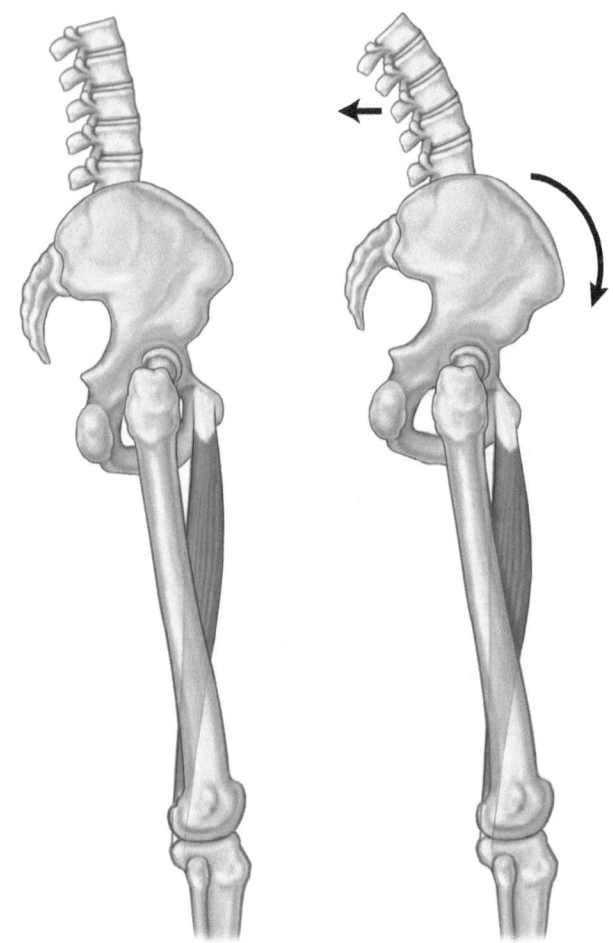

Fig. 76.13 Hip/spine balance. Flexion deformity of the hip rotates the pelvis forward and hyperextends the lumbar spine.

pressure between the acetabulum and the femoral head before and after cutting the acetabular labrum and transverse ligament. Simulating a single-limb stance, a peripheral distribution of load was seen in the intact acetabula.[150] This pattern was altered only minimally after removal of the transverse acetabular ligament, the labrum, or both. Conversely, Ferguson et al. checked the sealing effect of the acetabular labrum in vitro; they found a decrease in the intra-articular fluid pressure after labral resection, indicating the imperative sealing effect of the labrum.[151] Song et al. measured the resistance to rotation, which reflects articular cartilage friction, in five cadaveric hips joints during half, one, two, and three times body-weight cyclic loading in the intact hip and after focal and complete labrectomy.[64] Resistance to rotation was significantly increased after focal/partial labrectomy at one to three times body-weight loading and after complete labrectomy at all load levels.

Dynamic Imaging Studies

Studies on live subjects have the potential to be the most accurate methods for dynamic biomechanics studies. One option to perform those studies is to use an optical tracking system while the subjects perform different movements; the results are applied to a 3D model, which is based on the subject's MRI or CT images. Charbonnier et al. used an optical tracking device with a combination of 3D MRI to study the hip motions of 11 pairs of female ballet dancers with no morphologic abnormalities.[130] Based on the results, four dancing movements seemed to be potentially harmful for the hip joint, inducing significant stress in the hip joint, with a high frequency of impingement and femoroacetabular translations ranging from 0.93 to 6.35 mm. For almost all movements, the computed zones of impingement were mainly located in the superior or posterosuperior quadrant of the acetabulum. Martin et al. performed a study

investigating the efficacy of a combined high-speed, biplane radiography and model-based tracking technique to study hip joint kinematics and arthrokinematics. They compared their model-based tracking to the gold standard of radiostereometric analysis and concluded that model-based tracking of the hip provides an opportunity to study pathologic hip conditions noninvasively.[152]

Hip-Spine Relationship

The hip and spine are closely related. Reduced ROM in the hip may result in overuse of the lumbar spine, and vice versa (Fig. 76.13). Esola et al. examined the role of the low back and hip in forward bending in subjects with and without a history of back pain.[153] Mean total forward bending for all subjects was 111 degrees—41.6 degrees from the lumbar spine and 69.4 degrees from the hips. The lumbar spine had a greater contribution to early forward bending, the lumbar spine and hips contributed almost equally to middle forward bending, and the hips had a greater contribution to late forward bending. Patients with a history of back pain tended to move more at their lumbar spine during early forward bending and had a significantly lower lumbar/hip flexion ratio during middle forward bending. Additionally, hip disorders can cause back pain secondarily by creating an abnormal sagittal balance and irregular gait that places further strain on the spine.[154,155]

Recently Hellman et al. found that patients presenting with femoroacetabular impingement (FAI) may have a lower pelvic incidence (PI) than the general population. However, the clinical significance of a 5.7 difference in PI is unknown.[156] Gomez-Hoyos et al recently conducted a cadaveric study looking at the effect of IFI on lumbar facet joints. They concluded that limited terminal hip extension due to simulated IFI significantly increases L3 to 4 and L4 to 5 lumbar facet joint load when compared with non-IFI native hips.[157]

SUMMARY

Over the years the hip joint has been the subject of many anatomic and biomechanical studies. The anatomy of the hip joint seems simple on the basic level. However, more detailed inspection reveals that the hip joint is quite complex in anatomy and particularly biomechanics. The hip appears to be a ball-and-socket joint, but it functions more like a gimbal joint. Although plenty of biomechanical studies exist, more advanced study of hip biomechanics is needed. The current chapter aimed to review the most updated studies in those areas, offering fundamental tools for understanding of the various hip joint pathologies.

For a complete list of references, go to ExpertConsult.com.

SELECTED READINGS

Citation:
Safran MRLN, Zaffagnini S, Signorelli C, et al. In vitro analysis of periarticular soft tissues constraining effect on hip kinematics and joint stability. *Knee Surg Sports Traumatol Arthrosc.* 2012;21:1655–1663.

Level:
III

Summary:
This article pertains to an in vitro cadaveric study on the stability of the hip joint. The study showed that with hip motion, the femoral head is translating relatively to the acetabulum in all three planes. This translation increased with removal of the soft tissue around the joint, confirming its importance to hip stability.

Citation:
Lee MC, Eberson CP. Growth and development of the child's hip. *Orthop Clin North Am.* 2006;37(2):119–132.

Level:
III

Summary:
This review regards the growth and development of the hip, beginning with prenatal cellular development. The authors discuss the ossification centers and blood supply of the femur and acetabulum.

Citation:
Stops A, Wilcox R, Jin Z. Computational modeling of the natural hip: A review of finite element and multibody simulations. *Comput Methods Biomech Biomed Engin.* 2011;15(9):963–979.

Level:
III

Summary:
This article provides reviews on finite-element and multibody simulations of the hip. The former offers knowledge on contact pressures and the effects of musculoskeletal geometries, in particular cartilage and bone shapes, whereas the latter deals with the influence of gait patterns and muscle attachment locations on force magnitudes.

Citation:
Franz JR, Paylo KW, Dicharry J, et al. Changes in the coordination of hip and pelvis kinematics with mode of locomotion. *Gait Posture.* 2009;29(3):494–498.

Level:
III

Summary:
This article summarizes a biomechanical/kinematic study on 73 healthy adult runners who were running on a treadmill. The influence of pick hip extension during walking and running on pelvic tilt and lumbar lordosis is explored.

Citation:
Ferguson SJ, Bryant JT, Ganz R, et al. An in vitro investigation of the acetabular labral seal in hip joint mechanics. *J Biomech.* 2003;36(2):171–178.

Level:
III

Summary:
This article reviews a biomechanical study on the acetabular labrum and is one of the most cited articles on the subject. It is shown that hydrostatic fluid pressurization within the intra-articular space is greater with the labrum than without it, which may enhance joint lubrication. It is also shown that cartilage consolidation is quicker without the labrum than with it, because the labrum adds extra resistance to the flow path for interstitial fluid expression.

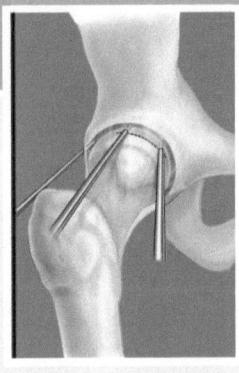

77

Hip Diagnosis and Decision-Making

Austin W. Chen, Benjamin G. Domb

OVERVIEW OF PATHOLOGIES

Understanding the differential diagnosis for hip pathology is necessary before collecting a history and performing a physical examination. This background allows the clinician to tease out important elements in the history to narrow the differential and provide a focus for the physical examination. An overview of hip pathology is presented in the following sections (Box 77.1).

Soft Tissue Injuries

Inflammation and pain originating from the trochanteric, ischial, iliopsoas, and iliopectineal bursae are common. Movement at bone and soft tissue interfaces leads to repetitive friction and inflammation in these areas. Trochanteric bursitis is frequently diagnosed but may be more accurately described as greater trochanteric pain syndrome (GTPS). Magnetic resonance imaging (MRI) findings for this diagnosis have shown frequent abductor tendinitis and tears with bursitis lacking in up to 80% of patients.[1] Nonetheless, patients with trochanteric bursitis describe lateral thigh pain that can be reproduced with palpation on examination. Ischial bursitis typically presents with pain upon sitting and can be reproduced by palpation over the ischial tuberosity (IT). The iliopsoas bursa lies between the iliopsoas muscle and pelvic brim.[2] Patients typically present with inguinal pain that is reproducible with provocative maneuvers such as the Thomas test. The iliopectineal bursa is adjacent to the iliopsoas bursa but lies over the iliopectineal eminence. Symptoms are similar to those of iliopsoas bursitis, although iliopectineal bursitis can be seen in conjunction with a snapping iliopsoas muscle over the iliopectineal eminence.[3]

Snapping hip syndrome, also referred to as *coxa saltans*, causes an audible or palpable "snap" with hip range of motion (ROM). The etiology of a snapping hip is classified as external, internal, or intra-articular.[4] An external snapping hip is caused by the iliotibial band (ITB) passing over the greater trochanter. An internal snapping hip is attributed to shifting of the iliopsoas tendon from medial to lateral over the femoral head, iliopectineal eminence, iliacus muscle, or lesser trochanter among others during hip flexion and extension.[3,5–7] An intra-articular snapping hip is related to labral tears, loose bodies, or osteochondral injuries.

Contusions involving the hip, thigh, and pelvis are frequently encountered in athletes and occur after low-energy trauma. An iliac crest contusion, or "hip pointer," results from a direct blow

to the iliac crest, and an overlying hematoma often develops. Quadriceps contusions typically involve a direct blow to the anterior thigh, which can result in hematoma formation and difficulty ambulating. A direct blow to the inner thigh may result in a groin contusion. Myositis ossificans can occur after a contusion and hematoma.[8] The hematoma organizes and calcifies, which can lead to pain and stiffness. Myositis ossificans can also be seen in the absence of trauma.

Muscle strains and ligamentous injuries around the hip can be quite debilitating. Strains typically involve tearing at the musculotendinous junction and often occur during an eccentric contraction.[9] Strains are classified by the affected muscle groups, including adductor, iliopsoas, external oblique, hamstring, and quadriceps. With significant force during athletics, or in the setting of trauma, the strong sacroiliac ligaments can be sprained. Pain typically originates in the lower back and radiates into the buttock or groin.

Hernias involve the extrusion of abdominal contents through a defect in the abdominal wall. A delay in diagnosis is common because hernias can mimic other conditions that cause groin pain with activity. Three hernias can present as hip or pelvic pain: inguinal, femoral, and sports hernias. Inguinal hernias involve the protrusion of abdominal contents through the deep inguinal ring or medial to the deep inguinal ring. Femoral hernias occur when a hernia sac protrudes through the femoral sheath to enter the anterior thigh. The "sports hernia" or athletic pubalgia is an increasingly recognized condition caused by posterior inguinal/abdominal wall weakness or tearing in athletes. No true protrusion of abdominal contents occurs, but patients experience chronic groin pain that is often difficult to diagnose.[10] The pain can also radiate to the perineum and origin of the adductors. Sports that require frequent pivoting and cutting such as ice hockey, soccer, and American football have the highest incidence of this injury. Athletes often lack symptoms with rest but experience pain with activity or sport that prevents them from playing to their potential.[11]

Bone Injuries

Sport-related trauma can involve significant energy resulting in fractures of the pelvis and femur. Pelvic ring injuries, acetabular fractures, femoral head and neck fractures, peritrochanteric fractures, and femoral shaft fractures lead to the acute onset of pain and difficulty or inability to weight bear or ambulate. Prompt recognition and treatment of fractures about the pelvis

BOX 77.1   Overview of Hip Pathology

Soft Tissue Injuries
Bursitis
  Trochanteric
  Ischial
  Iliopsoas
  Iliopectineal
Snapping hip syndrome
Contusions
  Iliac crest
  Quadriceps
  Groin
Myositis ossificans
Strains
  Adductor
  Iliopsoas
  External oblique
  Hamstring
  Quadriceps
Sacroiliac sprain
Hernias
  Inguinal
  Femoral
  Sports (athletic pubalgia)

Bone Injuries
Traumatic fractures
Dislocation

Stress fractures
  Pelvic
  Sacral
  Femoral neck
Osteitis pubis
Osteonecrosis

Degenerative Joint Disease
Nerve Entrapment Injuries
Sciatic
Obturator
Pudendal
Ilioinguinal
Femoral
Lateral femoral cutaneous

Intra-Articular Pathology
Labral tears
Femoral acetabular impingement
Loose bodies
Chondral injuries
Ruptured ligamentum teres

Infection
Pediatric Conditions
Avulsion fracture
Slipped capital femoral epiphysis
Legg-Calvé-Perthes disease

and femur are critical, as delay in diagnosis can result in long-term morbidity.

Stress fractures of the pelvis and femur occur in the setting of repetitive submaximal loading of bone. Pain that is aggravated by activity and subsides with rest is the hallmark feature of a stress fracture. Pelvic rami and sacral stress fractures are seen in athletes who participate in high-impact activities such as running and jogging. The pain is typically in the groin, buttock, or thigh when the ramus is involved and in the low back when the sacrum is the source.[12] Femoral neck stress fractures typically present with activity-related groin pain. The location of the stress fracture is critical to determining treatment. Tension-sided femoral neck stress fractures along the superior lateral neck require surgical treatment to prevent nonunion, avascular necrosis, or fracture displacement. Compression-sided femoral neck stress fractures occur along the inferior medial neck and are often amenable to nonoperative treatment.[13]

A stress injury of the pubic symphysis can lead osteitis pubis.[14] This is frequently secondary to a muscular imbalance between the rectus abdominis (pelvic elevator) and the adductor tendons (pelvic depressor) that attach to fibrocartilage plate of the pubic symphysis. The pain is typically insidious in onset and is located at the midline over the symphysis or referred to the groin. Degeneration of the symphyseal cartilage can be followed by boney lytic changes, sclerosis, and widening of the symphysis.[11]

Osteonecrosis, or avascular necrosis, of the femoral head is a cause of hip pain in young adults. Many conditions have been associated with osteonecrosis; however, the majority are related to corticosteroid use, trauma, alcohol abuse, and coagulopathy.[15] No cause is identified in 10% to 20% of cases, and this type of necrosis is termed "idiopathic avascular necrosis." Patients typically present with pain in the groin or buttock and often walk with a limp. Bilateral avascular necrosis has been found in 40% to 80% of patients.[15–17] Early identification may allow treatment that can prevent femoral head collapse and the need for arthroplasty.

Instability

Hip dislocations typically occur when significant force disrupts the soft tissue restraints of the hip joint.[18] However, low-energy injuries may also cause hip dislocations in the setting of femoroacetabular impingement (FAI) morphology (cam, pincer, acetabular retroversion). Clinical and basic science studies support the mechanism of the anterior impingement levering the femoral head posteriorly.[19] Hip dislocations are typically posterior, which leads to the patient having a shortened, internally rotated, and abducted hip. Less commonly, the dislocation will be anterior, which presents as an externally rotated and abducted hip. Expeditious recognition and reduction may be essential to prevent avascular necrosis.

Microinstability of the hip is a more recent, but increasingly recognized, cause of hip pain. Several predisposing factors have been identified and include: generalized ligamentous laxity, repetitive microtrauma, ligamentum teres (LT) injuries, varying degrees of acetabular dysplasia, and iatrogenesis. Soft tissue and dynamic stabilizers of the hip such as the capsule, labrum, LT, and tendinous structures such as the iliopsoas may all play a role in microinstability. The clinical presentation may be subtle and difficult to detect. Most patients complain of pain in the groin, buttock, or thigh, but some may note "giving way" or apprehension. The onset is insidious with gradual worsening of symptoms.[20,21]

Degenerative Joint Disease

Degenerative joint disease (DJD) results from the loss of cartilage in the hip joint and leads to progressive pain and stiffness. Many pathologic processes can lead to DJD, including but not limited to osteoarthritis, rheumatoid arthritis, avascular necrosis, infection, trauma, FAI, and dysplasia/instability. Although the process may be idiopathic, we now recognize that structural abnormalities of the hip are frequently associated with DJD.[22] The diagnosis is usually confirmed by observing joint space narrowing, subchondral cysts and/or sclerosis, and/or osteophyte formation on plain radiographs. Patients typically present with the insidious onset of hip pain that worsens with activity.

DJD is a spectrum and ranges in severity. While advanced DJD is usually obvious, milder forms of DJD may be more ambiguous. It is crucial to determine how much joint degeneration is present, as this can have dramatic implications on treatment and surgical outcomes.[23] In addition to plain x-rays, delayed gadolinium-enhanced magnetic resonance imaging of cartilage (dGEMRIC) can provide a helpful quantitative analysis of the articular cartilage health.[24] An algorithm (Fig. 77.1) helps stratify patients by degree of arthritis and the appropriate respective treatments.[23]

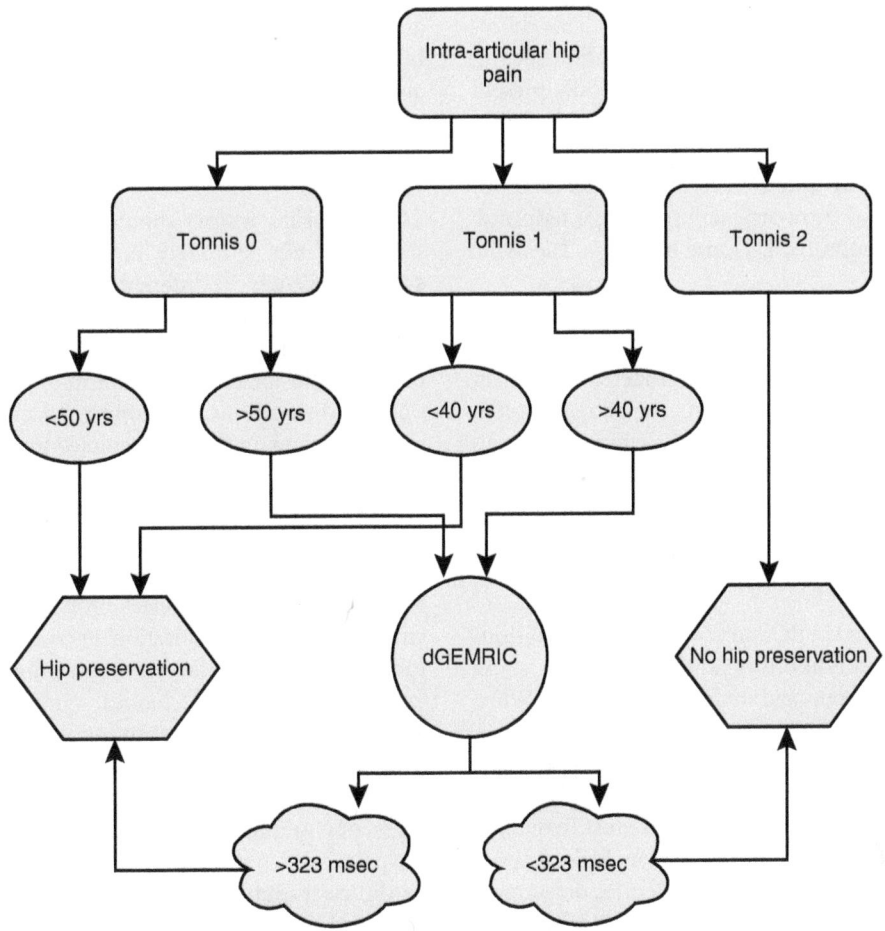

Fig. 77.1 Algorithm for patient selection for hip arthroscopy using radiographic and delayed gadolinium-enhanced magnetic resonance imaging of cartilage *(dGEMRIC)* parameters as a guide.

Nerve Entrapment Injuries

Nerve entrapment surrounding the hip can involve the sciatic, obturator, pudendal, ilioinguinal, femoral, and lateral femoral cutaneous nerve. Diagnosing and treating these conditions can be difficult and frustrating for the patient and clinician. The pain often has a burning quality and is confined to a nerve root distribution. Electromyographic nerve conduction studies are helpful in confirming the diagnosis and ruling out a lumbar radiculopathy. Sciatic nerve entrapment often presents with pain radiating down the buttock and posterior thigh. In some cases, this pain may be related to piriformis syndrome.[25] Obturator nerve entrapment causes pain in the medial thigh that can radiate toward the knee.[26] Prolonged compression during activities such as cycling can cause pudendal nerve entrapment.[27] Numbness and pain in the perineum and shaft of the penis are typical. Ilioinguinal nerve entrapment is a very rare cause of inguinal pain that often radiates into the groin. Pain over the anterior thigh can be caused by femoral nerve entrapment, and when severe, it may cause quadriceps weakness and difficulty with gait.[28] Lateral femoral cutaneous nerve entrapment, or *meralgia paresthetica*, causes anterolateral thigh pain and numbness that extends toward the lateral knee.[29]

Intra-Articular Pathology

Our understanding of intra-articular pathology has significantly expanded during the past few decades. Structural abnormalities of the hip joint seen in persons with dysplasia and FAI often lead to injury of the labrum and chondral surface. Hip dysplasia, or developmental dysplasia of the hip, results in a broad spectrum of disease. The underlying abnormality is inadequate acetabular coverage of the femoral head, which in severe forms can cause hip dislocations in children. Often the degree of undercoverage is mild or "borderline" and leads to pathology during adulthood because of the concentration of forces on a shallow acetabulum.[30] FAI is caused by abnormalities of the femur and acetabulum that lead to abnormal contact within the hip joint.[31] Deformity on the femoral side is termed *cam impingement* and is due to an aspherical femoral head commonly located at the anterosuperior head-neck junction. Deformity on the acetabular side is termed *pincer impingement* and occurs with excessive acetabular coverage of the femoral head. Most commonly, both abnormalities exist in the same hip joint, and this condition is termed *combined impingement*. Iliopsoas impingement is compression and damage to the underlying anterior acetabular labrum at the 3 o'clock position (right hip) by a tight iliopsoas tendon or an inflamed tendon adherent to the anterior capsulolabral complex causing a repetitive traction injury to the labrum. This differs from the typical 1 to 2 o'clock labral tear distribution seen in FAI.[32] Patients with intra-articular pathology typically present with groin, lateral hip, or buttock pain. Scrutinizing hip radiographs will often help the clinician identify morphologic abnormalities of the hip that may lead to intra-articular pathology.[14] Multiple other sources of intra-articular pathology have also been described, such as ruptured LT, loose bodies, and synovial disease.

Infection

Septic arthritis of the hip should always be considered in a patient who presents with the acute onset of pain. The patient is often febrile and lacks a history of trauma. Physical examination reveals pain with attempted passive ROM. Inflammatory markers are typically elevated. Prompt recognition and treatment are necessary to prevent long-term complications.[33]

Pediatric Hip Conditions

Skeletally immature patients often present with hip conditions that differ from the hip conditions of adults. Open physes and apophyses are areas of weakness and are frequently injured. When muscles are overloaded in children, failure can occur at the origin of the muscle, particularly when an apophysis is present.[34] This scenario causes an avulsion fracture at the muscle origin, which differs from the pathology seen in adults, who most frequently experience a soft tissue tear of involving the tendon. Males account for up to 86.7% of these injuries. Avulsion fractures occur most commonly at the anterior superior iliac spine (ASIS), anterior inferior iliac spine (AIIS), and IT, when the sartorius/tensor fasciae latae, rectus femoris, hamstrings, and iliopsoas muscles, respectively, are overloaded. Lateral and distal displacement of ASIS injuries can be misdiagnosed as AIIS avulsions. Patients with IT avulsions tend to be younger due to earlier ossification center formation and 12% will have a contralateral sided injury. Less common avulsion injuries include the iliac crest, pubic symphysis, and lesser trochanter with muscle forces from the abdominal muscles, adductors, and iliopsoas, respectively. If misdiagnosed or delayed in presentation, these injuries can lead to hip impingement or nerve irritation and exhibit the respective symptoms.[35]

Slipped capital femoral epiphysis (SCFE) is a disorder of the proximal femoral physis. The proximal femoral physis fails, leading to anterior superior displacement of the femur relative to the epiphysis.[36] This condition typically involves patients 11 to 14 years of age, often affects obese children, and may be seen in the setting of endocrine abnormalities. Displacement at the physis can frequently be identified with a frog-leg lateral radiograph. Duration of symptoms and stability at the physis is important for treatment and prognosis. Patients with an unstable slip are unable to weight bear and have approximately a 50% chance of AVN.[37] When SCFE is identified, surgical treatment is often indicated.

Legg-Calvé-Perthes disease (LCPD) is a childhood disorder that leads to ischemic necrosis of the growing femoral head. The process typically affects patients 5 to 8 years of age and predominantly involves boys. Like SCFE, there may also be an association with obesity.[38] Parents notice that the child is limping, but the patient often has only mild pain. Radiographs can identify abnormalities in the femoral epiphysis.

HISTORY

The goal of the history should be to (1) rule out any alarming sources of hip pathology, including malignancy, infection, or systemic disease; (2) differentiate true hip pain from back pain; and (3) narrow the differential diagnosis to perform a focused physical examination. Patient age and profession or sport, chief complaint, history, and mechanism of trauma—including previous hip dislocations, developmental or childhood hip-related conditions, and previously attempted treatment modalities should all be ascertained. These modalities often include analgesic or antiinflammatory medications, assistive devices, interaction with other physicians, injections, physical therapy, or previous surgery.[39] A history of acute onset or trauma is a better prognostic indicator than an insidious onset of symptoms.[40] Important pain characteristics include: location, intensity, quality, onset, duration, radiation, alleviating factors, aggravating factors, and associated factors (Fig. 77.2). Mechanical symptoms such as snapping, popping, locking, clicking, and subjective instability should also be elicited. Pain or catching during flexion and axial loading activities (e.g., rising from a seated position, walking up or down stairs, or entering and exiting a vehicle) also implies mechanical hip pain.[41] Patients may also admit to pain with sexual intercourse or difficulty putting on shoes or socks because of rotational force and complex hip movements.[42]

The remainder of the standard history should not be overlooked. A medical and surgical history may uncover recent or

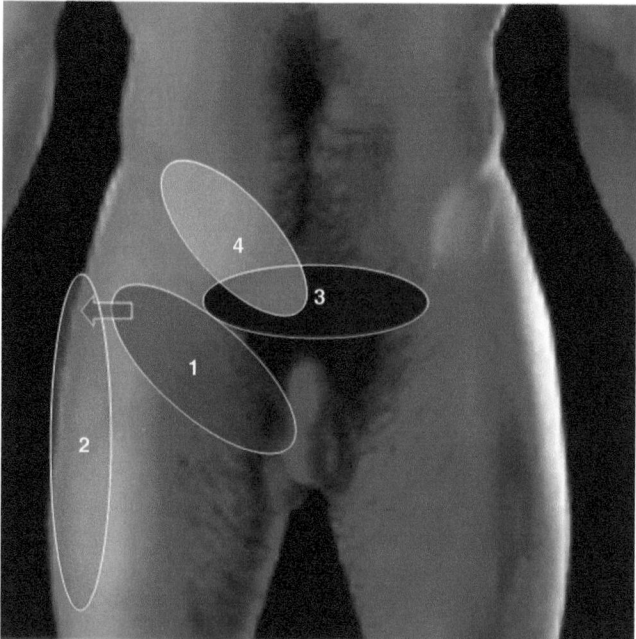

Fig. 77.2 The location of pain can aid in diagnosis. *1*, Intra-articular pain can be caused by osteoarthritis or labral pathology. *2*, Lateral hip pain can be caused by trochanteric bursitis or abductor contracture. *3*, Symphyseal pain can be caused by osteitis pubis. *4*, Abdominal pain can be caused by athletic hernias.

remote illness including malignancy, an immunocompromised state, tuberculosis or other infection, deep venous thrombosis, or hernia. A family history of cancer, systemic inflammatory arthritis, hip instability, or DJD is also useful. A social history detailing abuse of tobacco, alcohol, or illicit drugs is also important and may increase the index of suspicion for osteonecrosis of the femoral head or malignancy. Obtaining a sexual history as part of the social history can help evaluate the patient's risk of a sexually transmitted infection and associated septic arthritis. Pain with menses also should be noted. The social history should also include a review of the patient's activities of daily living, work activities, hobbies, athletic activities, and impairments to these activities that are a result of the chief complaint. Participation in running, basketball, soccer, ballet, hockey, golf, tennis, martial arts, or rugby is specifically associated with hip pathology.[43-45] A review of systems including recent fever, chills, malaise, night sweats, or unintended weight loss warrants further investigation.[46] The clinician should remember that genitourinary—including pelvic floor musculature, gastrointestinal, neurologic, or vascular pathology can also masquerade as hip pain.

When eliciting the history, the clinician should ask the patient what he or she believes is causing the pain. The patient's expectations of the encounter should be addressed, and he or she should be given a specific opportunity to ask questions or raise concerns. In addition, the patient may provide or recall more pertinent history during the physical examination, and thus the clinician must always listen attentively (Box 77.2).

PHYSICAL EXAMINATION

The physical examination of the hip consists of several steps, including inspection, symptom localization, measurements, ROM, and special maneuvers.

Inspection

Observation of stance and gait inspection are essential components of the physical examination. The patient's stance should be inspected for a flexed position of the hip or knee, which may be indicative of hip pathology. The patient's stance should also be inspected for gross atrophy, spinal malalignment, or pelvic obliquity. While sitting, the patient should be observed for leaning to the unaffected side to avoid excessive flexion. The gait should be observed in multiple planes and for six to eight strides in the frontal and sagittal plane.[47]

BOX 77.2 Information Obtained From Patient History

Character and location of pain
Mechanism of injury (be specific if possible)
Duration of symptoms
Activity-related pain (e.g., Does it subside with rest?)
Pain related to bowel or bladder activity or ingestion of food
Pain related to menses
Treatment history (injections, physical therapy, other physician evaluations)

Patients may present with one of several gait abnormalities, including an antalgic gait, a pelvic wink, a Trendelenburg gait, excessive pelvic internal or external rotation, or true or false leg length discrepancies.[39] The antalgic gait involves a limp to decrease the time of stance phase on the affected side and limit weight bearing through the affected hip. An antalgic gait could indicate pain anywhere along the affected lower extremity. A pelvic wink is greater than 40 degrees of rotation in the axial plane toward the affected hip during terminal extension and signifies a hip flexion contracture in the setting of lumbar lordosis or forward-stooping posture. A Trendelenburg gait, also known as an abductor lurch, involves leaning the trunk toward the affected hip. Abductors normally stabilize the pelvis when the contralateral leg is raised. If the abductor muscles or the nerves supplying those muscles are injured or not functioning, the patient will lurch to the ipsilateral side to prevent pelvic sagging. A Trendelenburg sign can be elicited by having the patient raise the contralateral leg. A pelvic sag of more than 2 cm on the ipsilateral side is a positive Trendelenburg sign, indicating abductor pathology. Internal or external rotation should be noted both during gait and in the sitting position, which stabilizes the pelvis. Decreased internal rotation is a sign of internal hip pathology.[48] Excessive internal rotation with decreased external rotation indicates increased femoral anteversion.[49] A short leg limp during gait may indicate a true or false leg length discrepancy, or the limp may be secondary to ITB pathology. Children with leg length discrepancy may present with a circumduction gait or a vaulting gait to clear the long leg.[50]

Snapping or clicking noises should be noted as the patient walks. These noises can indicate iliopsoas, ITB, or intra-articular pathology. Lateral snapping is more likely with ITB pathology and generally is easily visualized.[51] Audible anterior snapping is more likely a result of iliopsoas tendon pathology. Either etiology of snapping may be palpable and/or reproducible.

Symptom Localization

Numerous techniques can help localize symptoms. A simple tool involves asking the patient to localize his or her pain by using a single finger. This technique can narrow the differential. In addition, examination of this location can be reserved for the end of the examination, thus enhancing the patient's trust by not causing pain at the beginning of the examination. This pain location in conjunction with Hilton's law can help distinguish the cause of pain in the hip region. Hilton's law states that "the same trunks of nerves whose branches supply the groups of muscles moving a joint furnish also a distribution of nerves to the skin over the insertion of the same muscles, and the interior of the joint receives its nerves from the same source."[52] This law helps explain why muscle spasms and superficial pain accompany hip pathology. The L3 nerve predominantly innervates the hip joint, and thus pain down the entire L3 dermatome (the anterior and medial thigh crossing laterally to the knee) can accompany hip pain. This pain can be confused with compression of the lateral femoral cutaneous nerve, also known as meralgia paresthetica, which will cause pain or neuralgia in the L2 or L3 dermatome.[53-56]

Another useful observation is the C sign. The C sign occurs when a patient cups his or her hand above the greater trochanter

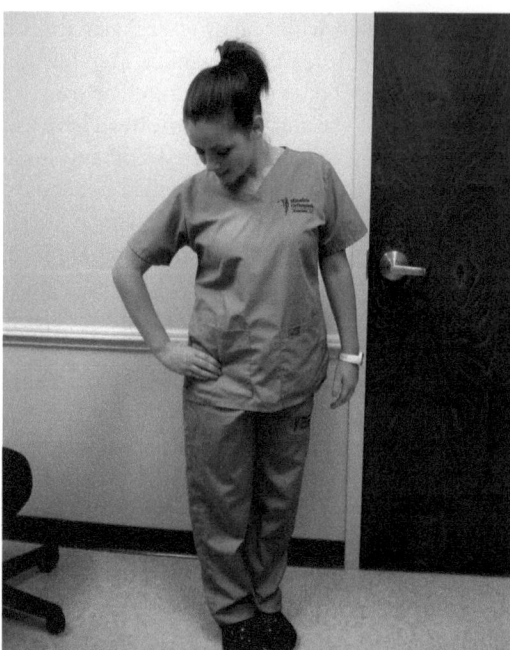

Fig. 77.3 The C sign. Cupping the thumb and the index finger around the lateral thigh indicates deep hip pathology.

when describing hip pain. The hand forms a "C" and is placed on the lateral hip, which may lead the clinician to mistakenly consider lateral hip pathology such as ITB or trochanteric bursitis (Fig. 77.3). However, this sign is most characteristic of deep interior hip pain.[42,57] When a C sign is observed, the clinician should ensure that the examination and subsequent testing include a complete evaluation for intra-articular hip pain.

Palpation can also assist in localization of symptoms in the hip, although not as much as in other joints. The clinician must be familiar with the superficial and deep anatomy of the hip region for palpation to be of assistance. Initial palpation of the abdomen to check for fascial hernias or masses is important to rule out gastrointestinal or genitourinary sources of pain. Palpation of the lumbar spine, sacroiliac joint, ischium, iliac crest, greater trochanter, trochanteric bursa, various muscle bellies, rectus femoris and iliopsoas tendons, the adductor tubercle, and the pubic symphysis can help distinguish the location of pain. Pubic symphysis pain can indicate fracture, calcification, or osteitis pubis. The clinician can also palpate the femoral nerve. A positive Tinel sign indicates a neurologic cause of pain. Identification of bursitis on examination is often extremely helpful in narrowing the differential and can be followed up with an injection of a local anesthetic to confirm the diagnosis. The addition of a steroid to the injection is often therapeutic as well.

A distal neurovascular examination should also be completed, including palpation of the dorsalis pedis and posterior tibial arteries, an assessment of capillary refill, and lymphatic return. A thorough motor and sensory examination can often be helpful in differentiating hip from lumbar pain. Strength testing of the iliopsoas, quadriceps, extensor hallucis longus, tibialis anterior, and gastrocnemius provides an assessment of the L2-S1 nerve roots. Any asymmetric weakness compared with the contralateral side may indicate a radicular component to the pain, and this finding should prompt further investigation into lumbar spine or peripheral nerve pathology. A thorough sensory examination will often help confirm radicular or peripheral nerve problems. When assessing numbness, the examiner should differentiate a radicular (L2-S1) pattern from a peripheral nerve pattern (femoral, peroneal) to provide a focus for additional testing. Intra-articular hip pain should not cause sensory disturbances or weakness in the foot. In the setting of injury, muscle testing also can be helpful. If the clinician believes that a specific muscle group has been affected, then resisted contraction can reproduce the patient's symptoms. Specifically, leg abductors (superior gluteal nerve L4-S1), leg adductors (obturator nerve L2-L4), knee extensors and hip flexors (femoral nerve L2-L4), hip extensors (inferior gluteal nerve L5-S2), and knee flexors and lower leg muscles (sciatic L4-S3) should be tested. The strength of patients with intra-articular pathology is often limited by pain, and the clinician should be aware that weakness in the iliopsoas or abductors may be a result of pain instead of being neurogenic. The algorithm in Fig. 77.4 is useful in the setting of hip-spine syndrome and an ambiguous diagnosis.[58] Diagnostic injections of the hip joint are invaluable in differentiating hip and lumbar pathology.[59,60] If possible, the patient should perform a symptom-aggravating activity, be examined prior to the injection, observed while the anesthetic takes effect, and finally, re-examined. Differences in pain scale, ROM, and special maneuvers should be documented. Injection of local anesthetic concurrently with an MR arthrogram is unreliable, as the contrast agent itself can be irritating.

Active ROM, passive ROM, and resisted ROM may reproduce hip pain. ROM examination can help differentiate muscle strains from intra-articular pathology. In general, passive ROM may reproduce hip pain but not pain from a muscle strain. A strain of the hip flexors can be detected with the active hip flexion but not passive hip flexion.

Measurements and Range of Motion

Several measurements are important during the hip evaluation. Ipsilateral measurements from the shoulder of the iliac crest or from the ASIS to the medial malleolus can detect a true leg length discrepancy. Degenerative changes and collapsed avascular necrosis frequently cause a leg length discrepancy. Preoperative templating and the physical examination are the keys to successfully restoring leg length at the time of reconstruction.

The measurement of thigh circumference can detect muscle atrophy from chronic conditions. It is important to choose the same level of the thigh for circumference measurements. For example, 10 cm above the patella is a typical location for this measurement. The contralateral side must be measured for comparison, and this measurement can be taken at subsequent visits to gauge response to treatment.

Hip ROM must be accurately and reproducibly measured during the physical examination of the hip (Table 77.1). ROM can indicate the extent of hip pathology and the response to treatment. Hip flexion is best tested in the supine position, and the normal range is up to 120 degrees.[61] Hip extension is best tested in the prone position, and the normal range is up to 15 degrees. Internal and external rotation should be tested with the

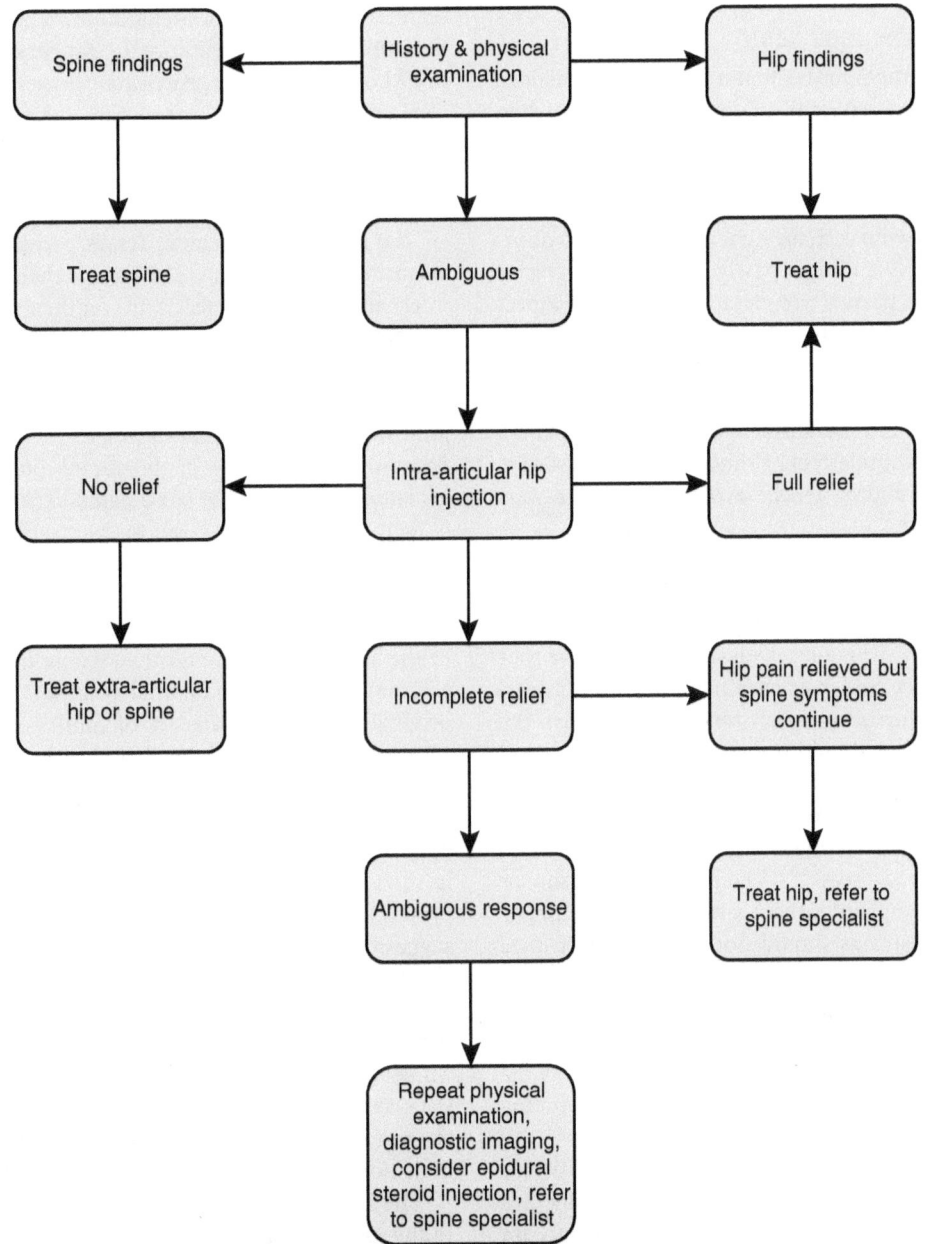

Fig. 77.4 Algorithm helping to differentiate hip and spine pain sources.

TABLE 77.1	Average Hip Range of Motion
Motion	**Degrees**
Flexion	115
Abduction	50
Adduction	30
Internal rotation	45
External rotation	45

hip flexed at 90 degrees, which is best accomplished in the seated position to stabilize the pelvis. Normal internal rotation is up to 45 degrees, and normal external rotation is up to 50 degrees.[61] Arthritis, effusion, SCFE, FAI, or muscle contractures can cause a decrease in internal rotation.[49,62] Abduction and adduction

should be measured with reference to the shaft of the femur at the midline of the pelvis. Normal abduction is 45 degrees, and normal adduction is up to 30 degrees.[61] An abductor contracture may decrease adduction ROM.[61] Differences between the normal and affected side can help detect hip pathology.[48] In patients with DJD, hip ROM is often globally decreased, with pain at the extremes of motion. Patients with dysplasia have shallow acetabuli and anterior superior undercoverage, which allows increased internal rotation with the hip flexed. Patients with FAI typically lack internal rotation in a flexed position because of the abnormal contact between the femoral head and neck with the acetabulum. After acetabular rim trimming and femoral osteoplasty, intraoperative ROM can be tested. Typically, as the impingement is relieved, the patient will gain internal rotation with the hip flexed.

Evaluation of Ligamentous Laxity

Testing for general ligamentous laxity is a good complement to the abduction–extension–external rotation examination when instability is suspected. Generalized laxity can be estimated by utilizing the Beighton criteria.[73] This gives the patient a numerical score out of a possible nine points, with one point assigned to each of the following with each right and left sides accounting for unique scores: small finger passive dorsiflexion greater than 90 degrees, thumb passive dorsiflexion to the flexor aspect of the forearm, elbow hyperextension greater than 10 degrees, knee hyperextension greater than 10 degrees, and palms flat on the floor with forward flexion and knees fully extended. A score of four or greater denotes generalized ligamentous laxity and a possible concern for an underlying connective tissue disorder. A referral for medical and/or genetic evaluation may be warranted in some patients.[45]

Special Maneuvers

Supine

The straight-leg raise (SLR) is a test to assess lumber nerve root pathology. With the knee held in extension and the contralateral pelvis stabilized, the clinician passively raises the leg. When the patient feels pain, the hip should be extended 10 degrees and the foot dorsiflexed to elicit radicular symptoms. Pain from 0 to 30 degrees suggests a compressed nerve root, pain from 30 to 60 degrees may suggest sacroiliac disease, and pain after 60 degrees suggests sacroiliac disease.[63,64] The pain should be similar to the patient's chief complaint rather than generalized stiffness. Stretching of the hamstrings should not be confused with a positive SLR test.

An SLR against resistance, also known as an active SLR, can indicate hip pain. Again, in the supine position, the patient flexes at the hip with the knee extended, but the clinician resists the flexion, thus generating force across the hip joint. Pain with the active SLR indicates hip pain.

The log roll test is the most specific test for intra-articular hip disease. The femur is gently rotated both internally and externally without motion of the pelvis or undue pressure on the surrounding muscles. Pain is specific but not sensitive for hip pathology. The heel strike and Stinchfield tests can be useful accompaniments to the log roll test. Striking the heel with the fist causes an axial load through the hip and can recreate hip pain. The Stinchfield test involves gradually increasing resisted flexion of the hip, with pain indicating either joint pain or iliopsoas pathology.[49] Plain radiographs or MRI will often confirm physical examination findings for intra-articular pain. If the history and physical examination findings are confusing, a diagnostic injection of local anesthetic in the hip joint can be helpful in ruling out extra-articular pain.

The anterior impingement test involves forced flexion, adduction, and internal rotation of the hip (FADIR). This test is the most sensitive maneuver to detect subtle hip pathology, including FAI. Because this maneuver may be uncomfortable in a normal hip, a comparison to the unaffected side is extremely important. This position of the hip loads the anterior superior aspect of the hip joint by bringing the femoral head and neck into contact with the anterosuperior acetabulum. When this test is positive, the clinician should scrutinize the patient's radiographs for signs of FAI or DJD. If no degenerative changes are observed, further workup with an MRI arthrogram may be helpful to further evaluate the hip joint. A positive anterior impingement test may also guide decision-making intraoperatively by leading the surgeon to treat anterior pathology identified during arthroscopy.

The lateral impingement test is performed with the hip in extension and abducted. The knee is then flexed and the hip is internally rotated. A lateral cam on the femoral head/neck will impinge the superior aspect of the acetabulum causing pain and a positive test. The Patrick test, also known as the flexion, abduction, and external rotation (FABER) test, can stress the sacroiliac joint or imply lateral impingement or iliopsoas pathology. A figure-of-four is made in the supine position by placing the ipsilateral ankle over the contralateral knee. The ipsilateral knee is then pressed down. Posterior pain indicates sacroiliac joint disease, lateral pain indicates lateral impingement, and groin pain indicates iliopsoas pathology.[49]

The McCarthy test involves bringing both hips in to full flexion in the supine position and then extending the affected hip in external rotation and internal rotation. Reproduction of the original pain during this arc of motion constitutes a positive McCarthy test and indicates labral pathology.[65–69]

The Scour test can help detect irregularities along the femoral head or acetabulum. The clinician flexes the hip and knee while pointing the knee to the shoulder. While taking the hip through its arc of motion, any bumps or catches should be noted. The presence of bumps or catches indicates a positive test and is suggestive of FAI.

The Thomas test determines the presence and degree of a flexion contracture (iliopsoas contracture) of the hip. The patient should flex the unaffected hip and draw the knee to the chest while lowering the affected leg to the table. A positive Thomas test occurs when the patient cannot lower the affected extremity to the table. Any popping or clicking during the Thomas test may indicate a labral tear.[46]

The Dial test of the hip can help detect hip capsular laxity. In the supine position, the patient's hip and knee are extended. The clinician places a hand on the femur and a hand on the tibia and internally rotates the entire lower extremity at the hip joint. The lower extremity is then released and allowed to externally rotate. External rotation less than 45 degrees with a firm end point constitutes a negative Dial test. Passive external rotation beyond 45 degrees constitutes a positive Dial test and is indicative of hip capsular laxity.[47]

The posterior apprehension test can detect posterior hip micro or macro instability. The hip is flexed to 90 degrees, adducted, and internally rotated. Next, a posteriorly directed force is applied to the knee. When positive, this results in posterior pain or sensation of instability.[70]

The LT test is performed with the hip flexed at 70 degrees and 30 degrees short of full abduction and the knee at 90 degrees of flexion. The hip is then maximally internally and externally rotated. Pain on either internal or external rotation is consistent with a positive test result. Pain should be relieved with rotation in the opposite direction and reproducible with rotation in the direction of pain again. The sensitivity and specificity of the test are reported to be 90% and 85%, respectively.[71]

The resisted internal rotation test is one of the senior author's tests for gluteus medius and minimus pathology. The patient's hip and knee are each flexed to 90 degrees. In this position, the tip of the greater trochanter is directed posteriorly causing the much of the abductor complex to become an internal rotator of the hip. The clinician then instructs the patient to actively internally rotate the hip. This is often best conveyed by passively demonstrating which direction the patient will be moving their leg and foot. The clinician then resists the patient's internal rotation force. Pain and/or weakness at the lateral aspect of the hip is considered a positive test.

Lateral

Several examinations may be performed to help evaluate the hip in the lateral position. Flexing and extending the hip while moving the abductor mechanism across the hip can recreate visual ITB snapping. However, the patient will usually be able to actively reproduce a snapping ITB better than the clinician.

Abductor testing can be performed from the lateral position. Hip abduction against gravity or resistance may reveal weakness or pain. When weakness is discovered, the cause may be neurologic or musculotendinous. If neurologic weakness is suggested, an electromyogram can be a useful test for differentiating lumbar radiculopathy from superior gluteal nerve pathology. Painful weakness may suggest gluteus medius tendinopathy, trochanteric bursitis, or a trochanteric fracture. Further imaging with plain radiographs or MRI can be helpful in this setting.

Impingement testing with the flexion, adduction, and internal rotation maneuver can also be accomplished in the lateral position. While standing behind the patient, the clinician places one hand under the knee for support and the other hand on the hip joint with the index finger anterior and the thumb pointing posterior. If flexion, adduction, and internal rotation cause discomfort, the test is positive.

Ober testing comprises three parts: extension, neutral, and flexion. The extension test may detect an ITB contracture, the neutral test may detect a gluteus medius contracture, and the flexion test may detect a gluteus maximus contracture. The extension Ober test consists of flexing the knee, extending the hip, abducting the hip, and then releasing the hip. A delay in return to adduction indicates ITB pathology. The neutral Ober test consists of flexing the knee with the hip in the neutral position, abducting the hip, and then releasing the hip. A delay in return to adduction indicates gluteus medius pathology. The flexion Ober test consists of rotating the torso so that the patient's shoulders are flat on the table with the legs still in the lateral position, flexing the hip, extending the knee, abducting the hip, and then releasing the hip. A delay in return to adduction indicates gluteus maximus pathology.[72]

Prone

The modified Thomas test and Ely test can differentiate between iliopsoas contracture and rectus femoris contracture. A positive modified Thomas test is simply an observation of the pelvis rising up in the prone position, which suggests an iliopsoas contracture.[61] The Ely test is performed by flexing the knee as far as possible with the patient prone. Upward motion of the buttocks and pelvis indicates a positive Ely test, which suggests a rectus femoris contracture because the rectus femoris crosses both the hip and knee joints.[45]

The posterior impingement test is performed with the hip in extension and the leg flexed up. The hip is then externally rotated to bring the femoral head and neck into the posterior acetabulum. A positive test can be a sign of posterior labral pathology, excessive acetabular anteversion, or degenerative changes. Again, this test can assist the surgeon preoperatively and intraoperatively by indicating when to address a posterior lesion. While performing this maneuver, an anteriorly directed force can be placed on the posterior greater trochanter to translate the femoral head anteriorly. Pain or apprehension in the groin or anterior hip can be a sign of anterior instability.[74]

The femoral nerve stretch test should also be conducted in this position by flexing the knee. Nerve type pain with this maneuver indicates femoral nerve pathology instead of hip joint pathology.

CONCLUSION

A thoughtful, systematic approach to the hip joint is necessary for the diagnosis and treatment of hip pathology. Because hip, back, and knee pain can easily be confused for one another, a consistent and careful history and physical examination are crucial to avoid misdiagnosis.[48] The physical examination maneuvers previously described as well as diagnostic injections should allow the clinician to narrow the differential diagnosis and help determine whether the patient's pain is intra-articular or extra-articular. These distinctions are important, given recent advances in imaging and treatment options for the hip.

ACKNOWLEDGMENT

Adam G. Brooks, MD—Contributing author of 4th edition; John Muir Health and Sutter Health, Antioch, California
John Redmond, MD—Contributing author of 4th edition; Southeast Orthopedic Specialists, Jacksonville, Florida
Brandon Walton, BS—Videographer and editor; American Hip Institute, Westmont, Illinois

For a complete list of references, go to ExpertConsult.com.

SELECTED READINGS

Citation:
Buckland AJ, et al. Differentiating hip pathology from lumbar spine pathology: key points of evaluation and management. *J Am Acad Orthop Surg.* 2017;25(2):e23–e34.

Level of Evidence:
V

Summary:
This article discusses the difficulty in differentiating hip and spine pathology. Keys in the history, physical examination, diagnostic tests, and differential are discussed.

Citation:

Flynn JM, Widmann RF. The limping child: evaluation and diagnosis. *J Am Acad Orthop Surg.* 2001;9(2):89–98.

Level of Evidence:

V

Summary:

This article provides a framework for evaluating a child with a painful hip. The history, physical examination, and additional studies are outlined.

Citation:

Parvizi J, Leunig M, Ganz R. Femoroacetabular impingement. *J Am Acad Orthop Surg.* 2007;15(9):561–570.

Level of Evidence:

V

Summary:

In this review article on femoroacetabular impingement, the pathophysiology, history, physical examination, and treatment are discussed.

Citation:

Lynch TS, et al. Athletic hip injuries. *J Am Acad Orthop Surg.* 2017;25(4):269–279.

Level of Evidence:

V

Summary:

This review article discusses the "sports hip triad," consisting of adductor strains, osteitis pubis, athletic pubalgia, or core muscle injury, often with underlying range-of-motion limitations secondary to femoroacetabular impingement.

Citation:

Domb BG, Brooks AG, Byrd JW. Clinical examination of the hip. *J Sports Rehab.* 2009;18:3–23.

Level of Evidence:

V

Summary:

This article provides a brief overview of the history, physical examination, and relevant imaging related to the athletic patient with hip pathology.

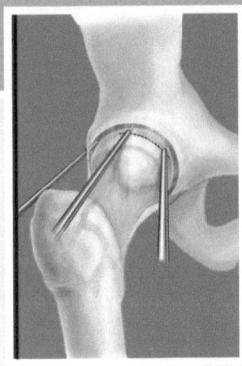

78

Hip Imaging

Brian Busconi, R. Tyler Huish, Erik Mitchell, Sean McMillan

A multitude of structural hip disorders can occur in athletes with hip pain. Although the history and physical examination play a critical role in determining the diagnosis, it is also important to have a systematic approach to help diagnose these disorders radiographically. This chapter describes the key imaging studies used when examining a skeletally mature patient with a pathologic hip, as well as a systematic approach to interpretation of these studies.

RADIOGRAPHIC TECHNIQUES

Traditionally the anteroposterior (AP) view of the pelvis demonstrates the acetabular version, whereas the lateral hip radiograph demonstrates details of the femoral neck and helps identify cam impingement pathology. Several radiographic views are important for proper evaluation of the hip. Among these, the most commonly referenced include the AP view of the pelvis (AP pelvic view),[1,2] a cross-table lateral view,[3] a 45-degree or 90-degree Dunn view,[4,5] a frog-leg lateral view,[6] and a false-profile view.[7] All views are technique dependent, and each demonstrates a different anatomic perspective of the hip joint. Descriptions of each view are provided in the following sections.

Standing Anteroposterior Pelvic View

A proper AP view of the pelvis should be taken with the patient standing. The x-ray tube-to-film distance should be approximately 120 cm, and the x-ray tube should be aimed perpendicular to the film. Both lower extremities should be internally rotated by 15 degrees to account for normal anatomic femoral neck anteversion. The crosshairs of the beam should be centered on a point half the distance between the superior border of the pubic symphysis and on a line drawn connecting the anterior superior iliac spine (ASIS).[8] The coccyx should be centered in line with the pubic symphysis. The radiographic teardrops, iliac wings, and obturator foramina should be symmetrical in appearance.[9] A 1- to 3-cm gap should be seen between the apex of the coccyx and the superior border of the pubic symphysis for proper pelvic inclination.[10] A standing rather than a supine AP radiograph is obtained because acetabular roof obliquity, center edge angle, and minimum joint space width may vary between weight-bearing and supine positions.[11]

The standing AP pelvis radiograph assesses (1) functional leg length inequalities, (2) neck shaft angle (NSA), (3) femoral neck trabecular patterns, (4) lateral center edge angle, (5) acetabular inclination, (6) joint space width, (7) lateralization, (8) head sphericity, (9) acetabular cup depth, and (10) anterior and posterior wall orientation (Figs. 78.1 and 78.2).[9]

Cross-Table Lateral View

For the cross-table lateral view radiograph, the patient should be supine on the x-ray table. The contralateral hip and knee should be flexed out of the way of the x-ray beam (typically >75 degrees). The hip of interest should be rotated internally 15 degrees to help accentuate the anterolateral surface of the femoral head-neck junction (Fig. 78.3). The x-ray beam should be parallel to the table and oriented at a 45-degree angle to the limb of interest, with the crosshairs aimed at the center of the femoral head.[8]

45-Degree or 90-Degree Dunn View

The Dunn view is commonly used for assessment of femoral head sphericity in patients believed to have cam-type femoroacetabular impingement (FAI). It was originally described as a technique to measure femoral neck anteversion in children.

The 90-degree Dunn view assesses the patient with 90-degree hip flexion, whereas the 45-degree Dunn view ("modified Dunn view") assesses the patient with 45 degrees of hip flexion (Fig. 78.4). For both views, the film cassette is placed beneath the pelvis and the tube is centered over the upper border of the pubic symphysis. Each leg should be abducted 15 to 20 degrees from the midline, and the pelvis and tibia should be parallel to the long axis of the body (neutral rotation).[4] The crosshairs of the beam should be directed at a point midway between the ASIS and the pubic symphysis, and the tube-to-film distance should be approximately 40 inches in a line directed perpendicular to the table.[8]

Frog-Leg Lateral View

To obtain the frog-leg lateral view, the patient should be positioned supine on the x-ray table with the hip of interest abducted 45 degrees, the ipsilateral knee flexed 30 to 40 degrees, and the ipsilateral heel resting against the contralateral knee (Fig. 78.5). The cassette is positioned so that the top of the film rests at the ASIS. The crosshairs of the beam are directed at a point midway between the ASIS and the pubic symphysis, with an x-ray tube-to-film distance of approximately 40 inches.[8]

This view permits assessment of another view of medial and lateral joint space width, femoral head sphericity, congruency, head-neck offset, alpha angle, and bone morphology.[9]

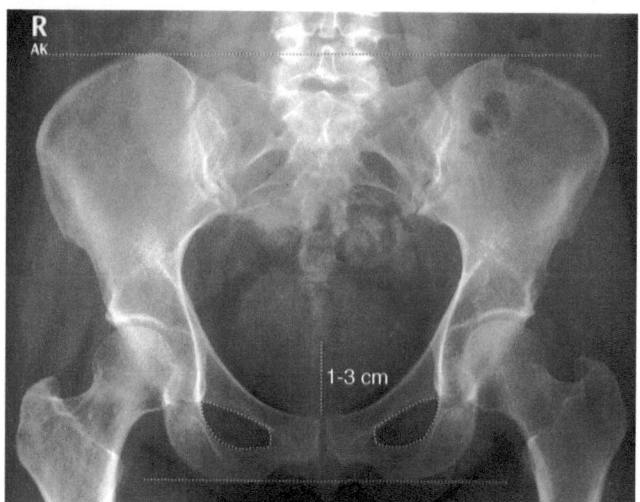

Fig. 78.1 The standing anteroposterior radiograph is obtained with the feet in neutral rotation and shoulder width apart. The coccyx should be centered in line with the pubic symphysis, and the iliac wings, obturator foramina, and radiographic teardrops should be symmetrical in appearance. If pelvic inclination is appropriate, a 1- to 3-cm gap should be seen between the superior border of the pubic symphysis and the tip of the coccyx. (From Martin HD. Clinical examination and imaging of the hip. In: Thomas Byrd JW, Guanche CA, eds. *AANA Advanced Arthroscopy: The Hip*. Philadelphia: Elsevier; 2010.)

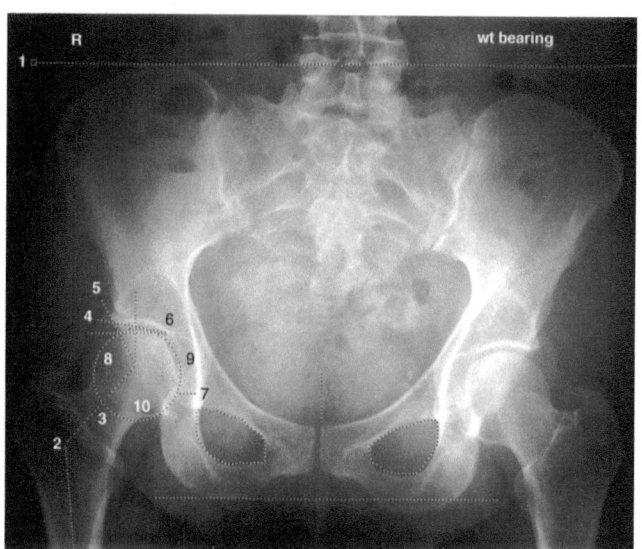

Fig. 78.2 The standing anteroposterior radiograph assesses the following characteristics: *1*, functional leg length inequalities; *2*, neck shaft angle; *3*, femoral neck trabecular patterns; *4*, acetabular inclination; *5*, lateral center edge angles; *6*, joint space width; *7*, lateralization; *8*, head sphericity; *9*, acetabular cup depth; and *10*, anterior and posterior wall orientation. (From Martin HD. Clinical examination and imaging of the hip. In: Thomas Byrd JW, Guanche CA, eds. *AANA Advanced Arthroscopy: The Hip*. Philadelphia: Elsevier; 2010.)

False-Profile View

The false-profile view is helpful for evaluation of the anterior acetabular coverage of the femoral head. The view is obtained with the patient standing, the affected hip against the cassette, and the pelvis rotated 65 degrees from the plane of the cassette (Fig. 78.6). The beam is centered on the femoral head and

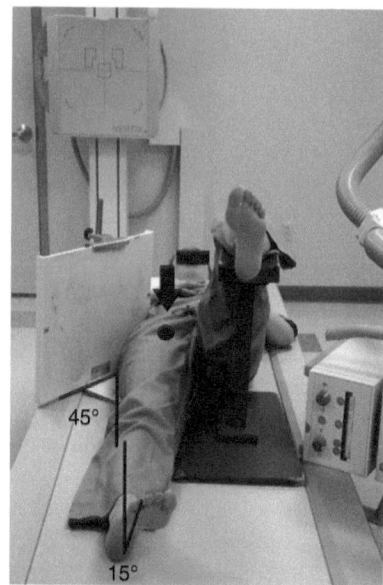

Fig. 78.3 The positioning for a cross-table lateral radiograph with the limb in 15 degrees of internal rotation. The *black arrow* points to the center of the femoral head *(black dot)*, the target for the crosshairs of the x-ray beam. (From Clohisy JC, Carlisle JC, Beaulé PE, et al. A systematic approach to the plain radiographic evaluation of the young adult hip. *J Bone Joint Surg Am*. 2008;90[suppl 4]:47–66.)

perpendicular to the cassette. The tube-to-film distance should be approximately 40 inches.[8]

INTERPRETATION OF PLAIN RADIOGRAPHIC IMAGES

Interpretation of both the AP pelvis and false-profile views generally helps to characterize the acetabular morphology, whereas the other views better describe the proximal femoral anatomy. By combining all views, one should be able to define the following parameters for each patient: leg length inequalities, NSA, femoral neck trabecular patterns, lateral and anterior center edge angles, acetabular inclination, joint space width, lateralization, head sphericity, acetabular cup depth, and anterior and posterior wall orientation.

Functional Leg Lengths

Functional leg lengths may be assessed on an AP pelvis radiograph by constructing a line horizontally off the superior most portion of the iliac crest. Ideally this line should be symmetrical to the contralateral hemipelvis. A discrepancy greater than 2.0 cm corresponds with a functional leg length discrepancy and can have an adverse effect on the kinematic function of the hip.[12]

Neck Shaft Angle

The NSA is defined by the angle formed by the longitudinal axes of the femoral neck and the proximal femoral diaphyseal axis.[13] One line is drawn down the anatomic axis of the femoral neck, and the other is drawn down the anatomic axis of the femur. The angle formed represents the NSA. This angle is normally between 125 and 140 degrees. An angle less than 125 degrees is classified as coxa varus. An angle greater than 140 degrees

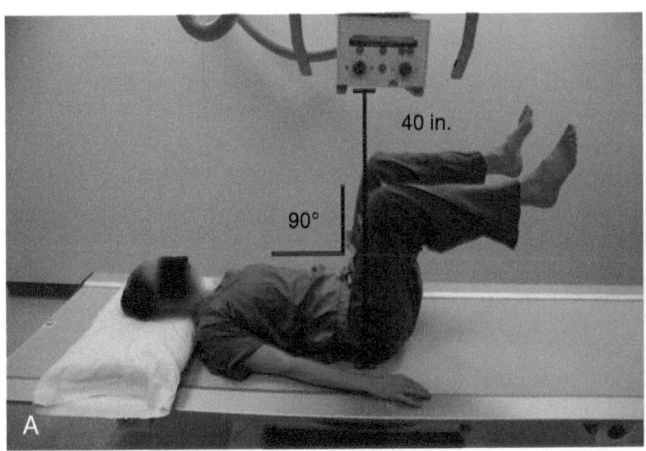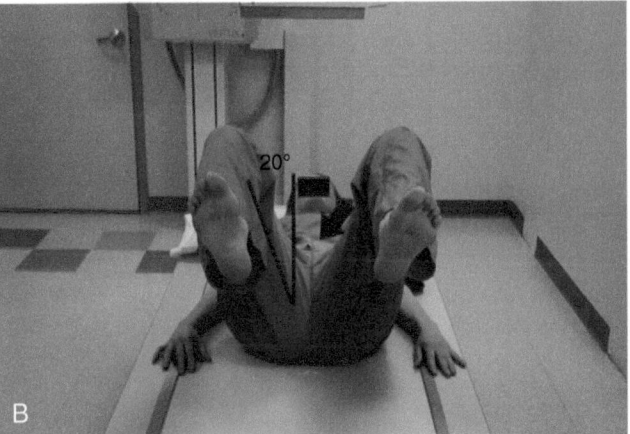

Fig. 78.4 (A and B) Positioning for a 90-degree Dunn view with the hips flexed and abducted 20 degrees. The *black arrow* (B) points to the crosshairs, centered at a point midway between the pubic symphysis and the anterior superior iliac spine. (From Clohisy JC, Carlisle JC, Beaulé PE, et al. A systematic approach to the plain radiographic evaluation of the young adult hip. *J Bone Joint Surg Am.* 2008;90[suppl 4]:47–66.)

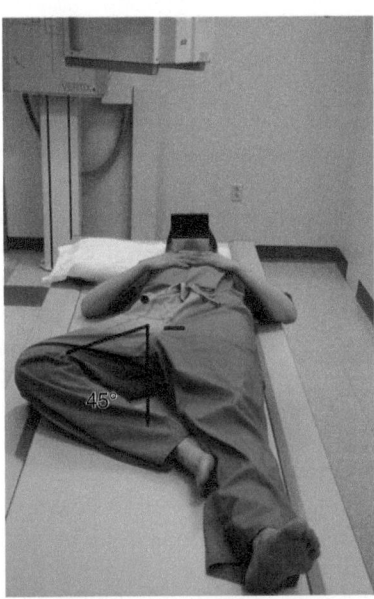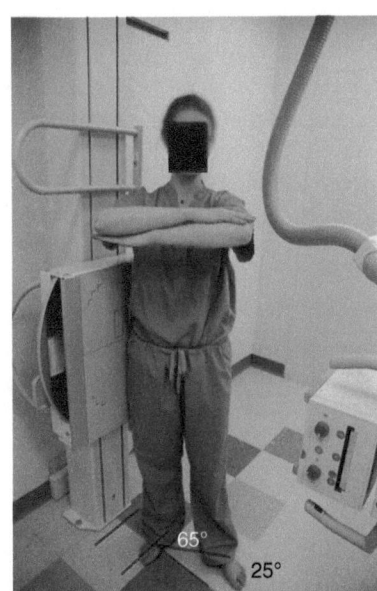

Fig. 78.5 The positioning for a frog-leg lateral view with the hip abducted 45 degrees and the crosshairs centered at a point midway between the anterior superior iliac spine *(black dot)* and the pubic symphysis *(black line)*. (From Clohisy JC, Carlisle JC, Beaulé PE, et al. A systematic approach to the plain radiographic evaluation of the young adult hip. *J Bone Joint Surg Am.* 2008;90[suppl 4]:47–66.)

Fig. 78.6 The false-profile view of the right hip is obtained with the pelvis rotated 65 degrees in relationship to the Bucky wall stand, with the foot on the affected side parallel to the radiographic cassette (shown in the *black lines*). (From Clohisy JC, Carlisle JC, Beaulé PE, et al. A systematic approach to the plain radiographic evaluation of the young adult hip. *J Bone Joint Surg Am.* 2008;90[suppl 4]:47–66.)

corresponds to coxa valgus. The NSA dictates the load transfer from the femur to the acetabulum.[9]

Trabecular Pattern

The trabecular pattern is influenced directly by the NSA and reflects the compressive and tensile forces within the femoral neck. For cases of coxa varus, tensile trabeculae are more prominent. For cases of coxa valgus, compressive trabeculae are more prominent.[14]

Lateral Center Edge Angles

The lateral center edge angles can be used to assess the superolateral coverage of the femoral head by the acetabulum.[15] The

lateral center edge angle is calculated by measuring the angle between two lines of an AP pelvis radiograph: (1) a line through the center of the femoral head, perpendicular to the transverse axis of the pelvis, and (2) a line through the center of the femoral head, passing through the most superolateral point of the sclerotic weight-bearing zone of the acetabulum.[8] Normal values range from 22 to 42 degrees in adults, although values less than 26 degrees may indicate inadequate coverage of the femoral head.[12]

Anterior Center Edge Angles

The anterior center edge angles are created through use of the false-profile view. This angle assesses the anterior coverage of the femoral head. It is calculated by measuring the angle between the vertical line through the center of the femoral head and a line connecting the center of the femoral head and the most anterior point of the acetabular sourcil.[16] Values of less than 20 degrees can be indicative of structural instability.[8]

Acetabular Inclination

Also known as the Tonnis angle, acetabular inclination is best appreciated on the AP view. It is formed by drawing a horizontal line and a tangent from the lowest point of the sclerotic zone of the acetabular roof to the lateral edge of the acetabulum. Acetabular inclination can be classified into three different groups based on degree of inclination[8,17]:

1. Normal = Tonnis angle of 0 to 10 degrees
2. Increased = Tonnis angle greater than 10 degrees, subject to structural instability (increased inclination)
3. Decreased = Tonnis angle less than 0 degrees, subject to pincer-type FAI (decreased inclination)

Joint Space Width

Joint space width is described as the shortest distance between the surface of the femoral head and the acetabulum. Joint space width is examined using the standing AP radiograph because the effects of position influence the joint space observed.[18] Evidence of joint space narrowing can be classified using the Tonnis grade for osteoarthritis.[13]

Hip Center Position

For hip center position, the distance between the medial aspect of the femoral head and the ilioischial line is measured. If the distance is greater than 10 mm, then the hip is classified as lateralized. The distance of 10 mm should serve as a general reference point, and film magnification and patient body habitus must be taken into account and may influence this measurement.

Head Sphericity

Assessment of head sphericity should be performed with both the AP and all lateral views because a patient may have an apparently spherical head on one view and not on the other. The femoral head is classified as spherical if the epiphysis does not extend beyond the margin of a reference circle by more than 2 mm. It is classified as aspherical if it extends beyond this reference circle by more than a 2-mm margin.[19,20] The margin of reference is known as a Mose template (concentric circles).[21]

Acetabular Cup Depth

The acetabular cup depth is a relationship between the floor of the fossa acetabula and the femoral head relative to the ilioischial line. If the floor of the fossa acetabula touches or is medial to the ilioischial line or the posterior wall extends lateral to the center of axis of rotation, the hip is classified as coxa profunda.[9] If the medial aspect of the femoral head is medial to the ilioischial line, the head is classified as protrusion.[15] In addition, the inner acetabular wall thickness, medial wall shape, and inferior cup orientation should be recognized.[9]

Acetabular Version

Normally the acetabulum is anteverted by approximately 20 degrees. Acetabular version can be defined as either being retroverted or anteverted by identifying the presence or absence of a crossover sign on the AP view of the pelvis.[1] The acetabulum is considered to be anteverted if the line of the anterior aspect of the rim does not cross the line of the posterior aspect of the rim before reaching the lateral aspect of the sourcil, and it is considered to be retroverted if the line of the anterior aspect of the rim does cross the line of the posterior aspect of the rim before reaching the lateral edge of the sourcil.[8] It is important to note that true acetabular retroversion is associated with a deficient posterior wall,[1] whereas a hip with a crossover sign but no posterior wall deficiency refers to anterior over-coverage—cranial acetabular retroversion or anterior focal acetabular retroversion.[8,22]

Head-Neck Offset

Head-neck offset can be evaluated from an AP pelvis, frog-leg lateral, Dunn view, or cross-table lateral radiograph, and is classified on the basis of the gross appearance of the relationship between the radius curvatures of the anterior aspect of the femoral head with the posterior aspect of the head-neck junction.[19] If the anterior and posterior concavities of the head-neck junction are symmetrical, then the head-neck offset is classified as symmetrical. If the anterior concavity has a radius of curvature greater than that at the posterior aspect of the head-neck junction, it is classified as having a moderate decrease in head-neck offset.[9] If the anterior aspect has a convexity, as opposed to a concavity, the head-neck junction is classified as having a prominence (cam-type FAI).[19]

Alpha Angle

The alpha angle is classically described for use with axial magnetic resonance imaging (MRI) scans; however, its use may be extrapolated to lateral radiographs. The angle is formed between a line connecting the center of the femoral head to the anatomic axis of the femoral neck and a second line running from the center of the femoral head to the prominence of the head-neck junction where the head sphericity ends. The angle between these two lines is known as the *alpha angle*. Values of more than 42 degrees are suggestive of head-neck offset deformity.[8]

COMPUTED TOMOGRAPHY EVALUATION OF THE HIP

Computed tomography (CT) is an ideal modality for characterization of the osseous structures in the area of the hip. Three-dimensional (3D) multiplanar reformatted CT images have been used to assess hip morphology and potential pathology. CT scans have been shown to be helpful in traumatic injuries and aid in a thorough evaluation of femoral head and neck, as well as acetabulum. It is often used to evaluate loose bodies caused by a hip dislocation after closed reduction. Although the CT images and the 3D reformatted images that they create are an excellent noninvasive method of demonstrating osseous morphology, the disadvantages of this technique are the utilization of ionizing radiation in the young patient population and the fact that CT does not allow direct visualization of intra-articular soft tissue structures.[23] As a result, the workup of a painful hip should progress to MRI evaluation, which is discussed in the following section.

MAGNETIC RESONANCE EVALUATION OF THE HIP

MRI is the best available imaging tool for hip evaluation. It allows for accurate identification of hip pathologies such as avascular necrosis, loose bodies, and labral pathologies. Magnetic resonance arthrography (MRA) of the hip has been used with increasing frequency to identify pathology of the hip such as FAI or developmental dysplasia of the hip (DDH). MRA also provides a minimally invasive method of assessing the extent of cartilage damage of the hip. Knowledge of the extent of damage—particularly of the cartilage—is essential in helping the surgeon to use sound judgment in determining the correct surgical procedure. More recent technologic advances in MRI, including 3Tesla MRI and delayed gadolinium-enhanced MRI of cartilage (dGEMRIC) biochemical imaging of the hip, have provided improved accuracy in diagnosing chondral injury.[54]

Labral Conditions

Labral pathology can often be stratified by patient age. In young patients, pathology is more likely to be caused by a traumatic mechanism, ranging from an acute twist injury of the hip during sport all the way to a hip dislocation. For middle-aged patients (<50 years), the mechanism is often FAI. More senior patients often experience degenerative tears associated with osteoarthritis.

Labral Variant

The acetabular labrum is a fibrocartilaginous rim that deepens the socket of the hip joint, although its role in hip stability remains unclear.[26] It encompasses approximately three-fourths of the circumference of the acetabulum and is absent along its inferior aspect. It is here where the transverse acetabular ligament extends from the anterior to the posterior aspect of this inferior acetabular fossa.

Several clinically insignificant labral variations have been described in asymptomatic patients. The posterior inferior sublabral sulcus should not be misinterpreted as a posterior labral tear on axial images.[27] In addition, an anterosuperior cleft may be seen as a normal variant in the presence of a normal lateral acetabular labrum. On anterior coronal or sagittal images, this cleft is seen as a partial undercutting of the labrum on a single image.[28] A transverse ligament labral junction sulcus is a normal sulcus found between the transverse ligament and the labrum either anteriorly or posteriorly. Finally, the perilabral sulcus resembles the normal space between the acetabular labrum and the capsule on coronal images (Figs. 78.7 and 78.8).

The shape of the labrum also varies among subjects. It most commonly has a triangular appearance (70% to 80%), although it may also be round, flat, irregular, or even absent (1% to 14%) in asymptomatic people.[28] An enlarged or hypertrophic labrum may occur in patients with mild DDH (Fig. 78.9).

An area located above the anterosuperior margin of the acetabular fossa on the coronal view may appear deficient in articular cartilage. It is often stellate or crease-like in appearance (Fig. 78.10). This variant is normal and should not be confused with an osteochondral lesion.

Occasionally contrast material may demonstrate tubelike intraosseous tracking within the posterior margin of the acetabular fossa (Fig. 78.11). This tracking is a common artifact that is posited to represent dilation of the nutrient foramina along the anterior and posterior margin of the acetabular fossa.[29]

Finally, another entity often viewed on the MR arthrogram with unknown clinical significance is the pectinofoveal fold (Fig. 78.12). This fold may resemble a hip plica and can have various appearances and attachment sites.[30]

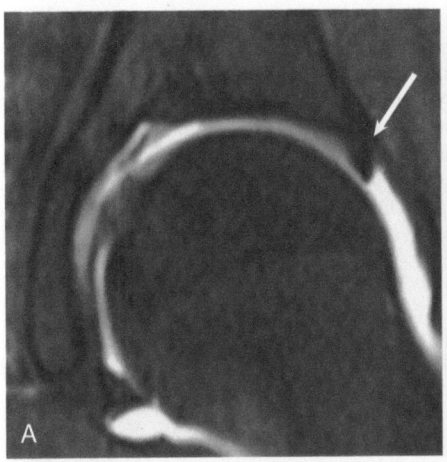 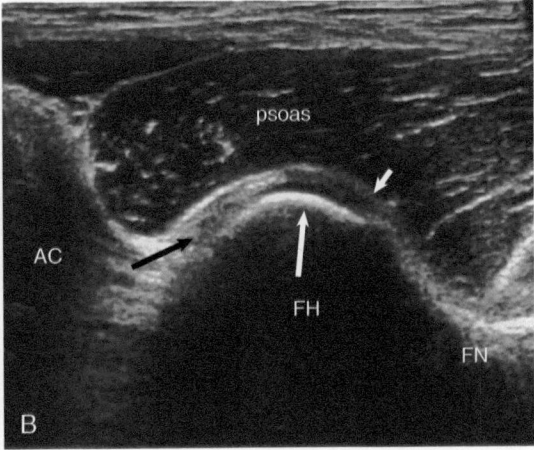

Fig. 78.7 (A) A coronal fat-saturated T1-weighted image shows a triangular-shaped superior labrum *(arrow)*. (B) An oblique sagittal ultrasound image shows the anterior labrum *(black arrow)*, femoral head *(FH)*, cortex *(large white arrow)*, anterior joint capsule *(small white arrow)*, femoral neck *(FN)*, iliopsoas muscle *(psoas)*, and acetabulum *(AC)*. (From Patel K, et al. Radiology. In: Busconi BD, Miller MD, eds. *Clinics in Sports Medicine: Sport-Related Injuries of the Hip*. Philadelphia: Elsevier; 2011.)

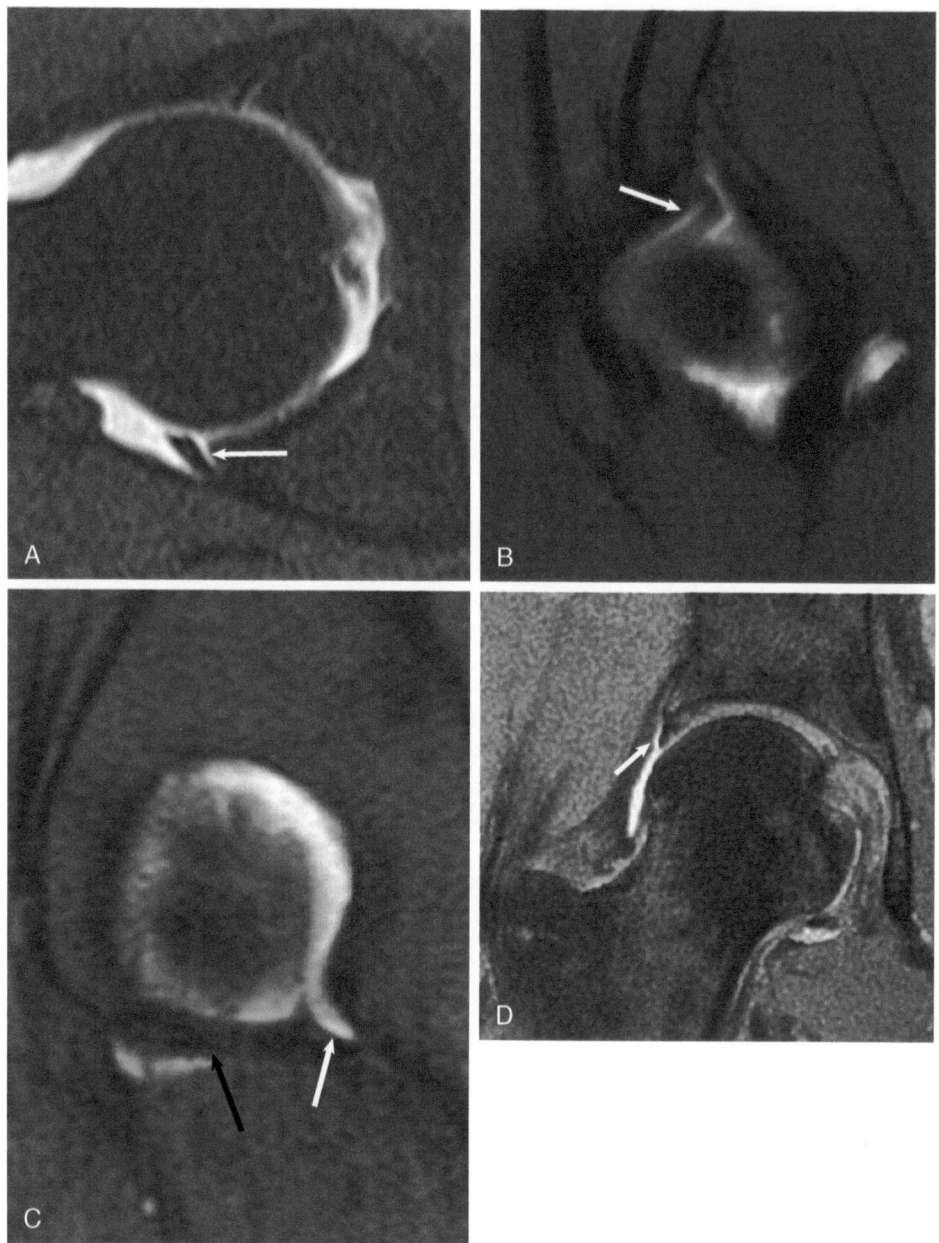

Fig. 78.8 (A) The posterior inferior sublabral sulcus or groove *(arrow)* does not extend completely underneath the labrum. (B) The anterosuperior cleft *(arrow)* partially undercuts the labrum on a single coronal image, which does not extend completely through the labrum. (C) A normal transverse ligament labral sulcus *(white arrow)* and transverse acetabular ligament *(black arrow)*, which extends from the anterior to the posterior aspect at the inferior acetabular fossa. (D) The perilabral sulcus *(arrow)*, a normal space between the capsule, lateral acetabular rim, and labrum. (From Patel K, et al. Radiology. In: Busconi BD, Miller MD, eds. *Clinics in Sports Medicine: Sport-Related Injuries of the Hip*. Philadelphia: Elsevier; 2011.)

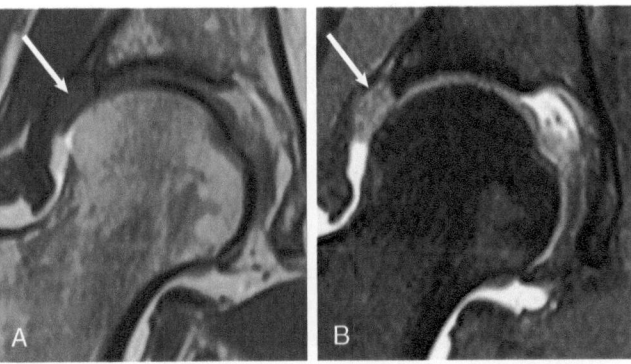

Fig. 78.9 (A) A coronal T1-weighted image shows a large hypertrophic superior labrum *(arrow)*. (B) A coronal proton density fat-saturated image shows increased signal intensity of hypertrophic labrum *(arrow)*, suggesting intralabral degeneration. (From Patel K, et al. Radiology. In: Busconi BD, Miller MD, eds. *Clinics in Sports Medicine: Sport-Related Injuries of the Hip*. Philadelphia: Elsevier; 2011.)

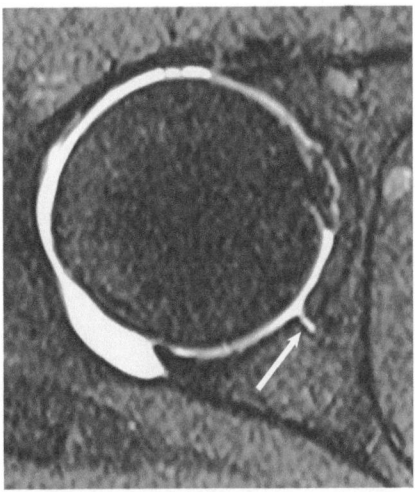

Fig. 78.11 An axial fat-saturated T1-weighted image shows tubular acetabular intraosseous contrast tracking *(arrow)* along the posterior margin of the acetabular fossa, which likely represents dilatation of the nutrient foramina. (From Patel K, et al. Radiology. In: Busconi BD, Miller MD, eds. *Clinics in Sports Medicine: Sport-Related Injuries of the Hip*. Philadelphia: Elsevier; 2011.)

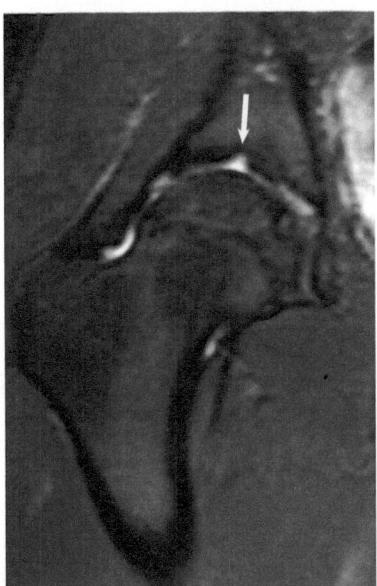

Fig. 78.10 The stellate crease *(arrow)* represents a bare area deficient in hyaline cartilage and not degeneration. (From Patel K, et al. Radiology. In: Busconi BD, Miller MD, eds. *Clinics in Sports Medicine: Sport-Related Injuries of the Hip*. Philadelphia: Elsevier; 2011.)

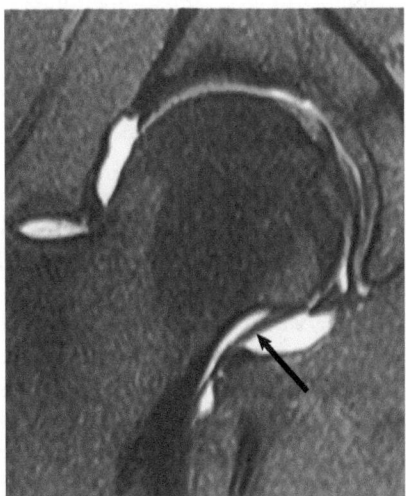

Fig. 78.12 A coronal fat-saturated T1-weighted image shows the pectino-foveal fold *(arrow)* arising from the medial aspect of the femoral neck, extending inferiorly to attach on the proximal femur. The relationship of this fold to internal impingement is not known. (From Patel K, et al. Radiology. In: Busconi BD, Miller MD, eds. *Clinics in Sports Medicine: Sport-Related Injuries of the Hip*. Philadelphia: Elsevier; 2011.)

Labrum Tear

MRA appears to be superior to conventional MRI for the diagnosis of acetabular labral tears.[31] Criteria for tears on an MRA include contrast material extending into the labrum or acetabular/labral interface, blunted appearance, and displacement/detachment from the underlying bone.[32] It is important to distinguish normal variants (described previously) from true pathologic entities. With all this in mind, it is important to consider the sensitivity and specificity of MRA for the diagnosis of labral tears. Studies comparing MRA with surgical findings have shown a range of sensitivity from 60% to 100%[33] and a specificity from 44% to 100%.[34] These studies demonstrate that a negative scan does not fully rule out a labral tear and that hip arthroscopy remains the gold standard.[35]

Most labral tears occur in the anterior superior labrum or posterior superior (which is more common in the younger population) and run along the base of the labrum or along the long axis (longitudinal tear).[28] The diagnosis of a labral tear is established when gadolinium is seen traversing or undercutting the labrum.

Labrum tears are frequently associated with developmental dysplasia, FAI, Legg-Calvé-Perthes disease, slipped capital femoral epiphysis, and degenerative hip disease. Traumatic tears may occur along the inner free margin with a radial flap, the most common type, or they may be unstable and displaced longitudinal tears (Fig. 78.13).[28] Overall the frequency of tears by location is

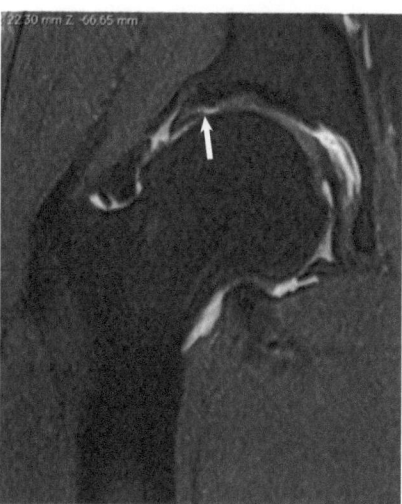

Fig. 78.13 A coronal fat-saturated T1-weighted image shows a longitudinal cleavage tear *(arrow)* of the hypertrophic anterior superior labrum. (From Patel K, et al. Radiology. In: Busconi BD, Miller MD, eds. *Clinics in Sports Medicine: Sport-Related Injuries of the Hip.* Philadelphia: Elsevier; 2011.)

as follows from most to least: anterosuperior, posterosuperior, anteroinferior, and posteroinferior.[36]

Chondral Injury

With the increasing developments in hip joint preservation surgery, accurate diagnosis and assessment of femoral head and acetabular cartilage status is becoming increasingly important. Traditional MRI lacks the ability to analyze the biological status of cartilage degeneration. The technique of dGEMRIC is sensitive to the charge density of cartilage contributed by glycosaminoglycans (GAGs), which are lost early in the process of osteoarthritis.[52,53] Cartilage imaging with dGEMRIC has been established as an accurate and reliable tool for assessment of cartilage status in the knee and hip joint. Fig. 78.14 illustrates an example of a dGEMRIC scan juxtaposed on the radiograph and fat suppressed T1-weighted MRI of a 42-year-old man with bilateral FAI.[51]

Femoroacetabular Impingement

FAI occurs when morphologic abnormalities result in abnormal contact between the femoral neck/head and the acetabular margin, causing tearing of the labrum and avulsion of the underlying cartilage region, continued deterioration, and eventual onset of arthritis.[37] It is a major cause of early osteoarthritis of the hip, especially in young and active patients.[16] Ganz et al.[16] described two distinct types of FAI based on the pattern of chondral and labral lesions observed during surgical dislocation of the hip: cam impingement and pincer impingement.

Cam impingement is more common in young active males. The mechanism is related to an abnormally shaped femoral head (nonspherical) that gets jammed into the acetabulum during normal motion and especially during flexion. Downstream effects of this mechanism include tearing of the labrum from this abnormally prominent femoral neck being jammed into the acetabulum. The labral tear may extend to involve the acetabular cartilage

and cause separation from the subchondral bone. The labral and chondral lesion is often observed in the anterosuperior area of the acetabulum.[38] The following triad of MRA findings has been described in patients with cam-type FAI: an abnormal alpha angle, an anterior/superior acetabular cartilage lesion, and an anterior/superior labral tear (Fig. 78.15).[39]

Pincer-type impingement is the acetabular cause and is more common in middle-aged and older women who engage in athletic activities. Abnormal contact occurs between the acetabular rim and the femoral neck. The femoral head in this situation may be normal, and the abutment is mostly a result of over-coverage of the femoral head in conditions such as coxa profunda[40] or acetabular retroversion.[1] The first structure to fail through this mechanism is usually the acetabular labrum, which often appears small but normally progresses to downstream degenerative changes in the labrum, intrasubstance ganglion formation, or ossification of the rim,[37] which may lead to further deepening of the acetabulum and worsening of the overcoverage. In persons with pincer-type impingement, the cartilage lesions are often seen along the posterior aspect of the acetabulum as a result of the countercoup type of injury because the femur abnormally touches the acetabular rim and the associated labral degeneration, and tears are most commonly found in the anterosuperior labrum (Fig. 78.16).[28]

Most patients (86%) have a combination of both forms of impingement, which is called *mixed pincer and cam impingement*; only a minority (14%) have the pure FAI form of either cam or pincer impingement.[15]

Hip Sprain and Dislocation

Hip sprain is an injury that occurs often in athletes, especially football players, when they fall onto a flexed and adducted hip. Radiographs often appear normal or may show a small posterior acetabular rim fracture. MRI may demonstrate pericapsular soft tissue edema and traumatic disruption of the iliofemoral ligament near its femoral attachment.[28]

Dislocation of the femoral head may occur during episodes of severe trauma. Hip dislocations represent approximately 5% of all dislocations and most frequently occur posteriorly (80% to 85%). This dislocation may result from a dashboard injury in which the flexed knee strikes the dashboard during a head-on automobile collision.[41] Radiographs typically demonstrate posterior acetabular rim fractures (Fig. 78.17). The MRI may show accompanying shear or compression fractures on the anterior and inferior portions of the femoral head (Fig. 78.18).[28]

Stress Injuries

Stress fractures, including both fatigue and insufficiency fractures, are common injuries and may account for as many as 10% of all injuries seen in sports medicine clinics.[42] Wolff[43] describes bone as a dynamic tissue in which normal stresses stimulate remodeling, allowing adaptation to a changing mechanical environment. Bone remodeling is stimulated by fatigue damage, and fatigue damage occurs in the form of microfracture.[44]

Fatigue fractures are more common in runners who have recently started a new and intensive physical activity or who have recently changed their training regimen.[45] The femoral neck

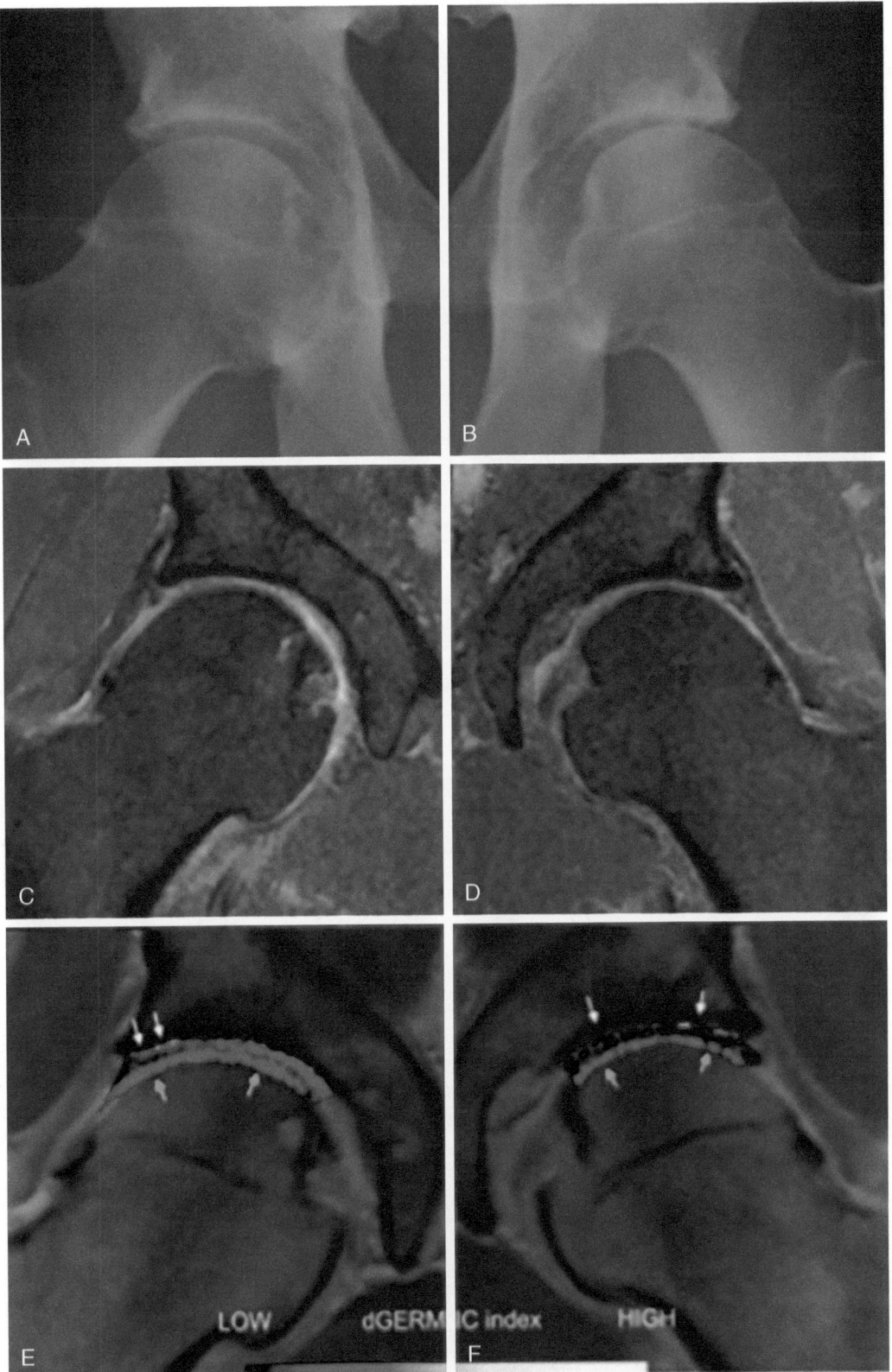

Fig. 78.14 An example of a delayed gadolinium-enhanced magnetic resonance imaging of cartilage (dGEMRIC) scan juxtaposed on the radiograph and fat suppressed T1-weighted MRI of a 42-year-old man with bilateral femoroacetabular impingement. (A and B) Demonstrates mild joint space narrowing on the left, with intact joint spaces on the right. (C and D) T1-weighted fat suppressed images after intravenous contrast injection. Demonstrates mild joint space narrowing in left hip with intact cartilage in right hip. (E and F) The dGEMRIC scan shows entire acetabular cartilage in left hip (F, *white arrows*) to have significant degenerative changes while the femoral head cartilage appeared to be less affected. The dGEMRIC scan of the right hip shows degenerative changes only in the acetabular cartilage at the labral–chondral junction (E, *white arrows*). Again, the femoral head cartilage is less affected (E, *blue arrows*). (From Jessel RH, Zilkens C, Tiderius C, et al. Assessment of osteoarthritis in hips with femoroacetabular impingement using delayed gadolinium enhanced MRI of cartilage. *J Magn Reson Imaging*. 2009;30[5]:1110–1115.)

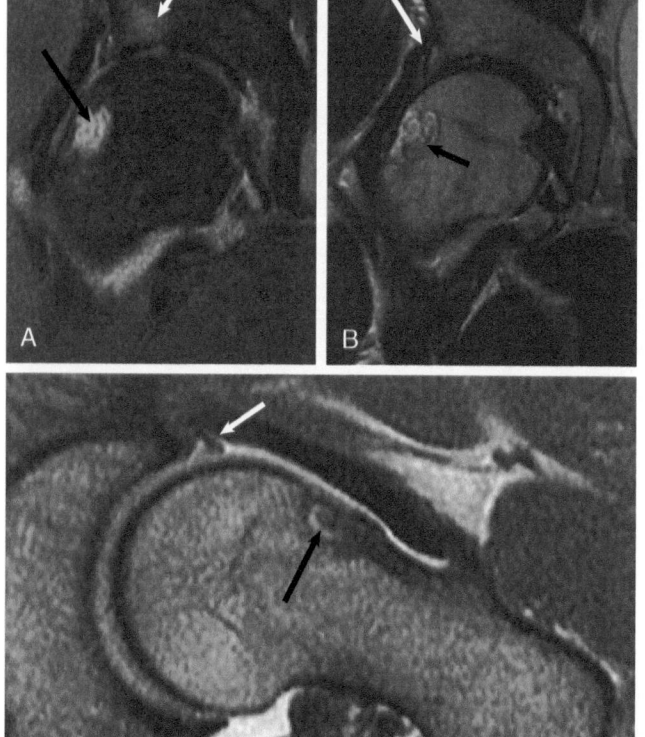

Fig. 78.15 (A) A coronal T1-weighted fat-saturated image shows anterior acetabular cartilage loss, subchondral edema *(white arrow)*, an osseous bump, and fibrocystic changes of the femoral head *(black arrow)*. (B) A coronal T1-weighted image shows absent labrum *(black arrow)* and an acetabular bone spur *(white arrow)*. (C) An oblique axial T1-weighted image shows a displaced anterior labrum tear *(white arrow)*, an osseous bump, and fibrocystic changes of the femoral neck *(black arrow)*. (From Patel K, et al. Radiology. In: Busconi BD, Miller MD, eds. *Clinics in Sports Medicine: Sport-Related Injuries of the Hip.* Philadelphia: Elsevier; 2011.)

is typically involved, and the other most common pelvic bones involved are the pubic rami and sacrum.[46]

Radiographs are the usual initial imaging modality because of their wide availability and low cost; however, they are notoriously insensitive for finding stress fractures and have a sensitivity approaching 0% for stress fractures of the posterior pelvis and sacrum.[46,47] Bone scintigraphy is more sensitive for stress injuries or fracture, and abnormal findings of a bone scan may be seen as early as 6 to 72 hours after the injury occurred.[28] However, these scans are not specific for stress fractures, and increased uptake may be seen with infection, a tumor, or an early stage of avascular necrosis.[28] MRI is reported to be as sensitive as scintigraphy for stress fractures, approaching 100%; however, it is much more specific as well, given its higher level of soft tissue and bone marrow contrast (Figs. 78.19–78.21).[46]

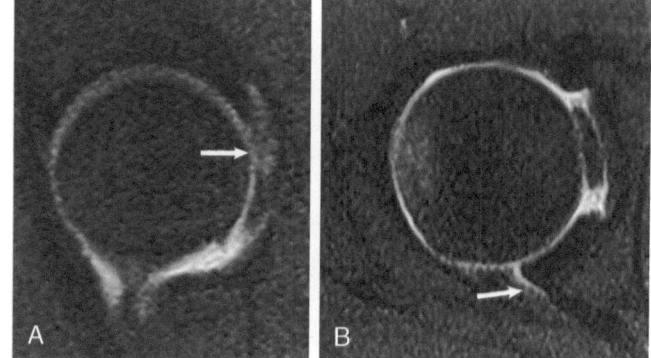

Fig. 78.16 Sagittal (A) and axial (B) T1-weighted fat-saturated images show a posterior labrum tear *(arrows)*. (From Patel K, et al. Radiology. In: Busconi BD, Miller MD, eds. *Clinics in Sports Medicine: Sport-Related Injuries of the Hip.* Philadelphia: Elsevier; 2011.)

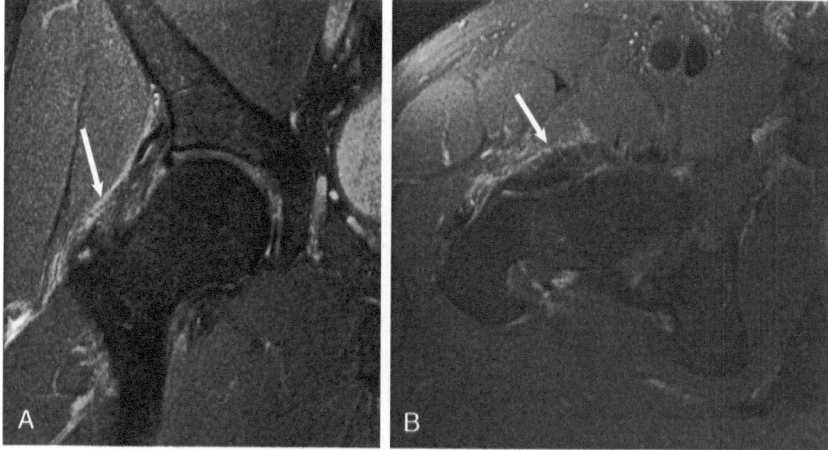

Fig. 78.17 Proton density, fat-saturated T1-weighted coronal (A) and axial (B) images show pericapsular edema and a partial-thickness iliofemoral ligament tear *(arrows)* after a right hip sprain. (From Patel K, et al. Radiology. In: Busconi BD, Miller MD, eds. *Clinics in Sports Medicine: Sport-Related Injuries of the Hip.* Philadelphia: Elsevier; 2011.)

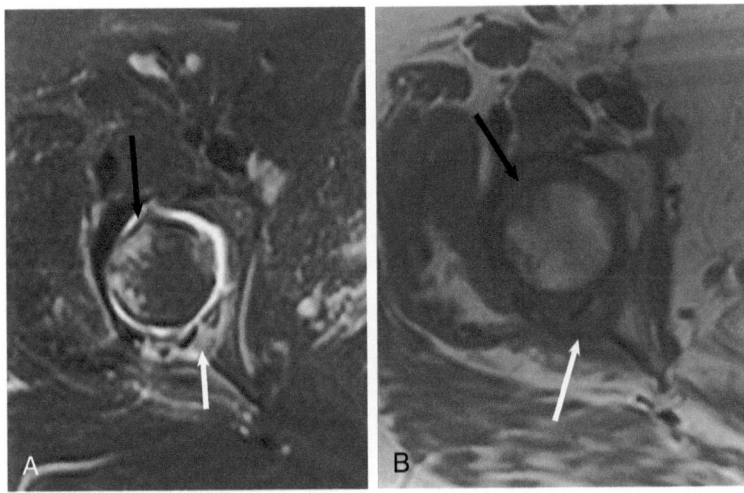

Fig. 78.18 An axial short-tau inversion recovery image (A) and an axial T1-weighted image (B) show a posterior acetabular rim fracture *(white arrows)* and compression injury of anterior femoral head *(black arrows)*. (From Patel K, et al. Radiology. In: Busconi BD, Miller MD, eds. *Clinics in Sports Medicine: Sport-Related Injuries of the Hip.* Philadelphia: Elsevier; 2011.)

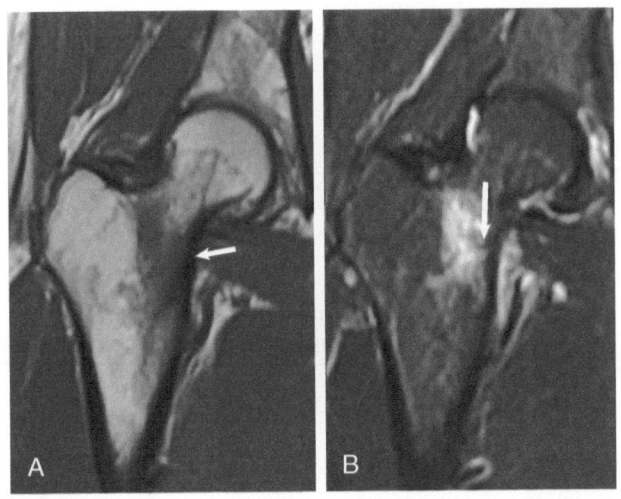

Fig. 78.19 (A) A coronal T1-weighted image shows medial femoral neck cortical thickening and edema *(arrow)*. (B) A coronal short-tau inversion recovery–weighted image shows an incomplete fracture line *(arrow)*. (From Patel K, et al. Radiology. In: Busconi BD, Miller MD, eds. *Clinics in Sports Medicine: Sport-Related Injuries of the Hip.* Philadelphia: Elsevier; 2011.)

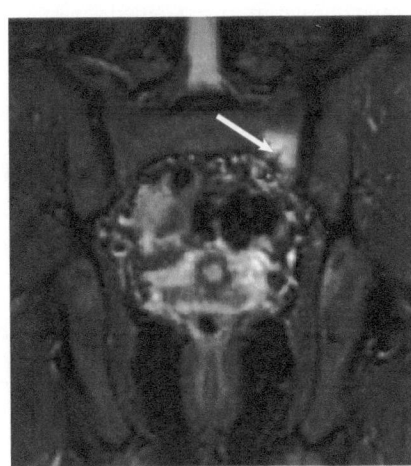

Fig. 78.21 A coronal short-tau inversion recovery–weighted image shows an incomplete stress fracture of the left sacral ala *(arrow)*. (From Patel K, et al. Radiology. In: Busconi BD, Miller MD, eds. *Clinics in Sports Medicine: Sport-Related Injuries of the Hip.* Philadelphia: Elsevier; 2011.)

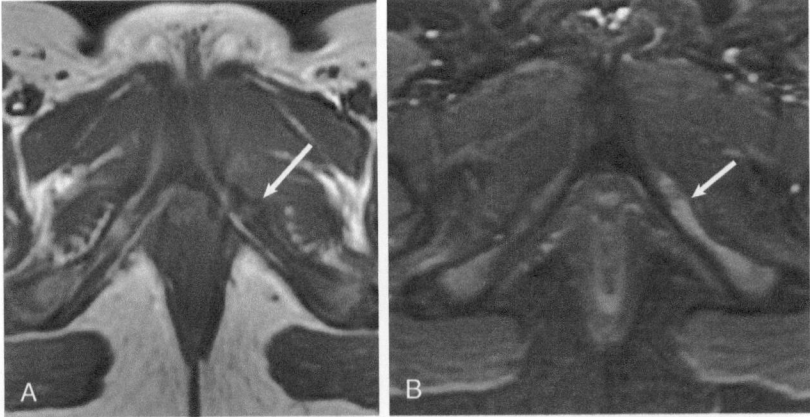

Fig. 78.20 A T1-weighted image (A) and short-tau inversion recovery–weighted image (B) show a left inferior pubic ramus stress fracture *(white arrows)*. (From Patel K, et al. Radiology. In: Busconi BD, Miller MD, eds. *Clinics in Sports Medicine: Sport-Related Injuries of the Hip.* Philadelphia: Elsevier; 2011.)

Ultrasound

Ultrasonography historically has had a limited role in the assessment of hip pathology due to the deep location of the hip joint and the use of more conventional radiologic studies.[48] However, as ultrasound units have become more readily available in the office setting, and as our knowledge of hip pathology increases, the role of hip ultrasonography has expanded. While MR is still considered the preferred modality for radiographic evaluation of intra-articular hip pathology, periarticular soft tissue, and bone marrow lesions, US can be particularly helpful in patients with prior hip replacements, as well as in other circumstances where MR might be contraindicated.[48]

Ultrasonography can be used for pathologic assessment as well as diagnostic and therapeutic interventional procedures surrounding the hip joint. Muscle injuries, tendinopathies, bursal pathologies, effusions, and cortical surface lesions can all be identified with the use of ultrasound.[48] Dynamic ultrasonography can also be performed to aid in the diagnosis of both internal and external snapping hip syndrome.[49] Guided aspirations and injections can also be help aid in the diagnosis as well as therapeutic intervention of intra-articular as well as extra-articular pathologies. This can help the clinician determine the best treatment options and also help better predict the patient's prognosis.[50]

For a complete list of references, go to ExpertConsult.com.

SELECTED READINGS

Citation:

Clohisy JC, et al. A systematic approach to the plain radiographic evaluation of the young adult hip. *J Bone Joint Surg Am.* 2008;90A(suppl 4):47–66.

Level of Evidence:

V

Summary:

This article describes a systematic algorithm for evaluating the young patient with hip pain. The techniques for obtaining proper radiographs are also discussed, and many supporting illustrations are provided.

Citation:

Martin HD. Clinical examination and imaging of the hip. In: Byrd TJ, ed. *AANA Advanced Arthroscopy: The Hip.* Philadelphia: Elsevier; 2010.

Level of Evidence:

V

Summary:

This chapter presents a broad overview of physical examination techniques for younger patients with hip pain.

Citation:

Parvizi J, et al. Femoroacetabular impingement. *J Am Acad Ortho Surg.* 2007;15(9):561–570.

Level of Evidence:

V

Summary:

This article describes the mechanism of femoroacetabular impingement (FAI) and helps the reader properly diagnose it through radiographic, clinical, and physical examination techniques. It also presents a good overview of surgical versus nonsurgical treatments for FAI.

Citation:

Patel K, et al. Radiology. In: Miller M, ed. *Clinics in Sports Medicine: Sport-Related Injuries of the Hip.* Philadelphia: Elsevier; 2011.

Level of Evidence:

V

Summary:

This chapter delves into magnetic resonance imaging analysis of the patient with hip pain. It includes several illustrations depicting common pathologic conditions within the hip.

Citation:

Smith T, et al. The diagnostic accuracy of acetabular labral tears using magnetic resonance imaging and magnetic resonance arthrography: a meta-analysis. *Eur Radiol.* 2011;21(4):863–874.

Level of Evidence:

IV

Summary:

This article compares the diagnosis of labral tears through MRI and MRA imaging and concludes that MRA appears to be superior to conventional MRI. It also describes the five etiologic causes of labral tears and physical examination techniques that can help the practitioner better diagnose these tears.

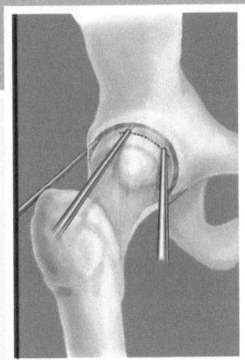

Hip Arthroscopy

Joshua D. Harris

The technique of hip arthroscopy has undergone a period of rapid evolution and growth. In its infancy, hip arthroscopy was mostly for diagnostic and limited therapeutic utility. It was "a technique looking for indications." Now, improved understanding of intra- and extra-articular hip disease has led to increased investigation of both non- and prearthritic hip disorders. The unique technical challenges to arthroscopic access imposed by the hip joint, different from that of the knee and shoulder, include its deep location surrounded by multiple musculotendinous and neurovascular structures, "ball and socket" type joint congruity requiring traction, and necessity of variable degrees of capsular incision for visualization and instrumentation. Improved equipment and technique has now permitted safer and easier arthroscopic and endoscopic access to virtually any musculoskeletal structure around the hip. Thus hip arthroscopy is now able to effectively diagnose and treat most hip pathology. This largely accounts for the proliferation in performance of hip arthroscopy in the United States and across the world.[1]

INDICATIONS

Indications for hip arthroscopy are based on a thorough history, physical examination, and imaging analysis. The Warwick Agreement defined femoroacetabular impingement (FAI) syndrome as a motion-related clinical disorder based on the triad of symptoms (history), clinical signs (physical examination), and imaging findings (plain radiographs and advanced imaging).[2] Symptoms typically are motion- or position-related hip and/or groin pain. Pain may also be experienced in the back, buttock, or thigh. Mechanical symptoms such as catching, clicking, locking, stiffness, loss of motion, or giving way may also be perceived. A variety of hip impingement tests may be used to elicit the patient's typical "chief complaint" pain. The flexion-adduction-internal rotation (FADIR) is the most common test for impingement. Restricted hip flexion and internal and/or external rotation are frequently observed. Orthogonal views of the pelvis, including an anteroposterior (AP) and one of many lateral views (e.g., Dunn, frog-leg, cross-table, false profile), are used to identify cam and/or pincer morphology. Confirmation of all three components of the triad during the medical decision-making component of the treatment algorithm for patients with hip pain, in most cases, warrants a trial of nonsurgical measures (rest, activity modification, education, oral nonnarcotic medications, physical therapy, selective intra-articular injections).[3]

In the event of failure of nonsurgical treatment, patient dissatisfaction with their current hip condition may indicate hip arthroscopy.

The primary indications for hip arthroscopy include FAI syndrome due to either cam and/or pincer morphology, labral injury, femoral head and/or acetabular articular cartilage injury, intra-articular loose bodies (e.g., synovial chondromatosis, localized focal pigmented villonodular synovitis), septic arthritis, and certain types of "extra-articular" impingement (e.g., anterior inferior iliac spine [AIIS] subspine impingement, iliopsoas impingement). Patient selection is critical in recognition of one or more of these indications that frequently coexist. Patient selection is even more critical in recognition of any contraindications that could portend an increased risk of failure, complications, reoperations, or conversion to total hip arthroscopy.

Contraindications

Contraindications to hip arthroscopy include advanced hip osteoarthritis, more than mild or borderline dysplasia (without concomitant simultaneous or staged periacetabular osteotomy), and patients with asymptomatic cam or pincer morphology. Patients with advanced joint space narrowing along the weight bearing sourcil (<2 mm) are at a significantly higher risk of failure of arthroscopy.[4,5] Other radiographic signs of advanced arthrosis include subchondral acetabular cyst formation,[6] osteophytes, subchondral sclerosis, and Tönnis 2 or 3 classification. These patients are better treated with either continued nonsurgical measures or arthroplasty. Patients with clinical and radiographic features of significant acetabular dysplasia include those with a lateral center edge angle (and anterior center edge angle) of less than 18 to 20 degrees, a Tönnis angle of greater than 15 degrees (acetabular index), a femoral head extrusion index greater than 25%, a broken Shenton's line, femoral head migration, percent medialization of the iliofemoral line,[7] and an elevated FEAR (Femoro-Epiphyseal Acetabular Roof) Index.[8] Although technically more challenging, patients with protrusio acetabuli (femoral head medial border is medial to the ilioischial line) pincer morphology are not contraindicated and may be successfully managed arthroscopically.[9] Given the high prevalence of cam (37%; 55% in athletes and 23% in nonathletes) and pincer (67%) morphology in asymptomatic individuals, surgeons must always remember to "treat the patient, not the x-ray."[10] There is no role for prophylactic arthroscopic hip preservation surgery in asymptomatic individuals.[11]

Learning Curve

A steep learning curve is associated with performance of hip arthroscopy. Surgeons must be aware of this learning curve and do as much as possible to reduce the risk of adverse events during the curve. This includes both observation and hands-on training with an experienced hip arthroscopist(s). Attendance at society, institutional, and/or industry cadaveric laboratory workshops are highly valuable in learning the techniques, equipment, and instrumentation. Patient-reported outcome scores,[12,13] reoperation rate,[12] arthroplasty conversion rate,[12] operative time,[13–15] complication rates,[13,14,16–18] failure rates,[15] and patient satisfaction[12,13] have all been shown to significantly improve with greater surgeon experience. Additionally, the rate of iatrogenic articular cartilage and labral injury during portal placement (the most common hip arthroscopy complication at the most likely time) has been shown to be reduced with greater surgeon experience.[13–16]

OPERATING ROOM SET-UP AND POSITIONING

Prior to entering the operating room theatre, the patient's correct site (hip) and side (right vs. left) are marked by the surgeon, and confirmed with the preoperative medical records and written informed consent form. A multimodal pain management protocol is begun in the preoperative holding area in order to reduce the need for postoperative narcotic use. The author's preferred "cocktail" includes oral acetaminophen 500 mg, celecoxib 400 mg, pregabalin 75 mg, famotidine 20 mg, and promethazine 12.5 mg; and transdermal postauricular scopolamine 1 mg patch. Upon entry into the operating room, intravenous antibiotic (cefazolin—first generation cephalosporin [1 g if <75 kg body weight; 2 g if 75 kg or greater] or clindamycin [600 mg] if allergic to penicillin or cephalosporin) is commenced within 30 minutes of anticipated skin incision.

Equipment and Instrumentation

Dedicated hip arthroscopy instrument sets are necessary to effectively perform hip arthroscopy. A variety of different arthroscopy towers exist to hold the camera system, camera light source, arthroscopy image/video data source and printer, arthroscopy fluid pump, arthroscopy suction canister and storage source, radiofrequency system, and shaver/burr power system (Fig. 79.1). The video monitor may be on the tower or on a separate ceiling or wall fixture, to visualize the arthroscopy video on one screen and fluoroscopy images on a separate screen. The arthroscopic fluid pump should be at a low pressure (40 to 50 mm Hg) with high flow in order to reduce the risk of fluid extravasation outside the hip joint, potentially into the pelvis, abdomen, retroperitoneum, or chest.[19,20] The instruments necessary to perform hip arthroscopy may be placed on the scrub technician's back table and at least one Mayo stand (Figs. 79.1 and 79.2A to C). The instruments used for hip arthroscopy, as opposed to knee or shoulder arthroscopy, must be longer in some circumstances. The deep location, thick muscular envelope, and sometimes adipose layer may make standard joint arthroscopy instruments too short to successfully reach the joint. Additionally, the congruent spherical nature of the joint makes curved and flexible instrumentation necessary.

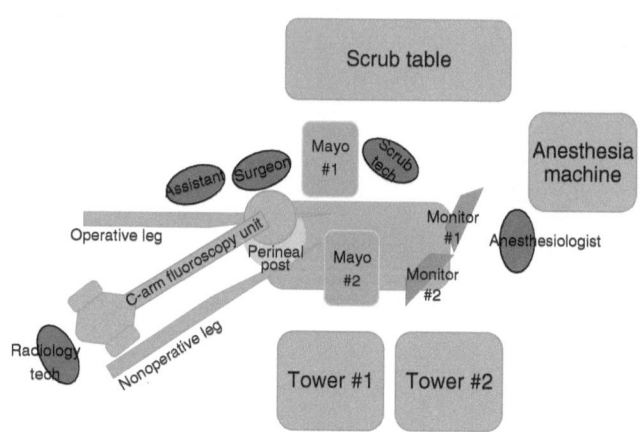

Fig. 79.1 Diagram illustrating room set-up for right-side hip arthroscopy. Note the eccentric positioning of the perineal post to increase the lateral vector upon distraction.

Supine Position

A variety of operating room tables may be used to successfully perform hip arthroscopy. These include fracture tables, joint replacement tables, and hip arthroscopy-specific traction tables. Although the author prefers the supine position, lateral decubitus is also a viable option. The author prefers the Advanced Supine Hip Positioning System with two Universal Hip Distractors and two Active Heel Traction Boots (Smith & Nephew, Andover, MA) and a well-padded perineal post (~25 cm diameter) between the legs. The table has a perineal post holder that is eccentrically located toward the operative side to increase the lateral vector during distraction and reduce pressure on the perineum. Each soft boot is securely placed and Velcro strapped in the Active Heel Traction Boot so that no creases, rivets, grooves, or bulges would cause excessive pressure on each foot or ankle. A self-adherent elastic bandage is placed over the soft boot to increase the surface friction once placed in the Active Heel Traction Boot to reduce the risk of the foot pulling out of the Active Heel Traction Boot.

Examination under anesthesia is performed. This includes measurement of bilateral hip flexion, abduction, and internal and external rotation at 90 degrees hip flexion. Assessment of external rotation recoil, dial testing (maximal limb internal rotation and permissive passive external rotation assessment for endpoint and greater than 45 degrees of external rotation), and traction testing (with or without fluoroscopic assistance) all evaluate capsular (especially the iliofemoral ligament) integrity. Fluoroscopic examination under anesthesia can be helpful to accurately identify trochanteric-pelvic and ischiofemoral impingement. Femoral head translation, in addition to rotation, may also be fluoroscopically observed if the head-neck junction levers on the acetabular fulcrum (microinstability) with or without the presence of a vacuum sign.[21–23]

Traction

General anesthesia with complete muscle relaxation paralysis reduces the force necessary to obtain sufficient distraction (<50 to 75 pounds) for atraumatic entry into the hip joint.[24,25] In the lateral position, for every pound increase in distraction

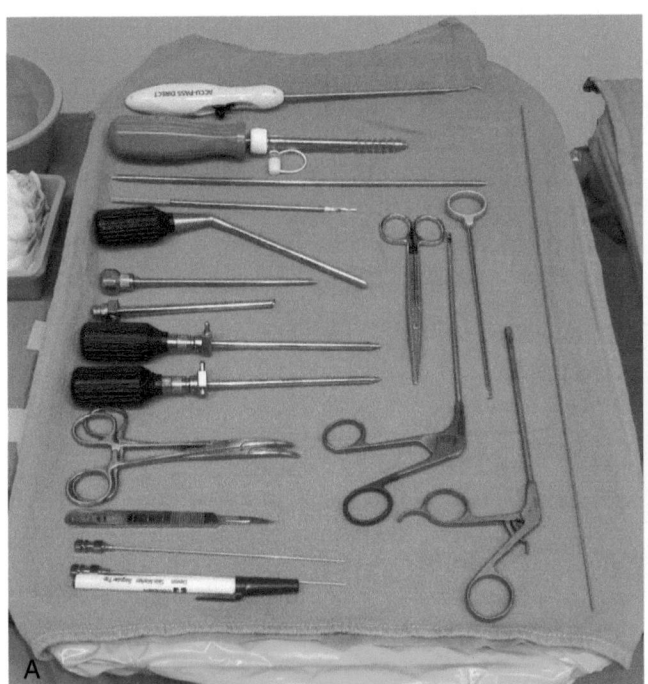
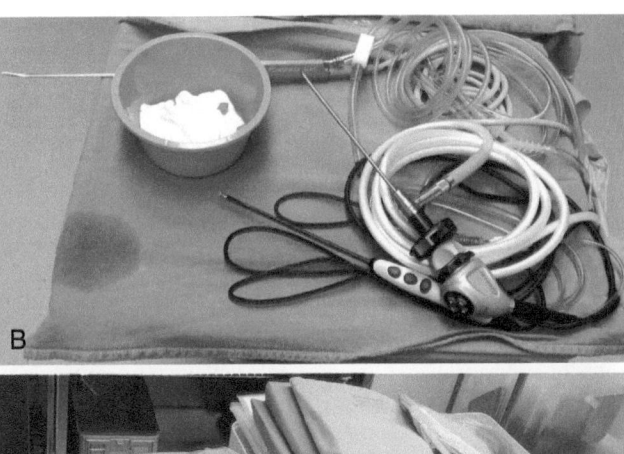
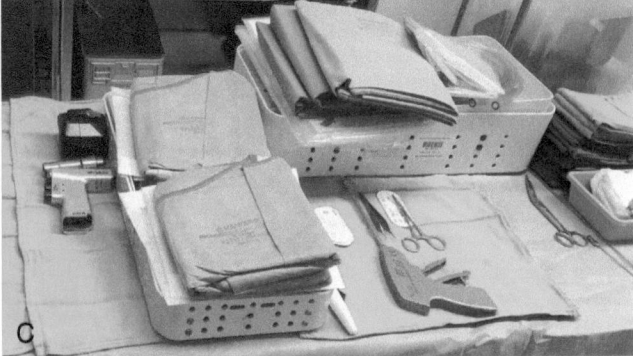

Fig. 79.2 (A) Mayo stand near the surgeon (Mayo #1 in Fig. 79.1) contains (from top to bottom on left side of stand) suture passing device (Accu-Pass Direct, Smith & Nephew, Andover, MA), 8.5 mm clear cannula, switching stick, beaver blade, slotted cannula, 5.0 mm obturator, 5.0 mm cannula, 5.0 mm cannulated obturator in cannula *(blue)*, 4.5 mm cannulated obturator in cannula *(green)*, two hemostats, #11 blade scalpel, two 17-gauge spinal needles, marker; and on right side of stand (from left to right) suture-cutting scissors, looped suture retriever, knot-pusher, arthroscopic suture cutter, and nitinol wire. (B) Mayo stand across table from surgeon (Mayo #2 in Fig. 79.1) contains (clockwise, from top) arthroscopic 4.5 mm curved shaver, arthroscopic fluid tubing, 70-degree arthroscope, radiofrequency wand, and moist lap sponge in fluid bowl. (C) Scrub technician back table contains sterile gowns and glove, two dedicated hip arthroscopy instrument sets, battery power pack for drilling (for suture anchor placement), "shower curtain" sterile adhesive hip arthroscopy drape, nonabsorbable 3-0 suture (for portal incision closure), and sterile towels.

force applied, there is a 4% increase in odds of an adverse nerve event.[25] While traction time has not been shown to influence the risk of a postoperative nerve palsy, the duration should be under 2 hours to reduce the risk of a compressive, ischemic "tourniquet-like" effect on the nerves in the perineum.[25,26] In order to reduce the risk of perineal injury secondary to traction, some authors have performed successful "postless" hip arthroscopy without a perineum or groin complication.[27,28] The most common complication of hip arthroscopy is iatrogenic articular cartilage and/or labral injury (0.4% to 3.8% and 0.7% to 18%, respectively), occurring primarily during portal placement.[29,30] Thus patient positioning and traction must optimize the ability to successfully place portals with a reduced, and potentially eliminated, risk of iatrogenic chondrolabral injury.[31–33]

Once the patient's feet are securely placed in the traction boots and all bony and soft tissue prominences padded (especially the perineum), distraction commences. A surgical pause "time-out" is performed prior to the initiation of distraction. The nonoperative limb is first placed in approximately 5 degrees of flexion, 45 to 60 degrees of abduction, and neutral rotation. A gentle axial longitudinal distractive pull is applied to provide a counter-traction lateral force to the operative side. The operative limb is placed in approximately 30 degrees abduction and 30

degrees of flexion in neutral rotation and a gentle axial longitudinal distractive pull applied. Next, in a slow, gentle application of zig-zagging hip extension-adduction, extension-adduction, extension-adduction moments, the operative limb is positioned in approximately 5 degrees flexion, 5 degrees adduction, and neutral rotation. The limb is then internally rotated to the degree of femoral anteversion (measured from preoperative imaging, either computed tomography [CT] scan or 3D biplanar fluoroscopy EOS) (if 20 degrees anteversion, then 20 degrees internal rotation). A minimum of 10 mm of distraction is necessary to safely proceed. The C-arm fluoroscopic unit is placed between the legs, roughly parallel with the nonoperative limb, and does not interfere with the surgeon or limb manipulation before or after traction application.

Preparation and Draping

Sterile preparation and draping of the limb with an Isolation Drape with Incise Film and Pouch (3M Health Care, St. Paul, MA) allows for quick and easy application of a surgical drape that protects the sterile field and covers the patient's body (Fig. 79.3). Using a sterile marker, a straight line is drawn connecting the anterior superior iliac spine and the patella. No portal should be established at or medial to this line. If posterior portals (posterolateral [PL] or accessory/modified PL) are to be established, the draping must ensure to not block out portal placement posteriorly.

PROCEDURE
Surface Landmarks

Tactile sensation of surface landmarks is used to assist in portal placement during hip arthroscopy. Given the deep constrained nature of the joint, even small errors in portal location can significantly limit access to intra- and extra-articular structures. The anterior superior iliac spine, greater trochanter (tip, anterior

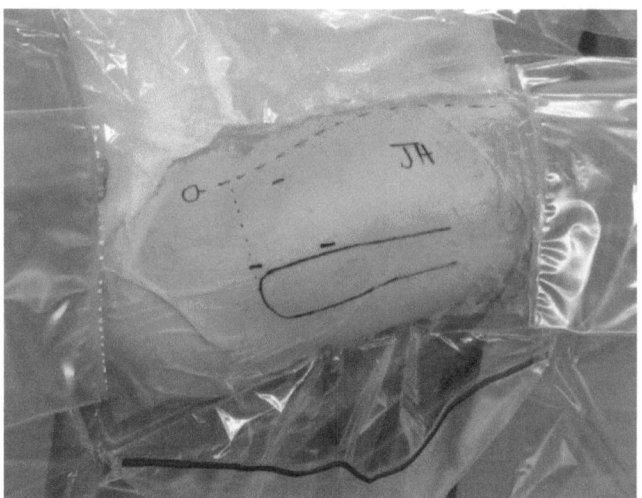

Fig. 79.3 Right hip arthroscopy with sterile preparation and draping. The anterior superior iliac spine is marked with a circle and connected (via *dotted line*) to the patella. No portal or incision should proceed medial to this line. The proximal femur is marked laterally. These surface landmarks are used to estimate the positions of the portals intended to be used.

and posterior margins), and patella are the primary landmarks used. These are reliably and accurately located in most patients' body habiti.[34] Traction and adduction may assist in further defining the anterior abductor margin. A 17-gauge spinal needle may be used to estimate the approximate starting point and trajectory of the initial portal placed, the anterolateral (AL) portal. Fluoroscopy is used to ensure correct placement. Over time, both fluoroscopy time and absorbed radiation dose significantly decrease over the first 100 cases of a surgeon's learning curve.[35]

Arthroscopic Portals
Anterolateral

The AL portal is the initial portal established. The closest structure to the portal is the superior gluteal nerve. However, the nerve is approximately 4.4 cm proximal to the portal.[36] A 17-gauge spinal needle is aimed to enter the joint at the 12:30 position on the acetabular clockface (in a right hip). This should roughly parallel the line of the sourcil. The sharp long end of the bevel should be away from the femoral head to avoid iatrogenic articular cartilage damage (Fig. 79.4A). Fluoroscopy is used to assist in AL portal placement. Seldinger technique over a nitinol guidewire is utilized to place a 4.5-mm cannula and introduce the 70-degree arthroscope. Alternatively, some authors recommend initial spinal needle entry into the joint with the bevel facing superiorly to reduce the risk of initial labral injury.[31,32] An air arthrogram is produced. The capsulolabral interval can sometimes be visualized on the arthrogram (see Fig. 79.4B). Then, the stylet is reinserted and the needle withdrawn to just outside the capsule. Joint venting increases the intra-articular pressure and allows relaxation of the labrum due to the loss of negative intra-articular pressure. The needle may then be reinserted with the bevel facing superiorly to avoid the labrum. As soon as the "pop" is felt, the bevel is rotated 180 degrees so that the bevel is facing inferiorly to reduce risk of iatrogenic femoral head articular cartilage injury. The stylet is removed, a nitinol wire inserted, and the needle removed, followed by dilation, cannulation, and arthroscope

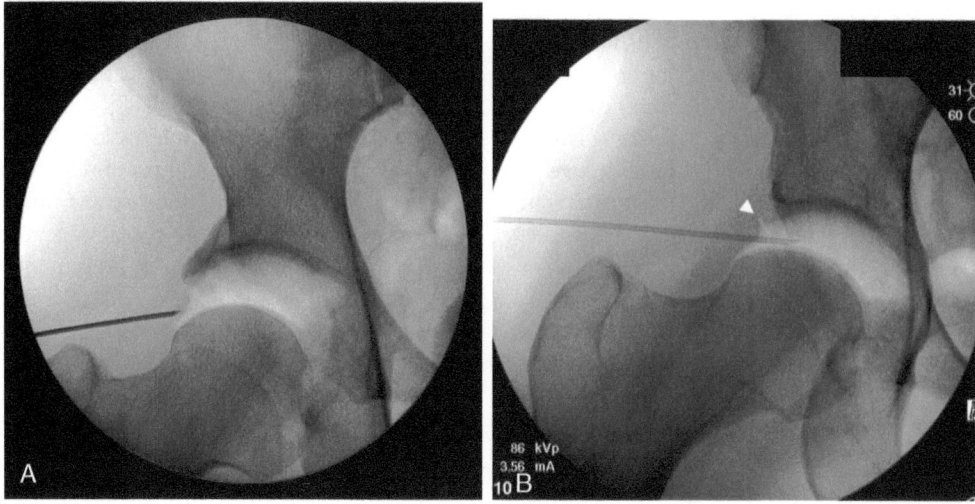

Fig. 79.4 (A) Right hip anteroposterior fluoroscopy image illustrating 17-gauge spinal needle with bevel sharp end away from the femoral head. (B) Right hip anteroposterior fluoroscopy image illustrating an air arthrogram with demarcation of the capsulolabral interval *(white arrowhead)*.

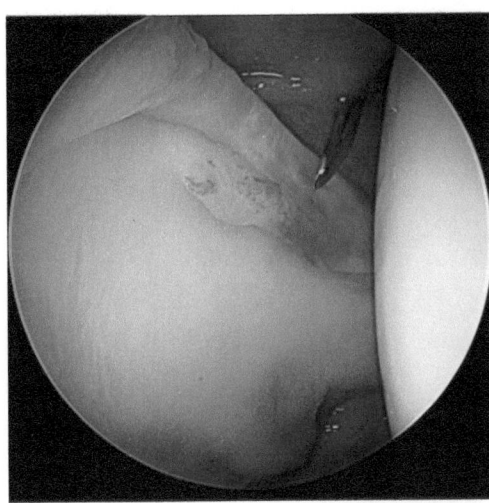

Fig. 79.5 Right hip arthroscopy, 70-degree arthroscope, viewing from anterolateral portal. Placement of spinal needle at approximately 3:00 on clockface for creation of modified mid-anterior portal.

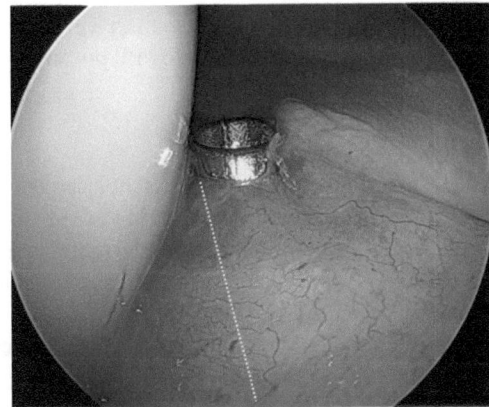

Fig. 79.6 Right hip arthroscopy, 70-degree arthroscope, viewing from modified mid-anterior portal. A 5.0 mm cannula is in the anterolateral portal. Given the known size of the cannula, the interportal capsulotomy can be placed a minimum of 5 to 6 mm from the labrum at the level of the anterolateral portal and move further away from the labrum (while carefully avoiding the femoral head) as it approaches the modified mid-anterior portal. Moving further away from the labrum ensures a sufficient cuff of tissue for interportal capsulotomy repair at the case conclusion.

insertion. This method has been shown to reduce the risk of iatrogenic chondrolabral injury to less than 1%.[31]

Modified Mid-Anterior

A modification of the original description of the anterior portal is used. The original anterior portal path is close to the lateral femoral cutaneous nerve (LFCN), within 3 mm.[36] Additionally, the portal is within 2 mm of terminal branches of the lateral femoral circumflex artery and within 4 cm of the femoral nerve. The modified mid-anterior portal (MMAP) is lateral and distal to the traditional anterior portal. A superficial skin incision, not penetrating deeply with the knife, is less likely to injure the LFCN. The MMAP is placed in the center of the anterior triangle (Fig. 79.5), entering the joint at approximately the 2:30 to 3:00 position on the clockface, while viewing from the AL portal. Interportal capsulotomy is then created using an arthroscopic beaver blade to connect the AL and MMAP (Fig. 79.6). This greatly enhances visualization and instrumentation in the central compartment.

Distal Anterolateral Accessory Portal

The distal anterolateral accessory (DALA) is placed approximately 4 cm distal to, and in line with, the AL portal. It is most frequently used for percutaneous suture anchor placement. During labral repair, suture anchors are placed in the acetabular rim. Angle of drill and anchor insertion is critically important in ensuring secure anchor placement and avoiding articular cartilage or psoas fossa penetration.[37–40] Anteriorly, at the 3 o'clock position, the acetabular rim angle is the smallest around the clockface and the amount of bone available is the smallest, making anchor placement challenging (Fig. 79.7).[41,42] Using the MMAP and a straight drill guide, there is a significantly greater chance of intraarticular penetration.[41] Thus a DALA portal may be used to improve the safety and effectiveness of anchor placement anteriorly to avoid articular cartilage damage. Alternatively, flexible drills and curved suture anchors may be used to circumvent this challenge.[43] Use of the DALA portal may be associated with

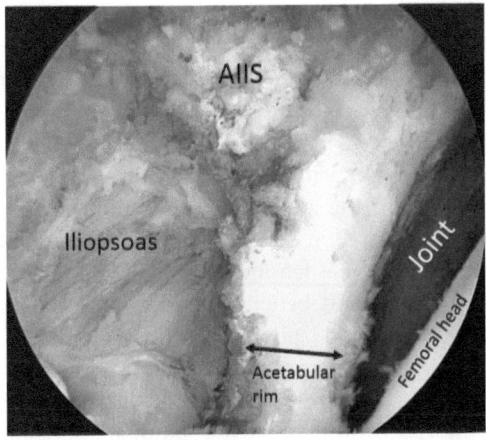

Fig. 79.7 Left hip arthroscopy in cadaveric specimen with labrum removed illustrating the thickness of acetabular rim at the 3 o'clock position. This can be a challenging location for anchor placement if guide starting position, angle of entry, or security of anchor are poor. *AIIS,* Anterior inferior iliac spine.

psoas tunnel perforation and persistent pain following labral repair due to the friction associated with the prominent anchor on the adjacent iliopsoas.[39]

Posterolateral

A PL portal is placed 1 cm posterior and 1 cm proximal to the posterosuperior tip of the greater trochanter, approximately parallel to the same trajectory of the AL portal. This portal may be used for posterior labral repair anchor placement, posterior acetabular rim trimming, or for inflow/outflow fluid management. Although external rotation of the limb moves the sciatic nerve further posterior, it also presents a block (greater trochanter) to proper portal placement. Although internal rotation of the limb moves the sciatic nerve further anterior, the greater trochanter moves out of the way for portal placement. Neutral limb rotation presents the optimal positioning for PL portal creation.

Technique
Central Compartment
Atraumatic technique during proper portal placement permits an optimally sized interportal capsulotomy to visualize the central compartment, containing the acetabular and femoral head articular cartilage, the fovea and ligamentum teres, the acetabular rim and labrum, and the AIIS. The interportal capsulotomy cuts the fibers of the iliofemoral ligament perpendicularly. The capsular cut should be made with an arthroscopic knife while carefully avoiding accidental articular cartilage injury while inserting the knife. The author does not typically extend the capsulotomy more anterior than 3:00, as this opens the potential for fluid extravasation into the iliopsoas tendon sheath to the pelvis and abdomen. Each case having different requirements, the length of the capsulotomy is variably 2 to 4 cm in length. Posterior to 12:00, the capsule becomes thin and largely deficient blending into the ischiofemoral ligament. From portal placement to interportal capsulotomy creation, the author prefers dry arthroscopy before fluid is introduced and the potential for a "red-out" is reduced. The lateral component of the interportal is made while viewing from the MMAP portal. The medial component of the interportal is made while viewing from the AL portal. After capsulotomy completion, gentle débridement of any frayed ligament fibers using a mechanical shaver or radiofrequency device improves visualization without aggressive capsulectomy. To assist with evaluation of the acetabular rim without capsulectomy, traction sutures placed in each limb of the capsule helps lift the capsule off the rim ("suspension technique"), visualize the capsulolabral interval, and better see and treat acetabular-sided pathology (pincer and subspine impingement).[44] While an increased length of interportal capsulotomy improves central compartment access and visualization,[45] it may significantly increase the risk of postoperative rotational and translational hip instability if left unrepaired.[46–49] The importance of capsular closure is illustrated by improved clinical outcomes with complete closure versus partial or nonclosure.[50,51] Thus the integrity of the capsule proximal to the interportal capsulotomy must be sufficient to sustain multiple sutures for repair.[52–54] This emphasizes making the interportal cut far enough away from the labrum (minimum of 8 to 10 mm) to hold the capsular repair: "the key to repairing the capsule is preparing the capsule."

Adequate exposure of the acetabular rim is necessary to properly address pincer and subspine impingement (Fig. 79.8) and labral tears. Anterior rim visualization (from 1 o'clock anterior to the anterior edge of the transverse acetabular ligament) is improved with use of the AL portal as the viewing portal. Posterior rim visualization (from 1 o'clock posterior to the posterior edge of the transverse acetabular ligament) is improved with use of the MMAP as the viewing portal. Upon identification and characterization of chondrolabral pathology, the decision to perform an acetabuloplasty rim trimming with or without labral takedown/detachment is made. If the labrum is taken down sharply (with a variety of instruments—Bankart elevator, arthroscopic beaver blade, radiofrequency device), rim trimming

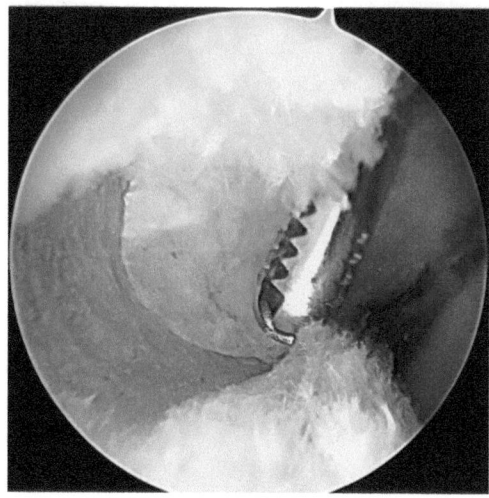

Fig. 79.8 Right hip arthroscopy, anterolateral portal viewing illustrating a completed 2 mm acetabuloplasty rim trimming for focal pincer impingement from 12:00 to 3:00 o'clock and a subspine decompression for a type III anterior inferior iliac spine.

may be visualized better and more precisely treated. This does leave the labrum more unstable than if left attached to the rim. Thus with labral repair/refixation after labral detachment, the potential for overcorrection and labral eversion (and possible suction seal loss) is greater than if left attached to the rim. If the labrum is left attached to the rim, although labral repair/refixation is technically easier and less likely to overly evert the labrum, acetabular rim trimming is more challenging to visualize and treat. Following arthroscopic hip preservation surgery, there is no difference in patient-reported outcome score absolute values or magnitudes of improvement between patients undergoing labral repair/refixation with or without labral detachment.[55]

Preoperative imaging can significantly help in determining the exact magnitude and location of acetabuloplasty rim trimming prior to labral treatment. Standing AP pelvis radiographs best illustrate the lateral center edge angle and standing false profile radiographs best illustrate the anterior center edge angle. There are two different techniques of measurement of these two angles: use of the lateral edge of bone versus the lateral edge of sourcil.[56] On average, the bone lateral center edge angle is 4 degrees greater than the sourcil lateral center edge angle. On average, the bone anterior center edge angle is 10 degrees greater than the sourcil anterior center edge angle. Thus the surgeon must be cognizant of the exact techniques of measurement pre- and intraoperatively. Once the decision is made to perform an acetabuloplasty, algebraic equations can assist in calculation of the anticipated change in lateral center edge angle (change in angle = 1.8 + [0.64 × rim reduction in millimeters]) based on rim resection at the 12:00 o'clock position.[57] One millimeter of resection equals 2.4 degrees of lateral center edge angle change and 5 mm of resection equals 5 degrees of change. A standard resection between 12:00 and 3:00 o'clock leads to an anterior center edge angle reduction 1.9 times the magnitude of the lateral center edge angle.[58] One millimeter of resection equals 2.0 degrees of anterior center edge angle change. The surgeon must be careful to not over-resect. Resection of 4 to 6 mm of rim can increase contact pressures at the base of the acetabulum by threefold.[59] Additionally, iatrogenic dysplasia can lead to postoperative instability (dislocation/subluxation).[60] After the magnitude of bony resection is determined, standard clockface nomenclature can help determine exact location via correlation of preoperative imaging with intraoperative arthroscopic management. The superior margin of the anterior labral sulcus (psoas-u) should be used as 3 o'clock for reference.[42] Based on this consistent easily identified arthroscopic landmark, the AIIS is typically found at 2:00 to 2:30 and the stellate crease at 12:30. Starting at the capsulolabral interval at the 2:00 to 2:30 position, from deep to superficial, the iliofemoral ligament medial limb (capsule) is first visualized, then iliocapsularis (inferior AIIS facet), and then direct head rectus femoris (superior AIIS facet). Thus if a subspine decompression is to be performed, the capsule necessarily needs to be elevated off the bone in order to visualize the AIIS inferior facet. If performing a subspine decompression, the surgeon must be careful to not inadvertently resect acetabular rim and create iatrogenic anterior undercoverage. Alternatively, a separate superficial to deep trajectory can be used and come on top of the capsule and manage the subspine with a burr from superficial to deep. The surgeon must be careful to not violate the rectus tendon if this latter technique is chosen.

After the rim is managed, the decision to perform labral repair versus débridement is made. The literature is clear that labral repair is better, with significantly greater subjective and objective outcomes.[61,62] The majority of suture anchors are drilled and placed behind the labrum in the capsulolabral interval. However, alternatively, the thin acetabular rim at the 3 o'clock position may make an internal (in front of the labrum) technique easier (Fig. 79.9). There are two primary techniques for repair available: a looped circumferential suture that goes around the entire substance of the labrum (Fig. 79.10A) or a pierced through-type labral base refixation technique (see Fig. 79.10B) that goes through the mid-substance of the labrum. In a cadaveric model, labral base through-type repairs are significantly better than looped repairs in restoring maximal negative pressure ("suction seal")

and maximal force to distract.[63,64] Although biomechanical evidence suggests that the suction seal is better retained with a pierced labral base refixation technique, the clinical outcomes between the latter and a looped circumferential repair technique are not significantly different.[65,66] If labral tissue is deficient (e.g., prior débridement), then a labral reconstruction can significantly improve hip biomechanics (suction seal and resistance to distraction) and patient-reported outcomes.[63,64,67] Segmental and complete reconstructions similarly improve without significant differences in outcome scores.[68] There is no difference in outcome improvements based on graft type.[68,69] The author prefers allograft peroneus longus because of the ease of size matching (approximately 5.5 to 6.5 mm diameter), the ease of manipulation in

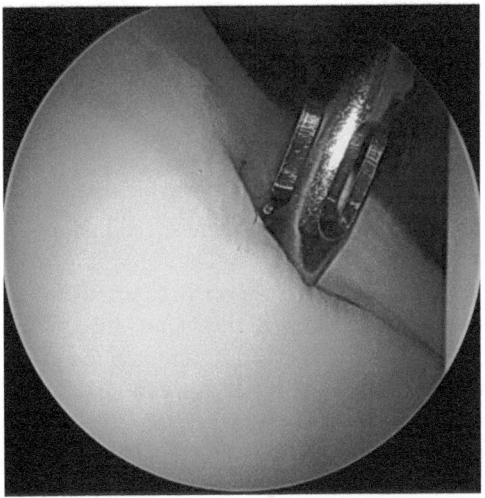

Fig. 79.9 Right hip arthroscopy, anterolateral portal viewing, drill guide for 1.8 mm anchor placement at the 3:30 position. Note guide position in front of the labrum, rather than the more frequently used capsulolabral interval position behind the labrum. The thin acetabular rim between 3:00 and 4:00 o'clock makes the internal position easier for visualization and safe anchor placement.

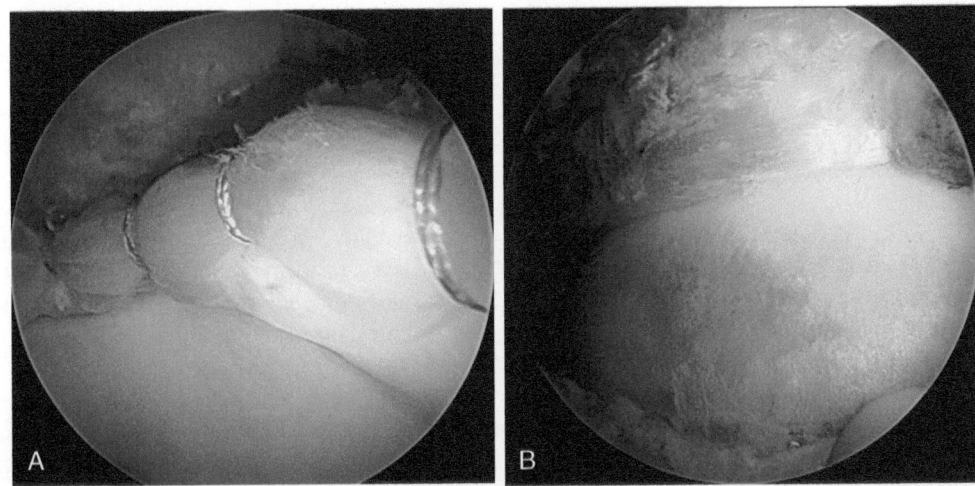

Fig. 79.10 (A) Left hip arthroscopy, anterolateral portal viewing, four suture anchor labral repair with a looped circumferential repair technique. (B) Left hip arthroscopy, modified mid-anterior portal viewing, illustrating the "suction seal" of a pierced through-type labral base refixation technique using four suture anchors.

the joint, the relative lack of swelling in comparison to other graft types, and the minimal preparation time needed.

Peripheral Compartment

Peripheral compartment disorders are managed without traction. Both interportal and T capsulotomies may be created and manipulated to completely visualize and treat all pathologies in the peripheral compartment. These primarily include cam morphology, loose bodies, and synovitis. The author prefers the T capsulotomy as it provides significantly better visualization of the peripheral compartment, with significantly greater cross-sectional area visualization than that of an 8-cm interportal capsulotomy.[45,70] A precapsular fat pad is frequently present over the fibers of the iliofemoral ligament and must be removed (with a mechanical shaver or radiofrequency device) to expose the interval for the capsulotomy (iliocapsularis [medial] and the gluteus minimus [lateral]).[71] A variety of instruments may be used to create the capsulotomy. The author prefers to view from the MMAP and use a 3.0-mm radiofrequency probe (Dyonics RF Hook 30° Probe; Smith & Nephew, Andover, MA) to create the capsulotomy, bisecting the intermuscular plane down the AL femoral neck to the intertrochanteric line. Traction sutures may be placed in each limb of the "T" to optimize visualization of the head-neck junction, the lateral ascending vessels, and the medial and lateral synovial folds. The author uses a SpeedStitch device (Smith & Nephew, Andover, MA) through the AL portal to place one traction suture in the lateral limb and through the DALA portal to place one traction suture in the medial limb of the "T" capsulotomy. This permits visualization behind the lateral ascending vessels posteriorly and beyond the medial synovial fold inferiorly.

The limb can be manipulated in any position necessary to accomplish a comprehensive cam correction. The author performs the majority of the cam correction in approximately neutral rotation, 5 degrees of flexion, and 10 to 20 degrees of abduction. Intraoperative cam correction should be patient- and hip-specific and based on preoperative imaging. Six intraoperative AP fluoroscopic views (3 views in hip extension [30 degrees external rotation, 30 degrees internal rotation, neutral] and 3 views in 50 degrees flexion [neutral, 40 degrees external rotation, 60 degrees external rotation]) may be used to optimize the correction as these correlate with preoperative 3D CT at the typical cam morphology location from 11:45 to 2:45.[72] The best intraoperative marker of resection depth is the hard, sclerotic, cortical cam bone. A 5.5 mm round arthroscopic burr is used to perform the cam resection. It is of critical importance to make the correction perfect (Fig. 79.11). A restoration of "ball and socket" mechanics is not achieved if either under- or over-correction occurs. Under-correction (residual cam morphology) is the most common reason for revision hip arthroscopy.[73] Over-correction is, in essence, a problem correctable only via arthroplasty. Thus meticulous technique with smooth transition from the proximal head to the head-neck junction, without sharp edges and "shark bites," is necessary. Both arthroscopic visualization during dynamic impingement maneuvering and fluoroscopic assessment can ensure a proper cam correction. Concurrent use of a 70-degree arthroscope and an AP fluoroscopic image can be challenging at

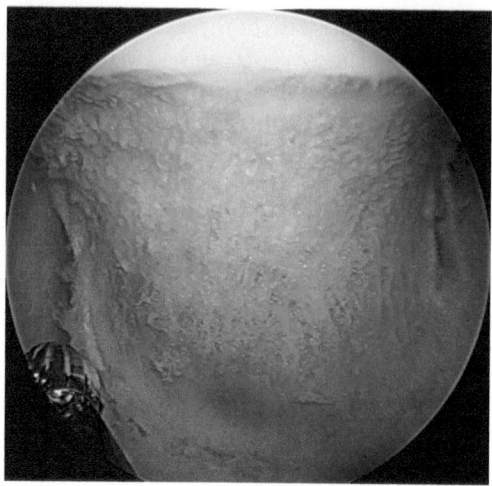

Fig. 79.11 Right hip arthroscopy, modified mid-anterior portal viewing, illustrating a comprehensive cam correction.

times. If bone resection is being performed and the fluoroscopic image is not changing, the solution is not to keep resecting bone. This is particularly important far laterally and posterolaterally, where the cam morphology is near the vessels and under the labrum. Hip extension and gentle distraction can bring these more proximal lateral cam morphologies into better view. If the osseous morphology extends far beyond the vessels posteriorly or into the vessels, an open surgical approach is indicated. The surgeon must be cognizant of the most proximal extent of the correction and be sure to not over-resect proximally along the entire radial arc of the anterior head-neck junction.[74] Additionally, distal anterior inferomedial cam is frequently problematic in hypermobile athletes, including dancers, gymnasts, and yogis.[75] This area must be scrutinized arthroscopically and corrected as this is an area that will mechanically conflict at the AIIS in these patients. The latter illustrates the merit of the T-capsulotomy, as it provides significantly improved visualization and correction in this location. At the conclusion of the cam correction, all bony debris should be evacuated from the joint to minimize the risk for postoperative heterotopic ossification.

Capsular closure commences from distal to proximal along the T capsulotomy. This is a ligament repair. The capsule is the iliofemoral ligament. Thus healing of the iatrogenically violated ligament (the T in parallel and the interportal perpendicular) and subsequent repair is the subject of controversy. The author repairs the capsule in nearly all patients, plicates in those at risk for instability (e.g., hypermobile, Ehlers-Danlos, ballet, borderline dysplasia), and leaves the interportal capsulotomy unrepaired in stiff, tight, male, large cam, Tönnis 1 hips. Both biomechanical and clinical outcomes of hip arthroscopy are significantly better with, rather than without, capsular repair.[50,76,77] Measurement of generalized joint hypermobility is highly predictive of capsular thickness and a Beighton score of less than four correlates with a capsular thickness of greater than or equal to 10 mm, while a Beighton score of greater than or equal to four correlates with a capsular thickness of less than 10 mm.[78] Thus in patients with a preoperative Beighton score greater than or equal to four, the author prefers to plicate, rather than side-to-side repair, the capsule.

Capsular closure is performed using nonabsorbable #2 suture. In the T limb, three or four sutures are typically used, with greater degrees of plication performed in those at risk for instability. In the interportal limb, two to four sutures are typically used, dependent on the size of the interportal capsulotomy made and the degree of inferior capsular shift.[54] Simple, non-mattress, full-thickness suture technique is used. For the T limb, the arthroscope is in the MMAP and the instrumentation and tying are via the DALA portal. For the interportal limb, the arthroscope is in the AL portal and the instrumentation and tying are via the MMAP. The T limb is closed using a 70-degree up SlingShot (Stryker Sports Medicine, Greenwood Village, CO) to perform a capsular plication. The SlingShot can secure approximately 1 to 2 cm of suture in its penetrating needle and retriever. The surgeon then passes the needle and suture through the lateral limb first (slightly thicker than medial) with an approximately 5- to 10-mm bite of tissue. The suture is deployed deep to the capsule and the needle removed and then repositioned over the medial limb. The needle then pierces and retrieves the suture through the medial limb at approximately 5- to 10-mm bite of tissue. The greater the potential of instability, the greater the plication performed. The author ties each suture, using an initial surgeon's knot, followed by three reversing half-hitches on alternating posts, sequentially, rather than passing all three sutures and then tying. The surgeon then places two to four sutures into the distal limb of the interportal capsulotomy via the DALA portal and each suture is secured with a single hemostat and marked. The arthroscope is then switched to the AL portal. Each distal interportal limb is retrieved through the MMAP and passed through the proximal interportal limb using a SpeedStitch (Smith & Nephew, Andover, MA), proceeding from medial/inferior to lateral/superior. Knots are tied sequentially, the same as the T capsular closure, rather than pass all suture first and then tie. Verification of capsular closure security (Fig. 79.12) is then performed with a dynamic motion examination and all arthroscopic

debris evacuated. A postoperative cocktail is placed over the capsule via each portal with a total of 30 mL of 0.5% ropivacaine, 10 mg morphine, and 30 mg ketorolac. Nonabsorbable monofilament suture is used to close the three arthroscopic portals and a sterile dressing applied.

A hinged hip brace (limited from 0 to 90 degrees hip flexion, 0 to 10 degrees abduction) and derotational boots are applied in the operating room. Cryotherapy and compression are recommended for the first 2 weeks. Continuous passive motion machine is recommended for the first two weeks from 0 to 90 degrees hip flexion up to 3 to 4 hours/day while awake. Crutch-assisted foot-flat weight bearing is recommended for 4 weeks postoperatively. Transition to full weight bearing as tolerated commences from week 4 to 6. Patients continue to ambulate with two crutches (without a one crutch transition) until they can successfully walk with a normal gait without a limp. Physical therapy begins preoperatively with patient education and commences postoperatively on day 1 following surgery.

For a complete list of references, go to ExpertConsult.com.

SELECTED READINGS

Citation:
Frank JM, Harris JD, Erickson BJ, et al. Prevalence of femoroacetabular impingement imaging findings in asymptomatic volunteers: a systematic review. *Arthroscopy*. 2015;31:1199–204.

Level of Evidence:
IV, systematic review of levels I-IV evidence

Summary:
In this systematic review of 26 studies (2114 asymptomatic hips; 57% male; mean age 25 years), the prevalence of cam morphology was 37% (55% in athletes; 23% in nonathletes), pincer morphology was 67%, and labral tear was 68%. This illustrates the high prevalence of abnormal imaging findings in an asymptomatic population, emphasizing the role of treating patients, not x-rays.

Citation:
Griffin DR, Dickenson EJ, O'Donnell J, et al. The Warwick Agreement on femoroacetabular impingement syndrome (FAI syndrome): an international consensus statement. *Br J Sports Med*. 2016;50:1169–76.

Level of Evidence:
Not applicable

Summary:
This international multidisciplinary consensus represented 22 panel members, 5 specialties, and 9 countries. It defined FAI syndrome as a motion-related clinical disorder of the hip with a triad of symptoms, clinical signs, and imaging findings. It encouraged usage of terminology "FAI syndrome," "cam morphology," and "pincer morphology" and discouraged usage of "asymptomatic FAI," "symptomatic FAI," "FAI morphology," "deformity," "lesion," or "abnormality" referring to cam or pincer morphology.

Citation:
Degen RM, Poultsides L, Mayer SW, et al. Safety of hip anchor insertion from the midanterior and distal anterolateral portals

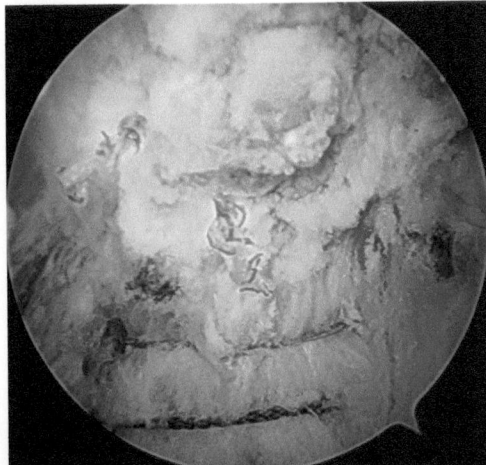

Fig. 79.12 Right hip arthroscopy, anterolateral portal viewing, illustrating a completed capsular closure with three sutures for the T capsulotomy and three sutures for the interportal capsulotomy.

with a straight drill guide: a cadaveric study. *Am J Sports Med.* 2017;45:627–35.

Level of Evidence:
Not applicable

Summary:
This cadaveric laboratory investigation of 16 pelvic specimens examined the safety of suture anchor insertion around the acetabulum (from 9 to 4 o'clock). It showed that anteriorly (2 to 4 o'clock), there is a higher rate of articular surface (4.5%) and psoas tunnel (7.7%) perforation from either the mid-anterior or distal anterolateral accessory portal than previously anticipated.

Citation:
Frank RM, Lee S, Bush-Joseph CA, et al. Improved outcomes after hip arthroscopic surgery in patients undergoing T-capsulotomy with complete repair versus partial repair for femoroacetabular impingement: a comparative matched-pair analysis. *Am J Sports Med.* 2014;42:2634–42.

Level of Evidence:
III, cohort study

Summary:
In this two-year follow-up comparative study of partial versus complete capsular closure by a single surgeon performing arthroscopic hip preservation, patients that underwent complete repair had significantly better sport-specific outcomes compared with those undergoing partial repair. There was a 13% revision rate in the partial repair group, while no patient needed a revision in the complete repair group.

Citation:
Philippon MJ, Trindade CA, Goldsmith MT, et al. Biomechanical assessment of hip capsular repair and reconstruction procedures using a 6 degrees of freedom robotic system. *Am J Sports Med.* 2017;45:1745–54.

Level of Evidence:
Not applicable

Summary:
This cadaveric laboratory investigation of 10 hip specimens examined range of motion for intact specimens, capsulotomy types (interportal and T), capsular repair, and capsular reconstruction. Both capsular repair and reconstruction may lead to improved patient-reported outcomes by improving rotational hip motion to more near normal in the early postoperative period.

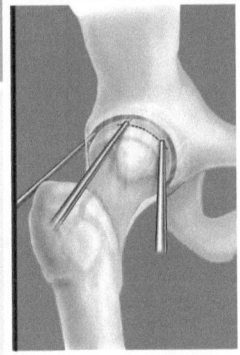

80

Femoroacetabular Impingement in Athletes

Shane J. Nho, Vignesh Prasad Krishnamoorthy, Drew Lansdown, Gift Ukwuani

The concept of hip impingement was first described in the medical literature in the 19th century,[1] and the idea that variations in hip morphology can contribute to secondary hip arthritis has been known for more than 100 years.[2] The first surgical description of treating femoral head and neck deformities appeared in 1913, with good results following resection.[3] The modern concept of femoroacetabular impingement (FAI) was formulated by Ganz et al.[4] in 1999, and the understanding that FAI can eventually lead to osteoarthritis of the hip was described by Ganz and colleagues in 2003.[5] This type of hip osteoarthritis was first described in adults in the 40- to 50-year age group. However, it is now recognized that FAI can cause serious joint damage among young athletes, even in their second and third decades.

FAI has been classically defined as an abutment between the proximal femur and the acetabular rim arising from morphologic abnormalities affecting the acetabulum, the proximal femur, or both.[6] This repetitive mechanical conflict occurs mainly during activities involving extreme flexion and internal rotation of the hip, which can lead to lesions of the acetabular labrum and the adjacent acetabular cartilage.[6] Two types of FAI have been classically described: a cam type (Fig. 80.1) and a pincer type (Fig. 80.2). Most cases of FAI are now recognized and classified as mixed cam-pincer impingement, as they usually involve both these mechanisms.[7]

Cam impingement is caused by an aspherical femoral head moving inside the acetabulum. This may be seen as an osseous bump at the femoral head-neck junction or as a reduced or absent offset between the femoral head and neck.[7] The osseous prominence on the femoral neck is similar to a cam, which is an eccentric part added to a rotating device,[7] hence the name. This type of altered proximal femoral morphology has been classically described as the "pistol grip" deformity,[8] best seen on anteroposterior (AP) pelvic radiographs; it may be due to a developmental disorder of the femoral head-neck junction (premature eccentric closure of the capital femoral physis),[9] resulting in the nonspherical shape of the femoral head. Carsen et al.,[10] in a cohort study of pediatric patients, followed pre- and postphyseal closure using magnetic resonance imaging (MRI); they showed that the cam morphology was present exclusively in the closed physeal group. This finding suggested that the deformity likely developed during the period of physeal closure. It was also postulated that increased physical activity during this period was associated with the development of the cam morphology.

The cam deformity has also long been recognized as a sequela of a slipped capital femoral epiphysis,[11] in which the posterior and inferior displacement of the capital epiphysis produces a prominence of the anterior and superior neck. It can also be associated with conditions like Legg-Calvé-Perthes disease[12] and epiphyseal dysplasias[13] and can be secondary to femoral neck fractures malunited in retroversion.[14] During flexion, the non-spherical, eccentric portion of the head slides into the antero-superior acetabulum, creating compression and shear stresses at the transition zone between the fibrous acetabular labrum and the hyaline articular cartilage and at the tidemark region of the articular cartilage. The labrum is pushed away from the joint and the articular cartilage is compressed and pushed centrally. With repetitive motion, this eventually results in separation of the cartilage from the labrum and from the subchondral bone of the acetabulum, creating the "carpet lesions" or chondral flap tears. Early in the disease process, persons with cam morphology develop more chondral pathology, with relative labral preservation. However, over time, the labrum also starts to fail, but only after the process is advanced on the articular surface. Cam impingement is typically seen in athletic men[13] and often presents with problems in young adulthood. Some studies[15] have reported a near 3 : 1 male predominance.

Pincer impingement is due to acetabular overcoverage and is caused by an overhanging anterolateral rim of the acetabulum, abutting on the femoral head-neck junction during hip flexion. This can occur due to overgrowth of the anterior edge of the acetabulum or the presence of a separate bony fragment at the anterior acetabular rim, referred to as an os acetabulum.[16] The bony fragment may be a nonfused ossification center or a stress fracture of the acetabular rim,[17] or it can be secondary to labral ossification.[7] This type of impingement can also be caused by acetabular retroversion,[7] which has been described as posterior orientation of the acetabular opening. Coxa profunda,[18] or a deep acetabular socket, and protrusio acetabuli can also predispose to pincer impingement[7] due to global overcoverage. The prominent anterior acetabular rim crushes the anterior labrum against the femoral head-neck junction during hip flexion and eventually leads to degeneration and failure of the acetabular labrum as a result of this repetitive microtrauma. A variable amount of damage to the articular cartilage of the acetabulum follows secondarily over time. This type of impingement is less commonly associated with severe anterior acetabular chondral damage as compared with the cam type, although "contrecoup" degeneration can occur

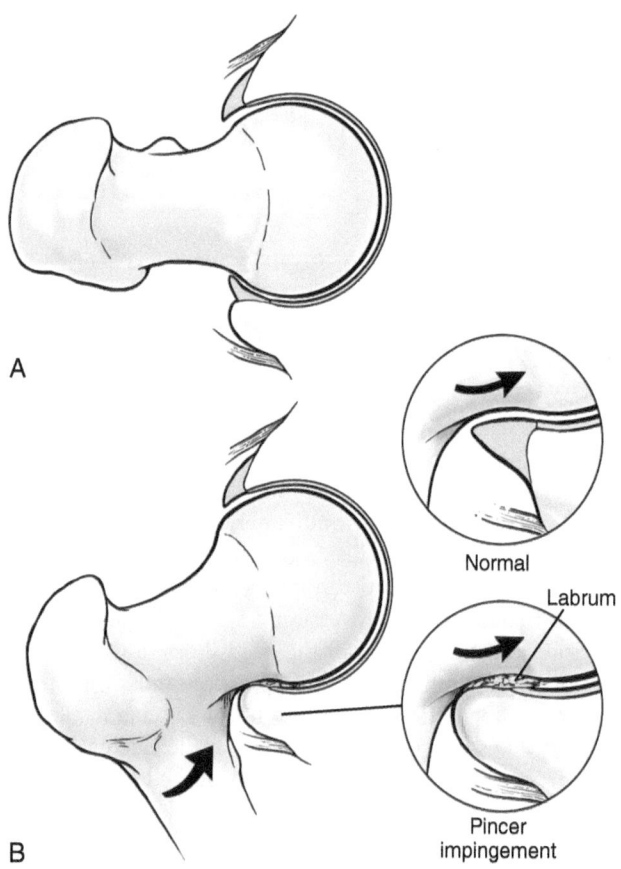

Fig. 80.1 Pincer-type femoroacetabular impingement is acetabular-based, with overcoverage of the socket on the femoral head.

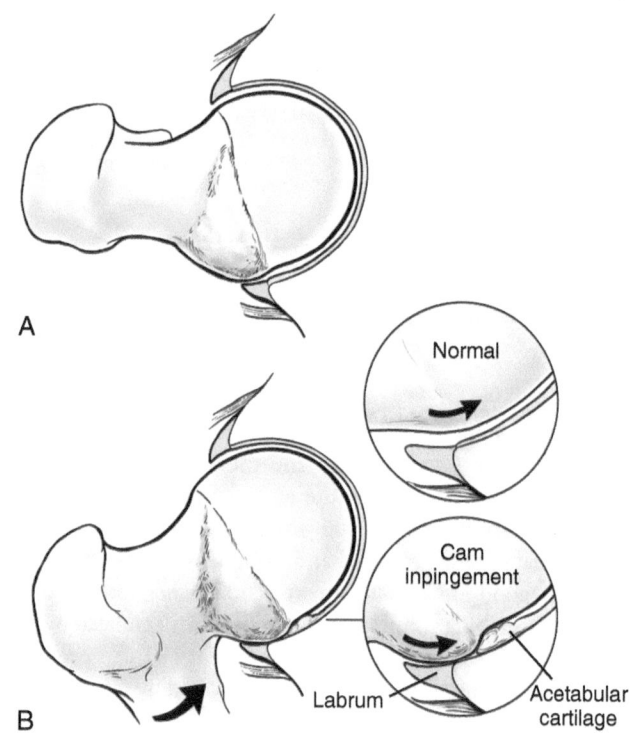

Fig. 80.2 Cam-type femoroacetabular impingement is the result of deformity at the femoral head-neck junction, leading to abutment of this region on the acetabular labrum and adjacent cartilage.

on the posterior and inferior aspect of the acetabulum owing to leverage of the femoral head and subsequent overloading of the posterior aspect of the joint.[7,19] The pincer type of FAI occurs more commonly in women,[13,19] with the onset of symptoms frequently in middle age. Dynamic pincer impingement can also occur in normal hips, as seen in gymnasts and dancers, who have greater range of motion (ROM) in the hip.[20]

Most cases of FAI have a combination of both these mechanisms,[7] and the demographics are intermediate between the pincer and cam forms. Patients typically present with features of both labral and chondral damage caused by the pincer and cam deformities, respectively. The pattern of damage to the articular cartilage is a combination of the two patterns of damage,[7] with the eventual outcome being influenced by the predominant type.

FAI has gained considerable attention in the last decade, ever since Ganz reported the vessel-sparing surgical dislocation (SD) of the hip joint[21] and later, in 2004, used it for the treatment of FAI.[22] In the past, these subtle deformities of the proximal femur and acetabulum were probably missed, and it is now believed by some surgeons that the majority of the cases of "primary" osteoarthritis are in fact, due to FAI morphology.[13] With the increasing recognition that cam and pincer deformities predispose the hip joint to chondral and labral damage and eventual joint destruction, particularly in young athletes and individuals with greater ROM of the hips, the number of patients being diagnosed and treated for FAI has increased. However, it should be

emphasized that these deformities are also commonly encountered in the pelvic radiographs of asymptomatic individuals in the general population.[23] Hence FAI is not a radiologic diagnosis alone but a condition associated with groin or hip pain (symptoms) and limited range of hip motion with positive impingement signs (clinical signs) along with abnormal imaging findings.[24]

CLINICAL PRESENTATION

The clinical presentation of patients with FAI can be variable, but most present with deep-seated intermittent hip or groin pain with hip rotation or during or after activity. The onset of the pain is usually insidious, but some athletes may report a specific injury or an acute precipitating event prior to the onset of symptoms.[25] Patients may have pain or associated discomfort in the lateral hip, buttock, thigh, or low back regions. Groin pain may be referred to the anterior or medial thigh[26] or to the symphysis pubis region in patients with anterior impingement. Byrd reported that athletes often demonstrate the "C-sign" in describing deep interior hip pain by cupping the hand above the greater trochanter with the fingers gripping into the anterior groin (Fig. 80.3).[27] Patients with posterior impingement may present with buttock pain or pain in the sacroiliac region.[28] With chronic degeneration, the symptoms may become more constant with activity and less intermittent.

Athletes are usually aware of their limited hip mobility long before symptoms begin.[29] However, they do not have major functional limitations, as the decreased ROM in the hip is compensated by increased pelvic and lumbosacral motion. These compensatory effects on the bony and soft tissue structures within the hip joint, hemipelvis, and the lumbosacral spine can lead to other conditions like athletic pubalgia, trochanteric or iliopsoas bursitis, sacroiliac joint dysfunction, and lower back problems, which usually coexist in patients with FAI.[30,31] On examination, these secondary findings may be more evident and obscure the underlying element of primary hip dysfunction; therefore hip disorders can go undetected for a protracted period. In one study, Clohisy reported that patients presented with ongoing pain that had lasted for 12 to 16 months.[32]

Mechanical symptoms like popping, locking, catching, snapping, and giving way have also been reported in patients with FAI.[25] Patients with severe impingement may have difficulties with activities like prolonged sitting, squatting, or climbing up stairs.[33] Patients with posterior impingement may have pain with

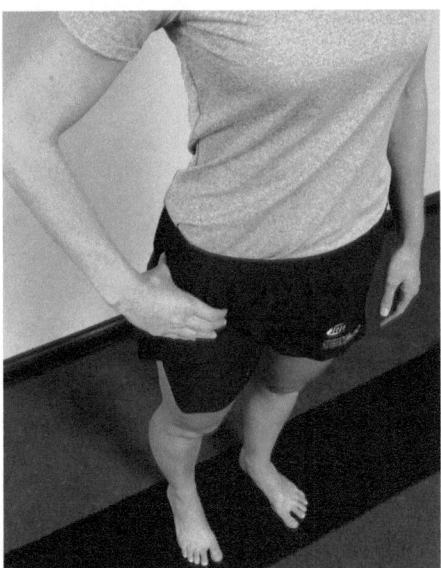

Fig. 80.3 The C-sign is a common finding in symptomatic femoroacetabular impingement, where the patient makes a C-shape with his or her hand at the affected hip to indicate the deep-seated location of the pain.

activities like walking downhill or fast walking, where the hip is repeatedly hyperextended.[28]

PHYSICAL EXAMINATION

A thorough physical examination is important to clarify the source of the patient's pain and potential associated conditions (Table 80.1). Physical examination may elicit tenderness in the groin or trochanteric region. On examination, almost all patients have diminished hip ROM, particularly flexion and internal rotation, caused by the altered bony architecture of the joint.[34] However, patients may demonstrate reduced internal rotation without pathologic impingement due to other causes, such as decreased femoral anteversion,[35] and some athletes with pathologic impingement may have normal or even increased internal rotation. Also, although only one hip may be symptomatic, the altered morphology is often present in both hips; thus the ROM must be examined in the other hip as well.

The FADIR (flexion, adduction, internal rotation) impingement test is a very sensitive test for FAI but not necessarily specific, as it can be positive in any irritable hip condition (Fig. 80.4).[36] With the hip in 90 degrees of flexion, the joint is progressively rotated from external to internal rotation while moving from abduction to adduction. To be considered positive, this maneuver should reproduce the patient's typical pain experienced with activities.[24] Using this maneuver, it is possible to identify the most likely position of impingement and the most likely area of the acetabular rim injury.[28] This exam test may be somewhat uncomfortable, so it is better to perform it on the asymptomatic side first and then compare with the symptomatic hip. The internal foot progression angle walking (FPAW) test is more specific though less sensitive than FADIR testing for the diagnosis of FAI. A positive internal FPAW test is the presence of hip pain on walking with the ipsilateral foot 15 degrees internally rotated from the baseline gait pattern.[37] The log-roll test, although not sensitive, is the most specific test for hip joint pathology independent of its etiology. Rolling the leg back and forth rotates only the femoral head in relation to the acetabulum without stressing any of the surrounding structures.[27] The Drehmann

TABLE 80.1	Physical Exam Maneuvers for the Evaluation of Femoroacetabular Impingement	
Physical Exam Test	**How to Perform**	**Definition of a Positive Test**
FADIR test	Hip flexed to 90 degrees and the femur rotated from external to internal rotation while adducting the thigh.	Maneuver reproduces patient's typical pain from impingement of femoral head on acetabular rim/labrum.
Internal foot progression angle	Observe foot position during gait.	Greater than 15 degrees of internal rotation relative to the contralateral side indicates dynamic limitation in ROM.
Log-roll test	With patient in supine position, the affected leg is rolled internally and externally.	Pain present in the hip region suggesting intra-articular hip pathology.
Drehmann sign	Observe rotational profile when passively flexing the hip.	Presence of obligate external rotation, indicating limitations in ROM.
Posterior impingement test	Hip placed in extension and external rotation.	Reproduces patient's typical pain from posterior-based FAI.
FABER test	Hip flexed to 90 degrees, abducted, and externally rotated.	Reproduces patient's typical pain; may indicate posterior impingement.
Trendelenburg sign	Patient stands on one leg.	Pelvis drops on contralateral side, indicating abductor weakness.

FABER, Flexion, abduction, external rotation; *FADIR*, flexion, adduction, internal rotation; *FAI*, femoroacetabular impingement; *ROM*, range of motion.

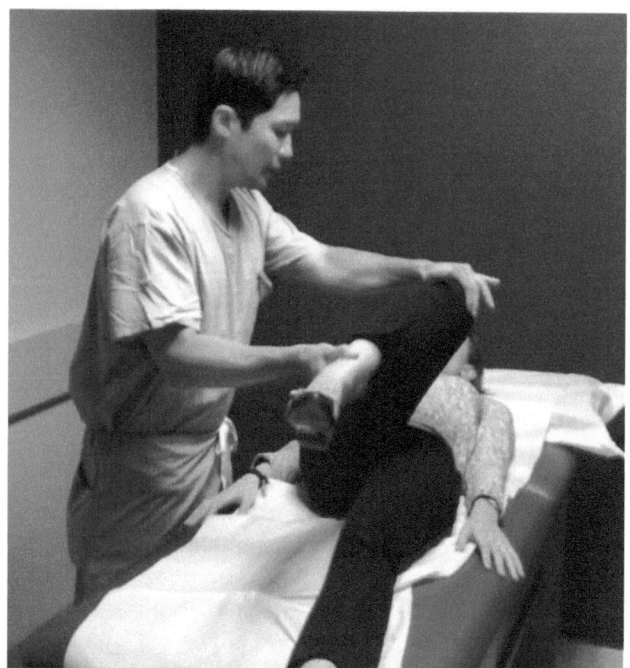

Fig. 80.4 The FADIR (flexion, adduction, internal rotation) maneuver is shown, with the examiner moving the symptomatic hip to 90 degrees of flexion, adduction, and internal rotation. A positive test results in this position reproducing the patient's typical pain in the hip region.

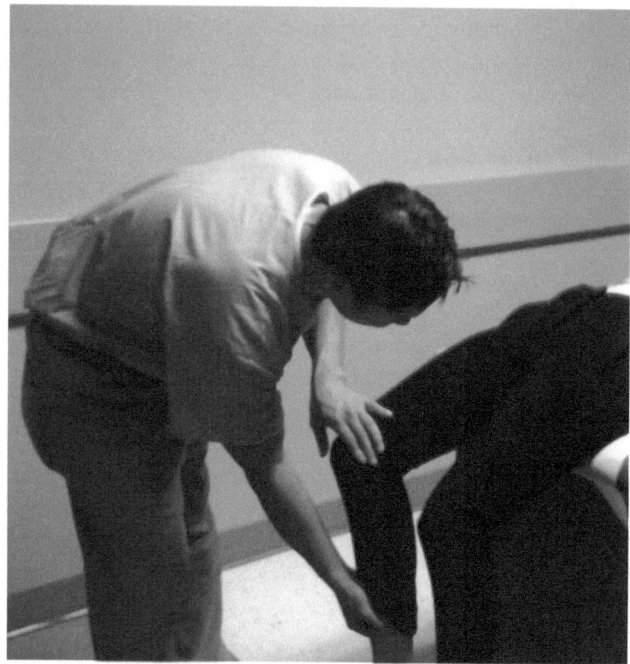

Fig. 80.5 The posterior impingement test is demonstrated. The patient is supine on the exam table, toward the end of the table with the hip resting in extension. The examiner externally rotates the hip, which will reproduce the pain if the symptoms are from posterior impingement.

sign may be seen in patients with FAI and is considered positive if there is an unavoidable passive external rotation of the hip when a hip flexion is being performed.[38] However, it can also be positive in slipped capital femoral epiphysis,[38] Legg-Calvé-Perthes disease, and avascular necrosis of the femoral head.

Posterior impingement may occasionally be encountered and is assessed by the "posterior impingement test," placing the hip in extension and external rotation (Fig. 80.5).[39] The test is considered positive if it reproduces the patients' typical pain or if there is decreased ROM. The FABER test places the hip in flexion-abduction-external rotation. Lateral-sided hip pain and increased distance between the lateral knee joint line and the examination table have been reported during the FABER test in patients with posterior impingement.[33]

Additional tests that should be part of a thorough hip examination include assessing the gait, straight-leg raise, single-leg control, and investigation of any secondary findings in the symphysis pubis, sacroiliac joints, lumbar spine, and the trochanteric region due to conditions commonly encountered in FAI as a result of the compensatory pathomechanics.

A mild to moderate limp is common, occurring in up to 71% of patients.[25] Abductor weakness is often seen on the affected side, with a positive Trendelenburg sign. The pelvis should be examined for any anterior tilt, which may be the cause of focal anterior overcoverage and pincer impingement. Patients may have exaggerated lumbar lordosis associated with the anterior tilt of the pelvis and also exaggerated lumbar spine mobility as a compensation for the reduced hip motion. They may also have limb-length discrepancy secondary to coxa vara, which has been associated with cam impingement or anterior tilt of the hemipelvis.

Lateral pain may be present from trochanteric bursitis, and posterior pain and tenderness may be present at the ischial tuberosity from chronic hamstring tendinopathy due to the adaptive posterior tilt of the pelvis seen in patients with FAI who are attempting to reduce anterior impingement.[31] Posterior tenderness may be present within the gluteal muscles from overfiring in an attempt to splint the joint. Posterior sacroiliac joint tenderness may be present from sacroiliac joint dysfunction, which is more common in patients with acquired FAI due to labral ossification.[40] The lower abdominal and adductor area must be carefully palpated to localize tenderness suggestive of athletic pubalgia. This tenderness can mimic or coexist with FAI. Pain with resisted hip adduction or situps should raise a suspicion for athletic pubalgia.[31]

DIAGNOSIS

Plain Radiographs

The radiologic assessment of any patient with hip pain and suspected FAI should begin with conventional radiography. Our preference for the initial radiographic evaluation of a patient with suspected FAI includes a well-centered AP pelvis view, a Dunn lateral view, and false-profile view of the affected hip (Fig. 80.6). These views allow for an initial assessment of the cam and pincer lesions associated with impingement while also evaluating other acute or chronic changes including secondary joint destruction.

It is important to maintain neutral pelvic tilt and rotation in AP radiographs, with the tip of the coccyx centered in the midline and the distance between the midportion of the sacrococcygeal joint and the upper border of the symphysis pubis between 32

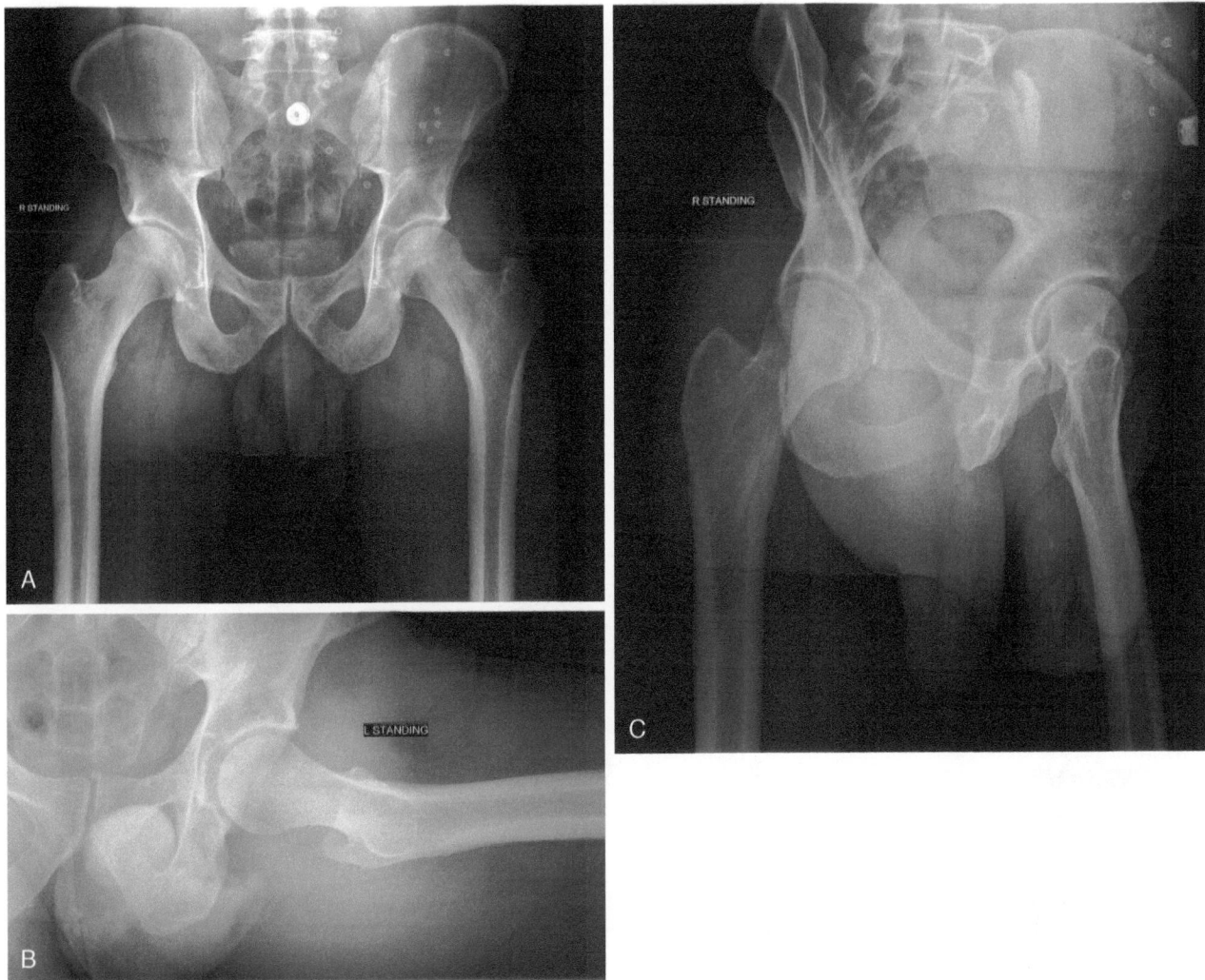

Fig. 80.6 A standard radiographic series is shown for the initial evaluation of a patient with potential femoroacetabular impingement. (A) A well-centered anteroposterior view, (B) a 90-degree Dunn lateral, and (C) a false-profile view.

and 47 m, to correctly identify pincer impingement.[41] Overcoverage of the anterior acetabulum, characteristic of pincer impingement, is evaluated by the presence of the crossover sign,[42] posterior wall sign,[42] and the prominent ischial spine sign.[43] The crossover sign is positive when the cranial part of the anterior acetabular wall is more lateral than the posterior wall, creating a figure-of-8 configuration indicative of focal acetabular retroversion (Fig. 80.7).[29,42] The posterior wall sign is positive when the posterior acetabular wall lies medial to the center of the femoral head (Fig. 80.8).[29,42] This indicates that the posterior wall is deficient and is usually associated with acetabular retroversion. It is important to recognize this, as it puts the patient at risk for iatrogenic posterior instability with isolated anterior wall decompression. A prominent ischial spine sign can be seen on an AP radiograph and is also indicative of acetabular retroversion (Fig. 80.9).

Global overcoverage may be associated with coxa profunda or protrusio acetabuli, both of which are accompanied by an excessive center-edge angle. Coxa profunda is present when the floor of the acetabular fossa is medial to the ilioischial line (Fig. 80.10).[7,18] Protrusio acetabuli is present when the femoral head overlaps the ilioischial line medially (Fig. 80.11).[7] The lateral center-edge angle (LCEA) can be used to assess lateral overcoverage, with values greater than 40 degrees indicative of pincer morphology (Fig. 80.12).[44] Other findings of rim impingement include rim fractures, a downsloping sourcil, Tönnis angle below 0 degrees,[44] presence of labral ossification causing the appositional bone sign,[29] os acetabuli and saddle-like callus formation at the impact area of the femoral neck.[45] A synovial herniation pit may be present in the region of the anterolateral femoral head-neck junction in patients with FAI,[5] seen on conventional radiographs as a region of decreased bone density with well-defined borders.[46] The 45-degree Dunn view,[47] frog-leg lateral view,[48] and the profile view in impingement position (PIP)[49] have also been used for assessment of the femoral cam morphology and quantification of the asphericity of the femoral head with the alpha angle (Fig. 80.13). Values greater than 50 degrees are indicative of cam deformity.[29]

Lequesne's false-profile view,[50] obtained with the patient in a standing position with the affected hip against the cassette and the pelvis rotated 65 degrees in relation to the wall stand, is used

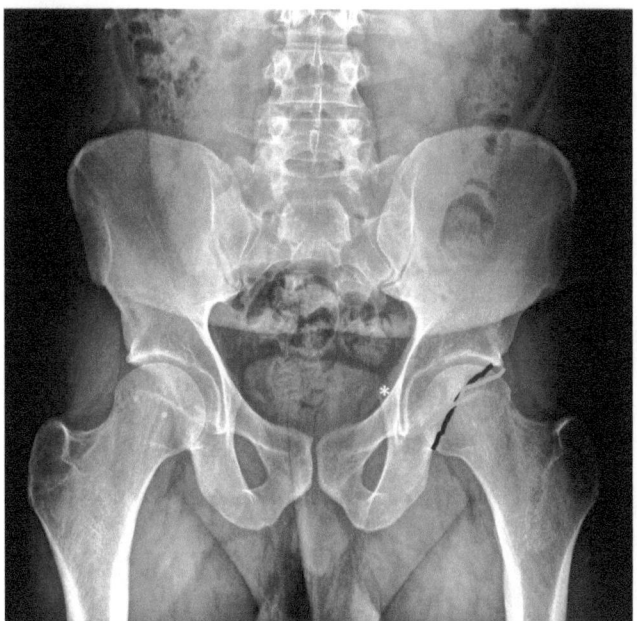

Fig. 80.7 An anteroposterior radiograph is shown with multiple features of acetabular overcoverage, including a prominent ischial tuberosity (*) and a crossover sign. The anterior acetabular wall is outlined in *light blue* and the posterior wall is outlined in *dark blue*, with a crossover present near the center of the femoral head, indicating relative retroversion.

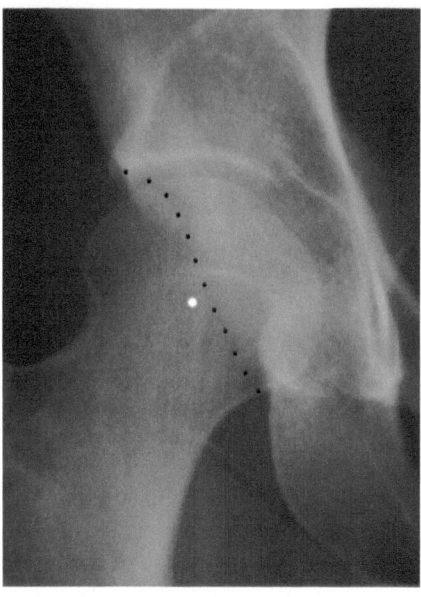

Fig. 80.8 The posterior wall sign is demonstrated on the radiograph of a patient with acetabular impingement. The posterior wall is located medial to the center of the femoral head.

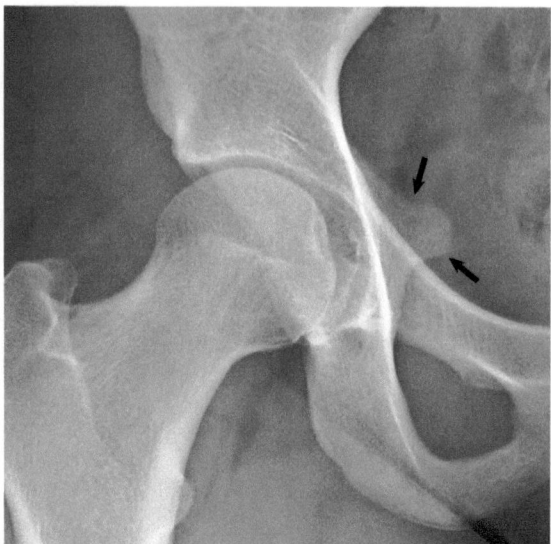

Fig. 80.9 A prominent ischial spine sign is seen on an anteroposterior radiograph of the right hip *(black arrows)*, which is suggestive of acetabular retroversion.

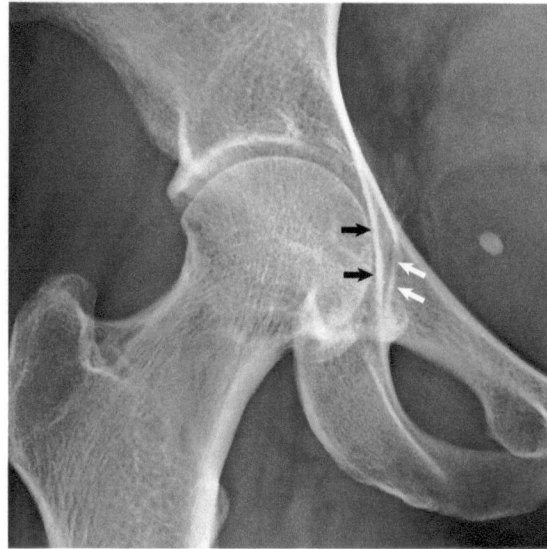

Fig. 80.10 Coxa profunda is defined by the floor of the acetabulum *(white arrows)* located medial to the ilioischial line *(black arrows)*.

to quantify anterior overcoverage. An anterior center-edge angle (ACEA) greater than 40 degrees indicates excessive anterior overcoverage.[44] This view is also used to assess the morphology of the anteroinferior iliac spine and contrecoup lesions seen in the posteroinferior part of the hip joint.

Nepple et al. utilized a clock-face technique (the superior femoral neck is 12 o'clock and the anterior neck is 3 o'clock) to correlate the position of the head-neck junction profiled on plain radiographs with radial oblique computed tomography (CT) reformats.[51] The 12 o'clock position is seen with the AP pelvis radiograph, 1 o'clock with the 45-degree Dunn view, 2 o'clock with the frog-leg lateral view, and 3 o'clock with the cross-table lateral view. Given the typical location of cam deformities at the anterolateral femoral head-neck junction (1 o'clock), the deformity is most readily identified on the 45-degree Dunn view, where the hip is abducted 20 degrees and flexed to 45 degrees.[51] Compared with the Dunn view, the frog-leg lateral view has greater specificity for detecting cam morphology.[51]

It is crucial that all radiographs be scrutinized for evidence of acetabular dysplasia, as acetabular dysplasia may coexist with FAI or be the primary pathology in a patient presenting with hip pain. Radiographic findings concerning for acetabular dysplasia include an LCEA below 25 degrees and a Tönnis angle

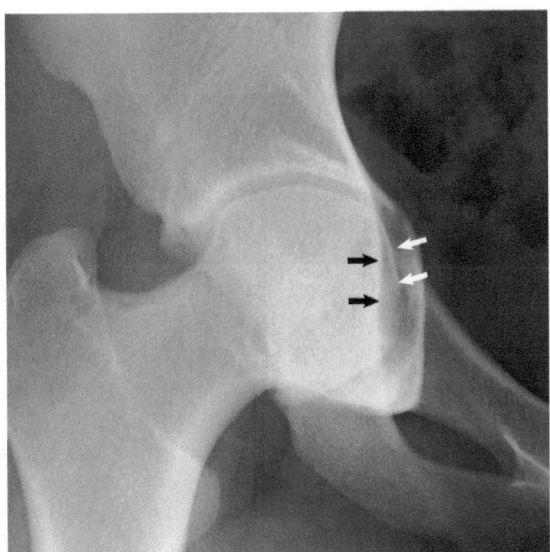

Fig. 80.11 Protrusio acetabuli is diagnosed when the femoral head *(white arrows)* lies medial to the ilioischial line *(black arrows).*

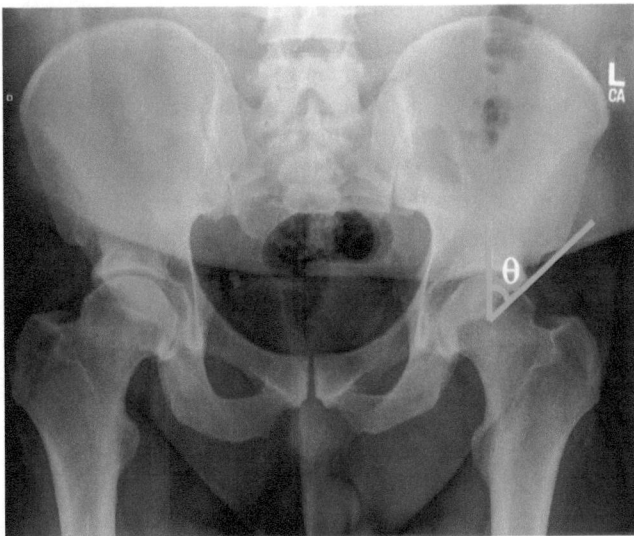

Fig. 80.12 An anteroposterior radiograph is shown for a patient with mixed-type femoroacetabular impingement and increased lateral over-coverage of the acetabulum. The lateral center-edge angle is measured with the vertex at the center of the femoral head. The vertical limb is perpendicular to a horizontal line across the base of the ischium of teardrops and the second limb across the lateral aspect of the acetabulum.

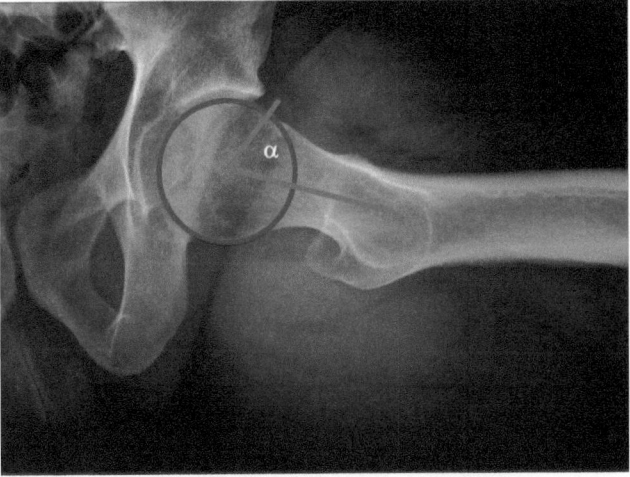

Fig. 80.13 A 90-degree Dunn lateral radiograph shows a patient with cam-type femoroacetabular impingement with depiction of the alpha angle. A circle is outlined over the femoral head, using the posterior aspect of the head to place the circle. The angle is drawn with the vertex at the center of the circle and one line down the femoral neck. The other line bisects the point where the femoral head-neck junction exits the round contour of the circle.

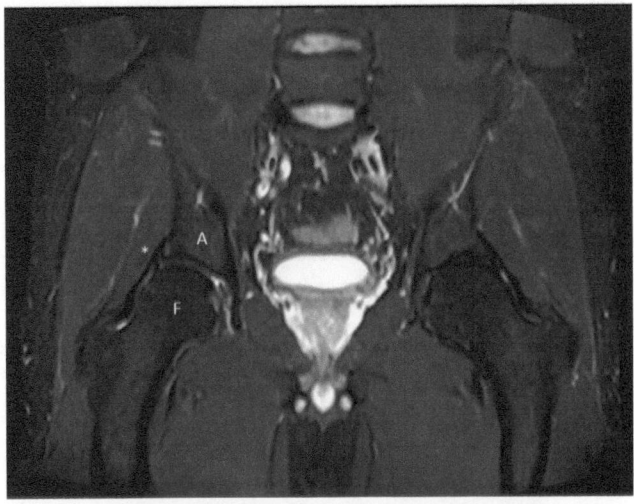

Fig. 80.14 A coronal fat-suppressed T2-weighted magnetic resonance image of the bilateral hips demonstrates an anterosuperior labral tear (*) at the right hip. The labral tear is visualized as a fluid cleft between the acetabular rim and the labral tissue. *A,* Acetabulum; *F,* femoral head.

greater than 10 degrees on the AP pelvic radiograph (see Fig. 80.5) and an ACEA below 20 degrees on the false profile view.[44]

Magnetic Resonance Imaging

MRI is useful in the assessment of osseous morphological abnormalities, labral lesions, cartilage status, and associated soft tissue injuries seen in patients with FAI as a result of compensatory mechanisms.[52] MRI is also useful in alpha-angle measurement and quantification of the cam deformity. If possible, all imaging should be performed using a high-resolution 1.5-Tesla or greater MRI scanner to allow for improved resolution in evaluating the articular cartilage, labrum, and surrounding soft tissues. Saied et al. showed that conventional MRI (cMRI) has better sensitivity for the detection of labral lesions (86%), than for chondral lesions (76%).[53]

Labral degeneration of pincer impingement manifests as increased signal within the labrum on fluid-sensitive MRI sequences, such as T2-weighted and short TI inversion recovery (STIR) sequences.[54] Labral tears are manifest as linear fluid signal intensity extending from the labral surface into the substance of the labrum (Fig. 80.14).[52] True labral tears are commonly seen in the anterosuperior labrum in patients with FAI and must be differentiated from naturally occurring clefts or sublabral recesses, which are usually seen in the inferior labrum and typically do not extend the full thickness of the labrum.[55] Labral hypertrophy can be indicative of underlying acetabular dysplasia.

Increased signal intensity in the anterior acetabulum on T2-weighted images is indicative of subchondral edema and suggests failure of the overlying articular surface (Fig. 80.15). Paralabral cysts and subchondral cysts (Fig. 80.16) are also indirect signs of labral and chondral injury, respectively.[52] Beaulé et al showed that radial images are more sensitive to the presence and size of the cam deformity than conventional oblique axial images and recommended that radial imaging be considered in patients with FAI.[56]

Magnetic Resonance Arthrography

Magnetic resonance arthrography (MRA) is MRI enhanced with intra-articular gadolinium contrast; it allows for the evaluation

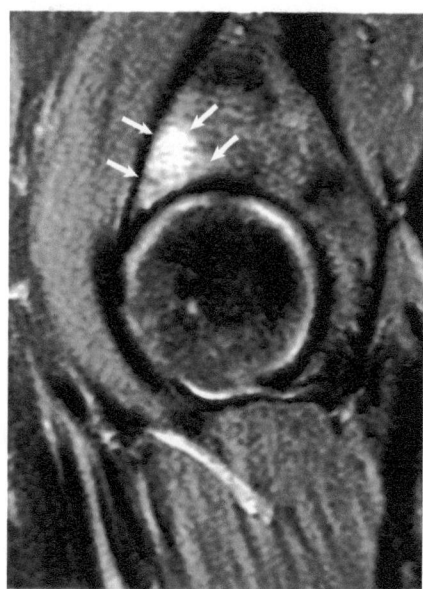

Fig. 80.15 A fat-suppressed, T2-weighted magnetic resonance image of the hip demonstrates subchondral edema (white arrows) in the acetabulum, indicative of insufficiency of the articular surface.

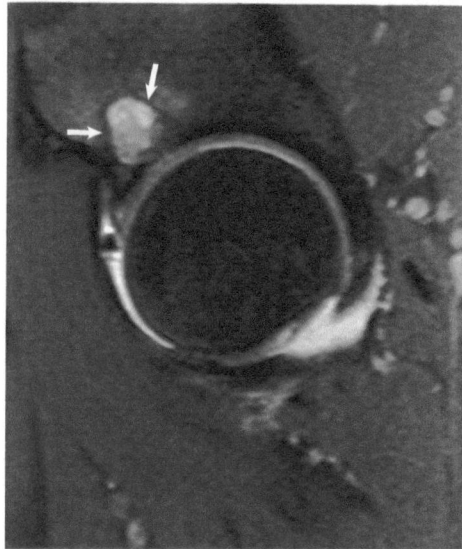

Fig. 80.16 A fat-suppressed, T2-weighted magnetic resonance image of the hip shows a subchondral cyst (white arrows), which may be seen as the result of a chondrolabral injury.

of intra-articular hip pathology.[57] MRA provides better visualization of the joint anatomy owing to easy differentiation of the joint surface and a higher soft tissue contrast obtained by intra-articular gadolinium dilution.[58] Contrast material may be introduced directly by intra-articular injection into the joint, as in direct magnetic resonance arthrography (dMRA), or indirectly by intravenous injection, as in indirect magnetic resonance arthrography (iMRA). The advantages of iMRA over dMRA are that it is simple, less time-consuming, and less invasive; hence it may be more accepted by patients.[53]

The addition of a long-acting anesthetic to the intra-articular gadolinium in dMRA can provide additional diagnostic value. The athlete is asked to perform pain-provoking activities, to generate pain prior to the intra-articular injection of diluted contrast material and local anesthetic agent, and postcontrast images are obtained after the injection. Temporary symptom relief after injection verifies an intra-articular source of pain. The drawback of dMRA as compared with cMRI is that it is invasive, with some patients experiencing postprocedural pain.[59]

Delayed gadolinium-enhanced magnetic resonance imaging of cartilage (dGEMRIC) is a newer imaging technique that involves intravenous gadolinium administration followed by a short period of exercise and subsequent imaging after 60 minutes. The distribution of gadolinium in the cartilage is inversely proportional to its glycosaminoglycan content. Areas of chondral degeneration with decreased glycosaminoglycan will therefore have increased gadolinium concentration.[52] This protocol can be a useful adjunct when there is a concern for articular cartilage degeneration, as preexisting chondral damage is a known risk factor for poor outcome following hip preservation surgery.[60] Hesper et al. recently reported that, with increasing concerns about the use of contrast agents, 3-Tesla MRI with noncontrast T2 mapping may be a useful alternative to dGEMRIC to assess cartilage damage at the chondrolabral junction.[61]

Computed Tomography

CT provides better information regarding the bony architecture than MRI, therefore it can be a useful adjunct in planning bone resection during arthroscopic hip preservation surgery. CT scans can be especially helpful in identifying focal rim lesions such as cephalad retroversion and differentiating these from true acetabular retroversion. They also permit direct quantification of acetabular version and depth. Werner et al.[62] reported that the equatorial-edge angle (EE angle) can be used to measure acetabular retroversion on CT scans and that this was the angle of the acetabular opening with the sagittal plane at the CT slice showing the maximum diameter of the femoral head. Three-dimensional (3D) reconstruction of CT images provides the best picture of the cam deformity (Fig. 80.17). Software programs can be applied to 3D CT images to model areas of impingement and plan the level and amount of bone resection needed.

Ultrasonography

Lerch et al. reported that ultrasound is as reliable as plain radiographs in the diagnosis of cam-type FAI and found no significant difference between the alpha angles on MRI, frog-leg lateral-view radiographs and ultrasound in patients with FAI.[63] However,

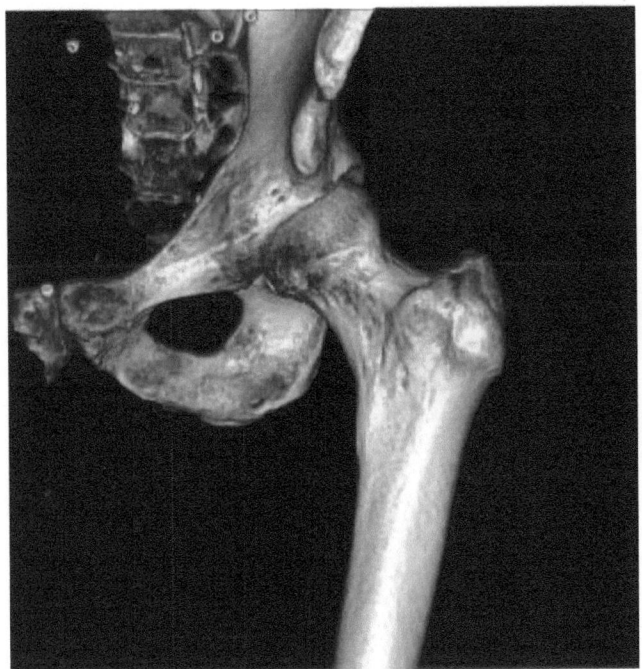

Fig. 80.17 A three-dimensional (3D) reconstruction from a computed tomography scan of a left hip. The 3D image is often used to better localize the bony impingement and determine surgical planning for precise cam resection.

musculoskeletal ultrasonography is considered to be operator-dependent, and hip ultrasound examination is not routinely included in the initial imaging of FAI.

DIAGNOSTIC INTRA-ARTICULAR INJECTION

Intra-articular injection of a local anesthetic agent is a useful adjunctive tool in the diagnosis of FAI. Corticosteroids can be added to the injection as a therapeutic measure. The injection can be performed under ultrasound or fluoroscopic guidance in the office setting or in combination with intra-articular gadolinium administration for MRA. Patients are instructed to perform pain-provoking activities after the injection. Significant or complete relief of pain with injection signifies an intra-articular source of pathology. Patients who have little or no pain relief after injection should be assessed for potential extra-articular sources of impingement, such as subspinal impingement or other pelvic or lumbar spinal pathology. Khan et al. reported that injections performed under ultrasound guidance were better tolerated than those performed under fluoroscopic guidance,[64] although both methods allow for confirmed introduction of the injection into the hip joint.

Management
Nonoperative Management
The mainstay of conservative management of FAI is the early recognition of the condition, identifying athletic activities that provoke pain/symptoms and modifying the activities, as would be appropriate for the patient's level of athletic participation. It includes symptomatic management with anti-inflammatory medications and also physical therapy.[65]

Since FAI and associated reduced hip ROM can result in compensatory mechanisms, with resultant injury to the surrounding musculature and bony structures, physical therapy directed toward improving mobility may provide symptomatic relief. Therapy should also be directed toward improving muscular strength around the hip joint and core muscle strength and, more importantly, should be customized to address the individual needs of patients and their athletic demands. Although a trial of physical therapy may be appropriate in the initial symptomatic management of FAI, there is no evidence to suggest that it will alter the natural history of the condition and the progression of degenerative changes. Also, to date, there are no randomized clinical trials comparing conservative and surgical interventions for FAI.

Operative Management
The decision to proceed with operative treatment is based on a combination of patient history, physical examination, imaging studies, failure of conservative management, and temporary relief with diagnostic intra-articular injection. Successful treatment outcome requires a comprehensive approach, addressing both the primary deformity and the resultant intra-articular damage.

Open Surgical Dislocation
Surgical treatment of FAI was first described utilizing an open vessel-sparing SD with a trochanteric osteotomy.[6] This method is still used in patients with severe deformities such as those secondary to Perthes disease and slipped capital femoral epiphysis, which are associated with relative femoral neck shortening. Distalization of the trochanteric osteotomy would lead to relative lengthening of the femoral neck in such cases.[66] Also, an open procedure may be applicable when a periacetabular or proximal femoral osteotomy is needed, as in cases associated with acetabular dysplasia or femoral neck deformities. Combined hip arthroscopy and a limited open approach for the treatment of cam-type impingement has also been reported.[67]

Hip Arthroscopy
Arthroscopic surgery for the treatment of FAI was first reported by Philippon et al. in 2005[68] and is currently the technique preferred by most surgeons. Patients treated with hip arthroscopy show a trend toward faster recovery.[69] However, incomplete decompression of the impinging lesion is common and is the leading cause of recurrent pain and revision surgery in patients undergoing hip arthroscopy.[60,70]

Hip arthroscopy is typically performed on a traction table, preferably in the supine position (Fig. 80.18), utilizing a minimum of two arthroscopic portals (Fig. 80.19 and Table 80.2). Distraction of the hip joint by at least 10 mm and the use of multiple accessory portals are important in gaining access and improving visualization of the hip joint. The procedure begins with fluoroscopic localization of the anterolateral portal, located 1 cm anterior and 1 cm proximal to the anterolateral border of the greater trochanter. This portal should enter the hip capsule at 12 o'clock. Next, the anterior portal is established under direct visualization, located 1 cm lateral to a vertical line drawn from the anterosuperior iliac spine (ASIS) and 1 cm distal to a horizontal

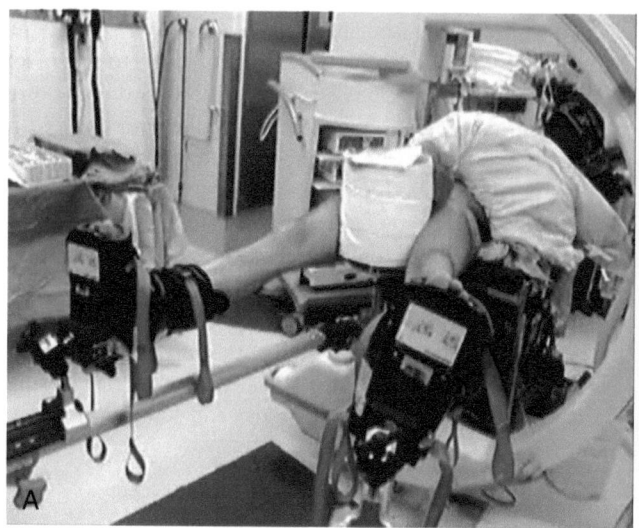
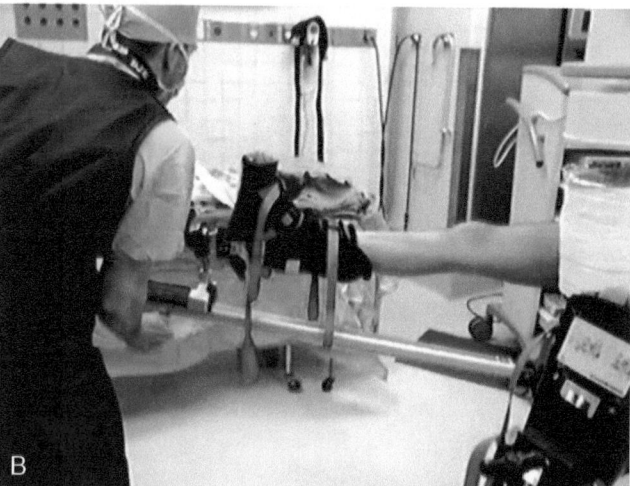

Fig. 80.18 For hip arthroscopy, the patient is positioned supine on a traction table with a well-padded perineal post. (A) The C-arm unit is positioned over the patient to permit intraoperative imaging for portal localization and determination of bony resection of the acetabular rim and femoral osteochondroplasty. (B) The operative leg is placed under traction to allow for access to the hip joint.

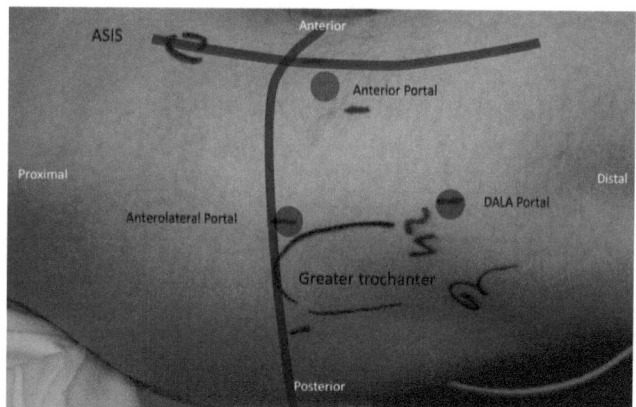

Fig. 80.19 Surface anatomy and preoperative skin markings are shown for a right hip prior to arthroscopy. The anterolateral, anterior, and distal anterolateral accessory *(DALA)* portals are shown in their typical locations relative to lines drawn in reference to the anterosuperior iliac spine *(ASIS)* and greater trochanter.

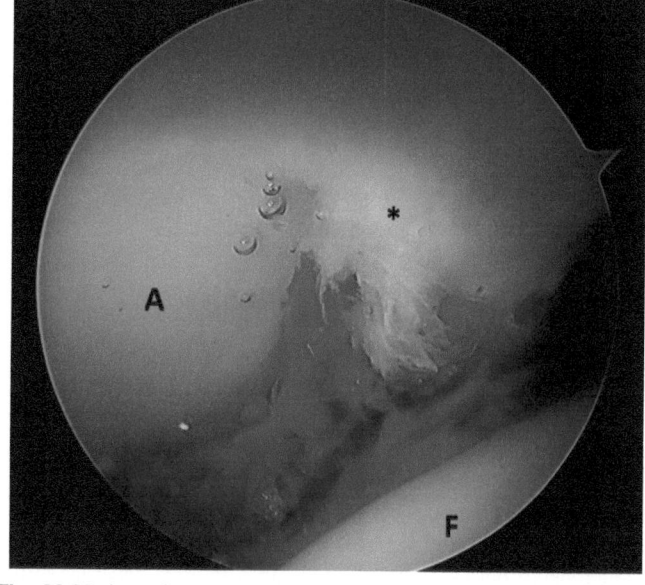

Fig. 80.20 An arthroscopic image is shown through the anterolateral viewing portal from a 70-degree arthroscope visualizing a typical anterosuperior labral tear (*). *A,* Acetabular cartilage; *F,* femoral head cartilage.

TABLE 80.2	Locations of Commonly Used Arthroscopic Portals for Femoroacetabular Impingement Surgery
Arthroscopic Portal	**Location of Portal**
Anterolateral portal	1 cm proximal and 1 cm anterior to the anterolateral border of the greater trochanter
Anterior portal	1 cm lateral to the longitudinal line from the ASIS and 1 cm distal to the horizontal line from the anterolateral portal
Distal anterolateral accessory portal	4–6 cm distal to the anterolateral portal
Posterolateral portal	1 cm proximal and 1 cm posterior to the posterolateral border of the greater trochanter

ASIS, Anterosuperior iliac spine.

line from the anterolateral portal, entering the capsule at 2 o'clock. An interportal capsulotomy can be performed between these portals to allow for improved visualization and access with instruments. Most pathology in the central compartment can be addressed with these portals, as the typical injury pattern is primarily anterior, although a posterolateral portal can be established 1 cm proximal and 1 cm posterior to the posterolateral border of the greater trochanter if access to the posterior joint is needed. The procedure typically begins by addressing the pathology in the central compartment (Fig. 80.20), including the pincer deformity as well as any chondrolabral injury. If a labral tear is identified, the acetabular rim is débrided with a motorized burr and suture anchors are placed to reattach the labrum. Once pathology in the central compartment has been fully addressed, traction is released. With a restored labrum, the suction seal can be visualized as the femoral head is reduced back into the acetabulum.

Then the arthroscope is advanced into the peripheral compartment for decompression of the cam deformity. A distal anterolateral accessory portal, established under direct visualization, may be made 4 to 6 cm distal to the anterolateral portal. The use of extensive capsulotomy (interportal, H-shaped, or T-shaped) has been described to improve access to pathology in both the central and peripheral compartments. The T-type capsulotomy with a short transverse interportal part and a vertical part along the femoral neck to the intertrochanteric line is preferred to avoid damage to the retinacular vessels. Capsular management continues to be an area of controversy in the management of FAI. Although some authors argue that anatomic closure is required to restore the stability of the hip, others do not. Nho and his colleagues reported improved sport-specific outcomes in patients with FAI who underwent complete closure of the T-capsulotomy as opposed to patients who had partial repair.[71] However, Domb et al. found no significant difference in patient-reported outcome scores between patients with repaired and unrepaired capsulotomies after controlling for various confounding variables.[72] Our preference is to perform a T-capsulotomy in most cases to allow for greater visualization and to routinely perform a capsular closure to limit the risk of postoperative iatrogenic instability.

Central compartment.

Pincer impingement. Acetabuloplasty or rim trimming involves removal of pincer impingement. This is usually done with labral detachment at the chondrolabral junction, which allows access to the acetabular rim for trimming, followed by refixation of the labrum with suture anchors (see Fig. 80.20). It can also be performed without labral detachment in patients with an intact chondrolabral junction. The extent of resection should be determined preoperatively from the baseline imaging studies, and intraoperative fluoroscopy helps to monitor the amount of resection. Care must be taken to prevent overresection and iatrogenic instability.

Labral injuries. The acetabular labrum is very important in providing stability and maintaining a suction seal at the hip joint. The characteristics of labral injury in FAI depend on the type and duration of impingement. In early cam impingement, the intra-articular damage is mainly caused by the sheer stress between the articular cartilage and the subchondral bone, and the labral pathology is minimal. In contrast, long-standing cam impingement and combined impingement typically lead to intrasubstance tearing and degeneration of the labrum, with insufficient labral tissue available for repair. In the setting of an irreparable labrum, options include selective labral débridement or labral reconstruction with either autograft or allograft tissue. In most primary cases, however, the labrum is repairable back to the acetabular rim with suture anchors (Fig. 80.21).

Chondral injuries. Chondral injuries associated with FAI can range from delamination to full-thickness loss of articular cartilage. Significant chondral injury is a poor prognostic factor and one of the important predictors of continued pain and

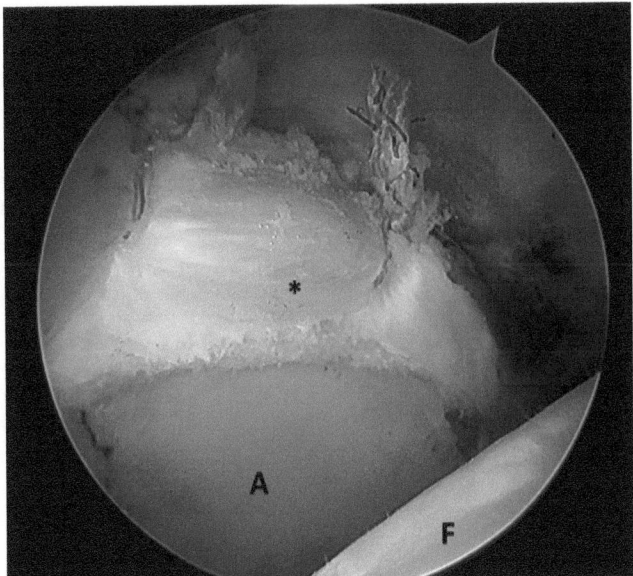

Fig. 80.21 An arthroscopic image through the anterolateral viewing portal shows fixation of the acetabular labrum (*) with two suture anchors, with simple sutures through the torn labrum. *A,* Acetabular cartilage; *F,* femoral head cartilage.

decreased postoperative function after FAI surgery. Detached and unstable flaps pose a clinical challenge. Treatment options include débridement, fixation of the chondral flap with fibrin glue, removal, and microfracture or mosaicplasty. Treatment of hip chondral injuries remains a challenging problem with no treatment yet that clearly produces predictable and successful outcomes.

Peripheral compartment.

The hip must be positioned from extension and internal rotation to flexion and external rotation to permit access to the cam deformity in the peripheral compartment. Effective management of cam impingement depends on proper understanding of the deformity, preoperative determination of the amount of resection, adequate visualization, and full access to the cam deformity during arthroscopy. An adequate resection is confirmed with intraoperative fluoroscopic and dynamic examination (Fig. 80.22). The resection (femoral osteochondroplasty) is typically performed with a high-speed burr (Fig. 80.23). Failure to address the cam deformity adequately, with a residual pistol-grip deformity, is a key factor contributing to treatment failure and necessitating revision hip arthroscopy.[60,73] A final view confirms full resection of the cam deformity, restoration of the suction-seal of the labrum, and reduction of the hip joint (Fig. 80.24).

Rehabilitation

Proper postoperative rehabilitation is a key component of the successful management of FAI. Immediately following surgery, patients are limited to partial weight bearing on the operative hip, allowing approximately 20 pounds of weight on that side. We prefer using a brace in the early postoperative period to prevent flexion past 90 degrees and extension past neutral. Supervised physical therapy starts immediately in the days following surgery. In the first phase over 3 weeks, the goal is to protect the surgical repair and prevent any irritation at the hip joint. Patients are instructed to begin gentle isometric strengthening, including the quadriceps, gluteus, and adductors, as well as light core exercises. Prone lying and stationary bicycle are incorporated to provide stretching, and a continuous passive motion (CPM) machine is prescribed for home use. The brace is discontinued at 3 weeks after surgery, and the patient may begin to wean off his or her crutches. From weeks 3 to 6 after surgery, restoration of a normal gait, balance, and proprioception are the

focus of the rehabilitation program. Hip flexion and gluteus medius strengthening is incorporated. End-range stretching is initiated after week 6, and hip flexor strengthening is advanced. We allow for light elliptical work beginning at week 6 (limited to 3 minutes), and for treadmill use to start at week 12. By week 20, patients may return to running and agility activities, with the addition of plyometrics and cutting activities over the next 4 weeks. In general patients should expect to return to sport at approximately 6 months after surgery. Throughout the

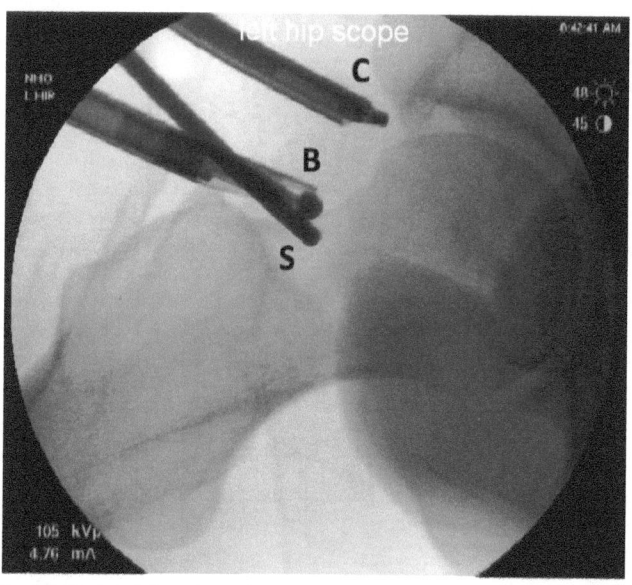

Fig. 80.22 An oblique lateral fluoroscopic view of a right hip while performing a femoral osteochondroplasty with the burr *(B)* along the femoral neck and the 70-degree arthroscopic camera *(C)* viewing the resection. A switching stick *(S)* is used to retract the capsule so as to permit complete access to the cam deformity.

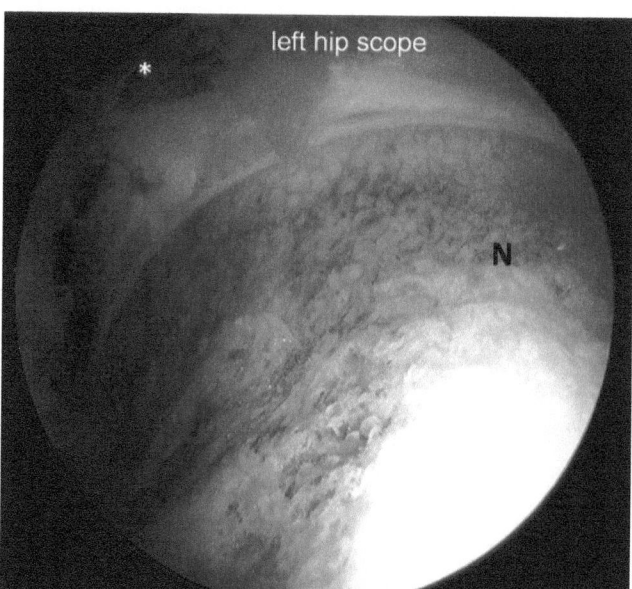

Fig. 80.24 A final arthroscopic image demonstrates complete cam resection with restoration of the femoral head-neck junction between the femoral head and neck *(N)*, repair of the labrum *(*)*, and restoration of the suction seal of the labrum on the femoral head.

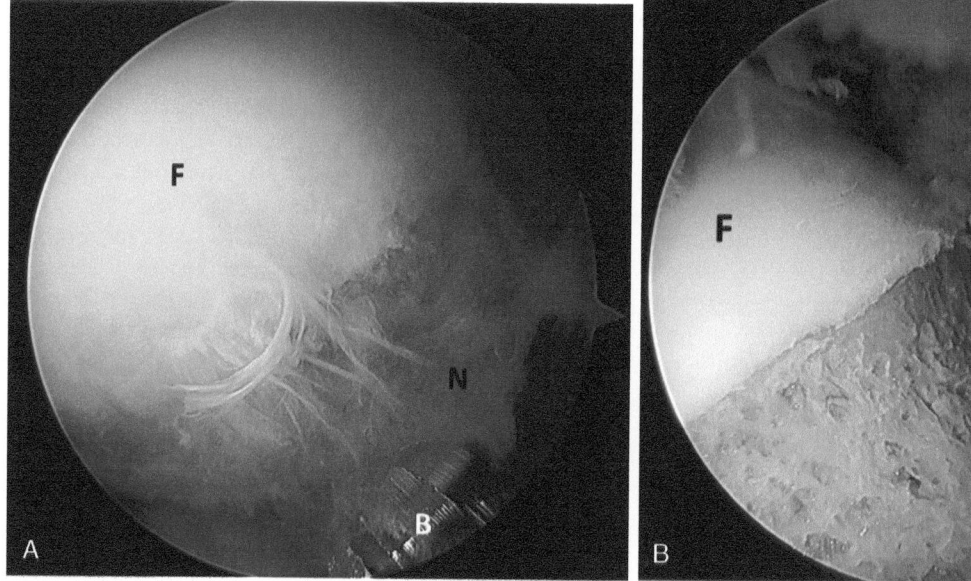

Fig. 80.23 A cam deformity viewed intraoperatively (A) in the peripheral compartment between the femoral head cartilage *(F)* and the transition to the femoral neck *(N)*. A burr *(B)* is used to perform the femoral osteochondroplasty. Following resection (B), there is a smooth transition from the femoral head cartilage to the femoral neck.

rehabilitation process, it is paramount to progress at a gradual pace to avoid inflammatory flares, which may prolong the recovery process.

Outcomes

Proper patient selection is critical for a successful outcome following operative treatment of FAI. Clohisy, in a systematic review on the surgical treatment of FAI, reported that improved hip function after surgery was noted in all studies.[74] Bizzini et al.[75] first published the results of open SD for the treatment of FAI in athletes, reporting that three of five professional hockey players (60%) returned to their previous level of competition. Naal et al.[76] reported that 19 of 22 (86%) professional athletes treated with surgical hip dislocation returned to their previous levels of sporting activity. The outcome of arthroscopic management of FAI among athletes was first published by Philippon et al. They reported on 45 professional athletes with 42 (93%) returning to professional competition and 35 (78%) remaining active in sport at an average follow-up of 1.6 years.[77] Nho et al.[78] reported that 78% of high-level athletes were able to return to competition at the same levels or better after arthroscopic treatment of FAI. Multiple gait studies demonstrate improved hip kinematics following corrective surgery for FAI.[79]

The long-term effect of hip arthroscopy and its potential to alter the natural history of FAI and prevent early degenerative joint disease remain to be determined. The presence of preoperative osteoarthritis (Tönnis grade ≥2) is the strongest predictor of poor outcome following hip arthroscopy. Other factors associated with a poorer outcome include older age, longer duration of symptoms, and worse preoperative pain and functional scores.[80]

COMPLICATIONS

The major complication rate following surgery for FAI ranges from zero to 20% with open dislocation, zero to 17% with the mini-open technique, and 0% to 5% with arthroscopic procedures.[81] Complications of open FAI surgery include osteonecrosis of the femoral head, trochanteric nonunion, symptomatic hardware, and trochanteric bursitis. Surgical hip dislocation is associated with higher morbidity due to the larger exposure of trochanteric osteotomy and its associated problems. Femoral neck fracture due to excessive resection of the cam lesion, inadequate osteochondroplasty, failure of labral refixation, postoperative hip instability, intra-abdominal fluid extravasation, transient neuropraxias, and injury to perineal structures due to the application of traction are complications reported with arthroscopic treatment. Heterotopic ossification limiting hip ROM as well as both superficial and deep wound infections can be encountered with both open and arthroscopic procedures.

CONCLUSIONS

Femoroacetabuluar impingement is a common condition that leads to pain and functional limitations. There have recently been great advances in hip arthroscopy, which is currently the mainstay for surgical treatment of FAI, with high rates of return to sport and normalization of hip joint kinematics.

For a complete list of references, go to ExpertConsult.com.

SELECTED READINGS

Citation:

Levy DM, Kuhns BD, Frank RM, et al. High rate of return to running for athletes after hip arthroscopy for the treatment of femoroacetabular impingement and capsular plication. *Am J Sports Med.* 2017;45(1):127–134.

Level of Evidence:

IV

Summary:

This study investigates a cohort of recreational and competitive runners who underwent hip arthroscopy for the treatment of femoroacetabular impingement by a single fellowship-trained surgeon and evaluates their ability to return to running postoperatively.

Citation:

Frank RM, Ukwuani G, Allison B, et al. High rate of return to yoga for athletes after hip arthroscopy for femoroacetabular impingement syndrome. *Sports Health.* 2018;1941738118757406.

Level of Evidence:

IV

Summary:

This study investigates a cohort of self-identified yoga participants who underwent hip arthroscopy for the treatment of femoroacetabular impingement by a single fellowship-trained surgeon and evaluates their ability to return to yoga practice postoperatively.

Citation:

Frank RM, Ukwuani G, Chahla J, et al. High rate of return to swimming after hip arthroscopy for femoroacetabular impingement. *Arthroscopy.* 2018;34(5):1471–1477.

Level of Evidence:

IV

Summary:

This study investigates a cohort of recreational and competitive swimmers who underwent hip arthroscopy for the treatment of femoroacetabular impingement by a single fellowship-trained surgeon and evaluates their ability to return to swimming practice postoperatively.

Citation:

Frank RM, Ukwuani G, Clapp I, et al. High rate of return to cycling after hip arthroscopy for femoroacetabular impingement syndrome. *Sports Health.* 2017;1941738117747851.

Level of Evidence:

IV

Summary:

This study investigates a cohort of recreational and competitive cyclists who underwent hip arthroscopy for the treatment of femoroacetabular impingement by a single fellowship-trained surgeon and evaluates their ability to return to cycling postoperatively.

Citation:

Kuhns BD, Weber AE, Batko B, et al. A four-phase physical therapy regimen for returning athletes to sport following hip arthroscopy for femoroacetabular impingement with routine capsular closure. *Int J Sports Phys Ther*. 2017;12(4):683–696.

Level of Evidence:

V

Summary:

This clinical commentary presents a four-phase rehabilitation protocol for returning to sport following arthroscopic correction of femoroacetabular impingement with routine capsular closure.

Citation:

Knapik DM, Sheehan J, Nho SJ, et al. Prevalence and impact of hip arthroscopic surgery on future participation in elite American football athletes. *Orthop J Sports Med*. 2018;6(2): 2325967117752307.

Level of Evidence:

III

Summary:

This study, using data from the National Football League (NFL) Combine database, examines the incidence and abnormalities treated with hip arthroscopic surgery as well the impact on future participation in American football athletes invited to the NFL Scouting Combine.

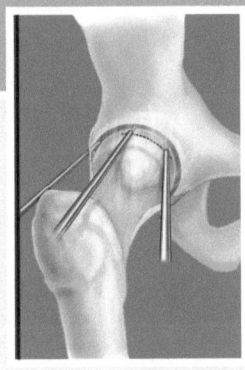

81

Hip Dysplasia and Instability

Jeffrey J. Nepple, John C. Clohisy

OVERVIEW OF PATHOLOGIES

Hip dysplasia, or developmental dysplasia of the hip (DDH), is a common cause of pain in young adults, including athletes. Hip dysplasia encompasses a wide spectrum of disease pathology, from severe dysplasia with hip subluxation/dislocation, to milder deformities often not recognized until adulthood. Several factors appear to play a role in the pathophysiology of hip dysplasia, including acetabular deformity (acetabular dysplasia), femoral deformity (femoral dysplasia), and soft tissue laxity. A thorough understanding of hip dysplasia is important for all clinicians because the history and physical examination of many patients with hip dysplasia can be very similar to other hip disorders, including femoroacetabular impingement (FAI). Hip dysplasia has a relatively clear natural history with progressive damage to the acetabular rim and eventual osteoarthritis. The periacetabular osteotomy (PAO) has become the accepted standard for treatment of acetabular dysplasia to alter the underlying structural hip instability. Good outcomes of PAO have been reported out to 20 years postoperatively. The PAO has undergone significant evolution in the past two decades to improve the recovery from the procedure, including successful return to sporting activities. Increased recognition of the role of labral and articular cartilage pathology in the dysplastic hip has increased the role of hip arthroscopy in this population. Isolated hip arthroscopy in the dysplastic hip is associated with high rates of failure, including some catastrophic complications, including hip dislocation and rapid progression of osteoarthritis. Hip arthroscopy appears to have a role in combination with PAO in patients with significant labral or cartilage pathology. Optimal acetabular correction and bony correction of any associated head-neck offset deformity appear to be important to avoid creating FAI after PAO. Symptomatic hip instability is increasingly recognized as a cause of hip pain in individuals with borderline hip dysplasia or atraumatic hip microinstability. The role of bony correction versus soft tissue plication remains to be better defined in future research. In absence of bony deformity, capsular plication appears to have a role in addition to treatment of labral pathology.

Hip Dysplasia

Hip dysplasia encompasses a complex and variable group of deformities of the hip. Acetabular dysplasia is the most commonly recognized and treated component of hip dysplasia. Classic acetabular dysplasia results from insufficiency of the anterosuperior acetabulum. This results in overload of the anterosuperior acetabular rim, which Klaue et al. termed "acetabular rim syndrome."[1] In the nondysplastic hip, the acetabular labrum functions to seal the hip joint rather than absorb direct load.[2-4] However, in the dysplastic hip, the labrum and acetabular rim are subjected to direct load, which contributes to the typical labrochondral pathology in these locations.[5] The increased forces seen by the anterosuperior labrum may play a role in the development of labral hypertrophy, which is generally but not uniformly present. The hypertrophic labrum may provide increased hip stability in the setting of acetabular dysplasia but also appears susceptible to ultimate overload and tearing.[6] The radiographic appearance of acetabular dysplasia is variable (Fig. 81.1).[7] Severe acetabular dysplasia, with associated hip dislocation or subluxation, is generally well recognized on plain radiographs, with a break in the Shenton line recognized as a simple radiographic marker of hip subluxation. Mild or borderline acetabular dysplasia requires a thorough assessment of hip morphology to avoid missing this diagnosis. The variability of acetabular version in the dysplastic hip and recognition of the variable patterns of deformity are increasingly noted. Nepple et al.[7] defined three common patterns of acetabular deformity in hip dysplasia based on low-dose computed tomography (CT). Anterosuperior, global, and posterosuperior insufficiency of the acetabulum were all fairly common (Fig. 81.2).

The femoral deformity in hip dysplasia is generally less severe and less commonly treated than the acetabular deformity, although in some cases femoral deformity may predominate.[8] Increased femoral anteversion is commonly present in the dysplastic hip and places additional stress on the anterior hip stabilizers. Normal femoral anteversion is approximately 5 to 15 degrees. In the setting of hip dysplasia, hips with anteversion more than 20 degrees above normal are relatively common, with severe increases in femoral anteversion greater than 35 degrees being less common. Coxa valga may be present in some dysplastic hips, although plain radiographic assessment of the femoral neck-shaft angle in high with increased femoral anteversion may give the appearance of more severe coxa valga than is truly present. Wells et al. reported the variability of femoral morphology in the dysplastic hip.[8]

The natural history of acetabular dysplasia has been fairly well defined, compared with other young adult hip disorders. However, this natural history is solely based on radiographic

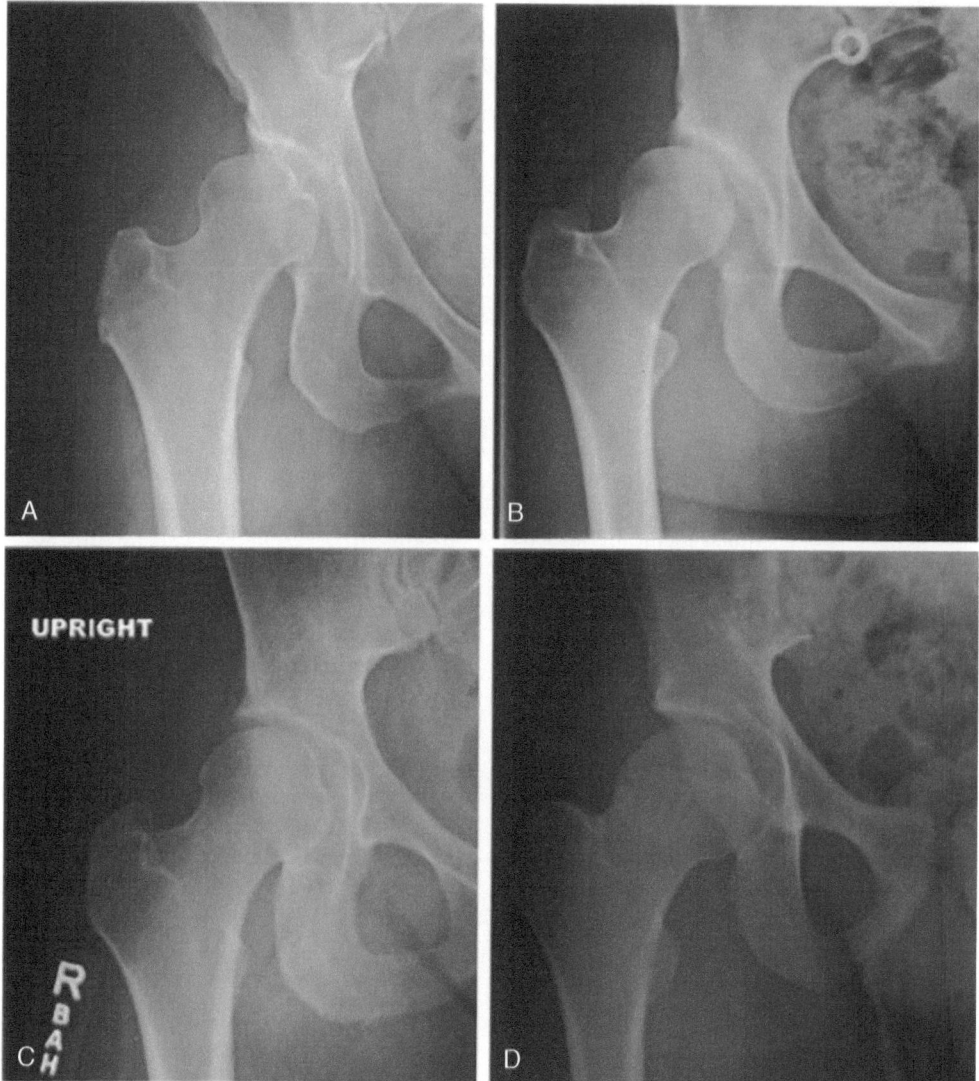

Fig. 81.1 Hip dysplasia variants. (A) Moderate hip dysplasia with associated break in the Shenton line. (B) Moderate hip dysplasia with intact Shenton line. (C) Mild hip dysplasia with normal femoral morphology. (D) Mild hip dysplasia with associated cam morphology of proximal femur. (Reprinted from Nepple JJ, Clohisy JC. The dysplastic and unstable hip: a responsible balance of arthroscopic and open approaches. *Sports Med Arthrosc.* 2015;23[4]:180–186.)

characterization of the lateral center edge angle. The role of other factors, including femoral version, sex, soft tissue laxity, and activity level, remains to be better defined. Wiberg described the lateral center edge angle in his 1939 study on hip dysplasia and suggested that a value less than 20 degrees was linked to osteoarthritis.[9] He reported a cohort of 18 such patients who all developed osteoarthritis at 4- to 29-year follow-up. This threshold appears to capture the lowest 5% of acetabular coverage within a population. It is important to note that deformities of acetabular dysplasia occur less commonly than those of FAI morphology, which are generally 10% to 25%. Cooperman et al.[10,11] subsequently demonstrated similar progression of osteoarthritis among a cohort of 20 hips. However, the rates of osteoarthritis development did not appear to correlate with the severity of dysplasia and are likely influenced by a number of other patient-specific factors. In another key study in 1986, Murphy et al.[12] reported the outcomes of the contralateral hip of 286

patients undergoing total hip arthroplasty for hip dysplasia. All hips with an lateral center edge angle (LCEA) less than 16 degrees developed osteoarthritis by the age of 65. However, not all studies have been in agreement on the link between hip dysplasia and osteoarthritis. Jacobsen et al.[13] followed 81 dysplastic hips over 10 years (compared with controls) and demonstrated no difference in joint space width in hips with dysplasia. Hips with mild dysplasia (LCEA 15 to 25 degrees) did not uniformly develop osteoarthritis during the 10-year period. Lane et al.[14] performed perhaps the best level of evidence in a prospective cohort study. They demonstrated that LCEA less than 30 degrees was associated with a 3.3 times increased risk of osteoarthritis at 8-year follow-up. This supports the potential increased risk for structural instability and hip osteoarthritis in hip with borderline dysplasia (LCEA 20 to 25 degrees). Li et al.[15] demonstrated the potential role of femoral anteversion in the dysplastic hip and found that hip osteoarthritis development was associated with increased

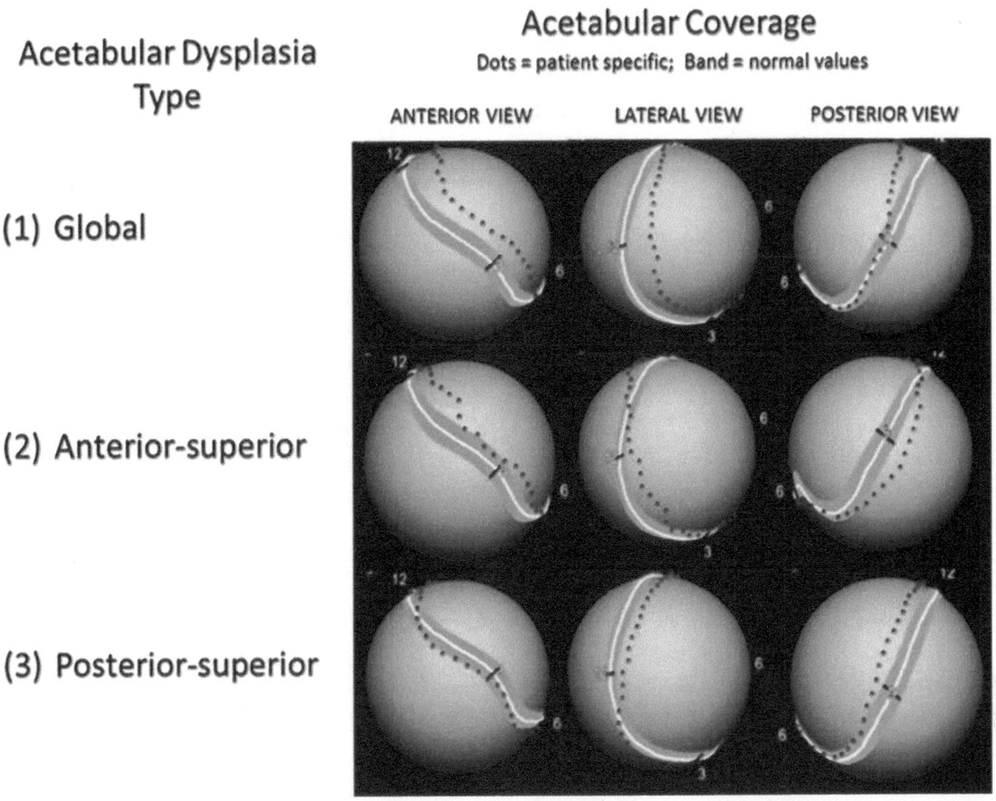

Acetabular Dysplasia Type

Acetabular Coverage
Dots = patient specific; Band = normal values

ANTERIOR VIEW   **LATERAL VIEW**   **POSTERIOR VIEW**

(1) Global

(2) Anterior-superior

(3) Posterior-superior

Fig. 81.2 Three subtypes of bony deficiency in the setting of acetabular dysplasia are common, including global, anterosuperior, and posterosuperior deficiency patterns. (Reprinted from Nepple JJ, Wells J, Ross JR, et al. Three patterns of acetabular deficiency are common in young adult patients with acetabular dysplasia. *Clin Orthop Relat Res.* 2017;475[4]:1037–1044. doi:10.1007/s11999-016-5150-3.)

femoral anteversion (osteoarthritis, mean femoral anteversion 18 degrees; compared with 15 degrees with no osteoarthritis). Combined acetabular and femoral anteversion appears to play a similar role. The authors recommended combined anteversion greater than 40 degrees or femoral anteversion greater than 20 degrees as risk factors for hip osteoarthritis. The natural history of dysplasia in males is less clear. Croft et al.[16] found no association of hip dysplasia (LCEA <25 degrees) with osteoarthritis in a study of 1516 pelvic radiographs.

HISTORY

As in all young adult hip disorders, a comprehensive history and physical examination plays an important role in arriving at a proper diagnosis. Patients with symptomatic acetabular dysplasia typically present with groin pain, although lateral pain secondary to abductor overload is also commonly present. In addition, more than 20% report a history of low back pain.[17] One study reported anterior groin pain in 72% of patients with hip dysplasia and lateral hip pain in 66%. Most patients describe activity-related pain with an insidious onset and gradual progression. Most commonly patients report a duration of symptoms of 1 to 3 years prior to any surgical treatment.[17] Pain is often worsened by prolonged walking or other activities, although in some cases it is worsened by sitting. Most patients report no history of childhood hip disease including DDH. A family history of hip dysplasia or osteoarthritis is present in many patients. Higher

activity level and greater dysplasia severity appear to result in pain development at a younger age.[18] Although definitely more common in females (constituting 72% to 83% in most studies),[17,19] hip dysplasia also occurs in males.

PHYSICAL EXAMINATION

The physical examination in the setting of hip dysplasia can be very similar to that of FAI in many patients. Pain with resisted straight and impingement tests is a marker of intra-articular hip pain, rather than being specific to FAI. Assessment of any abnormalities of gait, including alterations in foot-progression angle, are important to observe. The Trendelenburg sign is an important assessment of hip abductor weakness and is commonly positive in the dysplastic hip, although not specific to this pathology. Supine hip range of motion (ROM) should include assessment of hip flexion, abduction, and adduction, as well as rotational motion in 90 degrees of flexion (internal rotation in flexion [IRF], external rotation in flexion [ERF]). Increased IRF is generally a marker of underlying increased femoral anteversion, rather than the acetabular deformity. Decreased IRF or normal IRF (20 to 30 degrees) is present in many dysplastic hips with associated head-neck junction deformity or normal femoral version and does not rule out associated hip dysplasia. The apprehension test is a useful ancillary test for symptomatic anterior hip instability. This test is performed supine with the hip extended and then the hip is externally rotated. This can easily be accomplished over the side of the exam table or by moving the patient down to the end of the exam table. Pain or apprehension in this position should suggest underlying hip instability. Assessment of internal (psoas) hip snapping is also useful because this is commonly present in the setting of hip flexor overload. Prone examination of internal and external rotation and the Craig test (trochanteric prominence angle) are helpful to provide a clinical estimate of femoral version. Diagnostic hip injections performed under fluoroscopy or ultrasound can serve as a useful extension of the physical examination. Intra-articular injection of anesthetic followed by a repeat physical examination can be useful to localize pain to an intra-articular source.

IMAGING

Traditional classifications of hip dysplasia have focused on differentiating the relatively severe forms of hip dysplasia. The Crowe radiographic classification has classically been used to describe the severity of hip dysplasia, with grade 1 hips having superior subluxation of the femoral head less than 50%, grade 2 hips having subluxation 50% to 75%, grade 3 hips having subluxation 75% to 100%, and grade 4 hips having subluxation greater than 100%.[20] Hartofilakidis provided alternative classification as dysplastic, low dislocation, or high dislocation.[21] A dysplastic hip remains contained within the original acetabulum with varying degrees of subluxation. In low dislocations, there is overlap between the true and false acetabulum, whereas in high dislocations the femoral head is completely outside of the true acetabulum.

Although severe forms of hip dysplasia are commonly recognized at birth or in early childhood, milder forms of acetabular dysplasia commonly present in adolescence or young adulthood. A detailed assessment of the hip imaging is important to recognize milder forms of hip dysplasia. The anteroposterior (AP) pelvis radiograph is the standard for diagnosis of hip dysplasia and represents the historical standard used in studies investigating the natural history of hip dysplasia.[22] The AP pelvis radiograph is preferred over AP hip views, due to the differing appearance of acetabular coverage and version between these views due to the beam location. Recently, many clinicians have favored the standing AP pelvis over supine AP pelvis radiograph because it represents the functional position of the pelvis. Pelvic tilt is commonly variable in this population, with some patients demonstrating anterior pelvic tilt that may allow for more functional acetabular coverage.[23]

The LCEA is the most commonly used radiographic parameter of acetabular dysplasia. Measurement of the LCEA is fairly straightforward when done systematically and has been shown to be highly reliable.[24] Accurate measurement of the LCEA requires identification of the femoral head center, identification of the horizontal reference of the pelvis (using ischial tuberosities or teardrops), and identification of the lateral extent of the acetabular sourcil. The extent of the congruent acetabular sourcil should be used for measurement of the LCEA, rather than the most lateral extent of the entire acetabulum, which may overestimate the LCEA. LCEA measurements less than 20 degrees are generally defined as acetabular dysplasia, with measurements of 15 to 20 degrees representing mild acetabular dysplasia. LCEA values of

20 to 25 degrees define borderline acetabular dysplasia. Measurement of the acetabular inclination, or Tönnis angle, is also a useful adjunct to the LCEA and quantifies the obliquity of the weight-bearing acetabular surface. AI measurements greater than 15 degrees are indicative of dysplasia, whereas values of 10 to 15 degrees are viewed as borderline. Lateralization of the hip joint center is also commonly present even without hip subluxation and places additional stress of the abductor musculature. Assessment of an acetabular version on AP pelvis radiographs should be performed. Verification of normal pelvic rotation is important prior to assessing acetabular version. Similarly, an understanding of the underlying pelvic tilt is also important to take into context because it also alters the appearance of the acetabular rims. Acetabular retroversion has been shown to be present in one in six hips with acetabular dysplasia and appears to be more common in males.

The false profile radiograph was originally described by Lequesne as a useful assessment of anterior coverage of the acetabulum. The false profile radiograph is performed in the upright position with 65 degrees of pelvic rotation compared with the AP pelvis radiograph. The anterior center edge angle (ACEA), similar to the LCEA, is measured on this radiograph, with values less than 20 degrees indicating dysplasia. The relevance of head-neck offset deformities and asphericity is increasingly recognized in cases of combined FAI and dysplasia, as well as for FAI occurring after PAO (Fig. 81.3). Commonly used lateral radiographs most commonly include the 45-degree Dunn view and frog lateral radiographs. Assessment of head-neck junction morphology, including the alpha angle and head-neck offset ratio, is important in hip dysplasia. In addition, correction (or overcorrection) of the acetabular bony deformity may create FAI. The recognition of FAI after PAO was an important point that allowed Ganz and colleagues to refine the concept of FAI.

Magnetic resonance imaging (MRI) plays an important role in the assessment of intra-articular pathology in the setting of hip dysplasia. Similar to in other young adult hip disorders, MR arthrography (MRA) may optimally image the acetabular labrum and cartilage, although 3.0 Tesla scans may minimize the advantage of MRA. In the setting of hip dysplasia, the morphology of the acetabular labrum and its degree of hypertrophy are important to note. The hypertrophic labrum will commonly demonstrate significant intrasubstance degeneration in addition to detachment. The anterosuperior acetabular rim should be scrutinized for articular cartilage changes and associated acetabular rim edema or cyst formation. Similarly, edema in the femoral head is a worrisome finding that may indicate progressive end-stage disease. Particularly in the setting of hip dysplasia, delayed gadolinium-enhanced magnetic resonance imaging of cartilage may improve the assessment of the biochemical quality of articular cartilage compared with referenced standards.

CT represents the "gold standard" for assessment of bony morphology. However, radiation exposure from CT has traditionally limited the utilization of this technology to otherwise young, healthy populations. The development of low-dose CT protocols for hip imaging now allows for more routine utilization of low-dose CT for preoperative planning with a radiation exposure similar to three to four AP pelvis radiographs.[25] These

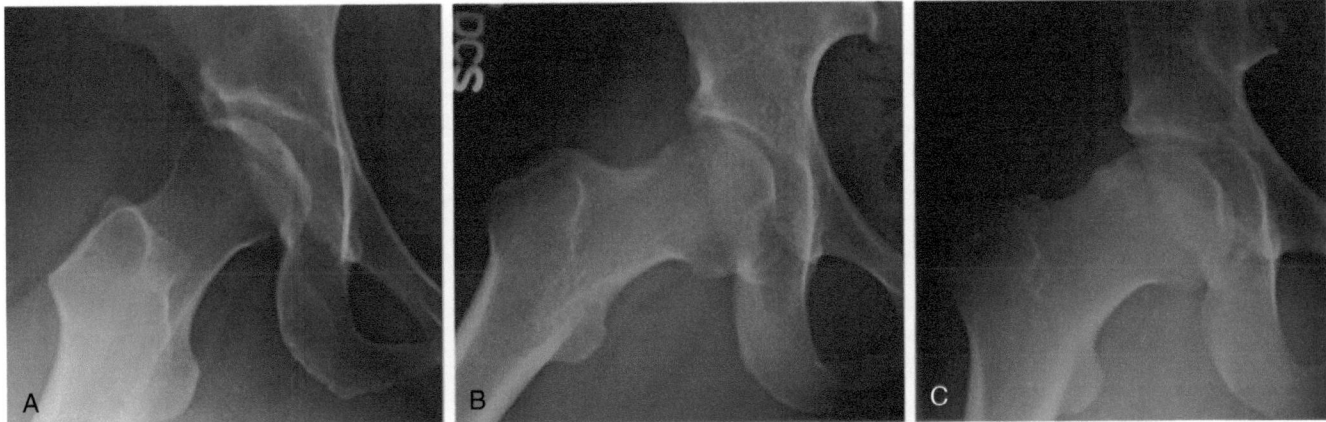

Fig. 81.3 Femoral morphology variants in hip dysplasia. (A) Dysplastic femoral morphology with associated asphericity. (B) Mildly decreased head-neck offset. (C) Severe cam morphology with convexity of head-neck junction in setting of acetabular dysplasia. (Reprinted from Nepple JJ, Clohisy JC. The dysplastic and unstable hip: a responsible balance of arthroscopic and open approaches. *Sports Med Arthrosc.* 2015;23[4]:180–186.)

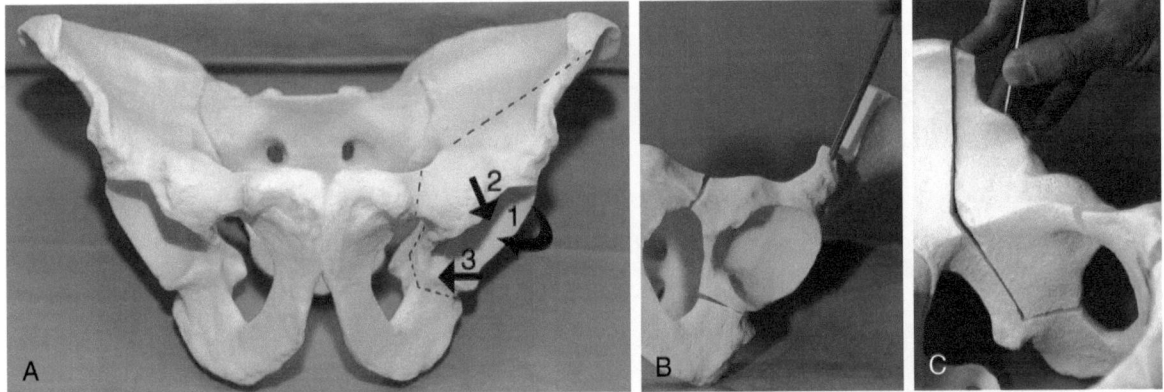

Fig. 81.4 Sawbones model of periacetabular cuts and acetabular reduction of dysplastic hip with PAO. The goal of reorientation is to enhance anterolateral femoral head coverage, to maintain or obtain acetabular anteversion, and to translate the hip center medially if indicated. (A) We perform the acetabular reduction with *(1)* internal rotation (lateral coverage and anteversion), *(2)* forward tilt or extension (anterior coverage), and *(3)* medial translation (medialization of joint center). (B, C) Periacetabular cuts are demonstrated. (Reprinted from Clohisy JC, Barrett SE, Gordon JE, Delgado ED, Schoenecker PL. Periacetabular osteotomy in the treatment of severe acetabular dysplasia. Surgical technique. *J Bone Joint Surg.* 2006;88[suppl 1, Pt 1]:65–83.)

low-dose CT protocols limit radiation exposure through optimization of dosing parameters (kV, mAs) and limiting the field of view (inferior sacroiliac joint to the lesser trochanters). Three-dimensional assessment via low-dose CT is increasingly used in the setting of hip dysplasia and can be particularly useful in the setting of complex or borderline deformity. Comprehensive characterization of the underlying deformity may play a role in improving the precision and accuracy of acetabular correction.

DECISION-MAKING

Hip Dysplasia

Surgical treatment of hip dysplasia most commonly involves correction of acetabular dysplasia through acetabular reorientation. A variety of pelvic osteotomies has been historically used in this population. In 1988 Ganz described the technique for a new Bernese PAO.[26] The PAO uses a modified Smith-Peterson approach to perform cuts of the ischium, pubis, ilium, and posterior column (Fig. 81.4). The posterior column cuts preserve

integrity of the posterior column and provides additional stability to the osteotomy. Since that time the PAO has become the gold-standard in North America for treatment of acetabular dysplasia in the skeletally mature patient. PAO techniques continue to evolve and minimize the recovery from this surgical procedure. Rectus-sparing techniques not requiring transection and repair of the direct head of the rectus tendon are now routinely used. Large multicenter cohort studies have demonstrated low complication rates of the PAO in the hands of experienced surgeon. Zaltz et al.[27] reported a major complication rate of 5.9% (grade 3 or 4 modified Dindo-Clavien classification) in the Academic Network of Conservational Hip Outcomes Research (ANCHOR) PAO cohort. Acetabular correction likely plays an important role in ultimate outcome of PAO, but the optimal outcome remains to be seen (Fig. 81.5). Recent studies have established normative data for acetabular coverage based on three-dimensional imaging.[28] Acetabular correction with residual anteversion or lateral undercoverage would tend to lead to residual hip instability, whereas acetabular correction with acetabular retroversion or lateral

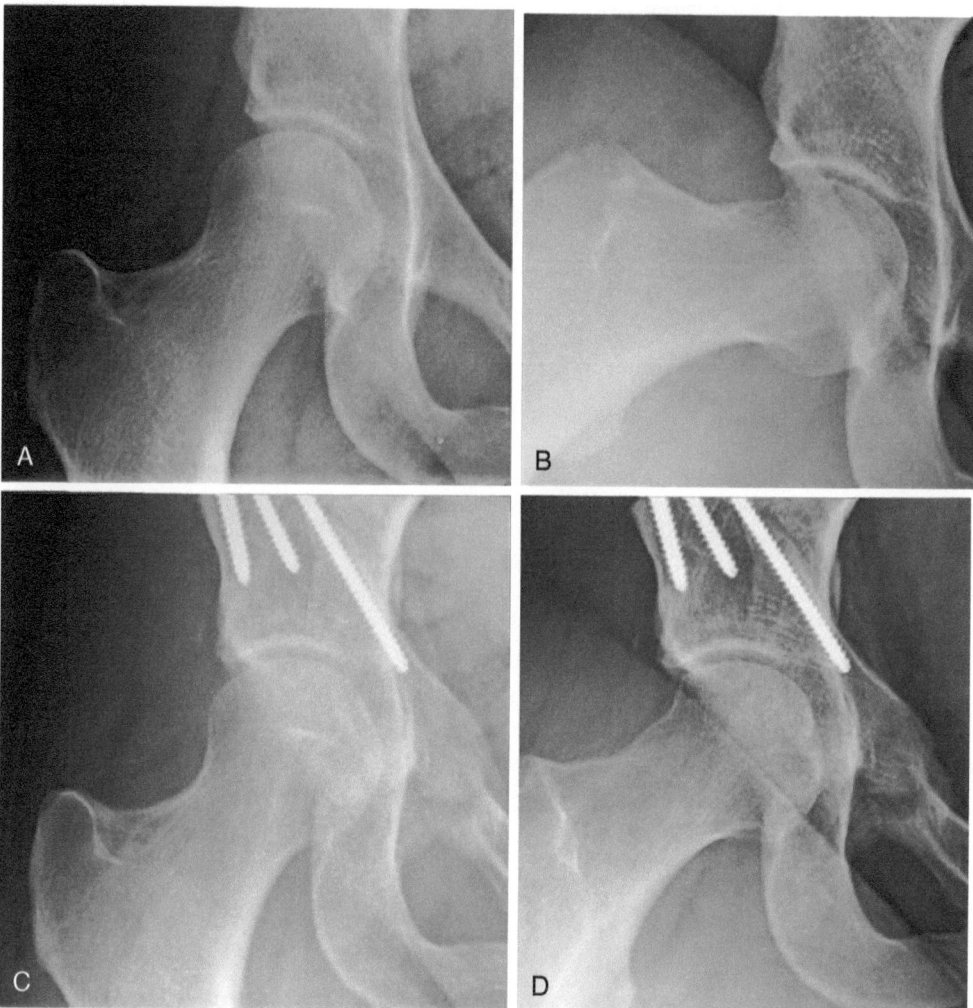

Fig. 81.5 Case example of mild/borderline dysplasia treated with periacetabular osteotomy (PAO). (A and B) Preoperative radiographs of a 23-year-old female patient with persistent right hip pain after previous hip arthroscopy with labral débridement, attempted osteoplasty, and unrepaired capsulotomy; (C and D) Postoperative radiographs 1 year after PAO with correction of underlying dysplasia and excellent clinical outcome.

overcoverage would tend to lead to FAI and ROM limitations. Fluoroscopic or plain radiographic assessment of correction before and after final fixation of the PAO is critical to optimize correction. It is important to ensure a horizontal reference of the pelvis is correct. In addition, it is important to understand the potential differences in acetabular wall projections between a fluoroscopic AP hip view and an AP pelvis view. The AP hip view will tend to make the acetabulum appear more anteverted than the AP pelvis view.

PAO is now commonly combined with other procedures in many patients in an attempt to optimize outcome. Significant labral and chondral pathology appears to be present in many, but not all, symptomatic dysplastic hips. Ross et al.[29] reported greater than 60% rates of labral and acetabular cartilage pathology requiring treatment in an early cohort undergoing hip arthroscopy and PAO. Increasing dysplasia severity was associated with more severe intra-articular pathology. Younger patients earlier in the disease pathophysiology may have pain secondary to dysplasia without developing structural damage to the labrum or articular cartilage. On the other hand, treatment of labral and chondral

pathology in addition to PAO may have a role in optimizing the outcomes of PAO. MRI (or MRA) is routinely used to screen for significant labrochondral pathology. In addition, the presence of sharp groin pain and mechanical symptoms should also raise concern for underlying intra-articular pathology. In cases of mild to moderate dysplasia, hip arthroscopy has a growing role in combination with PAO. Hip arthroscopy can be safely performed in the same setting as PAO. An efficient, central compartment arthroscopy can deal with labral and chondral pathology, while minimizing soft tissue extravasation of fluid that can make the PAO exposure more difficult. Although peripheral compartment work can be performed arthroscopically, we have found it more efficient to perform osteoplasty through the open incision. This approach minimizes additional fluid extravasation during this portion of the procedure and also allows for performance of the osteoplasty after the PAO correction. Hip arthroscopy combined with PAO in this manner appears to demonstrate no significant increase in complication rates compared with PAO alone. Performing the osteoplasty after the PAO correction allows for head-neck offset recontouring to be adjusted depending on the

ROM and minimize the risk of FAI after PAO. In the setting of severe acetabular dysplasia, hip arthroscopy can be more challenging and we prefer open arthrotomy to treat labral pathology.

The role of hip arthroscopy in the setting of acetabular dysplasia has evolved significantly over the past decade. In general, the use of hip arthroscopy for the treatment of young adult hip disorders has expanded rapidly during this period. Early reports of hip arthroscopy in the setting of acetabular dysplasia were encouraging. Byrd et al.[30] reported good results (80% with significant clinical improvement) in a cohort of 16 dysplastic hips and 32 borderline dysplastic hips at 2 years postoperatively (two patients undergoing total hip arthroplasty). However, subsequent reports demonstrated significant complications and inferior outcomes. Parvizi et al.[31] reported significant complications, including postoperative dislocation and rapid progression to osteoarthritis in a cohort of 34 patients. Larson et al.[32] reported a 32% failure rate among a series of 88 dysplastic or borderline dysplastic hips. With modern techniques including labral repair and capsular plication, the failure rate decreased to 18% but remains relatively high at short-term follow-up.

The midterm to long-term outcomes have been reported on the early experience of the PAO. At 20 years after PAO, survivorship is approximately 60%.[33] Compared with the available natural history studies, this would suggest an improvement associated with the PAO, although further studies will continue to establish the role of PAO in altering the natural history. The ANCHOR prospective multicenter cohort of PAO reported 2-year outcomes of 391 hips undergoing PAO, including 93% satisfaction with the procedure and major improvements in modified Harris hip score (23.6 point) and hip disability and osteoarthritis outcome score subscales (>20 points on all subscales including pain, activities of daily living, and sports/recreation).[34] In addition, data from our group document excellent long-term survivorship of 92% at 15 years.[44]

Several factors have been associated with inferior outcomes after PAO in these early cohorts. Advanced articular cartilage damage has been associated with inferior outcomes.[33] A post-PAO lateral center edge angle less than 30 or greater than 40 degrees has also been associated with poorer outcome.[35] Other studies have supported undercorrection (including persistent lateralization, extrusion index >20%t, excessive acetabular anteversion, and lateral center edge angle <22 degrees) to be associated with poorer outcome.[33,36,37] FAI after acetabular correction remains to be better defined.[37,38] Albers et al.[37] have demonstrated inferior outcomes and disease progression after PAO when FAI occurs. This included acetabular overcoverage, acetabular retroversion, and lack of head-neck junction osteoplasty in the setting of an aspherical femoral head-neck junction. A detailed assessment of ROM after final fixation of the PAO is important. Satisfactory ROM is generally considered at least 90 degrees of hip flexion and at least 15 degrees of IRF. Consideration of the functional ROM requirements of athletes is also important. In the setting of limited ROM an osteoplasty performed through an open arthrotomy allows for correction of FAI. The anterior inferior iliac spine has been increasingly recognized as a potential source of subspine impingement, which is also relevant to the post-PAO hip. The long-term effect of osteoplasty of outcomes after PAO remains to be seen.

Borderline Dysplasia

Borderline hip dysplasia is a commonly but poorly investigated condition. Several natural history studies indicate that the risk of osteoarthritis in hip dysplasia may extend up to an LCEA of 25 degrees or potentially higher. Borderline hip dysplasia is a commonly used term to refer to patients with LCEA between 20 and 25 degrees. Patients in this subgroup may have symptomatic hip instability, whereas others appear to have symptoms secondary to underlying FAI, or in some cases both instability and impingement. It is important to recognize that measurements in the borderline range are more common than those in the dysplastic range. For the female athlete, particularly in a high hip ROM sport, borderline acetabular coverage is extremely common. In a cross-sectional study of female collegiate athletes, 21% had evidence of dysplasia (LCEA <20 degrees) and an additional 46% had borderline dysplasia (LCEA 20 to 25 degrees).[39] In total, 67% had an LCEA of 25 degrees or less. In a similar study in male collegiate athletes, 7% demonstrated dysplasia and an additional 19% borderline dysplasia.[40] Together these studies emphasize that borderline acetabular dysplasia is present in approximately three times as many hips as true acetabular dysplasia. In this population, clinical decision-making remains challenging and requires a thorough understanding of all relevant patient-specific factors to choose the best treatment. Important factors in this population include sex, age, soft tissue laxity (Beighton score), ROM, femoral version, and head-neck morphology. Three-dimensional characterization of acetabular morphology may provide additional information in borderline cases to determine the optimal treatment.

The role of hip arthroscopy versus PAO in the setting of borderline acetabular dysplasia remains controversial. As previously mentioned, Larson et al. reported relatively high rates (greater than 30%) of failure of arthroscopy in the setting of dysplasia or borderline dysplasia.[32] Domb et al.[41] reported the outcomes of 22 patients with borderline acetabular dysplasia (study definition of 18 to 25 degrees) treated with hip arthroscopy and capsular plication at 2 years postoperatively. In this study, good/excellent short-term outcomes were reported in 80% of patients (one patient suffered dislocation postoperatively; none required total hip arthroplasty). Nevertheless, larger studies with longer follow-up that analyze all characteristics of hip instability and impingement are needed to clarify the best treatments in the borderline hip.

Atraumatic Hip Microinstability

The role of soft tissue laxity in the hip continues to be better defined. The role of soft tissue laxity in other joints, including the shoulder and knee, is well established, and only recently has it received significant attention in the hip. Gross hip instability can occur without major trauma but is exceptionally rare. Atraumatic hip microinstability is currently recognized as a clinical disorder. Capsular plication has emerged as a potential treatment. Initially, open capsular plication was used, but as arthroscopic techniques have improved, arthroscopic capsular plication emerged as a common treatment technique. Capsule closure appears to improve early outcomes compared with unrepaired capsulotomy in the setting of hip arthroscopy.[42] Arthroscopic capsular plication techniques are generally performed similar to those of capsular closure with larger bites of the capsular flaps used or with resection of some of the distal capsular flap. Capsular plication with an oblique capsular (distal medial to proximal lateral) shift has been advocated to maximize the effect of the plication.[41]

Early reports of the role of capsular plication in selected patients have been encouraging. Domb et al.[41] reported good results of capsular plication as part of the arthroscopic treatment of a cohort of patients with borderline hip dysplasia. Larson et al.[43] reported excellent outcomes of hip arthroscopy with capsular plication in a cohort of females with Ehlers-Danlos syndrome. Future studies will be important to determine the generalizability of these results. The longevity of capsular plication remains a concern, because recurrent instability from stretching out of plication appears to be an issue with other joint plications such as the shoulder.

For a complete list of references, go to ExpertConsult.com.

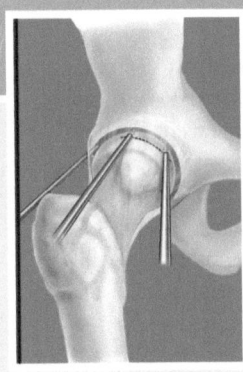

82

Iliopsoas Pathology

Christian N. Anderson

The iliopsoas musculotendinous unit is a powerful hip flexor that is important for normal hip strength and function; however, disorders of the iliopsoas can be a significant source of pain and disability in the athletic population. These conditions include iliopsoas bursitis, tendonitis, impingement, and snapping; they have been shown to be the primary cause of chronic groin pain in 12% to 36% of athletes and are observed in 25% to 30% of athletes presenting with an acute groin injury.[1–4] Acute trauma may result in injury to the musculotendinous unit or avulsion fracture of the lesser trochanter in skeletally immature patients. Athletes with differing iliopsoas pathologies often present with a similar constellation of symptoms and findings on physical exam. Consequently it is important to develop an understanding of the normal anatomy and function of the iliopsoas as well as the pathophysiology of these disorders to accurately determine the diagnosis and formulate an appropriate treatment strategy.

Iliopsoas Anatomy and Function

The iliopsoas tendon-muscle complex is composed of the iliacus, psoas major, and psoas minor muscles (Fig. 82.1).[5] The psoas major is a long fusiform muscle that originates on the T12 to L5 vertebrae and intervertebral disks[5,6] and is innervated by the ventral rami of L1 to L4.[5,7] The iliacus is a triangular fan-shaped muscle composed of the medial, lateral, and ilioinfratrochanteric bundles[5,6,8–10]; it originates from the ilium and sacral ala and is innervated by the femoral nerve (L1-L2).[5,6,8,9] The psoas major and iliacus muscles converge at the level of the L5 to S2 vertebrae to form the iliopsoas muscle.[10] Prior to this convergence, the psoas major tendon originates above the level of the inguinal ligament from within the center of the psoas major muscle.[10] As the tendon courses distally, it rotates clockwise (right hip) and migrates posteriorly within the muscle, lying immediately anterior to the hip joint, and inserts on the lesser trochanter (Fig. 82.2).[10–12] The iliopsoas bursa is positioned between the musculotendinous unit and the bony surfaces of the pelvis and proximal femur. It typically extends from the iliopectineal eminence to the lower portion of the femoral head, with an average length of 5 to 6 cm and width of 3 cm.[10] The psoas minor is a long slender muscle that originates from the vertebral bodies of T12 and L1 and is present in only 60% to 65% of individuals.[13,14] Distally it merges with the iliac fascia and psoas major tendon, and in 90% of specimens it has a firm bony attachment to the iliopectineal eminence.[14]

Significant variability in the iliopsoas musculotendinous unit has been reported in the literature.[6,10–12,15–17] In a cadaveric study, Tatu and colleagues[10] reported the presence of two tendinous structures—the psoas major and iliacus. The medial iliacus muscle bundle was shown to insert onto the iliacus tendon, which progressively converges with the larger and more medial psoas major tendon.[10] The lateral muscle bundle of the iliacus courses distally, without any tendinous attachments, and inserts on the anterior surface of the lesser trochanter and infratrochanteric ridge.[10] These findings were corroborated in a study by Guillin and colleagues[9] using ultrasound (US) to map the iliopsoas anatomy. Conversely, in a study utilizing magnetic resonance imaging (MRI) with cadaveric correlation, Polster and coworkers[15] noted the medial iliacus bundle merged directly into the psoas major tendon, whereas the medialmost fibers of the lateral iliacus bundle inserted on a distinct thin intramuscular tendon. Philippon et al.[6] examined 53 fresh frozen cadavers and demonstrated, at the level of the hip joint, the prevalence of a single-, double-, and triple-banded iliopsoas tendon was noted 28.3%, 64.2%, and 7.5% of the time, respectively. However, in the pediatric population, the presence of two distinct tendons was observed in only 21% of patients undergoing MRI.[16] Gómez-Hoyos and coworkers observed a double (psoas and iliacus) tendinous footprint in 70% and a single tendon in 30% of specimens, which inserted on the anteromedial tip of the lesser trochanter, occupying 19% of its total surface.[11] Conversely, in a separate study by Philippon and coworkers,[12] the iliopsoas insertion was described as having an inverted teardrop shape that occupied the entire posterior surface of the lesser trochanter. Although controversy exists regarding the number of tendons, the relative contributions of the different muscle fibers to each tendon, and the location of the insertion point on the lesser trochanter, the current literature challenges historical descriptions of a single common conjoint tendon.

Reports of communication of the iliopsoas bursa with the hip joint through a congenital defect between the iliofemoral and pubofemoral ligaments are also variable. Tatu and colleagues[10] reported no communication in 14 cadaveric dissections; however, others have observed a direct communication between the joint and bursa in 15% of patients.[18] It is important to consider this communication during diagnostic injections, as the anesthetic material can move between the intra-articular and bursal compartments, thus confounding the results of the test.

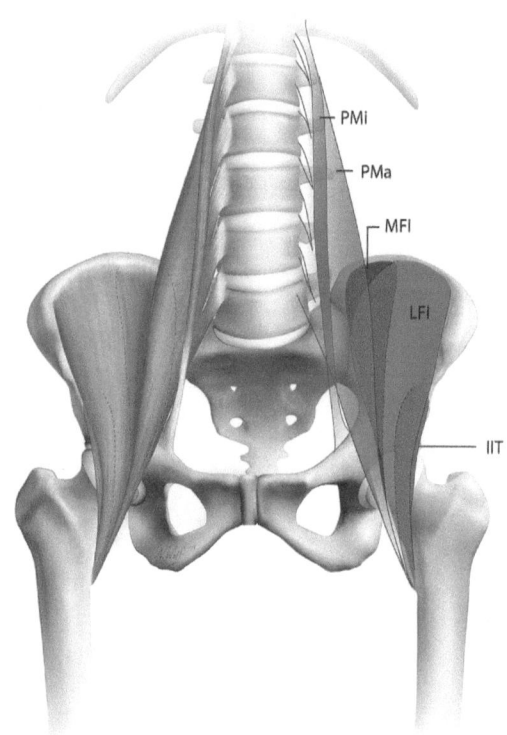

Fig. 82.1 Anteroposterior anatomy of the iliopsoas musculotendinous unit as described by Guillin et al[9] and Tatu et al.[10] *IIT*, Ilio-infratrochanteric muscle; *LFI*, lateral fibers of the iliacus; *MFI*, medial fibers of the iliacus; *PMa*, psoas major; *PMi*, psoas minor. (Copyright 2017, Nicole Wolf, all rights reserved.)

The iliopsoas unit functions primarily as a powerful hip flexor, but it also has important functions in femoral external rotation and with lateral bending, flexion, and balance of the trunk.[19–22] The iliacus and psoas major have been shown to have individual and task-specific activation patterns.[19,21] The iliacus is important for stabilizing the pelvis[17] and for early rapid hip flexion while running.[19] The psoas major is important for sitting in an erect position and for stability of the spine in the frontal plane.[21] Variable contributions of each muscle are observed during situps depending on the angle of hip flexion.[21] The exact function of the psoas minor has not been fully defined, but given its attachment to both the iliac fascia and bony pelvis, it has been hypothesized that it may assist in partially controlling the position and mechanical stability of the underlying iliopsoas as it crosses the femoral head.[14]

Iliopsoas Snapping

Iliopsoas snapping, also known as coxa saltans interna or internal hip snapping, is a disorder characterized by painful audible or palpable snapping of the iliopsoas during hip movement. In 1951, Nunziata and Blumenfled[23] first described the mechanism of internal coxa saltans as snapping of the iliopsoas tendon over the iliopectineal eminence of the pelvis. Since then, dynamic US has been used in several studies to confirm this mechanism as the primary source of iliopsoas snapping.[24–28] Most studies report a sudden "jerky" movement and audible or palpable snap of the

iliopsoas over the iliopectineal eminence as the hip is brought from a position of flexion, abduction, and external rotation (FABER) to extension and neutral. Even so, more recent studies have demonstrated a sudden flipping of the psoas tendon over the iliacus muscle as the source of snapping (Fig. 82.3A–C).[9,24,29] In these studies, dynamic US revealed that as the hip was placed in the FABER position, the iliacus became interposed between the psoas tendon and the superior pubic rami (see Fig. 82.3A). As the hip was brought to neutral, part of the medial iliacus muscle became trapped as the tendon follows a reverse path to its original position (see Fig. 82.3B). The trapped iliacus is suddenly released, resulting in an audible snap of the tendon against the pubic bone (see Fig. 82.3C). Contrary to the original mechanism described by Nunziata and Blumenfeld, the iliopectineal eminence was medial to the psoas tendon and not involved with the observed snapping phenomenon.[29]

Although abnormal movement of the tendon over the bony pelvis is commonly described as the source of the snapping phenomenon, alternative mechanisms have been proposed. Several studies have proposed that soft tissue abnormalities—such as an accessory iliopsoas tendinous slip,[29] a paralabral cyst,[29] and or stenosing tenosynovitis—are the source of snapping.[30] Other authors have determined the iliopsoas snapping occurs over a bony prominence other than the pelvis, such as the lesser trochanters[31] or femoral head.[32] Overall, the exact mechanism of snapping remains controversial, and the lack of consensus regarding the mechanism supports the possibility of several potential etiologies for iliopsoas snapping.

Iliopsoas Bursitis and Tendonitis

Iliopsoas bursitis and tendonitis have been shown to be closely associated with the repetitive pathologic movement of the tendon observed in symptomatic coxa saltans interna.[27,31,33,34] The irregular movement of the tendon during the snapping phenomenon is thought to cause irritation and inflammation of the underlying bursa.[35–37] Even so, some studies have demonstrated no objective abnormality of the bursa in patients undergoing open surgery for symptomatic snapping.[31,38] Nevertheless, these conditions coexist so frequently that Johnson and coworkers[33] suggested they be considered a single entity referred to as "iliopsoas syndrome." Correspondingly, the diagnostic workup and treatment for these conditions are the same.

Iliopsoas Impingement

Iliopsoas impingement (IPI) is a pathomechanical process whereby an excessively tight iliopsoas tendon impinges upon the underlying acetabular labrum, resulting in labral injury.[39,40] This phenomenon was first described by Heyworth and colleagues in 2007[39] in a study (LOE IV) on revision hip arthroscopy; there they noted IPI and corresponding labral injury in 7 of 24 patients. After iliopsoas release at the level of the acetabulum, they noted that the tendon no longer impinged on the anterior labrum during hip extension.[39] Domb and coworkers (LOE IV)[40] further defined the pathophysiology of IPI in a series of patients with direct anterior labral tears at the 3 o'clock position (right hip) in the absence of bony abnormalities. They noted that the labral injury occurred directly beneath the iliopsoas tendon at the

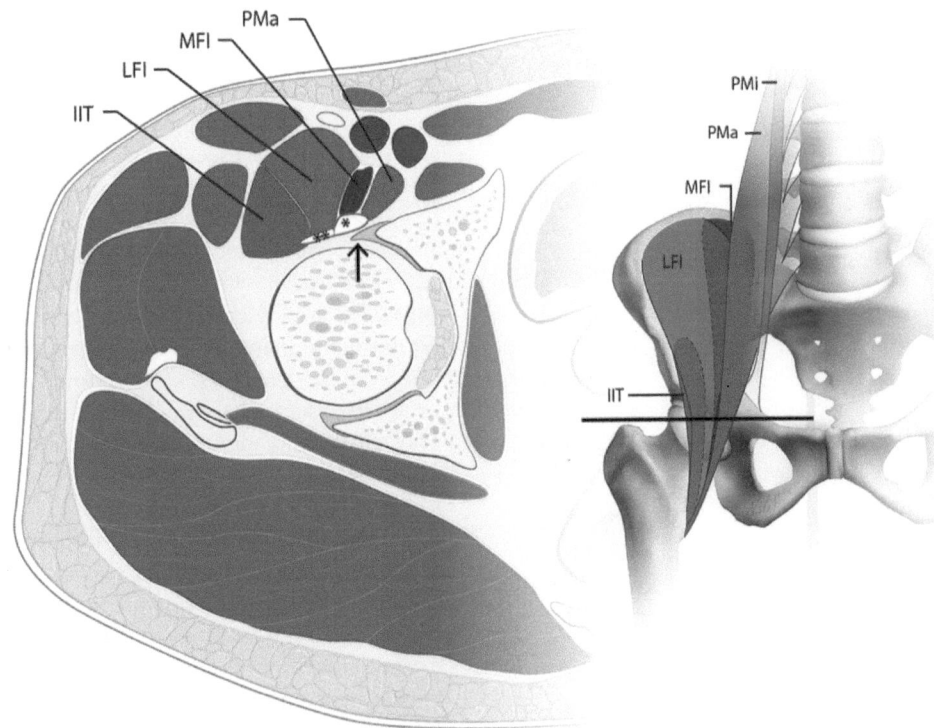

Fig. 82.2 Cross-sectional anatomy of the iliopsoas as described by Guillin et al[9] and Tatu et al.[10] The plane *(black line)* is through the hip joint, as demonstrated on the AP image. At this level, the iliacus *(**)* and psoas *(*)* tendons are posterior to the iliopsoas muscle bundles and anterior to the hip join and labrum *(arrow)*. *IIT*, Ilio-infratrochanteric muscle; *LFI*, lateral fibers of the iliacus; *MFI*, medial fibers of the iliacus; *PMa*, psoas major; *PMi*, psoas minor. (Copyright 2017, Nicole Wolf, all rights reserved.)

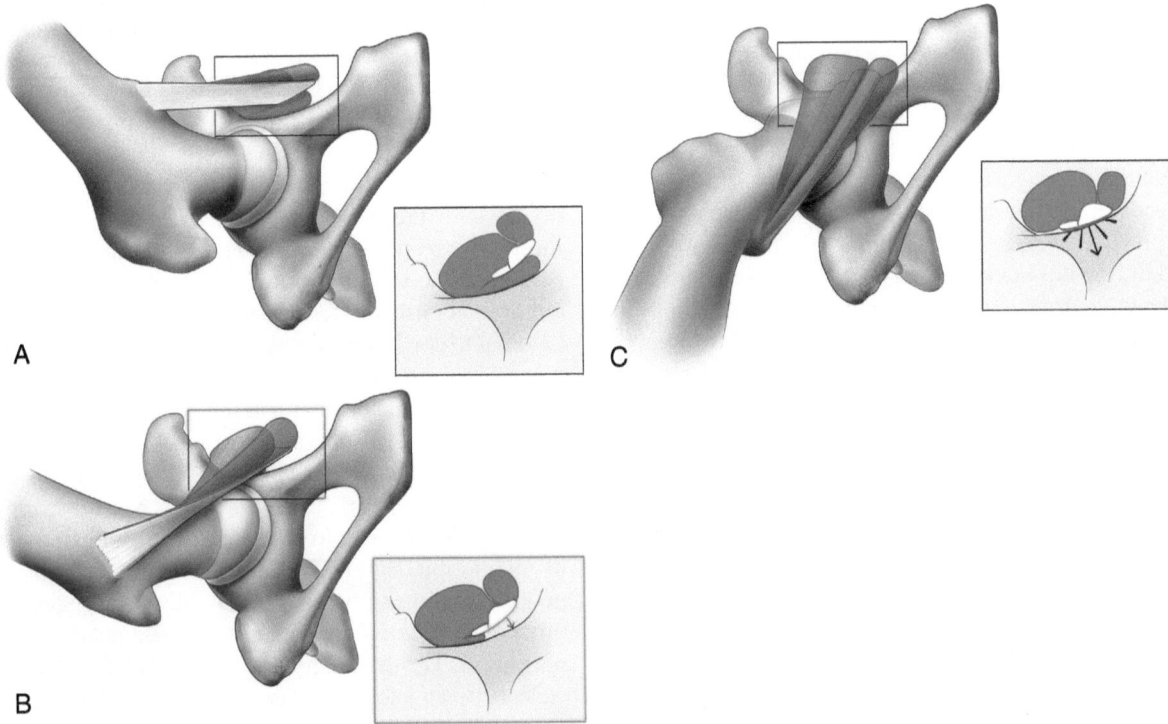

Fig. 82.3 Iliopsoas snapping mechanism as described by Deslandes et al.[29] With the hip flexed, abducted, and externally rotated, the iliacus muscle becomes interposed between the iliopsoas tendon and superior pubic ramus (A). When the hip is then brought to the neutral position, part of the iliacus muscle becomes trapped between the tendon and bone as the tendon follows a reverse path to its resting position on the pubic bone (B). As the hip is brought further into neutral, the trapped muscle suddenly releases, resulting in the tendon snapping against the adjacent pubic ramus (C). (Copyright 2017, Nicole Wolf, all rights reserved.)

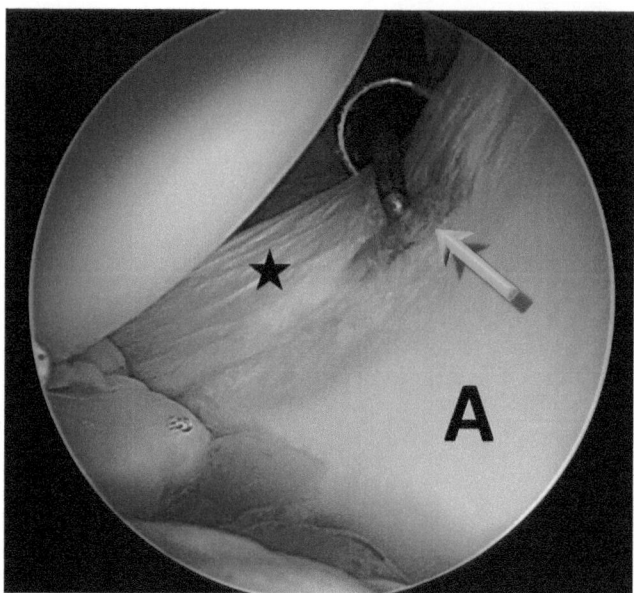

Fig. 82.4 Arthroscopic view from the posterolateral portal of a labral tear at the 3 o'clock position *(green arrow)* in a patient with iliopsoas impingement. The iliopsoas notch, anterior labrum *(star)*, and anterior acetabulum *(A)* are well visualized from this portal.

iliopsoas notch (Fig. 82.4), which significantly differs from the traditional 1 to 2 o'clock location observed in femoroacetabular impingement (FAI).[41,42] Pathologic findings at the time of arthroscopy included labral tearing, labral inflammation (referred to as the *IPI sign*), or adjacent tendinous inflammation and scarring of the tendon to the anterior capsule. The authors concluded that the labral injury was possibly the result of a tight iliopsoas impinging on the anterior labrum or a repetitive traction injury to the labrum from adherence of the tendon to the adjacent capsulolabral complex. Similar to the observations of Heyworth and colleagues, Domb and coworkers found that releasing the tendon decreased compression on the underlying labrum in all cases. A cadaveric study by Yoshio et al.[43] demonstrated that maximal pressure underneath the iliopsoas tendon occurs at the joint level during hip extension, supporting the possibility that excessive pathologic force from the iliopsoas possibly results in labral injury. Although the exact cause of the excessive tightening of the iliopsoas is unknown, Gómez-Hoyos and colleagues[44] observed that lesser trochanteric retroversion was significantly increased in patients with IPI compared with a control group. The authors postulated that because the iliopsoas tendon makes an obtuse angle as it crosses over the iliopectineal eminence, increasing retroversion of the lesser trochanter may elevate contact pressures underneath the tendon and contribute to impingement of the iliopsoas on the labrum.

HISTORY

Iliopsoas Snapping

The diagnosis of iliopsoas snapping begins with a thorough history. Patients often report painful snapping during sporting activities that require significant hip range of motion (ROM), such as dance, soccer, hockey, and football.[24,45] Symptoms can also occur during activities of daily living, such as climbing stairs

or standing from a sitting position.[46] The snapping sensation is accompanied by groin pain, which may radiate into the thigh or top of the knee. A history of acute trauma has been associated with the development of snapping in up to 50% cases.[25] However, patients may also have preexisting asymptomatic snapping that becomes painful after repetitive training activities involving high hip flexion angles.[45] Symptomatic snapping is more common in females than males,[47] and although the true prevalence of this disorder is unknown, symptomatic snapping has been observed in up to 58% of elite ballet dancers.[24] Even so, the prevalence of asymptomatic snapping in the general population has been shown to be as high as 40%.[9] Therefore careful assessment is important in order to determine whether the snapping is symptomatic before proceeding with a treatment plan.

Iliopsoas Impingement

Iliopsoas impingement occurs most frequently in young active females, many who participate in regular sports.[40,48–50] Patients typically present with anterior groin pain that worsens with athletic activities and activities of daily living, such as active hip flexion, prolonged sitting, and getting out of a car.[40,48,49] Iliopsoas snapping is less commonly observed in IPI but has been reported in up to 17% of cases.[48,49]

PHYSICAL EXAM

Iliopsoas Snapping

Physical examination should include a complete musculoskeletal evaluation of the hip and focused specialty tests specific for the suspected diagnosis. The "active iliopsoas snapping test" is the most commonly described examination maneuver for detecting internal hip snapping. This test is performed by having the patient actively move the hip from the FABER position to extension and neutral (Fig. 82.5A–C). The examiner's hand should be placed on the groin to palpate the iliopsoas snapping, which typically occurs with the hip between 30 and 45 degrees of flexion.[51] Iliopsoas strength is assessed by resisted hip flexion with the patient in the sitting position, which may result in groin pain but does not usually recreate snapping. Localized swelling of the inguinal region has been reported in up to 59% of patients with painful internal snapping.[27] Diagnostic US-guided injections of the iliopsoas bursa are useful in the evaluation of iliopsoas snapping (Fig. 82.6).[52] A pre- and postinjection examination can be performed to determine whether the patient experiences pain relief; if so, it supports the diagnosis of painful snapping.[53]

It is important also to evaluate patients for external snapping of the iliotibial band (ITB) over the greater trochanter, which may present in a similar manner to iliopsoas snapping. Patients often report a sensation of the hip dislocating during the snapping event. The examination is the most efficient way to distinguish between internal and external hip snapping. Our preferred exam technique—the "bicycle test"—for determining the presence of external hip snapping is performed by having the patient actively cycle the affected extremity from flexion to extension while lying in the lateral decubitus position (Fig. 82.7A and B). A palpable snap or clunk over the greater trochanter is confirmatory for this diagnosis.

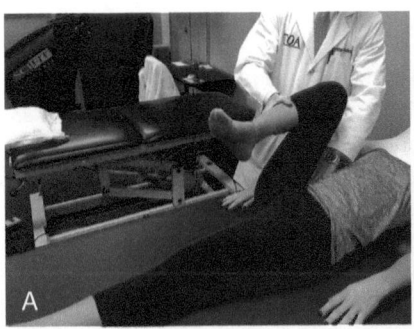
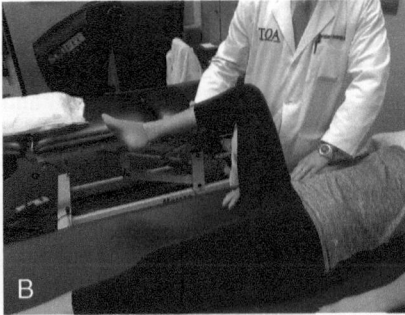
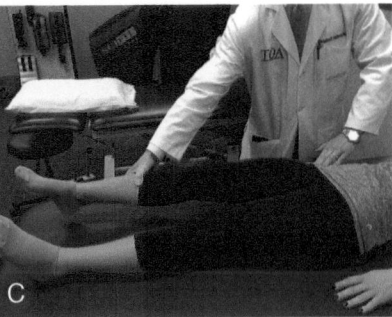

Fig. 82.5 The "active iliopsoas snapping test" for internal snapping of the iliopsoas. The patient actively moves the hip from flexion (A) to abduction and external rotation (B) and then to extension and neutral (C). A palpable clunk or pop is often felt with the examiner's hand placed over the hip.

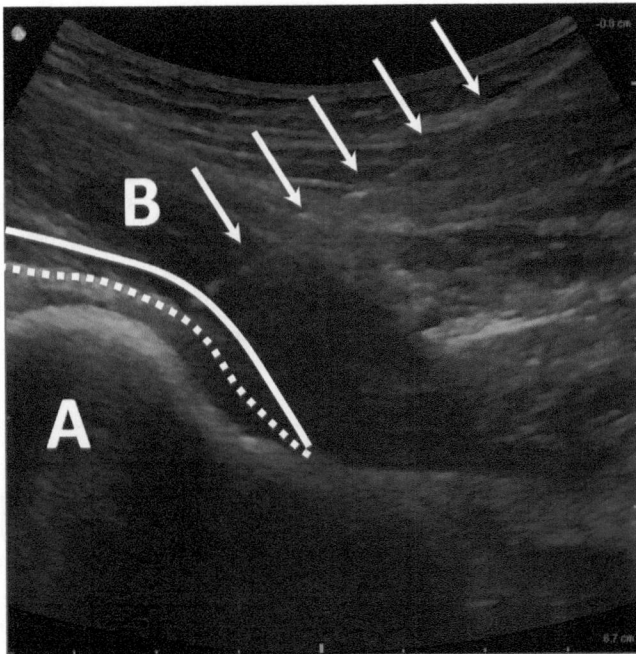

Fig. 82.6 Ultrasound-guided injection of the iliopsoas bursa. The needle trajectory *(arrows)* is toward the femoral head (A). The tip of the needle should penetrate through the iliopsoas muscle (B) into the iliopsoas bursa, which is located between the posterior surface of the iliopsoas *(solid line)* and the joint capsule *(dashed line)*.

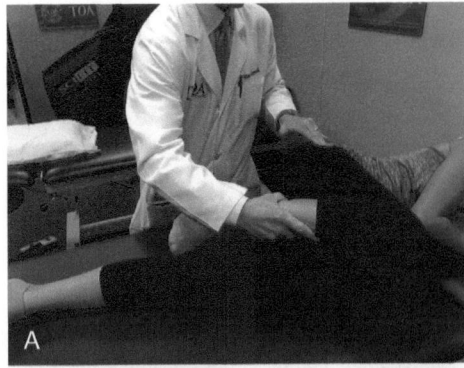
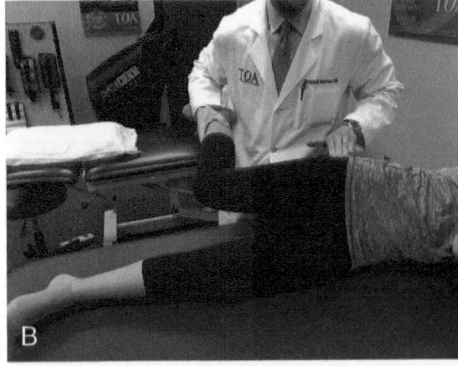

Fig. 82.7 The "bicycle test" for external snapping of the iliotibial band. In the lateral decubitus position, the patient actively flexes (A) and then extends (B) the hip. A palpable, audible, and/or visible clunk can be detected over the greater trochanter.

Iliopsoas Impingement

Patients with iliopsoas impingement typically have a positive impingement test (flexion, adduction, and internal rotation), scour sign (flexion, adduction, and axial compression), and tenderness with manual compression over the iliopsoas.[40,48,49] Approximately half of patients have pain with FABER and resisted straight leg raise testing.[48,49] Intra-articular injections have shown variable results, with some studies reporting transient improvement in 50% of patients[40] while others report improved symptoms in all patients undergoing injection.[48]

IMAGING

Although iliopsoas snapping is typically diagnosed with a thorough history and physical exam, imaging studies can be valuable for confirming the diagnosis and identifying concomitant hip pathology. Radiographic evaluation should begin with anteroposterior (AP) radiographs of the pelvis and lateral hip to rule out acute or chronic osseous abnormalities and evaluate for radiographic signs of FAI. In cases where the source of snapping is uncertain, dynamic US can be used to visualize the iliopsoas tendon or ITB during provocative maneuvers such as the active iliopsoas snapping and bicycle tests.[9,24–29,34] US is also useful in identifying joint effusions and synovitis, rectus femoris tendinopathy, and iliopsoas bursitis and tendonitis.[27,34] In addition to also being able to detect iliopsoas tendinitis and bursitis,[25] MRI is useful in diagnosing associated chondral and labral pathology, which is present in 67% to 100% of patients presenting

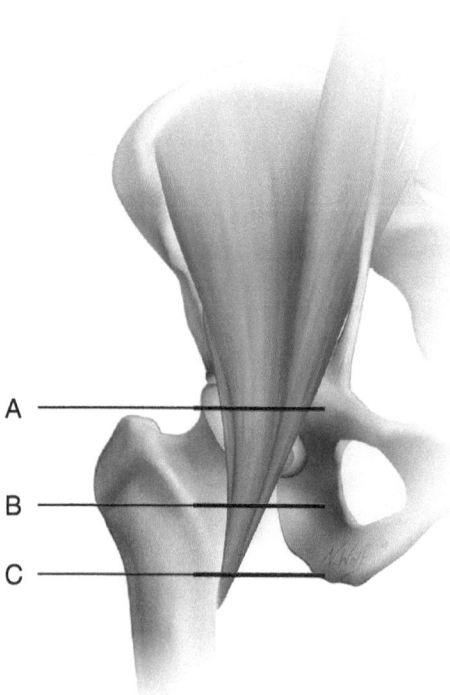

Fig. 82.8 The three described levels of iliopsoas release: central compartment *(A)*, peripheral compartment *(B)*, and lesser trochanter *(C)*. At these levels, the ratio of tendon to muscle is 40% tendon/60% muscle belly, 53% tendon/47% muscle belly, and 60% tendon/40% muscle belly, respectively.[71] (Copyright 2017, Nicole Wolf, all rights reserved.)

with painful iliopsoas snapping.[53–56] MRI can determine the pathologic reason for snapping in up to 100% of patients.[27] For patients with suspected IPI, plain film x-rays may show signs of FAI[49]; however, the most pertinent radiographic finding is a labral tear at or near the 3 o'clock position as seen on MRI.[48]

TREATMENT OPTIONS

The first line of treatment for both iliopsoas snapping and impingement is a conservative program including activity modification, physical therapy, nonsteroidal antiinflammatory drugs (NSAIDs), and corticosteroid injections. Surgical treatment is considered in patients who have failed a 3-month conservative course. The goal of surgical treatment is to lengthen the iliopsoas musculotendinous unit to prevent snapping or mechanical overpressurization of the underlying labrum. Iliopsoas lengthening can be performed by either an open or an arthroscopic approach. Arthroscopic release of the iliopsoas tendon has been described at three locations (Fig. 82.8)—in the central compartment (Fig. 82.9),[49,54,55,57] in the peripheral compartment (Fig. 82.10),[58,59] and at the lesser trochanter (Fig. 82.11).[53,56,60,61] Labral pathology associated with FAI or iliopsoas impingement is typically treated with correction of bony abnormalities followed by labral repair or débridement as indicated by tissue quality at the time of surgery.

POSTOPERATIVE MANAGEMENT

The postoperative rehabilitation program begins immediately after surgery and is a multiphase program that lasts for 25 weeks. The goals of therapy are to protect tissue repairs, preserve ROM, decrease inflammation and pain, and restore normal muscle strength and function. Phase I (0 to 2 weeks) consists of initial exercises, and patients are restricted to 20 lb foot-flat weight bearing with crutches. Passive ROM and stretching exercises are emphasized, with hip flexor stretching and hip extension limited to the neutral position to protect capsular repairs. Patients also begin active ROM, isometric strengthening, stationary bike with no resistance, and early proprioceptive exercises. Patients are advised to take naproxen 500 mg twice daily for 3 weeks to decrease the likelihood of heterotopic ossification and control inflammation during early rehabilitation.[64] In phase II (3 to 12 weeks), patients are weaned off crutches and advanced to intermediate exercises. Hip flexor exercises are started after 6 weeks to allow healing of the released iliopsoas tendon. Exercises include progression of balance and proprioceptive exercises, cardiovascular exercises (stationary bike with resistance and elliptical), and lower extremity strengthening. Phase III (13 to 16 weeks) consists of advanced exercises including plyometric progression, running, and agility drills. Last, patients are advanced to phase IV (17 to 25 weeks), which includes high-level activities such as multiplane agility and sport-specific drills.

RESULTS

Iliopsoas Snapping

Historically an open surgical approach was used for iliopsoas release; however, open surgery has been shown to be associated with increased morbidity and inferior results compared with arthroscopic techniques. In a systematic review of 11 studies, Khan et al.[65] found that patients undergoing open procedures had more postoperative pain, and recurrent snapping occurred in 23% of open compared to 0% of the arthroscopic surgeries. Furthermore, patients who underwent open surgery had a complication rate of 21% compared with 2.3% using arthroscopic techniques.[65] In addition to the lower rate of complications and recurrent snapping, the arthroscopic approach can be used to diagnose and treat concomitant intra-articular pathology. Treatment of associated intra-articular abnormalities in conjunction with iliopsoas snapping, relative to open procedures, may result in improved patient-reported outcomes. Currently, however, there are no direct comparative studies evaluating open versus arthroscopic techniques for iliopsoas lengthening.

Case series studies (LOE IV) evaluating arthroscopic iliopsoas release universally report good to excellent patient reported outcomes (PROs), low recurrence rates, and minimal complications.[53–59] In a study (LOE IV) evaluating athletes with painful iliopsoas snapping, Anderson and Keene[53] reported return to sport in all patients at an average of 9 months after release of the tendon at the lesser trochanter. In a randomized trial (LOE I) and a comparative study (LOE IV), Ilizaliturri and colleagues[66,67] found favorable results with iliopsoas release at either the lesser

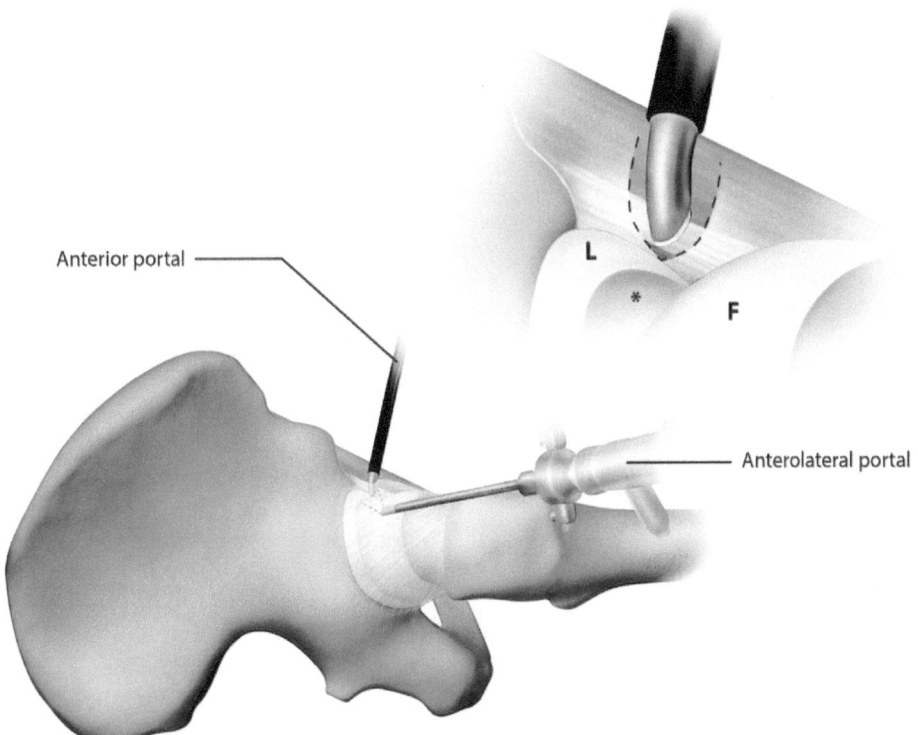

Fig. 82.9 Release of the iliopsoas tendon in the central compartment. With the hip under traction and a 70-degree arthroscope in the anterolateral portal, a banana blade is used to extend the interportal capsulotomy medially *(dashed line)* to expose the iliopsoas tendon, located just anterior to the iliopsoas notch at the 3 o'clock position on the acetabulum *(*)*. The tendon can then be released with the blade or an electrocautery device, taking care to leave the muscular portion of iliopsoas intact. This results in a fractional lengthening of the musculotendinous unit. *F,* Femoral head; *L,* labrum. (Copyright 2017, Nicole Wolf, all rights reserved.)

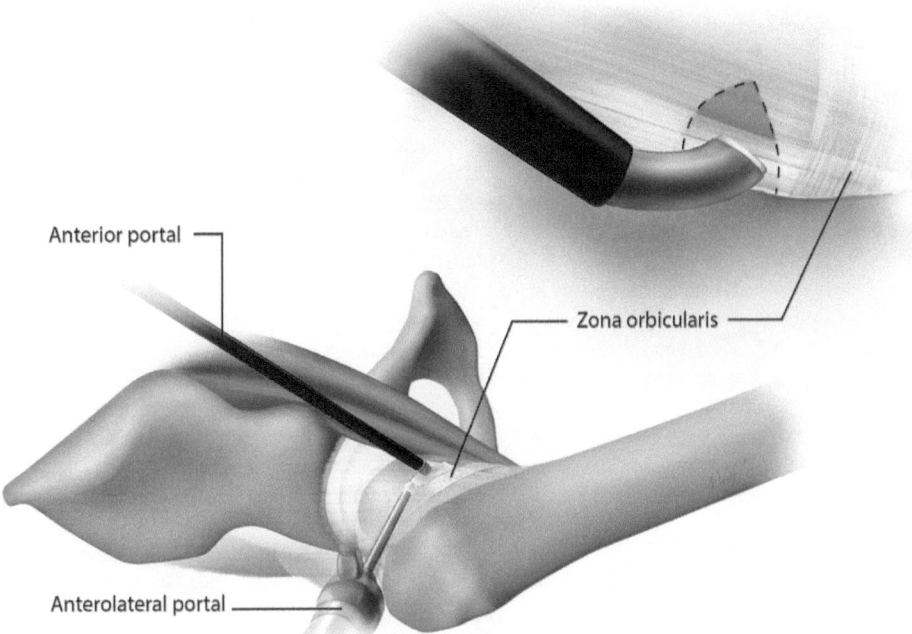

Fig. 82.10 Iliopsoas tenotomy in the peripheral compartment. To facilitate visualization, traction is released and the hip is placed in 30 degrees of flexion. A 30-degree arthroscope is placed in anterolateral portal and pointed anteriorly towards the joint capsule. A small (1 cm) transverse capsulotomy is made lateral to the medial synovial fold and just proximal to the zona orbicularis anteriorly. The tendon is identified through the capsulotomy and then divided with an electrocautery device or banana blade. (Copyright 2017, Nicole Wolf, all rights reserved.)

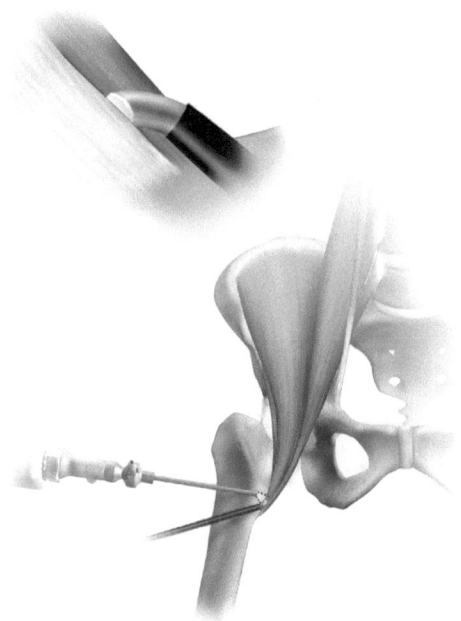

Fig. 82.11 Iliopsoas tendon release at the lesser trochanter. To access the lesser trochanter, the hip is flexed 30 degrees and externally rotated until the lesser trochanter is parallel to the coronal plane of the body and maximally visualized with fluoroscopy. A spinal needle is then advanced anterior and perpendicular to the femur until it reaches the lesser trochanter. A cannula is placed in this position and a second portal is made in a similar manner 5 to 7 cm distal to the first one. The 30-degree arthroscope is then placed in the proximal portal and an electrocautery is used in the distal portal to clear any soft tissues and release the iliopsoas tendon at its insertion on the lesser trochanter. (Copyright 2017, Nicole Wolf, all rights reserved.)

trochanter or in the central compartment, with no significant differences between the techniques. Fabricant and colleagues (LOE IV)[57] studied 67 consecutive patients undergoing iliopsoas release in the central compartment and determined that patients with high femoral anteversion (>25 degrees) had lower modified Harris hip scores (HHS) compared with patients who had normal/low (≤25 degrees) femoral anteversion. These investigators hypothesized that the iliopsoas may act as an important dynamic stabilizer given its anatomic location at the anterior aspect of the hip joint.[57] Even so, Chandrasekaran et al.[68] (LOE IV) demonstrated that although females had higher mean rates of femoral anteversion compared with male patients, they had greater improvements in their PROs. These investigators suggested that with appropriate restoration of other soft tissue constraints, such as the labrum and capsule, fractional lengthening of the iliopsoas can be performed without compromising outcomes.[68] Overall, additional research is necessary to determine predictors of functional and patient-reported outcomes and the best technique of iliopsoas release.

Iliopsoas Impingement

Surgical management of IPI with iliopsoas lengthening and treatment of concurrent labral pathology has demonstrated favorable results in LOE IV studies.[40,49,50] Domb and colleagues,[40] demonstrated that 95% of patients surveyed reported that their physical ability was "much improved" and none reported worse symptoms at an average of 21 months after arthroscopic tendon lengthening and either labral débridement or repair. HHS and hip outcome scores (HOS) were available in eight patients at final follow-up; these demonstrated significant improvements compared with preoperative scores.

 Author's Preferred Technique

Our preferred surgical technique for the treatment of iliopsoas disorders is an arthroscopic release in the central compartment. We typically correct bony abnormalities associated with FAI and treat labral pathology in the central compartment prior to performing release of the iliopsoas tendon to decrease the chance of intra-abdominal fluid extravasation.[62,63] The patient is positioned supine on the operating table against a well-padded perineal post. Both feet are placed in padded traction boots and the operative extremity is positioned in 10 degrees of flexion, 10 degrees of abduction, and neutral rotation. The contralateral extremity is placed in 45 to 60 degrees of abduction, neutral rotation, and neutral flexion and serves as countertraction to the operative leg. The C-arm is placed between the lower extremities. Traction is then incrementally applied to the operative leg and fluoroscopy is used to confirm that at least 1 cm of hip joint distraction has been obtained. Paralysis is used to allow adequate distraction of the hip during traction.

We prefer the use of three portals for access to the central compartment—the anterolateral, midanterior, and posterolateral portals (Fig. 82.12). The anterolateral portal is placed 1 cm anterior to the tip of the greater trochanter using the Seldinger technique. A 17-gauge spinal needle is introduced first, and an air arthrogram is performed to ensure that the needle is within the central compartment. Once central compartment access has been confirmed, a nitinol wire is introduced through the spinal needle and a cannulated trocar is then placed over the guidewire into the central compartment. A 70-degree arthroscope is

introduced into the hip and the pump is not turned on until the midanterior portal has been established. The midanterior portal is placed approximately 2 cm lateral and 2 cm distal to the junctional point formed between a horizontal line drawn medially from the tip of the greater trochanter and a vertical line drawn distally from the anterosuperior iliac spine (ASIS) (see Fig. 82.12). Viewing anteriorly with the arthroscope in the anterolateral portal, the midanterior portal is established under direct visualization by placing the spinal needle through the capsule midway between the labrum and the femoral head. The pump is then turned on and the camera is directed posteriorly to establish the posterolateral portal, which is placed 1 to 2 cm posterior to the greater trochanter. The arthroscope is then switched to the posterolateral portal and viewing anteriorly. A banana blade is used to make an interportal capsulotomy between the anterior and anterolateral portals. For patients with suspected iliopsoas impingement, the posterior portal allows excellent visual inspection of the labrum and chondrolabral junction at the psoas-U (see Fig. 82.4). A probe is introduced through the midanterior and anterolateral portals to allow complete inspection of the labrum and articular surface of the acetabulum. The camera is then switched to the anterolateral portal and, using the banana blade in the midanterior portal, the capsulotomy is extended medially toward the psoas-U. The blade is used with a controlled sawing motion, taking care to section only the joint capsule. It is important to note that the capsulotomy should be performed so that there is adequate tissue on the proximal and distal edges of the capsule to allow a repair at the end of

Author's Preferred Technique—cont'd

the procedure. The psoas tendon is visualized by its distinct glistening fibers and is located immediately anterior to the capsule at the 3 o'clock position on the acetabular clock face. A shaver is then used to resect the tenosynovium circumferentially from around the tendon. The tendon is then bisected using an electrocautery device or banana blade, leaving the muscle fibers intact. Since anatomic studies have shown that up to 72% of individuals may have more than one tendon slip,[6] we routinely search for additional tendons. If a smaller iliacus tendon is encountered first, the larger psoas tendon will be found medial to the iliacus tendon and should be sectioned in a similar manner. Once the tendons have been lengthened, the traction can be released and pathology in the peripheral compartment can be addressed. We routinely perform a capsular repair in the setting of iliopsoas release to minimize the chance of iatrogenic instability.

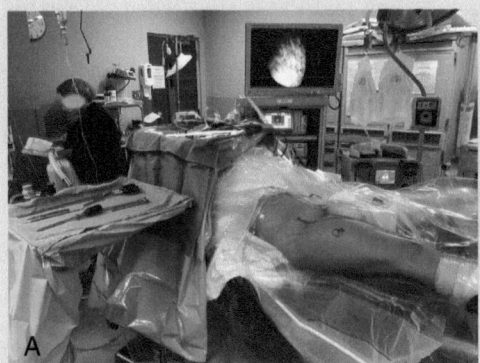 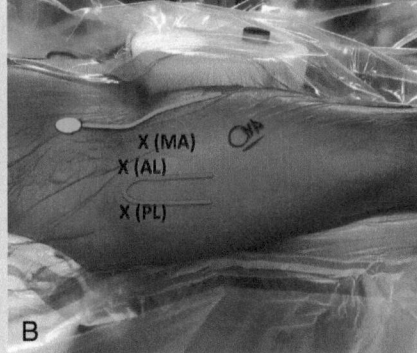

Fig. 82.12 (A) The operating room setup showing (B) the location of the arthroscopy portals. *AL,* Anterolateral; *ASIS,* anterior superior iliac spine; *blue line,* line drawn from the ASIS distally toward the center of the patella; *green oval,* ASIS; *MA,* midanterior; *PL,* posterolateral; *red line,* outline of greater trochanter.

In a case series of 16 patients with a minimum of 6 months of follow-up, Cascio and coworkers[50] demonstrated improvement in HHSs from a mean of 70 to 94 after tendon lengthening with or without labral repair. The authors noted, however, that one patient required revision surgery at 18 months for repair of a labral tear that was not addressed at the initial surgery. Nelson and Keene[49] reported good to excellent results (modified HHS ≥80 points) in 23 of 30 patients undergoing tendon release for IPI. Patients with lower final PROs had avascular necrosis (*n* = 1), progressive degenerative joint disease (*n* = 1), trochanteric bursitis (*n* = 2), or recurrent painful iliopsoas snapping (*n* = 3). Two of the three patients with recurrent symptomatic snapping underwent a second iliopsoas release at the lesser trochanter and subsequently demonstrated good to excellent outcomes 1 year after the revision surgery. Although these Level IV reports are encouraging, further studies with larger sample sizes and long-term follow-up are necessary to determine the optimal treatment for IPI.

COMPLICATIONS

Although the outcomes of iliopsoas release are generally good, several complications specific to this procedure have been reported. Postoperative hip flexor weakness[53,55,56,58,59,61,67,69] and atrophy of the iliopsoas on MRI[69,70] have been observed after tenotomy. There is consensus in the literature that significant weakness occurs in the early postoperative period but also controversy regarding whether this weakness resolves over time. Several studies evaluating posttenotomy iliopsoas strength using a standard 5-point manual muscle testing scale have demonstrated complete resolution of the weakness by 3 to 6 months after surgery.[53,55,56] Furthermore, studies by Ilizaliturri et al.[61,67]

and Hwang et al.[58] demonstrated "improvement" or "recovery" of strength by 8 to 10 weeks; however, no formal strength testing was performed. In contrast, Brandenburg and associates [69] (LOE III) used a dynamometer mounted to a custom test frame to demonstrate a 19% decrease in seated hip flexion strength and noted a 25% decrease in the iliopsoas volume measured on MRI reconstructions compared with the contralateral hip at a mean of 21 months post surgery. The reason for the discrepancy in postsurgical hip flexor strength between these studies is unclear but may involve the differing techniques of measuring strength (hand measurements vs. dynamometer). Interestingly, no significant differences in postoperative hip flexion strength have been observed with tendon release at the different described levels.[65–67] The latter observation can partly be explained by the similar ratio of muscle-to-tendon volume observed at these locations.[71] Consequently each technique results in a comparable volume of muscle fibers remaining intact within the musculotendinous unit, allowing similar forces to be generated for hip flexion.

Other reported complications after iliopsoas release include recurrent snapping,[17,54] fluid extravasation,[62,63,72] and gross hip instability.[73–75] Shu and Safran[17] (LOE V) reported a case of recurrent snapping due to a bifid iliopsoas tendon that was not recognized during release in the peripheral compartment. The recurrent snapping resolved after revision arthroscopy and release of the two tendinous slips. In a Level IV case series, Bitar and coworkers[54] noted that 18% of patients developed recurrent snapping after iliopsoas lengthening in the central compartment. Patients with recurrent snapping had no improvement in PROs and had lower satisfaction compared with those whose snapping had resolved.[54] Although the exact causes of recurrent snapping were not noted, the authors hypothesized that multiple tendon slips, scar tissue formation, or tightness in the muscular portion of the iliopsoas may have contributed.[54] These studies underscore the importance of assessing both preoperative MRIs and intraoperatively for the presence of multiple tendons.

Fluid extravasation is a rare but potentially life-threatening complication that can result in abdominal compartment syndrome.[72] A recent systematic review (LOE IV) of 14 studies by Ekhtiari and coworkers[72] demonstrated that the prevalence of symptomatic abdominal extravasation was 1.6%. They concluded that female sex was the only variable found to increase the risk of fluid extravasation and that iliopsoas tenotomy was not a risk factor.[72] However, in a study evaluating postarthroscopy CT scans, Hinzpeter et al.[62] (LOE IV) demonstrated intra- or retroperitoneal fluid extravasation in 47.5% of asymptomatic patients. In this study, iliopsoas tenotomy was associated with a nonstatistical increase in the mean volume of fluid extravasation.[62] Other risk factors for increasing extravasation were female sex and operative time.[62] Kocher and colleagues[63] performed a survey (LOE IV) for the Multicenter Arthroscopy of the Hip Outcomes Research Network (MAHORN) and determined that the prevalence of symptomatic intra-abdominal fluid extravasation was only 0.16%. In agreement with the study by Hinzpeter, they determined that along with fluid pump pressure, iliopsoas release was a risk factor for developing extravasation.[63] The authors determined that this complication was likely the result of fluid tracking along the iliopsoas sheath following iliopsoas tenotomy.[63] Consequently they recommended performing tendon release at the end of the procedure.[63] Symptoms of intra-abdominal fluid extravasation include abdominal pain, hypotension, hypothermia, abdominal distention, shortness of breath, and cardiopulmonary arrest.[63,76] Using clear arthroscopy drapes (Fig. 82.12), frequently palpating the abdomen, and monitoring the core body temperature are recommended to assist in the earlier detection of this complication.[72] If intra-abdominal extravasation is identified, immediate cessation of the procedure, diuresis, warming of the core temperature, and general surgery consultation are warranted.[72]

Gross hip instability is another rare but potentially devastating complication that has been reported after iliopsoas release.[73–75] A systematic review (LOE IV) by Duplantier and associates[73] determined that 3 of 11 reported cases of hip dislocation or subluxation reported in the literature after hip arthroscopy were associated with iliopsoas release. A labral débridement was performed in one of the three cases,[74] and capsular closures were not reported in any of them.[74,75] The iliopsoas has been hypothesized to function as a dynamic anterior stabilizer of the hip.[43,57] However, it is unclear what its overall contribution to hip stability is relative to the bony anatomy of the acetabulum and other soft tissue stabilizers, such as the capsule, labrum, and ligamentum teres. Given the multiple confounding variables associated with gross hip instability after arthroscopy, further research is needed to determine the role of iliopsoas release in the development of this complication.

FUTURE CONSIDERATIONS

The iliopsoas is an anatomically complex musculotendinous unit that functions primarily as a powerful hip flexor and secondarily as a femoral rotator and stabilizer of the lumbar spine and pelvis. Initial treatment of iliopsoas disorders generally consists of a combination of physical therapy, activity modification, NSAIDs, and corticosteroid injections. If conservative treatment fails, arthroscopic surgery to address the existing pathologic condition has demonstrated encouraging results mostly in Level IV studies. Further studies with higher levels of evidence and longer-term follow-up and studies utilizing validated strength measurement testing and PROs are needed to determine both positive and negative predictors of outcomes. Biomechanical studies are also needed to determine the exact role of the iliopsoas in acting as a dynamic stabilizer to the hip joint.

For a complete list of references, go to ExpertConsult.com.

SELECTED READINGS

Citation:

Philippon MJ, Devitt BM, Campbell KJ, et al. Anatomic variance of the iliopsoas tendon. *Am J Sports Med.* 2014;42(4):807–811.

Level of Evidence:

Descriptive laboratory study

Summary:

This article is an anatomic study of 53 cadavers in which single-, double-, and triple-bundled iliopsoas tendons were noted in 28%, 64%, and 8% of patients, respectively.

Citation:

Deslandes M, Guillin R, Cardinal E. The snapping iliopsoas tendon: new mechanisms using dynamic sonography. *AJR Am J Roentgenol.* 2008;190(3):576–581.

Level of Evidence:

Descriptive imaging study

Summary:

Dynamic US was used in this study to demonstrate that iliopsoas snapping occurs when the iliacus muscle becomes trapped between the iliopsoas tendon and the superior pubic ramus, then suddenly releasing as the hip is brought from FABER to neutral, resulting in the tendon snapping against the bony pelvis.

Citation:

Domb BG, Shindle MK, McArthur B, et al. Iliopsoas impingement: a newly identified cause of labral pathology in the hip. *HSS J.* 2011;7(2):145–150.

Level of Evidence:

IV

Summary:

This article defined the pathophysiology of iliopsoas impingement (IPI), determining that most individuals with IPI had labral tears or bruising at the 3 o'clock position on the acetabulum. Iliopsoas release resulted in decreased compression of the iliopsoas on the underlying labrum and improvements in validated outcome scores.

Citation:

Anderson SA, Keene JS. Results of arthroscopic iliopsoas tendon release in competitive and recreational athletes. *Am J Sports Med.* 2008;36(12):2363–2371.

Level of Evidence:
IV

Summary:
This study evaluated iliopsoas release at the lesser trochanter in 15 athletes with a history of painful iliopsoas snapping. Significant improvements were observed in mHHS and all patients returned to sport within 9 months after surgery.

Citation:
Bitar El YF, Stake CE, Dunne KF, et al. Arthroscopic iliopsoas fractional lengthening for internal snapping of the hip: clinical outcomes with a minimum 2-year follow-up. *Am J Sports Med*. 2014;42(7):1696–1703.

Level of Evidence:
IV

Summary:
This study evaluated 55 patients who underwent iliopsoas release in the central compartment and demonstrated that the majority of patients had resolution of snapping and improvement in validated outcome scores. Patients who did not have resolution of snapping (18%) had no significant improvement in outcomes.

83

Peritrochanteric Disorders

John W. Stelzer, Scott D. Martin

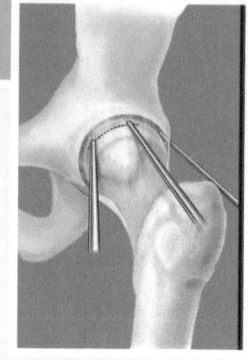

Peritrochanteric disorders often present with hip pain that is challenging for the clinician to diagnose and treat. Recently extra-articular disorders that generate pain throughout the hemipelvis have been defined more clearly as biomechanics and anatomic relationships have become better understood. Although nonoperative therapies are sufficient for the treatment of many peritrochanteric disorders, surgical intervention can be utilized in specific cases. Increasingly, the intra-articular advancements in arthroscopy have been applied to the peritrochanteric space and have shown positive surgical outcomes.[1–4] This chapter will allow the clinician to clearly identify common peritrochanteric disorders, review current treatment modalities, and consider the indications for the use of each treatment option.

GLUTEUS MEDIUS AND MINIMUS TEARS

History

Gluteus medius and minimus tears were first described in 1997 as the "rotator cuff tear of the hip."[5] The tears are commonly seen in aging individuals, with up to 25% of women in their 60s reporting abductor tendon tears.[6] Similar to rotator cuff tear repairs, the abductor tendon tear repairs were initially done with open surgical techniques, which have increasingly been replaced by endoscopic techniques in recent years. The gluteus medius and minimus span from the ilium to the greater trochanter and are innervated by the superior gluteal nerve. Functionally they serve to abduct the hip and stabilize the pelvis during gait.[2,7,8] The gluteus medius and minimus stabilize the pelvis by elevating the contralateral hemipelvis during the stance phase of gait, and if pelvic stabilization is not achieved, a Trendelenburg gait can be appreciated.[7,9] Ultimately proper ambulation and stability can be severely compromised if the gluteal tendons are weak or ruptured.

Physical Examination

Abductor tendon tears are classically insidious or due to trauma, causing avulsion of the tendon from its attachment on the greater trochanter. The patient may present with symptoms of hip abductor weakness, including a Trendelenburg sign, gait, and lurch, which may mimic a leg-length discrepancy from lack of pelvic stabilization. This pelvic instability, especially during the stance phase of gait, results in difficulty ambulating properly and without pain. In addition to pain during activity, the patient can present with lateral hip tenderness over the greater trochanter, with reports of tenderness to palpation or inability to lie on the affected side. Additional physical exam maneuvers that mimic those done in patients with rotator cuff pathology can support the diagnosis of gluteal tendon tears. The hip lag sign has been described with the patient's symptomatic hip passively put into extension and internal rotation with the knee flexed at 90 degrees while lying on their unaffected side. The patient's inability to maintain the position of the leg when the examiner stops supporting the limb could yield sensitivities and specificities for abductor tendon damage as high as 89% and 96%, respectively.[10]

Imaging

A clinical evaluation is paired with magnetic resonance imaging (MRI) findings for diagnosis of the condition (Fig. 83.1), since MRI findings alone may discover incidental gluteal tendon tears in elderly populations.[2,4,7] Radiographs are usually unremarkable, since they do not accurately visualize tendinous structures, and although ultrasound can detect inflammation and gluteal tendon tears, MRI is preferred.

Decision-Making Principles

Although trauma can elicit acute tears, gluteal tendon tears are often insidious in onset, making them difficult to diagnose. Due to their gradual progression of pain and functional limitation, abductor tendon tears are commonly mistaken for chronic processes within the hemipelvis, such as arthritis, bursitis, or radiculopathy from lumbar deterioration.[1,2,4,7–9] Further clinical evaluation and workup of abductor tendon tears can be found in Box 83.1.

Treatment Options

Since gluteal tendon tears can range from partial to full tears, treatment modalities span from conservative to surgical as well. Conservative management should be started in patients initially presenting with signs of abductor tendon weakness. Physical therapy, nonsteroidal antiinflammatory drugs (NSAIDs), and activity modification are preferred to limit inflammation and strengthen the remaining musculature and surrounding hemipelvis. Surgical repair is generally reserved for discrete gluteal tendon tears or tears that have failed previous conservative therapies. Of note, patients with the symptomology of abductor tendon rupture who simply suffer from chronic weakness accompanied by image-supporting muscle atrophy may not be surgical candidates.[2,9]

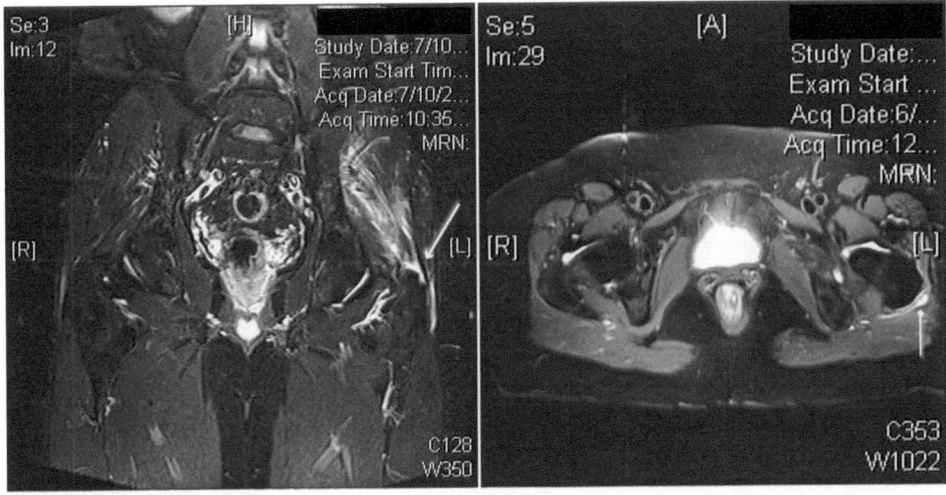

Fig. 83.1 Coronal *(left)* and axial *(right)* T2 magnetic resonance images revealing a gluteus medius tear of the left hip *(white arrows)*. Detachment can usually be seen with tendon retraction superiorly and posteriorly in the coronal and axial views, respectively. (Courtesy of Scott D. Martin, MD, Boston, MA.)

BOX 83.1   Presentation and Management of Gluteus Medius and Minimus Tendon Tears

History
- Lateral hip pain commonly associated with hip abduction weakness
  - Exacerbated by activity or lateral pressure
  - Gait alteration
- Insidious onset
- Increasing prevalence by middle age
- Higher prevalence in women

Physical Examination
- Pain upon palpation of greater trochanter
- Decreased hip abduction strength
- Trendelenburg gait—contralateral pelvic drop through stance phase
- Trendelenburg lurch—compensatory lean toward affected side to prevent pelvic drop
- Trendelenburg sign—inability to balance on affected leg with contralateral pelvic drop

- Hip lag sign—inability to maintain active internal rotation of the hip with slight hip extension

Imaging
- Radiographs often unremarkable
  - Dystrophic calcification
  - Cortical changes at insertion
- Ultrasound can identify tears and secondary inflammation
- MRI is diagnostic (91% accurate, 73% sensitive, and 95% specific)
  - Full- and partial-thickness tears, degree of tendon retraction, and fat atrophy
  - Secondary bursitis

Management
- Conservative management including physical therapy, NSAIDs, activity modification, and cautious anesthetic/corticosteroid injections
- Surgery if failed conservative management

MRI, Magnetic resonance imaging; *NSAIDs*, nonsteroidal antiinflammatory drugs.
See references 1, 2, 4, 8, and 9.

Authors' Preferred Technique

Prior to surgical repair, the anatomic attachments of the abductor tendons must be well understood to reestablish the native anatomy and abductor biomechanics. The complicated insertion sites are best described in relation to the following four facets of the greater trochanter: superoposterior, lateral, anterior, and posterior. The gluteus medius is composed of anterior, middle, and posterior fiber groupings, which attach to two facets on the greater trochanter. The anterior and middle fibers of the gluteus medius insert onto the lateral facet of the greater trochanter, and the posterior fibers insert onto the superoposterior facet.[1,2,4,8] The gluteus minimus, which travels deep to the gluteus medius, attaches at the lateral facet of the greater trochanter and joint capsule. The natural configuration of the attachments of gluteal tendon7 on the greater trochanter forms a tendon-free "bald spot" between the insertion sites.[2,8] The identification of these greater trochanteric landmarks is important in recreating the native anatomy during endoscopic repair (Fig. 83.2).

The peritrochanteric space is accessible with the patient in the lateral decubitus position, utilizing a bean bag or peg board, with the pelvis orthogonal to the floor. Slight abduction of the operative extremity is maintained with a padded bump between the legs and the hip in neutral rotation to reduce tension on the iliotibial band (ITB). The peritrochanteric space is injected with epinephrine-infused saline to further enable access to the space while also maintaining hemostasis. Viewing portals are established on the lateral aspect of the thigh approximately 3 to 4 cm proximal and distal to the greater trochanter. The portals are angled toward the gluteal tendon insertion sites at approximately 45 degrees. Fluoroscopic guidance is used to assist the surgeon with triangulation of the instruments toward the greater trochanter. Anterior and posterior accessory portals can be established by direct visualization upon completion of the placement of the lateral portal (Fig. 83.3).[11]

Once the space has been visualized endoscopically with a pump pressure of approximately 40 mm Hg, further anatomic orientation is possible. The peritrochanteric space is divided into superficial and deep regions. The superficial peritrochanteric space is bordered superficially by the subcutaneous tissue and deep by the musculotendinous sheath, which is made up of the ITB, tensor fascia

Continued

Authors' Preferred Technique—cont'd

lata, and gluteus maximus (Fig. 83.4).[14] The deep peritrochanteric space is accessed with advancement of the scope through the ITB and musculotendinous sheath, which serves as the ceiling to the deep space (Fig. 83.5). The floor of the deep peritrochanteric space is the greater trochanter of the femur. Noteworthy structures within the deep space include the proximally located gluteus medius and minimus tendons, the posteriorly located gluteus maximus muscle belly and tendon, the distally located origin of the vastus lateralis, and the trochanteric bursa.

The gluteus medius and minimus tendons, which retract posteriorly from their attachment sites in full-thickness tears, are identified within the deep peritrochanteric space (Figs. 83.6 and 83.7). Partial-thickness tears are technically more challenging to repair within the deep peritrochanteric space since tendon retraction is limited and the intact tendon crowds the available footprint for anchor placement (Fig. 83.8).

Once the torn structures have been identified and mobilized, the bony footprint is scarified for tendon attachment.[8,12] The senior author prefers a composite 4.75-mm SwiveLock (Arthrex, Inc., Naples, FL) anchor double-loaded with no. 2 FiberWire (Arthrex, Inc.) suture and no. 2 FiberTape (Arthrex, Inc.) for the proximal row of the transosseous equivalent technique. A composite 5.5-mm anchor can be used if bone quality is poor. The sutures are shuttled through the tear with a suture shuttle relay in a horizontal mattress configuration and pulled through a waiting portal. Next, FiberWire is passed through the tendon both anteriorly and posteriorly and put through a separate composite 4.75-mm SwiveLock anchor. The sutures are then tied down using a sliding knot with a Weston knot and multiple half hitches. The second row of anchors, placed at a "dead man's" angle of 45 degrees into the region of the vastus ridge, secure the limbs of the previously tied sutures. This technique provides a tension-free tendon repair (Figs. 83.9–83.13). A similar repair can be accomplished with the aid of a clever hook for passing sutures through the tendon.

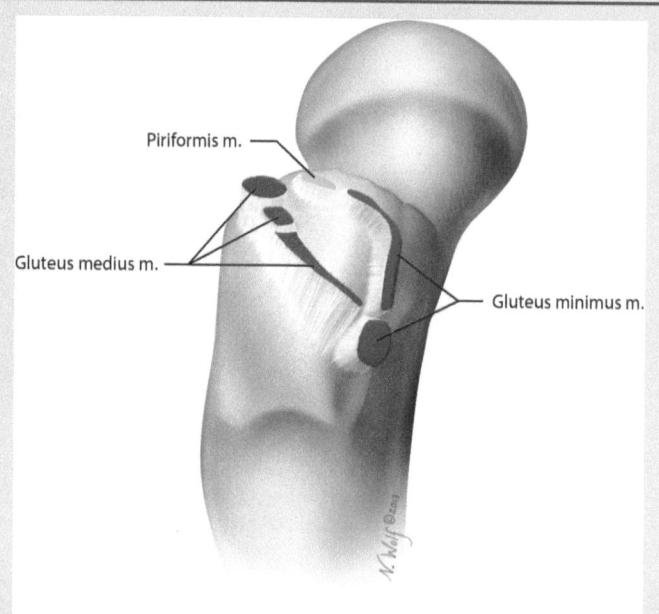

Fig. 83.2 Gluteal tendon insertion sites on the greater trochanter. The anterior and middle fibers of the gluteus medius attach to the lateral facet and the posterior fibers attach to the superoposterior facet *(purple)*. The gluteus minimus attaches on the anterior facet and joint capsule *(blue)*. *m*, muscle. (Illustration by Nicole Wolf, MS; ©2016. Reprinted with permission.)

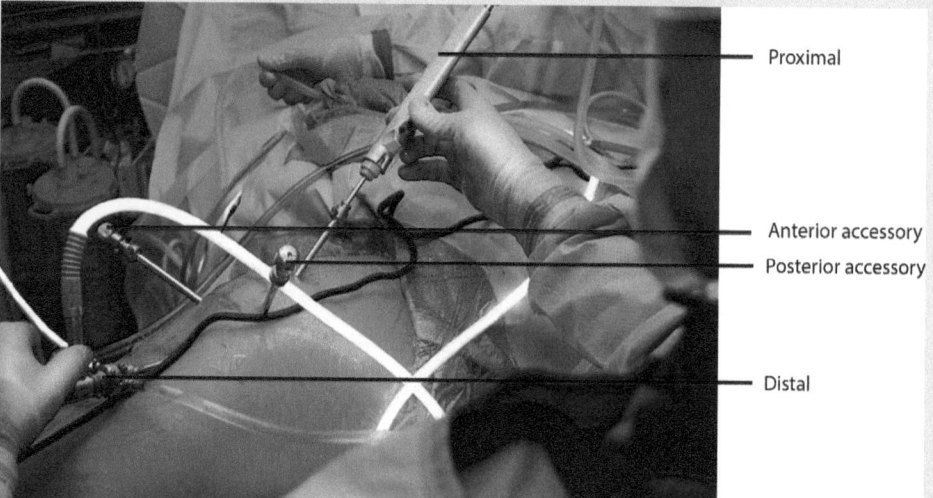

Fig. 83.3 Portal placement. In relation to the greater trochanter the portals are arranged as proximal and distal working portals as well as anterior and posterior accessory portals. (Illustration by Nicole Wolf, MS; ©2016. Reprinted with permission.)

Authors' Preferred Technique—cont'd

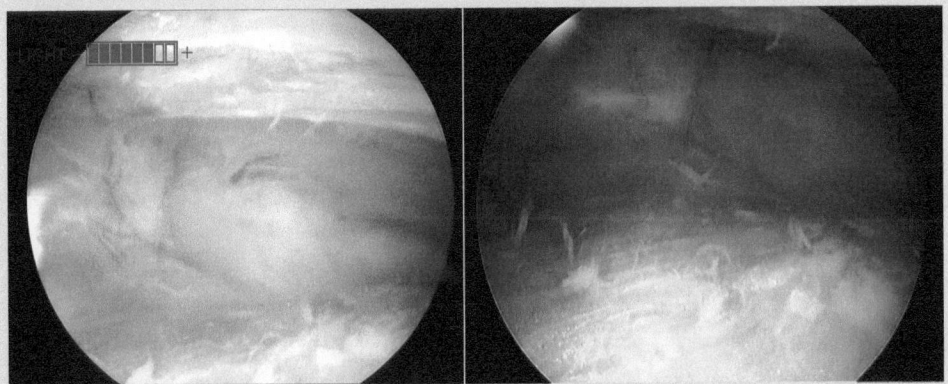

Fig. 83.4 Iliotibial band visualized as the floor of the superficial peritrochanteric space. (Courtesy of Scott D. Martin, MD; Boston, MA.)

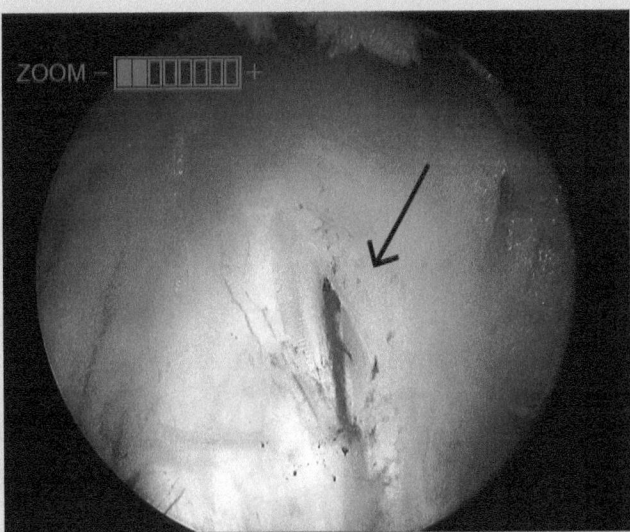

Fig. 83.5 Entry into the deep peritrochanteric space is performed with incision of the iliotibial band *(black arrow)*. (Courtesy of Scott D. Martin, MD, Boston, MA.)

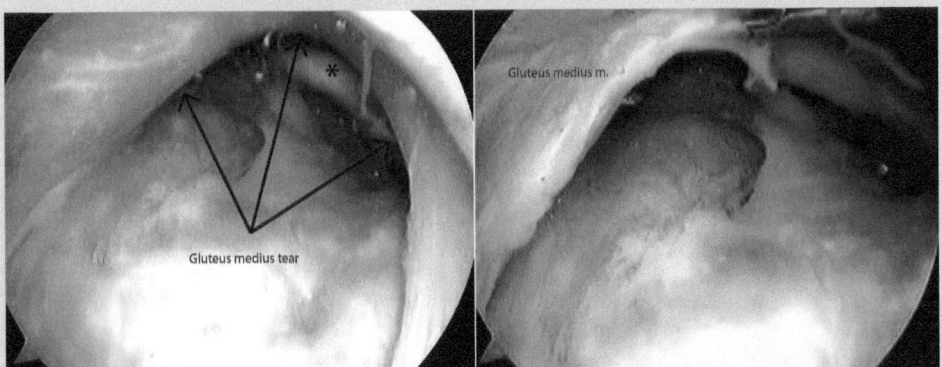

Fig. 83.6 Full-thickness tear of the gluteus medius *(left)* with the gluteus minimus tendon seen beneath it *(asterisk)* and gluteus medius tendon mobilized by a tissue grasper *(right)*. (Courtesy of Scott D. Martin, MD, Boston, MA.)

Continued

Authors' Preferred Technique—cont'd

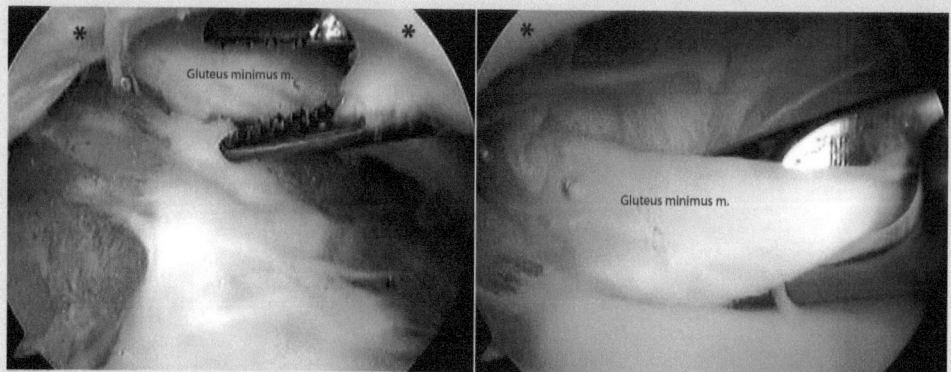

Fig. 83.7 Tissue grasper in position to mobilize the retracted gluteus minimus tendon *(left)*, which lies under the torn gluteus medius tendon *(asterisk)*. The gluteus minimus tendon is better visualized once it is pulled down into view *(right)*. (Courtesy of Scott D. Martin, MD, Boston, MA.)

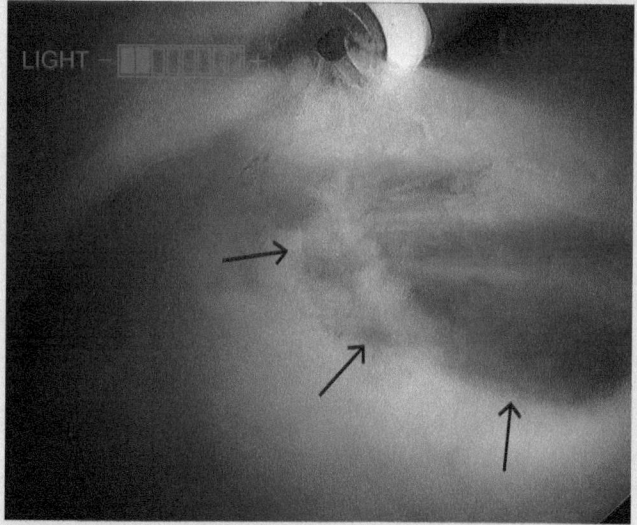

Fig. 83.8 Partial-thickness tear of the gluteus medius tendon *(black arrows)*. (Courtesy of Scott D. Martin, MD, Boston, MA.)

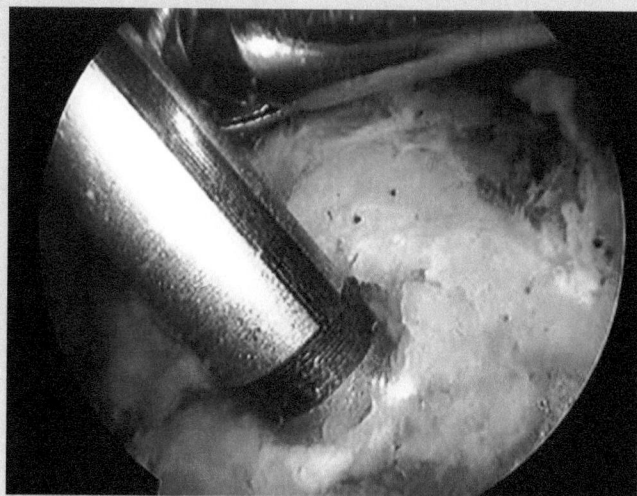

Fig. 83.9 Anchor placement at a "dead man's angle" into the gluteal tendon footprint. (Courtesy of Scott D. Martin, MD, Boston, MA.)

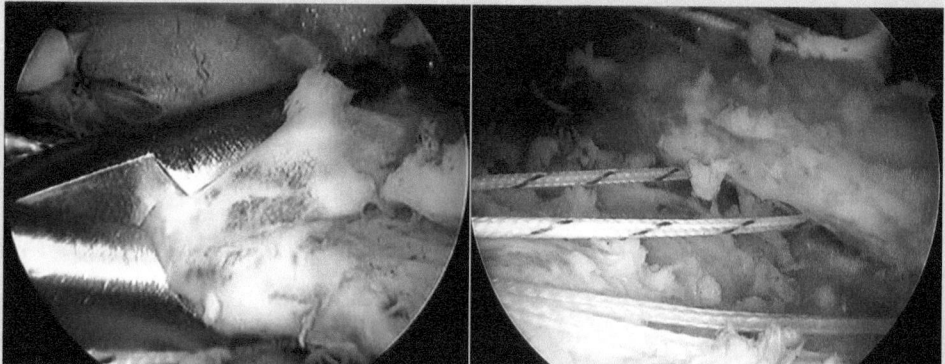

Fig. 83.10 A suture shuttle is used to pass the suture through the gluteal tendon *(left)*, and sutures are passed through the gluteal tendon prior to relocating it into its anatomic position *(right)*. (Courtesy of Scott D. Martin, MD, Boston, MA.)

📌 **Authors' Preferred Technique—cont'd**

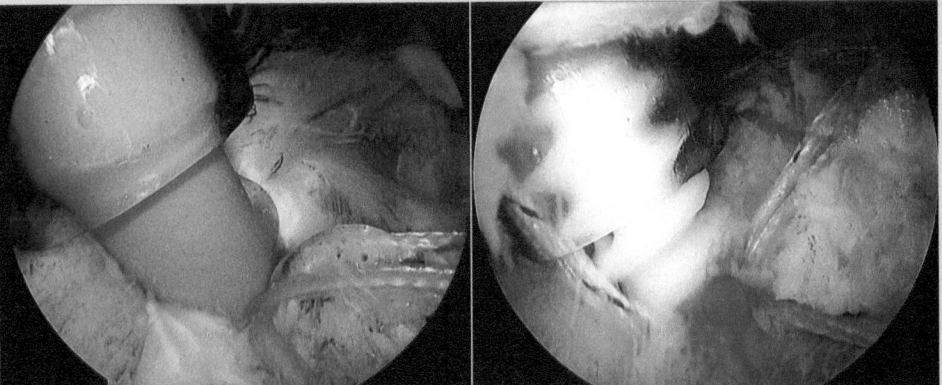

Fig. 83.11 Distal anchors are placed into the vastus ridge, securing the gluteal tendon into its native position and backing up the repair. (Courtesy of Scott D. Martin, MD, Boston, MA.)

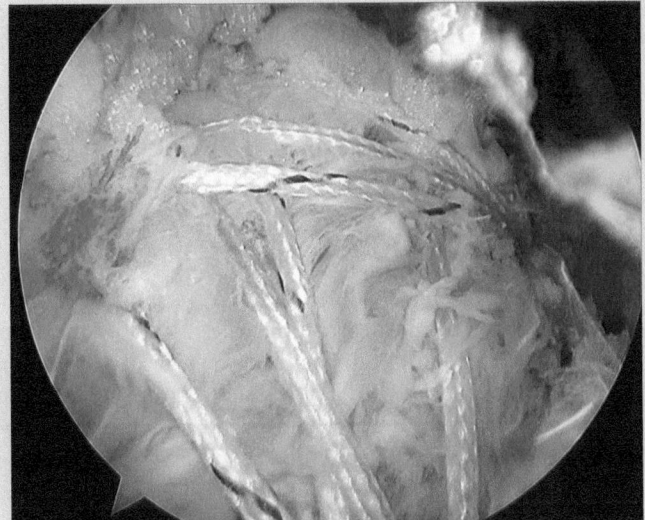

Fig. 83.12 Completed transosseous repair of the gluteus medius. (Courtesy of Scott D. Martin, MD, Boston, MA.)

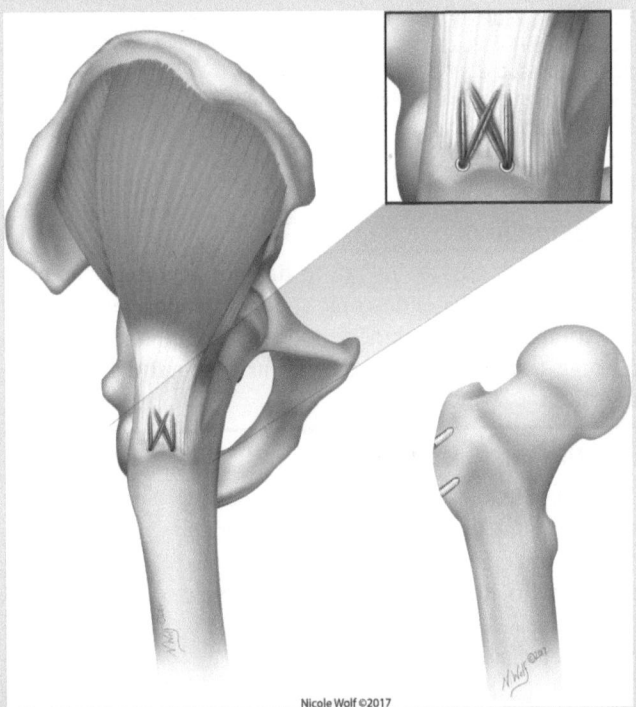

Nicole Wolf ©2017

Fig. 83.13 Completed gluteus medius and minimus repair, showing placement of suture and anchor. (Illustration by Nicole Wolf, MS; ©2016. Reprinted with permission.)

Postoperative Management

For the first 6 weeks postoperatively, crutches are used with a flat-footed gait, with weight bearing as tolerated. The patient is instructed to maintain a level pelvis without a limp or Trendelenburg lurch during ambulation, avoiding unnecessary tension on the tendon repair. Activity is progressively integrated, with strengthening beginning at 3 months after surgery. Physical therapy–guided strengthening can gradually improve the patient's gait toward normal after several months of targeted exercise.

Results

Outcomes of endoscopic abductor tendon tear repairs have been investigated in relatively small samples. This is partially because of the few patients who present themselves as surgical candidates and the relatively short time period within which endoscopy has been utilized for these repairs. Overall, endoscopic gluteal tendon repairs have shown remarkable improvements in functional outcome, with the benefit of very low complication rates (Table 83.1).[2,12–16]

TABLE 83.1	Outcomes and Complications of Endoscopic Abductor Tendon Repair					
Study, Year	Level of Evidence	Mean Age (y)	Operative Hips	Mean Follow-Up (mo)	Functional Outcomes (Preop to Postop)	Complications
Voos et al.,[13] 2009	IV	50.4	10	25.0	All 10 patients regained 5/5 strength postop mHHS: 94 postop; HOS: 93	NR
Domb et al.,[14] 2013	IV	58.0	15	27.9	RMC: 4.2–4.73; mHHS: 48.9–84.6; HOS-ADL: 47.47–88.1; HOS-SSS: 28.18–78.83; NAHS: 46.02–76.74	NR
McCormick et al.,[12] 2013	IV	65.9	10	22.6	HHS: 84.7; HOS-ADL: 89.1; HOS-SSS: 86.8	NR
Thaunat et al.,[15] 2013	IV	68.5	4	6.0	HHS: 35.7–74.0; NAHS: 38.3–83	NR
Chandrasekaran et al.,[16] 2015	IV	57.0	34	24.0	Statistically significant improvement in mHHS, NAHS, HOS-ADL, HOS-SS	No repair failures; 4 hips went onto total hip arthroplasty (11–16 months postop)

HOS, Hip outcomes score; *HOS-ADL,* hip outcomes score–activities of daily living; *HOS-SSS,* hip outcome score–sport-specific subscale; *mHHS,* modified Harris hip score; *NAHS,* nonarthritic hip score; *NR,* none reported; *Postop,* postoperative; *Preop,* preoperative; *RMC,* resisted muscular contraction score.
Data from references 12–16.

Complications

Although the current literature has not reported significant complications after endoscopic abductor tendon repair, potential complications include tendon retear, muscle herniation through the ITB, neurovascular injury, wound dehiscence, or infection.

Future Considerations

Like many tendinous repairs in orthopaedics, future considerations for gluteus tendon repair could benefit from the evolving field of biologics. The implementation of stem cell therapies may serve to augment the healing of these repairs, similarly to the research currently conducted on the use of biologics on rotator cuff tendon repairs.

COXA SALTANS

Coxa saltans (snapping hip syndrome) is a condition that involves a snapping in or around the hip. Extra-articular causes must be differentiated from intra-articular etiologies, such as labral tears, which commonly present with groin pain associated with mechanical catching and locking of the hip.[17] Extra-articular and intra-articular coxa saltans may present together; therefore careful evaluations of the patient's history and physical exam are necessary to distinguish the conditions. Two extra-articular etiologies of snapping hip that can be considered include internal and external coxa saltans.[17–20] Snapping hips are commonly benign; the prevalence in the general population is estimated to be as high as 10%. Active populations, however—including dancers, soccer players, and runners—have been shown to experience a higher prevalence due to repetitive movements involving the hip flexors.[1,18,21–25]

Internal Coxa Saltans
History

Internal coxa saltans is defined as a snapping of the iliopsoas in the anterior hip, most commonly over the iliopectineal eminence or femoral head.[17–19] The iliacus, which originates from the internal border of the iliac crest and upper iliac fossa, and the psoas major, which originates from the anterior transverse processes and lateral vertebral bodies of T12 to L5, run down deep to the inguinal ligament but superior to the femoral head. They insert on and directly below the lesser trochanter through the tendon sheath known as the iliopsoas tendon. These muscles serve as hip flexors and internal rotators, which can snap over prominent bone or implants deep to the tendon sheath when firing eccentrically. This phenomenon can occur naturally or can be seen after total hip arthroplasty with an oversized acetabular cup and anterior overhang. In this case internal coxa saltans can present because of snapping over the anteriorly projected implant component.[18]

Physical Examination

The snapping can be heard and reproduced with provocative movements but is not commonly visualized during the physical exam. The snapping often occurs when the hip is moved from a position of flexion, abduction, and external rotation to a position of extension, adduction, and internal rotation (Fig. 83.14). At times the snapping can occur with just hip flexion to extension; nevertheless the patient is likely familiar with the movements that produce the snapping.[17–19]

Imaging

Radiographs are unlikely to show any offending agent unless heterotopic bone or a prominent implant is the cause of the

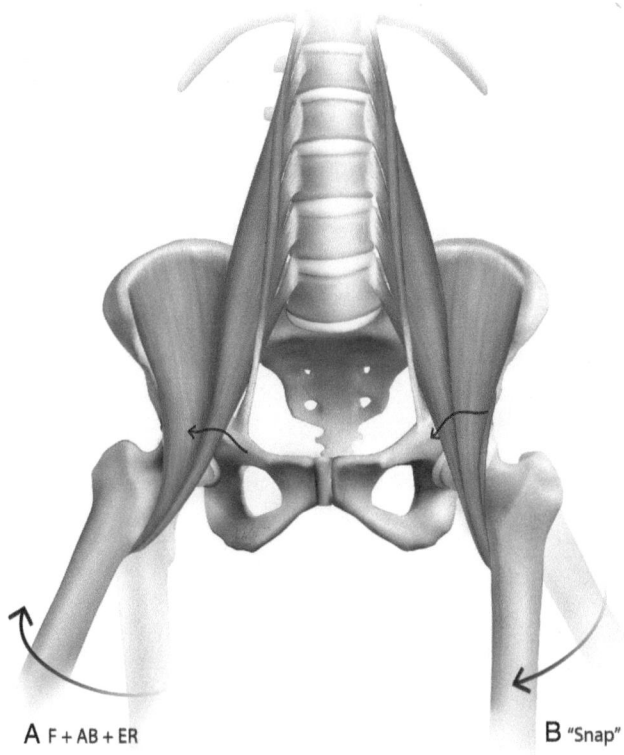

A F + AB + ER   B "Snap"

Nicole Wolf ©2017

Fig. 83.14 Internal coxa saltans is due to snapping of the iliopsoas tendon over the iliopectineal eminence. The snapping is reproduced when the hip is moved from (A) flexion abduction external rotation (F+AB+ER) to (B) extension adduction internal rotation. (Illustration by Nicole Wolf, MS; ©2017. Reprinted with permission.)

BOX 83.2   Presentation and Management of Internal Coxa Saltans

History
- Snapping or catching sensation over anterior hip
  - Often audible
- Insidious onset commonly resulting in overuse injury in active patients
- Can occur after THA with prominent anterior hardware

Physical Examination
- Symptoms recreated with hip flexion to extension while supine
- Symptoms recreated with hip flexion, abduction, external rotation to extension, adduction, internal rotation

Imaging
- Radiographs often unremarkable
  - Possible anterior bony prominence
  - Possible anterior hardware prominence
- Ultrasound may reveal snapping tendon with provocative movements
  - Inflammation, tendon thickening, secondary bursitis
- MRI often unremarkable, but may rule out alternate etiologies
  - Inflammation, tendon thickening, secondary bursitis

Management
- Benign, nonpainful findings do not require treatment
- Conservative management including stretching, physical therapy, NSAIDs, activity modification, and anesthetic/corticosteroid injections
- Surgical release of iliopsoas tendon if failed conservative management

THA, Total hip arthroplasty; *MRI,* magnetic resonance imaging; *NSAIDs,* nonsteroidal anti-inflammatory drugs.
See references 17–19, and 26.

internal snapping. Ultrasound can show the abnormal tissue movement over the hip and MRI can reveal local inflammation in the affected area.[18,19] Since ultrasound can show the snapping dynamically, MRI is often unnecessary, as it will reveal only inflammation and tendinous thickening in the iliopsoas region.[26]

Decision-Making Principles

The diagnosis can be elusive due to the adjacent conditions that cause catching or snapping around the hip joint. Symptomatic intra-articular conditions including labral tears seen in femoroacetabular impingement must be excluded, since iliopsoas dysfunction can occur secondary to gait changes from intra-articular sources of pain.[18,20] Further clinical evaluation and workup of internal coxa saltans can be found in Box 83.2.

Treatment Options

Since the condition is commonly asymptomatic, only symptomatic individuals experiencing painful snapping should be treated. Conservative treatment—such as physical therapy, NSAIDs, and activity modification—should be relied on initially. Anesthetic and corticosteroid injections have also been used successfully for pain relief and the reduction of inflammation.[27–29] If conservative treatment is ineffective, patients may be candidates for surgical intervention with iliopsoas tendon recession.

Postoperative Management

For the first 4 weeks postoperatively, crutches are used to aid in maintaining the normal gait pattern, with weight bearing as tolerated. Physical therapy can begin within the first week after surgery; however, aggressive strengthening of hip flexors should be delayed until 6 weeks after surgery. A slow progression of strengthening and range of motion can be continued, with resumption of full activity after 3 months.

Results

Outcomes of iliopsoas release procedures for the refractory internal snapping hip have shown positive results overall, with minor complications (Table 83.2). Atrophy and hip flexion strength have been reduced when iliopsoas tendon release was performed with hip arthroscopy compared with hip arthroscopy alone.[30] The majority of internal snapping hips were resolved; however, in isolated studies, a small portion of hips remained symptomatic.

Complications

Neurovascular injury can occur, since the femoral nerve, artery, and vein run anterior to the iliopsoas. Other complications of iliopsoas tendon release include heterotopic bone formation and loss of iliopsoas tendon integrity. If care is not taken during recession and the tendon is resected completely, hip flexion strength may be compromised.

Authors' Preferred Technique

Iliopsoas tendon recession is performed only in symptomatic patients who have intractable snapping hip pain after failing conservative treatment modalities. The iliopsoas tendon release can be done from an intra-articular approach or directly with endoscopic techniques. Intra-articularly, the tendon can be accessed medial to the anterior portal in the peripheral compartment between the zona orbicularis and the labrum at the level of the medial synovial fold. Extra-articular release of the tendon is performed endoscopically with two portals—one anteriorly at the level of the lesser trochanter, and the other 4 cm distal to the lesser trochanter, which functions as the utility portal. Electrocautery is used in a transverse plane to cut the psoas component of the tendon, partially releasing the iliopsoas, so as to avoid compromising its function (Fig. 83.15).

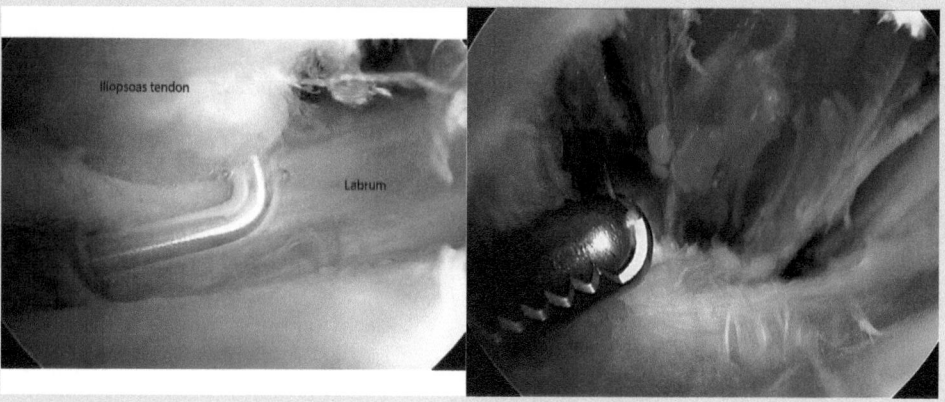

Fig. 83.15 While it is in the peripheral compartment, the iliopsoas tendon can be recessed with an electrocautery hook probe, working through the anterior portal *(left)*, until it is completely released *(right)*. (Courtesy of Scott D. Martin, MD, Boston, MA.)

TABLE 83.2   Outcomes and Complications of Endoscopic Iliopsoas Release

Study, Year	Level of Evidence	Mean Age (y)	Operative Hips	Mean Follow-Up (mo)	Functional Outcomes (Preop to Postop)	Complications
Flanum et al.,[29] 2007	IV	39.0	6 Released	12.0	All patients returned to preop jobs and activity; mHHS: 58–96	NR
Anderson et al.,[31] 2008	IV	25.0	15 Released	12.0	No recurrence of snapping; postop mHHS: 41–96 (competitive athletes), 44–97 (recreational athletes)	NR
Contreras et al.,[32] 2010	IV	33.6	7 Released	24.0	No recurrence of snapping; VAS: 7.7/10–2.4/8; mHHS: 56.1–87.9	NR
El Bitar et al.,[20] 2014	IV	28.2	55 Released	28.0	10 patients had recurrence of snapping; mHHS: 62.3–80.5; HOS-ADL: 60.9–81.8; HOS-SSS: 43.4–70.0; NAHS: 57.6–80.2	1 Superficial wound infection, 1 HO, 1 perineal numbness
Ilizaliturri et al.,[33] 2015	IV	29.3	28 Released	30.6	No recurrence of snapping; WOMAC: 39.0–73.6 (bifid tendon) & 47.2–77.9 (no bifid tendon)	NR
Hwang et al.,[34] 2015	IV	32.0	25 Released	24.0	VAS: 6–2; HHS:65–84; HOS-ADL: 66–87; HOS-SSS: 60–82; Activity was improved in 17, but remained the same in 8	1 reoperation due to refractory painful snapping

HHS, Harris hip score; *mHHS,* modified Harris hip score; *NR,* none reported; *Postop,* postoperative; *Preop,* preoperative; *VAS,* visual analog scale for pain; *WOMAC,* Western Ontario and McMaster Universities Osteoarthritis Index.
Data from references 20, 29, 31–34.

External Coxa Saltans

History

External coxa saltans is defined as a snapping of the ITB or gluteus maximus over the greater trochanter. The snapping is most commonly due to the ITB, but gluteus maximus snapping has also been described.[35] Like internal coxa saltans, external coxa saltans is rarely acute and often due to repetitive motion of the musculotendinous units over the greater trochanter.[4,19,36] Coxa vara is a proposed contributor to the external snapping hip due to the more prominent greater trochanter and decreased efficiently of abductor during external rotation, both of which cause increased tension within the ITB.[37] Additionally, postsurgical external snapping can been seen with prominent implants.[38]

Physical Examination

Snapping can be visualized or palpitated over the lateral hip when the symptoms are reproduced during hip flexion and extension.[1] Unlike internal coxa saltans, external snapping is not usually audible, but patients with external snapping hip are likely to be able to reproduce the snapping at will. Patients sometimes describe the external snapping as a feeling of hip "dislocation" because of their ability to see and feel the snap as it occurs. The secondary inflammation surrounding the ITB is the source of pain. While the hip is flexed, the ITB is anterior to the greater trochanter; however, when the hip is moved into extension, the ITB moves posteriorly over the greater trochanter (Fig. 83.16).[4,18,19]

Imaging

Radiographs are usually unremarkable unless they reveal a structural bony abnormality or prominent implant as the underlying cause of the lateral snapping. Dynamic ultrasound can show the tissue snapping over the greater trochanter, along with inflammation, yet MRI usually shows local inflammation and ITB thickening without gross structural abnormalities.[4,18,19,39,40]

Decision-Making Principles

Like internal coxa saltans, other causes of hip pain, catching, and snapping must be ruled out, since external coxa saltans symptoms may mimic or accompany intra-articular snapping. The lateral location of the external snapping makes misdiagnosis less likely as compared with internal coxa saltans, which occurs anteriorly, over the femoral head. Laterally, conditions such as gluteus medius injury must be ruled out. Overlap in the treatment options for external coxa saltans, ITB syndrome, and primary trochanteric bursitis do exist, making the initial steps of management more direct. Further clinical evaluation and workup of external coxa saltans can be found in Box 83.3.

Treatment Options

Treatment for symptomatic external coxa saltans begins with conservative modalities, including ITB stretching, NSAIDs, corticosteroid injections, and activity modification. It has been well established that activity modification with physical therapy–directed stretching and strengthening will improve the symptoms in the majority of patients.[18,41,42] In cases recalcitrant to conservative management, operative intervention can be considered. The ITB release procedures have evolved from the earliest open procedures, which date back to the 1920s, to current minimally invasive endoscopic techniques, but all focus primarily on partial recession of the ITB at the lateral hip.[43] Endoscopic ITB release reduces the tension of the ITB on the greater trochanter during

Nicole Wolf ©2017

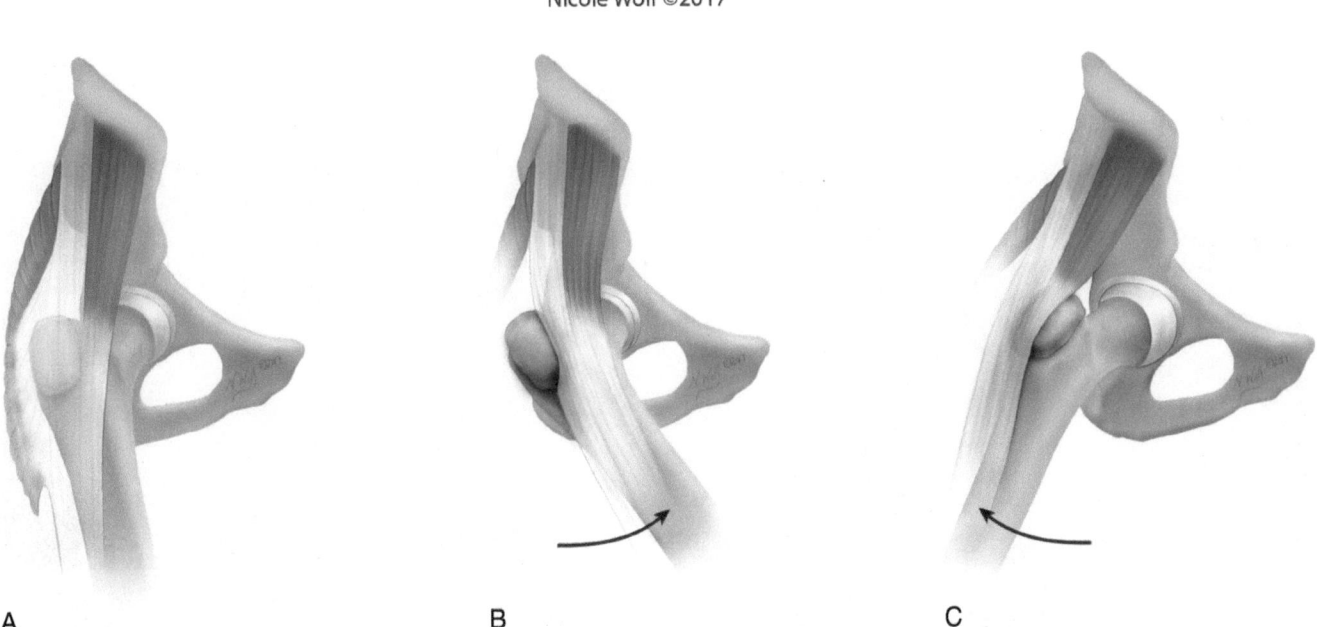

A   B   C

Fig. 83.16 External snapping hip is characterized by the movement of the iliotibial band (ITB) over the greater trochanter as the hip is flexed and subsequently extended (A→B→C). An overly taut ITB can cause local inflammation to the lateral hip, including the underlying trochanteric bursa. (Illustration by Nicole Wolf, MS; ©2017. Reprinted with permission.)

BOX 83.3   Presentation and Management of External Coxa Saltans

History

- Snapping or catching sensation over lateral hip
  - Often visible
  - May be described as hip "dislocation"
- Insidious onset commonly resulting in overuse injury in active patients

Physical Examination

- Symptoms recreated with hip flexion to extension
- Symptoms recreated with hip flexion, abduction, external rotation to extension, adduction, internal rotation
- Snapping tissue may be palpated on lateral hip during provocative movements

Imaging

- Radiographs often unremarkable
- Ultrasound may reveal snapping tendon over greater trochanter with provocative movements
  - Inflammation, tendon thickening, secondary bursitis
- MRI often unremarkable, but may rule out alternate etiologies
  - Inflammation, tendon thickening, secondary bursitis

Management

- Benign, nonpainful findings do not require treatment
- Conservative management including stretching, physical therapy, NSAIDs, activity modification, and anesthetic/corticosteroid injections
- Surgical lengthening of ITB if failed conservative management

See references 1, 4, 18, 19, 39, and 40.
ITB, Iliotibial band; *MRI*, magnetic resonance imaging; *NSAIDs*, nonsteroidal antiinflammatory drugs.

hip movement, allowing for a reduction in snapping and inflammatory symptoms.[1,9,18,19,36]

Postoperative Management

Postoperatively weight bearing for a maximum of 1 week is tolerated with the aid of a cane or crutch. Also, a home stretching program focusing on the ITB and lateral musculature is begun with progressive return to full activity after 1 month.

Results

Release of the ITB is a straightforward procedure that is predictable and effective when done correctly. Overall, endoscopic ITB release techniques have achieved favorable outcomes without serious complications (Table 83.3).

Complications

In addition to bleeding and neurovascular injury, serious complications specific to ITB release hinge upon the integrity of the ITB. The Z-plasty and H-plasty techniques are performed such that the ITB is not fully released. This allows the ITB to continue to function as a stabilizer during gait, aiding the lateral musculature of the hip in extension, abduction, and internal rotation. If the release is too aggressive, stabilization of the ITB can be compromised, making it difficult to regain function without surgical intervention.

Future Considerations

Since the understanding of the pathophysiology of internal and external snapping hips has been well established, clinicians can

Authors' Preferred Technique

The senior author's preferred ITB release technique is an endoscopic H-plasty ITB release. Two portals are established on the lateral aspect of the thigh approximately 3 to 4 cm proximal and distal to the greater trochanter and angled toward the greater trochanter at approximately 45 degrees. The superficial peritrochanteric space is accessed and visualization of the ITB is obtained. The ITB is recessed with a hook probe electrocautery device in an H-plasty technique.[1] Additionally, multiloculated trochanteric bursae can be visualized and removed during the ITB release. While still maintaining its function during gait stability, the ITB can expand and lengthen, which relieves tension over the greater trochanter and trochanteric bursa (Figs. 83.17 and 83.18).

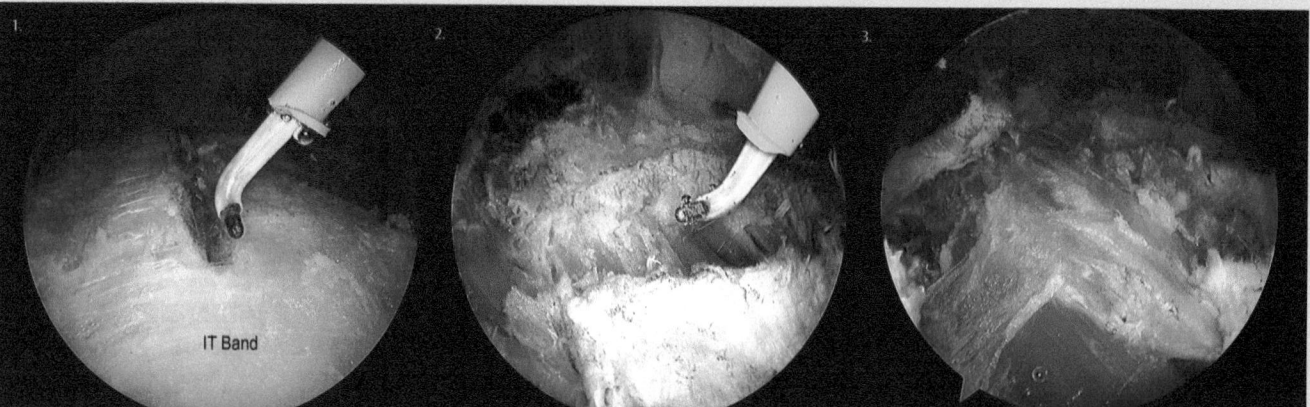

Fig. 83.17 Hook probe electrocautery is used to perform the H-plasty release of the iliotibial band *(ITB)* by first creating a longitudinal incision *(1)*. The electrocautery is working through the posterior accessory portal while being viewed through the distal portal. Once the longitudinal incision has been made, perpendicular incisions are created *(2)*, eventually leading to a completed H-plasty of the ITB *(3)*, allowing tension reduction over the trochanteric bursa and greater trochanter. (Courtesy of Scott D. Martin, MD, Boston, MA.)

Authors' Preferred Technique—cont'd

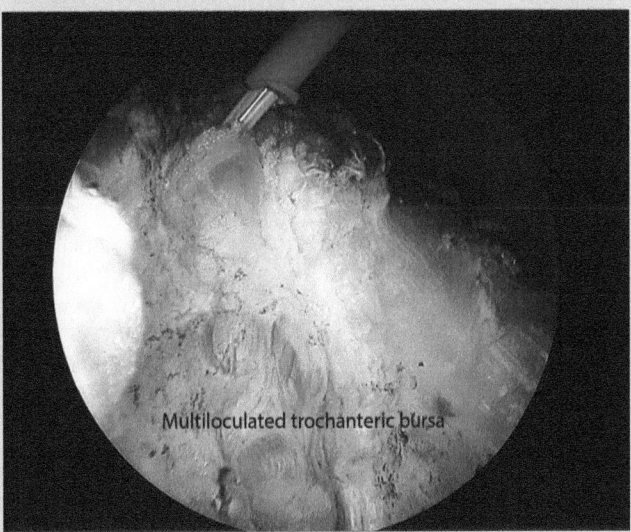

Fig. 83.18 Multiloculated trochanteric bursa mobilized and brought into view by a hook probe after initial longitudinal incision of the iliotibial band. (Courtesy of Scott D. Martin, MD, Boston, MA.)

TABLE 83.3 Outcomes and Complications of Endoscopic Iliotibial Band Release

Study, Year	Level of Evidence	Mean Age (y)	Operative Hips	Mean Follow-Up (mo)	Functional Outcomes (Preop to Postop)	Complications
Provencher et al.,[36] 2004	IV	25.6	9 Z-plasty	22.9	8/9 returned to full activity; No refractory snapping	1 persistent groin pain
Ilizaliturri et al.,[22] 2006	IV	26.0	11 Z-plasty	24.0	WOMAC: 81–94; all returned to full activity without pain; one had continued snapping	None
Farr et al.,[44] 2007	IV	43.5	2 Released	41.0	All returned to full activity without pain	None
Govaert et al.,[45] 2012	IV	NR	5 Released	1.5	VAS: 75–13 out of 100; WOMAC significantly improved	1 Hematoma requiring evacuation
Zini et al.,[46] 2013	IV	25.0	15 Released	33.8	VAS: 5.5–0.53 out of 10; postop mHHS: 97.5; TAS: 7.6–7.6; 60% were pain-free; all patients experienced relief of snapping; patient satisfaction: 9.3 out of 10	None
Drummond et al.,[47] 2016	IV	65.0	57 Released	20.7	VAS: 7.8–2.8 out of 10 Oxford Hip Score: 20.4–37.3 iHOT-33: 23.8–70.2	None

mHHS, modified Harris hip score; *NR,* none reported; *Preop,* preoperative; *Postop,* postoperative; *TAS,* Tegner activity level scale; *VAS,* visual analog scale for pain; *WOMAC,* Western Ontario and McMaster Universities Osteoarthritis Index.
Data from references 22, 36, 44–47.

more appropriately treat these conditions with nonoperative conservative techniques. Over the last decades the threshold of surgical intervention has fluctuated such that surgical releases of the iliopsoas and ITB seem to have become more prevalent. Although innovative and minimally invasive techniques should be explored for intractable snapping hips, conservative therapies should achieve symptom resolution in the majority of patients.

TROCHANTERIC BURSITIS

History

Primary trochanteric bursitis is rarely seen, as trochanteric bursitis is commonly secondary due to concurrent external coxa saltans or a tight ITB. More commonly lateral hip pain in the distribution of the trochanteric bursa is referred from alternate etiologies including arthritis, femoroacetabular impingement, abductor tendon tears, and lumbosacral disease. Frequently the symptoms of trochanteric bursitis are relieved when the inciting cause of the lateral hip pain is addressed.[1,4,48,49] The ITB is a musculotendinous unit derived from the gluteus maximus and tensor fascia lata, which crosses the hip laterally over the greater trochanter and inserts on the lateral condyle of the tibia. When this structure is excessively taut, it can catch on the lateral hip, thicken, and cause inflammation in the surrounding lateral hip, including the trochanteric bursa.[42,44,50-52]

Physical Examination

Patients classically have lateral hip pain over the area of the greater trochanter. The injury is rarely acute and usually presents in patients with overuse injuries or concomitant hemipelvic injury. Tenderness over the lateral hip is apparent on palpation. Tightness in the ITB band can be appreciated with the Ober test. With this maneuver the patient lies on the unaffected side while the clinician passively extends the hip slightly and abducts the thigh with the knee is flexed at 90 degrees. A positive test is appreciated if, due to the tight ITB, the thigh will not immediately relax into adduction once the thigh has been released by the clinician.

Imaging

If conservative treatment fails to provide relief, imaging may support a direct cause of lateral hip pain. Ultrasound may reveal ITB inflammation and thickening with a secondary bursitis, and MRI may reveal evidence of bursal edema, loculations, and thickening.[4,50-53]

Decision-Making Principles

Since primary trochanteric bursitis is rarely seen, the clinician must not jump to the diagnosis without first ruling out more serious underlying etiologies of lateral hip pain. Physical exam of the lumbosacral region and hip will guide the steps in management of lateral hip pain, which start with noninvasive therapies. Further clinical evaluation and workup of trochanteric bursitis can be found in Box 83.4.

Treatment Options

Once underlying conditions are excluded, trochanteric bursitis is treated conservatively with physical therapy focused on pelvic core strengthening and stretching.[41,49,52,54] In addition to a comprehensive strengthening and stretching program, at least two corticosteroid bursal injections can be used to decrease bursal inflammation. Once pain has proven to be recalcitrant to all conservative therapies, surgical intervention may be considered if alternative lateral hip pain etiologies have been excluded. Interventions including bursectomy, Z-plasty, or H-plasty—which was described previously in this chapter—have been shown to provide pain relief.[47,50-56]

PIRIFORMIS SYNDROME

History

The idea behind piriformis syndrome was first introduced by Yeoman in 1928, when he suggested that further attention be

---

> ### BOX 83.4   Presentation and Management of Trochanteric Bursitis
>
> **History**
> - Pain over lateral hip
>   - Exacerbated by lateral pressure
> - Insidious onset commonly resulting in overuse injury
>
> **Physical Examination**
> - Pain is reproduced upon palpation over greater trochanter
> - Ober test reveals ITB tightness
>
> **Imaging**
> - Radiographs often unremarkable
> - Ultrasound may reveal ITB inflammation and thickening with secondary bursitis
> - MRI often unremarkable, but may rule out alternate etiologies
>   - Secondary bursitis
>
> **Management**
> - Conservative management including stretching, physical therapy, NSAIDs, activity modification, and anesthetic/corticosteroid injections
> - Surgical lengthening of ITB if failed conservative management

See references 1, 4, 50–54.
ITB, Iliotibial band; *MRI,* magnetic resonance imaging; *NSAIDs,* nonsteroidal antiinflammatory drugs.

---

given to the piriformis muscle as a potential cause for extraspinal sciatica.[57] Years later, cadaveric studies showed anatomic variants of sciatic nerve location with respect to the piriformis muscle as it exited the pelvis, and it was proposed that the nerve could be compressed by the piriformis in certain anatomic variations. The anatomic variants that could clearly impinge the nerve—such as a Beaton class D variant, which describes the sciatic nerve exiting directly through a bifid piriformis muscle belly—was seen in less than 1% of cadavers.[58] The piriformis muscle lies deep to the gluteus maximus, originating from the sacrum and inserting on the greater trochanter as it passes through the greater sciatic foramen. It functions as an external rotator and is characteristically superficial to the sciatic nerve, although rare anatomic variations exist. In recent decades, piriformis pain syndrome has been increasingly diagnosed in patients presenting with unilateral buttock pain; however, its pathophysiology is still poorly understood, creating controversy within the medical community. The terminology surrounding entrapment syndromes of the sciatic nerve has recently evolved, as the term "piriformis syndrome" is being replaced by "deep gluteal syndrome" to include other potential sources of sciatic compression.[59-61]

Posttraumatic nerve entrapment caused by fibrosis or heterotopic ossification is an accepted cause of piriformis-like pain, which can be treated with surgical decompression; however, this etiology of gluteal pain is clearly a separate presentation as compared with chronic, nontraumatic piriformis pain syndrome.

Physical Examination

Symptoms of piriformis pain syndrome include chronic buttock pain, which may be accompanied by sciatica. Patients feel pain on deep gluteal palpation and have difficulty with activities that strain the deep gluteal region, such as prolonged sitting, walking, and internal hip rotation. The pain is insidious and sometimes associated with other pelvic pain, such as dyspareunia, dyschezia, and tenderness to piriformis palpation through the vaginal wall. Multiple physical exam tests have been described in relation to piriformis syndrome; these elicit hip flexion, abduction, and adduction to involve the deep gluteal muscles, which can produce both local buttock pain as well as shooting leg pain. Unfortunately many of the tests used for piriformis syndrome produce similar pain in patients with lumbosacral disease, making it difficult to differentiate the two conditions.[61-64]

Imaging

Radiographs are often unremarkable in chronic, nontraumatic piriformis pain syndrome. Ultrasound also does not give rise to definitive piriformis-related pathology but may show inflammation in the deep gluteal region. MRI may show local inflammation, fibrous adhesions, and heterotopic bone formation within the piriformis muscle in circumstances of posttraumatic nerve entrapment, but it is nonspecific in chronic piriformis syndrome.[62,65,66] If true nerve entrapment is suspected, electromyography and nerve conduction studies can be used to confirm sciatic impingement.

Decision-Making Principles

Piriformis syndrome is commonly a diagnosis of exclusion, since the vague symptomatology mimics and is often associated with lumbosacral disease rather than isolated piriformis impingement. When true nerve entrapment is present, pain and radiculopathy occur following a posttraumatic event that disrupts the deep gluteal anatomy. Therefore the patient's history of symptom duration, associated factors, and lumbosacral disease can help to further differentiate the etiology of deep gluteal pain. Further clinical evaluation and workup of piriformis syndrome can be found in Box 83.5.

Treatment Options

After negative lumbosacral workups are confirmed, management of a patient with symptoms of piriformis pain syndrome begins with conservative modalities, including physical therapy, stretching, and NSAIDs.[61-63] For sciatica symptoms, botulinum toxin and corticosteroid injections have led to the improvement of pain for short periods of time, although the etiology of pain in multiple studies is poorly differentiated in relation to piriformis-related pain and lumbosacral disease.[67,68] Surgical intervention with piriformis release or sciatic nerve decompression should be reserved only for true nerve entrapment confirmed by electromyography and nerve conduction studies.

Future Considerations

Additional research directed at the pathophysiology, diagnosis, and treatment of deep gluteal pain syndrome should be conducted in order to gain a better understanding of the condition and further options for treatment. The differentiation between piriformis-related and lumbosacral-related gluteal pain and radiculopathy is a challenging task in individuals without clear evidence of either on imaging. Although clinical improvements have been reported in limited studies following piriformis release

---

BOX 83.5 Presentation and Management of Piriformis Syndrome

History
- Pain in unilateral buttock associated with radiculopathy
  - Exacerbated by deep buttock pressure
  - Insidious onset
- Intolerance to sitting, walking, squatting
- Possible dyspareunia
- Possible dyschezia

Physical Examination
- Symptoms recreated upon palpation over greater sciatic notch
- Symptoms recreated with hip flexion, adduction, internal rotation
- Symptoms recreated with the following tests that stretch nerve roots and musculature of the lumbosacral and deep gluteal regions:
  - Freiburg test
  - Pace test
  - Beatty test
  - Straight-leg raise

Imaging
- Radiographs often unremarkable
  - Possible posttraumatic heterotopic ossification
- Ultrasound often unremarkable
  - Possible subgluteal inflammation
- MRI often unremarkable, but may rule out alternate etiologies
  - Possible posttraumatic heterotopic ossification, adhesions, fibrous tissue constricting the sciatic nerve
- EMG and nerve conduction studies may reveal evidence of nerve impingement

Management
- Conservative management including stretching, physical therapy, NSAIDs, and activity modification
- Anesthetic/corticosteroid/botulinum toxin injections for refractory pain
- Surgical decompression if no alternative source of pain is identified and structural nerve impingement is confirmed with EMG and nerve conduction studies

See references 61–64.
EMG, Electromyography; *MRI*, magnetic resonance imaging; *NSAIDs*, nonsteroidal antiinflammatory drugs.

---

in chronic piriformis syndrome, the threshold for surgical intervention remains controversial.[69,70]

ISCHIOFEMORAL IMPINGEMENT

History

Ischiofemoral impingement (IFI) was first described by Johnson in 1977 in three cases following total hip arthroplasty from failure to recreate the native offset.[71] Bony impingement in this area is rare, since the distance between the lesser trochanter and ischium ranges from approximately 18.6 ± 8 mm to 23.0 ± 7 mm in healthy populations.[72] The condition is classically associated with either structural impingement from implants following total hip arthroplasty or posttraumatic ossification of soft tissue following injury to the pubic rami, femoral neck, or intertrochanteric line. These conditions, which can cause an increased femoral neck inclination angle or femoral neck shortening, can cause encroachment into the native ischiofemoral space, resulting in posttraumatic IFI (Fig. 83.19).

The quadratus femoris, which originates on the ischial tuberosity and inserts on the intertrochanteric crest, can be impinged when the ischiofemoral space narrows, causing pain in the deep buttock and hemipelvis. The sciatic nerve can also be impinged upon in this area, causing radicular pain symptoms. Within the last decade, IFI has been diagnosed with increasing frequency in patients with chronic, nontraumatic presentations of gluteal pain.

Physical Examination

The population diagnosed with nontraumatic IFI is most commonly described as comprising middle-aged to elderly women, although the condition can be seen in men as well. Insidious pain is described in the hip, groin, or buttock, with radiation occasionally down the leg in a sciatica-like pattern.[61,73,74] As in the case of piriformis syndrome, many tests for diagnosis have been proposed, but proven maneuvers have yet to be accepted due to the inexplicit criteria for diagnosis. Pain can be accentuated during physical exam with movements that bring the lesser trochanter in closer proximity to the ischium, such as combinations of hip extension, adduction, and external rotation.[1,61,73,75–78]

Imaging

Weight-bearing anteroposterior and lateral radiographs may be normal and are not considered diagnostic for nontraumatic IFI,

as they can be with posttraumatic IFI.[79] The quadratus femoris muscle may show edematous signal enhancement and atrophy on MRI, with measurable narrowing between the lesser trochanter and ischium.[74] Although these MRI features are considered essential diagnostic criteria for IFI, the degree of ischiofemoral space narrowing is debated, as various studies have identified diagnostic cutoffs between 10 and 17 mm.[69,79–81]

Decision-Making Principles

Unlike posttraumatic structural IFI, the pathophysiology behind chronic, nontraumatic IFI is poorly understood, making this entity difficult to differentiate from other causes of deep gluteal pain. Therefore a comprehensive peritrochanteric workup should be performed to rule out conditions such as gluteal tears, which can cause dynamic IFI and deep gluteal pain (Figs. 83.20 and 83.21). Further clinical evaluation and workup of IFI can be found in Box 83.6.

Treatment Options

Operative management of IFI due to anatomic deformation has shown symptom improvement and is an accepted treatment modality within the orthopaedic community.[71] Due to the knowledge gaps within the pathophysiologic understanding and diagnostic criteria of chronic, nontraumatic IFI, treatment is poorly defined.[1,61,73] Treatment for nontraumatic IFI should begin with conservative measures including rest, physical therapy, and activity modification. Corticosteroid injections into the quadratus

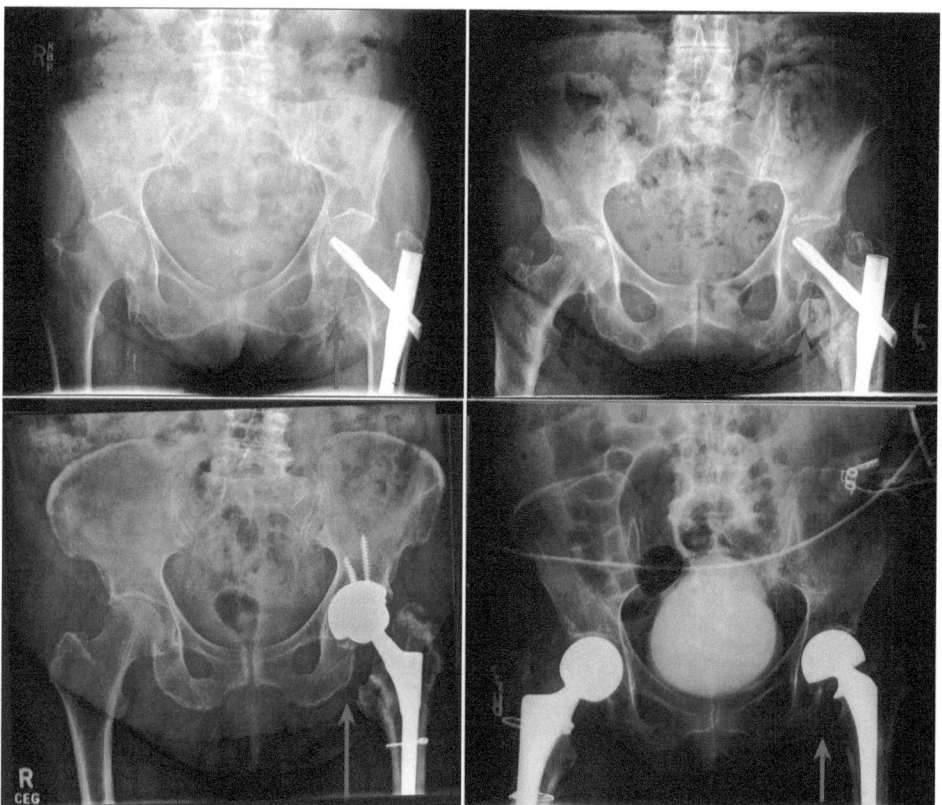

Fig. 83.19 Weight-bearing anteroposterior radiographs showing evidence of unilateral ischiofemoral space narrowing *(red arrows)* in examples of posttraumatic lesser trochanter displacement *(top)* and increased inclination angle post–total hip arthroplasty *(bottom)*. (Courtesy of Michael J. Weaver, MD, Boston, MA.)

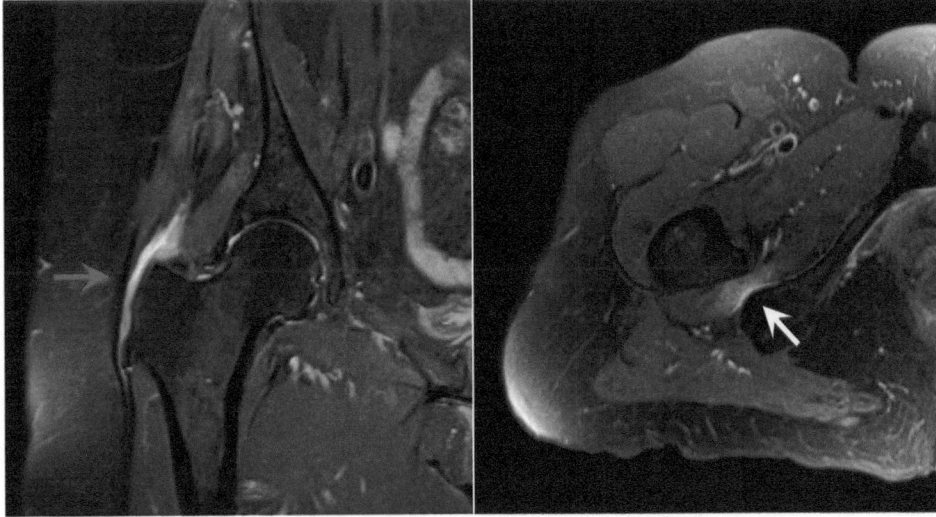

Fig. 83.20 Magnetic resonance imaging (MRI) showing concomitant right-sided ischiofemoral impingement (IFI) in a patient with a right-sided gluteus medius tear. Coronal T2 MRI *(left)* revealing a gluteus medius tear of the right hip *(red arrow)*, and axial T2 MRI *(right)* revealing evidence of right-sided dynamic IFI *(white arrow)*. (Courtesy of Scott D. Martin, MD, Boston, MA.)

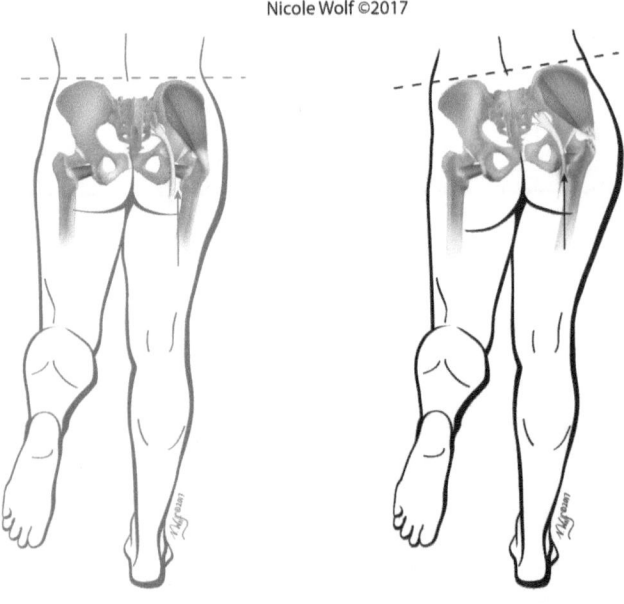

Nicole Wolf ©2017

Normal   Trendelenburg Sign

Fig. 83.21 The pathophysiology of dynamic ischiofemoral impingement is illustrated with a Trendelenburg gait, which could be due to an abductor tendon tear, narrowing the ischiofemoral space by bringing the ischium into closer proximity with the lesser trochanter. (Illustration by Nicole Wolf, MS; ©2017. Reprinted with permission.)

BOX 83.6 Presentation and Management of Ischiofemoral Impingement

History
- Pain in unilateral buttock, groin, hip ± radiculopathy
  - Insidious onset
- Possible hemipelvic weakness
- Increasing prevalence by middle/old age
- Higher prevalence in women

Physical Examination
- Symptoms recreated with combinations of hip extension, adduction, and external rotation
- Symptoms recreated with long-stride walking

Imaging
- Radiographs often unremarkable
  - Possible posttraumatic heterotopic ossification, femoral neck shortening, coxa valga, or malpositioned hardware
- Ultrasound often unremarkable
- MRI may reveal narrowing of the ischiofemoral space, edematous quadratus femoris muscle with fat atrophy, and/or peritrochanteric musculature atrophy
  - May rule out alternate etiologies
  - Possible posttraumatic bony impingement from heterotopic ossification, femoral neck shortening, coxa valga, or malpositioned hardware

Management
- Conservative management including stretching, physical therapy, NSAIDs, and activity modification
- Anesthetic/corticosteroid injections for refractory pain
- Surgical decompression if no alternative source of pain is identified and posttraumatic structural bony impingement is identified

See references 61, 73, 74,79–81.
MRI, Magnetic resonance imaging; *NSAIDs,* nonsteroidal antiinflammatory drugs.

femoris and surrounding deep gluteal region have allowed only short-term improvements of pain in a limited number of case reports.[79,82] Surgical interventions for nontraumatic IFI have been proposed, focusing on decompression of the ischiofemoral space by resection of the lesser trochanter, quadratus femoris, or ischium.[61,78,83–87]

Results

Surgical intervention for nontraumatic IFI, including variations of lesser trochanter and quadratus femoris resection, have shown improvements in patient-reported pain in isolated studies.[78,83] Unfortunately studies of the operative management of nontraumatic IFI are limited, mainly involving case reports and small case series without long-term follow-up.[61,78,83–87]

Complications

Although no serious complications have been reported, care should be taken during surgical management. Potential complications specific to resection of the lesser trochanter and quadratus femoris include vascular injury to the medial femoral circumflex artery, which can result in avascular necrosis of the femoral head as well as pelvic instability and weakness during hip flexion.[61,84]

Future Considerations

Chronic, nontraumatic IFI may be due to the dynamic impingement that occurs in the ischiofemoral space with concurrent lumbosacral or peritrochanteric disorders. If the peritrochanteric musculature sustains injury or atrophy due to traumatic, neurogenic, or iatrogenic causes, the muscles cannot support the hemipelvis, resulting in a Trendelenburg gait that narrows the ischiofemoral space by bringing the ischium into closer proximity to the lesser trochanter. Therefore treatment would have to address the underlying condition causing the dynamic IFI rather than surgically decompressing the native anatomy. Future research in this area will require larger, multicenter involvement to increase the understanding of the condition's pathophysiology, diagnosis, and treatment.

For a complete list of references, go to ExpertConsult.com.

SELECTED READINGS

Citation:
Byrd JW. Disorders of the peritrochanteric and deep gluteal space: new frontiers for arthroscopy. *Sports Med Arthrosc.* 2015;23(4):221–231.

Level of Evidence:
V

Summary:
This summary article focuses on the surgical interventions evolving in the area of peritrochanteric disorders.

Citation:
Voos JE, Rudzki JR, Shindle MK, et al. Arthroscopic anatomy and surgical techniques for peritrochanteric space disorders in the hip. *Arthroscopy.* 2007;23(11):1246, e1–5.

Level of Evidence:
V

Summary:
This summary article details surgical anatomy and techniques for the peritrochanteric space as well as the common indications for peritrochanteric endoscopy.

Citation:
Chandrasekaran S, Vemula SP, Gui C, et al. Clinical features that predict the need for operative intervention in gluteus medius tears. *Orthop J Sports Med.* 2015;3(2):2325967115571079.

Level of Evidence:
III

Summary:
This case-control study gives an overview of gluteus medius tears, evidence of when surgical intervention may be necessary, and indicators to accurately select surgical patients.

Citation:
Lustenberger DP, Ng VY, Best TM, et al. Efficacy of treatment of trochanteric bursitis: a systematic review. *Clin J Sport Med.* 2011;21(5):447–453.

Level of Evidence:
III

Summary:
This systematic review of studies from levels I to IV defines trochanteric bursitis, the indications for intervention, and the efficacy of treatments for the condition.

Citation:
Hernando MF, Cerezal L, Perez-Carro L, et al. Evaluation and management of ischiofemoral impingement: a pathophysiologic, radiologic, and therapeutic approach to a complex diagnosis. *Skeletal Radiol.* 2016;45(6):771–787.

Level of Evidence:
V

Summary:
This review article outlines the currently proposed pathophysiology, imaging, and potential therapies to address ischiofemoral impingement.

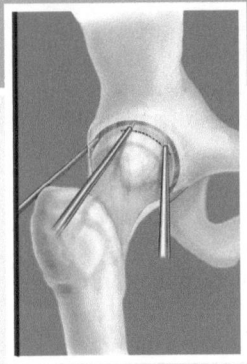

84

Athletic Pubalgia/Core Muscle Injury and Adductor Pathology

Christopher M. Larson, Jeffrey J. Nepple

Athletic pubalgia, or core muscle injury, is an umbrella term describing several anatomic injury patterns present in athletes with groin pain. The term *sports hernia* has fallen out of favor, as it is clearly a misnomer where no true hernia is involved. The correct diagnosis and treatment of this entity can be challenging.[1,2] However, increased recognition and surgical treatment of athletic pubalgia has increased dramatically in the last 20 years. Various terms—including *sports hernia, Gilmore's groin, osteitis pubis, slap-shot gut,* and *sportsman's hernia*—have been utilized to describe the condition.[2-5] There is growing recognition, however, that groin injuries in athletes comprise a complex set of injuries to the musculature of the abdominal wall, adductors, hip joint, pubic symphysis, and sacroiliac joint that can be a source of significant disability.[3,4,6,7] The term *core muscle injury* is also increasingly utilized as an alternative to *athletic pubalgia*. Athletic pubalgia most commonly involves the abdominal wall and adductors but may have significant overlap with conditions of the pubic symphysis (osteitis pubis) and motion-limiting conditions of the hip joint (femoroacetabular impingement).

Although our understanding of the pathophysiology of athletic pubalgia has improved significantly, considerable controversy still remains. Numerous methods of surgical treatment of athletic pubalgia exist, all generally with high rates of return to athletics and short recoveries noted in the literature. Combined treatment of adductor tendon pathology and underlying femoroacetabular impingement also vary. The pathophysiology of athletic pubalgia is most commonly theorized to involve (1) pathology of the rectus abdominis or rectus-adductor aponeurosis, (2) posterior inguinal floor defect, or (3) inguinal or genital neuropathy.[8]

Anatomy

Given the complexity of the anatomy of the hip joint, pelvis, pubic symphysis, and the associated abdominal wall, a thorough understanding of relevant anatomy is important for the clinician assessing an athlete with groin pain. This is particularly true for the anatomic considerations of athletic pubalgia. The pubic symphysis is perhaps the simplest structure relevant to athletic pubalgia and is a nonsynovial amphiarthrodial joint.[9] Static stability of the joint is provided by the disk and four ligaments. The arcuate or inferior ligament has attachments to the inferior articular disk, the inferior attachment of the rectus abdominis, and the adductor and gracilis aponeurosis. The superior ligament spans the space between the pubic tubercles. The anterior ligament blends with fibers of the external oblique and rectus

abdominis superficially. The deep portion of the anterior ligament attaches to the intra-articular disk. The posterior ligament is poorly developed. The term *pubic joint* was introduced by Myers and has been used to describe the complex biomechanics of the muscular envelope at the pubis symphysis. The pubic symphysis acts as the fulcrum for forces generated at the anterior pelvis. It represents the common attachment of the confluence of the rectus abdominis fascial sheath with the fascial sheath of the adductor longus; these merge anterior to the pubis to form a common sheath.[9-11] Pathology of other adductors, including the adductor brevis and pectineus, is less commonly seen in athletic pubalgia. Imbalance between the rectus abdominis and adductor muscular and pathology of the common attachment appears to be a major factor in athletic pubalgia.

The abdominal wall has a layered structure. From superficial to deep, the structures of the abdominal wall are skin, fascia, external oblique muscle/fascia, internal oblique muscle/fascia, transversus abdominis muscle/fascia, and transversalis fascia. The posterior fascia is deficient in the lower third of the rectus. Fibers from the rectus, conjoint tendon (fusion of the internal oblique and transversus abdominis fascia), and external oblique merge to form the pubic aponeurosis (also called rectus abdominis/adductor aponeurosis), which is confluent with the adductor and gracilis origin. The conjoint tendon inserts anterior to the rectus abdominis on the pubis (Fig. 84.1).[12]

Weakness of the floor of the posterior inguinal canal may play a role in athletic pubalgia. The inguinal canal is formed anteriorly by the external oblique aponeurosis; posteriorly by the transversalis fascia and conjoint tendon; superiorly by the transversalis fascia, internal oblique, and transversus abdominus; and inferiorly by the inguinal ligament (from the external oblique aponeurosis). The inguinal canal contains the spermatic cord (in males), round ligament (in females), genital branch of the genitofemoral nerve (which supplies motor function to cremaster muscle and sensory function to the scrotum), and ilioinguinal nerve (supplying sensory function to the groin). The role of nerve-mediated pain in athletes with groin pain remains somewhat poorly understood and controversial. Knowledge of the nerve anatomy of the groin is important in elucidating the potential role of each nerve in athletic pubalgia. One possible source of pain has been theorized to be the result of entrapment of the genital branch of the genitofemoral or ilioinguinal nerve.[13] Weakness of the posterior inguinal floor has been proposed to result in dynamic compression of the

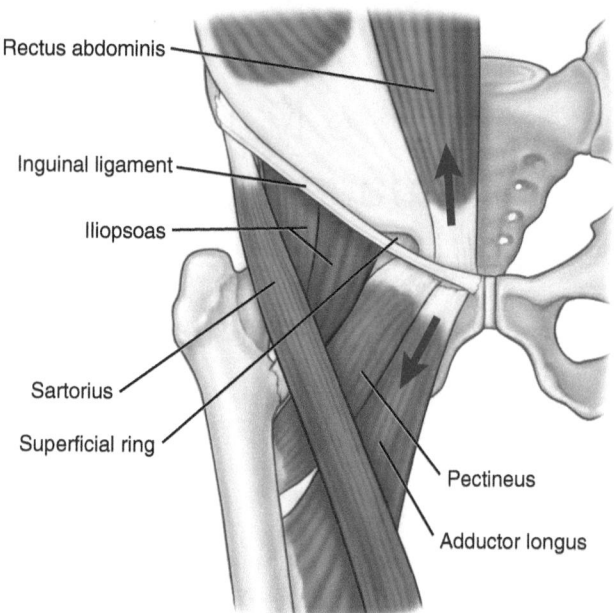

Fig. 84.1 Injury to the abdominal wall at the fascial attachments of the rectus and adductors onto the pubis is implicated in athletic pubalgia. (From Omar IM, Zoga AC, Kavanagh EC, et al. Athletic pubalgia and "sports hernia": optimal MR imaging technique and findings. *Radiographics.* 2008;28[5]:1415–1438.)

Labels: Rectus abdominis, Inguinal ligament, Iliopsoas, Sartorius, Superficial ring, Pectineus, Adductor longus

genital branch of genitofemoral nerve. The symphysis itself is innervated by branches of the pudendal and genitofemoral nerves.[9]

Historical Background

Groin injuries were discussed in the medical literature as early as 1932, when Spinelli reported on pubic pain in fencers.[16] Nearly 50 years later, in 1980, Gilmore recognized a "severe musculo-tendinous injury of the groin" in three professional soccer players. He identified a triad of pathology including injuries to the external oblique aponeurosis and conjoint tendon, avulsion of the conjoint tendon from the pubic tubercle, and dehiscence of the conjoint tendon from the inguinal ligament.[3] He later reported a 97% return to sport after surgical repair.[17]

In 1993, Hackney first used the term *sports hernia* to describe a syndrome of groin pain in athletes that had failed nonsurgical management. At surgery, he identified weakening of the transversalis fascia with separation of that fascia from the conjoint tendon, dilation of the inguinal ring, and one case of a small direct hernia. He treated all patients with a surgical repair of the posterior inguinal wall and obtained an 87% return to sport in 15 athletes.[18] Irshad et al. described "hockey groin syndrome" in 22 National Hockey League players in 2001.[19] They found tearing of the external oblique aponeurosis and entrapment of the ilioinguinal nerve. Meyers proposed that use of the term *athletic pubalgia*[4] would be more appropriate for the constellation of injuries to the abdominal wall, adductors, and pubic symphysis presenting with pubic area or inguinal pain than the more commonly used *sports hernia*.[2] He proposed that the primary pathology in athletic pubalgia was an imbalance between the strong adductors and the relatively weak abdominal muscles. More recently, the term *core muscle injury* has also been increasingly used to describe athletic pubalgia. Meyers describes 17 different variants of athletic pubalgia, the most common of which were multiple tears or detachment of the anterior and antero-lateral fibers of the rectus abdominis from the pubis and combined injuries to the rectus and adductors.[20]

Over the last two decades, treatment of athletic pubalgia has become increasingly common in high-level athletes involved in cutting/pivoting and acceleration/deceleration sports, including soccer, football, and ice hockey. Between 2012 and 2015, some 4.2% of athletes of the National Football League (NFL) had undergone surgical treatment of athletic pubalgia (most commonly defensive backs and wide receivers).[21]

As the understanding of intra-articular hip pathology has improved, there has been increasing recognition that acetabular labral pathology and femoroacetabular impingement can coexist with athletic pubalgia.[7,10] Significant overlap between athletes with athletic pubalgia and femoroacetabular impingement is seen in clinical practice but has only recently been recognized.[7,10] Feeley et al. described the "sports hip triad" of labral tears, rectus abdominis strain, and adductor strain.[22] The loss of internal rotation of the hip appears to play a role in the development of groin pain and osteitis pubis.[14] Based on these observations, Birmingham et al. performed a cadaveric study looking at the effect of femoroacetabular impingement on rotation at the pubic symphysis in a cadaveric model.[15] At higher torque values, motion through the symphysis was much greater in cadavers with simulated cam morphology than in the native hip state. This supports the previous hypothesis that the altered rotational profile seen in the setting of femoroacetabular impingement contributes to altered mechanics at the pubic symphysis through stress transfer. Limitations in range of motion (ROM) at one location can result in additional motion occurring at other locations.

Larson et al. reported the outcomes of surgical treatment in a subset of athletes with coexistent femoroacetabular impingement and athletic pubalgia.[7] Failure to treat both pathologies resulted in a low return to sport (25% if athletic pubalgia was addressed in isolation, and 50% if the intra-articular hip pathology was addressed in isolation). This prompted the development of a surgical protocol to address both etiologies under the same anesthesia when athletes present with both symptomatic athletic pubalgia and intra-articular hip disorders (FAI). Using this approach, these investigators achieved an 85% to 93% return to sport.[7]

In addressing the athlete with groin pain, it is therefore important to carefully investigate other potential sources of the athlete's pain. Intra-articular hip pathology and associated hip pathomorphology must be carefully screened for if symptomatic and limiting. This assessment should also take into account the high rates of potential asymptomatic labral pathology on magnetic resonance imaging (MRI) in this population. Additionally, it is important to be aware of the broader differential diagnosis of groin pain. Disorders of the gastrointestinal, genitourinary, or gynecologic systems must also be considered, with several authors identifying tumors, Crohn disease, and other pathologies in the evaluation of the athlete with groin pain.[2,21]

HISTORY

Athletic pubalgia is particularly common among those who participate in sports requiring repetitive twisting, pivoting, and cutting motions, as well as activity requiring frequent acceleration and deceleration. Trunk hyperextension and hip hyperabduction place significant stress across the pelvis, including the rectus abdominis and adductors. Soccer, football, ice hockey, and rugby have a particularly high incidence, with a lower incidence reported in basketball and baseball.[3,19,21] Meyers noted that in the 1980s, less than 1% of his patients with athletic pubalgia were female. Over the last two decades, however, that has changed dramatically, and female patients now represent 15% of patients presenting with athletic pubalgia.[20]

Athletes with athletic pubalgia may report an insidious onset of groin pain or less commonly have a more acute presentation. Most athletes report pain with athletic activities but not at rest. Although there is some variability in the location and characteristic of symptoms, Meyers et al.[6] found that all of their athletes reported lower abdominal pain with exertion, whereas 92% had minimal to no pain at rest. Forty-three percent developed bilateral symptoms and 67% developed adductor pain after the onset of lower abdominal pain. Pain may also radiate to the rectus, perineum, or testicular region.[7] Exacerbation typically occurs during activities involving kicking, acceleration, and pivoting.[6,22] Abdominal crunches or situps, coughing, or sneezing may also reproduce symptoms. Osteitis pubis presents in a similar fashion, with pubic pain that may radiate to the adductors and is typically exacerbated by weight bearing.[21] Intra-articular hip pathology from labral tears or femoroacetabular impingement typically presents with deep anterior groin pain that may radiate to the anterior thigh and lateral hip. There is considerable overlap between intra-articular hip symptoms and athletic pubalgia symptoms, which, when combined with high rates of potentially asymptomatic pathology of radiographs and MRI, increases the complexity of making an accurate diagnosis in this challenging patient population.

PHYSICAL EXAMINATION

Assessment for athletic pubalgia should begin with palpation of the pubic symphysis, insertion of the rectus abdominis, adductor origin, external and internal obliques, transverses abdominis, pectineus, gracilis and inguinal ring for areas of tenderness. Provocative testing can be useful to reproduce symptoms, including simulated coughing, Valsalva maneuver, resisted situps (46%), (Fig. 84.2), or resisted hip adduction.[6] With traditional assessment for inguinal hernia, there is no palpable hernia, but this should be ruled out. There is usually tenderness around the conjoint tendon, pubic tubercle (22%), adductor longus (36%), superficial inguinal ring, or posterior inguinal canal.[6,28,29] Detailed assessment of hip ROM including provocative testing is warranted given the interplay between athletic pubalgia and FAI.

Exam findings for osteitis pubis frequently overlap (or coexist) with athletic pubalgia and include tenderness of the pubic symphysis (67%), adductor origin tenderness (59%), pain with the

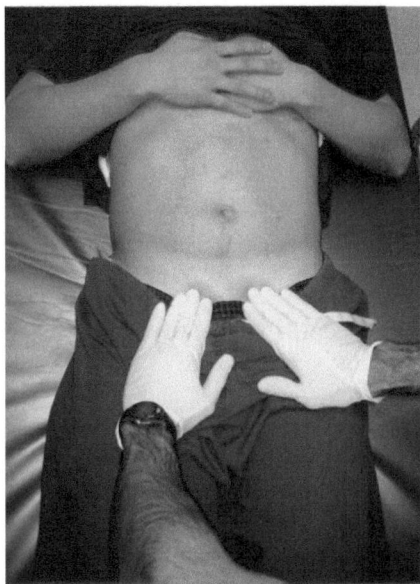

Fig. 84.2 Pubic and/or groin pain with resisted situps is associated with athletic pubalgia. (From Minnich JM, Hanks JB, Muschaweck U, et al. Sports hernia: diagnosis and treatment highlighting a minimal repair surgical technique. *Am J Sports Med.* 2011;39[6]:1341–1349.)

adductor squeeze test (96%),[5] and apprehension throughout the hip's ROM.[30] More severe cases of osteitis pubis may present with a classic waddling gait pattern.[28]

Diagnostic Injections

As indicated earlier, the symptoms of femoroacetabular impingement, athletic pubalgia, osteitis pubis, and adductor strain can present with overlapping symptomatology and physical examination findings. An intra-articular injection of local anesthetic into the hip followed by physical examination or by having the athlete perform activities that typically provoke the pain can be useful in the evaluation of this population as well as in the resultant decision-making. Pain that resolves or significantly improves with this injection can then be assumed to be related to intra-articular hip pathology and be treated accordingly.[7] Persistent pain the lower abdominal and proximal adductor regions after intra-articular injections is consistent with coexistent athletic pubalgia. Similarly, injection of the pubic symphysis may be useful for confirming the diagnosis of osteitis pubis. Radiocontrast dye can be used for the symphyseal injection, and extravasation of this dye up the rectus abdominis tract or down the adductor tract may indicate underlying pathology consistent with athletic pubalgia. Adductor pathology can be ruled in or out with an injection of anesthetic into the pubic cleft. Diagnostic injections can be used in the assessment of other pathology around the hip and groin as well. If psoas disorders are suspected, a diagnostic psoas bursal injection with anesthetic can be carried out. If impingement is suspected from the anterior inferior iliac spine, a subspinal injection can be carried out. Together these targeted diagnostic injections can be useful adjuncts to clinical assessment and aid in treatment decision-making, particularly in decisions regarding combined surgical treatments.

IMAGING

Radiographic Analysis

Plain radiographs are vital in the initial evaluation of the athlete with hip or groin pain. A number of pathologies including osteitis pubis, avulsion fractures, stress fractures, apophysitis, osteoarthritis, femoroacetabular impingement, and hip dysplasia may be identified on radiographs. It is essential to obtain good-quality, properly oriented images according to an established imaging protocol.[32]

The anteroposterior (AP) pelvic view (Fig. 84.3) may be used to evaluate the pubic symphysis for evidence of osteitis pubis, including sclerosis, fragmentation, and cyst formation within the pubic ramus as well as symphyseal widening. Most authors now favor performing this radiograph in the standing position to best simulate the functional position of the pelvis, which commonly differs from the supine position. In evaluating for femoroacetabular impingement, also assed are deformities of the femoral head neck and acetabular depth and version. In the adolescent athlete, the AP view can be useful to identify apophyseal avulsion injuries. Additionally, stress fractures of the femoral neck and pubic rami and sacroiliitis may be identified.[12]

In cases of possible pubic symphyseal instability associated with osteitis pubis, stress radiographs may be useful. The stability of the pubic symphysis can be determined on single-leg-stance AP views (the "flamingo view"). Symphyseal widening greater than 7 mm or vertical translation greater than 2 mm on a single-leg-stance view suggests instability of the pubic symphysis.[30]

Magnetic Resonance Imaging

MR arthrography has been used for the assessment of intra-articular hip pathology. More recently, noncontrast 3.0 Tesla MR has been evaluated and found to be sensitive for intra-articular pathology including articular cartilage injury and labral

pathology. The use of arthrography on MR is now dependent on the surgeon and institutional preference. Routine assessment of common sites of pathology in athletic pubalgia on hip MRI can be useful in athletes with groin pain, but dedicated protocols for pelvic MRI are optimal for visualization. Coronal oblique and axial oblique sequences through the rectus insertion and pubic symphysis should be obtained in addition to standard sagittal, coronal, and axial sequences. MRI is 68% sensitive and 100% specific for rectus abdominis pathology as compared with findings at surgery (the gold standard) and is 86% sensitive and 89% specific for adductor pathology. MRI is 100% sensitive for osteitis pubis.[33] Nonarthrographic studies may be preferred for in-season athletes to avoid the potential for irritation secondary to the administration of intra-articular contrast.

The MRI should be evaluated in a systematic fashion for pathology consistent with athletic pubalgia. The pubic bones should be evaluated for edema, subchondral sclerosis, and cysts suggestive of osteitis pubis (Fig. 84.4).[11,34] Evaluation of the tendinous insertions of the core muscles around the pubic symphysis should then be performed (Fig. 84.5). Frequent findings include fluid signal within the rectus abdominis or adductor origin, thickening of either structure, peritendinous fluid, or partial or complete disruption of either tendon. Most commonly there is a confluent fluid signal extending from the anteroinferior insertion of the rectus abdominis into the adductor origin, with corresponding fluid signal in the pubis.[33]

Dynamic Ultrasonography

Dynamic ultrasound has become a common form of diagnostic evaluation in patients with athletic pubalgia. Ultrasound takes advantage of the dynamic nature of the pathology in athletic pubalgia. Visualization of the structures muscular insertions at the pubis and the posterior inguinal canal can be performed at rest and with stress. A convex anterior bulge of the posterior inguinal canal is a common finding in the setting of posterior

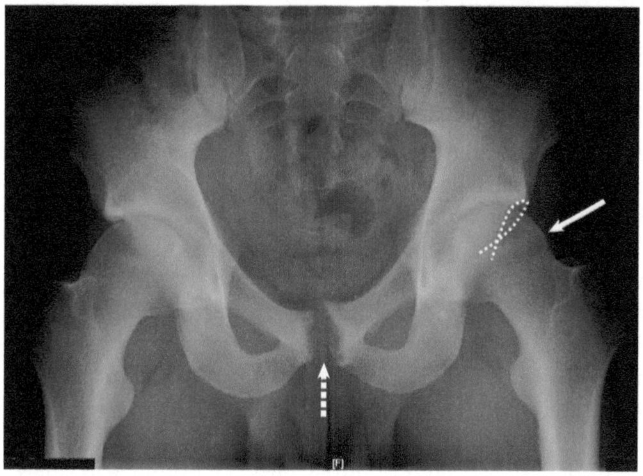

Fig. 84.3 Well-aligned anteroposterior radiograph of the pelvis. Note the coccyx centered over the pubic symphysis and a centimeter proximal. On this radiograph, there are finding consistent with osteitis pubis *(large arrow)*, including erosion, irregularity, and cyst formation. Additionally, there is a positive crossover sign, suggesting possible pincer impingement and a large cam lesion on the femoral head-neck junction *(small arrow)*.

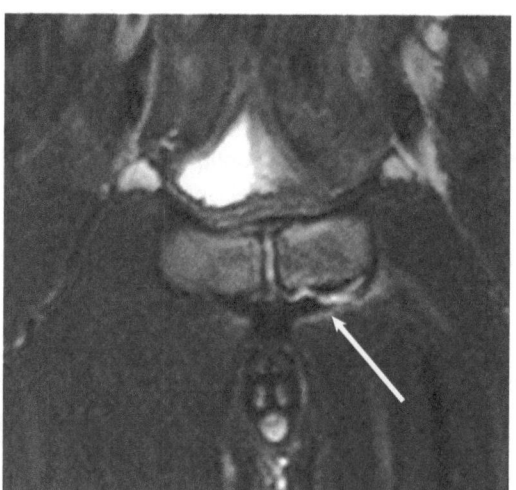

Fig. 84.4 Oblique axial fat-suppression T2 magnetic resonance image of the pubic symphysis. There is disruption of the left rectus aponeurosis as it inserts on the anterior aspect of the superior pubic ramus *(tip of the white arrow)*.

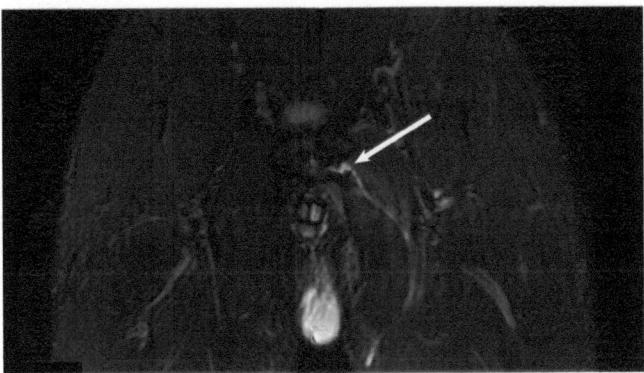

Fig. 84.5 Coronal fat-suppression T2 image of the pelvis demonstrating injury to the left adductor longus at its origin on the anteroinferior aspect of the superior pubic ramus. There is a fluid signal coursing linearly distally through the proximal muscle fibers *(tip of the white arrow).*

inguinal canal deficiency.[35] Ultrasound is dependent on the expertise and experience of the ultrasonographer and is most applicable to high-volume centers.

DECISION-MAKING PRINCIPLES

Treatment decisions must take into account a number of factors including the degree of limitation and ability to participate in the athlete's respective sport, duration of symptoms, pathology identified on physical examination and imaging, response to prior treatment modalities, and where the athlete is with respect to his or her training, sport season, and upcoming athletic events. The common locations of pain are the groin (FAI, athletic pubalgia, adductor), lower abdomen or pubic symphysis (athletic pubalgia, adductor longus), posterior hip (FAI, proximal hamstring, low back, sacroiliac joint, sciatic nerve entrapment disorders), or lateral thigh/hip (iliotibial band or gluteus medius/minimus). Conservative management should be attempted prior to surgical intervention. If no previous treatment has been attempted at presentation, a conservative trial should include rest, nonsteroidal antiinflammatory drugs (NSAIDs), physical therapy, and injections in select situations. Physical therapy is focused on restoring core muscle strength and correcting any underlying imbalance between core muscle groups. If the athlete continues to be symptomatic after 6 to 12 weeks of nonsurgical treatment, then surgery may be considered. The timing of the surgery depends on the degree of disability and the time point in the season. If the athlete must participate and he or she is productive and functional, a delay until after the season may be attempted. Surgery can then be performed at the end of the season if the athlete remains symptomatic. If the athlete is not able to compete at a reasonable level, then in-season or season-ending surgery can be considered. If there is a combined pathology such as FAI and athletic pubalgia, these can be surgically addressed at the same setting or staged in order to minimize postoperative rehabilitation time, total time lost from participation, and potential need for subsequent surgery. There is, however, no evidence to show that carrying out these procedures separately or in a staged manner, has any negative impact on outcome.[7]

TREATMENT OPTIONS

Adductor Strain

Adductor-related pain can present as an acute injury or a chronic condition. Muscle imbalance between the abductors and adductors does appear to contribute to injury of the adductors. Tyler et al. found that professional hockey players were 17 times more likely to sustain an adductor strain if their adductor strength was less than 80% of their abductor strength.[36] In a follow-up study, they were able to demonstrate a clinically and statistically significant decrease in adductor strains in the same population with institution of a preventative adductor strengthening program.[37] Recognition of at-risk athletes with such muscular imbalance thus may play an important role in injury prevention in this population.

Nonoperative Management

Treatment starts with a brief period of rest, judicious use of ice and NSAIDs, and the institution of core and lower extremity strengthening programs. Once the athlete is able to perform a pain-free concentric contraction of the adductor against resistance, the program can be progressed to core strengthening and adductor-specific exercises. Identification and treatment of any deficits or imbalances in the contralateral extremity is useful at this stage as well. It has been suggested the athlete can progress to sport-specific training when the adductor strength is 75% of the ipsilateral abductor and passive ROM is normal.[37,38]

One randomized clinical trial is available; it presents an 8- to 12-year follow-up after nonoperative management of adductor-related groin pain.[39] The initial study randomized 59 athletes to either (1) a passive rehabilitation protocol consisting of modalities and stretching or (2) an active rehabilitation protocol emphasizing strengthening of the core, abductors, and adductors.[39] In the initial study period, 23 of 29 patients treated with 8 to 12 weeks of active therapy had returned to sport by 4 months after initiating treatment.[38] In the passive therapy group, only 4 of 30 patients had returned to sport at the 4-month mark. At 8 to 12 years after treatment, 50% of the active rehabilitation group had no adductor pain with activity, no groin pain during or after activity, and were active in athletic activity at or one level below their previous level of athletic activity in the same sport, whereas only 22% of the passive therapy group met the same criteria.

The evidence for platelet-rich plasma (PRP) injections about the hip and pelvis, however, is lacking. There is one case report of injecting a complete tear of the adductor longus with PRP followed by a return to competitive soccer without surgery.[40] However, successful nonoperative treatment of this injury has been reported without PRP as well. Dallaudiere et al.[41] reported the clinical and ultrasound-based outcomes of 40 patients with chronic hip pain due to either the adductor or hamstring tendons. Improvements in WOMAC scores and decreased lesion size were noted at mean follow-up of 20 months.

Operative Management

Acute adductor injuries generally do not require surgical treatment. Schlegel et al. reported on 19 professional football players who sustained spontaneous rupture of the adductor longus. Twelve of 19 had groin or abdominal pain that preceded acute rupture. Of the 19 athletes identified, 14 were treated conservatively and 9 underwent surgical repair with suture anchors. The nonoperative group returned to play at an average of 6 weeks after injury with no noted strength deficits. The operative group returned to play at an average of 12 weeks after injury, and 20% experienced wound complications.[42] Given that there are minimal functional deficits after spontaneous rupture of the adductor at its origin, controlled release in the context of a surgical procedure might similarly have few long-term functional consequences.

Surgical treatment of chronic proximal adductor pain is indicated when an athlete has failed 3 to 6 months of conservative management. Successful outcomes of a variety of techniques—including complete proximal release, percutaneous partial release, or fractional lengthening—has been reported, although the degree of residual weakness may differ. Akermark and Johansson published a case series of 16 competitive athletes with long-standing (mean 18 months) and recurrent groin pain localized on physical exam to the adductor origin.[43] All athletes had failed conservative management with rest, stretching, NSAIDs, and corticosteroid injections. Surgical treatment involved open tenotomy 1 cm from the adductor origin. All patients were improved and able to resume sporting activities at some level. Ten of 16 patients were pain-free. The operated leg was weaker in adduction torque in all patients after full recovery, although not necessarily symptomatic. Atkinson et al. reported on 48 athletes who underwent 68 percutaneous adductor tenotomies for adductor strain. All patients were significantly restricted in their chosen sport preoperatively, and 54% were able to return to full sport at a mean of 18.5 weeks.[44] Proximal adductor release does appear to result in some persistent adductor weakness, although this has not been demonstrated to affect return to sport.[45]

Given the overlapping symptoms of core muscle injury, including adductor-related pain and athletic pubalgia, controversy exists on the optimal treatment or treatments. In athletes undergoing athletic pubalgia surgery, the combination of treatment of proximal adductor pathology in the presence of significant adductor symptoms may play a role in optimizing outcome. Some authors have also suggested that the treatment of adductor pathology may improve athletic pubalgia symptoms even in the absence of surgical treatment.

Athletic Pubalgia/Sports Hernia

Nonoperative Management

Generally a brief period of rest is indicated. Physical therapy should emphasize core strengthening and the identification and treatment of weakness and restricted motion in the musculature of the hip and pelvis. Ice and NSAIDs can be helpful for managing pain. Avoidance of heavy weight, deep hip flexion, low repetition, squats/lunges/cleans is advisable during this period of rehabilitation. As with adductor pathology, the role of PRP or other biologics remains to be defined. Case reports indicate that injection into the distal rectus insertion can have a good short-term outcome.

Operative Management

A variety of surgical procedures have been described in the literature for the treatment of athletic pubalgia, all with generally excellent reported outcomes. These procedures can be classified as involving primary repair, mesh-based repair, or minimal repair. Gilmore first described "Gilmore's groin" as a cause of chronic groin pain in athletes in 1980.[11] His repair involves plication of the transversalis fascia, reapproximation of the conjoint tendon to the inguinal ligament, and approximation of the external oblique aponeurosis. Utilizing this technique, the reported return to sport has been 96% to 97% within 10 to 12 weeks.[16,44] Hackney published his technique in 1993. On surgical exploration, weakness of the transversalis fascia with separation from the conjoint tendon and dilatation of the internal inguinal ring was identified. A direct repair was performed with the goal of reconstitution of the internal inguinal ring, plication of the transversalis fascia, and apposition of the conjoint tendon and internal inguinal ring.[17] Hackney presented a series of 15 patients with an average duration of groin pain for 20 months prior to surgical intervention. Postoperatively, swimming and cycling were allowed at 3 weeks, running at 4 to 5 weeks, and sport-specific exercise at 6 weeks. Eighty-seven percent of the athletes were able to resume full participation in sporting activities.

Meyers has published the largest cohorts on the treatment of athletic pubalgia utilizing a "pelvic floor repair."[6] This involves an open surgical approach with reattachment of the anteroinferior rectus abdominis to the pubis and a variation of an adductor release. In 276 athletes evaluated for groin pain, 157 had clinical symptoms and exam findings consistent with athletic pubalgia, subsequently undergoing primary pelvic floor repair. Imaging and intraoperative findings were somewhat variable and included unilateral or bilateral tearing or scarring of the rectus, tearing of the external oblique aponeurosis, and scarring of the adductor origin. Postoperatively, 152 were able to return to their preinjury levels of competition. In 2008, Myers reported on his experience of over 20 years and 5460 surgeries in a population that included 83% athletes (most commonly soccer, football, and ice hockey). He noted the evolving understanding of the pathophysiology of athletic pubalgia and associated treatments aimed at correcting the underlying pathology. This included performance of 26 different procedures and 121 combinations of these in the group. Overall, 95.3% of athletes were able to return to sports by 3 months postoperatively. Myers reported that athletes operated on more recently were following either a 3- or 6-week return-to-sport protocol, after which the majority were able to return to full participation.[18] Management of the genital branch of the genitofemoral nerve and ilioinguinal nerve remains controversial, with some surgeons advocating routine resection whereas others advise against this.

More recently a laparoscopic approach has been reported with the potential of allowing a more rapid recovery. Genitsaris et al. identified 131 athletes with groin pain who had failed 2 to 8 months of physical therapy. All patients underwent laparoscopic bilateral mesh repairs (transabdominal preperitoneal), with the mesh extending from the pubis to the anterosuperior iliac spine bilaterally. The peritoneum was closed over the mesh. All patients were able to return to full sports participation at 2 to 3 weeks postoperatively.[47]

Kluin et al.[48] identified 14 athletes with persistent groin pain despite 3 months of conservative management. During

Authors' Preferred Treatment

The authors prefer a fractional lengthening or recession of the adductor longus performed through a 2-cm incision (Fig. 84.6). The adductor tendon is released 3 to 5 cm distal to its origin, leaving the underlying muscle intact (Fig. 84.7). This may have less potential for longer-term adductor weakness. In the setting of significant degenerative tearing and tendinosis proximally, however, a proximal release near the origin is performed.

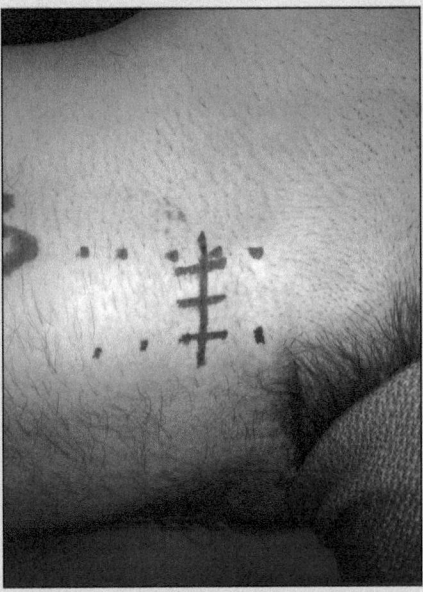

Fig. 84.6 Skin markings for the 2-cm incision utilized for open adductor tenotomy. Note the *dotted lines* marking the borders of the adductor tendon and the location of the incision 4 to 5 cm distal to the origin.

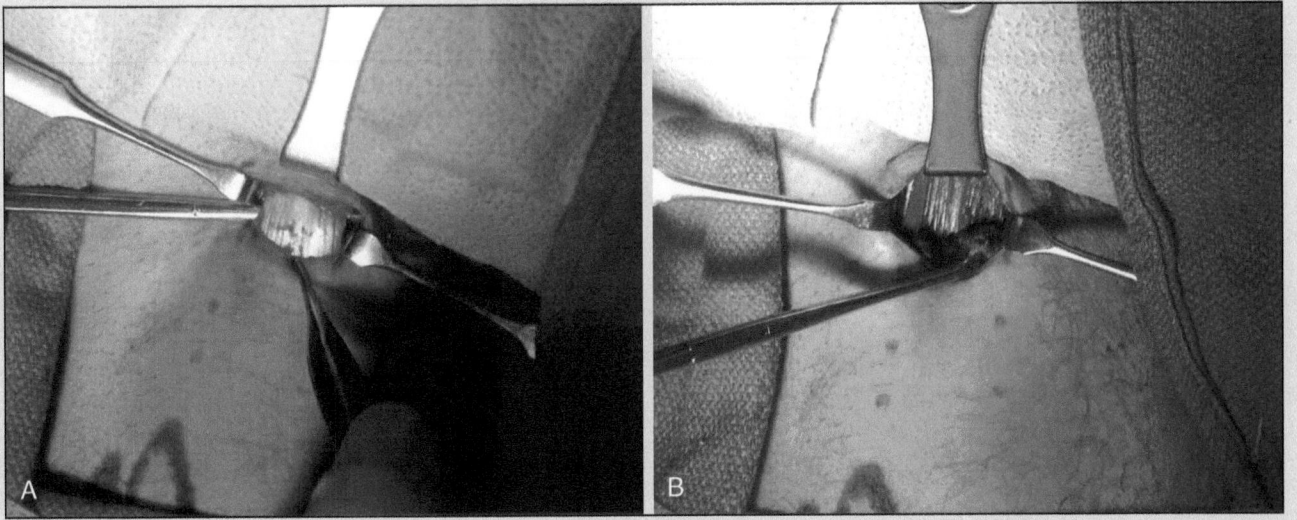

Fig. 84.7 (A) Intraoperative image of the exposed adductor longus tendon. (B) Intraoperative image of the underlying adductor muscle belly after release of the tendinous portion.

laparoscopic exploration, 9 occult inguinal hernias, 4 occult femoral hernias, and 3 preperitoneal lipomas were identified, among other pathology. Treatment was with laparoscopic tension-free mesh repair. Overall, 13 of 14 athletes were able to return to sport by 3 months. Ingoldby et al. compared traditional open and laparoscopic results in 28 athletes. Fourteen open procedures and 14 laparoscopic procedures were performed. Full training was resumed at an average of 5 weeks after the open procedures and 3 weeks after the laparoscopic procedures.[49]

Muschaweck and Burger developed a "minimal repair" technique in 2003 (Fig. 84.8).[50] They identified patients with athletic pubalgia on the basis of clinical history of groin pain radiating to the inner thigh, pubis, testicles, or scrotum. Findings on examination included tenderness on palpation of the internal inguinal

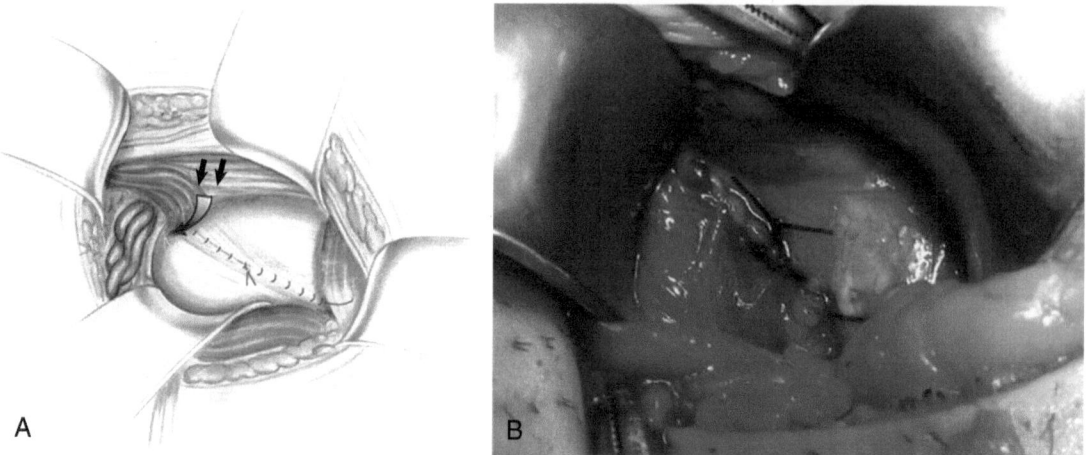

Fig. 84.8 (A) Illustration and (B) intraoperative image of tension-free repair of the defect in the posterior wall of the inguinal canal. (From Minnich JM, Hanks JB, Muschaweck U, et al. Sports hernia: diagnosis and treatment highlighting a minimal repair surgical technique. *Am J Sports Med.* 2011;39[6]:1341–1349.)

ring; ultrasound confirmed bulging of the posterior inguinal wall with Valsalva. The "minimal repair" that was subsequently implemented involved decompression (if intact) or resection (if damaged) of the genital branch of the genitofemoral nerve with a tension-free suture repair of any defect in the posterior wall of the inguinal canal. this procedure can be performed without general anesthesia. Return to sport generally occurred by day 14. A total of 132 such procedures were performed in 128 patients including 89 high-level athletes. Overall, 83.7% of the athletes were fully competitive in their sport at 28 days postoperatively. In a more recent cohort of 129 prospectively enrolled patients, similar outcomes were demonstrated with return to training at 7 days postoperatively.[51]

Paajanan et al. performed a prospective randomized controlled trial comparing nonoperative management to laparoscopic sports hernia repair. All athletes reported 3 to 6 months of symptoms prior to enrollment in the study. These patients were either professionals or high-level recreational athletes. The group randomized to nonoperative management underwent a period of rest followed by physical therapy, local injections of corticosteroids, and use of oral NSAIDs for a total of 8 weeks. At 1 month, 20% of athletes had returned to sport; by 3 months, 27% had returned to sport. At 6 months, 7 of 30 had elected to switch to the operative arm of the study. At 1 year, 15 had returned to sport and 14 reported complete relief of pain. Operative management consisted of a laparoscopic procedure with insertion of a preperitoneal mesh repair. Adductor tenotomy was performed in six patients who had adductor tenderness preoperatively. Of these, 67% had returned to sport at 1 month postoperatively and 90% had returned at 3 months. Twenty-nine of 30 athletes had returned to full participation and were pain-free at 1 year after surgery. Pain scores and patient satisfaction scores were better in the operative group at all points up to a year out from surgery.[52]

Osteitis Pubis
Nonoperative Management
Options for nonoperative management of osteitis include rest, use of therapeutic modalities, NSAIDs and corticosteroid injections,

and rehabilitation focusing on strengthening of the core and pelvic musculature. Currently all available studies of nonoperative management of osteitis pubis provide Level IV evidence.[53]

In a prospective cohort study, Verrall et al. identified 27 professional Australian-rules football players with chronic groin injuries diagnosed on history and physical exam. On MRI, these athletes had findings consistent with osteitis pubis. Treatment consisted of 12 weeks of non-weight bearing. Swimming and upper-body lifting activities were allowed initially. Cycling was allowed at 3 weeks, along with a core/pelvic strengthening program as long as this did not provoke pain. Stair stepping was initiated at 6 weeks, followed by a graduated running program at 12 weeks. With this protocol, 89% were able to return to sport by 1 year after initiation of treatment. By the second season, 100% of the athletes had returned and 81% were without symptoms.[13]

Rodriguez et al.[54] identified 44 professional soccer players with osteitis pubis on the basis of history, physical exam, radiographic findings including irregularity of the pubic symphysis and rami, and bone scan demonstrating increased uptake in the pubic rami. Thirty-five athletes underwent a conservative rehabilitation protocol that included multiple therapeutic modalities (electrical stimulation or ultrasound, ice massage, and infrared laser) for the first 14 days in conjunction with high-dose NSAIDs. Subsequently the athletes followed a gradual activity progression including stretching; strengthening of the adductors, abductors and abdominal muscles; running progression; plyometrics; and kicking progression. Athletes with mild symptoms returned to sport at an average of 3.8 weeks after initiation of treatment. Those with moderate symptoms returned to sport 6.7 weeks after initiation of treatment. No long-term follow-up was available.

There is some Level IV evidence in the literature to support the use of additional modalities including injection of corticosteroids into the pubic symphysis. O'Connell et al. found that 14 of 16 in-season athletes were able to return to sport within 48 hours of symphyseal injection of corticosteroid with significant pain relief. However, at 6 months, only 5 of 16 were pain-free, and 4 had required an additional period of rest before returning to full activity.[55]

Holt et al.[56] presented a case-control study of 12 athletes at the University of Wisconsin presenting with physical examination and radiographic findings consistent with osteitis pubis. In the initial arm, 9 athletes underwent 4 months of conservative management consisting of rest, NSAIDs, stretching, and a gradual return to sport-specific activities. After failure of this protocol to resolve symptoms, 8 athletes underwent symphyseal injection of corticosteroids. Of these, 7 were able to return to sport after one to three injections and an additional period of rest ranging from 4 to 24 weeks. In the second arm, three athletes with osteitis pubis were identified; they underwent 7 to 10 days of conservative management, and after failure of early treatment, underwent injection. All three were able to return to sport within 2 weeks and remained symptom-free at 1 year after injection. The authors advocated early consideration of corticosteroid injection after diagnosis of osteitis pubis, as it may allow early return to sport and sustained symptom relief.

Operative Treatment

Operative treatment of osteitis pubis is generally considered a salvage technique and used most frequently in the scenario of demonstrable instability on radiographic studies or failure of several months of conservative management. Techniques described in the literature include curettage of the symphysis,[57] wedge resection,[58] mesh reinforcement of the symphysis, and arthrodesis of the symphysis with bone graft and compression plating.[29]

Wedge resection of the pubic symphysis was first described by Schnute in 1961[59] in a case series. He reported that use of the wedge resection resulted in significant clinical improvement patients who were severely limited by pain. Grace et al.[58] reported on 10 patients who underwent wedge resection at an average of 32 months after onset of symptoms. Of these, 3 patients developed chronic pain and another required fusion of the sacroiliac joints for posterior instability that developed secondary to the wedge resection. Moore et al. reported two additional patients who developed sacroiliac instability after wedge resection.[60] No published study documents the use of this procedure in high-level athletes, and given the relatively high risk of developing late posterior sacroiliac instability, this technique should be used cautiously in the athletic population.

Williams et al. described fusion of the pubic symphysis with compression plating and bone grafting as a viable treatment option for chronic osteitis pubis.[30] They treated seven rugby players with chronic groin pain diagnosed as osteitis pubis on physical examination and radiographic findings. Surgical treatment involved excision of the articular surface of the pubis, cancellous bone grafting, and application of a compression plate. One athlete also underwent mesh repair by Gilmore after injuries to the external oblique aponeurosis and conjoint tendon were identified. Postoperatively the athletes returned to sport at around the 6 months. All seven athletes were able to return to sport and at an average of 52 months after surgery, all were pain-free.

In the largest published study of operative treatment of osteitis pubis in athletes, Radic et al. treated 23 patients with curettage of the pubic symphysis.[57] Surgical treatment involved curettage of the articular surface until all articular cartilage was removed and bleeding bone was encountered. No stabilization of the joint was performed. Initially, 70% were able to return to their previous level of activity at an average of 5.6 months after surgery. However, with longer follow-up, 39% remained asymptomatic and 26% experienced a one-time recurrence of their symptoms that resolved with rest. Yet 30% of their cohort were never able to resume their preinjury level of activity and did not consider the surgical procedure to have been worthwhile. Mesh reinforcement of the pubic symphysis was described by Paajanen et al. in 2005.[61,62] They identified 16 athletes with clinical histories suggestive of osteitis pubis and MRI demonstrating pubic bone marrow edema and a positive bone scan. Eight patients with more severe symptoms, who failed 6 months of conservative management, elected to undergo surgical intervention, which involved laparoscopic placement of mesh behind the pubis held in place with titanium tacks. Two athletes had concomitant adductor or gracilis release. Seven of eight operatively treated patients returned to sport at an average of 2 months postoperatively. At an average of 2.7 years after surgery, all surgically treated patients were competing at their preinjury levels of athletics. The authors also reported on eight patients with more mild symptoms who were treated nonoperatively. Four of eight conservatively managed patients were able to return to their preinjury level of activity after 1 to 1.5 years of conservative management and four were competing with some pain at one level below their preinjury level.[55] The authors felt that surgical management with mesh repair allowed their cohort to return more quickly to sport with better resolution of pain than with conservative management.

There has been one report of treatment of osteitis pubis with an endoscopic decompression of the pubic symphysis in a chronic case that occurred in association with FAI.[63] The FAI was also treated arthroscopically at the same sitting and the patient was improved with resolution of the presenting waddling gait. Matsuda et al.[64] reported a combined case series of seven patients treated with endoscopic pubic symphysectomy combined with arthroscopic treatment of FAI. Two patients demonstrated postoperative scrotal swelling, one to the size of a volleyball, which resolved with observation. Good outcomes were reported in five of seven patients without evidence of instability, whereas one patient required fusion due to persistent symptoms. Further studies are needed to clarify the role of endoscopic surgery for osteitis pubis.

Meyers initially excluded athletes with osteitis pubis from surgical treatment of athletic pubalgia.[6] However, as clinical experience improved, prior patients who had been diagnosed with osteitis pubis, in addition to athletic pubalgia, were reviewed after undergoing isolated surgical treatment of athletic pubalgia. Similar outcomes were seen in patients with and without adductor release. This reinforces the hypothesis that athletic pubalgia and osteitis pubis represent a spectrum of injuries caused by abnormal forces around the pubic symphysis.[19]

🏷 Authors' Preferred Treatment

It is the authors' experience that mild symphyseal instability can be the result of disruption of the central pivot or rectus abdominis adductor aponeurosis. A repair of the central pivot appears to stabilize the pubic symphysis in this situation. For greater degrees of instability or in recalcitrant cases despite a pelvic floor repair, more aggressive surgical stabilization with open reduction internal fixation and fusion may be warranted. However, we have not encountered the need for fusion in the athletic population. In the absence of athletic pubalgia, an open or endoscopic decompression may be warranted but further outcomes are necessary to better define the results after these procedures in an athletic population.

COMPLICATIONS

Athletic Pubalgia

The most common postoperative complaint after athletic pubalgia surgery is minor bruising or edema involving the abdomen, thighs, genitals, and perineum. Postoperative hematoma requiring reoperation occurred in 0.3% of patients, and the wound infection rate was 0.4%. Nerve dysesthesia of the ilioinguinal, genitofemoral, anterior or lateral femoral cutaneous nerve distribution occurred in 0.3% of patients. Penile vein thrombosis occurred in 0.1% of patients but all resolved.[19] There is also the potential for postoperative scar tissue and subsequent neural dysesthesias. The most common reason for reoperation was development of similar symptoms on the contralateral side. The second most common was for adductor release not carried out at the first surgery.[19] Another common reason for continued disability after surgical treatment results from failure to identify associated intra-articular hip pathology (i.e., FAI).[7,19]

Osteitis Pubis

Complications associated with curettage of the symphysis for osteitis pubis include hemospermia and intermittent scrotal swelling.[30]

Adductor Tenotomy

For proximal adductor procedures there is a potential for spermatic cord injury if dissection is carried medial to the gracilis origin on the pubis.[65]

FUTURE CONSIDERATIONS

The understanding of diagnosis and treatment of athletic pubalgia is constantly improving. Although it was formerly thought to be an isolated pathology, there is now evidence to suggest otherwise. As the understanding evolves, a more athlete-specific pathology targeted approach is emerging. Based on the evidence

supporting a link between athletic pubalgia and femoroacetabular impingement in athletes presenting with groin or pelvic pain, both FAI and athletic pubalgia should be considered. One important question is whether all athletes presenting with symptoms consistent with both intra-articular hip pathology and athletic pubalgia/require treatment of both entities initially. This is a challenging scenario as there is probably a transition point where addressing the FAI alone is inadequate because permanent injury has occurred to the anterior pelvic musculature, leading to athletic pubalgia. At this time there are no clear cut indicators as to when the athletic pubalgia symptoms/pathology are beyond a point where they can be relieved with restoration of hip ROM after FAI corrective procedures. When timing is an issue, both might be best treated at the same sitting.

More sensitive imaging modalities would be helpful in determining the exact location of subtle anatomic injuries for athletic pubalgia and FAI. This would give some conformity with respect to which athletic pubalgia surgical approach would be best indicated for a particular patient, since there are several variants. With future studies focusing on the variable anatomic pathology and specific approaches used to treat these entities, we may develop a better understanding of the best approaches for treating this challenging patient population.

For a complete list of references, go to ExpertConsult.com.

SELECTED READINGS

Citation:

Birmingham PM, Kelly BT, Jacobs R, et al. The effect of dynamic femoroacetabular impingement on pubic symphysis motion: a cadaveric study. *Am J Sports Med.* 2012;40(5):1113–1118.

Level of Evidence:

Controlled cadaveric laboratory study

Summary:

This is a cadaveric study looking a motion through the pubic symphysis in the native state and with a simulated cam lesion. The authors found that rotation was increased through the symphysis in the presence of dynamic femoroacetabular impingement caused by a cam lesion and hypothesized that this pathologic motion could contribute to the development of athletic pubalgia.

Citation:

Larson CM, Pierce BR, Giveans MR. Treatment of athletes with symptomatic intra-articular hip pathology and athletic pubalgia/sports hernia: a case series. *Arthroscopy.* 2011;27(6):768–775.

Level of Evidence:

IV, therapeutic case series

Summary:

In a retrospective review, the authors identified 31 athletes (37 hips) who presented with symptoms consisted with both femoroacetabular impingement and athletic pubalgia. Treating either entity in isolation resulted in low rate of return to sport (25% treated for athletic pubalgia alone and 50% treated for femoroacetabular impingement alone), leading the authors to treat both entities in a staged or concurrent fashion with 85% to 93% return to sports.

Citation:
Meyers WC, McKechnie A, Philippon MJ, et al. Experience with
   "sports hernia" spanning two decades. *Ann Surg.*
   2008;248(4):656–665.

Level of Evidence:
IV, retrospective review

Summary:
The authors present their experience with 8490 patients with the
   diagnosis of sports hernia, 5218 of whom underwent surgical
   treatment. The authors noted an increase in percentage of
   patients opting for surgical treatment and a changing patient
   demographic over the last 20 years.

Citation:
Zoga AC, Kavanagh EC, Omar IM, et al. Athletic pubalgia and the
   "sports hernia": MR imaging findings. *Radiology.*
   2008;247(3):797–807.

Level of Evidence:
IV, retrospective review

Summary:
The authors retrospectively reviewed the MRIs of 141 patients with
   symptoms with athletic pubalgia to determine the sensitivity and
specificity of imaging findings compared with the standards of
   surgical or physical examination findings. MRI was 68% sensitive
   and 100% specific for injuries to the rectus abdominis and 86%
   sensitive and 89% specific for adductor tendon injury.

Citation:
Holmich P, Nyvold P, Larsen K. Continuing significant effect of
   physical training as treatment for overuse injury: 8- to 12-year
   outcome of a randomized clinical trial. *Am J Sports Med.*
   2011;39(11):2447–2451.

Level of Evidence:
I, randomized controlled trial, 80% long-term follow-up

Summary:
In the initial randomized controlled trial, the authors compared an
   active physical therapy program, emphasizing core stability and
   eccentric strengthening, to a passive therapy program in the
   treatment of adductor related groin pain in athletes. At long-term
   follow-up, the active therapy group demonstrated sustained
   improvement in outcome scores compared with the passive
   therapy group.

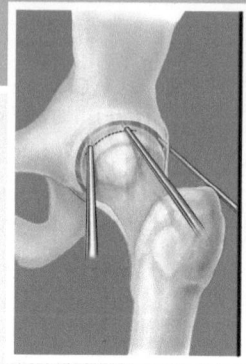

85

Posterior Hip Pain

Hal David Martin, Anthony Nicholas Khoury, Juan Gomez-Hoyos

Posterior hip pain can be a debilitating condition, and a structured physical examination is essential for a differential diagnosis in patients with a posterior hip complaint.[1] The examination incorporates the five levels of the hip: osseous, capsulolabral, musculotendinous, neurovascular, and the kinematic chain. To adequately develop a comprehensive treatment plan, diagnostic strategies require the interpretation of abnormal anatomy and biomechanics of each level. Utilizing a comprehensive approach will develop a detailed understanding of posterior hip complaint. The evaluation of a patient with posterior hip pain must rule out the lumbar spine and intrapelvic entrapment through magnetic resonance imaging (MRI), appropriate injections, and trained pelvic therapists. Any psychological impairment from chronic pain or long-term narcotic use may require psychological consult and rehabilitation. Isolated treatments of single layers may not provide the solution and will lead to frustration for both the patient and the physician. The use of a common language and techniques helps facilitate the understanding of each of these levels. The osseous contribution must also be understood in all three planes, considering the torsional alignment of the femur and acetabulum. The entire hip joint anatomy, surrounding structures, and the core physical examination must be understood in order to thoroughly evaluate the source of pain.

SCIATIC NERVE CHARACTERISTICS

Peripheral nerve fibers are arranged in widely variable numbers into bundles (fascicle) (Fig. 85.1). Each fascicle is surrounded by the perineurium, a multilayered epithelial sheath.[2] The space among the perineurium/fascicles is filled by connective tissue, including vessels. Finally, the nerve is surrounded by the epineurium, a thicker areolar tissue, which is highly vascular and provides a cushion for the nerves. While the endoneurium offers little mechanical support, the perineurium is dense, providing strength in tension and maintaining the pressurized blood-nerve barrier. The fascicular pattern is continually modified along the length of peripheral nerves with an interchange of nervous fibers among different fascicles.[3] Vascular considerations for peripheral nerves should not only include the in-flow, but also the out-flow, since varicosities can cause dilations within the nerve (Fig. 85.2).[4] The vascular supply of hip and thigh nerves is different from that of the upper body (Fig. 85.3).[5]

Peripheral nerves possess the ability to glide and stretch, accommodating normal joint biomechanics. The nerve is susceptible to mechanical compression as it courses around musculotendinous, osseous, and ligamentous structures. The neural and muscular biomechanics in the deep gluteal space must be closely monitored during the physical examination. The sciatic nerve maintains a unique movement pattern as it stretches and glides, accommodating strain or compression during hip joint movement. Recent investigations have provided significant insight to sciatic nerve mechanics. A proximal excursion of 28 mm is observed during hip flexion and straight leg raise with knee extension. There is a 6.6% increase in sciatic nerve strain relative to the extended hip.[6] Sciatic nerve strain does not remain consistent throughout the trajectory of length. Strain at the level of the hip joint is approximately 8% to 12%, whereas strain at the distal levels is 5%.[7] Strain greater than 10% or prolonged strain greater than 30 minutes results in decreased blood flow and neural activation.[8] Anatomic orientation of the femur has also been proven to affect normal nerve mechanics. Martin et al. studied the effect of femoral version during hip abduction and hip flexion, and concluded an 84.23% decrease in sciatic nerve strain during hip abduction to 40 degrees and terminal hip flexion, independent of femoral version due to premature coupling.[9] The authors described the trajectory of the nerve during hip flexion to have a "wrap-around" effect to the medial aspect.[9] Therefore an accurate and detailed understanding of the neural pathway and biomechanics is necessary.

Peripheral nerve entrapment syndromes comprise nerve dysfunction due to localized interference of microvascular function and structural changes in the nerve or adjacent tissues.[10] Acute and chronic nerve compression increase vascular permeability with edema formation, and consequently impair axonal transport.[11] Diabetes mellitus, other metabolic and unknown factors can increase the susceptibility to compression injuries or influence the treatment outcome.

General symptoms include a burning or lancinating pain to the area supplied by the nerve. Upon physical examination there may be evidence of impaired sensory perception of the nerve and pain relief by anesthetic injection to the site where pain occurs. However, vague and poorly localized symptoms can produce complex clinical presentations. Furthermore, peripheral nerve entrapments can occur at more than one point in the same nerve fiber, or can coexist with lumbosacral root compression.

This concept has been developed in the upper limb "double crush syndrome."[12]

3T MRI is the most used imaging method for the evaluation of peripheral nerve entrapment (Fig. 85.4). The findings include direct and indirect signs of nerve injury.[13] Hyperintensity on fluid-sensitive images, which is focal or similar to that of adjacent vessels, is more likely to be significant.[13] Abnormalities in nerve size, fascicular pattern, or blurring of the perineural fat tissue are suggestive of neural injury, although those features are

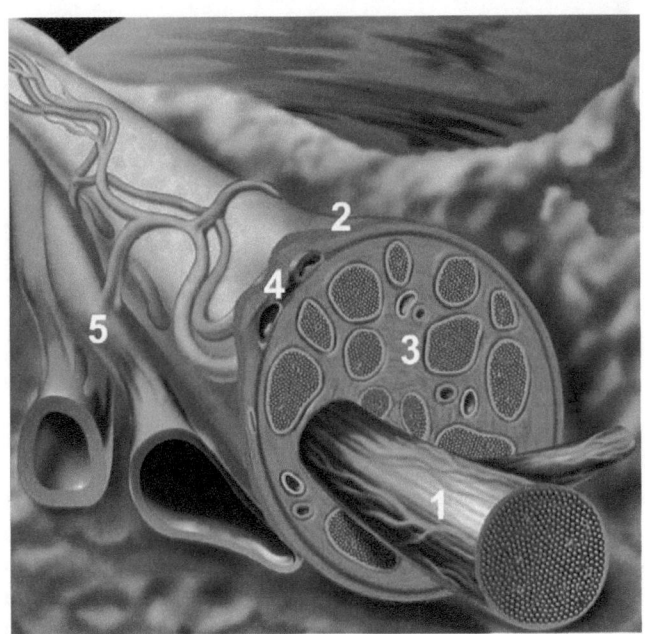

Fig. 85.1 Organization of a peripheral nerve: *1*, nerve fascicle with endoneurium, evolved by perineurium; *2*, epineural sheath enveloping the bundle of fascicles; *3*, connective tissue among the fascicles; *4*, epineural blood vessels; *5*, neighboring vasculature. (From Enneking FK, Chan V, Greger J, Hadzić A, Lang SA, Horlocker TT. Lower-extremity peripheral nerve blockade: essentials of our current understanding. *Reg Anesth Pain Med*. 2005;30(1):4–35.)

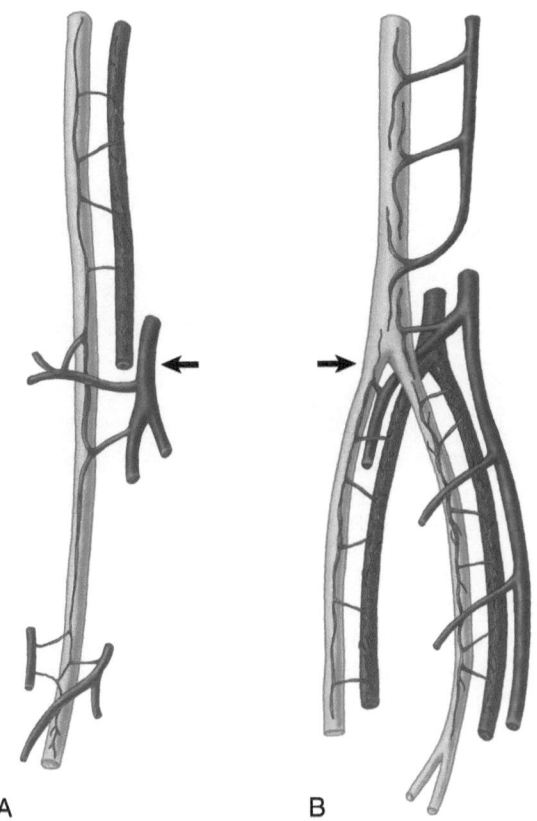

Fig. 85.3 Schematic diagram of the venous drainage of median and sciatic nerves. Arrows designate the level of the elbow and knee. From proximal to distal the dominant venous drainage of: (A) The median nerve is to the plexus around the brachial artery and via muscular veins in the arm. In the forearm the dominant venous drainage is provided by the median vein. (B) The sciatic nerve is via the perforators of the profunda system in the thigh and directly to the popliteal vein at the knee. In the leg, the anterior and posterior tibial nerves drain predominantly to the plexus around their accompanying arteries, as well as to the muscular veins. (From Del Pinãl F, Taylor GI. The venous drainage of nerves: anatomical study and clinical implications. *Br J Plast Surg*. 1990;43[5]:511–520).

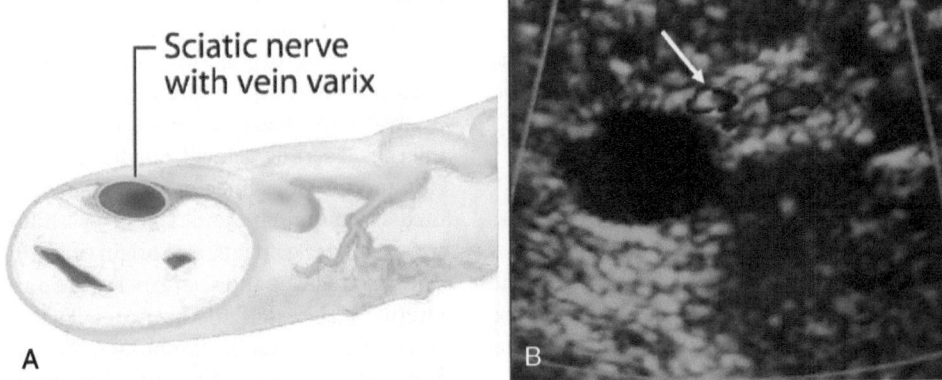

Fig. 85.2 Varicose veins within the sciatic nerve. (A) Schematic drawing of varicose veins within the perineurium and the sciatic nerve. (B) Sciatic nerve at midthigh with varicose veins within the nerve (*arrow*) in a patient who presented with pain and swelling. A larger refluxing vein is also seen in adhesion with the nerve. (From Labropoulos N, Tassiopoulos AK, Gasparis AP, Phillips B, Pappas PJ. Veins along the course of the sciatic nerve. *J Vasc Surg*. 2009;49[3]:690–696.)

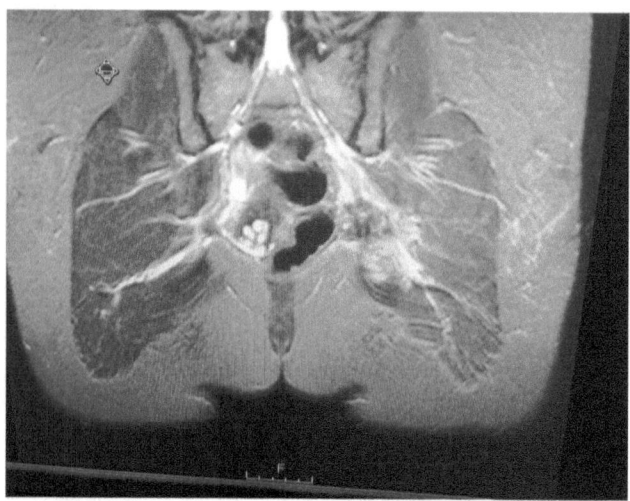

Fig. 85.4 Magnetic resonance imaging of a "double crush" sciatic nerve with venous dilatation distal to the entrapment.

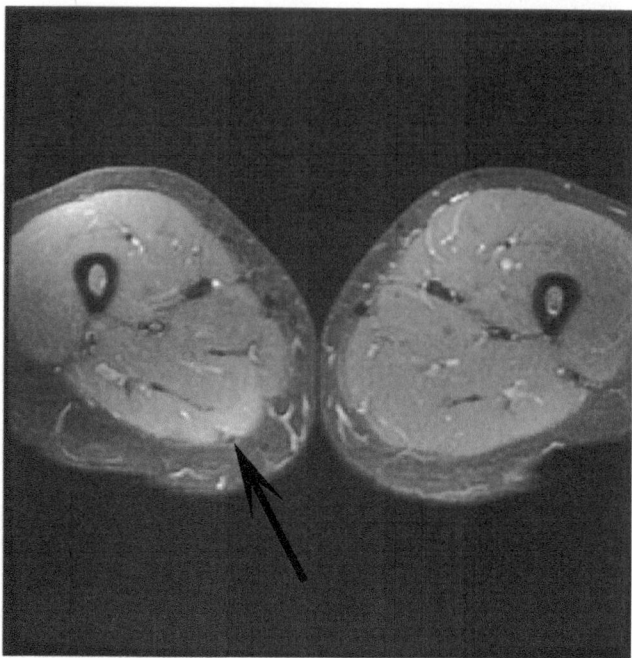

Fig. 85.5 Axial magnetic resonance imaging of the midthigh in a patient with entrapment of the sciatic branch to the semimembranous and extensor portion of the adductor magnus muscle. The arrow indicates a denervation hypersignal area in those muscles.

difficult to be noted in small diameter nerves.[13] The main indirect sign of nerve entrapment injury is the muscular denervation edema and vascular dilatation distal to the site of entrapment (Fig. 85.5).[14] Ultrasonography is an important method to guide nerve blocks and has been increasingly used for nerve evaluation, with the advantages of dynamic evaluation and Doppler assessment of nerve vessels.

Electrodiagnostic studies for lower extremity nerve entrapments are more complex than for the upper limb.[15] Obesity, edema, and age can impair the acquisition of sensory nerve action potentials in the lower limb, mainly in the proximally located nerves. Moreover, asymptomatic patients (usually elderly) often present neurogenic changes in the eletrodiagnostic studies.[15] These features may be problematic for the differential diagnosis between lumbosacral and peripheral entrapment.[15] However, electrodiagnostic assessment can be useful when associated with adequate physical examination and nerve block. Electrodiagnostic studies must be performed in the dynamic positions of entrapment (hip flexion/abduction/external rotation) to recreate the entrapment.

Conservative measures can control the symptoms in most patients and include the following: oral and topical analgesics; steroidal and nonsteroidal antiinflammatory drugs (NSAIDs); neuromodulation drugs, including tricyclic antidepressants, gabapentin, and pregabalin; physiotherapy; transcutaneous electric nerve stimulation (TENS); cryoablation; and nerve blocks.

DEEP GLUTEAL SYNDROME/SCIATIC NERVE ENTRAPMENT

Four main sources of extra-pelvic posterior hip pain present with similarities; however, each are subtly unique and must be differentiated[16]: (1) pain lateral and superior at the level of the external rotators or piriformis muscle along the sciatic tract—assessment of deep gluteal syndrome; (2) pain lateral to the ischium—evaluate ischiofemoral impingement (IFI), or ischial tunnel syndrome; (3) pain at the ischium—consider hamstring issues; and (4) pain medial to the ischium—rule out pudendal

nerve entrapment (covered in the next section). In the early 1900s the piriformis muscle was considered to be the source of sciatic nerve entrapment and was given the name "piriformis muscle syndrome."[17-19] However, in recent years, the identification of a number of etiologies of sciatic nerve entrapment has given rise to the nomenclature "deep gluteal syndrome."[8] Entrapment of the sciatic nerve is characterized by nondiscogenic, extrapelvic nerve compression presenting with symptoms of pain and dysesthesias in the buttock area, hip, or posterior thigh, and/or as radicular pain.[20-22]

Anatomy

The subgluteal space is anterior and beneath the gluteus maximus, and posterior to the posterior border of the femoral neck, the linea aspera (lateral), the sacrotuberous and falciform fascia (medial), the inferior margin of the sciatic notch (superior), and the hamstring origin (inferior), and is continuous with the peritrochanteric space laterally (Fig. 85.6). Within this region of great importance are the sciatic nerve, piriformis, obturator internus/externus, gemelli, quadratus femoris, hamstrings, superior and inferior gluteal nerves, lateral ascending vessels of the medial femoral circumflex artery, ischium, sacrotuberous and sacrospinous ligaments, and origin of the ischiofemoral ligament. The sacral plexus and sciatic nerve are anatomically close to the internal iliac vessels and branches. The superior gluteal vessels run either between the lumbosacral trunk (L4-L5 ventral rami) and first sacral ventral ramus or between the first and second sacral rami. Whereas the inferior gluteal vessels lie between either the first and second, or second and third, sacral rami. The sciatic nerve, formed by L4-S3 sacral roots, courses distally through the subgluteal space anterior to the piriformis muscle and

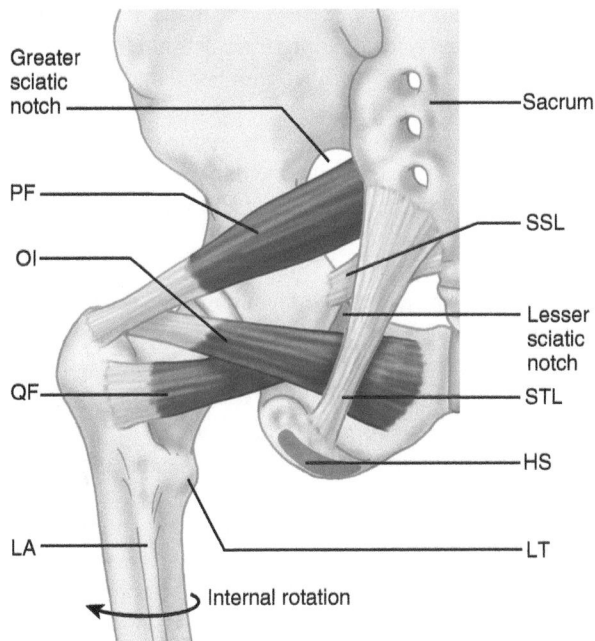

Fig. 85.6 Schematic of the deep gluteal space. *HS,* hamstring origin; *LA,* linea aspera; *LT,* lesser trochanter; *OI,* obturator internus; *PF,* piriformis; *QF,* quadratus femoris; *SSL,* sacrospinous ligament; *STL,* sacrotuberous ligament. (From Wilson TJ. *Operative Hip Arthroscopy.* 3rd ed. New York: Springer; 2013.)

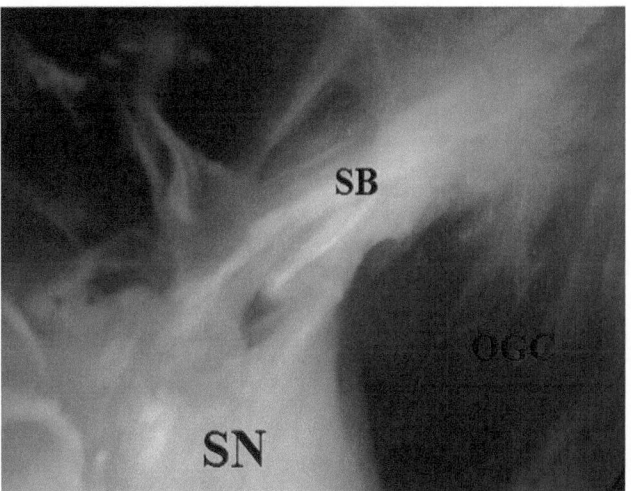

Fig. 85.7 Endoscopic view of scar bands secondary to open sciatic nerve decompression. *OGC,* obturator/gemelli complex; *SN,* sciatic nerve; *SB,* scar band.

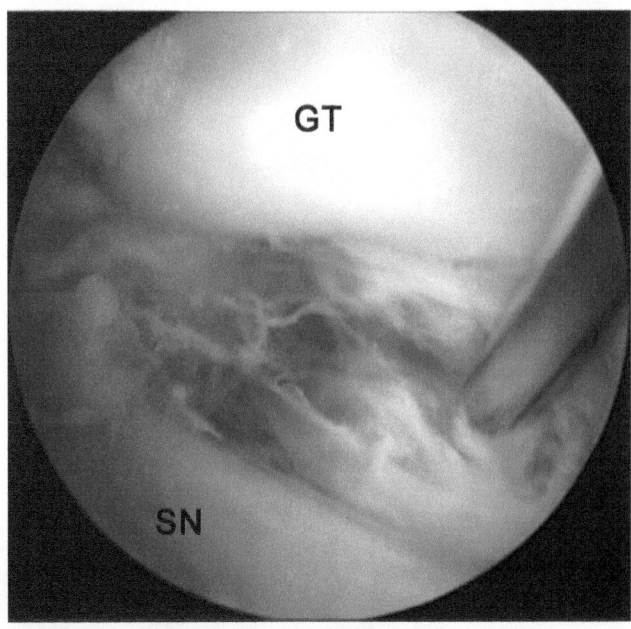

Fig. 85.8 Endoscopic view of the decreased space between greater trochanter *(GT)* and sciatic nerve *(SN)* in internal rotation. External rotation produces the compression of sciatic nerve between the GT and ischium tuberosity.

posterior to the obturator/gemelli complex and the quadratus femoris. Variations exist concerning the relationship between the piriformis muscle and the sciatic nerve. Six categories have been described,[23] which are important for the surgeon to recognize; however, the anomaly itself may not be the etiology of deep gluteal syndrome (DGS) symptoms. The prevalence of piriformis–sciatic nerve anomalies is 16% to 17%.[24] Age may have an effect on sciatic nerve kinematics. A detailed understanding of the anatomy and variations is critical.[4,6,8,21,25-32]

Etiology

Sources of sciatic nerve entrapment include the piriformis muscle,[20,21,27,32-39] fibrous bands containing blood vessels,[21,33,39] gluteal muscles,[8] hamstring muscles,[40,41] the gemelli-obturator internus complex,[42-44] ischial tuberosity,[45-47] and acetabular reconstruction surgery.[48] Also reported to cause sciatic nerve compression are vascular abnormalities,[4,22,37,49] prolonged surgery in the seated position,[50] after total hip replacement,[51] and secondary to space-occupying lesions.[34,35] Some lesser known sources of entrapment include boney entrapments by the greater trochanter (GT), lesser trochanter (LT), and ischium.

The piriformis muscle and tendon is the most common source of extrapelvic sciatic nerve impingement.[20,21,37] In many cases, a thick tendon can hide under the belly of the piriformis overlying the nerve.[21,37] Hypertrophy of the piriformis muscle has been attributed to sciatic nerve entrapment[20,27,37,52]; however, Benson and Schutzer found that only 2 of 14 cases had larger piriformis muscles on the symptomatic side and 7 appeared smaller than the unaffected side.[20] Atypical fibrovascular scar bands and greater trochanteric bursae hypertrophy have been reported in many cases of sciatic nerve entrapment.[21,39] Large

fibrovasular scar bands have existed, reaching from the posterior border of the GT to the gluteus maximus on to the sciatic nerve and up to the greater sciatic notch (Fig. 85.7).[21] The obturator internus/gemelli complex can also be a source of sciatica-like pain.[21,42-44] The sciatic nerve exits the sciatic notch anterior to the piriformis and posterior to the superior gemelli/obturator internus, which can cause a scissor effect between the two muscles, resulting in entrapment.[21,43,44] Distally at the ischium, the insertion of the hamstring tendon can be thickened due to trauma or hamstring avulsion and can involve the sciatic nerve.[21,53] Other sources of sciatic nerve entrapment include malunion of the ischium or healed avulsions, GT (Fig. 85.8), tumor, vascular abnormalities (Fig. 85.9),[22,37,49] gluteus maximus (from a prior iliotibial band release), or as a result of acetabular fracture or post hip reconstruction.[48,51]

Ischial tunnel syndrome or hamstring syndrome is described as pain in the lower buttock region radiating down the posterior thigh to the popliteal fossa, and is often associated with hamstring weakness. Common complaints include pain with sitting, stretching, and with exercise, primarily running (sprinting and acceleration).[40,54] Palpable tenderness is located around the ischial tuberosity in the proximal hamstring region. Puranen and Orava first reported on the surgical release of the sciatic nerve from adhesions in the proximal hamstring area.[40] At the lateral

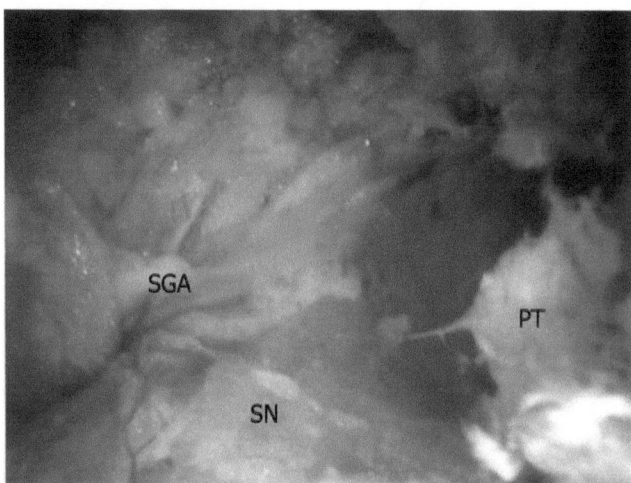

Fig. 85.9 Entrapment of the sciatic nerve (*SN*) by superior gluteal artery (*SGA*). A branch of the SGA is in diastole crossing the SN distal to the sciatic notch. The piriformis tendon *(PT)* is seen released to the right. (From Wilson TJ. *Operative Hip Arthroscopy.* 3rd ed. New York: Springer; 2013.)

insertion of the hamstring tendons to the ischial tuberosity, tight tendinous structures and adhesions were thought to be the result of scarring or a fibrotic band between the tendons and sciatic nerve.[8,40] To better clarify the location of this pathology, Young et al., have suggested this condition be named "proximal hamstring syndrome."[41] Pain associated with hamstring tears alone is located more distal in the muscle belly and commonly is accompanied by a palpable defect from the tear.[41] Clinical presentation has shown that the straight leg raise test (Lasègue test) is variable; there is no neurologic deficit, but there is marked weakness of the hamstring muscle at 30 degrees knee flexion, yet there is normal strength at 90 degrees knee flexion.[41] Hamstring avulsions, especially the semimembranosus, can lead to ischial tunnel syndrome involving the sciatic nerve by scarring around the sciatic nerve, or the formation of tight fibrotic bands in the area of the ischial tuberosity.[21,55,56]

Boney entrapments are not as common, but should be considered as a source of entrapment. Hip flexion with external rotation can cause GT impingement up on the ischium (see Fig. 85.8). Ischiofemoral impingement as an etiology of posterior hip pain has recently been reported,[46,47,57] and is described as a narrowing of the ischiofemoral space and an abnormal quadratus femoris muscle MR signal intensity.[46,47] The ischiofemoral space is defined as the smallest distance between the lateral cortex of the ischial tuberosity and the medial cortex of the LT. The quadratus femoris space is defined as the smallest space for passage of the quadratus femoris muscle defined by the superolateral surface of the hamstring tendons and the posteromedial surface of the iliopsoas tendon or LT. Normal ischiofemoral space has been reported to be 17 mm or greater, and normal quadratus femoral space is 8 mm or greater (Fig. 85.10).[47] Patients presenting with pain lateral to the level of the ischium with persistence in pain when sitting or with ambulation, consideration should be given for the possibility of IFI.[58,59] The clinical presentation of patients

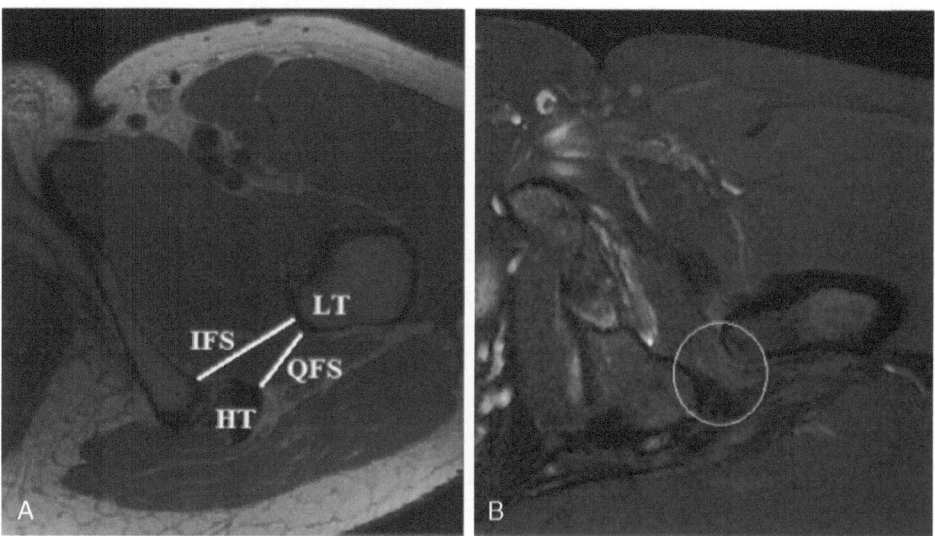

Fig. 85.10 Magnetic resonance imaging (MRI) of ischiofemoral impingement. (A) Left side MRI of a normal ischiofemoral space *(IFS)*. (B) MRI of a patient with ischiofemoral impingement showing a narrowed ischiofemoral space with edema in the quadratus femoris muscle *(circle)*. *HT*, hamstrings' tendons; *LT*, lesser trochanter; *QFS*, quadratus femoris space.

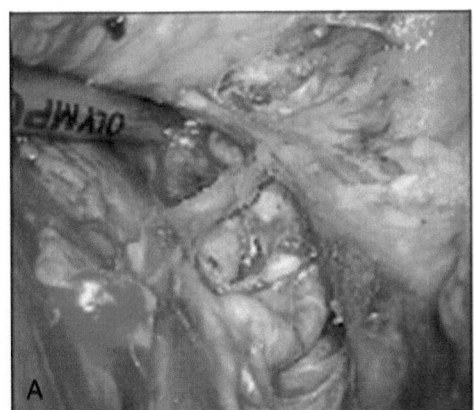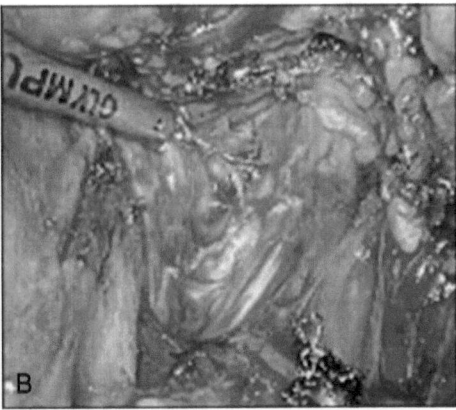

Fig. 85.11 Vascular intrapelvic sacral plexus entrapment. Vascular entrapment covering the entire distal sacral plexus and the sciatic nerve (right side). (A) Before decompression. (B) After decompression. (From Possover M, Schneider T, Henle KP. Laparoscopic therapy for endometriosis and vascular entrapment of sacral plexus. *Fertil Steril.* 2011;95:756–758).

with IFI can be confused with deep gluteal syndrome; however, there are aspects distinctly different from DGS pain, which must be recognized. Ischiofemoral impingement patients have pain with terminal hip extension at the posterolateral ischial region and will grab the source of impingement lateral to the ischium. Gait evaluation will reveal that the patient can walk with a short stride length quite adequately. However, if asked to extend the stride length toward terminal hip extension the pain is exacerbated and replicated. This is particularly evident in athletes who may be able to jog but increase their pace. There also may be a sciatic component with or without a hamstring tear at the level of the ischial tunnel. The radiographic criteria from even simple anteroposterior radiograph may demonstrate the diminished space at the ischiofemoral level and one can consider further assessment on an MRI. MRI assessment requires stabilization of the feet with tape in a neutral walking position between the proximal, axial, and distal assessment. Surgical treatment for IFI has included complete resection of the LT and partial resection or simple quadratus femoris resection of this region, and early results are promising.[59]

The exact etiology of sciatic neuropathy can be difficult to detect. Other sources of entrapment the examiner should be aware of are intrapelvic and vascular pathology. Sciatica can be caused by vascular entrapment of sacral neural roots (Fig. 85.11) or gynecologic conditions (Fig. 85.12); therefore intrapelvic sciatic pathology must be considered.[60] This condition is especially important to rule out with cyclic sciatic endometriosis. Some patients can feel sciatica without direct contact between the endometriosis tissue and the sacral plexus, and the suggested cause is the stimulation of the sacral plexus by inflammation of the retroperitoneum.[61] Gynecologic sciatica etiologies affect the right side in 70% of the patients. It is suggested that the sigmoid colon plays a role in prevention of pressure on or stimulation of the sacral plexus on the left side.[62] Varicosities associated with incompetent veins along the sciatic nerve have been reported to be the source of sciatic nerve symptoms.[4,63] These patients have pain while sitting, which is relieved when standing or walking. There are multilevel connections between the venous network

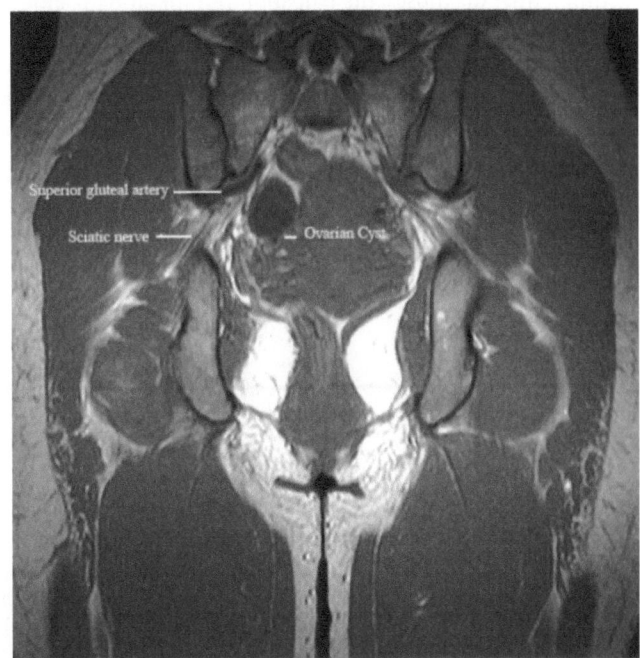

Fig. 85.12 Ovarian cyst close to the sacral neural roots on the right side.

surrounding the sciatic nerve and the veins inside the nerve. At these connection sites, a limited number of valves exist and there is an absence of valves within the sciatic nerve veins, which may allow for symptomatic dilation. Duplex ultrasonography can be used to identify reflux in the standing position with distal manual compression followed by sudden release.[4] Significant relief can be achieved by treatment of the varicosities and recurrence can be treated.[4,63]

Potential sources of entrapment involve each layer; thus a comprehensive physical examination, a detailed history, and standardized radiographic interpretation are paramount in evaluating hip pain.[21,64-66] In all cases of suspected nerve entrapment, the spine must first be ruled out by MRI and comprehensive history/physical examination. Clinical presentation often includes a history of trauma and symptoms of sit pain (the inability to sit for more than 30 minutes), radicular pain of the lower back or hip, and paresthesias of the affected leg.[20,21] As noted before, several etiologies of posterior extraarticular hip pain exist and these symptoms should be sorted by the physical examination. Some patients may present with neurologic symptoms of abnormal reflexes or motor weakness.[22] Symptoms related to nerves other than the sciatic nerve may be observed, such as weakness of the gluteus medius and minimus muscles (superior gluteal nerve), weakness of the gluteus maximus (inferior gluteal nerve), peroneal sensory loss (pudendal nerve), or loss of posterior cutaneous sensation (posterior femoral cutaneous nerve).[67]

PHYSICAL EXAMINATION

A comprehensive history and a physical examination are essential for a differential diagnosis in patients with hip pain.[1] To aid in the differential diagnoses, the palpation test for sit pain should be performed. The physician palpates in three positions of the gluteal area: the piriformis (lateral/superior), at the level of the external rotators, and lateral to the ischium (Fig. 85.13). If pain is localized at the ischium, rule out ischial tunnel syndrome, the hamstring bursa, or hamstring tears; and if the pain is lateral to the ischium, consider IFI. If pain is more medial, one should evaluate the pudendal nerve.

Six key physical examination tests will aid in the differentiation of posterior hip pain. The seated palpation test also can be performed during the seated piriformis stretch test (Fig. 85.14A), which is a flexion, adduction with internal rotation test performed with the patient in the seated position.[64,68] The examiner extends the knee (engaging the sciatic nerve) and passively moves the flexed hip into adduction with internal rotation while palpating 1 cm lateral to the ischium (middle finger) and proximally at the sciatic notch (index finger). A

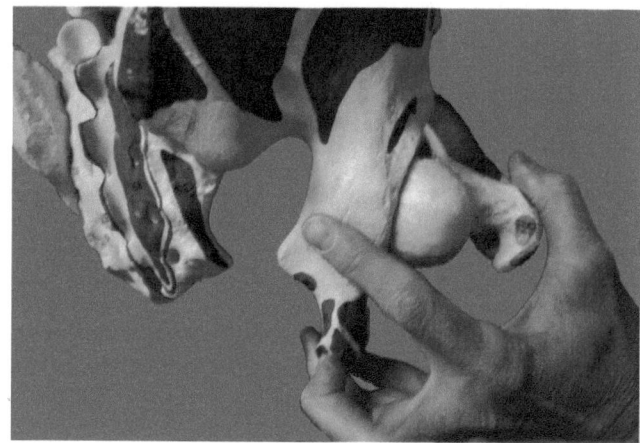

Fig. 85.13 Seated palpation test. The physician palpates the gluteal area: lateral/superior at the piriformis muscle/sciatic nerve *(index finger)*, ischium at the hamstring/hamstring tendinosis or avulsion *(middle finger)*, medial at the obturator internus/pudendal nerve *(ring finger)*. Pain lateral to the ischium, particularly with hip extension, may be ischiofemoral/ sciatic nerve.

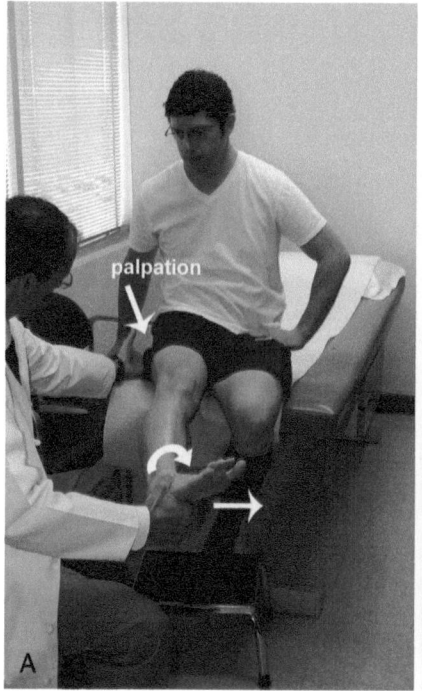
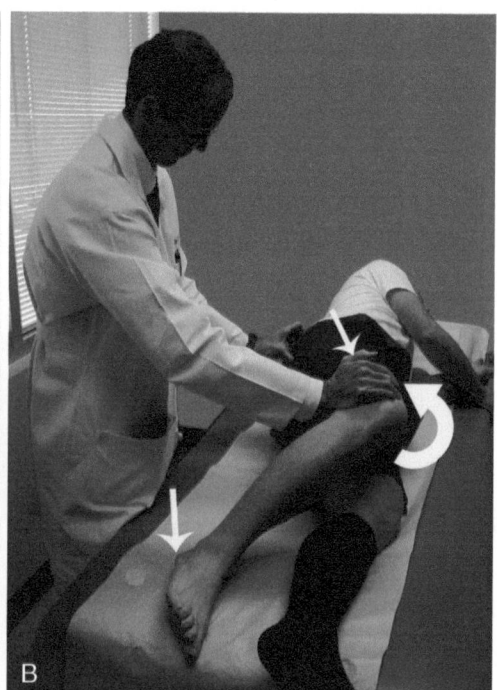

Fig. 85.14 Seated piriformis stretch test and active piriformis test. (A). The patient is in the seated position with knee extension. The examiner passively moves the flexed hip into adduction with internal rotation while palpating 1 cm lateral to the ischium *(middle finger)* and proximally at the piriformis *(index finger)*. (B) With the patient in the lateral position, the examiner palpates the piriformis. The patient drives the heel into the examining table, thus initiating external hip rotation while actively abducting and externally rotating against resistance. (From: AANA Advanced Arthroscopy, 2010, Martin HD, Byrd JWT [Ed].)

positive test is the re-creation of the posterior pain at the level of the piriformis or external rotators. An active piriformis test is performed by the patient pushing the heel down into the table, abducting and externally rotating the leg against resistance, while the examiner monitors the piriformis (see Fig. 85.14B). The use of both tests provides a sensitivity of 0.91 and a specificity of 0.80.[68] Active hamstring testing is performed in the seated position and in gait testing (Fig. 85.15A to C). A positive seated hamstring test with 30 degrees and/or 90 degrees of knee flexion is hamstring syndrome. Re-creation of pain with long-stride walking *with hip flexion* at heel strike also can be positive for hamstring tears.[69] Patients with IFI have re-creation of pain with long-stride walking *with hip extension*, which is relieved with short-stride walking (Fig. 85.16A). The IFI test

(see Fig. 85.16B) takes the hip into passive hip extension (lack of full extension range of motion [ROM]), and re-creation of the pain lateral to the ischium with the hip in neutral or slightly adducted is positive for IFI. Relief of pain and the full range of terminal hip extension motion will be achieved with the hip in abduction.[58]

Injection tests are utilized in supporting the diagnosis of DGS when the piriformis is involved. Pace and Nagle used a double injection technique of an anesthetic and corticosteroid toward the piriformis muscle, which relieved the pain in 41 of 45 patients.[70] Guided injections utilizing computed tomography (CT), fluoroscopy, ultrasound, or open MRI to the piriformis muscle have been used to assist diagnosis.[27] Patient positioning prior to imaging may affect MRI sensitivity and should be

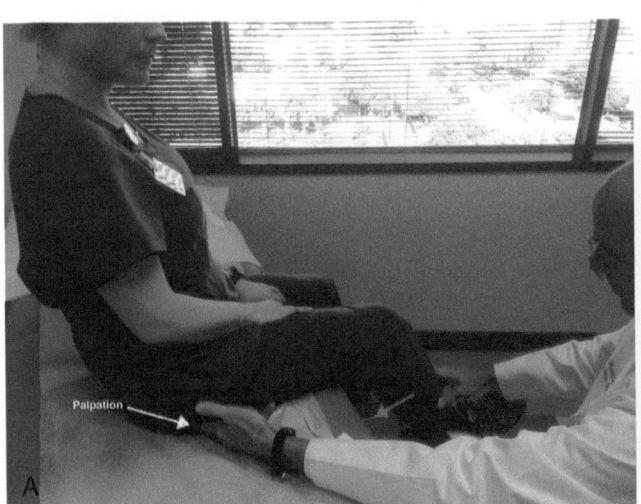
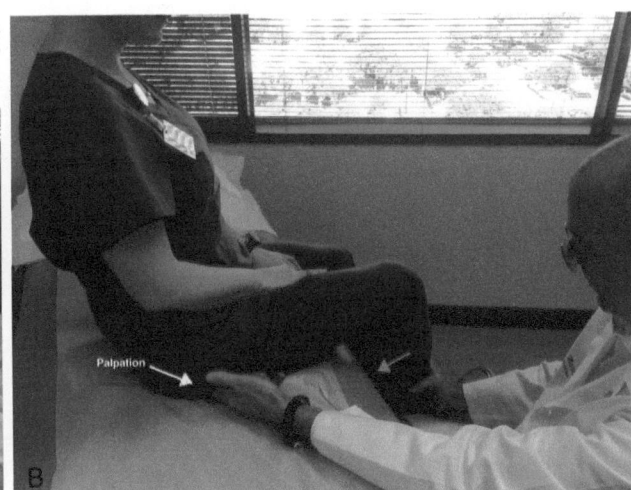
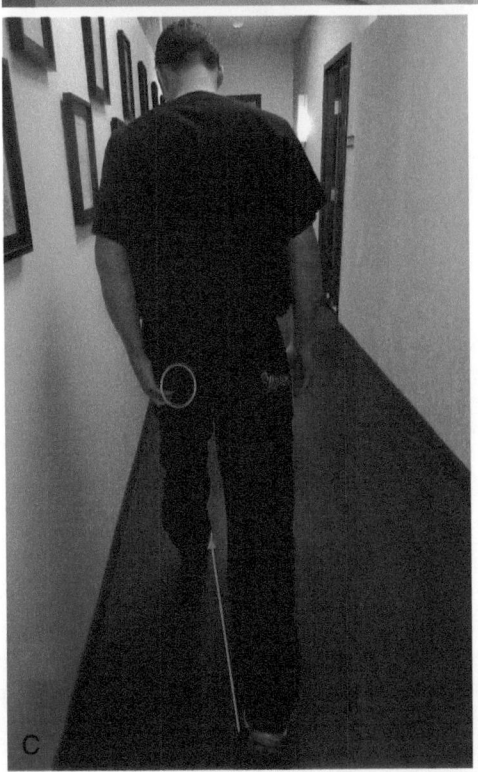

Fig. 85.15 Hamstring tests. (A) Active 30-degree hamstrings test. With the knee in 30-degree flexion, the examiner actively restricts knee flexion, while palpating the hamstrings origin. (B) Active 90-degree hamstring test. With the knee in 90-degree flexion, the examiner actively restricts knee flexion while palpating the hamstrings origin. (C) Long Stride Heel Strike (LSHS). The patient is instructed to perform long stride gait. The re-creation of pain both proximal and lateral to the ischium during hip flexion with heel strike is a positive examination.

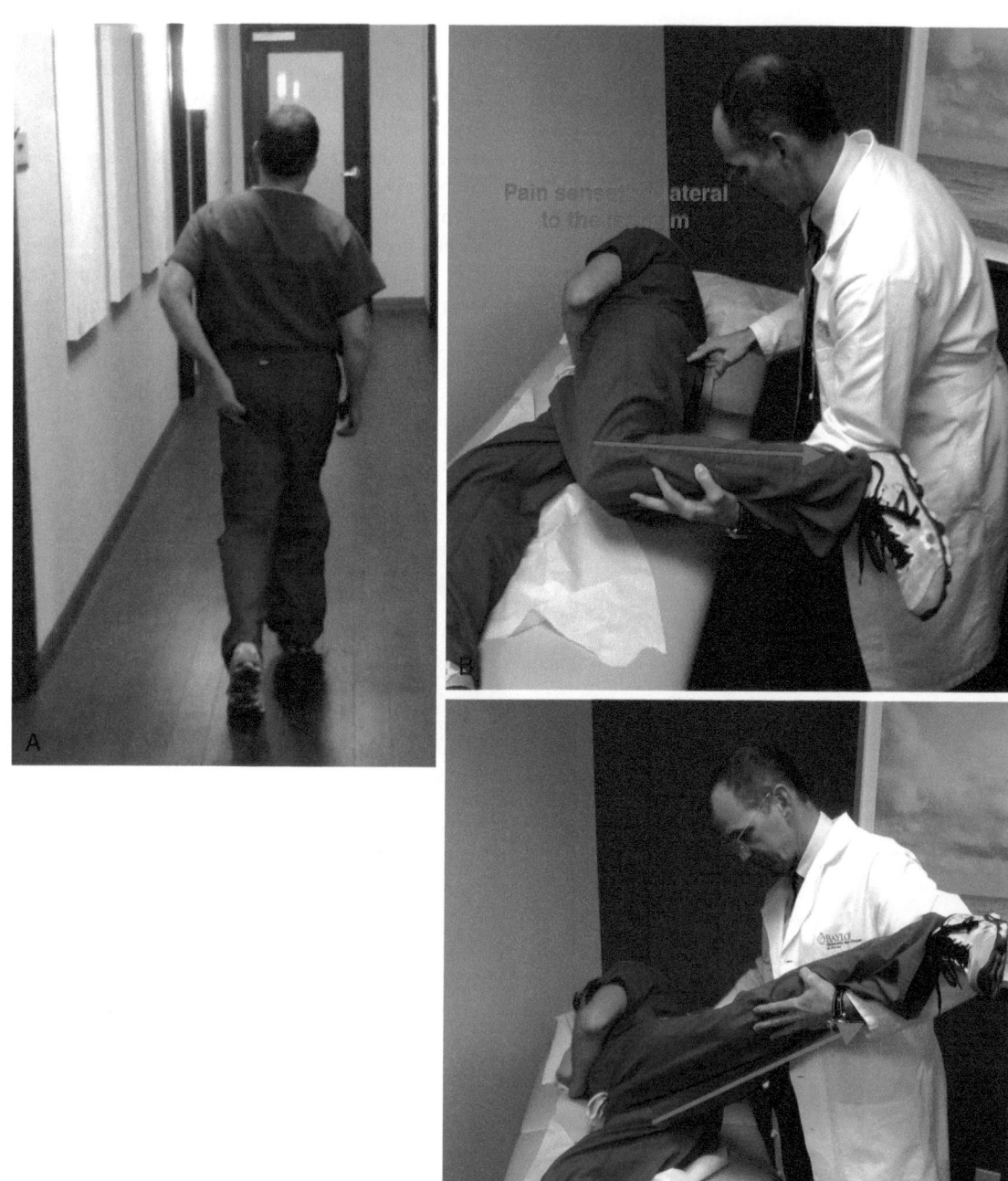

Fig. 85.16 Ischiofemoral impingement (IFI) tests. (A) Long Stride Walking (LSW) IFI test. (B) The examiner places the hip in passive hip extension, while palpating lateral to the ischium. (C) Pain is alleviated with hip abduction during passive hip extension.

controlled by standardization. Complementary diagnostic studies include electromyography (EMG) and nerve conduction studies, which can be beneficial to the diagnosis of deep gluteal syndrome when positive. Piriformis entrapment of the sciatic nerve is often indicated by H-reflex disturbances of the tibial and/or perineal nerves.[71,72] It is important to compare side to side and to perform a dynamic test with the knee in extension and the hip in adduction with internal rotation. Intra-articular and spinal pathologies are ruled out by physical examination, injection tests, and imaging.[21,27] Extrapelvic sciatic entrapment is suspected when the pudendal nerve, ischiofemoral syndrome, and hamstrings are ruled out. Strain parameters can change dynamically through the spine with hip flexion and extension due to premature coupling and secondary strain transfer.

PREOPERATIVE AND POSTOPERATIVE REHABILITATION

Nonoperative treatment for deep gluteal syndrome begins with a conservative approach addressing the suspected site of impingement. Impingement from a hypertrophied, contracted, or inflamed muscle (piriformis, quadratus femoris, obturator internus, superior/inferior gemellus) begins with rest, antiinflammatories, muscle relaxants, and physical therapy. The physical therapy program should include stretching maneuvers aimed at the external rotators. The piriformis stretch, or FAIR, involves placing the leg in flexion, adduction, and internal rotation (Fig. 85.17). Patients with cam impingement, anterior pincer impingement, or acetabular retroversion may not be able to stretch adequately into this position and should be evaluated and treated primarily as most will resolve with appropriate surgical intervention. In a seated position, the patient brings the knee into the chest and across midline and pulls the knee to the opposite shoulder. Gradually progress the stretching by increasing the duration and intensity until a maximal stretch is obtained. Greater trochanteric sciatic nerve mobilization is performed by (Fig. 85.18 inlay) hip circumduction with knee flexion, nerve glides, and the Ober stretch (see Fig. 85.18A to C) are performed under the limit of pain. A knee brace is used to avoid knee extension and to maintain a relaxed sciatic nerve during therapy. The utilization of the knee brace is dependent upon the strain of the sciatic nerve, which is influenced by the degree of femoral anteversion and the number of sites of entrapment. The knee is locked at 45 degrees for 3 weeks applying only nerve glides and circumduction. After 4 weeks, knee extension can increase up to 10 degrees every 2 weeks as tolerated. Increase ROM for hip flexion and adduction can be carefully applied, plus gentle nerve glides, and stretching maneuvers aimed at the external rotators. Standard physical therapy protocol can begin as early as 6 weeks, and be independently modified depending upon pathology. Again, a word of caution in cases of previous abdominal surgery and femoral retroversion as strain parameters will be a dependent factor, and the nerve may be impinged in more than one location. The therapist should be diligent in recognizing these potential outcome factors.

Additional physical therapy techniques that may be helpful include ultrasound and electrical stimulation. Injections of a muscle anesthetic or corticosteroid can provide pain relief in patients not responding to physical therapy. It is important to administer the injection to the correct site; technique options include fluoroscopic guidance (with or without a radiographic dye), CT, ultrasound, EMG, and MRI guidance. A trial of up to three injections has been recommended before opting for more aggressive therapy, taken on a case by case basis.[22,27,73] Most cases of deep gluteal syndrome/sciatic nerve entrapment will respond to conservative nonoperative measures.

Operative Treatment

Options for operative treatment include open and endoscopic techniques. The open transgluteal approach has been described to effectively perform piriformis muscle resection and neuroplasty of the sciatic and posterior femoral cutaneous nerves.[27,39] A number of case studies have been successful with an open approach, and the largest case series have reported good to excellent outcomes in 75% to 100% of the procedures.[20,27,41] Additionally, release of the hamstrings and neurolysis of the sciatic nerve at the hamstring origin has been performed, achieving satisfactory results with significant pain relief and increased hamstring strength.[41] Contrasting release is surgical repair, which is recommended early to avoid involvement of the sciatic nerve.[55,56] The surgical technique, indications, and contraindications for surgery have been outlined by Miller and Webb.[53] The concepts of treatment in this area continue to evolve.

Endoscopic Decompression

Endoscopy is an effective and minimally invasive approach to the treatment of deep gluteal syndrome. Dezawa et al. first reported on six cases of endoscopic piriformis muscle release.[36] Internationally, the endoscopic treatment of deep gluteal syndrome has shown similar success. Perez-Carro et al.[99] report 19/26 good to excellent outcomes with improved mHHS scores from 56 to 79. Polesello et al. and Cabrita et al. contribute to the success with 3- and 15-patient case series.[74,75] An international posterior hip study group is underway with a large patient cohort.

The supine technique is utilized and modified by positioning the table in maximal contralateral patient tilt. Nerve conduction and EMG is monitored intraoperatively and post release can demonstrate immediate improvement. Using a 70-degree long arthroscope and adjustable/lengthening cannulas the peritrochanteric space is entered through the anterolateral and posterolateral portals. A systematic inspection of the peritrochanteric

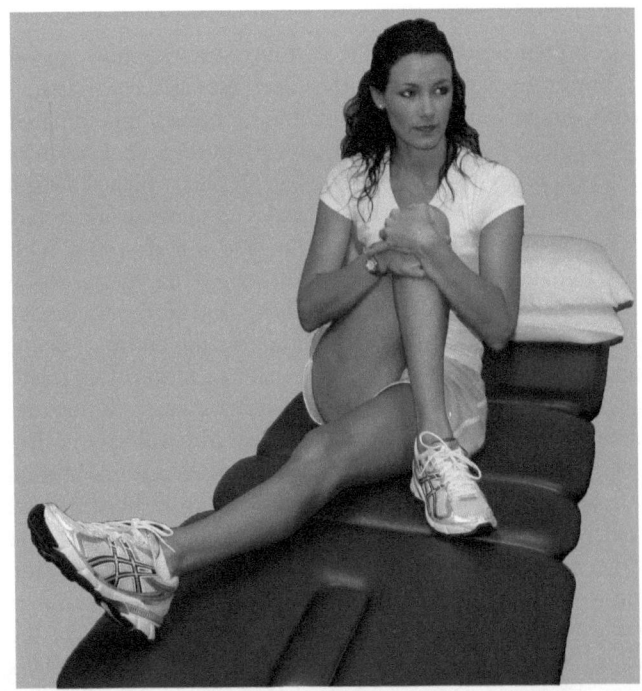

Fig. 85.17 Piriformis stretch. In a seated position, the patient brings the knee into the chest and across the midline, and pulls the knee to the opposite shoulder.

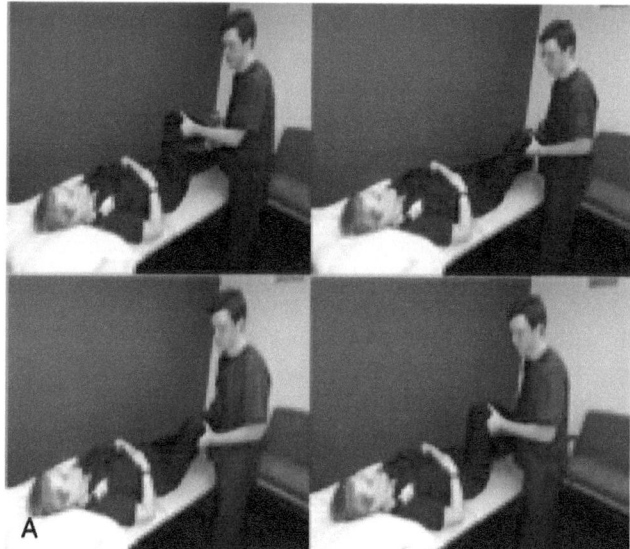

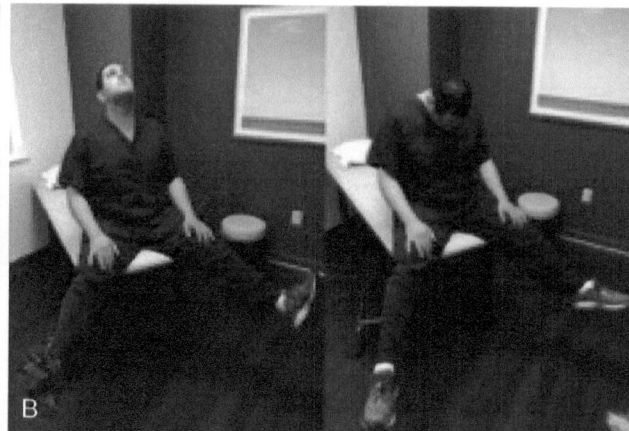

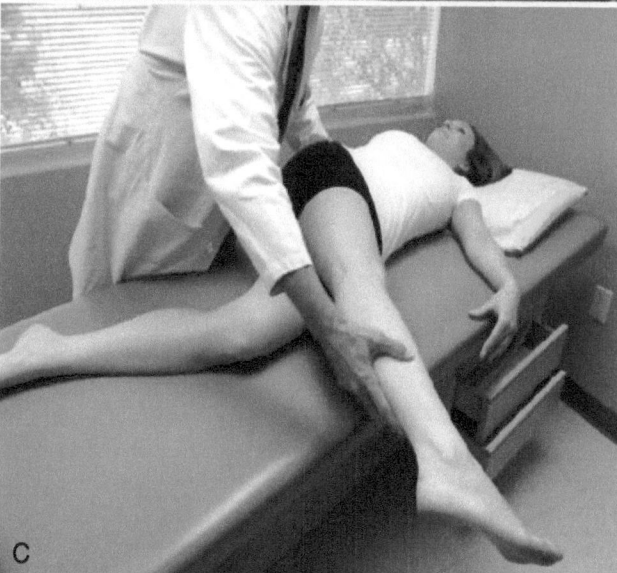

Fig. 85.18 Pre- and postoperative rehabilitation exercises. (A) Circumduction. (B) Nerve glides. (C) Ober stretch.

space is then performed.[76] The starting position is shown in Fig. 85.19A and once orientation has been established the arthroscope should be turned proximally, and bursectomy initiated. The auxiliary posterolateral portal is established 3 cm posterior and 3 cm superior to the GT (see Fig. 85.19B), which allows for better visualization of the sciatic nerve up to the sciatic notch.

Endoscopic piriformis tendonotomy is summarized in Table 85.1. Initiate bursectomy noting the extent of the fibrous bands and inspect the gluteus minimus, medius, and maximus muscles. Identify the quadratus femoris muscle at the entrance of the subgluteal space and inspect the kinematic excursion of the sciatic nerve by internal/external rotation with the leg in flexion and extension.[6,21] Normal sciatic nerve appearance will have noticeable epineural blood flow and epineural fat, and normal motion with internal/external rotation will glide along the border of the external rotator muscles. An abnormal sciatic nerve will appear white, resembling a shoestring; it will not move with rotation and will feel taught with probing. Release any fibrous bands at the level of the quadratus femoris. Inspect at the level of the ischial tunnel and sacrotuberous ligament, and release any fibers from the sciatic nerve. Turn the long scope proximally, then identify and inspect the obturator internus muscle and tendon. Move to the long scope to the auxiliary or posterolateral portal

TABLE 85.1   Endoscopic Piriformis Tendonotomy

1.	Establish anterolateral, posterolateral, and auxiliary portals.
2.	Perform bursectomy, and inspect gluteus minimus, medius, and maximus.
3.	Internally rotate the extremity, view the quadratus femoris at the entrance of the deep gluteal space.
4.	Free the sacrotuberous ligament/hamstring fibers from nerve distally.
5.	Turn the long scope proximally to inspect, then move the long scope to the posterolateral/auxiliary portal.
6.	Internally and externally rotate with hip flexion of 40–60 degrees.
7.	Identify the branch of the inferior gluteal artery, cauterize (or ligate) and release.
8.	Shave the distal border of the piriformis muscle.
9.	Use arthroscopic scissors for tendon release.
10.	Repeat hip motion and probe the sciatic nerve.

(Fig. 85.20). A branch of the inferior gluteal artery crosses the sciatic nerve in this region and must be cauterized (or ligated if large) and released before the inspection of the piriformis muscle and tendon (Fig. 85.21). Identify the piriformis muscle and shave the distal border if necessary to identify the tendon, which is often hidden under the belly of the muscle. Use arthroscopic scissors for tendon release, pulling the scissors toward you to ensure only the tendon is released (Fig. 85.22). Following tendon resection, shave the tendinous stump back 1 to 2 cm. Inspect nerve motion with hip flexion and internal/external rotation with probing. Cautiously probe the sciatic nerve up to the sciatic notch noting that the superior gluteal neurovascular structures exit the sciatic notch superior to the piriformis muscle. Using a curved probe, thoroughly probe the retrosciatic region to identify and release any ancillary musculotendinous branches that may be binding the nerve (Fig. 85.23).

Endoscopic sciatic neurolysis is summarized in Table 85.2. Probe the nerve while internally and externally rotating the hip.

TABLE 85.2	**Endoscopic Sciatic Nerve Neurolysis**
1.	Probe the nerve and move the hip.
2.	Assess the epineural blood and epineural fat.
3.	Assess the hamstring tendon and sacrotuberous ligament, releasing any involved fibers.
4.	Identify the posterior femoral cutaneous nerve, sciatic artery, and inferior gluteal nerve.
5.	Dissect fibrous bands at the sciatic notch.
6.	Confirm the location using fluoroscopy.
7.	Inspect nerve motion by probing, and assess ancillary tendons.
8.	Assess the obturator tendon and check nerve motion and nerve color.
9.	Perform retrosciatic dissection, releasing fibrous bands.

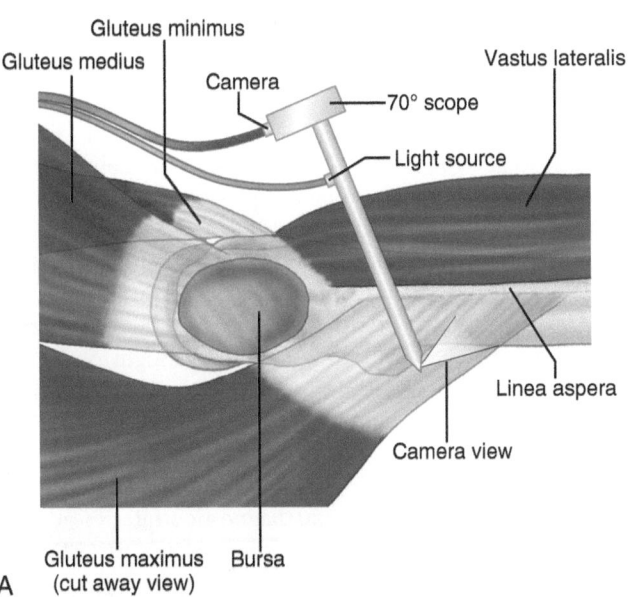

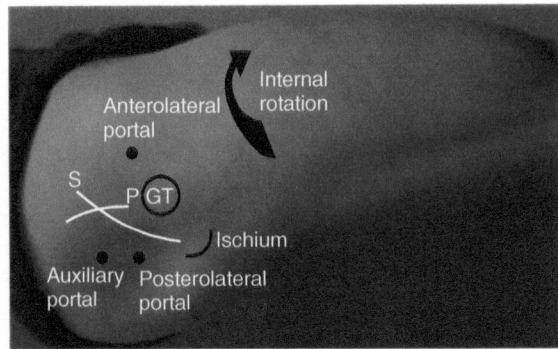

Fig. 85.19 Peritrochanteric space and portal placement. (A) Peritrochanteric space and anatomical landmarks with orientation of the arthroscope and light source. The scope is introduced into the PTS and turned around to introduce the auxiliary portal. (From Martin H. Diagnostic Arthroscopy. In: Kelly BT, Philippon MJ, eds. *Arthroscopic Techniques of the Hip: A Visual Guide.* Thorofare, NJ: Slack Inc.; 2009.) (B) The anterolateral portal placement is 1 cm anterior and 1 cm superior to the greater trochanter (GT). The posterolateral portal placement is 3 cm posterior to the GT and in line with the anterolateral portal. The auxiliary portal is positioned 3 cm posterior and 3 cm superior to the GT. The course of the sciatic nerve (S) and piriformis (P) are depicted in relation to the GT and ischium. (From Martin HD, Shears SA, Johnson JC, Smathers AM, Palmer IJ. The endoscopic treatment of sciatic nerve entrapment/deep gluteal syndrome. *Arthroscopy.* 2011;27:172–181.)

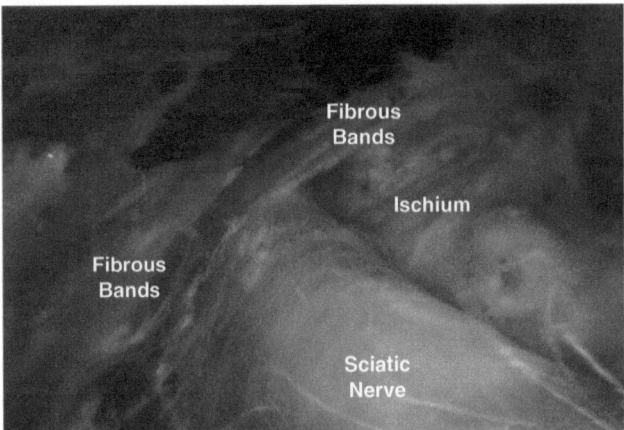

Fig. 85.20 Sciatic nerve decompression/inspection: distal to the quadratus femoris. Endoscopic view of the left hip through the posterolateral portal looking distal to the quadratus femoris. With internal and external rotation of the hip, inspect and release fibrous bands adjacent to the ischium and check the ischial tunnel. (From Wilson TJ. *Operative Hip Arthroscopy.* 3rd ed. New York: Springer; 2013.)

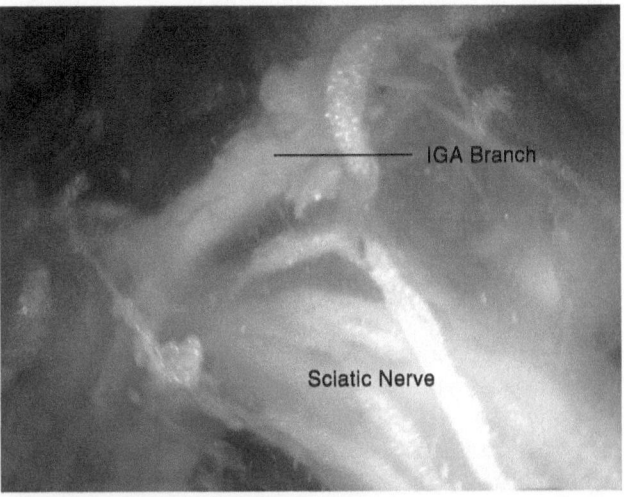

Fig. 85.21 A branch of the inferior gluteal artery crossing posterior to the sciatic nerve.

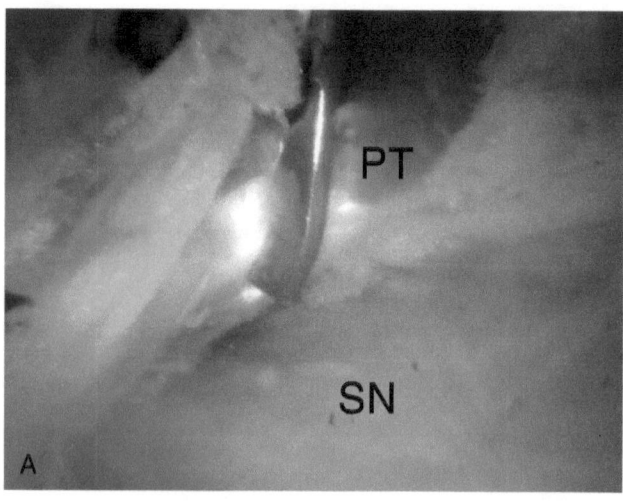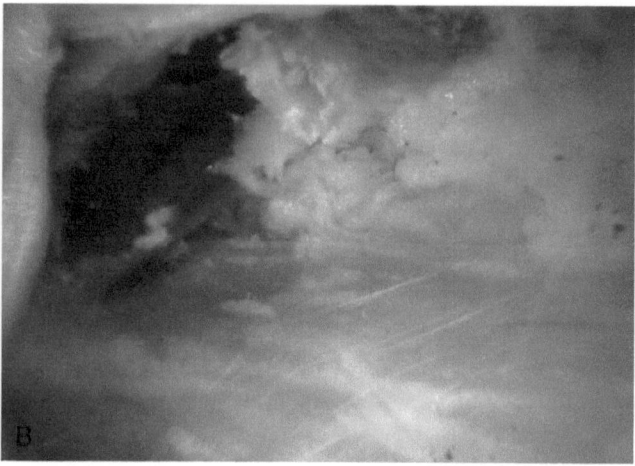

Fig. 85.22 Piriformis tendonotomy. (A) Before tendonotomy. (B) After tendonotomy. *PT*, piriformis tendon; *SN*, sciatic nerve.

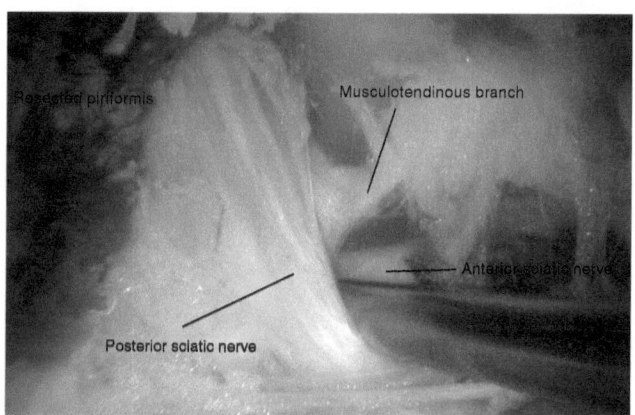

Fig. 85.23 Ancillary musculotendinous branch through the sciatic nerve.

Assess the epineural blood flow and fat. Identify the posterior femoral cutaneous nerve, sciatic artery, and inferior gluteal nerve. Dissect the fibrous band at the sciatic notch with a blunt probe, confirming the location with fluoroscopy. Internally and externally rotate the hip and probe around and underneath the nerve using a curved probe to identify any ancillary tendon involvement. At the level of the obturator internus, release any fibrous bands, then probe and check nerve color and motion. Perform a retrosciatic dissection of fibrous bands. Lastly, assess and dissect at the level of the hamstring tendons and sacrotuberous ligament to ensure adequate motion.

The endoscopic approach appears useful in detecting pathology and treatment, and further studies are underway. We reported on a case series of 35 patients presenting with deep gluteal syndrome.[21] The average duration of symptoms was 3.7 years with an average preoperative verbal analog score of 7, which decreased to 2.4 postoperatively. Preoperative mHHS was 54.4 and increased to 78 postoperatively. Twenty-one patients reported preoperative use of narcotics for pain; two remained on narcotics postoperatively (unrelated to the initial complaint). Eighty-three percent of patients had no postoperative sciatic sit pain (the inability to sit for >30 minutes).[21] Now, among 300 cases, complications

continue to be extremely low; however, poor outcomes seem to be related to femoral retroversion and previous abdominal surgery. It is very important to assess acetabular and femoral version, which has an effect on sciatic nerve biomechanics. In cases of sciatic nerve entrapment by the GT or the ischium, greater trochanteric osteoplasty or osteotomy may be a consideration. Complications have involved hematoma brought on by early postoperative use of NSAIDs with excessive postoperative activity. Concomitant pudendal nerve and sciatic nerve complaints are often resolved; however, in two cases the pudendal complaints worsened. By understanding the anatomy and biomechanics, and by applying clinical tests and diagnostic strategies, adequate treatment of all four layers can be obtained as a part of a comprehensive plan of treatment.

PUDENDAL NERVE ENTRAPMENT

The pudendal nerve arises from S2 to S4 ventral rami and exits the pelvis through the greater sciatic foramen and below the piriformis muscle. Accompanied laterally by the internal pudendal vessels, it crosses the sacrospinous ligament close to its insertion to the ischial spine, or passes over the ischial spine. The pudendal nerve then enters Alcock (pudendal) canal formed by the obturator fascia and sacrotuberous ligament (Figs. 85.24 and 85.25).[30,77] In 87 of 100 cadaveric hips, the sacrotuberous ligament was found to be composed of two parts: a ligamentous band and a membranous falciform process.[30] The sacrotuberous ligament is anatomically close to the pudendal nerve and this proximity is important in this nerve entrapment.[30] In the posterior part of the Alcock canal, the pudendal nerve gives rise to the inferior rectal nerve, the perineal nerve, and the dorsal nerves of the penis or clitoris (Table 85.3).[78]

Four main types of pudendal nerve entrapment are based upon the location of entrapment.[79] Type I: at the exit of the greater sciatic notch accompanied by piriformis muscle spasm. Type II: at the ischial spine, sacrotuberous ligament, and lesser sciatic notch entrance. Type III: at the entrance of the Alcock canal associated with the obturator internus muscle spasm. Type

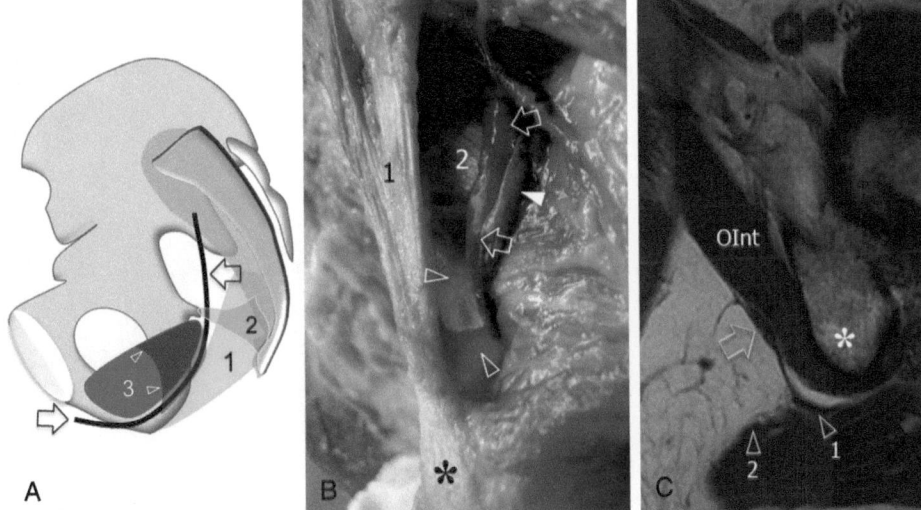

Fig. 85.24 Pudendal nerve course. (A) Schematic drawing of the pelvis illustrates the pudendal nerve exiting the pelvis through the lower part of the greater gluteal foramen and then entering the gluteal region again passing through the lesser sciatic foramen in close relationship with the sacrotuberous *(1)* and the sacrospinous *(2)* ligaments. After crossing the sacrotuberous ligament, the pudendal nerve *(arrow)* redirects its course anteriorly entering the Alcock canal, a restricted tunnel underneath the fascia *(arrowheads)* of the obturator internus muscle *(3)*. (B) Cadaveric dissection shows the sacrotuberous ligament *(1)* inserting into the ischial tuberosity *(asterisk)* and the pudendal nerve *(empty arrows)* and artery *(white arrowhead)* as they cross underneath it. Note the location of the falciform process *(empty arrowheads)* of the sacrotuberous ligament, which is a possible site for pudendal nerve entrapment. *(2)* Sacrospinous ligament. (C) Axial T1-weighted magnetic resonance image demonstrates the pudendal nerve *(arrow)* running close to the obturator internus muscle *(OInt)* in the Alcock canal. Note the position of the sacrotuberous *(1)* and the sacrospinous *(2)* ligaments and the ischial tuberosity *(asterisk)*. (From Martinoli C, Miguel-Perez M, Padua L, Gandolfo N, Zicca A, Tagliafico A. Imaging of neuropathies about the hip. *Eur J Radiol.* 2011;82[1]:17–26.)

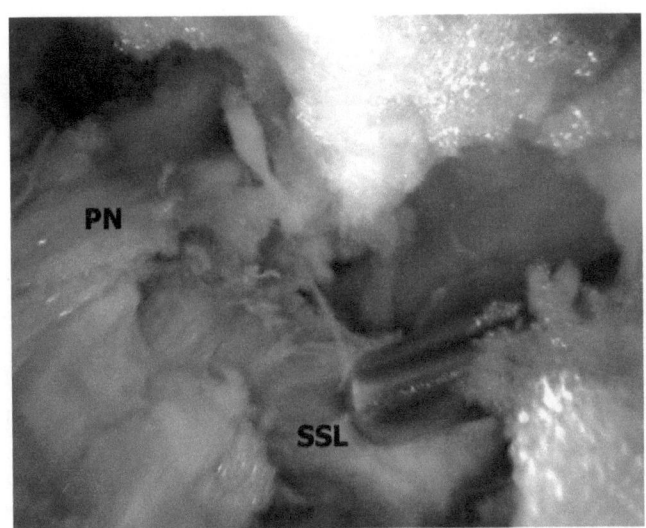

Fig. 85.25 Endoscopic view of a cadaveric sacrospinous ligament *(SSL)* and its relationship to the pudendal nerve *(PN)*. (From Wilson TJ. *Operative Hip Arthroscopy.* 3rd ed. New York: Springer; 2013.)

TABLE 85.3	Pudendal Nerve Function	
Nerve	**Motor Innervation**	**Sensory Innervation**
Pudendal Nerve		
Inferior rectal nerve	Inferior anal canal and circumanal skin	External anal sphincter
Perineal nerve	Scrotum, labium majus	Perineal muscles, external anal sphincter and levator ani
Dorsal nerve of the penis or clitoris	Corpus cavernosum	Penis or clitoris skin

IV: distal entrapment of terminal branches.[79] Antolak et al. has suggested that aberrant development and subsequent malpositioning of the ischial spine found in men with pudendal nerve entrapment could be associated with athletic injuries during their youth.[80] Cycling, endometriosis, previous pelvic surgery, and vascular sacral plexus entrapment also have been described as possible etiologies of pudendal nerve entrapment.[81,82] Pelvic biomechanics can influence the pudendal nerve through the sacrospinous ligament.

The diagnosis of pudendal neuralgia has been primarily clinical and empirical[83]; however, progress in clinical nerve imaging and injection techniques are aiding in the differential diagnosis of pudendal nerve entrapment.[79] In 2008, Labat et al. validated the Nantes Criteria with five essential diagnostic criteria: (1) pain in the anatomical territory of the pudendal nerve (Fig. 85.26), (2) worsened by sitting (relief when sitting on a toilet seat), (3) the pain does not wake the patient at night, (4) pain with no objective sensory impairment, and (5) pain is relieved by diagnostic pudendal nerve block.[83] Also defined in the report are complementary diagnostic criteria, exclusion criteria, and associated signs, including the diagnosis.[83] The physical examination is useful for the preliminarily sorting of patients into four categories: type I, sciatic notch tenderness only; type II,

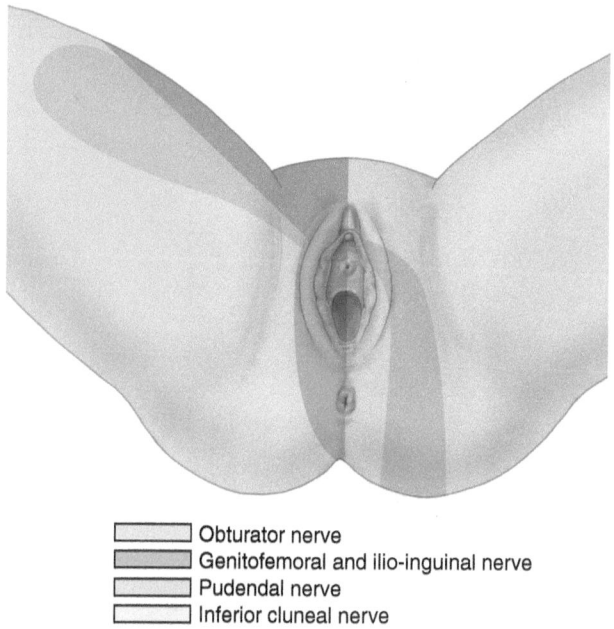

Obturator nerve
Genitofemoral and ilio-inguinal nerve
Pudendal nerve
Inferior cluneal nerve

Fig. 85.26 Innervation of the perineum. (From Labat JJ, Riant T, Robert R, Amarenco G, Lefaucheur JP, Rigaud J. Diagnostic criteria for pudendal neuralgia by pudendal nerve entrapment (Nantes criteria). *Neurourol Urodyn*. 2008;27[4]:306–310)

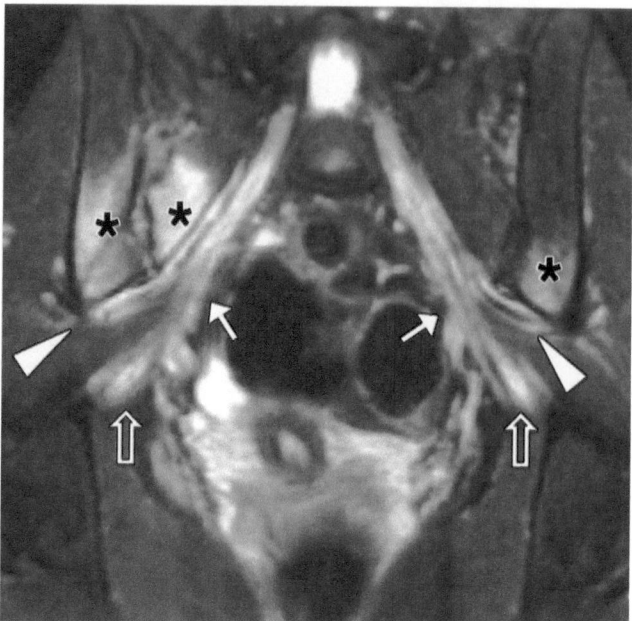

Fig. 85.27 Superior gluteal nerve neuropathy secondary to bilateral sacroiliitis. Coronal fat-suppressed T2-weighted magnetic resonance image (6100/80) shows increased signal intensity in both sacroiliac joints (*). The sciatic *(open arrows)* and superior gluteal *(arrowheads)* nerves and possibly the inferior gluteal nerves *(solid arrows)* have increased size and signal intensity. (From: Petchprapa CN, Rosenberg ZS, Sconfienza LM, Cavalcanti CF, Vieira RL, Zember JS. MR imaging of entrapment neuropathies of the lower extremity. Part 1. The pelvis and hip. *Radiographics*. 2010;30[4]:983–1000.)

midischial tenderness; type IIIa, obturator internus muscle tenderness only; type IIIb, obturator and piriformis muscle tenderness; and type IV, no palpable tenderness.

The conservative treatment is based on pain medications, physical therapy of the pelvic floor muscles, and guided nerve anesthetic blocks, including steroids.[84] The published outcomes of serial pudendal nerve blocks in controlling pain after 1 year range from 12% to 87%.[79,85] Surgical decompression may be considered when nonsurgical treatments have failed, and is traditionally performed through trans-gluteal open approaches.[79,86-88] One published randomized, controlled trial compared 16 surgically treated with 16 conservatively treated patients. At 12 months, 71% of the surgery group improved compared with 13% of the nonsurgery group.[88] In contrast to extrapelvic approaches, a laparoscopic intrapelvic decompression technique has been described in a case series including 18 patients, with 15 (83%) patients with significant pain relief with a mean follow-up of 21 months.[82]

SUPERIOR AND INFERIOR GLUTEAL NERVES

The superior gluteal nerve arises from L4, L5, and S1 ventral rami.[78,89] It leaves the pelvis for the deep gluteal space crossing the greater sciatic foramen above the piriformis, and is accompanied by the superior gluteal vessels. In the deep gluteal space, it runs between the gluteus medius and minimus, dividing into superior and inferior branches, although variation is possible. The inferior gluteal nerve arises from L5, S1, and S2 ventral rami[78] and accesses the deep gluteal space through the greater sciatic foramen, passing below the piriformis together with the inferior gluteal vessels. In the deep gluteal space, it gives off

TABLE 85.4   Function of the Gluteal Nerves

Nerve	Motor Innervation
Superior gluteal nerve	
Superior branch	Gluteus medius and occasionally minimus
Inferior branch	Gluteus medius, minimus, and tensor fasciae latae
Inferior gluteal nerve	Gluteus maximus

branches that enter the undersurface of the gluteus maximus muscle (Table 85.4).

The gluteal nerves are at risk of being damaged in lateral or posterior surgical approaches to the hip.[90-92] Abitbol reported abnormal EMG findings in over 77% of patients at 6 postoperative weeks, whether a posterior or a lateral approach was used.[90] Percutaneous iliosacral screws can entrap the superior gluteal nerve, as reported by Collinge in a cadaveric study, at a rate of 18%.[93] Bone calluses related to fracture and prominent osteophytes around the greater sciatic foramen can also entrap the superior gluteal nerve.[94] Sacroiliac inflammatory and infectious processes can cause gluteal nerves neuropathy due the anatomical proximity (Fig. 85.27).[13] Gluteal injections also have been described to cause superior gluteal nerve injury.[95]

Limp or gait pattern changes can be noted in patients with dysfunction of gluteal nerves.[92,96] Weakness of the abductor musculature and a positive Trendelenburg test are also found in superior gluteal nerve neuropathies. Usually, superior or inferior nerve entrapment does not cause obvious gait abnormalities.

Conservative treatment is usually indicated the gluteal nerves neuropathy. Surgical excision of bone or screw compression should be considered in some cases. Bos et al. suggested, in the lateral hip approach, limiting the proximal extension of the gluteal medius incision to 3 cm cranial to GT, aiming to prevent superior gluteal nerve damage.[97] Posterior approaches to the hip also have been associated with nerve damage. Therefore in order to avoid inferior gluteal nerve damage, Ling and Kumar proposed that gluteus maximus splitting of more than 5 cm from the GT towards the posterior superior iliac spine be avoided.[92] In cases of severe abductor dysfunction with good gluteus maximus function, gluteus maximus flap transfer should be considered.[98] Both the superior and inferior gluteal nerves can be easily visualized and assessed endoscopically.

CONCLUSION

A structured physical examination that incorporates the five levels of the hip: the osseous, capsulolabral, the musculotendinous, neurovascular, and kinematic chain, is essential for a differential diagnosis in patients with posterior hip pain. The five-level approach will help to avoid frustration for both the patient and the physician. An understanding of the osseous contribution is critical in all three planes as they affect the nerve biomechanics in a dynamic manner. The neurovascular layer can present a challenging condition, and utilizing the valid posterior hip physical examination tests will aid in the diagnosis. The use of a common language and technique will facilitate communication and the understanding of each level. In order to treat pathologic conditions of the posterior hip, a comprehensive treatment plan should address all levels of the hip.

For a complete list of references, go to ExpertConsult.com.

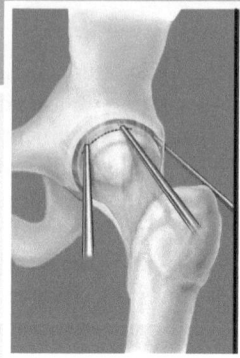

86

Hamstring Injuries

Kyle E. Hammond, Lee M. Kneer

INTRODUCTION

Hamstring injuries are common in athletic populations and can affect athletes at all levels of competition.[1-4] Several studies have shown that the rates of muscle strain in high school football (12% to 24%) and collegiate football (18.9% to 22.2%) are fairly high.[5-9] In one study, injury surveillance conducted by the National Football League identified 1716 hamstring strains among all players, with a range of 132 to 210 injuries per year, which accounts for an overall injury rate of 0.77 per 1000 athlete-exposures and a reinjury rate of 16.5%.[10] Hamstring injuries accounted for nearly one-fifth of all injuries sustained by elite track and field athletes, with males at twice the risk compared with their female counterparts.[11] One literature review identified previous hamstring injury as the greatest risk factor for reinjury, with age and male sex also increasing injury risk.[12] The injured muscle may have an altered compliance or deformation pattern, predisposing it to reduced tensility or higher muscle strain. Although some studies suggest that contact activities are the cause of hamstring injuries, most studies have shown that more than 90% of injuries occur without contact, with the classic injury being sustained by a water skier who gets pulled up by the boat, resulting in abrupt knee extension and hip flexion.[5,13]

The hamstring complex consists of the short and long heads of the biceps femoris, semitendinosus, and semimembranosus. The semitendinosus, semimembranosus, and long head of the biceps are biarticular and are innervated by the tibial portion of the sciatic nerve. The short head of the biceps is monarticular and innervated by the common peroneal nerve. These muscles work together to extend the hip, flex the knee, and externally rotate the hip and knee; they have significant overlap at the myotendinous junction.[12]

The proximal hamstring complex has a strong bony attachment on the ischial tuberosity (Fig. 86.1).[14] The ischial footprint is composed of the common proximal tendon of the semitendinosus and the long head of the biceps femoris as well as a distinct semimembranosus footprint. The semimembranosus passes anteriorly to the conjoined semitendinosus/biceps femoris tendon to its origin on the lateral ischium (see Fig. 86.1).

Biomechanically the hamstrings are subjected to high tensile load, given their extensive eccentric role. Hip and knee flexion during the initial swing phase requires simultaneous eccentric and concentric activity of the hamstrings. During terminal swing, the hamstrings continue to play a dual role of preventing knee hyperextension while opposing hip flexion.[15] The hamstrings work synergistically with the gluteal muscles to stabilize, decelerate, and propel the hip. During the propulsion phase, the medial hamstrings assist in decelerating hip external rotation, which maintains the gluteus maximus at an ideal length to act as an accelerator (along with the hamstrings) of the femur in the sagittal plane. The hamstrings along with the rectus abdominis are also decelerators of pelvic anterior tilt throughout stance. Given these functional relationships, it is conceivable that hamstring strain or rupture has its source in the inhibition and weakness of its closest synergists, the gluteal and abdominal muscles; these muscle groups have become targets for injury prevention and rehabilitation.[16]

Hamstring injuries most commonly occur proximally, as one study of 275 soccer players has demonstrated.[17] In this study of hamstring strains, purely tendinous injuries (7.9% of all hamstring strains) were relatively rare, with the proximal myotendinous junction, muscle belly, and distal myotendinous junction (36.1%, 32%, and 17.7%, respectively) implicated more frequently. The long head of the biceps femoris was most commonly (56.5%) implicated, whereas injuries to the short head of biceps femoris occurred only 5.6% of the time.[17]

Hamstring injuries occur on a continuum that can range from musculotendinous strains to avulsion injuries.[1,2] A strain is a partial or complete disruption of the musculotendinous unit.[1,4] A complete tear or avulsion, in contrast, is a discontinuity of the unit. Distal avulsion injuries are quite rare and not discussed in this chapter. Most hamstring strains do not require surgical intervention and resolve with a variety of modalities and rest. Differentiating the complete and partial tears from the muscle strain subgroup is of importance, as patients with complete or partial tears can experience more substantial disability.

HISTORY

The history of an acute injury classically involves a traumatic event with forced hip flexion and the knee in extension, as observed in water skiing, although studies have suggested that most injuries occur during high-speed running or moments of rapid change of pace.[2,18-23]

Commonly athletes with proximal hamstring tendon tears describe an acute popping or tearing sensation with associated function-limiting pain.[24,25] Although pain is typically the

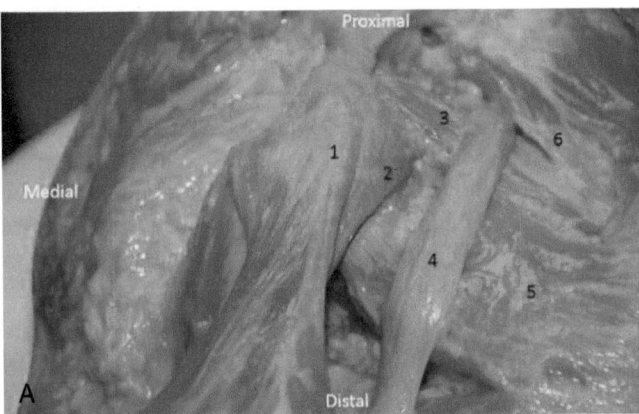
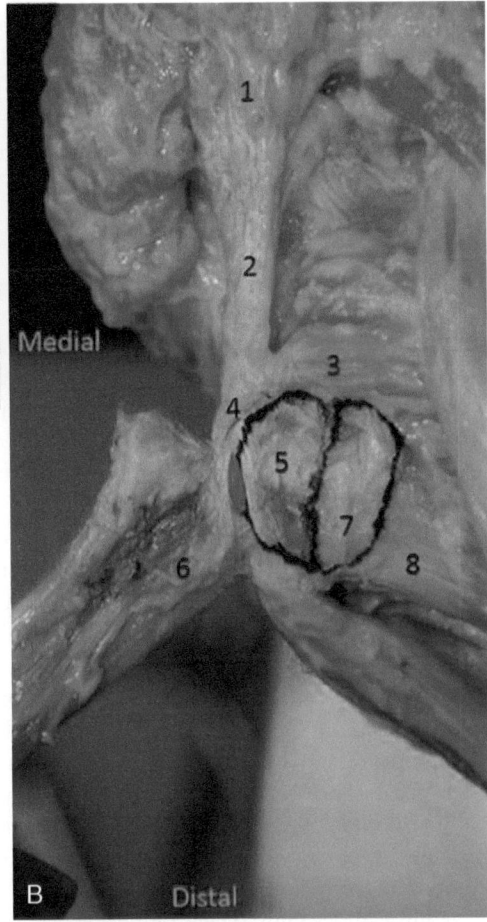

Fig. 86.1 Normal anatomy of the hamstring origin. (A) The posterior view of a cadaveric dissection of the ischium in a left hip. The conjoined semitendinosus/biceps femoris tendon (1) passes posteriorly to the semimembranosus tendon (2) to insert medially on the proximal hamstring footprint at the posterolateral ischium. The inferior gemellus (3), sciatic nerve (4), quadratus femoris (5), and piriformis (6) are closely associated with the proximal hamstring. (B) The footprint of the hamstring on the posterolateral ischium is composed of the conjoined tendon (5) medially and the semimembranosus (7) laterally. Structures near the hamstring footprint include the sacrum (1), sacrotuberous ligament (2), inferior gemellus (3), medial bony prominence (4), conjoined tendon (6), and quadratus femoris (8).

chief complaint, the patient may also complain of a sense of instability or gait incoordination.[22,25-28] Occasionally patients who present with hamstring tears may report altered sensation or pain in a dermatomal distribution much like that seen in radiculopathy.[22,25,27,29] This may be explained by acute nerve traction, the caustic effect of blood on the nerve, or compression from the associated hematoma. The patient may complain of a previous similar injury in the same leg, given the high risk of recurrence.[30]

PHYSICAL EXAMINATION

The examination is typically performed with the patient in the prone position. Maintaining the knee in a slightly flexed position will make the examination more comfortable for individuals with more severe injuries. Inspection and palpation of the posterior thigh may reveal fasciculations or muscle spasm. Ecchymosis may be observed if the fascial covering is also disrupted. Palpation of the entire posterior thigh is important to localize the

injury. Palpation should be performed systematically, starting at the broad insertion along the ischial tuberosity. Identification of a more proximal injury is important, as studies have shown a prolonged recovery course for injuries occurring more proximally, especially within the tendon.[31,32] Given the biarticular nature of the hamstring complex, it is important to examine the strength of both knee flexion and hip extension as well as range of motion (ROM). The authors suggest evaluating knee flexion in both relative extension (15 to 30 degrees flexion) and flexion at 90 degrees as well as hip extension with the knee fully extended and again at 90 degrees of knee flexion while the patient is prone. Eccentric testing of the hamstrings via resisted extension of the knee from 90 to 15 degrees may elicit pain with milder injuries. Careful note should be taken of side-to-side strength differences. Similarly, a decrement in painless ROM may be used to identify a more chronic hamstring injury, and several examination maneuvers have been described to assess for tendinopathic functional changes.[33] Our preferred test for proximal tendinopathy pain is a supine single-leg plank.

During examination, one must have a high index of suspicion for a tear. In less acute situations where the tear is several days old, it is possible that even a large defect may not be palpable clinically owing to the overlying hematoma. It is especially critical to assess these patients with imaging studies to delineate the type of tear that is present and to guide management.

IMAGING

No initial imaging is indicated for hamstring injuries involving no loss of strength and minimal to moderate pain, especially if discomfort is isolated to the muscle belly. If pain is more severe and located proximally, plain radiographs including an anteroposterior view of the pelvis and lateral image of the affected hip are warranted to rule out and characterize an avulsion injury. If a fracture is identified, computed tomography (CT) or magnetic resonance imaging (MRI) may assist in assessing the displacement and fracture configuration for possible surgical planning. Special consideration should be given to obtaining radiographs in the younger patient at risk for apophyseal injuries (Fig. 86.2).

MRI and ultrasound are the imaging modalities of choice to evaluate nonavulsion injuries resulting in weakness, gait abnormalities, or severe pain or in lesser injuries involving elite athletes.[34] MRI has been shown to be more accurate in evaluating tears, especially to deeper tissues or in patients with recurrent tears, as scar tissue can be more easily mistaken for acute injury with ultrasound. However, studies have not examined this in recent years, as ultrasonographic image resolution has greatly improved.[35] MRI findings, particularly the Peetrons classification and size of muscular edema, have been shown to be predictive of return to play (RTP) following grade 1 and 2 injuries.[36,37] Data support the use of MRI as the preferred tool for the evaluation of tendon retraction in the case of a complete tear as well, making it particularly helpful in surgical planning (Fig. 86.3). Incomplete tears without retraction often reveal a "sickle sign," as demonstrated by a curvilinear signal on T2-weighted images (Fig. 86.4).[23] One must be cautious in considering advanced

imaging, as partial hamstring tears have been detected in up to 15% of asymptomatic patients.[38,39]

Ultrasound is useful as a point-of-care examination tool; it allows for dynamic imaging and comparison to the contralateral limb; it is also far less expensive than MRI. Recent advances in technology have allowed for the development of portable units with resolution allowing for their use as sideline tools, and there are no considerations for patient mass, implanted devices, or claustrophobia. Ultrasound is highly user-dependent and not available universally. Moreover, the evaluation of pathology can

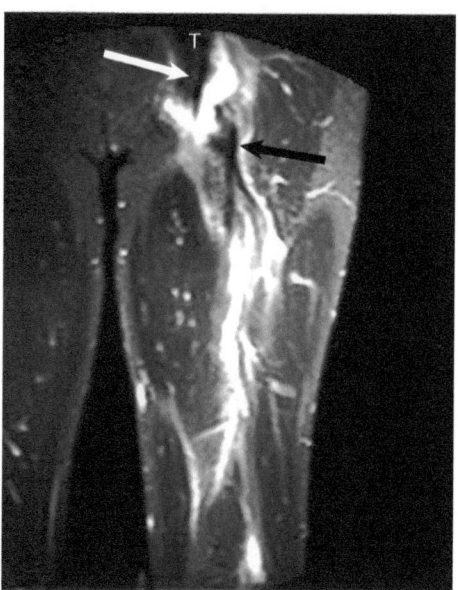

Fig. 86.3 A coronal T2-weighted magnetic resonance image of a complete three-tendon rupture of the proximal hamstring. The *black arrow* points to the common avulsed tendon. The *white arrow* identifies the tuberosity (*T*).

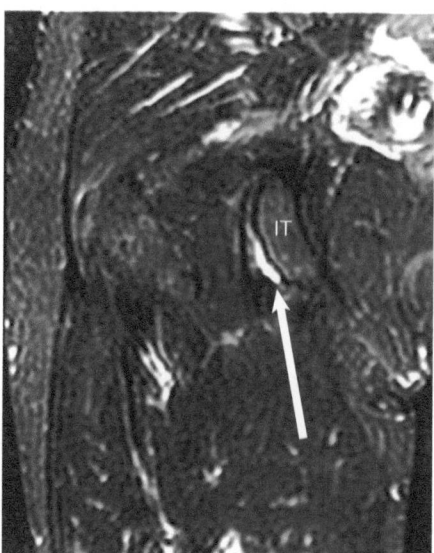

Fig. 86.4 A coronal T2-weighted magnetic resonance image of a right hip showing the sickle sign *(arrow)*, which indicates fluid within the ischial bursa. *IT*, Ischial tuberosity.

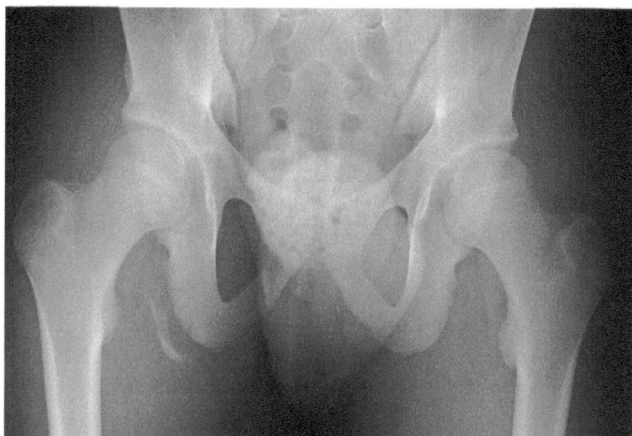

Fig. 86.2 An anteroposterior radiograph of the pelvis showing a bony avulsion of the right ischial tuberosity.

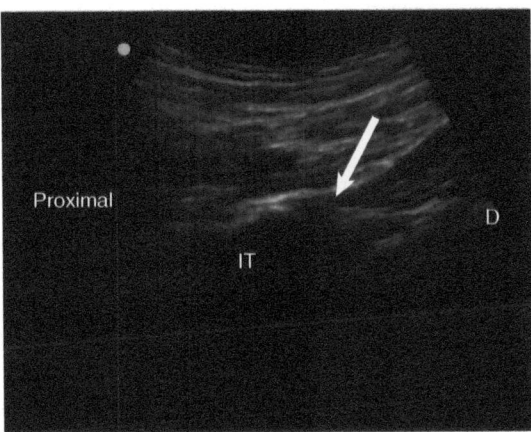

Fig. 86.5 Ultrasound image of the origin of the left hamstring *(arrow)*. *D*, distal; *IT*, ischial tuberosity.

be hindered by the presence of large hematomas, as is often common in hamstring tears (Fig. 86.5). Despite this, ultrasound has been shown to be highly accurate in the evaluation of partial tears and insertional tendinosis.[40]

DECISION-MAKING PRINCIPLES

Whether the surgical procedure is performed with an open approach or endoscopically, the indications are the same. The only certain indication for the open procedure is a large retracted tear with chronic atrophy as noted on MRI. In these cases, the procedure would more than likely require extensive mobilization and probably the use of a graft for reconstruction of the avulsed segment, which would have to be performed in an open fashion at this time, usually with a longitudinal incision. The first indication for surgery is an acute hamstring avulsion of at least two out of the three tendons in an active patient with greater than 2 cm of retraction. Some patients have a clinically evident partial hamstring avulsion involving the biceps/semitendinosus tendon, with refractory ischial pain and the inability to return to high-level sports. Finally, patients are also candidates for surgical intervention when they have a history of refractory ischial bursitis and no discernible tear and conservative treatment has failed, including at least 12 weeks of physical therapy and potentially ultrasound-guided ischial injections with corticosteroids and/or biologics.

TREATMENT OPTIONS

Nonoperative

Initial nonoperative treatment is warranted for the majority of hamstring injuries, with surgical management reserved for larger avulsions or large muscular tears. Tenets include active rest, the use of oral nonsteroidal antiinflammatory medications, and a physical therapy program consisting of gentle hamstring stretching and strengthening. As the initial inflammation resolves, core, hip, and quadriceps exercises can be added in association with a more aggressive hamstring injury prevention program.[41,42] In a recent randomized controlled trial, male soccer players showed a decrease in hamstring injuries with the implementation

of Nordic hamstring exercises as part of the standard conditioning program.[43] Progression then advances to sport-specific exercises, and full participation is allowed when the patient can perform these without symptoms.[12] If progress does not occur with this program, an ultrasound-guided corticosteroid injection may be used; this has been shown to be both safe and effective at providing significant relief and allowing a hastened (RTP).[40] Fader et al. showed that in patients with refractory chronic proximal hamstring tendinopathy, platelet-rich plasma injections can improve pain scores compared with other nonoperative means.[44] Patients who experience failure of nonoperative treatment for partial tears may benefit from surgical débridement and repair, similar to patients with other commonly seen partial tendon tears (i.e., the rotator cuff). As described further on, newer and less invasive endoscopic techniques are also an option for this problem.

Nonoperative treatment of complete ruptures of the proximal hamstring or those with more than 2 cm of retraction is less frequently recommended because surgical repair has resulted in the successful return of patients to a high level of function.[18,20,24,25,29,45-49] One study showed that up to 40% of patients with partial proximal hamstring tears and less than 2 cm of retraction go on to require surgical intervention, and other studies have shown similar results.[20,46] Partial hamstring injuries have been shown to be successfully treated with débridement and suture anchor placement after a period of failed conservative care; however, this approach is less effective in the treatment of complete tears or those treated acutely.[47]

Surgical Treatment

Open

Open techniques are still the standard of care and are most often described in the literature. The indications for surgical treatment of proximal hamstring ruptures include all acute complete three-tendon tears and two-tendon tears with retraction of 2 cm or more.[48] Acute surgical repair initially is not indicated for patients with a one- or two-tendon tear with less than 2 cm of retraction; they are treated surgically if nonoperative treatment is not successful. In addition, less active patients or patients who are unable to comply with the postoperative rehabilitation protocol should be managed nonoperatively. Patients with complete or partial tears for whom conservative management fails may be candidates for delayed repair.

A transverse incision in the gluteal crease inferior to the ischial tuberosity is used.[19,21,48,49] The tendon should be placed on the lateral aspect of the ischial tuberosity and should lie down flat to allow optimal bone healing as well as to prevent prominence (Fig. 86.6).

Endoscopic

Some surgeons have begun to utilize an arthroscopic approach.[50] With this technique, the patient is placed in the prone position after induction of anesthesia, with all prominences and neurovascular structures protected. The table is flat (as opposed to the slightly flexed position of the table in the open repair procedure) to help maintain the space between the gluteal musculature and the ischium.

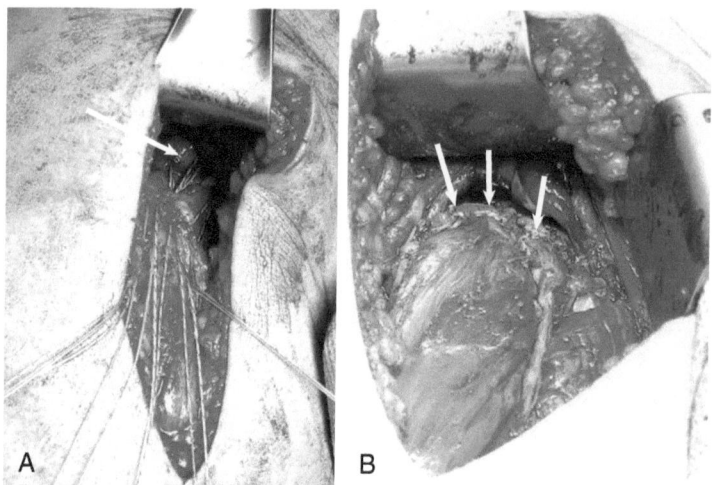

Fig. 86.6 Open repair of the proximal hamstring on the ischial tuberosity *(arrow)*. (A) The view is of a longitudinal incision in the left hip. Multiple sutures are in place, with the ischial tuberosity visualized in the wound. (B) Final repair of the hamstring, with multiple suture points visualized *(arrows)*.

Two portals are then created, one each 2 cm medial and lateral to the palpable ischial tuberosity (Fig. 86.7). The lateral portal is established first by using blunt dissection with a switching stick as the gluteus maximus muscle is penetrated and the submuscular plane is created. The medial portal is then established, taking care to palpate the medial aspect of the ischium. A 30-degree arthroscope is then inserted in the lateral portal and an electrocautery device is placed in the medial portal. The space between the ischium and the gluteus muscle is then developed, taking care to stay along the central and medial portions of the ischium to avoid any damage to the sciatic nerve. With the lateral aspect identified, the dissection continues anteriorly and laterally toward the known area of the sciatic nerve (Fig. 86.8). Very careful and methodical release of any soft tissue bands is then undertaken in a proximal-to-distal direction to mobilize the nerve and protect it throughout the exposure and ultimate repair of the hamstring tendon.

Once the nerve has been identified and protected, attention is directed once again to the area of the tendinous avulsion. The tip of the ischium is identified through palpation with the instruments. The tendinous origin is then inspected to identify any obvious tearing. With acute tears the area is obvious and the tendon is often retracted distally. In these cases, a large hematoma is occasionally present and must be evacuated. It is especially important to protect the sciatic nerve during this portion of the procedure because it is sometimes obscured by the hematoma.

Once the area of pathology has been identified (in persons with incomplete tears), an endoscopic knife can be used to longitudinally split the tendon along its fibers. The hamstring is then undermined and the partial tearing is débrided with an oscillating shaver. The lateral wall of the ischium is cleared of devitalized tissue and a bleeding bed is established in preparation for the tendon repair.

An inferior portal may then be created approximately 4 cm distal to the tip of the ischium and equidistant from the medial and lateral portals. This portal is used for insertion of suture

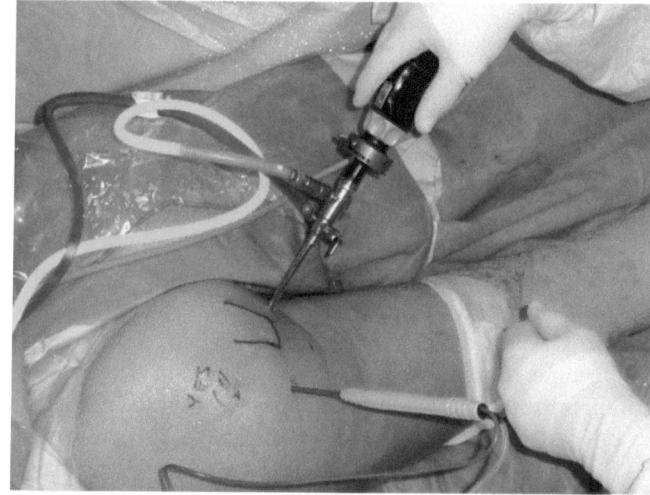

Fig. 86.7 Portals for the endoscopic approach. Note that the arthroscope is in the medial portal and the empty portal is the distal portal. The ablator is in the lateral portal.

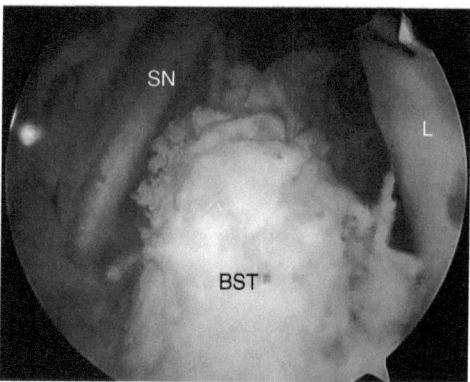

Fig. 86.8 Normal arthroscopic anatomy exposure in a left hip as viewed from the lateral portal. Note the tool entering from the medial portal. *BST,* common biceps/semitendinosus; *L,* lateral ischium; *SN,* sciatic nerve.

anchors as well as suture management. The principles are essentially the same as those used in arthroscopic rotator cuff repair. Once all of the sutures have been passed through the tissue of the avulsed hamstring, the sutures are tied and a solid repair of the tendon is completed.

POSTOPERATIVE MANAGEMENT

Rehabilitation

Assuming that hamstring strain or rupture has its source in the inhibition and weakness of its closest synergists, the gluteal and abdominal muscles, it is important to focus on both groups in the rehabilitation of these injuries, whether they are treated surgically or not. Because the gluteal muscles work in conjunction with the hamstrings to extend the hip, when the agonists (gluteal muscles) for hip extension are weak, an increased relative effort of the hamstrings is required to control trunk and hip flexion during the loading phase of running.[51] In one prospective evaluation, 24 athletes underwent rehabilitation in one of two protocols: either an isolated hamstring stretching and progressive strengthening protocol or a progressive agility and trunk stabilization protocol.[42] Follow-up at 2 weeks and 1 year revealed a significantly higher reinjury rate in athletes treated with the isolated hamstring rehabilitation protocol (54.5% vs. 0% and 70% vs. 7.7%, respectively). This finding suggests that strong neuromuscular control of the lumbopelvic region allows the lower extremity muscle to function at high velocity while maintaining a protected ROM for hamstring muscles.

Using the synergistic concept as the premise for the rehabilitation program, the patient ambulates non-weight-bearing on crutches with for the first 4 weeks, depending on the quality of tension on the repair. Weight bearing is advanced to full weight bearing by 6 weeks with continued use of crutches as needed until 8 weeks, as the knee brace is extended to neutral by 6 weeks.

Authors' Preferred Technique

The authors' preferred technique is to perform an outpatient open repair between 2 and 4 weeks postinjury in acute ruptures. With chronic full and partial ruptures that undergo surgical repair, there is no time constraint. Although primary repairs of acute ruptures can be successfully made up to 8 weeks postinjury, it is certainly easier to mobilize the tissue within 4 weeks of the injury. We like to pay close attention to their sciatic nerve examination, both preoperatively and postoperatively. We routinely decompress the sciatic nerve and perform a neurolysis in all cases to optimize the outcome for the nerve. We use a standard prone position with a table break at the patient's iliac crest, which will be flexed about 30 degrees to improve access at the gluteal crease (Fig. 86.9). We place pillows and pads underneath the knee down to the foot, so the knee is in flexed position of about 30 degrees. We utilize a gluteal crease incision for cosmesis and keep this incision as short as safely possible and centered over the lateral aspect of the ischial tuberosity (Fig. 86.10). We utilize a standard fascial layer approach, localize and protect the gluteal neurovascular structures, and then localize the sciatic nerve to perform a neurolysis and protect it throughout the remainder of the case (Fig. 86.11). We then decompress any seroma and/or hematoma and decorticate the footprint of the ischial tuberosity with a rongeur and currete. We then utilize five 3-0 biocomposite, single-loaded SutureTak anchors (Arthrex) in a clustered pattern to fill the footprint. Once this is completed, we begin to suture the tendon after it has been débrided and prepared using a locking stitch and single-pass stitch in a mattress fashion from each anchor. Once all anchors have been sutured, we tie down beginning with the proximal footprint and bringing the knee into 45 degrees of flexion. A layered closure with Vicryl is performed of the hamstring and gluteal fascia; then Monocryl and Dermabond are used for the skin closure. Postoperatively we use a standard hinged postoperative knee brace locked at 30 degrees and make the patient non-weight-bearing for 6 weeks. Partial chronic tears that require surgery are performed in the same manner, and chronic retracted tears are repaired utilizing an Achilles allograft with a longitudinal incision (Fig. 86.12). In the chronic technique, we will place a small bone block into the ischial tuberosity with a biocomposite interference screw and then add additional fixation around the bone block with suture anchors and soft-tissue fixation. We then attach the allograft to the native musculotendinous end of the hamstrings under tension and 90 degrees of knee flexion. Postoperatively, the knee is kept at 90 degrees for 6 weeks in the chronic repairs.

The postoperative protocol is similar for both arthroscopic and open techniques with similar expected outcomes. To date, there is no a study to our knowledge that compares outcomes for arthroscopic versus open techniques.

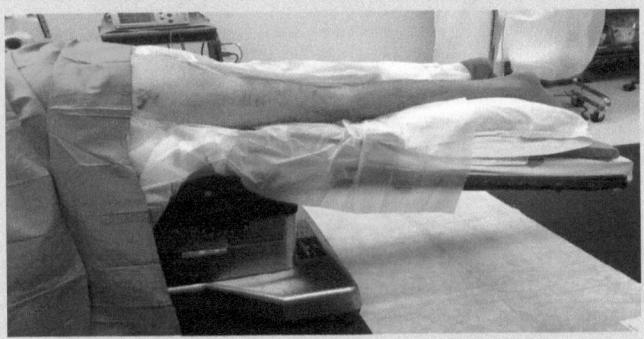

Fig. 86.9 The patient is positioned in the prone position with the break in the operative table flexed to 30 degrees to expose the gluteal fold.

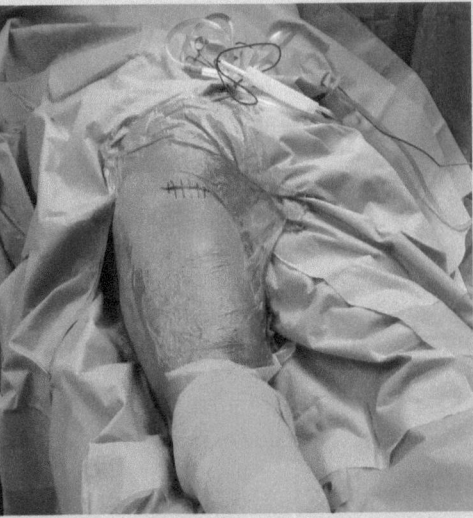

Fig. 86.10 The standard transverse incision is kept as small as possible to perform the surgery safely and adequately, as well as being placed directly in line with the subgluteal skin crease to maximize cosmesis.

Authors' Preferred Technique—cont'd

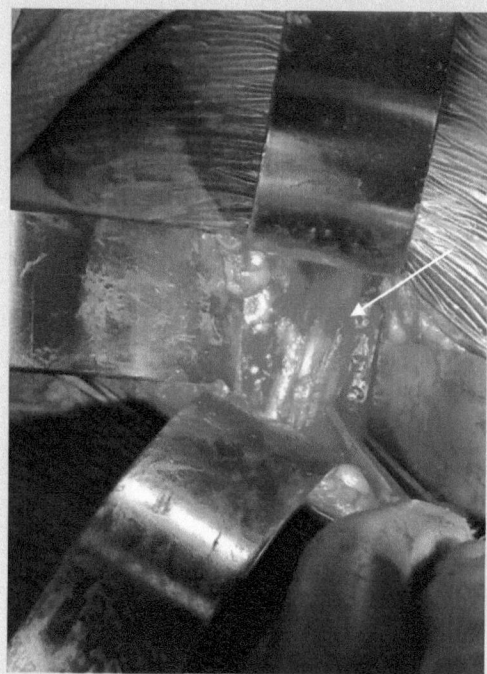

Fig. 86.11 The *white arrow* points to a sciatic nerve exposed and decompressed in a case of hamstring syndrome.

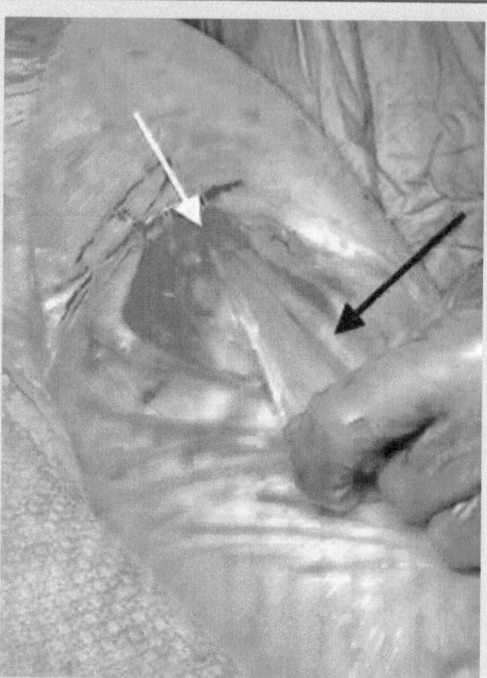

Fig. 86.12 The *white arrow* points to the ischial tuberosity, where the Achilles allograft *(black arrow)* has been fixed with an interference screw and suture anchor fixation.

The brace is removed around 8 weeks after surgery. Passive hip ROM is begun with a therapist at 2 weeks and active hip flexion is started at 4 weeks. Isotonic strengthening (at 6 weeks), isokinetic strengthening (8 weeks), and aqua therapy are initiated with progression of core pelvic and closed-chain exercises. Dry land training and sport-specific training are initiated at 12 weeks, with return to full sports participation 6 to 9 months after surgery.

RESULTS

In one study of 52 patients in which the open technique was used for both acute[52] and chronic[12] repairs, a 96% satisfaction rate was found with the use of subjective validated outcome scales and at an average of 27 months follow-up.[53] Lower Extremity Functional Scale results indicated that acute repairs had statistically significant greater outcomes than did chronic repairs ($P = .023$). Thirty-five patients (67%) reported that they could participate in strenuous activities at their latest follow-up. Mansour et al. showed that in the National Football League there was an initial 90% return to sport rate for one game after acute repair of a complete rupture, but only a 50% return to sport rate at the final follow-up; however, the sample size was small.[54]

Another study of eight patients with a similar suture anchor repair revealed postoperative Cybex testing at 88% of peak torque, with the ratio of hamstring-to-quadriceps strength being 0.55, which was not significantly different from the other side.[26] An analysis of 10 athletes with acute complete hamstring tendon tears revealed that the average peak torque was 82% and the hamstring-to-quadriceps strength ratio was 0.56.[27] Nine of ten patients returned to their previous level of professional sports activities. Three patients had acute sciatic nerve symptoms that were successfully treated with hematoma evacuation and neurolysis.

Most studies evaluating late surgical repairs have been in patients with chronic tears for complaints of pain while sitting, hamstring weakness, and sciatic nerve symptoms due to scarring, also known as hamstring syndrome.[24,48,55] These chronic tear repairs yield less consistent results, and the potential exists of scarring of the hamstring-avulsed tissue to the sciatic nerve, which necessitates a sciatic neurolysis. As a result of the inferior results, most surgeons experienced in proximal hamstring repair recommend early reattachment compared with delayed repair.[56] In the study by Sarimo et al., 41 athletes underwent surgical repair of either acute or chronic proximal hamstring injuries. The authors found that the odds ratio of having a moderate or poor result was 29-fold with a delay of surgical repair of greater than 3 months.[25] On the other hand, a more recent study comparing the acute versus chronic repair of complete tears showed that there were good functional and subjective results in both groups with no statistical difference in their outcome scores.[57] Subbu et al. showed a quicker return to sport in the acutely (within 6 weeks of injury) repaired group between 9 and 13 weeks, as well as fewer postoperative complications.[58] A recent systematic analysis showed both operative repair and nonoperative management to result in similar positive outcomes without a significant benefit in surgical repair.[59] However, as in most systematic reviews, there was heterogeneity of the included studies, thus limiting the ability to utilize these findings clinically.

For patients with chronic ruptures who undergo repair, an allograft may be necessary for reattachment to the ischial tuberosity.[56] The literature includes few results with regard to this procedure; however, Folsom and Larson[52] have reported on five patients who required Achilles tendon allograft reconstruction for repair of a chronic rupture. They found that reconstruction of chronic ruptures with an Achilles allograft appeared to restore function and strength at a level comparable with acute repairs.

For patients with high-grade partial insertional tears who fail to respond to nonoperative treatment, surgical repair is performed. The surgical approach is the same as previously described. Once the tendon is exposed, it is incised and released from the tuberosity with use of an elevator. It is then repaired using the same technique for complete tears with suture anchors. Treatment of partial tears has been reported by Lempainen et al., with 41 of 47 athletes returning to sport in average of 5 months.[60]

Chronic proximal hamstring tendinopathy with sciatic nerve symptoms has also traditionally been included in the generic term *hamstring syndrome*. In this specific injury, the tendon is traumatized from repetitive overuse injury. Theoretically the tendon undergoes repetitive stretch and mechanical overload and is unable to fully heal. The sciatic nerve can undergo similar types of stress, leading to scarring, adhesion, and impingement from the thickened tendon. In the cohort in the study by Lempainen et al.,[60] surgical treatment was performed with tenotomy of the thickened semimembranosus tendon and tenodesis to the biceps femoris with sciatic nerve release; 89% of the patients had good to excellent results.

COMPLICATIONS

Potential complications associated with proximal hamstring ruptures prior to surgical treatment are related to the mechanism of injury. The complications can be early or delayed. The early complications most commonly involve a neurapraxia injury to the sciatic nerve as a result of a stretch injury. Depending on the mechanism and force of the injury, the sciatic nerve can be damaged, leading to burning symptoms radiating down the leg and weakness of the foot. During the initial examination it is critical to determine if the sciatic nerve is functioning appropriately to document and ensure that no iatrogenic injury is present at the time of surgery. Fortunately neurapraxia injury most commonly resolves over time despite being troubling to the patient initially. Delayed complications of nonoperative treatment of proximal hamstring ruptures have been described by Puranen and Orava.[55] These complications include knee flexion and hip extension weakness, difficulty sitting, hamstring deformity, and the potential development of symptoms similar to those of hamstring syndrome as the tendons scar down to the sciatic nerve. Hamstring syndrome consists of local posterior buttock pain and discomfort over the ischial tuberosity. In

addition, the pain may worsen with stretching and during exercise (e.g., sprinting, hurdling, and kicking).

Surgical repair of proximal hamstring ruptures also has its inherent risks. Superficial and deep wound infections can occur, as with other surgeries; however, the location of the incision can potentially increase this risk because of the proximity of the incision to the perineum. Additionally, the three main nervous structures at risk of iatrogenic injury are the posterior femoral cutaneous, inferior gluteal, and sciatic nerves. The posterior femoral cutaneous nerve exits the sacral plexus and enters the pelvis through the greater sciatic foramen below the piriformis muscle. It then descends beneath the gluteus maximus with the inferior gluteal artery and runs down the back of the thigh beneath the fascia lata and over the long head of the biceps femoris to the back of the knee.[60,61] It provides sensation to the skin of the posterior surface of the thigh and leg as well as to the skin of the perineum. It can be injured during the surgical approach for repair if it is not protected. The inferior gluteal nerve is the major innervation of the gluteus maximus, which is the principal extensor of the thigh. This nerve can be injured with aggressive retraction of the gluteus during the surgical approach.[61]

The sciatic nerve is the longest and widest single nerve in the human body and provides innervation of the skin of the leg as well as the muscles of the posterior compartment of the thigh; it also provides the motor function of the calf and foot. The nerve is in close proximity to the ischial tuberosity as it runs along the lateral aspect. It may be injured from retraction during exposure of the tuberosity for repair.[25,29]

Other potential complications associated with proximal hamstring repair include repeat rupture, weakness, and sitting pain. According to the reports on hamstring repair, repeat ruptures are rare. In the cohort in the study by Sarimo et al., 3 of 41 patients failed surgical repair.[25] Upon a repeat operation, anatomic repair of the injury could not be achieved. The authors believe that the quality of the tendon can deteriorate with delays in surgical treatment, fatty degeneration, and muscle denervation from nerve injury.[25] Several studies have tested postoperative hamstring strength after repair. Recently Carmichael et al.[29] found that mean postoperative isotonic strength was 84% compared with the contralateral side; however, other studies have shown a return of strength ranging from 60% to 90% after repair.[21,26,45,49]

A concern unique to the endoscopic approach is that of fluid extravasation into the pelvis as a result of the fluid used in distending the potential space around the hamstring tendon. Every effort should be made to regularly check the abdomen for any evidence of abdominal distention.

One of the most important aspects in the treatment of proximal hamstring ruptures is early recognition and treatment. Early recognition of the injury allows for early repair of the acute injury, which is substantially easier to perform immediately after the injury occurs (within 4 weeks). Later recognition and delayed surgery lead to a more difficult repair that ultimately may result in increased surgical complications and poorer patient outcomes. Patients who undergo repairs of acute injuries have had better outcomes, as reported in the literature, than those who undergo repairs of chronic injuries.[24,25]

In summary, recognition of proximal hamstring ruptures allows early treatment with surgical repair. With proper treatment, good functional results can be achieved.

FUTURE CONSIDERATIONS

Few clinical studies have been conducted to test hamstring strength—to assist in determining a range of strength deficit if the tendon is not repaired—in patients who have undergone nonoperative treatment of acute ruptures.[24] As a result, in discussing the options of repair or conservative treatment with patients after a diagnosis of a complete proximal hamstring rupture, it is difficult to define the percentage of weakness that may be expected if the repair is not performed.

It will also be interesting to observe if more organized sporting teams begin to implement Nordic exercise programs or others that may be studied in the future to aid in the prevention of hamstring injury.

The emerging field of orthobiologics offers promise of improving outcomes in both the surgical and nonsurgical settings. However, despite its popularity, there is a paucity of high-level evidence to support the use of stem cells or platelet-rich plasma in either the clinical or surgical arena. Targets for research include optimizing injectate composition, stratification of appropriateness based on injury severity and location, and the development of postinjection rehabilitation protocols. Orthobiologics continues to be a popular topic within our societies and their validity should be studied at the highest level.

In addition, further development and refinement of the endoscopic technique is necessary, as at present it is clearly in its earliest phases. The extent to which this technique can be used in all tears remains to be seen. Further studies are necessary to document the outcomes of the technique and compare them with the traditional open procedures.

For a complete list of references, go to ExpertConsult.com.

SELECTED READINGS

Citation:
Elliott MC, Zarins B, Powell JW, et al. Hamstring muscle strains in professional football players: a 10-year review. *Am J Sports Med.* 2011;39:843–850.

Level of Evidence:
IV

Summary:
The authors of this article provide a summary of the types of strains and ruptures seen in the professional athlete.

Citation:
Miller SL, Gill J, Webb GR. The proximal origin of the hamstrings and surrounding anatomy encountered during repair. A cadaveric study. *J Bone Joint Surg Am.* 2007;89(A):44–48.

Level of Evidence:
Anatomic study

Summary:
The authors of this article provide a review of the pertinent surgical anatomy that delineates the appropriate anatomic areas that must be understood in approaching the area.

Citation:
Sarimo J, Lempainen L, Mattila K, et al. Complete proximal hamstring avulsions: A series of 41 patients with operative treatment. *Am J Sports Med.* 2008;36:1110–1115.

Level of Evidence:
IV

Summary:
This articles includes the largest series published, with a good summary of the mechanisms, treatment, and outcomes of the open procedure.

Citation:
Folsom GJ, Larson CM. Surgical treatment of acute versus chronic complete proximal hamstring ruptures: results of a new allograft technique for chronic reconstructions. *Am J Sports Med.* 2008;36:104–109.

Level of Evidence:
II

Summary:
In this article the surgical technique and indications for reconstruction of the hamstring in chronic rupture cases are described.

Citation:
Van der Made AD, Reurink G, Gouttebarge V, et al. Outcome after surgical repair of proximal hamstring avulsions: a systematic review. *Am J Sports Med.* 2015;43(11):2841–2851.

Level of Evidence:
Systematic review

Summary:
Surgical repairs resulted in slightly higher subjective outcomes vs. nonoperative treatments, but there were still deficits compared with baseline and the conclusion was that there was no significant improvement. Delaying repair, both as a primary repair or with an allograft, also showed good outcomes.

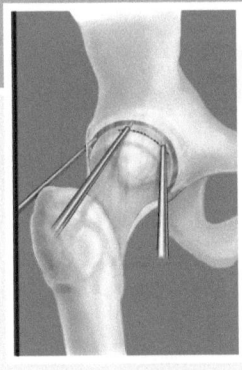

87

Hip and Thigh Contusions and Strains

Blake R. Obrock, Christopher P. Bankhead, Dustin Richter

CONTUSIONS

Contusions are the most common injuries to the hip, thigh, and pelvis. Collisions with other athletes and falls to the ground are the most common causes of contusions. Contusions can be superficial and limited to the subcutaneous tissue, or they can be deep, involving the bone, muscle, and ligaments. When they are associated with muscle involvement, contusions can result in slow bleeding with significant hematoma formation. Depending on the depth of the contusion and the extent of the injury, symptoms may occur immediately or after a 24- to 48-hour delay. Occasionally the force of the impact can cause a shearing of the connection between the muscle and subcutaneous tissue. Often, particularly with superficial contusions, treatment is of short duration and is based on the patient's symptoms. Patients generally have a rapid return to play (RTP). With the diagnosis of a deep contusion, however, the treatment period may be extended. Aside from icing, treatment should be delayed for 48 hours to ensure that all bleeding has stopped. After 48 hours, treatment with antiinflammatory drugs, heat, massage, and physical therapy is implemented. Rehabilitation should be aimed at maintaining flexibility and muscle mass. Range of motion (ROM) should be monitored because patients are prone to the development of myositis ossificans after sustaining deep contusions involving the muscle.

Iliac Crest Contusion

Iliac crest contusion, commonly known as a hip pointer, is an anterior pelvic contusion that often affects athletes involved in contact sports. These contusions result from either a direct fall onto the iliac crest or from a direct blow, as seen in football, hockey, and soccer (Fig. 87.1)[1,2]

History

The athlete will almost immediately note pain over the iliac crest and/or greater trochanter after a fall or collision. He or she will note an inability to ambulate without a limp and pain with side-to-side or attempted crossover movements.[3]

Physical Examination

Examination of the injured athlete will reveal an antalgic gait, pain with palpation of the pelvic brim, bruising, and swelling. Active ROM of the hip will be decreased. Strength testing will demonstrate a marked decrease in any or all of the following muscle groups, depending on the location of the contusion: the hip flexors, sartorius and rectus femoris, internal and external obliques, tensor fascia lata, gluteus medius, latissimus dorsi, and paraspinal muscles.[3,4]

Imaging

Diagnosis of a hip pointer is made primarily on the basis of the history and physical examination. Radiographs are used only to rule out further injury, such as a fracture (Fig. 87.2). Rarely, magnetic resonance imaging (MRI) or ultrasound are needed; however, some investigators have advocated their role in the evaluation of hematoma formation in an effort to quantify RTP.[3]

Treatment Options

Nonoperative treatment with protection, rest, ice, compression, and elevation (PRICE) is central to the treatment of hip pointers. Crutches may be used for the first few days. Ice, rest, and compression should be instituted for the first 48 hours to decrease the risk of hematoma formation. Antiinflammatory agents may also be used during the first 5 to 7 days. Beginning on day 3, the athlete may begin painless ROM activities. Some investigators have advocated delivery of a cortisone injection to the affected area to decrease pain and swelling; however, the risks of such injections must be weighed. Physical therapy may be initiated once a painless ROM has been established. Therapy should include stretches, sport-specific massage, and strengthening. Surgery is rarely indicated for hip pointer injuries; however, concomitant injuries such as sports hernias must be ruled out.[5]

📌 Authors' Preferred Technique
Iliac Crest Contusion

Our preferred technique is to initiate PRICE and use of crutches for the initial 24 h. A repeat physical examination in the office should be undertaken within 3–4 days of the injury. Provided that an avulsion fracture is not suspected, ROM exercises and gentle stretches are begun. A localized cortisone injection is considered for athletes who are not progressing as rapidly as anticipated. In those instances, activities are stopped for 48–72 h, after which rehabilitation is resumed in earnest. RTP is expected in 2–4 weeks once the athlete has completed strength testing and sport-specific drills.

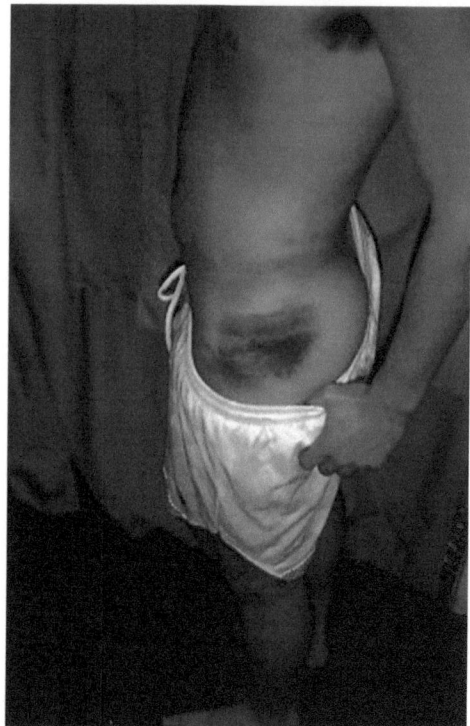

Fig. 87.1 Clinical photograph of a hip pointer in a soccer athlete.

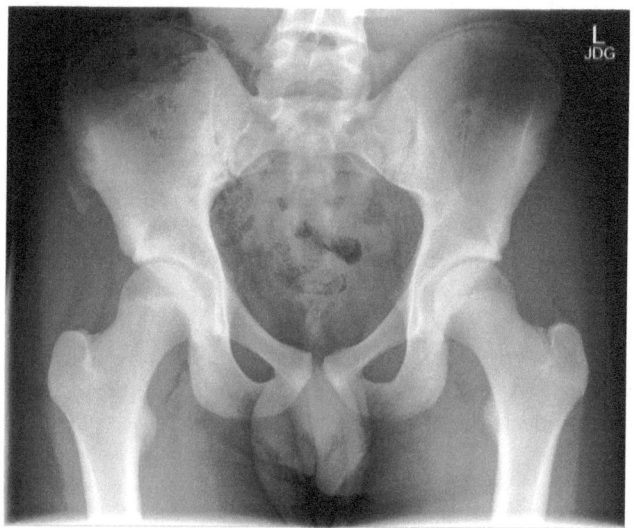

Fig. 87.2 Pelvic radiograph demonstrating an avulsion fracture of the anterosuperior iliac spine.

Return to Play

RTP is anticipated 2 to 4 weeks after the time of injury. Sport-specific drills and strength testing of the affected limb must be completed prior to resumption of competitive activities. Upon returning to activities, appropriate padding should be worn to prevent reinjury.[3,6]

Results

The treatment of hip pointers has yielded excellent results. Almost all athletes are able to return to their previous level of competition and performance once the injury has sufficiently healed.[3,4,7]

TABLE 87.1	Classification of Quadriceps Contusions
Grade	Range of Motion
Mild	>90 degrees
Moderate	45–90 degrees
Severe	<45 degrees

Complications

Complications after hip pointers are rare. Those most commonly seen include hematoma formation, cutaneous nerve injury, or myositis ossificans. Missed fractures or avulsions injuries are rare complications.[3,5,7] Occasionally, as a result of severe impact, there can be an internal degloving injury, known as a Morel-Lavallée lesion, whereby the subcutaneous tissue is stripped of its connection to the underlying fascia. The resulting hematoma can be painful and may expand to fill a large cavity. Untreated, this cavity can form a cystic lesion, allowing the fluid collection to recur, and the hematoma can even serve as a nidus for bacterial colonization and infection. In the acute setting, conservative management—with cold therapy, compression, early ROM, and observation—is appropriate. If symptoms worsen or persist, advanced imaging studies can be helpful in directing treatment options, which include aspiration and either percutaneous or open drainage. A high index of suspicion is necessary to diagnose this condition, which is rare but has been reported in National Football League (NFL) players after a direct blow or slide on the ground.[8-10]

Quadriceps Contusion

The quadriceps consists of the rectus femoris and the vastus musculature (medialis, lateralis, and intermedius). Quadriceps contusions are the result of a direct blow or trauma to the thigh. They typically occur in the anterior or lateral compartment and are most commonly associated with football, soccer, rugby, or high-speed traumas. The pathophysiology associated with quadriceps contusions involves microtrauma to the muscle fibers, with resultant swelling and edema. More significant contusions can also result in hemorrhage formation, myositis ossificans, and even tears.

Jackson and Feagin[11] established a classification system based on knee flexion. They describe the muscle contusion as mild, moderate, or severe. Forty-eight hours after injury, mild contusions are able to flex greater than 90 degrees; moderate contusions, from 45 to 90 degrees; and severe contusions, less than 45 degrees (Table 87.1). This classification helps guide counseling and treatment, and resolution occurs on days 6.5, 56, and 72, respectively. No corresponding MRI classification system has been developed. Persons with injuries classified as moderate to severe were significantly more likely to experience myositis ossificans than were those with mild contusions.[11,12]

History

Typically the patient will present on the field with a chief complaint of pain, lack of movement, or explosiveness and an antalgic gait. Twenty-four to 48 hours later, the patient may note similar or amplified symptoms, with noticeable limitations of knee ROM, thigh pain, loss of function, and swelling.[12] As previously stated, the mechanism of injury is usually collision with a helmet or a severe kick to the thigh.

Physical Examination

Physical examination begins by evaluating the gait of the patient as he or she walks. Typically an antalgic gait is noted in persons with a moderate to severe contusion. A localized physical examination will note a tender, swollen, and often ecchymotic thigh in the area corresponding to the blunt trauma that was sustained. The thigh should be compared with the contralateral side as well. Palpation of the affected thigh may yield a palpable defect in persons with severe contusions, indicating a partial or complete tear. In addition, a firm thigh compared with the contralateral side has been associated with longer recovery times.[13] However, the most important component of the physical examination is the ROM of the knee, because this component correlates with the severity of the injury and the anticipated return to activity.[12,13] Rarely, symptoms of an anterior thigh compartment syndrome can be identified on the basis of the physical examination.[13]

Imaging

Plain radiographs may be taken in the initial setting to rule out fracture; however, they typically have a low yield when a thorough history and physical examination is conducted. Radiographs, to evaluate for developing myositis ossificans, may have a more substantial role 2 to 4 weeks after injury if a firm mass is palpated.[14,15]

MRI and ultrasound may also be used to evaluate the extent of the muscular edema and hemorrhage (Fig. 87.3); however,

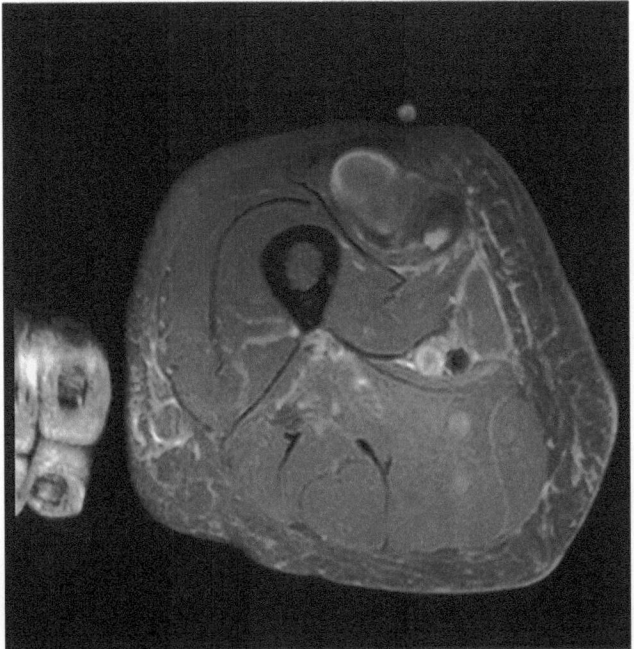

Fig. 87.3 Cross-sectional T2 magnetic resonance image of the thigh, demonstrating a developing hematoma in the body of the rectus femoris.

no level I studies have shown that imaging evaluations will accurately correlate with the severity of the contusion or predict RTP better than the Jackson and Feagin knee flexion classification.[11,13,16,17]

Treatment Options

Nonoperative treatment. The treatment of quadriceps contusions is usually managed in a nonoperative or conservative fashion. Depending on the severity of the injury, some athletes may be able to continue their activity and present for evaluation after competition or training. Based on military studies, knee immobilization with the knee flexed to 120 degrees for the initial 24 hours is recommended.[18] Severe contusions may benefit from flexion immobilization for up to 48 hours.[12,18] This can be achieved with either a hinged knee brace with locking capabilities, a compressive elastic wrap, or an anteriorly placed splint. Ice and compression should also be initiated in the first 24 to 48 hours, followed by elevation (the PRICE protocol). After the initial period of flexion, active, pain-free ROM exercises should be initiated. For severe contusions, crutches may be used until quadriceps control has returned. In these cases, physical therapy may be warranted, as well as the use of electrical stimulation. Ryan et al.[12] demonstrated a shortened recovery time for the moderate and severe groups from 56 to 19 days and from 72 to 21 days, respectively, via utilization of the aforementioned protocol. After return to pain-free motion, patients are allowed to return to noncontact sport-specific training. Return to contact sports is allowed after the thigh firmness has resolved and the muscle is not tender to palpation. If the patient is involved in a contact sport, a thigh pad with a ring should be recommended to minimize recurrence.[12,18]

Nonsteroidal antiinflammatory drugs (NSAIDs) are used initially to decrease pain and swelling, but their long-term use is discouraged. However, for persons with severe contusions or contusions with firm masses that do not dissipate in the initial 7 to 10 days, NSAIDs may be used to prevent heterotopic bone formation or myositis ossificans. Although randomized controlled studies have not been performed to examine the effectiveness of NSAIDs in the treatment of myositis ossificans, their presumed effectiveness is based on animal studies and reports of their use in patients who have had a total hip replacement.[18-20]

Operative treatment. Operative treatment of quadriceps contusions is primarily reserved for persons with compartment syndromes.[21-23] Aspiration or surgical decompression of a thigh hematoma has been reported; however, no literature is available to support the effectiveness of these treatments.[21] Aspiration of knee effusions associated with severe contusions may decrease painful ROM, but support of this treatment is anecdotal. Other surgical considerations are reserved for partial or complete quadriceps tears or avulsion off the patella. Operative treatment of myositis ossificans should be reserved for patients with symptomatic loss of motion, pain, and strength once bone maturation has been demonstrated on a three-phase bone scan. Such treatment usually is performed 12 to 24 months after the time of injury.[24-26]

Postoperatively, compressive dressings, ice, rest, elevation, and standard surgical site care should be instituted. Again, early ROM is critical to increase healing and decrease the risk of heterotopic bone formation.

Decision-Making Principles

The ROM classification system proposed by Jackson and Feagin[11] currently serves as the gold standard for the treatment and prognosis of thigh contusions. As a rule, nonoperative treatment should be pursued when possible provided compartment syndrome has not been identified. The aforementioned military studies have demonstrated the quickest return to activity, with immediate flexion of the affected knee to 120 degrees during the initial 24 to 48 hours from the time of injury. Subsequent passive and active ROM should follow to prevent heterotopic bone formation and increase rates of RTP.[12,14] Heterotopic bone formation should be managed with the previously outlined contusion rehabilitation protocol and may be monitored with triple-phase bone scans to evaluate for skeletal maturity. Surgical intervention should be considered for myositis ossificans only if loss of strength and ROM has not resolved during the ensuing months. Bony maturation must be identified prior to excision to prevent local recurrence.[26-28]

Authors' Preferred Technique
Quadriceps Contusion

Timely evaluation of the patient should be undertaken to assess the severity of the contusion and rule out more severe sequelae, such as compartment syndrome. Ice, knee flexion, and a gentle compressive wrap are instituted if assessment takes place on the field. For patients with moderate to severe contusions, we prefer to institute immediate knee flexion to 120 degrees with a locked, hinged knee brace. Use of ice and a compressive wrap or sleeve is also instituted with rest. The patient is reevaluated within 24–48 h by the treating physician or a therapist, and active ROM of the knee is begun, with a greater than 120-degree return to ROM desired as soon as possible. Electrical stimulation is added as warranted. If no contraindication exists, NSAIDs are begun at prescription-strength dosage for 5–7 days around the clock. However, they are discontinued if the patient cannot tolerate them. Noncontact training is permitted once quadriceps control and painless full ROM has returned, which is typically seen in 10–14 days. Full contact is permitted at the 3- to 4-week mark provided no further setbacks occur and if a thigh pad is worn. For patients who demonstrate worsening symptoms at the 14- to 21-day mark, radiographs are repeated and return to sporting activities is tabled.

Return to Play

A mild contusion may be managed symptomatically with ROM exercises and NSAIDs, thus allowing the athlete to continue in competition or training. For moderate or severe injuries, noncontact training is permitted once quadriceps control and painless full ROM has returned, which is typically seen in 10 to 14 days. Full contact is permitted at the 3- to 4-week mark provided that no further setbacks occur and a thigh pad is worn. The patient should be seen and cleared by a physician, and dedicated strength testing may be warranted to ensure the patient's safety.[11-13]

Results

With some exceptions, the literature on management and outcomes after thigh contusions is mostly based on case studies or anecdotal evidence. Nonetheless, most reports note good to excellent results, with almost all athletes retuning to play. Ryan et al.[12] demonstrated a shortened recovery time for the moderate and severe groups from 56 to 19 days and from 72 to 21 days, respectively, with utilization of immediate flexion of the knee to 120 degrees, followed by early ROM exercises. These findings were duplicated by Aronen et al.[18]

Myositis Ossificans

Myositis ossificans is heterotopic ossification in an area of muscle, soft tissue, or disrupted periosteum (Fig. 87.4). It is generally associated with a severe contusion and has a reported occurrence rate of 9% to 14%.[29-31] In their military studies, Ryan et al.[12] identified the greatest risk factors for myositis ossificans: knee flexion less than 120 degrees, sustaining the injury while playing football, having had a previous quadriceps injury, experiencing a delay in treatment greater than 3 days, and having an ipsilateral knee effusion.

Although this disease process can occur without a history of trauma, athletes can usually describe a sentinel event that caused a hematoma formation. The hematoma organizes, and calcium deposits are formed by the body. In a process that is not entirely understood, osteoblasts invade the formed hematoma and begin to make bony spicules.[36] This process tends to occur near joints and at tendon origins, but it can occur anywhere along the course of a muscle. The process can start as soon as 1 week after injury and can be detected on plain films a minimum of 3 weeks after injury. Patients present with a rapid enlargement within the soft tissues, decreased ROM, and significant pain 1 to 2 weeks after injury. The patient has swelling and warmth at the site as well as an increased erythrocyte sedimentation rate and serum alkaline phosphatase level.[26] Any treatment modalities implemented should not promote hematoma formation. Massage and manipulation should be avoided. Therapy should consist of active stretching and strengthening. Passive ROM should be delayed for at least

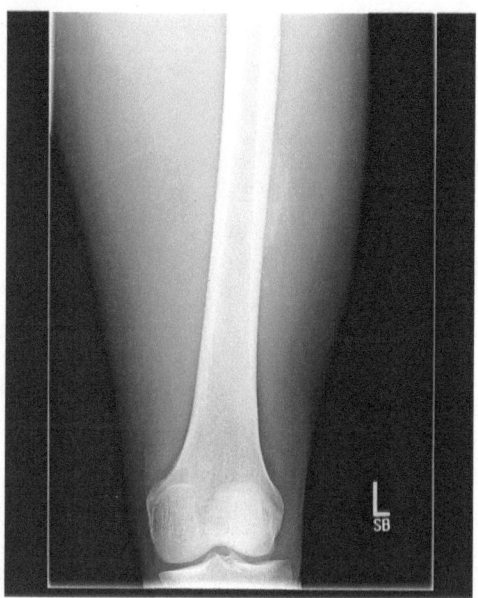

Fig. 87.4 Anteroposterior view of the femur demonstrating myositis ossificans.

3 to 6 months.[37] For patients with refractory loss of ROM, surgery should be considered. Surgery, if warranted, should be delayed for at least 9 to 12 months to allow the lesion to mature. A bone scan can help ascertain the maturity of the lesion. Patients and clinicians should be aware that the lesion may recur despite surgical removal.

Complications

Thigh compartment syndrome is a rare complication associated with quadriceps contusion, and treatment of this condition remains controversial. Most authors advocate emergent fasciotomies, but some reports in the literature advocate nonsurgical intervention, even when compartment pressure standards are met for a diagnosis of compartment syndrome.[21-23,32] The rationale for this proposal is derived from Robinson et al.[32] and others, who note that in cases of sports-related thigh compartment syndromes with pressures greater than 55 mm Hg, no adverse sequelae were identified at 1 year with a return to preinjury strength and ROM. Standard compartment syndrome measurement should be taken, and identification is made on the basis of one of the following criteria as identified in various studies: compartment pressures of 30 mm Hg, 45 mm Hg, or less than 30 mm Hg difference between compartment pressure and diastolic blood pressure.[33-35]

Future Considerations

Future consideration should be given to the pursuit of level I and II studies on the management of quadriceps contusions. Additionally, exploration of the nonoperative management of thigh compartment syndrome is also warranted.

Groin Contusions

Groin contusions involve the adductor musculature and usually occur from a direct blow to the inner thigh. They are often seen in soccer players and cyclists (Fig. 87.5). Aside from the standard contusion treatment of ice, NSAIDs, physical therapy, and gradual RTP, the treating clinician should be aware of the possibility that vascular complications may develop, such as phlebitis and thrombosis. Ultrasound is a useful noninvasive method of diagnosing vascular complications.

STRAINS

Muscle strains are among the most common athletic injuries, representing 30% to 50% of all injuries.[26,38,39] Most strains occur at the myotendinous junction in the fast-twitch type 2 muscle fibers of biarticular muscles undergoing eccentric contraction. Although most strains occur at this interface, muscle strains can occur anywhere along the length of the muscle.[40,41] Over a 10-year collection period in the NFL, Feeley and colleagues[42] noted that 41% of strains involved the hamstrings, 28% involved the quadriceps, and 17% involved the groin.

Classification

The clinical classification system describes the severity of the muscle injury: mild, moderate, or severe (Table 87.2). Mild (grade I) strains involve tearing of a few muscle fibers with mild pain and minimal loss of strength. Moderate (grade II) strains involve increased tearing of muscle fibers with some loss of strength. Severe (grade III) strains include tearing of the entire muscle with complete loss of strength.[43,44] Occasionally in adolescents and a small subset of adults, the tendons of origin or insertion may be avulsed these are classified as grade IIIB.

Quadriceps Strains

The only biarticular muscle in the quadriceps is the rectus femoris, but all muscles receive innervation from the femoral nerve. The direct head of the rectus femoris gives rise to a central tendon in the proximal thigh, allowing strains to occur proximal to the musculotendinous junction. The primary function of these muscles is knee extension.[18]

Quadriceps strains typically affect the rectus femoris. These strains can occur proximally or distally. The quadriceps is commonly affected for several reasons: it crosses two joints, has a high percentage of type II fibers, and has a complex musculotendinous architecture. Sudden forceful eccentric muscle contraction of the quadriceps is required during hip extension and

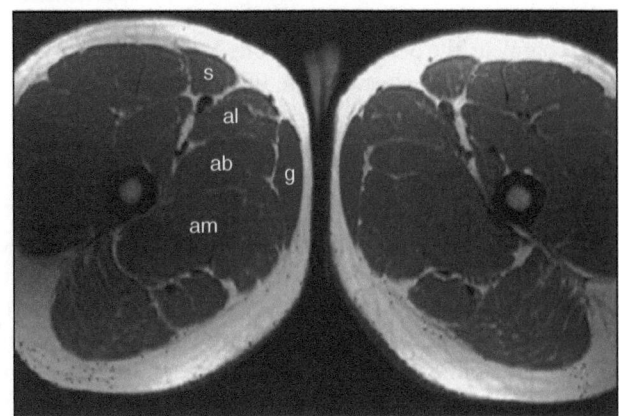

Fig. 87.5 Cross-sectional anatomy of the thigh on a T1-weighted axial magnetic resonance image. The musculature of the medial thigh includes the adductor longus *(al)*; adductor brevis *(ab)*; adductor magnus *(am)*; gracilis *(g)*; and sartorius *(s)*.

TABLE 87.2	Clinical Grading System for Strains			
Grade	Muscle Tearing	Strength Loss	Pain	Physical Examination: Muscle Defect
I	Mild	Minimal/none	Mild	Absent
II	Moderate	Moderate/severe	Moderate/severe	Possible palpable defect
IIIA	Severe	Severe	Severe	Frequent palpable defect (complete rupture of musculotendinous unit)
IIIB	Severe	Severe	Severe	Frequent palpable defect (avulsion fracture at the tendon's origin or insertion)

knee flexion and can lead to increased forces across the muscle-tendon interface, resulting in strain.[38,45-47]

History

Athletes with a quadriceps strain typically play sports that require cutting, jumping, or kicking, such as soccer, rugby, football, and basketball. A thorough history will tend to reveal the onset of anterior thigh pain either during the maximal extension phase of the thigh, after a sudden change in direction or during deceleration after a forceful kick.[48] Often patients will have an antalgic gait, loss of knee flexion, or an anterior thigh mass.[45,49-52] Most commonly quadriceps strains occur distally at the musculotendinous junction; however, they can also occur proximally or centrally.[51] Pain may be reported immediately after the injury has occurred, but often the athlete may be able to continue playing through a practice or game with the onset of symptoms occurring after a cooling-down period.[43,46,53]

Physical Examination

Initially physical examination is best carried out with the patient lying supine; it concludes with a prone examination. With the patient supine, a thorough palpation of the muscle should be undertaken to assess for tenderness, swelling, masses, or defects. Ecchymosis may occur 24 hours or more after the onset of injury, after which ROM of the knee and hip should be performed and the injured knee compared with the contralateral side. Next, evaluation of knee extension should be undertaken with the hip flexed to 90 degrees and then with the hip in extension. Weakness identified in hip flexion indicates injury to the rectus, whereas weakness in hip extension points toward a vastus injury. It should be noted that rectus injuries have a slower recovery time than do those that occur in the vastus.[24,54] Once the supine examination is complete, the patient is positioned prone and strength is retested, which can help to isolate the quadriceps for motion and strength evaluation. For moderate to severe strains, pain is usually felt with resisted knee extension.

Imaging

Imaging in quadriceps strains is typically used more as an adjunct than for diagnosis. Radiographs, ultrasound, and MRI may all be used and can provide information regarding the length of recovery. Radiographs are routinely normal; however, in the young athlete they can be particularly important in identifying avulsion fractures or stress fractures. Ultrasound and MRI are most beneficial in predicting recovery time. Finlay and Friedman[70] reported that ultrasound is a highly sensitive and specific method for evaluating acute quadriceps injuries. The use of dynamic ultrasound with the knee in flexion and extension can allow differentiation between hematoma and muscle tears; however, ultrasound is highly operator-dependent. MRI is still considered to be the gold standard for quadriceps evaluation (Fig. 87.6),[55-57] although its use in the initial evaluation phase is usually restricted to high-level or professional athletes to better predict a RTP. For recreational athletes, MRI is indicated if the symptoms do not improve after 2 to 3 weeks of rehabilitation or for evaluation of chronic (>8 weeks) strains.[40] Cross et al.[53] reported that MRI can estimate the size of the quadriceps strain

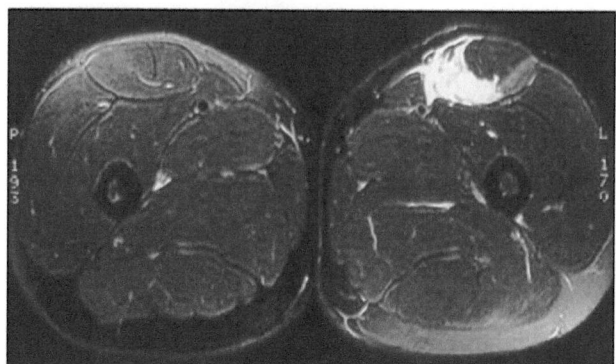

Fig. 87.6 A T2-weighted axial magnetic resonance image of the thighs showing increased fluid in the rectus femoris, indicative of a quadriceps strain.

Phase	Activity
I	RICE, NSAIDs
II	Isometric exercises
III	Isotonic exercises
IV	Isokinetic exercises
V	Running, plyometrics, jumping exercises
VI	Sport-specific training

TABLE 87.3   Treatment Protocol for a Quadriceps Strain

NSAIDs, Nonsteroidal antiinflammatory drugs; *RICE*, rest, ice, compression, and elevation.

and predict the duration of rehabilitation. Furthermore, involvement of the central tendon signifies a significantly longer rehabilitation interval.[53]

Treatment Options

Most quadriceps strains can be managed nonoperatively (Table 87.3). In the acute phase, the treatment of quadriceps strains begins with the standard PRICE protocol in an effort to decrease swelling and hematoma formation. Severe strains may require a short period of crutch use. Passive, pain-free stretching should also be initiated in the first 24 to 48 hours.[24,54] At the 3- to 5-day mark, the active rehabilitation phase may begin. First, isometric exercises and increasing movement within a pain-free arc of motion are begun. Eccentric contraction of the quadriceps should be avoided. As strength and ROM continue to improve, the patient is transitioned to isotonic training with increasing resistance as tolerated.[24] Once strength has improved, isokinetic exercises should focus on low resistance and high speeds. A progressive running and kicking program should then be initiated, starting with a slow jog and advancing to sprinting. When sprinting is tolerated, kicking may be started with a light ball over short distances, advancing to a normal-weight ball over longer distances.[53] Finally, sport-specific training should begin. The patient may RTP after completion of this training but should continue to work on a quadriceps rehabilitation program involving stretching, isokinetic strengthening, and conditioning.

Surgical intervention is reserved for total or near-total muscle tears, persistent pain with nonoperative treatment, reattachment

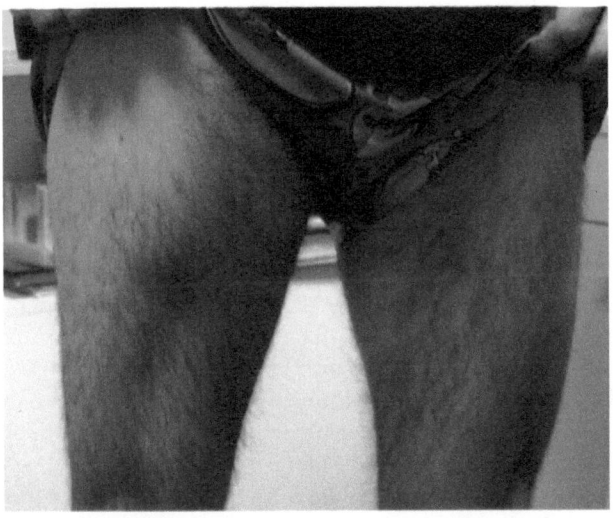

Fig. 87.7 Quadriceps rupture with retraction.

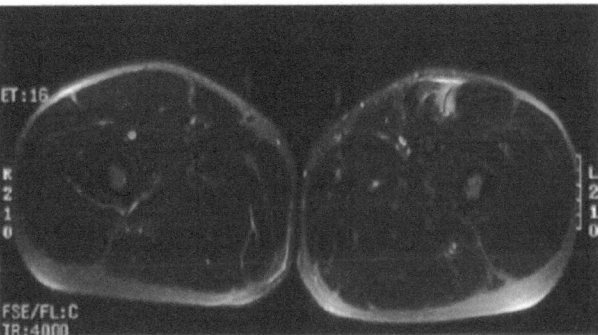

Fig. 87.8 An acute bull's-eye lesion.

of avulsion fractures, and large hematoma evacuation. Time until RTP after rectus reattachment surgery was noted to be 9 months in one report (Fig. 87.7).[24,48,58]

Decision-Making Principles

Nonoperative treatment should be pursued whenever possible for quadriceps strains. There are very few indications for surgical intervention. Moreover, controversy exists regarding the value of surgical decompression of large hematomas as well as the need for operative intervention for rectus avulsion injuries. Complete muscle tears, true fractures associated with quadriceps strains, or symptomatic mature myositis ossificans appear to be the only criteria for surgical intervention. However, based on some published reports, recalcitrant nonoperative treatment of severe quadriceps strains may also warrant surgical intervention.[48]

🔖 Authors' Preferred Technique
Quadriceps Strains

We prefer to use nonsurgical management. In the initial 24–72 h, PRICE, NSAIDs, and gentle ROM are begun. If sufficient progress is noted, the rehabilitation protocol is then begun at day 3–5, with a focus on pain-free motion. If at any point a setback is experienced, the protocol is backed down. Antiinflammatory modalities are also instituted by the trainer or physical therapist, along with ultrasound and electrical stimulation for moderate to severe strains. Operative intervention is considered only for avulsion fractures that are symptomatic for 12 months or more. Gentle passive ROM is begun 7–10 days after the surgery, with an emphasis on avoiding eccentric muscle contractions. Once patients can tolerate this gentle passive ROM, they may begin the aforementioned rehabilitation protocol.

Return to Play

A review of the literature by Orchard et al.[54] notes a lack of consensus for safe RTP after muscle strains. Despite this finding, certain criteria that appear in the literature seem to lower the risk of reinjury after a quadriceps strain. ROM of the knee should be equal to that of the contralateral leg. Isokinetic quadriceps

strength should fall within 15% of the contralateral side. Ideally, a sport-specific program should be completed, including observed straight-ahead sprinting and figure-eight cutting sprints. Most patients are able to RTP within 2 to 3 weeks while wearing a compressive thigh wrap and continuing a dedicated stretching and strengthening program.

Results

Good to excellent results have been reported with use of the phased treatment protocol for quadriceps strain. Recent articles suggest that higher-level athletes should resume play earlier with the understanding that the risk of reinjury is then higher. Stratification of the risk of reinjury can be aided by imaging, such as ultrasound or MRI, to quantify the severity of the initial injury.[54] Based on imaging, injuries involving greater than 15% of the rectus cross-sectional area have demonstrated a longer recovery phase (14.6 days vs. 8.9 days). Strains greater than 13 cm in length also resulted in a doubling of recovery time. Contrast enhancement around the central tendon, the so-called acute bulls-eye lesion, also revealed a significantly worse prognosis (26.8 days vs. 9.2 days) (Fig. 87.8).[41,45] Although many investigators have recommended surgical treatment for proximal avulsion fractures, Hsu and coworkers[58] treated two NFL kickers with a nonoperative regimen and noted that both were able to return to full practice after 3 to 12 weeks.

Limited data exist for surgical outcomes of quadriceps strains, with the majority of the information being case reports. Straw et al.[48] reported a full return of strength and return to competition after repairing a chronic proximal rectus avulsion in a semiprofessional soccer player. Similar reports exist in the literature, noting a return to previous activity level with nearly symmetric strength in athletes treated surgically for chronic rectus weakness.[58]

Complications

Complications associated with quadriceps strains include myositis ossificans, reinjury, residual weakness, and compartment syndrome. Risk stratification for reinjury is used only as a guide, further emphasizing the need for dedicated RTP criteria and a thorough warmup and stretching program. Residual weakness that persists for more than 12 months should warrant evaluation of surgical intervention. Myositis ossificans has previously been discussed in the contusion section, and urgent intervention in the initial 24 to 72 hours for severe strains is warranted.

Future Considerations

The future of quadriceps strains lies in identifying more rapid improved RTP criteria while limiting reinjury risk. Some have advocated removing the athlete from competition completely until all symptoms have resolved. However, others are advocating a RTP even before the full RTP criteria have been met. Anecdotally it is the physician's charge to protect the athlete and limit short- and long-term risk.

Adductor Strains

Adductor strains, which are the most common groin injuries in athletes, occur as a result of a forced push-off or side-to-side motion.[59,60] These injuries are seen more often in athletes who play soccer, hockey, rugby, martial arts, and football. Their reported incidence ranges from 13% to 43%.[61-64] Adductor strains are commonly the result of a forceful abduction of the thigh during an intentional adduction movement. The musculotendinous junction of the adductor longus is most commonly involved.[60,65] Inflexibility, previous injury, and strength imbalance between adductors and abductors have been implicated as risk factors for adductor strains.

Adductor strains can be graded from I to III. Mild (grade I) strains result in pain with minimal strength loss, moderate (grade II) strains result in strength loss and pain, and severe (grade III) strains result in complete functional and motor loss.

History

The athlete will typically present with a chief complaint of acute groin pain, tenderness, and swelling. The mechanism may be a sudden change in direction, or the athlete may note that he or she was attempting a forceful kick that was met with opposite resistance, such as an opposing player blocking the kick. Pain will be noted to be worse with side-to-side movement. Often the patient has a history of an adductor injury. A review of the literature suggests the need for a thorough history and examination because groin pain in 27% to 90% of athletes has more than one cause.[66,67] A differential of groin pain includes osteitis pubis, athletic pubalgia, hernias, femoroacetabular impingement, and stress fractures.

Physical Examination

Patients with moderate to severe injuries may display an antalgic gait; in rare instances they may not be able to bear weight on the affected limb. A complete examination with palpation of the medial groin should be performed to look for tenderness, swelling, ecchymosis, and defects. ROM and strength should also be assessed. Medial groin pain is accentuated with resisted hip adduction. In addition, the pubic rami and inferior abdominal wall should be inspected to rule out other causes of pain.

Adductor strains must be differentiated from other sources of groin pain. Tenderness to palpation at the pubis may result from osteitis pubis, athletic pubalgia, or avulsion injury of muscular origin.[68] Osteitis pubis results in tenderness over the pubic tubercle or inguinal ring and often can be differentiated because symptoms exacerbate with situps.[66,69] Persons with athletic pubalgia may have tenderness over the pubic tubercle, and this tenderness can

be reproduced with resisted situps or the Valsalva maneuver. An inguinal hernia examination should also be performed. Pain with provocative hip testing—as with the flexion, adduction, internal rotation (FADIR) maneuver—may indicate femoroacetabular impingement or hip labral tearing.

Imaging

Plain radiography with the patient standing on one leg is the initial imaging modality of choice. These radiographs are acquired less for diagnosis of adductor strains and more to rule out other pathology, such as avulsion fractures or osteitis pubis. A bone scan, MRI, and ultrasound have also been used to varying degrees (Fig. 87.9). An MRI is not routinely ordered and is used only as a guide in estimating the length of recovery. Much as with other strains of the thigh, involvement of greater than 50% of the cross-sectional area, tissue fluid collection, and deep muscle tears are predictive of a slower return to sport.[38] Ultrasound has been used to evaluate the musculotendinous junction and to aid in the differentiation of a strain from other conditions, including hernia.[70]

Treatment Options

Nonoperative. Adductor strains are managed similarly to quadriceps and hamstring strains. The majority of these injuries are treated nonsurgically. PRICE, NSAIDs, and a progressive rehabilitation program are initiated. Typically persons with grade I strains do not seek medical attention; however, if they do seek treatment, a 3- to 7-day course of progressive ROM and strengthening is recommended. Sport-specific drills should be performed and observed prior to clearance. For patients with more severe strains, early stretching sometimes has been noted to aggravate the injury. A gentle progression through isometric, isotonic, and

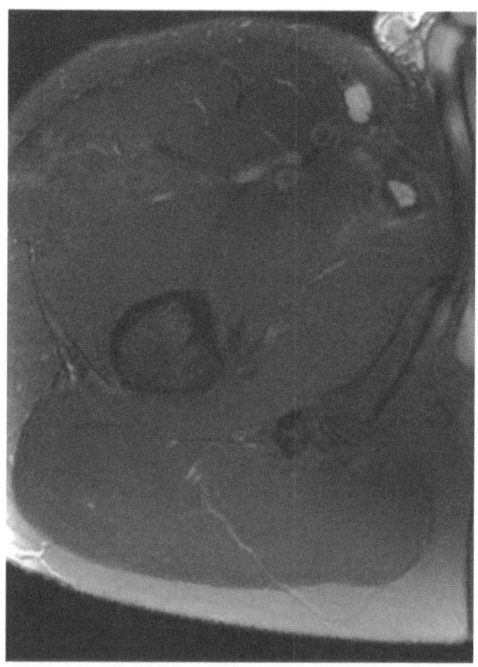

Fig. 87.9 Cross-sectional T2 magnetic resonance image of the pelvis showing a complete tear of the proximal adductor longus.

isokinetic exercises should be initiated, and the patient should be noted to be pain-free before advancing to sport-specific drills. Upper-body and core exercises may begin in phase II. Swimming and use of a stationary bike and elliptical machine may begin in phase III. Sports-specific drills may begin once the patient has ROM and adductor strength that is 75% of ipsilateral abductors. Emphasis should be placed on reinjury prevention via a focused stretching and strengthening program designed to create an adduction-to-abduction strength ratio of 0.8 or higher.[71] Corticosteroid injections and platelet-rich plasma (PRP) injections have yet to yield sufficient data to be considered first-line treatment options.

Operative. Surgical intervention is rarely required for adductor strains. Strains recalcitrant to conservative care with persistent pain and weakness may require tenotomy versus repair. The literature for surgical intervention is predominately based on case reports. Patients with complete avulsions who have had persistent symptoms for 6 months or longer may be treated with repair. For incomplete tears that are symptomatic, tenotomy may be best indicated.[60,72]

Decision-Making Principles

Nonoperative treatment is the overwhelming option of choice for adductor strains. Although a high reinjury rate applies, surgical intervention is very rarely warranted and has had mixed results. Proper education of the athlete and the trainer as to the rehabilitation course and future prevention is the key to a successful outcome. Surgical intervention is considered only for complete avulsions that hinder RTP for 6 months or more or for chronic partial tears that may require tenotomy after a similar length of time.

Authors' Preferred Technique
Adductor Strains

We prefer nonsurgical management, with an emphasis on normalizing abductor-adductor strength imbalance while rehabilitating the athlete. The athlete is initially treated with the standard PRICE protocol and a 5- to 7-day course of NSAIDs. Beginning on day 3, passive ROM and gentle isometric exercises are begun. Eccentric loading is avoided in phase I. Advancement to phase II is permitted once the athlete can adduct against gravity without pain. Phase II consists of isotonic exercises under supervision. Stationary biking and swimming are permitted, as is core and upper-body training. Stretching, which is typically avoided in phase I, is permitted to the level of discomfort without pain. Attention to abductor-adductor strengthening is begun. Progression to phase III occurs once the patient demonstrates pain-free strength against submaximal abduction-adduction resistance. In phase III, isokinetic training is incorporated, followed by sport-specific drills. A dedicated warmup and stretching program should be instituted to focus on reinjury awareness for the athlete. RTP is permitted once single-leg strength is demonstrated to be equal to the contralateral side in all planes and the adduction-to-abduction strength ratio is greater than 80%.

Return to Play

Return to competition is permitted once pain-free sport-specific movements can be performed with adductor strength within 20% of the contralateral side. Although most patients

RTP in 2 to 3 weeks, severe cases may take 8 to 12 weeks. Dedicated warm-up stretching should be emphasized, as should in-season strengthening. RTP prior to pain-free sport-specific training has been associated with chronic adductor strains.[71] Reinjury education and prevention is warranted as well. RTP after tenotomy for chronic adductor pain ranges from 8 to 12 weeks.

Results

Adductor strains treated with a dedicated rehabilitation program and injury prevention awareness have demonstrated excellent results. Tyler et al.[75] reported a greater than fourfold reduction in adductor strains in the National Hockey League after institution of a dedicated adductor strengthening and stretching program. Holmich et al.[76] noted that active therapy in persons with chronic adductor strains provided better results than those seen in patients treated with passive therapy programs. RTP rates after surgical tenotomy for chronic adductor strains have been demonstrated to range from 60% to 90%. Concomitant injuries, such as sports hernias and subsequent repair, have been shown to affect outcome.[73,74]

Complications

The most common complication of adductor strains is reinjury. Seward et al.[77] and Tyler and associates[75] report recurrence rates of 32% and 44%, respectively. The highest risk factor for adductor strain is an adductor-to-abductor strength of 80% or less.[71] Other complications include myositis ossificans, compartment syndrome, calcific tendinitis, and chronic groin pain.

Future Considerations

Currently there is significant interest in the treatment of muscle, tendon, and ligament injuries with PRP. This involves using a commercially available kit to centrifuge a blood sample in order to concentrate platelets and reduce red blood cells.[78] Platelets, the first cell type to arrive at the site of injury, possess high quantities of growth factors, which they release to stimulate tissue repair. PRP therefore is replete with growth factors and cell signaling molecules that may be key to the regulation of tissue healing.[79] Multiple small studies exist that attest to its safety, but they demonstrate inconsistent results. PRP has shown promise in treating hamstring injuries among NFL athletes within 24 to 48 hours of acute injury. Mejia and Bradley[80] have shown faster RTP in grade 1 and 2 injuries without recurrence, which resulted in a one-game difference in favor of PRP. On the other hand, deVos et al.,[81] in a randomized controlled trial, were unable to demonstrate improved pain or function in Achilles tendinopathy as compared with saline injection. These inconsistencies are confounded by variations in platelet and white blood cell (WBC) concentrations among the different kits, making it difficult to draw conclusions across studies.[78] Ultimately we are unable to recommend for or against the use of PRP in the treatment of hip and thigh muscle contusion or strain at this time but advocate for future level 1 studies, which may help to delineate its best use.

SPECIAL CONSIDERATIONS FOR THE PEDIATRIC AND ADOLESCENT ATHLETE

Avulsion injuries are uncommon in the pediatric and adolescent populations and are easily misdiagnosed as muscle strains or apophysitis without a high degree of clinical suspicion and vigilance. They occur during a forceful muscle contraction and result from failure through a secondary apophysis rather than a typical strain, which usually occurs at the myotendinous junction.[82,83] Most of these apophyseal ossification centers are closed by age 17 except for the Anterior superior iliac spine (ASIS), which can remain unfused until age 25.[84] The incidence reflects a gender bias, with males accounting for 66% to 86% of injuries. The most common sites affected are the anterior inferior iliac spine (AIIS) at 33%, ischial tuberosity at 31%, and ASIS at 25%.[85]

History

Athletes with avulsion fractures will typically be participating in a sport that requires sprinting, jumping, or kicking, such as football, basketball, or soccer.[82,83,86] Most are able to describe a distinct moment of injury accompanied by a pop or crack, followed by pain. This can be differentiated from apophysitis, which is a chronic overuse injury and presents with a more gradual onset.[87]

Physical Examination

The physical exam can be conducted in much the same way as with muscle strain. Observation of gait, palpation of the affected area, and neuromuscular exam are all key components of the clinical visit. Swelling and tenderness to palpation are typical of these injuries, as is muscle weakness and pain with passive stretch.

Imaging

Although it is understandable to want to limit radiation in this population, plain radiographs have been shown to diagnose avulsion fractures in 99% of cases and should be used, in preference to MRI or CT, if there is clinical suspicion.[88]

Treatment

The majority of these patients can be treated nonoperatively with a dedicated rehab protocol. Schuett et al.[88] showed that 86% of patients had complete resolution of pain at 3 months. A 5-stage protocol has been demonstrated to be consistently effective in the majority of these patients. This protocol begins with 1 week of non–weight bearing, ice, and NSAIDs, then 2 to 3 weeks of passive ROM and partial weight bearing. Full weight bearing and isokinetic strengthening are then initiated at 4 weeks after injury. Following this, some authors allow sport-specific activities, whereas others begin resistance training. A return to sport is allowed at 2 months after injury.[83,89] Operative treatment is typically reserved for failed nonoperative management. This includes persistent pain, symptomatic nonunion, or hip impingement after AIIS avulsion.

ACKNOWLEDGMENT

We would like to acknowledge the authors of the previous edition of this chapter: Drs. Sean McMillan, Brian Busconi, and Michael Montano. We would also like to thank Dr. Gary Mlady and Dr. Jennifer Weaver for assisting in the collection of new MRI and radiographic images for this book chapter and the video presentation.

For a complete list of references, go to ExpertConsult.com.

SELECTED READINGS

Citation:

Ryan JB, Hopkinson WJ, Wheeler JH, et al. Quadriceps contusions. West Point update. *Am J Sports Med*. 1991;19(3):299–304.

Level of Evidence:

II

Summary:

The authors of this article provide defining data for the appropriate management of quadriceps contusions, altering previous standards of care. Current treatment regimens are predicated on the findings presented in this article.

Citation:

Beiner JM, Jokl P. Muscle contusion injury and myositis ossificans traumatica. *Clin Orthop Relat Res*. 2002;403S:S110–S119.

Level of Evidence:

II

Summary:

The authors provide an analysis of the etiology, treatment, and outcomes of myositis ossificans.

Citation:

Orchard J, Best TM, Verrall GM. Return to play following muscle strains. *Clin J Sport Med*. 2005;15(6):436–441.

Level of Evidence:

III

Summary:

Consensus regarding return-to-play guidelines has been lacking in the literature. This article provides treatment parameters and offers a perspective on earlier return to competition.

Citation:

Beiner JM, Jokl P. Muscle contusion injury and myositis ossificans traumatica. *Clin Orthop Relat Res*. 2002;403S:S110–S119.

Level of Evidence:

III

Summary:

The authors provide a comprehensive review of hamstring injuries, treatments, and outcomes. Gaps within the literature on hamstring injury are also identified.

Citation:

Lovell G. The diagnosis of chronic groin pain in athletes: a review of 189 cases. *Aust J Sci Med Sport*. 1995;27(3):76–79.

Level of Evidence:

III

Summary:

The author provides a systematic review evaluating the effectiveness of exercise therapy for groin pain in athletes and also considers the treatment of this disorder.

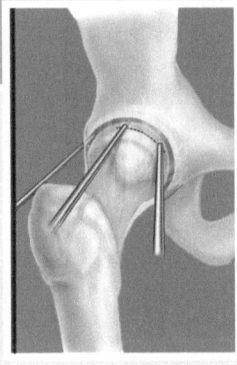

88

Hip Arthritis in the Athlete

Guillaume D. Dumont, Robert D. Russell

Hip arthritis is a common disease. One in four people may develop symptomatic hip osteoarthritis in their lifetime.[1] The treatment of arthritis in the active individual is challenging. The often intuitive recommendation of avoiding pain generating activities and sports seems unthinkable to the athlete. Our understanding of the hip joint has increased substantially in the past 2 decades, with the modern description of femoroacetabular impingement by Ganz and his colleagues and its suspected involvement in the development of osteoarthritis.[2,3] Corrective procedures for this disorder as well, and others such as acetabular dysplasia, have born the field of hip preservation. Though the efforts of hip preservationists have helped many athletes return to function, and hopefully stave off osteoarthritic changes, solutions for hip osteoarthritis short of arthroplasty remain distant. Hip arthroplasty has continued to evolve, and remains one of the most commonly performed orthopaedic surgeries performed.

HISTORY

Hip arthritis in the young and active patient can often be a challenging entity with regard to selecting appropriate treatment options. Making an accurate diagnosis is the first step in providing suitable treatment options for the patient.[4,5] Burnett et al. reported that a mean of 3.3 providers were seen prior to a definitive diagnosis being made.[6] This process can often lead to frustration. A structured history and physical exam can simplify the treating provider's approach to this sometimes complex problem.

Initial patient history should include a detailed description of the patient's current symptoms, including their time of onset, duration, and any inciting trauma or injury. Patients with arthritis often describe a gradual onset of pain, though some may remain asymptomatic until the later stages of disease and experience onset of pain after a particular injury or activity. Aggravating factors such as specific activities or positions should be noted, as should alleviating factors including any already attempted treatments. Patients typically report worsened pain with increased activity such as walking, standing, running, or playing a sport, and improved pain with rest. Sitting with the hip flexed, such as during an extended car or plane ride, or entering or exiting a low vehicle may also aggravate symptoms. The pain often worsens as the day progresses, and can persist as an aching pain at night. The physician's initial task should be to determine whether the patient's pain is indeed intra-articular in origin, as opposed to extra-articular. The location of pain is quite useful in beginning this differentiation. Intra-articular hip pain is often localized to the deep anterior groin. Patients often use the "C" sign when describing the location of their symptoms.[7] Though intra-articular pathologies can sometimes present as posterior hip pain, this is much less common. Posterior pain is worthy of considering musculotendinous strains, deep gluteal space syndrome, sacroiliac joint pathology, or lumbar spine pathology. Pain localized to the lateral hip is often the result of greater trochanteric pain syndrome (GTPS). The term GTPS was coined as a less specific but often more precise description for the etiology of lateral hip pain. It encompasses trochanteric bursitis, gluteus medius and minimus tendinopathy or tearing, and snapping iliotibial band or iliotibial band friction syndrome.[8] Anterior hip pain may also represent musculotendinous injuries, including to the hip flexor musculature, core muscle injuries (including injury to the rectus abdominis insertion and adductor longus origin), or pubic symphysis pathology such as osteitis pubis.[9] In the athlete, consideration should also be given to pelvic or proximal femoral stress fractures.[5,10-12]

Patients with hip arthritis often report associated stiffness. Substantial limitations in motion may be a sign of later stages of arthritis. Mechanical symptoms such as catching, clicking, or locking may be experienced, and may represent the presence of loose bodies or chondral injuries, or alternatively snapping of musculotendinous structures.

PHYSICAL EXAM

Examination begins with evaluation of the patient's gait. An antalgic gait is noted in patients with various hip pathologies, including intra-articular issues such as hip arthritis. The antalgic gait is hallmarked by a decrease in the duration of the stance phase of the ipsilateral hip. This effectively decreases the amount of time the patient is applying his weight through the affected hip. Another common gait abnormality is the Trendelenburg gait. This is seen in patients with abductor injuries, including those to the gluteus medius and gluteus minimus tendons. During the stance phase of the affected hip, the contralateral hemipelvis is noted to drop. A compensatory thoracolumbar lurch is noted toward the affected hip to maintain coronal balance.[13] In patients with hip arthritis, a decreased stride length may also be noted secondary to diminished range of motion (ROM) of the hip. Gait parameters have been shown to correlate highly with radiographic femoroacetabular impingement (FAI) morphology as well.[14] General observation of the patient may also offer some insight into the underlying cause of pain. The overweight or obese patient may understandably be predisposed to earlier arthritis in the hip due to increases in joint reactive forces, and this factor should be included in the overall assessment and treatment of the patient. The patient's sitting posture often reveals avoidance of deep hip flexion both in cases of nonarthritic intra-articular pain such as femoroacetabular impingement, or cases of hip arthritis.

Examination of the hip then begins with assessment of any skin lesions such as contusions or scars from previous surgical procedures. The log roll test is performed with the patient in the supine position. This simple maneuver consists of rolling the limb gently back and forth between internal and external rotation, avoiding drastic end range motions. This maneuver avoids stressing the musculotendinous structures that surround the hip, instead simply rotating the femoral head within the acetabulum. The test is not very sensitive, though it is specific for pain from intra-articular pathologies. Basic ROM measurements should then be performed. A standardized approach to this is important and leads to reproducible more measurements. Measurements can be performed in the supine position. Flexion, extension, internal rotation, and external rotation are noted. Internal and external rotation measurements are typically made with the hip flexed 90 degrees.[5,15,16] It is important to ensure that the patient's lumbar spine remains flat on the table, and that the pelvis is not rotating throughout this testing, as this can alter measurements obtained. Comparing ROM measurements to the contralateral side is valuable, as each patient has a unique normal baseline ROM. Patients with intra-articular pathology may show globally decreased ROM. Patients with femoroacetabular impingement tend to have decreased internal rotation.[17] More specifically, individuals with cam morphology of the femoral head-neck junction have more limited ROM than those without cam morphology.[18]

Palpation of bony landmarks and soft tissue structures about the hip and pelvis is a simple and useful part of the physical exam to help identify extra-articular sources of pain. A structured approach to this is simple and efficient and plays an important role in guiding treatment. Although both the patient and treating physician's focus often is directed at underlying joint disorders, including arthritis, identification, and improvement of associated soft tissue symptoms can be useful. The adductor longus origin is palpated in the groin with the patient in the supine position with the hip flexed to approximately 45 degrees, and externally rotated. Asking the patient to adduct the thigh against resist, thus contracting the adductor musculature, can increase the sensitivity of this test. Pain may be indicative of adductor longus tendinopathy, or sometimes adductor tendon partial or complete tearing. The pubic symphysis and pubic rami may also be palpated, and specific tenderness here may indicate osteitis pubis. With the patient still in the supine position, the rectus abdominis near its insertion at the superior pubic rami is palpated while the patient is asked to perform a resisted sit up. Tenderness elicited here may represent a core muscle injury. In the setting of hip arthritis, with limited motion of the joint, increased strain may be placed on the rectus abdominis–adductor

aponeurosis as the patients unknowingly compensate for limited joint motion with increased lumbopelvic and abdominal rotation. The proximal anterior thigh hip is palpated to screen for hip flexor strains. The patient is then asked to move to lateral decubitus position. The greater trochanter is palpated. Tenderness here is common and may represent isolated peritrochanteric symptoms or secondary symptoms often seen with intra-articular disorders. The patient's sacroiliac joint and lumbar spine is then palpated. If posterior pain is reported, palpation of the ischial tuberosity and hamstring origin can help narrow the differential diagnosis. Posterior hip pain presents a diagnostic dilemma, though more recent descriptions of deep gluteal syndrome, a nondiscogenic, extrapelvic entrapment of the sciatic nerve, has offered some guidance to the assessment of this group of patients.[19,20]

Strength testing is then performed. While in the supine position, hip flexion and adduction strength is tested. In the lateral decubitus position with the knee slightly flexed to relax the iliotibial band, abduction strength is tested. Muscle strength is graded using the traditional five-point scale. Patients with chronic hip joint pain have been reported to have reduced hip muscle strength in all muscle groups or the ipsilateral hip and to a lesser degree the contralateral hip.[21]

Multiple special tests exist that are helpful in identifying the etiology of pain about the hip. The "Impingement Test," performed by placing the hip in flexion, adduction, and internal rotation (FADIR), has been used to screen for femoroacetabular impingement. The motion brings the anterosuperior femoral-head junction in close proximity to the anterosuperior acetabular rim. In patients with pincer and/or cam morphology, or those with anterosuperior labral pathology, conflict between the acetabulum and femoral head-neck causes pain. The maneuver is not specific and may cause with a number of intra-articular hip pathologies, including hip arthritis. The contralateral side should also be examined, as an aggressive maneuver may cause some degree of discomfort in even a normal, asymptomatic hip. The FABER (flexion, abduction, external rotation) maneuver is the performed. The ipsilateral ankle may be rested on the contralateral knee while in the supine position, and gentle downward pressure applied to the ipsilateral knee. The maneuver may elicit symptoms in various regions, including the ipsilateral hip joint, ipsilateral posterolateral hip soft tissues, and the contralateral sacroiliac joint. Ipsilateral hip joint pathology typically causes deep anterior pain with this maneuver. It is important to note location of pain, as opposed to simply its presence. The posterior impingement test is performed by abducting, extending, and externally rotating the hip. Unlike the FADIR maneuver, it brings the posterolateral femoral head-neck junction in conflict with the posterior acetabular rim, potentially causing pain. It may also cause pain in a hip with limited ROM, or one with adhesive capsulitis. Patients with arthritis often have globally diminished ROM, and this maneuver may be painful.[5,13,16]

The Stinchfield test, a resisted straight leg raise performed at approximately 30 degrees of hip flexion with the patient supine, may cause deep anterior hip pain in patients with intra-articular pathology. However, this is not a specific test, as those with hip flexor strains or other musculotendinous injury will likely also have pain with it.

In summary, physical examination of the hip with arthritis can be expected to show globally diminished ROM; the patient may commonly have sites of tenderness to the extra-articular musculotendinous structures of the hip and pelvis; the log roll, FADIR, FABER, Stinchfield, and posterior impingement tests may elicit pain. The patient may present with an antalgic gait pattern.

IMAGING

Imaging of the hip begins with plain radiographs. In cases where the clinical presentation and plain radiographs fit the diagnosis of arthritis, further imaging beyond plain radiographs is often unnecessary. Pain radiographs of the hip should begin with a well centered anteroposterior (AP) view of the pelvis. This is most commonly obtained in the supine position, but may also be obtained in the standing position to provide information about the patient's functional sagittal pelvic tilt.[22,23] The coccyx and pubic symphysis should be in line, with the caudal tip of the coccyx between 2 and 3 cm from the pubic symphysis. The obturator foramen should be symmetric bilaterally (Fig. 88.1).[24] Variations in pelvic tilt, thus providing oblique views with characteristics of the inlet or outlet view, have been shown to skew interpretations of acetabular version. When the pelvis is tilted anteriorly, the acetabulum may appear falsely retroverted, and when the pelvis is tilted posteriorly, the acetabular may appear falsely anteverted. Rotation of the pelvis can similarly skew measurements of acetabular version as well as acetabular depth. On the anterosuperior measurement, general observation of any joint space narrowing should be assessed. The joint space should be measured, as the severity of joint narrowing has been inversely correlated with success after treatment with hip arthroscopy. Joint space of less than 2 mm has been reported as a lower limit, below which arthroscopy should be avoided for treatment. Measurements are routinely made in three locations: superomedially,

superiorly, and superolaterally. The presence of subchondral sclerosis of the acetabulum or femoral head should be noted, as should the presence of osteophytes. Subchondral cyst formation in the acetabulum or femoral head, when visible on plain radiographs, typically indicates more advanced degenerative changes. Fig. 88.2 demonstrates a hip with these advanced arthritic findings. Degenerative changes are often classified using the Tönnis grading system (Table 88.1).[25] The Lateral Center Edge Angle of Wiberg is then measured (Fig. 88.3). This provides a measurement of lateral acetabular coverage of the femoral head. A best fit circle of the femoral head is drawn, and an angle from its center with one limb directed superiorly and the other to the lateral margin of the acetabulum is drawn. Conventionally, acetabular dysplasia has been diagnosed when the lateral center edge angle is less than 25 degrees. More recently, a subcategory of "borderline" dysplasia has been described in patients with LCE measurements of 18 to 25 degrees. Acetabular dysplasia has important implications for treatment of hip pain, as patients with true dysplasia are typically not good candidates for hip arthroscopy, and may indeed require pelvic osteotomies to correct

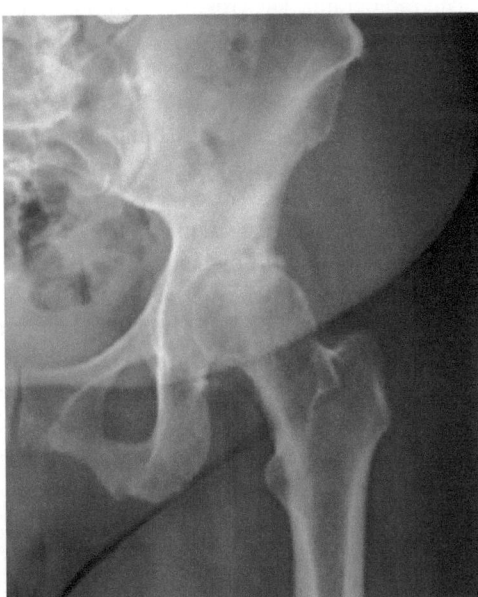

Fig. 88.2 An anteroposterior view of the left hip showing severe joint space narrowing, femoral and acetabular sclerosis, and subchondral cyst formation. These changes are consistent with Tönnis grade 3.

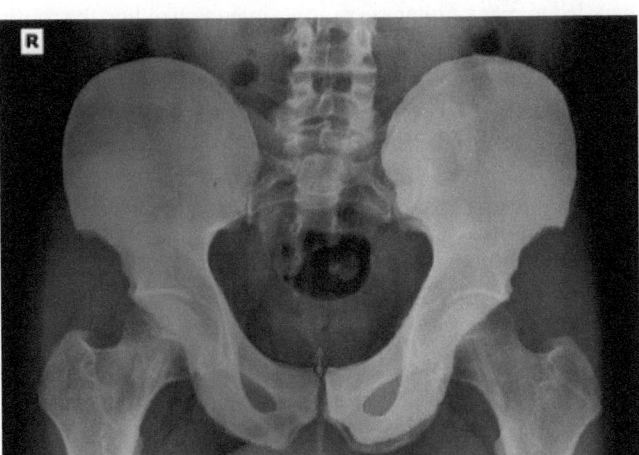

Fig. 88.1 Anteroposterior view of the pelvis. A well-centered view is important, including symmetry of the bilateral hemipelvic, obturator foramen, and a distance of 2 to 3 cm between the coccyx and pubic symphysis.

TABLE 88.1	Tönnis Classification of Osteoarthritis
Tönnis Grade	**Imaging Characteristics**
0	No signs of osteoarthritis
1	Slight narrowing of the joint space, slight osteophyte formation, and slight sclerosis of the femoral head or acetabulum
2	Small cysts in the femoral head or acetabulum, increased narrowing of the joint space, and moderate loss of sphericity of the femoral head
3	Large cysts, severe narrowing or obliteration of the joint space, severe deformity of the femoral head

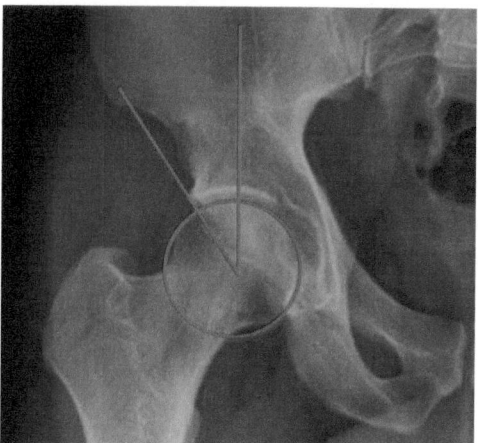

Fig. 88.3 The lateral center edge angle is used to measure lateral acetabular coverage of the femoral head.

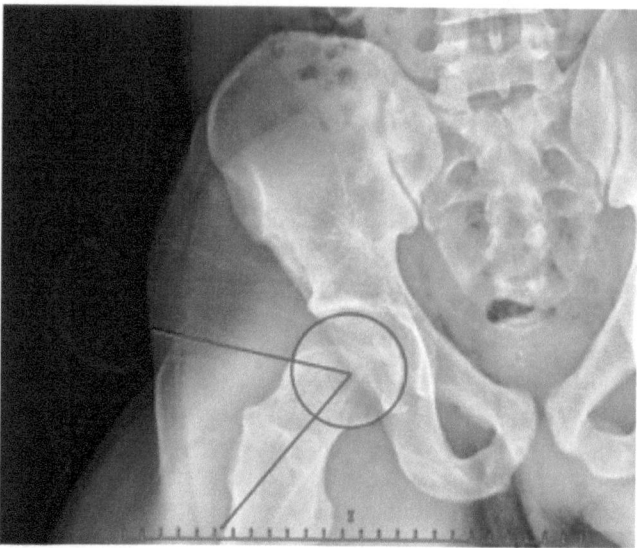

Fig. 88.4 The alpha angle is used to quantify the cam morphology at the femoral head-neck junction.

their underlying bony acetabular deficiency if substantial arthritis is not present.

The presence of an acetabular crossover sign is evaluated on the AP plain radiograph. The crossover sign is present when the anterior acetabular wall and posterior acetabular wall cross prior to their convergence at the lateral acetabular sourcil. This indicates some degree of retroversion of the acetabulum, sometimes a contributing factor in femoroacetabular impingement. The further distal/medial the point of crossover, the more substantial the retroversion.[26] The crossover sign can be quantified as a ratio of the distance between the lateral margin of acetabular sourcil and the crossover point to the diameter of the acetabulum altogether. The posterior wall sign is present when a point marked at the center of the femoral head lies lateral to the posterior wall of the acetabulum on the AP radiograph, and may indicate undercoverage of the posterior acetabulum, which can exist as part of a retroverted acetabulum or in the setting of global acetabular undercoverage.

Various lateral views of the hip exist. Commonly used examples include the frog-leg lateral, the cross-table lateral, and the Dunn 45-degree or Dunn 90-degree views. Each view may offer a slightly different angle and view of the femoral head-neck junction. The frog-leg lateral is a technically simple and easily reproducible. In many hip arthroscopy and preservation clinics, the Dunn 45-degree lateral view is utilized, given that it has been shown to be most sensitive for the presence of CAM morphology.[27] Regardless of which view is utilized, the presence or absence of CAM morphology should be noted, and when present it should be quantified. The CAM morphology can be quantified using the alpha angle. The alpha angle was classically described using axial magnetic resonance imaging (MRI) cuts, but can be extrapolated to lateral radiographic views.[28] This is measured by first drawing a best fit circle on the femoral head. At the center of this circle, an angle with one limb directed parallel to the femoral neck and the other directed to the point where the femoral head-neck exits the best fit circle (Fig. 88.4). Gosvig et al. classified alpha angle measurements as pathologic (>57 degrees), borderline (51 to 56 degrees), subtle (46 to 50 degrees), very subtle (43 to 45 degrees), or normal (≤42 degrees).[29] Commonly alpha angle

values greater than 50 degrees are generally regarded as abnormal, and represent CAM morphology.[30] Another available method of quantifying CAM morphology is the femoral offset. Again using the center of the femoral head on the lateral view, a line is drawn in the axis of the femoral neck. Two other parallel lines are drawn—one at the femoral neck and the other at the anterior-most border of the femoral head. A decreased offset is seen in patients with cam morphology. As an alternative to reporting the true offset, the offset ratio may be obtained by dividing the offset by the diameter of the femoral head, and may offer a more standardized value.[24]

MRI is commonly used to aid in the evaluation of the athlete with hip pain. It can be obtained with or without intra-articular contrast (arthrogram). Magnetic resonance arthrogram (MRA) has excellent sensitivity in identifying labral tears at the chondrolabral transition zone. Debate exists on the necessity of arthrogram for assessment of chondrolabral structures of the hip.[31,32] Improvements in MRI technology and the use of 3.0 T scanner have led to many hip preservation surgeons avoiding the routine use of the arthrogram. 3.0 T nonarthrogram MRI has shown excellent sensitivity and specificity in identifying arthroscopically proven labral tears.[33,34] In addition to assessment of the labrum, MRI is a sensitive imaging modality able to identify early degenerative changes, including subchondral edema and subchondral cyst formation. Acetabular and femoral head chondral irregularities, thinning, or delamination can be evaluated. The clinical relevance of this often depends on the degree of arthritis. One must take care to avoid focusing on the presence or absence of labral pathology. Subchondral edema may indicate early stages of degenerative disease, and may be masked by the stark contrast created by intra-articular contrast, thus offering an additional reason to consider nonarthrogram studies. In a study of 208 hip patients over 50 years of age, MR arthrogram identified some degree of labral pathology in 93% of patients and true labral tearing in 73% of patients (with no statistical correlation between labral tearing and presence/degree of arthritis).[35]

Patients with diagnosed labral tears may be quite determined that repair of this structure will rid them of their symptoms. Treatment of a torn acetabular labrum in the arthritic hip is unlikely to provide substantial mid to long-term improvement, and should be avoided. The ligamentum teres is also visualized, with surrounding synovium in the cotyloid fossa. Damage to the ligamentum teres or synovitis in the cotyloid fossa and diffusely throughout the joint may be seen. Loose osteochondral bodies may also be present in the setting of arthritis, and may be responsible for some mechanical symptoms.

Evaluation of the periarticular soft tissues may also yield important information about other extra-articular sources of pain. Correlation to the physical examination is important, as sites of musculotendinous edema, or even low grade partial thickness tearing, may not always be clinically relevant, and are commonly noted around the degenerative joint. Pathology of the gluteus medius or gluteus minimus tendons at the respective insertions at the greater trochanter should be evaluated, along with adjacent greater trochanteric bursitis. Tears of these abductor tendons are clinically significant when the patient's pain can be localized to the lateral hip at the greater trochanter, and in these cases should be treated. Peritrochanteric pathology and intra-articular pathology may be compensatory to each other; thus thoughtful assessment and treatment of the underlying cause of pain as well as associated symptoms may yield the best results. Femoral neck and acetabular stress fractures should be ruled out on MRI, and are especially common among longer distance runners and other impact activities. These may not be visible on plain radiographs but easily noted on MRI. They may be present concurrently in a runner with arthritis, but may cause acute chronic pain in the athlete with known arthritis of the hip.

Computed tomography (CT) is not usually necessary for diagnostic purposes around the hip in the setting of FAI or osteoarthritis. It does have a role for preoperative planning in patients who have an established diagnosis and are indicated for surgery. Two-dimensional radiographs also do have some limitations, and the use of the measurements such as lateral center edge angle and anterior center edge angle may not tell the whole story as it relates to acetabular coverage. Similarly, femoral head-neck convexities and irregularities exist in variations that two-dimensional radiographs do not fully represent. Three-dimensional reconstruction of CT imaging is now possible, providing easily manipulated imaged that morphology aberrances such as CAM or pincer morphology, thus guiding surgical treatment. Various commercially available software options exist that allow motion assessments of the hip, indicating areas of bony conflict between the acetabulum and femoral head in FAI.

DECISION-MAKING PRINCIPLES

In keeping with the typical goals of treating the active patient, the treatment of athletic patients with hip arthritis aims at minimizing pain or discomfort while keeping the patient active. Unlike many other conditions diagnosed and treated by sports medicine specialists, arthritis carries certain weight and implications for the patient. Many patients view it as an end to their ability to either compete in their sport or enjoy it recreationally. In general,

regardless of the severity of arthritis on imaging, treatments should be begin with noninvasive to minimally invasive measures, directed at reducing pain and limiting the progression of degenerative changes.

TREATMENT OPTIONS

Nonsurgical Measures

Nonsurgical treatment of hip arthritis includes the use of medications to relieve pain and physical therapy to optimize ROM and strength of the hip and pelvic musculature. Nonnarcotic analgesics such as acetaminophen or nonsteroidal antiinflammatory drugs (NSAIDs) can provide relief. Both categories of medications should be prescribed and taken with knowledge of dosing guidelines. Current guidelines recommend against the use of greater than 3000 mg of Tylenol per day to avoid hepatic injury. NSAIDs may need to be taken with gastroprotective agents, especially in patients with a history of gastroesophageal reflux, gastric ulcers, or upper gastrointestinal bleeding. Narcotics are avoided due to their potential for the development of dependency or addiction. The use of narcotics also is contraindicated while driving and operating machinery. Nationwide efforts to reduce the misuse of narcotics have also been launched, and an effort should be made to avoid prescribing them unless absolutely necessary. In cases of acute injury or pain, a period of relative rest may be useful. In recreational athletes, activity modification, including temporary or long-term transition from high impact activities such as running and jumping to lower impact activities such as cycling, elliptical treadmill, and swimming, should be attempted. Manual therapy with myofascial mobilization may be beneficial to improve soft tissue symptoms about the hip. Cryotherapy and/or heat therapy may also provide relief of soft tissue symptoms.

Injections may provide a useful adjunct to treatment, both from a diagnostic and therapeutic standpoint. The use of the ultrasound in musculoskeletal medicine has allowed for precise placement of injections, thus allowing clinicians to more reliably target areas or structures responsible for pain. Common injection sites include the hip joint itself, the iliopsoas bursa, the peritrochanteric bursa, the hamstring origin, the piriformis muscle/tendon, and the sacroiliac joint. In the patient with hip arthritis, intra-articular injections are useful to assess how much of the patient's pain is directly related to the degenerating joint versus the result of compensatory soft tissue dysfunction about the hip and pelvis. Injections are typically performed with a local anesthetic and a corticosteroid. Whereas the diagnostic utility of the local anesthetic is likely more relevant in the nonarthritic hip, the therapeutic benefits of the corticosteroid may be of the utmost importance in the arthritic joint. Ultrasound guided diagnostic injections tend to be less painful and more convenient for patients than those performed under fluoroscopic guidance.[36] Viscosupplementation has been utilized in the hip with some evidence of improved symptoms in hip osteoarthritis.[37,38] Though pain may be improved in the short term, the natural course of hip osteoarthritis has not been shown to be altered by viscosupplementation. More research will be necessary prior to broadly recommending such treatment.

SURGICAL TREATMENT

Hip Arthroscopy

The role of arthroscopy in treating disorders or the hip has greatly increased in recent years.[39,40] This increase is largely attributable to the understanding and more frequent treatment of femoroacetabular impingement. Despite this, arthroscopy has a limited role in the treatment of arthritis once it is present. Arthroscopy should not be viewed as a tool to treat hip arthritis. Short-term and now long-term studies have shown that patients with arthritis have poorer results after hip arthroscopy.[41-46] A study of patients undergoing hip arthroscopy including 43 patients with Tönnis grade 2 changes showed that those with grade 2 Tönnis changes had a 7.73 odds ratio of undergoing total hip arthroplasty (THA; compared to those with Tönnis grade 0 or 1 changes) at minimum follow-up of 2 years.[47] The role of arthroscopy lies in the treatment of irregularities thought to represent precursors to arthritis. Femoroacetabular impingement has been described as a predisposing lesion to hip osteoarthritis. The presence of CAM morphology leads to delamination of adjacent acetabular cartilage, thus beginning the cascade of arthritic changes. Pincer morphology may have a more important role as a precursor to labral pathology. The labrum has an important role as a regulator of fluid dynamics within the hip joint; when torn or resected, the negative pressure seal of the hip is compromised and increased joint reaction forces are noted, potentially leading to arthritis.[48] Fig. 88.5 shows an anterosuperior hip joint with disruption at the chondrolabral junction. Early adjacent chondromalacia is noted adjacent to the labral tear. Hip arthroscopy offers the ability to correct the bony irregularities in FAI, as well as stabilize the labrum and chondrolabral junction by repairing the labrum and resecting any unstable chondral flaps. Microfracture of the acetabulum chondral lesions in association with the treatment of FAI when necessary has also yielded promising results.[49-51] Though labral repair has been regarded as a superior option over labral débridement due to improved functional outcome scores at short term follow-up, focal/selective débridement remains a reasonable option when labral tissue is too friable and degenerated to allow for repair. Complete excision of the labrum to bone is not recommended, as this has shown worse patient reported outcomes.[52] Comparison of labral repair versus débridement has actually shown fairly similar outcomes at 10-year follow-up, with a slight advantage to labral repair. Capsular management has gained interest. Repair of capsulotomies has been associated with improved patient reported outcomes after hip arthroscopy, lending credence to the important role of fluid dynamics in the hip joint, and the important role of the thick capsular ligaments of the hip in preventing microinstability of the hip.[53,54] In patients with borderline acetabular dysplasia, capsular plication associated with labral preservation (repair) has been successful in the short term.[55] Longer term evaluation of the patient's hip will be important. In general, hip arthroscopy should be either avoided or entertained with extreme caution in patients with degenerative changes beyond Tönnis grade 1. Those patients with some degenerative changes that are treated with arthroscopy should be educated that their postoperative improvements may be less substantial, and that the rate of conversion to hip arthroplasty is higher. Endoscopic techniques have also evolved and now also allow the treatment of extra-articular disorders such as gluteus medius and minimus tears, proximal hamstring tendon pathology, and posterior deep gluteal space pathology.

Osteotomy

Hip arthroscopy should be avoided in patients with overt acetabular dysplasia. Whereas arthroscopic techniques allow surgeons to correct pincer and CAM morphology by removing excessive bone, bone cannot be added in cases of insufficient acetabular coverage. The Bernese periacetabular osteotomy (PAO) is utilized to treat acetabular dysplasia. This procedure is performed by making a single incision and several bony cuts in the innominate bone prior rotating the acetabulum to provide greater coverage of the femoral head and then fixed in its new position using screws.[56,57] As with arthroscopy, the technique is most successful in the absence of advanced arthritic changes. The procedure is typically performed by surgeons specializing in joint preservation, and is not without its complications. In the presence of chondrolabral injury or cam morphology of the femoral head-neck junction associated with acetabular dysplasia, arthroscopy for labral repair and femoroplasty has been described in the same setting as PAO, with good results.[58] Proximal femoral dysplasia requiring osteotomy represents a much smaller subset of the pathology encountered, but in certain cases may be beneficial.

Hip Resurfacing

Historically hip resurfacing was a preferred surgical option for young patients who wanted to remain active. The advantage to hip resurfacing is preservation of proximal femoral bone stock in the younger patient population to make subsequent revision less invasive. In 2006, the Birmingham Hip Resurfacing was approved by the FDA for use in the United States; however, use has recently fallen out of favor due to concerns associated with metal on metal bearing surfaces and failure rates. Moreover, recent studies have demonstrated no functional benefit to the Birmingham Hip Resurfacing over traditional THA.[59]

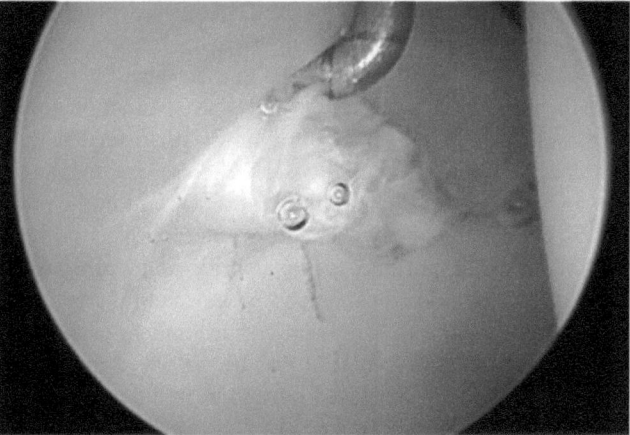

Fig. 88.5 Arthroscopic view of the anterosuperior chondrolabral junction in a patient with femoroacetabular impingement. There is early chondral fraying and softening adjacent to the area of labral tear.

Total Hip Arthroplasty

In a young and active patient, joint preservation remains the goal. However, when degenerative changes in the hip preclude preservation of the joint, THA is the gold standard treatment. THA is reserved for patients with end-stage degenerative changes of the hip joint (e.g., bone on bone articulation) that have failed all conservative measures, including nonsteroidal anti-inflammatories, formal physical therapy, intra-articular corticosteroid injections, and have pain affecting their daily activity. Previously THA was reserved for older and more sedentary patients; however, recent improvements in materials and implant fixation have expanded the indication for THA to younger patients. Studies have demonstrated that delaying THA in an appropriately indicated patient actually diminishes the chance of obtaining a satisfactory result.[60]

The most commonly used approaches for THA include the posterolateral approach, anterolateral approach, and direct anterior approach. The optimal surgical approach is at the discretion of the operating surgeon and should be tailored to each individual patient, taking into account factors such as retained hardware, abnormal anatomy, body mass index, and flexion contractures. There is evidence that the direct anterior approach has expedited recovery, including less time using assistive devices after surgery and lower dislocation rates even without hip precautions.[61]

Cementless fixation in THA is the gold standard in the United States, particularly in younger patients. The benefit of biologic fixation between the implant and bone provides a longer durability of the prosthesis and allows for bone remodeling. Excellent long-term outcomes have been demonstrated with these components. Selection of the bearing surface for young active patients undergoing THA is an important consideration. Factors to consider include wear characteristics, maximum head diameter, and potential complications from wear over time. Currently the bearing of choice for young patients for most arthroplasty surgeons is a ceramic head with a modern generation highly cross-linked polyethylene liner. Depending on the cost difference between a metal and ceramic head at any given institution, the use of a ceramic head becomes cost effective typically around the age of 65 years or younger.[62] Metal on metal THA has largely fallen out of favor for concerns with pseudotumor formation and metallosis. Ceramic on ceramic bearings have excellent wear characteristics; however, there have been cases of liner fracture as well as squeaking.

POSTOPERATIVE MANAGEMENT

Hip Arthroscopy

Rehabilitation after hip arthroscopy is widely variable depending on surgeon preference and physiotherapist experience. Most agree that early ROM, including circumduction of the hip, can help avoid stiffness and postoperative adhesions.[63] Structured rehabilitation protocols are typically broadly divided into four phases: (1) mobility and initial exercise, (2) intermediate exercise and stabilization, (3) advanced exercise and neuromotor control, and (4) return to activity.[64-67] Patient progression through these phases is highly variable, and most recommend progression based on individual symptoms and abilities. Return to running can be undertaken through a running progression program, with patients monitoring and categorizing their symptoms, and determining progression based on these symptoms. Functional abilities and the presence and degree of pain seem to be better regulators of the patient's ability to return to running than time from surgery.[68] In a survey of high-volume hip arthroscopy centers, 70% of surgeons recommended waiting 12 to 20 weeks before returning to sport. A total of 85% of surgeons recommended criteria of pain free running, jumping, lateral agility drills, and single-leg squats be used prior to returning to sport.[69]

Total Hip Arthroplasty

In general, the postoperative course after THA allows the patient to be full weight bearing immediately after surgery. There may be motion restrictions based on the approach; however, the direct anterior approach to THA results in no restriction. Patients typically graduate from ambulation with a walker to a cane as soon as they feel comfortable and then to no assistive device. Most surgeons limit high-impact activity, including heavy lifting, jogging, or running, for a period of time after the operation to allow for sufficient osseointegration of the implants. Many surgeons discourage running or jogging after THA to decrease the risk of early failure. This can be challenging, particularly in the young patient population; however, modern implants may be able to better withstand higher impact activity.

RESULTS

Several studies now exit showing very short-term outcomes after hip arthroscopy for treatment of labral tears and femoroacetabular impingement. Consider the 2009 systematic review by Clohisy et al., with 11 studies (nine level 4 and two level 3) with a mean follow-up of 3.2 years. Reduced pain and function was noted in all studies (range 68% to 96%). The study did note the need for longer term follow-up to determine survivorship of the procedure and the impact it could have on the natural progression toward osteoarthritis.[70] Outcomes of hip arthroscopy, specifically in athletes, have been examined and are shown to be excellent. Nho et al. revealed significant improvement in Modified Harris Hip Scores and Hip Outcome Scores in their series of 33 elite athletes and that 79% of patients had returned to play sports at 1 year, with 73% playing sports at 2 years postoperatively.[71] Philippon et al. published outcomes on hip arthroscopy for labral repair and treatment of FAI in professional hockey players, showing high satisfaction at 2 years postoperatively and improvement in the mean mHHS from 70 to 95.[72] Studies with longer term follow-up are fewer in number, but share present information. Byrd et al. reported the outcome of 26 patients treated for acetabular labral tears with 10-year follow-up. They reported a mean improvement in the mHHS of 29 points (from 52 preoperatively to 81 postoperatively). Perhaps the most valuable lesson is noted when the cohort was further divided into patients with and without arthritis. Among the 18 patients without arthritis, 15 (83%) continued to have substantial improvement at 10-year follow-up. Conversely, 7/8 (88%) of patients with preexisting arthritis were converted to THA at a mean of 63 months.[42] In a wider study of 52 patients undergoing hip arthroscopy for a wider range of diagnoses (labral pathology, chondral damage, synovitis, loose bodies), including those of the previous study, the authors again note that the presence of hip arthritis at the time of the index procedure was a poor prognostic factor.[73] Skendzdel et al. specifically examined preoperative hip joint space on plain radiographs as a predictor of outcomes. Their study examined 466 patients at a minimum of 5 years follow-up; 54/63 (86%) patients with joint space less than or equal to 2 mm were converted to THA, while only 63/403(16%) were converted to THA.[45] Philippon et al. assessed hip arthroscopy for FAI inpatients 50 years old or older. Patients with joint space greater than 2 mm fared well, while those with joint space narrowing had increased conversion rate to THA.[46] Menge et al. reported on a series of 154 patients with 10-year follow-up to compare the outcomes of labral débridement versus labral repair. Both groups showed significant improvements in outcome scores, though joint space less than or equal to 2 mm, increased age (>50 years), and acetabular chondral injury requiring microfracture were independently associated with increased hazard rate for THA.[41]

The midterm results of modern day THA are typically reported to be greater than 95% at 5 to 10 years, even in young patients.[74] However, in young patients, survivorship at follow-up of 13 to 15 years has been reported to drop as low as 54% with earlier generation implants.[75,76] Further studies with modern generation implants are needed to understand their long-term survivorship.

COMPLICATIONS

Hip arthroscopy is a challenging procedure. Several known complications exist, including traction related, neuropraxias, pudendal nerve neuralgia from compression of the perineal postoperative infection, retroperitoneal fluid extravasation, heterotopic ossification of the periarticular soft tissues, iatrogenic chondrolabral injury, bursitis, deep venous thrombosis, and postoperative femoral fracture. Conversion to hip arthroplasty is also commonly listed as a potential complication. Though in some instances this may be the case, in most this may be the natural progression of existing disease, and thus the importance of patient selection is highlighted. Using a national database study, Truntzer et al. reported the rate of conversion to THA within 1 year at 2.85%.[77] In a recent 10-year survivorship study of 154 hips by Menge et al., 34% of patients underwent THA.[41] Though age might contribute, most agree that joint space narrowing and the preexistence of arthritis at the time of arthroscopy are most predictive of conversion to THA.

Complications of THA in young patients are similar to those in the older patient population. Common causes of revision are bearing surface wear and aseptic loosening of the acetabular component. In patients with ceramic on ceramic articulation, component chipping or fracture is possible but rare. In a study of 102 THAs performed in patients with a mean age of 20 years, there was a 9% rate of complications resulting in a return to the operating room.[78] These complications included dislocation, periprosthetic fracture, peroneal nerve palsy, and arterial injury.

Authors' Preferred Technique

In the young patient with intra-articular hip pain that has been and some degree of arthritis, initial treatment comprises initial conservative measures including relative rest/activity modification, physical therapy or a home stretching program, and NSAIDs. Intra-articular injections to the hip can be utilized. If they provide extended relief, these are a reasonable option for the patient who is too arthritic for hip arthroscopy, and younger than preferable for THA. Our preference is to avoid hip arthroscopy in patients with less than or equal to 2 mm of joint space, or with osteophytes secondary to arthritis. We also avoid hip arthroscopy in patients that have notable subchondral edema or cyst formation. We prefer hip arthroscopy for patients with symptomatic FAI and/or labral pathology, without any substantial arthritic changes. We prefer labral repair over débridement if the labral tissue quality allows for this, though partial labral débridement remains a good option in patients with focal labral injuries and friable tissue not amenable to repair. Femoroplasty and acetabuloplasty are performed as needed to correct impingement morphology. Our preferred technique for capsular management involves utilizing an interportal capsulotomy connecting the anterolateral portal and anterior portals, which is repaired at the conclusion of the procedure. For young patients requiring THA, we prefer the direct anterior approach. The patient is placed supine on an operating table that allows manipulation of the extremity during the surgery. The interval between the sartorius and tensor fascia lata is developed. The rectus femoris is retracted medial, and no muscles or tendons are incised. A "T"-capsulotomy is performed and later repaired. Cementless implants are used on both the acetabular and femoral side. Screws are used if necessary through the acetabular component, and a highly cross-linked polyethylene is placed. A tapered design femoral stem is used that is proximally porous coated. A ceramic head is used, which is typically either a 32- or 36-mm diameter. Smaller femoral heads are favorable to allow for thicker polyethylene liner dimensions. Postoperatively the patients have no restrictions on weight bearing or ROM.

FUTURE DIRECTIONS

Hip arthritis is a difficult diagnosis to treat in the active adult. Recent innovations have helped us understand the link between femoroacetabular impingement and hip osteoarthritis, and have given us an opportunity to hopefully change the natural course of this disease. Unfortunately, once the hip has crossed into the realm of arthritis, options for hip preservation quickly narrow. History has shown us in the knee and shoulder that arthroscopy is not generally helpful in the arthritic joint, and this seems to hold true in the hip. Perhaps future developments in biologics will give us more options for restoring articular cartilage. As much as we have learned about femoroacetabular impingement and the possibilities hip arthroscopy offers, it may be that we are still just scratching the surface in this field that is still in its infancy. Arthroplasty generally offers reliable results for the arthritic hip, but certainly presents its own challenges in the younger, more active patient. Although the volume of young patients undergoing THA continues to increase, the long-term results of modern generation implants remain to be seen. The combination of earlier intervention of hip arthritis with THA and longer life expectancy will likely result in an increase in revision THA in the future. Careful surveillance of these patients with routine follow-up is necessary for early intervention.

For a complete list of references, go to ExpertConsult.com.

Knee

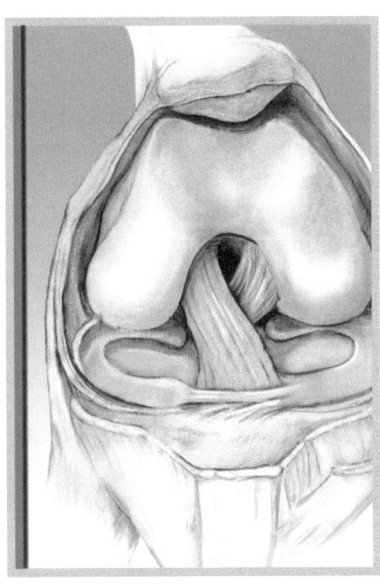

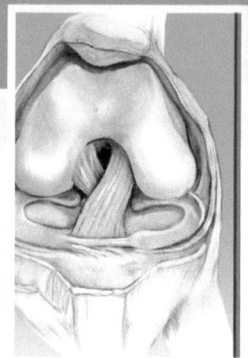

89

Knee Anatomy and Biomechanics of the Knee

Matthew J. Kraeutler, Jorge Chahla, Francesc Malagelada, Jordi Vega,
Pau Golanó, Bruce Beynnon, Fatih Ertem, Eric C. McCarty

KNEE ANATOMY

Superficial Anatomy

An understanding of the superficial anatomy is essential to explore the knee in a correct manner (Fig. 89.1).

When the knee is viewed from the anterior aspect, the presence of the patella is highlighted. It is located in the center of the joint, and on its anterior face, the entire perimeter of the patella can be palpated. The motion of the patella from lateral to medial and from proximal to distal can functionally vary based on the position of the knee and the contraction of the quadriceps femoris muscle. The more extended the knee and the more relaxed the quadriceps femoris muscle, the more mobile the patella will be, whereas as the knee flexes, the patella follows the femoral trochlear groove (patellar surface) and becomes more immobile. On the other hand, the normal superficial appearance of the patella can be altered by inflammatory processes that affect the prepatellar bursa, which can cause the typical morphologic appearance of the anterior knee to disappear.

On the superior border of the patella, the tendon of the quadriceps femoris muscle can be palpated, and on either side, the vastus medialis and lateralis, components of the same muscle, can be palpated. At the level of the apex of the patella, and directed distally, the patellar tendon can be identified as it descends to the tibial tuberosity, which is easily visible and palpable. This tuberosity continues distally with the anterior border of the tibia. Lateral to this anterior border, the muscle masses of the anterior compartment of the leg can be palpated, specifically the tibialis anterior muscle, and lateral and proximal to this tuberosity the anterior tubercle or Gerdy tubercle can be palpated, which constitutes the point of insertion for the iliotibial tract. Medial to the tubercle, palpation can lead to recognition of the insertion, on the medial aspect of the tibia, of the tendons of the sartorius, gracilis, and semitendinosus muscles, also known as the pes anserinus tendons. The most superficial structure corresponds to the sartorius muscle, and deep to this muscle, the tendons of the gracilis and semitendinosus muscles can be appreciated. At the upper limit of the pes anserinus, the cordlike tendon of the gracilis muscle can be palpated, which is located about 2 cm distal to the tibial tubercle. This understanding will prove useful during anterior cruciate ligament (ACL) reconstruction with use of autograft tendons from the pes anserinus (hamstring tendons).

Approximately two fingerbreadths proximal to the tibial tubercle, and on either side of the patellar tendon, the femoral condyles, medial and lateral, and the proximal region of the tibia or the tibial condyles can be palpated. The femoral and tibial condyles can be palpated most easily with the knee in 90 degrees of flexion. In this position, the space delineated between the femoral and tibial condyles forms a triangle on either side of the patellar tendon. This triangle, which by palpation corresponds to a soft spot, is where the anteromedial (AM) and anterolateral arthroscopic portals can be positioned. On the other hand, in cases of articular effusion, which is frequently associated with intra-articular pathology of the knee, the appearance of this triangular space can be more difficult to appreciate.

In the lateral region of the knee, distal to the lateral condyle of the tibia, the prominence of the fibular head can be observed. With the knee flexed to 90 degrees, and with varus articular force, one may palpate, and occasionally visualize, a cordlike structure that runs from the fibular head to the lateral condyle of the femur. This structure corresponds to the lateral collateral ligament (LCL). At the same level, but in the medial region, the medial collateral ligament (MCL) can be found, but because it is a flat structure, it is not possible to see or palpate it.

In the posterior region, osseous structures cannot be observed because they are covered with muscular structures. From a posterior view, with the knee in extension, a space that forms a rhombus can be appreciated; this space is called the popliteal fossa. This view is more easily defined when the patient actively flexes the knee. The popliteal fossa is traversed, in its medial zone, by a horizontal line that corresponds to the flexion crease of the knee. The edges of this rhombus correspond to the margins or limits of different muscle groups and the center of the popliteal fossa.

The inferior borders of the popliteal fossa correspond to the medial and lateral head of the gastrocnemius muscle, which are divergent at their origin but converge distally to reunite with the soleus muscle to form the calcaneal or Achilles tendon. The superomedial border corresponds to the tendons of the semitendinosus superficially and the semimembranosus deeply at their musculotendinous junction. With the knee flexed, these tendons are more easily appreciable, and they can even be pinched between one's fingers. In persons in whom the pes anserinus tendons have been used as an autograft for ACL reconstruction,

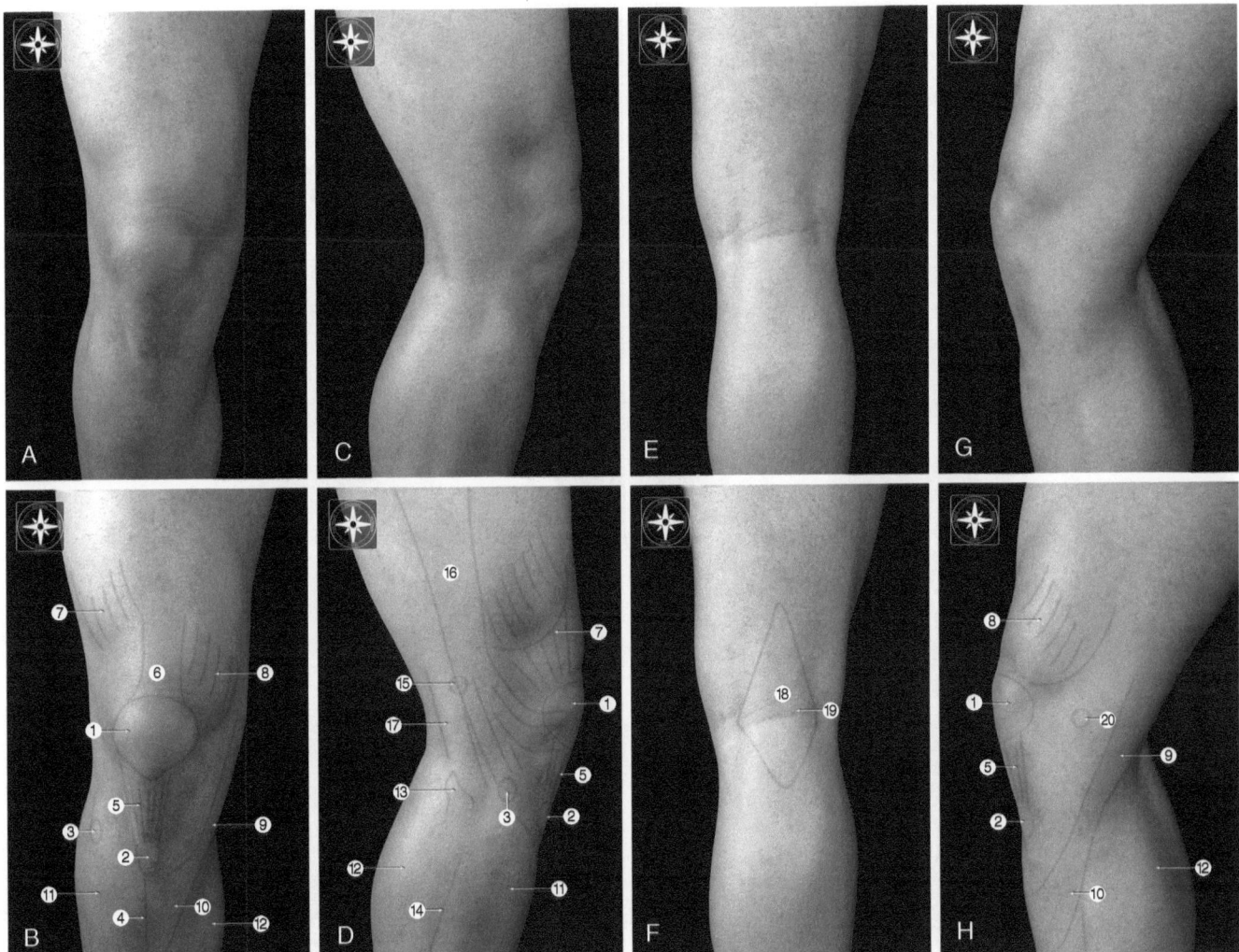

Fig. 89.1 Surface anatomy. (A and B) Anterior view. (C and D) Lateral view. (E and F) Posterior view. (G and H) Medial view. *1*, Patella. *2*, Tibial tuberosity. *3*, Anterior tubercle or Gerdy tubercle. *4*, Anterior border of the tibia. *5*, Patellar tendon. *6*, Quadriceps tendon. *7*, Vastus lateralis. *8*, Vastus medialis. *9*, Pes anserinus tendons. *10*, Pes anserinus area in the medial face of the tibia. *11*, Muscles of the anterior compartment of the leg. *12*, Muscles of the posterior compartment of the leg. *13*, Head of the fibula. *14*, Shaft of the fibula. *15*, Lateral epicondyle. *16*, Iliotibial tract. *17*, Biceps femoris muscle. *18*, Popliteal fossa. *19*, Flexion crease of the knee. *20*, Medial epicondyle. (Copyright Pau Golanó.)

this border may disappear or may appear altered. Finally, the superolateral border corresponds to the tendon of the biceps femoris, on its path to its insertion on the fibular head. At this level, one can begin to appreciate the thick iliotibial tract.

In the popliteal fossa, one can palpate diverse neurovascular structures: the tibial nerve, the common peroneal nerve, and the popliteal artery. The tibial nerve is encountered in the medial region of the popliteal fossa and can be recognized as a thick cordlike structure. One technique to highlight the nerve during exploration consists of placing the patient in the lateral decubitus position with the hip flexed to 90 degrees. In this position, one maintains the patient's knee slightly flexed with the ankle in dorsiflexion. Using the index finger, the hand can be passed from the inferior portion of the knee toward an anterior position and the nerve palpated. The common peroneal nerve can be localized in the lateral region of this fossa. With the knee in flexion, by

sliding the index finger laterally, one may palpate a cordlike structure that is much smaller than that of the tibial nerve. The popliteal artery can be localized medial to the tibial nerve and is easily recognizable by palpation of its pulse.

OSSEOUS ANATOMY

The knee contains three osseous components: the femur, the tibia, and the patella (Fig. 89.2). These three structures form the tibiofemoral and the patellofemoral articulations, which together comprise the knee joint. In the lateral region of the knee, a third articulation is encountered, the proximal tibiofibular joint, which does not truly participate in the flexion-extension movement of the knee but is involved in the lateral stability of the knee via the insertion of the LCL and the biceps femoris tendon onto the fibular head.[1]

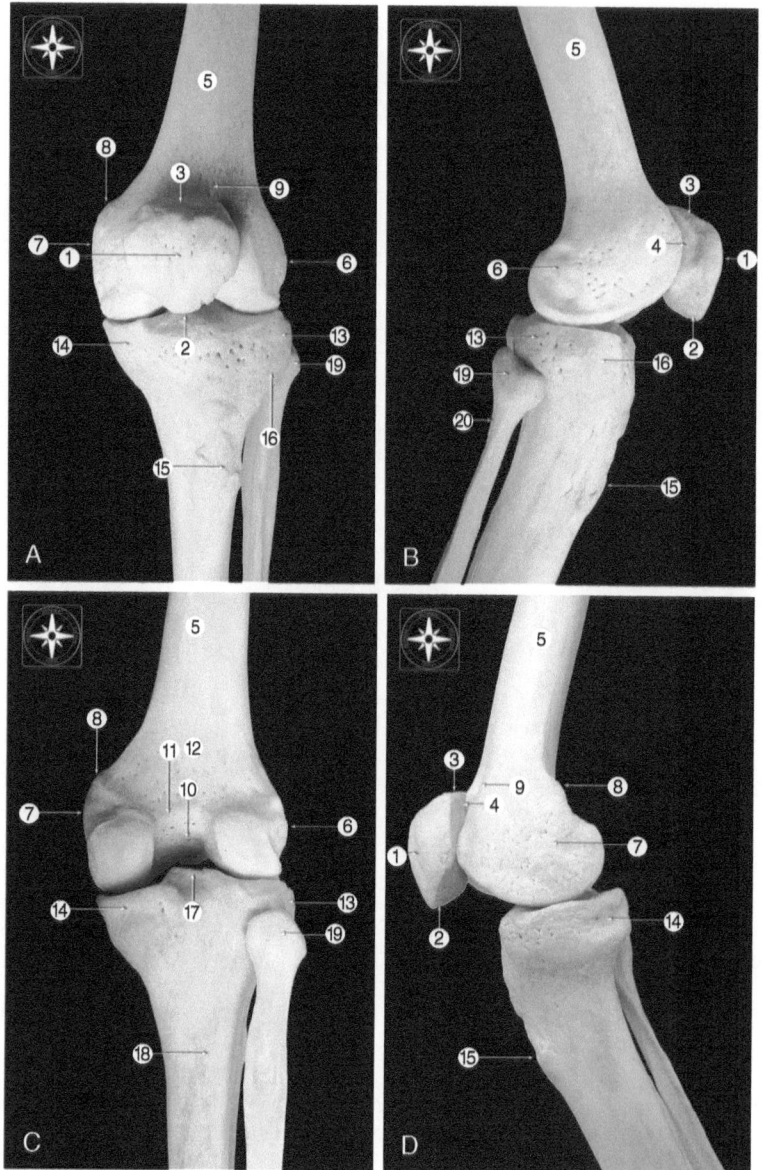

Fig. 89.2 Bony anatomy. (A) Anterior view. (B) Lateral view. (C) Posterior view. (D) Medial view. Patella: *1,* Anterior surface. *2,* Apex. *3,* Base. *4,* Articular surface. Femur: *5,* Shaft. *6,* Lateral condyle and lateral epicondyle. *7,* Medial condyle and medial epicondyle. *8,* Adductor tubercle. *9,* Supratrochlear fossa. *10,* Intercondylar notch. *11,* Posterolateral rim of the intercondylar notch. *12,* Popliteal surface. Tibia: *13,* Lateral condyle. *14,* Medial condyle. *15,* Tibial tuberosity. *16,* Anterior tubercle or Gerdy's tubercle. *17,* Intercondylar eminence. *18,* Soleal line. Fibula: *19,* Head and apex. *20,* Neck. (Copyright Pau Golanó.)

Femur

The distal region of the femur is formed by the two condyles, one medial and one lateral. A prominence named the *lateral epicondyle* is located on the lateral condyle, and the LCL inserts onto this prominence. At the level of the medial condyle is the adductor tubercle, and anterior and distal to this tubercle lies the medial epicondyle, the origin of the MCL.

Both femoral condyles, which are united at the anterior level by the femoral trochlear groove (patellar surface), are separated at the posterior level by a great notch—the intercondylar notch. The femoral trochlear groove permits the patella to slide during the movements of knee flexion and extension. The intercondylar

notch is the point of proximal insertion of the ACL and the posterior cruciate ligament (PCL). A wide zone on the medial wall of the notch constitutes the origin of the PCL, whereas the lateral wall has a flattened area that represents the proximal origin of the ACL. This area includes discrete bony prominences that are used as landmarks for the reconstructive surgery of the ACL. The prominences that are referenced for the correct positioning of the osseous tunnels are the lateral intercondylar ridge (LIR) and the lateral bifurcate ridge (BR).[2–4] The lateral BR is located perpendicular to the LIR, and in their posterior margin, an imaginary "T" is formed between them. The LIR is considered the anterior limit of the ACL, and the lateral BR represents the separation of the two bundles (AM and posterolateral [PL]) of the ACL.[4] Because of the confusion of the LIR with the posterolateral rim of the intercondylar notch during localization of the femoral tunnel for anterior ligamentoplasty, this prominence is now popularly called *resident's ridge* (Fig. 89.3).[5-7]

Tibia

The proximal epiphysis of the tibia forms two flattened surfaces, named the tibial plateaus or condyles. The medial tibial surface is larger and its shape is almost flat, whereas the lateral surface is more narrow and convex. Both present posterior declination of approximately 10 degrees with respect to the tibial diaphysis. At the posterior level, the lateral tibial condyle presents a flat and oval articulation with the fibula. In its most posterior zone, the medial tibial condyle presents a deep transverse groove for the insertion of the semimembranosus muscle (reflected tendon) and another medially for the insertion of the MCL.

The central region, located between the tibial plateaus, is occupied by the intercondylar eminences with the medial and lateral spines (medial and lateral intercondylar tubercle). Anterior and posterior to these eminences one can find the anterior and posterior intercondylar areas, respectively, which offer insertion for the cruciate ligaments and menisci.

The tibial tuberosity protrudes on the anterior face of the tibia, which corresponds to the insertion of the patellar tendon. Approximately 2 to 3 cm lateral to this tuberosity, the anterior tubercle or Gerdy tubercle is encountered, which constitutes the point of insertion for the iliotibial tract.

Patella

The patella is the largest sesamoid bone in the human body. It has a triangular shape, and we can highlight three edges, two surfaces, and one apex. The anterior surface is separated from the skin by the prepatellar bursa. The posterior or articular surface is divided by a central ridge into a medial articular surface and a larger lateral surface that occupies approximately two-thirds of the patella (Fig. 89.4).

The superior edge (base) of the patella is the location of insertion for the fibers of the tendon of the quadriceps femoris, principally the rectus femoris, vastus lateralis, and vastus intermedius. Most of the fibers of the vastus medialis insert on the medial edge; only a small portion insert along the superior edge. The fibers of the quadriceps femoris tendon envelop the anterior surface of the patella and merge at the level of the patellar vertex with the patellar tendon or ligament (Fig. 89.5).

MUSCULAR ANATOMY

The muscles that act on the knee joint may be divided schematically and with regard to their location into four groups (Fig. 89.6): anterior, posterior, medial, and lateral. In some anatomy texts these muscle groups are referred to as *dynamic elements* of the knee, but instead of following that discussion in this chapter, we only refer to them with regard to their origin and insertion and provide some anatomic detail that may prove useful to the reader.

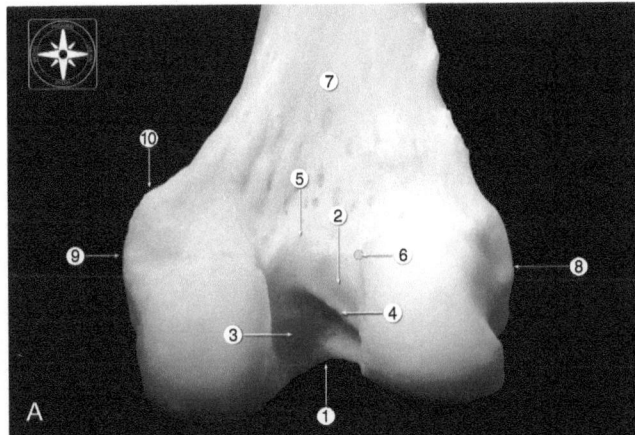
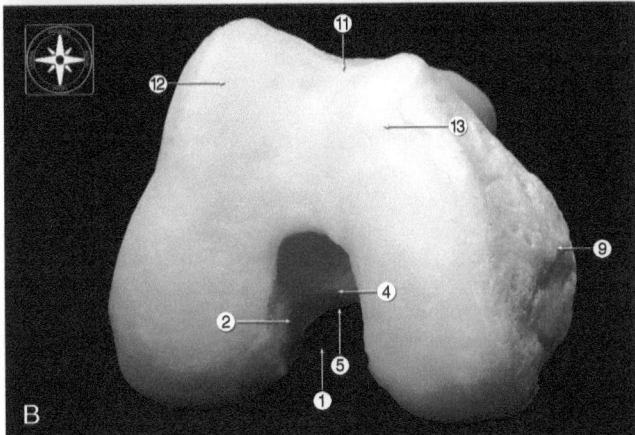

Fig. 89.3 Intercondylar notch morphology. (A) Posterior view of the distal epiphysis of the femur (knee in extension). (B) Distal view of the distal epiphysis of the femur (knee at 90 degrees of flexion). *1*, Intercondylar notch. *2*, Femoral footprint of anterior cruciate ligament. *3*, Femoral footprint of posterior cruciate ligament. *4*, Lateral intercondylar ridge or resident's ridge. *5*, Posterolateral rim of the intercondylar notch. *6*, Over the top. *7*, Popliteal surface. *8*, Lateral condyle and lateral epicondyle. *9*, Medial condyle and medial epicondyle. *10*, Adductor tubercle. *11*, Femoral trochlear groove (patellar surface). *12*, Lateral slope of the patellar surface. *13*, Medial slope of the patellar surface. (Copyright Pau Golanó.)

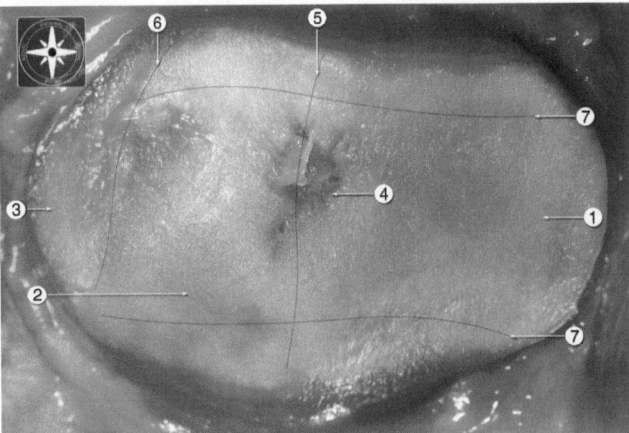

Fig. 89.4 Posterior (intra-articular) view of the patella. *1*, Lateral facet. *2*, Medial facet. *3*, Odd facet. This facet comes in contact with the femur only when the knee approaches full flexion. *4*, Articular cartilage lesion (grade III-IV Outerbridge classification). *5*, Central ridge, which corresponds to the femoral trochlear groove (patellar surface). *6*, Vertical ridge. *7*, Horizontal ridges. (Copyright Pau Golanó.)

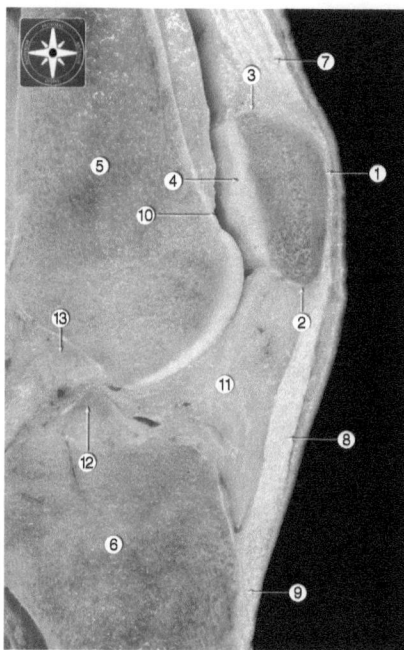

Fig. 89.5 Sagittal section of the knee joint. *1,* Anterior surface of patella. *2,* Apex of patella. *3,* Base of patella. *4,* Posterior or articular surface of patella. *5,* Femur. *6,* Tibia. *7,* Quadriceps tendon. *8,* Patellar tendon. *9,* Tibial tuberosity. *10,* Supratrochlear fossa. *11,* Infrapatellar fat pad (Hoffa's fat pad). *12,* Tibial insertion of anterior cruciate ligament. *13,* Femoral insertion of posterior cruciate ligament. (Copyright Pau Golanó.)

Anterior

The anterior group is formed by the quadriceps femoris muscle, which is the primary extensor of the knee joint. It is formed in turn by four muscular components, the rectus femoris (which also functions as a hip flexor), vastus intermedius, vastus lateralis, and vastus medialis. The insertion of this muscle at the level of the base of the patella has been described previously in the osseous anatomy section.

Posterior

In the posterior region of the knee and in its most proximal zone, three muscles belonging to the posterior muscle compartment of the thigh may be observed: the semimembranosus and semitendinosus (more superficial) muscles on the medial side and the biceps femoris muscle on the lateral side, all of which act as knee flexors. In the distal zone, the popliteus muscle and the gastrocnemius muscle, muscles of the posterior compartment of the leg, deep, and superficial, respectively, also have a flexor function.

The semimembranosus is one of the hamstring muscles. The distal semimembranosus tendinous insertions are important structures that contribute to the stability of the posterior medial corner of the knee.[8] The semimembranosus inserts at the posterior level of the knee joint through five tendinous expansions: the anterior or tibial expansion (the reflected expansion), the direct expansion, the inferior or popliteal expansion, the capsular expansion, and the oblique popliteal ligament. The anterior expansion extends anteriorly, passing under the posterior oblique ligament, and inserts in the medial aspect of the proximal tibia under the MCL. The direct expansion also has an anterior course, deep to the anterior arm, and attaches in the posterior medial

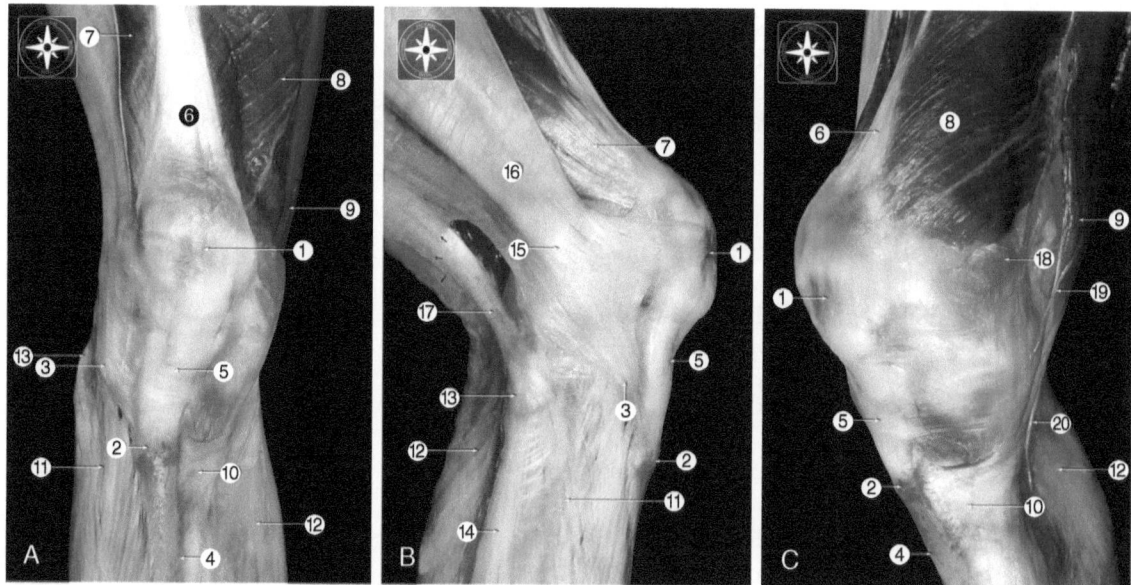

Fig. 89.6 Muscular anatomy. (A) Anterior view. (B) Lateral view. (C) Medial view. *1,* Patella. *2,* Tibial tuberosity. *3,* Anterior tubercle or Gerdy tubercle. *4,* Anterior border of the tibia. *5,* Patellar tendon. *6,* Quadriceps tendon. *7,* Vastus lateralis. *8,* Vastus medialis. *9,* Sartorius muscle. *10,* Pes anserinus area in the medial surface of the tibia. *11,* Muscles of the anterior compartment of the leg. *12,* Muscles of the posterior compartment of the leg. *13,* Head of the fibula. *14,* Shaft of the fibula (peroneus longus muscle). *15,* Lateral epicondyle. *16,* Iliotibial tract. *17,* Biceps femoris muscle (femoral fascia opened). *18,* Medial epicondyle. *19,* Infrapatellar branch (cut) of the saphenous nerve. *20,* Saphenous nerve (cut). (Copyright Pau Golanó.)

aspect of the tibia. The inferior expansion extends more distally than the anterior and the direct expansions. It passes under the distal tibial segments of the posterior oblique ligament and the MCL, inserting just above the tibial attachment of the MCL. The capsular expansion is adjacent to the posterior oblique ligament. The oblique popliteal ligament is a thin, broad lateral extension of the semimembranosus tendon that covers and blends with the posterior medial capsule and extends beyond the midline of the joint to intertwine its fibers with the arcuate ligament from the lateral posterior aspect of the knee (Fig. 89.7).[8,9]

The popliteus muscle originates on the posterior aspect of the tibia and inserts on the lateral femoral epicondyle. Because of its multiple attachments to other posterior and posterolateral structures, the popliteus muscle is an important structure that provides dorsolateral stability, stabilizes the lateral meniscus, and

balances the neutral tibial rotation.[10,11] This muscle possesses a tendon of some 2.5 cm in length that runs across a hiatus located in the segment medial and posterior to the lateral meniscus, making its visualization possible during arthroscopic exploration of the knee.

The gastrocnemius muscle comes from the lateral and medial femoral condyles through two heads of origin. Together with the soleus and plantaris muscles, they form the superficial posterior compartment of the leg.

Medial

The medial musculature of the knee includes two muscles, the sartorius muscle of the anterior compartment of the thigh and the gracilis muscle of the medial or adductor compartment of the thigh. These muscles act at the level of the knee as flexors and internal rotators of the leg. Their insertion on the medial region of the tibia is characteristic and, together with the insertion of the semitendinosus muscle, is known as the *pes anserinus* (see Figs. 89.6C and 89.8). Knowledge of the anatomy and

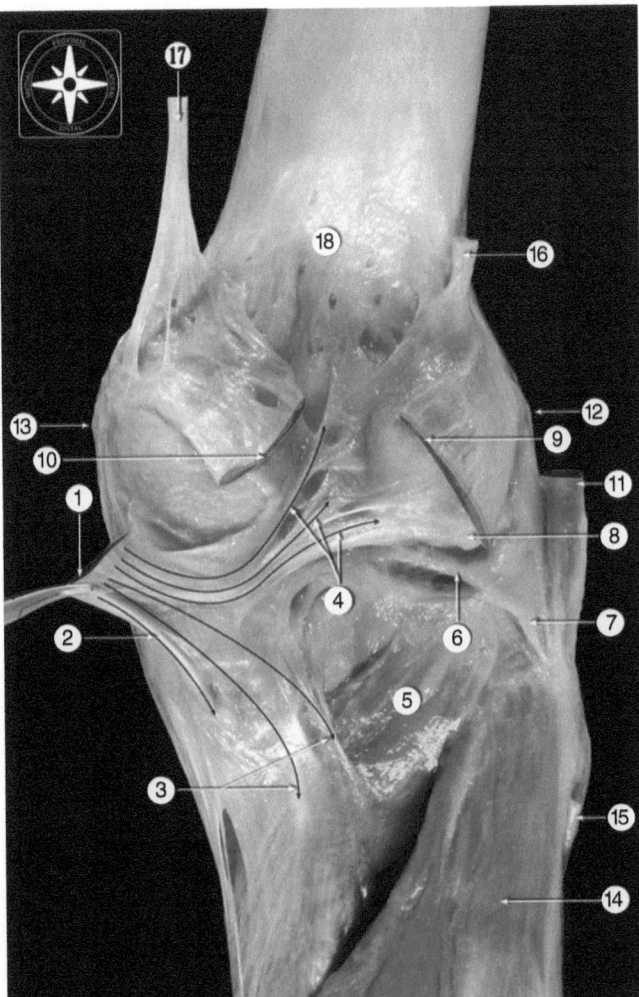

Fig. 89.7 Posterior view of the capsular structures of the knee joint. *1,* Semimembranosus tendon (cut). *2,* Direct expansion. *3,* Inferior or popliteal expansion. *4,* Oblique popliteal ligament. *5,* Popliteus muscle. *6,* Popliteus capsular extension. *7,* Fabellofibular ligament. *8,* Os fabella. *9,* Lateral head of gastrocnemius muscle (cut). *10,* Medial head of gastrocnemius muscle (cut). *11,* Biceps femoris tendon (cut). *12,* Lateral epicondyle. *13,* Medial epicondyle. *14,* Fibular origin of the soleus muscle. *15,* Common peroneal nerve (cut). *16,* Lateral intermuscular septum insertion (cut). *17,* Adductor magnus tendon insertion (cut). *18,* Popliteal surface. (Copyright Pau Golanó.)

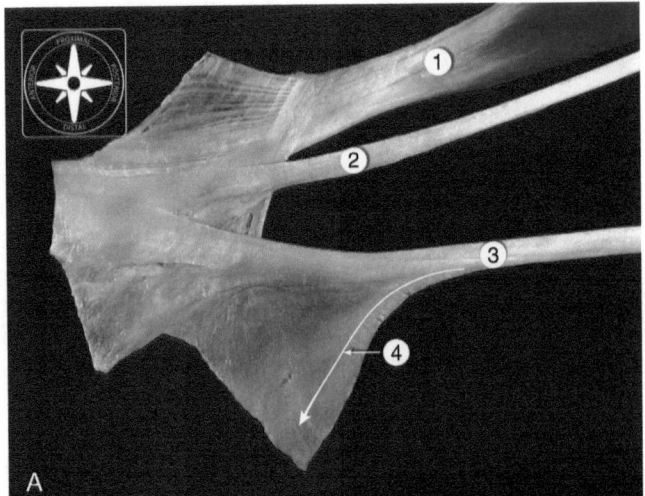

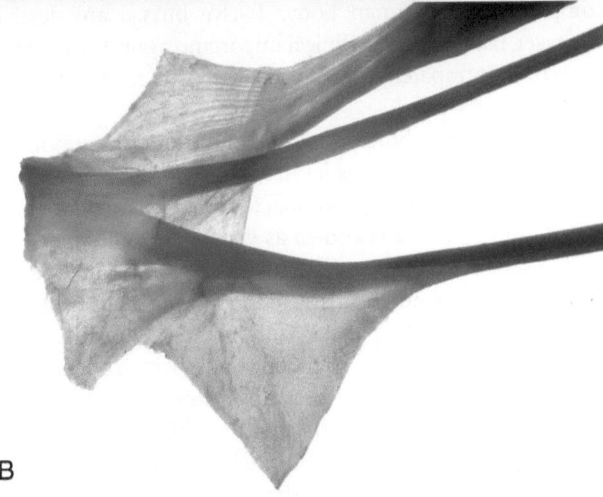

Fig. 89.8 Pes anserinus anatomy, deep view. (A) Anatomical dissection. (B) Anatomical dissection by transillumination. *1,* Sartorius tendon (superficial layer). *2,* Gracilis tendon. *3,* Semitendinosus tendon. *4,* Semitendinosus tendinous expansions directed toward the fascia of the medial head of the gastrocnemius muscle. (Copyright Pau Golanó.)

position of these tendons at the level of the pes anserinus is fundamental to correctly harvest autografts during reconstruction of the ACL or PCL.[12]

The pes anserinus insertion is, on average, 19 mm (range, 10 to 25 mm) distal and 22.5 mm (range, 13 to 30 mm) medial to the apex of the tibial tubercle, with an average width of 20 mm (range, 15 to 34 mm).[12] The sartorius inserts more anterior and superficially than the gracilis and the semitendinosus, and forms an aponeurotic fascia. On the superior margin of this fascia is a thickened band that can be confused with the tendon of the gracilis, which is immediately distal. This confusion at the moment of obtaining the graft would result in a tendon of smaller length and attached to a muscle belly. Posteriorly, and deep to the sartorius, lies the tendon of the gracilis at the proximal level and the tendon of the semitendinosus muscle at the distal level.[13] These last two tendons can be used for ACL reconstruction procedures. Both tendons (semitendinosus and gracilis) have tendinous expansions directed toward the fascia of the medial head of the gastrocnemius muscle[13] that need to be sectioned for correct harvesting of both tendons. If these expansions are not carefully freed from the tendons, the tendon stripper can inadvertently transect the main tendon, leaving the surgeon with a shortened graft (see Fig. 89.8).[12,14]

Lateral

The tendon of the biceps femoris muscle is the only tendon located at the lateral side of the knee. Its insertion is formed by three bands: one that is directed to the lateral part of the fibular head; another to the lateral condyle of the tibia, where it merges with the iliotibial tract; and finally a third one that comprises the deep fascia of the lateral part of the leg, where it coincides with the joint capsule of the knee. This muscle is a flexor at the level of the knee and an external rotator for the leg.

BURSAE

The knee has a system of bursae that is the most extensive and complex in the human body. Twelve bursae are described. However, based on their clinical importance, only the prepatellar, superficial infrapatellar, anserine, and gastrocnemius bursae are described.

The prepatellar bursa is located in the anterior region of the knee, at the subcutaneous level, anterior to the inferior half of the patella and to the superior half of the patellar tendon. Inflammation of this bursa is known as *housemaid's knee.*

The superficial infrapatellar bursa is also located in the anterior aspect of the knee and similarly in the subcutaneous plane, above the distal limit of the patellar tendon and the tibial tuberosity.

The anserine bursa is in the medial aspect of the knee. This bursa is located three fingerbreadths below the medial joint line and between the medial surface of the tibia, the MCL, and the tendons of the pes anserinus at the level of their insertion.

Two bursae are found in the posterior area, located deep between the heads of the medial and lateral gastrocnemius and the posterior joint capsule. The lateral subtendinous gastrocnemius bursa rarely communicates with the knee joint, but the medial bursa does so commonly. In certain occasions, the medial

subtendinous gastrocnemius bursa may enlarge and create a space known as a *Baker* or *popliteal cyst.*[15]

Menisci

The menisci, medial and lateral, are two half-moon–shaped fibrocartilage structures that cover the peripheral portion of the medial and lateral tibial condyles. In section, they are triangular with a peripheral base. Their superior surface is slightly concave, whereas the inferior is flat, adapting to the articular surface of the femoral and tibial condyles, respectively. Each meniscus is differentiated into 1) the center or meniscal body, 2) the meniscal ends or anterior and posterior horns, and 3) their attachment to the tibial surface, the meniscal roots (Fig. 89.9).

They are also inserted into the tibial condylar ridge through their capsular union or coronary ligament. In 50% to 90% of knees, the anterior horns are connected by a dense fibrous band named the anterior transverse ligament, anterior intermeniscal ligament, or anterior transverse geniculate ligament.[16–18] Both menisci slide with flexion and extension of the knee. The degree of this movement is larger for the lateral meniscus, with 9 mm, compared with 3 mm for the medial meniscus.[19,20]

Medial Meniscus

The medial meniscus possesses a semilunar or "C" shape. Because of its strong insertions at the level of the body and posterior horn, this meniscus is less mobile than the lateral and is exposed to a greater risk of injury. Anteriorly the meniscus does not have a connection to the capsular tissue or fat pad. Whereas in its medial portion it is firmly inserted into the deep capsular ligament, in its posterior body the meniscus is firmly fixed by the oblique popliteal ligament to blend with the joint capsule.

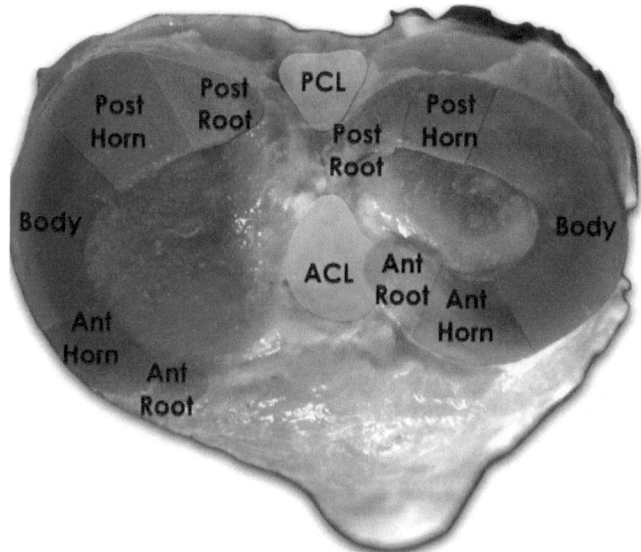

Fig. 89.9 Anatomic dissection demonstrating the shape of both menisci (medial and lateral). As seen in this left knee tibial plateau, the lateral meniscus has an "O" shape and the medial meniscus a "C" shape. The four zones of the meniscus are depicted (anterior and posterior roots [*Ant/Post Root*]; anterior and posterior horns [*Ant/Post Horn*]) and the body. The anatomic relationship to the anterior and posterior cruciate ligaments (*ACL* and *PCL*, respectively) is also shown.

Lateral Meniscus

The lateral meniscus is almost circular, with an "O" shape. Because of the poor union of the meniscus to the margin of the lateral tibial condyle and the absence of insertion in the zone where the popliteus tendon courses, the meniscus possesses a mobility that relatively protects it from injury. In 69% to 74% of knees, a dense fibrous band can be observed arising from the posterior meniscal horn and running upward and posteriorly to the PCL; it inserts on the medial femoral condyle, known as the posterior meniscofemoral ligament or the ligament of Wrisberg.[21-24] In approximately 50% to 74% of knees, another fibrous band can be observed arising from the posterior horn and passing upward and in front of the PCL, also terminating on the medial femoral condyle; it is named the anterior meniscofemoral ligament, or the ligament of Humphry (Fig. 89.10).[21,23-25]

Because many functions of the meniscus have been described, its resection can cause mechanical alterations that can lead to degenerative articular changes.[26] For this reason, avoidance of complete meniscal resection is advised. The degree of osteoarthritis (OA) and the time until OA onset are likely most dependent on the volume of meniscus taken at the time of surgery, as studies have shown that increasing meniscectomy size results in reduced contact area within the knee joint and thus greater contact pressures on the cartilage in the ipsilateral compartment.[27-32]

LIGAMENTS

Cruciate Ligaments
Anterior Cruciate Ligament

The ACL extends from the distal femur and attaches to the anterior medial portion of the tibia.[33] The average width of the midsubstance of the ACL is 10 to 11 mm, with a range of 7 to 17 mm

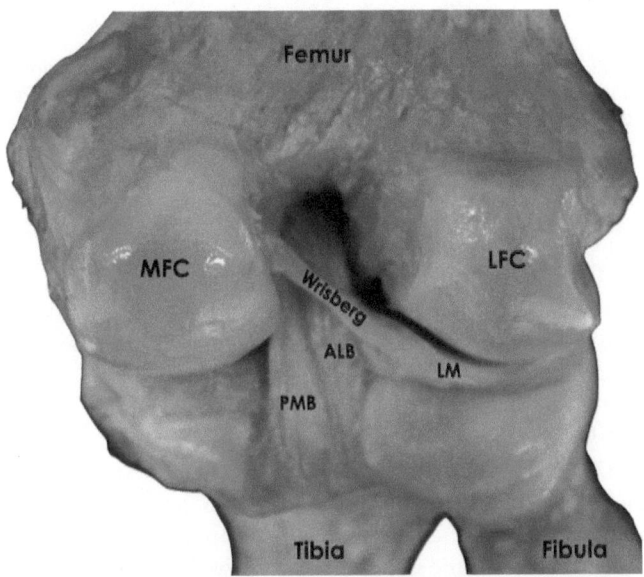

Fig. 89.10 Finely dissected posterior aspect of a right knee. The posterior meniscofemoral ligament (Ligament of Wrisberg) can be seen emerging from the posterior horn of the lateral meniscus *(LM)*. *ALB,* Anterolateral bundle of the posterior cruciate ligament; *LFC,* lateral femoral condyle; *MFC,* medial femoral condyle; *PMB,* posteromedial bundle.

and a thickness of 3.9 mm.[34,35] The isthmus (region of the ACL with the smallest cross-sectional area) is located an average 53.8% of the distance from the tibial insertion center to the femoral insertion center.[36] The cross-sectional area at the isthmus is smallest in extension and increases with flexion.[36] The ACL is formed by two bundles, the AM and PL, which are named according to their tibial insertion site. Each bundle comes into play at different points of knee flexion, as the ACL is not isometric. The load in the ligament shifts from bundle to bundle as the knee flexes throughout a normal range of motion (ROM).[37]

The LIR of the femur is present in 94% to 97% of human femora.[3,38] In an arthroscopic evaluation of 60 patients undergoing ACLR, Ferretti and associates[4] visualized the LIR in 100% of patients. The anterior margin of the ACL femoral attachment site is an average distance of 0.5 mm from the proximal part of the LIR.[38] The center of the ACL femoral attachment is an average of 1.7 mm proximal to the BR, with the AM bundle attachment center 4.8 mm proximal to the BR and the PL bundle attachment center 5.2 mm distal to the BR.[39]

The ACL is composed of thick sporadic bundles of collagen fibers encased in loose connective tissue. The random fiber arrangement gives the ligament a higher tensile strength than many other ligaments. The ACL is composed of two major types of fibers: one with a nonuniform diameter, which resists tensile forces, and one with a uniform diameter, which resists shearing forces.[40] The nonuniform diameter fibers account for 50.3% of the ACL and have a diameter ranging from 25 to 85 nm. The uniform diameter fibers account for 43.7% of the ACL and have a diameter of 45 nm. Elastic fibroblasts run between the larger fibers and account for the remaining 6% of ACL tissue.[40]

With the knee in extension, the femoral insertion site of the PL bundle is posterior and inferior to the AM bundle on the lateral femoral condyle (LFC).[41] Other studies have suggested that, approximately 2 to 3 mm from its femoral attachment, the AM and PL bundles connect to form a flat "ribbon" without a clear separation between the two.[42] At the tibia, the ACL inserts in an elliptical (51%), triangular (33%), or "C"-shape (16%).[43] The anterior lateral (AL) meniscal root inserts deeply beneath the ACL, with an average distance from the center of the ACL to the AL meniscal root attachment of 5.0 mm and an ACL-AL root overlap of 88.9 mm (Fig. 89.11).[2,44]

Posterior Cruciate Ligament

The PCL inserts in the posterior intercondylar area of the tibia and is directed to its attachment on the roof of the notch and the medial wall of the femoral intercondylar notch. As with the ACL, the presence of two different bundles has been described, the anterolateral (AL) and the posteromedial (PM).[45] In complete extension, the PM bundle of the ligament encounters more tension than the AL bundle, whereas during flexion, the PM fibers relax and the AL fibers are taut (Fig. 89.12).

Collateral Ligaments
Medial Collateral Ligament

The MCL, with a more or less triangular shape, is an intrinsic ligament that is intimately related to the medial meniscus and joint capsule, forming the medial meniscoligamentous complex.

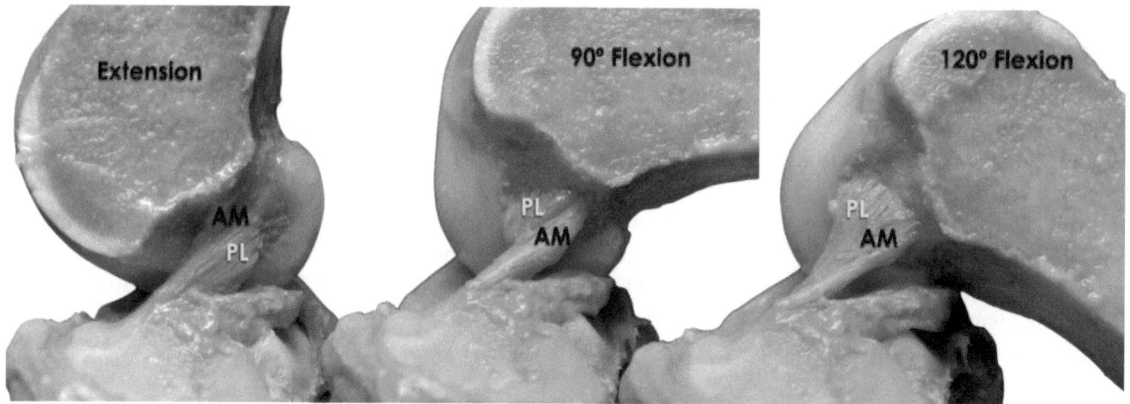

Fig. 89.11 Right knee dissection demonstrating the changes in shape and position of the *AM* (anteromedial bundle) and the *PL* (posterolateral bundle) of the anterior cruciate ligament. With the knee in extension, the femoral insertion site of the PL bundle is posterior and inferior to the AM bundle on the lateral femoral condyle.

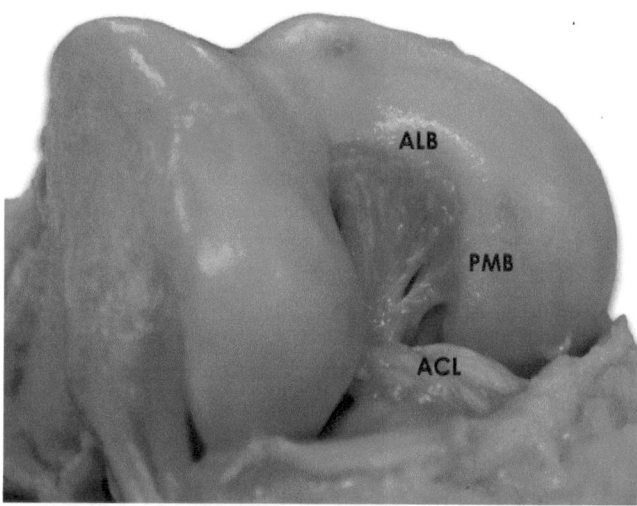

Fig. 89.12 Right knee dissection showing the *ALB* (anterolateral bundle) and *PMB* (posteromedial bundle) of the posterior cruciate ligament. Of note, the ALB travels almost vertically from the tibial PCL facet to the roof of the notch, adjacent to the cartilage. This bundle is more prominent than the PMB, which attaches more posteriorly (5 mm from the cartilage) in the medial wall.

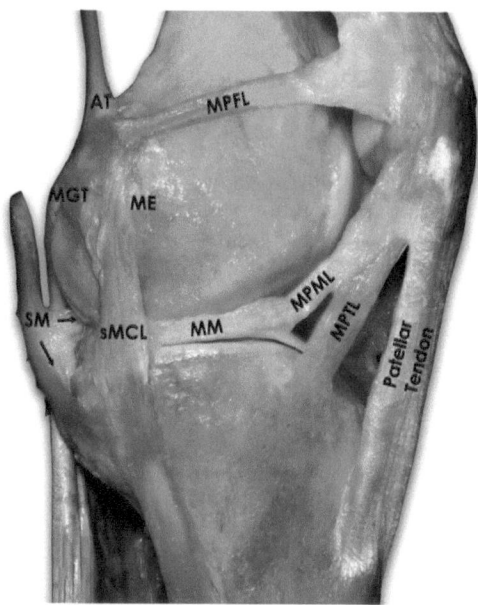

Fig. 89.13 Medial view of a left knee at 90 degrees of flexion demonstrating the attachment sites and orientations of the medial structures of the knee. *AT*, Adductor tendon; *ME*, medial epicondyle; *MGT*, medial gastrocnemius tendon; *MM*, medial meniscus; *MPFL*, medial patellofemoral ligament; *MPML*, medial patellomeniscal ligament; *MPTL*, medial patellotibial ligament; *SM*, semimembranosus; *sMCL*, superficial medial collateral ligament.

This ligament has two layers, one deep and the other superficial. The fibers of the deep layer extend from the medial femoral condyle to the medial tibial condyle. The fibers of the superficial layer extend like a fan from the medial epicondyle to the medial tibial condyle, posteriorly to the insertion of the pes anserinus, approximately 10 cm distal to the medial joint line. It then merges with the posterior joint capsule, where they form a strong capsular reinforcement known as the posterior oblique ligament (Fig. 89.13).[9,13]

Fibular Collateral Ligament

The fibular collateral ligament (FCL), a cordlike band, is considered an extrinsic capsular ligament between 5.5 and 7.1 cm in length[1] that extends from the LFC to the fibular head. At the proximal level, the ligament is closely related to the joint capsule, which is separated by fat, through which run the lateral inferior articular artery and veins at the level of the joint line.

Distally it attaches to the lateral aspect of the fibular head and has expansions anteriorly and posteriorly from the biceps femoris (Fig. 89.14).[1,46,47]

Anterolateral Ligament

In 1879, Paul Segond described an avulsion fracture (now known as a Segond fracture) at the anterolateral proximal tibia.[48] At the location of this fracture, Segond noted the presence of a "pearly, resistant, fibrous band that invariably showed extreme amounts of tension during forced internal rotation (of the knee)."[48] Although references to this ligament were occasionally made in the anatomy literature following Segond's discovery,[49] it was not until 2012 that Vincent and colleagues[50] named this ligament

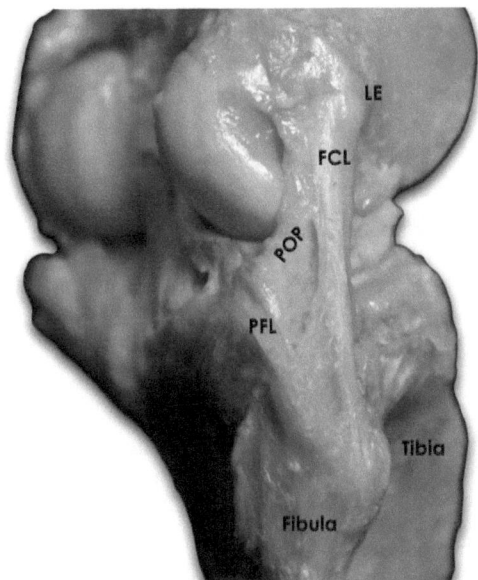

Fig. 89.14 Right knee dissection showing the posterolateral corner of the knee. In this picture, the fibular collateral ligament *(FCL)*, the *PFL*, (popliteofibular ligament) and popliteus tendon can be observed. Of note, the emergence of the FCL is slightly posterior and proximal to the lateral epicondyle. *LE*, Lateral epicondyle; *POP*, popliteus tendon.

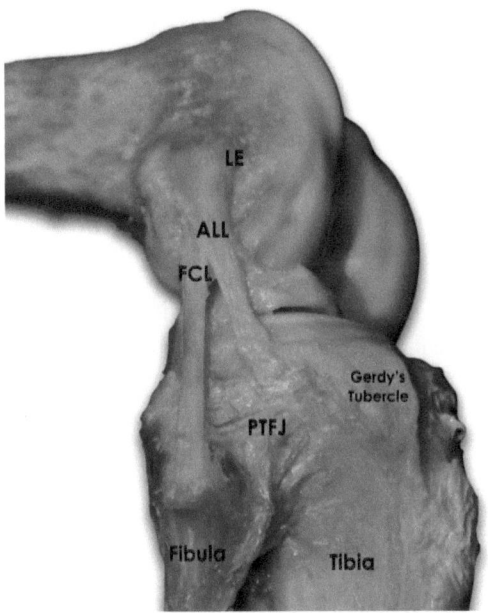

Fig. 89.15 Right knee dissection showing the relationship between the anterolateral ligament *(ALL)* and the fibular collateral ligament *(FCL)*. As seen in this picture, the ALL attachment on the femur is located almost 5 mm posterior and proximal to the center of the FCL.

what we know it as today, the anterolateral ligament (ALL). Interestingly, it was Claes in 2013 who has been given most credit for the "rediscovery" of the ALL following the publication of a detailed anatomical description of the ALL as found in a series of cadaveric knees.[48]

The ALL exists as a ligamentous structure that comes under tension during internal rotation at 30 degrees.[51] In the majority of specimens, the ALL can be visualized as a ligamentous structure, whereas in some cases it may only be palpated as bundles of more tense capsular tissue when internal rotation is applied.[52] The ligament originates on the femur and inserts on the tibia, with a mean length at full extension of 33 to 37.9 mm, a mean width of 7.4 mm, a mean thickness of 2.7 mm, and a mean cross-sectional area of 1.54 mm.[2,53–55] The ALL is not an isometric ligament.[54,56–58] The length of the ligament increases with knee flexion, which to a degree depends on the relationship of the femoral origin of the ALL and LCL.[56,57] The length of the ALL also increases with internal tibial rotation.[58]

The ALL originates on the femur either directly on the lateral epicondyle or posterior and proximal to the lateral epicondyle.[59,60] The ligament attaches to the femur in a fan-like shape with an average attachment area at its femoral origin of 67.7 mm.[2,51,59] The ligament may attach posterior and proximal or anterior and distal to the attachment site of the LCL.[51,53,57] The ALL overlaps with the LCL near its femoral origin. At the femoral origin, the mean diameter of the ALL is 11.85 mm.[59]

Between the femur and tibia, dense collagen fibers of the ALL insert onto the external surface of the lateral meniscus. The site of meniscal insertion is between the anterior horn of the lateral meniscus and the lateral meniscus body, with a mean attachment length of 5.6 mm.[61] Four types of meniscal attachment may be appreciated: complete, central, bipolar, or inferior-only.[62]

At the tibia, the ALL has an average attachment area of 53.0 to 64.9 mm[2] and attaches an average of 24.7 mm posterior to the center of Gerdy tubercle and 26.1 mm proximal to the anterior margin of the fibular head.[51,63] The tibial insertion site of the ALL can be found an average of 9.5 mm distal to the joint line and just proximal to the tibial insertion of the biceps femoris (Fig. 89.15).[51,63]

JOINT CAPSULE AND SYNOVIAL MEMBRANE

The knee has the most extensive joint cavity and synovial membrane of the human organism. The capsule extends from the patella and the patellar tendon anteriorly to the medial, lateral, and posterior expansions. Proximally it inserts on the femur, some three to four fingerbreadths above the patella, and distally it presents a circular insertion over the tibial ridge, except at the point where the popliteus tendon penetrates the joint traversing to its hiatus.

The capsule constitutes a fibrous membrane with a number of areas of thickening that act as reinforcement and are considered intrinsic ligaments (especially the medial and lateral patellofemoral ligaments). The capsule is reinforced posteriorly by the oblique popliteal ligament, an expansion of the semimembranosus that extends from medial and distal to proximal and lateral. The arcuate complex is found in the posterolateral corner.[11] These two structures contribute to the posterior stability of the knee. The popliteal oblique ligament is found in the floor of the popliteal fossa, the space for the popliteal artery and vein, and more superficially for the tibial nerve.

The synovial membrane not only covers the internal walls of the capsule but also surrounds the cruciate ligaments, the popliteus tendon, the coronal recesses situated beneath the menisci, and the infrapatellar fat pad (the Hoffa fat pad), situated behind the patellar tendon. The synovial folds are quite numerous, especially at the level of the suprapatellar pouch. Plicae are synovial folds and are considered vestigial synovial septae that were never reabsorbed during the developmental process of the knee. The three most frequent plicae or synovial folds are the infrapatellar (ligamentum mucosum), suprapatellar, and medial patellar plicae.[64–66]

The infrapatellar plica or ligamentum mucosum is encountered most frequently and is considered a normal structure in the knee joint (Fig. 89.16).[67] The medial patellar plica is the one that most frequently becomes symptomatic.[65]

The posterior synovial cavity communicates with the medial subtendinous bursa of the gastrocnemius muscle and can participate in the generation of a popliteal or Baker cyst.[15]

NEUROVASCULAR ANATOMY

Vascularization

The knee is vascularized by an extensive arterial plexus, superficial and deep, formed by seven arterial branches: five articular or genicular arteries, which are branches of the popliteal artery; the descending articular artery, a branch of the femoral artery; and the recurrent anterior artery, a branch of the anterior tibial artery.[68]

The superficial plexus forms a vascular circle around the patella.[69] The deep plexus is located between the inferior margin of the femur and the superior margin of the tibia. Of all the arteries that form the plexus, three require special attention for their contribution to the cruciate ligaments and the menisci: the lateral inferior genicular artery, the medial inferior genicular artery, and the middle genicular artery.

The blood supply of the menisci predominantly originates from the inferior medial and lateral genicular arteries.[70] Their

branches give off the parameniscal capillary plexus located on the peripheral ridge of the meniscus around its insertion on the posterior capsule. At the lateral side, the proximity of the articular genicular to the meniscal insertion to the capsule makes it susceptible to injury during lateral meniscal resection. On the medial side, the genicular artery lies some two fingerbreadths below the joint line and passes through a tunnel formed by the tibia and the MCL.

The vascularity of the cruciate ligaments is provided by the middle genicular artery and by a few branches of the inferior medial and lateral genicular arteries.[71–73] Although the medial genicular artery offers additional branches to the distal femoral epiphysis and to the proximal tibial epiphysis, the osseoligamentous junction of the cruciate ligaments does not significantly contribute to ligament vascularity. Although the ACL is capable of offering a vascular response after injury, spontaneous repair does not occur.[74]

Innervation

From a clinical point of view, it is worth mentioning the common peroneal nerve and the infrapatellar branch of the saphenous nerve.

- The common peroneal nerve is the terminal branch of the lateral sciatic nerve. It runs parallel and posterior to the tendon of the biceps femoris muscle in the posterolateral region of the knee until it reaches the fibular head.
- The infrapatellar branch of the saphenous nerve, a branch arising from the femoral nerve, runs through the medial and infrapatellar area of the knee, innervating the skin of the AM aspect of the knee. It can be injured when a medial knee incision is performed to obtain the gracilis and semitendinosus tendons, which are used for cruciate ligament reconstruction, MCL repair, or medial meniscus repair. Injury to this nerve can generate an anesthetic zone over the medial, anterior, and distal leg.[12,75–77]

BIOMECHANICS OF THE KNEE

The knee joint is the largest and most complex joint in the human body. The joint capsule and ligaments, which provide structural stability to the knee, are particularly vulnerable to injury by large moments that can be created through the forces acting along the long lever arms of the lower limb, and thus it is not surprising that the knee is one of the most frequently injured joints. An injury to the knee, such as disruption of the ACL, can result in an extensive disability because this injury may alter normal knee biomechanics and therefore locomotion. Knowledge of knee biomechanics provides an essential framework for understanding the consequences of injury and joint disorders; it aids in the intelligent planning of surgical procedures, serves as the basis for developing objective rehabilitation programs, and describes the effects of different types of orthoses on the knee joint.

The knee joint is composed of three independent articulations: one between the patella and femur, and the remaining two between the lateral and medial tibial and femoral condyles. The patellofemoral articulation consists of the patella, which

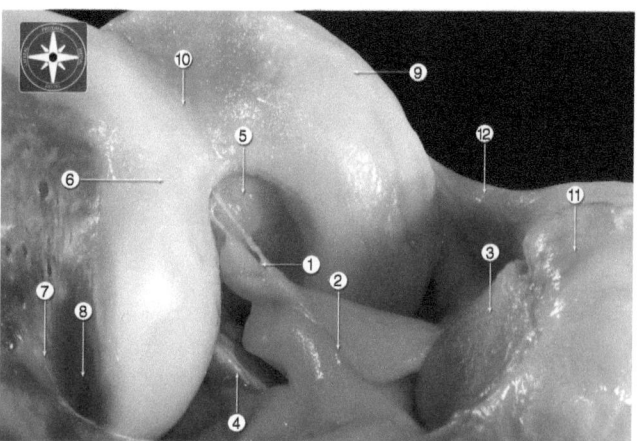

Fig. 89.16 Anatomic dissection of the anterior region of the knee joint showing the morphology and relationship of the infrapatellar plica or ligamentum mucosum. *1,* Infrapatellar plica. *2,* Infrapatellar fat pad (Hoffa's fat pad). *3,* Posterior surface or articular surface of patella. *4,* Anterior cruciate ligament. *5,* Femoral insertion of posterior cruciate ligament covered by a synovial fat pad. *6,* Lateral slope of the patellar surface. *7,* Epicondyle insertion of lateral collateral ligament. *8,* Popliteus tendon insertion. *9,* Medial slope of the patellar surface. *10,* Femoral trochlear groove. *11,* Deep surface of quadriceps tendon. *12,* Joint capsule. (Copyright Pau Golanó.)

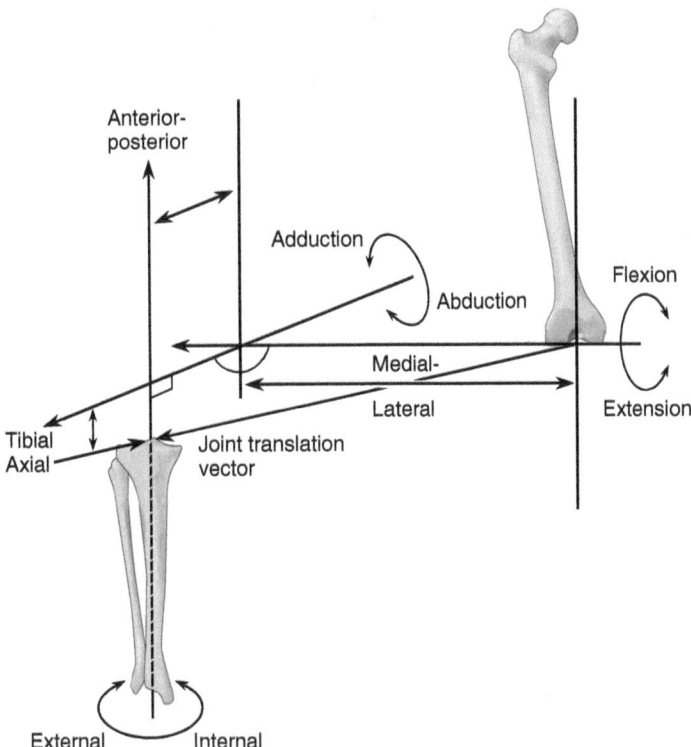

Fig. 89.17 Coordinate system for knee joint rotations and translations. Flexion-extension rotation is about the fixed femoral axis. Internal-external rotation is about a fixed tibial axis. Abduction-adduction is about an axis that is perpendicular to the femoral and tibial axes. The joint translations occur along each of the three coordinate axes. (From Hefzy MS, Grood ES. Review of knee models. *Appl Mech Rev.* 1988;41:1–13.)

has a multifaceted dorsal surface that articulates with the femoral trochlear groove. The tibiofemoral articulations consist of femoral condyles with saddle-shaped tibial condyles and interposing menisci. The posterior aspects of the femoral condyles are spherical in profile, whereas the anterior aspects of the femoral condyles are more elliptical. Thus in extension, the flat portions of the femoral condyles are in contact with the tibia, and in flexion, the spherical portions of the femoral condyles are in contact with the tibia.

To the untrained observer, the knee joint may appear to function as a simple pinned hinge (ginglymus), with flexion-extension rotation the only apparent motion between the femur and tibia. However, the motion characteristics of the knee joint are complex, requiring a full 6 degrees of freedom (three translations and three rotations) to completely describe the coupled, or simultaneous, joint motions (Fig. 89.17). An example of coupled motion is demonstrated with flexion rotation of the knee from the extended position. With this rotation, there is a coupled posterior movement of the femoral contact regions on the tibial surface in the sagittal plane and an internal rotation of the tibia relative to the femur in the transverse plane. By use of the Eulerian-based coordinate system described by Hefzy and Grood,[78] the translations and rotations can be described in anatomically referenced directions (see Fig. 89.17). Although many different types of coordinate systems have been used to describe three-dimensional knee motion, this system is appealing because it allows joint rotation to be expressed in terms familiar to the clinician. Grood and Noyes[79] have applied the three-dimensional coordinate system

to the interpretation of various clinical examination techniques and have developed a "bumper model" of the knee joint. This model is useful in describing the soft tissue restraints to anteroposterior translation and internal-external rotation of the knee joint. In addition, the model can be applied to demonstrate the types of tibiofemoral subluxations that may result when different soft tissue structures are disrupted. Application of this approach may aid in the examination of injuries to the knee ligaments and capsular structures.

This section assumes a working knowledge of the biomechanical terms essential to the description of knee function. For an introduction to basic knee biomechanics, the reader is encouraged to review the work of Mow and Hayes,[80] along with the definition of biomechanical terms as they apply to the knee presented by Noyes and coworkers.[81] A review of experimental studies of the tibiofemoral and the patellofemoral joints with associated contact morphometry studies is presented in this section.

DESCRIPTION OF BIOMECHANICAL TECHNIQUES

The American Society of Biomechanics has defined the term *biomechanics* as the study of the structure and function of biologic systems using the methods of mechanics. Specifically for the knee joint, this process involves modeling and experimental investigation techniques. Perhaps the most commonly described knee model is the crossed four-bar linkage called the *cruciate*

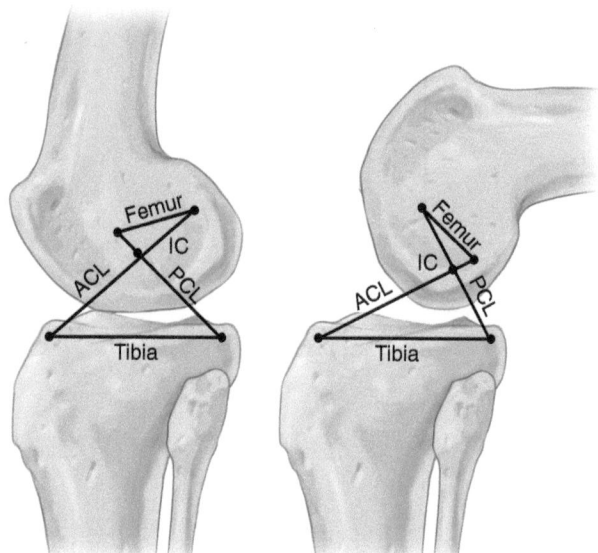

Fig. 89.18 The four-bar cruciate linkage model. The model includes two crossed bars, which represent the anterior and posterior cruciate ligaments (*ACL, PCL*). The remaining two bars represent the tibial and femoral attachments of the ligaments. *IC,* Instantaneous center of joint rotation. (From Hefzy MS, Grood ES. Review of knee models. *Appl Mech Rev.* 1988;41:1–13.)

linkage.[78,80,82–85] This approach has been used to study the interaction of the cruciate ligaments with the tibiofemoral joint (Fig. 89.18). The model consists of two crossed rods representing the cruciate ligaments and two connecting bars representing the tibial and femoral attachments of these ligaments. This approach has been used to describe the shape of both the tibial and femoral condyles, the path of the instantaneous center of knee joint rotation, and the posterior migration of the tibiofemoral contact point that occurs with knee flexion. The four-bar approach is based on rigid interconnecting cruciate linkages that are not allowed to elongate. Because the cruciate ligaments elongate and twist during normal joint articulation,[86–88] this technique may be inadequate for modeling the detailed interaction of the cruciate ligaments with the tibiofemoral joint.

Churchill and associates[89] described the knee in passive and active flexion, respectively, in three dimensions with use of a compound-hinge model. Flexion is described about the transepicondylar axis, and internal-external rotation is described about an axis parallel to the longitudinal axis of the tibia (Fig. 89.19). The model accounts for three-dimensional kinematics while allowing the axes to remain fixed in bone. Previous models use the concept of an instantaneous center of rotation, which accounts for femoral rollback by using a different center of rotation with each flexion angle.[90–92]

Coughlin and coworkers[93] characterized the 6 degrees of freedom of the tibiofemoral joint in terms of two rotations about the femoral epicondylar (FE) axis and an axis parallel to the anatomic tibial axis. The FE axis is defined as the line passing through the spherical centers of the medial and lateral condyles. In the midsagittal plane, the patella follows a circular arc with a constant radius of curvature. These axes remain nearly

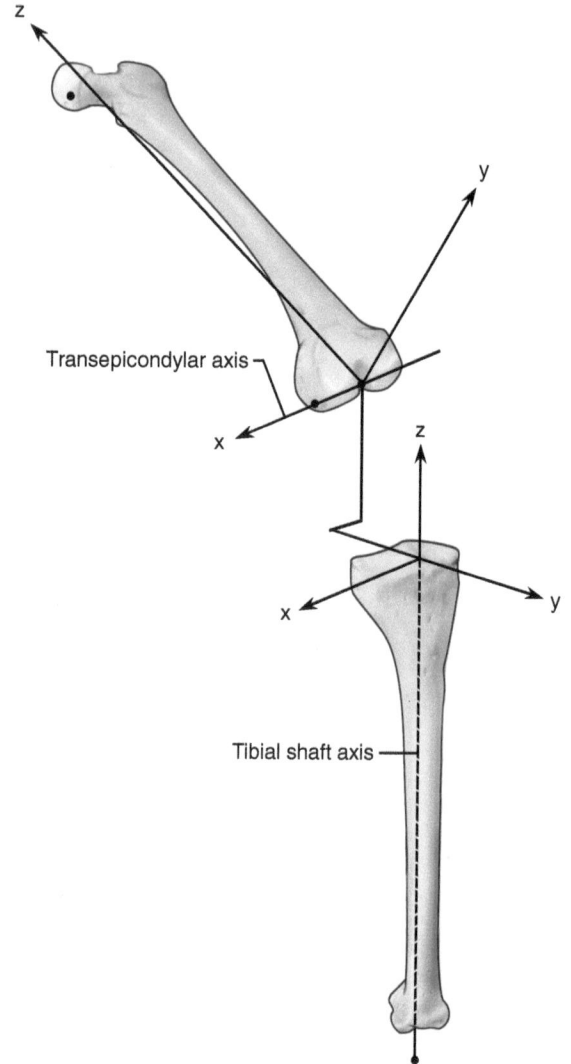

Fig. 89.19 The compound-hinge model describes the three-dimensional kinematics of the knee using two axes: the transepicondylar axis and an axis parallel to the longitudinal axis of the tibia.

perpendicular, with the patella tracking along a circular arc that can be described relative to the FE axis during flexion from 0 to 90 degrees. The authors suggest this model has clinical application in identifying the FE axis intraoperatively.[93]

TIBIOFEMORAL JOINT BIOMECHANICS

Force Measurement of Ligaments

Measurement of ligament or tendon force continues to be one of the biggest challenges in orthopedic biomechanics. To meet this challenge, Salmons[94] introduced the buckle transducer. The buckle transducer is a structure containing a beam over which the ligament is looped to create bending of the buckle frame. The beam is attached separately, and therefore transverse cutting of the ligament is not required. Lengthwise incisions are required, however, disrupting many ligament fibers and altering the normal function of the ligament by dissociating one group of fiber bundles from another.[95–97] Salmons[94] and other investigators[98–100] have applied this technique to various knee ligaments. This approach is limited to in vitro applications in which a knee ligament is instrumented with the transducer and then the knee joint is loaded, and the output from the buckle transducer is then directly recorded. After the tissue is tested in situ, it is dissected free from one of its bony attachments so that a known load can be applied to the tissue-buckle system and a calibration of the gauge–soft tissue system can be made. With use of this approach, the load can be determined for the tissue in situ.

Markolf and colleagues[101–104] have presented a direct approach to the measurement of ACL and PCL force in cadaveric knees. This technique involves isolating the tibial attachment of the cruciate ligament by creating a bone plug with a coring cutter and attaching a load sensor to the external portion of the bone plug. This approach facilitates the measurement of resultant cruciate ligament force. For example, the authors have used this approach to demonstrate that passive flexion-extension motion of the knee from 10 degrees to full flexion does not load the ACL, whereas loading of the quadriceps musculature (simulating active extension of the lower limb against gravity) developed ACL loading between the limits of 0 and 45 degrees. In later studies using human cadaver knees, Markolf and coworkers[105] demonstrated that hamstring loading has a greater effect on cruciate force than quadriceps loading. PCL force increases significantly with hamstring loading beyond 30 degrees of flexion.

Although direct force measurements of the cruciate ligaments are desirable, the current state-of-the-art force transducers allow the associated errors to fall within relatively large error bounds. Fleming and colleagues[106] reported mean errors ranging from 20% to 29% for the arthroscopically implantable force probe (AIFP), if it is calibrated after implantation. They noted that similar limitations have been reported for other force transducers that operate on the same principle, although the errors associated with other arthroscopic force transducers have not been reported. In addition, Fleming and colleagues[107] determined that the output of AIFPs is specimen dependent. When the force transducer was removed and reimplanted into the same location, the results were not repeatable, with errors ranging from 4% to 109%. Upon reimplantation into another location in the same ACL, the percentage errors ranged from 2% to 203%. These findings highlight a need for a more repeatable transducer that yields relative measurements of ACL stress in vivo. Because stress is directly related to strain, several investigators have chosen to measure strain in the ligaments. Beynnon and Fleming and coworkers[108,109] have shown that the accuracy associated with strain measurements in the ACL is on the order of 0.2% and 0.1% with use of the Hall-effect strain transducer and the differential variable reluctance transducer (DVRT), respectively.

Strain Measurement of Ligaments

Several investigators have measured ligament displacement, enabling the calculation of strain pattern, to understand the effect of knee joint position and muscle activity on ligament biomechanics.[110–115] Most of this work has been carried out in vitro, and the results are conflicting.

Edwards,[112] Kennedy,[113] Brown,[111] Berns,[116] Hull,[117] and their associates used mercury-filled strain gauges to measure the length of ligaments at various angles of knee flexion. Henning and colleagues[118] have constructed a device to measure displacement in the ACL in vivo.

Butler and associates[119] and Woo and colleagues[120] have developed optical techniques for mapping surface strains in various tissues. Butler and coworkers[119,121] used high-speed cameras to record the movements of surface markers and measured both midsubstance and insertion-site deformations of soft tissues. These techniques are ideal methods for monitoring surface strains, particularly during high-rate tests, but they are not useful for out-of-plane movements or for ligaments such as the cruciate ligaments that cannot be directly viewed. They also suffer from the theoretical disadvantage that the tissue of interest has to be exposed and therefore is not in a physiologic state.

Other investigators have calculated strain by measurement of the change of ligament attachment length under various applied joint loadings. For example, Wang and colleagues[115] measured the three-dimensional coordinates of pins stuck in a cadaveric joint at the palpated origin and insertion points of the major knee ligaments. They recorded the relationship between torque and angular rotation of the femur relative to the tibia. After excision of certain ligaments, the tests were repeated to determine the contribution of these elements to torsional restraint. In the most extensive and elegant studies, Sidles and associates[122] used a three-dimensional digitizer to compute ligament length patterns. In a slightly different approach, Trent and colleagues[123] used pins embedded in the ligament attachments and measured the displacement of one pin relative to the other. In addition, in this study they located the instant centers of transverse joint rotation. Warren and coworkers[124] also used pins placed at ligament origins but measured displacements with a radiographic technique.

The pins or other markers used as locators of ligament origin generally estimate average ligament strain. This technique may produce confusing results because of both the difficulty in choosing the center of a ligament insertion and the changes in strain from place to place within a ligament. For example, Covey and colleagues[125] demonstrated that the fiber anatomy across the PCL leads to differences in strain measurement among four geographically distinct areas of the ligament.

Previous work at the University of Vermont has focused on the measurement of ACL displacement in vitro by use of the Hall-effect strain transducer and, more recently, a DVRT, which allow for the calculation of strain.[110,114,126,127] This technique has been applied to the measurement of ACL strain in vivo.[86,87,109,126,128–130]

Ligament Biomechanics

The primary functions of the knee ligaments are to stabilize the knee, control normal kinematics, and prevent abnormal displacements and rotations that may damage articular surfaces. Ligaments are the most important static stabilizers and are primarily composed of type I collagen, the constituent that provides resistance to a tensile load developed along the length of the ligament; collagen fibers and their orientation within the tissue are responsible for the primary biomechanical behavior of these structures. The fibers of the large distinct ligaments are almost all arranged in parallel bundles, making them ideal for withstanding tensile loads, whereas capsular structures have a less consistent orientation, making them more compliant and not as strong in resisting axial loading. However, the fibers within ligaments do not act uniformly across a ligament during loading; using excursion filaments implanted in four distinct fiber regions of the PCL, Covey and associates[125] demonstrated the differential behavior of the fiber regions.

The ligament insertion sites are designed to reduce the chance of failure by distributing the stresses at the bone-ligament interface in a gradual fashion. This goal is accomplished by the passing of the collagen fibers from the ligament into the bone through four distinct zones: (1) ligament substance, (2) fibrocartilaginous matrix, (3) mineralized fibrocartilage, and (4) bone itself.[131] Despite the transitions, Noyes and colleagues[132] demonstrated that some strain concentration occurs near the ligamentous insertion sites. The knee ligaments can best control motion of the bones relative to each other if the motion takes place along the direction of the ligament fibers. For example, when the knee is loaded in valgus, the MCL develops a tensile stress in combination with a compressive force across the lateral compartment of the knee, and a resistance to medial joint opening is provided. Acting alone, ligaments cannot restrain the relative rotation associated with applied torques because the ligament would simply rotate about its bony insertion sites. A second force, usually developed through cartilage-to-cartilage compression, is required. For example, as the knee is loaded with an internal torque, a transverse rotation causes the femoral condyles to ride up the tibial spines (Fig. 89.20). This combination creates a compressive force across the tibiofemoral contact regions and an oppositely directed tensile force along the cruciate and collateral ligaments. This example may help demonstrate the mechanism by which the ACL interacts with tibiofemoral articular compression to resist an applied internal rotation to the knee joint.

The ability of a ligament to resist applied tensile loading may best be described through examination of the load-elongation curve produced during tensile failure testing of an ACL (Fig. 89.21). As a tensile load is applied, the ligament elongates; the slope of the measured load-displacement relationship represents the stiffness of the ligament. The steeper the slope of this curve, the stiffer the ligament. In the unloaded state, the ligament fibers are under minimal tension, and the collagen fibers have a wavy pattern. As a tensile load is applied, the wavy pattern begins to straighten. Initially little load is required to elongate the ligament, which is characterized by the relatively flat "toe" region of the curve. The change from the toe to the linear portion of the curve represents the change in stiffness that an examiner perceives during a clinical laxity examination when a ligament's end point is reached. As the tensile load continues to increase, all the collagen fibers are straightened, and the curve becomes nearly linear. This region of the curve characterizes the elastic deformation of the ligament until the yield point is reached. At this point, there is a sudden loss in the ability of the ligament to transmit load because some fibers within the ligament fail. If loading continues, a maximal or ultimate failure load is reached, and a sudden drop in load is recorded when many or all fibers fail, representing total failure of the ligament. The area under the load-deformation curve represents the amount of energy absorbed by a ligament during failure testing. Noyes

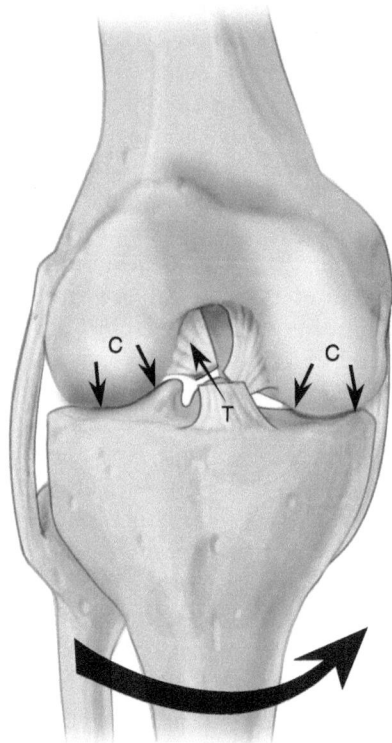

Fig. 89.20 Internal rotation of the tibia relative to the femur. The internal rotation causes the femoral condyles to ride up on the tibial spine, producing tension in the cruciate ligaments and a compressive force across the articular surfaces. *C,* Compressive force produced between the tibiofemoral articular surfaces; *T,* tensile load developed along the anterior cruciate ligament.

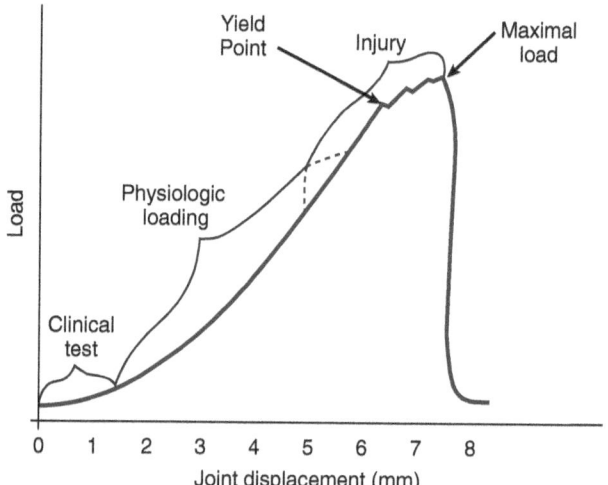

Fig. 89.21 Load-elongation curve for the tensile failure of the anterior cruciate ligament. (From Cabaud HB. Biomechanics of the anterior cruciate ligament. *Clin Orthop.* 1988;172:26.)

and associates demonstrated that the characteristics of the ACL's load-displacement curve are dramatically affected by variables such as age,[133] strain rate,[134] and duration of immobilization (disuse).[135] Young adults have a yield point that can be as much as three times greater than that of an older person.[133] In addition, Chandrashekar and coworkers[136] revealed sex-based differences in the material properties of the ACL. The female ACL withstood 8.3% lower strain at failure when evaluated in a tensile failure test, 14.3% lower stress, and 22.5% lower modulus of elasticity. Recent studies have revealed gender-based differences in joint laxity; Hsu and associates[137] found that the application of simultaneous tibial and valgus torque revealed 25% lower torsional joint stiffness in female knees as well as rotary joint laxity 30% higher than that for male knees.[137]

Most orthopaedic surgeons who operatively restore the function of the ACL perform an intra-articular reconstruction with autograft material.[138] Noyes and associates[132] characterized the relative strength of the various ligament replacement materials, demonstrating that a 14-mm wide bone–patella tendon–bone preparation was 168% as strong as the normal ACL, with the strength of all other autogenous replacements being less in comparison with the normal ACL. Woo and coworkers[139] have demonstrated that the normal tensile strength of the ACL may be as high as 2500 N rather than the original 1725 N standard presented by Noyes and associates.[132] This finding has led some surgeons to use combinations of autogenous graft material in an effort to increase the strength of the ACL replacement. Butler[140] used the primate model to demonstrate that maintaining a vascular supply to an ACL graft produces no material property differences in comparison with a similar free graft 1 year after implantation.

Papannagari and associates[141] demonstrated that bone–patellar tendon–bone autograft reconstruction does not restore normal knee kinematics under physiologic loading conditions. Three months after surgery, subjects displayed an additional 2.9-mm anterior translation of the tibia relative to the femur at full extension and 2.2-mm anterior translation at 15 degrees of flexion compared with the contralateral knee under weight-bearing conditions. Tashman and colleagues[142] developed a three-dimensional system to accurately assess dynamic joint motion, revealing abnormal kinematics in ACL-reconstructed knees during weight-bearing motion. A combination of radiographic targets inserted into bone to eliminate skin artifact for biplane imaging (radiographic stereophotogrammetric analysis) and subject-specific bone modeling revealed an additional 4-degree external rotation and 3-degree adduction in the tibiofemoral joint of the ACL-reconstructed knee compared with the contralateral normal limb during dynamic weight-bearing motion.[142]

Zantop and coworkers[143] assessed the role of the anteromedial bundle (AMB) and posterolateral bundle (PLB) of the ACL in tibial translation and rotary laxity. AMB transection significantly increased anterior tibial translation at 60 and 90 degrees, whereas isolated PLB transection resulted in increased tibial translation at 30 degrees of flexion in addition to increased combined internal-external rotation in response to internal-external rotary load. From these results, the investigators concluded that ACL reconstruction should include both bundles to restore normal translational and rotational kinematics. Mae and colleagues[144] examined the force sharing of AM and posterolateral grafts in "anatomic" two-bundle reconstruction in response to 134-N anterior tibial loading. They observed that this reconstruction technique yielded grafts that shared force similarly to the two bundles of the normal ACL.[144]

Function of the Cruciate Ligaments in Controlling Joint Biomechanics

The concept of primary and secondary knee stabilizers was introduced by Butler and colleagues,[145] who demonstrated that the ACL is a primary restraint to anterior translation of the tibia relative to the femur, providing an average restraint of 87.2% to the applied load at 30 degrees. With the knee at 90 degrees, this restraint was 85.1%. After ACL transection, the remaining intact ligamentous structures provided little restraint to anterior subluxation, leading Butler to describe the function of the remaining soft tissues as secondary restraints to this particular motion. The remaining ligament and capsular structures each contributed less than 3% to the total restraining force resulting from an applied anterior shear load. Butler and colleagues[145] demonstrated that the PCL is the primary restraint to posterior translation of the tibia relative to the femur, providing 94% of the restraining force at 90 and 30 degrees of knee flexion. None of the remaining ligamentous and capsular secondary structures contributed more than 2% of the total restraining force to an applied posterior shear load. Markolf and colleagues[146] compared posterior tibial translation after isolated transection of the PLB of the PCL and found small increases in laxity after transection at 0 and 10 degrees of flexion. Sectioning of the PLB had no significant effect at higher flexion up to 90 degrees. Force measurements of the anterolateral bundle remained unchanged with PM bundle sectioning, leading the authors to conclude that the anterolateral bundle was the primary restraint to posterior tibial translation.

Fukubayashi and associates[147] investigated the coupled behavior between anteroposterior shear loading and internal-external tibiofemoral rotation in human cadavers. They showed that interaction of the ACL with tibiofemoral geometry produces an internal tibial rotation with anterior-directed shear load applied across the tibiofemoral joint, whereas the PCL produces an external tibial rotation with applied posterior shear loading. The magnitude of tibial rotation, coupled with applied anteroposterior shear loading, decreased after transection of either cruciate ligament.

Gollehon and coworkers[148] investigated the role of the cruciate ligaments, LCL, and deep complex (arcuate ligament and popliteus tendon) in joint stability. This investigation showed that the PCL was the principal structure resisting posterior translation of the tibia relative to the femur. Isolated transection of the PCL did not affect varus or external rotation of the knee. Transection of the PCL, LCL, and deep complex was then performed to investigate the effects of a combined injury. This transection created a significant increase in varus rotation, posterior translation, and external rotation at all angles of knee flexion, suggesting that subjects with such a combined injury may have a functionally impaired joint. Combined sectioning of the ACL and the posterolateral structures produced a significant increase in internal-external rotation of the tibia, indicating that patients with this combined injury may also have compromised knee function.[148]

Similar methods were used by Markolf and coworkers, and their coupled-motion results are in agreement with those of Gollehon and colleagues. Markolf et al.[149] also measured force in the cruciate ligaments and found that the cruciate ligaments become load-bearing structures with the application of varus rotation after transection of the LCL and deep complex.[149] The same group measured force in the ACL and the PCL in the intact cadaveric knee under combined loading conditions.[104,150] They found that force in the ACL increases most in response to anterior directed forces applied to the tibia combined with internal tibial torque when the knee is near full extension. Force in the ACL was also increased when anterior tibial force was combined with a valgus moment at knee flexion angles greater than 10 degrees. The combination of posterior tibial force, varus moment, and internal torque produced the greatest forces in the PCL. In addition, they reported that the forces in the ACL were higher than the forces in the PCL in forced hyperflexion.[102,103,149] More recently, Withrow and coworkers[151] confirmed the results of Markolf and colleagues regarding the effect of valgus loading on the ACL. Peak strain in the AM aspect of the ACL increased 30% with the addition of valgus loading in combination with impulsive compression loading, leading the authors to suggest that minimizing valgus loading, or abduction, during impulsive compression may reduce ACL strain.

Grood and associates[152] investigated the role of the PCL and posterolateral structures (LCL, arcuate ligament, and popliteus tendon) in the control of knee joint biomechanics. Isolated sectioning of the PCL revealed that the amount of posterior tibial translation, measured relative to the femur, was twice as much at 90 degrees compared with that at 30 degrees of knee flexion. This amount of translation occurred without abnormal axial tibial rotation and varus-valgus rotation. The concurrent increase in posterior laxity with flexion of the knee was attributed to slackening of the posterior portion of the joint capsule, which provides a secondary restraint to posterior translation. The authors concluded that clinical examination of the PCL should be performed at 90 degrees of flexion, because at this degree the secondary restraints are less effective in blocking posterior tibial translation.[152] At this knee angle the clinician can gain a full appreciation of the PCL contribution to joint laxity. Removal of the posterolateral complex while leaving the PCL intact produced an increase in both external tibial rotation and varus rotation. The increase in external rotation was greatest at 30 degrees of flexion, at which point it was two times larger compared with that measured at 90 degrees. This finding demonstrated that the posterolateral complex provides the primary restraint to external rotation with the knee at 30 degrees. Therefore the authors recommend clinical examination of the posterolateral complex with the external rotation examination while the knee is between 20 and 40 degrees of flexion.[152] A significant increase in external tibial rotation with the knee flexed to 90 degrees required transection of both the PCL and the posterolateral complex. This finding suggests that in a clinical examination demonstrating a significant increase in external tibial rotation with the knee at 90 degrees of flexion, deficiencies in both the PCL and posterolateral complex may exist.

Several investigators have measured ACL displacement patterns, enabling calculation of strain pattern, to understand the effect of knee joint position and muscle activity on ligament biomechanics.[97,110,113,116,122,124,153] Most of this work has been carried out in vitro, and the results are conflicting. The results of in vitro studies do not capture the effects of muscle activity or the effects of body weight, soft tissues, and secondary stabilizers in the knee.

In vivo studies have used magnetic resonance imaging and three-dimensional computer modeling techniques to observe morphologic changes in ligaments, such as elongation, rotation, and twist.[88,154] Li and coworkers[154] demonstrated the elongation and rotation that the ACL undergoes during weight-bearing flexion. The ACL length decreased by 10% at 90 degrees flexion compared with full extension. At 30 degrees of flexion, the ACL exhibited a 20-degree internal rotation. At lower flexion angles, the ACL oriented 60 degrees vertically and 10 degrees laterally, leading the authors to suggest that the ACL may have a greater role in weight-bearing activities at lower flexion angles. Li and associates[88] used the same technique to demonstrate the reciprocal behavior of the ACL and PCL in vivo during weight-bearing flexion. The AMB of the ACL displayed a relatively constant length from full extension to 90 degrees of flexion, whereas the PLB shortened. Both bundles of the PCL elongated during flexion, leading the authors to highlight the reciprocal behavior of the ACL and PCL under weight-bearing flexion, rather than that of the two bands of the ACL.[88]

Beynnon and Fleming and colleagues[86,87,126,128,155] have measured the in vivo strain biomechanics of the ACL in humans. This work involved arthroscopic implantation of the Hall-effect strain transducer or the DVRT into the AMB of the ACL after the routine surgical procedure was complete. These subjects had normal ACLs and consented to have their surgery performed with use of local anesthesia, allowing them full control of the lower limb musculature. The objective of these studies was to provide invaluable data for the clinical management of patients with ACL ruptures.

It was revealed that anterior shear loads of 150 N applied at 30 degrees of flexion (the Lachman test) produced more strain within the normal AMB than did shear testing at 90 degrees (the anterior drawer test).[87,155] It was possible to predict AMB strain from anterior tibial translation at 30 degrees of flexion but not at 90 degrees of flexion.[155] These in vivo results[87] are in agreement with previously published studies that used either instrumented knee laxity testing or clinical impressions to assess the behavior of the ACL under clinical examination conditions and to confirm that the Lachman test is the clinical examination of choice to evaluate the integrity of the ACL.[156–161]

The in vivo study revealed that no significant change in ACL strain occurred during isometric quadriceps contraction when the knee was maintained at a flexion angle of 90 degrees.[87] At this flexion angle, the ACL remained unstrained as quadriceps activity increased. Isometric quadriceps strengthening should therefore be safe in the ACL-injured or reconstructed knee if the flexion angle is maintained at 60 and 90 degrees. At 15 and 30 degrees of knee flexion, isometric quadriceps activity produces a large increase in AMB strain and should be carefully controlled, especially during the early stages of rehabilitation after reconstruction in which soft tissue fixation may be tenuous.[87,162] The in vivo ACL strain study[87] indicated that the knee flexion angle at which isometric quadriceps activity produced an increase in ACL strain and may become unsafe for the injured or reconstructed

ACL was somewhere between 45 and 50 degrees. The model predictions presented by Nisell and coworkers[163] suggest that isometric quadriceps extension efforts at knee angles between 60 and 0 degrees may become unsafe for a newly reconstructed ACL, whereas this activity would be safe for a PCL reconstruction. Isometric quadriceps extension with the knee positioned between 60 degrees and full flexion may be unsafe for a PCL reconstruction, whereas this activity would be safe for an ACL reconstruction.

Fleming and coworkers[164] used in vivo strain measurement to demonstrate that the gastrocnemius muscle acts as an antagonist to the ACL. Gastrocnemius contraction produced greater strain on the ACL at 5 and 15 degrees of flexion than at 30 and 45 degrees. The authors proposed that development of rehabilitation programs should take into account knee flexor torque supported by the gastrocnemius when it is desirable to minimize strain on the healing ACL graft.[164]

In vivo strain measurement within the ACL when a seated subject performed an isotonic quadriceps contraction (active range of motion [AROM]) consistently revealed ACL strain between 10 and 48 degrees and an unstrained region between 48 and 110 degrees of flexion.[87] AROM rehabilitation programs may now be prescribed with these two flexion angle regions adapted to the clinician's requirements. In the unstrained region, quadriceps activity associated with AROM did not produce significantly different ACL strain values in comparison with the same knee motion without contraction of the leg musculature (flexion-extension motion of the subject's knee performed by an investigator and termed passive range of motion [PROM]).[87] This finding suggests that AROM between the limits of 50 and 100 degrees may be performed safely immediately after ACL reconstruction. The AROM activity may then move to flexion angles nearer full extension, when the ACL graft and fixation will tolerate greater levels of strain.[87] The maximal AROM strain values were greater (ranging between 4.1% and 1.5%) than the maximal PROM strain values.[87] Application of a 10-lb boot to a subject's foot during the AROM activity increased the ACL strain values compared with the same activity without a weighted boot.

ACL strain was also evaluated during open and closed kinetic chain exercises and revealed no significant differences between the two exercises evaluated.[126] This finding suggests that the specific closed kinetic chain exercise evaluated (squatting with and without resistance) is not necessarily "safer" than the open kinetic chain exercise tested (active flexion-extension). The results conflict with the results of some cadaveric studies, which conclude that closed kinetic chain activities are safer for the ACL than open kinetic chain activities.[101,165] In a separate study, our group reported strains of the same magnitude (about 2.7%) during stair climbing.[129] In addition, we investigated strain in the ACL during steady-state cycling and found the mean peak strain to be half of that experienced during closed kinetic chain exercises (squatting) or open kinetic chain exercises (active flexion-extension).[130] The results imply that cycling may be a safe method of rehabilitating the knee musculature without damaging a healing ACL.

Fleming and coworkers[166] evaluated strain in the ACL during flexor-extensor exercises against resistance torque with and without a compressive load applied at the foot. Application of a

compressive load did not reduce the peak strain measurement of the ACL. However, ACL strain did not increase with an increase in resistance while the compressive load was applied.[163] The same group later demonstrated that one-legged closed kinetic chain exercises did not produce more strain on the ACL than two-legged exercises.[167] Peak ACL strain values at 30, 50, and 70 degrees of flexion were similar during four exercises: single-leg step-up and step-down, lunge, and one-legged sit-to-stand. The strain values were greatest at 30 degrees of flexion across all exercises. These results led the investigators to suggest that closed kinetic chain exercises can be used with increased resistance to rehabilitate muscles without placing additional strain on the healing ACL graft.[166,167]

Our findings illustrate that both muscle activity and knee position determine ACL strain at rest and with joint motion.[87] A ranked comparison of the different activities evaluated in subjects with normal ACLs, ordered from high to low risk on the basis of peak strain values, has been used to develop rehabilitation programs after ACL reconstruction.[168]

In vivo strain measurement within the ACL for PROM between 110 degrees and full extension revealed that the ACL is strained as the joint is brought into extension, and measurement remains at or below the zero strain level between the limits of 11.5 and 110 degrees of flexion when distal leg support loading is used.[87] Therefore continuous passive motion of the knee within these limits should be safe for the reconstructed ACL immediately after surgery when the leg is supported throughout flexion-extension motion without applied varus or valgus loading, internal or external torques, or anterior shear forces. However, the limits of near extension (0 to 10 degrees) can cause small magnitudes of strain (1% or less).[87] We believe this should not be viewed as a constraint to bracing a patient's knee in the fully extended position (0 degrees) or to the use of continuous passive motion during a rehabilitation program.

The cruciate ligaments serve several functions as passive stabilizers of the knee. The cruciate ligaments guide the knee joint through normal biomechanics, as demonstrated by the four-bar linkage model. The anterior and PCLs are the primary restraints to corresponding anterior and posterior translation of the tibia relative to the femur and have a reciprocal relationship during weight-bearing flexion. The coupled internal and external tibial rotation that occurs with corresponding anterior and posterior shear loading is controlled in part by the cruciate ligaments and should be considered a significant aspect of the clinical examination. In addition, the cruciate ligaments act as secondary restraints to varus-valgus motion of the knee joint.

Medial and Lateral Collateral Ligaments and Their Function in Controlling Joint Biomechanics

Warren and associates[124] assessed the restraining action of the MCL complex in human cadaver specimens. They demonstrated that sectioning of the superficial long fibers of the MCL complex produced a significant increase in valgus rotation of the tibiofemoral joint in experiments performed at 0 and 45 degrees of knee flexion. Sectioning the posterior oblique or deep medial portions of the MCL complex had no significant effect on increasing valgus knee angulation.

Grood and colleagues[169] also investigated the medial ligament complex and presented results that support the findings of the Warren group.[124] More recently, Ellis and associates[170] demonstrated in cadaveric knees that ACL deficiency led to an increase in MCL insertion site and contact forces during anterior tibial loading and had no effect during valgus loading, indicating that the ACL does not play a role in valgus restraint. These results led the investigators to suggest that increased valgus laxity during clinical examination of an ACL-deficient knee would indicate MCL compromise.[170]

Grood and coworkers[169] demonstrated that the long superficial portion of the MCL complex provided 57% of the valgus restraint at 5 degrees, which increased to 78% at 25 degrees of flexion. The variable restraint behavior with valgus loading was attributed to the restraint provided by the posterior medial capsule, which decreased as the knee was moved from an extended into a flexed position. Haimes et al.[171] studied intact and MCL-deficient cadaveric knees and found that a coupled external rotation is associated with abduction in an MCL-deficient knee at extension, 15 degrees of flexion, and 30 degrees of flexion. In contrast, the intact knees studied had a coupled internal rotation associated with abduction. This finding (i.e., the presence of a coupled external rotation as opposed to a coupled internal rotation) may be used in physical examination for diagnosis of isolated MCL injuries.

Grood and coworkers[169] investigated the LCL complex. They demonstrated that in response to varus stress, this complex limits lateral opening of the joint. In response to varus loading, the LCL was found to provide 55% of the total restraint at 5 degrees and 69% at 25 degrees of knee flexion. An increase in the contribution of the LCL to the total varus restraint resulted as the knee was brought from an extended to a flexed position. This change was attributed to a decrease in resistive support provided by the posterior portion of the lateral capsule as the knee was flexed. With the knee joint in full extension, the investigators demonstrated that the secondary restraints (including the cruciate ligaments and the posterior portion of the joint capsule) block opening of the knee joint after the collateral ligaments have been cut.[172] Simulating the forces applied by the dynamic stabilizers (the iliotibial tract and biceps muscles) revealed their important contribution to varus stability of the knee in vivo.[169] The contribution of the dynamic stabilizers to overall laxity of the knee is difficult to assess because the actual muscle force magnitudes for a specific activity are unknown. In a later investigation, Gollehon and associates[148] studied the contribution of the LCL and deep ligament complex (popliteus tendon and arcuate ligament) to joint laxity. They demonstrated that the LCL and deep ligament complex function together as the principal structures resisting varus and external rotation of the tibia.[148] Höher and colleagues[173] conducted a cadaver study and concluded that the LCL and popliteus carry most of the force in PCL-deficient knees under a posterior load at high flexion angles. Further, they loaded the popliteus in tension to simulate muscle activation and found that the force in the popliteus complex was significantly greater than the force in the LCL at all flexion angles tested (0 to 90 degrees) in both intact cadaveric knees and PCL-deficient knees.

MENISCAL BIOMECHANICS

Function of the Meniscus in Load Transmission

Meniscal injury is thought to be the most common injury sustained by athletes.[174] The menisci were originally thought to be vestigial structures that served no significant function for the tibiofemoral joint.[175] The meniscus was thought to be an expendable structure; this perspective prompted many orthopaedists to treat meniscal tears by completely removing the meniscus.[176-180] As recently as 1971, Smillie[180] recommended complete removal of the meniscus even if the posterior horn was the only structure suspected of being damaged at the time of anterior arthrotomy. Conversely, as early as 1948, Fairbank[181] had suggested the load-transmission function of the meniscus and postulated that a complete meniscectomy frequently resulted in tibiofemoral joint space narrowing, flattening of the femoral condyles, and osteophyte formation. In long-term follow-up studies performed in the late 1960s and 1970s, several investigators confirmed Fairbank's observations, reporting a high incidence of unsatisfactory results after a complete meniscectomy was performed.[182-184] It was not until the mid-1970s that several biomechanical studies confirmed the clinical observations by measuring the load-transmission function of the meniscus.[172,185-192] These investigations predicted that between 30% and 99% of the load transmitted across the tibiofemoral joint passes through the menisci during weight-bearing activities.

Maquet and colleagues[187] used a contrast injection radiography technique to measure contact area in human cadaver specimens subjected to a physiologic compressive load. This study revealed a posterior translation of the medial and lateral contact areas as the knee was brought from an extended to a flexed position, along with a decrease in contact surface area with knee flexion. The contact area also decreased significantly with meniscectomy, leading Maquet and colleagues to postulate that the menisci transmitted a significant proportion of tibiofemoral compressive load.

Seedhom and Hargreaves[188,189] reported that 70% to 99% of the tibiofemoral compressive load is transmitted through the normal menisci and that all of the load is transmitted through the posterior horns of the menisci with joint flexion past 75 degrees. These investigators also revealed that partial removal of the meniscus decreased the compressive stress transmission of the joint to a lesser extent compared with removal of the entire structure, provided that the circumferential continuity of the meniscus was maintained. More recently, Zielinska and Donahue[193] used a three-dimensional finite element model to quantify changes in contact pressure in response to varying degrees of medial meniscectomy. The maximal contact pressure and contact area were linearly correlated with the proportion of the meniscus removed. The investigators revealed that removal of 60% of the medial meniscus increases the contact pressure on the remaining meniscus by 65% and by 55% on the medial tibial plateau.[193]

Krause and coworkers[186] reported an increase in stress across the knee joint of about three times in the canine model and two and one-half times in human cadaver knees after removal of both menisci. The investigators also measured the circumferential displacement of the medial meniscus with an applied axial compressive load, demonstrating the presence of "hoop," or tangential stress, acting at the outside fibers of the meniscus. This observation led Johnson and Pope[194] to demonstrate how the meniscus absorbs energy by undergoing circumferential elongation as a load is developed across the knee joint. As the joint compresses, fibers elongate. Thus the meniscus absorbs energy and reduces the impulsive shock loading that would otherwise be developed across the articular cartilage and subchondral bone.

Ahmed and Burke[195] directly measured the tibiofemoral pressure distribution using a microindentation transducer. They demonstrated that the medial and lateral menisci transmit at least 50% of the compressive load imposed on the tibiofemoral joint in the flexion range between 0 and 90 degrees. Removal of the medial meniscus caused a reduction in the contact area that ranged between 50% and 70%, with the latter reduction occurring at greater axial load. Because articular contact stress is inversely proportional to contact area, a 50% decrease in the contact area would cause a twofold increase in contact stress.

Allen and colleagues[196] determined the resultant load acting on the meniscus in human cadaver knees using an instrumented testing system. They found that the application of a 134-N anterior tibial load on an ACL-deficient knee significantly increases the resultant force acting on the medial meniscus compared with an intact knee at all flexion angles tested (0, 15, 30, 60, and 90 degrees). On the basis of the results, they suggest that ACL reconstruction contributes to the goal of preserving meniscal integrity.

These biomechanical investigations provide a basis for the concept of partial meniscectomy, which has been made possible with the technology provided by modern arthroscopic surgery. There can be no doubt that partial meniscectomy provides better results compared with total excision of that structure.[197]

Function of the Meniscus in Joint Stability

The menisci have been shown to provide increased geometric conformity to the tibiofemoral joint (thereby optimizing contact stress) and to share efficiently in the transmission of the tibiofemoral compressive load. Johnson and associates[183] and Tapper and Hoover[184] have performed postoperative clinical examinations in patients undergoing meniscectomy. Both studies revealed an increased varus-valgus and anteroposterior laxity in 10% to 25% of these patients, leading the investigators to conclude that the menisci provide some ability to stabilize the knee joint in connection with knee ligaments and bony geometry. The clinical follow-up study presented by the authors suggested a relationship between an increase in joint laxity after complete meniscectomy and sequelae of marginal spur formation and even degenerative changes.[183]

Bylski-Austrow and coworkers[198] subjected human cadaver knees to physiologic loads at three flexion angles and measured displacements of the menisci radiographically. The tibias were either loaded in the anteroposterior direction with 100 to 150 N or torqued to 10 to 15 Nm. In all cases, a 1000-N compressive load was applied to the tibiofemoral joint. Internal rotation caused the lateral meniscus to move 3 to 7 mm farther posteriorly than the medial meniscus moved anteriorly. Similarly, external rotation caused the medial meniscus to move posteriorly and

the lateral meniscus to move a greater distance anteriorly. In all cases, the menisci "stayed with the femur" as the tibia was moved. The authors suggest that increased or decreased meniscal displacement, caused by ligament injury, meniscal repair, or meniscal replacement, might increase the risk for meniscal injury.

Shefelbine and associates[199] performed an in vivo study of human knees using magnetic resonance imaging to demonstrate that meniscal translation was not affected by ACL deficiency, but bone kinematics were altered. With a 125-N compressive load applied at the foot, the femur in ACL-deficient knees translated, on average, 4.3 mm further anteriorly from 0 to 45 degrees flexion than observed in the healthy knees. At full extension, the contact area centroid was shifted posteriorly relative to the tibia in the ACL-deficient knee. Translation of the medial meniscus did not differ between ACL-deficient and normal knees, leading the authors to suggest that altered bone kinematics subsequent to ACL injury, coupled with lack of compensation in meniscal translation, may increase the risk for secondary meniscal injury. Von Eisenhart-Rothe and colleagues[200] revealed similar findings: magnetic resonance imaging revealed posterior translation of the medial femoral condyle relative to the tibia in ACL-deficient knees during isometric contraction of flexor and extensor muscles. Meniscal translation was the same across healthy and ACL-deficient knees.

Allen and colleagues[196] conducted a study to measure anteroposterior translation in intact cadaveric knees, ACL-deficient knees, and ACL-deficient knees that underwent a medial meniscectomy. Their findings agreed with those of Hsieh and Walker[201]: the anteroposterior laxity of the intact knee was significantly different from the anteroposterior laxity of both groups of ACL-deficient knees. Further, they found that the coupled internal rotation associated with the anterior tibial load was less for both groups of ACL-deficient knees than for the intact knees. In both loading scenarios, the ACL-deficient knee that underwent a meniscectomy was the most lax, followed by the ACL-deficient knee, indicating that both the ACL and the meniscus are important in preventing anteroposterior laxity in the knee.

Beynnon and associates[202] conducted in vivo testing to assess tibial movement relative to the femur during transition from non–weight-bearing to weight-bearing subsequent to ACL injury. Knees with ACL insufficiency demonstrated an average anterior tibial translation of 3.4 mm compared with 0.8 mm observed in the healthy, contralateral knee. The authors hypothesized that further translation is prevented by the posterior horn of the medial meniscus, which would experience greater strain during transition to weight-bearing after ACL injury.[202]

Hollis and colleagues[203] conducted testing similar to that performed by Allen and coworkers[196] in nine human cadaver knees. They loaded the tibia from 0 to 38 N in the anteroposterior direction while applying a 200-N axial force along the axis of the tibia and measured meniscal strains in cadaveric knees with intact ACLs, sectioned ACLs, and reconstructed ACLs. Their results showed that meniscal strains increase after the ACL has been sectioned. After ACL reconstruction, however, the meniscal strains return to levels observed in the ACL-intact state, suggesting that ACL reconstruction reduces the likelihood of meniscal damage. Conversely, Pearsall and Hollis[204] evaluated lateral and medial meniscal strain using DVRT strain gauges in eight cadaveric knees with intact PCLs, sectioned PCLs, and reconstructed PCLs. Strain in both menisci increased at 60 and 90 degrees of flexion in knees with sectioned PCLs. Similar to the results of Hollis and associates,[203] PCL reconstruction reduced meniscal strain to PCL-intact levels.[204]

Markolf and colleagues[103] evaluated the effect of meniscectomy on varus-valgus, and rotary knee laxity in human cadavers with an instrumented laxity-testing device. They observed that bicompartmental removal of the menisci increased anteroposterior joint laxity between 45 and 90 degrees of knee flexion, whereas only a minor increase in laxity occurred in the rotary and varus-valgus planes. In a later study, these researchers demonstrated that although bicompartmental meniscectomy made the unloaded knee looser, in the knees with a developed tibiofemoral compressive load, laxity measurements were little affected.[165] Bargar et al.[98] used the instrumented laxity-testing device to evaluate antero-posterior load-displacement and varus-valgus torque-rotation responses of a subject's knee joint in vivo. They demonstrated that medial meniscectomy alone does not create a measurable increase in varus-valgus laxity, whereas a trend of increased anteroposterior laxity was observed. A significant increase in anteroposterior laxity was observed in subjects with a combined medial meniscectomy and torn ACL.[98]

Levy and associates[205] used human cadavers to investigate the effects of isolated medial meniscectomy and to study the effects of medial meniscectomy in the ACL-deficient knee. They demonstrated that an isolated medial meniscectomy did not produce a significant change in the anteroposterior load-displacement response of the knee. This finding is corroborated by the previous works presented by Hsieh and Walker[201] and Bargar and associates.[98] In the ACL-deficient knee without a compressive joint load, Levy and coworkers[205] demonstrated that resection of the meniscus caused a significant increase in the anterior displacement of the tibia relative to the femur at 30, 60, and 90 degrees of knee flexion. This observation led these researchers to suggest that in the ACL-deficient knee, the posterior horn of the meniscus acts as a wedge between the tibiofemoral articular surfaces, resisting anterior excursion of the tibia relative to the femur. In a later study, this observation was confirmed by Sullivan and colleagues.[206] In this work, the medial ligament structures in an ACL-deficient knee with an intact meniscus were sectioned, revealing an increase in anterior tibial displacement relative to the femur in comparison with the knee in which only the ACL was cut. In the ACL-deficient knee with an intact medial ligament complex, the mechanism of anterior tibial restraint was demonstrated to be the wedging apart of tibiofemoral articular surfaces by the meniscus—a distraction resisted by the intact medial ligament complex and capsular structures—and the development of a tibiofemoral compressive load.[206] The authors hypothesized that this may be one of the mechanisms that produces posterior horn tears of the menisci in an ACL-deficient knee.[206]

Tienen and coworkers[207] demonstrated the relative immobility of the posterior horn of the medial meniscus with use of cadaveric knees. In the absence of tibial torque, the anterior horn moved further posteriorly and laterally than the posterior horn during flexion. Application of external torque revealed constrained posterior horn displacement during the first 30 degrees of flexion. Watanabe and associates[208] demonstrated that anterior tibial translation increases after two-thirds and complete resection of the posterior horn of the medial meniscus. In addition, applied varus torque increased external tibial rotation by 2.2 and 6.7 degrees after two-thirds and complete resection of the posterior horn, respectively.[208]

In a later study, Levy and coworkers[209] investigated the effect of lateral meniscectomy on the motion of the human knee joint without compressive joint loading. They determined that isolated lateral meniscectomy did not produce a significant change in the anteroposterior load-displacement behavior of the knee. In addition, these investigators revealed that the lateral meniscus does not act as a restraint to anterior translation of the tibia relative to the femur, leading the researchers to suggest that this structure may not behave like the medial meniscus in providing an effective posterior wedge to anterior translation.[209] It is important that the results of these investigations of the meniscus be applied to events that occur without a compressive joint load, such as the swing phase of gait, and not to activities that include compressive joint loading.

The menisci have also been thought to assist with joint lubrication, provide resistance to extreme joint flexion or extension, and aid in the damping of impulsive loads transmitted across the tibiofemoral joint. These functions are difficult to characterize biomechanically or to describe with clinical impressions.

PATELLOFEMORAL JOINT BIOMECHANICS

A study of patellofemoral joint biomechanics is necessary to understand the pathologic processes, develop rational treatment regimens, and understand the effects that various rehabilitation programs have on this joint. For example, an abnormally high compressive patellofemoral joint reaction (PFJR) force produces abnormally high stress across the articular cartilage and is thought to be one of the initiating factors of alterations in articular cartilage metabolism, chondromalacia, and subsequent OA.[210–213] In addition, morphometric abnormalities in the trochlear groove or the dorsal articular surface of the patella in combination with high lateral forces at the patellofemoral articulation have been thought to cause lateral subluxation or dislocation of the patella.[213–216]

Patellofemoral Contact Area

In the normal knee, the patellofemoral contact area is optimally designed to respond to the increase in PFJR load developed with knee flexion through a corresponding increase in contact area. This mechanism helps distribute the contact force while minimizing patellofemoral contact stress.

Goodfellow and colleagues[217] used the dye method to measure patellofemoral contact area in human cadaver knees subjected to simulated weight-bearing conditions. Area measurements were made at 20, 45, 90, and 135 degrees of knee flexion and are presented in (Fig. 89.22). Movement of the knee from full extension to 90 degrees revealed that the contact area on the dorsal aspect of the patella moves in a continuous zone from the inferior to the superior pole of the patella. Continued flexion of the knee to 135 degrees developed two separate contact regions: one on the "odd medial facet" and the other on the lateral aspect of the patella (see Fig. 89.22). Singerman and colleagues[218,219] calculated the center of pressure from a 6-degrees-of-freedom patellar transducer in human cadaver knees and reported that the center

of pressure translates superiorly and medially as the knee is flexed to 90 degrees. At flexion angles greater than 85 degrees, the results were somewhat variable, but the center of pressure always moved inferiorly with extension.[218] Huberti and Hayes[220] used pressure-sensitive film to measure the increase of patellofemoral contact area that occurs concurrently with knee flexion (Fig. 89.23). At a flexion angle of 10 degrees, contact between the dorsal surface of the patella and the trochlea is initiated. The length of the patellar tendon controls when patellar-trochlear contact occurs. In patients in whom the patellar tendon is too long, patella alta may be present, and flexion of the knee greater than 10 degrees may be required to seat the patella adequately in the trochlear groove. Von Eisenhart-Rothe and colleagues[221] used an open magnetic resonance system coupled with three-dimensional image postprocessing to evaluate kinematics and contact areas in the knee compartment in vivo. Patella tilt decreases during flexion from 30 to 90 degrees, coupled with an increase in lateral patellar shift. The femur rotates externally and translates posteriorly relative to the tibia in the same flexion range. These movements result in a significant increase in contact area.[221] With knee movement between extension and 90 degrees, the patella was found to be the only component of the extensor mechanism that contacts the femur, holding the quadriceps tendon away from the femur. With knee motion between 90 and 135 degrees, the quadriceps tendon contacts the femur.[222] Once the quadriceps tendon contacts the femur, the compressive PFJR force is divided between contact of the broad band of the quadriceps tendon with the femur and patellofemoral contact.

The interaction between the patellofemoral contact area and PFJR force can be demonstrated with the squatting activity. During this activity, as knee flexion increases, the PFJR force initially increases, whereas the patellofemoral contact area available for distributing the contact force also increases, effectively distributing the articular contact stress. Besier and colleagues[223] demonstrated that patellofemoral contact area increased on average by 24% during weight-bearing knee flexion in both female and male subjects. The opposite situation may occur with knee extension during weight-training programs that apply a weight to the distal aspect of the tibia with the athlete in a seated position. For this activity, the patellofemoral contact area decreases as the PFJR force increases; therefore the PFJR stress may become high even if light weights are applied to the distal aspect of the

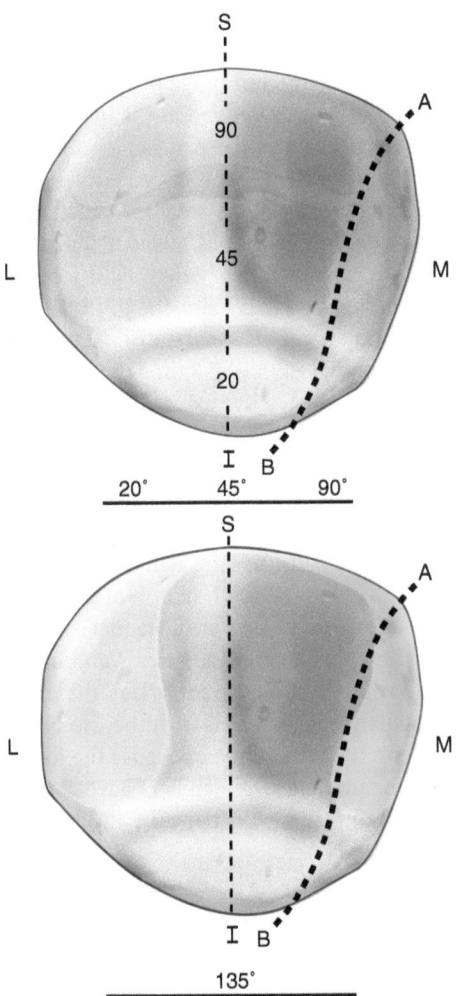

Fig. 89.22 Patellofemoral contact regions at different knee flexion angles. *I,* Inferior; *L,* lateral; *M,* medial; *S,* superior. (From Goodfellow J, Hungerford DS, Zindel M. Patellofemoral joint mechanics and pathology. *J Bone Joint Surg Br.* 1976;58:287–290.)

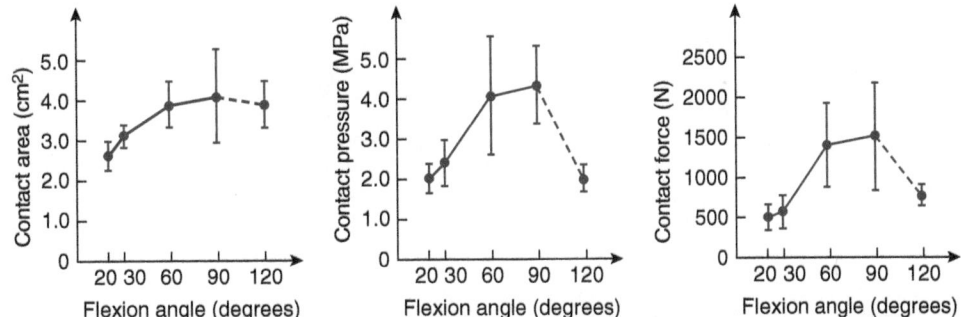

Fig. 89.23 Experimental measurement of patellofemoral contact made in human cadaver specimens for the squatting activity with a normal Q angle. Values between 90 and 120 degrees have been extrapolated. *Left,* Contact area; *middle,* contact pressure; *right,* contact force. (From Huberti HH, Hayes WC. Patellofemoral contact pressures: the influence of Q-angle and tibiofemoral contact. *J Bone Joint Surg Am.* 1984;66A:715–724.)

tibia. This example may help explain why isotonic or isokinetic exercises through a full ROM are not advised in the treatment of patellofemoral pain syndromes. Quadriceps exercises extending the knee only through the last 15 to 20 degrees of extension are more likely to be tolerated, as demonstrated by the decrease in PFJR force in Fig. 89.23.

Patellofemoral Force Transmission

The patella transmits force from the quadriceps muscle group to the patellar tendon while developing a large PFJR force. This mechanism serves to stabilize the knee against gravity when the joint is in a flexed position and assists in the forward propulsion of the body as the knee is extended during gait. Therefore the loads developed along the patellar tendon and the PFJR force are a function of both quadriceps force and knee flexion angle. A sagittal plane analysis can be used to demonstrate this concept. This analysis applies statics to describe the forces and moments required to maintain the knee joint in equilibrium. For example, with use of this technique, the quadriceps force (F_{Quads}), the PFJR force, and the patellar tendon force (F_{PT}) may be related at chosen knee flexion angles. Fig. 89.24 is a simplified sagittal plane static representation of the relation between the PFJR and the quadriceps muscle forces. The mass of the upper body (W), assumed to act at the hip joint, is supported by the F_{Quads} developed by the quadriceps muscle groups. The vertical line below the center of mass at the subject's hip joint represents the force vector due to upper body weight, which falls well behind the flexion axis of the knee. The distance from the center of mass force vector to the flexion axis of the knee is defined as the moment arm (c). The moment arm is relatively small, with the knee near extension. Therefore the support mechanism provided by the F_{Quads} and the developed PFJR are relatively small. In the right portion of Fig. 89.24, the knee is in a position of greater flexion with an associated increase in the moment arm (c'). To maintain the knee in static equilibrium, the new force (F_{Quads}) generated by the quadriceps must increase significantly. As a result of the

increased quadriceps force, the PFJR must also be larger. This model may help explain the mechanism by which both PFJR and F_{Quads} increase during squatting activities.

In the earlier force analysis studies, the patella-trochlea articulation was represented as a frictionless pulley.[210,214,224–230] This assumption was justified on the basis of the low coefficient of friction between the patellofemoral articular surfaces. With this approach, the forces developed by the quadriceps muscle group were assumed to be equal to the force developed along the patellar tendon throughout the full range of knee motion, with the direction of the PFJR force defined as the bisector of the angle between the quadriceps and the patellar tendon force vectors. Using the mechanics principle of static equilibrium, and with the assumption that the patella-trochlea articulation behaves like a frictionless pulley, Reilly and Martens[229] predicted a compressive PFJR force of 0.5 times body weight for level walking. For ascending and descending stairs, the PFJR was estimated to reach 3.3 times body weight.[229] Analysis of the squatting activity revealed that a maximal PFJR of 2.9 times body weight occurred at 90 degrees of flexion.[229] Active extension of the lower leg with a 9-kg boot while the femur was oriented in a horizontal position produced a peak PFJR at 36 degrees of flexion.[229] Maquet[231,232] questioned the frictionless pulley assumption and demonstrated with a lateral vector diagram of the patellofemoral articulation that the forces in the quadriceps mechanism and patellar tendon can differ and can also vary as a function of knee flexion angle. Several investigators have confirmed Maquet's findings.[233–238]

In later work performed by Huberti,[233] Van Eijden,[238] Buff,[236] Ahmed,[234] Singerman,[218] and their coworkers, the combined tibia, femur, and patella were evaluated with the use of both experimental and theoretical techniques. Because the force values F_{PT} and F_{Quads} are unequal, these researchers have chosen to report results by calculating the ratio between the two force values (F_{PT}/F_{Quads}) at selected knee flexion angles. Huberti's group simulated the squatting activity in human cadaver specimens while measuring F_{Quads} with a tensile load cell and the F_{PT} with a buckle

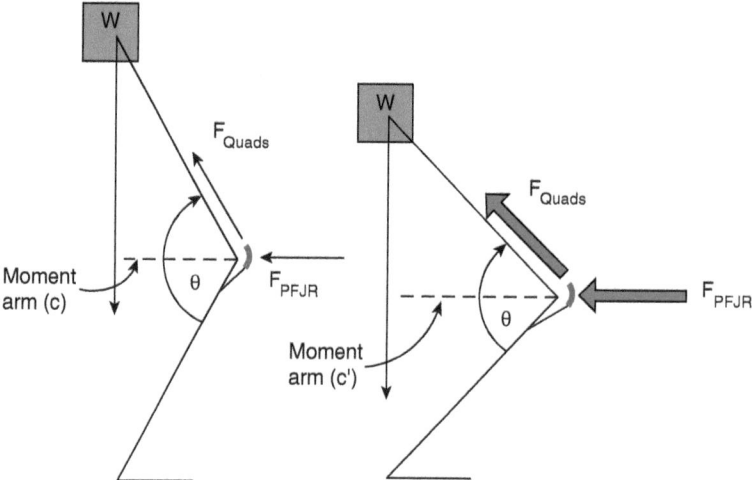

Fig. 89.24 Static model of the patellofemoral joint reaction force (F_{PFJR}) at two positions of knee flexion. With the knee in the flexed position (right), the values of F_{Quads} and F_{PFJR} are large, supporting the weight (W) of the upper body acting through a large moment arm (c'). The F_{Quads} and F_{PFJR} values are much less with the knee in a more extended position (left), in which the moment arm (c) is smaller.

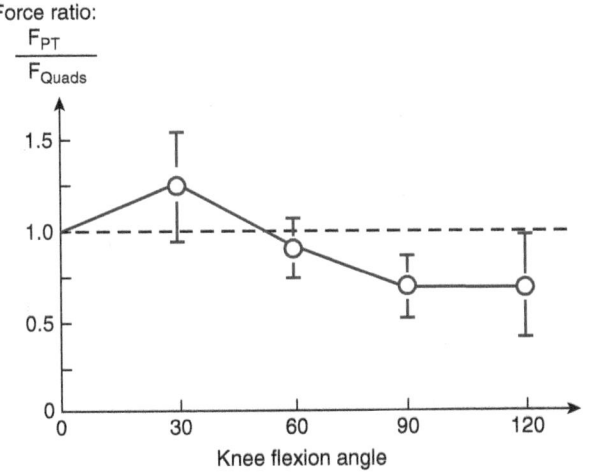

Fig. 89.25 The predicted force ratio F_{PT}/F_{Quads} for the knee positioned between 0 and 120 degrees of flexion. Between 0 degrees and 45 degrees, the force developed in the patellar tendon is greater than that developed by the quadriceps musculature, whereas from 45 to 120 degrees, the patellar tendon force is less. (From Huberti HH, Hayes WC, Stone JL, et al. Force ratios in the quadriceps and the ligamentous patellae. *J Orthop Res.* 1984;2:49.)

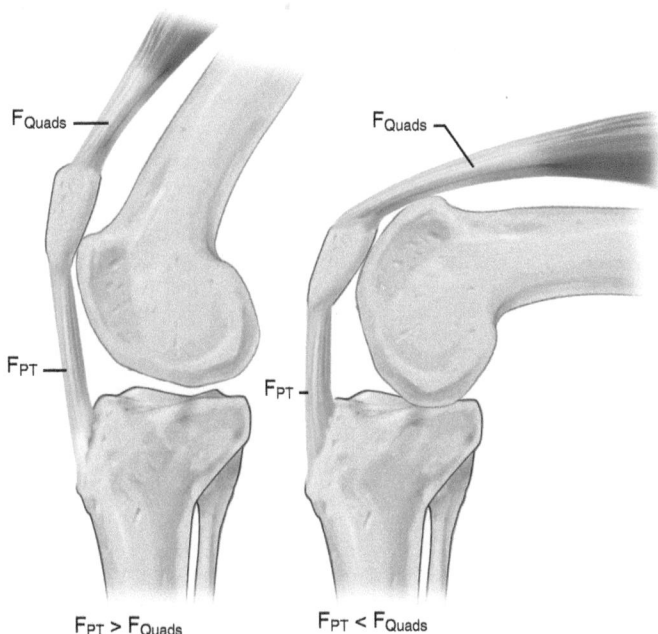

Fig. 89.26 The mechanical function of the patella as a lever and as a spacer to increase the patellar tendon moment arm. *Left,* With the knee near the extended position, the levering action of the patellar mechanism produces greater force values in the patellar tendon (F_{PT}) in comparison with those developed by quadriceps contraction (F_{Quads}). *Right,* With the knee in the flexed position, the levering action of the patella is decreased, and the force values developed in the patellar tendon are less than those developed by the quadriceps. (From Huberti HH, Hayes WC, Stone JL, et al. Force ratios in the quadriceps tendon and ligamentous patellae. *J Orthop Res.* 1984;2:49.)

transducer.[233] They demonstrated that for knee flexion between 0 and 45 degrees, the F_{PT} developed was greater than F_{Quads} (Fig. 89.25). With continued knee flexion to 120 degrees, the F_{PT} was consistently less in comparison with F_{Quads}. The authors suggested that not only does the patella function as a pulley that changes the magnitude and direction of forces in the quadriceps and patellar tendon, but the patella also has two distinct mechanical functions.[233] In the first and more classically described function, the anteroposterior thickness of the patella can be attributed to increasing the effective moment arm of the quadriceps muscles and patellar ligament, whereas in the second function, the patella acts as a lever (Fig. 89.26). Therefore the parameters that define the proximal and distal lever arms of the patella have a direct effect on the balance of forces in the quadriceps and patellar tendon. The researchers reasoned that the parameters were the length of the patella, the location of the patellofemoral contact area, and the angle between the quadriceps tendon and patellar tendon.[233] In a parallel experimental investigation of the squatting activity, Huberti and Hayes[220] estimated that the compressive PFJR force reached a maximal value of 6.5 times body weight. With knee flexion to 120 degrees, tendofemoral contact supported one-third of the compressive PFJR force.[217]

Van Eijden and associates[238] developed a mathematical model of the patellofemoral articulation and verified model predictions with experimental findings. Predictions of the F_{PT}/F_{Quads} ratio were similar to the experimental findings presented by Huberti,[233] Ahmed,[234] Buff,[236] and their coworkers. Van Eijden's group demonstrated that the PFJR is about 50% of the quadriceps force at full extension and increases to 100% of the quadriceps force with the knee positioned between 70 and 120 degrees of flexion (Fig. 89.27).[238]

These studies have important implications for knee rehabilitation programs that are designed to minimize patellar tendon forces, as in patellar tendinitis. In these programs, application of

the large isokinetic or isometric knee moments with the knee in positions between extension and 45 degrees should be avoided. In this flexion range, quadriceps activity actually produces forces of greater magnitude in the patellar tendon. This finding has been demonstrated by the work of Huberti and colleagues,[233] who showed that the F_{PT}/F_{Quads} ratio is greater than 1.0 for knee positions between extension and 45 degrees (see Fig. 89.25). It may be advisable to restrict rehabilitation programs for patellar tendinitis to flexion angles between 45 and 120 degrees, in which the F_{PT}/F_{Quads} ratio is less than 1.0. This constraint prevents an amplification of F_{PT}. This restriction would not apply to normal gait, in which the bending moments and therefore F_{Quads} are not high. Because of the changing relationship between developed F_{Quads} and resulting F_{PT} as the knee courses from extension through full flexion, the effectiveness of the quadriceps in developing an extension moment becomes substantially smaller at larger knee flexion angles, which also prevents the amplification of F_{PT}.

These studies also have important implications in the rehabilitation and surgical treatment of patellofemoral pain syndromes. Rehabilitation programs designed to minimize the PFJR but not the F_{Quads} should avoid large isokinetic, isotonic, or isometric moments with the knee positioned between 60 and 120 degrees of flexion. In this range, the predicted PFJR force is equal to the F_{Quads} (see Fig. 89.26).[238] With the requirement of minimizing the PFJR force, it may be advisable to restrict knee

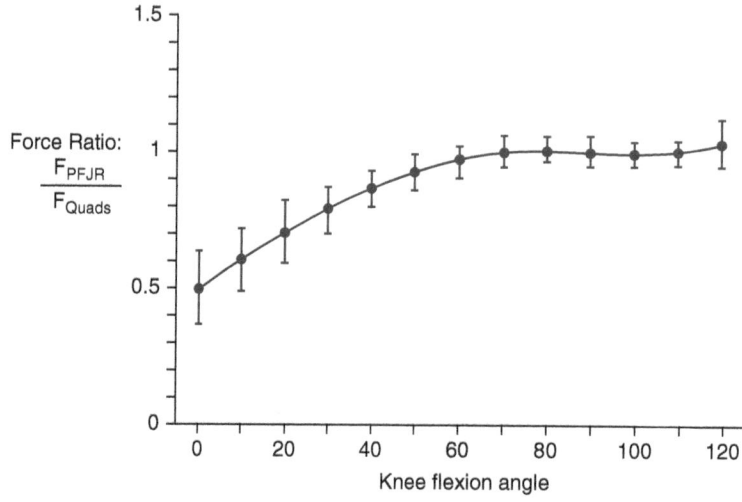

Fig. 89.27 The predicted force ratio patellofemoral joint reaction force/quadriceps force (F_{PFJR}/F_{Quads}) for the knee positioned between 0 and 120 degrees of flexion. Between 0 and 70 degrees, F_{PFJR} is less than that developed by quadriceps contraction, whereas from 70 to 120 degrees, F_{PFJR} is equal to F_{Quads}. (From van Eijden TM, Kouwenhoven E, Verburg J, et al. A mathematical model of the patellofemoral joint. *J Biomech.* 1986;19:219–288.)

rehabilitation to range between the limits of extension, when the PFJR is about 50% of the F_{Quads}, and 40 degrees, when the PFJR is 90% of the F_{Quads}.[238] Maquet[212] has investigated the surgical treatment of patellofemoral pain, demonstrating that by increasing the extensor moment arm by a 2-cm elevation of the tibial tubercle, a 50% reduction in the PFJR force occurred when the knee is flexed to 45 degrees. Ferguson and associates[239] investigated the effect of anterior displacement of the tibial tubercle on patellofemoral contact stress. In this study, the patella-trochlea interfaces of human cadaver specimens were instrumented with miniature force sensors to monitor the patellofemoral contact stress. They revealed that anterior displacement of the tibial tubercle decreased the patellofemoral contact stress between 0 and 90 degrees of flexion.[239] The largest decrease in contact stress was achieved with a 12.5-mm elevation of the tubercle; further elevation produced only a minimal decrease in contact stress.[239] This finding demonstrates the importance of the anteroposterior position of the patellar tendon and its role in controlling the extensor moment arm. In addition, the proximal-distal location of the patellofemoral contact point is critical to the function of the patella as a lever (as explained earlier).

In the frontal plane, the axis of the F_{Quads} forms an angle with the patellar tendon. This angle has been defined as the Q angle and is measured as the intersection of the center line of the patellar tendon and the line from the center of the patella to the anterior superior iliac spine.[237] The normal Q angle is reported to range between 10 and 15 degrees with the knee in full extension.[240,241] With knee flexion, the Q angle decreases because a coupled internal rotation of the tibia occurs relative to the femur.[214] Contraction of the quadriceps creates a bowstring effect that displaces the patella in a lateral direction, producing a contact force against the lateral margin of the femoral trochlear groove. Abnormal tracking of the patella, which allows lateral subluxation of only a few millimeters, markedly decreases the contact area, greatly increasing the local stress (force per unit area; Fig. 89.28).

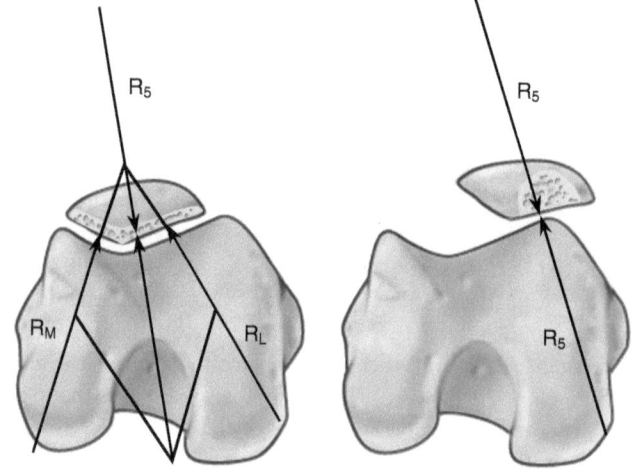

Fig. 89.28 Patellofemoral joint reaction forces for the normal knee *(left)*. The joint reaction force (R_5) is resisted by the lateral (R_L) and medial (R_M) components. In the knee with a lateralized patella *(right)*, the joint reaction force is resisted by the lateral component only (R_5). (From Maquet P. Mechanics and osteoarthritis of the patellofemoral joint. *Clin Orthop.* 1979;144:70.)

This mechanism may contribute to patellofemoral pain and degeneration of the patellar articular cartilage (chondromalacia). Other anatomic conditions can also contribute to abnormal patellar tracking. These conditions include hypoplasia of the trochlear groove, abnormal patellar articular configuration, underdevelopment of the vastus medialis, transverse plane rotational malalignment of the proximal tibia relative to the distal femur, and an abnormally high Q angle. Huberti and Hayes[220] studied the effect of different Q angles by simulating the squatting activity in human cadaver specimens while measuring patellofemoral contact pressure with pressure-sensitive film. They demonstrated that either an increase or a decrease in Q angle developed an increased peak patellofemoral pressure and the associated unpredictable patterns of cartilage loading. Cox[242] has presented a retrospective study of the Roux-Elmslie-Trillat procedure for realignment of the knee extensor mechanism and prevention of recurrent subluxation of the patella. An evaluation of 116 patients observed for at least 1 year demonstrated that this procedure is a satisfactory method for the prevention of lateral subluxation, with recurrence in only 7% of the cases. Careful attention to the medial transfer of the tibial tuberosity without a posterior displacement was emphasized as the key to successful long-term results.[242] Procedures resulting in some posterior transfer of the tibial tuberosity, such as that described by Hauser, decrease the patellar tendon moment arm and consequently increase the patellofemoral contact stress. Fulkerson and Hungerford[243] have reviewed the clinical and radiologic outcomes of the Hauser procedure and have presented evidence of progressive knee joint degeneration.

For a complete list of references, go to ExpertConsult.com.

SELECTED READINGS

Citation:
Farrow LD, Chen MR, Cooperman DR, et al. Morphology of the femoral intercondylar notch. *J Bone Joint Surg Am.* 2007;89A(10):2150–2155.

Level of Evidence:
V

Summary:
In this study the morphologic features of the femoral intercondylar notch are described. The posterolateral rim of the intercondylar notch is not well defined. Accurate placement of commercial femoral tunnel aiming guides may be difficult.

Citation:
Warren LF, Marshall JL. The supporting structures and layers on the medial side of the knee: an anatomical analysis. *J Bone Joint Surg Am.* 1979;61A:56–62.

Level of Evidence:
V

Summary:
In this study the anatomic structures in the medial side of the knee are described. This study is one of the most important works describing the medial side of the knee. Only minor variations in the overall anatomic pattern are found.

Citation:
LaPrade RF, Morgan PM, Wentorf FA, et al. The anatomy of the posterior aspect of the knee. An anatomic study. *J Bone Joint Surg Am.* 2007;89A:758–764.

Level of Evidence:
V

Summary:
In this study an anatomic detailed description of the posterior aspect of the knee is provided.

Citation:
LaPrade RF, Engebretsen AH, Ly TV, et al. The anatomy of the medial part of the knee. *J Bone Joint Surg Am.* 2007;89A:2000–2010.

Level of Evidence:
V

Summary:
In this study an anatomic description of the medial aspect of the knee is provided.

Citation:
Beynnon BD, Fleming BC. Anterior cruciate ligament strain in vivo: a review of previous work. *J Biomech.* 1998;31:519–525.

Level of Evidence:
IV

Summary:
The strain behavior of the anterior cruciate ligament (ACL) has been measured by arthroscopic implantation of the differential variable reluctance transducer while subjects are experiencing local anesthesia. Movement of the knee from a flexed to an extended position, either passively or through contraction of the leg muscles, produces an increase in ACL strain values. Isolated contraction of the dominant quadriceps with the knee between 50 degrees and extension creates substantial increases in strain. In contrast, isolated contraction of the hamstrings at any knee position does not increase ACL strain. With the knee unweighted, the protective strain shielding effect of a functional knee brace decreases as the magnitude of anterior shear load applied to the tibia increases. The approach used in this study is novel in that it can be used to measure an important portion of the ACL's strain distribution while clinically relevant loads are applied to the knee, subjects perform rehabilitation exercises, or in the presence of different orthoses such as functional knee braces.

Citation:
Beynnon BD, Fleming BC, Labovitch R. Chronic anterior-cruciate ligament deficiency is associated with increased anterior translation of the tibia during the transition from non-weightbearing to weightbearing. *J Orthop Res.* 2002;20:332–337.

Level of Evidence:
III

Summary:
Translation of the tibia relative to the femur was measured while a group of subjects with normal knees and a group with anterior cruciate ligament (ACL) tears underwent transition from non–weight-bearing to weight-bearing stance. A fourfold increase in anterior translation of the tibia for the knees with ACL tears compared with the contralateral side is a concern because it is substantially greater than the 95% confidence limits of the side-to-side differences in anteroposterior knee laxity measured from subjects with normal knees. This observation could explain, at least in part, one of the mechanisms that initiates damage to the meniscus and articular cartilage in subjects who have sustained an ACL tear.

Citation:
Beynnon BD, Johnson RJ, Naud S, et al. Accelerated versus nonaccelerated rehabilitation after anterior cruciate ligament reconstruction: a prospective, double-blind investigation evaluating knee joint laxity using roentgen stereophotogrammetric analysis. *Am J Sports Med.* 2011;39(12):2536–2548.

Level of Evidence:

I

Summary:

Rehabilitation with the accelerated and nonaccelerated programs administered in this study produced the same increase in the envelope of knee laxity. Most of the increase in the envelope of knee laxity occurred during healing when exercises were advanced and activity level increased. Patients in both programs had the same clinical assessment, functional performance, proprioception, and thigh muscle strength, which returned to normal levels after healing was complete. For participants in both treatment programs, the Knee Injury and Osteoarthritis Outcome Score assessment of quality of life did not return to preinjury levels.

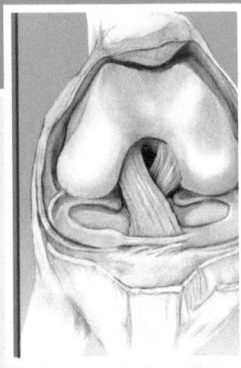

90

Knee Diagnosis and Decision-Making

Andrew J. Riff, Peter N. Chalmers, Bernard R. Bach Jr.

For the experienced practitioner, the history and physical examination remains the most efficient, sensitive, specific, accurate, and cost-effective method of establishing a diagnosis in patients with knee-related complaints. Several investigators have demonstrated that the history and physical examination have equivalent sensitivity and specificity to magnetic resonance imaging (MRI) for a variety of intra-articular pathologies, with an overall accuracy of 93%.[1,2] When taking a systematic approach to patients with knee-related concerns, assessing each structure in question sequentially for possible injury is critical.[2]

Developing an intuitive and comprehensive approach to the physical examination requires a detailed understanding of knee anatomy, in particular the relation of the surface skin to the underlying structures, to be able to relate tenderness to pathology. In-depth knowledge of knee pathology can be helpful so that the history and examination can be dynamically tailored. From an organizational standpoint, it is helpful to stratify knee pathology based on onset (acute injury versus insidious onset) and population affected (adult versus pediatric; Table 90.1). Common acute knee injuries in adults include ligament injuries (including anterior cruciate ligament [ACL] tear, posterior cruciate ligament [PCL] tear, medial and lateral collateral ligament injury, and posterolateral corner [PLC] injury), meniscal tears, patellar dislocation/subluxation, patellar or quadriceps tendon ruptures, and fractures (most commonly patellar or tibial plateau). Additional acute injures that warrant consideration in the pediatric patient include physeal and apophyseal injuries (including tibial eminence avulsion fracture, tibial tuberosity avulsion fracture, or patellar sleeve avulsion fracture).

Common causes of insidious knee pain in the adult include patellofemoral pain (including patellofemoral syndrome, lateral patellar tilt, patellar and quadriceps tendinitis/tendinopathy), iliotibial band syndrome, degenerative meniscal tears, pes anserine bursitis, medial plica syndrome, patellofemoral and tibiofemoral chondral and osteochondral defects, and osteoarthritis, rheumatologic conditions, septic arthritis, and pigmented villonodular synovitis. Insidious knee pain in the child may also be secondary to osteochondritis dissecans (OCD), discoid meniscus, Osgood-Schlatter disease, Sinding-Larsen-Johansson syndrome, juvenile rheumatoid arthritis, lyme arthritis, and hip pathology such as Perthes disease or slipped capital femoral epiphysis (SCFE).

HISTORY

Eliciting the history starts with the chief or primary complaint that leads the patient to present for an evaluation. We endeavor to record this complaint in the patient's own words, because he or she provides the first clues regarding the patient's reason for the office visit. Asking an open-ended question such as "What brings you to the office today?" is very helpful. Giving patients the opportunity to "tell their story" also allows them to develop a more significant and meaningful relationship with their physician.

Once the patient has completed his or her initial response, the surgeon can return to the beginning of the story as necessary to fill in gaps and collect more details. In particular, the examiner must determine the duration of symptoms and, if possible, the date of onset. Important details often can be gathered from the patient's recollection of the inciting event or trauma, should one exist. If the injury occurred during an athletic endeavor, the examiner should obtain a full account of the event, including whether this incident was a contact or noncontact injury and if it occurred during practice or during a competition. These details may provide the first clues as to the underlying pathology. For instance, a valgus stress suggests an injury to the medial collateral ligament (MCL), whereas a high-energy trauma such as a motorcycle accident may suggest a knee dislocation or multiligamentous injury. In comparison, noncontact ACL injuries usually occur in the context of stopping quickly, cutting sharply, and landing and changing direction with the foot planted. The mechanism of ACL injury in skiers is different—when skiers injure the ACL, they are moving out of control with the knee bent or extended. The uphill arm is back, the body is off balance, the hips are lower than the knees, and the weight is placed on the inside edge of the downhill ski. This mechanism of injury has been referred to as the "phantom foot" mechanism.[3] Recollection of an auditory pop or a tearing sensation may be present. Up to 66% of patients with an ACL injury describe such a sensation.[4,5] Swelling immediately after the event may also occur. Indeed, a hemarthrosis develops in most persons with ACL injuries within 3 hours of the initial tear (Table 90.2). It is often helpful to inquire about foot position during the injury. A fall onto a flexed knee may result in either a patellar fracture (if the ankle is dorsiflexed) or a PCL injury (if the foot is plantar flexed).

If no specific event can be recalled, the patient should be asked if he or she has had a recent change in activity, which

TABLE 90.1   Acute and Insidious Causes of Knee Pain in Adult and Pediatric Patients

	Traumatic	Atraumatic
Adult	• Ligamentous injury (ACL, PCL, MCL, LCL, PLC) • Meniscal tear • Patellar dislocation • Osteochondral fracture • Extensor mechanism rupture (patellar or quadriceps tendon) • Fracture (most commonly patella or tibial plateau)	• Patellofemoral syndrome • Lateral patellar tilt • Tendinitis (patellar/quadriceps) • Iliotibial band syndrome • Pes anserine bursitis • Degenerative meniscal tear • Osteochondral defect • Osteoarthritis • Rheumatologic condition • Septic arthritis • Pigmented villinodular synovitis • Osteochondritis dissecans (OCD) • Discoid meniscus • Osgood-Schlatter disease • Sinding-Larsen-Johansson syndrome • Juvenile rheumatoid arthritis • Lyme arthritis • Hip pathology (Perthes disease or slipped capital femoral epiphysis [SCFE])
Pediatric	• Tibial eminence fracture • Tibial tuberosity avulsion • Patellar sleeve avulsion	

ACL, Anterior cruciate ligament; *LCL,* lateral collateral ligament; *MCL,* medial collateral ligament; *PCL,* posterior cruciate ligament; *PLC,* posterolateral corner.

TABLE 90.2   Potential Etiologies for a Hemarthrosis of the Knee

Traumatic	Atraumatic
• Anterior cruciate ligament tear • Posterior cruciate ligament injury • Chondral fracture • Patellar dislocation • Meniscal tear • Intra-articular fracture • Tear in the deep portion of the joint capsule	• Pigmented villonodular synovitis • Hemangioma • Hemophilia • Sickle cell anemia • Charcot arthropathy • Pharmacologic coagulopathy • Thrombocytopenia

might suggest overuse. Commonly patients may have changed training techniques (e.g., increased frequency, increased distances, or a change in terrain or surfaces). A recent increase in running, particularly among marathon trainees or military recruits, may suggest a tibial stress fracture, patellofemoral syndrome, or iliotibial band syndrome. Acute changes from inactivity to activity may lead deconditioned patients to subject their knees to nonphysiologic kinetics as a result of loss of neuromuscular control.

The major symptoms on which to focus for a patient presenting with knee-related concerns include (1) pain, (2) instability, (3) mechanical symptoms, (4) swelling, and (5) stiffness. As with any patient encounter, the patient should be asked about the characteristics of pain, including onset (acute or insidious), location, duration, severity, quality, and radiation. The patient should be asked about the continued presence of pain and any change in character or severity of the pain. Use of visual analog scales can be helpful. Pain ratings based on a 0 to 10 scale can be used. It is helpful to hear whether the pain is constant, is only related to activities, or occurs after activity. Pain related to prolonged sitting or linear activities like stair climbing or running suggests a patellofemoral etiology, whereas pain with twisting or rotating activities (e.g., rolling over in bed or getting out of a car) is suggestive of meniscal pathology. Pain that arises at progressively earlier intervals into a run may be suggestive of iliotibial band syndrome.

Subjective instability should be explored, with attention paid to determining the frequency and inciting events or activities surrounding each instability event. For example, patients with an ACL tear often state that they experience instability with pivoting, twisting, or cutting activities. They may also describe a sensation of movement with their knees that they often explain by placing two fists together and moving one with respect to the other in what has been called the *two-fist sign.* In contrast, instability that is experienced linearly, as in walking on level ground or on stairs, is often associated with quadriceps weakness and deconditioning. Side-to-side instability on level ground may suggest valgus or varus laxity, whereas instability when descending a ramp may also be experienced by patients with damage to the PLC.

The presence of mechanical symptoms (catching and locking) is suggestive of a displaced intra-articular fragment, most commonly either a displaced meniscal tear or osteochondral loose body. A medial meniscal tear is more likely to promote mechanical symptoms while a lateral meniscal tear is more likely to present as pain in isolation. In addition, the presence of a bucket handle medial meniscal tear is suggestive of underlying ACL insufficiency until proven otherwise.

Although not universal, a knee effusion should heighten the examiners suspicion for a structural intra-articular abnormality. A knee effusion following an acute injury may be the result of a ligament injury, meniscal tear, chondral injury, or intra-articular fracture. The timing and size of the effusion are helpful clues to the diagnosis. Rapid onset (within 2 hours) of a large effusion is suggestive of an ACL tear injury or intra-articular fracture (e.g., tibial plateau) while a more gradual onset (24 to 36 hours) is more consistent with a meniscal tear. The presence of an effusion is also helpful in differentiating a patellofemoral chondral injury from patellofemoral syndrome.

The patient should be asked about any evaluation or treatment he or she received at the time of the injury or subsequent to the injury. It may also be helpful to know if weight-bearing restrictions were recommended. Knowledge of previous immobilization is also helpful, particularly if the patient has residual loss of range of motion (ROM). For any patient with a prior surgical intervention, the operative report and arthroscopy images can provide valuable information. Finally, the physician should ask which, if any, of these treatments have benefited the patient. These questions help guide the surgeon in creating a treatment plan that avoids the replication of prior failed treatments.

Once the history surrounding the present complaint is fully understood, the physician should collect general medical, surgical, and social histories. For athletes, a more complete understanding of their athletic history should be sought, including their current and past level of play; the number of hours per week that they play; and their skill level, potential, and athletic goals. These factors all play a role in surgical decision-making.[6] In particular, in the patient with an ACL tear who plans to return to category I hard cutting or pivoting sports such as basketball, football, rugby, volleyball, or mogul/black diamond skiing, the risk for reinjury with nonoperative treatment of an ACL tear is high.[6] The surgeon should also obtain an occupational history, because a patient who is reliant on the injured extremity for his or her livelihood likely requires a more aggressive treatment regimen.

A review of systems should always be collected as well. A particular focus should be placed on pain and swelling in other joints, eye disease, back pain, pain with urination, and skin disorders, all of which may hint at a diagnosis of an inflammatory arthropathy. Similarly, a history of fevers, night sweats, or drainage may lead the physician to suspect infection. A history of atraumatic knee pain with an associated mass with primarily nocturnal or constant pain may lead the physician to a neoplastic diagnosis. Pain out of proportion, hypersensitivity, and color and/or temperature changes to the knee should lead the physician to suspect a complex regional pain syndrome.

Finally, the physician must discuss goals and expectations with the patient. Expectations frequently need to be tempered. In athletes and former athletes presenting with a knee injury, it behooves the surgeon to come to a better understanding of whether the athlete would like to return to play (RTP) or simply desires a painless knee for activities of daily living. The patient is most likely to achieve a successful result if he or she understands the goals of the treatment program for the presumed diagnosis.

PHYSICAL EXAMINATION

Physical examination of the knee requires an in-depth understanding of the anatomic structures and the function of these structures, because each provocative test seeks to isolate the function of each structure. We often view the examination as a multistep process: (1) inspection; (2) palpation; (3) ROM and strength testing; (4) patellar testing; (5) meniscal testing; (6) ligamentous stability testing; (7) gait assessment; (8) evaluation of muscle weakness and imbalance (e.g., hamstring tightness, quadriceps tightness, or core weakness); and (9) assessment of the back, hip, and feet. We start by examining the noninjured extremity, which may provide important information regarding baseline abnormalities and also helps to relax the patient.

INSPECTION

A great deal of information can be gained from inspection of the patient before taking a history or performing a focused physical examination (Box 90.1). If possible, patients should be observed as they enter the examination room or at some other time when they do not know they are being observed.[7] Once the patient is in the examination room, the physician can gain insight into the patient's general mobility by observing his or her transfer from a chair to the examination table.

The periarticular skin should be carefully inspected for (1) any surgical scars, which may affect future surgical planning;

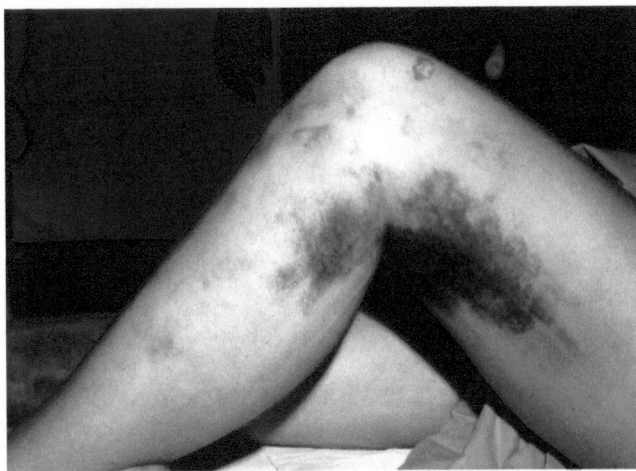

Fig. 90.1 Ecchymoses reflect a subcutaneous hemorrhage and may signal a capsular injury. These posterolateral hemorrhages raise suspicion for a posterolateral corner ligamentous injury.

(2) erythema, which should be demarcated with a skin-marking pen if it is believed to reflect an underlying cellulitis; (3) ecchymoses, which reflect subcutaneous hemorrhage that may signal a capsular injury (Fig. 90.1); and (4) abrasions, which may provide a clue to the direction of the primary trauma. For example, with a dashboard mechanism, a patellar abrasion is concerning for patellar fracture, while an anterior tibial abrasion should raise concern for a PCL injury because of the posteriorly directed force on the anterior tibia at the time of injury (Fig. 90.2). Attention should be directed to the presence or absence of effusion, any localized swelling, and muscle tone within the periarticular muscles—in particular the quadriceps and vastus medialis obliquus. The examiner should examine a patient with a suspected dislocation for the presence of any abnormal skin furrows or dimpling, which could signal buttonholing of the condyles through the capsule and the need for open reduction.[8,9] Although general inspection may reveal atrophy, the most sensitive measurement of atrophy is a comparison of thigh circumference with the contralateral knee (typically performed 15 cm proximal to the superior pole of the patella; Fig. 90.3).[10] This measurement can be used as a marker for the rehabilitation process after surgery. General inspection may reveal stigmata of other general medical conditions, such as signs of venous stasis, ulcerations, or prior amputations as a result of diabetic neuropathy or vascular insufficiency, as well as signs of chronic infections or abscesses. Predrawn knee schematics may be helpful for recording findings from visual inspection. Alternatively, obtaining a photograph at the time of presentation can be invaluable for comparison at a later date. Photographs can be entered into the electronic medical record. Serial examinations

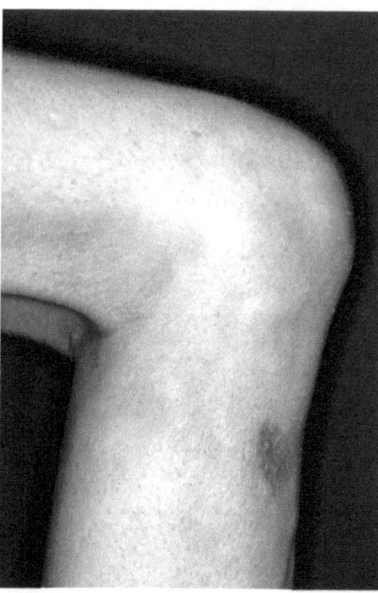

Fig. 90.2 An anterior tibial abrasion is shown with associated posterior subluxation of the tibia, suggesting a posterior cruciate ligament injury.

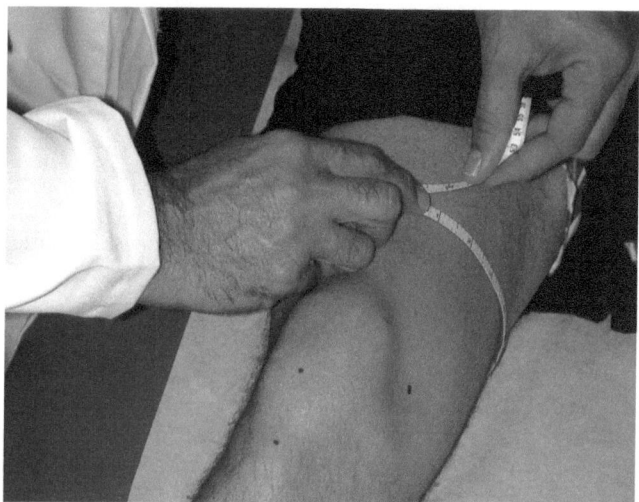

Fig. 90.3 Thigh circumference, which the examiner should always measure at the same distance proximal to the superior patellar pole, is a sensitive measure of quadriceps atrophy.

can be crucial for the determination of progression, especially in the acutely injured patient.

Patients should remove their shoes so that the entire limb can be inspected. Mechanical limb alignment should be visually estimated within the coronal, sagittal, and axial planes. The presence of genu varum, valgum, procurvatum, or recurvatum should be further evaluated radiographically. Specific attention should be directed to malrotation.[11] With the patient supine, the examiner should also visually inspect the height level of the patella for alta or baja. The physician may also want to measure limb length. Although the most accurate method for limb length measurement is the placement of sized standing blocks under the short leg until the pelvis is level, a rapid, rough estimation can be gained with a glance at the relative heights of the medial malleoli in the supine patient. The physician can also estimate the Q angle visually and measure it with a goniometer, although

this measurement can be affected by a variety of other deformities. Deformities within the foot should also be observed. For instance, pes planus may be a contributing factor to genu valgum or may be a sign of generalized ligamentous laxity. Gluteal strength can also be observed by asking patients to stand on one leg, perform a single-leg squat, or do repetitive single leg jumps. Inability to maintain a level pelvis, increased trunk lean, increased hip adduction, and excessive knee valgus during these activities is indicative of gluteal/core weakness that can indirectly contribute to patellofemoral symptoms.

The patient's gait should be observed. Although gait is a complex process requiring normal function of the foot, ankle, knee, hip, and lumbosacral spine, some gait abnormalities can also be referred to the knee. One should observe for varus and valgus thrusts, an antalgic gait with shortening of the stance phase for the affected limb, and the foot progression angle. Patients with ACL deficiency may exhibit a quadriceps avoidance gait, possibly to prevent excess anterior tibial translation.[12]

PALPATION

It should be noted that many patients in the acute postinjury phase have generalized inflammation with diffuse tenderness that tends to be nondiagnostic; as a result, the patient may need to return at a later date for a repeat examination.

The knee should be palpated for the presence or absence of an effusion. The examiner can milk fluid down from the suprapatellar bursa while holding the patella between the thumb and forefinger of the contralateral hand to assess for the ability to ballot the patella. Alternatively, the examiner can feel for swelling at the soft spots medial and lateral to the patellar tendon, where the capsule is fairly subcutaneous. The other area where the surgeon may be able to palpate synovial fluid is in a Baker cyst, which is most commonly posteromedial between the semimembranosus and the medial head of the gastrocnemius.

The quadriceps tendon and its patellar insertion can be palpated both for tenderness associated with quadriceps tendonitis and a gap associated with a quadriceps tendon tear. The patella should be palpated for prepatellar tenderness or fullness that may be a sign of prepatellar bursitis. The distal pole of the patella and the patellar tendon origin should be palpated for tenderness associated with patellar tendonitis (or Sinding-Larsen-Johansson syndrome in adolescents; Fig. 90.4), as well as for a gap associated with a patellar tendon tear. The tibial tubercle should be palpated (Fig. 90.5) for bony tenderness, which may be associated with Osgood-Schlatter syndrome.

On the medial side of the knee, the entire course of the MCL should be palpated for tenderness. The femoral and patellar attachments of the medial patellofemoral ligament should be evaluated for a palpable gap or tenderness. The medial tibial plateau should be palpated for tenderness because it might be associated with an acute fracture or stress fracture. The region just anteromedial to the patella should be assessed for a palpable tender band from plica syndrome (Fig. 90.6). The distal insertion of the sartorius, semitendinosus, and gracilis tendons should be palpated for pes anserine bursitis. The posteromedial joint line should also be palpated for a possible meniscal tear. Whereas

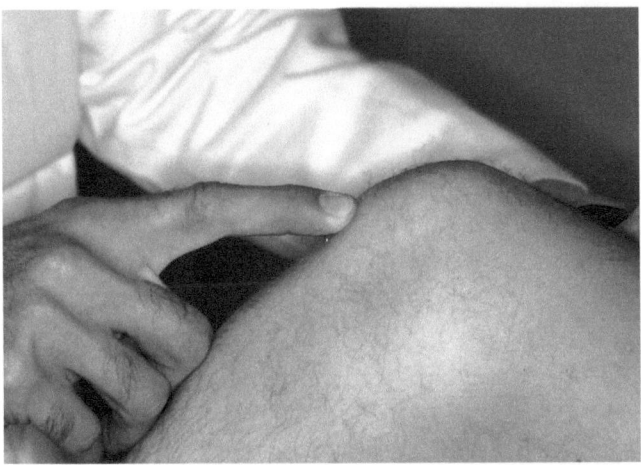

Fig. 90.4 Tenderness at the inferior pole of the patella suggests patellar tendonitis.

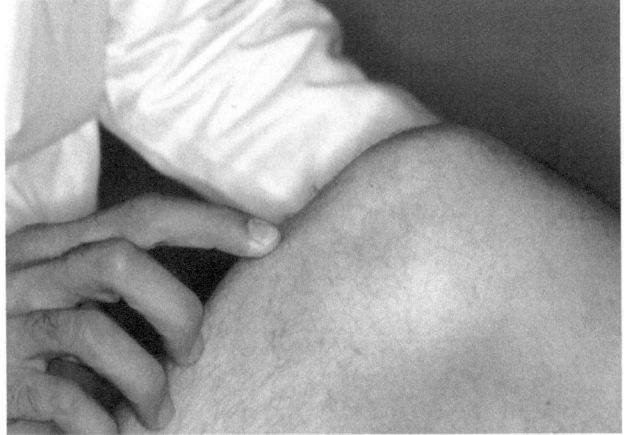

Fig. 90.5 Tenderness to palpation at the tibial tubercle suggests Osgood-Schlatter syndrome, fracture of the tibial tubercle, or possibly insertional patellar tendonitis.

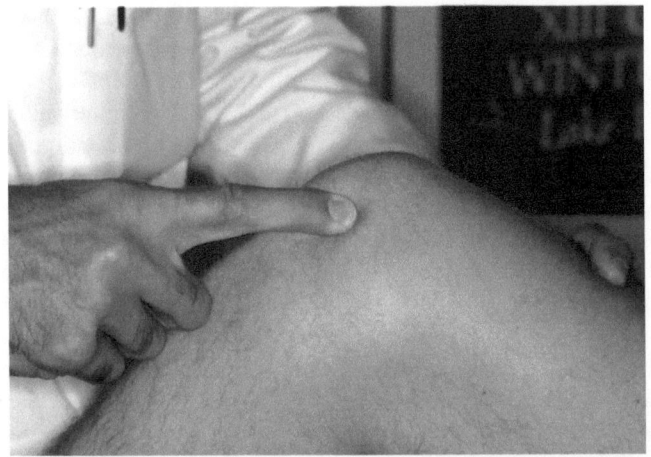

Fig. 90.6 A tender palpable band, which may snap back and forth over the medial femoral condyle, suggests medial plica syndrome.

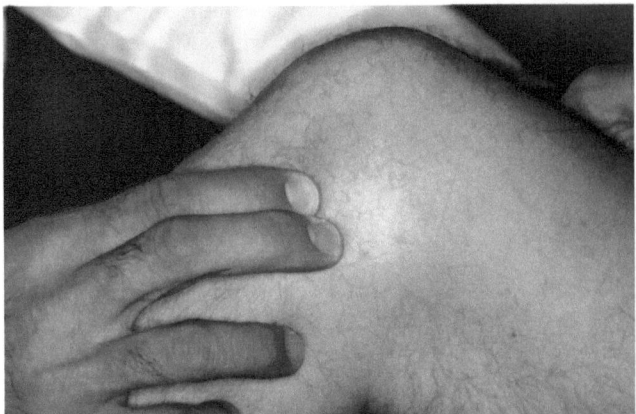

Fig. 90.7 Palpation for tenderness at the anterior medial joint line.

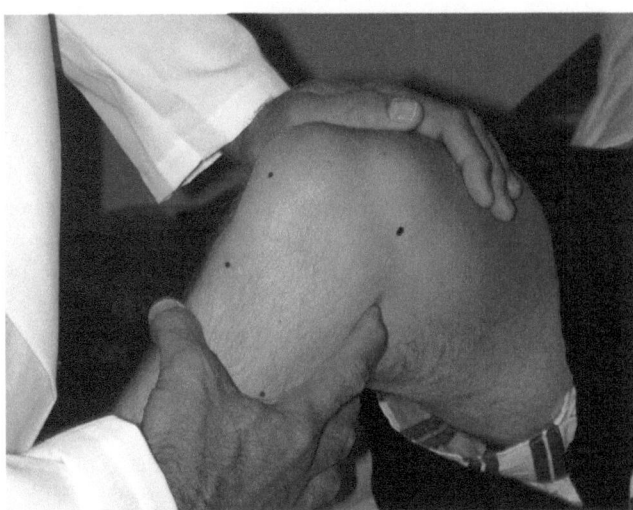

Fig. 90.8 Palpation for tenderness at the posterior lateral joint line.

anteromedial (Fig. 90.7) and medial joint line tenderness is often associated with plica syndrome or hypertrophic fat pad syndrome, displaced bucket handle meniscal tears characteristically have more tenderness anterior than the classic posteromedial location associated with most meniscal tears.

Similarly, the surgeon must also palpate the lateral structures. The lateral collateral ligament is best identified with the knee in the "figure-of-four" position, where varus stress makes the ligament taut and more easily palpable. The other structures of the PLC, such as the popliteus tendon and the popliteofibular ligament, can be more difficult to assess with palpation. The biceps tendon is most easily assessed as a cord at the posterolateral surface of the fibular head. Just anterior to the biceps tendon is the iliotibial band, which can be palpated as it passes over the lateral femoral condyle and at its tibial attachment at the Gerdy tubercle. The fibular head should also be assessed. The lateral tibial plateau should be palpated for tenderness, which might be associated with an acute fracture or stress fracture. The lateral joint line (Fig. 90.8) is palpated for a possible meniscal tear. While medial meniscal tears are more likely to manifest with tenderness over the posteromedial joint line, lateral meniscal tears tend to be more tender over the midbody or anterior horn of knee of meniscus. Anterolateral joint line tenderness can be associated with hypertrophic fat pad syndrome. Just distal to the fibular head, the examiner can commonly palpate the common peroneal nerve. In patients with suspected pathology of the peroneal nerve, the examiner should attempt to elicit a Tinel sign. Pain associated with common peroneal neuritis may be referred to the anterolateral proximal tibial region.

RANGE OF MOTION AND STRENGTH TESTING

ROM is a fairly sensitive predictor of intra-articular pathology and is critical for knee function. Normal knee ROM has been described as 0 to 120 degrees,[7,13] although the ROM actively used for gait is 10 to 120 degrees.[14] However, considerable variation exists. At terminal extension, many persons have up to 5 degrees of hyperextension, which, in combination with range from 0 to 10 degrees of flexion, may be useful for the "screw home" mechanism of internal rotation that tensions the cruciate ligaments and "locks" the knee at full extension. Many persons have additional passive flexion beyond their active range; in men this is commonly 140 degrees and in women it is 143 degrees, although in societies where kneeling is common, such as in Japan, India, and the Middle East, passive flexion to 165 degrees is common.[13] One hundred and twenty-five degrees of flexion are necessary to squat, whereas 110 degrees of flexion is required to descend stairs in normal fashion. The loss of as little as 10 degrees of flexion will affect running speed. The loss of as little as 5 degrees of extension can cause a limp with increased quadriceps activation during gait and resultant quadriceps strain and fatigue, as well as patellofemoral pain. Differences between passive and active ROM should be noted. A loss of both is considered a "contracture" and implies a block to motion, whereas a loss of active ROM with preserved passive ROM is considered a "lag" and implies a muscle tightness or imbalance.

Several methods may be used to test ROM. A goniometer can be placed on the lateral side of the knee with the proximal end pointed toward the greater trochanter and the distal end pointed toward the lateral malleolus. This method has high inter- and intraobserver reliability.[15] A more sensitive indicator of full extension and flexion is the measurement of the heel-height difference with the patient placed in the prone position (Fig. 90.9). Similarly, the heel-buttock distance can be measured in full flexion in the supine position. One centimeter correlates with approximately 1 degree.[14]

Restricted knee ROM must be understood in context. Postsurgical motion restriction is almost universally the result of either global or focal arthrofibrosis (e.g., cyclops lesion). Early studies suggested that up to 35% of patients undergoing ACL reconstruction experienced postoperative motion loss[16]; however, this has decreased to 0% to 4% with appropriate surgical timing, technique, and an accelerated rehabilitation program.[17–19] Risk factors for postsurgical motion loss following ACL reconstruction include acute reconstruction (<1 week following injury), improper graft placement or tension during ACL reconstruction, concomitant extra-articular procedures (meniscal repair, collateral ligament reconstruction), prolonged immobilization, infection, and complex regional pain syndrome.[14] Postinjury motion restriction in the acute phase may be the result of

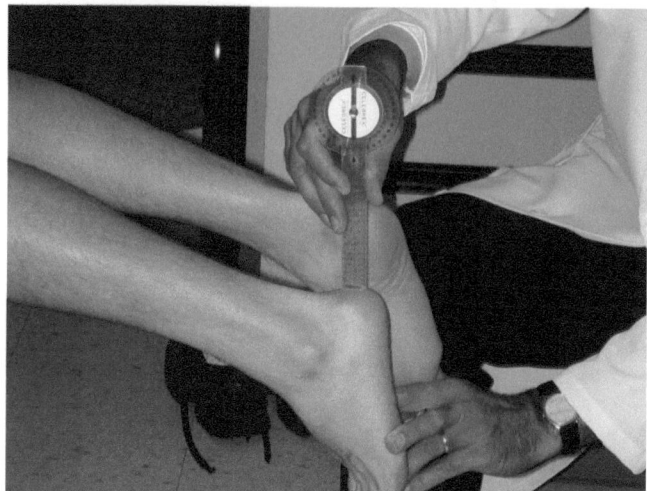

Fig. 90.9 The most sensitive way to measure extension deficit is to measure the heel-height distance difference with the patient in the prone position. A 1-cm difference roughly correlates with a 1-degree difference.

hemarthrosis or displaced intra-articular fragment (such as a displaced osteochondral fracture, ACL tissue flipped into the intercondylar notch, or displaced meniscal tear). In the acute phase, a displaced bucket handle meniscal tear is more likely to promote a more significant block to full extension (15 degrees or greater); however, after several weeks this may result in a subtle side-to-side difference (5 degrees or less).

ROM testing should also be performed on the ankle and hip joints and lumbar spine. We also commonly test for generalized ligamentous laxity, specifically by examining for elbow recurvatum, hyperextension at the metacarpophalangeal joint, the ability to abduct the thumb to meet the forearm, and excess external rotation of the humerus in adduction, all of which may signal a connective tissue abnormality. It should be noted that some confusion exists in the literature regarding the terms *laxity* and *instability*. *Laxity* is a term used to describe a finding on physical examination, whereas *instability* is a term used to describe a patient's subjective experience of this same entity. It is possible for a person to have generalized ligamentous laxity with no instability, and vice versa.

Several other structures can be assessed during ROM testing. For instance, if the patient reports lateral knee pain with a palpable snap, the examiner can flex the knee, internally rotate, and then extend the knee to elicit snapping of the biceps tendon over a prominent fibula head (Fig. 90.10).[20] This observation may not be detected with external or neutral tibial rotation. It is important to consider this entity because it can mimic an unstable lateral meniscal tear. More commonly, the patient should be assessed for hamstring tightness in the supine position with the examiner attempting to flex the hip with the knee extended. We grade hamstring flexibility in degrees from the examination table. In this same position, the patient should be assessed for the ability to perform a straight leg raise. The examiner may also wish to assess for iliotibial band tightness using the Ober test. In this test, the patient is placed in the lateral decubitus position with both hips and knees flexed to 90 degrees, so as not to flatten the lumbar spine. Concomitantly, the affected leg

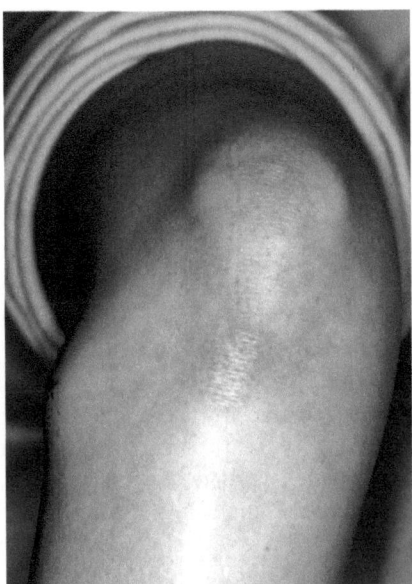

Fig. 90.10 Observation may reveal prominence of the fibular head, which may predispose to snapping of the biceps tendon with flexion/extension.

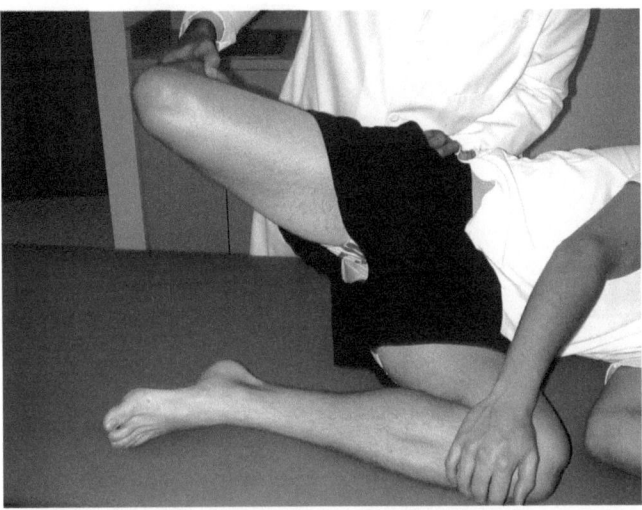

Fig. 90.11 To test for contracture of the iliotibial band, the examiner can use the Ober test, in which the patient is placed in the lateral decubitus position and the knee is flexed to 90 degrees while the hip is abducted to 40 degrees and fully extended, and an attempt is then made to adduct the hip. An inability to adduct past midline signifies tightness within the iliotibial band.

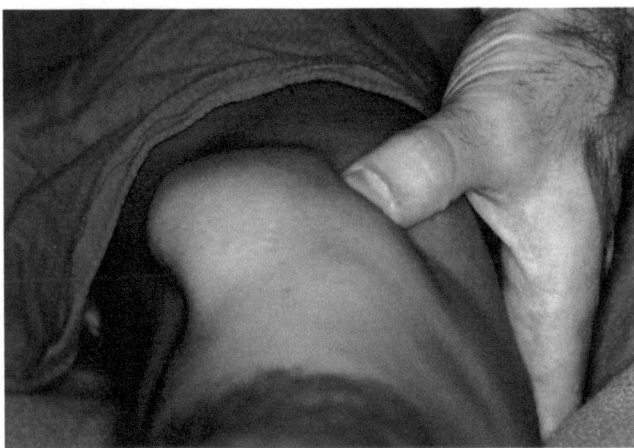

Fig. 90.12 Patellar mobility can be assessed in full extension to assess fibrosis within the retinaculum, capsule, and other peripatellar tissues.

is abducted to 40 degrees and fully extended, and an attempt is then made to adduct the hip. An inability to adduct past midline signifies an iliotibial band contracture (Fig. 90.11).

ROM testing is also an excellent time to assess muscular strength, including hip abduction, knee flexion and extension, ankle flexion and extension, foot eversion and inversion, and extension of the hallux. In a patient with demonstrable weakness, one must determine whether neuromuscular inhibition due to pain may be contributory. While testing distal strength, one should assess distal sensory function in the sural nerve at the lateral border of the foot, the saphenous nerve at the medial ankle, the superficial peroneal nerve over the dorsum of the foot, the deep peroneal nerve at the dorsal first web space, and the tibial nerve over the plantar surface of the foot. Patients with previous longitudinal anterior knee incisions should be assessed for residual numbness in the distribution of the infrapatellar branch of the saphenous nerve; any numbness would be lateral to any incision, because the nerve runs from medial to lateral. Whereas testing sensation to light touch is commonly sufficient for examination of the knee in the setting of a sports physician's office, testing with a 5.08 Semmes-Weinstein monofilament is the most sensitive method of testing for a sensory deficit in this region of the body and the preferred method in patients with suspected diabetic neuropathy.

The vascular status of the limb can be assessed with palpation of pulses at the posterior tibial artery at the posteromedial ankle, the dorsalis pedis artery over the proximal dorsal foot, and the popliteal artery at the posterior knee. Patients without palpable pulses require assessment with a Doppler device. This portion of the examination is crucial in the acute assessment of any patient with trauma to the knee, particularly patients with suspected or confirmed knee dislocations. These patients may require additional assessment with an ankle-brachial index, and any patient with an ankle-brachial index score of less than 0.8 requires further investigation with an angiogram or magnetic resonance angiogram.[21]

PATELLA

While many clinicians lump all anterior knee complaints as patellofemoral syndrome/chondromalacia, a targeted physical exam can help discern between patellofemoral syndrome, patellar tendinitis, lateral patellar tilt, medial plica syndrome, and hypertrophic fat pad syndrome. To assess the retinaculum and peripatellar capsular structures, the examiner can assess patella mobility with the knee in extension before it engages with the trochlea (Fig. 90.12). In anxious patients, the examiner may wish to repeat this portion of the examination with the patient in the prone position, which relaxes the quadriceps.[11] The knee can then be flexed to 30 degrees when the patella has fully engaged into the trochlea where the retinaculum is tightened. At this position, patellar tilt can be assessed and palpated by attempting to lift the lateral patella from the lateral trochlea. Furthermore, the examiner should palpate the lateral edge of the patella and determine if static lateral translation of the patella is present in relation to the lateral femoral condyle and whether this translation is correctable. The lateral edge of the patella can be palpated to determine if it overhangs the lateral femoral sulcus; if anatomically positioned, both structures are palpable. The apprehension sign can be elicited by pressing laterally on the medial border of the patella (Fig. 90.13). In a patient who has undergone a previous lateral release, a medially directed positive apprehension sign indicates an overzealous lateral retinacular release with subsequent medial instability. The examiner should also assess how far the patella can be translated laterally, which is then graded into quadrants. As a rule of thumb, the examiner should not be able to displace the patella more than half of its width laterally. The knee can then be taken through a flexion/extension cycle with the examiner's hand on the patella to feel for crepitus (Fig. 90.14), as well as any dynamic maltracking (Fig. 90.15). While observing patellar movement during ROM, one should determine whether the patella subluxes in extension or in flexion. Specifically the examiner should note the presence or absence of a "J sign" as the patella translates laterally out of the trochlea in terminal extension. Finally, with the knee in 60 to 90 degrees of flexion, the examiner can press with one hand on the patella and stabilize the ankle with the other hand while asking the patient to attempt to actively straighten his or her knee. If this maneuver elicits pain, the examiner should suspect patellofemoral pathology.[11] The degree of flexion of the knee at the time of the pain may signal chondral injury more proximally versus distally within the groove. However, even in healthy patients, synovium can become entrapped between the patella and the trochlea and cause pain with compression against the patella.

The Q angle should be observed with the knee between 70 and 90 degrees of flexion. It is also useful to assess the dynamic Q angle—the extent to which the Q angle increases with external rotation of the foot—as patients with patellar instability and an elevated dynamic Q angle may warrant consideration of tibial tubercle osteotomy. In a patient with a long-standing distal extensor mechanism reconstruction (e.g., Hauser procedure), the Q angle may be negative, with resultant posteriorization of the patellar force vectors. Arthroscopic assessment consequently will demonstrate severe medial patellofemoral arthritis as a result of this slingshot effect.

MENISCUS

A variety of meniscal examination maneuvers have been described. In a recent meta-analysis of numerous previously published studies examining the sensitivity, specificity, and accuracy of the various physical examination tests for meniscal pathology, joint line tenderness was found to be the most sensitive test overall, whereas the McMurray test is the most specific.[22] Joint line tenderness can be elicited with palpation as a sign of a meniscal tear, commonly posterior to the midaxial line in the sagittal plane, although a displaced bucket handle tear is more tender anteromedially or anterolaterally at the anterior apex of the "bucket."

The most commonly used provocative meniscal test is the McMurray test, which is performed with the patient supine. To

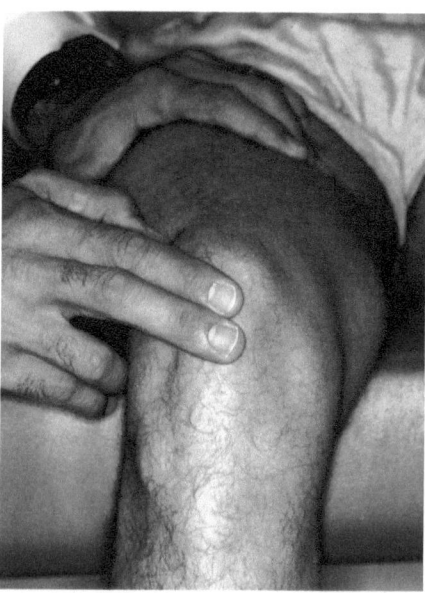

Fig. 90.14 Palpation of the patella during flexion/extension cycles allows the examiner to assess for crepitus and maltracking.

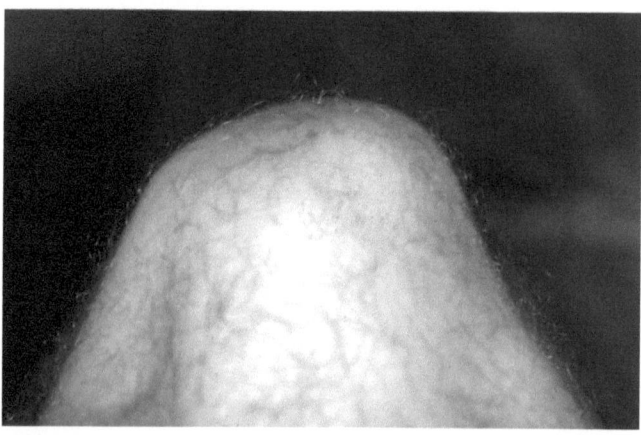

Fig. 90.15 Lateral patellar maltracking.

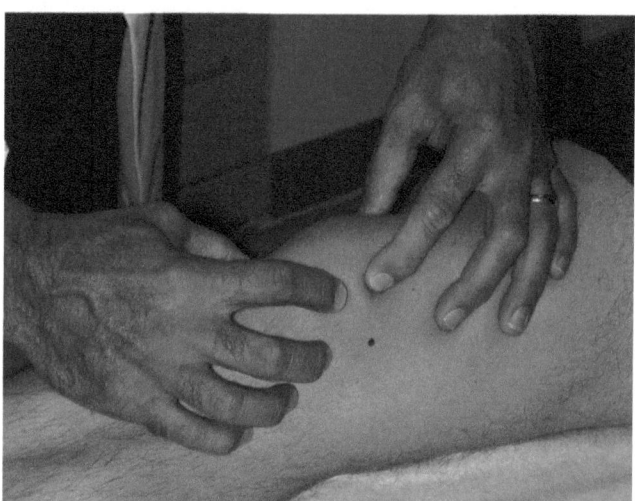

Fig. 90.13 Patellar apprehension, a sign of instability, is present if pressure laterally on the medial border of the patella causes pain or patient concern for impending dislocation or subluxation.

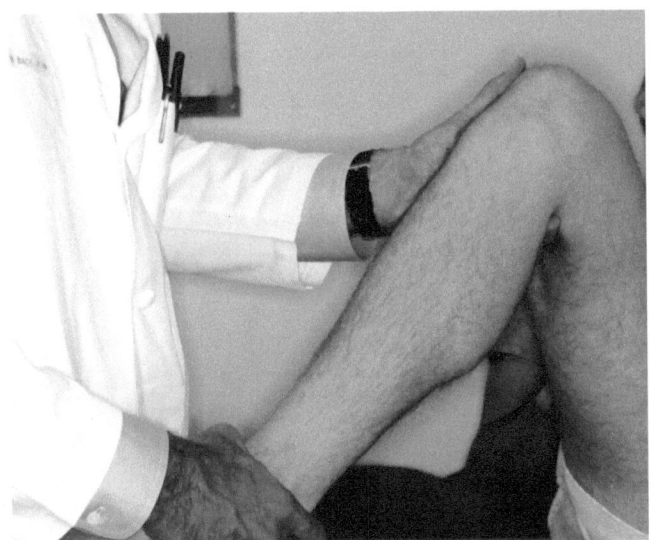

Fig. 90.16 The McMurray meniscal test involves flexion, external rotation, and either varus or valgus stress with either medial or lateral joint line palpation for tears within the medial and lateral menisci, respectively.

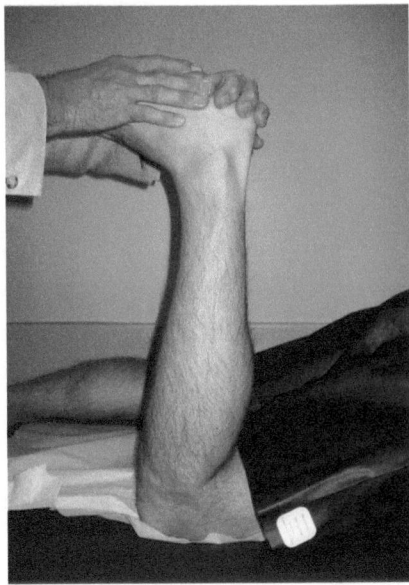

Fig. 90.17 The Apley meniscal test involves prone positioning, flexion of the knee to 90 degrees, axial compression, and then internal and external rotatory movements.

test the medial meniscus, the knee is flexed and brought into a varus stress and externally rotated and then slowly extended while palpating the medial joint for a mechanical click and asking the patient for any sensation of pain (Fig. 90.16). To test the lateral side, the aforementioned maneuver is performed with a valgus stress.[23] The senior author has not found the position of tibial rotation to be particularly sensitive; instead, we assess for pain referred to the affected compartment with hyperflexing, rotating, and extension maneuvers. The Apley test is performed with the patient in the prone position. The knee is brought into 90 degrees of flexion and then internally and externally rotated while applying an axial load (Fig. 90.17). A positive test occurs with the reproduction of pain or a catching or locking sensation. In addition, the test can be repeated in distraction across the joint, with continued pain and symptomatology signaling an articular cartilage lesion instead of a meniscal tear.[24] The bounce home test is performed with the patient supine with a flexed knee and the foot cupped in the examiner's hand. The knee is passively extended and allowed to bounce home into extension with a sharp endpoint. Inability to achieve full extension or the presence of a rubbery end-point is suggestive of an interposed meniscus or alternate loose fragment. The Thessaly test is performed with the patient's own weight causing the compression. In this test, the patient stands on the affected leg, supported with his or her outstretched hands by the examiner, and flexes the affected knee to 5 degrees while internally and externally rotating three times. The test is repeated in 20 degrees of flexion. In the original description of this test, the accuracy was 94% for medial meniscal tears and 96% for lateral meniscal tears, with all other tests having lesser accuracy—78% to 84% for the McMurray tests, 75% to 82% for the Apley test, and 81% to 89% for joint line tenderness.[25]

LIGAMENTOUS STABILITY

Ligamentous stability testing in the knee is among the most difficult to learn aspects of the physical examination and one of

the most important portions of the examination.[26,27] A variety of tests have been described for testing the ACL. The anterior drawer test is historically the oldest test but is the least sensitive. With this test, one attempts to anteriorly translate the tibia with the knee flexed to 90 degrees with the ankle stabilized. Generally this test is only positive with loss of not only the ACL but also the secondary restraints to anterior tibial translation such as the posterior horn of the medial meniscus (e.g., meniscal resection or an unstable peripheral meniscal tear). If the anterior drawer test is more positive than the Lachman test, one should suspect a PCL injury because the tibia is in a posterior resting position and is being translated to its neutral position. Increased antero-medial rotation of the tibia while flexed at 90 degrees is suggestive of a posteromedial corner injury.

The Lachman test is the most sensitive test for determining an ACL injury. The examiner attempts to anteriorly translate the tibia with the knee at 30 degrees of flexion (Fig. 90.18).[28,29] We perform this test with one hand stabilizing the distal femur and the other hand gripping the distal tibia such that a thumb is placed on the joint line and can palpate the translation of the tibia relative to the femur. This distance is then used to grade the test; grade 1 has 0 to 5 mm of translation, grade 2 has 5 to 10 mm of translation, and grade 3 has greater than 10 mm of translation (Fig. 90.19).[30] When compared with the opposite knee, the examiner should also assess for the true presence of a "soft" or "firm" end point. The sensitivity of the Lachman test is 94% to 98% in a patient who is awake.[31]

The most definitive test for assessing the functional integrity of the ACL is the pivot shift test, which characterizes the subluxation-reduction phenomenon of ACL deficiency. The goal of ACL reconstruction surgery is to eliminate the pivot shift regardless of the preoperative grade. Unfortunately, eliciting a positive pivot shift in the office can be difficult because patients are often apprehensive and guarding their knee. Furthermore, once a physician has elicited this sensation, subsequent efforts

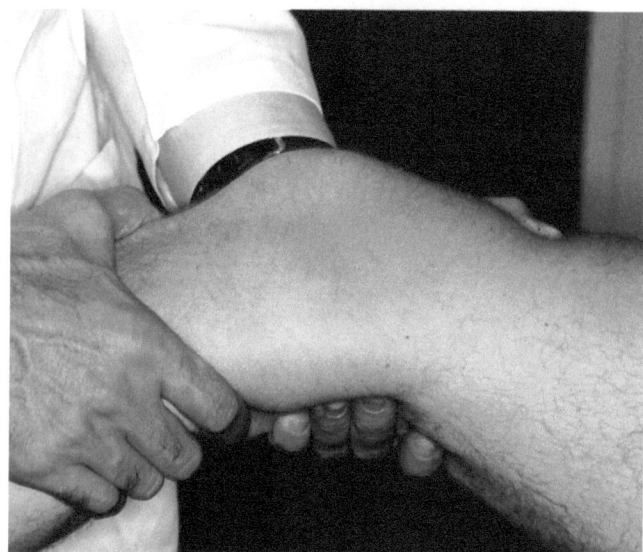

Fig. 90.18 Lachman testing, which is similar to anterior drawer testing but performed at 30 degrees of flexion.

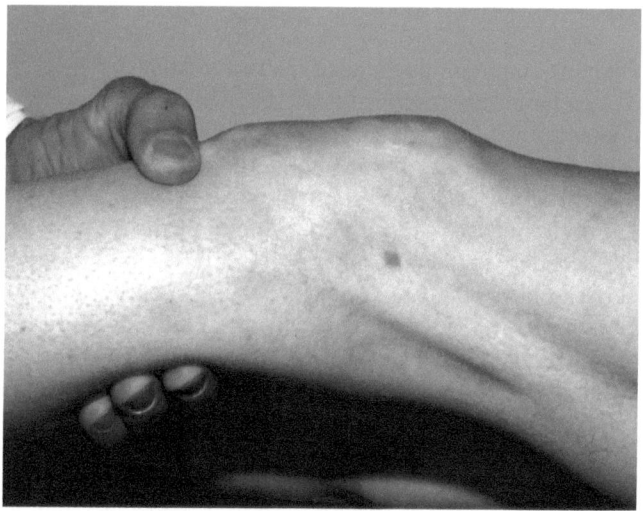

Fig. 90.19 A positive Lachman test with anterior subluxation of the tibia.

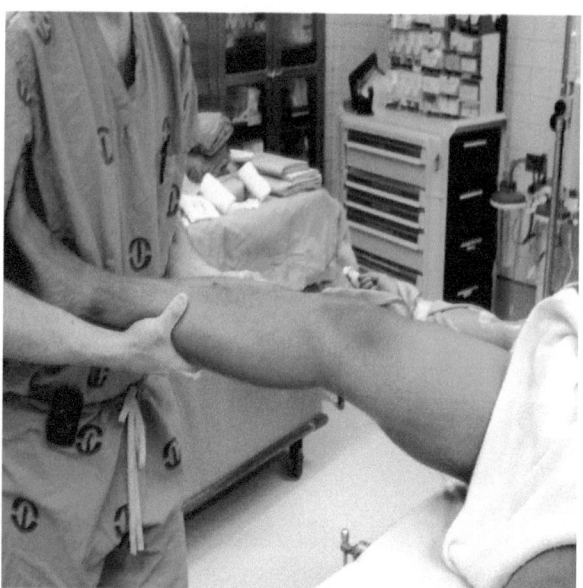

Fig. 90.20 Pivot shift testing, shown preoperatively after administration of an anesthetic. In this examination maneuver, the examiner applies an external rotation and valgus stress to the fully extended knee and then slowly flexes, feeling for a reduction "clunk" at 20 to 30 degrees of flexion.

the position of the thigh when tested (abduction vs. adduction), and tibial rotation (external vs. internal rotation) can affect the pivot shift phenomenon. Perfecting this examination is an art form that takes years to master. It is easily inadequately performed, interpreted improperly, or sadly, not performed as part of an examination with the patient anesthetized prior to arthroscopic evaluation. We have encountered many patients who have been informed that they have a partial ACL tear (as determined by MRI, physical examination, and/or arthroscopy) but who are found to have an obvious pivot shift phenomenon upon careful examination.

To perform the pivot shift maneuver as initially described, the physician exerts a valgus and internal rotation moment on the tibia with the knee extended and then slowly flexes the knee (Fig. 90.20). We also advocate abducting the hip (and externally rotating, not internally rotating, the tibia) to relax the IT band and eliminate its tenodesis effect. A positive result is a subluxing sensation at approximately 20 to 30 degrees of flexion.[33] The biomechanical explanation for this maneuver is that in the ACL-deficient knee the tibia subluxes anteriorly at full extension. Valgus stress traps the lateral condyle in this subluxed position. With increasing flexion, the periarticular soft tissues exert an increasing ligamentotaxis effect, pulling the tibia posteriorly. Eventually this force causes the posterior lip of the tibia to be pulled posteriorly over the convex femoral condyle, reducing the knee with a palpable clunk.[34] One modification of this test is the "pivot jerk" maneuver in which the knee is brought from flexion to extension with a similar valgus and internal rotation force, with the clunk experienced as the reduced tibia subluxes anteriorly.[7]

Several grading scales have been proposed for the pivot shift test. In the most commonly used scale, grade I is a gliding sensation without a palpable clunk, grade II is a palpable and

are usually met with patient guarding. In the office, we prefer to note that the patient is guarding on pivot shift maneuvers rather than stating that the test is negative. It is of interest that after reconstruction, if the ACL is functionally stable, the patient will allow the physician to perform multiple pivot shift attempts without apprehension. The pivot shift phenomenon is a complex combination of subluxation, rotation, and reduction motions. It is most easily conceptualized as a subluxation of the tibia in extension and a reduction with knee flexion. The pivot shift, as described by Galway (the Hughston "jerk test") and Noyes ("flexion rotation drawer"), as well as the Losee test, the Slocum test, and the Bach-Warren test, are all subtle modifications of this phenomenon.[32] An excellent overview of the various described maneuvers has been presented by Lane et al.[32] It is critical to recognize that axial load and valgus force can have an impact on the grade of the pivot shift phenomenon. Incarcerated ACL stumps, displaced meniscal fragments, meniscal deficiency, associated ligamentous patholaxity (e.g., MCL), knee stiffness, arthritis, sometimes audible clunk or jump, and grade III is a locked knee. Transient locking is usually observed with associated meniscal deficiency. In 1987, Jakob and colleagues[35] proposed an alternate grading scale in which a grade I pivot is "trace"—that is, only elicited with the patient anesthetized; a grade II pivot is positive in internal rotation and neutral; and a grade III pivot is positive in external rotation and less obviously so in internal rotation. Conversely, Bach and colleagues[30] noted improved sensitivity of the pivot shift test with hip abduction and tibial external rotation, an effect believed to be due to the tenodesis effect of the iliotibial band. The iliotibial band is one of several structures that can affect the ability of the ACL-deficient knee to pivot; with an MCL injury, valgus stress no longer causes a compressive force across the lateral compartment, and a flexion contracture of bucket handle meniscal tear prevents making full extension. Conversely, several injuries can accentuate the pivot further; injury to the PLC increases the examiner's ability to externally rotate the tibia and thus increase the pivot. A prior medial meniscectomy can also result in increased anterior tibial translation and an increased pivot shift.

Unfortunately, the pivot shift maneuver is subject to poor interobserver reliability because of the vast variation in force applied by the examiner during the maneuver.[34] In addition, because of patient anxiety and guarding, these rotatory instability tests may be difficult to elicit. Any patient scheduled to have a surgical knee intervention should undergo repeat ligamentous testing once general anesthesia has been induced. Sensitivity of the pivot shift maneuver without use of an anesthetic has been described to be as low as 32% to 40%, rising to 97% to 100% with use of an anesthetic.[32] The senior author can recall only a single patient in 30 years who, when examined after inducement of anesthesia, had a negative pivot shift despite complete ACL disruption. Authors of other studies have described sensitivities as high as 89% with the pivot shift maneuver.[36] Almost all studies have described specificities for the anterior drawer, Lachman, and pivot shift tests in excess of 95%.[36,37]

The most important examination for PCL diagnosis is the posterior drawer test. The knee is flexed to 90 degrees and a posteriorly directed force is placed on the tibia while the examiner feels and observes for posterior translation. Similar to the anterior drawer and Lachman tests, this test is commonly graded I for 0- to 5-mm translation, II for 5- to 10-mm translation, and III for 10- to 15-mm translation compared with the opposite knee (Fig. 90.21).[1] Differentiating between grades has important prognostic significance.[27,38,39] A grade III injury may only be possible with concomitant injury to the PLC, capsule, and/or MCL and should cause the examiner to examine closely for such a combined injury.[26,40] The posterior drawer test is the most sensitive and specific test for PCL injury, although in combination, these clinical examination tests have an accuracy of 96%, a sensitivity of 90%, and a specificity of 99%.[41] In the quadriceps activation modification, the knee is brought to 70 degrees of knee flexion and the patient is asked to actively extend at the knee while the ankle is stabilized, while the examiner watches for anterior tibial translation (≥2 mm), which signifies an abnormally posterior resting tibial position. Normally the anterior medial tibial plateau extends 10 mm anterior to the medial femoral

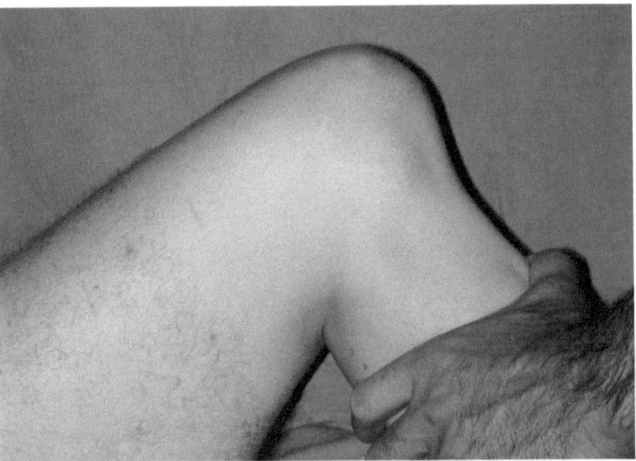

Fig. 90.21 A positive posterior drawer test demonstrates posterior subluxation of the tibia relative to the femur.

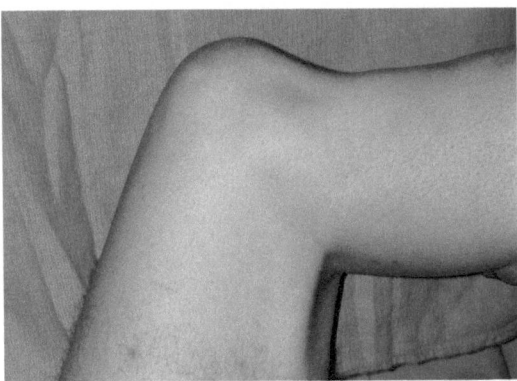

Fig. 90.22 The posterior sag test is similar to the posterior drawer test but allows gravity to provide the subluxation force. This tibia demonstrates posterior subluxation.

condyle. In a knee with a PCL injury, this step-off is reduced. In a grade I PCL injury, the tibial plateau sits ~5 mm anterior to the femoral condyles, in a grade II injury the tibia may be flush with the femoral condyle, and with a grade III injury the tibia sits posterior to the femoral condyles (Fig. 90.22).[27] The presence of a *posterior sag sign* is 100% specific for a PCL injury.[37]

Testing of the MCL starts with palpation, as previously described, with which the examiner may be able to specify whether injury occurs at the proximal or distal end of the ligament.[42] This differentiation may have prognostic clinical significance because proximal MCL injuries have been demonstrated to have a slower recovery of full ROM than distal MCL injuries.[43] The integrity of the MCL can be tested clinically with the patient in the supine position and the ankle cradled between the torso and the elbow while the examiner's hand on the lateral side of the knee exerts a valgus stress and the hand on the medial side of the knee rests with fingers at the joint line to measure the tibiofemoral separation. Similar to tests for the ACL and PCL, this test is commonly graded I for 0- to 5-mm separation, II for 6- to 10-mm separation, and III for greater than 10-mm separation.[30,44] This test should be performed at both full extension and 30 degrees of flexion (Fig. 90.23). Although an isolated MCL injury will cause valgus laxity at 30 degrees, no laxity is observed at

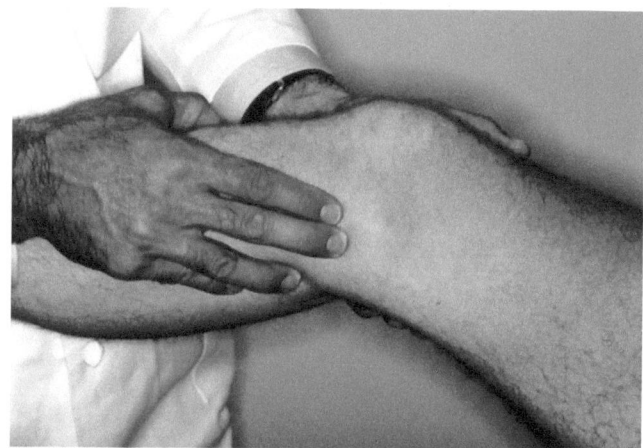

Fig. 90.23 Valgus stress testing performed at 30 degrees of flexion to assess the medial collateral ligament. Note the examiner's fingers on the medial joint line to assess tibiofemoral separation.

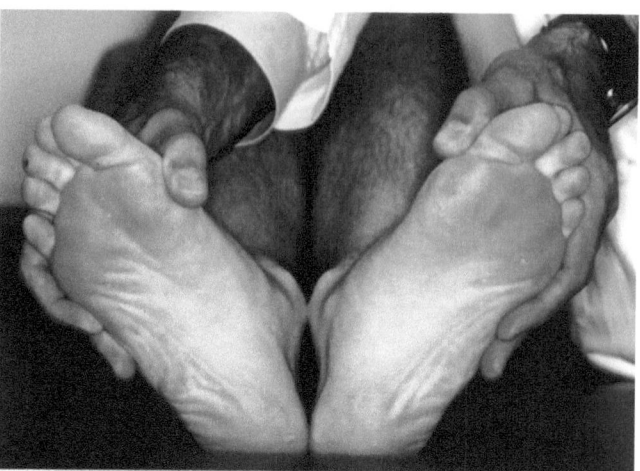

Fig. 90.25 Dial testing performed with the patient supine at 30 degrees of flexion. The side-to-side difference in the angle between the foot and the axis of the tibia denotes degree of laxity of the posterolateral corner.

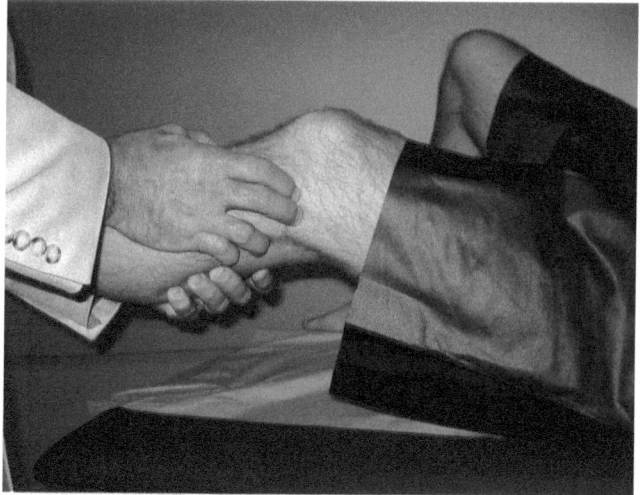

Fig. 90.24 Varus stress testing performed at 30 degrees of flexion. Again, note the position of the examiner's fingers on the lateral joint line.

full extension without injury to the secondary restraints such as the cruciate ligaments, posterior capsule, or posterior oblique ligament.[44,45] These tests must be interpreted in combination to determine the degree of injury (which, it should be noted, is separate from the grade of the valgus stress test), with first-degree injuries exhibiting tenderness without instability, second-degree injuries exhibiting laxity to valgus stress but with a firm end point, and third-degree injuries exhibiting laxity to valgus stress with no end point.[42,44]

We commonly conclude with testing of the structures of the PLC. Similar to the medial side, the examiner can examine for tibiofemoral separation with varus stress at both full extension and 30 degrees of flexion (Fig. 90.24), the latter of which tests the lateral collateral ligament. Also similarly, this test is commonly graded I for a 0- to 5-mm opening, II for a 5- to 10-mm opening, and III for a 10- to 15-mm opening.[30] Similar to valgus stress testing, a positive result at 30 degrees suggests an injury to the lateral structures, whereas a positive result at 0 degrees suggests concomitant injury to the secondary stabilizers

in addition to the lateral collateral ligament, cruciate ligaments, and posterior capsule.[45] However, to fully test the remainder of the structures, the physician must also perform rotatory testing. The most commonly used rotatory test is the dial test, in which the physician attempts to maximally externally rotate both tibia at both 30 and 90 degrees of flexion (Fig. 90.25). Side-to-side testing is crucial, and a side-to-side-difference of less than 10 degrees is considered a mild injury, whereas 10 to 20 degrees is considered moderate and greater than 20 degrees is considered severe. In general, an abnormality at 30 degrees of knee flexion is considered to be an isolated PLC injury, whereas abnormality noted at both 30 and 90 degrees requires injury to both the PLC and PCL.[46] Of note, a complete MCL injury may also allow excess external rotation (because of anteromedial rotation of the tibia).[44,47] The dial test can also be performed in the supine or seated position, again with the examiner assessing for asymmetric thigh-foot angles.

Several additional rotatory tests have been described, many of which describe overlapping functions of the PLC and PCL.[48] For instance, in the recurvatum test, the examiner holds the knee extended by the hallux in the supine and relaxed patient, and observes for asymmetric and excess recurvatum and external rotation (Fig. 90.26).[49] Similarly, with the patient at 90 degrees of flexion and the ankle stabilized, the examiner can test the ability of the tibia to abnormally spin posterolaterally (also described as the external rotation drawer test), a finding most likely to be positive with both PCL and PLC injuries. In addition, a reverse pivot shift maneuver has been described in which the knee is held flexed and a valgus and external rotation stress is placed as the knee is extended, feeling for a reduction "clunk" at 30 to 40 degrees of flexion. In this maneuver, the tibia begins in a posteriorly subluxed position and is forced to reduce anteriorly with increasing extension.[35] Although this test is most likely to be positive with both PLC and PCL injuries, it can also be positive with isolated injuries to either ligamentous structure. These tests have varying sensitivity; the posterolateral external rotation spin test has a sensitivity of 76%, and the external rotation recurvatum test has a sensitivity of 73%.[50]

It should be noted that although these tests are not highly specific to any single structure within the PLC, the examiner may be able to gather some idea of which structures are injured based on the physical findings. Category A injuries have increased external rotation with injury to the popliteofibular ligament and popliteus tendon. Category B injuries have increased external rotation and opening to varus stress of 5 mm at 30 degrees of flexion with injury to the category A structures, as well as attenuation of the lateral collateral ligament. Category C injuries have increased external rotation and opening of 10 mm at varus stress at 30 degrees with injury to the category A structures, as well as tears of the lateral collateral ligament, lateral capsule, and possibly the cruciate ligaments.[8] LaPrade and Terry[50] found that a positive reverse pivot was associated with injuries to the lateral collateral ligament, popliteus, and mid third lateral capsular ligaments, whereas a positive spin test was associated with lateral collateral ligament and lateral gastrocnemius injuries, and a positive varus stress test was associated with injury to the posterior arcuate ligament. Patients with these injuries must be closely examined for injuries to the peroneal nerve as well.

SYNTHESIS AND DECISION-MAKING

A busy office setting often requires one to perform an efficient and focused physical examination. Although experience remains the most valuable tool that will inform which questions to ask and which examination maneuvers to perform in a given patient, we have attempted to synthesize the information provided in this chapter into useful algorithms (Figs. 90.27 and 90.28) that

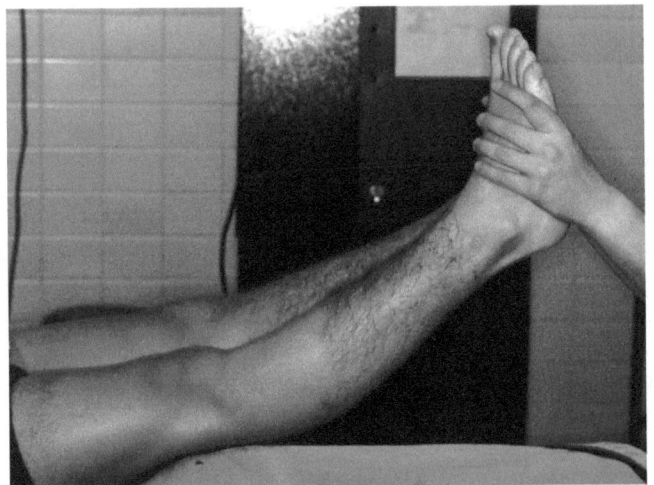

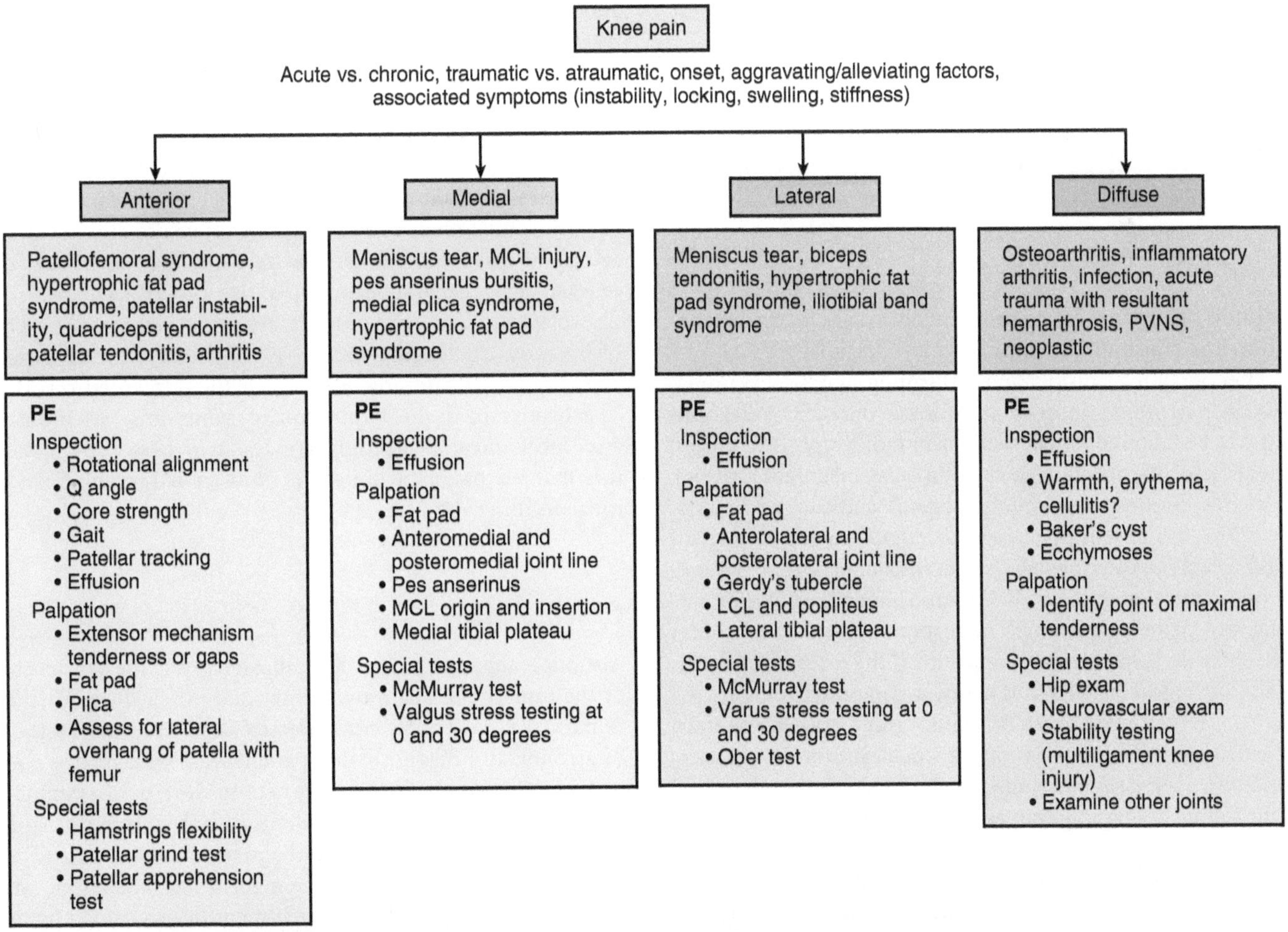

Fig. 90.26 External recurvatum testing performed preoperatively after administration of an anesthetic.

Fig. 90.27 Algorithm for the evaluation of knee pain. *LCL*, Lateral collateral ligament; *MCL*, medial collateral ligament; *PE*, physical examination; *PVNS*, pigmented villonodular synovitis.

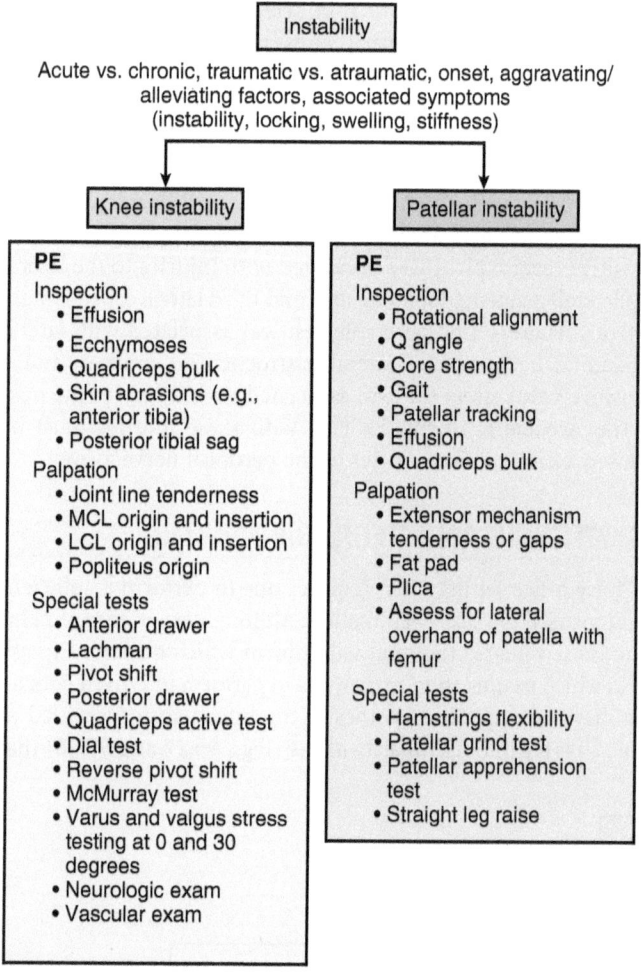

Fig. 90.28 Algorithm for the evaluation of knee instability. *LCL,* Lateral collateral ligament; *MCL,* medial collateral ligament; *PE,* physical examination.

can guide physicians with respect to performing a focused examination and efficiently reaching a clinical diagnosis.

After obtaining a history and performing a physical examination, the practitioner must form a working differential diagnosis that is to be followed initially with plain radiographs. We suggest that all new patients undergo standing bilateral anteroposterior, 30-degree flexion posteroanterior, lateral, and sunrise views of the knees. In the setting of varus or valgus malalignment, 3-ft standing anteroposterior views are also recommended to evaluate the mechanical axis. When ligamentous, meniscal, and/or cartilaginous pathologic features are suspected, we routinely order MRI scans to help elucidate and confirm the diagnosis. Finally, in the setting of patellar instability, a computed tomography scan can be obtained to assess the distance between the tibial tuberosity and the deepest point of trochlear groove on superimposed axial images. Computed tomography can also be helpful in the setting of revision ligamentous surgery to assess for tunnel osteolysis.

Although most sports-related knee conditions are initially treated with a trial of nonoperative treatment consisting of physical therapy, medications, and bracing, certain conditions require early surgical intervention. These conditions include displaced bucket handle meniscus tears (isolated or in the setting of a concomitant ligamentous injury), irreducible knee dislocations, multiligament knee injuries with associated vascular injury, acute PCL osseous avulsions, acute displaced osteochondral injuries, patellar dislocations with a loose osteochondral fragment causing mechanical symptoms, extensor mechanism tear, and intra-articular sepsis. The decision to proceed with immediate surgical care can only be made with an accurate diagnosis that, once again, is dependent on a systematic and focused history and physical examination.

The physiologic age of the knee is also an important factor to consider in the decision-making process. A patient in his or her 50s may have a healthy knee with no degenerative changes, whereas another person in his or her 30s may present with a knee with posttraumatic arthritis. We believe that the chronologic age of the patient should not necessarily influence who is offered surgical reconstruction. Other factors to consider when deciding between forms of treatment include a patient's activity level, occupation, off-season timelines, and as previously outlined, his or her expectations and goals.

Although an individualized treatment plan should be tailored according to the aforementioned patient factors, certain findings from the history and clinical examination can be used to guide treatment, as well. For example, patients with acute ACL tears who have an effusion and quadriceps inhibition should not undergo surgical reconstruction until ROM and quadriceps function have been optimized. Associated injuries must also be taken into account. A patient with an ACL injury who has a coexisting bucket handle meniscal tear will be treated more emergently than a patient with an isolated ACL tear. A patient's mechanical axis alignment can also influence decision-making regarding the knee. Significant varus or valgus malalignment may require corrective osteotomies in the setting of ipsilateral compartmental pathology, as in the case of cartilage regenerative or reparative procedures, meniscus transplantation, or early unicompartmental osteoarthritis. One of the most challenging patients is the person who has degenerative joint disease and meniscal pathology noted on MRI. The history of a short duration of symptoms (<3 months) and mechanical symptoms are the two best prognosticators that the patient will benefit from an arthroscopic partial meniscectomy.

CONCLUSION

Although they are difficult to master given the complexity of the underlying anatomy, history and physical examination remain the most safe, cost-effective, and accurate methods of arriving at a diagnosis in a patient with knee-related complaints. We encourage practitioners to develop a systematic approach when evaluating patients, which is important not only to efficiently arrive at a diagnosis but also to prevent missing conditions that require emergent intervention or associated injuries that can affect treatment decision-making and prognosis.

For a complete list of references, go to ExpertConsult.com.

SELECTED READINGS

Citation:

Karachalios T, Hantes M, Zibis AH, et al. Diagnostic accuracy of a new clinical test (the Thessaly test) for early detection of meniscal tears. *J Bone Joint Surg Am.* 2005;87(5):955–962.

Level of Evidence:

I, diagnostic

Summary:

This large prospective review of several physical examination tests for meniscal injury demonstrates excellent diagnostic accuracy for the Thessaly test and for joint line tenderness.

Citation:

Kocher MS, Steadman JR, Briggs KK, et al. Relationships between objective assessment of ligament stability and subjective assessment of symptoms and function after anterior cruciate ligament reconstruction. *Am J Sports Med.* 2004;32(3):629–634.

Level of Evidence:

II, diagnostic

Summary:

The retrospective correlation between postoperative physical examination findings and clinical outcome after anterior cruciate ligament reconstruction demonstrates a significant association between the pivot shift examination and a variety of functional outcomes, without a similar relationship between instrumented laxity or the Lachman test.

Citation:

Lane CG, Warren R, Pearle AD. The pivot shift. *J Am Acad Orthop Surg.* 2008;16(12):679–688.

Level of Evidence:

Not applicable

Summary:

This article provides an excellent recent summary of the biomechanics, anatomic features, modifications, mitigating and aggravating factors, and clinical evidence surrounding the pivot shift maneuver.

Citation:

LaPrade RF, Terry GC. Injuries to the posterolateral aspect of the knee. Association of anatomic injury patterns with clinical instability. *Am J Sports Med.* 1997;25(4):433–438.

Level of Evidence:

I, diagnostic

Summary:

This large prospective examination of the correlation between a variety of physical examination maneuvers is designed to assay the structures of the posterolateral corner and the intraoperative pathologic findings.

Citation:

Rubinstein RA, Shelbourne KD, McCarroll JR, et al. The accuracy of the clinical examination in the setting of posterior cruciate ligament injuries. *Am J Sports Med.* 1994;22(4):550–557.

Level of Evidence:

I, diagnostic

Summary:

This prospective, randomized, controlled examination of a variety of examination maneuvers in patients with isolated posterior cruciate ligament tears, isolated anterior crucial ligament knees, and normal knees demonstrates that the posterior drawer test is the most sensitive and specific test for isolated injuries to the posterior cruciate ligament.

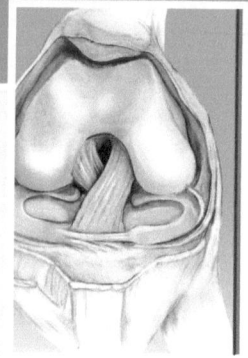

91

Imaging of the Knee

Nancy Major, Christopher Coleman

BACKGROUND

Imaging plays an important role in diagnosing knee joint pathology. There are a variety of imaging techniques that allow visualization of abnormalities that can affect the bones as well as directly visualizing articular cartilage. In addition, after treatment intervention, imaging can assess interval change. The most common pathologic processes affecting the knee joint are traumatic and degenerative in nature and can be major causes of morbidity.

IMAGING

Radiographs are often an important first step in imaging. Fractures, malalignment, joint effusion including lipohemarthrosis, and soft tissue mineralization are some of the important findings that can be identified on radiographs and can also be correlated with findings of advanced imaging. Standard radiographic series includes a frontal projection, with or without a flexed weight-bearing image, lateral view, and a patellofemoral view (Fig. 91.1). The latter can be a merchant view, in which the beam is directed along the patellofemoral articulation with 45 degrees of flexion. Alternatively, the sunrise view can be utilized, for which the patient lies prone and flexes 90 degrees. The beam is directed retrograde toward the patellofemoral articulation. In the setting of acute trauma, a cross table lateral is used in place of the true lateral. Internal and external oblique projections are used to carefully profile the medial and lateral tibial plateau, and are often employed in the setting of trauma. A fracture is seen in only 5% of emergency department radiographs. However, per the American College of Radiology (ACR) Appropriateness Criteria, radiographs should be the first study obtained if there is a twisting injury or fall with focus tenderness, inability to bear weight, or a discernible suprapatellar effusion on exam.[1]

Computed tomography (CT) also plays a role in knee joint imaging. It is employed as a second imaging technique to assess fractures and identify mineralization that is not clearly detected on conventional x-rays. CT without contrast can be performed if a radiographically occult fracture is suspected clinically, such as in the setting of a lipohemarthrosis. Alternatively, known fractures can be further characterized, such as when measuring the degree of displacement of fracture fragments or more accurately determining articular step off of a depressed tibial plateau fracture. Comminuted or complex fractures are often further characterized with CT when planning for open reduction internal

fixation (ORIF). Surface rendered sagittal and coronal reformats and three-dimensional reconstruction are helpful to visual complex fracture patterns in an orientation that simulates what will be encountered in surgery. CT angiography can replace conventional angiography in certain cases of posterior dislocation and concern for lower extremity arterial injury.[2] CT can also be useful for evaluation of bone and soft tissue tumor matrix. Matrix assessment is beyond the scope of this chapter. In brief, cartilaginous tumors such as enchondromas have calcified chondroid oriented in rings and arcs matrix. Tumors such as osteosarcoma have osteoid, or fluffy/cloudlike matrix, and lesions like fibrous dysplasia or non-ossifying fibromas have ground glass matrix (Fig. 91.2).

CT with sagittal and coronal reformatting as well as 3D reconstruction is valuable for preoperative planning for total knee arthroplasties. The shape of the glenoid is demonstrated for the surgeon that will allow for presurgical planning and sizing the prosthesis.[3]

CT arthrography can be a useful alternative in patients with contraindications for MRI, such as certain types of pacemakers and debilitating claustrophobia. Iodinated contrast (20 to 30 mL), often diluted to 50% strength with a combination of anesthetic and normal saline, is injected into the knee joint under fluoroscopic guidance. At our institution, the patients are placed supine with 20 to 30 degrees of flexion. A 45-degree caudocranial trajectory is taken to land the 22-gauge, 3.5-inch needle on the mesial aspect of the medial femoral condyle. A lateral or medial approach to the patellofemoral articulation can alternatively be used.

Ultrasound plays an adjunct role in imaging of the knee. A fluid collection in the popliteal recess, a.k.a. Baker cyst, can be a source of posterior knee pain. Ultrasound is also the preferred method for identifying and characterizing deep venous thrombosis (DVT) of the popliteal, peroneal, and posterior tibial veins. Targeted ultrasound can also be used to evaluate high-grade injuries to the Achilles, quadriceps, and patellar tendons, although these are often quite apparent clinically. Ultrasound can determine if intact tendon fibers remain attached to their respective insertions. Recent research has suggested that ultrasound can identify characteristics in the medial meniscus, which can be associated with the onset and progression of osteoarthritis.[4] Ultrasound can be shown in some cases, showing sensitivity and specificity for diagnosing meniscal tear of 85% and 86%, respectively.[5] However, it has been our experience that the evaluation of the

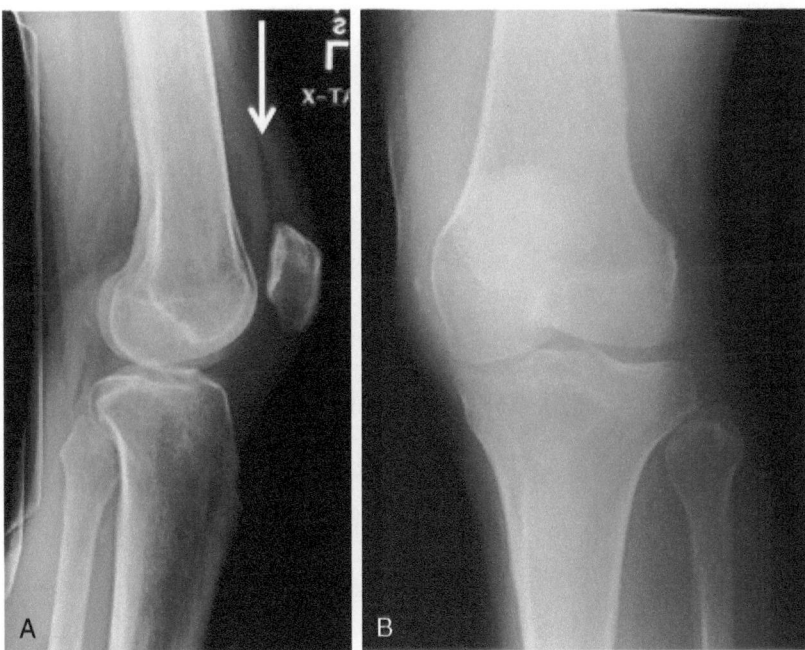

Fig. 91.1 Lateral radiograph (A) demonstrates the straight line between the layering radiolucent fatty component and the more radiodense fluid/cellular component of a knee joint lipohemarthrosis *(white arrow)*. Oblique frontal radiograph (B) fails to show the fracture.

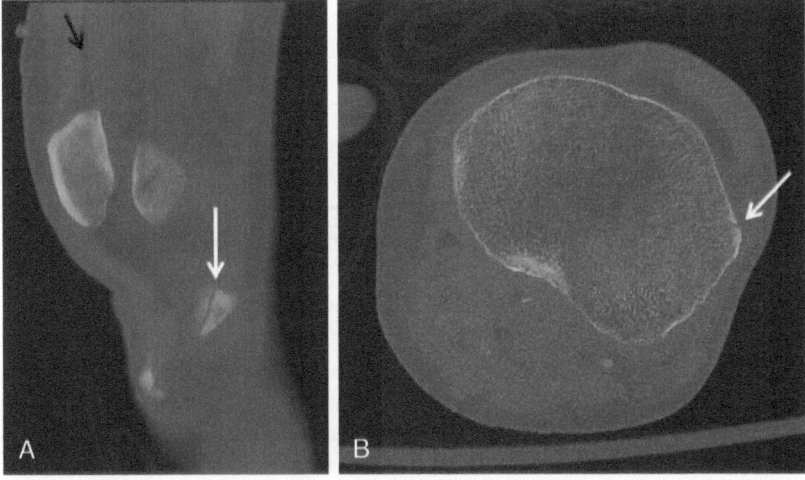

Fig. 91.2 Sagittal (A) and axial (B) computed tomography images of same patient as Fig. 91.1 show the nondisplaced lateral tibial plateau fracture *(white arrows)*. The lipohemarthrosis is again noted in A *(black arrow)*.

free edge as well as the posterior root attachments are extremely limited in even the most experienced hands (Fig. 91.3).

MAGNETIC RESONANCE IMAGING

Magnetic resonance imaging (MRI) is the mainstay of knee joint imaging. The ideal MRI is performed on a high field strength magnet (1.5 Tesla or greater), using a dedicated knee surface coil to improve signal to noise ratio (SNR). At least one sequence should be performed in the axial, coronal, and sagittal planes. Some sequences should be performed with fat-suppression (FS) to accentuate abnormal signal from fluid and/or edema. At least one T1-weighted sequence should be used to look for hypointense

fracture lines and assess the signal of red and yellow marrow distribution. Proton density (PD) weighting is the workhorse for the knee joint because of its ability to distinguish subchondral bone from cartilage from joint fluid. Emphasis is placed on keeping the echo time (TE) of the sagittal PD FS images at or below 20 ms to ensure that abnormal signal from subtle meniscal tears can be appreciated.

A variety of advanced imaging techniques has been developed for articular cartilage imaging in the knee joint; these are not routinely employed with knee imaging and largely remain areas of research, development, and investigation. Delayed gadolinium-enhanced magnetic resonance imaging of cartilage (dGEMRIC) is based on the increased delayed uptake of the negatively charged

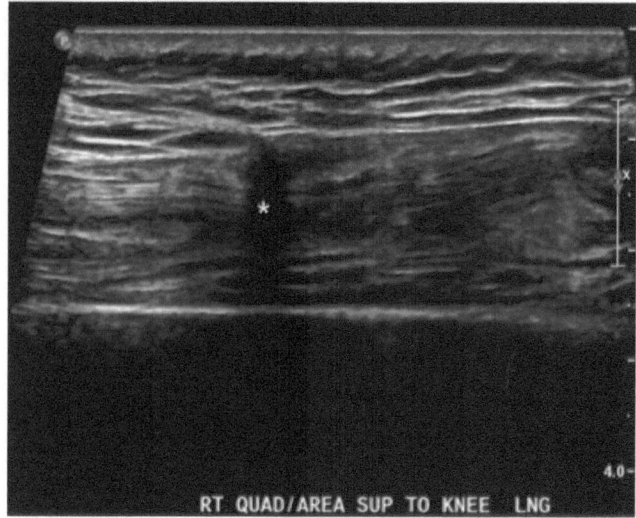

Fig. 91.3 Long-axis grayscale ultrasound image of quadriceps tendon show a focal full or near full thickness tear *(asterisk)*.

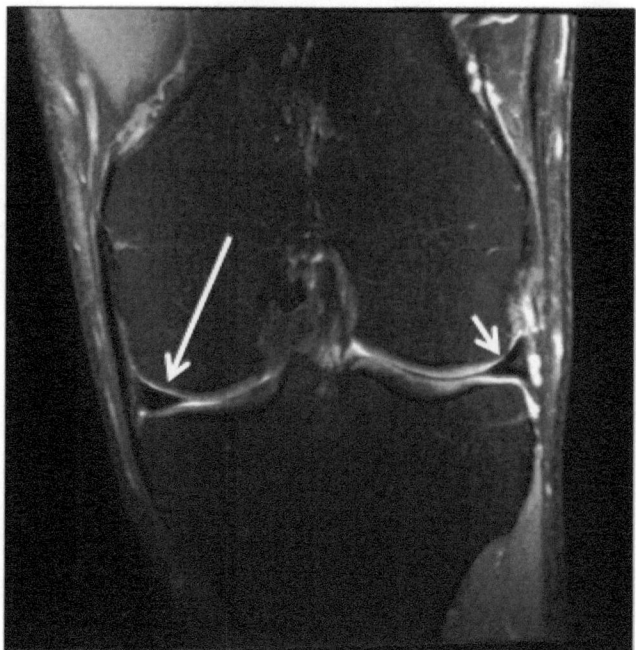

Fig. 91.4 Coronal proton density fat saturation image shows a normal medial meniscus *(long arrow)* and lateral meniscus *(short arrow)*.

gadolinium-based contrast agent (GBCA) in areas of damaged cartilage, which contain abnormally low amounts of negatively changed glycosaminoglycans (GAGs) compared with healthy cartilage.[6] This increased uptake of GBCA shortens the T1 relaxation times, allowing detection of cartilage damage on the structural level before morphologically apparent thinning can be identified by unenhanced MRI. T2 mapping assesses the suprastructure of cartilage. Healthy cartilage has a stratification of the both the organization and water content moving from the subarticular bone plate to the lamina splendens. This organization is lost in chondromalacia.[7] Sodium MRI imaging is another technique that serves to quantify the amount and organization of remaining GAGs.[8] Other techniques including T1 Rho have also been researched.

The remainder of this chapter will be presented by anatomic structure. An overview of anatomy will be followed by useful radiographic signs of injury, variety of pathology, and MR imaging findings of each. Emphasis will be placed on the ideal sequence and imaging plane for each structure.

MENISCI

The medial and lateral menisci are curvilinear fibrocartilaginous structures that cover the medial and lateral tibial plateau, respectively. When viewed in the axial plane, the lateral meniscus is a more well-formed "C," with the anterior and posterior root attachments positioned more centrally along the anteroposterior axis of the tibial plateau. The medial meniscus resembles a semicircle, with the anterior and posterior attachments close to the anterior and posterior margin of the plateau, respectively. The deep fibers of the medial collateral ligament (MCL) attach to the medial meniscal body in the form of the meniscofemoral and meniscotibial attachments. The posterior horn of the medial meniscus is attached to the joint capsule by the meniscocapsular ligaments, while the posterior horn of the lateral meniscus is attached to the adjacent popliteus tendon by the meniscopopliteal fascicles. The meniscus is best evaluated on sagittal images. The

body of the meniscus is uniformly low in signal (black) and resembles a rectangle or slab of meniscal tissue. There are typically a couple of body segments if using a 4 mm slice thickness (Fig. 91.4). The anterior and posterior horns are triangular in shape and low in signal when normal (Fig. 91.5). The lateral meniscus has anterior and posterior horns that are similar in size, while the medial meniscus posterior horn is two times the size as the anterior horn. These relationships are important to remember when evaluating the meniscus to identify different types of tears.

Radiographs can play a role in identifying chondrocalcinosis, which can be seen most commonly in the lateral meniscus. Chondrocalcinosis may reflect calcium pyrophosphate arthropathy or sequelae of age.

Meniscal tears are best identified as abnormal signal on PD sequences. Abnormal signal that violates the articular surface on two consecutive images is necessary for diagnosis. Amorphous, ill-defined intrameniscal signal that does not violate an articular surface is often related to meniscal contusion in young patients, and mucoid degeneration/chondrocalcinosis in older individuals. Meniscal tears can be broadly separated into longitudinal and radial types. Longitudinal tears follow the long axis of the meniscus. They can be either vertical or oblique tears. Oblique tears ultimately propagate through the superior or inferior surface, rather than the true free edge. The central half of the cross-sectional area of meniscal tissue is known as the "white zone," since it is avascular. Tears isolated to this region are unlikely to heal. Treatment is either meniscectomy or nonsurgical. Conversely, tears involving the peripheral half, or "red zone," are often repaired arthroscopically. Care should be taken to look on MRI for a flap tear in which the inferior/peripheral portion of the body of the meniscus is displaced in the inferior gutter, deep to the MCL, as this can be difficult to identify during arthroscopy,

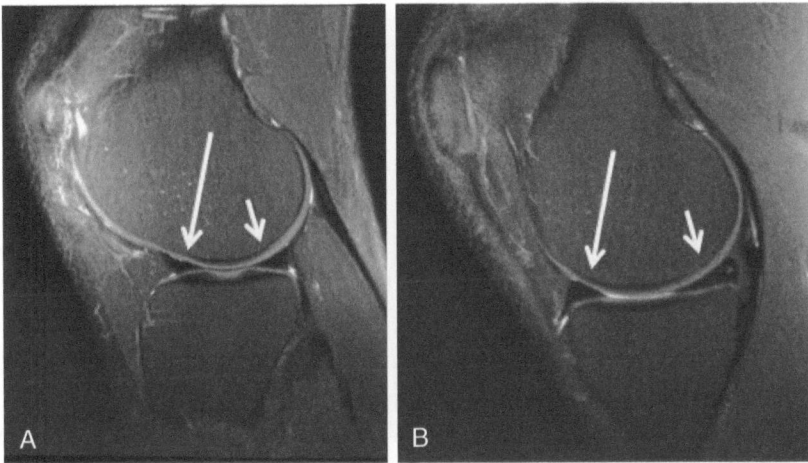

Fig. 91.5 Sagittal proton density fat saturation images in the lateral compartment (A) and medial compartment (B) show normal anterior and posterior horns (*long arrow* and *short arrows*, respectively).

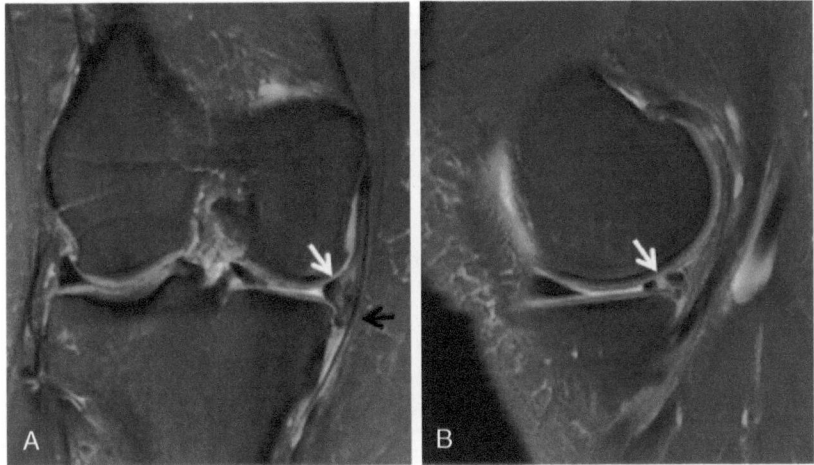

Fig. 91.6 Coronal (A) and sagittal (B) proton density fat saturation images demonstrate a medial meniscal tear *(white arrows)*. A fragment is flipped into the inferior gutter (*black arrow* in A).

and can lead to persistent pain postoperatively if not addressed. One way to recognize is by assessing the body segments. Typically the meniscus is not rectangular in shape, nor does it resemble a "slab" of meniscal tissue, as a portion of the undersurface is absent (Fig. 91.6).

Vertical, longitudinal tears usually extend from the superior to inferior articular surface of the meniscus. A subset is the bucket handle tear, where a portion of white (or sometimes white and red) zone tissue is flipped away from the body of the meniscus centrally, anteriorly, or posteriorly. Depending on where the tear begins and ends, this can result in the double posterior cruciate ligament (PCL) sign, or the double delta sign of the anterior horn of the meniscus (Fig. 91.7). The double PCL sign is unique to medial meniscus, as the ACL prevents central flipping of the bucket handle when the lateral meniscus demonstrates tears in this fashion.

Radial tears extend through the cross section of the meniscus, orthogonal to the long axis. On MRI these tears are recognized as blunting of the anterior or posterior horn on sagittal imaging and will demonstrate loss of the low signal on coronal images (vertical intermediate signal; Fig. 91.8). These can be partial, as in free edge tearing, or a complete radial tear (resembling a fractured meniscus). A posterior root disruption is a subtype of complete radial tear. They are recognized on MRI as loss of the low signal (or slightly increased signal) at the root attachment (Fig. 91.9). Often the meniscus will be extruded into the gutter. When this finding is recognized, attention should be paid to the signal of the root of the meniscus. These tears are unlikely to heal spontaneously. There is also disruption of the hoop stress resistance, one of the most important functions of the meniscus that leads to the extrusion. This often leads to accelerated osteoarthrosis in the affected compartment. Surgical repair is usually necessary.

Meniscal cysts are an often encountered abnormality and can be intrameniscal or parameniscal in location. Intrameniscal cysts cause swelling of the meniscus and are increased in T2 signal. They are most often not fluid signal in their appearance (Fig. 91.10). The origin of this abnormality is not well understood, but many feel it is a result of intrinsic meniscal degeneration that leads to local necrosis accumulation of abnormal signal within the substance of the meniscus.[9] Intrameniscal cysts are not always associated with meniscal tears, and a careful search

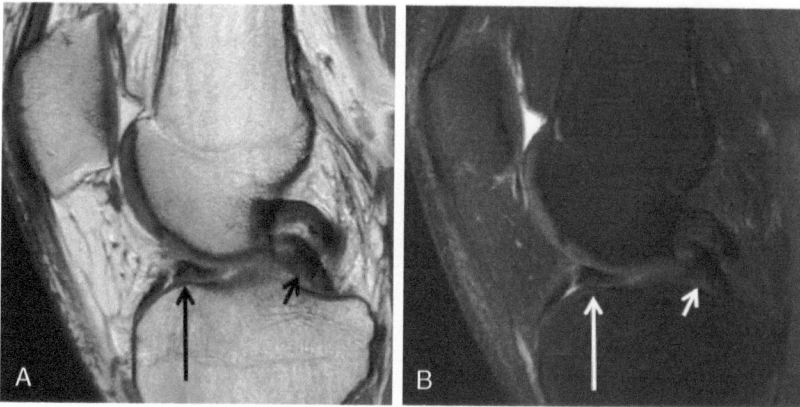

Fig. 91.7 SAG PD (A), PD FS (B) images demonstrate the double delta *(long arrows)* and double posterolateral corner *(short arrows)* signs of a bucket handle tear of the medial meniscus.

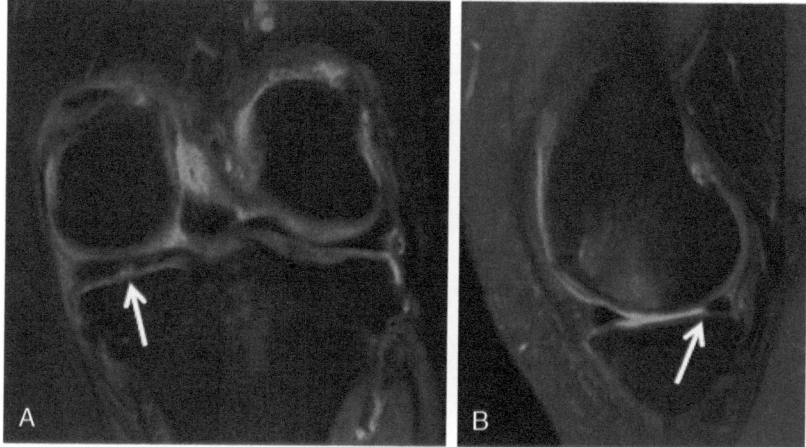

Fig. 91.8 Coronal proton density fat saturation (PD FS) image (A) image demonstrates increased signal in the posterior horn of the medial meniscus *(arrow)*. Sagittal PD FS MR image (B) demonstrates corresponding blunting of the free edge on lateral view *(arrow)*. Findings represent partial thickness radial tear.

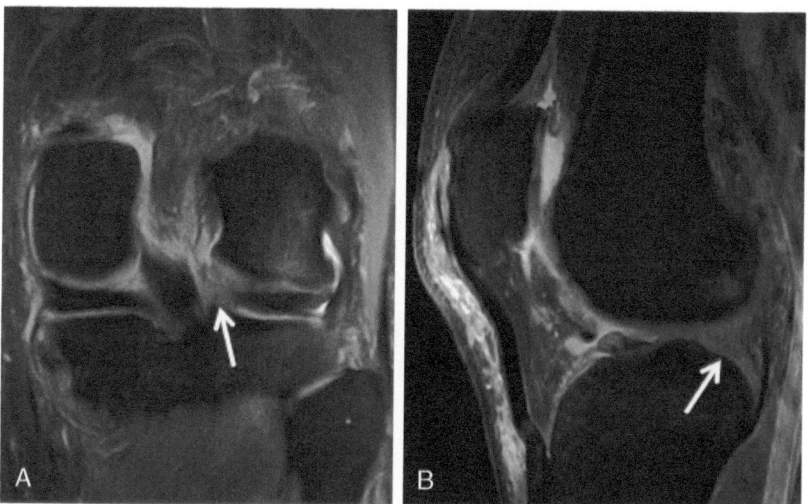

Fig. 91.9 Coronal proton density fat saturation (PD FS) image (A) demonstrates a complete posterior root tear of the lateral meniscus *(arrow)*. Sagittal PD FS (B) image demonstrates the "ghost meniscus" *(arrow)*.

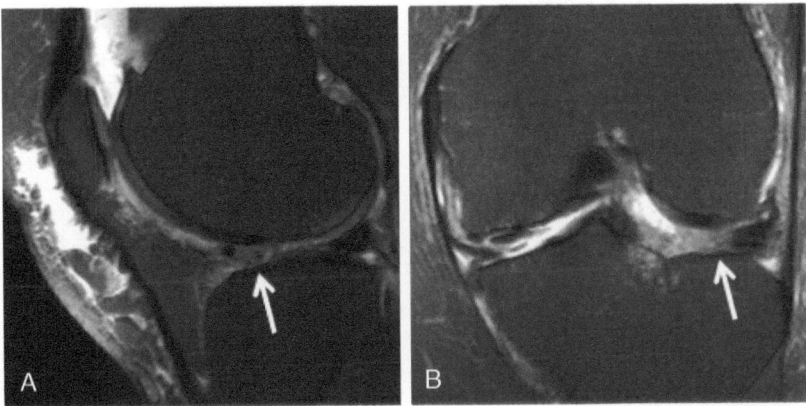

Fig. 91.10 Sagittal (A) and coronal (B) T2 fat saturation images demonstrate an intrameniscal cyst *(arrows)* in the lateral meniscus. No tear is present.

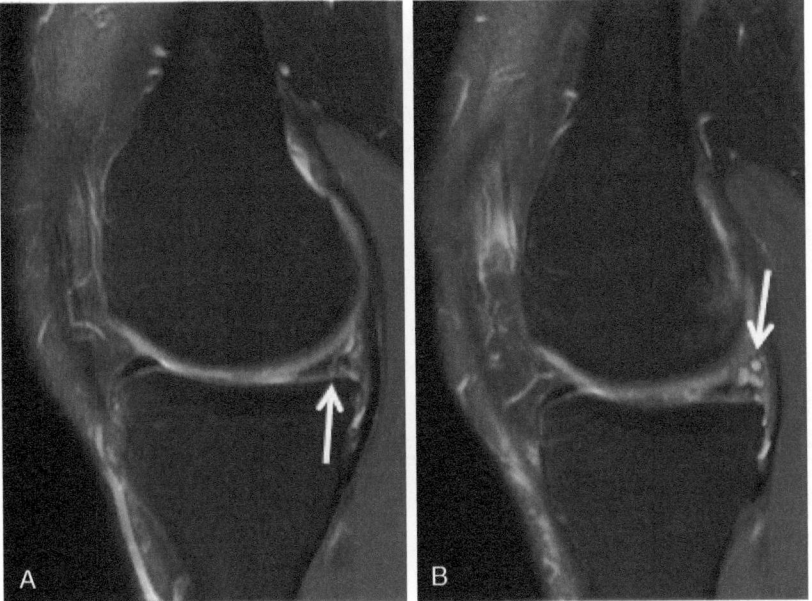

Fig. 91.11 Sequential sagittal proton density fat saturation (A and B) images demonstrate a posterior horn medial meniscal tear *(arrow in A)* communicating with a parameniscal cyst *(arrow in B)*.

of the superior and inferior surface of the meniscus should be taken to identify an associated tear.

Parameniscal cysts, on the other hand, do demonstrate fluid signal on T2-weighted imaging. These cysts have a communication to the meniscus and that communication must be identified before the diagnosis of a parameniscal cyst can be made (Fig. 91.11). Parameniscal cysts are most often confused for a bursa on imaging. This error can be avoided if the neck of the cyst is identified originating from the meniscus. The parameniscal cysts can be located anywhere around the periphery of the meniscus and articular surfaced tears are not always present. Formal decompression of a parameniscal cyst is considered unnecessary during partial meniscectomy.[10]

In the setting of advanced osteoarthrosis, complex tears of the meniscus with radial and oblique components are often present. Root tears, extrusion, or flipped fragments should be sought carefully.

Prior partial meniscectomy can be indistinguishable from fraying, and surgical history is valuable in making a proper diagnosis.

PITFALLS

The posterior horn of the lateral meniscus should be examined carefully. Normal anatomy of the meniscofemoral ligaments and the popliteus tendon as it traverses the struts of the posterior horn of the lateral meniscus cause a normal intervening, vertical focus of increased signal in the posterior horn of the lateral meniscus (Fig. 91.12). This is not to be confused with a peripheral tear and can be verified, as the meniscofemoral ligaments and popliteus tendon can be followed on consecutive sagittal images. In addition, prior partial meniscectomy can make identification of a superimposed tear difficult. Comparison with prior imaging is quite useful. Finally, in the setting of an ACL tear, the posterior

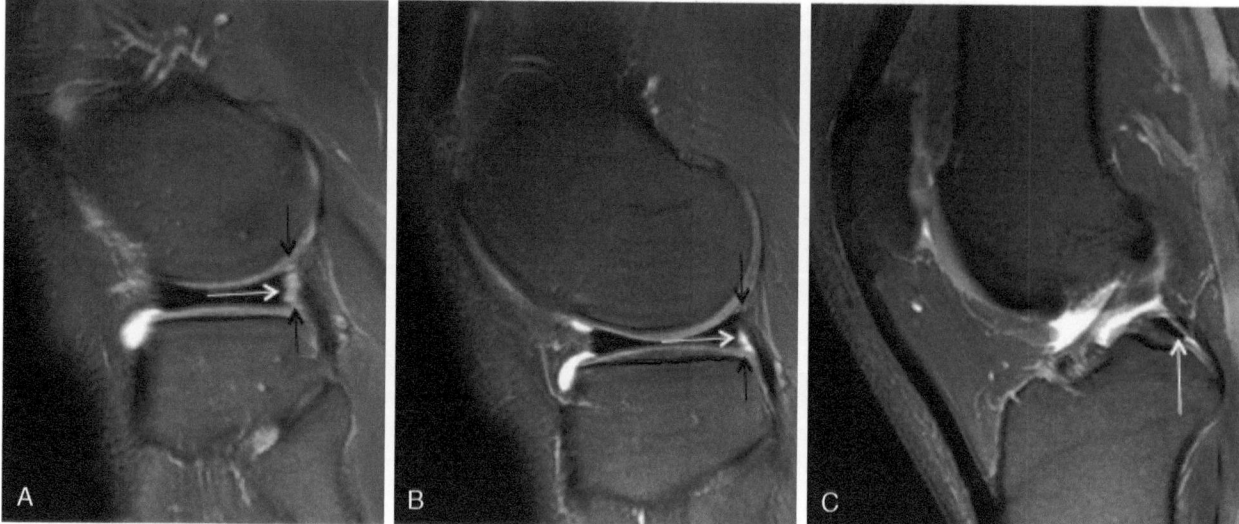

Fig. 91.12 Sequential sagittal proton density fat saturation images lateral to medial (A–C) demonstrate the normal increased signal posterior to the posterior horn lateral meniscus (*white arrow* in A and B), bordered superiorly and inferiorly by the meniscopopliteal fascicles (*black arrows* in A and B). The medial-most image (C) demonstrates the takeoff of the meniscofemoral ligament of Humphrey *(arrow)*. Incidental note is made of a discoid configuration to the lateral meniscus, a relatively common variant.

horn of the lateral meniscus often is associated with a peripheral, radial tear of the posterior horn of the lateral meniscus, but is often overlooked. Abnormal signal in this region in the setting of an ACL should be diagnosed as a tear (making sure that the popliteus tendon and meniscofemoral ligaments have been reconciled).

MUSCULOTENDINOUS STRUCTURES

In addition to the ligaments and menisci, multiple muscles and tendons help stabilize the knee. The vastus medialis, vastus lateralis, and vastus intermedius coalesce with the rectus femoral to form the quadriceps and patellar tendon, ultimately inserting on the tibial tubercle. These structures are discussed in the extensor compartment section below. The Sartorius, gracilis, and semitendinosus cross the knee joint medially, and their tendons form the pes anserine, inserting on the tibial tubercle. The adductor tubercle of the medial condyle provides the insertion of the adductor magnus. The semimembranosus attaches at the posterior/medial aspect of the medial femoral condyle. Just lateral to this is the medial head of the gastrocnemius. In between these structures is the popliteal recess, where popliteal cysts can form. The lateral head of the gastrocnemius arises from the lateral femoral condyle posteriorly. The popliteus originates from the popliteal hiatus of the lateral femoral condyle, sweeps laterally across the posterior joint, and is part of the posterolateral corner, discussed later.

Tendon anatomy is best illustrated with T1-weighted MRI, while pathology is diagnosed on T2 WI, particularly when fat suppression is applied. Musculotendinous injury manifests as increased T2 signal within the fibrils of the tendon or the surrounding soft tissues, representing grade I strain. Grade II is partial disruption of hypointense fibers identified as increased T2 signal or fluid signal. The tendon may also demonstrate increased thickness or be attenuated in its appearance. A grade

III injury is a complete disruption, often with retraction of tendon ends. T1 images are useful to demonstrate associated hematoma, as well as fatty atrophy of the muscle bellies. Both processes demonstrate T1 hyperintensity. Atrophy is seen in long-standing injury or denervation. Most myotendinous injuries are best identified on coronal or sagittal planes, where the feathery edema tracks along the long axis of the muscle. Measuring tendon gap in full thickness tears is also easiest in those planes and may have implications in treatment.

The plantaris is a thin muscle that arises from the lateral supracondylar ridge of the femur, just superior to the lateral head of the gastrocnemius. Its tendon extends inferomedially to insert on the Achilles tendon. The plantaris assists in foot plantar flexion. "Tennis leg" can be caused by rupture of either the plantaris or the medial head gastrocnemius. MRI shows abnormal increased T2 signal edema and increased T1 signal hematoma tracking deep to the gastrocnemius muscle belly (Fig. 91.13) and often torn, retracted plantaris tendon fibers. Treatment is supportive.

LIGAMENTS

The anterior cruciate ligament (ACL) runs from the mesial aspect of the lateral femoral condyle and inserts on the anterior tibial plateau, blending with the anterior horn of the lateral meniscus. It consists of two bundles: the anteromedial band and the stronger, posterolateral band. The sagittal T2-weighted images are best to evaluate the integrity of the ACL. There is often heterogeneously increased intrasubstance signal because of fiber organization. This can be a source of false positives for partial tear to the untrained eye. Sprains and partial tears are seen as ill-definition and increased signal, often affecting one of the two bands to a greater degree. Laxity or alteration in thickness of the ligament are additional signs of a partial tear or sprain. Full thickness tears can be anywhere along the length of the ligament

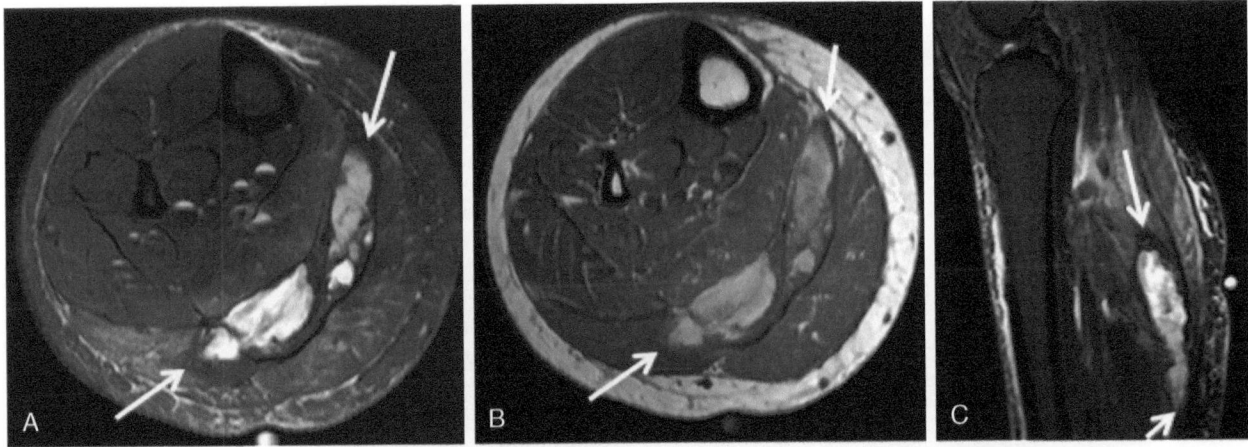

Fig. 91.13 Axial T2 fat saturation (A), T1 (B) images demonstrate heterogeneous hematoma/edema in the expected region of the plantaris *(arrows)*. Sagittal short-tau inversion recovery image (C) demonstrates tracking of the collection craniocaudally *(arrows)*.

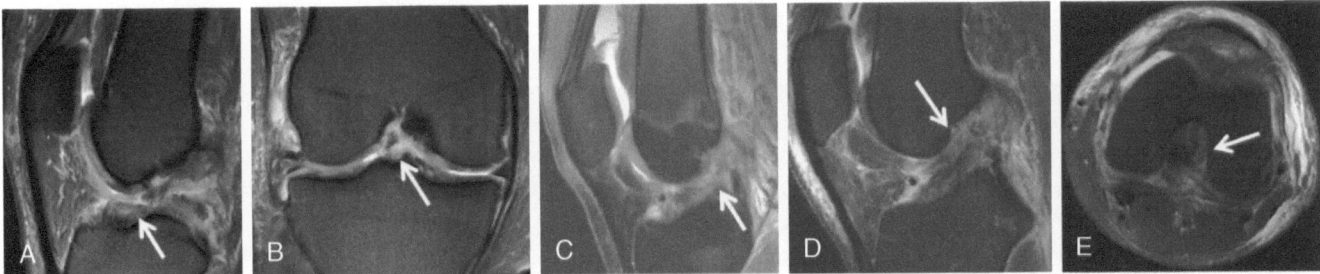

Fig. 91.14 Sagittal (A), coronal proton density fat saturation (PD FS) (B) images demonstrate a complete anterior cruciate ligament (ACL) tear at the tibial attachment *(arrows)*. Sagittal PD FS image (C) in a second patient demonstrates a midsubstance ACL tear. Sagittal (D), axial T2 FS (E) images in a third patient demonstrate ACL tear from the femoral attachment *(arrows)*.

(Fig. 91.14). The coronal and axial images can be used to confirm integrity or tear of the ACL. Coronal plane provides great visualization of the tibial attachments, while the axial view is helpful to evaluate the femoral origin. Mucoid degeneration within the substance of the ACL can simulate injury. Increased signal is identified throughout the ligament and the ligament is enlarged, but the fibers within the ACL are still identified, and have taken on the appearance likened to a celery stalk (Fig. 91.15).

Several secondary signs can support a diagnosis of ACL injury. The radiologic anterior drawer sign represents anterior translation of the tibia with respect to the femur in the setting of an incompetent ACL. The Segond fracture, an often curvilinear fragment lateral to the lateral tibial plateau, is thought to represent an avulsion fracture from the lateral capsular attachment (Fig. 91.16). A lateral femoral notch greater than 2 mm has been proposed as an additional indirect sign of ACL tear.[11] A curvilinear bone avulsion of the fibular head (arcuate sign) is also a conventional radiographic sign of ACL injury. Bone contusions identified on fluid sensitive sequences are typically in the lateral femoral condyle, with or without the additional involvement of the posterior lateral tibial plateau. These have been referred to as kissing contusions. The presence of these contusions is indicative of an ACL tear. The only exception to that is in adolescents. This population typically has more flexibility to the ligament and can have a pivot shift injury resulting in bone contusion pattern without tearing the ACL.[12]

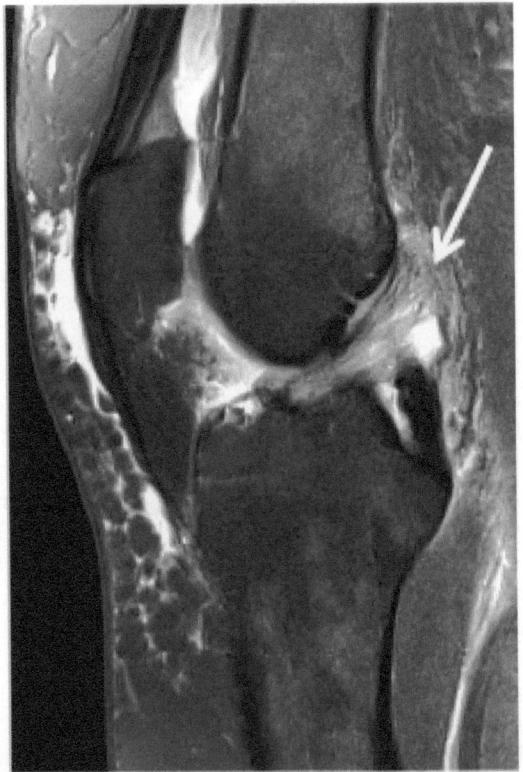

Fig. 91.15 SAG PD FS image demonstrates mucoid degeneration of the anterior cruciate ligament *(arrow)*.

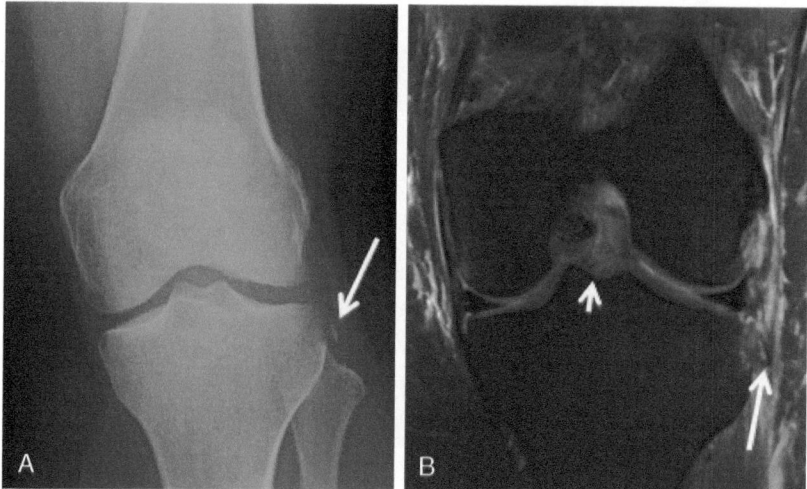

Fig. 91.16 Frontal radiograph (A) demonstrates a curvilinear fragment of mineralization adjacent to the lateral tibial plateau consistent with a Segond fracture *(arrow)*. Coronal proton density fat saturation image (B) demonstrates the Segond fracture *(long arrow)* with edema in the fracture and host bone. The anterior cruciate ligament tear is partially visualized *(short arrow)*.

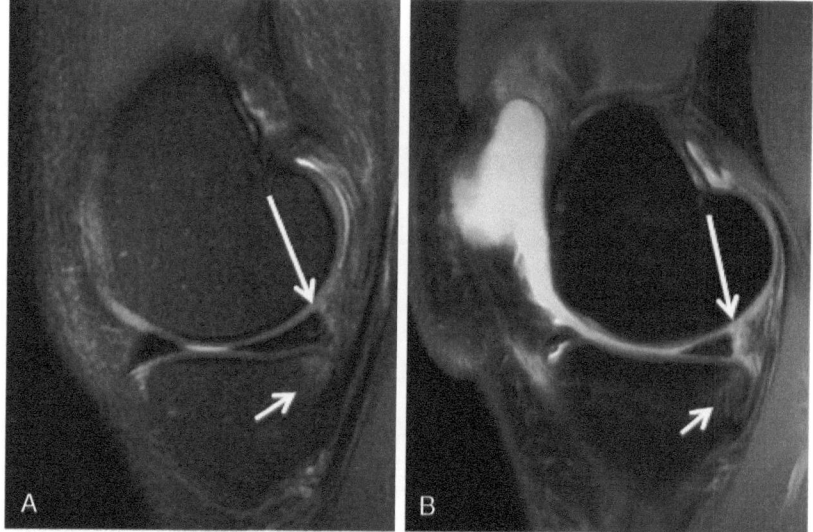

Fig. 91.17 Sagittal proton density fat saturation (PD FS) image (A) demonstrates meniscocapsular contusion without separation *(long arrow)*. Medial tibial plateau edema also presents *(short arrow)*. Sagittal PD FS image in a different patient (B) shows meniscocapsular separation *(long arrow)* with medial tibial plateau edema *(short arrow)*. Both cases had complete anterior cruciate ligament tears (not shown).

Contrecoup contusion patterns occur on the medial femoral condyle and medial tibial plateau as a result of relocation of the pivot shift mechanism. The presence of medial contusions indicates a more significant injury. In addition, a careful search for a meniscocapsular separation should be sought. The presence of posterior medial tibial plateau contusion has a high association with meniscocapsular injuries as evidenced as fluid signal between the meniscus and capsule (separation) or contusion (abnormal increased signal at the meniscocapsular interface; Fig. 91.17).[13]

The normal appearance of the posterior cruciate ligament on MRI is a curved low signal structure arising from the notch in the medial femoral condyle and inserts on the lateral tibial spine. It is best evaluated on a short TE image (the same images used to evaluate the meniscus). On radiographs and sagittal MRI, the radiographic posterior drawer sign can often be identified

and represents posterior translation of the tibia with respect to the femur in the setting of an incompetent PCL (Fig. 91.18).

In contradistinction to the ACL, the findings in PCL tears are much subtler. Any intrasubstance signal should raise concern for injury on the short TE images. A T2-weighted image will often demonstrate low signal, making the observation of a PCL tear easy to overlook. The thickness of the ligament also increases and can be a subtle finding. The subtle increase in signal on the short TE images (PD) and the increase in thickness of the ligament provide MRI evidence of a PCL tear. Even high-grade injury may produce no complete disruption of the ligament. Because of the PCL's intrinsic strength, usually only severe injury produces PCL tears, and additional injury should be sought carefully. Particular attention should be paid to the posterolateral corner (PCL), discussed later. Unlike the contusion pattern noted

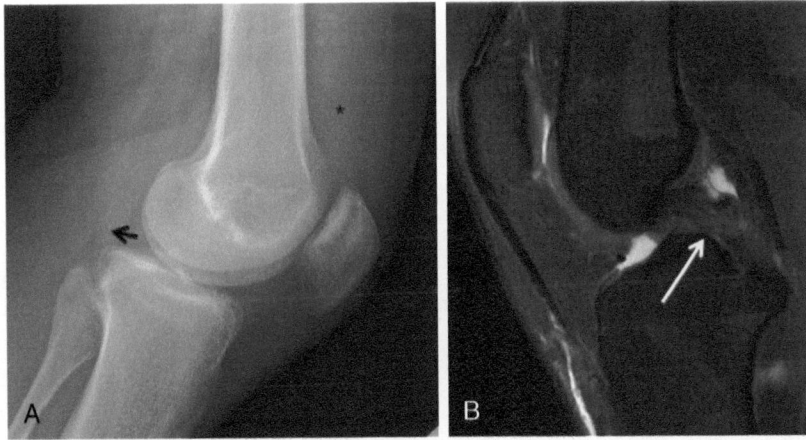

Fig. 91.18 Lateral radiograph (A) shows posterior translation of the tibia with respect to the femur *(arrow)* and moderate joint effusion *(asterisk)*. Corresponding sagittal proton density fat saturation image (B) shows complete posterior cruciate ligament tear *(arrow)*.

with ACL tears, there is no consistent contusion pattern associated with PCL tears. However, the presence of a contusion of the anterior tibial plateau should warrant careful inspection of the PCL on the short TE images.

The MCL originates from the adductor tubercle and inserts on the medial tibial metadiaphysis, caudal to the joint line. On MRI it is uniformly low in signal intensity and taught in appearance. The deep layer of the MCL is adherent to the peripheral medical meniscus. The MCL can be injured by direct blow, or more commonly valgus stress. The latter is seen in football clipping injuries and can be associated with the "terrible triad" of ACL and medial meniscal disruption. Radiographs can show focal soft tissue swelling/stranding in the expected region of the MCL. Widening of the medial joint line is a secondary sign of MCL incompetence.

A three-point grading system is often used to classify MCL tears. Grade I is seen as increased signal on fluid-sensitive sequences superficial and deep to the MCL. Grade II is partial disruption, with at least some fibers clearly visualized intact along their length. Grade III is complete disruption, often with retraction (Fig. 91.19). Any associated femoral avulsion fracture can be identified radiographically and by MRI, similar to the Segond fracture discussed above. In the setting of remote injury, dystrophic mineralization can be seen near the femoral attachment—the so-called Pelligrini-Stieda lesion, which may be easier to identify on conventional radiography than on MRI, unless there is signal from the mineralization (ossification; Fig. 91.20).

The iliotibial (IT) band, a continuation of the IT tract, crosses the knee laterally to insert on Gerdy tubercle of the anterior, lateral tibia. It is uncommonly torn and has an MR appearance compatible with previously discussed ligamentous injuries. IT band friction syndrome is characterized by abnormal signal deep and superficial to the band at the level of the joint line. Thickening of the band may also be seen with ITB friction syndrome. An adventitial bursa can form superficial to the Gerdy tubercle, appearing as fluid signal collection, often with surrounding inflammation and/or edema.

The posterolateral corner is a complex group of ligaments and tendons that provide posterolateral stability. The fibular collateral ligament originates from the lateral femoral condyle

before blending with the biceps femoris tendon to form the conjoined insertion on the fibular head. The popliteus tendon originates from the popliteal hiatus. The popliteus musculotendinous complex consists of the popliteofibular, fabellofibular, and arcuate ligament. The arcuate ligament is a "Y"-shaped structure that connects the fibular styloid to the oblique popliteal ligament and the posterior joint capsule.

PLC injuries are often present in association with ACL and/or PCL injuries and can be subtle and difficult to identify on physical exam due to pain and swelling of the knee. Axial and coronal fluid-sensitive sequences are often best to demonstrate these injuries. Generalized increased T2 signal in the region of the PLC should raise concern for injury. The fibular collateral ligament and conjoined tendon should be plainly visible on T1 and fluid-weighted sequences. If a bare area is identified in the hiatus, a popliteal origin injury should be suspected. A fibular head avulsion can simulate a PLC injury on radiograph. Careful correlation should be performed with T1-weighted sequences and, if available, radiographs (Fig. 91.21).

EXTENSOR MECHANISM

The extensor mechanism consists of the confluence of the quadriceps tendons, which ultimately insert on the tibial tubercle after running along the patella. The patellofemoral articulation is also supported by the medial patellofemoral ligament (MPFL) and retinaculum. On axial MRI, the muscle belly of the vastus medialis becomes confluent with the MPFL as a supporting structure. Distal to this, the medial retinaculum takes over. The lateral patellofemoral ligament (LPFL) and retinaculum provide similar support laterally. There are three definable fat pads that should be recognized on conventional radiography. The prefemoral, suprapatellar, and Hoffa fat pads are easily recognized on lateral radiography. The density differences intervening between the prefemoral and suprapatellar fat pads provide the soft tissue contrast, which allows visualization of suprapatellar effusion on lateral radiographs.

Sagittal T2FS as well as the corresponding axial sequences are best to evaluate the quadriceps and patellar tendons on MRI.

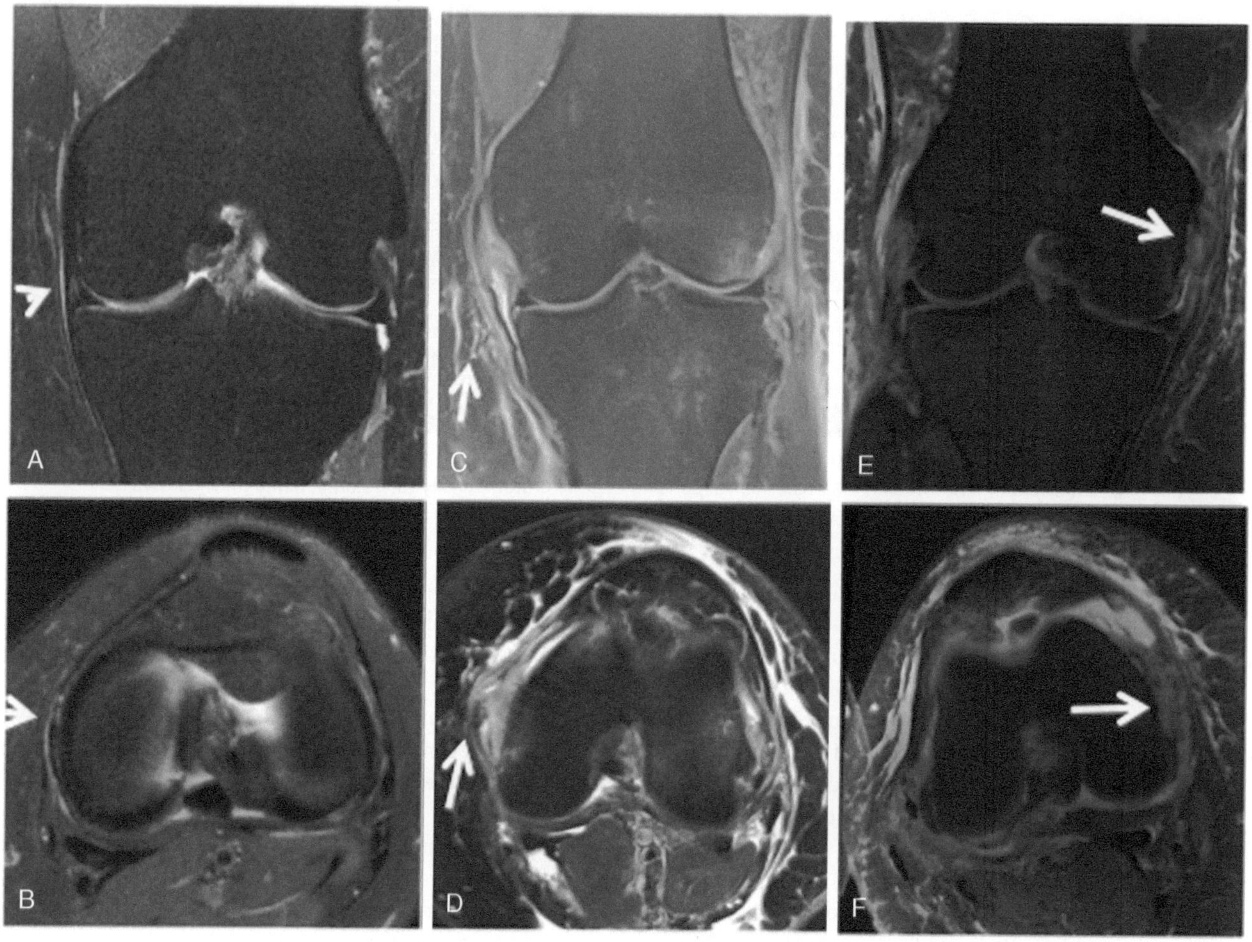

Fig. 91.19 Coronal (A) and axial proton density fat saturation (PD FS) (B) images demonstrate increased fluid signal superficial and deep to the medial collateral ligament (MCL) *(arrows)*, consistent with grade I injury. Coronal (C) and axial PD FS (D) images in a second patient demonstrate partial disruption of the MCL fibers *(arrows)*, consistent with grade II injury. Coronal (E) and axial PD FS (F) images in a third patient show complete MCL disruption *(arrows)*, consistent with grade III injury.

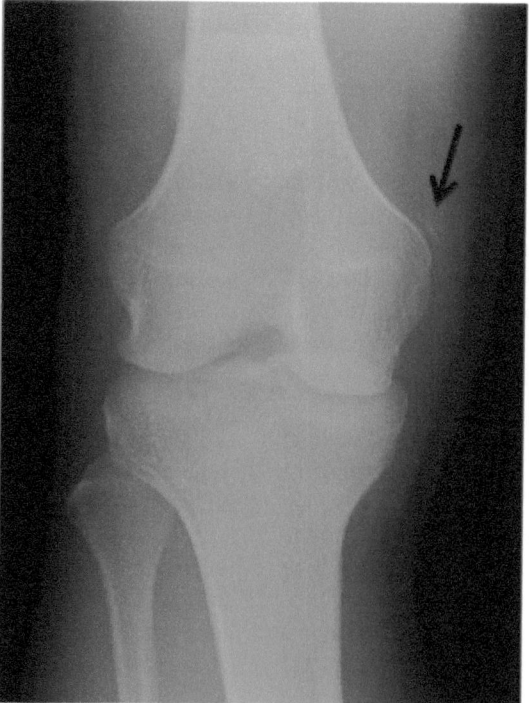

Fig. 91.20 Frontal radiograph demonstrates heterogeneous ossification in the region of the medial collateral ligament origin *(arrow)* consistent with a Pelligrini-Steida lesion.

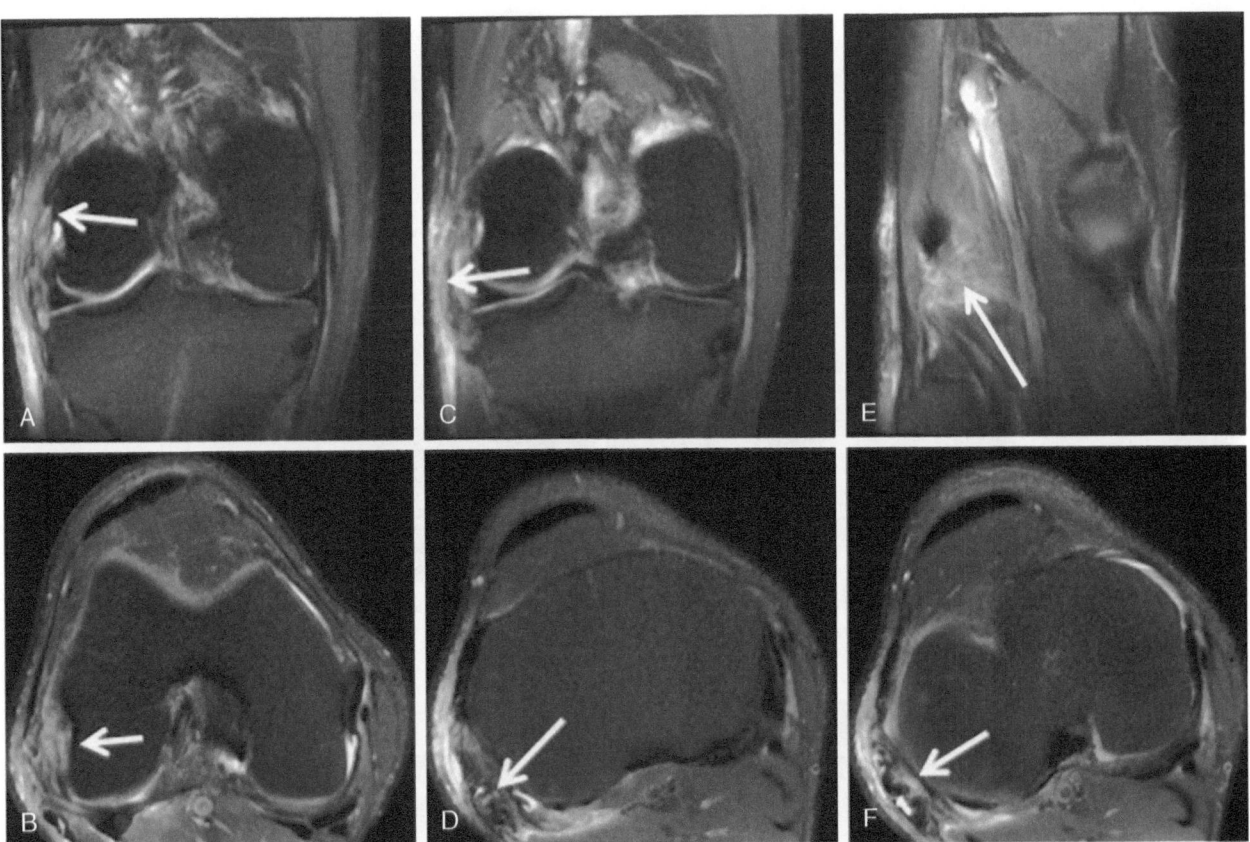

Fig. 91.21 Coronal (A) and axial proton density fat saturation (PD FS) (B) images demonstrate a fibular collateral ligament complete tear *(arrows)*. Coronal (C) and axial PD FS (D) images demonstrate biceps femoris insertion partial tear *(arrows)*. Coronal (E) and axial PD FS (F) images demonstrate arcuate ligament tear *(arrows)*.

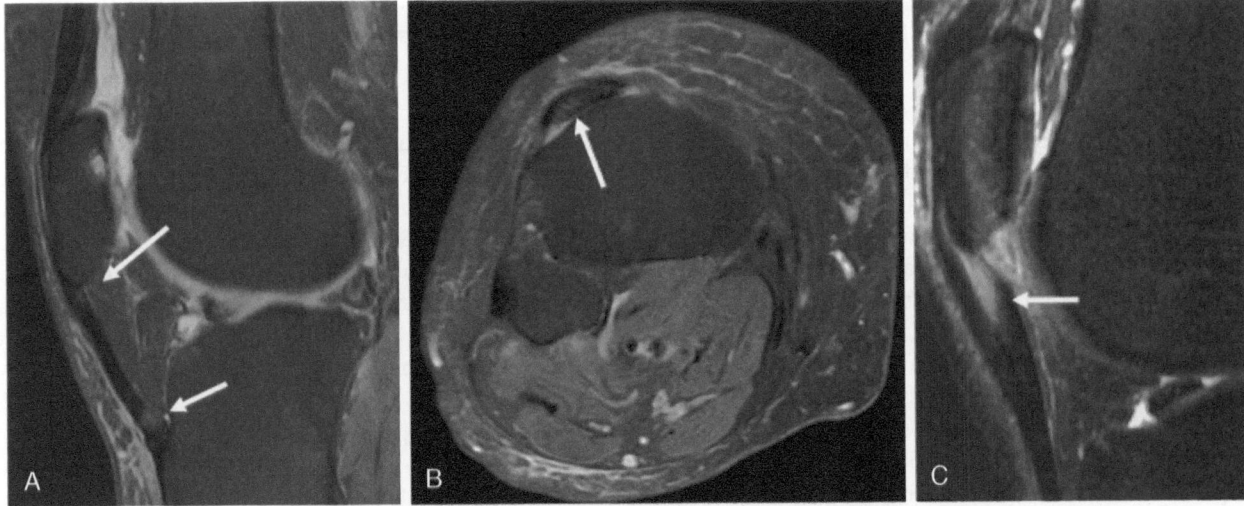

Fig. 91.22 Sagittal proton density fat saturation (PD FS) (A) and axial (B) images increased signal in the proximal and distal patellar tendon consistent with patellar tendinosis *(arrows)*. Sagittal PD FS image (C) in a different patient demonstrates a more striking signal abnormality in the proximal patellar tendon *(arrow)* in a patient with jumper's knee.

Normal striations are seen in the distal quadriceps tendon. The patellar tendon should be essentially devoid of signal unless injured such as with tendinopathy (a.k.a., jumper's knee). Patellar tendon disease often manifests as globular high signal on fluid-weighted sequences (Fig. 91.22). Complete rupture of the quadriceps or patellar tendon results in inferior (patella baja) or superior (patella alta) patellar translation, respectively (Fig. 91.23).

Transient patellar dislocation is a common entity. A shallow trochlear groove, patella alta, and prior patellar dislocation can predispose to dislocation. A persistently dislocated patella is quite

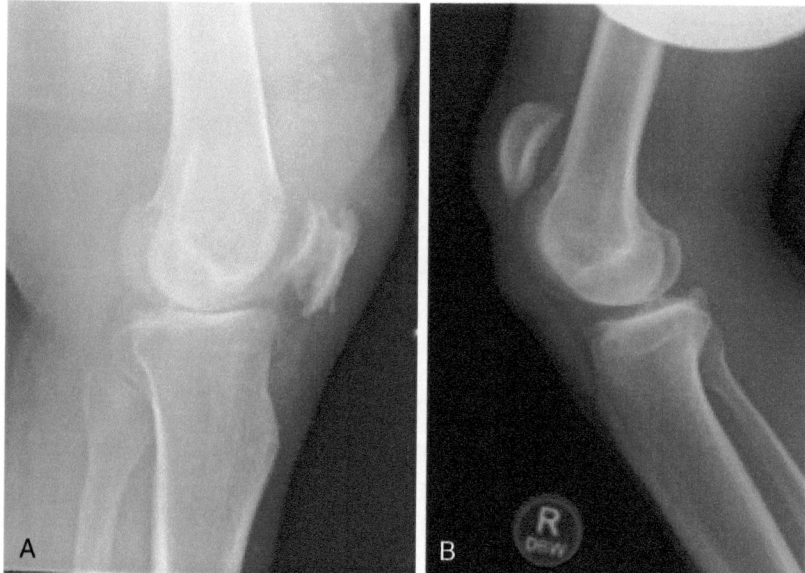

Fig. 91.23 Lateral radiograph (A) demonstrates patella baja with quadriceps rupture. Lateral radiograph (B) in a second patient shows patella alta and patellar tendon rupture.

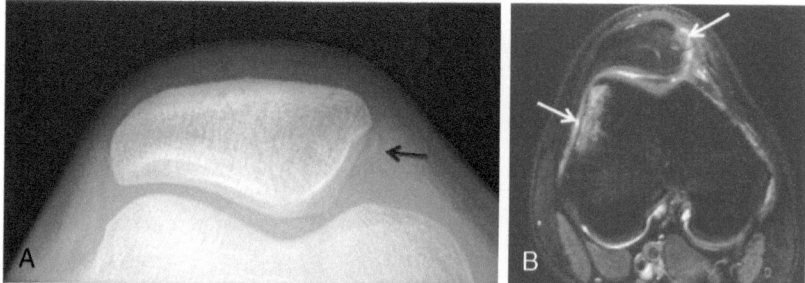

Fig. 91.24 Patellofemoral radiograph (A) demonstrates an avulsion fracture from the medial patellar facet. Axial T2 fat saturation image (B) shows the contusion pattern in the medial patellar facet and lateral femoral trochlea *(arrows)*.

obvious clinically. However, relocation has often occurred by the time of presentation. Conventional radiography will demonstrate a large joint effusion. It is also possible to identify impaction fractures of the patella or lateral femoral condyle. A loose body may be present secondary to a displaced osteochondral lesion (OCL). MRI demonstrates characteristic findings associated with patellar dislocations. Marrow edema, cartilage injury, and torn medial patellar retinaculum are present. The impaction between the medial or odd patellar facet and the anterior, lateral femoral results in characteristic bone marrow edema pattern noted on the fluid sensitive sequence (Fig. 91.24). Fractured and displaced cartilage and/or osseous fragments are often present and should be searched for carefully. The usual donor sites include the most lateral aspect of the lateral trochlea, as well as the medial to apex of the patellar cartilage. A joint effusion is often large, which facilitates the search for free fragment. All three planes should be used to search for free fragments (Fig. 91.25).

MRI is also useful to evaluate anatomic causes of patellar maltracking. Femoral trochlear depth can be directly evaluated on axial images, as can tibial tubercle-trochlear groove distance (TTTG). Focally increased T2 signal in the superolateral corner of the Hoffa fat pad can be seen in patellar tendon lateral femoral condyle friction syndrome, also known as Hoffa fat pad impingement syndrome (Fig. 91.26). Sagittal and axial T2FS are best used to identify this finding. Measurements of the TTTG can be obtained on MRI and a measurement of greater than 15 mm is suspicious for maltracking. Recognizing the associated chondral loss from the lateral facet of the patella and lateral trochlear groove is supportive evidence of excessive lateral pressure and patellar maltracking.

OSSEOUS STRUCTURES AND CARTILAGE

A variety of distal femoral and proximal tibial/fibular fractures can occur. Many have been discussed elsewhere in this chapter. Put simply, fractures manifest as linear T1/T2 hypointensity with surrounding increased T2 signal. MRI is useful for evaluation of the overlying cartilage, which is often disrupted in intra-articular fractures such as tibial plateau fractures. Coronal sequences are best for femur, tibia, and fibula fractures, while sagittal sequences best evaluate the patella.

A lipohemarthrosis occurs when an intra-articular fracture allow marrow to seep into the joint. If allowed to settle, there will be layering of the lower density fatty elements atop the

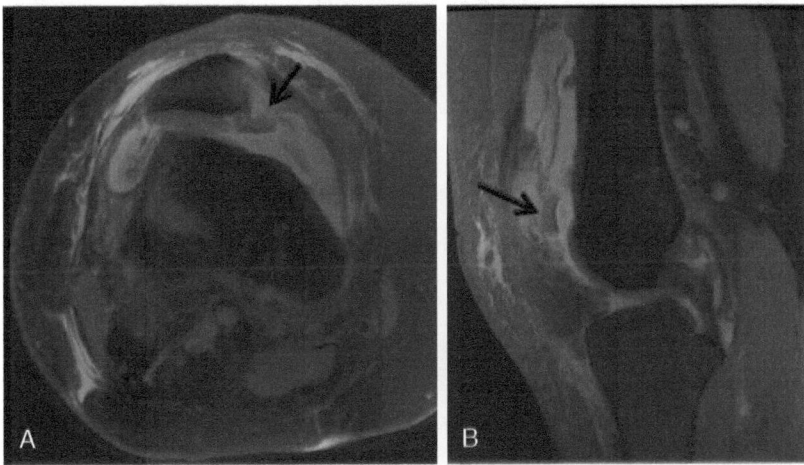

Fig. 91.25 Axial (A) and sagittal proton density fat saturation (PD FS) (B) images demonstrate transient patellar dislocation with a 14 mm displaced osteochondral lesion from the medial patellar facet *(arrows)*.

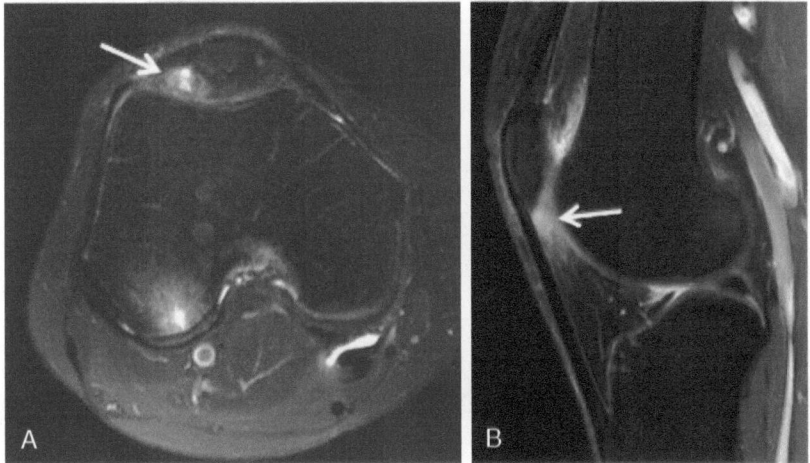

Fig. 91.26 Axial T2 fat saturation (A) and sagittal proton density fat saturation (B) demonstrate focal edema in the superolateral aspect of Hoffa fat *(arrows)*, consistent with superolateral Hoffa fat pad impingement.

remaining fluid. On true lateral radiographs, the lucent fat is demarcated by a straight horizontal line. On MRI, the nondependent fluid will be hyperintense on T1-weighted sequences and will lose signal when fat suppression is applied (Fig. 91.27).

An entity previously known as spontaneous osteonecrosis of the knee (SONK or SPONK) is now thought to represent a subchondral insufficiency fracture. A focal area of subchondral bone, often medial femoral condyle, demonstrates low T1/T2 signal, parallel to the articular surface, surrounding increased T2 marrow signal is often robust. Little to no antecedent trauma is reported. Over time, the area will sclerose and become hyperdense on radiographs. Remodeling of the articular surface can occur (Fig. 91.28). Meniscal body extrusion and varus alignment may contribute to worsening of the sclerosis and remodeling, as well as the secondary osteoarthrosis that follows.[15]

Cartilage lesions are best evaluated with PD FS imaging or gradient-recalled echo (GRE) imaging. Coronal and sagittal imaging are best for the femorotibial compartments. Sagittal imaging is best for the trochlea, and axial imaging is best for the patella. The Outerbridge classification is commonly used to grade cartilage injuries. Grade I chondromalacia is essentially

occult on MRI, but may manifest as increased signal without significant thinning. Grade II and III damages involve lesions of less than or greater than 50% of cartilage thickness, respectively. Grade IV chondromalacia is a full thickness lesion, often associated with subchondral marrow edema or cystic change.

OCLs are focal abnormalities in the bone and overlying cartilage. In adults, these lesions are often posttraumatic or degenerative. On MRI, fluid-sensitive sequences demonstrate focal marrow edema and/cystic change present with overlying cartilage damage. Unstable fragment is suggested by a thin rim of fluid undercutting the lesion. When displaced, OCLs become intraarticular loose bodies. Eventually, the donor site fills in with granulation tissue. If a defect in a chondral surface appears to be filled in with amorphous, intermediate T2 signal, a careful search should be performed for loose bodies, as previously described.

Several of the bursa or areas of common fluid accumulation around the knee have already been mentioned. Popliteal recess is most common. Fluid escapes the joint and gets trapped in the recess. A ruptured cyst can be identified with MRI at the time of internal derangement evaluation and is seen best on axial

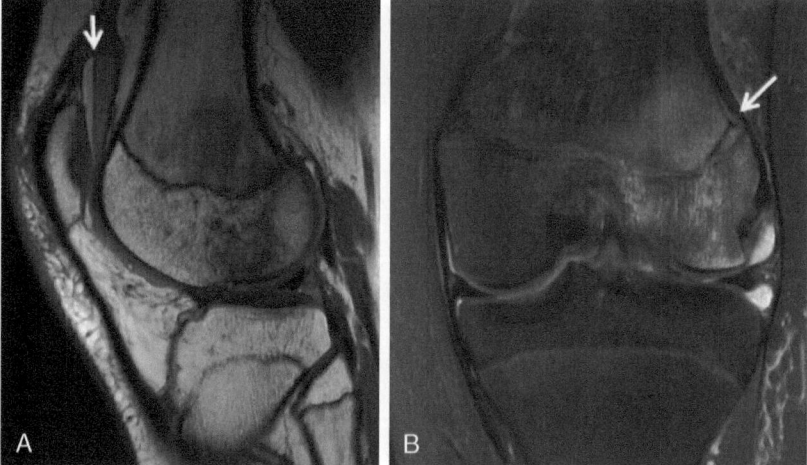

Fig. 91.27 Sagittal T1 image (A) demonstrates fat-fluid level *(arrow)* in the suprapatellar recess. Corresponding coronal proton density fat saturation image (B) demonstrates the Salter-Harris type II fracture of the lateral femoral condyle *(arrow)*. Distal femoral physeal injuries are rare, representing only 5% on physeal injuries.[14]

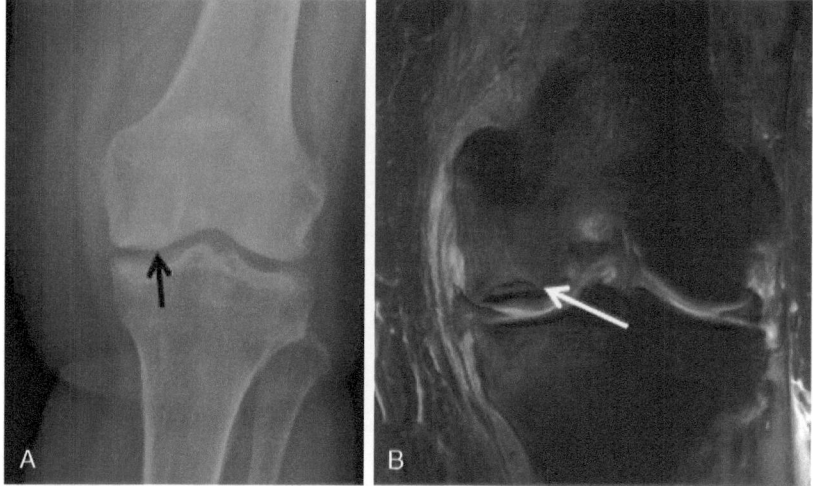

Fig. 91.28 Frontal radiograph (A) demonstrates flattening of the medial femoral condyle *(arrow)*. Coronal proton density fat saturation image (B) demonstrates hypointense subchondral fracture line *(arrow)* and surrounding marrow edema.

T2FS as hyperintense fluid tracking along the medial head of the gastrocnemius. A small residual collection often remains in the recess. Additional bursa that can mimic as medial meniscal tears clinically are the pes anserine bursa and the semimembranosus-tibial collateral ligament (SMTCL) bursa. The space between the medial (a.k.a. tibial) collateral ligament and the semimembranosus is a potential space that can fill with bursal fluid. This bursa has a characteristic appearance on fluid sensitive sequences, resembling a "comma" shape as it drapes over the semimembranosus (Fig. 91.29). SMTCL bursa can be confused for a parameniscal cyst. The origin of a parameniscal cyst should be identified arising from the medial meniscus before that diagnosis is made (see Fig. 91.7). The SMTLC bursa is to be distinguished from the pes bursa, which is more distal and anterior, though the treatment is the same for both. Adventitial bursae can form at any point of friction between adjacent structures. The most common place is beneath the IT band. Adventitial bursa appear as fluid signal collections, often surrounding by hazy, mildly increased T2 signal.

POSTOPERATIVE IMAGING

Imaging the postoperative knee can be challenging. Complete discussion warrants its own chapter. Several highlights will be touched upon here. Hardware creates susceptibility artifact on MRI. Several techniques can reduce this artifact, including using 1.5 T MRI instead of 3.0 T. On CT, the metal creates streak artifact. Total knee arthroplasty often contains the metallic femoral and tibial components, and the plastic patellar components and the polyethylene linear. The latter two are relatively radiolucent. Radiographs can demonstrate periprosthetic lucency, fracture, or migration of components. The threshold for calling lucency is generally 2 millimeters in thickness. It can indicate loosening or infection. Anterior tilt of the stem of a tibial component can also suggest an abnormality (Fig. 91.30). The patellar component and the polyethylene liner can displace, often producing subtle findings on radiograph. Multiple tiny metallic densities indicate particle disease.

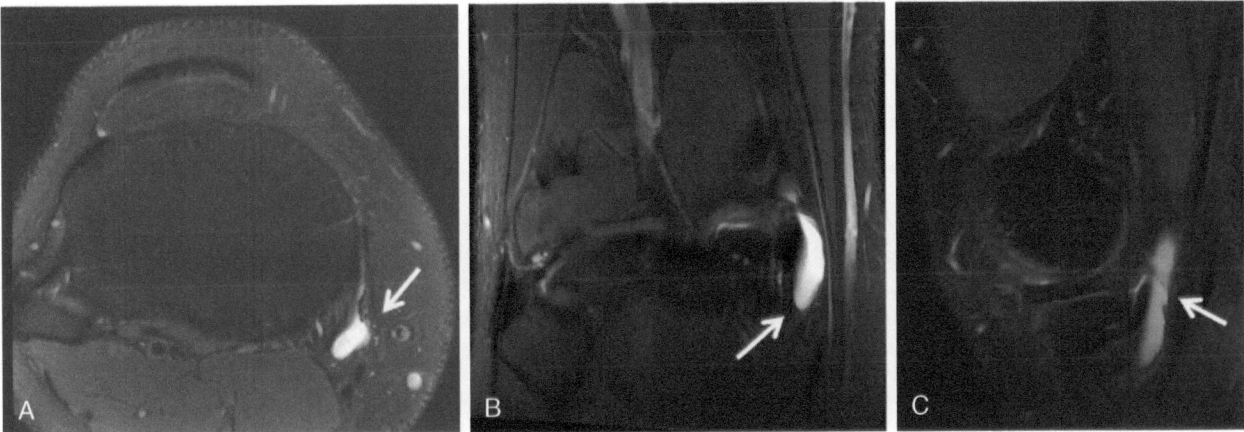

Fig. 91.29 Axial (A), coronal (B), sagittal proton density fat saturation (C) images demonstrate semimembranosis-tibial collateral ligament bursal fluid with the characteristic comma shape *(arrows)*.

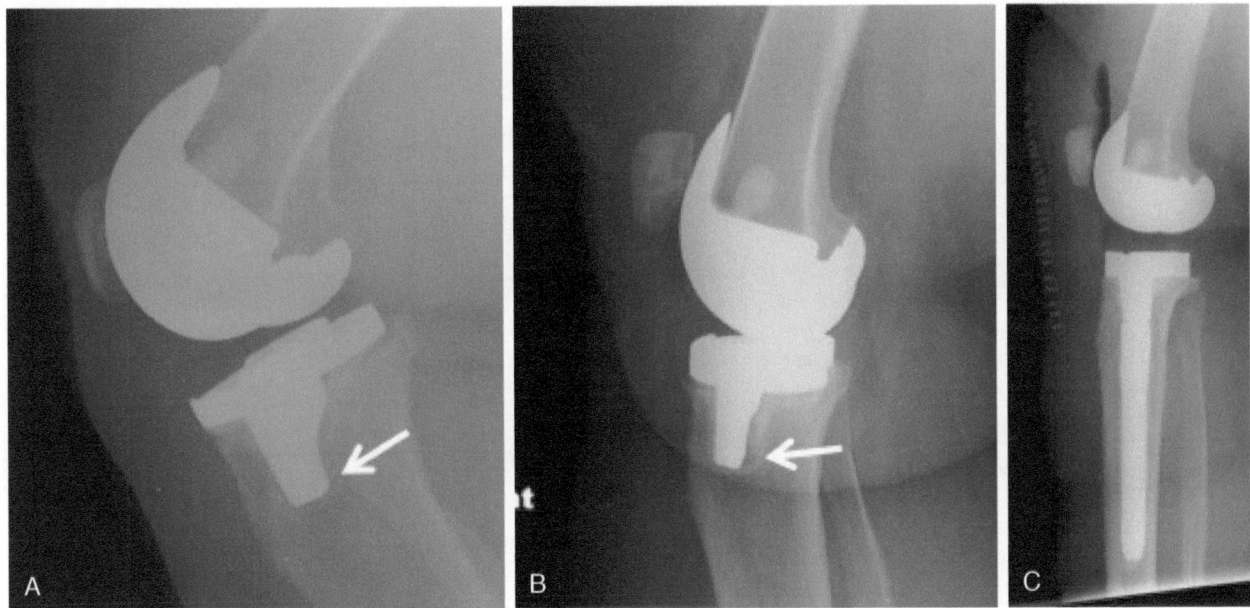

Fig. 91.30 Two subsequent lateral radiographs (A and B respectively) demonstrate a right knee TKA with worsening anterior tilt of the tibial component *(arrows)*. Lateral radiograph following revision arthroplasty (C).

ACL reconstruction, using either a patellar bone-tendon-bone graft or hamstrings graft, is a common procedure. Radiographs can be useful to follow patients with ACL reconstructions. The Blumensaat line should approximate the normal course of the graft. Widening of the femoral or tibial tunnels suggests micromotion and may suggest failure. On MRI, evaluation technique is similar to that of the native ligament. The graft should approximate the Blumensaat line. The extra osseous portion of the graft should be straight. Redundancy of the graft suggests laxity. Complete disruption of graft fibers is often accompanied by anterior translation of the tibia with respect to the femur. Focal scarring can occur anterior to the graft, known as focal arthrofibrosis, or cyclops lesion. Occasionally after graft repair, a fibrocartilaginous mass can form in the notch that may lead to graft failure. This abnormality should be searched for when follow-up imaging is performed. These can cause decreased range of motion and rarely pain. Many of the other tendinous and

ligamentous structures of the knee can be repaired or reconstructed, and the same principles apply.

In the setting of severe meniscal injuries in young patients, cadaver meniscal transplantation can be performed. Allograft meniscal tissue can be anchored to bony attachments, which are then placed into corresponding artificially created defects in the host tibia. Alternatively, suture anchors can be used to affix the transplant to the host tibia through tibial tunnels. Evaluation on MRI can be quite challenging, and comparison with any posttransplant imaging is essential. Incorrect sizing can be seen by incomplete coverage of the articulating femur and tibia, or transplant tissue hanging over the margins of the bone. Re-tears can be subtle unless significantly displaced. Dislodgement of the bone plugs or radial tears results in displacement of the tissue, often into the gutters (Fig. 91.31). Interestingly, meniscal transplant subluxations have been shown to not be associated with extrusions of the native meniscus.[16]

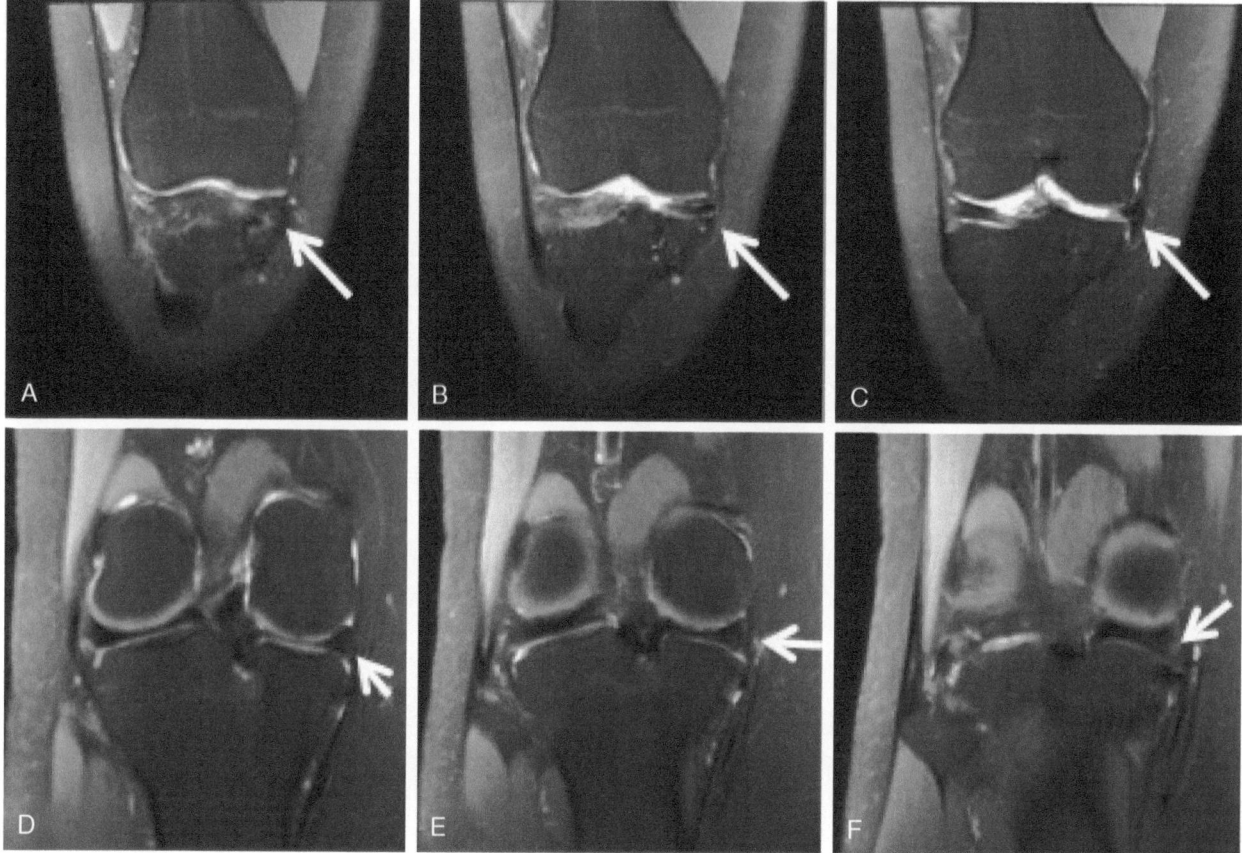

Fig. 91.31 Sagittal proton density fat saturation series demonstrates anterior (A–C) and posterior attachment (D–F) of a medial meniscal transplant *(arrows)* that is frayed but not completely torn.

In summary, radiographic assistance to management of orthopedic ailments can be performed through a variety of techniques. Excellent communication between the radiologist and ordering physician can provide the best outcome for the patient, as the proper study, appropriate views, and cross-sectional imaging with proper protocols can be implemented. This chapter was not designed to be all-inclusive, but instead to assist with an awareness of anatomy and pathology that are commonly encountered.

For a complete list of references, go to ExpertConsult.com.

SELECTED READINGS

Citation:
Tuite MJ, Kransdorf MJ, Beaman FD, et al. ACR Appropriateness Criteria acute trauma to the knee. *J Am Coll Radiol.* 2015;12(11):1164–1172.

Level of Evidence:
V

Summary:
Decision support for choosing the appropriate imaging in cases of trauma to the knee.

Citation:
Miller TT. Common tendon and muscle injuries: lower extremity. *Ultrasound Clini.* 2007;2(4):595–616.

Level of Evidence:
V

Summary:
Description of technique and ultrasound appearance of musculotendinous pathology around the knee with a focus on the extensor mechanism.

Citation:
Helms CA, Major NM, et al. *Musculoskeletal MRI.* Philadelphia: Saunders; 2001:353–383.

Level of Evidence:
V

Summary:
Overview of the MRI appearance of a variety of surgical and nonsurgical pathology of the knee aimed at the radiologist.

Citation:
McAdams TR, Mithoefer K, Scopp JM, et al. Articular cartilage injury in athletes. *Cartilage.* 2010;1(3):165–179.

Level of Evidence:
V

Summary:
Overview of the treatment options for cartilage injuries in athletes and an algorithm based on lesion characteristics.

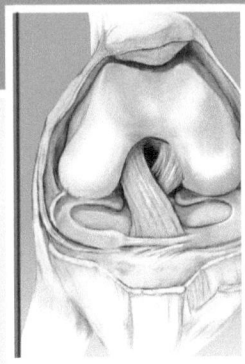

92

Basics of Knee Arthroscopy

Stephen R. Thompson, Mark D. Miller

Few areas in orthopaedic surgery have grown as rapidly as knee arthroscopy. Arthroscopy often can be performed more quickly and with increased accuracy, lower complication rates, decreased hospitalization time, and shorter recovery periods, compared with many more open operative techniques. The effective use of arthroscopy is based on the understanding of the benefits and indications for arthroscopy, as well as its limitations.

The knee was the first joint to be examined arthroscopically, and many of the fundamental principles of arthroscopy were developed for the knee.[1] The first knee arthroscopy was performed in Europe and was advanced significantly by Japanese surgeons (Takagi and Watanabe).[1] Applications continue to expand, and the future scope of arthroscopic applications is limited only by the imagination of the arthroscopist.

PREOPERATIVE EVALUATION

Indications for knee arthroscopy continue to expand at a rapid rate. Each patient's unique anatomy must be considered before initiating arthroscopy. Systematic evaluation of the entire knee includes a thorough physical examination and history. Additional studies including radiographs and advanced imaging should be reviewed, and proper documentation must be performed.[2] Preoperative consultation with appropriate medical specialties and an anesthesiologist help reduce perioperative complications.[3] Postoperative prophylaxis for deep vein thrombosis (DVT) should be considered in at-risk patients. Local, regional, and general anesthetic considerations should be reviewed with the patient and the anesthesia team.

INDICATIONS

Arthroscopy has diverse application in various forms of knee disease. Diagnostic arthroscopy helps confirm suspected knee injuries.[4] An arthroscopic synovectomy can be useful for synovial biopsies to aid in the diagnosis of rheumatologic disorders, to remove diseased synovium and loose bodies, and to resect synovial folds or plicae. Arthroscopic treatment of septic arthritis of the knee has increased in frequency. Treatment of meniscal disease is perhaps the most common application of arthroscopy. Meniscal tears and repairs account for about half of knee injuries that require surgery. Osteochondral lesions commonly are addressed arthroscopically. Microfracture, autologous

chondrocyte implantation, and osteochondral plug transfers are also performed arthroscopically.

Injuries to the cruciate ligaments can be diagnosed easily with arthroscopy and subsequently treated. Arthroscopic-assisted reconstruction of these ligaments is one of the most common orthopaedic procedures today.[5] Other procedures that sometimes are aided with arthroscopy include tibial plateau fracture reduction, reduction and fixation of tibial eminence fractures, loose body removal, anterior fat pad débridement, and lateral release for patellar malalignment.[3]

Contraindications for knee arthroscopy must be considered as well. One such consideration includes local skin infections over the portal sites. In addition, alternative treatments should be considered for patients who have too high a risk for surgery and those who are not expected to be compliant with postoperative rehabilitation.[6]

POSITIONING

Two different forms of positioning are commonly used for knee arthroscopy. The patient can be positioned supine on the operating table, and a lateral post can be used for countertraction. Alternatively, the operative leg can be positioned in a commercially available leg holder (Fig. 92.1). The operative leg is allowed to hang freely over the end of the operating table, and the opposite leg is positioned in a well-padded leg holder, taking care not to compress the peroneal nerve.

PORTAL PLACEMENT

Landmarks, including the inferior pole of the patella and the joint line, are marked. Portal incisions are typically vertical, 1 cm in length, and made with a no. 11 blade while the knee is flexed.[4] A spinal needle can be used for localization of the anteromedial portal (Fig. 92.2). Portal placement is key to successful knee arthroscopy. Standard arthroscopic portals for knee arthroscopy have traditionally included a superomedial or superolateral portal for fluid inflow and outflow, and inferomedial and inferolateral portals positioned just above the joint line on both sides of the patellar tendon for arthroscopy and instrumentation (Fig. 92.3).[7] Typically the inferolateral portal is used for arthroscopic visualization and the inferomedial portal is used for instrumentation, although alternating instrumentation between the medial and lateral portal is often necessary to reach certain structures

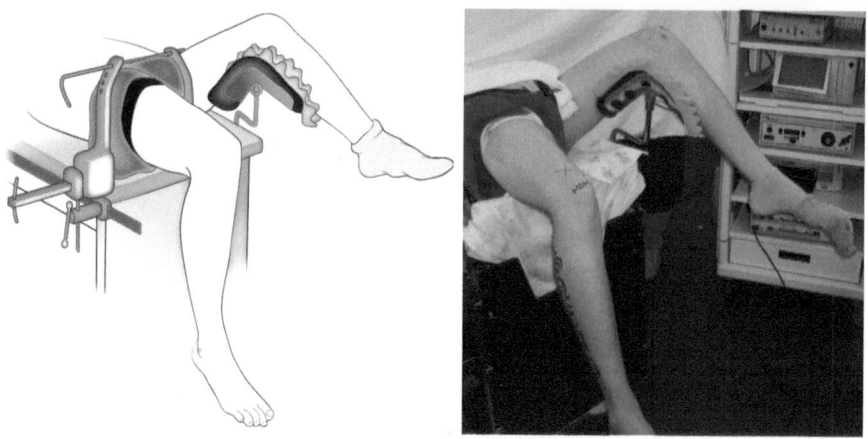

Fig. 92.1 The patient is positioned supine with use of a leg holder on the lateral post. (From Miller MD, Chhabra AB, Safran MR. *Primer of Arthroscopy*. Philadelphia: Elsevier; 2010.)

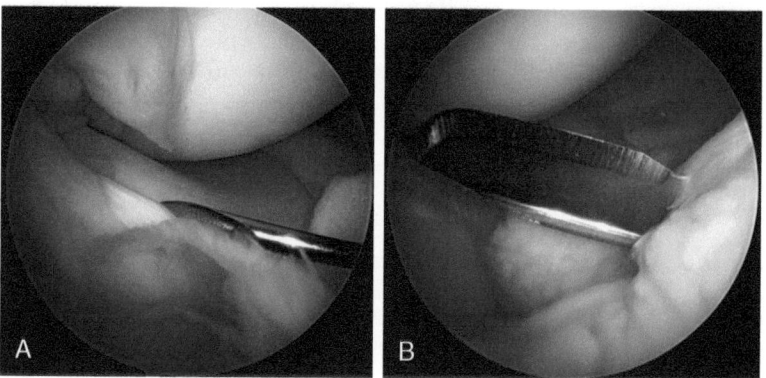

Fig. 92.2 Anteromedial portal localization. (A) The arthroscope is turned toward the anteromedial capsule. A spinal needle is inserted and positioned until it is just above the meniscus and its trajectory is satisfactory for intra-articular work. (B) The spinal needle is carefully removed, and a no. 15 or no. 11 blade is inserted blade-side up.

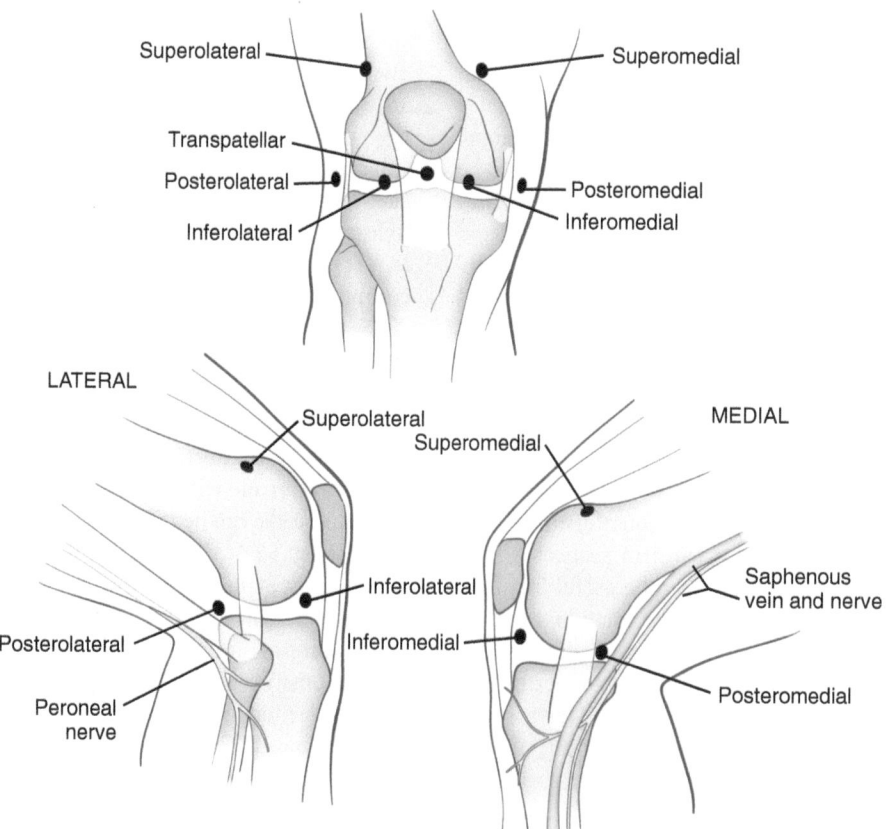

Fig. 92.3 Portal placement for knee arthroscopy. (From Miller MD, Chhabra AB, Safran MR. *Primer of Arthroscopy*. Philadelphia: Elsevier; 2010.)

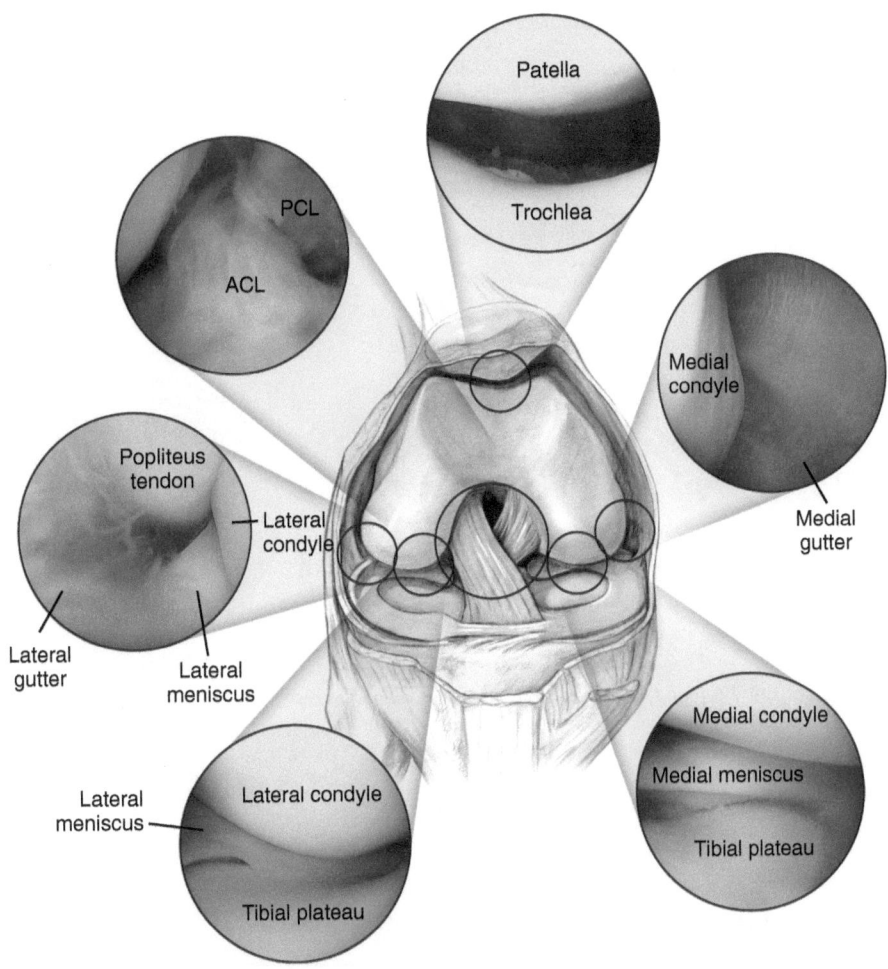

Fig. 92.4 Visualization during diagnostic arthroscopy. *ACL,* Anterior cruciate ligament; *PCL,* posterior cruciate ligament. (From Miller MD, Chhabra AB, Safran MR. *Primer of Arthroscopy.* Philadelphia: Elsevier; 2010.)

(Fig. 92.4). Newer arthroscopic fluid control systems have now made the use of superior outflow portals optional. The use of a far proximal superior portal can still be helpful for the visualization of patellar tracking (see Fig. 92.3).

Accessory portals for the knee include the posteromedial, posterolateral, far medial and lateral, and proximal superomedial portals. The posteromedial portal is often helpful for visualizing the posterior cruciate ligament and the posterior horn of the medial meniscus (Fig. 92.5).[8] The posterolateral portal, located just posterior to the lateral collateral ligament between the iliotibial band and the biceps tendon, sometimes is helpful, but extreme care should be taken to ensure that the portal is anterior to the biceps tendon to avoid injury to the peroneal nerve (Fig. 92.6). An accessory medial portal has been developed for obtaining access to the appropriate angle for anatomic femoral tunnel placement in anterior cruciate ligament (ACL) surgery.[9] Other portals include the midpatellar portal, far medial and lateral portals (which are sometimes helpful for instrument placement in hard-to-reach areas), and the proximal superomedial portal, located 4 cm proximal to and in line with the medial edge of the patella (for assessment of patellar tracking).

DIAGNOSTIC ARTHROSCOPY

As with any joint, systematic examination of the knee is appropriate. Before positioning the patient, a complete examination is conducted after induction of anesthesia to assess instability in all planes. An arthroscopic cannula is placed in the superomedial or superolateral portal for inflow and outflow (although the use of these superior portals is now optional with many of the new pump systems), and the obturator and sheath are introduced into the inferolateral portal after incision with the knee flexed at 60 to 90 degrees, angled toward the notch. As the knee is brought into extension, the obturator and sheath are advanced into the suprapatellar pouch and the obturator is replaced by a camera for visualization. The anteromedial portal can be made at the outset of the case or created under visualization with the spinal needle (see Fig. 92.2). Although many examination sequences are possible, it is important to visualize the suprapatellar pouch, patellofemoral joint (Fig. 92.7), medial and lateral gutters, medial and lateral compartments (meniscus and articular cartilage), and intercondylar notch (cruciate ligaments) in all patients.[4] Surgeons differ with regard to fat pad excision for visualization and therapeutic purposes.

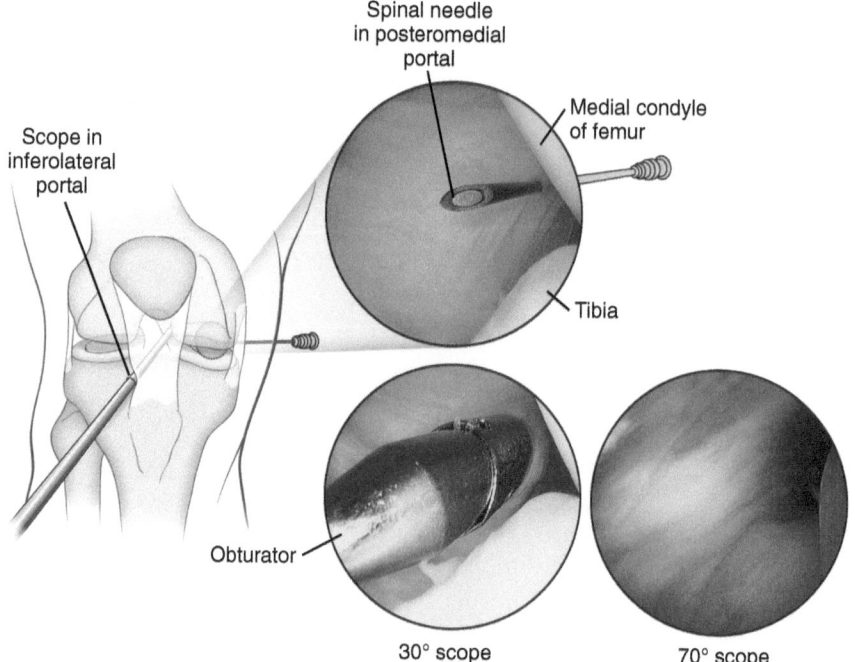

Fig. 92.5 View of the intercondylar notch from the posteromedial portal. (From Miller MD, Chhabra AB, Safran MR. *Primer of Arthroscopy.* Philadelphia: Elsevier; 2010.)

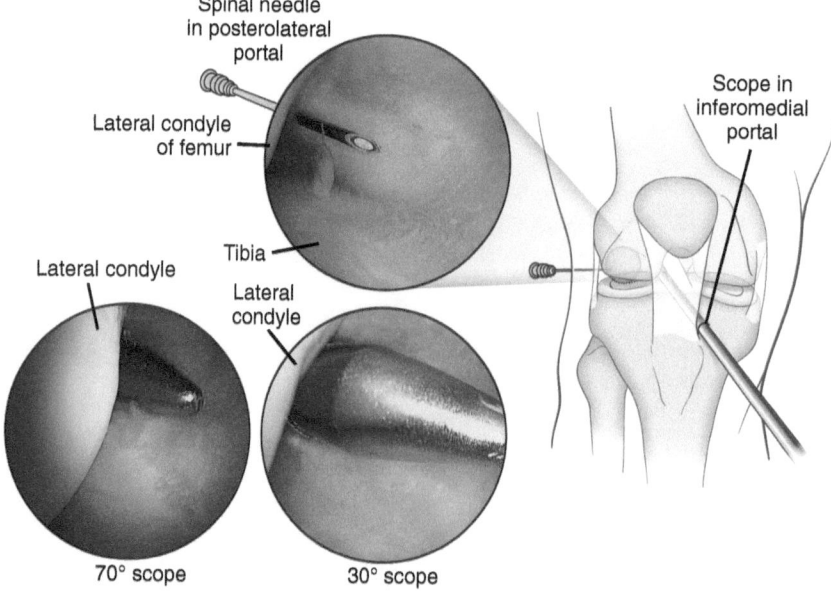

Fig. 92.6 View of the intercondylar notch from the posterolateral portal. (From Miller MD, Chhabra AB, Safran MR. *Primer of Arthroscopy.* Philadelphia: Saunders; 2010.)

The patellofemoral joint is inspected and articulation is examined, including the patella facets and trochlea. Engagement should be full at 40 degrees. The gutters are examined for loose bodies. The knee is flexed and the scope is brought down into the intercondylar notch. The ACL is inspected by directing the scope to view it laterally and by probing the ligament (Fig. 92.8). The ACL is composed of the two separate bundles that are often not distinct but can occasionally be recognized. The posterior cruciate ligament is also evaluated, although often only the femoral side is examined, with the remainder hidden by the ACL.[10] The

medial compartment is then visualized with valgus stress and extension using an assistant or with the surgeon resting the ankle on his or her hip. The foot can be externally rotated to improve access. The meniscus and articular surfaces are examined. Once all lesions are characterized, the lateral compartment is visualized in the same fashion in the figure-of-four position.

Accessory viewing portals are established as necessary if other areas need to be evaluated. A posteromedial portal can be helpful whenever medial meniscus pathology is suspected but is unable to be identified from the anterior portals. This portal is established

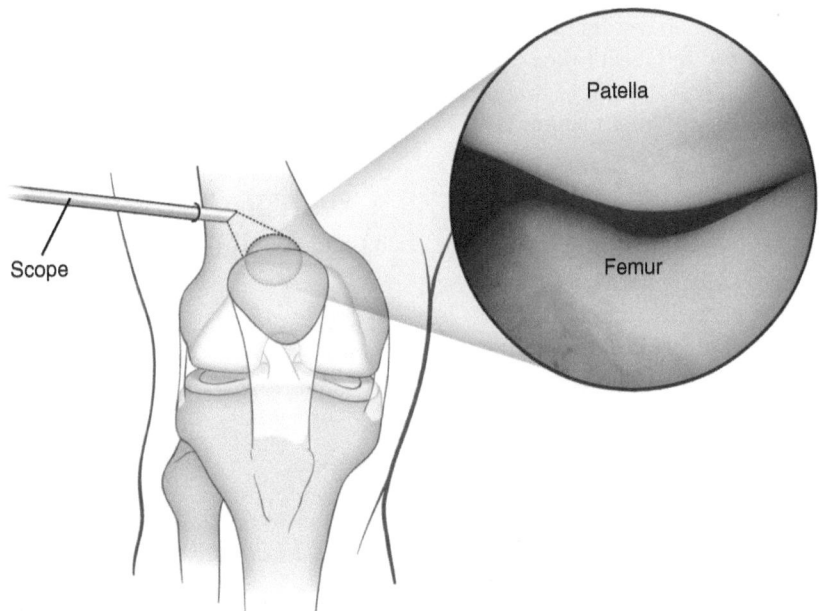

Fig. 92.7 Visualization of the patellofemoral joint. (From Miller MD, Chhabra AB, Safran MR. *Primer of Arthroscopy*. Philadelphia: Elsevier, 2010.)

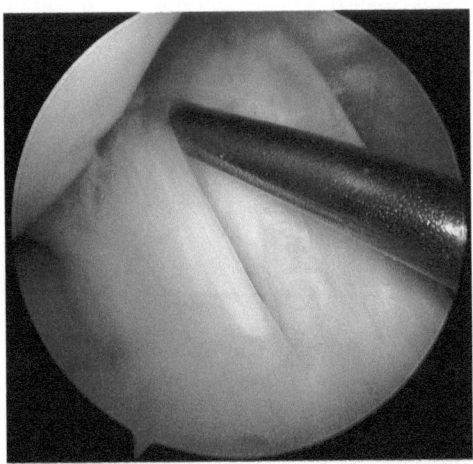

Fig. 92.8 Arthroscopic appearance of the two bundles of the anterior cruciate ligament. (From Miller MD, Chhabra AB, Safran MR. *Primer of Arthroscopy*. Philadelphia: Elsevier; 2010.)

by introducing the arthroscopic cannula into the back of the knee by directing it from anterior to posterior on the notch side of the medial femoral condyle. Care must be taken to avoid the saphenous nerve and vein. A spinal needle is used to establish the position of the portal. Next, a small incision is made in the skin only, followed by spreading with a blunt instrument down to the capsule. Once the arthroscope is in the posterior aspect of the knee, the posterior horn of the medial meniscus can be visualized. Use of a 70-degree scope may be helpful. After a complete evaluation of the joint is performed, all surgical pathology is addressed accordingly.

INSTRUMENTATION

A 30-degree arthroscope is most commonly used, although a 70-degree scope may be helpful in the posterior corners.[8] An arthroscopic probe can be used and provides a sense of touch to the arthroscopist. Instruments angled upward, including biters, are best for the medial compartment, whereas straight instruments often work best in the lateral compartment. Arthroscopic shavers are available in both large and small sizes and should be chosen on the basis of the dimensions of the compartment.[5]

POSTOPERATIVE CARE

Upon completion of the procedure, the fluid is evacuated from the joint and the instruments are removed. Typically nonabsorbable monofilament is used to close the portals and is removed 10 to 14 days after surgery. In some centers, portals are routinely left open, because it is believed that open portals permit easier fluid extravasation and reduce postoperative swelling and pain.[11] A local anesthetic can be injected at the end of the surgery into the skin only. Although the weight-bearing status may differ depending on the surgery performed, most patients require crutches for some period of time. Postoperative pain medicines are typically prescribed for a short period for most patients undergoing knee arthroscopy.

COMPLICATIONS

Postoperative complications can include infection, arthrofibrosis, nerve and vessel injury, iatrogenic cartilage injury, compartment syndrome, collateral ligament injury, and DVT or pulmonary embolism.[6,12] Perhaps the most common complication is inadvertent damage to the intra-articular structures.[12] This risk is inversely proportional to the surgeon's experience and the care with which the surgeon performs the procedure. Proper portal placement, use of a gentle technique, and attention to detail are crucial. The exact prevalence and long-term sequelae of iatrogenic cartilage lesions are unknown, but studies involving second-look arthroscopy and animal models have shown that this is a true risk and that the lesions do not tend to fill with time. Nerve or vessel injury can result from improper placement of the portals.[7] For this reason, a thorough knowledge of local anatomy is necessary before performing arthroscopy.

Tourniquet paresis can be reduced with use of a wide cuff and by limiting tourniquet time whenever possible. Positioning devices (e.g., leg holders) can have a tourniquet effect, even when the tourniquet is not inflated. Fluid extravasation has been reported, although the incidence of this complication can be reduced with careful placement of inflow cannulas and proper use of inflow pumps. Synovial fistula formation is a rare complication of arthroscopy and is usually remedied by 7 to 10 days of immobilization and, occasionally, delayed closure. Infection is an extremely rare complication of arthroscopy with less than a 1% occurrence rate and is usually the result of a break in sterile technique. High-dose antibiotics and arthroscopic irrigation and débridement may be indicated in severe cases. Hemarthrosis can occur as well, although it can be avoided with meticulous technique and care after procedures such as a lateral release.[5]

Arthrofibrosis is unusual after knee arthroscopy, although it can occur with procedures such as ACL reconstruction and multiligamentous knee reconstructions. Attainment of full motion preoperatively and early motion postoperatively are key to avoiding such an outcome.

An unusual but potentially life-threatening complication of knee arthroscopy is the development of a postoperative DVT or pulmonary embolism. Although the risk for these events is low, careful screening of risk factors must be performed to identify patients who require routine prophylaxis.[3,6] These risk factors include immobilization, increased body mass index, personal or family history of clotting disorder, and advancing age.

SUMMARY

Knee arthroscopy is effective in treating a number of intra-articular knee pathologies. Proper evaluation and management are key to successful patient outcomes. Results vary based on the underlying etiology, but they do appear to help patients in the symptomatic management of intra-articular disorders.

For a complete list of references, go to ExpertConsult.com.

SELECTED READINGS

Citation:

Hoogeslag RA, Brouwer RW, van Raay JJ. The value of tourniquet use for visibility during arthroscopy of the knee: a double-blind, randomized controlled trial. *Arthroscopy.* 2010;26(suppl 9):S67–S72.

Level of Evidence:

I

Summary:

In this randomized controlled trial, significantly improved visibility during routine knee arthroscopy was demonstrated with use of a tourniquet.

Citation:

Jameson SS, Dowen D, James P, et al. The burden of arthroscopy of the knee: a contemporary analysis of data from the English NHS. *J Bone Joint Surg Br.* 2011;93B(10):1327–1333.

Level of Evidence:

II

Summary:

In this article a prospective, large-volume registry analysis of knee arthroscopies occurring in the United Kingdom National Health Service is provided. The overall rate of complications was less than 1%.

Citation:

Sikand M, Murtaza A, Desai VV. Healing of arthroscopic portals: a randomised trial comparing three methods of portal closure. *Acta Orthop Belg.* 2006;72(5):583–586.

Level of Evidence:

II

Summary:

In this article a prospective randomized controlled trial comparing suture closure of arthroscopy portals with Steri-Strip application or no closure whatsoever is described. Swelling was significantly lower in the two groups without suture closure. Patient satisfaction with regard to final scar appearance was higher in the two groups without suture closure.

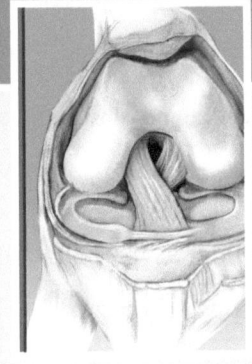

93

Arthroscopic Synovectomy of the Knee

Mick P. Kelly, Charles A. Bush-Joseph

The synovial lining is a specialized mesenchymal tissue that is integral to the normal functioning of a joint. Synovial disorders can involve varying amounts of the synovium. Rheumatoid arthritis shows total joint involvement, whereas on the other end of the spectrum, plica syndrome is caused by an isolated synovial lesion.

Volkman performed the first synovectomy in 1855 for tuberculous synovitis. Although the indications and technique have changed over time, the procedure is still performed, and the objective of removing the diseased synovium remains the same.[1] Compared with open procedures, arthroscopic techniques have enabled surgeons to perform a synovectomy without a large arthrotomy, decreasing the risk of postoperative arthrofibrosis. Arthroscopy also serves as an effective technique to remove synovium in the posterior compartment and allows viewing of synovial lesions that may be missed with open procedures. Arthroscopic synovectomy can be used in the surgical treatment of rheumatoid arthritis, pigmented villonodular synovitis (PVNS), hemophilic synovitis, plicae, synovial hemangioma, synovial osteochondromatosis, and degenerative synovitis.

As with all orthopedic conditions, a complete workup including a thorough history and physical examination and complete imaging analysis is needed to evaluate these patients. In addition, a trial of medical management should be performed before initiation of surgical treatment. Surgical treatment consists of arthroscopically removing varying amounts of synovium, the amount of which is based on the underlying disease process.

History

A complete history is important in the evaluation of patients with synovial disorders. The presence of other affected joints, chronicity of symptoms, exacerbating factors, and the amount of disability experienced by the patient on a daily basis are important pieces of information. Patients with rheumatoid arthritis may have more systemic complaints, including morning stiffness and other affected joints, particularly the small joints of the hands and feet. PVNS is typically a monoarticular process that affects adults in the third or fourth decade of life. Symptoms are mechanical in nature and may be similar to those seen in patients with meniscal tears.[2] Clinically patients have the insidious onset of localized warmth, swelling, and stiffness with occasional locking and a palpable mass. Plica syndrome is a finding in patients with anteromedial knee pain. Patients experience tightness, snapping, giving way, and pain with repetitive activities. Clinically it is difficult to distinguish plica syndrome from other causes of knee pain such as meniscal tears, patellar tendinitis, or patellofemoral pain syndrome.

Physical Examination

Other joints may be affected in patients with rheumatic or autoimmune disorders, and these joints should be evaluated. Patients with rheumatoid arthritis often have a flexion contracture and quadriceps atrophy in the knee region.[3] The skin should be examined, as well as previous incisions and subcutaneous nodules. Knee examination includes overall alignment, range of motion (ROM), the presence of an effusion, warmth, tenderness, crepitus, strength, meniscal integrity, and stability. Collateral ligament instability or bony malalignment suggests more severe articular loss, and patients with these conditions are poor candidates for a synovectomy.

The physical examination for PVNS is often nonspecific. An effusion is associated with diffuse involvement. Palpation of the joint may show warmth and tenderness. Aspiration of the joint fluid may show a dark-brown fluid that is a result of recurrent bleeding into the joint. Cytologic studies of the aspirate may show hemosiderin pigment and multinucleated foreign body giant cells, but often the findings of these studies are normal.[4] Ligamentous instability is uncommon in persons with PVNS.

Plica syndrome begins insidiously. Tenderness over the medial parapatellar region is common. A plica may sometimes be directly palpated and rolled under the finger, recreating the patient's symptoms. If the medial border of the patella is palpated while pushing the patella medially with one hand and the other hand produces a valgus stress with external rotation of the tibia, pain may be elicited, suggesting plica syndrome.[5] An effusion is not typically present in persons with plica syndrome.

Imaging

Patients with rheumatoid arthritis may have periarticular erosions and osteopenia. Cervical spine flexion and extension views should be obtained in preoperative patients to rule out cervical instability. Radiographs in patients with PVNS can show erosive, cystic, and sclerotic lesions of the articular surface. If enough synovium that contains hemosiderin is present, soft tissue masses may be seen, but often the findings of the films are normal with well-maintained joint spaces. Magnetic resonance imaging is considered to be the most diagnostic study for PVNS. It may show nodular intra-articular masses of low signal intensity on

T1- and T2-weighted images and also allows for the evaluation of the location and extent of disease.

DECISION-MAKING PRINCIPLES

A full rheumatologic workup should be completed for patients with systemic diseases, and appropriate laboratory tests should be up to date. Patients with hemophilia require a consultation with a hematologist. If surgical treatment is to be pursued, it is essential to have a well-thought-out plan for perioperative management of clotting factors.

In disorders associated with a localized lesion, such as a localized PVNS (Figs. 93.1 and 93.2) or plica, arthroscopic intervention can remove the pathology in its entirety. Persons with diffuse conditions such as rheumatoid arthritis (Figs. 93.3 through 93.6) or hemophilia can undergo surgery to decrease the severity of disease symptoms once conservative measures have been exhausted.

Treatment Options

Treatment options vary based on etiology. Recently medical management of rheumatoid arthritis has improved significantly. The goals of medical treatment include reducing the number

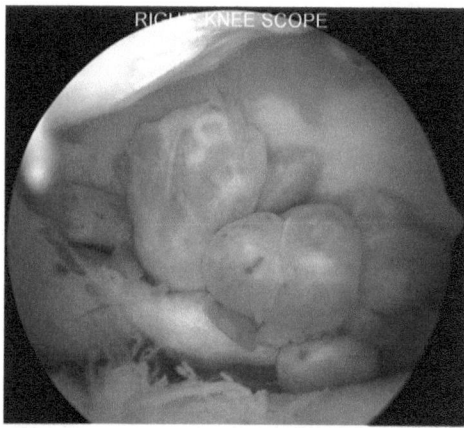

Fig. 93.1 Arthroscopic appearance of localized pigmented villonodular synovitis.

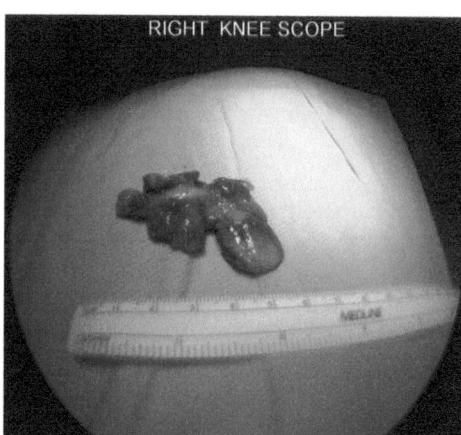

Fig. 93.2 Gross view of the localized pigmented villonodular synovitis specimen from Fig. 93.1.

of painful and swollen joints, suppressing the acute phase response, decreasing the rheumatoid factor titer, and slowing radiographic progression of the disease. Medical management should consist of a combination of disease-modifying antirheumatic drugs, nonsteroidal antiinflammatory drugs, an appropriate physical therapy regimen, activity modification, and intra-articular steroid injections.[6] A patient with rheumatoid arthritis and minimal degenerative changes on radiographs would be a candidate for arthroscopic synovectomy after the failure of approximately 6

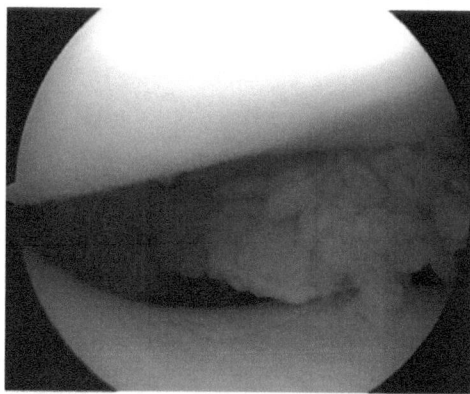

Fig. 93.3 The patellofemoral joint of a left knee in a 39-year-old patient with rheumatoid arthritis. Despite conservative treatment, the patient experienced a flexion contracture with uncontrolled swelling and elected to undergo arthroscopic synovectomy.

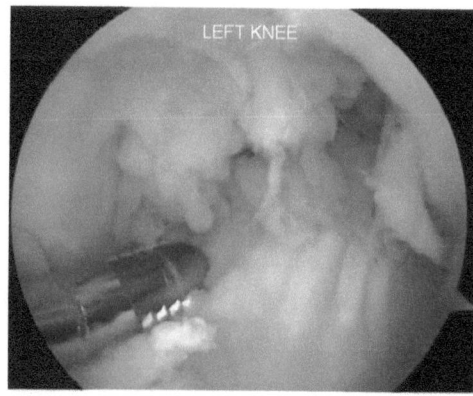

Fig. 93.4 The arthroscopic view of the notch before débridement in the left knee of the patient in Fig. 93.3.

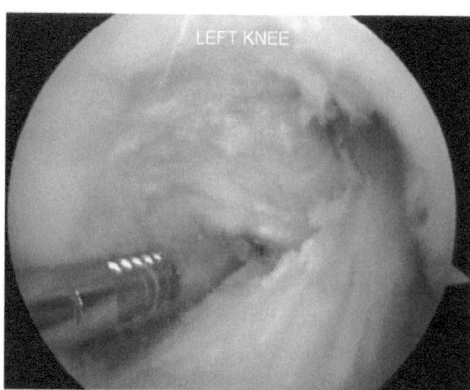

Fig. 93.5 The arthroscopic view of the notch after débridement in the same patient shown in Fig. 93.3.

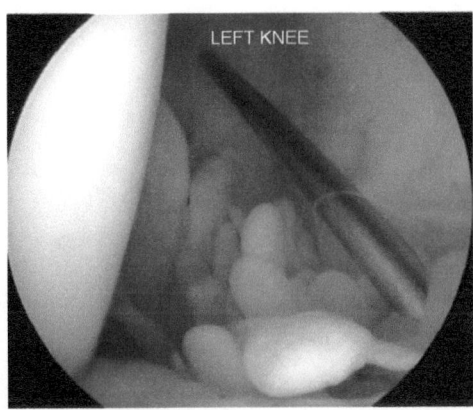

Fig. 93.6 The arthroscopic view of the posteromedial compartment of the patient shown in Fig. 93.1. The spinal needle is used to localize the ideal portal location.

months of medical management. Significant joint space narrowing or mechanical malalignment is a relative contraindication to synovectomy for inflammatory synovial knee disorders, and a total knee arthroplasty is recommended.

Hemophilic synovitis can also be associated with significant joint destruction and has shown favorable improvement in symptoms with synovectomy.[7–9] Radiosynovectomy is indicated as the first procedure in persons with hemophilic synovitis, with satisfactory results in 80% of patients.[10] No more than three radiosynovectomies can be performed per year. If the three radiosynovectomy procedures fail to relieve symptoms, an arthroscopic synovectomy is indicated.[10] Although joint deterioration is not preventable, a synovectomy can reduce recurrent hemarthrosis and maintain ROM. A hemophilic synovectomy requires an inpatient stay for coordinated management of clotting factors with the patient's hematologist.

In PVNS, arthroscopic synovectomy is the treatment of choice for localized disease, but open synovectomy may be required for diffuse-type PVNS and recurrence of local tumors. Adjuvant therapies including intra-articular radiotherapy or moderate-dose external beam radiotherapy further reduce likelihood of recurrence with advanced forms and recurrent disease.[11]

> ### Authors' Preferred Technique
>
> Arthroscopic synovectomy requires the use of multiple portals to access all spaces in the knee joint; therefore detailed preoperative planning and patient setup is essential for a successful operation. General anesthesia is recommended, and the use of a Foley catheter should be considered. An epidural can be used if required for medical reasons and may also help with postoperative pain relief.

Examination After Inducement of Anesthesia

Both knees are examined for an assessment of the ROM, ligamentous stability, patellar mobility, patellar tracking, and the presence of an effusion.

Positioning

The patient is placed supine on the operating room table. The well leg is appropriately padded and secured in a well leg holder after placement of a compressive stocking and sequential compression device. A leg holder is not used on the operative leg because it may interfere with the use of the superomedial and superolateral portals. The foot of the operating table is dropped and the mid portion of the table is flexed to avoid hip hyperextension. A well-padded thigh tourniquet is placed high on the operative leg.

Surgical Steps
Anterior Compartments

After standard prepping and draping is performed, the extremity is exsanguinated and the tourniquet is inflated to 300 mm Hg. The tissue obtained from the synovectomy should be collected and sent for pathologic evaluation. The anterior aspect of the knee is addressed first. A superomedial outflow portal is created, and the outflow cannula is placed here. Standard inferolateral and inferomedial portals are created. The arthroscope is placed in the inferolateral portal, and an initial diagnostic arthroscopy is performed. The synovectomy then proceeds with the use of an arthroscopic shaver. While viewing from the inferolateral portal with the knee in extension, the shaver is used in the superolateral and inferomedial portals to remove all synovial tissue, but avoiding injury to surrounding muscle, tendon, and fascia (Table 93.1).

Posterior Compartments

The anterior compartment should now be finished, and attention is turned to the posterior compartments, beginning with the posteromedial compartment. Typically the posterior compartments can be visualized with a 30-degree scope; however, a 70-degree scope can be used if difficulty is encountered. The arthroscope must first be placed in the posterior compartment. The blunt-tipped trocar is placed in the arthroscopic sheath and inserted into the inferolateral portal. The trocar is directed toward the medial femoral condyle, and when it is contacted, the trocar is carefully advanced posteriorly through the interval between the medial femoral condyle and the posterior cruciate ligament, raising the hand with insertion to match the slope of the tibia. If this maneuver proves difficult, a central and vertically oriented patellar tendon portal may provide easier access to the posterior compartment. The arthroscope is inserted, and the posterior portion of the medial femoral condyle and the posterior horn of the medial meniscus should be visible (see Fig. 93.6). While looking medially, a spinal needle is inserted anterior to the medial head of the gastrocnemius into the posteromedial compartment. The needle is used to ensure that all areas in the posterior knee that are in need of synovectomy can easily be reached. Once the ideal portal location has been determined, a longitudinal incision is made in the skin. A hemostat is used to bluntly dissect and then penetrate the capsule, and a cannula is placed. The shaver is placed through the cannula, and the synovium in the posteromedial compartment is resected.

The posterolateral compartment is accessed in a manner similar to the posteromedial compartment. A blunt-tipped trocar is placed in the arthroscopic cannula in the inferomedial portal between the lateral femoral condyle and the anterior cruciate ligament. The hand is gently raised and advanced posteriorly,

TABLE 93.1	Steps for Performing an Arthroscopic Synovectomy of the Knee		
Step	Area of Synovial Resection	Camera Portal/Leg Position	Instrument Portal
1	A. Suprapatellar pouch B. Lateral gutter	Inferolateral/extension	Superolateral
2	A. Begin medial gutter B. Medial aspect suprapatellar pouch C. Intercondylar notch	Inferolateral/extension	Inferomedial
3	A. Finish medial gutter B. Medial suprapatellar pouch	Inferolateral/flexion	Superomedial
4	A. Retropatellar space B. Inferolateral gutter	Superolateral/extension	Inferolateral
5	A. Retropatellar space B. Inferomedial gutter	Superolateral/extension	Inferomedial
6	A. Posteromedial compartment	Inferolateral/flexion	Posteromedial
7	A. Posterolateral compartment	Inferomedial/flexion	Posterolateral

taking care not to violate the posterior capsule, which could put the neurovascular structures at risk. The arthroscope replaces the trocar, and the posterior lateral femoral condyle and the posterior horn of the lateral meniscus are viewed. Again, a spinal needle is used to make a posterolateral portal under direct visualization. Placing the needle in the soft spot, anterior to the biceps femoris muscle and posterior to the iliotibial band, helps protect the common peroneal nerve. The needle should be inserted posterior to the fibular collateral ligament and anterior to the lateral head of the gastrocnemius. Once it is determined that the spinal needle is placed so that all areas that require synovectomy can be reached, the skin is incised and a hemostat is used to dissect to the posterior capsule. The capsule is then punctured under direct visualization and a cannula is placed. The shaver is placed through the cannula, and the posterolateral compartment synovectomy is performed.

After the synovectomy is complete, the tourniquet is deflated and an electrocautery device is used to achieve hemostasis. It is common to use a suction drain for 24 hours to help minimize hemarthrosis. Ice, elevation, and a light compressive dressing are used to minimize swelling, and early motion is encouraged.

Postoperative Management

The patient can bear weight as tolerated after surgery. Physical therapy is begun on postoperative day 1 after drain removal and concentrates on closed chain exercises. The most immediate goals are regaining knee extension and quadriceps function. A continuous passive motion machine can be used for the first few days after surgery.

RESULTS

Goetz et al.[12] evaluated 32 knees at 14-year follow-up after combined arthroscopic and radiation synovectomy for rheumatoid arthritis. These investigators concluded that combined arthroscopic and radiation synovectomy led to a stable improvement of knee function for a minimum of 5 years, but repeat surgery was frequent, with 56% of patients having another operation by 10 years.[12] If total knee arthroplasty was considered the end point, the joint survival rate was 88.5% at 5 years, 53.9% at 10 years,

and 39.6% at 14 years.[12] Carl et al.[13] studied 11 patients with rheumatoid arthritis who were undergoing a synovectomy. These investigators found that a synovectomy led to an overall reduction of acute inflammatory infiltrates by 82.1% and of chronic inflammatory infiltrates by 62.5%.[13]

A meta-analysis of 630 patients with PVNS who underwent arthroscopic, combined anterior arthroscopic, and posterior open synovectomy, or open synovectomy had an overall recurrence rate of 21% (137/630).[11] A multivariate analysis of recurrence showed no difference between surgical approaches for localized disease, and low-quality evidence of significant reduction by open (OR = 0.47; 95% CI 0.25 to 0.90; $P = .024$) or combined (OR = 0.19; 95% CI 0.06 to 0.58; $P = .003$) synovectomy versus with arthroscopic surgery. Rates of wound complications and reoperation were similar between groups, but the open synovectomy group had significantly increased postoperative stiffness (10.5%, 37/354) versus the combined group (2.7%, 1/37) and the arthroscopic synovectomy group (2.1%, 5/239).[11]

Although few follow-up data are available regarding synovectomy in patients with hemophilia in general, Verma et al.[14] suggest that the primary predictor of outcome in hemophiliacs is the degree of intra-articular preexisting degenerative changes. In more severe cases, the results of arthroscopic synovectomy are less predictable, and total joint arthroplasty should be considered.

Complications

After synovectomy, a recurrent hemarthrosis may occur. The fluid can often be aspirated with a large-bore needle, but an arthroscopic washout may be needed. Joint stiffness and loss of extension are also possible. Performing aggressive and early ROM exercises, using extension boards, and dynamic bracing may help with these symptoms. A septic joint or neurovascular injury can also occur. With use of careful technique, these complications can be minimized.

FUTURE DIRECTIONS

Future directions include adjuvant therapies to reduce likelihood of recurrence of disease following arthroscopic synovectomy. For example, PVNS tumors are stimulated by the overexpression of macrophage colony-stimulating factor (M-CSF) by synovial fibroblasts. Tyrosine kinase inhibitors, such as imatinib, have been shown to reduce tumor progression and may become an effective treatment for advanced form and recurrent disease.[15]

For a complete list of references, go to ExpertConsult.com

SELECTED READINGS

Citation:
Goetz M, et al. Combined arthroscopic and radiation synovectomy of the knee joint in rheumatoid arthritis: 14-year follow-up. *Arthroscopy*. 2011;27(1):52–59.

Level of Evidence:
IV, therapeutic case series

Summary:
The authors evaluated the outcome of 32 knees treated with combined arthroscopic and radiation synovectomy of the knee joint in early cases of rheumatoid arthritis in terms of knee function and the need for repeat surgical intervention. At an average of 14 years of follow-up, with any repeat surgical intervention as the end point, the survival rate was 32%, challenging the long-term benefit of the procedure.

Citation:
Carl HD, et al. Site-specific intraoperative efficacy of arthroscopic knee joint synovectomy in rheumatoid arthritis. *Arthroscopy*. 2005;21(10):1209–1218.

Level of Evidence:
III

Summary:
The authors assessed site-specific intraoperative reduction of inflammatory infiltrates achieved with arthroscopic knee synovectomy in patients with rheumatoid arthritis using preoperative and postoperative synovial tissue samples. They concluded that arthroscopic synovectomy reduces acute and chronic inflammatory infiltrates in patients with rheumatoid arthritis. However, this reduction appears to depend on the anatomic region of the joint.

Citation:
Mollon B, Lee A, Busse JW, et al. The effect of surgical synovectomy and radiotherapy on the rate of recurrence of pigmented villonodular synovitis of the knee. *Bone Joint J*. 2015;97-B(4):550–557.

Level of Evidence:
IV, therapeutic study

Summary:
The authors performed a meta-analysis of 630 patients who underwent surgical synovectomy of the knee for PVNS. The overall rate of recurrence was 21.8% (137/630). Open synovectomy and combined arthroscopic/open synovectomy had lower recurrence rate than arthroscopic synovectomy for diffuse PVNS, but not for localized disease. Perioperative radiotherapy reduced recurrence of diffuse PNVS. Complication rates were similar except for significantly increased post-operative stiffness in the open and combine arthroscopic/open synovectomy groups.

Citation:
Kim TK, et al. Neurovascular complications of knee arthroscopy. *Am J Sports Med*. 2002;30:619–629.

Level of Evidence:
IV, review article

Summary:
The authors summarize causes and frequencies of complications related to arthroscopic procedures, including anterior and posterior compartment synovectomy. Complication management and medicolegal implications are reviewed.

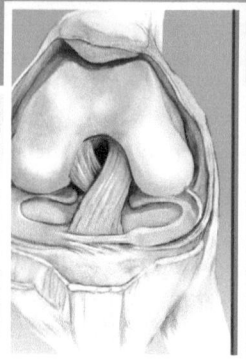

94

Meniscal Injuries

Joseph J. Ruzbarsky, Travis G. Maak, Scott A. Rodeo

HISTORY OF THE MENISCUS

One of the earliest descriptions of the menisci was recorded by Bland-Sutton in 1897. At that time, the menisci were thought to be vestigial tissue and were depicted as "the functionless remnants of intra-articular leg muscles."[1] Further advances in our understanding of the menisci have demonstrated that they provide mechanical support and secondary stabilization, localized pressure distribution and load sharing, lubrication, and proprioception to the knee joint.[2,3]

In 1936, King[4,5] initially documented meniscal healing at the meniscosynovial junction in a canine model. He also documented minimal healing of intrasubstance tears. Significant articular chondral degeneration was documented in the setting of partial or complete meniscectomy. These data suggested that the available vascular supply may serve a crucial role in meniscal healing and that the menisci may have a role in chondroprotection.[4,5]

Fairbank substantiated this chondroprotective role in 1948 using radiographic evaluation of patients after a total meniscectomy. This study documented specific radiographic "Fairbank changes" including formation of an anteroposterior ridge extending from the femoral condylar margin, marginal flattening of the femoral articular surface, and joint space narrowing. These radiographic findings were identified as early as 5 months after a complete meniscectomy and demonstrated time-dependent progression. These observations led to the conclusion that the menisci may have a function during weight bearing and that a complete meniscectomy may contribute to intra-articular degenerative changes. This awareness, in conjunction with further substantiating data,[6–8] increased the focus on meniscal preservation through limited partial meniscectomy, meniscal repair, biologic stimulation procedures, and an advanced algorithm to guide the effective use of these treatment options.

MENISCUS ANATOMY AND STRUCTURE

The menisci are fibrocartilaginous structures that are semilunar in shape and wedge-shaped in cross-section. Two menisci (medial and lateral) exist between the femoral and tibial articulation. The femoral articulating meniscal surface is concave, whereas the tibial articulating surface is convex. These surfaces conform to the convex and concave opposing chondral surfaces, respectively. The conforming articulation provides perfect congruency between the femoral condyle, meniscus, and tibial plateau, which establishes the foundation for the biomechanical function of the menisci.

The medial and lateral menisci are significantly different in shape largely because of the structural differences between the medial and lateral femoral condyles and tibial plateau (Fig. 94.1). Both the macroscopic and microscopic anatomy of the menisci determine their function. The medial and lateral menisci are two C-shaped fibrocartilaginous structures attached anteriorly and posteriorly to the tibial plateau. The medial meniscus is longer in the anteroposterior direction compared with the lateral meniscus. The anterior horn of the medial meniscus is smaller in sagittal cross-section compared with the posterior horn. The anterior and posterior horns of the lateral meniscus, on the other hand, are similar in size. Approximately 50% of the medial tibial plateau is covered by the medial meniscus, compared with 59% coverage of the lateral tibial plateau by the lateral meniscus.[9]

Anchoring of the menisci occurs through insertional fibers and ligament attachments. Insertional fibers anchor both menisci to the subchondral bone at their anterior and posterior horns. The intermeniscal ligament also directly attaches the anterior horns of both menisci in most patients. The medial meniscus is continuous with the deep fibers of the medial collateral ligament and medial joint capsule, rendering it less mobile than the lateral meniscus. Nevertheless, the posterior horn of the medial meniscus remains mobile up to 5 mm to accommodate femoral rollback with knee flexion.[2,10] The lateral meniscus, on the other hand, has significantly fewer capsular and ligamentous attachments and thus is more mobile. Normal lateral meniscal excursion has been documented up to 11 mm and may partially explain the reduced frequency of lateral meniscal injuries.[10] The intra-articular portion of the popliteus tendon can be identified at the popliteal hiatus located between the posterolateral border of the lateral meniscus and the posterior knee capsule. This area of potential hypermobility is stabilized by the superior and inferior popliteomeniscal fasciculi that secure the posterolateral meniscus to the popliteus and posterior joint capsule (Fig. 94.2).[11] Fascicular injury can produce lateral meniscus hypermobility and may require meniscocapsular repair to reestablish meniscal stability.

In addition to the fasciculi, additional lateral meniscal stability may be achieved through accessory meniscofemoral ligaments in up to 66% of patients. Two accessory ligaments are frequently encountered: the ligament of Humphrey and the ligament of Wrisberg. Although uncommon, a Wrisberg ligament variant may also exist in the setting of a discoid lateral meniscus, in which

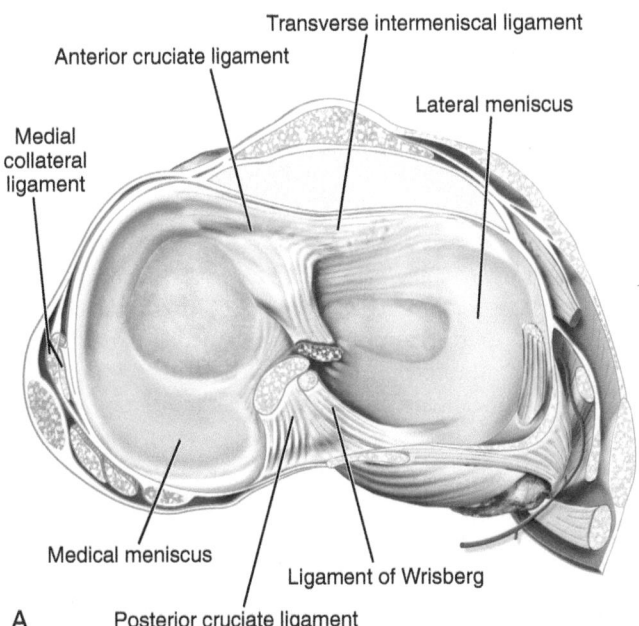

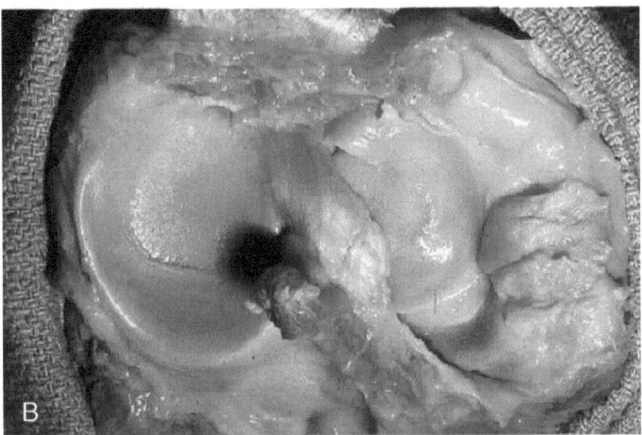

Fig. 94.1 Superior schematic (A) and cadaveric dissection (B) views of meniscal axial anatomy demonstrate the structural differences and specific attachment sites of the anterior and posterior horns of the medial and lateral meniscus. (Modified from Pagnani MJ, Warren RF, Arnoczky SP, et al. Anatomy of the knee. In: Nicholas JA, Hershman EB, eds. *The Lower Extremity and Spine in Sports Medicine*. 2nd ed. St Louis: Mosby; 1995.)

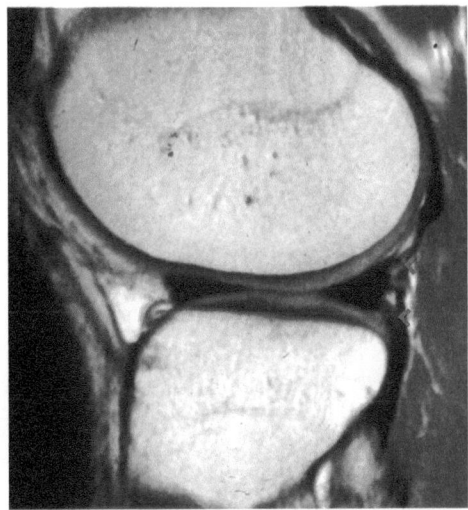

Fig. 94.2 A sagittal magnetic resonance imaging scan demonstrating the anatomic relationship of the superior and inferior popliteomeniscal fasciculi of the lateral meniscus *(red arrowheads)*.

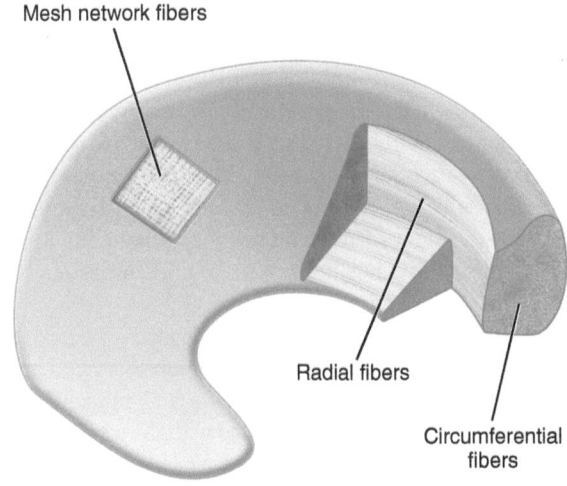

Fig. 94.3 Meniscal microstructure. (From Bullough PG, Munuera L, Murphy J, et al. The strength of the menisci of the knee as it relates to their fine structure. *J Bone Joint Surg Br*. 1970;52B:564–567.)

there is deficiency of the meniscocapsular attachments, with only a stout Wrisberg ligament stabilizing the posterior horn (see Figs. 94.1 and 94.2). The ligament of Humphrey extends from the medial femoral condyle to the posterior horn of the lateral meniscus and courses anterior to the posterior cruciate ligament (PCL). The ligament of Wrisberg and Wrisberg's variant have similar attachments but course posterior to the PCL.

Histologically, dense fibrocartilage is composed of collagen fibers that are arranged circumferentially (to disperse compressive loads or "hoop stresses") with some radial fibers as well (to resist longitudinal tearing). At the surface, collagen fibers are arranged randomly to disperse shear stress associated with flexion and extension of the knee joint (Fig. 94.3).[2] Proteoglycan macromolecules hold and retain water, which is paramount to the

compressive, shock-absorbing properties of the menisci, and augments its ability to aid in lubrication of the knee joint.

The blood supply of the menisci originates at the periphery in the perimeniscal capillary plexus, which are tributaries of the medial and lateral geniculate arteries. Importantly, only the peripheral 25% to 30% of the meniscus is vascularized (Fig. 94.4).[12] The gradient attenuation in vascularity from the periphery to the central portion of the menisci is gradual, but the need for ease of clinical classification led to the designation of three vascular "zones." The outer third is known as the "red–red zone" because of its relatively high concentration of vascular channels. In this zone, bleeding at the site of injury promotes fibrovascular scar formation and migration of anabolic cells in response to cytokines released during the inflammatory response. As a result, tears in this zone have the highest healing potential. The middle vascular zone is termed the *red–white zone*. This zone

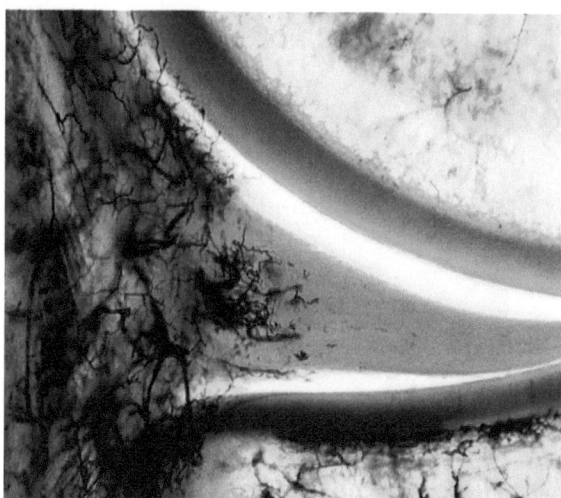

Fig. 94.4 Adult meniscal microvasculature.

has intermediate vascularity, which leads to a less predictable result with regard to healing of meniscal tears. If a repair is attempted in this zone, ancillary techniques such as synovial abrasion, vascular access channels, and a fibrin clot may be used to increase local blood flow and maximize healing potential. The red–red and red–white zones combine to form the outer 4 mm of the meniscus.[13] The remainder of the meniscus is avascular in adults and is therefore called the *white–white zone*. Nutrition of this tissue is achieved solely from the synovial fluid via passive diffusion, which is aided by motion of the knee joint. Consequently, injury in the white–white zone of the meniscus does not stimulate a healing response, and the prognosis for healing after attempted repair is poor.

Meniscal neuroanatomy and vascular anatomy are extremely similar both in density and location. The periphery and anterior and posterior horns of the menisci have a significantly higher density of neural components compared with the central regions.[2,8] Both mechanical and sensory fibers have been identified in these locations and may contribute to pain and proprioception during knee range of motion (ROM). Dye et al.[14] substantiated these basic science data through a clinical study with use of neuro-sensory meniscal mapping. This study documented significant neural activity at the meniscocapsular junction and meniscal periphery, compared with limited activity in the central region. These data suggest that mechanical loading of the peripheral meniscal rim and the meniscocapsular junction may be responsible for most of the pain experienced after a meniscal injury.

MENISCUS BIOMECHANICS AND FUNCTION

The medial and lateral menisci function to provide mechanical support and secondary stabilization, localized pressure distribution and load sharing, lubrication, and proprioception to the knee joint.[2,3] Mechanically, the menisci also transmit at least 50% to 75% of the axial load in knee extension and up to 85% with the knee in 90 degrees of flexion (Fig. 94.5).[15] The femoral and tibial radii of curvature are significantly different and thus are poorly congruent at the point of articulation. The menisci provide the congruency necessary for both load transmission

and knee stability. They decrease the peak contact stresses at the articular surface by 100% to 200%.[16–18] Removal of the menisci during partial or total meniscectomy results in increased point contact loading at the femorotibial articulation and significantly increased contract stresses focused in a small area. A biomechanical study by Lee[19] highlighted this function by documenting increased contact stress with incrementally increasing meniscectomy in a dose-response fashion. Resection of 75% of the posterior horn can increase contact stresses similar to those present after a total meniscectomy.[16,19] Furthermore, complete tears of the posterior horn of the medial meniscus are the functional equivalent to meniscal root avulsions, disturbing the ring continuity of the meniscus and therefore significantly increasing the contact pressures seen in the medial compartment.[20]

Meniscal injury or dysfunction is particularly notable in the lateral compartment because of its specific anatomic differences. The femoral and tibial articulation is a convex-convex articulation that is buffered by the lateral meniscus, which covers up to 70% of the tibial surface area. This articulation is in direct contrast to the convex-concave femorotibial articulation in the medial compartment. For this reason, partial or complete removal of the lateral meniscus results in greater contact stresses and increased risk for progression of osteoarthrosis compared with the medial compartment.[17,21]

The menisci perform a crucial role in shock absorption in addition to contact stress distribution. The meniscal collagen ultrastructure is organized in a circumferential fashion with radial linking fibers, thereby allowing conversion of axial loads to horizontal "hoop" stresses. This shock absorption is also aided by the reduced meniscal cartilage stiffness, increased elasticity, and biphasic structure. Prior data have demonstrated that total meniscectomy results in a 20% decrease in shock absorption, and thus preservation of meniscal integrity is crucial to minimize chondral damage.[22]

The role of the meniscus as a secondary stabilizer of the knee has also been well documented. Bedi et al.[23] noted that transection of the anterior cruciate ligament (ACL) and meniscectomy resulted in nearly double the anterior tibial translation in both Lachman and pivot shift testing compared with that of the ACL alone, as measured with knee-specific computer navigation software. The secondary stabilizing effect is primarily due to the posterior horn of the medial meniscus in resisting anterior tibial translation as demonstrated during a Lachman maneuver.[23,24] Prior data have demonstrated that deficiency of the posterior horn of the medial meniscus in the setting of primary ACL reconstruction is associated with a higher risk of graft elongation and recurrent joint laxity.[25] In this setting, the posterior horn of the medial meniscus functions as a wedge buttress to inhibit anterior tibial translation. Prior data have documented a 58% increase in anterior tibial translation with medial meniscectomy in the flexed ACL-deficient knee.[26]

The biomechanical stabilizing effect of the lateral meniscus has also been well documented. Lateral meniscal deficiency may significantly reduce knee stability, specifically with tibial internal rotation (and subsequent pivot shift).[27] Musahl et al.[28] used computer-assisted navigation in a cadaveric model to document a significant 6-mm increase in anterior tibial translation after a

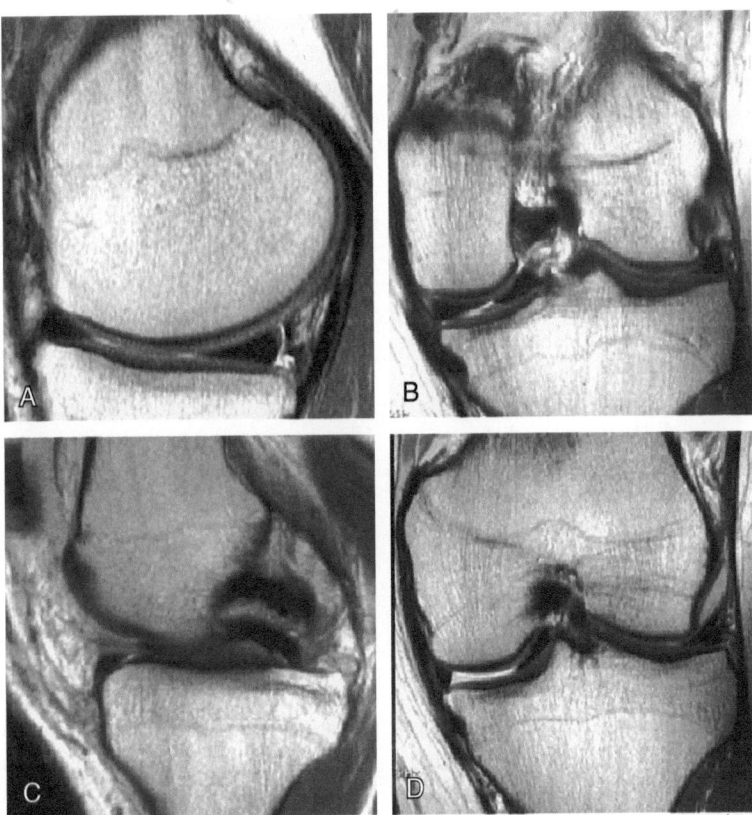

Fig. 94.5 Magnetic resonance imaging of the medial and lateral menisci. (A) A sagittal image demonstrates increased signal within the peripheral rim of the posterior horn of the medial meniscus, indicating a peripheral vertical meniscal tear. (B) A coronal view demonstrates a complex medial meniscal tear. (C) A double posterior cruciate ligament sign indicates a bucket handle meniscal tear displaced into the notch. (D) A coronal view demonstrates an absent posterior horn due to a displaced bucket handle tear that can be visualized in the notch.

lateral meniscectomy in ACL-deficient knees during the pivot shift but not the Lachman maneuvers. These data demonstrate the importance of the lateral meniscus as a stabilizer during axial, rotatory loading of the knee.

EPIDEMIOLOGY

Acute and chronic tears of the menisci are very common orthopaedic injuries that affect patients of various ages and activity levels. Meniscal injury often causes pain and physical impairment, and clinical symptoms, such as pain, catching, locking, and decreased ROM, may frequently require surgical intervention for relief. The treatment for meniscal tears has evolved over the course of several decades with both technological and intellectual advances in orthopaedic surgery.

Since 1936, when total meniscectomy was the treatment of choice,[4] abundant research has led to the understanding that meniscal tissue should be retained whenever feasible.[29,30] For this reason, recent measures have attempted to preserve as much of the meniscus as possible. These measures have evolved from open total meniscectomy to open partial meniscectomy and finally to arthroscopic partial meniscectomy or repair. Meniscal injury was noted to be the most common musculoskeletal injury, occurring with a frequency of 23.8/100,000 per year.[31] The American Academy of Orthopedic Surgeons estimates that arthroscopy

procedures of the knee total nearly 1,000,000 cases per year in the United States as of 2006.[32] Within this cohort, arthroscopic treatment of meniscal injury is among the most common procedure performed, accounting for up to 50% of all arthroscopic surgeries.[32]

Improved understanding of the etiology, management, and outcomes for meniscal injury has been obtained from epidemiologic data regarding gender, age, activity level and type, and patient comorbidities.[33–39] Men are up to four times more likely than women to sustain a meniscal tear.[2,33] Cutting and pivoting sports requiring knee flexion at high activity levels generate the highest risk for meniscal injury, including basketball, soccer, gymnastics, wrestling, football, and skiing. Additionally, lateral meniscal tears are less common than medial meniscal tears for most of these activities and all age groups.[33,36,39]

Recent advances in radiology including magnetic resonance imaging (MRI) have significantly improved the diagnosis of meniscal injury. However, improved imaging has also demonstrated the frequency of incidental meniscal pathology that does not necessarily correlate with clinical symptoms. Prior data have documented a 5.6% incidence of asymptomatic meniscal tears in a young patient population (mean age: 35 years).[40] Abnormal signal characteristics were also identified in the posterior horn of the medial meniscus in 24% of patients. These incidental findings significantly increase with age, with a 76% prevalence of meniscal tears in asymptomatic older patients (mean age: 65 years).[41]

Advanced imaging techniques have also aided in diagnosing meniscal pathology in the setting of concomitant ligament injury. Injury to the ACL has been associated with a significantly increased risk of lateral and medial meniscal tears due to the mechanism of acute ACL injury and secondary stabilizing effects in chronic ACL tears, respectively. Prior data have documented a 60% to 70% prevalence of meniscal tears in the setting of acute ACL injury.[42] Lateral meniscal tears more commonly occur as a result of the rotational and translational mechanism of injury.[42,43] Previous data in a young population with acute ACL ruptures documented a 57% and 36% prevalence of concomitant lateral and medial meniscal tears, respectively.[42] However, medial meniscal tears are more commonly identified in the setting of chronic ACL tears.

MENISCAL INJURY: CLASSIFICATION

Multiple types of tears have been described, including vertical (longitudinal or circumferential), radial, horizontal (transverse or cleavage), degenerative, complex tears, and horn detachment (Fig. 94.6). Vertical, oblique, and longitudinal patterns are most common in the younger population, whereas complex degenerative tears are more often seen in patients older than 40 years. Numerous authors have observed that tear type and configuration were predictive of outcome, with complex unstable tears (i.e., those with >3-mm displacement upon examination with an arthroscopic probe) faring worse than simple vertical-longitudinal tear types.[44,45]

Vertical (longitudinal or circumferential) meniscal tears are frequently due to a traumatic etiology such as an ACL tear. These tears are also termed *bucket handle tears* when they are large (>1 cm), displaced, and unstable. Bucket handle tears may frequently cause mechanical symptoms, including locking and the inability to fully extend the knee. They more frequently occur in the medial meniscus because of the limited motion afforded by the strong peripheral meniscocapsular attachments. Smaller, incomplete vertical tears more commonly occur and are frequently identified at the time of arthroscopy. These incomplete tears may not require intervention in the setting of concomitant ACL injury if they are determined to be stable when manually probed.[46,47]

Oblique (parrot beak or flap) tears commonly occur at the junction of the posterior and middle body of the meniscus. These unstable tears frequently cause mechanical symptoms including locking and catching during knee motion that may or may not produce pain. The associated pain has been hypothesized to be associated with irritation of the meniscocapsular junction and surrounding synovium. This tear type is not typically amenable to repair because it most commonly occurs in the white–white meniscal region. Excision of the unstable fragment is effective in addressing the mechanical symptoms.

Radial tears are oriented perpendicular to the circumferential fibers and are commonly identified in the lateral meniscus after an acute ACL rupture. Again, variability exists in the length of these tears, which range from small to large tears that extend from the white–white zone through to the periphery. A small radial tear involving less than 60% of the meniscus does not significantly influence compartment biomechanics, whereas a large radial tear that extends through more than 90% of the meniscus to the periphery results in a significant increase in peak compartment pressures.[48] Partial tears preserve the crucial peripheral circumferential fibers and thus the load distribution ability of the meniscus. This radial tear subtype can be débrided to a stable edge in most circumstances. Complete tears, on the other hand, result in complete circumferential fiber disruption, which not only compromises the function of the meniscus but also increases the biomechanical tendency for repair diastasis with axial load. Although diastasis significantly impairs healing, repair of this tear type should be attempted, because the only alternative treatment is effectively a near-total meniscectomy. Although further data are required to understand the role of mechanical load on meniscus healing, most recommend an initial period of avoidance of weight-bearing after repair of complete radial tears to reduce the potential for tear diastasis.

Horizontal tears often develop from variable shear stress between the superior and inferior meniscal regions in the early stage of meniscal degeneration. This tear type can occur in young patients but is more commonly a degenerative tear and may be associated with meniscal cyst formation that may communicate with the periphery. These latter tears have been commonly identified on MRI; however, their presence is not necessarily linked to clinical symptoms.[49] The treatment philosophy of these lesions continues to evolve over time. Some older data suggest that cyst

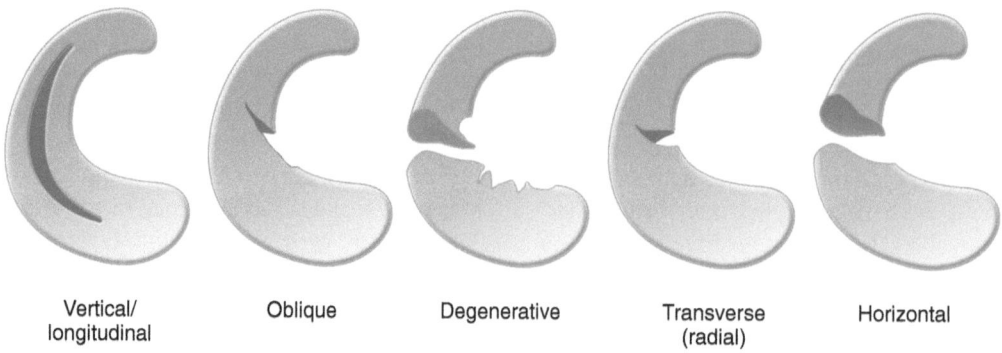

Vertical/longitudinal   Oblique   Degenerative   Transverse (radial)   Horizontal

Fig. 94.6 A descriptive classification of meniscal tears. (Modified from Ciccotti MG, Shields CL, El Attrache NS. Meniscectomy. In: Fu FH, Harner CD, Vince KG, eds. *Knee Surgery*. Baltimore: Williams & Wilkins; 1994.)

aspiration and suture repair of the horizontal tear may obviate the need for meniscectomy,[50] but for most of the last decade the prevailing philosophy for most horizontal tears, including associated flaps, is treatment with a partial meniscectomy. A recent systematic review[51] reports a 78% success rate in repairing these lesions in a young population. Given this high success rate and the benefits of meniscal preservation, repair of such horizontal cleavage tears should be attempted in the younger cohort of patients as this can restore tibiofemoral contact pressures to levels similar to that of the native meniscus.[52] If repair is not possible, preserving the superior leaflet of the horizontal tear offers the best preservation of tibiofemoral load sharing.[53] In the older cohort of patients with suspected degenerative tears, careful evaluation and exhaustion of conservative measures should be performed before proceeding to surgery as the results of surgery in this patient population may not be durable.[54]

Complex tears of the meniscus occur in a stellate pattern and propagate through multiple planes, although the horizontal cleavage plane is most common. These tears most commonly occur at the posterior root, are degenerative in nature, and should be treated with partial meniscectomy if surgical management is indicated.

A meniscal tear zone classification has been documented and divides each meniscus into three radial and four circumferential zones. This classification system permits improved clinical documentation and comparison of outcomes (Fig. 94.7).[55]

HISTORY

Meniscal tears can be either traumatic or degenerative. Degenerative tears have been closely associated with osteoarthritis. Acute tears are often related to trauma, most frequently as a result of a twisting motion. Early diagnosis and treatment of acute meniscal tears can significantly affect the short-term meniscal viability and subsequent long-term articular chondral protection. This treatment is particularly critical in a younger population

given the high incidence of acute, traumatic meniscal tears, and the importance of joint preservation in younger patients.

A carefully completed history, physical examination, and diagnostic imaging evaluation facilitates efficient and accurate diagnosis, and guides appropriate treatment. The aforementioned epidemiology should aid in guiding the patient history with regard to age, mechanism of injury, activity level, concomitant pathology, and previous ipsilateral injury or surgery. Additionally, fundamental questions should also be asked, including the location and duration of symptoms, exacerbating activities, and alleviating mechanisms, including medication and activity modification.

Patients may or may not be able to recall a single traumatic event. These events typically include twisting or hyperflexion with or without a mild effusion that may be noticed the day after injury. Notably, this effusion is not specific for meniscal pathology. Pain is often localized to the joint line and is usually intermittent. Constant pain or pain at rest usually indicates separate or additional pathology, such as osteoarthritis. Mechanical symptoms may also herald an unstable flap or bucket handle meniscal tear; these symptoms include catching, locking, popping, pinching, or the feeling of having to move the knee through a specific ROM to "reset" the joint. Locking due to an incarcerated torn meniscal fragment will most often present with an inability to achieve full extension. Unlike traumatic tears, degenerative, chronic meniscal tears are atraumatic and are rarely associated with an acute effusion. Instead, patients may describe mild intermittent effusions, infrequent mechanical symptoms, and generalized joint-line pain. These tears more commonly affect an older, less active population and may exist with concomitant osteoarthrosis.

PHYSICAL EXAMINATION

Physical examination of the patient with a possible meniscus tear should include an evaluation of gait, standing alignment, ROM, and strength testing of the hip and knee, ligament stability testing, and a careful inspection and palpation of the knee with particular attention directed to the joint line. Additional specialized tests including the McMurray and Apley grind tests may also be included.[56–61] The contralateral extremity also should be examined for comparison because of the variability and patient-specific nature of these physical examination findings.

Physical examination may reveal an antalgic gait with varus or valgus alignment. The patient with a medial meniscus tear should be observed for a varus thrust. This alignment may prove to be pertinent to the etiology and treatment of the meniscal tear. Displaced tears may present with a mechanical block to ROM that is also associated with distinct pain at that end point. Pain with deep knee flexion is nonspecific but is common for posterior horn injuries. Cruciate and collateral ligament stability should then be evaluated. A visible knee effusion may also exist that can be exaggerated with "milking" or manipulation of the suprapatellar pouch to maximize the size of the effusion inferiorly. At this time, palpation for point tenderness should be performed with a focus on ligamentous and tendinous origins

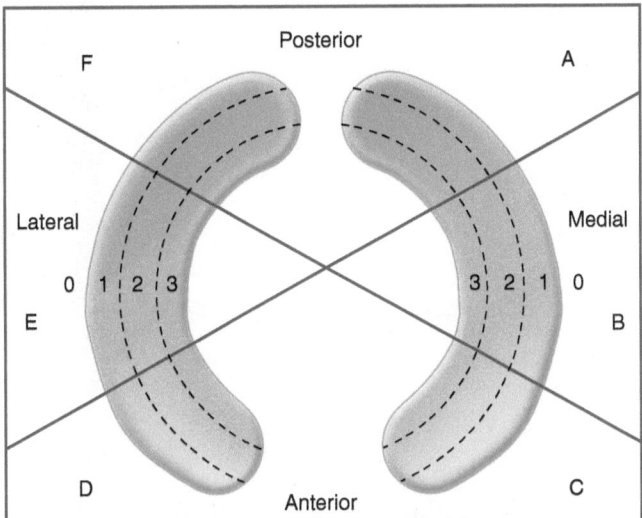

Fig. 94.7 Classification of a meniscal tear according to the anatomic position and vascularity. (Modified from Cooper DE, Arnoczky SP, Warren RF. Arthroscopic meniscal repair. *Clin Sports Med.* 1990;9:589–607.)

and insertions and the joint line. We prefer to perform the palpation component of the examination with the patient in a supine position with the hip externally rotated and the knee flexed to 90 degrees. Notably, palpable joint-line tenderness has been repeatedly identified as the most sensitive and specific physical examination finding for meniscal pathology.[43,56,59,62] However, joint-line tenderness is significantly less accurate for identifying meniscal pathology in the setting of an ACL injury.[60]

Provocative maneuvers that cause meniscal fragment impingement between the femoral and tibial surfaces have also been described. The McMurray test is performed on the medial meniscus by flexing the knee, creating a varus stress by internally rotating the tibia, and bringing the knee into full extension. Reproducible pain with a palpable mechanical click or pop indicates a positive examination. Conversely, the lateral meniscus is tested with an applied valgus stress and external tibial rotation. Another commonly performed test is the Apley grind test, in which an axial load is created with concurrent internal and external rotation ("grind") with the patient positioned prone and the affected knee flexed to 90 degrees. A positive examination is defined as pain at the medial and/or lateral joint line. Another test, termed the *Thessaly test,* has been used to increase the diagnostic accuracy of the physical examination for meniscal tears by dynamically reproducing the load transmission in the knee joint at 5 and 20 degrees of knee flexion. The Thessaly test is performed with the examiner holding the patient's outstretched hands while he or she performs a single leg stance flat-footed on the affected extremity and axially rotates three times with the knee in 5 degrees and then 20 degrees of flexion. A positive test is documented with the presence of medial or lateral joint-line pain and possible mechanical symptoms. When this test is performed in 20 degrees of flexion, a 94% and 96% accuracy has been documented for medial and lateral meniscal tears, respectively, with low false-positive and false-negative results.[61]

IMAGING

Isolated meniscal pathology can be accurately diagnosed in more than 90% of patients with history and physical examination alone. Nevertheless, diagnostic imaging, including plain radiographs and MRI, is critical to confirm clinical suspicions, evaluate alignment, and identify concomitant pathology. Imaging is particularly useful when concomitant chondral or ligament pathology exists because the history and physical examination are far less accurate in this setting.

Plain radiographs should be the first-line radiographic study but are not sensitive or specific to meniscal pathology. Weight-bearing anteroposterior, lateral, and 45-degree flexed posteroanterior views should be obtained. A Merchant patellar view allows evaluation of patellofemoral pathology. Standing knee alignment can be assessed and correlated with meniscal pathology and, if a significant concern exists for abnormal alignment, a full-length, standing, long cassette, anteroposterior hip to ankle view of both lower extremities should be obtained. Degenerative joint disease may indicate a degenerative meniscal tear, but acute tears have no specific radiographic findings.

MRI is the ideal radiographic study for visualizing soft tissue pathology, including injury to the meniscus, capsule, ligaments, and articular cartilage. Arthrography was historically used prior to MRI to identify meniscal tears and may be considered in the setting of a contraindication to MRI. MRI is a noninvasive study that is performed without exposure to ionizing radiation and is able to image in multiple planes, thereby providing a three-dimensional depiction of soft tissue and osseous structures. Previous studies have documented a very high accuracy for MRI identification of meniscal abnormalities.[63,64]

We routinely obtain MRI imaging for the evaluation of meniscal pathology using both fat-suppressed and diffusion-weighted fast spin-echo (cartilage sensitive) axial, coronal, and sagittal images (Fig. 94.8). Normal meniscal architecture is demonstrated by uniform low signal intensity on both fast spin-echo and fat-suppressed images. A high signal within the meniscal substance but not extending to the articular surface frequently exists as a result of intrasubstance degeneration. This signal may lead to an overinterpretation of a meniscal tear. Grading of the meniscal high signal can minimize this overinterpretation (see Fig. 94.8).[65] Grade I is characterized by a nonfocal intrasubstance high signal without articular extension. Grade II is a focal linear high-signal region without articular extension. Grade III is a focal linear high-signal region located at the free edge of the meniscus with superior or inferior articular extension. A grade III signal that is identified on two or more MRI images has 90% sensitivity for representing a true meniscal tear.[65] Nevertheless, careful evaluation of the surrounding structures, including the meniscofemoral and intermeniscal ligaments and popliteus tendon, should be conducted because they may mimic a meniscal tear.

Sagittal meniscal windows may aid in identifying acute, vertical meniscal tears and bucket handle tears, whereas coronal images are most helpful for the identification of horizontal degenerative tears. Axial imaging may further confirm the existence of radial

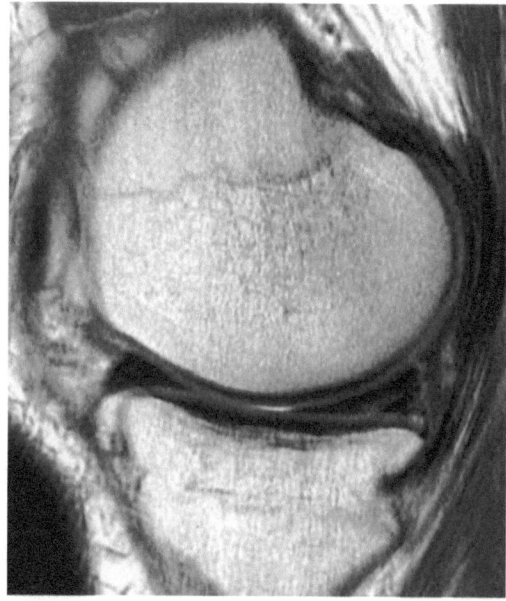

Fig. 94.8 A sagittal fat-suppressed magnetic resonance imaging slice demonstrates a grade III linear signal communicating with joint space through the inferior surface of the meniscus.

and flap tears. Bucket handle tears should be carefully evaluated at the intercondylar notch with the classic double PCL sign where the displaced medial meniscal tissue may be identified as a second low-signal line parallel and anterior to the PCL.

Despite the high sensitivity and noninvasive attributes of MRI, significant limitations exist, including higher cost and technical errors in both imaging technique and interpretation. Multiple studies have shown a high percentage of asymptomatic meniscal tears on MRI examination ranging from 36%[66] to 76%.[41] This percentage increases significantly with patient age.[67] Prior MRI data from asymptomatic patients older than 65 years documented a 67% prevalence of meniscal tears.[41] This prevalence increased to 86% in the setting of symptomatic osteoarthritis. For this reason, it is important to correlate MRI findings with the history and physical examination and, when indicated, findings on arthroscopy.

TREATMENT OPTIONS

Nonoperative Management

Nonoperative management of meniscal tears is not designed to facilitate healing of the tear, but rather is directed at symptom management. Although prior data have documented spontaneous healing of stable, isolated peripheral meniscal tears, this outcome is a rare exception. Most unrepaired meniscal tears will not progress to healing,[68] and therefore nonoperative management must be directed at reducing symptoms in carefully selected patients. Our experience suggests that most symptomatic meniscal lesions in the absence of significant concomitant osteoarthrosis do not respond well to nonoperative management, especially in the setting of mechanical symptoms, despite some evidence that symptom resolution may occur with this approach.[68] However, nonoperative treatment is frequently used in the setting of associated medial or lateral compartment osteoarthrosis with concomitant meniscal tears and the absence of mechanical symptoms.

Nonoperative management should include rest, use of ice and nonsteroidal antiinflammatory medications, and activity modification for 6 to 12 weeks. Intra-articular injections of corticosteroids, analgesic medications (e.g., lidocaine or bupivacaine), and viscosupplementation may also be used if concomitant osteoarthrosis is present. We do not suggest this treatment approach in the absence of osteoarthrosis, and it should be noted that corticosteroids may impair meniscal healing and that bupivacaine may lead to chondral damage.[69–71] It is important to note that nonoperative management of an unstable, repairable meniscal tear may also result in tear propagation, thereby producing an irreparable tear that must be excised.

Operative Management
Surgical Indications

The definitive treatment of meniscal tears involves either repair or excision of the pathologic tissue. Surgery is indicated in patients who have persistent mechanical symptoms and/or pain and have not responded to a course of nonoperative treatment. The indications for arthroscopy include (1) symptoms of meniscal injury that affect activities of daily living, work, and/or sports participation such as instability, locking, effusion, and pain; (2) positive

physical findings of joint-line tenderness, joint effusion, limitation of motion, and provocative signs such as pain with squatting, a positive pinch test, or a positive McMurray test; (3) failure to respond to nonsurgical treatment, including activity modification, medication, and a rehabilitation program; and (4) ruling out other causes of knee pain identified by patient history, physical examination, plain radiographs, or other imaging studies.[72,73]

Timing of the injury and surgical management must also be considered. Acute tears have a higher rate of successful healing compared with chronic ones; it is documented that repairs of tears less than 8 weeks old heal more frequently compared with older tears.[74] Additionally, patients undergoing repairs of traumatic meniscal tears have better 6-year functional results than do persons with degenerative meniscal tears.[75,76] However, the majority of these studies combine traumatic meniscal tear and concomitant injury. Stein et al.[77] compared long-term outcomes after arthroscopic meniscal repair versus partial meniscectomy for traumatic meniscal tears and documented no difference in function score. However, the meniscal repair group demonstrated a higher rate of return to preinjury and sporting activity levels. Additionally, only 40% of the meniscal repair group demonstrated osteoarthritic progression at 8-year follow-up compared with 81% of the partial meniscectomy group. For these reasons, a recent traumatic history should be considered a good prognostic factor for meniscal healing within the meniscal repair algorithm.

The influence of patient age on meniscal repair outcome has been well documented. Prior data have documented a reduced cellularity and healing response in patients older than 40 years.[78] Increased repeat tear rates have also been documented in patients older than 30 years,[79] although failure occurred later in older patients.[80] The association between increased age and worse outcome seems to be negated in the setting of avascular tears and meniscal tears with concomitant ACL rupture. No difference between younger patients and older patients (>40 years) has been found with regard to clinical success after meniscal repairs performed for tears with relative avascularity.[81,82] Kalliakmanis et al.[83] documented no difference in repair failure between patients older or younger than 35 years of age in the setting of a concomitant ACL tear. Although prognostic factors, including avascular tears, concomitant ACL rupture, and continued ligamentous instability, seem to play identical roles in younger patients,[84] the consequence of postmeniscectomy arthritis remains significantly greater.

From the aforementioned variables, one may synthesize surgical indications for meniscal repair that can predict healing prognosis. Contraindications for repair include older or sedentary patients or patients who are unable to perform the necessary postoperative rehabilitation. Additionally, isolated inner third white–white tears with a remaining rim greater than 6 mm should not be repaired. Borderline tears including middle third white–white tears should only be considered for repair if extension exists into the red–white or red–red region. Degenerative or stable longitudinal (<12 mm in length) tears should also not be repaired. Meniscal tears with a peripheral rim less than 4 mm should be considered for repair, because removal of this large tear will result in biomechanical alterations similar to a total meniscectomy.[85] Particular consideration should be given in this circumstance to patients younger than 40 years of age and those with active lifestyles. Meniscal repair is ideal in younger patients with acute traumatic tears. The adverse sequelae of meniscectomy are most marked after a lateral meniscectomy in young, active women, with some patients demonstrating a relatively rapid progression to lateral compartment arthrosis. Thus aggressive attempts should be made to repair the lateral meniscus in this setting.

Arthroscopy

Arthroscopy can be used both to confirm the diagnosis and to treat meniscal pathology. Careful evaluation of the meniscal tear configuration should aid in preoperative planning regarding potential meniscectomy, meniscal repair, or even transplantation. Nevertheless, a complete diagnostic arthroscopy with careful probing of all intra-articular structures remains the gold standard for diagnosis of meniscal injury and should be conducted to confirm the preoperative diagnosis and identify other potential intra-articular pathology.

Special Circumstances

Meniscal root tears. Diagnosis and treatment of a tear in the anterior or posterior root of the medial or lateral meniscus is extremely important because of the biomechanical role that these attachments play in meniscal stability. These tears often occur with concomitant ligamentous injury, including ACL ruptures and multiligamentous knee injury. Unstable posterior root tears of the lateral meniscus may be identified with high-energy acute ACL tears because of the translation and impaction of the posterolateral meniscus and the tibial plateau that occur during the traumatic pivot shift.[86]

Anterior or posterior root tears can be repaired through an arthroscopic approach. Bone tunnel and suture anchor repairs have been described with good success. Both techniques should include preparation of the anatomic insertion site with osseous abrasion to stimulate a vascular footprint. The first step of the bone tunnel repair requires passing nonabsorbable sutures through the anterior or posterior root tissue. An arthroscopic guide can then be used to facilitate the creation of a bone tunnel from the anterior tibial cortex to the meniscal root footprint. The nonabsorbable sutures should then be retrieved through the tunnel and secured at the anterior tibial aperture over a bone bridge or other preferred cortical fixation device. The suture anchor repair is performed by placing a suture anchor in the footprint of the meniscal root followed by passing the loaded sutures through the meniscal root and subsequent reduction and fixation. A posteromedial or posterolateral accessory portal is required to place the suture anchor in the correct position for posterior horn tears.

Lateral meniscus fascicular tears. Tears of the fascicular attachments to the lateral meniscus represent a unique injury to the lateral meniscus. Stabilization of the lateral meniscus differs from the medial meniscus because of the intra-articular position of the popliteus tendon. For this reason, direct meniscocapsular attachment is not possible in this region. Two popliteomeniscal fasciculi that anchor the lateral meniscus to the popliteus tendon have been described.[11] Fascicular tears can produce an unstable

posterolateral meniscus and mechanical symptoms. Repair of these anchoring fasciculi can be achieved using an inside-out or all-inside repair because of the vascular nature of these peripheral attachments. Incarceration of the popliteal tendon should be avoided during suture placement.

Meniscal cysts. Meniscal cysts may also be identified in conjunction with an adjacent meniscal tear. Meniscal tears may lead to the formation of meniscal cysts, likely because of a one-way valve mechanism that allows extravasation and capture of synovial fluid. This mechanism is particularly prevalent with horizontal cleavage tears in the anterior meniscal region. Prior data have suggested that cysts are up to seven times more common in the lateral compartment, but MRI data have documented an equivalent prevalence.[87,88]

Treatment of both the cyst and the associated meniscal tears is important to effectively address the one-way valve mechanism by which the cyst likely occurred. Arthroscopic partial meniscectomy and débridement remove the one-way valve mechanism created by the opposing flaps and provide access to and decompression of the associated cyst. Intra-articular extravasation of the cyst fluid may be observed during the arthroscopic débridement and can serve as a confirmatory sign of effective management. Open cystectomy may also be performed in rare cases with no associated meniscal pathology or an unusually large fluid collection. Both surgical techniques have been associated with good outcomes.[89–92] Ultrasound-guided aspiration of the cyst is rarely a definitive treatment, because the fluid in the cyst may reaccumulate.

Discoid meniscus and meniscal variants. Young[93] first identified the discoid meniscus during a cadaveric dissection in 1889. This variant likely occurs as a congenital anatomic variant but has been previously thought to occur because of abnormal embryologic apoptosis of the central meniscus during development. The prevalence of the discoid meniscus variant is approximately 5% but appears to be increased in the Asian population.[94–100] Both medial and lateral discoid menisci have been described, but the lateral side is much more common.[96,98,101] Bilateral discoid menisci may also occur in up to 20% of cases.

Three main lateral discoid meniscal variants exist according the classification system described by Watanabe et al.[102] This system was developed from arthroscopic observations of the lateral meniscus and its tibial attachments (Fig. 94.9). Type I is an incomplete variant that has intact peripheral attachments but does not fully cover the tibial plateau. Type II is a discoid variant that fully covers the lateral tibial plateau and also has intact peripheral attachments. Type III, or the Wrisberg ligament type, is lacking the normal posterior meniscal attachments and is posteriorly anchored solely by the meniscofemoral ligament of Wrisberg. For this reason, this type has increased mobility of the posterior meniscal body and subsequent clinical instability. This instability has been termed *snapping-knee syndrome.* Fortunately, this unstable variant has a low prevalence of between 0% and 33%.[95,103,104] Notably, the posterior meniscal instability has been most commonly identified in younger patients with complete discoid morphology.[97] Absence of capsular attachments of the anterior aspect of a discoid meniscus with resultant instability of this portion of the meniscus has also been described.[105]

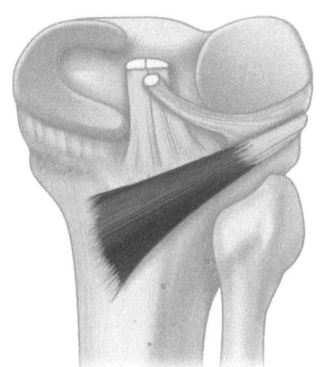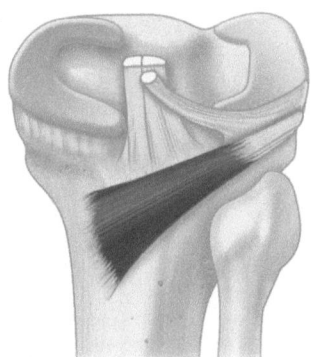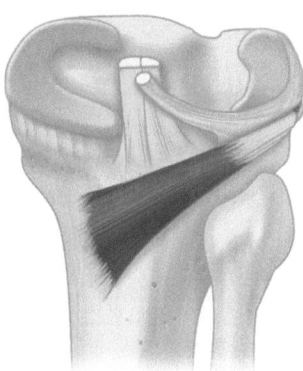

Watanabe classification for discoid lateral menisci

Fig. 94.9 The Watanabe classification for discoid lateral menisci. (From Kocher MS, Klingele K, Rassman SO. Meniscal disorders: normal, discoid, and cysts. *Orthop Clin North Am* 2003;34:329–340.)

Other classification systems also exist that attempt to provide a more specific description of the stability and structure and may prove more useful in guiding treatment.[106] The majority of discoid menisci are incidentally identified and asymptomatic and thus do not require treatment; however, some discoid menisci require operative intervention because of symptomatic tears that occur from high intra-articular sheer stress. Common symptoms include mechanical snapping or clicking with type III discoid menisci or tears in previously stable type I or II variants. These mechanical symptoms may be associated with lateral joint-line pain and swelling. The patient may or may not be able to recall a specific traumatic event that was associated with the symptoms. Joint-line palpation may reveal focal tenderness at the location of the tear with or without a palpable click during motion. Diagnostic imaging should be performed, including plain radiographs, which can demonstrate lateral joint space widening and tibial plateau concavity, a flattened lateral femoral condyle, tibial spine hypoplasia, meniscal calcification, and concomitant lateral femoral condyle osteochondritis dissecans.[107,108] MRI evaluation should also be used to specifically evaluate the morphology of the meniscus and identify any tears. An absent "bow-tie" sign may be identified, demonstrating meniscal continuity between the anterior and posterior horns in three or more consecutive 5-mm sagittal images (Fig. 94.10). Although this sign can be easily used to identify type I and II discoid variants, it is less effective for the type III variant. The type III variant can only be identified by the absence of small peripheral capsular attachments because of the otherwise normal meniscal morphology.[107,109] Diagnostic arthroscopy should be used to confirm a clinical suspicion in this case.

Symptomatic type I and II variants should be treated with arthroscopic "saucerization" or partial meniscectomy with contouring to mimic normal meniscal morphology (see Fig. 94.9).[104,110–112] A motorized shaver or arthroscopic biter can be used to resect the abnormal central tissue and other associated torn or degenerative tissue. A peripheral 6- to 8-cm meniscal rim should be maintained and contoured to avoid potential repeat tearing. Careful technique should be used to avoid iatrogenic chondral injury, because the discoid meniscus is frequently associated with a tight, narrow joint space and thickened meniscus.

The techniques previously described for partial meniscectomy should also be applied in this case. If a large meniscal tear that extends to the periphery or an unstable peripheral detachment is present, the surgeon should consider repair and stabilization according to the techniques described in the meniscal repair section.

The combination of saucerization and peripheral repair is particularly suited for treatment of a symptomatic, unstable type III discoid lateral meniscus. Careful evaluation of the stability of the peripheral rim should be performed to confirm an adequate repair and stabilization, because this variant can be significantly unstable. We suggest using an inside-out repair technique for these cases because of the young age and significant instability of this variant. Nevertheless, continued improvements in all-inside implants may increase the utility of the all-inside technique in this setting.

A total meniscectomy should be avoided, if possible, because of the clear association with early compartmental arthrosis.[113–117] Long-term data after a total meniscectomy have documented increased compartmental degeneration and arthrosis. Saucerization and repair, on the other hand, have been correlated with good to excellent early clinical results[104,110,118–120]; however, the mid- to long-term radiographic results in those treated with saucerization have not been as promising. Two recent case series[121,122] reported on long-term follow-up on cohorts of patients undergoing mostly saucerization with or without stabilization for symptomatic discoid menisci. At an average of 4.7 and 8 years of postoperative follow-up, respectively, both studies report a maintenance of good to excellent patient-reported outcomes, but an 11% and 40% rate of early radiographic findings of osteoarthritis. This high rate of radiographic arthritis is alarming in a young patient population, but early degenerative changes may be the natural history of discoid menisci. A recent case-control study[54] observed more tibiofemoral varus alignment and both arthroscopic and radiographic signs of tibiofemoral compartment arthritis in patients over the age of 40 with previously untreated discoid menisci compared to age-matched controls without discoid menisci undergoing arthroscopy for meniscal tears.

Unfortunately, in the discoid population a total meniscectomy is required in some circumstances because of significant tissue

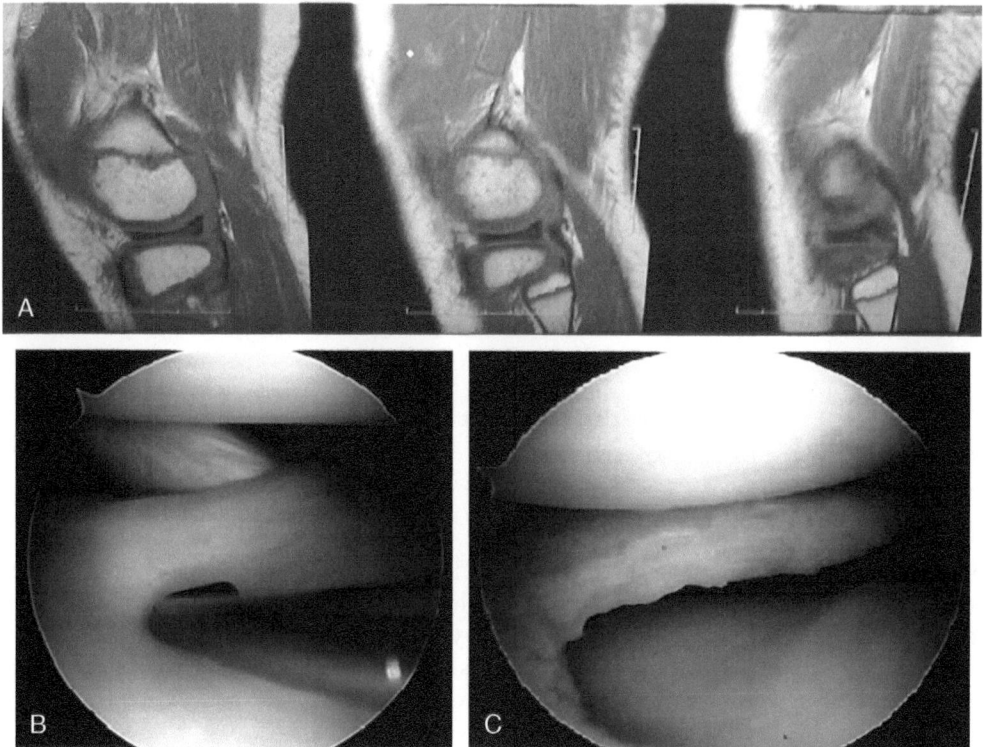

Fig. 94.10 Discoid lateral meniscus. (A) Diagnostic magnetic resonance imaging scans demonstrate absence of the classic "bow-tie" appearance of the lateral meniscus in three successive 5-mm cuts. (B) The arthroscopic view of a complete discoid lateral meniscus. (C) The arthroscopic view of a final saucerization procedure.

degeneration or tearing without the possibility of repair. Patients in whom total meniscectomy is required should be observed carefully for early signs and symptoms of meniscal deficiency (i.e., early arthrosis) to optimize the potential for a future meniscal transplant when indicated.

Meniscal allograft transplantation. Although recent improvements in the understanding of meniscal biomechanics and pathology and advancement in surgical techniques have resulted in more focused attempts to preserve the meniscal integrity and structure, this goal is not possible in many cases. Severe cases may require total meniscectomy or segmental meniscal excision with subsequent chondral deterioration and osteoarthrosis. This degeneration can result in significant pain, activity limitation, and functional impairment. In these circumstances, a meniscal allograft transplant has been used as a surgical management option. Clinical and radiographic evaluation, surgical indications and techniques, and postoperative management for meniscal allograft transplantation are discussed in detail in another chapter in this book.

DECISION-MAKING PRINCIPLES

We believe that the history and physical examination are the most important components for optimizing the management of a patient with meniscal pathology. The specific age, activity level, occupation, and sport-specific requirements must be carefully considered when developing an individualized treatment plan.

We routinely obtain an MRI for any patient with potential meniscal pathology. Noncontrast cartilage-specific MRI is used to carefully evaluate the menisci, ligaments, and articular cartilage. MRI can provide confirmation of a meniscal tear or identify mimicking pathology such as an articular chondral injury. Tailored nonoperative management or preoperative planning can be carefully constructed on the basis of these diagnostic imaging data. A concomitant articular chondral injury may also be identified and, when indicated, addressed at the time of surgery.

We believe that early diagnosis and management of a meniscal injury optimize the biologic and clinical outcome. This early intervention is particularly important for younger patients. Meniscal surgery procedures are done on an outpatient, ambulatory basis with use of a regional anesthetic. We typically use the anteromedial and anterolateral portals for most meniscal procedures but may create accessory posteromedial or posterolateral portals for improved visualization and instrumentation. We do not routinely use a superomedial or superolateral outflow portal because it is rarely required for visualization and can unnecessarily injure the quadriceps muscle.

We use synovial abrasion for partial-thickness tears and stable, vertical tears less than 10 mm in length. The remaining repairable tears undergo formal repair. Improvements in instrumentation have allowed a transition to an all-inside technique for most vertical posterior and midbody tears. We currently use the FasT-Fix suture system (Smith & Nephew, Andover, MA) but other implants may also be used. We continue to use the formal inside-out technique for isolated repair of a large bucket-handle tear in an ACL-intact knee, for tears with marginal vascularity, and for unstable type III discoid variants. Optimal repair may require a combination of techniques. For example, we may use an all-inside technique for the posterior component of a tear followed by the use of inside-out and outside-in techniques for anterior tear extension. We only consider repairing meniscal tears in the avascular zone in young patients who have a large fragment, particularly in the setting of concomitant ACL reconstruction.

Partial meniscectomy is reserved for irreparable tears, including radial, horizontal, oblique, and degenerative tear configurations. The basic principle is to limit the meniscal resection to only that which is necessary to maintain a stable remaining construct. Both ipsilateral and contralateral portals are used to maximize visualization and instrument access. A motorized shaver is used for final contouring of the meniscectomy. We prefer to use a curved shaver because the shaving edge can be easily mobilized with rotation and it provides excellent access to the posterior meniscal tissue.

The most important surgical decision regarding a meniscal injury is whether to excise or repair the lesion. This decision is directly dependent on the aforementioned vascular supply of the meniscal region in which the tear occurs: red–red, red–white, or white–white zones. Vertical tears are particularly amenable to repair if they occur at the meniscal periphery in the red–red zone. Repair of a centrally located red–white tear, on the other hand, is less successful because of the more limited vascular supply. Nevertheless, meniscal repair may be considered in this region depending on the tear type. White–white tears, on the other hand, have a low likelihood for successful healing, and thus a partial meniscectomy should be performed in this region.[55,123–128]

Surgical Techniques
Meniscectomy

Surgical meniscectomy should be performed after arthroscopic confirmation of an irreparable, unstable meniscal tear. The size of the tear should be carefully delineated using an arthroscopic probe to ensure that meniscal tissue is maximally preserved and all unstable fragments are removed. Fragments that can be displaced above or below the stable meniscal body or into the compartment should be removed (Fig. 94.12).

Resection of meniscal tears can be performed efficiently using arthroscopic instruments including meniscal biters, punches, or motorized shavers. The position of the meniscal tear should be considered prior to instrument selection. Posterior horn tears of the medial meniscus may be easily viewed from the anterolateral portal, whereas an up-going punch can be placed through the anteromedial portal for resection. This arrangement should be reversed for posterior horn tears of the lateral meniscus, and a straight biter may prove more useful given the convexity of the lateral tibial surface. Care should be taken during meniscectomy to minimize iatrogenic chondral injury that can occur with intra-articular instrument introduction and movement within the joint. Positioning of the extremity can assist in minimizing this injury by increasing the space within each specific compartment. Applying a valgus force with concomitant flexion or extension can widen the medial compartment joint space. The "figure-of-four" position is used to provide a varus force to increase the lateral compartment joint space, again with concomitant

✒ Authors' Preferred Technique
Meniscal Repair

Careful preoperative surgical planning and setup will enable improved efficiency, intraoperative ease, and postoperative outcome. Most arthroscopic meniscal surgeries are ambulatory using a general, regional, or local anesthetic. The patient is placed in the supine position with the use of a thigh-level leg holder or lateral post to provide lateral resistance to allow the application of valgus loading and to improve medial compartment visualization. This method reduces the risk of medial compartment iatrogenic chondral injury and improves access and visualization of the posterior meniscus. However, excessive valgus loading can lead to iatrogenic injury of the medial collateral ligament and should be avoided if possible.

Standard surgical instrumentation includes an arthroscopic cannula system with inflow and outflow cannulae. A 30-degree arthroscope is sufficient for addressing most meniscal pathology, although a 70-degree arthroscope may be used if necessary. Excision instrumentation includes straight, up-going, and side-directed duckbill meniscal punches, as well as a motorized shaver to facilitate fragment excision and meniscal rim contouring. A curved 4.5-mm shaver is very helpful for posterior meniscectomy in the standard knee, and a curved 3.5-mm shaver may be used in a tight compartment to minimize chondral damage.

Each arthroscopic procedure should include a systematic diagnostic evaluation. This technique ensures that all pathology is effectively identified and addressed. Careful probing of the menisci aids in identifying tears that may be difficult to visualize. Peripheral vertical tears or meniscocapsular detachments may also be identified by meniscal hypermobility and subluxation. Undersurface horizontal cleavage tears may only be visualized by lifting the superior flap to view the inferior undersurface. The probe should also be used to discriminate between stable and unstable meniscal tears. Meticulous evaluation of the posterior rim and root should be completed, because injuries in this region may be subtle.

Posteromedial and posterolateral visualization can be accomplished by passing the arthroscope between the PCL and the medial femoral condyle or the ACL and the lateral femoral condyle, respectively (Fig. 94.11). Alternatively, posteromedial and posterolateral portals can be established to improve visualization and instrumentation in these regions if necessary. Surgical familiarity with these techniques allows complete and effective diagnosis and management of all meniscal pathology.

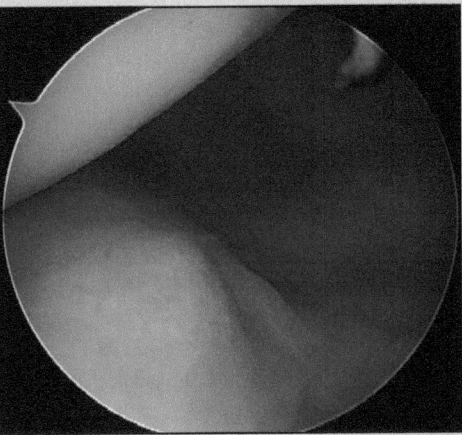

Fig. 94.11 An arthroscopic view in the posterior compartment of the knee with visualization of the posterior horn of the medial meniscus and the meniscotibial attachments.

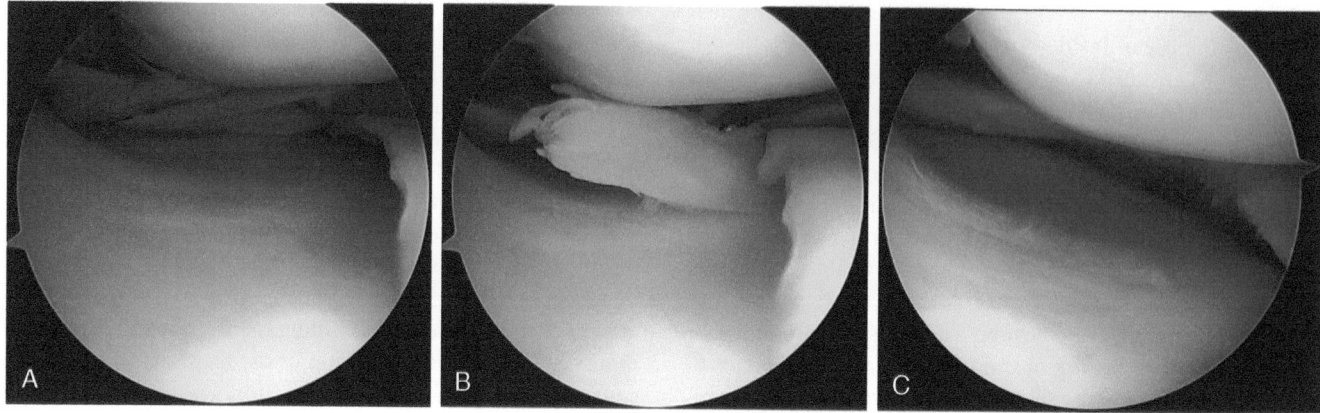

Fig. 94.12 A complex meniscal tear with an unstable, parrot's beak tear. The flap is reduced (A) and presented (B) with an arthroscopic probe. (B) The appearance after a partial meniscectomy. Meniscal tissue should be preserved when possible, and resection should be limited to only unstable parts of the meniscus. Careful contouring of the remaining meniscus may minimize the risk of a repeat tear.

flexion or extension as necessary. Lastly, other surgeons have used radiofrequency probes for meniscectomy and meniscal contouring[128,129]; however, we prefer not to use this technique because of the potential undesired meniscal and chondral damage that may occur as a result of thermal injury.

Meniscal Repair: The Basics

The first reported meniscal repair was performed in an open fashion in 1885.[130] This procedure was infrequently used until the importance of the meniscus was appreciated within the past 30 years. Recent advances in arthroscopic techniques have replaced open meniscal repair and include inside-out, outside-in, and all-inside arthroscopic repairs. Careful arthroscopic evaluation of the tear should be performed, including probing to identify the location, configuration, and extent of the meniscal tear. These factors, in combination with the patient history, should then be considered in determining the potential for meniscal healing. The synovial fringe and healing bed should be stimulated on both sides of the tear using a combination of meniscal rasps and a small, 3.5-mm shaver. This technique should optimize the vascular response and subsequent healing potential. All frayed edges of the meniscal tear should be removed to minimize mechanical prominences surrounding the repair. After the site has been adequately prepared, the tear can be repaired using crossing sutures or appropriate implants. Vertical mattress sutures provide optimal biomechanical strength because of the capture of longitudinally oriented collagen fibers and should be used whenever possible.[129–131]

Meniscal Repair: Inside-Out

The inside-out technique was initially described in 1986 by Scott et al.[132] as a minimally invasive substitute for open meniscal repair. Double-limbed sutures are passed using arthroscopic assistance through the meniscus and capsule and are then retrieved through a small, extracapsular counter incision. Meticulous positioning of the incision and instrumentation is crucial for the inside-out repair. The neurovascular structures including the peroneal and saphenous nerves and popliteal artery should be protected throughout the procedure because injury to these

structures may occur during surgical dissection and suture placement, especially during repair of posterior horn meniscal tears. Meniscal tears that occur in the anteriormost location are difficult to repair with use of this technique because placement of the arthroscopic guide is limited by the posteriorly directed angle.

The inside-out repair is best performed with the patient in the supine position and the operative knee flexed to 90 degrees for access to the lateral compartment and just slight flexion for the medial compartment. This position optimizes visualization while providing access to the posterior aspect of the knee. This access is required for the counter incision and suture retrieval. We use a lateral post that is placed in an elevated position to allow buttressing of the lateral thigh. A footrest may also be used to provide hands-free extremity positioning. After confirmation of the tear location and size, the arthroscope should be placed in the ipsilateral anterior portal. The arthroscopic needle guide is then placed in the contralateral portal to ensure that the needles are not angled directly posterior. This position minimizes the risk of neurovascular injury and facilitates needle recovery through the counter incision. A variety of needle-guide cannulas are available, including single- and double-barreled, curved, and straight cannulas. Vertical mattress sutures are used whenever possible.

Careful placement of the posteromedial or posterolateral counter incision and exposure of the joint capsule are crucial for easy, safe suture passage and knot placement (Fig. 94.13). A 3- to 4-cm incision should be placed posterior to the mid axis, and it should be 2 to 3 cm distal and 1 cm proximal to the joint line. The medial dissection proceeds to the anterior margin of the sartorius fascia, which is longitudinally incised. Blunt dissection should then be used to define and posteriorly retract the sartorius, gracilis, and semitendinosus. Care to avoid injury to the saphenous nerve is necessary. The medial head of the gastrocnemius is then exposed and should be elevated from the underlying posteromedial capsule and retracted posteriorly. A Henning or popliteal retractor should be placed between the gastrocnemius and posteromedial capsule to protect the infrapatellar branch of the saphenous nerve posteriorly and facilitate suture retrieval.

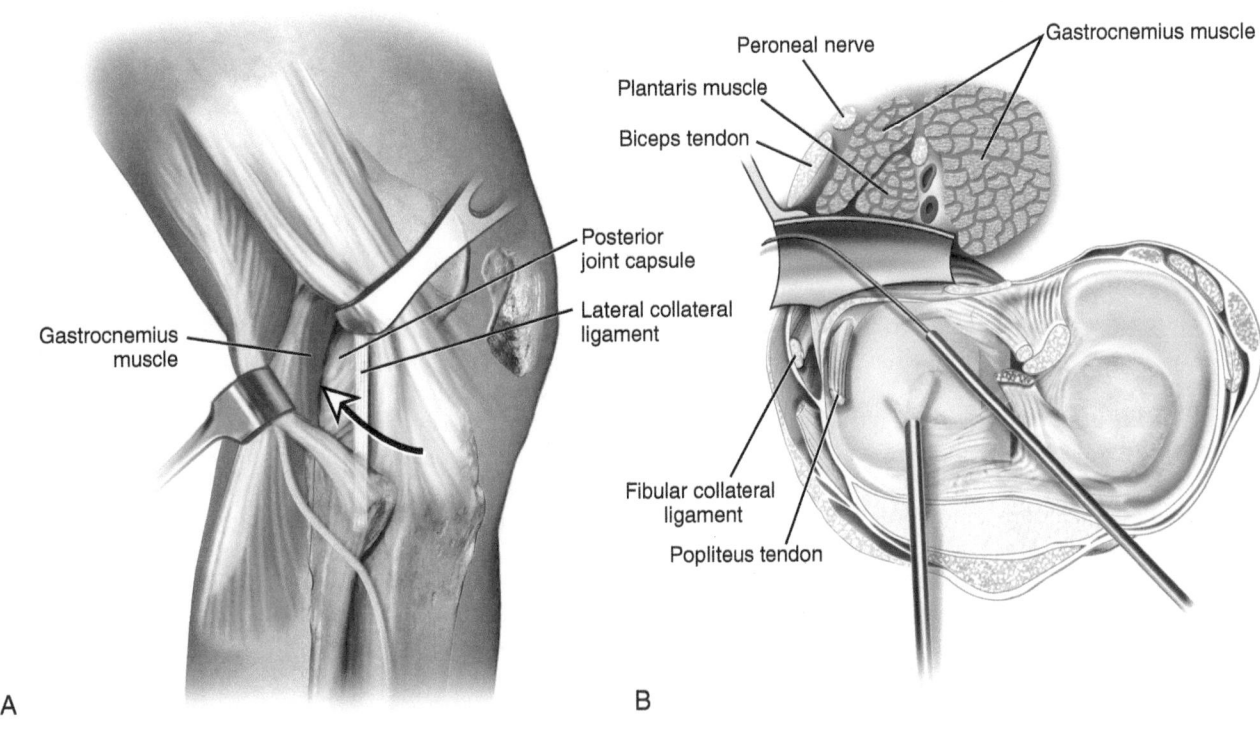

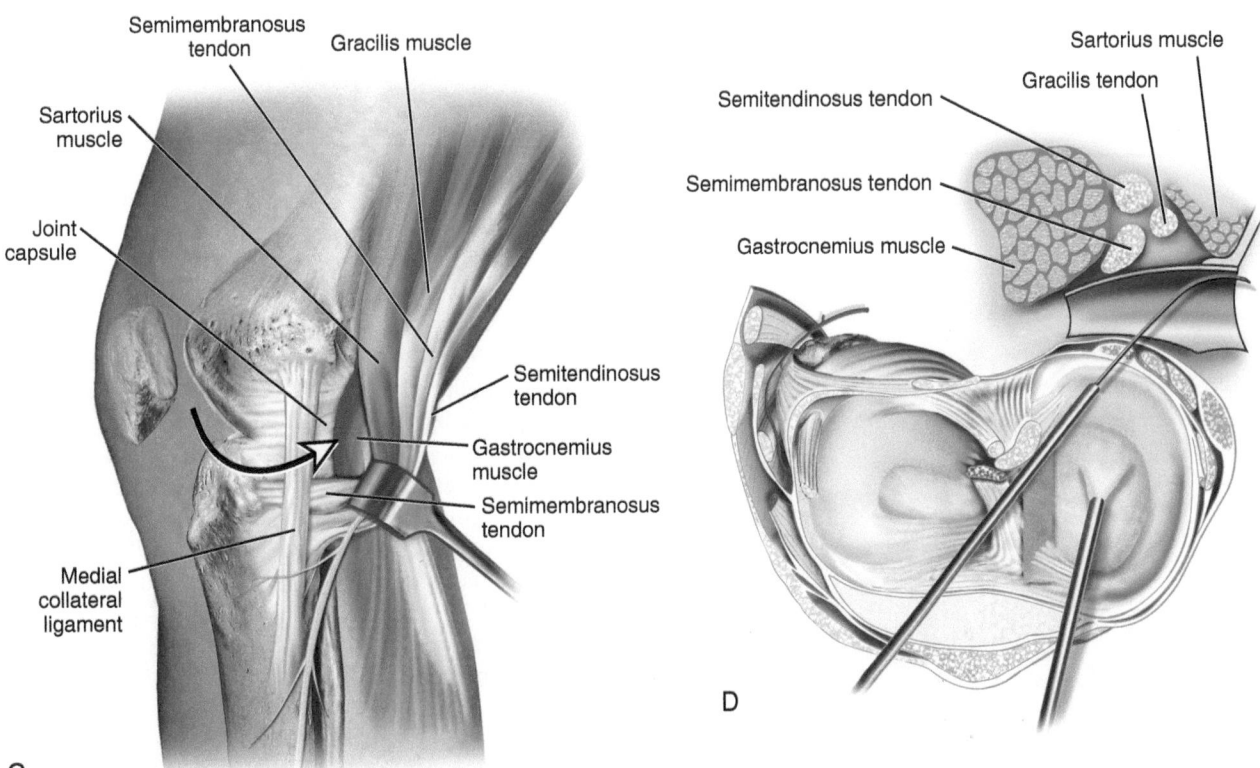

Fig. 94.13 A schematic representation of the inside-out lateral (A and B) and medial (C and D) meniscal repair with the counter incision and subsequent surgical exposure. (Modified from Noyes FR, Barber-Westin SD, Rankin M. Meniscal transplantation in symptomatic patients less than fifty years old. *J Bone Joint Surg Am.* 2005;87:149–165.)

Joint-line positioning of the incision is similar for the lateral counter incision. The dissection plane is between the iliotibial band and biceps femoris. The posterior margin of the iliotibial band is incised longitudinally, and the interval between these structures is developed. Care should be taken to retract the biceps femoris posteriorly, thereby protecting the peroneal nerve, which is located posterior to the biceps tendon. The lateral head of the gastrocnemius can then be visualized and should be posteriorly mobilized from the underlying posterolateral capsule. The afore-mentioned preferred retractor should then be placed in the interval between the gastrocnemius and capsule to protect the posterior neurovascular bundle and facilitate suture retrieval. Care needs to be taken to avoid injury to the lateral inferior geniculate artery.

The surgical ease of suture passage and retrieval for the inside-out approach directly depends on the intra-articular visualization and extra-articular capsular exposure (Fig. 94.14). Double-limbed 2-0 absorbable or nonabsorbable sutures attached to flexible long needles are used for repair. The surgeon should focus on guide cannula placement, arthroscopic visualization, and suture passage while an assistant retrieves the sutures through the counter incision. The guided needle can be used to pierce a single limb of the meniscal tear and then functions as a joystick to guide the optimal capsular placement. The needle should then be advanced through the capsule until it encounters the protecting

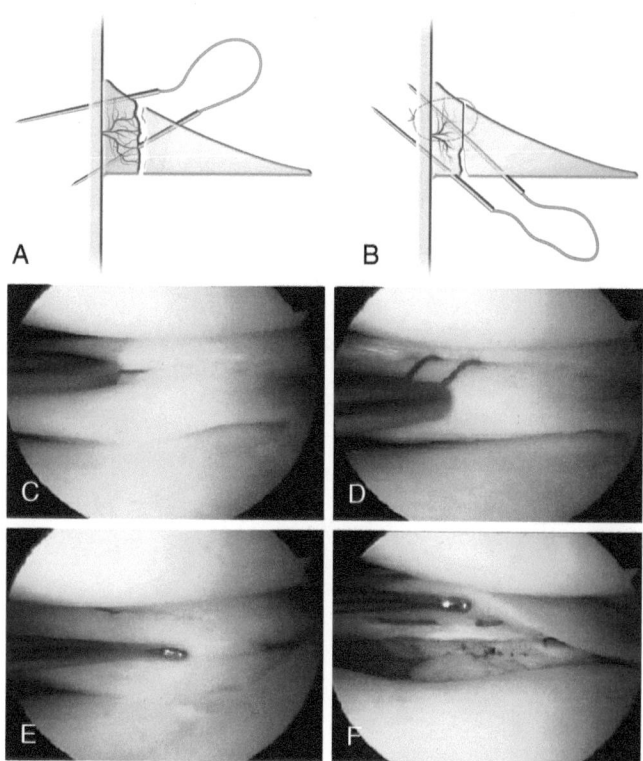

Fig. 94.14 Inside-out meniscal repair. A schematic representation of vertical mattress suture placement into the superior (A) and inferior (B) surfaces. (C–F) Arthroscopic images demonstrate the needle guide, suture placement, and final construct. (From Rubman MH, Noyes FR, Barber-Westin SD. Arthroscopic repair of meniscal tears that extend into the avascular zone: a review of 198 single and complex tears. *Am J Sports Med.* 1998;26:87–95.)

posterior retractor and is then retrieved through the counter incision. The needle from the second limb of the suture can then be passed in a similar fashion to position and reduce the opposing meniscal tissue. This sequence should be repeated with suture spacing at approximately 3- to 5-mm increments until the entire tear is fully repaired. Ideally, sutures should be placed on the superior and inferior aspects of the meniscus to improve rigid meniscal fixation. After all sutures have been placed, the knee should be flexed to 15 to 20 degrees and the sutures can be directly tied to the extra-articular side of the capsule under direct visualization.

Although the basics of the inside-out meniscal repair are straightforward, a few surgical tips may improve efficiency and avoid complications. First and foremost, careful positioning of the counter incision and retractor placement significantly mini-mizes the risk of neurovascular injury and difficulty with suture retrieval. If the needle is not easily visualized during passage and the posterior retractor is not encountered, the surgeon should reposition the retractor. Frequently, the incision and subsequent retractor placement is too proximal and the retractor should be replaced into a distal, inferior position. Initial tear reduction also may be difficult and can be aided by placement of the first suture pair into the middle of the tear along the superior flap of the meniscus, which facilitates accurate reduction of most tears.

Meniscal Repair: Outside-In

Rodeo and Warren[133,134] described the outside-in technique in an attempt to minimize the incidence of neurovascular injury that was associated with the inside-out repair. Repair of tears of the anterior third of the meniscus and anterior meniscal allograft fixation are also more easily performed with use of this technique. This technique also can be used to produce any desired suture configuration allowed by spinal needle insertion, and thus dif-ficult meniscal tears including radial and flap tears may be more easily and successfully addressed in this manner.[126] However, the outside-in technique can prove difficult for repairs of the pos-terior third of either meniscus because it is difficult to start far enough posteriorly to avoid an oblique needle orientation across the tear. There is also some risk due to the close proximity of the neurovascular structures.

The outside-in surgical technique uses an 18-gauge spinal needle as a guide for suture passage and retrieval with an arthroscopic grasper under direct arthroscopic visualization. The spinal needle is introduced percutaneously and is advanced through the meniscus on each side of the tear. The needle should exit through the central aspect of the desired superior or inferior meniscal leaf. An arthroscopic probe or grasper can be used for meniscal positioning prior to needle puncture to optimize final suture fixation and repair position. These instruments can also provide counter pressure during passage of the needle. A second spinal needle is placed in a similar fashion at the desired position. After needle placement, one 0-0 or 2-0 polydioxanone (PDS) suture is passed through each spinal needle and retrieved with a grasping device through the contralateral portal. Early techniques used mulberry knots that were tied on each end of the sutures to reduce the meniscal tear with tension placed against the meniscus at the knot-meniscal interface (Fig. 94.15). A small

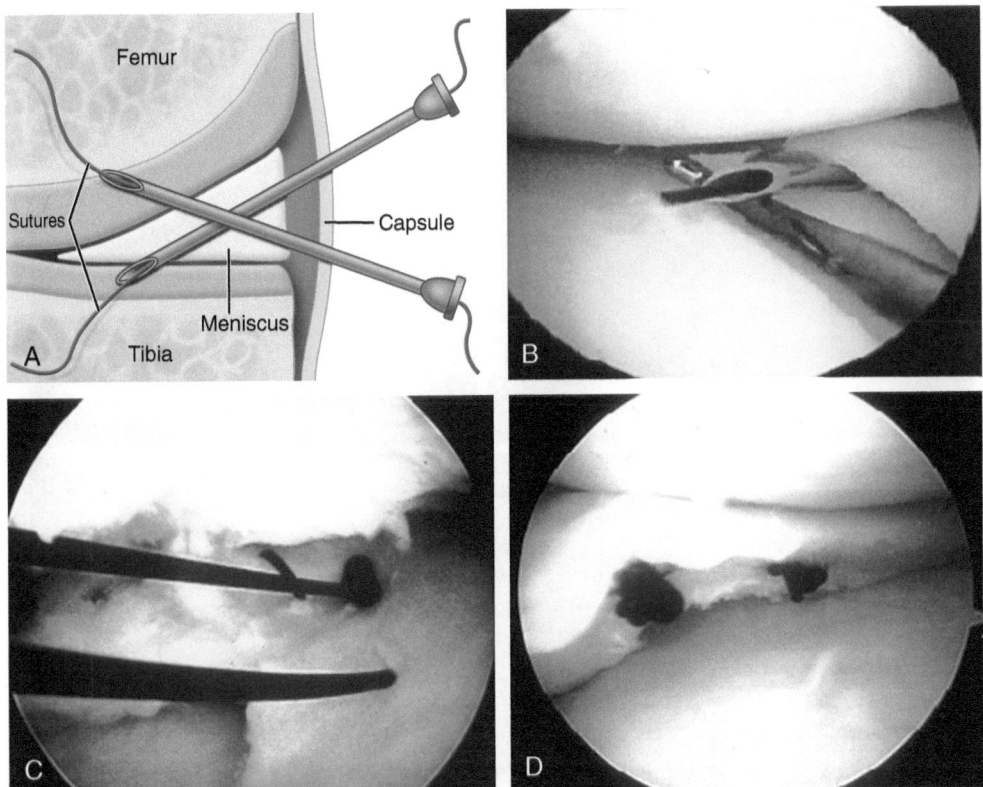

Fig. 94.15 Outside-in meniscal repair. (A) A schematic representation of spinal needle and suture placement through the superior or inferior meniscus. (B) An arthroscopic view demonstrates spinal needle placement through the inferior meniscal margin and polydioxanone suture introduction. (C) Suture shuttled through the working portal. (D) The final construct using intraarticular mulberry knots.

incision was then used to retrieve the extracapsular suture ends, which are then tied over the capsule. We prefer to use a modified technique in which the initial sutures are used as shuttle sutures to pass a single PDS or nonabsorbable braided suture in an inside-out direction. These sutures are then tied over the capsule in a similar fashion. This modification eliminates the necessity for mulberry knots and also offers the possibility of placing spanning sutures across the meniscal tear. This technique is particularly useful during placement of horizontal mattress sutures to approximate a displaced radial tear. The outside-in technique has been used to effectively repair anterior meniscal tears with excellent results in up to 90% of patients.[133,134]

Meniscal Repair: All-Inside

Early techniques for all-inside meniscal repairs used shuttling devices and arthroscopic knot tying to complete the meniscal repair. These techniques were technically challenging and required posterior accessory portals for posterior horn repairs. In many circumstances, this technique was more challenging than the aforementioned options.

Recent technical advances and improved implants have attempted to reduce the incidence of complications associated with early implants and the aforementioned technical challenges. Additionally, newer implants have improved the strength and healing rates of the meniscal repair (Fig. 94.16). Currently used devices include the Omnispan (Mitek, Westwood, MA), FasT-Fix 360 (Smith & Nephew, London, UK), the Crossfix II (Cayenne

Medical, Scottsdale, AZ), the NovoStitch Plus (Ceterix Orthopaedics, Freemont, CA) and the Knee Scorpion and SpeedCinch (Arthrex, Naples, Florida). Previous biomechanical data have demonstrated that many of the all-inside constructs have strength equivalent to inside-out vertical mattress sutures, which persists even with cyclic loading.[135-140]

BIOLOGIC STIMULATION

Despite the many technical and implant-related advances, meniscal healing continues to rely on the biologic healing response that occurs after repair. For this reason, extensive research has been directed toward stimulating and maximizing this biologic meniscal healing response. Early attempts to augment healing included trephination, synovial abrasion, and fibrin clot augmentation. In the past decade the focus has shifted to alternatives, such as platelet-rich plasma (PRP), meniscal scaffolds, and directed modifications of the growth factor/cytokine milieu.

Trephination

Trephination is designed to theoretically introduce vascular access channels into an avascular region of the meniscus to aid in stimulating a proliferation of fibrovascular tissue into the repair site. This technique is performed arthroscopically by repeatedly passing a spinal needle or small trephine in an outside-in fashion through the desired meniscal tissue. The resultant channels should theoretically allow for neovascularization and tissue ingrowth.

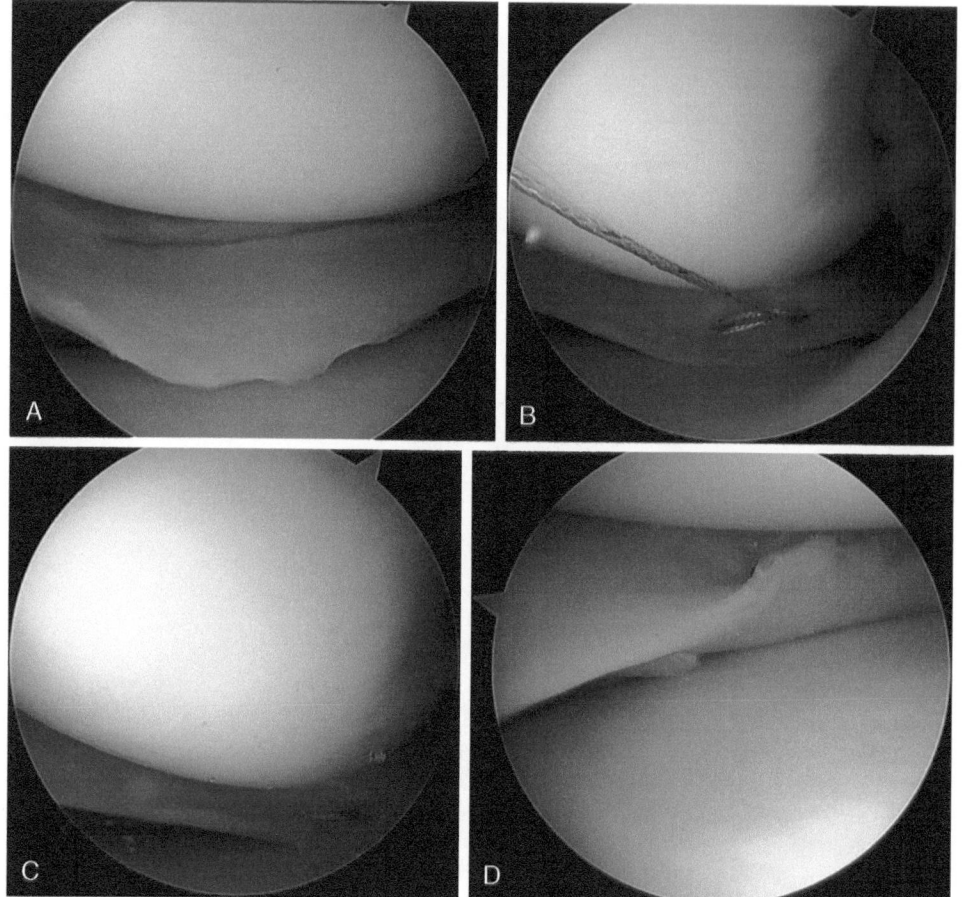

Fig. 94.16 All-inside meniscal repair. Arthroscopic views demonstrate identification and delineation of a vertical tear, red–white zone, and medial meniscus (A); tensioning the suture of the all-inside repair using a FasT-Fix 360 device (B); two perspectives of the final suture construct (C and D).

Although trephination can be easily performed in an arthroscopic fashion, there exists some risk of permanent disruption and fragmentation of the meniscal tissue during this process. This risk directly increases with the caliber of the horizontal channels.

Synovial Abrasion

Synovial abrasion is also easily accomplished with the use of a motorized shaver or arthroscopic rasp. This technique is also designed to stimulate a fibrovascular pannus that should creep from the synovial periphery into the tear site and aid in a reparative response. The shaver or rasp is used under direct arthroscopic visualization to abrade the synovial tissue adjacent to the desired repair site to stimulate visible bleeding and subsequent repair.[141]

Fibrin Clot Augmentation

Fibrin clot augmentation was initially described in an animal model by Arnoczky et al.[123] This technique was designed to introduce an exogenous fibrin clot into the tear site to serve as a reparative scaffold and to provide a chemotactic and mitogenic stimulus. The surgical technique requires drawing blood from a peripheral vein followed by hemoagitation to produce a semisolid clot. The clot is introduced directly between the flaps of the meniscal tear with the goal of facilitating a local proliferation of fibrovascular tissue to aid in the healing process.

Prior data have documented improved healing of meniscal tears with tenuous vascularity when they were treated with fibrin clot augmentation.[125,126,142,143]

Platelet Rich Plasma

PRP has been used for a variety of applications[144] throughout orthopaedics most commonly to augment a healing response in a difficult to heal tissue. Theoretically, since platelets are a reservoir of several important growth factors including transforming growth factor β (TGF-β), platelet-derived growth factor (PDGF), insulin-like growth factor (IGF I, II), fibroblast growth factor (FGF), epidermal growth factor (EGF), vascular endothelial growth factor (VEGF), and endothelial cell growth factor (ECGF), delivery of PRP to a specific site leads to supraphysiologic concentrations of these different factors in the local environment of injection. Although the exact interplay amongst all of these molecules is incompletely understood, it is hypothesized that the locally high concentrations create an anabolic environment to facilitate the healing process. It is not surprising that the meniscus has been a focus of PRP therapy. Early in vitro and in vivo animal model research has demonstrated increased tissue bonding, fibrochondrocyte proliferation, and extracellular matrix molecule deposition in a rabbit meniscal tear model with PRP augmentation.[145] Conversely, human studies[146,147] have reported mixed results for its use in meniscal repair. However, some types of tears, including the horizontal cleavage variety, may have better healing rates when augmented with PRP.[146] Adding a source of stem cells to PRP has the potential for creating a robust healing response in addition to regenerating tissues, but there is currently very little information available about the effect of PRP on stem cell differentiation. Pak et al. combined PRP with adipose-derived stem cells and injected the combination into human joints, demonstrating that this process was safe with no reported infections or tumors.[148] These early data require further investigation to evaluate efficacy in meniscal repair. One problem of published PRP data is the lack of a standard formulation. There is tremendous variability in different PRP formulations, with different platelet concentrations, differential inclusion of white cells, and variables related to how and when the PRP is activated. Considering the lack of details on the composition of PRP and the myriad preparations used in most of these clinical studies referenced, it is difficult to glean any significant conclusions from the current evidence base.

Cell-Based Approaches

Cell-based approaches for augmentation of meniscal repair have recently begun to be evaluated after demonstrating success in various animal models. Mesenchymal stem cells (MSCs) from a variety of origins including synovium,[149,150] fat,[151] bone marrow,[152] and embryos[153] in addition to terminally differentiated cells of cartilaginous origin (articular, costal, meniscal, nasal)[153] have all been used for the purpose of augmenting meniscal repairs. A simple intra-articular injection of synovial tissue-derived MSCs resulted in the formation of neomeniscal tissue that was both a higher quality and quantity than that of controls in a rabbit model.[149,150] The injected cells were found to occupy areas of injury and remained localized to the joint for 28 days. Similarly, in another rabbit in vivo model it was confirmed that the injected adipose-derived MSCs localized to the site of meniscal injury. Additionally, those joints injected with MSCs were found to have decreased levels of proinflammatory cytokines including MMP-1 and tumor necrosis factor-α (TNF-α), thus suggesting that these cell-based therapies can function both as precursors for direct tissue repair and act as modulators of the intra-articular cytokine environment, another important target for augmenting meniscal healing. Ng et al.[154] used a different stem cell delivery modality, a decellularized meniscus hydrogel embedded with human MSCs which was then implanted into injured rat menisci. These authors found that the MSCs in a hydrogel led to more meniscal regeneration than MSCs embedded in a collagen scaffold or those in the control group. Finally, Scotti et al.[155] demonstrated that terminally differentiated cells rather than stem cells have some meniscal regenerative capabilities in the appropriate medium and environment. They found that harvested articular chondrocytes embedded in a fibrin glue hydrogel when sandwiched between two sleeves of pig meniscal tissue led to the development of continuous fibrocartilaginous tissue at the interface, while none was seen in the control arm.

Despite a substantial evidence base in the aforementioned cell-based methods for augmenting meniscal repairs in the animal models, there is a relative paucity of evidence in the form of human trials. Vangsness et al.[156] studied an intra-articular injection of allogenic MSCs in patients having undergone partial meniscectomies in a randomized controlled trial (RCT). Two year follow-up MRIs demonstrated not only increased meniscal volume in the MSC groups but also decreased signs of osteoarthritis, suggesting either a direct effect on the articular cartilage or a more global cytokine milieu-modifying capability. The results of the trial by Whitehouse et al.[157] were not as promising. Although three of the five total patients who had MSCs embedded in a collagen scaffold inserted at the site of meniscal repair in the avascular zone demonstrated MRI evidence of meniscal healing, the other two patients had failures at follow-up requiring meniscectomies. So although several animal and human studies have demonstrated promise for cell-based methods of meniscal repair augmentation, there are many issues that need to be resolved, including the ideal cell type, the timing of implantation with respect to injury or surgery, the quantity of implanted cells required, and the optimal delivery mechanism.

Cytokine and Growth Factor Modulation

An improved understanding of the local environment of cytokines and growth factors with the knee joint following meniscal injury has led to new targets for enhancement of meniscal repair and articular cartilage preservation as these factors certainly influence the healing response. Liu et al.[158] demonstrated that in the setting of meniscal injury, the total activity levels of proinflammatory cytokines, including MMPs and prostaglandins, were 25 and 290 times higher than those of normal knees, respectively. Determining which cytokines and their respective cascades contribute to healing and which ones are detrimental is a challenge and still requires further understanding to identify optimal and promising therapeutic targets. Animal and in vitro studies have demonstrated the beneficial effects of basic-fibroblast growth factor (bFGF),[159] TGF-β,[159,160] and insulin-like growth factor-1 (ILGF-1)[161] for meniscal anabolism, whereas interleukin-1 (IL-1), platelet-derived growth factor-BB (PDGF-BB),[162] and TNF-α have had the converse effect, acting to inhibit meniscal repair processes.[163] Similarly to the application of PRP, the limited understanding of the complex interplay between the various cytokines and growth factors has limited the translation to clinical trials. However, given that many exogenous factors and inhibitors are available, improved understanding may lead to eventual clinical application.

Meniscal Scaffolds

Scaffolds are another area of active area of research that may improve the treatment of meniscal injuries. They offer the potential for filling small defects as well as for bulk meniscal replacement. Earlier generations of scaffold engineering focused primarily on the structural properties of the scaffold itself including pore size, biocompatibility, and its biomechanical profile. Many animal tissue-based (i.e., collagen[164]) and synthetic or polymer-based varieties (i.e., silk[165] or polyurethane[166]) have been created and tested in vivo.[153] The chemical and microarchitectural details are still being worked out for many of these designs.[167,168] More recently, newer methods for engineering nanofiber-based scaffolds and optimizing pore sizes has allowed for increased cell affinity for the scaffold and a microenvironment more conducive to extracellular matrix deposition.[168] However, despite these advancements, few of these designs have proceeded to human trials. Current indications for clinical trials include (1) young patients, (2) significant meniscal tissue deficiency, (3) ligamentous stability, and (4) absence of malalignment.[153] Warth et al.[169] recently systematically reviewed the use of collagen-based, resorbable meniscal scaffolds in humans. Although most of the studies were small retrospective case series (10/14 studies included), there was some evidence in comparative studies that implantation of a collagen-based scaffold resulted in slightly better early clinical and radiographic results when compared to partial meniscectomies alone.[170] An acellular polyurethane-based synthetic meniscus, Actifit (Orteq, UK), has been evaluated for use in humans.[171–173] This implant is designed to slowly degrade while being replaced gradually by neomeniscal tissue populated from the vascularized meniscus rim and possibly synovial cells.[172] Early clinical studies demonstrated positive results in terms of safety, patient-reported outcome measures, preservation of neighboring articular cartilage, and even histologic evidence of colonization by chondrocytes and fibrochondrocytes as evidenced by biopsy.[173] Despite the promising early data, the recent long-term follow-up data on this implant reveal more modest results: a failure rate of over 20% and persistence of abnormal meniscal signal on MRI, indicating persistence of the implant and/or neomeniscal tissue with abnormal microstructure and composition. However, the durability of improved pain and patient-reported outcomes have endured.[172] Continued follow-up on the initial cohorts treated with this implant will be necessary to test its long-term durability, to understand the kinetics of tissue formation, and to determine the ideal candidates for its use.

Although preclinical and clinical trials using acellular scaffolds have demonstrated excellent safety and good preliminary results, recent preclinical trials have begun to augment these scaffolds with cells and/or growth factors. An early study using a large animal model demonstrated improved vascularization, scaffold remodeling, and greater production of extracellular matrix components in a collagen-based scaffold seeded with autologous fibrochondrocytes as compared to the acellular scaffold alone.[164] Furthermore, even a polymer-based scaffold, polyglycolic acid, seeded with allogenic fibrochondrocytes and implanted in a rabbit knee maintained shape and size in addition to histologic characteristics more similar to native menisci compared to an acellular scaffold after 36 weeks.[174] A recent systematic review[175] identified at least 20 additional studies that examined the in vivo characteristics of cell-enriched meniscal scaffolds. The cell types implanted included chondrocytes (articular, auricular, costal), fibrochondrocytes, bone marrow-derived MSCs, synovium-derived MSCs, and myoblasts.[175] Finally, although most research has focused on first building a scaffold and then implanting cells, a scaffold-free meniscus approach was recently developed. Chondrocytes and fibrochondrocytes are seeded into a mold and cultivated.[176] Under appropriate conditions these cell networks synthesize their own extracellular matrix, which have material properties similar to scaffold-based designs by biomechanical testing.[176] Although none of these cellular scaffolds have been tested in humans, it is likely that cellular augmentation of acellular scaffolds will have an impact on meniscus regeneration and repair, just as other homologous designs, such as articular chondrocyte-embedded matrices[177] have impacted the treatment of articular cartilage defects.

POSTOPERATIVE MANAGEMENT

We divide our postoperative rehabilitation after meniscal repair into three distinct phases. This protocol is designed to maximize early healing and to protect the healing meniscus during the remodeling phase. These protocols are carefully individualized with regard to the tear configuration and location, repair type, concomitant procedures, and patient activity. Immediate ROM is initiated for all patients and continues throughout the rehabilitation program. We may limit knee flexion to 90 degrees for the first 4 weeks after repair of radial or complex tears. Progressive weight bearing is allowed, beginning with toe-touch ambulation. Early weight bearing with the knee in full extension is encouraged after repair of vertical or bucket handle tears because it provides a compressive load across the repair site that may facilitate healing. Weight bearing after repair of radial and complex tears, on the other hand, may create a distraction force at the repair and thus is more restricted. We allow toe-touch ambulation for the first 4 to 6 weeks followed by progressive ambulation in persons who have undergone repair of such tenuous tear types.

Phase 1 of our rehabilitation protocol is initiated immediately postoperatively and continues for approximately 6 weeks after surgery. Progression through these phases depends primarily on patient recovery and ability, whereas the time-specific guidelines function solely as rough estimates. Immediate passive and active-assisted ROM is initiated with a motion goal of full extension to 90 degrees of flexion prior to progression to phase 2. We may restrict flexion to 90 degrees in the setting of posterior horn repairs in an attempt to minimize the shear and distraction forces that occur at the posterior meniscocapsular junction during deep flexion. Weight bearing is allowed in the aforementioned fashion according to repair type. A nonantalgic gait is required prior to discontinuation of assisted ambulation. We also immediately initiate quadriceps strengthening with straight leg raises and isometric exercises to minimize postoperative quadriceps atrophy.

Phase 2 typically occurs during weeks 6 to 14 and is focused on progressing ROM to achieve a normal arc and initiating muscle strengthening and proprioception. Strengthening exercises should be delayed until a full, normal ROM is obtained. Postoperative bracing is discontinued during phase 2 when functional quadriceps control is demonstrated. We frequently use pool and bicycle therapy during this phase to facilitate a return to functional activities while improving ROM and strength.

Phase 3 typically occurs during weeks 14 to 22 and is designed to facilitate strengthening and to initiate functional sports-specific activities. Core muscle strengthening is also important during this phase. Running begins early in this phase, followed by agility and sport-specific exercises. Isokinetic and plyometric training are introduced, with deep flexion and pivoting activities incorporated in the later stages of this phase.

RETURN TO PLAY

Successful return to play (RTP) occurs after completion of phase 3 of our rehabilitation protocol. Although no data exist regarding strict RTP criteria, we have identified some tests that have proven useful. Full ROM, absence of mechanical symptoms, and strength greater than 80% of the strength of the contralateral extremity are required prior to RTP. We also use the single-leg hop and crossover hop tests because they both require significant proprioception and ipsilateral strength. For this reason, patients may RTP if they can demonstrate less than a 15% deficit during these strenuous tests. Most patients are able to return to sporting activities at approximately 6 months, but this time frame is dependent on the patient's progress.

RESULTS

Long-term data are available regarding the impact of surgical and demographic variables on the end result of removal of meniscal tissue.[72] A great deal of data have supported the hypothesis that increased meniscal resection predicts worse radiographic and functional long-term status.[178–182] Obesity[183,184] and advanced age[185,186] have been shown to be further predictive of even poorer functional and clinical results after resection of meniscal tissue. Data regarding medial versus lateral arthroscopic partial meniscectomy are mixed. Although in vitro computer modeling suggests that lateral partial meniscectomy may lead to more degenerative changes when compared with medial partial meniscectomy,[187] in vivo studies have shown no significant clinical differences.[185] Short- and medium-term analyses of outcomes regarding gender differences at 8.5 to 14.5 years after surgery demonstrate no difference in surgical outcome between men and women.[181,188,189] Nevertheless, 15- to 22-year follow-up data indicate that symptoms and functional limitations are worse in women who have undergone meniscectomy compared with men,[186] and osteoarthritis tends to develop more frequently in women.[183] Radiographic osteoarthritis is accelerated in patients with malalignment, likely due to greater articular cartilage stresses in the affected compartment.[188] Therefore meniscal preservation is important whenever possible, and a substantial body of research has identified predictors of improved prognosis after meniscal repair.

Meniscal repair has generally been associated with good outcomes and is considered preferable to meniscectomy in the setting of a repairable meniscal tear, such as those in the red–red or red–white vascular zone. Long-term success has been documented with use of an inside-out meniscal repair technique. Success rates up to 92% have been reported with complete resolution of symptoms and an 80% return to previous activity.[132] Second-look arthroscopy demonstrated complete healing in 61.8%, and incomplete, stable healing in 16.9% of patients. The long-term fate and function of incompletely healed meniscus tears is currently unknown. Healing rates were notably increased after repairs

of narrow (<2 mm) peripheral tears or repair with concomitant ACL reconstruction. Other series have substantiated these results.[190,191]

Meniscal vasculature and the specific vascular zones also play an important role in healing after repair. Prior outcome data regarding the repair of meniscal tears in the central avascular zone demonstrated an 80% rate of complete resolution of symptoms at a mean of 42 months after surgery.[81] However, second-look arthroscopic evaluation demonstrated complete healing in only 25% of tears and incomplete healing in 38% of tears. Noyes and Barber-Westin[82] have suggested that improved healing rates may be accomplished in the avascular zone in a subset of patients younger than 20 years. This study documented a 75% rate of clinical success in 71 meniscal repairs. These indications were then extended to patients older than 40 years who had meniscal tears that also extended into the avascular zone. An 87% successful clinical outcome was observed as measured by the absence of symptoms at a mean 33-month follow-up.[82] Nevertheless, the excellent clinical outcomes that have been reported after repair of avascular meniscal tears may not correlate with complete meniscal healing. Fortunately, these healing rates significantly increase with repair of tears in the vascular zones with similarly good clinical outcomes. Theoretically, the risk of a repeat meniscal tear may be higher in the setting of incomplete healing, and thus we favor the use of partial meniscectomy in all but a limited subset of patients with avascular tears, including young, active persons with tear extension from the vascular zone into the avascular zone.

COMPLICATIONS

Complications after meniscal repair include chondral injury, implant failure, postoperative joint-line irritation, nerve injury, arthrofibrosis, persistent or recurring effusion, infection, deep venous thrombosis (DVT), and pulmonary embolus.[192,193] When all these complications are included, they occur in approximately 2.5% of knee arthroscopies and 1.2% of meniscal surgeries.[194] Bleeding or pseudoaneurysms have been reported after meniscal surgery, but are primarily associated with posterior horn resection and not meniscal repair.[195,196] The incidence of infection after knee arthroscopy is less than 0.1%, with increased risk in patients who have longer surgeries, undergo multiple procedures, have had prior surgery, and are given corticosteroids intraoperatively. Although DVT has been documented in up to 18% of knee arthroscopies, fatal pulmonary embolism remains an extremely rare event. Nevertheless, risk factors for DVT include obesity, advanced age (>40 years), a history of DVT, tobacco use, and oral contraceptive use. We frequently prescribe enteric-coated aspirin for many patients during the perioperative period in an attempt to minimize this risk.

Nerve injury has also been documented with meniscal repair techniques. Medial meniscal repair has been associated with injury to the saphenous nerve, producing transient neuropraxia, but permanent injury has only been identified in 0.4% to 1% of documented cases.[194,197,198] Peroneal nerve injury is a rare but devastating injury that may occur during lateral meniscal repair. A carefully dissected posterolateral safety incision with proper retractor placement significantly reduces this risk.[199] Overall, for meniscal repairs, the most commonly encountered complications were saphenous neuropathy (7%) and arthrofibrosis (6%).[192]

FUTURE CONSIDERATIONS

This chapter has outlined many areas in which improvements in basic science and operative management are necessary to move the field forward. Implant improvements have allowed the use of the all-inside technique with excellent results, but research continues to produce new, improved implants and techniques. Two principal areas of improvement were also identified, including management of avascular meniscal tears and tears in younger patients with significant meniscal tissue deficiency. Current research and development efforts are aimed at addressing these two areas. Cellular and acellular meniscal repair and regeneration techniques have been developed with some preliminary data now available. These techniques are designed to stimulate and maximize meniscus healing and/or to function as a scaffold to support new meniscal tissue regeneration. Scaffolds are already demonstrating efficacy in other regions in the knee, which address deficiencies of the ACL [198] and articular cartilage.[177] Although significant obstacles remain regarding the ideal regenerative meniscal scaffold, we believe that advances in tissue engineering, biomaterials, and understanding of basic meniscus cell biology and the function of progenitor cells hold great potential to lead to innovative approaches for the treatment of meniscal injuries.

CRITICAL POINTS

The roles of the menisci in force transmission and chondral protection within the knee have been well documented. Knowledge of the gross and microscopic meniscal anatomy, biomechanical function, and role in articular congruity and shock absorption is important for diagnosis and treatment. The range of repairable meniscal tears is expanding because of recent augmentation techniques and improved understanding of meniscal healing. Clinical and radiographic identification of repairable meniscal tears is crucial to healing success and improved outcomes. Careful consideration should be given to the factors that may contribute to or inhibit meniscal healing, including tear location, tear type, tear etiology, concomitant injury, and patient profile. Treatment of all identified repairable meniscal tears should be carefully managed to maximize the healing potential after repair. Focus should be placed on optimizing the biologic environment and mechanical stability of the repaired meniscus to maximize healing. Careful surveillance should be performed after a total meniscectomy in the young patient to identify potential candidates for meniscal allograft transplantation, because the outcomes may be optimized if this procedure is performed prior to the onset of articular cartilage degeneration. Finally, the outcomes of meniscal repair and transplantation should be reported to aid the current understanding of meniscal healing and to improve this crucial process.

For a complete list of references, go to ExpertConsult.com.

SELECTED READINGS

Citation:

Arnoczky SP, Warren RF. Microvasculature of the human meniscus. *Am J Sports Med*. 1982;10(2):90–95.

Level of Evidence:

V, cadaveric study

Summary:

In this study 20 cadaver specimens were histologically evaluated regarding the meniscal microvascular blood supply. These data demonstrated the presence of a perimeniscal capillary plexus that supplied the peripheral 10% to 25% of the menisci.

Citation:

Burks RT, Metcalf MH, Metcalf RW. Fifteen-year follow-up of arthroscopic partial meniscectomy. *Arthroscopy*. 1997;13:673–679.

Level of Evidence:

IV, case series

Summary:

This study is a large cohort retrospective case series with 14.7-year follow-up of 146 patients after a partial meniscectomy. The data demonstrated an 88% rate of good to excellent results in knees with stable ligaments and suggested that valgus alignment was protective after a partial medial meniscectomy.

Citation:

Dienst M, Greis PE, Ellis BJ, et al. Effect of lateral meniscal allograft sizing on contact mechanics of the lateral tibial plateau: an experimental study in human cadaveric knee joints. *Am J Sports Med*. 2007;35(1):34–42.

Level of Evidence

V, cadaveric study

Summary:

In this study the effect of allograft sizing on the contact mechanics of the lateral tibial plateau was evaluated. Oversized allografts resulted in increased contact forces compared with undersized allografts, and 10% size variability above or below normal was demonstrated to have mechanics similar to those of intact knees.

Citation:

Lee SL, Aadalen KJ, Malaviya P, et al. Tibiofemoral contact mechanics after serial medial meniscectomies in the human cadaveric knee. *Am J Sports Med*. 2006;34(8):1334–1344.

Level of Evidence:

V, cadaveric study

Summary:

In this study 12 cadaveric knees were evaluated after serial medial meniscectomies. Incrementally increased contact pressures were documented after each meniscectomy, with the greatest effect demonstrated after removal of the posterior and peripheral zones.

Citation:

Rubman MH, Noyes FR, Barber-Westin SD. Arthroscopic repair of meniscal tears that extend into the avascular zone: a review of 198 single and complex tears. *Am J Sports Med*. 1998;26(1):87–95.

Level of Evidence:

IV, retrospective case series

Summary:

In this study 198 meniscal tears were evaluated at a mean 42 months after repair of a major central avascular segment with partial extension into the vascular zone. Eighty percent of tears were asymptomatic and 20% required revision meniscectomy. Ninety-one repairs were evaluated arthroscopically and demonstrated a 63% rate of partial or full healing.

Citation:

Shoemaker SC, Markolf KL. The role of the meniscus in the anterior-posterior stability of the loaded anterior cruciate-deficient knee: effects of partial versus total excision. *J Bone Joint Surg Am.* 1986;68:71–79.

Level of Evidence:

V, cadaveric study

Summary:

In this study the biomechanical effect of the menisci on the anterior cruciate ligament-deficient knee was evaluated. A 10% increase in anteroposterior laxity was demonstrated after total medial meniscectomy, with an additional 10% increase after subsequent removal of the lateral meniscus.

Citation:

Tenuta JJ, Arciero RA. Arthroscopic evaluation of meniscal repairs: factors that effect healing. *Am J Sports Med.* 1994;22(6):797–802.

Level of Evidence:

IV, case series

Summary:

In this study 54 meniscal repairs were arthroscopically evaluated at a mean of 11 months after repair in an attempt to identify factors that affect healing. Notably, patients with simultaneous meniscal repair and anterior cruciate ligament reconstruction had a significantly higher healing rate (84%), whereas patients with an intact meniscal rim width greater than 4 mm had a 0% healing rate.

Citation:

Leroy A, Beaufils P, Faivre B, et al. Actifit polyurethane meniscal scaffold: MRI and functional outcomes after a minimum follow-up of 5 years. *Orthop Traumatol Surg Res.* 2017;103(4):609–614.

Level of Evidence:

IV, case series

Summary:

In this study the results of 13 patients who had undergone implantation of the Actifit polyurethane meniscal scaffold were reported on at a mean follow-up of 6 years. There were persistent improvements from baseline in reported pain, IKDC scores, and quality-of-life components of the KOOS score. There were 3/13 patients that were deemed failures and magnetic resonance imaging performed at 5 years revealed that the implant still had an abnormal signal.

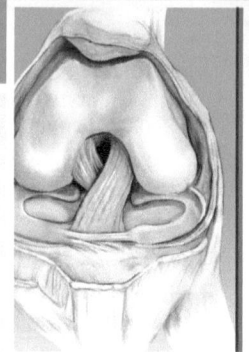

95

Meniscal Transplantation

Frank B. Wydra, Derek P. Axibal, Armando F. Vidal

INTRODUCTION

Our understanding of the role of the meniscus has evolved over many years. Dating back to 1948, Fairbank et al. described changes to the knee joint such as narrowing of the joint space, squaring of the femoral condyle, and ridge formation following meniscectomy.[1] This led to his conclusion that a simple meniscectomy is not "wholly innocuous" and it leads to changes in joint mechanics that can be detrimental.

Through the years, extensive research has improved the understanding of meniscal anatomy, biology, mechanics, function, and pathology. This knowledge has adapted our treatment approaches. Prior to Fairbank's work, total meniscectomies were thought to be the ideal choice for knee pain due to a meniscal injury.

Starting in the 1980s, multiple publications identified the benefits of a partial meniscectomy over a total meniscectomy. These benefits included lower contact pressures, less long-term degenerative changes on radiographs, and improved patient satisfaction.[2–5] Since this research, trends toward meniscal preservation developed including partial meniscectomy or meniscal repair.[6]

Even with all the advances made over the years, there are still complex situations when meniscal preservation is not possible. For these difficult scenarios, meniscal transplantation may be an option. Dating back to 1989 when the first series of meniscal transplantations was published, there has been an increasing acceptance of meniscal allografts used for situations where the meniscus is nonfunctional, symptomatic, and irreparable.[7] This chapter offers a comprehensive review of meniscal transplantation including preoperative workup, indications, techniques, and outcomes.

HISTORY

A thorough history is imperative for accurate diagnosis and reasonable treatment recommendations. A detailed understanding of a patient's pain including duration, quality, location, description, and alleviating and aggravating factors can give a valuable insight into their ailment. Other important factors include locking, catching, or swelling that indicates there is a mechanical issue with the knee. Reports of instability with increased joint line tenderness localized to the involved compartment are sometimes seen with meniscu deficiency. Intermittent swelling may also be present, specifically with an increased level of activity. Emphasis should be placed on reports of increasing pain in a particular compartment, because this pain may be associated with increased compartment loading and risk for progressive chondral damage.

Respecting patients' goals of therapy is also important and can help guide the aggressiveness of treatment. Their age and activity level should be taken into consideration as this can alter the optimal treatment strategies for patients. A thorough surgical history regarding the knee can make future surgical procedures more difficult but also allow the surgeon to understand what state the knee is currently in. It is helpful to obtain prior operative reports as well as arthroscopy images if available to gain a better understanding of the status of the knee.

PHYSICAL EXAMINATION

The physical exam is key to determining the location of patients' symptoms. Correlating symptoms with the location of the affected compartment is critical to a successful result.

Additionally, assessment of the patient with meniscal deficiency and/or articular cartilage damage must occur in the context of the alignment, stability, and meniscal status (Fig. 95.1).[8] The physical exam and imagining should focus on understanding the entire context of these factors.

Inspecting the standing alignment of the leg and assessing for varus or valgus angulation is essential to understanding the biomechanical context in which a patient's meniscal deficiency exists and should be substantiated with appropriate imaging. Assessment of range of motion (ROM) is helpful in differentiating the arthritic knee from the healthy knee. Significant motion loss is a contraindication to joint-preserving procedures. The presence or absence of an effusion is also a critical "vital sign" for how the knee is behaving. Joint effusions can be due to many etiologies including trauma, systemic diseases, infection, and mechanical irritation. A knee that is actively delaminating cartilage often presents with recurrent effusions and therefore large effusions can be indicative of progressive articular cartilage loss in this setting.

Focal tenderness along the joint line is also helpful in correlating symptoms in the affected compartment.[9] Although there are a variety of provocative physical exam maneuvers described for detecting meniscal pathology, they are better suited to detecting meniscal tears rather than meniscal deficiency.[10] A comprehensive ligamentous exam is essential, as untreated instability is a contraindication to meniscal reconstruction.[11]

Lastly, since the vast majority of these patients have had prior surgery, assessment of prior incisions on the knee is key to consider as this may limit or alter the surgical plan.

IMAGING

The history and physical exam should guide further workup of the patient, which in most cases entails additional imaging.

Radiographs

A complete radiographic evaluation should include standing anterior–posterior and 45-degree flexed posterior–anterior views as well as lateral and skyline views of the affected knee. Full-length standing x-rays of both legs is important to assess the overall alignment of the limb and evaluate for genu varum or valgum.

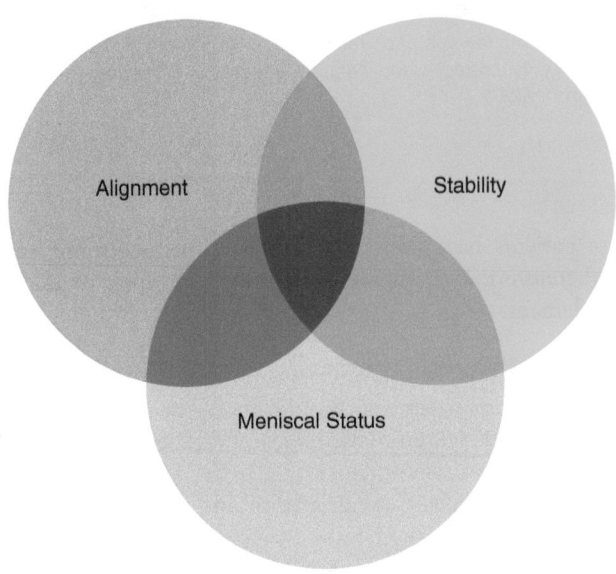

Fig. 95.1 Venn diagram of the key components of the physical exam.

Magnetic Resonance Imaging

Magnetic resonance imaging (MRI) is a valuable tool in the workup of these patients. It allows the physician to evaluate the soft tissue structures of the knee including the meniscus, cartilage, and ligaments, which are all important to consider when formulating a treatment plan. The MRI can also help assess the integrity and amount of residual meniscus (Fig. 95.2).

Bone Scan

Bone scans are sometimes helpful and often underutilized. In view of other normal studies such as an MRI, an increased uptake on a bone scan may suggest compartment overload and impending chondral damage, thus increasing the importance of attempting to restore the compartment load-sharing through meniscal allograft transplantation (MAT), realignment osteotomy if indicated, or both.

DECISION-MAKING PRINCIPLES/INDICATIONS

Decision-making in joint preservation must consider patient factors, the pathophysiology, and any other contributing factors. The knee should be viewed holistically as an organ. Understanding the mechanical alignment, stability, and articular cartilage status is key for a successful outcome.

Patient

Ideally, meniscal transplantation is best reserved for younger patients with compartment-specific knee pain who are meniscal deficient from prior near-total or total meniscectomy, but who still have preserved articular cartilage. It is ideally suited for patients who would like to remain active and have minimal to no arthritic changes.[12]

Pathophysiology

The joint should be evaluated holistically when considering a patient for a meniscal transplant. There is conflicting evidence

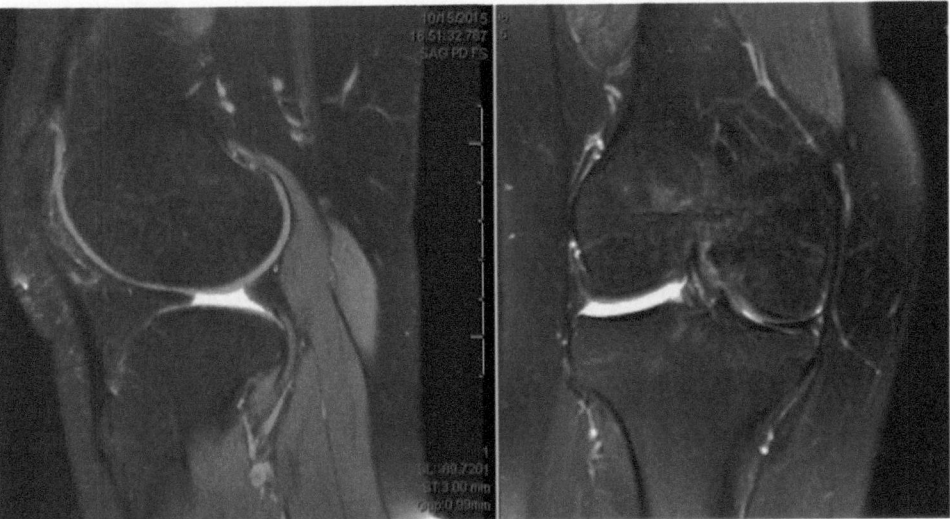

Fig. 95.2 T2-weighted magnetic resonance imaging of an 18-year-old female with right knee lateral meniscal deficiency.

regarding how arthritic changes may affect the outcome of a meniscal transplant. Some believe that arthritic degeneration precludes patients from meniscal transplantation; however, other studies have shown pain relief in patients even with Outerbridge grade III and IV lesions as long as they are isolated.[8,13,14] These higher-degree lesions can and should be addressed at the time of surgery through various methods such as microfracture, osteochondral allografts, articular cartilage paste grafting, or autologous chondrocyte implantation.[8,14,15] Bony changes such as flattening or osteophyte formation commonly seen with advancing osteoarthritis may alter the shape of the condyle and lead to poor outcomes with meniscal transplantation.[16] Instability of the knee should also be taken into account for meniscal deficient patients and should be addressed either in a staged or concomitant fashion. Anterior cruciate ligament (ACL) reconstruction at the time of meniscal transplant is an acceptable treatment approach and shows similar outcomes to patients who underwent an isolated meniscal transplant.[11] In addition to its load-sharing and articular cartilage preservation role, the stabilizing effect of the medial meniscus should not be overlooked. The posterior horn of the medial meniscus is an important contributor of secondary stabilization to anterior translation of the tibia relative to the femur in the ACL deficient and ACL reconstructed states.[17] This secondary stabilization is an important factor to consider when assessing the ACL deficient patient, particularly in the revision setting.[18]

Contributing Factors

Limb alignment is one of the most important issues to evaluate when considering meniscal transplantation. As discussed previously, full-length x-ray can highlight joint deformities such as genu varum or valgum, which increases joint pressures through the respective compartment of the knee.[19] Realignment procedures such as high tibial or distal femoral osteotomies can be performed concomitantly or prior to meniscal transplantation to decrease contact pressures through the compartment (Fig. 95.3).[16,20] Although patients who undergo concomitant procedures have favorable outcomes, it is still unclear if these procedures should ideally be performed concomitantly or in a staged fashion if osteotomy alone is insufficient to relieve symptoms. If done in a staged fashion, the osteotomy should be performed first and consideration of meniscal transplantation should be reserved for the persistently symptomatic patient.

Contraindications

While meniscal transplantation can be beneficial when applied to the above indications, there are several contraindications including prior or current joint infection, advanced osteoarthritis, obesity, synovial disease, or rheumatoid arthritis.[12]

TREATMENT OPTIONS

A young patient with symptomatic meniscal insufficiency is a challenging clinical scenario. Options vary and considerations must take into account multiple factors such as patient goals, prior surgeries, and status of the residual meniscus. Most of

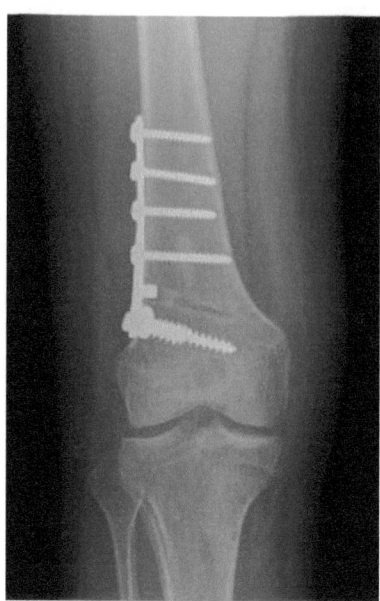

Fig. 95.3 Anterior–posterior radiograph status after a distal femoral osteotomy to correct genu valgum effectively unloading the lateral compartment.

these patients have had prior sub-total meniscectomies and are therefore not candidates for a meniscal repair or further débridement.

Nonoperative Management

Conservative management should always be attempted first in patients with symptomatic meniscal deficiency. A course of nonsteroidal antiinflammatories, rest, ice, and elevation can help calm down acute inflammation and reduce pain. Some may benefit from strengthening, stretching, or formal physical therapy.[21] Unloader bracing is an effective way to reduce pressures unilaterally across the knee joint and enhance stability; however, compliance among patients is universally poor.[22,23] Steroid injections in younger meniscal deficient patients should be used sparingly as recent studies have shown that use may be deleterious to hyaline cartilage.[24]

Operative Management

Young patients with symptomatic meniscal deficiency have limited options. These patients have already undergone a complete or near complete meniscectomy, so further débridement or repair is not an option. Operative considerations should look to address a combination of factors in these patients. Instability and malalignment must be corrected either before or concomitant to the meniscal transplant as these factors place the transplant at risk of failure.[11,16,20] In patients who have malalignment, often osteotomy alone is sufficient to decrease loads across the compartment and meniscal transplantation is not necessary. Unicompartmental or total knee arthroplasty is an alternative option for meniscal deficient patients; however, this may limit younger patients' activities and likely subject them to a revision surgery in their lifetime.[25]

Positioning and Diagnostic Arthroscopy

The patient is positioned supine on the operative table. An exam under anesthesia is performed to confirm full knee passive ROM and a thorough ligamentous examination of both knees is performed to confirm knee stability.

The operative knee is positioned with a lateral thigh post, as well as a foot post to hold the knee in 90 degrees of flexion. A tourniquet is placed, but only inflated if necessary. Standard anterolateral and anteromedial portals are created and a diagnostic arthroscopy is performed to diagnose any associated injuries, confirm knee stability, and rule out any advanced arthritic disease.

If the patient is a candidate for meniscus transplant given the above stated factors, the procedure is continued on and the graft is open and thawed.

Lateral

For lateral meniscal transplantation, the author prefers an all soft tissue technique. The graft is prepared, rinsed, and threaded with three sutures: one in each root and one at the posterior horn–body junction. The graft and all sutures are thoroughly irrigated using antibiotic impregnated normal saline. Intra-articular preparation is performed by removing the remaining meniscus down to a thin rim at the capsule (Fig. 95.4). Ideally a rim of native meniscus should be preserved to minimize the risk of meniscal allograft extrusion. Confirmation of circumferential capsular bleeding is obtained.

An approximate 3-cm incision is made parallel to and immediately posterior to the lateral collateral ligament (LCL), one-third

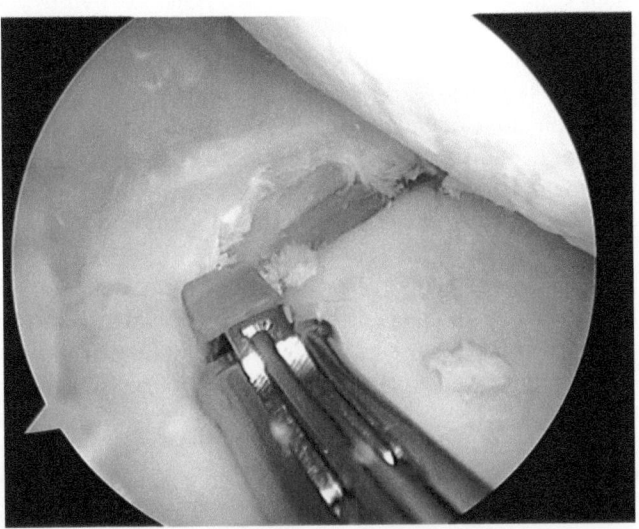

Fig. 95.4 Preparation of remaining meniscus.

above and two-thirds below the joint line. The internervous plane between the biceps femoris and iliotibial band is identified. The lateral head of the gastrocnemius is identified and elevated off of the posterolateral capsule. A Henning retractor is then placed in the posterolateral aspect of his knee.

The posterior root for the lateral meniscus is then drilled. A low-profile multiuse marking (Arthrex) hook is placed through the medial portal. An approximate 3-cm incision is made over the anteromedial tibia. Under direct visualization, a 6-mm Flip-Cutter (Arthrex) is advanced. Once in the anatomic position of the root, a curved curette is placed over it to protect the ACL and the posterior neurovascular structures. A 5-mm blind socket is created in that location to accommodate the posterior root. A passing stitch is placed through that tunnel. In a similar fashion, an additional passing stitch is placed using an inside-out technique just lateral to the popliteus. This correlates to two of the three sutures previously placed in the graft: one in the posterior root and one at the popliteal hiatus.

A 5-cm arthrotomy is made in line with the lateral portal. With the scope in the medial portal, the passing stitches from the root and popliteal hiatus are passed through the previously placed passing stitches in the transplant and the meniscal allograft is reduced. The root is held in place using tension, and numerous vertical mattress sutures are used with zone-specific cannulas in an inside-out fashion. These are alternated between the superior and inferior aspects of the meniscus and spaced approximately 3 to 5 mm apart. The allograft is tied to any remaining remnant of the native meniscus.

Once all sutures are passed, the anterior root footprint is identified and drilled directly through the arthrotomy. A small Beath pin is advanced into the anterior root insertion and then over-reamed with a 4.5-mm drill to create a small bleeding surface. The sutures from the anterior root are passed through the anteromedial tibia with a free needle. Suturing of any remaining anterior portion of the graft is completed using a freehand #2 FiberWire (Arthrex) suture through the arthrotomy.

All of the peripheral meniscus sutures are tied down. The knee is cycled through a full ROM to confirm meniscus stability as well as absence of catching or irregularity of the meniscus. A small area in the anteromedial tibia is cleared and a 4.5-mm screw with a washer (Synthes) is placed as a post and the two meniscal root sutures are secured down over the post.

Arthroscopic visualization is used to confirm coverage of the lateral plateau and stable roots. The entire allograft is probed. The knee is once again cycled through full ROM to confirm stability.

Medial

For medial meniscal transplantation, the author prefers a two bone-plug technique. The graft is prepared with two separate bone plugs of the desired diameter and length (the author prefers 6 mm in diameter and 5 mm in depth). Two sutures are prepassed through the allograft to aide in meniscal delivery and reduction—one through the posterior root and the other through the meniscus at the posterior horn–body junction.

Once again, the compartment is first prepared by removing the remaining meniscus, leaving a thin rim at the capsule and confirming capsular bleeding. The knee is brought into 90 degrees of flexion and a notchplasty is performed. The medial tibial spine is débrided, if necessary, for access to the posterior medial meniscus root. This is performed below the posterior cruciate ligament (PCL) taking great care to protect the PCL fibers at all times.

An ACL guide or multiuse marking hook (Arthrex) is placed in the center of the posterior root of the medial meniscus. A small anteromedial incision is made and the guide pin is advanced through the anteromedial aspect of the tibia up into the footprint of the posterior horn of the medial meniscus. A 6-mm FlipCutter (Arthrex) is advanced and a 5-mm blind socket is created. A passing stitch is placed through that tunnel.

An inside-out repair technique is preferred for suturing the meniscus to the capsule and meniscal rim. A standard exposure for an inside-out meniscal repair is performed. A Henning retractor is placed in the posteromedial aspect of the wound for suture retrieval.

A Hewson suture passer is passed through the bone tunnel in the posterior root. The medial portal incision is extended and a small medial arthrotomy is performed. The suture passer is retrieved through the medial arthrotomy and used to shuttle a passing stitch through a posterior root tunnel to aid in reducing the meniscus.

With the scope in the medial incision, a zone-specific cannula is used at the junction of the posterior horn and midbody segment and a Nitinol wire with a free loop is passed and retrieved through the posteromedial incision. This will serve to shuttle the prepassed suture at the posterior horn–body junction in the transplant.

The sutures for the posterior root are shuttled using the passing suture in the posterior root tunnel. The stitch placed at the junction of the posterior horn and midbody segment is then passed through the Nitinol wire with the loop and shuttled through the capsule.

The knee is then brought into flexion and valgus. Gentle traction is applied to the stitches and using a blunt trocar, the meniscus is reduced. Anatomic placement is confirmed.

Using zone-specific cannulas, sutures are placed at the periphery of the graft. The posterior horn and body sutures are performed using an inside-out approach, while the anterior sutures are performed using an outside-in approach or directly through the arthrotomy. These are all placed in vertical mattress fashion.

The anterior root is similarly drilled through the arthrotomy. A Beath pin is drilled in the anterior root site and reamed to a depth of about 15 mm. Using a free needle, the two sutures placed in the anterior root are passed directly through the bone. The bone plug is manually reduced and tapped down so that it is flush with the articular surface. The root sutures can then be tied down over a bone bridge anteriorly or to a button or post.

The knee is cycled through a full ROM to confirm meniscus stability as well as absence of catching or irregularity of the meniscus (Fig. 95.5). Arthroscopic visualization, including a Gillquist portal, is used to confirm coverage of the medial plateau and stable roots. The entire allograft is probed. The knee is once again cycled through full ROM to confirm stability.

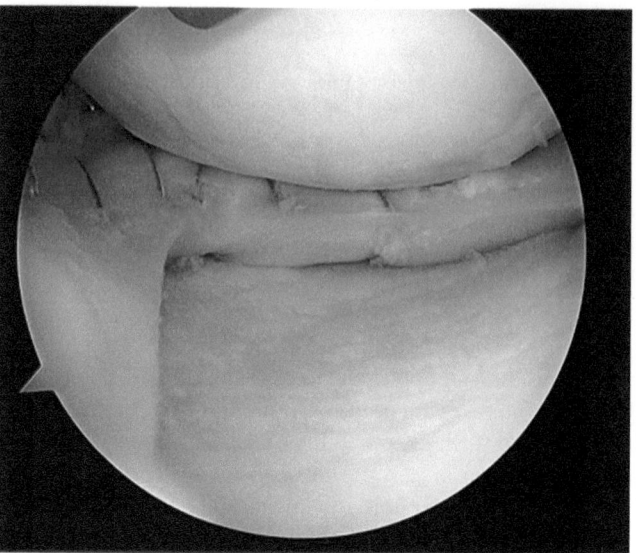

Fig. 95.5 Well-reduced meniscal allograft with sutures in place.

Single Bone Plug and Trough

MAT on the lateral side can also be performed with a single rectangular bone block and trough as described by Goble et al.[26]

The lateral meniscus allograft is prepared with a single rectangular bone block connecting the anterior and posterior horns. Various guide sutures are preinserted into the allograft. Goble et al. describes the critical suture placement as the posterolateral corner, the edge of the anterior horn (15 mm lateral to its insertion), and two sutures in the common bone block (10 cm apart). The bone block is prepared until it matches a chosen sizing block (8, 9, or 10 mm). A silicone template is then trimmed to match the allograft bone block. The silicone template is inserted, and the trough is made using a power burr (beginning 1 cm posterior to the anterior edge of the lateral tibial plateau and progressing posteriorly). Using an ACL tibial guide, two transosseous holes are placed 10 mm apart in the middle of the trough (matching the single bone block sutures) and exiting the tibia anteriorly. The meniscal allograft is inserted and the two sutures in the bone block are pulled through their respective transosseous hole. A spinal needle and suture are inserted outside-in through the posterolateral corner of the knee, and the preinserted suture in the posterolateral edge of the allograft is then pulled through. A combination of pulling on the three guide sutures, gently placing the graft into the trough, and varus stress on the knee will anatomically reduce the allograft. Guide sutures are tied, and any other additional peripheral sutures are placed.[26]

The technique for a single bone plug for the medial meniscus is similar to the lateral meniscus technique, with a few exceptions. The medial meniscus horns are farther apart compared to those of the lateral meniscus, and therefore the single bone block connecting the two horns is much longer. The medial trough is performed starting at the anterior margin of the tibial plateau below the fat pad, and the bone is débrided in line with the medial tibial spine axis. Lastly, it is frequently necessary to strengthen the single bone block with a 1/16″ guide wire through the center of the bone plug.[26]

POSTOPERATIVE MANAGEMENT

There is significant variability in surgical rehabilitation protocols for postoperative management after MAT. In their systematic review, Rosso et al. found full weight-bearing was allowed at an average of 6.2 weeks, while full ROM was allowed at an average of 6.3 weeks. A total of 43% of studies (24 of 55) reported the use of a brace, while 16% (9 or 55) reported the use of a continuous passive motion (CPM) machine.[27]

In the literature's largest case series of meniscal allograft transplantation (included in the systematic review above), Kim et al. describes his postoperative protocol. Isometric strengthening exercises begin immediately after surgery. A CPM device is used postoperative day 1, 0 to 60 degrees for the first 3 weeks, up to 120 degrees during weeks 4 to 6, with full flexion allowed during weeks 8 to 12. The patient is non-weight-bearing for 3 weeks, partial-weight-bearing at 4 weeks, and full-weight-bearing at 7 weeks.[28]

The author's postoperative protocol consists of non-weight-bearing for 6 weeks. The patient is allowed to toe touch when standing still, but not for ambulation. The patient is limited from 0 to 90 degrees for the first 3 weeks and is progressed thereafter. The patient initiates a CPM device starting on postoperative day 1, starting from 0 to 30. The patient is instructed to increase by 5 degrees per day up to 90 degrees for the first 3 weeks. Thereafter, the patient will start progressing until they reach 120 degrees.

RESULTS

MAT outcomes are confounded by differences in surgical fixation, surgeon technique, and concomitant procedures.[29]

Most literature report an improvement in pain, function, and patient satisfaction. Rosso et al. included 55 papers in his systematic review of MAT, with an average follow-up of 53 months. The weighted average Lysholm score improved from 56 preoperatively to 83 and the weighted average Visual Analogue Scale (VAS) pain score improved from 6.4 to 2.4, although some authors described a worsening of the results over time. Rosso et al. found an 82% average patient satisfaction.[27] Elattar et al. included 44 studies (352 grafts) in his systematic review. The average preoperative Lysholm score improved from 44 to 77, the mean Tegner activity score improved from 3 to 5, and the overall VAS went from 48 to 17. These authors also noted the improvement in these scores tended to gradually decline over time. Elattar et al. found an 89% average patient satisfaction.[30] Hergan et al. reported on 14 studies in his systematic review. The authors noted improvements in objective and subjective outcome measures in relatively young patients without instability, malalignment, or substantial cartilage damage. The authors concluded MAT may alleviate knee pain, improve knee function, and have good patient satisfaction if done on the optimal candidate.[31]

One of the most important outcomes for MAT is its influence on preventing or delaying the onset of osteoarthritis. It is unclear at the current time if MAT successfully alters the natural history of the meniscus-deficient knee. González-Lucena et al. studied 33 patients with a mean follow-up of 6.5 years. The authors

observed no significant joint space narrowing between the preoperative (mean 3.19 mm) and postoperative periods (mean 3.21 mm).[32] In the Hommen et al. study of 20 MAT, 10 of 15 allografts revealed significant radiographic joint space narrowing, and 12 allografts showed progression of degenerative joint disease in the transplanted compartment. Of the seven patients who received MRIs, all grafts had moderate meniscus shrinkage and five had grade III signal intensities.[33] Saltzman et al. reported on six patients evaluated with radiographs at a mean last follow-up of 8.5 years. The authors reported preservation of joint space narrowing in two patients, minor-to-mild joint space narrowing in two patients, and progression of joint space narrowing with mild-to-moderate change in two patients.[34] Although some have suggested MAT may prevent the progression of osteoarthritis, this effect has not been definitively demonstrated and therefore no final conclusions can be drawn.

Few studies compare bone plugs and suture-only fixation. In the Abat et al. study of 33 suture-only grafts and 55 performed with bone plug fixation, a higher percentage of extruded meniscal tissue was seen in the suture-only group compared to the bone plug method ($P < .001$). However, there was no difference in functional score between the two groups.[35] In the Hommen et al. report of 13 suture-only grafts and 6 fixed with bone plugs, the two methods yielded similar postoperative Lysholm results ($P = .3228$) and postoperative pain scores ($P = .7653$).[33] The literature is scarce in comparing suture-only techniques and bone plug fixation, with the existing data reporting no difference in functional outcomes or pain scores between the two, although the suture-only technique has a higher rate of extrusion.

COMPLICATIONS

The definitions of failure vary within the literature, likely resulting in differing survival times and survival rates. Noyes et al. reported on 72 consecutive medial and lateral MATs, defining failure as reoperations related to the transplant, signs of meniscal tear on clinical examination, loss of joint space in the involved tibiofemoral compartment on 45 degrees weight-bearing posteroanterior (PA) radiographs, or grade 3 signal intensity or extrusion greater than 50% of the meniscus transplant width on MRI. The estimated probability of survival was 85% at 2 years, 77% at 5 years, 45% at 10 years, and 19% at 15 years.[36] In the Verdonk et al. study of 100 consecutive MATs, failure was defined as moderate or severe occasional or persistent pain or as poor knee function. The mean cumulative survival time (11.6 years) was identical for the medial and lateral allografts. The cumulative survival rate for medial transplants was 86.2% at 5 years, 74.2% at 10 years, and 52.8% at 14.5 years. The cumulative survival rates for lateral allografts was 90.2% at 5 years, 69.8% at 10 years, and 69.8% at 14.5 years. These did not differ significantly ($P = .733$).[13] van Arkel et al. reported on the outcomes of 63 consecutive MATs, defining allograft failure as persistent pain, an unsuccessful knee assessment scoring system (KASS) result, a poor Lysholm score, or a detached allograft. The mean survival time for the lateral allografts was 111 months versus 69 months in the medial allografts. The cumulative survival rate of the lateral allografts was 76% versus 50% in the medial allografts ($P = .004$).[37]

In their systematic review of 55 studies, Rosso et al. found 176 complications in 1666 grafts, with a complication rate of 10.6%. The most common complication was an allograft tear (105 cases, 60% of all complications). Synovitis or effusion was reported in 54 cases (31% of all complications), superficial infections were reported in 11 cases (6% of all complications), a decrease in ROM was reported in five cases (3% of all complications), and deep infection was reported once.[27]

CONCLUSION/FUTURE CONSIDERATIONS

Although technically challenging, meniscal allograft transplantation is a viable option in a young patient with a symptomatic, meniscal-deficient knee. Appropriate patient selection is key to a successful outcome. The patient's symptoms should be localized to the affected compartment and the knee should be absent of or have minimal arthritic changes. Knee stability should be assessed and accounted for if it is compromised. Malalignment should be evaluated and corrected in a staged or concomitant fashion if indicated, as uncorrected malalignment results in increased forces through the respective compartment and a suboptimal environment for allograft survival.

Although MAT's ability to improve pain and function has been established with high overall patient satisfaction, there is still much to be determined. With complication rates reported up to 10% and early failure rates as high as 15%, further study is necessary to establish how to prevent these undesirable outcomes. A standardized definition of MAT failure is needed to better establish complication and failure rates and to enable comparison of surgical techniques. Lastly, the ideal outcome of meniscal reconstruction is chondroprotection and the prevention of osteoarthritis. Further refinement of techniques, added study of the role of concomitant procedures, and the role of biologics are all areas of future interest and exploration to achieve this ultimate outcome.

For a complete list of references, go to ExpertConsult.com.

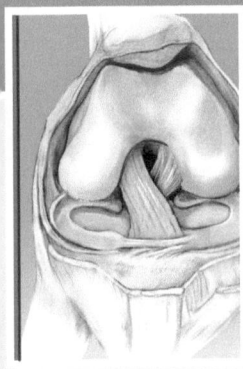

96

Articular Cartilage Lesions

Michael S. Laidlaw, Kadir Buyukdogan, Mark D. Miller

Articular cartilage lesions are a key concern in orthopaedic surgery because cartilage has an extremely poor capacity to heal. Treatment of these lesions aims to restore an articular surface that matches the biomechanical properties of normal hyaline cartilage and to prevent the progression of focal cartilage injury to end-stage arthritis.

A cartilage defect has a very limited ability to recover spontaneously due to its unique characteristics. It is avascular, aneural, alymphatic, and composed of just one cell type—the chondrocyte. That is why no surgical technique has ever been completely successful in stimulating articular cartilage repair and regeneration. Conventional surgical techniques to repair cartilage defects such as microfracture or drilling lead to poor subchondral bone regeneration and fibrocartilage tissue, thus mechanical competence and structural organization is significantly inferior to hyaline cartilage. Osteochondral transfers are viable options as well and attention continues toward the development of biological methods such as third-generation autologous chondrocyte implantation (ACI) to enhance regeneration of native cartilage, to decrease the degenerative condition of joints, and improve clinical outcomes.

Besides the biology of cartilage repair techniques, improved outcomes after cartilage repair depend on the patient and lesion-specific variables such as age and comorbidities, as well as location, size, and chronicity of lesion and concomitant pathologies of the affected knee.

The purpose of this chapter is to review the clinical evaluation of articular cartilage lesions and summarize the current treatment modalities for the management of these injuries. Subsequently, we will discuss our preferred methods in more detail.

RELEVANT ANATOMY AND BIOMECHANICS

Articular cartilage is highly specialized tissue and provides a bearing surface with a minimum-low friction. Due to absence of vascular, neural, and lymphatic components, articular cartilage has a limited capacity for self-repair. It has been generally accepted that partial-thickness defects/injuries, which do not penetrate subchondral bone, are not repaired by the body, whereas those that extend past the depth of the subchondral plate initiate migration of marrow cells to fill the defect with a predominance of fibrocartilage. Unfortunately, fibrocartilage has inferior biomechanical properties and eventually progresses to symptomatic degeneration at the defect size.

Symptomatic articular cartilage lesions of the knee encompass a growing burden to the daily practice of orthopaedic surgeons. Curl et al. reviewed 31,516 knee arthroscopies and found that articular cartilage lesions were encountered in at least 1 of every 100 knee arthroscopies.[1] Another large study reported similar findings after reviewing 25,124 knee arthroscopies and found that chondral lesions existed in 60% of the patients.[2] In consecutive knee arthroscopy series, focal chondral or osteochondral defects were found in 11% to 19% of the patients. The medial femoral condyle and the patellar articular surface were the most frequent localization of the cartilage lesions with an average defect area of 2.1 cm.[2–4] It has been suggested that patients under the age of 40 years may benefit more than older patients after cartilage repair surgeries. Patients under the age of 40 with localized high-grade chondral lesions comprised of 5% to 11% of all analyzed patients in these large series.[1–4] Although the natural history of these defects is largely unknown, several studies showed that, if left untreated, these defects caused a deterioration in the affected knee and may progress to symptomatic degeneration of the joint.[5–7]

Damage to the articular cartilage occurs for a variety of reasons, including chronic mechanical overload, developmental or genetic predisposition, and traumatic impact.

Trauma is one of the most common inciting events for cartilage injury with 61% of patients who underwent knee arthroscopy relating their current knee problem to a previous trauma.[4] The majority of lesions are found concomitantly with meniscal and anterior cruciate ligament (ACL) injuries.[8,9] Additionally, mechanical malalignment of the extremity and maltracking of the patella may lead to or aggravate cartilage defects when they both occur within the same joint.[10] So before undertaking a cartilage repair procedure, condition of the menisci and ligaments, instability of patella, and alignment of the extremity must be considered regardless of the chondral defect treatment technique.

It is obvious that restoration of a neutral biomechanical environment is the single most important factor for the success of any cartilage repair procedure.[11] In normal knee alignment, the medial compartment bears more than 60% of the physiologic load and in flexion an increasing amount of stress is transmitted through the medial side. Furthermore varus malalignment of the lower extremity disrupts this load distribution and even a 4% to 6% increase in varus malalignment increases the load in the medial compartment by up to 20%.[12] In a cadaveric model it has been demonstrated that loading is nearly equally distributed between the medial and lateral compartments for alignments of 0 degrees to 4 degrees of valgus.[13] Achieving more valgus after osteotomy results in unloading of the entire medial compartment; however, athletes and high-demand patients cannot tolerate such degrees of overcorrection. Therefore when performed simultaneously with cartilage repair procedures, osteotomy should restore neutral alignment rather than overcorrection.

If patellar or trochlear lesions occur with patellar maltracking or instability, these extensor mechanism pathologies should be corrected prior to or concomitantly with the cartilage repair procedures. In a similar concept, patellar malalignment or maltracking with an increased Q angle can lead to overloading of the lateral cartilage and increase the contact pressures.[14] With tibial tubercle osteotomies, realignment of the extensor mechanism and relief of patellofemoral contact stresses can be achieved.[15] A distal realignment with anteromedialization of the tibial tubercle by 10 mm can reduce the pressure applied to lateral patellar cartilage without overloading medial cartilage.[16] Recently a systematic review was performed to determine whether a difference exists in outcomes of combined ACI and osteotomy versus isolated ACI with a minimum 2 years follow-up. Both groups showed improvements but when individual studies were compared, significantly greater clinical outcomes in subjects undergoing ACI combined with osteotomy were observed.[17]

A high incidence of articular cartilage lesions associated with ACL injuries is well recognized, where the chondral injury is attributed to the actual, acute traumatic ACL injury.[18] Articular cartilage is exposed to high shear forces either from the initial trauma to the knee or due to chronic instability secondary to the ACL tear. An increased risk of cartilage degeneration over the medial tibial plateau and patella has been shown if this ligamentous disruption is not treated properly.[18] Furthermore, several studies have reported increasing incidence and severity of cartilage lesions with a delay in ACL reconstruction.[19,20] This highlights the importance of ligament stability in patients undergoing cartilage repair procedures regardless of the technique used.

The knee meniscus protects the articular cartilage by both increasing the joint congruity and contact area and preventing the focal concentration of stresses.[21] Complete or partial loss of a meniscus can have deleterious effects on a cartilage leading to a progression of osteoarthritis.[22] Therefore meniscal repair should be the preferred option for patients with a meniscal lesion. Unfortunately, meniscectomy is unavoidable in the lesions that are not amenable to repair. In selected symptomatic patients with previous total or subtotal meniscectomy, meniscal transplantation can be a viable treatment option. Indications for meniscal transplantation are still being defined and the ideal candidate should be a young patient with joint line pain correlated with previous meniscectomy in a well-aligned and stable knee. Despite the fact that meniscal allograft transplantation is utilized as a salvage procedure in a majority of studies, the reported early and midterm results after meniscal allograft transplantations are encouraging with a survival rate of 75% to 87.8% at 5 years.[23,24] Furthermore, when combined with articular cartilage repair procedures, improvements in both objective and subjective outcome measures were comparable to results of these procedures performed in isolation.[25] However, there is insufficient literature reporting on the long-term outcomes of allograft meniscal transplantation. In a recently published prospective study high rates of failure have been detected due to deleterious remodeling of allograft. Authors suggested that preoperatively, patients should be counseled about the need for potential additional surgeries in the future given these findings.[26]

CLASSIFICATION

With regard to the macroscopic evaluation of the cartilage surface, routinely performed at the time of surgery by arthroscopic or open means, the two most commonly used cartilage classification systems are the Outerbridge and International Cartilage Repair Society (ICRS) (Table 96.1).[27] Different from radiographic classifications, which are numerous, these two classification systems standardize and take into account the ability of the surgeon to physically palpate the chondral surface and grade the cartilage quality.

HISTORY

Many times, distinct differences exist with the patient's presentation of focal chondral lesions and more global knee chondromalacia and arthrosis. Careful listening to the patient's descriptive history can provide guidance as to the potential underlying pathology. Whether it is the timeline of symptom onset, a recounting of previous traumatic injury, or even the detailing of prior surgical procedures, all of these details can provide important information. Activity-related pain in the knee with associated

TABLE 96.1 Classification Systems for Cartilage Lesions

Grade of Lesion	Outerbridge Classification	ICRS Classification (With Subclassifications)
Grade 0	Normal cartilage	Normal cartilage
Grade 1	Cartilage with softening and swelling	(a) Softening or fibrillations (b) Superficial fissuring
Grade 2	Partial-thickness defect with fissures on the surface that do not reach subchondral bone or exceed 1.5 cm in diameter	Less than one-half cartilage depth
Grade 3	Fissuring to the level of subchondral bone in an area with a diameter more than 1.5 cm	More than one-half cartilage depth (a) Not to the calcified layer (b) To the calcified layer (c) To the subchondral bone (d) Blisters
Grade 4	Exposed subchondral bone	Osteochondral lesion violating the subchondral plate

ICRS, International Cartilage Repair Society.
Excerpt from Farr J, Gomoll AH. *Cartilage Restoration: Practical Clinical Applications*. New York, NY: Springer-Verlag; 2013:42, Table 4.1.

swelling, and possibly focal throbbing and aching after cessation of the activity, is commonly reported. This can be more pronounced with higher-impact activity such as sports participation and running and less noticeable with low impact-activities such as walking. Large chondral defects with associated displaceable flaps or even unstable chondral segments with associated loose bodies can become interposed within the joint surfaces, thus not only causing pain but also progressive damage to other initially uninvolved cartilage segments. These symptoms could also manifest as mechanical locking, giving way, crepitus, and sharp, lancinating pain.

PHYSICAL EXAMINATION

Just as it is absolutely paramount to listen to the patient's history to guide a thought process as to the potential etiology and chronicity of their presenting pathology, it is also just as important to carefully perform a physical exam to elicit even the most-subtle of physical exam findings. Many times, this can help guide your treatment regimen even prior to considering additional diagnostic imaging if indicated. Unless in an acute presentation, an acute hemarthrosis is unlikely. Typical findings can include mild soft tissue swelling with variable joint effusion size, joint line tenderness upon palpation and possible focal tenderness to the femoral condyle or patellar facets, possible varus/valgus pseudo-laxity depending upon how much unicompartmental chondral loss is present, standing varus or valgus malalignment, positive findings for patellar maltracking of J sign or excessively tight lateral retinaculum, possible quadriceps atrophy from an inhibitory mechanism, and also an antalgic gait to the symptomatic side.

IMAGING

While basic information can be obtained with a normal 3-view study of the knee (anteroposterior [AP], lateral, and merchant view), the most information can be obtained from a weight-bearing Rosenberg view (45-degree flexion posterior–anterior view) as well as weight-bearing both limb full-length alignment films. These two weight-bearing films help to not only quantify the amount of joint space narrowing and relative chondral involvement to include potential subchondral sclerosis or collapse but also the weight-bearing axis of the affected limb in question. Computed tomography (CT) scans can also be helpful but of limited utility for everyday use. CT scans, to include CT arthrograms, can be useful in the setting of evaluating subchondral and osseous lesions, displaced osteochondral segments, assessments of the sequelae of prior surgical cartilage restoration procedures performed, and for patients unable to obtain magnetic resonance imaging (MRI) secondary to medically related contraindications. MRI is truly the workhorse of not only the in-office evaluations of articular cartilage but also in the research setting. The improvement in many cartilage-specific imaging protocols has dramatically improved the visualization and quantification of chondral and osteochondral lesions. T1-rho imaging, from a research perspective, is quite useful as an indirect way of evaluating the water content and glycosaminoglycan (GAG) content of articular cartilage, as well as its ability to review other

biochemical markers for chondral health.[28,29] While stronger MRI magnets have become more prevalent and can provide better resolution, it is the desired image sequences that are of importance when reviewing the cartilage as well as the remaining knee structures, such as meniscus, ligaments, tendons, and even bone. While there are many radiographic-based scoring systems to assess the structural outcomes from cartilage restoration procedures, still none of these to date correlate with the clinical outcomes of these procedures.[30] CT and MRI scans, combined, can also provide valuable information for defining patellofemoral pathology as it pertains to chondral-based lesions and the potential for underlying maltracking. Both the tibial tubercle trochlear groove (TTTG) and the tibial tubercle posterior cruciate ligament (TT-PCL) measurements can be obtained on each. More often, the TTTG is used. The normal range for the TTTG is less than 15 mm, whereas an elevated distance is defined as greater than 20 mm. CT-based measurements have been shown to be more reproducibly accurate than MRI-based assessments, with the latter resulting in discrepancies in measurements by up to 4 mm.[31] These measurements can be helpful in guiding treatment measures should specific patellar facet chondral lesions exist in the setting of an elevated TTTG.

DECISION-MAKING PRINCIPLES

Indications for Cartilage Restoration

Presuming there is no gross block to range of motion (ROM) or loose osteochondral fragment from either an acute injury or from chronic repetitive trauma, conservative care is the mainstay for initial treatment of articular lesions and defects. Physical therapy, to include activity modification and pain modalities, and adjuncts are important, but also a global picture of body habitus and weight reduction is vital if applicable. Injection therapy has shown equivocal results in the literature. While the heterogeneity of viscosupplementation molecular weights and processing as well as the stage of arthritis reported in the literature adds to these equivocal results, a recent systematic review reported a positive benefit for younger patients with early chondromalacia treated with intra-articular hyaluronic acid injection therapy.[32] Surgical treatment is indicated in grade III or IV full-thickness chondral lesions after conservative nonoperative treatment measures have failed to provide adequate symptom relief. At this point, not only is it important to discuss with the patient what their expectations are moving forward, but also the expectations of what the surgical procedure can yield in terms of outcomes and longevity of symptom relief.

Contraindications

Inflammatory arthropathies, tricompartmental arthrosis, coronal malalignment, meniscal deficiency, collateral or cruciate ligament laxity, smoking, and obesity (BMI >35) are all considered contraindications to cartilage restorative procedures unless corrected prior to or during the surgery, if applicable. While tricompartmental arthrosis is considered a strict contraindication, in young patients with intolerable symptoms and no other available treatment options cartilage restoration procedures can still be considered.

Treatment Algorithm

There are multiple factors that interplay to determine what cartilage restoration procedure would be best served to address the patient-specific symptomatic complaints at hand. Having said that, the lesion location and size are the two main considerations when determining a treatment strategy. More commonly, the medial femoral condyle and the patellofemoral joint are the main locations where focal chondral lesions occur. Given the tibiofemoral and patellofemoral compartments see drastically different forces directed throughout their arc of motion, compression versus shear respectively, different surgical treatment modalities should be considered for each.

Osteochondritis Dissecans Lesions

Treatment decisions in osteochondritis dissecans (OCD) lesions are based on the presence of open growth plates, size, stability, and displacement of the fragment. Stable OCD lesions in juvenile patients with an open physis should be treated nonoperatively because these lesions have a greater tendency toward resolution and healing. However, if the fragment is displaced, every attempt should be made to reduce and fix the unstable fragment in patients with either open or closed physis. Headless compression screws and bioabsorbable pins can be used for fixation with satisfactory union rates.[33] In some cases, fragments are not amenable to fixation due to comminution or inadequate subchondral component of the fragment. Removal of unstable fragments as a sole procedure is reserved for patients with low functional demands or those who are unable to follow rehabilitation protocols after repair. In long-term follow-up studies radiographic evidence of early degenerative joint disease was found in 65% to 71% of patients who underwent excision of OCD without any cartilage repair techniques.[34,35] A recently published randomized trial has compared the outcomes of osteochondral allograft transplantation (OAT) and microfracture procedures for the treatment of OCD in young active athletes at an average of 10 years follow-up. The OAT technique allowed for a higher rate of return to and maintenance of sports (75%) at the preinjury level compared with microfracture (37%).[36] Another multicenter study revealed functional improvement and pain relief in 85% of patients after ACI despite the complexity and severity of the osteochondral lesions.[37] Fresh OAT is another option for treatment for OCD lesions of the femoral condyle with 70% good or excellent results.[38]

Patient Age and Defect Chronicity

The age-dependent outcomes of marrow stimulation techniques are still continuing to be reported today. Cell numbers and their metabolic activity decline over time resulting in poor healing response in older patients. As a result, the clinical success rate of microfracture has been most consistent in patients under the age of 40 years.[39,40] However, failure rates of other cartilage restoration techniques in older patients, such as ACI, OATs, and osteochondral allografting, are comparable with rates reported in younger patient groups.[41] Depth of injury is also found to be age-related. Adolescents tend to develop osteochondral lesions, whereas adults have a tendency to get pure chondral lesions, possibly because of the well-developed and matured calcified zone.[42] Time since onset of symptoms is an essential variable that should be taken into account because delayed treatment tends to result in less-predictable outcomes whereas significant improvements in the clinical scores were more frequent with a preoperative duration of symptoms of less than 12 months.[40,43]

TREATMENT OPTIONS

Before planning a treatment procedure, patient-specific and lesion-specific variables must be taken into consideration. Physical condition and readiness of the patient for an extended rehabilitation program, concomitant knee pathologies, and limb alignment hold the key for success or failure in cartilage repair.[44] There are several techniques described for the management of cartilage lesions. Examples of current attempts at cartilage restoration include marrow stimulating techniques, osteochondral autografts, autologous chondrocyte transplantation, particulated juvenile cartilage allograft, and OAT.[45] Débridement and lavage is one of the most basic options and indicated for low-demand older patients with small lesions.[46] Although symptomatic relief from this technique is not likely predictable, arthroscopic débridement can reduce pain in more than half of the patients; however, this benefit generally diminishes after 1 year.[47] Additionally, unstable chondral flaps and loose bodies that cause mechanical symptoms can be removed with a very short recovery time and can be repeated if needed. Currently this technique is reserved for small lesions found incidentally during arthroscopy or low-demand patients who could not adjust to activity or weight-bearing restrictions postoperatively.

Marrow Stimulation

Biological rationale behind marrow stimulation techniques is that direct stimulation of mesenchymal stem cells (MSCs) in the subchondral bone could direct these cells to the chondrogenic pathway to initiate a healing response. Marrow stimulating techniques have been used to treat cartilage defects since 1959 when Pridie introduced subchondral drilling with K-wires.[48] Later Johnson described the abrasion of sclerotic lesion with a burr to expose vascularity, providing a tissue bed for blood clot attachment.[49] Finally Steadman introduced the microfracture technique to avoid heat necrosis from drilling. In his technique, the bone plate is not completely destroyed in comparison to an abrasion chondroplasty.[50] Microfracture involves débridement of loose and unstable cartilage back to a stable rim. Then specially designed awls are used to make multiple perforations, or microfractures, into the subchondral bone plate. Perforation of subchondral bone results in the influx of marrow elements with the formation of blood clot in the defect. It is important to create a well-contained lesion because rims will support the fibrin clot within lesion. As noted it is crucial to breach the calcified cartilage layer to gain better access to the bone marrow stroma.[51] This calcified layer appears to be at least 6 mm beneath the surface of the articular cartilage. Thus a routine awl will not be sufficient to breach this calcified layer in most knees, and it has been suggested that nanofracture technique will allow for deeper drilling to overcome this obstacle.[52] Histologic findings showed that drilling to a depth of 6 mm had superior results in an animal model compared with drilling to 2 mm, without a deleterious effect on the subchondral bone.[53,54] Over time this blood clot is slowly remodeled into primarily fibrocartilage rather than normal hyaline articular cartilage. Mature fibrocartilage is predominantly type I collagen with minimal amounts of type II collagen, resulting in a less-durable construct with inferior wear characteristics. The advantages of marrow stimulation techniques include their minimal invasive nature with low technical demands and favorable cost-effectiveness ratio. On the other hand, they require a prolonged restricted weight-bearing period of 4 to 6 weeks and use of a continuous passive motion (CPM) device for 6 to 8 hours per day, for 6 weeks.[55]

Osteochondral Autograft Transfer

Osteochondral autograft transfer technique involves transfer of one or more cylindrical osteochondral plugs into the cartilage defect. The lesions should be small to medium-sized (0.5 to 4 cm^2) because the amount of donor tissue available is limited.[56,57] Single or multiple small osteochondral plugs can be harvested to match the lesion's diameter. Traditionally plugs are harvested from less-weight-bearing areas of articular surface, such as the periphery of the trochlea and the intercondylar notch. The lesion is prepared with a punch to create a recipient socket that matches the plugs. Both preparing the socket and harvesting plugs require tubular cutting instruments such as OATS (Arthrex, Naples, FL), mosaicplasty (Smith and Nephew, Andover, MA), or COR (Depuy Mitek, Raynham, MA) to place plugs orthogonal to the articular surface to avoid graft obliquity. Multiple plugs can be used to fill larger defects, but it could be difficult to match the contour of the defective articular surface to the donor plug.[58] Elevated angled grafts relative to articular surface result in elevated contact pressures, so it is suggested to leave an edge slightly sunk rather than elevated.[59] Thus ideal locations for osteochondral autograft transfer are the convex surfaces of the femoral condyles rather than the patellofemoral joint and tibia with their varying surfaces, which make plugs more difficult to fit in place.[60] It is crucial to place grafts in a press-fit fashion for maintaining stability until osseous integration of the plug and socket occurs. This procedure offers several advantages over microfracture or chondrocyte implantation techniques, including the ability to perform the procedure in a single-stage operation, transplanting an autogenous living hyaline cartilage, decreased cost, and relatively brief rehabilitation period.[61] Major limitations of this procedure include donor site morbidity and the limited availability of grafts. Residual gaps between plugs may affect the quality of healing and there is an inherent risk for cartilage or bone collapse. The postoperative recovery requires a short period of non-weight bearing and the use of a CPM for up to 6 weeks.

Autologous Chondrocyte Implantation

The rationale behind ACI is to cover the cartilage defect with autologous chondrocytes, which have been cultured in vitro. This technique was first described by Brittberg et al. in 1994 and is one of the first tissue engineering techniques for articular cartilage regeneration.[62] ACI is currently a two-stage procedure. First a cartilage biopsy (weight 200 to 300 mg) is taken from a non-weight-bearing area of the affected joint and transferred to a laboratory. The chondrocytes are isolated from the cartilage tissue by enzymatic digestion and then expanded in monolayer culture. The optimal density of the cells during reimplantation remains debated. Generally, a final concentration of 2 to 3×10^7 chondrocytes/mL is recommended for medium-sized defects, but the number of available cells is limited by the amount of cartilage that can be collected.[63] This expansion amplifies the total number of cells for implantation, allowing the surgeon to fill the cartilage defect. The cell suspension is returned to the defect during the second stage of the procedure and held in place with a periosteal patch or membrane. ACI can be performed for high-demand patients who have failed arthroscopic débridement or microfracture. The technique is indicated for larger (2 to 10 cm^2) symptomatic lesions involving the femoral condyles, trochlea, and the patella.[64] The primary theoretical advantage of ACI is to provide hyaline-like cartilage rather than fibrocartilage, resulting in better long-term outcomes and durability of healing tissue. Clinical results are encouraging and overall the patients are satisfied.[65,66] This technique is however not without its limitations. These include technical complexity and cost of the two surgical procedures, de-differentiation of chondrocytes during in vitro expansion and periosteal graft delamination, and late periosteal hypertrophy.[67–69] Also, previous marrow stimulation techniques have a strong negative effect on outcomes of subsequent cartilage repair with ACI, limiting its use as a salvage procedure.[70] Second-generation ACI procedures involve use of collagen sheets to replace periosteal flaps. These collagen matrices avoid graft harvesting and donor site morbidity and using cell-free collagen sheets dramatically eliminated adverse events related to graft hypertrophy and delamination.[71] In the third generation of ACI the cultured chondrocyte cells are seeded directly onto a biodegradable porcine type I/III collagen scaffold. Matrix Autologous Chondrocyte Implantation ([MACI] Genzyme, CA) method has been in clinical use for a number of years in Europe and is now approved by the Food and Drug Administration (FDA) and available in the United States.[72] This enables three-dimensional (3D) culture of chondrocytes, aiming to prevent de-differentiation and loss of phenotype. Uneven distribution of chondrocytes within the defect and the potential for cell leakage from the defects that often lack intact cartilage rims can be prevented through using scaffolds.[73] Additionally, the scaffolds used may act as a barrier to fibroblast invasion.[74] Outcomes of these techniques have been promising and are at least equivalent to those achieved with ACI, with reported good clinical medium-term results.[72,75] The postoperative treatment is broadly similar to marrow stimulation techniques while time periods are generally extended. Rehabilitation should focus on maintaining muscle function and joint flexibility, with the use of CPM. Full weight bearing is avoided for 8 to 12 weeks.

Particulated Juvenile Cartilage Allograft

In the past, allograft transplants were limited to osteochondral grafts because it has been generally accepted that graft incorporation to host tissue was only possible at the bone level.[76] The concept that cartilage could be transplanted without its underlying bony component is a fairly new and innovative approach. Particulated juvenile cartilage allograft technique DeNovo NT (Zimmer, Warsaw, IN) uses human juvenile allograft articular cartilage minced into small pieces. Mechanical mincing of cartilage into 1- to 2-mm pieces was crucial for successful cartilage repair. This promotes chondrocytes escaping from the extracellular matrix (ECM), multiplying and migrating to surrounding tissues to form a new hyaline-like cartilage tissue matrix that integrates with the surrounding host tissue.[77–79] Cartilage is retrieved from the femoral condyle of donors aged 0 to 13 years. Because juvenile chondrocytes are capable of producing greater amounts of ECM compared with mature chondrocytes, these cells also do not stimulate an immunogenic response in vivo.[80,81] DeNovo NT has an average 40-day shelf life similar to a fresh osteochondral allograft. During surgery, fragments are mixed with fibrin glue to make a putty-like structure to fill the osteochondral defect so that no sewing of a patch is needed.[79] Each package contains 30 to 200 particles and fills defects up to 2.5 cm^2, so multiple packets can be used for larger lesions. The use of DeNovo NT has the advantage of being a single-stage procedure and offers unlimited graft material for large lesions. At postoperative period patients are limited in weight-bearing for 2 weeks for small lesions, and 6 weeks for larger lesions.[78] Although the preliminary clinical reports show encouraging results, clinical data are still limited.

Osteochondral Allograft Transplantation

Fresh OAT entails the transfer of size-matched cadaveric osteochondral graft into the cartilage defect. After standardizations had been established for graft storage in the late 1990s, fresh osteochondral allografts became commercially available from tissue banks and thus accelerated the more widespread use of these tissues.[82] This type of transplantation offers some advantages over other cartilage repair techniques for treatment of wide and deep osteochondral lesions given its ability to replace medium to large osteochondral defects in all locations and contours. Additionally, the cartilage defect is replaced with articular cartilage rather than fibrocartilage in a single-stage operation. In most treatment algorithms, OAT is the only current biologic salvage option when previous treatments have failed. Another advantage is that failure does not preclude other reconstructive procedures, such as a second graft procedure or arthroplasty.[83] Historically, bulk allografts resulted in collapse at the osseous part of the graft, rather than failure at the articular cartilage itself. The subchondral bone and marrow components of the graft may elicit a strong immune response resulting in incomplete osseous integration due to the slow process of creeping substitution.[84] Therefore OAT with cartilage-bone composite thicknesses of only 6 to 8 mm yields the best result in the management of shallow lesions.[76] The disadvantages include graft availability, limited shelf life, accurate size matching, technical difficulties, cost, and concerns with possible disease transmission. However, small risk of disease transmission has been minimalized with stringent screening of donors and modern serologic and microbiologic clearance testing. Postoperative rehabilitation is tailored according to type of surgery and stability of allograft used and includes non-weight bearing for 6 to 8 weeks and the use of a CPM machine.

POSTOPERATIVE MANAGEMENT

Rehabilitation is a key factor to achieve greater success regardless of which type of cartilage restoration technique is applied. The primary goal for rehabilitation following cartilage restoration is the provision of an optimal environment for the functional recovery and adaptation of the chondral healing tissue.[85] However, treatment goals may differ between professional athletes and recreational players. Considering the short duration of professional careers, athletes desire to return to their previous high-demanding activity level in a very short recovery time whereas pain relief can be adequate for nonathletic patients. Besides biology of repair technique, patient- and lesion-specific variables should be considered when planning a rehabilitation program. Thus an individualized rehabilitation should be performed for every patient.[86] In general, current rehabilitation protocols can be divided into three phases aiming at protection of the graft by a gradual increase in weight bearing and active ROM.[87] The first phase is a proliferation period that covers the first 6 weeks after the surgical procedure. The main goal in this phase is graft protection and that patients limit their weight bearing during this period. To prevent muscle atrophy and joint stiffness, low-resistance isometric strengthening exercises should be introduced as soon as the patient can tolerate. During this phase, a CPM machine is used for 6 to 8 hours per day to reduce adhesions. Separate rehabilitation protocols are required for the patellofemoral and tibiofemoral joints due to differences in joint kinematics. Generally patellofemoral lesions demonstrate a slow advance in ROM but allow a faster progression of weight bearing when compared to lesions located in femoral condyles.[85] Weight bearing can be modified to the type of surgery performed. In contrast to marrow stimulation techniques and ACI, early weight bearing could be tolerated in osteochondral autograft or allografting procedures. Furthermore size of the lesion and stability of graft, as well as the procedures performed for concomitant pathology, such as ligamentous reconstruction, meniscal repair, and osteotomies, govern how early weight bearing can be introduced. After this initial phase, rehabilitation is followed by a transitional phase with increased load bearing and progressive ROM exercises. Together with closed-chain and gentle strengthening exercises, proprioceptive training is introduced in this period as well if the patients tolerate. The final remodeling phase of rehabilitation generally begins 3 months after surgery. In this phase, patients are gradually introduced back to normal daily activities and allowed to perform light sporting activities. However, they need to continue with muscle, proprioceptive, and sports-specific rehabilitation exercises.[88] The rehabilitation periods after cell-based therapies such as ACI and microfracture tend to be more conservative and longer than osteochondral transfer and transplant procedures. Recently a randomized study compared the traditional approach (12 weeks) of postoperative weight-bearing rehabilitation with the accelerated approach (8 weeks) in patients who underwent

MACI to the femoral condyles. While the visual analog scale (VAS) demonstrated significantly less frequent pain at 5 years in the accelerated group, there were no other significant differences between the 2 groups. Outcomes of this randomized trial demonstrate a safe and effective accelerated rehabilitation protocol that provides comparable clinical outcomes.[89] Overall, the rehabilitation period is a complex process and requires a multidisciplinary approach to understand postoperative symptoms as they occur and address them in a timely fashion. So, a stepwise and systemic rehabilitation is recommended for an individualized protocol. This allows not only the best chances at recovery and a return to sports at the preinjury level but also to continue professional careers and reduce the risk for reinjury or joint degeneration.[86]

Return to Play

Return to previous levels of athletic activity is the main goal for athletes who undergo cartilage restoration procedures. Before returning to sports participation, athletes should have a pain-free and stable extremity with full ROM. Athletes should fully understand that high-impact activities jeopardize the repair tissue. High-impact and pivoting activities should be delayed until a stable, healed tissue is obtained. Return to play (RTP) is generally influenced by several factors such as athlete's age, preoperative duration of symptoms, level of play, lesion size, and repair tissue morphology.[90] Rate for return to sports is higher for younger and more competitive athletes.[91] A comprehensive review of 2549 patients, treated with different surgical techniques, revealed an overall 76% return to sport rates at 2 years postoperatively, with the highest rates of return after osteochondral autograft transfer (93%), followed by OAT (88%), ACI (82%), and microfracture (58%). The same study also showed the fastest return to sports was at 5.2 months and was achieved with osteochondral autograft transfer compared to 9.1 months for microfracture, 9.6 months for OAT, and 11.8 months for ACI.[92] Age ≥25 years and preoperative duration of symptoms ≥12 months negatively affected the ability to return to athletic activity.[93]

 Authors' Preferred Method

Articular Cartilage Lesion

Previous algorithms have been developed that not only take into account patient activity and demand levels, but also guide a decision-making process with regard to the defect size and location in the knee (Fig. 96.1).[94]

In the following section we discuss five commonly used current techniques for the treatment of chondral and osteochondral lesions in our clinical practice.

Marrow Stimulation

Marrow stimulation/microfracture is a prevalent procedure and is performed most commonly through an arthroscopic approach. The setup for a basic knee arthroscopy is performed and the patient is positioned per routine. Should posterior articular lesions be anticipated, then it is important that maximal knee hyperflexion be attainable during the procedure and a knee positioner can be useful.

Approach and Defect Preparation

After completing the diagnostic arthroscopy and confirming the presence of the chondral defect, it is important to débride all loose chondral flaps by shaver or curette while at the same time establishing stable vertical shoulders to the chondral lesion. The importance of this step at creating vertical shoulders cannot be overstated. This can be done with varying curettes or even an 11 blade or Beaver blade (Fig. 96.2). Next, remove the calcified cartilage layer by curette.

Marrow Stimulation

After thorough preparation of the defect, a microfracture awl or K-wire on power can be used to create multiple holes. It is important to remain orthogonal to the defect surface, either by changing the flexion of the knee, changing portals, using different angled awls, or by creating new portals as needed. It is vital to not place the holes too close to each other to avoid fracturing the subchondral plate and creating an unstable subchondral segment. Doing this properly and routinely allows roughly 3 to 4 holes to be placed in a 1 cm² area (Fig. 96.3). Placement of holes directly at the shoulder edges improves the fibrocartilage cap transition to the native cartilage. Turning the arthroscopic inflow off and critically evaluating for punctate bleeding or fatty marrow content egress is required to ensure an adequate depth has been reached during the procedure (Fig. 96.4). It is the senior author's recommendation that should this technique be employed, it is recommended to start at the peripheral shoulder edge of the lesion and then work centrally.

Wound Closure

Routine closure of the arthroscopy portals is performed and full range of motion (ROM) is allowed. Fifty percent partial weight bearing and immediate ROM is instituted, possibly with use of a CPM, to help protect and sculpt the fibrocartilage cap as it formalizes for the first 6 weeks.

Osteochondral Autograft Transplantation

Osteochondral autograft transplantation can be used as either an open or arthroscopic procedure. Many times this can be dictated based upon the osteochondral lesion location, size, or surgeon's preference. A basic knee arthroscopic setup is performed with the use of a tourniquet to help with visualization from both the open graft harvest and transplantation. Once again, a knee positioner can be useful to provide adequate hyperflexion of the knee should the articular lesion be in the posterior condyles.

Approach, Graft Harvest and Defect Preparation

The chondral/osteochondral lesion is identified by arthroscopic visualization. Additional arthroscopic portals are made as needed, after localizing with spinal needle, to ensure the defect preparation and graft placement is orthogonal to the lesion's surface. An arthroscopic ruler (Fig. 96.5), sizing rod, or probe can be used to measure the defect size, taking into consideration any undermined and delaminated cartilage flaps at the periphery of the lesion that might need to be resected prior to sizing the lesion.

Potential donor locations for graft harvest include the lateral or medial trochlea as well as the intercondylar notch. A maximum of three large osteochondral plugs can be obtained, up to 8 mm each, from the far lateral trochlea, which is the senior author's preferred location (Fig. 96.6).

Continued

📌 Authors' Preferred Technique

Articular Cartilage Lesion—cont'd

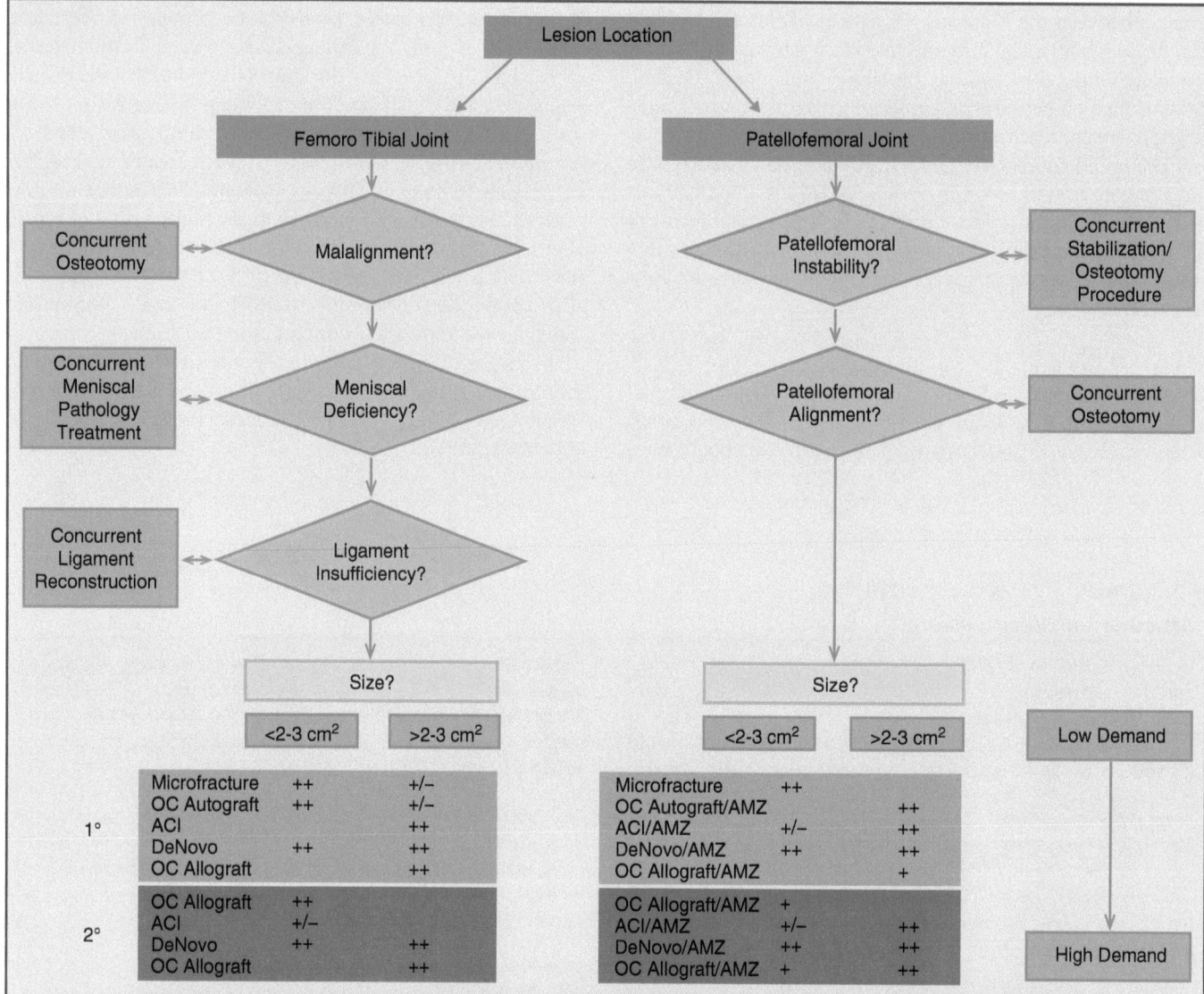

Fig. 96.1 Knee chondral and osteochondral lesion algorithm addressing location, size and treatment options. (Modified from Alford JW, Cole BJ. Cartilage restoration, part 2: techniques, outcomes, and future directions. *Am J Sports Med.* 2005;33[3]:443–460.)

Sometimes, arthroscopic harvest of the osteochondral plugs can be performed; however, it is more reproducible to gain access by a small 2- to 3-cm parapatellar incision and arthrotomy in order to visualize the donor site. While many proprietary systems are available, we routinely use a system that has a coring reamer with a serrated tooth at its end. This allows for a clean cut at the end of the transplantation plug and easier retrieval. Each plug is harvested to a depth of at least 10 to 12 mm while remaining completely orthogonal to the articular surface. The definitive size and depth of the osteochondral plug are measured and the graft placed on the back table still in the harvester tube.

Next the recipient chondral lesion site is prepared. This can be done arthroscopically if the lesion is in the other compartment of the knee or through the arthrotomy site if it is ipsilateral to the harvest location. Now knowing the size and depth of the autograft plug, the defect is drilled line to line and to the same depth taking into consideration the cartilage cap height (Fig. 96.7). While drilling the lesion, consideration for any slight obliquity of the donor plug can be adjusted for with the drill at that time so that it can be matched to the recipient site articular curvature as best as possible.

The harvester tube with the plug is then inserted at the same angle (either arthroscopic or open), the plug is gently moved into place by a plunger, and final adjustments are made with a size-appropriate tamp (Fig. 96.8).

Great care is taken to ensure the graft is flush, if not slightly recessed, and not proud (Fig. 96.9). This process is repeated step by step, with graft harvest, recipient site preparation, and graft placement, until the articular lesion is effectively treated. Multiple smaller plugs can be used for a mosaicplasty or two larger plugs in a "snowman" configuration can be placed to treat more oval shaped defects. The donor site can be either backfilled with synthetic graft, allograft, or left unfilled. Final arthroscopic images are obtained to critically evaluate the overall transplantation construct.

Wound Closure

Routine closure of arthroscopic portals is performed and the parapatellar arthrotomy is closed in successive layers. Fifty percent partial weight bearing with 0 to 90 degrees ROM is allowed for the first 6 weeks. It is important to monitor for a postoperative hemarthrosis that can significantly limit range of

Articular Cartilage Lesion—cont'd

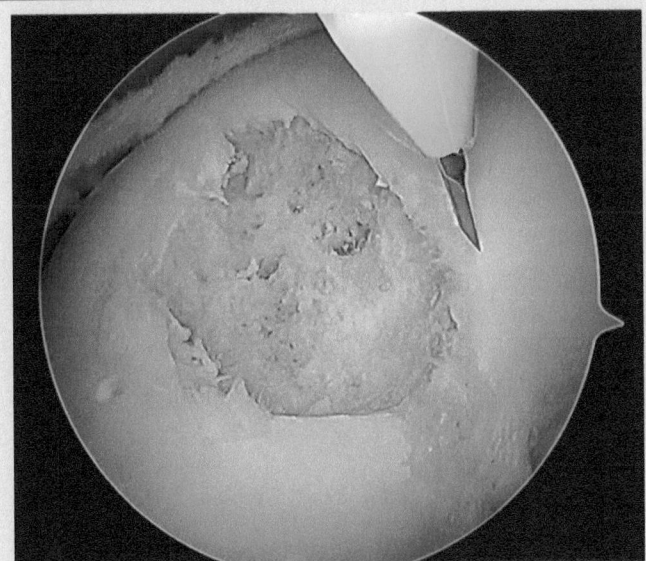

Fig. 96.2 Note the vertical shoulders created by the beaver blade at the periphery of the lesion.

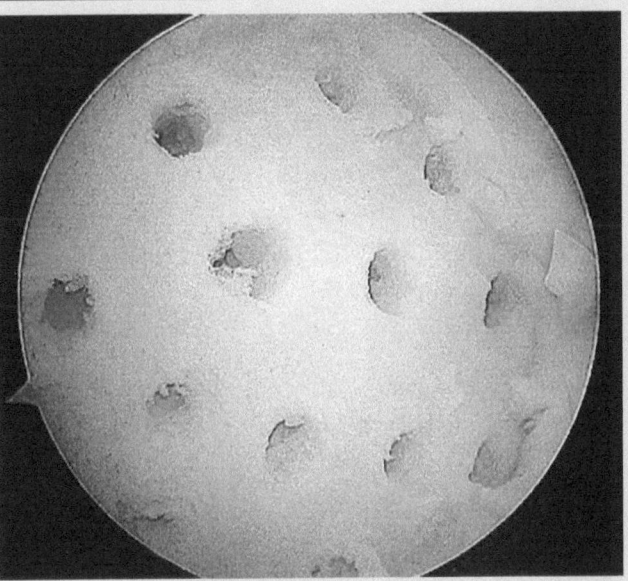

Fig. 96.3 Microfracture awl is used to create multiple punctate trans-subchondral plate perforations.

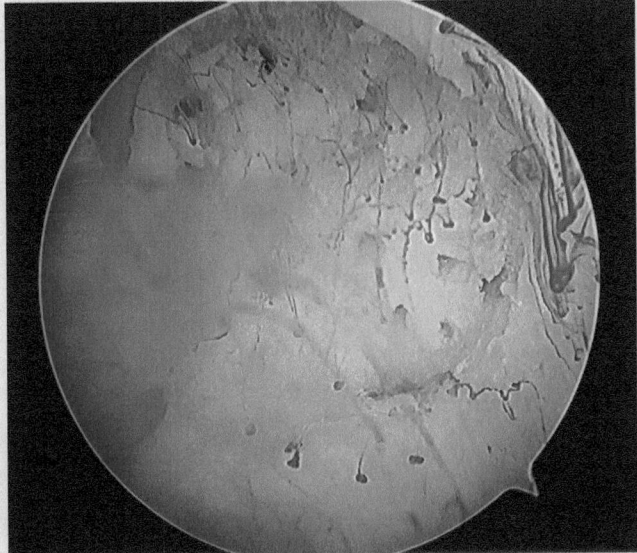

Fig. 96.4 Note the marrow element egress from the microfracture perforations.

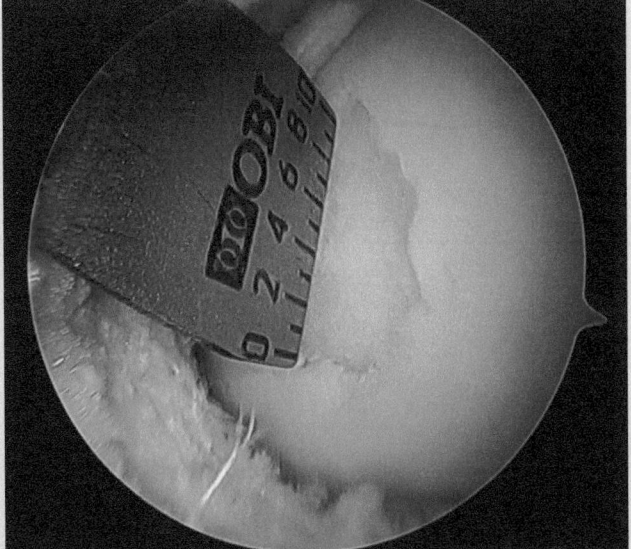

Fig. 96.5 Arthroscopic measurement of chondral defect.

motion or cause quadriceps inhibition. Sterile serial aspirations can be performed as needed.

Autologous Chondrocyte Implantation

Once the arthroscopic cartilage biopsy has been completed and the culture finalized, usually taking 6 weeks, the cell suspension is ready for implantation. Standard patient positioning for an open knee procedure can be used; however, a knee positioner can be useful for far posterior lesions, which helps with maintaining deep knee flexion throughout the case. Should the surgeon wish to use a periosteal patch, then it is important to drape out to the level of the mid tibia or to at least include the surgical site of choice.

Approach and Defect Preparation

Compartment-specific paramedian incisions with parapatellar arthrotomies can be used for isolated single lesions; however, a standard utilitarian midline incision with medial parapatellar arthrotomy can be used to gain access to multiple lesions of the knee. Possible fat pad retraction/resection might be necessary for visualization. A bent Homann is placed into the intercondylar notch for patellar retraction. As per any cartilage restoration procedure, it is vital to create a recipient site conducive to healing for the procedure to succeed. Débridement of devitalized tissue and creation of vertical shoulders at the defect's articular edges is performed. It is the senior author's recommendation, though, that if excessive resection were to turn a contained lesion into an uncontained lesion,

Continued

Authors' Preferred Technique
Articular Cartilage Lesion—cont'd

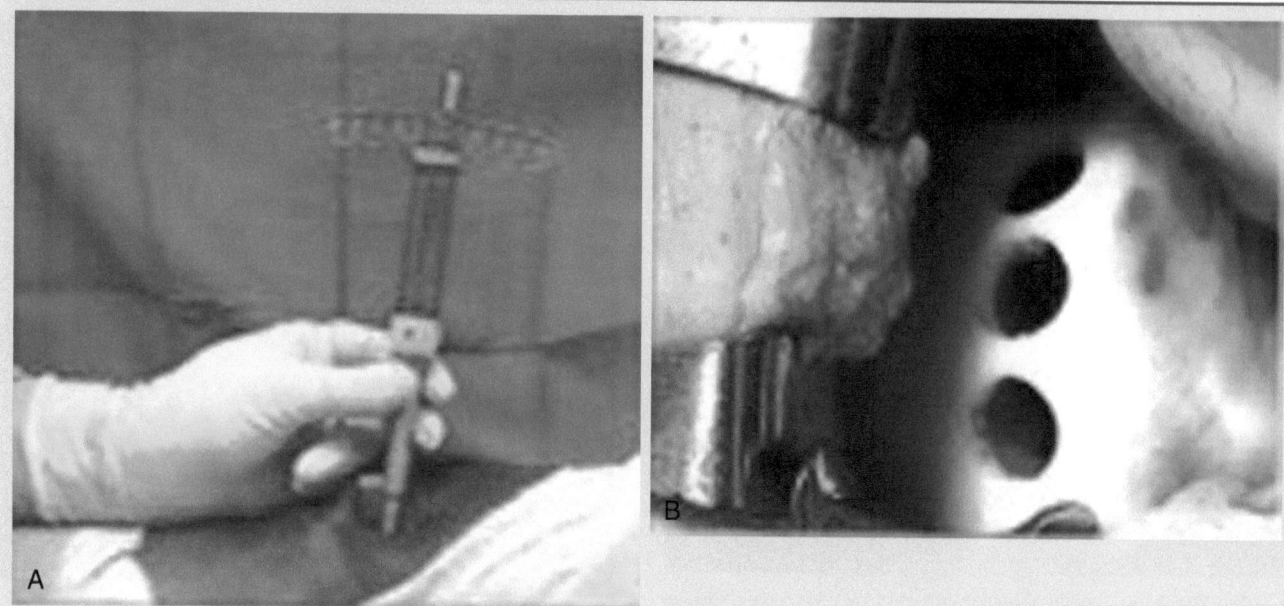

Fig. 96.6 (A) and (B), Note the orthogonal position of the harvester to the articular surface, not the extremity.

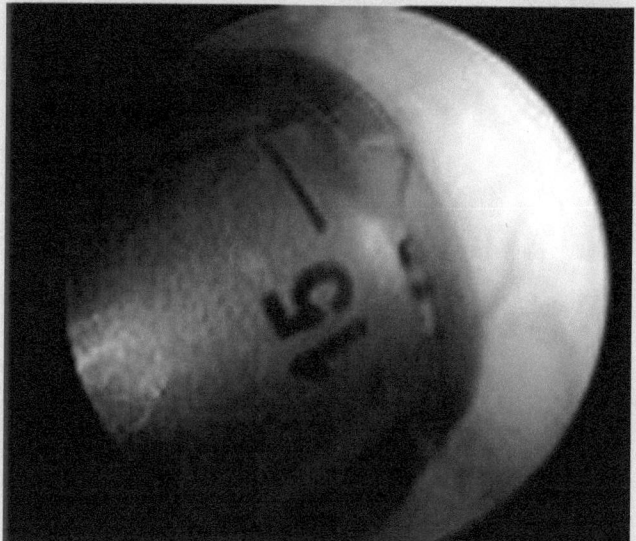

Fig. 96.7 Lesion is drilled to the same depth as the measured osteo-chondral plug.

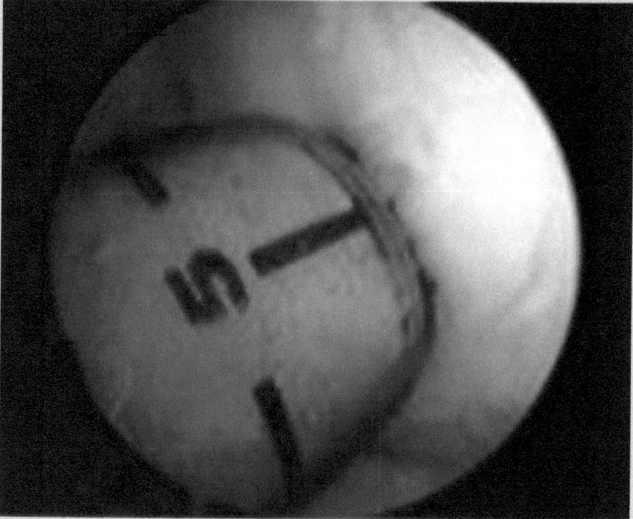

Fig. 96.8 Critical to ensure same angle of insertion as the defect was drilled (see Fig. 96.6) and to monitor the transplanted chondral surface depth in relation to the native cartilage surface so that it is flush or slightly recessed.

then it would be best served to leave a slight rim of degenerative cartilage tissue present to suture to than to be faced with needing other forms of patch fixation to maintain the implanted cells. It is important to maintain the subchondral plate/bone layer. Should previous failed surgical procedures from OAT or marrow stimulation techniques be present, a sharp curette or burr can be used to gently freshen and decorticate the bone without breaking the subchondral plate. If bleeding from the defect base is encountered, then very minimal amounts of thrombin or fibrin glue can be considered for use. Once the defect has been prepared for implantation, the size is measured with glove paper. Should a periosteal flap be used, this should be oversized by approximately 2 to 3 mm given it will shrink slightly upon its harvesting. This will also allow an adequate suture line to be placed to the

articular cartilage, lessening the tension on the repair. Some surgeons prefer to use an artificial membrane or collagen I/III bilayer patch, however, currently this is off-label use in the United States and should always be discussed with the patient preoperatively.

Periosteal Harvest
Should a periosteal patch be desired, the most reproducible location for harvesting is the proximal medial tibia, just distal to the pes anserinus. The skin incision can either be extended distal past the sartorial attachment or an additional

Authors' Preferred Technique
Articular Cartilage Lesion—cont'd

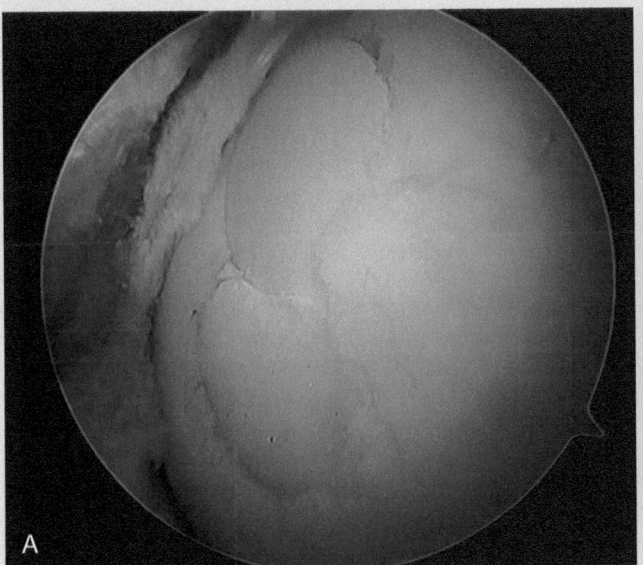
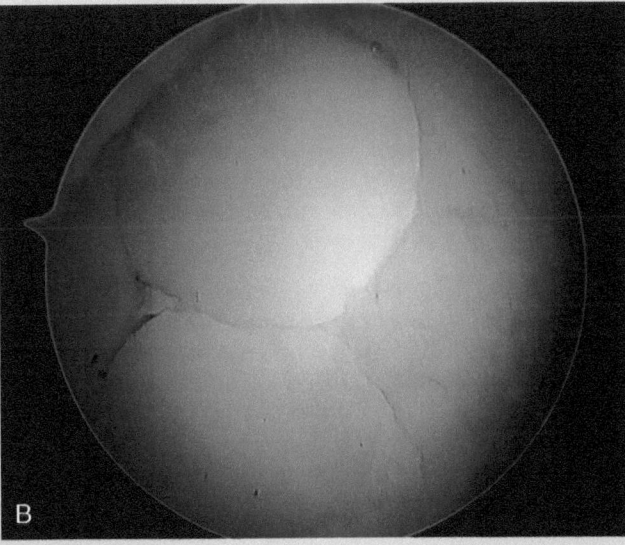

Fig. 96.9 (A) and (B), Note the flush contour of the osteochondral plug placement to native articular chondral curvature.

incision can be made, approximately 3 cm distal to the pes, which can usually be palpated with the hamstring insertions as a landmark or it can be measured roughly at 5 cm distal to the medial joint line. After satisfactory soft tissue dissection to the tibial periosteum, the glove paper template is used to mark and incise the periosteum with a fresh 15 blade. Great care should be used when teasing the patch off the bone and can be done so with a sharp periosteal elevator. Once procured, immediately spread out the patch on a moist ray-tec. This helps to avoid its desiccation and shrinkage.

Patch Fixation
Once the defect has been prepared, the patch is placed over the lesion with the cambium layer down against the defect and stretched out with nontoothed forceps. Should a collagen patch be used, the glove paper template is used and it is usually cut dry and then hydrated. The collagen patch will sometimes increase in size upon rehydration and so minimal resections might be necessary for final fit and placement. Approximately a 1- to 2-mm rim should still be maintained at the patch periphery to help with the suture placement interface. Using a 6-0 Vicryl or Biosyn on a P-1 cutting needle immersed in mineral oil to help with smooth passage, the sutures are placed through the patch and then the articular cartilage, attempting to exit roughly 3 mm away from the defect's articular edge. This will nicely evert the edge and provide a better seal against the defect shoulder. Routinely sutures are initially placed at the 3, 6, 9, and 12 o'clock positions and tension is placed so that the patch is centralized. All of these steps limit further trimming, limit suture cut through, and allow the patch to sag into the defect. The knots are tied on the patch side below the articular edge. Additional sutures are placed circumferentially to seal the patch; however, a small defect is left at the most superior aspect to allow an angiocath to be introduced for cell implantation. The seal can be tested prior to cell implantation by injecting saline using a tuberculin syringe and an angiocatheter. Any residual leakage can be corrected with additional suture placement or with fibrin glue if it is small enough. The saline is aspirated by angiocatheter once the seal is confirmed to dry the bone bed for implantation.

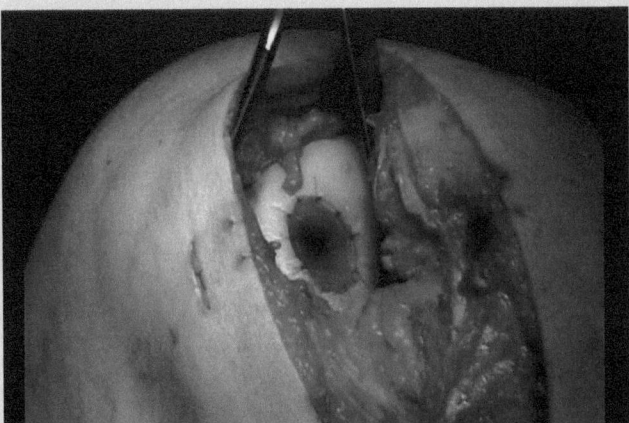

Fig. 96.10 Note the completed Matrix Autologous Chondrocyte Implantation method (MACI) procedure with sutured and sealed borders after cell implantation.

Cell Implantation
After resuspending the cultured cells, a 16 g needle on a tuberculin syringe is used to aspirate the suspension. Exchanging to at least an 18 g angiocatheter, the tip is inserted into the superior patch defect and placed into the inferior-most aspect of the patch. While retracting the tip, the suspension is injected into the defect and careful watching of the patch fill is performed. Final sutures or fibrin glue are used to seal the superior patch defect once the cells have been implanted (Fig. 96.10).

Wound Closure
The arthrotomy is closed in successive layers per routine. Given the nature of the procedure, a drain is not recommended as it could potentially damage the recipient site. Protected weight bearing is allowed with 0 to 90 degrees range

Continued

Authors' Preferred Technique

Articular Cartilage Lesion—cont'd

of motion for the first 6 weeks; however, for patellofemoral lesions, progressive increases in ROM at 30-degree intervals are allowed every 2 weeks given the more shear-force nature of that cartilage location.

Juvenile Particulate Allograft Cartilage Transplantation

Approached through an open arthrotomy more commonly than by arthroscopic means, this procedure can be used as either an independent procedure or in combination with a routine diagnostic arthroscopy, where the arthroscopy can better delineate the lesion prior to grafting.

Defect Preparation and Graft Application

A paramedian incision with parapatellar arthrotomy can be used to gain access to all lesions throughout the knee. Similar to marrow stimulation and ACI, stable vertical shoulders are paramount as well as débriding all devitalized tissue and the calcified cartilage layer by either curette or blade (Fig. 96.11). It is important to resect any undermined or delaminated chondral surface that would "peel away" and not provide a stable transition zone or interface with the graft. While keeping the lesion base dry, a thin layer of fibrin glue is applied. Next, at least 1 vial per 2.5 cm² is used to layer/fill the defect. Great care is taken to limit excessive filling of the defect so as to not allow a prominence of cartilage irregularity. A final thin coat of fibrin glue is then placed over the defect to seal the allograft cartilage transplant. Again, great care is taken to not place so much graft material and fibrin glue in a single location that there is a gross elevation of the grafted surface relative to the native articular surface curvature (Fig. 96.12).

Wound Closure

Gentle irrigation of the knee joint is performed after the fibrin glue has cured and the arthrotomy is closed in successive layers per routine. Given the technique employed, a drain is not recommended as it could damage the grafted defect site. Fifty percent partial weight bearing is allowed with 0 to 90 degrees ROM for the first 6 weeks; however, for patellofemoral lesions, progressive increases in ROM at 30-degree intervals are allowed every 2 weeks given the more shear-force nature of that cartilage location.

Osteochondral Allograft Transplantation

OAT is reserved for large, isolated chondral and osteochondral lesions. The patient is positioned supine on a well-padded operating room table with a knee positioner if far posterior condylar work is to be performed, which allows for knee hyperflexion. A tourniquet can be useful for visualization while preparing and reaming the lesion site. A mega-OAT procedure will be described for both cylindrical and oblong-shaped lesions.

Approach and Defect Preparation (Mega-Osteochondral Allograft Transplantation)

Although a utilitarian midline incision with a medial parapatellar arthrotomy can be used, paramedian skin incisions can also be utilized with a lesion location-compartment specific arthrotomy performed. Some surgeons prefer a subvastus or mid vastus quadriceps sparing approach given the potential for accelerated postoperative rehabilitation. The senior surgeon recommends using a medial paramedian or a lateral paralateral incision specific to the involved condyle. The patella is retracted with a bent Homann, which is placed carefully into the intercondylar notch. Retraction and/or resection of Hoffa's fat pad can help with visualization.

After identification of the lesion, the abnormal cartilage is measured (Fig. 96.13). It is important to attempt to reconstitute the articular surface congruity with the allograft transplant segment. A cannulated trephine reaming system can be used to size the defect initially. Sometimes this can be accomplished with a single plug, but sometimes two plugs in a "snowman" configuration might be needed to repair the defect if it is oblong in nature. However, more recently, the senior surgeon has been using an oblong-shaped graft procurement system to address these more asymmetric lesions and this will be described below. From a technical perspective, the symmetric cylindrical lesions routinely are prepared first and the graft is then obtained, whereas for the asymmetric oblong-shaped lesions, the system requires you to procure the graft first, with measured depth of graft obtained, and then prepare your lesion site.

For symmetrically contained lesions within a cylindrical shape, the lesion is measured with a reamer sized to adequately resect the lesion. After placing a

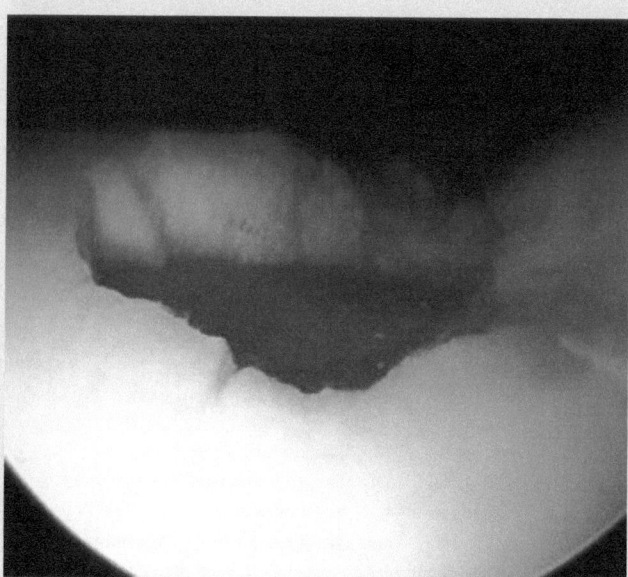

Fig. 96.11 Note the vertical shoulder of the trochlear lesion once prepared.

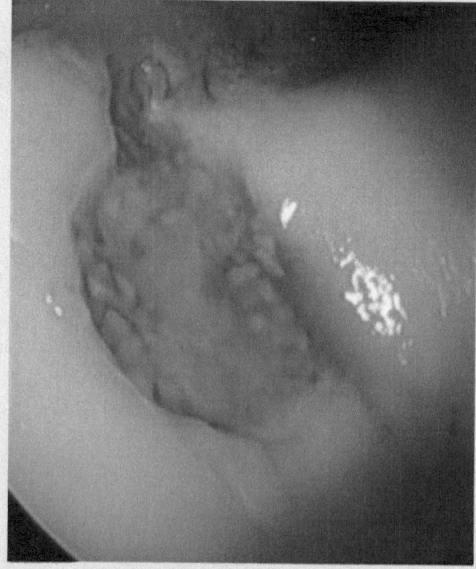

Fig. 96.12 Note the particulate graft material layered into the lesion defect with fibrin glue layer placed superficially.

Authors' Preferred Technique
Articular Cartilage Lesion—cont'd

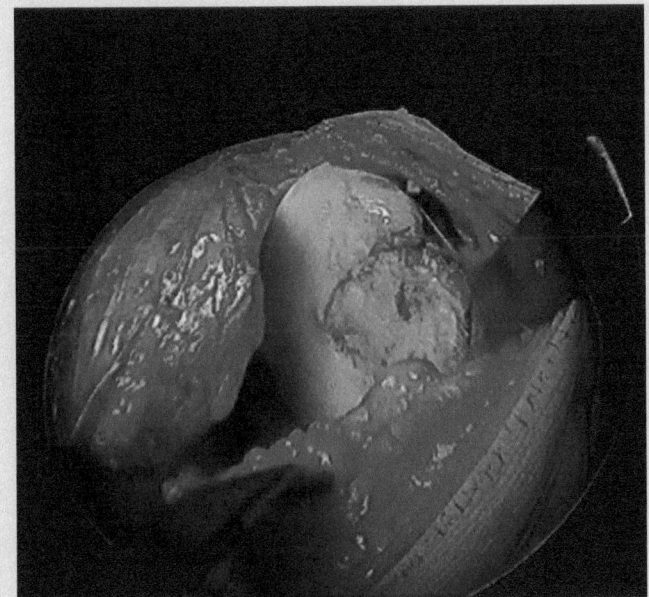

Fig. 96.13 Note the more cylindrical-shaped lesion on the lateral femoral condyle. (Courtesy Dr. Eric Carson.)

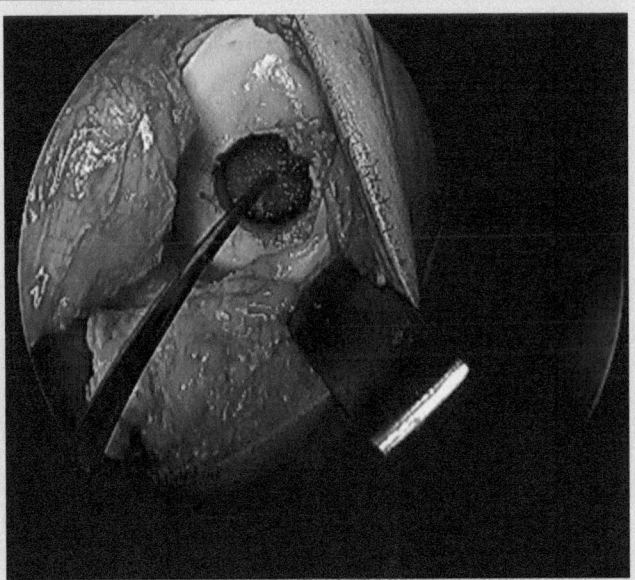

Fig. 96.14 Appropriately sized trephine reamer is selected and adequate osteochondral resection performed of the diseased articular segment in Fig. 96.13. (Courtesy Dr. Eric Carson.)

guidewire in the center of the lesion, a 6- to 8-mm deep recipient socket is usually created with a cannulated reamer (Fig. 96.14).

In an attempt to limit thermal necrosis, great care is taken to use irrigant at the lesion site as it is prepared and reamed, especially if there is sclerotic bone. After cylindrically reaming the lesion and confirming the depth of the recipient site, drill holes can be placed in the site's floor to help promote healing. Should significant cysts be encountered, then it is the senior author's recommendation to backfill these defects, after débriding the cyst's walls to healthy bleeding bone, with autologous bone graft.

Graft Procurement and Placement
After securing the allograft hemicondyle on the back table, the same-sized line-to-line cylindrical coring reamer is selected. It is imperative to recreate the same articular arc, and so the coring reamer is placed directly over the corresponding articular graft segment desired. This is done by direct visualization and palpation. The cylindrical graft is extracted from the reamer and its depth trimmed on the back table to what was measured during the lesion site preparation. This helps to ensure adequate depth upon placement so that the grafted surface is flush with the native articular surface. It is also marked for correct orientation prior to placement. Final preparation of the recipient site with a calibrated dilator can be used as needed and the allograft can then be press-fit with manual pressure and ranging the knee so that the graft reduces. This is completed to satisfaction

until it is deemed stable and the articular surface is flush (Fig. 96.15). Should additional fixation be needed if concern exists for stability, then absorbable headless screws can be used.

For asymmetric lesions contained within an oblong shape, selecting the appropriate oblong sizer to cover the native lesion is performed. It is then used to confirm the location of the correct area on the allograft that will become the procurement donor site. This reproducibly allows the articular congruity and arc of the procured graft segment to match the native articular curvature. Securing the graft to the workstation, the corresponding oblong cutter is used to obtain the graft and oscillating saw with jig is used to cut it at the correct depth transversely. Next the recipient site is prepared by proprietary system techniques of a scoring device, cylindrical reamers, and box cutter to remove final remnants of bone. The site is cleared of debris, a dilator used, the graft is placed by hand, and a tamp is used for gentle, final impaction/adjustments (Fig. 96.16). Should fixation be a concern, then once again headless bioabsorbable screws can be used as needed.

Wound Closure
Satisfactory irrigation followed by layered arthrotomy closure is to be performed with drain use as per the surgeon's preference. Protected weight bearing is allowed and 0 to 90 degrees for the first 6 weeks is allowed to protect graft incorporation.

Continued

Authors' Preferred Technique

Articular Cartilage Lesion—cont'd

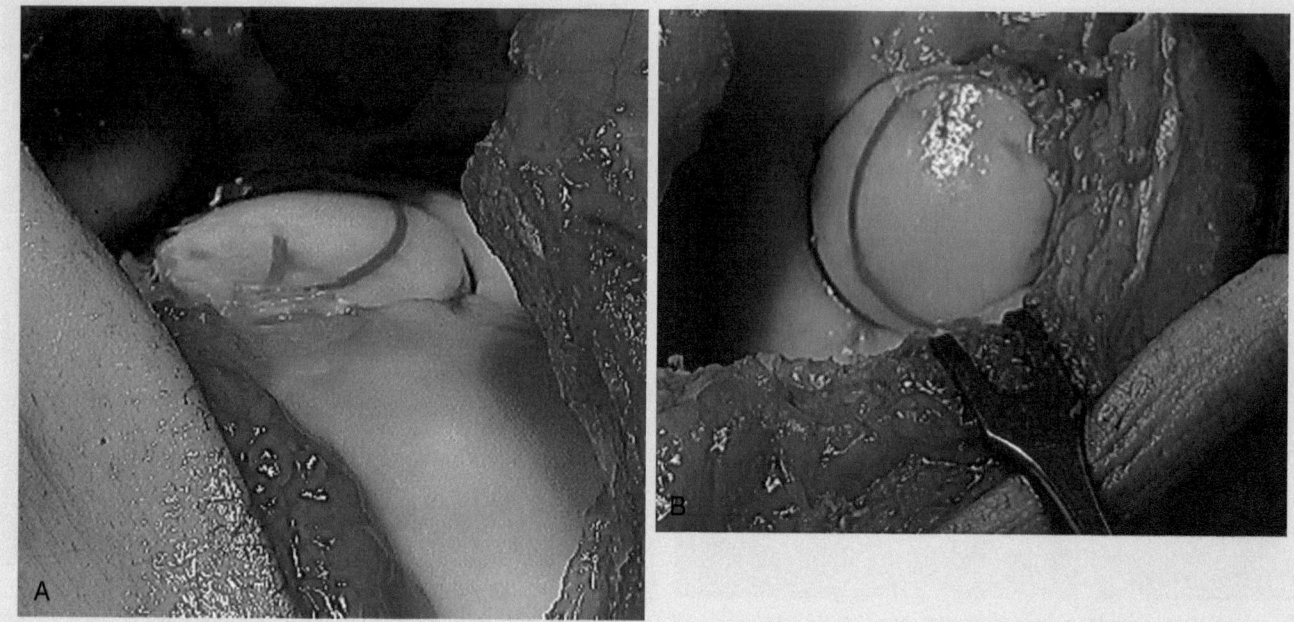

Fig. 96.15 (A) and (B), Note the articular surface congruity with satisfactory placement of the osteochondral allograft segment. (Courtesy Dr. Eric Carson.)

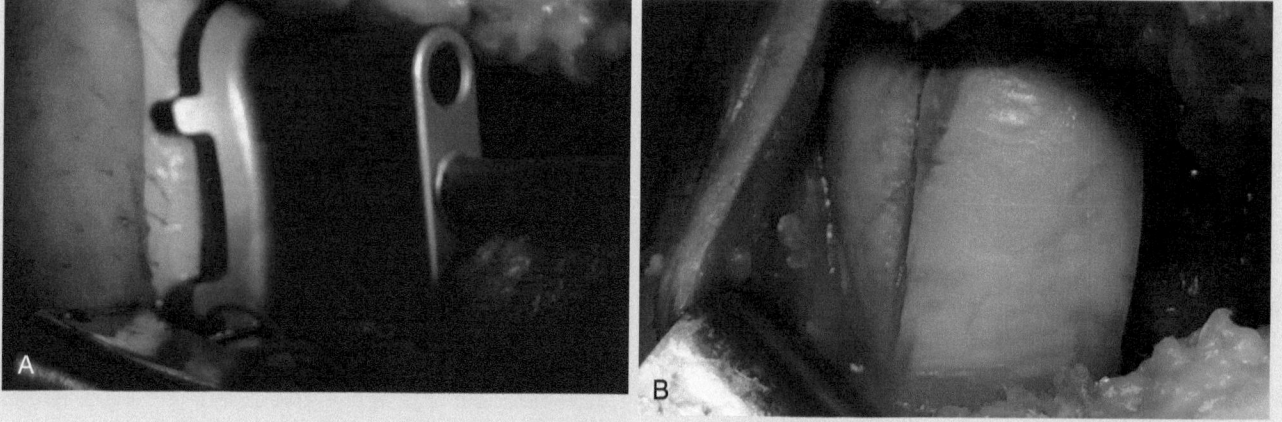

Fig. 96.16 (A) and (B) Oblong defect measured with sizer and final allograft placement after harvest. Again, note the articular congruity and satisfactory placement.

SURGICAL TECHNIQUE RESULTS

Marrow Stimulation

Marrow stimulation/microfracture techniques result in the formation of an intralesional collection of MSCs and blood products. This has the potential to formalize into a fibromyxoid tissue layer, with the predominant type of cartilage being type I cartilage, or fibrocartilage. Focal contained lesions less than 4 cm² in athletically active patients less than 40 years of age were found to have demonstrated G/E outcomes in 70% of patients.[95] However, long-term follow-up has revealed a decrease in sports participation and decrease in symptom relief associated with this procedure.[95] Recent literature comparing marrow stimulation to autograft OAT procedures in athletes showed a higher rate of return to sporting activity and maintenance of sporting activity compared to preoperative status in OAT patients as well as cost benefit analyses suggesting a lower cost to RTP in patients undergoing OAT procedures over marrow stimulation.[36,96] Longer-term 10-year outcome data, reviewed in a meta-analysis recently, have also revealed that the OAT procedure may achieve a higher activity level and a lower risk of failure for lesions even greater than 3 cm² compared to microfracture and that the risk of failure with microfracture was 2.4 times that seen with OAT.[97] Additional study findings have also implicated marrow stimulation procedures with complicating secondary cartilage restoration procedures, such as ACI, with inferior clinical results and higher associated failure rates.[70,98] Recent reports also highlighted the risks associated with microfracture; that disruption of the subchondral plate could predispose the bone to the development of subchondral cysts and fragile bone subsequently accelerating osteoarthritis.[52,99] Optimal outcomes are achieved in the following setting: age less than 40 years old, body mass index less than 30, no prior cartilage surgery, symptom duration less than 12 months, lesion size less than 4 cm^2, preoperative Tegner score greater than 4, and postoperative MRI evidence of lesion fill greater than 66%.[40,100] The drawback of this technique is the high recurrence rate of symptoms in long-term follow-ups.[101] Given the type of cartilage produced at the lesion site with marrow stimulation, the long-term viability and durability is currently the concern with this procedure as is evident in its longer-term outcomes when compared to other cartilage restoration procedures.

Osteochondral Autograft Transfer

The osteochondral autograft transfer procedure advantage is that it uses local articular cartilage. Seventeen-year clinical results in an athletic population, with lesions measuring 1 to 4 cm^2, reported G/E outcomes in 91% of condylar lesions, 86% in treated tibial lesions, and 74% in trochlear lesions.[56,57] Slight deterioration of results was noted at the 9.6-year follow-up time point for this athletic population. Additional long-term reported outcomes at 10- to 14-year follow-up, state 40% poor outcomes, defined as later knee arthroplasty or a Lysholm score of 64 or lower. These poor outcomes were associated with female gender (61%), patient age greater than 40 years (59%), and a defect larger than 3 cm^2 (57%).[102] Subset analysis of those patients who were younger than 40 years and had an articular cartilage lesion less than 3 cm^2 showed a failure rate of only 12.5% and a favorable Lysholm score of at least 82. Conversely, for women over the age of 40 years with a chondral lesion over 3 cm^2, the failure rate was 83%.[102] Additional prognostic risk factors resulting in a favorable outcome have been reported as male gender, medial femoral condyle defects, OCD, deep, small defects, and the shortest time delay to surgery.[103] A prospective randomized study in young active athletes under the age of 40 has also shown significant superiority of mosaicplasty over microfracture for the repair of articular cartilage defects in the knee. At an average of 6.5 months, 93% of OAT patients returned to sports activities at the preinjury level. On the other hand, 52% of microfracture athletes could return to sports at the preinjury level.[104] Current evidence suggests that OAT is a viable option to be considered for chondral lesions measuring less than 3 cm^2, however, the clinical results do have the potential to start decreasing at roughly the 10-year point and that preoperative risk factors of age, gender, lesion location, lesion size, and chronicity can play a role in longer-term outcomes.

Autologous Chondrocyte Implantation

Long-term studies have demonstrated good to excellent results after ACI. Favorable factors for ACI include younger patients with fewer than two previous procedures on the same knee, a less than 2-year history of symptoms, a single defect, and a defect

on the trochlea or lateral femoral condyle.[44] Depth of lesion is also reported as a risk factor for failure. Some authors suggest grafting the bony defect before application of ACI if the depth of the lesion is greater than 8 to 10 mm.[105] Long-term outcome studies have shown favorable results for ACI treating condylar lesions with graft survivorship rates of 71% at 10-year follow-up and nearing 75% improved functional status.[106,107] Subgroup analysis revealed that concurrent high tibial osteotomy had a protective effect and increased graft survivorship.[107] A recent study with 4-year follow-up data treating patellar lesions with ACI has shown statistically significant improvements in clinically assessed physical outcome scales with 86% rating their knees as G/E at final follow-up.[108] A previous randomized controlled trial comparing ACI to microfracture clearly found that while no gross differences existed between the two procedures at 5 years with regard to clinical improvement or progression of radiographic arthrosis, subgroup size analysis did reveal that lesions greater than 4 cm^2 did poorly with microfracture and that ACI results demonstrated no correlation with lesion size.[109] As alluded to earlier, prior marrow stimulation procedures not only have been found to have a deleterious effect on outcomes, with a markedly higher graft implantation failure rate of 26% in patients undergoing ACI after marrow stimulation compared to an 8% failure rate of ACI as an index procedure, but have also shown inferior clinical outcomes associated with ACI after marrow stimulation procedures.[70,98] Ten-year results of a prospective randomized study comparing ACI and OAT for symptomatic articular cartilage lesions, mean size 4 cm^2, of the knee reported graft failure in 17% of patients in ACI group and 55% of patients in OAT group. Of note, the functional outcome of those patients with a surviving graft was significantly better in patients who underwent ACI compared with OAT.[110] Recent evidence suggests that neither lesion size nor location affects return to low or moderate sport athletic participation or even return to work rates; however, return to high-stress elite-level athletic participation is unlikely following ACI.[111]

One commonly reported complication found postoperatively at the 7- to 9-month point with the use of a periosteal patch is patch hypertrophy resulting in symptomatic clicking and popping, which can be a cause of subsequent surgery after ACI and which has been reported up to 36%.[41,112,113] While using a type I/III collagen patch has dramatically reduced this potential risk for hypertrophy to 5%, this is still off label use for the knee without FDA approval as of yet.[114]

While still not approved in the United States, MACI has 15-year reported outcome data overseas showing improved and maintained patient reported outcome measures compared to preoperative levels.[115] A prospective randomized trial compared the efficacy of MACI with microfracture for patients with symptomatic focal cartilage defects ≥3 cm^2. Clinical outcomes from baseline to 2 years were significantly more improved with MACI than with microfracture.[116] Additional research has also reported no significant implication of preoperative subchondral edema and MACI outcomes at 5 years with regard to patient outcomes for pain and symptoms or MRI-based cartilage assessments.[117] Unfortunately, there is recent literature that still focuses on the potential graft hypertrophy in MACI with rates that approach what was seen with periosteal patch ACI use.[118]

Particulated Juvenile Cartilage Allograft

Limited data exist for particulated juvenile cartilage allograft technique because this system was regulated as a minimally manipulated human allograft tissue and no clinical outcome data were provided during the approval process. However, short-term preliminary clinical reported data show encouraging results.[76,119] Recent 2-year follow-up revealed significant improvements in patient-reported outcomes, MRI T2 data showing a return of cartilage signal to near normal articular cartilage, and histologic evaluation detailing a mixture of hyaline and fibro-cartilage with more type II collagen than type I with excellent transition zones.[120] Improved patient outcomes have also been reported in the treatment of grade IV patellar lesions with corresponding near normalization of cartilage signal as seen on MRI with this treatment modality.[121] Further research and longer-term outcome data will be of interest to review as it is presented in the coming years.

Osteochondral Allograft Transplantation

Short-term follow-up data have revealed overall patient satisfaction rates of 86% at 58-month follow-up points in patients of a mean age younger than 40 years and a mean lesion of 6.3 cm^2 in size.[122] Additional studies have reported on the outcomes of OAT as the primary treatment for cartilage injury in patients with no previous surgical treatment. The majority of patients (86%) were extremely satisfied and survivorship was 89.5% at 5 years and 74.7% at 10 years.[123] A recent long-term mean 22-year follow-up study reporting on fresh OAT for patients younger than 50 years with unipolar condylar lesions greater than 3 cm^2 revealed graft survival at 10, 15, 20, or 25 years of 91%, 84%, 69%, and 59%, respectively.[124] Additional studies detailing OAT in the patello-femoral joint have not shown as reliable of graft survivorship, with rates approaching between 50% and 75% in studies reporting on a mean of 8- to 10-year follow-up data.[125,126] Overall, poorer results have been reported in older patients, bipolar and patellofemoral lesions, and corticosteroid-induced osteonecrosis when treated with OAT.[127–130]

COMPLICATIONS

Routine knee arthroscopy as well as open knee procedures carry the inherent risks of bleeding and infection, with the potential for their relative increase in risk compounded by comorbidities. With open procedures, an increased risk of infection, arthro-fibrosis, and injury to the infrapatellar branch of the saphenous nerve with parapatellar arthrotomy is always of concern. With additional procedures performed either open or arthroscopic, there is the potential for peroneal nerve and popliteal artery injury, although this is rare. Tourniquet-related compression/ischemia and peripheral regional nerve analgesia also carry an inherent risk with their use. Some previous complications directly attributable to the specific procedure performed have been mentioned already but in general, subchondral plate fracture or subchondral cyst formation with collapse in association with

marrow stimulation procedure, osteochondral autograft and allograft transfer with graft instability potentially requiring additional fixation or failure of union or fragmentation, and juvenile particulate allograft transplantation as well as ACI with the potential for graft hypertrophy and resultant abundance of scar tissue requiring subsequent surgery for resection or lysis of adhesions.

FUTURE CONSIDERATIONS

In the attempt to provide histologically normal-appearing cartilage with the hopes that this will translate into functionally viable and durable cartilage in the long term, the advancement of cartilage restoration procedures continues to evolve. Current clinical trials in the United States are under way comparing marrow stimulation techniques to NOVOCART 3D (Aesculap Biologics, Breinigsville, PA). This treatment modality of third-generation matrix-based ACI has been implemented in Europe already with reported follow-up data. These 3D scaffolds are seeded with autologous chondrocytes from a previous operation, where osteochondral plugs were harvested, and ultimately implanted. Bone marrow edema (BME) has been associated with these third-generation ACI techniques with possible influences on clinical outcomes. A recent study reviewing 3-year follow-up data using NOVOCART 3D found overall significant clinical improvements throughout and that the occurrence of BME did not correlate to clinical outcomes.[131] An additional short-term follow-up study has also shown the clinical benefits and radiographic improvements of NOVOCART 3D for large focal chondral and osteochondral defects.[132] However, just as with other ACI predecessors, graft hypertrophy still is a potential complication, with specific focus detailing NOVOCART 3D in more acute injuries such as acute chondral trauma or OCD, where these etiologies are at risk for developing graft hypertrophy as evidenced with 2-year follow-up data.[133]

A newer technology is porous osteochondral allograft material Cartiform (Osiris, Columbia, MD). With its cryopreserved, viable chondrocytes, chondrocyte growth factors, ECM, minimal bone thickness, and porosity, this implantable device when combined with a marrow stimulation technique allows for marrow elements to penetrate the graft during formalization of the intralesional mesenchymal clot. No studies have been performed on this implantable allograft material to date and there are no results to report as to its efficacy.

Finally, the harvesting of nasal chondrocytes for autologous cartilage tissue implantation into the knee for post-traumatic femoral chondral defects, 2 to 6 cm^2 in size, is a novel idea in the continued efforts to address intra-articular chondral lesions of the knee. In 10 patients, these nasal chondrocytes were then embedded into an ECM rich in GAG and type II collagen with frozen section analysis revealing the constructs maintained at least 70% viable chondrocyte cells. Histologic assessments also found viable type II collagen to be present as well as type I collagen at the construct periphery of the implantable tissue. While second look biopsy did not show typical architectural organization of articular cartilage, it did show at least 50% of tissue cells were round, surrounded by lacunae in ECM, which stained significantly for type II collagen and GAGs with only faint type I and X collagen. At 24-month follow-up, patient International Knee Documentation Committee (IKDC) scores and Knee Injury and Osteoarthritis Outcome Scores (KOOS) all significantly improved compared to preoperative levels. This study is still ongoing and it will be interesting to see if additional research in the future includes a controlled clinical trial.[134]

CONCLUSION

Cartilage restoration procedures are powerful tools and techniques whose potential benefit can be transformative for patients who meet their strict indications. It is paramount to consider the focal nature of the lesion, the overall limb alignment, status of the meniscus and ligament competency, size of the lesion, and the overall patient demand. While taking into account the patient's expectations is important when weighing which procedure might be of most benefit, it is also of vital importance to have upfront discussions with the patient to help manage overall long-term expectations as well.

For a complete list of references, go to ExpertConsult.com.

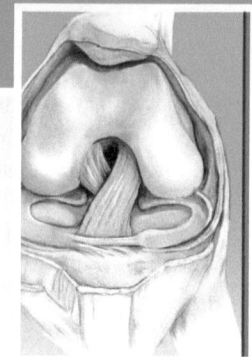

97

Frontiers in Articular Cartilage Treatment

Rachel M. Frank, Armando F. Vidal, Eric C. McCarty

Articular cartilage defects in the knee (Fig. 97.1) are common and often result in pain and dysfunction. Over the past several decades, research efforts have focused on better understanding how to diagnose and treat these lesions. Comprised predominately of type II collagen, articular cartilage is relatively avascular, depending on diffusion to obtain nutrients and oxygen, making spontaneous healing of articular cartilage defects exceedingly difficult.[1,2] Importantly not all defects are symptomatic, as many are simply incidental in nature, found on diagnostic imaging studies or during diagnostic arthroscopies being performed for other diagnoses, such as anterior cruciate ligament (ACL) tears. In fact, such defects are found in more than 60% of patients undergoing arthroscopy of the knee.[3-5] One of the first challenges, therefore, is determining which lesions should be treated, and which can simply be managed with "benign neglect."

For most patients, the combination of a thorough history, focused physical examination, imaging studies, and if necessary, a diagnostic arthroscopy, can determine if a given cartilage injury is symptomatic and warrants treatment. Once the diagnosis is made, a variety of treatment options are available. The optimal management for a given cartilage lesion varies based on lesion location (femoral condyle, tibial plateau, patella, trochlea), size, containment/stability, chronicity, and associated knee pathologies, including meniscus deficiency, ligament insufficiency, and/or malalignment. Bipolar "kissing" lesions (i.e., corresponding lesion on medial femoral condyle and medial tibial plateau, or on the patella and trochlea) are especially difficult to manage. In addition, factors unique to the patient, including age, activity level, expectations, body mass index, history of prior treatment, and ability to comply with rehabilitation, may influence the treatment decision. The goals of the patient are especially important to consider, as these may impact decision-making. For example, treatment for a high-level athlete hoping to return to the same (or better) level of play may differ from treatment for a weekend warrior who has already undergone multiple procedures and is hoping to manage activities of daily living without pain and swelling. Finally, surgeon- and facility-specific factors, including surgeon experience and the availability of treatments/products, will impact clinical decision-making. In most areas within the United States, for example, allograft tissue is readily available and can be considered as part of the treatment algorithm, whereas in many countries around the world, allografts are unavailable, and thus treatment for two very similar patients with two very similar defects can vary simply based on location.

Treatment for articular cartilage defects includes both nonoperative and operative options. Nonoperative options include activity modification, physical therapy with a focus on quadriceps and core strengthening, cryotherapy, oral nonsteroidal anti-inflammatory medications, and a variety of injectable agents, including corticosteroids, hyaluronic acid, and more recently, biologics. Biologic therapies have recently emerged as a potential treatment for a wide variety of orthopedic pathologies, including articular cartilage lesions, and can be administered both in the outpatient clinic setting as well as in the operating room. Biologic therapies, including platelet-rich plasma (PRP) and mesenchymal stem cell injections such bone marrow aspirate concentrate (BMAC), can be given either as isolated treatments, or combined with a surgical procedure. Surgical procedures for articular cartilage defects have historically been broken down into palliative (débridement, chondroplasty), reparative (marrow stimulation including microfracture), and restorative (autologous chondrocyte implantation, osteochondral autograft/allograft) procedures.[6-23] This chapter will focus on emerging surgical techniques for articular cartilage treatment. The advantages, disadvantages, outcomes, and complications associated with newer reparative techniques, including enhanced/augmented microfracture, as well as emerging reconstructive techniques, including matrix-associated autologous chondrocyte implantation, minced cartilage products, and off-the-shelf osteochondral allograft products, will be discussed in detail.[24-49] It should be noted that several of these emerging technologies and products have only recently been introduced in the United States, with many are unavailable unless the patient is enrolled in a clinical trial. The majority of such products have been introduced and studied in Europe and/or Asia prior to becoming available in the United States, and even then, products must be considered "minimally manipulated" or intended for "homologous use" in order to bypass the US Food and Drug Administration approval process.

SURGICAL MANAGEMENT

For any patient undergoing surgical management of an articular cartilage defect, it is critical to (1) discuss goals/expectations and (2) treat any associated malalignment, meniscus insufficiency, and/or ligament insufficiency.[50] Patients must understand the unclear natural history of articular cartilage lesions and sometimes unpredictable nature of articular cartilage lesion treatment, especially with respect to returning to high-level athletics. In

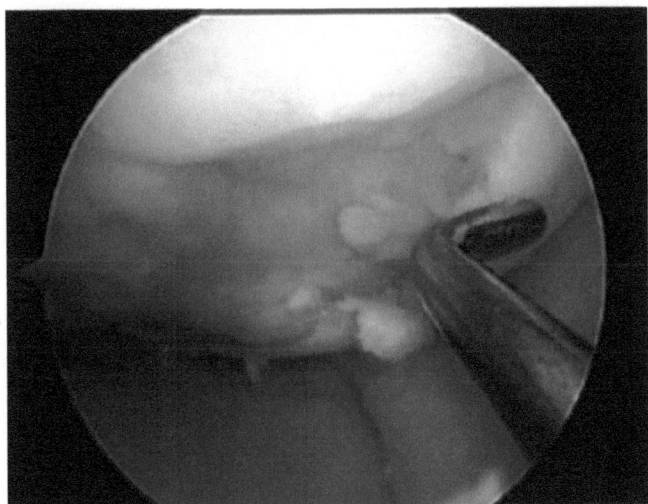

Fig. 97.1 Intraoperative example of a full thickness focal chondral defect of the medial femoral condyle (right knee).

addition, even with the most sophisticated articular cartilage treatments, unaddressed concomitant knee pathology is likely to result in failure of cartilage treatment, particularly in the setting of malalignment, as this may lead to overload of the newly treated cartilage lesion. While beyond the scope of this chapter, in some cases, isolated realignment osteotomy may be the ideal definitive solution for an articular cartilage lesion in a young patient with malalignment.

Palliative

Arthroscopic débridement, lavage, and chondroplasty continue to be viable treatment options for many patients with symptomatic, focal chondral defects who have failed nonoperative treatment. This approach is considered palliative as the goals are not to "regenerate" or replace cartilage, but rather to remove any flaps of loose cartilage that may be irritating to the patient and causing mechanical symptoms, and to stabilize the rim of the defect, decreasing the risk of further cartilage delamination. During the procedure, it is critical to débride the lesion down to the level of the subchondral bone, without violating the subchondral bone layer, taking care to maintain vertical walls around the lesion. Similar to a tire rolling over a pothole that is uniform and smooth along its rim, it follows that a well-performed chondroplasty will result in a defect with a uniform and smooth rim that is less likely to cause mechanical symptoms during loading and range of motion. Advantages of this technique include its technical simplicity, ability to be performed arthroscopically for defects in nearly any location (condyle, tibia, trochlea, patella), ability to perform other concomitant procedures such as meniscus surgery or ligament reconstruction, low overall cost, and ease of postoperative rehabilitation.[7] The obvious disadvantage is that this procedure does not have any ability to replace the missing cartilage, and thus the patient may remain symptomatic. Chondroplasty has historically been considered an acceptable first-line treatment for low-demand patients with small articular cartilage lesions; however, this may also be appropriate for elite, high-demand patients who seek a minimally invasive approach with

a quick rehabilitation process and relatively early timeline for return to play.

Reparative

Another viable first-line treatment for patients with focal chondral defects is marrow stimulation. This approach is considered reparative, as the goals are to fill the cartilage defect with actual cartilage, as opposed to débriding the defect and leaving it "empty" as during chondroplasty. Marrow stimulation techniques include drilling/abrasion arthroplasty and microfracture (Fig. 97.2), widely considered the gold-standard surgical procedure for small, isolated focal chondral defects. As reported in a 2014 epidemiology study by McCormick and colleagues,[51] surgical procedures for articular cartilage defects in the knee are increasing by approximately 5% on an annual basis in the United States, and of all coded procedures, microfracture remains the most common. The advantages of microfracture are similar to those of chondroplasty, including its technical simplicity, ability to be performed arthroscopically in a single-stage in a minimally invasive fashion, ability to perform other concomitant procedures such as meniscus surgery or ligament reconstruction, low overall cost, and different from chondroplasty, its ability to "fill" the defect with a cartilage product.[52-57]

From a biologic standpoint, microfracture and other marrow stimulation techniques induce an influx of marrow substrates to "fill" the cartilage defect, ultimately resulting in a fibrocartilage plug composed primarily of type I collagen. Importantly, fibrocartilage repair tissue lacks many of the intrinsic biochemical and viscoelastic properties of normal hyaline cartilage, is more stiff, and thus does not possess same shock absorption and force distribution capabilities as normal hyaline cartilage. When considering the pothole analogy described earlier, while the fibrocartilage produced by microfracture "fills" the defect, and may be superior to leaving the defect empty, the long-term efficacy of microfracture remains unclear due to the lack of hyaline-type cartilage (type II collagen) filling the void.

Recently efforts have been made to improve traditional microfracture techniques by using matrices and/or scaffolds to stabilize the mesenchymal clot produced by marrow stimulation, and to improve mesenchymal stem cell (MSC) differentiation into hyaline-type cartilage as opposed to fibrocartilage. Described "augmented microfracture"[58,59] techniques include including Bio-Cartilage (Arthrex, Inc., Naples, FL), autologous matrix-induced chondrogenesis (AMIC), BST-CarGel (Smith and Nephew Inc., Andover, MA), GelrinC (Regentis Biomaterials Ltd., Or-Akiva, Israel), and Chondrotissue (BioTissue AG, Zurich, Switzerland). The AMIC technique involves performing microfracture followed by the application of a porcine collagen I/III matrix (ChondroGide, Geistlich, Pharma AG) fixated with either autologous or allogeneic fibrin glue.[60-64] The BST-CarGel technique involves performing traditional microfracture followed by the application of the product, which is a bioscaffold containing liquid chitosan and autologous whole blood.[65,66] The GelrinC technique involves performing microfracture followed by the application of a hydrogel composed of polyethylene glycol di-acrylate (PEG-DA) and denatured fibrinogen, at which time the materials are exposed to UV light, forming a semisolid biodegradable scaffold for

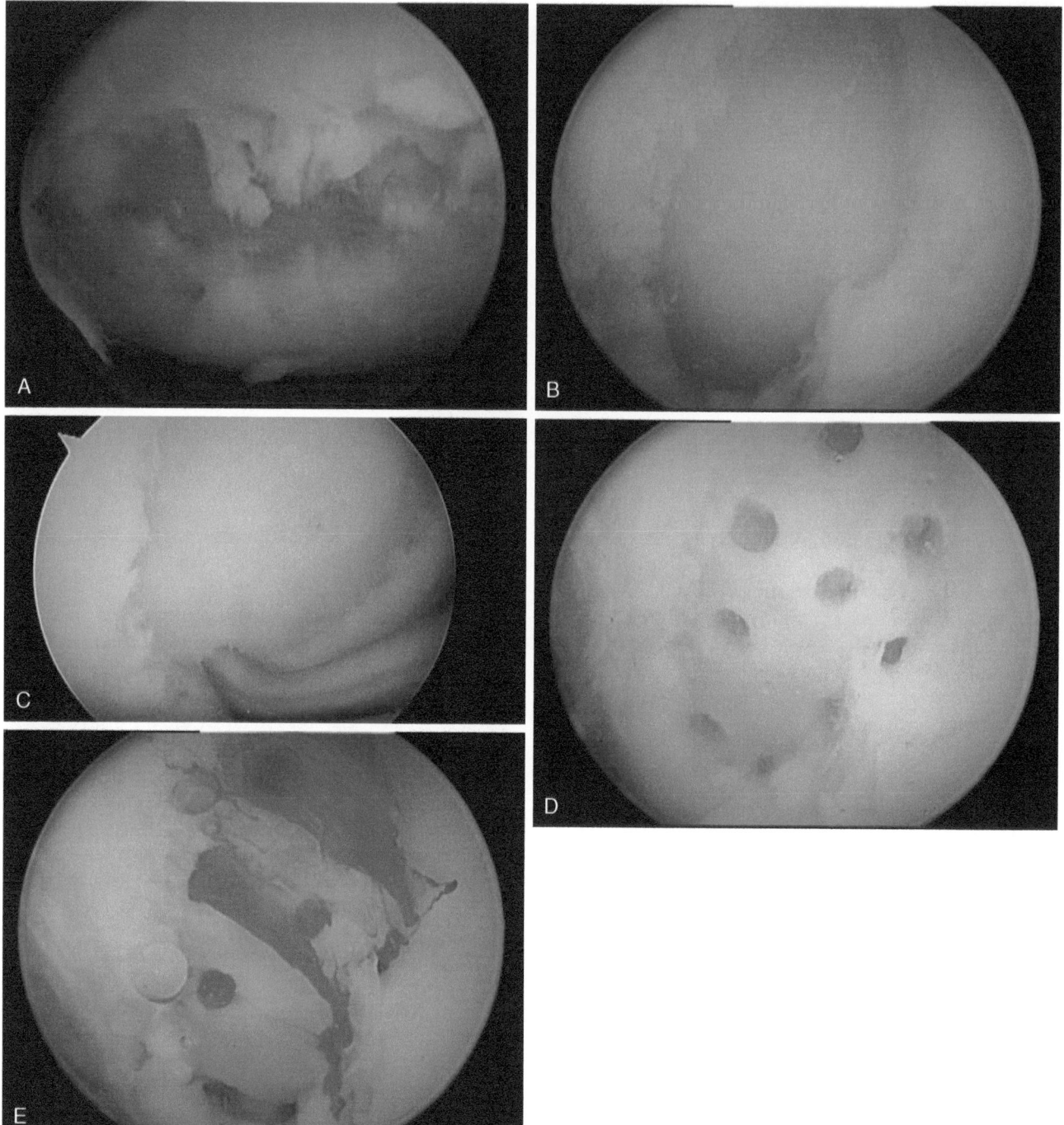

Fig. 97.2 Intraoperative example of a full thickness focal chondral defect of the lateral femoral condyle (right knee) undergoing microfracture including (A) defect, (B) débridement to stable vertical walls, (C) microfracture with an awl, (D) microfracture holes evenly spaced 3 to 4 mm apart, 3 to 4 mm deep, and (E) marrow products flowing into defect.

mesenchymal stem cells.[67] The Chondrotissue technique involves performing microfracture followed by application of a scaffold composed of polyglycolic acid (PGA) and hyaluronic acid (HA) immersed with PRP. Different from the aforementioned enhanced microfracture techniques/products, as of the time of publication of this text, BioCartilage (Fig. 97.3) is available for routine use in the United States. The BioCartilage technique involves performing microfracture followed by the application of 1 mL of

dehydrated, micronized allograft articular cartilage extracellular matrix combined with 1 mL of autologous PRP.[48,49]

Each of these enhanced microfracture techniques are advantageous in that they are performed in the same general way as traditional microfracture, utilizing a single-stage, minimally invasive approach, and offer the theoretical benefit of improving the stability and biology of the defect repair site. These techniques can be performed either arthroscopically or through a mini-open

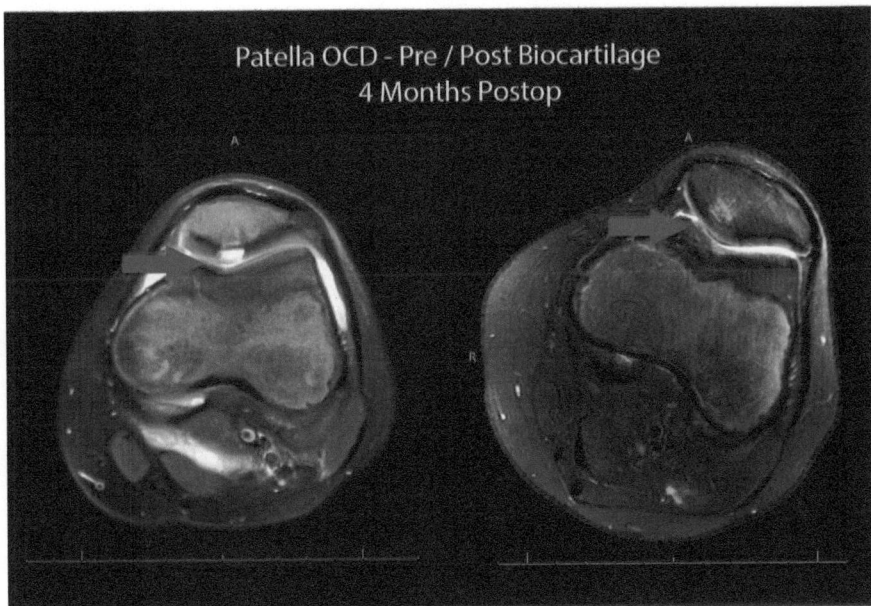

Fig. 97.3 MRI images pre- and post-BioCartilage procedure to the patella (4 months postoperative).

arthrotomy, depending on the ability to fully visualize and treat the lesion.

Restorative

For larger lesions, for lesions involving both the subchondral bone in addition to the cartilage, as well as for revision procedures, cartilage restoration surgery can be performed. A variety of restorative procedures are available, including autologous chondrocyte implantation (ACI), matrix-associated ACI (MACI), minced cartilage techniques, stem cell-scaffold techniques, osteochondral autograft transfer (OATS), surface allograft transplantation with "off-the-shelf" allograft products, and osteochondral allograft transplantation (OCA). These techniques are considered restorative, as they aim to treat the cartilage defect by restoring hyaline-type articular cartilage to entire defect site, either with or without subchondral bone. While many of the restorative techniques can be performed in a single-stage and through arthroscopic techniques, some require two separate procedures in a staged fashion, and some cannot be performed arthroscopically and require a small arthrotomy. The advantages of these procedures include their ability to treat large lesions as well as lesions that have failed prior attempts at cartilage repair, the presence of hyaline-type cartilage (as opposed fibrocartilage), and their ability to treat the subchondral bone in addition to the cartilage (for the osteochondral grafting procedures; Fig. 97.4). Disadvantages include the potential high cost associated with allograft tissue, the relatively long recovery period needed for graft incorporation, the potential safety concerns with allografts (for allograft procedures), and the need for two procedures instead of a single surgery in some cases (for ACI and MACI procedures). As ACI, MACI, minced techniques, OATS, and OCA were covered in the previous chapter, the following section of this chapter will focus on emerging articular cartilage techniques, including stem cell-scaffold techniques, novel minced techniques, and off-the-shelf surface allograft transplantation.

Mesenchymal Stem Cells With Three-Dimensional Matrices

Recently several unique products combining MSCs with three-dimensional scaffolds have been introduced in an effort to provide an alternative option to ACI for the management of focal chondral defects that, unlike ACI, can be performed in a single operation. Similar to ACI, the aim of these techniques is to treat the defect by restoring the surface with durable hyaline-type cartilage. Described products in this category include Hyalofast (Anika Therapeutics, Bedford, MA), which utilizes autologous MSCs, and Cartistem (Medipost Co., Ltd., Korea), which utilizes allogeneic MSCs. The thought process behind these techniques is that the scaffold with create an environment that is biologically favorable for MSC differentiation into hyaline-type cartilage.

Hyalofast, which is not currently available in the United States, is performed in a single stage by shaping/sizing the hyaluronan scaffold (HYAFF11 scaffold) to the defect shape/size, soaking the scaffold in the patient's BMAC, and then securing the scaffold to the defect with 6-0 PDS suture and/or fibrin glue.[68] BMAC is most often harvested from the patient's iliac crest, and contains adult MSCs, platelets, cytokines, bone morphogenic protein (BMP) 2 and 7, and a variety of growth factors, including PDGF and TGFβ. The cells, proteins, and growth factors are thought to establish a favorable biologic environment for cartilage restoration due to their anabolic and anti-inflammatory properties. While clinical data is limited, Gobbi and colleagues have found that at 5 years, patients undergoing treatment with Hyalofast compared with microfracture had better rates of returning to preinjury activity levels, despite microfracture patients having better return rates at 2 years following treatment.[68]

Similar to Hyalofast, Cartistem is also performed in a single stage and combines MSCs with a three-dimensional scaffold. In contrast, Cartistem utilizes allogeneic stem cells, specifically culture-expanded human umbilical cord blood derived

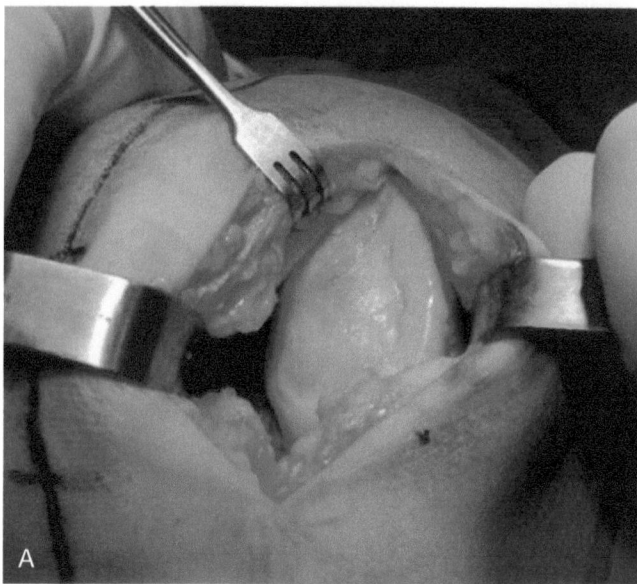 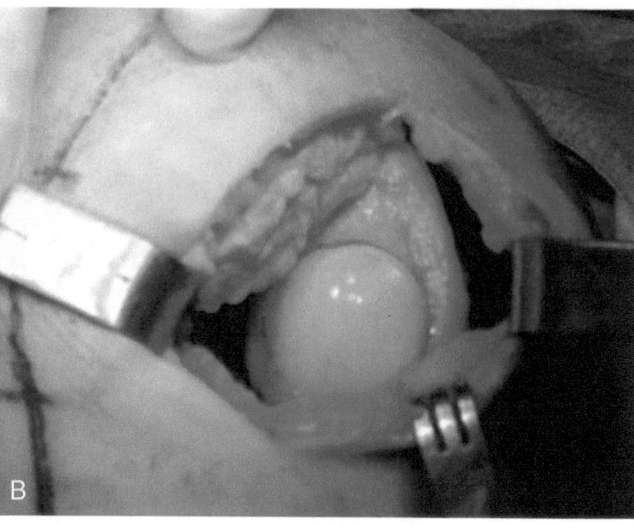

Fig. 97.4 Intraoperative example of (A) a full-thickness focal chondral defect of the medial femoral condyle (right knee) undergoing (B) osteochondral allograft transplantation.

mesenchymal stem cells (hUBC-MSCs), which avoids the donor-site morbidity associated with BMAC harvest. In this technique, the hUBC-MSCs are combined with a sodium hyaluronate scaffold and inserted implanted into the defect site. Preliminary outcomes from a clinical trial out of Korea including seven patients undergoing Cartistem are encouraging, though certainly further research is warranted.[69]

Several other stem cell-matrix combinations for the treatment of focal chondral defects have recently been described, and are currently in the initial phases of clinical testing. Specifically, the implantation of adipose derived stem cells (ADSCs) combined with scaffolds and bioactive factors have been reported by several groups.

Minced Cartilage Techniques

While the DeNovo Natural Tissue (DeNovo NT, Zimmer Biomet, Warsaw, IN) cartilage restoration technique was discussed in the previous chapter, at least two other emerging minced cartilage techniques have been reported, including Cartilage Autograft Implantation System (CAIS) and CartiONE. In brief, minced (or particulated) cartilage restoration techniques involve the placement of either autologous or allogeneic hyaline cartilage into the cartilage defect, combined with a scaffold delivery system, and secured with fibrin glue. The cartilage is minced into 1 to 2 mm³ fragments, which is theorized to allow chondrocytes to escape the extracellular matrix and produce hyaline-type cartilage and, ultimately, integrate with the patient's normal/healthy surrounding cartilage.[43-47]

DeNovo NT (see previous chapter for details; Fig. 97.5) is similar to BioCartilage, as both products utilize minced juvenile allograft cartilage, but is different in that the technique does not involve violation of the subchondral bone (no associated microfracture). Cartilage Autograft Implantation System (CAIS; DePuy Mitek, Raynham, MA) is another single-stage minced cartilage technique, but unlike DeNovo NT, CAIS utilizes autologous stem

cells harvested from the patient's intercondylar notch or trochlear border. Following harvest, the cells are minced into 1 to 2 mm³ fragments, combined with a scaffold of polycaprolactone (35%) and polyglycolic acid (65%) with PDO mesh, and fixed to the defect using biodegradable anchors. While preliminary outcomes following the use of CAIS were promising, due to expense and poor patient enrollment, trials involving CAIS in the United States were discontinued.

CartiONE (Orteq Ltd., London, United Kingdom) is another restorative technique involving minced cartilage that can be performed as a single operation. In this technique, autologous cartilage is harvested from the periphery of the patient's trochlea (nonarticulating portion) or intercondylar notch, minced, treated with a patented cell-isolation technology, combined with BMAC, added to a scaffold, and implanted into the defect site. Early clinical outcomes, including histologic outcomes, imaging outcomes, and clinical outcomes, from the INSTRUCT trial utilizing this product have been promising.

Off-the-Shelf Surface Allograft Transplantation

The utilization of osteochondral autografts and allografts was discussed in detail in the previous chapter. Among many reasons, both osteochondral autografts and allografts are advantageous, as they are composed of hyaline cartilage with associated bone and are thus are ideal for restoration of articular cartilage defects (especially those with symptomatic bone marrow edema), can be used to treat large defects, and can be used as a revision treatment solution for defects that have failed prior treatment. The main disadvantages of osteochondral autografts include their associated donor-site morbidity and their limited ability to treat large lesions. The main disadvantages of osteochondral allografts include their cost, potentially limited availability (especially outside the United States), and concerns regarding disease transmission. In an effort to provide an osteochondral solution that maintains the benefits but eliminates the disadvantages,

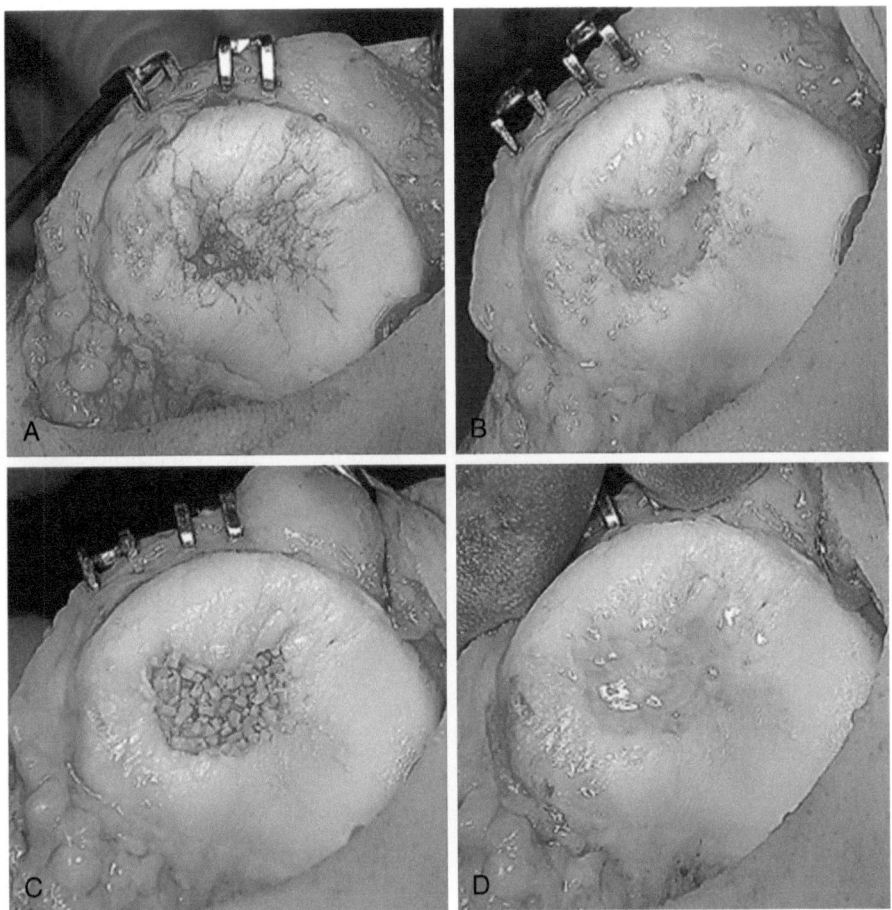

Fig. 97.5 Intraoperative example of a full-thickness focal chondral defect of the patella undergoing DeNovo NT transplantation including (A) defect, (B) preparation of defect with stable vertical walls, (C) transplantation of cells, and (D) covering of defect with fibrin glue.

several off-the-shelf surface allograft products have been developed. Surface allografts available in the United States include Chondrofix (Zimmer Biomet, Warsaw, IN) Cartiform (Arthrex Inc., Naples, FL), and ProChondrix (AlloSource, Denver, CO).

In 2012, Chondrofix was introduced as an off-the-shelf osteochondral allograft for single-stage treatment of full thickness articular cartilage lesions. This product was described as a preshaped, cylindrical, sterile, decellularized bone-cartilage construct with a shelf life of 24 months. The graft is precut to 10 mm in length, and comes in either 7, 9, 1, or 15 mm diameters. Preliminary data on 32 patients undergoing treatment with Chondrofix was reported by Farr et al. in 2016, and unfortunately failures were noted in 72% of the cohort (23 knees) at an average follow-up of 1.29 years (range, 0.11 to 2.8 years).[41,42] The average defect size of the cohort was 2.9 ± 2.0 cm², and a median of 2 allografts were implanted per knee (range, 1 to 5 grafts).

Cartiform and ProChondrix are two more recently described off-the-shelf osteochondral allograft products available in the United States. Unlike Chondrofix, which does not contain any viable chondrocytes, both Cartiform and ProChondrix do contain viable chondrocytes. Cartiform (Fig. 97.6) is described as a cryopreserved, viable osteochondral allograft composed of full-thickness articular cartilage and a thin layer of subchondral bone, with a 24-month shelf-life (stored at −80°C), and

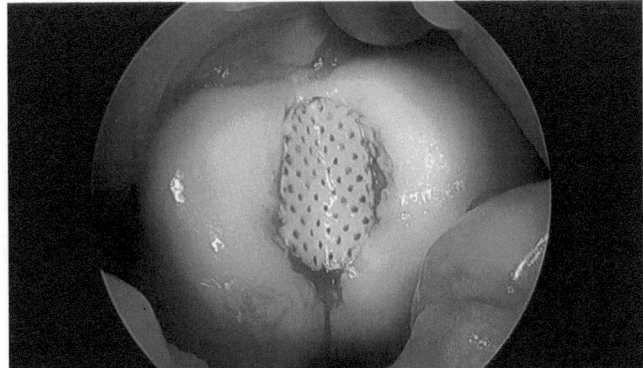

Fig. 97.6 Intraoperative example of a full-thickness focal chondral defect of the trochlea undergoing Cartiform cartilage restoration.

comes in four sizes (10 mm diameter, 20 mm diameter, 12 × 19 mm and 20 × 25 mm). The graft contains full-thickness pores/perforations that allow the cryopreservation solution to bathe the entire graft and preserve cell viability during storage, and also allows for graft flexibility during implantation. ProChondrix is described as a cellular 3D fresh osteochondral allograft composed of viable chondrocytes, matrix, and growth factors, with a 35-day shelf life (stored at 4°C), and comes in 5 sizes

(11, 13, 15, 17, and 20 mm diameter). The depth of the graft can be customized intraoperatively based on the depth of the osteochondral defect. As both of these off-the-shelf osteochondral allograft products are relatively new, clinical outcomes in patients undergoing treatment with these products are currently unavailable.

SUMMARY

Focal chondral lesions of the knee, especially those involving the weight-bearing surfaces of the medial or lateral femoral condyles as well as those involving the patellofemoral joint, often result in pain, effusions, mechanical symptoms, and ultimately dysfunction and disability. For appropriately indicated patients, surgical intervention is helpful in reducing pain, improving function, and restoring normal joint mechanics. Emerging techniques including augmented microfracture, scaffold and matrix-associated constructs, minced cartilage transplantations, MACI, and off-the-shelf osteochondral allograft transplantations, have been described, and warrant additional research and comparison to more "conventional" techniques, including standard chondroplasty, traditional microfracture, ACI, OATS, and OCA.

For a complete list of references, go to ExpertConsult.com.

SELECTED READINGS

Citation:

Crawford DC, DeBerardino TM, Williams RJ 3rd. NeoCart, an autologous cartilage tissue implant, compared with microfracture for treatment of distal femoral cartilage lesions: an FDA phase-II prospective, randomized clinical trial after two years. *J Bone Joint Surg Am.* 2012;94(11):979–989.

Level of Evidence:

I

Summary:

Results from a Phase II RCT comparing the safety of autologous cartilage tissue implantation with NeoCart to traditional microfracture surgery.

Citation:

Farr J, et al. High failure rate of a decellularized osteochondral allograft for the treatment of cartilage lesions. *Am J Sports Med.* 2016;44(8):2015–2022.

Level of Evidence:

IV

Summary:

Case series demonstrating a high failure rate following implantation of preshaped, cylindrical sterilized and decellularized osteochondral allografts.

Citation:

Frank RM, et al. Do outcomes of osteochondral allograft transplantation differ based on age and sex? A comparative matched group analysis. *Am J Sports Med.* 2018;46(1):181–191.

Level of Evidence:

III

Summary:

Cohort study demonstrating that osteochondral allograft transplantation is a safe and reliable treatment option for osteochondral defects in patients aged ≥40 years. Male and female patients had similar outcomes.

Citation:

Frank RM, et al. The utility of biologics, osteotomy, and cartilage restoration in the knee. *J Am Acad Orthop Surg.* 2018;26(1):e11–e25.

Level of Evidence:

V

Summary:

Review of the latest evidence over the use of biologics, osteotomies, and cartilage restoration.

Citation:

Gille J, et al. Outcome of autologous matrix induced chondrogenesis (AMIC) in cartilage knee surgery: data of the AMIC Registry. *Arch Orthop Trauma Surg.* 2013;133(1):87–93.

Level of Evidence:

IV

Summary:

Prognostic study demonstrating that AMIC is an effective and safe method of treating symptomatic chondral defects of the knee, but that a longer term is needed to determine if grafted area will maintain quality and integrity over time.

Citation:

Moran CJ, et al. Restoration of articular cartilage. *J Bone Joint Surg Am.* 2014;96(4):336–344.

Level of Evidence:

V

Summary:

Review of the latest evidence techniques for articular cartilage restoration.

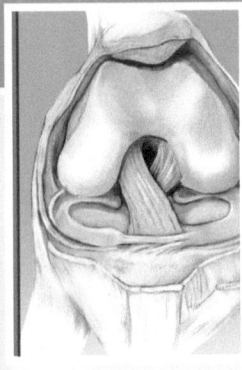

98

Anterior Cruciate Ligament Injuries

Edward C. Cheung, David R. McAllister, Frank A. Petrigliano

HISTORY

The anatomy and injury of the anterior cruciate ligament (ACL) has been well-documented in history for centuries, but it was not until the mid-1800s that reports of surgical treatment of ACL injuries began to appear in surgical literature.[1] Although there are some reports of success with early repair, surgeons realized that a more robust reconstruction was necessary to provide adequate knee stability. Ernest William Hey Groves was one of the first to report on ACL reconstruction in the early 1900s. He used a fascia lata graft placed through femoral and tibial tunnels and sutured it to the periosteum.[2] Over time, Hey Groves' original idea of intra-articular ACL reconstruction has evolved with a number of different simultaneous advancements, including early proponents of extra-articular reinforcements like that described by MacIntosh, which used an iliotibial band around the anterolateral aspect of the knee.[3] Additional attempts to use synthetic grafts such as GORE-TEX or polypropylene were used in the early stages of ACL reconstruction. Due to high failure rates, stretching and fragmentation, resultant knee effusions, pain, and instability, these were quickly replaced by tendon autografts and allografts.[1,4]

With the development of fiber optics and miniature television cameras in the 1970s arthroscopic assisted ACL surgery became more mainstream.[5] Initially, femoral and tibial tunnels were drilled independently through a two-incision technique, and the grafts were fixed on the anterior tibia and lateral femur. However, in the early 1990s, a single-incision ACL reconstruction in which the femoral tunnel was drilled through a tibial tunnel became popular. In some instances, this approach resulted in a relatively vertical femoral tunnel. As arthroscopic instrumentation and imaging modalities like computed tomography (CT) and magnetic resonance imaging (MRI) continued to improve, more biomechanics research was performed, and a heightened understanding of ACL anatomy and its influence on knee kinematics and stability showed that a femoral tunnel placed in the center of the native femoral footprint might convey a biomechanical advantage.[6–8]

ANATOMY AND BIOMECHANICS

The ACL originates on the tibial articular surface, just lateral and anterior to the medial intercondylar spine. Proximally, it courses posteriorly as well as laterally and inserts on the posteromedial wall of the lateral femoral condyle. Two functional bundles are present, the anteromedial (AM) and the posterolateral (PL), which are named for their tibial insertion sites (Fig. 98.1).[8,9] The ACL provides rotational stability and resists anterior tibial translation, varus stress, and valgus stress.[10]

The position of the AM and PL bundles varies with flexion and extension of the knee. In extension, the AM and PL bundles are parallel, but as the knee flexes, the bundles cross and the PL bundle moves anteriorly. The AM bundle is tight in flexion and the PL bundle is tight in extension.[11] The tibial origin of the ACL is oval and is approximately 136 mm^2 in size. The femoral attachment is circular and spans an average area of 113 mm^2. ACL fibers do not pass anterior to the cruciate ridge (also referred to as the lateral intercondylar ridge), which runs proximal to distal on the lateral femoral condyle.[12,13]

Indirect comparison from various studies suggests that ACL strength decreases with age.[14] Under normal walking conditions, the ACL experiences forces of approximately 400 N, whereas passive knee motion only produces 100 N. High-level activities such as cutting, accelerating, and decelerating are estimated to produce forces up to 1700 N, which approaches the average maximal tensile strength of the ligament, 2160 ± 157 N.[15] Despite this narrow window, the ACL works in concert with other stabilizing structures in the knee to resist translational force and rotational torque, and usually requires a high load to rupture.[16] Many other structures in the knee can be injured in conjunction with an ACL rupture, including the menisci, collateral ligaments, articular cartilage, and joint capsule.[17–19]

Though a complete discussion of anatomic structures that influence and/or are affected by ACL injury is beyond the scope of this chapter, the anterolateral ligament (ALL) and the proximal tibial slope (PTS) deserve mention as both have gained newfound interest. Though the specific anatomic description of the ALL location varies slightly by author, the consensus is that it courses from the lateral femoral condyle to an area near the anterolateral meniscus.[20–22] Human cadaveric and biomechanic studies show that the ALL contributes to internal rotatory stability of the knee.[23–29] With the resurgence of interest in the anterolateral region of the knee, modifications of early extra-articular ACL reconstructions are being performed in conjunction with modern intra-articular ACL reconstructions, with mixed early results.[30–33] Further study is needed to clarify if and when these reconstructions are appropriate.

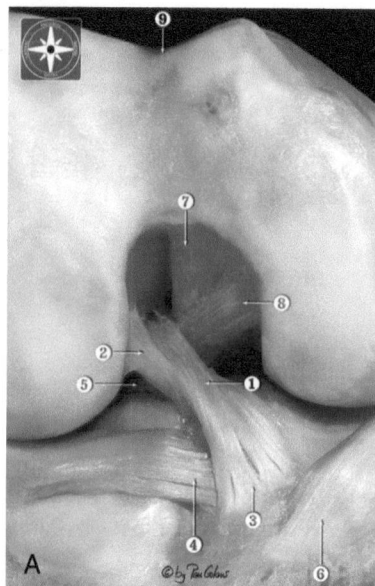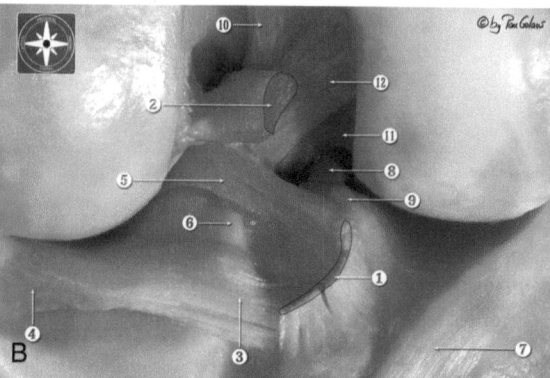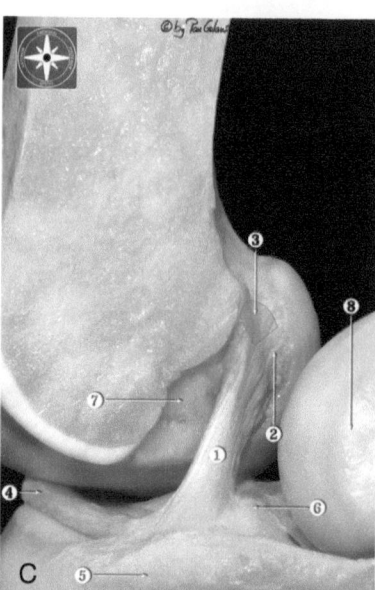

Fig. 98.1 Functional bundles of anterior cruciate ligament (ACL) in a cadaveric specimen. (A) The anterior view with the knee in 90 degrees of flexion. *1*, The anteromedial bundle of the ACL; *2*, the posterolateral bundle of the ACL; *3*, the tibial insertion of the ACL; *4*, the anterior horn of the lateral meniscus; *5*, the posterior horn of the lateral meniscus; *6*, the anterior horn of the medial meniscus; *7*, the femoral insertion of the posterior cruciate ligament; *8*, the anterior meniscofemoral ligament (Humphrey ligament); and *9*, the femoral trochlear groove. (B) The anterior view of the intercondylar notch with the ACL midsubstance resected. *1*, The ACL tibial footprint; *2*, the ACL femoral stump; *3*, the anterior horn of the lateral meniscus; *4*, the body of the lateral meniscus; *5*, the posterior horn of the lateral meniscus; *6*, the lateral tibial spine; *7*, the anterior horn of the medial meniscus; *8*, the posterior horn of the medial meniscus; *9*, the medial tibial spine; *10*, the anterolateral bundle of the posterior cruciate ligament; *11*, the posteromedial bundle of the posterior cruciate ligament; and *12*, the anterior meniscofemoral ligament (Humphrey ligament). (C) The sagittal view of the intercondylar notch and ACL. *1*, The ACL midsubstance; *2*, the anteromedial bundle of the ACL; *3*, the posterolateral bundle of the ACL; *4*, the body of the lateral meniscus; *5*, the anterior horn of the medial meniscus; *6*, the medial tibial spine; *7*, the medial wall of the lateral femoral condyle; and *8*, the medial femoral condyle. (Copyright Pau Golanó.)

The bony morphology of the proximal tibia can also influence ACL injury. When the knee is axially loaded with an increased PTS, sheer forces are directed anteriorly, which place increased stress on the ACL.[34–36] With the ACL being the main restraint to anterior translation, the increased PTS is thought to be an anatomic risk factor for injury. The influence of the medial and the lateral tibial slope is currently being investigated, with some studies showing that the medial slope has a greater influence,[37] some showing that the lateral slope has a greater influence,[34,38–40] and some showing no association with slope and ACL injury.[41] More research is needed to more clearly define the role of tibial bony anatomy and its influence on ACL injury and ACL reconstruction.

BASIC SCIENCE

Microanatomy

The ACL is composed of longitudinal collagen fibrils that range in diameter from 20 to 170 μm. The fibrils are composed primarily of type I collagen but also contain type III collagen.[42] They are arranged to form a unit called the *subfascicular unit*, which is surrounded by a layer of connective tissue called the *endotendineum*. These units combine to form the fasciculus,

which has an outer layer called the *epitendineum*. The fasciculus is ensheathed by the paratenon, forming the largest ligamentous unit. The microscopic architecture changes to a more fibrocartilaginous appearance near the bony attachments on the tibia and femur.[43,44]

The blood supply to the ACL comes primarily from branches of the middle geniculate artery and secondarily from branches of the inferior medial and lateral geniculate arteries, the infrapatellar fat pad, and synovium. The proximal portion of the ACL has better vascularity because the middle geniculate artery gives rise to ligamentous branches proximally and courses distally along the dorsal aspect of the ACL. The largest ligamentous branch is the tibial intercondylar artery, which arises proximally and bifurcates distally at the tibial spine to supply the tibial condyles.[45,46]

Nerve fibers have been found in all regions of the ACL. These fibers primarily run parallel with the vasculature in a longitudinal manner, but also incorporate freely into the connective tissue. The proximity of the nerve fibers and vasculature suggests a role in vasomotor control. However, the diameter of the nerve fibers in the connective tissue suggests a role in pain or reflex activity.[46] This role is supported by findings of altered proprioception in patients with capsuloligamentous injury and partial restoration of this function with ligamentous reconstruction.[47]

Anterior Cruciate Ligament Biology

The ACL is an intra-articular structure encased by a thin soft tissue envelope formed by the synovial lining. Rupture of the ligament usually causes disruption of this synovial lining and hematoma formation throughout the joint space with very little local reaction. Extra-articular ligaments, such as the medial collateral ligament (MCL), are contained within a robust soft tissue envelope. Injury to these ligaments causes formation of local hematoma and fibrinogen mesh that allows for invasion of inflammatory cells, resulting in healing with granulation tissue and eventually organized fibrous tissue.[48]

Epidemiology

ACL injuries comprise 40% to 50% of all ligamentous knee injuries, primarily as a result of sporting activity.[25,49] Injury to the ACL is most common in young athletes and disproportionally high in female athletes during their adolescent years.[50] Sports in which athletes are particularly prone to ACL injury are skiing, soccer, basketball, and football.[51] Over 70% of ACL injuries occur in noncontact situations.[52] Some studies have shown that the maximum strain on the ACL occurs with the knee near extension and a valgus force applied with internal tibial rotation and anterior tibial translation.[53] Females have a higher risk of ACL injury, which many have suggested is the result of difference in ACL geometry, pelvic tilt, generalized joint laxity, hormonal influences, and differences in muscle reaction time.[54–56] However, the exact reasons are currently unknown.

The number of ACL reconstructions has increased over the years. Currently, it is estimated that 200,000 ACL reconstructions are performed annually in the United States with a 5% to 15% failure rate.[57,58] Failure can occur early or late, with early failure occurring within 6 months of reconstruction and late failure occurring after 6 months. Failure can be due to recurrent trauma, nonanatomic placement of tibial or femoral tunnels, and lack of graft incorporation.[59]

CLINICAL HISTORY

A detailed patient history, including the injury mechanism and symptoms, is the first step in diagnosing an ACL rupture. The initial presentation often includes a history of a noncontact, low-velocity, twisting injury with or without an audible pop or snap and immediate knee swelling.[60] Though many patients may be unable to recall the exact mechanism of injury, some studies have demonstrated that as high as one out of every two patients with an acute hemarthrosis has an ACL injury.[61,62] A large proportion of patients with an ACL rupture experience immediate pain, swelling, and a feeling of instability. Most are unable to return to sport.

A severe knee effusion soon after injury is an indication of an intra-articular pathology. Early arthroscopic studies demonstrated that nearly 75% of patients with acute hemarthrosis of the knee after injury had some degree of disruption of the ACL.[62,63] Rupture of the ligament disrupts the blood supply and causes this hemarthrosis. Though a high proportion of hemarthroses can be attributed to ACL injuries, it is important to consider other intra-articular pathology such as meniscal or osteochondral injuries, fractures, or posterior cruciate ligament (PCL) ruptures. Additionally, the lack of a large hemarthrosis should not rule out an ACL injury.

PHYSICAL EXAMINATION

Physical examination is very important in diagnosing an ACL injury. Together with the patient history, the physical examination can often provide enough information for a definitive diagnosis. It is critically important to examine both the affected and unaffected knee to get a baseline measure for each patient. Examining the unaffected knee first can calm the patient, set expectations, and help the patient to relax, which will be important when testing for ligamentous stability of the injured knee.

Examination of an acutely injured knee should start with inspection. An effusion can be an obvious clue to injury. The patient's skin should be examined for cuts or abrasions or bruising. The affected knee will often be held in flexion which can relieve intra-articular pressure due to a hemarthrosis. If several days or weeks have passed since the injury occurred, the quadriceps may be atrophied compared with the contralateral leg.[64]

Following inspection, examiners should palpate the knee for warmth, a more subtle effusion, crepitus, and local tenderness. A large majority of acutely injured knees have tenderness to palpation either medially, laterally, or on both sides.[63] Local swelling or tenderness over the lateral or medial aspects of the knee suggests injury to the medial or lateral collateral ligament (MCL or LCL). Focal joint-line tenderness could indicate meniscal or chondral injury. Osteochondral injury or the presence of loose bodies may present with crepitus on knee range of motion (ROM) testing although this is rare with most ACL injuries.[64]

Knee ROM is often restricted in patients with acute ACL injuries. Apprehension and guarding are common, and physical examination findings can be more revealing after aspiration or local intra-articular injection.[64] Although it is not commonly performed, aspiration can also provide clues to the diagnosis because a hemarthrosis suggests ligamentous injury, whereas the presence of fat globules suggests a bony injury. Both active and passive ROM should be tested to determine if there is injury to the extensor mechanism or if there is a mechanical block from a meniscal tear, loose body, or ACL fragment that is obstructing motion.

Ligamentous Laxity

There are various physical exam maneuvers that can help examiners diagnose ACL injuries. The Lachman test for anterior laxity testing of the knee is performed by translating the tibia anteriorly while stabilizing the femur at 20 to 30 degrees of knee flexion. The anterior drawer test is performed at 90 degrees of knee flexion but is of little diagnostic value. In a recent meta-analysis comparing physical examination maneuvers in the diagnosis of ACL injuries with and without anesthesia, examination under anesthesia had a higher sensitivity than examination without anesthesia. Without anesthesia, the anterior drawer had a sensitivity and specificity of 38% and 81% compared to a sensitivity and specificity of 81% and 81% for the Lachman test.[65] The ACL not only provides anterior stability, but also provides rotational stability for the knee. The pivot shift test is performed using a combination of valgus stress with rotatory and axial loading during knee flexion. A positive test is marked by a palpable clunk produced by reduction of the subluxed lateral tibial plateau by the iliotibial band as the knee moves from full extension into flexion.[66] The sensitivity and specificity of the pivot shift test in diagnosing an ACL tear without anesthesia is 28% and 81%, and increases to 73% and 98% with anesthesia.[65] In all circumstances (with or without anesthesia, and in the acute or chronic setting), a 2006 study showed that the Lachman test is the most reliable test when considering combined sensitivity and specificity.[67]

Instrumented testing systems such as the KT-1000 and the KT-2000 can be used as an adjunct to manual maneuvers like the Lachman and anterior drawer tests, but are not necessary to diagnose ACL ruptures. They have sensitivities and specificities at maximal manual force of 93% and 93%.[65] These instrumented systems are most commonly used for research purposes.

IMAGING

Imaging studies should include standard anterior-posterior and lateral radiographs of the knee. These images can help exclude associated injuries such as loose bodies, tibial eminence avulsion fractures in younger patients, degenerative changes, and acute fractures of the proximal tibia or distal femur. Radiographic evidence of a lateral proximal tibia fracture, commonly known as a Segond fracture, is pathognomonic for an ACL injury. Recent literature suggests that the Segond fracture is an avulsion of the ALL.[20,22,68]

MRI is the imaging gold standard for diagnosing an ACL injury because it is both highly sensitive and specific in detecting ACL tears (Fig. 98.2).[69] The majority of ACL tears occur in the mid-substance of the ligament and are visualized on MRI as increased signal intensity with discontinuity of the ligamentous

fibers. Hemarthrosis is common. The presence of a bone bruise is observed on MRI in 84% of patients with an ACL rupture, with the highest incidence on the lateral tibial plateau and lateral femoral condyle, at 73% and 68%, respectively. Additionally, the LCL, which is oblique in orientation and typically not visualized in its entirety, may be seen from its origin to insertion on a single coronal image. MRI is also useful for evaluating meniscal injury and osteochondral defects. In patients with ACL rupture, injury is observed to the menisci in 51% of patients with injury to the medial meniscus at a rate of 13.9%, to the lateral meniscus in 24.9% of patients, and injury to both menisci observed in 13.1% of patients.[70] MCL injury is observed in 23% of patients with an ACL rupture.[71–73]

DECISION-MAKING PRINCIPLES

Operative Versus Nonoperative Treatment

The desired activity level of the patient must factor into the decision about whether to pursue nonoperative management of an ACL rupture or ACL reconstruction. The most common complaint of patients with a deficient ACL is recurrent instability, "giving way," and difficulty with cutting sports.[74] No large prospective trials have been conducted to demonstrate the natural history of ACL deficiency and the risk for further injury and osteoarthritis. There have been smaller studies showing that patients treated without ligament reconstruction after ACL tear have a higher risk of meniscal tears, arthritis, and knee arthroplasty compared to normal controls without ACL injury.[75] In patients with ACL injuries treated operatively and nonoperatively, there is a lower risk of secondary meniscal injuries after ACL reconstruction compared to those patients managed conservatively.[76] Although ACL reconstruction may protect the meniscus, it does not completely guard against rerupture, nor does it prevent subsequent osteoarthritis.[77]

Age

Age is an important factor when considering treatment options for patients with ACL injuries. As reported in a cohort study looking at more than 21,000 patients undergoing primary ACL reconstruction, the 5-year risk of revision was 9% in patients less than 21 years of age, 8.3% in those between 20 and 40, and 1.9% in those greater than 40 years of age.[78] The higher rate of revision may be due to the higher activity levels of younger patients.

As youth become more active, there is an increasing frequency of ACL injuries in the skeletally immature. In New York state, one study showed that there has been a threefold increase in ACL reconstruction from 1990 to 2009 in patients less than 20 years old.[50] Historically, skeletally immature patients with ACL injuries were treated nonoperatively. However, a better understanding of the risks of nonoperative management, along with the development of new techniques, has supported a trend for earlier surgical treatment of pediatric patients.[79]

Overall, patients between 20 and 40 years of age do well with ACL reconstructions. Though some argue that nonoperative means should be attempted first,[80] many have attempted to categorize patients with ACL injuries into the copers and the

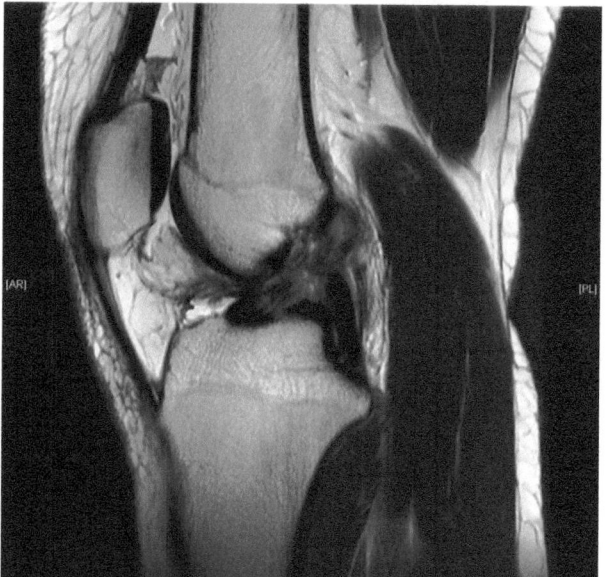

Fig. 98.2 A sagittal magnetic resonance imaging scan of the anterior cruciate ligament showing complete rupture.

noncopers. Those who are unable to return to high-level sporting activities, or those with symptomatic instability are those who are categorized as noncopers. Those who are able to return to sport and activity are categorized as copers.[81]

The success of ACL reconstruction is age independent, with 91% of patients older than 40 years reporting excellent or good results at 2-year follow-up, compared with 89% for patients younger than 40 years.[82] Nonoperative management with activity modification produces good to excellent results in 57% of patients older than 40 years.[82] Older patients often have more social and professional obligations that may prevent them from proceeding with ACL reconstruction and successfully completing a rehabilitation program, which highlights the importance of stratifying patients by activity level to determine the indication for ACL reconstruction. The use of an allograft instead of an autograft in the older population decreases morbidity and has been shown to produce comparable results.[83] Ultimately, physiologic age and activity level seem to be more important than chronologic age when deciding between operative and nonoperative management.

Gender

Female athletes are at a two- to eightfold greater risk for ACL injury compared with their male counterparts.[84] Many studies have looked at high school and collegiate athletes in soccer, basketball, and volleyball. The majority of injuries occurred as a result of noncontact mechanisms, which led to investigation and speculation about gender differences that can account for this significant disparity.[85,86] Possible etiologies have centered on hormonal and neuromuscular differences, environmental conditions, and differences in anatomy, such as alignment or joint laxity.[87]

Anatomic differences that have been evaluated include Q angle, the size and shape of the intercondylar notch, the size of the ACL, material properties of the ACL, foot pronation, body mass index, and generalized ligament laxity.[88] None of these differences alone places females at a greater risk of ACL injury. A study of West Point cadets produced a logistic regression model that could predict risk for noncontact ACL injury in 75% of cases, based on anatomic characteristics such as a narrow femoral notch, a high body mass index, and generalized joint laxity.[89] Some studies have shown that hormonal changes during the menstrual cycle affect the material and mechanical properties of the ACL, which could make it more vulnerable to injury during specific phases of the cycle.[90] However, this effect has not been shown definitively and requires further investigation.[91]

Partial Anterior Cruciate Ligament Tears

Diagnosis of a partial ACL tear can be challenging and requires close evaluation of the history, physical examination, and MRI findings. The gold standard for diagnosis is arthroscopy.[92] Partial tears comprise 10% to 28% of all ACL tears, and if left untreated, 42% will proceed to complete rupture. In addition, a large majority of patients with partial tears are unable to return to their preinjury activity level.[93] Decision-making regarding treatment of partial ACL tears should include evaluation of the patient's desired activity level, the degree of laxity, and symptomatic

instability. Options for conservative management include rehabilitation, focusing on hamstring (HS) strengthening, activity modification, and brace wear during activity. Proposed operative treatments include augmentation, partial (selective) ACL reconstruction, or traditional ACL reconstruction.[94] Well-designed prospective clinical trials are needed to accurately compare treatment regimens for partial ACL injuries.

Associated Injuries

Rupture of the ACL can be associated with injury to other structures in the knee, including the medial and lateral menisci, MCL and LCL, chondral surfaces, PL corner structures, and fracture of the distal femur and/or proximal tibia.[95] Many years ago, the phrase "unhappy triad" was coined by O'Donoghue to refer to the constellation of ACL rupture, MCL injury, and tearing of the medial meniscus.[17] Subsequent studies have shown that lateral meniscal tears are equally common with ACL rupture.[73] A recent review demonstrates that increased time from injury to ACL reconstruction increases the risk of intra-articular pathology, which included the trochlea, lateral femoral condyle, medial tibial plateau, and meniscus across all age ranges included.[96] Therefore surgical timing should be considered when deciding to pursue operative reconstruction to reduce associated injuries.

All associated meniscus injuries should be evaluated individually to form an overall management plan. There is some evidence that stable lateral meniscus tears, or partial thickness lateral meniscus tears, may respond particularly well to nonoperative management.[97–99] Injury to the medial meniscus should be addressed aggressively, and it has been shown that repair of stable peripheral tears decreases the risk of postoperative pain and the need for subsequent partial meniscectomy.[62]

MCL injuries are common in the setting of ACL rupture, occurring in approximately 23% of cases.[73] A consensus of ACL reconstruction and nonsurgical management of grade I and II MCL injuries is accepted; however, there is controversy in the management of grade III MCL injuries in the setting of ACL injury.[100] It was previously thought that high-grade MCL injuries may need to be treated operatively in the setting of ACL rupture. However, recent data have shown that nonoperative bracing of MCL injuries after ACL reconstruction results in equivalent clinical outcome as tested by anterior tibial displacement, function, participation in sporting activities, strength, and one-leg–hop testing.[101] However, in some persons with severe combined ligamentous injuries, MCL repair may be indicated, and there is no consensus on the timing of surgical management or reconstruction of the MCL in relation to the ACL.[102]

Revision Anterior Cruciate Ligament

As the number of ACL reconstructions increases, so does the total number of failures. These failures can typically be categorized as biologic, technical, or traumatic. The majority of failures in the past were due to technical errors, such as improper graft placement, inadequate notchplasty, inadequate graft fixation, improper graft tensioning, use of a graft with inadequate tensile strength, or failure to correct other causes of instability in the knee.[103] However, more recent data have shown that traumatic reinjury, which occurs in 32% of patients, is the primary mode of failure.[104] The technical approach to revision ACL reconstruction has been refined during the past 10 to 20 years; however, the results of revision surgery are worse than those for primary reconstruction.[105,106] The risk of chondral damage in the lateral compartment and patellofemoral space is increased with revision ACL reconstruction.[107] Moreover, risk of chondral lesions at revision reconstruction increases in the presence of a previous partial meniscectomy.[108] Patients must be counseled regarding the limitations of revision surgery and the potential for future failures.

TREATMENT OPTIONS

Nonoperative Options

In a 2016 Cochrane review analyzing current research comparing operative and nonoperative treatment of ACL injuries, the authors concluded that there was insufficient evidence to recommend ACL reconstruction based on patient-reported outcomes alone.[109] Some authors in the past have advocated for conservative treatment in lower demand patients.[110] Others have tried to determine if patients will be copers or noncopers to help guide treatment.[74] Conservative management can lead to recurrent instability and meniscal injury in athletes.[111,112] For this reason, ACL reconstruction is recommended in patients who are active, have symptomatic instability, have failed conservative management, or require the ability to cut or pivot during physical activity.

Persons older than 40 years can do well with a conservative training program but should be advised that a return to their previous activity level is unlikely.[113] Patients should not make a decision whether or not to pursue surgical management based on their age alone, because studies have shown equivalent outcomes in patients younger and older than 40 years.[114,115] In a randomized controlled trial of young, active adults, early reconstruction versus rehabilitation with the option of delayed reconstruction was evaluated. Patients undergoing delayed reconstruction had outcomes similar to those receiving early reconstruction, and the majority of patients assigned to the rehabilitation group elected to continue with nonoperative management.[116]

Operative Options

Timing

The timing of when to reconstruct ACL injuries has been debated in the past, with many studies recommending delayed reconstruction as some patients are able to cope with their injuries with rehabilitation.[74] Additionally, some have argued that there is a risk of arthrofibrosis with early reconstruction within the first month.[117,118] If postoperative stiffness occurs, loss of terminal extension is the primary difficulty encountered, and patient satisfaction is greatly influenced by stiffness and restricted ROM.[119] Patients who have an effusion, swelling, inflammation, and stiffness beyond 4 weeks after the injury was sustained, and who undergo ACL reconstruction, have an equal likelihood of experiencing arthrofibrosis, suggesting that it is the amount of effusion, stiffness, and inflammation present at the time of surgery that results in an increased risk of the development of arthrofibrosis.[120] The risk of arthrofibrosis with early treatment is concerning, with one study suggesting that operative treatment should wait

for 2 to 6 weeks when motion returns.[121] Preoperative loss of motion has a significant correlation with postoperative loss of motion. Sixty-seven percent of patients who have restricted ROM after surgery had limited ROM at the time of reconstruction.[117]

Other studies have argued for early reconstruction. They cite cost savings and improved quality adjusted life years (QALYs) with early reconstruction within 10 weeks of injury, compared to rehabilitation and optional delayed reconstruction.[122] Additionally, a meta-analysis of the current literature found no difference in knee stiffness when reconstruction was performed between 1 and 20 weeks.[123] We believe that the best approach is to allow time for the swelling to resolve and wait for the patient to regain good preoperative ROM prior to surgery. The amount of time for this to occur varies considerably from patient to patient.

Graft Selection

When choosing the appropriate graft for ACL reconstruction, it is important that the graft exhibits material properties similar to the native ACL, allows for secure fixation, incorporates into the bone tunnels, and limits donor-site morbidity.[124,125] All autografts including bone patellar tendon bone (BPTB), quadruple HS, and quadriceps tendon (QT) have greater tensile strength and stiffness compared with the native ACL.[126,127] This also holds true for BPTB allografts. Synthetic devices are no longer used in the United States because of an unacceptably high rate of complications, including failure and persistent effusion.[128] HS and BPTB autografts are popular, but the choice of graft should be discussed with the patient. It has been shown that though there is no clear consensus on the "best" graft, there are advantages and disadvantages of each, and ultimately, patients rely heavily on their surgeons to guide their decision on a graft choice.[129]

The first step in decision-making is choosing between an autograft and an allograft. An autograft incorporates into bone earlier, matures more rapidly, and avoids the risk of a host immune reaction, as well as disease transmission. Conversely, the use of an allograft is associated with less morbidity and requires a shorter surgical time.[130,131] A meta-analysis of BPTB autografts versus allografts showed that patients treated with an autograft had a lower incidence of graft rupture and performed better on hop testing. However, return to preinjury activity level and a decrease in anterior knee pain were significantly in favor of allografts.[132] In the same study, there was a three-fold increase in failure of BPTB allografts compared to autografts. Patients who underwent allograft reconstruction more commonly reported a final International Knee Documentation Committee (IKDC) score of A (normal knee). However, if a good result was defined as an IKDC score of A or B, no difference existed between the groups.[133] Recent evidence suggests a higher failure rate of ACL allografts in young, active patients.[134] A retrospective cohort study found that patients 25 years and younger undergoing ACL reconstruction had a 29.2% failure rate with allograft tissue compared with an 11.8% failure rate with BPTB autografts.[135] Patients in a large, young, active cohort, comprised of members of the United States Military Academy, were more likely to experience clinical failure if they underwent ACL reconstruction with allograft.[136]

Sterilization and preservation techniques can alter allograft tissue structure. Allografts sterilized with radiation or ethylene oxide are significantly weakened. The current technique of cryopreservation maintain the biomechanical properties of tendon allografts.[137,138] Disease transmission from tendon allografts has been reported, but the incidence is infrequent, occurring on average in less than one patient per year. Stringent guidelines have almost eliminated the risk of hepatitis C or human immunodeficiency virus (HIV), but there is still a theoretical risk of transmission. These risks fall between 1 in 173,000 and 1 in 1 million for HIV and approximately 1 in 421,000 for hepatitis C.[139] A few reports of bacterial infection from donor grafts have been reported in the past 10 years.[140] A large retrospective cohort examining greater than 1400 patients demonstrated no difference in infection between BPTB allograft or autograft with an infection risk of 0.5% and 0.6%. For HS autografts, there was an infection risk of 2.5%, which was higher than HS allograft.[141]

BPTB and HS tissues are most commonly used for ACL reconstruction. There are advantages and disadvantages to each graft choice. Numerous studies have compared BPTB and HS autografts and have found that BPTB autograft has a greater improvement of instability symptoms than HS autograft, without differences in clinical knee scores,[142–145] or rate of failure.[143,145–147] The use of the patellar tendon is not without potential complication. Compared to the HS group, greater number of patients in the BPTB group reported anterior knee pain (17.4% vs. 11.5%) and required manipulation under anesthesia for lysis of adhesions (6.3% vs. 3.3%).[148] Additionally, the risk of patellar tendon rupture, patellar fracture, and quadriceps weakness is increased with a BPTB autograft. The morbidity with HS autograft includes pain from hardware prominence or HS weakness. There is a higher rate of hardware removal (5.5% vs. 3.1%) for HS autografts versus BPTB, and though there is increased HS weakness associated with HS autograft, this weakness generally resolves within 1 year.[148,149] A systematic review of current literature found that no single graft source is clearly superior to others.[150] There may be early postoperative anterior knee pain with BPTB autograft, and early ROM limitations,[151] but at long-term follow-up, there do not appear to be differences in patient ROM or osteoarthritis compared to HS autografts. Those patients with BPTB were more likely to be participating in sport on a weekly basis compared to HS autograft patients.[152]

QT has been proposed as another source of autograft tissue. Recently, there has been some resurgence in interest in QT grafts. In a survey of orthopaedic surgeons, only 1% of orthopaedic surgeons utilize the QT for ACL reconstruction.[153] Biomechanically, QT autograft has been shown to be equivalent to quadrupled HS tendon.[154] When compared to BPTB, early results show equal postoperative laxity with a KT-1000, less anterior knee pain, and less loss of sensation. At 1 to 2 years follow-up, there were no differences in IKDC scores.[155] A systematic review of the literature on QT autograft versus other graft options and showed similar outcomes in terms of patient satisfaction, Lachman, pivot shift, instrumented laxity, and IKDC scores, with less donor site morbidity with QT autograft.[156]

We prefer using autografts rather than allografts in most patients having an index procedure because of the lower failure rate with autografts and the slight risk of disease transmission with allografts. Our preferred choice for an autograft in patients who place a high demand on their knees is BPTB because of earlier incorporation of the bone plugs into the tibial and femoral tunnels and excellent clinical results. We reserve the use of allografts for patients who place a lower demand on their knees, in the revision setting, or in cases of specific patient preference.

Graft Harvest

Harvesting of each type of tendon provides unique technical challenges. Patellar tendon autografts require harvesting bone from the patella and tibial tubercle, which can increase the risk of fracture and damage the articular cartilage of the patella.[124] Many surgeons prefer repairing the paratenon to improve glide and prevent scarring to the overlying tissue.[157] HS harvest requires elevating the sartorius to access the semitendinosus and gracilis and can put the superficial branch of the saphenous nerve at risk. Amputating the tendon prematurely during the harvest is also a risk. The QT is another autograft option.[124] If bone QT is taken, there is a risk of patella fracture as well as possible quadriceps rupture.

Graft Tension and Fixation

Graft tension is influenced by the amount of force placed on the graft, as well as the amount of knee flexion and rotation. The graft needs enough tension to stabilize the knee, but too much tension can stretch the graft and lead to failure of the graft itself or failure of fixation. It has also been suggested that grafts should be preconditioned prior to implantation to prevent creep. There has been cadaveric research examining the effect of multiple pretensioning protocols, but none have shown superiority, with pretensioning ranging from 80 to 500 N.[158] Previously, cadaveric studies have advocated for pretensioning between 40 and 60 N.[159,160] It has been shown that physicians are unable to reproduce the same graft tension utilizing a one-handed pull, and that intra-articular graft tension is different than extra-articular graft tension.[161,162] There is disagreement as to whether pretensioning the graft has an effect on knee laxity after ACL reconstruction.[163,164] Some authors recommend providing tension with the knee in full extension, whereas other authors argue that it is best to provide tension with the knee in 20 to 30 degrees of flexion.[165] Evaluation of outcome is complicated because most surgeons provide tension manually and in various knee positions, so comparison between studies is difficult. Graft-tensioning boots are used by some surgeons because they eliminate the need for manual provision of tension and allow the surgeon to use both hands for tibial fixation. Further trials are required to provide more comprehensive data regarding provision of graft tension.

Graft fixation should be strong enough to withstand closed-chain exercises for at least 12 weeks until the bone or tendon is able to incorporate into the bone tunnels. Closed-chain exercises produce on average 200 N of force but can produce up to 500 N of force.[166] Poor fixation can cause the graft to slip or the fixation to fail altogether.[166] Interference screw fixation of patellar bone blocks has the highest stiffness and fixation strength, ranging from 423 N to 558 N. Screw placement parallel to the bone block is optimal for maximum pull-out strength, whereas divergence greater than 30 degrees has increased risk of failure from pullout.[167] Screw diameter and length also influence fixation strength.[168,169] The use of tibial dilators has no effect on fixation strength, nor does the use of bioabsorbable instead of metallic screws.[170,171]

Many graft fixation devices are commercially available. Soft-tissue grafts can be secured with use of interference screws, suture posts, screw and washer constructs, and staples on the tibial side. Similar fixation can be used on the femoral side in addition to cross-pins and buttons.[124] Cross-pins, screw and washer constructs, and buttons all provide indirect fixation, meaning the graft is suspended within the bony tunnel. All others provide direct fixation, which compresses the graft against the side of the bone tunnel. It should be noted that the clinical implications of most biomechanical fixation pull-out studies are limited because they were performed on porcine and bovine specimens at time zero.

Graft Healing

A successful ACL reconstruction relies on incorporation of the graft into the surrounding bone, as well as ligamentization and revascularization of the graft. Bone-to-bone healing is stronger and faster than soft tissue healing to bone. BPTB allografts and autografts heal in a process similar to fracture healing.[124] With soft-tissue grafts, the tendon takes 12 weeks to incorporate into the surrounding bone through remodeling of a cellular and fibrous layer formed at the tendon-bone interface. At 12 weeks, collagen fibers form an attachment to bone that resembles Sharpey fibers.[172] At 12 months after ACL reconstruction, all histologic markers of ligamentization and revascularization, including fiber pattern, cellularity, and degree of metaplasia, resemble those of a native ACL. Vascularity and fiber pattern demonstrate no maturation after 6 months, suggesting that tendon autografts may be mature enough at 6 months to proceed with more aggressive rehabilitation and possible return to sport.[173]

Patellar tendon autografts incorporate faster than allografts and have stronger mechanical properties at 6 months. Allografts have a prolonged inflammatory response, decreased strength, and a slower rate of incorporation and tissue remodeling at the 6-month time point.[130]

Extra-Articular Augmentation

There have long been discussions regarding contributions to extra-articular structure for secondary rotatory stability of the knee. The iliotibial band has historically been proposed, and Segond in 1897 discussed a "pearly fibrous resistant band" that was under tension in severe internal rotation.[174] Claes suggested that the classic avulsion of the proximal lateral tibial plateau is actually an avulsion of the bony attachment of the ALL in 2014.[68] Since then, there has been a recent resurgence of interest in the anterolateral capsule of the knee or ALL providing secondary external rotatory stability in the knee. Though there have been various anatomic descriptions in the literature, an expert consensus group has decided that (1) the ALL is a distinct ligament on the anterolateral side of the knee, (2) that the femoral attachment is posterior and proximal to the lateral epicondyle, (3) that the tibial attachment lies between Gerdy's tubercle and the fibular

head, and (4) that the ALL has a constant attachment to the lateral meniscus.[25] Biomechanical and clinical studies have shown that the anterolateral structures of the knee provide significant secondary rotatory stability and when ruptured lead to a higher pivot shift grade.[26,27,175] Various methods of ALL reconstruction have been described.[30,176,177] Some authors argue for concomitant ALL and ACL reconstruction in selective patients. Though there is an increased interest in the ALL and its role in rotatory stability of the knee in the setting of ACL injury, more definitive evidence is needed to determine how to select patients that could benefit most from combined ALL and ACL reconstruction.

Role of Tibial Slope

The role of tibial slope on the risk of ACL injury has gained increased popularity in the literature.[36,178,179] Though there is some debate in biomechanical studies about the effect of increased tibial slope on anterior tibial translation, it appears that increased tibial slope leads to increased anterior tibial translation, which places more strain on the ACL.[34,36] Clinical studies suggest that increased posterior tibial slope is a risk factor for ACL rupture and rerupture after reconstruction.[39,180,181] There has been some suggestion regarding proximal tibial osteotomy in combination with ACL reconstruction in the setting of a previously failed ACL reconstruction,[182,183] but further research is needed to better examine the efficacy of these procedures and how to best select patients.

Revision Options

Determining the cause of failure is the key to successful revision ACL reconstruction. Physicians and patients should discuss the expected outcomes and the anticipated postoperative activity levels. Planning for a revision ACL reconstruction should involve all the steps of a primary reconstruction, including evaluation for associated injuries. In addition, thought should be given to correcting any technical error from the primary surgery and graft selection for revision. The same graft options in primary ACL reconstruction exist for revision surgery, although reharvesting previously harvested graft tissue is not advised.

In one recent study, it was reported that only 54% of patients returned to their preinjury activity level after revision surgery.[184] Patellar tendon autografts and allografts used for revision ACL reconstruction have produced equivalent clinical results and ligamentous stability on arthrometer testing.[185] Overall, revision ACL reconstruction should be viewed largely as a salvage procedure, and patients should be aware that they may never return to their preinjury function and activity level.

POSTOPERATIVE MANAGEMENT

Rehabilitation

Advancements in surgical technique and graft fixation have enabled patients to participate in early postoperative rehabilitation, focusing on ROM and progressing to patellar mobilization and strengthening. Patients can bear weight on the affected limb immediately. Early weight bearing and rehabilitation do not compromise ligamentous stability and result in a lower incidence of anterior knee pain compared with non–weight bearing.[188,189]

⚑ Authors' Preferred Technique

Primary Anterior Cruciate Ligament Reconstruction

A single-bundle ACL reconstruction uses one large graft that is fixed in place at the insertion site of the ACL on the tibia and femur (the so-called footprints of the ACL).

Positioning and Setup

The patient is positioned supine on the operating table. After administration of an appropriate anesthetic, both the operative and uninvolved legs are examined, including ROM and anterior drawer, Lachman, and pivot-shift tests. Special attention is given to varus, valgus, and posterolateral instability because those structures are not assessed arthroscopically. A post is placed proximally and laterally against the thigh to allow for valgus stress on the knee and visualization of the medial compartment.

Graft Harvest

If examination of the anesthetized patient confirms the diagnosis of an ACL tear, we proceed directly to harvesting of the graft. We most commonly use a BPTB autograft. The incision is marked 1 cm medial to the inferior pole of the patella, extending longitudinally 1 cm medial to the tibial tubercle (Fig. 98.3). The skin is incised and sharp dissection is carried down through the skin and subcutaneous tissue to the level of the patellar tendon paratenon. The paratenon is incised at the midline and separated from the underlying tendon with use of a scalpel. The knee is slightly flexed and a scalpel is used to harvest the central portion (usually 9 to 10 mm) of the patellar tendon. An oscillating saw is used to make the bone cut on the tibial side. Our goal is to make the tibial bone plug 20 to 25 mm in length and trapezoidal in shape, which is achieved by making a cut perpendicular to the surface of the bone medially and a lateral cut that is angled 20 degrees toward the medial cut. The distal cut is made last, and the bone plug is extracted by hand with use of a 0.5-inch curved osteotome (Fig. 98.4).

The knee is then placed into extension with the inferior two thirds of the patella exposed. The patellar bone cut should be 20 to 25 mm in length and triangular in shape, which is achieved by making medial and lateral bone cuts angled 45 degrees from the bone surface with an oscillating saw. The cuts should be made to a depth of 10 to 12 mm and should meet, allowing for easy extraction.

Graft Preparation

The bone plugs are shaped to fit into a 10-mm tunnel, and any excess bone is reduced to morsels for bone grafting of the patellar defect (Fig. 98.5). Because loss of fixation is more likely in the tibial tunnel, the patellar bone plug (which has a denser architecture) is placed into the tibial tunnel to maximize purchase with the interference screw. Two perpendicular 2-mm drill holes are made at the distal one third of the patellar bone plug, and two drill holes are placed in the tibial bone plug. Heavy nonabsorbable suture is loaded onto a Keith needle and passed through each hole. The bone-tendon junction is marked with a sterile marker to allow for visualization during graft passage. The tendinous portion of the graft is measured with a sterile ruler.

Portal Placement and Diagnostic Arthroscopy

The AM, anterolateral, and superolateral arthroscopic portals are established. The suprapatellar pouch, patellofemoral joint, medial and lateral gutters, medial and lateral compartments, and femoral notch (Fig. 98.6) are evaluated for concomitant intra-articular pathology. Meniscal injuries in the poorly vascularized white zone are débrided. Meniscal tears in the red-red or red-white zones are repaired whenever possible using an inside-out or all-inside technique.

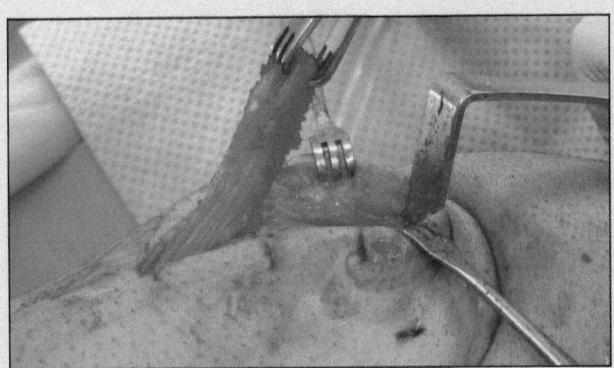

Fig. 98.4 Harvesting of the patellar tendon.

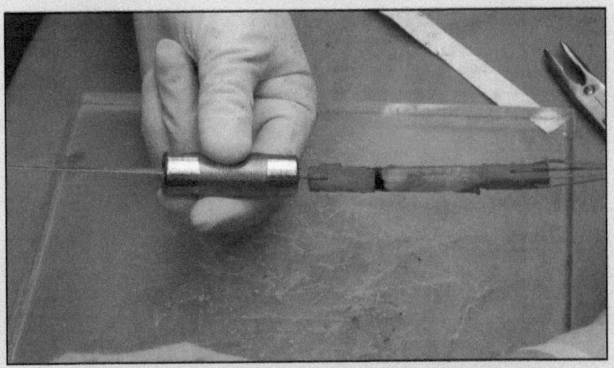

Fig. 98.5 Sizing of the patellar tendon autograft.

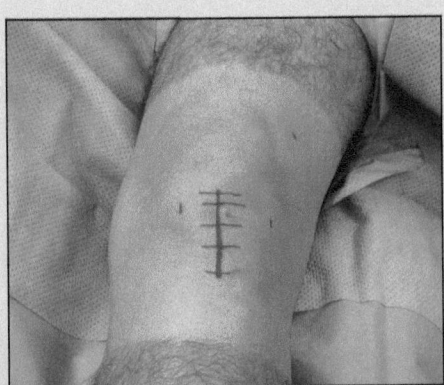

Fig. 98.3 Superolateral, anteromedial, and anterolateral portal sites and the patellar tendon graft incision.

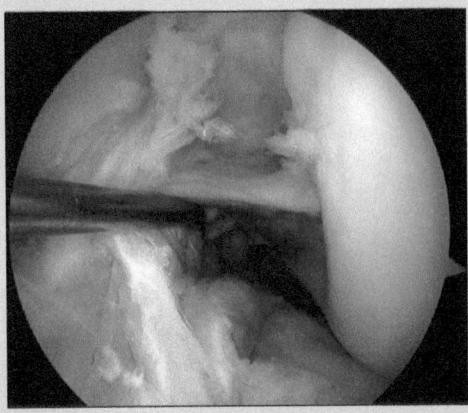

Fig. 98.6 The arthroscopic view of a torn anterior cruciate ligament.

Continued

📌 Authors' Preferred Technique—cont'd

Tunnel Placement

The precise positions for both femoral and tibial tunnel placement remain a matter of debate. The definition of an "anatomic reconstruction" has not been consistently described, and accordingly, we avoid this nomenclature. However, the available literature suggests that (1) the graft should be placed in an oblique position to resist rotational laxity and (2) the femoral and tibial tunnels should be placed within the native footprint of the ACL to achieve this goal.[186] We typically use a motorized shaver to débride the torn ACL down to the footprint on both the femur and tibia. A small portion of the footprint is left intact to permit identification of the native ACL origin and insertion. Enough tissue should be débrided from the lateral and superior aspects of the notch to allow for visualization of the over-the-top position (Fig. 98.7). A motorized burr is used to perform a small notchplasty as needed to prevent impingement of the graft and to visualize the periosteum on the posterior aspect of the lateral condyle.

The center of the femoral footprint is then marked with an awl or curette. This position is typically 6 to 7 mm anterior to the back wall and midway between the lateral edge of the PCL and the articular cartilage of the lateral femoral condyle. The angle on the tibial drill guide is set to N+7, in which N is the length (mm) of the tendinous portion of the graft.[187] The guide arm is oriented so the path of the guide pin points from the ACL footprint on the tibia to the footprint on the lateral condyle of the femur. The drill should penetrate the center of the tibial footprint, which is typically located in line with the posterior aspect of the anterior horn of the lateral meniscus (Fig. 98.8). The length of the tunnel is measured from the tibial drill guide and should be at least 2 mm longer than the soft tissue portion of the tendon graft based on the N+2 rule if using a BPTB graft.[115] If the proposed tunnel length is too short, it can be lengthened by increasing the angle on the guide. After the proper tibial tunnel length is confirmed, the guidewire is advanced and the tibial tunnel is created with use of a cannulated drill. A large curette is used to control the guide pin and protect the articular cartilage during drilling. The reamings are collected and used later for bone grafting of the patellar defect. A rasp is used to smooth out the surface of the tibial tunnel, and a shaver is used to remove soft tissue around the tibial tunnel entrance.

A Beath pin is placed through the tibial tunnel and directed toward the previously marked spot at the center of the femoral footprint. The pin is advanced through the femur and out the anterolateral thigh. This maneuver is referred to as the *transtibial technique* because the femoral tunnel is established through the tibial tunnel. A cannulated reamer is advanced to a depth of 10 mm and the posterior wall is visualized to confirm adequate positioning and bone tunnel integrity (Fig. 98.9). If the tunnel position is adequate, the tunnel is drilled to a depth of 30 mm.

In some cases, it is not possible to reach the appropriate position in the femoral notch via a transtibial approach. In these cases, the femoral tunnel can be drilled through the AM portal with a straight reamer or flexible reamer system. Commercially available flexible reamers permit reaming through the AM portal with knee flexion of 100 to 110 degrees. When using a flexible reamer system, a flexible guidewire is introduced through the AM portal with a cannulated guide to position the guidewire in a superior and lateral position prior to advancing the wire into the femoral footprint and out the anterolateral thigh. A flexible 10-mm reamer is placed over the guidewire under direct visualization to avoid damaging the medial femoral condyle. Another approach to achieving the appropriate position of the femoral tunnel is to use a straight reamer introduced through an AM portal. In these cases, it is important to hyperflex the knee during femoral tunnel reaming to avoid creating a short tunnel or violating the back wall of the femoral tunnel. Finally, an outside-in or two-incision technique can be used to ream the femoral tunnel. In these instances, a femoral aiming guide is placed through a second incision over the anterolateral femur and reamed from outside-in.

Graft Placement and Fixation

If the femoral tunnel was made transtibially, the eyelet of the pin is loaded with the suture from the graft and the graft is gently pulled into the femoral and tibial tunnels. If the femoral tunnel was created via AM portal reaming, a suture is placed through the eyelet of the guide pin and the pin is passed through the femoral tunnel. A probe is used to retrieve the suture loop through the tibial tunnel. Suture on the tibial tubercle bone plug (intended for the femoral tunnel) is placed through the loop of suture and the graft is passed through the tunnels. When an AM reaming portal is used, the femoral bone plug is often shortened

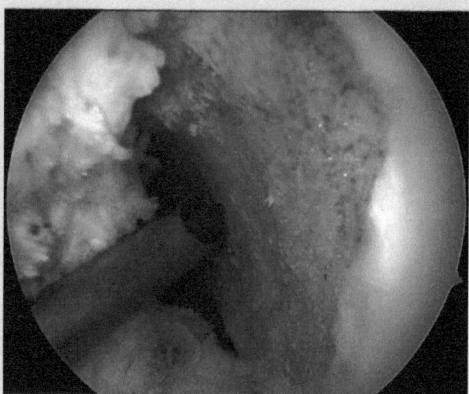

Fig. 98.7 An anteromedial guidewire placed in the center of the femoral anterior cruciate ligament footprint.

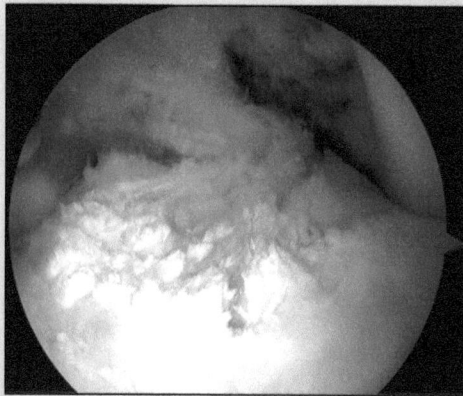

Fig. 98.8 The tibial footprint of the anterior cruciate ligament (ACL). The insertion of the ACL remains as a guide for positioning of the tibial tunnel.

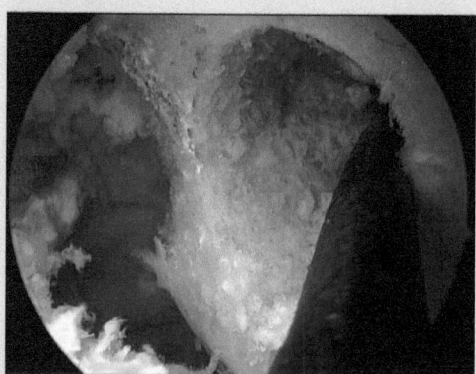

Fig. 98.9 The intact back wall after flexible anteromedial reaming.

Authors' Preferred Technique—cont'd

to 20 mm to facilitate passage of the graft through the acute angle between the tibial and femoral tunnels. The bone plug is then oriented in the femoral tunnel with the cancellous side facing anteriorly. The bone plug is left slightly proud on the articular surface to allow for placement of the interference screw guidewire. A guidewire is introduced through the AM portal and placed anteriorly between the graft and tunnel (Fig. 98.10). The graft is advanced so it is flush with the surrounding bone and a 7 × 20-mm or 25-mm cannulated metal interference screw is inserted over the guidewire (Fig. 98.11). The interference screw should be flush with the bone block, and care should be taken to avoid damaging the tendon with the threads of the screw. The knee should be ranged under visualization to evaluate for impingement of the graft on the femoral notch.

The knee is cycled 10 times with approximately 10 lb of tension with use of the sutures in the distal bone plug to create tension. The graft should tighten (shorten) over the terminal 30 degrees of each cycle. Tibial fixation is performed with the knee in 0 to 30 degrees of flexion. Grafts fixed closer to extension will avoid excessive tension on the graft in extension. A guidewire is placed between the bone plug and tunnel wall. Manual tension should be maintained while a 9 × 20-mm or 25-mm tibial interference screw is placed over the guidewire. We do not apply a posterior drawer force on the proximal tibia during fixation. The Lachman test is performed to ensure adequate fixation and elimination of anterior laxity.

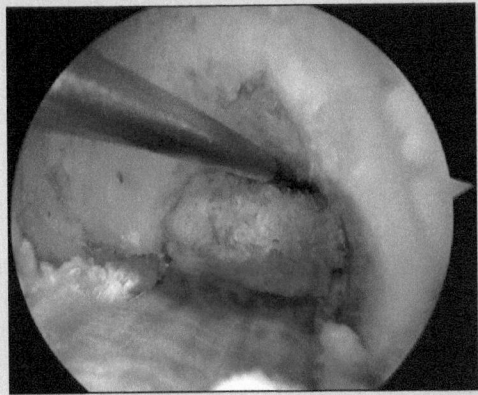

Fig. 98.10 Tibial bone block docking in the femoral tunnel. A guidewire is placed for later interference screw fixation.

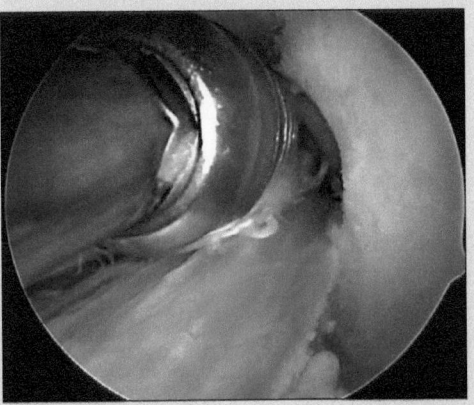

Fig. 98.11 Femoral interference screw placement.

A survey conducted by the American Orthopaedic Society for Sports Medicine reported that 63% of surgeons who perform ACL reconstructions use functional bracing postoperatively.[190] The advantage of bracing is that it can improve patient confidence, reduce tibiofemoral motion by normalizing translational, rotatory, and valgus loads across the knee.[191] The potential disadvantages are that it can cause altered gait if worn inappropriately, there is an increased risk for muscle atrophy, and braces have increased cost.[192–194] A 2007 systematic review of level 1 randomized controlled trials found no evidence that braces provided added benefit to postoperative recovery.[195] A 2017 systematic review of the literature looking at level I and II trials as well as a retrospective comparative study demonstrated mixed results. Some studies demonstrated improved knee kinematics and gait with bracing, with decreased quadriceps activation and ROM, while others showed no differences between those with and without braces.[196] There is no definitive evidence if functional bracing is beneficial in the immediate postoperative period.

The goal during rehabilitation in the early postoperative period is to preserve full extension and work on gaining 10 degrees of flexion every day. Several systematic reviews have demonstrated moderate evidence that there is no added benefit to a continuous passive motion (CPM) machine.[197,198] Though a CPM machine can be used to supplement early active and passive ROM, although we do not routinely use this machine.

Muscle Training (Open and Closed Kinetic Chain)

Quadriceps strength correlates with functional stability and correlates with self-reported function of the knee postoperatively and has been the focus of many postoperative training programs.[199,200] However, biomechanical studies of quadriceps and HS contraction showed that HS contraction decreases strain on the ACL through a posterior force on the proximal tibia during knee flexion.[201] Analysis of forces during knee flexion showed that force of contraction between the quadriceps and HS is balanced at a flexion angle of 22 degrees. At flexion angles greater than 22 degrees, the quadriceps, HS, and gastrocnemius muscle groups work together to unload the ACL.[202]

Debate in postoperative rehabilitation protocols has focused on open versus closed kinetic chain exercises. In the early postoperative period, closed-chain exercises are thought to be safer than open-chain exercises. Closed kinetic chain exercises are performed with the foot fixed in place in constant contact with the ground. Examples of closed kinetic chain exercises are squats and the leg press, which require activation of multiple muscle groups for stabilization and also distribute ground reaction force to all lower limb joints (Fig. 98.12A). During open kinetic chain exercises, such as leg extension, the limb is free to move and the joint reactive force is focused on the knee (Fig. 98.12B). In a study by Kvist and Gillquist, it was found that tibial translation

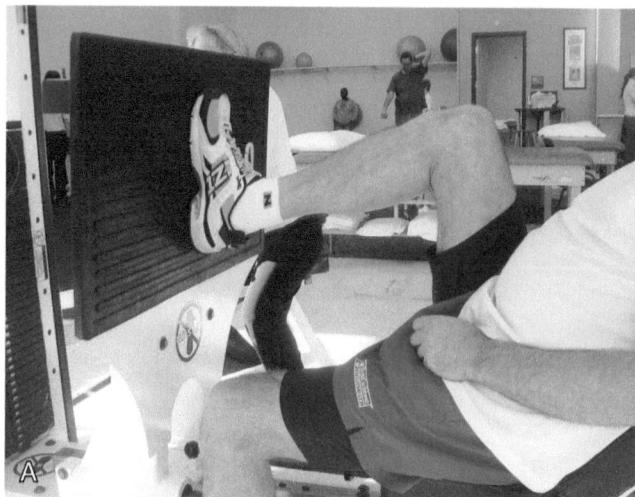
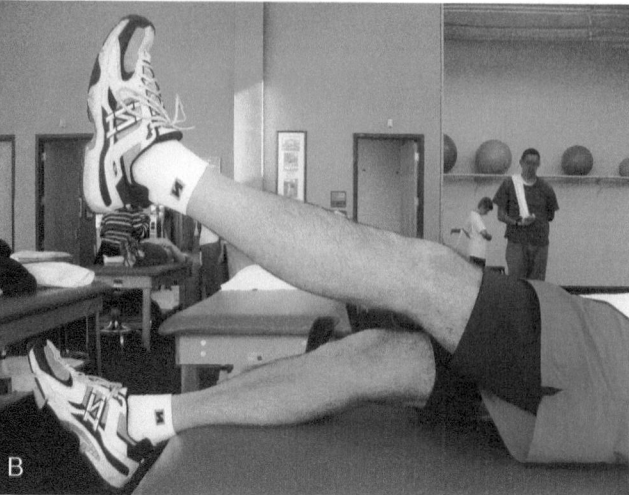

Fig. 98.12 Closed-chain (A) and open-chain (B) kinetic exercises after anterior cruciate ligament reconstruction.

is less in closed-chain exercises (between 10 and 40 degrees of knee flexion) but is greater at knee flexion greater than 70 degrees. These investigators also found that squats with the center of gravity behind the feet result in the least amount of tibial translation.[203] A prospective randomized trial of patients participating in open versus closed kinetic chain exercises after ACL reconstruction showed superior results with closed-chain exercises. Early results show that open-chain exercises lead to a 9% increase in laxity compared to closed-chain exercises.[204] Another prospective randomized controlled trial showed that compared to an open-chain group, patients performing closed-chain exercises postoperatively had greater knee stability, less patellofemoral pain, and greater overall satisfaction and return to activity. Ninety-five percent of patients in both groups regained full ROM.[205]

Other reviews of current literature suggest that a combination of open and closed kinetic chain exercises should be considered, especially in patients who require strengthening of the quadriceps muscle. Some show no difference in laxity, pain, and function after open- and close-chained rehabilitation.[206] Proponents of integrating open-chain exercises argue that the exercises can be modified to minimize strain on the ACL and decrease stress on the patellofemoral joint.[201] Functional outcomes are similar in patients participating in open versus closed kinetic chain exercises in the first 2 to 6 weeks after surgery.[207] However, patients who participate in open kinetic chain exercises plus closed kinetic chain exercises starting 6 weeks after surgery increase their quadriceps torque and return to sports 2 months earlier compared with patients who performed closed-chain exercises alone.[208] The literature supports a combination of closed- and open-chain rehabilitation, but the timing of each exercise during the postoperative period is not yet defined.

Electrical Stimulation, Biofeedback, and Proprioception

The use of electrical stimulation in the rehabilitation protocol is controversial because it has not produced consistent results. However, all studies have shown that it is safe, and when combined with volitional exercises, it can result in a more normal gait pattern and stronger quadriceps muscle activity.[209] A review of eight randomized controlled trials found that neuromuscular electrical stimulation may be more effective than exercise alone in restoring quadriceps strength after ACL reconstruction. The effect on functional performance was inconclusive, and overall analysis was complicated by inconsistencies in electrical stimulation protocols.[210]

Muscle strength depends on neural signaling, motor unit activation, and muscle contraction. Although electrical stimulation addresses muscle contraction, it does not require initiation of the movement or a sustained effort by the patient to maintain muscle contraction. Electromyographic biofeedback has been used to help patients monitor the quality of muscle contraction during a voluntary contraction. This modality is more effective than electrical stimulation in restoring peak torque in the quadriceps extensor mechanism after ACL reconstruction.[211]

The importance of proprioception has been described by several studies that have examined the neural anatomy of the ACL and how disruption of the sensory system can lead to decreased functional stability. Johansson and colleagues[212] showed that the ACL has a sensory system and mechanoreceptors that detect stretching at moderate loads, which signals to modify muscular stiffness around the knee. Knee proprioception is impaired for 6 to 12 months after ACL reconstruction, and improved proprioception correlates well with improved functional outcome and patient satisfaction after surgery.[213,214] These findings suggest that restoring mechanical stability alone is insufficient for optimizing functional outcome. Because proprioception does not return for up to 1 year after reconstruction, patients should incorporate proprioception training exercises throughout the rehabilitation process.

Functional Training

Rehabilitation programs have advanced to incorporate proprioception and neuromuscular control. Focus is placed on ankle, knee, and hip ROM, functional exercises to re-establish confidence, working on form, posture and dynamic joint stability, resistance, sensorimotor training, and neuromuscular training.[215]

In addition to restoring basic proprioception, it is important to emphasize neuromuscular control when the dynamic stabilizers are fatigued, especially in athletes, who require endurance and muscle stabilization at the end of exercise. Sensorimotor training places patients on uneven surfaces in a controlled manner to help regain muscle reaction and provide more stability. Low-resistance exercises such as stair climbing, cycling, use of an elliptical machine, and slide boards are safe repetitive activities that can be used at the end of a training session to encourage dynamic stabilization.[216]

Techniques to Limit Pain and Swelling

Cryotherapy has been used to lower the temperature of the knee joint and surrounding tissue, which can provide pain relief and shorten the recovery period after ACL reconstruction. Improved pain relief allows for more aggressive early rehabilitation, which is thought to result in better long-term results.[217] However, a meta-analysis of all studies on cryotherapy showed that it is effective for pain control but does not influence long-term outcome.[218] Martimbianco compared outcomes for cryotherapy versus ice pack, no treatment, or placebo and demonstrated that cryotherapy is better at controlling pain postoperatively than placebo in the immediate postoperative period.[219]

Rehabilitation Protocol

Our patients who undergo primary and revision ACL reconstruction are allowed to bear weight on the surgical extremity with crutches after surgery with a hinged knee brace locked in extension. Physical therapy begins immediately, with an initial emphasis on ROM and progressive patellar mobilization and strengthening. Use of the brace is discontinued 1 to 2 weeks after surgery. Stationary cycling begins when the patient is out of the brace. Associated meniscal injuries that were repaired at the time of ACL reconstruction do not change the rehabilitation program. Studies have shown that no difference exists in the failure rate of meniscal repair in patients who underwent ACL reconstruction and immediate postoperative rehabilitation compared with the published rate for meniscal repair alone.[220]

Return to Play

No standard or objective criteria are currently available to determine when a patient is ready to return to competitive sport or unrestricted activity after ACL reconstruction. In a systematic review looking at return to play (RTP) criteria, Harris et al. demonstrated that 40% to 65% of articles included did not have specific criteria for RTP.[221] In a meta-analysis, Ardern et al. demonstrated that 81% to 82%, 63% to 65% and 44% to 55% of patients following ACL reconstruction returned to any sport, previous level of competition and competitive sports, respectively.[222] Historically, a major consideration to deciding when to return to sport was the amount of time since ACL reconstruction. There has been a movement towards more specific criteria and functional testing to determine RTP criteria. Some suggestions have included quadriceps size, patient-reported outcome measures, single-leg stance and hop tests, and sport specific tests.[223] To date, there is no consensus on a standard RTP criteria.

With our patients, if ROM, strength, and balance have returned, we allow patients to begin running in a straight line at 3 months after surgery and return to full sport without restrictions 8 to 9 months after surgery.

RESULTS

Good overall results have been achieved with ACL reconstruction using BPTB and HS grafts. Patient satisfaction rates are greater than 90%, and 95% of patients report normal to near-normal knee function at long-term follow-up.[224]

Graft Type

Current level I evidence from randomized controlled trials shows no overall difference in outcome between BPTB and quadrupled HS grafts in postoperative laxity, clinical outcome, return to sport, one-leg–hop test, ROM, anterior knee sensory deficit, patellofemoral crepitus, osteoarthritis, or thigh muscle circumference.[149] A systematic review of patients after ACL reconstruction found greater anterior knee pain and kneeling pain in the BPTB group but equivalent patient-recorded outcomes and clinical assessments in both groups.[149,225]

Single Versus Double Bundle

It is currently unclear if the native ACL bundles function independently of one another. Double-bundle reconstruction has been advocated by some authors because it more closely mimics the normal anatomy of the ACL. However, clinical studies of conventional anatomic single-bundle and anatomic double-bundle ACL reconstruction have shown mixed results. Some studies have shown increased rotatory laxity on pivot-shift examination after single-bundle reconstruction but no difference in clinical outcome, return to sports, or functionality between the single-bundle and double-bundle groups.[149] Other studies have shown no difference in anterior laxity or rotatory stability in patients treated with double-bundle versus single-bundle reconstruction.[226,227] Most studies have failed to show a difference in clinical outcome as measured by Lysholm scores, IKDC scores, or other outcome measures.[228,229] Therefore further randomized studies are required to show superiority of the double-bundle repair.

Complications

The most severe complications of ACL reconstruction are infection and graft failure. Fortunately, infection is rare occurring between 0.3% and 1.7% of the time.[230] The graft failure rate is around 5% and is generally due to improper tunnel placement, repeat traumatic rupture, or failure to diagnose concurrent injuries to other structures in the knee.[231] Loss of ROM is the most common complication and can be minimized by regaining full ROM prior to surgery and being diligent with postoperative rehabilitation under supervision.[232] Patellar fracture and patellar tendon rupture can occur with BPTB autograft reconstruction but are rare occurrences. Between 30% and 50% of patients report anterior knee pain with BPTB reconstruction.[233] However, the pain improves with time and usually does not prevent high-level athletic activity.[222] Injury to the saphenous nerve is a concern with harvesting of the HS and can result in decreased sensation but is rarely a concern in the long term.[234] Osteoarthritis develops in many patients who rupture their ACL, but evidence is lacking to show that ACL reconstruction protects patients from the development of osteoarthritis.

Tunnel widening is a known radiographic complication of ACL reconstruction. Two separate studies of patients who underwent ACL reconstruction with HS versus BPTB showed a significant increase in tibial and femoral tunnel diameters in the HS group, although the two groups had similar clinical outcomes.[235]

FUTURE CONSIDERATIONS

Soft-tissue grafts have a slower rate of healing and incorporate into the bone tunnel later than bone grafts (BPTB). Many techniques for accelerating the healing process have been explored, including the use of growth factors, mesenchymal stem cells (MSCs), and periosteum augmentation. Platelet-derived growth factor and transforming growth factor β-1 have shown some promise in increasing the density of collagen fibrils.[236,237] Bone morphogenic protein-2 has been used to accelerate bone growth around the graft.[238] Periosteum has been used to enhance soft tissue and bone-graft incorporation into the surrounding bone tunnel. A prospective clinical trial using HS autograft enveloped with autologous periosteum found decreased femoral tunnel widening after reconstruction.[239] With the popularity of platelet rich protein (PRP), there is increased interest to see if it could have a role in ACL healing and graft incorporation. A recent systematic review demonstrated that there is still a paucity of clinical trials looking at the effect of PRP on clinical outcomes, bone-graft integration, and prevention of bone tunnel enlargement.[240]

Attempts have also been made to create ligaments in vitro through tissue engineering. However, further efforts are required to make this process a reality. A study by Vavken and colleagues demonstrated comparable biomechanical results with bioenhanced ACL repair using a collagen-platelet composite compared with ACL reconstruction in a large animal model.[241] However, this technique is still under investigation and has not been introduced into clinical practice.

For a complete list of references, go to ExpertConsult.com.

SELECTED READINGS

Citation:
Anderson MJ, Browning WM 3rd, Urband CE, et al. A systematic summary of systematic reviews on the topic of the anterior cruciate ligament. *Orthop J Sports Med.* 2016;4(3): 2325967116634074.

Level of Evidence:
IV, systematic review

Summary:
A comprehensive review of the anterior cruciate ligament (ACL) literature. The authors discuss ACL anatomy, epidemiology of ACL injuries, prevention strategies, associated injuries, the diagnosis of ACL injuries, operative versus nonoperative treatment, graft choice, surgical techniques including fixation methods, rehabilitation advancements, outcomes of operative and nonoperative treatments, and complications related to surgical reconstruction.

Citation:
Beynnon BD, Johnson RJ, Abate JA, et al. Treatment of anterior cruciate ligament injuries, part 1. *Am J Sports Med.* 2005;33(10): 1579–1602.

Level of Evidence:
III, retrospective cohort

Summary:
The authors of this article provide a review of the current knowledge regarding anterior cruciate ligament (ACL) injuries, focusing on biomechanics of the ACL, prevalence of injury and risk factors, natural history of ACL-deficient knees, associated injuries, indications for treatment, and management.

Citation:
Beynnon BD, Johnson RJ, Abate JA, et al. Treatment of anterior cruciate ligament injuries, part 2. *Am J Sports Med.* 2005;33(11): 1751–1767.

Level of Evidence:
III, retrospective cohort

Summary:
The authors of this article provide a review of the technical aspects of anterior cruciate ligament reconstruction, bone tunnel widening, graft healing, rehabilitation, and the effect of age, sex, and activity level on outcome.

Citation:
Maletis GB, Chen J, Inacio MC, et al. Increased risk of revision after anterior cruciate ligament reconstruction with bone-patellar tendon-bone allografts compared with autografts. *Am J Sports Med.* 2017;363546517690386.

Level of Evidence:
III, retrospective cohort

Summary:
The authors of this article examine a large anterior cruciate ligament (ACL) registry and identify risk of revision surgery after an ACL reconstruction with bone patellar tendon bone (BPTB) autografts versus BPTB allografts. They find that BPTB allografts have a 4.5 times higher risk of revision compared to BPTB autograft.

Citation:
Bottoni CR, Smith EL, Shaha J, et al. Autograft versus allograft anterior cruciate ligament reconstruction: a prospective, randomized clinical study with a minimum 10-year follow-up. *Am J Sports Med.* 2015;43(10):2501–2509.

Level of Evidence:
I, randomized controlled trial

Summary:
Ninety-nine active military patients were randomized to hamstring autograft versus tibialis posterior allograft anterior cruciate ligament (ACL) reconstruction and followed for 10 years. There were 4 autograft and 13 allograft failures. The authors conclude that at a minimum of 10 years following ACL reconstruction, 80% of all grafts were intact with good stability, but allografts failed at a rate 3 times higher than autografts.

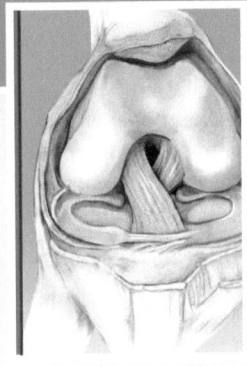

Revision Anterior Cruciate Ligament Injuries

Joseph D. Lamplot, Liljiana Bogunovic, Rick W. Wright

As the number of primary anterior cruciate ligament (ACL) reconstructions performed annually continues to increase, the number of revision procedures is also projected to increase.[1,2] A larger number of patients returning to high-demand sports and activities following primary reconstruction has resulted in an increased number of revision and repeat revision reconstructions.[3,4] Failure of primary ACL reconstruction, defined by recurrent laxity or graft failure, has been reported in 2.9% to 44% of patients, with higher failure rates in younger patients and following allograft reconstruction.[5-15] It is estimated that between 1.7% and 7.7% of patients who underwent primary ACL reconstruction will undergo revision reconstruction.[1,16-20] As approximately 175,000 to 200,000 primary reconstruction procedures are performed in the United States annually, it is estimated that approximately 3000 to 13,000 patients will undergo revision ACL reconstruction each year. This group is typically composed of a young, active population that desires a return to their previous activities.[21,22]

Revision ACL reconstruction is a challenging procedure with technical issues that can include retained hardware, incorrect bone tunnel placement and dilation, and limited graft choices.[3,23-26] This procedure requires proficiency with multiple techniques and flexibility when encountering unexpected obstacles to a successful revision reconstruction. Furthermore, patients undergoing revision ACL reconstruction have a lower rate of return to sport, an increased incidence of meniscal and chondral injuries, and inferior clinical outcomes compared with primary reconstruction.[8,9,11,21,27-29] Although excellent results can be achieved following a well-executed revision ACL reconstruction, patients must be counseled regarding expectations following this procedure.

Epidemiology

Recurrent instability is defined as failure of the reconstructed ligament to provide adequate anterior and rotatory stability to the knee. Recurrent instability or graft failure necessitating revision most commonly affects patients in the third decade of life.[8,22,30,31] Risk factors for graft failure include male gender, return to sports involving pivoting or jumping, contact sports, allograft, and age younger than 25 years.[14,21,29,32-35] Although patients in their 20s comprise the highest absolute number of revision ACL reconstructions, those aged 10 to 19 have the highest incidence of graft failure, and each 10-year decrease in age has been shown to increase the odds of graft failure by 2.3-fold.[14] This is likely attributable to a higher activity level among younger patients

with ACL injuries, as well as a higher likelihood of premature return to activities prior to adequate rehabilitation.[35] Although females have a higher rate of tearing an intact contralateral ACL, males are more likely to tear the reconstructed graft within the first 2 years following ACL reconstruction[21]; 55% to 70% of revision reconstructions are performed in male patients.[11,21,22,33,36-39] Although the reasons for higher rates of revision reconstructions among males have not been elucidated, males may have an increased propensity to return to high-risk activities that put the graft at risk.

Approximately 90% of revision reconstructions are first-time revision procedures.[22] Seventy percent of patients report a noncontact injury resulting in rerupture, with 40% occurring during cutting and 30% during jumping activities. Three-quarters of patients report an injury while playing sports, with most occurring during soccer and basketball. The mean time from prior reconstruction to revision is greater than 2 years in approximately 66% of patients, 1 to 2 years in 20% of patients, and less than 1 year in 15% of patients.[22] Of all patients undergoing revision ACL reconstruction, autograft was found to be used in the prior reconstruction in approximately 70% of cases and allograft in 30% of cases.[22]

HISTORY

ACL graft failure should be considered in the setting of objective sagittal (anteroposterior [AP]) or rotatory knee laxity, subjective knee instability, knee pain following prior ACL reconstruction, extensor mechanism dysfunction, and infection.[29] Knee pain should be distinguished from instability.[28] A complete history should be obtained, including mechanism of injury, quality of symptoms (swelling, giving way, locking, catching, crepitus, gait changes), symptom duration, previous injuries and surgical interventions including ligamentous, meniscal, and articular cartilage injuries, graft type and source, and graft fixation.[28,29] If the patient describing recurrent instability is unable to recall a causative traumatic episode, this may suggest technical or biologic reasons for graft failure. The patient should be asked to describe the postoperative course following the previous reconstruction, detailing the time course to rehabilitation milestones and return to activity/sport. Failure to return to the same level of activity postoperatively may suggest a technical error or inadequate rehabilitation.[29] Inadequate postoperative rehabilitation resulting in poor proprioception, deconditioning, stiffness, and pain may be unimproved after a revision reconstruction.[28,29,40,41] Such patients benefit from preoperative rehabilitation. Previous operative notes, clinic notes, therapy notes, imaging studies, and intraoperative arthroscopic images should be reviewed. Associated intra-articular injuries, including meniscal and chondral injuries, diagnosed at the time of the previous reconstruction must be considered in the setting of patient dissatisfaction following a previous reconstruction.[42]

PHYSICAL EXAM

Physical exam begins with assessment of lower extremity alignment, gait, muscle tone, specifically evaluating the bulk of the vastus medialis obliquus (VMO), and the location of previous incisions.[29] Range of motion (ROM) should be measured, assessing for a flexion contracture or extensor lag, and prone heel height examination may identify a subtle flexion contracture not appreciated while supine.[29] The ACL should be evaluated with the Lachman test to determine anterior laxity, and a pivot shift exam should be attempted to determine rotatory instability, with both exams compared with the uninjured contralateral leg.[40,43] However, approximately 32% of autograft-reconstructed knees may have positive findings on a Lachman test and 22% positive findings on the pivot-shift test, suggesting that postoperative laxity may exist in a large number of patients after reconstruction despite satisfactory subjective outcomes.[28] Conversely, despite normal findings on Lachman and pivot shift examination, some patients may describe the subjective perception of knee instability, with an inability to trust their knee during pivoting and twisting activities. In equivocal cases, the KT-1000/2000 arthrometer (MEDmetric, San Diego, CA) may be used to provide a more objective measurement of AP laxity.[28,29,44] A greater than 3-mm side-to-side difference correlates with failure of the native ACL, and multiple studies have used this criterion to quantify failure of a reconstructed ACL.[45-51] Other studies have defined graft failure as a greater than 5 mm side-to-side difference.[24,52-57]

In addition to these ACL-specific examination tests, a complete knee exam should be performed including examination of the posterior cruciate ligament (PCL), medial collateral ligament (MCL) and lateral collateral ligament (LCL), posterolateral corner, and menisci. As described later in greater detail, associated injury to other ligamentous and soft tissue structures may contribute to instability following ACL reconstruction.[58]

IMAGING

A complete weight-bearing series of knee radiographs, including AP in extension, flexion posteroanterior (PA) (Rosenberg), lateral, and axial (sunrise or merchant) views should be obtained in the setting of pain or instability following ACL reconstruction (Fig. 99.1). If there is concern for coronal malalignment or instability, full-length standing AP radiographs should also be obtained. Radiographs should be used to assess tunnel location, tunnel expansion and associated bone loss, osteoarthritis (OA) progression, coronal or sagittal malalignment, and the presence of hardware or implants that may affect revision surgical planning. A full extension lateral with the ankle supported to allow hyperextension can assess tibial tunnel position in relation to Blumensaat line.

Radiographic Tunnel Positioning

A malpositioned femoral tunnel is typically either too anterior and/or too vertical, and a malpositioned tibial tunnel is typically too anterior. On a lateral radiograph, the tibial plateau and Blumensaat line may be divided from anterior to posterior into four equal quadrants.[59] The tibial tunnel should enter the joint in the posterior third of the second quadrant, and the femoral tunnel should enter in the most posterior quadrant.[59,60] Taking 0% as the anterior and 100% as the posterior extent of Blumensaat line, a femoral tunnel more than 40% anteriorly along Blumensaat line is considered excessively anterior.[60] Femoral tunnels located at least 60% posteriorly along Blumensaat line and tibial tunnels at least 20% posteriorly along the tibial plateau have

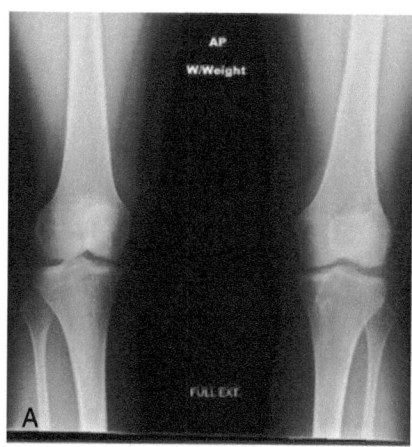
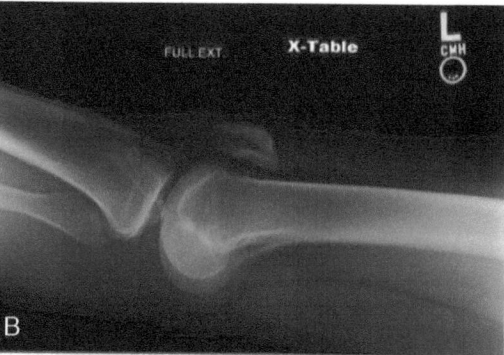

Fig. 99.1 Preoperative radiographs. (A) Standing anteroposterior radiographs demonstrate varus malalignment of the left knee in setting of prior anterior cruciate ligament (ACL) reconstruction. Full-length standing anteroposterior radiographs may be obtained in this setting to plan for concomitant high tibial osteotomy (HTO), which may be performed prior to or during revision ACL reconstruction. (B) Full extension lateral radiograph with ankle supported to allow hyperextension may be used to assess tibial tunnel position in relation to Blumensaat line. Notice knee hyperextension in setting of prior failed ACL reconstruction.

demonstrated improved clinical outcomes,[61] whereas those with more anterior femoral or tibial tunnels are associated with increased failure rates and inferior clinical outcomes.[62] Outcomes following revision for excessively anterior femoral tunnel malpositioning primary are improved compared to revision for another cause.[63]

Femoral tunnel malpositioning in the coronal plane can also contribute to graft failure. On an AP or PA radiograph, fixation along the anterior rather than lateral cortex may indicate a "vertical" femoral tunnel (Fig. 99.2).[64] A double-blinded study assessing the results of high and low femoral wall position showed improved International Knee Documentation Committee (IKDC) scores for the low position group.[65] The tibial tunnel should penetrate the articular surface at the midpoint of the plateau on an AP or PA radiograph. A cadaveric study using landmarks to determine anatomic tunnel location demonstrated the sagittal tibial

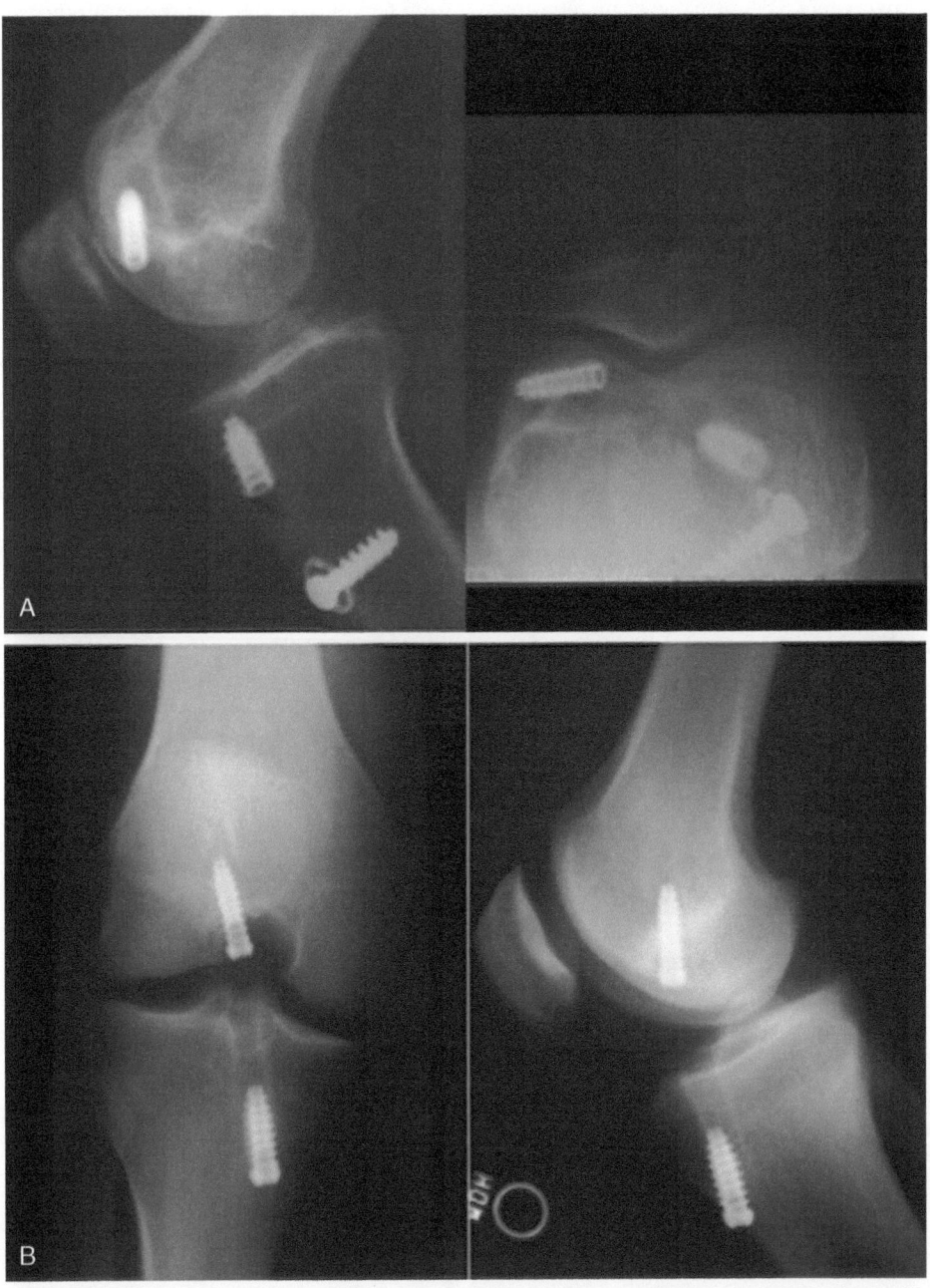

Fig. 99.2 Examples of incorrect tunnel placement. (A) Excessively anterior femoral and tibial tunnels. Taking 0% as the anterior and 100% as the posterior extent of Blumensaat line, a femoral tunnel more than 40% anteriorly along Blumensaat line is considered excessively anterior. The tibial tunnel should enter the joint in the posterior third of the second quadrant of the tibial plateau, and the femoral tunnel should enter in the most posterior quadrant of Blumensaat line. (B) Vertical femoral tunnel placement, best visualized on antero-posterior or posteroanterior (PA) radiograph. On a PA radiograph, fixation along the anterior rather than lateral cortex may indicate a "vertical" femoral tunnel. Lateral view also demonstrates anterior femoral and tibial tunnel placement.

tunnel angle to be 75 degrees and the coronal angle to be 65.7 degrees.[66] A tibial tunnel angle greater than 75 degrees in the coronal plane may result in a loss of flexion and increased sagittal (AP) laxity.[74,75]

Graft Impingement

A hyperextension lateral radiograph is the best method to assess for anterior graft impingement,[67] which is associated with increased rates of effusion, lack of extension, and increased failure rates.[68-71] The Multicenter ACL Revision Study (MARS) group demonstrated that approximately 51% of patients undergoing revision reconstruction had no graft impingement, 47% had some degree of impingement, and 2% had complete impingement with the tibial tunnel completely anterior to Blumensaat line.[60] A study defined the distance posterior to the anterior edge of the tibia that minimizes the risk of anterior graft impingement,[72] and if the center of the tibial tunnel at the articular surface was at least 22 to 28 mm posterior to the anterior edge of the tibia, then no graft impingement resulted.[73] Another study demonstrated that if the tibial tunnel is positioned in the posteromedial portion of the native ACL footprint, then graft impingement does not occur.[67]

Advanced Imaging

Computed tomography (CT) may be obtained to provide a more detailed assessment of existing tunnel location, tunnel dilation, and bone quality (Fig. 99.3). Excessively posterior femoral tunnel placement may result in posterior wall blowout, limiting fixation options at the time of revision surgery to those relying on lateral cortical fixation or necessitating bone grafting followed by staged ACL reconstruction.[76,77] The authors routinely obtain magnetic resonance imaging (MRI) preoperatively to assess for concomitant meniscal, chondral, and ligamentous injury, and it can also be useful to assess graft integrity and tunnel dilation. The authors routinely obtain MRI preoperatively. However, its utility may be compromised by artifact if metallic implants were used for fixation during the prior reconstruction.[77]

DECISION-MAKING PRINCIPLES

Causes of Failure of Anterior Cruciate Ligament Reconstruction

Instability following ACL reconstruction may be categorized into early (less than 6 months postoperative) or late (greater than 6 months postoperative) instability. Early laxity generally results from technical errors, failure of graft incorporation, loss of graft fixation, premature return to activity/sport, overly aggressive rehabilitation, or a combination of these factors.[11,28,78-80] Late instability generally results from traumatic rerupture and less often from technical errors.[32] A less common cause of late instability is failure to address concomitant ligamentous pathology at the time of primary reconstruction.[77,81] With appropriate surgical technique and rehabilitation, primary ACL grafts are at no greater risk of rupture compared with the contralateral uninjured ACL.[14,32,82]

Patients undergoing revision reconstructions report trauma resulting in recurrent instability in approximately 55% to 70% of cases, most often from a noncontact injury during sports.[22] However, at the time of revision, the MARS surgeons have deemed the cause of failure to be traumatic in only one-third of cases, technical error in approximately one-quarter of cases, biologic failure (lack of graft incorporation) in 7% of cases, and multifactorial in 31%.[22] Up to 53% of patients undergoing revision reconstruction have some degree of technical error contributing to graft failure,[29,83] and among these patients, 80% have femoral tunnel malposition. Injury resulting in rupture of a well-positioned and well-fixed graft is nearly as frequent as failure due to incorrect femoral tunnel placement.[22,33,55,63,84] Interestingly, two decades ago, failure due to malpositioned tunnels was two to three times more likely than traumatic rerupture of

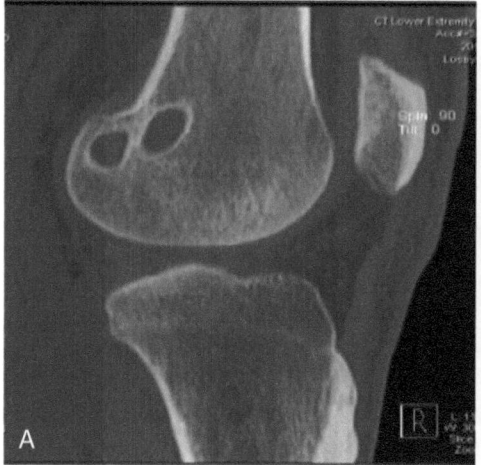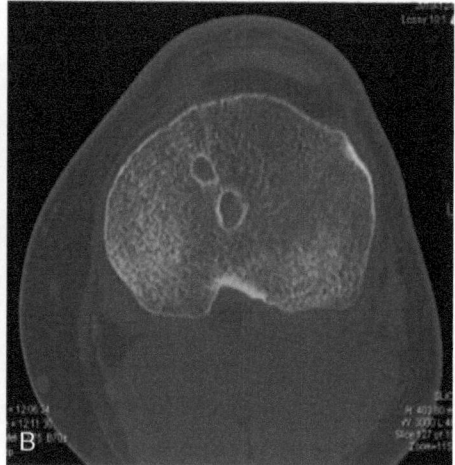

Fig. 99.3 Preoperative computed tomography scan may be obtained to assess tunnel location, size and bone quality. (A) Selected sagittal cut of lateral femoral condyle demonstrates two femoral tunnels occupying large portion of proximal lateral intercondylar notch. (B) Selected axial cut redemonstrates femoral tunnels. In this case a two-stage revision was performed in which these femoral tunnels were bone grafted prior to revision reconstruction. The large size and location of the existing femoral tunnels prevented the placement of a new, properly placed revision femoral tunnel.

a well-positioned, well-healed graft. These differences may be attributable to higher-demand patients expecting a return to their previous activity level, overaggressive rehabilitation protocols that may prevent adequate graft healing, and improved surgical techniques resulting in more consistently accurate tunnel placement during primary reconstruction.[63,85,86]

Tunnel Malpositioning

Tunnel malpositioning is the most common technical error during primary and revision ACL reconstruction and can result in excessive graft forces and strain resulting in inadequate graft incorporation, graft loosening, and atraumatic graft failure.[21,63,84,87,88] Occurring three times more frequently than tibial tunnel malpositioning, excessively anterior placement of the femoral tunnel is the most frequent technical error.[29,84] This is, in part, due to difficulties in visualizing the native femoral footprint[89,90] and results in a short graft with excessive graft tension in flexion and an initial loss of knee flexion.[63,84] During rehabilitation and return to sport, recurrent stretching of the graft leads to laxity and eventual failure.[29,63,84,91] Conversely, excessively posterior femoral tunnel placement results in excessive graft tension in extension with laxity in flexion.[84] A vertical femoral tunnel may provide sagittal (AP) stability but will result in rotational instability.[92]

An excessively anterior tibial tunnel results in graft impingement against the intercondylar notch with loss of terminal extension.[69,70,93-95] Excessively posterior tunnel placement results in graft impingement against the PCL and a vertical graft. This initially results in a loss of terminal flexion, with eventual graft laxity if full flexion is achieved.[84,96] Errant placement of a tibial tunnel too far medially or laterally can also result in graft impingement on the intercondylar notch, potentially causing articular cartilage injury.[97]

Untreated Ligamentous Laxity

Of patients undergoing revision ACL reconstruction, 3% to 31% of patients may have had unrecognized collateral ligament instability or malalignment contributing to graft failure.[6,24,29,33, 49,51-54,56,57,61,91,98-100] Untreated varus malalignment can result in varus thrust and graft attenuation.[81] Similarly, untreated posterolateral or posteromedial corner injuries may result in excessive forces within the graft and early failure; these injuries should be addressed before or during revision ACL reconstruction.[25,81,100] In the setting of combined ACL and PCL injury, reconstruction of the ACL prior to addressing PCL insufficiency will predictably lead to ACL failure.[58] As the medial meniscus is a secondary constraint to anterior tibial translation, the graft within a medial meniscus-deficient knee experiences increased forces that contribute to early failure.[63,77] Meniscal transplant should be considered in these patients.[11,21]

Primary Reconstruction Graft Choice

Numerous studies and meta-analyses of primary hamstring and patellar tendon autograft ACL reconstructions have demonstrated average failure rates of 3.6%, with no difference in failure rates between these autografts.[10,34,137-142] However, allograft reconstructions have a three- to five-times higher likelihood of graft failure compared with autograft.[48,101-103] This may be attributable, in part, to patients having relatively less postoperative pain and a more rapid postoperative rehabilitation following allograft reconstruction, thereby returning to a higher activity level prior to adequate graft healing.[34,104] Allograft processing may also increase the risk of graft failure, as irradiated grafts have demonstrated a significantly higher failure rate compared with nonirradiated grafts.[103,105]

Concomitant Intra-Articular Pathology

Knees undergoing revision ACL reconstruction have a higher incidence of chondral injuries and meniscal tears compared to primary reconstruction.[24,28,52,106,107] In one study, 90% of knees undergoing revision reconstruction had a meniscus or chondral injury and greater than 50% demonstrated both.[22] Similarly, MARS group reported modified Outerbridge grade 2 or higher lesions in 73% of patients undergoing revision, with concurrent meniscal and cartilage damage in 57%.[22]

Meniscus Injury

Although is it known that the medial meniscus plays a critical role in limiting anterior tibial translation in an ACL-deficient knee, it remains unknown if there is a critical amount of medial meniscus that, if removed, predisposes the reconstruction to failure.[21,108] Previous partial meniscectomy, but not meniscal repair, is associated with a higher incidence of articular cartilage lesions at the time of revision.[21,106] The MARS group demonstrated an overall 74% incidence of meniscal injury at the time of revision reconstruction,[22] similar to that at the time of primary reconstruction.[109-111] The prevalence of medial meniscus tears at the time of revision is 40% to 46%, higher than at the time of primary reconstruction.[8,22,112] Conversely, there is actually a decreased incidence of new, untreated lateral meniscal tears at revision compared with primary reconstruction.[11] Thus patients undergoing revision due to recurrent instability appear to be continuing to put the medial meniscus at risk for further injury.

Articular Cartilage Injury

Inferior patient-reported outcome scores have been reported following revision ACL reconstruction compared with primary reconstruction, and this is associated with an increased incidence and severity of chondral lesions at the time of revision.[6,53] Although it is unlikely that these lesions affect stability in the reconstructed knee, increased chondrosis at the time of revision may have detrimental effects on clinical outcomes despite appropriate surgical technique, graft healing, and adequate clinical laxity.[29] Even when controlling for meniscus status (prior meniscectomy versus no prior meniscectomy), there is an increased risk of lateral and patellofemoral compartment chondrosis at the time of revision compared with primary reconstruction.[11] There is a strong association between ACL deficiency and acceleration of degenerative changes,[23,113,114] and the status of the articular cartilage at the time of revision reconstruction may be one of the most important predictors of a successful clinical outcome.[33] Patients undergoing delayed revision reconstruction (greater than 6 months following onset of symptomatic instability) have a markedly higher incidence of articular cartilage degeneration compared with earlier revisions (53% vs. 24%), and the prevalence of advanced degenerative changes is also significantly higher in the delayed group.[23] Early restoration of stability may lead to reduced secondary articular cartilage damage and a return to previous activity levels,[7,23,115] and it has been suggested that revision reconstruction should be performed within 6 months of graft failure to minimize the risk of degenerative changes and arthritis progression.[23,53,116]

TREATMENT OPTIONS

Several factors must be considered in the setting of revision ACL reconstruction, including graft selection, incision locations, tunnel locations, tunnel sizes and need for bone grafting, previous fixation type and need for removal, method of revision fixation, and postoperative protocol. The revision reconstruction often must be adapted to the technique previously used.[91] The revising surgeon must be proficient with a variety of techniques to address such issues as retained implants, malpositioned tunnels, bone loss, and expanded tunnels. Additional knee pathology, including meniscus or ligamentous injury, may be addressed at the time of revision ACL reconstruction or staged, with the revision ACL reconstruction often the final procedure. Although most revisions are performed as single-stage procedures, specific situations in which two-stage procedures should be considered are patients with incomplete ROM requiring lysis of adhesions, malalignment requiring corrective osteotomy, significant tunnel widening necessitating bone graft, and infection.[91]

Evaluation of Tunnels

Prior tunnel placement may be categorized in one of three ways: (1) accurate and not requiring redirection, (2) completely inaccurate in a location that will not interfere with new tunnel creation, or (3) overlapping, such that the prior tunnel and a properly placed tunnel will partially overlap.[76] Partially overlapping tunnels are generally the most challenging of these three because they require the surgeon to adjust his or her technique due to enlarged tunnels. The scope should be inserted into each tunnel to assess tunnel size and the quality of the surrounding bone to determine the need for grafting and the best method of fixation.[91] The tibial tunnel can be viewed by placing the scope directly into the tunnel through the previously made tibial skin incision. The femoral tunnel can be visualized by placing the scope through the previous anteromedial portal.

Prior Fixation

Bioabsorbable implants are generally difficult to remove and may be left in place and overreamed after guide pin placement. However, metal interference screws must be removed if interfering with the planned tunnel location. In the rare case that properly placed tunnels can be made independent of prior tunnels and metallic implants, the implants may be left in place (Fig. 99.4). If metallic hardware is removed, the size and location of the resulting defect must be considered. The defect may necessitate grafting, either as part of a single-stage of two-stage revision, or the use of larger bone blocks with a patellar tendon autograft or various bone block allograft options.

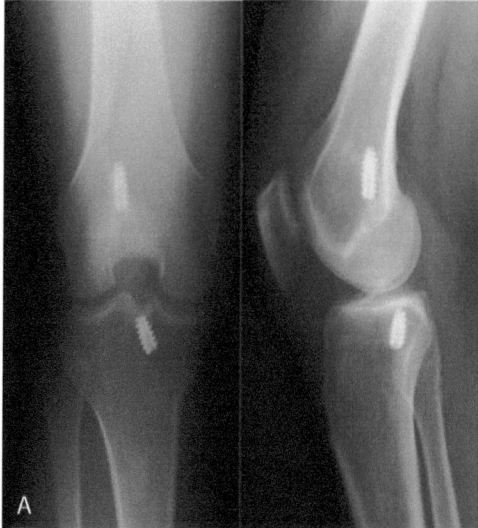

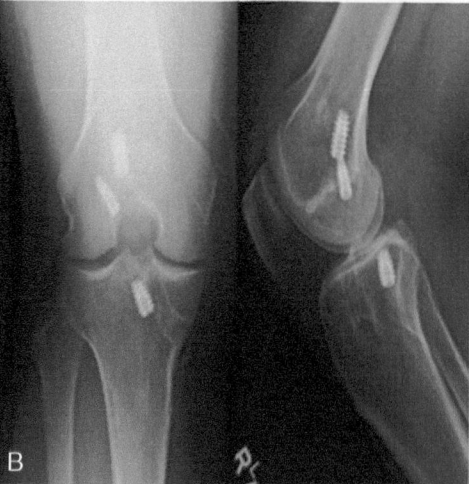

Fig. 99.4 Correction of femoral tunnel malpositioning. (A) Preoperative radiographs with fixation from prior failed anterior cruciate ligament (ACL) reconstruction demonstrate excessively posterior tibial tunnel and vertical femoral tunnel. (B) Postoperative radiographs following revision ACL reconstruction with new tibial tunnel anterior to Blumensaat line and less vertical femoral tunnel at approximately 1030 position.

Tunnel Grafting

Bone grafting of existing tunnels should be strongly considered when expanded tunnels measure more than 15 mm, because ACL graft options are limited and fixation may be compromised in tunnels this large.[76] Bone grafting may be performed at the time of revision ACL reconstruction or as a staged procedure, with staged reconstructions generally performed for larger defects (Fig. 99.5). Of all patients undergoing revision ACL reconstruction, approximately 9% undergo tibial tunnel grafting and 8% undergo femoral tunnel grafting as a staged procedure prior to revision reconstruction.[22] Conversely, concomitant revision reconstruction and bone is performed in only 3% of patients.[22] In the setting of a two-stage procedure, serial radiographs should be obtained to confirm complete graft incorporation prior to the second-stage procedure, which generally follows grafting by approximately 6 months.[76]

Prior to grafting, a thorough débridement of any prior graft and fixation material must be performed to facilitate new graft

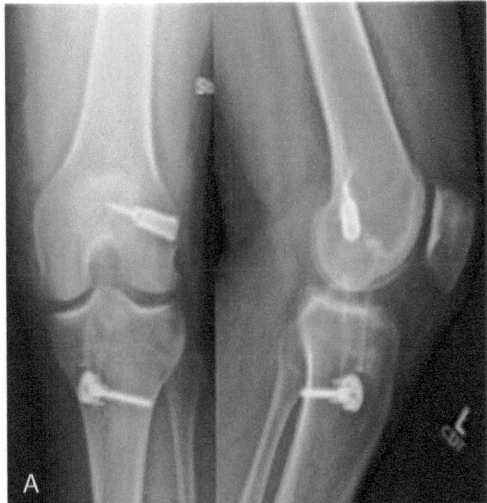

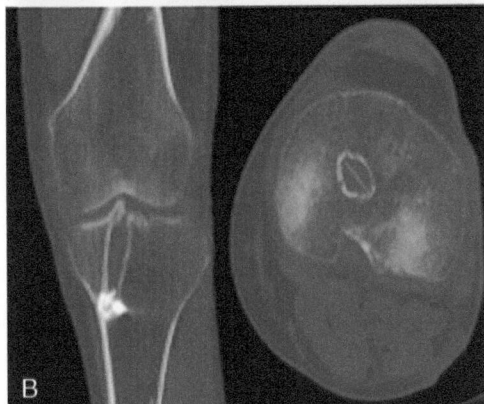

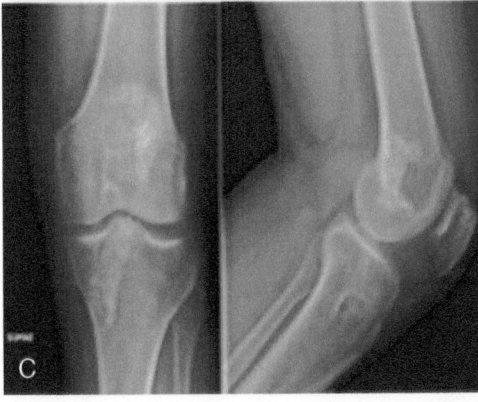

Fig. 99.5 Tunnel expansion in revision anterior cruciate ligament (ACL) reconstruction. (A) Preoperative radiographs prior to revision ACL reconstruction demonstrate fixation from prior failed ACL reconstruction. Tunnels are in a position that would overlap with planned revision ACL tunnels. (B) Computed tomography obtained prior to revision ACL reconstruction demonstrates expansion of tibial tunnel, with tunnel diameter measuring approximately 17 mm. Tunnel expansion would preclude a single stage procedure. (C) Revision ACL reconstruction was performed in staged manner, with allograft dowel plugs used to fill previous tunnels 6 months prior to revision ACL reconstruction.

healing to native bone. Autograft may be harvested from Gerdy tubercle, distal femur, or in the setting of larger defects, the iliac crest. Cancellous allograft can be used alone or in combination with autograft. Alternative autograft sources, including single or multiple press-fit osteochondral autograft transplantation (OAT)

plugs harvested from the iliac crest or medial tibial metaphysis,[118,119] allograft dowel plug grafting (which may allow for larger diameter plugs), and calcium phosphate putties have been described as well, but no long-term results of biologic incorporation in the setting of revision ACL reconstruction are available at this time.[120] Expanded tibial tunnels may be filled with graft placed in an inferior to superior direction directly through the tibial skin incision using a small tamp. When grafting the femoral side, dry arthroscopy may be useful to prevent washing out graft. During femoral tunnel grafting, a small arthroscopic cannula or skid can be placed through an accessory medial portal made in line with the previous femoral tunnel. Allograft dowels may be sized to fit the dilated tunnel size and impacted into place.[121]

Tunnel Preparation

Revision ACL reconstruction is typically performed using a single-bundle technique with tunnels placed in the center of the anatomic footprints.[76] In the setting of overlapping tunnels, in which the previous and newly planned tunnels will overlap, the new femoral or tibial tunnels may be created using the concept of divergent tunnels.[87] Although the previous and new tunnels may converge as they approach the intracondylar notch, the tunnels should separate as they progress further away from the joint, and the new tunnel should sufficiently diverge from the previous tunnel to provide a cylinder of native bone for adequate graft fixation.[76] In the setting of tunnel overlap, an expanded tunnel may also be created by progressively reaming until a uniform cylinder results. Following this, depending on defect size, a custom autograft or allograft plug may be sized to fill the entire defect.[83,122]

Femoral Tunnel

Transtibial drilling of the femoral tunnel limits the position from which the femoral footprint can be accessed. Other options that can be used to access the femoral footprint in an anatomic trajectory include outside-in femoral tunnel creation using a rear-entry technique or using an accessory anteromedial portal, both of which allow creation of an independent femoral tunnel. Notchplasty in the revision setting may result in inferior patient-reported outcomes and should not routinely be performed unless deemed necessary at the time of surgery.[123] For the outside-in rear-entry technique, an incision is made over the lateral aspect of the distal femur, splitting the iliotibial band to allow introduction of a drilling guide (Fig. 99.6). Care should be taken to avoid prior tunnels by using a more horizontal trajectory. Allowing for creation of a completely new femoral tunnel, this technique can provide an excellent way to obtain a new fixation point in the revision setting. Alternatively, an accessory anteromedial portal can be made using arthroscopic visualization with a spinal needle, as varying inferior and medial portal positioning provides a variety of angles to approach the femoral footprint. The knee should be hyperflexed to optimize the length and anterior direction of the newly created tunnel, thereby helping to prevent posterior condyle blowout and peroneal nerve injury.[124] A guide pin may then be placed through this newly created accessory medial portal, directed into the femoral footprint, and driven

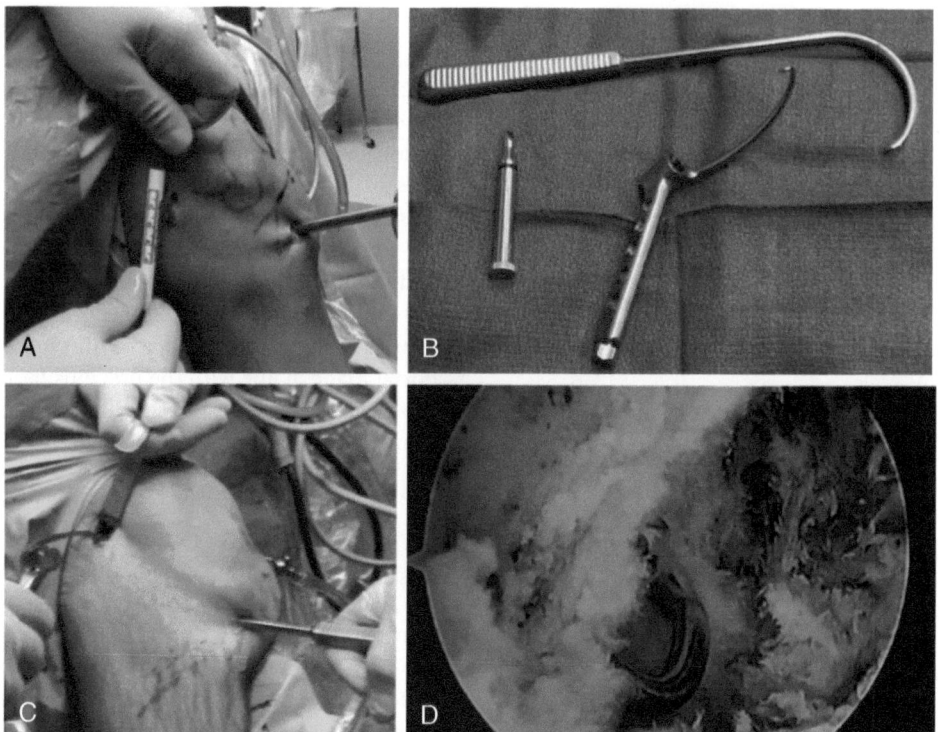

Fig. 99.6 Outside-in rear-entry femoral tunnel preparation. (A) Lateral thigh incision for outside-in rear-entry technique. (B) Guides for rear-entry femoral approach. (C) Rear entry guide pulled through anterolateral portal into notch with curved hook. (D) This technique allows the ability to place guide and drill tunnel at desired location within the intercondylar notch—here femoral tunnel is placed low in notch.

through the lateral cortex of the femur. The guide pin should exit above the level of the superior pole of the patella and anterior to the midline of the femur. With the knee remaining hyperflexed and the surgeon taking care to avoid iatrogenic articular cartilage damage, the guide pin should be overreamed to complete creation of the new femoral tunnel. Use of a unipolar or low-profile reamer may decrease the risk of iatrogenic articular cartilage damage. Following creation of the femoral tunnel, a motorized shaver may be used to remove debris.

Tibial Tunnel

Tibial tunnel management is generally less challenging than on the femoral side because the tibial tunnel is directly accessible through a prior open incision. A variable-angle drilling guide should be directed to enter the tibial articular surface in an anatomic and, if possible, a distinct location from the prior tunnel in order to facilitate adequate fixation. The angle of the new tunnel may be adjusted to create a longer tunnel, if necessary. An excessively posterior tibial tunnel presents a challenge in that the new, more anterior tunnel may overlap with the previous tunnel. Analogous to a blocking screw, a bioabsorbable screw or allograft bone dowel may be placed posteriorly to fill the previous tunnel and facilitate new graft placement in a more anterior position.

Graft Fixation

Prior to graft insertion and fixation, the new tunnel diameters, bone quality, and graft size must be carefully evaluated to ensure

an environment that is adequate for graft fixation and healing. If tunnel expansion is anticipated or occurs following tunnel creation, soft tissue grafts should be used with caution. If 2 to 3 mm of graft-tunnel mismatch occurs, a stacked-screw technique may be used.[76] Alternatively, a bone-patellar tendon-bone (BPTB) autograft with appropriately sized blocks to fill the mismatch may be used. In the setting of larger graft-tunnel mismatch, allograft with affixed bone block (Achilles tendon, BPTB) with appropriately large bone plugs should be prepared taking into account the mismatch. Synthetic dowels and allograft bone plugs have also been used to provide supplemental interference fixation within tunnels.[83,122] In the setting of a loss of tunnel integrity, such as femoral tunnel blowout, or if the bone quality is poor, alternative methods of fixation besides inference screws should be considered. Laterally based bioabsorbable cross-fixation pins and arthroscopic buttons can provide improved fixation on the intact lateral cortex in this setting. Stay sutures may also be inserted through the graft and fixed to a femoral post, with a supplemental post placed on the lateral femur or anterior tibia. Recently, the MARS group has demonstrated improved results with metal screw fixation, and, although the reasons for these results are not yet understood, this should be taken under consideration.[123]

Double-Bundle Reconstruction in Revision Setting

Although double-bundle reconstruction has gained popularity in the past decade,[125-127] there are no absolute indications for this technique in the setting of primary or revision ACL reconstruction.[76,128,129] A failed double-bundle primary reconstruction may present specific challenges because prior tunnel placement with two separate tunnels and soft tissue grafts often interferes with planned tunnels at the time of revision. Although it has been described as feasible, there is currently no evidence that double-bundle reconstruction provides improved stability or clinical outcomes compared to single-bundle reconstruction in the revision setting.[130,131] In addition, conversion from a single- to a double-bundle reconstruction may require staged procedures, with initial bone grafting followed by revision reconstruction, which may unnecessarily delay revision reconstruction, increasing the likelihood of progressive chondrosis.[23]

In the setting of a vertical graft with an excessively posterior tibial tunnel that provides adequate sagittal plane stability but inadequate rotatory stability, an augmentation procedure may be considered in which the previous vertical graft is left intact.[131] A second graft may be placed anterior to the excessively posterior tibial tunnel into a femoral tunnel site located within femoral footprint of the posterolateral bundle. No long-term outcomes following this procedure have been reported, and due to a lack of available data at this time, we cannot recommend the use of any double-bundle reconstruction technique in the revision setting.

Graft Choice

Multiple factors impact the choice of graft in revision ACL reconstruction, including age, sex, previous graft choice, ACL revision number, concurrent ligamentous repair, surgeon preference, and the surgeon's opinion of the prior failure.[132] Although graft choice may impact outcomes in the revision setting, the ability to choose a graft may be limited by a number of other factors.

Factors Affecting Graft Choice

Graft choices for revision reconstruction include semitendinosus and gracilis (hamstring autograft), BPTB, quadriceps tendon, and various allograft choices.[91,138] If autograft is chosen, it should be harvested only after determining that all of the technical steps of the revision reconstruction can be successfully performed.[91] In 2010 the MARS group investigated graft choice at the time of revision ACL reconstruction and found that autograft was used in 45% of cases and allograft in 54%; 64% of autografts 55% of allograft were BPTB. Hamstrings graft made up 29% of autografts and only 5% of allografts.[22] More recently, the MARS group reported that autograft was used in 48% of revision reconstructions and allograft in 49%, with 3% using a combination of both.[132] Surgeon preference was found to be the most important factor in determining revision graft choice. Other factors affecting graft choice were prior graft type and patient age. If an autograft was used previously, an allograft was 3.6 times more likely to be chosen for the revision. It is well established that there is a higher rate of allograft failure in young, active athletes following primary reconstruction,[34] and recent data suggest higher rates of reoperation following prior reconstruction with allograft.[133] The surgeon's opinion of the failure has also been shown to impact graft choice at the time of revision, and a belief that an allograft failed for biologic reasons leads to a higher likelihood of using autograft.

Comparison Among Graft Choices

The use of autograft hamstring, BPTB, and combinations of hamstring, BPTB, and quadriceps tendon autograft has yielded results similar to those reported after primary reconstruction in terms of objective laxity.[51,53,55,56,91,116] The MARS group reported improved patient-reported outcome scores and sports function following autograft revision reconstruction compared with allograft.[134] Furthermore, autograft resulted in a decreased risk of graft failure at 2-year follow-up, and these patients were 2.78 times less likely to undergo subsequent revision reconstruction compared with allograft. No studies have demonstrated differences in terms of graft failure or patient-reported outcomes comparing soft tissue and BPTB autografts. Key factors predisposing to allograft failure appear to be patient age, activity level, and the method of graft processing.[34,135] Irradiation of allograft likely adversely affects graft laxity, predisposing to reconstructions failure.[49,136]

In the setting of graft failure without evidence of technical error from the original procedure, the contralateral or ipsilateral patellar tendon may be the preferred graft source. The contralateral hamstring tendon may be considered as a graft choice if the primary procedure was performed with ipsilateral hamstring autograft.[29] Allograft should be given considering when tunnel expansion precludes the use of autograft alone.

Two-Stage Revision Anterior Cruciate Ligament Reconstruction

Two-stage revision reconstruction is often performed to avoid overlap between tunnels used at the time of revision ACL reconstruction and those made during the previous reconstruction.[24] Because increased time to revision correlates with a higher incidence of meniscal and chondral lesions,[23,53] the revising surgeon must be judicious when deciding whether a two-stage procedure is necessary or a single-stage procedure will suffice. A two-stage procedure generally requires a 6-month window between procedures in which the patient may continue to have instability.[24] When possible, preference should be given to a single-stage procedure as long as appropriate tunnel placement and graft fixation can be achieved. A two-stage revision should be reserved for cases in which tunnel expansion precludes a single-stage procedure.

POSTOPERATIVE MANAGEMENT

Principles of Rehabilitation

The principles of postoperative management following revision ACL reconstruction are similar to primary reconstruction.[143] However, although specific protocols describing the goals and timing for rehabilitation following primary reconstruction are well described,[143-145] there are limited data on rehabilitation following revision surgery. Rehabilitation and eventual return to sport are generally slower than primary reconstruction,[146] especially in the setting of allograft reconstruction in which graft incorporation may take longer.[147,146] Overaggressive rehabilitation may result in early graft failure or late-onset laxity.[29] As previously mentioned, revision patients are more likely to have concomitant intra-articular pathology addressed at the time of

Authors' Preferred Technique

General Principles

As previously mentioned, surgical options may be limited in the revision setting by what was done during the previous reconstruction, as well as based on the etiology of graft failure. Prior graft selection may limit choices in the revision setting. The location and size of previous tunnels may dictate whether graft is necessary and whether the procedure may be successfully completed in one or two stages. The authors use a single-stage procedure unless tunnel dilation exceeds 15 mm, in which case the tunnels are grafted and the revision reconstruction performed in a staged fashion, typically approximately 6 months following tunnel grafting and complete graft incorporation. The second stage procedure is then performed similar to a primary ACL reconstruction but generally rehabilitated more slowly, as described later.

When possible, the authors use autograft, even if the contralateral extremity needs to be used. The authors use a rear-entry two-incision technique unless the locations of prior incisions prohibit this. A rear-entry two-incision approach allows femoral tunnel drilling to be performed independent of the tibial tunnel position, thereby allowing more flexibility in the revision setting. What remains most critical is creating tunnels in a fashion that the surgeon is comfortable with while allowing for adequate fixation. We describe our preferred technique for single-stage, single-bundle revision ACL reconstruction.

Diagnostic Arthroscopy

Standard diagnostic arthroscopy is performed, generally using prior portal incisions. Any additional intra-articular pathology may be treated prior to beginning revision ACL reconstruction. The remnant ACL is débrided and prior tunnel locations identified and assessed. The location of planned tunnels should be compared with the existing tunnels. Hardware is removed if it will affect the revision.

Tunnel Preparation

An incision over the planned tibial tunnel site is made, usually using or extending the prior incision used for tibial tunnel preparation. The exit point of the planned tibial tunnel should lie at the anatomic insertion of the native ACL. If the exit point of the existing tibial tunnel is appropriate, then the newly planned tunnel may be designed to converge with the existing tunnel at the articular surface. If this approach is used, care must be taken to ensure that the two tunnels diverge as they move away from the joint to prevent excessive tunnel dilation. Alternatively, if the previously drilled tunnel is in an appropriate location without excessive tunnel dilation, any hardware interfering with fixation may be removed and the same tunnel used.

Next, the femoral tunnel is prepared. The native femoral insertion should be identified and any graft stump débrided from this location. An accessory anteromedial tunnel is created or extended using a prior incision. Care must be taken not to violate the posterior condylar wall if the newly planned tunnel lies posterior to the previously drilled tunnel. If the previously drilled tunnel enters the joint appropriately at the native insertion, then converging tunnels may be used, as described previously for the tibia. Alternatively, if the previous drilled tunnel is in an appropriate, anatomic position, it may be used in a similar fashion as described for the tibia.

Graft Insertion

Following tunnel preparation, the graft is passed from the distal aspect of the tibial tunnel and pulled through the femoral tunnel similar to a primary reconstruction. The authors generally use interference screw fixation in both the primary and revision setting.

---

surgery, which can also slow rehabilitation depending on which specific structures are injured or repaired.[84,148,149]

Rehabilitation Protocol

Phase 1: Acute Postoperative Phase (0 to 4 Weeks)

The patient is allowed weight bearing as tolerated beginning immediately postoperative as long as there are no contraindications due to other intra-articular injuries. Similar to previous findings in primary ACL reconstructions, recent data demonstrated no improvement from a rehabilitative brace or knee immobilizer (Wright et al., 2017, unpublished data). Crutches are provided for assistance. Patients begin quadriceps activation with active knee ROM and gentle assist on postoperative day 1, with a goal of at least 90 degrees of knee flexion and full extension. Elevation, compression, and icing should be used to minimize effusion.[150] Specific exercises in the acute postoperative phase include quadriceps sets, straight-leg raises, and hamstring activation (heel slides, standing knee flexion). Gait training may begin during the later stages of this first phase.[149] Closed kinetic chain (CKC) exercises, including heel raises and mini-squats, may also commence late in the first stage.

Phase 2: Subacute Postoperative Phase (2 to 8 Weeks)

As the knee joint effusion and pain levels decrease over the first postoperative month, the ability to weight bear without assist and achieve greater motion will also improve. Exercises to improve motion including supine wall slides, active-assisted heel slides, and prone/standing hamstring curls.[149] Aggressive passive knee flexion should be avoided. Patients who have advanced through the first phase may progress to limited open kinetic chain (OKC) exercise (limited isometric knee extension from 45 to 90 degrees), additional CKC exercises through a greater ROM (terminal extension with TheraBand, split squat, hip dominant squat, leg press, step-ups), core strengthening, more advanced gait training, balance exercises, and low-level cardiovascular conditioning including stationary bike.[149,151-154] Aquatic therapy may also be implemented.

Phase 3: Neuromuscular Conditioning (6 Weeks to 8 Months)

Knee ROM should be full extension to greater than 120 degrees of flexion and a normal gait achieved by approximately 12-weeks postoperative. Strengthening and cardiovascular exercises may be intensified. Until approximately 3 months postoperative, CKC exercises predominate, including body-weight squatting, lunges, and leg press.

At 3 months postoperative, patients should not yet be progressed to agility training, instead focusing on an increased intensity of both OKC and CKC exercises, along with progression of core exercises. At approximately 5 to 6 months postoperative, complex movement training reflecting the patient's demands should be implemented. To begin these exercises, which often impart rotational forces about the knee, the patient must have sufficiently progressed in terms of strength and ROM. Cardiovascular training may include progression to jogging and careful incorporation of form running drills, with change of direction drills introduced late in the phase as indicated by patient progression.[149]

Phase 4: Return to Activity (8 Months to 1 Year)

Critical assessment of patient-specific demands in the context of rehabilitation milestones must take place prior to return to full activity. Requisite neuromuscular control and endurance must be achieved to safely meet their sport/activity-specific demands. Functional testing may be performed, including single-hop tests, vertical leap, agility tests, and functional performance testing.[149,155] Reaction drills may be also implemented.[156] Once all deficiencies have been addressed and the patient is psychologically prepared for return to preinjury level of activity, they may be cleared for full a return.[157,158] Recent data suggest that the use of an ACL derotation brace at the time of return to sport may improve patient-reported outcome scores among patients undergoing revision reconstruction and thus should be considered (Wright et al., unpublished data 2016).

RESULTS

Results following revision ACL have been repeatedly demonstrated as inferior to those after primary reconstruction. Although objective rotatory and sagittal laxity can be restored to similar levels as those seen after primary reconstruction, failure rates following revision are three to four times higher than after primary reconstruction.[9] Clinical outcomes scores are also significantly worse compared with primary reconstruction, with lower Cincinnati, Lysholm, Tegner, Marx activity, IKDC, and multiple Knee injury and Osteoarthritis Outcomes Score (KOOS) subscale scores.[9,28,76,159] However, these measures are all significantly improved compared with before revision reconstruction.[3,6,29,87] Approximately 40% of patients undergoing revision ACL reconstruction do not return to the same level of sport or competition.[6,33,54,57,91,98,116,160]

An increased incidence of meniscal and chondral injuries plays significant role in the inferior outcomes compared with primary reconstruction.[6,53] Multiple studies have demonstrated inferior outcomes in patients undergoing revision reconstruction when chondral lesions or meniscal tears are present at the time of revision.[6,53] One study found lower subjective and objective IKDC scores in patients who had undergone prior meniscectomy or were found to have significant cartilage damage at the time of revision ACL reconstruction.[6]

Multiple Revisions

Repeat revision ACL reconstruction restores AP and rotational graft stability while improving the functional outcomes in patients who have failed prior revision reconstruction. However, most patients do not return to the same level of activity following repeat revision.[3,21,117] Although the most common cause of first-time recurrent laxity is a traumatic noncontact injury, multiple-revision patients tend to have recurrent instability without a traumatic injury.[21] This suggests that there may be fundamental differences in how ACL grafts fail in the multiple-revision setting. There is also an increased rate of chondral injuries both within the medial and patellofemoral compartments, suggesting that medial compartment degeneration may be an important factor in recurrent graft injury.[21]

There have been limited reports of multiple revisions, with failure rates ranging from 0% to 13%.[3,117] Repeat revision for recurrent instability without an identifiable traumatic event, the presence of International Cartilage Repair Society (ICRS) grade 3 or 4 chondrosis, and obesity have been associated with inferior outcomes following multiple revision reconstruction.[3,117] In one study, technical error (most often tunnel malposition) was more common in the multiple-revision group than the first-time revision group. Furthermore, staged bone grafting is performed 22% of the time in the multiple-revision knee, double the rate of first-time revision, suggesting that the remaining host tibial and femoral bone is limited after two or more ACL reconstructions. These data also suggest that femoral tunnel malpositioning should be corrected at the time of first revision to lower the risk of recurrent failure.

COMPLICATIONS

Revision ACL reconstruction has a higher complication rate than primary reconstruction, but overall numbers are still relatively low.[7,21,29,61,161] The types of complications following revision reconstruction are similar to those following primary surgery, including infection, stiffness, and venous thromboembolism. Deep surgical site infections occur in 0.5% to 0.8% of patients undergoing revision reconstruction and venous thromboembolism in less than 0.5%.[21,162]

FUTURE CONSIDERATIONS

Revision remains a challenging clinical scenario that requires the widest skill set of any sports procedure including hardware removal, bone grafting, and meniscal and chondral work, along with consideration of alignment and graft choices. The challenge remains to return patients to their previous activity and prevent future injury. Continued evaluation by large prospective cohorts will hopefully continue to elucidate subtle issues contributing to failure and worse outcomes. The MARS group embarked upon a 10-year follow-up with onsite evaluation that may show new findings not found with questionnaire-based follow-up.

For a complete list of references, go to ExpertConsult.com.

SELECTED READING

Citation:
Wright RW, Gill CS, Chen L, et al. Outcome of revision anterior cruciate ligament reconstruction: a systematic review. *J Bone Joint Surg Am.* 2012;94(6):531–536.

Level of Evidence:
IV, systematic review of level I-IV studies

Summary:
This systematic review evaluates 21 eligible studies reporting outcomes of revision ACL reconstruction at minimum 2-year follow-up. The authors report that ACL reconstruction results in a worse outcome compared with primary ACL reconstruction and a dramatically elevated failure rate, 3-4 times higher than primary ACL reconstruction.

Citation:

Group MARS, Wright RW, Huston LJ, et al. Descriptive epidemiology of the Multicenter ACL Revision Study (MARS) cohort. *Am J Sports Med*. 2010;38(10):1979–1986.

Level of Evidence:

II, cross-sectional study

Summary:

This study describes the formation of the prospective MARS cohort and reports patient demographic and clinical features of this group of patients. This comprises the largest revision ACL reconstruction cohort in the literature.

Citation:

MARS Group. Effect of graft choice on the outcome of revision anterior cruciate ligament reconstruction in the Multicenter ACL Revision Study (MARS) cohort. *Am J Sports Med*. 2014;42(10): 2301–2310.

Level of Evidence:

II, prospective cohort study

Summary:

This multicenter prospective study of 1205 patients demonstrates improved sports function and patient-reported outcomes decreased risk of graft rerupture after use of autograft compared with allograft in revision ACL reconstruction.

Citation:

Borchers JR, Kaeding CC, Pedroza AD, et al. Intra-articular findings in primary and revision anterior cruciate ligament reconstruction surgery: a comparison of the MOON and MARS study groups. *Am J Sports Med*. 2011;39(9):1889–1893.

Level of Evidence:

II, prospective cohort study

Summary:

This study compares meniscal and articular cartilage injuries found at the time of primary and revision ACL reconstruction using two of the largest available prospectively collected patient cohorts. The authors report a significantly higher incidence of lateral and patellofemoral compartment chondrosis in the revision setting, with a higher incidence of articular cartilage damage following prior meniscectomy.

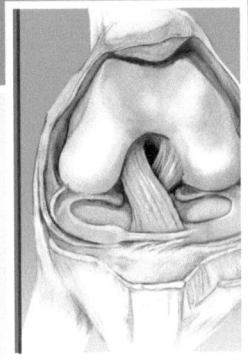

Posterior Cruciate Ligament Injuries

Frank A. Petrigliano, Evan E. Vellios, Scott R. Montgomery, Jared S. Johnson, David R. McAllister

The treatment of posterior cruciate ligament (PCL) injuries is a controversial topic in orthopaedic surgery. In contrast to anterior cruciate ligament (ACL) injuries, for which an abundance of basic science and clinical data is available, the PCL has only recently become a topic of intense investigation. PCL injuries are less common compared with ACL injuries, and thus studies on outcomes are underpowered, making it difficult to draw definitive conclusions regarding management. However, recent biomechanical and clinical data have highlighted the importance of the PCL in knee stability and function. Injury to the PCL, which acts as the primary restraint to posterior tibial translation, may lead to instability, pain, diminished function, and eventually arthrosis.

The purpose of this chapter is to discuss the evaluation, diagnosis, and management of PCL injuries and to present the relevant historic and recent literature on these topics. After a brief review of the pertinent components of the history, physical examination, and imaging modalities, we discuss important considerations in decision-making and treatment options in patients with PCL injuries, as well as our preferred surgical technique and outcomes of surgical management of PCL injuries. Decision-making in this patient population is largely dependent on the grade of PCL injury and the presence or absence of concomitant ligamentous injuries in the knee. We also focus on the latest evidence regarding transtibial versus the tibial inlay technique, single- versus double-bundle methods of reconstruction, and the outcomes of these various surgical treatment options.

HISTORY

The true incidence and prevalence of PCL injuries are unknown and difficult to estimate because many of these injuries, particularly prior to the introduction of magnetic resonance imaging (MRI), were not diagnosed.[1] The reported incidence of PCL injuries has differed depending on the population studied. The incidence is as low as 3% in the outpatient setting[2] and as high as 37% in the traumatic setting.[3] Traumatic injuries and sports-related injuries account for the majority of PCL injuries. A prospective analysis of patients presenting with acute hemarthrosis of the knee and diagnosed with a PCL injury demonstrated that 56.5% of patients were trauma victims, whereas 32.9% had a sports-related injury.[3] Yet isolated PCL injuries were infrequent in this cohort, with 96.5% being part of a multiligamentous

injury. Similarly, in a retrospective cohort of 494 patients with PCL insufficiency, Schulz et al.[4] found traffic accidents (45%) and athletic injuries (40%) to be the most common causes of injury. Among specific sports, the incidence of PCL injury tends to be greater in those involving contact, such as football, soccer, and rugby. In the cohort reviewed by Schulz and colleagues,[4] skiing and soccer were the sports with the highest incidence of PCL injuries. Overall, the incidence of PCL injury has been estimated to be relatively low in athletes across a variety of sports.[5-8]

Important information can be obtained from the history of the patient presenting with acute knee pain or trauma. Any patient with knee pain and swelling with a high-energy mechanism of injury should be suspected of having a PCL injury, another capsuloligamentous injury, or both. Patients commonly report the inability to bear weight, instability, and decreased knee range of motion (ROM). In contrast to ACL injuries, which often result from a noncontact event, PCL injuries are typically due to external trauma. The classic "dashboard injury" pattern results from a posteriorly directed force on the anterior aspect of the proximal tibia with the knee in a flexed position. In patients with a higher energy mechanism of injury, it is possible that a knee dislocation occurred at the time of the injury even if the knee is reduced at the time of the evaluation.

In athletics, the typical mechanism of isolated PCL injury is a direct blow to the anterior tibia (Fig. 100.1A) or a fall onto the knee with the foot plantar flexed. When the foot is in a position of dorsiflexion, the force is transmitted to the patella and distal femur, decreasing the risk of injury to the PCL (Fig. 100.2). Noncontact mechanisms of injury, although less common, have also been reported. Most commonly, this mechanism of injury occurs via forced hyperflexion of the knee (see Fig. 100.1B).[9] In a small cohort reported by Fowler and Messieh,[9] these injuries would often lead to incomplete tearing of the PCL with the posteromedial (PM) fibers intact. Knee hyperextension has also been described as a mechanism of injury, which is usually combined with a varus or valgus force that results in multiple ligament injury (see Fig. 100.1C). Isolated injuries may have more subtle presentations, with patients reporting stiffness, swelling, and pain located in the back of the knee or pain with deep knee flexion (squatting and kneeling). In contrast to acute ACL tears, a "pop" is not usually reported with acute isolated PCL injuries and athletes are often able to continue to play. Reports of anterior knee pain, difficulty ascending stairs, and instability

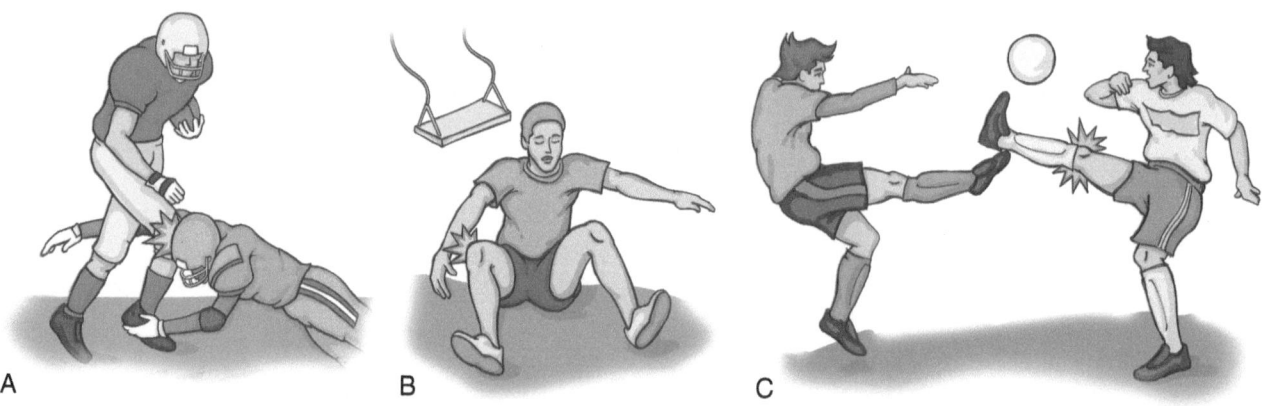

Fig. 100.1 Posterior cruciate ligament injuries are most frequently the result of a blow to the front of the flexed knee.

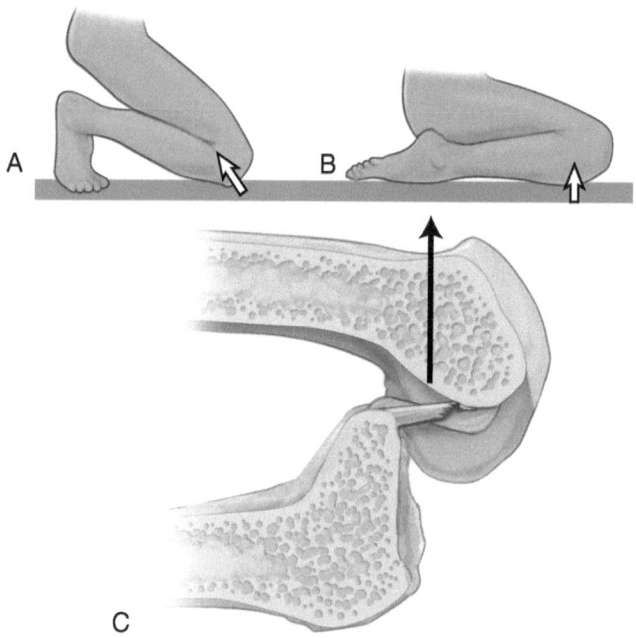

Fig. 100.2 (A) Falling on a flexed knee with the foot in a dorsiflexed position spares injury to the posterior cruciate ligament (PCL) by transmitting the force to the patellofemoral joint. (B) Landing with the foot in a plantar flexed position injures the PCL because the posteriorly directed force is applied to the tibial tubercle. (C) Hyperflexion of the knee without a direct blow is a common mechanism of PCL injury in athletes.

are common when patients present in the chronic phase of an isolated PCL injury.[10]

PHYSICAL EXAMINATION

Posterior Drawer Test

The posterior drawer test was described initially by Hughston et al.[11] in 1976 and later by Clancy et al.[12] in 1983 and is considered the most accurate clinical test to assess the integrity of the PCL, with a sensitivity of 90% and 99% specificity.[13,14] The results of this examination also guide treatment recommendations. A posteriorly directed force is placed on the proximal tibia

with the patient lying supine and the knee flexed to 90 degrees. This test can be performed with the tibia in neutral, external, and internal rotation. It is important to remember that with a PCL injury, the tibia subluxes posteriorly. Thus it is important to first apply an anteriorly directed force to reduce the posterior subluxation before applying the posteriorly directed force (Fig. 100.3). In cases of isolated PCL tears, a decrease occurs in posterior tibial translation with internal tibial rotation.[15] The superficial medial collateral ligament (MCL) and posterior oblique ligament act as a secondary restraint with the tibia in internal rotation.[16] Translation is measured as the change in distance of step-off between the medial tibial plateau relative to the medial femoral condyle. It is critical to examine the contralateral knee, because the normal relationship between the medial tibial plateau and medial femoral condyle is variable, with the plateau normally resting on average 1 cm anterior to the condyle. Understanding this relationship is also critical in avoiding a false-positive anterior drawer test. The presence or lack of a firm end point should also be noted.

The amount of posterior translation observed during the posterior drawer test is used to grade the PCL injury. In grade I injuries, 0 to 5 mm of increased posterior translation is observed compared with the contralateral knee, but the anterior step-off of the plateau relative to the condyle is maintained. Grade II injuries are defined as those with 6 to 10 mm of posterior translation, which results in the plateau being flush with, but not posterior to, the medial femoral condyle. In both grade I and II injuries, the PCL is usually partially torn. With grade III injuries, posterior translation exceeds 10 mm and the medial tibial plateau displaces posterior to the medial femoral condyle during the posterior drawer test. This finding usually represents a complete tear of the PCL and could also represent a combined PCL and posterolateral corner (PLC) injury.

Posterior Sag Test (Godfrey Test) and Quadriceps Active Test

The posterior sag test may be positive in patients with complete PCL tears or partial tears. The patient lies supine with the hip and knee flexed to 90 degrees and the limb supported at the foot by the examiner. The anterior aspect of the proximal tibia

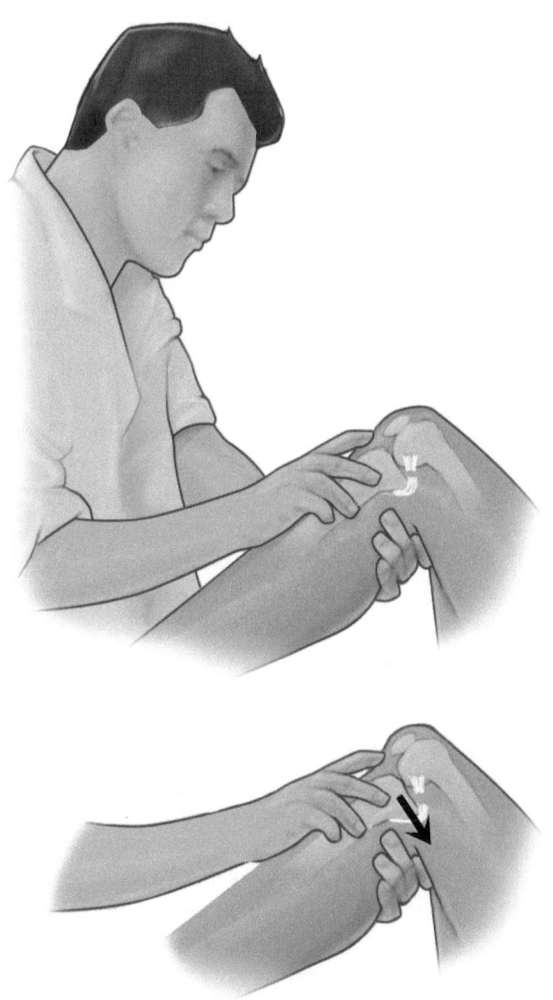

Fig. 100.3 Assessing the tibial step-off before performing the posterior drawer examination. (Modified from Miller MD, Harner CD, Koshiwaguchi S. Acute posterior cruciate ligament injuries. In: Fu FH, Harner CD, Vince KG, eds. *Knee Surgery*. Vol. 1. Baltimore: Williams & Wilkins; 1994.)

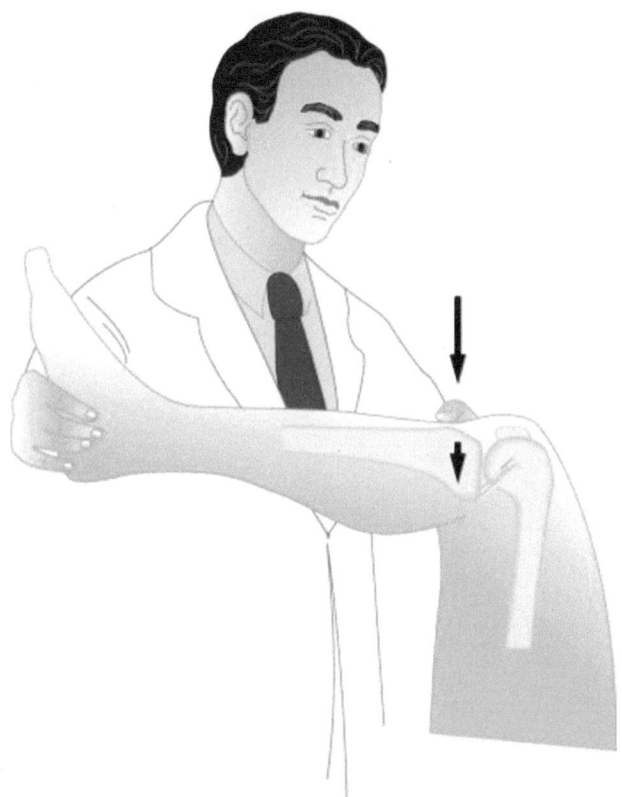

Fig. 100.4 A positive Godfrey test. (Modified from Miller MD, Harner CD, Koshiwaguchi S. Acute posterior cruciate ligament injuries. In: Fu FH, Harner CD, Vince KG, eds. *Knee Surgery*. Vol. 1. Baltimore: Williams & Wilkins; 1994.)

is viewed from the side and compared with the uninjured, contralateral knee. Gravity displaces the tibia posterior to the femur in the case of a complete tear (Fig. 100.4). The quadriceps active test can aid in the diagnosis of complete tears. With this test, the patient lies supine and the knee is placed at 90 degrees of flexion. While the examiner stabilizes the foot, the patient is asked to contract the quadriceps isometrically. In the presence of a complete tear of the PCL (grade III), the patient will achieve dynamic reduction of the posteriorly displaced tibia.

External Rotation of the Tibia (Dial Test)

The dial test is performed to evaluate for concomitant injuries to the PLC, which will affect decision-making and treatment options because these patients are more likely to require surgery. The dial test is performed with the patient positioned prone or supine, while an external rotation force is applied to both feet with the knee positioned at 30 degrees and then 90 degrees of flexion. The degree of external tibial rotation is measured by comparing the medial border of the foot with the axis of the femur. It is essential to compare the results with the contralateral

side because wide variability of external rotation is possible at these positions.[18,19] More than a 10-degree side-to-side difference is considered abnormal.[20] At all degrees of knee flexion, the popliteus complex portion of the PLC is the primary restraint to external rotation, but its effect is maximal at 30 degrees. An increase of 10 degrees or more of external rotation at 30 degrees of knee flexion, but not at 90 degrees, is considered diagnostic of an isolated PLC injury.[21] Increased external rotation at both 30 and 90 degrees of knee flexion suggests a combined PCL and PLC injury.

Reverse Pivot-Shift Test

The reverse pivot-shift test is also used to assess combined injuries and is performed with the patient supine. The knee is passively extended from 90 degrees of flexion with the foot externally rotated and a valgus force applied to the tibia. A positive result is observed when the posteriorly subluxed lateral tibial plateau is abruptly reduced by the iliotibial band at 20 to 30 degrees of flexion. A positive test typically indicates injury to the PCL and another capsuloligamentous structure, usually the PLC.[22]

Collateral Ligament Assessment

Varus and valgus stress tests are used to assess the lateral collateral ligament (LCL) portion of the PLC. The tests are performed with the knee in full extension and in 30 degrees of flexion. Although an isolated PCL injury does not significantly affect varus or valgus stability, increased varus opening at 30 degrees of knee flexion indicates an injury to the LCL and possibly the popliteus complex. If a significant degree of varus opening is noted at full extension, a combined injury of the PLC, PCL, and/or ACL is likely present.[24,25]

Gait and Limb Alignment

The evaluation of gait and limb alignment is particularly important for persons with chronic injury of the PCL or the PLC. In these patients, varus alignment, external rotation, and varus thrust may be observed. Compromised function of the stabilizers of the lateral knee can lead to excessive posterolateral rotation and varus opening (or thrust) in the stance phase of gait.

IMAGING

Radiography

In the acute setting, plain radiographs of the knee should be performed, including bilateral standing anteroposterior, flexion posteroanterior 45 degrees with weight bearing, and Merchant patellar and lateral radiographs. These views are evaluated for posterior tibial subluxation, avulsion fractures, posterior tibial slope, and tibial plateau fractures. Tibial plateau fractures often indicate a high-energy injury with multiligament involvement. Bony avulsion fractures can be seen at the insertion of the PCL and at the fibular head, medial tibial plateau (medial Segond fracture), or the tibial tubercle.[26] Identification of bony avulsion injuries of the PCL, when recognized acutely, may be repaired primarily with superior results compared with late reconstruction.[26,27] Identification of tibial tubercle fractures is also critical. The unopposed pull of the hamstrings causes posterior tibial subluxation in this scenario, which can become fixed within a short time, requiring open reduction. Medial Segond fractures represent a medial capsular avulsion in PCL injuries that may be associated with a peripheral medial meniscus tear.[28,29] Lastly, long leg hip-to-ankle views are critical to evaluate overall lower extremity alignment, particularly varus, in chronic or revision cases.

Stress radiographs are not necessary to diagnose a PCL injury but may be helpful to differentiate between complete and partial PCL tears. However, these radiographs are most commonly used for research purposes. In a retrospective review of 21 patients with partial or complete PCL tears, Hewett and colleagues[31] found that stress radiographs were more accurate than KT-1000 measurements in diagnosing PCL tears. With the knee flexed to 70 degrees and an 89-N weight suspended from the tibia at the level of the tibial tubercle, a lateral radiograph was taken. The mean translation of the medial tibial plateau was 12.2 mm in the presence of a complete tear compared with 5.2 mm seen with a partial tear as confirmed with diagnostic arthroscopy. The magnitude of posterior tibial translation during stress radiography has been correlated with the presence of combined ligament injury. In a cadaveric study by Sekiya et al.,[32] the authors demonstrated that greater than 10 mm of posterior tibial translation on stress radiography correlated with the presence of a PLC injury in addition to a complete disruption of the PCL. It should be noted that the accuracy of stress radiography may be decreased by patient guarding and partial reduction of the tibia

with quadriceps activation; in addition, this infrequently performed examination is operator dependent. Stress radiographs can also be influenced by tibial rotation, and thus some authors have concluded that physical examination may be equally sensitive to stress radiographs in determining the presence and extent of a PCL tear.[33]

Magnetic Resonance Imaging

MRI has become the imaging modality of choice for confirming the presence of an acute PCL tear and to diagnose associated injuries with a sensitivity of up to 100%.[14,34,35] The location and physical characteristics of the tear can also be assessed with MRI and may have implications for prognosis and treatment.[36,37] MRI may be less sensitive in the diagnoses of chronic tears. The normal PCL appears dark on T1- and T2-weighted sequences and is curvilinear in appearance.[38] In contrast, chronic tears of the PCL can heal and assume the aforementioned curvilinear appearance; thus MRIs are much less sensitive for chronic PCL tears, and the appearance of a normal shape of the ligament should not be used as a criterion for a normal PCL.[39,40]

Lastly, MRI provides important information on the status of the menisci, articular cartilage, and other ligaments in the knee, because concomitant injuries affect treatment decision-making and prognosis.[41] Bone bruises have been found in 83% of grade II and III PCL injuries on MRI, but in contrast to the bone bruise associated with ACL tears, the location is variable.[42] The utility of MRI for the diagnosis of associated injuries to the PLC has previously been evaluated. With use of thin-slice coronal oblique T1-weighted images through the entire fibular head, LaPrade and colleagues[43] were able to identify injury to the posterolateral structures with an accuracy of 68.8% to 94.4%, depending on the structure. Similarly, Theodorou et al.[44] found that MRI has an accuracy of 79% to 100% for the diagnoses of posterolateral injuries confirmed with arthroscopy.

Bone Scan

Although a bone scan is not frequently used, it can be useful in the evaluation and management of chronic PCL injuries. In particular, patients with these injuries are predisposed to early medial and patellofemoral compartment chondrosis.[12,45,46] In the setting of an isolated PCL-deficient knee with medial or patellofemoral compartment pain and normal radiographs, a bone scan to assess these compartments may be indicated. Increased uptake suggests that surgical intervention may be beneficial,[47] although this supposition has not been proven definitively.

DECISION-MAKING

Decision-making in the treatment of PCL injuries is dependent on the natural history of the disease, with most treatment recommendations made on the basis of symptoms, activity level, grade of the injury, and associated injuries. As with any orthopaedic ailment, operative intervention should be chosen only if it results in superior outcomes compared with nonsurgical management. Controversy exists regarding PCL treatment because the extent to which posterior laxity causes symptoms or accelerates the development of degenerative joint disease (DJD) is unclear.

However, a computational knee kinematic study by Kang et al. suggests that PCL deficiency leads to significantly increased contact forces on the patellofemoral joint as well as PLC structures during normal gait.[48] Furthermore, it is unknown whether reconstruction sufficiently mitigates laxity to result in clinical improvement and slow the development of DJD. Reducing posterior laxity with reconstruction may improve long-term outcomes in patients with PCL injuries, and yet residual laxity is common even after reconstruction.[49,50] Some investigators propose that isolated PCL tears follow a benign course in the short term without reconstruction[1,9,47,51] but that diminishing results may be seen at a later point.[52] To date, no study has demonstrated that PCL reconstruction can prevent the development of DJD.[53]

Controversy remains regarding indications for nonoperative versus operative management because few clinical studies have sufficient sample sizes and duration of follow-up to draw definitive conclusions. Additionally, a variety of PCL reconstructions are currently used, and the treatment of isolated PCL injuries is often reported in conjunction with combined injuries, such as PLC injuries, making outcome studies relatively heterogeneous. Currently most studies are retrospective in nature and use various outcome measurements, which make comparisons difficult. Until randomized prospective clinical trials are conducted, this debate will likely continue. The next section reviews the results of nonoperative management of PCL injuries and conclude the section with our decision-making rationale.

Nonoperative Treatment

Many studies have found favorable outcomes when isolated PCL injuries are treated conservatively. Parolie and Bergfeld[1] evaluated patient satisfaction in 25 persons with isolated PCL tears that had resulted from sporting injuries at a minimum of 2 years of follow-up. These investigators found that 68% of patients returned to their previous level of activity and 80% were satisfied with their knee function. They evaluated laxity and found no correlation with DJD. More recently, Shelbourne and Muthukaruppan[54] prospectively evaluated 215 conservatively treated patients with isolated PCL tears. Their study focused on patients with grade II laxity or less. These investigators found that subjective scores did not correlate with the degree of laxity and mean scores did not decrease with time from injury. They were unable to identify any risk factors that would predict which patients would have a decline in knee function over time. Patel et al.,[55] in another recent retrospective review of 57 patients with grade A or B PCL tears, a grading system proposed by MacGillivray and colleagues[56] also found that functional scores did not correlate with the degree of PCL laxity. Lysholm knee scores were excellent in 40% and good in 52%. Patel et al.[55] found grade I medial compartment osteoarthritis (OA) in seven knees, grade II in three knees, and mild patellofemoral OA in four knees at an average of 6.8 years of follow-up. They concluded that most patients with acute, isolated PCL tears do well with nonoperative management at intermediate follow-up. Furthermore, a more recent study by Shelbourne and colleagues showed that at an average of 14.3 years follow-up 89% (39/44) of individuals with isolated grade I or II PCL injuries treated nonoperatively showed full ROM, good quadriceps strength, and minimal OA.[57]

Other investigators have also found good initial clinical outcomes with nonoperative treatment but have found deterioration at extended follow-up. Boynton and Tietjens[52] observed 38 patients with isolated tears for a mean of 13.4 years. Of these patients, eight had subsequent meniscal injuries and surgery. Of the remaining 30 patients with normal menisci, 24 (81%) had occasional pain, 17 (56%) had occasional swelling, and a positive increase in articular cartilage degeneration was seen on radiographs over time. Fowler and Messieh[9] prospectively followed up 13 patients with acute isolated PCL tears that were confirmed by arthroscopy and treated with physiotherapy. All patients had a good subjective functional score according to the Houston criteria, but objective scores were good in only 3 patients and only fair in the other 10 patients.

Although relatively good results have been observed with nonoperative treatment, it should be noted that many of the patients in these series had grade II laxity or less and not all patients achieved a normal outcome, especially patients with grade III injuries. The benign course observed may be due to the integrity of the secondary restraints and various portions of the PCL complex remaining intact in persons with less serious injuries. Tibial slope may also affect the stability of the PCL deficient knee. In a cadaveric study, increasing the posterior tibial slope decreased the static posterior instability of the PCL/PLC-deficient knee, whereas decreasing the tibial slope increased posterior instability and the magnitude of the reverse pivot-shift test.[58]

Despite acceptable clinical results with nonoperative treatment, it is well understood that PCL deficiency alters knee kinematics and the distribution of load during activity. In an uninjured knee, numerous biomechanical studies have shown that the PCL plays a significant role in tibiofemoral joint stability throughout an active and passive ROM especially in the presence of a posteriorly directed tibial force, while it has been shown that the PCL-deficient knee experiences increased contact pressures in the patellofemoral and medial compartments.[48,59,60] Logan et al.[59] evaluated the effect of PCL rupture on tibiofemoral motion during squatting with use of MRI. They concluded that PCL deficiency is similar to a medial meniscus resection and results in a "fixed" anterior subluxation of the medial femoral condyle (posterior subluxation of the medial tibial plateau). This subluxation changes the kinematics of the knee and may explain the increase in medial compartment OA seen in PCL-deficient knees. Currently more attention is being placed on additional injuries that are commonly associated with grade III tears that lead to greater instability and more severely altered biomechanics.

Although it is known that the kinematics of the knee are altered in the presence of a PCL injury, specific prognostic factors that predict outcome have proven elusive. In many studies the time from injury and objective instability have not correlated well with final outcome and radiographic changes. Surgical reconstruction is not recommended for isolated grade I injuries. Because many patients with isolated grade II posterior laxity only improve to grade I laxity with reconstruction, we agree with other authors that operative intervention in these patients may not offer improved outcome when compared with nonoperative treatment.[49,54] The treatment of acute isolated grade III PCL injuries is controversial. In these patients, some surgeons favor a more aggressive approach involving PCL reconstruction, whereas others recommend nonsurgical treatment. In cases with greater than 10 mm of abnormal posterior laxity, the clinician should remember to have a high index of suspicion for a combined ligamentous injury involving the PLC.

Level I evidence does not currently exist to support strong recommendations on the management of PCL injuries. However, based on the previously described data, we recommend nonoperative management for the treatment of acute and chronic isolated grade I and II PCL injuries (Figs. 100.5 and 100.6). Operative management is reserved for chronic isolated grade III PCL injuries with symptoms of pain or instability when an adequate course of conservative treatment has failed. In addition, surgical treatment is usually recommended for acute and chronic combined ligamentous injuries. The treatment of acute grade III PCL tears is controversial, with some surgeons recommending PCL reconstruction and others recommending nonoperative treatment. Lastly, open reduction and internal fixation are recommended for acute avulsion fractures at the PCL tibial attachment site.

TREATMENT OPTIONS

Nonoperative Treatment

As discussed in the previous section, nonoperative treatment is recommended in patients with acute, isolated grade I or II PCL tears.[1,45] Nonoperative management is aimed at counteracting the forces of gravity and the hamstring muscles, which act to sublux the tibia posteriorly on the femur. Pierce and colleagues[62] have recently reviewed the literature on rehabilitation protocols for nonoperative and operative treatment of PCL injuries. Based on the finding of the reviewed studies, a three-phase rehabilitation

protocol was recommended. We follow a similar protocol at our institution.

In the first 6 weeks after injury (phase I), rehabilitation is focused on partial weight-bearing, hamstring and gastrocnemius stretching to reduce the posterior pull on the tibia, quadriceps strengthening and prone ROM exercises. In this initial phase, a number of immobilization techniques have been described to decrease stress on the healing ligament. These techniques include bracing the knee locked between 0 and 60 degrees of knee flexion,[63] use of a cylindrical leg cast with a posterior support to prevent posterior displacement of the tibia,[64] and use of a brace with a dynamic anterior drawer to apply an anterior force on the posterior proximal tibia.[65,66] In phase II, 6 to 12 weeks after injury, the focus is on progressive strengthening, reestablishment of full ROM, and improving proprioception. In phase III, 13 to 18 weeks after the injury occurred, the patient is allowed to begin running and to perform sports-specific exercises, with return to sports allowed 4 to 6 months after the initial injury, assuming quadriceps strength is comparable to that of the contralateral leg. It is important to note that this time frame can be significantly accelerated in the case of elite athletes with potential return to sport as early as 6 to 8 weeks but with the expected risk of increased residual joint laxity.[61]

Operative Treatment

A number of surgical techniques for PCL reconstruction can be considered. Current surgical treatment options include transtibial and tibial inlay reconstruction techniques with single- or double-bundle reconstruction and a variety of fixation methods. Several biomechanical and anatomic studies have been published recently investigating the benefits and pitfalls of these techniques.

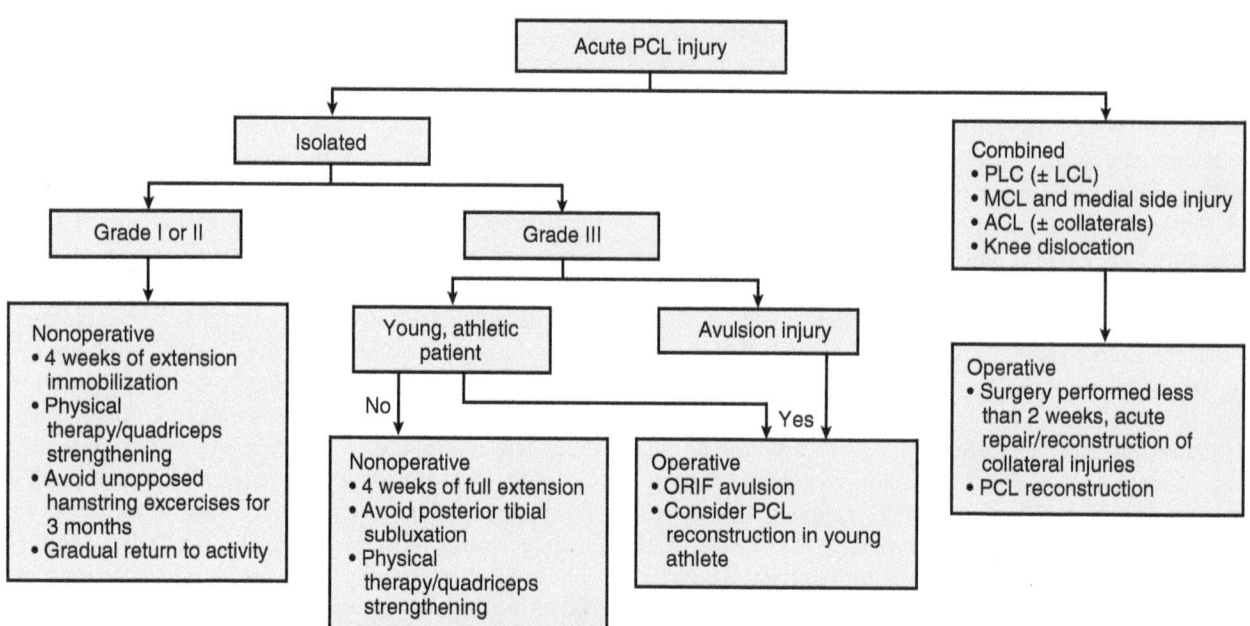

Fig. 100.5 Treatment recommendations for acute injuries of the posterior cruciate ligament *(PCL)*. *ACL,* Anterior cruciate ligament; *LCL,* lateral collateral ligament; *MCL,* medial collateral ligament; *ORIF,* open reduction, internal fixation; *PLC,* posterolateral corner.

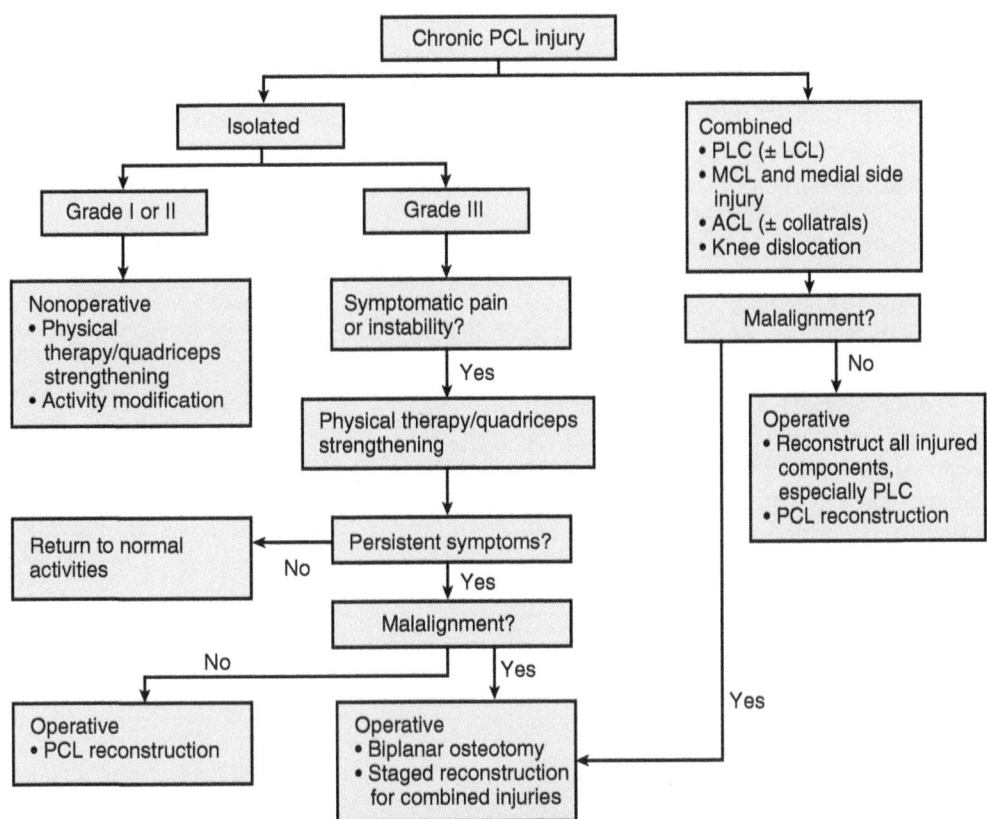

Fig. 100.6 Treatment recommendations for chronic injuries of the posterior cruciate ligament *(PCL)*. *ACL,* Anterior cruciate ligament; *LCL,* lateral collateral ligament; *MCL,* medial collateral ligament; *PLC,* posterolateral corner.

However, no consensus currently exists on the best method of PCL reconstruction.

Transtibial Tunnel Versus Tibial Inlay Techniques

The transtibial technique is a commonly used method of PCL reconstruction. In this technique, the tibial and femoral tunnels are drilled and the graft must make a sharp turn around the "killer turn" as it surfaces from the tibial tunnel and changes direction before entering the knee joint. This acute turn has been implicated as the cause of graft abrasion with subsequent thinning of the graft and eventual graft rupture or excessive laxity.[65] The residual posterior knee laxity observed clinically after traditional transtibial PCL reconstruction techniques may be related to this acute turn. To address the concern of graft attenuation resulting from this tunnel, the tibial inlay technique was developed and reported by Jakob and Ruegsegger,[67] as well as by Berg.[68] In this technique, direct fixation occurs at the tibial attachment site of the PCL, preventing an acute turn as the graft passes from the tibia to the femoral tunnel.

A number of cadaveric biomechanical studies have compared the transtibial and tibial inlay techniques. Although McAllister et al.[69] found no significant differences in mean knee laxities between the tibial tunnel and tibial inlay techniques at time zero, increased laxity was observed with this technique after cyclic loading. Bergfeld et al.[70] assessed anteroposterior laxity in cadaveric knees undergoing tunnel reconstruction or inlay reconstruction. Minimal differences in anteroposterior laxity were observed

in the inlay group when compared with the tunnel group from 30 to 90 degrees of knee flexion and after repetitive loading at 90 degrees of knee flexion. However, evaluation of the grafts after testing demonstrated evidence of graft thinning and attenuation in the tunnel group but not in the inlay group. In a detailed cyclic loading analysis, Markolf and colleagues[71] also evaluated cadaver knees with tibial inlay and transtibial reconstruction. Ten of 31 grafts in the tunnel group failed at the acute angle before 2000 cycles of testing could be completed, whereas all 31 grafts that had been fixed to the tibia with use of the inlay method survived the testing intact. In addition, a significant increase in graft thinning and stretching out was observed in the remaining tunnel grafts that survived testing compared with the inlay grafts.

Thus in vitro analyses comparing the transtibial technique with tibial inlay suggest that although initial knee stability is equivalent, posterior laxity increases with cyclic loading with the transtibial technique when compared with the tibial inlay technique. Attempts have also been made to decrease the effects of the killer turn by reducing the sharp edge at the tibial tunnel exit, but this technique has only been attempted in an animal model.[72] Weimann and colleagues[72] found that rounding the sharp edge of the tibial tunnel decreased graft damage associated with the killer turn in a porcine model of PCL reconstruction. To date, retrospective studies comparing patients undergoing transtibial versus tibial inlay procedures[56,73] have not shown significant differences in subjective outcome or knee laxity measurements.[74,75] Thus although the tibial inlay technique may have some biomechanical advantages when tested in a cadaveric model, these advantages have yet to be realized in the clinical setting.

Single-Bundle Versus Double-Bundle Reconstruction

Controversy also exists regarding the utility of single- versus double-bundle techniques of PCL reconstruction. The native PCL can be divided into an anterolateral (AL) and a PM bundle (Fig. 100.7). The AL bundle is tight in knee flexion and becomes lax in extension, whereas the PM bundle is tight in knee extension and becomes lax in flexion. The AL bundle is larger in cross-sectional area and thus is most commonly reconstructed in single-bundle procedures (Fig. 100.8). Double-bundle PCL reconstructions were proposed to more closely reproduce the anatomy and biomechanical properties of the intact PCL. Biomechanical studies have indicated that the two bundles demonstrate reciprocal tightening during knee ROM and both are active in reducing posterior tibial translation and external tibial rotation, suggesting that both are required for normal knee kinematics.[76,77]

Single- versus double-bundle PCL reconstruction have been compared in several biomechanical studies, and some investigators have suggested improved biomechanics with double-bundle reconstruction.[78,79] Milles et al.[80] compared single-bundle versus double-bundle reconstruction in cadaveric human knees using five different surgical techniques and found increased stiffness and decreased laxity in double-bundle reconstructions at numerous flexion angles. Tsukada et al.[81] compared single AL bundle reconstruction, single PM bundle reconstruction, and double-bundle reconstruction in cadaveric human knees at different angles of knee flexion. The double-bundle reconstruction resisted posterior tibial load better than the AL single bundle at 0 and 30 degrees of knee flexion and better than the PM single bundle at 30, 60, and 90 degrees of knee flexion under the posterior

tibial load, leading the authors to conclude that double-bundle reconstruction reduces laxity in extension.

Additional studies have demonstrated potential drawbacks of double-bundle reconstruction, and some studies have been unable to demonstrate a benefit. Whiddon et al.[82] compared single- and double-bundle tibial inlay reconstruction in a cadaver

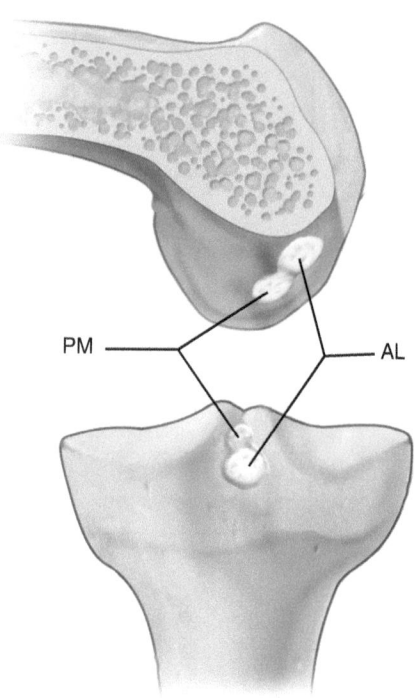

Fig. 100.7 Femoral and tibial insertion sites of the posteromedial *(PM)* and anterolateral *(AL)* bundles of the posterior cruciate ligament. (From Chahla J, Nitri M, Civitarese D, et al. Anatomic double bundle posterior cruciate ligament reconstruction. *Arthrosc Tech.* 2016;5(1):149–156.)

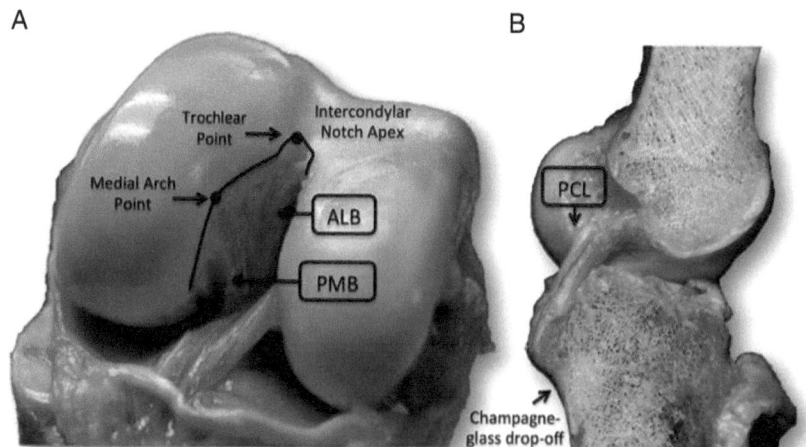

Fig. 100.8 (A) Left knee showing both bundles: anterolateral bundle *(ALB)* and posteromedial bundle *(PMB)*. The trochlear point is easily identifiable on the distal aspect of the trochlea. The more anterior aspect of the ALB is noted by the trochlear point, whereas its more inferoposterior aspect is delineated by the medial arch point. Likewise, the PMB is located along the wall of the notch and distal to the medial arch point. (B) Profile view of a hemi-sectioned left knee showing the tibial and femoral insertion of the posterior cruciate ligament *(PCL).* (From Chahla J, Nitri M, Civitarese D, et al. Anatomic double-bundle posterior cruciate ligament reconstruction. *Arthrosc Tech.* 2016;5[1]:e149–e156. Elsevier, Inc.)

model and found that the double-bundle technique improved rotational stability and posterior translation in knees with a concomitant PLC injury. However, no advantage was seen with a double-bundle reconstruction when compared with a single-bundle reconstruction with regard to posterior translation with the PLC intact. In addition, excessive rotational constraint was observed at 30 degrees. Wiley and colleagues[83] also observed that although posterior laxity was reduced compared with single-bundle reconstruction, overconstraint at 30 degrees of flexion was seen with double-bundle reconstruction. In a comparison of single-bundle AL reconstruction with double-bundle reconstruction in cadaver knees, Markolf and colleagues[84] found that the addition of a PM bundle reduced laxity from 0 to 30 degrees of flexion but at the expense of increased PCL graft forces. Bergfeld et al.[85] compared single- and double-bundle tibial inlay reconstruction in cadaveric knees using Achilles tendon grafts. No differences in translation between the single- and double-bundle reconstruction were observed at any flexion angle.

A number of clinical studies have shown no significant differences in subjective and objective results between single- and double-bundle PCL graft reconstructions.[86–88] Jain and colleagues performed a retrospective review of 40 patients, 18 of which underwent double-bundle PCL reconstruction and 22 of which underwent single-bundle PCL reconstruction and looked at clinical, functional, and radiologic outcomes at 24 months postoperatively.[8] KT-1000 measurements showed an average side-to-side difference in the double-bundle group of 1.78 mm and 2.4 mm in the single-bundle group ($P < .04$). Stress radiographs showed increased posterior tibial translation in the single-bundle group as compared to the double-bundle group. However, both double-bundle and single-bundle groups showed significant functional improvement in Lysholm and IKDC scores with no statistically significant difference between the groups themselves. Furthermore, Hatayama et al.,[88] in a retrospective clinical study comparing arthroscopic single-bundle and double-bundle PCL reconstruction showed that at 2-year follow-up of 3/10 patients who underwent double-bundle PCL reconstruction showed rupture of the PM bundle at second-look arthroscopy.[89] Based on the literature to date, we believe evidence is lacking to support the routine use of double-bundle reconstruction. However, this type of reconstruction remains a topic of interest and is undergoing continued investigation in the treatment of PCL injuries.

Graft Choice and Fixation

Graft choice and fixation techniques are also important considerations when discussing treatment options for surgery. Both autograft and allograft tissues have been used for PCL reconstruction. Bone–patellar tendon–bone, hamstring, and quadriceps tendons are common autograft sources. The Achilles tendon, as well as anterior and posterior tibial tendons, are frequently used allografts. Among autografts, bone–patellar tendon–bone grafts have the advantage of bone-to-bone healing in the bone tunnel. In comparison, the tendon portion of the quadriceps graft and both ends of hamstring grafts require tendon-to-bone healing in the bone tunnel, which may have inferior biomechanical properties.[90] Weakening of the quadriceps tendon, which acts

synergistically with the PCL to prevent posterior tibial translation, is a concern with this graft option, as is the variable length of the tendinous portion.[91] Lin et al.[92] performed a retrospective review of 59 patients with isolated PCL injuries who either underwent arthroscopic transtibial single-bundle PCL reconstruction using autologous patellar tendon or hamstring tendon grafts looking for differences in clinical outcomes. At an average of 4 years follow-up, patients who underwent single-bundle PCL reconstruction using bone–patellar tendon–bone grafts demonstrated significantly more kneeling pain, anterior knee pain, squatting pain, posterior drawer laxity, and osteoarthritic change on radiography. Allograft tissue has the advantage of avoiding donor-site morbidity, reducing operating time, and offering improved graft diameter with greater collagen tissue when Achilles and tibialis anterior tendons are used. Pitfalls of allografts include a small risk of disease transmission, cost, and availability. In a survey of orthopaedic surgeons, Dennis et al.[93] reported that allograft Achilles tendon was the most commonly used graft for acute (43%) and chronic (50%) PCL reconstructions. For the reasons previously discussed, we favor the use of Achilles tendon allografts for PCL reconstruction.

A number of biomechanical studies have investigated various graft fixation constructs used in PCL reconstruction. Most recently, Lim et al.[94] compared cross-pin fixation in a porcine model with bone blocks, interference screw fixation with bone blocks, cross-pin fixation of soft tissue with backup fixation, and interference screw fixation of soft tissue with backup fixation on the tibial side using Achilles allograft PCL reconstruction. Although cross-pin fixation with backup fixation had a higher maximum failure load and stiffness, tendon graft displacement was increased compared with bone-block fixation. Gupta and colleagues compared bioabsorbable to metallic screws for inlay fixation and found no difference in failure load or linear stiffness.[95] Markolf and colleagues[96] demonstrated the importance of bone-block position and orientation within the tibial tunnel; they found that positioning the bone–patellar tendon–bone graft flush with the posterior tunnel opening with the graft oriented so the bone block faced anteriorly in the tibial tunnel was the position with the best biomechanical properties. Margheritini et al.[97] found that combining distal and proximal tibial fixation resulted in significantly less posterior tibial translation and more closely restored intact PCL in situ forces at 90 degrees than did reconstruction with distal fixation.

High Tibial Osteotomy for Chronic PCL Injuries

A chronic isolated PCL injury results in posterior translation of the tibia and external rotation of the tibia in relation to the femur. These anatomic changes result in increased forces and subsequent development of OA in the medial and patellofemoral compartments.[98–100] Additionally, a chronic combined PCL and PLC injury can result in chronic posterolateral instability and varus malalignment associated with bony deformity, lateral soft tissue deficiency, and hyperextension and external rotation as a result of PLC deficiency (i.e., triple varus).[101] In cases of chronic PCL or combined PCL/PLC injury with resultant varus malalignment and posterior or posterolateral instability, soft-tissue procedures alone may be insufficient, whereas performance of a high tibial osteotomy (HTO) prior to soft-tissue reconstruction may improve outcomes by decreasing forces across the lateral supporting structures of the knee.

A medial opening wedge HTO can improve alignment and decrease instability by addressing both coronal and sagittal malalignment. In addition to correcting varus malalignment, a medial opening wedge osteotomy with the anteromedial gap equal or larger than the posterior medial gap increases the posterior tibial slope[102] and thus decreases the posterior resting position of the tibia.[103] In contrast, a lateral closing wedge osteotomy may decrease posterior tibial slope, consequently increasing the posterior resting position of the tibia,[104] and thus may not be appropriate in the knee with a PCL injury. Several investigators have demonstrated a concomitant increase in posterior tibial slope with opening wedge HTO.[105,106] Specifically, Noyes et al.[102] calculated that for each increase of 1 mm in the anterior gap, an increase of 2 degrees occurs in the posterior tibial slope. In the coronal plane, in the absence of medial compartment OA, the osteotomy should result in the mechanical axis crossing the center of the knee. If medial compartment joint space narrowing is present, some authors have recommended valgus hypercorrection with the mechanical axis crossing lateral to the center of the knee.[101]

Although satisfactory long-term outcomes have been observed in patients undergoing HTO for medial compartment OA,[106] studies reporting results of HTO specifically for chronic PCL deficiency or combined PCL/PLC insufficiency are limited and heterogeneous in patient population, duration of follow-up, and outcomes. In a case series of 17 HTOs for symptomatic hyperextension varus thrust that included four patients with isolated PCL injuries and seven with combined PCL and posterolateral ligament injuries, improved subjective activity scores were observed postoperatively at a mean follow-up of 56 months.[105] Similarly, Badhe and Forster[107] reported the results of HTO with or without ligament reconstruction in 14 patients with knee instability and varus alignment, including nine patients with PLC or combined PCL injury. The mean time from injury to HTO was 8.3 years. Although the mean Cincinnati Knee Score improved from a mean preoperative score of 53 to a mean postoperative score of 74, no patients were able to participate in competitive sports, and more than 30% had continued knee pain at follow-up. Thus although biomechanical studies suggest that HTO may improve alignment and stability in patients with chronic PCL insufficiency or combined PCL/PLC injury with varus malalignment and instability, data on outcomes in this patient population are currently minimal.

 Authors' Preferred Technique

Posterior Cruciate Ligament Reconstruction

As discussed previously, many techniques have been described for PCL reconstruction. We prefer the tibial inlay method of reconstruction with an Achilles tendon allograft. The tibial inlay approach avoids the "killer turn" that may predispose the graft to stretch out and failure. We also believe that the acute angle of the graft as it enters the notch in the transtibial technique can make tensioning more difficult. Some surgeons are concerned that the posterior approach to the tibia needed for the open inlay procedure, which may involve a change to the prone position, is more technically demanding. We believe that with experience these challenges are easily overcome and that this technique leads to better biomechanical stability.

Previous studies have demonstrated that the AL bundle is the most important component of the native PCL. The AL bundle has a higher cross-sectional area and is stronger than the PM bundle. Therefore the goal of a single-bundle reconstruction is to recreate the native AL bundle. However, it should be remembered that the footprint of the native PCL is much larger than the typical drill used to create the femoral tunnel, and thus the surgeon must choose which portion of the PCL to reconstruct. Clinical studies comparing single- versus double-bundle reconstructions have not found any significant differences in patient outcome scores. Multiple options are available for graft tissue, and no study has conclusively demonstrated a superior graft. We use an Achilles tendon allograft for most of our PCL reconstructions. We prefer to use the Achilles tendon because of its size, strength, and versatility. For the aforementioned reasons, we prefer to use a single-bundle tibial inlay technique with use of an Achilles allograft for PCL reconstruction. This procedure is described in the following sections.

Graft Preparation

The soft-tissue portion of the Achilles allograft is sized for a 10-mm bone tunnel. The bone plug is then fashioned into a trapezoidal shape 25 mm in length and 13 mm in width. The bone plug is predrilled and tapped for a 6.5-mm cancellous screw. The bone plug is drilled with a 4.5-mm drill from the cancellous to cortical surface to protect the soft tissue and is then tapped with a 6.5-mm tap. A 6.5-mm cancellous screw, approximately 35 mm in length, and a metal washer are then placed into the bone plug from the soft tissue/cortical surface to the cancellous surface. The screw is placed so that the tip is 5 mm past the cancellous surface to facilitate later tibial fixation. A running locking stitch is then placed along approximately 30 mm of tendon using a no. 2 braided polyester suture, which tabularizes the graft to aid in passage through the femoral tunnel.

Arthroscopy/Femoral Tunnel

For the arthroscopic portion of the case, the patient is laid supine on the operative table. We recommend that the patient be intubated to protect the airway during position changes. A complete examination is performed after inducement of anesthesia prior to placement of a tourniquet. It is very important to evaluate for both PCL and associated capsuloligamentous injuries at this time. A thigh tourniquet is then placed but not inflated. A routine diagnostic arthroscopy is performed, and any meniscal or chondral injuries are treated at this time. The ACL may appear lax because of posterior tibial subluxation and should tighten with an applied anterior drawer. The PCL is then examined, and often, the ligament is lax or stretched out rather than frankly torn (Fig. 100.9). Once incompetence of the PCL has been confirmed, the residual PCL tissue is removed with a shaver and hand-operated punches. If the ligaments of Humphrey and Wrisberg are present, they are preserved if possible. The native footprint is preserved as a guide for femoral tunnel placement. Our goal of reconstruction is to restore the AL bundle of the PCL. The tunnel is placed in the distal and anterior portion of the native PCL footprint. A small medial incision is made through the skin and then through the medial retinaculum, which facilitates optimal drill-guide placement with the tunnel oriented slightly posteriorly. The medial articular margin is used as a landmark for the guide. An outside-in arthroscopic guide is used to establish the tunnel position, and a femoral guide pin is placed. The femoral tunnel is created with a cannulated drill over the guide pin (Fig. 100.10).

Authors' Preferred Technique

Posterior Cruciate Ligament Reconstruction—cont'd

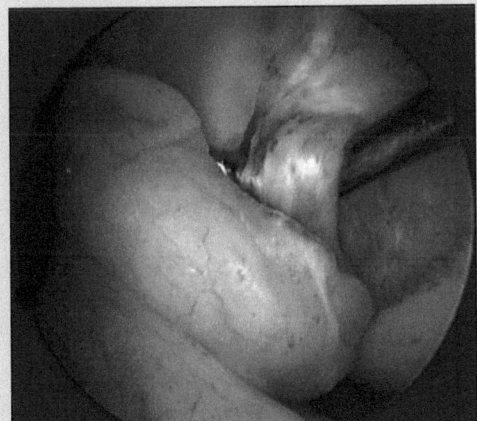

Fig. 100.9 An arthroscopic view of a posterior cruciate ligament tear.

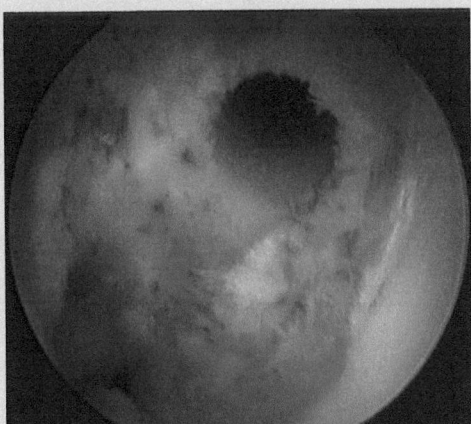

Fig. 100.10 An arthroscopic view of the femoral tunnel created in the footprint of the native anterolateral bundle with a cannulated drill over a guide pin.

The drill size is determined by the size of the graft and is typically 10 mm in width. An 18-gauge wire loop is passed through the femoral tunnel from the outside and positioned in the posterior notch to be retrieved later for graft passage.

Tibial Inlay

The patient is then rotated into the prone position in a sterile fashion in preparation for the tibial inlay portion of the case. The extremity is exsanguinated and a tourniquet is inflated. The PM exposure to the tibia, as described by Burks,[108] is then performed. The skin incision is a gentle curve with a horizontal end at the medial popliteal crease and vertical limb overlying the medial aspect of the gastrocnemius. Dissection is carried down the investing fascial layer, which is incised over the medial head of the gastrocnemius. The medial sural cutaneous nerve can be at risk but typically perforates the fascia distal to the horizontal limb of the incision. The medial border of the medial gastrocnemius is identified. The interval between the medial gastrocnemius and semimembranosus tendon is developed. Blunt dissection is performed down to the joint capsule. The medial head of the gastrocnemius is then retracted laterally with a blunt-tipped retractor, which protects its motor branch and neurovascular structures. At this point the posterior proximal tibia and posterior femoral condyles are palpated and a vertical incision is made through the posterior capsule. The posterior notch and tibial attachment of the PCL should now be exposed and the tibial insertion site of the native PCL is prepared for placement of the graft. Typically two prominent processes are found on the medial and lateral borders of the PCL that can be palpated. The insertion site is resected using osteotomes, a rongeur, and/or a burr. A graft recipient site is created that will anatomically accommodate the previously prepared graft. The bone graft is then placed into the site and secured with a 6.5-mm cancellous screw and washer (Fig. 100.11). The sutures in the tendinous portion of the graft are shuttled through the femoral tunnel using the previously placed wire loop. After the sutures are passed, the capsule is repaired. The tourniquet is deflated and hemostasis is achieved. The wound is irrigated and closed in layers.

Graft Tensioning

After wound closure the patient is again returned to the supine position in a sterile fashion. The arthroscope is placed back into the knee and the graft is inspected, entering the femoral tunnel (Fig. 100.12). The knee is cycled several

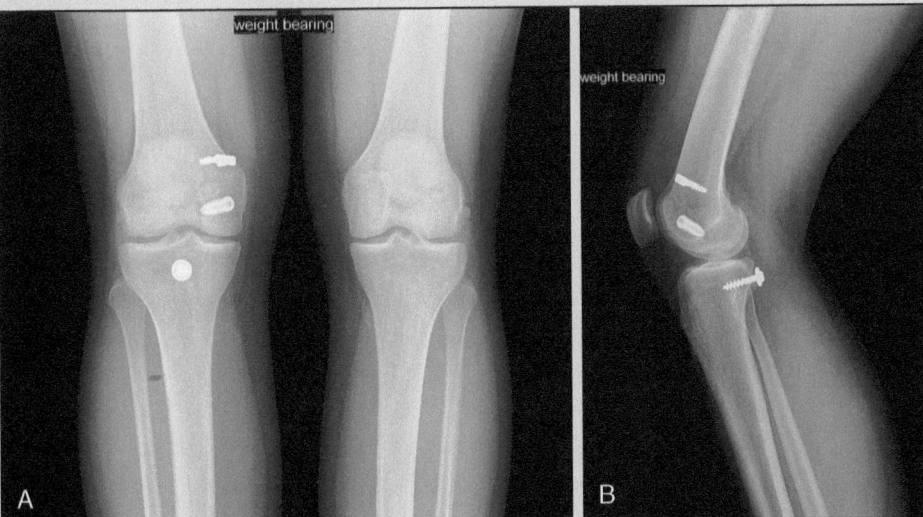

Fig. 100.11 (A) Anteroposterior and (B) lateral radiographs of the knee after completion of single-bundle posterior cruciate ligament reconstruction.

🖈 Authors' Preferred Technique

Posterior Cruciate Ligament Reconstruction—cont'd

times, which allows the surgeon to evaluate ROM and helps apply tension to the graft. Tension is applied to the graft in 70 to 90 degrees of flexion with an anterior drawer force placed on the proximal tibia. A 9 × 25-mm soft-tissue interference screw is then used to fix the graft in the femoral tunnel. A staple is then placed over the soft tissue portion of the graft into the medial femoral condyle to augment fixation. The arthroscopic portals and the incision for the femoral tunnel are closed in the standard fashion.

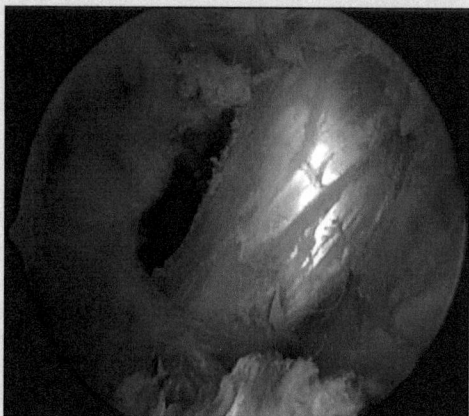

Fig. 100.12 An arthroscopic view of a completed posterior cruciate ligament reconstruction.

Transtibial Technique and Double-Bundle Reconstruction

Alternatively, PCL reconstruction can be achieved via an arthroscopic transtibial technique. The patient is positioned supine. A detailed examination is performed after inducement of anesthesia followed by arthroscopic assessment of the knee joint to confirm the extent of the injury and to assist with the repair or reconstructive procedure. The tibial footprint is prepared via an accessory anteromedial portal, and occasionally with use of a 70-degree arthroscope. A tibial tunnel is then created from the anteromedial tibia and directed posteriorly to the native PCL tibial attachment (Fig. 100.13). If a single-bundle procedure is performed, care is taken to place the single guidewire in the center of the tibial footprint via direct visualization and/or radiographic guidance with use of a guide. If a double-bundle reconstruction is performed, two guidewires are placed and confirmed radiographically, with the AL guidewire being more lateral and distal and the PM guidewire being more medial and proximal. The tunnel(s) is (are) reamed under power to the posterior cortex and then completed by hand with direct visualization.

After the tibial tunnels are completed, attention is focused on creating the femoral tunnels. The femoral insertion site anatomy is identified, and the appropriate tunnel position is marked for a single-bundle reconstruction or double-bundle reconstruction. The lateral portal is enlarged, and the knee is hyperflexed to drill the femoral tunnel(s) (Fig. 100.14A). One or two grafts are used depending on whether a single-bundle or double-bundle reconstruction is being performed. These grafts are passed anterograde through the tibial tunnel (Fig. 100.15) and subsequently retrograde into the femur. The grafts are fixed on the femoral or tibial side and then tension is applied to the other side of the graft and it is fixed. Tension is applied to the AL bundle and it is fixed at 90 degrees of flexion, whereas tension is applied to the PM bundle and it is fixed at 30 degrees of flexion.

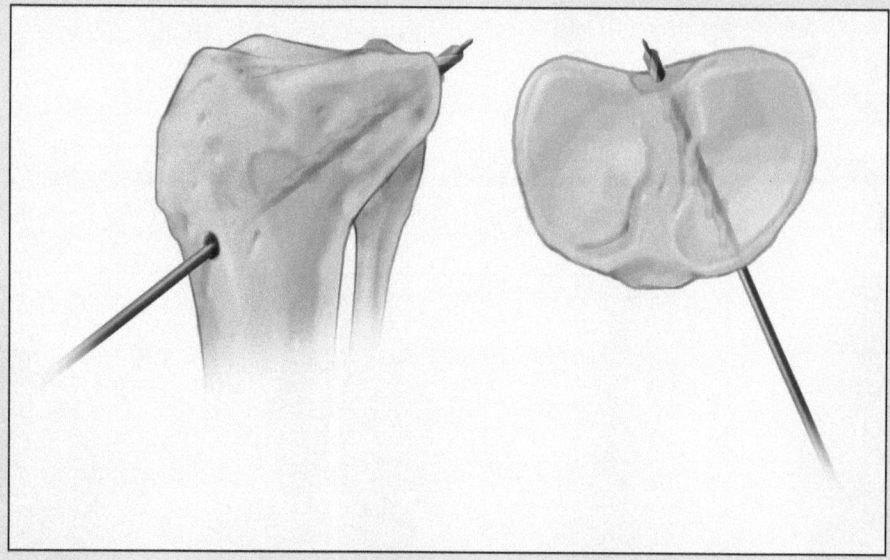

Fig. 100.13 Posterior cruciate ligament tibial guidewire placement and drilling. (Modified from Miller MD, Harner CD, Koshiwaguchi S. Acute posterior cruciate ligament injuries. In: Fu FH, Harner CD, Vince KG, eds. *Knee Surgery*. Vol. 1. Baltimore: Williams & Wilkins; 1994.)

Authors' Preferred Technique

Posterior Cruciate Ligament Reconstruction—cont'd

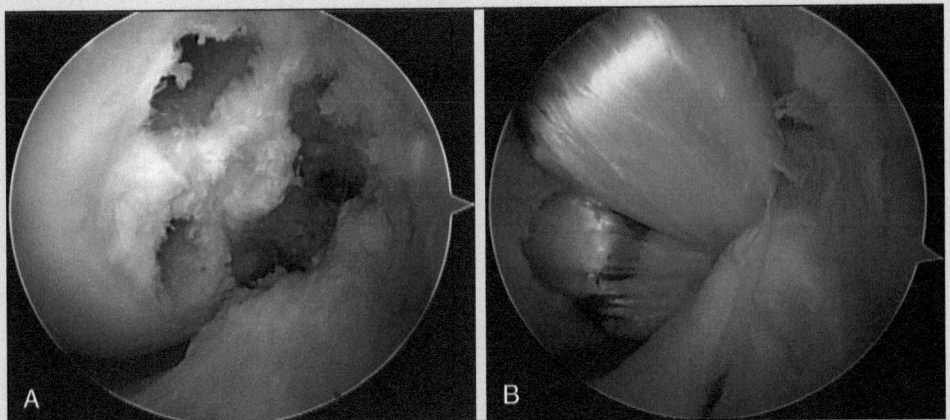

Fig. 100.14 Positioning of femoral tunnels for double-bundle reconstruction. (A) Femoral tunnel position for anterolateral and posteromedial bundles. Note that the anterolateral bundle is more anterior. (B) Double-bundle reconstruction with tibialis anterior allografts.

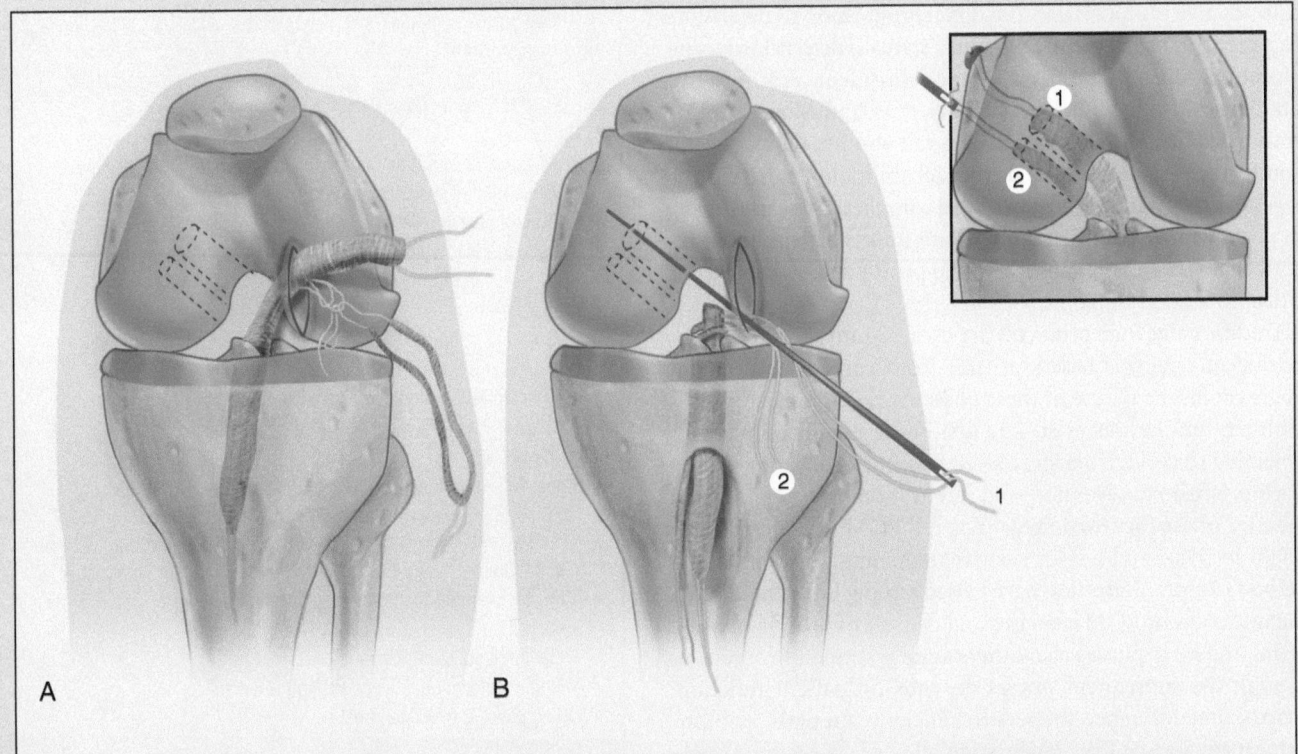

Fig. 100.15 Graft placement. (A) The graft for the anterolateral bundle (inset, *1*) and a second graft for the posteromedial bundle (inset, *2*) are passed in anterograde fashion through the tibial tunnel. (B) The grafts are then fixed to corresponding femoral tunnels. (Modified from Petrie RS, Harner CD. Double bundle posterior cruciate ligament reconstruction technique: University of Pittsburgh approach. *Op Tech Sports Med.* 1999;7:118–126.)

POSTOPERATIVE MANAGEMENT

Although rehabilitation after ACL reconstruction has been investigated by numerous authors, postoperative management after PCL reconstruction has been studied less extensively. Because PCL reconstruction has not been as successful as ACL reconstruction in restoring objective stability, many surgeons recommend a more conservative postoperative course. No level I studies have been performed to compare different protocols, and in a recent review of the literature, Pierce et al.[61] found that currently no consensus exists regarding a set of optimal guidelines. In general, rehabilitation should focus on quadriceps strengthening and regaining ROM while avoiding posterior tibial translation, which places stress on the graft. These goals are usually achieved by initial immobilization and avoidance of active hamstring forces, limited ROM, and progressive weight bearing and strengthening based on the time from surgery and the patient's progress.

The aim of reconstruction and rehabilitation is to help the patient return to previous levels of function. The goal of most protocols is to achieve this goal around 9 months after surgery. Postoperative protocols use functional progression to determine the patient's advancement. Functional status is determined using a combination of subjective patient assessment and objective data. These data include joint stability, ROM, effusion, proprioception deficits, muscle strength, and gait abnormalities. Careful monitoring of these factors during rehabilitation can help the surgeon identify and manage potential complications early during the postoperative course. It is important for the patient to understand that strict compliance with the postoperative protocol is critical to a good outcome.

Traditionally, PCL protocols are divided into specific phases, and advancement is based on time from surgery and patient progression. The nature of these phases varies among surgeons, but many similarities exist. The first phase usually emphasizes protecting the graft from stress, ROM within limits, non–weight bearing, effusion prevention, and reactivation of the quadriceps. The next phase focuses on regaining full ROM, advancement of weight bearing, and low-impact strengthening. The length and method of immobilization have varied among different studies. The initiation of ROM exercises and degrees of motion allowed during the early phases also differs among studies. Progression through the subsequent phases depends on patient function. Factors that influence progression include strength, stability, endurance, and agility. Patients are allowed to return to play when they regain appropriate quadriceps strength and painless active ROM, which, as previously stated, is usually at around 9 months after surgery.

To regain strength and proprioception, most protocols include open and closed kinetic chain exercises. For this reason it is important that open- and closed-chain exercises be part of the PCL rehabilitation program. Open-chain knee flexion resulting from hamstring contraction causes significant posterior translational forces across the tibia and should be avoided during early phases of rehabilitation.[109] Open-chain knee extension can protect the graft by producing anteriorly directed shear forces across the tibia, and most investigators advocate that these forces

be initiated early.[61,109] Closed kinetic chain exercises at low arcs of motion have also been shown to decrease posterior shear forces and are included in PCL rehabilitation. We use the following protocol.

RESULTS OF OPERATIVE TREATMENT

Isolated Posterior Cruciate Ligament Injuries

The results of isolated PCL reconstruction have been evaluated in many published studies. Although most patients demonstrate

---

📌 Authors' Preferred Technique
Postoperative Management

A   Acute Immediate Postoperative Phase (Early Protection Phase)
- Bracing: After surgery, the hinged brace is locked at zero
- ROM: passive ROM (initiated after 2 to 3 weeks of immobilization in extension)—patient-assisted tibial lift into flexion (0 to 70 degrees) with passive knee flexion
- Exercises:
  - Quadriceps isometrics, straight leg raise—adduction, abduction proximal weight

B   Acute Phase (Maximal Protection Phase)
- Goals:
  - Minimize external forces to protect the graft
  - Prevention of quadriceps atrophy
  - Control postsurgical effusion
- Weight bearing: weight bearing as tolerated with an assistive device
- ROM: as tolerated to 90 degrees
- Exercises:
  - Continue isometric exercises and quadriceps strengthening
  - Closed kinetic chain mini-squat, shuttle, bike
  - Open kinetic chain knee extension (60 degrees to 0 degrees)
  - Proprioception training
  - Weight shifts
- Brace: Fit with a functional brace at 4 to 6 weeks after surgery

C   Progressive Range of Motion/Strengthening Phase
- Weight bearing: weight bearing as tolerated without an assistive device
- ROM: as tolerated to 125 degrees flexion
- Exercises:
  - Continue quadriceps strength training
  - Begin isotonic quadriceps strength exercises
  - Leg press (0 to 60 degrees)
  - Step-ups
  - Sport-cord progression program
  - Rowing, NordicTrack
  - Initiate closed kinetic chain terminal knee extension

D   Functional Activity Phase
Few scientific data are available to help determine the best method of rehabilitation as the patient transitions into functional stages, and thus progression at this level is determined by the patient's tolerance to exercise and level of function. The evaluation of power and endurance that have been used for ACL programs should theoretically measure total length, strength, and endurance and can be used for the PCL reconstructed knee. As previously stated, the anticipated return to previous activity after PCL reconstruction is anticipated to take approximately 9 months.

improvement, some patients report persistent knee symptoms and have residual laxity that may inhibit return to preinjury-level activities.[56,65,88,89,110–122] The main limitation of these studies is the low incidence of isolated PCL injury requiring reconstruction, which results in a small sample size. Many of these studies are also retrospective case series that differ in operative technique, outcome measurements, and postoperative treatment, making direct comparison between studies difficult. A summary of these studies can be found in Table 100.1.[112,120,121,123–130]

Hermans et al.[112] evaluated 25 patients who underwent isolated AL bundle PCL reconstructions at an average follow-up of 9.1 years. They used an arthroscopic transtibial, single-bundle approach with use of various graft types. The final International Knee Documentation Committee (IKDC), Lysholm, and functional Visual Analog Scale scores were significantly better than preoperative scores, but only 41% of patients had normal or near-normal clinical findings according to the IKDC guidelines. This finding was mostly attributed to residual laxity with a mean side-to-side difference of 4.7 mm by Telos stress radiographs at final follow-up. Preoperative symptomatic instability greater than 1 year and chondrosis at the time of surgery correlated with poorer subjective outcomes. These findings confirm that although isolated PCL reconstruction often results in improved functional outcome, many patients have residual laxity. Lahner et al.[121] prospectively followed up on 33 patients with chronic symptomatic PCL injuries who underwent isolated single-bundle transtibial reconstruction. These patients were followed up over 2 years, and during this time, their IKDC scores improved from 41.8 to 69.5, and 72.8% regained normal to near-normal knee function. In this study, nine patients (27.4%) showed no improvement in knee function postoperatively. Chen and Gao[120] evaluated a transtibial double-bundle reconstruction using a suture suspension technique at a minimum follow-up of 2 years. In their series of 19 patients, 78.9% regained normal knee function and 15.8% regained near-normal knee function. These rates are significantly higher than those reported in other studies and may be attributable to higher preoperative scores. The patients in this series had an average preoperative IKDC score of 65.6 and less posterior laxity compared with subjects in other studies.

Transtibial Versus Tibial Inlay

Several case series have compared the outcomes of transtibial and tibial inlay methods of PCL reconstruction. No significant difference in clinical outcome scores between the two techniques have been identified. The details of these studies are outlined in Table 100.2. MacGillivray et al.[56] evaluated 20 patients who underwent reconstruction of an isolated PCL injury. The mean follow-up was 5.7 years. Thirteen patients underwent transtibial reconstruction and seven underwent tibial inlay, all with a single-bundle graft. These investigators found that the posterior drawer improved in 57% of patients in the inlay group and in 38% in the transtibial group. No significant difference in Tegner, Lysholm, or American Academy of Orthopaedic Surgeons knee scores was found between the two groups. The investigators concluded that neither method predictably restores original laxity and that there was no difference in outcome scores.

Seon and Song[73] retrospectively reviewed 21 isolated transtibial and 22 tibial inlay reconstructions. They found a significant improvement in Lysholm knee scores in both groups but no intergroup differences. Postoperative Tegner scores were also improved in both groups. Final follow-up found normal or grade I laxity on posterior drawer in 19 patients in the transtibial group and in 20 patients in the inlay group. Mean side-to-side differences were also improved, with no significant difference between the two groups. The authors concluded that the transtibial and inlay techniques resulted in relatively good clinical and objective outcomes and are both satisfactory options for reconstruction. Kim et al.[115] compared three different PCL reconstruction techniques. Twenty-nine patients underwent single- or double-bundle arthroscopic tibial inlay reconstruction or transtibial single-bundle reconstruction. These investigators found a significant difference in postoperative posterior tibial translation when the double-bundle tibial inlay group was compared with the single-bundle transtibial group, with less translation in the former. Although they noted a difference in translation, they found no significant difference in postoperative Lysholm scores or ROM. Song and colleagues retrospectively reviewed 36 isolated transtibial and 30 isolated tibial inlay reconstructions at an average follow-up of 148 months. Both groups showed no significant differences in terms of Lysholm knee scores, Tegner scores, or residual posterior laxity. Knees from both groups demonstrated development of OA on radiograph with no significant difference in prevalence.[75]

Single Versus Double Bundle

A number of in vivo studies have compared single-bundle and double-bundle PCL reconstructions. Yoon et al.[131] prospectively followed up 53 patients who underwent single- or double-bundle reconstruction. All reconstructions were performed with a transtibial approach using Achilles tendon allograft and had a minimum of 2-year follow-up. At final follow-up, patients were evaluated for ROM and posterior stability using stress radiography and by subjective knee scoring. The authors found no significant difference in ROM, Tegner activity scores, Lysholm scores, and IKDC evaluation. The only difference that could be identified was in posterior laxity. Both groups had improved stability postoperatively; however, the double-bundle group had less posterior translation with a difference of 1.4 mm, which was statistically significant. Although they did have less instability on objective testing, the patients' clinical outcomes as measured by subjective scoring were the same in both groups. These findings were later corroborated by a study by Li et al. who prospectively followed 46 patients who underwent single- or double-bundle PCL reconstructions using tibialis allograft via a transtibial approach. In this study, the authors found no significant difference in Lysholm scores, or Tegner activity scores but the double-bundle group showed a statistically significant difference in residual posterior laxity compared to the single-bundle group (2.2 mm vs. 4.1 mm).[132]

Several studies to date have shown no significant differences in subjective or objective results between single- and double-bundle PCL graft reconstructions. Wang et al.[127] prospectively compared single- and double-bundle PCL reconstruction using

TABLE 100.1   Results of Isolated Posterior Cruciate Ligament Reconstruction

Study	No. of Patients	Age (Years)	Follow-up (Years)	Chronicity/Grade	Graft Type	Surgical Technique
Lahner et al. (2012),[114] prospective	33	32.5	2	Chronic 13 grade II 20 grade III	Hamstring autograft	Transtibial, single bundle
Hermans et al. (2009),[105] retrospective	25	30.8	9.1	7 acute, 18 chronic, grade II or more	9 BPTB autograft 7 quadrupled hamstring autograft 8 double hamstring autograft	Transtibial, single bundle
Chen and Gao (2009)[113]	19	39	Minimum of 2	Unknown Average time 14 months 15 grade II 4 grade III	8-strand hamstring autograft	Transtibial, double bundle
Chan et al. (2006),[116] prospective	20	29	3.3	Unknown Average time 4 months All grade III	Quadrupled hamstring autograft	Transtibial
Sekiya et al. (2005),[117] retrospective	21	38	5.9	5 acute 16 chronic All grade III	Achilles allograft	Transtibial
Ahn et al. (2005),[118] retrospective	Group I: 18	30	2.9	All chronic 11 grade II 7 grade III	Hamstring autograft	Transtibial
	Group II: 18	31	2.3	10 grade II 8 grade III	Achilles allograft	Transtibial
Jung et al. (2004),[119] retrospective	12	29	4.3	Unknown Average time 5.4 months Range 1–10 months	Patellar tendon autograft	Tibial inlay
Wang et al. (2003),[120] retrospective	30	32	3.3	13 acute 17 chronic All grade III	Mixed	Transtibial
Deehan et al. (2003),[121] prospective	27	27	3.3	All chronic (16 patients 4–12 months after injury, 11 patients >1 year) Grade II and III injuries	Hamstring autograft	Transtibial
Chen et al. (2002),[122] retrospective	Group A (quad tendon): 22	29	2.5	All grade III 12 acute 10 chronic	Quadriceps tendon autograft	Transtibial
	Group B (hamstring tendon): 27	27	2.2	16 acute 11 chronic	Quadrupled hamstring autograft	
Mariani et al. (1997),[123] retrospective	24	26	2.2	All chronic	Patellar tendon autograft	Transtibial

A, Abnormal; *bio,* biologic; *BPTB,* bone–patellar tendon–bone; *IKDC,* International Knee Documentation Committee; *IS,* interference screw; *KT,* KT-1000 testing; *N,* normal; *NA,* not available; *NN,* near-normal; *OAK,* Orthopädische Arbeitsgruppe Knie; *SA,* severely abnormal.

Fixation	Subjective Outcome	Instrumented Laxity	Posterior Drawer	Miscellaneous
Tibia: bio IS + button Femur: FlippTack	IKDC: 69, 72.8% N/NN Tegner: 5.9	Telos radiograph: 5 mm	Grade I: 25 Grade II: 8	Minor extension deficit 3–5 degrees in only 2 patients
Tibia: IS Femur: IS	IKDC: 65 Lysholm 75 Tegner 5.7	KT posterior drawer: 4.7 mm Side-side difference: 2.1 mm	Grade 0: 2 Grade I: 15 Grade II: 5	11 patients with residual positive quadriceps active test IKDC N to NN in only 41% Poorer results in chronic injuries
Suture suspension	Lysholm: 92.1 IKDC: 92.1, 78.9% N, 15.8% NN	KT posterior drawer: 9.4 preoperative to 1.0 postoperative Stress radiograph: 2.0	Grade 0: 17 Grade I: 1 Grade II: 1	Average preoperative IKDC score 65.6
Tibia: bio IS + screw and washer Femur: bio IS + washer	Lysholm: 93 Tegner: 6.3 IKDC: 85% N/NN	Average postoperative KT posterior drawer: 3.8 mm	Grade I: 16 Grade II: 3 Grade III: 1	18/20 showed no radiographic deterioration 3 patients had stiffness
Tibia: screw and washer Femur: metal IS	IKDC knee function: 57% N/NN, 43% A/SA IKDC activity level: 62% N/NN, 38% A/SA	KT posterior drawer: 4.5 mm KT side-side difference: 1.96 mm	IKDC acute/subacute: 75% N/NN Chronic: 40% N/NN	Acute/subacute group had significantly better IKDC and KT-1000 than chronic group
Femur: IS and screw and washer Tibia: IS and screw and washer	Lysholm: 90 IKDC: 16 N/NN, 2 A	Telos stress radiograph posterior displacement: 2.2 mm	NA	No difference in outcome between groups
	Lysholm: 85 IKDC: 14 N/NN, 3 A, 1 SA	2.0 mm	NA	
Femur: IS Tibia: screw and washer	OAK score: 92.5; 7 excellent, 4 good IKDC: 11/11 were N/NN	Stress radiographs: 3.4 mm side-side difference; KT side-side difference, 1.8 mm	NA	
Femur: IS; tibia: screw and post	Lysholm: 92 (24 excellent/good, 6 fair/poor) Tegner: 4.5	NA	Grade I: 16 Grade II: 12 Grade III: 3	Significant correlation between poor results and more chronic injuries
Femur: IS Tibia: IS	Lysholm: 94 IKDC: 25 N/NN, 2 A/SA	KT side-side difference <2 mm: 17 patients 3–4 mm, 6 patients	Grade 0/I: 23 Grade II: 1	No correlation between time from injury to surgery and outcome
Tibia: suture and post Femur: metal IS	Lysholm: 90.63 IKDC: 18 N/NN, 4 A/SA	Average postoperative KT posterior drawer: 3.72 mm	NA	1 patient had stiffness 86% had normal radiographs
Tibia: screw and washer Femur: screw and washer	Lysholm: 91.44 IKDC: 22 N/NN, 5 A/SA	Average postoperative KT posterior drawer: 4.11 mm		1 patient had stiffness 92% had normal radiographs
Tibia and femur: metal IS	Lysholm: 94 Tegner: 5.4 IKDC: 19 N/NN, 5 A/SA	KT side-side differences: 6, 0–2 mm 13, 3.5 mm 3, 6–10 mm 2, >10 mm	NA	Significant correlation between poor results and more chronic injuries

TABLE 100.2 Results of Isolated Posterior Cruciate Ligament Reconstruction: Transtibial Versus Inlay

Study	No. of Patients	Age (Years)	Follow-up (Years)	Chronicity/Grade	Graft Type	Surgical Technique	Fixation	Subjective Outcome	Instrumented Laxity	Posterior Drawer	Miscellaneous
Kim et al. (2009),[108] retrospective	Group T (transtibial): 8	32.4	3.9	Average time to surgery, 9.4 months; all grade III	Achilles allograft in all cases	Transtibial single bundle	Tibia: bio IS Femur: bio IS	Lysholm: 86.9	Telos side-to-side difference: 5.6 mm	NA	Significant difference in posterior translation between groups T and I2
	Group I1 (inlay): 11	31.9	I1: 3.0	all grade III		AS inlay single bundle	Tibia: bio IS and washer Femur: bio IS	Lysholm: 79.7	4.7 mm		No significant difference in Lysholm scores
	Group I2 (inlay): 10	33.6	I2: 2.5			AS inlay double bundle	Tibia: bio IS and washer Femur: bio IS	Lysholm: 84.3	3.6 mm		
Seon and Song (2006),[71] retrospective	Group A (transtibial): 21	29.1	2.6	All chronic; all grade II or greater	Hamstring autograft	Transtibial	Tibia: bio IS Femur: anchor screw	Lysholm: 91.3 Tegner: 5.6	Telos side-side difference: 3.7 mm	19 normal/grade I 2 grade II	No significant differences between groups
	Group B (tibial inlay): 22	29.4	3.0		Patellar tendon autograft	Tibial inlay	Tibia: screw and washer Femur: bio IS screw	Lysholm: 92.8 Tegner: 6.1	Telos side-side difference: 3.3 mm	20 normal/grade I 2 grade II	
MacGillivray et al. (2006),[55] retrospective	Group I (transtibial): 13	29	6.3	All chronic 5 grade II 8 grade III	Mixed	Transtibial	Tibia: IS Femur: IS	Lysholm: 81 Tegner: 6	KT posterior drawer: 5.9 mm	3 grade I 6 grade II 4 grade III	Neither method restored anteroposterior stability to the knee
	Group II (tibial inlay): 7	31	4.8	3 grade II 4 grade III		Tibial inlay	Tibia: screw/washer Femur: IS	Lysholm: 76 Tegner: 6	KT posterior drawer: 5.5 mm	3 grade I 3 grade II 1 grade III	
Song et al. (2014),[6] retrospective	Group I (transtibial): 36	37	1	Unknown/All grade II or greater	Mixed	Transtibial	Tibia: IS Femur: ligament anchor screw	Lysholm: 89.9 ± 9.7 Tegner: 5.9	KT posterior drawer: 83.3% Grade I, 16.7% Grade II	IKDC Guidelines 16.7% Grade C	
	Group II (tibial inlay): 30	35	1.1	Unknown/All grade II or greater		Tibial inlay	Tibia: two screws/washers Femur: IS	Lysholm: 92.1 ± 10.4 Tegner: 6	KT posterior drawer: 86.7% Grade I, 13.3% Grade II	IKDC Guidelines 10% Grade C	

AS, Arthroscopic; bio, biologic; IKDC, International Knee Documentation Committee; IS, interference screw; KT, KT-1000 testing; NA, not available.

hamstring autograft. No significant differences were observed between the two groups with regard to functional score, ligament laxity, and radiographic changes of the knee. Hatayama and colleagues[88] were also unable to detect a difference in posterior tibial translation between patients treated with single- compared with double-bundle PCL reconstruction. Similarly, in a comparison of bone–patellar tendon–bone in one femoral tunnel compared with hamstring autograft in two tunnels, Houe and Jorgensen[87] found no difference in postoperative laxity or Lysholm and Tegner scores. Finally, a study by Deie and colleagues showed that after a mean follow-up of 12.5 years there was no significant difference in Lysholm scores, stress radiography measurements, or knee arthrometry between patients who underwent single-bundle or double-bundle PCL reconstruction with hamstring allograft.[133]

COMPLICATIONS

The complications of PCL reconstruction include the more common problems that occur with orthopaedic surgery, such as infection and stiffness. In addition, some complications are associated with the specific nature of the procedure. One of the most common problems after PCL reconstruction is persistent posterior laxity. Hermans et al.[112] found that 11 patients in a case series of 25 patients had a positive quadriceps active test after surgery. In addition, four patients required hardware removal because of soreness, and one patient required open capsular release for postoperative arthrofibrosis and decreased ROM. The exact incidence of complication after PCL reconstruction is unknown.

Vascular injury during PCL reconstruction is rare but is a known complication. Nemani et al.[113] reported on a case involving a popliteal venotomy that occurred during PCL reconstruction in the setting of a previous popliteal artery bypass graft. In this case the patient had sustained a knee dislocation with vascular injury. During the PCL reconstruction, the popliteal vein was found to be adherent to the PCL remnant, and a venotomy was noted after débridement. The authors recommend caution in the setting of previous surgery because the relationship of the neurovascular structures can be altered. Although complications appear to be uncommon, the clinician should have a frank discussion with the patient preoperatively to discuss the potential risks associated with the procedure.

FUTURE CONSIDERATIONS

The optimal treatment for the PCL-deficient knee remains unclear. Future studies will help to better define the indications for the different treatment options. These studies will attempt to overcome the limitations of prior investigations. A need exists for randomized and prospectively designed studies with controlled variables that will allow clinicians to draw definitive conclusions. The difficulties encountered in PCL study design have been discussed, but small sample size due to low incidence is probably one of the most significant. Multicenter trials will likely be required to achieve the necessary power to derive treatment recommendations. Conducting multicenter trials is difficult because of

different surgical indications and methods of reconstruction that would need to be controlled. Future efforts should focus on overcoming these limitations and thus providing data that could help elucidate the best treatment recommendations for PCL injuries.

For a complete list of references, go to ExpertConsult.com.

SELECTED READINGS

Citation:
Markolf KL, Zemanovic JR, McAllister DR. Cyclic loading of posterior cruciate ligament replacements fixed with tibial tunnel and tibial inlay methods. *J Bone Joint Surg Am.* 2002;84A(4): 518–524.

Level of Evidence:
Biomechanical study

Summary:
Markolf and colleagues performed a cadaveric study comparing posterior cruciate ligament reconstruction fixed with tibial tunnel and tibial inlay techniques. Knees were subjected to 2000 cycles of tensile force of 50 to 300 N. The authors found that the inlay technique resulted in less graft failure and graft thinning.

Citation:
McAllister DR, Petrigliano FA. Diagnosis and treatment of posterior cruciate ligament injuries. *Curr Sports Med Rep.* 2007;6(5):293–299.

Level of Evidence:
Review

Summary:
McAllister and Petrigliano reviewed current concepts in the diagnosis and treatment of posterior cruciate ligament injuries.

Citation:
Yoon KH, Bae DK, Song SJ, et al. A prospective randomized study comparing arthroscopic single-bundle and double-bundle posterior cruciate ligament reconstructions preserving remnant fibers. *Am J Sports Med.* 2011;39(3):474–480.

Level of Evidence:
II

Summary:
Yoon and colleagues compared single- and double-bundle posterior cruciate ligament reconstruction in a prospective, randomized study. Although a small benefit was observed with regard to posterior laxity in the double-bundle group, no difference was seen with subjective outcome measures.

Citation:
Song EK, Park HW, Ahn YS, et al. Transtibial versus tibial inlay techniques for posterior cruciate ligament reconstruction. *Am J Sports Med.* 2014;42(12):2964–2971.

Level of Evidence:
IV, cohort study

Summary:
Song and colleagues compare transtibial and tibial inlay PCL reconstruction techniques at an average long-term follow-up of 148 months. Clinical and radiographic outcomes were

comparable between the two methods with a significant number of patients demonstrating worsening arthritis.

Citation:

Fanelli GC, Edson CJ. Posterior cruciate ligament injuries in trauma patients: part II. *Arthroscopy*. 1995;11(5):526–529.

Level of Evidence:

IV

Summary:

Fanelli and Edson offer one of the few studies on the incidence of PCL injuries in trauma patients with acute hemarthrosis of the knee. More than 200 acute knee injuries with hemarthrosis were reviewed. PCL injuries occurred in 38% of acute knee injuries; 56.5% were trauma patients, and 32.9% were sports related.

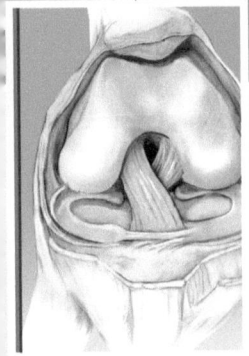

Medial Collateral Ligament and Posterior Medial Corner Injuries

M. Christopher Yonz, Brian F. Wilson, Matthew H. Blake, Darren L. Johnson

Medial ligament injuries of the knee are often assumed to be only medial collateral ligament (MCL) injuries. However, the medial ligament includes not only the MCL but also postero-medial structures that play a vital role in the stability of the knee. The work of LaPrade and colleagues[1,2] has demonstrated that the posterior oblique ligament (POL) is an important valgus and rotational stabilizer of the knee. The management of the MCL has evolved during the past 30 years. Most isolated MCL injuries are treated conservatively, with a rare role for surgical intervention. However, the treatment of MCL sprains with anterior cruciate ligament (ACL) injury (or any other concomitant ligamentous injury for that matter), along with the timing of ACL reconstruction, continue to be controversial. This chapter describes the anatomy of the medial knee (including the increasingly important posteromedial corner), the evaluation of the knee, the treatment of medial ligament injuries, and the role of rehabilitation.

HISTORY

The history will depend on whether the injury is witnessed by the physician on the sidelines or elicited from the patient in the clinic. Most of these injuries present in the office setting as potentially chronic conditions. A description of the mechanism of injury should be elicited in as much detail as possible. It is important to ascertain when the patient was hurt and how. Typically, the injury is the result of a blow to the lateral aspect of the leg or lower thigh. Up to 70% of MCL injuries in athletes are from contact mechanisms.[3,4] The mechanism may be the result of a clipping injury in football or a noncontact injury from cutting, pivoting, or twisting. Skiers are prone to medial side injuries, with 60% of skiing knee injuries affecting the MCL.[5,6] The majority of medial-sided knee injuries occur in competition rather than practice.[4,7] In addition, it is important to ask the patients about pain, onset of swelling, ability to ambulate, the sensation of a "pop," and the presence of a deformity necessitating a reduction, such as patellar dislocation or a more severe knee dislocation. In addition, a history of knee injuries or surgeries should be elicited because they can cloud an acute knee injury examination.

PHYSICAL EXAM

Ideally, the examination of the knee should occur at the time of injury before the onset of muscle spasm. However, most of these injuries are examined in the office setting after some time has elapsed after the injury. A thorough knee examination includes observation of the patient's gait, documentation of the neuro-vascular status, palpation of the knee for tenderness, swelling, and ecchymosis, and assessment of stability. The physician should follow some basic principles: (1) assess the ligaments and muscles while the patient is as relaxed as possible, (2) perform the physical examination as gently as possible, and (3) examine the uninjured knee before assessing the injured knee.

The patient's gait should be observed as the patient walks into the room or at some point during the examination. However, gait may be misleading because patients with a complete MCL tear may walk with a barely perceptible limp. Hughston and colleagues[8,9] found that 50% of athletes with grade III injuries could walk into the office unassisted, and reported that a complete disruption of the medial compartment can occur "without subsequent significant pain, effusion, or disability for walking." However, patients with an MCL tear may exhibit a vaulting-type gait in which the quadriceps are activated, allowing stabilization of the medial-sided structures during gait. This gait differs from that of a patient with an ACL or meniscus tear who may walk with a bent knee gait because of pain or an effusion. As with any orthopaedic injury, the neurovascular status of the limb should be assessed. Pedal pulses should be palpated and sensation should be assessed over the dorsum, plantar, and first web space of the foot. If a knee dislocation is a possibility, ankle brachial indices should be performed to evaluate for vascular injury. Compartments should be examined to rule out compartment syndrome. The ability to passively and actively dorsiflex and plantarflex the ankle and great toe should be assessed.

On the skin, the physician should look for edema, effusion, and ecchymosis to help localize the site of injury. It is important to differentiate between localized edema and an intra-articular effusion. Isolated MCL injuries usually have localized swelling. Hemarthrosis of the knee may indicate intra-articular pathology, such as an ACL or peripheral meniscal tear. Severe medial complex injuries with an ACL tear frequently show no evidence of effusion because the capsular rent is large enough to allow extravasation of fluid and blood. If hemarthrosis is present, the examiner should exclude other injuries such as a torn cruciate, patellar dislocation, an osteochondral fracture, and a peripheral meniscal tear. Along with assessment of swelling, palpation of the anatomic sites of attachment can provide clues to the diagnosis. The entire course of the MCL should be palpated from proximal to distal.

Pain at the medial femoral epicondyle signifies injury at the femoral insertion of the MCL. With tibial-sided injuries, patients have pain along the proximal tibia around the pes anserine adjacent to the tibial tubercle. Midsubstance tears result in pain at the joint line, and such pain may also present with a medial meniscal injury, posing a diagnostic dilemma. Hughston and colleagues[8] showed that point tenderness can accurately identify the location of injury in 78% of cases, and localized edema can identify a tear in the medial meniscus 64% of the time. A valgus injury that disrupts the MCL may also result in lateral meniscus tears or osteochondral fracture to the lateral femoral condyle or lateral tibial plateau. Therefore a thorough examination of the lateral knee should also be performed.

Valgus stress testing at 30 degrees of knee flexion is still the gold standard for assessing isolated injury to the MCL. This test should be performed with the foot in neutral rotation because increased laxity will be noted if the knee moves from internal to external rotation. To relax the hamstrings and quadriceps muscles, the thigh should rest on the examination table and the foreleg should move freely off the edge of the table at 30 degrees of flexion. The examiner then grasps the ankle and applies a valgus stress with the other hand resting on the medial side of the knee to assess the amount of opening and the quality of the end point compared with the uninjured side. The laxity of the MCL can be recorded based on a grading system or the amount of opening. The American Medical Association Standard Nomenclature of Athletic Injuries uses the following grading system[10]: grade I, localized tenderness without laxity; grade II, increased tenderness and gapping but with an endpoint signifying a partial tear; and grade III, laxity without an endpoint indicating a complete tear. Other classification systems are based on the amount of opening with grade I, 0 to 5 mm laxity; grade II, 6 to 10 mm laxity; and grade III, over 10 mm of laxity.[11] As described by Noyes, 5 to 8 mm of medial opening signifies a significant collateral ligament injury with "impairment of the ligament's restraining effect."[12] There is no consensus on which grading system is best. It is important to compare findings to the contralateral knee. After assessing the degree of opening, a repeat valgus stress should be performed with the examiner palpating the medial meniscus to assess if it subluxates in and out of the joint, indicative of injury to the meniscotibial ligament.[13]

In addition to valgus testing in flexion, opening of the medial joint should be assessed with the knee in full extension. The cruciate ligaments, POL, posteromedial capsule, and MCL all contribute to knee stability in full extension. Asymmetric joint opening in extension compared with the contralateral side should alert the physician to the possibility of a combined MCL/POL injury with a cruciate tear. If any increased laxity is observed in full extension compared with the uninvolved knee, it is unlikely that an isolated MCL injury is present; rather, it is likely that the patient has a concomitant injury to the posteromedial capsule and POL in addition to the MCL lesion. The ACL should be assessed with the Lachman test because the pivot shift is difficult to perform as a result of guarding and the loss of the pivot axis with medial instability. In addition, the posterior cruciate ligament and lateral ligamentous structures should be examined. Along with cruciate injury, patellar instability and tearing of the

vastus medialis oblique are associated with laxity in full extension. Hunter and colleagues[14] found 18 of 40 laterally displaceable patellae on stress radiographs in patients with medial-sided injuries and a 9% to 21% incidence of damage to the extensor mechanism with medial ligament injury. In addition to valgus testing at 30 and 0 degrees, the Slocum modified anterior drawer test and an anterior drawer test in external rotation should be performed to assess for medial-sided injuries (Table 101.1). Finally, varus stress testing and dial tests at 30 and 90 degrees should be performed to evaluate for lateral and posterolateral-sided knee injuries. However, it is important to note that dial testing can appear positive in patients with severe medial sided knee injuries.[15] In this case, it is important to determine the direction of rotational instability of the tibial plateau in relation to the femoral condyles to distinguish if the positive result is due to a posterolateral knee injury or from anteromedial rotatory instability.[10]

IMAGING

Radiography, arthrography, magnetic resonance imaging (MRI), and arthroscopy can provide information regarding knee injuries. Radiography with anteroposterior (AP), lateral, and sunrise views should be performed for both knees. These radiographs should be evaluated for occult fractures, the lateral capsular sign (Segond fracture), ligamentous avulsions, old Pellegrini-Stieda lesions (i.e., an old MCL injury) (Fig. 101.1), and loose bodies. Stress x-rays must be performed in skeletally immature patients who have medial knee pain associated with a normal x-ray to rule out physeal injury.

In addition to ruling out physeal injuries in skeletally immature patients, stress radiography can be used to evaluate the severity of medial-sided knee injuries as well as the presence of concomitant ligament injuries. LaPrade and colleagues have noted that stress radiographs allow better objective measurements of knee instability than traditional physical exam maneuvers.[16] However, this modality is often limited by pain in the acute setting and may be more beneficial for the evaluation of chronic injuries. Previous studies have demonstrated that normal, intact knees may have side-to-side gapping differences of up to 2 mm.[17] Cadaveric sectioning studies have provided guidelines for expected medial gapping with stress radiographs based to the severity of injury in comparison to the contralateral knee: (1) isolated superficial MCL tear, 3.2 mm gapping at full extension and 20 degrees flexion; (2) superficial MCL and POL injury, 6.8 mm and 9.8 mm gapping at full extension and 20 degrees flexion; (3) complete medial side injury and ACL tear, 8.0 mm and 13.8 mm gapping at 0 and 20 degrees; (4) complete medial side injury and posterior collateral ligament tear, 11.8 mm and 12.6 mm gapping at 0 and 20 degrees; and (5) complete medial side injury and tears to both cruciates, 21.6 mm and 27.6 mm of gapping at 0 and 20 degrees.[16]

MRI without contrast is the imaging study of choice for evaluating MCL tears because it is less invasive than other studies and provides detail including location of tear, meniscal injury, superficial MCL, POL, posteromedial complex, and semimembranosus tendon (Fig. 101.2). MRI can reveal a Stener-type lesion

TABLE 101.1   Methods for Examining the Medial Collateral Ligament

Examination	Technique		Grading	Significance
Valgus stress at 0 and 30 degrees	Valgus force applied to tibia while stabilizing the femur; this should be done at 0 and 30 degrees of flexion and compared with the opposite leg		Grade I: 0- to 5-mm opening, firm end point Grade II: 5- to 10-mm opening, firm end point Grade III: 10- to 15-mm opening, soft end point	Opening at 30 degrees occurs from isolated MCL injuries; valgus stress at 0 degrees is associated with other ligament tears (anterior cruciate ligament, posterior collateral ligament, or posterior oblique ligament).
The Slocum modified anterior drawer test	Valgus force in 15 degrees of external rotation and 80 degrees of flexion		This test is positive if there is a noticeably increased prominence of the medial condyle compared with the other side.	The disruption of the deep MCL allows the meniscus to move freely and allows the medial tibial plateau to rotate anteriorly, leading to an increased prominence of the medial tibial condyle.
Anterior drawer test in external rotation	Anterior drawer test at 90 degrees of knee flexion with an external rotation applied to proximal tibia		This test is positive if a noticeably increased anterior translation of the medial condyle is present.	A disruption of the MCL alone should not lead to an increased anteromedial translation; an increased anteromedial translation indicates an anteromedial rotatory instability that involves an injury of the posteromedial structures.

MCL, Medial collateral ligament.

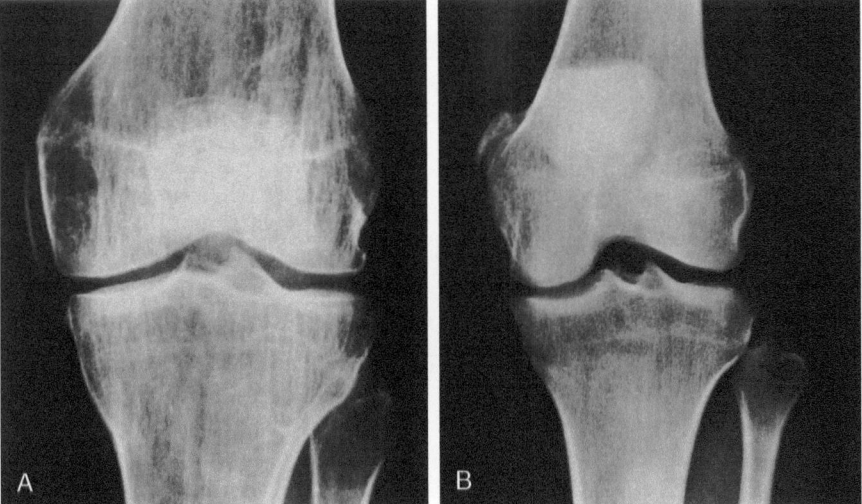

Fig. 101.1 (A) and (B) A Pellegrini–Stieda lesion. (From Pavlov H. Radiology for the orthopedic surgeon. *Contemp Orthop.* 1993;6:85.)

of the distal MCL with the distal MCL retracted superior to the pes tendons or into the knee joint. In addition, MRI is beneficial in assessing injuries to anterior and posterior cruciate ligaments and osteochondral structures. A 45% incidence of bruising of the lateral femoral condyle of lateral tibial plateau has been identified in isolated medial knee injuries.[18] Loredo and associates[19] showed that intra-articular contrast may help to highlight and to better define the structures of the posteromedial complex, but still concluded that the assessment of the posteromedial

complex was difficult. They found that the posteromedial complex was best visualized on coronal and axial images. In addition, increased T2 signal extending beyond the posterior border of the superficial MCL may indicate a posteromedial corner injury.[11] Indelicato and Linton[20] stated that MRI can provide advantages in four circumstances: (1) when the status of the ACL remains uncertain despite physical examination; (2) when the status of the meniscus is in question; (3) when surgical repair of the MCL is indicated and localization of the tear will help limit the

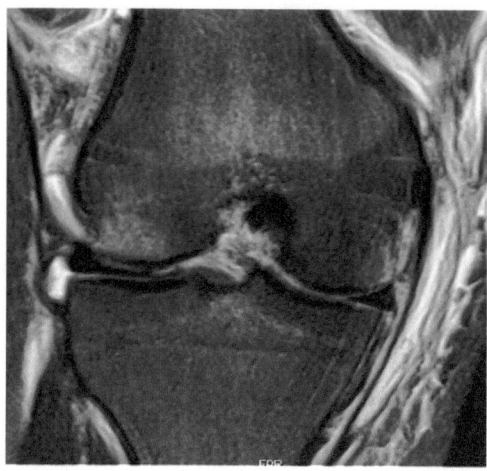

Fig. 101.2 Magnetic resonance image showing a medial collateral ligament tear.

exposure; and (4) when an unexplainable effusion occurs during rehabilitation.

However, MRI does not always provide concrete diagnosis, and the clinical examination becomes the deciding factor. Examination after administration of an anesthetic is another tool the physician can use to assess the injury pattern in patients who present long after an injury has occurred or in patients for whom the office examination and MRI do not provide a diagnosis. Final confirmation and planning must occur at the time of diagnostic arthroscopy, which confirms under direct vision zone of injury as well as amount of opening. Upon examination with use of an anesthetic, Norwood and coworkers[21] found that 18% of patients had anterolateral rotatory instability that was not suspected preoperatively. In addition to MRI, arthrograms can be used to evaluate meniscal disease and capsular tearing with extravasation of contrast material. Kimori and colleagues[22] found arthrography to be more useful than arthroscopy in diagnosing tears of the meniscotibial and meniscofemoral ligaments.

With the increased use of MRI, arthroscopy is used infrequently as a diagnostic tool. ACL and meniscal tears may be identified on MRI. Also, it is rare to find an intrasubstance medial meniscal tear in an isolated MCL rupture because meniscocapsular separation occurs, and thus the fulcrum to load the medial compartment and tear the medial meniscus is lost. However, a series by Ra et al. demonstrated a 27% incidence of medial meniscus posterior root tears in patients with acute, severe medial knee instability.[23] Over 30% of those injuries were not diagnosed on MRI and were found only during arthroscopy.

DECISION-MAKING PRINCIPLES

When considering treatment of the MCL, one must remember that the majority of MCL injuries heal reliably with conservative management, and treatment decisions should involve the functional demands of the knee. It is also imperative to determine the involvement of the POL in patients with MCL injuries. If the medial sided injury extends past the MCL, involving the POL and the posterior capsule, rotational laxity occurs. While the majority of people, as well as high-performance athletes, can

tolerate small amounts of valgus laxity, rotational laxity is not well tolerated.

The debate continues regarding nonoperative versus surgical treatment for primary repair of the MCL/POL with concomitant ACL injury. With most MCL injuries, clinical outcomes will be satisfactory after a period of immobilization and recovery of motion and strength, followed by progressive activities. In the small subset of patients with continued pain, instability, or impaired performance, surgical management must be considered. Surgical treatment should be provided to patients with chronic symptomatic valgus instability, an MCL that is incarcerated in the joint, a distal tibial MCL avulsion that is interposed in the pes tendons (a Stener lesion), and a grade III MCL tear with rotational instability or with grade III valgus laxity in full extension resulting from a complete POL tear.[1,2,24,25] Surgical management of chronic laxity of the medial structures can be quite difficult, and therefore anatomic repair of the medial support structures in the acute setting is preferred when indicated.

A review of literature for nonoperative versus operative treatment of complete isolated MCL injuries does not delineate the site of injury. The site of injury may have a role in the functional recovery of patients who place a high demand on their knees. In our practice, caring for Division I collegiate athletes, several complete soft tissue avulsions of the MCL/POL complex off the tibial insertion failed to heal reliably with nonoperative treatment. After recovery, athletes may have varying amounts of valgus knee instability preventing return to competitive sports and resulting in dysfunction in activities of daily living. Most MCL sprains should be treated nonoperatively. Complete avulsions of the superficial and deep MCL from the tibia with disruption of the meniscal coronary ligament have a poorer prognosis with nonoperative treatment and may be optimally managed with acute surgical repair for improved valgus stability of the knee.

Before proceeding with a treatment plan, it is essential to know the extent of injury. Initially we perform a thorough history and physical examination. With MCL injuries, we assess the grade of injury of the MCL and any associated ligamentous, meniscal, posteromedial corner, or patellar injuries. We obtain radiographs as a routine diagnostic tool to rule out fracture or any signs of chronic medial insufficiency (Pellegrini-Stieda lesion) and chronic ACL deficiency (the deep femoral notch sign, peaked tibial spines, or a cupula lesion). The use of MRI is dependent on the grade of the MCL lesion and associated injury posteriorly. Isolated grade I or II injuries can be diagnosed with clinical examination and do not require MRI. However, in a grade I or II injury with an indeterminate cruciate examination and effusion, we order an MRI. We also obtain MRI for all grade III injuries because the site of involvement—tibia or femur—is important in our decision-making, particularly the extent of injury to the POL and posteromedial capsule. With grade III laxity in full extension and complete involvement of the POL and capsule, avulsion of the posterior horn of the medial meniscus root may be seen (Fig. 101.3) and demands surgical intervention. In addition, most grade III lesions are associated with concomitant ligamentous injuries. Our treatment algorithm is outlined in Fig. 101.4.

Management of grade III injuries is controversial. Even with physical examination and advanced imaging, it remains difficult to gauge the extent of damage to the POL and the posteromedial capsule in combined injuries. The treatment of grade III MCL sprains has significantly evolved. The general consensus has been to treat isolated grade III injuries conservatively. Generally agreed upon operative indications include: tibial-sided MCL injury with a Stener lesion, joint entrapment of the MCL, a medial meniscal tear requiring repair, persistent instability following a nonoperative trial, and persistent medial instability after ACL reconstruction.[26] We believe that the treatment of grade III injury is dependent not only on the specific location of the MCL rupture but also on the degree of laxity on physical examination, as well as the degree of the arthroscopic drive-through sign. It is the posterior extension of the medial-sided injury into the POL and posterior capsule that is critically important in the decision-making in the athletically active patient. Nonoperative management of these

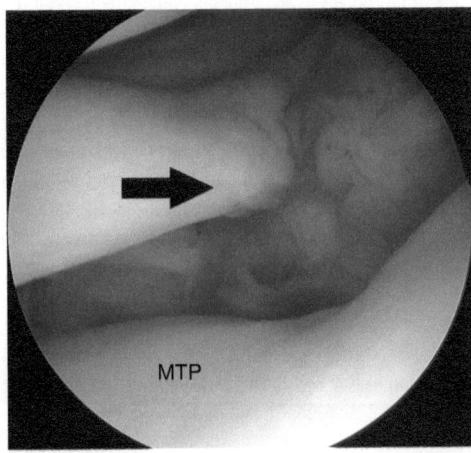

Fig. 101.3 Arthroscopic image of the medial compartment of the knee. The *arrow* points to the posterior horn of the medial meniscus avulsion injury. *MTP,* Medial tibial plateau.

injuries is inferior in this setting and may lead to a rotational instability in addition to valgus laxity, which is not well tolerated by athletes involved in pivoting sports.[27,28]

TREATMENT OPTIONS

Management of the MCL and medial-sided knee injuries can be divided into operative and nonoperative approaches. Numerous factors, including the timing, severity, location, and associated injuries such as an ACL tear need to be considered when formulating a treatment plan. The MCL has the greatest capacity to heal of any of the four major knee ligaments because of its anatomic and biologic properties.[29,30] As a result of multiple biomechanical, clinical, and functional studies, the trend has been toward a conservative, nonsurgical method for the majority of MCL injuries.

Grade I and II isolated tears of the MCL generally respond well to nonoperative management. Partial tears are treated routinely with temporary immobilization and protected weight bearing with crutches. Once the swelling subsides, range of motion (ROM), resistive exercises, and progressive weight bearing are initiated. Nonsteroidal antiinflammatory drugs can be used to help with pain and swelling. Studies have shown no deleterious effect of nonsteroidal drugs on ligament healing.[31]

Management of grade III injuries remains much more controversial. Even with physical examination and advanced imaging, it remains difficult to gauge the extent of damage to the POL and posteromedial capsule in combined injuries. Nonoperative management of these injuries may lead to a rotational instability in addition to valgus laxity, which is not well tolerated by athletes involved in pivoting sports. Grade III injuries not only involve complete disruption of its fibers but also are frequently associated with additional ligamentous injuries. Posteromedial corner injuries have been recognized as a separate entity from MCL

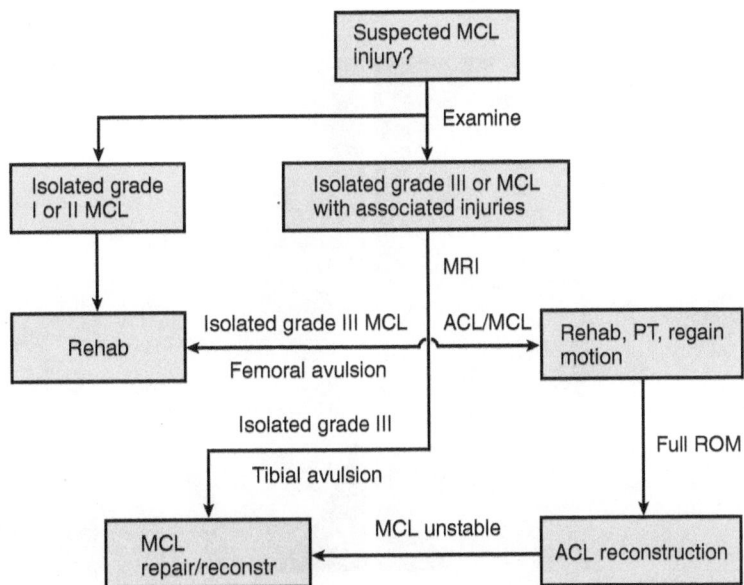

Fig. 101.4 Algorithm for treatment of medial collateral ligament *(MCL)* injuries. *ACL,* Anterior cruciate ligament; *MRI,* magnetic resonance imaging; *PT,* physical therapy; *ROM,* range of motion.

injuries and may need to be addressed more aggressively because of rotational laxity and instability that can result from their injury.[1,2,24]

In the last 5 years, multiple surgical techniques have been described for treating Grade III injuries. Surgical options include direct repair,[32–34] repair augmented with tendon reconstruction[35] or suture,[36] and anatomic reconstruction.[2,37,38] The most described reconstruction techniques in the literature include (1) triangular reconstruction of the superficial MCL and POL[37,39,40]; and (2) the use of two separate grafts and four tunnels to re-create the medial-sided structures.[2] For grade III injuries requiring surgery, the reconstruction techniques addressing the POL offer improved clinical stability, restoration of knee mechanics, and lower failure rates.[1,39,41–43]

⚑ Authors' Preferred Technique

Medial Collateral Ligament Injury

We treat isolated grade I and II MCL injuries conservatively. In the first 48 hours, we encourage rest and the use of ice, compression, and elevation to help reduce swelling. In addition, we have all patients use a hinged knee brace and provide crutches for protected weight bearing. If patients have significant pain and valgus laxity, initially we lock the brace in extension. Once the swelling subsides and pain is improved, we encourage aggressive range-of-motion (ROM) exercises and straight leg raises with quadriceps exercises. Once the patient has regained full ROM and ambulation without a limp, the use of crutches and the brace can be discontinued. Stationary bicycle and progressive resistive exercises are instituted as tolerated. Once full ROM and 80% strength of the opposite side have been achieved, closed-chain kinetic exercises and jogging are allowed. Once athletes have achieved 75% of the maximal running speed, sport-specific training is allowed. Return to sports is permitted after the patient has strength, agility, and proprioception equal to the other side. We recommend a functional brace for contact or high-risk sports.

Patients with grade I sprains usually return to sports in 10 to 14 days; because immobilization is temporary, these patients regain strength and motion quickly. However, return to play (RTP) after grade II sprains is much more variable. With grade II sprains, the period of immobilization can be up to 3 weeks to allow the pain to dissipate. Therefore patients can lose more strength and motion with an increased time of immobilization compared with patients with grade I sprains. Patients are allowed to RTP when they have equal strength of both knees and no pain is experienced with valgus stress.[44]

The treatment of grade III MCL sprains has significantly evolved during the past 20 years. The general consensus has been to treat isolated grade III injuries conservatively. We believe that the treatment of grade III injury is dependent not only on the specific location of the MCL rupture but also the degree of laxity on physical examination, as well as the degree of the arthroscopic drive-through sign. The extent of injury and laxity of the injury to the POL and posterior capsule is instrumental in our decision-making.

Diagnostic arthroscopy is performed initially to evaluate intra-articular injuries. A valgus force is placed on the knee while the knee is flexed at 30 degrees of flexion with the arthroscope viewing from the anterolateral portal. Tibiofemoral widening with valgus stress, which allows the arthroscope to be easily "driven through" to the posteromedial aspect of the knee, is called the "medial drive-through" sign. This indicates a medial sided injury. One can easily assess, when performing this maneuver, if the MCL injury is primarily based on the femur or tibia, and where it will be necessary to operate and perform a repair. For femoral-sided MCL injuries, the medial meniscus remains reduced with the tibia upon valgus opening (i.e., a gap forms above the medial meniscus). On the other hand, tibial-sided MCL injuries demonstrate that the medial meniscus remains reduced with the femur on valgus opening (i.e., a gap forms between medial meniscus and tibia, with the medial meniscus lifting off the tibia). If the medial meniscus elevates off the tibia, the coronary ligament, which attaches the meniscus to the tibia, is torn and should be repaired. An injury with extension to the POL and posterior capsule can also avulse the medial meniscus root from its attachment site. This also is critical to recognize and repair.

With valgus opening of the knee during arthroscopic examination, it may be observed whether the knee opens posteriorly to the medial meniscus, particularly as the knee is slowly extended with valgus load. If the capsule is exposed with this maneuver posteriorly, the patient has an injury of the POL and posterior medial capsule, which needs to be addressed at the time of surgical correction (Fig. 101.5).

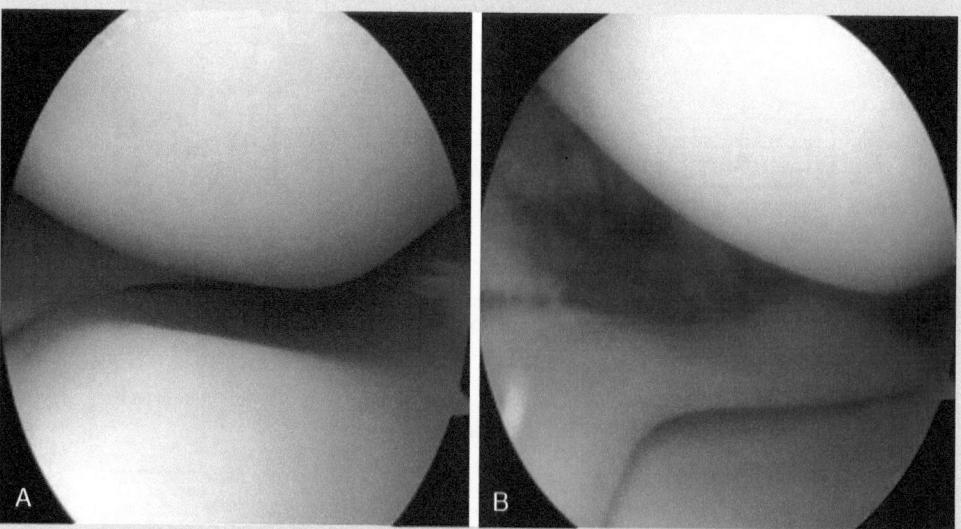

Fig. 101.5 A normal appearing medial joint space (A) is actually shown (B) to have a positive medial drive through sign upon valgus stress and tearing of the posterior medial capsule.

Authors' Preferred Technique
Medial Collateral Ligament Injury—cont'd

If the injury is acute, less than 14 days old, primary medial repair is attempted. In this setting particularly in the young athlete, repair is generally successful in the majority of cases with tibial based avulsions. For chronic injuries, the medial structures are repaired and augmented or can be primarily reconstructed.

For acute repair, the origins and insertions of the deep and superficial MCL are evaluated. Typically, the lesion is on the tibial side. Isolated femoral-sided lesions often heal reliably without surgical repair.

The surgical approach is a fairly easy one in that the incision is similar to a hamstring harvest incision, except the length of the incision is longer in the proximal direction. The surgical incision is longitudinal between the tibial tubercle and the medial aspect of the knee. This exposure is carried from the inferior margin of the superficial MCL and may be taken proximally to the femoral insertion if required. The sartorial fascia is incised to expose the MCL. The hamstrings are retracted for dissection to the distal MCL insertion on the tibia.

The initial approach is made from the inferior aspect of the lesion by placing grasping tension sutures in the entire MCL structure. Careful dissection is performed while lifting it off the tibia with a scalpel or periosteal elevator, following its course superiorly and posteriorly. Following the MCL structures superior to the medial joint line and exposing the insertion of the deep MCL results in further dissection.

Repair of the deep MCL and coronary ligament that attaches the medial meniscus to the tibia is performed by placing multiple suture anchors from posterior to anterior along the tibial joint line; four anchors with double-loaded nonabsorbable sutures are typically used.

Sutures are then passed through the deep and superficial MCL structures and tied down to the tibia while maintaining tension on the grasping sutures placed at the start of dissection. Tying of sutures to the tibial insertion is performed at 30 degrees of flexion with a varus load applied to the knee. The tibial insertion of the superficial MCL is often secured to the tibia with a large fragment screw and spiked-washer construct 6 cm distal to joint line with the grasping sutures.

Posteriorly to the repaired MCL structures, the POL and capsular tissue are reefed from multiple posterior to anterior directed sutures, typically figure of 8 sutures or horizontal mattress sutures. The objective is to take the laxity and slack out of the medial POL, which helps tighten the rotational instability caused from the injury.

Chronic medial-sided injuries are also initially assessed with arthroscopy. As previously described, the liftoff test is performed in a valgus maneuver to the knee. If the medial meniscus lifts off the tibia with valgus stress to the knee, we approach reconstruction of the tibial side. If the medial meniscus stays to the tibia with valgus stress to the knee, it is a more femoral-based injury. Surgical exposure and approach are the same as stated previously in the acute repair.

For chronic MCL injury reconstructions, if postoperative stiffness is not a concern or if the patient has an isolated MCL injury, an autograft hamstring tendon is harvested in the same surgical incision. Otherwise, the allograft tendon is used for reconstruction.

The deep MCL structures and capsule are repaired to the anatomic origin and insertion of the femur and tibia with suture anchors that are double-loaded with nonabsorbable sutures, as described previously for the acute injury repair. The tissue is reefed to remove laxity and slack in the injured structures. Augmentation with the autograft or allograft is performed once this maneuver is complete.

To augment the repair, autograft semitendinosus hamstring is harvested with an open-ended tendon stripper, leaving the distal attachment intact to the tibia at the pes anserine. The muscle tissue is cleaned from the semitendinosus tendon proximally with a large periosteal elevator, and a nonabsorbable whipstitch suture is placed in the free end of the tendon. All accessory attachments of the semitendinosus distally are carefully freed. A Kirschner wire is inserted at the medial epicondyle. The tendon is looped over the wire and the isometry of the tendon is evaluated with the knee in flexion and extension. If the excursion is more than 2 mm, the wire is moved to a position of isometry. Once isometry is confirmed, a large fragment screw and spiked washer are placed provisionally in the femur without fully setting the head at that isometric position of the medial femoral epicondyle. A bone trough is made around the screw shank. The tendon is looped around the screw. The screw is then tightened to the femur with the knee in 30 degrees of flexion, and varus stress is applied to the knee.

A right-angled hemostat is used to create a window in the direct head semimembranosus tendon attachment of the femur posteriorly. The free end of the semitendinosus tendon autograft is then directed posterior and obliquely and pulled through this window, recreating the central arm of the POL. The autograft is sutured to the semimembranosus tendon with use of a nonabsorbable suture.

If an allograft tendon is used, the aforementioned technique is modified, with attachment of the tibial limb of the allograft augment secured to the tibial insertion of the superficial MCL with another large fragment screw and spiked washer fixation.

A case example is that of a 16-year-old high school football player who sustained a contact MCL and ACL injury that was treated operatively in a staged fashion (Figs. 101.6–101.8). After treatment, he was allowed full return to contact sports 1 year from injury. Although most femoral-sided tears can be treated successfully with conservative methods, complete tibial-sided avulsions of the deep and superficial MCL, although rare, often heal with residual laxity.[24] In athletes who participate in level I sports, we frequently favor operative repair of these tibial-sided complete avulsions that display retraction of the deep or superficial MCL on MRI (Fig. 101.9). Figs. 101.9 and 101.10 highlight a case example of a Division I football player with an isolated tibial-sided complete MCL avulsion with gross laxity and an impressive arthroscopic drive-through sign that was treated surgically.

Our rehabilitation protocol for grade III lesions is placement in a long-leg hinged knee brace locked in extension with weight bearing as tolerated on crutches for 2 weeks. After approximately 2 weeks we unlock the brace during weight bearing. In the first 4 weeks, our goal is to have the patient attain nearly full ROM and normal gait pattern with full weight bearing in a hinged knee brace, and begin quadriceps and hamstring strengthening.

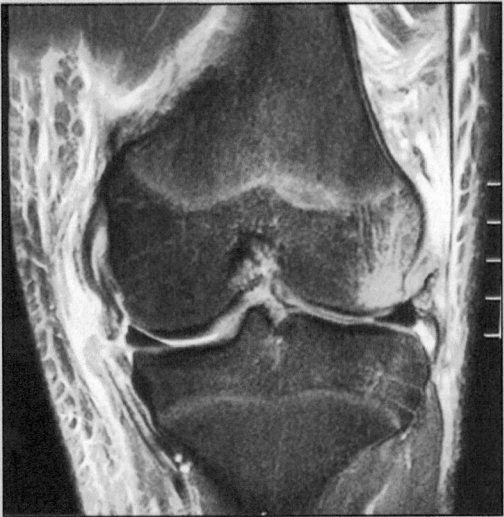

Fig. 101.6 Coronal magnetic resonance image shows complete avulsion of the superficial and deep medial collateral ligament with an unattached medial meniscus.

Continued

📌 Authors' Preferred Technique
Medial Collateral Ligament Injury—cont'd

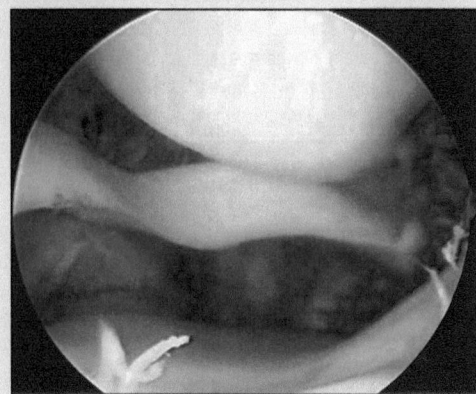

Fig. 101.7 Arthroscopy confirms gross laxity of the medial compartment with complete disruption of medial support structures and a free-floating meniscus.

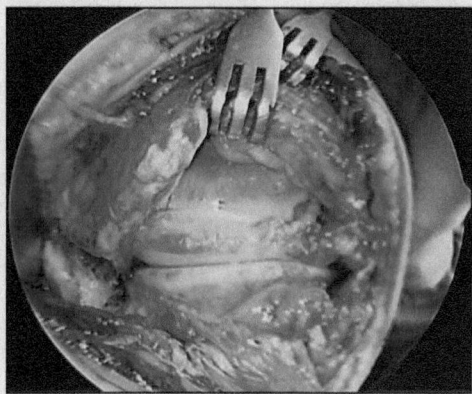

Fig. 101.8 Open surgery confirms complete avulsion of the medial collateral ligament from the tibia with a free-floating, unattached medial meniscus between the articular cartilage of the medial femoral condyle and the tibial plateau.

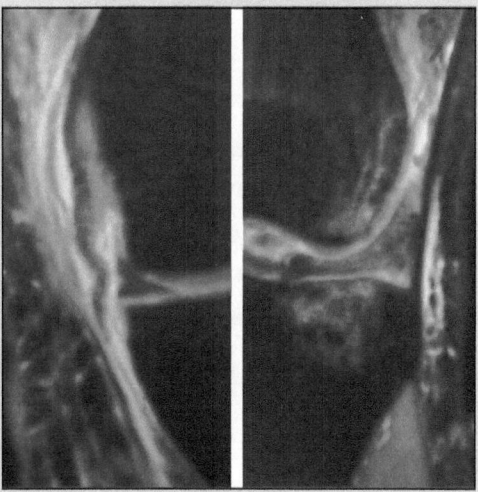

Fig. 101.9 A coronal magnetic resonance image shows tibial-sided avulsion of the medial collateral ligament with retraction and a contrecoup bipolar bone bruise lesion laterally, which suggest a high-energy injury pattern.

In contrast, patients who undergo a repair of the MCL follow a different protocol. Postoperatively, a hinged knee brace is locked from 30 to 90 degrees for 3 weeks, followed by unlimited motion. Weight bearing is limited for 3 weeks with crutches and then progressed to full weight by 4 to 6 weeks. Bracing is discontinued at 6 weeks and nonimpact conditioning is allowed, with running started by 3 months.

Chronic laxity of the medial support structures after nonoperative management is difficult to treat. A firefighter we treated after nonoperative management of his grade III medial lesion had chronic medial instability, which for him was a significant safety issue for performance of his professional duties. Fig. 101.11 shows medial reconstruction of his POL and MCL using allograft tissue and performed anatomically as an isolated procedure for chronic medial stability.

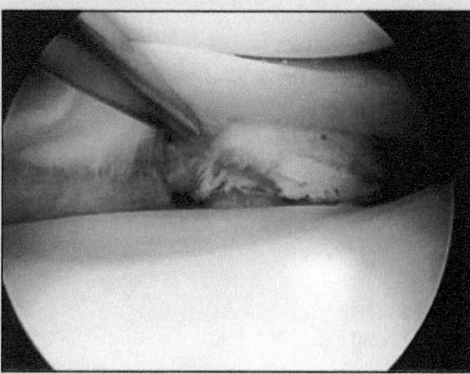

Fig. 101.10 Arthroscopy confirms a drive-through sign with liftoff of the medial meniscus from the tibia, requiring open repair of medial structures.

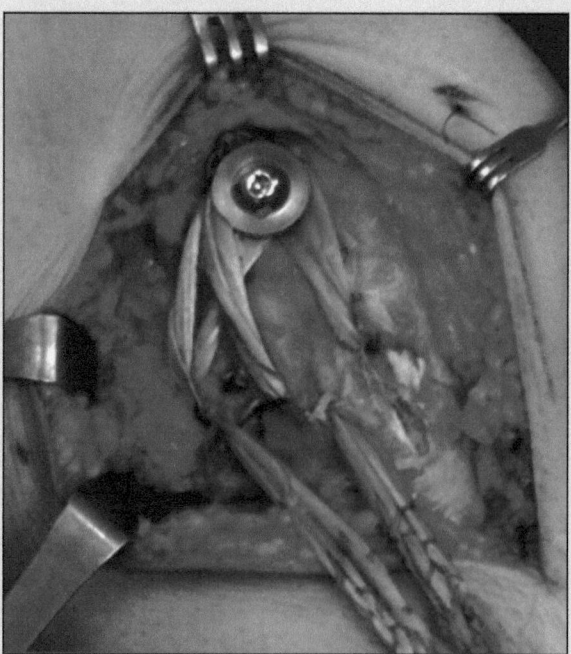

Fig. 101.11 The medial side of the knee illustrating medial reconstruction of the medial collateral ligament and posterior oblique ligament using allograft tissue and performed anatomically.

POSTOPERATIVE MANAGEMENT

The treatment of MCL injuries initially promotes nonoperative management; thus rehabilitation is pivotal and is the primary modality for treatment. No one perfect rehabilitation protocol exists that will work for every athlete. Upon reviewing the literature, no apparent consensus exists regarding the most efficacious rehabilitation protocol, and protocols are usually based on surgeon preference and experience. Steadman,[45] Bergfeld,[46] O'Connor,[47] and Cox[48] have had excellent success with their individual protocols for treatment of MCL injuries. To effectively treat MCL injuries, the grade of the injury must be determined because the parameters of rehabilitation are based on the degree of injury. Table 101.2 shows the general principles for rehabilitation of MCL injuries.

Isolated grade I sprains are treated with rest, ice, compression, and elevation for the first couple of days to help reduce swelling. Patients are allowed weight bearing as tolerated with the use of an assistive device if pain is experienced with walking. The only exception is patients with significant valgus deformity, because they will place more stress on the MCL, affecting healing. In these patients, it may be safer to allow partial weight bearing for a couple of weeks. With grade I MCL tears, immobilization in a brace is rarely required, and if patient compliance is of concern, a short-leg hinged brace is used to control valgus and rotational stresses. ROM is begun immediately to prevent arthrofibrosis and stiffness. In addition, quadriceps strengthening and closed chain exercises are started. Once the patient regains full ROM, resistive exercises are begun along with sport-specific drills.

Isolated grade II injuries are treated similarly to grade I injuries with rest, ice, elevation, and compression. Because grade II injuries involve a greater degree of damage to the ligament with increased valgus instability, a long-leg hinged brace is usually needed. Patients are allowed to progressively bear weight as tolerated in the brace; however, if the patient is having significant pain, the brace can be locked in extension until the pain subsides, usually in 1 week. Assistive devices are used until the patient has a nonantalgic gait. Active ROM exercises are started immediately. During the early period, quadriceps strengthening is performed in a nonweight-bearing fashion with straight leg raises, quadriceps-setting exercises, and electrical stimulation. Once the patient has achieved full ROM and functional strength, proprioceptive and agility drills can be initiated.

Isolated grade III injuries usually involve disruption of both the superficial and the deep fibers. Therefore the rehabilitation process is slower, and a longer period of immobilization is required.

The treatment of grade III injuries can be divided into stages. In the first phase (for about 4 weeks), the patient should wear a brace locked in extension, and progressively increase weight bearing to attain a normal gait pattern. Also, the patient needs to perform ROM exercises with eccentric strengthening of the quadriceps and hamstrings. Failure to perform ROM exercises and prolonged immobilization results in increased ligament creep and poorer cellular metabolism.[50] In phase II, which lasts 4 to 6 weeks, the patient continues to attain full ROM, unlocks the brace, and achieves quadriceps and hamstring strengthening. After 6 weeks, the brace can be discontinued if the patient has a nonantalgic gait and has regained quadriceps strength for daily ambulation. Phase III starts after 6 weeks and includes squatting, light jogging with agility drills, and continued strengthening to return to sports.

After surgical repair of an isolated MCL, the brace is locked at 30 degrees and the patient is allowed to perform toe-touch weight bearing for 3 weeks. The patient is encouraged to continue ROM from 30 to 90 degrees. The patient also continues strengthening of the quadriceps and hamstring while wearing a brace. If possible, we prefer to add a compression cryotherapy device (such as a Game Ready, Concord, Georgia, USA) as ACL studies have demonstrated improved knee ROM and functional scores with the use of compression cryotherapy compared to cryotherapy alone.[51] After 3 weeks, the patient is allowed to progress to full weight bearing with full-time brace wear to continue to protect the repair. The brace can be worn unlocked to allow free ROM, as well as valgus and rotational stability. From 3 to 6 weeks, the goal is to restore full ROM along with continued strengthening with closed kinetic chain exercises. After 6 weeks, the patient continues to progressively increase activities with resistive and sport-specific exercises.

Combined injuries of the MCL and ACL require additional steps compared with the rehabilitation of isolated MCL tears. Upon reviewing the literature on ACL and MCL injuries, as stated previously, conservative treatment of MCL injuries followed by surgical reconstruction of the ACL is the favored management in most patients. Initially the protocol focuses on the severity of the MCL injury. For example, a grade I MCL injury with an ACL injury will proceed with the protocol presented earlier for grade I injuries. The patient will quickly regain ROM and functional strength, and then the surgeon can proceed with reconstruction of the ACL. Conversely, the patient with a grade III injury with an ACL injury will take much longer to heal because of the slower protocol for type III injuries. Regaining ROM and functional strength training may take 8 to 10 weeks, and therefore it will take longer to proceed with ACL reconstruction with a type III injury. The ACL is reconstructed accompanied by conservative treatment of the MCL, following the rehabilitation protocol for an ACL reconstruction. After a combined ACL reconstruction

TABLE 101.2 Principles for Rehabilitation of the Medial Collateral Ligament

Phase	Goals	Criteria for Progression
Maximal protection phase	Early protected ROM	No increase in instability
	Decrease effusion and pain	No increase in swelling
	Prevent quadriceps atrophy	Minimal tenderness
		Passive ROM at least 10 to 100 degrees
Moderate protection phase	Full painless ROM	No instability
	Restore strength	No swelling or tenderness
	Ambulation without crutches	Full painless ROM
Minimal protection phase	Increase strength and power	

ROM, Range of motion.

and medial-sided repair, the knee is braced in full extension, and a standard ACL protocol is followed with protected weight bearing. In a combined ACL and MCL injury, it is important to remember that ACL rehabilitation takes precedence over medial-sided repair.

For RTP guidelines, see Box 101.1.

RESULTS

Numerous authors have shown excellent results with nonoperative treatment of grade I and II MCL tears.[44,52–54] Ellsasser and associates[52] looked at 74 knees in professional football players and achieved a 98% success rate with a nonoperative protocol. They had strict inclusion criteria to ensure an isolated MCL injury was present: (1) up to grade II laxity with a firm end point in flexion, (2) no instability to valgus stress in extension, (3) no significant rotatory or AP subluxation, (4) no significant effusion, and (5) normal stress radiograph findings. In this series, patients were treated with crutches, no brace, and progressive weight bearing. Based on their experience, Ellsasser and associates concluded that by 1 week, patients should progress to full extension, have no effusion, and perceive decreased tenderness. The players returned to football in 3 to 8 weeks. The only failure occurred in a patient with an osteochondral fracture that was found at later follow-up.

Derscheid and Garrick[44] performed a prospective study that examined 51 grade I and grade II MCL injuries in college football players. They used a nonoperative rehabilitation protocol with a knee immobilizer initially. Players with a grade I injury returned to full participation at an average of 10.6 days, and players with a grade II injury returned at an average of 19.5 days. At long-term follow-up, these patients showed slight increases in medial instability. Injured knees had a higher incidence of reinjury than did control knees, but this finding was not statistically significant. Bassett and associates[53] and Hastings[54] studied the use of a cast brace in treating isolated MCL ruptures. In both studies, early return to athletics was found with the use of the cast brace. Nonoperative treatment varies from casting to functional bracing to no bracing, and good outcomes occur with all three forms of treatment.

Fetto and Marshall[55] found an 80% incidence of concomitant ligamentous injuries with a grade III MCL tear, with 95% of the associated injuries being an ACL tear. Early authors recommend primary repair for grade III injuries. O'Donoghue[56]

stressed the importance of immediate repair of complete tears of the MCL. Hughston and Barrett[57] supported primary repair of all medial structures, including the superficial MCL and POL. They believed that repair and advancement of the POL was key to restoring medial stability. Their results were good to excellent in 77% to 94% of patients. Muller[58] reported 65% good and 31% excellent results in the repair of isolated grade III MCL injuries. He repaired the superficial MCL avulsion with screws and washers and intrasubstance tears with a combination of approximation and tension-relieving sutures. Hughston and Barrett,[57] O'Donoghue,[56] Muller,[58] Collins,[59] Kannus,[60] LaPrade and Wijdicks[1,2] have written that surgical intervention is necessary for complete ruptures of the MCL.

Although good results have been demonstrated with surgical repair of the MCL, many studies have focused on the nonoperative management of grade III MCL injuries. Fetto and Marshall[55] were among the first to assess outcomes after nonoperative treatment of grade III MCL injuries. They studied 265 MCL injuries and found that patients with grade II injuries did much better than patients with grade III injuries (97% compared with 73%). Initially, in their study, all patients with grade III injuries underwent operative intervention. However, some patients with grade III injuries did not have an operation because of skin lesions and infection. At follow-up, patients with operative treatment of isolated MCL ruptures had no improved outcome compared with the nonsurgical group. This incidental finding led the way for more prospective studies to investigate the role of nonoperative treatment in patients with isolated grade III MCL injuries.

Indelicato[61] prospectively compared operative and nonoperative treatment of isolated grade III ruptures. All patients underwent examination with the use of an anesthetic and arthroscopy to rule out any other pathology, such as ACL and meniscal tears. Indelicato[61] found objectively stable knees in 15 of 16 patients treated operatively and in 17 of 20 patients treated nonoperatively. Both groups followed a rigid rehabilitation protocol including casting at 30 degrees of flexion for 2 weeks and then 4 weeks longer in a cast brace with hinges that allowed motion from 30 to 90 degrees. Subjective scores were higher in the nonsurgical group, with good to excellent results for 90% in the nonsurgical group and 88% in the surgically repaired group, suggesting that surgical intervention offered no benefit. Indelicato also showed that patients treated with early motion returned to football 3 weeks earlier than did immobilized patients. A subsequent study by Indelicato and associates[62] showed that a conservative approach in patients with complete MCL ruptures was successful in collegiate football players. All players were managed with a functional rehabilitation program, and 71% had good to excellent results.

Similar to Indelicato, both Reider and colleagues[63] and Jones and associates[64] found excellent outcomes in athletes with isolated grade III medial ligament injuries who were treated conservatively and agreed that nonoperative treatment of these lesions is justified. Reider and colleagues studied 35 athletes who were treated with early functional rehabilitation for isolated grade III tears. Of these 35 athletes, 19 returned to full and unlimited activity in less than 8 weeks. At an average follow-up of 5.3 years, outcomes based on subjective and objective measurements were comparable with earlier investigations using a surgical repair.

In 1986, Jones et al. reported results for 24 high school football players who returned to competition at an average of 34 days. Management consisted of 1 week of immobilization followed by gradual ROM and strengthening. The knee was tested weekly with valgus stress, and instability was reduced to grade 0 or 1 by 29 days. No increased incidence of reinjury was found the following spring.

Although Indelicato,[61] Fetto and Marshall,[55] Jones et al.,[64] and Reider et al.[63] found excellent results with nonoperative treatment, Kannus[60] studied 27 patients with grade III lesions at an average 9 years of follow-up. Patients were found to have poor outcomes (an average Lysholm score of 66) and degenerative changes on radiographs. Kannus concluded that early surgical repair would prevent deterioration. A careful review of the patients showed that 16 of 27 had greater than a 2+ Lachman score, and 10 of 27 had anterolateral instability. Thus this study did not show that nonoperative treatment has poor outcomes but that associated injuries, such as ACL injuries, need to be addressed to prevent poor long-term outcome.

In the last decade, anatomic restoration of the medial knee structures has been found to provide satisfactory outcomes. Lind et al.[37] described a technique to reconstruct the MCL and POL. The clinical results they published showed that 98% of their patients treated with this technique had normal or near normal International Knee Documentation Committee (IKDC) measures at follow-up of more than 2 years.

LaPrade and associates[2] reported their technique and follow-up at an average of 1.5 years for reconstruction of the MCL and POL. Their outcomes showed improved IKDC measures and decreased valgus opening on stress radiographs.

Several cadaveric studies of anatomic MCL reconstruction have been recently performed. Wijdicks and associates[35] performed a cadaveric biomechanical study comparing augmented repair versus reconstruction of a completely transected superficial MCL. The MCL was reconstructed via the LaPrade method.[2] Compared to the transected state, augmented repair and reconstruction both decreased medial gapping. However, the authors noted that neither technique reproduced the stability of the intact ligament. Gilmer et al.[36] performed a cadaveric analysis comparing a repair of the MCL and POL versus a repair with internal bracing versus LaPrade's allograft reconstruction technique. They found that the mean moment to failure was highest in the intact ligament. Augmentation with internal bracing improved moment to failure and valgus angle at failure compared to repair alone, and was similar in comparison to allograft reconstruction. Finally, Omar and colleagues[65] performed a biomechanical analysis of fixation techniques for use in augmented repair. Spiked polyetheretherketone washers (PEEK) reinforced with polyester sutures provided the best results with regard to elongation during cyclic loading and load to failure.

Combined injury to the MCL and ACL represents a completely different entity than an isolated MCL injury. The ACL is a primary restraint to anterior displacement and acts as a secondary stabilizer to valgus stress, especially in full extension. Conversely, the MCL is the primary restraint to valgus stress at 30 degrees of flexion. Therefore injury to the MCL and ACL results in both anterior and valgus instability and can significantly compromise

knee function. Even though the apparent consensus is that a solitary MCL rupture can be treated nonoperatively, the optimal treatment for a concurrent ACL and MCL injury is debated. The extent of involvement of the posteromedial capsule and POL may help to guide treatment strategies.

The management of combined ACL and MCL injuries has been a controversial topic in the literature. The first issue pertains to the various surgical options available for managing these injuries. Three principal surgical options exist: (1) surgical reconstruction and repair of both ligaments; (2) ACL reconstruction and nonoperative MCL management; and (3) operative management of MCL with nonoperative ACL treatment. ACL reconstruction with nonoperative management of the MCL remains the most popular option. The second controversial issue regarding combined injuries is whether early or late ACL reconstruction provides better functional and long-term results.

In years past, authors recommended surgical intervention for both ligamentous structures in concomitant ACL and MCL ruptures.[55,66,67] Fetto and Marshall[55] had 79% unsatisfactory outcomes in patients treated operatively for ACL and MCL tears. Even though studies have shown that operative repair of all ligaments results in stable, functional knees, a high incidence of knee stiffness was found.[68–70] Other authors have stated that isolated operative MCL repair and nonoperative ACL reconstruction leads to good results. Hughston and Barrett[57] reported that 94% of their patients with combined ACL and MCL injury who were treated with only MCL reconstruction returned to their preinjury levels of athletic performance. They stated that the key to obtaining excellent results was reconstruction of the POL and posteromedial structures. Noyes and Barber-Westin[71] criticized the method used by Hughston and Barrett to report results, and stated that the results may have been overly optimistic. However, Hughston[72] continued to report good results at 22 years of follow-up. In addition to Hughston, Shirakura and associates[73] reported excellent results in 14 patients with combined lesions but reconstruction of the MCL only; however, they did not report AP instability. Conversely, Frolke and coworkers[74] reported poor results with solitary MCL repair. They performed arthroscopically guided repair of the MCL, which led to functional stability in 68% of knees, but clinical testing of all 22 knees showed abnormal or severe abnormal examination findings. More recently, Pandey and associates[75] found higher IKDC scores, higher Lysholm scores, and fewer complaints of instability in patients with combined injuries who underwent repair of the MCL and POL as well as ACL reconstruction compared to patients who underwent repair of medial sided structures only.

Most authors suggest that nonoperative treatment of the MCL with reconstruction of the ACL provides good to excellent results. Shelbourne and Porter[76] demonstrated good to excellent results in 68 patients with ACL reconstruction and nonsurgical management of an MCL tear. They also showed that these patients achieved a greater ROM and more rapid strength gains than did patients with surgical reconstruction and repair of both ligaments. Similarly, Noyes and Barber-Westin[71] demonstrated a higher incidence of motion problems when MCL and ACL were treated operatively, and they recommend arthroscopic reconstruction of the ACL with nonoperative management of the MCL after recovery of

ROM and muscle function. In a prospective randomized study, Halinen and associates[77] treated 47 consecutive patients with combined ACL and grade III MCL injuries. All patients underwent early ACL reconstruction within 3 weeks of injury. The MCL was treated operatively in 23 patients and nonoperatively in 24 patients. All patients were available for follow-up at a mean of 27 months. The nonoperative treatment of the MCL led to results similar to those obtained with operative treatment with respect to subjective function, postoperative stability, ROM, muscle power, return to activities, and Lysholm score. Halinen and colleagues concluded that MCL ruptures did not need to be treated operatively when the ACL was reconstructed early.

In a retrospective study, Millett and colleagues[78] reported on 19 patients with a complete ACL injury and a minimal grade II MCL tear who underwent early ACL reconstruction and nonoperative treatment of the MCL. At the 2-year follow-up, subjective evaluation showed a Lysholm score of 94.5 and a Tegner activity score of 8.4. Clinical examination revealed good ROM and strength. None of the patients experienced graft failure or required subsequent surgery.

More recently, there has been increased interest in anatomic repair or reconstruction of combined injuries. Piatkowski et al.[32] examined the primary repair of grade III MCL injuries with delayed reconstruction of ACL tears. Good to very good outcomes were achieved in 63% based on IKDC scores, and good outcomes were achieved in 74% based on the Lysholm scale. They noted that patients over 40 years of age were less likely to have good outcomes. Blanke et al.[33] presented a case series of patients who underwent screw and suture repair of grade II MCL injuries at the same time as ACL reconstruction. The chronicity of the injuries was not reported. At the 9-month follow-up, all five patients had grade A IKCD medial instability and postop instability scores. The average Lysholm score was 94.6. Zhang et al.[79] also examined simultaneous ACL reconstruction and MCL reconstruction. The patients in their series had a mean time from injury to surgery of 7.6 months. At 40 months follow-up, they noted significant decreases in valgus laxity with normal to near normal mean gapping on stress radiographs. The presence of anteromedial rotatory instability decreased from 71% preoperatively to 0% postoperatively. Patients' IKDC scores improved postoperatively to a mean of 87.7. One patient had loss of flexion over 15 degrees.

Dong and colleagues[39] performed a randomized, controlled trial comparing anatomic ligament repair to triangular reconstruction in patients with acute grade III MCL injury and concomitant ACL tears. No significant differences in valgus instability, knee ROM, return to sport, functional scores, or flexion/extension deficit were noted between groups. The reconstruction group had significant decreases in anteromedial rotatory instability (9.4% vs. 34%). The primary repair group had a nonstatistically significant increase in medial knee pain, four ACL re-ruptures, and two patients undergoing revision for continued medial instability. One patient in the reconstruction group underwent revision reconstruction of the MCL secondary to hardware failure, and another patient underwent surgical release for arthrofibrosis.

Dong et al.[80] also retrospectively reviewed outcomes of triangular ligament reconstruction in patients with isolated grade III MCL injuries and those with concomitant ACL injuries who had failed 6 months of nonoperative treatment. In both groups of patients, medial instability and the presence of anteromedial rotatory instability significantly improved. A total of 58.9% of patients had Grade A IKDC scores and 35.7% had grade B IKDC scores. However, patients with concomitant MCL and ACL reconstruction were more likely to have extension deficits at final follow-up.

Finally, in a systematic review of MCL and posteromedial corner techniques, Delong and associates[34] report that 76% of MCL repair cases in the literature had a concomitant ACL reconstruction. A total of 75% of cases in the systematic review had medial laxity less than grade I at final follow-up, and the average Lysholm score was 91.6.

Another controversial issue regarding combined ACL and MCL injury is whether early or late ACL reconstruction provides optimal return of function and long-term results. Based on animal studies, MCL healing is adversely affected by ACL insufficiency,[81] and therefore it has been proposed that early ACL reconstruction will improve healing of the MCL. Both Halinen and colleagues[77] and Millett and associates[78] showed good subjective scores and minimal loss of motion complications with early ACL reconstruction (within 3 weeks). Conversely, Petersen and Laprell[82] demonstrated poorer results with early ACL reconstruction compared with late ACL reconstruction in combined injuries. All patients underwent nonoperative treatment of MCL injury, with early ACL reconstruction performed within 3 weeks of injury and late ACL reconstruction after a minimum of 10 weeks. The late reconstruction group had a lower rate of loss of motion and higher Lysholm scores compared with the early reconstruction group.

The literature supports nonoperative treatment of the MCL tear with surgical reconstruction of the ACL, and most surgeons are currently following this protocol. However, early versus late reconstruction continues to be a subject of debate, with studies supporting both points of view. Other factors, such as preoperative and postoperative rehabilitation protocol along with bracing, may need to be further analyzed to help assess whether early or late reconstruction is more beneficial.

COMPLICATIONS

Complications of MCL ruptures are rarely reported in the literature. Failure to diagnose associated ligament injuries, such as ACL, can lead to long-term instability and degenerative problems.[12,60] Failure to recognize and repair all injured medial and posteromedial structures can also lead to residual instability.[12,13] In addition, missed associated meniscal tears and articular cartilage defects can lead to continued pain. Atrophy and arthrofibrosis are rare complications given the aggressive rehabilitation protocols with early motion and strengthening.[13] Infection is a rare complication with surgical reconstruction. Persistent pain and Pellegrini–Stieda lesions can occur after MCL sprains, usually near the femoral origin in the region of the medial epicondyle.[83] Treatment consists of a local injection or antiinflammatory medication, and resection of the lesion may be required for relief. In addition to pain, patients with femoral-sided lesions are more prone to have loss of motion and associated stiffness.[13,83]

FUTURE CONSIDERATIONS

As with most topics within orthopaedic surgery, basic science knowledge is ever increasing. The avenues for future research are vast in the areas of chemistry, biology, and biomechanics. Our understanding of cellular processes allows us to alter the progression of injury or speed up the restoration of health.

Collagen healing is currently being investigated for the ligaments of the knee. Enzymatic processes in the inflammatory process of ligament injury and healing are plentiful. Research into the MCL and ACL response to a procollagen growth factor and transforming growth factor-β1 is ongoing.[84] In addition, newer research has explored different expressions of lysyl oxidases in ACL and MCL tissue in response to transforming growth factor-β1 and TNF alpha.[84,85] This research is furthering the investigation into the role of procollagen processes of ligament healing.

The past decade has seen an increase in anatomic and biomechanical studies of the structures of the knee. Data from these and future studies will continue to influence surgical techniques. Finally, the majority of the literature consists of studies level 3 or below in evidence.[86,87] Future level 2 and higher studies would help provide answers to many of the controversies regarding medial-sided knee injuries.

For a complete list of references, go to ExpertConsult.com.

SELECTED READING

Citation:
Wijdicks CA, et al. Structural properties of the primary medial knee ligaments. *Am J Sports Med.* 2010;38(8):1638–1646.

Level of Evidence:
Cadaveric study

Summary:
The two tibial attachments of the superficial medial collateral ligament (MCL) sustain clinically important loads, as do the central arm of the posterior oblique ligament and the deep MCL. Anatomic medial knee reconstructions may allow recreation of the unique stabilizing characteristics of these structures.

Citation:
Marchant MH Jr, et al. Management of medial-sided knee injuries, part 1: medial collateral ligament. *Am J Sports Med.* 2011;39(5):1102–1113.

Level of Evidence:
V, clinical review

Summary:
In this article the anatomy and biomechanics of medial-sided knee injuries are reviewed. Superficial medial collateral ligament and combined anterior cruciate ligament injuries are reviewed.

Citation:
Tibor LM, et al. Management of medial-sided knee injuries, part 2: posteromedial corner. *Am J Sports Med.* 2011;39(6):1332–1340.

Level of Evidence:
V, clinical review

Summary:
In this article the anatomy and biomechanics of medial-sided knee injuries are reviewed. Posteromedial corner and combined posterior cruciate ligament injuries are reviewed.

Citation:
DeLong JM, Waterman BR. Surgical techniques for the reconstruction of medial collateral ligament and posteromedial corner injuries of the knee: a systematic review. *Arthroscopy.* 2015;31(11):2258–2272.e2251.

Level of Evidence:
IV, systematic review

Summary:
The authors provide a review of outcomes from MCL reconstruction in the literature. Included is a review of the most common reconstruction techniques reported.

Citation:
Dale KM, et al. Surgical management and treatment of the anterior cruciate ligament/medial collateral ligament injured knee. *Clin Sports Med.* 2017;36(1):87–103.

Level of Evidence:
V, clinical review

Summary:
The authors discuss the management of combined ACL/MCL injuries, including operative and nonoperative treatment.

Citation:
LaPrade MD, et al. Anatomy and biomechanics of the medial side of the knee and their surgical implications. *Sports Med Arthrosc Rev.* 2015;23(2):63–70.

Level of Evidence:
V, clinical review

Summary:
The authors review the anatomy and biomechanics of key medial knee structures. The article also reviews stress radiography for medial knee injuries.

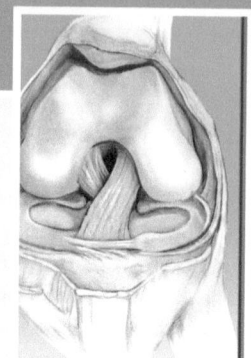

Lateral and Posterolateral Corner Injuries of the Knee

Ryan P. Coughlin, Dayne T. Mickelson, Claude T. Moorman III

As understanding of the posterolateral corner (PLC) has increased, its significance to overall knee function and biomechanics has become clearer. Although it is a relatively uncommon injury, PLC injuries can have severe consequences for overall knee stability and function. Missed injuries may affect the outcome of surgeries to correct concomitant injuries. This chapter reviews the epidemiology, relevant anatomy, biomechanics, presentation, examination, imaging, and treatment of PLC injuries. Rehabilitation, potential complications, and future considerations for the management of these serious injuries are also discussed.

Isolated PLC injuries are relatively rare and have been reported to range from 1.6% to 7% of all knee injuries in persons who present for evaluation.[1-6] However, the true incidence is not fully known, because these injuries are believed to be underreported or often missed at the time of evaluation. In a review of 68 persons with PLC injuries, Pacheco et al. found that 72% were not correctly diagnosed at time of presentation to the hospital and 50% were still misdiagnosed by the time they were referred to a knee specialist.[7] This misdiagnosis may in part be due to the fact that understanding of the PLC has only recently improved. With recent advances, physicians are developing a better understanding of the anatomy, biomechanics, and mechanism of these injuries. In addition, the effects of chronic deficiency on gait, level of activity, natural progression, and impact on the management of other injuries are becoming clearer. Finally, surgical techniques continue to evolve as the best way to treat these injuries continues to be debated.

ANATOMY

An understanding of the PLC begins with an understanding of the relevant anatomy of the region. This anatomy is among the most complex around the knee. The PLC has been characterized by dynamic and static restraints, anatomic layers, and various structures with multiple names in the literature, thus making the use of consistent nomenclature difficult.

Layers of the Lateral Side of the Knee

Seebacher et al.[8] described the structures on the lateral side of the knee in three anatomic layers. The most superficial layer, layer 1, consists of the lateral fascia, iliotibial (IT) band, and the superficial portion of the biceps femoris tendon. The peroneal nerve, located posterior to the biceps, is located in the deepest aspect of layer 1. The intermediate layer, layer 2, consists of the retinaculum of the quadriceps and the proximal and distal patellofemoral ligaments. The deep layer, layer 3, includes the lateral part of the joint capsule, the lateral collateral ligament, the fabellofibular ligament, the coronary ligament, the popliteal tendon, and the arcuate ligament. Even when described in layers, Seebacher et al.[8] found anatomic variations within their dissected specimens.

Individual Structures

Recent descriptions have focused more on specific anatomic structures and their relation to the posterolateral knee, including the IT band, lateral collateral ligament, popliteus tendon, long and short heads of the biceps femoris, and several smaller structures (Fig. 102.1).

Iliotibial Band

The IT band, or IT tract, is composed of different layers and has at least four separate attachments at the knee.[9-12] The main component, the superficial layer, which covers much of the lateral side of the knee, has a wide attachment to Gerdy tubercle. In addition, it has an anterior component attaching to the patella called the iliopatellar band, which influences patellar tracking. The deep layer, a structure found on the medial aspect of the superficial layer, attaches to the lateral intermuscular septum of the distal femur. Distal to the lateral epicondyle of the femur, the deep layer blends with the superficial layer and attaches to the Gerdy tubercle.[12] The capsular-osseous layer, beginning at the lateral intermuscular septum of the femur, receives contributions from the lateral gastrocnemius and biceps femoris before inserting on Gerdy tubercle. This layer also has attachments to the patella and can influence patellar tracking.[12] When viewed as a whole, the IT band is the first structure encountered during exposure for PLC reconstruction and serves as a stabilizer of the lateral side of the knee.

Fibular Collateral Ligament

With attachments on the fibular head and distal femur, the fibular collateral ligament (FCL; also known as the lateral collateral ligament) is a primary restraint to varus stress on the knee. Its fanlike attachment on the femur is in a bony depression 1.3 to 1.4 mm proximal and 3.1 to 4.6 mm posterior to the lateral epicondyle, but it does not actually attach to the epicondyle.[13,14] With an average length of 6.3 to 7.1 cm, it traverses distally deep to the superficial layer of the IT band and attaches to the

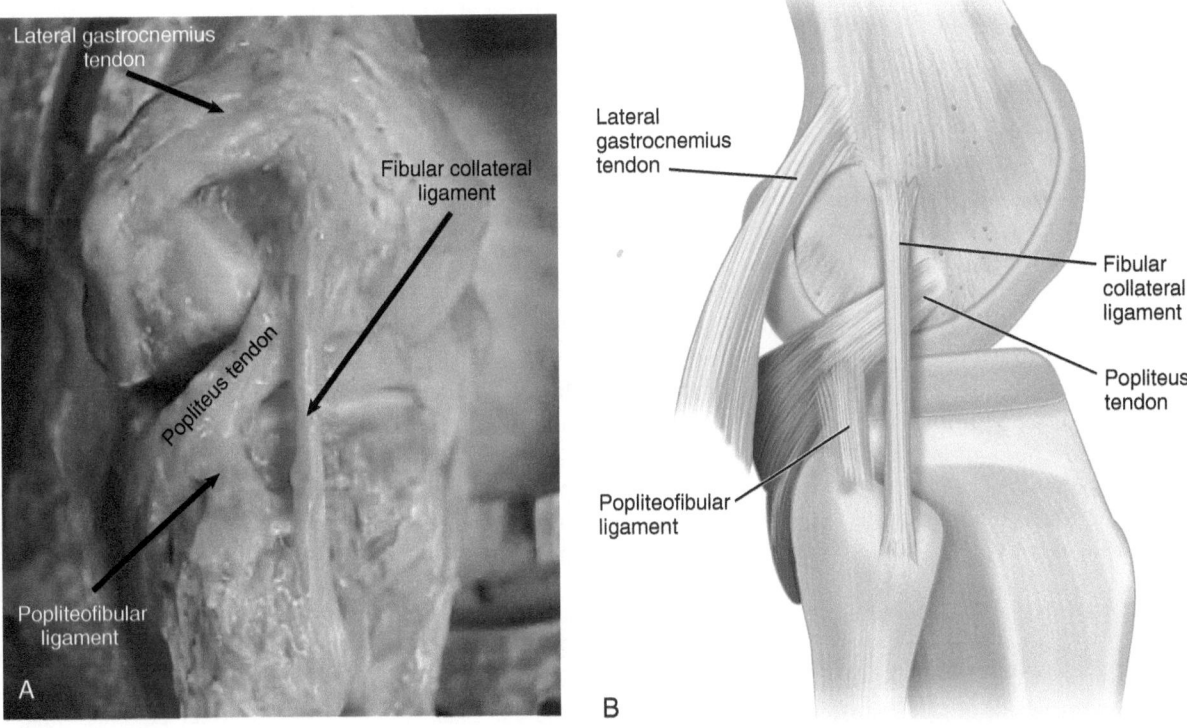

Fig. 102.1 Image (A) and illustration (B) of the anatomy of the posterolateral corner and the relationships of individual structures to each other. (From LaPrade RF, Ly TV, Wentorf FA, et al. The posterolateral attachments of the knee: a qualitative and quantitative morphologic analysis of the fibular collateral ligament, popliteus tendon, popliteofibular ligament, and lateral gastrocnemius tendon. *Am J Sports Med.* 2003;31:854–860.)

fibular head.[15-18] The tendon narrows as it courses distally to its narrowest point midway between the femoral and fibular attachments, where it measures 3.4 mm in an anteroposterior (AP) plane and 2.3 mm in a medial to lateral plane.[16] It then expands into its fanlike attachment on the lateral aspect of the fibular head, covering 38% of the width of the head, and is located 8.2 mm posterior and 28.4 mm distal to styloid process.[13,15,16] An understanding of FCL anatomy is essential to anatomic surgical reconstruction for both fibular and femoral tunnel placement.

Popliteus Tendon Complex

The popliteus begins on the posteromedial aspect of the tibia and courses proximally to insert in the popliteal sulcus on the lateral femoral condyle. At the level of the popliteal fossa, the muscle gives rise to the popliteus tendon, which then inserts into the popliteal sulcus. It is at this musculotendinous junction that the popliteofibular ligament attaches the popliteus to the fibula.[13] The tendon becomes intra-articular and runs medial to the FCL. It then inserts onto the femur typically 9.7 mm distal and 5.3 mm posterior to the lateral epicondyle,[14] which represents a distance of 18.5 mm between the femoral attachments of the two structures, a concept to take into consideration when planning a reconstruction.[13] In addition to its attachments on the femur and tibia, the popliteus contains popliteomeniscal fascicles that extend to the lateral meniscus, as well as attachments to the posterior capsule.

The popliteofibular ligament, originating at the musculotendinous junction of the popliteus, travels distally and laterally to insert on the fibular head.[13,17] With anterior and posterior divisions, the ligament provides a strong connection between the fibula and the popliteus.[19] The smaller anterior division attaches to the anteromedial aspect of the fibular styloid 2.8 mm from the tip of the styloid, whereas the larger posterior division attaches to the posteromedial aspect of the fibular styloid 1.6 mm distal to the tip of the styloid.[13] The true role of the popliteofibular ligament to overall stability has been debated. Some investigators propose that it is a primary stabilizer to varus stress, external tibial rotation, and posterior tibial translation.[20,21] However, others have found that it serves purely as a secondary stabilizer, serving a purpose if the FCL is transected.[22]

Biceps Femoris Muscle

Long head. The long head of the biceps femoris muscle, originating at the ischial tuberosity, travels distally to the knee and forms two tendinous portions, the direct and anterior arms, with the direct arm attaching to the posterolateral fibular head and the anterior arm crossing lateral to the FCL and attaching to the lateral fibular head.[19] The anterior arm is separated from the FCL by the FCL-biceps bursa. This bursa, typically measuring 8.4 by 18 mm, is consistently found between the two structures and serves as a surgical landmark for identifying the FCL attachment to the fibular head.[18] In addition, the long head has three fascial attachments, the reflected arm and the lateral and anterior aponeurosis. The reflected arm travels superficial to the short head of the biceps femoris and inserts on the posterior aspect of the IT tract.[10,19]

Short head. The short head of the biceps femoris, originating from the femur, travels distally at a 45-degree angle to the femur, where it splits into six components, including attachments to the long head of the biceps, the posterolateral aspect of the joint capsule, and the IT tract.[19] The attachment to the capsule (the "capsular arm") forms a large fascial sheath that includes the fabellofibular ligament.[17] In addition, further distal, the short head attaches just lateral to the tip of the fibular styloid and a separate anterior arm travels proximal to the fibular styloid and medial to the FCL to attach posterior to the Gerdy tubercle.[17] The final component, the lateral aponeurotic expansion, attaches to the posteromedial aspect of the FCL.[19]

The long and short heads of the biceps femoris are innervated by different components of the sciatic nerve. The long head is innervated by the tibial component and the short head by the common peroneal nerve.

Fabellofibular Ligament

The fabellofibular ligament represents the most distal aspect of the capsular arm from the short head of the biceps femoris.[17] Originating from the fabella or fabella-analog, it courses distally to attach to the fibular styloid. It is thought to provide stability to the knee once it has reached close to full extension.[17]

Arcuate Ligament Complex

The arcuate ligament complex (also referred to as the *arcuate popliteal ligament* or *arcuate complex*), one of the more inconsistently referenced structures in the knee, is a Y-shaped structure consisting of medial and lateral limbs. Both limbs originate on the fibular styloid process. The lateral limb ascends proximally along the lateral joint capsule to insert on the lateral femoral condyle at the posterior joint capsule, whereas the medial limb courses over the musculotendinous junction of the popliteus, blends with the oblique popliteal ligament (ligament of Winslow), and then inserts variably onto the fabella, if present, or the posterior joint capsule.[8,19,23,24] The arcuate ligament complex, when present, is believed to be more accurately described as a variable confluence of several structures, including the posterior oblique, popliteofibular, fabellofibular, and short lateral ligaments, with the final appearance of a Y-shaped ligament complex.[25] It has been shown to contribute to the prevention of varus instability.[26]

Lateral Gastrocnemius Tendon

The lateral gastrocnemius tendon originates at the musculotendinous junction of the lateral gastrocnemius muscle and then courses proximally, first attaching to a fabella or fabella-analog before blending into the meniscofemoral portion of posterior capsule.[17] It ultimately attaches to the femur at the region of the supracondylar process 13.8 mm posterior to the fibular collateral attachment and 28.4 mm from the popliteus tendon attachment.[13]

Mid-Third Lateral Capsular Ligament

The mid-third lateral capsular ligament, a thickening of the lateral capsule of the knee, originates on the femur in an area around the lateral epicondyle and then travels distally and provides a capsular attachment to the lateral meniscus before inserting on the tibia between the Gerdy tubercle and the popliteal hiatus.[17,27] It is composed of meniscotibial and meniscofemoral ligaments. Clinically, the meniscotibial ligament is responsible for the Segond fracture, an avulsion of the lateral tibial plateau.[28,29] A Segond fracture can easily be seen on radiographs and magnetic resonance imaging (MRI) and is indicative of ligamentous injury to the knee.[27,29]

Neurovascular Structures

The peroneal nerve is intimately related to the structures of the PLC. As a result, the nerve is injured in 13% of PLC injuries.[26] In the popliteal fossa, the sciatic nerve splits to form the tibial and common peroneal nerves. The peroneal nerve courses distal and lateral to emerge from under the biceps femoris and then passes behind the fibular neck, ultimately passing deep to the peroneal longus.[30] The nerve is located approximately 15 mm from the joint capsule.[31]

The inferior lateral genicular artery is the main artery associated with the PLC. Originating from the popliteal artery, it is found along the posterior joint capsule proximal to the lateral meniscus. It continues laterally and passes anterior to the fabellofibular ligament and posterior to the popliteofibular ligament before traveling within the lateral capsular ligament along the lateral meniscus.[17]

Biomechanics

With its complex anatomy and its association with the function of other ligaments, the biomechanics of the PLC have proven difficult to determine and remain difficult to understand. In its most basic terms, the PLC serves to resist varus angulation, external tibial rotation, and posterior tibial translation. Through cadaveric sectioning studies, the role of individual structures has become clearer. Previous studies have identified the lateral collateral ligament, popliteus tendon, and popliteofibular ligament as being the key structures contributing to PLC function and stability.[32-36] In addition, the PLC structures affect the function and loads seen on the cruciate ligaments (Fig. 102.2).

Role of Posterolateral Corner Structures to Varus Motion

The FCL is the primary restraint to varus stress. Sectioning of the FCL causes increases in varus motion in all degrees of knee flexion.[37] As long as the FCL remains intact, minimal change occurs in varus translation regardless of what other structures may be torn.[38] However, isolated sectioning of the popliteus tendon has shown small but significant increases in varus motion, but to a much smaller degree than isolated sectioning of the FCL.[39] Varus stress produces the greatest load on the FCL with the knee in 30 degrees of flexion, and the load subsequently decreases once the knee reaches 90 degrees of flexion, with an ultimate maximum tensile load of 295 to 309 N.[40-42] Once the FCL is torn, secondary structures assume the main restraint to varus motion, including the posterior cruciate ligament (PCL), popliteofibular ligament, posterior capsule, mid-third lateral

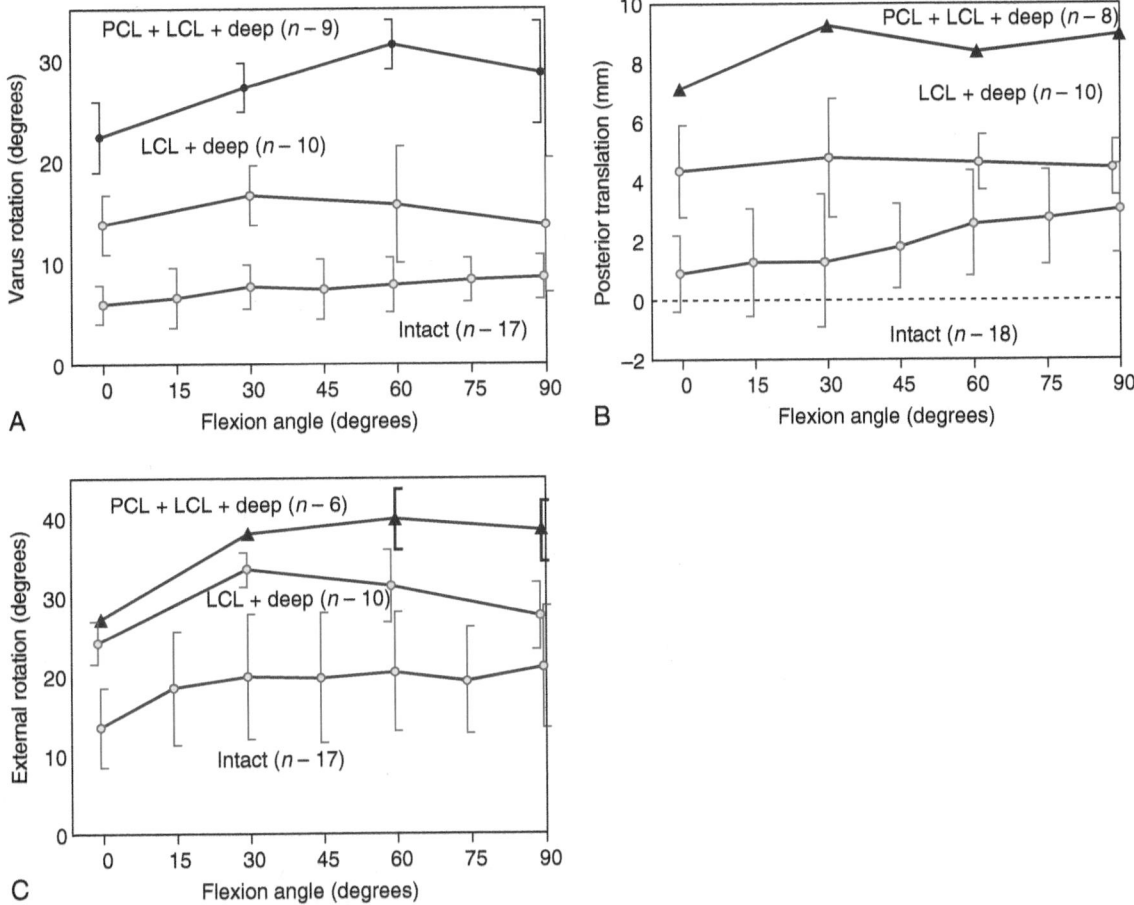

Fig. 102.2 Sectioning studies showing motion versus knee flexion angle relative to contribution of the posterolateral structures and posterior cruciate ligament with respect to varus rotation (A), posterior translation (B), and external rotation stability (C). *LCL,* Lateral collateral ligament; *PCL,* posterior cruciate ligament; *deep,* popliteus-arcuate ligament complex. (Modified from Gollehon DL, Torzilli PA, Warren RF. The role of the posterolateral and cruciate ligaments in the stability of the human knee: a biomechanical study. *J Bone Joint Surg Am.* 1987;69:233–242.)

capsule ligament, IT band, and popliteal tendon.[22,39,43,44] This primary function of the FCL is essential to consider during reconstruction to recreate the main contributor to varus stability in the knee.

Role of the Posterolateral Corner Structures in Preventing External Rotation

The popliteus tendon and the popliteofibular ligament are the primary restraints to external rotation.[20-22] Isolated sectioning of the popliteus leads to significant increases in external rotation, and conversely, a reconstructed popliteus demonstrates significantly decreased external rotation compared with a sectioned specimen.[39] However, the FCL appears to have a greater contribution to external rotation stability than previously thought, especially at 30 degrees of knee flexion where the maximal load from external rotation forces is greater on the FCL than on the popliteus and popliteofibular ligament.[40] Consequently, it appears that the FCL plays a primary role in external rotation restraint when the knee is closer to full extension, and the popliteus and popliteofibular ligament assume responsibility with increasing degrees of knee flexion.

The PCL also affects external rotation resistance. The PLC and PCL work in concert to resist external rotation stresses. Isolated sectioning of the PCL does not affect external rotation motion of the knee if the PLC is intact.[38,43] As noted, the PLC experiences greatest external rotation moments at 30 degrees of knee flexion.[38,43] The PCL does not experience external rotation loads until 80 to 90 degrees of knee flexion, when it becomes a secondary stabilizer to external rotation, thus explaining why in the dial test, decreased external rotation at 90 degrees compared with 30 degrees of knee flexion suggests an intact PCL and an isolated PLC injury.[45]

Role of the Posterolateral Corner Structures in Preventing Anterior/Posterior Tibial Translation

Injured PLC structures have little effect on total anterior tibial translation if the anterior cruciate ligament (ACL) is intact.[36,38,43] The FCL, popliteus, and popliteofibular ligament each experience negligible force when subjected to an anterior drawer test in a knee with a competent ACL.[40] This finding is significant during the physical examination. In persons with an isolated PLC injury, findings of the Lachman test and anterior drawer test will be mostly normal because of the minimal impact of the PLC on anterior tibial translation. Slight differences in total translation may be found because sectioning the popliteus can cause up to a 2.6-mm increase of anterior translation.[39] However, the test should have a firm end point and very minimal clinical difference, although if the ACL is also torn, the combined ACL/PLC injury leads to significantly increased anterior tibial translation. Combined sectioning of the PLC and ACL causes an additional 7 mm of anterior translation,[34] which may lead to a more pronounced Lachman test during the physical examination.

Isolated PLC injuries can cause increased posterior tibial translation, even in the setting of an intact PCL.[36,38,43] This increase is small but significant, with the greatest increase occurring in the first 45 degrees of knee flexion. In the knee with a deficient PCL, the PLC assumes a major stabilizing role, with increases in force load of six to eight times that of the knee with an intact PCL, especially at higher degrees of knee flexion.[46] Total posterior tibial translation increases significantly, up to 20 to 25 mm, when both the PCL and PLC are torn and no longer resist posterior tibial translation.[38,47] Clinically, this finding is manifested in a more pronounced posterior drawer test than is found with isolated PCL tears, with a minimum of at least a grade 3 posterior drawer in the combined injury setting.[47]

Recent biomechanical studies have focused on the reconstruction of the cruciate ligaments in the setting of concomitant PLC injury to better explain the higher failure rate seen after cruciate ligament reconstruction in the knee with multiple ligament injuries. Graft rupture after ACL reconstruction has been reported to range from 1.8% to 10.4%, with an average rate of 5.8% reported in a recent review.[48] It is becoming increasingly clear that missed PLC injuries may contribute to a higher failure rate.[49-51] In response to varus load, ACL graft forces are increased with isolated FCL sectioning, and this force is further increased with varus and external rotation loads.[49] In addition, concomitant reconstruction of the ACL and PLC decreases instability by allowing less anterior tibial translation, and instability was the major reason cited for poor subjective outcomes by patients with residual PLC injury after ACL reconstruction.[50,52]

In the setting of PCL injury, concomitant injury to the PLC is the most frequently associated injury and occurs in up to 60% of all PCL injuries.[53] A missed PLC injury can affect the success of PCL reconstruction.[53] In an isolated PCL injury, forces on the PCL graft resulting from external rotation loads, posterior tibial loads, or combined posterior and external rotation loads are similar to the native PCL. However, in the setting of residual PLC injury, forces acting on the PCL graft are increased during all loading conditions, with increases as much 150% on the reconstructed graft.[54] The increased load may predispose the PCL reconstruction to failure.

Classification

Classification systems have been created on the basis of the amount of instability and the location of the injury (Table 102.1). The American Medical Association initially standardized ligamentous injuries into grades I, II, and III based on the extent of injury and subsequent motion.[55] Hughston et al.[56] were the first to classify lateral side instability and

TABLE 102.1	Classification Systems to Describe Posterolateral Corner Injuries
System/Grade	**Description**
AMA	*Injury Severity*
I	Minimal tearing of ligament fibers, no increased motion
II	Partial tear of ligament, slight to moderate abnormal motion
III	Complete tear of ligament, loss of function and marked abnormal motion
Fanelli	*Structures Injured*
A	Popliteofibular ligament and popliteus tendon
B	Popliteofibular ligament, popliteus, and fibular collateral ligament
C	Popliteofibular ligament, popliteus, fibular collateral ligament, lateral capsule avulsion, and cruciate ligament disruption
Hughston	*Amount of Instability*
1+	Opening of 0–5 mm to varus stress
2+	Opening of 5–10 mm to varus stress
3+	Opening of 10+ mm to varus stress

identified six types of lateral compartment instability based on physical examination tests: anterolateral rotatory instability, posterolateral rotatory instability, combined anterolateral and posterolateral rotatory instability, combined anterolateral and anteromedial rotatory instability, combined posterolateral, anterolateral, and anteromedial rotatory instability, and straight lateral instability. These types were graded on the basis of various clinical exams as 1+, or minor, if the joint surfaces separated 5 mm or less; 2+, or moderate, if they separated 5 to 10 mm; and 3+, or severe, if they separated 10 mm or more. A classification system was developed by Fanelli and Feldmann[11] based on the location of the injury. Finally, injuries can be classified more simply as either stable or unstable, because it is instability that dictates surgical management.

HISTORY

Most PLC injuries are sustained during athletic competitions, motor vehicle accidents, and falls.[6,57-60] In one study, 65% of injuries were sports related, with 26% from motor vehicle accidents and 9% from falls.[7] A typical mechanism is a posterolaterally directed force to the anteromedial tibia, which leads to hyperextension and a varus force. Additional mechanisms include knee hyperextension or severe tibial external rotation in a partially flexed knee, and both contact and noncontact mechanisms have been reported.[61] An emerging mechanism that is increasing in frequency is injury during low-energy knee dislocation in obese persons. Azar et al.[62] reported on 17 obese persons with "ultra–low-velocity" knee dislocations, of which 50% had documented injury to the lateral-sided structures. In the United States alone, 35.7% of adults are considered obese, which is not only a major risk factor identified for these ultra–low-velocity knee dislocations but also increases the risk of limb-threatening neurovascular injury during dislocation.[62,63]

Concomitant Injury

PLC injuries are rarely isolated and are associated with concomitant injuries in 43% to 87% of patients.[2,3,35,26,60,64] These associated injuries commonly include ACL and PCL tears, as well as tibial plateau fractures. In the study by Gardner et al.[65] of operative tibial plateau fractures, 29% of the fractures had a complete FCL tear and 68% had injuries to the popliteofibular ligament and/or the popliteus tendon. Given that PLC injuries can occur in the setting of knee dislocations, in the case of multiple ligamentous injury, high clinical suspicion should be maintained for spontaneously reduced knee dislocation and subsequent neurovascular injury.

PHYSICAL EXAMINATION

In the acute setting, patients present after some form of trauma[6,57-60] and report pain, typically at the posterolateral aspect of the knee and at the fibular head.[2,61] They will have varying degrees of effusion. In a prospective study, LaPrade et al.[3] reported that 9.1% of patients presenting with a knee hemarthrosis had a PLC injury. Initially, depending on the degree of trauma, the basics of trauma care should be followed. First, a thorough primary survey consisting of airway, breathing, and circulation should be performed. During the secondary survey, a more detailed musculoskeletal examination can be completed. Gross deformity may suggest a knee dislocation. Recognizing a vascular injury is of paramount importance, and failure to do so can lead to amputation. In an acute setting, a detailed neurovascular examination should be performed. An ankle-brachial index score should be obtained, and any abnormal finding warrants additional workup and consultation. A thorough neurologic examination is necessary because of the high incidence of peroneal nerve injuries associated with PLC tears.[26] Particular attention should be given to peroneal nerve sensation, as well as ankle dorsiflexion, eversion, and great toe extension.[59]

In the chronic setting, patients often report pain at the medial joint line and/or lateral joint line, as well as at the posterolateral aspect of the knee.[26,59] However, with time, swelling and pain subside and instability becomes a primary complaint. This instability is most evident with the knee in extension and often presents as a varus or hyperextension-varus thrust during the stance phase of gait.[66] Patients experience difficulty ascending and descending stairs, may be seen walking with the knee in slight flexion or the ankle in equinus to alleviate these symptoms, and report having difficulty with twisting, pivoting, and cutting exercises.[35] One must also be mindful of the potential for a steppage gait if a foot-drop occurs from a concomitant peroneal nerve injury.[59]

For both chronic and acute cases, the physical examination should begin with an evaluation of the entire extremity, looking for areas of tenderness, ecchymosis, and deformity. As stated earlier, a detailed neurovascular examination is essential to evaluate for neurovascular injury. Overall limb alignment should be evaluated because it is important to identify varus malalignment. This malalignment may not only exacerbate the instability but may also predispose a reconstruction to increased risk of failure.[57,67-69]

Next, examinations specific for ligamentous injury of the knee should be performed, which includes assessing for ACL, PCL, and medial collateral ligament (MCL) injuries. A thorough evaluation of the PLC is then pursued. In the series by DeLee et al.,[2] all patients had tenderness and swelling diffusely over the posterolateral joint. Point tenderness is often found at the fibular head.[2,61] Varus stress examination is paramount to a basic physical examination. This test should be performed with the knee in both full extension, as well as at 30 degrees of flexion. Varus instability in full extension is suggestive of a PLC injury and a PCL injury, whereas isolated instability at 30 degrees of flexion is more suggestive of an isolated PLC injury.[56] One must be sure that when testing at 30 degrees of flexion, a pure varus directed force is applied without external rotation of the tibia, which could contribute to false-positive examinations.[2] In a the series of PLC injuries to the knee reported by DeLee et al.,[2] the most sensitive examination technique was varus instability with the knee at 30 degrees of flexion. The frog-leg maneuver is a newly described clinical test for identifying posterolateral knee instability. With the patient lying supine, both knees are abducted and flexed to 90 degrees, bringing the soles of the feet together (frog-leg position). A varus stress is applied, and the index or middle fingers of each hand are used to palpate the lateral joint lines to assess for lateral compartment gapping. When combined with the frog-leg test, the sensitivity of the conventional varus stress test has been found to increase from 83.3% to 90.0%.[70]

Other more specific tests for a PLC injury exist, including the posterolateral drawer test, the external rotation recurvatum test, the dial test, the standing apprehension test, and the reverse pivot shift.

The posterolateral drawer test has been described by having the physician flex the hip to 45 degrees and the knee to 80 degrees. The tibia is held in mild external rotation (approximately 15 degrees). With the examiner's thumbs on the tibial tubercle (Fig. 102.3), a posterior directed force on the proximal tibia will cause the tibial plateau to rotate posterolaterally on the femur.[2] The examiner should feel the posterolateral rotation.

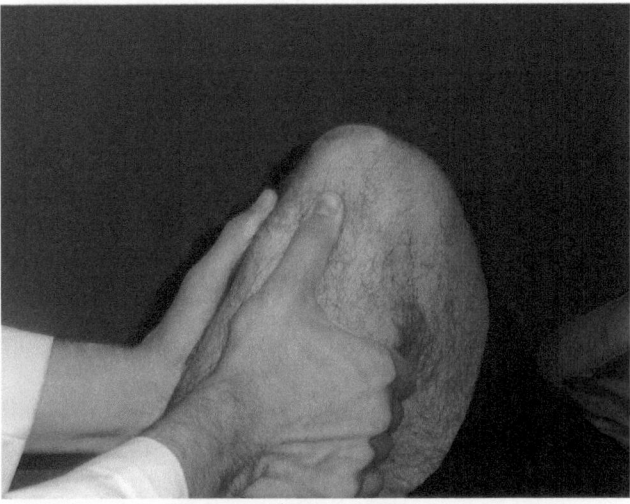

Fig. 102.3 Posterolateral drawer test.

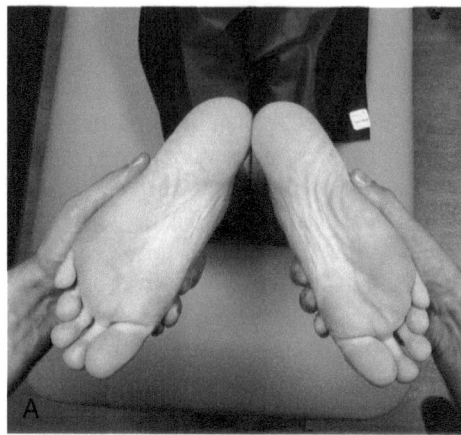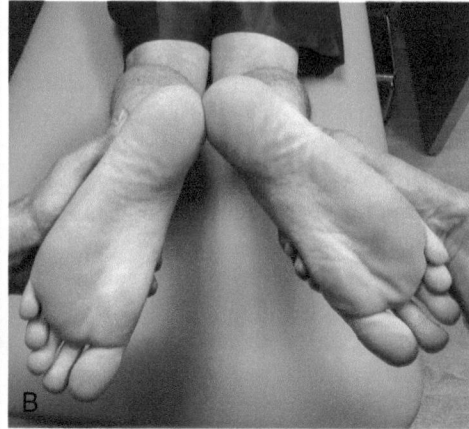

Fig. 102.4 Dial test performed in the prone position. (A) Test performed with knees bent at 90 degrees showing symmetric external rotation. (B) Test performed with knees bent at 30 degrees showing increased external rotation on the right side consistent with a posterolateral corner injury.

The dial test is performed by positioning the patient either prone or supine with the knee at the edge of the examination table. If the patient is supine, an assistant must stabilize the knees to hold the patella in line.[71] The knees are flexed to 30 degrees, and both feet are externally rotated. The same maneuvers are then performed at 90 degrees of knee flexion. A difference in external rotation of 10 to 15 degrees or more compared with the contralateral side is a positive test.[72] Increased external rotation at 30 degrees of flexion indicates an isolated PLC injury (Fig. 102.4).[72] A positive examination finding at both 30 degrees and 90 degrees of flexion raises suspicion for a PCL injury in addition to the PLC injury.[72] Tibial positioning during testing is important because reduced tibial external rotation will be found on the dial test with a posteriorly subluxated tibia.[73,74] Therefore when performing the dial test, an anterior force should be applied to the tibia if a concomitant PCL injury is suspected.[73,74] This full reduction of the tibia will allow for a more accurate estimate of tibial external rotation with dial testing.

The external rotation recurvatum test, described by Hughston and Norwood,[75] is performed by lifting the great toe of a patient in the supine position to observe the quantity of genu recurvatum (Fig. 102.5). The amount of recurvatum can be measured with a goniometer or the distance from the heel to the examination table.[26] One should also note differences in varus alignment and tibial external rotation.[71] The external rotation recurvatum test is less sensitive for PLC injuries because it has been proposed that the intact anteromedial bundle of the ACL provides some stability with this maneuver.[2] For this reason, this test can be useful in identifying PLC injury with an ACL tear.[13,75] For identifying combined ACL/PLC injuries, this test has sensitivity of 100% but specificity of 30%.[13] One must be aware that this test has a high rate of false-negative findings in the setting of PLC injuries with intact ACLs.[13] It is seldom useful for isolated PLC injuries or combined PLC/PCL injuries.[76] Finally, an important consideration is that the posterolateral drawer test demonstrates instability in flexion, whereas the external rotation recurvatum test demonstrates instability in extension.[75]

The standing apprehension test (Fig. 102.6) is performed by having the patient stand with the knee at almost full extension.

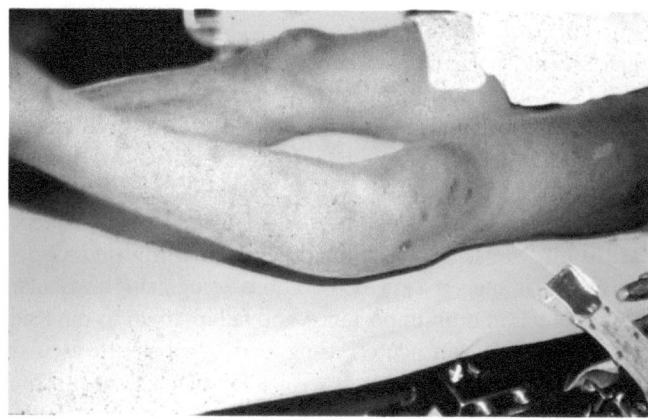

Fig. 102.5 An example of the external rotation recurvatum test showing severe posterolateral corner injury.

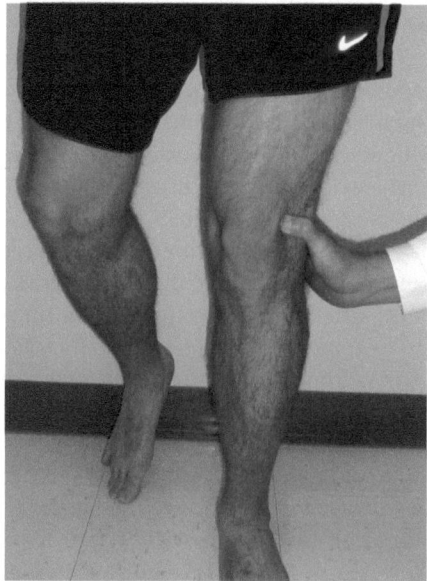

Fig. 102.6 The standing apprehension test. As force is directed medially, the patient experiences instability and the examiner can feel the femur rotate on the tibia.

A force is the directed medially across the anterolateral femur.[59] To consider this test positive, the patient must feel an unstable sensation and rotation of the femur on the tibia must occur.[6] The utility of this examination should be placed in context with the remainder of the history and examination because it has the potential to be nonspecific.

The reverse pivot shift is another specific test for the PLC that is specific for the FCL, mid-third lateral capsular ligament, and popliteus complex.[26] To perform this maneuver, the knee is flexed to 45 degrees with a valgus stress transmitted through the externally rotated foot.[26] With subsequent extension of the leg, a subluxation is felt at approximately 25 degrees of flexion.[59] Biomechanically, the posteriorly subluxated lateral tibial plateau reduces at 20 to 30 degrees of flexion because the IT band changes from knee flexor to extensor.[35,77] False-positive rates have been reported to be as high as 35%, and thus careful comparison with the unaffected limb is essential.

Gait examination is more useful in the chronic injury setting. During ambulation, the patient may have the appearance of a varus thrust with a lateral tibial shift. These findings can be attributed to external rotation of the tibia during full extension in the stance phase of the gait cycle. Previous authors liken this gait examination to a standing external rotation recurvatum test.[35] Furthermore, a hyperextension thrust gait can be present when loading the lower extremity during the early stance phase.[59] For this reason, some patients walk with a flexed knee.

The physical examination is critical in the detection of PLC injuries. Although modern imaging modalities are highly accurate for detecting injury to these structures, it is believed that they may be oversensitive for these injuries. In addition, imaging cannot replace the physical examination for assessing clinical instability resulting from injury. Therefore the physical examination is the most important part of the workup to determine the need for operative intervention of PLC injuries. In essence, the examiner should trust the physical examination during the decision-making process.

IMAGING

Radiographs

Imaging initially begins with radiographs and may include standard AP, lateral, sunrise, and posteroanterior-flexion views. Radiographs are helpful in identifying tibial plateau fractures, Segond fractures, and avulsions of the fibular head. In addition, they may reveal proximal tibiofibular joint dislocations, widening of the lateral joint surface, and arthritis. Evaluating for medial compartment arthritis is especially useful in the chronic setting. The "arcuate sign" refers to the radiographic finding of avulsion of the fibular styloid where the popliteofibular, fabellofibular, and arcuate ligaments attach, or it can represent a larger avulsion involving more of the fibular head that results from the pull of the biceps femoris and FCL, and it may be seen on a radiograph or MRI (Fig. 102.7).[78] Stress radiographs have been shown to aid in the diagnosis of PLC injuries.[79,80,81] Specifically, varus-stress radiographs with increased lateral joint space widening of 4.0 mm suggest isolated grade III PLC injury, widening of 6.6 mm suggests a combined PLC and ACL tear, and widening of 7.8 mm suggests PLC, ACL, and PCL injuries.[81] In a separate clinical

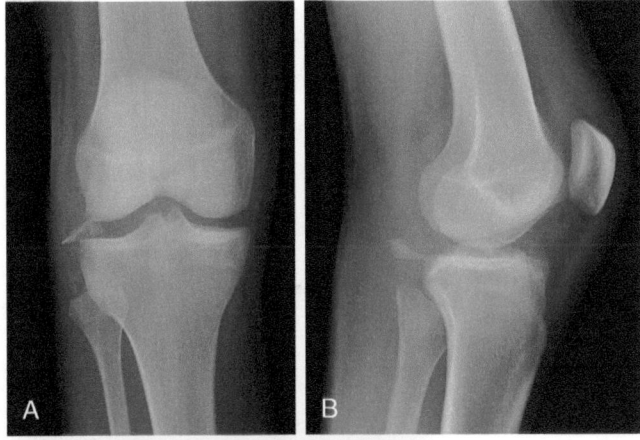
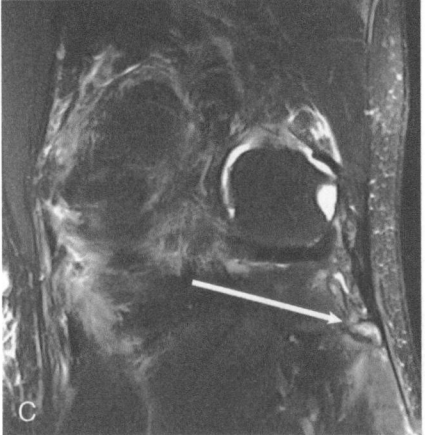

Fig. 102.7 The arcuate sign as seen on anteroposterior (A) and lateral (B) radiographs. (C) The arcuate sign (arrow) seen on coronal magnetic resonance imaging.

study, lateral widening from varus stress totaled 18.6 mm for a complete injury and an average of 12.8 mm in partial injuries.[82] Therefore side-to-side comparisons can provide evidence of clinical laxity and warrant further clinical correlation to determine the need for surgical reconstruction. In addition, in the chronic setting, AP full-leg radiographs (hip to ankle) should be obtained to evaluate for varus malalignment.

Magnetic Resonance Imaging

MRI allows visualization of individual components of the PLC, including the IT band, FCL, biceps femoris tendon, and popliteus (Fig. 102.8).[23,83] LaPrade et al.[84] found that the accuracy of identifying torn individual structures ranges from 68% for the popliteofibular ligament to 95% for the FCL. Other studies have reported an ability to detect PLC injuries in 80% to 100% of the cases, especially if the MRI is performed in the acute setting.[8,85,86] MRI also identifies concomitant injuries such as tears of the cruciate ligaments, because isolated tears of the PLC are rare and most often occur in the setting of additional ligamentous injury (Fig. 102.9).[3] In addition, similar to other ligamentous injuries, characteristic bone bruise patterns have been reported with PLC injuries, with the most common location being the anteromedial femoral condyle.[87] Although the complex anatomy of the PLC is better visualized on MRI, it remains difficult to determine clinically significant instability based on MRI

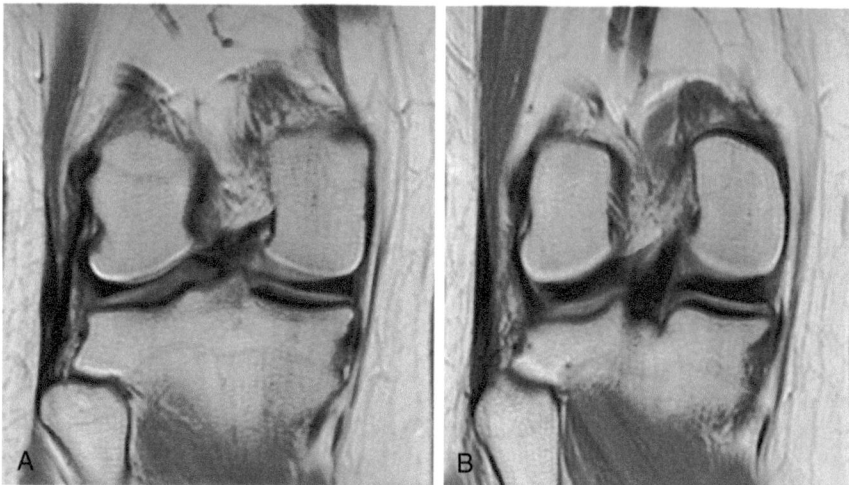

Fig. 102.8 Coronal magnetic resonance imaging of the fibular collateral ligament and biceps femoris inserting on the fibula (A) and the popliteus and biceps femoris (B).

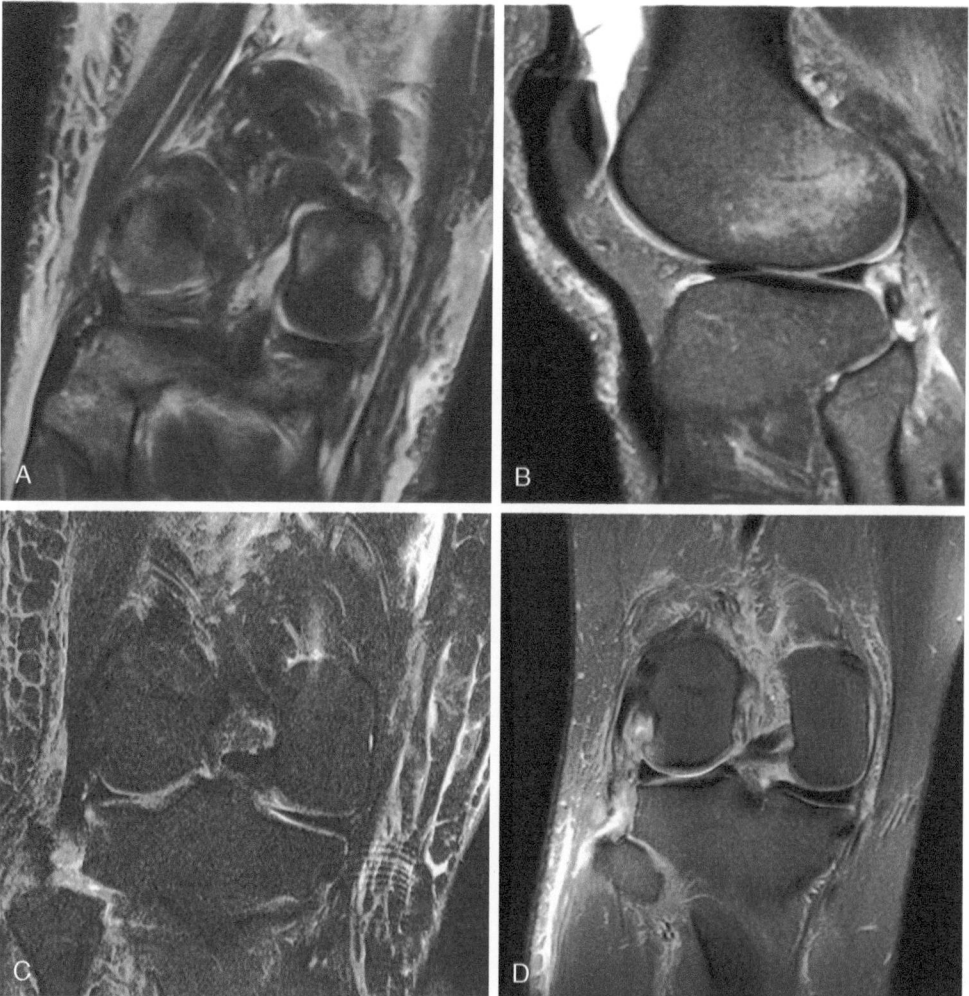

Fig. 102.9 (A) A tear of fibular collateral ligament near its femoral attachment with retraction of the ligament. (B) The popliteus is torn and retracted. (C) A tear of the biceps femoris. (D) The fibular collateral is torn from its fibular insertion.

findings alone. In an effort to simplify this diagnosis, it has been suggested that MRI evidence of injury to at least two structures, especially the popliteus, FCL, or posterior lateral joint capsule, is indicative of posterolateral rotatory instability and warrants a thorough clinical evaluation.[88]

Ultrasound

Ultrasound has emerged as an additional imaging modality for the evaluation of PLC injuries. This technique, which can be performed quickly and is noninvasive and inexpensive, has been shown to be useful in identifying the structures of the PLC.[89,90] Static ultrasound imaging has an overall sensitivity of 92% and a specificity of 75%, and dynamic ultrasound testing revealing greater than 10.5 mm of total lateral joint line width has sensitivity of 83% and a specificity of 100%.[91] In addition, ultrasound has the ability to visualize dynamic processes and oblique structures, which are sometimes poorly visualized on MRI.

DECISION-MAKING PRINCIPLES

The decision on how to ultimately treat a particular PLC injury depends on a number of factors, including the timing of the diagnosis, the extent of the injury, and the degree of subsequent instability.

Timing of Diagnosis

PLC injuries are classified as either acute or chronic. Typically, acute refers to treatment within 3 weeks from the time of injury, but some investigators include up to 6 weeks. Studies have shown that efforts should be made to treat PLC injuries acutely, assuming the patient and the knee are in a suitable condition for surgery, because acutely treated injuries have better outcomes than do chronically managed injuries.[6,35,59,64,80,92] Within the acute stage, structures are more easily visualized, scarring is not as prominent, and the tissue is more amenable to repair, if primary repair is to be attempted. However, as reconstructive techniques continue to improve, the timing of treatment is becoming less important, because reconstruction can effectively be performed in both the acute and chronic settings.

Nonoperative Management

The decision to treat a PLC injury nonoperatively must take into consideration the extent of the injury and the overall stability of the joint.

Grade I Injuries

Isolated grade I injuries are stable, and nonoperative treatment consistently produces good results.[6,57,61,64,93,94] The true outcome of these injuries is difficult to determine, because it is likely that many people do not seek treatment for isolated grade I injuries. These injuries are treated symptomatically. Physical therapy directed at quadriceps strengthening and range of motion (ROM) exercises can begin almost immediately.

Grade II Injuries

The decision of how to treat grade II injuries is more difficult. Isolated grade II injuries with only mild abnormal joint motion typically respond well to nonoperative management but may result in some degree of residual instability.[6,57,61,64,93,94] For stable grade II injuries, management is similar to grade I injuries, and they are treated symptomatically. A similar physical therapy protocol may be used, but the patient should progress more slowly. For more severe grade II injuries and grade II injuries with concomitant ligamentous injuries, surgical intervention should be considered, which includes cases with concomitant ACL or PCL reconstruction because of the increased failure rate of these reconstructions in the setting of untreated PLC injuries.[49,50,52]

Grade III Injuries

Grade III injuries (those with significant instability) have universally inferior outcomes when treated conservatively compared with those treated surgically.[93-95] In each of these studies, conservatively managed grade III injuries were reported to have persistent instability, only fair outcomes, and increased rates of osteoarthritis. Similar to grade II injuries, concomitant cruciate ligament reconstructions have inferior outcomes in conservatively managed grade III PLC injuries.[49,50,52] For this reason, as in severe grade II injuries, surgical treatment is recommended to produce a more stable knee.

Repair Versus Reconstruction

Historically, it had been believed that primary repair within the acute setting produced good results and should be the primary treatment.[2,6,64,96] Repair consisted of identifying individual structures and securing avulsed structures to bone or performing side-to-side repair. However, recently, studies have started to cast doubt on the benefits of primary repair. Stannard et al.[97] found a 37% failure rate in acutely repaired knees. Levy et al.[98] identified a 40% failure rate of repair compared with 6% for reconstruction, and Geeslin and LaPrade[99] found superior results of combined repair and reconstruction. It has also been shown that the FCL and popliteus tendon have little healing potential, thus making primary repair less likely to be successful.[95] As a result, attempts at primary repair should be limited to the acute setting for structures with easily identified avulsions from bone without evidence of midsubstance injury and that are easily anatomically reduced with the knee in full extension.[57,100] Otherwise, reconstruction should be performed. Proponents of acute reconstruction also point out the ability for accelerated therapy and ROM exercises compared with the need for longer immobilization for the repaired structures to heal.

TREATMENT OPTIONS

Treatment is determined by the timing of the diagnosis, the extent of the injury, and the degree of subsequent instability.

Nonoperative Management

The decision to treat PLC injuries conservatively is based on the extent of injury and the presence of instability. Unstable joints warrant surgical intervention. Truly stable joints, which are based on examination after administration of an anesthetic, may be treated nonoperatively.

Surgical Considerations

The timing of surgery and the appropriate procedure for operative PLC injuries have long been debated. Treatment options consist of primary repair and reconstruction, whether "anatomic" or "nonanatomic" reconstruction techniques are used.

Diagnostic Arthroscopy

Diagnostic arthroscopy may assist in the diagnosis of PLC injuries, as well as any concomitant injuries in the knee. Arthroscopy is successful at identifying most injuries to the popliteus, coronary ligament, lateral meniscus, mid-third lateral capsular ligament, articular cartilage, and the cruciate ligaments, but it has less capability of identifying injuries to the popliteofibular ligament.[101,102] However, not all injuries to the popliteus identified during open dissection were visualized during arthroscopy.[102] Various arthroscopic findings have been described to suggest PLC injuries. The "lateral gutter drive-through" sign, signified as the ability to advance the arthroscope into the posterolateral compartment between a lax popliteus tendon and the lateral femoral condyle, suggests an avulsion of the popliteus off the femur.[103] The "drive-through sign," signified as greater than 10 mm of lateral compartment joint opening (Fig. 102.10), also suggests injury to the PLC.[101] The visualization of torn structures on diagnostic arthroscopy or the presence of either the drive-through sign or the lateral gutter drive-through sign should prompt close examination of the PLC to avoid missing subtle injuries.

Primary Repair

Debate continues over the merits of primary repair of structures. Historically, primary repair has been shown to be adequate for acute PLC injuries if performed in the first 3 weeks after an injury is sustained.[64,92] In this technique, avulsed structures are repaired directly to bone using suture anchors, nonabsorbable suture, bone tunnels, screw and washer constructs, or other fixation devices. However, recent studies have found that repair carries significantly inferior results compared with reconstruction, with up to a 40% failure rate in the setting of isolated repair.[97,98] Some experts advocate repair only if the injury is truly an isolated avulsion and no evidence is found of midsubstance injury.[100] In addition, repair of avulsed structures can help to augment the reconstruction procedures.[99]

Repair Techniques

For acute avulsions of the popliteus or FCL from their insertion on the femur (Fig. 102.11), repair may be performed by the recess procedure.[92] Originally described by Hughston, this technique uses small bone tunnels drilled at the anatomic insertion site of the avulsed structure. Initially, the structure is freed of adhesions, and its ability to be anatomically reduced is confirmed. Its proximal end is prepared with suture, which is then passed through the bone tunnel and tied on the medial side of the femur. Various techniques may be used for suture passing through bone, including cruciate ligament guides, Beath needles, or freehand drilling. A second incision is made medially, and the suture is tied over a button and against the medial cortex of the femur. For concomitant injury, care must be taken to avoid interfering with cruciate ligament reconstruction tunnels.[104]

A similar technique may be used to repair structures back to their insertion on the fibular head. Whether the biceps femoris, the popliteus, or the FCL, the structure's insertion is initially identified and anatomic reduction is confirmed. Bone tunnels or suture anchors are used to secure the structure into its anatomic position. The popliteofibular ligament may be primarily repaired if the popliteus or FCL is uninjured.[100] For fibular head fractures, anatomic reduction and fixation is performed, addressing any concomitant avulsion injuries at the same time.

Reconstruction Techniques

Biceps tenodesis. Initially described by Clancy, the biceps tenodesis attempts to recreate the FCL and popliteofibular ligament and to reinforce the posterolateral joint capsule.[105,106] A 12-cm lateral incision is made from 6 cm proximal to the lateral epicondyle down past the Gerdy tubercle. The lateral epicondyle is palpated, and the IT band is split longitudinally over the epicondyle. The biceps tendon is freed of attachments to the lateral

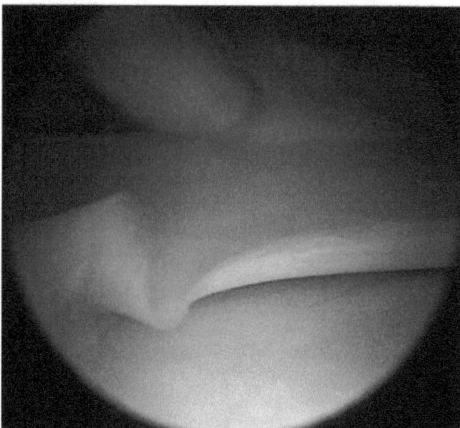

Fig. 102.10 The lateral compartment "drive-through sign" consistent with a posterolateral corner injury. An opening greater than 10 mm is present between the tibia and femur (the femoral condyle is not visualized).

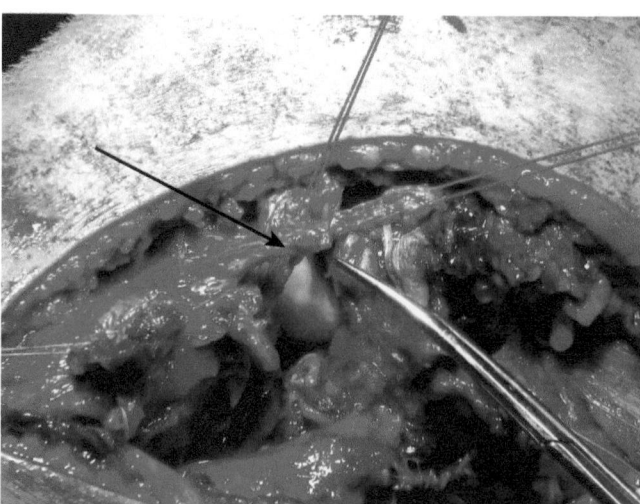

Fig. 102.11 Preparing the fibular collateral ligament (arrow) for primary repair back to the femoral condyle. (Courtesy Dean Taylor, MD.)

gastrocnemius muscle. Distally, the peroneal nerve is identified and freed of attachments to the biceps tendon to prevent tethering once the biceps is rerouted. Proximal excess muscle is removed from tendon to create a 6-cm tendinous portion at the level of the epicondyle. The lateral epicondyle is freed of soft tissue. The origin of the FCL is identified. A trough is made in the bone, and a point 1 cm anterior to the lateral epicondyle is selected for drilling.[105,106,107] A 3.2-mm drill hole is made, and a 6.5-mm screw and washer construct is selected. The proximal biceps tendon that had been freed of muscle is brought under the IT band and placed around the screw. The screw and washer are tightened to attach the tendon to the lateral femoral condyle. It is important to plan bone tunnels appropriately in the setting of multiligament reconstruction.[104] This nonanatomic technique requires that the distal biceps attachment to the fibula remains intact for tensioning purposes.

Split biceps tendon transfer. In a modification to the technique described by Clancy, a portion of the biceps tendon is rerouted and attached via tenodesis to the epicondyle. This technique requires a stable proximal tibiofibular joint and an intact attachments between the biceps tendon and the posterolateral capsule, and, as previously described, the biceps attachment to the fibular head remains intact.[108] A lateral-based incision is made for exposure from the lateral epicondyle down to the fibular head. The peroneal nerve is identified, freed of adhesions, and protected throughout the repair. The IT band is split longitudinally over the epicondyle to expose the origin of the FCL and popliteus. The long head of the biceps is isolated, and the anterior two-thirds of the tendon is separated. This portion of the tendon is detached proximally, freed of excess muscle, brought medial to the IT band, and attached via tenodesis to an area 1 cm anterior to the lateral epicondyle using a screw and washer construct similar to that previously described. Tendon remaining after the tenodesis can be secured to the fibular head for additional reinforcement. The posterolateral capsule is then incised and attached to the newly rerouted tendon to augment the reconstruction with a posterolateral capsular shift.

Posterolateral corner sling procedure. The PLC sling procedure, using autograft or allograft, creates an extraarticular sling extending from the posterior tibia to an area anterior and superior to the lateral femoral epicondyle.[109] With the knee flexed 45 degrees, an incision is made along the IT band from mid femur to a point distal to the Gerdy tubercle. The peroneal nerve is identified and protected. A plane between the lateral head of the gastrocnemius and the FCL is created, and the gastrocnemius is retracted posteriorly. The popliteus and joint capsule are then identified, and the popliteus is mobilized and retracted posteriorly. A retractor is placed along the posterolateral aspect of the tibia. A 6- to 8-mm bone tunnel is created 1 to 1.5 cm below the articular surface of the tibia and medial enough to avoid violating the proximal tibiofibular joint. An allograft or autograft is passed through this tunnel from anterior to posterior and secured. The graft is brought proximal and secured to a point 1 cm anterior to the lateral femoral epicondyle using bone tunnels, suture anchors, or screw and washer constructs to complete the sling. An all-arthroscopic sling reconstruction of the popliteus tendon has been described.[110]

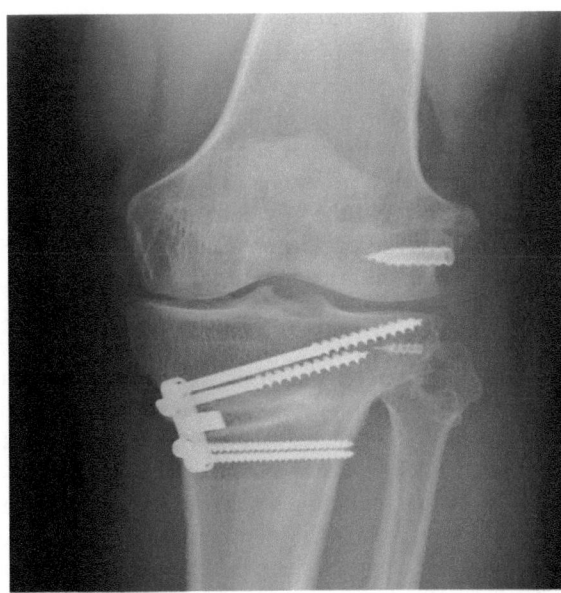

Fig. 102.12 After presenting because of a failed posterolateral corner reconstruction, a proximal tibial osteotomy was performed and no additional reconstruction was required.

Proximal tibial osteotomy. In the setting of genu varum and a chronic PLC injury, a proximal tibial osteotomy (Fig. 102.12) has been shown to improve stability and, in the right patient population, can serve as the primary treatment for chronic posterolateral instability.[111] In addition, it may serve as the initial procedure to correct malalignment in a two-stage approach to reconstruction. Both opening and closing wedge osteotomies have been described.[111,112] The goal of the osteotomy is the restore the mechanical axis to neutral or a slightly valgus position. Standard osteotomy techniques are used based on the surgeon's preference and experience. Arthur et al.[111] found that correction of the varus malalignment was sufficient to restore stability in 38% of their total study population (patients with PLC and other ligamentous injuries) and 67% of patients with isolated PLC injury, and thus a secondary procedure was not necessary.

Proximal tibial osteotomy has the potential to not only correct coronal malalignment but can also influence tibial slope (sagittal alignment). An osteotomy to change coronal alignment has been used in the ACL- and PCL-deficient knee to affect stability. However, the impact of altering tibial slope to treat PLC injuries and instability remains controversial. It has been reported that, in the combined PCL- and PLC-deficient knee, increasing tibial slope better stabilizes the joint and decreases forces on the PLC structures.[113] However, a biomechanical study showed that increasing the tibial slope in a knee with a combined PCL and PLC injury had no impact on stability during dial testing at 30 and 90 degrees and did not alter the reverse pivot shift test.[114]

Anatomic Reconstructions

Isolated structure reconstruction. Various techniques have been described for reconstructing individual structures, including the FCL, popliteus tendon, and popliteofibular ligament. In each case, an autograft or allograft may be used. Each procedure relies on a precise understanding of the anatomy of the PLC to accurately reconstruct the injured structure. A standard exposure is performed. The peroneal nerve is identified and protected. For the popliteus, the femoral origin of the popliteus is identified and cleared of soft tissue. A bone tunnel is created, and an interference screw is used to secure the graft into the femur. The graft is passed distally to the posterolateral aspect of the tibia. Similar to the sling procedure previously described, an anterior-to-posterior bone tunnel is made in the tibia and the popliteus is passed from posterior to anterior and secured with interference screws. For the FCL, the femoral origin for the FCL is identified, a bone tunnel is created, and the graft is secured with an interference screw. A bone tunnel is then made in the proximal fibula (while protecting the peroneal nerve) and the graft is passed through this tunnel and brought back up to the femoral origin of the graft for additional fixation. The popliteofibular ligament can be reconstructed by extending the graft used to reconstruct the FCL through the same tibial tunnel that would be made for popliteus reconstruction after it exits the fibular tunnel.[115,116] When securing grafts in a fibular tunnel, the leg is placed in 30 degrees of knee flexion and a slight valgus stress is applied during fixation. Grafts in the tibial tunnel are secured with the knee in 60 degrees of flexion and with a similar valgus load applied.

Anatomic Reconstruction Technique

The anatomic reconstruction technique has been popularized by LaPrade et al.[116,117] In the orthopaedic literature, the "anatomic" technique has come to mean the inclusion of a tibial tunnel. After an initial lateral hockey stick incision is made, dissection is carried down to the IT band and the long head of the biceps femoris. The peroneal nerve is identified, and a neurolysis performed. A small incision is made through the anterior arm of the biceps femoris and dissection is carried down to the FCL, and its anatomic attachment to the fibula is identified and cleared from the bone. With use of a cruciate ligament tunnel guide, a 7-mm tunnel is made in the fibular head while protecting the peroneal nerve. The tibial tunnel is then drilled by first identifying relevant landmarks, including the starting point, which is an area just medial and distal to Gerdy tubercle and the exit point of the tunnel, which is a small sulcus on the posterolateral tibial plateau at the level of the musculotendinous junction of the popliteus.[117] With use of a cruciate ligament tunnel guide and a guide pin, the tibial tunnel is drilled while protecting neurovascular structures. The IT band is then split over the lateral epicondyle of the femur. Dissection is carried down to the femoral attachment of the popliteus and FCL. Guide pins are placed through the attachment sites of each structure, and 9-mm tunnels are reamed. Previous prepared grafts with bone plugs are passed into these tunnels by using a passing stitch in the guide pin and bringing the pins out medial, and the plugs are secured with interference screws. The tendinous portion of the grafts have been tubularized and prepared for passage through the tunnels. One graft is then passed along the anatomic path of the popliteus and brought through the tibial tunnel in a posterior-to-anterior fashion. The second graft is passed along the anatomic path of the FCL and brought through the femoral tunnel from lateral

to medial and then through the tibial tunnel from posterior to anterior. Interference screws are used for fixation in the tibia and fibula.

Fibula-based reconstruction. The focus of the fibula-based technique is reconstruction of the lateral collateral ligament and the popliteofibular ligament. This technique offers several advantages, including needing only a single hamstring autograft tendon, allowing for remaining native tissue to be preserved and incorporated into the reconstruction, and avoiding tunnels that could threaten a femoral tunnel created for ACL reconstruction in cases of concomitant injury. In addition, it is relatively easy to perform and can be used in all settings of PLC injuries, including instances of associated tibiofibular dislocation. In this case, the tibiofibular joint is simply stabilized prior to proceeding with reconstruction. The fibula-based reconstruction is described in the Authors' Preferred Technique section.

POSTOPERATIVE MANAGEMENT

A four-phase rehabilitation protocol is used (Table 102.2). In phase I, typically in postoperative weeks 0 to 8, the goals are to protect the reconstructed structures, decrease inflammation and swelling, and carefully advance ROM of the joint. Initially, the patient performs only toe-touch weight bearing for at least 6 weeks. The extremity is protected in a hinged knee brace locked in extension for 2 weeks. After 2 weeks, passive ROM is begun as symptoms allow. Quadriceps sets are allowed, and patella mobilization is performed. Hamstring contractions and stretching are avoided. Precautions are taken to specifically prevent tibial external rotation and varus stress. After 8 weeks, the brace is unlocked and active and passive ROM is advanced as tolerated.

In phase II, typically during postoperative weeks 9 to 12, attempts are made to eliminate inflammation and swelling, obtain full ROM, restore normal gait, and improve lower extremity strength. During this phase, more aggressive ROM exercises are performed until full ROM is achieved, which includes the use of a stationary bicycle. Closed kinetic chain quad strengthening begins, and cross-training machines may be used for conditioning. Gait mechanics are restored and proprioceptive exercises are performed.

In phase III, typically during postoperative weeks 13 to 24, attempts are made to increase strength to at least 85% of the contralateral limb, improve aerobic endurance, initiate plyometric exercises, and begin a running program. Modalities include using a spin bike, Cybex training, agility drills, and advanced proprioception exercises. Strengthening is continued. A return to running is initiated, initially using a treadmill, and is advanced to level, outdoor surfaces.

Phase IV is started once the extremity has reached greater than or equal to 85% of the strength of the contralateral limb and has results of a single-leg hop test greater than or equal to 85% of the contralateral limb, when no pain is experienced with forward running, agilities, jump training, or strengthening, and when the patient demonstrates good knee control with single-leg dynamic proprioceptive activities. This phase attempts to return the patient to full sport activities, to create equal strength, balance,

Authors' Preferred Technique

For injuries that produce an unstable joint based on physical examination, we prefer a fibula-based reconstruction technique in both the acute and chronic settings.[118] The procedure is performed with the patient supine on the operating table. Initially, an examination is performed after administration of an anesthetic to confirm the diagnosis and recognize concomitant ligamentous injury. A tourniquet is placed on the upper thigh. A diagnostic arthroscopy is performed and intra-articular pathology is addressed, including articular cartilage injuries and meniscus tears. Typically, cruciate ligament reconstruction is performed at this time. After arthroscopy, the extremity is exsanguinated and the tourniquet is inflated. A semitendinosus tendon is harvested and prepared on the back table by tubularizing it and preparing each end with no. 2 nonabsorbable suture to facilitate graft passage.

A longitudinal incision is made on the lateral side of the knee centered on the lateral epicondyle proximally and between Gerdy tubercle and the fibular head distally (Fig. 102.13). The incision is carried down to the IT band with thick soft-tissue flaps preserved. The peroneal nerve is identified behind the biceps femoris, marked with a vessel loop, and protected throughout the procedure.

Next, exposure of the deep structures is performed through the three windows described by Terry and LaPrade.[19] In an acute injury, primary repair of individual structures can then be performed before proceeding with reconstruction with the use of direct sutures to bone, suture anchors, or screws and washers.

The femoral attachment of the FCL and the insertion of the popliteus are visualized. A point equidistant between these two structures is identified, and the soft tissue in this area is elevated off of bone (Fig. 102.14). A 6.5-mm screw and an 18-mm washer construct is used as an anchor and drilled appropriately. A countersink attached to the drill removes additional soft tissue and creates a bleeding bone bed to facilitate healing. An 18-mm washer is specifically chosen to help maintain the anatomic relationship of the femoral attachments of the popliteus and FCL, because they are 18.5 mm apart.[13] The screw, usually 30- to 35-mm long, is inserted until just enough protrudes to allow graft passage.

The peroneal nerve is then identified distally, and a neurolysis is performed if necessary. It is protected with retractors, and a tunnel is drilled anterior to posterior through the fibular head using a 6- to 7-mm acorn reamer over a guidewire 1 to 1.5 cm distal to the proximal tip of the fibular head (Fig. 102.15). The prepared semitendinosus graft is passed through this tunnel. A posterior limb is passed under the biceps femoris and under the IT band up to the screw on the femur. The anterior limb is passed under the IT band and up to just below the screw. The anterior limb does not pass around the screw so as to avoid excess soft tissue causing a more prominent screw and washer. The anterior limb is sutured to soft tissue just distal to the screw. The posterior limb is made longer than the anterior limb. The knee is flexed 30 degrees, valgus and internal rotatory forces are placed on the knee, and the screw and washer are tightened. The posterior limb is passed back through the tunnel in the fibular head. The passing sutures are then tied to each other and the graft limbs are sewn together for additional support.

The area is copiously irrigated. The tourniquet is let down and hemostasis is maintained. The incisions in the lateral capsule and IT bands are closed. The skin is closed, and a bandage is applied. A hinged knee brace, locked in extension, is applied.

Surgical Pearls

- Use an 18-mm washer to restore the anatomic arrangement of the popliteus and FCL on the femur.
- In case of tibiofibular joint instability, drill a fibular tunnel for a graft before stabilizing the joint to avoid cutting the fixation device with the drill through the fibula.
- Minimize the amount of the graft under the washer to avoid prominent hardware.
- For obese patients, consider external fixation for added stability in the early postoperative period.
- When drilling for a femoral screw, dropping the hand slightly toward the ankle to allow a proximally directed screw will limit interference with ACL tunnels.
- Protection of the peroneal nerve is imperative during fibular tunnel preparation.

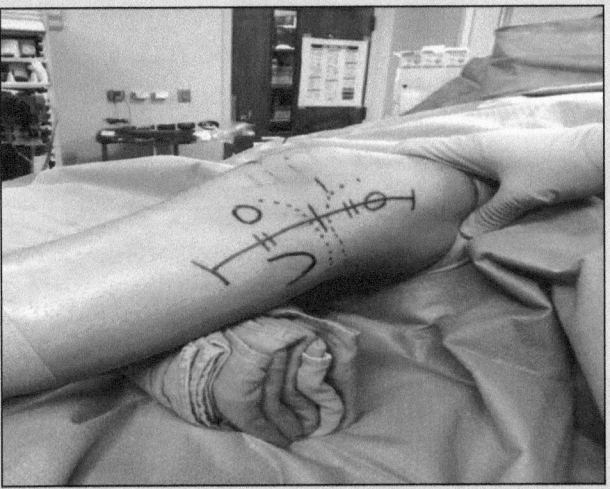

Fig. 102.13 Surface anatomy for planning the incision to perform a posterolateral corner reconstruction on a left knee.

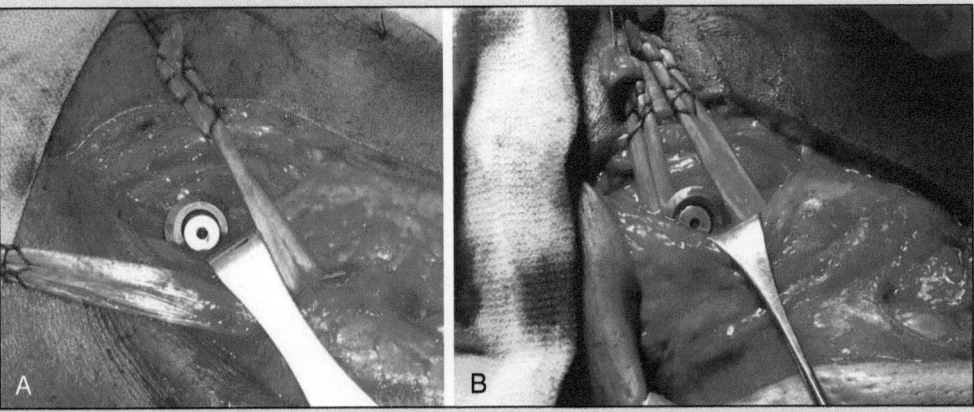

Fig. 102.14 (A) Graft passage through the fibular tunnel. (B) Graft passage around the femoral washer.

Continued

Authors' Preferred Technique—cont'd

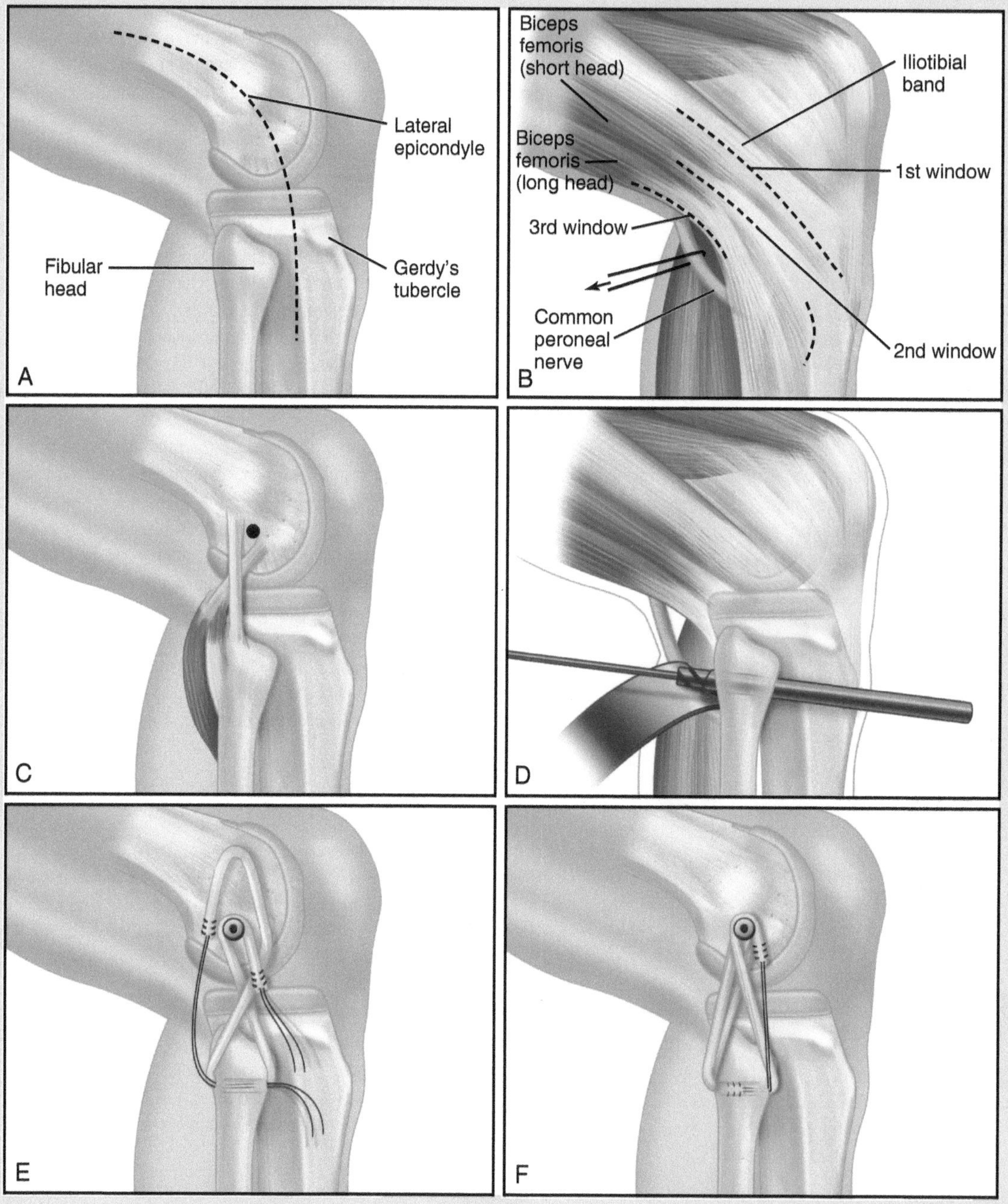

Fig. 102.15 (A) The longitudinal skin incision crosses the lateral epicondyle proximally and bisects the Gerdy tubercle and the fibular head distally. (B) The lateral side of the knee is exposed through the three windows. (C) The position of the femoral drill hole is at "ground zero," which is a point equidistant from the femoral attachment of the lateral collateral ligament and the insertion of the popliteus tendon. (D) A 7-mm tunnel is drilled through the fibular head 1 to 1.5 cm from the proximal tip and superior to the point where the peroneal nerve crosses the neck of the fibular. (E and F) The graft is passed through the fibula and around the washer and back through the tunnel (if length allows). (From Larson MW, Moinfar AR, Moorman CT, III. Posterolateral corner reconstruction: fibular-based technique. *J Knee Surg.* 2005;28[2]:163–166.)

📌 Authors' Preferred Technique
Proximal Tibial Osteotomy

In the setting of chronic varus malalignment, we perform an opening wedge osteotomy for deformity correction. Similar to the findings of Arthur et al.,[111] we have found that osteotomy alone can restore stability and PLC reconstruction is not always necessary (Fig. 102.16).

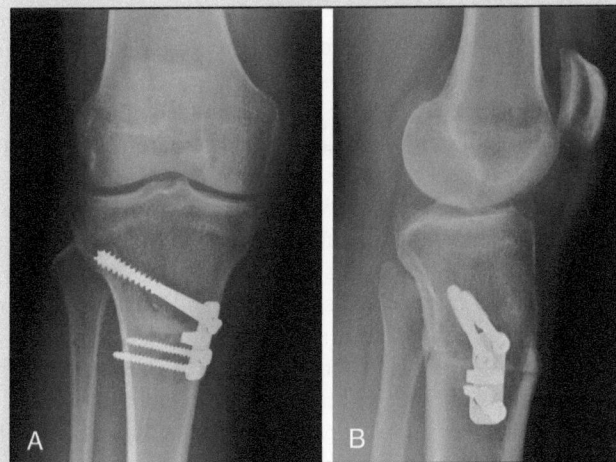

Fig. 102.16 Final anteroposterior (A) and lateral (B) radiograph appearance of a completed high tibial osteotomy.

📌 Authors' Preferred Technique
Proximal Tibiofibular Joint Instability

Proximal tibiofibular joint instability should be considered in the setting of PLC injury. Acute anterolateral dislocation, the most common form of instability, is frequently associated with injury to the FCL and biceps femoris tendon and results from injury to the anterior and posterior capsular ligaments.[119,120] The diagnosis can be made clinically and radiographically, with various tests and radiographic measures described.[120]

Proximal tibiofibular joint instability does not prevent a fibula-based reconstruction. The key is to identify the injury and stabilize the joint. Various techniques have been described throughout the literature. We use a suture fixation device technique for stabilization (Fig. 102.17). The incision created for PLC reconstruction is used. Dissection is carried down to the peroneal nerve. The nerve is identified and protected throughout. The suture device is passed across the fibula and into the tibia and finally deployed on the medial side of the tibia. It is tightened to the appropriate tension and tied over the fibula. A second device is deployed in a similar fashion. The knots are buried in soft tissue to avoid irritation of the peroneal nerve, or newer knotless devices may be used.

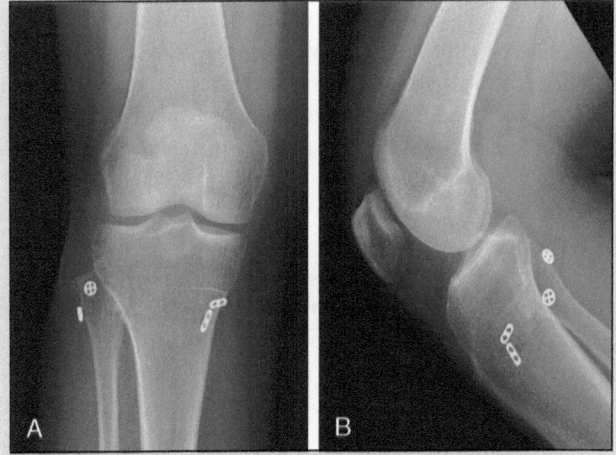

Fig. 102.17 Anteroposterior (A) and lateral (B) radiographs showing proximal tibiofibular joint stabilization.

TABLE 102.2	Four-Phase Rehabilitation Protocol Used After Posterolateral Corner Reconstruction		
Phase 1 (Weeks 0–8)	**Phase 2 (Weeks 9–12)**	**Phase 3 (Weeks 13–24)**	**Phase 4 (Weeks 24+)**
Restricted motion to promote healing (knee locked in extension for 2 weeks and then passive ROM 0–90 degrees with therapy after 2 weeks)	Obtain full knee ROM	Improve aerobic endurance, initiate plyometric exercises	Begin sport-specific functional motions
Toe-touch weight bearing for 6 weeks, and then gradual progression of weight-bearing status	Restore normal gait, initiate proprioception exercises	Initiate running program on level surfaces	Obtain equal balance and proprioception, gradually increase level of participation in sports
Quadriceps strengthening/patella mobilization	Continue strengthening, including closed kinetic chain exercises	Increase strength to at least 85% of the contralateral limb	Obtain equal bilateral lower extremity strength
Avoid hamstring stretches and external rotation/varus stress on the tibia	Eliminate residual swelling/inflammation	Have no pain with running, agility exercises, jumping, or strengthening	Pass all sport-specific functional screens and activities

ROM, Range of motion.

proprioception, and power bilaterally, and to achieve a 100% global function rating. Exercises started in phase III are advanced, with a gradual increase in the level of participation in sport-specific activities, and the patient progresses to running on all surfaces without restriction.

RETURN TO PLAY

Once the athlete has progressed to stage IV of the rehabilitation protocol, he or she begins sport-specific rehabilitation, conditioning, and training. Minimal data exist on PLC injuries in elite athletes, given their rare diagnosis.[121-123] In a retrospective review of National Football League players, Bushnell et al.[121] found that nine players over a 10-year period were diagnosed with isolated grade III FCL tears, and the four who underwent operative treatment and the five who were treated nonoperatively all returned to play in the NFL. In general, it may take at least a year for an athlete to return to a preinjury level of play. Extensive rehabilitation is required, and clearance from the treating physician must be obtained before returning to competitive training and sports. This decision is based on functional screening measures, strength testing, the knee's ROM, absence of swelling, and painless sport-specific activities. Preoperatively, it is important to discuss the expected time frame for returning to sporting activities so the athlete has realistic expectations during the rehabilitation process.

RESULTS

Numerous studies demonstrating the results of various techniques used to treat PLC instability have been published. Without a standardized outcome measure, it is difficult to truly compare these various techniques. In addition, the length of follow-up varies between the different studies, which can make one technique appear superior to another. Also, authors often use similar descriptive terms for techniques but offer a modification to a previously described technique of the same name. For example, within the literature, multiple authors describe an anatomic reconstruction, but great variability exists between the different anatomic techniques. In Tables 102.3[116,124-128] and 102.4,[67,93,97,98,111,129-136] studies indicating "fibular based" imply isolated tunnels in the fibula and femur, whereas studies indicating "anatomic" imply an additional tibial tunnel.

COMPLICATIONS

Complications may be separated into two categories: those resulting from the injury and those resulting from the surgery. As with any surgery, the risk of bleeding, infection, deep venous thrombosis, and prominent/painful hardware are associated with reconstruction of PLC injuries. Because injuries to the PLC more commonly occur with additional ligamentous injuries, they are often seen in the setting of knee dislocations and therefore may carry many of the same risks. In the setting of significant soft tissue injury or open wounds, infection and soft tissue healing can become a problem, and infection occurs in up to 43% of open knee dislocations.[139] With its close proximity to the lateral joint capsule, common peroneal nerve injury is common and has been documented in 13% of patients with PLC injuries.[26,140] The rates of nerve recovery for complete disrupted injury, complete stretched injury, and partial injury are found to be 0%, 50%, and 100%, respectively, with an overall rate of recovery of 50%.[141] Nerve injury appears to be related to disruption of the distal attachment of the biceps tendon to the fibular head, causing the nerve to be displaced into an abnormal position, thus making it vulnerable to injury.[142] In the chronic setting, the risk of iatrogenic peroneal nerve injury may be increased because of the presence of more scar tissue, and subsequently, a more difficult neurolysis procedure (Fig. 102.18). Vascular injury, which requires immediate recognition and treatment, has been reported to occur in 12% to 64% of knee dislocations.[143,144] The presence of normal distal pulses cannot completely rule out arterial injury due to collateral circulation. The ankle-brachial index (ABI) is a reliable, noninvasive screening tool for diagnosing vascular injury

TABLE 102.3	Biomechanical Studies of Posterolateral Corner Reconstruction			
Study	Year	No. of Knees	Technique	Outcome
Kang et al.[127]	2017	3D-computational model	TBR vs. mFBR vs. cFBR	Cruciate ligament forces greatest in cFBR model, with no difference between the TBR and mFBR models; joint contact stresses of the three surgical models were greater than those of the intact model
Plaweski et al.[128]	2015	8 cadaveric knees	mFBR	Restoration of external varus rotation in extension and translation of the lateral tibial plateau at 90-degree flexion similar to intact knee
Rauh et al.[124]	2010	10 cadaveric knees	Fibula based vs. anatomic	No difference in stability observed between either reconstruction technique
Apsingi et al.[125]	2009	10 cadaveric knees	Fibula based vs. anatomic	No difference in stability observed between either reconstruction technique
Nau et al.[126]	2005	10 cadaveric knees	Fibula based vs. anatomic	No difference in stability observed between either reconstruction technique
LaPrade et al.[116]	2005	10 cadaveric knees	Anatomic	No difference in external rotation stability between intact knee or reconstructed knee

3D, Three-dimensional; *cFBR,* conventional fibular-based; *mFBR,* modified fibular-based; *TBR,* tibial-based.

TABLE 102.4   Results of Various Techniques for Posterolateral Corner Reconstruction

Study	Year	N	Mean Follow-Up and Range (Months)	Mean Age and Range (Years)	Technique	Outcome
Kannus[93]	1989	23	99 (72–126)	34 (14–61)	Nonoperative management	Grade I and II: 82% returned to preinjury level of activity; Grade III: 25% returned to preinjury level of activity
Levy et al.[98]	2010	10	34 (24–49)	Not reported	Repair (acute)	40% failure rate
Stannard et al.[97]	2005	57	24 (24–59)	33 (17–57)	Repair (acute)	37% failure rate
Arthur et al.[111]	2007	21	37 (19–65)	32 (18–49)	High tibial osteotomy (chronic)	38% of patients stable after high tibial osteotomy only (no reconstruction needed)
Yoon et al.[137]	2011	32	35 (24–63)	35 (20–54)	Fibular sling (chronic)	Mean postoperative Lysholm and IKDC 86.4 and 75.3, respectfully; 1 failure with persistent laxity
Zorzi et al.[136]	2013	19	38 (–)	29 (17–41)	Fibular sling (chronic)	Mean postoperative IKDC 86; 11% persistent laxity
Ibrahim et al.[156]	2013	20	44 (24–52)	26 (18–48)	Fibular sling (acute)	Mean postoperative Lysholm 90; 6% persistent laxity
Fanelli et al.[135]	2014	34	32 (24–84)	27 (15–53)	Sling; capsular imbrication (chronic)	Mean postoperative Lysholm 91.8; 1 patient with persistent laxity
Kim et al.[106]	2003	46	40 (24–93)	35 (16–62)	Biceps tenodesis (chronic)	17% with loss of stability at final follow-up
Yoon et al.[129]	2006	21	22 (12–41)	34 (21–64)	Anatomic (acute and chronic)	19% with greater than 1+ excess laxity
LaPrade et al.[130]	2010	64	53 (24–86)	32 (18–58)	Anatomic (chronic)	Mean postoperative IKDC 62.6; 5% recurrent instability requiring revision surgery
Jakobsen et al.[131]	2010	27	46 (24–86)	28 (13–57)	Anatomic (chronic)	5% with rotatory instability and 5% varus instability
Gormeli et al.[134]	2015	21	40.9 ± 13.7	31.1 ± 9.2 years	Anatomic (chronic)	Mean postoperative Lysholm, IKDC and Tegner 80, 64, and 4, respectfully. No differences between isolated PLC and multi-ligament reconstruction
Kim et al.[138]	2013	65	34 (–)	37.2 (16–64)	Anatomic (chronic)	Mean postoperative Lysholm 86.3; 18% failures on varus stress radiographs
Camarda et al.[67]	2010	10	28 (18–40)	27 (16–47)	Fibular based (chronic)	0% loss of stability, 10% overconstrained compared with uninjured side
Schechinger et al.[132]	2009	16	30 (24–75)	30 (19–61)	Fibular based + capsular shift (chronic)	Mean postoperative Lysholm and IKDC 89.9 and 81.3, respectively; No functional instability, 25% with 1+ varus laxity
Khanduja et al.[133]	2006	19	67 (24–110)	30 (21–47)	Fibular based (chronic)	26% with "residual minimal posterolateral instability" but not further defined

IKDC, International Knee Documentation Committee; PLC, posterolateral corner.

following knee dislocations. An index greater than 0.90 was found to have a 100% negative predictive value of arterial injury, and in this situation the patient can be monitored with serial clinical examinations.[145] However, an ABI less than 0.90 requires further investigation with either an arterial duplex ultrasound or CT angiography. A detailed neurovascular examination is imperative, not only to identify limb-threatening emergencies, but to also identify neurologic deficit prior to surgical intervention, given the proximity of the peroneal nerve to the surgical field. Posttraumatic joint space narrowing after PLC reconstruction was reported to occur in 29% of patients followed up 4 years postoperatively, with most of those patients having evidence of early chondrosis at the time of initial surgery.[146] Joint stiffness, or arthrofibrosis, may also occur after these injuries and their reconstruction. Some period of immobilization is required to promote healing, which places the knee at risk for the development of arthrofibrosis. This risk can be decreased by determining, intraoperatively, a safe degree of flexion to allow in the early postoperative period and to perform patellar mobilization.[59] Iatrogenic fracture of the fibular head can occur during bone tunnel preparation if the guide pin is not appropriately placed prior to reaming. Painful hardware has been a problem with the tibial screw and washer construct in the past. Lower profile hardware may minimize this concern.

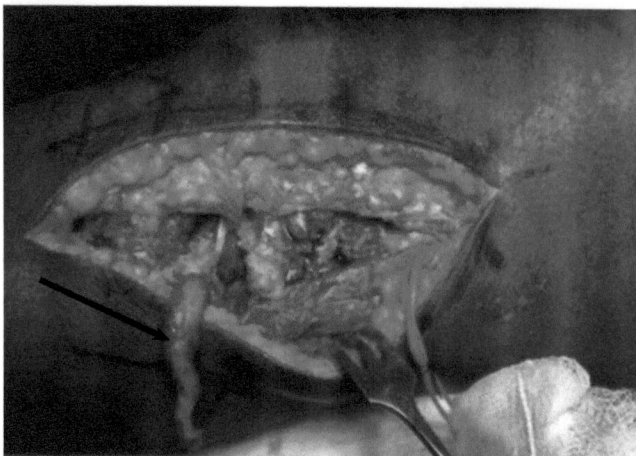

Fig. 102.18 A peroneal nerve avulsion injury *(black arrow)* after a posterolateral corner injury. (Courtesy Katherine Coyner, MD.)

FUTURE CONSIDERATIONS

Pediatric Posterolateral Corner Injuries

As the number of children playing sports increases and as more demands and expectations are placed on these adolescent athletes, the rate of injury is going to increase and may include a higher incidence of PLC injuries. Purely ligamentous injury is uncommon in the pediatric population, which is most often attributed to the ligament being stronger than the adjacent growth plate.[147,148] PLC injuries appear to be especially rare. In a review of 39 adolescents undergoing ACL reconstruction, despite 67% having concomitant injuries, none were diagnosed as having PLC injuries.[149] Case series have described isolated avulsions of the popliteus tendon and injuries to both the popliteus and FCL.[150-154] Von Heideken et al.[154] identified 23 reported cases of isolated pediatric PLC injuries in the literature, with most involving avulsion fractures at the femoral attachment of the popliteus and FCL. However, no extensive report on pediatric PLC injuries was found in the literature.

Given its rare incidence, treatment of isolated pediatric PLC injuries is not clear. Kannus and Jarvinen[155] reported on the nonoperative treatment of 33 adolescents with grade II and III ligament injuries, including five grade II and two grade III FCL injuries. The findings, which were not just specific to the LCL injuries, resembled those found in adults, with the grade II injuries doing well and the grade III injuries having poor results and persistent instability. It was recommended that the grade III injuries be treated surgically. However, the best way to surgically treat these injuries remains unclear. In addition, surgical treatment in adolescents poses the additional risk of operating around the physis and risking growth disturbance. Complicating this situation is the fact that the one patient in the case series by Von Heideken et al.[154] who was treated nonoperatively was the only patient in whom a growth disturbance and angular deformity of the injured extremity developed. More research is necessary to better determine the best way to treat these rare injuries.

For a complete list of references, go to ExpertConsult.com.

SELECTED READINGS

Citation:

Larson MW, Moinfar AR, Moorman CT III. Posterolateral corner reconstruction: fibular-based technique. *J Knee Surg.* 2005;18(2):163–166.

Level of Evidence:

IV

Summary:

The fibula-based technique for both acute and chronic posterolateral corner reconstruction is a successful way to restore stability, preserve native tissue to incorporate into the reconstruction, and minimize bone tunnels during combined reconstructions, and it is relatively easy to perform. The technique is thoroughly described.

Citation:

LaPrade RF, Ly TV, Wentorf FA, et al. The posterolateral attachments of the knee: a qualitative and quantitative morphologic analysis of the fibular collateral ligament, popliteus tendon, popliteofibular ligament, and lateral gastrocnemius tendon. *Am J Sports Med.* 2003;(31):854–860.

Level of Evidence:

Cadaveric study

Summary:

The femoral and tibial attachments for the major structures of the posterolateral corner have a consistent anatomic relationship to each other with consistently measurable distances between the various structures. It is important to consider these relationships and restore this anatomic relationship during reconstruction techniques.

Citation:

Levy BA, Dajani KA, Morgan JA, et al. Repair versus reconstruction of the fibular collateral ligament and posterolateral corner in the multiligament-injured knee. *Am J Sports Med.* 2010;38(4):804–809.

Level of Evidence:

III

Summary:

Comparing the acute repair of structures with the reconstruction of the posterolateral corner revealed a much higher failure rate in the acute repair group, in which 40% failed compared with 6% in the reconstruction group. Reconstruction should be considered, even in the acute setting, because of the much higher rate of failure in the primary repair group.

Citation:

LaPrade RF, Resig S, Wentorf F, et al. The effects of grade III posterolateral knee complex injuries on anterior cruciate ligament graft forces. *Am J Sports Med.* 1999;27(4):469–475.

Level of Evidence:

Cadaveric study

Summary:

Untreated grade III posterolateral corner injuries lead to significantly higher forces on the anterior cruciate ligament. Therefore in the setting of combined injury, untreated grade III posterolateral corner injuries contribute to ACL graft failure because of this higher force experienced by the graft.

Citation:

LaPrade RF, Wentorf FA, Fritts H, et al. A prospective magnetic resonance imaging study of the incidence of posterolateral and multiple ligament injuries in acute knee injuries presenting with a hemarthrosis. *Arthroscopy*. 2007;23: 1341–1347.

Level of Evidence:

II

Summary:

Out of 331 patients with acute knee injuries presenting with a hemarthrosis, 9.1% of the entire group and 16% of the group diagnosed with ligament tears were found to have a posterolateral knee injury, and in more than 50% of these injuries, more than one posterolateral corner structure was involved. Posterolateral corner injuries may be more common than previously reported, and when present, they are usually associated with additional ligamentous injury.

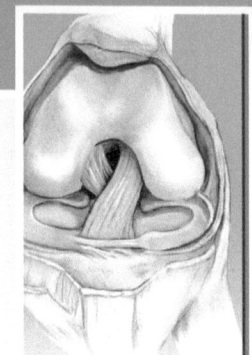

103

Multiligament Knee Injuries

Samantha L. Kallenbach, Matthew D. LaPrade, Robert F. LaPrade

Knee ligaments are responsible for providing the static stability of the knee, control of kinematics, and prevention of abnormal rotation and/or displacement that may damage the articular surfaces or the menisci. Knee dislocations are rare and are estimated to account for 0.02% to 0.2% of orthopaedic injuries[1]; however, it is generally accepted that multiligament injuries may occur at a higher rate because some knees spontaneously reduce before presentation.[2,3] These injuries may spontaneously reduce or may present as an acutely dislocated knee requiring reduction. The diagnosis and management of multiligament injuries pose unique challenges to orthopaedic surgeons, and a wide spectrum of injury exists, ranging from two-ligament injuries such as a cruciate and collateral ligament rupture to a grossly unstable knee that requires spanning external fixation. Although the immediate concerns should be to determine the integrity of the neurovascular structures, other essential concepts include accurate identification of all injured structures, repair versus reconstruction, management of acute versus chronic injuries, single- versus two-stage surgery, and postoperative rehabilitation. During the past three decades, clinical outcome studies along with anatomic and biomechanical investigations have greatly improved the management of these complex injuries.

HISTORY

In evaluating a patient who presents with knee pain or instability, the clinician must obtain a careful history of symptom onset, mechanism of injury, history of prior knee injuries, and previous operative and nonoperative treatments. Multiligament injuries associated with sports are considered low-energy and are often isolated to the involved extremity, whereas those associated with automobile or motorcycle crashes are considered high-energy[4] and may be combined with other life-threatening injuries.

Acutely injured patients may be unable to ambulate because of swelling, pain, and instability. Determination of the time since the injury occurred is crucial in patients who present with persistent dislocation because of the possibility of vascular injury and limb ischemia. Patients with chronic injuries may report mechanical symptoms, including clicking, catching, or locking or they may report instability on uneven ground, with cutting motions, and during activities of daily living. Neurologic deficits may be reported, including the presence of paresthesias in the common peroneal nerve distribution and a foot drop. Synthesis of this information will guide the clinician in the physical examination and selection of imaging studies.

PHYSICAL EXAMINATION

Examination of a patient with a suspected multiligament injury in the acute setting must include the assessment of vascular status. If an arterial injury is suspected, an ankle-brachial index score should be determined; a score of less than 0.9 is an indication that advanced arterial imaging should be obtained.[5] Serial neurovascular examination and selective computed tomography angiography has been recommended; "hard signs" of ischemia warrant emergent vascular consultation.[6]

The neurologic status must also be assessed. The common peroneal nerve supplies motor innervation to the anterior (deep peroneal) and lateral (superficial peroneal) compartments of the leg, as well as the extensor hallucis brevis and extensor digitorum brevis (deep peroneal) on the dorsum of the foot. A 25% to 35% nerve injury rate has been reported in the population with high-velocity knee dislocations.[7] In a series of acute isolated or combined posterolateral corner (PLC) knee injuries in an orthopaedic sports medicine referral practice, 4 of 29 patients had a complete palsy of the common peroneal nerve and an additional 7 of 29 had a partial motor/sensory deficit.[8] A recent study by Moatshe et al. found that peroneal nerve injury was significantly associated with vascular injury; thus injury to the peroneal nerve should raise suspicion of a vascular lesion.[2] Tibial nerve injuries may also occur in knee dislocations; although these injuries occur less frequently.

Physical examination of knee stability is a repeatable method of predicting intra-articular pathology but may be more difficult in patients with acute injuries. It is important to examine both legs to assess for pathologic instability versus physiologic laxity. Multiligament injuries are not subtle on examination; however, attention to subtle findings will aid the clinician in determining which specific structures are injured. Anteroposterior (AP) stability should be assessed with the Lachman, pivot shift, and posterior drawer tests. The posterior sag and quadriceps active tests also aid in the evaluation of the posterior cruciate ligament (PCL).

Lateral and posterolateral knee injuries are typically combined with an injury to one or both of the cruciate ligaments.[8-10] In acute injuries, the patient may have tenderness upon palpation of the fibular head. Examination maneuvers should include varus stress[11] at 0 and 20 degrees, reverse pivot shift, external rotation recurvatum,[12] and the dial test at 30 and 90 degrees. In a patient with a positive varus stress test at 30 degrees and negative findings at 0 degrees, an isolated fibular collateral ligament (FCL) tear is suspected. However, with multiligament injuries, the varus stress test will also be positive at 0 degrees. A positive dial test at both 30 and 90 degrees suggests a combined PCL and PLC injury.[13,14] A positive posterolateral drawer test reinforces findings consistent with a PLC injury but must be interpreted with caution, as discussed further on.

Medial structures are evaluated with the valgus stress test at 0 and 20 degrees of flexion[15]; instability at full extension is indicative of a combined cruciate ligament injury. Assessment of medial compartment gapping at 20 degrees under a valgus stress primarily isolates the superficial medial collateral ligament (MCL). Evaluation of associated rotational abnormalities is assessed with anteromedial tibial rotation at 90 degrees of flexion and the dial test at 30 and 90 degrees of flexion.[16] Increased anteromedial rotation suggests a more extensive knee injury that includes the superficial MCL as well as the posterior oblique ligament (POL) and deep MCL. The examiner must be careful to differentiate anteromedial from posterolateral tibial rotation during the dial test by palpation and visualization of tibial subluxation with the patient in the supine position.[16]

Gait assessment is an important component of the physical examination but may be compromised because of pain in persons with acute injuries. In subacute or chronic injuries, a varus thrust gait or foot drop may be observed in patients with combined lateral injuries. Patients with medial knee injuries may demonstrate a valgus thrust during the stance phase of gait, but this manifestation is less common and usually occurs in patients with genu valgus alignment.

IMAGING

Radiographic examination for patients with a suspected multiligament knee injury should include standard AP and lateral views (Fig. 103.1) as well as weight-bearing flexion (Rosenberg)

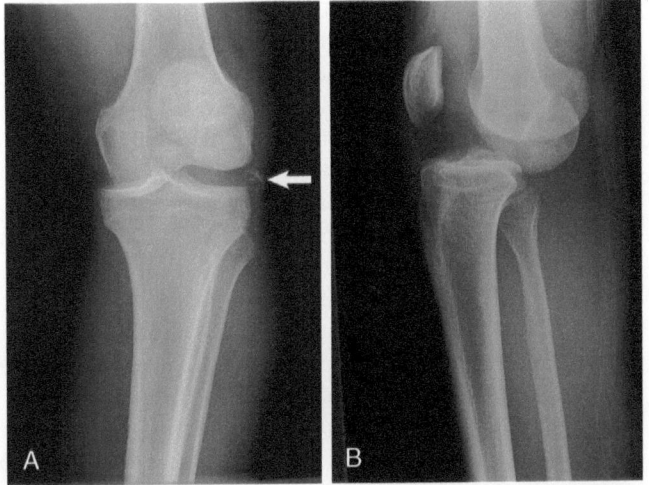

Fig. 103.1 Anteroposterior (A) and lateral (B) radiographs demonstrating an acute left knee dislocation. An arcuate fracture is also visible on the anteroposterior radiograph *(arrow)*.

views.[17] These views allow visualization of tibial plateau, femoral condyle, or osteochondral fractures. Segond[18] and/or arcuate[19] fractures may be visualized with lateral/posterolateral injuries, and calcification near the MCL origin (Pellegrini-Stieda ossification) may be visualized in chronic medial-sided injuries. Baseline bilateral standing long-leg radiographs allow the clinician to determine the mechanical axis of the injured and contralateral extremities, which may have a significant impact on treatment decisions for chronic multiligament injuries.[20,21]

Preoperative stress radiographs provide quantitative objective information on the stability to valgus and varus stress and should also be routinely obtained postoperatively. Biomechanical studies were performed to objectively quantify the amount of joint opening with varus[11] and valgus[15] stress; radiographic techniques were developed and tested by sequential sectioning in cadaveric knees with intact cruciate ligaments. Isolated sectioning of the FCL (simulating a grade III injury) resulted in an increase of 2.7 mm of lateral joint gapping at 20 degrees of flexion when compared with the contralateral knee. Sectioning of the FCL, popliteus tendon (PLT), and PFL (simulating a complete grade III PLC injury) was associated with lateral joint gapping of 4 mm at 20 degrees of flexion. Isolated sectioning of the superficial MCL (simulating a grade III injury) resulted in 3.2 mm of increased medial joint gapping at 20 degrees of flexion when compared with the contralateral knee. Increased medial joint gapping of 6.5 and 9.8 mm at 0 and 20 degrees of flexion, respectively, was associated with sectioning of the superficial MCL, deep MCL, and POL (simulating a complete medial knee injury).

Several imaging techniques have been developed to allow quantitative assessment of the integrity of the PCL; these are especially useful in persons with chronic injuries. Stress radiographs have been described using the kneeling knee technique[22] and Telos device (Telos GmbH, Marburg, Germany)[23]; these two techniques have been reported to allow the quantification of posterior displacement of the tibia and are superior to a physical examination and use of the KT-1000 arthrometer.[24]

Magnetic resonance imaging (MRI) has become part of the standard of care for the evaluation of knee instability, especially in persons with acute injuries for whom examination may be limited by pain and swelling (Fig. 103.2). With high sensitivity and accuracy, MRI allows visualization of the cruciate and collateral ligaments, posteromedial corner and PLC,[25] bone marrow edema,[9,26,27] meniscal injuries, and cartilage lesions. Anteromedial femoral condyle bone bruises should alert the physician to a possible PLC injury.[9] In addition, lateral-sided tibial or femoral bone bruises have also been associated with MCL injuries.[28]

It is important to recognize common imaging findings associated with multiligament knee injuries. Plain radiographs may be negative in the acute setting if the patient is lying supine, and it may be difficult to obtain weight-bearing films. In chronic injuries, weight-bearing films may reveal varus or valgus gapping or loss of joint space and early findings of degenerative disease. Stress radiographs are especially useful to quantitatively assess stability of the PCL, medial complex, and posterolateral complex. In patients with acute injuries, MRI will usually reveal the status of the cruciate ligaments and allow assessment of the collateral

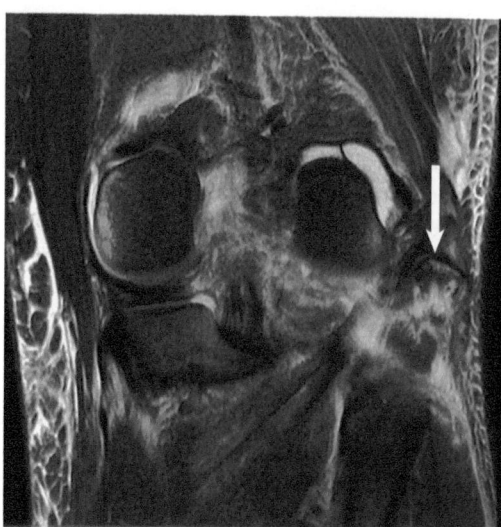

Fig. 103.2 A coronal magnetic resonance image of a left knee injury with bicruciate rupture and a complete posterolateral corner injury including arcuate fracture (arrow) and grade III injury of the fibular collateral ligament, popliteus tendon, and popliteofibular ligament.

structures if appropriate cuts and slice thicknesses are obtained. Classic bone bruises associated with ACL ruptures may be seen, as well as those associated with PLC injuries.

DECISION-MAKING PRINCIPLES

Patients with multiligament injuries are a heterogeneous group and may present with a variety of skin, bony, neurovascular, and ligamentous injuries. Although several general treatment algorithms have been developed, individualized treatment for the patient's specific knee injuries and concomitant injuries is necessary. Meniscus injuries should ideally be repaired, especially in the young patient, but this may require a partial meniscectomy. Management of vascular injuries, open injuries, skin coverage, fracture treatment, and meniscus injuries is not specifically discussed here. Important considerations for the treatment of multiligament injuries include operative versus nonoperative treatment, surgical timing, single- versus two-stage cruciate ligament reconstruction techniques, and repair versus reconstruction of collateral structures.

Knee ligament injuries have historically been classified with the use of a grading scale that assesses sagittal (AP) and coronal (varus/valgus) plane[16,29] stability. Rotational stability does not have a formal classification system, although many injury types have been described.[30-32] Treatment must be based on the extent of injury to individual structures and the number of structures injured. Knee ligament injuries are often subjectively classified according to the original American Medical Association guidelines, rated as grade I, II, or III.[33] An additional classification system is based on the number and location of torn ligaments.[34]

Nonoperative Versus Operative Treatment

It must be recognized that multiligament knee injuries are rare and that few studies have been conducted that compare treatment strategies with a high level of evidence. Current literature favors surgical management of multiligament knee injuries,[35-37]

whereas in early reports nonoperative treatment was often recommended for "uncomplicated" cases (i.e., absence of vascular injury or fracture).[38,39] A recent review indicates improved outcomes in multiple subjective and objective facets for patients treated with an operation compared with those treated conservatively with immobilization.[37]

Surgical Timing

Several studies have evaluated the impact of surgical timing. However, interpretation of outcomes of surgically treated multiligament injuries is difficult because of the wide range of pathology within individual studies.[36] Irreducible knee injuries, open injuries, and popliteal vascular injuries necessitate emergent management. If the multiligament injury is associated with a high-energy trauma, the patient's overall medical status and serious concomitant extremity, torso, and head injuries may delay definitive treatment. Overlying skin injuries and associated plateau or femoral condyle fractures may necessitate delayed ligament reconstruction. These complicating factors are not specifically evaluated; rather, the focus here is on single-extremity multiligament injuries without concomitant injuries.

Timing of surgery is typically divided into one of the following three categories: acute (often defined as surgery within 6 weeks), chronic (often defined as surgery after 6 weeks), or staged (the index procedure is performed within 3 to 6 weeks of injury and second-stage surgery is delayed).[36] Harner et al.[40] reported improved subjective outcomes in acutely treated patients and no ultimate difference in range of motion (ROM); however, 4 of 19 patients with acutely reconstructed knees required manipulation for loss of flexion. Fanelli and Edson[41] reported on 35 patients with multiligament injuries and found no subjective differences (according to Tegner, Lysholm, and Hospital for Special Surgery knee ligament rating scales) or objective differences (according to use of the KT-1000 arthrometer) between the acute and chronic cohorts.

A recent systematic review of surgical treatment for multiligament injuries found increased anterior instability for patients treated acutely but no difference in posterior, varus, or valgus instability when compared with chronically treated injuries.[36] Additionally, flexion loss (>10 degrees) as well as the need to undergo a subsequent repeat operation for stiffness were more frequent in acutely treated patients; no difference was found for extension. Last, patients treated with staged reconstructions had more "excellent" or "good" outcomes than did those treated acutely. As described later in this chapter, these findings may be difficult to interpret because many of these patients were treated with acute PLC repairs (which have been found to frequently fail) rather than reconstructions.

Patients with chronic multiligament injuries may present to the orthopaedic surgeon because of a failed index procedure, failed nonoperative management, or concomitant injuries that precluded acute surgical management of the multiligament injury. These patients may have varus malalignment, and a high-tibial osteotomy may be required to correct the mechanical axis prior to ligament reconstruction because a failure to correct varus malalignment with a chronic PLC injury has been reported as a cause of PLC reconstruction graft failure.[42,43]

Cruciate Ligament Reconstruction

It is widely accepted that cruciate ligament injuries in patients with multiligament injuries require reconstruction. A biomechanical study by Veltri and colleagues[44] demonstrated the importance of reconstructing the cruciate ligaments in multiligament injuries. Options for anterior cruciate ligament (ACL) reconstruction in multiligament injuries include transtibial versus transportal drilling for femoral tunnels and autograft versus allograft; no known studies recommend double-bundle ACL reconstruction in these patients. The debate regarding the best PCL reconstruction technique to use in persons with multiligament injuries is similar to the debate for isolated injuries; graft fixation techniques, single- versus double-bundle technique, and transtibial tunnel versus tibial inlay technique. Few studies have been performed to compare cruciate ligament reconstruction techniques in the multiligament injury patient population; therefore surgeons must apply the principles used for the reconstruction of isolated cruciate ligament injuries to this unique patient group.

Collateral Structures

Until recently it was believed that PLC structures could be successfully repaired if treated acutely. This practice has been challenged by outcomes studies that compared repairs versus reconstructions.[45,46] It has been biomechanically demonstrated that a deficient PLC leads to increased ACL[47] and PCL[48,49] graft forces; interestingly, Mook et al.[36] reported that more patients treated acutely for multiligament injuries underwent repairs rather than reconstructions of the PLC and suggest that repairs may have been insufficient to protect the ACL graft during healing. These findings may provide clinical evidence that reinforces the biomechanical principles of secondary stabilization between cruciate and collateral ligaments and may support the trend toward acute reconstruction rather than repair of PLC structures.[50] As discussed later in this chapter, a gradual trend has occurred from local tissue transfers and acute repairs toward several different autograft or allograft tissue reconstruction techniques.

A well-defined and successful treatment algorithm for isolated grade III MCL injuries and those combined with ACL ruptures includes a short period of rest and edema control followed by physical therapy.[16] However, treatment of MCL injuries associated with bicruciate injuries is less well defined. Some authors advocate delayed cruciate reconstruction while the medial structures are protected with a brace and allowed to potentially heal. Other authors recommend acute repairs or reconstruction of medial structures, although a higher risk of arthrofibrosis is reported.

Graft Choice

Graft choice in multiligament injury reconstruction is determined by injury pattern, graft availability, and surgeon preference. Often surgeons prefer to use allografts when treating multiligament injuries because of multiple graft size options and the ability to avoid the increased operative time and donor site morbidity associated with harvesting the patellar and hamstring tendon and possibly quadriceps tendon grafts. Because of the heterogeneity of multiligament injuries, no conclusive studies are available to recommend a particular graft choice. Several techniques are discussed in the Treatment Options section, further on, along with graft choices.

Special Considerations

Pediatric patients with multiligament injuries require special consideration because of their open physes and the potential risk of growth alteration with traditional ligament reconstruction. Physeal sparing techniques for ACL[51] and PCL[52] reconstruction have been described. Recently a modified physeal sparing technique was described for PLC/FCL injuries in pediatric patients.[53] Lateral and medial structures may be repaired via augmentation or recess procedures[8] or with use of suture anchors.

A recently defined type of knee dislocation described by Azar and colleagues has been termed *ultra–low velocity*.[54] These injuries are sustained by patients with a high body mass index as a result, for example, of falling from a standing height or tripping on an object. Patients who sustain ultra–low velocity multiligament knee injuries have higher rates of neurovascular injuries as well as a higher incidence of postoperative complications compared with patients who suffer low- or high-velocity multiligament injuries.[55] Their treatment must be individualized based on medical comorbidities, patient expectations, preinjury activity level, and ability to comply with rigorous rehabilitation.

Conservative therapy with immobilization may be the only treatment suitable for elderly patients with multiligament injuries who have preinjury medical comorbidities.[56] Additionally, the presence of arthritis is a relative contraindication to multiligament reconstruction; in fact, most studies exclude patients with preexisting arthritis.

TREATMENT OPTIONS

Treatment recommendations for specific ligament injuries in this patient population are limited by the lack of comparative studies. No known studies have evaluated the impact of a specific cruciate ligament reconstruction technique on the outcomes of multiligament injuries. Repair versus reconstruction of collateral ligaments has been debated, but specific reconstruction methods have not been directly compared in clinical studies.

Acute Management

Every multiligament knee injury is unique, and a wide range of pathology exists. Most injuries are adequately stabilized in a knee immobilizer. However, some knees associated with a high-energy injury may remain subluxed in a knee immobilizer and require a spanning external fixator to achieve stability in the acute setting.

Anterior Cruciate Ligament

Although ACL reconstruction is recommended, the specific technique receives relatively little discussion in the context of multiligament injuries. Many authors have described single-bundle reconstruction using an allograft or autograft with femoral tunnels created via a transtibial technique. Levy et al.[45] prefer to use a tibialis anterior allograft, Strobel et al.[57] recommended use of a hamstring autograft. Engebretsen et al.[1] initially preferred allografts for ACL reconstruction but changed their graft choice to a bone–patellar tendon–bone autograft. Harner et al.[40] prefer allograft bone–patellar tendon–bone but use an anteromedial portal drilling technique for ACL femoral tunnels rather than the transtibial technique as utilized by previous authors.

Posterior Cruciate Ligament

A review of treatment options for addressing PCL insufficiency in this patient population follows. It is generally accepted that PCL tears should be reconstructed in these patients, although the optimal technique has not yet been defined. A review of the causes of failure of a series of PCL reconstructions identified the importance of tunnel positioning and addressing concomitant collateral ligament instability.[21] However, investigators have not yet determined the role for the single- versus double-bundle technique and for transtibial versus tibial inlay graft placement.

Some studies have demonstrated that double-bundle PCL reconstructions restore native biomechanics[48,58]; however, relatively few studies have specifically described the detailed technique and associated outcomes of double-bundle PCL reconstructions in the multiligament injury population. Spiridonov et al.[59] recently described a double-bundle PCL reconstruction in 7 patients with isolated PCL ruptures and 32 with multiligament injuries. Their technique includes two femoral tunnels and a single transtibial tunnel to anatomically reconstruct the anterolateral bundle (ALB) and posteromedial bundle (PMB). Because of the morbidity of graft harvest and the need for large collagen volume, the authors used allografts, specifically Achilles tendon, for the ALB and a semitendinosus tendon for the PMB.

Several authors have described single-bundle PCL reconstructions in patients with multiligament injuries. Fanelli and Edson[41] recommended a single-bundle transtibial PCL reconstruction and reported using either an autograft or allograft. Engebretsen et al.[1] described a single-bundle transtibial PCL reconstruction; during the time of data collection, the investigators changed their graft source from allograft to hamstring autograft. Chhabra et al.[60] reported that approximately one-third of patients with an acute multiligament injury have an intact PMB and menisco-femoral ligaments. They attempted to preserve these bundles and performed a reconstruction of the ALB using an Achilles tendon allograft via a transtibial tunnel. In patients with complete ruptures of the entire PCL and those with chronic injuries, the authors recommend double-bundle PCL reconstruction using an Achilles tendon allograft for the ALB and a tibialis anterior allograft for the PMB.

A recent systematic review on the topic of transtibial versus tibial inlay technique for PCL reconstruction revealed a paucity of comparative outcomes studies and recommended surgeon preference as a reasonable consideration in technique choice until further evidence is available.[61] Biomechanical studies have compared the two techniques but it is difficult to apply their results to the multiligament injury population. Some investigators have recommended that the tibial inlay technique not be used for patients with multiligament injuries; however, this evidence is level V.[62] Stannard et al.[63] described a technique for double-bundle PCL reconstruction with a tibial inlay technique in patients with multiligament injuries. Their technique requires a single Achilles

tendon allograft, split longitudinally, to reconstruct the ALB and PMB. Cooper and Stewart[64] described a single-bundle tibial inlay PCL reconstruction using either a bone–patellar tendon–bone autograft or allograft to reconstruct the ALB.

Medial/Posteromedial Structures

In a recent review, LaPrade and colleagues[16,65] underscored the importance of completely evaluating and treating the three main structures of the medial/posteromedial knee: the superficial MCL, deep MCL, and POL. When associated with multiligament injuries, most authors agree that grade III MCL injuries require treatment, often repair or reconstruction. A systematic review reported an absence of sufficient studies to allow formulation of evidence-based recommendations for the treatment of MCL injuries in the multiligament injury population.[66] A general trend has been noted in the literature toward repair and/or reconstruction of medial knee injuries, which may be due to a better understanding of the anatomy and availability of biomechanically validated reconstruction techniques.

In early reports, Fanelli et al.[67] compared valgus stability in patients with bicruciate ruptures and medial-sided injuries. Bicruciate reconstructions were performed in all patients; two acutely presenting patients were treated with primary surgical repair of the MCL tears and seven were treated with bracing to allow the MCL injury to heal with nonoperative treatment followed by subsequent bicruciate ligament reconstruction. More recently, Fanelli and Edson[41] describe an anterosuperior shift of the posteromedial capsule for the repair of MCL injuries; when lesions are not amenable for repair, an autograft semitendinosus or allograft is used to reconstruct the superficial MCL and is accompanied by a capsular shift.

Lind et al.[68] described a rerouting of the ipsilateral semitendinosus tendon to reconstruct the superficial MCL and posteromedial structures in patients with multiligament injuries. The semitendinosus tendon was identified and harvested proximally but left intact at the pes insertion. A blind femoral tunnel, located at the isometric point of the MCL insertion, was created with a diameter equal to the size of the double-looped tendon. Additionally, a transtibial tunnel exiting 10 mm below the tibial plateau and posterolateral to the semimembranosus was drilled through the medial tibial plateau from anterior to posterior and reamed to the diameter of the semitendinosus tendon. The double-looped tendon was secured using interference screw fixation in the femur, pulled through the tibial tunnel, and secured with an additional interference screw.

LaPrade and colleagues[65] described an anatomically based and biomechanically validated[69] reconstruction of the medial knee structures.[70] Their technique reconstructs the POL and both the proximal and distal divisions of the superficial MCL. Two femoral and two tibial tunnels are created, and grafts are fixed in the tunnels with use of interference screws.

In a series of patients with knee dislocations, Harner et al.[40] described repair or reconstruction of MCL injuries. Avulsions and midsubstance injuries were repaired with suture anchors and nonabsorbable sutures, respectively. Chronic injuries were treated with a reconstruction of the MCL using a semitendinosus autograft or Achilles tendon allograft.

Lateral/Posterolateral Structures

In contrast to the extra-articular medial structures, it is well recognized that grade III PLC injuries do not heal with bracing and, without operative treatment, can lead to significant morbidity. Recently reconstruction rather than repair of PLC injuries has been emphasized because of results of comparative outcomes studies. Early investigators reported good results with acute anatomic repair of PLC injuries; however, these patients were immobilized in a cast for 6 weeks postoperatively, and subjective outcomes scoring tools were not available.[71-73]

More recently, Stannard et al.[46] and Levy et al.[45] performed a mix of single- and dual-stage operations and found lower failure rates with reconstructions when compared with repairs of the PLC. Stannard et al.[46] performed a modified two-tailed technique with a tibialis anterior or posterior allograft for PLC reconstructions. This technique uses a single femoral tunnel at the isometric point along with a single fibular and tibial tunnel.

Levy et al.[45] used a fibula-based technique with an Achilles tendon allograft, along with an anterodistal shift of the posterolateral capsule, to reconstruct the PLC.

LaPrade and colleagues recently reported on the acute[8] and chronic[20] treatment of isolated and combined PLC injuries. All PLC and concomitant cruciate ligament tears were treated with a single-stage surgery. Acute avulsions of PLC structures were repaired with suture anchors or recess procedures; however, most acute PLC injuries were not amenable to repair and were treated with a complete anatomic PLC reconstruction of the FCL, PLT, and/or PFL. A minority of the patients in the chronic PLC injury study were found to have varus malalignment and required an opening wedge proximal tibial osteotomy to correct the mechanical axis before undergoing a soft tissue reconstruction. The remainder of the patients were treated with an anatomic reconstruction of the PLC with single-stage reconstruction of coexistent cruciate ligament tears.

⚡ Authors' Preferred Technique

Ligamentous Injuries

Our preferred technique for the treatment of multiligament injuries is an anatomic single-stage reconstruction of the cruciate ligament(s) with concurrent treatment of medial/posteromedial and lateral/posterolateral supporting structures with anatomically based and biomechanically validated techniques. Grade III injuries to the medial and lateral structures require surgical treatment for patients with multiligament injuries with a repair and/or reconstruction when indicated. A repair of some structures may be possible in acute injuries with avulsions directly off bone; however, a reconstruction is required for acute injuries with midsubstance tears or inadequate tissue quality and for chronic injuries. It is the preference of the senior author to operate on patients with acute injuries within 3 weeks of injury so as to allow identification of injured structures and repair of meniscal pathology and extra-articular structures.

Preoperative Planning

Preoperative planning for the treatment of multiligament injuries is critical because of the inherent complexity of these procedures. The injury history, physical examination, and imaging studies will allow the surgeon to plan the details of the operation. The surgeon must be certain that all required equipment is available, including surgical instruments and any required allograft materials. Standard cruciate ligament reconstruction instruments including cannulated drill guides, eyelet-tipped passing pins, suture anchors, and cannulated interference screws (metallic or bioabsorbable) will be necessary. Appropriate graft harvesting instruments will be needed if the surgeon plans to use autografts; a graft preparation station will also be needed. A standard arthroscopic setup with 30- and 70-degree arthroscopes will be necessary for the evaluation and treatment of intra-articular injuries.

Patient Positioning

The patient is placed supine on the operating table and, after administration of an anesthetic, an examination is performed to confirm the suspected ligamentous pathology. A leg holder is placed to allow sufficient access to the medial and lateral aspect of the injured extremity. A well-padded proximal thigh tourniquet is set in place. The operative leg is prepped and draped free in the usual sterile fashion.

Extra-Articular Injury Identification and Treatment

We recommend that open dissection for lateral and/or medial injuries be performed prior to arthroscopic examination, which will allow the identification of injuries and assessment of tissue quality prior to arthroscopic fluid extravasation.

Lateral and Posterolateral Knee

An incision in a hockey-stick shape centered over the posterior to midportion of the iliotibial band is used to expose the lateral/posterolateral knee. The incision is positioned more posteriorly in patients with a planned autogenous patellar tendon graft harvest for a concurrent ACL reconstruction to maintain a minimum of 6 cm between the two incisions. This incision is continued down through the skin and superficial tissues to the superficial layer of the iliotibial band. Posteriorly, the long and short heads of the biceps femoris are identified; palpation approximately 2 to 3 cm distal to the long head will usually allow identification of the common peroneal nerve. A neurolysis is then performed to release the nerve from scar tissue entrapment and safely isolate it from the surgical site (Fig. 103.3).

Avulsions of the biceps tendon are repaired with use of suture anchors with the knee in full extension. Arcuate avulsion fractures may be repaired with No. 5 nonabsorbable sutures passed through the proximal tendon and bony fragment and tied through drill holes in the fibula.[8]

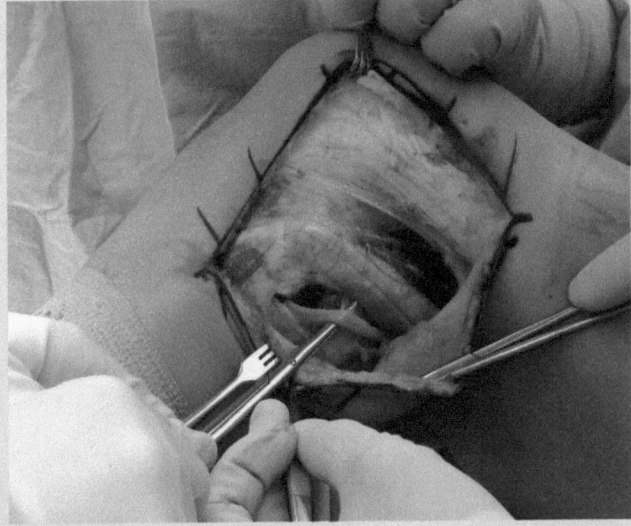

Fig. 103.3 The open surgical approach to the posterolateral aspect of a left knee. The common peroneal nerve is elevated by the Metzenbaum scissors.

Continued

Authors' Preferred Technique

Ligamentous Injuries—cont'd

Blunt dissection between the soleus and the lateral head of the gastrocnemius muscle will expose an interval through which the posteromedial aspect of the fibular head can be palpated. In this region the popliteofibular ligament (PFL) and musculotendinous junction of the PLT are found.

Next, an incision 1 cm proximal to the fibular head is made through the anterior arm of the long head of the biceps and the underlying biceps bursa. The distal aspect and insertion of the FCL can be identified through this incision, and a traction stitch is placed for upcoming identification of the proximal aspect of the ligament. Acute avulsions of the FCL directly from bone without intrasubstance stretch injuries, which usually occur in skeletally immature patients, may be repaired with use of suture anchors; however, the majority of FCL injuries are not amenable to repair and require a ligament reconstruction. A fibular tunnel is drilled with use of a cruciate ligament aiming guide. The desired trajectory for anatomic graft placement is from the FCL attachment site of the lateral aspect of the fibular head to the posteromedial downslope of the fibular styloid. A retractor is placed medially to prevent iatrogenic injury to deep structures, and a guide pin is advanced; the tunnel is overreamed with a 7-mm reamer, and the entry and exit apertures are chamfered with a rasp.

Next, a tibial tunnel is created for passage and fixation of the PFL and PLT reconstruction grafts. The anterior tunnel aperture is located at the flat spot between Gerdy's tubercle and the tibial tubercle; an elevator is used to release the soft tissues from this region. The posterior tunnel aperture is located at the posterolateral aspect of the proximal tibia, slightly distal to the plateau. The previously identified popliteus musculotendinous junction, located 1 cm medial and 1 cm proximal to the fibular head reconstruction tunnel, is the landmark for the posterior aperture of the reconstruction tunnel. A cruciate ligament reconstruction aiming guide is used to create this tunnel; a retractor is placed posteriorly to protect against an erroneously placed guide pin. Accurate placement of the guide pin is confirmed by palpating posteriorly while cross-referencing with a blunt probe placed through the fibular tunnel.

Tension is then applied to the traction stitch in the FCL remnant to identify and evaluate the FCL femoral origin.[74] To allow direct visualization of the FCL and PLT attachment sites on the femur and prepare for potential tunnel drilling, a splitting incision is placed through the superficial layer of the iliotibial band from a point proximal to the lateral epicondyle and extended distally to Gerdy's tubercle. Next, a vertical incision through the lateral capsule allows identification of the femoral insertion of the PLT. Avulsions of the PLT directly from the femur without intrasubstance stretch injury or musculotendinous avulsion may be amenable for a recess procedure performed with the knee in full extension.[75] The creation of femoral tunnels for reconstruction of the FCL and PLT requires a thorough understanding of the anatomy (Fig. 103.4)[74] and is performed according to previously described techniques.[76] With use of a collateral ligament aiming guide, two eyelet-tipped guide pins are aimed anteromedially to the adductor tubercle from the FCL and PLT attachment sites and advanced in a parallel fashion; tunnel orientation is important to avoid collision of the PLC tunnels with ACL reconstruction tunnels. The tunnels are then overreamed to a depth of 20 mm and a diameter of 9 mm (Fig. 103.5).

A split Achilles tendon allograft is prepared for the two limbs of the PLC reconstruction, and the grafts are secured in their femoral tunnels with 7- by 20-mm cannulated interference screws (Fig. 103.6). The FCL graft is passed through the fibular tunnel, but final fixation is delayed until the end of the procedure. Treatment of associated PLC structures is performed when indicated. Popliteomeniscal fascicle and coronary ligament tears are repaired with mattress sutures. Bony (Segond)[18] or soft tissue avulsions of the tibial attachment of the lateral capsular ligament[25] are repaired with suture anchors.[8]

Medial and Posteromedial Knee

The treatment of combined ACL/MCL injuries is well defined and is not specifically discussed here. The focus of this discussion is our preferred treatment of severe grade III medial ligamentous injuries combined with PCL or bicruciate ruptures as well as possible associated lateral injuries. Surgical treatment is delayed until knee swelling decreases; medial tissues may be amenable to repair with augmentation, or a reconstruction may be required. Concurrent, rather than staged, cruciate ligament reconstruction is performed in all patients.

Exposure of the medial knee is performed via an anteromedial incision that extends distally from the region between the medial border of the patella and the medial epicondyle to the region overlying the pes anserine tendons.[70] Next, the gracilis and semitendinosus tendon attachments are identified by incising the anterior border of the sartorial fascia. The semitendinosus tendon is removed with use of a standard tendon harvester and sectioned to create grafts of 16 and 12 cm for reconstruction of the superficial MCL and POL, respectively. Nonabsorbable sutures are used to tubularize each end, and the tendons are sized for 7-mm tunnels.

Within the pes anserine bursa, the superficial MCL distal tibial attachment is identified. Next, the superficial MCL is followed distally, and the tibial attachment is identified at the anteromedial proximal tibia. The superficial MCL has both proximal and distal tibial attachments; the distal attachment is approximately 6 cm distal to the joint line.[65] The tendon of the sartorius muscle is retracted distally, and the largest portion of the POL, the central arm, is identified. The tibial attachment site of the POL central arm, with an underlying small bony ridge, can be found near the direct arm of the semimembranosus tendon.

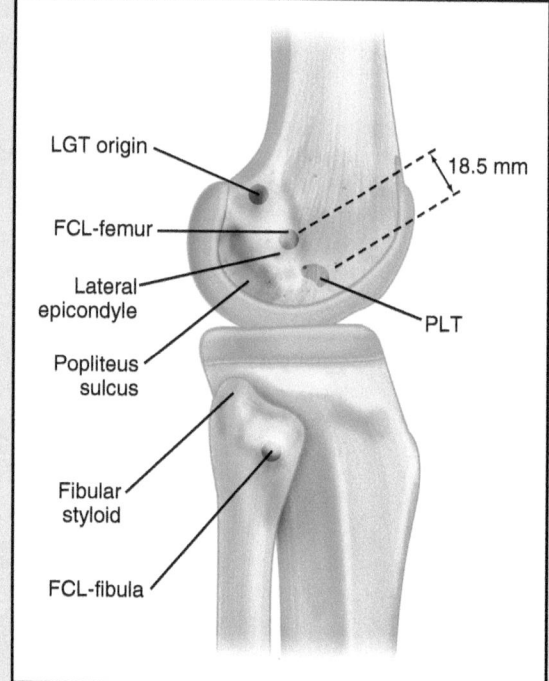

Fig. 103.4 Attachments of key posterolateral knee stabilizing structures and associated bony landmarks. *FCL*, Fibular collateral ligament; *LGT*, lateral gastrocnemius tendon; *PLT*, popliteus tendon.

📌 Authors' Preferred Technique

Ligamentous Injuries—cont'd

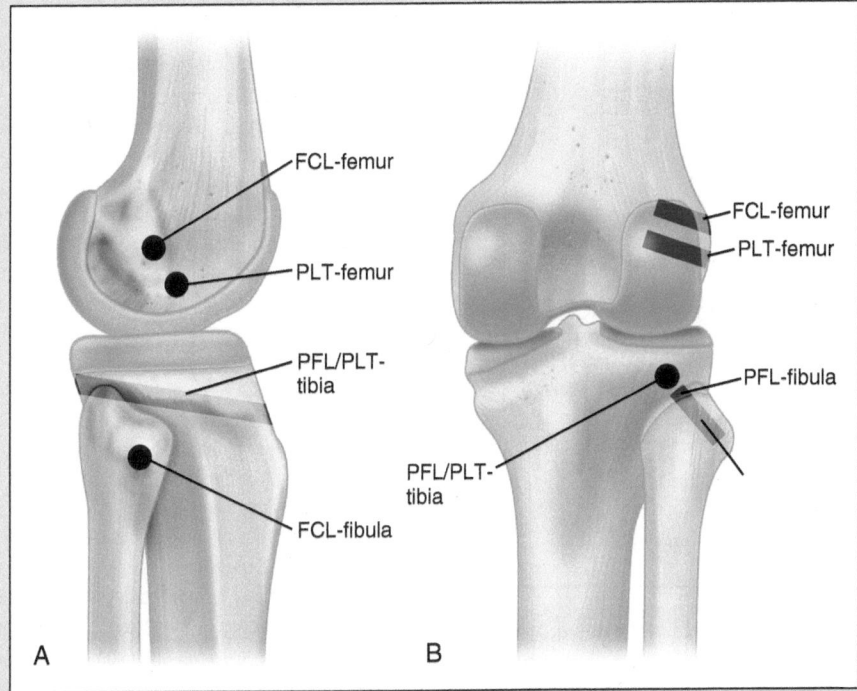

Fig. 103.5 Lateral (A) and posterior (B) aspects of the knee demonstrating the position of bone tunnels for a complete reconstruction of the posterolateral corner of the knee. *FCL,* Fibular collateral ligament; *PFL,* popliteofibular ligament; *PLT,* popliteus tendon.

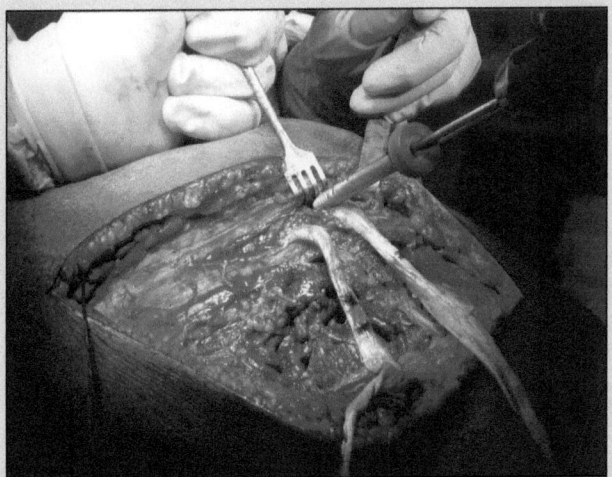

Fig. 103.6 The intraoperative posterolateral aspect of the right knee demonstrating fixation of the posterolateral corner grafts in the femoral tunnels. An iliotibial band–splitting incision is visualized and an interference screw is advanced into the popliteus tendon femoral tunnel.

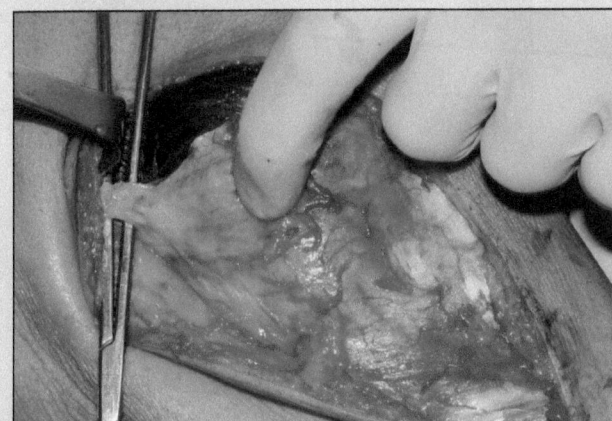

Fig. 103.7 The open surgical approach for the medial aspect of a left knee. The adductor tendon is elevated by the hemostat and a gloved finger is shown palpating the medial epicondyle. The vastus medialis obliquus muscle is also visible.

Identification of the femoral attachments of the medial knee structures is often difficult because the bony and soft tissue landmarks are not as obvious as those on the posterolateral knee. The initial step is to identify the adductor magnus tendon and its distal attachment to the adductor tubercle (Fig. 103.7). The senior author calls the adductor magnus tendon "the lighthouse of the medial aspect of the knee." This step will allow the surgeon to more accurately identify the medial epicondyle, the gastrocnemius tubercle, and the anatomic attachment sites of the superficial MCL and the POL (Fig. 103.8). The femoral attachment of the superficial MCL is approximately 12 mm distal and 8 mm anterior to the adductor tubercle, and the POL femoral attachment is approximately 11 mm posterosuperior to the superficial MCL.[65] After identification of the femoral and tibial attachments of the superficial MCL and POL, guide pins are inserted and overreamed with a 7-mm cannulated drill and advanced to a depth of 30 mm. Allografts or semitendinosus autografts are prepared (16 cm for the superficial MCL and 12 cm for the POL) and are fixed into the femoral tunnels using 7-mm bioabsorbable interference screws. Graft fixation in the tibial tunnels is delayed until the end of the procedure.

Continued

📌 Authors' Preferred Technique

Ligamentous Injuries—cont'd

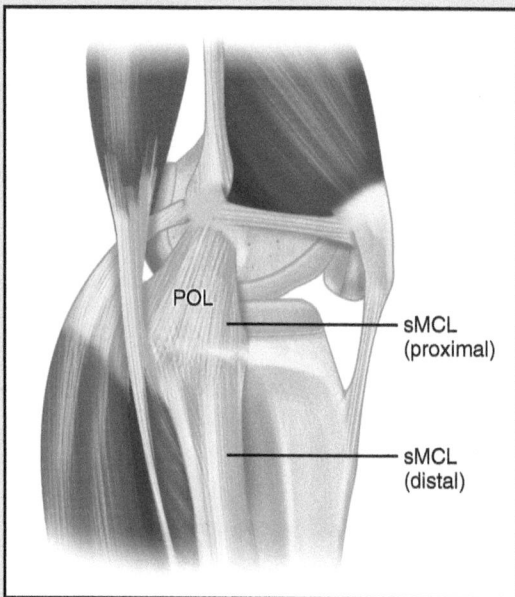

Fig. 103.8 Anatomy of the medial aspect of the left knee. The posterior oblique ligament *(POL)* and superficial medial collateral ligament *(sMCL)* are demonstrated. (From Coobs BR, Wijdicks CA, Armitage BM, et al. An in vitro analysis of an anatomical medial knee reconstruction. *Am J Sports Med.* 2010;38[2]:339–347.)

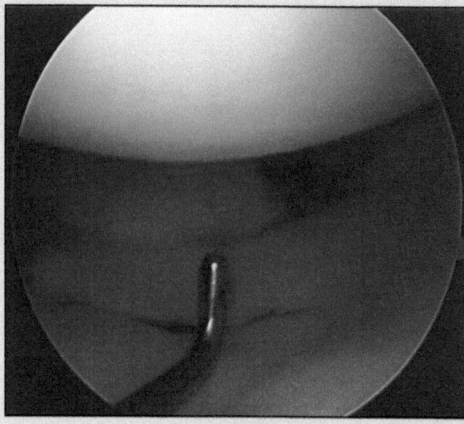

Fig. 103.9 A lateral compartment "drive-through sign" is seen in this arthroscopic photograph in a patient with a posterolateral corner knee injury.

Intra-Articular Injury Identification and Treatment

The arthroscopic portion of the surgery is delayed until after open dissection and injury identification to prevent arthroscopic fluid extravasation. Vertical inferomedial and inferolateral parapatellar portals are created and a standard arthroscopic assessment of the knee is performed. Varus and valgus stress is applied and the lateral and medial compartments, respectively, are observed for gapping (Fig. 103.9). The articular cartilage surfaces are examined for lesions, and the meniscal roots and bodies are similarly assessed; meniscal tears are repaired if possible. Cruciate ligament injuries are addressed as discussed in the following sections.

Posterior Cruciate Ligament

An endoscopic double-bundle PCL reconstruction is preferred in patients with multiligament injuries. An Achilles tendon allograft is used for the ALB reconstruction and a tibialis anterior allograft is used for the PMB reconstruction. The femoral attachments of these two bundles are identified with an arthroscopic coagulator. An additional portal is created through the posteromedial capsule to allow evaluation and debridement of the PCL tibial attachment. Debridement is continued until the popliteus muscle fibers are visualized. With use of a PCL guide, a guide pin is drilled from the anteromedial tibia, approximately 6 cm distal to the joint line, and exits at the PCL tibial attachment approximately 1 cm distal to the joint line at the PCL bundle ridge; pin placement is verified with intraoperative radiographs or fluoroscopy.

Femoral tunnel creation for the PCL reconstruction is performed according to previously described techniques.[59] The ALB is positioned so that the aperture edge is adjacent to the articular cartilage margin at the top of the intercondylar roof and along the anterior aspect of the medial femoral condyle. An 11-mm tunnel is drilled to a depth of 25 mm. Similarly, a 7-mm PMB tunnel is created at the previously described location and reamed to a depth of 25 mm; a minimum 2-mm bone bridge is maintained between the two tunnels.

After creation of the femoral tunnel, the tibial tunnel is reamed. The previously placed tibial guide pin is used to advance a 12-mm headed reamer to create a complete tunnel exiting at the posterior tibia. The posterior tissues are protected against iatrogenic injury via retraction with a large curette placed through the posteromedial portal. To minimize the potential for cyclic graft failure due to friction against the tibial tunnel aperture, a "smoother" is passed through the tibial tunnel and out the anteromedial portal and cycled several times to clean out the posterior tibial aperture.

The grafts are then passed into their respective femoral tunnels endoscopically via the anterolateral arthroscopic portal. A 7-mm titanium screw is used to fix the ALB graft bone plug into its femoral tunnel, and a 7-mm bioabsorbable interference screw is used to fix the PMB soft tissue graft into its femoral tunnel. The ALB and PMB grafts are then pulled distally through the tibial tunnel, and the knee is cycled; tibial graft fixation is delayed until the end of the procedure.

Anterior Cruciate Ligament Reconstruction

A single-bundle anatomic ACL reconstruction is preferred for patients with multiligament injuries. A bone–patellar tendon–bone autograft or allograft is chosen based on the preference of the patient/surgeon and availability. The tibial attachment is identified, and residual tissue is debrided with the shaver. Next, the femoral attachment is similarly identified and debrided to identify the lateral intercondylar ridge. A burr hole is made to mark the midpoint of the ACL femoral attachment between the anteromedial and posterolateral bundles.

The femoral tunnel is created via the anteromedial portal technique. This closed socket femoral tunnel is created with a low-profile reamer prior to tibial tunnel reaming. This sequence allows for identification of the important regional anatomy of this tunnel prior to significant fluid extravasation from the joint. If there was no concurrent medial knee reconstruction incision or if an allograft was used, a 2-cm anteromedial tibial incision is centered approximately 35 mm distal to the joint and 10 mm anterior to the MCL. An ACL reconstruction guide is placed into the joint and centered over the native ACL attachment site; a guide pin is then advanced and the tunnel is reamed. The ACL graft is passed and fixed in the femoral tunnel. Tibial fixation is delayed until the end of the procedure.

Final Graft Fixation

The order of final graft fixation is important. To restore the central pivot of the knee, tibial fixation of the PCL grafts is performed according to previously defined techniques[59] once all associated ligament reconstruction grafts have been fixed

Authors' Preferred Technique
Ligamentous Injuries—cont'd

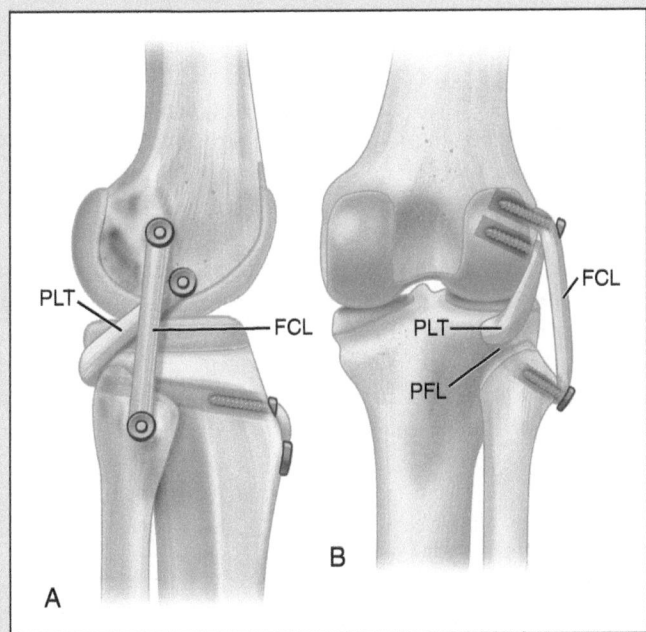

A   B

Fig. 103.10 The lateral (A) and posterior (B) views of a posterolateral corner knee reconstruction are demonstrated in this illustration. The fibular collateral ligament *(FCL)*, popliteus tendon *(PLT)*, and popliteofibular ligament *(PFL)* grafts are shown.

in their femoral tunnels. PLC grafts are secured next; care is taken to avoid overreducing the knee in patients with an associated medial knee injury. The FCL graft is passed through the fibula and fixed in its reconstruction tunnel at 20 degrees of knee flexion, in neutral rotation, and with a valgus reduction force on the knee. Next, the PLC grafts are passed anteriorly through the tibial tunnel, slack is removed from the grafts, and fixation of the PLT and PFL grafts is performed at 60 degrees of knee flexion, in neutral rotation, and with traction applied to the grafts (Fig. 103.10).

ACL graft tibial fixation is performed once the PLC grafts have been secured because of biomechanical evidence that fixation of the ACL graft prior to the PLC grafts can result in an external rotation deformity of the knee.[77] An interference screw is used in the tibial tunnel for fixation.

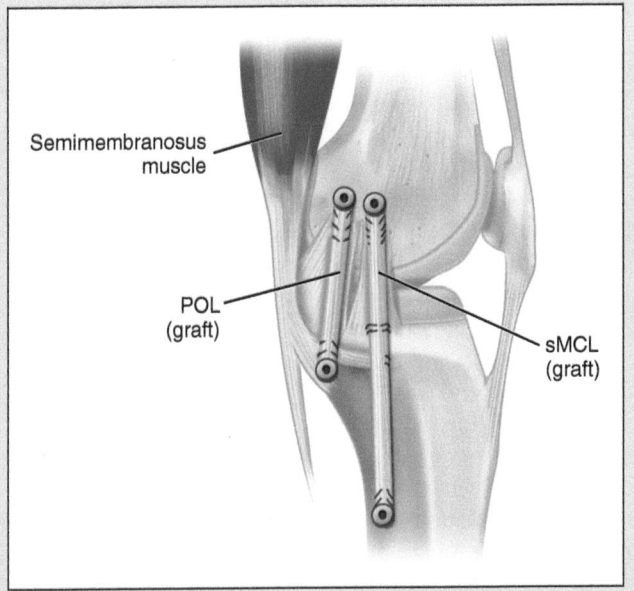

Fig. 103.11 The medial aspect of the left knee with reconstruction grafts fixed in the femoral and tibial tunnels with interference screws. *POL,* Posterior oblique ligament; *sMCL,* superficial medial collateral ligament. (From Coobs BR, Wijdicks CA, Armitage BM, et al. An in vitro analysis of an anatomical medial knee reconstruction. *Am J Sports Med.* 2010;38[2]:339–347.)

Graft fixation in the tibial tunnels is performed next for patients who underwent reconstruction of medial knee injuries (Fig. 103.11). The superficial MCL graft is passed into the tibial tunnel and tension is held while a varus moment is applied with the knee flexed to 20 degrees and in neutral rotation. At this position, the superficial MCL graft is secured with the interference screw. In a similar fashion, tension is applied to the POL graft via traction in full knee extension. The interference screw is inserted as a varus moment is applied with the knee held in extension and neutral rotation. A suture anchor is then used to recreate the proximal tibial superficial MCL attachment.

POSTOPERATIVE MANAGEMENT

An important consideration in the treatment of multiligament injuries is postoperative rehabilitation and eventual return to play. These topics have received great attention for isolated ligament injuries, but less information is available for patients with multiligament injuries; therefore principles from the former must be applied to the latter. Two general approaches to postoperative care in multiligament injuries are immobilization versus early mobilization. A balance must be achieved between immobilization aimed at preventing the development of instability and early mobilization to minimize scar tissue and resultant range-of-motion deficits. Although a full discussion of various rehabilitation protocols is beyond the scope of this chapter, the basic preferences of several investigators are described here.

Noyes and Barber-Westin described a program of early protected ROM in an attempt to limit arthrofibrosis.[78] They prescribed active assisted motion from 10 to 90 degrees six to eight times daily along with patellar mobilization for the first 4 weeks postoperatively. Between therapy sessions, the patient's knee was immobilized in a split cylinder cast to protect the reconstructed structures. After 4 weeks, the cast was changed to a hinged-brace and gradual increase in motion along with progression of weight bearing was then allowed.

A recent review of rehabilitation after the reconstruction of multiligament injuries recommended complete immobilization with the knee locked in extension for the first 5 weeks after surgery.[79] For the first 6 weeks, the authors allow the patients to bear full weight while standing statically on both legs, but they must use crutches for ambulation and abstain from bearing weight on the operative leg. From postoperative weeks 5 to 10, the brace is unlocked and patients are allowed to perform passive knee flexion; isolated hamstring strengthening is strictly avoided during this period.

Harner et al.[40] also described their preferred surgical treatment and rehabilitation for patients with multiligament injuries. For the first 4 weeks, the knee is held in full extension via a locked knee brace except during passive ROM exercises at up to 90 degrees of flexion. Isolated hamstring contraction is avoided until 6 weeks after surgery. Partial weight bearing is allowed with the brace in full extension for the first 4 to 6 weeks and progresses thereafter.

In a recent systematic review, Mook et al.[36] evaluated the impact of postoperative rehabilitation on multiligament injury outcomes. Their findings indicate that early mobilization in acutely treated patients is associated with less posterior instability, varus/valgus laxity, and ROM deficits as compared with immobilization after surgery. The apparent influence of early mobilization underscores the importance of a strong anatomic repair and/or reconstruction of posterolateral structures.

Wilkins[80] provided a detailed description of rehabilitation principles based on work by LaPrade and colleagues and describes early-phase rehabilitation (0 to 12 weeks) and late-phase rehabilitation (4 to 12 months). Similar to other authors, Wilkins recommends non–weight bearing for the first 6 weeks postoperatively, with occasional toe-touch weight bearing during showering and dressing activities; weight bearing is thereafter increased according to the protocol. For the first 2 weeks the brace is locked in full extension with the exception of therapy sessions, where the patient is allowed knee motion within the "safe zone" as defined intraoperatively. ROM is then increased to 90 degrees until 4 weeks postoperatively and thereafter gradually progressed to the goal of greater than or equal to 125 degrees. Because of posterior tibial translation associated with increasing flexion, isolated hamstring exercises are avoided for the first 4 months. Late-phase rehabilitation focuses on high-level balance training, sport-specific drills, and plyometric exercises and is initiated at approximately 4 months after surgery, when the patient has regained full active ROM, has resumed a normal gait, and has no signs of swelling.

RESULTS

No level I studies are available on the topic of treatment and associated outcomes of surgical reconstruction of multiligament injuries. Most available studies are level III or IV, and unfortunately evaluation of the results of some studies is limited by the heterogeneous patient mix. Often isolated injuries were included in the analysis with multiligament injuries, and high-energy injuries in polytrauma patients may be reported along with low-energy injuries associated with sports. A summary of selected literature is provided in Table 103.1.

COMPLICATIONS

Complications can be discussed within the context of the initial injury or those associated with treatment. Vascular injuries are not infrequent in the setting of multiligament injuries, and although the reported incidence varies, a commonly referenced number is 32%.[81] Urgent vascular surgery consultation is required for suspected large vessel injury because prolonged ischemia

may necessitate limb amputation. Peroneal nerve injuries are also common with multiligament injuries, especially when they are combined with PLC injuries, and are estimated to occur at a rate of 25% to 35%.[7] A poor prognosis is associated with complete lesions, whereas most persons with incomplete nerve palsies can often be expected to recover. Treatment options include physical therapy with an ankle-foot orthosis, neurolysis, primary nerve repair, nerve grafting, and tendon transfers.[82] With high-energy injuries, infection and skin compromise may also occur; inevitably definitive surgery will be delayed while skin concerns are addressed.

Complications may also be associated with treatment, whether nonoperative or operative. In both cases, persistent pain and instability may occur. If the initial treatment was nonoperative, the treatment is deemed a failure, and if the patient is a candidate, a chronic reconstruction may be required. If the initial treatment was operative, the patient may require revision reconstruction of all failed components.

Infection and bleeding can also occur with operative treatment. Incision and debridement with antibiotics and staged reconstruction may be necessary for infected cases. Bleeding may be the expected result of a difficult exposure, but attempts at adequate hemostasis must be obtained prior to closure. Bleeding may also occur because of iatrogenic injury to large vessels such as the popliteal artery that necessitates immediate intervention by a vascular surgeon. Iatrogenic injury to the common peroneal nerve may occur during neurolysis or as a failure of an adequate neurolysis prior to ligament reconstruction. However, adequately exposed and carefully handled nerves may still be associated with foot drop if the initial injury was severe. As with any surgery, deep venous thrombosis may occur; adequate prophylaxis is essential, especially in older and obese patients.

General causes of ligament reconstruction failure may include lack of incorporation of allografts, unrecognized or untreated ligament lesions, or technical concerns due to the repair technique or reconstruction tunnel placement. A persistent postoperative effusion may occur in some patients and will necessitate delaying progression of the rehabilitation protocol.

FUTURE CONSIDERATIONS

Because of the rarity of multiligament injuries and the variation of severity and presence of concomitant injuries, studies with a high level of evidence are limited. Additional clinical studies are necessary to make definitive recommendations on operative timing, surgical technique, and rehabilitation. Level I studies with randomization of surgical treatment may seem impractical because of the complexity of these injuries and the treatment preferences of particular surgeons. However, prospective multicenter studies with treatment outcomes assessed by a standardized method with validated subjective evaluations and unbiased objective measurements of stability and function would significantly benefit the multiligament injury evidence base.

In the past one to two decades, several ligament reconstruction techniques have been developed and tested in persons with isolated ligament injuries. However, few studies address the biomechanics of multiligament injuries and subsequent ligament

TABLE 103.1 Summary of Selected Recent Literature on Multiligament Knee Injuries

Study	Year	No. of Knees	Male (%)	Years of Follow-Up, Average (Range)	Timing: No. of Patients (Time to Surgery)	Average Age (Years)	Injury Type (Schenck Classification)	Knee Function (Average Scores)	Physical Examination (Stability)
Levy	2010	28	Not given	Repair: 2.8 (2–4.1) Reconstruction: 2.3 (2–3.4)	Repair: 10 (5–33 days) Reconstruction: 18 (17–731 days)	*	KD I: 12 KD III: 10 KD IV: 44 KD V: 1	4/10 repairs failed 1/18 reconstructions failed IKDC: 79 (repair), 77 (reconstruction) Lysholm: 85 (repair), 88 (reconstruction)	IKDC objective at final follow-up: 0 repairs and 2 reconstructions had 1+ laxity to varus stress at 30 degrees All patients were stable with the dial test at 30 and 90 degrees
Engebretsen	2009	85	53	5.3 (2–9.9)	A: 50 (<2 week) C: 35 Average: 14 months	35.2	KD II–III: 88% KD IV: 12%	Lysholm: 83 IKDC 2000: 64	Lachman: 57% normal, 33% 1+ Pivot shift: 90% normal, 4% 1+ Posterior drawer: 26% normal, 57% 1+ Dial test: 86% normal, 11% 1+ Valgus: 60% normal, 30% 1+ Varus: 67% normal, 25% 1+
Strobel	2006	17	76	(2–5.5)	C: 17 (5–312 months)	30.7	KD III: 17	IKDC: 71.8	Posterior drawer: 88% grade I or II, 12% grade III Lachman: 94% grade I or II, 6% grade III Posterolateral instability: 88% normal or nearly normal; 12% with residual instability
Stannard	2005	57	63	2.8 (2–4.9)	35 patients qualified for repair and were treated within 3 wk; 22 patients were chronic or had nonrepairable acute injuries	33	44 multiligament 13 isolated	Mean Lysholm, IKDC subjective repair success: 88.2, 59.8 Failed repair, s/p revision: 86.8, 63.6 Reconstruction success: 89.6, 56.1 Failed reconstruction, s/p revision: 92, 64.4	13/35 repairs failed; 12 underwent successful revision reconstruction 2/22 reconstructions failed IKDC objective: PLC repair success: 4 A, 14 B, 2 C, 1 D PLC repair failure: 3 A, 4 B, 4 C, 0 D PLC reconstruction success: 7 A, 9 B, 2 C, 2 D PLC reconstruction failure: 0 A, 1 B, 1 C, 0 D
Harner	2004	31	*	3.7 (2–6)	A: 19 (within 3 week) C: 12 (5 week–22 months)	28.4	Acute: KD I: 3 KD II+: 16 Chronic: KD II: 7 KD III–L: 2 KD III–M: 3	Lysholm A: 91; C: 80 KOS ADL A: 91; C 84 Sports Activities Scale: A: 89; C: 69 Meyers: 10 excellent, 13 good, 5 fair, 3 poor	Lachman: 48% normal, 52% 1+ Posterior drawer: 71% 1+, 29% 2+ Varus stress: 30 degrees: 29% 1+, 6% 2+ Valgus stress 30°: 16% 1+, 13% 2+
Fanelli	2002	35	74	(2–10)	A: 19 (<8 week) C: 16 (3–26 months)	*	KD II: 1 KD III–L: 19 KD III–M: 9 KD IV: 6	Lysholm: 91.2 HSS: 86.8	Lachman and pivot shift: 94% normal Posterior drawer: 46% normal, 54% 1+ Posterolateral stability: normal in 24%, "tighter than normal" in 76%

*Not given.
A, Acute; C, chronic; HSS, Hospital for Special Surgery; IKDC, International Knee Documentation Committee; KD, knee dislocation; KOS ADLA, Knee Outcome Survey Activities of Daily Living Scale; PLC, posterolateral corner; s/p, status postoperative.

reconstruction. Additionally, laboratory and clinical studies may evaluate the role of biologic treatments such as the use of stem cells and applied growth factors including platelet-rich plasma therapy in the setting of multiligament reconstruction.

For a complete list of references, go to ExpertConsult.com.

SELECTED READINGS

Citation:
Mook WR, Miller MD, Diduch DR, et al. Multiple-ligament knee injuries: a systematic review of the timing of operative intervention and postoperative rehabilitation. *J Bone Joint Surg Am.* 2009;91A(12):2946–2957.

Level of Evidence:
III

Summary:
Mook and colleagues performed a systematic review of the literature on multiple-ligament knee injuries to assess the impact of surgical timing and postoperative rehabilitation. The study included 24 retrospective studies and revealed several findings regarding the impact of these two factors on subjective and objective outcomes, which are discussed, with the associated limitations.

Citation:
Engebretsen L, Risberg MA, Robertson B, et al. Outcome after knee dislocations: a 2-9 years follow-up of 85 consecutive patients. *Knee Surg Sports Traumatol Arthrosc.* 2009;17(9):1013–1026.

Level of Evidence:
IV

Summary:
Engebretsen and colleagues report outcomes and surgical technique for 85 patients after knee dislocation. At final follow-up, the median Lysholm score was 83, knee function was found to be lower in patients who sustained high-energy compared with low-energy trauma, and 87% of injured knees had Kellgren and Lawrence grade 2 or higher compared with 35% of the uninjured knees.

Citation:
Harner CD, Waltrip RL, Bennett CH, et al. Surgical management of knee dislocations. *J Bone Joint Surg Am.* 2004;86A(2):262–273.

Level of Evidence:
III

Summary:
The authors describe their surgical technique and associated outcomes for 33 patients with multiligament knee injuries. Importantly, they found that acutely treated patients had higher subjective scores and improved objective knee stability.

Citation:
Fanelli GC, Edson CJ. Arthroscopically assisted combined anterior and posterior cruciate ligament reconstruction in the multiple ligament injured knee: 2- to 10-year follow-up. *Arthroscopy.* 2002;18(7):703–714.

Level of Evidence:
III

Summary:
Surgical technique and associated outcomes for 35 patients with multiligament injuries are reported. Nineteen patients were treated within 8 weeks and 16 were treated chronically; no significant subjective or objective differences were found between the two groups.

Citation:
Stannard JP, Brown SL, Farris RC, et al. The posterolateral corner of the knee: repair versus reconstruction. *Am J Sports Med.* 2005;33(6):881–888.

Level of Evidence:
II

Summary:
Stannard and colleagues performed a cohort study comparing posterolateral corner (PLC) repair versus reconstruction in combination with treatment of multiligament knee injuries. The failure rate for repairs of the PLC was significantly higher than for reconstructions.

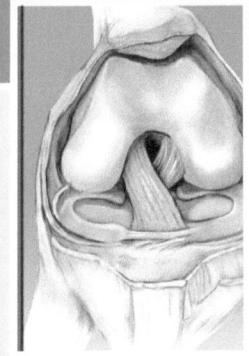

104

Knee Arthritis

Catherine Hui, Stephen R. Thompson, J. Robert Giffin

Knee osteoarthritis (OA) is an extremely common cause of disability. The etiology is multifactorial, but joint injury is a prevalent cause of OA in the knee.[1,2] Studies have shown that meniscal injury requiring a meniscectomy alters knee biomechanics and leads to gonarthrosis.[3] Anterior cruciate ligament (ACL) rupture, a frequently seen and often devastating injury, is characteristically associated with meniscal and chondral injuries.[4] Further deterioration of the joint related to multiple subluxation episodes over time leads to gonarthrosis, which typically affects the medial compartment and results in varus deformity.[5–9]

HISTORY

A thorough history will rule out systemic causes of pain, such as rheumatoid or other inflammatory arthritides, as well as referred hip pain or radiating pain resulting from degenerative disk disease. Patients with knee OA usually present with pain. Other symptoms include catching, locking, swelling, and decreased motion.[1,10,11] Instability is a frequent complaint, but in general it represents quadriceps weakness rather than true ligamentous instability.[12] Patients with chronic ACL deficiency in whom medial compartment gonarthrosis with subsequent varus deformity has developed may experience pain and/or instability. However, in these patients pain is the most common presenting symptom, and instability may not be present as a result of the constraint acquired through the degenerative process and the development of a "cupula" from posteromedial tibial wear.[8] Table 104.1 outlines key questions for patients presenting with knee OA.

PHYSICAL EXAMINATION

A systematic approach to the physical examination of the knee includes inspection, palpation, range of motion (ROM), and special tests when appropriate. A comparison of the affected and nonaffected limbs, an examination of the joints above and below the affected knee, and an assessment of the patient's distal neurovascular status are routine components of the physical examination.[13,14]

The inspection begins with an evaluation of limb alignment both while the patient is standing and walking. Varus, valgus, or neutral alignment is noted, as well as an antalgic or Trendelenburg gait or a thrust (i.e., a dynamic change in the deformity with weight bearing).[13,15] If possible, the patient should perform a full squat and the duck walk (Childress sign). Pain with either

or both of these activities suggests a meniscal tear.[16] Any previous incisions should be noted.

With the patient seated and his or her knees flexed over the edge of the table, patellar position and quadriceps asymmetry, if present, are determined. Quadriceps reflex inhibition due to knee injury and effusion frequently leads to quadriceps atrophy.[17,18]

An effusion, which is characterized by asymmetry in the peripatellar groove on either side of the patella, is confirmed with the swipe test. This test is performed with the patient in the supine position with his or her legs extended and relaxed. The examiner strokes the medial side starting just below the joint line and moves toward the suprapatellar pouch and then does the same on the lateral side while observing for a fluid-wave bulge medially. The presence of a fluid wave indicates a positive swipe test and confirms a small to medium intracapsular effusion.[14]

The patellar ballottement test identifies a moderate to severe effusion. With the knee in full extension, the examiner compresses the patella toward the trochlea and then releases it. If fluid is present, the patella will feel as if it were floating.[14]

Palpation of the knee structures is performed in a methodical fashion and guided by the suspected diagnosis. The temperature of the knee to touch is compared with that of the opposite knee. Increased warmth suggests the presence of inflammation. It is important to determine the point of maximal tenderness. Generally the area anticipated to be most tender is palpated last, so that the patient will not be guarding during the remainder of the examination.[14]

ROM compared with the contralateral knee is measured. Patellar tracking during ROM is palpated, as well as crepitus (a palpable grating sensation) during flexion and extension, with particular attention to its specific location.[14] Finally, the patient is asked to perform a straight leg raise to assess quadriceps strength and extensor mechanism function.[14]

Special tests are then performed, including an assessment of cruciate and collateral stability (see Chapter 90). These tests are particularly important to detect the presence of a chronically deficient ACL.

IMAGING

Radiographs taken during weight bearing are the gold standard for imaging any knee condition, especially OA. The standard radiographic knee series includes the following views: bilateral standing anteroposterior (AP), bilateral standing 45-degree posteroanterior

TABLE 104.1   Key Questions for Patients Presenting With Knee Osteoarthritis

Question	Patient Response
Identification	Age, occupation
Chief complaint	Pain/clicking/locking/swelling/decreased motion/instability
History of presenting illness	Pain history
	W: Where is most of the pain located? (point with finger)
	W: When did it start?
	Q: Quality of the pain; does it radiate?
	Q: Quantity of pain
	A: Aggravating factors
	A: Alleviating factors
	A: Associated symptoms
	Associated trauma or injury
	Mechanism of injury
	Date
	Treatment
Treatments to date	Analgesics, NSAIDs, bracing, physiotherapy, injections, surgery
Functional status	Walking tolerance (no. of blocks) as limited by knee symptoms
	Sleep disturbance
	Pain at rest
	ADLs
	Sports
Expectations	Return to physical work
	Return to sports and activities
	Level of competition
	High-impact versus low-impact activities

ADLs, Activities of daily living; *NSAIDs,* nonsteroidal antiinflammatory drugs.

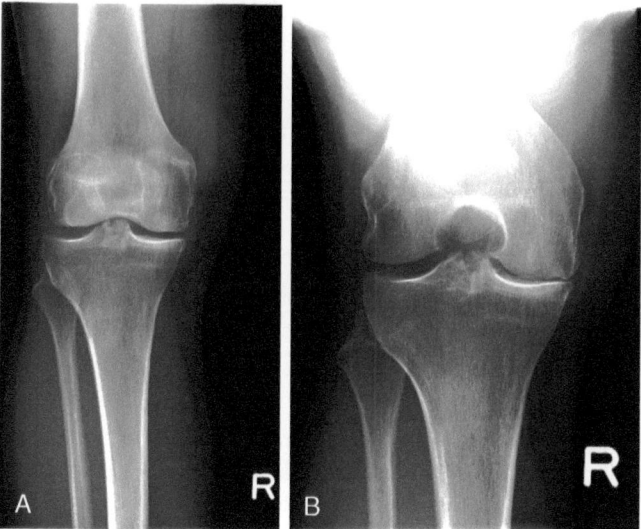

Fig. 104.1 (A) A conventional standing anteroposterior radiograph of the right knee with no visible joint space narrowing. (B) A "Rosenberg view" of the same knee shows evidence of joint space narrowing and osteoarthritis.

(PA) flexion, and lateral and skyline of the affected knee. The specific purpose of the two standing films is to identify joint space narrowing compared with the nonaffected knee.[19–21]

The weight-bearing 45-degree PA flexion radiograph was first described by Rosenberg et al.[21] in 1988 and is often referred to as the *Rosenberg view* (Fig. 104.1). The authors noted that some patients for whom no joint space narrowing was visible on standing full-extension AP views often were found to have areas of significant cartilage wear at the time of arthroscopy. As the knee is flexed during the stance phase of gait, the femorotibial contact area moves posteriorly and decreases in size, so that force per unit area loading of the knee is increased. Therefore the flexed knee is much more susceptible to chondral damage and subsequent OA. Furthermore, in patients with ACL deficiency, the altered knee biomechanics lead to increased posteromedial wear, particularly on the tibia. For these reasons, the Rosenberg view has better sensitivity and specificity than the conventional standing AP radiograph in detecting joint space narrowing and OA.[20,21]

If joint space narrowing is observed on the standard knee series, a standing hip to ankle radiograph should be obtained to assess limb alignment (Fig. 104.2). This view is critical for decision-making and surgical planning.[22–24] A line from the center of the hip to the center of the ankle defines the mechanical axis in the coronal plane.[25] This line generally passes through the

center of the knee in a neutrally aligned limb. Any deviation from this point is considered malalignment. If the line falls toward the medial side of the knee, the limb is in varus alignment; if the line falls toward the lateral side of the knee, the limb is in valgus alignment.[26]

Sagittal plane alignment is determined by measuring the posterior tibial slope. This angle is defined by a line perpendicular to the mid-diaphysis of the tibia and the posterior inclination of the tibial plateau on a lateral radiograph.[27]

Radiographs also identify signs of OA and its severity (e.g., osteophytes, joint space narrowing, subchondral sclerosis, and subchondral cysts), which areas of the knee are affected, limb alignment, posterior tibial slope, patellar height, previous fracture, deformity, and previous surgery as well as previous implants used and the location of the implants.

Magnetic resonance imaging (MRI) is a commonly ordered investigation in patients who present with knee conditions. However, most of the information required for decision-making in patients with knee OA can be gathered from a proper history, physical examination, and the aforementioned radiographs.[19] Bhattacharyya et al.[28] reviewed radiographs and MRI images in 154 patients (men ≥45 years; women ≥50 years) with symptomatic and asymptomatic knee OA. The groups were similar in age. However, patients in the symptomatic OA group had significantly higher body mass index (BMI) scores. The authors found that meniscal tears were highly prevalent in both asymptomatic (76%) and symptomatic (91%) cases of knee OA. Increased radiographic evidence of OA was associated with an increased rate of meniscal tears. No significant difference in pain and function was found on a visual analog scale or the Western Ontario and McMaster Universities Osteoarthritis Index (WOMAC) scores between patients with and without a medial or lateral meniscal tear in the osteoarthritic group. Ultimately the etiology of pain in patients with knee OA is multifactorial and can include cartilage lesions, synovial inflammation, and periarticular muscle strains. The

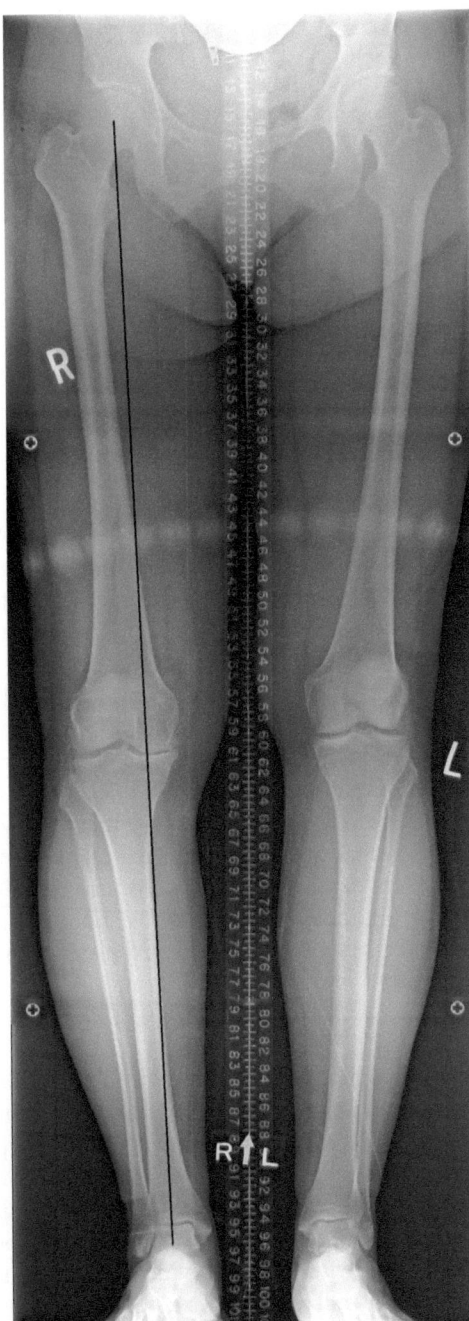

Fig. 104.2 This standing hip-to-ankle radiographic view is critical in decision-making and surgical planning. A line from the center of the hip to the center of the ankle defines the mechanical axis in the coronal plane. In a neutrally aligned limb, this line passes through the center of the knee. Any deviation from this point is considered malalignment. Here the line falls toward the medial side of the knee, indicating varus alignment of the limb.

investigators concluded that there is no indication for the routine use of MRI in the evaluation and management of patients with OA of the knee.[28]

TREATMENT OPTIONS

Fig. 104.3 shows possible treatment options, from least to most invasive.

Nonoperative Treatment Options

Education and Activity Modification

The natural history of OA is a waxing and waning course, with days when symptoms are manageable and days when symptoms seem to worsen. Patients should be educated about self-management techniques, including lifestyle and activity modification. Encouraging patients to take responsibility for their condition allows them to actively participate in their care and has been shown to improve symptoms.[29,30]

Weight Loss

Patients with symptomatic knee OA who have a BMI score of more than 25 kg/m^2 should be encouraged to lose weight through diet and exercise. Studies have shown an improvement in overall clinical function in the WOMAC function subscale with weight loss.[29,30] Other studies have shown that weight reduction decreases the knee joint load per step at a ratio of 1 lb lost to a 4-lb reduction in knee-joint load per step.[31,32] Weight loss not only has a beneficial effect on the symptoms of knee OA but also provides whole-body health benefits that cannot be overlooked.

Low-Impact Exercise

Multiple studies have shown that low-impact exercise—such as walking, biking, and using an elliptical trainer—has the beneficial effects of decreasing pain and disability in patients with knee OA.[29,30] The American Geriatrics Society recommends a minimum of 20 to 30 minutes of physical activity per day two to five times per week for persons with OA.[33]

Analgesic Medications

Patients who have a symptomatic osteoarthritic knee should be encouraged to use acetaminophen for pain relief. Studies comparing the use of acetaminophen (≤4 g/d) with a placebo have shown significant benefit in pain relief without any significant adverse effects.[29,30] In 2011, the US Food and Drug Administration (FDA) recommended that the dose of acetaminophen be changed to 3 g/day due to the risk of severe liver injury.[34]

Additionally, ketorolac (Tramadol) has been shown to have some benefit in the relief of pain and stiffness and improvement in function in patients with knee OA and may be considered.[35]

Nonsteroidal Antiinflammatory Drugs

In patients who have no risk factors for gastrointestinal disease, nonsteroidal antiinflammatory drugs (NSAIDs) may be prescribed for pain relief. Studies have shown a statistically significant favorable clinical response with the use of NSAIDs versus acetaminophen. Consideration for additional gastroprotective medication along with nonselective NSAID medication or cyclooxygenase-2 inhibitors is recommended. Topical NSAID medication has been shown to improve pain, stiffness, and function and should also be considered.[29,30]

Braces

The use of an unloader knee brace may be a cost-effective adjunct to treatment and a reasonable option to help decrease symptoms and increase function in patients with knee OA.[36,37] This type

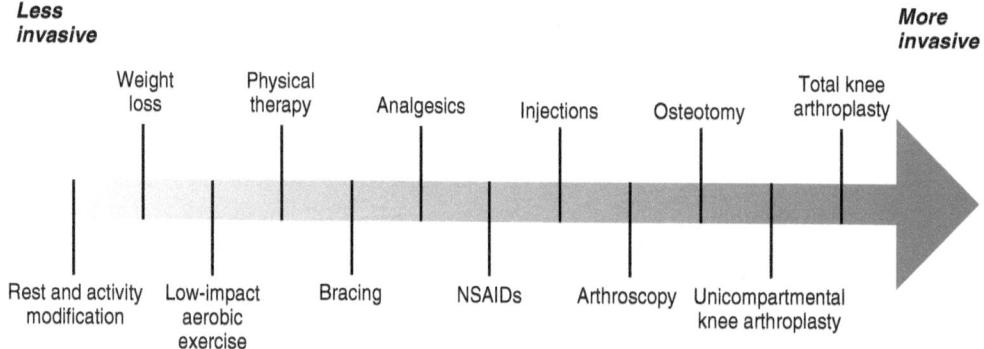

Fig. 104.3 Treatment options from least to most invasive for patients with symptomatic osteoarthritis of the knee. *NSAIDs,* Nonsteroidal antiinflammatory drugs.

of brace functions by helping to transfer the weight-bearing forces from the worn to the unworn part of the knee. Although it can be used for either varus or valgus deformities, it has been primarily studied in patients with medial compartment OA (MCOA). In a study by Kirkley et al.,[37] a varus unloader brace was shown to have significant benefit compared with a neoprene sleeve or medical management alone in decreasing pain and improving function. The authors recommended its use in patients with symptomatic unicompartmental OA who have a correctable deformity and an average-sized leg.[37] Also, the use of an unloader brace may help to determine whether the patient will have any benefit from a limb realignment procedure. A further advantage of bracing relates to proprioception. Studies have shown that patients with knee OA have decreased proprioception. Kirkley et al.[37] report that knee braces offer a proprioceptive benefit. The disadvantages to bracing are compliance, difficulty in obtaining a proper fit, and cost.

Physical Therapy
Quadriceps-strengthening exercises have been shown to provide a significant benefit for symptomatic pain relief. The use of ROM and stretching exercises has not been studied extensively and their clinical effect is unknown. However, flexibility and motion exercises appear to have no adverse effects and offer many health benefits.[38–40]

Injections
Corticosteroid. Intra-articular corticosteroid injections may be prescribed for the short-term relief of acute pain due to an arthritic "flareup." Studies have shown that the mean duration of the effect of a corticosteroid injection is 1 week.[41–43]

Viscosupplementation. Recent studies suggest that there is no benefit to viscosupplementation injections with hyaluronic acid in patients with symptomatic knee OA. A meta-analysis did demonstrate a statistically significant benefit of hyaluronic acid injections with regard to WOMAC pain, stiffness, and function, but these outcomes did not meet the clinically important improvement thresholds. In addition, meta-analysis in meaningfully important difference (MID) units demonstrated a low likelihood of patients achieving clinically important benefits from these injections. Based on these findings, we recommend against the use of hyaluronic acid injections in symptomatic knee OA.[35]

Platelet-rich plasma. Platelet-rich plasma (PRP) is derived from a patient's own blood. Therapeutic injections of PRP involve concentrating the levels of platelets in the plasma through ultra-high-speed centrifugation. Platelets secrete growth factors and proteins that stimulate tissue healing, and it is believed that this can help to alleviate the symptoms of knee arthritis. At present there is a paucity of evidence supporting the use of PRP in knee arthritis and it should be used with caution.[44]

Stem cells. Mesenchymal stem cells from bone marrow are the most common cells used in stem cell injections for OA. It is believed that these cells have the best potential for developing into cartilage cells that can repair damaged cartilage, decrease the rate of cartilage degeneration, suppress inflammation, and therefore decrease pain. Similar to PRP injections in knee OA, there is little evidence supporting the use of stem cell injections at present and they should be used with caution.[45]

Treatment Not Recommended
Several treatment options such as glucosamine and/or chondroitin, lateral heel wedges, and needle lavage have historically been prescribed as nonoperative treatment options for patients with symptomatic OA of the knee. However, a sufficient number of high-quality studies have shown that glucosamine hydrochloride and/or chondroitin sulfate have no clinical benefit compared with placebo.[35,46] Likewise, no good evidence exists to support the prescription of lateral heel wedges for MCOA of the knee.[47] Last, studies recommending needle lavage have been of poor quality, and the procedure has not been shown to have any lasting benefit.[48,49]

Operative Options
Arthroscopy
Arthroscopic lavage, débridement, and/or meniscectomy are not recommended in patients whose primary symptom is pain. In 2002 Moseley et al.[50] conducted the first of two randomized controlled studies of the effect of arthroscopic surgery in patients with OA of the knee who presented with knee pain. They compared arthroscopic surgery with arthroscopic lavage and "sham" surgery in 180 patients and found that results of arthroscopic surgery were no better than those of sham surgery at a follow-up of 2 years.[50] In 2008 Kirkley et al.[1] conducted another randomized controlled trial with 188 patients in which arthroscopic

surgery was compared with optimized physiotherapy and medical management. These investigators specifically addressed several weaknesses of the study by Moseley et al.,[50] which included the use of a nonvalidated outcome measure and the lack of generalizability of their results. This study also showed no difference among the three groups in WOMAC or Short Form (SF)-36 scores at 2 years after surgery. Dervin et al.[51] studied the ability of two groups of surgeons to independently predict the outcome of arthroscopic débridement based on clinical symptoms, signs, and plain radiography. A total of 126 patients were followed for 2 years subsequent to failure of medical management and arthroscopic débridement. Of these, 56 patients (44%) reported a clinically important reduction in pain on the WOMAC pain scale. Furthermore, the investigators found that physicians correctly predicted outcome only 59% or less of the time.[1]

Arthroscopic surgery is not recommended in patients with documented knee OA. Expert opinion suggests that arthroscopy should be considered only in cases where mechanical symptoms rather than pain are the chief complaint.[52]

Osteotomy

An osteotomy is a bone realignment procedure for unicompartmental arthritis of the knee. The biomechanical principle of osteotomy is to redistribute the weight-bearing forces from the worn to the unworn compartment of the knee to relieve pain and slow disease progression.[53–58] The most frequently seen deformity is varus alignment due to MCOA, with isolated lateral compartment OA one-eighth as common as isolated MCOA. The majority of osteotomies are performed on the proximal tibia to treat MCOA. Biopsy and second-look arthroscopic and other open procedures have shown that there is regrowth of fibrocartilage in the worn medial compartment with a predilection for the ulcerated regions of wear in the weight-bearing portion of the medial femoral condyle.[59–62] Box 104.1 outlines the indications for an osteotomy.

Medial compartment osteoarthritis. Both medial opening wedge high tibial osteotomy (HTO) and lateral closing wedge HTO have been used to successfully treat MCOA (Fig. 104.4).

The advantages and disadvantages of each technique are outlined in Table 104.2.

Medial opening wedge high tibial osteotomy. Historically, along with the points shown in Table 104.2, the concerns with medial opening wedge HTO have been prolonged immobilization and restricted weight bearing, both of which have a significant impact on the patient's quality of life. Recent improvements in implant technology have led to the development of locking plates for HTO. These devices are much stronger than previous nonlocking implants and allow weight bearing as early as 2 weeks after surgery with no loss of correction of the osteotomy and no delayed union or nonunion.[63,64] Another concern with medial opening wedge HTO is the morbidity associated with the harvesting of iliac crest bone graft required to fill the osteotomy. However, several recent studies have reported that an autograft, an allograft, and even no graft for corrections of 8 mm or less have produced good results, with union occurring by 12 weeks after surgery.[65,66]

Lateral closing wedge high tibial osteotomy. Coventry[67] first described the technique of lateral closing wedge HTO in 1965. Advantages and disadvantages are described in Table 104.2. Currently our only indication for this procedure is a previous successful lateral closing wedge HTO in the contralateral limb.

Other techniques. Less commonly used tibial osteotomy techniques include the dome osteotomy and external fixation. These techniques are recommended for deformities greater than 25 degrees as well for those that require gradual rather than acute correction, as in skeletally mature patients with Blount disease or in younger patients with idiopathic genu varum.[68–71]

BOX 104.1 Indications for an Osteotomy

Malalignment + Arthrosis
Malalignment + Instability
Malalignment + Arthrosis + Instability
Malalignment + Meniscal/Cartilage Transplant ± Instability

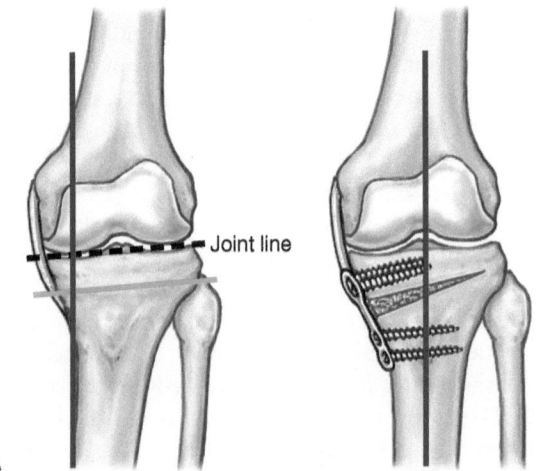

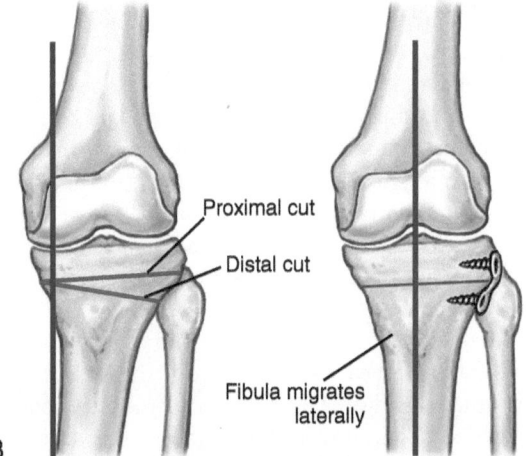

Fig. 104.4 Basic principles of opening wedge (A) and closing wedge (B) high tibial osteotomies.

TABLE 104.2	Medial Opening Wedge Versus Lateral Closing Wedge High Tibial Osteotomy	
	Advantages	**Disadvantages**
Medial opening wedge	The procedure is technically easier to perform (requiring just one bone cut). It provides the ability to achieve a predictable correction in coronal and sagittal planes. It can be combined with other procedures such as ligamentous reconstruction with relative ease. It restores bone stock.	Healing in distraction leads to more potential problems with delayed and nonunion. The tibial slope may be difficult to maintain.
Lateral closing wedge	Healing in compression leads to fewer problems with delayed and nonunion. It provides favorable alterations in the tibial slope to treat chronic anterior cruciate ligament deficiency.	The procedure is technically more difficult for inexperienced surgeons. • Peroneal nerve • Proximal tibiofibular joint It decreases bone stock. It makes future total knee arthroplasty more technically challenging.

Lateral compartment osteoarthritis. Lateral compartment OA can be caused by pathology on the femoral or tibial side of the knee. The osteotomy should be performed at the site of the cause of the deformity.

Proximal tibial osteotomies. The results of proximal tibial varus osteotomies have not equaled those of proximal tibial valgus osteotomies. A concern remains that proximal tibial osteotomies for lateral compartment OA will cause joint-line obliquity greater than 10 degrees, leading to lateral subluxation of the tibia. Another concern is that medial collateral ligament (MCL) laxity occurs if the wedge is taken above the MCL insertion. However, a role still exists for proximal tibial osteotomy in the valgus knee. This role includes small corrections of 12 degrees or less that avoid excessive joint line obliquity in persons with posttraumatic OA for whom the deformity is primarily at or below the joint. If the deformity is primarily in the femur or the correction is greater than 12 degrees, a distal femoral osteotomy should be considered.[72,73]

Distal femoral osteotomies. A distal femoral varus osteotomy is an appropriate procedure for patients with valgus deformity of the femur, such as a hypoplastic lateral femoral condyle, or if the required correction is greater than 12 degrees.[23] Again, this procedure can be a medial closing wedge or a lateral opening wedge osteotomy. The advantages and disadvantages of each procedure are similar to those listed for opening and closing wedge proximal tibial osteotomies in persons with MCOA (see Table 104.2). One additional advantage of a lateral opening wedge distal femoral osteotomy is that the correction can be tailored to the desired amount of varus. On the other hand, the medial closing wedge technique using a 90-degree blade plate typically results in a tibiofemoral angle correction of 0 degrees and a mechanical axis correction of 6 degrees varus.[72] Whether tailoring the correction with a lateral opening wedge technique is superior to using the medial closing wedge technique with regard to long-term outcome has yet to be determined.

Knee instability. Knee instability can be due to both bony and soft tissue factors. Ligamentous causes are the most common. However, altered tibial slope in the sagittal plane occurring in isolation as a result of a tibial physeal arrest or in combination with ligamentous insufficiency can also cause anteroposterior

instability. In such cases, the condition must be corrected to create a stable joint before ligamentous reconstruction, and a combined ligamentous and bony procedure should be considered to decrease the risk of graft failure.[5,8,74] Normally the posterior tibial slope is 10 degrees ± 3 degrees.[27] A posterior tibial slope greater than 13 degrees results in anterior tibial translation and altered joint biomechanics, as well as meniscal load sharing, leading to increased chondral wear. Similarly, a posterior tibial slope of less than 7 degrees (relative decreased slope) is also considered abnormal and leads to posterior translation of the tibia, which may have a similar outcome.[75] When these conditions are symptomatic, they should be addressed with an osteotomy to improve the bony stability. Osteotomies for sagittal plane deformities are usually approached anteriorly with either an anterior closing wedge osteotomy for increased tibial slope or an opening wedge osteotomy for decreased slope.[76]

Combined instability and pain. Patients with chronic ligamentous deficiency may present with pain, instability, or both. Patients most commonly have chronic ACL deficiency. However, posterior cruciate ligament and posterolateral corner insufficiency may also be present. It has been shown that in patients with instability and malalignment, soft tissue ligamentous reconstruction may fail because of the malalignment.[5,74] Therefore an osteotomy to correct the malalignment followed by simultaneous or staged ligamentous reconstruction should be considered.[8]

In patients for whom the primary symptom is instability with mild or moderate medial compartment degeneration, an osteotomy alone may not prove beneficial. Although ligament reconstruction alone has been shown to be successful,[9,77,78] it does not address the malalignment, predictably alleviate any symptoms of pain, or offer any chondroprotection to the damaged medial compartment. In these patients, an osteotomy to address pain combined with a simultaneous or staged soft tissue procedure to address ligament deficiency should be considered.

In patients presenting with chronic ACL deficiency, treatment options include lateral closing wedge osteotomy or combined HTO and ACL reconstruction. A lateral closing wedge osteotomy favorably decreases the tibial slope, which helps to improve instability related to ACL deficiency. A medial opening wedge osteotomy tends to change tibial slope in an unfavorable direction; therefore combined procedures should be considered.[53,55,79] Previous studies have described combined HTO and ACL reconstruction as simultaneous or staged procedures, with the osteotomy usually performed first.[74,80] Simultaneous medial opening wedge HTO and ACL reconstruction allows for biplanar correction of the knee deformity with restoration of ligamentous support in one operation and results in improvements in both bony and soft tissue support, which in theory leads to improved overall knee joint function.[6,81–83]

Return to sport after an osteotomy. The true benefit of an osteotomy is that is allows unrestricted activity while preserving the knee joint. Multiple studies have shown that HTO affords young, active patients with OA the ability to return to recreational sports and maintain an active lifestyle.[84,85] Van Raaij et al.[86] found that HTO postpones primary total knee arthroplasty (TKA) for a median of 7 years in this group of patients.

Patient satisfaction after high tibial osteotomy. With careful patient selection, satisfaction after HTO is very high. Hui et al.[87] showed that at a mean follow-up of 12 years, 85% of a cohort of 397 patients who underwent lateral closing wedge HTO were enthusiastic or satisfied and 84% would have the same surgery again. Similarly, at a mean of 6.5 years after surgery, Tang and Henderson[88] reported patient satisfaction of 76%, with 90% of patients saying they would choose the same surgery again.

Arthroplasty

Medial compartment osteoarthritis. For many years, unicompartmental knee arthroplasty (UKA) has been performed to treat isolated MCOA. The potential benefits of UKA compared with TKA are lower perioperative morbidity, less blood loss, maintenance of normal knee kinematics, and quicker patient rehabilitation and recovery.[89] Controversies remain regarding a fixed bearing versus mobile bearing implant design, but both have shown good long-term success.[90–92] However, concern remains regarding the durability of UKA in younger patients.[93]

Tricompartmental osteoarthritis. In patients presenting with severe tricompartmental osteoarthritis, the gold standard is a TKA. This procedure offers long-term, predictable pain relief. TKA for symptoms other than pain, such as stiffness, swelling, or instability, has unpredictable outcomes and is not recommended.[94]

Combined instability and pain. Historically, ACL insufficiency has been a contraindication to UKA because of concerns relating to increased anterior tibial translation and altered knee biomechanics with subsequent increased lateral compartment arthrosis and polyethylene wear resulting from posterior loading of the implant and ultimate prosthesis failure. Recently combined UKA using the Oxford prosthesis (Biomet, Oxford, UK) and ACL reconstruction has been performed to address both instability and pain related to MCOA. However, controversy remains regarding implant survival in this subgroup.[95,96] Lateral UKA is contraindicated in patients with ACL insufficiency because of increased lateral compared with medial compartment mobility, which leads to even more abnormal contact pressures and a potentially higher rate of failure.[97]

Return to sport after arthroplasty. Parratte et al.[93] reviewed data for 31 patients who underwent UKA at a mean age of 46 years (range, 41 to 49 years) and who were allowed unrestricted activity after surgery (data for a total of 35 knees were reviewed). At a mean follow-up of 9.7 years (range, 5 to 16 years), 75% had returned to manual work at the same level as before surgery, 60% had returned to the same level of participation in sports, and 30% were participating in sports at a lower level. Ten percent were unable to return to their sport. The authors acknowledge that revision for polyethylene wear remains the main concern.[93] In a biomechanical study, Kuster[98] previously demonstrated that running and jumping produces surface loads that exceed the limits of polyethylene resistance. The general recommendation for return to sport after an arthroplasty is low-impact activities such as cycling, bowling, swimming, scuba, golf, skating, cross-country skiing, weight lifting, dancing, and walking.[99]

DECISION-MAKING PRINCIPLES

Management of patients with knee OA should be individualized. Physiologic rather than chronologic age should be considered, along with the patient's goals and expectations. Patient education is paramount to the successful management of these patients. Fig. 104.5 outlines the treatment algorithm for patients presenting with knee OA. Management always begins with nonoperative treatment and progresses from less invasive to more invasive options (see Fig. 104.3).

Medial Compartment Osteoarthritis

Several factors must be considered in deciding on the best surgical treatment for patients with isolated MCOA of the knee for whom conservative management has failed. Table 104.3 outlines the indications for HTO versus UKA versus TKA in these patients.

TABLE 104.3 Indications for Surgery in Patients With Medial Compartment Osteoarthritis of the Knee

	HTO	UKA	TKR
Age[a]	≤65 years	≥55 years	≥65 years
Activity level	High	Low	Low
Body mass index	Any	<30	<30
Malalignment	5–20 degrees	0–5 degrees	Any
AP instability	Any	None[b]	Any[c]
ML instability	≤Grade II	None	Any[c]
ROM	Arc ≥120 degrees	Arc ≥90 degrees	Any
MCOA	Any	Any	Any
PFOA	≤Grade II[d]	≤Grade II[d]	Any
LCOA	Any	Any	Any

[a]Physiologic age should be considered here.
[b]Long-term results of combined ACL reconstruction and UKA have not been established.
[c]Increasing instability requires increased component constraint.
[d]For MCOA, the patient may have up to grade II PFOA if no patellofemoral symptoms are present.
AP, Anteroposterior; *HTO,* high tibial osteotomy; *LCOA,* lateral compartment osteoarthritis; *MCOA,* medial compartment osteoarthritis; *ML,* mediolateral instability; *PFOA,* patellofemoral osteoarthritis; *ROM,* range of motion; *TKR,* total knee replacement; *UKA,* unicompartmental knee arthroplasty.

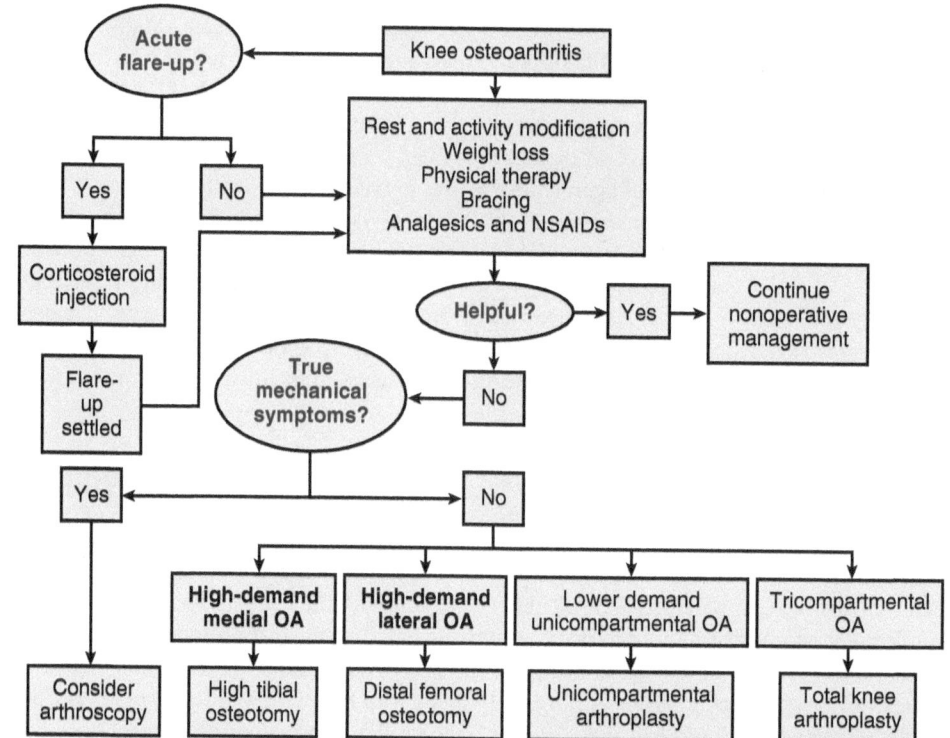

Fig. 104.5 A treatment algorithm for patients with knee osteoarthritis *(OA)*. *NSAIDs,* Nonsteroidal antiinflammatory drugs.

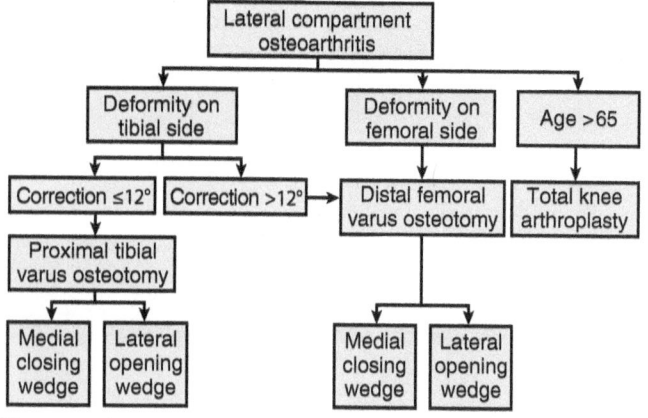

Fig. 104.6 A treatment algorithm for patients with lateral compartment knee osteoarthritis.

Lateral Compartment Osteoarthritis

In general, lateral compartment OA is better tolerated than MCOA. The treatment algorithm for patients with symptomatic lateral compartment OA of the knee for whom conservative management has failed is shown in Fig. 104.6. The lateral compartment UKA procedure remains controversial and is not recommended until longer-term results are reported.

Chronic Anterior Cruciate Ligamentous Insufficiency

Fig. 104.7 outlines the treatment algorithm for patients who present with symptomatic instability and pain caused by chronic ACL insufficiency. Use of UKA in patients with chronic ACL insufficiency with or without combined ACL reconstruction is controversial and is not recommended.

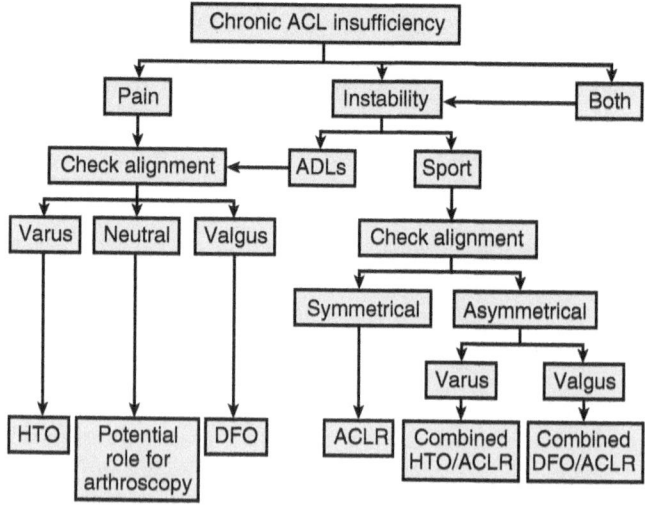

Fig. 104.7 A treatment algorithm for patients with chronic anterior cruciate ligament *(ACL)* insufficiency and osteoarthritis. *ACLR,* Anterior cruciate ligament reconstruction; *ADLs,* activities of daily living; *DFO,* distal femoral osteotomy; *HTO,* high tibial osteotomy.

⚐ Authors' Preferred Technique
Medial Collateral Osteoarthritis

Our preferred technique for physiologically young patients with medial compartment osteoarthritis who place a high demand on their knees is a medial opening wedge high tibial osteotomy. We use a modification of the technique previously described by Puddu and Franco.[100] Preoperative planning is critical to osteotomy surgery and begins with a determination of limb alignment in both the coronal and sagittal planes.

🔖 Authors' Preferred Technique

Medial Opening Wedge High Tibial Osteotomy

Preoperative Planning

1. Obtain the following radiographs of both limbs: standing anteroposterior (AP) in full extension, standing 30-degree posteroanterior, lateral, skyline, and standing hip to ankle.
   - Assess lateral and patellofemoral osteoarthritis (OA).
   - Measure patellar height.
   - Measure the posterior tibial slope.
2. Plan the osteotomy. We typically use the technique previously described by Dugdale et al. (Fig. 104.8).[101]
   - Measure the width of the tibial plateau.
   - Determine the correction point at 62.5% across the plateau from the medial edge. This point lies slightly lateral to the tip of the lateral tibial spine and equates to 3 to 5 degrees of mechanical valgus (see Fig. 104.8A).
   - Draw a line from the center of the femoral head to the 62.5% correction point (ȧ) and another line from the center of the ankle to this point (b) (see Fig. 104.8B).
   - Draw the intended osteotomy from the junction of the proximal tibial metadiaphysis (~4 cm from the top of the medial tibial plateau) to the top of the fibular head (ė) and measure the length of the osteotomy (see Fig. 104.8C).

- Transpose the intended osteotomy line (ė → ë) over the top of line b (see Fig. 104.8D).
- Draw a line (l) perpendicular to the top of line ë across to line ȧ. Measure the length of this line. This line serves as the base of an isosceles triangle and is the intended wedge size of the osteotomy (see Fig. 104.8E).

Diagnostic Arthroscopy

1. Examine the lateral and patellofemoral compartments.
   - If Ahlbäck grade II or III degeneration is present in the lateral compartment, consider correcting the weight-bearing line to 50% the distance across the width of the tibial plateau rather than to the 62.5% point.
   - If Ahlbäck grade IV degeneration is present in the lateral compartment, abandon the osteotomy and consider total knee arthroplasty at a later date.
   - If Ahlbäck grade IV degeneration is present in the patellofemoral joint, consider a concomitant tibial tubercle osteotomy (TTO).
2. Perform any meniscal work or débridement as required.
3. A 5-cm longitudinal incision is made starting 1 cm distal to the medial joint line midway between the tibial tubercle and the posteromedial border of the tibia (Fig. 104.9A).

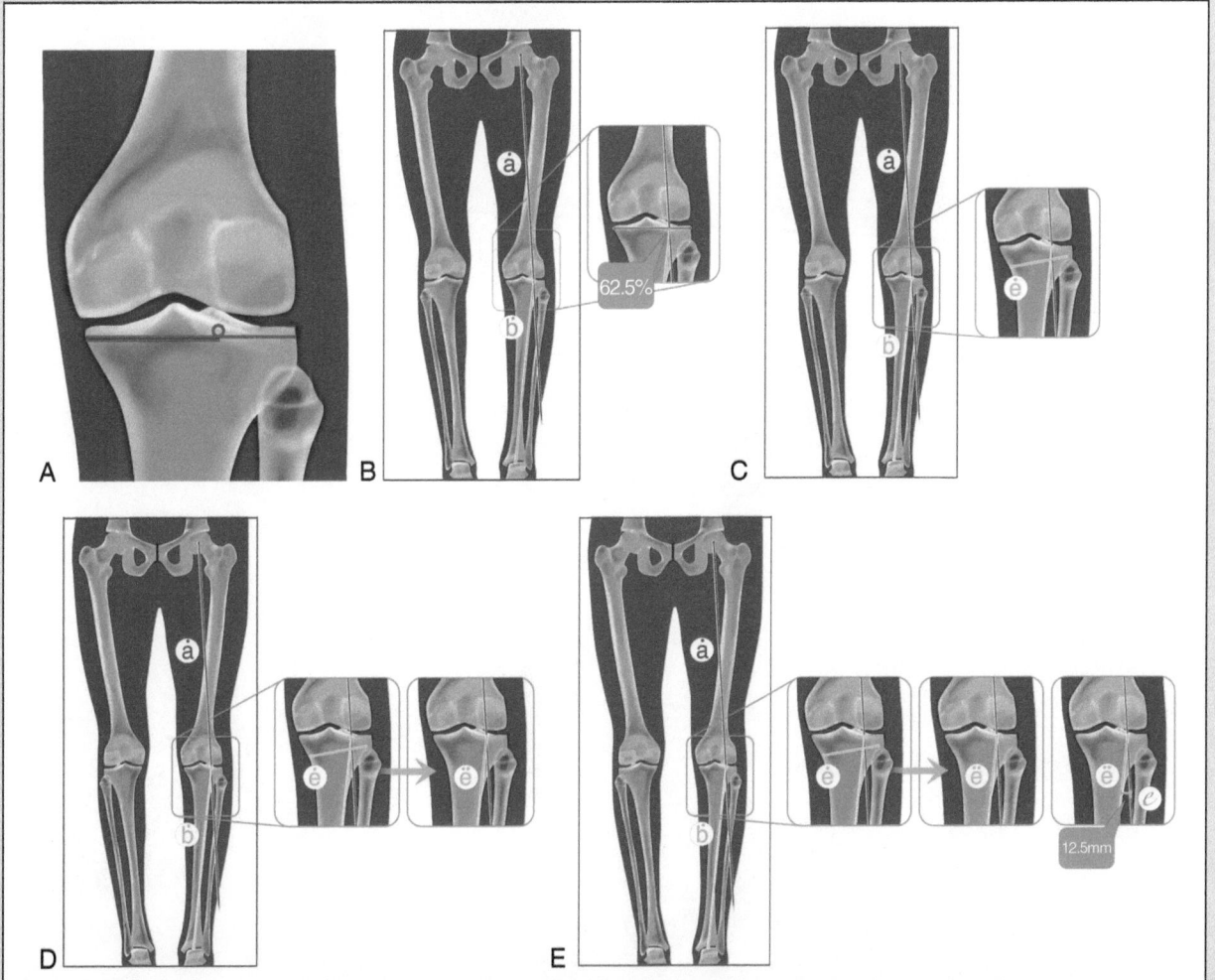

Fig. 104.8 The trigonometric method for planning the osteotomy size for an opening wedge high tibial osteotomy.

Continued

Authors' Preferred Technique—cont'd

Medial Opening Wedge High Tibial Osteotomy—cont'd

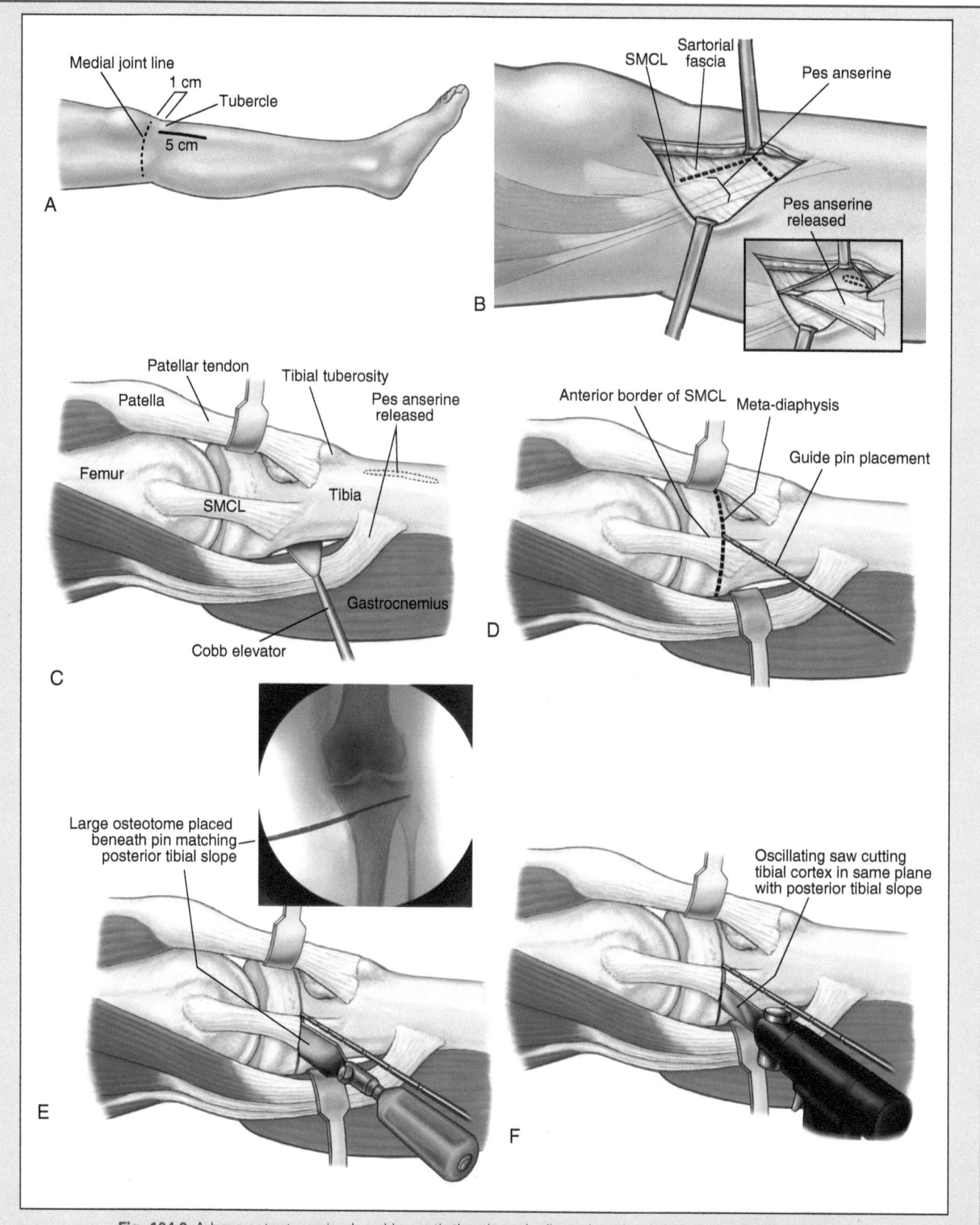

Fig. 104.9 A large osteotome is placed beneath the pin and adjusted so that it is in line with the posterior tibial slope on an anteroposterior image of the knee. With the knee and the osteotome in plane with the posterior tibial slope on the fluoroscopic image of the knee, the plane of the osteotomy will match the posterior tibial slope of the patient. This step is critical. *SMCL,* Superficial medial collateral ligament.

Authors' Preferred Technique—cont'd
Medial Opening Wedge High Tibial Osteotomy—cont'd

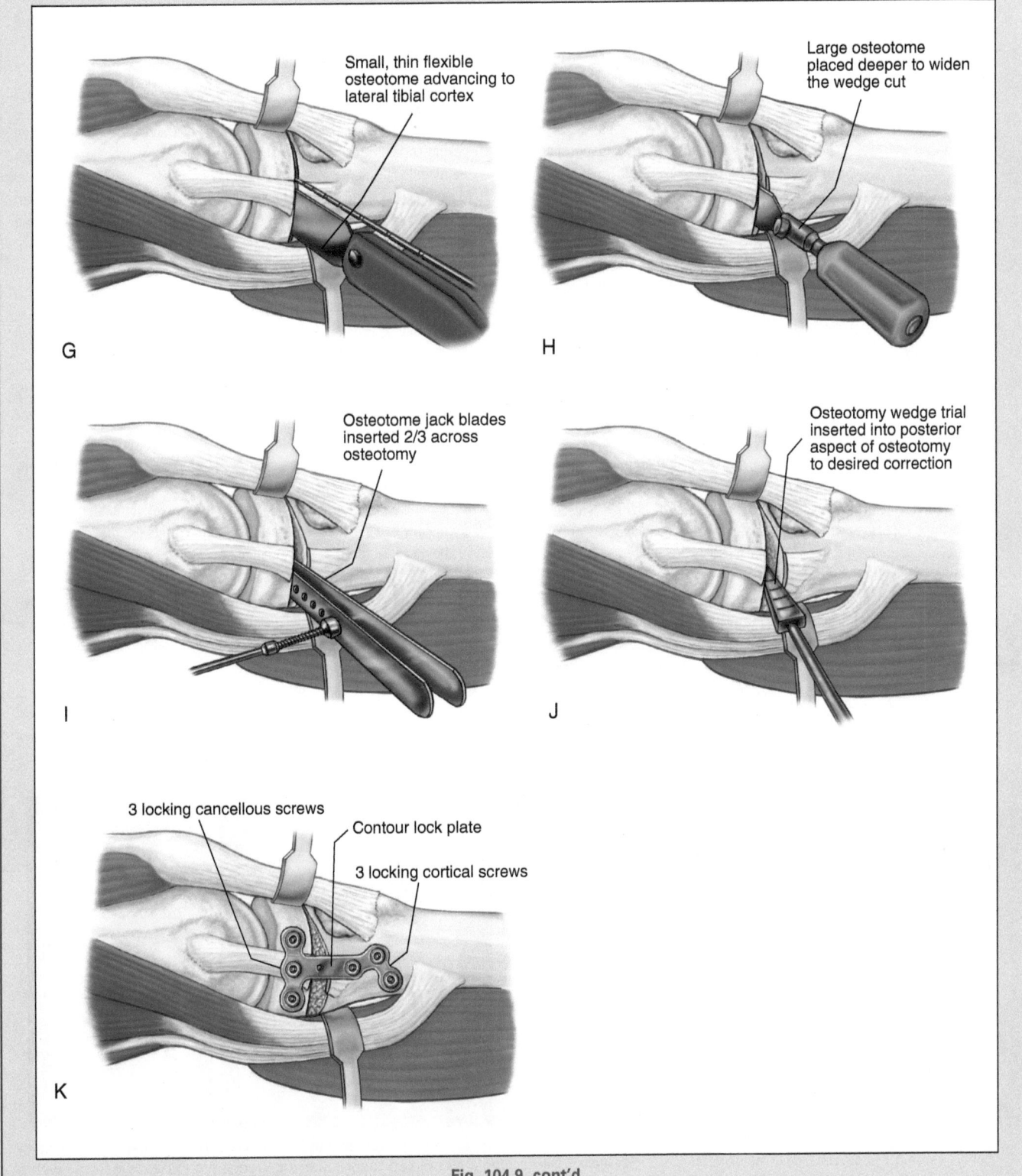

Small, thin flexible osteotome advancing to lateral tibial cortex

G

Large osteotome placed deeper to widen the wedge cut

H

Osteotome jack blades inserted 2/3 across osteotomy

I

Osteotomy wedge trial inserted into posterior aspect of osteotomy to desired correction

J

3 locking cancellous screws

Contour lock plate

3 locking cortical screws

K

Fig. 104.9, cont'd

Continued

Authors' Preferred Technique—cont'd

Medial Opening Wedge High Tibial Osteotomy—cont'd

4. Expose the sartorial fascia and open it at the top of the pes anserine. Retract the pes tendons distally. Sharply release the pes from its insertion onto the tibia to expose the superficial medial collateral ligament (MCL) (see Fig. 104.9B).

5. Identify the posteromedial border of the tibia and, using electrocautery, make a 1- to 1.5-cm longitudinal incision along this border in line with the fibers of the superficial MCL.

6. Using a Cobb elevator, bluntly lift the gastrocnemius off the posterior aspect of the tibia, making sure to stay on the bone (see Fig. 104.9C).

7. Insert a finger into this interval to ensure that the dissection has been carried out across the entire width of the tibia and insert a blunt retractor to protect the neurovascular structures.

8. Next, identify the medial border of the patellar tendon and the interval between the tibia and patellar tendon bursa. Place a retractor into this interval.

9. Obtain an AP image of the knee in line with the posterior tibial slope (at approximately 10 degrees of knee flexion).

10. Place a guide pin along the anterior border of the superficial MCL at the junction of the metadiaphysis of the proximal tibia. Under fluoroscopy, direct the pin toward the top of the fibular head to a point approximately 1 cm below the lateral joint line (see Fig. 109.4D).

11. Place a large osteotome beneath the pin and adjust it so that it is in line with the posterior tibial slope on an AP image of the knee. With the knee and the osteotome in plane with the posterior tibial slope on the fluoroscopic image of the knee, the plane of the osteotomy will match the posterior tibial slope of the patient. This step is critical (see Fig. 104.9E).

12. Mark the position of the osteotome with a marking pen followed by electrocautery (see Fig. 104.9D). If a TTO is required, mark the osteotomy line 1 cm short of the tibial tubercle (see the section titled "Concomitant Tibial Tubercle Osteotomy" in this box for details).

13. Cut the tibial cortex with a small oscillating saw blade between the tibial tubercle and the posteromedial tibial border (see Fig. 104.9E). It is imperative that the angle of the saw blade be in plane with the posterior tibial slope, similar to the osteotome in step 11. The osteotomy is made below the guide pin to avoid proximal migration of the osteotomy into the joint.

14. The osteotomy is advanced toward the lateral tibial cortex using small, thin, flexible osteotomes (see Fig. 104.9F).

15. Graduated solid osteotomes are then used, starting with the broadest, which is usually advanced to two-thirds the width of the osteotomy. A narrow osteotome is then used along the posterior tibial cortex and is advanced to approximately 1 cm from the lateral tibial cortex under fluoroscopic guidance. Again, it is critical for the plane of the osteotomy to mimic the posterior tibial slope (see Fig. 104.9G).

16. Check the mobility of the osteotomy by applying a valgus force across the osteotomy. It should open easily. If it does not open easily, step 15 should be repeated until the osteotomy opens without difficulty to the desired wedge size.

17. Insert both blades of an osteotome jack approximately two-thirds across the osteotomy and gradually open the jack to the desired correction (see Fig. 104.9H).

18. At this point, check that the osteotomy is trapezoid in shape (i.e., narrower anteriorly and wider posteriorly because the tibia is a triangular-shaped bone). A rectangular-shaped osteotomy indicates that the posterior tibial slope has been altered.

19. Insert the osteotomy wedge trial to the desired correction and confirm that the limb is in valgus alignment (see Fig. 104.9I).

20. With the wedge trial holding the osteotomy open, insert the plate into the osteotomy site. Bend the plate as required to fit the shape of the tibia. Once the plate has been inserted, remove the wedge trial.

21. Secure the plate with three locking cancellous screws above and three locking cortical screws below. The screws should be directed away from the osteotomy (see Fig. 104.9J).

22. Mix corticocancellous allograft bone chips with 1 g of vancomycin powder. Insert and pack the mixture into the osteotomy with a bone tamp. Note that bone grafting is optional for corrections of 7.5 mm or less (Fig. 104.10).

23. Repair the pes anserine over the top of the plate.

24. Insert a drain to exit separately from the incision.

25. Close the skin over the top of the drain.

26. Apply a hinged knee brace locked in full extension.

Concomitant Tibial Tubercle Osteotomy

Indications for a concomitant TTO are (1) large corrections greater than 12.5 mm and (2) severe patellofemoral osteoarthritis.

1. If a TTO is required, mark the osteotomy line 1 cm short of the tibial tubercle in step 12. It is important that the thickness of the TTO be 1 cm proximally to avoid fracture.

2. From this point, mark a line exiting the anterior tibial cortex approximately 3 cm distally using electrocautery. For a larger correction, the length of the TTO should be extended to allow enough room for adequate fixation because the tubercle will translate superomedially with the opening of the osteotomy.

3. After the osteotomy cut has been made, make a flat TTO cut along the previously marked line with the small oscillating saw from medial to lateral. It is important that the cut be flat to allow appropriate translation of the tubercle when the osteotomy is distracted.

4. Proceed with steps 14 to 22 as previously outlined.

5. Just before closure (step 23), secure the TTO with one or two 4.5-mm cortical screws from an anterior-to-posterior direction. It is important to countersink these screws to avoid screw prominence anteriorly.

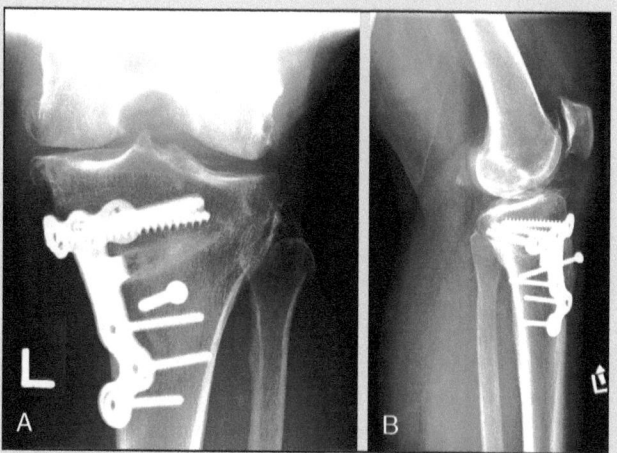

Fig. 104.10 Anteroposterior (A) and lateral (B) radiographs demonstrating a completed medial opening wedge high tibial osteotomy with a tibial tubercle osteotomy.

POSTOPERATIVE MANAGEMENT

The most important aspect of rehabilitation after an HTO is ROM. Early postoperative knee ROM exercises promote healing and articular cartilage nourishment as well as lower limb neuromuscular function. Normal weight bearing is encouraged as soon as possible to help with bone turnover and healing.[102] With the advent of locking-plate technology, partial weight bearing can commence at 2 weeks after surgery; full weight bearing is usually achieved by 6 weeks. Several recent studies have shown that early weight bearing with locking plates does not negatively affect limb alignment, loss of correction, and delayed/nonunion.[63,64]

Table 104.4 outlines our rehabilitation protocol after uncomplicated medial opening wedge HTO using a locking plate. Each phase in this regimen builds on the previous one, and every patient should be treated on an individual basis based on the type of surgery he or she underwent. For example, if concomitant procedures such as ligament reconstruction, microfracture, or meniscal transplant are performed, the rehabilitation program should be altered with these procedures in mind. If a nonlocking plate is used, the approximate time lines must be adjusted accordingly.

Return to sport and activity is permitted when radiographic and clinical evidence shows bone healing and the patient has regained muscle bulk and control of the newly aligned limb. Timing of return to play (RTP) depends on the individual patient, his or her type of surgery, and his or her sport or activity. RTP can occur in as few as 6 months or as many as 18 months after surgery. Most patients are able to return to the sport they previously played. However, some patients may never be able to return at the same level.[84,85]

RESULTS

The mid- and long-term outcomes of HTO for MCOA of the knee have been well established and are shown in Table 104.5.[87,88,103–108] Fewer, smaller studies reporting the outcomes of distal femoral osteotomies for lateral compartment OA of the knee are available (Table 104.6).[109–118] Lateral compartment OA is less common than medial compartment disease; frequently patients with lateral compartment OA have an inflammatory arthropathy that precludes realignment procedures.

Although numerous large long-term studies of closing wedge proximal tibia and distal femoral osteotomies have been performed, fewer studies of the opening wedge osteotomy exist. Hernigou et al.[108] published the largest study on medial opening wedge HTO in 1987 with a mean follow-up of 11.5 years. Outcomes of lateral opening wedge distal femoral osteotomies have been reported in small case series with short-term follow-up periods.[109,110]

Complications

Complications of HTO can be categorized as intraoperative, early postoperative, or late postoperative. Table 104.7[71,119–121] outlines the most common complications and their management. Complications after a distal femoral osteotomy are very similar to those that occur after a proximal tibial osteotomy.

TABLE 104.4   Postoperative Rehabilitation Guidelines After a Medial Opening Wedge High Tibial Osteotomy

Phase	Approximate Time Line	Guidelines	Restrictions
1 (Immediate postoperative)	Day of surgery to 2 weeks	Manage pain and swelling Start ROM exercises (may come out of brace) Activate quadriceps	Brace is worn full time except during exercises (locked in extension) Feather/touch weight bearing
2 (Early postoperative)	2–6 weeks	Regain full ROM (especially extension) Gait retraining → progress to WBAT Stationary bike with low resistance Core/proximal muscle/quadriceps strengthening	Brace is worn full time except during exercises (fully unlocked)
3 (Muscle strengthening and control)	6 weeks–3 months	Normal gait—no limp Continue strengthening Stretching and flexibility Increase cardiovascular fitness with low-impact exercise Balance and proprioception exercises (e.g., wobble board) Pool work (e.g., water running)	Brace is off Low-impact activities
4 (Neuromuscular retraining and return to normal function)	3–6 months	Begin neuromuscular training exercises Continue strengthening Progress to resistance on gym equipment and maintain cardiovascular fitness May ride normal bicycle	
5 (Return to sport and activities)	9–12 months	Progress to neuromuscular training exercises May progress to higher-impact activities Gradual return to all activities, including sports	No restrictions

ROM, Range of motion; *WBAT*, weight bearing as tolerated.

TABLE 104.5   Long-Term Outcomes of a High Tibial Osteotomy for Medial Compartment Osteoarthritis

Study	Year	No.	Mean Follow-Up (Years) (Range)	Mean Age (Years)	Technique	Outcomes
Hui et al.[87]	2011	455 patients	12 (1–19)	50	LCW	95% survival 5 years 79% survival 10 years 56% survival 15 years
Saragaglia et al.[103]	2011	110 patients (124 knees)	10.4 (8–14)	53.3	MOW	88% survival 5 years 74% survival 10 years
DeMeo et al.[104]	2010	20 patients	8.3 (2–14)	49.4	MOW	70% survival 8 years
Akizuki et al.[105]	2008	132 patients	16 (16–20)	63	LCW	98% survival 10 years 90% survival 15 years
Gstöttner et al.[106]	2008	111 patients (132 knees)	12 (1–25)	54	LCW	80% survival 10 years 66% survival 15 years
Tang and Henderson[88]	2005	67 knees	6.5 (1–21)	49	LCW	75% survival 10 years 67% survival 15 years
Naudie et al.[107]	2004	85 patients (106 knees)	14 (10–22)	55	LCW	95% survival 5 years 80% survival 10 years 65% survival 15 years
Hernigou et al.[108]	1987	184 patients (250 knees)	11.5 (10–13)	60.3	MOW	90% good/excellent 5 years 45% good/excellent 10 years

LCW, Lateral compartment wedge; *MOW*, medial opening wedge.

TABLE 104.6   Long-Term Outcomes of a High Tibial Osteotomy for Lateral Compartment Osteoarthritis

Study	Year	No.	Mean Follow-Up (Years) (Range)	Mean Age (Years)	Technique	Outcomes
Sternheim et al.[109]	2011	41 patients (45 knees)	13.3 (3–25)	46.2	MCW	90% survival 10 years 79% survival 15 years 21.5% survival 20 years
Puddu et al.[110]	2009	30 patients	– (4–12)	52	LOW	82% good/excellent
Das et al.[111]	2008	12 patients	74 months[a] (51–89)	52	LOW	58% good/excellent
Backstein et al.[112]	2007	38 patients (40 knees)	10 (3–20)	44	MCW	82% survival 10 years 45% survival 15 years
Wang and Hsu[113]	2006	30 patients	8 (5–14)	53	MCW	87% survival 10 years
Gross and Hutchison[114]	2000	20 patients (21 knees)	11 (5–20)	56	MCW	83% survival 4 years 64% survival 10 years
Marti et al.[115]	2000	15 patients	– (1–14)	59	MCW	73% good results
Finkelstein et al.[116]	1996	20 patients (21 knees)	11 (8–20)	59	MCW	64% survival 10 years
Healy et al.[117]	1988	21 patients (23 knees)	4 (2–9)	56	MCW	83% good/excellent
McDermott et al.[118]	1988	24 patients	4 (2–11.5)	52	MCW	92% good results (most improvement in pain)

[a]Telephone follow-up of functional Hospital for Special Surgery and Lysholm score.
LOW, Lateral opening wedge; *MCW*, medial compartment wedge.

SUMMARY

Knee OA is a common condition encountered by all physicians. Arthritis in an athlete can be particularly difficult to treat, given the high demands that athletes place on their bodies. Because opening wedge osteotomies have emerged as the preferred method of surgical management, future studies should focus on determining the long-term outcomes in larger numbers of patients. Additionally, better defining the success of early weight bearing after locking-plate HTO will be vital.

Conservative management should be the first line of therapy. Surgical intervention is considered in patients who have exhausted conservative therapies. Joint-preserving osteotomy procedures are recommended in active persons with unicompartmental OA.

TABLE 104.7   Complications Associated With High Tibial Osteotomy Surgery

Complication	Osteotomy	Frequency (%)	Management
Intraoperative			
Intra-articular fracture	MOW	7–18.2	Determine if additional fixation required
			Consider changing weight-bearing status postoperatively
Fracture of opposite cortex	MOW	4.3	No additional procedure required (MOW)
	LCW		Additional fixation required (LCW)
Peroneal nerve injury	LCW	2–16	Most commonly neurapraxia—monitor and consider NCS and EMG 6 weeks after surgery if no sign of improvement
			Tag ends of nerve and consult plastic surgeon if patient has direct nerve injury
Vascular injury	All	0.4	Gain proximal and distal control of vessel if possible
			Call vascular surgeon
Early Postoperative			
Undercorrection/overcorrection	All	—	Revision osteotomy
Hematoma	All	10.2	Preventable with insertion of drain
			Irrigation and débridement if associated with prolonged drainage
Infection	All	2.3–81	Antibiotic therapy
			Regular pin site care with external fixator
VTE	All	1.3–9.8	No routine prophylaxis required—encourage mobilization
			Consider prophylaxis with LMWH in high-risk patients
			Prophylaxis with 6 weeks of warfarin (Coumadin) in patients with known history of VTE
Stiffness	All	3	Preventable with early ROM
			Physiotherapy
			Consider manipulation with the patient anesthetized once the osteotomy has united
			Consider arthrolysis if severe
Compartment syndrome	All	2–2.6	Emergent compartment release
Late Postoperative			
Delayed union	MOW	4.3	Rule out infection
			Bone graft osteotomy site
Nonunion	MOW	0.7–4.4	Rule out infection
			Bone graft osteotomy site
Pseudoarthrosis	MOW	0.7–4.4	Rule out infection
			Bone graft osteotomy site
Hardware irritation	All	4.3	Implant removal
Loss of correction	All	4.4–15.2	Revision osteotomy
Failure of fixation	All	4.4–16.4	Revision osteotomy
Patella baja	All	7.6–8.8	Consider simultaneous TTO for MOWHTO corrections ≥12.5 mm
			Early ROM

EMG, Electromyography; LCW, lateral closing wedge; LMWH, low molecular weight heparin; MOW, medial opening wedge; MOWHTO, medial opening wedge high tibial osteotomy; NCS, nerve conduction study; ROM, range of motion; TTO, tibial tubercle osteotomy; VTE, venous thromboembolism.
Data from references 71, 119, 120, and 121.

TKA is a successful procedure reserved for less active persons or those with tricompartmental arthritis.

For a complete list of references, go to ExpertConsult.com.

SELECTED READINGS

Citation:

Bhattacharyya T, Gale D, Dewire P, et al. The clinical importance of meniscal tears demonstrated by magnetic resonance imaging (MRI) in osteoarthritis of the knee. *J Bone Joint Surg Am.* 2003;85A(1):4–9.

Level of Evidence:

I

Summary:

Meniscal tears are highly prevalent in both asymptomatic and clinically osteoarthritic knees of older persons. Because osteoarthritic knees with a meniscal tear are not more painful than those without a tear and the meniscal tears do not affect functional status, magnetic resonance imaging should not be routinely ordered for patients with osteoarthritis of the knee.

Citation:

Coventry M. Osteotomy of the upper portion of the tibia for degenerative arthritis. *J Bone Joint Surg.* 1965;47:984–990.

Level of Evidence:

IV

Summary:

In this classic article, Coventry describes his original lateral closing wedge high tibial osteotomy technique and his encouraging results in a case series of 32 patients with varus osteoarthritis of the knee.

Citation:

Dugdale TW, Noyes FR, Styer D. Preoperative planning for high tibial osteotomy. The effect of lateral tibiofemoral separation and tibiofemoral length. *Clin Orthop Relat Res.* 1992;274:248–264.

Level of Evidence:

IV

Summary:

This article describes how to preoperatively plan the correction required during high tibial osteotomy surgery to restore the weight-bearing line (center femoral head to center tibiotalar joint) to a point 62.5% across the width of the tibial plateau.

Citation:

Felson D, Zhang Y, Anthony J, et al. Weight loss reduces the risk for symptomatic knee osteoarthritis in women: the Framingham study. *Ann Intern Med.* 1992;116(7):535.

Level of Evidence:

IV

Summary:

This report on a large case series with long-term follow-up shows that weight loss reduces the risk for symptomatic osteoarthritis in women.

Citation:

Hernigou P, Medevielle D, Debeyre J, et al. Proximal tibial osteotomy for osteoarthritis with varus deformity. A ten- to thirteen-year follow-up study. *J Bone Joint Surg Am.* 1987;69A(3):332–354.

Level of Evidence:

IV

Summary:

This article includes the longest published follow-up of patients undergoing opening wedge high tibial osteotomy for varus osteoarthritis of the knee and shows good success at a mean of 11 years after surgery.

Citation:

Kirkley A, Birmingham TB, Litchfield RB, et al. A randomized trial of arthroscopic surgery for osteoarthritis of the knee. *N Engl J Med.* 2008;359(11):1097–1107.

Level of Evidence:

I

Summary:

This article reports that arthroscopic surgery for osteoarthritis of the knee provides no additional benefit to optimized physical and medical therapy.

Citation:

Moseley JB, O'Malley K, Petersen NJ, et al. A controlled trial of arthroscopic surgery for osteoarthritis of the knee. *N Engl J Med.* 2002;347(2):81–88.

Level of Evidence:

I

Summary:

This article reports that the outcomes after arthroscopic lavage or arthroscopic débridement were no better than those after a placebo procedure in patients with knee osteoarthritis.

Citation:

Richmond J, Hunter D, Irrgang J, et al. Treatment of osteoarthritis of the knee (nonarthroplasty). *J Am Acad Orthop Surg.* 2009;17(9):591–600.

Level of Evidence:

I

Summary:

This article provides American Academy of Orthopaedic Surgeons–approved evidence-based clinical practice guidelines for the appropriate nonoperative treatment of knee osteoarthritis.

Citation:

Rosenberg TD, Paulos LE, Parker RD, et al. The forty-five-degree posteroanterior flexion weight-bearing radiograph of the knee. *J Bone Joint Surg Am.* 1988;70A(10):1479–1483.

Level of Evidence:

IV

Summary:

This article reports that posteroanterior weight-bearing radiographs with the knee at 45 degrees of flexion were more accurate, more specific, and more sensitive than conventional extension weight-bearing AP radiographs.

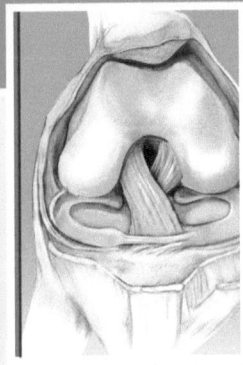

105

Patellar Instability

Seth L. Sherman, Betina B. Hinckel, Jack Farr

Patellar instability is a broad topic that encompasses a continuum of patellar abnormalities. To address this complex topic, it is important to first define several terms. During the normal knee flexion cycle, the patella tracks in the center of the femoral trochlea. *Maltracking* occurs when the patella deviates from the bony constraints of the trochlear groove during the range of motion (ROM) arc. The term *subluxation* is used to describe a specific episode in which the patella partially leaves the trochlear groove. When the patella displaces completely from the trochlear groove, it is considered a *dislocation. Recurrent patellar dislocation* refers to occurrences of two or more dislocations. *Chronic patellar dislocation* describes the rare situation in which the patella remains dislocated for months or years. Patients with abnormal skeletal anatomy, defined as *malalignment*, are predisposed to maltracking and instability. Similar to maltracking, malalignment implies a deviation from normal biomechanics or anatomy, but does not always result in patellar instability.

Patellar dislocations represent 2% to 3% of all knee injuries and are the second most common cause of traumatic knee hemarthrosis.[1,2] The annual risk of a first-time patellar dislocation is 5.8 per 100,000.[3] Although most people who experience a first-time dislocation will have no further instability, the literature reports a recurrence rate of 15% to 60% and an annual risk of recurrence of 3.8 per 100,000.[3–7] Patient demographic (i.e., young age, open physis) and morphologic (i.e., patella alta, trochlea dysplasia) risk factors have been shown to increase the relative risk of recurrent instability following an index dislocation event.

Great variability in patient symptoms and underlying bony and soft tissue pathology makes it difficult to form strict guidelines for treatment recommendations. A thorough understanding of the specific patellar abnormalities, the level of functional disability, and the patient's desired activity level must be taken into account when evaluating and assessing a patient with patellar instability. Identification and correction of anatomic and biomechanical risk factors form the basis for developing successful individualized nonoperative and operative treatment strategies.

HISTORY

In the assessment of a patient with patellar instability, it is imperative to determine the mechanism of injury. Sports-related activities account for 61% to 72% of first-time dislocations.[3,8] Patellar instability may result from direct trauma to the medial knee or, more frequently, an indirect injury, such as when the leg rotates around a planted foot (Fig. 105.1). In most cases of patellar dislocation, the patella will spontaneously reduce when the knee is extended. Often, patients will report feeling the knee "give way" and the kneecap "pop" or "clunk" in or out of place. They may describe an abnormal shape to the inside of the knee, often confusing the prominent medial femoral condyle for what they mistakenly think is a medially dislocated patella. Patients may state that the patella reduced when they extended their knee or that they pushed it back into place. Swelling will develop soon after the injury in most patients unless their patella is very unstable and multiple episodes have occurred; in those cases, subsequent swelling and pain may be minor or absent. The dislocation and reduction can occur so rapidly that the patient cannot recognize the dislocation, but only the abrupt pain and swelling or hemarthrosis. This is particularly important in children who more often are unable to provide details of the event. Patellar dislocation is the most frequent cause of hemarthrosis in children[9] and therefore should be suspected in any children with traumatic hemarthrosis.

It is important to distinguish pain secondary to patellar instability from that of other patellofemoral disorders. Patellofemoral pain syndrome (PFPS) is the most common cause of anterior knee pain and can be confused with patellar instability. Furthermore, it is not uncommon for patients with instability to also experience PFPS. Patients with PFPS typically describe anterior knee pain exacerbated by prolonged sitting or when descending the stairs. The pain may be bilateral, or it may change from one knee to the other over time. In addition, the patients may feel like the knee is "unstable," but when questioned carefully, they do not describe the same mechanisms of injury that would result in frank instability or they do not experience episodes in which the patella actually leaves the trochlear groove. Distinguishing between the two clinical entities is imperative because isolated PFPS is rarely treated successfully by surgical means.

Cartilage lesions are very common in patients with patellar instability and may be symptomatic. Joint swelling, although not specific to cartilage disease, is more suspicious for a cartilage etiology than pain alone. Identifying the cartilage defect as the sole source of pain is particularly difficult in patients with recurrent patellar instability. In these patients, the presence of biologic effusion between episodes of instability suggests that cartilage damage is at least a component of the symptomology.

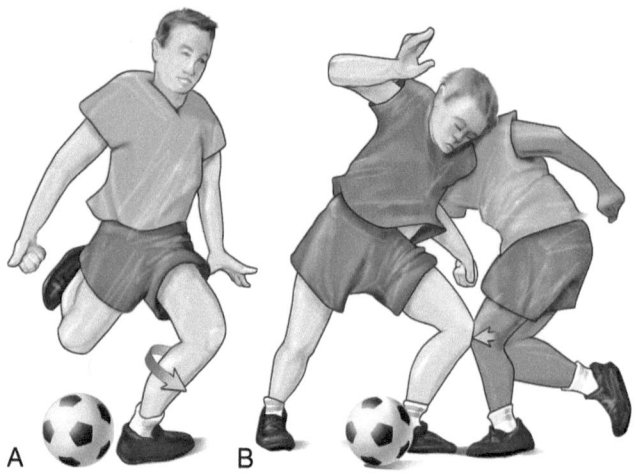

Fig. 105.1 Mechanisms of acute patellar dislocation. A noncontact dislocation occurs by external rotation of the lower leg relative to the body (A), whereas contact injuries are caused by a direct blow to the medial side of the knee (B). (Modified from The Cleveland Center for Medical Art & Photography, Copyright 2008.)

PHYSICAL EXAMINATION

Pertinent Bony Anatomy

Lower extremity alignment is determined primarily by the relationship between the femur and tibia. Abnormalities in the position and relationship of these bony structures result in malalignment that can predispose patients to patellar instability. Normally, the knee has an anatomical tibiofemoral angle of approximately 5 to 7 degrees of valgus.[10,11] With excess knee valgus, or genu valgum, the mechanical pull of the quadriceps muscle changes, increasing the normal laterally directed force vector on the patella. The rotation of the femur and tibia also influences patellar stability. Normally, the femoral neck has 7 to 20 degrees of anteversion and the tibia has 15 degrees of external rotation (Fig. 105.2).[12,13] Increases in femoral anteversion and external tibial torsion will further increase the laterally directed forces on the patella. Increased rotation between the femur and tibia also results in malalignment of the extensor mechanism, as the trochlear groove internally rotates and the patellar tendon insertion externally rotates.[14] The bony anatomy of the tibia and foot also affect patellar instability. Further lateralization of the tuberosity relative to the center of the patella will result in an increase in the laterally directed force on the patella. In addition, hindfoot valgus and excessive pronation of the foot place a valgus force on the knee, which also increases the laterally directed force on the patella.[15]

Under normal conditions, the patella "engages" in the trochlea at 10 to 20 degrees of flexion. The lateral trochlear ridge, which is typically larger, more proximal, and more anterior than the medial trochlear ridge, helps keep the patella centered in the trochlea by resisting pathologic lateral patellar excursion.[16] Trochlear dysplasia decreases the resistance to lateral patellar translation. Patients with a relatively longer patella tendon, called patella alta, have less osseous stability because more knee flexion is required before the patella is "engaged" and stabilized by the

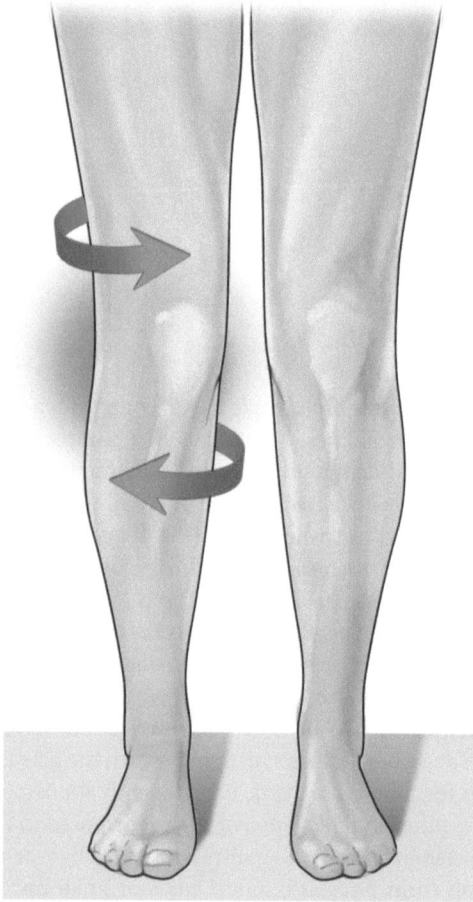

Fig. 105.2 Torsion of the femur and/or tibia. (Modified from The Cleveland Center for Medical Art & Photography, Copyright 2008.)

bony constraints of the trochlear groove. In addition, patients with patella alta have a decreased patellofemoral contact area compared with patients who have knees of normal patellar height.[17–19]

Pertinent Soft Tissue Anatomy

The quadriceps complex, consisting of the rectus femoris, vastus lateralis, vastus intermedius, and vastus medialis muscles, is the most important dynamic stabilizer of the patella (Fig. 105.3). All four muscles converge in the distal thigh and insert through the quadriceps tendon at the proximal pole of the patella. Each of the individual muscles contributes a different force vector based on its angle of insertion. The vastus medialis and lateralis muscles provide additional connections to the tibia through attachments to the medial and lateral patellar retinacula, respectively. The vastus medialis oblique (VMO) is a distinct part of the vastus medialis muscle that originates off of the lateral intermuscular septum and inserts at a high angle, up to 65 degrees, on the proximal third of the medial border of the patella.[20] The VMO is an important medial patellar stabilizer that counterbalances the pull of the vastus lateralis muscle.[21,22] In addition, the VMO may exert a force on the medial patellofemoral ligament (MPFL), adding additional medial stability to the patella.[23,24] Atrophy, hypoplasia, and impaired motor control of the VMO

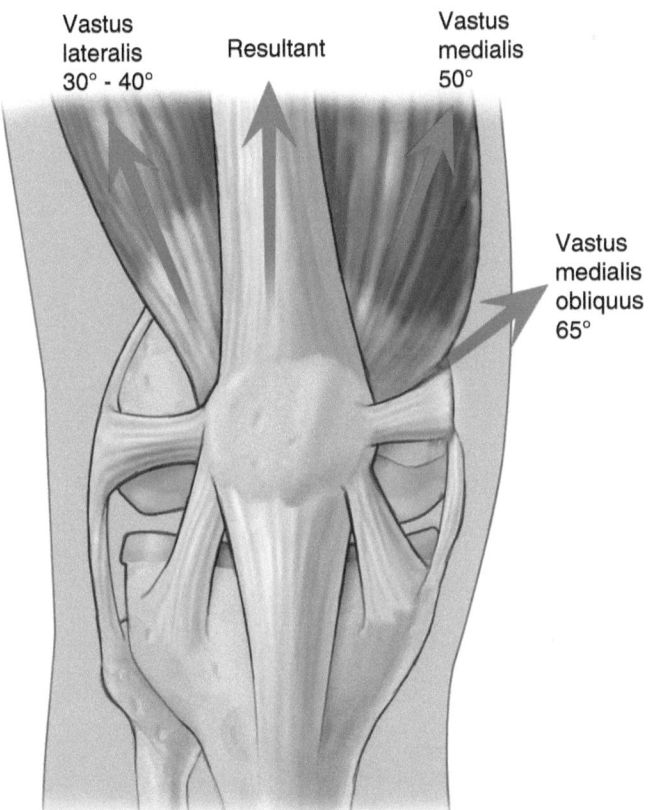

Fig. 105.3 Quadriceps musculature. (Modified from The Cleveland Center for Medical Art & Photography, Copyright 2008.)

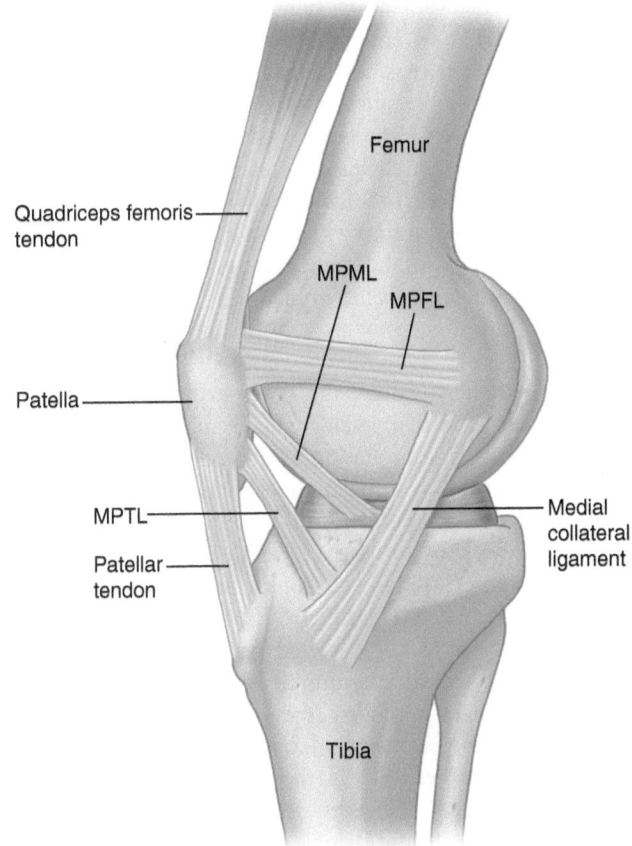

Fig. 105.4 Medial patellofemoral ligaments *(MPFL). MPML,* Medial patellomeniscal ligament; *MPTL,* medial patellotibial ligament. (Modified from The Cleveland Center for Medical Art & Photography, Copyright 2008.)

will therefore result in decreased opposed activity of the vastus lateralis muscle, producing increased lateral patellar displacement.[25] The dynamic muscular stabilizers can compensate to some degree for anatomic bony and soft tissue deficiencies that predispose to patellar instability. Conversely, weakness of the dynamic stabilizers may predispose athletes to patellar instability episodes during athletic activities even if they have "normal" anatomy and tracking under less stressful circumstances.

The primary medial soft tissue static stabilizers of the patella are the patellofemoral (MPFL), patellotibial (MPTL), and patellomeniscal ligaments (MPML) (Fig. 105.4). Studies have shown that the MPFL is the primary passive soft tissue restraint on the medial side of the patella, contributing 50% to 60% of the total restraining force against lateral patellar displacement in extension or first degrees of flexion.[26–29] However, contributions of the MPTL and MPML, as a unit, against lateral translation increase from 26% in extension to 46% at 90 degrees of flexion.[30] Additionally, the MPTL and MPML at 90 degrees of flexion are responsible for 72% of patellar tilt and 92% of patellar rotation.[30] The MPFL inserts between the adductor tuberosity and medial epicondyle on the femur and in the proximal two thirds of the medial border of the patella and the distal quadriceps tendon.[31] Its length is mean 56.9 mm (range, 46 to 75 mm), its width is mean 17.8 mm in the substance (range, 8 to 30 mm), mean 26 mm in the patella insertion (range, 14 to 52 mm), and mean 12.7 mm in the femur (range, 6 to 28.8 mm).[32] Close to the patella, extensions from the MPFL insert in the quadriceps tendon,

forming a medial patellofemoral complex that has an attachment of 30.4 ± 5.5 mm, on average.[33,34] The MPTL inserts in the proximal tibial about 13 to 14 mm distal to the tibial plateau, and in the distal third of the patella close to its distal border.[35] Its length is between 36 and 46 mm and width between 7 and 9 mm. The MPML inserts in the anterior horn of the medial meniscus and in the distal third of the patella.[35] Its length is between 33 and 43 mm.

The lateral soft tissue complex is composed of the iliotibial band, the vastus lateralis, the lateral patellofemoral ligament, and lateral patellotibial ligament, with tight connections between those structures.[36–40] The complex has superficial longitudinal fibers (superficial fibers of iliotibial band) and deep transverse fibers (deep fibers of the iliotibial band, vastus lateralis, lateral patellofemoral ligament, and lateral patellotibial ligament).[36–40]

EXAMINATION OVERVIEW

Acute Patellar Instability Episode

Clinical assessment of a patient who has recently sustained an episode of patellar instability can be difficult. Knee ROM is usually limited because of soft tissue swelling and joint effusion, and patients have difficulty relaxing for examination because of pain and fear. Aspiration of a joint effusion is occasionally indicated for comfort. The ligamentous, bony, and muscular structures of the knee should be systematically examined. Palpation along the course of the quadriceps, VMO, medial retinaculum, and whole MPFL helps to localize site of injury. Competence of the extensor mechanism should be confirmed by asking the patient to extend his or her knee against resistance from a flexed position. Concomitant injury to the collateral or cruciate ligaments or meniscus can be determined with use of the standard ligamentous and meniscal tests. Resolution of acute pain and swelling allows for a more comprehensive examination.

Static Standing and Gait Examination

With the patient standing, the lower extremity is inspected. Malalignment abnormalities, including genu valgum, pes planus, hindfoot valgus, and pronation of the foot, may be identified. Patients with rotational malalignment profile can have in-toe or out-toe posture. Toe in results in an increased lateral pull from the quadriceps. Quadriceps angle (Q-angle), formed between the anterosuperior spine, center of the patella, and tibial tuberosity, can be evaluated (Fig. 105.5). A larger Q angle theoretically results in a greater laterally directed force on the patella on contraction of the quadriceps muscle. Normal Q-angle in males and females ranges from 8 to 16 degrees and 15 to 19 degrees, respectively, in the supine position and 11 to 20 degrees and 15 to 23 degrees, respectively, in the standing position.[41–43] It is important to note that persistent patellar subluxation or dislocation may have falsely low Q angles due to lateral positioning of the patella. Gait observation provides insight into the dynamic factors influencing patellar tracking. In addition, core (spine, abdominal, hips and pelvis, and proximal lower limb muscles) strength testing is performed. A single-leg squat test is used to assess core control by requiring the patient to slowly lower the body over a single planted foot.[44] Poor control results in trunk lowering of the ipsilateral pelvis and increase in knee valgus, with a compensatory trunk movement.

Sitting Examination: Dynamic Change in Q Angle and J Sign

The Q-angle change can be evaluated during flexion and extension of the knee. The distance is normally greatest during terminal knee extension, in part because of the "screw home mechanism," where the tibia externally rotates on the femur, and smaller in flexion.[45–47] One should notice the Q-angle values and if it is greatly altered in flexion versus extension.

The J sign refers to the shape of inverted J of the patella tracking as the knee extends from a flexed position. As the patient extends the knee from 90 degrees of flexion, the patella will move laterally as it disengages from the proximal trochlea at near full extension. In patients with patella alta, it occurs earlier (i.e., at a greater flexion angle). A mild and smooth lateralization close to extension may be normal, especially if seen bilaterally in asymptomatic patients. In patients with patellar instability, a positive J sign has been associated with trochlear dysplasia, patella alta, lateral retinacular tightness, and/or medial retinacular insufficiency.[5,15] A "clunk" or abrupt change in tracking is associated with the presence of a trochlear "bump" or "spur."

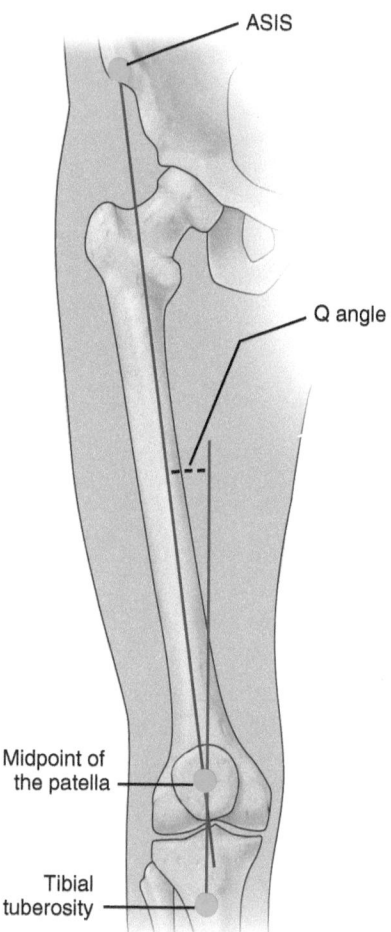

Fig. 105.5 The quadriceps angle *(Q angle)* formed by the intersection of a line from the anterior superior iliac spine *(ASIS)* to the midpoint of the patella, with a line from the midpoint of the patella to the midpoint of the tibial tuberosity. (Modified from Livingston LA, Mandigo JL. Bilateral Q angle asymmetry and anterior knee pain syndrome. *Clin Biomech [Bristol, Avon].* 1999;14[1]:7–13.)

Supine Examination: Muscle Balance and Special Tests

Muscle balance: Tone, strength, and tightness of the core (spine, abdominal, hips and pelvis, and proximal lower limb muscles) quadriceps, hamstrings, and gastrocnemius, should be evaluated.

Active extension subluxation: Proximal and patellar lateral translation during active quadriceps contraction with the knee fully extended. This indicates large quadriceps vector with medial soft tissue insufficiency.

Patellar tilt test: With the knee fully extended and the quadriceps relaxed, the examiner lifts the lateral border of the patella to evaluate the lateral soft tissue restraints (Fig. 105.6). Elevation between 0 degree (patella parallel to the floor) and 20 degrees is normal, whereas less than 0 degrees indicates tightness of the lateral retinaculum, and greater than 20 degrees indicates laxity.[48]

Patellar glide test: With the knee in full extension and the quadriceps relaxed, the patella is translated medially and laterally

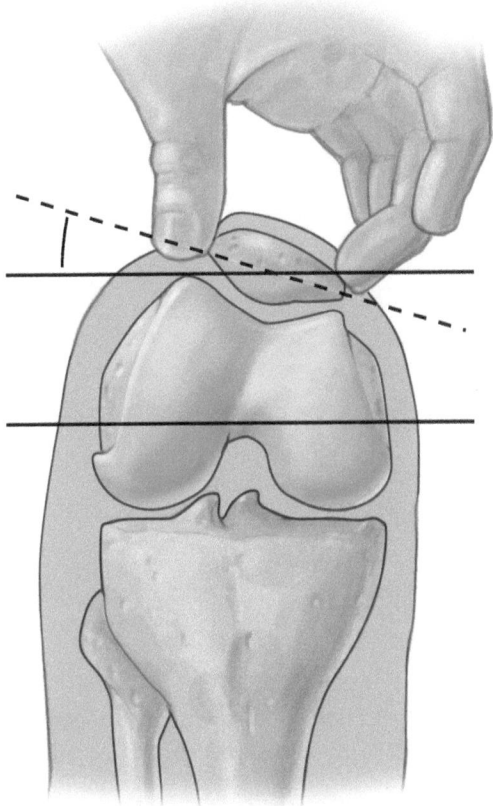

Fig. 105.6 Patellar tilt test. (Modified from The Cleveland Center for Medical Art & Photography, Copyright 2008.)

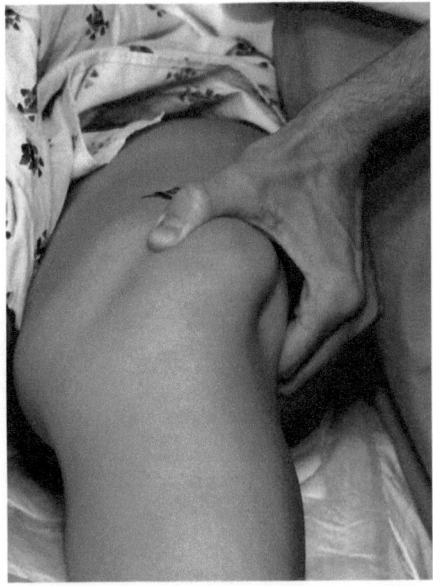

Fig. 105.7 Patellar glide test. Note that the patella is displaced laterally.

(Fig. 105.7). Using the width of the patella divided into quadrants, the amount of patellar glide is reported as the number of quadrants the patella translates. With a laterally directed force, a patellar glide more than 3 may suggest a deficiency in the medial soft tissue patellar restraints. A medial translation of one quadrant or less suggests tightness of lateral

TABLE 105.1   Different Indices of Patellar Height

Measurement	Normal	Alta	Baja
Insall-Salvati[86]	1.0	>1.2	<0.8
Modified Insall-Salvati[87]	—	>2.0	—
Blackburne-Peel[88]	0.8	>1.0	<0.5
Caton-Deschamps[89]	<1.2	>1.2	<0.6
Labelle-Laurin[90]	Visual	Visual	—

structures and more than 3 suggests lateral soft tissue insufficiency.[49] However, the clinician should compare the patellar mobility to the asymptomatic knee, when present, because increased patellar glide bilaterally is more indicative of generalized hyperlaxity. Repeat with progressive knee flexion. Lateral glide with deeper degrees of flexion suggests patella alta, trochlear dysplasia, or both.

Patellar apprehension test: The patella is manually translated laterally while the quadriceps is relaxed with the knee from 0 to 30 degrees of flexion. The test is positive if the patient has a feeling similar to a subluxation or dislocation episode.[48] Importantly, it is the apprehension, not the presence of pain alone, that makes the test positive. Although lateral patellar instability is more common, medial patellar instability may occur, especially in the setting of previous patellar realignment surgery.

Prone Examination

Femoral anteversion is measured using Craig's test.[50] The patient is placed prone, and the knee is flexed to 90 degrees. While the greater trochanter is palpated, the leg is rotated until the greater trochanter is positioned as far laterally as possible, placing the head into the center of the acetabulum. The angle between an imaginary vertical line and the axis of the tibia is the amount of femoral anteversion present.

IMAGING

Radiographs

The standard series of conventional radiographs includes standing anteroposterior (AP), lateral at 30 degrees of flexion, and Merchant views. These views may reveal fractures, arthritis, patellofemoral morphology, and alignment. The AP radiograph is useful for examining the tibiofemoral alignment and joint space in addition to identifying bipartite patella and patellar fractures. The axial radiograph is most useful for identifying positioning of the patella in relation to the trochlear groove and morphology of the trochlear groove. The Merchant view is obtained with the knee flexed 45 degrees over the end of the table and the x-ray beam angled 30 degrees downward.[51]

Patellar height is best assessed on a lateral radiograph obtained with the knee flexed to 30 degrees. Various methods of assessing relative patellar height have been described (Table 105.1),[52–56] including the Insall-Salvati,[57] modified Insall-Salvati,[58] Blackburne-Peel,[59] Caton-Deschamps,[60] and Labelle-Laurin[61] indices.

Trochlear dysplasia is best evaluated on a true lateral radiograph.[29,62–64] In a normal knee, the Blumensaat line continues anteriorly as the trochlear groove line, which should stay posterior

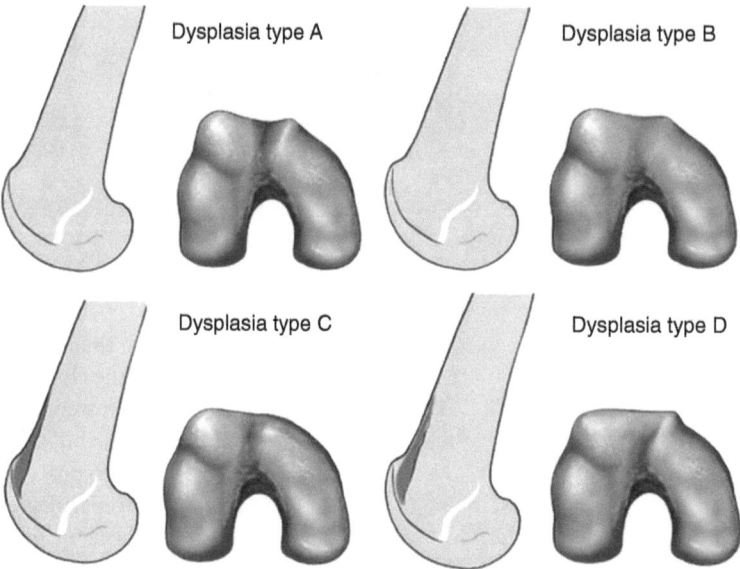

Dysplasia type A   Dysplasia type B

Dysplasia type C   Dysplasia type D

Fig. 105.8 Dejour's classification of trochlear dysplasia. *Type A*: crossing sign (flat or convex trochlea). *Type B*: crossing sign and supratrochlear spur. *Type C*: crossing sign and double contour. *Type D*: crossing sign, supratrochlear spur, double contour, and sharp step-off of the trochlea. (Modified from Grelsamer RP, Dejour D, Gould J. The pathophysiology of patellofemoral arthritis. *Orthop Clin North Am.* 2008;39[3]:269–274.)

to the projection of the femoral condyles (facets). However, when the lines of the lateral trochlear facet, medial trochlear facet, and trochlear groove coincide, this "crossing sign" indicates that those landmarks are at the same height and that the trochlea is flat.[63] Dejour et al.[63] reported the presence of the crossing sign in 96% of patients with history of a true patellar dislocation compared with 3% in the control group. The supratrochlear spur (or "bump" or "boss") was defined as the distance between a line drawn tangential to the anterior femoral cortex and the highest point of the trochlea.[65] The double contour is when the line of the hypoplastic medial condyle is posterior to the lateral facet line (continuing below the crossing sign). In the Merchant view, the sulcus angle is measured as the angle between two lines originating from the deepest part of the femoral trochlea to the highest points of the medial and lateral condyles. Values greater than 145 degrees suggest trochlear dysplasia.[66]

A classification of trochlear dysplasia has been developed using information from the lateral and axial computed tomography (CT) or magnetic resonance imaging (MRI) views (Fig. 105.8).[67] Type A dysplasia: crossing sign is present on lateral view. On the axial view, the trochlea is shallower than normal, but is still symmetrical and concave. Type B dysplasia: crossing sign and supratrochlear spur are present on lateral view. On axial view, the trochlea is flat or convex. Type C dysplasia: crossing sign and double contour are present on lateral view. On axial view, the lateral facet is convex. Type D dysplasia: crossing sign, supratrochlear spur, and double contour are present on lateral view. On the axial view, the trochlear facets are asymmetrical with a cliff between them.

Computed Tomography

One major limitation of radiographs is the inability to obtain axial images of the patellofemoral joint at angles from 20 degrees of knee flexion to full extension.

Two important additional measurements can be performed. Patellar tilt is measured as the angle between a line going through the patellar axis and a line tangential to the posterior condyles. Angles greater than 20 degrees are considered abnormal.[62,63] The tibial tubercle–trochlear groove (TT-TG) distance can be performed by superimposing an axial CT image of the tibial tuberosity and the trochlear groove. The TT-TG distance is that between the center of the tuberosity and the groove in a line parallel to the posterior femoral condyles (Fig. 105.9). A TT-TG distance of more than 15 to 20 mm is associated with patellar instability.[63,68–70]

CT imaging also allows for three-dimensional reconstructions to be performed, providing a better spatial understanding of the knee anatomy. Furthermore, dynamic CT has been used to assess patellar tracking, allowing visualization of the patellofemoral joint through clinically relevant ranges of motion.[71–73] Although studies of patellar instability using dynamic imaging modalities to date have been limited, this imaging protocol has become more widespread in the clinical setting and will likely enhance our understanding of the static and dynamic properties of the patellofemoral joint and guide therapeutic recommendations.

Magnetic Resonance Imaging

MRI provides additional imaging details not seen on conventional radiographs and CT imaging. MRI allows assessment of the articular cartilage, trochlear geometry, and soft tissue structures, including the MPFL.[74–76] The classical MRI findings after an acute episode of patellar instability include impaction injury to the lateral femoral condyle, osteochondral damage to the medial patella facet, and disruption of the medial retinaculum and MPFL (Fig. 105.10).[77] MRI is 85% sensitive and 70% accurate in detecting injury to the MPFL.[78] The same measurements made on radiographs and CT can be performed on the MRI;

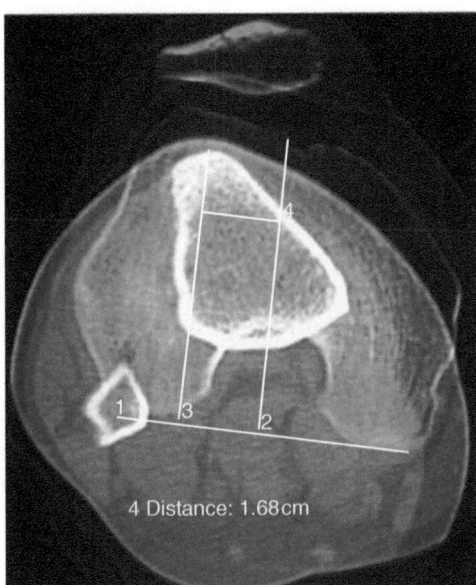

Fig. 105.9 A computed tomography scan showing the technique of measuring the tibial tuberosity–trochlear groove distance (TT-TG). The image of the trochlear groove is superimposed on the image of the tibial tuberosity using the digital radiology software. A line parallel to the posterior femoral condyles is drawn *(line 1)*. A perpendicular to line 1 is then taken through the central portion of the trochlea *(line 2)* and through the tibial tuberosity *(line 3)*. The difference between line 2 and line 3 (i.e., *line 4*) is the TT-TG. In this case, it is 1.68 cm. (Modified from Bicos J, Fulkerson JP, Amis A. Current concepts review: the medial patellofemoral ligament. *Am J Sports Med.* 2007;35[3]:484–492.)

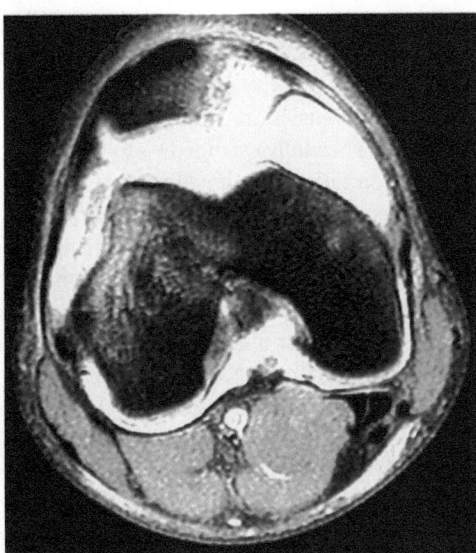

Fig. 105.10 An axial magnetic resonance imaging scan after acute lateral patellar dislocation shows knee effusion, bony bruising of the lateral femoral condyle and medial patellar facet from impaction, and disruption of the patellar attachment of the medial patellofemoral ligament.

however, thresholds of abnormalities may not be the same.[79–81,84] The tendinous-cartilaginous measure of the TT-TG can be performed between the deepest point in the trochlear cartilage and the center of the patellar tendon insertion.[82–84] Additional useful measurements described for MRI are the lateral trochlear inclination,[85] ventral trochlear prominence,[86] trochlear depth,[86] and tibial tuberosity to posterior cruciate ligament distance (TT-PCL). The lateral trochlear inclination is the angle between the posterior condyles and the lateral trochlear facet.[85] It is considered abnormal when less than 11 degrees, with good sensitivity and specificity.[85] The ventral trochlear prominence is measured as the distance between the line paralleling the femoral anterior cortical line and the most anterior cartilaginous point of the trochlea.[86] The range in control patients without trochlear dysplasia is between 0 and 10.5 mm; greater than 8 mm is considered abnormal.[86] The trochlear depth is calculated using the maximal AP distance of the medial femoral condyle (distance a) and lateral femoral condyle (distance b), and the minimal AP distance between the deepest point of the trochlear groove and the line paralleling the posterior outlines of the femoral condyles (distance c) according to the following formula: $([a + b]/2) - c$. A value less than 3 is considered abnormal.[86] The TT-PCL gives an independent measure of the position of the tibial tuberosity in the tibia. The measure is the distance from the medial border of the PCL and the center of the patellar tendon in lines parallel to the posterior tibial plateaus. Rotational alignment can be evaluated by CT or MRI.[14] Femoral anteversion is defined as the angle formed between the axis of the femoral neck and distal femur. Knee rotation of the femorotibial joint is given by the rotational angles between the distal femur and the proximal tibia and tibial torsion is assessed by measuring the rotational angle of the proximal tibia relative to the distal tibia. Kinematic MRI has been used to evaluate patellofemoral tracking.[87–92] The use of kinematic MRI in the clinical setting remains limited as a result of a lack of availability.

DECISION-MAKING PRINCIPLES AND TREATMENT OPTIONS

Treatment of patellar instability must be patient-specific. Historically, a plethora of rehabilitation regimens and surgical procedures have been described.[17,67,93–101] Important details from the history, physical examination, and imaging studies will help the clinician determine which treatment options are most suitable for each patient.

Acute Patellar Instability Episode

During the acute phase after a patellar injury, regardless of whether it is a first-time or recurrent injury, the immediate goals of management are to provide relief of symptoms. Relative rest, light compression, and elevation are the initial interventions. Most patients benefit from the use of crutches to assist weight bearing. Pain is generally well controlled with cryotherapy and over-the-counter analgesic medications. A knee immobilizer may be used transiently for patients who are particularly unstable or uncomfortable, followed by a more functional hinged or patellar brace within the first few days as symptoms allow. Knee aspiration is helpful in relieving pain for patients with a tense hemarthrosis. Heel slides and quadriceps activation exercises may be initiated within days of the injury, depending on the severity of pain, soft tissue swelling, and effusion. Conventional radiographs and MRI should be obtained to look for fractures or large osteochondral or chondral loose bodies. Formal referral to a physical therapist allows for a supervised functional progression back to activities of daily living in days to weeks and to athletic activities in weeks to months.

Subacute, First-Time Patellar Instability Episode

Nonsurgical treatment remains the mainstay of therapy for most first-time episodes of patellar instability.[2,102] Protocols vary, ranging from a simple period of immobilization to those that involve rapid rehabilitation. While immobilization facilitates healing of the torn MPFL it also leads to muscle atrophy and stiffness that can increase the risk of arthritis.[97] In most cases, it is appropriate to use rigid immobilization for ambulation and to avoid falls, only until the patient regains quadriceps control. Non–weight-bearing ROM exercises can be initiated as soon as swelling decreases. Rehabilitation protocols typically include strengthening of the quadriceps, gluteal, and core muscles. Recurrence rates after nonoperative treatment from 15% to 60% have been reported.[3–7,97]

Well-accepted indications for surgical intervention in the acute setting are irreducible patellar dislocation, large osteochondral or chondral lesions, and associated injuries that require surgical treatment.[2] While controversial, consideration can be given for concomitant repair or reconstruction of the MPFL if surgery was indicated after a first-time dislocation for other reasons.

Some authors have advocated surgical stabilization, by repair or reconstruction of the MPFL, after a first-time dislocation without the previously mentioned surgical indications,[2,4,5,7,94,103–107] but the benefit remains unclear. To date, few studies have compared nonoperative versus operative treatment in persons with first-time patellar dislocations.[2,4,5,7,94,103–107] In most studies that evaluate MPFL repair or procedures other than MPFL reconstruction, no major differences were found in postoperative episodes of instability, activity level or function, or subjective patient measures. However, MPFL reconstruction resulted in higher Kujala outcome scores and lower rates of recurrence in an RCT versus nonoperative treatment.[94] Additional high-quality studies are needed to delineate the role of primary surgical stabilization in the treatment of first-time episodes of patellar instability.[108]

Subacute, Recurrent Patellar Instability Episode

For patients with recurrent patellar instability, surgical stabilization is recommended.

History, physical examination, and imaging studies guide a patient-specific surgical plan. The goal of surgical intervention is to "individualize, customize, and normalize" a solution tailored to the unique pathologic condition that is leading to the recurrent instability.[93]

The MPFL is the essential lesion of patella instability and is always repaired or reconstructed. Other procedures can be added, as indicated, for soft tissue balance or bony realignment.

Procedures for soft tissue balance.

- *MPFL reconstruction:* Often the primary procedure indicated for patella instability. There are many techniques described, using the quadriceps tendon, patellar tendon, and hamstring autografts.[94,109,110] Allografts can also be utilized.

- *Lateral retinaculum lengthening:* Should be performed when the lateral retinaculum is tight. Indicators include: on physical exam, medial glide test is decreased (<1 quadrant of the patella) and tilt is increased and not reducible (lifting of the lateral edge of the patella does not reach zero degrees—parallel to the femoral axis); on imaging of an axial view of CT or MRI, tilt measurement is increased (>20 degrees). Additionally, lack of reduction of tilt with progressive flexion (clinically or imaging study) and similar tilt in a contralateral affected knee also suggest lateral retinaculum tightness.[49] The lateral retinaculum is sharply divided into a superficial layer of oblique fibers from the anterior iliotibial band and a deep layer of transverse fibers. These two layers must be identified separate from the articular capsule. The superficial layer is sectioned close to the patella and the deep layer as posteriorly as necessary and possible. Typically, 15 to 20 mm of lengthening can be achieved.[49]

- *Medial plication:* When the medial soft tissue has good quality it can be repositioned to reduce the slack. The goal should be not to constrain the medial side, but only to reinforce the MPFL within its limits.

- *MPTL reconstruction:* Many techniques are described for the MPTL reconstruction combined with the MPFL.[111–114] Based on anatomy and biomechanical studies the MPTL and MPML are more important in two moments during knee ROM: terminal extension, when it directly counteracts quadriceps contraction,[112,115] and deeper flexion, when it tightens and its contribution to lateral translation restraint increases.[30] It also improves kinematics of patellar tilt and rotation throughout ROM, especially in deep flexion.[30] Indications for this procedure include[113,114,116,117]: active extension subluxation (defined by patellar lateral translation during active quadriceps contraction with the knee fully extended)—to restrain lateral and superolateral translation, specifically opposing proximal and lateral quadriceps muscle pull[115]; flexion instability (obligatory patellar dislocation and lateral glide during flexion)—to restrain lateral translation in higher knee flexion angles, as the MPTL tightens with increasing knee flexion[30,118,119]; children with an excessive number of anatomic risk factors (trochlear dysplasia, large quadriceps vector, and patella alta)—to add additional support during extension and flexion when there is the risk of complications when doing bony procedures due to open physes[118,120–122]; and knee hyperextension associated with generalized laxity—to add additional support to functional patella alta and large quadriceps vector during hyperextension.[118,123]

Procedures for bone realignment.

- *Tibial tuberosity osteotomy (TTO):* Can be performed for medialization, distalization, or combination of both. Medialization is indicated when there is a malalignment between the trochlear groove and the tibial tuberosity, with the latter being relatively lateral, resulting in an increased lateral quadriceps vector. This is recognized on physical exam by a large Q-angle (>15 to 20 degrees)[41–43] and on imaging by an increased TT-TG (>15 to 20 mm)[63,68–70] and increased TT-PCL (24 mm).[124] Distalization is indicated when there is patella alta (Table 105.1). Associated anteriorization is not performed to treat instability; however, it can be associated to unload the compartment when treating concomitant cartilage pathology.

- *Trochleoplasty:* Many techniques are described such as proximal open grooveplasty,[125] deepening trochleoplasty V-shaped by Dejour,[126] U-shape by Bereiter (open[127] or arthroscopic[128]), and resection wedge Goutallier technique.[129] These procedures are indicated in patients with high-grade trochlear dysplasia types B, C, and D of Dejour classification. In those patients, trochleoplasty, along with other procedures including MPFL reconstruction, decrease the rate of dislocation compared with MPFL reconstruction alone (2.1% vs. 7%, respectively).[130]

- *Femoral osteotomy:* Another less common approach has been to address malalignment using femoral osteotomies.[131–135] Excessive femoral anteversion can be corrected in the proximal shaft by derotation osteotomy, most frequently in the pediatric population. Excessive valgus alignment can be corrected through distal femoral osteotomies. Both varus and derotation osteotomy can decrease the lateral quadriceps vector, changing the proximal component of the vector. Although femoral osteotomies have the advantage of directly correcting femoral malalignment, they should be recommended selectively.

Authors' Preferred Technique
Medial Patellofemoral Reconstruction

Injury to the MPFL is considered the essential lesion in recurrent lateral patellar dislocations.[26,74,136,137] MPFL reconstruction is the primary stabilization procedure performed for patients without marked bony malalignment. Alternatively, it is also performed as an adjunct to realignment osteotomy/trochleoplasty in patients with significant bony deformity. In either situation, the MPFL acts as a check-rein to lateral translation of the patella in early flexion. The MPFL cannot be used to "pull" the patella medially. If the patella cannot be centered on the trochlea in early flexion, consideration for lateral soft tissue lengthening, distal realignment, or both, may be necessary. These concomitant procedures should be performed prior to MPFL reconstruction. A variety of techniques have been described using different graft sources and a multitude of fixation techniques.[94,99,100,138–143] While overall success rates remain high, initial enthusiasm has been tempered somewhat by recent descriptions[144–146] of complications related to the surgical technique.

Surgical Technique
Positioning and Preparation
- Supine position, fluoroscopy from the operative side
- Lateral post and trauma bump can be useful
- Tourniquet applied, but not inflated throughout the case. Compressive stocking or sleeve on nonoperative limb
- General anesthesia plus adductor (sensory only) block
- Intravenous (IV) antibiotic prior to incision
- Careful examination under anesthesia comparing operative to nonoperative limb and grading competency of the medial and lateral soft tissue restraints (e.g., MPFL laxity/endpoint/symmetry, lateral patella tilt/lateral retinacular tightness), assessing patella tracking, and the ability to maintain patella centered on trochlea throughout ROM

Diagnostic Arthroscopy
- Complete joint assessment to rule out and treat concomitant pathology (e.g., meniscus tears)
- Patellofemoral evaluation including inspection for patulous medial soft tissue structures, tight or incompetent lateral structures, trochlea and patella morphology, presence and location of chondral lesions (i.e., patella, trochlea, lateral femoral condyle), and/or loose bodies
- Dynamic assessment of patella tracking in extension and flexion
- Treatment of chondral disease (e.g., chondroplasty for unstable flaps, sizing lesion for future cartilage restoration, biopsy for possible future matrix-induced autologous chondrocyte implantation [MACI], etc.) and synovectomy performed as indicated
- Following diagnostic arthroscopy, concomitant procedures should be performed as indicated. These include medialization or distalization TTO, lateral retinaculum lengthening, or rarely, trochleoplasty. MPFL reconstruction is typically the final procedure to be completed.

Graft Preparation
- In general, soft tissue allograft is our preferred graft choice for MPFL reconstruction although techniques for hamstring/quadriceps autograft have been described. Gracilis allograft is typically selected although other tendinous allografts of similar length and width may be utilized. Allografts should be nonirradiated and within 10 years of the patient age.

Soft Tissue Dissection
- If concomitant procedures are performed, extensile midline approach may be utilized from the tibial tuberosity to just above the patella. For isolated MPFL reconstruction, limited longitudinal medial incisions may be made at the level of the medial border of the patella and near the adductor tubercle.
- The medial retinaculum layer and native MPFL layer is incised from the medial patella. Careful dissection is performed leaving the medial capsular layer intact. An Allis clamp is utilized to assess the native MPFL, which is often patulous with poor tissue quality.

Patellar Preparation
- The bony insertion of the MPFL is prepared to a healthy bleeding bed with use of a burr and flat rasp (Fig. 105.11). Alternatively, a small medial patella trough can also be established.
- Anteroposterior (AP) fluoroscopy and direct palpation are utilized to locate the anatomic insertion of the MPFL on the patella. In general, suture anchors are utilized for patella MPFL graft fixation, although alternative methods such as transosseous tunnels or soft tissue only fixation (e.g., quadriceps tendon) have been described. The first point of fixation is located midway between the anterior cortex and the articular surface at a point just proximal to the patella equator. The second point of fixation is in the same AP plane but more proximal, equidistant from the proximal aspect of the patella and the first point of fixation (Fig. 105.12).
- These positions are confirmed with fluoroscopy and suture anchors are placed. In general, the smallest and shortest suture anchor with adequate strength is selected. Care is taken not to violate the articular surface.

Femoral Preparation
- The anatomic insertion of the femoral MPFL should be identified and confirmed using a combination of several techniques, and a guide pin should be placed (Fig. 105.13):
  - Anatomy, by palpation (insertion between the medial epicondyle and adductor tubercle).[31]

Continued

📌 **Authors' Preferred Technique**

Medial Patellofemoral Reconstruction—cont'd

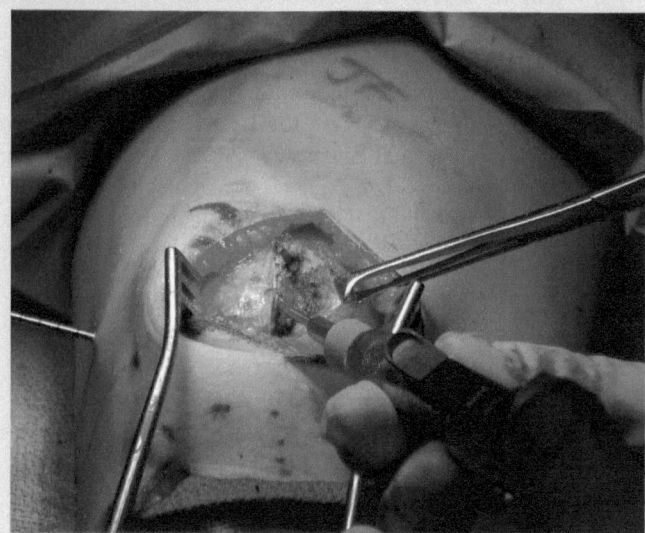

Fig. 105.11 Bony insertion of the medial patellofemoral ligament at the patella is prepared to a healthy bleeding bed with use of a burr and flat rasp.

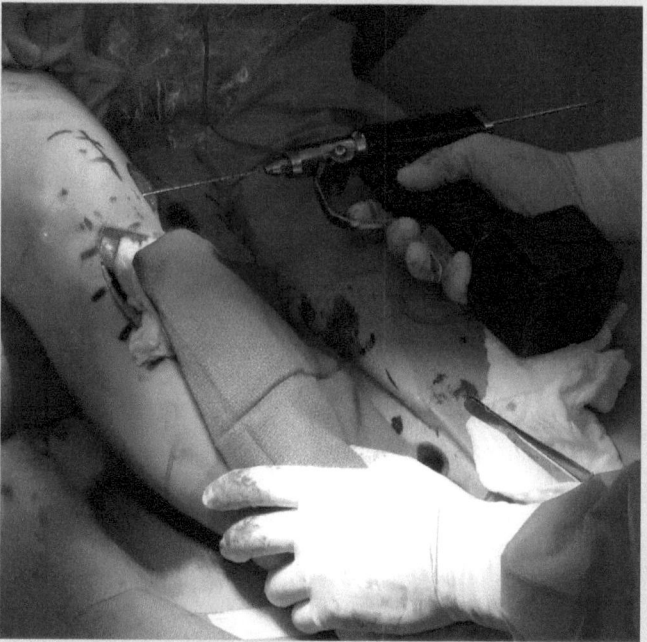

Fig. 105.13 The anatomic insertion of the medial patellofemoral ligament femoral attachment should be identified and confirmed using a combination of several techniques (including anatomy, fluoroscopy, and isometry), and a guide pin should be placed.

- Fluoroscopy, a point just anterior to the posterior cortex extension line and between the posterior origin of the medial femoral condyle and the posterior point of the Blumensaat line on a lateral radiograph[147] (Fig. 105.14).
- Isometry, testing using the femoral guide pin and sutures from the patella shuttled between the previously dissected layers to the femoral origin. The MPFL graft should either be mostly isometric or anatomometric (tight in extension, loose in flexion) (Box 105.1). If the sutures tighten in flexion, the guide pin should be moved, often distal and posterior until a favorable isometry profile is achieved.
- The looped end of the MPFL graft is docked at the femoral insertion site with proprietary fixation of choice (e.g., suture anchor, tenodesis screw, suspensory device, etc.).
- The graft is shuttled between the layers back towards the patella insertion for final fixation.

Final Fixation
- With the knee at 20 to 30 degrees and the patella centered on the trochlea, the MPFL graft is fixed to the patella using sutures from the suture anchor. The graft is fixed at a set resting length that has been predetermined by early steps. The MPFL is not "tensioned," but instead acts as a tether with specific length changes with ROM. Knee ROM and patella translation are assessed to ensure appropriate graft characteristics (Fig. 105.15).
- The native medial retinacular and MPFL layer are repaired over the graft with absorbable suture (Fig. 105.16).
- Final fluoroscopic images are taken and saved to the PACS system.
- Standard wound closure is performed. TENS unit, compressive ice machine, and hinged knee brace in extension are placed.

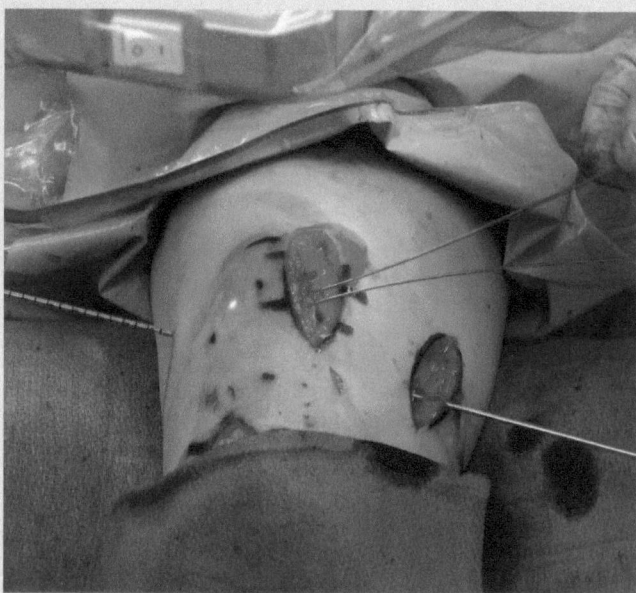

Fig. 105.12 Anteroposterior fluoroscopy and direct palpation are utilized to locate the anatomic insertion of the medial patellofemoral ligament patellar attachment. The first point of fixation is located midway between the anterior cortex and the articular surface at a point just proximal to the patella equator. The second point of fixation is in the same anteroposterior plane, but more proximal, equidistant from the proximal aspect of the patella and the first point of fixation.

Authors' Preferred Technique

Medial Patellofemoral Reconstruction—cont'd

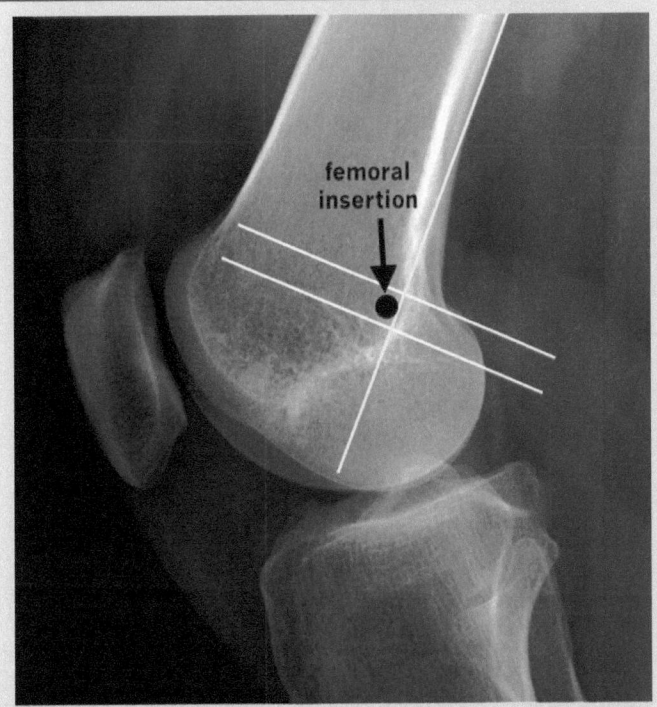

Fig. 105.14 Lateral radiograph of a right knee. The femoral insertion point is just anterior to the posterior cortex extension line and between the posterior origin of the medial femoral condyle and the posterior point of the Blumensaat line.

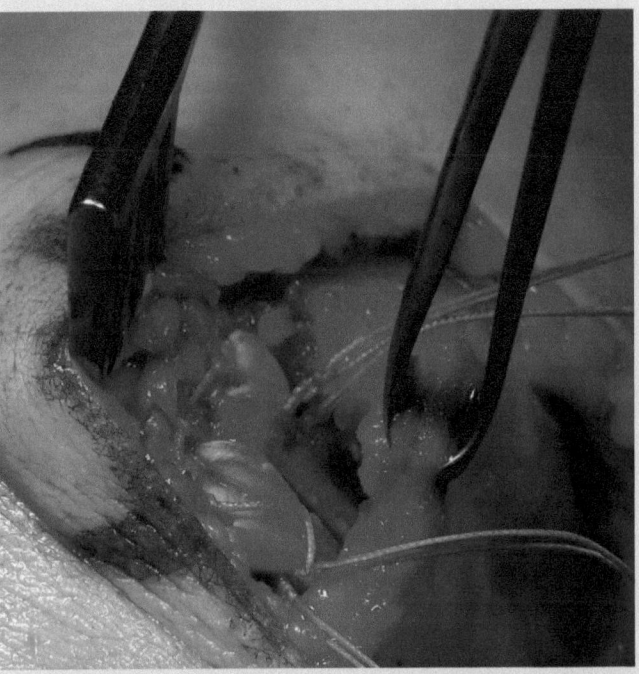

Fig. 105.15 With the knee at 20–30 degrees and the patella centered on the trochlea, the medial patellofemoral ligament (MPFL) graft is fixed to the patella using sutures from the suture anchor. The graft is fixed at a set resting length that has been predetermined by earlier steps. The MPFL is not "tensioned," but instead acts as a tether with specific length changes with range of motion (ROM). Knee ROM and patella translation are assessed to ensure appropriate graft characteristics.

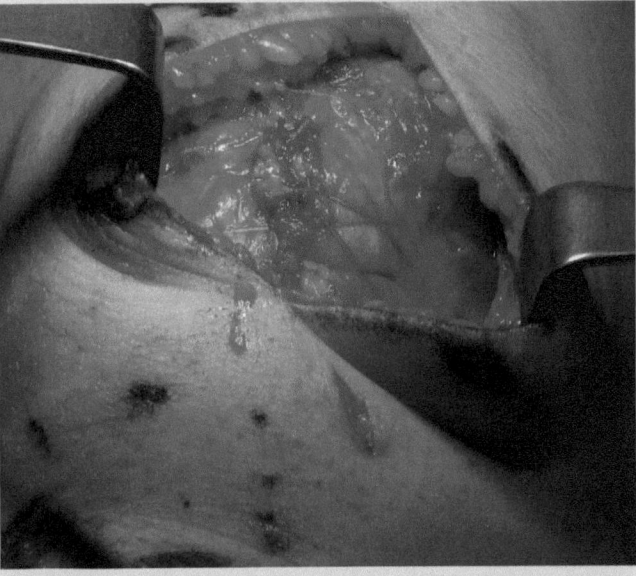

Fig. 105.16 The native superficial medial retinaculum, layer 1, and the patient's medial patellofemoral ligament, layer 2, are repaired over the graft with absorbable suture.

POSTOPERATIVE MANAGEMENT

- Patients are discharged with crutches and allowed to weight-bear as tolerated with the brace locked in extension once their nerve block wears off. They are instructed to perform isometric quadriceps sets, short arc quadriceps, and ankle pumps. Gravity-assisted ROM as tolerated may begin immediately out of the brace. Continuous passive motion (CPM) may be utilized per surgeon discretion.
- Formal physical therapy is initialized following the first post-operative visit. This is typically 2–3×/week for several months. Typical progression includes discontinuing crutches and hinged brace for a J-brace or sleeve once they have adequate quadriceps strength (often by 6 weeks), regaining full ROM between 6 and 8 weeks, low-impact activities (bike, elliptical) within the first several months, jogging by 3 months, criteria-based progression towards return to sport any time after 4–6 months.
- Concomitant procedures (e.g., TTO, cartilage restoration) will alter the rehabilitation guidelines and timeframe for recovery.

RESULTS

Studies have shown that MPFL reconstruction has a success rate of 70% to 100%, with very few cases of recurrent subluxation or dislocation.[138,139,142,143,146,148–152] Despite seemingly excellent results, most of the outcome data on MPFL reconstruction are limited by small sample sizes and short-term follow-up.[138] In addition, the population characteristics (with regard to risk factors) in which isolated MPFL reconstruction is performed and the various surgical techniques employed makes generalization of outcomes difficult. Therefore grade of recommendation on when to perform or not perform associated procedures is inconclusive.[153]

COMPLICATIONS

In a systematic review,[154] a total of 164 complications occurred in 629 knees (26.1%). These adverse events ranged from minor to major including patellar fracture, failures, clinical instability on postoperative examination, loss of knee flexion, wound complications, and pain. Twenty-six patients returned to the operating room for additional procedures. Complications can be minimized by decreasing technical error such as fixation malpositioning and inadequate graft tension. Malpositioning of the femoral (Fig. 105.17) or patellar tunnels or excessive graft tension are associated with serious potential complications, including medial patellofemoral articular overload, iatrogenic medial subluxation, and recurrent lateral instability.[93,144,145,155] The use of fluoroscopy, anatomy, and careful assessment of isometry can help minimize malpositioning. In addition, confirmation of full knee ROM before and after graft fixation can help ensure that the graft is not too tight, particularly in flexion, or too loose (Box 105.1).

Postoperative Management

- Drain is removed within 24 hours. Deep vein thrombosis (DVT) prophylaxis is considered.

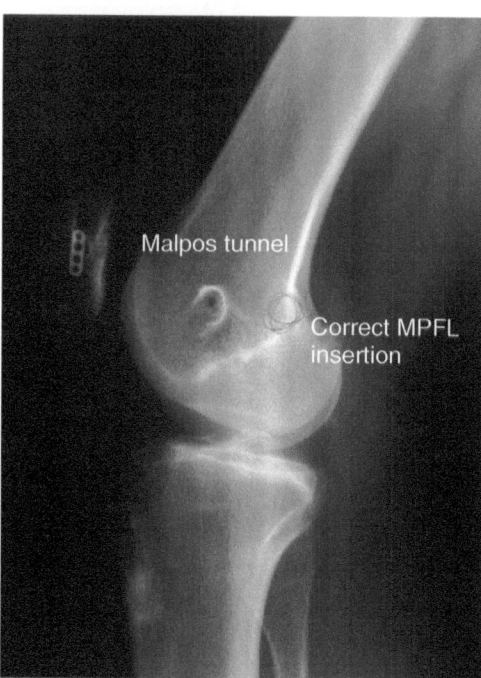

Fig. 105.17 A lateral radiograph showing an anteriorly and proximally positioned femoral tunnel in a 20-year-old woman after an autograft medial patellofemoral ligament *(MPFL)* reconstruction. Recurrent lateral instability developed. *Malpos,* Malpositioned. (From Bollier M, Fulkerson J, Cosgarea A, et al. Technical failure of medial patellofemoral ligament reconstruction. *Arthroscopy.* 2011;27[8]:1153–1159.)

BOX 105.1 Pearls for Setting Appropriate Medial Patellofemoral Ligament Graft Length

1. In full extension, the patella may not be centered in the trochlear groove and estimating correct MPFL graft length is difficult.
2. Have an assistant hold the patella in the groove in approximately 30 degrees of knee flexion while the graft is placed at proper length. This prevents overtightening of the MPFL graft.
3. While fixing the graft, keep the graft at length taking care not to tension it.
4. With the desired length, before final fixation, verify that the patella medial-lateral mobility is adequate (one to two quadrants of displacement).
5. The goal is to not overtighten the MPFL graft. The MPFL graft should guide the patella into the trochlear groove during early knee flexion. The patella should engage and center in the trochlear groove at 20–30 degrees of knee flexion (when the attachment distances are farthest apart; in deep flexion the distance between the attachment sites are closer, thus allowing more laxity in the graft as desired).

MPFL, Medial patellofemoral ligament.

- Patients are discharged home with crutches and are toe-touch weight bearing with the brace locked in extension for 4–6 weeks. CPM and/or gravity-assisted ROM is initiated as tolerated immediately. Isometric quadriceps sets and ankle pumps are performed.
- Patients may progress to full weight bearing at 6 weeks, unlock and then discontinue the brace when adequate quadriceps control is achieved. Full ROM should be achieved at this time.
- Low-impact activities are initiated within the first 3 months. Jogging and sport-specific drills may be initiated between

Authors' Preferred Technique

Tibial Tuberosity Osteotomy

Tibial tuberosity osteotomy changes the distal insertion of the patellar tendon, which leads to realignment of the extensor mechanism and can improve patellar tracking, change patellofemoral contact pressures, and/or correct the patellar height index.[67] Depending on the type of malalignment present, various transfer procedures have been described.[156–159] Isolated medialization of the tibial tuberosity, known as the Elmslie-Trillat procedure, is performed to medialize the patellar tendon. It is indicated for patients with a history of recurrent instability and excessive lateralization of the tuberosity, but minimal articular cartilage damage. Anteromedialization (AMZ), best known as the Fulkerson osteotomy, is indicated in patients with recurrent instability, a lateralized tuberosity, and chondral damage over the lateral and/or distal patellofemoral joint.[160] The goal of the surgical procedure is to correct excessive lateral forces and to unload joint surface areas that have been damaged. Distalization of the tibial tuberosity may be used to correct for instability believed to be related to patella alta.[161,162]

Surgical Technique
Positioning and Preparation
- Supine position, fluoroscopy from operative side if concomitant MPFL surgery
- Lateral post and trauma bump can be useful
- Tourniquet applied, but not inflated, throughout the case. Compressive stocking or sleeve on nonoperative limb
- General anesthesia plus adductor (sensory only) block
- IV antibiotic prior to incision
- Careful examination under anesthesia comparing operative to nonoperative limb and grading competency of the medial and lateral soft tissue restraints (i.e., MPFL laxity/endpoint/symmetry, lateral patella tilt/lateral retinacular tightness), assessing patella tracking, and the ability to maintain patella centered on trochlea throughout ROM

Diagnostic Arthroscopy
- Complete joint assessment to rule out and treat concomitant pathology (e.g., meniscus tears)
- Patellofemoral evaluation including inspection for patulous medial soft tissue structures, tight or incompetent lateral structures, trochlea and patella morphology, presence and location of chondral lesions (i.e., patella, trochlea, lateral femoral condyle), and/or loose bodies
- Dynamic assessment of patella tracking in extension and flexion
- Treatment of chondral disease (e.g., chondroplasty for unstable flaps, sizing lesion for future cartilage restoration, biopsy for possible future MACI, etc.) and synovectomy performed as indicated

Exposure
- Incision is made just lateral to midline extending approximately 6 cm distal to the insertion of the tibial tuberosity, just lateral to the anterior tibial crest.
- The medial and lateral borders of the patella tendon are exposed. The fat pad is reflected proximally and not violated.
- Contents of the anterior compartment are dissected from the anterolateral border of the proximal tibia and neurovascular structures protected with gentle retraction.
- The medial border of the tibial tuberosity pedicle is defined using sharp dissection and elevation of the medial periosteum.

Shingle Preparation
- A 6-cm tibial tubercle cutting guide is placed and secured with K-wires. The guide should be closer to the anterior tibial cortex distally.
- For medialization TTO, 0-degree guide angle (parallel to the floor) is selected.

- For AMZ, a 45- to 60-degree angle is selected based on preoperative template of desired amount of anteriorization and medialization.

Osteotomy
- An oscillating saw is used for initial osteotomy using copious irrigation.
- Longitudinal osteotomy is completed from medial to lateral with osteotomes leaving a periosteal hinge distally.
- The patellar tendon is retracted and proximal transverse cut is made with osteotome from medial to lateral under direct visualization.
- Osteotome is used to cut the lateral cortex from the lateral aspect of the proximal transverse osteotomy to the proximal aspect of the lateral longitudinal osteotomy.
- Gentle prying motion is used to mobilize the tibial tuberosity pedicle without fracturing the distal hinge.
- If distalization is indicated, the hinge is detached completely. The distal aspect of the tibial tuberosity pedicle is carefully measured and oscillating saw is used to remove distal bone enough to normalize the Caton-Deschamps ratio, per preoperative template. This resected distal bone may be placed proximal to the patella tendon insertion if desired.

Shingle Fixation
- A trauma bump is placed just proximal to the knee joint so that the neurovascular structures are not pressed against the posterior tibial cortex.
- Preliminary fixation is achieved with K-wire and/or clamp stabilization. Measurements are made with ruler to correct malalignment based on preoperative template. Patella tracking is assessed throughout a ROM arc.
- 2 or 3 bicortical screws are placed using lag technique under fluoroscopic guidance. Screw length and position are carefully assessed. Care is taken to ensure that screw heads are not prominent.
- Bone graft is often not needed for medialization/AMZ or distalization. Consideration can be made for smoothing off medial overhanging bone and/or transferring some prominent bone to the lateral side. Addition of bone marrow aspirate concentrate (BMAC) to augment healing can be considered.

Concomitant Procedures
- Following distal realignment fixation, attention is turned to proximal soft tissue balancing. Tight lateral retinaculum may be treated with lateral lengthening as indicated through an extensile exposure. MPFL reconstruction is performed either through extensile approach or through separate proximal medial based incisions.
- If cartilage restoration is to be performed, the tibial tuberosity pedicle is not fixed until after the cartilage procedure to facilitate easy joint access. After cartilage repair, the osteotomy is fixed and soft tissue balancing is performed as indicated.

Closure
- The periosteum over the medial tibial crest is repaired with absorbable no. 0 suture.
- The anterior compartment fascia is loosely repaired to anterolateral tibia with absorbable no. 0 suture.
- A drain is placed deep to the fascia within the anterior compartment for 24 hours to prevent compartment syndrome.
- Standard wound closure techniques are utilized.
- Sterile dressing, cryotherapy unit, TENS unit, compressive dressing, and hinged knee brace locked in extension are applied.

4 and 6 months. Patients may utilize criteria-based progression with return to play by 6 to 8 months. Concomitant procedures (i.e., cartilage restoration) may alter the rehabilitation timeframe.

Results

Excellent to good outcomes have been reported in 80% to 95% of patients.[160,163–167] Long-term studies have shown maintenance of patellar stability with rates of recurrent patellar instability between 8% and 15%.[167–170] However, some patients appear to have a high rate of postoperative patellofemoral pain and arthritis.[171,172] Pidoriano et al.[160] showed that the pattern of preoperative chondral damage correlated with clinical results after antero-medialization of the tibial tuberosity. As expected, patients with distal and lateral lesions improved after surgery, whereas patients with medial, proximal, or diffuse lesions did poorly. To our knowledge, no randomized controlled studies have been performed to examine the efficacy of TTO compared with alternative stabilization techniques.

Complications

A variety of complications have been described with TTO including delayed wound healing, infections, skin necrosis over the tuberosity (only seen with the Maquet procedure),[158,173,174] tuberosity fractures, proximal tibial fractures, delayed union of the osteotomy, and the need for later hardware removal.[164,175–178] Excess anteriorization may increase the risk of incisional breakdown. Compartment syndrome has been reported, and surgeons must remain vigilant for this potentially catastrophic complication.[179,180] Pulmonary emboli[180] and deep venous thrombosis[164] have also been reported, although the role for chemoprophylaxis in these patients remains unclear. Arthrofibrosis, potentially requiring arthroscopic lysis of adhesions and/or manipulation under anesthesia,[156,175,179] can also occur. Early motion[181] is imperative to prevent this complication, and in selected situations, a continuous passive motion machine can be helpful.[164] Because the osteotomy site can serve as a stress riser, a period of restricted weight bearing is critical to avoid proximal tibial fractures.[164,181] Nonunion at the osteotomy site is rare at 3.7% because of compressive interfragmentary fixation.[182,183]

FUTURE CONSIDERATIONS

The diagnosis and treatment of patellar instability remain a complex challenge. Each patient with patellar instability is unique, and his or her specific abnormality must be identified so that treatment plans can be individualized to produce the best outcomes. Despite numerous studies examining the treatment of patellar instability, high-quality outcome data are limited and lacking. Randomized controlled studies and studies with larger sample sizes and long-term follow-up are needed to delineate the role of nonoperative and surgical management. Additional biomechanical studies should provide insight regarding the surgical procedures that will best correct patellar instability and unload damaged articular surfaces. Finally, surgical techniques must be standardized to make studies comparable.

ACKNOWLEDGMENT

The current authors would like to acknowledge the previous authors of this chapter, Dr. Eric W. Tan and Dr. Andrew J. Cosgarea, who provided an excellent road map for creation of the current chapter. We appreciate the opportunity to add to their exemplary work.

For a complete list of references, go to ExpertConsult.com.

SELECTED READINGS

Citation:

Ridley TJ, Bremer Hinckel B, Kruckeberg BM, et al. Anatomical patella instability risk factors on MRI show sensitivity without specificity in patients with patellofemoral instability: a systematic review. *J ISAKOS: Jt Disord Orthop Sports Med.* 2016;1(3):141–152.

Level of Evidence:

III

Summary:

A systematic search of current literature with meta-analysis reveals wide variation of patellofemoral instability (PFI) imaging measurements used for clinical decision-making within the controls and PFI groups. This systematic review demonstrates that appropriate abnormality thresholds of anatomic patella instability imaging factors exist for the PFI group, indicating sensitivity. The wide variation in the majority of measurements, especially in the control group, suggests poor specificity in these measurements.

Citation:

Aframian A, Smith TO, Tennent TD, et al. Origin and insertion of the medial patellofemoral ligament: a systematic review of anatomy. *Knee Surg Sports Traumatol Arthrosc.* 2017;25(12):3755–3772.

Level of Evidence:

IV

Summary:

The MPFL is an hourglass-shaped structure running from a triangular space between the adductor tubercle, medial femoral epicondyle, and gastrocnemius tubercle and inserts onto the superomedial aspect of the patella.

Citation:

Buckens CFM, Saris DBF. Reconstruction of the medial patellofemoral ligament for treatment of patellofemoral instability: a systematic review. *Am J Sports Med.* 2010;38(1):181–188.

Level of Evidence:

II

Summary:

In this review of 14 articles, generally excellent outcomes are shown for medial patellofemoral ligament reconstruction. However, conclusions are limited by small sample sizes, short-term follow-up, use of various adjunct procedures, and lack of standardization of reconstructive surgical procedures.

Citation:

Vavken P, Wimmer MD, Camathias C, et al. Pagenstert g. Treating patella instability in skeletally immature patients. *Arthroscopy*. 2013;29(8):1410–1422.

Level of Evidence:

IV

Summary:

A systematic review of the treatment of immature and adolescent patients with acute and chronic patellar instability. Best evidence does not support the superiority of surgical intervention over conservative treatment in an acute patellar dislocation. However, anatomic variations and their effect on healing should be considered and included in decision-making. In recurrent patellar instability in pediatric and adolescent patients with normal or restored knee anatomy, reconstruction of the MPFL is the most effective treatment option and can be done safely, together with extensor realignment as needed.

Citation:

Farr J, Covell DJ, Lattermann C. Cartilage lesions in patellofemoral dislocations: incidents/locations/when to treat. *Sports Med Arthrosc*. 2012;20(3):181–186.

Level of Evidence:

IV

Summary:

PF dislocations are frequently associated with chondral injury. Chondral and osteochondral lesions are often associated with traumatic (high-energy) PF dislocations, whereas atraumatic (low-energy) PF dislocations in patients with significant PF risk factors have a much lower incidence of osteochondral damage. This article provides overview of the incidence and when to treat those lesions.

Citation:

Sherman SL, Erickson BJ, Cvetanovich GL, et al. Tibial tuberosity osteotomy: indications, techniques, and outcomes. *Am J Sports Med*. 2014;42(8):2006–2017.

Level of Evidence:

IV

Summary:

TTO is a well-described treatment option for a broad range of patellofemoral joint disorders, including patellofemoral instability, patellar and trochlear focal chondral lesions, and patellofemoral arthritis. The purpose of this article is to review the evolution of the TTO procedure, from the original Hauser procedure to the current anteromedialization procedure, as well as discuss the pertinent anatomy and radiographs that accompany this procedure. The article highlights the surgical techniques for some of the more commonly performed TTO procedures and discusses the outcomes of the various TTO techniques. Complications, as well as clinical pearls to avoid these complications, are also included.

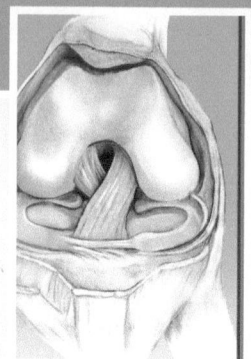

106

Patellofemoral Pain

Meagan McCarthy, Eric C. McCarty, Rachel M. Frank

Patellofemoral pain is common, with an incidence as high as 50% in some populations.[1] Often referred to as anterior knee pain, patellofemoral pain can be challenging for both patients and clinicians, as it can often be difficult to determine the underlying etiology responsible for the pain. Some patients with patellofemoral pain have no definable pathology. This process has been described by different names, including patellofemoral pain syndrome (PFPS) and idiopathic anterior knee pain. It is important to note that these terms to some extent are diagnoses of exclusion and should not be used to mislabel a definable disease process. It is also a misnomer to attribute all patellofemoral pain to "chondromalacia," because in many cases, no true chondral pathology exists.

ANATOMY

The anterior aspect of the knee has several unique properties that serve as a predisposition for pain. The patellofemoral joint itself is a sliding articulation with six degrees of freedom. Patellar tracking is defined by translation (medial/lateral), glide (superior/inferior), and tilt (medial/lateral). During initial knee flexion, the patella translates approximately 4 mm medially to engage the trochlear groove at approximately 20 degrees of knee flexion. With progressive flexion, the patella translates approximately 7 mm laterally by the time the knee reaches 90 degrees of flexion, associated with approximately 7 degrees of lateral tilt. Maximum contact between the trochlear groove and the patella occurs at 45 degrees of knee flexion.[126]

In addition to the bony anatomy described above, there are both passive and dynamic restraints that contribute to the stability of the patellofemoral joint. Passive restraints include the osseous morphology, the medial patellofemoral ligament (MPFL), the medial patellomeniscal ligament, and the lateral retinaculum. Dynamic restraints include the vastus medialis oblique (VMO) and the vastus lateralis. A thorough understanding of these structures allows for a better ability to understand the common clinical problems associated with the patellofemoral joint as it attempts to meet its contradictory demands of providing both mobility and stability.[122-127] Any imbalance to this complex network of structures can result in pain, instability, or both.

The patella serves to improve the mechanical leverage of the quadriceps muscle by increasing the lever arm and transmitting the tensile forces generated by the quadriceps to the patellar tendon. There is a delicate interplay of forces acting on the patella, which sees an incredible amount of force.[121] In particular, the patellofemoral joint experiences joint reaction forces that become higher as the knee flexion angle increases (Fig. 106.1).[2] Squatting and jumping, for example, have been reported to create forces 7.6-times and 12-times body weight, respectively.[3,4]

The anterior aspect of the knee also provides significant sensory feedback. In a 1998 study by Dye et al., in which SF Dye (first author of that study) underwent bilateral knee arthroscopies without anesthesia in an effort to determine conscious neurosensory characteristics of the knee, the authors described the highest subjective pain sensations in the anterior synovium, fat pad, and joint capsule.[5] Interestingly, structures that commonly require intervention (e.g., the menisci, articular cartilage, and ligaments) were much less sensitive.[5] Dye and colleagues[5] also reported accurate spatial localization to palpation in the anterior structures (Fig. 106.2), which correlates with previous findings about the relatively high concentration of type IVa afferent nerve fibers in the patellar ligament and retinaculum.[6]

Malalignment is a commonly proposed mechanism for patellofemoral pain.[10,11] Overall limb malalignment can cause or exacerbate patellofemoral joint disorders. The lines of action of the quadriceps and the patellar tendon are not collinear—the angular difference between them is called the quadriceps (Q) angle (Fig. 106.3). The Q-angle is an angle formed from a line drawn from the anterior superior iliac spine to the middle of patella, and from the middle of the patella to the tibial tuberosity on a full-length weight-bearing radiograph. A normal Q-angle in males is 13 to 14 degrees and 17 to 18 degrees in females.[120] Because of this angle, the force generated by the quadriceps both extends the knee and pulls the patella laterally. The relative magnitude of this laterally directed force is proportional to the Q-angle. External rotation of the tibia, internal rotation of the femur, and increasing knee valgus each result in an increase in Q-angle and an associated increase in the laterally directed force within the patellofemoral joint. While patella maltracking as a result of any of the above-listed factors can cause substantial pain and dysfunction, some authors have questioned the link between malalignment and patellofemoral pain.[12-14] The common occurrence of pain at rest in patients with patellofemoral pain is an argument against malalignment as a major component of anterior knee pain.[15] Dye[12] proposed that pain is from a loss of tissue homeostasis. Increased intraosseous pressure in the patella with resultant tissue ischemia has also been proposed.[16] Other studies suggested altered vascular flow (arterial and venous) and

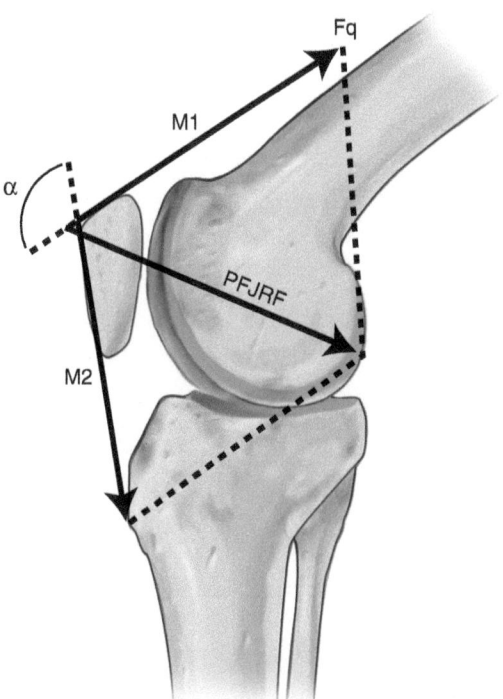

Fig. 106.1 The patellofemoral joint reaction force *(PFJRF)* becomes higher as the knee flexion angle increases. In complete extension, *M1* and *M2* are in opposite directions, but in the same plane; the resultant PFJRF is almost zero. As flexion increases, M1 and M2 converge, and the vector PFJRF increases. (From Scott WN, ed. *Insall & Scott Surgery of the Knee.* 5th ed. Philadelphia: Elsevier; 2012.)

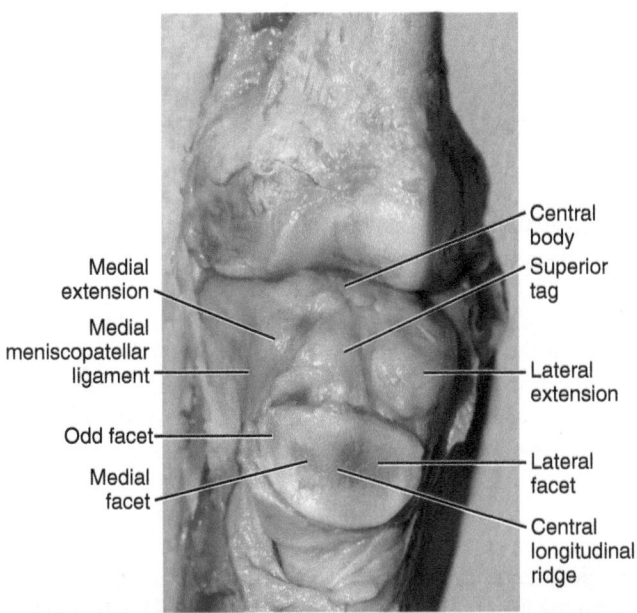

Fig. 106.2 Posterior anatomy of the patella with adjacent capsular thickenings and fat pads with the medial and lateral meniscopatellar ligaments. (From Noyes FR, ed. *Noyes' Knee Disorders: Surgery, Rehabilitation, Clinical Outcomes.* Philadelphia: Elsevier; 2010.)

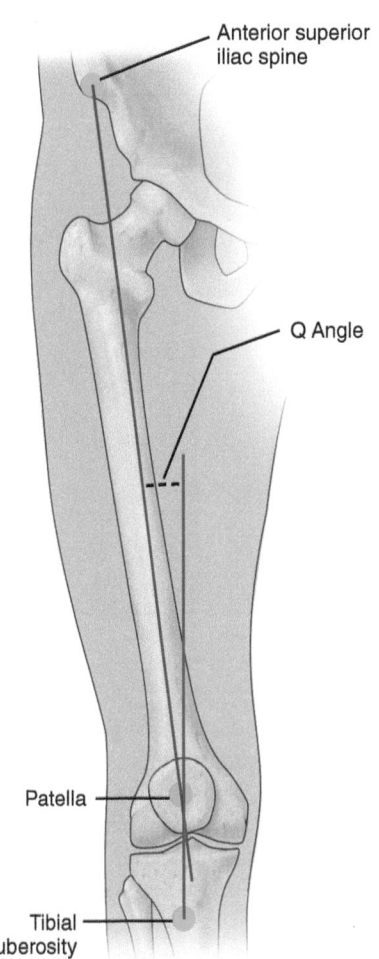

Fig. 106.3 Q angle. (Modified from Livingston LA, Mandigo JL. Bilateral Q angle asymmetry and anterior knee pain syndrome. *Clin Biomech [Bristol, Avon].* 1999;14[1]:7–13.)

concomitant degenerative conditions as being associated with symptoms generation in patellofemoral syndrome.[17–19]

PATIENT EVALUATION

History

A comprehensive history is critical to evaluation of patients presenting with patellofemoral pain. The first distinction is determining if the patient is presenting with pain or if the patient is complaining of patellar instability. While in many cases, patients have both of these complaints, when asked about their primary complaint, patients will often endorse either a chief complaint of instability with reasonable pain resolution after an acute incident, or significant pain with no symptoms of true instability. Many of the diagnoses associated with acute traumatic injuries (e.g., extensor mechanism disruption, patellar fractures, and patellar instability) are addressed in other chapters. Chronic, activity-related anterior knee pain is a common clinical complaint that occurs in a variety of knee disorders and is associated with a broad differential diagnosis (Table 106.1).

Patients should be asked about activities that cause pain, if pain occurs at rest and/or during sleep, and if the pain is

TABLE 106.1	Differential Diagnosis of Patellofemoral Pain	
Acute Pain	**Chronic Pain**	**Constant Pain**
• Extensor mechanism disruption	• Idiopathic (patellofemoral pain syndrome)	• Complex regional pain syndrome
• Patellar instability (dislocation, subluxation)	• Malalignment	• Neuroma
• Patella fracture	• Muscular imbalance/atrophy	• Oncologic process
• Chondral injury	• Overuse injury	
• Osteochondral injury	• Patella chondromalacia	
• Loose body	• Synovial fat pad impingement	
• Infection	• Symptomatic plica	
• Hip pathology (referred pain)	• Intraosseous hypertension of the patella	
• Slipped capital femoral epiphysis (referred pain)	• Lateral patella compression syndrome	
• Lumbar spine referred pain	• Osteoarthritis	
	• Inflammatory arthritis	
	• Iliotibial band syndrome	
	• Patellar tendonitis	
	• Osteochondritis dissecans	
	• Osteochondroses	
	• Osgood-Schlatter	
	• Sinding-Larsen-Johansson	

associated with swelling and/or mechanical symptoms. A history of effusions often is associated with an intra-articular problem, such as a chondral lesion, whereas the absence of effusions may suggest an extra-articular etiology of pain. Details on prior successful, as well as unsuccessful treatments, including activity modification, physical therapy, injections, and/or surgeries, should be documented. In the setting of chronic, activity-related anterior knee pain without a history of trauma, patients will often complain of discomfort while ascending or descending stairs, during deep squats, or after sitting for prolonged periods. In addition, it can be common for patients to complain of symptoms bilaterally.[20] An onset of patellofemoral pain is also common during sudden periods of increased activity, such as during high-intensity training with military recruits.[21]

Physical Examination

Similar to a comprehensive history, a thorough physical examination is essential in the evaluation of patients with patellofemoral pain. Notably, it is important to appreciate that many variations exist with respect to patellofemoral anatomy. These variations can become evident during examination, and while for some patients, they may be responsible for patellofemoral pain, in other cases, they may simply be "normal" for that particular patient. The examination findings are a portion of the complex clinical picture commonly encountered in the patient with anterior knee pain.

General

Patients presenting with anterior knee pain should undergo a standard physical examination of both knees, including an assessment of gait and alignment, range of motion (ROM), strength, generalized ligamentous laxity, stability, and neurovascular status. In addition, the clinician should examine the ipsilateral hip, particularly in pediatric and adolescent patients, as primary hip pathology can often present as knee pain.

Inspection

While there are many different techniques for performing a physical examination of the knee, it can be efficient to begin with the patient standing, then seated, and then supine (and prone, if desired). The critical aspect is ensuring that all components of the examination are completed for every patient. If beginning with the patient standing, the clinician can assess limb alignment, rotation profile, and gait. Patients with increased femoral anteversion, genu valgum, and pes planovalgus may be at an increased risk for patellofemoral pain. In addition, patients with external tibial torsion and foot pronation may experience increased patellofemoral pain. Monitoring the patient's gait as well as observing a single-leg squat can be helpful in the assessment of patellar tracking and general core strength.

Once seated with the legs hanging off the end of the examination table, an evaluation of patellar tracking and an assessment of the Q-angle can be performed. Techniques for assessing Q-angle are variable, and can be performed with the patient in the standing, seated, or supine position. In addition, Q-angle measurements can be performed statically (static Q-angle) with the quadriceps contracted or with the quadriceps relaxed, as well as in a dynamic-fashion (dynamic Q-angle). It is important to appreciate that the Q-angle value may be affected by the relationship of the proximal femur and the amount of knee flexion (Figs. 106.4 and 106.5), as well as by the method in which the assessment is performed. The Q-angle assessment with the knee in flexion may be more accurate than with the knee extended, as in flexion the patella is well-seated in the trochlear groove, whereas in extension, a laterally translated patella may falsely result in a "normal" Q-angle. Some authors have suggested a dynamic Q-angle evaluation may be of more utility than a static measurement in the evaluation of patients with patellofemoral pain, though this is controversial.[21a] An elevated Q-angle may predispose the patient to anterior knee pain, although significant variability exists. In the seated position, asking the patient to

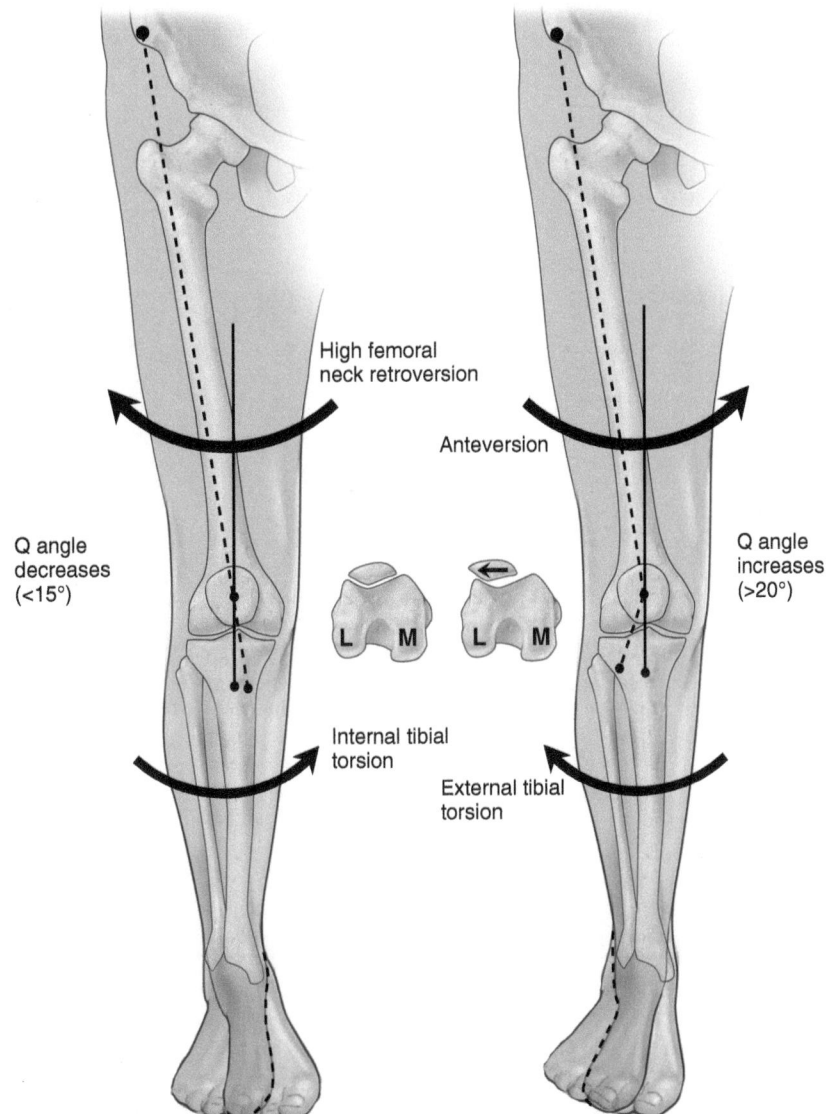

Fig. 106.4 High femoral neck retroversion rotates the distal end of the femur externally. In combination with internal tibial torsion, the Q angle is decreased. Patellar tracking is improved, and patellofemoral sulcus alignment is normal. High femoral neck anteversion rotates the distal end of the femur internally. In combination with external tibial torsion, the Q angle is increased. Patellar tracking is compromised, and the patella tends to track laterally. (From Tria Jr AJ, Klein KS. *An Illustrated Guide to the Knee.* New York: Churchill Livingstone; 1992.)

actively flex and extend his/her knee will allow for an assessment of patellar tracking. A J-sign is noted when the patella deviates laterally when the knee reaches terminal extension; the Q-angle may be less accurate in full extension in a patient with a positive J sign.

At any point during the inspection portion of the examination, the clinician should assess for muscular atrophy, particular with respect to the vastus medialis obliquus (VMO), prior surgical incisions, and the presence/absence of an effusion.

Palpation

Many of the structures about the knee that may be pain generators can be directly palpated, including the patella itself, the infrapatellar fat pad, quadriceps and patellar tendon attachments

on the patella, retinaculum/patellofemoral ligaments, tibial tubercle, iliotibial band, joint lines, and femoral condyles (among other structures). Palpating these structures can be helpful in determining an underlying anatomical source of pain, if one exists. In addition, palpating the patella during knee flexion/extension allows for an assessment of crepitus. In one study, 98% of adolescent patients with patellofemoral pain experienced pain with palpation over the MPFL.[23] Notably, larger body habitus as well as guarding can make the palpation portion of the examination more difficult.

Range of Motion and Strength

Knee ROM can be assessed in the seated, supine, or prone positions. Regardless of the position used, it is important to compare

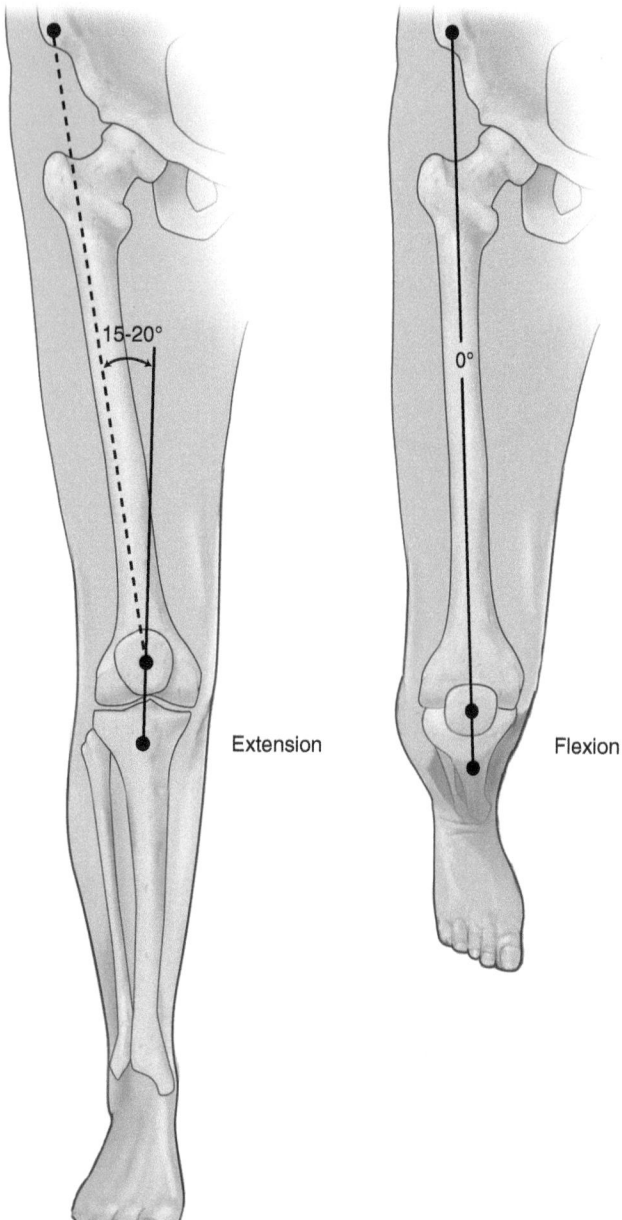

Fig. 106.5 Flexion of the knee decreases the Q angle as the result of internal tibial rotation. (From Tria Jr AJ, Klein KS. *An Illustrated Guide to the Knee*. New York: Churchill Livingstone; 1992.)

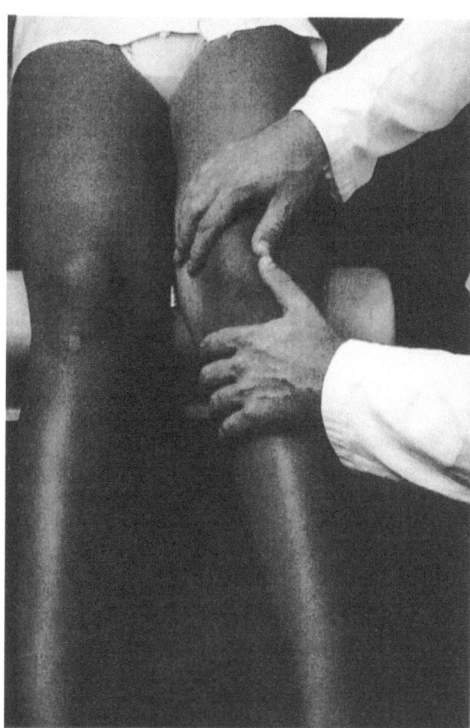

Fig. 106.6 The patellar compression test. With the knee flexed slightly to engage the patella in the femoral trochlea, direct compression is applied to the patella. (From Scott WN, ed. *Insall & Scott Surgery of the Knee*. 5th ed. Philadelphia: Elsevier; 2012.)

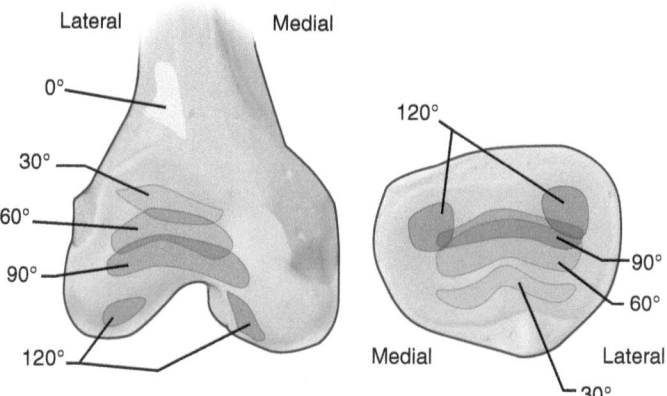

Fig. 106.7 The patellofemoral joint contact areas according to the knee flexion angle. (From Scott WN, ed. *Insall & Scott Surgery of the Knee*. 5th ed: Philadelphia: Elsevier; 2012.)

the symptomatic knee to the uninvolved knee, and to assess for baseline hyperextension. During ROM assessment, strength to resisted knee flexion and extension can also be assessed and compared side to side.

Provocative Tests

Provocative tests about the patella generally fall into two categories: tests to elicit pain, and tests to provoke instability. A variety of different tests have been described in which pressure is applied to the patella, including the patellar grind test, patellar compression test, and Clarke sign.[25,26] These tests involve some variation of applying pressure on the superior aspect of the patella with the examiner's thumb, often while asking the patient to contract

their quadriceps muscle. If pain occurs, these tests are considered positive for retropatellar chondral pathology. A more gently applied posterior force to the patella during flexion and extension may elicit crepitus and pain in patients with retropatellar chondral pathology (Fig. 106.6). This test may help identify the location of pathology, because a more distal lesion will be painful in early flexion as the patella engages the trochlea, whereas a more proximal lesion will be painful at greater degrees of knee flexion (Fig. 106.7).

Patellar instability testing is discussed in detail in Chapter 105. The patellar apprehension test is performed by application of a laterally directed pressure to the medial aspect of

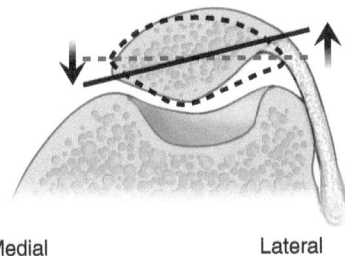

Medial   Lateral

Fig. 106.8 The passive patellar tilt test. In full extension, the transverse axis of a normal patella tilts beyond the horizontal. The inability to perform this maneuver may indicate an excessively tight lateral retinaculum. (From Scott WN, ed. *Insall & Scott Surgery of the Knee.* 5th ed. Philadelphia: Elsevier; 2012.)

the patella with the knee in approximately 20 to 30 degrees of flexion. The test is positive if the patient experiences apprehension that the patella may dislocate laterally. If the patient experiences no apprehension but his/her patella is able to be subluxated or substantially translated laterally, the patient may have baseline ligamentous laxity and the clinician should examine the opposite knee for similar findings. Notably, while patients with patellofemoral pain may experience pain during apprehension testing, pain itself does not represent a positive test for instability. Manipulation of the patella in the transverse plane may reveal a tight retinaculum, as evidenced by a lack of motion (Fig. 106.8). The patellar tilt test should also be performed as an assessment for a tight retinaculum and may have some utility in determining possible interventions.[28] The Ober test is useful to assess for iliotibial (IT) band tightness that can contribute to anterolateral knee pain as well as patellar maltracking.[128]

Diagnostic Studies

Imaging studies, including radiographs, computed tomography (CT), and magnetic resonance imaging (MRI) can be helpful in the valuation of patients with patellofemoral pain. Radiographs, including anterior-posterior (AP), lateral, and axial (merchant or sunrise), are useful for evaluating the osseous morphology of the patellofemoral and tibiofemoral joints, as well as for identifying signs of arthritis. The lateral radiograph is perhaps the most useful in the evaluation of the patellofemoral joint, as it is useful for determining patellar height (Fig. 106.9) as well as trochlear dysplasia. Patella height can be determined via several different techniques, including the Caton-Deschamps index, Insall-Salvati ratio, Blackburne-Peel ratio, and the relationship of Blumensaat line to the inferior pole of the patella at 30 degrees of knee flexion. Patients with patella alta may have a predisposition to instability, whereas patients with patella baja may encounter increased patellar load and the subsequent risk of degenerative conditions. The lateral view is also helpful for identifying abnormal trochlear morphology according to the Dejour classification system.[28a,28b] In the Dejour system, trochlea dysplasia is classified as types A, B, C, or D (most severe), depending on if a crossing sign, supratrochlear spur, and/or double contour are present. Axial views such as the Merchant view (Fig. 106.10)[29] can help determine sulcus angle as well as the depth of the groove. Murray

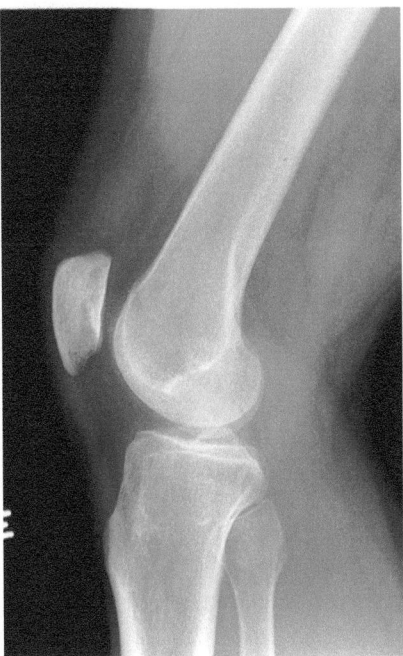

Fig. 106.9 Lateral radiograph of the knee.

et al.[30] demonstrated that the lateral and axial views are the most useful views for evaluating instability and noted a high sensitivity of the lateral view for detecting prior dislocation; thus a normal lateral radiograph can help rule out instability as a component of anterior knee pain in some patients. The axial view is also useful for evaluating patellar tilt and subluxation. Different parameters have been defined, and the clinical utility of these parameters remains uncertain (Fig. 106.11). When evaluating axial radiographs, it is important to note that the sulcus of the trochlea lies lateral to the midline of the femoral condyles and is not completely centered as previously thought.[31] Interestingly, articular congruity may exist on magnetic resonance arthrogram (MRA) imaging, even when osseous incongruity appears on plain radiographs.[32]

Advanced imaging with CT can be very helpful given its ability to analyze the three-dimensional relationships of the patellofemoral joint. Data from CT imaging can help identify patellar tilt and tibial tuberosity–trochlear groove (TT-TG) value. Notably, indications for CT imaging in patients without patellar instability are limited, as patellar tilt and TT-TG measurements are most useful in the evaluation of patients experiencing patellar subluxation or dislocation events (see Chapter 105 for details on these measurements).

MRI is the imaging modality of choice for evaluating the articular cartilage and underlying subchondral bone and soft tissue structures such as the MPFL (Fig. 106.12). One study demonstrated that edema in the superolateral fat pad on MRI correlates with other anatomic parameters (e.g., trochlear morphology and patellar alignment) suggestive of patellar maltracking or impingement in the young, symptomatic patient.[33] Data points helpful for evaluating patellar instability, including TT-TG (originally described on CT scan) and TT-posterior cruciate ligament (TT-PCL), can be taken on MRI. In addition, lateral trochlear

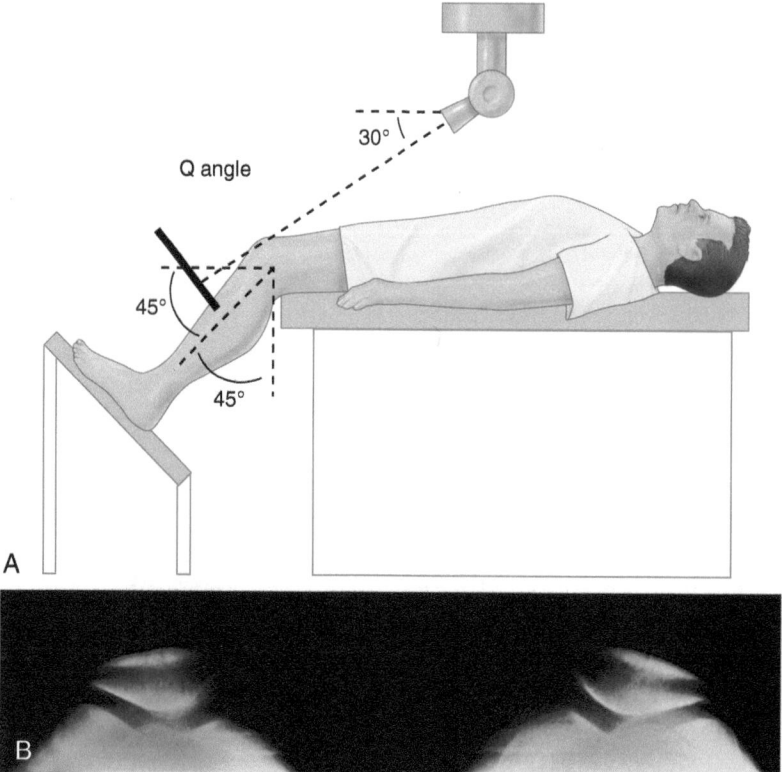

Fig. 106.10 Merchant view. (A) Technique. (B) A normal Merchant view. Patellofemoral alignment is normal bilaterally, and the osseous structures and articular cortices are normal. (From Scott WN, ed. *Insall & Scott Surgery of the Knee.* 5th ed. Philadelphia: Elsevier; 2012.)

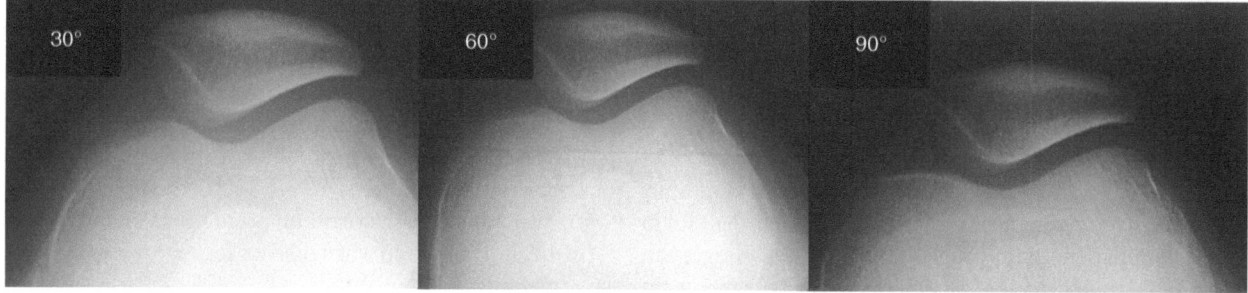

Fig. 106.11 Axial views performed at 30, 60, and 90 degrees of knee flexion. Note how the trochlear shape changes as flexion increases and the medial facet seems bigger. It is not necessary to routinely perform 60- and 90-degree flexion radiographs in common patellofemoral disorders. (From Scott WN, ed. *Insall & Scott Surgery of the Knee,* 5th ed. Philadelphia: Elsevier; 2012.)

inclination and medial trochlear inclination measurements can be taken on MRI, which may be more accurate than the sulcus angle in identifying abnormal trochlea morphology.

SPECIFIC CONDITIONS

Idiopathic Anterior Knee Pain/Patellofemoral Pain Syndrome

As mentioned throughout this chapter, as well as many other chapters in this text, a variety of factors contribute to anterior knee pain. As such, the differential diagnosis for anterior knee pain is broad (see Table 106.1). Many of the specific pathologies described in Table 106.1 have been discussed in detail throughout this text. Many patients have no identifiable lesion responsible

for their patellofemoral pain, and the remaining portion of this chapter will focus on those pathologies. This type of condition is often referred to as PFPS. In patients with PFPS, the practitioner may find some potentially predisposing factors on physical examination or imaging, including malalignment (lower limb or patella), muscular imbalance and/or atrophy, and overuse. In a prospective study, patients with a hypermobile patella had a higher incidence of anterior knee pain, and in a separate study this examination finding correlated with a worse prognosis for patients with patellofemoral pain.[34,35] However, these findings can be common in patients without anterior knee pain. Overall, this is a diagnosis of exclusion, and the lack of objective, diagnostic criteria make it challenging for determining optimal treatment options.

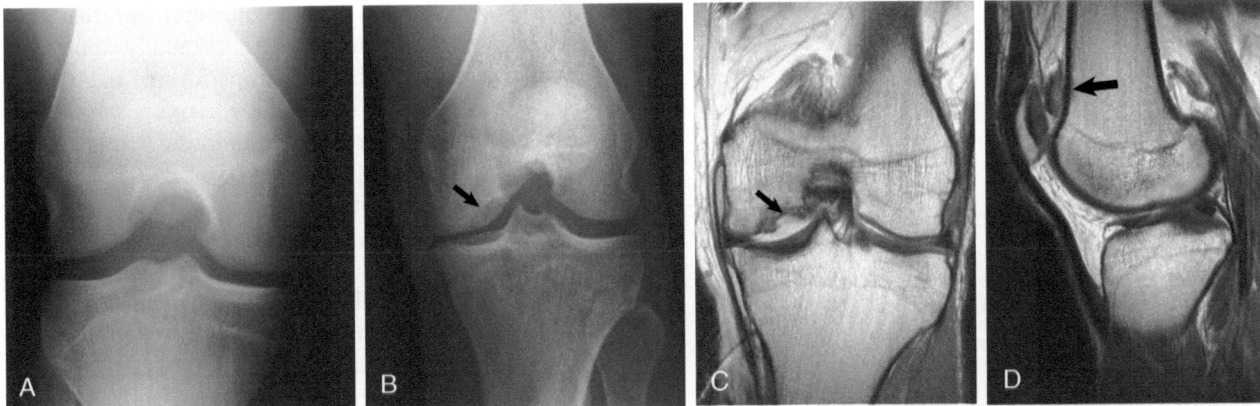

Fig. 106.12 Tunnel view. (A) A normal tunnel view demonstrates the posterior aspect of the femoral condyles, the tibial spines, the articular surfaces of the tibial plateau, and the intercondylar notch. (B) A tunnel view from a different patient demonstrating an ovoid area of lucency at the inner margin of the medial femoral condyle *(arrow)* that is suspicious for osteochondritis dissecans. Coronal (C) and sagittal proton density (D) magnetic resonance imaging confirms the large osteochondral defect *(arrow)* with a completely displaced osteochondral fragment located in the suprapatellar joint recess *(arrow)*. (Case courtesy the Hospital for Special Surgery, New York. From Scott WN, ed. *Insall & Scott Surgery of the Knee.* 5th ed. Philadelphia: Elsevier; 2012.)

The treatment of idiopathic PFPS focuses on primarily activity modification, physical therapy and muscular strengthening, bracing/taping, orthotics, electrotherapy, and pharmacotherapy. A systematic review of exercise therapy for patellofemoral pain demonstrated that exercise therapy showed little benefit with respect to pain reduction when compared to no exercise therapy.[37] In addition, another systematic review of the use of therapeutic ultrasound for treating PFPS failed demonstrate any clinically important effect on pain relief.[129] Furthermore, Callaghan et al. reviewed the use of patellar taping for PFPS in adults and found that there was limited evidence to suggest that taping can significantly improve outcomes compared to other exercise-based interventions not incorporating taping.[130] One study looking at military recruits with no history of anterior knee pain who were prospectively divided into a bracing group (dynamic patellofemoral brace) and a non-bracing group during basic training showed an almost 20% decrease in anterior knee pain symptoms in the bracing group (18.5% experienced pain versus 37% in the non-bracing group).[131] Another study showed that patients with a pronated foot type and poorer footwear motion control properties who wore a foot orthoses were associated with reduced anterior knee pain during the single-leg squat and improvements in the number of pain-free single-leg rises from sitting.[132] A systematic review of pharmacotherapy for the treatment of anterior knee pain found that there is only limited evidence for the effectiveness of nonsteroidal antiinflammatory drugs (NSAIDs) for short-term pain reduction.[38] Bizzini et al. analyzed the quality of randomized controlled trials for treatment of patellofemoral pain and showed that acupuncture, quadriceps strengthening, the use of a resistive brace, and the combination of exercises with patellar taping and biofeedback were effective in decreasing pain and improving function.[133] Overall, there is mixed evidence regarding the success of nonoperative treatment for the management of patellofemoral pain.

For patients who have significant disability despite use of nonoperative treatment modalities for a minimum of 6 months,

arthroscopy can be considered for diagnostic and therapeutic reasons, including assessment of potential chondral lesions (please see Chapters 96 and 104 on patellar cartilage disorders). It can be helpful before performing arthroscopy to attempt a diagnostic intra-articular injection with local anesthesia (with or without corticosteroid); if such an injection does not provide even temporary relief, the benefits of an arthroscopy are less predictable. Patellar denervation has been described using electrocautery[39] and can be accomplished via an anterolateral, anteromedial, and superior portal (either medial and lateral). This procedure should be applied sparingly, and the authors strongly urge the clinician to search for other diagnoses before labeling a condition as idiopathic anterior knee pain or PFPS.

Synovial Impingement Syndromes

Impingement is a common cause of patellofemoral pain. The offending structures are typically a plica or the infrapatellar fat pad. The plicae are embryologic remnants that are normal anatomic structures. Differentiating between pathologic and normal plica is difficult.[40] The medial plica is most commonly symptomatic (Fig. 106.13).[41] This plica was shown to be present in approximately 80% of the population in one study series.[42] Patients with synovial plica syndrome (SPS) often describe activity-related pain that worsens with flexion and is relieved with extension. With a hypertrophic plica, a thick palpable cord may be palpable on physical examination. Both flexion and extension tests have been described to aid in the diagnosis of pathologic plicae, but they are of limited utility.[43] MRI may detect a prominent plica, but no study has demonstrated a role for determining pathologic versus normal plicae. Chondral pathology of the medial femoral condyle has been noted in cases of severe plicae, and this pathology may be appreciated on MRI.[44] The treatment of symptomatic plicae should begin with nonoperative options, including activity modification, NSAIDs, and if needed, intra-articular corticosteroid injections. For patients who do not respond to nonoperative treatment, arthroscopy with plica excision is a

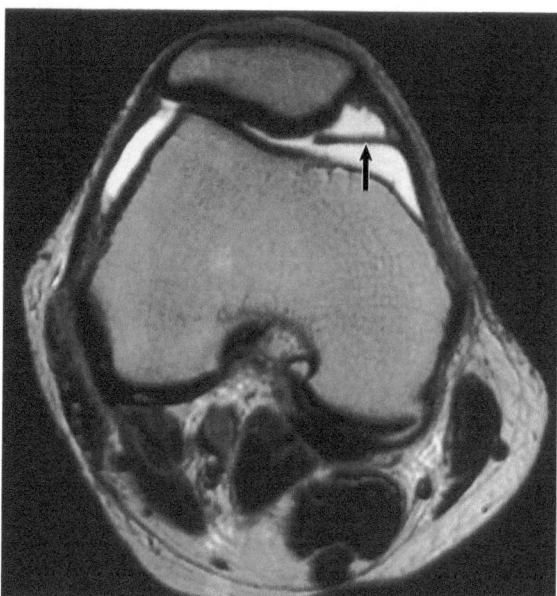

Fig. 106.13 An axial magnetic resonance image with a low-signal, thick medial patellar plica *(arrow)* that is highlighted by the large effusion. (From Scott WN, ed. *Insall & Scott Surgery of the Knee.* 5th ed. Philadelphia: Elsevier; 2012.)

relatively straightforward option with low associated morbidity, and in patients with associated cartilage degeneration, midterm results support plica excision.[46] If proceeding to arthroscopy, the surgeon should include a thorough evaluation for associated concomitant knee pathology.

The infrapatellar fat pad was implicated in anterior knee pain by Hoffa[47] in 1904. As previously described, this area has a rich innervation and can result in substantial anterior knee pain, associated with superficial swelling and tenderness to palpation. The Hoffa maneuver involves applying pressure just medial and lateral to the patellar tendon (separately) and extending the knee, which may elicit either pain or apprehension. While the diagnosis is primarily clinical, some evidence indicates that MRI may aid in the diagnosis, and use of MRI may become more relevant with the utilization of MRIs with stronger magnets.[33,48] The treatment of fat pad impingement is similar to the initial treatment for symptomatic plica, including nonoperative strategies. For patients who do not respond to conservative modalities, surgical excision of the fat pad has been described.[48–50] The authors recommend this treatment only when the patient has exhausted all nonoperative modalities and have excluded any other factor that may contribute to the patient's symptoms (alignment, muscle imbalance, etc.).

Intraosseous Hypertension of the Patella

Increased intraosseous pressure has been described in the femur and tibia of painful knees by Arnoldi and colleagues.[51] These investigators later correlated knee pain with increased pressure in the patella. It has been suggested that this phenomenon may be related to decreased venous outflow based on intraosseous phlebography.[52] The diagnostic criterion for patellar hypertension is an increase in intraosseous pressure of greater than 25 mm Hg with sustained knee flexion. Schneider and colleagues[53,54] reported

on a series of patients with patellofemoral pain that failed to respond to conservative measures. After administration of a local anesthetic a "provocation test" was performed (i.e., the reproduction of symptoms by raising the intraosseous pressure), and patients underwent intraosseous drilling and decompression. At 1-year follow-up, 88% of subjects had an objective decrease in pressure measurement.[53] A subsequent publication demonstrated improved clinical outcome scores (the visual analog scale score decreased from 7.6 to 2.1) with this treatment protocol at 3 years postsurgery.[55] While overall this diagnosis is somewhat controversial, several series have demonstrated that patellar drilling and decompression may benefit patients who fail to respond to nonoperative treatment for patellofemoral pain. It remains unclear if this diagnosis is the primary pathology or if it is secondary to other disease processes (including lateral patella compression syndrome).

Lateral Patella Compression Syndrome

Ficat[56] originally described lateral patellar compression syndrome, and the underlying etiology is thought to be attributed to a tight lateral retinaculum. Patients typically report pain (without instability) while ascending or descending stairs and may have a positive theatre sign (i.e., pain with prolonged sitting). As the condition progresses, chondral wear can occur, and symptoms including effusions, locking, clicking, catching, and/or giving way may occur. On examination, patients will have pain with patellar compression testing, particularly along the lateral aspect. Notably, patients will not exhibit excessive patellar mobility as the retinaculum is tight, and the examiner may have difficulty everting the lateral patellar edge above parallel to the floor. These patients may also have subtle findings of an increased Q-angle, a tight iliotibial band (IT band, seen with a positive Ober test[128]), and increased foot pronation. Axial radiographs or axial CT scans will demonstrate increased lateral patellar tilt and a decreased lateral patellofemoral angle. The treatment of lateral patellar compression syndrome should primarily focus on nonoperative modalities to decrease inflammation, including the use of NSAIDs, activity modification, and physical therapy. Modalities to help loosen the lateral retinaculum and IT band are useful adjuncts. For patients who fail to respond to nonoperative treatment and continue to have pain and dysfunction, surgery can be considered. This condition remains one of the few indications for an isolated lateral release. Certainly, if performing a lateral release, it is important to ensure the release is not too aggressive to avoid the development of iatrogenic medial patellar instability.[57] If any evidence of patellar hypermobility exists, then an open lateral retinacular lengthening procedure can be considered.

Complex Regional Pain Syndrome

Reflex sympathetic dystrophy was suggested as a cause of some anterior knee pain by Merchant[10] in 1988. Specific to anterior knee pain, scintigraphy has been demonstrated to aid in the diagnosis of sympathetically mediated pain, and a sympathetic blockade may be a useful treatment modality.[120] The discussion of complex regional pain syndrome is beyond the scope of this chapter, but it is an important consideration in the differential diagnosis for chronic patellofemoral pain.

ACKNOWLEDGMENT

The author and editors gratefully acknowledge the contributions of the previous authors, Brett W. Mccoy, Waqas M. Hussain, Michael J. Griesser, and Richard D. Parker.

For a complete list of references, go to ExpertConsult.com.

SELECTED READINGS

Citation:
Dye SF. The pathophysiology of patellofemoral pain: a tissue homeostasis perspective. *Clin Orthop Relat Res.* 2005;436:100–110.

Level of Evidence:
V

Summary:
In this article, the authors evaluate the perspective that tissue homeostasis such as intraosseous hypertension is the etiology of patellofemoral pain in contrast to structural abnormalities.

Citation:
Dye SF, Vaupel GL, Dye CC. Conscious neurosensory mapping of the internal structures of the human knee without intraarticular anesthesia. *Am J Sports Med.* 1998;26(6):773–777.

Level of Evidence:
V

Summary:
In this article, the authors report the case of a physician who underwent knee arthroscopy without use of an anesthetic, and the degree of noxious stimulus in various locations is noted.

Citation:
Kodali P, Islam A, Andrish J. Anterior knee pain in the young athlete: diagnosis and treatment. *Sports Med Arthrosc.* 2011;19(1):27–33.

Level of Evidence:
V

Summary:
In this review article, the various etiologies and treatments of anterior knee pain are discussed.

Citation:
Pihlajamaki HK, Visuri TI. Long-term outcome after surgical treatment of unresolved Osgood-Schlatter disease in young men: surgical technique. *J Bone Joint Surg Am.* 2010;92A(suppl 1 Pt 2):258–264.

Level of Evidence:
IV

Summary:
In this article, a case series is described with follow-up of patients with Osgood-Schlatter disease who did not respond to conservative management and subsequently underwent operative intervention. In this series, 87% of subjects had no activity limitation with activities of daily living and 75% returned to their preoperative athletic level.

Citation:
Witvrouw E, Lysens R, Bellemans J, et al. Intrinsic risk factors for the development of anterior knee pain in an athletic population. A two-year prospective study. *Am J Sports Med.* 2000;28(4):480–489.

Level of Evidence:
II

Summary:
In this description of a prospective cohort study, 282 athletic patients were followed up to evaluate risk factors for anterior knee pain. The authors noted a significant correlation between the incidence of patellofemoral pain and patients with a shortened quadriceps muscle, an altered vastus medialis obliquus muscle reflex response time, decreased explosive strength, and a hypermobile patella.

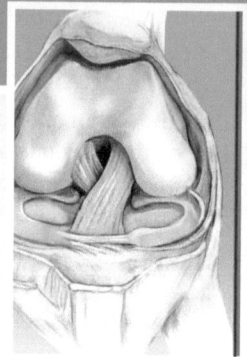

107

Extensor Mechanism Injuries

Matthew Bessette, Drew Toftoy, Richard D. Parker, Rachel M. Frank

The patellar and quadriceps tendons along with the patella make up the extensor mechanism of the knee. Disease of the extensor mechanism tendons ranges from tendinopathy to complete rupture. Tendinopathies commonly affect healthy athletes secondary to chronic overuse, but they can also occur in the presence of systemic diseases and endocrinopathies as well as in conjunction with certain medications and hormonal supplements. Ruptures commonly occur in the setting of preexisting tendinopathy. The patella is subject to additional patterns of injury including fracture, maltracking, and dislocation.

Advances in imaging assist in the evaluation and treatment of extensor mechanism disorders. In combination with clinical findings, these studies not only confirm pathology but also provide prognostic information, direct therapeutic approaches, and facilitate surgical planning. Operative and nonoperative treatment plans can be tailored based on patient characteristics, sport-specific demands, and imaging findings. An effective physician must understand the options and indications for both.

ANATOMY

The extensor mechanism is composed of the quadriceps, quadriceps tendon, patella, and patellar tendon. The patellar tendon has also been referred to as the patellar ligament. To minimize confusion, the structure is referred to as the *patellar tendon* throughout this chapter, as the patella is a sesamoid bone found within the extensor mechanism. Pathology and disability can be derived from any of these structures or any adjacent anatomy, such as the patellofemoral articulation.

The patella has multiple static stabilizers including the quadriceps and patellar tendons, the osseous congruence of the patella within the trochlear groove, the medial and lateral retinaculum, and multiple associated ligaments including the medial patellofemoral (MPFL) and patellomeniscal ligaments.[1] The patella is also surrounded by dynamic stabilizers including the rectus femoris, vastus lateralis, vastus intermedius, and vastus medialis (including the vastus medialis obliquus). Each of these muscles is innervated by the femoral nerve, which is composed of the posterior divisions of the second, third, and fourth lumbar spinal nerves. The direct head of the rectus femoris originates at the anteroinferior iliac spine, whereas the reflected head begins superior to the acetabulum.[2,3] It therefore crosses both the hip and knee joints and can serve to flex the thigh and extend the lower leg. The remaining three muscles of the quadriceps femoris

include the vastus lateralis, which originates from the lateral lip of the linea aspera and lateral surface of the greater trochanter; the vastus intermedius, which originates from the anterior aspect of the femoral shaft; and the vastus medialis, which originates from the medial lip of the linea aspera and the distal aspect of the intertrochanteric line. These muscles function as extensors of the knee.

The quadriceps tendon is a layered confluence of the individual insertions from the previously described muscles and attaches to the proximal pole of the patella, enveloping this area of the patella as it advances from proximal to distal. Arteries from the descending branches of the lateral femoral circumflex, the descending geniculate, and the medial and lateral superior geniculate arteries provide the tendon with nourishment,[4] although there is a relatively avascular portion of the tendon just proximal to the patella that measures approximately 1.5 × 3 cm. The patellar tendon is a continuation of the quadriceps tendon beyond the distal pole of the patella and inserts on the tibial tuberosity.[5] The blood supply of the patellar tendon is not as rich as that of the quadriceps tendon. It is carried by vessels from the infrapatellar fat pad as well as the inferomedial and lateral geniculate arteries (Fig. 107.1). The proximal and distal aspects are relatively avascular and thus more susceptible to injury.

The patella itself is the largest sesamoid bone in the body. It ossifies from a single center that usually appears in the second or third year of life, though notably its appearance may be delayed until the sixth year. Rarely, the bone ossifies from two adjacent centers. Ossification is completed around the age of puberty, and incomplete ossification may result in a bipartite patella. The incidence of bipartite patella ranges between 2% and 8%, most commonly involving the superolateral aspect of the patella; when present, it is found approximately 50% of the time on the contralateral side.

The patella is a flat triangular bone with a thick superior border that provides an attachment for the quadriceps tendon. The apex is pointed distally and provides an origin for the patellar tendon. The posterior articular surface is divided by a vertical ridge and then again into thirds by two horizontal prominences. The lateral facet is larger than the medial facet. The lower facets engage with the trochlear groove in early flexion followed by the middle and then the upper facets with increased knee flexion. In full flexion, the most medial aspect of the patellar articular surface, the crescentic or odd facet, is the main contact point. Patellofemoral contact is initiated at about 20 degrees of flexion,

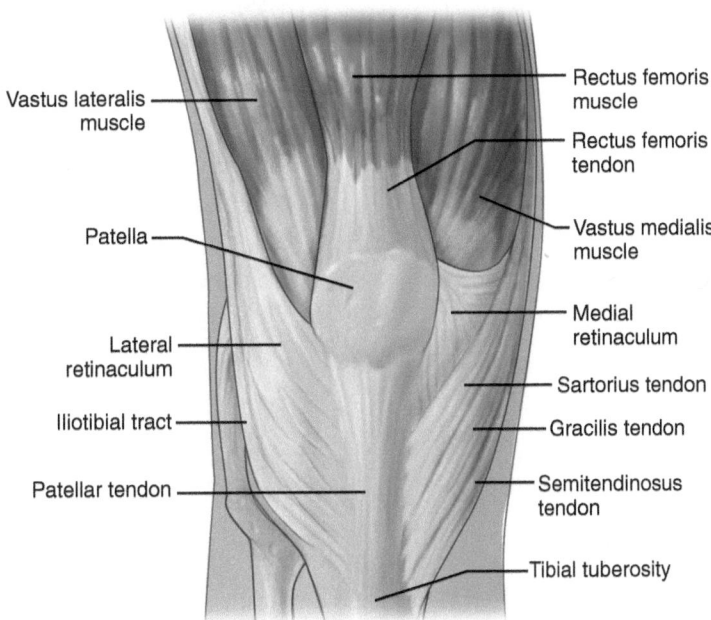

Fig. 107.1 Normal anatomy of the extensor mechanism of the knee. (Modified from Matava MJ. Patellar tendon ruptures. *J Am Acad Orthop Surg.* 1996;4[6]:287–296.)

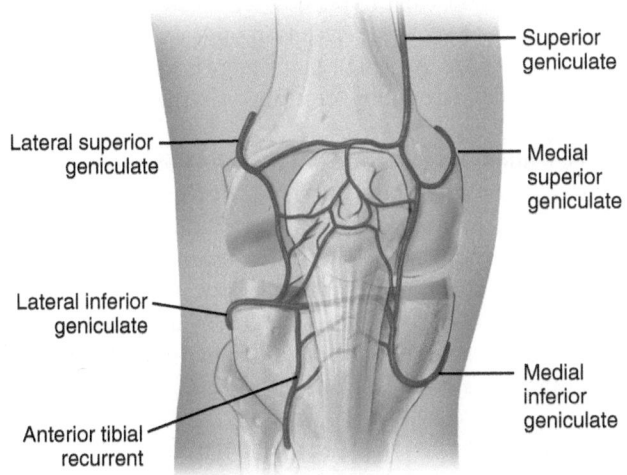

Fig. 107.2 Schematic arterial blood supply to the patella.

and the patella undergoes approximately 7 cm of excursion in relation to the femur from full extension to flexion. The forces generated across the patellofemoral joint are tremendous, ranging from half of the total body weight for normal walking to nearly eight times the body weight for jumping from a small height.[6] The articular surface of the patella is the thickest in the body so that it may counteract these forces, reaching thickness of more than 1 cm in depth.

The blood supply to the patella is from a vascular anastomotic ring lying in a thin layer of loose connective tissue covering the rectus expansion (Fig. 107.2). The main vessels contributing to this anastomotic ring are the descending genicular artery, the four medial and lateral superior and inferior geniculate arteries,

and anterior tibial recurrent artery. Nutrient vessels pass obliquely into the anterior surface of the patella from this complex network in a retrograde fashion from the distal and middle thirds of the patella.[7] Disruption of this supply by injury or surgical dissection can result in avascular necrosis. Rates of 3.5% to 24% have been reported after patellar fracture.[8]

BIOMECHANICS

The knee consists of three compartments: the medial tibio-femoral, lateral tibiofemoral, and the patellofemoral. The patella increases the extensor moment arm of the knee extensors by transmitting the longitudinal contractile force at a greater distance from the knee axis of rotation (Fig. 107.3). The efficiency of the extensor mechanism increases 1.5 times through this advantage. Patellofemoral contact shifts distally to proximally with increasing degrees of flexion (Fig. 107.4). Ascending stairs can create forces within the patellar tendon that are 3.2 times the body weight, and the greatest forces on this structure as well as the quadriceps tendon occurs at about 60 degrees of knee flexion.[9,10]

Huberti and colleagues[11] described the *extensor mechanism force ratio*, which compares the forces on the patellar tendon and the quadriceps tendon at various knee flexion angles. The ratio is greater than 1.0 (indicating more force on the patellar tendon) when the knee is in less than 45 degrees of flexion and the distal pole of the patella articulates with the trochlear groove, thus providing a mechanical advantage for the quadriceps tendon because of a relatively larger moment arm due to the added length of the proximal, nonarticulating patella. Conversely, with knee flexion angles greater than 45 degrees, the ratio drops below 1.0.

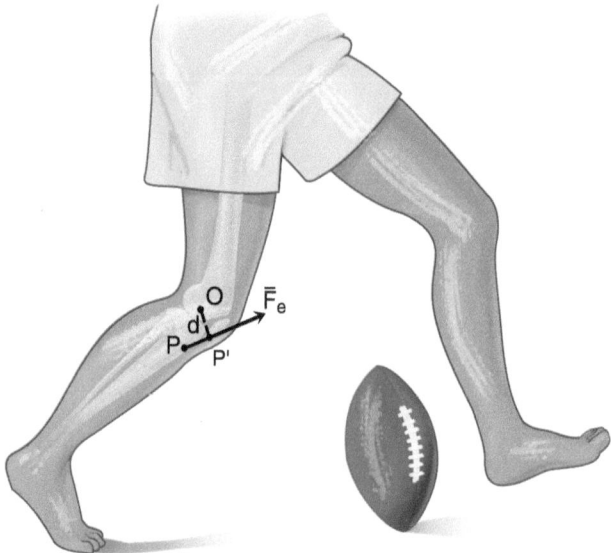

Fig. 107.3 Patellar biomechanics.

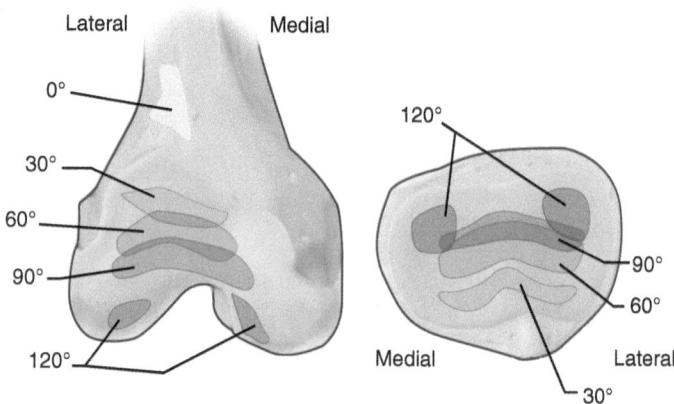

Fig. 107.4 Patellar contact areas according to degrees of knee flexion. (From Scott WN, ed. *Insall & Scott Surgery of the Knee*. 5th ed. Philadelphia: Elsevier; 2012.)

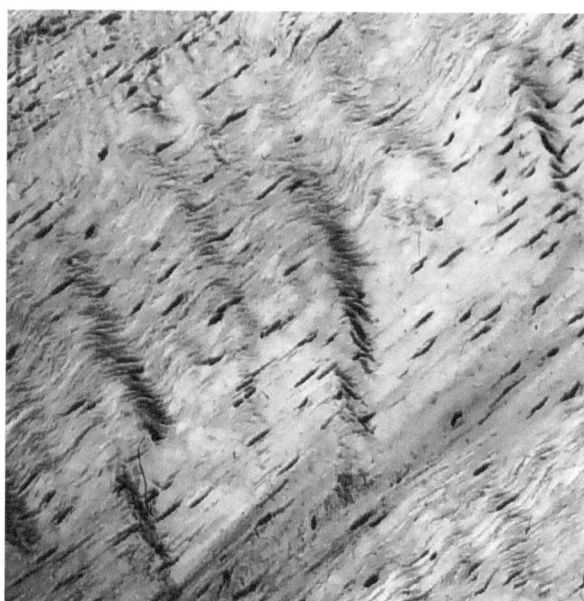

Fig. 107.5 Histologic features of a normal patellar tendon with the typical collagen crimp pattern.

PATELLAR AND QUADRICEPS TENDON STRUCTURE

A tendon is a complex material consisting of collagen fibrils embedded in a matrix of proteoglycans. Both quadriceps and patellar tendons are mainly composed of water in the extracellular matrix. The predominant cell type found within tendons is the fibroblast. This cell is present in the space between the parallel collagen bundles (Fig. 107.5).[9] The tendon is composed primarily of type I collagen and contains a high concentration of glycine, proline, and hydroxyproline. The secondary structure is the arrangement of each chain in a left-handed configuration, the tertiary structure involves three collagen chains combined into a collagen molecule, and the quaternary structure is related to the organization of collagen molecules into a stable, low-energy biologic unit based on the association of its amino acids with adjacent molecules. This quarter-stagger arrangement of adjacent collagen molecules results in oppositely charged amino acids being aligned. A great deal of energy is required to separate these molecules, accounting for the overall strength of this structure (Fig. 107.6).

The tendon possesses one of the highest tensile strengths of any soft tissue in the human body for two reasons. First, it is composed of collagen, which is one of the strongest fibrous proteins in the body. Second, tendon collagen fibers are arranged parallel to the direction of the tensile force. The elastic modulus of human tendon ranges from 1200 to 1800 megapascals (MPa), the ultimate tensile strength ranges from 50 to 105 MPa, and the ultimate strain ranges from 9% to 35%.[9]

EXTENSOR MECHANISM DISORDERS

Patellar and Quadriceps Tendinopathy

Patellar tendinopathy is the result of tendinosis of the patellar tendon or degeneration of the tendon itself, with inadequate restorative capabilities. Colloquially, it is known as "jumper's knee" owing to its prevalence in athletes participating in jumping sports. It can be the result of extrinsic causes, such as repetitive mechanical overload, as well as intrinsic causes, such as anatomic abnormalities and imbalances of the surrounding static and dynamic stabilizers.[12] Tendinosis is commonly found in the posterior and proximal patellar tendon adjacent to the inferior patellar pole.[13] Diagnosis and management of this disorder can be challenging, and our understanding continues to evolve. *Quadriceps tendinopathy* is much less commonly described, although it likely shares many pathologic attributes with patellar tendon disease.

The nomenclature associated with tendon pathology can be somewhat confusing given the variability of descriptions of

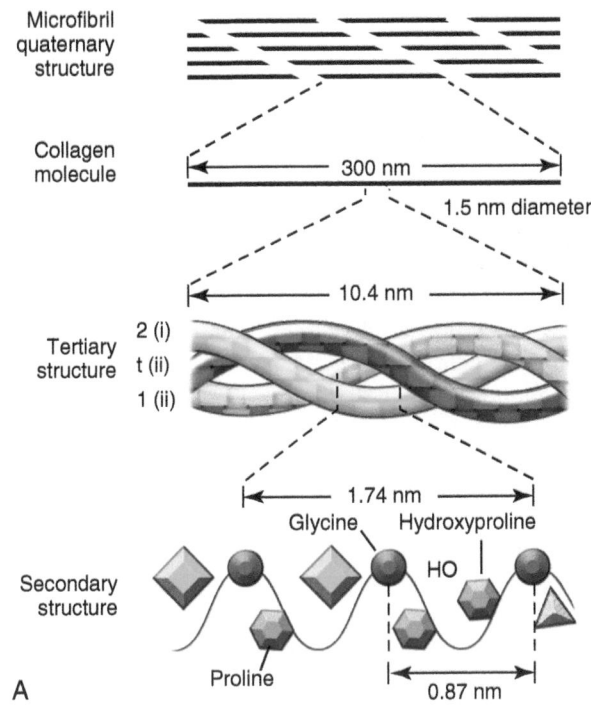

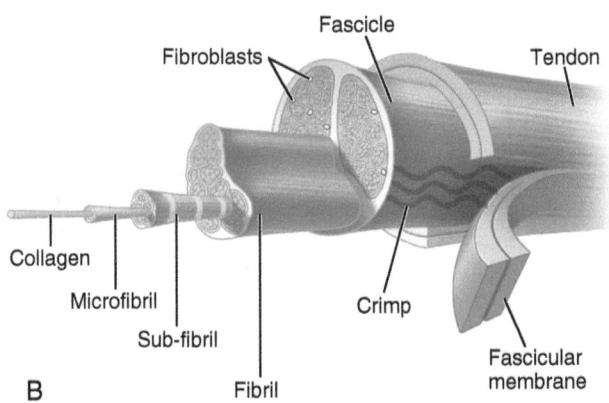

Fig. 107.6 Schematic drawings of the structural organization of collagen into the microfibril. (Modified from Woo SL, An KN, Arnoczky SP, et al. Anatomy, biology, and biomechanics of tendon and ligament. In: Buckwalter JA, Einhorn TA, Simon SR, eds. *Orthopaedic Basic Science: Foundations of Clinical Practice*. Rosemont, IL: American Academy of Orthopaedic Surgeons; 2007.)

different disease processes in the literature. Maffulli and colleagues recommended use of the term *tendinopathy* as a generic descriptor of a range of tendon pathology.[14,15] *Tendinitis* refers to the presence of inflammatory cells on histologic evaluation. In patellar tendinopathy, early pathologic alterations in the presence of repetitive microtrauma to the patellar tendon include inflammatory cell invasion, tissue edema, and fibrin exudation in the paratenon but not the tendon itself, referred to as *paratenonitis*. Continued microtrauma can overwhelm reparative capabilities, leading to chronic inflammation. The development of patellar tendinosis is thought to result from chronic peritendinitis and is characterized by histopathologic findings of mucoid degeneration, tendolipomatosis, calcifying

tendinopathy, and neovascularization but not the presence of inflammatory cells.[16-18]

Yuan et al.[19] and Cook et al.[20] presented evidence that the earliest identifiable morphologic changes in tendinosis occur in tenocytes and not collagen fibers. Microscopic evaluations of degenerative tendons demonstrate a paucity of inflammatory cells, changes in tenocyte morphology and density, accumulation of glycosaminoglycans, and collagen fiber thinning and disarray with or without neurovascular proliferation.[20-23] Lian et al.[21] studied biopsy specimens in patients with patellar tendinopathy and found increased cellularity compared with controls as well as a higher number of apoptotic cells. On a molecular level, an increased expression of cyclooxygenase-2, transforming growth factor β-1, glutamate, and prostaglandin E2 can be found in the presence of tendinopathy, indicating an abnormal healing response.[24-30]

Cyclic tensile loading of tendons is required to maintain normal tendon health. This process is referred to as *mechanotransduction* and couples tendon stretch with a cellular biologic response. Excessive mechanical stretch stimulates an anabolic response, whereas normal stimuli promote a catabolic response. Continued loading in the face of a weakened tendon can lead to an accumulation of injury, thus inhibiting the healing capacity and resulting in an overuse injury.[31]

Patellar and Quadriceps Tendon Ruptures

Tendons can become injured as a result of direct trauma, such as laceration or contusion, or indirect trauma through tensile overload. It is generally accepted that healthy tendons do not rupture in the setting of physiologic forces. When tensile overload of an otherwise healthy extensor mechanism occurs, it more commonly results in a transverse fracture of the patella rather than failure of the adjacent tendons.[32] Zernicke et al.[33] estimated that a force of 17.5 times body weight is required to cause rupture in healthy patients, supporting the notion that normal tendons do not tear. No widely accepted classification system exists for patellar tendon or quadriceps tendon ruptures. Clinically it is helpful to group them based on the location, configuration, and chronicity of rupture.

Ruptures of the patellar tendon are thought to occur less frequently than ruptures of the quadriceps tendons.[34] They are usually seen in patients younger than 40 years and are more commonly associated with healthy, active patients with underlying tendinopathy,[35] whereas quadriceps tendon ruptures are more common in patients older than 40 years and are often associated with underlying systemic medical conditions, such as diabetes mellitus. Both are more common in males.

When tendon ruptures do happen, they typically occur within the context of preexisting tendon pathology. Kannus and Jozsa[16] studied specimens from spontaneously ruptured tendons in 891 patients and compared them to age- and sex-matched controls. Under light and electron microscopy, all ruptured tendons demonstrated abnormal findings, with a majority demonstrating signs of degenerative changes. Two-thirds of the unruptured tendons demonstrated no pathology, whereas the remainder showed findings similar to those seen in the ruptured cohort. Characteristic histopathologic patterns in the ruptured tendons included combinations of hypoxic degenerative tendinopathy, mucoid degeneration, tendolipomatosis, and calcifying tendinopathy.

Mechanical testing performed on the patellar tendon has shown tensile strains to be less at the midbody than at the origin and insertion sites on the patella and tibial tuberosity. At peak load just prior to tendon failure, the end-region strain at the insertion site is three to four times than that seen in the midbody.[9] Thus healthy tendon rarely fails within its substance; if this occurs, the physician must consider external factors such as metabolic derangements (Box 107.1).

Metabolic abnormalities have been shown to influence the physiologic status and biomechanical function of tendons. These conditions can be innate, induced, or iatrogenic. Diabetes mellitus, for example, can compromise the blood supply and limit the reparative abilities. Rheumatoid arthritis, gout, renal failure, hypothyroidism, and chondrocalcinosis can also lead to tendinopathy and ruptures.[36-41] Local and systemic corticosteroid injections have been shown to limit the inflammatory phase of healing,[42] and tendon ruptures have been documented after the administration of these agents.[43] Fluoroquinolone antibiotics, such as levofloxacin and ciprofloxacin, have been shown to alter the extracellular matrix in tendons and can influence healing after injury.[44,45] Ciprofloxacin also induces interleukin-1β–mediated matrix metalloproteinase-3 release.[15] Matrix metalloproteinases are a family of proteolytic enzymes that have the ability to degrade the extracellular matrix network and facilitate tissue remodeling.[46-48] Fluoroquinolones can also inhibit tenocyte metabolism, reducing cell proliferation and collagen and matrix synthesis.[44,49] Additionally, investigations have noted decreased biomechanical properties of healing patellar tendon with administration of anti-inflammatory drugs compared with acetaminophen and controls.[50] Anabolic steroid use is also associated with an increased risk for tendon ruptures.[51-53] Polymorphisms in genes coding for collagen may be implicated in tendon rupture. Galasso et al.[54] described a case report of a patient with collagen type V α-1 polymorphism who incurred spontaneous, simultaneous quadriceps tendon ruptures.

Patellar Fractures

Patellar fractures are relatively uncommon, comprising approximately 1% of all skeletal injuries.[55] A recent epidemiologic study noted a bimodal distribution of injuries, with young males and elderly females more commonly injured.[56] The mechanism of injury is either a direct blow to the patella or an indirect force transmitted to the patella through the extensor mechanism.[57] Fracture patterns are usually representative of the injury mechanism as well as patient characteristics, such as bone density. Indirect forces typically produce nondisplaced or minimally displaced transverse fractures of the central or distal third and, uncommonly, a vertical fracture. Blunt injury to the patella either from a direct blow or from a fall onto the flexed knee produces a comminuted stellate fracture pattern. These fractures can be broadly divided into displaced and nondisplaced fractures. In the setting of a clearly displaced fracture, a concomitant retinacular injury should be suspected.

PATIENT EVALUATION

History

Patellar and Quadriceps Tendinopathy

Isolated quadriceps tendinopathy has not been well described in the contemporary literature and is often mentioned in the context of bilateral involvement due to underlying medical comorbidity. A few reports have been made of sequelae due to calcific tendinitis leading to chronic enthesopathic changes and, in some cases, bilateral tendon rupture.[58] The majority of publications describing extensor mechanism tendinopathy focus on the patellar tendon. Patellar tendinopathy is essentially an overuse injury and is commonly seen in athletes who participate in sports that involve jumping, such as volleyball and basketball.[59] Commonly, patients report discomfort in the distribution of the proximal patellar tendon and distal patellar pole. Pain usually starts without a clear traumatic etiology but can be related to an increase in activity. It may be present only after activity in mild cases and progress to continuous symptoms in more advanced cases.[13]

Zwerver et al.[60] noted in nonelite athletes that the prevalence of jumper's knee varied between 2.5% and 14.4% for different sports and that males were twice as likely to be affected. They also identified sport-specific loading characteristics, higher body weight, taller stature, and younger age as risk factors for the development of patellar tendinopathy. Lian et al.[61] studied the prevalence of jumper's knee among elite athletes from various sports. Cyclists were unaffected, whereas male basketball and volleyball players demonstrated a prevalence of 32% and 44%, respectively. Players routinely exhibited symptoms lasting longer than 2 years, and affected athletes had significant pain and functional impairment. Hägglund et al.[62] studied professional male soccer players and found that 1.5% of all reported injuries were patellar tendinopathies and that each season 2.4% of players were affected. The investigators noted no significant differences with regard to prevalence or incidence between play on artificial versus natural turf.

Ferretti et al.[63] demonstrated a linear relationship between training volume and the prevalence of tendinopathy among volleyball players. They also demonstrated a higher prevalence of tendinopathy among players who trained on a harder surface. Backman and Danielson[64] showed a correlation between low ankle dorsiflexion and an increased risk of patellar tendinitis in junior elite basketball players, likely due to more compensatory energy absorption by the patellar tendon. A systematic review by van der Worp et al.[65] found limited evidence that weight, body mass index, waist-to-hip ratio, leg-length difference, arch height, quadriceps and hamstrings flexibility, quadriceps strength, and jump performance were possible risk factors for the development of patellar tendinopathy. Symptoms may occur in young adults undergoing a rapid phase in growth. In these cases, a relative discrepancy in tendon length may be found compared with adjacent bony structures. This finding occurs when the tendon does not lengthen as quickly as the adjacent bone.[59]

Patellar and Quadriceps Tendon Ruptures

The mechanism of injury associated with patellar and quadriceps tendon rupture is typically involves forced knee flexion accompanied by a strong knee extensor muscle contraction. Patients with often describe a pop or tearing sensation accompanied by intense and immediate pain. Immobilization of the extremity in extension provides pain relief.[66] In a study of patellar tendon ruptures in National Football League (NFL) players, nearly half reported antecedent symptoms, which can implicate underlying tendinopathy as a preceding injury.[67]

Patellar Fractures

Patellar fractures result from either an indirect force applied through strong contraction of the extensor mechanism against a flexed knee or from a direct force, such as a fall or blunt trauma to the anterior knee. The subcutaneous location of this bone places it at risk for injury from direct impact. Traumatic separation of a bipartite patella can also occur,[68] and patients with this condition may have an antecedent dull ache or pain prior to the traumatic episode. Patients with patellar fractures usually present with a painful, swollen knee after either direct trauma or a fall in which an attempt is made to stop suddenly. Weight bearing is painful and, depending on the competence of the medial and lateral retinacula, the patient may or may not be able perform a straight leg raise.

Physical Examination

Patellar and Quadriceps Tendinopathy

A patient may have tenderness over the patellar tendon and signs of inflammation, such as redness, swelling, warmth, and crepitation secondary to paratenonitis. Pain is often centered on the distal patellar pole and the proximal part of the patellar tendon. Tenderness to palpation may be present with the knee in extension and absent with the knee in flexion. The patient may have a feeling of "bogginess" centered over the tendon itself and may also have pain with resisted extension and with full passive flexion.[59] The decline squat test involves a single-leg squat to 30 degrees on the affected extremity, which elicits symptoms by increasing the load on the patellar tendon.[69]

Blazina et al.[70] established a classification for patellar tendinopathy (Table 107.1). In stage 1, pain is present only after activity. In stage 2, pain is present at the beginning of activity, disappears after a warm-up, but may reappear with fatigue. In stage 3, pain is constant, both at rest and with activity. In stage 4, the patellar

TABLE 107.1 Classification of Tendon Disorders

New	Old	Definition	Histologic Findings	Clinical Signs and Symptoms
Paratenonitis	Tenosynovitis Tenovaginitis Peritendinitis	Inflammation of only the paratenon whether or not it is lined by synovium	Inflammatory cells in paratenon or peritendinous areolar tissue	Cardinal inflammatory signs: warmth, swelling, pain, crepitation, local tenderness, and dysfunction
Paratenonitis with tendinosis	Tendinitis	Paratenon inflammation associated with intratendinous degeneration	Same as above, with loss of tendon, collagen fiber disorientation, and scattered vascular ingrowth but no prominent intratendinous inflammation	Same as above, often with a palpable tendon nodule, swelling, and inflammatory signs
Tendinosis	Tendinitis	Intratendinous degeneration due to atrophy (e.g., aging, microtrauma, or vascular compromise)	Noninflammatory intratendinous collagen degeneration with fiber disorientation, hypocellularity, scattered vascular ingrowth, occasional local necrosis, or calcification	Often a palpable tendon nodule that may be asymptomatic but may also be point tender; swelling of the tendon sheath is absent
	Tendon strain or tear	Symptomatic overload of the tendon with vascular disruption and inflammatory repair response	Three recognized subgroups: each displays variable histologic characteristics from purely inflammation with acute hemorrhage and tear to inflammation superimposed on preexisting degeneration, to calcification and tendinosis changes in chronic conditions; in the chronic stage, it may be (1) interstitial microinjury, (2) central tendon necrosis, (3) frank partial rupture, or (4) acute complete rupture	Symptoms are inflammatory and proportional to vascular disruption, hematoma, or atrophy-related cell necrosis; symptom duration defines each subgroup: A: Acute (<2 weeks) B: Subacute (4–6 weeks) C: Chronic (>6 weeks)

tendon is completely ruptured. The Victorian Institute of Sport Assessment Questionnaire (VISA) is a validated patient-reported outcome measure commonly utilized to assess and follow patients with patellar tendinosis and is frequently reported in research on the matter.[71]

Patellar and Quadriceps Tendon Ruptures

Physical examination of a tendon rupture presents with a triad of pain, inability to actively extend the knee, and a palpable gap.[66,72] Patients are unable to actively extend the knee but may be able to maintain extension against gravity through an intact retinaculum. Clinicians must take care to thoroughly examine the knee in someone with a suspected patellar or quadriceps tendon rupture, particularly in patients who can exhibit some extensor mechanism function. Knee aspiration with an intra-articular local anesthetic can relieve pain, permit an adequate physical examination, and allow for an accurate diagnosis. A gap or palpable depression adjacent to the patella is pathognomonic for tendon rupture (Fig. 107.7). Despite their superficial nature, patellar and quadriceps tendon ruptures can frequently be over-looked or missed. Siwek and Rao[35] performed a retrospective analysis of 36 quadriceps and 36 patellar tendon ruptures and found that 38% of these injuries were initially misdiagnosed. Diagnosis may be more difficult when the injury is accompanied by hemarthrosis, which can mask the presence of a gap.[66] Intense pain may limit willingness to comply with examination. Diagnostic failure rates of 10% to 50% have been reported, and delays in diagnosis have ranged from days to months.[35,72-74]

Patellar Fractures

Localized tenderness, soft tissue swelling, and a hemarthrosis are typically present. It is important to examine the skin around the knee for abrasions and lacerations. Because of the superficial position of the bone, signs of an open or impending open fracture must be explored and ruled out.[57] With a displaced fracture, a gap between the two fragments may be palpated. The integrity of the extensor mechanism also needs to be evaluated. Sometimes an accurate exam may be limited by pain. Similar to patellar or quadriceps tendon ruptures, aspiration of the hemarthrosis followed by an injection of intra-articular local anesthetic can be performed to allow for a more accurate exam and verify the status of the surrounding retinaculum.

Imaging Studies
Patellar and Quadriceps Tendinopathy

Imaging is not routinely necessary for the initial treatment of patellar or quadriceps tendinosis. Standard radiographs, however, are commonly obtained upon initial evaluation in the clinic setting. Findings can be normal or may include traction osteophytes at the distal pole of the patella, tendon calcification, and even decreased bone mineral density at the sites of attachment.

Ultrasound and magnetic resonance imaging (MRI) are more sensitive modalities and are commonly employed when nonoperative treatment fails to provide relief or the diagnosis is in question. Ultrasound evaluations can localize tendinosis as a hypoechoic signal within the fibers of the patellar tendon. Other findings include tendon thickening, paratenon irregularity, intra-tendinous calcifications, neovascularization, and patellar pole errosions.[75] Warden et al.[76] performed MRI and gray-scale and color Doppler ultrasound on 30 patients with clinically diagnosed patellar tendinopathy and 33 activity-matched asymptomatic control subjects. These investigators concluded that ultrasonography was more accurate than MRI in confirming clinically diagnosed patellar tendinopathy. They added that the combination of gray-scale and color Doppler ultrasound best confirms clinically diagnosed patellar tendinopathy because of the high sensitivity of gray scale and the strong likelihood that symptomatic persons would demonstrate a positive color Doppler test (Fig. 107.8).

Sagittal MRI may demonstrate thickening of the patellar tendon, especially on the posterior, central, or medial aspects (Fig. 107.9).[77,78] MRI may also demonstrate foci of abnormal signal intensity in the posterior portion of the proximal patellar tendon (Fig. 107.10). The severity of findings on imaging has not been clearly correlated with the severity of reported symptoms,[79] although the presence of structural findings in asymptomatic athletes may predict a greater chance of future symptoms.[80] Edema in the inferior patellar pole marrow or the infrapatellar fat pad can portend inferior functional results and

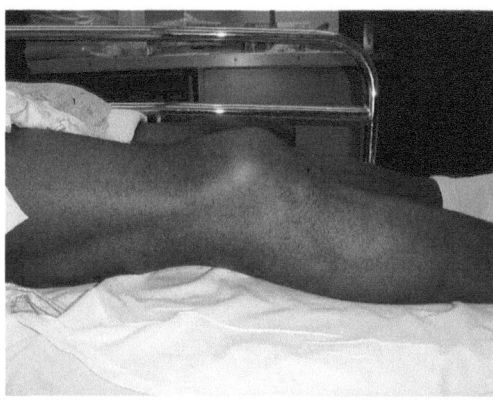

Fig. 107.7 A patient with a rupture.

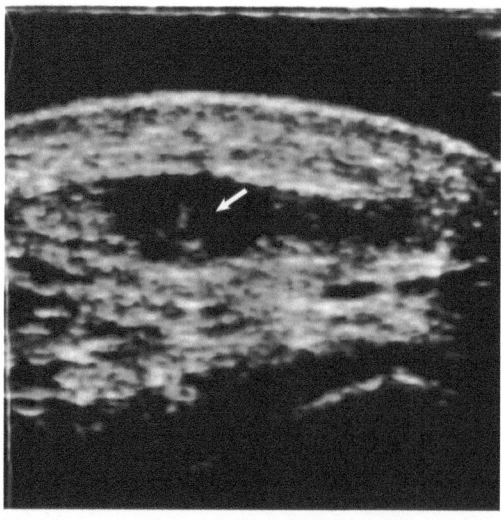

Fig. 107.8 Ultrasound of a knee and patellar tendon. The *arrow* points to a hypoechoic region of the patellar tendon.

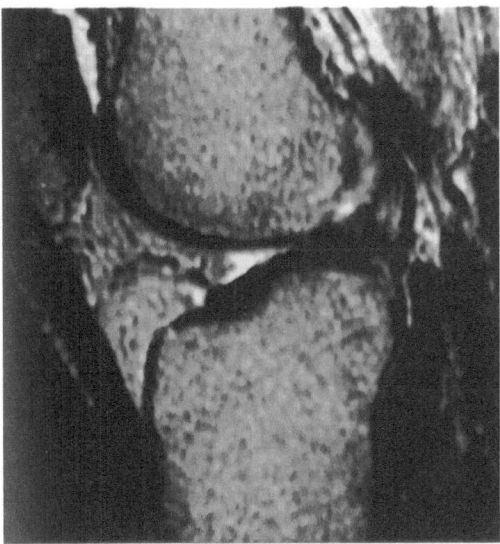

Fig. 107.9 A magnetic resonance image of the knee showing thickening of the patellar tendon.

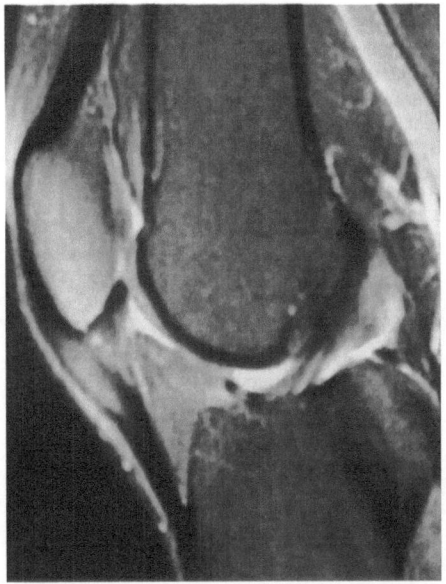

Fig. 107.10 A magnetic resonance image of the knee showing high signal intensity within the tendon.

slower recovery in patients undergoing operative treatment for patellar tendinopathy.[81]

Patellar and Quadriceps Tendon Ruptures

Although mostly a clinical diagnosis based on history and physical examination, various imaging modalities may be useful in the diagnosis of patellar and quadriceps tendon ruptures. Findings on radiographs may include the obliteration of the quadriceps or patellar tendon shadows, calcific densities at the proximal or distal patellar poles that may be avulsed, and patellar height alterations due to the tethering effect of the uninjured end of the tendon. In the case of patellar tendon ruptures, increased density of the infrapatellar fat pad as well as loss of sharp margins and waviness of the patellar tendon are consistently seen in addition to patella alta.[82]

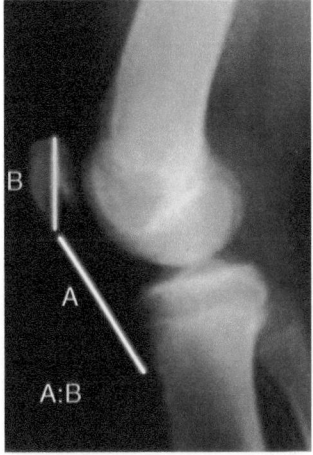

Fig. 107.11 The Insall-Salvati ratio.

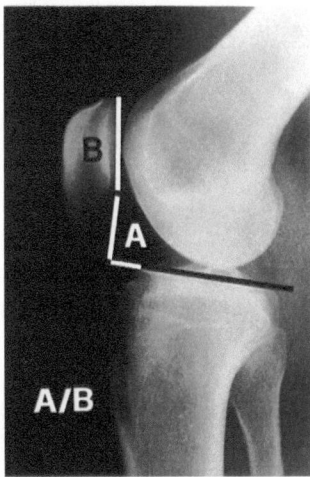

Fig. 107.12 The Blackburne-Peel method of measuring patellar height.

The Insall-Salvati ratio is a commonly used method for measuring patellar height, although it has high intra- and interobserver variability. This ratio is calculated by dividing the patellar tendon length by the greatest diagonal distance of the bony patella and is normally between 0.8 and 1.2 (Fig. 107.11). The Blackburne-Peel method has higher interobserver reliability and is less affected by knee position.[83,84] A line is drawn perpendicular to the tibial plateau extending to the inferior articular margin of the patella. The length of this line is divided by the length of the articular surface of the patella. Normal values for males and females are 0.805 and 0.806, respectively (Fig. 107.12), with values greater than 1.0 representing patella alta. Patellar tendon ruptures result in higher ratios (Fig. 107.13), whereas quadriceps tendon ruptures result in lower ratios and, in some cases, anterior tilt of the patella away from the trochlear groove (Fig. 107.14). Other techniques for measuring patellar height, including the Caton-Deeschamps index and the relationship of the Blumensaat line to the inferior pole of the patella at 30 degrees of knee flexion, are also helpful.

High-resolution ultrasonography has been shown to be an effective means of evaluating both the patellar and quadriceps tendons in acute and chronic tendon injuries. MRI is the most sensitive test available to evaluate the injured tendons.[34] It also provides accurate information about the location of injury, presence of additional injuries, such as concomitant meniscal tears; in addition, it can help with surgical planning (Fig. 107.15).

Patellar Fractures

Most patellar fractures can easily be diagnosed with standard radiographs (Fig. 107.16). The anteroposterior view is used to assess for fragmentation, but visualization can be difficult because of overlap of the distal femur. The lateral view best reveals the degree of comminution or separation between the fragments. Some vertical and osteochondral fractures may be best seen on tangential or Merchant views. Osteochondral, marginal, and chondral injuries are more accurately evaluated with MRI. In addition, MRI can diagnose occult, nondisplaced fractures that are not seen on standard radiographs. Bone scans have also been reported to be helpful in evaluating patellar stress fractures in athletes.[85] Computed tomography (CT) has been shown to improve the ability to detect fracture comminution and to frequently alter surgical planning when utilized.[86]

Importantly, a bipartite patella can be confused with an acute fracture and must be considered when radiographs reveal a small fragment separated from the main portion of the patella. In most cases these secondary ossification centers are located in the superolateral pole. The separation is minimal, and the borders are usually smooth.

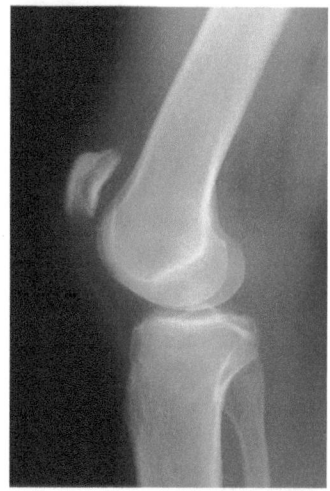

Fig. 107.13 A lateral radiograph of a patellar tendon rupture.

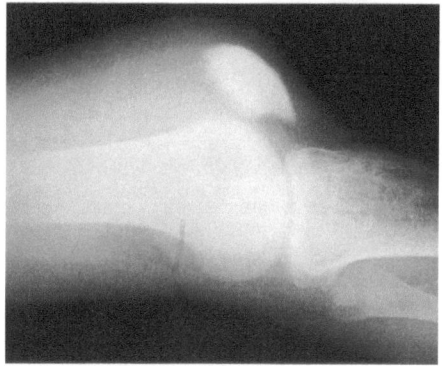

Fig. 107.14 A lateral radiograph of a quadriceps tendon rupture.

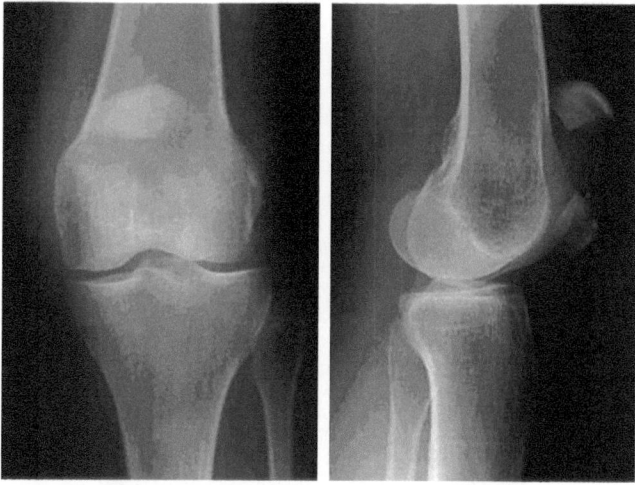

Fig. 107.16 A significantly displaced patellar fracture with disruption of the extensor retinaculum.

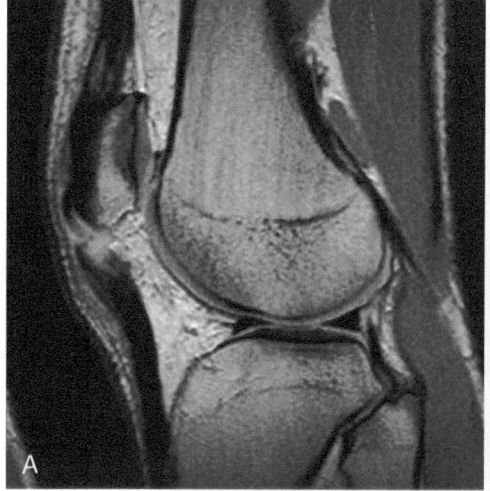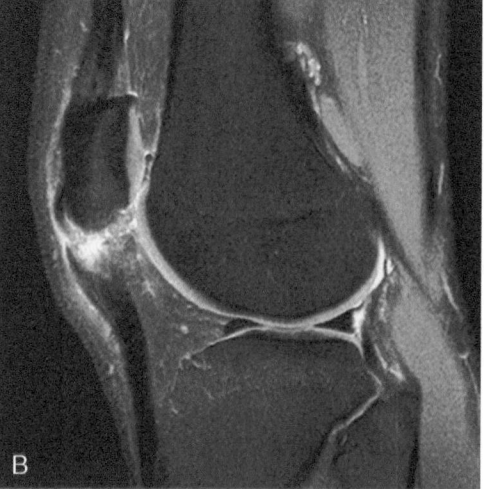

Fig. 107.15 (A and B) Magnetic resonance images of patellar tendon disruption.

DECISION-MAKING PRINCIPLES

Patellar and Quadriceps Tendinopathy

The initial treatment of patellar and quadriceps tendinopathy is nonoperative, with an emphasis on focused rehabilitation. Bahr et al.[87] performed a randomized controlled trial comparing surgery and eccentric training for patellar tendinopathy in 35 patients (40 knees) with grade 3 patellar tendinopathy. No advantage was demonstrated for operative treatment compared with eccentric exercise. The authors concluded that eccentric training should be initiated for 12 weeks before an open tenotomy was considered. When patients present with a history and physical examination consistent with patellar tendinosis, plain radiographs of the knee are obtained and scrutinized for coexisting pathology. In cases of severe or prolonged symptoms, an MRI may be useful. These images help determine prognosis, which can be helpful for managing patient expectations. After the initiation of physical therapy, a clinical reevaluation at 6 weeks is routine for patient reassurance and evaluation of compliance with the treatment regimen. Correspondence with the physical therapist assists in making subsequent recommendations. Improvement at 6 weeks is a good indicator of future clinical success, but failure to improve offers no insight. A full 3 months of therapy should be completed, as previously outlined, to improve symptoms.

Patellar and Quadriceps Tendon Ruptures

Except in the setting of illness or other situations that would preclude adequate anesthesia, complete ruptures of the patellar and quadriceps tendons require repair to restore extensor mechanism function. Due to pain, functional difficulties, and technical concerns regarding the ease of repair, these are generally done shortly after injury in a nonurgent manner in an inpatient or outpatient setting. Partial injuries amenable to immobilization alone are rare.

Patellar Fractures

Decision-making principles should be based on appropriate interpretation of the fracture pattern and preservation of the patella. Driving factors in decision-making include whether there is displacement or articular step-off greater than 2 mm, whether the retinaculum and extensor mechanism are intact, the quality of the patient's bone stock, and the patient's overall physiologic status.

TREATMENT OPTIONS

Nonoperative Treatment of Tendinopathy

Initial management should include activity modification, physical therapy, the use of anti-inflammatory medications, and the administration of cryotherapy. In addition, bracing, injections and shock-wave therapy have also been described, with varying degrees of success. Physical therapy, with a focus on core and eccentric strengthening exercises, is the mainstay of nonoperative treatment for patellar tendinopathy. Eccentric exercises are thought to induce remodeling of the diseased tendon,[13,88] and their efficacy is supported by high-level evidence.[89] Heavy, slow resistance training is an alternative therapy program that has shown promise as an effective treatment regimen.[90] For in-season athletes who wish to continue with competition, isometric and isotonic exercises can provide symptom relief without increasing pain.[91] Treatment of asymptomatic athletes with prophylactic eccentric training is helpful for patients without abnormalities on ultrasound, but this increases the risk of injury for players with positive ultrasound findings.[92] Bracing with patellar tendon straps is a common practice and is thought to alter tensile forces on the tendon from the knee extensors as well as patellofemoral biomechanics.[93] This can provide short-term symptom relief, although there may be a substantial placebo effect.[94]

Multiple injection therapies for patellar and quadriceps tendinopathy have been studied. Corticosteroid injections can be very effective in the short term; however, the results are not durable and the use of such injections is accompanied by the risk of iatrogenic tendon rupture.[95] Platelet-rich plasma has been utilized for its potential to induce structural and biochemical healing.[96] Although high-level evidence is lacking, it appears to be effective in accelerating recovery in conjunction with therapy without a major risk of adverse events.[97,98] Injections with sclerosing agents, such as polidocanol, are thought to inhibit neovascularization, which is present in a majority of symptomatic patients. Short-term results have been promising, but long-term results have not been as impressive and adaptation has not been widespread.[25,99] Ultrasound-guided injections with sclerosing agents have also been explored as investigative options for treating bilateral quadriceps tendinopathy.[100] Extracorporeal shock-wave therapy (ESWT), initially used for the management of kidney stones, has found multiple musculoskeletal applications in the treatment of various tendinopathies. Overall there are conflicting results regarding its efficacy in the treatment of patellar tendinopathy. Although it can serve as an adjunct to a comprehensive treatment program,[101,102] multiple randomized controlled trials have shown no benefit in addition to standard therapy.[103,104]

Nonoperative Treatment of Tendon Ruptures

Incomplete ruptures of quadriceps and patellar tendons may be treated nonsurgically in cases where the retinaculum remains intact and patients can perform a straight leg raise with no patellar maltracking and no extension lag. Reports are rare in the literature, as complete ruptures are more common than partial ruptures.[105] Accurate diagnosis is essential, and immobilization in extension for 3 to 6 weeks is recommended.[66] Gradual knee flexion after this initial period of immobilization is advocated once the patient achieves good quadriceps muscle control and is able to perform a straight-leg raise without discomfort.

Nonoperative Treatment of Patellar Fractures

As mentioned previously, the indications for nonoperative management of patellar fractures include non- or minimally displaced fractures with maintained articular congruity. The patient should have minimal displacement of fracture fragments (<2 to 3 mm) (Fig. 107.17) and minimal articular step-off. Patients must also demonstrate a preserved extensor mechanism. The retinaculum should be intact, as evidenced by the patient's ability to maintain extension against gravity without a lag. Overall health status is also an important factor to be considered before surgery.

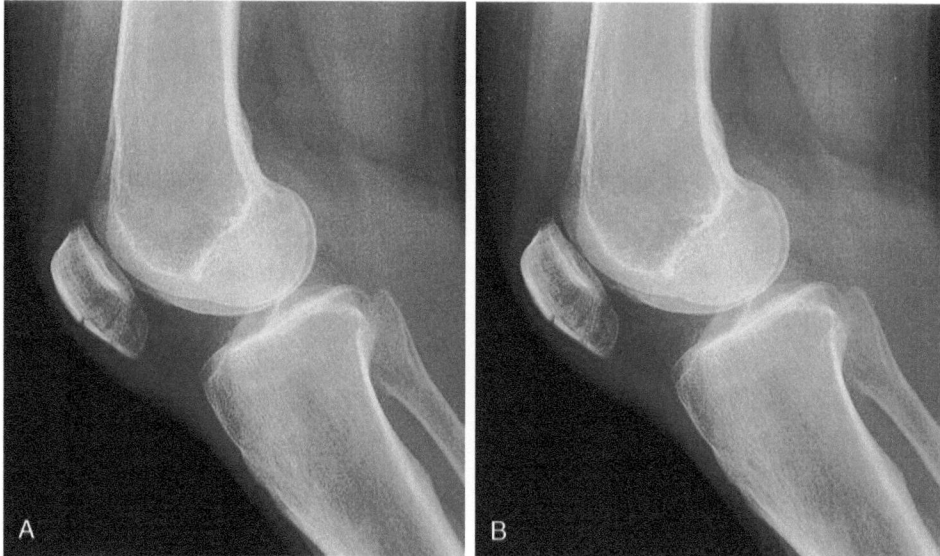

Fig. 107.17 A nondisplaced fracture amenable to nonoperative treatment.

Nonoperative treatment consists of casting in extension for up to 6 weeks. Weight bearing as tolerated is allowed, and performance of isometric quadriceps exercises is encouraged to limit atrophy. A loss of terminal extension or persistent lag is not uncommon. Resistance exercises are not started for at least 6 weeks, but gentle range of motion (ROM) exercises can be started earlier to preserve motion.

Operative Treatment of Tendinopathy

Although a majority of patients with patellar tendinopathy will respond to nonoperative treatment, patients with refractory symptoms and structural pathology on MRI or ultrasound are candidates for surgical treatment. Surgery can be accomplished through an open or arthroscopic approach and involves excision of abnormal tendon and stimulation of a healing response from the adjacent patella.

Open excision involves a longitudinal incision over the patellar tendon. The paratenon is incised in line with the skin incision, and the tendon is opened in line with its fibers. The degenerative, gelatinous tendon is exposed through this split and débrided. The distal pole of the patella is then perforated or partially resected to expose bleeding bone to the excision site. The tendon is then closed with absorbable suture.

Arthroscopic surgery starts with identification of the inferior pole of the patella and removal of synovial tissue and the adjacent fat pad. Degenerative tendon is identified and resected, and a burr is used to remove the inferior tip of the patella to stimulate healing. Additional portals and a 70-degree arthroscope can be helpful for visualization and instrumentation.[106]

Operative Treatment of Tendon Ruptures

Complete ruptures of quadriceps and patellar tendons that meet the aforementioned criteria warrant operative intervention. A delay in surgery can lead to complications and compromised outcomes. Surgical intervention for acute ruptures involves suture repair of the tendon with or without a reinforcing cerclage of nonabsorbable suture, tape, cable, or wire. Although midsubstance

tears are less common, they can usually be repaired through reapproximation of the tendon edges with heavy nonabsorbable suture. More commonly the disruption occurs at either the superior (quadriceps tendon rupture) or inferior (patellar tendon rupture) pole of the patella. In this situation suture fixation is obtained in the distal quadriceps or proximal patella, commonly with a series of Krackow stitches.[107] A small bony groove or trough is created at the adjacent, exposed patellar pole to allow the tendon to settle into a bleeding bony bed. The sutures can then be passed through drill holes created in the patella and tied together for fixation. An ACL guide may be used to facilitate accurate tunnel placement. Care should be taken to restore normal anatomy as closely as possible, especially in the repair of patellar tendons to avoid patella baja. Distal patellar tendon ruptures can be repaired back to the tibial tuberosity using suture anchors.

Neglected (chronic) and recurrent quadriceps and patellar tendon ruptures are more difficult to manage. Scar tissue and contractures make restoring native position and mobility difficult and releases may be required. Augmentation with fascia lata, Achilles tendon, or hamstring tendons has been advocated when the remaining tendon is unsuitable for direct repair (Figs. 107.18 and 107.19).[34] The use of bone–patellar tendon–bone grafts has also been described to reconstruct patellar tendons.[108] Chronic quadriceps tendon ruptures present challenges in achieving adequate length to reapproximate the injured tendon. The Codivilla technique involves an inverted-V flap that is turned down from the proximal quadriceps tendon in order to gain length needed to closed a gap and can be combined with synthetic augmentation devices.[109]

In both acute and chronic tendon repairs, synthetic augmentation can be employed utilizing heavy nonabsorbable suture, cable, or wire. This can encircle the repair through soft tissue or pass through transverse tunnels drilled in the patella and tibial tubercle in the case of patellar tendon repairs. Advantages of reinforcing the repair include the ability to initiate more aggressive rehabilitation in terms of motion while reducing the risk of disrupting the repair site.[110] Disadvantages include the need for hardware removal, irritation from subcutaneous hardware, and restrictions to motion.

More recently, several authors have studied the use of suture anchors as opposed to bone tunnels for fixation. Biomechanical studies have shown less gap formation and higher ultimate failures loads when suture anchors are used in the case of quadriceps[111,112] and patellar tendon repairs.[112] Purposed advantages of this technique aside from superior strength characteristics include lower operative time and incision size, although clinical trials are lacking.

Operative Treatment of Patellar Fractures

When operative treatment is indicated, the goal should be an anatomic reduction and rigid internal fixation, allowing early motion whenever possible. Comminution and poor bone quality can preclude secure fixation. Treatments options include tension-band fixation, cerclage wiring, external fixation, and plate-and-screw constructs, with no method demonstrating clear superiority in all situations.[113] In the case of significant comminution, consideration can be given to partial or total patellectomy, but the goal is to maintain as much viable portions of the patella as possible.

In preparing for surgery for a patellar fracture, skin integrity is an important consideration. Abrasions and lacerations should be closely scrutinized. Open fractures should be treated with immediate irrigation and débridement followed by operative fixation. Postoperative swelling can also present problems because of the lack of soft tissue coverage over the patella. Skin and subcutaneous necrosis due to swelling can result in a need for skin grafting or flap coverage. Meticulous skin-handling techniques and postoperative extremity elevation should be used to help prevent these complications.

Both transverse and longitudinal incisions have been used for exposure and repair of the patella and retinacula. A midline longitudinal incision allows excellent exposure and does not compromise subsequent surgical approaches. A concomitant retinacular injury usually allows excellent visualization of the articular surface during exploration, or the lateral retinaculum can be incised longitudinally to allow for better exposure.[114] Digital palpation of the chondral surface during reduction and fixation can confirm anatomic reduction of the articular surface.

Stabilization of bony fragments can be accomplished by cerclage wire, tension-band techniques, or interfragmentary lag-screw fixation. Circumferential cerclage wiring can reduce bone fragments through compression as tension is applied to the wire; this can be helpful in cases of extensive comminution. The Arbeitsgemeinschaft Osteosynthesefragen (AO) group has advocated the tension-band wiring technique whereby two Kirschner wires are passed longitudinally through the patella. A heavy-gauge wire is applied in a figure-eight fashion behind the wires and tightened over the anterior surface of the bone.[116] Biomechanical evaluation has found that this configuration produces a compression effect on the articular surface with knee flexion.[117]

Lag-screw fixation of larger fragments can be used alone or in conjunction with the tension-band techniques. Berg[118] described the use of cannulated screws through which a wire is passed and then secured in a figure-eight fashion. This technique has the advantage of applying compression through both the lag screws and wires via the tension-band technique while maintaining a low profile. Biomechanical analysis has shown greater resistance to displacement with this technique.[119] In comparing tension-band constructs utilizing wires or cannulated screws, Hoshino et al.[120] found an overall low incidence of hardware failure in both groups, but there was a trend toward more

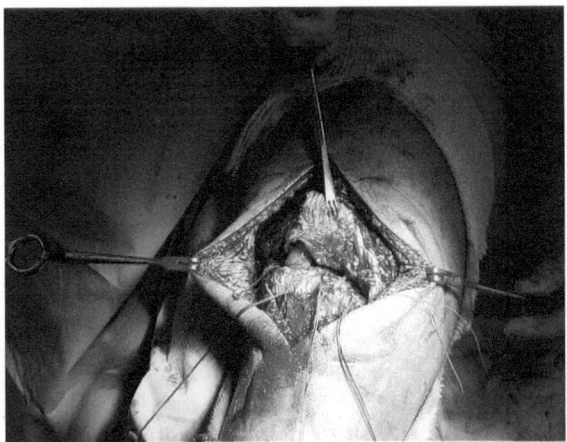

Fig. 107.18 Quadriceps tendon rupture repair.

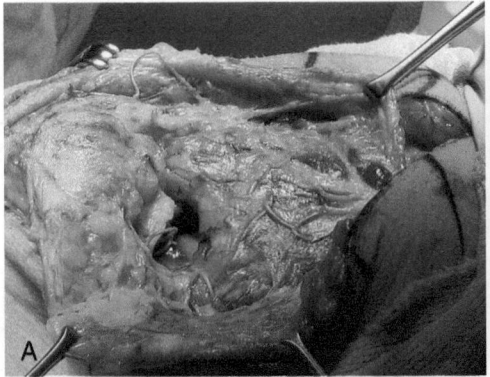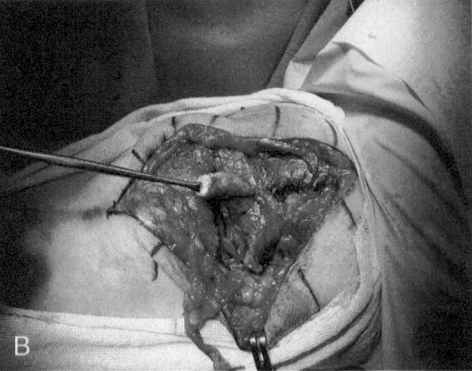

Fig. 107.19 Recurrent quadriceps tendon rupture. (A) Recurrent quadriceps rupture. (B) The Codivilla method of quadriceps tendon lengthening and repair.

frequent failure in the screw cohort (3.5% vs. 7.5%, P = .065). Removal of hardware was almost twice as common in the wire cohort (23% vs. 37%). In a retrospective review, Tian et al.[121] found better fracture reduction, lower implant migration, and lower rates of hardware removal when screws were used rather than wires.

To avoid prominent symptomatic hardware, heavy-gauge suture has been advocated as an alternative to wire or cable. Tension-band techniques using heavy sutures have demonstrated similar biomechanical properties to traditional wire,[122,123] with satisfactory clinical outcomes[124] and greatly reduced rates of subsequent hardware removal.[125] Low-profile cable and pin systems have shown promising results in comparison with traditional tension-band techniques.[121] The use of biodegradable wires and screws has not compared favorably with conventional fixation.

With respect to plates, Thelen et al.[126] also studied the use of polyaxial 2.7-mm fixed-angle plates for fracture stabilization in a synthetic model and concluded that both the plate fixation and cannulated screws with tension wiring maintained better reduction than did traditional tension-band wiring. In the laboratory, locked plating has compared favorably with tension-band fixation in resisting gap formation and in ultimate strength.[127,128] Multiplanar fixation with a low-profile mesh plate was shown by Lorich et al.[129] to result in better patient-reported outcome scores and lower rates of anterior knee pain as compared with tension-band techniques.

Fractures involving the distal pole of the patella can be treated with internal fixation of the fragment or by excision and reattachment of the patellar tendon. Veselko and Kastelec[130] compared osteosynthesis with a basket plate against distal pole resection. Internal fixation allowed for early mobilization, weight bearing, and overall better results than did distal pole excision. Patella baja was associated with poor outcomes. Excision and suture fixation, however, may result in fewer hardware-related complications.[131]

When the fracture is significantly fragmented, all attempts should be made to conserve the patella. After patellectomy, extensor lag, weakness, malalignment, and restricted motion are common problems. Quadriceps strength is reduced by 20% to 60% and tibiofemoral forces can increase up to 250%, leading to early degeneration of the tibiofemoral joint.[132] Contoured metal mesh plates have demonstrated excellent results and may be helpful for fracture patterns not amenable to more traditional fixation methods.[133] If the outcome is expected to be poor, partial or total patellectomy should be considered, because early intervention results in better outcomes than delayed treatment.[134] If a total patellectomy is performed, one should consider advancing the vastus medialis obliquus muscle over the closed defect for improved outcomes.[135]

Finally, external fixation is not commonly employed but can result in good outcomes. Liang and Wu[115] reported good or excellent results in 26 of 27 patients treated with an external compression fixator attached by transverse percutaneous pins. No osteomyelitis developed, and 80% of patients regained knee motion equal to that on the uninjured side.

Authors' Preferred Technique

Patellar Tendinopathy
If nonoperative interventions fail to produce clinical improvement, a discussion outlining surgical options and the risks and benefits of each procedure is appropriate. Our preferred treatment of refractory patellar tendinitis is to perform an open excision, the extent of which is based on preoperative advanced imaging. The remaining tendon and paratenon is closed with absorbable suture.

Patellar and Quadriceps Tendon Ruptures
We prefer to use a standard longitudinal anterior incision to allow full exposure of the affected segments of the extensor mechanism. Commonly ruptures occur adjacent to the patella, which enables the use of a locking Krackow-type nonabsorbable suture (no. 2 FiberWire, Arthrex, Naples, FL) in the residual tendon with free sutures exiting at the tear site. A bony trough is created in either the distal pole for patellar tendon ruptures or proximal pole of the patella for quadriceps tendon rupture to allow the tendon stump to lie adjacent to a bleeding base. The sutures are passed through three longitudinal drill holes in the patella and tied on the opposite side of the patella.

Patellar Fractures
Our preferred treatment is based on the configuration of the fracture patterns. Preservation of patella is preferred to excision when appropriate. We prefer rigid, strong fixation and favor a compression screw and tension-band construct whenever possible. We are aggressive in terms of surgical fixation because of the desire for early motion and rehabilitation.

POSTOPERATIVE MANAGEMENT

Patellar Tendinopathy

Postoperative management consists of early mobilization with full weight bearing after excision of involved portion of the patellar tendon. Strengthening is gradually introduced as pain and muscular control improves. Full return to sports typically is not possible until at least 3 months, and patients must demonstrate pain-free function comparable to the contralateral extremity. For in-season athletes, return to full participation is usually not possible until the following season.

Patellar and Quadriceps Tendon Ruptures

Rehabilitation from an extensor tendon repair involves a complex balance between protecting the repair and restoring knee motion. Knee motion is typically either restricted to full extension or to a small degree of flexion that is verified in the operating room to not cause any gapping at the repair site. Weight bearing is allowed in full extension, and isometric quadriceps and hamstrings exercises can be commenced shortly after surgery. Following a period of full or relative immobilization, gradual motion is introduced over the course of 6 weeks. Strengthening is begun slowly at 6 weeks, and full recovery is generally expected to take between 4 and 6 months. Rehabilitation protocols should be customized to each patient and should take into account the integrity of the repair with knee flexion in the operating room and the utilization of augmentation devices. The use of a cerclage wire after patellar tendon repair may allow patients to forego strict immobilization early in the recovery period without greatly increasing the risk of adverse events.[136]

Langenhan et al.[137] published a study of 66 quadriceps tendon repairs comparing rehabilitation including touch-down weight bearing and limited motion with full weight bearing and progressive flexion as tolerated. The investigators concluded that early mobilization with full weight bearing after primary repair is safe and does not lead to inferior outcomes or more complications. In addition, the authors postulated that the more permissive protocols were beneficial in the prevention of thromboembolic events and provided a superior environment for tendon healing and joint biomechanics.

Patella Fractures

For nondisplaced fractures, the knee is immobilized in a locked extension brace and the patient can bear weight on crutches for 6 weeks. Quadriceps exercise is continued during this period, after which the knee is mobilized to regain its ROM.

Intraoperatively during internal fixation, the knee is flexed to determine the safe degree of motion that does not disrupt the fixation construct. A hinged brace is applied and the patient is allowed to bear weight as tolerated. The knee is mobilized through the predetermined ROM twice a day. Both quadriceps and hamstring muscles are continuously strengthened throughout the recovery period.

Athletes are permitted to return to play (RTP) when healing of the bone is complete and they have achieved appropriate ROM and approximately 90% of strength compared with the uninjured side. Most are able to RTP within 6 to 9 months. Despite improved surgical techniques and rehabilitation protocols, athletes often have a difficult time returning to their preinjury levels of competition.[138]

CLINICAL OUTCOMES

Patellar and Quadriceps Tendinopathy

Numerous studies have examined the effects of both nonsurgical and surgical management of patellar tendinopathy. Panni et al.[139] performed a cohort study of 42 patients with patellar tendinopathy. After 6 months of treatment with therapy and antiinflammatory medications, 33 patients (79%) showed symptomatic improvement and were able to return to sports. Nine patients with Blazina stage 3 tendinopathy underwent open surgery. Good to excellent results were noted in all patients regardless of treatment, but patients with stage 2 tendinopathy fared better with nonoperative treatment than those with stage 3 disease.

Kon et al.[140] published a prospective study of 20 male athletes with an average of 20.7 months of symptoms and noted no adverse reactions and improved pain and activity levels after three weekly platelet-rich plasma (PRP) injections in and around the proximal patellar tendon. Gosens et al.[141] showed that patients treated with PRP had a better response if they had not been previously treated with other modalities including cortisone, ethoxysclerol, or surgery. Dragoo et al,[97] compared therapy and dry needling with and without PRP. VISA scores were better in the PRP group at 12 weeks, but no difference was found at 26-week follow-up. In a randomized trial of 46 patients comparing PRP to ESWT, better VISA and subjective outcomes were found in the PRP group at 6- and 12-month follow-up, although

no controls were used.[142] Despite some positive results, overall concerns for lack of standardization among study protocols, delivery mechanisms, and separation techniques have generated mixed reviews regarding the efficacy of this treatment.[143]

Hoksrud and Bahr[144] investigated the effects of sclerosing treatments for patellar tendinopathy at a mean of 44 months after injection. Twelve of 29 patients underwent subsequent knee surgery, although VISA scores showed significant and durable improvements in the cohort that did not undergo further treatment. Following this investigation, Hoksrud et al.[99] performed an additional prospective trial investigating sclerosing treatment in 101 patients. Subjects with clinical symptoms of tendinopathy and neovascularization evident on power Doppler ultrasound received up to a maximum of five ultrasound-guided injections of polidocanol at 4- to 6-week intervals. Although significant improvements in the VISA–Patellar Tendon were seen in the overall cohort, 36% of the cohort was noted to have poor results and the authors stated that reduced function and pain 2 years after treatment was common.

Clarke et al.[145] investigated injections of laboratory-amplified tenocyte-like cells for the treatment of patellar tendinopathy. They studied 60 patellar tendons with refractory symptoms and compared injections of collagen-producing cells derived from dermal fibroblasts suspended in plasma with plasma alone. There were statistically significant differences between the groups in terms of improvements on their VISA scores and time to improvement, although absolute differences between the groups were less substantial.

Panni et al.[139] treated nine patients with Blazina stage 3 tendinopathy with open surgical excision of degenerative tendon, placement of multiple longitudinal tenotomies, and drilling of the distal pole of the patella. At a mean of 4.8 years, clinical results were good to excellent in all patients. Shelbourne et al.[146] performed a similar study investigating 16 elite athletes with 22 symptomatic and MRI-documented cases of patellar tendinopathy who did not respond to nonoperative management. These patients underwent open excision of the diseased tissue with additional longitudinal cuts made the tendon to stimulate healing. Results were noted to be excellent for 11, good for 3, and fair for 2 patients. Of the 16 patients, 14 (87.5%) returned to sport at the same level of intensity at an average of 8.1 months.

Arthroscopic débridement of the patellar tendon, inferior patellar pole, and paratenon has demonstrated success in recent literature (see Fig. 107.20 for a treatment algorithm).[147,148] Pascarella et al.[149] noted that although open surgery is typically recommended for persons who have not responded to nonsurgical management, arthroscopy may be considered a safe and effective option. They studied 73 knees in 64 patients (including 27 professional athletes) who underwent arthroscopic débridement of the Hoffa fat pad as well as abnormal tendon and excision of the distal pole of the patella. The International Knee Documentation Committee (IKDC), Lysholm, and VISA-P scores all improved significantly at 1- and 3-year follow-up. Of 27 professional athletes. 19 returned to the same level of competition. All patients were able to return to sports within 3 months, although almost 10% were deemed failures due to a recurrence of symptoms with sports. Maier's cohort of 35 athletes undergoing arthroscopic

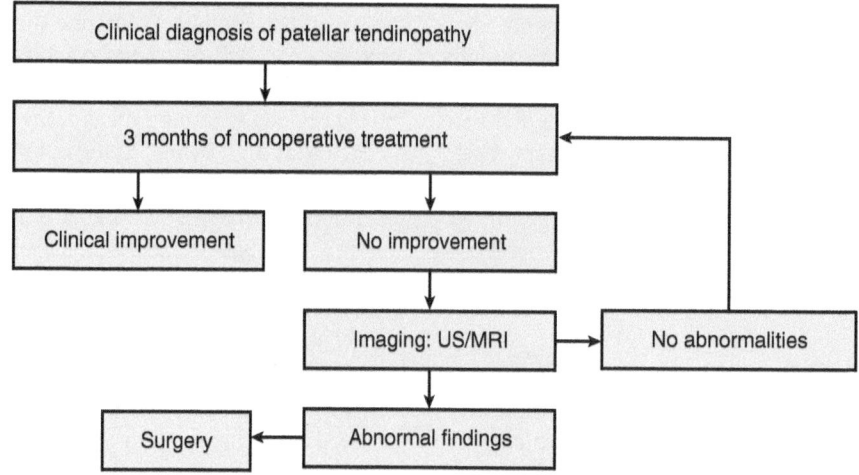

Fig. 107.20 Treatment algorithm for patellar tendinopathy. *MRI*, Magnetic resonance imaging; *US*, ultrasound.

patellar débridement demonstrated excellent symptomatic and functional improvement at over 4 years of follow-up, with 77% returning to full sport participation in 4.4 months.[150] Compared with sclerosing polidocanol injections in a 2011 randomized trial, patients undergoing arthroscopic surgery demonstrated less pain, greater satisfaction, and a faster return to sport.[151] In 2015, Brockmeyer et al.[152] published a systematic review of surgical treatment for patellar tendinosis. Although both open and arthroscopic treatment resulted in high rates of success (87% and 91%, respectively), RTP was much faster for patients undergoing arthroscopic treatment (3 vs. 8 to 12 months).

Patellar and Quadriceps Tendon Ruptures

Most patients who undergo a primary repair of patellar or quadriceps tendon ruptures relatively soon after the injury can expect good to excellent results, although some degree of weakness and lack of motion are common.[34,66] Timing of the repair does appear to correlate with overall outcome, and many advocate a 1-week time frame as optimal for performing the repair.[35]

Konrath et al.[73] studied 51 quadriceps tendon repairs in 39 patients. Of these, 84% returned to work and 51% returned to preinjury recreational activities. Just over half of this cohort had persistent quadriceps strength deficits at final follow-up. O'Shea's cohort of 19 patients demonstrated a higher return to preinjury activity level (18 of 19) as well as no strength or motion deficits.[153] Acute patellar tendon repairs also tend to have favorable outcomes in 80% or more with regard to strength and ROM.[35] Even with cerclage augmentation, rehabilitation focused on gaining motion can result in relatively normal knee function.[136]

Temponi et al.[154] reported a series of seven patients who underwent reconstruction of chronic patellar tendon ruptures with contralateral patellar tendon autograft at an average of 16 months after injury. Although significant improvements were noted from pre- to postoperative evaluation, IKDC, Lysholm, and Tegner scores were well below normal and quadriceps wasting was evident in all patients at an average of 16 months after surgery. No complications were encountered. Karas et al.[155] described the use of allograft patellar tendon or Achilles tendon for chronic

extensor mechanism injuries. Although outcome scores were improved but again below-normal, the authors concluded that this was an effective salvage procedure without a clearly superior alternative. Maffulli et al.[156] reported 14 of 19 patients as very satisfied at an average follow-up of almost 6 years after ipsilateral hamstrings reconstruction for chronic patellar tendon ruptures.

In their review of the available literature, Gilmore et al.[157] concluded that augmented primary repairs offered the best outcome in the case of acute ruptures, whereas chronic tears are optimally addressed with autogenous grafts as opposed to primary repair. The type of repair construct did not make a difference in outcomes. Clinical outcomes of contemporary suture-anchor constructs are currently unavailable.

Most patients who undergo a primary repair of patellar or quadriceps tendon ruptures relatively soon after the injury can expect good to excellent results even without augmentation. No relationship appears to exist between the configuration of the rupture, method of repair, and clinical outcome.[34,66] The timing of repair likely correlates with overall outcome, and most authors advocate a 1-week time frame as optimal for performing the repair. Although not reported by all, strength and functional deficits are not unexpected.

Boublik et al.[67] studied patellar tendon repairs in National Football League players. The investigators identified 24 ruptures in 22 players over a 10-year period. Three were associated with a concomitant ACL rupture, and players with 19 of the 24 injuries were able to RTP for at least one National Football League game. Of the players who returned, more were selected earlier in the draft, and the average number of games played totaled 45.4, ranging from 1 to 142. The authors concluded that although this injury may end a player's season, repair of isolated ruptures may allow for RTP the following season.

Patellar Fractures

Lebrun et al.[158] studied functional outcomes after operatively treated patella fractures in a cohort of trauma patients with a mean follow-up of 6.5 years. These investigators concluded that significant symptomatic complaints and functional deficits persisted. In addition to a disruption of the extensor mechanism, these cases also represent an intra-articular fracture of the patellofemoral joint. The investigators suggested that surgeons counsel patients on expectations for long-term pain and function and underscore current limitations in fracture management.

Lazaro et al.[159] prospectively followed 30 patients for 1 year after patellar fractures treated operatively. There was one case of wound dehiscence and one refracture. Eleven patients elected to undergo removal of hardware, 17 had patella baja on radiographs, and 24 described anterior knee pain with activity. Objective strength testing demonstrated significant deficits compared with the contralateral knee even at 1 year after injury.

Malik et al.[160] reported on 30 patients treated with tension-band wiring through 4.0-mm cannulated screws. Average time to union was 10.7 weeks, and final total ROM was nearly 130 degrees. No losses of reduction or hardware failures were noted. Although some authors have noted improved outcomes with fixation of distal fractures in comparison with partial patellectomy, other studies have shown the two treatments to be equivalent in terms of functional and patient-reported outcomes as well as complications.[161]

COMPLICATIONS ASSOCIATED WITH EXTENSOR MECHANISM INJURIES AND TREATMENT

Patellar Tendinopathy

Complications after injections include tendon rupture, particularly after corticosteroid injection. Bowman et al.[162] reported on three patients presenting with pain after PRP injections. Clinical and radiographic findings included worsening pain and function, tendon thickening; in one case there was osteolysis of the distal patella. Complications related to surgery are infrequent, although some studies have noted a recurrence of symptoms. Postoperative stiffness can be prevented with diligent rehabilitation.

Patellar and Quadriceps Tendon Ruptures

The most common complications after patellar and quadriceps tendon repairs and reconstructions are diminished quadriceps strength and loss of knee flexion, which can lead to diminished function. Rerupture is also a concern and compliance with postoperative instructions should be emphasized. Heterotopic ossification is not uncommon around the repair site. Other complications that can be encountered with surgery relate to the risks of the procedure itself, including infection, bleeding, recurrent rupture, wound dehiscence, deep venous thrombosis, myocardial infarction, and stroke.[163] Cases of stress fractures of the patella have been reported following the use of transosseous tunnels for suture fixation.[164]

Patella Fractures

Symptomatic hardware is perhaps the most common adverse outcome after fixation of patellar fractures and can affect up to 60% of patients.[113] Removal of symptomatic or failed implants is a frequent indication for subsequent surgery, especially when Kirschner wires are utilized. Persistent stiffness is also common. Prevention through rigid fixation that allows for early motion is the best defense. Patella baja can occur after prolonged immobilization or excision and advancement of distal pole fractures. Early ROM of the knee reduces this occurence.[165] Arthrofibrosis can also be reduced with early mobilization. Surgical site infections may occur in open injuries or as a result of skin necrosis. Wound débridement with appropriate soft tissue coverage and intravenous antibiotics often proves successful in eradicating the infection. A stable construct in the milieu of an infection should be left in situ until union occurs. Skin necrosis and tissue loss can be managed with a local medial gastrocnemius flap or a free muscle flap.

A study of 40 patients who underwent fixation of patellar fractures revealed a 20% incidence of an extensor lag greater than 5 degrees.[158] Mehdi et al.[166] reported an 8.5% rate of patellofemoral arthritis at 6-year follow-up, whereas Sorenson found that arthritis was present at over twice the rate seen in the contralateral knee in longer-term follow-up.[167] A meta-analysis of studies reporting on open reduction and internal fixation of 737 patellar fractures revealed a reoperation rate of 33.6%, 3.2% infection rate, and a 1.3% nonunion rate.[168] Nonunions are best treated with revision fixation, as when symptoms are present results are improved in comparison with observation.[169]

A history of cerebrovascular accident or diabetes has been shown to increase the risk of complications following operative treatment.[170] A study of nonoperative treatment of patellar fractures displaced by more than 1 cm in elderly patients treated without surgery revealed satisfactory outcomes in 9 of 12 patients; however one-third of the original cohort in this study died before final follow-up.[171]

FUTURE CONSIDERATIONS

Refining current nonoperative modalities for the treatment of tendinopathy, with a focus on injectable agents, will likely continue. Pulsed magnetic fields, direct current, laser therapy, radiofrequency ablation, administration of cytokines and growth factors, gene therapy, bone morphogenic protein–12, gene transfers, and tissue engineering with mesenchymal stem cells are all potential future avenues for research endeavours.[15] Future research and considerations in tendon and bone repair will likely focus on biologic enhancement or augmentation. Forthcoming clinical outcome trials associated with modern suture-anchor constructs may alter standard methods of fixation in the case of tendon ruptures, although cost will be an important factor to consider. For patellar fractures, recent studies on traditional or mesh plate-and-screw constructs may alter clinical practice in certain fracture patterns if more stable fixation and superior outcomes can be reliably achieved.

For a complete list of references, go to ExpertConsult.com.

SELECTED READINGS

Citation:

Dragoo JL, Wasterlain AS, Braun HJ, et al. Platelet-rich plasma as a treatment for patellar tendinopathy: a double-blind, randomized controlled trial. *Am J Sports Med.* 2014;42(3):610–618.

Level of Evidence:

I

Summary:

Twenty-three patients with symptomatic patellar tendinopathy and MRI findings were randomized to receive ultrasound-guided dry needling and standardized exercises with and without an injection of leukocyte-rich platelet-rich plasma. Differences in VISA scores favored the PRP group at 12 weeks ($P = .02$), but not at more than 26 weeks ($P = .66$). Lysholm scores were similar at 12 weeks ($P = .81$) and favored the control group at more than 26 weeks ($P = .006$). No adverse events were reported.

Citation:

Brockmeyer M, Diehl N, Schmitt C, et al. Results of surgical treatment of chronic patellar tendinosis (jumper's knee): a systematic review of the literature. *Arthroscopy.* 2015;31(12):2424–9.e3.

Level of Evidence:

IV

Summary:

Both open and arthroscopic treatment of patellar tendinosis are highly effective; however, arthroscopic treatment can lead to a significantly shorter return to activities.

Citation:

Garner MR, Gausden E, Berkes MB, et al. Extensor mechanism injuries of the knee: demographic characteristics and comorbidities from a review of 726 patient records. *J Bone Joint Surg Am.* 2015;97(19):1592–1596.

Level of Evidence:

IV

Summary:

A review of 726 patient records after surgical treatment for extensor mechanism injuries revealed that patellar fractures (58.8%) were more common than quadriceps tendon ruptures (28.9%), whereas patellar tendon ruptures (12.3%) were the least commonly encountered injury. Females with tendon injuries were likely than males to have an underlying medial comorbidity (96% vs. 68%, $P = .008$).

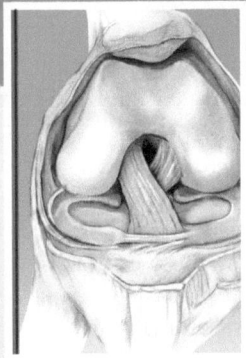

108

Loss of Knee Motion

K. Donald Shelbourne, Heather Freeman, Tinker Gray

Full range of motion (ROM) in the knee joint is critical for optimal function. A slight loss of knee motion can limit function and cause pain, and a more severe loss will lead to significant impairment and disability. For optimum function, the knee should have ROM and strength that is symmetric to the opposite, normal knee. When something causes a loss of normal knee motion, a cascade of events often follows, beginning with relative disuse of the involved lower extremity, increased pain, and subsequent loss of strength.

Loss of knee motion can occur for many reasons, including acute knee injury, lack of appropriate rehabilitation after a surgical procedure or injury, arthrofibrosis (which commonly occurs after anterior cruciate ligament [ACL] reconstruction or lower extremity fractures), relative disuse due to injury or degenerative joint disease, displaced bucket-handle meniscus tears, or mucoid degeneration of the ACL or posterior cruciate ligament (PCL). Clinicians should be vigilant about detecting loss of ROM of the knee in any patient with knee pain or injury because by restoring normal, symmetric knee motion first, followed by restoring symmetric strength, many symptoms may subside or abate, negating the need for further surgical intervention. Use of this proactive approach helps patients avoid problems in the short term after a knee injury or surgery, and some evidence indicates that it may also prevent long-term problems, including knee osteoarthritis.[1-3]

Early intervention for ROM loss requires early detection. To identify loss of knee motion, the opposite, normal knee must also be examined to establish a baseline for comparison, and the examination must include an assessment of knee hyperextension. Unfortunately this step is sometimes overlooked. A recent study found that in patients who were seeking a second opinion for their knee problem, only 37% reported having their opposite, normal knee physically touched during the physical examination.[4]

This chapter provides an overview of the diagnosis and treatment for loss of ROM of the knee. The reasons for loss of knee motion and thus the treatments are wide ranging. However, common themes regarding effective treatment remain the same regardless of the specific cause of loss of knee motion. Most cases of loss of knee motion can be effectively treated without surgery if proper rehabilitation is performed. In some cases, such as arthrofibrosis or displaced bucket-handle meniscus tears, surgical intervention is necessary to remove a mechanical block to knee ROM. The surgical treatment for arthrofibrosis after ACL reconstruction is outlined in detail in this chapter. The principles of rehabilitation for loss of knee motion remain the same whether or not surgical intervention is a part of the treatment plan, and these rehabilitation principles are also discussed.

HISTORY

Patients with loss of knee motion may present with varying subjective histories. It is important to determine how long the ROM loss has been present. This information can be difficult to elicit because patients are often unaware that their ROM is lacking, so we ask them how long they have felt that they had a bad knee. Generally speaking, the longer the ROM loss has been present, the more slowly it may respond to treatment. However, long-term ROM loss does not always mean that more aggressive forms of treatment are necessary; rather, it is important for both the clinician and patient to understand that progress may occur at a slower pace.

In patients who have had previous knee surgery, it is important to obtain pertinent details about the surgical procedure. When loss of motion is present, it is perhaps even more important to ascertain what, if any, pre- and postoperative rehabilitation was performed. In our experience, many patients with persistent pain after a knee arthroscopy or other knee surgery have loss of knee motion that was likely present before surgical intervention but was overlooked and not treated.

In patients who have not had a previous knee surgery, a careful subjective history can often identify a precipitating injury that may not have seemed significant at the time but may have led them to begin favoring their knee. When patients favor a knee, they stand with their weight shifted away from the involved lower extremity, holding the knee slightly bent. Over time, this habit slowly leads to increasing amounts of knee extension loss. Without full terminal knee extension, it is not comfortable to stand with the body weight shifted toward the involved knee because the ability to "lock out" the knee is lost, and therefore the quadriceps muscles cannot be relaxed during stance as it is for the opposite, normal knee. This scenario feeds the vicious cycle of disuse, increased pain, and further loss of strength.

Other times the subjective history reveals a significant injury to which the patient can attribute the ROM loss with certainty. A displaced bucket-handle meniscus tear blocks the intercondylar notch, resulting in the inability to fully extend the knee. Although this scenario may not always be caused by a specific injury, patients can usually identify exactly when this mechanism occurred and report that the involved knee feels "locked."

When a patient does not have a history of a specific injury, the ROM loss may be associated with degenerative joint disease. Another potential cause of ROM loss is mucoid degeneration of the cruciate ligaments, most commonly the ACL. This pathology presents as a gradual loss of knee flexion combined with posterolateral knee pain. An effusion is usually not present.

PHYSICAL EXAMINATION

The physical examination for any knee problem should include a careful assessment of the knee ROM of both knees, including an assessment of knee hyperextension. The uninvolved knee should always be examined before the involved knee; this examination is important to establish a baseline of what the ROM should be for the involved knee. It is also important that both knees be fully exposed (to the level of the midthigh) for the examination.

Knee extension (including hyperextension) is assessed in two ways. First, the examiner performs a passive assessment of hyperextension (Fig. 108.1). The examiner stabilizes the thigh on the examination table with one hand while the other hand passively lifts the heel off the table, assessing the amount of movement available and the quality of the end feel. When ROM is limited, the patient should be asked if the discomfort is perceived posteriorly or anteriorly when a stretch is applied. Posterior discomfort indicates capsular and soft tissue tightness, whereas anterior discomfort may indicate an intra-articular mechanical blockage. Second, knee extension should be measured with the patient lying supine, with both heels propped up on a 6- to 8-inch bolster, allowing the knees to fall into hyperextension. This position allows for visual assessment of knee extension symmetry as well as goniometric measurement of knee extension.

It is important to note that knee hyperextension is normal. DeCarlo and Sell[5] studied a group of healthy young athletes and found that 95% of males and 96% of females have some degree of knee hyperextension. The mean knee hyperextension was 5 degrees for males and 6 degrees for females. Therefore treatment to restore normal knee ROM should include restoration of hyperextension when it is present in the opposite knee.

Knee flexion is assessed with the patient lying supine or in a long-sitting position. The patient should be asked to grasp the front of his or her ankle with both hands (or use a towel looped around this area if necessary) and to pull the heel as far as possible toward the buttocks. Goniometric measurement can be made once maximal flexion is reached. Another method for assessing knee flexion is to ask the patient to sit on his or her heels (Fig. 108.2). Patients with full flexion of both knees are able to comfortably sit back onto their heels without any pelvic tilt. Knee flexion loss leads to minor to severe tilting of the pelvis away from the involved extremity. This method of assessing flexion is also very helpful for patients in self-assessing their knee flexion and adjusting their activity levels accordingly.

For the purposes of this chapter, we focus on the examination for ROM deficits, but a full knee examination should also be performed, including observation of gait, observation for disuse of the lower extremity in arising from a chair or with habitual standing postures, observation of patella alignment and mobility, palpation for crepitus, assessment for a joint effusion, and special testing for meniscal pathology and ligamentous laxity.

IMAGING

Bilateral radiographs—including weight-bearing posteroanterior, lateral, and Merchant[6] views—are routinely obtained. Again, even in the absence of bilateral symptoms, it is important to obtain bilateral radiographs to provide a baseline for comparison with the involved knee.

When osteoarthritis is suspected, we also recommend obtaining an anteroposterior view. A study by Rosenberg and colleagues[7] showed that the posteroanterior view is more sensitive for detecting joint space narrowing of the tibiofemoral joint. This view is more sensitive because it is taken with the knees bent to a 45-degree angle, allowing for weight bearing with the tibiofemoral joint aligned in a position where more cartilage degeneration is likely. The anteroposterior view is not as sensitive for detecting

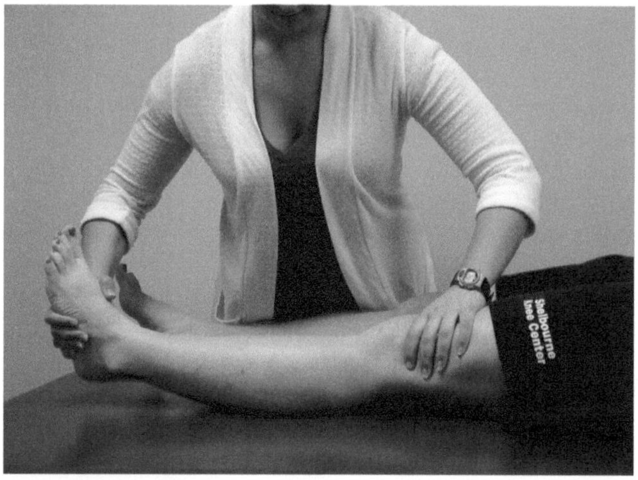

Fig. 108.1 Passive assessment of knee hyperextension.

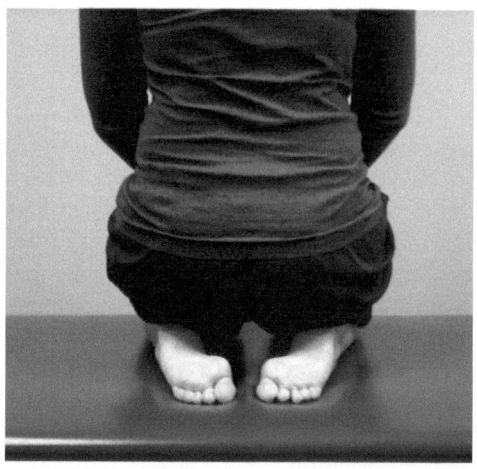

Fig. 108.2 Full knee flexion can be assessed by asking the patient to sit on his or her heels. If knee flexion is lacking in one knee, the patient shows a lateral pelvic tilt away from the involved knee.

joint space narrowing but provides information regarding the amount of joint space remaining when the knee is in a fully extended position.

In cases of long-standing ROM loss, the Merchant view radiograph can provide useful information through a visual comparison of the bone density of the patellae. When a patient has been favoring one knee for any considerable length of time, disuse osteopenia is evident on the Merchant view (Fig. 108.3).

In patients with severe ROM loss, it is important to observe for signs of patella baja on the lateral-view radiographs. Again, comparison with the opposite knee is important to determine the height of the patella compared with Blumensaat's line and the apparent length of the patellar tendon based on measurements from the inferior pole of the patella to the tibial tubercle. Although normal ranges have been established for each of these measurements, what is normal for each patient varies and should be based on the measurements for the uninvolved knee.

Magnetic resonance imaging (MRI) is useful when arthrofibrosis is present. In patients with arthrofibrosis types 1 or 2, the MRI can help identify the presence of a cyclops lesion, which is commonly present in patients with arthrofibrosis after ACL reconstruction. In persons with arthrofibrosis types 3 or 4, the MRI provides valuable insight about the extent of scar tissue formation in the fat pad.

DECISION-MAKING PRINCIPLES

Despite the wide range of pathologies that can cause limited knee ROM, a vast majority of cases of limited knee motion can be effectively treated with a directed rehabilitation program. One exception to this is in the case of a displaced bucket-handle meniscus tear, which would need to be arthroscopically reduced and removed or repaired.

Another condition to consider is arthrofibrosis, particularly in patients who have had previous knee surgeries, including ACL reconstruction, but also fractures around the knee. Arthrofibrosis is an abnormal proliferation of fibrotic tissue in the knee joint. The fibrotic tissue is commonly found in the extrasynovial space anteriorly in a fibrotic fat pad or near the intercondylar notch, presenting as a cyclops lesion at the base of the reconstructed ACL. Arthrofibrosis can cause a loss of knee extension alone, or knee extension and flexion may both be limited. Shelbourne et al.[8] developed a classification for arthrofibrosis to help guide treatment (Table 108.1). Most patients with type 1 arthrofibrosis respond to nonoperative rehabilitation and do not need surgery, but most cases of types 2, 3, or 4 require a combination of rehabilitation and operative treatment to achieve satisfactory results. In these patients, pre- and postoperative rehabilitation is a vital component of the treatment process. In nearly all other cases of knee ROM loss that were not caused by a previous surgery, a directed rehabilitation program completed under the supervision of a well-trained knee therapist can resolve significant deficits and provide a corresponding improvement in function.

Not all rehabilitation programs are designed the same way, but the foundation of a rehabilitation program for limited knee motion should be to work on regaining symmetry in three distinct, sequential phases: (1) knee extension, (2) knee flexion, and (3) knee strength. Our experience has shown us that these phases of rehabilitation should not overlap; rather, one should focus on only extension ROM until symmetry is restored, and then shift toward working on flexion ROM while maintaining full extension. Finally, once full ROM symmetry has been achieved, unilateral strengthening exercises should be initiated until strength symmetry is restored. This rehabilitation program is described in greater detail in the "Authors' Preferred Technique" and "Postoperative Management" sections, further on.

If ROM progress plateaus before symmetric knee extension is achieved, surgical intervention may be needed to remove a mechanical blockage to extension. When degenerative joint disease is present, the mechanical blockage may be caused by an osteophyte on the anterior tibia or near the intercondylar notch.

Mucoid degeneration of the ACL is a rare condition but presents with a classic history. Patients with this condition are typically middle aged and report an insidious onset of gradual loss

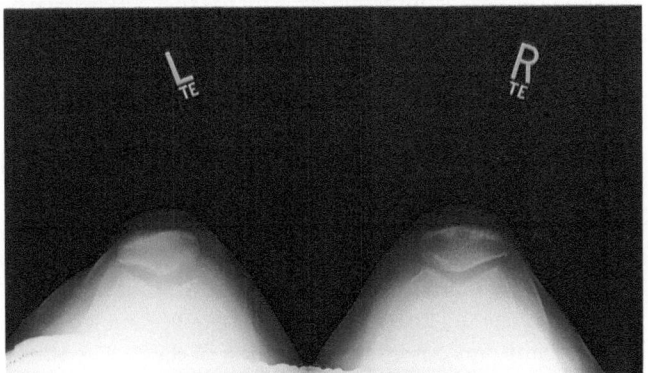

Fig. 108.3 A Merchant view radiograph showing disuse osteopenia of the right patella after relative disuse of the right lower extremity for an extended period.

TABLE 108.1	Classification of Arthrofibrosis		
Type	Knee Flexion	Knee Extension	Other Features
1	Normal	≤10-degree deficit[a]	Able to fully extend with overpressure
2	Normal	>10-degree deficit[a]	Unable to fully extend with overpressure
3	≥25-degree deficit[a]	>10-degree deficit[a]	Decreased medial/lateral patellar mobility
4	≥30-degree deficit[a]	>10-degree deficit[a]	Patella infera evident on radiographs

[a]All range of motion (ROM) deficits are based on comparison with the ROM of the normal, uninvolved knee.
From Shelbourne KD, Patel DV, Martini DJ. Classification and management of arthrofibrosis of the knee after anterior cruciate ligament reconstruction. *Am J Sports Med.* 1996;24:857–862.

of knee flexion accompanied by posterolateral knee pain. Some loss of knee extension may be present, but it is usually mild and easily resolves with rehabilitation using either a towel stretch or a passive knee stretch device (Ideal Stretch, Park City, UT) (Fig. 108.4). The appearance on MRI is often described as a "celery stalk" feature, with a striated appearance on T2-saturated images indicating fluid between the ACL fibers. An enlarged, bulbous area is usually present proximally (Fig. 108.5). Literature on this topic is sparse and mostly includes case reports regarding débridement or resection of the ACL, but residual instability has been an undesirable aftereffect of this procedure.[9,10] We have found that this condition responds favorably to oral or injected steroids and rehabilitation using the principles described in detail later in this chapter.

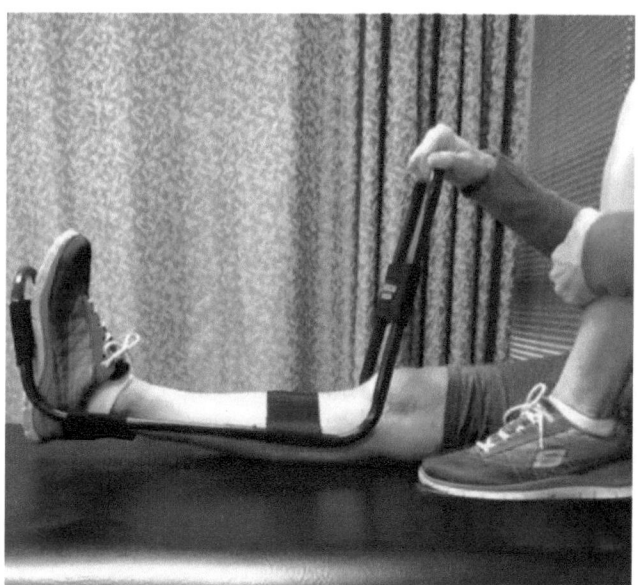

Fig. 108.4 A passive knee stretch device is used when limitation of knee extension is mild (with 5 degrees of neutral).

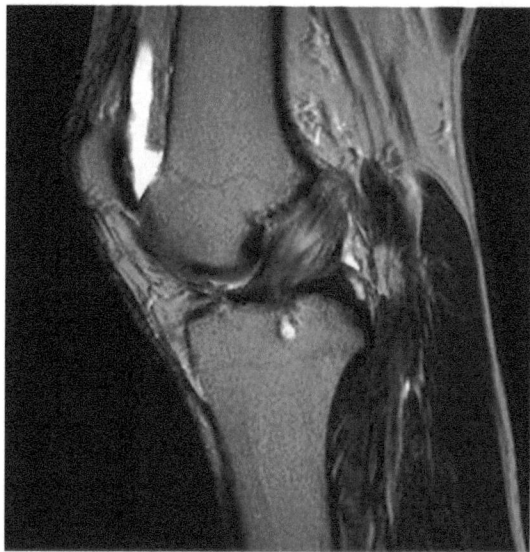

Fig. 108.5 A magnetic resonance image showing mucoid degeneration of the anterior cruciate ligament.

TREATMENT OPTIONS

Nonsurgical treatment with a carefully planned rehabilitation program is the first line of treatment for most patients with loss of knee ROM. As discussed in the previous section, surgery may be necessary in some cases to allow full, symmetric ROM to be regained, particularly in cases of type 2, 3, or 4 arthrofibrosis after an ACL reconstruction or when a bucket-handle meniscus tear becomes displaced and is blocking the intercondylar notch.

The following surgical interventions have been described for loss of knee motion: anterior interval release,[11] notchplasty and/or removal of a cyclops lesion,[12] posterior capsular release,[13,14] peripatellar release, and manipulation with the patient under anesthesia.[15]

The anterior interval is defined as the space posterior to the patellar tendon and extending to the anterior tibia and transverse meniscal ligament. Trauma to the infrapatellar fat pad can lead to fibrotic formation in this area of the knee, limiting both knee extension and flexion. This presentation is most commonly seen in patients who have undergone arthroscopic ACL surgery, with fat pad trauma occurring as a result of repeatedly passing instruments through the fat pad. Although arthroscopic ACL surgery is believed to be less traumatic for the patient, the trauma to the fat pad is underestimated. Fat pad trauma can lead to fat pad fibrosis; in its most severe form, fibrosis in this area can lead to infrapatellar contracture syndrome, which further limits patellar mobility and knee flexion.[16] If full knee flexion is not emphasized immediately after surgery, patellar mobility decreases and permanent flexion deficits may occur. Anterior interval release can be performed arthroscopically with use of a 30-degree scope and portals that are slightly farther away from midline than usual to allow for better visualization of this area.[11] Abnormal tissue may be removed with a basket forceps, meniscal shaver, or electrothermal probe.

Under normal circumstances, the ACL and PCL fit perfectly within the intercondylar notch, completely occupying this space when the knee is in terminal extension. Occasionally after ACL reconstruction, a mismatch occurs between the size of the graft and the width of the intercondylar notch, or a cyclops lesion[17] forms, blocking full knee extension. A cyclops lesion is a fibrous nodule that forms on the anterior aspect of the ACL graft (Fig. 108.6). We theorize that this complication can be prevented after ACL reconstruction by ensuring that full, symmetric knee extension is restored prior to and immediately after surgery. These lesions can be carefully excised during arthroscopy until terminal extension is regained. If the intercondylar notch width is not adequate to handle the size of the ACL graft and the PCL, a notchplasty can also be performed.

When knee extension has been lacking for a longer duration of time, the posterior capsule becomes tight. Arthroscopic release of the posterior capsule has been described by LaPrade et al.[13] and Mariani.[14] Another option is to use a more aggressive approach to rehabilitation that focuses on knee extension by using a passive knee extension device (Elite Seat, AKT Medical, Inc., Noblesville, IN) (Fig. 108.7). Use of a long-duration stretch of 10 to 15 minutes per session several times each day can

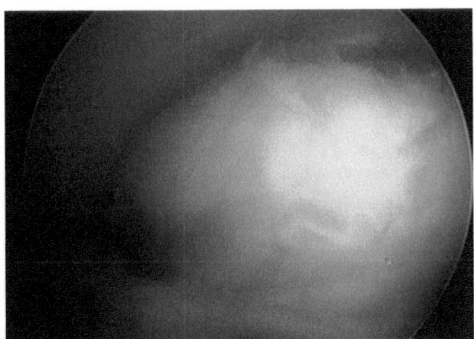

Fig. 108.6 An arthroscopic view of a cyclops lesion on the anterior aspect of the anterior cruciate ligament graft.

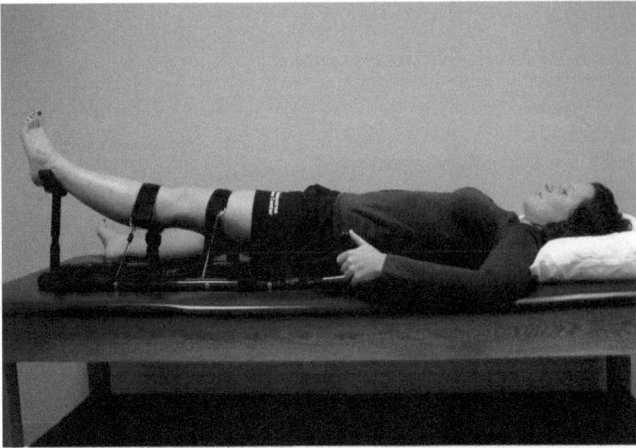

Fig. 108.7 A passive knee extension device is used to restore symmetric knee extension, including hyperextension. The patient lies supine and controls the intensity of the stretch with a handheld crank. The stretch is performed at least two to three times per day for 10 to 15 minutes per session.

eventually improve posterior capsular mobility and restore full knee extension compared with the opposite knee.

Decreased patellar mobility has been treated with release of the medial and/or lateral retinaculum and the suprapatellar pouch.[18,19] Care must be taken to provide adequate release without overreleasing these structures and inducing patellar instability.[18]

Manipulation with the patient under anesthesia has been described to regain knee extension and/or knee flexion.[15] Manipulation of the knee can effectively improve knee motion, but it does not directly approach the knee problem selectively, and

there is a risk of supracondylar femur fracture, patellar tendon rupture, and neurologic or vascular injury.

Many surgeons use more than one of these techniques in combination based on the location of the adhesions and the degree of ROM limitation that is present.

Authors' Preferred Technique

Loss of Knee Motion

It is important to emphasize that surgical treatment is only one part of the process for treating loss of knee ROM and that surgical intervention is not always needed. For optimal results, patients must first maximize their knee ROM with a directed rehabilitation program. Then, if surgery is needed, a focused postoperative rehabilitation program is used to further maximize knee motion. In fact, we now require all patients undergoing surgery for arthrofibrosis to use a passive knee extension device (see Fig. 108.4) several times daily before and after surgery to maximize results. In past years, extension casting was used on the operating room table and followed by serial extension casting on an outpatient basis to provide a low-load, long-duration stretch; however, this treatment was difficult to implement because of the postoperative hemarthrosis that developed and the frequency of outpatient visits required for serial casting. Instead, we now have the patient perform several stretching sessions each day in the passive knee extension device and have found that this technique is highly effective and more cost- and time-efficient.[20]

When surgical intervention is needed to treat arthrofibrosis, the lead author uses a stepwise process to address the specific areas of fibrosis that have developed in the knee. This section addresses the surgical treatment of arthrofibrosis, specifically arthrofibrosis that develops after ACL reconstruction. This approach is based on the classification of arthrofibrosis shown in Table 108.1 and has been previously described.[8]

Arthroscopy is performed after general anesthesia is induced and after the knee is injected with 20 mL of 0.25% bupivacaine and epinephrine. Knee ROM and patellar mobility are evaluated once general anesthesia is achieved and are reassessed throughout the surgical procedure to determine if additional surgical steps are needed to remove mechanical blockages to knee extension and flexion.

To improve visibility of the anterior aspect of the knee joint, standard medial, and lateral portals are used, but the position of the portals is adjusted to be more proximal and slightly farther medial and lateral, respectively.

The first step is to examine the area anterior to the proximal tibia. If extrasynovial scar tissue has formed in this area, a blunt trocar is used to loosen the scar between the posterior aspect of the patellar tendon and the anterior aspect of the tibia. A basket forceps and meniscal shaver may be used to excise scar tissue in this area. One should ensure that the entire area from the anterior horns of the medial and lateral menisci down to the upper tibia is free of extrasynovial scar tissue. Patients with type 2, 3, or 4 arthrofibrosis often have scar formation in this area of the knee (Fig. 108.8).

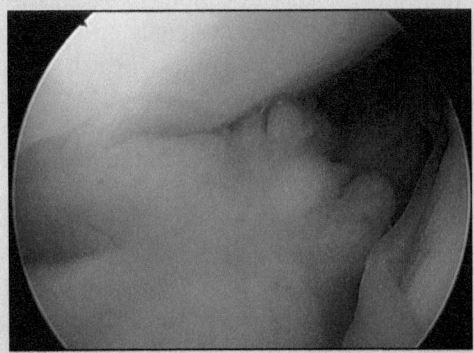

Fig. 108.8 An arthroscopic view of anterior scar tissue extending into the medial compartment.

Continued

Authors' Preferred Technique

Loss of Knee Motion—cont'd

Second, the intercondylar notch is examined for signs of impingement, including the base of the ACL where a cyclops lesion may form (see Fig. 108.6). In patients with type 1 arthrofibrosis, this area is typically the only area of mechanical blockage causing ROM loss; this lesion is located inside the synovium and is not part of the fat pad (Fig. 108.9). The knee must be placed through a ROM into full terminal extension to determine if the ACL fits into the intercondylar notch without any sign of impingement (Fig. 108.10). Excision or ablation can be used to remove scar tissue that has formed in this area. If needed, a notchplasty may be performed to allow the ACL to fit within the intercondylar notch; thus the remaining knee extension that needs to be regained after surgery can be achieved with the passive knee extension device.

Fibrosis of the infrapatellar fat pad and/or the joint capsule is usually associated with type 3 or 4 arthrofibrosis. After using a blunt probe to establish a plane between the patellar tendon and the scar tissue, the scar tissue should be removed distally to the level of the upper tibia and anteriorly to the horns of the menisci. When the joint capsule is fibrotic, excision of the fibrotic capsule can be performed up to the insertion of the vastus medialis oblique and vastus lateralis muscles, which improves mobility of the patella and patellar tendon.

Patients with type 4 arthrofibrosis are not likely to regain full, symmetric knee flexion because of the shortening of the patellar tendon. However, in patients with type 3 or 4 arthrofibrosis, a manipulation is performed to maximize knee flexion. We do not recommend forceful manipulation for knee extension because most of the knee extension loss is due to either mechanical blocks that can be selectively removed and/or posterior capsular tightness that can be slowly stretched out during the course of postoperative rehabilitation.

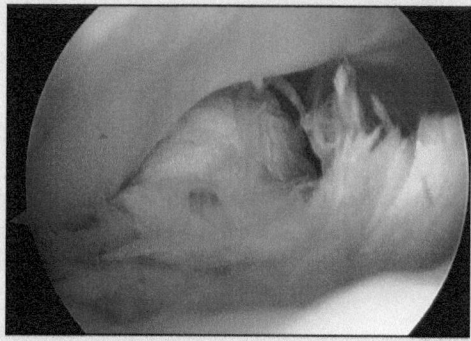

Fig. 108.9 An arthroscopic view of the same knee depicted in Fig. 108.7, showing the intercondylar notch area with the knee in about 30 degrees of flexion. Scar tissue that is visible anterior to the ACL graft gets impinged when the knee is placed in full extension. *ACL*, Anterior cruciate ligament.

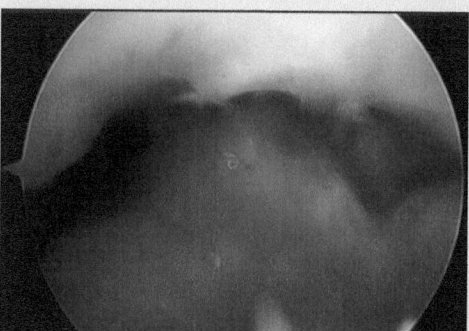

Fig. 108.10 An arthroscopic view after débridement of scar tissue (in the same knee as depicted in Figs. 108.7 and 108.8) shows a good fit of the anterior cruciate ligament graft in the intercondylar notch.

POSTOPERATIVE MANAGEMENT

The primary goals of postoperative treatment are to prevent a hemarthrosis and achieve/maintain full terminal extension symmetric to the opposite knee. Once the mechanical block to extension has been removed, immediate emphasis on full knee extension is needed to stretch the posterior capsule and allow the patient to regain full symmetric knee extension. To regain knee ROM, we have found that it is best to work only on knee extension first until symmetry is restored and then switch the focus of rehabilitation to knee flexion exercises during the next phase.

Patients remain in the hospital overnight as a 23-hour stay after surgery. Continuous intravenous administration of ketorolac is used for pain control and prevention of swelling. Antiembolism stockings and a cold/compression device (Cryo/Cuff, DJO Inc., Vista, CA) are used at all times starting immediately after surgery to prevent a hemarthrosis. The knee is placed in a continuous passive motion (CPM) machine set from 0 to 30 degrees, but the primary purpose of the CPM is to elevate the knee above the level of the heart (Fig. 108.11).

Knee extension exercises are performed three to four times per day to ensure that full terminal knee extension is maintained.

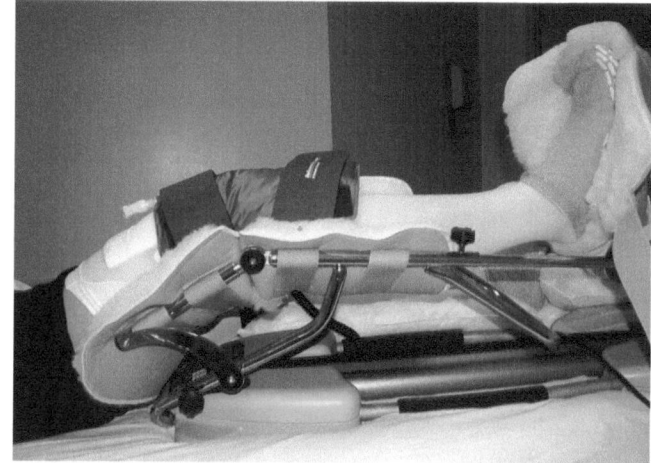

Fig. 108.11 A continuous passive motion machine is used in the early postoperative phase to help prevent a hemarthrosis by keeping the knee above the level of the heart. A cold/compression device is also applied to the knee.

When the knee is in full terminal extension, the intercondylar notch is completely filled by the ACL and PCL, which prevents formation of fibrotic tissue near this notch. Knee extension exercises consist of using either the passive knee stretch device (see Fig. 108.4) or the passive knee extension device (see Fig. 108.7), towel stretch (Fig. 108.12), active heel lift (Fig. 108.13), heel prop stretch, and straight-leg raises. The active heel lift and straight-leg raise exercises are used to improve quadriceps muscle control and active terminal knee extension, which is important for long-term maintenance of full, symmetric knee extension.

Patients are discharged home but continue to follow the previously outlined protocol for the first 5 postoperative days. Patients are instructed to remain lying down with the knee elevated in the CPM machine and to use the cold/compression device at all times except when ambulating to and from the bathroom. This component of the protocol is vital to prevent the development of a hemarthrosis. Prevention of a hemarthrosis allows good quadriceps muscle control, which helps regain/maintain full knee

extension and consequently allows for knee flexion deficits to be addressed sooner.

After the first postoperative week, patients continue to focus on the same rehabilitation goals but may gradually begin to return to normal daily activities. They are encouraged to use the cold/compression device at least three times a day for 30 minutes or more frequently if necessary to control swelling. During this phase of rehabilitation, it is important to educate patients about habits they need to work on to use the involved knee normally throughout the day and encourage full knee extension during daily activities. We call these *extension habits*. For the sitting extension habit, patients are advised to sit with the knee fully extended and the heel propped up on their other foot, allowing the knee to fall into full extension. The standing extension habit involves having the patient shift his or her weight onto the involved lower extremity, locking the knee out straight. This exercise encourages full knee extension and normal use of the involved lower extremity during activities of daily living. In addition, it maintains the newly achieved posterior capsular stretch and full contact of the femur, tibia, and ACL in terminal extension.

The speed at which each patient is ready to progress to the next phase of rehabilitation varies considerably based on the chronicity and extent of knee motion loss present. Once full, symmetric knee extension is regained and the patient can easily perform an active heel lift, knee flexion exercises are begun. In cases of more severe knee flexion loss, we begin with a wall slide exercise (Fig. 108.14). Heel-slide exercises are the primary exercise used to improve knee flexion, with a 5-second hold and 10 to 15 repetitions performed per exercise session. Full knee flexion is achieved when the patient can sit on his or her heels without tilting the pelvis laterally (see Fig. 108.2). Patients must be instructed regarding ways to monitor knee extension closely, and knee flexion exercises should be put on hold if any loss of knee extension occurs.

Low-impact exercise using a bike or elliptical machine may be slowly introduced at this point. We recommend starting without any resistance and gradually increasing the time of the workout by 2 to 3 minutes according to the ability of the patient.

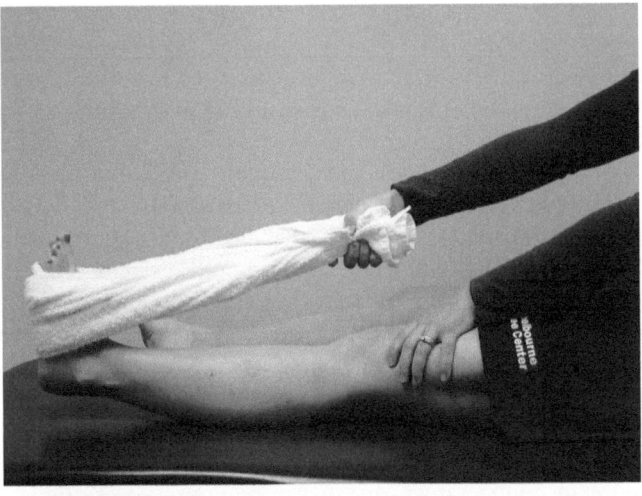

Fig. 108.12 The towel-stretch exercise for knee extension.

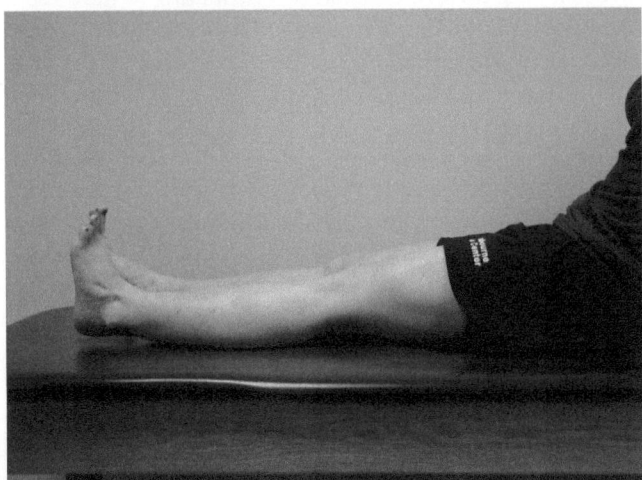

Fig. 108.13 The active heel lift exercise consists of having the patient contract his or her quadriceps muscle group to actively raise the heel off the table, achieving active terminal knee extension.

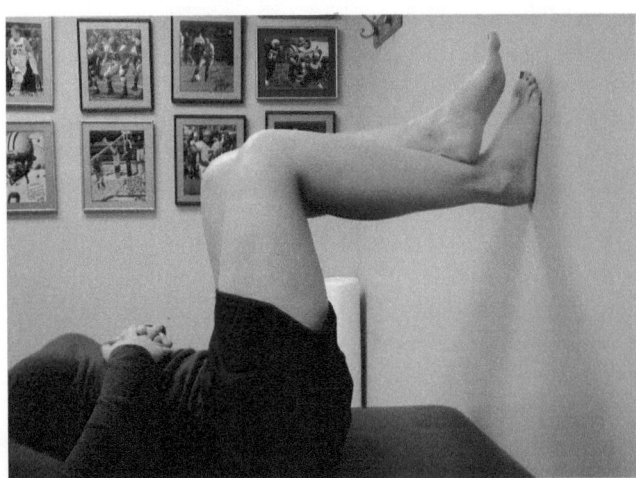

Fig. 108.14 The wall slide exercise is helpful for regaining knee flexion in patients with more severe loss of knee flexion.

ROM must be closely monitored and low-impact exercise should be stopped if the patient begins to lose motion.

Once full, symmetric knee flexion and extension are achieved and maintained, the rehabilitation focus shifts to a unilateral strengthening program to restore strength symmetry. We have found that trying to work on strength in the knee before full extension and flexion have been achieved is difficult because strengthening exercises frequently cause swelling and loss of ROM when they are performed on a stiff knee, thus defeating the purpose of the early phases of rehabilitation.

Loss of knee motion is often associated with significant strength deficits as a result of disuse. We recommend performing isokinetic testing of the quadriceps muscle group to quantify the amount of strength loss compared with the noninvolved knee. We consider strength to be symmetric when it is within 10% of the opposite, normal knee. We recommend using a high number of repetitions and low resistance for single leg press, single knee extension, and step-down exercises to achieve this goal. As with the other phases of the rehabilitation program, care must be taken to ensure that ROM loss does not occur once strengthening exercises commence. If the patient begins to lose knee motion, one should back off from the strengthening exercises until full ROM is restored and then slowly introduce strengthening exercises again.

Patients who are treated nonoperatively for knee ROM loss follow the same rehabilitation program and progression except for the surgery-specific measures such as the use of a CPM, antiembolism stockings, and a period of relative bed rest. We are finding that in a large number of patients who come to us for a second opinion, their knee ROM loss was overlooked and not treated by the previous physician and/or therapist. By carefully examining both knees and using the previously outlined treatment principles, many cases of anterior knee pain or generalized knee pain can be addressed effectively without surgery.

RETURN TO SPORTS

Participation in impact activities, such as running and jumping, is not encouraged until full ROM and strength symmetry are restored. Once these goals are reached, impact activities may be gradually introduced on an every-other-day basis. We recommend using a functional sports progression in which speed and change of direction are gradually increased based on the patient's tolerance. After the patient is comfortable performing individual speed and agility drills, individual sport-specific drills are introduced, followed by drills against a defender, and finally scrimmage and game situations are permitted. Close monitoring of knee extension and knee flexion must be performed on a daily basis to detect any loss of motion early and adjust activity levels accordingly. Patients should be instructed to monitor their own ROM by assessing end feel of the towel stretch exercise and sitting on their heels.

RESULTS

Because arthrofibrosis is a difficult complication to treat, prevention of this problem is the best treatment. The lead author coauthored a published series of 33 patients treated with the previously outlined protocol for arthrofibrosis.[20] The study group included 19 women and 14 men, with a mean age of 31 years. All of these patients were seen in our center after arthrofibrosis developed following knee surgery performed elsewhere, and 27 of these patients experienced arthrofibrosis after an ACL reconstruction. The mean preoperative ROM was 0-8-117 degrees (hyperextension-extension-flexion) for the involved knee compared with 5-0-147 degrees for the uninvolved knee. At a mean of 8.6 months after surgery, the mean involved knee ROM improved to 3-0-134 degrees. The mean subjective scores on the International Knee Documentation Committee (IKDC) survey improved from 45.3 to 67.1 ($P < .01$), and the patients who achieved normal ROM according to IKDC criteria (knee extension within 2 degrees and knee flexion within 5 degrees of the opposite knee) also had the highest subjective scores. Although these patients showed significant improvement after treatment, the results were still not nearly as good as they could have been if this ROM problem had been prevented and arthrofibrosis had not developed.

Another study looked at patients who did not have arthrofibrosis but were diagnosed with a deconditioned knee, including at least 5 degrees of extension loss compared with the opposite knee.[21] This group included 25 men and 25 women with a mean age of 53.2 years. Osteoarthritis was the underlying pathology in 41 of the 50 patients, and 7 had undergone previous arthroscopy without rehabilitation. All patients were treated nonoperatively with the previously described rehabilitation program. After 3 months of rehabilitation and a guided home exercise program, the mean side-to-side deficit in knee extension improved from 10 to 3 degrees ($P < .01$), and the mean side-to-side deficit in knee flexion improved from 19 to 9 degrees. Correspondingly, the IKDC subjective scores increased as ROM improved, with a mean at initial evaluation of 34.5 points, improving to 70.5 points 12 months later. This study shows that severe loss of ROM in nonoperative patients can be improved greatly with rehabilitation; correspondingly, subjective scores and function also improve. Without carefully examining each patient with knee pain, slight ROM loss that is contributing to the patient's knee symptoms can be overlooked, and unnecessary knee surgery may be performed.

COMPLICATIONS

As mentioned earlier, a vast majority of patients with knee ROM loss can be treated nonoperatively, especially when the ROM loss is detected early. Very few complications are associated with nonoperative treatment methods. An increased risk of complications is found in cases that are more advanced and require surgical intervention. As with any surgical procedure, the risk exists for infection, wound-healing problems, deep venous thrombosis, nerve injury, vascular injury, iatrogenic chondral injury, and development of a hemarthrosis. Manipulation is associated with a risk for supracondylar femur fracture or neurovascular injury. The risk of these complications can be minimized with careful surgical techniques, appropriate portal placement, and closely supervised perioperative care and rehabilitation.

FUTURE CONSIDERATIONS

We believe that the detrimental effects of knee ROM loss have been underestimated. In the short term, patients with loss of knee ROM might feel fine, but this condition can lead to problems in the future, just as a patient with high blood pressure or high cholesterol may feel fine now, but without early identification and treatment of these medical issues, more serious problems are known to occur with time. We believe that restoration of full, symmetric knee ROM is critical after any knee surgery. Secondarily, any loss of knee ROM must be identified early and proper treatment initiated. As a medical community, we are just beginning to understand the potentially devastating consequences of loss of knee ROM on long-term function.

Several studies have found a link between loss of normal knee motion and osteoarthritis after ACL reconstruction.[2,3,22,23] The development of osteoarthritis after ACL reconstruction is often attributed to meniscal damage or articular cartilage damage associated with the ACL injury, and evidence exists to support this association.[3,24–33] However, the results of recent studies indicate that the loss of normal knee ROM is associated with lower subjective scores and an increased incidence of radiographic arthritic changes. The impact is even greater when ROM loss is combined with meniscal or articular cartilage damage.[2,22,23] Shelbourne et al. reported results of 423 ACL reconstructions at a mean of 22 years after surgery. They found that the predictive factors related to the development of OA in the long term were older surgery age, medial meniscectomy, and any loss of normal knee extension, to include hyperextension.

One reason that loss of motion may have been overlooked in the past is that a long-term follow-up of at least 5 to 10 years is required for these trends to become evident in the data, and many studies in the orthopedic literature do not include follow-up times that are long enough to detect these long-term changes. Another potential reason that this factor may not be as well recognized in the literature is that precise measurements of knee ROM must be made and compared with the opposite, normal knee to detect smaller side-to-side differences that may still be significant enough to affect function but could easily be overlooked with a cursory evaluation of knee ROM.

Outside the context of ACL reconstruction, several other studies have found a relationship between ROM loss and abnormal findings of radiographs.[34–36] Although these studies were not designed to determine cause and effect, they interpreted loss of motion to be an indication of the extent of osteoarthritis. Current clinical reasoning seems to be that the presence of osteoarthritis leads to a loss of ROM, but is it possible that the loss of knee ROM could predispose the joint to arthritic changes? Another common thought seems to be that it is not possible to improve ROM in the arthritic knee. However, our experience and research have shown us that although the progress may occur more slowly, knee ROM can be improved in arthritic knees and is often accompanied by improvements in pain and function.[21] Further research is needed in this area, but careful assessment of every patient and early recognition and treatment of knee ROM loss can prevent long-term deficits that would be detrimental to the patient's functional outcome.

For a complete list of references, go to ExpertConsult.com.

SELECTED READINGS

Citation:

Biggs-Kinzer A, Murphy B, Shelbourne KD, et al. Perioperative rehabilitation using a knee extension device and arthroscopic debridement in the treatment of arthrofibrosis. *Sports Health*. 2010;2:417–423.

Level of Evidence:

IV

Summary:

This article provides a case series report of 33 patients who underwent arthroscopy and a perioperative rehabilitation program for the treatment of arthrofibrosis. Details of the pre- and postoperative rehabilitation are clearly described.

Citation:

Kim DH, Gill TJ, Millett PJ. Arthroscopic treatment of the arthrofibrotic knee. *Arthroscopy*. 2004;20(suppl 2):187–194.

Level of Evidence:

V

Summary:

This article provides a comprehensive description of the many potential causes of range of motion loss in the knee and a detailed, systematic approach to arthroscopic treatment based on the specific area(s) of pathology.

Citation:

Lintz F, Pujol N, Boisrenoult P, et al. Anterior cruciate ligament mucoid degeneration: a review of the literature and management guidelines. *Knee Surg Sports Traumatol Arthrosc*. 2011;19:1326–1333.

Level of Evidence:

IV

Summary:

This article provides a systematic review of the current literature on mucoid degeneration of the anterior cruciate ligament, describing the clinical features of this disease, epidemiology, appearance on imaging studies and arthroscopic examination, and treatment options.

Citation:

Shelbourne KD, Freeman H, Gray T. Osteoarthritis after ACL reconstruction: the importance of regaining and maintaining full range of motion. *Sports Health*. 2012;4(1):79–85.

Level of Evidence:

IV

Summary:

This article provides a review of the current literature with regard to the association between range of motion (ROM) loss and osteoarthritis after anterior cruciate ligament (ACL) reconstruction and discuss the potential long-term benefits of achieving and maintaining full symmetric ROM early after ACL surgery.

Citation:

Shelbourne KD, Wilkens JH, Mollabashy A, et al. Arthrofibrosis in acute anterior cruciate ligament reconstruction: the effect of timing of reconstruction and rehabilitation. *Am J Sports Med.* 1991;19:332–336.

Level of Evidence:

IV

Summary:

The effects of timing of surgery and rehabilitation programs (accelerated vs. nonaccelerated) used in conjunction with anterior cruciate ligament reconstruction were investigated in this retrospective review of 169 patients. A lower incidence of arthrofibrosis was found when surgery was delayed by at least 3 weeks from the time of injury.

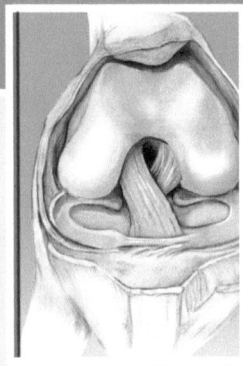

109

Vascular Problems of the Knee

Peter Lawrence, Kyle Rosen

The most common sources of pain and dysfunction in the lower limb of an athlete are musculoskeletal in origin; however, vascular pathology may also present with similar symptoms. Sports that involve frequent repetitive joint motion or high-impact collisions have the highest incidence of symptoms or injury due to vascular pathology.

Vascular issues in athletic patients may be difficult to diagnose for several reasons. First, most athletes are young and otherwise in good health, making vascular disease an unlikely concern in the differential diagnosis. Second, an injured athlete's signs and symptoms may have other plausible musculoskeletal etiologies, which could present in an identical fashion. Provocative testing and appropriate imaging are therefore often required for the diagnosis of underlying vascular pathology. Third, a clinician may not be entirely familiar with the typical presentation of vascular pathology in the lower limbs, details of the vascular physical examination, and diagnostic criteria for vascular disease in the differential diagnosis.

Underlying vascular issues should be suspected in any athlete who presents with limb pain, early-onset fatigue, limb swelling, limb discoloration, or skin color changes.[1] Familiarity with provocative physical examination maneuvers and imaging modalities is essential to confirm most vascular diagnoses. Moreover, simulation of an athlete's sport-specific positioning, motions, and level of exertion during vascular testing can uncover underlying pathology and can mean the difference between confirming or missing the diagnosis.

Vascular pathology that remains undetected for a prolonged period may have serious consequences for the athletic patient, including retirement, loss of limb function, or even limb amputation. Consequently it is important for the clinician to be familiar with the spectrum of traumatic and nontraumatic vascular knee injuries so as to facilitate early detection, diagnosis, and treatment and provide the athletic patient with a clear prognosis. The intent of this chapter is to review common vascular knee injuries in athletes and provide sports medicine practitioners with a reference for the presentation, evaluation, and clinical management of lower extremity sports-related vascular injuries, including a guide for return to sports when appropriate.

KNEE DISLOCATIONS

Tibiofemoral knee dislocation is a severe injury with the potential for limb-threatening vascular compromise. Although historically traumatic knee dislocations have been considered to be rare injuries, in recent years they have been reported more often.[2-4] The popliteal vessels—which cross the popliteal fossa and are anchored above and below the joint by the adductor hiatus and the soleus muscle, respectively—are particularly vulnerable to injury from knee dislocation (Fig. 109.1). Such dislocations are defined in terms of the tibial displacement with respect to the femur and can be characterized as anterior, posterior, lateral, and rotatory.

Anterior Knee Dislocations

Anterior dislocations are the most common, constituting 50% to 60% of all knee dislocations.[2,4,5] Forced hyperextension is the primary mechanism of injury causing anterior dislocation. In his 1963 landmark study, Kennedy[3] reproduced anterior knee dislocations using cadaver knee specimens subjected to various degrees of hyperextension and found that the vascular trauma occurred during forced hyperextension. Rupture of the popliteal artery occurs at an average of 50 degrees of hyperextension. However, at angles below the threshold of arterial rupture, stretching that results in injuries to the tunica intima, contusion, laceration, transection, or avulsion of the popliteal vessels may still occur. Intimal tearing increases the likelihood of arterial occlusion and thrombosis.[2] The poor collateral circulation surrounding the knee joint, as well as the soft tissue injury, further increases the risk for ischemia due to acute popliteal occlusion.[6,7] Damage to the popliteal artery occurs in 40% of anterior knee dislocations.[2,5,8] Moreover, stretching of the tibial nerve within the popliteal fossa may cause paresthesia in the lower leg, which is often a finding associated with knee dislocation and popliteal artery injury.

Posterior Dislocation of the Knee

Posterior dislocation of the tibia on the femur accounts for approximately 33% of knee dislocations and may also be a source of potential neurovascular injury.[8] Kennedy's hallmark study revealed that much greater forces are required to induce posterior knee dislocations compared with anterior knee dislocations,[3] such as those that occur in the classic "dashboard car injury."

Injury to collateral ligaments in association with damage to the posterior cruciate ligament (PCL) results in posterior dislocation and multidirectional instability that increases the likelihood of damage to the neurovascular structures within the popliteal fossa. Green and Allen[8] reported that 44% of posterior dislocations had

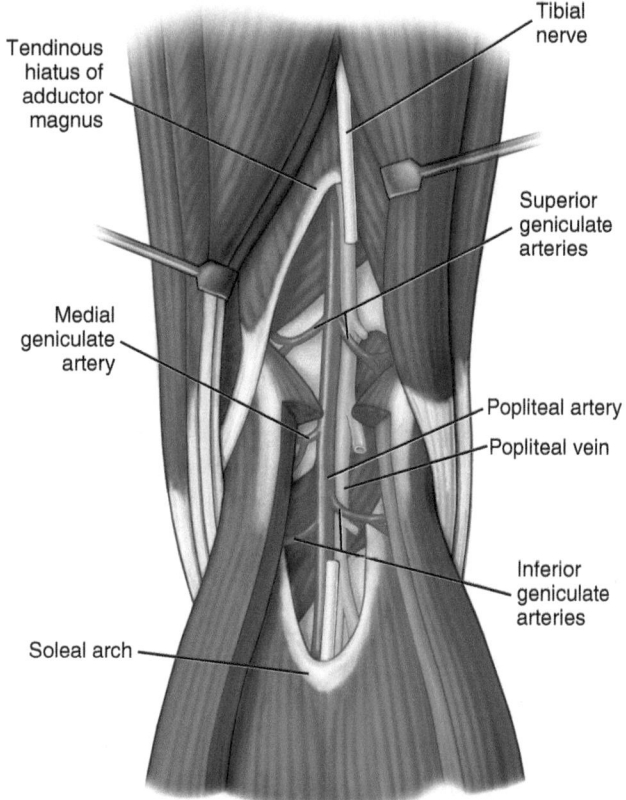

Fig. 109.1 Anatomy of the popliteal artery. The popliteal artery crosses the popliteal fossa and is anchored above by the adductor hiatus and below by the soleus muscle.

TABLE 109.1 Indicators of Popliteal Vessel Compromise During the Vascular Physical Examination

Type of Sign	Indicator
Hard	Pulse deficits in pedal pulses with an ankle brachial index <0.5
	Distal ischemia (pain, paresthesia, pallor, and other symptoms of acute ischemia)
	Active hemorrhage and pulsatile bleeding
	Expanding hematoma
	Evidence of compartment syndrome
Soft	Small hematoma that does not change in size
	Hemorrhage that has ceased
	Reduced ankle pressure <0.9 but >0.5
	Neural deficits from injury to the tibial nerve

associated injury to the popliteal vessels. Posterior displacement of the tibia directly translates force onto the popliteal artery and vein, with a high likelihood of vessel transection.

Vascular Injury From Knee Dislocation

When knee dislocation is diagnosed or suspected, one of the primary jobs of the clinician is to determine if concomitant injury to the popliteal artery and/or vein has occurred. Failure to recognize popliteal artery injury and restore vessel continuity after knee trauma is a potential cause of lower extremity amputation. Consequently early recognition of vascular injury remains paramount for limb salvage. During a knee dislocation, the popliteal vessels are at risk for injury because of their anatomic location (see Fig. 109.1). The superficial femoral artery traverses the tendinous hiatus of the adductor magnus muscle and continues as the popliteal artery. Small collateral vessels branch off of the popliteal artery as it crosses the knee joint within the popliteal fossa; these are the medial and lateral superior geniculate, middle geniculate, and medial and lateral inferior geniculate arteries. The popliteal artery exits the popliteal fossa anchored below the knee joint by the soleal arch before dividing into the anterior and posterior tibial arteries. The genicular arteries form an intricate network of collateral vessels surrounding the contiguous ends of the femur and tibia. This circumpatellar network is divided into superficial and deep plexuses. The superficial plexus is located between the fascia and skin and forms three

well-defined arches, one above the upper border of the patella and two below the patella. The deep plexus forms a close network of vessels that surround the articular surfaces of the femur and tibia. The network of genicular anastomoses provides the leg with collateral circulation, which is abundant in number but small in vessel caliber; frequently the collateral vessels are injured or disrupted in conjunction with the popliteal artery during knee dislocation as a result of soft tissue injury.

The anterior and posterior tibial veins converge to form the popliteal vein at the lower border of the popliteus muscle. Occasionally the popliteal vein is duplicated and present on both the medial and lateral aspects of the popliteal artery. Proximal to the popliteal fossa, the popliteal vein traverses the adductor hiatus and continues as the femoral vein.

Clinical Presentation

Injury to the popliteal artery has been reported to occur in approximately 30% of all complete knee dislocations.[8-11] Types of arterial damage sustained during dislocations of the knee may include injury to the tunica intima, avulsion injury, occlusions, aneurysm generation with secondary thrombosis, embolization, rupture, and transection. Although trauma to the popliteal vessels is easily detected in cases of open knee injuries, identification of neurovascular injury as a result of blunt knee dislocation or instability may be delayed or missed entirely. Clinical indicators of vascular trauma after knee dislocation are classified as hard or soft signs (Table 109.1). Hard signs demand immediate vascular repair and include pulse deficits, acute limb ischemia, active hemorrhage, and pulsatile hematoma.[12] Hallmark signs of acute limb ischemia include pain, paresthesia, loss of sensation or motor function, pallor, and pulselessness in the distal extremity of the affected limb. In the presence of these hard signs, a diagnosis of vascular injury is strongly suggested, and treatment should involve immediate vascular repair. Alternatively, soft signs of injury to the popliteal artery after knee dislocation warrant further diagnostic evaluation and monitoring. These signs include small hematomas, reduced pedal pulses and ankle pressures, neural deficits from injury to the tibial nerve or its branches, and early hemorrhaging that has ceased. When soft signs are present, imaging of the popliteal vessels is required to assess the extent of vascular trauma.

Vascular injuries associated with knee dislocations result from excessive stretching or transection of the popliteal vessels (Fig. 109.2). Common vascular injuries following anterior knee dislocations include intimal tears and the formation of intimal flaps. In such patients, blood flow through the artery may not be appreciably altered; consequently patients may present without any hard signs of vascular trauma. Nevertheless, the presence of intimal tears and flaps increases the risk of thrombosis and embolization. Moreover, extensive intimal injuries accelerate vessel wall damage over time, and patients who initially lack symptoms of vascular compromise may begin to exhibit diminished popliteal flow. Some authors suggest that posterior knee dislocations more commonly result in transection of the popliteal artery, with resultant acute limb ischemia.[13] Blood flow through the popliteal artery becomes significantly diminished (Fig. 109.3),

and patients present with immediate hard signs of vascular injury such as active hemorrhage, expanding hematoma, bruits in the distal arterial circuitry, and signs of acute ischemia such as pain, paresthesia, poikilothermia, pallor, and pulselessness. These signs indicate significant vascular compromise that demands immediate operative intervention and vascular repair.

Physical Examination and Testing

The high rate of popliteal artery injury associated with knee dislocations, combined with the possibility of delayed presentation of symptoms of vascular trauma as a result of knee dislocation, demands that diagnostic evaluation for vascular integrity be performed for all patients suspected of having a knee dislocation. The diagnosis of knee dislocation itself is based on the mechanism of injury obtained from the history, physical examination, and radiographic findings. Frequently patients may present with the knee already reduced.[5] Because the risk for arterial injury is the same in both the reduced and dislocated knee,[10] clinical suspicion of popliteal artery damage should remain high in such patients. Absence of hemarthrosis in patients suspected of having had a knee dislocation does not decrease the risk for vascular injury.

Diagnostic evaluation of vascular integrity in the lower limb is critical to determining a method of treatment (Fig. 109.4). Serial measurements of pulse quality in both the posterior tibial and dorsalis pedis arteries should be performed because the pulse may be diminished or absent after an upstream arterial injury. Studies reveal that clinical evaluation of peripheral pulses accurately identifies the existence of vascular lesions after knee dislocation with a specificity of 91%.[14,15] Although the presence of pulse abnormalities is sufficient to rule in the existence of vascular lesions, a low sensitivity of 79% means that vascular injury may exist in the absence of peripheral pulse deficits.[15,16] In addition to digital pulse evaluation, serial measurements of the ankle-brachial index (ABI) enable the clinician to qualitatively

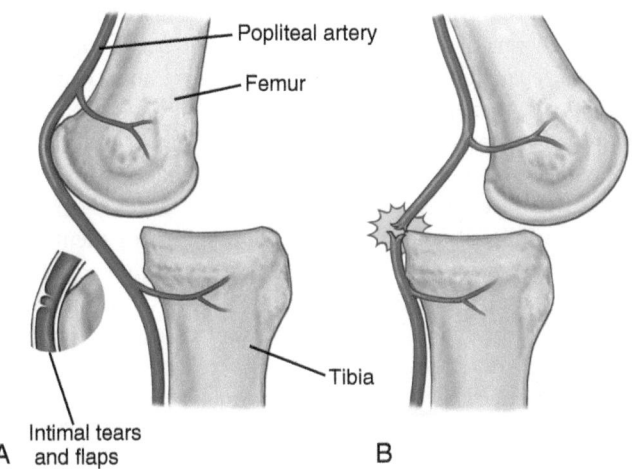

Fig. 109.2 Mechanisms of popliteal artery injury after knee dislocation. Posterior knee dislocations (A) and anterior knee dislocations (B) stretch the popliteal artery.

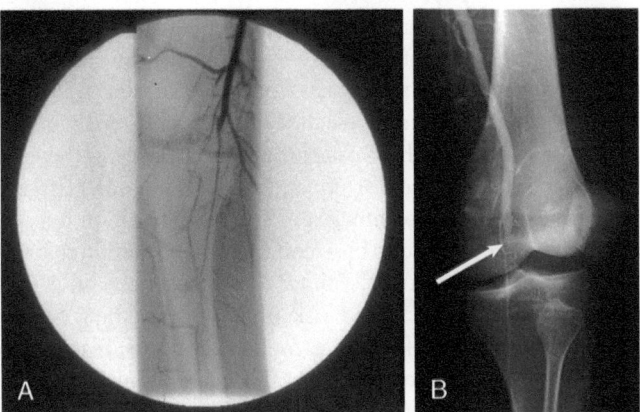

Fig. 109.3 Arterial injury after a knee dislocation. (A) Anterior dislocation of the knee causes occlusion at the popliteal-tibial artery junction. (B) A coronal view of the lower extremity angiogram after posterior knee dislocation reveals an occluded popliteal artery *(arrow)*. ([A] From Seroyer ST, Musahl V, Harner CD. Management of the acute knee dislocation: the Pittsburgh experience. *Int J Care Injured*. 2008;39:710–718. [B] From Kapur S, Wissman RD, Robertson M, et al. Acute knee dislocation: review of an elusive entity. *Curr Probl Diagn Radiol*. 2009;38:237–250.)

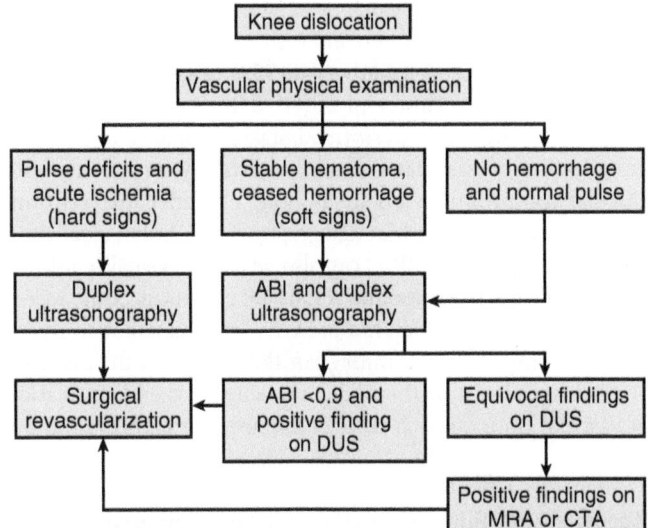

Fig. 109.4 Algorithm to determine the extent of vascular pathology associated with knee dislocations. *ABI,* Ankle brachial index; *CTA,* computed tomographic angiography; *DUS,* duplex ultrasonography; *MRA,* magnetic resonance angiography.

assess deficits in distal perfusion induced by vascular trauma. ABI values less than 0.9 indicate the presence of vascular injury requiring surgical intervention with 95% to 100% sensitivity and 80% to 100% specificity.[17]

Imaging

In patients presenting with pulse abnormalities and associated ischemia, surgical intervention and revascularization is the primary priority, and imaging may be performed to determine the location and severity of vascular compromise. In this context, imaging aids in determining the surgical approach and should be performed in the operating room to minimize warm ischemia time. Previous studies have found that approximately 3 hours are saved when arteriographic imaging is performed in the operating arena.[18] In patients with pulse abnormalities in the absence of ischemia, imaging is mandatory to determine if intervention and vascular repair are required.

Historically arteriography has served as the gold standard for symptomatic vascular lesions after knee dislocation. This form of imaging allows the examiner to identify the location and extent of injury and the presence of intimal flap tears within both the popliteal artery and its distal branches. However, the invasive nature of angiography has led to a trend in recent years toward less invasive and safer imaging modalities. Moreover, arteriography is not fully reliable as an imaging tool. Studies have reported 1% to 6% false-negative rates, which can delay patient treatment, and 2.4% to 7% false-positive rates, which can result in unnecessary surgical intervention.[14,19,20] In the Lower Extremity Assessment Project study, it was reported that patients with hard signs of vascular injury can be treated effectively without arteriographic imaging before surgery.[21]

In recent years, duplex ultrasonography has become a mainstay of the rapid evaluation of vascular pathology resulting from suspected popliteal artery injury; duplex ultrasound can be used to analyze flow through the popliteal vessels in real time in the emergency department or operating room (see Fig. 109.4). Studies assessing the diagnostic value of duplex scanning as a means of noninvasive imaging in persons with lower limb trauma have reported a diagnostic sensitivity of 95%, a specificity of 99%, and a diagnostic accuracy of 98%.[22] The rapidity with which duplex scanning can be performed makes it an ideal tool for the visualization of vascular trauma, particularly in patients with vascular compromise who are awaiting operative intervention.

Computed tomographic angiography (CTA) and magnetic resonance angiography (MRA) can also be used to visualize intimal tears when duplex ultrasound results are equivocal. Some recent studies challenge the usefulness of CTA imaging in patients with lower extremity vascular injury. For these patients, the presence of hard signs has a 100% predictive value for the identification of vascular injury, which reduces the need for CTA evaluation.

Treatment Options

Warm ischemia time remains the single most important variable determining functional outcome in patients with a popliteal artery injury resulting from knee dislocation.[21] Prompt diagnostic evaluation, including imaging to determine the extent of vascular injury, and operative intervention to restore adequate distal perfusion in the hypoperfused patient are essential for successful treatment and limb salvage. Warm ischemia times greater than 6 hours can cause irreversible neurologic injury and muscle necrosis distal to the site of blood flow obstruction, and the rate of amputation in patients who experience a delay in arterial reconstruction exceeding 8 hours has been reported to be 85%.[5,11] Consequently any delay of imaging and immediate intervention in cases of limb ischemia increases morbidity and worsens patient prognosis.

Immediate surgical repair is obligatory as soon as vascular trauma is confirmed. The principles of surgical intervention in patients with popliteal artery injuries include (1) rapid restoration of arterial blood flow to the distal extremity, (2) removal of thrombus in the distal artery, and (3) alleviation of acute compartment syndrome, which may exacerbate distal ischemia. Whether vascular or orthopaedic reconstruction should be performed first remains an area of debate, with the appropriate sequence of repair depending on the time course of injury and the severity of the ischemia. If the patient presents with prolonged warm ischemia time or severe deficits in distal perfusion, prompt vascular repair and restoration of arterial flow is indicated before orthopedic management. In such cases, however, secondary orthopedic procedures may damage newly repaired vascular structures. Consequently the order of repair should be determined on a case-by-case basis, with special consideration given to the extent and severity of ischemia in the presenting patient.

Reconstruction of the popliteal artery can be achieved through either posterior or medial approaches. The posterior approach allows for greater visualization of structures within the popliteal fossa and is more ideally suited for the treatment of lesions of the midpopliteal artery, whereas the medial approach allows easier access to distal structures of the popliteal fossa. The type of surgical repair performed depends on the extent of vascular injury and may include lateral repair of the artery, end-to-end arterial repair with interposition vein graft, repair of intimal injury by vein patch, or bypass by saphenous vein grafting.[13] The majority of popliteal artery repairs that result from knee dislocations require venous grafting. Venous patches are used to provide structural integrity in cases of intimal tears and flaps, and greater saphenous vein grafts from the contralateral leg are used for extensive arterial resection. End-to-end repair of the popliteal artery through a posterior approach requires the least dissection of the popliteal artery and surrounding soft tissue. If the popliteal vein is also damaged after knee dislocation, venous repair is required; this can be accomplished by lateral repair or interposition vein grafts.[13,23] Failure to repair venous injuries is associated with an increased risk of lower extremity edema, thrombosis, and embolization as well as limb loss. If ischemia has been present for more than 2 hours, a fasciotomy is mandatory to prevent compartment syndrome. Fasciotomy is required in the treatment of 50% to 80% of patients with injury to the popliteal artery and is associated with a significant improvement in the rate of limb salvage.[18,24] Primary amputation is rarely indicated and is used only when extensive muscle necrosis is present in the distal extremity. Typically warm ischemia times exceeding 6 hours are associated with a dramatic increase in the rate of eventual limb amputation.[21]

Although historically all popliteal artery injuries resulting from knee dislocations have been repaired through open surgical methods, endovascular techniques have become an increasingly popular form of treatment for blunt popliteal artery injuries and acutely ischemic distal lower extremities. Endovascular repair is a minimally invasive alternative to open surgery and is associated with a more rapid recovery time and decreased pain.[61] Proponents of endovascular repair in cases of blunt popliteal artery injury cite the usefulness of a percutaneous approach in cases where extensive soft tissue damage to the surrounding structures of the popliteal fossa may complicate open repair. In addition, through endovascular repair, hemostasis can be achieved in locations where distal and proximal control is difficult to obtain.[62] Furthermore, endovascular techniques allow for the visualization of the injury site, removal of any associated thrombus, protection against distal embolization, and repair of an intimal lesion. Authors have reported that there are no significant differences regarding early patient outcomes between endovascular and open repair in the management of traumatic lower extremity arterial injuries.[63] However, the primary criticism of endovascular repair in patients sustaining traumatic injuries originates from concerns regarding technical success. Rates of complication after embolization of injured peripheral vessels, stent grafting, or both range from 0% to 25%; the authors presume that this large range is indicative of the discrepancies in endovascular procedures performed in different institutions.[61]

More recently, the use of hybrid approaches, which combines the benefits of open vascular surgery and endovascular interventions, has become increasingly prevalent. Recent estimates suggest that 19% to 22% of revascularization procedures are done as hybrid procedures.[64] Hybrid procedures are associated with improved limb salvage and decreased length of hospitalization; their primary and secondary patency rates are comparable to those of the open procedures.[64]

Postoperative Management

Postoperative follow-up should include focused physical examinations with special attention to distal perfusion. Ankle pressures, ABI measurements, and duplex scanning should be performed to assess blood flow through the reconstructed artery within the popliteal fossa. Use of other imaging modalities such as CT/CTA and MRA are generally not recommended unless symptoms of graft occlusion or diminished blood flow reappear. Follow-up should be scheduled within 4 to 6 weeks after surgery and twice annually within the first year. In subsequent years, annual follow-up is recommended to ensure graft patency.

Complications

Postoperative complications after popliteal artery repair are centered on evaluation for delayed compartment syndrome, graft patency, maintenance of tension-free healing, and prevention of postsurgical deep venous thrombosis (DVT). Antiplatelet medications are typically prescribed for patients to prevent postsurgical graft thrombosis. Patency of the vein graft may be compromised by stenosis at the sites of venous graft-artery interface.

⚑ Authors' Preferred Technique
Popliteal Artery Repair in Knee Dislocation

I. Initial examination.
   A. Patient history and physical examination are completed.
   B. Pedal pulses on both the affected and contralateral limb are examined.
   C. Bilateral ankle brachial indexes are measured.
   D. The popliteal space is imaged using duplex ultrasonography.
II. In patients presenting with hard signs of vascular injury, no further imaging is required and immediate surgical intervention is warranted.
III. In patients presenting with soft signs of vascular injury or if the duplex scanning yields equivocal results, further imaging via magnetic resonance angiography and computed tomographic angiography is necessary to establish treatment protocol.
IV. Open surgical intervention.
   A. With the patient lying prone, an S-shaped incision is made in the popliteal region.
      • The posterior approach is preferred over the medial approach because it facilitates greater access to the neurovascular structures of the popliteal fossa with the least amount of soft tissue dissection and sparing of the saphenous vein.
   B. Skin flaps are raised to expose underlying deep fascia, which is then transected longitudinally.
      • Care should be taken to avoid transection of the median cutaneous sural nerve.
   C. The tibial nerve is encountered first and mobilized.
   D. The popliteal vein passes through the medial and lateral heads of the gastrocnemius muscle deep in the popliteal fossa.
   E. The popliteal artery lies deeper in the popliteal space and can be followed distally.
V. Arterial reconstruction is required if evidence of significant intimal injury, stenosis, occlusion, thrombosis, or laceration is observed.
   A. A short interposition vein graft is placed; it is usually harvested from the ipsilateral lesser saphenous vein or contralateral saphenous vein.
   B. An alternative is a short venous bypass graft with exclusion of the occluded artery to avoid thromboembolism.

Postsurgical follow-up should include physical examination and imaging via duplex ultrasonography to ensure graft patency and appropriate healing.

POPLITEAL ARTERY ENTRAPMENT SYNDROME

Popliteal artery entrapment syndrome (PAES) is characterized by the extrinsic compression of the popliteal vessels by the musculotendinous structures of the popliteal fossa. Anomalies in the embryologic development and migration of the medial head of the gastrocnemius muscle generate anatomic variants that entrap the popliteal vessels and tibial nerve.[27] PAES is usually a congenital abnormality, with estimates of its frequency reported between 0.62% and 3.5% of the population,[28,29] but functional PAES may occur in the absence of any embryologic or anatomic abnormality. In persons with functional PAES, the popliteal vessels become impinged from physiologic hypertrophy of the gastrocnemius, soleus, plantaris, or semimembranosus muscles.[30,31] Functional PAES is particularly prevalent in well-conditioned athletes.

History

Entrapment of the popliteal artery was first documented by 1879 by Anderson Stuart, an Edinburgh medical student, who described an abnormality in the course of the popliteal artery in the amputated limb of a patient with gangrene.[32] Nearly 50 years later, Louis Dubreuil-Chambardel described separation of the popliteal vessels by an accessory gastrocnemius muscle in a patient.[33] Although entrapment of the popliteal artery has been documented for more than a century, it was not until the mid-1960s that the term *popliteal artery entrapment syndrome* was first used by Love and Whelan[27] to define a clinical presentation. In 1985, Rignault et al.[30] presented the first case report of functional entrapment syndrome caused by hypertrophy of the gastrocnemius in an "intensively trained athlete."

After these initial reports, numerous publications documented the clinical progression of PAES in further detail. Studies have estimated that approximately 60% of young patients who present with intermittent claudication have PAES.[34]

Classification

Originally Insua et al.[35] presented the first classification system for PAES based on variations of the course of the popliteal artery in relation to the medial head of the gastrocnemius muscle. A simplified classification scheme for PAES, provided by Delaney and Gonzalez,[36] was proposed and consisted of four subtypes. Modifications to the Delaney scheme by Rich et al.[37] in 1979 yielded a five-subtype system that included impingement of both the popliteal artery and vein (Fig. 109.5). Last, with the documentation of functional PAES by Rignault and colleagues[30] in 1985, a sixth subtype was added to facilitate the classification of patients presenting with symptoms of PAES in the absence of any overt anatomic variation or developmental abnormality. The current six-subtype classification system is the most widely accepted system among clinicians.

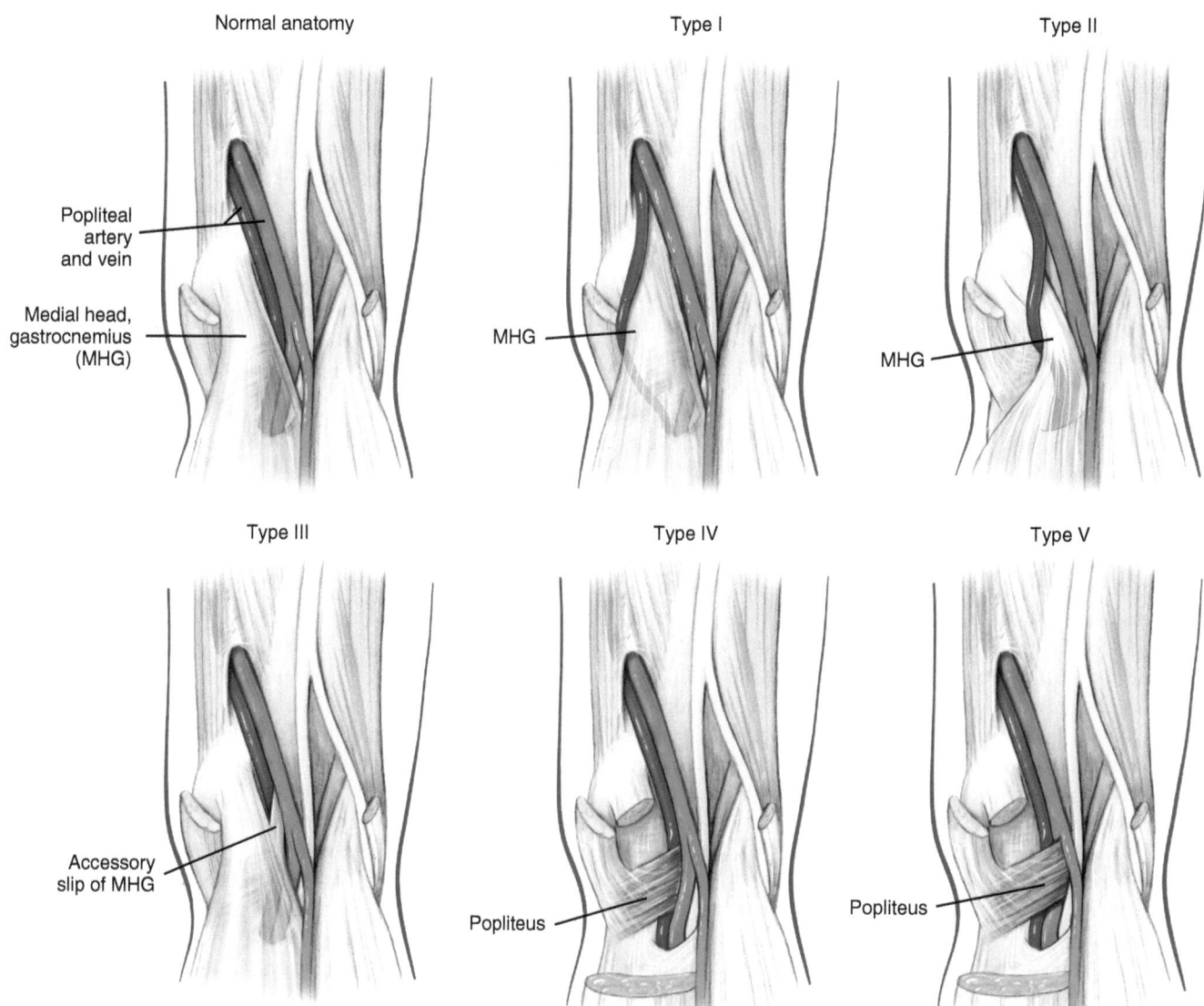

Fig. 109.5 Popliteal artery entrapment syndrome (PAES) classification scheme. Normal anatomy of the popliteal fossa and the classification types of PAES are shown.

Type I: Type I is the most common variant of PAES and is characterized by a significant medial shift of the popliteal artery with normal positioning of the medial head of the gastrocnemius muscle.[38] This type of arterial entrapment occurs when the popliteal artery completes its development before the embryologic migration of the medial head of the gastrocnemius muscle. Consequently, as the medial muscle head completes its migration, it sweeps the popliteal artery medially.[39]

Type II: In type II popliteal artery entrapment, the popliteal artery is shifted medially to a lesser degree than its type I counterpart, and the medial head of the gastrocnemius expresses variable attachment to either the lateral aspect of the medial femoral condyle, the intercondylar area, or the lower femur superior to the condyle.[38] Type II entrapment occurs when the distal popliteal artery forms prematurely and temporarily arrests the migration of the medial head of the gastrocnemius. Consequently the popliteal artery is medially displaced relative to an abnormally positioned medial head of the gastrocnemius.

Type III: Type III popliteal entrapment results from abnormal mature muscle slips or fibrotendinous bands that branch off the medial head of the gastrocnemius muscle, slip between the popliteal artery and vein, and attach to either the medial or lateral femoral condyle. These accessory tissues are derived from the embryologic remnants of the migrating medial head; in the adult, they persist posterior to the popliteal artery. As a result, the popliteal artery becomes separated from the popliteal vein and entrapped between the two layers of musculotendinous tissue.

Type IV: Type IV popliteal entrapment occurs when the axial artery, the embryologic precursor of the tibial arteries, persists as the mature distal popliteal artery. Consequently the artery remains in its embryologic position and is compressed as it passes deep to the popliteus muscle or associated fibrous bands.

Type V: Type V popliteal entrapment can occur via any of the aforementioned mechanisms but is unique in that both the popliteal artery and vein are entrapped and compressed. Impingement of both popliteal vessels is estimated to occur in 10% to 15% of all cases of popliteal entrapment.[39-41]

Type VI: Functional popliteal entrapment occurs in patients in the absence of any anatomic or developmental abnormality. Although the exact mechanism of popliteal entrapment in this subtype remains to be elucidated, it is believed that hypertrophy of the medial head of the gastrocnemius compresses the posteromedial aspect of the popliteal artery, resulting in physiologic occlusion of the artery during plantarflexion or extension.[30,31,38] Some investigators have proposed that a more lateral attachment of the medial head of the gastrocnemius within physiologic normal limits may predispose a person to functional popliteal entrapment upon hypertrophy of the gastrocnemius as a result of lower limb exercise.[38,42]

Clinical Presentation

The hallmark of PAES is a young, active, and otherwise healthy person with intermittent claudication of the calf and foot.

Approximately 60% of patients with symptoms of PAES are younger than 30 years, and the syndrome has a significant predilection for the male sex, with approximately 80% of all reported cases occurring in men.[1,41] In more than a fourth of all cases, PAES is simultaneously present in both lower extremities.[38] Participation in sports such as basketball, football, rugby, and martial arts is most commonly associated with popliteal entrapment.

Intermittent claudication of the calf or foot is the most common symptom and is reported to occur in 69% to 90% of patients with PAES.[34,43,44] In rare cases, symptoms may present in an atypical fashion, such as the onset of claudication after standing or walking, which improves with running.[45,46]

In addition to claudication, patients may present with symptoms such as coldness, pallor, or loss of sensation in the lower extremities. Because the tibial nerve travels adjacent to the popliteal artery through the popliteal fossa, all cases of PAES may potentially impinge the nerve and result in paresthesia in the distal extremity. In fewer than 10% of patients with PAES, concomitant symptoms of critical limb ischemia (CLI) may exist.[39,47] Signs and symptoms of CLI include paresthesia, pallor of the foot and toes, ischemia, pain upon resting, and tissue necrosis. Importantly, PAES results from the extrinsic compression of the popliteal artery rather than intrinsic occlusion from atherosclerosis, as observed in patients with peripheral arterial disease. Consequently the patient with PAES who has signs and symptoms of CLI will lack the diffuse atherosclerosis observed in patients with end-stage peripheral arterial disease. Acute limb ischemia is rare in patients with PAES.[39] A patient with PAES who has venous involvement may also report calf and ankle swelling.

In most cases, pedal pulses are palpable and normal at rest in a patient with PAES provided that compression of the popliteal artery has not progressed to a state of chronic occlusion. Blood flow through the lumen of the popliteal artery is significantly attenuated upon compression. Stress maneuvers such as active plantarflexion or dorsiflexion of the foot against resistance temporarily stenoses the otherwise patent lumen of the popliteal artery in the patient with PAES and results in diminished pedal pulses.[38] Left untreated, the constant compressive stimuli may compromise the structural integrity of the popliteal artery and cause chronic occlusion.

In approximately 12% of cases, poststenotic dilatation of the popliteal artery may occur after compression.[39] In such patients, degeneration of the popliteal artery increases the likelihood of aneurysm formation; popliteal aneurysms in these otherwise young and healthy persons can be a source of distal embolization. Studies report that between 20% and 30% of patients with popliteal artery aneurysm in conjunction with PAES experience an embolic event in the absence of intervention.[40,48] Alternatively, distal emboli may also result from focal thrombus formation secondary to arterial degeneration in a normal-caliber entrapped artery.[42]

Physical Examination and Testing

In most diagnostic cases, a detailed patient history and thorough physical examination are sufficient to include or exclude PAES as a differential diagnosis. If popliteal entrapment is suspected,

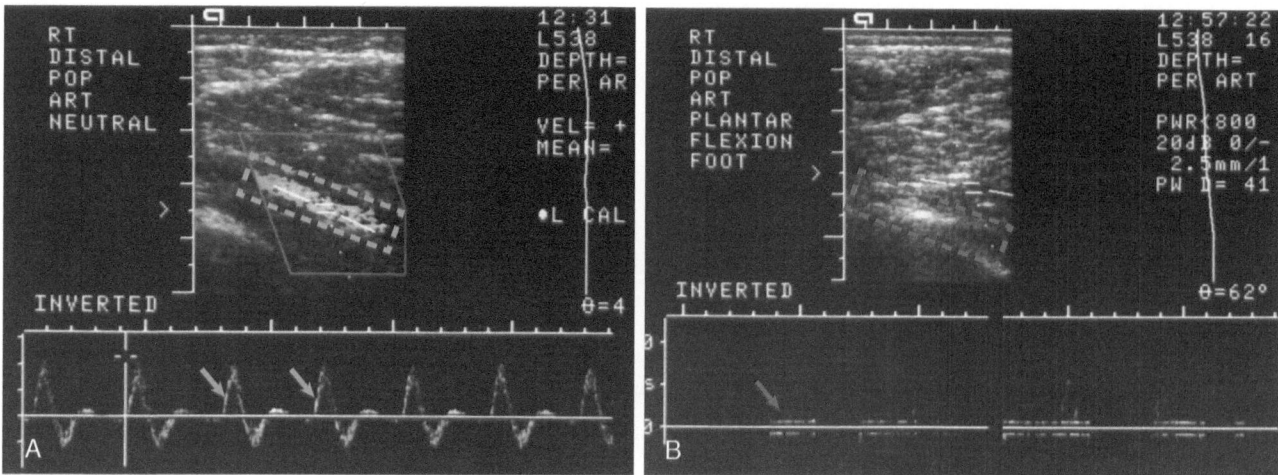

Fig. 109.6 Duplex ultrasonography (DUS) in a 49-year-old man with right popliteal artery entrapment syndrome. (A) DUS of the right popliteal fossa with the leg in neutral position shows a normal triphasic waveform *(arrows)*. (B) DUS obtained with plantarflexion of the right foot shows compression of the popliteal artery and diminished flow *(arrow)*. (From Macedo TA, Johnson CM, Hallett JW Jr, et al. Popliteal artery entrapment syndrome: role of imaging in the diagnosis. *AJR Am J Roentgenol.* 2003;181[5]:1259–1265.)

provocative testing and noninvasive diagnostic evaluations should be performed to both confirm the diagnosis and determine the severity of the entrapment. Initial testing includes a thorough assessment of the pulses in the femoral, popliteal, posterior tibial, and dorsalis pedis arteries in both the affected and contralateral limbs. Because PAES is characterized by intermittent claudication, pulses should also be qualitatively evaluated as the patient performs dynamic provocative maneuvers. Traditionally these maneuvers include active plantarflexion and dorsiflexion of the ankle against resistance with the knee in full extension.[47] In the late stages of PAES, a collateral network gradually develops as a result of extrinsic popliteal artery occlusion; thus the foot appears normal even when pulses are absent.

Resting and postexertional ABIs help confirm the diagnosis of PAES. An ABI value greater than 1 is considered normal; thus an ABI value less than 0.9 suggests arterial stenosis/occlusion. In persons with PAES, claudication typically develops in the lower limbs after exercise or exertion. ABI values should reflect this phenomenon and may be normal at rest but less than 0.9, with a reduction of greater than 0.15 upon stress testing.

In conjunction with examining the arterial circulation, a thorough venous evaluation should also be performed in the patient suspected of having PAES. Signs of venous obstruction in the popliteal fossa include swelling, cyanosis, and distention of the superficial veins of the distal extremities of the lower limbs. The presence of these signs supports the diagnosis of PAES, specifically type V.

Imaging

In addition to physical examination and provocative testing, imaging is an important diagnostic tool used to confirm a definitive diagnosis of PAES. Both noninvasive and invasive imaging protocols may be used in the evaluation of a patient with PAES. Noninvasive imaging modalities include duplex ultrasonography, CTA, and MRA.

Duplex Ultrasonography

Duplex scanning allows real-time visualization of the popliteal artery (Fig. 109.6). It is obtained as the patient performs dynamic provocative maneuvers and provides a qualitative measure of the degree of stenosis. A 50% decrease in the peak systolic velocity through the popliteal artery during active plantarflexion is considered diagnostic of PAES.[47] Although a positive duplex test upon provocative maneuvers supports the diagnosis of PAES, further imaging studies should be performed before undertaking surgical intervention. Studies measuring peak systolic velocities through the popliteal artery have reported high rates of compression (53% to 72%) in healthy patients without PAES.[41,49,50] Such high rates of false-positive results suggest that duplex testing overestimates the actual rate of popliteal artery compression. Consequently positive findings on duplex scanning should raise clinical suspicion of PAES but warrant the use of other imaging modalities.

Magnetic Resonance Imaging and Magnetic Resonance Angiography

In recent years the MRI/MRA modalities have emerged as highly accurate and minimally invasive tools for the diagnosis and evaluation of PAES. Similar to CT/CTA, MRI/MRA imaging allows for the visualization of anatomic and functional relationships between structures within the popliteal fossa. Also analogous to CT, MRI is noninvasive and able to differentiate between anatomic abnormalities with similarly presenting pathologies. Studies have demonstrated the superiority of MRI over ultrasound and CT-based imaging modalities in the diagnosis of PAES because it better facilitates visualization of the muscular anatomy (Fig. 109.7). Most studies suggest that MRI/MRA should be used as the principal diagnostic tool for the evaluation of young patients who present with symptoms of PAES.[51] As with all of the other imaging modalities, MRI/MRA for PAES should

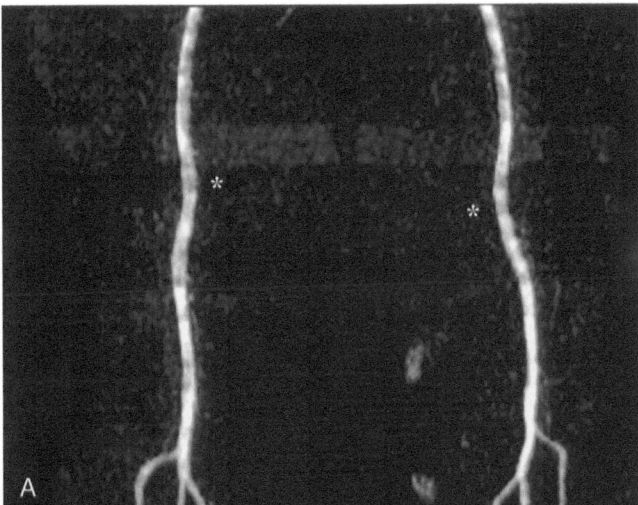
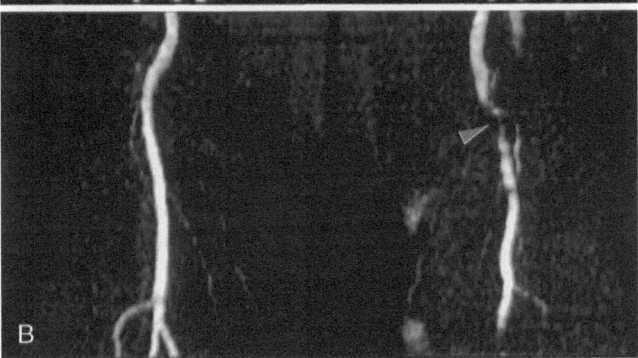

Fig. 109.7 Imaging in a patient with popliteal artery entrapment syndrome. (A) Time-of-flight magnetic resonance angiography (MRA) of the popliteal arteries in the neutral position shows normal arterial flow. Medial deviation along the path of both popliteal arteries is observed *(asterisks)*. (B) Time-of-flight MRA of the popliteal arteries with active plantarflexion of the feet shows near occlusion *(arrowhead)* of the left popliteal artery and no change in the right leg.

be performed in both resting conditions and under active plantarflexion against resistance (see Fig. 109.7). In this way, subtle popliteal entrapment that would otherwise be overlooked on neutral imaging may be identified.

Computed Tomography and Computed Tomographic Angiography

CT/CTA currently plays an alternative role as a diagnostic tool in the evaluation of patients suspected of having PAES. CT also allows for the visualization of the many structures within the popliteal fossa, specifically revealing the anatomic relationships between the popliteal artery and surrounding bony, tendinous, and muscular structures. In addition to elucidating relationships between structures in the popliteal fossa, CT/CTA can be used to reveal focal sites of arterial stenosis, occlusion, thrombosis, or degeneration (Fig. 109.8). As with the other imaging modalities, CT/CTA studies should be obtained while the patient is in both a neutral state and during active plantarflexion against resistance. In contrast to duplex ultrasonography and angiography, both limbs can be evaluated simultaneously with CT/CTA, thereby eliminating concern about the possibility of bilateral entrapment.[52-55] Lastly, CTA can be used to differentiate chronic vascular pathologies with otherwise similar clinical presentations, such as adventitial cystic disease and a popliteal artery aneurysm.

Angiography

Historically, contrast angiography has served as the gold standard in diagnosing PAES. As with noninvasive imaging modalities, provocative maneuvers are required in performing angiography to reveal the popliteal entrapment. In the absence of provocative testing, angiography has a low sensitivity for PAES and may indicate that a popliteal artery is healthy despite underlying pathology. Diagnosis of PAES on the basis of angiography is

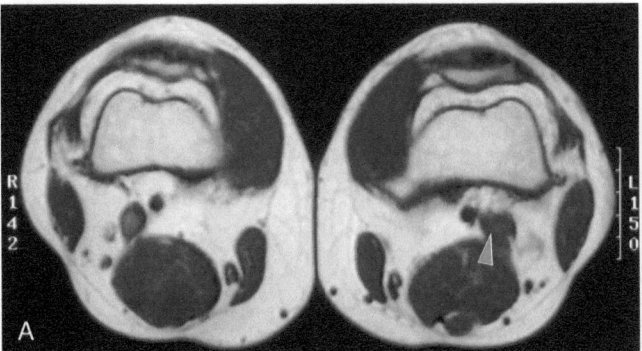
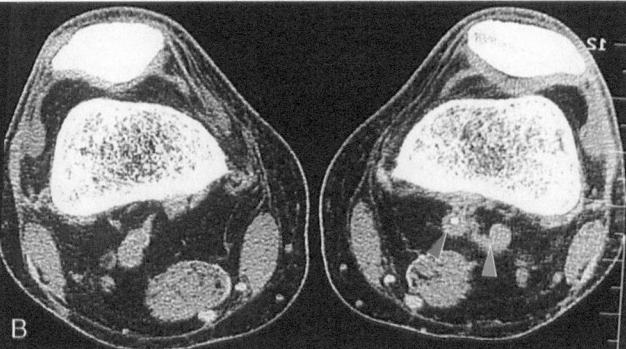

Fig. 109.8 Axial magnetic resonance imaging (MRI) and computed tomography (CT) in patients with popliteal artery entrapment syndrome. (A) T1-weighted MRI reveals abnormal muscle slip *(orange arrowhead)* between popliteal vessels. The contralateral image shows normal anatomy. (B) Bilateral CT angiography of the lower extremities shows an abnormal muscle band *(orange arrowhead)* from the medial head of the gastrocnemius muscle with significant occlusion of the right popliteal artery *(blue arrowhead)*. The contralateral extremity shows normal anatomy.

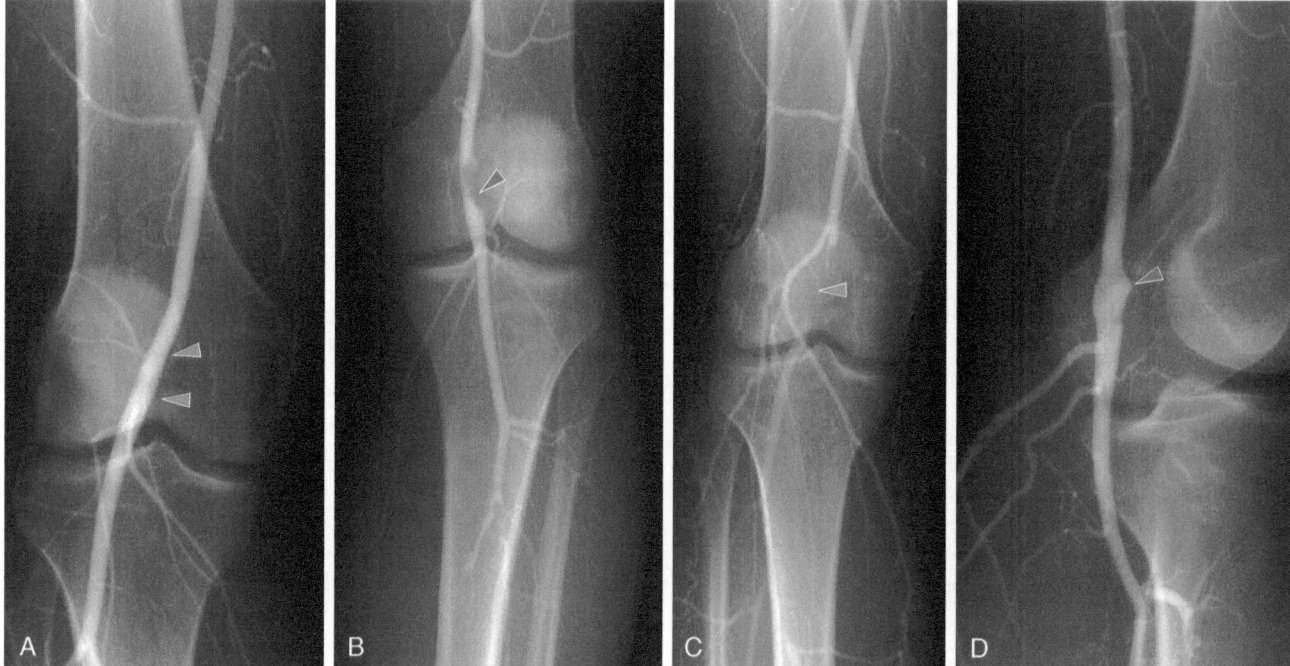

Fig. 109.9 Angiographic findings encountered with popliteal artery entrapment syndrome (PAES). (A) The angiogram of a 34-year-old woman with PAES shows medial deviation of the popliteal artery *(orange arrowheads)*. (B) The angiogram of a 21-year-old man with PAES shows nonocclusive acute thrombus of the popliteal artery *(blue arrowhead)* with embolization to the distal tibial artery. (C) The angiogram of a 34-year-old woman with PAES shows occlusion of the popliteal artery *(orange arrowhead)*. (D) The angiogram of a 37-year-old man with PAES shows a popliteal artery aneurysm *(blue arrowhead)*.

indicated when at least two of the following imaging features are present (Fig. 109.9)[39]:

1. Medial displacement of the proximal popliteal artery
2. Segmental stenosis of the midpopliteal artery
3. Poststenotic dilatation of the popliteal artery

Contrast angiography also allows for visualization of the tibial artery and is useful in cases of embolization resulting from popliteal aneurysm or a thrombogenic popliteal artery caused by entrapment.

Although angiography is an effective diagnostic tool for the evaluation of patients suspected of having PAES,[38,56] many concerns have been raised with regard to this imaging modality. Angiography is a fundamentally invasive procedure; as such it carries an increased risk of complications from arterial catheterization. Although in healthy persons the dye is cleared with relative ease, it may be a source of significant morbidity in patients with renal insufficiency. Angiography also does not evaluate muscular abnormalities. With the advent of CTA and MRA imaging methods, angiography is no longer used as a staple for the diagnosis of PAES; rather, these higher-specificity and less invasive imaging modalities are now favored.[51] Angiography is used in conjunction with treatment, however, as when thrombolysis of distal emboli is performed.

Treatment Options

Surgical intervention is the primary treatment option for symptomatic PAES and is warranted in almost all cases. The basic goals of surgical intervention in the treatment of PAES are threefold: (1) to relieve the neurovascular structures from entrapment,

(2) to restore normal blood flow and distal perfusion, and (3) to restore normal anatomy.[41]

The degree of surgical complexity in an individual patient depends on the anatomy within the popliteal fossa and the integrity of the popliteal vessels. At an early clinical stage, the popliteal artery, although entrapped, remains physiologically normal. In the absence of arterial disease, surgical therapy limited to musculotendinous release is sufficient to restore normal anatomy and blood flow through the popliteal vessels. Musculotendinous release is achieved by myotomy of the medial head of the gastrocnemius muscle as well as by excision of any abnormal muscle slips and tendinous bands that contribute to the entrapment (Fig. 109.10). Symptomatic patients with PAES who have normal popliteal vessels and are treated with surgical myotomy have been shown to return to prior levels of athletic activity, to not require additional intervention, and to maintain popliteal artery patency throughout a 10-year follow-up.[38]

A posterior or medial surgical approach may be used to perform musculotendinous release and decompression of the popliteal artery, although the posterior approach is more widely used and provides the surgeon with greater operative flexibility and a wider window for identification of anatomic abnormalities.[57] The approach is performed by making an S- or Z-shaped incision over the popliteal fossa in the prone patient. Once the neurovascular structures of the popliteal fossa and the anomalous anatomy are identified, the medial head of the gastrocnemius and any contributing muscle flaps and tendinous bands are released from their attachments. Reattachment of the medial muscle head after myotomy is usually not necessary because

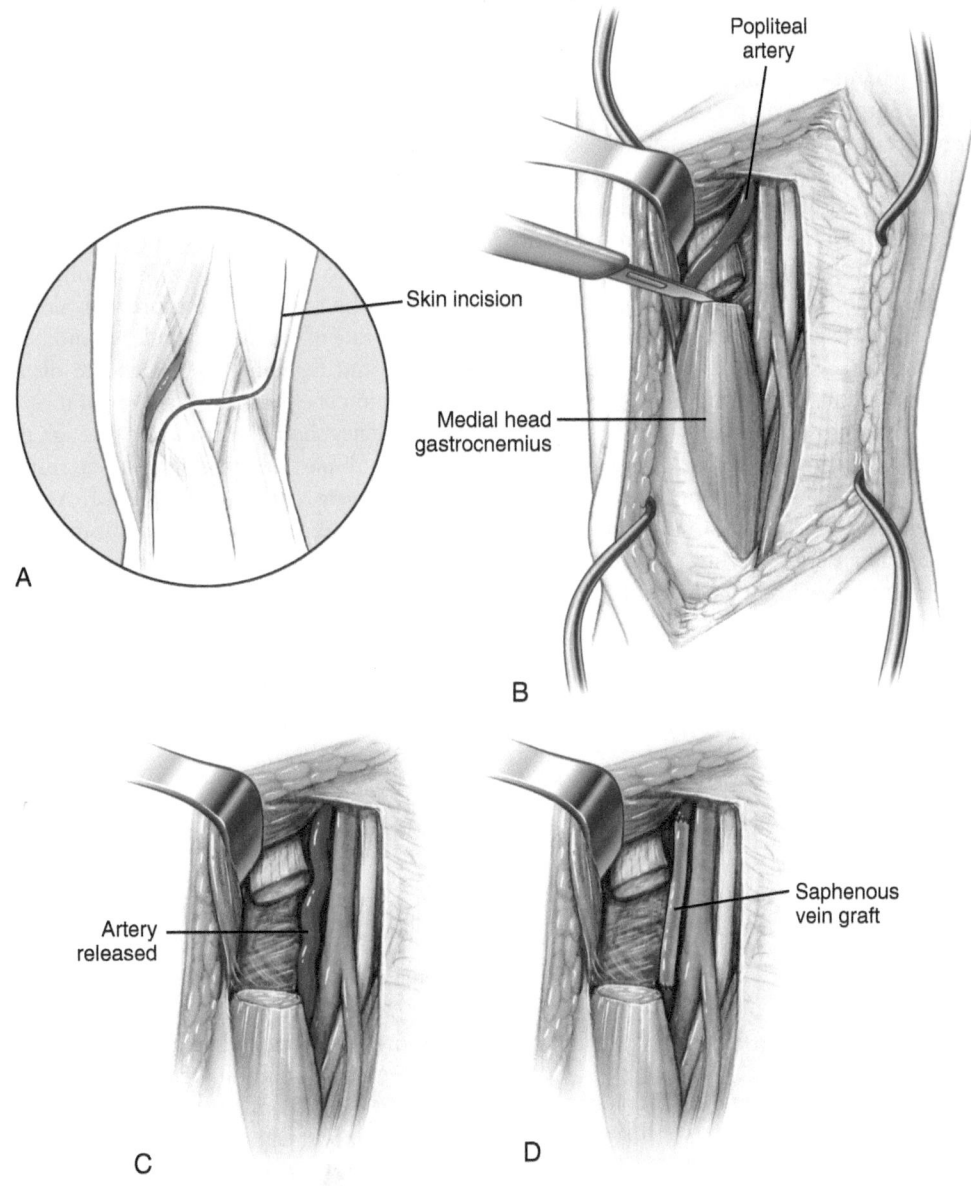

Popliteal artery

Skin incision

Medial head gastrocnemius

A

B

Artery released

Saphenous vein graft

C

D

Fig. 109.10 The operative approach for treating popliteal artery entrapment syndrome. (A) An S-shaped incision for the posterior surgical approach to the popliteal fossa. (B) Operative exposure showing type I popliteal artery entrapment and subsequent sharp division of the medial head of the gastrocnemius. (C) Successful release of the undamaged popliteal artery (the muscle will not have to be reattached). (D) Successful saphenous vein bypass of the injured popliteal artery after myotomy (if indicated by imaging and operative investigation).

no measurable postsurgical loss of strength is observed after its release.[58]

The major advantage of the medial calf approach is a more rapid postsurgical recovery compared with the posterior approach. Proponents of the medial approach highlight its utility in long-segment occlusions of the popliteal artery.[58] However, the medial approach has significant disadvantages that limit its applicability. Specifically, identification and adequate exposure of the various anatomic structures of the popliteal fossa are more difficult to accomplish through the medial approach. Accordingly the medial approach is associated with a higher rate of missed entrapment and recurrent entrapment.[39]

The natural history of PAES involves progressive popliteal arterial degeneration and fibrosis with eventual thrombosis and occlusion. Marked thickening of the arterial wall at the site of entrapment or poststenotic dilatation and aneurysm formation are additional signs of chronic arterial compression. In the presence of such findings, operative intervention must include, in addition to entrapment release, arterial resection and bypass using a saphenous vein graft. Once a popliteal artery has become occluded, dilated, or thrombosed, it should be resected and replaced with an autogenous conduit.[39,41] The posterior approach is useful in cases requiring popliteal artery reconstruction.

Type VI functional popliteal entrapment results from hypertrophy of the medial head of the gastrocnemius muscle and can, in time, cause arterial degeneration as a result of chronic entrapment. In a symptomatic patient with functional PAES, surgical intervention is indicated. Surgical decompression involves transection of the compressive portion of the medial head of the gastrocnemius muscle and should be performed through a posterior approach. Release of the entire tendon from its attachment is usually not necessary because these patients lack an anatomic abnormality.

Endovascular therapies for the treatment of PAES have limited value because of their inability to alter the extrinsic muscle compression in the popliteal fossa. Some studies report the use of initial endovascular intervention via balloon angioplasty and thrombolysis followed by myotomy several weeks later.[59] However, benefits of this approach are largely speculative. An inability to relieve the underlying source of popliteal compression raises the risk of reocclusion after endoluminal therapy. Consequently open surgery remains the gold standard for correcting anatomic abnormalities and restoring arterial flow in the patient with PAES.

⚡ Authors' Preferred Technique
Popliteal Artery Entrapment Syndrome

I. Patient evaluation and exposure of soft tissue structures of the popliteal fossa are achieved as described earlier, in the Authors' Preferred Technique box in the Knee Dislocation section.
II. Decompression of the popliteal entrapment via myotomy.
    A. Types I to V:
       • Divide the medial head of the gastrocnemius from its posterior attachment to the femoral condyles.
       • Resect any accessory muscle or tendinous tissue contributing to popliteal artery entrapment.
       • It is not necessary to reattach the muscle.
    B. Type VI:
       • Excision of the segments of the medial head of the gastrocnemius muscle that are compressing the popliteal artery, with preservation of the tendinous attachment to the posterior femoral condyle.
III. Popliteal artery reconstruction is required if evidence of chronic high-grade stenosis, occlusion, or thrombosis is found. The options include the following:
    A. Resection of degenerated and thrombosed artery.
    B. Placement of a short interposition vein graft, usually harvested from the ipsilateral lesser saphenous vein.
    C. A short venous bypass graft can be performed as an alternative with exclusion of the occluded artery to avoid thromboembolism.
    D. If poststenotic dilatation/aneurysm is present, arterial resection must be followed by a vein graft, since replacement is mandatory to avoid the later development of an aneurysm.

Postoperative Management

In the absence of arterial occlusion or signs of vessel degeneration, musculotendinous release and decompression are sufficient to alleviate claudication and restore adequate blood flow.[38] Postoperative recovery is based primarily on wound healing, and as mentioned earlier, it is more rapidly achieved with the medial surgical approach. Reports suggest that patients who begin postoperative physical therapy early and within an appropriate time frame experience better outcomes compared with patients who do not participate in physical therapy.[60] Patients can be discharged from the hospital once they are ambulatory with crutches, usually 1 to 2 days after surgery.

Criteria for Return to Play

A return to a full level of athletic activity can be achieved after treatment of PAES. Patients who require arterial reconstruction in addition to decompression have longer recovery times than do those who undergo decompression alone. Factors that determine the rate of recovery include wound healing, return of limb strength and flexibility, and adequate distal perfusion. Before the athlete can return to play, restoration of blood flow and vessel patency should be evaluated through physical examination, ABI, and duplex ultrasonography at rest and as provocative maneuvers are performed. CTA, MRA, and angiography are usually not necessary unless symptoms of claudication persist or recur. Recovery commonly takes 6 to 8 weeks, after which moderate strengthening exercises may be initiated. Once an initial strengthening regimen has been completed, preoperative levels of activity and strength training may be resumed. Once full return to physical activity is achieved, follow-up should be performed every 4 to 6 months for the first year and annually thereafter.

Complications

Postoperative complications are usually minimal after myotomy alone with decompression of the entrapped artery, and patients typically return to prior levels of athletic activity without requiring additional interventions. Patients with popliteal occlusion, degeneration, or aneurysm as a result of chronic compression require arterial resection and replacement in addition to a myotomy. Such patients have a higher risk of potential complications. Patients for whom arterial reconstruction is performed should be treated with antiplatelet drugs, such as aspirin. The potential for postsurgical graft failure and acute graft thrombosis also exists and is a potential source of postoperative morbidity. Because stenosis of the vein graft at the proximal and distal anastomoses also may occur, patients should be followed up closely with physical examination, ABI testing, and duplex ultrasonography to monitor the integrity of the graft. When vein graft stenosis is symptomatic or greater than 60%, balloon angioplasty is indicated.

For a complete list of references, go to ExpertConsult.com.

SELECTED READINGS

Citation:
Perlowski AA, Jaff MR. Vascular disorders in athletes. *Vasc Med.* 2010;15(6):469–479.

Level of Evidence:
II, prognostic studies

Summary:
Physical examination and imaging of an athlete suspected of sustaining a vascular injury should be performed with the patient

in both neutral and provocative positions specific to the suspected vascular injury to fully expose underlying pathology. Proper use of noninvasive diagnostic studies such as duplex ultrasonography, computed tomography, and magnetic resonance imaging can ensure prompt and accurate diagnosis. A multifaceted approach to the diagnosis and treatment of an athlete affected by vascular disease allows for faster recovery and a return to previous levels of activity.

Citation:

Green NE, Allen BL. Vascular injuries associated with dislocation of the knee. *J Bone Joint Surg Am.* 1977;59A(2):236–239.

Level of Evidence:

I, prognostic/therapeutic study

Summary:

A combined retrospective and prospective study of 245 cases reveals a high incidence of injury to the popliteal artery as a result of knee dislocation. Vascular intervention and repair must be performed within 6 hours from the time of injury to prevent ischemic injury and avoid amputation. In 95% of cases in which patients did not receive prompt treatment, either amputation was necessary or ischemic changes occurred.

Citation:

Varnell RM, et al. Arterial injury complicating knee disruption. Third place winner: Conrad Jobst award. *Am Surg.* 1989;55(12):699–704.

Level of Evidence:

I, diagnostic study

Summary:

A retrospective study of 30 patients with either knee dislocation or severe knee ligamentous disruption revealed no significant difference in the frequency of major or minor vascular abnormalities between the two groups. Doppler pressure measurements were highly predictive of major arterial trauma in both groups. Arterial injury can occur with both dislocation and ligament injury of the knee, and Doppler flow measurements should be assessed in all cases of suspected vascular injury.

Citation:

Bynoe RP, et al. Noninvasive diagnosis of vascular trauma by duplex ultrasonography. *J Vasc Surg.* 1991;14(3):346–352.

Level of Evidence:

I, prognostic/diagnostic study

Summary:

In a prospective evaluation of a large number of patients with potential vascular injury in the neck and extremities, duplex ultrasonography had more than 90% sensitivity, specificity, and overall accuracy in detecting vascular pathology. Duplex ultrasonography has no interventional risks and is a rapid and cost-effective method of screening patients with suspected vascular trauma in the neck and extremities.

Citation:

Levien LJ, Veller MG. Popliteal artery entrapment syndrome: more common than previously recognized. *J Vasc Surg.* 1999;30(4):587–598.

Level of Evidence:

I, therapeutic study

Summary:

A retrospective analysis of patients with unequivocal evidence of popliteal artery entrapment syndrome suggests that surgical intervention is required in all confirmed cases of popliteal entrapment (types I, II, III, and IV). Approximately 50% of the normal population may display transient popliteal compression in the extremes of limb movement. Consequently surgical decompression in patients with functional popliteal entrapment is indicated only if discrete and typical symptoms are present. If the patient has significant degeneration or occlusion of the popliteal artery, complete replacement with a vein graft is indicated.

Citation:

di Marzo L, Cavallaro A. Popliteal vascular entrapment. *World J Surg.* 2005;29(suppl 1):S43–S45.

Level of Evidence:

II, prognostic/therapeutic studies

Summary:

Signs and symptoms of claudication in a young patient should always raise suspicion of popliteal artery entrapment. The higher specificity and sensitivity of computed tomography and magnetic resonance imaging in evaluating the popliteal vessels represents a valid alternative to the more invasive digital angiography. Current studies encourage the identification of patients with popliteal artery entrapment syndrome at an early stage. The only parameter influencing the long-term outcome of patients with popliteal artery entrapment is age at presentation.

Leg, Ankle, and Foot

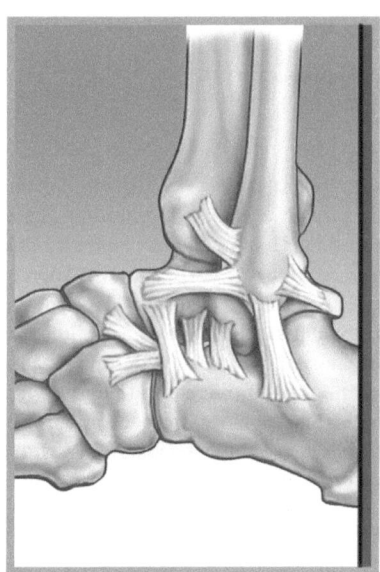

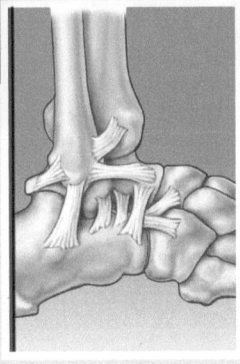

110

Foot and Ankle Biomechanics

Andrew Haskell

The relationship between the joints, ligaments, tendons, and fascia of the foot, ankle, and lower extremity allows weight-bearing athletes to perform extraordinary feats of power, speed, and endurance. In this chapter, motion of various foot and ankle segments (kinematics) and the forces experienced by the lower extremity (kinetics) are explored over the gait cycle. Special attention is given to the biomechanical mechanisms by which the components of the foot and ankle interact. The biomechanics of walking are compared with running, and clinical correlations are made throughout the chapter.

GAIT CYCLE

Gait consists of a cyclical series of whole body motions incorporating pelvic sway and rotation, hip and knee swing, tibia rotation, and ankle flexion and extension. A single iteration of the gait cycle is often described as occurring between initial ground contact of one step and the initial ground contact of the same foot on the subsequent step. A single cycle can be divided into a stance phase and a swing phase (Fig. 110.1). The stance phase of walking can also be divided into three intervals: the first interval extends from initial ground contact (typically heel strike) to the foot lying flat on the floor; the second interval occurs as the body passes over the flat foot; and the third interval extends from the moment the heel rises from the floor to when the toes lift from the floor. These intervals may also be referred to as rockers.

Changes in the gait cycle during running are illustrated in Fig. 110.2. During walking, the stance phase contains periods of double- and single-limb support, with one foot always in contact with the ground. As the speed of gait increases, a transition occurs with incorporation of a float phase, during which both feet leave the ground. As the speed of running increases, the duration of the stance phase, both in real time and in percentage of the gait cycle, decreases and the duration of the float phase as a percentage of the gait cycle increases.

WHOLE BODY KINEMATICS

Kinematics describes the motion of body segments. The coordinated motion of the pelvis, hip, knee, ankle, and hindfoot is well preserved between individuals, although factors such as age, gender, body mass index, leg length, speed, training, and fatigue may alter its characteristics.[1-3]

The rhythmic vertical displacement of the body is a necessary component of bipedal locomotion. The center of gravity of the body moves in a smooth sinusoidal path with amplitude of approximately 4 to 5 cm and reaching its peak immediately after passage over the weight-bearing leg.[4,5] Minimizing vertical displacement of the body's center of gravity during gait minimizes energy expenditure and is an important aspect of whole body biomechanics. As the foot strikes the floor, the knee flexes against an eccentric contraction of the quadriceps muscle, the ankle plantar flexes against an eccentric contraction of the anterior tibial muscle, and the hindfoot pronates. Next the center of gravity moves upward as the body moves over the stance leg. The stance leg functionally elongates through knee extension and plantar flexion of the ankle as the heel rises from the floor and the foot supinates.

Lateral and axial translation and rotation are also components of whole body motion during gait. The body shifts laterally over the weight-bearing leg, with each step creating a sinusoidal displacement of approximately 4 to 5 cm. The degree of lateral translation of the body's center of gravity is related to the degree of lateral deviation of foot placement from the central line. A series of axial rotations begin in the pelvis and traverse the femur and tibia. The tibia rotates internally during swing phase and into the beginning of stance phase and externally during the later period of stance. The degree of these rotations is subject to marked individual variations, with an average of 19 degrees and ranging between 13 and 25 degrees during a gait cycle.[6]

KINETICS OF GAIT

The functions of the ankle, subtalar, transverse tarsal, and metatarsophalangeal joints interrelate closely to fulfill the varying requirements of the foot during walking and running. At initial ground contact, a complex set of energy absorption mechanisms helps to lessen the shock wave that propagates up the axial skeleton. Later in stance, passive and active mechanisms alter the structure of the foot to provide the body with a stable platform and to functionally elongate the stance limb, allowing for a greater stride length. During walking, the toes are lifted from the floor, whereas in athletics, forceful push-off facilitates rapid acceleration and deceleration, directional change, and jumping.

The stresses applied to the joints of the foot and ankle vary greatly from normal walking to athletics. The stresses can be repetitive, as in a long-distance runner, or impulsive, as occurs

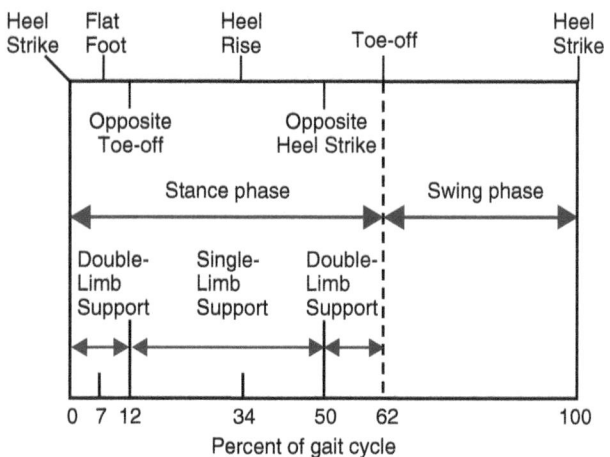

Fig. 110.1 The walking cycle. The gait cycle during walking is divided into stance and swing phases. The stance phase constitutes periods of double-limb support and single-limb support. (From Haskell A, Mann RA. Biomechanics of the foot and ankle. In: Coughlin MJ, Saltzman CL, Anderson RB, eds. *Mann's Surgery of the Foot and Ankle*. 9th ed. Philadelphia: Elsevier; 2014.)

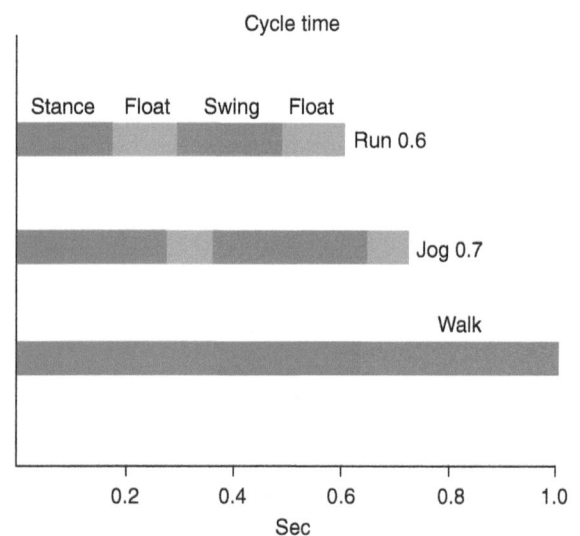

Fig. 110.2 Variations in the gait cycle. The stance phase of walking is greater than 50% of the total gait cycle. As the transition to jogging is made, a float period is incorporated during which neither foot is in contact with the ground. As running speed increases, stance phase decreases and the float phase increases. In the illustration, the walking pace is 16 minutes per mile, jogging is 9 minutes per mile, and running is 5 minutes per mile. (From Haskell A, Mann RA. Biomechanics of the foot and ankle. In: Coughlin MJ, Saltzman CL, Anderson RB, eds. *Mann's Surgery of the Foot and Ankle*. 9th ed. Philadelphia: Elsevier; 2014.)

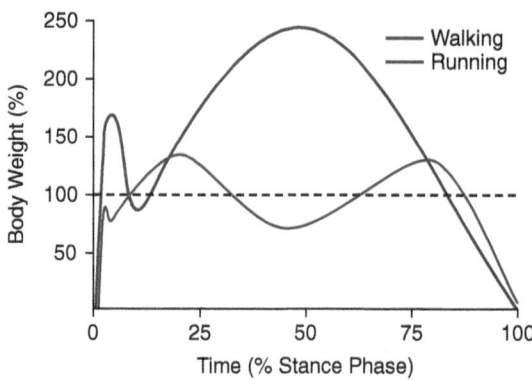

Fig. 110.3 Comparison of vertical ground reaction force for walking (*blue line*) versus jogging (*red line*). The horizontal axis is scaled as a percentage of the total time in the stance phase for walking (0.6 seconds) and running (0.24 seconds). The vertical axis is shown as a percentage of body weight.

in the push-off foot of a shot-putter. The whole-body vertical force involved in running is 2 to 2.5 times body weight compared with 1.2 times body weight in walking[7] and can be higher for many sports with extreme push-off, such as a football lineman engaged in blocking or a basketball player engaged in rapid accelerating and jumping activities (Fig. 110.3). The force applied across the ankle joint during walking is approximately 4.5 times body weight.[8] This maximum stress occurs during the flat foot portion of the stance phase as the body moves over the stance limb. If this force were extrapolated to running, in which the ground reaction force is more than double that of walking, we would see stress across the ankle joint that approaches 10 times body weight. Training and modification of running technique can affect these parameters.[9]

The foot and ankle complex must be supple enough to absorb impact and rigid enough to transmit muscle forces, or injuries such as sprains, strains, stress fractures, and fascial tears may result. Dysfunction of the foot and ankle complex may result in an altered gait pattern, declining athletic performance, and compensatory changes in the knee and hip joints. Athletic training can help to attenuate these forces and minimize the risk of injury.[10] The ankle and hindfoot joint complex function as a universal joint, linking pelvic, thigh, and leg rotation to hindfoot motion and longitudinal arch stability, which allows the ankle joints to compensate for some degree of dysfunction in the hindfoot and vice versa. However, athletics require maximum performance from these systems, and dysfunction of ankle and foot mechanics often leads to pain, injury, and loss of performance.

Stresses about the foot and ankle are measured in a variety of ways, including static modalities such as the Harris-Beath mat or a standing pressure sensitive grid, and dynamic modalities such as force plate analysis or a thin film pressure transducer placed in a shoe.[11,12] The nature of these stresses depends on the activity and includes vertical force, fore and aft shear, side-to-side shear, and torque. A measurement method should be chosen based on the type of data required, such as static versus dynamic, whole body versus discrete point, and barefoot versus in shoe.

KINEMATICS AND BIOMECHANICS OF THE ANKLE JOINT

During the gait cycle, the ankle joint's sagittal plane motion spans 20 degrees of dorsiflexion to 50 degrees of plantar flexion, with marked variability between individuals, along an axis running between the tips of the malleoli. The trochlear surface of the talus rotates around this axis, as would a section from a cone whose apex is most frequently described as based medially (Fig. 110.4),[13] although data from CT scans suggest may be based laterally.[14] Two series of dorsiflexion and plantar flexion occur

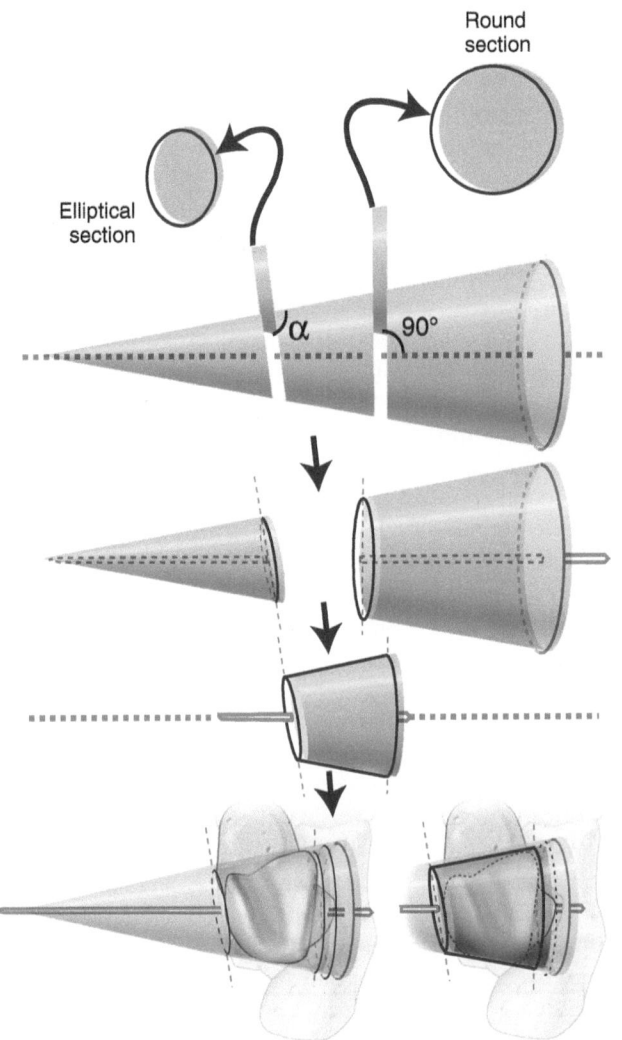

Fig. 110.4 The trochlear surface of the talus is a section from a cone. The apex of the cone is directed medially, and the open end is directed laterally. (From Stiehl JB, ed. *Inman's Joints of the Ankle*. 2nd ed. Baltimore: Williams & Wilkins; 1991.)

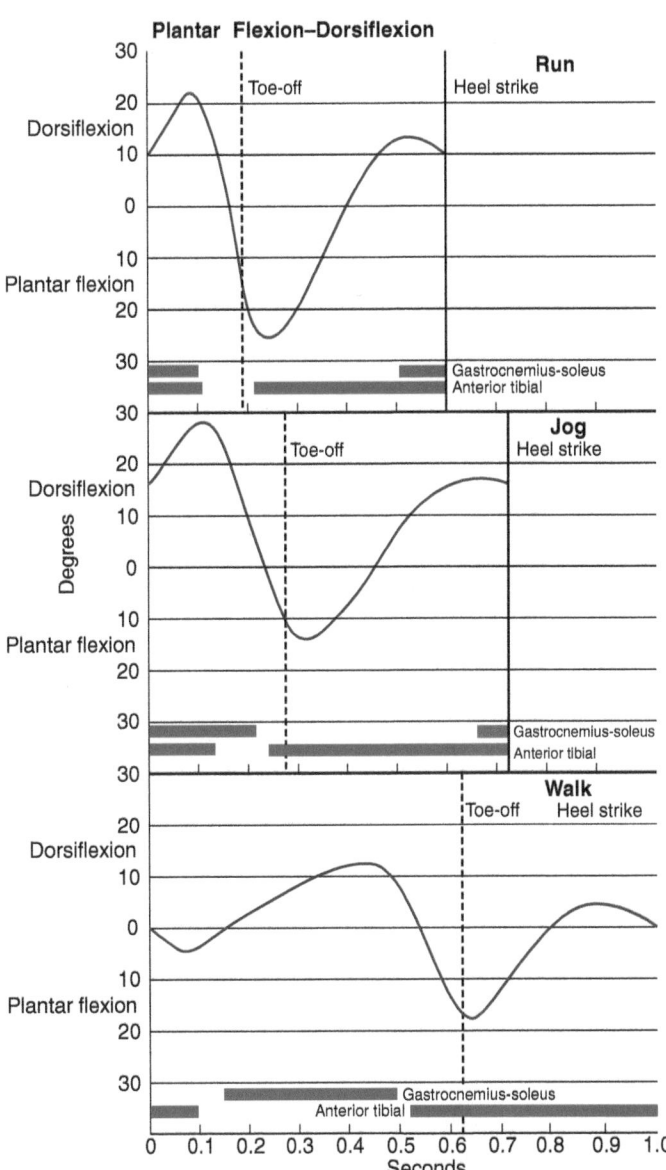

Fig. 110.5 Ankle joint range of motion for walking, jogging, and running. The muscle function of the anterior and posterior compartment is noted on the bottom of the graph. (From Mann RA. Biomechanics of running. In: American Academy of Orthopaedic Surgeons. *Symposium on the Foot and Leg in Running Sports*. St. Louis: CV Mosby; 1982.)

during the gait cycle when walking. At heel strike, the dorsiflexed ankle rapidly plantarflexes. This motion ends with the foot flat on the floor, after which progressive ankle dorsiflexion occurs as the body moves over the fixed foot. Dorsiflexion reaches a maximum at 40% of the walking cycle, when ankle plantar flexion begins as the heel rises, and continues until toe-off, when dorsiflexion occurs again during the swing phase (Fig. 110.5).

The talus is stabilized within the ankle mortise by bony and soft tissue restraints. The congruity of the ankle mortise leads to considerable inherent bony stability.[15,16] Ligament support includes the deltoid ligament medially and three separate ligamentous bands laterally: the anterior and posterior talofibular ligaments and the calcaneofibular ligament.[17–19] The anterior talofibular ligament is taut with the ankle joint in plantar flexion, and the calcaneofibular ligament is taut with the ankle joint in dorsiflexion (Fig. 110.6).[13,20] The anterior talofibular ligament is injured most frequently during ankle sprains, in part because the ankle has less intrinsic bony stability in plantar flexion when

this ligament is under tension.[21] Injuries to the calcaneofibular ligament are frequently seen in conjunction with anterior talofibular ligament sprains.

Muscle control of the ankle joint can be divided based on the anterior and posterior leg muscle compartments and the phases of the gait cycle. The lateral compartment muscles function with the posterior compartment. During normal walking, the anterior compartment muscles become active late in the stance phase and in the swing phase to bring about dorsiflexion of the ankle joint by a concentric (shortening) contraction (see Fig. 110.5).[22] This muscle group remains active after heel strike to control the rapid plantar flexion of the ankle joint that occurs by an eccentric (lengthening) contraction. This eccentric contraction during plantar flexion helps to dissipate the forces on

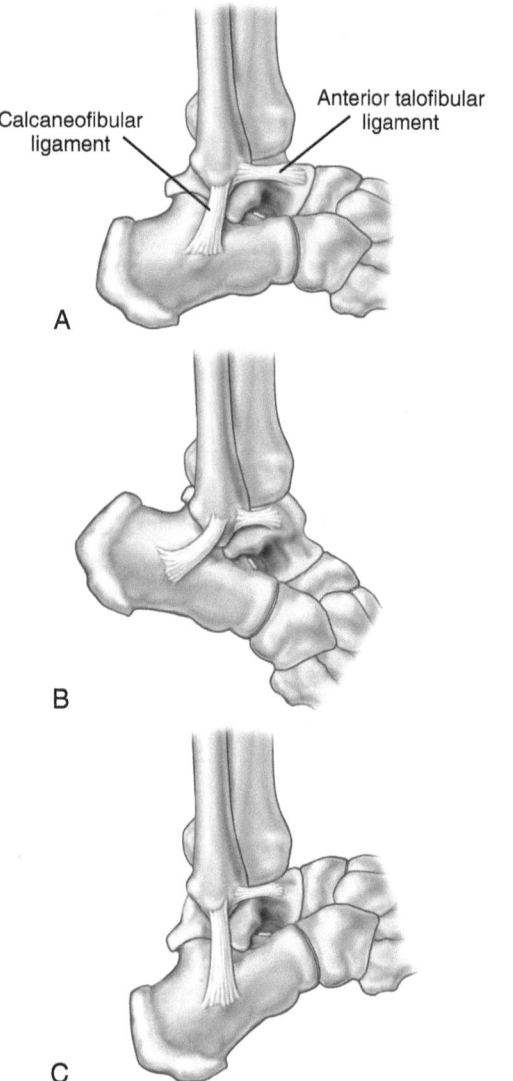

Fig. 110.6 Calcaneofibular (A) and anterior talofibular (B) ligaments. (A) In plantar flexion, the anterior talofibular ligament is in line with the fibula, thereby providing most of the support to the lateral aspect of the ankle joint. (B) When the ankle is in neutral position, both the anterior talofibular and the calcaneofibular ligaments support the joint. The obliquely placed structure depicts the axis of the subtalar joint. It should be noted that the calcaneofibular ligament parallels the axis. (C) When the ankle joint is in dorsiflexion, the calcaneofibular ligament is in line with the fibula and supports the lateral aspect of the joint. (Modified from Stiehl JB, ed. *Inman's Joints of the Ankle.* 2nd ed. Baltimore: Williams & Wilkins; 1991.)

the limb at initial ground contact. The anterior compartment ceases contraction by the time the foot is flat on the floor.

The posterior compartment muscles are active after the foot is flat (15% to 20% of gait cycle), during which time the ankle joint is undergoing dorsiflexion, and they remain active until approximately halfway through the cycle, at which time approximately 50% to 60% of ankle joint plantar flexion has occurred.[23] This muscle group initially undergoes an eccentric contraction slowing forward movement of the tibia over the foot, then a concentric contraction when plantar flexion begins. The posterior calf group ceases contraction before full plantar

flexion has occurred as the opposite limb accepts weight bearing, indicating that the last portion of plantar flexion is a passive phenomenon.

As the speed of gait increases to running and sprinting, and a period of double-limb support gives way to a period void of limb support, several changes occur. Most notably, at heel strike when running, the other foot is not in contact with the ground, and as running speed increases, the duration of stance phase reduces significantly. The ankle joint starts in slight dorsiflexion and, at heel strike, remains dorsiflexed (see Fig. 110.5). Rather than the ankle plantarflexing after heel strike as is seen in a walking gait, the foot-flat position is achieved while the ankle remains dorsiflexed by the tibia moving forward over the foot. The anterior compartment muscle contraction still begins late in stance and continues through swing, but during running it lasts through approximately the first third of the stance phase. The posterior calf muscle groups show a significant change in activity; they begin to contract late in the swing phase and remain active until approximately halfway through ankle joint plantar flexion.[24] This increased activity in the posterior calf musculature probably serves to stabilize the ankle joint at the time of initial ground contact.

Understanding the kinematics of running is important for maximizing performance and minimizing risk of injury. Sprinters fastest start times are recorded when they orient their ground reaction force toward a horizontal inclination, partially by increasing dorsiflexion of the ankle.[25] Kinematics patterns differ between recreational and elite runners, with parameters such as pelvic tilt, knee flexion, and ankle eversion in late stance adapting to improve performance.[26] Injury risk in collegiate cross-country runners over a season is associated with preseason peak external knee adduction moment (KAM) and peak ankle eversion velocity.[27] Age older than 40 years is associated with diminished angular motion of the ankle, knee, and pelvis compared with younger runners.[28] Increasing speeds in these runners is explained by increased hip angular displacement, which may put added stress on the hamstring and Achilles tendons.

Midfoot and forefoot strike patterns during running, more amenable to bare feet or shoes with minimal heel padding, alter kinematics and kinetics of the ankle compared with a heel-strike running pattern.[29,30] Running in shoes with less heel padding or barefoot favors the foot contacting the ground with more plantar flexion at the ankle, initially striking either the midfoot or forefoot.[31] Midfoot or forefoot strike patterns are associated with shorter stride length and higher stride frequency.[30,32] Flatter foot placement at touchdown correlates with lower peak heel pressures but significantly higher leg stiffness during the stance phase.[32,33] Tibial internal rotation excursion is similar.[34] Posterior compartment muscle force output is greater in forefoot striking than in rearfoot striking and in barefoot than in shod running, although Achilles tendon strain is lower while running barefoot than while running when wearing a standard shoe.[35] As speed of running increases in shoes with minimal heel padding, work is redistributed from the knee to ankle compared with shoes with more heel padding.[36]

Running with forefoot and rearfoot strike patterns requires similar oxygen uptake and internal mechanical work, with slight increased metabolic demand in shod runners explained by an approximately 1% increase in metabolic demand for each 100 g of added shoe weight.[32,35,37] Despite no difference in internal work, an increase in external and total mechanical work occurs in forefoot strike runners, which perhaps is explained by higher storage and release of energy in the elastic structures of the lower leg.[32,38] Another way to look at this is that traditional shoes with padded heels attenuate the foot-ground impact, which may decrease the capacity for storage and restitution of elastic energy by the leg, resulting in lower net efficiency in shod running compared with minimal-shoe running.[32,35]

Although runners will fervently defend their strike pattern, objective demonstration of practical differences remains elusive. There is no association between strike pattern and race time during marathons, although a large number of runners switched from a midfoot pattern at 10 km to a heel strike pattern at 32 km, perhaps related to fatigue or pace.[39] In a study of 52 middle- and long-distance collegiate runners, those with rearfoot strike patterns (two-thirds of the group) had approximately twice the rate of repetitive stress injuries than did runners who habitually had a forefoot strike, although a number of other covariates were present, including gender, race distance, and average miles per week; traumatic injury rates were not significantly different between the two groups.[40] Anecdotal reports suggest forefoot striking may help people with chronic exertional compartment syndrome,[41] but it may be associated with the development of metatarsal stress fractures.[42]

Clinically relevant conditions may also benefit from an understanding of their associated biomechanics. Patients with insertional Achilles tendinopathy do not have diminished non–weight-bearing dorsiflexion or isometric plantar flexor strength. Instead, altered ankle biomechanics during stair ascent produce greater symptom severity and likely contribute to decreased function.[43] Achilles tendon stiffness after repair may contribute more to loss of plantar flexion power than tendon elongation.[44] When we speak of ankle joint dorsiflexion and plantar flexion, only approximately half of this motion comes from the ankle joint; the remainder comes from the movement occurring within the subtalar and transverse tarsal joints.[45] If motion of the ankle joint is diminished, perhaps from an anterior impingement, osteoarthritic changes, or surgical fusion, the subtalar and transverse tarsal joints compensate for the lost motion.[46] If degenerative changes occur within the subtalar or transverse tarsal joints, any loss of ankle joint motion is magnified. This compensatory increase in motion of the neighboring joints is nonphysiologic and often leads to pain, loss of function, increased energy expenditure, and degenerative changes over time.[47,48]

KINEMATICS AND BIOMECHANICS OF THE SUBTALAR JOINT

The terms *pronation* and *supination* describe a coordinated series of movements linking the tibia, ankle joint, subtalar joint, transverse tarsal joints, metatarsophalangeal joints, and plantar aponeurosis. It is this linked series of movements that enable the athlete to absorb the forces of impact, yet create a rigid platform from which to push off (Table 110.1).

TABLE 110.1 Comparison of Foot Characteristics Based on Foot Position

	FOOT POSITION	
	Pronation	**Supination**
Joint position	Ankle dorsiflexion	Ankle plantarflexion
	Subtalar eversion	Subtalar inversion
	Transverse tarsal abduction	Transverse tarsal adduction
Arch stiffness	Supple	Rigid
Gait cycle	Heel strike	Flat foot to toe-off
Function	Energy absorption	Energy transfer to ground

The subtalar joint permits inversion and eversion. The axis of the subtalar joint varies between athletes but is approximately 42 degrees to the horizontal plane and passes from medial to lateral at approximately 23 degrees (Fig. 110.7).[8,49] The range of motion of the subtalar joint spans approximately 30 degrees of inversion to 15 degrees of eversion, although measurement of subtalar joint motion is difficult. Although the pattern of motion appears to be consistent between individuals over the gait cycle, the magnitude of motion varies considerably.[50]

The subtalar joint, which is stabilized primarily by the complex joint configuration of the anterior, middle, and posterior facets and by the interosseous talocalcaneal ligament, is less constrained than the ankle.[51,52] When the long axis of the tibia passes medial to the obliquely placed subtalar joint axis, subtalar joint eversion ceases because of the configuration of the joint surfaces and the interosseous ligament. When the weight-bearing line is lateral to the subtalar joint axis, inversion stability depends on lateral ligament support and active muscle function.

The subtalar joint has been likened to an oblique hinge that functions to translate motion between the transverse tarsal joint distally and the ankle joint and leg proximally (Fig. 110.8).[53–55] At the time of initial ground contact during walking, the slightly inverted subtalar joint undergoes rapid eversion, the tibia undergoes internal rotation, the transverse tarsal joints become supple, and the medial longitudinal arch flattens. These passive movements combine to help dissipate the energy imparted to the foot during heel strike.

This linkage is also important for efficient energy transfer during heel rise and toe-off, which involves both passive and active mechanisms. During the flatfoot phase, the subtalar joint undergoes progressive inversion, which reaches a maximum at toe-off. This movement increases the stability of the transverse tarsal joints and medial longitudinal arch, stiffening the foot and allowing it to act as a rigid extension of the leg. Pelvis rotation causes an external rotation torque, which is transmitted from the lower extremity across the ankle joint and is translated by the subtalar joint into hindfoot inversion. The plantar aponeurosis mechanism and the oblique metatarsal break enhance the inversion, as will be described later.

To best appreciate how various muscles affect the subtalar joint, examine the size and location of the muscles in relation to the subtalar joint axis (Fig. 110.9). In general, tendons passing medial to the axis produce inversion, whereas tendons passing laterally produce eversion, although these functions are affected

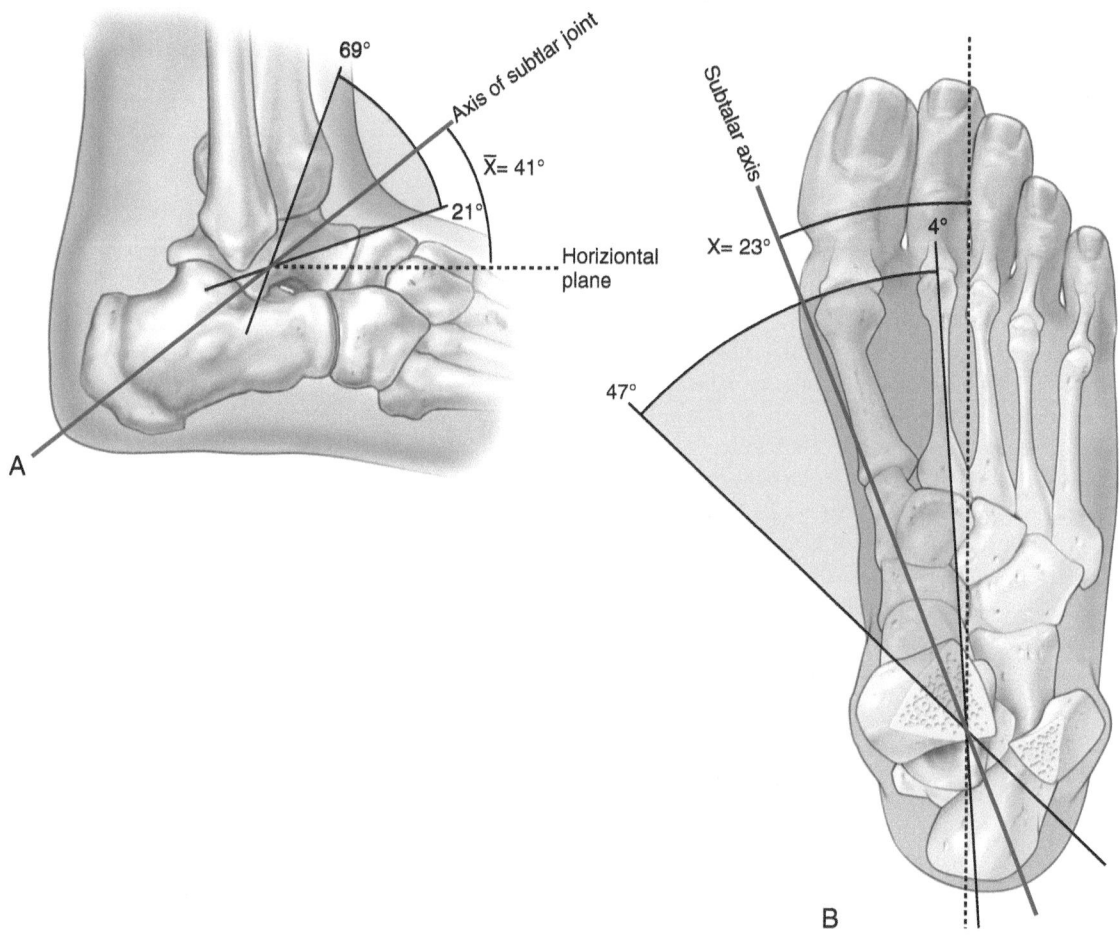

Fig. 110.7 Variations in the subtalar joint axes. In the horizontal plane (A), the axis approximates 45 degrees and (B) passes approximately 23 degrees medial to the midline. ([A] and [B], Modified from Isman RE, Inman VT. Anthropometric studies of the human foot and ankle. *Bull Prosthet Res.* 1969;10:97.)

by the starting position of the subtalar joint. The main inverters are the tibialis posterior and the gastrocnemius-soleus complex, and the main everter is the peroneus brevis and, to a lesser extent, the peroneus longus, which is mainly a plantar flexor of the first metatarsal. The tibialis anterior lies close to the subtalar joint axis and provides little influence on the neutral subtalar joint. However, it is the only functioning muscle at heel strike and may resist eversion of the initially inverted subtalar joint. The patient who lacks posterior tibial tendon function cannot initiate standing on tiptoe but can maintain the position when it is achieved. It may be concluded that posterior tibial tendon function is necessary to initiate inversion and that the gastrocnemius-soleus complex is necessary to maintain it. During running, the posterior calf muscles become active late in swing phase and remain active through most of stance (see Fig. 110.5). Besides providing stability to the ankle joint, these muscles contribute to inversion of the subtalar joint before initial ground contact.

If the motion in the subtalar joint is restricted, its ability to translate rotation proximally and distally is impaired, placing increased stress on the ankle and transverse tarsal joints. For example, talocalcaneal coalition can lead to a spastic peroneal flatfoot or ball-in-socket ankle because of the lack of subtalar motion. The degree of ankle joint dorsiflexion and plantar flexion

also is affected, and the ankle can become arthritic from the abnormal stresses.[56]

Foot morphology plays a role in hindfoot motion and force attenuation during the gait cycle.[57] For instance, people with flat feet have increased eversion of the subtalar joint during stance (Fig. 110.10). This eversion translates to increased tibial internal rotation, which can affect knee alignment, patellofemoral tracking, or the hip in selected cases. The theory behind orthotic use for many conditions involving the foot, ankle, knee, hip, and back is the effect they have on the linkage system within the lower extremity. The use of a medial heel wedge, whether built into the shoe or within an orthotic device, may influence the rotation of the subtalar joint,[58] which may decrease the degree of internal rotation or adduction moment transmitted to the lower extremity, which in turn may have a beneficial effect on the forces across the ankle, knee, and hip.[59] For instance, a runner with chronic anterior knee pain may be helped by an orthotic device that limits eversion of the calcaneus, which in turn diminishes internal rotation of the tibia and affects patellofemoral tracking.[60] However, reliable data to support this theory are lacking[61]; the benefit may in part be psychological,[62] and soft orthoses and compliant shoe material may simply help to absorb the impact of initial ground contact.

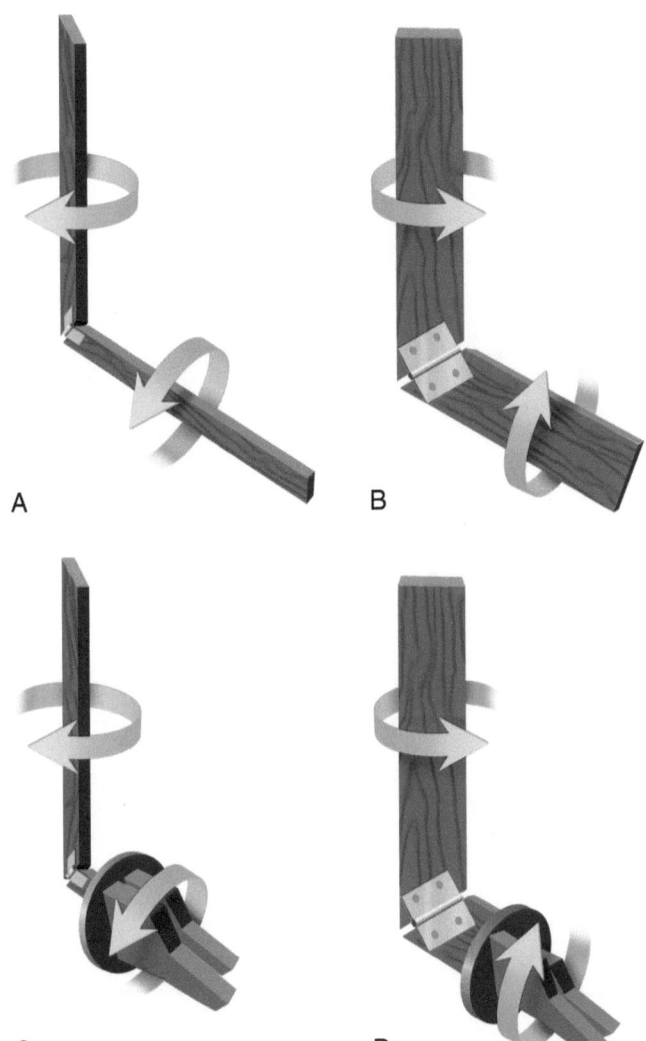

A

B

C

D

Fig. 110.8 The mitered hinge effect of the subtalar joint. The subtalar joint acts as a mitered hinge, linking motion between the calcaneus below and the tibia above (A and B). The model also demonstrates flattening and elevation of the longitudinal arch. Flattening of the longitudinal arch occurs at the time of heel strike with eversion of the calcaneus and internal rotation of the tibia (A and C). Elevation and stabilization of the longitudinal arch are associated with the outward rotation of the tibia, causing inversion of the calcaneus and locking of the transverse tarsal joint (B and D). (Modified from Mann RA, Haskell A. Biomechanics of the foot and ankle. In: Coughlin MJ, Mann RA, Saltzman CL, eds. *Surgery of the Foot and Ankle.* 8th ed. Philadelphia: Elsevier; 2007.)

Other clinical conditions may also benefit from shoe inserts that control hindfoot motion or attenuate impulsive forces. Laterally based heel wedges reduce KAM in patients with varus knee arthritis, regardless of walking speed.[63] Material that helps to absorb impact can also be beneficial for persons engaged in repetitive sports, such as long-distance running, especially if the athlete is having problems such as heel pain, metatarsalgia, or shin splints. However, softer material paradoxically can lead to greater vertical load when landing from jumps as the athlete stiffens the limb in an attempt to improve balance and stability.[64]

KINEMATICS AND BIOMECHANICS OF THE TRANSVERSE TARSAL JOINTS

The transverse tarsal joint, consisting of the talonavicular and calcaneocuboid joints, lies distal to the subtalar joint and is influenced strongly by subtalar position.[65] The function of the plantar aponeurosis, the transverse metatarsal break, and the muscles of the leg and foot further guide these joint motions. The transverse tarsal joint moves in adduction and abduction and is measured with the calcaneus in a neutral position of slight valgus and the forefoot parallel to the floor. Normal motion spans approximately 20 degrees of adduction to 10 degrees of abduction. The forefoot may also rotate into supination (forefoot varus) or pronation (forefoot valgus) through the transverse tarsal joints. Normally, forefoot rotation is neutral with the hindfoot held in a neutral position of slight valgus, but it may become fixed in a rotated compensatory position in people with long-standing planovalgus or cavovarus deformities.

The functional stability of the transverse tarsal joint is largely determined by subtalar joint position. When the calcaneus is in an everted position, the axes of the transverse tarsal joint are parallel, permitting motion to occur about this joint system. During normal walking, this phenomenon occurs at heel strike, creating a flexible foot to absorb the energy of initial ground contact. When the calcaneus is inverted, the axes of the transverse tarsal joint are nonparallel, limiting motion and creating a stable joint system (Fig. 110.11).[65] This situation occurs at heel rise and toe-off, creating a rigid foot to effectively lengthen the limb, and during running to assist in propulsion. An alternative description of transverse tarsal joint stability is one of constant compliance but with bimodal seating based on hindfoot station and longitudinal loading, with similar functional results.[66]

Impairment of the transverse tarsal joint impairs subtalar joint motion because, for subtalar motion to occur, rotation must occur about the talonavicular and calcaneocuboid joints. If an isolated arthrodesis of the talonavicular joint is carried out, most subtalar joint motion is lost.[67] When performing arthrodeses in the area of the hindfoot, sparing the talonavicular joint when appropriate usually results in a more functional foot.

WINDLASS MECHANISM, METATARSAL BREAK, AND FIRST METATARSOPHALANGEAL JOINT

The function of the plantar aponeurosis during gait is often described by comparing it with the mechanics of a windlass. The plantar aponeurosis arises from the tubercle of the calcaneus and inserts into the base of the proximal phalanges (Fig. 110.12). After heel rise, the metatarsophalangeal joints dorsiflex, tightening the plantar aponeurosis, as would a rope pulled around a windlass. This mechanism depresses the metatarsal heads, elevates and stabilizes the longitudinal arch, and helps bring the calcaneus into an inverted position (Fig. 110.13).[68,69] The inverted calcaneus causes the transverse tarsal joint axes to diverge, helping to stabilize the midfoot at toe-off.

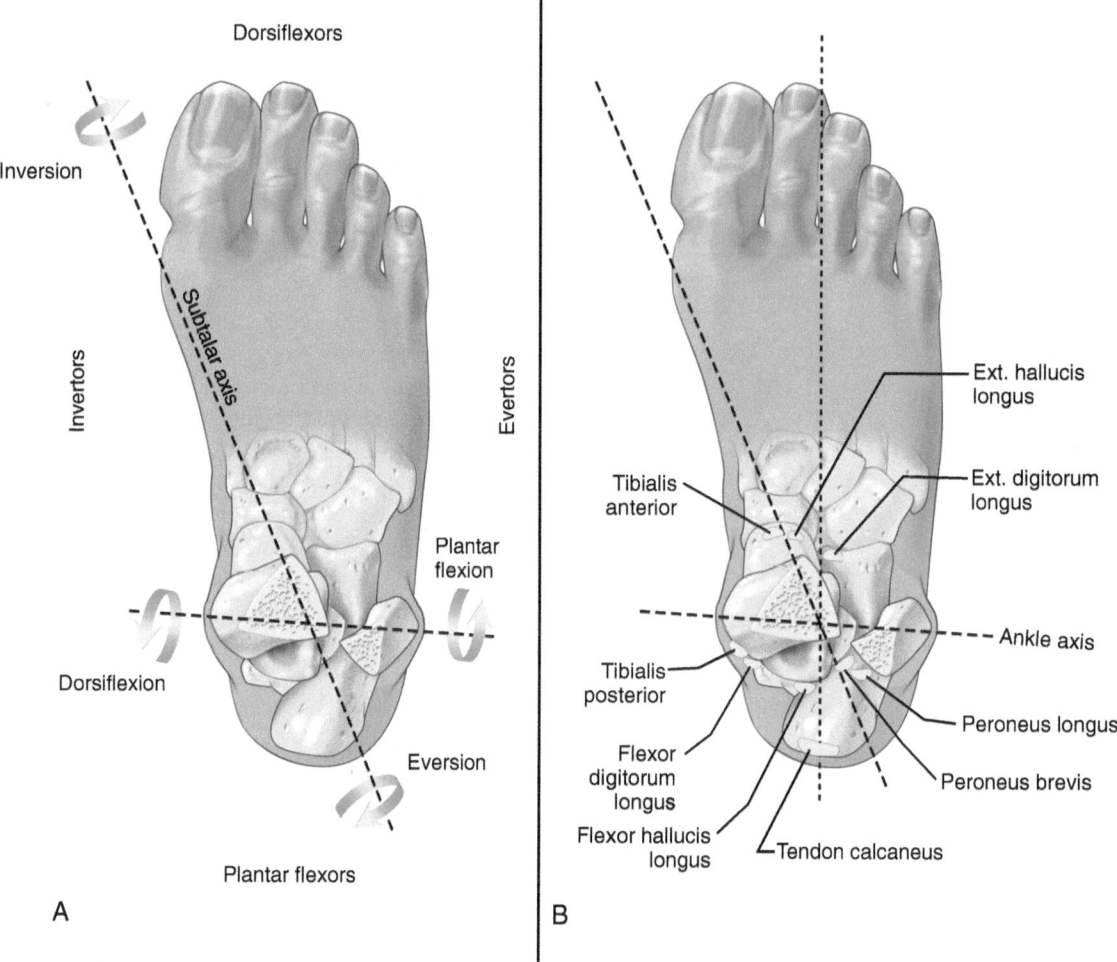

Fig. 110.9 (A) The location and the types of rotation that occur about the ankle and the subtalar axes. (B) The relationship of the various extrinsic muscles about the subtalar and ankle joint axes. *Ext,* Extensor. (From Haskell A, Mann RA. Biomechanics of the foot. In: American Academy of Orthopaedic Surgeons. *Atlas of Orthoses and Assistive Devices*. Philadelphia: Elsevier; 2008.)

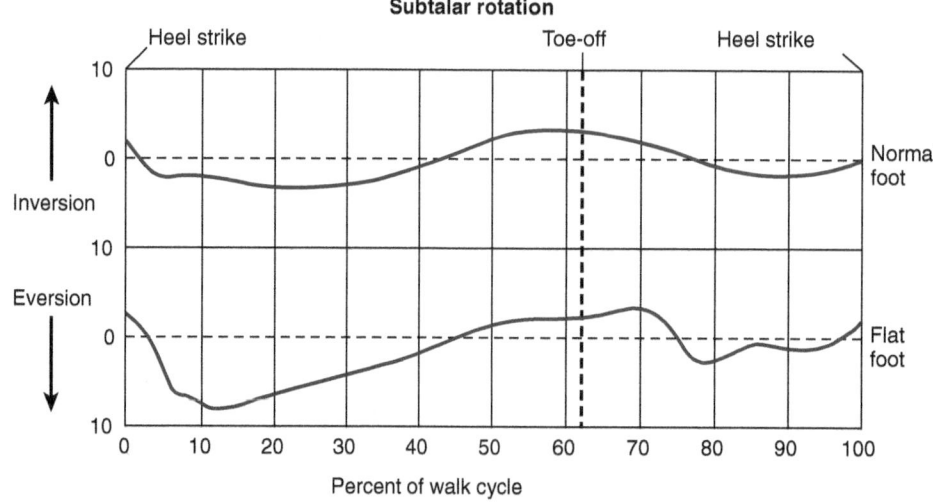

Fig. 110.10 Subtalar joint motion in a person with a normal foot and in a flat-footed person. (Data from Wright DG, Desai ME, Henderson BS. Action of the subtalar and ankle joint complex during the stance phase of walking. *J Bone Joint Surg Am*. 1964;46A:361.)

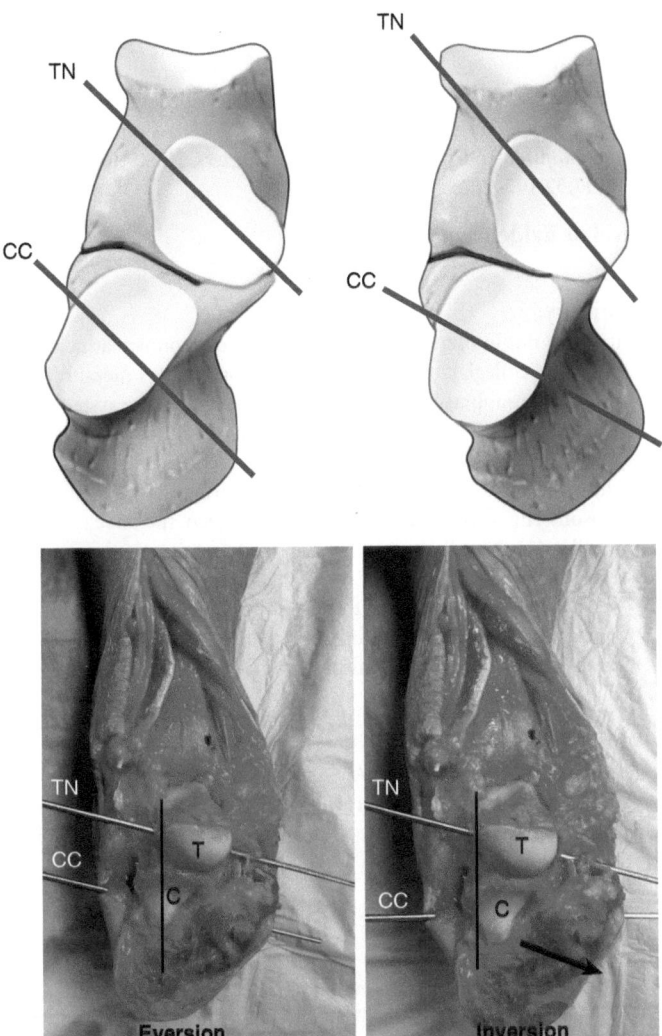

Fig. 110.11 The function of the transverse tarsal joint as described by Elftman. When the calcaneus is in eversion, the resultant axes of the talonavicular *(TN)* and calcaneocuboid *(CC)* joints are parallel or congruent. When the subtalar joint is in an inverted position, the axes are incongruent, giving increased stability to the midfoot. *C,* Calcaneal articular surface of the CC joint; *T,* talar articular surface of the TN joint. (Modified from Haskell A, Mann RA. Biomechanics of the foot and ankle. In: Coughlin MJ, Saltzman CL, Anderson RB, eds. *Mann's Surgery of the Foot and Ankle.* 9th ed. Philadelphia: Elsevier; 2014.)

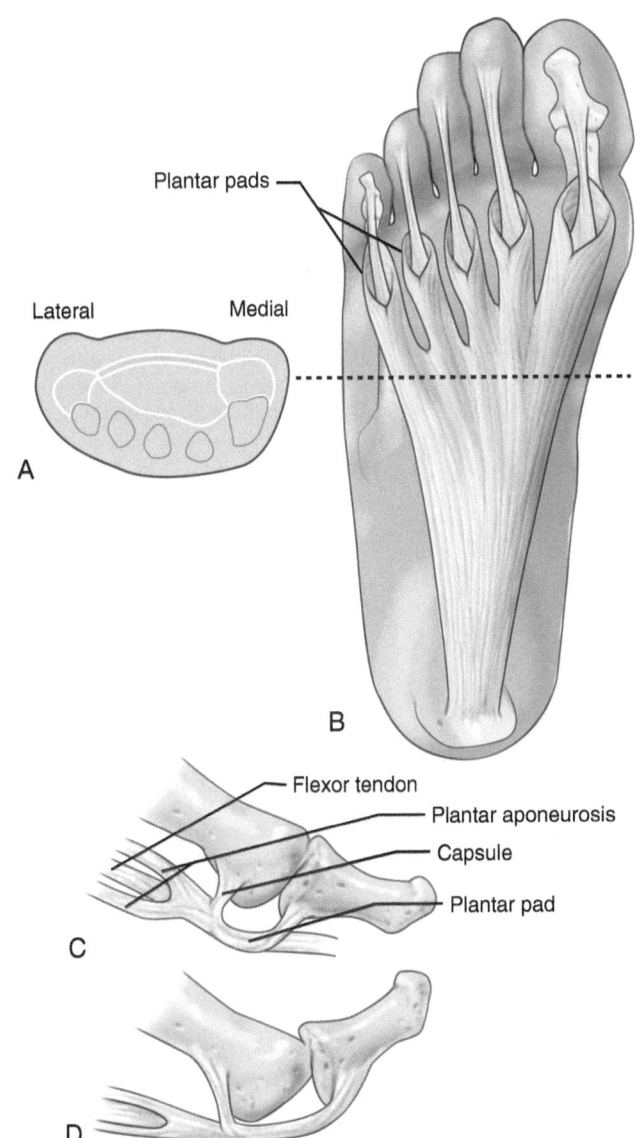

Fig. 110.12 Plantar aponeurosis. (A) Cross-section. (B) The plantar aponeurosis originates from the tubercle of the calcaneus and passes forward to insert into the base of the proximal phalanges. The aponeurosis divides, permitting the long flexor tendon to pass distally. (C) Components of the plantar pad and its insertion into the base of the proximal phalanx. (D) Extension of the toes draws the plantar pad over the metatarsal head, moving it into plantar flexion. (From Mann RA, Haskell A. Biomechanics of the foot and ankle. In: Coughlin MJ, Haskell A, Saltzman CL, eds. *Surgery of the Foot and Ankle.* 8th ed. Philadelphia: Elsevier; 2007.)

The oblique metatarsal break is created by the lateral slope formed by the increasingly proximal position of metatarsophalangeal joints two through five (Fig. 110.14).[35] This oblique line creates a camlike action after heel-rise as the body weight is brought over the metatarsal heads, inverting the hindfoot, and further enhancing external rotation of the lower extremity.

Turf-toe injuries are common in athletes and can lead to stiffness in the first metatarsophalangeal joint from arthrofibrosis or hallux rigidus, a degenerative arthritis of the first metatarsophalangeal joint. Loss of first metatarsophalangeal joint dorsiflexion prevents normal function of the windlass mechanism and metatarsal break. This situation frequently leads to external rotation of the foot during gait to relieve the stress across the involved area and can cause compensatory changes throughout the lower extremity.

Hallux valgus also alters the biomechanical function of the first ray and may contribute to altered kinematics and gait parameters throughout the lower extremity. The function of the first ray in with hallux valgus may be improved with taping.[70] Unfortunately, gait parameters and whole limb kinematics may not be improved after hallux valgus surgery.[71]

SUMMARY

A complex coordinated series of movement and energy transfer involving the foot, ankle, and lower extremity allows for walking

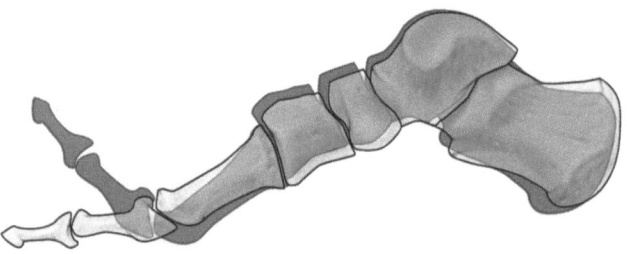

Fig. 110.13 The function of the plantar aponeurosis. The black outline shows the medial column with the foot at rest. The red figure shows the medial column with the first ray dorsiflexed. Note that dorsiflexion of the metatarsophalangeal joints tightens the plantar aponeurosis, which results in depression of the metatarsal heads, elevation and shortening of the longitudinal arch, inversion of the calcaneus, and elevation of the calcaneal pitch.

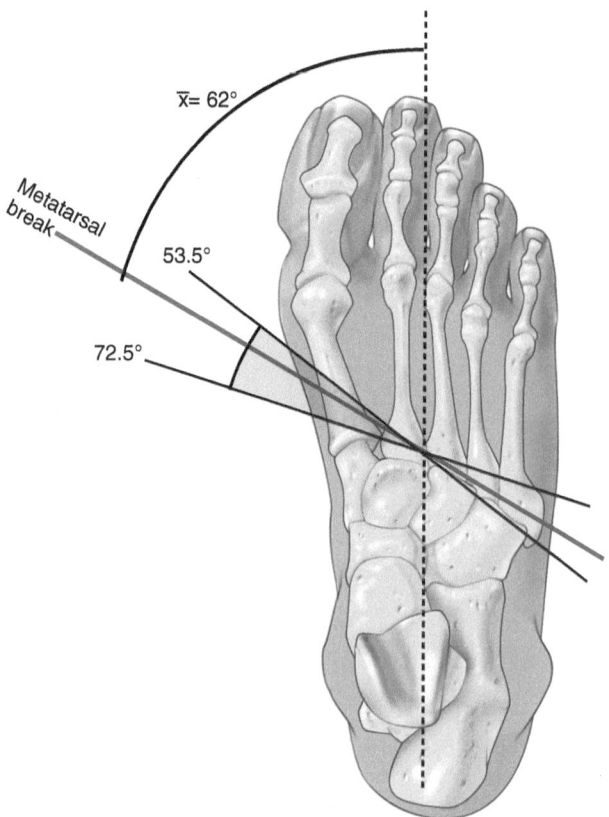

Fig. 110.14 The metatarsal break passes obliquely at an angle of approximately 62 degrees to the long axis of the foot. (Modified from Isman RE, Inman VT. Anthropometric studies of the human foot and ankle. *Bull Prosthet Res.* 1969;10:97.)

and running such that energy expenditure is minimized and stress applied to body segments is lessened. Over the gait cycle, a period of double-limb support during walking gives way to a float period with no limb support during running. Ankle, hindfoot, and forefoot mechanics combine to absorb impact at initial ground contact and provide stability as weight is borne on the forefoot. Alterations in the biomechanics of these systems can lead to reduced performance and injury.

For a complete list of references, go to ExpertConsult.com.

SELECTED READINGS

Citation:

Dudley RI, Pamukoff DN, Lynn SK, et al. A prospective comparison of lower extremity kinematics and kinetics between injured and non-injured collegiate cross country runners. *Hum Mov Sci.* 2017;52:197–202.

Level of Evidence:

I

Summary:

Thirty-two noninjured, NCAA Division 1, cross-country athletes on the same collegiate team had kinematic parameters measured during running using a nine-camera motion capture system and force plate prior to the season. Incidence of running-related injury (RRI) throughout the season was recorded. Twelve athletes developed RRI, for an incidence 38.7% during the 14-week season. The most common sites of injury were the knee (33.3%) and leg (25.0%). Runners who sustained an injury had a greater external knee adduction moment (KAM) and peak ankle eversion velocity when compared with uninjured runners. Incorporating strategies to reduce KAM and ankle eversion velocity into training and shoe modifications may help to prevent RRI in long distance runners.

Citation:

Almeida MO, Davis IS, Lopes AD. Biomechanical differences of foot-strike patterns during running: a systematic review with meta-analysis. *J Orthop Sports Phys Ther.* 2015;45(10):738–755.

Level of Evidence:

I

Summary:

In a systematic review with meta-analysis designed to determine the biomechanical differences between foot-strike patterns used when running, electronic databases searches revealed 16 studies that compared the biomechanical characteristics of foot-strike patterns in distance runners. At initial ground contact, a forefoot-strike pattern is associated with plantar-flexion of the ankle and a flexed knee position, compared with a dorsiflexed ankle and an extended knee position for the rearfoot strikers. Midfoot strikers have greater ankle dorsiflexion range of motion and decreased knee flexion range of motion compared with rearfoot strikers. Rearfoot strikers have higher vertical loading rates compared with forefoot strikers. Understanding these characteristics may help clinicians and trainers to advise runners on technique to minimize and manage running injuries.

Citation:

Squadrone R, Gallozzi C. Biomechanical and physiological comparison of barefoot and two shod conditions in experienced barefoot runners. *J Sports Med Phys Fitness.* 2009;49:6–13.

Level of Evidence:

I

Summary:

Eight experienced barefoot runners ran on a treadmill barefoot, with minimal running shoes, and with traditional running shoes while biomechanical and physiologic measurements were taken. When running barefoot, the foot strikes with more plantar flexion at the ankle, which was associated with reduced impact forces, shorter stride length and contact times, and greater stride frequency.

Citation:

Hof AL, Elzinga H, Grimmius W, et al. Speed dependence of averaged EMG profiles in walking. *Gait Posture.* 2002;16:78–86.

Level of Evidence:

I

Summary:

Twenty subjects walked on treadmills at varying speeds while electromyographic (EMG) data were collected from many muscles. The EMG activity of a muscle or functional muscle group can be described by a linear equation representing a fixed component and a component that varies with speed. This finding supports the concept of a central pattern generator for human locomotion.

Citation:

Hreljac A. Determinants of the gait transition speed during human locomotion: kinematic factors. *J Biomech.* 1995;28:669–677.

Level of Evidence:

I

Summary:

Twenty subjects walked and ran on treadmills at varying speeds while biomechanical measurements were made. Preselected parameters were tested against predefined criteria as possible determinants of why runners transition from walking to running. Maximum ankle angular velocity met the criteria most closely, followed by maximum ankle angular acceleration. The authors hypothesize that gait transition from walking to running is made to protect the ankle dorsiflexors, which are functioning at near-maximum capacity during fast walking.

Citation:

Nilsson J, Thorstensson A, Halbertsma J. Changes in leg movements and muscle activity with speed of locomotion and mode of progression in humans. *Acta Physiol Scand.* 1985;123:457.

Level of Evidence:

I

Summary:

Twelve subjects walked and ran at preset speeds on a treadmill while biomechanical measurements were made. The peak amplitude of the vertical ground reaction force in walking increased from 1.0 to 1.5 times body weight and during running increased from 2.0 to 2.9 times body weight as speed increased. Running has a shorter support phase duration and increased vertical peak force compared with walking.

111

Leg, Ankle, and Foot Diagnosis and Decision-Making

Anish R. Kadakia, Amiethab A. Aiyer

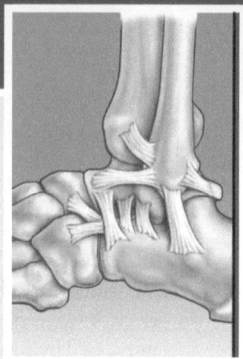

OVERVIEW OF PATHOLOGIES

Evaluation of conditions of the foot and ankle is facilitated by the relative subcutaneous location of the major bony, tendinous, and neurovascular structures. This ease of palpation is offset by the complex anatomy of the foot and ankle that transmits up to four times body weight during running and must act as a stable platform during gait. This difficulty is exemplified by a patient with a report of heel pain, in which case one would presume that the ease of palpation of the calcaneus and adjacent structures would facilitate the diagnosis. However, in the case of a chronic Achilles tendon rupture, the patient may have no tenderness with a focal examination, and the diagnosis may only be made by obtaining an appropriate history combined with findings of increased passive dorsiflexion and weak plantar flexion compared with the contralateral lower extremity. The goal of this chapter is to provide a framework for approaching cases of foot and ankle pain commonly seen in athletes.

Chronic exertional compartment syndrome is a condition that occurs in athletes and persons involved in repetitive exertional/loading activities. It is most commonly seen in the lower extremities of distance runners. The pain worsens over the course of the activity and requires premature cessation of exercise, followed by resolution after rest. The underlying cause of the pain has not been definitively determined. The presumed etiology is increased osmotic pressure and edema that results in increased intracompartmental pressure, causing occlusion of the microvasculature and ischemic pain. In contrast to acute compartment syndrome, this condition is not a surgical emergency.

Athletes may experience chronic lower limb pain, which may be attributable to peripheral nerve entrapment. Compared with other problems of the lower limb, this entity is quite rare, with a heterogeneous group of nerve disorders that present with often vague and diffuse locations of pain. The difficulty of properly understanding the entire spectrum of peripheral nerve entrapments may lead to misdiagnosis or underdiagnosis. Adequate treatment of peripheral nerve entrapment requires a proper understanding of the anatomic course, the possible causes, precise identification of the involved nerve, and a clear determination of the location of compression.

Acute ankle ligament injuries are very common; an ankle sprain occurs in an estimated 1 in every 10,000 persons each day. The lateral ligamentous complex is the most commonly injured. In addition to a simple lateral ankle sprain, a multitude

of ligamentous injuries can occur in the foot and ankle, and failure to recognize and appropriately identify these entities may lead to significant morbidity for these patients. With respect to the ankle, this includes syndesmotic injuries (high ankle sprains) and medial (deltoid) ligament injuries. Ankle and subtalar dislocations are not solely caused by high-energy injuries and can occur simply from sliding into a base while playing baseball. A diagnosis of a "foot sprain" is not sufficient to initiate treatment given that some injuries require operative intervention. Sprains of the hindfoot can be associated with fractures of the anterior process or disruption of the stability of Chopart joint. Both of these injuries respond poorly if aggressive treatment is begun, as is common for a lateral ankle ligament injury. Lisfranc injuries involve disruption of the stabilizing ligaments of the midfoot and are commonly associated with American football or soccer. Any patient who presents with midfoot pain and swelling after an injury should be presumed to have an injury to the tarsometatarsal joint complex, and all efforts should be made to rule out the diagnosis before functional nonoperative treatment is initiated. Rupture of the stabilizing plantar ligaments of the great toe, known as turf toe, can be particularly disabling and has the potential to end the career of a high-level athlete.

Injuries to the tendons that cross the ankle joint range from simple tendonitis to frank rupture. Along the anterior aspect of the ankle, the anterior tibial tendon is most commonly involved, with the extensor hallucis longus and extensor digitorum longus typically involved only in the setting of a traumatic laceration. Anterior tibial tendonitis most commonly involves the insertion of the tendon at the medial cuneiform, with a rupture occurring both at midsubstance or at the insertion. Unlike patients with injuries to the Achilles tendon, patients with rupture of the anterior tibial tendon do not commonly present acutely, and this delayed presentation creates difficulty with surgical reconstruction. Sports that involve explosive push-off are popular both with youth and patients who are older than 30 years and are a common inciting factor in ruptures of the Achilles tendon. Repetitive high-energy loading of the ankle as experienced during running or jumping may lead to excess strain on the both the Achilles and posterior tibial tendons. In these cases, the subcutaneous nature of the tendons greatly facilitates the diagnosis because localized swelling in the area of the foot and ankle is rarely a benign process. In the setting of posterior tibial tendon disease, patients may also note the presence or worsening of a flatfoot deformity. The flexor hallucis longus (FHL), in contrast, is the deepest tendon within the posterior ankle and may not present with subcutaneous swelling. The association with repetitive plantar flexion and injuries to the FHL should guide the examiner to perform more provocative testing to obtain the diagnosis after eliciting this history.

Osteochondral lesions of the talus and tibia (OLTs) can be particularly difficult to treat in the athletic population. To make an accurate diagnosis, knowledge of the functional consequence of the OLTs is required. These lesions may present with a sense of instability or giving way for the patient that can be easily confused with chronic ankle instability. Persons with OLTs commonly have additional pain and swelling between episodes, in addition to possible episodes of locking of the ankle joint. Given that plain radiographs may not clearly demonstrate an OLT, eliciting an accurate history and performing a thorough physical examination are crucial in determining the next most appropriate step in the care of the patient. Articular injuries are not isolated to the talus or tibia and commonly occur in the second metatarsal, known as *Freiberg infraction*. However, focal cartilage defects may also occur in the third metatarsal head and the first metatarsal head. Failure to recognize these conditions may lead to continued pain for the athlete and inability to play, in addition to possibly accelerating articular injury, leading to arthrosis. Pain and swelling of the joints without a clearly defined radiographic etiology raises the likelihood of this diagnosis.

Heel pain is a frequent complaint in athletes. Although heel pain rarely leads to surgical intervention, it can be very disabling and can be successfully treated if the correct diagnosis is made. Many patients with plantar heel pain may have tenderness over the plantar fascia, but this finding in and of itself does not complete the examination and permit a diagnosis to be made. In some cases, a concomitant calcaneal stress fracture, fat pad atrophy, or compression of the first branch of the medial plantar nerve may exist, requiring alteration of the treatment. Such alteration is most crucial in patients who fail to experience relief after a reasonable period of nonoperative treatment. The practitioner should always question the initial diagnosis in the setting of persistent pain to minimize the risk of pursuing an inappropriate treatment course.

Pain within the lesser forefoot is termed *metatarsalgia*; however, metatarsalgia is a descriptive term of the location of the pain and does not offer any true diagnostic information. Metatarsalgia may be the result of multiple etiologies, ranging from instability of the first tarsometatarsal to Freiberg infraction, Morton neuroma, plantar plate rupture, or an equinus contracture. Complicating the diagnosis is that multiple factors may contribute to the pain and each one must be addressed to achieve success. Pain within the sesamoid complex should be aggressively treated nonoperatively because an early stress fracture is difficult to differentiate from sesamoiditis at initial presentation. In this case, the clinical symptom of sesamoid pain is easy to make given the subcutaneous position of the bone; however, the underlying root cause is more difficult to determine even with advanced imaging. Therefore aggressive treatment, although cumbersome, can minimize the risk of long-term pain and discomfort, which is extremely disabling for the athlete.

HISTORY

Obtaining a thorough history not only provides information regarding the cause of the complaint but also aids in constructing a focused physical examination that maximizes the information gathered given the time constraints of the practitioner. The location of the complaint is one of the most useful aspects of the history in determining the cause. Having a patient use a single digit to locate the point of maximal tenderness and/or swelling greatly facilitates determination of the correct diagnosis. A working knowledge of the subcutaneous anatomy of the foot and ankle is required to gain the most information from this maneuver. The inability to localize a specific site also provides valuable information that the underlying cause may be neurologic, autoimmune, or medication related. Pain over the entire lateral aspect of the foot, for example, is more likely related to the sural nerve than the peroneal tendons or the fifth metatarsal. The concomitant sensation of a "pop" or the sense that something is moving out of place along with the painful episodes is associated with FHL stenosing synovitis (posterior), peroneal subluxation (lateral), or posterior tibial subluxation (medial).

When obtaining the history, rather than using a repetitive list of questions, the questions should be adapted to the patient's responses. For example, when inciting factors are elicited and the patient reports onset during exercise, the examiner should consider exertional compartment syndrome, with follow-up questions to determine if the severity increases with duration of exercise, if pain ceases after rest, and if pain is not present during activities of daily living to corroborate the diagnosis. Pain after a period of immobility is common in persons with inflammatory etiologies, such as tendonitis, arthritis, and plantar fasciitis. Persons with stress fractures, on the other hand, have minimal pain after immobility; in contrast, the pain gets worse over time, and the pain does not cease with rest as would occur with exertional compartment syndrome.

Clearly defining the exact activity that causes the pain is helpful. For example, many dancers experience foot and ankle pain, and determining whether they are ballet dancers engaging in en-pointe activity (leading to FHL synovitis) or ballroom dancers (who often have sesamoiditis) leads the examiner toward the most likely etiology. Not only is the particular activity critical in determining the diagnosis, it also plays an important role in determining the timing and type of surgical intervention that would be appropriate. In the case of ballet dancers, for whom maximum mobility is critical to their career, hallux valgus surgery is avoided and more minimally invasive techniques involving arthroscopy should be used to minimize stiffness. Conversely, in athletes for whom stability is more critical than flexibility, retention of hardware for syndesmotic and tarsometatarsal injuries is considered.

Initiation of a new activity or modification of activity such as an increase in intensity or duration is commonly noted in the setting of tendonitis and stress fractures. Additionally, alteration of shoe wear can be temporally related and may contribute to the cause of the discomfort, especially given the rise in the popularity of minimalist shoes and their association with metatarsal stress fractures. Stress fractures and acute tendonitis are also commonly seen in runners who are training for a marathon as they increase their duration to gain endurance. Regardless of the length of time patients have participated in the activity, they can still experience overuse injuries as a result of a deformity such as a cavovarus foot or biologic factors such as osteopenia or vitamin D deficiency. Pain associated with activity on uneven surfaces such as grass or gravel is related to the subtalar and transverse tarsal joints and is commonly noted in patients with sinus tarsi syndrome. Increased pain with use of stairs, particularly with descent, is noted in patients with Achilles tendon disease, given the strain placed across the tendon during the eccentric contraction needed to stabilize the body. In patients with plantar fasciitis or fat pad atrophy, running on a rubber surface may be preferable to running on a hard surface such as asphalt or concrete, as opposed to patients with stress fractures, who would not note a significant difference.

In addition to pain and swelling, the presence of mechanical symptoms must be determined. A sense of instability or frank episodes of giving way may be related to a multitude of causes. Paroxysmal instability that occurs without cause is most likely the result of an OLT or a loose body. Locking or catching of the ankle is indicative of a loose body or unstable osteochondral flap. A sense that the ankle feels loose associated with episodes of giving way is more likely related to laxity of the lateral collateral ligaments. Peroneal tendon disease can lead to instability because the role of these tendons as a secondary stabilizer is compromised. In these cases, however, the complaint is commonly associated with pain and swelling along the posterolateral aspect of the ankle. These conditions may occur concomitantly, and therefore even when a positive response is elicited for one diagnosis, the practitioner must further question the patient regarding other additional causes.

In cases of trauma, determining the mechanism of injury greatly facilitates the diagnosis; however, many patients are unable to recall the details of the injury. Although no mechanism creates the same injury in all cases, a common pattern does exist. For example, an inversion injury of a plantar-flexed foot without external force most commonly disrupts the lateral collateral ligaments of the ankle, creating an ankle sprain. Getting struck with an axial force by another player while the foot is in a plantar-flexed position increases the risk of a tarsometatarsal (Lisfranc) injury. Disruption to the syndesmosis occurs with an external rotation force coupled with axial loading to a dorsiflexed and externally rotated foot. This mechanism may be seen in sports that require frequent alteration of direction at high speeds such as basketball, American football, and soccer. Explosive push-off as seen in tennis or basketball is associated with a rupture of the Achilles tendon. Additionally, patients may state that they heard an audible pop or gunshot-type sound and felt as if they were kicked in the back of the leg. Hyperdorsiflexion of the great toe is directly linked to turf-toe injuries.

Neurologic reports of numbness, tingling, or burning should be elicited. Radiating pain from proximal to distal or less commonly from distal to proximal (the Valleix phenomenon) can occur as a result of nerve entrapment and is less likely to be the result of a musculoskeletal etiology. Transient numbness or even foot drop with exercise may occur in patients with exertional compartment syndrome. The transient nature of the symptom and the direct correlation to activity differentiate these symptoms from nerve entrapment, with which the symptom is present at rest. A prior history of surgery will guide the practitioner to examine the incisions carefully to determine possible iatrogenic causes of the neurologic symptoms. Failure to obtain relief with antiinflammatory medication is common in patients with nerve disorders.

Patients, often unknowingly, modify footwear habit in order to minimize symptoms prior to seeking professional advice. Teasing this information out of the patient can assist the practitioner towards accurate diagnosis. In presence of hallux valgus and lesser toe deformities, patients often have symptom relief with wide toe box or open toed footwear. Stiff-soled footwear is helpful in patients with arthritic or overload stress injuries. For example, hallux rigidus, midfoot arthritis, and metatarsal/calcaneal stress overload symptoms are minimized with stiff-soled footwear by limiting range of motion (ROM) and transferring less stress to the foot. On the contrary, ambulating bare foot or in footwear with thin soles (i.e., flip-flops) will make hallux rigidus, midfoot arthritis, and metatarsal/calcaneal stress overload symptoms worse. Cushioned footwear may provide comfort in patients with metatarsal/calcaneal stress overload or with heel fat pad atrophy. Footwear with wedge platform or built in heel lift is preferred by patients with noninsertional Achilles or posterior tibial tendon pathology. This essentially offloads tension by preventing the last few millimeters of stretch tendons endure during normal ambulation. Boots that come proximal to the ankle joint mimic function of an Arizona brace and are preferred by patients with hindfoot and/or ankle arthrosis.

Obtaining a complete history includes not only a detailed discussion of the chief complaint but must include a review of the patient's medical and surgical history in addition to current medications and prior thrombosis or thrombosis in family members. Clearly, a patient with an autoimmune disease requires alteration of the treatment plan because medical management must be optimized before considering any surgical intervention. Current fluoroquinolone use, although common knowledge to the medical community, may not be recognized by the patient and is associated with tendonitis, particularly of the Achilles tendon. Diffuse musculoskeletal pain or muscle tenderness may be related to the use of cholesterol-lowering statin medications and should be considered in cases without a clearly identifiable cause. Patients with diabetes should be examined for sensory neuropathy and may require prolonged periods of non–weight bearing compared with persons who are not diabetic. In patients with a history of thrombosis, consideration of the use of antithrombotic medication is critical when proposing immobilization for acute injuries.

PHYSICAL EXAMINATION

The examination should begin with the patient seated, with exposure of both lower extremities distal to the knee. Visual inspection for swelling quickly guides the examiner to possible areas of pathology. The location of the swelling is correlated with common disease processes. For example, posteromedial

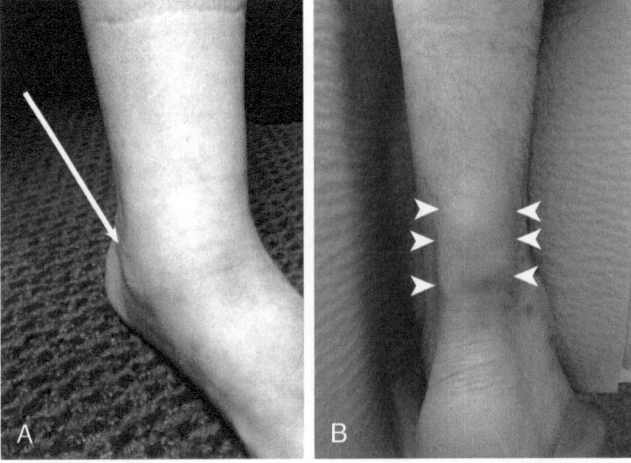

Fig. 111.1 (A) Posteromedial swelling *(arrow)* in a patient with acute posterior tibial tendonitis. Note the loss of contour of the medial malleolus. (B) Swelling and thickening of the posterior aspect of the heel *(arrowheads)* that is consistent with Achilles tendinosis.

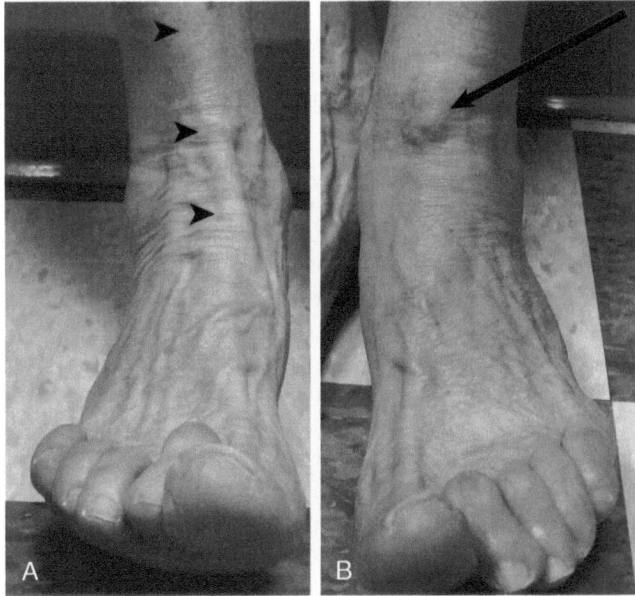

Fig. 111.2 (A) Patient with a chronic rupture of the left anterior tibial tendon. He was referred for a "mass" on the left ankle (B; *arrow*). The clear asymmetry from the intact anterior tibial tendon (A; *arrowheads*) with attempted dorsiflexion is consistent with an anterior tibial tendon rupture.

swelling is related to the posterior tibial tendon; swelling that is directly posterior is related to the Achilles tendon; posterolateral swelling relates to the peroneal tendons; swelling in the dorsal medial midfoot relates to the anterior tibialis; and swelling of the central forefoot can be attributed to a stress fracture (Fig. 111.1). In the setting of trauma, if the patient can be examined quickly after the injury, the focal area of swelling helps to determine the site of the injury. However, in a delayed presentation more than 24 hours after the injury, the swelling is typically diffuse, limiting the effectiveness of this finding. Asymmetric circumferential swelling of the leg after an injury or surgery may indicate the presence of a thrombosis and should be further evaluated, because the injury itself typically does not cause circumferential edema of the entire leg. The presence of any abnormal bony or soft tissue prominences should be noted. Although such prominences can be the result of a benign or malignant tumor, in some cases a posttraumatic deformity may be the cause. Classically, this posttraumatic deformity can be seen after a rupture of the anterior tibial tendon, and patients may present with a "pseudotumor" along the anterior ankle as a result of proximal migration of the tendon (Fig. 111.2). Further motor examination will clearly determine the diagnosis and avoid an inappropriate workup.

The presence of ecchymosis typically correlates with the area of injury. Plantar midfoot ecchymosis is highly indicative of a Lisfranc injury (Fig. 111.3). However, the presence of ecchymosis can be difficult to interpret in the delayed setting because blood tracks through the subcutaneous tissue after injury, as is commonly seen with distal forefoot ecchymosis after an ankle sprain. In the setting of an Achilles tendon rupture, bruising is commonly noted along the posterior superior calcaneus and not directly at the site of rupture given the dependent position of the limb. An understanding of this phenomenon can guide the examiner to look for a more proximal site of injury after identifying distal ecchymosis, such as with a Thompson test in this case. Further inspection for prior surgical scars can identify possible sites of nerve injury or entrapment. Although more relevant

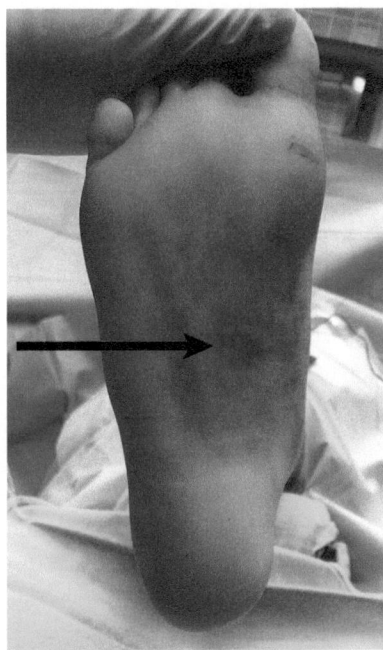

Fig. 111.3 Plantar ecchymosis *(arrow)* in the setting of a midfoot injury should raise the suspicion of a Lisfranc injury.

when examining for deformity, the presence of a callus formation notes an area of focal overload. In the athlete, a callus over the fifth metatarsal base and head is suggestive of a cavovarus deformity and is important to consider when treating ankle sprains, instability, fifth metatarsal fractures, and peroneal tendon disease. Diffuse callus formation over the plantar forefoot may suggest an equinus contracture, which must be addressed when treating patients with metatarsalgia.

Although evaluation of gait and alignment is important, this evaluation can be deferred in the setting of acute trauma to prevent further injury and decrease patient discomfort. The presence of a cavovarus deformity with an elevated longitudinal arch with hindfoot varus and a plantar-flexed first ray must be recognized and addressed when treating the previously described associated conditions to decrease the risk of recurrence (Fig. 111.4). The presence of pes planus with collapse of the longitudinal arch and hindfoot valgus may be seen as a normal condition, resulting from posterior tibial tendon dysfunction or chronic Lisfranc injuries. Comparison with the contralateral lower extremity is critical to help identify subtle differences, especially in cases in which the patient may already have congenital pes planus (Fig. 111.5). Abnormal gait patterns can clearly indicate the pathologic process. Steppage gait with increased knee and hip flexion during the swing phase occurs as a result of foot drop and may be seen with an anterior tibial tendon rupture or peroneal nerve palsy. A calcaneus gait pattern with increased dorsiflexion during heel strike occurs with triceps surae weakness after a chronic Achilles rupture. Pain with weight bearing results in an antalgic gait with a shortened stance phase on the affected limb.

To minimize the discomfort of the patient, palpation for the site of maximum tenderness in addition to provocative testing is deferred until the end of the examination. Tactile examination begins with a vascular evaluation to assess the dorsalis pedis and posterior tibialis pulses. Although this evaluation can become routine, special attention is required after severe trauma such as an ankle or hindfoot dislocation and in any patient who may require surgical intervention. A sensory examination of the five peripheral nerves that innervate the foot should follow. These nerves include the deep peroneal nerve (first web space), superficial peroneal nerve (dorsal foot), saphenous nerve (medial ankle), sural nerve (lateral foot), and tibial nerve (plantar foot; Fig. 111.6). After acute ankle sprains, decreased sensation over the course of the superficial peroneal nerve is not uncommon as a result of traction injury. If neuroma is a concern, provocative testing of the suspected nerve can be performed. Compression of the nerve at the suspected site of injury should reproduce the patient's symptoms. To adequately test the nerve, the compression should be held for 30 seconds. In the setting of a postsurgical neuroma, the site of injury is clearly identified by the scar. However, in suspected atraumatic neuroma formation, knowledge of the common sites of compression guide the examination: the distal third of the anterolateral tibia, superficial peroneal nerve; the tarsal tunnel, the tibial nerve; the dorsal hindfoot and midfoot, the deep peroneal nerve; and the second or third web space, the interdigital nerves. Compression of the abductor hallucis muscle increases the pressure on the first branch of the lateral plantar nerve and is important to perform when evaluating heel pain.

Motor testing involves assessment of individual muscles and can provide information regarding the status of tendon integrity and neurologic innervation. Isolated weakness of a single muscle is most likely related to a discontinuity of the tendon (Fig. 111.7). Neurologic causes of muscle weakness involve more than muscle groups and may be associated with a concomitant sensory deficit.

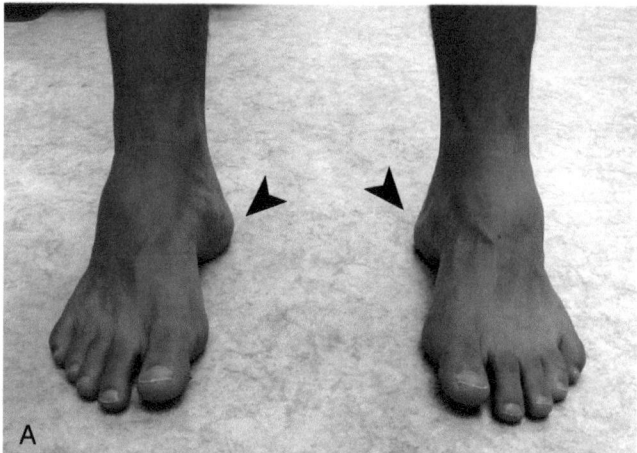
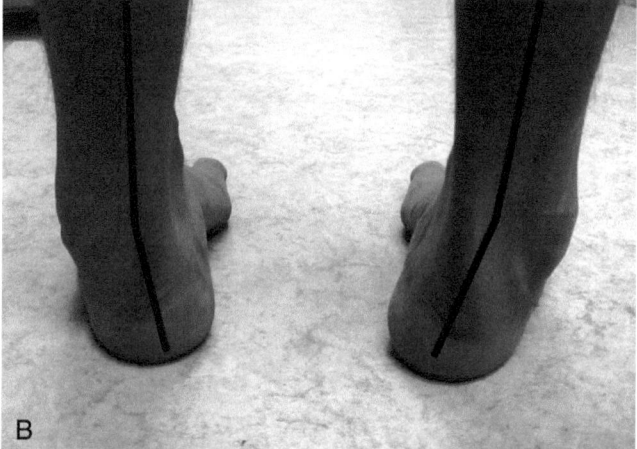
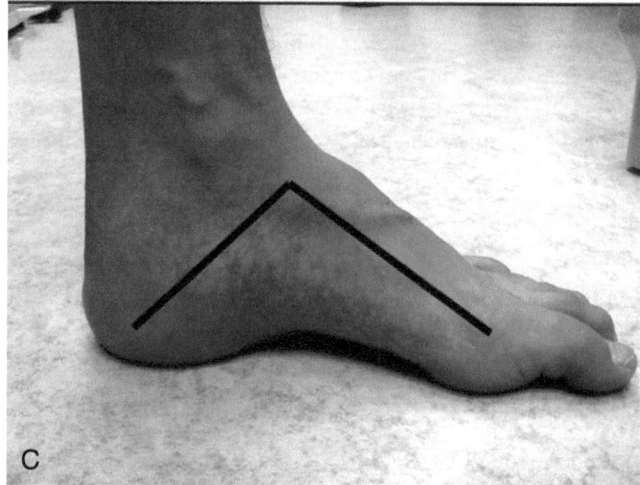

Fig. 111.4 (A) Frontal view of a patient with a cavovarus deformity. In patients with this deformity, the posteromedial aspect of the heel *(arrowhead)* is clearly visible. The varus hindfoot deformity can be viewed from the posterior aspect (B), and in severe cases, none of the lesser toes is visible. From the medial aspect (C), the cavus aspect of the deformity can be visualized.

Given that most of the tendons of the foot and ankle cross distal to the ankle joint, an isolated tendon injury may not result in complete loss of active mobility. Relative weakness compared with the contralateral limb is very useful to determine subtle weakness. In the setting of a complete rupture of the Achilles

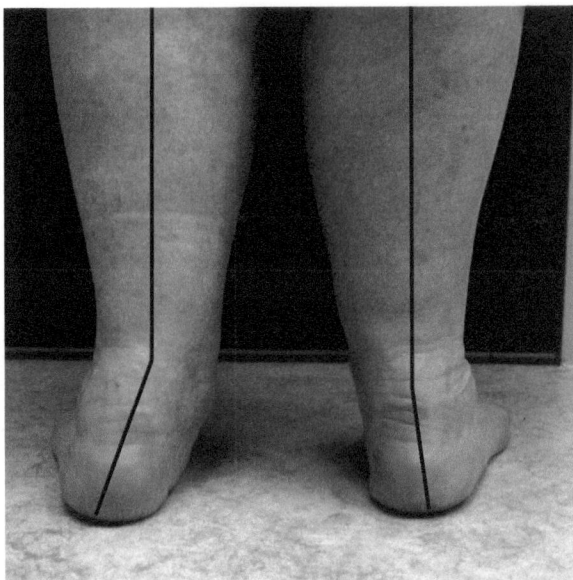

Fig. 111.5 This patient has a history of bilateral pes planus but presented with increased pain in the left lower extremity. The increased severity of the valgus on the left leg is clearly demonstrated when compared with her unaffected right leg. This finding is consistent with posterior tibial tendon dysfunction in most cases.

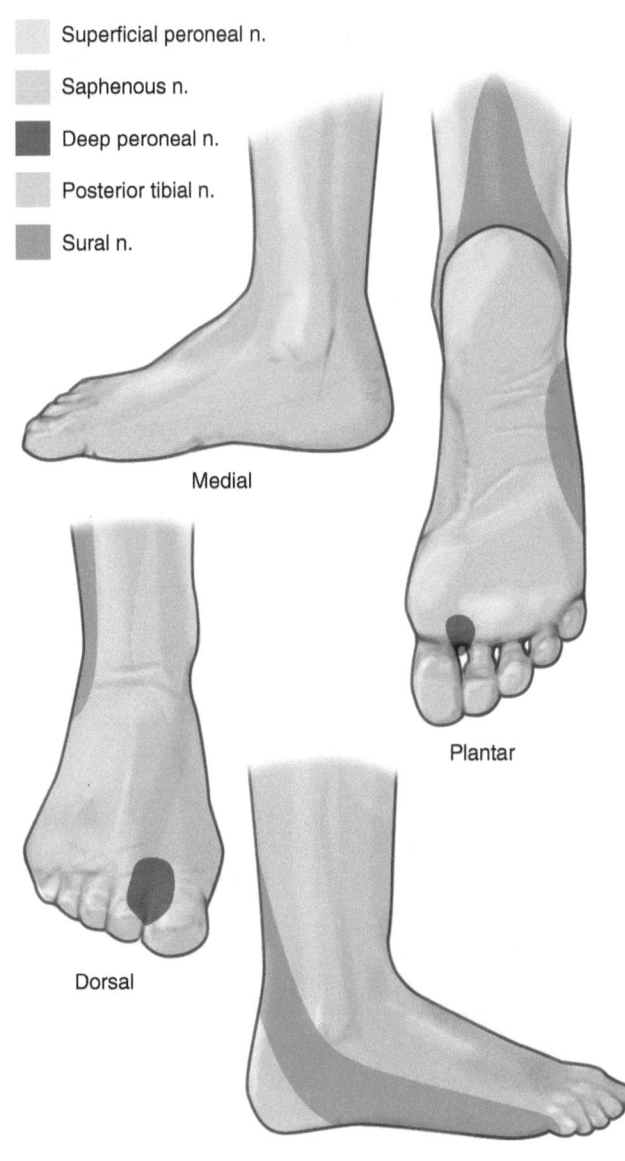

Superficial peroneal n.

Saphenous n.

Deep peroneal n.

Posterior tibial n.

Sural n.

Medial

Plantar

Dorsal

Lateral

Fig. 111.6 Sensory nerve distribution of the ankle.

tendon, plantar-flexion power to resistance (4 to 5) may still be present as a result of the multiple tendons that cross posterior to the ankle joint. Having the patient push against resistance with the contralateral hand palpating for the tested tendon can determine continuity and additionally assess for tendon disease if the patient reports pain during the maneuver. Subtle weakness may be difficult to discern with a manual resistance examination because of the strength of the lower extremity. Fatigue testing is useful in these cases, such as the repeated single-limb heel rise for the evaluation of the posterior tibial tendon (Fig. 111.8). The single-limb heel rise examination is also valuable when assessing strength in the setting of a chronic Achilles tendon rupture. Subtle anterior tibial tendon weakness may be tested with heel walking.

Both passive and active ROM should be compared with the contralateral side. Combining active ROM with a motor examination minimizes repetition. The rate of variability of normal motion of the joints of the foot and ankle is high, with no defined absolute normal. Asymmetry between extremities or pain at the extremes of motion is more relevant than the absolute value. Typically, dorsiflexion is evaluated with an interest in the amount of restriction of motion resulting from a gastrocnemius or Achilles contracture (Fig. 111.9). Importantly, however, increased motion is just as valuable, because this finding is seen with a chronic Achilles tendon rupture and may be the primary clue to the diagnosis (Fig. 111.10). Maximal ROM of the ankle is 10 to 23 degrees of dorsiflexion and 23 to 48 degrees of plantar flexion (Fig. 111.11). Maximal range of subtalar inversion is 5 to 50 degrees and eversion is 5 to 26 degrees (Fig. 111.12). Maximal ROM for the first metatarsophalangeal joint (great toe) is 45 to 90 degrees of dorsiflexion and 10 to 40 degrees of plantar flexion

(Fig. 111.13). Although active ROM after trauma may be significantly restricted, passive ROM should be present, although reduced. In the case of a severe restriction of motion or a locked joint, the risk of a dislocation or subluxation is present and must be evaluated with further imaging. Pain, grinding, or crepitus during passive ROM testing is consistent with articular cartilage degeneration from loose bodies or arthritis. Triggering during passive stretching of the tendon is a result of stenosing tenosynovitis that is associated most commonly with the FHL in the foot and ankle.

Palpation for the sites of tenderness can quickly provide information for diagnosis in cases of trauma, tendon disorders, and arthritis. However, palpation may cause significant pain for the patient if it is performed at the beginning of the examination, preventing the completion of a proper evaluation. Additionally, although palpation may be an easy way to determine the diagnosis in many cases, it is not extremely helpful in the evaluation

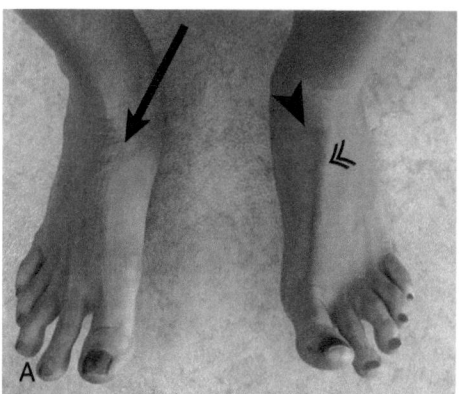
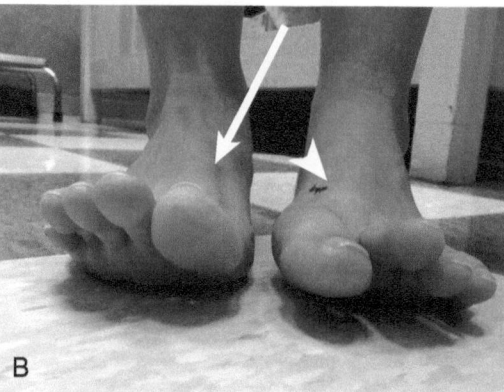

Fig. 111.7 (A) Chronic rupture of the anterior tibial tendon on the left lower extremity. The lack of function of the tendon is clearly seen *(black arrowhead)* when compared with taut anterior tibialis *(black arrow)* on the right leg. Additionally, the function of the extensor hallucis longus (EHL; *black double arrow*) and extensor digitorum longus rule out the possibility of a proximal neurologic etiology. The extensor recruitment allows the patient to perform active dorsiflexion. A follow-up examination with heel walking will demonstrate fatigue of the left leg compared with the right. (B) Traumatic laceration to the dorsum of the foot with a lack of function of the EHL *(white arrowhead)*, which is made more clear when compared with the normal contralateral foot *(white arrow)*.

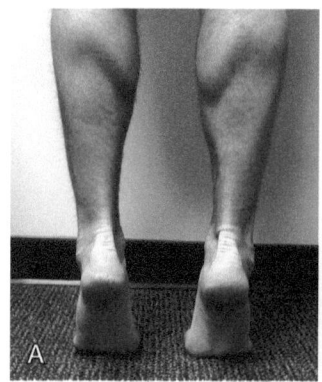
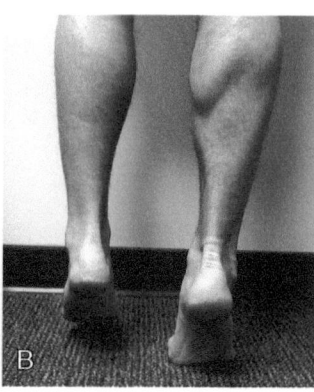

Fig. 111.8 Strength testing of the posterior tibial tendon with a double-limb heel rise (A) will be unable to detect dysfunction because the patient can compensate with the unaffected limb. To isolate the affected posterior tibial tendon, the patient must elevate the unaffected limb and perform the maneuver with only the affected extremity (B). This test is valid only for function of the posterior tibialis if the Achilles tendon is intact.

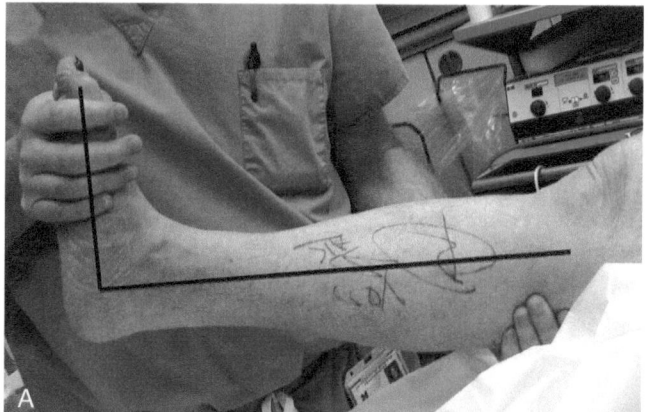
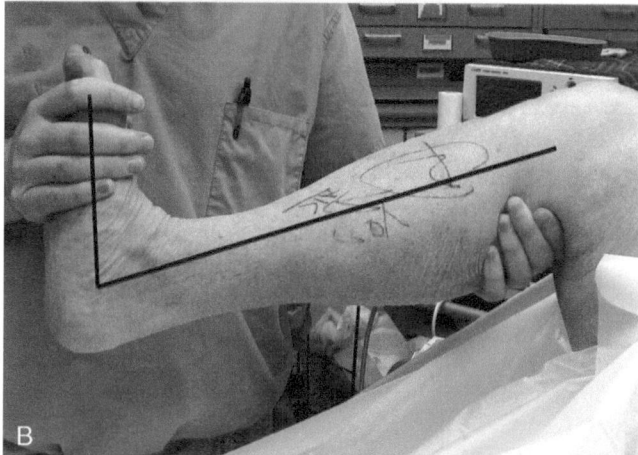

of instability, chronic tendon ruptures, exertional compartment syndrome, and neurologic disorders. A thorough knowledge of the subcutaneous anatomy of the foot and ankle greatly facilitates the usefulness of the examination. When evaluating patients with a suspected injury, such as an ankle sprain, palpation should be performed in a centripetal fashion to identify other areas of concomitant injury. Additionally, the amount of pressure used should be minimal to avoid harm and discomfort to the patient. In contrast, when performing the examination for chronic conditions, deeper palpation may be required to identify the areas of concern. Comparison with the contralateral lower extremity is crucial because many areas are tender to palpation in a normal patient, and a relative increase in discomfort provides more valuable information. The sinus tarsi is a particularly sensitive

Fig. 111.9 (A) Dorsiflexion of the ankle with the knee in extension does not achieve flexion past neutral. (B) With knee flexion the contribution of the gastrocnemius is eliminated, with a resultant increase in dorsiflexion, which is consistent with an isolated gastrocnemius contracture. If no increase in motion occurs, both the gastrocnemius and soleus are contracted, and lengthening of the Achilles tendon is required for correction.

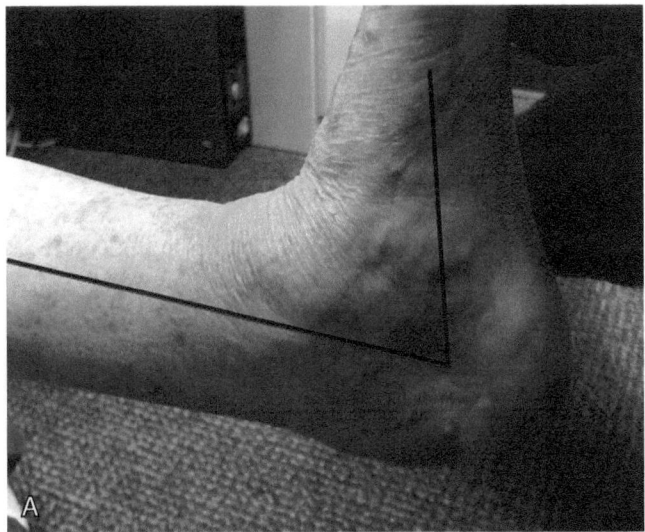

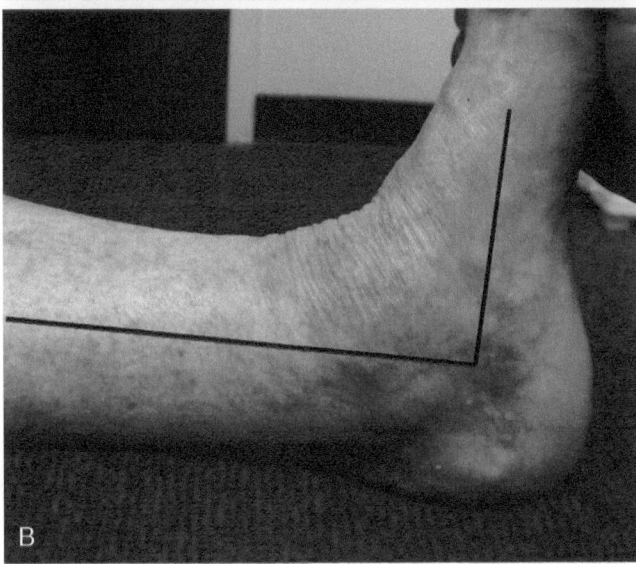

Fig. 111.10 This patient presented with heel pain and difficulty walking on stairs with the affected lower extremity. Note the hyperdorsiflexion of the affected ankle (A) compared with the uninjured side (B). Given the chronicity of the presentation, no clear defect may be palpable in these cases. Follow-up testing with manual strength examination and single-limb heel testing is appropriate to demonstrate weakness and thus corroborate the diagnosis of a chronic Achilles rupture.

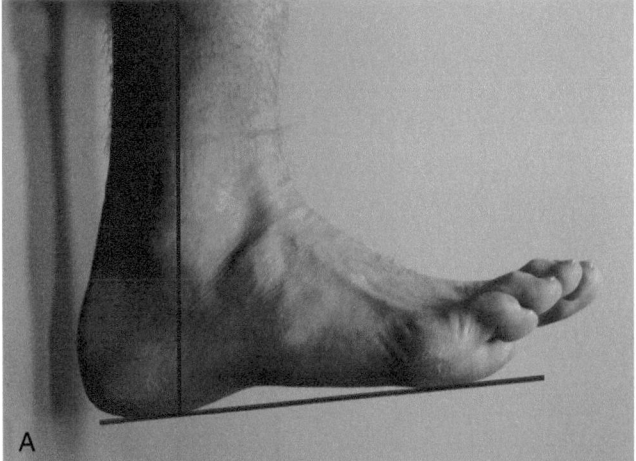

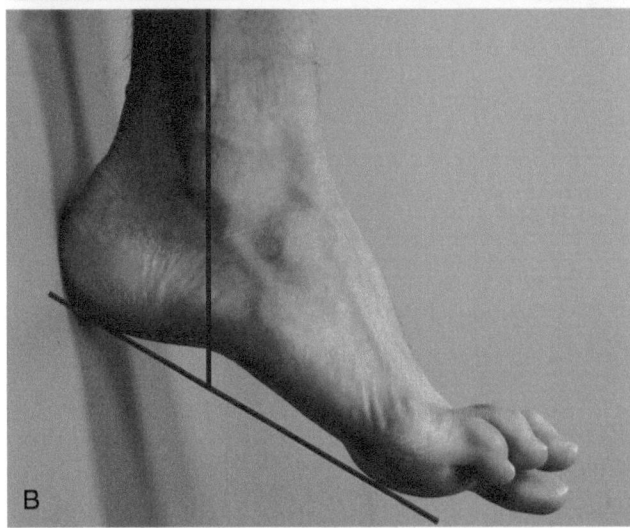

Fig. 111.11 Dorsiflexion of the ankle (A) is typically 25% to 50% the magnitude of plantar flexion (B). This difference partially accounts for why a small decrease in the absolute dorsiflexion is implicated in many pathologic conditions of the foot and ankle. A 5-degree loss of motion may result in a 50% loss of functional dorsiflexion for the patient.

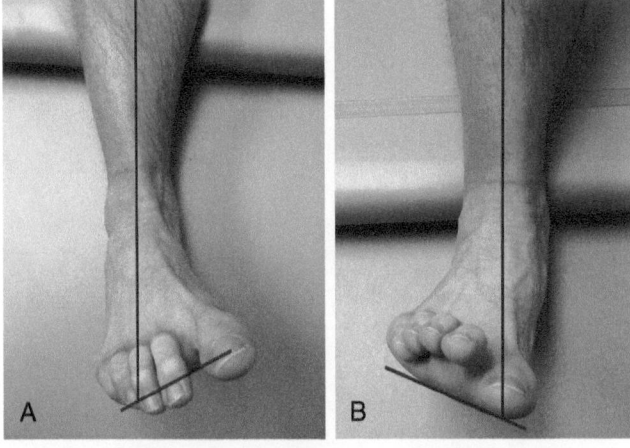

Fig. 111.12 Inversion of the hindfoot (A) is greater than eversion (B). This asymmetry partially accounts for why a pes planus deformity is better tolerated than a pes cavus deformity, because the foot has limited eversion capacity to compensate for hindfoot varus.

spot, and unless both extremities are examined and compared, the presence of pain with palpation is a nondiagnostic finding.

Stability of the lateral ankle ligaments can be assessed with the anterior drawer and varus talar tilt tests. The anterior drawer test is performed with anterior pressure on the hindfoot with the ankle in plantar flexion, which evaluates the anterior talofibular ligament (Fig. 111.14). The varus stress test is performed with inversion of the ankle in dorsiflexion to evaluate the calcaneofibular ligament (Fig. 111.15). Signs of ligamentous laxity should be tested, because these signs guide surgical treatment (Fig. 111.16). Stability testing is not isolated to the ankle and can also be performed for the hindfoot, midfoot, and forefoot joints. Stabilization of the hindfoot with dorsiflexion and plantar-flexion stress placed on the first metatarsal subjectively evaluates

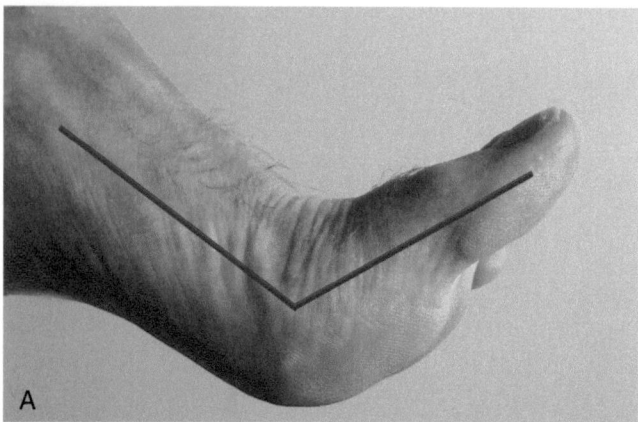

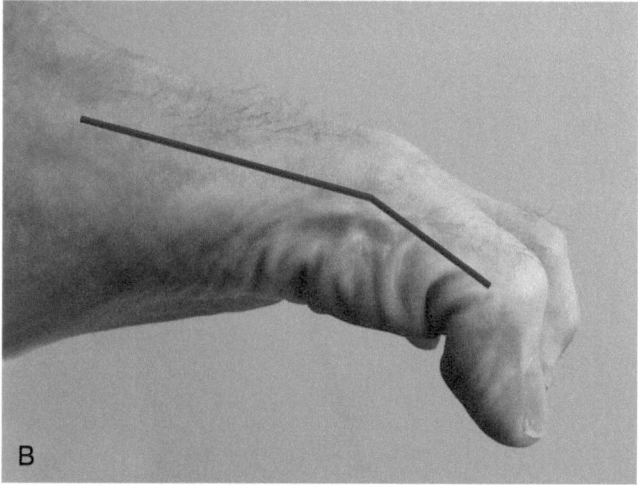

Fig. 111.13 Dorsiflexion of the first metatarsophalangeal (MTP) joint (A) is greater in magnitude and more critical to function than is plantar flexion of the first MTP joint (B).

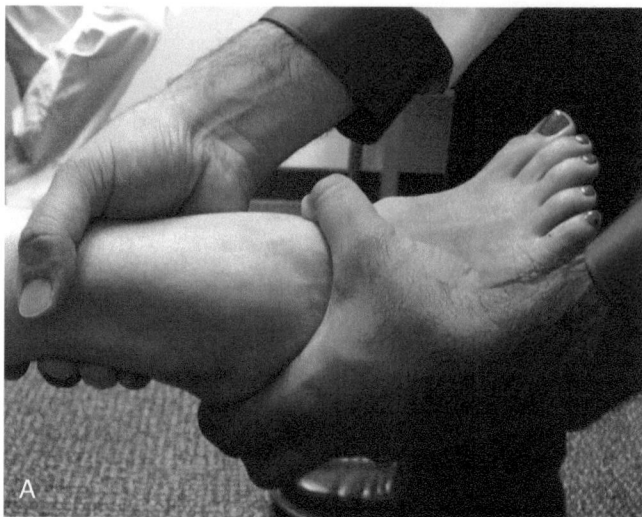

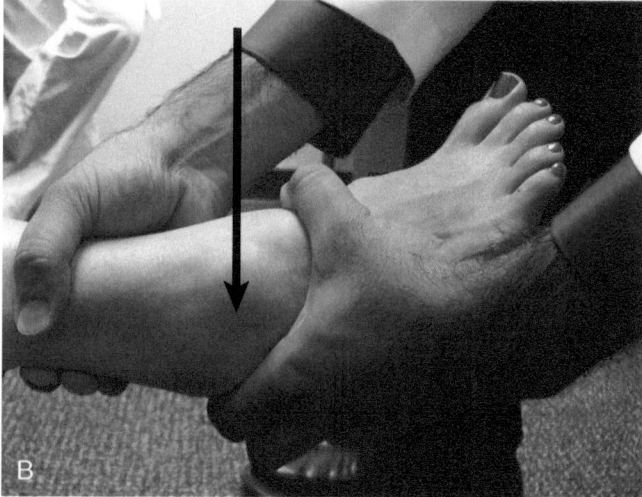

Fig. 111.14 To perform the anterior drawer test, one hand stabilizes the anterior distal tibia while the other is cupped around the posterior calcaneus (A). The heel is translated anteriorly with respect to the tibia, and any subluxation should be noted (B). Note the sulcus that is created over the anterolateral ankle with an unstable ankle (arrow).

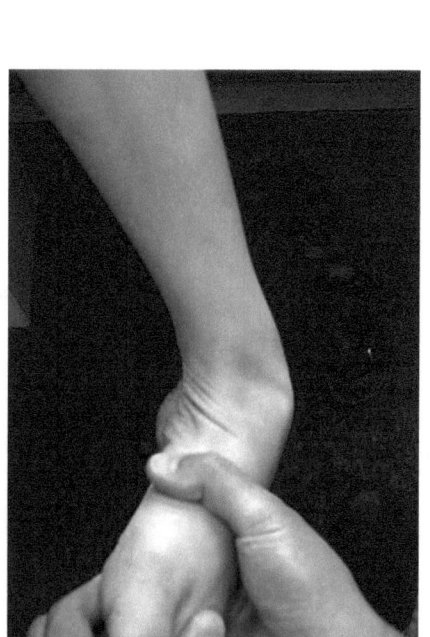

Fig. 111.15 The inversion stress test in a patient with severe laxity of the calcaneofibular ligament.

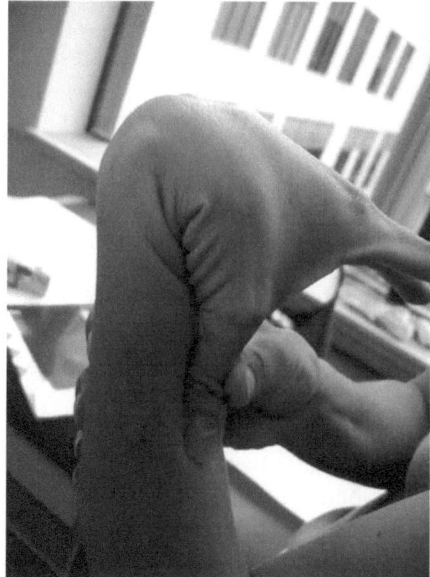

Fig. 111.16 Patients with hyperlaxity are easily able to flex the wrist and place the thumb on the volar forearm.

the first tarsometatarsal. The "vertical Lachman" test for lesser metatarsophalangeal instability is important to perform in the setting of forefoot pain. The hindfoot is difficult to examine for stability given the amount of mobility that is normally present; however, use of fluoroscopy during the examination for suspected instability of the subtalar or Chopart joints increases the yield from stress testing because subluxation of the joints can be directly visualized.

After a thorough physical examination of the lower extremities is conducted, further provocative testing (covered in detail in other chapters in this section) can be performed to evaluate specific suspected conditions. For example, a midcalf compression test and external rotation stress testing may be required to evaluate for a possible syndesmotic injury in a patient with lateral ankle swelling and pain after trauma. This specific test would not be indicated if midfoot swelling and pain were present, in which case stress testing of the midfoot along with a single-limb weight-bearing examination would be performed for evaluation of a Lisfranc injury. When evaluating a patient with a foot and ankle complaint, in many cases, a thorough history and physical examination is sufficient to determine the diagnosis without the need for further imaging.

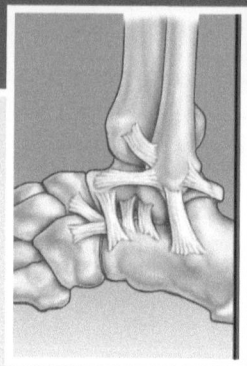

112

Imaging of the Foot and Ankle

Anish R. Kadakia, Amiethab A. Aiyer

RADIOGRAPHS

Radiographs are often the initial imaging study performed for any patient presenting with a problem related to the foot and ankle. Radiographs are clearly beneficial when evaluating for suspected arthritis, osteonecrosis, tumors, nonunion, or trauma. In addition, the alignment of the ankle and foot may contribute to the presenting complaint even if the radiographs being viewed are free of pathologic abnormalities. To appropriately evaluate the osseous structures and alignment of the foot, the radiographs should be obtained with weight bearing in all cases, except when a fracture may be suspected (Figs. 112.1–112.3). Specifically, in the setting of a suspected Lisfranc injury, if the initial non–weight-bearing radiographs are negative, follow-up weight-bearing films should be ordered to evaluate for diastasis of the tarsometatarsal joints.

COMPUTED TOMOGRAPHY

The most current generation of multidetector computed tomography (CT) scanners are capable of providing high-resolution images in all imaging planes and are superb for evaluating the extent and location of intra-articular fractures in the area of the ankle and hindfoot. Given the difficulty in assessing joint congruity in the hindfoot, follow-up CT imaging is recommended in this setting to better appreciate the fracture pattern and joint congruity. Cystic osteochondral defects of the talus are excellently visualized with this modality to accurately calculate the size of the lesion and guide preoperative planning. It is also an excellent method of assessing bony healing, including evaluation of fractures and arthrodeses. Sufficient data are available to suggest that determination of the percentage of bony trabeculation across an arthrodesis site in the ankle and hindfoot is grossly underestimated with plain radiography. The administration of intra-articular contrast material followed by CT imaging through the ankle (CT arthrography) is an accurate means of assessing internal derangement in patients who have a contraindication to magnetic resonance imaging (MRI). CT technology has now evolved into obtaining weight bearing scans of the lower extremity which can provide the surgeon with functional information regarding joint biomechanics. This technology can be extremely useful in situations where radiographs are not able to provide information due to overlap of bones. For example, in patients with midfoot arthrosis, weight-bearing CT is able to isolate each joint in the midfoot and assess for bone-on-bone apposition during weight bearing. It also provides accuracy and ease of assessing syndesmotic alignment as well as degree of subfibular impingement in hindfoot valgus deformity.

ULTRASOUND

The primary advantage of ultrasound compared with MRI is the ability to evaluate the tendinous structures in a dynamic fashion.[1] Ultrasound is the imaging modality of choice for the evaluation of peroneal tendon subluxation. The evaluation for tendon apposition in the setting of an Achilles tendon rupture or for evaluation of flexor hallucis longus (FHL) stenosing tenosynovitis are examples of when the ability to perform a dynamic examination is critical. Advantages include a relative cost saving compared with MRI and improved localization of soft tissue structures for injection. A limitation of ultrasound is that visualization of the affected structure may prove more difficult in patients with a high amount of subcutaneous fat.[2] Additionally, the clinician is reliant upon the interpretation of the radiologist and the skill of the ultrasonographer for the determination of the pathologic findings. Good communication between the clinician and the radiologist is critical to ensure that the radiologist has an understanding of the exact clinical concern so the examination can be tailored appropriately.

MAGNETIC RESONANCE IMAGING

MRI is well accepted as the primary noninvasive imaging modality for providing a global assessment of the foot and ankle and is very accurate for the evaluation of cartilaginous, tendon, ligament, and bony abnormalities. MR arthrography of the ankle can be used to obtain a more precise evaluation of articular cartilage injuries to the talar dome or tibial plafond.[3] T1-weighted fat-saturated images are key to evaluate the gadolinium contrast material in the joint. These images show the contrast to the greatest advantage. Because evaluation of bone marrow is also critical, T1-weighted non–fat-saturated images are also essential. T1-weighted images in general are superior to evaluate the anatomy, bone marrow, hemorrhage, masses, fat, and fatty infiltration of muscles. Proton density or intermediate images are high resolution and therefore important in the evaluation of ligaments, tendons, and small structures such as cartilage.[3] T2-weighted images are the best sequence to evaluate for fluid,

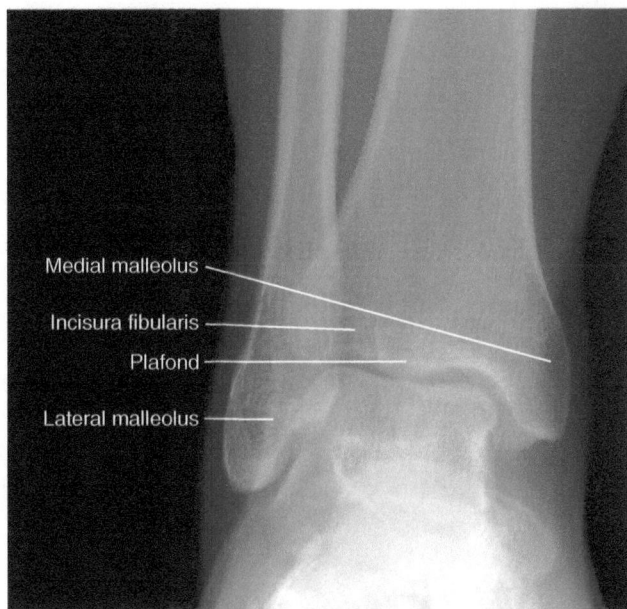

Fig. 112.1 An anteroposterior standing radiograph of the ankle. (From Miller M, Hart J, MacKnight J, eds. *Essential Orthopaedics*. Philadelphia: Elsevier; 2008.)

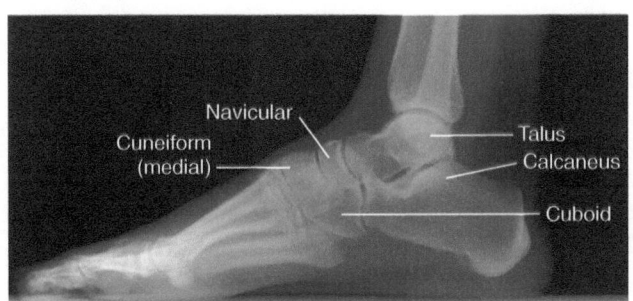

Fig. 112.2 A lateral standing radiograph of the foot. (From Miller M, Hart J, MacKnight J, eds. *Essential Orthopaedics*. Philadelphia: Elsevier; 2008.)

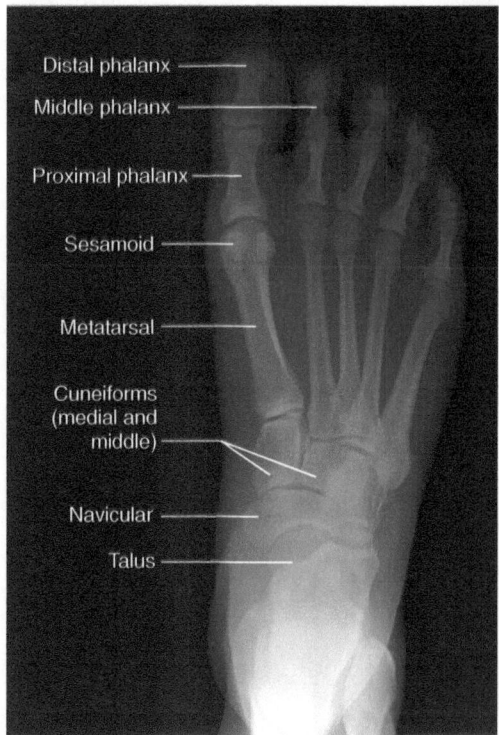

Fig. 112.3 An anteroposterior standing radiograph of the foot. (From Miller M, Hart J, MacKnight J, eds. *Essential Orthopaedics*. Philadelphia: Elsevier; 2008.)

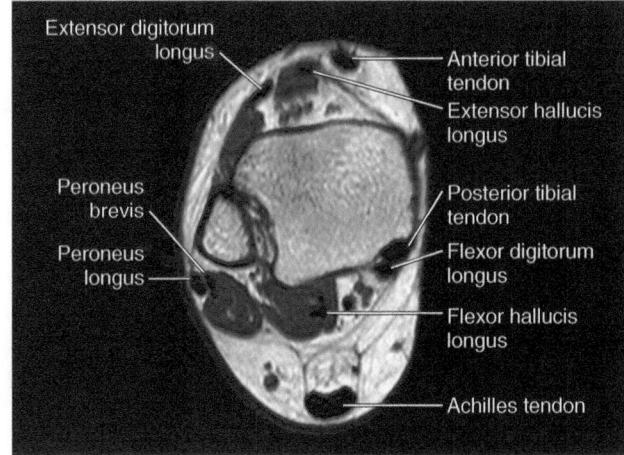

Fig. 112.4 An axial T1-weighted magnetic resonance image of the distal leg. The tendons at this level are denoted.

edema, joint effusions, muscle, and soft tissue injuries. Fluid sensitivity is increased with use of fat saturation.[4]

Dedicated foot and ankle coils or smokestack coils are critical in obtaining high-quality imaging of foot and ankle disorders. Images are performed in the sagittal, axial, and coronal imaging planes. When ordering an MRI, the specific area of concern should be communicated to the radiologist. Given that the smallest field of view optimizes image quality, an MRI scan that captures the entire foot and ankle will compromise the quality of the foot images. Additionally, specific protocols may exist for the forefoot versus the hindfoot, and therefore the specific site of the pathologic condition should be stated to ensure that the appropriate MRI protocol is used.

IMAGING OF TENDONS

Given a tendon's lack of fluid, a normal tendon has low signal intensity on all imaging sequences (Fig. 112.4). Axial cuts are the most useful to determine the presence and extent of tenosynovitis and tendinosis. Coronal imaging, although complementary,

provides the least information. An area of focal thickening is not a normal finding.

Achilles Tendon

Disorders of the Achilles tendon are diagnosed with relative ease as a result of the subcutaneous nature of the tendon. The presence of tendinosis is noted by focal thickening of the tendon that moves in conjunction with the tendon, as opposed to paratenonitis. The primary utility of MRI is to determine the precise location and affected volume of the tendon for preoperative planning. Increasingly, with nonoperative management of Achilles tendon ruptures demonstrating good results with functional rehabilitation, MRI

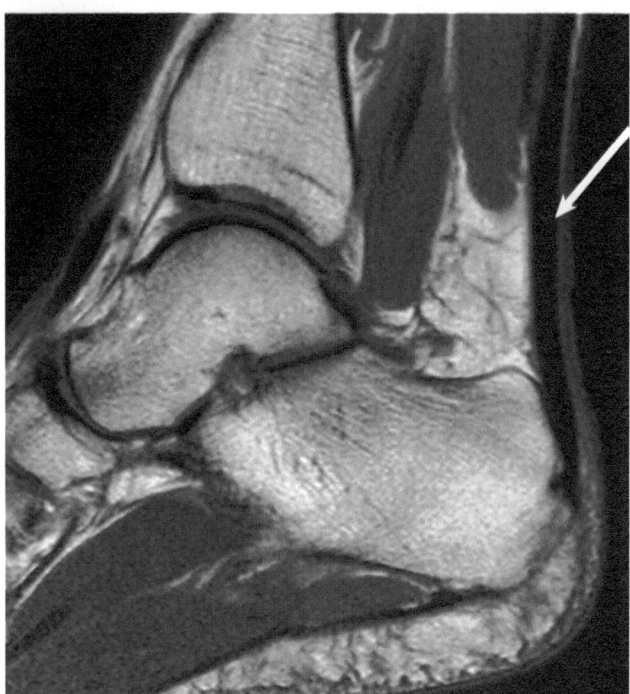

Fig. 112.5 A T1-weighted image of a normal Achilles tendon. Note the uniform thickness and the low signal intensity of the tendon *(arrow)*. (From Joos D, Tran N, Kadakia AR. Achilles tendon disorders. In: Miller MD, Sanders TG, eds. *Presentation, Imaging and Treatment of Common Musculoskeletal Conditions*. Philadelphia: Elsevier; 2011.)

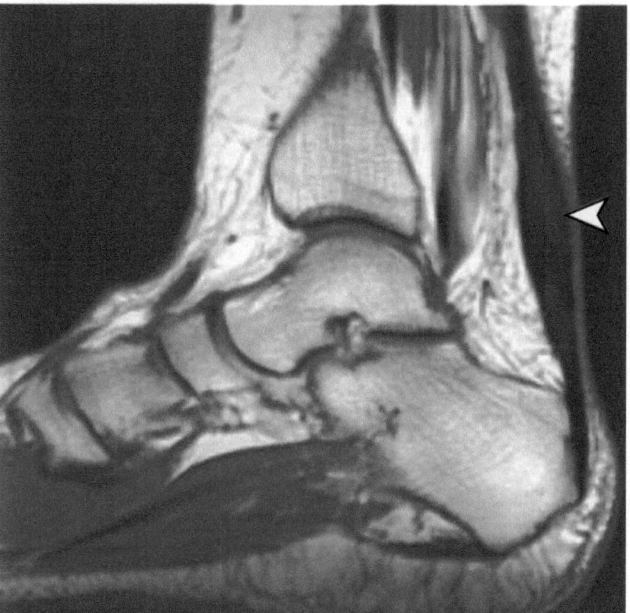

Fig. 112.6 A T1-weighted magnetic resonance image of a patient with noninsertional Achilles tendinosis. Note the intermediate signal intensity and fusiform thickening of the tendon *(arrowhead)*. (From Joos D, Tran N, Kadakia AR. Achilles tendon disorders. In: Miller MD, Sanders TG, eds. *Presentation, Imaging and Treatment of Common Musculoskeletal Conditions*. Philadelphia: Elsevier; 2011.)

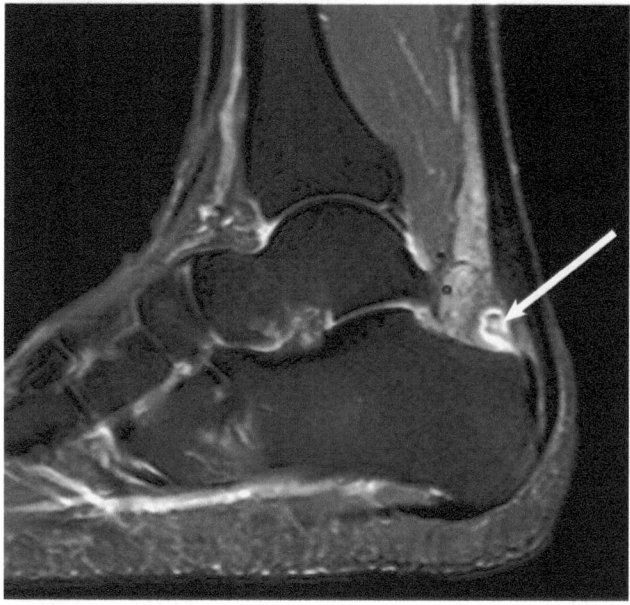

Fig. 112.7 A T2-weighted fat-saturated image with a teardrop high signal intensity immediately anterior to the Achilles at the level of the calcaneus is consistent with retrocalcaneal bursitis *(arrow)*. (From Joos D, Tran N, Kadakia AR. Achilles tendon disorders. In: Miller MD, Sanders TG, eds. *Presentation, Imaging and Treatment of Common Musculoskeletal Conditions*. Philadelphia: Elsevier; 2011.)

is very useful to determine if adequate apposition is obtained with plantar flexion of the ankle after the cast has been placed as an alternative to ultrasonography.

Normal Appearance

The primary evaluation of the Achilles tendon is performed with use of a combination of T1- and T2-weighted axial and sagittal images. The tendon has a near uniform thickness and flattens out distally as it inserts into the calcaneus. The tendon should be taut and parallel when comparing the anterior and posterior margins of the tendon (Fig. 112.5). A flat or concave anterior margin is normal. The normal anteroposterior diameter on axial or sagittal imaging is 7 mm.

Direct Magnetic Resonance Imaging Signs of Disease

Intermediate or high signal intensity on either a T1- or T2-weighted image with continuity of the tendon is indicative of Achilles tendinopathy. Fusiform thickening of the tendon noted on T1-weighted sagittal imaging is diagnostic of Achilles tendinosis (Fig. 112.6). High signal intensity on a T2-weighted image that is as bright as fluid is suggestive of a more acute process and is sometimes referred to as a "partial tear." Calcification of the Achilles insertion is easily visualized on T1-weighted sagittal images and is diagnostic of insertional Achilles tendinopathy. A teardrop fluid signal (high intensity) anterior to the Achilles tendon at the level of the calcaneus is suggestive of retrocalcaneal bursitis (Fig. 112.7). Fluid signal (high intensity) posterior to the Achilles tendon itself is suggestive of retro Achilles bursitis. A fluid signal defect (high intensity) within the Achilles

tendon on both T1- and T2-weighted fat-saturated images is indicative of an acute rupture (Fig. 112.8).

Indirect Magnetic Resonance Imaging Signs of Disease

High signal intensity on T1- or T2-weighted fat-saturated imaging of the Kager fat pad is suggestive of paratenonitis. A wavy or

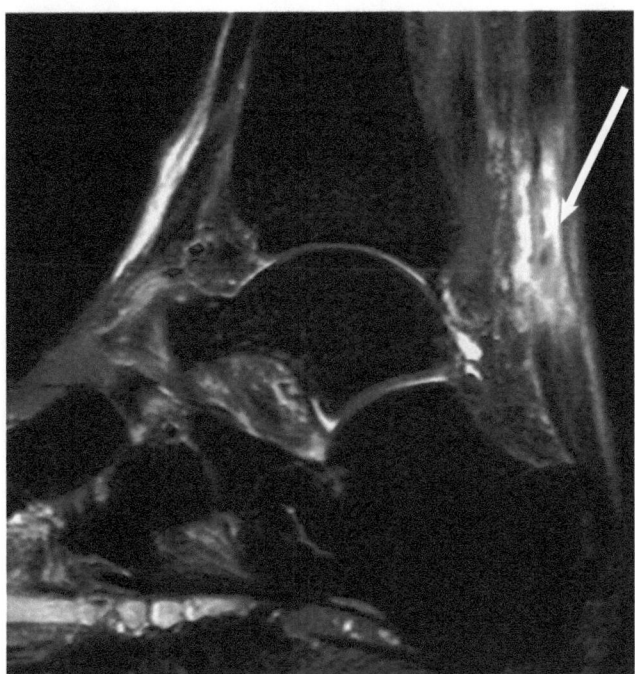

Fig. 112.8 A T2-weighted magnetic resonance image of an acute Achilles rupture. Note the high signal intensity *(arrow)* that completely disrupts the low signal of the Achilles tendon. (From Joos D, Tran N, Kadakia AR. Achilles tendon disorders. In: Miller MD, Sanders TG, eds. *Presentation, Imaging and Treatment of Common Musculoskeletal Conditions.* Philadelphia: Elsevier; 2011.)

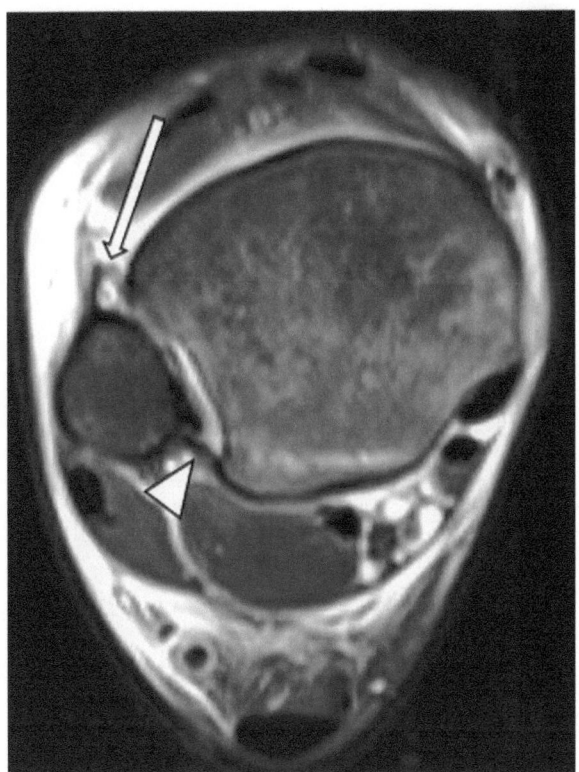

Fig. 112.9 A T2-weighted magnetic resonance image of acute syndesmotic injury. Anteroinferior tibiofibular ligament *(arrow)* is disrupted with surrounding high signal intensity. Posteroinferior tibiofibular ligament *(arrowhead)* is intact with associated nondisplaced posterior distal tibial fracture signifying a high-grade syndesmotic injury. (From Joos D, Sabb B, Tran NK, et al. Acute ankle ligament injuries. In: Miller MD, Sanders TG, eds. *Presentation, Imaging and Treatment of Common Musculoskeletal Conditions.* Philadelphia: Elsevier; 2011.)

retracted appearance of the tendon on T1- or T2-weighted fat-saturated imaging is highly suggestive of an Achilles rupture.

Pitfalls

A small amount of increased signal intensity near the insertion of the Achilles tendon represents interposed fat and is normal; it should not be confused with insertional tendinosis. The plantaris tendon can be intact in the presence of an Achilles rupture and should not be confused with a partial tear or intact Achilles tendon.

Posterior Tibial Tendon

Routine use of advanced imaging to determine of the presence of posterior tibial tendon disease is not required. Given the associated flatfoot deformity and subcutaneous position of the tendon, physical examination plays the major role in the diagnosis. However, in cases of suspected tenosynovitis or posttraumatic or sudden-onset flatfoot, and in patients in whom possible debridement and retention of the tendon is being considered, MRI is an excellent adjunct. Isolated debridement and retention of the tendon is typically considered only in the setting of tenosynovitis without intrinsic disease. In the setting of tendinosis, retention of the posterior tibial tendon with an associated tendon transfer will improve the postoperative inversion strength but carries the risk of persistent pain and should be performed with caution.

Magnetic Resonance Imaging

Normal appearance. Axial cuts are the most useful in evaluating the posterior tibial tendon. Ideally the patient should be positioned prone with the foot plantar flexed to place the tendons in a more linear position and reduce the "magic angle" effect. The posterior tibial tendon should be of uniform thickness throughout its length (Fig. 112.9).

Direct magnetic resonance imaging signs. The presence of fluid (high signal intensity) adjacent to the posterior tibial tendon on T2-weighted imaging is sensitive for tenosynovitis (Fig. 112.10). This finding is not specific and is seen in 22% of asymptomatic persons. A focal area of increased signal on T2-weighted images, known as a *punctate signal*, corresponds to a small intrasubstance tear. A focal area of increased signal intensity within the substance of the tendon that extends to the tendon surface on T1-weighted imaging and corresponding high signal intensity on T2-weighted imaging is consistent with a tear.[5] Complete absence of the posterior tibial tendon or replacement of the normal tendon location with high signal intensity on T2-weighted imaging indicates a rupture. Replacement or infiltration of the normally low signal intensity of the tendon with intermediate (gray) signal is consistent with tendinosis (Fig. 112.11). A small tendon caliber (smaller diameter than the flexor digitorum longus) is consistent with atrophic tendinosis and can be seen on any axial imaging sequence.

Indirect magnetic resonance imaging signs. Periretinacular soft tissue edema and thickening of the flexor retinaculum on

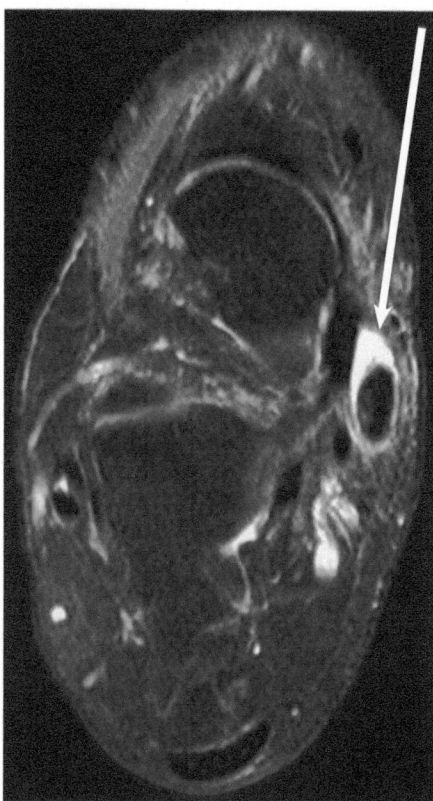

Fig. 112.10 An axial T2-weighted image of a patient with tenosynovitis of the posterior tibial tendon. Note the high signal intensity *(fluid)* adjacent to the tendon *(arrow)*. (From Joos D, Kadakia AR. Flexor tendon disorders. In: Miller MD, Sanders TG, eds. *Presentation, Imaging and Treatment of Common Musculoskeletal Conditions*. Philadelphia: Elsevier; 2011.)

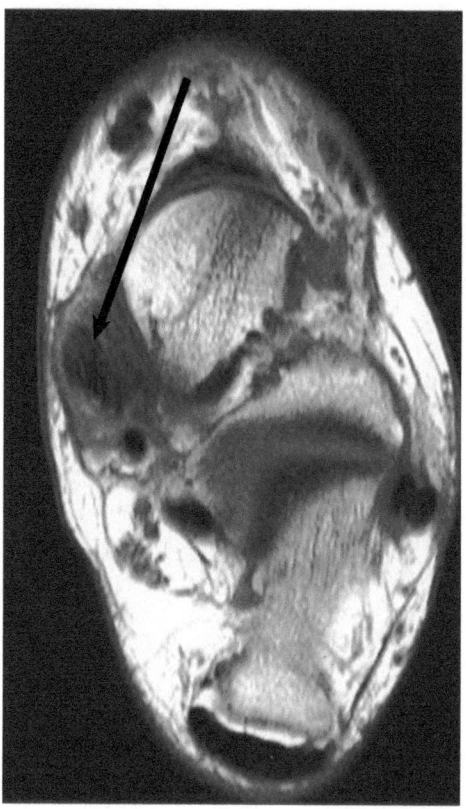

Fig. 112.11 An axial T1-weighted image with infiltration of the normally low signal intensity of the posterior tibial tendon with intermediate *(gray)* signal *(arrow)*. (From Joos D, Kadakia AR. Flexor tendon disorders. In: Miller MD, Sanders TG, eds. *Presentation, Imaging and Treatment of Common Musculoskeletal Conditions*. Philadelphia: Elsevier; 2011.)

any imaging sequence is suggestive of disease. Soft tissue edema adjacent to the flexor retinaculum can be seen on T2-weighted imaging. High signal intensity within the medial malleolus without a prior history of trauma may also be seen. High signal intensity noted on T2-weighted imaging within the accessory navicular can be present.

Pitfalls

A small amount of fluid within the tendon sheath can be normal; correlation with intrasubstance increased signal intensity is more specific for tendon disease.

Flexor Hallucis Longus

FHL tendinopathy has classically been described as a disorder in female ballet dancers, in whom constant ankle hyper plantar flexion can cause FHL irritation at its entrance to the flexor retinaculum. Recently it has been noted to affect other patients with chronic foot or ankle pain who often initially were diagnosed with other foot or ankle pathologic conditions. Ultrasound can be effective in determining the presence of dynamic entrapment of the FHL within the fibro-osseous tunnel. MRI is also particularly useful to evaluate for synovitis, the extent of tendon degeneration, and edema within the os trigonum, which can be associated with this condition.

Magnetic Resonance Imaging

Normal appearance. Sagittal cuts are a useful adjunct when evaluating the FHL as it passes under the sustentaculum tali to the forefoot. Ideally the patient should be positioned prone with the foot plantar flexed to place the tendons in a more linear position and reduce the "magic angle" effect. The tendon has a very low-lying muscle belly that is normally present at the level of the ankle.

Direct magnetic resonance imaging signs. MRI findings of tendinosis as outlined previously, with increased signal intensity within the tendon or tears of the tendon, are rarely seen in the FHL. The presence of fluid (high signal intensity) on T2-weighted imaging is diagnostic of FHL tenosynovitis. The most common location is posterior to the talus within the fibro-osseous tunnel (Fig. 112.12). However, it can also occur in the midfoot at the knot of Henry or distally at the level of the first metatarsophalangeal joint as it passes between the sesamoids. Careful inspection of the entire length of the FHL should be performed from the ankle to the insertion into the distal phalanx because compression can occur in the ankle, midfoot, and forefoot. The presence of fluid proximal and distal to the tendon at the level of the fibro-osseous tunnel posteriorly is diagnostic of stenosing tenosynovitis.[6] The severe compression limits the fluid from entering the tunnel.

Indirect magnetic resonance imaging signs. High signal intensity within the os trigonum on T2-weighted imaging should

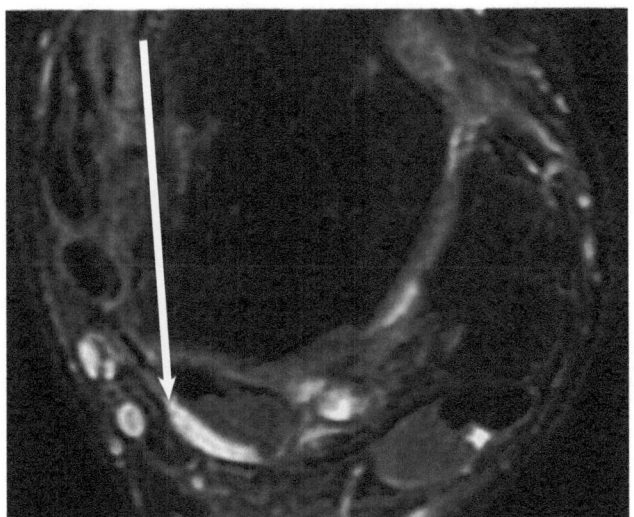

Fig. 112.12 An axial T2-weighted image with high signal intensity *(arrow)* adjacent to the flexor hallucis longus at the posterior aspect of the talus. (From Joos D, Kadakia AR. Flexor tendon disorders. In: Miller MD, Sanders TG, eds. *Presentation, Imaging and Treatment of Common Musculoskeletal Conditions.* Philadelphia: Elsevier; 2011.)

prompt close inspection of the FHL because both FHL synovitis and os trigonum syndrome can occur simultaneously.

Pitfalls

Failure to inspect the entire length of the tendon can lead one to miss the less common but symptomatic compression of the FHL within the knot of Henry and sesamoid complex.

Peroneal Tendons

Intrinsic disorders of the peroneal tendons include tenosynovitis, tendinosis, tendon tears, and painful os peroneum syndrome. Additionally, symptomatic subluxation or intrasheath subluxation may be present, producing pain in addition to instability. Chronic subluxation of the tendons increases the risk of developing degenerative tears of the tendons as a result of the mechanical trauma from the posterolateral fibrocartilaginous ridge of the fibula. Ultrasound can be a very effective tool for examination of the peroneal tendons, specifically in the setting of intrasheath subluxation, where subjective "snapping" may be the only appreciable finding. MRI is very useful when considering operative intervention to determine the presence of synovitis, tendinosis, tears, a low-lying muscle belly of the brevis, and a peroneus quartus, in addition to visualizing the concavity of the fibular groove.

Magnetic Resonance Imaging

Normal appearance. The primary evaluation of the peroneal tendons is performed using a combination of T1- and T2-weighted axial images. The peroneus quartus is a normal muscle variant encountered in 13% to 26% of patients. It will appear as a third tendon within the peroneal tendon sheath (Fig. 112.13). The common insertion is the calcaneus, although multiple variants have been noted. A flat or convex fibular groove is associated with peroneal tendon disorders, but a flat groove is seen in more than two thirds of normal persons.

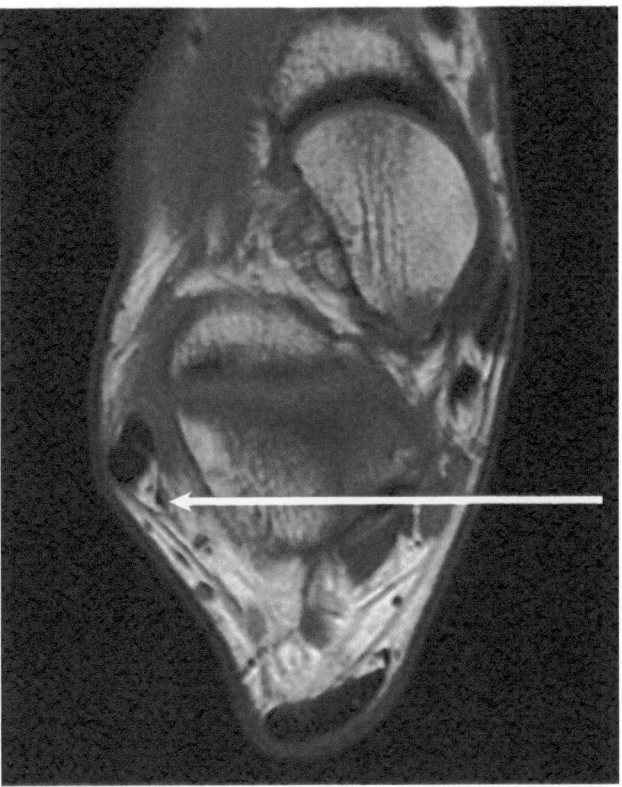

Fig. 112.13 A T1-weighted axial image of the ankle highlighting the presence of a peroneus quartus *(arrow).* The tendon is a small-caliber low signal intensity structure located posterior within the peroneal retinaculum. Proximally the tendon has its own muscle belly and typically will insert on the calcaneus. (From Joos D, Kadakia AR. Peroneal tendon disorders. In: Miller MD, Sanders TG, eds. *Presentation, Imaging and Treatment of Common Musculoskeletal Conditions.* Philadelphia: Elsevier; 2011.)

Direct magnetic resonance imaging signs. As measured on axial imaging, abnormal thickening of the peroneal tendon is noted if the tendon has a larger diameter than the posterior tibial tendon. Intermediate signal intensity within the peroneal tendons noted on three consecutive T1-weighted proton density–weighted images is 92% sensitive for the detection of clinically relevant peroneal tendon disorders (Fig. 112.14).[7] Fluid within the peroneal tendon sheath noted on T2-weighted imaging is a nonspecific finding that can be seen commonly in asymptomatic persons. However, the presence of circumferential fluid within the peroneal tendon sheath of greater than 3 mm in width is highly suggestive of clinically relevant peroneal tenosynovitis. The presence of a bisected or split peroneus brevis on either T1- or T2-weighted imaging is diagnostic of a tear (Fig. 112.15). A split that does not extend across the full width of the tendon is a partial tear.

Indirect magnetic resonance imaging signs. Irregular contour of the tendons on either T1- or T2-weighted imaging is suggestive of a peroneal tendon tear. The presence of a "C-shaped" peroneus brevis with the arms extending posteriorly around the peroneus longus is consistent with a tear. Thickening or attenuation of the lateral collateral ligaments warrants careful examination of the peroneal tendons because the two conditions commonly coexist. A peroneal tubercle that is greater than 5 mm

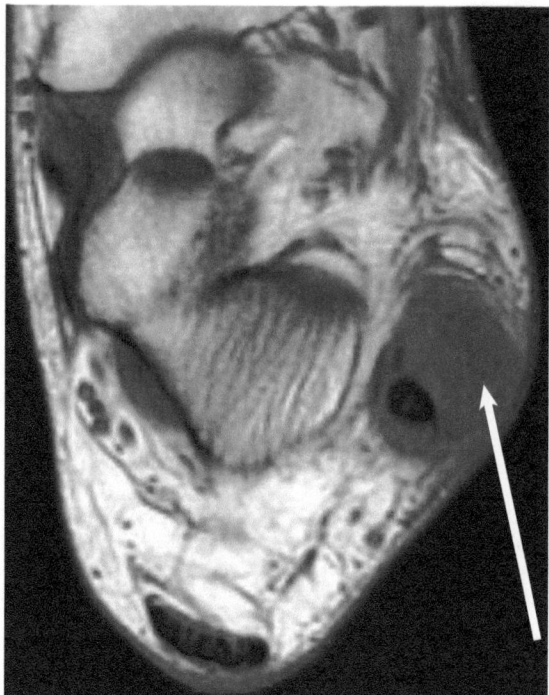

Fig. 112.14 A T1-weighted axial image with intermediate signal intensity in the location of the peroneus brevis. This finding was noted on multiple axial images, consistent with severe tendinosis of the peroneus brevis *(arrow)*. Obvious thickening of the tendon is also noted. The normal peroneus longus is noted posterior to the pathologic brevis. (From Joos D, Kadakia AR. Peroneal tendon disorders. In: Miller MD, Sanders TG, eds. *Presentation, Imaging and Treatment of Common Musculoskeletal Conditions.* Philadelphia: Elsevier; 2011.)

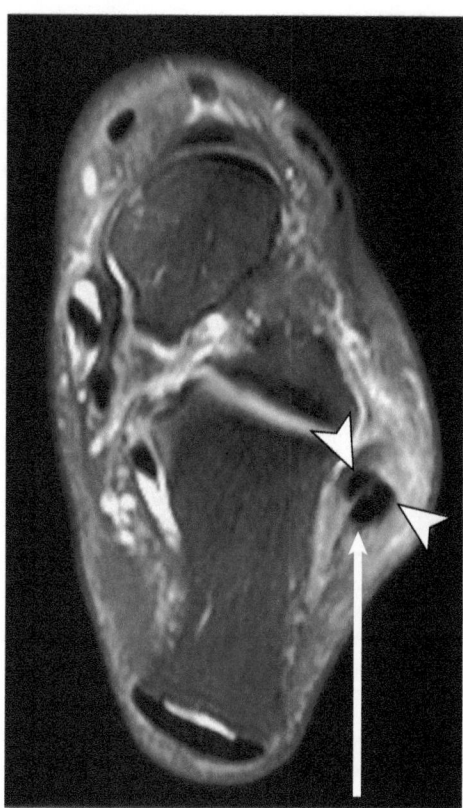

Fig. 112.15 A T2-weighted axial image of a longitudinal split tear of the brevis *(arrowheads)*. The normal peroneus longus *(arrow)* lies posterior to the split brevis. (From Joos D, Kadakia AR. Peroneal tendon disorders. In: Miller MD, Sanders TG, eds. *Presentation, Imaging and Treatment of Common Musculoskeletal Conditions.* Philadelphia: Elsevier; 2011.)

is an uncommon finding in normal persons and can be associated with peroneus longus synovitis and rupture. A "low-lying" muscle belly of the peroneus brevis is associated with peroneal tendon disease. Although the muscle belly can extend to the tip of the fibula in one third of normal persons, it rarely extends 1 cm past the fibular tip.

Pitfalls

Increased fluid signal within the tendons can be noted as they course around the distal fibula and is termed the *magic angle phenomenon*.[8] This signal is normal and should not be confused with a pathologic finding. The presence of intermediate signal intensity or fluid is a very common finding in healthy persons. MRI alone is specific for the diagnosis of peroneal tendon disease and must be used only as an adjunct with a good clinical examination to prevent misdiagnosis. The presence of a peroneus quartus should not be mistaken as a split tear of the peroneal tendons. The tendon has its own muscle mass, and the tendon structure of the longus and the brevis will be normal. Bifurcated or trifurcated tendon slips can be differentiated from a tear by the presence of the slip within the muscle proximal to the ankle joint.

Anterior Tibial Tendon

MRI and dynamic ultrasound are the two most common imaging studies used to confirm the diagnosis of a rupture of the tendon. MRI is excellent to determine the extent of disease in a patient

with insertional tendinosis. If the clinical situation is obvious based on the history and physical examination, further imaging is not necessary. However, if surgical intervention is planned, these studies are useful for preoperative planning.

Magnetic Resonance Imaging

Direct magnetic resonance imaging signs. Discontinuity of the tendon is consistent with a complete tear of the tendon (Fig. 112.16). Intermediate signal intensity within an extensor tendon noted on consecutive T1-weighted proton density–weighted images with an increased tendon diameter is sensitive for tendinosis (Fig. 112.17).[9] Tendon thickness of greater than 5 mm within the distal 3 cm of the anterior tibial tendon is 94% sensitive in the diagnosis of tendinosis. Increased signal intensity on both T1- and T2-weighted imaging without discontinuity of the tendon is diagnostic of a partial tear.[9]

Indirect magnetic resonance imaging signs. Dorsal osteophyte formation along the midfoot or hindfoot can be associated with an attritional anterior tibial tendon tear.

Pitfalls

Review of only T1-weighted imaging may lead to a misdiagnosis of a ganglion as tendinosis, because it will appear as intermediate signal intensity. This appearance is easily differentiated from tendinosis on T2-weighted imaging by the high signal intensity (fluid) of the ganglion that is not seen with tendinosis.

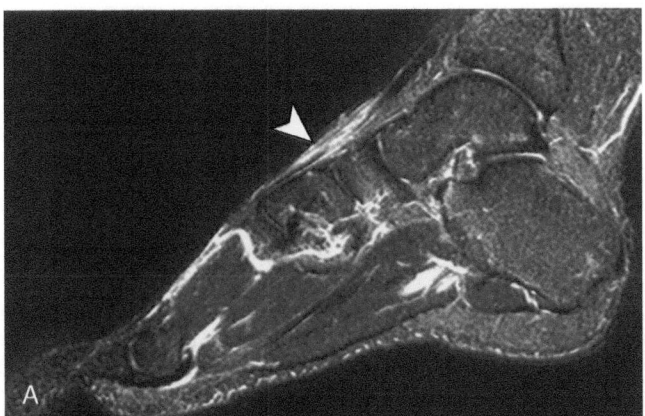

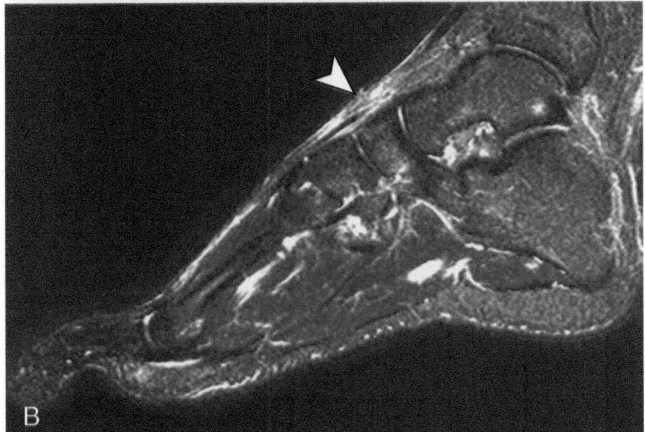

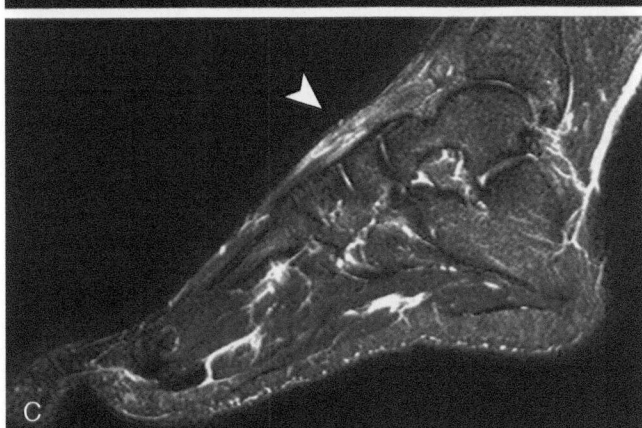

Fig. 112.16 Three consecutive sagittal T2-weighted images in a patient with a laceration of the extensor hallucis longus *(EHL)*. The EHL distal stump is identified (A, *arrowhead*). (B) The site of rupture *(arrowhead)*; note the rounding off of the cut edge. (C) Edema *(arrowhead)* and lack of the tendon that has retracted proximally. (From Joos D, Kadakia AR. Extensor tendon disorders. In: Miller MD, Sanders TG, eds. *Presentation, Imaging and Treatment of Common Musculoskeletal Conditions.* Philadelphia: Elsevier; 2011.)

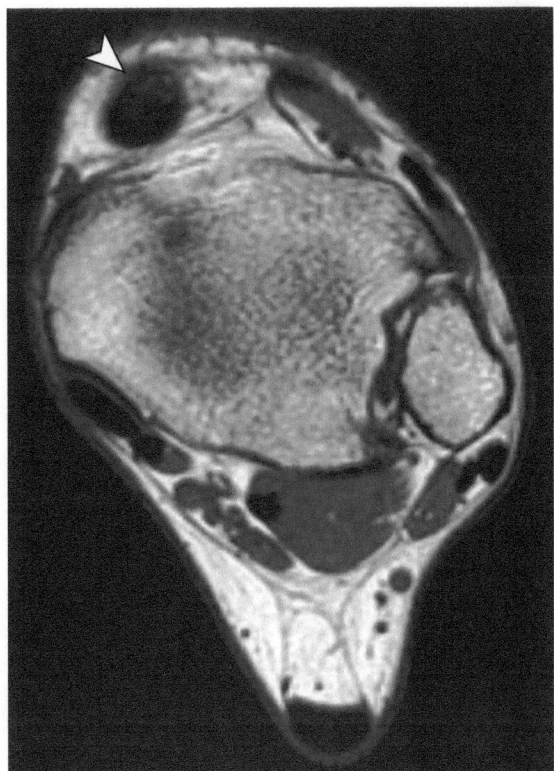

Fig. 112.17 An axial T1-weighted image of a patient with severe tendinosis of the anterior tibial tendon *(arrowhead)*. The tendon is thickened with significant intermediate signal present that is obliterating the normal architecture of the tendon. (From Joos D, Kadakia AR. Extensor tendon disorders. In: Miller MD, Sanders TG, eds. *Presentation, Imaging and Treatment of Common Musculoskeletal Conditions.* Philadelphia: Elsevier; 2011.)

IMAGING OF LIGAMENTS

Magnetic Resonance Imaging

Normal Appearance

The ankle ligaments are uniformly low in signal intensity on all imaging sequences. The anterior talofibular ligament is best seen in the axial plane on proton density and proton density fat-saturated images as a thin linear structure (Fig. 112.18). The calcaneofibular ligament (CFL) is well visualized in the axial and coronal planes. The syndesmotic ligaments are best seen in the axial plane. The deltoid ligament is best seen in coronal plane.

Direct Magnetic Resonance Imaging Signs

Acute ligamentous injuries are classified by MRI as grade I, II, or III. Grade I injuries will demonstrate edema (but not discrete fluid) around the ligament. Grade II injuries will have increased signal within the ligament, consistent with a partial-thickness tear. Fluid can also be present around the ligament. In the setting of a grade III injury, complete disruption of the ligament will be noted by the absence or discontinuity of the ligament. Avulsion fractures may be seen at the site of ligament insertion.

Remote or chronic ligament injuries, sprains, and tears have characteristic appearances on MRI. The previously injured ligament may be increased in signal, wavy, thickened, and attenuated or absent (see Figs. 112.7 and 112.8).[10] Typically no soft tissue edema surrounds the remotely torn ligament, which helps one distinguish between an acute and chronic injury.

Not only is MRI accurate at evaluating the ankle ligaments, but it can also help rule out or occasionally rule in other pathologic conditions. Osteochondral lesions of the talus (OLTs) and syndesmotic injuries can be difficult to distinguish from post-sprain instability. MRI is quick to identify most of these confounding processes.

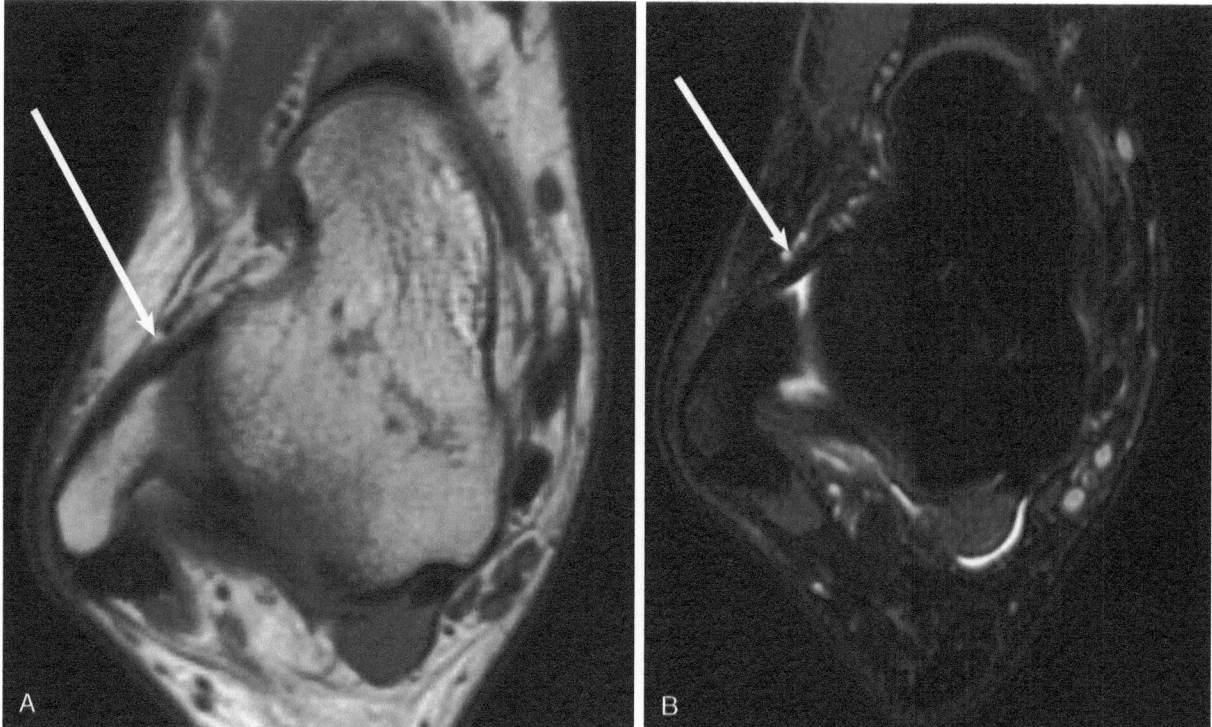

Fig. 112.18 Axial T1-weighted (A) and T2-weighted fat-saturated (B) images demonstrating the anterior talofibular ligament *(arrow)*. The ligament is low in signal intensity, of uniform thickness, and taut. (From Joos D, Sabb B, Tran NK, et al. Acute ankle ligament injuries. In: Miller MD, Sanders TG, eds. *Presentation, Imaging and Treatment of Common Musculoskeletal Conditions.* Philadelphia: Elsevier; 2011.)

Acute syndesmotic injury will demonstrate high signal intensity on T2-weighted imaging around or in the ligament with possibility of ligament disruption. Presence of high signal on T2-weighted imaging at origin of posterior inferior tibiofibular ligament indicates high-grade injury. Chronic injury may demonstrate wavy or curved ligamentous disruption with the possibility of irregular thickening without high signal intensity on T2-weighted imaging.

Indirect Magnetic Resonance Imaging Signs

Indirect syndesmotic injury may be noted by a linear fluid signal 1.25 cm/1.5 cm on T2-weighted fat-saturated images consistent with injury. This finding is not pathognomonic but is highly suggestive in the setting of trauma. The presence of an ankle effusion, especially when joint fluid leaks out of the joint capsule, is indicative of a tear of the anterior talofibular ligament. Bone marrow edema of the distal fibula or talar insertion of the anterior talofibular ligament can be present. Bone marrow edema of the medial malleolus and talar insertion of the deltoid ligament may also be seen.

Pitfalls

Fluid in the peroneal tendon sheath can be a secondary sign of CFL injury; however, peroneal tenosynovitis can incite surrounding edema (peritendinitis) and result in the appearance of a CFL sprain (a pseudosprain of the CFL). A couple of important exceptions exist to the rule that the ligaments are dark on all conventional MRI sequences. In particular, the deltoid ligament and the posterior talofibular ligament are usually intermediate to bright on T2-weighted fat-saturated images. This normal appearance can be misinterpreted as an acute or chronic ligament

sprain. Meniscoid lesions can be easily overlooked on imaging studies. One must be vigilant and systematic in the evaluation of the imaging to correctly establish this diagnosis by imaging. The lesion can be a source of pain for the patient and should be debrided if surgical intervention is performed.

OSTEOCHONDRAL LESIONS

OLTs may be visualized on plain radiographs as a result of an associated fracture of the subchondral bone or a cystic defect. However, these findings are not universally present and thus in cases of chronic injuries with mechanical symptoms, such as locking or giving way, or a feeling of instability of the ankle joint, in addition to pain and persistent swelling, MRI is the imaging modality of choice to visualize the articular surface and subchondral bone. However, caution is necessary because the presence of abnormal findings on MRI, especially within the medial talar dome, may not be the causative factor for the patient's complaint. Combining the information from the history and physical examination along with the MRI findings is critical prior to recommending surgical intervention for an OLT.

Magnetic Resonance Imaging
Normal Appearance

The talus is normally bright on T1-weighted images and is dark on the T2-weighted fat-saturated images. Because the cartilage of the talus is thin, it is sometimes difficult to see on conventional MRI sequences. However, when an osteochondral lesion is present, the effect on the subchondral bone is very apparent. MRI allows multiplanar imaging of the talus for localization and

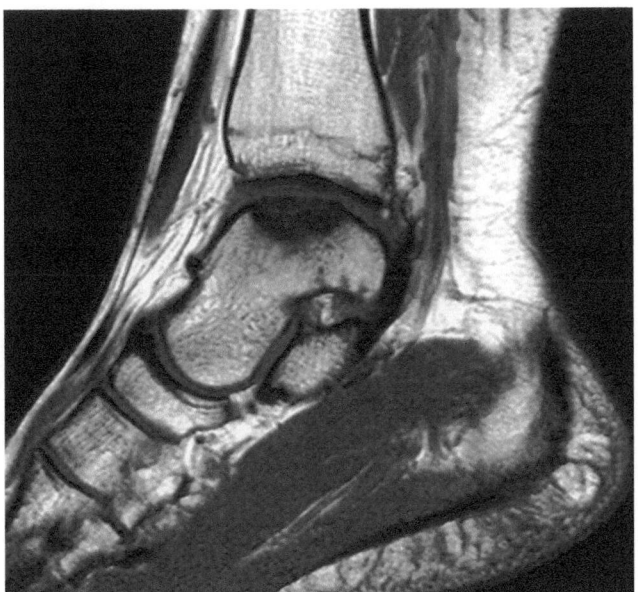

Fig. 112.19 Sagittal magnetic resonance imaging demonstrating the most common central location of osteochondral lesions. The lesion has the typical dark appearance on T1-weighted imaging. (From Joos D, Sabb B, Kadakia AR. Osteochondral lesions. In: Miller MD, Sanders TG, eds. *Presentation, Imaging and Treatment of Common Musculoskeletal Conditions*. Philadelphia: Elsevier; 2011.)

characterization of OLTs. MRI has been proven itself sensitive and specific in the diagnosis of OLTs.

Direct Magnetic Resonance Imaging Signs

The lesions can be located anywhere in the talar dome (but most often in the lateral or medial aspect of the talus, in its midportion from anterior to posterior; Fig. 112.19). The lesions are typically dark on T1-weighted images and variable on T2-weighted fat-saturated images. Signs of instability include fluid undercutting the lesion, a cystic lesion, or a high-intensity T2-weighted fat-saturated signal at the interface between the lesion and the underlying talus and partial or complete separation of the fragment from its normal location (Fig. 112.20).[11] Cystic lesions appear as a bright fluid-filled area beneath the subchondral bone on T2-weighted imaging.

Indirect Magnetic Resonance Imaging Signs

Intra-articular bodies must be scrutinized, and one would have to assess for talar dome donor sites. One of earliest signs of OLT is decreased T1-weighted signal, often without significant increased T2-weighted fat-saturated signal or any cartilage defect.[11]

Pitfalls

Early OLT may only appear as low T1-weighted signal intensity and should not be confused with posttraumatic edema or early osteoarthritis (OA). OA can also result in osteochondral abnormalities in the talus. This process is separate and occurs by a different mechanism. One pitfall is to have a patient with OA mistakenly diagnosed as having OLT; the treatment of osteochondral lesions in OA is not the same as the treatment of OLT in a younger nonarthritic patient. One way to help make the distinction is to evaluate the joint for overall changes of OA, including osteophyte, joint space narrowing, and changes of the associated tibial plafond.

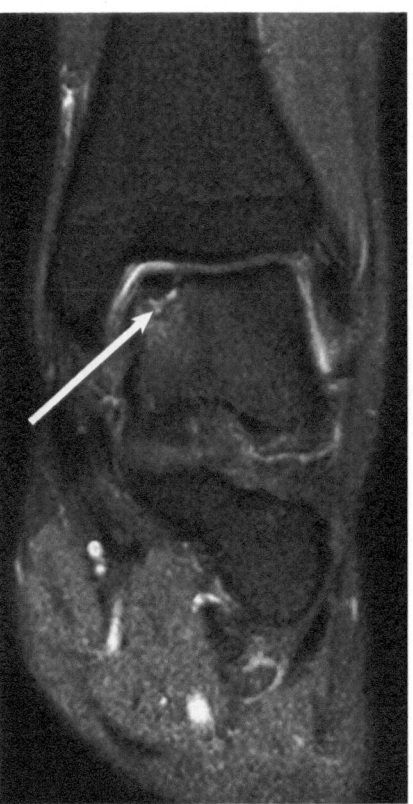

Fig. 112.20 A patient with an unstable osteochondral lesion of the talus. The bright fluid undercutting the lesion is well visualized on the fluid-sensitive T2-weighted fat-saturated image *(arrow)*. Fluid interposing between the osteochondral lesion of the talus and the talus is an excellent indicator of instability. (From Joos D, Sabb B, Kadakia AR. Osteochondral lesions. In: Miller MD, Sanders TG, eds. *Presentation, Imaging and Treatment of Common Musculoskeletal Conditions*. Philadelphia: Elsevier; 2011.)

NERVE ENTRAPMENT

Entrapment or compression of the peripheral nerves at the foot and ankle are common and often unrecognized causes of pain and disability. These disorders are diagnosed primarily by clinical examination and adjunctive nerve testing if such testing is believed appropriate. The use of ultrasound has been advocated by some authors in the diagnosis and as a localizing aid for injection of Morton neuromas. The primary role of MRI in the treatment of nerve compression disorders is to rule out a mass-occupying lesion, most commonly in the setting of suspected tarsal tunnel. Routine use of MRI in the evaluation of nerve disorders is not advocated.

Magnetic Resonance Imaging: Interdigital Nerve
Normal Appearance
The nerve should appear circular and less than 3 mm in width.

Direct Magnetic Resonance Imaging Signs
Coronal T1-weighted imaging is most useful for evaluation of the presence of a Morton neuroma. Use of contrast-enhanced T2-weighted imaging can be used to ensure that the mass is a neuroma, differentiating it from other lesions. The neuroma should appear as an ovoid or dumbbell-shaped plantar mass (inferior to the intermetatarsal ligament) between the metatarsal heads (Fig. 112.21). Neuromas will appear with low to

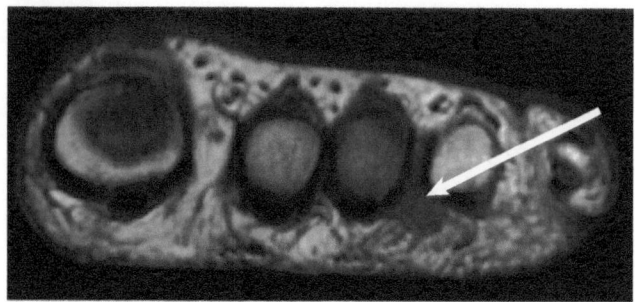

Fig. 112.21 A coronal T1-weighted image of a Morton neuroma *(arrow)*. Note that the neuroma is pear shaped and is plantar to the intermetatarsal ligament. (From Seybold J, Kadakia AR. Nerve entrapment syndromes. In: Miller MD, Sanders TG, eds. *Presentation, Imaging and Treatment of Common Musculoskeletal Conditions.* Philadelphia: Elsevier; 2011.)

intermediate signal intensity on T1- and T2-weighted imaging. Although MRI can aid in the diagnosis of a neuroma, the sensitivity has been reported as 76% to 87% with surgical confirmation as the gold standard. Surgically confirmed neuromas have been shown to have a high association with widths greater than 5 mm.

Indirect Magnetic Resonance Imaging Signs
The neuroma must be visualized directly to be diagnosed.

Pitfalls
Intermetatarsal bursitis is differentiated from a neuroma by its small size (<3 mm) and high signal intensity on T2-weighted imaging, consistent with fluid.

Magnetic Resonance Imaging: Tarsal Tunnel
Normal Appearance
The normal appearance of the tarsal tunnel should demonstrate the contents of the tarsal tunnel without any evidence of a mass-occupying lesion. The normal contents of the tarsal tunnel will be noted with a thin overlying flexor retinaculum. Axial imaging provides the most information (Fig. 112.22).

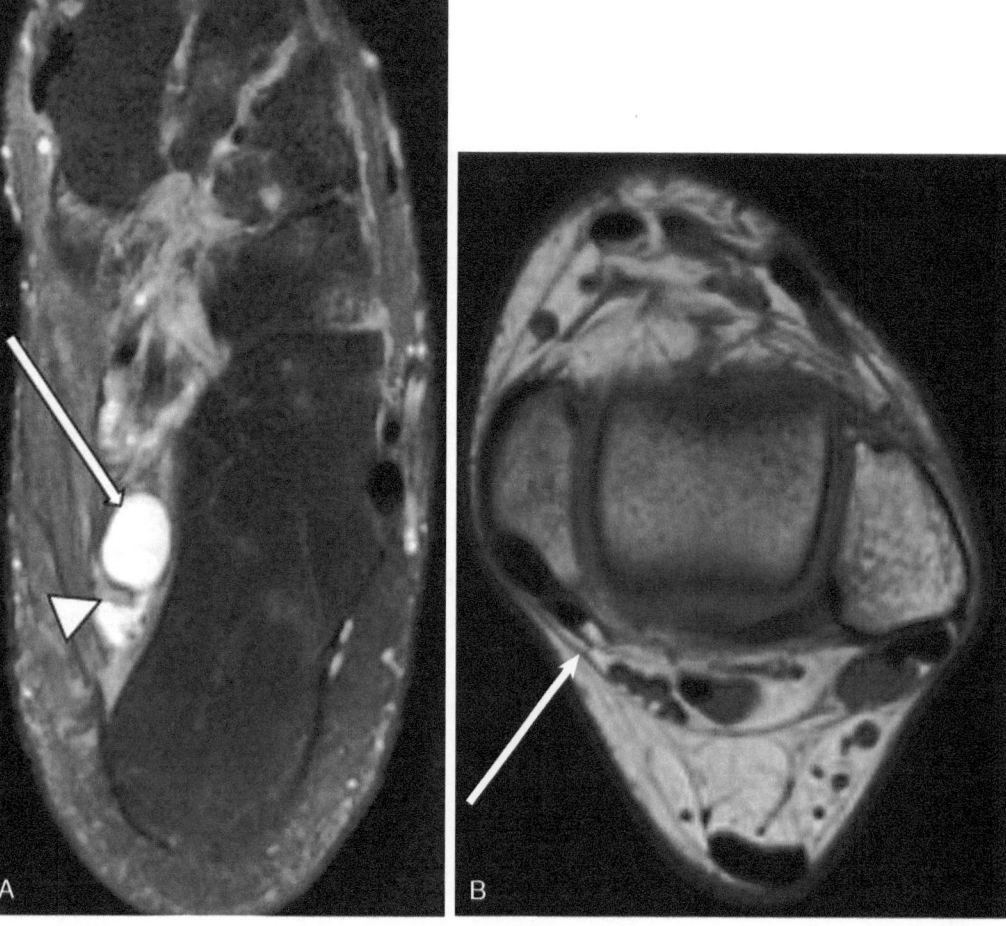

Fig. 112.22 (A) T2-weighted fat-saturated image of ganglion cyst *(arrow)* in tarsal tunnel compressing tibial nerve *(arrowhead)*. (B) An axial T1-weighted image of a normal tarsal tunnel. The flexor retinaculum can be visualized *(arrow)* as a thin hypoechoic band. The contents of the tarsal tunnel are easily visualized without any mass-occupying lesion. (From Seybold J, Kadakia AR. Nerve entrapment syndromes. In: Miller MD, Sanders TG, eds. *Presentation, Imaging and Treatment of Common Musculoskeletal Conditions.* Philadelphia: Elsevier; 2011.)

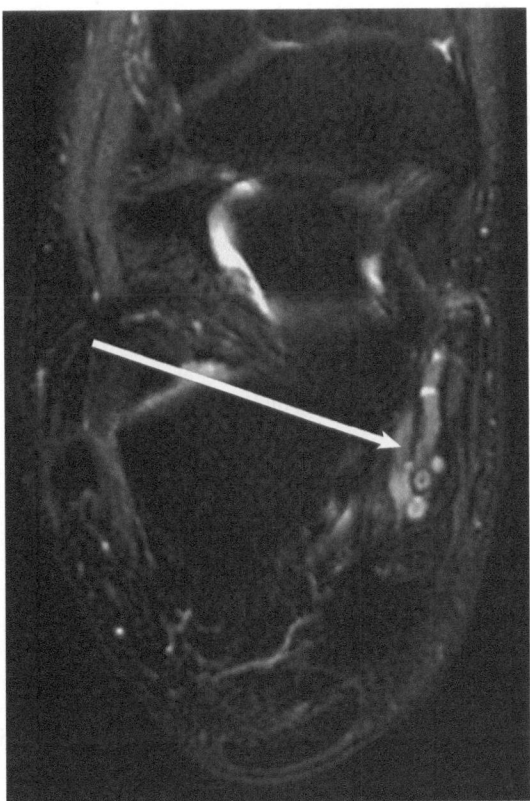

Fig. 112.23 An axial T2-weighted fat-saturated image of venous varicosities *(arrow)* within the tarsal tunnel. These varicosities appear as torturous high signal intensity structures. (From Seybold J, Kadakia AR. Nerve entrapment syndromes. In: Miller MD, Sanders TG, eds. *Presentation, Imaging and Treatment of Common Musculoskeletal Conditions*. Philadelphia: Elsevier; 2011.)

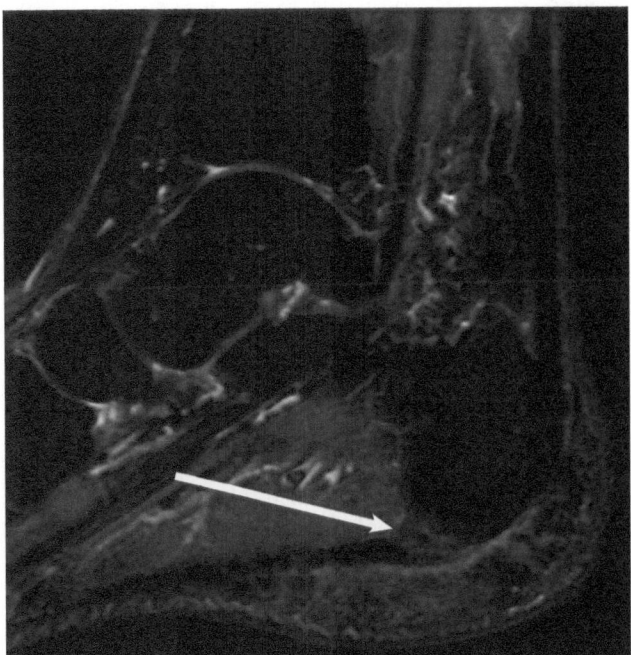

Fig. 112.24 A sagittal T2-weighted image demonstrating increased signal at the origin of the plantar fascia *(arrow)* in a patient with plantar fasciitis. (From Seybold J, Kadakia AR. The plantar fascia. In: Miller MD, Sanders TG, eds. *Presentation, Imaging and Treatment of Common Musculoskeletal Conditions*. Philadelphia: Elsevier; 2011.)

Direct Magnetic Resonance Imaging Signs

The most common MRI finding in the setting of tarsal tunnel is a mass-occupying lesion. These lesions include neurofibrosarcoma, neurilemoma, ganglion (see Fig. 112.22A), hemangioma, venous varicosities or dilated posterior tibial veins (Fig. 112.23), FHL tenosynovitis with fluid within the tendon sheath, and hypertrophy of the abductor hallucis.

Indirect Magnetic Resonance Imaging Signs

Flattening of the tibial nerve suggests tarsal tunnel syndrome, and a mass-occupying lesion should be sought.

PLANTAR FASCIITIS

MRI is not required to obtain the diagnosis of either planar fasciitis or fibromatosis. The primary use is to rule out other conditions such as a calcaneal stress fracture, plantar fascia rupture, neoplasm, and Baxter neuritis.

Magnetic Resonance Imaging
Normal Appearance
Sagittal and coronal imaging is superior for visualization of the plantar fascia. The ligament should appear hypoechoic on all sequences, and the maximum thickness is no greater than 4 mm.

Direct Magnetic Resonance Imaging Signs

Thickening of the plantar fascia (7 to 8 mm) at the insertion is seen with fasciitis. Increased signal intensity at the insertion of the fascia is seen best on T2-weighted or short tau inversion recovery sequences (Fig. 112.24). Plantar fascia rupture is noted by high signal intensity (fluid) at the proximal aspect of the plantar fascia with complete discontinuity from the calcaneal origin. Plantar fibromatosis can be identified by a single or multiple subcutaneous nodules that are not commonly greater than 3 cm in diameter.

Indirect Magnetic Resonance Imaging Signs

Increased signal intensity at the calcaneal insertional site is suggestive of plantar fasciitis, along with surrounding subcutaneous edema. With plantar fibromatosis, no reactive edema is usually noted.

For a complete list of references, go to ExpertConsult.com.

SELECTED READINGS

Citation:
Recht MP, Donley BG. Magnetic resonance imaging of the foot and ankle. *J Am Acad Orthop Surg*. 2001;9:187–199.

Level of Evidence:
V

Summary:
The authors provide an excellent overview of the normal and pathologic findings noted with magnetic resonance imaging of

the foot and ankle. The inclusion of excellent figures aids in the usefulness of this review.

Citation:

Feighan J, Towers J, Conti S. The use of magnetic resonance imaging in posterior tibial tendon dysfunction. *Clin Orthop.* 1999;365:23–38.

Level of Evidence:

III

Summary:

The authors present an excellent review of the appropriate technique and abnormalities noted on magnetic resonance imaging of posterior tibial tendon dysfunction. Supplemental cases provide additional clarification.

Citation:

Lo LD, Schweitzer ME, Fan JK, et al. MRI imaging findings of entrapment of the flexor hallucis longus tendon. *AJR Am J Roentgenol.* 2001;176:1145–1148.

Level of Evidence:

III

Summary:

The authors provide a retrospective review of the variable imaging findings noted in patients with flexor hallucis longus tendon entrapment. The authors provide a thorough discussion of the multiple causes for this disorder and their relevant imaging findings.

Citation:

Kijowski R, De Smet A, Mukharjee R. Magnetic resonance imaging findings in patients with peroneal tendinopathy and peroneal tenosynovitis. *Skeletal Radiol.* 2007;36:105–114.

Level of Evidence:

III

Summary:

The authors of this excellent study compare the magnetic resonance imaging findings of patients who have peroneal disease with the findings of persons who do not have any pathologic abnormality. The authors were able to conclude that intermediate signal was required on three consecutive images to be consistent with disease and that circumferential fluid of greater than 3 mm in maximal width is sensitive for peroneal tenosynovitis.

Citation:

Mengiardi B, Pfirrmann CW, Vienee P, et al. Anterior tibial tendon abnormalities: MR imaging findings. *Radiology.* 2005;235:977–984.

Level of Evidence:

III

Summary:

The authors of this excellent study compare the magnetic resonance imaging findings in patients who have known disease of the anterior tibial tendon with findings in age-matched control subjects. The authors concluded that thickening of greater than or equal to 5 mm and diffuse signal intensity abnormality within 3 cm of the insertion is consistent with anterior tibial tendinosis.

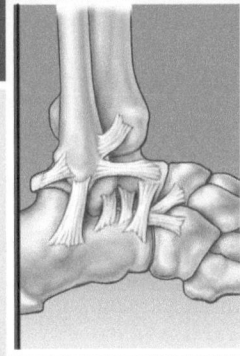

113

Leg Pain and Exertional Compartment Syndromes

Christopher Hogrefe, Michael Terry

Exertional leg pain (ELP) is a common problem encountered in recreational and competitive athletes. Although its incidence in the general population is unknown, ELP is thought to affect between 12.8% and 82.4% of athletes.[1] Specifically, at least 45% of runners will experience such pain, with running more than 40 miles per week serving as a significant risk factor.[2,3] Defined as pain distal to the knee and proximal to the talocrural joint, ELP can be a disabling condition whose specific cause can present a diagnostic challenge to even the most astute physician.[4] One aspect of this conundrum rests in the associated broad differential, which is detailed in Table 113.1. Another difficulty in pinpointing the cause of ELP is that the aforementioned differential components can coexist in the same athlete. Although each of these ELP etiologies is noteworthy, this chapter will focus on the musculoskeletal causes, specifically chronic exertional compartment syndrome (CECS).

Activity-induced compartment syndrome of the leg was first suggested in 1943 when Vogt described "march gangrene."[5] The description of this condition and its association with military training continued to evolve in the 1950s.[5-7] Mavor was the first to detail CECS in sport when he reported the case of a professional soccer player noted to have recurrent anterior leg pain and muscle herniation.[8] This player was treated with a fasciotomy and fascia lata grafting, resulting in complete resolution of his symptoms and a subsequent similar surgery on the other anterior leg. The athlete returned to his previous high level of function without documented complications. Through a review of the current understanding of the anatomy implicated in CECS, patient presentation highlights, optimal diagnostic evaluation, and treatment options, the goal is to return patients to activity just as Mavor reported doing more than 50 years ago.

EPIDEMIOLOGY

The true incidence of ELP is unknown, with reports attempting to address this issue varying widely. This variation likely stems from the difficulty in making a firm diagnosis and the potential for symptom overlap between the numerous causes of ELP. With that said, medial tibial stress syndrome (MTSS) and CECS account for the majority of the cases of exercise-induced leg pain. MTSS is thought to represent between 13.6% and 42.0% of these cases.[9,10] Meanwhile, CECS is reported to account for 14% to 33%.[11-13]

Identifying the typical population affected by CECS can assist in making the diagnosis. This condition is most common in

athletes and individuals involved in repetitive exertional/loading activities. It has been reported that 87% of patients with CECS are involved in sports, with 69% of these cases occurring in runners.[4] On the other hand, it can occur in a wide variety of other sports as well, including basketball, skating, and soccer.[14-16] However, nonathletes can also be affected by this condition. For instance, in one study, 90% of patients without vascular etiologies for ELP were found to have CECS.[17] Men are thought to be affected at the same rate as women, with the mean age of presentation between 26 and 28 years old.[18-20] Detmer et al. reported that in the 100 cases that they assessed the mean time to diagnosis was 22 months. In this population the diagnosis of CECS was present bilaterally in 82 patients.[18] It is worth noting that, although CECS is present in the lower leg 95% of the time, it can also be found in the forearm, thigh, and foot.[21-23]

ANATOMY

There are four muscle compartments in the lower extremity (Fig. 113.1). In addition, the deep posterior compartment may also contain a fifth compartment, which houses only the tibialis posterior.[24] It is important to remember this potential anatomic variation because it can serve as a cause for a delayed diagnosis and/or a failed surgical intervention.[25] Regardless, each compartment is bound by bone and sits within its own investing fascia. In CECS the most common compartment involved is the anterior compartment (45% to 60%), followed by the deep posterior compartment (32% to 60%). In a significant portion of these cases, both the anterior and posterior compartments can be symptomatic simultaneously. The lateral compartment (12% to 35%) and superficial posterior compartment (2% to 20%) are much less likely to be affected.[26-29]

Each compartment (aside from the fifth compartment) contains one or more muscles and one major neurovascular structure (Table 113.2).

There are a couple of noteworthy anatomic considerations herein. As indicated previously, the anterior compartment is most commonly implicated in CECS, likely due to its high vulnerability to injury and relatively limited compartment compliance. Meanwhile, due to the very thin, pliable fascia, the superficial posterior compartment is the least likely to be the source of CECS. Lastly, the superficial peroneal nerve exits the fascia of the lateral compartment adjacent to the intramuscular septum (IMS), approximately 11 cm proximal to the inferior aspect of

TABLE 113.1   Differential Diagnosis of Exertional Leg Pain in Athletes

Musculoskeletal
Medial tibial stress syndrome (MTSS)
Tibial bone stress injury (previously stress fracture)
Chronic exertional compartment syndrome
Muscle strains
Fascial herniation
Tendinopathy
Vascular
Popliteal artery entrapment syndrome
Arterial endofibrosis
Intermittent claudication
Venous insufficiency
Neurologic
Spinal stenosis
Peripheral or central nerve entrapment/impingement
Referred pain from proximal joints (e.g., hip, knee)
Tumor
Infection

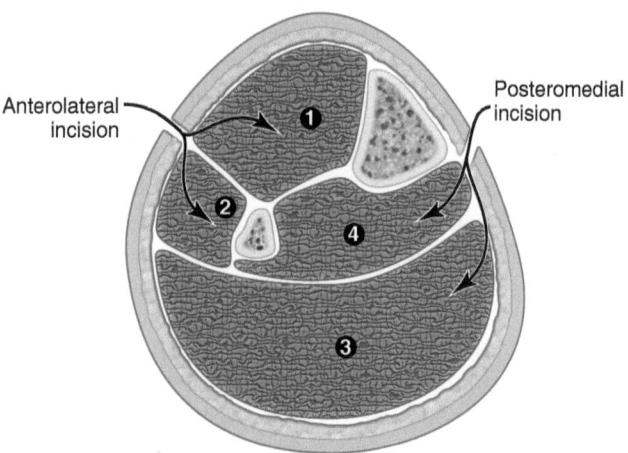

Fig. 113.1 A cross-sectional diagram of the leg demonstrating the compartments and the location for medial and lateral fascial incisions. *1,* Anterior compartment; *2,* lateral compartment; *3,* superficial posterior compartment; *4,* deep posterior compartment

the lateral malleolus. This anatomic landmark is particularly relevant because this is where herniations may occur, resulting in CECS symptoms and/or nerve entrapment.

PATHOPHYSIOLOGY

The pathophysiology resulting in pain attributed to CECS is not known. During exercise, normal muscle will increase by a volume of up to 20%.[30,31] Even in asymptomatic individuals intracompartmental pressures will increase.[32] The increase was initially attributed to thickened compartment fascia with a subsequent decrease in fascial compliance; however, this theory is currently questioned.[33–35] Other potential theories to explain the increase in compartment pressure with exertion include stiff connective tissue, vascular congestion, reduced microcirculatory capacity, and increased muscle mass within a compartment.[17,33,36,37] Furthermore, the rationale for why increased intracompartmental pressures produce pain has not been elucidated. Current speculation includes muscle and/or nerve deoxygenation, direct stimulation of fascial and/or periosteal sensory nerves, or the release of local kinins being the cause.[38–41] Some have even questioned if the increased pressure in CECS is a consequence of the underlying physiologic process rather than the cause of the associated pain.[42]

There are additional factors or associations that may shed light on the pathophysiology of CECS. Anabolic steroids and eccentric exercises induce muscular hypertrophy, increase intracompartmental pressures, and decrease fascial elasticity, all of which may predispose one to developing CECS. Creatine supplements have been shown to increase anterior compartment pressure as well.[43–46] Posttraumatic soft tissue inflammation, myofascial scarring, and venous hypertension all may also contribute to the pathophysiology of CECS.[47] In addition, sympathetic blockade has been shown to reduce the pain of CECS, inferring that there may be some vascular spasm secondary to sympathetic stimulation.[48] Regardless of the cause or mechanism for inciting pain, once the intracompartmental pressure exceeds the ability of the compartment to accommodate the change, pathologic pressure changes occur and result in CECS.

CLASSIFICATION

Compartment syndromes may be classified as either acute or chronic. Acute compartment syndromes represent a surgical

TABLE 113.2   Lower Leg Compartments and Their Respective Components

Anterior	Deep Posterior	Lateral	Superficial Posterior	"Fifth"
Tibialis anterior (M)	Flexor hallucis longus (M)	Peroneus longus (M)	Soleus (M)	Tibialis posterior (M)
Extensor digitorum longus (M)	Flexor digitorum longus (M)	Peroneus brevis (M)	Gastrocnemius (M)	
Extensor hallucis longus (M)	Tibialis posterior (M)	Superficial peroneal (N)	Plantaris (M)	
Peroneus tertius (M)	Popliteus (M)		Tibial artery (branch) (V)	
Anterior tibial artery (V)	Posterior tibial artery (V)		Tibial vein (branch) (V)	
Anterior tibial vein (V)	Posterior tibial vein (V)		Sural (N)	
Deep peroneal (N)	Peroneal artery (V)			**Key:**
	Peroneal vein (V)			Muscles (M)
	Tibial (N)			Vessels (V)
				Nerves (N)

emergency that can lead to devastating injury with loss of function and potentially the loss of a limb. Although the vast majority involve men (91%, with an average age of 32 years old), they are typically associated with trauma (36% involve tibial diaphyseal fractures) or an ischemic event.[49] They have also been described in the setting of exercise (e.g., untrained individuals who initiate a training program), with increases or changes in a training program, or with athletic injuries.[50–52] The immediate management of these injuries involves wide surgical decompression to avoid serious and long-term sequelae.

Conversely, exertional compartment syndromes are less severe. They are symptomatic only during exercise and typically slowly resolve upon stopping the associated activity. Exertional compartment syndromes generally do not require acute surgical decompression. However, they can progress or convert to an acute compartment syndrome.[53]

No classification system has been associated with the diagnosis of CECS. In general, the specific compartments involved are simply described. Of note, there is a high incidence of bilateral involvement, which occurs in up to 82% of cases.[18] With that said, the identical compartments may not be affected in each limb.[54,55]

HISTORY

A key in teasing out the diagnosis of CECS from the larger category of ELP lies in the clinical history. Patients classically describe leg pain that occurs after a specific volume of exertion (i.e., duration, distance, or intensity), often times following a change in training.[11,18] It typically occurs after a stereotypic exercise duration or intensity.[12,56,57] In addition, changes in footwear or training surface have also been implicated.[58] Pain at rest should alert the clinician to search for other causes. And because the vast majority of cases occur bilaterally, unilateral lower leg involvement should prompt the treating physician to consider other causes of ELP and/or biomechanical abnormalities.

The pain is often described as a pressure, fullness, burning, or cramp-like sensation. Sometimes the patient will note a sharpness of the pain with continued activity.[11,18] If the athlete continues to exercise at the same or an increased intensity level, the pain typically progresses. Inevitably, most athletes will not be able to continue at this level of exercise. Occasionally, decreased performance may be reported the day after the symptomatic exercise is performed.[59]

Patients may also complain of paresthesias and in some cases weakness related to compression of the nerve passing through the affected compartment. These symptoms typically occur in a sensorimotor distribution.[59] These key features can often help to differentiate CECS from MTSS and tibial bone stress injury, two other common causes of ELP. However, the astute physician should note that such neurologic symptoms may accompany other causes of ELP, including popliteal artery entrapment syndrome.[24]

An important feature of CECS is that the associated pain abates with decreased intensity, or more likely cessation of the provocative activity. Athletes can often predict the point or intensity at which symptoms will occur. However, over time the necessary recovery time may increase.[60] Symptoms typically return with subsequent exercise sessions that are of similar intensity or duration.[12,56,57] In extreme circumstances when the athlete continues to compete through the pain, acute compartment syndrome and rhabdomyolysis can occur.[50,61]

PHYSICAL EXAMINATION

Unlike MTSS and tibial bone stress injury, the physical examination at rest in CECS is completely normal.[60] For example, there is generally no tenderness to palpation of the lower leg. In such cases, further examination after engaging the athlete in the provocative activity is mandatory. Subsequently, diffuse tenderness to palpation of the affected compartment/muscle group may be present. After exercise, passive stretching of the involved muscle groups may precipitate pain as well.[62] Swelling or increased tissue tension may be detectable. Muscle herniations are not uncommon, especially at the exit site of cutaneous nerves.[63] Lastly, the patient may exhibit neurologic impairments in the sensorimotor nerve distribution of the affected compartment.

Recollection of the nerve distributions and functions can sometimes assist in the diagnosis of CECS. For instance, when the anterior compartment is involved, compression of the deep peroneal nerve can occur. This can result in dysesthesias over the dorsum of the foot (particularly the web space of the great toe), a foot drop, or the sensation of loss of ankle control.[64] When the lateral compartment is affected, there may be weakness of foot eversion and/or loss of sensation over the anterolateral shin and dorsum of the foot. With deep posterior compartment involvement, there may be weakness of the foot muscles and loss or abnormal sensation along the plantar aspect of the foot.

DIAGNOSTICS/IMAGING

If the patient's presentation and physical examination do not clearly point toward CECS, further imaging may be beneficial. One might consider plain films, bone scans, and/or magnetic resonance imaging (MRI) modalities. Because they should be normal in the setting of CECS, the value of these images lies in identifying or excluding other etiologies of ELP (e.g., tibial bone stress injury). In addition, vascular studies may be valuable. An example is ankle-brachial index (ABI) testing with ankle provocation maneuvers, which can assist in ruling in or out popliteal artery entrapment syndrome.[65] Computed tomography (CT) scans with angiography and MRI with or without angiography may be similarly beneficial in this context.

Attempts have been made to identify imaging or other modalities that might verify the diagnosis of CECS. Functional imaging modalities (e.g., thallium scintigraphy, thallium single-photon emission CT, methoxyisobutylisonitrile, ^{99m}Tc-tetrofosmin single-photon emission CT, and functional MRI) have all been studied to assess their utility in this regard but have not been shown to be clinically useful at this juncture.[66] Preliminarily, ultrasound may have a role in aiding with diagnosing CECS. One study showed its efficacy in detecting a significant increase in anterior compartment thickness in CECS. However, more research appears necessary to validate its use.[34] Some studies have demonstrated promise for near-infrared spectroscopy, which can detect decreased tissue oxygenation and delayed reoxygenation postexercise in CECS.[38,67] Early research indicates that this modality may approach the same diagnostic accuracy as intracompartmental pressure testing, but more studies are needed.[67-70] Nerve conduction studies following provocative activity have been assessed for this purpose but are not diagnostic of CECS.[71,72] However, there is a report that an absent extensor digitorum brevis F wave was identified in a patient with anterior compartment CECS.[73] This modality requires further evaluation before it is adopted clinically.

There remains current debate about the utility of the postexertion MRI in diagnosing CECS. Increased T2 signal intensity in the affected compartment that resolves with rest has been appreciated in some studies.[60,74-78] It is thought that the increased signal is secondary to the recruitment of muscle fibers during activity that results in increased interstitial water content, independent of vascular patency (Fig. 113.2).[76] Yet, there are only two studies that have produced a validated technique for diagnosing anterior compartment CECS with MRI.[76,77] Again, more research in this realm is warranted.

DECISION-MAKING PRINCIPLES

Ultimately, CECS, like acute compartment syndrome, continues to be a clinical diagnosis. First described in 1962, intracompartmental pressure testing remains the primary means by which

to further cement a clinical suspicion for CECS.[79] Numerous devices, techniques, and protocols have been used to this end.[80] Studies have monitored pressures at rest and during and after exercise.[47,80,81] However, the difficulty of measuring pressures during exercise makes it impractical in most settings. The most widely cited criterion for the diagnosis of CECS comes from Pedowitz et al.[19] (Table 113.3). Only one of the criteria is necessary to make the diagnosis of CECS. Preexercise pressures greater than 15 mm Hg and 1-minute and 5-minute postexercise pressures greater than 30 mm Hg and 20 mm Hg, respectively, are considered abnormal.

There are at least two literature reviews evaluating studies on compartment pressure testing and the referenced criteria that note important limitations.[47,81] Both reviews point out a general

TABLE 113.3 **Modified Pedowitz Criteria for the Diagnosis of Chronic Exertional Compartment Syndrome via Intracompartmental Pressure Testing**[a]
Preexercise pressure ≥15 mm Hg
1-minute postexercise pressure ≥30 mm Hg
5-minute postexercise pressure ≥20 mm Hg

[a]Only one abnormal measurement is needed to suggest chronic exertional compartment syndrome.

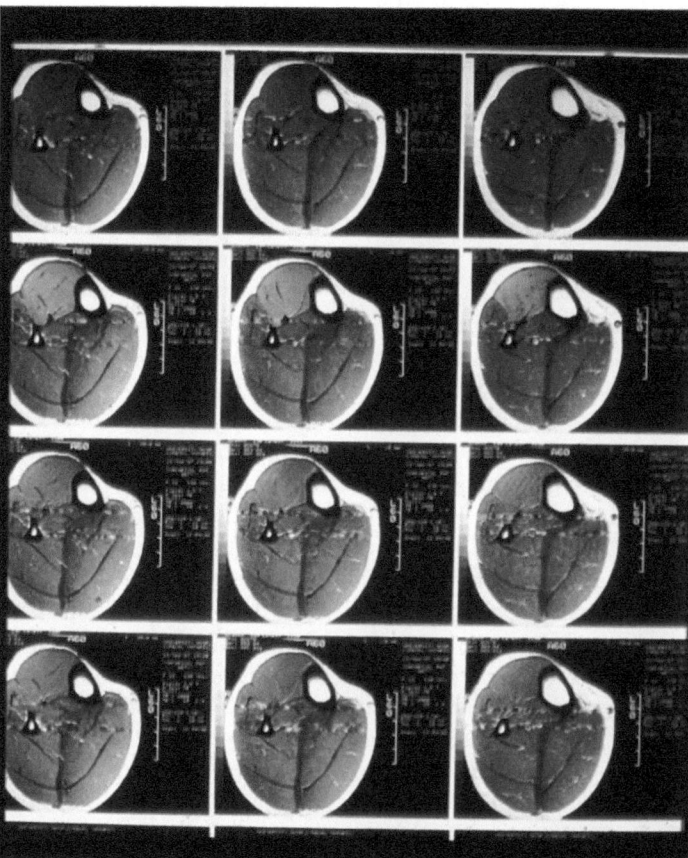

Fig. 113.2 Magnetic resonance imaging findings in a person with chronic exertional compartment syndrome involving the anterior compartment musculature before exercise *(top row)*, 5 minutes after exercise *(second row)*, 10 minutes after exercise *(third row)*, and 15 minutes after exercise *(fourth row)*.

lack of protocol standardization, an absence of validated control groups, and a significant degree of overlap in pressures recorded between control groups and symptomatic groups. Based on a systematic review, Aweid et al. propose that the only time point where there was no significant overlap between the symptomatic and control groups is 1-minute postexercise. At that point, pressures greater than 27.5 mm Hg are highly suggestive of CECS.[47] Recently, it has been suggested that further modifying the Pedowitz criteria may improve the sensitivity and specificity of intracompartmental pressure testing for diagnosing CECS. Roberts et al. report that this could be achieved by lowering the preexercise threshold to 14 mm Hg, increasing the 1-minute postexercise cutoff to 35 mm Hg, and increasing the 5-minute postexercise diagnostic threshold to 23 mm Hg (Table 113.4).[82]

An important related issue with intracompartmental pressure testing is the specific exercise protocol used to secure these values. At this time there is no clear exercise protocol for intracompartmental pressure testing. Some have suggested that patients exercise until the symptoms can no longer be tolerated, at which point postexercise testing should be performed.[83] The lack of standardization of this aspect of the assessment for CECS has called into question the applicability of the criteria established by Pedowitz and colleagues. Specifically, if a patient does not exercise similarly to the participants in the study that generated the criteria it may invalidate the subsequent results.[47,81] More research into this issue is needed moving forward.

COMPARTMENT TESTING

Compartment pressures can be reliably measured using the Stryker Intra-Compartmental Pressure Monitor (STIC; Stryker Orthopaedics, Mawah, NJ). This device has been validated with in vitro models possessing known pressures.[84] The STIC can be used for continuous monitoring but is more commonly used for intermittent monitoring with percutaneous needle penetration into the compartment. Various types of catheters or needles can be used (e.g., wick catheters, slit catheters, side port needles, and straight needles). Although there has been debate as to which of these options provide the most accurate results, evidence suggests that the slit catheter, side port needle, and straight needle all function with similar accuracy.[85] Practically, an international survey found that the side port needle was most commonly used for intracompartmental pressure testing.[47,55]

Currently there is no validated protocol regarding intracompartmental pressure testing, specifically as it pertains to the position, depth, and angle of the needle or catheter used.[47] The following protocol recommendations stem from a combination of the current available evidence on the topic and the authors' preferences.

The patient should be placed supine on a table for the pressure measurements (except the superficial posterior compartment, which should be measured with the patient prone). Positioning the knee at 10 degrees of flexion with the ankle at neutral or slight plantar flexion can help to avoid artificially raising or lowering the compartment pressures.[86] The location for the measurements to be taken should be marked on the skin with indelible ink. To identify the optimal sites of entry, visualize or draw a line around the junction of the proximal and middle thirds of the lower leg. The needle placement can then occur within 3 cm of this line in the appropriate compartment. Further recommendations regarding the optimal entry site, depth of insertion, and means to confirm proper placement can be found in Table 113.5.

Prior to measuring the intracompartmental pressures, the skin should be anesthetized with local anesthetic and prepped in an aseptic fashion. The monitor device should be held horizontally and zeroed before each pressure reading. No standard angle of entry has been agreed upon, but an angle of 45 degrees to the skin is reproducible, minimizes discomfort, and permits a reasonable depth.[80] The compartments can then be tested individually at a needle/catheter insertion depth as suggested previously (see Table 113.5). With each pressure measurement a small amount of fluid is injected and the reading is recorded. Care should be taken not to depress the syringe too quickly because this may create an artificially elevated reading. In addition, avoid pulling back on the syringe while it is inserted, as this may result in a piece of tissue becoming lodged in the needle/catheter. To

---

TABLE 113.4 Proposed Adjustments to the Modified Pedowitz Criteria for the Diagnosis of Chronic Exertional Compartment Syndrome via Intracompartmental Pressure Testing[a]

Preexercise pressure >14 mm Hg
1-minute postexercise pressure >35 mm Hg
5-minute postexercise pressure >23 mm Hg

[a]Only one abnormal measurement is needed to suggest chronic exertional compartment syndrome.

TABLE 113.5 Suggested Compartment Entry Sites and Depths for Intracompartmental Pressure Testing[a]

Compartment	Entry Site	Depth	Confirmed By
Anterior	1 cm lateral to the anterior tibia border	1–3 cm	Plantarflexion or dorsiflexion of the foot
Deep posterior	Posterior to the medial tibia border	2–4 cm	Toe extension Ankle eversion
Lateral	Anterior to the posterior border of the fibula	1–1.5 cm	Foot/ankle inversion
Superficial posterior	3–5 cm on either side of the vertical middle of the calf	2–4 cm	Dorsiflexion of the foot

[a]All points of entry should occur at the junction of the proximal and middle thirds of the lower leg.

further verify the placement of the needle in a given compartment, certain movements can be performed that should increase the pressure reading (see Table 113.5). Consideration should be given to testing both lower legs given the high incidence of bilateral involvement in CECS.

As a related aside, the role and impact of ultrasound guidance in intracompartmental testing has been analyzed. Wiley and colleagues have shown that ultrasound-guided insertion allows for a safe, reliable, and reproducible method for proper needle placement in the deep tibialis posterior compartment.[87] Despite this evidence, it does not appear that ultrasound guidance is necessary for routine deep and superficial posterior leg compartment pressure testing. The accuracy in testing both types of compartments is similar, regardless of the experience of the investigator.[88]

TREATMENT OPTIONS

The treatment of CECS can include either conservative or surgical measures. Among the conservative treatment options is the avoidance of the offending activity or activities that cause pain. Understandably, this option may not be satisfactory for some patients, and in those instances other options should be considered.

The modification of extrinsic factors may be of some benefit. Assessing for possible changes to the training surface, choice of footwear, and/or the training program itself could lead to a decrease in ELP. In addition, nonoperative treatments such as physical therapy, antiinflammatory medications, stretching, and orthotics can be used in the initial management of suspected CECS. Physical therapy, focusing on stretching and strengthening programs, can address potential mechanical factors related to the lower limb and core.

One may also pursue gait modifications to alter the biomechanical forces traveling through the affected compartment.[89] A specific gait modification that has shown some promise is forefoot running. Diebal and colleagues found that such a running technique was effective in treating anterior compartment syndrome. Patients in these studies experienced decreased symptoms and decreased intracompartmental pressures. Also of note, surgical intervention was avoided in these patients.[90,91]

Other nonoperative methods used have included deep tissue massage, myofascial release, and ultrasound. A newer treatment option features the injection botulinum toxin A into the musculature of the involved compartment(s). Reported in two case series, this treatment was shown to be effective in the treatment of anterior and lateral compartment CECS.[92,93] There are (at least) two noteworthy considerations for this potential treatment. First, a reduction of strength was reported in one study, which may limit its applicability in some patients.[93] Second, repeat injections may be necessary because reinnervation takes place over 6 to 9 months following such a treatment.[24]

If the response to the aforementioned conservative measures does not allow the athlete to return to the desired level of activity, operative treatment should be considered. An adequate trial of conservative measures is generally considered to be in the range of 3 to 6 months.[18,26,56,94]

Surgical treatment entails an open or endoscopic fasciotomy, with or without fasciectomy, and resection of any fascial bands. No direct comparison with fasciotomy or between open and endoscopic procedures exists.[95] When a fascial herniation is present it must be included in the release to avoid recurrent symptoms that can occur if neglected. When surgery is pursued, all symptomatic compartments should be addressed with surgical release. Previously, those individuals with anterior symptoms had anterior and lateral compartments released. Schepsis and colleagues found that, in patients with complaints isolated to the anterior compartment, isolated release of the anterior compartment produced results equal to a combined anterior and lateral compartment release.[94] It is now generally accepted that surgical release should be performed only on the symptomatic compartments.

The current trend is for limited incision techniques with a rapid return to weight bearing, motion, and resumption of activity. Initially, success rates were reported to be in the 80% to 90% range.[95–105] However, the success for deep posterior compartment surgical release has been shown to be between 30% and 65%, possibly due to the presence of the fifth compartment and/or the complex nature of this particular surgery.[106] In addition, a more recent study in a military population was less optimistic on the success of surgical fasciotomies for CECS. In this study, 44.7% of patients experienced symptom recurrence and 27.7% of patients were unable to return to full activity.[20] It is worth noting that surgical complication rates have been reported to be as high as 16%.[18,20]

POSTOPERATIVE CARE

Weight bearing is initiated immediately after surgery, with crutches discontinued as tolerated, generally within the first week. Early passive and active range of motion (ROM) exercises are implemented postoperatively immediately.[12,26,56,107] During the first 2 days, patients follow a PRICE (protection, rest, ice, compression, and elevation) protocol, as well as anterior and posterior stretching (toe pointing) three to six times per day. Postoperative compressive dressings should be left in place for the first 2 to 10 days, depending on the extent of swelling. If patients swell without compression, this intervention should be continued. From the third-day to the tenth-day follow-up visit, patients perform aggressive anterior and posterior compartment stretches three times per day and increase their walking distance as tolerated without provoking swelling. Once they are weaned from crutches, nonimpact activities such as hydrotherapy, stationary cycling, and elliptical training are initiated as soon as the wounds are appropriate. Low-impact stationary bicycling, treadmill or track walking, and/or hydrotherapy can be started initially.[108] When strength and control of the ankle and foot are regained, functional training can begin, usually by 3 to 4 weeks. At that point, running may be implemented as tolerated. We govern progression based on swelling. If nonimpact activities are tolerated without swelling, impact can begin. If swelling occurs, nonimpact exercises should be continued until swelling abates. After impact activities are initiated and tolerated, speed and agility drills are added.[12,26,107]

Authors' Preferred Technique

Anterior and Lateral Compartment Release

Single- and double-incision techniques are available to release the anterior and lateral compartments of the leg.[105] We prefer to use a single-incision technique because it is simple. The IMS is usually palpable digitally by placing firm pressure over the anterior lateral leg and moving in a horizontal motion midway between the anterior crest of the tibia and the fibula. A vertical incision is based over the palpated IMS or centered between the anterior tibial crest and the fibula if the IMS is not easily found. This incision should be centered vertically between the fibular head and the lateral malleolus and should extend approximately 3 cm. Soft tissue dissection should then be completed carefully until the fascia is identified and exposed. Once the fascia is exposed, the IMS is usually easily visually and palpably identifiable. After the IMS is identified, the fascia should be bluntly separated from the subcutaneous tissue in the superior and inferior directions. We prefer doing this with blunt mayo or Metzenbaum scissors with the tips pointed toward the fascia and pressure placed downward on the fascia. Run the tips of the scissors along the fascia away from the incision, with the blades closed, and then open them and bring them back toward the incision. After this is completed both superiorly and inferiorly, a small rent should be created in the fascia approximately 5 mm anterior to the IMS. The fascia is then separated from the underlying muscle in a similar fashion but with the tips of the scissors inside the fascia, with the tips facing anterior and with pressure anterior against the fascia. The scissors are advanced along the fascia with the tips closed. The tips are then opened at the end of the desired fasciotomy and brought back towards the opened rent. Once the fascia has been separated from the overlying subcutaneous tissue and the underlying muscle, it is divided superiorly and inferiorly. This is done by opening the tips of the scissors creating a 2 mm gap between the tips. The fascia is placed between the tips at the superior end of the previously created rent in the fascia, and the scissors are pushed proximally to the desired extent of the fasciotomy and then withdrawn. The inferior fascia is opened in a similar fashion, and then the lateral compartment is addressed using the previous steps through a rent created 5 mm posterior to the IMS. It is strongly urged to thoroughly separate the fascia from the underlying and overlying tissue prior to dividing it and to remove the scissors after the fasciotomy without closing the blades. Digital palpation after the fasciotomy can ensure that it was done in a complete fashion. The fasciotomy should extend distally to the superficial extensor retinaculum but not beyond. Superiorly, the lateral compartment release should stop well before the peroneal nerve (if palpable) or 4–5 cm distal to the fibular head (if the nerve is not palpable).

Posterior Compartment Release

We use a single-incision technique for the release of the superficial and deep posterior compartments as well. The incision is located 1–2 cm posterior to the posterior subcutaneous border of the tibia. It is centered at the level of the gastrocnemius musculocutaneous junction and is 3–4 cm long (Fig. 113.3A). The long saphenous nerve and vein are usually in the center of the field and are identified on the posteromedial border of the tibia during soft tissue dissection, which is carefully undertaken down to the level of the fascia. A small vertical incision is created in the fascia adjacent to the tibia after the fascia is separated from the subcutaneous tissue proximally and distally as outlined previously for the anterior and lateral releases. A small incision is made just posterior to the tibia, and the posterior compartment is entered. Separate the fascia from the underlying muscle as outlined previously, and then release the fascia in a similar fashion to what was described for the anterior and lateral compartments. The soleus will be encountered in the proximal one-third of the tibia at the soleus bridge. Complete release of this structure is necessary because it also represents the proximal confluence of the flexor hallucis longus (FHL) and flexor digitorum longus (FDL) fascia. This releases the deep posterior compartment. An elevator can then be used to release the tibialis posterior muscle off the tibia, completing the release of the tibialis posterior from the tibia (see Fig. 113.3B). Remaining on the posterior aspect of the tibia throughout the release ensures safety of the posterior tibial neurovascular bundle, which is posterior to the tibialis posterior and FDL. Digitally palpate the entire compartment to ensure that the release is completed adequately. The gastrocnemius can be identified through the medial incision and proximal to it. This muscle can be released in a similar fashion. Following the releases, the tourniquet is relaxed, if used, and hemostasis is obtained. The subcutaneous tissues and skin are closed and dressed in the preferred fashion, and a compressive dressing is applied.

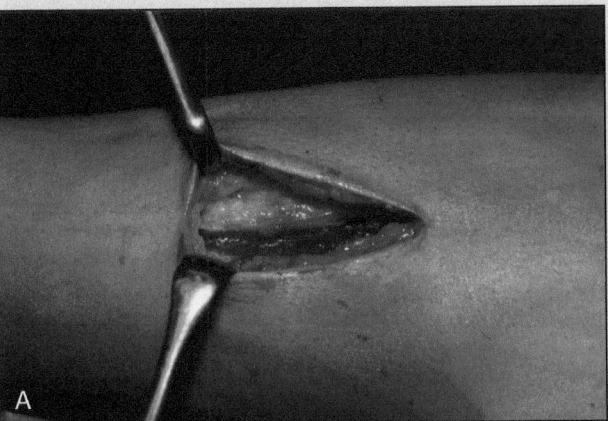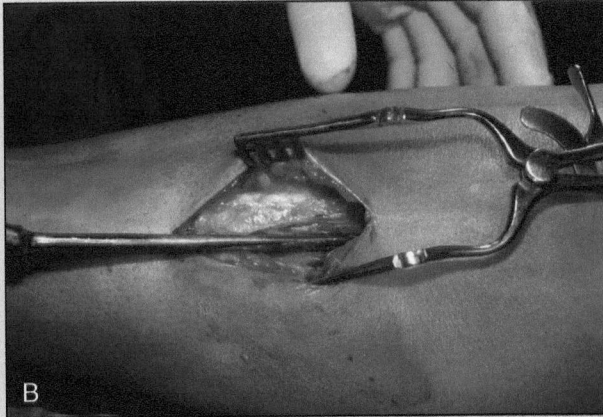

Fig. 113.3 (A and B) Fascial incisions for posterior compartment releases. The muscle fascia is taken directly off the posteromedial border of the tibia.

RETURN TO PLAY

There are no objective criteria for return to play (RTP) following fascial release for CECS. The RTP is based on satisfactory completion of the progression outlined in the preceding section. In summation, the athlete should be nearly pain-free, have demonstrated acceptable strength and endurance, and be able to replicate the demands of practice and play in the therapy sessions without swelling or any neurologic symptoms. A general guideline for full return to athletic activities is 6 to 12 weeks after surgical intervention.

RESULTS

Studies regarding the outcome of the surgical treatment of CECS have shown varying results. Most surgical procedures report a high rate of satisfaction and return to unlimited physical activity, with 60% to 100% rates of relief.[95–105,109–111] Beck et al. looked at pediatric patients with a mean age of 16.4 ± 1.38 years and found an 89.5% rate of return to sport. There was an 18.8% reoperation rate, which was 3.4 times more common if only the anterior and lateral compartments were released.[109] That study was in contrast to a study by Gatenby et al., which evaluated 36 legs in 20 patients in an adult population. This study showed a 90% return to sport, an 8.64 satisfaction rate, a reduction in Visual Analog Scale from 8.17 to 1.74, and a 2.8% conversion to a four-compartment release after a release of only the anterior and/or lateral compartments.[110] Campano et al. performed a meta-analysis of 204 papers and included 24 primary studies in their report. They described successful outcomes in approximately two-thirds of their patients and an 84% satisfaction rate with a 13% complication rate.[111] De Fijter and colleagues reported a 96% return to unlimited exercise in 118 military personnel following a percutaneous fasciotomy, with an average follow-up of 62 months.[99] Raikin and colleagues reported bilateral simultaneous releases in 16 patients; 16 months after surgery 14 patients were pain-free and all returned to sports an average of 10.7 weeks after surgery.[104] Moushine and coworkers detailed 18 consecutive athletes treated with a two-incision fasciotomy technique, all of whom returned to full sporting activity at the 2-year follow-up, with an average return to sporting activity of 25 days.[103]

Howard and colleagues reported slightly less favorable results of 68% pain relief. However, when stratified by compartment, patients treated with an anterior release had 81% relief, whereas a posterior release yielded 50% relief.[101] Slimmon and associates also had less favorable outcomes using a single-incision technique. They reported 60% good or excellent results in patients undergoing a single operation, with 58% of patients exercising at a lower level than before the development of symptoms.[95] Hutchinson and coworkers demonstrated incomplete releases with a single-incision technique, which may account for the less favorable outcomes.[112] Although Schepsis and colleagues found that releasing only the involved compartments versus both the anterior and lateral compartments yielded identical results, the release of both compartments resulted in a delay of return-to-sport by more than 3 weeks, on average (11.4 vs. 8.1

weeks).[97] In conclusion, minimally invasive, percutaneous, and single- and double-incision techniques are all currently used. There is evidence that single-incision techniques yield inferior results compared with double-incision techniques.[95]

Overall, there is a high rate of satisfactory outcome and return to sporting activities with a relatively low complication rate with surgical treatment of CECS. When an accurate diagnosis of CECS has been made, the patient wishes to undergo surgical treatment, and modification of activity is unacceptable, fasciotomy of the affected compartments may be recommended. In this context relative to CECS, excellent results can be achieved if the procedure is performed properly.

COMPLICATIONS

Complications reported have included hematoma or seroma formation (9%), superficial peroneal nerve injury (2%), anterior ankle pain (5%), and recurrence of symptoms (2%).[99] There have been theoretical concerns in the vascular surgery literature regarding the function of muscles and their compartments in the return of fluids in dependent limbs. This, in turn, raised the possibility of venous insufficiency after fascial release. However, there have not been any documented cases to date with clinically significant findings.[113]

Recurrence after fasciotomy for CECS has been reported in several studies. Schepsis and coauthors have described recurrence and subsequent retreatment of exertional compartment syndrome. In this situation, careful dissection, release of nerve entrapment, and fasciectomy are essential, and the results are not as predictable as the primary surgery.[114]

◼ SUMMARY POINTS

The history upon presentation is the key to narrowing the differential diagnosis for patients with ELP. For CECS, the onset of symptoms is consistently reproducible with a similar amount of exercise and is relieved by rest.

Compartment pressure testing can aid in confirming the diagnosis and both preexercise and postexercise criteria exist in this regard. However, CECS remains largely a clinical diagnosis.

A period of 3 to 6 months of conservative treatment (e.g., addressing extrinsic factors, physical therapy, gait modification with forefoot running, and/or botulinum toxin A injections) is recommended prior to pursuing a surgical intervention.

If surgery is performed, single- or double-incision techniques are both widely used.

Dissection between the subcutaneous tissue and fascia is performed bluntly using the fingers or the blunt tips of the dissecting scissors.

Early ROM and weight bearing are encouraged postoperatively to avoid secondary scarring after the fasciotomy. Crutch use is as needed and is generally discontinued after swelling abates.

Specific RTP guidelines for CECS do not exist. A gradual progression of activity, ending in full sport-specific activities, is recommended with a typical postoperative return occurring between 6 and 12 weeks.

For a complete list of references, go to ExpertConsult.com.

SELECTED READINGS

Citation:
Rajasekaran S, Finnoff JT. Exertional leg pain. *Phys Med Rehabil Clin N Am.* 2016;27:91–119.

Level of Evidence:
V

Summary:
This article provides an excellent analysis of the differential for exertional leg pain, including chronic exertional compartment syndrome (CECS). Specifically, the article details the pertinent anatomy of CECS, key historical and physical examination findings, important aspects of making the diagnosis, salient management options, and some of the highlights of the postoperative course.

Citation:
Pedowitz RA, Hargens AR, Mubarak SJ, et al. Modified criteria for the objective diagnosis of chronic compartment syndrome of the leg. *Am J Sports Med.* 1990;18(1):35–40.

Level of Evidence:
III

Summary:
As a retrospective analysis, this study features a review of 131 patients who were referred for evaluation of chronic exertional leg pain. The authors were able to utilize those patient evaluations to develop intramuscular compartment pressure criteria for the purpose of diagnosing CECS. The criteria include pressure measurements before exercise, 1-minute postexercise, and 5-minutes postexercise.

Citation:
Peck E, Finnoff JT, Smith J, et al. Accuracy of palpation-guided and ultrasound-guided needle tip placement into the deep and superficial posterior leg compartments. *Am J Sports Med.* 2011;39(9):1968–1974.

Level of Evidence:
III

Summary:
The intent of this study is to determine if ultrasound-guided superficial and deep compartment needle tip placement is more accurate than a palpation-guided technique. Twenty adult lower limb cadaveric specimen were injected via both palpation and ultrasound guidance, with each technique performed by both a sports medicine fellow and an attending physician. The investigation revealed similar accuracy rates for needle tip placement regardless of the use of ultrasound and/or the level of provider experience.

Citation:
Waterman BR, Laughlin M, Kilcoyne K, et al. Surgical treatment of chronic exertional compartment syndrome of the leg: failure rates and postoperative disability in an active patient population. *J Bone Joint Surg Am.* 2013;95(7):592–596.

Level of Evidence:
IV

Summary:
This study represents the largest known cohort with CECS (611 total patients who underwent 754 elective fasciotomies). The authors sought to assess the outcomes after elective fasciotomy. They report the majority of military personnel in the study returned to active duty (67%), but 44.7% of the soldiers had symptom recurrence. In this analysis 21.8% of individuals experienced unsuccessful surgical management.

Citation:
Winkes MB, Hoogeveen AR, Scheltinga MR. Is surgery effective for deep posterior compartment syndrome of the leg? A systematic review. *Br J Sports Med.* 2014;48(22):1592–1598.

Level of Evidence:
III

Summary:
The authors of this investigation assess seven level III studies to determine the efficacy of surgical interventions for CECS of the deep posterior compartment. The success rates are modest (30% to 65%), and no single surgical procedure appears to be superior. Overall, the conclusion states that the evidence for this intervention is poor, and there is a general need for prospective, controlled or randomized studies to help optimize this surgical procedure.

Citation:
Campano D, Robaina JA, Kusnezov N, et al. Surgical management for chronic exertional compartment syndrome of the leg: a systematic review of the literature. *Arthroscopy.* 2016;32(7):1478–1486.

Level of Evidence:
IV

Summary:
This systematic review features 24 studies and 1596 patients to evaluate the outcomes of surgical management for CECS. Given this information it appears that surgical intervention is successful in approximately two-thirds of young athletes, and 84% of the patients are satisfied with their outcome. The authors could not determine if an open fasciotomy is more efficacious compared to newer endoscopic or other minimally invasive techniques.

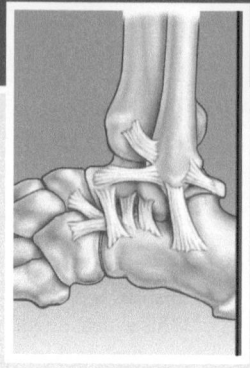

114

Peripheral Nerve Entrapment Around the Foot and Ankle

Norman Espinosa Jr., Georg Klammer

INTRODUCTION

Athletes may suffer from chronic lower limb pain, which could be caused by peripheral nerve entrapment. Compared with other problems of the lower limb, this entity is quite rare, with a heterogeneous group of nerve disorders and multiple, sometimes very complex, etiologies and clinical presentations. Even for a perceptive clinician, distinction between the different medical causes may be difficult, given that many of their presenting features overlap. The difficulty of properly understanding the entire spectrum of peripheral nerve entrapments may lead to mis- or underdiagnosis, with an inherent risk of potential patient mismanagement. This can be frustrating for both the athlete and the treating physician. However, the approach to the problem can be facilitated by means of a structured algorithm. Adequate treatment of peripheral nerve entrapment requires a proper understanding of the anatomic course, the possible causes, precise identification of the involved nerve, and clear determination of location of compression. When adhering to the presented diagnostic rules, an optimal treatment strategy can be formulated, which should always be tailored to the athlete's pathology and needs. The current chapter attempts to provide the reader with an overview of the most important peripheral nerve entrapment syndromes found around the foot and ankle, with specific focus on athletes.

SURAL NERVE ENTRAPMENT

Introduction

Because of its use in reconstructive surgery as a nerve graft, the sural nerve has become a well-investigated peripheral human nerve.[1-5] In 1974 Pringle and coworkers were first to report on the entrapment neuropathy of the sural nerve and its clinical sequelae.[6] This pathology may affect running athletes but also other individuals dedicated to sports[4,7] The sural nerve is purely sensory and provides sensation to the posterolateral part of the distal one third of the leg and the lateral border of the foot, including the lateral aspect of the heel and the fifth toe (Fig. 114.1).[8,9] Communicating branches may expand the region of sensible innervation, extending it up to the third and fourth webspace. Anatomically, in 80% of cases, it arises from the distal union of the medial sural cutaneous branch of the tibial nerve and the peroneal communication branch of the common peroneal nerve. In 20% of individuals, the peroneal communicating

branch is missing.[10,11] In those cases the sural nerve arises as a branch from the medial sural cutaneous nerve. The medial sural nerve runs between the heads of the gastrocnemius muscle and penetrates its deep aponeurosis halfway up the leg. Anatomically the peroneal nerve anastomoses with the sural nerve. The sural nerve progresses down the border of the Achilles tendon. First it runs in midline with the calf; then approximately 10 cm above the calcaneal tuberosity, it crosses the Achilles tendon and is positioned laterally (Fig. 114.2). Then the sural nerve runs approximately 1.5 cm posterior and inferior to the tip of the fibula to end up at the lateral side to the fifth metatarsal.[8]

Sural nerve entrapment may happen anywhere on its course. Common sites include the lateral aspect of the heel or foot.[12] Trauma plays a significant role as risk factor for sural nerve entrapment. Recurrent ankle sprains can cause stretching of the nerve and result in structural damage.[4] General edema after trauma can cause external compression and impair nerve function. In addition, fractures of the base of the fifth metatarsal or ganglions of the peroneal sheaths or calcaneocuboid joint can cause nerve injury.[13-15] Prior surgery at the posterior calf, Achilles tendon repair (especially percutaneous),[15] posterolateral portals of arthroscopy (Fig. 114.3),[16,17] calcaneal osteotomies, ankle ligament reconstructions,[18] peroneal tendon repairs,[19] exposure for subtalar fusion, traction, and any scar are felt to be risk factors resulting in lesion or entrapment of the sural nerve. Less commonly, sural nerve entrapment within the gastrocnemius has been reported in the literature.[20]

History

Patients may note radiating and tingling symptoms. Chronic burning, numbness, paresthesia, or aching along the course of the sural nerve specifically at the posterolateral aspect of the leg may be present, which might worsen during night or with physical activity (e.g., running).

Physical Examination

Occasionally the spot of maximum pain allows identification of entrapment. For this purpose, examination of the entire course of the sural nerve must be performed. Local tenderness and a positive Tinel sign are identified. Inspection for possible scars from previous surgeries is mandatory. Local anesthetic injections at suspected areas help to establish the diagnosis.

S1-S2 nerve root impingement should be evaluated with a thorough lumbosacral assessment. Exertional compartment

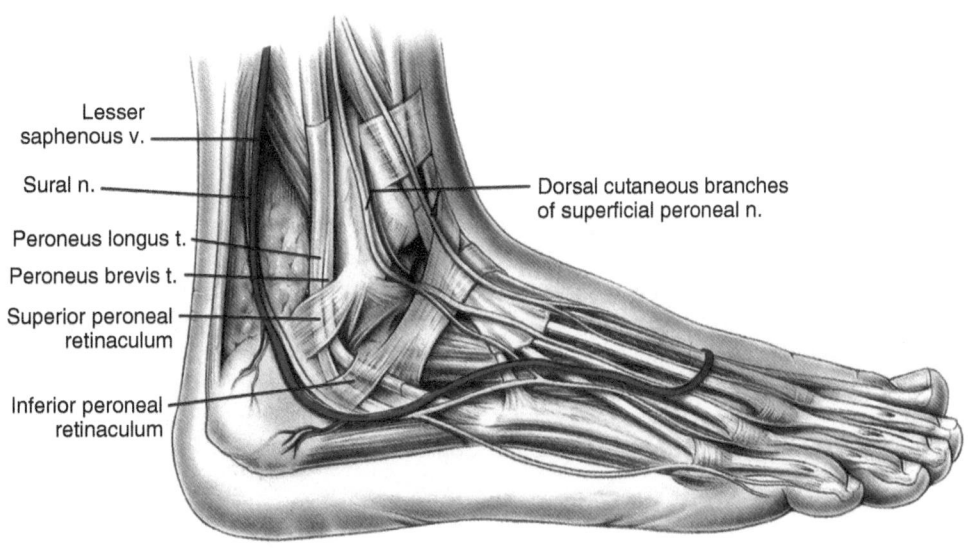

Fig. 114.1 Depicted is an artistic drawing presenting the anatomy of the lateral aspect of the foot and ankle. (From Ferkel RD, Weiss RA. Correlative surgical anatomy. In: Ferkel RD, Whipple TL, eds. *Arthroscopic Surgery. The Foot and Ankle*. Philadelphia/New York: Lippincott-Raven; 1996:90, Fig. 5.7, with permission.)

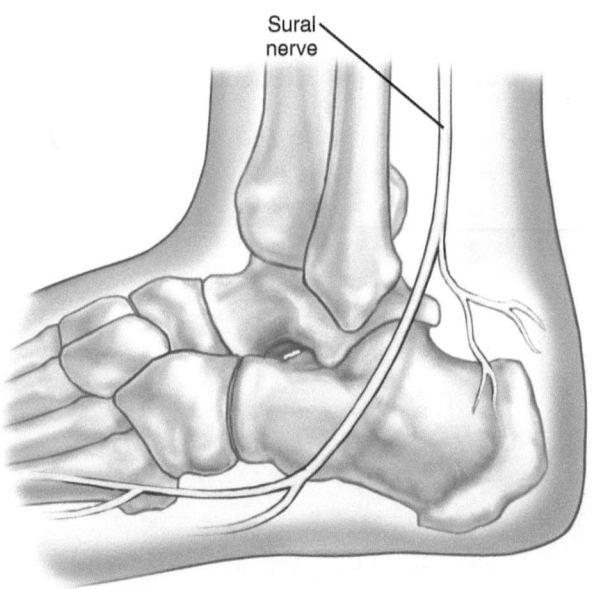

Fig. 114.2 The image shows the course of the sural nerve. For details, see text.

syndrome, popliteal artery entrapment, ankle sprains and Achilles tendon pathology can mimic neural entrapment.[21-23]

Imaging

Plain radiographs may rule out an osseous malformation that can result in compression of the nerve (e.g., hypertrophic callus formations after fracture). Some authors recommend stress views in the presence of hyperlaxity or chronic lateral ankle instability; however, the large variability in tibiotalar and anterior drawer values in both injured and non-injured ankles mitigates their value for routine use.[24] Magnetic resonance imaging (MRI) is

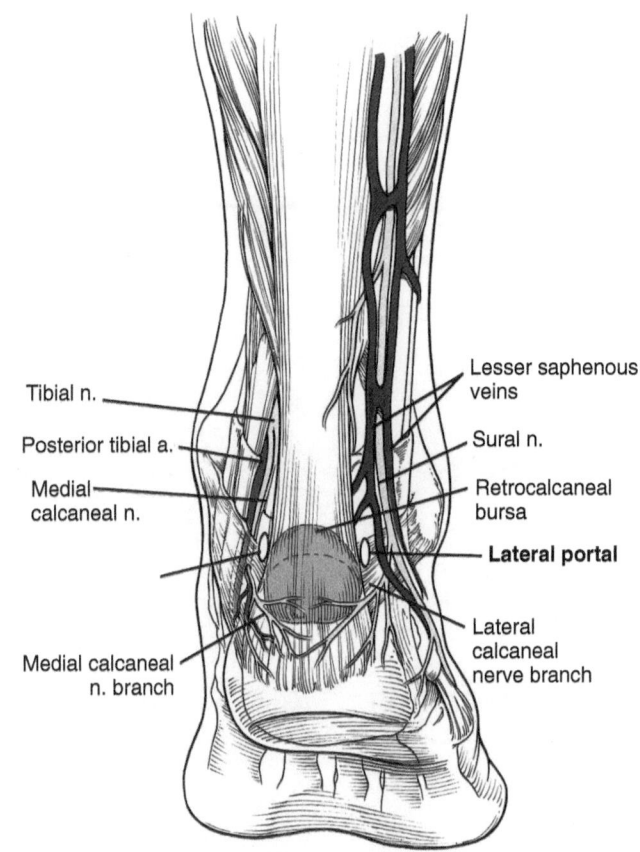

Fig. 114.3 Illustrated is the posterior anatomy of the hindfoot with regard to arthroscopic portals. The sural nerve can be injured when inserting the scope through the posterolateral portal. (From Ferkel RD, Weiss RA. Correlative surgical anatomy. In: Ferkel RD, Whipple TL, eds. *Arthroscopic Surgery. The Foot and Ankle*. Philadelphia/New York: Lippincott-Raven; 1996:314, Fig. 16.9A, with permission.)

useful to evaluate the nerve tissue and to identify a space-occupying mass.[25] Although computed tomography provides less detail in terms of soft tissue contents, it can be a useful adjunct when physical examination suggests an osseous structure is contributing to impingement or compression of a peripheral nerve or neurovascular bundle.[26]

Treatment Options
Conservative Treatment
Conservative measures should be fit according to the underlying pathomechanism. Chronic ankle instability can be addressed by bracing or application of orthotics. When using those measures, it is important to ensure that no external compression applied to the nerve. In case of external compression as, for example, chronic lymphatic edema, this should be treated first.

Isolated sural neuralgia might respond to vitamin B_6, nonsteroidal antiinflammatory drugs (NSAIDs), gabapentin, tricyclic antidepressants, lidocaine patches, and/or topically applied analgesic creams.[4]

Surgical Treatment
Surgical treatment is warranted when conservative measures have failed. The surgical options include sural neurolysis or neurectomy. In case of revision nerve surgery, neurectomy with burial into healthy soft tissues or bone might be preferred rather than pure neurolysis. However, patients must be counseled about the limited results obtained in revision nerve surgery. Incisions vary according to the presence of previous incisions, the location of neuroma or entrapment, and the type of possible additional operation performed.

Authors' Preferred Technique

The patient is placed in the lateral decubitus or prone position. Both positions allow adequate access to the entire course of the sural nerve. A 10 cm skin incision is made over the area of maximum tenderness (which should be assessed prior to surgery without anesthesia). The sural nerve is identified, and the compressive structure released and/or removed. Do not perform excessive soft-tissue resection. Avoid resection of fat away from the sural nerve, as this would lead to excessive scarring and thus to a potential recurrence of entrapment.

When considering neurectomy, the nerve should be identified and dissected further distally and proximally. Then the nerve can either be stripped or transected (Fig. 114.4A to C). The stump can be buried into soft-tissue as, for example, muscle or into bone. Burial into bone can be difficult. To facilitate, two small unicortical drill holes (2.5 mm) are made through the cortex of the bone (e.g., fibula) perpendicular to each other. The nerve stump is inserted into one end of the bone, while a suction is placed into the other drill hole. By so doing, the nerve is drawn into the bone. It is now possible to suture the epineurium onto the periosteum. Ensure that there is no tension on the nerve, while moving the ankle up and down together with simultaneous observation of the structures involved.

The author does not use vein wrapping procedures in case of sural nerve entrapment because of the reasonable results obtained with neurectomy.

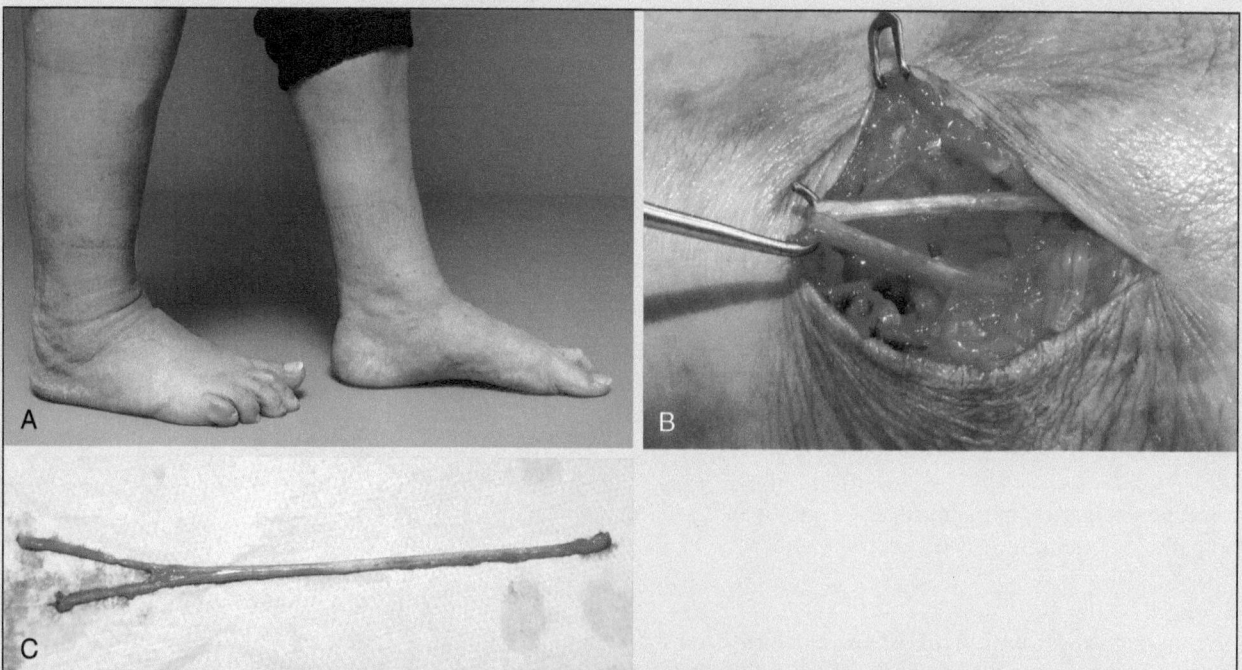

Fig. 114.4 (A) Illustrated is the right foot and leg of a 55-year-old patient who has previously been treated by means of a calcaneal osteotomy. Unfortunately, he developed therapy-refractory pain along the course of the sural nerve. (B) The nerve has been approached over its point of maximum tenderness. Intraoperative findings revealed that the bifurcation has been entrapped and damaged. (C) Intraoperative photograph of the resected sural nerve.

Postoperative Management

The lower limb is put into a cast for 1 week. The cast should be put in neutral position. Walking with crutches is recommended for 1 week. After that time period, gradual resumption of weight bearing in a boot for 3 weeks as tolerated is allowed. Physical therapy, including range of motion (ROM) exercises and wobble-board training, are begun. Full athletic training can be resumed 4 to 6 weeks postoperatively. In case of extensile surgery affecting a joint or including complex osteotomies, a boot should be worn for 4 weeks and training not resumed before 8 weeks postoperatively.

Results

In case of space-occupying lesions, resection yields satisfactory symptomatic relief. Decompression of the sural nerve by ganglia excision with neurolysis could be curative.[7] Posttraumatic bony impingement for sural nerve entrapment can be addressed by restoring anatomy. Gould and Trevino described three cases of fractures of the base of the fifth metatarsal with dorsal displacement of the fracture fragment and tenting of the sural nerve. After reduction of the fracture fragment and neurolysis, all patients improved within several months.[13] In a study performed by Fabre et al., 13 athletes (18 limbs) were treated due to sural nerve entrapment. Nine limbs showed an excellent result, eight limbs a good result, and one limb a fair result at time of follow-up. Ten patients had cessation of calf pain.[7] However, in patients in whom prior surgical scarring or injury was the cause, the results of nerve release are less predictable, and may ultimately require resection and burial despite not having a true neuroma. In the presence of a neuroma, resection of the damaged nerve and burial into healthy tissue (muscle, bone) can improve symptoms. In cases of ankle instability, lateral ankle ligament reconstruction without nerve release could be enough to help the patients reduce pain and discomfort and is reasonable to perform if no neuroma is present.[27]

SAPHENOUS NERVE ENTRAPMENT

Saphenous nerve entrapment is rare.[4] The saphenous nerve is the longest sensory branch of the femoral nerve arising from the L1,2,3 nerve roots. The nerve leaves the femoral triangle to enter the adductor canal (or subsartorial canal of Hunter) together with the femoral artery and vein. The walls of the canal comprise vastus medialis and adductor longus muscle and the membrane of the vastus and adductor bridges the roof. The sartorius muscle covers the proximal portion of the canal and also covers the two terminal branches of the saphenous nerve—the infrapatellar branch and the descending branch. The infrapatellar branch supplies the sensation to the medial portion of the knee joint and the overlying anteromedial skin. The descending branch accompanies the saphenous vein to supply the skin of the medial leg and foot (Figs. 114.5 and 114.6).[10,11,28]

Entrapment occurs at the subsartorial fascia just proximal to the femoral condyle.[29,30] Local trauma can damage the nerve. Harvesting the saphenous vein for cardiac or vascular surgery can potentially lead to damage to the saphenous nerve.[31] Other etiologies include angulation, stretch, pressure, and friction.

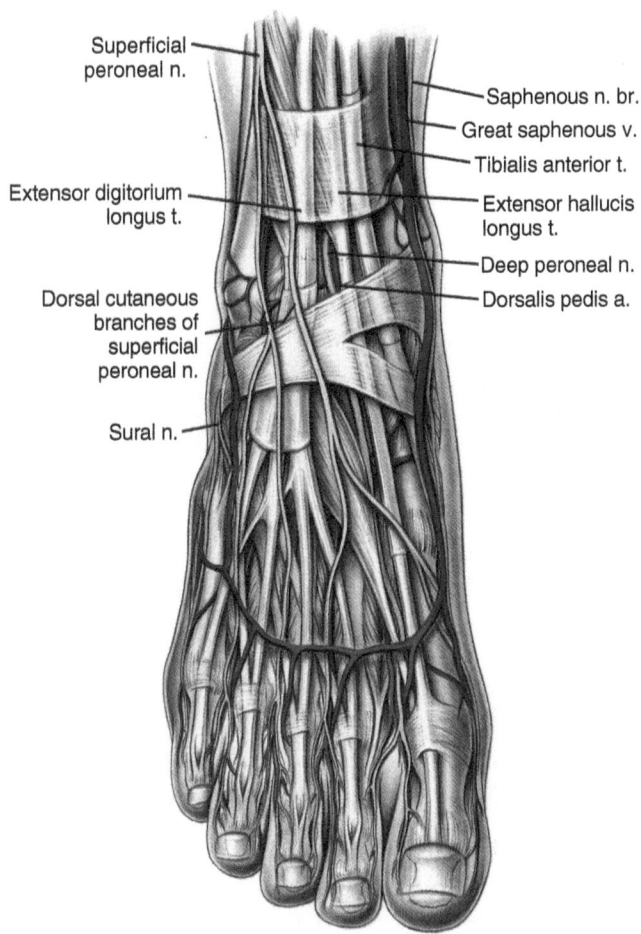

Fig. 114.5 Illustrated is an artistic drawing of the anatomy of the dorsum of the foot. (From Ferkel RD, Weiss RA. Correlative surgical anatomy. In: Ferkel RD, Whipple TL, eds. *Arthroscopic Surgery. The Foot and Ankle.* Philadelphia/New York: Lippincott-Raven; 1996:89, Fig. 5.6, with permission.)

History

Saphenous nerve entrapment can present itself in a variety of different symptoms. As a rule, symptomatology depends on site of entrapment. Proximal involvement of the saphenous nerve, (i.e., the infrapatellar branch) could result in atypical or refractory knee pain.[29] Flexion of the knee joint might worsen the symptoms. Some patients receive incorrect knee treatment by application of a constricting brace due to missed or neglected saphenous nerve entrapment and report pain. Patients may report claudicant or exercise-related medial leg or knee pain. This syndrome has been observed in cyclists and rowers. With distal involvement of the saphenous nerve patients may feel pain, numbness, or paresthesias localized to the medial side of the leg or foot (typically proximal to the first metatarsophalangeal [MTP] joint).

Physical Examination

The nerve should be palpated along its anatomic course starting proximally from the medial condyle of the femur and traced

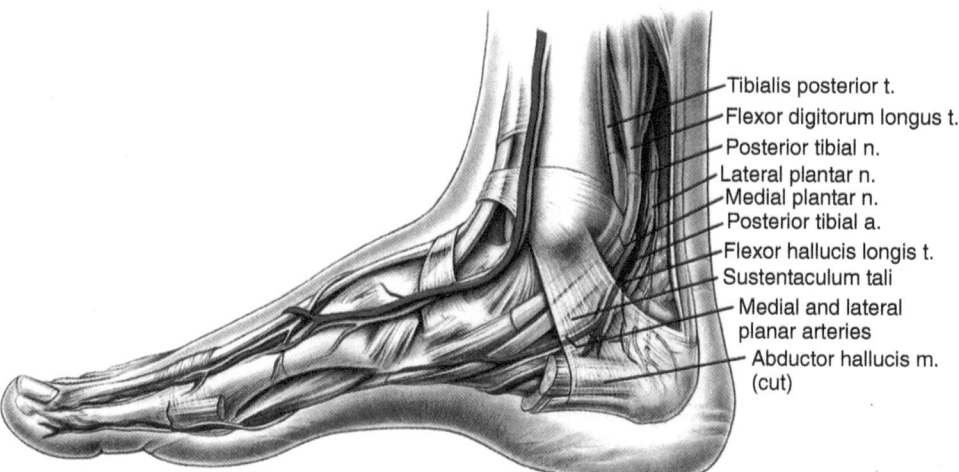

Fig. 114.6 Depicted is an artistic drawing presenting the anatomy of the medial aspect of the foot and ankle. (From Ferkel RD, Weiss RA. Correlative surgical anatomy. In: Ferkel RD, Whipple TL, eds. *Arthroscopic Surgery. The Foot and Ankle*. Philadelphia/New York: Lippincott-Raven; 1996:90, Fig. 5.8, with permission.)

down the medial side of the leg and the foot. Tenderness to palpation along the course of the nerve is the hallmark of diagnosis. Tenderness at the subsartorial fascia might be found. It might be associated with a reproducible Tinel sign at the site of entrapment.[32] Relief of pain with injection of a local anesthetic suggests localization of a more precise site of entrapment.

It is possible to use nerve conduction studies to assess the main branch of the saphenous nerve or the terminal branches.[33] However, routine testing may not yield useful results in patients with significant subcutaneous adipose tissue or swelling of the extremity.[34]

Electromyography for suspected saphenous nerve impingement should include testing of the adductor longus and quadriceps muscles. While electromyography is expected to be negative in saphenous nerve entrapment, it could be helpful to assess the presence of radiculopathy.[35]

Imaging

Conventional radiographs help identify posttraumatic and primary impingement on the nerve. Advanced diagnostic studies such as MRI or CT are not routinely indicated but can be considered to more clearly elucidate bony structures surrounding the course of the nerve (CT) or for preoperative planning and more precise localization of impingement in cases refractory to conservative measures.

Treatment Options
Conservative Treatment

Nonoperative treatment encompasses removal of any extrinsic factors that could lead to saphenous nerve entrapment. Activity modifications and physical therapy (strengthening exercises and proprioception) may help reduce pain. NSAIDs, topical analgesics, and systemic nerve modulators have been recommended in presence of saphenous nerve entrapment syndrome.[32] Local injections of anesthetics with or without steroids could alleviate

pain. Romanoff et al. reported an 80% success rate after a series of injections in 30 patients without application of steroids.[30] However, if all those measures do not improve the symptoms, surgery should be considered.

Surgical Treatment

Surgical treatment includes decompression, neurectomy, and neurolysis. Decompression is preferred and can be achieved by release of the anterior aspect of Hunter's canal and dissection of the saphenous nerve fibers from the surrounding sartorial fascia. Local nerve release may be necessary for more distal entrapments.

The best management for the transected proximal nerve is to bury and secure the nerve within an adjacent muscle belly. The nerve can also be compressed as it travels between the sartorius and gracilis muscles near their insertion. The nerve can either be released or divided in this region. Probably the most frequently seen problem in the sporting population is a neuroma of the infrapatellar branch. This can be irritated by repetitive movement of the knee or by direct pressure producing symptoms from the neuroma. Surgical treatment is simple. A straight incision is made over the neuroma, which is then excised, dividing the infrapatellar branch fairly proximally. In the author's experience, simple transection and placing it into muscle is all that is necessary.

Results

A reduction or elimination of pain can be expected in 60% to 80% of cases.[34] However, a large number of patients might still require neurectomy. There is an ongoing debate on whether neurolysis of the nerve or neurectomy achieves the best results. The chief problem with division of the saphenous nerve is the resulting distal anesthesia, with subjective discomfort in some patients. In the other hand, simple neurolysis includes complete fascial band release around the saphenous nerve with potential scar tissue formation, which could itself lead to new entrapment of the nerve. Worth et al. were able to show that in 15 patients suffering from saphenous nerve entrapment, complete relief was achieved in 13 knees after neurectomy. The authors concluded that neurectomy gave a more predictable result than neurolysis.[36] Neurectomy should be best performed proximal to the fascia in the canal between the vastus medialis and adductor magnus.[34]

Two patients in a study by Koppel and Thompson had relief of symptoms 24 hours after decompression. However, they were not followed up for a longer time. As such interpretation of those results is maximally limited. Dellon et al. reported the results of neurectomy in 70 patients. Of these, 62 patients were treated by neurectomy of the infrapatellar branch. Eighty-four percent revealed improvement of pain (Visual Analogue Scale).

TARSAL TUNNEL SYNDROME

Introduction

First described by Keck and Lam in 1962, tarsal tunnel syndrome is an entrapment neuropathy involving the tibial nerve. It is relatively uncommon in athletes and thus may go mis- or undiagnosed. While nonathletic patients are often middle-aged to elderly and an equal distribution among males and females is found, in athletes the patients are younger with a tendency to female preponderance.[37-39]

The tibial nerve arises from the sciatic nerve. The tarsal tunnel is located behind the medial malleolus (see Fig. 114.6). Its borders are created by the tibia anteriorly, the posterior process of the talus and calcaneus laterally, and the flexor retinaculum medially.

The flexor retinaculum is confluent with the sheaths of the posterior tibial tendon, the flexor hallucis longus tendon, and the flexor digitorum longus tendon. The flexor retinaculum and the abductor hallucis both are frequent sites of compression.[11] More recently, Singh et al. were able to demonstrate three well-defined, fascial septae in the sole of the foot.[40] Two of these septae represented potential sites of compression of the posterior tibial nerve and its branches and were distinct when compared with the classic entrapment sites. In most of the cases (93%), the tibial nerve splits into three major branches within the tarsal tunnel: the medial plantar nerve, the lateral plantar nerve, and the medial calcaneal branch. The medial calcaneal branch arises from the tibial nerve in 75% to 90% of cases and in 10% to 25% from the lateral plantar nerve, and it originates proximal to the tarsal tunnel in 39%, within the tarsal canal in 34%, and distal to the tunnel in 16%. In 21% of patients, multiple calcaneal branches are found (Fig. 114.7).[41,42]

Etiologies

A specific cause can be identified in approximately 60% to 80% of patients.[4,34,43] Table 114.1 provides a synopsis of the possible causes according to the work of Cimino.[44] Engorged varicose veins,[45] systemic diseases,[46] neurilemmoma (benign nerve sheath tumor),[47] pigmented villonodular synovitis,[48] lipomas, synovial cysts, intraneural degenerative cysts, ganglion cysts (flexor hallucis longus tendon sheaths), and accessory muscles[49] all can result in tibial nerve entrapment.

Postural deformities or mechanical abnormalities may contribute to the development of tarsal tunnel syndrome.[2,44,50-57]

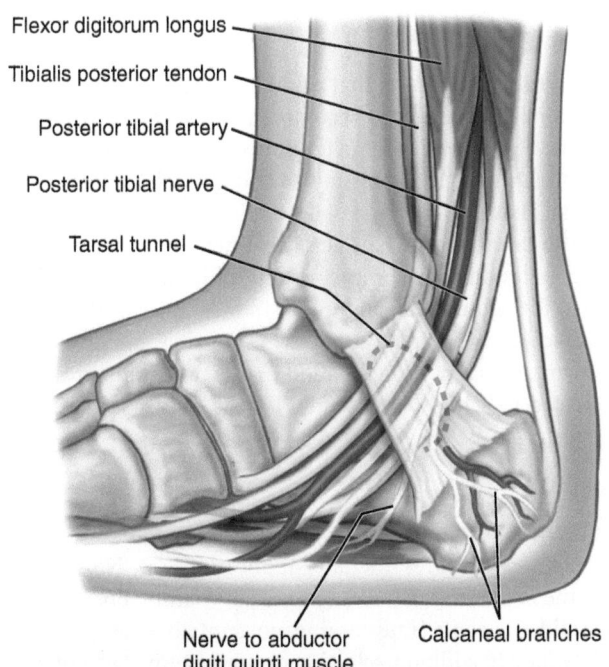

Flexor digitorum longus
Tibialis posterior tendon
Posterior tibial artery
Posterior tibial nerve
Tarsal tunnel
Nerve to abductor digiti quinti muscle
Calcaneal branches

Fig. 114.7 The image shows the course of the tibial nerve and its branches in the distal aspect of the lower limb and ankle.

Causes	Cases
TABLE 114.1 Causes of Tarsal Tunnel Syndrome	
Idiopathic	25
Traumatic	21
Varicosities	16
Heel varus	14
Fibrosis	11
Ganglion	10
Diabetes	3
Obesity	3
Tight tarsal canal	3
Hypertrophic abductor hallucis	3
Rheumatoid arthritis	3
Lipoma	2
Anomalous artery	1
Acromegaly	1
Ankylosing spondylitis	1
Regional migratory osteoporosis	1
Flexor digitorum accessorius longus	1
Subtotal	**122**
Causes not reported	**64**
Total	**186**

Work of Cimino WR, who summarized 24 studies.
From Cimino WR. Tarsal tunnel syndrome: review of the literature. *Foot Ankle.* 1990;11(1):47–52.

Hindfoot valgus (8% of cases) and deltoid ligament insufficiency can result in stretching of the tibial nerve and compression—as does hindfoot hyperpronation, which is typically appreciated in runners during dynamic examination of gait.[58] More frequent hindfoot varus (11%) with a hyperpronated forefoot is often associated with tarsal tunnel syndrome.[59] Rosson et al. found that pronation and plantar flexion significantly increased pressures in the medial and lateral plantar tunnels, to levels sufficient to cause chronic nerve compression; that a tunnel release and septum excision significantly decreased those pressures; and compared with cadaver pressures, patients had similar tarsal tunnel pressures but higher lateral plantar tunnel pressures in some positions.[60] Preexisting chronic nerve damage, (e.g., in patients with diabetic neuropathy) may have a lower threshold for developing tarsal tunnel syndrome, when other sites of nerve compression are involved (double crush phenomenon).

Direct trauma may lead to the formation of a painful neuroma, and even scarring following an ankle sprain involving the deltoid ligament can compromise the tarsal tunnel, causing tarsal tunnel syndrome.[61-63]

History

Symptoms can range from burning and shooting sensations, followed by paresthesia, disturbances in temperature perception, to mild loss of sensation or tingling over the heel and sole of the foot.[59] Athletes presenting with tarsal tunnel syndrome often report plantar pain and discomfort at the medial ankle, both being aggravated during sprinting, jumping, and certain martial sports. The symptoms are usually worse during activities and improve only slowly while resting (afterburn). This is in contrast to plantar fasciitis, where pain is worst within the first steps in the morning and remits with continued activity.[43] Some patients report pain during the night. Weakness or atrophy of intrinsic muscles will usually occur at late stage of disease.[64]

Physical Examination

Because of their implications regarding selection of treatment, any postural deformity should be ruled out (e.g., hindfoot valgus or varus). The entire course of the tibial nerve and its branches must be carefully palpated, and irritability, tingling, as well as any other discomfort are sought. Occasionally the Valleix phenomenon can be reproduced (tenderness proximal and distal to the entrapment site). Focusing on sensory examination alone is not sufficient because patients frequently do not suffer from sensory loss at the plantar aspect of the foot.[43] Sensory testing of distal sensory branches using the Semmes-Weinstein monofilaments or two-point discrimination can reveal tibial nerve deficits. Motor weakness is difficult to evaluate, especially when assessing the intrinsic muscles. At times, and in case of chronic tarsal tunnel syndrome, there might be weakness of the abductor hallucis and abductor digiti quinti muscles as reflected by atrophy. Moving the ankle into maximum dorsiflexion or heel into eversion may increase symptoms due to increased tension on the tibial nerve.[65]

Electrodiagnostic Studies

Electrodiagnostic studies (nerve conduction studies; amplitude measurement; motor-evoked potential; fibrillation potentials;

sensory conduction velocities) are recommended to confirm a clinically suspected tarsal tunnel syndrome and to rule out any other neuropathy in the foot. Of all electrodiagnostic studies, the sensory nerve conduction velocity is thought to be the most accurate study. The sensitivity is reported to range about 90%.[56,65-69] Electromyography (EMG) studies of intrinsic muscles yield high rates of false positive results (10% to 43%), especially in patients older than 60 years of age.[35,70,71] Be aware that in the presence of positive history and physical exam, a normal electrodiagnostic study does not exclude the diagnosis of tarsal tunnel syndrome.[64,72]

Imaging

Conventional radiography (including weight-bearing anterior-posterior views of the ankle, dorso-plantar and lateral views of the entire foot) may help to detect possible osseous alterations that could predispose to tarsal tunnel syndrome (e.g., malunited fractures of the hindfoot, coalitions, etc.). Hindfoot alignment views help estimate the amount of deformity and help prepare for any corrective intervention (e.g., supramalleolar or calcaneal osteotomies).[73,74]

If there is any suspicion of a space-occupying lesion, then MRI should be taken into consideration. In a study done by Frey and Kerr in 88% of patients with suspected tarsal tunnel syndrome, a pathologic condition could be found.[75] However, although imaging signs of direct tibial nerve dysfunction can sometimes be found, it is more likely that the tibial nerve will appear normal on imaging when no specific focal masses are present.[76]

Ultrasound (US) examination offers the possibility to visualize even smaller nerve branches and allows detection of nerve thickening with higher spatial resolution; however, it remains highly examiner dependent.[76,77]

Decision-Making Principles

In the absence of any lesion that could lead to nerve entrapment, nonoperative measures are recommended as the first line of treatment. If, despite adequate nonoperative measures, no improvement is found, then simple tarsal tunnel release may be warranted. However, in the presence of a space-occupying lesion within the tarsal tunnel, surgical treatment is preferred. The identifiable lesion that compresses the tibial nerve should be evaluated for and the mass removed. In case of a specific deformity or adjacent pathology that is responsible for any tarsal tunnel symptoms, this should be addressed and be either resected or corrected to achieve realignment of the hind- and forefoot, respectively.

Treatment Options

Conservative Treatment

Nonoperative measures include applications of NSAIDs to reduce the inflammatory response, oral vitamin B6, and tricyclic antidepressants (imipramine, nortriptyline, desipramine, amitriptyline). In addition, selective serotonin reuptake inhibitors (sertraline, paroxetine, duloxetine) or antiseizure drugs (gabapentin, topiramate, pregabalin, carbamazepine) can be used to improve symptoms.[59]

Neuropathic pain does not respond to NSAIDs; however, they may reduce the inflammatory response (i.e., tenovaginitis) and therefore the soft-tissue volume within the tarsal tunnel.[78]

Tricyclic antidepressants (amitriptyline, nortriptyline, desipramine, or imipramine) have a low number needed to treat (3.6) to achieve at least moderate pain reduction. They are well established and low priced; however, they have a high rate of side effects. Starting dosage should be low (10 to 25 mg/d administered in the evening because somnolence is one of the potentially encountered side effects). Daily intake can be increased weekly by 25 mg; however, success should not be judged until 2 weeks after the last rise. Do not exceed a maximal dosage of 100 mg/d (or 75 mg/d in the elderly) due to risk of cardiac arrhythmias and sudden cardiac death.[58]

Good evidence exists—and therefore this kind of treatment is often advised as first-line medication—for anticonvulsants such as gabapentin (starting at 3 × 100 mg/d [first dose at night], target dose 1200 to 2400 mg/d [max 3600 mg/d]) and pregabalin (starting at 1 × 25 to 50 mg/d [at night], target dose 150 to 300 mg/d [max 2 × 300 mg/d]).[58,78]

For local therapy, lidocaine patches (5%; 1 to 3/d) are recommended as second-line treatment due their good safety profile and tolerance.[58,78] The alternatives are capsaicin patches (8%; 1 to 4/3 months) with good evidence. However, concerns exist with sensation disturbances during long-term use.[58]

For opioids, a third-line recommendation is given. Usually the drugs are recommended in patients with contraindications to anticonvulsants or tricyclic antidepressants. Only in case of a positive response should the therapy be extended over more than 3 months.[58]

When feeling uncomfortable with administration of those medications, the patient may be referred to a neurologist. Physical therapy (including desensitization therapy and nerve mobilization) is useful and might serve to break up scar tissue within the tunnel to assist in mobilization of the constricted nerve. Stretching exercises should be avoided because they could aggravate tibial nerve symptoms.[79]

Local steroid injection into the area of the tibial nerve to reverse intraneural edema, stirrup-braces, night splints, off-the-shelf boot braces, or a short-leg walking cast may be successful means to treat tarsal tunnel syndrome. In case of any postural abnormality, orthotics could be used to place the foot in a more plantigrade position and to unload the medial longitudinal arch.[56,59,80]

Surgical Treatment

🔖 Authors' Preferred Method

The patient is placed in the supine position. A thigh tourniquet is used and inflated up to 280 mm Hg. Alternatively, no tourniquet can be used. The advantage is that veins and arteries can easily be visualized during surgery, and thus proper hemostasis performed.

A curved incision starting 10 cm proximal to the tip of the medial malleolus and 2 cm posterior to the tibial margin is done and directed distally crossing the course of the posterior tibial tendon to end up over the midportion of the abductor hallucis longus muscle (Fig. 114.8A). The flexor retinaculum is exposed bluntly to avoid injury of calcaneal nerve branches. Then the retinaculum is released. In the distal aspect of the tarsal tunnel, the retinaculum becomes dense and taut. Therefore a curved clamp can be inserted and the retinaculum incised, while protecting underlying neurovascular structures from inadvertent injury. After release of the retinaculum, the tibial nerve is explored proximally by blunt dissection and traced distally until reaching the bifurcation of branches. The medial plantar nerve is followed distally around the medial malleolus and beneath the abductor hallucis muscle belly (see Fig. 114.8B). At this point, there is a fibrous tunnel or septum that needs to be split to release the nerve branch. Be careful because large veins accompany the nerve on its course distally into the foot. The lateral plantar nerve is traced distally and slightly posterior to the medial malleolus. Quite frequently the nerve can be identified at the edge of

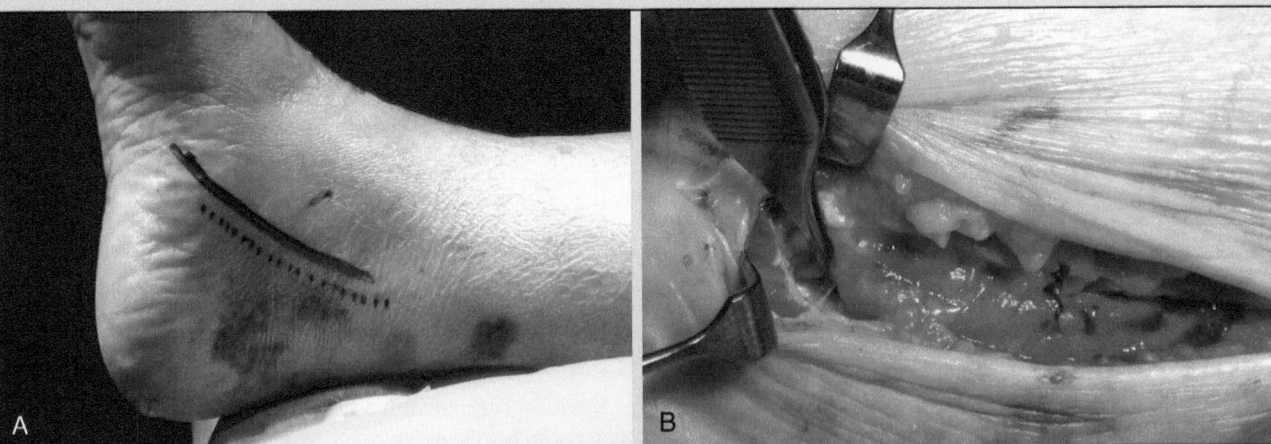

Fig. 114.8 (A) The surgical approach to the tarsal tunnel is outlined. Depending on the nerve, branches involving a slightly more anterior or posterior position of the skin incision should be chosen. In this case, it has been chosen a little bit more anterior to release the main tibial nerve. (B) The same patient is depicted as mentioned in (A). The tarsal tunnel has been released and the tibial nerve decompressed.

Continued

📌 | **Authors' Preferred Technique—cont'd**

the abductor hallucis. The superficial fascia over the muscle is released. The abductor is reflected plantarly and the deep fascia of the abductor released to relieve the first branch of the lateral plantar nerve. The lateral plantar nerve provides the nerve to the abductor digiti minimi muscle. Frequently, this nerve leaves the lateral plantar nerve before the latter passes under the abductor hallucis muscle belly. The medial calcaneal branch is identified (originating most often from the posterior tibial nerve but in 10% to 21% from the lateral plantar nerve).[41,42] Any constricting tissue should be released. When there is additional hindfoot malalignment, then this should be corrected (Fig. 114.9A and B). Take the tourniquet down prior to closure and obtain meticulous hemostasis to prevent new compression.

In case of so-called adhesive neuralgia (pain from a nerve scarred to surrounding tissue), a revision nerve release should be done first. This is a very delicate procedure, as the nerve could be tethered very closely to the scar and thus be damaged during preparation. The saphenous vein is harvested and its small side branch vessels tied off. Usually the entire saphenous vein must be harvested up to the knee. The ends of the vein are tied and the vein filled with a Marcaine and saline solution. Afterward, the vein is cut longitudinally and wrapped around the nerve. The inner lumen should be placed to the nerve's side. Each turn is secured by means of a simple suture using 7-0 Vicryl. After wrapping, the surgeon must ensure that there is no binding of the wrap and nerve.

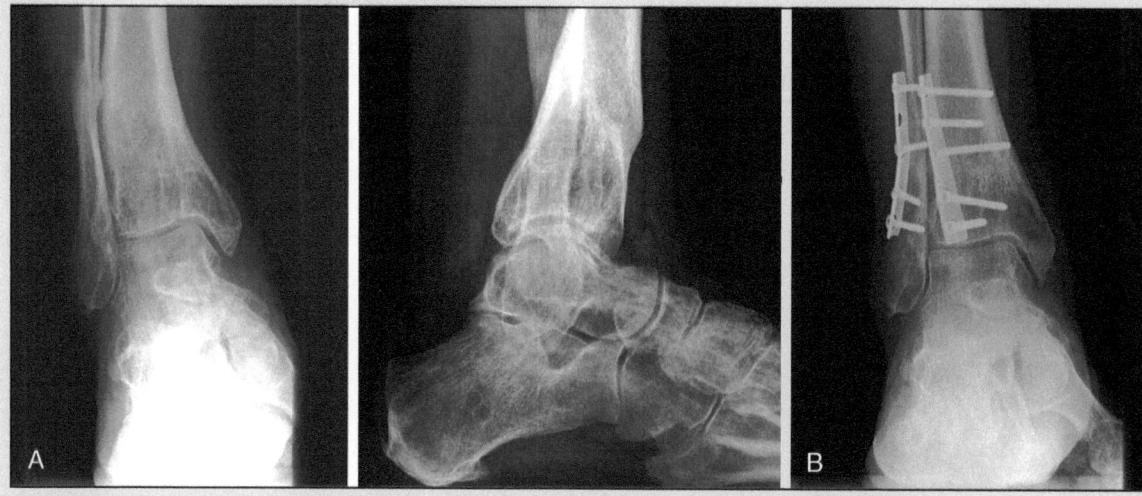

Fig. 114.9 (A) Illustrated is a case of a 64-year-old male patient who suffered from both posttraumatic ankle arthrosis and tarsal tunnel syndrome. To compensate for the clearly visible varus deformity, the patient exerted too much eversion at the subtalar joint, with subsequent stretching of the tibial nerve. (B) Depicted are the postoperative radiographs of the same patient as presented in (A). A supramalleolar osteotomy has been performed together with a tarsal tunnel release. One year after surgery, the patient was completely pain-free and very satisfied. Realignment resulted in unload of the ankle as well as subtalar joint.

Postoperative Management

After complete decompression of the tibial nerve, a non-weight-bearing short leg cast should be applied in neutral position for 2 weeks. Afterward, the cast is removed and the patient encouraged returning to activities of daily living without having any rehabilitation. Return to sports activities is allowed 3 months after the operation.

Results

When a well-localized lesion is present (e.g., lipoma, a ganglion, etc.), the clinical results are quite satisfactory in terms of symptomatic relief. Simple tarsal tunnel release is successful in approximately 75% of these patients. Twenty-five percent obtain little or no relief. However, considering all cases of tarsal tunnel syndrome, there are many studies in the literature proving the unpredictable character of surgically performed tarsal tunnel release.[52,81-83] The presence of a positive Tinel sign was attributed a positive predictive value of outcome after surgical release.[84]

In a review of 24 articles, including 122 patients, Cimino was able to show that in 91% of all cases, tarsal tunnel release achieved a good and improved result.[44] Seven percent showed poor results, and in 2% a recurrence had been found. Kinoshita treated 41 patients and found no functional deficit after a minimal follow-up of 24 months.[51] The same author presented the results after tarsal tunnel release in athletes after a mean follow-up of 59 months. Twenty-two percent (4/18 patients) were not able to return to their preoperative athlete level.[52] Sammarco and Chang presented their results of 62 patients. The duration of symptoms averaged 31 months. After a mean time interval of 9 months, the patients were able to return to their former activity level.[85] Release performed less than 10 to 12 months after onset of symptoms was associated with better outcomes.[85,86] Kim et al. have performed one of the largest studies on this topic. After a mean follow-up time of 33 years, 135 cases have been reviewed. Among them, 94 cases included tibial nerve lesions without discontinuity, which were treated by neurolysis.[87] Eighty-one percent (76 patients) of those patients had a good-to-excellent result. Similar results have been presented by Carrel and coworkers in a series of 200 patients.[88]

In summary, the likelihood of a satisfactory surgical result is increased in patients presenting well-defined lesions, a positive Tinel sign, and symptom interval less than a year of duration.[89]

LATERAL PLANTAR NERVE ENTRAPMENT

Introduction

One of the problems with lateral plantar nerve entrapment (including the calcaneal branches) is that it can mimic "nonspecific heel pain" and subsequently mislead treating physicians.[90] The diagnosis is mainly based on clinical findings. Among all patients who suffer from chronic unresolving heel pain, up to 20% are thought to have an entrapment of the first branch of the lateral plantar nerve. Although it is often termed the "inferior calcaneal branch" or the "Baxter's nerve," the nerve may arise directly from the tibial nerve.[64] There is no predominance regarding the activity level of the affected individuals. Most frequently, runners and joggers are affected by this kind of pathology, with a young and male preponderance (80% to 90%).[91] Other sports activities related to the problem include soccer, dance, baseball, basketball, and tennis.

Anatomically, the first branch of the lateral plantar nerve runs between the fascia of the abductor hallucis muscle and the quadratus plantae in an oblique direction. The first branch then divides into three branches that innervate the periosteum of the medial process of the calcaneal tuberosity, the flexor digitorum brevis muscle, the plantar ligament, and the abductor digiti minimi muscle.[10] Note that no sensory cutaneous innervation is present.[64]

Przylucki and Baxter both located the site of entrapment of the first branch of the lateral plantar nerve between the fascia of the abductor hallucis muscle and the medial plantar margin of the quadratus plantae.[92] Excessive pronation can cause stretching of the nerve branch. An edema within the abductor hallucis muscle as a result to repetitive stress or inflammation from chronic pressure can augment pressure within the compartment and compromise the nerve as it courses underneath the plantar ligament or at the osseous canal between the calcaneus and the flexor digitorum brevis. Other causes encompass hypertrophy of the quadratus plantae muscle, accessory muscles, and abnormal bursae and phlebitis within the venous system (see Fig. 114.7).[90,93-95]

History

More proximal and distal nerve entrapments must be excluded. Patients report chronic heel pain, which is aggravated during walking and running. Patients may recall heel pain in the morning when taking their first few steps, as plantar fasciitis may be concomitant. However, typically pain is progressively increasing through the day, possibly due to engorgement of the veins accompanying the first branch of the lateral plantar nerve.[96] The pain radiates from the medial inferior aspect of the heel proximally into the medial area of the ankle, or laterally and plantar into the foot.[34,59] In contrast to patients with plantar fasciitis, whose pain is more directly plantar, the presence of a more medial location of pain is typical for this condition.

In case of calcaneal nerve entrapment, the diagnosis is a little bit more difficult to establish because there is variation regarding location, origin, and course. Despite this, physicians are confronted with the fact that sometimes a medial calcaneal nerve branch might arise from the medial plantar nerve.

Physical Examination

Tenderness (reproducible symptoms and radiation of pain proximally and distally of the spot) over the first branch of the lateral plantar nerve deep to the abductor hallucis muscle on the medial heel is highly suspicious for the presence of lateral plantar nerve entrapment. Patients may also have pain over the origin of the plantar fascia, which does not rule out concomitant compression of the first branch of the lateral plantar nerve.

In medial calcaneal branch entrapment, loss of sensation at the medial heel can be noted; however, sensibility may be normal even in severe nerve compression if branching of the nerve has occurred above the flexor retinaculum.[64]

Imaging

The same imaging techniques as presented for the tarsal tunnel syndrome could be applied. Selective muscle edema in the more acute setting or fatty atrophy with chronic denervation may be observed in the abductor digiti minimi, possibly extending to the quadratus plantae and the short toe flexors.[97] However, it should be pointed out that clinical examination is crucial in order to establish the correct diagnosis.

The differential diagnosis in patients with this entrapment includes:

- Plantar fasciitis
- Fasciitis or tendinitis of the origin of the abductor hallucis muscle
- Periostitis
- Stress fracture of the calcaneus
- Tarsal tunnel syndrome
- Systemic arthritides

Decision-Making Principles

The problem of lateral plantar nerve entrapment is that it often goes mis- or undiagnosed. Many patients are treated for plantar fasciitis instead of the nerve disease. Thus the delay until proper treatment can be initiated may be long (up to 2 years). In case of a highly suspicious clinical finding or in patients who have not responded to nonoperative management after 6 to 12 months, surgery might be warranted.

Treatment Options
Conservative Treatment

Similar to the treatment strategies presented for tarsal tunnel syndrome, nonoperative measures in order to improve the conditions in athletes suffering from lateral plantar nerve entrapment include rest, NSAIDs, contrast baths, ice massage, physical therapy, and steroid injections. A shock-absorbing heel pad could help diminish inflammation and pressure. Excessive pronation can be inhibited by means of orthotic devices. Conservative treatment should be followed for 12 to 18 months because more than half of the patients require more than 6 months until achieving maximum improvement.[4]

Surgical Management

Authors' Preferred Method (Fig. 114.10)

The patient is placed in the supine position. The author uses a tourniquet. A 5-cm skin incision is made along the course of the lateral plantar nerve (on the medial heel over the abductor hallucis muscle). Subcutaneous dissection is followed by incision and splitting of the superficial fascia of the abductor hallucis muscle. The abductor hallucis muscle is reflected plantarly by means of a small retractor. By so doing, the deep fascia can be visualized and released. The muscle is then reflected superiorly and the rest of the deep fascia (where the nerve gets entrapped) released. Sometimes the medial aspect of the plantar fascia must be released to identify the proper fascial plane between deep abductor fascia and plantar fascia.

In case of calcaneal nerve entrapment, the lateral plantar nerve needs to be traced deep and distally into the heel. The calcaneal nerve branches are located superficial to the abductor muscle. The large nerve branch ramifies into the skin of the medial and plantar aspect of the heel. Accessory muscles need to be resected at their bulky portion.

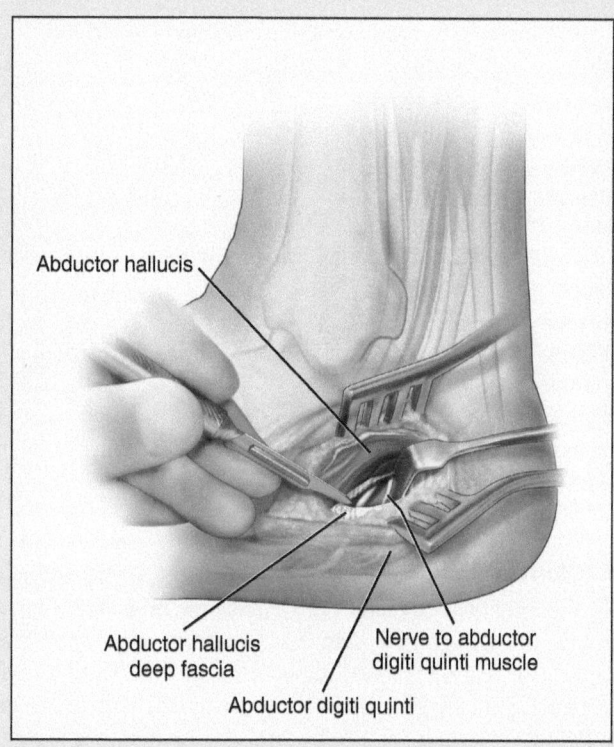

Fig. 114.10 The image shows the surgical approach to the lateral plantar nerve and its branches.

Postoperative Management

The operated foot is placed in a cast in neutral position for 2 weeks and kept non-weight-bearing for 14 days. The sutures are removed 2 weeks postoperatively, and the patient is then allowed to bear weight as tolerated. Return to sports might be possible 10 to 12 weeks postoperatively.

Results

Baxter et al. reported excellent and good results in 89% and complete resolution in 83%.[98] Watson and coworkers presented similar results (88% good-to-excellent) but in conjunction with a partial plantar fasciotomy. In their study, 7% reported fair results and the rest a poor outcome.[99] The mean time until resumption of sports activities was found to average 3 months for athletes.[4]

There is limited information available in the literature regarding surgical treatment of entrapped calcaneal nerve branches. However, Schon and Gould reported good-to-excellent results in 75% of cases.[43,100]

Complications

There are notable complications reported in the literature. Inadvertent transection of the medial calcaneal nerve results in numbness along the medial and plantar aspect of the heel and—in the worst case—could promote the development of a painful neuroma. However, although potential nerve injuries can occur, the overall rate is low. In the study presented by Watson et al., one wound dehiscence (1%) has been found and one (1%) developed a deep vein thrombosis.[99]

MEDIAL PLANTAR NERVE ENTRAPMENT

Introduction

The incidence or demographic predilection of medial plantar nerve entrapment is not known. Among athletes, joggers are mostly affected. This is how this pathologic entity also found its eponym: Jogger's foot. Dancers and gymnasts may also suffer from medial plantar nerve entrapment.

Anatomically, the medial plantar nerve courses underneath the flexor retinaculum and then deep to the abductor hallucis muscle, where the nerve might gets entrapped under its fascia of origin.[40] In most cases its course distally is along the medial side of the medial septum (a dorsal extension of the medial margin of the plantar fascia); however, it may cross underneath the septum and get compressed.[40] It then runs on the plantar surface of the flexor digitorum longus muscle while traversing the knot of Henry. Along the tendon of the flexor digitorum longus tendon, it spreads into its branches.[11]

Henry's knot is the typical site of compression and entrapment. Hyperpronation or excessive valgus while walking or running stresses the region of Henry's knot. In addition, external compression through medial arch supports could compress the medial plantar nerve.[34,41]

History

Patients often report shooting pain along the medial longitudinal arch, sometimes radiating into the medial three toes and proximally into the ankle, often worsened when running. At times, especially after exercise, sensation can be impaired.

Physical Examination

Inspection allows judging any postural abnormality as for example hindfoot valgus. Palpation along the medial plantar nerve may reproduce medial arch pain possibly associated with radiation, dysesthesia, and/or paresthesia to the medial three toes and the medial half of the fourth toe. Sometimes it may be difficult to distinguish between neuralgia and tendinitis. Heel rise or eversion of the heel tightens the adductor hallucis brevis muscle and aggravates symptoms.

Imaging

The reader is referred to the paragraph of tarsal tunnel syndrome. MRI may show fatty infiltration of the abductor hallucis or flexor hallucis brevis due denervation.[101]

Decision-Making Principles

Following the current leading opinions of experts in this field, once medial nerve entrapment has been diagnosed, it should be treated surgically rather than conservatively.

Treatment Options

Conservative Treatment

Measures include removal of disturbing or compressive orthotic devices and adjusting the training of the athlete.

Surgical Treatment

The patient is placed in a supine position. A 6 to 10 cm skin incision is made plantar to the talonavicular joint and parallel to the floor. The superficial fascia of the abductor hallucis muscle is split and the muscle reflected plantarly, followed by release of the deep fascia. The knot of Henry needs to be exposed and the naviculocalcaneal ligament released.

Postoperative Management

The operated foot is placed in a cast in neutral position for 2 weeks and kept non-weight-bearing for 14 days. The sutures are removed 2 weeks postoperatively, and the patient is then allowed to bear weight as tolerated. Return to sports might be possible 10 to 12 weeks postoperatively.

SUPERFICIAL PERONEAL NERVE ENTRAPMENT

Introduction

Entrapment of the superficial peroneal nerve is rare condition and was first described by Henry in 1945.[102,108] The typical athlete affected by superficial peroneal nerve entrapment is a runner with an average age of less than 30 years. There is no gender preponderance between males and females. Superficial peroneal nerve entrapment may also occur in persons doing stop-and-go sports activities. Approximately, 25% of patients reveal a traumatic event before commencing of symptoms (most often ankle sprain).[103]

The superficial peroneal nerve is a branch of the common peroneal nerve. It provides motor innervation to the peroneus longus and brevis muscles along its course within the anterolateral compartment. Approximately 10 cm above the tip of the fibula, the nerve pierces the fascia and becomes subcutaneous. It then divides into two branches (the intermediate and the medial dorsal cutaneous nerves), which provide sensation to the dorsum of the foot (including the medial distal aspect of the greater toe to fifth toe) (see Figs. 114.1 and 114.5).[104]

The site where the superficial peroneal nerve exits, the fascia is a typical location of entrapment (Fig. 114.11).[105] In addition, chronic ankle sprains could lead to stretching of the superficial peroneal nerve and induce a focal lesion.[106] The presence of exostoses or osteochondromas may result in impingement anywhere along the course of the nerve. Other causes include entrapment within scar tissue after previous anterior compartment fasciotomy,

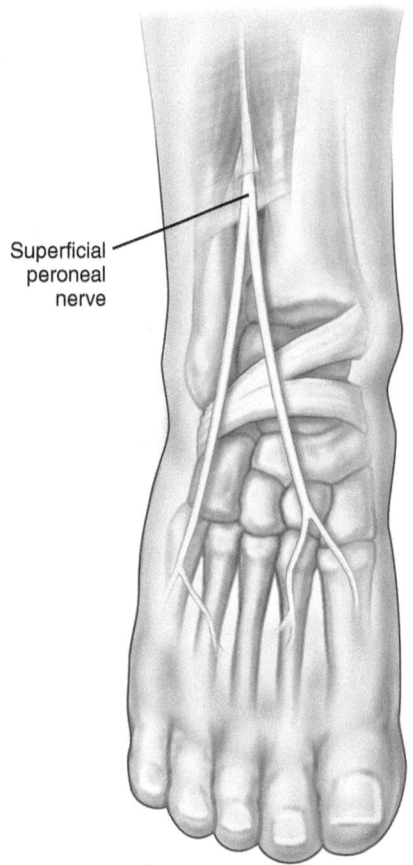

Fig. 114.11 A very frequent site of superficial peroneal nerve entrapment is the spot where the nerve pierces the fascia in order to become anteriorly.

Superficial peroneal nerve

direct hit by blunt trauma, ganglion formations, fibular fractures (including iatrogenic damage to the nerve due to surgery), exertional compartment syndrome, fascial defects,[102] syndesmotic sprains, lower extremity edema, neoplasia, and idiopathic causes.[4] Postural deformities, as for example hindfoot varus, result in greater risk to sustain ankle sprains or may predispose to chronic ankle instability.

History

Affected individuals report a long-standing history of pain, similar to an ankle sprain that failed to resolve, which is found over the anterolateral border of the shank (mid to distal third) and might radiate down over the dorsum of the foot. The latter can be a single symptom without the presence of pain at the anterolateral border of the shank. Approximately one third of patients report numbness and paresthesias along the course of the superficial peroneal nerve. Pain is often aggravated with physical activity as, for example, jogging; walking; running; kneeling; and squatting. Twenty-five percent of patients have a positive history of prior ankle sprains or chronic ankle instability.[107]

Physical Examination

Before assessing the lower limb, examination of the lumbar spine is required to rule out any spinal disorder that could be responsible for leg pain (e.g., disc herniation). The lower leg should be inspected for any varus deformity or scar that could indicate a potential site of nerve entrapment. Proximal entrapment of the common peroneal nerve is examined by palpating the subcapital region of the fibular head. To identify any entrapment at the fascial exit of the superficial peroneal nerve, the examiner palpates the anterolateral region of the calf approximately 10 cm proximal to the tip of the fibula. Paresthesia and numbness following external compression are suggestive for entrapment. In addition, three tests to identify possible superficial nerve entrapment could help to assess[108] (1) active dorsiflexion and eversion against resistance while the nerve impingement site is palpated; (2) plantar flexion and inversion against resistance without pressure over the nerve; and (3) plantar flexion and inversion against resistance with pressure along the course of the nerve.[105,109-111]

Localized injection of anesthetic at the site of maximal tenderness could be a diagnostic and therapeutic measure.

Nerve conduction studies in the superficial peroneal nerve are performed in a standardized fashion, and positive results are obtained in nearly 98% of patients. Nerve conduction studies should be reserved for situations where the diagnosis is in question. However, studies have shown reproducible and consistent changes to conduction velocity in the superficial peroneal nerve in case of impingement. Other studies have shown increased latencies and attenuation of action potentials. Be aware that normal nerve conduction studies do not rule out superficial peroneal nerve involvement and must be seen as an adjunctive tool in establishing the diagnosis.

Imaging

A standardized workup includes anteroposterior and lateral views of the entire lower leg to assess bony impingement secondary to injury or prior fracture. A CT scan may provide more detailed information if bony involvement in the impingement is suspected following plain radiography. MRI can be useful to define soft tissue involvement, and might be used to examine the passage of the nerve through the crural fascia or to assess nerve compressing soft tissue lesions. US can be helpful to identify a cystic mass impinging on the nerve. Because the superficial peroneal nerve does not have an accompanying vascular structure, it can be difficult to localize with MRI or US without a good appreciation of its expected anatomic course.

Decision-Making Principles

The superficial peroneal nerve is less responsive to conservative treatment than the deep peroneal nerve. However, once entrapment of the superficial peroneal nerve is diagnosed, nonoperative measures should be tried first before embarking on surgical treatment. There are no recommendations regarding how long conservative measures should be tried. It is the author's experience that at least 6 months should be awaited before deciding whether surgery is warranted or not.

Treatment Options
Conservative Treatment

Nonoperative measures include strengthening exercises of the peroneal muscles and should focus on ROM. To prevent inversion of the ankle, a supportive ankle brace or lateral heel and sole wedges in the shoe could be applied and reduce the varus thrust. Occasionally dorsiflexion night-splints can be of benefit. Cortisone injections, with or without the addition of local anesthetics, may help reduce symptoms. However, the latter can never be seen as causal cure.[3,4,103,107,108]

🔖 Authors' Preferred Method

The patient is placed in the lateral decubitus or supine position. The more distally and anterior the site of entrapment is found, the more supine the patient is placed. A 10-cm skin incision is done over the area of maximum tenderness (which should be assessed prior to surgery without anesthesia). The nerve is identified and the compressive structure released and/or removed (Fig. 114.12A and B). The author always releases the fascia—a common site of entrapment or compression—to decompress and provide relief to the nerve.

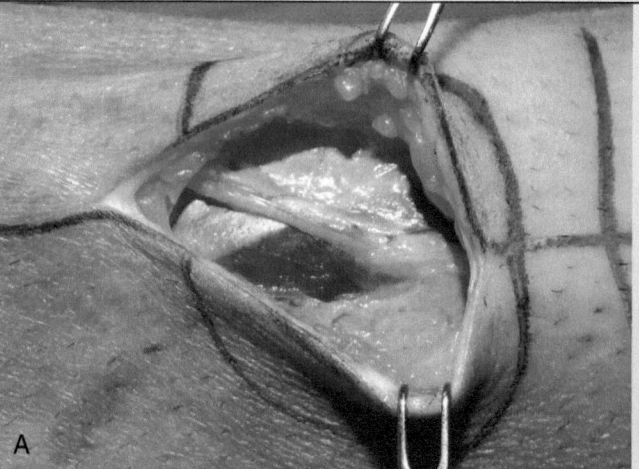 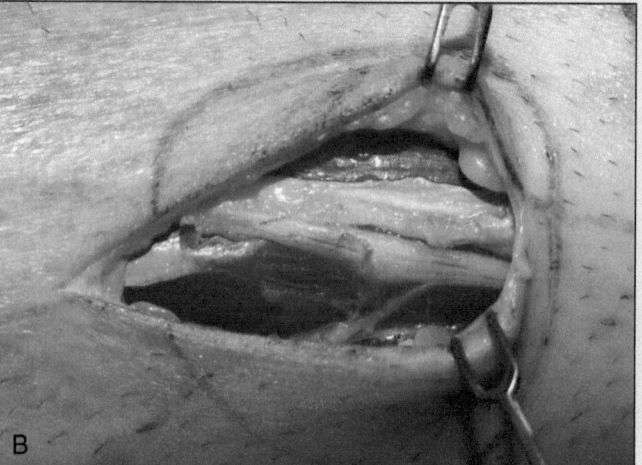

Fig. 114.12 (A) Depicted is a fascial entrapment of the superficial peroneal nerve within a scar that has developed due to previous surgery (endoscopic compartment release). (B) Illustrated is the intraoperative photograph after release of the scar tissue, fasciotomy, and careful mobilization of the nerve.

Surgical Treatment

If conservative treatment fails, surgery is warranted. In such a case, superficial nerve release is performed. Release of the nerve is done at its site of entrapment. Therefore no specific type of surgery can be proposed in this chapter. However, the author describes his technique of nerve decompression.

Postoperative Management

The patient wears a compressive wrap or splint for 2 weeks until the sutures are removed. The patient is allowed to ambulate as tolerated 3 to 4 days after surgery. Three weeks postoperatively, activities can be resumed. Return to sports may take up to 8 and 12 weeks.

Results

Although decompression of the superficial nerve yields improvement in 75% of patients, the results are less predictable for athletes. Styf reported that only 9 of the 19 in their series were completely satisfied with the procedure. It appears that there can be chronic irreversible damage to the nerve in this condition. In case of persisting symptoms after release, reexploration and transection and burial into muscle should also be considered.[108]

DEEP PERONEAL NERVE ENTRAPMENT

Introduction

Historically, Kopell and Thompson first described entrapment of the deep peroneal nerve in 1960.[112] Marinacci termed the pathology "anterior tarsal tunnel syndrome" with involvement of either the motor or sensory component.[113] Typically runners are the affected population.[3,114,115]

The course of the deep peroneal nerve is complex and deserves specific attention. As a branch of the common peroneal nerve, it tracks within the proximal third of the calf and lies between the muscle bellies of the tibialis anterior and extensor digitorum longus muscles. The anterior tibial artery accompanies the nerve. When entering the distal third of the calf nerve runs between extensor hallucis and extensor digitorum longus (5 cm above joint line), secondary to the oblique path of the extensor hallucis longus (EHL) tendon that travels medially. The deep peroneal nerve provides motor innervation to the tibialis anterior, the extensor digitorum communis, and the EHL muscle. At level of the ankle joint, the nerve sends a branch to the extensor digitorum brevis muscle, while the other sensory branch delivers sensation to the first webspace (see Fig. 114.5).[10,11,116]

Most commonly, the sensory branch of the deep peroneal nerve gets entrapped underneath the inferior extensor retinaculum (Fig. 114.13). This is the site of the so-called anterior tarsal tunnel syndrome. Entrapment may also occur at the superior edge of the inferior extensor retinaculum and at a location where the EHL tendon crosses the nerve. Osteophytes at the talonavicular joint, pes cavovarus, improper footwear (tight ski boots), and trauma (repetitive ankle sprains) are possible causes for deep peroneal nerve entrapment.[117-125]

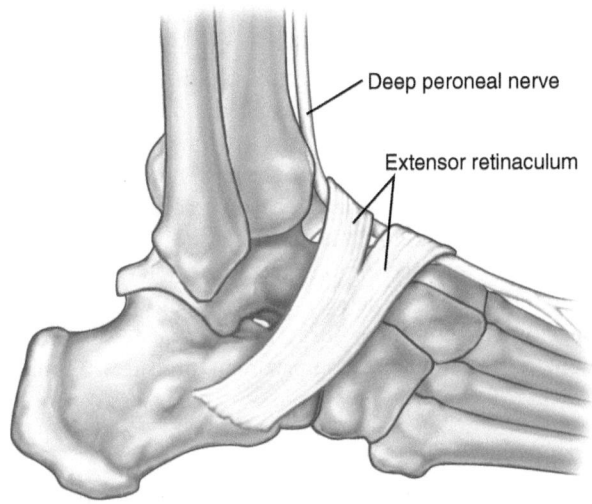

Fig. 114.13 The deep peroneal nerve can become entrapped under the inferior extensor retinaculum.

History

In general, the patients report dorsal foot pain and disturbances of sensation at the first webspace. The classic anterior tarsal tunnel syndrome is characterized by pain or burning sensations over the dorsum of the foot and may result in atrophy and weakness of the extensor digitorum longus muscle. Patients may report paresthesias in the first dorsal webspace, although this is less common. Symptoms may be aggravated by physical activity, especially with the foot held in plantar flexion, a position that places stretch on the nerve and compresses the contents of the anterior tarsal tunnel against the dorsal aspect of the talonavicular joint. Patients may note resolution of pain with rest as well as nighttime symptoms.[119] These symptoms can also be seen in patients with exertional anterolateral compartment syndrome, and this condition can be an underlying cause of nerve compression exacerbated with activity.[126] Pain might be associated with specific footwear or a specific activity.

Physical Examination

Palpation along the course of the deep peroneal nerve may reveal the spot of highest nerve irritation and identifies any alteration of sensation. In addition, the presence of osteophytes and other foot abnormalities should be evaluated.[34] The proximal course of the nerve near the fibular neck should also be examined, as tenderness is often elicited to percussion (Tinel sign) at the site of entrapment or along the course of the nerve distally. Forceful plantar flexion and inversion of the ankle places the nerve on stretch and decreases the available space in the anterior tarsal tunnel, resulting in compression of the nerve against the floor of the tunnel. This maneuver may provoke symptoms over the dorsum of the foot.[121,127] As previously mentioned, careful motor examination is also important. The subtle weakness caused by decreased or loss of innervation to the extensor digitorum brevis is often difficult to discover. Palpating the extensor digitorum brevis during active dorsiflexion of the toes may detect loss of the contribution of this muscle.

Electrodiagnostic studies may be useful in diagnosing deep peroneal nerve entrapment and to determine involvement of the extensor digitorum brevis (indicating a lesion proximal to the inferior retinaculum).[128] Electrodiagnostic studies are able to reveal increased latency and reduced motor recruitment of the extensor digitorum brevis muscle. However, these findings should be interpreted with caution; in a study performed by Rosselle et al., abnormal signals have been found in approximately 76% of asymptomatic individuals, as well as decreased extensor digitorum brevis motor recruitment in 38% of asymptomatic individuals. In patients in whom an exercise-induced compartment syndrome is suspected, exercise testing, with or without measurement of compartment pressures, should be considered.

Imaging

Plain radiographs are able to demonstrate the presence of dorsal osteophytes (on the lateral view of the foot), particularly at the talonavicular joint, which could impinge against the nerve or lead to space-obliteration in the anterior ankle compartment. Conventional radiographs can also help detect fractures, bone fragments, or soft tissue swelling near the course of the nerve. MRI has a limited role in diagnosis of the condition, but becomes important when the problem is felt to be secondary to impingement from an adjacent mass.[25,76,129]

Treatment Options

Conservative Treatment

The goal is to reduce pressure or to eliminate compressive forces at the dorsum of the foot that could harm the deep peroneal nerve. Usually conservative treatment includes proper footwear adaptation (accommodative, avoiding any external pressure over the nerve). NSAIDs, vitamin B6, tricyclic antidepressants, gabapentin, Lidocaine patches, or analgesic creams (Capsaicin) can modulate nerve pain. Corticosteroid injections have been reported to be useful to reduce nerve irritation. Sometimes orthotics should be considered to correct flexible flatfoot deformities.[103,130]

Surgical Treatment

> ### ✒ Authors' Preferred Method
>
> The patient is placed in a supine position on the operating table. Before surgery, the maximum point of tenderness should be assessed and marked out with a pen to decompress the correct spot. A 5- to 10-cm skin incision is made. In case of "classic anterior tarsal tunnel syndrome," the retinaculum is released, with emphasis on release at the site of compression. Extensive release could lead to bowstringing of the anterior tibial or other extensor tendons. A Z-shaped incision of the retinaculum allows lengthening and tension-free closure. Any bony exostosis must be removed. In case of hindfoot deformity, this should be corrected. In addition, if there is ankle instability, ankle ligament reconstruction combined with a lateralizing calcaneal osteotomy should be considered. In case of anterior compartment syndrome, a fasciotomy should be done. If the extensor hallucis brevis is the cause of nerve entrapment, a segmental resection of the muscle belly is needed, along with release of the deep fascia in the midfoot.

Postoperative Management

The lower limb is put into cast for 1 week. The cast should be hold in neutral position. Walking with crutches is recommended for 1 week. After that time period, gradual resuming of weight bearing as tolerated is allowed. Training can be resumed 4 to 6 weeks postoperatively. In case of extensive surgery, a boot should be worn for 4 weeks and training resumed 8 weeks postoperatively.

Results

Surgical decompression might yield excellent and good results in approximately 80%. However, there are still 20% who do not improve at all.[131] However, structural nerve damage is related to poor outcomes, and simple decompression may not be enough. In the latter case, nerve resection might be an option. Resection and translocation of the nerves into the anterolateral compartment yields excellent results in more than 80% of patients. Segmental resection of the extensor hallucis brevis together with a transfer to the EHL yields good-to-excellent pain relief more than 6 months postoperatively. Liu et al. have reviewed 10 patients who have been treated for deep peroneal nerve entrapment or its branches, and have studied the anatomy of the tunnel in 25 adult feet. Operative decompression in nine feet of eight patients gave successful results at 1.5 and 4 years follow-up.[125]

INTERDIGITAL NEURALGIA (MORTON NEUROMA)

Introduction

The clinical symptoms of interdigital neuroma were first described by Civinni in 1835 and thereafter by Durlacher.[132] Morton, for whom the eponym of the condition is given, mistakenly attributed the etiology to a pathologic fourth MTP joint, and noted relief of symptoms with resection of the fourth metatarsal head. The term "neuroma" is incorrect and—according to the author's opinion—the pathology should rather be called *interdigital neuralgia*. The nerve is the structure that suffers due to perineural fibrosis. Interdigital neuralgia is a common pathology found in daily orthopaedic practice with the potential of becoming very debilitating and impairing quality of life. Its incidence has been calculated to be 50.2 for men and 87.5 for women with regard to the annual age standardized rates per 100,000 of new presentations in primary care. Interdigital neuromas are frequently found unilaterally. In 15% there is a bilateral occurrence. In only 3% there is a simultaneous development of two adjacent interdigital neuromas in the same foot. There are twice as many neuromas found in the third webspace than in the second webspace. Interdigital neuromas in the fourth webspace are rare.

Although there are many studies that support the hypothesis of entrapment neuropathy beneath the transverse metatarsal ligament, other factors are also able to promote the formation of a primary interdigital neuroma, leaving uncertainty about its etiology. Thus a multifactorial process must be considered more likely. Anatomic, traumatic, and extrinsic causes all have been discussed to promote the development of an interdigital neuroma. In addition, there are conditions that could mimic symptoms, as seen in patients with interdigital neuroma.[133,134] Therefore before embarking on any treatment, it is important to identify the exact cause of a symptomatic interdigital neuroma. This is even more important and complex in the presence of recurrent interdigital neuroma.

Pathomechanism and Etiologies

The hypothesis of intrinsic nerve pathology beyond simple compression by the intermetatarsal ligament is well accepted.[135] On an ultrastructural level, the nerve undergoes the following alterations: thickening of the perineurium and deposition of amorphous eosinophilic material built up by filaments of tubular structures, demyelinization and degeneration of nerve fibers without signs of wallerian degeneration, local initial hyperplasia of unmyelinated nerves followed by degeneration, and intraneural fibrosis and sclerohyalinosis and increase of elastic fibers within the stroma. Those changes are induced either by anatomic, traumatic, or extrinsic factors, which will be discussed in detail.[136,137]

Anatomic factors include variants with communicating branches within the third webspace connecting the lateral plantar nerve and medial plantar nerve that result in a thickening of the common digital nerve. However, the frequency of such communicating branches has only found to be about 28%.[138,139] As such, it cannot be the solitary explanation for interdigital neuroma. In addition, the degree of mobility of the first medial three rays in relation to the lateral two rays also plays a role in the development of an interdigital neuralgia. Similar to the hand, the mobility for the lateral two rays is greater when compared with the medial three rays that are firmly attached to the cuneiforms. The greater mobility between the fourth and third ray could result in higher strains and stresses within the nerve and underneath the intermetatarsal ligament. Nevertheless, this kind of theory is negated by the fact that interdigital neuralgia could also be found in the second webspace.[140] Hyperextension of the toes leads to increased plantar depression of the metatarsal heads. The nerve is tethered and squeezed underneath the intermetatarsal ligament. Patients with excessive hyperextension at the MTP joints show an 8 to 10 times higher incidence of interdigital neuroma. Other factors include traumatic ones, which might occur in runners, dancers, and other sports athletes. The increased incidence in those athletes is explained by exposure to repetitive stresses exerted to the metatarsal region.[141] Besides this acute trauma, crush injuries or direct penetration of the forefoot by a sharp object must be included into the differential diagnosis.

Besides anatomic and traumatic factors, extrinsic causes should be discussed. A mass below or above the ligament can employ abnormal pressures on the common interdigital nerve. Such a mass encompasses an inflamed bursa, a ganglion, or synovial cyst that arise from the MTP joint and a lipoma from the plantar aspect of the foot.[135] Degeneration of the MTP joint can result in a local inflammatory response. In addition, the capsule attenuates and the proximal phalanx of the third toe deviates medially. As a result, the third metatarsal head is pushed laterally against the fourth metatarsal head, compressing the bursa and obliterating the third webspace. MTP joint instability itself can exert traction on the capsule and the nerve inducing pain in approximately 10% to 15% of patients.[142] Ultimately, the intermetatarsal ligament itself is thickened.

Athletes who have sustained a fracture of the metatarsal head and/or neck region that resulted in malunion and altered pressure distribution of the forefoot could also suffer from interdigital neuralgia.

History

In general, a thorough history helps perform a proper clinical examination and achieve the correct diagnosis. Most of the patients complain about plantar pain that is increased when walking (92%) but relieved when either resting (89%) or removing footwear (70%). The pain usually is characterized as burning, tingling, or electric with radiation into the involved toes (62%). Numbness is less frequently reported (40%).[140]

Physical Examination

The foot is grasped with both hands and the plantar interspaces palpated starting proximal to the metatarsal heads and proceeding more distally. Reproducible pain and paresthesias are highly suspect for the presence of an interdigital neuroma. Mulder's click sign consists of milking the small mass of nerve and bursal tissue between the involved metatarsal heads with alternating thumb and forefinger pressure while simultaneously compressing these same metatarsal heads.[143] The "mini-Lachmann" test is performed to evaluate the MTP joints for possible instability.[144]

Local injection of 1 to 2 mL of local anesthetic into the affected webspace may provide pain relief. But the finding should be interpreted with caution, as a positive result does not habitually reflect the presence of an interdigital neuralgia. Other abnormalities as, for example, inflammatory processes, MTP joint instability, or degeneration of the plantar plate and/or joint capsule can mimic symptoms like interdigital neuralgia. The result of local injection must therefore always be correlated to the clinical and radiographic findings.

Electro-diagnostic studies are only indicated where a peripheral neuropathy or radiculopathy is suspected.

Imaging

Conventional radiography (standing and weight-bearing dorsoplantar and lateral views of the foot) is often normal but serves to identify any osseous abnormality, subluxation or dislocation of the MTP joints, degenerative or arthritic changes within the MTP joints, or possible evidence of a foreign body (fracture fragments etc.).[145]

It is still debated whether ultrasonography or MRI should be used in order to diagnose interdigital neuralgia.[146] US is user dependent and may result in lower sensitivities and specificities when performed by inexperienced personal. However, in experienced hands, US yields a high sensitivity (91% to 100%) and specificity (83% to 100%).[147] More recently, Symeonidis and coworkers were able to demonstrate that US could lead to overdiagnosis with a high rate of incidental findings in an asymptomatic population having interdigital nerve enlargement. The authors concluded that US is unreliable unless it is correlated with an equivocal clinical examination, and that clinical examination alone remains the gold standard in assessing interdigital neuralgia.[148]

MRI is the primary diagnostic tool to assess interdigital neuralgia and is often used to identify or to exclude other pathologies in the forefoot. Recently, Lee and coworkers presented a retrospective analysis to compare the diagnostic accuracy of both ultrasonography and MRI for the assessment of primary interdigital neuroma.[149] The data were correlated with the surgical and pathologic findings. The detection rate of primary Morton neuroma was 79% for ultrasonography and 76% for MRI. However, even MRI can lead to misinterpretation of the results. Zanetti and coworkers were able to demonstrate a 30% prevalence of interdigital neuromas in an asymptomatic population. Comparing their results with a symptomatic group, they concluded that a mass—suggestive of interdigital neuroma—greater than size 5 mm could be seen as a true interdigital neuroma. Thus even in the presence of highly sophisticated imaging technology, only the combination of symptoms and positive imaging can help establish the correct diagnosis.[150-152]

Decision-Making Principles

In general, only symptomatic athletes should undergo treatment. It is the author's preferred algorithm of treatment to start with a conservative (i.e., nonoperative) treatment, which should be continued for at least 6 months. In case of failure of conservative measures, surgical resection should be considered. Generally speaking, smaller sized lesions are more amenable to conservative treatment, while larger ones may be treated rather surgically.

Treatment Options

As mentioned earlier, conservative and surgical treatment strategies attempt to resolve pain. Usually the nonoperative management should be continued for at least 6 months before embarking on surgery. Although many patients are successfully treated by conservative measures, approximately 70% elect surgical treatment over time because the symptoms interfere with their quality of life. When selecting surgery, patients must be primed since most reports agree that resection rarely exceeds a 90% success rate.

Conservative Treatment

The goal of nonoperative treatment is to alleviate the pressure underneath the metatarsal heads (i.e., to achieve proper decompression within the affected webspace). This is best achieved by means of footwear modifications, including fitting the foot into wide, soft, laced shoes. Soft-heeled shoes are preferred. A metatarsal bar or pad elevates the metatarsal heads and reduces the forefoot pressure. Local injection of a mixture containing Lidocaine and corticosteroids may be added after shoe modifications have been started. The effect of combined shoe adaptation and local injections of local anesthetics and steroids is better than the sole use of shoe modifications. However, side effects of corticosteroid injections must be kept in mind; these include subcutaneous tissue atrophy and discoloration of the skin, risk of wound breakdown, and disruption of the MTP joint capsule with consecutive joint instability. In case that surgery is considered, it should not be performed within 4 weeks after local injection of steroids.

Radiofrequency ablation and alcohol injections have been reported to be less traumatic, but the literature remains inconclusive. The use of ethanol injection in the treatment of symptomatic interdigital neuralgia remains inconclusive. Recent studies presented more than 90% of patients having a partial or total symptomatic relief after US-guided injections with alcohol (70% Mepivacaine-adrenaline and 30% ethylic alcohol).[153-155] Another study showed a high failure rate after local alcohol injections without US guidance. The authors concluded that nonguided alcohol injections are not efficacious and have abandoned their use in their clinic.[132]

Surgical Treatment

Nerve resection. An interdigital neuroma can be excised through either a plantar or dorsal approach. A more recent investigation found no statistically significant differences between plantar and dorsal approaches in terms of outcomes or complications. However, supporters of the dorsal approach claim that there are lesser problems observed with scar formation. If a keloid develops from any plantar incision, the symptoms can become very difficult to treat.[156,157] The author prefers the dorsal approach in order to treat primary intermetatarsal neuralgia. In cases of revision surgery, sometimes a plantar approach is needed, as this allows for extensile exposure of the nerve proximally. In the case of revision, the risk of a painful plantar scar is outweighed by the need to ensure adequate resection of the nerve.

Postoperative Management

The patients are allowed to ambulate in a postoperative and stiff-soled shoe for 2 weeks. The sutures are removed 2 weeks postoperatively. After 3 to 5 weeks postoperatively, the patient could start to work on active and passive ROM exercises. Return to sports might take up to 6 weeks.

Results

Mann and Reynolds reported 71% essentially asymptomatic, 9% significantly improved, 6% marginally improved, and 14% failures, in their series of nerve resections for interdigital neuralgia.[140] Coughlin and Pinsonneault reported an average good-to-excellent satisfaction of 85%, but 65% were pain free with minor or major footwear restrictions.[158] Akermark et al., Giannini et al., and Benedetti et al. have reported similar results.[156,159] Akermark and coworkers did not find any difference between a plantar or dorsal approach.

Complications

In patients who have received multiple steroid injections before surgery, soft-tissue conditions can be critical, raising the risk of possible wound-healing problems and infection. Resection of adjacent web space neuromas could lead to vascular compromise or deprivation resulting in increased risk of frostbite in the winter. In case of excessive soft-tissue resection during surgery, vascular compromise could theoretically result in necrosis of the involved toe, needing amputation. A few patients might suffer from complex regional pain syndrome type 2 after resection of the neuroma.

When using the plantar approach, the incision must strictly be kept between the metatarsals. An improper incision placement is unforgiving. The incision is carried out through the

📌 Authors' Preferred Technique

The author almost always uses the dorsal approach. An incision is made in the dorsal aspect of the foot, starting in the web space over the affected common interdigital nerve. The length of the incision varies, but averages 3 cm. The dorsal digital nerves are avoided. The incision is deepened through the subcutaneous tissue. The innominate fascia is explored and incised. Afterwards, a laminar spreader is placed beneath the metatarsal heads (Fig. 114.14A). After spreading, the transverse metatarsal ligament becomes taut and can be split. The spreader

is placed a little deeper beneath the metatarsal heads. The nerve is exposed at its proximal aspect. The nerve is traced proximally until it enters intrinsic musculature. Then the common digital nerve is cut proximal to the metatarsal heads. The nerve is then dissected out distally past the bifurcation and excised (see Fig. 114.14B). Make sure to remove any accessory branch to the either the common or interdigital nerves. The nerve specimen should be sent for histologic examination.

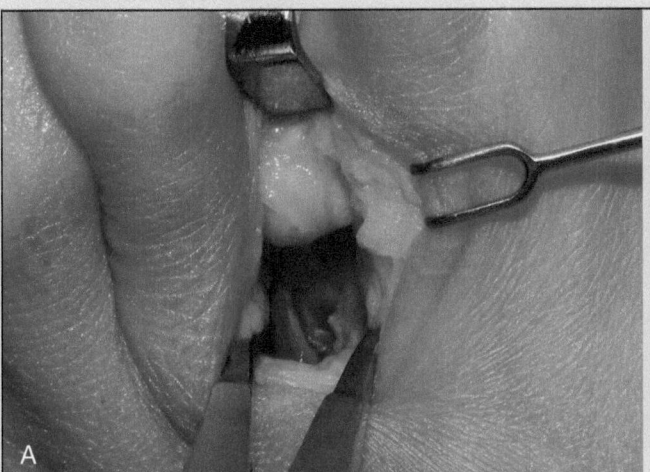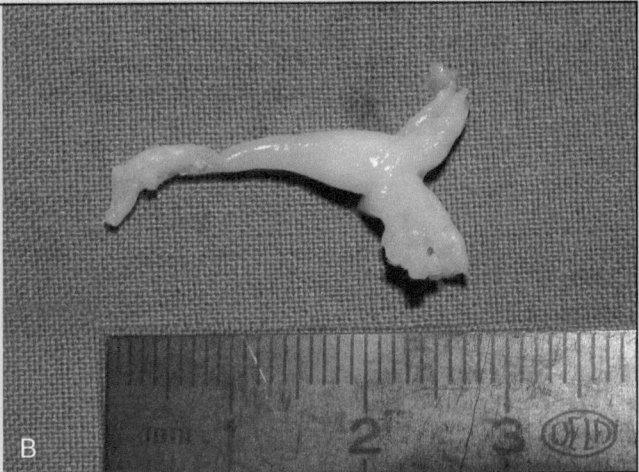

Fig. 114.14 (A) Depicted is the dorsal approach to the intermetarsal webspace. A 3 cm skin incision is done. After transection of the innominate fascia and the transverse ligament, the enlarged interdigital nerve appears. To improve visualization, a laminar spreader is inserted. (B) This is an intraoperative picture of the resected nerve. On the left side, the common interdigital nerve stump can be appreciated. On the right side, the bifurcation is visible.

subcutaneous tissue. The common digital nerve is exposed and traced down to the bifurcation. The nerve branches are cut and the specimen sent to pathology.

Surgical neurolysis offers an alternative to nerve resection. It can be performed endoscopically or open. Okafor noted that 72% of patients had complete resolution of pain. In combination with forefoot deformity, the results appeared to deteriorate. Further investigations are needed to judge the true value of neurolysis. However, given that recurrence rates up to 77% have been reported in the literature, neurolysis is not currently recommended by the authors.[160]

For a complete list of references, please go to ExpertConsult.com.

SELECTED READINGS

Citation:
Akermark C, Crone H, Saartok T, et al. Plantar versus dorsal incision in the treatment of primary intermetatarsal Morton's neuroma. *Foot Ankle Int.* 2008;29(2):136–141.

Level of Evidence:
III, retrospective, comparative study

Summary:
No matter whether a dorsal or plantar approach is chosen for the surgical treatment of painful Morton neuroma, the clinical and patient satisfaction was comparable among the groups. The authors found significant differences in favor of plantar incisions regarding residual sensory loss and number of complications.

Citation:
Espinosa N, Seybold JD, Jankauskas L, et al. Alcohol sclerosing therapy is not an effective treatment for interdigital neuroma. *Foot Ankle Int.* 2011;32(6):576-580.

Level of Evidence:
IV, retrospective case series

Summary:
In the clinical setting without ultrasound-controlled guidance, alcohol injections for the treatment of painful intermetatarsal Morton neuroma are not effective.

Citation:
Kim DH, Ryu S, Tiel RL, et al. Surgical management and results of 135 tibial nerve lesions at the Louisiana State University Health Sciences Center. *Neurosurgery.* 2003;53(5): 1114–1124.

Level of Evidence:
IV, retrospective case series

Summary:
In 33 years of clinical and surgical experience with tibial nerve lesions, the authors were able to demonstrate excellent outcomes after surgical exploration and repair. Best results were obtained in patients with recordable nerve action potentials treated by external neurolysis, while patients with larger nerve lesions in

continuity or reoperations due to tarsal tunnel syndrome did less well.

Citation:
Sammarco GJ, Chang L. Outcome of surgical treatment of tarsal tunnel syndrome. *Foot Ankle Int.* 2003;24(2):125–131.

Level of Evidence:
IV, retrospective case series

Summary:
After an average follow-up of 5 years, 108 ankles were reviewed considering surgical treatment of tarsal tunnel syndrome. Patients who suffered from symptoms less than 1 year before surgery showed higher outcome scores than those with long-standing symptoms.

Citation:
Zanetti M, Ledermann T, Zollinger H, et al. Efficacy of MR imaging in patients suspected of having Morton's neuroma. *AJR American J Roentgenol.* 1997;168(2):529–532.

Level of Evidence:
II, prospective, diagnostic study

Summary:
Thirty-two patients were prospectively enrolled into the study. In 16 of the 32 patients, additional surgical evaluation of the intermetatarsal spaces was done. The authors concluded that MRI is accurate in diagnosing Morton neuroma and to assess correct localization.

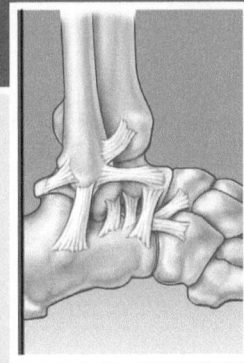

115

Ankle Arthroscopy

Niall A. Smyth, Jonathan R. Kaplan, Amiethab A. Aiyer,
John T. Campbell, Rachel Triche, Rebecca A. Cerrato

Historically, the ankle joint was believed to be unsuitable for arthroscopy because intra-articular access of this joint is narrow.[1] Tagaki[2] and later Watanabe[3] described techniques and pioneered the use of arthroscopy in the examination of the ankle. Compared with open arthrotomy, arthroscopy has recognized benefits of shortened recovery times and limited surgical morbidity. Today, arthroscopy of the foot and ankle has evolved from simply a diagnostic tool to a versatile treatment modality for a variety of pathologies.

It is important to understand the surface and superficial anatomy in the area of the ankle to minimize the risk of damage to the surrounding structures when performing ankle arthroscopy. Important landmarks to identify include the tibialis anterior tendon, the peroneus tertius tendon, the level of the joint line, the superficial peroneal nerve and its branches, and the great saphenous vein. It is also important to understand the location of the deep peroneal nerve and dorsalis pedis artery as they cross the anterior ankle joint. The branches of the superficial peroneal nerve are most commonly injured during this procedure.[4] These branches can be identified and marked prior to the procedure by plantar flexing and inverting the foot.

The anteromedial, anterolateral, and posterolateral portals are most commonly used for ankle arthroscopy. Anterior portal options include the anteromedial, anterolateral, anterocentral, and accessory anteromedial and anterolateral portals. The anteromedial portal is made just medial to the tibialis anterior tendon at the level of the joint line. Confirmation of planned portal placement is recommended with use of an 18-gauge needle to localize and insufflate the joint with approximately 10 mL of saline solution before creating the portal. All portals should be created by making a small incision with a scalpel through the skin only and then using a blunt instrument such as a mosquito clamp to spread the soft tissue down to the capsule. Once the soft tissue is safely cleared, the capsule can be penetrated with a blunt instrument, such as the blunt trocar, with care being taken to prevent injury to the articular cartilage. This technique helps minimize the risk of damage to overlying structures. An accessory anteromedial portal can be created 1 cm anterior and 0.5 to 1 cm inferior to the medial malleolus.

The anterolateral portal is created under direct visualization once the arthroscope has been introduced through the anteromedial portal. A needle is once again used to confirm portal placement at or just above the level of the joint lateral to the peroneus tertius tendon. This helps to avoid injury to the intermediate dorsal cutaneous branch of the superficial peroneal nerve. The needle can be used to confirm that the portal will allow adequate access to the area being treated before making the skin incision. An accessory anterolateral portal can be placed 1 cm anterior to and at the level of the tip of the distal fibula.

The anterocentral portal carries an increased risk of neurovascular damage and thus is not commonly used.[5] It is located between the extensor digitorum tendons, with the deep peroneal nerve and dorsalis pedis artery just medial to this portal, coursing between the extensor hallucis and extensor digitorum communis tendons.

Posterior portal options include posterolateral, trans Achilles, and posteromedial (Fig. 115.1). A posterolateral portal is placed just lateral to the Achilles tendon approximately 1 to 1.5 cm proximal to the tip of the distal fibula. This portal can be established under direct visualization if anterior arthroscopy is being performed. If hindfoot endoscopy is being performed, this portal should be established first, followed by the posteromedial portal. The trans Achilles portal can be established at or just below the joint level through the midportion of the tendon but is less favored because of Achilles tendon morbidity and increased difficulty with instrument manipulation. The posteromedial portal risks damage to the posterior tibial artery and tibial nerve, as well as the calcaneal nerve and branches. If used, it is placed medial to the Achilles tendon at the joint level after establishing the posterolateral portal. After a small skin incision is made, a blunt instrument, such as a mosquito, is directed toward the arthroscope and "walked down," maintaining contact with the arthroscope until bone is palpated. The lens of the arthroscope is directed laterally to protect it until the mosquito reaches the bone, at which point the lens can be turned medially to visualize the introduction of an instrument, usually a motorized shaver, through the newly established portal.

SOFT TISSUE CONDITIONS AMENABLE TO ARTHROSCOPY

It is estimated that 3% of all ankle sprains lead to anterolateral impingement.[6] Wolin et al.[7] were the first to describe the pathology. They described a mass of hypertrophied fibrocartilaginous scar tissue that originated from the anterior talofibular ligament and rested in the lateral gutter. They coined the term *meniscoid lesion* because of its similar appearance to a knee meniscus. Bassett et al.[8] described another cause of impingement after an inversion

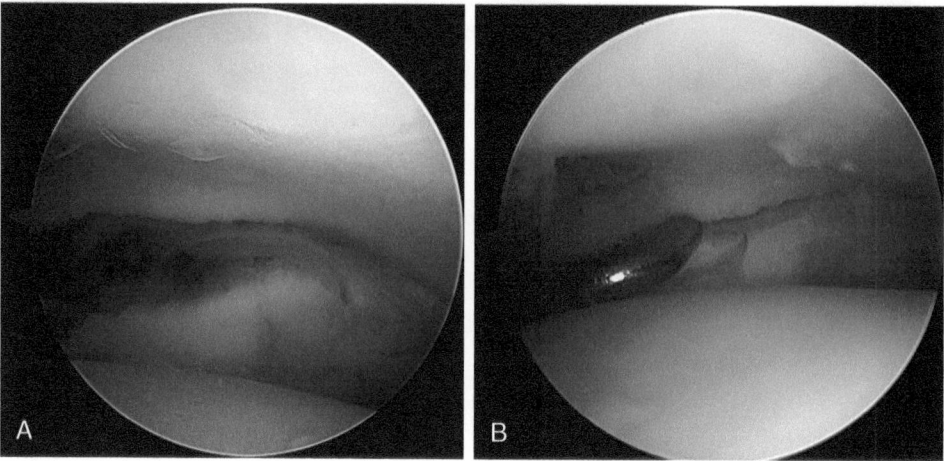

Fig. 115.1 Arthroscopically assisted ankle fracture open reduction with internal fixation. (A) The view of the medial malleolar fracture before reduction. (B) The view of the medial malleolar fracture after reduction.

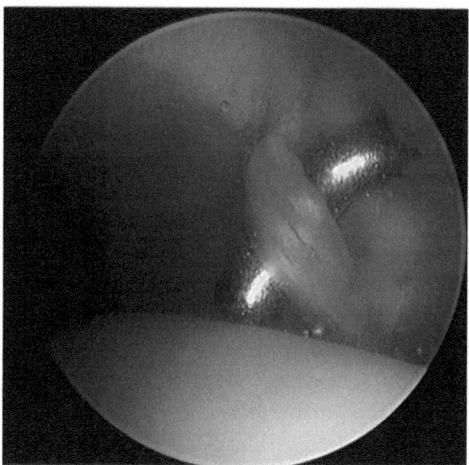

Fig. 115.2 An anterolateral soft tissue impingement lesion.

sprain. The distal fascicle of the anteroinferior tibiofibular ligament can impinge on the talus when it becomes thickened or scarred from an injury (Fig. 115.2).

Proposed causes for anteromedial impingement include injury to the deltoid ligament and capsule, resulting in scarring and hypertrophy of the synovium,[9] repetitive capsular traction resulting in "traction spurs,"[10] and repetitive dorsiflexion of the ankle.

With a syndesmotic injury, the anteroinferior tibiofibular ligament can become scarred and hypertrophied. Chronic synovitis can occur at the tibiofibular joint, resulting in a soft tissue lesion impinging on the talus.

Plicae have been well described in the knee. The origin of these lesions in the ankle is not well understood, but theories include congenital and traumatic causes. As with the knee, these fibrous cords typically can be found across the anterior ankle joint and have been implicated as a source of ankle pain, clicking, and occasional locking. *Plicae syndrome* refers to the painful impairment of joint function in which the only finding that helps explain the symptoms is the presence of thickened plicae. When encountered during an arthroscopic procedure, the thickened plicae are routinely excised.

Posterior ankle impingement can be caused by overuse or trauma. The overuse group comprises ballet dancers and athletes in sporting activities that involve forced plantar flexion of the foot. Repetitive plantar flexion results in swelling, partial rupture, and fibrosis of the posterior ankle capsule, synovium, and posterior ligamentous structures. A prominent posterior talar process or os trigonum can produce the syndrome. Dancers or athletes who often go *en pointe* may have hypertrophy of the flexor hallucis longus (FHL) muscle belly resulting in further impingement of these tissues posteriorly.

The role of arthroscopy in the treatment of a patient with an inflammatory arthritic condition such as rheumatoid arthritis is limited. A patient with painful synovitis that is recalcitrant to conservative therapies may benefit from an arthroscopic complete synovectomy. The synovial lining is typically proliferative and thickened.

Pigmented villonodular synovitis (PVNS) is a benign neoplastic process of the synovium. It is most common in the knee but also can be seen in the ankle and hindfoot.[11,12] It is seen in two forms: generalized synovitis and a localized form. Localized lesions respond well to arthroscopy, but recurrence is common with the generalized form.

Septic arthritis of the ankle is amenable to treatment with arthroscopic lavage and débridement; however, only two case series have focused on arthroscopic treatment of ankle septic arthritis, and both included various joints in the study.[13] Despite the paucity of literature regarding the use of ankle arthroscopy in the management of septic arthritis, this practice is widely accepted.

Synovial chondromatosis is a benign condition in which the synovial lining of joints, bursae, or tendon sheaths undergoes metaplasia and ultimately forms cartilaginous loose bodies. Milgram[14] described three stages of the process. Stage I is the active synovial phase, without the presence of loose bodies. Stage II is the transitional phase, with both active synovial disease and chondral loose bodies. Stage III describes the burnout phase, with no further synovial activity and residual loose bodies.

Lateral ankle ligament injuries are the most common injuries that occur in sports and recreational activities (refer to Chapter

117 for full details regarding this pathology). Recently, arthroscopic and arthroscopically assisted reconstruction of the lateral ligament complex has been reported either by autograft reconstruction,[15] anchor fixation techniques,[16–18] and thermal shrinkage.[19–21]

Pain and disability from ankle arthritis may be treated with arthroscopy. In mild cases without significant loss of cartilage and in active patients for whom a fusion or replacement is not reasonable, arthroscopic débridement provides a low-risk alternative. In cases of end-stage arthritis, ankle arthrodesis may be indicated to relieve pain at the tibiotalar joint when prior conservative treatment has failed. Since the first description of arthroscopic ankle arthrodesis in 1983, this procedure has gained popularity. Contraindications include significant extensive bone loss, active infection, a neuropathic joint, and ankle fusion nonunion.

Arthroscopy of an acute ankle fracture can assist in the anatomic reduction of some fractures, diagnose syndesmotic instability, and assist in the treatment of concomitant osteochondral and chondral injuries. Direct visualization can confirm articular congruency and identify other fracture lines/fragments not seen on preoperative radiographs (see Fig. 115.1A and B). Arthroscopy in the setting of chronic fractures can assist in the diagnosis and management of postfracture pathology. The indication for arthroscopy in the treatment of chronic ankle fractures (>3 months) is persistent joint pain that is unresponsive to conservative management.

History

Patients with anterolateral impingement typically report pain with weight-bearing activities after an inversion ankle injury that has not resolved. They can describe a feeling of instability, even without true mechanical instability, if the intermittent pain causes a feeling of giving way. Anteromedial impingement presents with anteromedial ankle pain with activities that place the ankle in a dorsiflexed position, such as running, kicking, or climbing stairs. The clinical presentation of syndesmotic impingement is similar to that of anterolateral impingement, with pain upon weight-bearing activities, variable swelling, and the feeling of locking or clicking of the ankle with range of motion (ROM).

Patient presentation can vary widely with synovial chondromatosis, with ankle pain, swelling, limited ROM, and palpable nodules at the joint line.

Patients with posterior ankle impingement report pain toward the posterior aspect of the talus, mainly with plantar-flexion maneuvers.

Physical Examination

The diagnosis of anterolateral impingement is clinical, based on the physical examination. Molloy et al.[22] reported a sensitivity of 94.8% and specificity of 88% on special physical examination testing for impingement.[22] Patients exhibit palpable tenderness along the anterolateral corner of the ankle, along with anterior syndesmosis. Occasionally, asymmetric fullness along the anterolateral corner can represent scar tissue. Pain often can be elicited with passive dorsiflexion of the ankle, either while it is unloaded or with weight bearing. Tenderness at the sinus tarsi may be present but should be mild compared with the anterolateral

ankle. An injection of a local anesthetic can confirm the diagnosis of soft tissue impingement when excellent pain relief is achieved.

Examination reveals anteromedial ankle joint tenderness and pain with dorsiflexion either while the ankle is loaded or with no weight bearing in patients with anteromedial impingement.

Patients with syndesmotic impingement have a more variable examination than do those with anterolateral or anteromedial impingement; findings can range from significant tenderness at the distal syndesmosis to no pain elicited on palpation. In chronic cases, examination of syndesmotic disruption (the squeeze test and external rotation test) may not be painful.

Patients with PVNS present with nonspecific findings such as a swollen, warm, diffusely tender ankle that is painful with activity. During the workup, aspiration of the joint can produce dark, serosanguineous fluid.

Palpation of the posterior talar process performed posterolaterally between the peroneal tendons and the Achilles tendon will reproduce the pain in patients with posterior impingement. The passive forced plantar-flexion test is executed with repetitive quick passive hyper-plantar-flexion movements with the patient sitting and his or her knee flexed at 90 degrees. van Dijk described application of a rotational movement at the point of maximal plantar flexion and stated that a negative test rules out posterior impingement.[6] The diagnosis is supported by relief of the pain with plantar flexion upon infiltration of an anesthetic.

Imaging

In the setting of anterolateral impingement, radiographs are often normal but can demonstrate anterior tibial and talar neck spurring. Standard anteroposterior and lateral radiographs may not detect the presence of all osteophytes, specifically off the medial aspect of the tibia and talus. van Dijk et al.[23] described an oblique anteromedial impingement view (a 45-degree craniocaudal radiograph with 30-degree external rotation of the leg and the foot in plantar flexion). The anteromedial impingement view improves diagnosis of both talar and tibial anteromedial osteophytes.[24] Radiographs may reveal ossification along the syndesmosis in the setting of syndesmotic impingement, and in cases in which instability is a concern, fluoroscopic external stress imaging is necessary to determine the presence of laxity. Radiographs can appear normal in stage I and early stage II cases in patients with synovial chondromatosis, whereas multiple calcific nodules within the anterior and posterior aspects of the ankle clearly indicates the diagnosis.

Plain radiographs may reveal an os trigonum or Stieda process in the setting of posterior impingement.

Magnetic resonance imaging (MRI) is the most valuable modality for evaluating soft tissue pathology. The reported sensitivity for an MRI scan in the diagnosis of anterolateral impingement varies from 39% to 100%, and its specificity varies from 50% to 100%.[25,26] MR arthrography with diluted gadolinium solution increases the sensitivity in diagnosing ankle impingement.[27] Although not required for the diagnosis of impingement, it is helpful in excluding other ankle pathologies, such as osteochondral defects. MRI can also identify soft tissue edema, bone edema involving an os trigonum/Stieda process, tenosynovitis of the FHL, and loose bodies when evaluating patients with posterior impingement. In the setting of PVNS, MRI scans typically reveal swollen synovial tissue and hemosiderin deposits. Computed tomography (CT) and MRI have been useful tools in the diagnosis of synovial chondromatosis. Depending on the extent of calcification and synovial proliferation, the appearance may vary.

Decision-Making Principles

A wide variety of pathologic conditions can be treated by means of routine anterior ankle arthroscopy. Diagnostic ankle arthroscopy without a preoperative diagnosis has limited value.[28] Relative contraindications for ankle arthroscopy include moderate degenerative joint disease and joint disease with severely reduced joint space, vascular disease, and severe edema. Absolute contraindications include severe degenerative joint disease not amendable to arthroscopic arthrodesis and a localized soft tissue infection.

Although septic arthritis can be treated effectively with arthroscopy, infection involving the soft tissue envelope around the ankle is best treated with an open débridement. In the early phases of synovial chondromatosis, with active synovial disease, a synovectomy with loose body removal is indicated. For patients with stage III disease, only removal of loose bodies is indicated.

When considering whether to perform an arthroscopy ankle arthrodesis, the surgeon should understand that this technique is an in situ fusion and that significant deformity in any plane is considered a contraindication. Coronal plane deformities greater than 15 degrees are not appropriate for an arthroscopic approach. Additionally, in the setting of osteoporosis or loss of bone stock of the talar body, an open approach with plate fixation should be considered to ensure adequate fixation.

With regard to posterior ankle arthroscopy, a systematic review was published assessing the current level of evidence supporting its use for certain pathologies. The article concluded that posterior ankle impingement syndrome, subtalar arthritis, and retrocalcaneal bursitis have the strongest recommendation in favor of treatment.[29]

Nonoperative Management

Initial management involves rest, activity modification, use of oral antiinflammatory medications, ice, corticosteroid injections, orthoses, heel lifts, and physical therapy. Patients with chronic symptoms who fail to respond to conservative treatment after 3 to 6 months are appropriate surgical candidates. Surgery may be considered more urgently if the patient notes mechanical symptoms, such as catching or locking, which may suggest a loose body or cartilaginous flap tear.

General Surgical Technique: Ankle Arthroscopy
Arthroscopic Equipment
A range of arthroscope sizes are available, with the 2.7-mm size being the most versatile for the ankle and allowing visualization in the reduced space available in the medial and lateral gutters. The smaller sized arthroscopes are designed for smaller joints and include a shorter lever arm, which affords increased control over the instrument in a small joint and is preferred to prevent articular cartilage injury during the procedure. A 30-degree arthroscope is recommended for most ankle arthroscopic procedures

because it increases the field of view (compared with a 0-degree scope) without the disadvantage of a central blind spot (as with the 70-degree scope). Occasionally a 70-degree arthroscope can be helpful, particularly when it is necessary to see around a corner, such as into the posterior ankle, but its use is accompanied by a learning curve. When performing hindfoot endoscopy, a 4.0-mm arthroscope is commonly used because the size and anatomic constraints are not as limiting as in anterior ankle arthroscopy.

As is the case with the arthroscope itself, a line of small joint instruments has also been developed; these instruments are smaller in diameter and have shorter lever arms. Availability of a probe, graspers, punches, curettes, and baskets is important. Other instruments now available include osteotomes designed for arthroscopic ankle arthrodesis, awls for microfracture, small joint drill guides and targeting devices, and small radiofrequency probes. A range of options are available for disposable arthroscopic shavers and burrs as well, ranging in aggressiveness and sizes from 2.0, 2.9, to 3.5 mm. Generally a 3.5-mm shaver is recommended; the smaller options can be quite useful in certain circumstances, such as in tighter joints or in the gutters, although they do tend to reduce efficiency.

Inflow/Outflow

A two-portal or three-portal system (usually with use of the posterolateral portal for inflow) with gravity or a pump system can be used. A two-portal system is most commonly used for both anterior ankle arthroscopy and hindfoot endoscopy, along with a pump to improve flow and visualization. Frequently, if a soft tissue procedure, such as a lateral ligament reconstruction is planned, a pump system is not used to minimize the amount of soft tissue fluid extravasation.

Positioning

For anterior ankle arthroscopy, the patient is positioned supine on the operating table. A beanbag can be used underneath the patient and positioned so that the ipsilateral hip is slightly elevated, and the remaining part of the beanbag is gathered under the thigh to hold the patient in position if distraction is applied. This area needs to be well padded. Alternatively, a padded leg holder or thigh support can be used and serves to position the limb and provide support to keep the patient in position when distraction is used. A nonsterile tourniquet can be placed on the thigh and inflated if necessary or according to the surgeon's preference. The patient should be positioned toward the end of the table to ease access and surgeon comfort while allowing enough room for the distraction setup to effectively apply a force.

For hindfoot endoscopic procedures, the patient is positioned prone. A small bolster or support under the operative leg will allow for adequate ankle motion. Again, a thigh tourniquet should be applied; it may be used more often in these procedures than during anterior ankle arthroscopy.

Distraction

Initially, distraction was described using the placement of pins in the calcaneus and distal tibia to allow the application of a distractive force.[30] Although this technique provides excellent

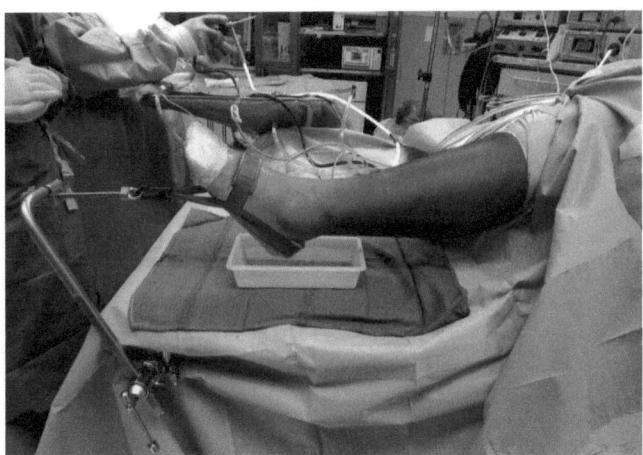

Fig. 115.3 Noninvasive distraction. The foot is attached to a disposable harness that is attached to the distractor along the side of the operating table.

distraction, disadvantages include risk of fracture, pin site infection, and neurovascular injury. Therefore noninvasive distraction has become the more favored option. Noninvasive distraction is performed using a disposable strap that passes over the dorsal foot and around the posterior aspect of the heel. This strap is attached to a sterile distractor that connects to the table rail (Fig. 115.3). To minimize the risk of

neurovascular injury for either method of distraction, it is recommended that the distractive force be applied for a maximum of 90 minutes.

Anesthesia

Inducement of regional anesthesia with use of a popliteal nerve block can be very effective in managing postoperative pain and minimizing the need for general anesthetics. Administration of a popliteal nerve block can be performed with use of a nerve stimulator or ultrasound guidance. We recommend the use of a popliteal nerve block in conjunction with general anesthesia to facilitate distraction and the use of a tourniquet if needed.

Tourniquet

A well-padded thigh tourniquet should be applied prior to patient positioning at the start of the case. Depending on the surgeon's preference and anticipated bleeding, the use of the tourniquet may or may not be necessary. Commonly the case can be performed without a tourniquet, but if bleeding becomes problematic, it can be inflated. A randomized, controlled trial assessing the use of a tourniquet versus no tourniquet for anterior ankle arthroscopy demonstrated that there was no difference in surgical time, visualization, and functional scores between the two groups. However, it was noted that there was statistically less pain in the early postoperative period for the nontourniquet group.[31]

⚑ Authors' Preferred Technique

Anterior Arthroscopic Débridement

Patients are placed in the supine position with a thigh tourniquet (inflation is optional). The patient's leg is secured on a nonsterile thigh holder. Before preparing the area, the course of the superficial peroneal nerve is identified by plantar flexing and inverting the foot. The path of the nerve is marked with a surgical marking pen. For use of noninvasive distraction, the foot strap harness is placed and distraction is applied to the foot. It is important to avoid excessive use of distraction. With longer procedures (more than 90 minutes) consideration should be given to relaxing some of the tension on the distraction device. Palpation of the joint line, anterior tibialis tendon, and peroneus tertius is performed. As previously described, the anteromedial and anterolateral portals are marked. At the marked anteromedial portal, sterile normal saline solution is infused through a 22-gauge needle. A knife with a no. 11 blade is then used to make a small vertical incision through the skin only. Blunt dissection through the subcutaneous tissue is made with use of a mosquito clamp. The blunt trocar with the attached arthroscope cannula (a 4.0- or 2.7-mm scope) is carefully introduced through the ankle capsule into the joint. The arthroscope (typically 30 degrees) is exchanged for the blunt trocar, and the inflow side post is opened to infuse normal saline solution. For most procedures, the inflow is set up to gravity pressure only, or a pressure pump set to small joints. A 22-gauge needle is inserted at the anterolateral portal into the ankle joint and visualized with the scope. The position of this portal can be adjusted on the basis of the location of the ankle lesion. Using the same technique as with the anteromedial portal, the anterolateral portal is established. Sequential examination of the ankle is performed as previously described. A posterolateral portal can be established for inflow or visualization if necessary. For many anterior impingement lesions, visualization of the anterior compartment is maximized with minimal distraction and dorsiflexion of the ankle.

After the diagnostic examination, débridement with use of various arthroscopic tools and shavers is performed. Débridement includes removal of inflamed synovium, thickened adhesive bands and ligamentous tissue, osteophytes, and loose bodies. Typically the postfracture ankle and the arthritic ankle are contracted and challenging to navigate. Iatrogenic injury to the already traumatized articular surface should be avoided. Osteophytes are first débrided of soft tissue, capsule, or adhesions. An arthroscopic burr, pituitary rongeur, and small osteotome can be introduced through both anterior portals to completely remove the spurs. The goal for adequate resection is to establish an angle of 60 degrees with lines tangential to the talar neck and anterior tibia. Chondral lesions are débrided of loose fragments with a motorized shaver. Full-thickness lesions are débrided, and the subchondral base is drilled, similar to the technique described for microfracture/abrasion arthroplasty for talar osteochondral defect.

For anterolateral lesions, the diseased tissue may extend superiorly to the syndesmotic ligaments. For medial lesions, the arthroscope is placed in the anterolateral portal with instruments passed through the anteromedial portal. Care is taken to preserve the deep deltoid ligament. For cases of syndesmotic impingement, before preparing the limb, the stability of the syndesmosis is evaluated with stress radiographs obtained with the use of an anesthetic.

Gravity inflow should be used in the setting of an acute ankle fracture to avoid excessive fluid extravasation into the soft tissues. Hemarthrosis, fibrinous debris, and chondral/osteochondral fragments are removed or repaired. Fracture reduction is performed with a Freer elevator, arthroscopic probe, or reduction tenaculum. Fracture fixation is performed based on the pattern of injury, and the arthroscope is used to confirm an anatomic reduction.

The portals are closed with use of nylon suture in a vertical mattress pattern.

Authors' Preferred Technique

Posterior Impingement

Patients are placed in a prone position, with placement of a thigh tourniquet. With the ankle in a neutral position, the posterolateral portal is made at the level of the tip of the lateral malleolus, just lateral to the Achilles tendon (Fig. 115.4). A vertical incision is made using a no. 11 blade through skin only. A mosquito clamp spreads the subcutaneous layer and is directed anteriorly in the direction of the interdigital web space between the first and second toe. Once the clamp touches bone, it is exchanged for a 2.7- or 4.0-mm 30-degree arthroscope. The camera is directed laterally. The posteromedial portal is made at the same level. Once the skin incision is made, a mosquito clamp is directed to the arthroscope shaft. When the mosquito clamp touches the arthroscope

shaft, the clamp moves anteriorly toward the ankle joint, touching the arthroscope the entire way. The arthroscope is slightly pulled back, visualizing the tip of the clamp. An arthroscopic shaver is exchanged for the clamp, and the fatty tissue and synovium overlying the posterior ankle and subtalar joint are débrided. The posterior tibiofibular and talofibular ligament are identified. The posterior talar process, os trigonum, and FHL are identified. Care is taken to stay lateral to the FHL to prevent injury to the medial neurovascular bundle. Excision of an os trigonum or hypertrophic posterior talar process requires partial detachment of the posterior talofibular ligament, flexor retinaculum, and posterior talocalcaneal ligament (Fig. 115.5). After débridement, the skin portals are closed with nylon suture in a vertical mattress pattern.

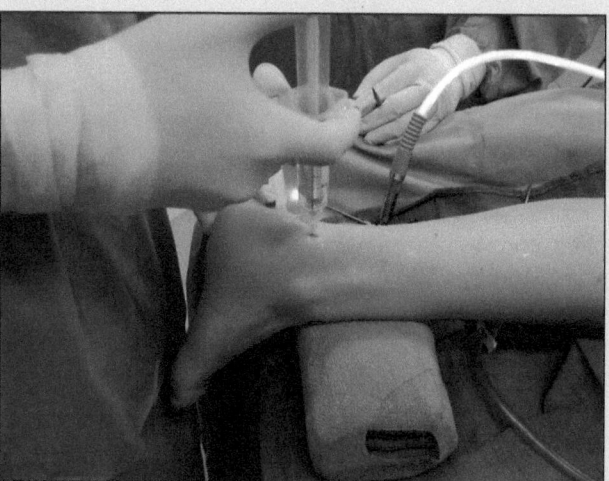

Fig. 115.4 The setup for posterior ankle endoscopic procedures. The needle is placed at the posterolateral portal, directed to the first web space, and placed parallel to the weight-bearing axis of the foot.

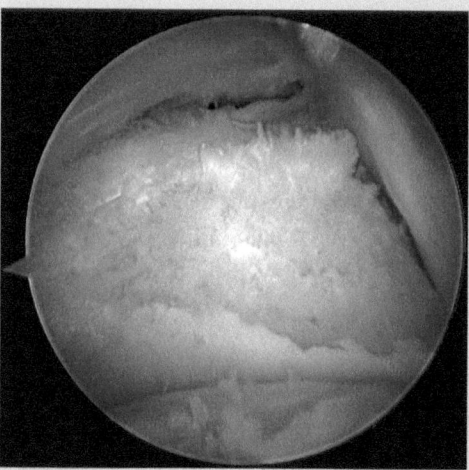

Fig. 115.5 The view of the posterior ankle/subtalar joint after excision of an os trigonum.

Authors' Preferred Technique

Lateral Ankle Ligament Reconstruction

Position, equipment, distraction, and portal placement were outlined previously for a standard anterior ankle arthroscopy approach. After a complete diagnostic arthroscopy of the ankle and treatment of accompanying lesions, lateral ankle instability can be visually confirmed with talar tilt and anterior drawer maneuvers. The lateral gutter is débrided of all scar tissue, and the periosteum is removed off the anterior aspect of the fibula (immediately distal from the anterior-inferior tibiofibular ligament). With the suture-anchor technique, a suture anchor is delivered through the anterolateral portal and placed into the prepared surface of the fibula. An accessory anterolateral portal is made 1 to 2 cm in front of the tip of the distal fibula. The sutures are pulled through the accessory anterolateral portal, and deep stitches with the sutures are made in the lateral ligament complex. The knot is tightened with the foot held in eversion and with a slight posterior drawer force. With the thermal energy technique, the thermal electrode is passed through the anterolateral portal and serially swept across the area of the anterior talofibular ligament (and calcaneofibular ligament posteriorly) with the foot placed in an everted position.

Arthroscopic Examination

The ankle can be divided into the anterior, central, and posterior compartments. Ferkel[4] has described the 21-point examination, including 8 points in the anterior compartment, 6 in the central compartment, and 7 in the posterior compartment. The anterior compartment examination includes the deltoid ligament, medial gutter, medial talus, central talus, lateral talus, talofibular articulation, lateral gutter, and anterior recess (see Fig. 115.3). The central compartment focuses on the tibiotalar articulation, examining the medial, central, and lateral aspects of this articulation, as well as slightly posteriorly looking at the posteroinferior and transverse tibiofibular ligaments and the reflection of the FHL tendon. The posterior compartment examination is performed while viewing from the posterolateral portal and includes the deltoid ligament, medial gutter, posteromedial talus and tibial plafond, central and lateral talus, posterior talofibular articulation, lateral gutter, and posterior recess.

Authors' Preferred Technique
Arthroscopic Ankle Arthrodesis

As previously described, two- or three-portal arthroscopy is performed. Non-invasive or invasive distraction facilitates exposure. Good visualization may require the removal of anterior scar tissue and osteophytes. The joint often has a large distal tibial and talar neck osteophyte that must be débrided not only for exposure but also to achieve adequate apposition of the joint surfaces. All remaining articular cartilage is removed with use of an arthroscopic shaver, straight and angle curettes, and osteotomes. The posterior talus and posterior malleolus are best approached from the posterolateral portal. After removal of all residual cartilage, the subchondral surface is prepared with a motorized abrader, removing a 1- to 2-mm layer of bone to the level of viable bleeding bone (Fig. 115.6). After débridement, the distractor is removed and the foot is positioned. The ideal position for fusion is 0 to 5 degrees of valgus, neutral dorsiflexion, and external rotation matching the contralateral ankle (typically 0 to 5 degrees). Internal fixation is performed with 6.5- or 7.0-mm cannulated, partially threaded screws. Two-screw fixation includes one placed from the medial malleolus toward the lateral process of the talus and a second screw placed lateral traversing the fibula into the talus. Three-screw fixation includes a final screw placed laterally, either anterior or posterior to the fibula. Final fluoroscopic views of the ankle are taken to confirm screw length and placement, as well as reduction and compression of the joint.

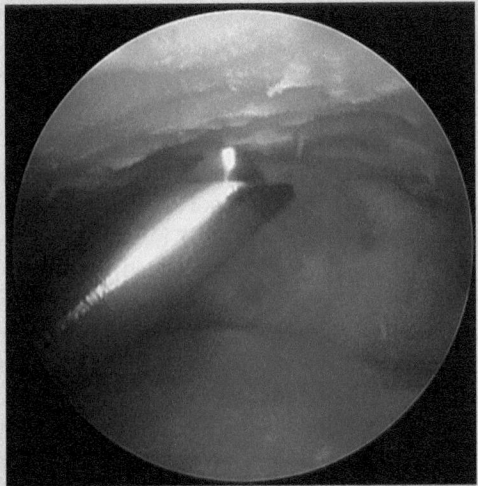

Fig. 115.6 Arthroscopic preparation of the tibiotalar joint; the subchondral surface is débrided with use of a motorized burr.

Postoperative Management

We prefer the use of a well-padded below-knee splint as the initial surgical dressing. This splint protects the limb, diminishes pain, and helps control swelling. The splint is removed around 10 to 14 days after surgery, and sutures are removed. For most conditions, a removable fracture boot is used to permit early motion exercises. The patient also increases weight bearing as allowed by pain and swelling of the limb. Formal physical therapy may also assist in facilitating the patient's rehabilitation and recovery. Patients typically perform therapeutic exercises without restrictions except if a lateral ligament reconstruction is performed; in that instance, limitation of inversion for the first 4 to 6 weeks can assist in early ligament healing. Discontinuation of the boot brace occurs around 4 to 6 weeks, followed by use of a lace-up ankle brace for patients with ligament reconstruction.

An exception to this general protocol is in cases of arthroscopic ankle arthrodesis; patients who have undergone this procedure are typically immobilized in a below-knee cast and restricted from weight bearing for approximately 6 to 8 weeks followed by progression of partial weight bearing to full weight bearing in a boot over another 4 to 6 weeks. Final discontinuation of the boot immobilization occurs once clinical and radiographic healing is confirmed.

Return to play in cases of loose body removal, synovectomy, and débridement of anterior or posterior impingement lesions is variable, but in most cases it is permissible 10 to 12 weeks after surgery. This time frame allows resolution of pain and edema along with advancement of the patient's rehabilitation and conditioning. Later phases of recovery focus on return to running, cutting and lateral movements, jumping, agility training, and sport-specific drills. Return to aggressive sports is, of course, very limited in cases of ankle arthrodesis, with many patients able to participate in light sporting activities but not in sports that entail heavy running or cutting.

Results

Most studies on ankle impingement are level IV case series, and rates of good to excellent patient outcomes are reported in more than 80% of cases.[13] Scranton and McDermott[32] compared open resection and arthroscopic resection of osteophytes in a retrospective study (level III). Length of stay and time to recovery were shorter in the arthroscopic group. In several prospective studies (level II), the success of arthroscopic débridement was reported as being between 73% and 96%.[33–35] One prospective, randomized (level I) study compared arthroscopic treatment of patients with a chronic syndesmotic injury both with or without medial instability.[36] The authors found no significant outcome difference between the two groups and reported an overall satisfaction rate of 90%. Long-term studies assessing the outcomes of ankle arthroscopy for anterior impingement are lacking, however Parma et al. published a study with a mean follow-up of 104.6 months. The authors concluded that while the postoperative American Orthopaedic Foot and Ankle scores (AOFAS) were still significantly improved at final follow-up compared to the preoperative assessment, chondral lesions, advanced age, and previous trauma were negative prognostic factors.[37]

Most studies involving the benefits of posterior ankle endoscopy involve level IV research.[38–41] Morag et al.[38] and Ogut et al.[39] reported on the results of endoscopic treatment of several pathologies in their patients, including Haglund deformity, peroneal tendonitis, and Achilles pathologies. Another series reviewed the outcomes of 55 patients treated for posterior ankle impingement with hindfoot endoscopy.[40] Symptoms were caused by trauma in 65% of patients and by overuse in 35% of patients. Postoperative AOFAS improved, with patients in the overuse group more satisfied than those in the posttraumatic group.[40] Willits et al.[41] reported their results for 23 patients treated for posterior ankle impingement. All patients showed satisfactory scores on all outcome measures and a high rate of return to sports. Smyth et al. published a systematic review assessing the outcomes of arthroscopic management of posterior ankle impingement. The authors noted that the overall complication rate of the procedure was 6.2%, with the most common being sural nerve dysthesia.[42]

A further indication for ankle arthroscopy for treating impingement is in patients who develop the symptoms following total ankle arthroplasty (TAR). In a study assessing the outcomes following TAR, the authors noted that 12 patients suffered from anterior, anteromedial, medial, lateral gutter, or posterior impingement. Following ankle arthroscopy, eight patients reported good pain relief, while the remaining patients reported minimal benefit.[43] As the number of TAR being performed increases each year,[44] the role of ankle arthroscopy for treating postoperative complications will likely grow.

With regard to arthroscopic management of ankle instability, only level IV studies for both plication and anchor fixation techniques are available at the time of the writing of this chapter.[15–21] Despite the debate over the effects of thermal energy on ligamentous tissue, the existing studies have demonstrated good results. Nery et al.[18] reviewed 38 patients treated with arthroscopic Broström-Gould repairs who were followed up an average of 9.8 years. Postoperative AOFAS scores were graded as excellent and good in 94.7% of patients. The Ankle Instability Group published a systematic review assessing the evidence of arthroscopic surgical management of ankle instability. They noted that the highest recommendation that good be given is grade C (poor-quality evidence) for the use of arthroscopic repair and arthroscopic reconstruction.[45] Prospective, randomized, controlled trials are needed to compare this approach with the standard open procedure.

Outcomes of degenerative ankles with arthroscopy have paralleled the experience of arthroscopic débridement of other joints. The treatment of specific degenerative pathology, such as impinging osteophytes, loose bodies, and limited chondral lesions, improves the chance of a good result.[46] Ogilvie-Harris and Sekyi-Out[47] reported on the arthroscopic débridement of 27 arthritic ankles and found that two-thirds of patients had symptomatic relief (level IV). Amendola et al.,[48] in a level IV study, found uniformly poor results with arthroscopic débridement in 11 arthritic ankles. Patients with anterior tibiotalar osteophytes and loose bodies have demonstrated better outcomes after arthroscopic débridements.[49] The consensus in the literature is that arthroscopic ankle débridement for degenerative joint disease is only appropriate in select cases and should be reserved for persons with early-stage disease.

Arthroscopic ankle arthrodesis has demonstrated faster rates of union, decreased complications, reduced postoperative pain, and shorter hospital stays.[50–54] Myerson and Quill[50] compared patients who underwent open and arthroscopic arthrodesis in comparative studies (level III). Both groups demonstrated similar fusion rates, with a shorter time to union in the arthroscopic group. O'Brien et al.,[53] in another retrospective study (level III), noted that both the open and arthroscopic groups had a similar fusion rate; however, the arthrodesis group demonstrated shorter operating room times, tourniquet time, and hospital stays. In the study with the longest term of follow-up, Glick et al.[51] followed up 34 patients for an average of 7.7 years after arthroscopic ankle fusions. A 97% rate of fusion success was reported, with clinical results reported as excellent and good in 86%.[51] The

results of open versus arthroscopic ankle arthrodesis has been compared in a large database study, noting that there was no difference in consequent revision arthrodesis between the two techniques. In addition, arthroscopic arthrodeses will likely become more popular, with a significant increase over a 12-year period being reported in the literature.[55]

Two level I studies were conducted to compare ankle fracture treatment with open reduction and internal fixation (ORIF) with and without arthroscopy.[56,57] In the smaller study with 19 patients, Thordarson et al.[56] showed similar outcomes at 21-month follow-up. Takao et al.[57] compared 72 patients and found that the arthroscopic group had statistically higher AOFAS scores.

van Dijk et al.[28] compared the results of arthroscopic débridement in postfracture patients who had impingement symptoms with the results of those who had more diffuse ankle complaints (level II). At 2-year follow-up, the impingement group reported better pain relief with 86% satisfaction compared with the patients with grade II osteoarthritis, who had a satisfaction rate of 70%.[28] Utsugi et al.,[58] in a prospective case series (level IV), performed an arthroscopic débridement in 33 ankles at the time of removal of their ankle fracture hardware. These investigators recognized a negative correlation between the presence of arthrofibrosis and joint function. They stated that arthroscopic débridement resulted in functional improvement in 89% of the patients.[58]

Complications

The average complication rate of ankle arthroscopy in the literature ranges from 3.5% to 10.3%.[59–61] Neurologic injury is the most common complication reported, comprising almost half of all complications. Neurovascular injury can be contributed to incorrect portal placement, prolonged or inappropriate use of distraction, or use of a tourniquet. Anterolateral portal nerve injury can result in hypersensitivity or paresthesia over the intermediate branch of the superficial peroneal nerve. During noninvasive distraction, the foot strap has been implicated in the development of midfoot dysesthesias.[60] Overly aggressive anterior débridement can potentially result in hemarthrosis or deep peroneal nerve injury, although these complications are rare. Nonneurologic complications included wound complications, deep venous thrombosis, tourniquet complications, articular cartilage damage, compartment syndrome, and complex regional pain syndrome.[59]

Future Considerations

Given the small number of evidence-based studies that are available, it is difficult to determine the role of arthroscopic reduction internal fixation or arthroscopy-assisted ORIF in the management of ankle fractures. The incidence of cartilaginous injury associated with these fractures has been documented to be from 20% to 88% and may support routine arthroscopic techniques with future studies.[62–65]

SUBTALAR ARTHROSCOPY

Arthroscopy of the subtalar joint was described by Parisien[66] in 1986 with the advent of improved arthroscopic technology and techniques, along with experience in ankle arthroscopy. Arthroscopy of the subtalar joint offered the ability to diagnose and treat intra-articular pathology that previously could only be addressed with open arthrotomy.[66,67] Early reports focused on portals located to allow access to the posterior facet of the subtalar joint, while acknowledging that visualization of the anterior and middle facets is prevented by the contents of the sinus tarsi and tarsal canal.[66,67] These descriptions included anterolateral and posterolateral portals for use with small-diameter arthroscopes. An anatomic study investigated the proximity of these portals to nearby neurovascular structures and found relative safety, with the sural nerve and its branches approximately 4 to 8 mm away from these sites.[68] These portals also allowed access to more than 90% of the posterior facet.[68]

History
Pathologic conditions of the subtalar joint produces pain, swelling, and stiffness that can present medially and laterally in the hindfoot. Patients particularly note difficulty ambulating on uneven ground. Symptoms are usually proportionate to the individual's level of activity.

Physical Examination
Careful physical examination can localize tenderness to the sinus tarsi and subtalar joint rather than the ankle joint. Inversion-eversion motion of the joint should be determined along with any obvious findings of crepitus. Examination of nearby structures may also help rule out other potential sources of pain, including

the peroneal tendons. A diagnostic injection with a local anesthetic can prove useful but may require the inclusion of radiopaque dye to allow radiographic confirmation that the injection is intra-articular and does not extrude into the ankle joint or peroneal tendon sheath, which may confound the test.[69]

Imaging
Standard weight-bearing radiographs of the foot and ankle are obtained to identify the presence of subtalar arthritis and assess overall alignment of the foot. CT and MRI can be obtained to identify occult pathology such as a focal cartilage abnormality or osteochondral defect, soft tissue inflammation, and the early presentation of arthritis.[70] However, these modalities may not fully evaluate the joint, and arthroscopy may ultimately provide so-called "gold standard" diagnostic assessment.[70]

Decision-Making Principles
Regardless of etiology, initial treatment focuses on nonoperative modalities. The use of antiinflammatory medications may relieve pain and swelling. Custom orthotic insoles can assist in improving hindfoot alignment and relieving impingement of the joint, and a lace-up ankle brace limits painful inversion and eversion. The benefit of physical therapy for subtalar conditions remains unclear but may be attempted for a short period. Corticosteroid injection of the subtalar joint can be performed to relieve inflammation and pain, although the duration may be temporary in most cases. Surgery is typically recommended when symptoms fail to respond to these measures after 4 to 6 months.

⚑ Authors' Preferred Technique
Arthroscopic Subtalar Débridement

For standard subtalar arthroscopy, the patient is placed in a lateral[70,71] or semilateral decubitus[72,73] position on the operating table. Noninvasive distraction may facilitate visualization of the joint, although in some cases simply positioning the limb on a bump may allow the joint to fall into varus.[71] Standard portals for subtalar arthroscopy include anterolateral, anterior or middle accessory, and posterolateral portals (Fig. 115.7).[67,88] The anterolateral portal is established 1 cm inferior and 2 cm distal to the tip of the lateral malleolus[67,68,70–73] in the palpable soft spot at the angle of Gissane. The portal can be localized by a needle inserted approximately 40 degrees in the semicoronal plane and aimed slightly cephalad, with insufflation of the joint capsule with normal saline solution. The anterior accessory portal is placed immediately anterior to the tip of the lateral malleolus and aiming horizontally in a medial direction,[67,68,71–73] with intra-articular confirmation performed with the arthroscope in the anterolateral portal. The posterolateral portal is located 1 cm above the level of the tip of the lateral malleolus and immediately lateral to the Achilles tendon.[67,68,71–73] A spinal needle can be placed to visually confirm the position again from the anterolateral portal prior to incision of the posterolateral skin. All portals are carefully created by incising only the skin with a scalpel blade to avoid injury to nearby nerves, followed by spreading of the subcutaneous tissues with a hemostat clamp and entry into the joint with a blunt trocar and cannula.

  The use of small joint arthroscopes and instruments is necessary for subtalar arthroscopy. A 2.5- or 2.7-mm 30-degree arthroscope[67,88,70–72] is used along with 2.5- or 3.5-mm power shaver blades. A 2.7-mm 70-degree arthroscope may be

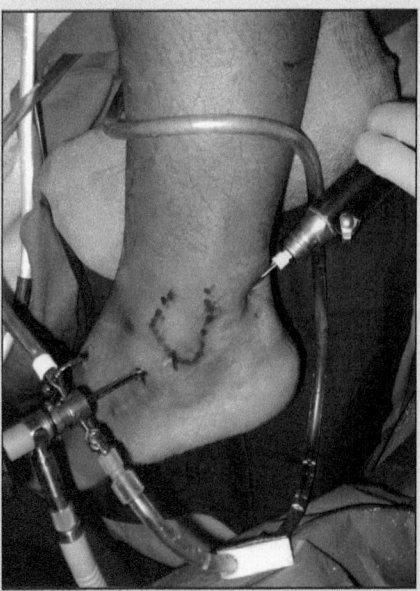

Fig. 115.7 Subtalar arthroscopy portals. The arthroscope is in the anterolateral portal and the shaver is in the posterolateral portal.

Continued

📌 Authors' Preferred Technique—cont'd

Arthroscopic Subtalar Débridement—cont'd

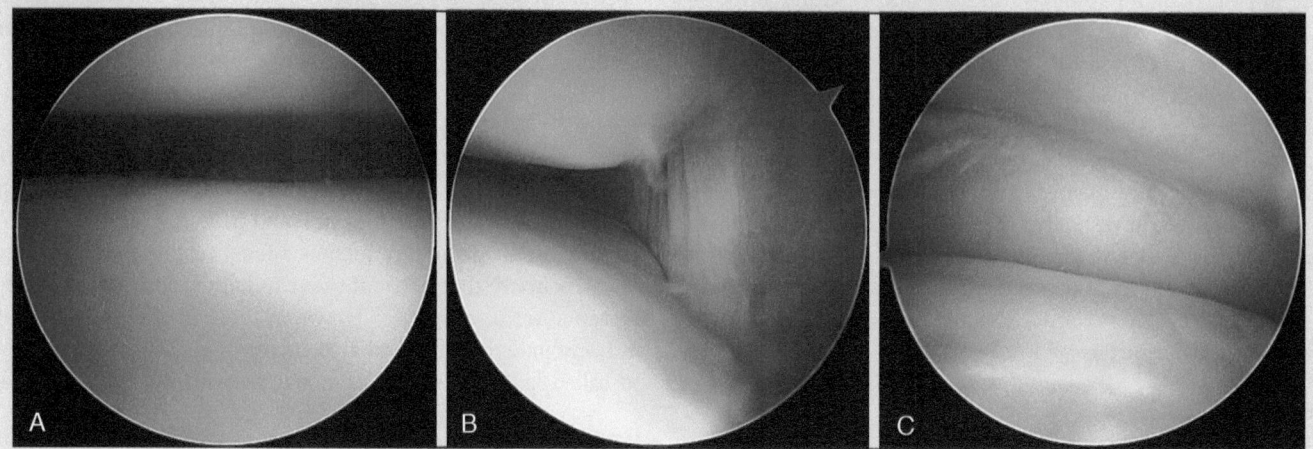

Fig. 115.8 Views of subtalar arthroscopy. (A) The posterior facet joint surface is visualized from the antero-lateral portal. (B) The view of the lateral recess beneath the lateral malleolus. (C) The view of the posterior joint surface from the posterolateral portal.

useful in some instances to improve visibility. The use of specialized small joint basket forceps, probes, and grabber devices is appropriate. Soft tissue pathology, such as synovitis, fibrosis, and chondral lesions are addressed with basket forceps and both fine and aggressive power shaver blades; bony lesions are débrided with small joint arthroscopic chisels and motorized burrs.

Visualization of the joint is performed by alternating placement of the arthroscope in the different portals, with instruments placed in the remaining portals. Inspection of the subtalar joint includes the interosseous ligaments anteriorly, the lateral recess inferior to the lateral malleolus, the chondral surfaces of the calcaneus and talus, and the posterior joint space (or pouch) (Fig. 115.8).[86]

Arthroscopy of the subtalar joint was initially described for débridement of soft tissue lesions or impingement (Fig. 115.9). Indications include the removal of loose bodies[70,71,73] along with the treatment of joint synovitis,[70,71,73] sinus tarsi syndrome,[71,72] cartilage flap tears,[70,71,73] and subtalar adhesions.[71,73] Indications have expanded to include the removal of osteophytes[73] and the treatment of arthritis.[71,73]

Subtalar arthroscopy also has been used to treat sequela of calcaneal fractures. Patients often have subtalar adhesions, contracture, and joint stiffness after an intra-articular calcaneal fracture,[74,75] manifesting as pain, stiffness, and difficulty walking on uneven ground.[74,75] Subtalar arthroscopy has been used to débride the sinus tarsi, intra-articular adhesions, and inflammation and fibrosis in the lateral recess and posterior joint space.[74,75]

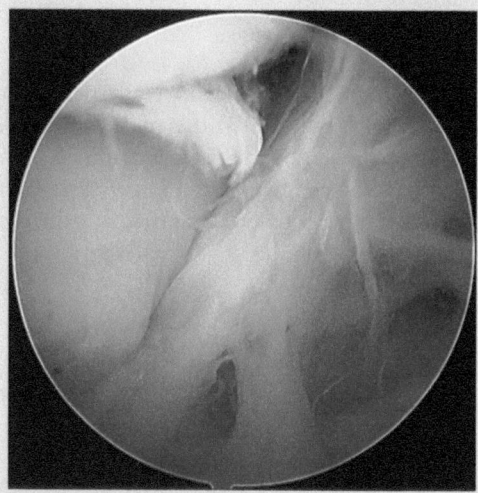

Fig. 115.9 A view of torn subtalar interosseous ligaments before débridement.

📌 Authors' Preferred Technique

Arthroscopic Subtalar Arthrodesis

Arthroscopic subtalar arthrodesis is indicated in the same instances as open arthrodesis, namely the treatment of end-stage posttraumatic arthritis, osteoarthritis, inflammatory arthritis, hindfoot deformity, or tarsal coalition.[76–78] Arthroscopic subtalar arthrodesis may result in less pain and morbidity than open arthrodesis[76,77]; older studies also suggested a shorter postoperative hospitalization,[76] although in contemporary practice subtalar fusion is commonly performed on an outpatient basis. Arthroscopic fusion may also result in less disruption of the osseous blood supply, which may facilitate bony healing.[77,79] Contraindications to arthroscopic subtalar fusion include hindfoot deformity of greater than 5 degrees of varus or 15 degrees of varus,[77,79] which may preclude effective arthroscopy and joint preparation. Significant bone loss, collapse, or osteonecrosis may also be contraindications.[79]

Early descriptions of arthroscopic subtalar arthrodesis used a supine position with a bump under the ipsilateral hip.[76,77] An anterolateral portal is created 1 cm distal and 1 to 2 cm anterior to the lateral malleolus, with an accessory portal placed immediately anterior to the malleolus.[76,77] A posterolateral portal is localized just adjacent to the Achilles tendon at the level of the posterior facet, which can be identified under fluoroscopy.[76,77] More recently, case series have discussed the advantages of prone positioning to allow better visualization of the posterior facet with little risk to the neurovascular bundle.[78,79] Initially, the prone approach was performed with three portals, but newer reports suggest excellent exposure with two portals.[78,79] The posterolateral portal is created as previously described. A posteromedial portal is made just medial to the Achilles tendon, and the blunt trocar is aimed laterally to touch the arthroscope.[78,79] The instrument

📌 Authors' Preferred Technique—cont'd
Arthroscopic Subtalar Arthrodesis—cont'd

is then carefully directed toward the posterior joint, staying lateral to the FHL tendon to avoid iatrogenic injury to the neurovascular structures.[78,79] Distraction of the joint can be performed with a soft tissue strap and clamp system similar to ankle arthroscopy.[77] The use of invasive pin fixation with an AO distractor is of historical interest only.[76] A blunt trocar can also be inserted into the joint via an anterolateral accessory portal to separate the joint surfaces and help exposure.[79]

Débridement of the sinus tarsi soft tissues and the interosseous ligaments is carried out with a motorized shaver from an anterior or posterior portal.[76] This débridement allows access to the anterior and middle facets, which can be débrided with a curette, although some authors believe that this procedure is not necessary.[78,79] The remaining cartilage of the posterior facet is then removed with curettes, motorized shavers, and power burrs, working through the various

portals to access the joint.[78,79] Fixation is readily performed, especially when the patient is positioned prone. The use of one or two 6.5-, 7.0-, or 7.3-mm screws has been described.[78–79] The authors prefer the use of two cannulated 6.5-mm compression screws directed from the calcaneal tuberosity across the fusion into the talar dome and neck, respectively. To augment biologic healing of the fusion, the use of demineralized bone matrix,[76] autologous tibial or iliac crest bone graft,[77] allograft cancellous bone,[79] or synthetic bone substitute[79] can be considered based on the surgeon's preference and patient risk factors. Postoperatively, the limb is immobilized for 2 weeks in a padded splint followed by the use of a below-knee cast for 4 weeks while the patient is non–weight bearing.[76,78,79] After 6 weeks, the patient can begin partial weight bearing in a walking cast or removable boot brace and is typically able to resume wearing shoes by 10 to 12 weeks if radiographic healing has been achieved.[76,78,79]

📌 Authors' Preferred Technique
Arthroscopically Assisted Treatment of Calcaneal Fractures

Treatment of comminuted intra-articular calcaneal fractures with ORIF has a high rate of soft tissue complications, including wound necrosis, dehiscence, and infection.[80,81] Extensile exposure can also cause significant soft tissue contracture and stiffness, compromising clinical outcomes. Recently, a trend has emerged favoring minimal incision or percutaneous fixation techniques when permitted by the fracture pattern to minimize such complications. Several authors have recommended concomitant use of subtalar arthroscopy to assist in the removal of joint debris and confirm appropriate fracture reduction intraoperatively.[80,81] This technique is appropriate in two-part calcaneal fractures (type II Sanders classification), particularly tongue-type patterns; it is contraindicated in more severely comminuted fracture patterns (types III and IV).[80–82] The patient is placed in a lateral decubitus position on the operating table, and a tourniquet is applied

to the thigh.[80–82] A combination of anterolateral, middle lateral accessory, and posterolateral portals is used.[80–82] A 2.0- or 2.7-mm arthroscope is used along with small joint instruments.[80–82] A partially threaded Schanz screw is inserted percutaneously into the displaced tongue fracture fragment or tuberosity to allow manipulation and reduction of the joint surface.[80–82] This maneuver can also be facilitated by a percutaneous elevator to disimpact and elevate the joint fragment along with Kirschner wires to act as a joystick.[80,82] Fine tuning of the reduction can be carried out based on the appearance of the congruity of the joint surface, which often appears reduced on fluoroscopy but still malreduced arthroscopically.[80–82] Provisional fixation is carried out with Kirschner wires followed by percutaneous lag or cannulated screw fixation.[80–82]

Postoperative Management

The patient is initially managed in a well-padded below-knee splint for 10 to 14 days, at which point the dressing is removed and the sutures are withdrawn. In débridement procedures, the goal is to commence early ROM and progressive weight bearing in a fracture boot orthosis. The patient then weans out of the boot as tolerated once pain and swelling subside. Formalized physical therapy can assist in the individual's transition toward functional recovery.

In patients treated for calcaneal fractures, non–weight bearing is maintained for approximately 8 to 10 weeks depending on the surgeon's confidence in the quality of fixation and the patient's bone stock. Early motion exercises, muscle stimulation, and strengthening are critical to prevent stiffness and atrophy after these types of fractures. As radiographic healing becomes apparent, weight bearing advances in a boot brace and then the patient progresses to wearing shoes.

Patients undergoing subtalar arthrodesis are non–weight bearing in a below-knee cast for a period of 6 to 8 weeks, again depending on fixation strength, bone quality, and progressive healing demonstrated on radiographs. This period is followed by progressive weight bearing in a removable boot orthosis until radiographic fusion is demonstrated. The patient then resumes use of comfort shoe wear, often by 12 to 14 weeks.

Results

Débridement procedures performed arthroscopically have been described in numerous level IV series. One report of 12 patients treated with subtalar arthroscopy indicated its utility in providing an accurate diagnosis, often more effectively than with radiographs or MRI scanning.[70] These authors indicated better results in patients treated for loose bodies or chondral tears, with worse results noted for patients with synovitis or arthritis.[70] A second series of 45 patients who underwent subtalar arthroscopy yielded 94% excellent or good results, even though 54% of the patients had Workers' Compensation claims.[71] The authors described a low complication rate, with three neurapraxias, one infection, and one portal fistula. They also found various pathologies during arthroscopy for so-called *sinus tarsi syndrome*, including interosseous ligament tears, arthrofibrosis, and subtalar arthritis; the authors recommended that this term be dropped in favor of more accurate diagnoses discovered during arthroscopy.[71] The authors of another series of 33 cases reached the same conclusion about the term *sinus tarsi syndrome* being vague and diagnostically inadequate.[72] These patients demonstrated interosseous ligament tears (88%), synovitis (55%), cervical ligament tears (33%), fibrosis (24%), and soft tissue impingement lesions (21%) upon arthroscopic evaluation. After débridement, patients had improvement in the Pain Visual Analogue Scale of 7.3 to 2.7

points, and 88% had excellent or good outcomes.[72] A comprehensive study of 115 patients treated with subtalar arthroscopy for débridement of soft tissue lesions, subtalar arthritis, calcaneal or talar fractures, and talocalcaneal coalitions produced overall 59% excellent, 38% good, and 3% poor results with the use of the AOFAS Ankle-Hindfoot Scoring instrument.[73] Of the subgroup of patients with a preoperative diagnosis of "sinus tarsi syndrome," the authors found interosseous ligament tears, arthritis, loose bodies, osteochondral lesions, and fibrosis due to tarsal coalition.[73]

One level IV report demonstrated 82% pain relief in 17 patients treated for posttraumatic stiffness, with the remaining patients ultimately requiring subtalar arthrodesis for continued symptoms.[75] The authors noted that better results with arthroscopy occurred within a year of the initial fracture and with lower grades of cartilage damage or arthritis.[75] Surgeons have also reported successful arthroscopic treatment of subfibular impingement due to lateral calcaneal abutment after a calcaneal fracture.[83–85] Arthroscopy was performed after patients failed to respond to nonsurgical treatment with medications and injections.[83] The authors also believed that arthroscopic treatment allowed improved visualization and assessment of the joint cartilage compared with open arthrotomy.[83] These reports describe débridement of the lateral calcaneal exostosis due to the fracture with use of anterolateral, posterolateral, and middle accessory portals.[83–85] Initially, fibrosis is resected with use of a motorized shaver followed by removal of the calcaneal prominence with use of a burr to decompress the subfibular space.[83–85] In a retrospective series with limited numbers of patients, it was reported that pain relief was achieved in roughly 80% of cases, with the remainder needing subtalar fusion.[83,84] Clearly this technique warrants further study, but it may offer a less invasive option for these posttraumatic conditions.

Outcomes of arthroscopic subtalar arthrodesis are generally excellent. Scranton[76] retrospectively compared 12 patients who underwent open fusion versus 5 patients who underwent arthroscopic fusion. He noted a slightly longer operative time in the arthroscopic group but a 100% union rate compared with a 92% union rate in the open group. A prospective series of 41 arthroscopic fusions in 37 patients had a mean follow-up of 55 months.[77] Mean surgical time was 75 minutes. The authors noted delayed unions in the first three cases but subsequently had a 100% union rate by 11 weeks after initiating cast immobilization postoperatively. Amendola et al.[79] reported on 11 fusions in 10 patients treated with prone arthroscopic subtalar arthrodesis. Nine patients were very satisfied, one was satisfied, and one was dissatisfied because of a nonunion. The fusion rate was 91% by 10 weeks. No infections or nerve injuries occurred; one patient required hardware removal. Another series of 16 patients treated with prone arthroscopic subtalar arthrodesis had a follow-up of 72 months.[78] The operative time averaged 72 minutes. The authors realized a 94% union rate by 11 weeks with one nonunion; 81% had a good result, with 13% having a fair result and 6% having a poor result. Complications included one infection but no nerve injuries or deep vein thromboses. Rungprai et al. published one of the largest series, comparing open versus arthroscopic subtalar arthrodesis. The authors concluded that while the union and

complication rate were not significantly different, the arthroscopic groups time to union was shorter. In addition, the arthroscopic group returned to work and athletic activities at an earlier time point.[86] Arthroscopic subtalar arthrodesis appears to offer excellent clinical outcomes with few complications and a high union rate. This appears to be true, regardless of the etiology of subtalar pathology. There is evidence in the literature that suggests that the outcomes of arthroscopic subtalar arthrodesis show comparable results whether performed for posttraumatic arthritis or adult-acquired flatfoot deformity.[87] However, because of the technical difficulty, most authors agree that this procedure should be performed by experienced arthroscopists to minimize complications and optimize outcomes.

The management of calcaneal fractures by arthroscopically assisted reduction and fixation has been studied. Level IV case series have described outcomes with this technique in small numbers of patients. An early report discussed the utility of subtalar arthroscopy in calcaneal fractures in three ways.[81] A cohort of 28 patients who had previously undergone ORIF subsequently returned for hardware removal. At the time of that procedure, they underwent subtalar arthroscopy to assess the intra-articular reduction. The authors found that 23% had greater than a 2-mm step-off or Outerbridge grade III chondral damage, whereas another 23% had greater than a 1-mm step-off or grade II chondral changes. Only 53% had a congruent reduction.[81] A second cohort of 55 patients underwent ORIF with arthroscopic assessment of the quality of joint reduction; 22% of these patients still had residual step-off despite fluoroscopic evaluation that suggested good reduction.[81] A final group of 18 patients underwent arthroscopically guided percutaneous reduction and fixation of type II calcaneal fractures. Fifteen patients had a follow-up of 15 months, with 80% of patients pain free. Patients returned to work an average of 11 weeks after surgery.[81] Another study detailed results with arthroscopically assisted percutaneous reduction of type II calcaneal fractures.[82] The authors treated 22 patients with a follow-up of 33 months. They found correction of Bohler's angle postoperatively, which held up over time.[82] Further, patients showed clinical improvement as measured by a Visual Analogue Pain Scale, the AOFAS Ankle-Hindfoot score, and the Short-Form 36 instrument; these results continued to improve up to 2 years after surgery.[82] In a similar study of 33 patients, improvements were found in AOFAS scores, with low rates of residual pain and maintained correction of Bohler's angle, which reinforced the results of prior reports.[80] Although this technique is indicated for a small subset of persons with calcaneal fractures, and evidence-based studies are limited, the technique appears promising and will likely prove useful with additional study.

Complications

Complications after subtalar arthroscopy are uncommon. Most series report a low incidence of complications, although the retrospective nature of the vast majority of these reports potentially affects the reported incidence. Infection rates after subtalar arthroscopy have been reported to be from 0% to 1.1%.[71,73,79,88] A persistent sinus tract or fistula is rare, with reports of this phenomenon occurring in 0% to 2% of patients.[71,78] Nerve injuries including transient numbness or neurapraxia are the most frequent complication, ranging from 0% to 6%.[71–73,78,79] Authors of one large series of 186 patients treated with posterior ankle, subtalar, and hindfoot arthroscopy discovered an overall complication rate of 8.5%.[88] They did not find a correlation between complications and the surgeon's experience, or the use or type of distraction used.[88] Neurologic complications were most common with a 3.7% incidence, including transient tibial neurapraxia, sural neurapraxia, and complex regional pain syndrome.[88] These complications were treated with oral gabapentin and subsequent neurolysis when necessary; whereas complex regional pain syndrome was addressed with gabapentin, physical therapy, and anesthetic injections. Emphasizing prevention, the authors recommended meticulous surgical technique, including careful portal placement, incision of the skin, spreading of the subcutaneous tissues, and minimizing the frequency of withdrawal and reinsertion of instruments through the portal sites to avoid nerve injury.[88] They also commented specifically on posterior subtalar and ankle arthroscopy, emphasizing the need to remain lateral to the FHL tendon to avoid iatrogenic nerve injury to the medial neurovascular structures.[88]

ENDOSCOPIC HAGLUND RESECTION/ CALCANEOPLASTY

Pain in the posterior superior aspect of the calcaneus can be related to several factors that can be present in isolation or more commonly in combination. Retrocalcaneal bursitis, prominence of an enlarged superior calcaneal tuberosity (Haglund deformity), insertional Achilles tendinosis, or inflammation of an adventitial bursa between the Achilles tendon and posterior skin can all cause pain in this area. A difference in outcomes between Achilles tendinosis and retrocalcaneal bursitis with Haglund deformity has been noted, though the two often coexist.

Anatomically, the Achilles tendon inserts on the calcaneus between 10 to 13 mm distal to the superior aspect of the tuberosity with a crescent-shaped insertion that extends 3.5 mm anterior medially and 1.0 mm laterally on average from the most posterior point of the tuberosity.[89,90] The retrocalcaneal bursa is located between the Achilles tendon and the calcaneal tuberosity. It is a disk-shaped bursa that covers the posterosuperior angle of the calcaneus.[91] Mechanical irritation can lead to inflammation of the bursa, as well as hypertrophy of the tissue.

The sural nerve runs lateral to the Achilles tendon, and the plantaris tendon runs medially. The blood supply to the posterior calcaneus is from the medial and lateral branches of the posterior tibial artery and the peroneal artery.

History

Patients report posterior heel pain that is exacerbated by walking and climbing stairs. Often they note stiffness and pain upon arising from bed or after prolonged sitting. Some patients note swelling or enlargement of the posterior heel as well. These symptoms may wax and wane over time but generally worsen.

Physical Examination

On examination the posterior heel may appear swollen, or an enlargement of the posterior calcaneus may be present. The Achilles tendon is palpated for tenderness and any nodularity, which may signify tendinosis. The retrocalcaneal bursa is immediately anterior to the tendon and may be tender or boggy if inflamed. Direct pressure over the insertion point on the calcaneus may reveal tenderness along with painful spur formation.

Imaging

Calcification of the Achilles tendon noted on lateral radiographs as extensive calcification (>50%) in the tendon is a contraindication to endoscopic resection, and open resection should be recommended in that case. An MRI scan is frequently recommended to assess the tendon itself and also to confirm the presence of retrocalcaneal bursitis. Extensive tendinosis, splitting, or tearing seen on an MRI scan may be a contraindication to endoscopic débridement because open tendon débridement and repair will be necessary to fully address the pathology.

Decision-Making Principles

Most patients respond to nonoperative management including rest, activity modification (cross-training with low-impact activities), use of antiinflammatory medication and ice, and possible injection into the retrocalcaneal bursa, although a diagnostic injection with lidocaine is preferred to cortisone with lidocaine even in the bursa, given the risk of tendon weakening and rupture. Use of heel lifts, open-backed shoes, and Achilles pads can also be helpful. Occasionally a fracture boot or short leg cast may be used in patients with very active symptoms. Surgical intervention is considered when nonoperative treatment has failed after a recommended minimum of 6 months. Endoscopic and open techniques have both been described and have been demonstrated to be effective, although less morbidity is associated with endoscopic débridement.[92,93]

 Authors' Preferred Technique

Endoscopic Haglund Resection

Positioning

The patient can be positioned either supine or prone with the foot and ankle free at the distal end of the operating table. This positioning allows for dorsiflexion and plantar flexion at the ankle with use of pressure from the surgeon's chest, leaving both hands free for manipulation of the instruments. In the supine position, a bump or well leg holder should be used to allow adequate working space. We prefer to use a prone position, with the ankle located just at the edge of the operating table. The procedure can be performed with use of a regional or general anesthetic. A well-padded thigh tourniquet should be placed because the bony resection can result in bleeding.

Continued

📌 **Authors' Preferred Technique—cont'd**

Endoscopic Haglund Resection—cont'd

Portal Locations

Two portals are generally used—one medial and one lateral—although single medial portal use has been described as well.[92] The portals are located just medial or lateral to the Achilles tendon at the level of the superior aspect of the calcaneus. The lateral portal is often established first by making a vertical skin incision followed by blunt dissection to minimize the risk of injury to the sural nerve. A blunt trocar is then introduced, followed by the 4.0-mm 30-degree arthroscope (a 2.7-mm arthroscope can also be used in smaller patients). A needle is then used to localize the medial portal and is advanced in a lateral direction until it is visible. A vertical skin incision is then created followed by blunt dissection with a hemostat clamp. A 3.5- or 4-mm motorized shaver is then inserted, and resection of inflamed bursa and soft tissue will allow adequate visualization.

Retrocalcaneal Bursectomy

Resection of the retrocalcaneal bursa is performed once the portals have been established, allowing adequate visualization of the posterior calcaneus and anterior surface of the Achilles tendon. A 4-mm power shaver can be used to resect the inflamed bursal tissue. The use of an electrocautery device can also be helpful to remove the soft tissue and periosteum on the calcaneus.

Haglund's Resection

The goal of débridement of Haglund deformity is to resect enough bone to eliminate the mechanical irritation of the tendon and bursal tissues. The resection needs to be carried down to the insertion of the Achilles both medially and laterally, which can be performed with the aid of intraoperative fluoroscopy to confirm adequate bony resection. A combination of a shaver, a burr, and a reciprocating rasp can be used (Fig. 115.10). The Achilles tendon is protected by maintaining the closed portion of the instrument against the Achilles while working on the resection. The edges can then be smoothed using a curette and bone rasp.

Achilles Tendon Débridement

The Achilles tendon is then visualized and inspected for diseased tissue. A diseased tendon can be resected with the shaver. An anatomic study had shown that as much as 50% of the tendon can be débrided safely if necessary.[94] However, actual repair of the tendon in the presence of partial tearing is difficult and likely requires an open procedure.

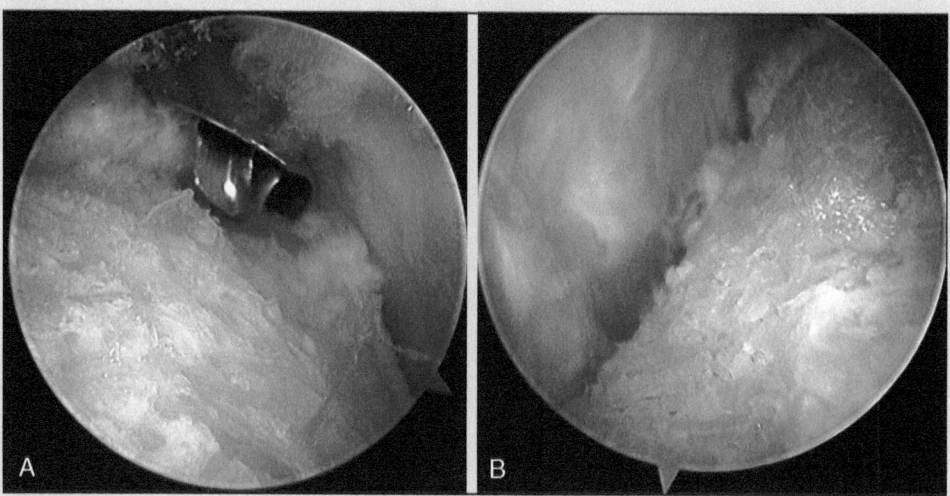

Fig. 115.10 (A) Endoscopic resection of Haglund process with motorized burr. (B) A view of the superior calcaneus after débridement.

Postoperative Management

Initially the patient is non–weight bearing and wears a padded below-knee splint to provide compression and minimize soft tissue tension that may affect wound healing. After 7 to 10 days, the splint is removed and the sutures are discontinued. The patient then advances to a removable fracture boot orthosis and can commence weight bearing. Physical therapy can assist in regaining ROM and ankle strength and proprioception. Return to running and other sports typically occurs at 3 months after the procedure.

Results

Endoscopic treatment of Haglund deformity and retrocalcaneal bursitis has been shown to be safe and effective.[93,95,96] van Dijk et al.[95] reported excellent or good results in 19 of 20 patients treated with endoscopic débridement. A retrospective study of 81 patients demonstrated excellent or good results in 75 patients (93%).[93] The authors did note a learning curve, with improved operative times after gaining more experience with the procedure.[93] In another retrospective series, excellent or good results were reported in 29 of 30 patients after 35 months of follow-up.[96] One patient did sustain a complete rupture of the Achilles tendon that required open repair.[96] A prospective study comparing open and endoscopic treatment in 17 and 33 patients, respectively, demonstrated similar outcomes with AOFAS Ankle-Hindfoot scores, a similar recovery time, and a faster operative time in the endoscopic group.[92] The endoscopic group also had fewer complications than the open group, including fewer instances of wound infection, nerve injury, and scar tenderness.[92]

Complications

Potential complications include wound infection, delayed portal healing, incisional tenderness, sural nerve injury, heel numbness, incomplete pain relief, and Achilles tendon rupture. Most of these complications can be prevented with careful surgical technique, as previously detailed. Incomplete relief of symptoms may be due to improper patient selection in the setting of insertional calcification or extensive tendinosis; these patients may have better results with open procedures.

For a complete list of references, go to ExpertConsult.com.

SELECTED READINGS

Citation:
Beimers L, Frey C, van Dijk CN. Arthroscopy of the posterior subtalar joint. *Foot Ankle Clin.* 2006;11:369–390.

Level of Evidence:
V

Summary:
The authors provide an excellent overview regarding the diagnostic and therapeutic indications for this technique. Additionally, the anatomy and technique of the procedure are explained in detail.

Citation:
van Dijk CN. Hindfoot endoscopy. *Foot Ankle Clin.* 2006;11: 391–414.

Level of Evidence:
V

Summary:
The author provides a review of hindfoot endoscopy and its relevance in posterior tibial tenosynovectomy, diagnosis of a peroneus brevis length rupture, peroneal tendon adhesiolysis, flexor hallucis longus release, os trigonum removal, endoscopic treatment for retrocalcaneal bursitis, endoscopic treatment for Achilles (peri)tendinopathy, and treatment of ankle joint or subtalar joint pathology.

Citation:
van Dijk CN. Anterior and posterior ankle impingement. *Foot Ankle Clin.* 2006;11:663–683.

Level of Evidence:
V

Summary:
The author provides a review of the etiology and clinical features of ankle impingement. Additionally, a detailed explanation of the surgical technique and results are presented.

Citation:
van Dijk CN, Scholten PE, Krips R. A 2-portal endoscopic approach for diagnosis and treatment of posterior ankle pathology. *Arthroscopy.* 2000;16:871–876.

Level of Evidence:
IV

Summary:
The authors describe a two-portal endoscopic approach of the hindfoot with the patient in the prone position. They describe the case of a professional ballet dancer with chronic flexor hallucis longus tendinitis and posterior ankle impingement syndrome caused by an os trigonum of both ankles.

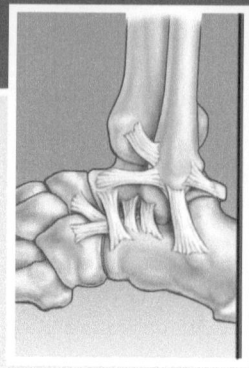

116

Sports Shoes and Orthoses

Nicholas LeCursi

SPORTS ORTHOSES

Foot orthoses—also commonly called orthotics, arch supports, and inserts—have been applied to the treatment of pathologic musculoskeletal conditions for more than a century.[1] The term *foot orthosis* refers to any orthotic device that is distal to the ankle. This naming convention was introduced in the early 1970s by the Committee on Prosthetic-Orthotic Education.[2]

A foot orthosis may be as simple as a prefabricated arch support available over the counter at the local pharmacy or as complex as a custom-designed device incorporating multiple supportive elements. Whatever the type, the beneficial effects of a foot orthosis are determined by its relative shape, stiffness, and compressibility with respect to the weight-bearing foot.

Although research suggests that foot orthoses are efficacious in the treatment of pathologic musculoskeletal conditions, outcome studies point to considerable variation in the reliability and effectiveness of orthotic treatment.[3] Clinical methodologies have been developed in an attempt to standardize treatment and improve the predictability of the clinical outcome.[4] Still, the results achieved by clinicians often differ, and interpractitioner variability appears to play a major role in the biomechanical response to orthotic intervention.[5,6] There is little objective evidence regarding *how* foot orthoses achieve favorable therapeutic results.[7] In spite of this, a growing body of objective evidence suggests that foot orthoses often produce positive clinical outcomes.[8-17] The potential benefits of a conservative, cost-effective treatment modality arguably justifies the continued prescription of foot orthoses and interest in orthotic-related research. An improved understanding of the mechanisms of action of foot orthoses is necessary to enhance clinical methodologies and better inform their prescription.

Research

Historically the focus of research has been the response of the lower extremity to the mechanical influence of an orthosis. Many studies have attempted to isolate the passive response of the limb by studying patients with neuropathy or utilizing cadaveric specimens.[18-20]

Study designs have attempted to isolate variables of interest and to measure the discrete mechanical influence of orthotic supportive elements such as base materials, interface materials, and metatarsal/scaphoid pads. Biomechanical studies suggest that foot orthoses are capable of altering plantar pressure distribution, foot and ankle kinetics/kinematics, and knee kinetics.[14,21-28]

Brodtkorb et al. found that the thickness of a metatarsal pad was more significant than its positioning in load shielding the metatarsal heads and that the maximum load-shielding effect occurred distal to the apex of the pad.[23]

Kogler et al. isolated the mechanical effects of arch supports as well as full-foot and forefoot wedges on plantar fascial strain. These cadaveric studies demonstrated the load-sharing effect of arch supports with the plantar fascia.[18,29,30] The medial column of the foot approximated the arch support's boundaries (Fig. 116.1).

Tsung et al. investigated the effect of arch supports on plantar pressure distribution in patients with sensory neuropathy. In this study, the method of casting determined the shape of the arch support for patients with neuropathy and strongly influenced the plantar pressure distribution. Foot shape was captured with the subjects in non–weight bearing, semi–weight bearing, and full weight-bearing conditions. In their study, the authors found that casting the foot in what they termed semi–weight bearing, with the subject standing with equal body weight on both feet, resulted in an orthotic shape with the least mean plantar pressure. The control of orthotic shape by the magnitude of the physiologic load produced orthoses with predictable, plantar pressure distributions.[28]

Guldemond et al. investigated the effects of metatarsal pads, arch supports, and full foot wedges on plantar pressure distribution in patients with neuropathy. The orthotic elements were added to a basic insole to alter its relative shape at the medial longitudinal arch and transverse arch.[20] This study revealed that the plantar pressure distribution could be altered in a predictable fashion and that the load-shielding effects of the various elements were additive (Fig. 116.2).

More recent studies suggest that in addition to their direct mechanical influence, foot orthoses can also evoke a neuromotor response that may play a significant role in their function.[31,32] Evidence suggests that tactile stimuli may, under certain conditions, affect foot and ankle posture.[25,26] Several authors have investigated the influence of comfort and surface texture on the biomechanical effectiveness of foot orthoses.[31,33,34]

Ritchie et al. found that plantar sensory feedback influenced midfoot pronation. The addition of mild, non–mechanically supportive surface features plantar to the medial arch elicited active arch elevation in walking subjects.[35]

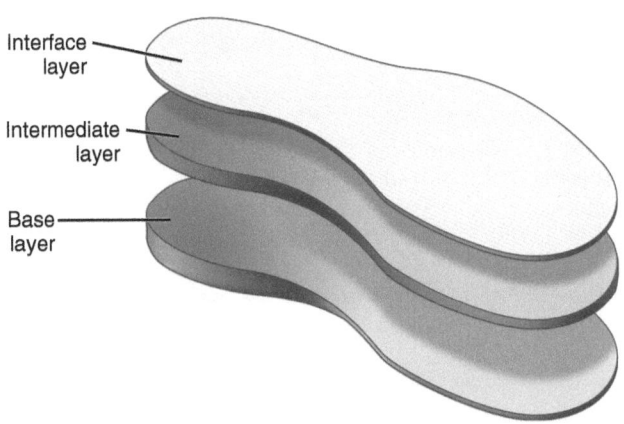

Fig. 116.1 Foot orthosis construction.

Interface layer

Intermediate layer

Base layer

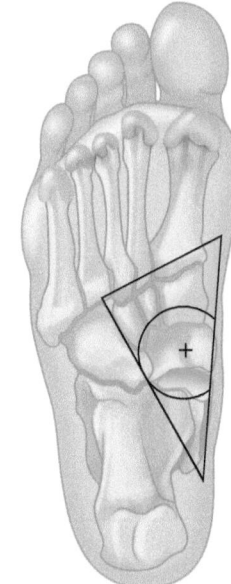

Fig. 116.2 Plantar aspect of the bones of the right foot showing primary support region for the longitudinal arch support mechanism of a foot orthosis. Partial circle indicates the position of the vertices of the orthotic support. (From Kogler GF, Solomonidis SE, Paul JP. Biomechanics of longitudinal arch support mechanisms in foot orthoses and their effect on plantar aponeurosis strain. *Clin Biomech [Bristol, Avon]*. 1996;11[5]:243–252.)

Mundermann et al. found that foot and ankle kinematics were related to orthotic comfort.[31] In these studies, orthotic use also significantly changed muscle activity.[31,36]

The evidence suggests that the neuromotor response to orthotic stimuli may play a significant role in the orthotic influence on biomechanical function.[32,33,37] Some manufacturers have even begun incorporating tactile elements in products based on this evidence. At this writing, the orthotic action upon a sensate, volitional foot appears to comprise a complex combination of direct mechanical action and the neuromotor response to the orthotic stimulus.[6,31,33,35]

Further exploration of the tactile response to orthotic mechanical action and the individual and combined mechanisms of action of functional elements in foot orthoses may help to enrich our understanding of the complex nature of foot orthosis design.

An improved understanding of these functional elements may ultimately also enhance communication for clinical collaboration and research.

Clinical Applications

Injuries of the lower extremities are extremely common in runners,[38] and the majority of running injuries are associated with overuse.[39] Although training distance and history of previous injury are primary risk factors, a significant contributing factor is biomechanical abnormality of the lower extremity.[14,38] At this writing, there is evidence to suggest that foot orthoses may be efficacious in the treatment of metatarsalgia, plantar fasciitis, tendinopathies, stress fractures, compartment syndrome, and shin splints.[12-14,21,22,39-43] Foot orthoses may also be efficacious in the treatment of posterior tibial syndrome and foot pain secondary to postural pes planus and pes cavus.[9,10,44,45]

The complexity of the action of foot orthoses in treating foot pathology derives from the complexity of foot and ankle biomechanics and the neuromotor response to orthotic action. The clinician's initial approach to orthotic design is mechanically focused. The process of orthotic design typically begins with identification of the nature and severity of the patient's biomechanical deficits. Orthotic supportive elements are selected with the intent of providing a mechanical influence that may beneficially affect the biomechanical deficits.

The delivery of orthotic care is an iterative process of optimization of the orthotic design based on both subjective and objective clinical indicators. Patient comfort is an important clinical indicator utilized by most clinicians during orthotic fitting and optimization. Comfort in this sense implies not just the tactile feel of the orthosis but also the beneficial change in biomechanical variables associated with orthotic treatment of the pathology.[31] It is difficult to predict the response of a specific foot to orthotic support, which may account for some of the variability in patient satisfaction that occurs when the same condition is treated with a similar orthotic design. Despite having acquired an appropriately prescribed orthosis, many patients require multiple adjustments to achieve pain relief, and such adjustments are critical to ensuring the patient's satisfaction. Some basic guidelines that may serve as a starting point for the prescription of orthoses in the treatment of sports-related injuries are shown in Table 116.1. Note that these guidelines are intended to serve only as a starting point.

It is helpful to consider the focal influence of discrete orthotic supportive elements when foot orthoses are being prescribed to treat pathologic musculoskeletal conditions. There is some evidence, for example, suggesting that a simple flat insole added to a shoe may alter the comfort, pressure distribution, friction, or resistance to bacterial growth within the shoe.[24,46-49] Polyurethanes and elastomers such as Poron and Spenco, respectively, are examples of resilient insole materials that may enhance a shoe's comfort. Although cushioned insoles influence pressure distribution, it should be noted that there is evidence to suggest that they appear to have a questionable influence overall on shock attenuation.[50] Leather, vinyl, and silver-impregnated fabrics such as X-Static® are examples of interface layers that may influence friction and discourage bacterial growth.

TABLE 116.1   Guideline for the Orthotic Treatment of Sports-Related Pathologies

Pathology	Elements of Orthotic Support in Foot Orthoses
Sesamoiditis with no other postural abnormality	• Dancer pad—well out for the sesamoids. • P-cell foam insole with relief over first metatarsal head. • Addition of a reverse Morton extension may sometimes provide additional symptomatic relief. This stiffens the forefoot while minimizing the pressure over the sesamoids.
Metatarsalgia	• The height of the pad may be more effective than its placement in relieving metatarsal head pressure. • Having the pad placed immediately plantar to the metatarsal head may actually increase pain. • Additional use of a Morton extension may decrease pain secondary to elimination of the metatarsal pad extension.
Morton neuroma with no other postural abnormality	• Metatarsal pad added to native shoe insole with apex of pad at neuroma. • Metatarsal pad added to prefabricated orthosis with apex of pad at neuroma.
Plantar fasciitis with mild pes planus	• Consider relative height of orthosis arch support with respect to the weight-bearing foot. • Full support, with soft interface may be most effective at decreasing plantar fascia strain. • Addition of pressure relief with a cushioned heel for calcaneal pain may provide symptomatic relief.
Mild pes planus	• Three-quarter-length or full-length prefabricated insole with a supportive arch.
Moderate to severe pes planus	• Full-length orthotic with hindfoot inversion and medial arch support. • Consider planal dominance and nature of postural abnormality when selecting and balancing support for hindfoot, midfoot, and forefoot.
Pes cavus	• Soft custom orthosis may provide symptomatic relief by reducing plantar fascial strain. • In some cases it may be beneficial to provide full arch support where there is discomfort due to rigid pes cavus.
Diabetes	• Full-length accommodative orthotic fabricated from Plastozote.

The addition of discrete pads to the native shoe insole may enhance the support or comfort of a shoe. Metatarsal pads and bars, arch pads, lifts, and wedges are support elements that are available in various materials including felt, elastomers, and polyurethanes. Felt is typically supportive, whereas elastomers and polyurethanes are typically more resilient and conformable. Several examples of orthotic materials, pads, and their applications are shown in Table 116.2.

The decision whether to prescribe prefabricated or custom foot orthoses involves consideration of the posture of the weight-bearing foot. The inclusion of supportive elements in the design of the orthosis that are intended to treat biomechanical deficits should also be considered. Comfort may associate with the blending of the supportive elements with the anatomical contour, and this may best be achieved using custom devices.

The primary application of prefabricated foot orthoses is the enhancement of medial longitudinal arch support. The shape of these orthoses is designed to fit the average foot; therefore their application is most often limited to feet with normal arch height.

Custom foot orthoses fall into two categories, accommodative and corrective. The basis for the orthotic design of custom foot orthoses is an anatomic model produced by casting, foam impression, contact, or optical scan of the patient's foot.

The shape of the patient's foot in weight bearing determines the shape of an accommodative foot orthosis. Most commonly these orthoses are designed to redistribute focal pressure or to minimize the mean plantar pressure. Rigid deformities of the foot such as posttraumatic pes planus and arthrosis from a Lisfranc injury are best treated with an accommodative orthotic, as any attempt to realign the foot will create increased focal pressure and pain. Diabetic foot orthoses are another example of an accommodative type.[51]

The shape of corrective foot orthoses is also anatomic, but with the inclusion of intentionally incongruous contours termed *modifications*. Examples of anatomic mold modifications used to create orthotic supportive elements are enhanced or reduced medial longitudinal arch supports, metatarsal pads, medial or lateral heel wedges, and medial or lateral forefoot wedges. The intent of these modifications is the seamless incorporation of supportive elements into the anatomic contour. These elements are often intended to influence foot and ankle kinetics and kinematics by redistributing plantar pressure. The Functional Foot Orthosis and the University of California Biomechanics Laboratory (UCBL) orthosis are two examples of corrective types.

Materials selection is an important aspect of foot orthosis design. Most foot orthoses comprise multiple layers, including a base and intermediate and interface layers. The use of multiple layers offers the combined benefits of their individual properties (Fig. 116.3). Firm base materials such as ethylene vinyl acetate (EVA), with compressibility like that of shoe outsoles, are typically used for the base layer of what are termed *soft foot orthoses*. Rigid base layers employ materials such as polypropylene, copolymer, and fiber glass or carbon lamination. Laminated foot orthoses typically offer the highest stiffness while taking up the least room in the shoe.

Soft, resilient, and conformable intermediate-layer materials include polyurethane foams, polyethylene foams, and elastomers. The intermediate layer helps to disperse plantar pressure and improve comfort.

TABLE 116.2   Common Foot Orthoses, Pads, and Materials

Component	Example	Intended Application	References
Foam-cushioned insole	Polyurethane, ªPoron EVA, ªP-cell polyethylene, ªPlastozote	• Decrease impulse • Enhance comfort • Decrease focal plantar pressure	Mills et al.[46] Paton et al.[49] Chiu and Shiang[24]
Antifriction insole	Leather interface	• Decrease shear • Reduce callus formation (diabetic applications)	Yavuz et al.[77] Lu[48]
Antibacterial insole Metatarsal pad	Silver-impregnated fabric, ªX-Static®	• Discourage bacterial/fungal growth • Decrease metatarsal head plantar pressure	Sedov et al.[47] Brodtkorb et al.[23] Guldemond et al.[20]
Cushioned heel cup		• Decrease focal plantar heel pressure	Perhamre et al.[25]
Medial/lateral heel wedge		• Influence center of pressure at heel • Influence varus/valgus moment at heel • Influence rate of change of inversion/eversion at heel • Influence varus/valgus moment at knee	Huerta et al.[26,27] Leitch et al.[78] Bonanno et al.[79]
Full-foot medial/lateral wedge	Cork, EVA, or polyurethane Preformed wedge material	• Influence varus/valgus moment at knee • Influence plantar fascial strain	Shelburne et al.[80] Kogler et al.[30]
Arch support (scaphoid pad)		• Influence plantar fascial strain • Influence plantar pressure distribution • Influence joint angles of the weight-bearing foot	Kogler et al.[18,29] Tsung et al.[28] Kitaoka et al.[19]

EVA, Ethylene vinyl acetate
ªAcor Orthopaedics, Inc. Cleveland, OH; www.acore.com

The interface layer of a foot orthosis is typically leather, vinyl, or foam; it may enhance the durability and hygiene of the orthosis or alter the friction between the foot and the orthosis. Polyethylene foam such as Plastozote may enhance moisture control, friction, or pressure distribution of the interface layer. Fabrics may enhance the comfort, moisture control, or odor control of the orthosis.

One or more of the supportive elements may be incorporated into the orthotic design by casting or scanning, modification of the anatomic model, and materials selection for fabrication. The function of the orthosis is evaluated during its fitting and optimized for the patient's comfort.

SPORTS SHOES

Because early humans were largely dependent on hunting, one can postulate that the earliest footwear was used in running. With civilization's advancement and socialization, shoes took on symbolic functions.[52] Papyrus sandals for religious ceremonies and jeweled sandals for high-fashion gatherings have been

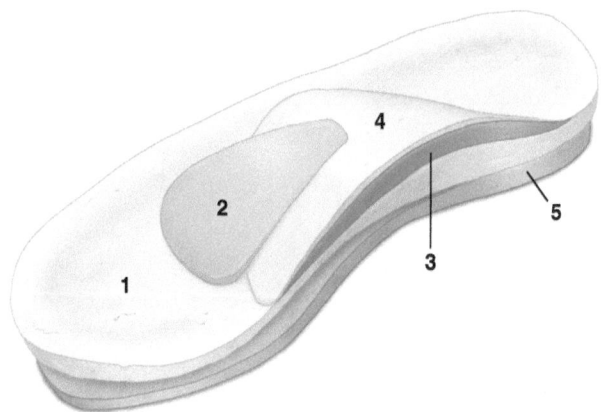

Fig. 116.3 Right angular front view of basic insole with components. *1*, Basic insole; *2*, metatarsal dome; *3*, "normal" arch support; *4*, "extra" arch support; and *5*, wedge (medial). (From Guldemond NA, Leffers P, Schaper NC, et al. The effects of insole configurations on forefoot plantar pressure and walking convenience in diabetic patients with neuropathic feet. *Clin Biomech [Bristol, Avon].* 2007;22[1]:81–87.)

discovered at the burial sites of Egyptian pharaohs.[53] Although these have little to do with sports shoes, they do foreshadow the current specialization and fashionable designs of athletic footwear. A shoe designed for sports alone did not come into existence until the latter half of the 19th century. The croquet sandal known as the *sneaker* had a fabric upper, rubber sole, and laces.[52,54,55] Further sports shoe development followed in the late 1800s with the demand for durable but lightweight shoes. It is from these developments that the multibillion-dollar athletic shoe industry evolved in an explosion of sport-specific footwear. Today's casual and professional athletes may select from a broad range of shoes designed for sprinting, running, cross training, volleyball, basketball, hiking, dance, and bowling, among other activities.

Over the last half century, significant progress has been made in the design, materials, and methods used to fabricate athletic shoes. Manufacturers have flooded the market with stylish models. These shoes are packed with inventive features ranging from mesh uppers to directionally siped soles. New features tend to fall in and out of fashion, however, suggesting that the consumer's selection of athletic shoes for sports activities may at times be more about form than function. In reality, the design and performance of the modern athletic shoe has dramatically improved. Manufacturers and independent researchers have performed studies to demonstrate the biomechanical influence of shoe features. While there is evidence that many of these features influence biomechanical variables, their efficacy in the prevention of sports injuries or in the enhancement of performance is less clearly understood. Although it remains difficult to identify specific aspects of design that will reduce sports injuries for a given athlete, fit and comfort appear to play a significant role in injury prevention.[56,57]

Clinicians have understandably been reluctant to recommend specific footwear for their patients. This reluctance is warranted given the almost overwhelming number of shoe models available, the pace of new product introduction, and the highly individualized nature of shoe fit and comfort. It is beneficial that consumers have a broad selection of shoe models from which to choose. To assist the clinician in helping to guide their patients in their selection, the next section describes some of the features designed into the modern sports shoe and their intended application.

Anatomy of the Sports Shoe

In simplest terms, the shoe can be broken down into the bottom and the upper. The bottom protects the foot, interfaces with the floor, and comprises the outsole, wedge, midsole, and insole. The upper covers the foot, supports the ankle, and comprises the toe box, tongue, closure, collar, and heel counter (Fig. 116.4). Each of these parts plays a role in the form, function, and fit of the shoe. Material properties play a major role in shoe performance, support, and durability.

Outsole

Advanced manufacturing methods have been developed to give modern athletic shoe sole materials unique physical properties. The primary function of the shoe outsole is to grip the running surface and resist wear. Shoe outsoles may be made of carbon rubber, the same material used for car tires. Carbon rubber is extremely durable, with exceptional wear resistance. Greater hardness imparts greater wear resistance and may distribute the contact forces from the outsole to the midsole more effectively. An outsole that is too hard, however, may impart a "stiff feel" to the shoe. Conversely, an outsole that is too soft may reduce the stability of the shoe.[58] Blown rubber is another example of an outsole material that is sometimes used for the forefoot section of a sports shoe. This material is more flexible and light in weight than carbon rubber but is less durable.

The coefficient of friction (COF) for shoe outsoles may range from 0.1 to 0.34 or higher but is heavily dependent upon the contact surface and is strongly influenced by moisture.[59,60] Research has shown that sole friction is time- and temperature-dependent as well; it also depends on tread design, even on hard flat surfaces.[60] Shoe manufacturers have employed outsole materials with friction properties suitable for specific sports applications. The nonmarring soles used for volleyball and high-friction outsoles for hiking are two examples.

Midsole

As stated previously, one function of the outsole is distribution of the compressive load to the midsole. Shoe midsole design has received much attention from shoe manufacturers. Because this is the primary dynamic element of the shoe sole, shoe designers have added ever more creative features to the midsole in an effort to improve stability, attenuate shock, and even enhance motor activation.

Shoe midsoles are most typically made of EVA, polyurethane, or some blend of thermoplastic elastomers (TPEs).[61] Advanced methods have been developed to vary the properties of midsole materials during manufacture. For example, manufacturing methods have been developed that facilitate the selective modification of midsole density along the sole contour, creating regions with different mechanical characteristics.[62] Research has shown

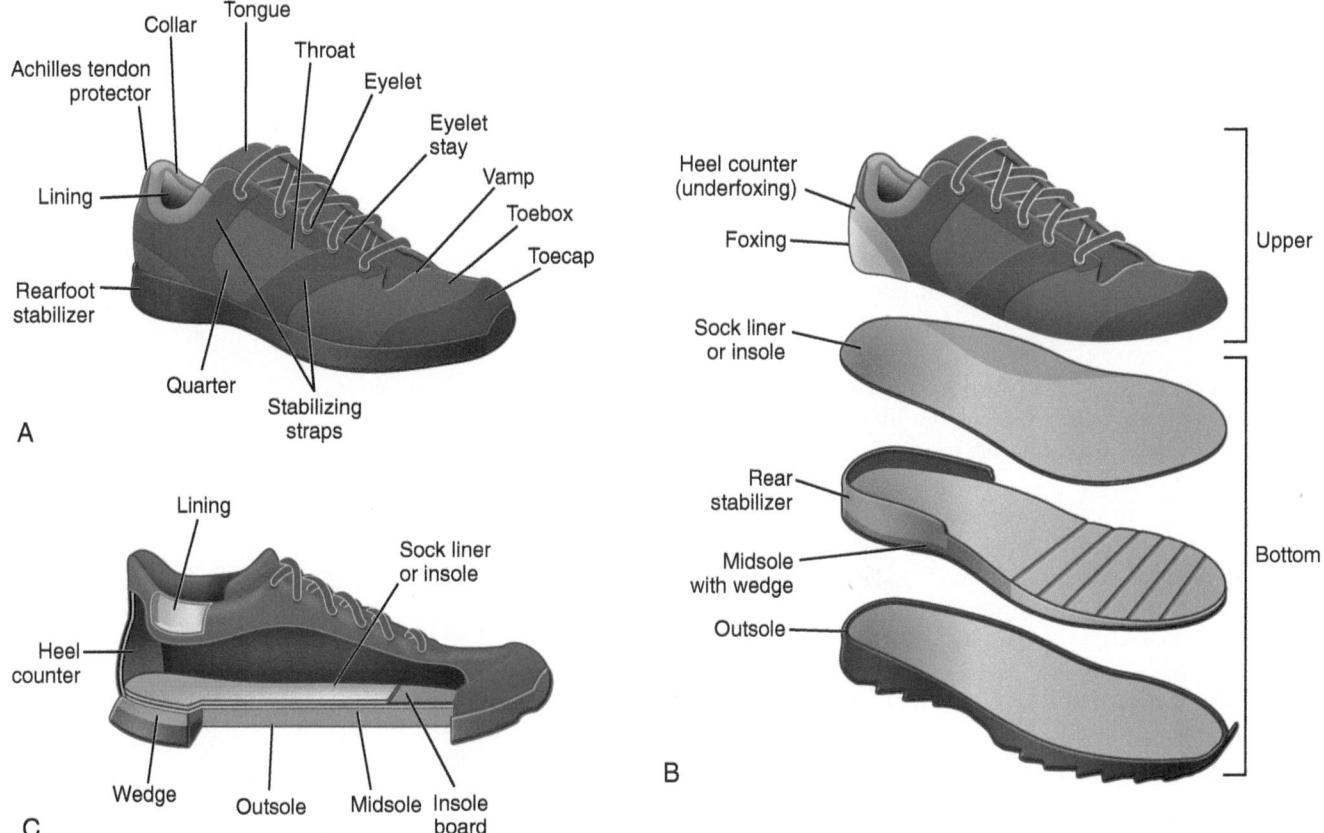

Fig. 116.4 Illustrations of athletic shoes. (A) Overview of external appearance. (B) Separation of shoe into component parts. (C) Sectional view of interior of shoe.

that the mechanical characteristics of midsole materials deteriorate significantly under normal use.[61] Thicker materials may deteriorate at a higher rate than thinner materials as well.[61] The rule of thumb is to replace athletic footwear after every 4 to 6 months of regular use.

The geometry of the midsole has also received much attention from shoe designers. Frequently incorporated into the modern athletic shoe midsole is sparse structure and open cantilever or honeycomb structures intended to vary mechanical characteristics and reduce weight.[63] These geometric features are intended to influence the compressibility, energy return, and flexibility of the midsole. Midsole geometry may also incorporate corrugations of various shapes, sipes, and other features to create directionally oriented flexion characteristics in the shoe sole.[64,65] More recently, some manufacturers have begun adding composite structures in the wedge or midsole to enhance mediolateral stability of the heel, midfoot, or forefoot of the shoe. One example of this approach is New Balance Rollbar Technology.

Any discussion of athletic shoe soles would be incomplete without mention of heel and forefoot rockers. There is considerable evidence to support the role of these features in influencing the kinematics and kinetics of the lower extremity. One recent study found that running with rocker soles may lower mechanical loading on the Achilles tendon; however, loading on the knee joint was found to be increased.[66]

Insole

The shoe insole connects the midsole to the foot. This layer is fabricated using resilient materials like polyurethanes. The geometry of the insole may also be designed to support the medial longitudinal arch. Arch support provided by the insole may vary depending on manufacturer and on the intended application of the shoe. For example, cross trainers may in general have less arch support than running shoes. Many athletic shoes are designed with removable insoles to simplify cleaning and accommodate custom foot orthoses. It should be noted, however, that the interface layer deep to the insole plays a significant role in the overall postural support of a custom arch support. In fact, the fit and function of flexible custom orthoses is typically adjusted by grinding the bottom surface of the insert. This fitting method alters the contour of the insert with respect to the shoe to influence the postural support of the foot.

Upper

The modern athletic shoe upper is fabricated by weaving, stitching, molding, and gluing operations. The shoe is assembled over a "last," a foot-shaped model that defines the interior shape of the shoe. Standards have been established to define the shapes of shoe lasts. More recently, some authors have proposed expanding these standards to better accommodate a broader range of foot shapes.[67] Manufacturers customize their lasts to meet the design specifications of their product line, sometimes employing the same last in the fabrication of different models of shoes.

The toe box, shoe collar, and heel counter protect the foot and provide postural support to the ankle. High-top uppers, for example, have been shown to decrease ankle inversion during cutting movements, and collar height may play a more significant role than counter stiffness in mediolateral stability.[68,69] More recently tactile elements have been developed that may find their way into the native shoe insole and upper with the goal of eliciting active arch elevation through the neuromotor response.[70]

High-top uppers are typically used for basketball shoes with designs that wrap around the malleoli but they are lower posteriorly to permit free plantarflexion.

Selection and Fitting of Sports Shoes

Some authors have recently proposed two new paradigms for running shoe selection, including the "preferred movement path" and the "comfort filter." The authors identify studies showing that shoes and inserts can significantly affect the incidence of injury, raising questions regarding previously accepted predictors of injury such as pronation and impact forces. On the basis of prior data indicating that shoes and/or shoe insoles did influence the range of skeletal movement, the authors propose that a "good running shoe" would be one that facilitates the individual runner's "preferred movement path." Furthermore, the authors acknowledge that shoe comfort is associated with a lower frequency of movement-related injury as well as lower oxygen consumption. Last, they propose that the runner automatically selects the shoe that facilitates his or her "preferred movement path" as the one that is most comfortable.[57]

The approach to orthotic treatment whereby the clinician considers both objective and subjective clinical indicators is consistent in this approach. The clinician familiar with the patient's history of orthotic use and fitting preferences can leverage the individual's awareness of shoe models and orthotic designs to help him or her find the most suitable athletic footwear and achieve a comfortable fit.

Perhaps those with greatest familiarity of sports shoe models and their features are the sales representatives at athletic shoe stores. These representatives may be skilled in helping their customers identify the subtle differences between sports shoe brands and models. The athlete should be encouraged to consult these specialty stores regarding options and features but cautioned that there is little objective evidence to associate sports shoe features with injury prevention.

When shoes are being fitted, a useful starting point to determine shoe size is measurement of foot length using the Brannock device.[72] This device was invented by Charles Brannock in 1927 and is the standard of measure for the world's footwear industry. Brannock devices are available at most shoe stores. It is important to note that although shoes are sized by the length of the longest toe on the longest foot, a more useful measure may be arch length. To measure the foot, place the patient's longest foot on the Brannock device and ask the patient to stand with the heel against the heel cup. Read the foot length by the longest toe.

TABLE 116.3	Guideline for the Selection of Sports Shoe Features
Pathology	Shoe Feature
Sesamoiditis with no other postural abnormality	• Cushioned insole • Rigid forefoot • Distal sole rocker
Metatarsalgia	• Cushioned insole • Rigid forefoot • Distal sole rocker
Morton neuroma with no other postural abnormality	• Cushioned insole • Rigid forefoot • Distal sole rocker
Plantar fasciitis with mild pes planus	• Cushioned heel • Supportive arch • Rigid forefoot • Distal sole rocker
Mild pes planus	• Supportive arch • Rigid forefoot • Distal sole rocker
Moderate to severe pes planus	• Supportive arch • Rigid forefoot • Distal sole rocker
Pes cavus	• Supportive arch • Rigid forefoot • Distal sole rocker • Surgical opening
Diabetes	• Extra depth • Wide last • Cushioned insole • Rigid forefoot • Distal sole rocker

Then measure the arch length by aligning the arch length pointer with the first metatarsal head. To determine the shoe size, use the larger of the two measurements and add one shoe size to the measurement. It should be noted that this measure is only a starting point for shoe selection.

The American Orthopaedic Foot and Ankle Society (AOFAS) offers suggestions for selection of athletic footwear.[71] The AOFAS recommends purchasing athletic shoes from a specialty shoe store at the end of the day or after a workout when the feet are swollen. They recommend that shoes be sized while wearing the type of socks to be worn with the shoe, that there should be room for the toes and no slip of the heel, and finally that the shoe should feel comfortable at the first fitting while walking and running and during simulated activities that most closely approximate the sports activity.[71]

If the athlete participates in the sport three or more times per week, the AOFAS recommends purchase of a sports-specific shoe. It is important to note, however, that different manufacturers may build contradictory features into the same type of sports-specific shoe; therefore this selection criterion should be used with caution.

If there are specific pathologic musculoskeletal conditions, the clinician and athlete may find Table 116.3 a helpful guideline to aid in the selection of the best type of orthosis.

For a complete list of references, go to ExpertConsult.com.

SELECTED READINGS

Citation:
Guldemond NA, Leffers P, Schaper NC, et al. The effects of insole configurations on forefoot plantar pressure and walking convenience in diabetic patients with neuropathic feet. *Clinical Biomechanics.* 2007;22(1):81–87.

Level of Evidence:
II

Summary:
The effect of medial longitudinal arch pads, metatarsal pads, and full-foot wedges on the plantar pressure distribution of a foot orthosis were investigated in neuropathic patients. The effect of medial longitudinal and metatarsal pads appeared to be additive in decreasing pressure at the central and medial forefoot with less pressure relief at the lateral forefoot.

Citation:
Kogler GF, Solomonidis SE, Paul JP. Biomechanics of longitudinal arch support mechanisms in foot orthoses and their effect on plantar aponeurosis strain. *Clin Biomech (Bristol, Avon).* 1996;11:243–252.

Level of Evidence:
II

Summary:
The effect of medial longitudinal arch supports on plantar fascial strain was investigated in cadaveric specimens. Foot orthoses were fabricated using foot molds created by elevating the medial longitudinal arch; these decreased plantar fascial strain more than prefabricated and functional foot orthoses.

Citation:
Mundermann A, Nigg BM, Humble RN, et al. Orthotic comfort is related to kinematics, kinetics, and EMG in recreational runners. *Med Sci Sports Exerc.* 2003;35(10):1710–1719.

Level of Evidence
II

Summary:
The effects of foot orthosis posting and molding on lower extremity kinematics, kinetics, electromyography, and perceived comfort were investigated in recreational runners. There appeared to be a significant correlation between the perceived comfort of foot orthoses and measured biomechanical variables.

Citation:
Mills K, Blanch P, Chapman AR, et al. Foot orthoses and gait: a systematic review and meta-analysis of literature pertaining to potential mechanisms. *Br J Sports Med.* 2010;44(14):1035–1046.

Level of Evidence:
II

Summary:
A systematic review of the effects of foot orthosis posting and molding on lower extremity kinetics and kinematics in normal individuals. Foot orthosis posting reduced peak hindfoot eversion and tibial internal rotation, molding attenuated shock. The neuromotor influence of foot orthoses remained unclear.

117

Ligamentous Injuries of the Foot and Ankle

Paul Rothenberg, Eric Swanton, Andrew Molloy, Amiethab A. Aiyer, Jonathan R. Kaplan

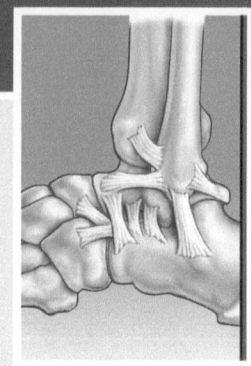

The ankle is a highly specialized joint that allows us to propel ourselves in an efficient manner during multiple activities. The mortise shape facilitates transmission of 1.5 times the body weight when walking, and up to four times the body weight when running.[1] Activities such as standing and walking and all athletic ability require stable, strong foot and ankle function to provide a stable platform for propulsion and yet allow adaptation for uneven surfaces and changes in speed and direction. This chapter covers the pathology, history, examination, investigation, treatment, and rehabilitation of ligament injuries of the foot and ankle.

LATERAL ANKLE SPRAIN

Ankle sprains are one of the most common soft tissue injuries affecting athletes of all sporting levels and account for nearly 40% of sports injuries.[1-8] Athletes in sports such as basketball, football/soccer, running, and volleyball have a higher incidence of ankle injuries.[8-13]

The lateral ligament complex, consisting of the anterior talofibular ligament (ATFL), the posterior talofibular ligament (PTFL) and calcaneofibular ligament (CFL), is most commonly involved. The injury results from an inverted, plantar-flexed foot with an internally rotated hindfoot and an externally rotated leg.[2,3,9,14,15] The medial side is rarely injured.[16] These injuries can lead to chronic instability, which can cause significant public health issues in persons who do not participate in sports, and can have a profound effect with regard to the time it takes to return to sports in athletes. The incidence of chronic ankle instability after an acute ankle sprain has been reported to be between 5% and 70%.[4,17-20]

Lateral ankle sprains comprise 85% of all ankle sprains.[13] The most commonly injured structure is the ATFL (Fig. 117.1). The strain in the ATFL increases as the ankle moves from dorsiflexion into plantar flexion. The ATFL demonstrates lower maximal load and energy to failure values under tensile stress compared with the PTFL, CFL, and anterior inferior tibiofibular ligament (AITFL),[21,22] which may explain why the ATFL is the most frequently injured lateral ligament.[23] The CFL is the second most common ligament to be injured, followed by the PTFL.[24] Injury of the ATFL causes increased internal rotation of the hindfoot and stress on the remaining ligaments.

Risk factors for lateral ankle sprains include a previous sprain, greater height and weight, limb dominance, pes cavus, a larger foot size, the use of inappropriate footwear, generalized joint laxity, ankle flexor strength asymmetry, decreased slow eccentric inversion strength, increased fast concentric plantarflexion strength, reduced hip extension strength, and reduced muscle reaction time due to neuromuscular control.[2-4,25-34]

History and Physical Examination

Persons with acute injuries have a preceding traumatic event that involves an inversion mechanism of injury with associated swelling, ecchymosis, and difficulty with weight bearing. The findings are frequently the same in persons with acute and chronic injuries. However, persons with chronic injuries have a history of recurrent instability, which frequently occurs with less severe trauma. One must be careful to inquire about whether the patient has adapted his or her lifestyle to minimize injury, such as via cessation of regular sporting activities, avoidance of uneven ground, and not wearing high-heeled shoes. In persons with chronic instability, the overall severity of the injury is less and therefore patients tend to have less swelling and bruising, together with a diminished effect on the ability to fully bear weight after each episode.

Palpation should be specific with regard to tenderness over the course of the ligamentous structures, namely the ATFL, CFL, and AITFL, to aid in the diagnosis. Bony structures including the distal fibula, anterior process of the calcaneus, lateral process of the talus, and base of the fifth metatarsal should be palpated specifically to assess for possible osseous injuries. One should also specify if tenderness of the peroneal myotendinous units is present from just superior to the metaphyseal flare of the distal fibula to the insertion point at the base of the fifth metatarsal. Tenderness to palpation within the ankle joint itself may suggest the presence of synovitis, occult fracture, or osteochondral lesion. Although rare, dislocation of the hindfoot may occur, and limited passive motion should raise suspicion of this injury.

The anterior drawer test should be performed, along with talar tilt stress testing. The anterior drawer test assesses the integrity of the ATFL, whereas the talar stress test assesses the CFL, although it is sometimes difficult to identify specific ligaments from the examination of an acute injury, and the stress test is not very accurate.[3,35]

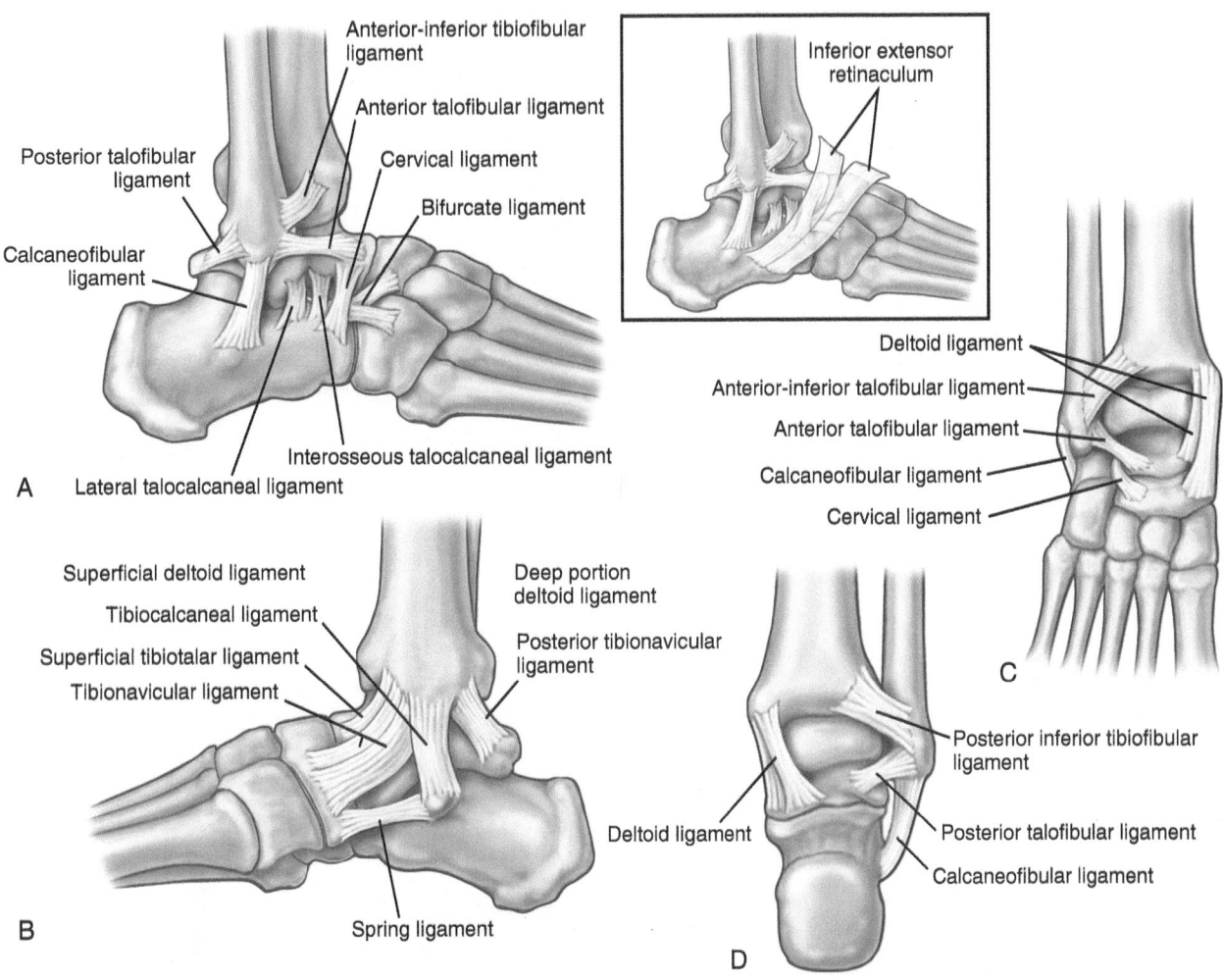

Fig. 117.1 Compendium of the foot and ankle ligaments. (A) The lateral view of the foot and ankle demonstrating the anterior talofibular ligament, calcaneofibular ligament, posterior talofibular ligament, anterior-inferior tibiofibular ligament, lateral talocalcaneal ligament, inferior extensor retinaculum, interosseous talocalcaneal ligament, cervical ligament, and bifurcate ligament. (B) The medial view of the foot and ankle demonstrating the superficial deltoid ligament, including the tibionavicular, spring ligament, tibiocalcaneal, and superficial tibiotalar components. (C) The anterior view of the ankle and hindfoot demonstrating the deltoid ligament with its superficial and deep components, the anterior-inferior tibiofibular ligament, the cervical ligament, the anterior talofibular ligament, and the calcaneofibular ligament. (D) The posterior view of the ankle and hindfoot demonstrating the deltoid ligament with its superficial and deep components, the posterior-inferior tibiofibular ligament, the posterior talofibular ligament, and the calcaneofibular ligament.

The anterior drawer test is performed with the patient seated and the distal tibia stabilized with one hand of the examiner while the other hand grasps the heel and the foot is anteriorly translated. The ankle is positioned into plantarflexion while testing. The presence of anterior subluxation of the foot should be compared to the contralateral side. In persons with a complete ATFL tear, the talus subluxates anteriorly and a dimple forms on the anterolateral joint area (the "sulcus sign") (Fig. 117.2).[36]

In isolated lateral ligament injuries, the medial-sided static stabilizers may prevent anterior translation during the anterior drawer test. For this reason a modification of the anterior drawer test, called the anterolateral drawer test, was developed. Similar to the anterior drawer test, one hand stabilizes the distal tibia and the other provides an anterior translational force. However, in this test the examiner does not constrain rotation of the talus

and also directly palpates movement on the talus by placing a thumb along the lateral joint line between the talus and the distal fibula. This allows the examiner to directly assess translation and rotation of the talus.[37,38]

In the acute setting, if it is difficult to examine the patient because of pain, infiltration of a local anesthetic and reexamination of the patient provides a more accurate test result for the anterior drawer test.[39] However, it is more common in our practice to reexamine the patient a few days after the injury to avoid use of this invasive maneuver.

The talar tilt test is performed with the patient seated and the leg secured with the examiner's hand while the heel is grasped with the opposite hand and an inversion force is administered to cause talar tilt (Fig. 117.3). Results are compared with those of the other side to assess differences in the tilt. The CFL is tested

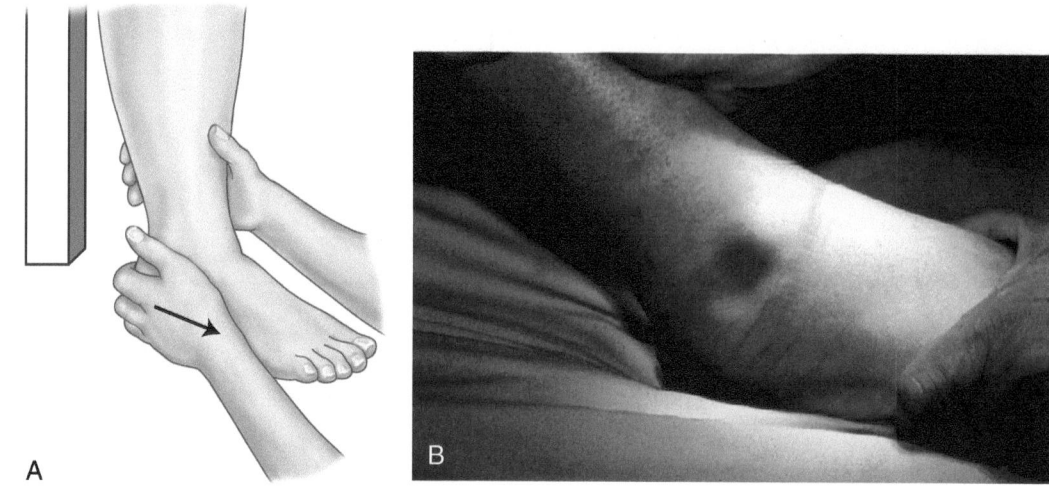

Fig. 117.2 (A and B) The anterior drawer test of the ankle. Note the skin dimple consistent with a positive test.

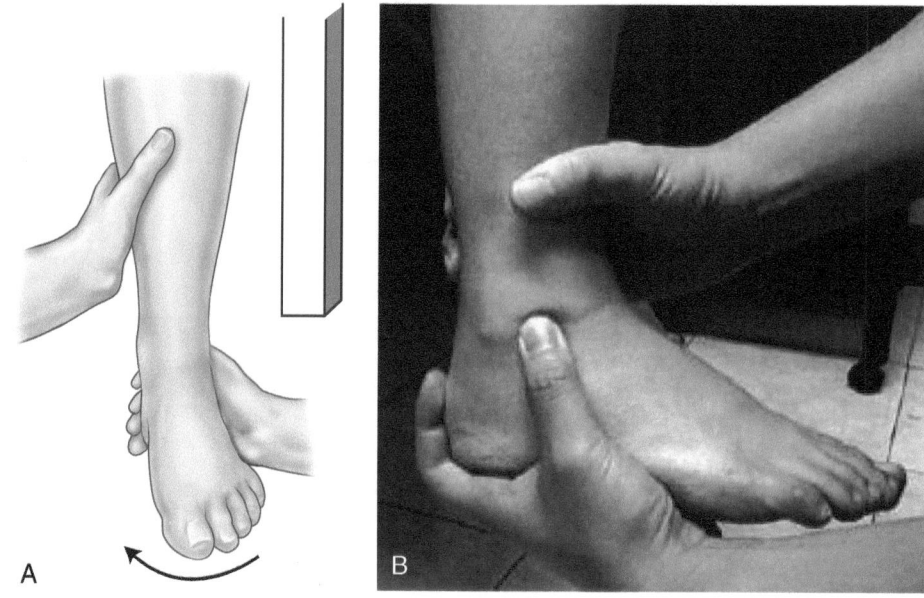

Fig. 117.3 (A and B) The talar tilt (inversion stress) test of the ankle.

in neutral, whereas the ATFL is tested in plantar flexion, but once again this testing can be difficult to perform because the contribution of the subtalar joint sometimes can cause false-positive results.[40,41]

The examination is completed with checking of proprioception and joint hyperlaxity by calculating the Beighton score as shown in Table 117.1. A score of 4 or higher is indicative of hyperlaxity.

Imaging

Radiographs to assess ligamentous injuries include standard weight-bearing anteroposterior (AP), lateral, and mortise views, as well as anterior drawer and talar tilt stress views, which can

TABLE 117.1	Beighton Scoring Method
Testing	**Points**
Able to extend the little finger beyond 90 degrees	1 point for each side (maximum: 2)
Able to bend the thumb and touch the volar forearm	1 point for each side (maximum: 2)
Able to hyperextend the elbow beyond 10 degrees	1 point for each side (maximum: 2)
Able to hyperextend the knee beyond 10 degrees	1 point for each side (maximum: 2)
Able to lean forward and touch the ground with the knee straight	1 point

A score of ≥4 indicates hyperlaxity.

be obtained either manually or mechanically. The anterior drawer should measure less than 10 mm or within 3 to 5 mm of the opposite side. The talar tilt can range from 5 to 23 degrees, although the literature suggests that an absolute value of more than 10 degrees or more than 5 degrees when compared with the other side could be diagnostic.[3,41–43] The degree of tilt is calculated by measuring the difference in angle between the distal tibial articular surface and the dome of the talus (Fig. 117.4).

Magnetic resonance imaging (MRI) is the most accurate noninvasive modality; however, it is often positive for ATFL tears even in asymptomatic individuals.[44] Therefore it is not usually required in the setting of a routine ankle sprain and should be reserved for suspicion of a syndesmotic injury, osteochondral defect, or peroneal tendon injury, or after failure of conservative management.

Multiple classifications and grading of ankle sprains exist, although none is superior. Maffulli classified them as grades I to III, but for sports injuries, Malliaropoulus further subdivided these grades to take into account the anterior drawer radiographs.[11,45] The classification is shown in Table 117.2. This grading is performed after 48 hours of rest and treatment with ice,

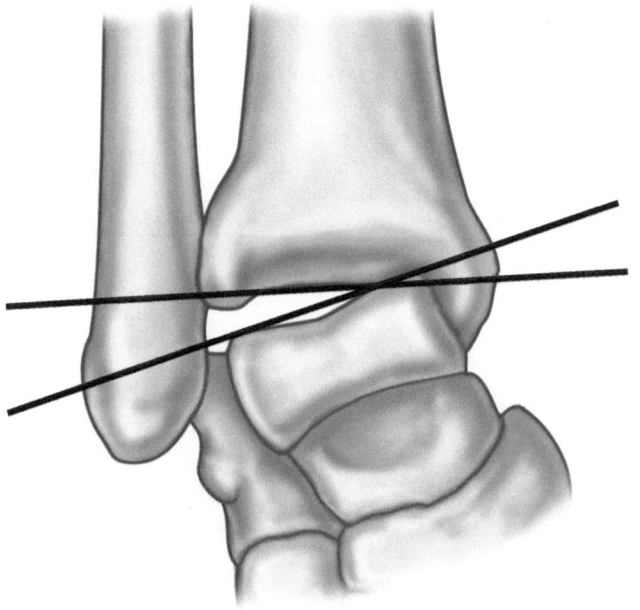

Fig. 117.4 The talar tilt (inversion) as it would be seen on a stress radiograph. The talar tilt angle refers to the angle between two lines drawn to the tibial plafond and the talar dome.

TABLE 117.2	Classification of Ankle Sprains		
Grade	**I**	**II**	**III**
Injured structures	Partial	ATFL	ATFL and CFL
Decrease in range of movement	<5	5–10	>10
Edema	≤0.5 cm	0.5–2 cm	>2 cm
Stress radiographs	Normal	Normal	>3 mm laxity

ATFL, Anterior talofibular ligament; *CFL,* calcaneofibular ligament.

compression, and elevation (RICE), together with gentle early range-of-motion (ROM) exercises.

One must be mindful of associated injuries that can be seen in the setting of acute ankle sprains. These include but are not limited to fractures of the lateral malleolus, lateral talar process, os trigonum, cuboid, and fifth metatarsal, as well as peroneal tendon tears/subluxations, intra-articular osteochondral lesions of the talus or tibia, medial ankle sprains, and syndesmotic injuries.[46] Patient history, physical examination, and imaging should be scrutinized to correctly diagnose these injuries in this setting.

Decision-Making Principles

Prevention is better than cure, but evidence supporting the use of proprioception exercises to prevent first-time sprains is limited, and no evidence exists to support the use of braces for the prevention of first-time sprains.[11,47] The natural history of ankle sprains is that by 2 weeks after the injury, most patients experience rapid improvement of their pain, followed by a further 2 weeks when the pain subsides much more slowly. Rates of reinjury can range between 3% and 54%; this can be as high as 29% in athletes, based on the severity of the injury.[18,48]

At 1 year, most patients have been noted to have some residual symptoms with pain and instability. Long-term follow-up at 3 years has revealed that as many as 34% of patients have had a repeat sprain, and 36% to 85% have had a full recovery. Therefore the appropriate treatment of sprains is imperative to guide early recovery and facilitate the prevention of future sprains.

Treatment
Conservative

The initial treatment of any acute sprain includes RICE, early ROM, progressive weight bearing, and physiotherapy. Treatment modalities include nonoperative and operative ones; the former involving casting, bracing, and early functional rehabilitation. The treatments depend on the severity of the injury and the patient's choice; however, multiple studies have demonstrated that nonoperative management is as successful as operative treatment in the acute setting. Presently, no evidence exists to support one treatment regimen over another.[3,49–51]

The CAST trial showed that casting relieves pain in the initial period and is as effective as an Aircast splint (DJO Incorporated, Vista, CA), but it is better than Tubigrip (i.e., an elastic bandage) alone.[52] Casting is usually implemented for 3 weeks followed by 12 weeks of proprioceptive rehabilitation. Complications, such as deep vein thrombosis, have been reported, and most studies have shown that functional management is the nonsurgical treatment of choice and that casting is not routinely used.[9,53,54]

Functional management is classified as an early mobilization program with use of bracing and early rehabilitation. Multiple studies indicate that functional management of these injuries is recommended in contrast to other conservative treatment modalities such as immobilization. Authors of multiple articles and reviews have all come to the same conclusion.[4,9,17,53,55–57] The purpose of rehabilitation exercise is to improve muscle strength, range of movement, and sensorimotor control, which are commonly impaired after an ankle sprain.

In most studies, functional treatment involved RICE for 48 hours followed by early supervised mobilization under the guidance of a physical therapist and progression to full weight bearing. Early isometric muscle strengthening may be initiated within a week, progressing to isokinetic strengthening after 1 week based on the patient's ability to tolerate the treatment. Furthermore, proprioception and peroneal strengthening begun be instituted concomitantly. As pain subsides, the therapy should be gradually expanded to include muscle strength and endurance exercises. Some series include adjuvants, such as cryotherapy, although no definite evidence has demonstrated their effectiveness. The use of braces or aids to support the ankle is recommended in functional treatment, and has been proved to decrease the rate of reinjury.[3,47,50,53,55,58–60] Numerous ankle braces are available; we recommend using braces that lace up and have a strap that "locks" the ankle to prevent inversion, which could injure the healing of laterally based ligaments. Functional treatment should be performed for a minimum of 6 weeks.

Surgical Treatment

Operative treatment is reserved for persons for whom conservative treatment has failed, where the primary complaint is chronic instability. Operative intervention is typically not indicated for acute instability events. Isolated ankle pain, without persistent instability should prompt further investigation. It is important to identify the quality of the rehabilitation the patient is undergoing. If it is deemed to be insufficiently robust or if the patient has had issues with compliance, he or she should be referred for physical therapy. The aim of the program is to improve strength and speed of firing of the peronei, as well as proprioception. We have found it helpful to refer patients to physical therapists who specialize in the treatment of foot and ankle disorders. The incidence of patients who have residual functional instability ranges from 5% to 70%.[4,17–20] For patients with persistent ankle instability and/or ankle pain despite adequate functional rehabilitation, further imaging (i.e., an MRI) should be obtained.

Two forms of surgical treatment can be performed: anatomic and nonanatomic reconstructions. Anatomic repairs are more commonly performed in primary surgery. The seminal work on these repairs was carried out by Broström.[61] He described an end-to-end repair or an advancement of the torn end of the ATFL into the distal anterior fibula (Fig. 117.5). A total of 72% of patients were asymptomatic at 2.9 years, with 82% of those examined having a normal examination. Gould et al.[62] described a modification of this technique, with excision of part of the scarred ATFL, ligament repair, and reinforcement with a ligamentous flap and the inferior extensor retinaculum (Fig. 117.6). Excellent results were again achieved. Karlsson et al.[63] described a further modification in which both the ATFL and CFL were advanced into a bony trough in the fibula together with reinforcement from a periosteal flap.

The use of a synthetic tape has been reported as a method to augment the Broström repair.[62–64] Direct suture repair or the use of suture anchors alone has been shown to have a significantly inferior strength to the intact ATFL in a cadaveric model.[65] The use of a synthetic tape (Fibertape; Arthrex Inc., Munich, Germany) to augment the repair can produce an initial construct that is

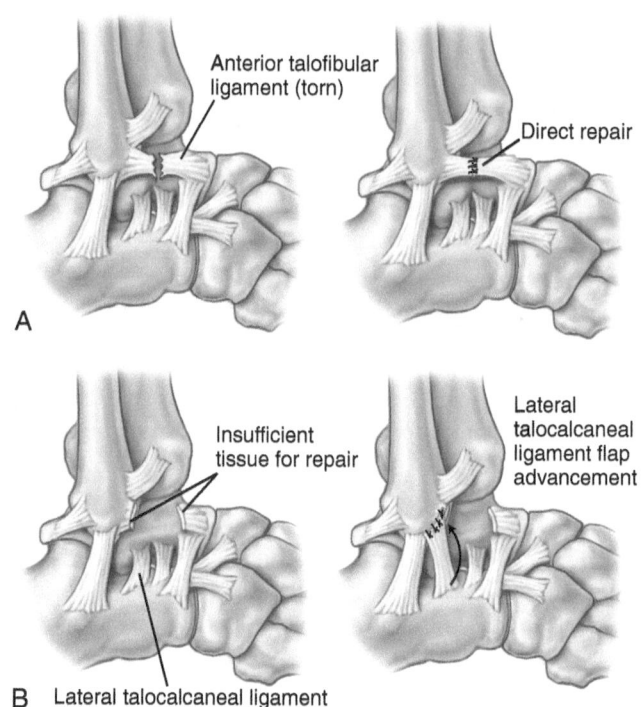

Fig. 117.5 The repair of a chronic lateral ankle ligament rupture as described by Broström. (A) A chronic anterior talofibular ligament rupture and direct repair. (B) A chronic anterior talofibular ligament rupture with insufficient tissue for simple direct repair and reconstruction with advancement of the flap of the lateral talocalcaneal ligament into the fibula. (Modified from Broström L. Sprained ankles. VI. Surgical treatment of "chronic" ligament ruptures. *Acta Chir Scand*. 1966;132:551–565.)

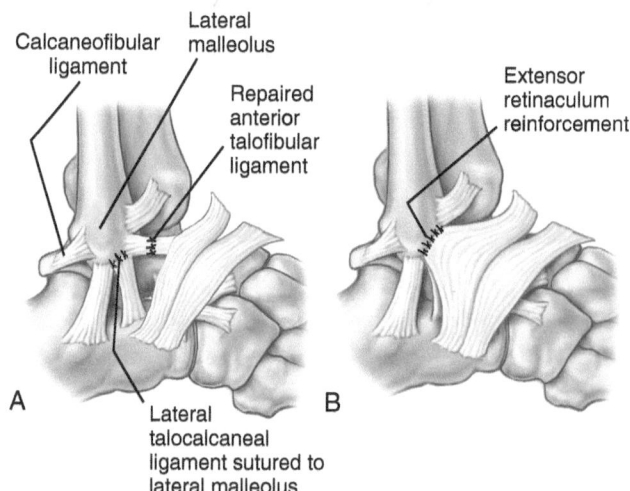

Fig. 117.6 Gould modification of the Broström technique. After repair of the anterior talofibular or calcaneofibular ligament, reinforcements with the lateral talocalcaneal ligament (A) and extensor retinaculum (B) are made.

at least as strong as the native ATFL,[63,64] and can potentially allow a quicker recovery time.[62]

Some authors have advocated the simultaneous use of arthroscopy, which allows full evaluation of the ankle joint and treatment of any other pathologic conditions that are found, such as loose bodies, soft tissue or bony impingement, and osteochondral defects.[64,65] Although proponents of routine arthroscopy have demonstrated the presence of intra-articular pathologic features in a high percentage of patients, no clear evidence is available to indicate that routine arthroscopy affords a superior clinical result. The best indication for arthroscopy is the presence of ankle pain in addition to instability, or the presence of radiographic intra-articular pathologic conditions.

More recently, authors have advocated performing the ligamentous repair arthroscopically as well.[66,67] Proponents of arthroscopic repair believe it has quicker recovery, decreased morbidity, and the ability to address intra-articular pathology with the same approach.[68] A recent systematic review stated that both open and arthroscopically repaired ankles did well, based on patient satisfaction and American Orthopedic Foot and Ankle scores (AOFAS),[69] although with a 15% surgical complication rate versus 8% in the open group. The most common complication in the arthroscopic group was superficial peroneal nerve neuritis, but this did not impact the patient satisfaction score.[69]

However, another systematic review from the same year stated there was insufficient evidence to make a high-grade recommendation for minimally invasive surgery for chronic ankle instability.[70]

Nonanatomic repairs include the Evans procedure and the Watson-Jones procedure, in which the peroneus brevis tendon is transferred to act as a lateral tie bar to prevent instability and inversion. Chrisman and Snook[71] described using a split peroneus brevis transfer along a more anatomic course to recreate the ATFL and CFL. Although good results were achieved—even at 10 years—moderate restriction in subtalar movement was still present.[72] Ligamentous reconstructions should be reserved for revision cases given the restriction of physiologic movement and are not recommended for use as the index procedure. Many authors have described free tendon grafts with use of the fascia lata, semitendinosus, and gracilis; however, these grafts are best used in cases of revision or ligamentous laxity given the excellent results achieved with primary repair.[73–76]

🖈 Authors' Preferred Technique

Lateral Ankle Sprain

1. The patient is positioned supine with the leg placed in an ankle distractor. Arthroscopy is performed with use of standard anteromedial and anterolateral portals. Any incidental pathology is then treated arthroscopically.
2. The patient is then placed in a lateral position. A longitudinal incision is performed over the distal fibula and the soft tissues distal to it. The subcutaneous tissues are dissected from the lateral ligament complex. Careful inspection for any branches of the superficial peroneal nerve should be performed. Care is taken to preserve the inferior extensor retinaculum for the later Gould modification.
3. A U-shaped incision is made in the lateral ligament complex 0.5 cm distal to the fibula. The incision extends from just superior to the origin of the anterior talofibular ligament (ATFL) to just posterior to the origin of the calcaneofibular ligament (CFL).
4. A subperiosteal flap is raised off the fibula for approximately 1.5 cm. Rongeurs are used to remove the lateral and distal cortex (Fig. 117.7). A suture anchor is placed at each of the positions of the origin of the ATFL and CFL.
5. The sutures are then used to draw the distal flap onto the distal fibula, and they are tied off. The edge of this distal flap is then sutured to the base of the subperiosteal flap. The subperiosteal flap is then sutured distally to lateral soft tissues to act as a double-breasted reinforcement (Fig. 117.8).
6. As an alternative to the use of suture anchors, a pants-over-vest technique is also very effective. The ATFL and CFL are transected 1 mm distal to the tip of the fibula. Bleeding of the cancellous bone of the distal cortex of the fibula is created with a rongeur. In this case, no subperiosteal proximal flap is created. The distal flap is then secured to the proximal soft tissue in a pants-over-vest fashion, taking care to perform an adequate imbrication to decrease the laxity; typically, two or three knots are required. The suture is begun on the distal flap, which allows the knot to be placed distally and away from the skin, and is then reinforced with a figure of 8, number 0 absorbable suture after completion of the pants-over-vest imbrication.
7. The extensor retinaculum is then identified and sutured to the reconstruction and the periosteum of the fibula, with the hindfoot and ankle held in a neutral position and dorsiflexion.
8. The wound is closed in layers. The leg is placed into a below-knee backslab cast in dorsiflexion and eversion.

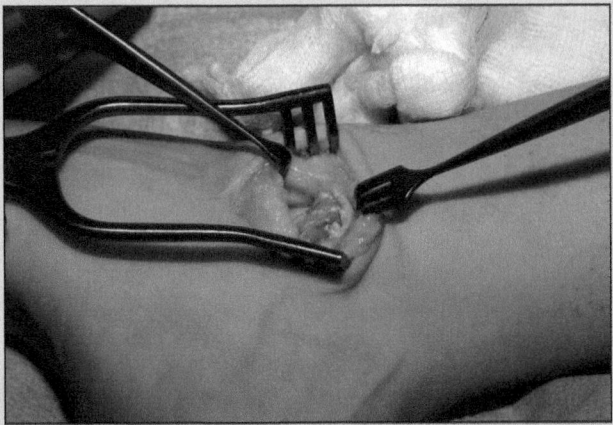

Fig. 117.7 Intraoperative image showing cortical débridement of the fibula after a subperiosteal flap has been raised.

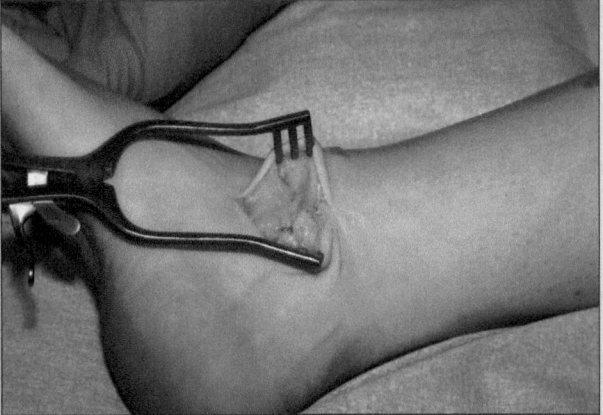

Fig. 117.8 Intraoperative image showing the completed anatomic imbrication of the lateral ligament complex.

Postoperative Management

The patient wears a splint and is non–weight bearing for 2 weeks. At this stage the sutures are removed and the patient is allowed to bear weight in a locked ROM walker boot.

At 4 weeks the ROM walker is unlocked and physical therapy is begun. For the next 2 weeks this therapy consists of ankle ROM exercises that are isolated to dorsiflexion and plantar flexion only, and swelling management.

At 6 weeks the patient is weaned into a semirigid functional brace. The intensity of physical therapy can be increased, with more robust ROM exercises (except forced inversion), early cardiovascular work, ankle-strengthening exercises, and proprioception exercises. Usually by 9 weeks the patient is being weaned out of the brace and is starting more sport-specific exercises, with progression to return to activity. The rehabilitation regime is obviously altered if other significant pathologic conditions were present in the ankle and addressed arthroscopically (e.g., an osteochondral defect).

Results

In isolated lateral ankle sprains without instability, the vast majority of athletes are able to return to their previous level of play without significant time missed from sport. In a large epidemiologic study, Roos et al. found that there were almost 2500 ankle sprains amongst all NCAA sports over a 5-year period. Among those, 44% were able to return to their sport within 24 hours while only 3.6% required more than 3 weeks before returning.[8] Maffulli et al. reported long-term outcomes of 42 athletes who underwent Broström repair for chronic lateral ankle instability. Sport at the preinjury level was still being practiced by 58% of the patients; 16% had changed to lower level sports, but were still active; and 26% had abandoned sport, but were still active.[77] White et al. reported their experience with 42 professional athletes who underwent modified Broström repair. The indication for surgery was confirmed as acute grade III lateral ligament injury on MRI and instability on physical examination. Those with isolated ATFL and CFL injuries returned to training and sport at an average of 63 and 77 days, respectively. Those who had concomitant injuries returned to training and sport at 86 and 105 days, respectively. No patient had developed recurrent instability at 2 years, and all had returned to their preinjury level of professional sport.[78]

Complications

Patients can have persistent pain and can have recurrent instability. With persistent long-term significant instability, the risk of posttraumatic osteoarthritis is undoubtedly increased. Most studies have shown that a small chance of recurrent instability exists in the long term. Our preferred method for dealing with cases of long-term instability is a nonanatomic lateral ligament reconstruction (i.e., Chrisman Snook).

MEDIAL ANKLE SPRAINS

Medial-sided ankle sprains, typically involve the deltoid ligament. They are quite uncommon and represent 4% to 5% of all ankle sprains.[79–82]

The deltoid ligament is made up of the superficial and deep layers. The superficial layer originates from the superficial margin of the anterior part of the medial malleolus and attaches to the dorsal talus, navicular, and sustentaculum. The deep deltoid layer is made up of two parts—the deep anterior and deep posterior tibiotalar ligaments—which arise from the deep margin of the posterior colliculus and attach to the medial talus while blending with the medial capsule of the ankle joint.[83–85] The deep deltoid resists posterior and lateral translation in addition to valgus angulation of the talus. The superficial structures of the deltoid complex resist external rotation of the talus relative to the tibia and valgus stress. The flexor retinaculum and the posterior tibial tendon sheath also contribute to the medial ligament complex stability.

Medial sprains are graded I for a ligament stretch injury, II for a partial tear, and III for a complete tear. Hintermann developed an anatomical classification based on whether the injury was a proximal avulsion or tear (grade I), midsubstance (grade II), or a distal avulsion or tear (grade III).[86]

History and Physical Examination

The deltoid ligament injury occurs when the hindfoot is in valgus and the forefoot is everted. The main risk factor for this type of injury is being a male athlete, with a possible link to pes planus deformity.[79,86] These injuries tend to be relatively high-impact injuries as opposed to simple "giving way" because of the relative strength and surface area of this ligament, as well as the higher inherent osseous stability of the ankle joint on the medial side.

A patient with an acute injury presents with medial-sided pain and swelling with ecchymosis. The patient may report hearing a "pop" on the medial part of the ankle before the onset of pain and usually has difficulty with weight bearing. Repeated episodes of giving way are uncommon with chronic injuries. Patients with chronic injuries tend to have residual pain together with a lack of trust in the ankle or a sense that "it just doesn't feel right."

After an appropriate focused physical examination is performed, the patient should be asked to lower himself or herself to a squatting position with the feet flat on the floor. In more significant cases of deltoid insufficiency (usually chronic cases), the medial malleolus becomes overtly prominent compared with the other ankle (a positive medial malleolar pointing sign). It should also be noted whether pes planovalgus is present.

Examination of the superficial deltoid is performed with the patient seated with mild ankle plantar flexion. The heel is cupped in the examiner's hand and brought forward while the tibia is stabilized with the opposite hand. In the case of superficial deltoid insufficiency, enhanced external rotation of the talus is observed in comparison with the contralateral side. In acute superficial deltoid ligament injuries, the anterior portion of the medial malleolus is normally painful to palpation, but this sign may be absent in athletes with chronic instability.[83]

The deep deltoid ligament is assessed by examining the posterior translation of the talus from the tibia, which is best done with the patient prone with the legs hanging off the table. The degree of translation is compared with the other side.

Muscle function should be assessed. The main muscle to be tested is the tibialis posterior muscle. Patients should be asked to perform the double-heel raise test. The heel should smoothly swing from a valgus position to around 10 degrees of varus. The patient also should be asked to perform the single-leg raise test (except in the most acute settings). The patient should be able to perform this test with equal numbers and to an equal height on both legs.

If a valgus, pronated deformity of the foot corrects with single-heel raising, this finding indicates that the patient has a purely ligamentous injury (deltoid and spring ligament) with sparing of the tibialis posterior.[80]

Imaging

Radiographs to assess ligamental injuries include standard weight-bearing AP, lateral, and mortise views. An AP hindfoot alignment view (Salzmann or Cobey view) is also indicated. Translational deformities can be assessed from the radiographs (Figs. 117.9 and 117.10).

Stress radiographs under fluoroscopy have some use, particularly with the valgus stress test on an AP film bilaterally. A finding of more than 2 to 3 degrees of valgus is considered positive. Widening of the medial clear space by 6 mm on AP/mortise radiographs of the affected ankle is also suggestive of a medial injury.[83,87]

An MRI can be helpful to evaluate the deltoid ligaments in detail.[88] However, the position of the foot may influence the visualization of the relevant anatomy because the tibionavicular and anterior tibiotalar parts are best seen with the foot in plantar flexion, whereas the tibiocalcaneal and posterior tibiotalar parts are best seen in dorsiflexion.[89]

Decision-Making Principles

The primary decision is whether the ligaments have discontinuity, because this factor has the largest influence on potential treatments. One must ensure that the syndesmosis, spring ligament, and tibialis posterior are intact. Although clinical acumen is pivotal in this decision, further imaging is essential when a partial or complete tear of the deltoid ligament is suspected. Normally, operative treatment is indicated only with failure of conservative treatment unless additional pathologic conditions need to be addressed concomitantly.

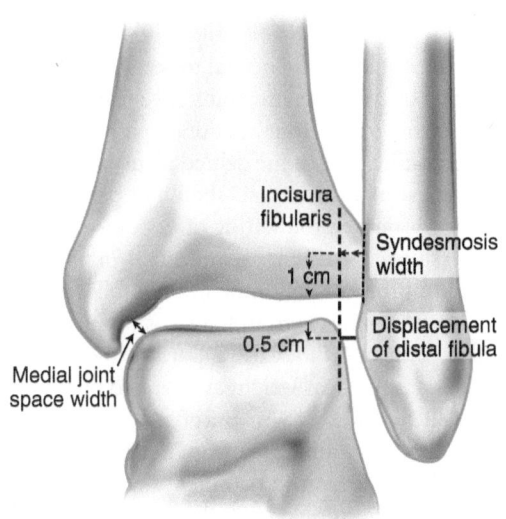

Fig. 117.9 Techniques of measuring the lateral displacement of the lateral malleolus (mortise view) and the width of the syndesmosis (mortise view) and medial joint space (anteroposterior view). (Modified from Harper MC. The deltoid ligament: an evaluation of need for surgical repair. *Clin Orthop.* 1988;226:156–168.)

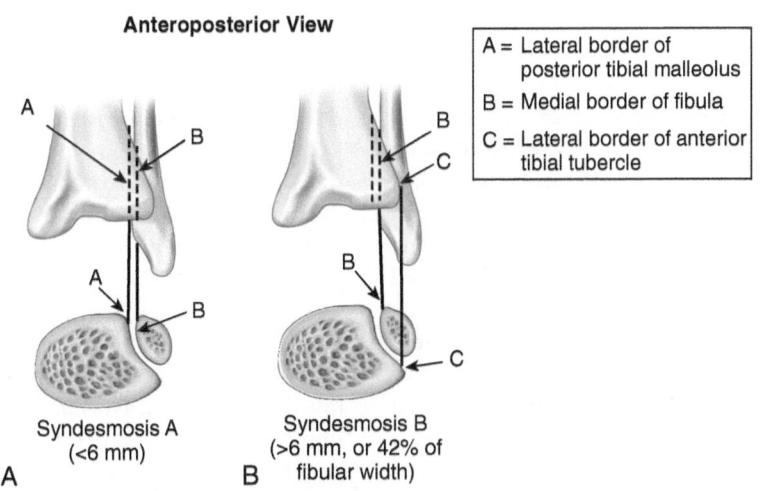

Fig. 117.10 Syndesmotic radiographic criteria. (A) The syndesmosis clear space as depicted on the anteroposterior view and by coronal section. The tibiofibular clear space is the distance between the lateral border of the posterior tibial malleolus (point *A*) and the medial border of the fibula (point *B*) on the anteroposterior radiograph. This space is normally less than 6 mm. (B) The syndesmosis overlap as seen on the anteroposterior view and by coronal section. The tibiofibular overlap is the distance between the medial border of the fibula (point *B*) and the lateral border of the anterior tibial prominence (point *C*) on the anteroposterior radiograph. This space is normally greater than 6 mm, or 42% of the fibular width. (Modified from Stiehl JB. Complex ankle fracture dislocations with syndesmosis diastasis. *Orthop Rev.* 1990;14:499–507.)

Treatment

Grade I (Sprain)

Strains can be treated with a semirigid brace that allows ankle plantar flexion and dorsiflexion but prevents inversion and eversion. Elevation and cold therapy are also indicated for the first week. A structural rehabilitation program is indicated and should initially focus on proprioception and maintenance of ROM. Return to sport is achieved in a graduated fashion as dictated by symptoms, but normally occurs within 3 weeks, with the use of a laced ankle brace for another 3 weeks.

Grades II (Partial Tear) and III (Complete Tear)

An MRI scan should be performed to see if any evidence exists of an avulsion or complete intrasubstance tear of the deltoid, as well as any of the other aforementioned pathologic conditions. If complete insufficiency of the deltoid is suspected, an examination with the use of an anesthetic should be performed. Surgical repair is appropriate in the setting of documented instability.

If conservative treatment is indicated, initial immobilization is used to promote anatomic healing followed by physical therapy. Our preference is to initially treat patients in a locked ROM walker with an orthotic to support the medial longitudinal arch. The patient can bear weight as tolerated but must keep the boot on at all times except for purposes of hygiene. At 4 to 6 weeks the boot can be unlocked from 5 degrees dorsiflexion to 30 degrees plantar flexion to commence early mobilization. At 6 weeks the boot is completely unlocked and can be removed during physical therapy for ROM, proprioception, and ankle and inversion strength exercises. The patient is gradually weaned out of the boot into a functional ankle brace and undergoes a graduated return to sport-specific exercises with return to play (RTP) in a brace for a further 6 weeks.

Surgical treatment is reserved for those with documented instability or failure of conservative management. This involves either deltoid ligament repair or reconstruction if there is insufficient residual deltoid tissue. Nonunited avulsion fragments or heterotopic ossification can produce localized osseous impingement at the medial gutter. They can also produce a local prominence that can rub against footwear. It is prudent to obtain a preoperative MRI to check for a medial osteochondral defect whose symptoms can be masked by the presence of these fragments. These can be removed either through a deltoid-splitting incision or, for larger areas of ossification, by detaching the deltoid and re-attaching using suture anchors.

Surgical repair or reconstruction an acute deltoid ligament is uncommon; however, currently, it may be more routinely performed in the setting of ankle fractures with documented syndesmotic injury. In high-level athletes, MRI findings of a complete superficial and deep deltoid disruption, operative management can be considered. Given the paucity of literature on this injury, the decision in this patient population is based on the discussion between the surgeon and the player, weighing the benefit of a quicker RTP against those of wound complications and potential stiffness.

It is difficult to compare results in patients undergoing deltoid repair versus reconstruction because the pathologic entities are often very different. An adequate amount of deltoid remaining for repair is often the result of chronic instability, and when there is very little repairable tissue it is often the result of an end-stage flatfoot deformity.[90] Therefore reconstruction techniques are out of the scope of this text.

📌 Authors' Preferred Technique
Medial Ankle Sprain

If the ankle is unstable upon examination with use of an anesthetic, then surgical exploration can be indicated.

1. A medial longitudinal incision is performed from the medial malleolar metaphyseal flare down to the level of the talonavicular joint. The subcutaneous tissues are dissected off the deltoid ligament with careful inspection for any branches of the saphenous nerve in the superior margins of the wound.

2. If a superior avulsion is present, the torn ends of the ligament are dissected free. The cortex is removed with the use of rongeurs. One to three suture anchors (depending on strands of suture and size of tear) are then used to reattach the ligament. Alternatively, bone tunnels can be used to anchor the ligament.

3. If an intrasubstance tear is present, the subperiosteal flap should be raised and suture anchors used as in the surgical technique for lateral ligament insufficiency.

4. The wound is closed in layers. The patient's ankle is placed in a backslab in dorsiflexion and inversion. The postoperative regimen is similar to that for conservative treatment once the patient progresses to a locked ROM walker with an orthotic at 2 weeks.

Results

In a prospective series of 52 patients with chronic anterior deltoid incompetence, pain in the medial gutter was found in all ankles (100%), pain along the posterior tibial tendon was found in 14 ankles (27%), and pain along the anterior border of the lateral malleolus was found in 13 ankles (25%). Repair of the deltoid ligament was performed in all 52 patients, repair of the spring ligament was performed in 13 patients (24%), repair of the lateral ligaments was performed in 40 patients (77%), and an additional calcaneal-lengthening osteotomy was performed in 14 patients (27%). At a mean follow-up of 4.4 years (range: 2.0 to 6.6 years), the AOFAS hindfoot score had improved from 42.9 points preoperatively to 91.6 points. The clinical result was considered good to excellent in 46 cases (90%), fair in four cases (8%), and poor in one case (2%).[91]

Complications

Two possible local complications can arise from isolated deltoid injuries. Nonunited avulsion fragments or heterotopic ossification can produce localized osseous impingement at the medial gutter. They can also produce a local prominence that can rub against footwear. It is prudent to obtain a preoperative MRI scan to check for a medial talar osteochondral defect—the symptoms of which can be masked by the presence of these fragments. These fragments can be removed either through a deltoid-splitting incision or, for larger areas of ossification, by detaching the deltoid and reattaching it with suture anchors or bone tunnels (Figs. 117.11 and 117.12).

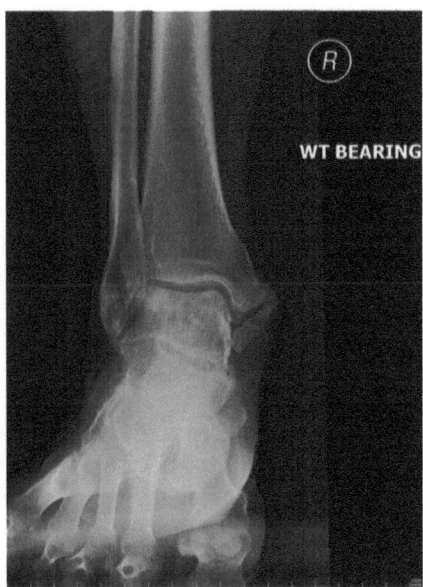

Fig. 117.11 Radiograph showing a chronic heterotopic ossification after a deltoid ligament avulsion injury.

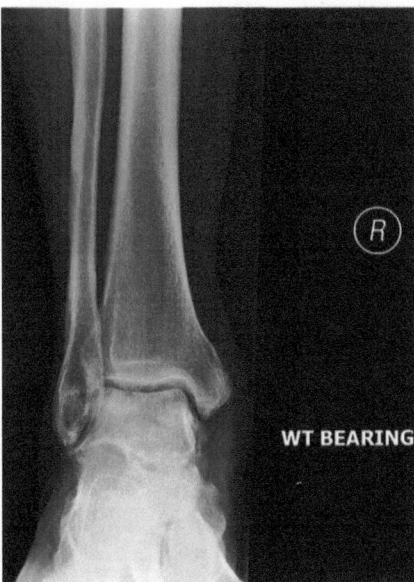

Fig. 117.12 Postoperative radiograph 6 weeks after débridement of heterotopic ossification and reattachment of the deltoid ligament.

Chronic instability is the second complication and is most commonly due to insufficiency of the superficial deltoid. Hintermann et al.[92] described three types of this instability. Type I is due to a chronic avulsion from the medial malleolus, and type II is a chronic intrasubstance tear. They are treated as outlined in the section on acute injuries. Type III lesions are from the distal insertion of the deltoid. These lesions are repaired with nonabsorbable sutures into the spring ligament, as well as a suture anchor into the superior edge of the navicular tuberosity if additional insufficiency of the tibionavicular part of the superficial deltoid is present. With use of this treatment algorithm, the authors managed to achieve a 90% rate of excellent results at 4 years.

Chronic instability of the deep deltoid ligament is an extremely challenging condition. Many different choices of graft and graft fixation have been attempted with equivocal results.

SYNDESMOSIS SPRAIN

The incidence of ankle syndesmosis injuries, or high ankle sprains, is around 15 per 100,000 in the general population and is much higher in the athletic population. These injuries can represent between 1% and 11% of all ankle injuries.[93,94]

The distal tibiofibular syndesmosis is composed of the anterior inferior and posterior inferior tibiofibular ligaments (AITFL and PITFL) and the interosseous membrane with its corresponding ligament. The PITFL is further divided into superficial and deep components, with the deep component (also referred to as the transverse ligament) in one cadaveric study only being present 70% of the time.[95]

The interosseous tibiofibular ligament is the strongest connection between the tibia and fibula and runs from the lateral distal tibia to the medial distal fibula. It is in continuation with the interosseous membrane proximally.[96]

The AITFL provides 35% of the resistance to diastasis stress of the syndesmosis, whereas the PITFL contributes 40% to 45%, and the remainder comes from the interosseous ligament.[97] All components of the syndesmosis also contribute to rotatory stability to the ankle. Clanton et al. performed a biomechanical study, sequentially sectioning components of the syndesmosis in cadavers. They found that sectioning the AITFL resulted in a 24% decrease in resistance to external rotation, compared to a 17% decrease in resistance with isolated sectioning of the superficial and deep PITFL.[98]

The AITFL is the first and most commonly injured ligament in a syndesmosis sprain, and the PITFL is the last ligament injured.

The syndesmosis, along with the deltoid ligament, prevents diastasis of the joint and maintains function. During non–weight-bearing plantar flexion, the distal fibula moves anteriorly and inferiorly and medially rotates after the internal rotation of the talus, whereas in dorsiflexion, the distal fibula glides in a posterosuperior direction and rotates laterally with the talus, which explains the mechanism of injury.[99]

History and Examination

The mechanism of injury is usually an externally rotated and dorsiflexed foot and axial loading,[100,101] which places stress on the ligaments. The AITFL fails first as noted, and the PITFL tries to stabilize the syndesmosis. With continued external rotation and/or abduction, the entire system fails and results in a diastasis.

Usually, in most complete disruptions, associated injuries are found, such as Weber B or C fracture, Maisonneuve fracture, plus deltoid disruption and medial malleolar fracture, depending on the pattern of injury. Diastasis without fracture can occur but is extremely rare.

The clinical features that are in keeping with a syndesmosis injury classically are pain over the anterior and posterior tibiofibular ligaments. Often patients can point to this area where they have maximal tenderness. As the severity of the injury increases, the tenderness moves proximally to the anteromedial part of the fibula where the interosseous membrane is attached. The distance of the most proximal extent of the tenderness to the distal tip of the fibula is called the "tenderness length," and has been correlated with increased time to RTP.[102]

In addition to palpation of the syndemosis, many provocative tests are available for the diagnosis of a syndesmotic sprain. These tests include the squeeze test, dorsiflexion compression test, external rotation test, manual stability test, cross-leg test, and heel thump test. The squeeze test and the external rotation test are those most frequently performed.

The squeeze test is performed with the patient at the end of the examination table with the knee bent at 90 degrees. A compressive force is applied between the fibula and tibia superior to the midpoint of the calf. A positive test will elicit pain distally in the region of the syndesmosis.[103]

The external rotation test is performed with the patient seated, the hip and knee flexed, and the foot and ankle in the neutral position. With the knee facing forward, a gentle external rotation is applied to the foot. The test is positive if the pain is reproduced at the anterior syndesmosis.

A recently published report found that the most sensitive test is syndesmotic tenderness (92%); the most specific is the squeeze test (88%); and the highest diagnostic accuracy is the external rotation test (66.7%). They concluded that clinicians should not rely on one test alone to make a diagnosis.[104]

Multiple classification systems for isolated syndesmotic injuries currently exist without clear consensus. Almost all involve grades between I and III, with grade I being a mild injury requiring only conservative treatment, and III being severe and generally requiring operative intervention. Where most differ is on grade II injuries, some consider these stable, while other consider these unstable.[103] We prefer to use the West Point Ankle Grading system, which is one of the more commonly used classification systems.[105]

A grade I injury is characterized by a stable syndesmotic joint that has mild tenderness at the distal tibiofibular joint. This injury involves the anterior deltoid ligament and the distal interosseous ligament, but without tearing the more proximal syndesmosis or the deep deltoid ligament. Grade I injuries are stable because no diastasis is present on radiograph.

A grade II injury is defined as partial syndesmotic ligament disruption with normal radiographic findings and has a positive external rotation and squeeze test on examination.

Grade III injuries include complete injury to the syndesmotic ligaments. On plain radiography there will be clear widening of the medial clear space and/or syndesmosis. All clinical tests are typically positive.[103]

In an effort to simplify the classification to aid clinical decision-making, the Ankle and Foot associates of the European Society of Sports Traumatology, Knee Surgery and Arthroscopy (ESSKA), issued a consensus statement in 2016. They recommended classifying syndesmotic injuries as acute (<6 weeks), subacute (between 6 weeks and 6 months), and chronic (>6 months). Acute syndesmotic sprains were then further subdivided as stable and unstable. Unstable injuries were defined as frank diastasis on pain radiographs or latent diastasis, which would need to be assessed either with stress radiographs, MRI, or arthroscopically. They recommended that stable injuries undergo conservative management, while unstable injuries undergo operative management.[106]

Imaging

Radiographs should include AP, mortise, and lateral views, including the entire tibia and fibula if a syndesmotic injury is suspected, to rule out a high fibula fracture or a Maisonneuve injury. Ideally a weight-bearing view is preferred, but in a person with an acute injury, obtaining such a view may not always be possible. The three measurements that may help in diagnosing syndesmosis injuries are tibiofibular clear space, medial clear space, and tibiofibular overlap.

Recent data demonstrate that basing treatment of syndesmotic injuries on previously reported radiographic criteria can lead to unnecessary operative intervention or failure to treat.[107] The mean tibiofibular overlap is 8.3 mm on the AP and 3.5 mm on the mortise view; whereas the mean clear space is 4.6 mm on the AP and 4.3 mm on the mortise view. The least amount of overlap on the AP view was 1.8 mm. On the mortise view, a subset of patients had a complete lack of overlap (<0 mm), with the greatest gap noted to be 1.9 mm. The greatest clear space on the AP view was 8 mm, and on the mortise view it was 7.6 mm. The problem with relying on absolute values is that significant variations exist in the patient population, which may lead to misdiagnosis; therefore comparison with the contralateral lower extremity provides a more reliable "normal" measurement on which to base treatment. The clear space on the mortise view radiograph has been proved to be relatively independent of rotation, and 95% of patients have a less than 2 mm side-to-side difference.[108] If the initial radiographs are still not helpful, stress radiographs with the leg in external rotation may help assess for diastasis (Fig. 117.13).

If the diagnosis is still in doubt, further testing is indicated, including standing bilateral axial computed tomography (CT) imaging, MRI, and diagnostic arthroscopy. Although CT has been proven to show smaller diastases from 1 mm, MRI currently seems to be the more favored modality because of its high sensitivity and specificity, and because it helps show the injured anatomy and may aid in surgical planning (Fig. 117.14).

Decision-Making Principles

A chronic, unstable, untreated syndesmosis injury can predispose the patient to further injury, degenerative changes, chronic pain, and osteochondral lesions.[109] Therefore the key principle in the treatment of a syndesmotic injury is to maintain a high suspicion of the injury. Any evidence of widening of the syndesmosis, clear space, or fracture requires operative intervention.

Treatment

Grade I injuries are stable and can be treated nonoperatively. Rehabilitation with use of the RICE method with initial non–weight bearing in a boot and early mobilization is indicated. Serial radiographs may be indicated to ascertain that the injury has not progressed. The treatment is tailored to the athlete's progress. Once the swelling and pain have improved, early mobilization (between 3 and 6 weeks) is initiated. At this time, patients may still need some external support so they can start their

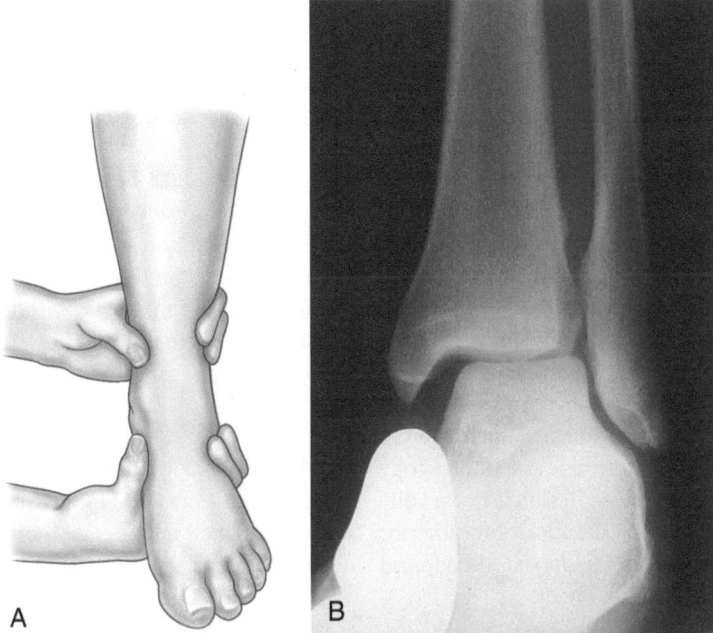

Fig. 117.13 (A) The direct eversion maneuver is accomplished with the patient in a seated and relaxed position. The examiner gently secures the leg and foot as a direct eversion or abduction force is applied across the ankle. Increased translation compared with the contralateral ankle is a positive result. (B) A positive stress radiograph showing increased translation. ([A], Modified from Stiehl JB. Complex ankle fracture dislocations with syndesmotic diastasis. *Orthop Rev.* 1990;19:499–507.)

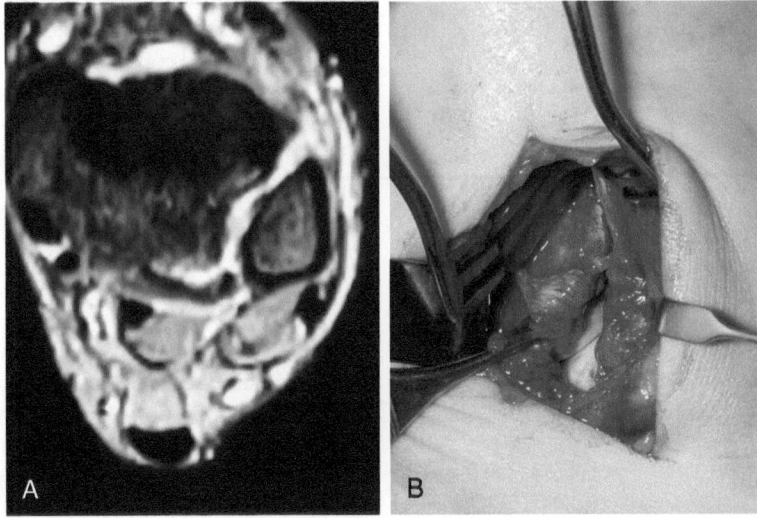

Fig. 117.14 (A) A magnetic resonance image demonstrating a complete tear of the anterior inferior tibiofibular ligament and a partial tear of the posterior inferior tibiofibular ligament. (B) Open treatment of a syndesmotic rupture.

rehabilitation program, starting with ROM exercises and increasing to strengthening exercises as tolerated.

Grade II and III injuries are unstable and require surgical treatment. Historically the most common method of syndesmotic fixation is with trans-syndesmotic screw(s). This method uses either one or two 3.5 or 4.5 mm screws inserted from lateral to medial through both fibular cortices and then through either one or two tibial cortices. Based on a national survey, most surgeons insert the screw between 2.1 and 4 cm proximal to the tibial plafond.[110] Biomechanical studies have differed in their recommendation for ideal screw placement, with one advocating

for 2 cm proximal to the plafond,[111] and the other recommending between 3 and 4 cm.[112] There is no consensus on the appropriate screw size or the number of cortices to engage.[105] Although it appears that the majority of surgeons routinely remove trans-syndesmotic screws,[110] the literature is in disagreement, and there is still no consensus on this topic.[105]

Recently there has been a surge in the use of sutures with an Endobutton—the most common device being the TightRope system (Arthrex; Naples, FL). The idea behind flexible fixation is that it stabilizes the syndesmosis without abolishing physiologic motion. Also, because of its low profile, it would not require routine removal.[113] Numerous recent studies have been published demonstrating no difference in outcomes, the ability to reduce the syndesmosis, or the ability to restore rotational stability.[114–118] However, longer term outcome data and more uniform outcome reporting are still needed.[119] There is also concern about its ability to restore sagittal stability.[105] Currently there is no consensus on the number of suture button devices that should be used. In fact, some surgeons will use one tight rope and one syndesmotic screw, to prevent theoretical widening of the syndesmosis once the syndesmotic screw is removed.[113]

Regardless of the technique used, anatomic reduction of the syndesmosis is the most critical, and malreduction has been associated with poor outcomes.[120] Intraoperatively, an assessment of reduction can be made with fluoroscopy, intraoperative CT scans, or direct visualization. However, standard fluoroscopy often can be unreliable and intraoperative CT scan is not readily available at most institutions.[113] Direct visualization of the inferior tibiofibular joint through an anterolateral incision has been found to be an effective method to assess reduction.[120]

Postoperative Management

Patients are non–weight bearing in a cast or a removable controlled ankle motion walker for 6 weeks. Patients then graduate to using an unlocked ROM walker boot or a semirigid brace for

---

 Authors' Preferred Technique

Syndesmosis Sprain

1. A longitudinal incision is made over the distal fibula. All branches of the superficial peroneal nerve are identified and protected.
2. The anterior inferior tibiofibular ligament (AITFL) is carefully inspected. If an avulsion fragment is present, a decision is made about whether it can be fixed anatomically. Occasionally the ligament still has reasonable quality and a direct repair can be performed at the end of the procedure.
3. All extraneous fibrous tissue and any ossification is removed. Fibular reduction can be done either with a large reduction clamp or manual reduction with the thumb. Historically, a large reduction clamp has been utilized; however, if it is not placed in the anatomic axis of the syndesmosis, a malreduction may occur with rotational and translational malalignment. The use of the thumb/manual reduction has shown to result in similar if not superior reduction compared to the large reduction clamps. If it is irreducible or if significant force is required to achieve reduction, soft tissue may be interposed in the medial gutter. A separate medial incision is performed and the tissue is removed. Care is taken to prevent excessive pressure with the clamp as this can result in over-reduction of the syndesmosis with associated complications related to this.
4. Fixation of the syndesmosis is performed with use of two tricortical 3.5-mm screws through a   tubular plate. These screws are inserted at 90 degrees to the joint line under fluoroscopic control. In the setting of a concomitant fibular fracture that has been anatomically reduced, the use of a suture button device may be considered and as discussed previously, has excellent radiographic and clinical outcomes. If the fibula is not stabilized, as in a Maisonneuve fracture pattern, isolated suture button fixation is not appropriate as the length cannot be maintained and malunion will likely occur.
5. The integrity of the deltoid ligament is then assessed both clinically and under fluoroscopic control. If it is found to be insufficient, a repair is performed as described in the deltoid ligament section. If possible, repair of the AITFL is then performed.

---

another 6 weeks. If screw removal is planned, patients are limited to nonimpact activity until removal of the hardware to minimize the risk of screw fracture. The rehabilitation program should then be carried out as for conservatively treated syndesmosis injuries.

Screws should be removed no earlier than 3 months after surgery. Removal between 4 and 5 months from the time of the injury allows increased time for the soft tissue healing to occur but increases the risk of hardware failure. One should consider later removal in patients with chronic injuries or in very heavy patients. Patients should be counseled that it will take at least 6 months for symptoms to resolve and that some patients will have a permanent decrease in function.

Results

Return to sport takes longer in persons with syndesmotic injuries compared with persons with ankle sprains. Nussbaum et al. reported on a series of 60 collegiate athletes with clinically diagnosed syndesmotic injuries without diastasis on radiographs. With conservative management they had an average RTP of 13.4 days.[121] Similarly, Miller et al. separately looked at clinically diagnosed, stable syndesmosis injuries in 20 college football players. Among those 20 with clinical syndesmotic injuries, 10 also had evidence of an interosseous membrane tear on ultrasound. They reported an average RTP of 15.5 days.[122] Calder et al. looked at professional athletes with complete tears of the AITFL on MRI and stratified them into stable and unstable groups. The stable group was treated conservatively with an average RTP of 45 days. The unstable group was treated with tightrope fixation with an average RTP of 64 days.[123]

Chronic or lingering symptoms are common with syndesmotic injury. Taylor et al.[124] showed that at 47 months, 23% of subjects had chronic ankle pain, 36% had ankle stiffness, and 18% had persistent swelling.

Complications

Patients should be counseled that a significant minority (up to 20%) will have some degree of permanent symptoms. The most common complication being stiffness. Patients with higher-grade injuries almost certainly have an increased chance of the development of posttraumatic osteoarthritis. Greater age at the time of injury has been associated with increased risk for chronic pain and dissatisfaction with surgery.[125]

Patients should have regular weight-bearing radiographs after surgery and for some months after the removal of the metalwork because of the risk of recurrent diastasis. In the event of these complications, surgical strategies are available. Techniques of syndesmosis reconstruction have been described with the use of autograft or allograft tendons, along with isolated syndesmosis fusion.

BIFURCATE LIGAMENT SPRAIN/FRACTURE OF THE ANTERIOR PROCESS OF CALCANEUM

The bifurcate ligament is a Y-shaped ligament composed of the calcaneonavicular and calcaneocuboid arms that originates from the anterior process of the calcaneum and attaches to the navicular and cuboid, respectively. It lies distal and anterior to the inferior lip of the fibula, and superior and proximal to the base of the fifth metatarsal. The bifurcate ligament is commonly damaged by forceful inversion and plantar flexion of the foot, which can either cause a bifurcate ligament sprain or a fracture of the anterior process of the calcaneum.[126,127]

The anterior process of calcaneus fractures can be caused by tension, compression, or shear forces. Tension injuries cause avulsion fractures such as those seen with a plantar-flexed inverted foot. Shear fractures are caused by forefoot abduction with the heel fixed to the ground and forced dorsiflexion. Compression fractures are caused by dorsiflexion eversion injuries, which tend to cause intra-articular fractures.

Degan classified these fractures into three types. Type I is an undisplaced fracture, type II is displaced fracture without intra-articular involvement, and type III is a displaced fracture involving the calcaneocuboid joint.[128,129]

History and Physical Examination

The history can be variable, but an inversion plantar flexion injury should lead one to look for this condition. However, this injury is not normally isolated, because ankle sprains, particularly on the lateral side, can be present along with the bifurcate sprain.[130] The patient may have felt a pop or a snap with acute onset of pain followed by ecchymosis and swelling.

Examination confirms diffuse swelling over the lateral hindfoot and midfoot. The pain may be localized over the course of the ligament, which is normally separate from the ATFL, which is the other ligament that is often damaged with this mechanism of injury. Inversion and plantar flexion reproduces the pain. Broström suggested that the way to distinguish ATFL pain from bifurcate pain is to manipulate the heel to produce lateral-sided pain, whereas forced forefoot motion with the hindfoot stabilized will elicit bifurcate pain.[128]

Imaging

Routine AP, lateral, and oblique views of the foot and ankle are obtained. In persons with a bifurcate sprain, the radiographs are likely to be normal, but may show an anterior process of a calcaneum fracture. The normal series may not always show the fracture, and therefore an oblique radiograph with the central ray directed 10 to 15 degrees superior and posterior to the middle of the foot is often useful because this technique projects over the process over the talus and makes visualization of the fracture much easier.[131] CT is the preferred choice to assess fractures but is not useful for bifurcate sprains, for which MRI is superior.[126]

Decision-Making Principles

The treatment of bifurcate sprains is initially conservative. The only exception to this approach is the presence of a large or displaced anterior process fracture that may be amenable to surgical treatment. If such a fracture is suspected on plain radiographs, a CT scan should be performed to delineate the size of the fragment, whether it extends into the calcaneocuboid joint, and whether it is multifragmentary, which will determine the appropriateness of early surgery.

Treatment

Acute sprains are initially treated with RICE followed by ROM and protected weight bearing. They can be initially supported with a short removable boot, a walking cast, or a functional brace. Physical therapy emphasizes subtalar flexibility, motor function, and coordination.[131] The rehabilitation program starts with simple ROM exercises, as well as isometric exercises. As the acute phase subsides, more aggressive therapies can be introduced, starting with closed-chain activities and graduating up to sport-specific exercises, followed by a graduated RTP. Søndergaard et al.[132] reported excellent results, with the time to return to sports averaging 21 days.

Chronic sprains can be treated similarly to acute sprains, but steroids also can be injected either intralesionally or intra-articularly at the calcaneocuboid level under fluoroscopic guidance. If symptoms do not diminish, operative treatment should be considered, which can be in the form of an open or arthroscopic procedure. However, operative treatment is rarely required.

Authors' Preferred Technique
Bifurcate Ligament Sprain

1. A lateral incision is made from just distal to the tip of the fibula toward the base of the fourth metatarsal. Care is taken not to damage any branches of the superficial peroneal nerve in the superior margins of the wound.
2. The extensor digitorum brevis is raised as a flap off the lateral border of the calcaneus, leaving a small cuff of tissue for later repair.
3. The sinus tarsi is identified as far distally as the superior aspect of the calcaneocuboid joint. Inflamed and fibrotic tissue is débrided with rongeurs. If a small malunited or nonunited fracture of the anterior process of the calcaneus is present, it is excised. If the procedure is acute and a large fracture is to be fixed, the fracture site is cleared, reduction is performed with a wire, and a headless compression screw is used for fixation.
4. Stress views of the hindfoot and ankle should then be performed to determine if any residual instability is present to help determine the postoperative regimen of mobilization.
5. The wound is closed in layers and a splint is applied.

Postoperative Management

The splint is kept in place for 2 weeks. A semirigid ankle brace is applied, and the patient is then allowed to bear weight. The same rehabilitation program is then used as outlined in the section on conservative treatment.

If any residual instability was present at the time of the operation, the patient's ankle is mobilized in a ROM walker boot with the range of movement gradually increased over a period of 4 to 6 weeks. The patient then undergoes rehabilitation according to the more standard postoperative regimen. It should be noted that, unfortunately, symptoms can occasionally be protracted.

RESULTS

No peer-reviewed articles are available that delineate the expected results from this injury.

Complications

The main complication is nonresolving pain with or without instability. Steroid injections with a further rehabilitation program can often be successful in relieving symptoms. In the rare cases in which pain persists, an arthrodesis may be required. Isolated calcaneocuboid fusion can be performed; however, union may be difficult to achieve. Arthrodesis of the triple-joint complex has a higher rate of union but imparts a significant loss of hindfoot motion.

LISFRANC SPRAINS

Lisfranc sprains or midfoot sprains occur at the Lisfranc joint, which is the second most common area in the foot to be injured in athletes after the metatarsophalangeal joint.[133,134] This area of the midfoot is named after Jacques Lisfranc, the French Napoleonic surgeon.

The incidence of midfoot sprains is around 4%. A Lisfranc sprain is a sprain of the midfoot due to a low-impact injury, whereas a Lisfranc fracture dislocation is the result of a high-impact injury.[135]

The Lisfranc joint is the articulations between the three cuneiform bones and the cuboid bone with the five metatarsals. The shape of the articulating surfaces with the metatarsal bases provides primary stability, with the second tarsometatarsal joint acting as a keystone and providing stability in both the longitudinal and transverse arches.

These joints also classify the columns in the foot. The medial column is made up of the first ray and medial cuneiform bone, the middle column is made up of the second and third rays, and the middle and lateral cuneiform bones, and the lateral column is made up of the fourth and fifth rays with the cuboid bone. The rigidity of the medial and middle column is important to the function of the foot, and the Lisfranc ligament provides the rigid connection between the columns.[136]

Numerous ligaments in the Lisfranc joint provide the secondary stabilization. Dorsal and plantar ligaments are present, with the plantar ligaments being stronger than the dorsal ligaments.[137] The most important structure is the Lisfranc ligament, which is the plantar ligament running between the medial cuneiform and the base of the second metatarsal.[138]

History and Physical Examination

The mechanism of injury can be either direct or indirect.[139] Direct-force injuries as described by Myerson et al.,[140] and entail an axial-directed force acting on the dorsum of the foot, causing tension on the plantar surface and leading to injury. These injuries are usually higher energy injuries in an industrial setting. Because of the mechanism of injury, open fractures and compartment syndrome are more common in this setting than in indirect injuries.

The more common indirect-force injuries are usually low-energy injuries, which occur when a weight-bearing hyper-plantar-flexed foot with a rotational or bending force is applied to the foot, or when the plantigrade foot is kept fixed to the floor (e.g., upon stamping in soccer) with the body rotating over the top

of the foot. The severity of these injuries depends on the force and mechanism of injury.

In 2002 Nunley and Vertullo[141] classified Lisfranc injuries into three stages on the basis of radiographic and clinical findings and bone scan results. Stage I is a nondisplaced injury in which the patient may be able to bear weight but cannot return to sports. Stages II and III show displacement and require operative intervention. This classification has more relevance in low-energy injuries such as midfoot sprains.

Myerson and colleagues[140] classified Lisfranc injuries based on the classification performed by Hardcastle and colleagues.[142] Unfortunately, the classification systems do not significantly aid in determining treatment and outcome. A descriptive analysis of the involved joints, the presence of a fracture, and articular comminution is more useful than any particular classification scheme.

Associated injuries include a stress fracture of the base of the second metatarsal, particularly in female dancers with low-energy injuries, a nutcracker fracture of the cuboid, and compartment syndrome, particularly in high-energy injuries.

Clinical examination of the entire foot and ankle is performed to evaluate for other concomitant injuries. Patients usually present with pain and swelling and—depending on the extent of injury—may not be able to bear weight. Any ecchymosis present in the center of the plantar aspect of the foot is highly indicative of a Lisfranc injury.

Stability is tested in the sagittal plane if possible. With the midfoot secured with one hand and the other hand holding the first metatarsal, a dorsiflexion force is applied and abnormal translation and pain is noted compared with the normal foot on the other side. In the frontal plane, stability is tested with abduction and adduction forces. Myerson and colleagues described the pronation–abduction test, which is positive if it elicits pain and reproduces the patient's symptoms.[143] Pain with single-limb weight bearing is also suggestive of a Lisfranc injury and should be performed after obtaining appropriate imaging to ensure that no fractures have occurred.

Imaging

The best plain films are weight-bearing bilateral AP, lateral, and oblique views; however, based on the severity of injury, patients may not be able to tolerate weight bearing radiographs. Non-weight-bearing radiographs miss up to 50% of Lisfranc injuries and sprains.[135] Normal foot anatomy and congruency of the joints in all views should be assessed, and abnormal findings, such as fracture and diastasis, should be sought. Particular attention should be directed to looking for a "fleck sign" at the medial base of the second metatarsal, which is indicative of a cortical avulsion of the Lisfranc ligament (Fig. 117.15).

One should beware of normal appearances of non–weight-bearing radiographs when a high clinical index of suspicion exists. In this scenario, we recommend further imaging or conservative treatment until full weight-bearing films can be obtained. Single-limb weight-bearing views of the affected foot may also demonstrate subtle instability because patients shift weight to the unaffected extremity with a double-limb weight-bearing view.

The patient must be examined for Lisfranc variants with intercuneiform instability or disruption of the naviculocuneiform

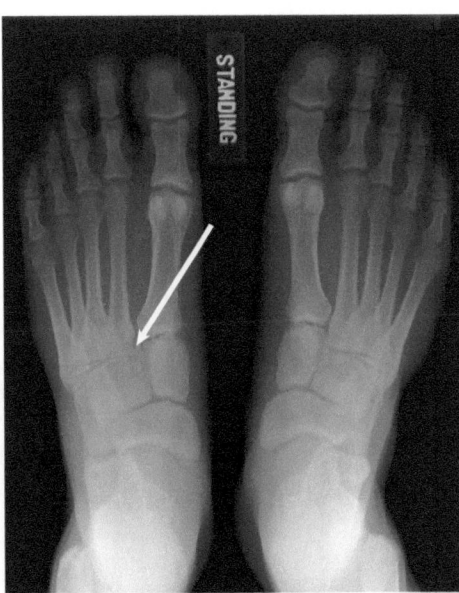

Fig. 117.15 A patient with a Lisfranc injury identified by the "fleck sign" *(arrow)*. In this case, the ligament itself remained intact and the injury occurs by avulsion of the ligament from the base of the second metatarsal. The function of the ligament is compromised, and operative intervention is indicated.

joint with an impaction fracture of the navicular. Stress radiographs are not routinely performed in the office because they cause extreme pain, and patient guarding limits their utility. Examination with use of an anesthetic is typically required to determine the instability of the midfoot with manual stress testing. Pronation abduction and adduction stress testing is performed, and the joint is assessed with imaging.[135,144]

Bone scintigraphy has a very limited role. CT scanning can be helpful, particularly in demonstrating fracture patterns and the presence of any occult fractures. CT scans are particularly useful in assessing high-energy injuries. MRI assessment of soft tissue is excellent and may be helpful, particularly with sprains and low-energy injuries; ligamentous anatomy and disruption can be examined when the diagnosis is in doubt.[144]

Decision-Making Principles

In cases with midfoot pain after an injury, the diagnosis of a Lisfranc injury is presumed. Nonoperative management is considered in cases with normal weight-bearing radiographs and/or corroborative MRI findings of an intact Lisfranc ligament. Biweekly weight-bearing radiographs for the first 6 weeks and a follow-up radiograph at 3 months are recommended to ensure that no displacement occurs. Any evidence of displacement or bony fracture requires operative reduction and stabilization.

Treatment

Stage I sprains can be treated conservatively with initial immobilization in a non–weight-bearing cast for 6 weeks. If the athlete is asymptomatic at this stage, a semirigid orthosis can be applied and the patient can be mobilized. If the patient still has symptoms, the use of an ankle foot orthosis for an additional 4 weeks may be required.[134,138,141]

ROM can usually be initiated at around 8 weeks, but full weight bearing should not be initiated until 3 months after the injury. Supportive heel cushions may be needed once the athlete returns to training. Repeat imaging must be performed to ensure lack of displacement. Any diastasis or change in the alignment should be corrected with surgical intervention.

Patients with stages II and III injuries are treated with surgery. The goal of surgery is to reduce the joints in an anatomic position and maintain this reduction until healing occurs. For this reason Kirschner wires should not be used because of the high incidence of recurrence of deformity. Usually the joints that need to be treated can be determined preoperatively, but fluoroscopic stress views should be carefully obtained intraoperatively to ensure that no residual instability is present.

The injuries can be addressed with screw or plate fixation. Reduction needs to be anatomic. The use of a bridging plate minimizes further articular injury because no screws cross the affected joints, and in cases of hardware failure, no intra-articular hardware will be present. However, during hardware removal, a large incision is required. In a prospective randomized study, Ly and Coetzee[145] found that patients who underwent primary fusion rated their postoperative activity level at 92% compared to 65% in their open reduction internal fixation (ORIF) group. They noted their belief that better results could be achieved with the use of primary fusion instead of fixation in all Lisfranc injuries except those with minimal or no displacement. However, Henning et al. in a similar prospective randomize trial found no difference between the two groups at any point in terms of postoperative SF-36 and Short Musculoskeletal Function Assessment scores or patient satisfaction scores.[146] A recent meta-analysis comparing primary fusion to ORIF, noted there were no significant differences in outcomes between the two groups, but there was a higher rate of hardware removal in the ORIF group.[147] Although they noted a lack of high quality research. Currently, there are insufficient data to recommend primary arthrodesis over ORIF for ligamentous Lisfranc injuries. In cases with articular comminution, arthrodesis is preferred, given the high likelihood of posttraumatic arthrosis. The use of suture button devices is being utilized by some surgeons; however, given the lack of data with this technique, this should be considered with caution at this time.

Postoperative Management

Patients are kept non–weight bearing for 6 weeks. This period is extended if high levels of comminution are present. The patient is then allowed to bear weight in a ROM walker with an orthotic to support the medial longitudinal arch. Although no exact consensus exists with regard to the timing of hardware removal, it should be removed no earlier than 3 months after the procedure. Delaying hardware removal in obese patients and laborers may decrease the rate of late failure but increases the rate of hardware fracture. Removal of hardware from between 4 and 5 months offers a good compromise between ligamentous healing and hardware failure. The foot continues to be supported orthotically for a further 3 months. With the advent of bridge plating, hardware retention of the middle column is more common given the limited motion of these joints. In laborers, or athletes that require stability over agility, this may be considered. Given the

Authors' Preferred Technique

Lisfranc Sprain

1. In minimally displaced injuries in patients with good bone stock, a percutaneous reduction may be attempted. Stab incisions are made over the lateral part of the base of the second metatarsal and the medial side of the medial cuneiform. A large reduction clamp is applied. Careful fluoroscopic examination is undertaken. If a perfect reduction is achieved, a 4.0-mm cannulated screw is inserted from the base of the second metatarsal into the medial cuneiform. The fluoroscopic examination is repeated along with stress views to see if any other joint requires stabilization. If so, they are addressed in a similar fashion. If this technique is to be used, it is essential that anatomic reduction be achieved. If any doubt exists about the possibility of anatomic reduction, conversion to an open operation should take place.

2. If percutaneous reduction is not indicated or is unsuccessful, then an open procedure is performed. Different approaches are available to expose the midfoot. Traditionally, a longitudinal incision is made between the first and second metatarsals, extending proximally to the naviculocuneiform joint. The neurovascular structures are carefully retracted. This surgical approach allows the exposure of the first and second TMT joints; however, it does require exposure of the neurovascular bundle and does risk injury to the first dorsal interosseous artery. An alternative option is to approach the first TMT through a medially based approach, and the second TMT through a more centrally located dorsal approach immediately medial to the third TMT joint. Although two incisions are required, the ease of visualization and diminished risk of injury to the neurovascular bundle does offer significant benefit. Any interposed soft tissue or loose osseous fragments are removed. Reduction is performed from proximal to distal and from medial to lateral. Therefore the intercuneiform should be stabilized, followed by the first tarsometatarsal, which creates a stable corner into which the second metatarsal can be reduced. In the setting of a naviculocuneiform variant, reduction of the intercuneiform joint allows for the reduction of the impaction fracture of medial navicular. Fixation is then performed with the same cannulated screws or a bridging locking plate depending on bone quality and if associated fractures are present. If the third tarsometatarsal joint is involved, this condition is best addressed through a second incision (if a 1 to 2 TMT incision is used) based on the medial aspect of the fourth metatarsal, which also allows exposure of the cuboid if needed (Fig. 117.16).

3. Normally the fourth and fifth metatarsals reduce and remain stable. If this is not the case, Kirschner wires are used for 6 weeks because it is important to maintain high levels of flexibility in these joints.

4. Primary arthrodesis is reserved for the most severe injuries. This procedure is performed in a fashion similar to that performed for primary osteoarthritis. It is obviously complicated by the lack of bone stock, and bone grafting is often necessary.

5. The wounds are closed in layers. The foot is protected in a splint.

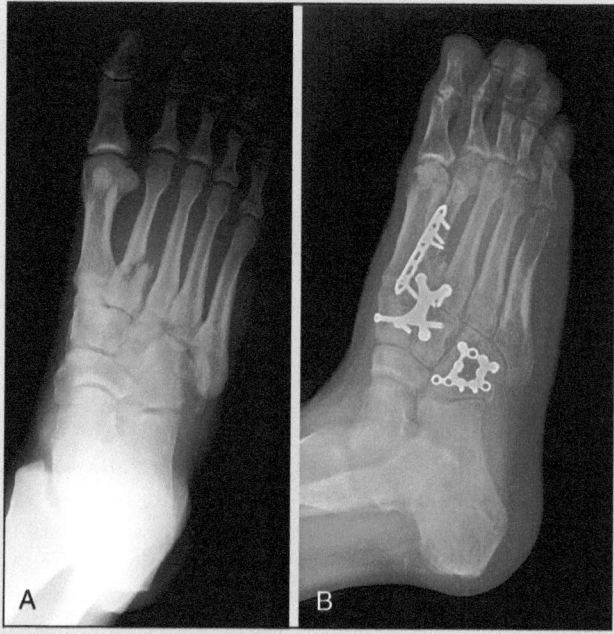

Fig. 117.16 (A and B) A combination of screw and plate fixation was used to maintain the reduction in a patient with a high-energy Lisfranc injury. Plate fixation is very useful in the setting of fractures of the base of the metatarsals that prevent adequate purchase for a screw. The patient also had a cuboid fracture that required plate fixation.

lack of trans-articular hardware, there is no risk of iatrogenic damage to the articular surface. Physical therapy prior to hardware removal focuses on ankle and hindfoot movement, as well as low-impact cardiovascular work (e.g., the use of an exercise bike). A graduated rehabilitation program can be undertaken after hardware removal.

Results

Athletic Lisfranc injuries occur from lower energy mechanism that the nonathletic variant. Therefore results for treatment of this injury should be viewed in the correct context. Chilvers et al.[155] reported on Lisfranc injuries in elite female gymnasts. There is not a tremendous amount of published literature on outcomes of stable and unstable Lisfranc injuries in athletes. Although the results that are available show that stable Lisfranc injuries treated conservatively typically do well, with full return to sport within 11 to 20 weeks.[148–150] Deol et al. shared their results of operative fixation of 17 unstable Lisfranc injuries in professional soccer and rugby players. Only one athlete retired and the remainder returned to full training and competition at an average of 20.1 weeks and 24.1 weeks, respectively.[151] In a similar paper looking at 28 NFL players with Lisfranc injuries found that 90% were able to RTP with an insignificant drop in performance.[152]

These results are in contrast to those who sustain a non–sport-related Lisfranc injury. Their AOFAS scores are around 70 at medium-term follow-up for open reduction with internal fixation.[153,154] The most significant factor for optimum results is the accuracy of reduction.

Complications

The most significant complications are stiffness, residual pain, and posttraumatic arthritis. An arthrodesis is performed as a pain-relieving operation, although it may not improve the overall sporting function of the patient. If a primary arthrodesis is performed, nonunion, and stress fractures are reported complications. Complex regional pain syndrome is also widely reported. It is therefore necessary that soft tissues be handled as gently as possible during operative treatment.

For a complete list of references, go to ExpertConsult.com.

SELECTED READINGS

Citation:

Gould N, Seligson D, Gassman J. Early and late repair of lateral ligament of the ankle. *Foot Ankle.* 1980;1:84–89.

Level of Evidence:

III

Summary:

In this seminal article on operative treatment of chronic instability, the authors outline a description of a modification of the Broström technique.

Citation:

Hintermann B, Knupp M, Geert IP. Deltoid ligament injuries: diagnosis and management. *Foot Ankle Clin.* 2006;11:625–637.

Level of Evidence:

IV

Summary:

The authors provide an overview of medial ligament injuries, a classification, an algorithm based on the classification, and the results of this algorithm.

Citation:

Rammelt S, Zwipp H, Grass R. Injuries to the distal tibiofibular syndesmosis: an evidence-based approach to acute and chronic lesions. *Foot Ankle Clin.* 2008;13(4):611–633.

Level of Evidence:

IV

Summary:

In this article both acute and chronic injuries are reviewed and the authors' results for treatment of chronic injuries are detailed.

Citation:

Degan TJ, Morrey BF, Braun DP. Fractures of the anterior process of the calcaneus. *J Bone Joint Surg Am.* 1982;64A:519–524.

Level of Evidence:

III

Summary:

The authors classify fractures of the anterior process of the calcaneus, as well as treatment options and outcomes.

Citation:

Myerson MS, Fisher RT, Burgess AR, et al. Fracture dislocations of the tarsometatarsal joints: end results correlated with pathology and treatment. *Foot Ankle.* 1986;6:225–242.

Level of Evidence:

III

Summary:

In this seminal article the authors outline the etiology, classification, treatment algorithm, and outcomes of Lisfranc injuries.

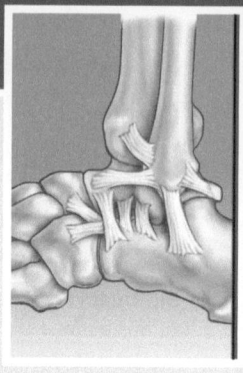

118

Tendon Injuries of the Foot and Ankle

Todd A. Irwin

ANTERIOR TIBIAL TENDON INJURIES

Acute injuries to the anterior tibial tendon are uncommon and are often the result of open injuries or lacerations.[1] Chronic ruptures are decidedly more common, but they usually occur in an older population either as a result of minor trauma or with an insidious onset.

History

Open injuries or lacerations to the anterior ankle should elicit suspicion of an acute injury to the anterior tibial tendon. Often, other structures may be injured concomitantly, including the extensor hallucis longus (EHL), the extensor digitorum longus (EDL), the superficial peroneal nerve, and the anterior neurovascular bundle.[2] Hockey players are at added risk because of the potential for boot-top lacerations from the hockey skate.[3]

Chronic ruptures are frequently missed initially because of the history of minor trauma that results in forced plantar flexion of the foot, sometimes with acute pain and the feeling of a "snap." Once the initial swelling and symptoms resolve, patients may notice a painless mass in the anterior ankle as a result of retraction of the proximal tendon. Often the diagnosis does not become apparent until the patient or a family member notices difficulty with walking or using stairs, a high-stepping gait, or weakness with dorsiflexion. Although chronic ruptures are not typically athletic injuries, several chronic ruptures have been reported after sporting activities such as cross-country skiing and fencing.[4,5] The differential diagnosis should include foot drop as a result of peroneal nerve palsy or L5 radiculopathy.

Physical Examination

In the chronic setting, swelling in the anterior ankle is a common finding. A mass (pseudotumor) may be palpable in the supramalleolar region as a result of retraction of the proximal tendon and is more commonly the presenting complaint in persons with chronic ruptures. Weakness to resisted dorsiflexion is expected but is isolated to the anterior tibialis with normal sensory findings, clearly differentiating this presentation from a radiculopathy or peroneal nerve palsy. High-stepping gait with recruitment of the toe extensors is likely (Fig. 118.1). If the patient has a chronic rupture, secondary claw toe formation may occur as a result of extensor recruitment. Walking on the heels demonstrates loss of dorsiflexion of the affected side.

Imaging

Magnetic resonance imaging (MRI) and dynamic ultrasound are the two most common imaging studies used to confirm the diagnosis. If the clinical situation is obvious based on the history and physical examination, further imaging is not necessary. However, if surgical intervention is planned, these studies may be useful for preoperative planning. Sagittal MRI scans provide the best view of the amount of retraction and subsequent gapping at the rupture site.

Decision-Making Principles

Surgical repair of an acute open injury should be performed. In the chronic setting, the patient's activity and lifestyle should be considered when determining whether operative or nonoperative treatment is appropriate. In a sedentary patient or a patient with multiple medical comorbidities who is a high surgical risk, nonoperative treatment is appropriate. In these patients the need for pain-free ambulation is easily resolved with the use of an ankle-foot orthosis. Patients who lead active lifestyles or refuse to use long-term bracing are best treated with surgical intervention in all cases. Use of age as a criterion is no longer appropriate because it has been clearly documented that older patients do very well with surgical intervention. The presence of a gastrocnemius contracture should be evaluated in all patients, and a gastrocnemius recession should be performed when such a contracture is present to increase range of motion (ROM) and decrease strain on the repair.

Treatment Options

Acute ruptures should be treated with an end-to-end repair. When a laceration is the cause of the rupture, exploration of the wound is important to evaluate and repair concomitant tendon or neurovascular injuries. Timing, location of the rupture, and residual tendon quality are also important considerations. In the subacute setting (i.e., <6 to 8 weeks), primary repair may still be possible, but the surgeon should be prepared to use an autogenous or allogeneic graft if necessary. In the chronic setting, delayed reconstruction is often necessary and is usually achieved with either interpositional grafts or a tendon transfer. Interpositional autograft options include plantaris, EHL, EDL, peroneus tertius, and Achilles tendon.[6] The most common tendon transfer uses the EHL into the medial cuneiform, followed by the EDL.[7,8] Lengthening the anterior tibial tendon utilizing a sliding autograft or half-thickness transposition has also been described.[9,10] When

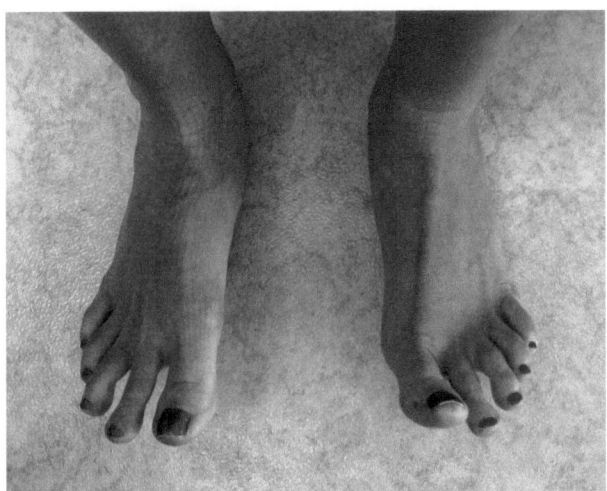

Fig. 118.1 A patient with insertional rupture of the anterior tibial tendon. Note that with attempted dorsiflexion of the ankle, the extensor hallucis longus (EHL) and extensor digitorum longus (EDL) are recruited to allow for ankle dorsiflexion on the left side. The right side is normal and no EHL or EDL recruitment is needed. (From Joos D, Kadakia AR. Extensor tendon disorders. In: Miller MD, Sanders TG, eds. *Presentation, Imaging and Treatment of Common Musculoskeletal Conditions: MRI-Arthroscopy Correlation*. Philadelphia: Elsevier; 2012.)

the rupture occurs at the insertion of the tibialis anterior on the medial cuneiform, direct repair to the medial cuneiform can be achieved with use of suture anchors or an interference screw if the quality of the tendon is good. If the quality of the tendon is poor, tendon transfer or allograft reconstruction is preferred.

Postoperative Management

The patient's ankle is typically immobilized with a splint or cast and the patient is restricted from weight bearing for at least 2 to 4 weeks. For more complex or tenuous repairs, this period of nonweight bearing may be extended to a total of 6 to 12 weeks at the discretion of the surgeon. Patients are typically transitioned to a removable boot at 6 weeks, and weight bearing is started. Gentle ROM may be initiated; however, passive plantar flexion past neutral is avoided until 12 weeks after surgery. At 12 weeks most patients can be weaned from the boot and strengthening can be started. Athletic activities and high-impact activities are avoided for 6 months.

Results

One study showed comparable outcome scores between patients treated operatively and nonoperatively. However, an age bias

---

Author's Preferred Technique

Anterior Tibial Tendon Injury

The incision is centered over the course of the anterior tibial tendon; preoperative MRI or ultrasound may facilitate location of the proximal stump and guide incision length. The incision should be carried proximal to the site of the rupture to visualize the proximal stump. Distally the incision must be carried down to the proximal aspect of the distal stump. Exposure can be achieved through one long incision or two separate proximal and distal incisions to minimize morbidity and preserve the extensor retinaculum, depending on the severity and the ability to visualize the tendon stumps.[11] In cases of insertional rupture, this maneuver requires exposure of the medial cuneiform. Preservation of the superior extensor retinaculum should be attempted to minimize adhesions. Débridement of abnormal and diseased tendon should be performed prior to repair; this presentation is more likely to be seen in the older population. The amount of débridement may be significant enough to preclude end-to-end repair of the tendon, and the surgeon should be prepared to perform a graft reconstruction or tendon transfer in each case.

Intratendinous Rupture

In the setting of an acute intratendinous rupture, the proximal and distal stumps are prepared with a locking whipstitch. My preference is no. 0 nonabsorbable suture. Tension is placed on both the proximal and distal stumps, and the tendon should be apposed at neutral dorsiflexion of the ankle. In cases of late presentation, the proximal stump is contracted and direct apposition may not occur immediately. By placing traction on the proximal stump for 10 to 15 minutes, the muscle can be relaxed and end-to-end repair may be possible, mitigating the need for graft reconstruction. Placing additional suture crossing at the rupture site minimizes gapping of tendon under tension; this reinforcement can be performed with multiple figure-of-8 sutures on the anterior and posterior aspects of the tendon. The tendon should not demonstrate any gapping with intraoperative plantar flexion of the ankle.

Chronic intratendinous ruptures or cases in which débridement has created a tendon gap cannot be repaired with end-to-end fixation. For the reconstruction to be successful, the proximal muscle belly of the anterior tibial tendon must be healthy and viable. Critical aspects of the procedure are exposure of the muscle with release of any scar tissue and ensuring that elasticity is present. If the muscle is fibrotic and nonviable, a tendon transfer should be performed as described later in this chapter. Anterior tibial tendon or hamstring allograft, or hamstring autograft, can be used to bridge the gap in this case.[12] A doubled or quadrupled hamstring graft should be used given the cross-sectional diameter of the normal anterior tibial tendon. Side-to-side tenodesis or placement of the graft through a soft tissue tunnel using the Pulvertaft weave technique within the proximal and distal stump of the tendon can be performed. Fixation to the proximal stump can be performed initially. Distal fixation can be performed either with a side-to-side tenodesis to the distal stump or through bone tunnel fixation into the medial cuneiform if the soft tissue quality of the distal stump is questionable. The use of fluoroscopy in conjunction with a guide wire facilitates placement of the bone tunnel. The ankle should be held in neutral dorsiflexion with maximal tension placed on the proximal limb. Fixation is then completed distally with multiple nonabsorbable sutures (my preference is no. 0) to the distal stump. In the setting of a bone tunnel through the medial cuneiform, an appropriately sized interference screw based on the circumference of the graft can be used, or the graft can be sewn upon itself. The use of a soft tissue button on the plantar aspect of the foot is a useful adjunct to fixation to further decrease the risk of pullout. After fixation, the sheath of the anterior tibial tendon is closed to prevent bowstringing of the reconstruction.

An alternative option to the use of a graft is an EHL transfer to reconstruct the anterior tibial tendon. An additional incision is made distally at the level of the first metatarsophalangeal joint, exposing both the EHL and extensor hallucis brevis. The EHL is affixed by tenodesis to the extensor hallucis brevis with the

Continued

Author's Preferred Technique
Anterior Tibial Tendon Injury—cont'd

interphalangeal (IP) joint held in 20 degrees of dorsiflexion. The EHL is then sectioned immediately proximal to the tenodesis. The EHL is then passed through the medial cuneiform through a bone tunnel, and fixation can be performed with an interference screw or the tendon can be sewn back onto itself. The foot should be held in neutral with maximum tension placed on the tendon. Proximally, the stump of the anterior tibial tendon is secured to the EHL in a side-to-side fashion with moderate tension. Given the decreased power of the EHL relative to the Achilles tendon, an EHL transfer is more successful in the setting of a proximal tenodesis to increase the power that can be generated for dorsiflexion.

In the setting of a completely nonviable proximal anterior tibialis muscle belly, an isolated EHL transfer is unlikely to return full function. In this setting, transfer of the peroneus brevis or the posterior tibial tendon (PTT) may be required to provide sufficient dorsiflexion power.

Insertional Rupture
Insertional ruptures require a different approach relative to intratendinous ruptures. The lack of an adequate distal stump precludes tendon-to-tendon fixation. In these cases, fixation to the medial cuneiform with the aid of suture anchors is the most effective method. To maximize pullout, two suture anchors should be used and placed 45 degrees relative to the line of pull of the tendon, with the tip of the anchor angled proximally. Given the broad insertion of the tendon, one anchor can be placed within the medial cuneiform and the second anchor can be placed within the navicular or proximal aspect of the first metatarsal depending on the anatomy of the tendon and directed from plantar medial to dorsolateral. In the setting of a chronic rupture, use of a graft or an EHL transfer can be performed as previously described (Fig. 118.2).

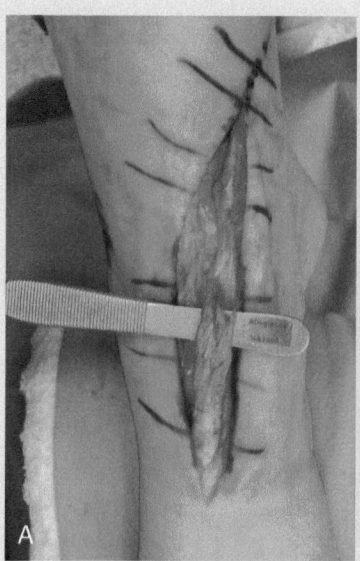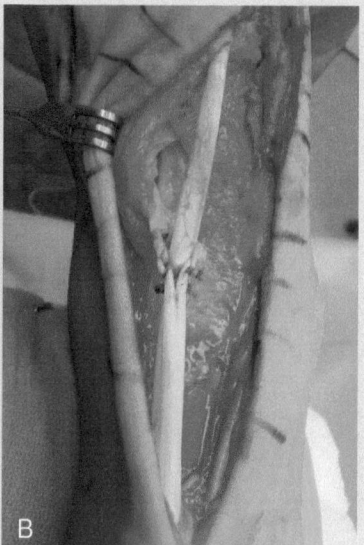

Fig. 118.2 (A) Intraoperative photograph of chronic insertional anterior tibial tendon rupture prior to débridement. (B) After looped semitendinosis allograft reconstruction with insertion into the medial cuneiform and lateral cuneiform.

was present and recognized by the authors, as elderly patients were treated nonoperatively and younger active patients were treated operatively. The authors still recommended surgical repair or reconstruction in younger patients with an active lifestyle.[13] Four recent studies examined the results of surgical repair or reconstruction in both acute and chronic ruptures.[6–8] A total of 56 anterior tibial tendon ruptures were included in the four studies. Seventeen ruptures were repaired primarily and reconstruction was delayed for 39 ruptures, including 12 EHL tendon transfers, 3 EDL tendon transfers, and 24 interposition autogenous grafts. The four studies all showed improved outcome scores and high patient satisfaction. Although dorsiflexion strength was noted to be weaker compared with the nonoperative side, primary repair compared with delayed reconstruction showed no difference in dorsiflexion strength. To decrease the morbidity of autograft harvest or tendon transfer, there is a trend toward the use of interpositional allograft reconstruction as opposed to tendon transfer, especially in those cases with large (>4 cm) gaps. One recent study utilizing primarily anterior tibial tendon and semitendinosis allografts showed this technique to be a safe and

reliable alternative with satisfactory strength, good patient reported outcomes and no allograft-associated complications.[12] The importance of a healthy anterior tibial muscle belly free of fatty infiltration or fibrosis cannot be overstated when utilizing this allograft technique.

Complications
Complications of nonoperative treatment include a flat, pronated foot, decreased ankle motion, and Achilles contracture.[13] Operative complications were rare but included wound dehiscence, tendon adhesion to the extensor retinaculum, superficial peroneal nerve entrapment, and early failure requiring revision of interpositional autograft and tendon transfer operations.[6,12]

POSTERIOR TIBIAL TENDON

Acute injuries to the PTT are relatively uncommon. The most common acute injury is a closed anterior dislocation of the tendon after disruption of the flexor retinaculum of the ankle; many of these injuries occur as a result of sporting activity. Most of the literature available regarding this injury is in the form of case reports, although recent systematic reviews of the literature suggest that these injuries are more prevalent than originally thought.[14,15] Acute PTT ruptures are also relatively rare, although the majority occur in association with ankle fractures.[16,17] Posterior tibial tendinitis is relatively common in the athletic population and is usually associated with either a normal arch or pes planus. When this entity becomes chronic, it is termed *PTT dysfunction* (PTTD) and may ultimately lead to a progressive loss of arch. Johnson and Strom[18] developed the most used classification system for PTTD (also commonly referred to as *adult acquired flatfoot deformity*), and Myerson[19] added a fourth stage. Stage I is described as a tenosynovitis of the PTT without deformity. Stage II refers to tendon dysfunction leading to a flexible flatfoot deformity that is correctable. Stage III is a rigid flatfoot deformity, and stage IV refers to a stage III deformity with associated valgus ankle alignment. In the athletic population, stages I and II are by far the most common and are discussed later in this chapter.

History

Acute dislocations of the PTT usually occur after forced dorsiflexion and inversion of the ankle in the setting of a violent contraction of the posterior tibial muscle. The diagnosis is often missed initially, which leads the patient to report medial ankle pain or possibly a snapping sensation. Patients with tendinitis also report medial ankle pain and swelling that gets worse with activity. In athletes this pain may be debilitating because of the inability to run properly or perform any athletic activity that requires a strong push-off action.[20] The athlete may note worsening pain with elevating on the toes. In the chronic setting of any of the aforementioned entities, patients may report a progressive collapse of the arch with associated valgus position of the heel.

Physical Examination

Tenderness with or without swelling at the medial aspect of the ankle along the course of the PTT is a hallmark of any PTT disease. The tenderness may be primarily in the retromalleolar region, at the insertion of the tendon on the navicular, or along its entire course. In the setting of an acute or chronic dislocation, the tendon may be palpated as a cordlike structure anterior to the posteromedial ridge of the medial malleolus, although this finding is not always present. Resisted inversion of the foot with dorsiflexion or plantar flexion may elicit instability of the tendon, although again this finding is uncommon. A high degree of clinical suspicion is necessary to accurately diagnose acute or chronic PTT dislocation because these pathognomonic findings are variable. Resisted inversion of the foot while the ankle is plantar flexed should be tested. The ability to perform a single-limb heel raise should be tested because this maneuver isolates the PTT and is associated with inversion of the heel (Fig. 118.3). Patients who report medial ankle pain when attempting the single-limb heel raise or who are unable to perform this test should be suspected of having a pathologic condition of the PTT. The presence of an asymmetric pes planus deformity and hindfoot valgus is an indication that chronic PTTD is present. ROM of the hindfoot in inversion and eversion, as well as adduction and abduction of the transverse tarsal joints, should be tested to determine the flexibility of the deformity.

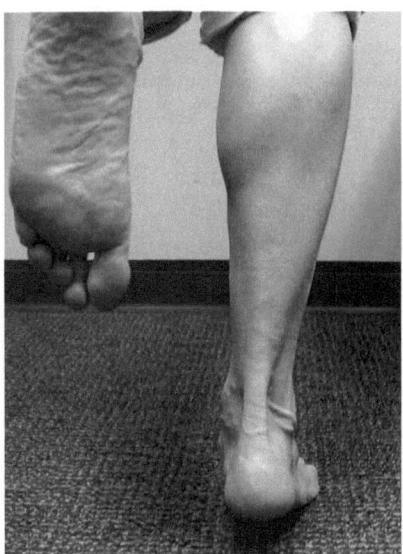

Fig. 118.3 This patient is able to perform a single-limb heel rise, indicating the intact function of the posterior tibial tendon. Patients with stage I disease can perform this test, but it is very painful to do so. (From Joos D, Kadakia AR. Flexor tendon disorders. In: Miller MD, Sanders TG, eds. *Presentation, Imaging and Treatment of Common Musculoskeletal Conditions: MRI-Arthroscopy Correlation.* Philadelphia: Elsevier; 2012.)

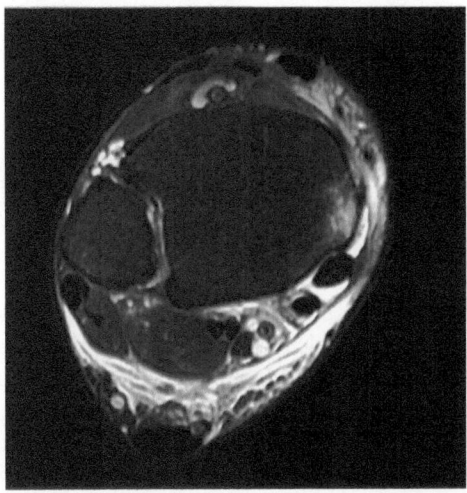

Fig. 118.4 An axial T2-weighted magnetic resonance image of a subacute ankle injury. Note the posteromedial tibial bone edema, fluid within the posterior tibial tendon sheath, and the anterior false pouch where the posterior tibial tendon previously dislocated.

Imaging

Radiographs, MRI, and ultrasound are commonly used to confirm or diagnose pathologic conditions of the PTT. In the setting of PTT dislocation, standard ankle radiographs may show a chip fracture of the medial aspect of the medial malleolus, representing disruption of the flexor retinaculum. Axial MRI scans may show the dislocated PTT sitting anterior to the disrupted flexor retinaculum, as well as the depth of the retromalleolar groove. However, if the tendon is appropriately located, bone edema present in the posteromedial aspect of the medial malleolus may be an indication that an injury occurred to the flexor retinaculum with associated tendon instability (Fig. 118.4). In these cases, dynamic ultrasound can be extremely useful to visualize the subluxation or dislocation of the PTT over the ridge of the medial malleolus. Associated tendon tears and excessive fluid in the tendon sheath can be visualized with either MRI or ultrasound. In the chronic setting, standing foot radiographs may demonstrate a pes planus deformity through an apex plantar lateral talo-first metatarsal angle, plantar gapping at the naviculocuneiform or first tarsometatarsal joint, or increased talonavicular uncoverage on the anteroposterior (AP) view. Hindfoot alignment views can also delineate the extent of hindfoot valgus that is present.[21] Debate exists about whether ultrasound or MRI provides a better evaluation of the extent of PTT disease in the chronic setting.[22,23]

Decision-Making Principles

Early diagnosis of PTT dislocation is difficult, which often leads to late presentation. If clinical suspicion is high and early diagnosis is achieved, it is reasonable to attempt conservative treatment with immobilization as long as the tendon is reliably located in the retromalleolar groove. However, because most cases have a delayed presentation, persistent symptoms are best treated with surgical intervention.

Acute PTT ruptures are most common in association with ankle fractures.[16,17] When an acute rupture is identified during fracture fixation, primary repair should be performed in the same setting.

Posterior tibial tendinitis is almost exclusively treated conservatively initially because most patients, in particular younger patients and athletes, respond to nonoperative treatment. In the patient who does not respond to physical therapy, bracing modalities, and immobilization, surgical intervention is an option.[24]

PTTD is an often-discussed and sometimes controversial topic. Initially, stage I PTTD should be treated conservatively. Most cases abate or resolve, although rarely, surgical intervention is warranted despite no progressive loss of arch. With progressive degeneration and failure of the PTT, ligament failure occurs, leading to the flexible flatfoot deformity described in stage II. The spring (calcaneonavicular) ligament attenuates, leading to the collapse of the talonavicular joint, and the interosseous ligament of the subtalar joint becomes involved, leading to a hindfoot valgus deformity.[25] Initially stage II PTTD should also be treated conservatively, because many patients subjectively and functionally improve.[26] However, if symptoms do not improve, surgical intervention should be considered prior to the development of a rigid deformity. This process can take many years; however, the surgical reconstruction of a rigid deformity (usually a triple arthrodesis) has significantly more morbidity than the joint-sparing procedures used to reconstruct a flexible flatfoot.

Treatment Options

Delayed presentation of a PTT dislocation commonly leads to surgical intervention based on persistent symptoms. The hallmark of surgery is retinaculum repair (if the tissue is amenable to repair) versus reconstruction. If advanced imaging shows evidence of a shallow retromalleolar groove, a groove-deepening procedure should be considered.[14,15,17,27] Evaluation for concomitant injuries, such as a deltoid ligament tear, flexor digitorum longus (FDL) tear, or intra-articular ankle disease, should also be conducted, and these injuries should be addressed if they are identified.

Conservative treatment for posterior tibial tendinitis first involves ankle bracing and physical therapy. If a pes planus deformity is present, orthotics with a longitudinal arch support with medial heel posting may provide some relief. If the pain is moderate to severe with even limited activity, immobilization in a walking boot is appropriate. When conservative treatment fails, surgical options include an open surgical release of the tendon sheath, tendoscopy, and/or possible FDL tendon transfer. Open release of the tendon sheath involves excision of scar tissue, a partial tenosynovectomy, and possibly intratendinous débridement if degenerative lesions are present (Fig. 118.5).[28] Tendoscopy is a less invasive option that has gained in popularity in recent years, and can be utilized both for diagnostic purposes and to perform tenosynovectomy, release of adhesions, and débridement of partial tears.[29–31] If the tendon is excessively degenerated and is deemed to be insufficient, an FDL tendon transfer may be necessary and is the most commonly performed procedure for this problem.[32] In all surgical cases, evaluation for a possible gastrocnemius contracture should be undertaken and surgical release should be performed if such a contracture is present. Additionally, a concomitant medial slide calcaneal osteotomy can be considered in the setting of an FDL transfer despite lack of clinical deformity to prevent late recurrence.

The surgical options for stage II PTTD depend on the extent of the patient's dysfunction, as well as certain specific components of the developed deformity. Many patients with PTTD have a concomitant gastrocnemius contracture, and when such a contracture is present, a gastrocnemius recession should be performed. Second, the PTT should be evaluated and an FDL tendon transfer is performed to reconstruct the dynamic function of the tendon. The extent of PTT disease can vary from a mildly thickened tendon to severe degeneration with longitudinal and

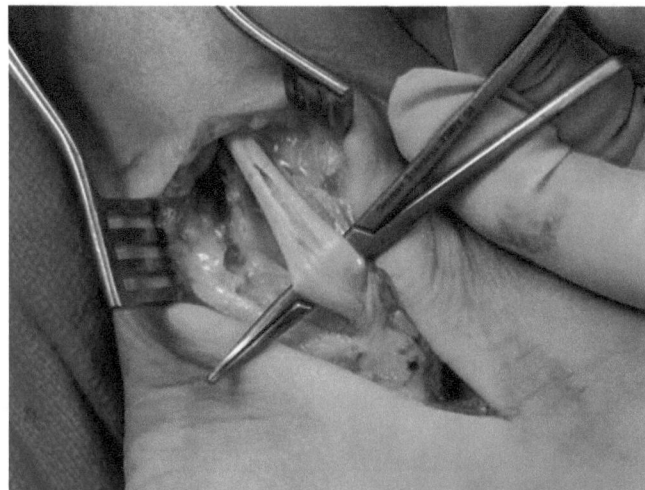

Fig. 118.5 A longitudinal split tear in the posterior tibial tendon can be seen in stage I disease. This tear should be treated with débridement and tubularization of the tendon. If any evidence is seen of hindfoot valgus, excision and tendon transfer with the addition of a calcaneal osteotomy should be considered. (From Joos D, Kadakia AR. Flexor tendon disorders. In: Miller MD, Sanders TG, eds. *Presentation, Imaging and Treatment of Common Musculoskeletal Conditions: MRI-Arthroscopy Correlation.* Philadelphia: Elsevier; 2012.)

sometimes complete ruptures. In the case of moderate to severe degeneration of the tendon, the diseased tendon is resected, leaving the distal stump on the navicular. In the case of mild degeneration of the tendon, some surgeons opt to leave the PTT in place, whereas others choose to excise the tendon regardless of the extent of disease. Either way, an FDL tendon transfer is nearly always performed to augment the function of the damaged tendon. Third, because stage II PTTD implies a hindfoot valgus deformity, a medial displacement calcaneal osteotomy is usually performed to translate the weight-bearing portion of the heel back underneath the mechanical axis of the leg.[33,34] These three procedures account for a high proportion of the surgical treatment options in a patient with stage II PTTD. However, for a more advanced disease process that is not yet rigid, other options

are available. The spring ligament should always be evaluated and either repaired or reconstructed if it is torn or insufficient. With significant forefoot abduction (evidenced by significant talonavicular uncoverage on the AP foot radiograph), a lateral column-lengthening procedure can be performed.[35] Options for lateral column lengthening are either through the anterior process of the calcaneus or through a calcaneocuboid distraction arthrodesis, although most surgeons today prefer to use the anterior process of the calcaneus. With midfoot collapse of either the first tarsometatarsal or naviculocuneiform joint, an associated arthrodesis of the involved joint helps to stabilize the medial column. This procedure also corrects a residual forefoot varus deformity, as does a plantar flexion osteotomy through the medial cuneiform.[36]

Author's Preferred Technique

Posterior Tibial Tendon Injury

Flexor Retinaculum Reconstruction

A curvilinear medial approach just posterior to the medial malleolus is made along the course of the PTT. The PTT and its sheath are evaluated for a possible false pouch anterior to the medial malleolus. A U-shaped flap consisting of retinaculum and medial malleolus periosteum is developed and cut anteriorly so that it is left attached to the posterior portion of the retinaculum. A trough is created at the anterior ridge of the retromalleolar groove using a small burr and is smoothed down with a rasp followed by bone wax. The retinaculum-periosteal flap is then passed into the trough from deep to superficial using intraosseous nonabsorbable sutures that lie posteriorly, minimizing soft tissue irritation. After imbrication of the retinaculum, the tendon should be stably located within the groove through all ROM of the ankle.

Posterior Tibial Tendoscopy

In a supine position without a hip bump, anatomical references including the navicular tuberosity, medial malleolus, and PTT are marked. The first portal is established about 2 cm distal to the medial malleolus along the course of the PTT sheath. A 2.7 mm arthroscope with saline inflow is used with a 30-degree inclination angle. The second portal is established about 2 to 4 cm proximal to the medial malleolus. A third portal can be established about 7 cm proximal to the medial malleolus for visualization of the myotendinous junction if necessary. The second portal typically serves as a working portal for blunt probe and shaver. Diagnostic evaluation is performed, with tenosynovectomy, release of adhesions, and possible tendon débridement as needed (Fig. 118.6).[29–31]

Posterior Tibial Tenosynovectomy and Débridement

The tendon is approached as previously described, the PTT sheath is incised, and the tendon is evaluated. Diseased synovium is excised, with the incision extended as needed to ensure adequate débridement. Degenerative portions of the tendon are identified by the thickened and amorphous appearance (smooth with a lack of striations). The diseased portion is incised longitudinally, the nonviable portion is excised, and the longitudinal rent is repaired with running 3-0 Prolene sutures. Care is taken to avoid creating a full-thickness disruption of the tendon, resulting in discontinuity. The tendon sheath is then closed to prevent subluxation. If more than 50% of the tendon has been débrided, a concomitant FDL tendon transfer is indicated.

Flexor Digitorum Longus Tendon Transfer

The same approach to the PTT is used, extending it distal along the medial border of the foot. In these cases, the severity of tendon degeneration does not allow

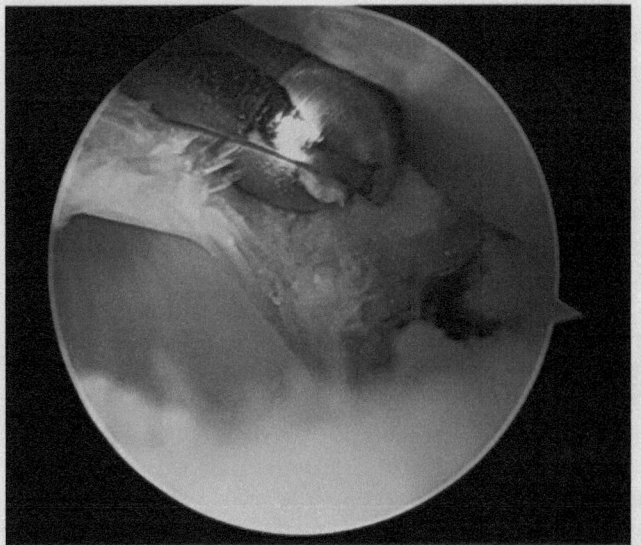

Fig. 118.6 View of posterior tibial tendoscopy showing débridement of tenosynovitis using arthroscopic shaver, with fibrotic band around the tendon.

for repair and therefore it is resected, leaving a 1-cm stump on the navicular tuberosity for fixation. Securing the tendon to this distal stump theoretically allows the FDL to restore the stabilizing effect to the plantar midfoot through the multiple distal connections of the PTT. Isolated reconstruction to the navicular does not allow for restoration of this critical function of the PTT. The FDL tendon sheath is incised in the floor of the PTT sheath, inferior to the medial malleolus, and opened to a point 2 to 3 cm distal to the navicular tuberosity. The FDL tendon is dissected from its attachments to the flexor hallucis longus (FHL; master knot of Henry) and transversely cut as far distal as possible. Distal tenodesis can be performed at this point to help restore the function of the FDL; however, given the lack of gait disturbance, it is not required and is not routinely performed in my practice. A more proximal transection of the FDL, proximal to the knot of Henry, preserves the interconnections between the FDL and FHL but results in less tendon length for reconstruction. A 4.5-mm drill hole is created in the medial navicular tuberosity from dorsal to plantar, using fluoroscopy as a guide for placement of the hole. While holding the foot in 20 degrees of inversion and 20

Author's Preferred Technique

Posterior Tibial Tendon Injury—cont'd

degrees of plantar flexion, the FDL is delivered through the drill hole from plantar to dorsal, an appropriately sized interference screw is placed typically from dorsal to plantar, and any residual tendon is sutured to surrounding periosteum and the PTT stump using size 0 nonabsorbable suture. Tensioning is critical and the foot should not be able to evert past neutral after repair. Alternatively, especially in the setting of a short segment of FDL, the tendon can be sutured directly to the stump of the PTT or fixed to the navicular with dual suture anchors. No clinical superiority of fixation has been demonstrated.

Medial Displacement Calcaneal Osteotomy

To perform a medial displacement calcaneal osteotomy, make an incision posterior and inferior to the course of the peroneal tendons along the lateral hindfoot at 45 degrees to the plantar border of the foot. Dissect through subcutaneous tissues while avoiding sural nerve branches. Sharply incise through periosteum along the line of the incision and elevate 2 to 3 mm of periosteum dorsally and plantarly.

Check the position of the planned osteotomy by inserting a small Kirschner (K) wire or saw blade and assessing the position under fluoroscopy with a lateral and axial heel alignment view. Adjust as needed and perform the osteotomy using a larger saw blade, being careful to just perforate the far cortex to avoid injury to medial neurovascular structures; alternatively, the medial cortex can be perforated with an osteotome. Mobilize the posterior fragment using a wide osteotome or elevator, taking care not to crush the soft cancellous bone. Use of a wide elevator can minimize this complication. Translate the posterior tuberosity medially from 8 to 10 mm. Place one 6.5-mm partially threaded cannulated screw and check its position using lateral and axial fluoroscopy. Given the medial translation, the screw should be inserted relatively lateral on the tuberosity so that it remains with the distal calcaneus. Plates have also been developed for fixation, but given the low cost of the implant and high clinical success rate of screw fixation, they are not routinely used in my practice. Minimally invasive techniques have also recently been described and are gaining in popularity.[37]

Postoperative Management

Patients who have undergone a flexor retinaculum reconstruction have a splint placed postoperatively and are instructed not to bear weight. After 2 weeks, a short leg cast or walking boot is applied and weight bearing is initiated. Six weeks after surgery an ankle lace-up brace is applied and ROM is initiated and progresses over the next 6 weeks. Physical therapy can be started for ROM and strengthening.

For patients undergoing posterior tibial tendoscopy, early motion is important. Patients can either be placed in short leg splint for 7 to 10 days or into a weight-bearing tall boot immediately. Early ROM exercises are initiated including active inversion and eversion, depending on the severity of the tendon disease seen intraoperatively. Patients are transitioned into an ankle lace-up brace at 4 to 6 weeks postoperatively, with consideration for formal physical therapy.

Patients who have undergone a tenosynovectomy for posterior tibial tendonitis are treated initially with a splint for the first 2 weeks, followed by the use of a removable walking boot for 4 weeks. Early ROM exercises are initiated and physical therapy can be considered, especially in athletes who are trying to return to play. At 6 weeks an ankle lace-up brace is worn, and full activity is allowed at between 6 and 8 weeks. For each of the aforementioned procedures, full return to sporting activity is variable but is expected at around 3 to 4 months after surgery. Use of an over-the-counter full-length arch support is encouraged to minimize recurrence.

Reconstructions for flatfoot deformity entail a longer recovery period. Patients wear a splint for the initial 2 weeks with the foot in an inverted and plantar-flexed position. A short-leg non-weight-bearing cast or controlled ankle motion boot is then used for 4 weeks, followed by weight bearing in a tall walking boot for 4 to 6 weeks. Physical therapy can be initiated about 8 to 10 weeks after surgery with an emphasis on inversion strengthening, with concomitant use of a lace-up ankle brace for a further 3 months. Sporting activity usually cannot be resumed until about 6 to 9 months postoperatively with the use of an over-the-counter orthotic to minimize stress on the reconstruction.

Results

Lohrer and Nauck[14] performed a systematic review of the literature regarding PTT dislocations and noted a higher prevalence than originally thought. Nearly 60% of the injuries were induced by sport. Of the 61 cases reported, only 10 were treated conservatively. Surgical treatment included a variety of retinaculum reconstruction techniques, direct suture repair, and retromalleolar groove deepening combined with reconstruction or repair. Results were rated as excellent in 80%, good in 13%, and fair in 7%. No comparison between surgical and conservative treatment could be performed.[14]

Most of the studies evaluating posterior tibial tendoscopy report good results with low complication rates, albeit with relatively low patient numbers.[29–31,38] One study showed good results when treating pathologic vincula and synovitis associated with rheumatoid arthritis, but release of adhesions was less successful.[38] The most recent study showed significant improvement in functional outcome scores and a potential improvement in diagnostic accuracy compared to MRI.[31] Further studies are needed, but tendoscopy is a promising tool that allows for fewer wound problems, less morbidity, and earlier mobilization and recovery compared to open procedures.

Tenosynovectomy for posterior tibial tendinitis has generally good results. McCormack et al.[24] published a series on tenosynovectomy in young competitive athletes. Twenty-two months after surgery, seven of eight patients had returned to full sports participation without difficulty. Teasdall and Johnson[39] reported results on 19 patients treated with synovectomy and débridement for stage I PTTD. Complete relief was reported by 74% of patients, whereas 16% had minor pain, 5% had moderate pain, and 5% had severe pain. Only 10% required conversion to a subtalar arthrodesis for progressive deformity and pain.

As the treatment of PTTD has evolved, so have the reported results in the literature. Alvarez et al.[26] reported the result of a structured nonoperative management protocol for stage I and stage II PTTD involving the use of a short-articulating ankle-foot orthotic and an aggressive physical therapy protocol including a home program.[26] Their patients had successful subjective and functional outcomes 83% of the time, whereas only 11% did not respond to conservative treatment and required surgery. Surgical intervention has also been shown to be beneficial in patients who do not respond to nonoperative treatment. Combining FDL transfer with a medial displacement calcaneal osteotomy has been shown to restore functional inversion and provide excellent pain relief and patient satisfaction, with variable radiographic and patient-perceived arch correction.[33,34]

Complications

The most common complication of PTT dislocation is missed diagnosis leading to delayed presentation, because 53% of patients in a systematic review were initially misdiagnosed.[14] Low complication rates are reported for posterior tibial tendoscopy, with the most common being persistent pain as indications are still being evaluated.[30] Tenosynovectomy for posterior tibial tendonitis is well tolerated with few reported complications, although if the tendon dysfunction is more chronic than originally thought, progression of the deformity may require further surgical intervention. Complications of PTTD correction include undercorrection with persistent pain, overcorrection resulting in varus hindfoot, and rarely, neurovascular injury either at the calcaneal osteotomy site or the FDL harvest site.[34]

Future Considerations

The treatment of PTT injuries and dysfunction will likely continue to evolve. Tendoscopy techniques offer promise as appropriate indications are determined and instrumentation is improved. The importance of the spring ligament in both acute injuries and chronic PTTD has been demonstrated.[25,40] Determining which patients will benefit from spring ligament repair or reconstruction and what effect this will have on the overall treatment algorithm is an area of current research. Novel rehabilitation protocols and early diagnosis may also lead to improved outcomes and more refined surgical protocols.

FLEXOR HALLUCIS LONGUS INJURIES

Although lacerations to the FHL tendon have been reported, the most common pathology related to the FHL is tenosynovitis.[41,42] The FHL arises from the posterior aspect of the fibula and interosseous membrane. It then courses distally through a fibro-osseous tunnel posterior to the ankle joint, crosses deep to the FDL at the master knot of Henry in the midfoot and between the sesamoid bones in the forefoot, and inserts onto the base of the distal phalanx of the hallux. Symptoms can occur anywhere along this course, although the most common presenting complaint is posterior to the ankle. Both athletes and non-athletes may report symptoms consistent with FHL tenosynovitis, although the highest prevalence is seen in classical ballet dancers.[42–44] Stenosing tenosynovitis is a related clinical entity that is discussed. Posterior impingement of the ankle, often as a result of a large os trigonum, is commonly seen in association with FHL tenosynovitis and is often treated concurrently.[45]

History

The most common presenting complaint is pain in the posteromedial ankle that is worsened with activity. Chronic repetitive plantar-flexion activities such as en pointe dancing tend to exacerbate the symptoms. Triggering of the hallux may also be present in patients in whom a stenosing tenosynovitis has developed.[46,47] Triggering occurs as a result of a bulbous thickening of the FHL that causes the hallux to lock as the FHL attempts to pass through the fibro-osseous tunnel with plantar flexion or dorsiflexion of the ankle. Patients may also report limited dorsiflexion of the hallux, again as a result of stenosis at the proximal level of the fibro-osseous tunnel. Other less common complaints include pain medial and deep to the medial band of the plantar fascia in the midfoot and pain plantar to the first metatarsal.

Physical Examination

Pain associated with extreme plantar flexion of the ankle is the first indication that a pathologic condition is present posterior to the ankle. Although this pain may be an indication of posterior impingement, further examination is required to isolate the FHL. Pain with resisted plantar flexion of the hallux is the hallmark of FHL tenosynovitis. Symptoms may worsen with dorsiflexion of the ankle as the musculotendinous junction is delivered into the fibro-osseous tunnel. Swelling may be present in the posteromedial ankle, and tenderness and crepitus may be present with palpation of the FHL while moving the hallux. The Tomassen sign is the finding of decreased passive dorsiflexion of the hallux with the ankle in neutral dorsiflexion, which is improved with plantar flexion of the ankle.[48] However, upon forcible active contraction of the FHL, a snap or pop is noted in the posterior medial region of the ankle, and the patient is then unable to extend the IP or metatarsophalangeal joints of the great toe. Subsequent passive extension of the IP joint produces a painless snap or pop posterior to the medial malleolus with subsequent freeing of motion in the great toe.

The master knot of Henry is another potential area where the FHL can be symptomatic. Deep palpation just medial to the medial border of the plantar fascia that worsens with moving of the great toe can elicit pain. Pain with palpation of the plantar aspect of the first metatarsal, between the sesamoids and with motion of the great toe, can indicate distal entrapment of the FHL.

Imaging

The findings of standard foot and ankle radiographs are often normal, although lateral ankle radiographs may demonstrate an os trigonum or prominent posterior talar process. If suspicion of posterior impingement or FHL tenosynovitis is high, or for confirmation of the diagnosis, an MRI scan is often performed. In one study, 82% of patients suspected of FHL tenosynovitis had positive MRI findings in the form of excessive fluid in the FHL tendon sheath posterior to the ankle (Fig. 118.7).[44] Ultrasound has also gained in popularity and can dynamically visualize the FHL, which may be helpful in confirming a stenosing tenosynovitis or in guiding an injection.[49]

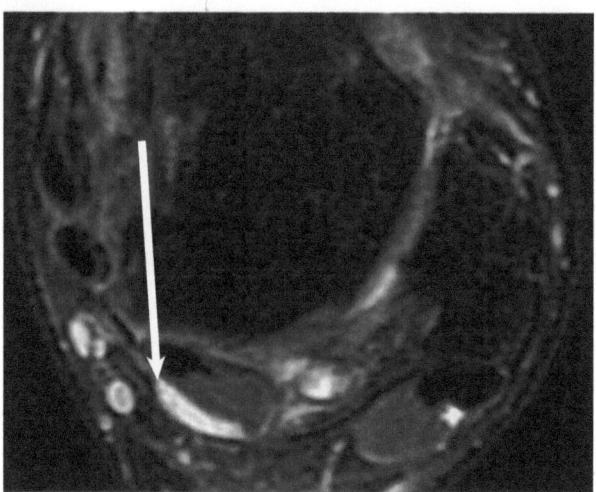

Fig. 118.7 An axial T2-weighted image with high signal intensity *(white arrow)* adjacent to the flexor hallucis longus at the posterior aspect of the talus. (From Joos D, Kadakia AR. Flexor tendon disorders. In: Miller MD, Sanders TG, eds. *Presentation, Imaging and Treatment of Common Musculoskeletal Conditions: MRI-Arthroscopy Correlation.* Philadelphia: Elsevier; 2012.)

Decision-Making Principles

Conservative treatment is the appropriate initial step in the management of both FHL tenosynovitis and stenosing tenosynovitis. If conservative treatment fails, symptoms have been present for longer than 3 months without relief, or the patient is a high-level athlete or performer who is unable to execute the desired activities, surgical intervention can be considered. It is important to determine the presence of posterior impingement, FHL tenosynovitis, or both, because this information may help to determine the appropriate approach and intervention. Some authors argue that the presence of triggering is an indication for earlier operative intervention.[50,51] Interestingly, Hamilton et al.[42] have reported the potential morbidity related to surgical intervention in the dancer population, both medically and professionally. They noted the competitive environment and stigma associated with having an injury as reasons professional dancers may elect to not have surgery, as well as reasons why amateur dancers may have been prevented from having a professional

career. For this reason, understanding the patient's social situation is exceedingly important during a discussion of treatment options in this patient population.

Treatment Options

The initial treatment for FHL tenosynovitis should include formal physical therapy including an FHL-specific stretching program, as well as the use of antiinflammatory medication. Trial periods of bracing or boot immobilization are used if the pain is significant. Activity modification should also be instituted, in particular avoiding repetitive plantar-flexion activities such as dancing en pointe.

When conservative treatment fails, surgical intervention is an option. The great majority of patients who require surgical intervention have posterior ankle symptoms, although release of the FHL at the knot of Henry and between the sesamoids has been described.[44] Surgical techniques that have been described include addressing the FHL tenosynovitis alone or in combination with a suspected posterior impingement.[42,45,52] The treatment of choice for FHL tenosynovitis is release of the tendon sheath. In the case of stenosing tenosynovitis and triggering, the integrity of the tendon should be evaluated, and if tears or nodules are present, they are addressed with repair or débridement. The traditional surgical approach is through a medial approach to mobilize the neurovascular bundle, although posterolateral and posteromedial approaches have also been described.[42,44] If posterior impingement alone is being addressed, a straight posterolateral approach can be used to débride the impingement and remove the os trigonum if it is present. Access to the FHL fibro-osseous tunnel may be difficult, although by making the incision just lateral to the Achilles tendon and dissecting anterior to it, this difficulty may be minimized. Incising just medial to the Achilles tendon is another option to address both clinical problems and also minimizes manipulation and exposure of the tibial nerve.

Alternatively, posterior hindfoot endoscopy techniques have evolved and significantly increased in popularity in the past decade.[53–57] While many of these procedures are performed for posterior ankle impingement, with or without clinical evidence of FHL tenosynovitis, FHL pathology can be definitively treated with this technique.[55,57] If extensive débridement or repair of the FHL is required, conversion to an open procedure may be necessary.

 Author's Preferred Technique
Posterior Hindfoot Arthroscopy

The patient is placed in the prone position, with the foot placed on two blankets slightly past the edge of the bed. Instruments required include a 4.0-mm arthroscope with 30-degree angle, 4.0- to 5.5-mm shavers, as well as arthroscopic curettes, periosteal elevators and osteotomes. Twenty milliliters of normal saline solution is injected into the posterior ankle starting just lateral to the Achilles tendon. A lateral portal is created just lateral to the Achilles tendon, slightly superior to the level of the tip of the fibula. Dissection is performed with a straight hemostat, being careful to direct the dissection straight anteriorly. The 4.0-mm arthroscope is introduced, aiming straight anterior or towards the second toe. The medial portal is made just medial to the Achilles tendon, at the same level, and dissecting slightly lateral toward the arthroscope tip. A 5.5-mm shaver is introduced and soft tissue débridement is performed. It is very important to

stay lateral until visualization is improved with insufflation of the fluid to avoid iatrogenic damage to the neurovascular bundle. Continue débridement medially until the FHL tendon is visualized (Fig. 118.8). The neurovascular bundle should be protected as long as the dissection stays lateral to the FHL. Use a combination of the shaver, curette, periosteal elevator, grasper, and possibly the osteotome to remove the os trigonum or posterior talar process if it is deemed an inciting factor. Flex and extend the great toe to evaluate the FHL along its course. The arthroscope can be advanced relatively far distally into the fibro-osseous tunnel for further visualization. A shaver and biter can be used to débride the tendon and release the FHL tendon sheath. Conversion to an open posteromedial approach may be necessary if further débridement or repair of the FHL is necessary or if the sheath is unable to be adequately released.

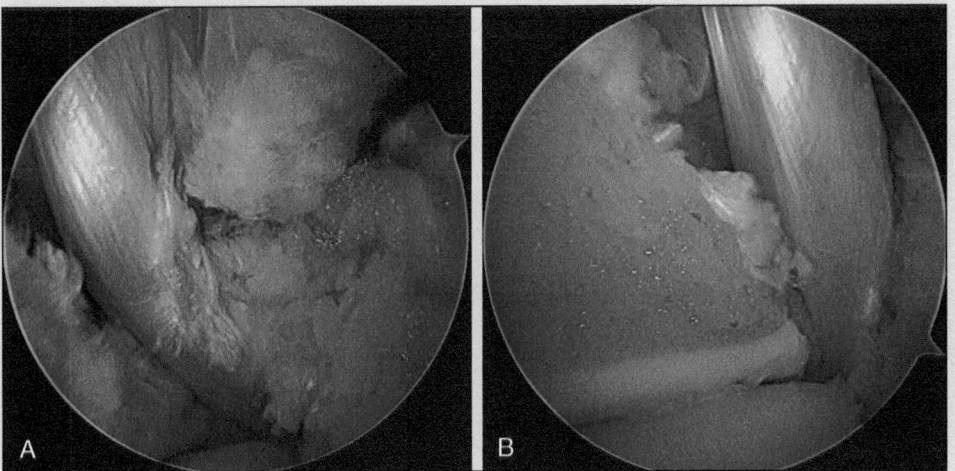

Fig. 118.8 (A) Posterior arthroscopic view of the flexor hallucis longus (FHL) tendon with incomplete longitudinal tear and surrounding synovitis. (B) A view of the FHL after débridement of the surrounding synovitis and excision of impinging posterior talar process (note the fresh cancellous bone).

Postoperative Management

After posterior hindfoot endoscopy, most patients are placed in a tall CAM walking boot with partial to full weight bearing for the first 2 weeks. Early ankle, subtalar, and great toe ROM is initiated and encouraged.[53,56] Transition to regular shoe wear with an ankle lace-up type brace as needed occurs at 2 to 4 weeks postoperatively. For open procedures, it is reasonable to immobilize the ankle for 2 weeks to allow for wound healing, followed by a short course of boot immobilization for 2 to 4 weeks. Early ROM is initiated when the wounds have healed.

Return to sporting activities averages approximately 3 to 6 months. A formal physical therapy program can be initiated at 2 weeks postoperatively and may help shorten this time.[58] For dancers, achieving the en pointe position can be critical and may take a prolonged period depending on the severity of the preoperative condition. While debatable, more recent studies indicate the endoscopic approach allows a shorter return to previous level of sporting activity compared to open procedures.[52–54,56]

Results

Successful outcomes using nonoperative treatment alone have been reported to be as high as 64%.[44] The most common treatment used was an FHL-stretching regimen, in particular in patients with evidence of entrapment at the posteromedial ankle or limited dorsiflexion of the hallux.

Surgical outcomes have been promising in the more recent literature. In the series by Hamilton et al.[42] 28 of 34 professional dancers had good or excellent results after an open procedure, whereas only 2 of 6 amateur dancers had equally successful outcomes. Kolettis et al.[50] reported that 11 of 13 ballet dancers were able to return to full dancing participation without restrictions after 5 months after an open medial release of the FHL. Marotta

and Micheli[45] reported the results of 12 ballet dancers (15 ankles) who underwent excision of the os trigonum, through a lateral approach, for treatment of posterior impingement. At follow-up, 2 years after surgery, 8 (67%) still had occasional discomfort, but all 12 dancers returned to unrestricted dance activity.[45] In the review by Michelson and Dunn,[44] only 23 of the 81 patients with FHL tenosynovitis required surgical intervention, although each surgical outcome was deemed successful. Patients had significant subjective improvement after 6 weeks.[44] Similar good results have been seen after posterior hindfoot arthroscopy. Scholten et al.[53] reported an increase in the American Orthopaedic Foot and Ankle (AOFAS) hindfoot score from 75 to 90 at 3-year follow-up, although they did note that the patients with overuse injuries were more satisfied than were the patients with post-traumatic injuries. Willits et al.[54] reported a postoperative AOFAS hindfoot scale score of 91 in 15 patients (16 ankles). At an average 5.8 months, 14 of 15 patients were able to return to their pre-injury level of athletics, while the average return to work was 1 month. Smyth et al. reported similar improvement in functional outcome scores, while all 19 patients who competed in sports were able to return to their previous level of competition at mean 12 weeks.[56] Interestingly, only 5 out of 15 patients in the Willits et al. study had FHL tenolysis performed, while all 22 patients in the Smyth et al. study had evidence of FHL tenosynovitis with subsequent FHL arthroscopic tenosynovectomy as part of the procedure.[54,56]

Complications

Typical postoperative complications such as wound healing problems and minor infections have been reported, although at low rates. Complications specific to an open approach for FHL tenosynovectomy include scar dysesthesias and rare transient nerve neuropraxias.[42,45] The largest retrospective review of posterior hindfoot arthroscopy procedures showed an 8.5%

complication rate, including 2% with plantar numbness, 1.6% with sural nerve dysesthesias, and 2% with Achilles tendon tightness.[59]

Future Considerations

Higher clinical suspicion in the nondancer population should lead to increased awareness and earlier diagnosis. In one study evaluating arthroscopic FHL release and tenosynovectomy, none of the 27 patients were professional athletes or ballet dancers, 18 were worker's compensation cases, and all related their symptoms to an ankle sprain.[55] The development of more refined therapy protocols and further outcome studies may help decrease the need for surgical intervention. There is a definite trend toward treating FHL pathology arthroscopically, which will likely continue with continued improvement in instrumentation and techniques. Further studies will need to confirm shorter return to work/play and rehabilitation time.

PERONEAL TENDON INJURIES

Peroneal tendon injuries are a common and increasingly recognized diagnosis, especially in the athletic population. Persistent lateral ankle symptoms after an ankle "sprain" should elicit suspicion of a peroneal tendon injury. Although most patients present with chronic injuries, acute tears of the peroneus brevis and less commonly the peroneus longus do occur. Peroneal subluxation or dislocation is another clinical entity that may be recognized acutely or chronically, and is often associated with peroneal tendon tears. Disruption of the superior peroneal retinaculum (SPR), usually as a result of a forced contraction of the peroneals in a dorsiflexed position, can lead to peroneal instability. Chronic instability of the tendons can then lead to peroneal tendon tears, often of the peroneus brevis as it rubs over the posterolateral ridge of the fibula.[60] Finally, snapping of the tendons without evidence of subluxation or dislocation indicates an intrasheath peroneal subluxation.[61]

History

Patients with acute tears of the peroneal tendons may report a sharp pain and acute "pop" at the lateral aspect of the ankle. However, most patients present several weeks or months after an acute injury and report lateral ankle pain or discomfort that worsens with activity. The pain may radiate proximally along the lateral aspect of the leg and may be associated with a snapping or popping sensation. Repeated episodes of ankle instability should raise suspicion of peroneal tendon involvement. Forced dorsiflexion of the ankle, such as when skiers quickly decelerate and stop, should alert the examiner to a subluxation or dislocation episode.[62,63] An accurate history can be extremely helpful in determining the true nature of the peroneal pathology.

Physical Examination

Swelling along the peroneal tendons in the posterolateral ankle, as well as distal and anterior to the tip of the fibula, is a consistent finding in persons with peroneal tendon disease. Tenderness to palpation along the retrofibular groove—or distally along the cuboid groove in the case of the peroneus longus—may indicate peroneal tendon tearing. Eversion and external rotation strength should be tested both from a contracted and lengthened position. Complete peroneal tendon ruptures are uncommon; most tearing occurs in a longitudinal fashion. Therefore peroneal tendon strength is often intact, although resisted contraction of either the peroneus brevis or longus may elicit pain. Pain with resisted eversion of the foot can indicate either peroneus brevis or longus involvement, although pain with resisted plantar flexion of the first ray (counterpressure at the plantar aspect of the first metatarsal head) indicates peroneus longus involvement. To evaluate for peroneal instability, resisted dorsiflexion and eversion should be tested while gently palpating the fibular ridge and feeling for tendon subluxation (Fig. 118.9).[64] Repeated circumduction of the foot can also elicit peroneal instability. If a palpable snapping or clicking of the tendons occurs with

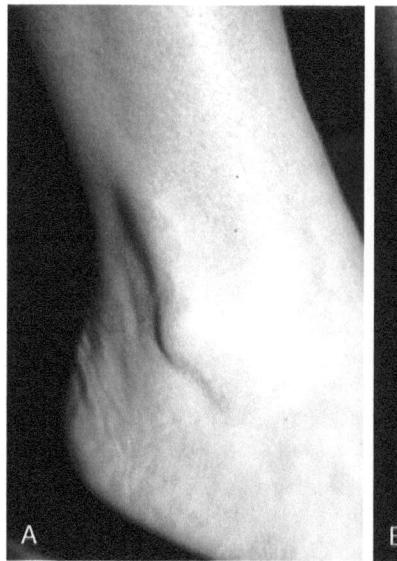 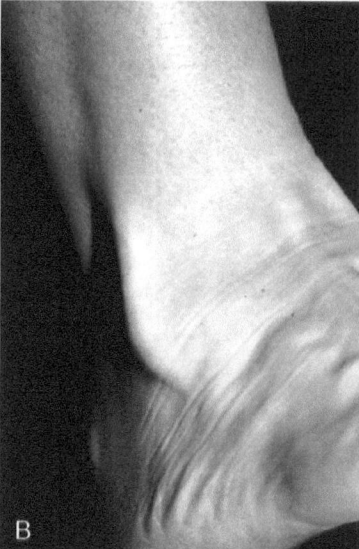

Fig. 118.9 (A) Normal appearing peroneal tendons in the retromalleolar groove. (B) Dislocation of the peroneal tendons with dorsiflexion and eversion.

circumduction, but without evidence of subluxation or dislocation over the ridge of the fibula, intrasheath subluxation may be present. Finally, hindfoot and forefoot alignment should always be checked during examination while the patient is standing. The presence of cavovarus alignment increases the risk of peroneal tendinopathy and/or instability. A Coleman block test should be performed to determine if the varus hindfoot is the result of a plantar-flexed first ray alone or if it occurs in combination with a fixed varus heel deformity.[65]

Imaging

Standing foot and ankle radiographs should be performed as an initial assessment. Evidence of a hypertrophied peroneal tubercle may be a source of peroneal disease. The presence of an os peroneum, an accessory bone located just lateral to the cuboid and seen best on the oblique foot radiograph, is present in 10% to 20% of persons and is completely enveloped by the peroneus longus tendon.[66] An elongated or fractured os peroneum may indicate either chronic or acute disruption of the peroneus longus, respectively. A chip fracture identified just lateral to the lateral malleolus is an indication of an avulsion of the SPR and is likely associated with peroneal subluxation or dislocation.[67]

Advanced imaging most commonly involves either ultrasound or MRI. The advantages of ultrasound are not only that it is a noninvasive and inexpensive method, but that it allows dynamic evaluation of the peroneal tendons throughout their ROM and with provocative maneuvers. Sensitivity, specificity, and accuracy of ultrasound in diagnosing peroneal tendon tears has been shown to be 100%, 85%, and 90%, respectively.[68] Comparison with the unaffected side is another advantage.

MRI is likely the most common modality ordered for suspected peroneal disease, especially considering the propensity for ordering MRIs in the primary care population. Axial images provide the best cut for peroneal evaluation proximal to the inferior tip of the fibula.[69] Torn tendons may appear thickened or nodular or they may have increased intrasubstance signaling, and excessive fluid within the tendon sheath usually indicates peroneal tendon disease (Fig. 118.10). The specificity of MRI to diagnose peroneus brevis tears, longus tears, or both has been shown to be 80%, 100%, and 60%, respectively.[70] Another study reported the sensitivity, specificity, and positive predictive value of MRI to diagnose peroneal tendon pathology was 90%, 72%, and 76%, respectively, as confirmed by tendoscopy.[71] However, both false-positive and false-negative results have been reported with one study showing peroneal tendon pathology in 35% of asymptomatic patients.[72,73] Diagnosis and decisions about management should be made primarily by the history and physical examination, with advanced imaging used for confirmation or in unclear cases.

Decision-Making Principles

Because acute peroneal tendon tears (or at least the recognition of them) are relatively uncommon, primary repair of the tendon tear is not always necessary unless it is diagnosed in a high-level athlete. Conservative treatment can almost always be tried initially, and decisions for surgical management can be made on the basis of the response to treatment. Peroneal tendinitis is

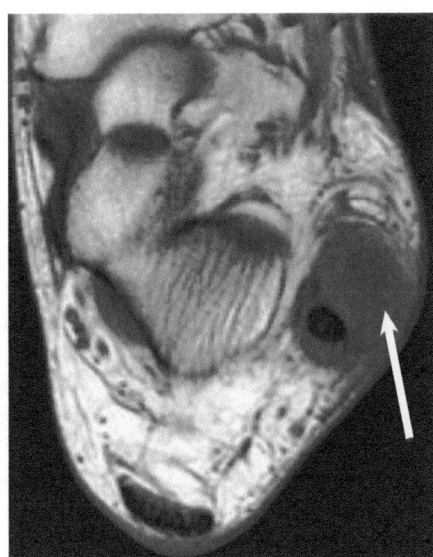

Fig. 118.10 A T1-weighted axial magnetic resonance image with intermediate signal intensity in the location of the peroneus brevis *(arrow)*. This was noted on multiple axial images, consistent with severe tendinosis of the peroneus brevis. Obvious thickening of the tendon is also noted. The normal peroneus longus is noted posterior to the pathologic brevis. (From Joos D, Kadakia AR. Peroneal tendon disorders. In: Miller MD, Sanders TG, eds. *Presentation, Imaging and Treatment of Common Musculoskeletal Conditions: MRI-Arthroscopy Correlation.* Philadelphia: Elsevier; 2012.)

almost always managed well with conservative treatment. Even mild degenerative tears of the peroneal tendons often respond to conservative treatment. Hindfoot alignment is important to consider because a simple orthotic may add significant benefit to the treatment protocol.

Peroneal tendon tears that are recalcitrant to conservative treatment likely benefit from surgical intervention. The extent and location of the tear are important determining factors with regard to the appropriate surgical option. Krause and Brodsky[60] based the method of surgical treatment on the cross-sectional area of tendon involvement. If 50% or more of the tendon remained after débridement of the damaged portion (grade I tear), they repaired the tendon. If less than 50% remained (grade II), proximal and distal tenodesis of the peroneus brevis tendon to the longus tendon was performed.[60] This rule is a good general guideline, although often multiple splits are present and the decision must be individualized. Peroneus brevis tears usually occur around the retrofibular groove. When a concomitant SPR disruption is present, reconstruction or repair of the SPR should be performed. Distal peroneus brevis tears are significantly less common. If the patient does not respond to conservative treatment, surgical débridement with reattachment to the base of the fifth metatarsal may be required.[74] Peroneus longus tendon tears occur less often than do brevis tears and are more likely distal to the tip of the fibula either at the peroneal tubercle or in the cuboid notch. In addition, in one study, 82% of peroneus longus tendon tears were associated with a cavovarus hindfoot position.[75] A similar approach to tendon débridement and/or repair can be used for the peroneus longus, although complete ruptures may be seen through the os peroneum or just distal or proximal to the os. In these cases, if direct repair is not possible, transfer into the cuboid is an option.[74] Tears seen in both the peroneus longus and peroneus brevis concomitantly are even less common, although they present a challenge when they are seen.[72]

Acute or chronic dislocating peroneal tendons, especially in the athletic population, should be treated surgically. Conservative treatment of dislocating tendons, either acute or chronic, has generally shown poor results.[76–79] The depth of the fibular groove has been recognized as a potential contributing factor to peroneal tendon instability, and fibular groove deepening is a common procedure to address flat or convex fibular grooves in the setting of peroneal instability.[80–82] However, one recent study demonstrated no significant difference in shape of the groove based on MRI in patients with and without peroneal dislocation.[83] If chronic ankle instability is present, a lateral ankle ligament reconstruction also should be performed.[84] In the presence of a varus hindfoot or cavovarus deformity, cavovarus reconstruction should be considered.[65] Finally, when a low-lying peroneus brevis muscle belly or peroneus quartus is identified, appropriate débridement should be performed.[85,86]

Treatment Options

Conservative treatment includes the use of nonsteroidal antiinflammatory drugs; physical therapy focusing on ROM, peroneal strengthening, and proprioception; bracing with an ankle lace-up-type brace; or sometimes boot immobilization if symptoms are acute or severe.[74] In patients with a varus heel or cavovarus deformity, a simple lateral heel wedge or custom orthotic with lateral heel posting and a depressed first ray can be effective.

Surgical management of peroneal tendon tears most commonly involves open exploration of the tendon to determine the extent of tearing. When tenosynovitis is encountered, it should be débrided. As mentioned earlier, the tear can be débrided alone, débrided and repaired, or in severe cases, attached by tenodesis to the intact tendon (Fig. 118.11). In severe cases, the author has used the concept of "restoring at least one functioning tendon" via tenodesis of any remaining viable tendon. In the athlete, every attempt should be made to repair the tendons if possible.[74]

Peroneal tendoscopy is an alternative treatment option that has gained traction, though experience with advanced arthroscopic and endoscopic techniques are recommended.[71,87] The location of the peroneal tendon pathology will dictate the location of the portals, with most procedures utilizing two or three portals proximal and distal to the tip of the fibula. While diagnostic tendoscopy with débridement of tenosynovitis is relatively simple, more advanced techniques including tendoscopic groove deepening, tendon repair, and SPR repair have been described.[87–89]

Peroneal tendon dislocation should be treated with reconstruction of the SPR. Eckert and Davis[67] came up with a classification system to define the injury to the SPR. In grade I injuries, the retinaculum and periosteum were elevated from the lateral malleolus, and the tendons lay between the periosteum and the bone. In grade II injuries (33% of their patients), the distal 1 to 2 cm of the fibrocartilaginous ridge was elevated along with the retinaculum, and in grade III injuries (16% of their patients), a thin cortical rim of bone was avulsed along with the retinaculum, the fibrous lip, and the periosteum. Oden[63] described

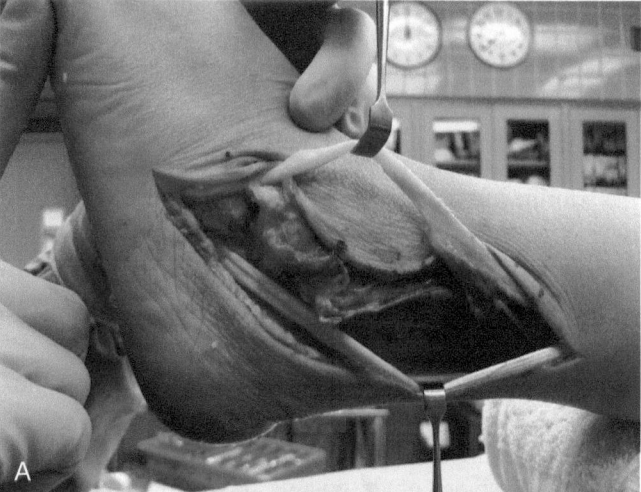

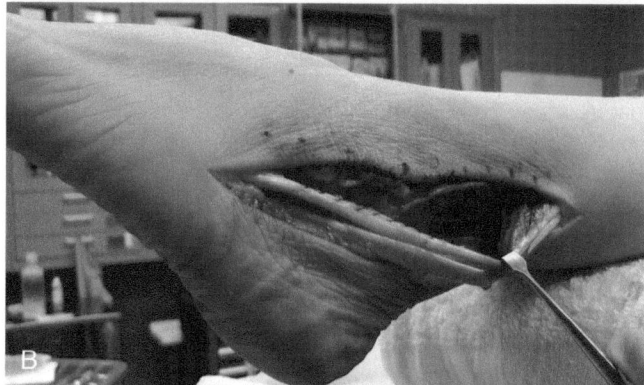

Fig. 118.11 Intraoperative photographs of a patient who had a peroneus brevis tear in association with synovitis. (A) Appearance of the tendons after excision of the synovitis. (B) Tubularization of the peroneus brevis with a running nonabsorbable suture. (From Joos D, Kadakia AR. Peroneal tendon disorders. In: Miller MD, Sanders TG, eds. *Presentation, Imaging and Treatment of Common Musculoskeletal Conditions: MRI-Arthroscopy Correlation.* Philadelphia: Elsevier; 2012.)

a similar classification scheme based on 100 cases but defined a type II injury as a tear rather than an elevation of the retinaculum from the fibula, and added a type IV injury—an avulsion of bone from the posterior rather than anterior fibular insertion site. Several procedures have been described to treat the SPR insufficiency, including direct reattachment, reconstruction using either local or free grafts, rerouting the calcaneofibular ligament, and bone-block procedures.[67,78,90–92] When the peroneal tendons dislocate anteriorly to the fibula, a false pouch is often created that must be closed as part of the reconstruction. Multiple options for groove deepening have also been described. Direct groove deepening involves raising osteoperiosteal flaps with excavation of bone followed by laying back down the smooth osteoperiosteal surface.[93] Indirect groove deepening involves reaming out the posterior intramedullary fibula with the use of a cannulated drill from the tip of the fibula and then tamping the intact periosteal surface to create a deeper groove.[81,82] Finally, endoscopic fibular groove deepening also has been described.[89]

Associated pathologic conditions should also be addressed when present. Chronic lateral ankle instability can be treated with a modified Broström-Gould procedure, although in the presence of a peroneus brevis tendon tear, a modified Broström-Evans procedure is a useful alternative.[94] This procedure involves transferring the anterior one-half to one-third of the peroneus brevis into the distal fibula as an augmentation to the standard Broström procedure. If a varus heel is present, a lateralizing calcaneal osteotomy should be performed with the use of either a standard oblique lateral-based wedge or a Z-shaped osteotomy.[95,96] When a hypertrophied peroneal tubercle is present, it should be excised.[66] In the case of intrasheath peroneal subluxation, groove deepening has been described as an effective treatment option.[61]

Postoperative Management

Patients wear a short-leg, non–weight-bearing splint in the immediate postoperative period. After 2 weeks, a tall removable boot is worn and weight bearing is allowed. For most peroneal tendon procedures, it is important to initiate early ankle ROM exercises to limit adhesion of the tendons. The patient can perform these exercises at home or with formal physical therapy. Inversion past 10 degrees from neutral is avoided until approximately 10 weeks after surgery to facilitate complete tendon healing. If concomitant osteotomies are performed to correct a cavovarus

alignment, weight bearing is delayed until 6 weeks after surgery. At 6 weeks, most patients transition into an ankle lace-up–type brace, and activities progress. A realistic return to sporting activity is 4 to 6 months after surgery. Generally straight-ahead running is allowed at 3 months and cutting activities are allowed at 4 months, although this schedule is extremely variable.

Results

Outcomes of peroneal tendon repairs have mostly been reported in retrospective reviews and case reports. Bassett and Speer[98] reported that eight college-level athletes were able to return to full athletic activity after repair of five peroneus longus tendons and three peroneus brevis tendons, although the time frame was not discussed. AOFAS scores at medium-term follow-up after peroneal tendon repairs have been shown to be 82 to 85, with good to excellent patient-reported outcomes and normal to moderate peroneal strength in more than 90% of patients, although with prolonged time to maximum function.[72,99] In a recent study it was reported that the average return to activity was 3.2 months in an athletic population who underwent peroneal tendon repair and SPR reconstruction for symptomatic peroneal tendon subluxation.[100] However, Steel and DeOrio[70] reported that only 46% of 30 patients treated surgically for peroneal tendon

---

🏃 Author's Preferred Technique

Peroneal Tendon Injury

Peroneal Tendon Repair

A curvilinear lateral approach is made over the peroneal tendons. If the SPR is intact, be careful to preserve a cuff lateral to the fibrocartilaginous ridge for later repair when incising through the retinaculum. Distal to the fibula, be sure to identify and release the separate sheaths in which the peroneus brevis and longus run, separated by the septa that attach to the peroneal tubercle. If the peroneal tubercle appears hypertrophied or is suspected of contributing to symptoms, have a low threshold to excise it. All tenosynovitis present is débrided. Evaluate the extent of the tendon tear and excise any degenerated tendon; if more than 50% of viable tendon remains, the tendon is repaired using a running, 3-0 or 4-0 nonabsorbable suture. If the tendon is irreparable (i.e., generally <50% is viable, although this general rule can be modified), tenodesis to the intact tendon (longus or brevis) proximal and distal to the rupture site is performed with use of 0 or 2-0 nonabsorbable suture. Ensure that the tenodesis is performed both proximal and distal to the fibular groove to avoid fibular impingement.[97] In all cases, preservation of the function of the peroneus brevis is more critical than the function of the peroneus longus.

Chronic Peroneal Tendon Dislocation

In the setting of peroneal subluxation or dislocation, the tendons are explored and synovectomy along with appropriate treatment of peroneal tendon tears are performed as previously described. The fibular groove should be deepened. While using either the direct groove deepening technique with a cortical window or the indirect technique described earlier are reasonable options, the author's preferred technique is a direct approach using an oval burr on the posterior aspect of the fibula to deepen the groove. The deepening should extend from the proximal aspect of the fibular metaphysis to the tip of the fibula, including the medial side of the fibula while keeping the lateral fibular rim intact. Use of a rasp to smooth the surface followed by bone wax creates a very smooth surface. This procedure negates problems with the cortical bone "popping" back into its original place as can occur in the traditional direct groove deepening technique.

The tendons should lie within the groove without subluxation with gentle dorsiflexion and plantar flexion of the ankle. The SPR is then imbricated to the fibula through drill holes within the posterolateral border of the fibula (Fig. 118.12). The fibrocartilaginous ridge can also be used for fixation as an alternative to drill holes in the distal aspect of the fibula. The use of nonabsorbable no. 0 suture in a horizontal mattress fashion with the knot located on the SPR imbricates the tissue and prevents the knot from being placed in a subcutaneous location that can be irritating to the patient.

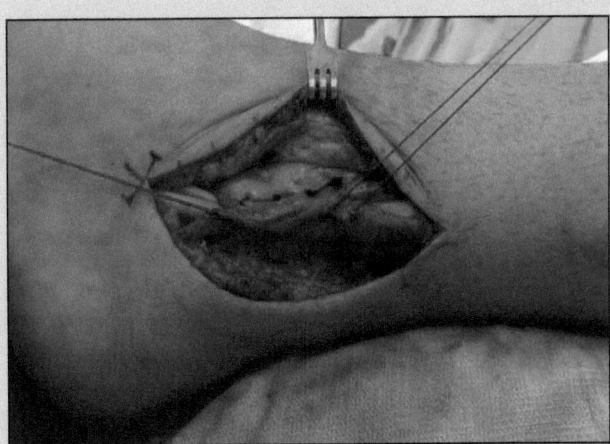

Fig. 118.12 Repair of the superior peroneal retinaculum (SPR) is performed through drill holes in the fibula to imbricate the SPR to the deep aspect of the lateral fibula. It is critical to ensure that the SPR is placed to the underside of the lateral fibular ridge. (From Joos D, Kadakia AR. Peroneal tendon disorders. In: Miller MD, Sanders TG, eds. *Presentation, Imaging and Treatment of Common Musculoskeletal Conditions: MRI-Arthroscopy Correlation.* Philadelphia: Elsevier; 2012.)

tears were able to successfully return to sports. Tendoscopic procedures have shown good functional outcomes, though most of these procedures involved débridement of tenosynovitis or partial débridement of small tears.[71,88] Larger tendon tears were typically converted to open or mini-open techniques.

Results of SPR reconstruction vary by the technique described. Eckert and Davis[67] reported only a 4% redislocation rate after SPR reattachment, although with only a 6-month follow-up. Maffulli and colleagues[101] performed anatomic repairs of the SPR on 14 patients with chronic, recurrent peroneal tendon subluxations. At follow-up of 38 months, none had experienced recurrent subluxations, and all had returned to their normal activities.[101] Poll and Duijfjes[92] reported on 10 patients in whom the insertion of the calcaneofibular ligament was mobilized and lifted with a cancellous bone block from the calcaneus. The peroneal tendons were then brought under the ligament, and the bone block was replaced and fixed with a small cancellous screw. They reported excellent results in all 10 patients and recommended the procedure because it precluded scarring and adhesions of the peroneal tendons to the surrounding structures.[92] Groove-deepening procedures have had similar good results. Zoellner and Clancy[93] reported on 10 patients using their technique and stated that the results were excellent at an average follow-up of 2 years. Porter et al.[102] modified their technique and accelerated the rehabilitation program and found no recurrent dislocations, minimal symptoms, and an average return to sports at 3 months after a 3-year follow-up. Ogawa et al.[81] reported good clinical outcome scores and no recurrence of instability in 15 patients treated with the indirect groove-deepening method. Not surprisingly, the patients who had concomitant peroneal tendon tears had worse outcomes than those treated for instability alone. Finally, Vega et al. reported on seven patients who underwent tendoscopic groove deepening without formal SPR reconstruction for patients with chronic peroneal subluxation. No patients experienced recurrent subluxation, and the AOFAS outcome score improved from 75 preoperatively to 93 at final follow-up.[89]

Complications

Failure to diagnose the peroneal tendon tear or subluxation is likely the most common complication. Recurrent pain may be caused by inadequate débridement or failure to recognize and excise associated disease such as a low-lying muscle belly, peroneus quartus, or hypertrophied peroneal tubercle. Tendon adhesions and decreased mobility are another common cause of pain and dysfunction, especially after tenodesis is performed.[74] Recurrent tendon instability may be the result of persistent chronic lateral ankle instability and the subsequent strain on the SPR repair, as well as a failure to recognize and correct a subtle cavovarus alignment. The most common complications after peroneal tendoscopy include injury to the peroneal tendons during portal placement and damage to the sural nerve and its branches.[88]

Future Considerations

Prospective studies are needed to determine the best and most appropriate SPR reconstruction method. Synthetic or specially processed allograft tissue may offer alternatives to local tissue

when it is insufficient. The true benefit of groove-deepening procedures needs to be elucidated with higher level studies. As advanced imaging techniques improve, we may be able to better detect both peroneal tendon tears and subtle instability of the tendons and the fibulae that require groove deepening. Tendoscopy offers typical advantages of endoscopic techniques including smaller scars, less pain, and often higher patient satisfaction. Advancements in tendoscopic instrumentation and further studies evaluating these techniques are needed to potentially expand the indications for tendoscopy for peroneal tendon pathology.

ACHILLES TENDON INJURIES

The Achilles tendon is a common source of complaints in the orthopaedic surgeon's practice, especially in the athletic population. Acute Achilles tendon ruptures remain a very common injury and are prevalent in elite-level athletes, weekend warriors, and older patients. Surgical versus conservative treatment for acute Achilles tendon ruptures has followed a cyclical path in history and remains somewhat controversial. Chronic Achilles tendon dysfunction has been labeled many ways, including tendinitis, tendinosis, paratenonitis, and peritendinitis. Because these descriptions can be misleading, the preferred term as described by Maffulli and colleagues[103] is *Achilles tendinopathy*. Most conditions are then further categorized into insertional versus noninsertional tendinopathy. Retrocalcaneal bursitis and Haglund deformity (pump bump) are additional clinical entities that are associated with insertional disease.

History

Acute Achilles ruptures usually present after a traumatic event in which the patient feels as if he or she has been kicked or struck on the back of the ankle above the heel with subsequent weakness and difficulty with ambulation. This event is often the result of an explosive sporting maneuver, such as jumping for a rebound in basketball, but can be less significant and symptomatic if some intrinsic tearing was present. Although most patients seek immediate treatment, it is not uncommon for patients to disregard the initial event if the symptoms are mild and eventually seek treatment as a result of an altered gait, swelling, or heel walking.

Achilles tendinopathy causes chronic posterior ankle and heel pain that is worsened with activity. Runners show the highest incidence of noninsertional Achilles tendinopathy, which manifests as aching pain above the insertion of the Achilles, sometimes with associated swelling.[104] In the early stages, the pain occurs only with prolonged running, but as the disease progresses, pain may occur even at rest. Insertional Achilles tendinopathy is seen in the athletic population but is more common as patients age and tendon degeneration occurs. Patients commonly localize their pain to the midline at the insertion of the Achilles on the calcaneus, although sometimes the pain is localized to the medial or lateral side. Exercise, stair climbing, and running on hard surfaces tend to exacerbate the pain. Symptoms may occur initially with strenuous activities alone, but often progress to pain being present at rest.[105]

Physical Examination

Prone examination of both lower extremities provides all the information needed to determine the presence of an acute Achilles rupture. The resting tension of both Achilles tendons is evaluated by asking the patient to bend both knees and then inspecting the stance of the foot. Normal stance shows the foot plantar flexed about 20 degrees. Decreased stance (loss of plantar flexion) or asymmetry indicates a lengthened tendo-Achilles complex. A palpable gap and associated tenderness is often present at the rupture site, though these symptoms can be subtle if the injury is subacute. The most common site for rupture is 2 to 6 cm above the insertion on the calcaneus, thought to be secondary to an avascular zone.[106,107] The entire length of the gastrocsoleus complex should be palpated because ruptures can occur anywhere from the musculotendinous junction to the insertion on the calcaneus. The Thompson test is the classic and most sensitive way to determine a disruption in the Achilles tendon: with the knee flexed, squeeze the calf and inspect the motion of the foot.[108] If the foot plantar flexes, the Achilles is intact; if no motion occurs, discontinuity is present (Fig. 118.13).

Noninsertional Achilles tendinopathy classically presents with tenderness to palpation and swelling in the region proximal to the insertion of the Achilles tendon on the calcaneus. Similar to ruptures, this tendinopathy commonly occurs about 2 to 6 cm proximal to the calcaneal insertion (Fig. 118.14). Often a fusiform thickening of the tendon is palpated and tenderness is present. Assessment of lower extremity alignment is important, including limb-length inequality and the presence of cavus versus planus feet.

Insertional Achilles tendinopathy presents with the focus of tenderness on the posterior aspect of the insertional ridge of the calcaneus where the Achilles tendon inserts. Although not specific, midline tenderness tends to correlate with insertional tendinopathy, whereas lateral and less frequently medial tenderness tends to correlate with retrocalcaneal bursitis. Often a large prominence is noted on inspection either enveloping the entire posterior heel or predominantly laterally. When the bony prominence is isolated to the superolateral aspect of the calcaneal tuberosity, it is commonly referred to as a *Haglund deformity* (or pump bump). Testing for gastrocnemius tightness with the Silverskiöld examination should be performed for all patients suspected of having Achilles tendinopathy.

Imaging

Standard ankle radiographs should be performed in most cases of Achilles tendon ruptures and all cases of Achilles tendinopathy. For ruptures it is important to evaluate whether a distal avulsion of the calcaneus is present, although this presentation is less common, and suspicion should be raised on the examination. Soft tissue thickening or calcifications can be visualized in patients with noninsertional tendinopathy, whereas insertional disease may show a large bony spur at the insertional ridge, a prominent Haglund deformity, or intratendinous calcifications. The width of the soft tissue shadow also can give an indication of tendon degeneration.

Ultrasound and MRI have become useful tools in identifying Achilles tendon disease, although neither is necessary to make the diagnosis in the great majority of cases. Ultrasound is the modality of choice to determine the proximity of the tendon edges in an acute Achilles rupture.[109] The dynamic nature of the test allows measurement of the gap present with the foot at neutral versus 20 degrees of plantar flexion, which can have treatment implications. Although MRI can be useful in unclear cases or cases of chronic Achilles rupture, a recent study showed that physical examination findings were more sensitive in diagnosing acute Achilles ruptures than was MRI.[110]

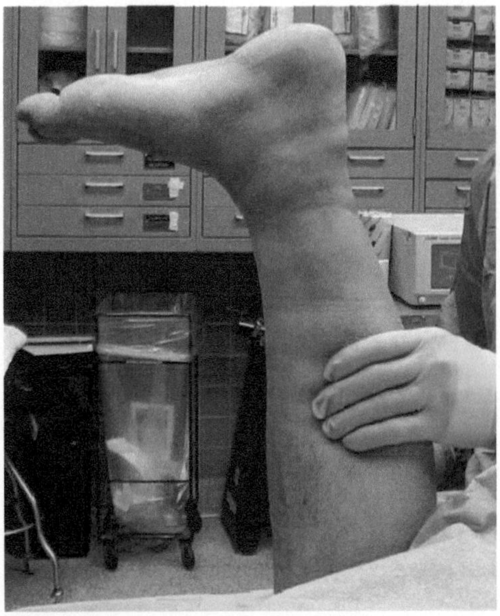

Fig. 118.13 A positive Thompson test with a lack of plantar flexion with calf squeeze. (From Joos D, Tran N, Kadakia AR. Achilles tendon disorders. In: Miller MD, Sanders TG, eds. *Presentation, Imaging and Treatment of Common Musculoskeletal Conditions: MRI-Arthroscopy Correlation.* Philadelphia: Elsevier; 2012.)

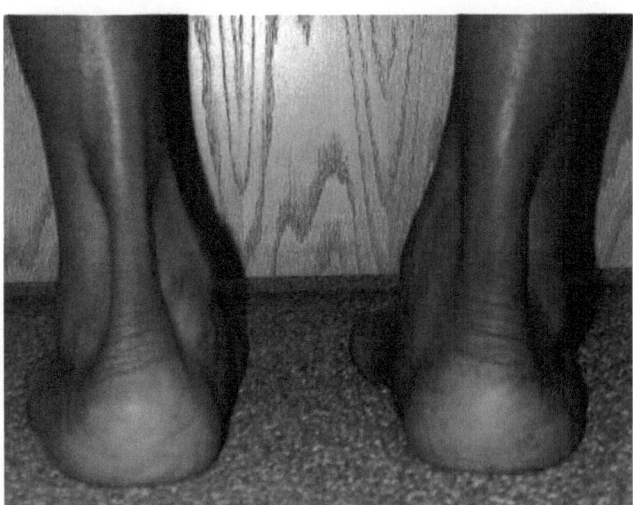

Fig. 118.14 A patient with right Achilles tendinosis. Note the thickening of the tendon on the affected right leg compared with the normal left leg. (From Joos D, Tran N, Kadakia AR. Achilles tendon disorders. In: Miller MD, Sanders TG, eds. *Presentation, Imaging and Treatment of Common Musculoskeletal Conditions: MRI-Arthroscopy Correlation.* Philadelphia: Elsevier; 2012.)

For Achilles tendinopathy, ultrasound can be used to better delineate the presence of neovascularization in the tendon, which is a part of the degeneration process.[111] MRI can be used to better classify the degree of degeneration present in the tendon, as well as to distinguish intratendinous pathology from peritendinous pathology (Figs. 118.15 and 118.16). MRI has also been shown to help predict the response to nonoperative treatment in persons

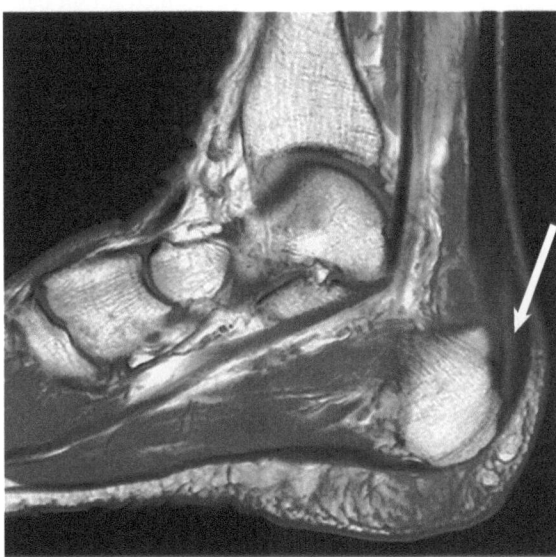

Fig. 118.15 A T1-weighted magnetic resonance image of a patient with insertional Achilles tendinosis. Note the intermediate signal intensity and thickening of the tendon at the insertion of the Achilles tendon into the calcaneus *(arrow)*. (From Joos D, Tran N, Kadakia AR. Achilles tendon disorders. In: Miller MD, Sanders TG, eds. *Presentation, Imaging and Treatment of Common Musculoskeletal Conditions: MRI-Arthroscopy Correlation.* Philadelphia: Elsevier; 2012.)

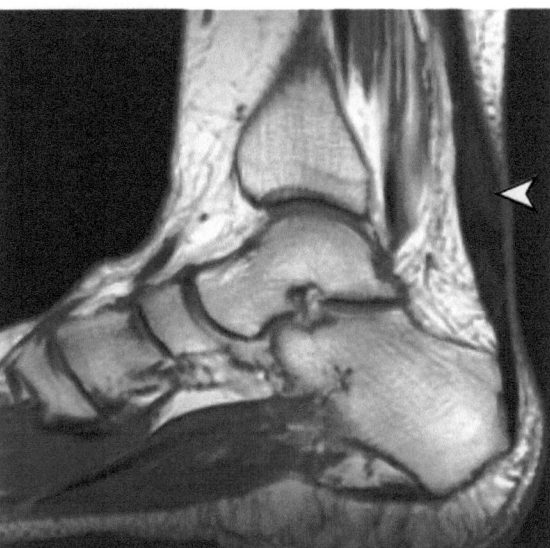

Fig. 118.16 A T1-weighted magnetic resonance image of a patient with noninsertional Achilles tendinosis. Note the intermediate signal intensity and fusiform thickening of the tendon *(arrowhead)*. (From Joos D, Tran N, Kadakia AR. Achilles tendon disorders. In: Miller MD, Sanders TG, eds. *Presentation, Imaging and Treatment of Common Musculoskeletal Conditions: MRI-Arthroscopy Correlation.* Philadelphia: Elsevier; 2012.)

with insertional Achilles tendinopathy.[112] Both modalities can be used to assess response to treatment and for preoperative planning.

Decision-Making Principles

The debate between operative and nonoperative treatment for acute Achilles tendon ruptures has evolved with both improved surgical techniques and improved rehabilitation protocols.[113] Multiple historical studies have compared the results of conservative versus surgical treatment.[114–120] However, rehabilitation protocols allowing motion and protected weight bearing earlier in the recovery period are now commonly used both during conservative treatment and after surgery with significant functional improvements.[121–127] The benefits and risks to both treatment options remain the same, although with these new rehabilitation protocols, the difference is not as stark. The advantage of nonoperative treatment is avoiding the risks (or disadvantages) of surgery: wound-healing problems, scar, and cost. The disadvantage of nonoperative treatment has historically been a higher repeat rupture rate and decreased strength and endurance compared with surgical treatment. Using a modern rehabilitation protocol, multiple recent studies reexamined the question of operative versus nonoperative treatment. Willits et al.[124] showed equivalent repeat rupture rates and no clinically important difference in measured outcomes between operative and nonoperative groups, with increased complication rates in the operative group (18% vs. 8%). However, at the extreme plantar-flexion strength level measured (240 degrees/s), the surgical group showed a significant increase compared with the nonoperative group when measured as a ratio (affected/unaffected side). It was not stated how this measurement correlates clinically. Nilsson-Helander et al.[125] reported no difference in functional outcome scores between operative and nonoperative groups 12 months after surgery, with a 4% repeat rupture rate in the operative group and a 12% repeat rupture rate in the nonoperative group (the finding did not reach significance). Although a high rate of deep vein thrombosis (DVT) was found in the entire group (34%), all of the other complications reported were in the surgical group, mostly related to the scar. Two more recent randomized controlled trials again showed no significant difference between the operative and nonoperative groups using two different Achilles-tendon-specific outcome scores, though surgical wound infections were seen in both operative groups. Interestingly, the rerupture rate in the nonoperative group was 10% and 14% in the two studies, versus 0% and 3% in the operative group, respectively.[126,127] Furthermore, Lantto et al. reported improved calf muscle strength in the operative group at 18 months.[127] A systematic review of randomized controlled trials demonstrated a significantly reduced repeat rupture rate (3.6% operative vs. 8.8% nonoperative) and increased surgical complications with surgical treatment; however, no conclusion regarding return of strength could be made.[128] Nevertheless, a recent meta-analysis of randomized trials showed equal rerupture rates between operative and nonoperative groups when functional rehabilitation was employed, with a risk increase of 15.8% in the operative group for complications other than rerupture.[129] Although support has increased regarding the effectiveness of nonoperative treatment in Achilles tendon ruptures in the general population, most surgeons agree that in the athletic population, surgical repair is the most predictive method of restoring strength and ability to return to high-level sports. A frank discussion should be held with each patient to discuss the benefits and risks of both treatment options.

Conservative treatment is always the first-line option in Achilles tendinopathy. If patients do not respond to the initial treatments, such as rest, activity modification, footwear modification, and eccentric physical therapy, both invasive and noninvasive intermediate treatments are available and should be individualized to the patient. Noninvasive treatments for noninsertional tendinopathy include ultrasound, low-level laser therapy, shock-wave therapy, and glyceryl trinitrate patches.[104] Invasive treatments include platelet-rich plasma injections, prolotherapy, and aprotinin injections. Similar treatments have been described for insertional tendinopathy including shock-wave therapy and sclerosing injections.[105] Corticosteroid injections are not recommended based on the catabolic effect and subsequent risk of rupture.[130] Based on the limited literature available for most of these treatment options, insufficient evidence exists to support recommendation of these procedures, but the noninvasive treatments are relatively safe and may benefit some patients.

Surgical management can be considered for both insertional and noninsertional Achilles tendinopathy when nonoperative treatment fails. Because multiple surgical options exist, determining the appropriate procedure can be difficult. In general, for noninsertional tendinopathy, less invasive surgical treatments, such as percutaneous longitudinal tenotomy and minimally invasive stripping procedures, are appropriate for mild to moderate focal lesions, whereas open procedures including débridement, tenosynovectomy, and possibly FHL transfer are appropriate for moderate to severe tendinopathy.[131–134] Similarly, surgical management of insertional Achilles tendinopathy is dependent on the extent of degeneration of the Achilles tendon. Open retrocalcaneal decompression with Achilles tendon débridement and the use of the Haglund excision have been used effectively for patients with persistent pain but minimal degeneration of the Achilles tendon, whereas an extensive débridement, reattachment of the Achilles tendon, and possible FHL transfer are more appropriate for patients with more extensive disease.[135–139] Finally, isolated gastrocnemius recession may be an option for patients with either insertional or noninsertional tendinopathy and gastrocnemius tightness.[140]

Treatment Options

Conservative treatment of an acute Achilles tendon rupture should be managed with a modern rehabilitation program. As outlined by Willits et al.[124] and Tan et al.[141] this protocol includes initial equinus immobilization for 2 weeks, followed by progressive weight bearing with heel lifts and ROM with dorsiflexion blocks during the next 4 to 6 weeks. A physical therapy program is then initiated, including transition to footwear with a heel lift, open-chain exercises with a focus on eccentric strengthening, and eventual resistance exercises at about 10 weeks (Table 118.1).

Surgical options include primary open repair versus a "minimally invasive" or limited incision technique. The approach to primary open repair is usually performed just medial to the Achilles tendon, although central and lateral approaches can be

TABLE 118.1 Protocol for Nonoperative Management of Acute Achilles Tendon Ruptures

Timing	Treatment
Initial evaluation	Ultrasound or magnetic resonance imaging examination demonstrating less than 5 mm of gap with maximum plantar flexion or less than 10 mm of gapping with the foot in neutral position with greater than 75% of tendon apposition with the foot in 20 degrees of plantar flexion
Initial management	Cast with foot in full equinus with dorsiflexion block; non–weight bearing
2-week evaluation	Transition to a removable cast or cast boot with the foot in 20 degrees of plantar flexion with two 1-cm wedges in the cast boot; can bear weight as tolerated; the boot is to be worn 24 h/day
4-week evaluation	Clinical examination: able to palpate continuity of the tendon; recommend repeat ultrasound or magnetic resonance imaging to verify that tendon edges are apposed without evidence of gapped ends; if tendon edges are not apposed, recommend surgical consideration; the boot is removed 5 min/h when awake to perform active dorsiflexion to neutral with passive plantar flexion
6-week evaluation	Clinical examination to document continuity of the tendon; removal of one 1-cm wedge; continue active dorsiflexion to neutral with passive plantar flexion; initiate a physical therapy program to begin proprioception and non-weight-bearing muscle strengthening out of the boot
8-week evaluation	Clinical examination to ensure tendon continuity and evaluation with ultrasound or magnetic resonance imaging to document continued tendon apposition; if the patient has a lack of tendon healing or continuity, consider operative intervention; if the tendon is in continuity, recommend transition of the boot to daytime wear only, without the use of a wedge; continue a formal physical therapy program
10-week evaluation	Discontinue use of the boot and use a 1-cm heel wedge for 3 more months; may start to ride a stationary bike and progress with the physical therapy program with weight bearing as tolerated with a lift in the shoe; no sprinting or running is allowed until the use of the heel wedge is discontinued

used. Krackow, Bunnell, and Kessler suture configurations are all options, although one study showed that the Krackow technique was stronger than the others.[142] Two-strand versus four-strand repairs can be used, with four-strand repairs being biomechanically superior.[143] Percutaneous and limited incision techniques have increased in popularity since Ma and Griffith[144] reported their results in 1977. Multiple studies have now reported their results using specially designed devices to decrease the risk of sural nerve injury and to ensure placement of the sutures within the paratenon.[145–148] Currently neither treatment can be recommended over the other, although most surgeons would recommend an open repair in the elite-level athlete.

The conservative and surgical options for Achilles tendinopathy are listed in the section "Decision-Making Principles." Endoscopic decompression of the retrocalcaneal space has also been described for insertional tendinopathy. Good clinical outcomes have been reported, although the ability to débride the tendon and remove any calcifications is limited.[149–151]

Postoperative Management

Acute repair of Achilles tendon ruptures follow the same accelerated rehabilitation protocol as that used for nonoperative treatment (see the brief description in the "Treatment Options" section). Early motion and early weight bearing (after 2 weeks of immobilization) have been shown to significantly increase functional outcomes and health-related quality of life.[122,152] Patients are generally progressed into a shoe with a heel lift at 8 to 10 weeks after surgery. Straight-ahead running is allowed at 3 months, and cutting exercises are allowed at 4 months. Return to full athletic activity is usually achieved by 9 months.

A similar postoperative course is followed in the patient undergoing débridement and repair of a noninsertional Achilles

---

 Author's Preferred Technique

Achilles Tendon Rupture

An open repair technique for acute Achilles ruptures in the athletic population is preferred to ensure excellent tendon apposition and restoration of tension (Fig. 118.17). The patient is positioned prone, with the incision just medial to the Achilles tendon. Alternatively, the patient can be placed supine with the affected leg externally rotated using a medial approach to access the tendon. Although this technique can be used routinely, it is excellent for obese patients with respiratory compromise or patients with a compromised airway. One should sharply incise through skin, subcutaneous tissue, and paratenon to avoid devascularization of the skin edges. Identify the rupture and gently débride it of hematoma; do not débride frayed tendon edges. Place a Krackow locking stitch using no. 2 polydioxanone suture (PDS) in the proximal and distal tendon stumps. Larger nonabsorbable no. 5 suture or newer no. 2 suture that has the strength of traditional no. 5 nonabsorbable suture is also frequently used. Four to five passes through both the medial and lateral column should suffice. Typically I use a four-strand repair with the second two strands passed orthogonal to the first (i.e., one in the coronal plane and one in the sagittal plane). Sutures are tied while holding the tendon edges apposed with the other suture limbs with the foot in about 20 to 30 degrees of plantar flexion. Near maximal tension is the goal of suture repair, as some stretch occurs during rehabilitation. Epitendon suture is placed using 3-0 PDS in running fashion. The paratenon is carefully closed and a splint in 20 degrees of plantar flexion is applied to maximize perfusion to the posterior skin.

Noninsertional Achilles Tendinopathy: Tendon Débridement With Longitudinal Repair

For tendon débridement with longitudinal repair, a prone approach is used with a medial incision carried down through the paratenon. A longitudinal incision of the thickened, degenerative portion of the tendon is performed. Sharp débridement of all degenerative-appearing tendon, essentially shelling out the inner core of the tendon, is carried out, taking care not to create a discontinuity (Fig. 118.18). Longitudinal repair is performed with tubularization of the healthy tendon edges and additional closure of the paratenon if possible.

Insertional Achilles Tendinopathy: Achilles Débridement, Haglund Excision, Flexor Hallucis Longus Transfer (if >55 Years Old), and Tendon Reattachment

The longitudinal midline approach is carried down through the paratenon, and the creation of paratenon flaps for later closure is undertaken. A longitudinal incision is made through the midline of the Achilles tendon, and detachment of

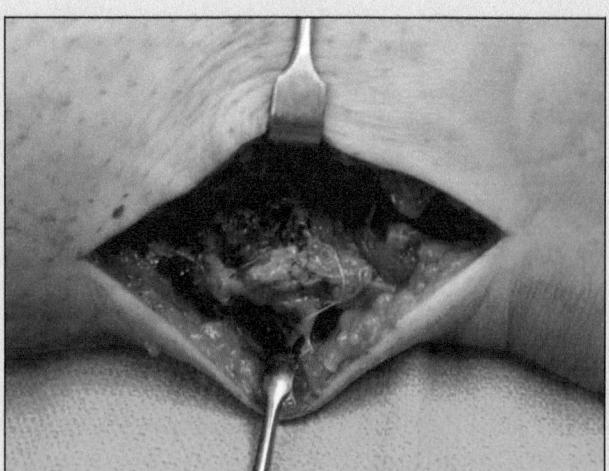

Fig. 118.17 Intraoperative photograph of the Achilles tendon after repair. The tendon ends should be completely apposed without any gapping. (From Joos D, Tran N, Kadakia AR. Achilles tendon disorders. In: Miller MD, Sanders TG, eds. *Presentation, Imaging and Treatment of Common Musculoskeletal Conditions: MRI-Arthroscopy Correlation.* Philadelphia: Elsevier; 2012.)

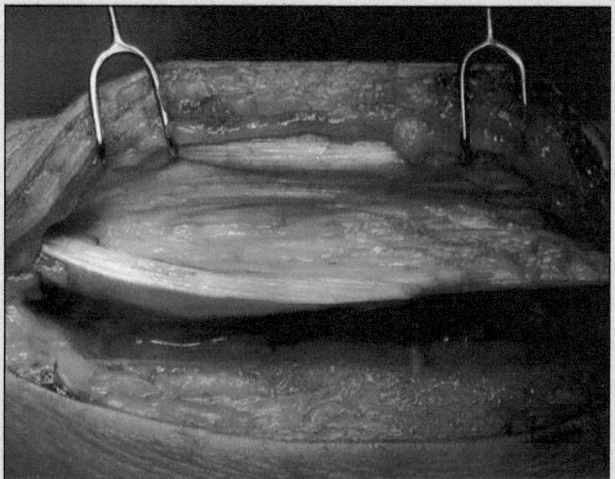

Fig. 118.18 An intraoperative photograph demonstrating resection of the central diseased portion of the Achilles tendon. (From Joos D, Tran N, Kadakia AR. Achilles tendon disorders. In: Miller MD, Sanders TG, eds. *Presentation, Imaging and Treatment of Common Musculoskeletal Conditions: MRI-Arthroscopy Correlation.* Philadelphia: Elsevier; 2012.)

Author's Preferred Technique
Achilles Tendon Rupture—cont'd

the middle 75% of the Achilles insertion from the calcaneal ridge is performed. An attempt is made to preserve the far medial and lateral Achilles tendon attachments. Sharp débridement of all degenerative Achilles tissue is performed. Resection of the posterior superior prominence of the calcaneus (Haglund deformity) is undertaken with a saw or osteotome from distal posterior to proximal anterior. Fluoroscopy is used to ensure that an adequate amount of bone has been resected to prevent further impingement. Excessive resection of the tuberosity is not required and may make reconstruction more difficult by minimizing the amount of bone for tendon fixation. Reattach the detached limbs of the Achilles tendon onto the calcaneus using two suture anchors placed distal to the FHL transfer, one medial and one lateral. Alternatively, a 4-anchor knotless construct can be utilized that potentially creates greater cross-sectional area for the insertional Achilles to heal to the cut surface of the calcaneus, while minimizing knot irritation. Repair the midline tenotomy using size 0 or no. 1 nonabsorbable suture.

Carefully close the paratenon, subcutaneous tissue, and skin, and apply a splint in 20 degrees of plantar flexion.

Flexor Hallucis Longus Transfer (if Necessary)
Divide the deep posterior fascia and identify the FHL muscle belly. Release the FHL tendon from its medial fibro-osseous tunnel and sharply divide as far distal as possible. Place tag suture using size 0 nonabsorbable suture. Note that the tibial nerve is located immediately medial to the tendon and must not be violated. Measure the diameter of the tendon and place a long Beath needle in the midline of the cut calcaneus through the plantar surface of the foot, again using fluoroscopy as a guide. Ream through the calcaneus using an appropriately sized reamer, slightly larger than the diameter of the measured tendon. Deliver the FHL through the reamed hole and place an interference screw in maximal tension with the foot held in 5 degrees of plantar flexion.

---

tendon lesion. For insertional Achilles tendon procedures, the postoperative course depends on the extent of surgery. If possible, the insertional attachment should be preserved in the athletic population. Weight bearing is delayed until 4 weeks after surgery in patients who undergo an FHL transfer. When Achilles reattachment is required, boot immobilization is maintained until 12 weeks to facilitate improved tendon to bone healing. Return to full sporting activities is generally delayed until about 12 months after surgery.

Results

Recent studies comparing nonoperative and operative treatment for acute Achilles tendon ruptures are discussed in the section "Decision-Making Principles." In 1998, Speck and Klaue[153] prospectively evaluated the clinical outcomes of 20 patients who had 6 weeks of early full weight bearing in a removable ankle-foot orthosis after an open repair of a torn Achilles tendon. All 20 patients reached their preoperative level of sports activity and had no significant side-to-side difference in ankle mobility and isokinetic strength. No repeat ruptures occurred. In a larger prospective study, Mortensen and colleagues[123] randomly assigned 71 patients who had repairs of acute Achilles tendon ruptures to either conventional postoperative management (i.e., a cast for 8 weeks) or early restricted motion of the ankle in a below-the-knee brace for 6 weeks. They found that patients who engaged in early motion had a smaller initial loss in ROM and returned to work and sports activities sooner than did patients managed with a cast. No repeat ruptures occurred in either group. In 2007, Twaddle and Poon[122] found that the common denominator between operative and nonoperative treatment was early motion. They found no differences in the outcomes of operative and nonoperative treatment in patients who were treated with early motion controlled with a removable orthosis. It is clear from these studies that early motion or an accelerated functional rehabilitation protocol, as well as early weight bearing, leads to improved functional results in both operative and nonoperative cases. The controversy regarding difference in strength and repeat rupture rate between operative and nonoperative treatment

remains, although most investigators would agree the elite-level athlete should undergo surgical treatment. However, the definition of "elite" is debatable.

Limited incision techniques also have shown good results. Recent studies have evaluated devices designed to enhance the limited open repair. Davies et al. reported excellent Achilles Tendon Rupture Scores (ATRS) and no reruptures in 143 patients at a mean 25 months after surgery, though two patients had sural nerve entrapment.[148] Vadala et al. reported 33 of 36 professional athletes were able to return to their preoperative sports activity level by 10 months, with no reruptures or sural nerve injury.[154] However, they did report decreased endurance of 6.78% at the 28-month follow-up. Hsu et al. compared traditional open versus mini-open techniques in a large single-center study. The overall complication rate for the entire group of 270 operatively treated patients (101 mini-open, 169 open) was 8.5%, with no reruptures. Importantly, there were no significant differences in rate of complications between the mini-open and open groups, though a greater number of the mini-open group returned to baseline activity by 5 months (98% vs. 82%).[155]

Eccentric exercises have demonstrated improved results in the nonoperative treatment of noninsertional Achilles tendinopathy compared with other therapies, primarily because of decreased pain.[156–158] Platelet-rich plasma injections have gained notoriety in recent years, but no comparison studies have been able to prove their efficacy in treating noninsertional Achilles tendinopathy.[159,160] Longitudinal tenotomies have shown good results in the running population.[131] Success rates greater than 80% have been obtained from open procedures with tenosynovectomy and tendon débridement.[133,161] Isolated gastrocnemius recession can provide significant and sustained pain relief, though power and endurance were less than matched controls.[140] Improved rates of pain, functional outcomes, and patient satisfaction also have been reported with use of FHL tendon transfers in severe cases of chronic Achilles tendinopathy.[134,162]

Surgical interventions for insertional Achilles tendinopathy have elicited similar patient satisfaction and good functional outcomes. Yodlowski et al.[136] reported that 90% of patients had complete or significant relief of symptoms after open retrocalcaneal decompression. Endoscopic calcaneoplasty has demonstrated sustained improvement at 5 years with AOFAS scores improving from 52.6 to 98.6.[151] Maffulli et al.[163] and McGarvey et al.[164] displayed good clinical results through a medial approach and a central tendon-splitting approach, respectively. Some factors that negatively affected outcomes included presence of intratendinous calcifications and age greater than 55 years.[135,164] When adding an FHL transfer, Den Hartog[138] reported significant improvement in AOFAS scores and an 88% rate of patient satisfaction. Similarly, Elias et al.[139] showed 95% patient satisfaction and no loss of plantar-flexion strength or power with the use of a similar technique.[139] Hunt et al. compared insertional Achilles reconstruction with and without FHL transfer in a prospective randomized study. They found no differences in outcome scores or patient satisfaction between groups, though the FHL group demonstrated improved ankle plantarflexion strength at 6 months and 1 year.[165]

Complications

Nonoperative treatment of Achilles tendon ruptures may lead to weakness and an elevated repeat rupture rate, though the current literature remains unclear regarding the rate of rerupture in operative versus nonoperative groups.[128,129] However, nonoperative treatment avoids the surgical complications associated with open repair, which was found to increase absolute risk by 15.8% for complications other than rerupture.[129] A meta-analysis reported a deep infection rate of 2.36%, whereas noncosmetic scar complaints were reported in 13.1% in the surgical group. The most significant reported complication from limited open approaches for Achilles tendon repair is sural nerve injury, which was present in 13% of cases in one early study.[166] Improved designs using a jig to ensure placement of the suture within the paratenon have significantly decreased rates of sural nerve injury.[145,147,148,154,155] Rates of DVT after Achilles tendon ruptures have been reported to be as high as 34%, although a recent large review of a health care management database revealed DVT rates of 0.43% and pulmonary embolism rates of 0.34%.[125,167]

Postoperative complications were reported in 11% of patients in one large retrospective series of patients undergoing surgery for chronic Achilles overuse injuries.[168] These complications included skin edge necrosis, infections, sural neuritis, DVT, and sensitive or hypertrophic scars. Achilles tendon ruptures or avulsions also have been reported, albeit rarely.[135,169,170] Cock-up deformity and medial plantar nerve transection have been reported after FHL transfers.[171,172]

Future Considerations

The debate regarding operative versus nonoperative treatment for acute Achilles tendon ruptures continues, though in the high-level athlete the possibility of increased rerupture rates and especially decreased strength favors operative treatment. Further prospective studies are needed to determine the efficacy of limited open approaches for acute Achilles tendon ruptures, especially in the athletic population. Improved designs may permit stronger repairs, with the added benefit of decreased wound healing complications. The advancement of invasive, nonsurgical techniques

for Achilles tendinopathy, with the utilization of orthobiologics or autologous products, such as platelet-rich plasma, may allow for improved results with less morbidity.

For a complete list of references, go to ExpertConsult.com.

SELECTED READINGS

Citation:

Huh J, Boyette DM, Parekh SG, et al. Allograft reconstruction of chronic tibialis anterior tendon ruptures. *Foot Ankle Int.* 2015;36(10):1180–1189.

Level of Evidence:

IV, therapeutic

Summary:

Eleven chronic tibialis anterior tendon ruptures were treated with intercalary allograft reconstruction. Good functional outcomes with mean dorsiflexion strength of 4.8/5 was achieved without the morbidity of autograft or tendon transfer.

Citation:

Lohrer H, Nauck T. Posterior tibial tendon dislocation: a systematic review of the literature and presentation of a case. *Br J Sports Med.* 2010;44:398–406.

Level of Evidence:

III, therapeutic

Summary:

The authors performed a systematic review of the literature and evaluated 61 cases of posterior tibial tendon dislocations, including clinical presentation, treatment, and outcomes. More than half of the cases were missed initially and 83% were fixed surgically, of which 80% were judged to have excellent results.

Citation:

Michelson J, Dunn L. Tenosynovitis of the flexor hallucis longus: a clinical study of the spectrum of presentation and treatment. *Foot Ankle Int.* 2005;26:291–303.

Level of Evidence:

IV, therapeutic

Summary:

The clinical presentation and results of treatment in 81 patients with symptomatic flexor hallucis longus tenosynovitis were retrospectively evaluated. Nonoperative treatment was successful in 64% of patients, whereas successful outcomes were reported for all 23 patients treated surgically (the majority with flexor hallucis longus decompression and synovectomy at the posterior ankle).

Citation:

Scholten PE, Sierevelt IN, van Dijk CN. Hindfoot endoscopy for posterior ankle impingement. *J Bone Joint Surg Am.* 2008;90(12):2665–2672.

Level of Evidence:

IV, therapeutic

Summary:

The authors provide a retrospective review of 55 patients treated for posterior ankle impingement with posterior hindfoot endoscopy for both traumatic and overuse injuries. Outcome scores significantly improved and return to sports occurred at an average of 8 weeks, although patients in the overuse group fared slightly better than did those in the traumatic group.

Citation:
Krause JO, Brodsky JW. Peroneus brevis tendon tears: pathophysiology, surgical reconstruction, and clinical results. *Foot Ankle Int.* 1998;19:271–279.

Level of Evidence:
IV, therapeutic

Summary:
Twenty patients with peroneus brevis tendon tears were evaluated and a new classification system was determined that defined tears as greater than or less than 50% of the cross-sectional area. Grade 1 tears were treated with débridement and repair, grade 2 tears were treated with tenodesis to the peroneus longus, and good to excellent results were achieved in the majority of patients, although with a prolonged return to maximum function.

Citation:
Eckert WR, Davis EA Jr. Acute rupture of the peroneal retinaculum. *J Bone Joint Surg Am.* 1976;58:670–672.

Level of Evidence:
IV, therapeutic

Summary:
Seventy-three skiers with acute peroneal tendon dislocations were evaluated and three grades of injury to the superior peroneal retinaculum were identified based on the location of disruption of the SPR on the posterolateral fibula. Surgical repair was deemed very successful, with only three cases of recurrent dislocation.

Citation:
Willits K, Amendola A, Bryant D, et al. Operative versus nonoperative treatment of acute Achilles tendon ruptures: a multicenter randomized trial using accelerated functional rehabilitation. *J Bone Joint Surg Am.* 2010;92A:2767–2775.

Level of Evidence:
I, therapeutic

Summary:
The authors report a randomized, controlled trial comparing operative versus nonoperative treatment of acute Achilles tendon ruptures in 144 patients with use of an accelerated functional rehabilitation protocol in both treatment groups. Outcome scores and clinical findings showed no clinically important differences between the groups, and the repeat rupture rates were equivalent, but complications were slightly higher in the operative group.

Citation:
Hsu AR, Jones CP, Cohen BE, et al. Clinical outcomes and complications of percutaneous Achilles repair system versus open technique for acute Achilles tendon ruptures. *Foot Ankle Int.* 2015;36(11):1279–1286.

Level of Evidence:
III, therapeutic

Summary:
Two hundred and seventy patients treated operatively for Achilles tendon ruptures were reviewed, comparing traditional open treatment (169 patients) versus a percutaneous (or mini open) technique with a jig (101 patients). The overall complication rate for the entire group was 8.5% with no reruptures and no significant difference in complication rate between the two groups. A greater number of the percutaneous group reached baseline activity level at 5 months postoperatively (98% vs. 82%, respectively).

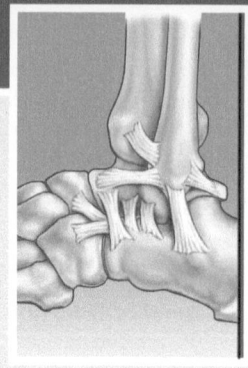

119

Articular Cartilage Injuries and Defects

David R. Richardson, Jane C. Yeoh

OSTEOCHONDRAL INJURIES AND DEFECTS IN THE FOOT AND ANKLE

Osteochondroses of the foot and ankle are found in multiple locations, including the talus, tibia, metatarsals, navicular, cuneiforms, and calcaneus. The cause of osteochondrosis is varied and complex, and has been described as traumatic, constitutional, idiopathic, and hereditary. Most investigators now believe that numerous factors are responsible for these changes. For example, excessive physical demands during athletic activity may incite osteochondral changes in growing bone made vulnerable by constitutional factors. Once the process has begun, repetitive trauma or pressure may prolong recovery or contribute to deformity. Osteochondroses often heal and defects are filled with fibrocartilage, but treatment may be required to relieve pain or prevent residual deformity. Treatment of any osteochondritic condition of the foot and ankle must be individualized to facilitate a rapid, safe return to activity and to minimize sequelae of the condition.

OSTEOCHONDRAL LESIONS OF THE TALUS

History

The incidence of osteochondral lesions of the talus (OLT), at least in military recruits, has been steadily rising during the past 10 years and is 27 per 100,000 person-years.[1] Most lesions are unilateral, but 10% of patients may have bilateral OLT.[2] Patients with acute injuries usually present with swollen and painful ankles or feet, limiting the specificity of physical examination. Patients with chronic injuries generally report mechanical symptoms, such as locking, catching, or giving way, or a feeling of instability of the ankle joint, in addition to pain and persistent swelling. Pain may occur only with certain ankle movements during sport or strenuous activity. An OLT should be considered in any patient who presents with a history of a "persistent ankle sprain."

Chondral injuries are frequent in patients with chronic ankle instability and ankle fractures. Chondral injuries have been found in 25% to 95% of ankles with chronic ankle instability.[3-6] Taga and associates[5] found cartilage lesions in 89% of acutely injured lateral ankle ligaments and in 95% of ankles with chronic lateral ligament instability. They concluded that the longer the time from the initial injury, the more severe the associated cartilage lesions. No correlation has been found between the amount of cartilage damage and the severity of the lateral ligament injury.

In their prospective study, Stufkens and colleagues[7] performed ankle arthroscopies in 288 consecutive patients with ankle fractures; they found talar cartilage lesions in 65%, tibial lesions in 50%, and fibular lesions in 39%. Deep lesions (>50% depth) at the anterior and lateral talus significantly increased the odds of poor long-term clinical outcome as measured by the American Orthopaedic Foot and Ankle Society (AOFAS) ankle-hindfoot scale.[7]

Physical Examination

Visual inspection of the foot and ankle should be performed to identify areas of swelling and ecchymosis, which are critically important in the acute setting. Alignment should be inspected from both the anterior and posterior aspects with the patient standing to determine if he or she has distal tibial varus or valgus or hindfoot varus or valgus, which may need to be corrected to improve the long-term outcome. The ankle and foot should be palpated to identify locations of tenderness; the medial and lateral corners of the talar dome should be palpated with the ankle maximally plantar flexed. A careful neurovascular examination is essential. Range of motion (ROM) in the involved foot and ankle should be compared with that of the contralateral extremity. Stability of the ankle should be evaluated with an anterior drawer test with the ankle plantar flexed and dorsiflexed, with a talar tilt test, and with inversion and eversion stress testing. Other soft-tissue or bony causes should be ruled out.

Imaging and Diagnosis

Weight-bearing anteroposterior, mortise, and lateral views of the ankle are essential. Oblique and plantar flexed radiographic views that avoid tibial overlap can show the lesion more clearly than plain films. If clinical examination or radiographs are suggestive but not diagnostic of OLT, three-dimensional (3D) imaging such as computed tomography (CT) or magnetic resonance imaging (MRI) provides more definitive information. In a study comparing MRI and CT, MRI demonstrated 96% sensitivity and 96% specificity, whereas CT demonstrated 81% sensitivity and 99% specificity, although the differences were not statistically significant.[8] Axial and sagittal cuts can help determine the location of the lesion (anterior, medial, or posterior), as well as its depth and size (Fig. 119.1). MRI can show other soft-tissue structures around the foot and ankle that can be injured concurrently with OLT, specifically the lateral and medial ankle ligaments and the peroneal tendons. In addition, MRI demonstrates bony

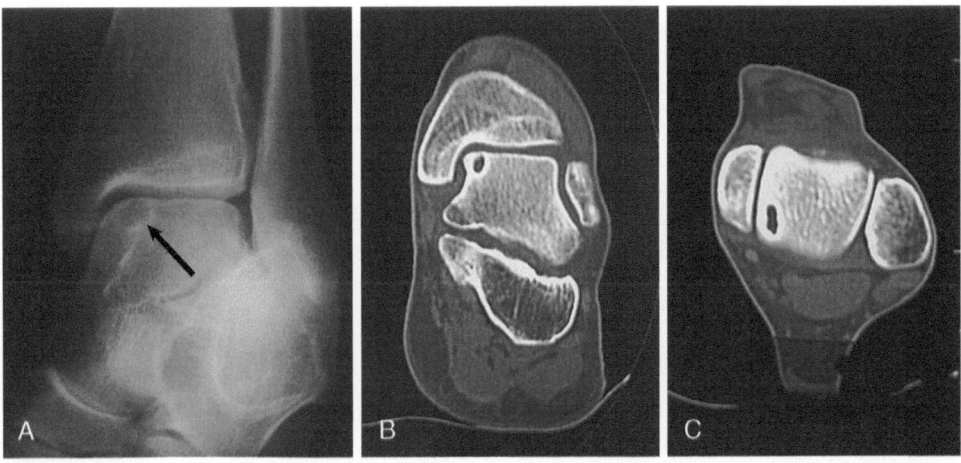

Fig. 119.1 (A) A posteromedial osteochondral lesion of the talus *(arrow)*. (B) A coronal plane computed tomography (CT) image. (C) An axial plane CT image. (From Richardson DR. Sports injuries of the ankle. In: Azar FM, Beaty JH, Canale ST, eds. *Campbell's Operative Orthopaedics*. 13th ed. Philadelphia: Elsevier; 2017.)

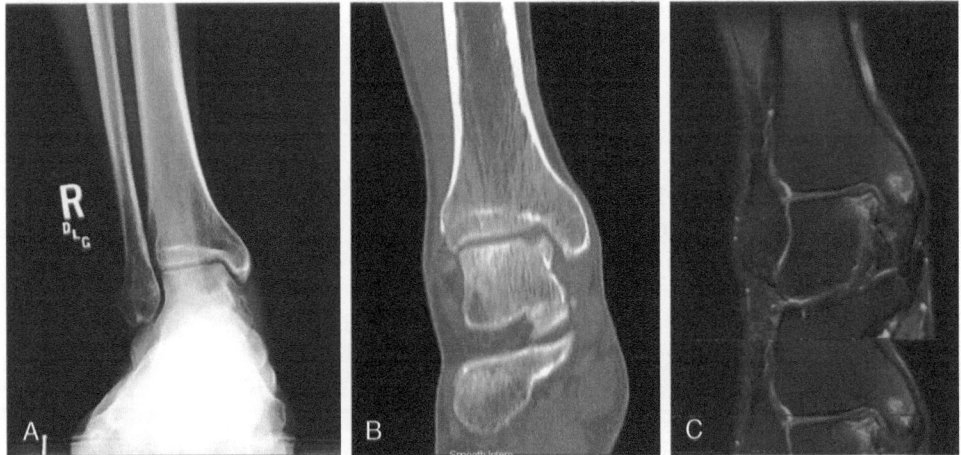

Fig. 119.2 (A) Plain radiographs, (B) computed tomography, and (C) magnetic resonance imaging appearance of a displaced (stage 4) osteochondral lesion of the talus. Note the bone marrow edema visible on the talus and tibia on magnetic resonance imaging.

edema not demonstrated by CT.[8] MRI is useful for both preoperative evaluation and postoperative follow-up and has become the standard in noninvasive diagnostics. Anderson and colleagues[9] demonstrated that low-signal intensity in T1-weighted images is an early and definitive sign of even stage 1 lesions. A high-signal rim between the osteochondral fragment and the talar bed is considered indicative of instability of the fragment, and joint fluid or fibrous granulation tissue is present as a result of the mobility of these fragments. Anderson and colleagues[9] noted that the diameter of the lesion measured on MRI was significantly larger than that indicated on plain radiographs, which is an important factor in preoperative planning. We recommend MRI evaluation to detect changes that provide information about the detachment and viability of the fragment and help with decision-making for surgical treatment (Fig. 119.2). MRI also may be useful for preoperative planning because it delineates the lesion more accurately than either plain radiography or CT.[8] OLT that have a high-signal rim on T2-weighted images are most likely unstable.[8] In a study of 22 ankles with OLT, Higashiyama and associates[10] found that the low- and high-signal rims present

before surgery disappeared in 100% and 77% of ankles, respectively. A decrease in or disappearance of the signal rim correlated well with clinical results; no patient in whom the signal rim persisted had a good result.[10] It has been demonstrated that helical CT, MRI, and diagnostic arthroscopy are significantly better than history, physical examination, and standard radiography for detecting or excluding OLT.[8] Single-photon emission CT (SPECT-CT) can evaluate OLT to help determine if the OLT was incidental or symptomatic.[11] SPECT-CT identifies scintigraphic osteoblastic activity to combine biologic information with anatomic information. Based on these SPECT-CT images, three independent, blinded orthopedic surgeons changed their treatment plan in 52% of the 25 cases.[11] By providing information on the subchondral plate and lesion depth, SPECT-CT may have additional diagnostic value.[12] Verhagen and colleagues[8] also examined the sensitivity and specificity of diagnostic arthroscopy, demonstrating 100% and 97%, respectively. In their study, diagnostic arthroscopy incorrectly identified 2 OLT (false positives), which were in fact cartilage softening caused by underlying degenerative changes.[8] In general, diagnostic arthroscopy should not be used as the initial method for diagnosing OLT because of its invasiveness and because noninvasive 3D imaging allows for preoperative preparation.

Decision-Making Principles

The choice of surgical or nonsurgical treatment depends largely on the patient's symptoms, age, physical demands, level of dysfunction, and the size of the OLT. Asymptomatic or incidental osteochondral lesions should not be treated operatively. Klammer and associates[13] concluded that asymptomatic or minimally symptomatic OLT in patients who wished to be treated nonoperatively do not clinically or radiographically worsen over time with conservative management. The mean follow-up of the 43 ankles in 41 patients in their study was 50 months.[13] Diagnostic injections into the ankle joint can help delineate true ankle pain from other causes in the differential diagnosis. Mechanical symptoms, such as locking, clicking, catching, or functional instability, often require operative intervention. Chronic lateral instability in an ankle with an OLT should be surgically treated concurrently, which has been demonstrated to have good outcomes.[14] Surgical treatment should not be limited to young patients or athletes only. Choi and associates[15] demonstrated no difference in the age groups when comparing outcomes in 173 ankles with OLT treated arthroscopically. Patients were stratified into six age groups (<20, 20–29, 30–39, 40–49, 50–59, and >60 years).[15] All age groups had statistically significant improvements in postoperative clinical outcomes at an average of 70.3-month follow-up.[15] Even though surgical treatment has shown benefit in all age groups, some studies have shown increasing age to be correlated with poorer outcomes.[16–18] In a study by Cuttica and associates,[16] age influenced outcomes until the age of 33; after the age of 33 years, age was not correlated with worse outcomes.

The choice of surgical procedure depends on the size of the OLT, the location of the lesion, and whether initial nonoperative management has failed. Generally, larger OLT have been associated with worse outcomes. Uncontained lesions and lesions larger than 1.5 cm^2 have been associated with poor clinical outcomes and may need to be treated with an initial procedure more extensive than arthroscopic débridement and bone marrow stimulation (BMS).[16] Although some studies use an area of greater than 1.5 cm^2 to indicate a "larger" OLT, more recent evidence indicates that an area of greater than 1 cm^2 or diameter of greater than 1 cm is a poor prognostic indicator in OLT treated with BMS. A 2017 systematic review concluded that an area greater than 107.4 mm^2 or a diameter greater than 10.2 mm is a poor prognostic indicator, and BMS is appropriate for lesions smaller than this size.[19]

Location of the OLT also dictates surgical management. Most OLT occur in the centromedial (zone 4, 24%[1] to 53%[20]) and centrolateral (zone 6, 26%[20] to 49%[1]) zones of the talus (Fig. 119.3). It is important to identify posteriorly oriented OLT because they may require arthroscopic transmalleolar approaches, posterior ankle arthroscopy, or open malleolar osteotomy (Fig. 119.4). Careful history taking and review of operative reports can help determine the patient's surgical history and previous procedures. In patients with OLT and failed primary arthroscopic BMS treatment, osteochondral autologous transplantation (OATS) is a better choice than repeat arthroscopic BMS procedures.[21] Postoperative

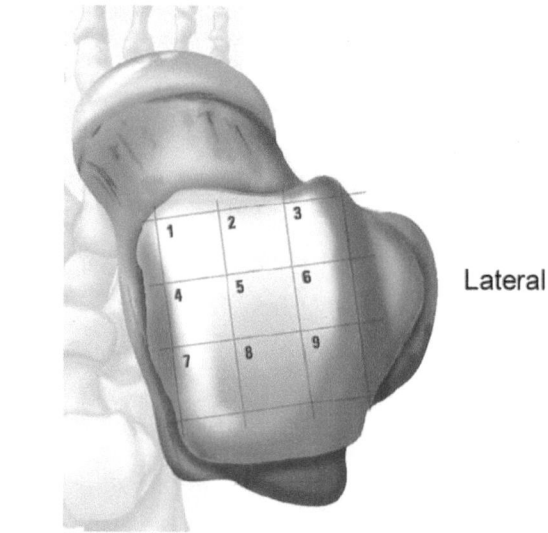

Fig. 119.3 Zones of osteochondral lesions of the talus based on a grid scheme. (From Raikin SM, Elias I, Zoga AC, et al. Osteochondral lesions of the talus: localization and morphologic data from 424 patients using a novel anatomical grid scheme. *Foot Ankle Int.* 2007;28:154–161.)

visual analog scale (VAS) and AOFAS ankle-hindfoot scales were statistically superior at 24 and 12 months, respectively, in the OATS group at an average of 48 months.[21]

Treatment Options
Nonoperative

Although it is reported to be successful in only about half of the patients,[22–26] nonoperative treatment generally should be attempted first in patients with acute nondisplaced lesions and cystic lesions (determined by CT) with or without communication to the ankle joint. In skeletally immature patients, nonoperative treatment may be tried for chronic nondisplaced surface lesions as well. Nonoperative treatment is not recommended in adult patients with chronic symptomatic nondisplaced or in any patient with a displaced lesion.[24]

Nonoperative treatment of acute, nondisplaced OLT generally involves an initial period of non–weight bearing with cast immobilization, followed by progressive weight bearing and mobilization to full ambulation by 12 to 16 weeks. The recommended duration of nonoperative treatment varies, with some authors recommending 6 months[23] and others up to 12 months[22] before operative treatment is undertaken. In patients with nondisplaced acute or traumatic OLT and MRI stage 1 or 2 OLT, we continue cast immobilization and non–weight bearing for 6 to 10 weeks. In patients with cystic or nondisplaced OLT, we prefer to try 3 to 6 months of nonoperative management before proceeding to operative treatment. Major contraindications to nonoperative management of OLT in both adults and children are acute, displaced OLT.[27]

Based on the results of nonoperative treatment of 35 chronic cystic OLT, Shearer and colleagues[24] concluded that (1) nonoperative management of chronic cystic OLT is a viable option with little or no risk for the development of significant osteoarthritis;

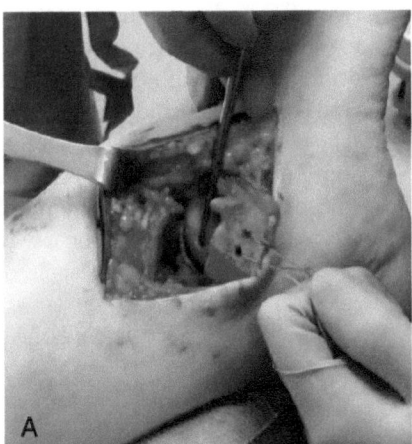 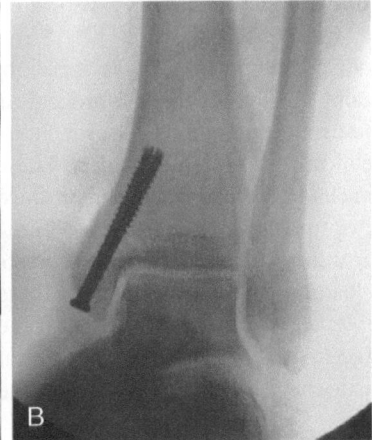

Fig. 119.4 Medial or lateral malleolar osteotomy often is necessary for treatment of posteriorly oriented osteochondral lesions of the talus (OLT) or large OLT (treated with osteochondral autologous transplantation or bulk allograft). The authors' preferred medial malleolar osteotomy is a chevron osteotomy (A) fixed with two 4.0-mm partially threaded cannulated screws (B).

(2) most lesions remain radiographically stable; (3) poor correlation exists between changes in lesion size and clinical outcome, although few patients with lesions that decrease significantly in size tend to do well, and those with lesions that increase significantly in size tend to do poorly; (4) the development of mild radiographic changes of osteoarthritis does not correlate with clinical outcome; (5) the general course of chronic cystic OLT is benign, with more than half of the patients improving to good or excellent results with nonoperative management; (6) lateral lesions tend to do better than medial ones; and (7) adult-onset lesions tend to do better than juvenile-onset lesions. Contrary to earlier reports, however, more recent investigations have determined that patient age is not an independent predictor of surgical results.[15] Alexander and Lichtman[28] suggested that a delay in treatment does not affect outcome, but more recent studies have questioned this suggestion.[17,29,30] Lesions presenting more than 1 year after injury or the onset of symptoms may have a poorer prognosis.[29]

Operative

Options for open or arthroscopic treatment of OLT generally are based on one of three specific goals: (1) stimulating the bone marrow by débridement and drilling or microfracture, with or without loose body removal; (2) stimulating the development of hyaline or hyaline-like cartilage; (3) placing osteochondral autograft or allograft; or (4) securing an acute OLT to the talar dome so that it will heal in place (Box 119.1). The choice between open and arthroscopic management depends on the comfort and skill level of the surgeon, as well as the nature and location of the OLT. More specifically, techniques include excision, débridement, curettage, drilling, and microfracture; internal fixation for acute lesions and bone grafting; osteochondral autograft or allograft procedures; autologous chondrocyte implantation (ACI); and retrograde drilling. The advent of orthobiologic and synthetic therapies has increased the treatment possibilities for OLT, but currently most have lower quantity and/or lower quality evidence (level IV and V).

Lavage, débridement, and excision and bone marrow stimulation (curettage, drilling, and microfracture). First-line

---

BOX 119.1 Surgical Treatment of Osteochondral Lesions of the Talus

Approaches
- Arthroscopic
  - Anteromedial and anterolateral portals
  - Posterior portal for posteriorly oriented lesions
  - Transmalleolar drilling techniques
- Open
  - Anterior (anterior, anterolateral, anteromedial) arthrotomy
  - Medial or lateral malleolar osteotomies for posteriorly oriented lesions

Surgical Treatments
- Débridement, loose body removal
- Bone marrow stimulation
  - Chondroplasty
  - Antegrade or retrograde drilling
  - Microfracture
- Internal fixation
  - Headless screws, bioabsorbable devices, or Kirschner wires
- Osteochondral autograft (including osteochondral autologous transplantation system)
  - Single plug
  - Double or multiple plugs (mosaicplasty)
- Osteochondral allograft (bulk allograft)
- Autologous chondrocyte implantation (traditional ACI, CACI or MACI)
- Particulated juvenile articular cartilage

Adjunctive Treatments
- Adjunctive hyaluronic acid with bone marrow stimulation
- Adjunctive platelet-rich plasma with bone marrow stimulation
- Other orthobiologic and adjunctive treatments (see text)

ACI, Autologous chondrocyte implantation; *CACI,* collagen-covered ACI; *MACI,* matrix- or membrane-induced ACI.

treatment for most smaller, chronic, symptomatic lesions includes arthroscopic lavage, débridement, and BMS. Arthroscopic lavage and débridement alone may benefit by removing catabolic cytokines and loose bodies from the ankle; however, this combination alone is no longer recommended since the addition of BMS with curettage, drilling, and microfracture has been associated with better results.[25,31]

Marrow-inducing reparative techniques, such as abrasion, drilling, and microfracture, aim to stimulate chondroprogenitor cells within the underlying marrow. Penetration of the subchondral plate allows the release of these cells into the defect. These stem cells populate the fibrin clot in the talar defect and produce a fibrocartilaginous matrix composed of chondroblasts, chondrocytes, fibrocytes, and an unorganized matrix that protects the surface from excessive loading. The disadvantage of these reparative techniques is the weaker mechanical properties of the type I collagen fibrocartilage matrix, which lacks the normal biomechanical and viscoelastic characteristics of type II hyaline cartilage.[32]

Fair grade evidence (grade B recommendation) supports BMS as a first-line treatment for the index procedure for chondral and osteochondral lesions or as a repeat procedure after failed arthroscopic management.[27,33] Recent evidence supports superior results of OATS procedures instead of repeat arthroscopic procedures with BMS after failed initial arthroscopic management.[21] Most authors use a less than 1.5-cm diameter as the boundary for a small OLT[27]; however, this boundary varies from 0.8 cm to 2.0 cm.[32] Other authors use an area of greater than 1.5 cm² to define a large OLT.[16,34] Arthroscopic results appear to be superior to those of open procedures.[27] A 2017 systematic review reported treatment with BMS had an 82.1% success rate in 10 studies (1053 patients)[19]; this was consistent with a 2010 systematic review that included 18 studies (388 patients) reporting an 85% success rate (range 46% to 100%).[26] OLT associated with cyst formation have been successfully treated with BMS alone (without bone grafting), achieving good to excellent results in 74% of patients.[35] The authors also noted no difference in postoperative AOFAS ankle-hindfoot scales between cystic and noncystic small OLT.[35] When the overlying cartilage is intact, antegrade or retrograde drilling can effectively stimulate a response. Fair

(level IV) evidence with consistently positive results is available to warrant a grade B recommendation for antegrade or retrograde drilling of OLT with intact overlying cartilage.[27] Although antegrade (transtibial) and retrograde (transtalar) drilling are technically easy, both can result in cartilage damage and osseous necrosis. Some authors advocate retrograde drilling of symptomatic OLT with the cartilage and subchondral bone intact.[36,37]

Internal fixation. Fixation devices include permanent or bioabsorbable low-profile pins, nails, or headless screws (Fig. 119.5). Acute OLT do markedly better after fixation than do chronic lesions. Lesions need to be larger than 8 mm to allow secure internal fixation.

Restoration of articular hyaline cartilage. Restorative techniques usually are recommended for defects larger than 1.5 cm².[16,38] These techniques can include osteochondral autograft and allograft, ACI (including traditional ACI, collagen-covered ACI, and matrix-induced ACI), arthroscopic allograft or autograft implantation, and fresh osteochondral graft. Platelet-rich plasma (PRP), stem cell-mediated implants, and scaffolds also aim to restore hyaline or hyaline-like cartilage. These procedures are described in more detail later in the chapter. These procedures are generally contraindicated in bipolar (kissing) lesions that involve both the tibia and the talus, as well as in patients with advanced generalized arthritis.[39,40]

Osteochondral autograft and allograft. Osteochondral autografting procedures such as OATS or mosaicplasty (multiple OATS plugs) require the harvest of grafts from a donor site, such as the lateral supracondylar ridge or intercondylar notch of the femur, for insertion into the OLT. These techniques generally are used for moderate to large grade III or IV lesions. Concerns about donor site morbidity have prompted graft harvest from sites other than the distal femur (e.g., the anterior talar dome) and the use of allografts.

Fresh-frozen allografting (bulk talar osteochondral allograft) is another option for large OLT, especially shoulder lesions and

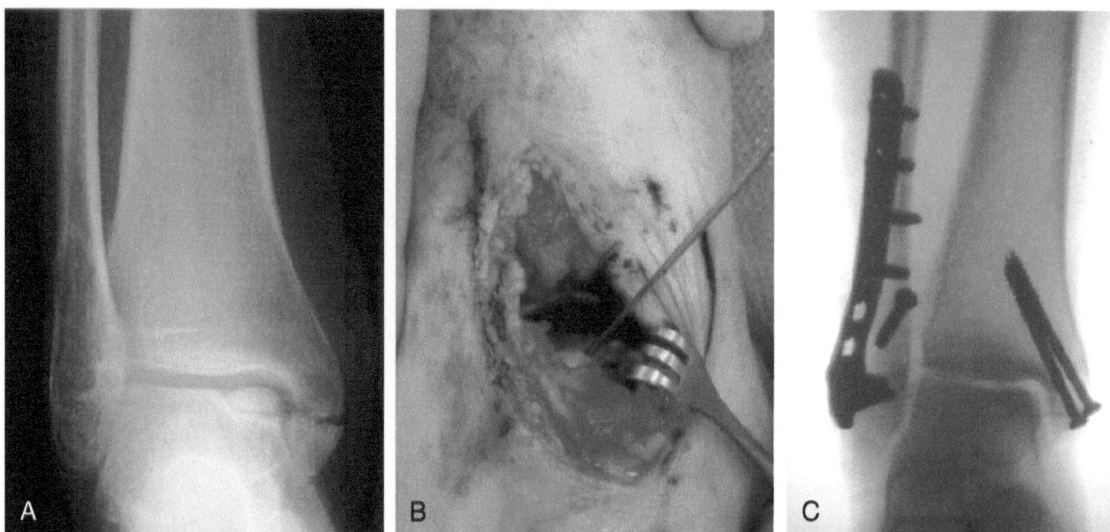

Fig. 119.5 (A) An acute osteochondral lesion of the talus associated with an ankle fracture. (B) Kirschner wire was used to predrill for placement of an absorbable pin. (C) Completed fixation. (From Richardson DR. Sports injuries of the ankle. In: Azar FM, Beaty JH, Canale ST, eds. *Campbell's Operative Orthopaedics*. 13th ed. Philadelphia: Elsevier; 2017.)

lesions with morphology that is difficult to duplicate using non-talar grafting.[41] Another benefit of this technique includes avoiding donor site morbidity. Gross and colleagues[42] listed as their indication for this procedure a lesion at least 1 cm in diameter and 5 mm deep that could not be internally fixed. Hahn and colleagues[43] listed as the following indications for a fresh-frozen allograft procedure: (1) greater than 1 cm size on one dimension on MRI, (2) greater than 6 months from last operative treatment, (3) little or no degenerative changes in the ankle, (4) functional ROM, and (5) skeletally mature patient. The average size of fresh frozen allografts implanted by Hahn et al. was 1.9 cm × 1.4 cm (2.7 cm^2); in another study the average size was 3.6 cm^2.[44] Chondrocyte viability is a primary concern, and it is essential that the graft be harvested within 24 hours of the donor's death and be stored at 4°C. One study found a minimal decrease in viability after 14 days of storage in a serum-free modified culture medium, but after 28 days, viability was significantly decreased.[45] Because most tissue banks require a 21-day screening process to minimize the risk of disease transmission and the grafts are not released for 3 days after screening is complete, the minimal time to implantation is 24 days. Other considerations, such as scheduling, can delay implantation even longer. Fortunately, the biomechanical properties of these allografts do not appear to deteriorate even after 28 days from procurement. Recent studies have suggested that, compared with current protocols, the storage of osteochondral allografts at higher temperatures (25°C and 37°C) can increase the window of opportunity for implantation of optimal tissue from 14 to 42 days after disease-testing clearance.[46,47]

Other less common autografting procedures (osteoperiosteal bone graft and free vascularized autograft). Large, chronic OLT are traditionally treated with OATS or fresh-frozen osteochondral allograft procedures. However, some authors have described surgical treatment of larger OLT with osteoperiosteal bone grafts from the distal medial tibia[48] and treatment of larger shoulder OLT with free vascularized bone grafts from the medial condyle of the femur.[49] These autograft options that are reported infrequently do not restore hyaline cartilage to the OLT.

Autologous chondrocyte implantation or transplantation traditional or matrix-induced. ACI is best suited for large and well-contained stage 3 or 4 defects, large lesions with extensive subchondral cystic changes, and lesions in which previous operative treatment has failed. According to Ferkel and Hommen,[40] the ideal patient for ACI is between 15 and 55 years old and has no malalignment, degenerative joint disease, or instability of the joint. First-generation, traditional ACI involves harvesting 200 to 300 mg of autologous chondrocytes from the distal femur, growing the cells in vitro for 2 to 5 weeks, and then implanting them into the defect. An autologous periosteal flap is harvested and sewn over the implanted cells and sealed with fibrin glue.[50] First-generation ACI (traditional ACI, periosteal ACI) is technically challenging, involves periosteal harvest, and has complications including periosteal hypertrophy, delamination, and graft failure.[51,52] Second-generation, collagen-covered ACI (CACI) involves a bioabsorbable collagen membrane.[52] Like traditional ACI, CACI involves an open procedure. Finally, third-generation, matrix- or membrane-induced ACI (MACI), involves harvesting,

seeding, and proliferating chondrocytes on type I/type III collagen membranes and implanting the membranes into OLT. Other types of matrix have been used in MACI techniques, including a mixed thrombin and fibrin gel matrix.[53]

Because of concerns about donor-site morbidity after harvest from the distal femur,[54,55] other donor sites have been suggested. Giannini and associates[41] and Kreulen and associates[56] used detached talar osteochondral and chondral fragments, while Lee and associates[53] used the cuboid surface of the calcaneocuboid joint as a source of chondrocytes.

Newer orthobiologic or synthetic therapies. Newer orthobiologic and synthetic therapies include particulated juvenile allograft cartilage (PJAC) implantation; allograft cartilage extracellular matrix (ECM); autologous matrix induced chondrogenesis (AMIC); BMS with adjunctive hyaluronic acid (HA), PRP, platelet-derived growth factor (PDGF), bone marrow aspirate (BMA) or cells, or mesenchymal stem cells (MSCs); and synthetic bone graft substitute or plugs.

PJAC implantation (*DeNovo* NT Natural Tissue Graft, Zimmer, Warsaw, IN) is a single-step procedure that is ideal for younger patients (<50 years old) with large (>1 cm^2) OLT and OLT that has failed previous microfracture.[57] The technique for PJAC involves preparing and drying the OLT bed (Fig. 119.6A), placing a fibrin glue layer (see Fig. 119.6B), laying particulated juvenile cartilage (see Fig. 119.6C), and sealing with another layer of fibrin glue (see Fig. 119.6D and E).

Allograft cartilage ECM (BioCartilage, Arthrex, Naples, FL) contains components of cartilage, including type II collagen, proteoglycans, and growth factors. Authors who have reported using allograft cartilage ECM in small OLT describe a single-step arthroscopic technique where they microfracture the OLT and then place the allograft cartilage ECM.[58]

The technique for AMIC for treatment of OLT involves microfracture, placement of a porcine collagen type I/III matrix (chondro-Gide, Geistlich Surgery), and securing the collagen matrix in place with fibrin glue (Tisseel, Baxter, Deerfield, IL).[59,60]

Adding adjunctive HA to BMS has been postulated to improve clinical outcomes and quantitative MRI findings because of its high viscosity and joint protective properties.[61–64] Adding PRP after BMS has the theoretical effect of inducing mitogenic, chemotactic, angiogenic, and differentiation platelet functions at the OLT.[62,63] Adding BMA to a scaffold boasts the advantage of a single-step, arthroscopic procedure by introducing autologous, live, iliac crest bone marrow cells to OLT.[65–67] Adding MSCs to BMS introduces cadaver-donor MSCs to aid in healing OLT by MSC differentiation into chondroblasts and osteoblasts.[68,69] Adding recombinant human PDGF with β-tricalcium phosphate carrier (rhPDGF/β-TCP) and sealing with fibrin glue after BMS theoretically induces mitogenic, chemotactic, osteoblastic, and chondroblastic activity in treating OLT.[70] There is very sparse evidence at present for rhPDGF/β-TCP in the treatment of OLT.[70]

There is inadequate evidence to support synthetic bone graft substitutes or plugs such as Tru-fit (Smith & Nephew, Andover, MA), which is made of calcium triphosphate bone substitute with poly DL-lactide-coglycolide cartilage substitute.[71]

Although the advent of these orthobiologic and synthetic therapies has increased the possibilities in the treatment of OLT,

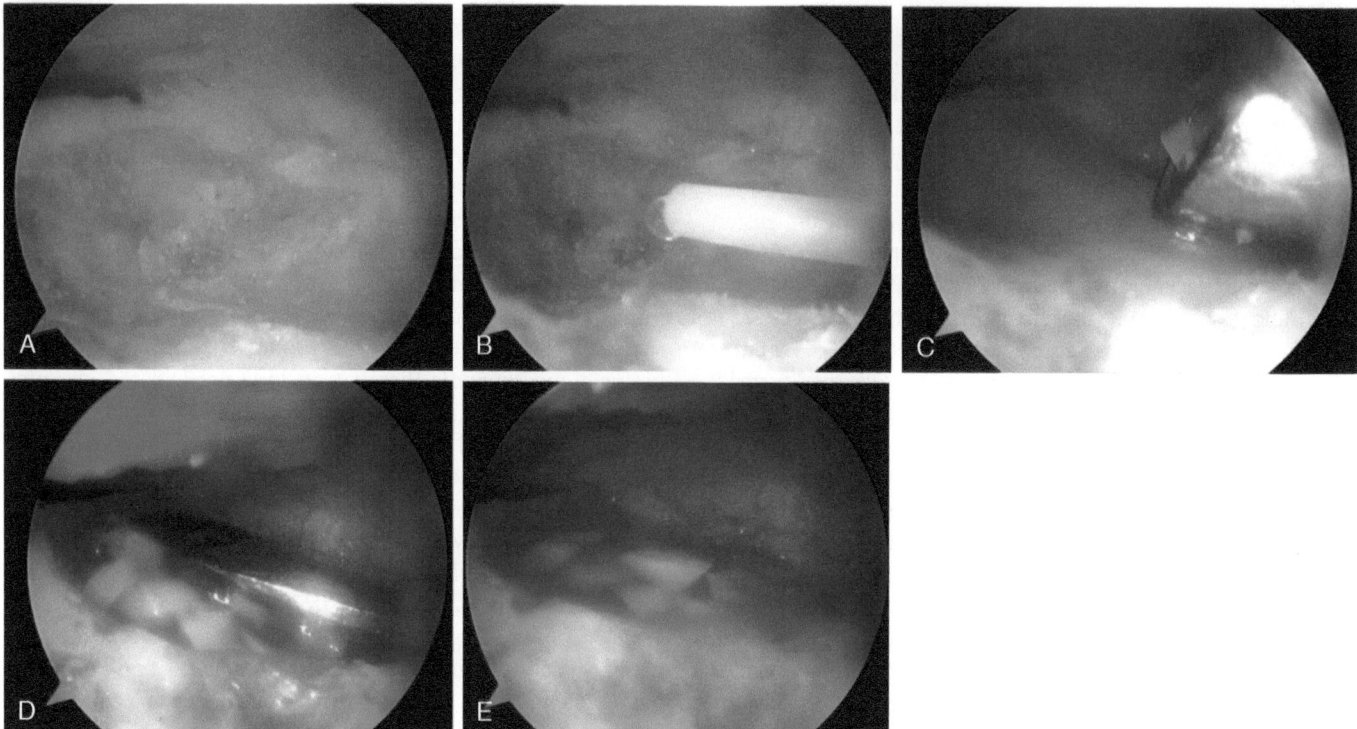

Fig. 119.6 Technique for arthroscopic particulate juvenile articular cartilage implantation. (A) The bed of the osteochondral lesion is prepared with usual débridement and curettage. The joint is cleared of arthroscopy fluid and the bed of the osteochondral lesion is dried. (B) The base fibrin glue layer is placed at the bony base of the osteochondral lesion. (C) The particulated juvenile cartilage is delivered through a cannula. (D) The cartilage layer is smoothed and spread with a Freer elevator or appropriate tool. (E) The particulated juvenile cartilage is sealed with another layer of fibrin glue and allowed to set.

there are few studies with higher quality evidence supporting these treatments in the current literature.

Results

Most of the OLT literature consists of case series (level IV evidence) and retrospective cohort studies (level III evidence), with few prospective cohort studies or randomized controlled studies (level I and II evidence). For some of the techniques, the numbers are too small and the follow-up is too short to make definitive recommendations. There also are variations in the techniques used to measure the size of OLT, and CT and MR images will result in different-sized measurements of OLT. This should be taken into consideration when reading and interpreting studies related to OLT.

Noninvasive follow-up after cartilage repair techniques such as microfracture, OATS, or ACI has become more common. To avoid the use of ambiguous terms, postoperative cartilage changes have been described in the literature with use of the magnetic resonance observation of cartilage repair tissue (MOCART) scoring system.[72] This scoring system describes the hyaline and fibrocartilage structure, the degree of defect filling, and the native border integration, as well as characteristics of the subchondral lamina and bone (Box 119.2).

Conservative or Nonoperative Management

Shearer and colleagues[24] reviewed the results fot nonsurgical management of 35 OLT and concluded that nonsurgical

---

BOX 119.2   Variables in Magnetic Resonance Observation of Cartilage Repair Tissue

- Degree of defect repair and filling of defect (complete, hypertrophy, incomplete)
- Integration to border zone (complete, incomplete)
- Surface of repaired tissue (intact, damaged)
- Structure of repaired tissue (homogenous, inhomogenous)
- Signal intensity
- Subchondral lamina (intact, not intact)
- Subchondral bone (intact, not intact)
- Adhesions (absent, present)
- Effusion (absent, present)

See original article cited for full description.
From Marlovits S, Singer P, Zeller P, et al. Magnetic resonance observation of cartilage repair tissue (MOCART) for the evaluation of autologous chondrocyte transplantation: determination of interobserver variability and correlation to clinical outcome after 2 years. *Eur J Radiol.* 2006;57:16–23.

management of chronic cystic (stage 5) OLT is a viable option with little or no risk for the development of osteoarthritis. Their clinical results were good or excellent in 54%, fair in 17%, and poor in 29%.[24] Shelton and Pedowitz[73] reported just 25% satisfactory results after nonoperative treatment of stage 2 and 3 lesions. Klammer and colleagues[13] reported 43 minimally or nonsymptomatic OLT with a minimum size of 4 mm in patients who elected nonoperative treatment. The average size of the lesions at initial MRI was 9.6 mm width × 15.6 mm length × 8.6 mm depth.[24] The authors concluded that these OLT did not enlarge in size and the ankles did not show progression of arthritis.[24] A systematic review of 14 studies with a total of 201 patients showed only a 45% success rate of nonsurgical treatment of stage 1 and 2 and medial grade 3 OLT, and nonoperative treatment of chronic lesions had a success rate of 56%.[25]

Operative Management

Lavage, débridement, and excision, and bone marrow stimulation (curettage, drilling, and microfracture). In their systematic review, Verhagen and colleagues[25] concluded the highest success rate was obtained with excision, curettage, and drilling, followed by excision and curettage, and subsequently followed by curettage alone. Excision alone had an overall success rate of 38%, with a range of 30% to 100% in individual studies. Excision and curettage had a success rate of 76% (range, 53% to 100%). Excision, curettage, and drilling or BMS had a success rate of 85% (range, 33% to 100%). Arthroscopic procedures had a higher success rate (84%) than did open procedures (63%). Good to excellent results after BMS have been reported in 28% to 93% of patients. Ferkel and Hommen[40] reported 72% excellent or good results in 64 patients; Taranow and coworkers[37] reported an 81% success rate in 16 patients with retrograde drilling at an average of 24 months follow-up; and Becher and Thermann[74] reported 83% excellent and good results and 17% satisfactory results in 30 patients at an average follow-up of 2 years after microfracture. A 2017 systematic review assessed 1868 ankles with OLT in 25 studies treated with BMS[19] and determined that BMS for treatment of OLT generally improves postoperative outcomes. Fourteen studies demonstrated an improvement of AOFAS ankle–hindfoot scale from 62.4 preoperatively to 83.9 postoperatively; 10 studies reported an 82.1% successful outcome at an average 56-month follow-up.[19]

Polat and colleagues[75] reported the long-term results (average 121.3 months follow-up, range 61 to 217 months) of arthroscopy and microfracture in 82 patients with OLT with an average size of 1.7 ± 0.7 cm². The patients had sustained improved postoperative results of AOFAS ankle–hindfoot scales (85.5) and VAS (1.8). The authors documented no grade 4 arthritis; however, 32.9% of patients had one grade progression of arthritis.

To determine whether the presence of a subchondral cyst affected the results of arthroscopic microfracture or abrasion arthroplasty, Han and colleagues[35] compared the results in 20 defects that included cysts with those in 18 defects that did not include cysts and found no differences in the clinical results. They concluded that small cystic lesions can be successfully treated by arthroscopic microfracture or abrasion arthroplasty. At an average follow-up of 48 months, Lee and associates[76] found no functional or radiographic differences in outcomes in 102 cystic and noncystic smaller OLT (<2.0 cm²) treated with arthroscopy and BMS. The average size of the cystic and noncystic OLT was 100.9 mm² and 99.3 mm², respectively. No OLT were treated with bone grafting.

Lesion size may play a role in microfracture outcomes. Choi and associates[77] reported that lesions larger than 150 mm², as calculated on MRI, have a statistically significant increased risk of clinical failure (80% failure rate vs. 10.5% failure of lesions smaller than 150 mm²). Cuttica and colleagues[16] also reported that patients with OLT larger than 1.5 cm² had worse outcomes (odds ratio, 1.4). A 2017 systematic review concluded that lesions larger than 107.4 mm² or larger than 10.2 mm in diameter is a poor prognostic indicator, and BMS is more appropriate for OLT smaller than this size.[19]

Savva and coworkers[78] described repeat arthroscopic débridement without drilling or microfracture in 12 of 215 patients who had arthroscopic treatment of OLT; at an average 6-year follow-up, results were good in all 12 patients, and 8 had returned to their preinjury levels of sports.

Autologous cancellous bone grafting. Saxena and Eakin[79] treated stages 2 through 4 OLT in 26 ankles with microfracture techniques and 20 stage 5 OLT with corticocancellous autologous bone grafting from the medial malleolus. Overall, 96% of patients had excellent or good results, and no difference was found between the groups with regard to the percentages of those who returned to sports and postoperative AOFAS ankle–hindfoot scales. In patients participating in high-demand sports, stage 5 OLT treated with bone grafting required a longer time to return to activity than did stages 2 to 4 OLT treated with microfracture. Patients with anterolateral lesions had the fastest return to activity and the highest AOFAS ankle-hindfoot scales. Draper and Fallat[80] retrospectively compared the results of 14 patients with larger OLT treated with bone grafting with those of 17 patients with smaller OLT treated with curettage and drilling. At almost 5-year follow-up, patients who had bone grafting had better ROM and less pain. The studies by Saxena and Eakin[79] and Draper and Fallat[80] were both retrospective and admittedly their results are confounding because the groups treated with bone grafting had different OLT (in stage or size) than the BMS alone group. Not all authors have experienced such good results with bone grafting. Kolker and colleagues[81] reported that 6 of 13 patients required further surgery after open antegrade autologous bone grafting and concluded that autologous bone grafting alone should not be used as primary treatment for patients with symptomatic advanced OLT and deficient or absent overlying cartilage.

Few studies have been performed on the retrograde drilling of OLT. Techniques vary widely from fluoroscopy-controlled to computer-guided systems with fixed bony referencing. Anders and colleagues[82] demonstrated improved AOFAS ankle-hindfoot scales and decreased VAS after retrograde drilling in 41 OLT with intact cartilage at a mean follow-up of 29 months; however, disrupted surface integrity resulted in poorer outcomes. Gras and coworkers[83] showed an 86% decrease in surgical time using a Fluoro-Free navigation procedure.

Osteochondral autografts (osteochondral autologous transplantation system, mosaicplasty). Scranton and associates[84] reported 90% good to excellent results in 50 patients with stage 5 OLT at an average 3-year follow-up after osteochondral autograft transplantation using a single, arthroscopically-harvested graft from the distal femur. Of their 50 patients, 32 (64%) had at least one previous operation that failed to relieve symptoms. Hangody and colleagues[85] described good to excellent results in 34 of 36 patients 2 to 7 years after mosaicplasty. Kreuz and coworkers[86] used mosaicplasty procedures for the treatment of 35 OLT after failure of arthroscopic excision, curettage, and drilling. The osteochondral graft was harvested from the ipsilateral talar facet, and a malleolar or tibial wedge osteotomy was used to access central or posterior lesions. Although no nonunions of the osteotomies occurred, patients with small osteochondral lesions accessible through an anterior approach without additional osteotomy had the best results. Haleem and associates[87] showed no difference in functional outcomes and MOCART in 14 patients treated with double-plug OATS procedures compared to a matched cohort of 28 patients treated with single-plug OATS procedures at a mean follow-up of 85 months. The double-plug OATS procedure was indicative of larger-sized OLT (average 208 ± 54 mm^2). Liu and coworkers[88] treated 16 acute stages 3 and 4 osteochondral fractures of the talar dome associated with ankle fractures with OATS at the time of fixation of the ankle fracture. They reported excellent postoperative AOFAS ankle-hindfoot scales of 95.4, no posttraumatic arthritis, and 93.7% osteointegration on MRI at the 3-year average follow-up. Liu and coworkers[88] recommended OATS for acute, mostly cartilaginous, comminuted, unstable OLT at the time of ankle fracture fixation. Improved results also have been correlated with normal integration or minor incongruity of the transplant on follow-up MRI.[89]

Osteochondral allografts. Although several studies have reported good results with osteochondral allografts in the knee, the literature includes smaller, retrospective studies of osteochondral allografts in the ankle. Gross and associates[42] reported that six of nine allografts remained in situ with a mean survival rate of 11 years; three patients required ankle arthrodesis because of graft resorption and fragmentation. Hahn and coworkers[43] reported 4-year average follow-up of 13 patients with larger OLT (>1.0 cm in one dimension) treated with fresh allografts. The OLT averaged 1.9 cm (A/P) × 1.4 cm (M/L) in size. The authors reported five reoperations. However, there were significant improvements in functional outcomes; all patients returned to activities at 1 year; all patients would have the procedure again; and 11 of 13 patients returned to high impact activities. Görtz and colleagues[44] reported that, at 3-year follow-up, 10 of 12 fresh osteochondral allografts (average 3.6 cm^2; range, 1.7 to 6.0 cm^2) had incorporated, 1 patient eventually required arthrodesis, and there was overall improvement in functional outcome scores.

Lesions on the talar shoulder are challenging to treat because of cartilage geometry and loss of articular buttress. Allografts may be considered in these situations when other traditional treatment options would be difficult.[90–92] Adams and associates[90] reported eight patients who, at the 48-month follow-up, had decreased pain and increased function after undergoing an osteochondral allograft. Half required an additional procedure, but none required ankle arthrodesis or arthroplasty even though five had radiographic lucencies at the graft-host interface. Raikin[91] reported good or excellent results in 11 of 15 patients treated with allografts for large-volume cysts (a mean of 6059 mm^3) in the talar dome at an average 54-month follow-up. A systematic review by VanTienderen and associates[92] reported on 91 patients (90 ankles) in five studies that were treated for large OLTs (average 3751 mm^3) with bulk fresh-frozen osteochondral allograft. This systematic review

highlights the challenging nature of treating large OLT; 25.3% of patients underwent reoperation and 13.2% of cases were considered failures (requiring eventual arthrodesis or arthroplasty).

Autologous chondrocyte implantation or transplantation. Koulalis and colleagues[93] reported excellent to good results at 17-month follow-up in all eight of their patients treated with traditional, first-generation ACI. Whittaker and associates[94] described traditional ACI in 10 patients, 9 of whom were "pleased" or "extremely pleased" with their results at 4-year follow-up; however, 1 year after surgery, Lysholm knee scores had returned to preoperative levels in only 3 patients, suggesting donor-site morbidity in the other 7 patients. Baums and coworkers[39] reported 12 patients with traditional ACI of the talus for defects that averaged 2.3 cm^2. At the 63-month follow-up, 7 had excellent results, 4 had good results, and 1 had a satisfactory result. The mean AOFAS ankle-hindfoot scales improved from 43.5 before surgery to 85.5 after surgery. Six patients who had been involved in competitive sports were all able to return to their full activity levels. However, a more recent large retrospective case series suggests that patients tend to modify their return to play (RTP) by decreasing their participation in contact and high-impact sports.[95]

Second-generation CACI has not become as popular as traditional ACI and MACI. Lee and coworkers[53] reported 38 patients treated with ACI harvested from the cuboid surface of the calcaneus and implanted with fibrin-matrix mixed gel-type ACI, a second-generation technique. They reported a significant improvement in postoperative VAS and functional outcomes (AOFAS ankle-hindfoot scales and HSS score) at the 12- and 24-month follow-ups, but mixed results on re-look arthroscopy and complications associated with medial malleolar osteotomy (9/31 cartilage damage, two delayed unions, one nonunion). The AOFAS ankle-hindfoot scale was not associated with International Cartilage Repair System score on re-look arthroscopy.

Several small studies reported improvement in outcomes with third-generation, matrix-induced ACI (MACI) when looking at markers of outcome preoperatively compared to postoperatively. Kreulen and colleagues[96] described nine patients with OLT treated with MACI at a follow-up of 7 years, and demonstrated improvement in AOFAS ankle-hindfoot scales, short form-36 (SF-36) physical function, and pain. Dixon and coworkers[97] reported 27 patients with 28 grafts at a mean follow-up of 3.7 years, concluding that younger patients had better outcomes. Specifically, after MACI procedures, younger patients had less moderate/daily pain on the AOFAS ankle–hindfoot scale, were less likely to be impaired from recreational activities (36% ≤ 40 years vs. 78% >40 years), were more likely to return to running (82% ≤ 40 years vs. 23% >40 years), and to have improved MOCART assessments. The authors reported three graft failures (detachment of graft) confirmed by MRI, one medial malleolar osteotomy, one reflex sympathetic dystrophy (RSD), three graft overgrowths treated with arthroscopy, one wound issue, two implant removals, and two patients with very low AOFAS scores (one of which was the RSD patient). Anders and associates[98] described sustained improvement of AOFAS ankle–hindfoot scales, VAS, Tegener activity level, and MOCART scores in 22 patients with full-thickness cartilage lesions an average of 63.5 months after treatment with MACI (MOCART scores improved until 2 years, and then plateaued).

The authors reported no major complications. Apprich and colleagues[99] compared 10 ankles treated with microfracture to 10 treated with MACI in matched patients with similar demographics and AOFAS ankle-hindfoot scales. Using MOCART scores on 3-Tesla MRI, repaired tissue treated with MACI was more similar to healthy articular cartilage than repaired tissue treated with microfracture.

A 2012 meta-analysis of 16 studies reporting the use of ACI for OLT led to inconclusive results.[100] The meta-analysis included PACI and MACI procedures. All studies were level IV case studies and failed to show a superiority or inferiority of ACI compared with microfracture or other surgical techniques.

Newer Orthobiologics, Adjuncts, and Future Considerations

A prospective, randomized, level I study in 57 patients suggested that improved pain and function scores were obtained if microfracture was supplemented with a postoperative HA injection.[61] Another study by Shang and associates[64] supported the use of adjunctive HA with microfracture, reporting statistically significantly improved AOFAS ankle-hindfoot scales (87.6 vs. 80.8), VAS (2.1 vs. 3.1), and quantitative MRI outcomes in the microfracture with adjunctive HA group compared to microfracture alone in 35 patients.

Orthobiologic techniques continue to be developed; however, the evidence demonstrating benefit remains variable. PRP has been used in multiple orthopedic indications, including the treatment of OLT. In a level II study of 30 OLT, Mei-Dan and coworkers[63] showed better AOFAS ankle-hindfoot scales, short-term pain reduction (6 months) and less stiffness after PRP injection compared to HA in the nonoperative treatment of OLT. The exact indications for the use of PRP, as well as its many different proprietary concentrations and configurations, have not yet been well established. In a nonblinded study of 35 patients, Guney and associates[101] reported better AOFAS ankle-hindfoot scales, Foot and Ankle Ability Measure (FAAM), and VAS in patients with OLT treated with microfracture and PRP compared to microfracture alone at an average of 16 months after surgery. One group of authors has published several articles about bone marrow-derived cell transplantation[66,67,102] as a one-step arthroscopic option for treatment of OLT. In their most recent description of 49 patients with 4-year follow-up, they reported a peak improvement of AOFAS ankle-hindfoot scales at 24 months, and then a slight decline at 36 and 48 months;

MOCART scores improved postoperatively and did not correlate with clinical outcome.[67]

Kim and colleagues[68,69] compared the use of MSCs with BMS to BMS alone and found statistically significant better postoperative AOFAS ankle–hindfoot scales, VAS, Roles and Maudsley score, Tegner score, and MOCART score in the group treated with adjunctive MSCs. One study by Kim and associates[68] looked at an older cohort (>50 years old) only. Interestingly, another study by Kim and coworkers[69] found a correlation between MOCART scores and functional outcomes.

Coetzee and associates[103] reported outcomes of 24 ankles in 23 patients treated with PJAC; at an average follow-up of 16.2 months, 78% had AOFAS ankle–hindfoot scales greater than 80 (good or excellent) and a mean VAS of 24. There was one graft delamination and six reoperations, including implant removal, treatment of impingement, and arthroscopic débridement. In a systematic review (33 ankles) and report of a case series of six patients treated with PJAC, Saltzman and colleagues[104] showed short-term postoperative benefits in pain and function.

Ahmad and Maltenfort[58] described primary treatment of 30 small (≤1.5 cm^2) OLT with allograft cartilage ECM (BioCartilage, Arthrex, Naples, FL). Allograft cartilage ECM contains components of cartilage, including type II collagen, proteoglycans, and growth factors. At an average of 20.2 months after arthroscopic microfracture and allograft ECM, there were improvements in VAS and FAAM scores. The study does not compare the use of microfracture and allograft cartilage ECM to microfracture alone.

Two studies by Usuelli and colleagues[59] and D'Ambrosi and colleagues[60] reported short-term results (24-month follow-up) of AMIC. Both studies describe arthroscopic treatment of OLT with microfracture and placement of a porcine collagen type I/III matrix, which was secured in place with fibrin glue. Usuelli and colleagues[59] examined 37 patients with average OLT size of 153.5 mm^2 on MRI, while D'Ambrosi and colleagues[60] examined 11 young patients (average 17.9 years old) with average OLT size of 132.2 mm^2. Both studies demonstrated postoperative improvements in VAS, AOFAS ankle–hindfoot scales, SF-12, and cross-sectional imaging. Neither study compared AMIC to another method of treatment.

To our knowledge, PDGF has yet to demonstrate benefit in OLT; one study discussed proof of concept of PDGF in OLT.[70] Other novel or lesser known surgical techniques, including osteoperiosteal cylinder autografts,[48] vascularized bone grafting,[49] and computer-assisted retrograde drilling,[36,83] have yet to become mainstream in the treatment of OLT.

Authors' Preferred Techniques
Osteochondral Lesions of the Talus

Arthroscopy, Débridement, and Bone Marrow Stimulation
For a stage 1 or 2 OLT, non–weight bearing in a cast or boot is first tried for 6 to 10 weeks, depending on the size of the lesion. If this strategy fails to relieve symptoms, arthroscopic excision, curettage, and BMS (microfracture or drilling) is performed as follows:
- View anterolateral lesions through an anteromedial portal, with instrumentation for drilling, excision, or pinning inserted through an anterolateral portal, changing portals as necessary for optimal viewing and fixation.

- Posteromedial lesions can be more difficult to view and treat. With noninvasive distraction (Fig. 119.7A) and use of a small, 2.7-mm arthroscope (see Fig. 119.7C) in the anterolateral portal, most posteromedial lesions can be treated through anteromedial and posterolateral portals (see Fig. 119.7B).
- Other helpful instruments are curved and open-ended curettes (see Fig. 119.7C and D), a small 2.7-mm full-radius resector, and a small 2.7-mm burr.
- Use a small, curved curette to débride the OLT and/or a curved microfracture awl to make perforations in the subchondral bone.

Continued

Authors' Preferred Technique

Osteochondral Lesions of the Talus—cont'd

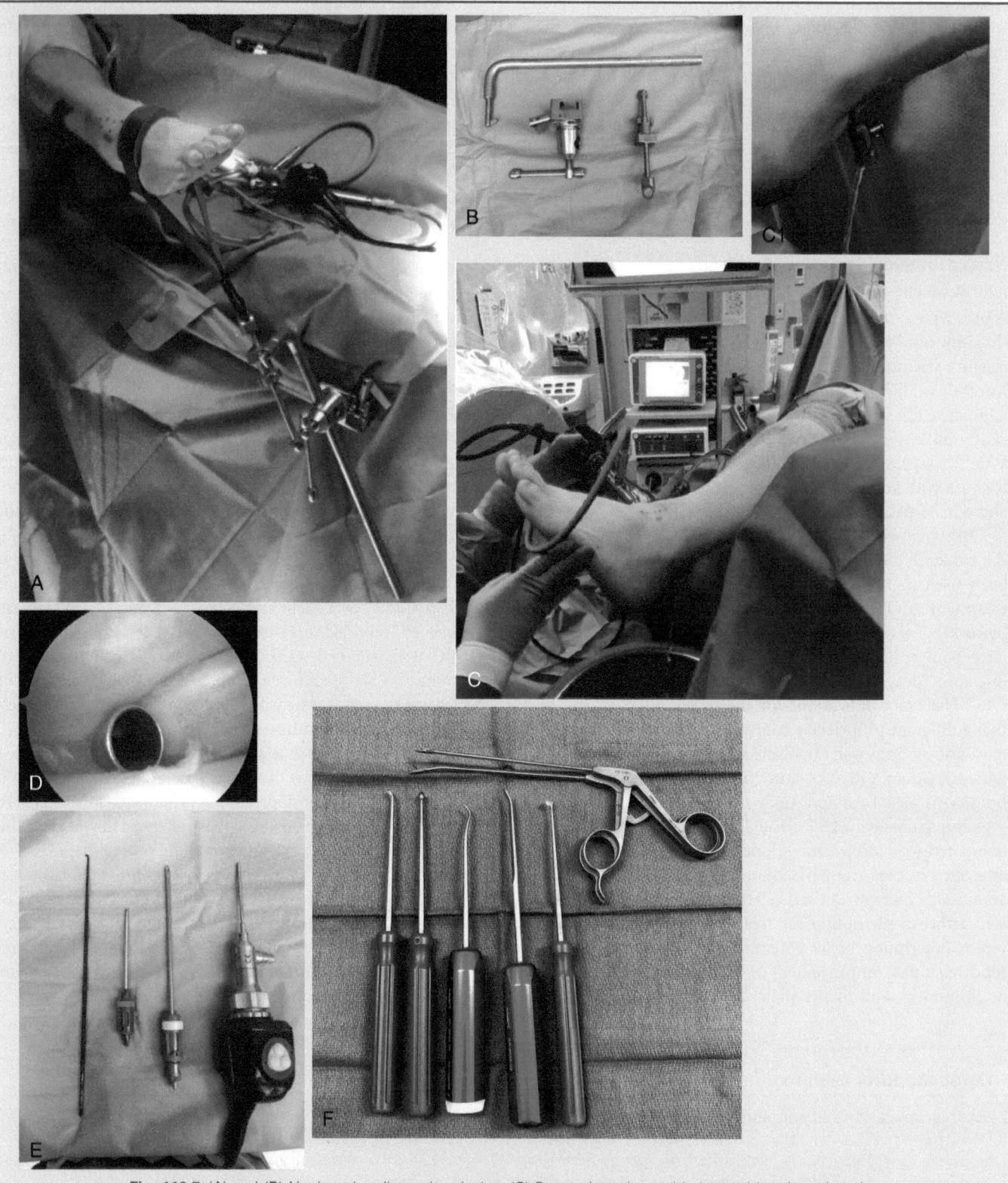

Fig. 119.7 (A) and (B) Noninvasive distraction device. (C) Posterolateral portal is located just lateral to the lateral edge of the Achilles tendon at the level of the ankle joint. Arthroscopy and fluoroscopy are helpful to confirm proper placement of the portal. (D) Anterior intra-articular view of posterolateral portal. Small-joint instrumentation for ankle arthroscopy includes (E) probe, 3-mm shaver, 3-mm burr, and small-joint 2.9-mm, 30-degree arthroscope and (F) ring curettes and picks.

Authors' Preferred Technique

Osteochondral Lesions of the Talus—cont'd

- If needed, make a small bony trough on the anteromedial tibia to improve access to posterior lesions.
- If the lesion still is not accessible, use a guide to place a Kirschner wire through the medial malleolus (transmalleolar approach) for drilling of the lesion (Fig. 119.8).
- A malleolar osteotomy may be required for open treatment of larger lesions.
- For lesions with intact overlying cartilage, use a retrograde drilling technique. This technique can be used for lesions of both the talus and the tibial plafond.
  - Identify the lesion arthroscopically and with the use of fluoroscopy.
  - Through a separate portal, insert a targeting drill guide similar to those used in ACL reconstructions but smaller and made specifically for ankle arthroscopy and direct it at the lesion. This procedure allows precise placement of the guidewire up to, but not through, the intact cartilage of the lesion. Place a drill over the guidewire with the use of fluoroscopy and pass it through the sclerotic zone, using a "loss-of-resistance" technique. Take care not to perforate the chondral surface.
- The use of a noninvasive ankle distractor will help with visualization of posterior lesions.
- If the lesion is associated with a large cyst, use a bone graft to fill the void (Fig. 119.9). Some experts advise bone grafting for cysts greater than 6 mm,[105] but a more recent article by Lee and colleagues[76] suggests that BMS alone in small OLT resulted in no difference between cystic and noncystic OLT.

Osteochondral Autologous Transplantation and Mosaicplasty Procedure

- For stage 3 or 4 OLT in skeletally mature patients, arthroscopic microfracture or drilling is the first choice, and good results have been obtained in about 90% of our patients (Fig. 119.10). If this option fails to relieve symptoms, an

OATS (for lesions <1.5 cm²; Table 119.1) or osteochondral allograft (for lesions >1.5 cm²) is used, as follows[43,91,106,107]:

- After administration of general anesthesia, prepare the affected lower extremity from the ankle to the knee. Examine the ankle arthroscopically to further delineate the chondral lesion.
- OATS are made for lesions 5 to 11 mm (larger sizes also are available) and mosaicplasty technique may be used for larger lesions.
- The approach for autograft insertion in OATS is determined by the size and location of the lesion. Lesions in the anterior third of the talus can be reached through a standard anterior approach with a plafondplasty and maximal plantar flexion of the ankle. An anterior approach avoids osteotomy of the medial malleolus or fibula; however, an approach through a malleolar osteotomy allows more direct access to central and posterior lesions.[106]
- Approach lateral lesions through an anterolateral incision and perform a medial malleolar osteotomy for medial lesions. Rarely, a lateral malleolar osteotomy will be needed to access posterolateral lesions.
- Use a commercially available recipient sizer and harvester to create a recipient hole for the donor osteochondral plug. Extract the plug to a depth of 10 mm (Fig. 119.11A and B). Place the harvester perpendicular for dome lesions and at 45 degrees for talar shoulder lesions.
- Drill multiple holes into the subchondral bone of the recipient OLT hole.
- Obtain a graft from the ipsilateral knee, arthroscopically from the medial femoral condyle or from the lateral femoral condyle through a small incision. For talar shoulder lesions, obtain a graft from the lateral trochlea.
- Use the specially designed donor harvester to obtain osteochondral grafts that measure 5 to 11 mm in diameter and 10 to 12 mm in depth (slightly deeper than the recipient hole) (see Fig. 119.11C and D).

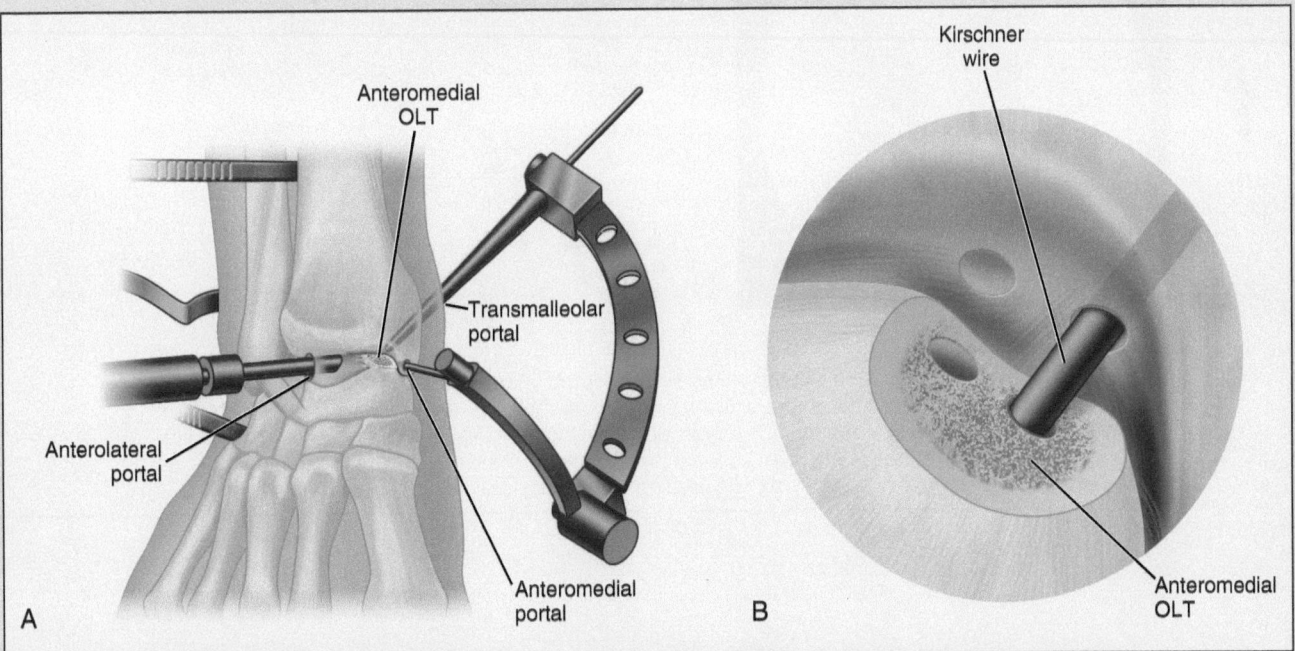

Fig. 119.8 (A) Transmalleolar drilling of an osteochondral lesion of the talus (*OLT*) using a guide. The scope is in the anterolateral portal, and inflow is through the posterolateral portal. (B) Holes are drilled through the medial malleolus into the talus down to areas of bleeding bone. (From Ferkel RD. Arthroscopy of the ankle and foot. In: Mann RA, Coughlin MJ, eds. *Surgery of the Foot and Ankle.* 8th ed. Philadelphia: Elsevier; 2006.)

Continued

📌 **Authors' Preferred Technique**

Osteochondral Lesions of the Talus—cont'd

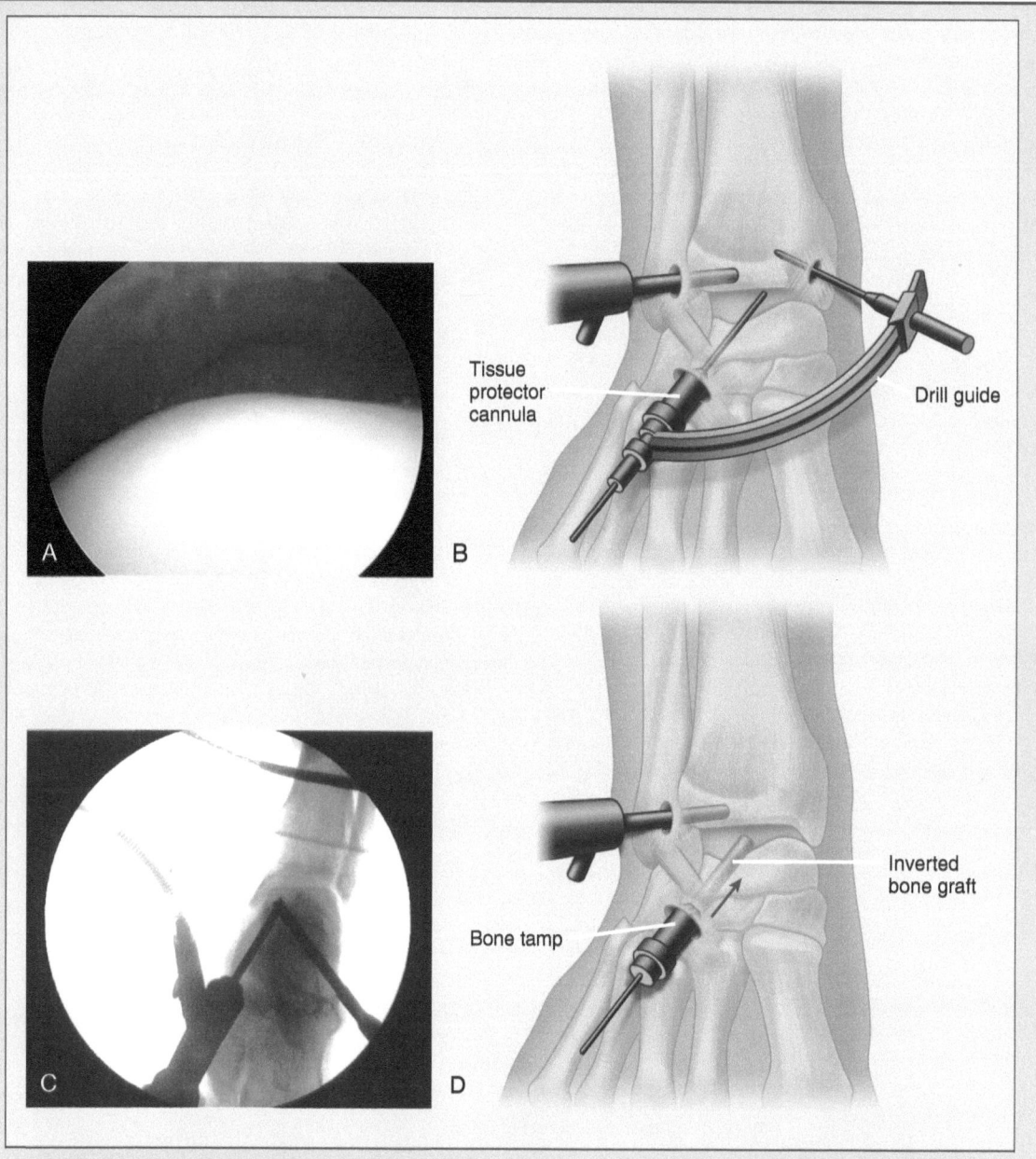

Fig. 119.9 Retrograde drilling of an osteochondral lesion. (A) Intact articular cartilage is confirmed arthroscopically. (B) A guide pin is placed through the sinus tarsi with use of modified ligament guide. (C) A subchondral lesion is drilled in a retrograde fashion. (D) A graft is placed into the channel and gently compressed into position with a tamp and mallet. ([B] and [D], From Richardson DR. Sports injuries of the ankle. In: Canale ST, Beaty JH, eds. *Campbell's Operative Orthopaedics.* 12th ed. Philadelphia: Elsevier; 2013.)

📌 Authors' Preferred Technique

Osteochondral Lesions of the Talus—cont'd

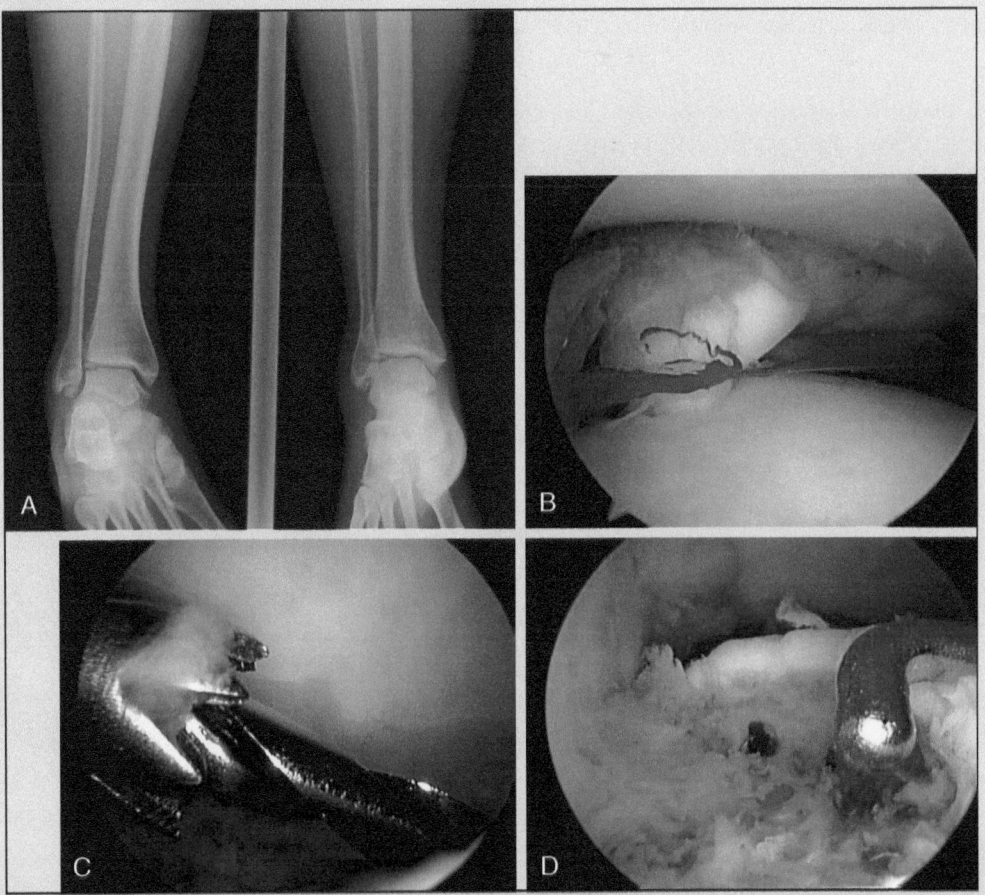

Fig. 119.10 (A) A stage 4 osteochondral lesion of the talus. (B) An arthroscopic view of a displaced osteochondral fragment. (C) Arthroscopic excision and drilling. (D) Note vascular channels created in the defect.

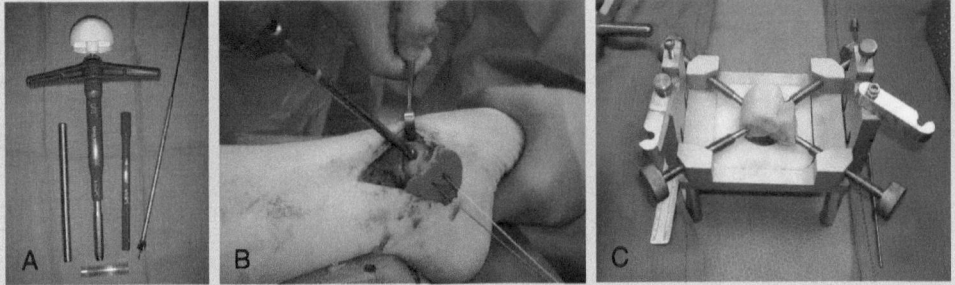

Fig. 119.11 Osteochondral autograft and allograft transplantation. (A) Instrumentation for osteochondral autologous transplantation including *(from left)* harvester and drill guide pin with cannulated headed reamer. (B) Cannulated headed reamer. A plug 10 to 12 mm deep is removed from the recipient site. (C) Donor graft in the harvester.

Continued

🔖 Authors' Preferred Technique

Osteochondral Lesions of the Talus—cont'd

- Insert the cylindrical grafts carefully into the recipient hole using the designed extruder or collared pin through the donor harvester (see Fig. 119.11E and F).
- Do not remove the OATS harvester before completion of full graft extrusion, and do not allow the harvester to deviate from the insertion angle; either maneuver may cause fracture of the donor core.
- Use the sizer-tamp to gently tamp the core flush with the surrounding cartilage. Flush graft placement is important to restore near-normal joint contact pressure. An elevated graft significantly increases contact pressure at the graft site, and a recessed graft transfers excess pressure from the graft to the native cartilage rim.[107]
- In mosaicplasty, these steps are repeated until the OLT is filled (see Fig. 119.7G).
- Test ROM of the ankle to ensure that the graft is well seated and secured.
- The malleolar osteotomy is secured with two partially threaded cancellous screws (holes are predrilled before the osteotomy) (see Fig. 119.7H and I).

- Close the incision and secure the osteotomy in the usual fashion. Place one drain in the knee and apply a compressive dressing to the ankle. Apply a posterior splint with strips.

Bulk Osteochondral Allograft Procedure

- For very large lesions (more than 3 cm³), bulk allografts can be harvested from an ipsilateral donor talus (see Fig. 119.7J).
- After direct access is obtained, resect, measure, and template the defect to allow a matched resection from the talar allograft.
- Graft any remaining cystic lesions with cancellous bone chips before allograft placement.
- Insert the allograft into the resected area to recreate the native morphology.
- Fixation of the allograft with headless screws[91] or bioabsorbable pins[43] is required for these bulk osteochondral allografts.

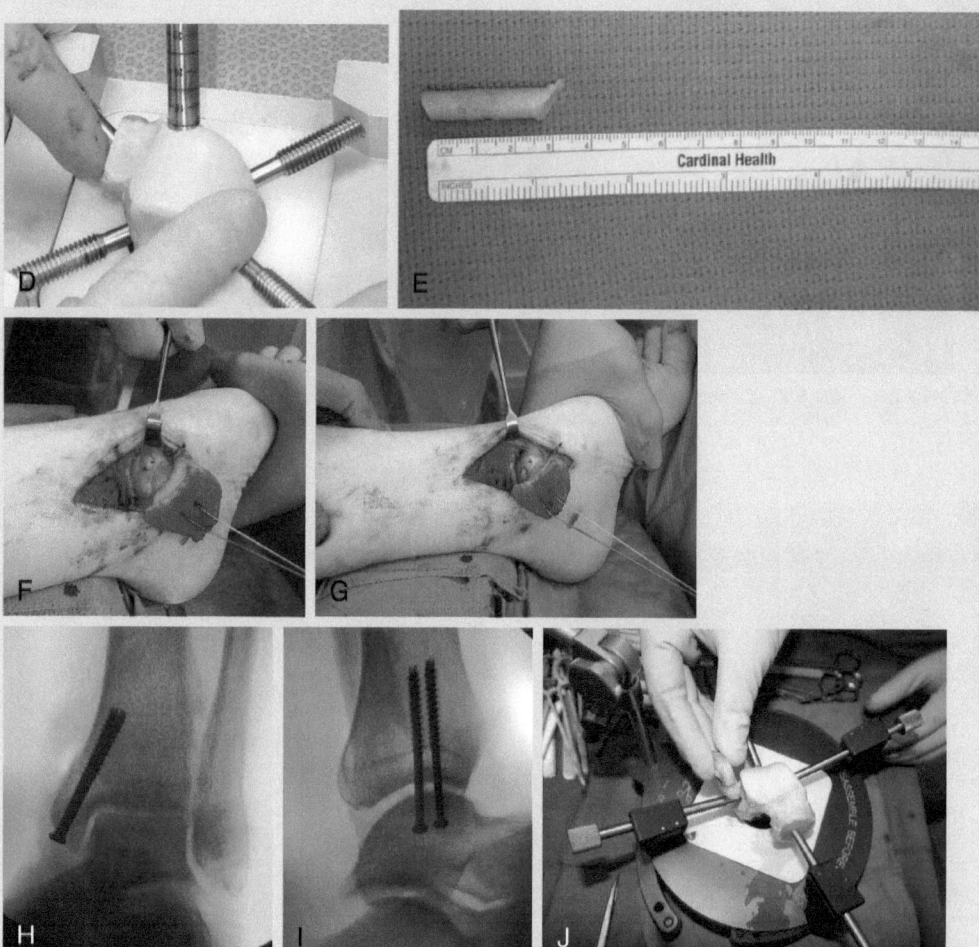

Fig. 119.11, cont'd (D) Obtain osteochondral grafts that measure 5 to 11 mm in diameter and 10 to 12 mm in depth (slightly deeper than the recipient hole). (E) and (F) The graft is placed in the recipient hole. Note the blue marks made to place the graft in the correct orientation. (G) In mosaicplasty, these steps are repeated until the osteochondral lesions of the talus is filled. (H) and (I) The malleolar osteotomy is secured with two partially threaded cancellous screws (holes are predrilled before the osteotomy). (J) Bulk osteochondral allograft.

📌 Authors' Preferred Technique

Osteochondral Lesions of the Talus—cont'd

TABLE 119.1	Authors' Preferred Treatment of Osteochondral Lesions of the Talus		
MRI Stage (Hepple et al., 1999)	**Conservative Treatment**	**Primary Operative Treatment**	**After a Failed Primary Procedure**
1 Articular cartilage damage only	• Ankle brace for 3 months	• Arthroscopic excision, microfracture/drilling	• Damaged surface and <1.5 cm²: osteochondral allograft transplant • Damaged surface and >1.5 cm²: bulk osteochondral allograft
2 Cartilage injury with underlying fracture with or without underlying bony edema	• Cast or boot, non-weight bearing for 6–8 weeks	• Non-damaged surface: arthroscopic transtalar drilling +/– bone graft, internal fixation if amenable • Damaged surface: microfracture/drilling	• As above
3 Detached but undisplaced fragment	• Acute injury (<10 weeks) or skeletally immature: cast or boot, non–weight bearing for 6–10 weeks • Skeletally mature or chronic injury: proceed to operative treatment	• Minimally damaged surface: arthroscopic transtalar drilling, internal fixation if amenable • Damaged surface: microfracture/drilling	• As above

4 Detached and displaced fragment	• No role for conservative treatment	• Minimally damaged surface:
		  • <1 cm²: excise fragment, microfracture/drilling
		  • >1 cm² and acute (<10 weeks): internal fixation
		• Damaged surface: microfracture/drilling
			• As above

5 Subchondral cyst formation	• Cast or boot, weight bearing as tolerated for 6–10 weeks • Ankle brace for 6 months	• Cyst <1.5 cm: as above + bone graft + micronized allograft cartilage as needed • Cyst >1.5 cm: bulk allograft	• As above

MRI, Magnetic resonance imaging.
MRI stage from Hepple S, Winson IG, Glew D. Osteochondral lesions of the talus: a revised classification. *Foot Ankle Int.* 1999;20(12):789–793.

Postoperative Management/Return to Play

- After arthroscopic excision, curettage, and BMS, the patient is non–weight bearing in a boot for 4 weeks and then progresses to weight bearing in the boot during physical therapy. Active motion is begun at 12 days after surgery.
- After OATS or internal fixation of an osteochondral allograft, the patient is non–weight bearing in a cast for 8 weeks and then progresses to weight bearing in a boot for 4 weeks during physical therapy.
- A brace is then worn during a gradual return to activities as dictated by symptoms.
- An athlete may RTP when he or she (1) has minimal or no symptoms and minimal swelling; and (2) is participating in physical therapy without wearing the boot.
- After internal fixation, OATS, or cartilage replacement, a brace must be worn while participating in sports for 6 months after the procedure.

OSTEOCHONDRAL LESIONS OF THE DISTAL TIBIAL PLAFOND

Osteochondral lesions of the distal tibial plafond (OLTP) are much less common than those of the talus and are less frequently reported in literature. The incidence of OLTP is approximately 1 OLTP for every 14 to 20 OLT.[108] Symptoms may include pain, stiffness, swelling, locking, and instability. Mologne and Ferkel[109] reported that 11 of 17 patients recalled an inversion injury to the ankle. "Mirror image" or "kissing" lesions of the talus and distal tibia also have been described.[110,111] Radiographs may or may not be helpful, but MRI and CT can identify the lesion (Fig. 119.12). Ross and associates[112] reported that the most common locations for OLTP are centromedial (23%) and anteromedial (19%) based on a grid scheme. In contrast, another study reported no predilection for location using the same grid scheme.[113] Treatment is similar to that of OLT: débridement and curettage of the lesion,

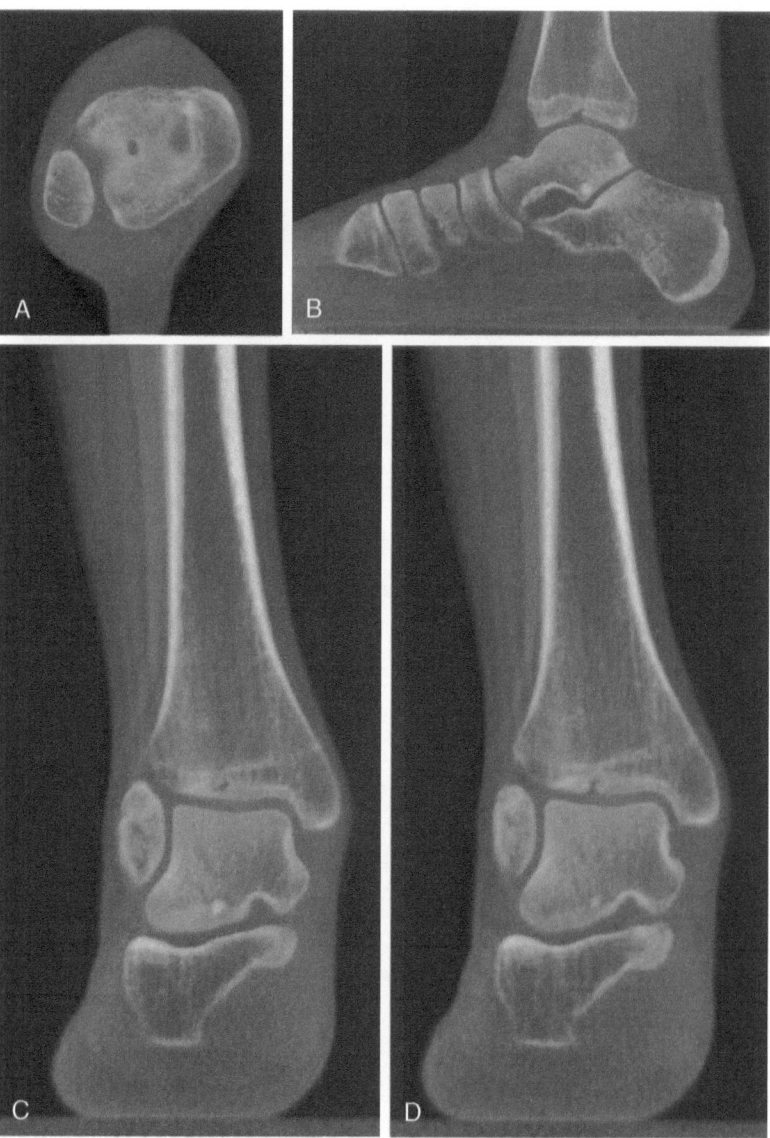

Fig. 119.12 An osteochondral lesion of the distal tibial plafond in a 16-year-old male with persistent ankle pain. (A) Axial, (B) sagittal, and (C) and (D) coronal computed tomography (CT) show a central lesion and small subchondral cyst.

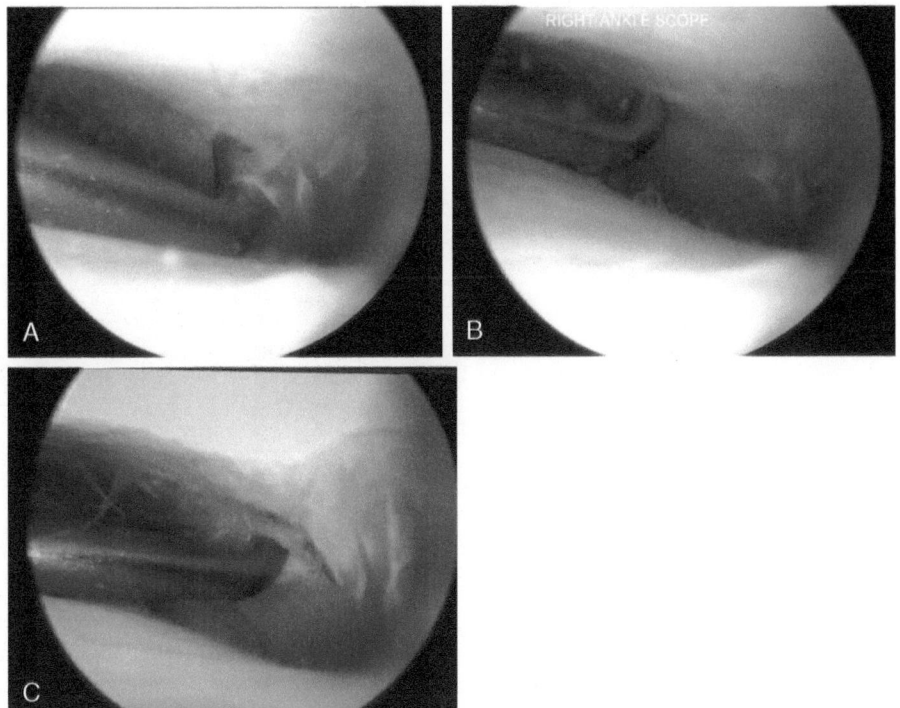

Fig. 119.13 (A)–(C), Arthroscopic probing and microfracture of an osteochondral lesion of the distal tibial plafond (same lesion as in Fig. 119.12).

abrasion of the defect to subchondral bone, and BMS (drilling or microfracture) of the subchondral bone (Fig. 119.13) Ross and associates[112] described functional and MRI outcomes in 31 OLTPs treated with arthroscopic microfracture, antegrade transmalleolar drilling (two ankles), OATS (one ankle), or concomitant lateral ligament repair (four ankles). At an average follow-up of 44 months, Foot and Ankle Outcome Scores (FAOS) and SF-12 had improved. Postoperative MOCART assessment demonstrated that 7 of 23 OLTPs had less than 50% fill or subchondral bone exposed.[112] Patients took an average of 6.3 months to return to activity.[112] Mologne and Ferkel[109] reported excellent or good results in 14 of 17 patients an average of 44 months after débridement, curettage, abrasion, and drilling or microfracture. Cuttica and colleagues[108] described 13 patients with OLTP treated with ankle arthroscopy and BMS (microfracture or antegrade drilling if cartilage cap intact) with bone allograft if cystic. The authors reported an improvement in postoperative modified AOFAS ankle-hindfoot scale; however, four patients (30.8%) had poor outcomes.[108] The authors warned of more frequent inferior outcomes in OLTP compared to OLT.[108] If an antegrade approach is unsuccessful, a retrograde osteochondral autograft or allograft transfer procedure can be performed[114,115]; instrumentation has been developed to make this process easier.

OSTEOCHONDRAL LESIONS OF THE FIRST METATARSAL

Osteochondral lesions (OCL), osteochondral injury, or osteochondritis dissecans of the first metatarsal is distinct from hallux rigidus because of the isolated nature of the defect. OCL of the first metatarsal are thought to be incited by trauma. OCL of the first metatarsal can occur concurrently with hallux rigidus or can eventually lead to hallux rigidus and degeneration.[116] First metatarsal OCL can be treated open or arthroscopically. BMS (drilling or microfracture) techniques (Fig. 119.14) and OATS have been described in the surgical treatment of first metatarsal OCL. Kim and associates[116] reported the largest series of first metatarsal OCL in patients with a mean age of 38.9 years, comparing 14 consecutive patients treated with subchondral drilling to 10 consecutive patients treated with OATS at an average follow-up of 25.1 months. The authors recorded significant improvement in VAS in both groups with no difference at final follow-up. However, patients treated with OATS had better AOFAS ankle–hindfoot scales at final follow-up (81.5 vs. 73.2) and more "excellent" Roles and Maudsley scores at final follow-up (9/10 vs. 5/14). Furthermore, large defects (>50 mm²) in the drilling group had poorer VAS and AOFAS ankle-hindfoot scales; thus the authors concluded that larger first metatarsal OCL had better results when treated with OATS.

COMPLICATIONS

Sequelae of nonoperatively treated osteochondral lesions in the foot and ankle include ongoing symptoms and progression of degenerative arthritis. In a systematic review, nonoperative treatment was successful in only 45% of stage 1, 2, and 3 OLT.[25] Of 35 patients, 13 (37%) with stage 5 (cystic) OLT treated nonoperatively had evidence of degenerative arthritis at least 2 years after the onset of their diagnosis.[24]

Current operative treatments for OLT include BMS (curettage, drilling, and microfracture), osteochondral autograft (OATs and mosaicplasty), osteochondral allograft, ACI, and other newer

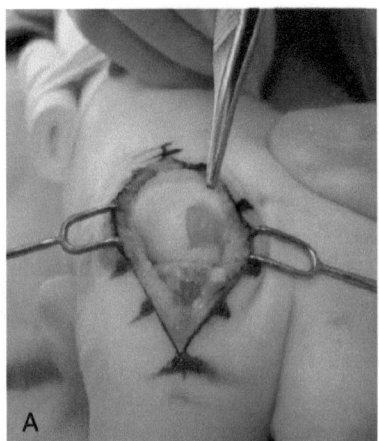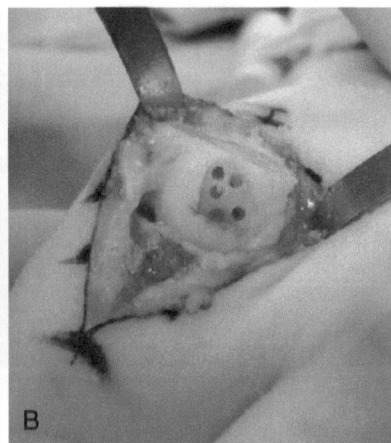

Fig. 119.14 (A) and (B) First metatarsal osteochondral lesion treated with open débridement and bone marrow stimulation with drilling. This patient had a cheilectomy at the time of treatment of the osteochondral lesion.

orthobiologic and synthetic therapies. All surgical treatment options of OLT also can be complicated by ongoing symptoms and progression of arthritis. In one study, one-third of patients (32.9%) with OLT treated with BMS (microfracture) had documented one grade progression of arthritis.[75] Osteochondral autograft procedures can cause donor site morbidity, typically at the knee or distal femur donor site. A study of second-look arthroscopy after OATs procedures reported fibrous adhesions, anterior impingement, synovitis, incongruent grafts, and uncovered areas between plugs.[117] Complications of bulk or large osteochondral allograft procedures of OLT include graft nonunion, graft resorption, and ongoing symptoms requiring eventual ankle arthrodesis or arthroplasty.[92] ACI-specific complications include detachment of the ACI graft,[96] hypertrophy of the ACI graft,[51,52,97] periosteum donor-site related symptoms (in first-generation ACI),[52] and theoretically, chondrocyte harvest-related donor site morbidity at the knee.

Complications of operative treatment of OLT can also be associated with approach: arthroscopic, open or malleolus osteotomy. Complications of ankle arthroscopy include neurovascular injury, infection, neuroma, reflex sympathetic dystrophy, and distraction-related complications.[118] The most common neurologic injury related to ankle arthroscopy is superficial peroneal nerve injury.[118] If a medial malleolus osteotomy is performed, complications can include medial malleolus nonunion,[53,97] delayed union,[53] medial malleolar cartilage damage,[53] or hardware irritation.[97]

Complications of operative treatment of OLTP are generally similar to those of OLT. Studies specific to operative treatment of the OLTP have reported complications including ongoing pain,[108] subchondral cysts,[108,112] superficial peroneal nerve injury,[112] deep vein thrombosis,[112] and tourniquet-related neurapraxia.[109]

Complications of nonoperatively and operatively treated osteochondral lesions of the first metatarsal head include ongoing pain and degenerative arthritis or hallux rigidus. General risks of surgical treatment of the first metatarsophalangeal (MTP) joint include infection, neurovascular damage, and joint stiffness. Only one study comparing microfracture to OATs in the treatment of osteochondral lesions of the first metatarsal head reported on outcomes and degenerative arthritis, but the study did not report other complications of treatment.[116] Small series and case reports have published studies on arthroscopic microfracture of osteochondral lesions of the first metatarsal head.[119,120] Proponents of arthroscopic treatment of the first MTP joint report that arthroscopy may result in less scar fibrosis[120] and potentially less stiffness than open surgery.

For a complete list of references, go to ExpertConsult.com.

SELECTED READING

Citation:
Kraeutler MJ, Chahla J, Dean CS, et al. Current concepts review update: osteochondral lesions of the talus. *Foot Ankle Int.* 2017;38:331–342.

Level of Evidence:
V

Summary:
The authors provide an extensive review of the causes, diagnosis, and treatment of osteochondral lesions of the talus, with an emphasis on the outcomes of operative treatment.

Citation:
Zengerink M, Struijs PA, Tol JL, et al. Treatment of osteochondral lesions of the talus: a systematic review. *Knee Surg Sports Traumatol Arthrosc.* 2010;18:238–246.

Level of Evidence:
IV, systematic review that included randomized controlled trials to case series

Summary:
This is a systematic review of treatments of osteochondral lesions of the talus (OLT), searching databases from 1966 to 2006. Treatments that were evaluated included casting, excision of fragment, excision and curettage, excision and bone marrow stimulation (BMS), cancellous bone graft, internal fixation of the OLT fragment, antegrade drilling, retrograde drilling, osteochondral autologous transplantation, and autologous chondrocyte implantation. After exclusions, 53 articles were evaluated. The authors summarize the evidence of the available mainstream treatments of OLT.

Citation:

Chao J, Pao A. Restorative tissue transplantation options for osteochondral lesions of the talus: a review. *Orthop Clin North Am.* 2017;48:371–383.

Level of Evidence:

V

Summary:

Review of the restorative tissue transplantation techniques for the treatment of osteochondral lesions of the talus, including osteochondral autologous transplantation, osteochondral allograft transplantation, autologous chondrocyte implantation, particulated juvenile allograft cartilage, and autograft–allograft combination. The authors present descriptions of and recent evidence for these treatments.

Citation:

Giannini S, Buda R, Faldini C, et al. Surgical treatment of osteochondral lesions of the talus in young active patients. *J Bone Joint Surg Am.* 2005;87(suppl 2):28–41.

Level of Evidence:

IV

Summary:

The authors present their approach to treatment of osteochondral lesions of the talus (OLT) in young active patients based on a case series of 80 consecutive patients treated between 1996 and 2001. All patients were examined and results obtained at 12 months and 4 years postoperatively. Authors give a sensible approach and written and pictorial descriptions of treatments based on acuity and chronicity of lesion, cartilage condition, and size of the OLT.

Citation:

Cuttica DJ, Smith WB, Hyer CF, et al. Osteochondral lesions of the talus: predictors of clinical outcome. *Foot Ankle Int.* 2011;32(11):1045–1051.

Level of Evidence:

IV

Summary:

This article describes a retrospective series of 130 patients with osteochondral lesions of the talus (OLT) treated operatively with bone marrow stimulation techniques. Using logistic regression analysis, authors determined that larger lesions greater than 1.5 cm^2 and uncontained lesions had worse outcomes. This was in agreement with a previous study by Choi and colleagues (2009), which also determined that OLT greater than 1.5 cm^2 were poor prognostic indicators.

Citation:

Berndt AL, Harty M. Transchondral fracture of the talus. *J Bone Joint Surg Am.* 1959;41:988–1029.

Level of Evidence:

IV

Summary:

This classic article by Berndt and Harty is of historical interest and has significant current value because it is the first major article describing traumatic osteochondral lesions of the talus in the form of transchondral fractures (osteochondritis dissecans) of the talus. Authors reviewed 214 fracture cases and described a cadaver experiment, ultimately proposing a classification system and mode of failure of these medial and lateral transchondral fractures. Berndt and Harty described clinical results, anatomic studies, radiographic findings, and histologic assessments in a study that was at the forefront of their time.

Citation:

D'Ambrosi R, Maccario C, Ursino C, et al. Combining microfractures, autologous bone graft, and autologous matrix-induced chondrogenesis for the treatment of juvenile osteochondral talar lesions. *Foot Ankle Int.* 2017;38:485–495.

Level of Evidence:

IV

Summary:

This study describes treatment of osteochondral lesions of the talus (OLT) with autologous matrix induced chondrogenesis in young patients. Since our chapter does not discuss OLT in the pediatric or juvenile population in detail, we recommend this paper by D'Ambrosi and associates (2017), which summarizes their review of the literature of OLT in the young population in a tabulated form.

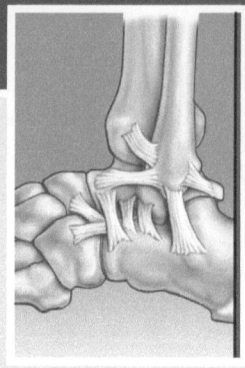

120

Heel Pain and Plantar Fasciitis: Hindfoot Conditions

Anish R. Kadakia, Amiethab A. Aiyer

POSTERIOR HEEL PAIN

Pain in the posterior, superior portion of the calcaneus may be multifactorial, ranging from retrocalcaneal bursitis, enlargement of the superior bursal prominence of the calcaneus, insertional Achilles tendinosis, to inflammation of an adventitious bursa between the Achilles tendon and the skin (Fig. 120.1).[1-6] Each of these entities may exist as an isolated condition or may be part of a symptom complex. Careful analysis of the patient's subjective complaints and objective findings are required to arrive at the correct diagnosis. Disorders of the Achilles tendon are covered in Chapter 118 and are not reviewed in detail here.

Retrocalcaneal bursitis may occur as an isolated entity but is more commonly associated with the prominent posterior superior bursal portion of the calcaneus, or Haglund deformity. When Achilles tendinosis occurs concomitantly with this condition, it is generally located in the area of the Achilles tendon just at or above the insertion of the Achilles tendon at the posterior portion of the os calcis. Retrocalcaneal pain syndrome is commonly associated with a high-arched cavus foot and a varus heel.[1] The combination of these factors tends to produce a foot that does not dorsiflex as readily as a normal foot. The heel is prominent and is more susceptible to increased pressure from the tendons and the counter of the shoe.

History

The history is generally that of slow onset of dull aching pain in the retrocalcaneal area aggravated by activity and certain footwear. Footwear with a narrow heel counter is most commonly associated with this condition. Pain that starts after sitting or when arising from bed in the morning is commonly reported. At times, the patient may have a history of the acute onset of pain, which is sometimes associated with a traumatic incident. When this history is reported, a rupture of the Achilles tendon or disruption of calcific tendinosis must be considered.

Physical Examination

Physical examination reveals swelling in the area of the retrocalcaneal bursa between the Achilles tendon and the calcaneus.[3,4] A prominence is generally present in the area of the superior portion of the heel. The swelling in the retrocalcaneal bursa will be found just anterior to the Achilles tendon. By palpating medially and laterally at the same time, and with the aid of ballottement, one can sometimes feel fluid within the bursa (Fig. 120.2).

With careful and discrete palpation, one can generally differentiate between swelling in the Achilles tendon and swelling in the retrocalcaneal bursa. The swelling of the Achilles tendon associated with retrocalcaneal bursitis is usually at the level of the tendon at or just proximal to the insertion. Dorsiflexion of the foot usually increases the pain in the area. A great deal of swelling and inflammation on examination may indicate involvement of both the retrocalcaneal bursa and the Achilles tendon. Redness and swelling may be present between the Achilles tendon and the skin, usually as a result of an adventitious bursitis produced by pressure of the shoe counter against the Achilles tendon. Periostitis may be present, which is a discrete localized area of tenderness of the os calcis, usually on the lateral side of the posterior portion of the os calcis and produced by pressure of the shoe counter. A "squeeze test," in which the palms of both hands apply moderate compression to the tuberosity, should be performed to rule out the presence of a stress fracture. If the patient reports pain with this examination, a high suspicion for a stress fracture should be noted.

Imaging

A lateral view of the foot is taken with the patient standing, which allows biomechanical evaluation of the foot and evaluation of the specific points of the os calcis. The points of the os calcis are identified as the posterior margin of the posterior facet, the superior bursal projection, the tuberosity indicating the site of the Achilles tendon insertion, the medial tubercle, and the anterior tubercle.[7] The shape and appearance of the superior bursal prominence are noted. Evaluation of the lateral radiograph may be performed using the method described by Fowler and Philip, which measures the posterior calcaneal angle (Fig. 120.3).[8] Fowler and Philip consider the bursal projection prominent if the angle is greater than 75 degrees. Some authors have concluded that a combination of the Fowler angle and the angle of calcaneal inclination is more effective in correlating the radiographic appearance with symptomatology than the Fowler and Philip angle alone, with the combined angle being greater than 90 degrees in patients with symptomatic Haglund disease.[9,10]

Parallel pitch lines have been used by Heneghan and Pavlov[3] to determine the prominence of the bursal projection (Fig. 120.4). The base line is constructed by placing a line along the medial tuberosity and the anterior tubercle, and a parallel line from the posterior lip of the talar articular facet. The bursal prominence is considered abnormal if it extends above this line.

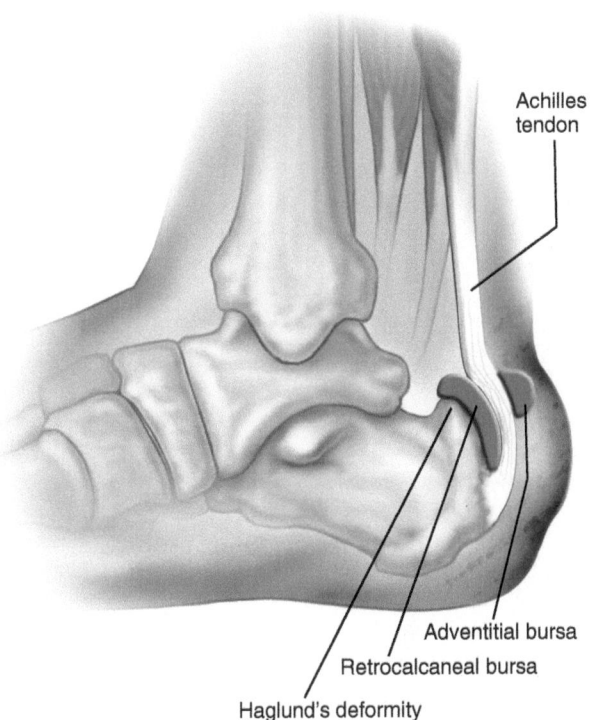

Fig. 120.1 Haglund deformity with a retrocalcaneal bursa between the Achilles tendon and the superior bursal prominence, and an adventitious bursa between the Achilles tendon and the skin.

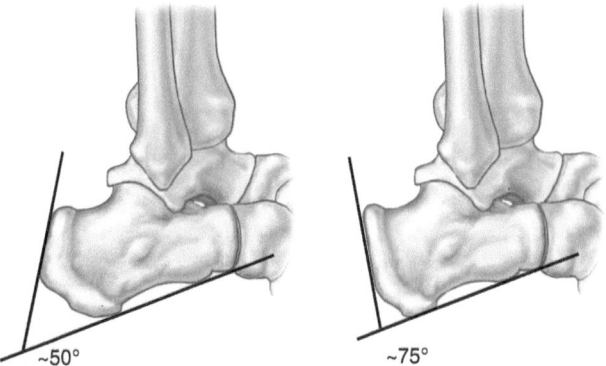

Fig. 120.3 Measurement of the Fowler and Philip angle. The normal angle is shown on the left, and an abnormal angle is shown on the right. The upper level of normal is considered to be 69 degrees. The drawing at the right indicates an abnormal angle of 75 degrees.

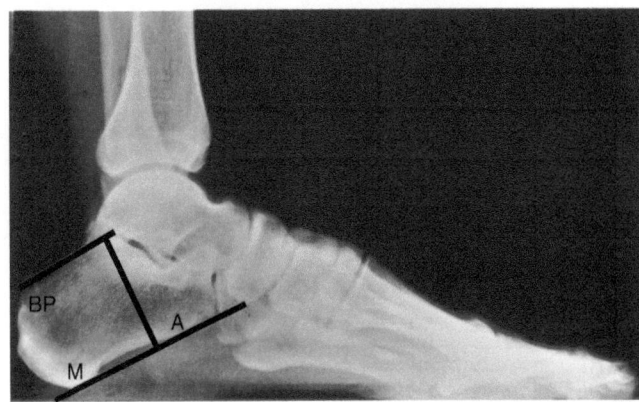

Fig. 120.4 Parallel pitch lines used to determine the prominence of the bursal projection. A line is drawn along the medial tuberosity *(M)* and the anterior tuberosity *(A)*. A parallel is constructed from the superior prominence of the posterior facet. If the bursal projection *(BP)* is above the superior line, the projection is considered abnormally large. (From Pavlov H, Heneghan MA, Hersh A, et al. The Haglund syndrome: initial and differential diagnosis. *Radiology* 144[1]:83–88, 1982.)

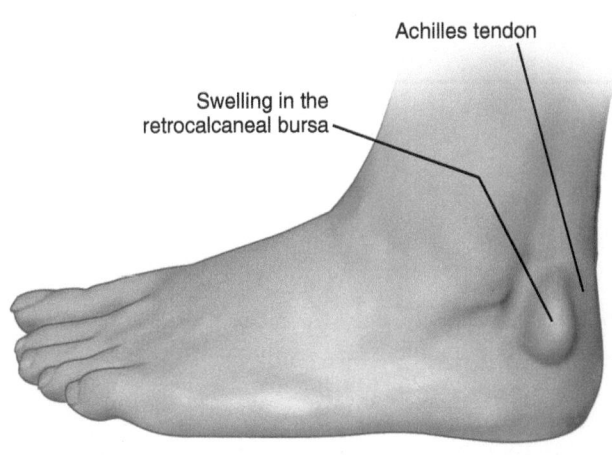

Fig. 120.2 The area of the swelling; retrocalcaneal bursitis with swelling is anterior to the Achilles tendon.

Magnetic resonance imaging (MRI) has provided clearer insight into the anatomic abnormalities associated with posterior heel pain.[11-14] The imaging allows visualization of the Achilles tendon and the bursa, as well as demonstrating any bony abnormalities in the posterior superior calcaneus. In patients with a suspected stress fracture of the calcaneus, an MRI scan can be ordered to delineate the diagnosis in an expeditious manner so that the most appropriate treatment may be initiated. In patients refractory to nonoperative treatment, a preoperative MRI will define which anatomic structures need to be addressed

(Fig. 120.5). The degree of tendinosis present in the Achilles tendon is easily visualized and distinguished from isolated bursitis.

Decision-Making Principles

Nonoperative treatment is successful at alleviating posterior heel pain regardless of cause in most patients. Adventitious bursitis is generally treated conservatively by softening the heel counter with use of a small U-shaped pad to relieve the pressure of the shoe or counter against the inflamed area; in addition, antiinflammatory medications are used. Surgical intervention performed solely for adventitious bursitis is unusual and carries a risk of wound slough, and thus it should be avoided if possible.

Retrocalcaneal bursitis and Haglund deformity are generally managed by conservative measures consisting of antiinflammatory medication, decreased activity, padding to prevent pressure on the affected area, orthoses or heel lifts, and strengthening and stretching exercises. If the condition does not respond to these modalities, then surgical intervention may be considered. Surgery generally consists of excision of the exostosis and the

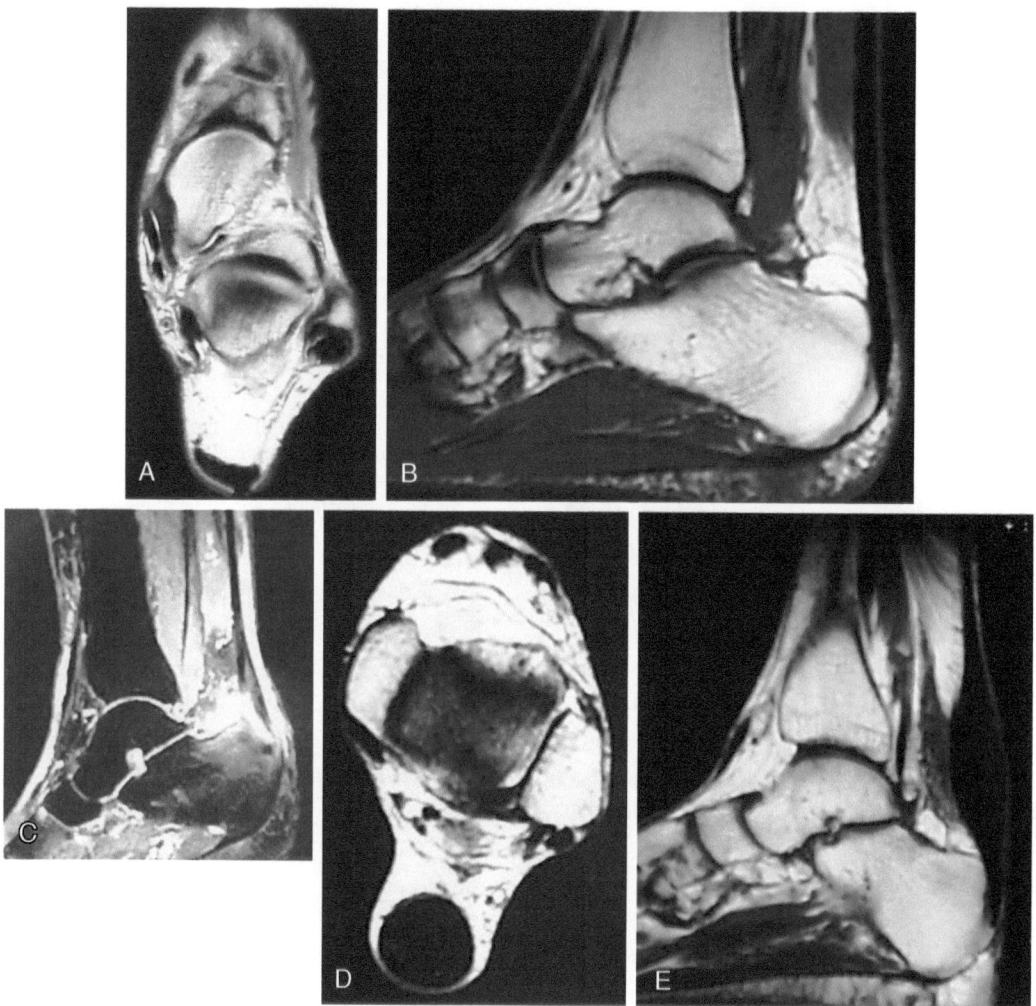

Fig. 120.5 (A) Axial magnetic resonance imaging (MRI) of a normal Achilles tendon showing the normal shape of the Achilles tendon. (B) A sagittal MRI scan of a normal Achilles tendon showing the normal shape of the Achilles tendon. (C) A sagittal MRI scan showing increased signal in the insertion of the Achilles tendon consistent with tendinosis. Increased fluid is present, demonstrating an inflamed bursa surrounding Haglund deformity. (D and E), Axial and sagittal MRI scans demonstrating chronic tendinosis of the Achilles with marked fusiform swelling of the tendon.

retrocalcaneal bursa and, at times, the adventitious bursa, if present, along with correction of the Achilles tendon disease with tendon transfer if necessary. Although good results after surgery are reported in most series, in the athlete, this condition may present a serious threat to continued full activity, even after surgical intervention.

Treatment Options
Nonoperative Therapy
Initial goals of the treatment of patients with retrocalcaneal bursitis are to control pain and attempt to allow the patient to return to normal function and activity. Rest, particularly soon after the onset of symptoms, can be helpful. The duration of rest may be prolonged, depending on the increasing duration of symptoms.[15,16] Cross-training with low-impact exercises, such as an elliptical machine, swimming, or biking, may prevent deconditioning in the athlete. Modified regimens may be suggested for an athlete who is unwilling to cross-train.[16-18] In patients with exquisite tenderness, immobilization in a controlled ankle

motion (CAM) boot or short-leg walking cast may be helpful.[17,19] Immobilization should be used cautiously in athletes, because patients can have resultant tendon and muscle atrophy, degeneration, and decreased blood supply.[18,20]

Nonsteroidal drugs that are administered orally or delivered locally in the form of a patch may decrease local inflammation.[20-22] Cryotherapy and ice can decrease pain, swelling, and inflammation as well.[20-22] Corticosteroids that are taken orally, injected locally, or applied topically have been used.[23] Injections must be used cautiously because they can lead to a higher incidence of tendon ruptures and tendinopathy.[24,25] Animal model studies with intratendinous injections have been shown to result in localized tendon necrosis and decreased mechanical strength. If used, the steroid injection must be placed anterior to the tendon, in the area of the retrocalcaneal bursa.[20,21] The patient is immobilized in a CAM walker for 3 to 4 weeks to minimize the risk of tendon rupture after injection into the retrocalcaneal bursa.

Orthoses may help these patients by providing a heel lift function, correcting hyperpronation, or minimizing leg length discrepancies.[20,21] Care must be exercised when correcting hindfoot pronation deformities, because overcorrection can result in inflexibility of the hindfoot with decreased shock absorption.[21] Heel cups can decrease the strain on an Achilles tendon and elevate a prominent superior calcaneal tuberosity away from the tendon. High heels, clogs, open-back shoes, gel braces, and horseshoe pads can also provide symptomatic relief for the patient.[19,26]

If retrocalcaneal bursitis is present with a normal Achilles tendon, conservative therapy is implemented until the patient has been asymptomatic for 4 to 6 weeks. The patient may then return to sports participation starting with limited activity and working up to full activity within 4 to 12 weeks, assuming that they have recovered full strength and mobility without pain. If retrocalcaneal bursitis is associated with degeneration of the Achilles tendon, nonoperative treatment should be used until the patient is asymptomatic; a gradual increase in activity is then allowed over a 6- to 12-week period.

Operative Therapy

If the patient does not respond to these modalities, then surgical intervention may be considered. Surgery generally consists of excision of the exostosis, the retrocalcaneal bursa, and at times the adventitious bursa, if present, along with correction of the Achilles tendon disease with tendon transfer if necessary. Although most authors report good results after surgery, in the athlete this condition may present a serious threat to continued full activity, even after surgical intervention.

🏃 Authors' Preferred Technique

Posterior Heel Pain

Surgical procedures are usually performed for retrocalcaneal bursitis associated with the superior bony prominence. The retrocalcaneal bursa and the superior bursal prominence are excised. The adventitious bursa is excised if it is prominent. If the adventitious bursa is excised, the surgeon must take care to excise it carefully and meticulously to avoid adversely affecting the blood supply or the skin overlying this area, because a skin slough can result in significant morbidity for the patient.

A medial or lateral incision, or a combination of incisions 1.5 cm anterior to the Achilles tendon, is made as determined by the location and width of the bony prominence (Fig. 120.6). Alternatively, a central posterior Achilles splitting approach can be used. Prone positioning can be used with all of the aforementioned incisions. A medial incision may be carried out with the patient supine and minimizes the risk of damage to the sural nerve, but the superior calcaneal

exostosis is typically lateral, which may make excision slightly more difficult. Given the elimination of sural nerve injury and simplified positioning, this is the author's preferred technique in these cases. If the patient has concomitant tendinosis of the Achilles tendon, the central posterior tendon splitting approach is used.

After incision of the central aspect of the posterior skin, the incision is carried directly to the level of the paratenon, and dissection is performed at this level to maintain full-thickness skin flaps to avoid skin loss. Attention should be given to the calcaneal branch of the sural nerve on the lateral side and the medial calcaneal nerve on the medial side. The Achilles tendon is inspected to confirm the presence and degree of tendinosis. Regardless of the surgical approach, the retrocalcaneal bursa is now excised. An exostosectomy is performed, removing the bone from the area of insertion of the Achilles tendon to the superior portion of the posterior facet of the os calcis (Fig. 120.7). Adequate bone is removed, and the edges are smoothed with a rasp. If greater than 50% of the insertion of the Achilles tendon is elevated from the calcaneus, repair with suture anchors is recommended to avoid rupture. In the case of a concomitant tendinosis, a flexor hallucis longus transfer may be required if a significant portion (>50%) of the Achilles tendon is excised as described in Chapter 118. The split in the Achilles tendon is repaired with an absorbable monofilament number 0 suture. The subcutaneous tissue and skin are closed after the procedure. Compressive dressings and plaster splints are applied to maintain 15 degrees of ankle plantar flexion to maximize perfusion to the posterior skin.

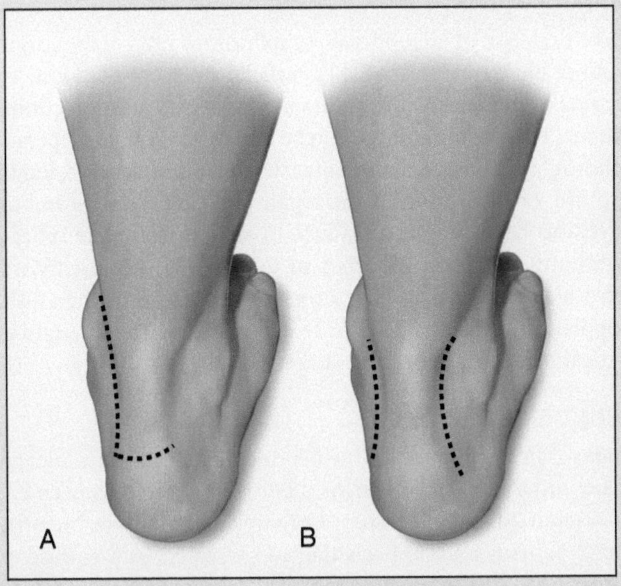

Fig. 120.6 Surgical incisions for retrocalcaneal bursitis. (A) The medial approach with J extension as described by Schepsis and Leach. (B) Medial and lateral approach incisions as described by Jones and James. ([A] From Schepsis AA, Leach RE. Surgical management of Achilles tendinitis. *Am J Sports Med.* 1987;15[4]:308–315 and [B] from Jones DC, James SL. Partial calcaneal osteotomy for retrocalcaneal bursitis. *Am J Sports Med.* 1984;12[1]:72–73.)

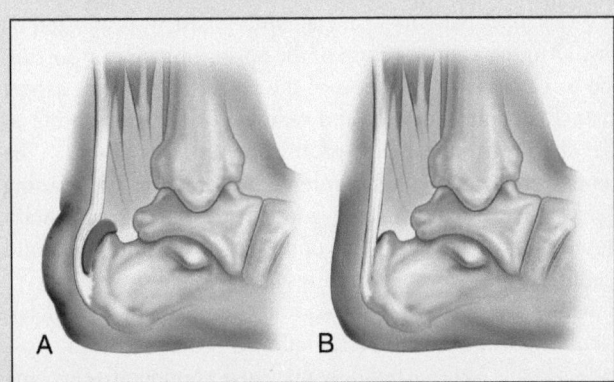

Fig. 120.7 (A) Haglund deformity with prominence of the posterior superior portion of the os calcis. (B) The appearance of os calcis after surgical resection of a posterior superior prominence for symptomatic Haglund deformity.

Postoperative Management

In cases in which the Achilles tendon is not involved, the patient is seen at 2 weeks for stitch removal, the lower extremity is placed into a removable CAM walker with the ankle at neutral position for an additional 4 weeks, and weight bearing is begun. A rehabilitation program for non-weight-bearing strengthening and range of motion (ROM) is begun at this initial visit. Six weeks after surgery, the walking boot is removed and the patient is allowed to weight bear with a   -inch heel lift during this time for 4 to 6 weeks. Therapy is continued and graduated to weight-bearing exercises. Patients are then advanced to regular footwear and continue to follow a strengthening program at home with a Theraband. Athletic activity is restricted for 3 months after surgery.

If surgery has been performed on the tendon in combination with excision of the retrocalcaneal bursa and exostosectomy, immobilization is continued for 8 weeks, but active (ROM) is begun at 3 weeks. Strengthening and stretching exercises are started at 6 to 9 weeks. Increased activity according to tolerance can be started at 12 weeks, and return to strenuous activity is allowed at 4 to 6 months if local symptoms have resolved.

Results

Ippolito and Ricciardi-Pollini[27] described three patients with invasive retrocalcaneal bursitis who had a large bursa and invasion of the os calcis. Pathologic examination revealed lymphoplasma cellular infiltrates containing proportionately more plasma cells than lymphocytes. Removal of the bursa provided clinical relief, and systemic rheumatic disease did not develop in later years.

Keck and Kelly[5] reported on 13 patients with 20 symptomatic heels that were treated surgically. In 17 heels, the superior bursa was excised, and in three heels a dorsally based closing wedge osteotomy was performed. Good results were reported for 15 of the heels treated. The initial results were good in all but two patients, whose pain recurred as a manifestation of generalized rheumatoid arthritis. An osteotomy was used to reduce the posterior prominence, and results were rated good in two heels—fair in one heel, and poor in two heels. The authors believed that too few osteotomies were performed in this series to evaluate this method. A disadvantage of the osteotomy was that a longer convalescence was required.[5]

A series of 65 patients with Haglund disease was reported by Ruch[9]; 17 underwent resection of the posterior superior portion of the os calcis, with resection of the posterior superior aspect both medially and laterally and removal of sufficient bone to render the previous palpable prominence entirely absent.[9] The patients were evaluated 6 months to 5 years after undergoing surgery. Fifteen demonstrated good to excellent results with elimination of symptoms. Three of the patients required a second procedure to obtain the desired result.

Schepsis and Leach[28] reported that the majority of athletes, particularly runners, who presented with acute or chronic posterior heel pain were successfully managed nonoperatively using a combination of (1) a decrease in or cessation of the usual weekly mileage, (2) temporary termination of interval training and workouts on hills, (3) a change from a harder bank surface to a softer surface, (4) a 0.25- to 0.50-inch lift inside the shoe or added to the shoe, and (5) a program designed to stretch and strengthen the gastrocnemius-soleus complex.[28] These measures were combined with use of oral anti-inflammatory medications and an occasional injection of corticosteroid into the retrocalcaneal bursa. Postural abnormalities were treated with orthotics. The authors retrospectively studied 45 cases of chronic posterior heel pain that were treated surgically in 37 patients. All but two of these patients were competitive long-distance runners who ran an average of 40 to 120 miles per week prior to the onset of symptoms. Their ages ranged from 19 to 56 years.

The surgical approach used by Schepsis and Leach[28] was a longitudinal incision 1 cm medial to the Achilles tendon that was continued transversely to form a J-shaped incision if necessary. A cast was applied and worn for 2 to 3 weeks, with weight bearing permitted after 1 week. When disease within the tendon required excision and repair, immobilization was continued for 1 to 2 weeks longer. (ROM) exercises were emphasized. A graduated program of swimming and stationary bicycling combined with isometric, isotonic, and isokinetic strengthening of the calf muscles was prescribed. Jogging was permitted after 8 to 12 weeks, but rarely sooner. Full return to a competitive level of sports activity usually required 5 to 6 months.

The patients were divided into three groups—those with Achilles tenosynovitis-tendinitis, those with retrocalcaneal bursitis, and those with a combination of both. In the 14 patients with retrocalcaneal bursitis, seven (50%) had excellent results, three (21%) had good results, and four (29%) had fair results. In the group with a combination of both conditions, five (71%) had excellent results and two (29%) had good results. It was noted that four of the six unsatisfactory results occurred in the group with retrocalcaneal bursitis.

Complications

More than half of all reported complications involve the surgical wound. Skin edge necrosis, superficial or deep infection, and seroma or hematoma formation are the most common complications. These complications can be minimized with postoperative splinting in 20 degrees of plantar flexion. Sural neuritis, tendon rupture, or disruption of the repair and deep vein thrombosis have also been reported. Failure to achieve complete relief of symptoms has been reported in up to 29% of patients with retrocalcaneal bursitis. Given the high demands of the athletic population, appropriate counseling regarding the outcomes is critical prior to performing surgery.

Future Considerations

Endoscopic techniques for the débridement of the retrocalcaneal space and the posterosuperior tuberosity of the calcaneus have been reported in the literature. Ortmann and McBryde[29] reported on 28 patients and 30 heels that were treated with endoscopic surgery; 86.67% of patients reported excellent results, with one major complication of an Achilles tendon rupture.[29] The medial column of the Achilles tendon, the sural nerve, and the plantaris tendons are at risk with use of this technique.[30] Despite these risks, the purported benefits of lower morbidity and recovery time make this procedure an excellent option for surgeons familiar with endoscopy.

PLANTAR FASCIITIS

In reviewing the literature, it is apparent that many different theories exist about the cause of subcalcaneal pain, and hence many different methods of treatment have been suggested.[31-43] It has been said that although this condition is familiar to all orthopaedic surgeons, it is probably fully understood by none.[36]

Snook and Chrisman[44] noted that conflicting literature exists on this subject with regard to two salient points: that there is no accepted explanation of the cause of the condition, and that no generally approved method of treatment exists. These investigators thought that the basic cause might lie in the subcalcaneal pad, which in some unknown manner lost its compressibility, either by local loss of fat with thinning or by rupture of the fibrous tissue septa. Ali[45] stated that "the painful heel is due to a fibrotic response, similar to plantar fibromatosis and not to the spur of bone, which is the end result of recurrent strain on the plantar fascia." Tanz[46] thought that "inferior heel pain is often due to irritation of a branch of the medial calcaneal nerve." Similarly, Baxter and Thigpen[31] and Przylucki and Jones[47] advanced the thought that the heel pain is due to an entrapment neuropathy that involves the branch of the lateral plantar nerve to the abductor digiti quinti. It has been noted that this branch passes more proximally than is shown in most anatomic studies and is in the area of the heel spur.[31,48]

Heel spurs may be present or absent, and may or may not be the primary pathologic entity in persons with heel pain. However, they must be considered in the context of the entire syndrome. Laboratory studies in most patients with subcalcaneal pain syndrome are normal. When the subcalcaneal pain syndrome is present, and especially if it is persistent and severe, consideration must be given to the diagnosis of a systemic disorder such as seronegative arthropathy. In patients with the subcalcaneal pain syndrome, it has been reported that the incidence of the subsequent development of a systemic arthritic disorder may be as high as 16%.[36]

History

The history usually reveals a slow but gradual onset of pain along the inside of the heel.[35-37] Occasionally the pain may be associated with a twisting injury of the foot, producing an abrupt onset of pain.[48] However, the clinical course is generally similar regardless of the onset. The location of the pain is generally described as along the medial side of the foot at the bottom of the heel. The pain is worse upon first arising in the morning and then decreases with increased activity. However, it may increase after prolonged activity. Periods of inactivity are generally followed by an increase in pain as activity is started again. Numbness of the foot is not present. When severe pain is present, the patient is unable to bear weight on the heel and will bear weight on the forepart of the foot.

Physical Examination

Specific examination of the foot reveals acute tenderness along the medial tuberosity of the os calcis along its plantar aspect. This tenderness may be at the origin of the central slip of the plantar fascia, or it may be deep, in which case it probably represents a deep inflammation, perhaps with involvement of the nerve to the abductor digiti quinti. The plantar fascia is palpated to determine whether the plantar fascia is tender just at its origin or throughout its course. The plantar fascia is also palpated for nodules, the presence of which suggests plantar fibromatosis. The plantar fascia is palpated both with the toes flexed so that it is supple and with the toes extended, which places tension on the plantar fascia. Careful examination of ankle ROM is essential to identify any concurrent gastrocnemius or soleus contractures.

Common conditions in the differential diagnosis of heel pain should be ruled out. Tarsal tunnel syndrome may generate pain in the distribution of the calcaneal branch and first branch of the lateral plantar nerve, and is typically elicited with palpation on the plantar medial aspect of the hindfoot, not directly under the foot. The associated sensory and motor changes are likewise not seen with plantar fasciitis (PF). Fat pad atrophy will often cause pain more posterior to the plantar tuberosity, directly under the calcaneus. Applying a squeeze around the calcaneus will elicit pain in patients with calcaneal stress fractures.

Imaging

Standing, full weight-bearing roentgenograms of the heel, including the foot, are taken in the anteroposterior and lateral standing projections. Roentgenograms taken in this manner will provide information about the osseous structures of the foot and specific details of the os calcis. Such radiographs will also help classify the foot as normal, flat, or cavus. The presence of a spur or calcification along the medial tuberosity will also be shown (Fig. 120.8). Axial non-weight-bearing views of the os calcis may be taken to provide information about the os calcis in a second plane.

Although much discussion has occurred about the relationship of the calcaneal heel spur to subcalcaneal pain, the relationship has not been definitely established. Tanz[46] stated that a heel spur is located in the origin of the short toe flexors and not in the plantar fascia. He noted that 15% of normal asymptomatic adult feet have subcalcaneal plantar spurs, whereas about 50% of adult feet with plantar heel pain have spurs. Tanz thought that heel spurs contributed to the plantar heel pain, although many patients with plantar heel pain did not have spurs. Snook and Chrisman[44] agreed with this supposition. In their report on 27 patients with subcalcaneal pain, they noted that 13 had a calcaneal spur and 11 did not have such a spur. Mann[49] stated

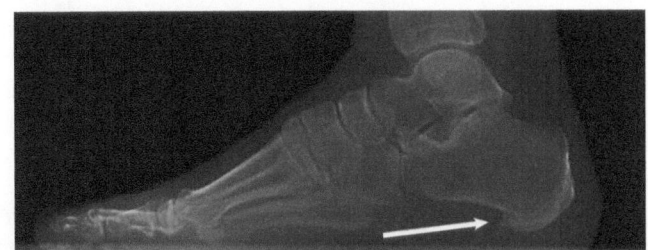

Fig. 120.8 An inferior plantar spur *(arrow)* commonly seen in patients with plantar fasciitis.

that "over a long period of time, proliferative bony changes at the origin of the fascia may lead to the formation of a spur."

Shmokler and colleagues[50] reviewed 1000 patients at random with radiographs of the foot. They found a 13.2% incidence of heel spurs. Only 39% of those with heel spurs (5.2% of the total sample) reported any history of subcalcaneal heel pain. Shmokler and coworkers[50] believed that these statistics tended to support the premise that the presence of a heel spur did not mandate pain.

Intenzo and colleagues[51] studied 15 patients reporting chronic heel pain who underwent three-phase technetium-99m methylene diphosphonate bone scintigraphy. Ten patients demonstrated abnormal scan findings consistent with PF, with uptake only in the early soft tissue phase, and they had responded to conventional therapy. Two patients were found to have calcaneal stress fractures, and one patient demonstrated a calcaneal spur that required no treatment. The remaining two patients had normal scans and did not appear to have PF clinically. These investigators found the three-phase bone scan useful in diagnosing PF and in distinguishing it from other causes of the painful heel syndrome.

Grasel et al.[52] evaluated various MRI signs of PF to determine if a difference exists in these findings between clinically typical and atypical patients with chronic symptoms resistant to conservative treatment.[52] These investigators found signs on MRI that included occult marrow edema and fascial tears. Patients with these manifestations seemed to respond to treatment in a manner similar to that of patients in whom MRI revealed more benign findings. MRI is not required to make the diagnosis of either PF or fibromatosis. The primary use is to rule out other conditions such as calcaneal stress fracture, plantar fascia rupture, neoplasm, and Baxter neuritis.

Decision-Making Principles

Operative treatment for PF is reserved for patients with moderate to severe symptoms who have not responded to at least 6 months (or more conservatively 12 months) of nonoperative management. Currently no prospective, randomized controlled trials exist that support any specific operative intervention for treatment of PF. Open techniques for plantar fascia release provide complete visualization of the fascia and allow the fascia to be incised in a controlled fashion. In addition, the first branch of the lateral plantar nerve can be decompressed with an open technique. Opponents of an open technique note a higher incidence of wound complications, infection, and postoperative pain, and a longer return to work. Endoscopic plantar fascia release for treatment of PF has been suggested to reduce complications and provide an earlier return to work and activity. However, endoscopic techniques are limited by a small field of view and may result in inadequate resection of the plantar fascia. In addition, the lateral plantar artery and first branch of the lateral plantar nerve is not exposed during this technique, and injury may occur.

In a patient with a tight gastrocnemius with a positive Silfverskiöld test, a gastrocnemius recession may relax the tension on the plantar fascia, relieving the pain. Successful relief of plantar foot pain after gastrocnemius recession has recently been demonstrated. Further research is required to validate these results.

Treatment Options
Nonoperative Therapy

Management of subcalcaneal heel pain should initially begin with nonoperative treatment. Although consensus does not exist on the efficacy of any particular conservative treatment regimen, it is agreed that nonsurgical treatment is ultimately effective in approximately 90% of patients. Because the natural history of PF has not been established, it is unclear how much of symptom resolution is in fact due to the wide variety of commonly used treatments. Activities are restricted according to the patient's symptomatic tolerance.

The mainstay of treatment is to stretch both the Achilles and plantar fascia. Simple plantar fascia stretching exercises are certainly the least expensive and easiest modality for patients to initiate. Plantar fascia–specific stretching has demonstrated superior success compared with isolated Achilles stretching (Fig. 120.9).

Nighttime dorsiflexion splints have demonstrated fair success in multiple randomized studies and are especially useful for relieving "start-up" pain in the morning. Resolution of symptoms has been reported as early as 12 weeks and may improve significantly even after 1 month of splint use.

Orthotics have demonstrated similar results to nighttime splints with better patient compliance. No conclusive evidence exists to support the use of a prefabricated versus a custom-molded orthotic. The use of a silicone heel pad is a simple and cost-effective method in patients without deformity.

Oral nonsteroidal antiinflammatory drugs have demonstrated trends toward improved patient pain and function but no statistically significant difference from placebo when used with other conservative modalities.

Localized administration of corticosteroids, either through injection or iontophoresis, has demonstrated reliable short-term relief but no significant long-term benefit. The risk of plantar fascia rupture or fat pad atrophy must be weighed against the limited short-term benefit of corticosteroid injections, and repeat

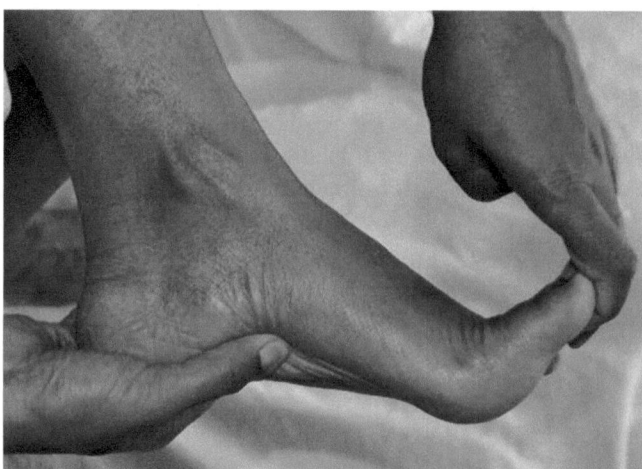

Fig. 120.9 A plantar fascia–specific stretch is performed with the leg in a figure four position. The contralateral hand is used to dorsiflex the hallux and ankle. The ipsilateral hand is used to palpate the plantar fascia to ensure that it is taut.

injections should be avoided. Iontophoresis may be a safer option but requires an increased time commitment and may be impractical in the typical clinic setting.

Cross-training activity is important. The patient should avoid repetitive impact activities such as running or use of a treadmill and instead cross-train with a bicycle or elliptical trainer. These options assist in maintaining conditioning and increasing flexibility while avoiding cyclic loading.

Once the patient has become asymptomatic without tenderness and has maintained this status for 4 to 6 weeks, a gradual increase in activity may be allowed. Use of the orthotic is continued for several months. After several months, use of the orthotic is discontinued unless the patient has a biomechanical abnormality of the foot, such as a flatfoot or cavus deformity. If the patient has a flatfoot deformity, a device designed to correct the biomechanical abnormality, support the foot, and prevent the abnormal biomechanical stresses along the plantar fascia and the medial side of the heel is used. If the patient has a cavus deformity, a soft orthotic designed to decrease the shock and increase the weight-bearing area may be used indefinitely, depending on the patient's symptoms. When a patient has a deformity and has had a significant episode of subcalcaneal pain requiring treatment, use of the orthotic can be continued permanently. Although the over-the-counter type of heel cup can be used initially to try to provide some symptomatic relief, in a patient with a true biomechanical abnormality, a specific orthosis should be used.

Postoperative Management

The patient is kept non-weight-bearing for 2 weeks and then can bear weight in a short-leg cast for 2 more weeks; increased activity is started at 12 weeks. This operation is used only for patients with recalcitrant conditions. It carries with it the expectation that the patient will probably, but not certainly, be able to return to his or her preinjury status.

Results

In 1986 Lutter[43] outlined the decision-making process in athletes with subcalcaneal pain. He described 182 patients with heel complaints related to sports injuries; most of the patients were runners (76%). Approximately 20% of these patients required 3 to 4 months of conservative treatment before returning to sports activity. Five percent had chronic heel pain and did not recover within 9 to 12 months. For these patients, a surgical approach was considered. The procedure used in these patients depended on the preoperative diagnosis and varied from release of the nerves to release of the fascia to complete exploration of the posterior tibial nerve and its branches, and release of the plantar fascia. Cycling or swimming was begun 2 weeks after the operation. Gentle walk-dash run training and a gradual escalation up to running was allowed approximately 6 weeks after surgery. Patients were asked to refrain from walking until they were pain free and had no tenderness. If pain occurred with increasing activity, the workup was cut by 50% until the patient could tolerate the workup without pain.

Shock wave therapy has been examined in the treatment of chronic PF in athletes who run. Rompe et al.[54] demonstrated that after 6 months of treatments three times a week with shock wave therapy, the treatment group experienced greater relief than the sham treatment group.

Baxter and Thigpen[31] performed 34 operative procedures in 26 patients with recalcitrant heel pain. The procedure consisted of isolated neurolysis of the nerves supplying the abductor digiti quinti muscle as it passed beneath the abductor with release of the deep fascia of the abductor hallucis longus and removal of

 ## Authors' Preferred Technique

Plantar Fasciitis

In the athlete, the least amount of surgery commensurate with high likelihood of a good result should be performed. In the athlete with recalcitrant subcalcaneal pain syndrome who desires to continue athletic activity, the exact site of the abnormality is evaluated carefully by means of differential blocks using a long-acting anesthetic such as bupivacaine hydrochloride. This evaluation allows more precise localization of the exact area of the pathologic condition. If clear evidence exists of an isolated gastrocnemius contracture without evidence of tarsal tunnel or Baxter neuritis, an isolated gastrocnemius recession is considered.

Prior to surgery, nerve conduction and electromyographic studies are considered in patients in whom a tarsal tunnel syndrome is possible. Laboratory studies are performed to exclude systemic arthritis or spondyloarthropathies. Bone scans with technetium-99m may be considered if one suspects a fatigue fracture, or if the exact location of the pain is not clear.

For partial release of the plantar fascia, the patient is positioned supine with a small bump placed under the contralateral hip to increase the external rotation of the affected limb. A tourniquet should be used to minimize the bleeding to ensure appropriate identification of the neurovascular structures. In all cases, the tourniquet is released and appropriate hemostasis is obtained prior to closure to minimize the risk of a hematoma and irritation of the nerves that may compromise the end result. A medial oblique incision along the heel is made as described by Schon (Fig. 120.10).[53] Loop magnification may be used. The sensory

branch of the medial calcaneal nerve is located, inspected, and preserved. If entrapment of the medial calcaneal nerve occurs as it comes through the fascia, this entrapment is explored and released. Subcutaneous fat is carefully dissected and retracted to expose the superficial fascia of the abductor hallucis, which is then incised. The abductor hallucis muscle is then retracted inferiorly, and the deep fascia of the muscle is released to decompress the first branch of the lateral plantar nerve. The abductor is then retracted superiorly to visualize the plantar fascia. The medial one third of the plantar fascia is released under direct visualization, and a 1-cm square segment is excised.

Any prominent calcaneal spur may be identified deep in the wound and carefully débrided back to a smooth, low-profile base. Removal of the spur is not required and may increase the risk of plantar fascia rupture and injury to the lateral plantar nerve. No specific criteria exist on which to base excision of the spur; only that "large" spurs should be excised.

After copious irrigation and hemostasis, the incision is closed with a nylon mattress suture and a short-leg cast is applied. The patient should not bear weight for 4 to 7 days. Weight bearing in a cast or an over-the-counter brace is maintained for 14 more days. At 3 weeks, weight bearing with a shoe is permitted. Running is started at 6 to 12 weeks, and activity is then allowed as tolerated. If the patient has a biomechanical foot abnormality, an orthotic device is used after the operation.

Continued

Authors' Preferred Technique

Plantar Fasciitis—cont'd

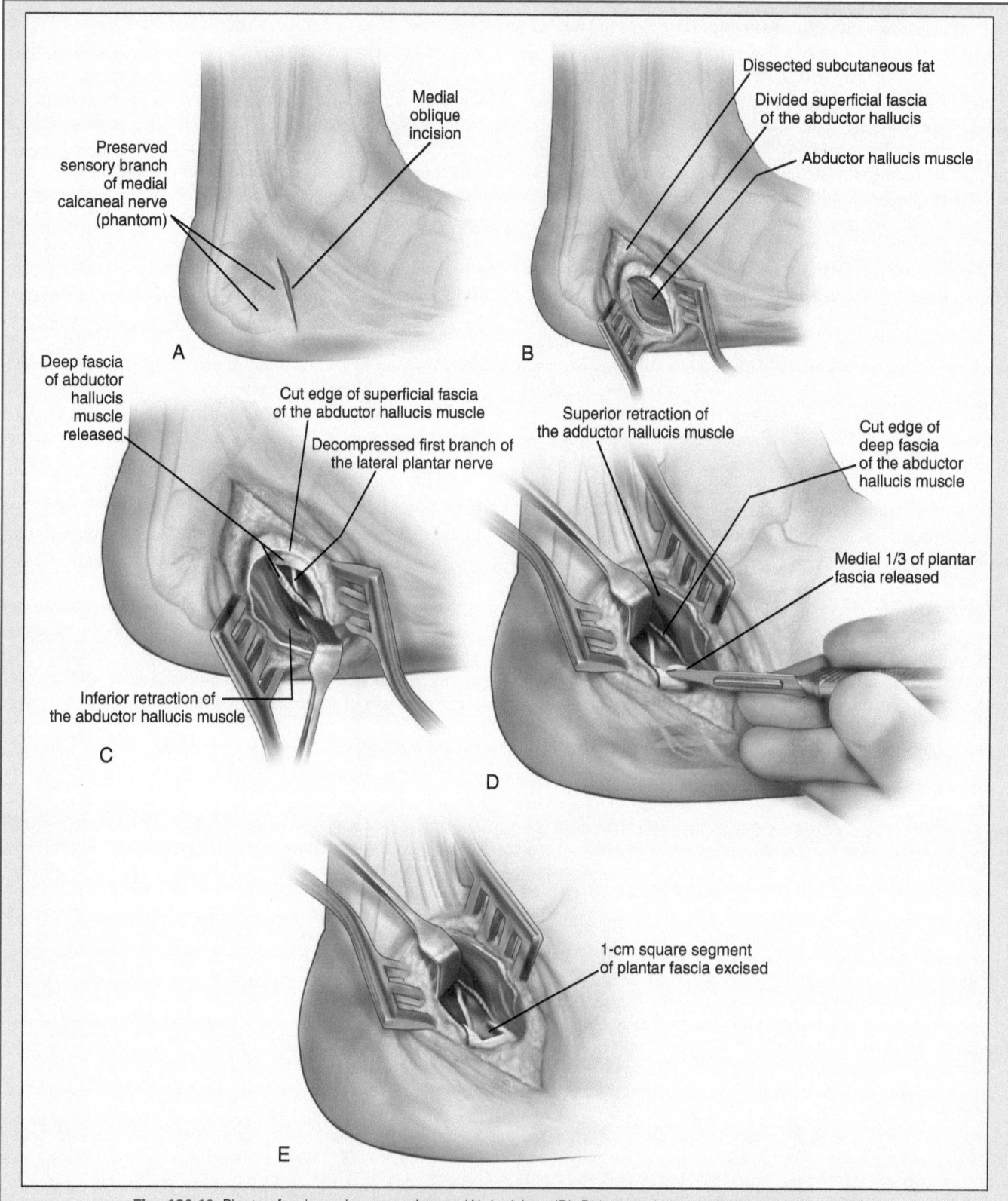

Fig. 120.10 Plantar fascia and nerve release. (A) Incision. (B) Release of the abductor hallucis muscle. (C) The abductor hallucis muscle is reflected proximally. (D) The abductor hallucis is retracted distally. (E) Resection of a small medial portion of the plantar fascia.

the heel spur if it impinged on or produced entrapment of the nerve.[31] Among the 34 heels operated on, 32 had good results and 2 had poor results.

Clancy[39] treated patients with a medial heel wedge and flexible leather support, heel cord stretching, and rest for 6 to 12 weeks, with a gradual return to running while wearing the orthotic and the medial heel wedge for 10 weeks. In patients who failed to respond to this treatment, surgery consisting of release of the plantar fascia and the fascia over the abductor hallucis longus was recommended. The 15 patients in whom surgery was performed returned to running within 8 to 10 weeks.

Henricson and Westlin[55] described 11 heels in 10 athletes who had chronic heel pain for which conservative therapy did not provide relief. The pain was due to compression of the calcaneal branches of the tibial nerve. Entrapment of the anterior calcaneal branch occurred where the nerve passed between the tight and rigid edges of the deep fascia of the abductor hallucis and the medial edge of the os calcis. Surgery consisted of identifying and releasing the tibial nerve and both calcaneal branches, and releasing the deep fascia of the abductor hallucis. Follow-up for 58 months after surgery revealed that 10 of the 11 heels were asymptomatic. The patients had resumed athletic participation after an average of 5 weeks.

Leach and coworkers[56] described 15 competitive athletes in whom 16 operations were performed. Surgery consisted of release of the plantar fascia at the insertion of the os calcis, making the incision along the medial aspect of the heel. In one instance, the medial calcaneal nerve was involved in the inflammatory process. One patient returned to running at 6 weeks; the majority returned to running 9 weeks after surgery. Most patients continued to improve up to 6 months after the surgical procedure. Of the 15 operations, 14 were entirely successful in that the athletes returned to their previous level of activity. One failure occurred in a marathon runner who improved but was unable to train at the level he desired. No complications were reported.

In 1984 McBryde[57] reported that in his running clinic, PF comprised 9% of the total running disorders seen. The conservative (nonoperative) approach of McBryde and his group consisted of (1) ice massage for 2 minutes four to six times daily, including before and after runs, (2) heel cord stretching for 3 to 5 minutes three to four times daily, (3) posterior tibial and peroneal strengthening, (4) heel cushioning and control, and (5) use of antiinflammatory medication. This regimen was usually successful in treating runners with PF who were seen within the first 8 weeks. In runners with symptoms lasting longer than 6 weeks, a period of absolute rest with use of a cast was usually required. Orthoses were used. Five percent of the patients in the series underwent surgery, consisting of plantar fascial release through a short 1-inch longitudinal incision in the medial arch. All returned to a successful running program 6 to 12 weeks after surgery. Overall, among the 100 patients with PF, 82 recovered with a conservative approach, 11 stopped running, 5 underwent surgery (all of whom returned to running), and 2 refused surgery and continued to be symptomatic.

Snider and colleagues[58] reported 11 operations for plantar fascial release for chronic fasciitis in 9 distance runners who had had symptoms for an average of 20 months and had not responded to nonsurgical treatment. The results of the operations were excellent in 10 feet and good in 1 foot, with an average follow-up time of 25 months. Eight of nine patients returned to their desired level of full training at an average time of 4.5 months.

Rask[59] reported a medial plantar neurapraxia that he termed *jogger's foot*. Three cases were reported in which there was probable entrapment of the medial plantar nerve behind the navicular tuberosity in the fibromuscular tunnel formed by the abductor hallucis; the inciting factor was eversion of the foot. All three patients were treated successfully with conservative measures, including a change in the running posture of the foot, antiinflammatory medication, and proper footwear.

In 2004, Saxena[60] reported on 16 athletes with intractable heel pain for whom conservative care had failed. Most of these athletes were runners. These patients were treated surgically with a uniportal endoscopic plantar fasciotomy. Saxena found that runners were able to return to athletic activity on average 2.6 months after surgery. Five poor results were found in patients with a body mass index greater than 27.

Complications

Acute complications after plantar fascia surgery are rare. Although few case series exist to determine reliable complication rates, the most commonly reported include wound dehiscence or infection. The most common complications reported after operative treatment for PF include further tearing or injury to the plantar fascia, collapse of the medial longitudinal arch, iatrogenic injury to the first branch of the lateral plantar nerve or neuroma formation, complex regional pain syndrome, and persistent pain. Complete excision of the plantar fascia has been associated with lateral column syndrome that presents a pain with weight bearing focused at the lateral border of the foot along the calcaneocuboid joint and fourth/fifth tarsometatarsal joints. In addition, recurrence rates after subtotal plantar fasciectomy have been reported as being approximately 10% in multiple studies.

Future Considerations

Increased focus on the role of a tight gastrocnemius complex and the effect on the function of the foot have begun to alter the surgical treatment for PF. With further research on biomechanical and clinical effect of a gastrocnemius release in patients with PF, the need for direct release of the plantar fascia may decrease. Although neither operation can be considered benign, patients with lateral column syndrome or injury to the lateral plantar nerve are severely limited without a good surgical recourse. Although injury of the sural nerve may occur, resection and burial can be performed, yielding an adequate result that does not preclude sporting activity.

For a complete list of references, go to ExpertConsult.com.

SELECTED READINGS

Citation:

Yu J, Park D, Lee G. Effect of eccentric strengthening on pain, muscle strength, endurance, and functional fitness factors in male patients with achilles tendinopathy. *Am J Phys Med Rehabil.* 2013;92(1):68–76.

Level of Evidence:

II

Summary:

The authors describe a prospective comparative study of 32 patients with Achilles tendinopathy who were placed into two treatment groups. One group underwent concentric strengthening and one underwent eccentric strengthening for an 8-week period. The authors were able to demonstrate a significant improvement in pain, balance, agility, and endurance in the patients who underwent eccentric strengthening. This article reinforces the critical nature of ensuring that therapy instructions are appropriately written for this disease process to focus on eccentric strengthening.

Citation:

Kearney R, Costa ML. Insertional achilles tendinopathy management: a systematic review. *Foot Ankle Int.* 2010;31(8):689–694.

Level of Evidence:

III

Summary:

The authors provide a systematic review of the literature regarding both operative and nonoperative management of insertional Achilles tendinopathy. Significant evidence favored conservative management, including both eccentric strengthening and shock wave therapy. The paucity of quality literature regarding operative intervention resulted in an inconclusive decision on the efficacy of surgery.

Citation:

Digiovanni BF, Nawoczenski DA, Malay DP, et al. Plantar fascia-specific stretching exercise improves outcomes in patients with chronic plantar fasciitis. A prospective clinical trial with two-year follow-up. *J Bone Joint Surg Am.* 2006;88(8):1775–1781.

Level of Evidence:

II

Summary:

The authors of this very significant article definitively demonstrate that plantar fascia–specific stretching is the critical component in the nonoperative treatment of plantar fasciitis. Efficacy was noted 2 years after the initiation of treatment with a 92% satisfaction rate.

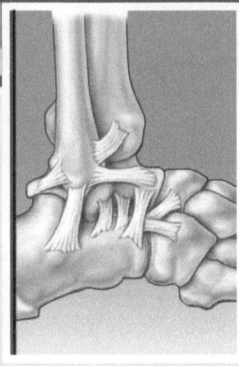

121

Forefoot Problems in Sport

Ben Hickey, Lyndon Mason, Anthony Perera

Great caution must be exercised in dealing with forefoot problems, particularly in athletes. Although the outcomes are the same as in nonathletes, even a small decrease in performance may prove to be very significant for an athlete. Therefore with certain exceptions, forefoot surgery should be considered only when conservative management has failed and the athlete is no longer able to play through the pain/dysfunction.

TURF TOE

Metatarsophalangeal (MTP) joint injuries are commonly the result of hyperextension. They are increasingly common and can be characterized by a significant delay in return to sporting activities.[1-4] Turf toe is more likely to occur on third-generation artificial surfaces versus grass, and is more than 13 times more likely to occur during a game as opposed to training.[5] Analysis of the National Collegiate Athletic Association (NCAA) Injury Surveillance System for Turf Toe in Intercollegiate Football found an overall incidence of 0.062 per 1000 athlete-exposures.[5] In a series of 20 male cadaveric feet, the first MTP joint was dorsiflexed to varying degrees and subsequently dissected to identify objective evidence of injury to the sesamoid complex, including tear in the soft tissue or avulsion fracture (deemed clinically relevant). Using binomial regression, a hallux dorsiflexion angle of 78 degrees had a 50% risk of first MTP joint sprain.[6]

History

Players may report localized pain, swelling, and pain with range of motion (ROM) and ambulation; in addition, periarticular swelling and ecchymosis are typically present. Push-off is impaired with running, and it may be difficult to crouch with the MTP joint extended.[7,8] Some patients, particularly elite footballers, may not present with an acute history and severe symptoms but may have an impending turf toe, so they should have early imaging.[9]

Physical Examination

Clinical evaluation should include evaluation of hallux alignment, including clinical MTP joint reduction, or the presence of an intrinsic-minus posture (i.e., MTP extension and interphalangeal flexion), suggesting disruption of the flexor hallucis brevis (FHB) tendon insertion. Palpation of plantar (including the individual sesamoids), medial, lateral, and dorsal structures for focal tenderness should be performed. Assessment of joint stability with respect to dorsoplantar and varus/valgus stress is

critical. Weakness in plantarflexion strength of the hallux may indicate loss of integrity of the plantar plate or the FHB.[10] Point tenderness over the plantar aspect of the first MTP joint that worsens with passive extension of the toe is indicative of injury.

Imaging

Bilateral weight-bearing anteroposterior (AP) views can identify proximal migration of the sesamoids. A forced dorsiflexion lateral view assists in the diagnosis of failure of distal sesamoid migration and diastasis of a bipartite or fractured sesamoid. The normal diastasis of a dominant foot bi- or multipartite sesamoid is on average 0.79 mm; it has been suggested that the sesamoid interval of more than 2 mm on AP radiograph of the foot is abnormal, with no statistically significant difference between gender, age, laterality of sesamoid, or foot dominance.[11] Weight bearing and stress radiographs of both feet are useful to document relative proximal migration of the sesamoids on the injured foot.[10] Magnetic resonance imaging (MRI) plays a crucial role in early and accurate diagnosis of structures involved in "turf toe" injuries.[12] Systematic assessment of the MRI can detail the integrity of the paired confluent metatarsosesamoid (MT-S) ligaments, paired sesamoid-phalangeal (SP) ligaments, the intersesamoid (IS) ligament, medial and lateral collateral ligaments, accessory collateral ligaments to the sesamoids, tendinous insertions and confluences with the plantar capsule, as well as the sesamoids, cartilage and alignment.[13] It is important to focus MR imaging on the first MTP joint during the assessment of turf toe by using an extremity coil with the joint at its isocenter as opposed to imaging the entire foot or forefoot.[13]

MRI can be used to evaluate the presence and extent of capsular or plantar plate disruption[14] and also osseous or articular damage in the presence of normal radiographs.[15] Rodeo and coworkers[16] have proposed a classification of first MTP joint injury, as shown in Box 121.1.

Decision-Making Principles

Operative intervention is rarely necessary in acute grade I and II injuries.[8] Management is usually centered on conservative methods because surgery can be associated with a restricted ROM. However, up to 25% to 50% of patients will have residual pain and limited dorsiflexion despite 6 months of rehabilitation[17]; some authors have therefore recommended surgical treatment of type III injuries.[18] On average, ligamentous turf toe results in a mean 9.1 days lost from play, whereas sesamoid fracture

BOX 121.1   **Classification of First Metatarsophalangeal Joint Injuries**

Grade 1: Acute Sprain of the First Metatarsophalangeal Joint Plantar Capsule
Localized tenderness, swelling, and pain with dorsiflexion
Normal radiographs
Conservative treatment

Grade 2: Acute Sprain of the First Metatarsophalangeal Joint With Significant Plantar Capsule Disruption
Ecchymosis, painful dorsiflexion, and loss of motion
Diastasis of a partite sesamoid or joint instability on radiographs
No degenerative first metatarsophalangeal joint changes
Conservative or surgical treatment

Grade 3: Chronic Symptoms Involving the First Metatarsophalangeal Joint Resulting From Previous Injury
Loss of motion
Degenerative joint disease, hallux rigidus, or malalignment on radiograph
Treatment is often surgical

BOX 121.2   **Sesamoid Function**

Protects the tendon of the flexor hallucis longus
Absorbs most of the weight bearing on the medial aspect of the forefoot
Increases the mechanical advantage of intrinsic musculature of the hallux
Elevates the first metatarsal head

results in a mean of 42 days lost.[5] Some patients will be out of elite-level competition for almost 6 months.[9]

Treatment Options

Nonoperative

A recent algorithm for the management of turf toe was suggested by Hong et al. in 2016. Grade 1 injuries can be treated with taping of the toe in slight plantarflexion for 3 weeks followed by a carbon fiber orthotic for 6 to 8 weeks. Grade 2 injuries are treated with a walking boot and crutches for 2 to 4 weeks and then, again, with a carbon fiber turf toe orthotic for 6 to 8 weeks. It is suggested that grade 3 injuries need surgical repair. Surgery should also be considered for sesamoid retraction or fracture, traumatic hallux valgus, first MTP joint instability, intra-articular loose bodies, or failed conservative treatment.[19] Ice, compression, and nonsteroidal anti-inflammatory drugs may be used.[1,7,20,21] However, activity should be restricted in athletes with more severe injuries and significant discomfort. The patient can continue to participate in athletics if pain is minimal. A rigid forefoot insole[1,7,20] to stiffen the shoe and taping of the toe to compress the joint and limit dorsiflexion motion all help reduce pain. For grade III injuries, immobilization and a period of restricted weight bearing is usually required for up to 8 weeks.

Return to sport depends on the severity of the injury, the resolution of symptoms, and the athlete's sport or position. Ideally, painless 60-degree dorsiflexion will be achieved in the first MTP joint before running or explosive activities are attempted. Serial examinations are important because deformity can progress with athletic activity.[21]

Operative

Less than 2% of cases require operative treatment.[5] Operative treatment is necessary in more severe injuries with joint instability, retraction of the sesamoids, diastasis of a bipartite

sesamoid or sesamoid fracture, traumatic hallux valgus, or the presence of a loose body or chondral injury. Arthroscopy is helpful in evaluating the injury, but an open approach (plantar medial with extension across the MTP joint if required) is most helpful; however, care must be taken with the plantar-medial nerve. Repair of the plate distal to the sesamoid can be achieved with suture anchors into the base of the proximal phalanx.[9] Care must be taken to avoid overtightening this repair. Despite open repair and direct visualization of the lateral sesamoid, it is recommended that intraoperative imaging may help the surgeon ensure that the plantar plate is tensioned adequately.[9] Similar techniques can be used for diastasis of a bipartite sesamoid. Postoperatively, patients are often placed into cast, boot, or splint for 4 to 6 weeks, followed by a resistive ROM program and running at 18 weeks.[10] Return to full participation in collegiate football can take 6 months.[10]

Postoperative Management

Postoperative management must balance soft tissue healing with early ROM of the MTP joint.[18] Immobilization in a removable splint (a toe spica splint in 5 to 10 degrees of plantarflexion with slight varus) with restricted weight bearing continues for 4 weeks.[21] Seven to 10 days after surgery, passive ROM is begun. At 4 weeks, weight bearing and active ROM are initiated in a walking boot. Wearing of modified footwear (i.e., a shoe with a stiff sole modified with a turf toe plate) is allowed at 8 weeks, with return to full sport at 3 to 4 months.

Results

Contrary to the common perception, evidence points to good outcomes when appropriate treatment is instigated. Most athletes with grade I and II injuries (53 of 56 in a series by Clanton et al.[1]) returned to sport within 3 weeks with careful conservative management. Even with grade III injuries, Anderson found that seven of nine players returned to sport; two failed to resume playing because of pain and degeneration.[18]

Complications

After a turf toe injury, athletes can experience persistent pain with toe-off and stiffness of the first MTP joint (Table 121.1). Instability, deformity, and degeneration can occur if the injury fails to heal well.

SESAMOID DYSFUNCTION

The sesamoid complex of the first MTP joint plays a significant role in the function of the great toe (Box 121.2). Sesamoid dysfunction is uncommon; however, it can occur with arthritis,[22–26]

Authors' Preferred Technique
Turf Toe

The patient is positioned supine with the heels at the end of the operating table. Dual incisions are recommended to repair a grade III turf toe (Fig. 121.1). A longitudinal medial incision is centered at the first metatarsophalangeal joint to access the medial sesamoid.

Care is taken during dissection to leave a cuff of joint capsule for closure at the conclusion of the case. The medial plantar digital nerve lies adjacent to the sesamoid and should be protected. A longitudinal plantar incision is commonly used for the lateral sesamoid. The lateral plantar digital nerve is at risk during this approach and must be identified and protected to prevent neuroma formation.

The plantar plate is then repaired from lateral to medial with use of nonabsorbable or slow-absorbing suture. Care must be taken to avoid damage to the flexor hallucis longus. In the absence of tissue along the proximal phalanx, use of a suture anchor to secure the plantar plate has been described. Fracture of both sesamoids should be treated with cerclage of the sesamoids to restore continuity of the flexor hallucis brevis and avoid a cock-up toe deformity. If one of the two sesamoids has severe articular damage, excision can be performed. However, in no case should both sesamoids be excised. Standard closure should be performed.

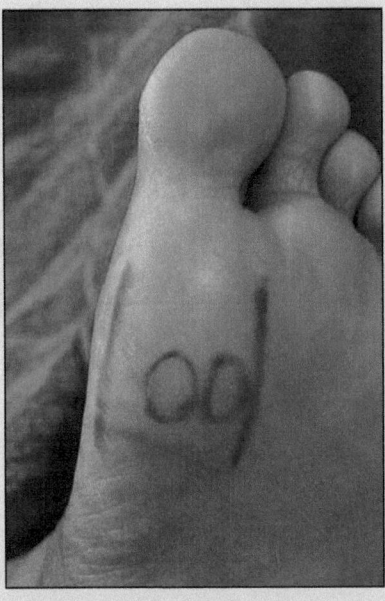

Fig. 121.1 Dual incisions are required to repair a turf toe. Each individual incision can also be used for an isolated sesamoidectomy. Care must be taken to protect the plantar digital nerve during dissection. (From Kadakia AR. Disorders of the hallucal sesamoids. In: Miller MD, Sanders TG, eds. *Presentation, Imaging and Treatment of Common Musculoskeletal Conditions*. Philadelphia: Elsevier; 2011.)

trauma,[22,24,27–36] osteochondritis,[29,37–39] infection,[40–44] or sesamoiditis.[23,38,39,45] Abnormalities and complaints regarding the sesamoids of the hallux are much more common in professional athletes than in others because of the stresses the first MTP joint is subjected to during athletic activities.[46,47]

The medial sesamoid is more commonly injured than is the lateral sesamoid because it bears greater force during normal gait.[48] The plantar lateral and plantar medial digital nerves are located adjacent to the lateral and medial sesamoids. Impingement

of either one of these branches may be a source of pain in the area of the sesamoids. Osteoarthritis of the sesamoids has been reported[22,23,25,37,49] in association with hallux valgus, hallux rigidus, and rheumatoid arthritis and as an isolated occurrence. When it is associated with a high-arched or cavus type of foot, a plantarflexed first ray may be the cause of the callus formation. When a sesamoid is involved, a more localized or concentric lesion is usually present.

History

The most frequent subjective symptoms are pain and discomfort in the toe-off phase of gait located directly plantar to the sesamoids.

Physical Examination

A cavus foot or gastrocnemius contracture increases forefoot loading and therefore should be specifically assessed. A plantar keratosis beneath either the tibial or fibular sesamoid may occasionally accompany a symptomatic sesamoid. Another method to support the diagnosis of sesamoiditis is the use of the passive axial compression test.[50] This is performed with the patient supine. After the sesamoids have been isolated, the hallux is maximally dorsiflexed at the MTP joint, which will cause distal migration of the sesamoids. The examiner's index finger is used to apply compression just proximal to the sesamoids. The patient's symptoms are reproduced with passive plantarflexion of the MTP joint as the sesamoids are compressed against the metatarsal head and phalanx.

Imaging

Often the most useful radiograph is the axial sesamoid view (Fig. 121.2). Fragmentation of a sesamoid in persons with osteochondritis may be seen on the axial radiograph. Radiographs are frequently normal despite subjective symptoms (sesamoiditis). MRI is one of the best methods for diagnosing disease of the sesamoids. Osteochondritis can be visualized very early, usually before any abnormality is seen on plain radiography. It is also useful in visualizing soft tissue abnormalities of the sesamoid mechanism.[51,52]

Decision-Making Principles

Most sesamoid problems in the athlete can be treated effectively without surgery. If conservative treatment has been unsuccessful, several surgical options are available depending on the pathologic condition. When surgical intervention is being considered, a concomitant deformity such as a gastrocnemius contraction or cavus foot alignment must be addressed.

Treatment Options
Nonoperative

Activity and footwear modification, use of insoles, and treatment of the callosities are all helpful. In patients with sesamoid pain, a stiff insole or a rocker-bottom sole reduces metatarsal joint motion and can relieve pain with ambulation. The use of a dancer's pad, which is designed with a concavity for the sesamoids, is extremely useful in nearly all cases.

TABLE 121.1   Anatomic Classification of Turf Toe

ANDERSON CLASSIFICATION[127,128]

Type of Injury	Grade	Description
Hyperextension (turf toe)	I	Stretching of plantar capsular ligamentous complex
		Localized tenderness, minimal swelling, minimal ecchymosis
	II	Partial tear of plantar capsular ligamentous complex
		Diffuse tenderness, moderate swelling, ecchymosis
		Restricted movement with pain
	III	Frank tear of the plantar capsular ligamentous complex
		Severe tenderness, marked swelling, and ecchymosis
		Limited movement with pain, plus vertical Lachman test
		Possible associated injuries:
		Medial/lateral injury
		Sesamoid fracture/bipartite diastasis
		Articular cartilage/subchondral bone bruise
Hyperflexion (sand toe)		Hyperflexion injury to hallux MTP or IP joint
		May involve injury to lesser MTP joints as well
Dislocation	I	Dislocation of the hallux with the sesamoids
		No disruption of the intersesamoid ligament
		Frequently irreducible
	IIA	Associated disruption of the intersesamoid ligament
		Usually reducible
	IIB	Associated transverse fracture of one or both sesamoids
		Usually reducible
	IIC	Complete disruption of intersesamoid ligament with fracture of one of the sesamoids
		Usually reducible

IP, Interphalangeal; *MTP*, metatarsophalangeal.

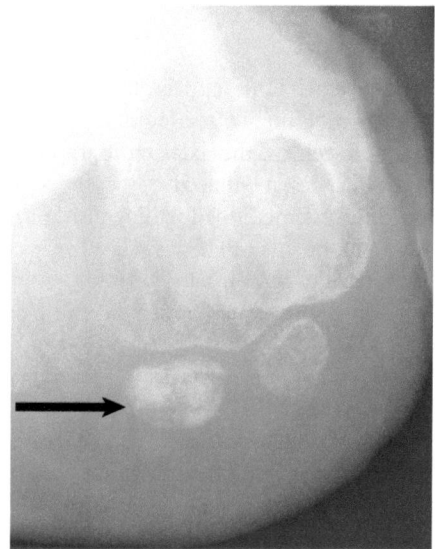

Fig. 121.2 Sesamoid views allow visualization of the metatarsal-sesamoid articulation. This view clearly demonstrates sclerosis *(arrow)*, flattening, arthritis, and fracture. (From Kadakia AR. Disorders of the hallucal sesamoids. In: Miller MD, Sanders TG, eds. *Presentation, Imaging and Treatment of Common Musculoskeletal Conditions.* Philadelphia: Elsevier; 2011.)

Operative

Surgical treatment includes a tibial or fibular sesamoidectomy as well as sesamoid shaving. Excision of a single sesamoid does not usually lead to deformity as long as careful operative technique is used.[52] Removal of both tibial and fibular sesamoids is rarely

indicated because it predictably results in the development of a cock-up and intrinsic-minus deformity of the hallux. Arthrodesis of the MTP joint with excision of the sesamoid may alleviate arthritic symptoms and provides a stable medial buttress to the first ray but it will severely compromise function in an athlete. Although a sesamoidectomy is occasionally necessary for cases of intractable plantar keratosis (IPK), surgical shaving of the involved sesamoid may preserve function in the athlete and facilitate a more rapid recovery (Fig. 121.3).[51,52] Sesamoid shaving or resection in the presence of a plantarflexed first ray is associated with a high rate of recurrence of the keratotic lesion.[53,54]

📌 Authors' Preferred Technique

Sesamoid Dysfunction

Excision of the affected sesamoid with use of the previously described incisions is the treatment of choice except in the case of an intractable plantar keratosis. Care must be taken to avoid damage to the flexor hallucis brevis and flexor hallucis longus. The soft tissue defect must be repaired to avoid iatrogenic deformity.

Postoperative Management

After sesamoid excision, a soft compression dressing is used and the patient is allowed to ambulate in a postoperative shoe. Weight bearing on the heel is recommended to minimize soft tissue trauma to the forefoot and promote healing of the incision. Return to play after surgical intervention for sesamoid dysfunction is typically between 2 and 4 months after surgery. When

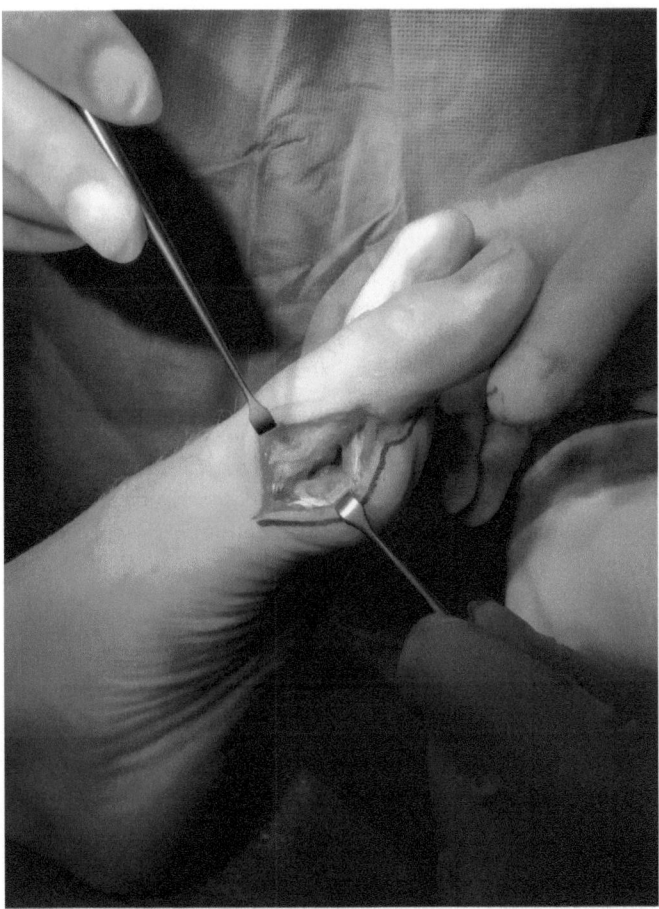

Fig. 121.3 Plantar medial incision to tibial sesamoid.

shaving of the tibial sesamoid is performed, the athlete is allowed to resume running about 6 weeks after surgery.

Results

Sesamoidectomy has not been described as a treatment for acute fractures or nonfragmented nonunions of the sesamoids. However, it has been described for sesamoiditis. Saxena and Krisdakumtorn reported a mean average return to activity between 7.5 and 12 weeks in 26 patients.[55] Eleven professional/varsity athletes returned to sports at a mean of 7.5 weeks, whereas 13 "active" patients returned to sporting activity at a mean of 12 weeks.

Complications

Saxena and Krisdakumtorn reported two cases of hallux valgus, one case of hallux varus, and two cases of postoperative scarring with neuroma-type symptoms in their series, representing a 19% complication rate.[55] Transfer metatarsalgia may also occur.

METATARSALGIA

The term *metatarsalgia* is defined as pain of the plantar forefoot beneath the second, third, and fourth metatarsal heads.[56,57] It is an umbrella diagnosis incorporating many etiologic origins. A key aspect in managing metatarsalgia is to assess the biomechanical factors involved.[58] Metatarsalgia can be subdivided into primary, secondary, and functional categories along with pathologic conditions that arise during the stance and propulsive phases of gait.[57,59] Primary metasarsalgia is due to anatomic abnormalities of the metatarsal lengths, tightness of the gastrocnemius, or hindfoot abnormality resulting in forefoot overload.[58] The first ray bears 40% of the weight distribution of the forefoot, with the lesser four rays sharing the remaining 60%.[60] Bearing in mind that the first, fourth, and fifth metatarsal-tarsal articulations allow considerable flexibility compared with the more rigid second and third metatarsal-tarsal articulations,[61] any factor that lessens the ground force of the first metatarsal can increase the pressure applied to the lesser metatarsal heads. Metatarsal length discrepancy can similarly cause overload of one or more of the metatarsal heads. The most common pathology is the presence of an excessively long second metatarsal.[62] Static metatarsalgia is often due to metatarsal slopes, whereas propulsive metatarsalgia is related to abnormal lengths.[58] During gait, the pressure center transfers under the metatarsal heads when the knee is extended and the ankle is in neutral dorsiflexion, between the 60th and 90th percentiles of the stance phase. In this critical phase, the knee is extended and gastrocnemius tightness may overload the forefoot, resulting in metatarsalgia.[63] Hyperextension of the lesser toe MTP joint during gait can produce a dynamic plantar protrusion of the metatarsal head as the toe is extending and the metatarsal head is forced plantarward.[57]

An IPK is a localized callosity occurring on the plantar aspect of the foot.[64] A generalized callus can develop in the forefoot of an athlete as a result of increased pressure, and it is normal for a moderate amount of callus to form; in contrast, an IPK is a well-localized keratotic lesion. DiGiovanni et al. studied a population of patients presenting with forefoot pain and found the incidence of gastrocnemius contracture to be 65% (out of 34 patients).[65] Many authors have emphasized the importance of gastrocnemius tightness in producing forefoot symptoms and the positive effect on the gait pattern when such tightness has been overcome.[66,67]

History

Barouk emphasized the distinction between stance and propulsive metatarsalgia and advocated different treatments for these conditions.[59] It is thus important to obtain a thorough history of the aggravating and relieving factors of the pain to try to discern between the two conditions. Athletes often report increased symptoms with specific activities or footwear. In persons with IPK, pain is usually directly under the callus.

Physical Examination

Physical examination first entails careful evaluation of the alignment of the foot when standing. The position of the hindfoot, the arch, and any great toe or lesser toe deformity should be noted. When a pes cavus deformity is suspected, a Coleman block test should be performed to determine if a fixed flexion deformity of the first metatarsal is present.[68] The plantar aspect of the foot should be carefully evaluated because the location of callosities can indicate the underlying problem. Stance-phase metatarsalgia generates proximal localized callosities or pain, whereas propulsive-phase metatarsalgia generates distal pain and a linear-type callosity.[59] Trimming of the callosity usually reveals a well-circumscribed keratotic lesion. Solitary keratotic lesions are sometimes difficult to distinguish from a wart; however, keratotic lesions occur directly under a bony prominence, and unlike warts, they are avascular.

A discrete IPK caused by a prominent metatarsal head lateral condyle can be seen on the lateral side of the metatarsal head, typically under the fourth metatarsal. Identification of this IPK is important because it is amenable to simpler surgical correction with a quicker rehabilitation and recovery and is a more predictable procedure than is a metatarsal osteotomy.

With suspected stance-phase metatarsalgia, the foot should be evaluated for abnormal plantar flexion of the lesser metatarsals. Elevation of the first metatarsal pushes the entire load of the second rocker onto the second metatarsal, resulting in isolated keratosis underneath the second metatarsal head.[57] Propulsive keratosis, however, occurs during the third rocker of the gait cycle when external rotation of the lower limb results in a shearing force. This produces a more rounded appearance of the callosity, which extends distally toward the toe.[57] Hypermobility of the first ray should be evaluated along with midfoot mobility, because an unstable first ray can overload the lesser metatarsals.[69]

Each MTP joint should be palpated to assess for position, synovitis, and joint stability because instability of the lesser toe MTP joints is a common but often under recognized cause of metatarsalgia.[70] The plantar flexion power of a lesser toe can be assessed using by the paper-pull test, where the patient tries to resist a strip of paper from being pulled from beneath the terminal phalanx. Inability to resist the paper being pulled from beneath is positive and may suggest a plantar plate tear.[70] The plantar plate provocation test can be used to differentiate plantar plate tears from Morton neuroma. In this test, the patient is seated with the foot hanging freely, and the examiner extends the toe, placing a plantar-directed force to the proximal phalanx to stress the plantar plate. If this causes pain, it is shown to correlate with subsequent findings of plantar plate injury on MRI.[71] Pain at the second metatarsal head, a positive drawer test, and edema have high sensitivity, whereas previous first ray surgery or crossover toes have high specificity.[72]

Each intermetatarsal web space should be palpated to assess for tenderness of the interdigital nerves. The Silfverskiöld test is performed to evaluate for contracture of the gastrocnemius and the gastrocnemius-soleus complex; the foot is maintained in an inverted position to avoid dorsiflexion movements at the midtarsal joints.[57,73,74]

Imaging

Evaluation includes weight-bearing dorsoplantar and lateral views of the foot. Sesamoid views are included, depending on the location of the pain. The length of each metatarsal (MT) is assessed. Maestro et al. described the "harmonic parabola" where, in gait analysis studies, they considered the lateral sesamoid of the first MTP joint as a pivot.[62] They also emphasized the longitudinal axis of MT2; the line passing through the center of the lateral sesamoid and bisecting a line perpendicular to the MT2 longitudinal axis is termed the Maestro line.[59] This line must pass through the center of the MT4 head to provide metatarsal harmony. Another method for assessing the relative lengths of

MT1 and MT2 was described by Hardy and Clapham, whereby a line is drawn along the axis of MT2 to bisect a transverse tarsal line drawn along the posterior articular surface of the cuboid. From this intersection, arcs are drawn at the level of the MT1 and MT2 articular surfaces, and the difference is assessed in millimeters. In an asymptomatic foot, MT1 has been shown to be between 2 and 4 mm longer than MT2 (mean 2 mm) using this method.[75] The kinetographic effects of a relative short MT1 with overload of the MT2 head and subsequent hypertrophic changes have been well described by Morton.[76] The slope of each MT and the difference in diaphyseal inclination between MT1 and MT2 are assessed on the lateral view. It is important to assess the oblique radiographs also to determine whether an apparently short metatarsal is truly short or whether it is apparently short due to increased plantar obliquity of the ray.[77] Radiographic evaluation may contribute to the diagnosis of a subluxated or dislocated MTP joint. Careful attention is given to bony abnormalities that may be responsible for areas of increased pressure. If the IPK is large, then ultrasonography can be helpful because dermoid inclusion cysts have been reported.[78]

An extended sesamoid view of the metatarsal heads end-on with the toes dorsiflexed out of the way is useful in identifying a prominent metatarsal head lateral condyle and abnormalities in the transverse arch.

Decision-Making Principles

If a keratotic lesion continues to be symptomatic and significantly impairs athletic function, surgical intervention is considered. Because of the lengthy postoperative recovery time and the possibility of restricted MTP motion, recurrence, or the development of a transfer lesion, a rigorous trial of trimming, padding, and orthotic management should be carried out before surgery is performed. Surgical release of a gastrocnemius contracture must be considered with great caution in athletes because a gastrocnemius recession may result in the weakening of push-off. However, more recently, interest in performing a proximal medial gastrocnemius recession has increased. Abbassian et al. have demonstrated that medial head release at the knee can be performed safely with use of a local anesthetic followed by immediate loading, and most importantly, the power loss is minimal.[79]

If all conservative efforts to treat metatarsalgia fail, then surgery is necessary. The goal of surgery is to distribute pressure evenly along the forefoot, thus reducing high-pressure areas. It is therefore essential to consider the clinical examination, pressure distribution, and x-ray evaluation to carefully plan a metatarsal osteotomy if this procedure is required. One should plan to correct metatarsal length to harmonize the parabola and elevate prominent heads to offload them.

Treatment Options
Nonoperative

The initial treatment of an IPK of any cause involves trimming the lesion to reduce the keratotic buildup. Trimming a callus also helps in differentiating it from a wart.

When the callus has been trimmed, a soft metatarsal pad is placed proximal to the keratosis to redistribute the pressure more uniformly. The use of a soft insole can alleviate the pressure

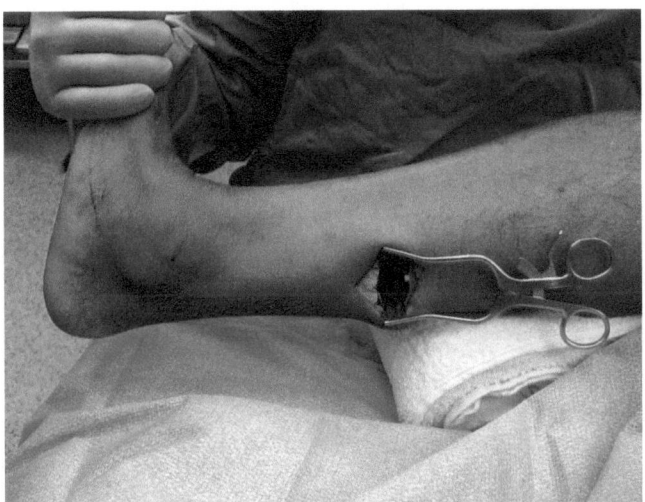

Fig. 121.4 After release of the gastrocnemius fascia, improvement is noted in the dorsiflexion range of motion of the ankle with the knee extended.

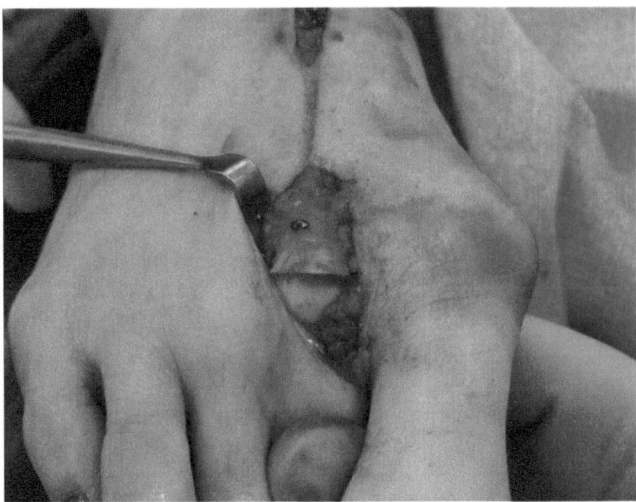

Fig. 121.5 Intraoperative appearance of the metatarsal head after fixation with a 2.4-mm screw. Note the dorsal overhanging bone that must be removed to allow for appropriate articulation. (From Seybold J, Kadakia AR. Claw and hammer toes. In: Miller MD, Sanders TG, eds. *Presentation, Imaging and Treatment of Common Musculoskeletal Conditions.* Philadelphia: Elsevier; 2011.)

further in athletes.[80] Athletic footwear should provide a wide toe box and a soft sole to lessen impact when running. A Plastazote orthosis can be fabricated to relieve pressure beneath the IPK and provide correction for a postural deformity. Patients with tightness of the calf, be it gastrocnemius or the gastrocnemius-soleus complex, are taught stretching exercises to lengthen the muscles and thereby decrease pressure at the forefoot. Rocker-bottom shoes may also be helpful in reducing symptoms of metatarsalgia.[58]

Operative

In all cases, the presence of a gastrocnemius contracture is treated with surgical release if the patient has persistent pain after engaging in a regimented nonoperative program (Fig. 121.4). In a series of 73 patients, some as young as 18 years of age (mean 50 years), gastrocnemius recession using Strayer technique was performed as an isolated primary procedure. All patients had positive Silfverskiöld test prior to surgery, and 38% ($n = 28$) had metatarsalgia preoperatively. Of these, only half reported excellent or good results, with visual analog scale pain scores decreasing from a mean of 5.6 preoperatively to 2.3 postoperatively at a mean follow up of 45 months.[81] Fair evidence (grade B) supports gastrocnemius recession for the treatment of isolated foot pain due to midfoot-to-forefoot overload syndrome in adults.[82] Mann and DuVries proposed that a small, discrete, IPK is caused by a prominent fibular condyle on the plantar aspect of the metatarsal head.[83] DuVries described a plantar condylectomy to correct this deformity.[84] Mann and Mann recommend removal of 20% to 30% of the condyle through a dorsal incision.[64] This procedure was later modified by Mann and DuVries, who performed an MTP arthroplasty, removing about 2 mm of the articular surface along with the plantar condylectomy.[83] After MTP joint arthroplasty, MTP joint motion is diminished by 25% to 50%. Although stiffness does not always affect function in a sedentary person, a competitive athlete typically requires more normal motion; if so, an MTP arthroplasty is contraindicated.

Elevation of the metatarsal head can be achieved with use of a vertical chevron procedure.[83,85,86] A distal oblique osteotomy,[87–92] capital oblique (Weil) osteotomy,[57,59,93,94] and three-step (Maceira) osteotomy[57,95] are designed to both shorten the metatarsal and elevate the metatarsal head (Fig. 121.5). These procedures are best used in the treatment of propulsive-phase metatarsalgia. It is believed that elevation of about 3 mm is necessary for adequate decrease of pressure beneath the symptomatic metatarsal head.[96] Hansen described midshaft segmental osteotomy in which two parallel cuts are made in the bone, which is subsequently fixed with a four-hole plate.[97] Galluch et al. reported good results with this osteotomy in 95 patients. A 99.2% union rate was reported, and transfer lesions developed in 5 patients.[98]

Postoperative Management

A compressive dressing is applied at the time of surgery, and the patient is allowed to bear weight in a postoperative shoe. After a metatarsal osteotomy, adequate time must be allowed for healing. Premature athletic activity may lead to failure of fixation, displacement of an osteotomy, or nonunion. In general proximal metatarsal osteotomies require 6 to 12 weeks for osseous union to occur. A vertical chevron osteotomy performed with a thin oscillating saw blade heals in about 6 weeks. After an MTP joint arthroplasty and condylectomy, about 6 weeks is necessary for adequate healing to occur at the MTP joint.

Once adequate healing has occurred (generally in 4 to 6 weeks), gentle ROM is initiated at the MTP joint to diminish postoperative stiffness. When radiographs demonstrate bony union, aggressive walking activity is initiated. Taping of the forefoot or the use of soft metatarsal pads helps to alleviate symptoms with athletic activity during recovery from surgery. About 4 weeks after the initiation of walking, jogging is initiated, followed by running activities as pain permits.

⚡ Authors' Preferred Method
Metatarsalgia

When a competitive athlete requires a more normal motion, a distal metatarsal osteotomy is generally considered the osteotomy of choice. A number of osteotomies have been described in both treatment of stance-phase and propulsive-phase metatarsalgia, although distal osteotomies are generally used to treat propulsive metatarsalgia.

The distal metatarsal is approached dorsally, between the metatarsals if two are to be operated on. The collateral ligaments are released in order to release the plantar tissues in case of a hammer-toe deformity; if the toe is subluxed/dislocated, the plantar plate is likely to be torn and will require repair. The collateral ligaments may require reefing in case of coronal plane deformity. The most important step in a distal metatarsal osteotomy is to make the cut as parallel to the weight-bearing axis of the foot as possible to ensure that shortening does result in plantar flexion of the metatarsal head. Next, a parallel slice of the metatarsal is removed according to the amount of shortening/elevation that is required. This osteotomy is fixed with a screw and is performed under image intensifier control to assess the metatarsal parabola (Fig. 121.6).

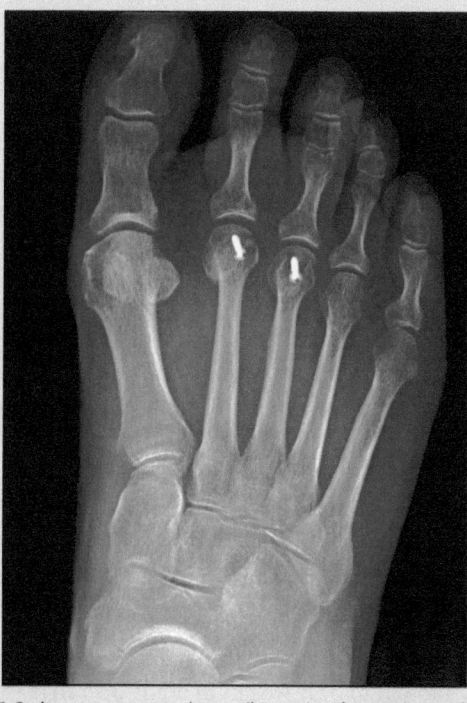

Fig. 121.6 An anteroposterior radiograph of a patient after Weil osteotomy of the second and third toes. The normal cascade of the foot is preserved, with the third toe slightly shorter than the second. Maintaining this cascade is critical to prevent iatrogenic metatarsalgia. (From Seybold J, Kadakia AR. Claw and hammer toes. In: Miller MD, Sanders TG, eds. *Presentation, Imaging and Treatment of Common Musculoskeletal Conditions.* Philadelphia: Elsevier; 2011.)

Decreased ROM is a significant risk after MTP arthroplasty as well as after a distal metatarsal osteotomy. In the postoperative follow-up, one should pay close attention to any impending deformity or stiffness; it will be easier to start passive stretching or manipulation with use of a block or anesthetic earlier rather than later. In athletes, plantarflexion is very important. Full return to athletic activity is expected when bony healing occurs. Usually between 6 and 12 weeks after surgery, aggressive walking is initiated. Walking is advanced to jogging after 4 weeks as permitted by pain and swelling. The athlete then increases running activities as tolerated, gradually returning to sport between 3 and 6 months after surgery.

Results

In the treatment of an IPK, Winson and coworkers found that 53% of their patients had significant postoperative symptoms, including transfer lesions in 32%, nonunion in 13%, and an overall recurrence of an IPK in 50% of patients.[92] In 66 of the 124 feet, major postoperative complaints were noted. The authors stressed that in either a cavus or a rigid foot, a distal oblique sliding osteotomy was contraindicated.

In the treatment of propulsive stance metatarsalgia, the Weil-type or triple-step osteotomy is becoming the most accepted practice. Good to excellent long-term results have been noted in 70% to 100% of patients treated with a Weil-type osteotomy.[99–101] The three-step osteotomy was introduced to try to reduce complications observed with a Weil osteotomy. Espinosa et al. reported that joint stiffness and floating-toe deformities were rarely seen with this type of osteotomy.[57] Pérez-Muñoz et al. reported on 82 patients treated with a Weil or three-step osteotomy; they found recurrence of metatarsalgia in 4.3%, moderate joint stiffness in 60.2%, floating toes in 4.3%, and delays in bone healing in 7.5%. All delayed unions occurred in the triple osteotomy group and were presumed to be a result of the decreased stability of the osteotomy.[102]

Mann and DuVries evaluated 100 patients with discrete IPKs and noted a recurrence rate of 17.6% after MTP arthroplasty. Of these recurrences, 5% were found under the symptomatic metatarsal. A transfer lesion developed in 13% of cases. Despite these results, 93% of the patients were satisfied with their outcome.[83]

Complications

Complications reported with a Weil-type osteotomy include joint stiffness, floating-toe deformity, and transfer metatarsalgia. Stiffness may be caused by morphologic alterations of the MTP joint postoperatively, fibrosis, reaction to osteosynthesis material, or biomechanical alterations of the intrinsic musculature.[57,99,103] Beech et al. noted that postoperative joint ROM was reduced in most cases.[94] Floating-toe deformity has been reported in up to 30% of cases.[104]

A 5% rate of complications was found after condylectomy and MTP arthroplasty for discrete IPK, which included fracture of the metatarsal head, avascular necrosis, drift of the involved toe, and cock-up of the involved toe.[83]

Future Considerations

With further study of the effect of a gastrocnemius contracture on the incidence of forefoot pain, a shift away from bony correction of the foot pathology may occur if the outcomes are favorable. The morbidity from forefoot surgery as described is a major detriment to performing these operations in the athlete, and the possibility of a soft tissue correction without subsequent loss of athletic function would be very desirable.

HALLUX RIGIDUS

History

Typical presenting symptoms of hallux rigidus are pain overlying the MTP joint from cartilage degeneration possibly combined with mechanical shoe pain as a result of a dorsal bony prominence. The pain worsens over time with activity and typically improves with rest and elimination of restrictive footwear. Athletes will report a reduction in motion when crouching or during push-off. Once pain at night or at rest is noticed, the degeneration within the joint is generally widespread. Plantar pain suggests degeneration in the inferior surfaces of the MTP joint or the MT-S joints and is a relative contraindication for cheilectomy.[105,106]

Examination

Hallux rigidus is a restriction of motion due to degenerative changes in the first MTP joint. The MTP joint may demonstrate a plantarflexed position with a dorsal prominence (Fig. 121.7). Tenderness typically starts dorsolaterally on the joint line and is worse at the extremes of motion. With increased severity, the patient may have pain with the "grind test," in which the examiner impacts the phalanx on the first metatarsal head in the central ROM. A positive test is consistent with end-stage arthritis, denoting that a simple cheilectomy will not be effective. Compression of the first MTP joint during assessment of ROM can help the clinician decide whether the articular surface glides freely and indicate intact cartilage.[106]

Hallux rigidus should be considered clinically as either functional or structural, and it is essential to examine the ROM at the first MTP joint during both non–weight bearing and weight bearing to assess the influence of gastrocnemius tightness. Patients who have good passive dorsiflexion range when non–weight bearing but a reduction during weight bearing are considered to have functional hallux rigidus. In these patients osteotomies should enable a change in functional arc of motion and improve symptoms. Functional hallux rigidus is assessed with the patient supine and upward pressure placed on the first metatarsal head

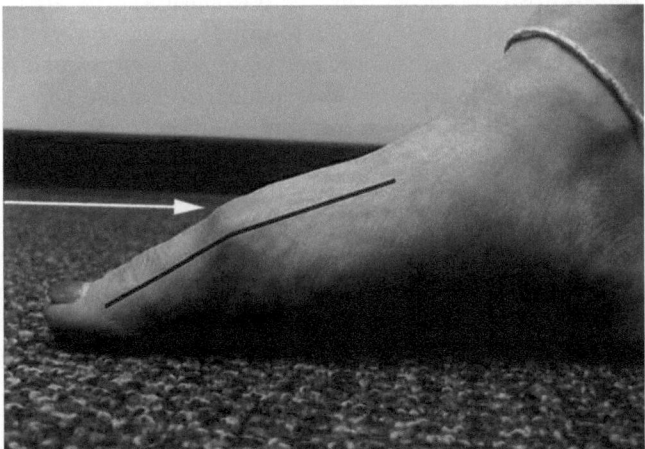

Fig. 121.7 A patient with hallux rigidus with a fixed flexion deformity of the hallux. Note the large dorsal prominence *(arrow)*. (From Seybold J, Sabb B, Kadakia AR. Arthritides of the foot and ankle. In: Miller MD, Sanders TG, eds. *Presentation, Imaging and Treatment of Common Musculoskeletal Conditions.* Philadelphia: Elsevier; 2011.)

to simulate weight bearing and bring the ankle to neutral position. The first MTP joint should have at least 60 degrees dorsiflexion in this position. When dorsiflexion is applied to the first MTP joint in this position, the movement should occur at the first MTP joint. If the ankle plantarflexes to achieve the ROM at the MTP joint, this is considered functional hallux rigidus.[107] If patients have restricted ROM during both non–weight bearing and weight bearing (i.e., structural hallux rigidus), arthrodesis or arthroplasty is preferred.[108]

Imaging

Radiologic classification systems have been proposed but do not correlate well with clinical features.[109] Narrowing of the joint, dorsal spurs from the metatarsal and phalanx, and loose body formation are common findings.

Decision-Making Principles

Although the clinical and radiographic severity of hallux rigidus can be classified according to Coughlin and Shurnas, ranging from stiffness with normal radiograph to stiffness and pain throughout the first MTP joint range with more than 50% joint space narrowing and severe dorsal osteophytes, it must be remembered that the natural history of hallux rigidus is inconsistent.[109,110] Conservative measures must always be tried in the first instance for all athletes; thus the real decision-making lies in the choice between joint-sparing and joint-loss procedures. Clearly sporting requirements must be considered, but some key clinical features will aid in the decision-making. For instance, pain at night or at rest, crepitation upon passive motion, or a positive grind test suggests a widespread problem that will not respond to a joint-sparing option and instead requires either fusion or a motion-sparing salvage procedure. As long as patients understand that outcomes may be reduced, cheilectomy can be considered even in the presence of radiographic degeneration provided that there is no significant bone loss.[106]

Similarly, sesamoid pain will not be alleviated by an MTP cheilectomy. On the other hand, a smooth arc of motion (albeit reduced) and pain at the end of the range suggest that a cheilectomy is feasible.

The issue becomes difficult in cases of a failed cheilectomy or when the choice between cheilectomy and fusion is not clear-cut; in these cases, radiographic findings and visualization of the joint (arthroscopy is better than MRI) is helpful in determining whether the joint is salvageable.

In patients with symptomatic functional hallux rigidus, distally based metatarsal osteotomies such as the Watermann-Green, Youngswick, and oblique distal metatarsal osteotomy are useful. All of these options result in shortening of the MT1 and therefore are best performed in cases of an elongated first ray, where shortening is desirable. The Watermann-Green is versatile and enables rotation of the distal bone to redirect intact plantar cartilage to a more dorsal position. However, it has been suggested that if this is not done with caution, symptoms may occur at the MT-S joint due to increased contact pressures. The Youngswick osteotomy is similar but the plantar limb is at 60 degrees rather than 135 degrees to the dorsal cut and is more reproducible, resulting in shortening and depression of the metatarsal head. Both osteotomies are inherently stable. Another option is the oblique distal osteotomy, which is at 30 degrees to the saggital plane and allows shortening and depression of the metatarsal head but has no scope for realignment of the articular surface. For this reason it is best used if the articular surface does not need realignment. In practice, all of these procedures are combined with a cheilectomy.[108] When there is functional hallux rigidus with an elevated first ray but no arthritis of the first MTP joint, a proximal plantarflexion osteotomy has been advocated.[108] Clinical heterogeneity of outcome studies with small numbers of study participants makes it impossible to draw definitive conclusions as to which osteotomy is superior.[111]

Treatment Options

Nonoperative

Surgery is not advised for asymptomatic functional hallux rigidus.[107] Certain activities such as dancing or sprinting demand a high degree of dorsiflexion. These cases are difficult to manage conservatively other than to treat the patient with intra-articular corticosteroid injections and nonsteroidal anti-inflammatory drugs. However, in a recent questionnaire study of patients who underwent corticosteroid injection for hallux rigidus, although 20 of 22 (91%) of patients reported a benefit, only 3 (14%) reported benefit that lasted more than 3 months. In view of this, corticosteroids have a limited role in management of hallux rigidus.[112]

Because injections are likely to accelerate the wear within the joint, they must be used judiciously. The mainstay of conservative treatment is stabilization of the first MTP. Taping and orthotics can be very useful in pain control, but these measures, of course, reduce the joint's motion.[109] A double-blind clinical trial of patients with hallux limitus, comparing custom-made in-shoe orthotics that elevated the first MTP joint versus the same orthotic without elevation, found a significant increase in maximal dorsiflexion in the intervention group or 22.2 degrees as compared with the control group, which increased range by 5.65 degrees. However, this study excluded patients with first MTP joint pain or radiographic osteoarthritis.[113]

Operative

Joint-sparing procedures should be performed for athletes if at all possible. If such procedures are not appropriate, joint-destructive but motion-sparing procedures (e.g., an osteotomy or interposition arthroplasty) should be considered. However, metallic or Silastic joint replacement has no role in the athlete. Ultimately fusion surgery is a durable and long-term solution that allows robust activity.

Cheilectomy.   A cheilectomy is the first line in surgical management. Impingement always starts dorsally and spreads downward except in traumatic lesions, which start centrally; thus a cheilectomy is not appropriate for this group. Removal of the dorsal 25% of the joint and the osteophyte is very successful at removing the footwear irritation and the end-of-range impingement pain. It does not usually improve the ROM but prolongs the athlete's career, even though it does not slow down the rate of progression (Fig. 121.8). In a recent single-surgeon study of 179 patients who underwent open cheilectomy, 58 patients were

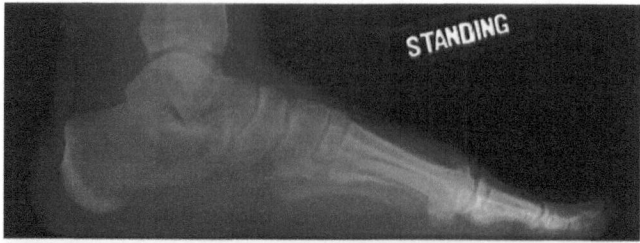
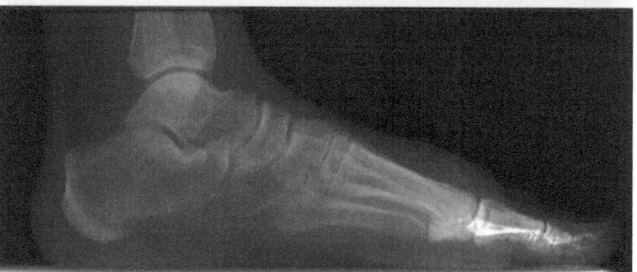

Fig. 121.8 Preoperative and postoperative radiographs of a patient with grade II hallux rigidus who underwent a cheilectomy. The postoperative radiograph demonstrates removal of the dorsal osteophytes from both the metatarsal and the phalanx. The final appearance of the metatarsal reveals colinearity, with the metatarsal shaft indicating adequate bony resection. (From Seybold J, Sabb B, Kadakia AR. Arthritides of the foot and ankle. In: Miller MD, Sanders TG, eds. *Presentation, Imaging and Treatment of Common Musculoskeletal Conditions.* Philadelphia: Elsevier; 2011.)

followed up at a mean follow up of 7.14 years (33.5% response rate). The mean percentage improvement in pain score was 87.71%, with 88% returning to normal function, including exercise. Overall, 95% of patients stated that they would undergo the procedure again whereas 88% reported either no pain or occasional pain.[114] Approximately 3% of patients required subsequent first MTP joint arthrodesis.[114]

Arthroscopic treatment of hallux rigidus.   Arthroscopic cheilectomy is preferred when the articular surfaces require direct inspection, for example when the radiographic findings do not correlate with symptom severity.[106] Fusion is also possible arthroscopically[115] and consent should include the intraoperative decision to convert to fusion if the joint has severe degeneration. For arthroscopic cheilectomy, the osteophyte can be marked with Kirschner wires under fluoroscopic imaging to penetrate the articular surface; then resection is completed arthroscopically with reference to these.[115] Other authors do not use wires to mark resection for arthroscopic cheilectomy but resect until 50 to 70 degrees of passive dorsiflexion is achieved.[106]

Minimally invasive treatment of hallux rigidus.   Minimally invasive first MTP joint fusion, using high-speed burr under radiographic imaging, enables patients to mobilize full weight bearing postoperatively, with 90% achieving clinical union at 6 weeks of follow-up and 85% having radiographic evidence of fusion at 1 year.[116] Minimally invasive cheilectomy results in significant reductions in pain at a minimum follow-up of 1 year.[105]

Osteotomy.   Moberg osteotomy is used in young active patients with moderate to severe hallux rigidus (Hattrup and Johnson grades II and III), to augment cheilectomy where conservative treatment has failed.[117] The Moberg procedure dorsiflexes the proximal phalanx, enabling greater movement through the third rocker before the MTP joint must engage; thus it results in a

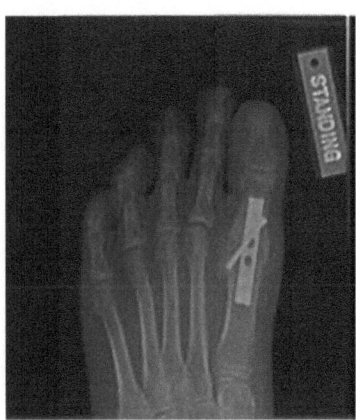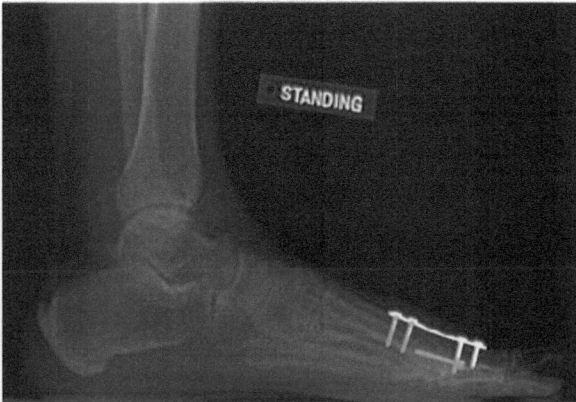

Fig. 121.9 A first metatarsophalangeal arthrodesis using a dorsal plate and lag screw for fixation. (From Seybold J, Sabb B, Kadakia AR. Arthritides of the foot and ankle. In: Miller MD, Sanders TG, eds. *Presentation, Imaging and Treatment of Common Musculoskeletal Conditions*. Philadelphia: Elsevier; 2011.)

functional increase in the dorsiflexion of the joint and can also decompress the joint.[118] A dorsal closing wedge is performed in combination with a cheilectomy; it is very stable and heals rapidly. If the joint has poor plantarflexion, the toe may be too elevated, causing problems with footwear in stance. Rehabilitation is similar to that for a cheilectomy. An important preoperative consideration for performing the Moberg procedure is to determine whether the patient has adequate first MTP joint plantarflexion preoperatively, which will be lost after the procedure. The patient should be counseled for this and also for the intraoperative decision to proceed with arthrodesis if the joint is found to have severe arthritis.[117]

Two metatarsal osteotomies can be considered, especially in the athlete with advanced degeneration who runs. In the long or elevated metatarsal, a shortening/plantarflexing osteotomy (the chevron type is the most stable) can be performed and is straightforward to plan, execute, and fix. If the metatarsal length is normal, then a dorsally rotating distal oblique osteotomy can be performed.

Motion-sparing procedures in advanced degeneration. Resection or interposition arthroplasty, although not joint sparing, can provide excellent pain relief while maintaining motion and may be preferable to arthrodesis in certain athletes for whom dorsiflexion is important, such as dancers or runners. Cosmesis may be poor with a short, elevated toe, but the range of movement may be excellent. Recently synthetic cartilage hemiarthroplasty of the first MTP joint using polyvinyl alcohol (PVA) hydrogel was found to result in functional outcomes and pain relief comparable to first MTP joint fusion, with the benefit of maintaining motion. However, the long-term outcomes and results in athletes are currently not known.[119–121] Resection or Keller arthroplasty is not recommended in a young active population, although the Valenti procedure—which resects the dorsal metatarsal head and dorsal phalangeal base and maintains length and plantar loading—can obviate some of these issues.[122]

Metatarsophalangeal arthrodesis. MTP arthrodesis remains the gold standard of pain relief and function.[123] Although it comes at the cost of sacrificing any remaining movement, generally very little movement is left in persons with late-stage disease

anyway. However, in athletes who require dorsiflexion or who have a short great toe, it should be used with caution. Care should also be taken in the person who has significant motion of the interphalangeal joint with uncovering of the phalangeal head and loading of the head. Loss of motion at the MTP joint will increase the loading on the phalangeal head in these cases, and this situation can be very difficult to manage.

The joint should be fused in 10 to 15 degrees of dorsiflexion relative the weight-bearing position of the foot to maximize the third rocker without setting the toe too high, in which case it may rub on the toe box (Fig. 121.9). We assess this simulated weight-bearing position intraoperatively with a footplate and ensure that the pulp of the hallux is approximately 1 cm off the plate. This position may also be achieved by placing a fingertip under the hallux pulp in the simulated weight-bearing position. This has been shown to equate a first MTP joint extension angle of between 1 and 10 degrees relative to the ground and is well tolerated clinically.[124] Fusion angles of less than this may place the interphalangeal joint at risk of subsequent degenerative change. Use of normal footwear can be resumed at 6 weeks after weight bearing on the heel in a protective shoe from the time of surgery. Participation in sports can generally be resumed 3 to 4 months after surgery. Nonunion mandates further surgery, but the rates with current implant techniques are very low.

Results

In appropriate cases, cheilectomy has excellent outcomes, and rehabilitation is rapid. Approximately 70% of patients obtain excellent relief, 10% obtain modest relief, and 20% get no relief.[126] Microfracture of lesions below the level of the osteotomy or of isolated central lesions has an unreliable outcome.

Percutaneous and arthroscopic techniques appear to improve the rate of rehabilitation, but few data are as yet available on this subject, with no studies comparing open versus arthroscopic treatment of hallux rigidus.[115] Arthroscopy allows visualization of the joint and therefore may be preferable. It is generally at least 8 weeks before running sports can be commenced, although cycling and swimming can be commenced earlier. It takes 3 to 4 months to achieve maximum outcome.

Authors' Preferred Technique

Hallux Rigidus

Cheilectomy is the mainstay of treatment of the athlete. The joint is approached dorsally and the collaterals are released to allow full visualization; it is important to free up the sesamoids and plantar plate because they are frequently adherent to the underside and can restrict movement. After removal of the dorsal 25% of the head, it is refashioned to make it rounder and more congruent. One should attempt to achieve at least 80 degrees of dorsiflexion; if this degree of dorsiflexion is not achieved, a dorsiflexing osteotomy of the proximal phalanx (a Moberg osteotomy) may be considered. Patients are able to bear weight and start gentle active motion immediately and can begin full rehabilitation once the wound has healed.

MTP fusion remains the gold standard in terms of pain relief and longevity, but if movement is important, our preferred motion-sparing option is the interposition arthroplasty.[125] A cushion of soft tissue is made from periosteum, attached fat, and tendon and stabilized by suturing to the plantar capsule. Alternatively, regenerative tissue matrix may be used as the interposition material. Implant arthroplasty has no role in the athletic population.

Complications

A cheilectomy can work very well, even in persons with radiologically advanced disease. However, a significant number of patients will have ongoing pain and stiffness that can limit participation in sports, and a small number may have significant arthrofibrosis that can prevent return to sport. This group is best served with revision to a fusion, although a course of intraarticular steroids may be of some benefit.

With modern fixation techniques, outcomes from fusion are reliable. Shortening of the big toe can cause rubbing on the end of the second toe, but this problem can readily be treated. A more difficult issue is the case with painful loading on the proximal phalangeal head, which occasionally requires conversion of a fused MTP joint into an interposition arthroplasty.

For a complete list of references, go to ExpertConsult.com.

SELECTED READINGS

Citation:
Anderson RB. Turf toe injuries of the hallux metatarsophalangeal joint. *Tech Foot Ankle Surg.* 2002;1(2):102–111.

Level of Evidence:
III

Summary:
The author provides an excellent review of turf toe injuries combined with an algorithm of treatment from the surgeon's extensive experience.

Citation:
Hong CC, Pearce CJ, Ballal MS, et al. Management of sports injuries of the foot and ankle: an update. *Bone Joint J.* 2016;98-B(10):1299–1311.

Level of Evidence:
III

Summary:
The authors provide an excellent contemporary review of turf toe injuries.

Citation:
Kadakia AR, Molloy A. Current concepts review: traumatic disorders of the first metatarsophalangeal joint and sesamoid complex. *Foot Ankle Int.* 2011;32(8):834–839.

Level of Evidence:
II

Summary:
The authors provide a comprehensive review regarding the diagnosis and treatment of injuries to the metatarsophalangeal (MTP) joint and sesamoids. The review covers the current level of evidence and grades of recommendation for the treatment of first MTP capsuloligamentous injury and sesamoid pathology.

Citation:
Cychosz CC, Phisitkul P, Belatti DA, et al. Gastrocnemius recession for foot and ankle conditions in adults: evidence-based recommendations. *Foot Ankle Surg.* 2015;21(2):77–85. http://doi.org/10.1016/j.fas.2015.02.001.

Level of Evidence:
IV

Summary:
In this topical review, the authors provide an up-to-date summary of the evidence for gastrocnemius recession.

Citation:
Mann RA, Mann JA. Keratotic disorders of the plantar skin. *J Bone Joint Surg Am.* 2003;85(5):938–955.

Level of Evidence:
III

Summary:
The authors of this excellent review cover the possible etiologies and discuss how to address the specific pathologic condition accordingly.

Citation:
Seibert NR, Kadakia AR. Surgical management of hallux rigidus: cheilectomy and osteotomy (phalanx and metatarsal). *Foot Ankle Clin.* 2009;14(1):9–22.

Level of Evidence:
III

Summary:
The authors provide a comprehensive review regarding hallux rigidus, with a focus on joint-sparing procedures. The technique and results of multiple operations are discussed.

Spine and Head

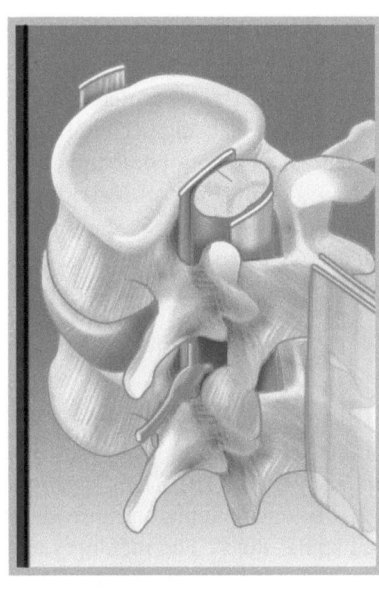

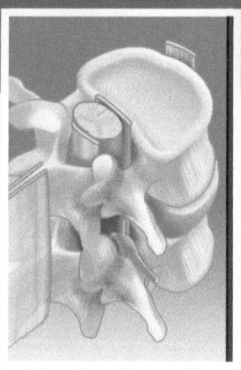

122

Head and Spine Anatomy and Biomechanics

Colin B. Harris, Rachid Assina, Brandee Gentile, Michael J. Vives

INTRODUCTION

The complexity of the central nervous system (CNS) as well as the bones and soft tissues that provide its protection present special challenges when treating the injured athlete. A thorough understanding of the normal anatomy and biomechanics of the brain and spine are necessary in order to identify pathologic states or unstable injuries and treat them appropriately. The following chapter presents a review of the anatomy of the head and spine, as well as the biomechanics of both normal and injured states. Despite the complexity of this topic, it is possible to identify common patterns that allow an improved understanding of head and spine anatomy that serves as a solid foundation for diagnosing and treating these injuries in the athlete.

ANATOMY

The relationships between the rigid bony structures that surround and protect the brain (skull), the spinal cord, and the nerve roots (cervical, thoracic, lumbar, and sacral-coccygeal vertebrae) as well as the intervening soft tissues that provide dynamic stability are outlined below. Athletic injuries can damage these structures by either sudden, high-energy trauma, such as a direct blow or whiplash type injury, to repeated loading within a more physiologic range that nevertheless can cause pain or disability. Spine and brain injuries are greatly feared by athletes in a variety of sports due to their potential catastrophic nature, such as traumatic brain injury (TBI) and spinal cord injury (SCI), which can have life-altering and often irreversible consequences. The following overview of the relevant anatomy is meant to provide a background for understanding the biomechanics of the head and spine as well as the pathologic states that can lead to these potentially devastating injuries.

SKULL (CRANIUM)

To best understand how concussions and other brain injuries occur, it is important to fully understand and appreciate the anatomy involved. The anatomy covered within this chapter is a brief overview, which begins with the most external parts and then works through internally. The cranium is the skeleton of the head, a union of functional components combined to form a single skeletal formation. The basic functional component is to house and protect the brain. The skull consists of 22 bones;

8 of which protect the brain—4 singular bones centered along the midline (frontal, ethmoidal, sphenoidal, and occipital) and 2 sets of bones occurring as bilateral pairs (temporal and parietal), with the remaining 14 bones comprising an individual's facial structure[1] (Fig. 122.1A). They are essentially fixed, immovable joints, which are connected along multiple suture lines. The only independent movement of the skull occurs at the temporomandibular joint.

BRAIN

The cranial meninges are the covering of the brain that lies immediately within the skull (see Fig. 122.1B). Their function is to protect the brain, provide the blood supply, and provide a space for the flow of cerebral spinal fluid[1]. The meninges are composed of three distinct layers: the dura mater, the arachnoid mater, and the pia mater[2]. Each layer has a specific role in the protection of the CNS. The dura mater is the outer-most layer of the meninges and is a tough, thick, bilaminar membrane that adheres to the internal surface of the skull. It is additionally comprised of three layers, which include the periosteal, meningeal, and dural sinus. The periosteal layer lines the skull and the meningeal layer lines the periosteal layer, except when separated by the dural sinus. The dural sinus forms the major venous drainage pathways from the brain, predominantly to the internal jugular veins. The dura mater has an extensive framework of blood supply to itself and provides significant blood supply to the skull through multiple branches of different arteries. The dura mater is also pain sensitive due to being innervated by branches of the trigeminal nerve.[1,3]

The arachnoid mater is avascular and not attached to the dura mater, but is held in place by the cerebrospinal fluid (CSF). The arachnoid mater is directly above the subarachnoid space, which is a cobweb-like structure housing CSF. The pia mater is the inner most layer of the meninges. It is a highly vascularized structure directly under the subarachnoid space and adheres to the brain by following its contours.

The brain is composed of the cerebrum, cerebellum, and brainstem (see Fig. 122.1D). When the skull and the dura are removed, the gyri, sulci, and fissures are made visible through the arachnoid and pia layers. The cerebrum is what makes up the major portion of the brain and is divided into two major parts: the right and left cerebral hemispheres, which are separated by the great longitudinal fissure. The two hemispheres can then

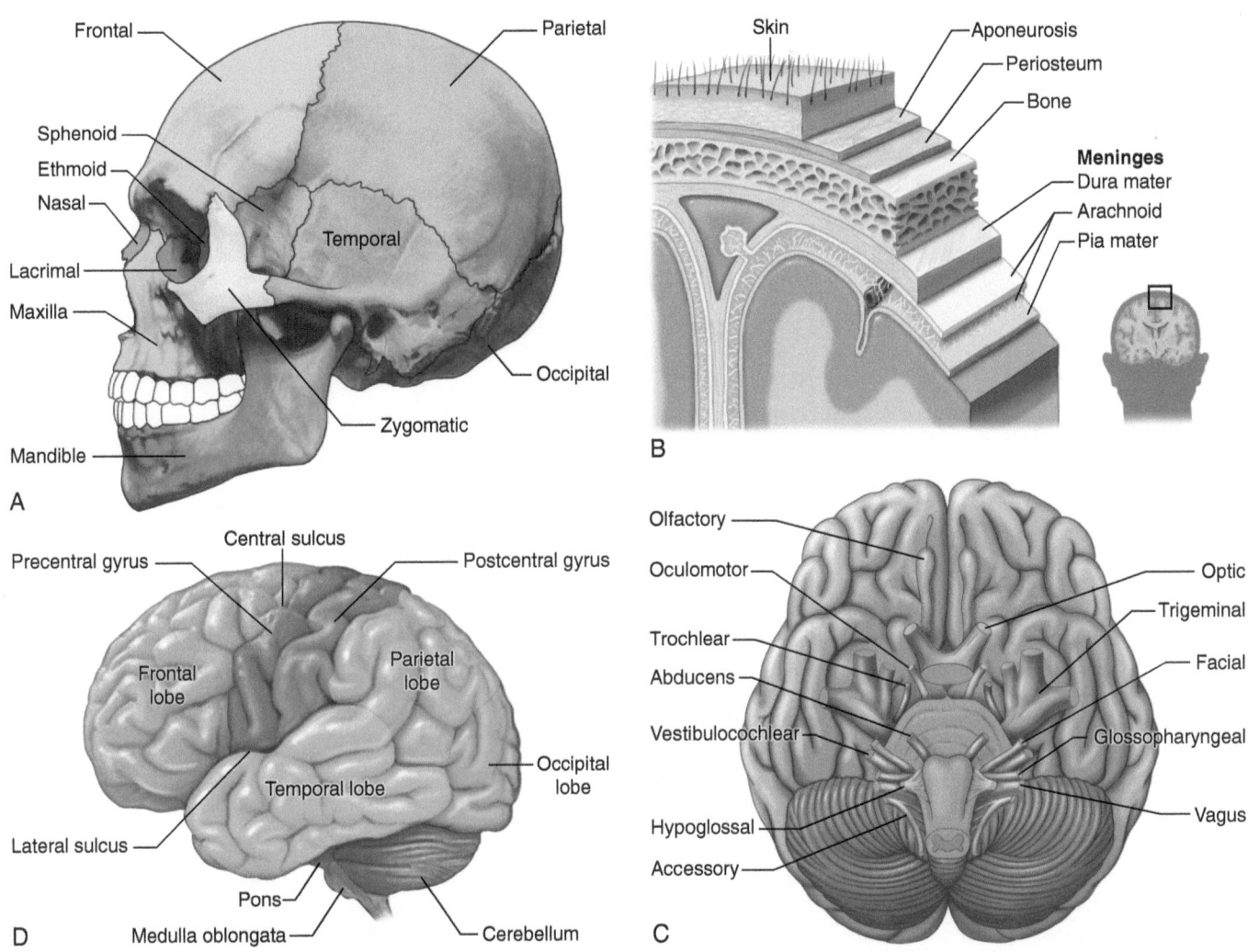

Fig. 122.1 (A) Sagittal view demonstrating the bones of the skull (https://en.wikipedia.org/wiki/Meninges#/media/File:Meninges-en.svg). (B) Coronal cross-section demonstrating the layers of the skull and meninges (https://en.wikipedia.org/wiki/File:Human_skull_side_simplified_(bones).svg). (C) The brain and brainstem (https://en.wikipedia.org/wiki/Lobes_of_the_brain#/media/File:Blausen_0101_Brain_LateralView.png). (D) View of the inferior surface of the brain demonstrating the cranial nerves (https://en.wikipedia.org/wiki/Cranial_nerves#/media/File:Brain_human_normal_inferior_view_with_labels_en-2.svg).

be subdivided into the frontal, parietal, temporal, and occipital lobes. Each lobe of the brain roughly correlates with the same location as the skull bone by the same name. The two hemispheres of the brain are conjoined by the corpus callosum, which allows the two hemispheres to continually deliver messages to the other. The cerebellum lies posterior to the pons and medulla oblongata. The cerebellum receives afferent information concerning voluntary movement from the cerebral cortex and from the muscles, tendons, and joints.[1] The brainstem consists of the medulla oblongata, pons, and midbrain. This area is crucial for cranial nerve (CN) function, excluding those associated with olfaction and vision, as well as sympathetic and parasympathetic autonomic functions. The brainstem also serves as the location for efferent and afferent pathways to cross between the cerebrum and cerebellum.

The CN are motor or sensory fibers that innervate muscles or glands. An injury can occur to the CN through injury to the skull, excessive movement of the brain, or tumors. There are 12

CN pairs that originate from the brain and penetrate through the dura. They are responsible for a variety of functions and are vulnerable to injury; a detailed review is out of the scope of this chapter (see Fig. 122.1C).

HEAD INJURIES

Head injuries are any injury to the scalp, the skull, or the brain and can range from minor bruising to severe TBI. Head injuries can be classified as closed, in which case the skull remains intact, or open where there is a breakdown of the scalp and/or fracture of the skull. Common head injuries include scalp wounds, skull fractures, concussions, contusions, and hemorrhages.

The skull is composed of outer and inner tables with an intermediate vascular diploic space. Skull fractures occur as a direct head trauma and may involve the cranial vault or the base of the skull. Cranial vault fractures can be open or closed, and can be linear (Fig. 122.2A) or depressed (see Fig. 122.2B). Skull

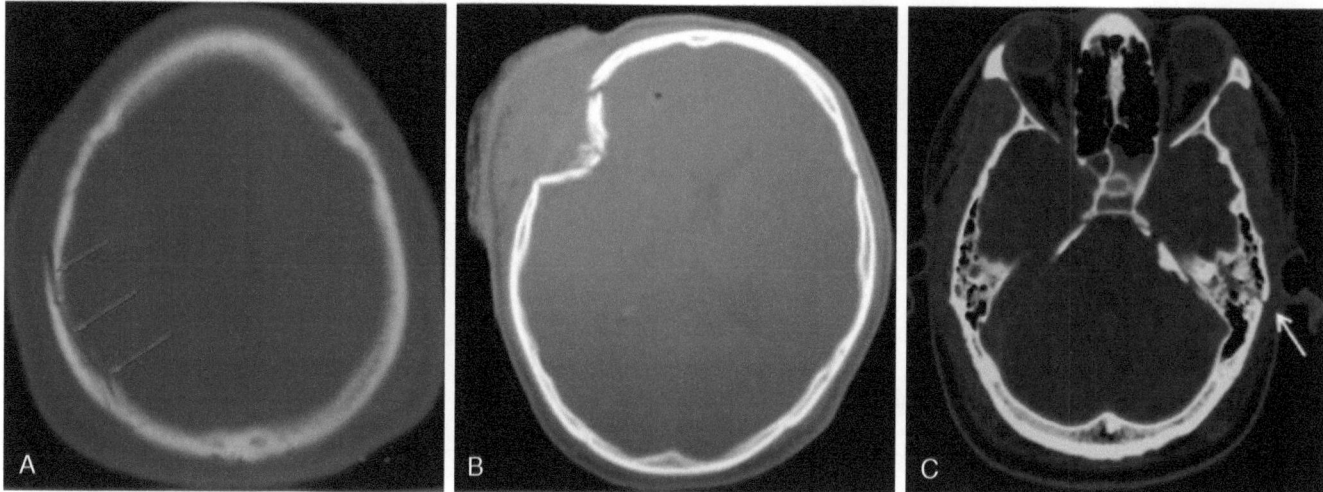

Fig. 122.2 Axial computed tomography images demonstrating a linear cranial vault fracture at the parietal bone as indicated by arrows (A), depressed cranial vault fracture at the frontal bone (B), and linear skull base fracture through the petrous portion of the temporal bone (arrow pointing to left temporal bone illustrates fracture line) (C).

base fractures are typically linear and may be associated with CN damage, dural laceration, and possible CSF leak from the nose (rhinorrhea), or the ear (otorrhea) (see Fig. 122.2C).

Traumatic intracranial hemorrhages occur when a blood vessel within the skull is damaged. Hemorrhage can occur at the epidural, subdural, arachnoid spaces or within the brain matter. A subdural hematoma is the most common hemorrhage after traumatic head injury. It is a brain bleed that has created its own space between the dura mater and the arachnoid mater. It is typically the result of a blow to the head that causes the brain to thrust back and forth within the skull; most often tearing a superior cerebral vein as it enters the superior sagittal sinus. It also can be caused by the rupture of a subdural artery. This type of hemorrhage follows the contour of the brain in a concave shape (Fig. 122.3A). An epidural hematoma is also typically the result of a blow to the head. However, this type of bleed is different from a subdural hematoma in that it is most commonly arterial in origin and occurs when blood from a torn branch of the middle meningeal artery collects between the skull and the dura mater. This can cause compression of brain tissue, requiring surgical evacuation. Epidural hematomas are usually associated with a lucid interval; which is a temporary improvement of the patient's condition after a TBI. The patient lapses into unconsciousness after recovery from the initial concussive force when the continued bleeding causes expansion of the hematoma past the brain's ability to compensate. The hemorrhage expands along the epidural space, but it does not cross the suture lines, forming a concave shape (see Fig. 122.3B). Cerebral contusions are another type of brain bleed that can occur after head trauma, and is a bruise of the brain tissue. It is associated with multiple diffuse or localized microhemorrhages from ruptured veins or arteries. It commonly occurs in coup injuries where the brain is bruised directly under the area of impact, and/or contrecoup injuries in which the brain is injured on the side opposite to the impact. The brain is easily bruised near sharp ridges of the inside of the skull under the frontal and temporal lobes, making the frontal and temporal lobes the most common contused areas

of the brain (see Fig. 122.3D). A subarachnoid hemorrhage is an arterial bleed into the subarachnoid space and may occur as a result of a head injury, the most common, or spontaneously, from a ruptured cerebral aneurysm or an arteriovenous malformation (see Fig. 122.3C).

CONCUSSION

A concussion is a temporary loss of brain function after a head trauma. It is also known as minor head trauma or mild traumatic brain injury. It is the most common type of TBI. The patient may or may not experience a temporary loss of consciousness, and intracranial hemorrhage or skull fracture may or may not be present. Therefore concussion is usually a diagnosis of exclusion and is considered a complex neurobehavioral syndrome with a multi-faceted clinical dilemma. A concussion is caused by a rapid acceleration or deceleration of an individual's brain within their skull, caused by either a direct or indirect blow to their head. This can occur in either a linear or rotational fashion; which then causes intracranial imbalances and metabolic changes to occur.[4] According to the Centers for Disease Control and Prevention, the number of emergency department, sports recreation-related traumatic brain injury (SRR-TBI) treatments increased between 2001 and 2012. During that time, there were approximately 3.42 million emergency room visits for children between the ages of 0 and 19 for the treatment of SRR-TBI.[5] Activities associated with the SRR-TBI varied by age and gender. There are many factors believed to play a role in how an individual is able to diffuse the impact sustained from a possible concussive force. Musculoskeletal strength as well as the musculoskeletal weakness of the individual—specifically the core and neck musculature, the levels of CSF of the individual, and the self-awareness of either a direct or indirect impact—are all believed to be possible factors in one's ability to defuse a possible concussive hit. For instance, the role of the CSF inside the cranium may play a role in decreasing concussions. If the forces exerted are not great enough to exceed the threshold needed to force

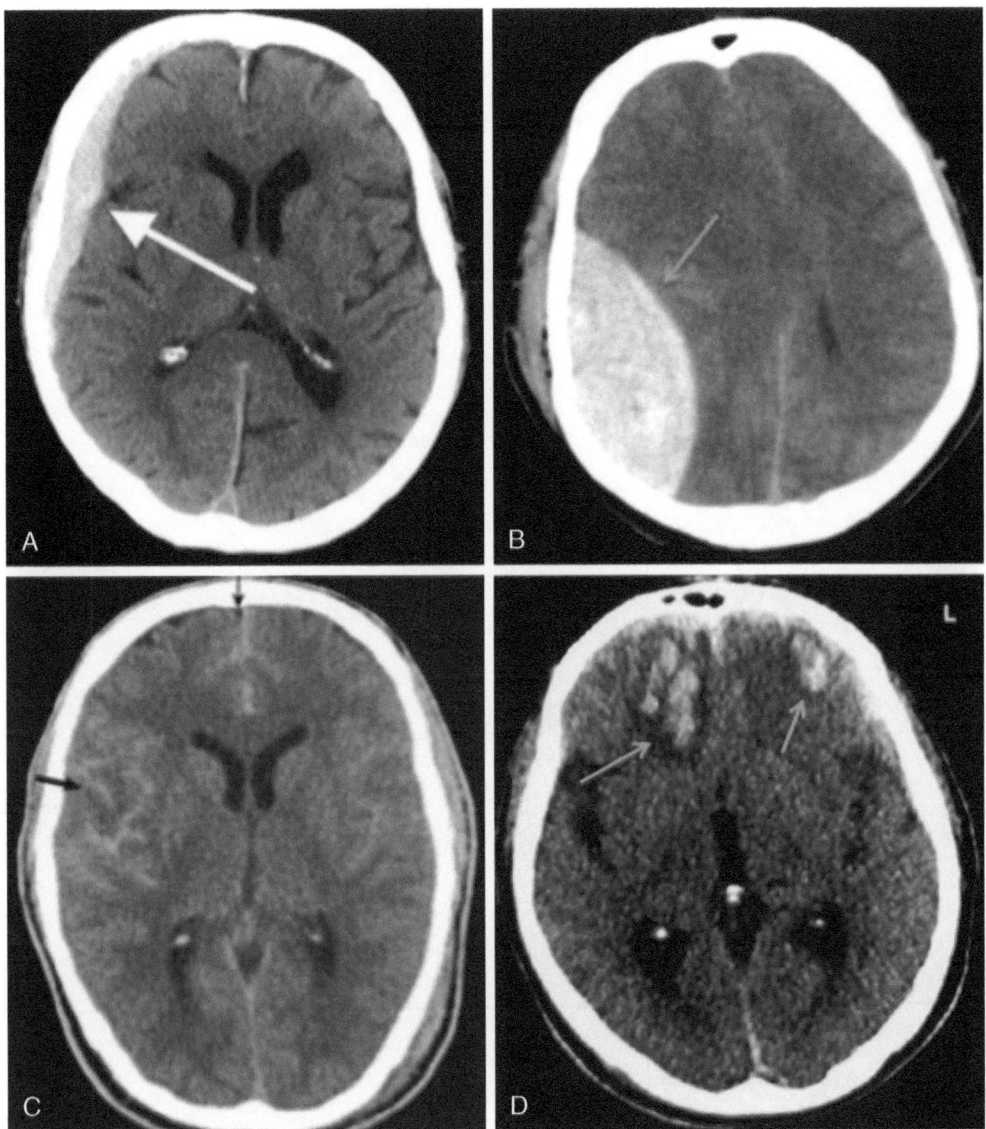

Fig. 122.3 Axial computed tomography scans demonstrating intracranial hemorrhages. (A) Acute right subdural hematoma *(arrow)* following the contour of the brain. Note the concave shape. (B) Acute right epidural hematoma *(arrow)* confined between the coronal and lambdoid sutures. Note the convex shape. (C) Acute traumatic right frontal and temporal subarachnoid hemorrhage *(arrow)*. (D) Bilateral frontal basal contusion *(arrow)* where the brain interfaces with the rough base of the anterior cranial fossa.

the brain to impact the interior of the skull, an injury may not occur.[6] A linear acceleration/deceleration action can occur in multiple different ways. For instance, a top-of-the-head type impact or anterior-to-posterior type injury can cause a coup or a coup-countrecoup-type mechanism of injury. A coup-countrecoup type of injury occurs on the side of the impact, as well as on the opposite side due to the rebounding of the brain inside the cranium, whereas a coup injury occurs only at the site of impact. Rotational acceleration impacts are thought to be more likely the cause of loss of consciousness in concussions rather than linear/translational acceleration types of impacts.[6] This is likely due to the location of the injury. It is believed that the rotational acceleration impact causes shearing and tensile strains of the cerebrum about the brainstem. Since one of the functions of the brainstem is consciousness, one could

hypothesize that if the brain stem were affected, consciousness could be as well.

The mechanical etiology of concussions and brain injury, as well as their neurologic consequence, are complex and continue to be researched. Concussions represent a clinical dilemma for sports medicine professionals. Understanding the anatomy, biomechanics, and varied symptoms is essential in furthering the understanding and advancement in the course of their treatment.

SPINE

The adult spine is composed of 33 vertebrae, or bony blocks, which protect the spinal cord and nerve roots, and support the cranium. The typical arrangement is 7 cervical, 12 thoracic,

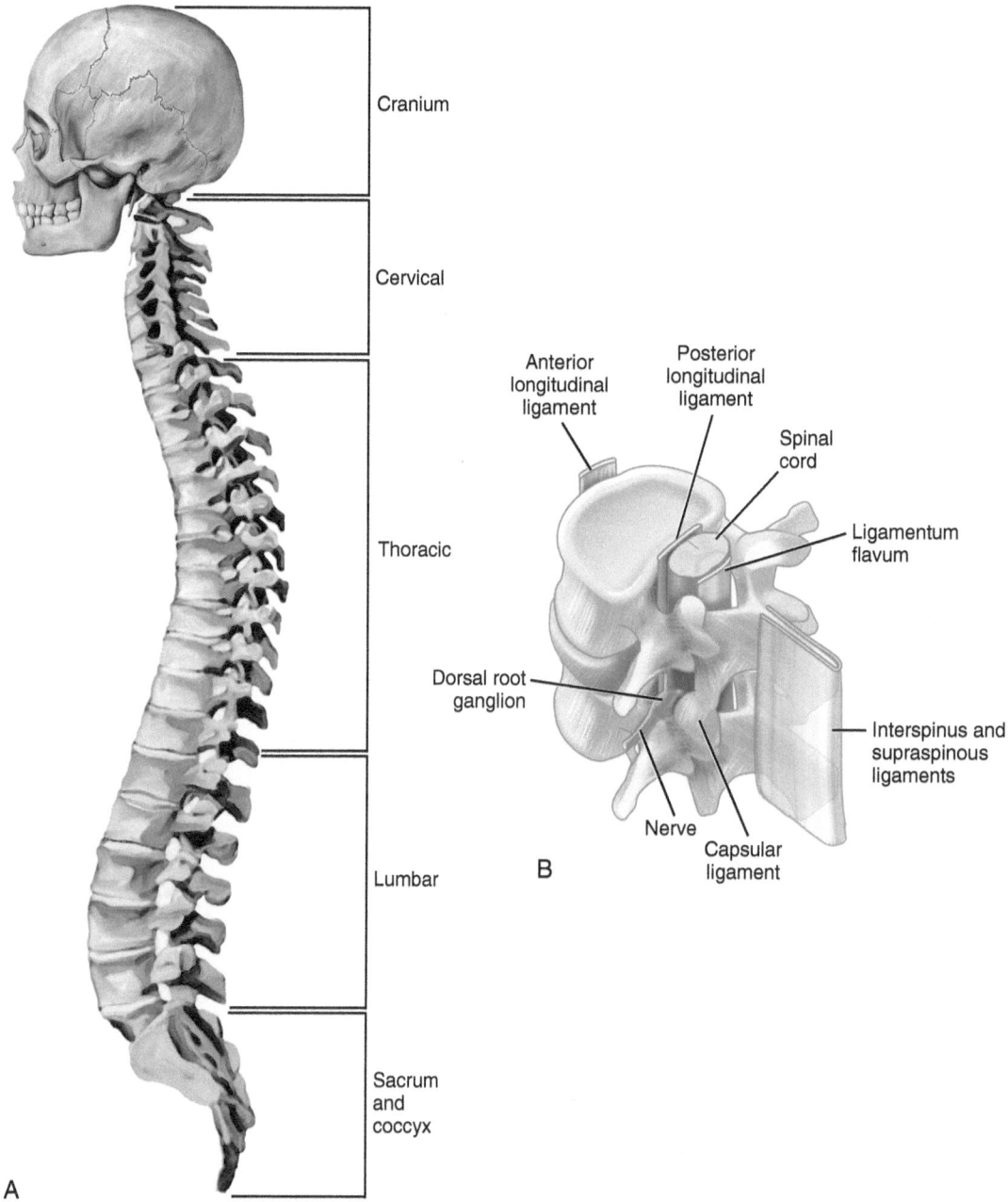

Fig. 122.4 The lateral view of the skull and spine (A). Detailed view of a spinal motion segment consisting of two vertebrae and the intervertebral disk, ligaments, and neural tissues (B).

5 lumbar, and 3 to 5 fused sacral and coccygeal vertebrae (Fig. 122.4A), although numerous variations in normal anatomy exist in up to 10% of the population.[7] Each vertebra from the second cervical (C2) to the first sacral (S1) is connected anteriorly by an intervertebral disc, and posteriorly by paired diarthrodial (facet) joints in addition to supporting ligamentous structures (see Fig. 122.4B). There is variation in size and alignment of the facet joints when moving from cranial to caudal segments, with size increasing more distally in the thoracolumbar and lumbar segments, and the facet joints being more coronally oriented in the thoracic spine, and more sagittally oriented in the lumbar spine.[8] The three-column concept of spinal stability as described by Denis remains important in describing spinal injuries of all mechanisms including those from athletic injuries.[9] According to Denis, the anterior column is composed of the anterior two-thirds of the vertebral body, disk, and anterior longitudinal ligament; the middle column is composed of the posterior third of the vertebral body, disk, and posterior longitudinal ligament; and the posterior column is composed of the facet joints, facet capsules, ligamentum flavum, and interspinous and supraspinous ligaments. When at least two of the three columns are disrupted, the result is a potentially unstable spine that may require surgical stabilization.

The cervical and lumbar spines are lordotic, while the thoracic spine and sacrum are naturally kyphotic (see Fig. 122.4A). Normal thoracic kyphosis is 10 to 40 degrees, and normal lumbar lordosis is 40 to 60 degrees, noting that an approximate difference of 30 degrees between thoracic kyphosis and lumbar lordosis will place most patients into good sagittal plane balance.[10]

The cervical spine is composed of seven vertebrae, including C1 (the atlas), C2 (the axis), and five subaxial (below C2) vertebrae, which share similar characteristics. The atlas has no vertebral body but consists of a bony ring containing lateral masses that lie between the superior and inferior articular processes, which articulate with the occiput and C2 (axis), respectively. Synovial condylar joints are present at the occiput–C1 articulation, whereas the C2–C3 vertebrae and all subaxial vertebrae are connected by an intervertebral disc anteriorly, and by paired diarthrodial (facet) joints posteriorly, along with supporting ligaments. The intervertebral disc primarily resists axial loads and acts as the "shock absorber" of the spine, while the posterior elements, including the facet joints, provide rotational stability and resist extension forces.[11] The second cervical vertebra contain a peg-shaped odontoid process (dens) that articulates with the anterior C1 ring and accounts for approximately 50% of cervical rotation, while the occiput–C1 junction accounts for approximately 50% of flexion and extension.[12] There is a complex interplay of ligaments at the craniocervical and atlantoaxial junctions, which allow for a physiologic range of motion (ROM) of the cervical spine. The anterior longitudinal ligament runs anterior to the vertebral bodies; the posterior longitudinal ligament is contiguous with the tectorial membrane; and the apical and transverse ligaments stabilize the atlantodental and atlantoaxial motion segments, respectively (Fig. 122.5A). One unique feature of the cervical spine is the presence of the uncovertebral joints of Luschka, allowing a bony articulation at the lateral edge of each disc space. The paired facet joints at the posterolateral aspect of each motion segment contain synovial fluid between the articular cartilage segments contained by a ligamentous capsule, and provide stability to torsional and bending loads.[13] The vertebral artery arises from the subclavian

artery and enters the spine at the transverse foramen at C6 in most cases, providing blood supply to the posterior cerebral circulation via the basilar artery. It can be vulnerable to injury in cervical spine trauma due to its close confines as it passes proximally from the C6 transverse foramen to the C1 foramen (V2 segment) and then passes along the posterior superior C1 ring (V3 segment) until it reaches approximately 1 cm from the midline and then enters the dura (V4 segment).[14] The cervical spine attaches to the thoracic spine and rib cage at the cervicothoracic junction, where the seventh cervical lateral mass articulates with the superior articular facet of the first thoracic vertebra and first rib. The cervical spine is the segment most prone to catastrophic injury in sports as it lacks the inherent stability of the rib cage at the thoracic levels, and contains the cervical spinal cord that is critical for upper and lower extremity motor and sensory function in addition to bowel and bladder control.

The kyphotic thoracic spine contains smaller vertebral bodies than those in the cervical spine, and has facets that are oriented in a more coronal plane. The transverse processes are longer and contain several articulations with the adjacent rib head. Rather than lateral masses containing the superior and inferior articulating facets, as in the cervical spine, the thoracic and lumbar spine contain a pars region, which is a narrow, lateral extension of the lamina that acts as a bridge between the superior articulating and inferior articulating facets. This area is especially prone to injury at the C2 and L5 levels due to regional anatomic variations, (elongation at C2, and thin medial to lateral dimension at L5).[15] In the lumbar spine, the vertebral bodies are larger in order to support the trunk and greater forces in this region, and the facet joints are more sagittally oriented, which allows for more flexion and extension. As noted previously, anatomic variations are present in approximately 10% of spines, commonly consisting of segmentation anomalies (sacralization of L5, rudimentary rib at L1), spina bifida occulta (absence of a portion or all of the lamina) and pars defects.

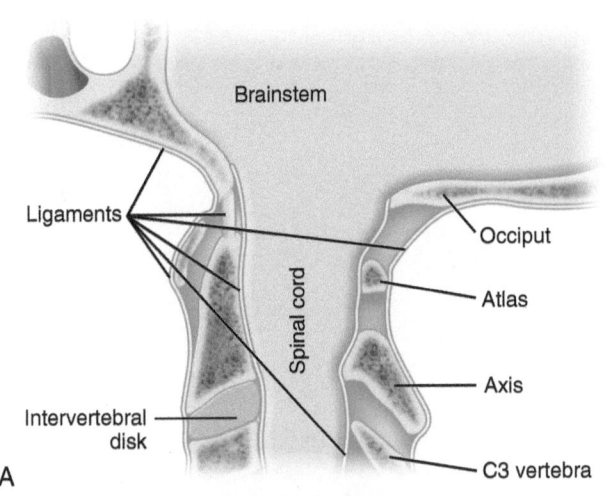
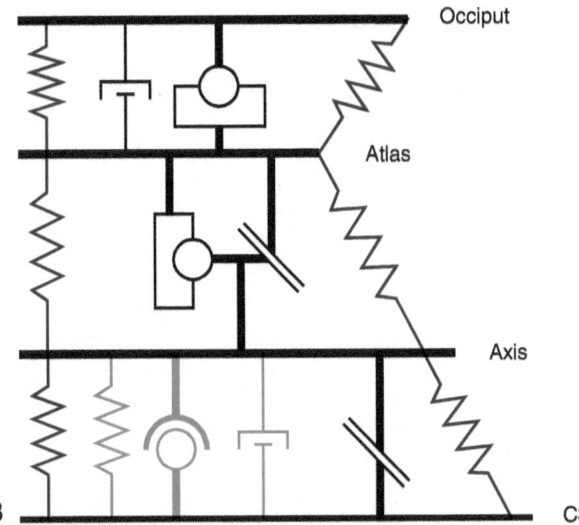

Fig. 122.5 The major anatomic tissues of the upper cervical spine (A) and the matching mechanical analogues for biomechanical modeling using a free-body diagram (B). A ligament can be modeled by a spring; and a disk by a spring and dashpot.

INTERVERTEBRAL DISK

The intervertebral disk is a fibrocartilaginous structure that forms the mobile articulation between adjacent vertebrae in the anterior and middle columns from the C2 to S1 levels. In an adult, the disk is avascular and receives its nutrients through diffusion from the cartilaginous endplates. It displays both viscoelastic and time-dependent properties, and contains a soft, inner core (the nucleus pulopsus) and a more rigid, outer ring containing concentric lamellae (annulus fibrosus).[16,17] The annulus is a ring containing type I collagen arranged in concentric lamellae approximately 65 degrees from the spinal axis, while the nucleus is an amorphous gel of type II collagen and proteoglycans, composed of almost 90% water in a young, healthy person.[18,19] The outer layers of the annulus fibrosus are innervated by sensory nerve structures, whereas the inner annulus and nucleus lack innervation. This is important in that intervertebral disk herniations can become painful when pathologic or repeated physiologic stresses affect the structural integrity of the annulus.[20] The nucleus pulposus is able to distribute and transfer compressive loads through its attachments to the surrounding annulus fibrosus, and loss of this normal physiologic process leads to increased load transfer to the facet joints and posterior structures.[20-23] Disc degeneration occurs as water content is lost and annular fissuring occurs; this is most common clinically at the L4–L5 and L5–S1 levels as well as the lower cervical spine.[24-26]

LIGAMENTS

As noted previously, the middle and posterior columns of the spine contain various ligaments that connect each vertebra to the adjacent vertebrae. Although the upper cervical spine has a different and more complex arrangement, the subaxial cervical spine, thoracic and lumbar spines share a common ligamentous structure. This includes the anterior and posterior longitudinal, ligamentum flavum (yellow ligament), interspinous, supraspinous, and bilateral facet capsules with their associated ligaments (see Fig. 122.4B). The upper cervical spine includes ligamentous attachments between the occiput, the atlas (C1) and the axis (C2), including the transverse, apical, alar, and accessory ligaments in addition to the anterior and posterior longitudinal as well as the ligamentum nuchae, a dense fibrous band contiguous with the supraspinous ligament extending from the occipital protuberance to the C7 spinous process. Ligaments throughout the spine are richly innervated and can provide proprioceptive feedback on head and neck position, and assist in stabilizing the cervical spine.[27,28] Ligaments are frequently involved in sports injuries to the spine given their important role in providing stability, and loss of innervation can result in significant rehabilitation demands on the injured athlete. Generally speaking, spinal ligamentous injuries are slower to heal than bony injuries and can lead to late instability if unrecognized at an early stage. A comprehensive review of ligamentous injury and strain are beyond the scope of this chapter, and more information can be found elsewhere in this edition.

MUSCLES

The majority of body weight is located anterior to the spinal column, so strong muscle groups are necessary to stabilize the spine and allow physiologic movement without compromising structural integrity. There are three basic groups of spinal muscles, the superficial, intermediate (both extrinsic), and deep (intrinsic). The superficial extrinsic muscles include the trapezius, latissimus dorsi, levator scapulae, and rhomboids, and primarily connect the upper limbs to the trunk.[1] The intermediate extrinsic muscles are comprised of the serratus posterior and serve as accessory respiratory muscles. The deep (intrinsic) muscle layer itself includes superficial, intermediate, and deep layers, and plays a role in providing an extensor moment to the spine as well as rotation and side bending, with innervation from the dorsal primary division of the spinal nerves. Lumbar flexion is accomplished primarily by the "core" abdominal muscles consisting of the internal and external obliques in addition to the transversus abdominus. Spinal muscles can be injured creating pain and dysfunction, in addition to loss of important stabilizing forces leading to further injury of vertebrae, ligaments, and discs if not addressed.

NEUROLOGIC TISSUES

The spinal cord and paired nerve roots are the neurologic structures that must be protected by the bones, ligaments, disc, and supporting muscles. The spinal cord originates proximally at its junction with the brainstem at the foramen magnum and ends in most adults at L1 or at the L1–L2 disc space level. The spinal cord ends more distally in children, and conditions such as tethered cord or spine bifida occulta can create aberrant neurologic anatomy. The spinal cord contains a central H-shaped gray matter composed of the cell bodies of interneurons and motor neurons, and a surrounding white matter composed of ascending and descending myelinated tracts (Fig. 122.6). The blood supply of the spinal cord is derived from a median ventral anterior spinal

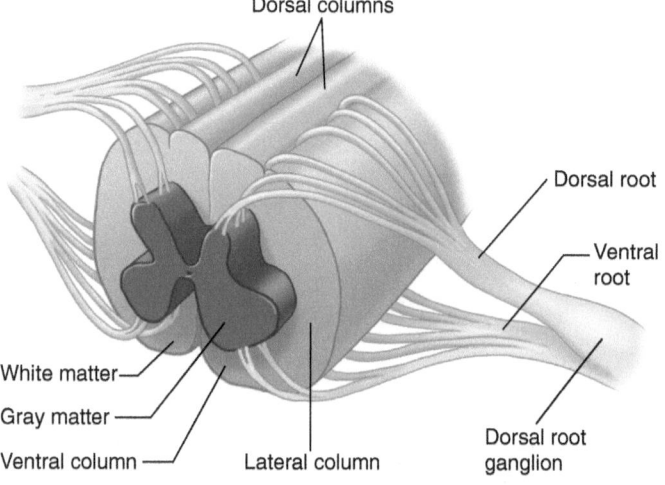

Fig. 122.6 Cross-section of the spinal cord demonstrating the relationship between the gray and white matter, the nerve root, and the dorsal root ganglion.

artery and two smaller dorsolateral spinal arteries.[29] Nerve roots exit the spinal canal at each level from the occiput-C1 articulation to the sacrum, and the distal spinal cord (conus medullaris) becomes the cauda equina ("horse's tail") distal to L1, which terminates at the S5 level. The spinal cord is surrounded by meninges that include the dura mater, arachnoid mater, and pia mater (moving from superficial to deep, analogous to the meninges surrounding the brain). Both anterior and posterior nerve roots extend from the spinal cord at each level, with the anterior and posterior primary rami forming the spinal nerve as it exits the neural foramen between the pedicles superiorly, the disc anteriorly, and the facet capsules posteriorly (see Fig. 122.4B). The spinal canal is bordered by the posterior vertebral body and disc anteriorly, the pedicles laterally, and the laminae dorsally. The dorsal root ganglion is located within the neural foramen and transmits important somatosensory information. This structure is very sensitive to external compression and is found distal to the dorsal and ventral roots, but proximal to the spinal nerve (see Fig. 122.6).[30] Afferent (sensory) fibers generally travel more dorsally within the spinal cord, whereas motor units travel more ventrally, leading to various SCI patterns depending on which anatomic section of the cord is damaged (e.g., anterior cord syndrome leading to motor impairment from ventral pathology including anterior spinal artery compromise). Medial branches of the dorsal primary ramus innervate the facet joints and are sometimes implicated in facet-mediated pain syndromes, while the disc is innervated posteriorly by the sinuvertebral nerve as discussed previously in this chapter.

BIOMECHANICS

As described earlier, the spinal column is a complex mechanical structure with multiple articulations. These articulations permit substantial motion in multiple planes both at the individual functional spinal unit and on a more regional basis. The biomechanical performance of the spine depends on several factors, including the material and constitutive properties of the involved tissues, the magnitude and direction of the applied loads, the rate and duration of applied loading, and the position of the head/spine at the time of loading.[31] The study of spinal biomechanics has utilized in vivo and cadaveric models as well as computational analysis to understand both the normal and the injured conditions.

NORMAL/PHYSIOLOGIC BIOMECHANICS

The unique anatomy of the craniocervical junction (occiput-atlas-axis) results in distinct biomechanics from the remainder of the cervical spine (see Fig. 122.5A). The occipital-axial complex can rotate up to 50 degrees in flexion-extension and 90 degrees in axial torsion, which represents approximately 50% of the motion of the entire cervical spine in these directions. However, the upper cervical anatomy permits only limited lateral bending (+/− 10 degrees). The subaxial levels are therefore the main contributors to the total cervical lateral bending range (20 to 45 degrees).[32,33] On a segmental basis, the ROM in the subaxial cervical region is similar at each level ranging from 4 to 23

degrees of sagittal plane motion.[34,35] Due to the complex anatomic shape of the vertebrae, movement of the functional spinal unit along one (primary) axis is accompanied by movement along a coupled (secondary) axis. This coupled motion is commonly cited in the subaxial cervical spine, where lateral bending occurs concomitantly with axial rotation in the same direction due to the orientation of the facet articulations.[36] The stabilizing effect of the ribcage limits the motion of the thoracic spine. The coronally oriented facets further limit flexion-extension. The upper thoracic spine displays coupled motion in lateral bending and axial rotation, whereas coupling in the lower thoracic spine is less pronounced.[37] The more sagittally oriented facets of the lumbar spine permit greater flexion-extension than the thoracic region, averaging 12 degrees at L1–L2 up to 17 degrees at L5–S1.

Despite regional differences, the general biomechanical responses of the subaxial (C2–C7) cervical, thoracic, and lumbar regions are similar. The intervertebral disk, ligaments, and bilateral facet joints limit and guide the relative motions of adjacent vertebrae, which leads to highly nonlinear load-displacement relationships (Fig. 122.7).[38] These relationships are characterized by curves featuring two main zones: the neutral zone and the elastic zone. These two zones together constitute the ROM of a vertebral segment (see Fig. 122.7).[38] In the neutral zone, the vertebral motion segment is highly flexible, permitting a great amount of motion for very small applied loads. In the elastic zone, the spinal tissues begin to individually engage and undergo loading, with increasing stiffness as load increases. Such a stiffening behavior results from the viscoelastic properties of the intervertebral disk and of the ligaments as they deform inhomogeneously and nonlinearly with an applied load. The disk absorbs and distributes a compressive load and is mechanically comparable to a spring in parallel with a viscous damper (see Fig. 122.5B). Ligaments are like cables and can only resist tensile loading; as such, the posterior spinal ligaments tighten during spinal flexion and the anterior ligaments tighten during extension. These tissues are mechanically analogous to springs (see

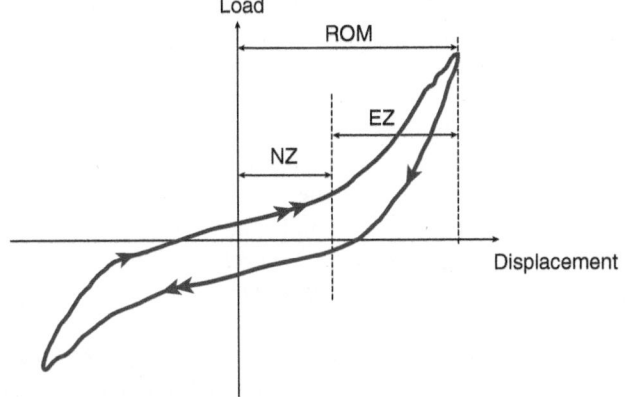

Fig. 122.7 A representative load-displacement curve for a motion segment showing the nonlinear relationship between the segmental displacement (translation or rotation) and load (force or moment) generated. The difference between the loading (*double arrow*) and unloading (*single arrow*) indicates hysteresis. The elastic (*EZ*) and neutral (*NZ*) zones are defined, and together comprise the total range of motion (*ROM*).

Fig. 122.5B). The cervical neural arch and the facet joints also transfer and support 3% to 25% of a compressive load and limit the motion between adjacent vertebrae, especially in the extremes of extension and anterior translation.[39-41] Although the orientation of the cervical facet joints, with respect to both the coronal and sagittal planes, increase moving caudally, the ROM in the subaxial cervical spine is similar at each level, ranging from 4 to 23 degrees in human voluntary and cadaveric studies of sagittal bending.[32,34,35]

As the primary axial stabilizing structure of the head and trunk, the spinal column is subjected to large loads during daily activities. The vertebral bodies can bear compressive forces of up to 1700 N, 4000 N, and 8000 N in the cervical, thoracic, and lumbar regions, respectively.[33] Not surprisingly, the lumbar vertebrae, which are required to sustain more of the body's weight, can support a greater axial load. Because of the different loading patterns and vertebral structures, the spinal ligaments also exhibit a wide range of failure strengths that range from 76 to 436 N in the upper cervical spine, with the cruciate, alar, and anterior longitudinal ligaments being the strongest. In the subaxial cervical spine, the capsular ligaments and ligamentum flavum are the strongest, with failure strengths ranging between 47 and 264 N. The anterior and posterior longitudinal ligaments in the lumbar spine are the strongest, with failure strengths reported from 100 to 510 N. Similarly, the maximum compressive load that the intervertebral disk can withstand also increases from the cervical to lumbar spines: 74, 1800, and 5300 N in the cervical, thoracic, and lumbar regions, respectively. Intervertebral disks are weaker in shear and can only resist shear loads of 20 N in the cervical spine and 150 N in the thoracic region. Without protection from the facet joints, the intervertebral disks can only resist 1.8 and 31 Nm of torsion in the cervical and lumbar spines, respectively.[33] While unaccounted in most cadaveric biomechanical studies, muscle activation not only stabilizes the spine and helps to protect it from excessive motion, but also it can produce loading to individual ligaments beyond their threshold for injury.[42,43]

The anatomic structures of the spine can fail when mechanical loading is outside a physiologic range. Injurious loads can result from a variety of scenarios: the combination of different loads, the application of physiologic loads in extreme spinal positions, and/or even from repetitive loading (fatigue) within the normal range.[44-47] The ensuing structural failures of the vertebrae, disk, and/or ligaments depends on the magnitude of the loads, their direction, and the rate of loading. For example, the neutrally aligned cervical spine is lordotic, and energy inputs can be dissipated to some extent by the intervertebral disks and paraspinal muscles. Numerous biomechanical studies have suggested that with flexion of approximately 30 degrees, the straightened cervical spine assumes the physical characteristics of a segmented column. Axially applied force is directly transmitted to the spinal structures. When the threshold vertical compression is reached, the cervical spine fails and buckles in a flexion mode with anterior column failure and possible facet subluxation or dislocation.[48-50]

Other examples of this phenomenon are the injuries sustained by quarterbacks or rugby players when they are sacked from behind. At a high rate of loading, the instantaneous axis of rotation (IAR) of a vertebra relative to its subadjacent vertebra moves upward into the top moving vertebra from its normal location during physiologic motions under the intervertebral disk. As a consequence, the inferior facets of the superior vertebra have an impact on the superior facets of the inferior vertebra instead of gliding posteriorly on them.[51,52] Such an extreme compression can produce facet joint hemarthrosis, cartilage fissures, and even facet fracture.[53,54] Given the complementary stabilizing effects of the discoligamentous structures, isolated injury may result in varying degrees of instability. For instance, in a cadaveric study, both the ROM and neutral zone have been shown to significantly increase by 50% to 60% in flexion after transection of the spinal ligaments (except the posterior longitudinal ligament) at the C5–C6 level.[55] In contrast, an annular cut of the C5–C6 intervertebral disc does not destabilize the segment until after facet capsule transection.[55] Similarly, a unilateral locked C5–C6 facet joint reduces segmental ROM by up to 3.6 degrees in all directions except ipsilateral torsion.[56] Major damage and failure of the osseous and ligamentous spinal tissues can result in serious neurologic pathologies.[57,58] Because the spinal cord and neural elements are no longer protected in such cases, they can be subjected to injurious loading (e.g., compression and shear) by the surrounding tissues. However, subtle and undetected structural failures of tissue can also occur and can lead to acute and chronic neurologic pathologies. Minor tissue damage can render the spine unstable and lead to nonphysiologic loading of the neurologic tissues in particular locations. For instance, subfailure stretching of the cervical capsular ligament in experimental in vivo animal studies has been shown to produce microstructural collagen fiber realignment and laxity, which can lead to central sensitization.[59,60] In addition, neurologic and vascular tissues can be loaded under nonphysiologic conditions even when the soft tissues of the spine only sustain minor damage. For instance, a transient reduction of the spinal canal diameter is induced by altered vertebral kinematics during high loading rates and can lead to spinal cord contusion.[51] While the unique architecture of the intervertebral disk enables it to act as a major stabilizing structure of the spine, degenerative changes may have significant effects on this function. In a cadaveric study, lumbar motion segments with increasing degrees of disc degeneration were found to have erratic excursions of the IAR, vertical translation of the center of rotation, and abnormal distribution across the disc space with lower pressures in the region of the nucleus and pressure spikes in the annular region.[61] The result is an unstable functional spinal unit and potentially increased risk of flare ups of back pain with routine daily or sporting activities.

Integration of Biomechanical Considerations for Treatment

The application of spinal biomechanics to the context of sports injury remains challenging, despite an abundance of research in this field. While some broad injury mechanisms, such as axial load, torsion, flexion, and extension, can be applied across all sports injuries to the spinal column, there is a great variability between how these injuries occur among different sporting activities. This is further complicated by the age of the athlete and any pre-existing degenerative changes that are present; the ability of the surrounding musculature to support or withstand non-physiologic forces; and the individual athlete's prior exposure or injuries.

As discussed previously, the function of the human spine is to support body weight, protect the neural elements, and to maintain posture as well as resist external forces. Despite the ability of the spine to function well under a variety of loading scenarios, athletic activities can cause damage through either repetitive physiologic loading mechanisms or through load to failure if enough force is applied in a specific manner, such as catastrophic cervical SCI through tackling in football.

The regions of the spine most vulnerable to injury generally include the cervicothoracic and thoracolumbar junctions (transitional zones between the mobile cervical and lumbar spines, and the rigid thoracic spine and accompanying rib cage), although any spinal level can sustain injury if the ability of the supporting structures in that area are compromised. Spine injury patterns in sports remain sport-specific to a large degree, and this information can be found elsewhere in this text in further detail.

▌ SUMMARY

The spinal column is composed of bone, disc, ligaments, and the surrounding muscles that serve to protect the neural elements and maintain posture as well as to resist and respond to various external loads. TBI and spinal cord injuries are among the most feared of all sports injuries due to their potential catastrophic and permanent nature. A greater understanding of spinal biomechanics has been helpful in revising the rules of play in various sports (e.g., the banning of spear tackling in American football), and in improving the design of protective equipment. Despite the use of the protective equipment, the cervical spine remains the most vulnerable to injury, and these injuries often have the most devastating consequences.

The CNS has limited healing potential once an injury occurs; therefore prevention is the best method of minimizing brain and spine injuries in sports. As the pathologic mechanisms associated with spine and brain injuries in sports remain incompletely understood, further research is needed to minimize their effects, especially in the realm of SCI. In rare cases, neurologic injury can occur despite no obvious bony or ligamentous injury, and observation of the head and trunk position to determine the mechanism of injury does not always offer useful information. All on-field personnel should be well trained to handle brain and spine injuries and to assume the worst-case scenario (an unstable spine) when caring for or transporting the athlete off the field.

For a complete list of references, go to ExpertConsult.com.

SELECTED READING

Citation:
Denis F. The three-column spine and its significance in the classification of acute thoracolumbar spinal injuries. *Spine*. 1983;8(8):817–831.

Level of Evidence:
IV

Summary:
Retrospective study of 412 thoracolumbar injuries, defining the concept of an anterior, middle, and posterior column osteoligamentous complex injuries. Mechanistic descriptions are applied to four basic injury patterns forming the basis for modern spinal injury classification systems.

Citation:
Panjabi MM. The stabilizing system of the spine. Part II. Neutral zone and instability hypothesis. *J Spinal Disord*. 1992;5(4):390–397.

Level of Evidence:
V, review

Summary:
Elegant hypothesis of the concept of spinal stability as it relates to passive and active stabilizers, normal (physiologic) function of the spinal motion segment, and pathologic spinal motion leading to dysfunction or pain. Neural and muscular adaptive mechanisms are discussed.

Citation:
Jaumard NV, Welch WC, Winkelstein BA. Spinal facet joint biomechanics and mechanotransduction in normal, injury and degenerative conditions. *J Biomech Eng*. 2011;133(7):071010.

Level of Evidence:
V, review

Summary:
Thorough review of the zygapophyseal (facet) joint anatomy and biomechanics with a focus on differences between normal, injury, and degenerative states. The authors provide a review of the biomechanical data on capsular strain, the response to load and mechanotransduction, and the use of finite element models.

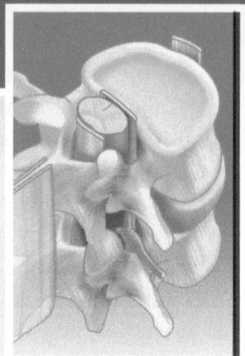

123

Head and Spine Diagnosis and Decision-Making

Rabia Qureshi, Jason A. Horowitz, Kieran Bhattacharya,
Hamid Hassanzadeh

HEAD

Anatomy and Biomechanics

Head injuries have multiple mechanisms, which include the injuries from an impact of the brain against the inside of the skull (Fig. 123.1). A coup injury occurs when the brain strikes the inner skull on the same side of impact of an object and typically occurs when a moving object comes into contact with a patient's stationary head. A countrecoup injury occurs when the brain strikes the inner side of a skull on the opposing side of impact of an object, which generally occurs when a mobile patient's head strikes a stationary object. The brain is suspended in cerebrospinal fluid (CSF), a fluid denser than the brain itself. In the cases of countrecoup injuries, the denser CSF moves towards the site of impact, likely displacing the brain in the opposite direction.[4] The mechanisms behind coup and countrecoup injures are only relevant when there is no skull fracture present, because any such displacement to the skull would cause the bone to directly damage brain tissue upon an impact.

Damage to the brain from a head injury may result from three types of applied forces: compressive, tensile, and shearing. Compression force involves squeezing of brain tissue, and tensile force is the opposite of compression and involves stretching of brain tissue. When rotational forces are applied to the brain, shearing stress results from areas where rotational motion of the brain is hindered, such as at rough, irregular contacts between the brain and skull. In severe traumatic brain injuries, brain tissue experiences compression, tension, and shearing. Compressive and tensile forces are handled relatively well by the head because CSF is able to absorb and convert focal shock into a more widely distributed stress throughout the head. However, shearing stresses are less tolerated by the brain, with the most vulnerable parts being the brainstem and corpus callosum due to their highly anisotropically oriented axons.[7]

Pathophysiology

Head injuries are found in a wide variety of sports. Concussion is the most commonly sustained head injury in athletes. However, it is poorly defined, and treatment modalities vary greatly and are dependent on a multitude of factors. Intracranial hemorrhage is the leading cause of death from head injury in athletes; four types exist—epidural, subdural, intracerebral, and subarachnoid. Intracranial hemorrhage is a focal brain injury that results from a ruptured blood vessel within the skull and leads to dangerous increases in intracranial pressure. Other severe, although less common, injuries include skull fractures, mild and severe traumatic brain injuries, CSF leaks, craniofacial injuries, and cranial nerve injuries.

As mentioned previously, concussions are the most common head injuries occurring in athletes. They have previously been defined as low-velocity injuries resulting in "brain shaking," and clinical symptoms that may not necessarily be related to the initial pathologic injury ensue.[8] The most recent (2012) Conference on Concussion in Sport differentiated concussion from a minor traumatic brain injury (mTBI) and considers the concussion to instead be its own subset of TBI.[8] Concussions can be the result of low-velocity impact to the head, face, neck, or anywhere else in the body that can transmit "impulsive" force to the head. For adults, this is most commonly seen is vehicular collisions and falls, but for children, the most common causes are bicycle and sporting accidents.[9] Concussions from vehicular collisions are likely to be much more severe and may include loss of consciousness (LOC) as compared with those concussions resulting from sporting accidents. Although concussions commonly occur in athletes, they are considered to be grossly underreported.[10,11] There are a variety of reasons for which this can occur: a player might believe that reporting a concussion might curtail his player career; a team or organization might not want to report injuries so as not to harm its public relations. Nevertheless, it is important that players, teams, and families fully understand the ramifications of concussions, and it has been demonstrated that an increased knowledge of concussion symptoms is associated with an increase in concussion reporting.[12,13]

At the time of injury, impairment of neurologic function can occur, although this is not necessary for diagnosis and impairment can appear hours after initial insult. Symptoms of a concussion typically resolve spontaneously. However, the course of recovery is variable, with some concussion patients experiencing symptoms weeks to months after acute injury. Concussions may or may not result in an LOC. In addition, if LOC does occur, it bears no effect on severity of concussion or recovery time. In some cases, concussions can result in the inability to remember new events (antegrade amnesia) or events immediately preceding the concussion (retrograde amnesia). Retrograde amnesia usually resolves spontaneously, although antegrade amnesia from concussions can be permanent.[14] Because the acute clinical symptoms

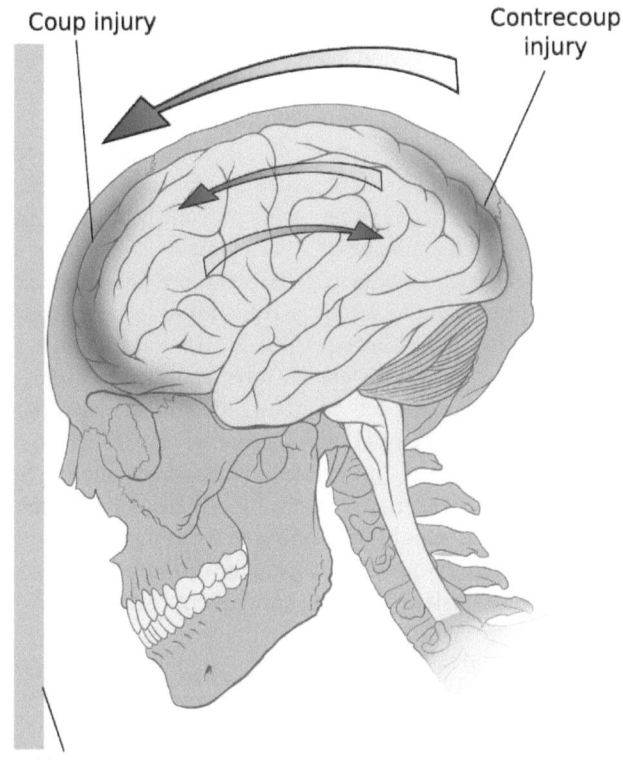

Coup injury

Contrecoup injury

Fixed object

Fig. 123.1 Coup and contrecoup injuries. (By Patrick J. Lynch, medical illustrator [CC-BY-SA-3.0 (http://creativecommons.org/licenses/by-sa/3.0/)], via Wikimedia Commons.)

of a concussion reflect functional dysregulation instead of structural injury, concussion cannot be diagnosed with computed tomography (CT) or magnetic resonance imaging (MRI).[8,15] However, imaging is used to rule out more serious injury, mainly hemorrhage.

History

Detailed history is imperative in patients sustaining head injury. Physicians should first determine whether further emergent neuroimaging is needed to rule out more severe brain injuries. Moreover, it is important to asses a patient's mental status and any changes since the initial injury. In many cases, it may be necessary to obtain a medical history from parents, friends, teammates, and coaches. In patients with concussions specifically, initial presentation may include a variety of symptoms and with differing severity. Physical symptoms can include headache, nausea, vomiting, issues with balance, photophobia, numbness and tingling, dizziness, and tinnitus. Cognitive symptoms may include depression, fatigue, irritability, sadness, nervousness, memory problems, and difficulty concentrating.[8,10] Furthermore, it is important to note if patients have sustained previous head injury or concussions because a prior concussion is a significant risk factor for subsequent concussions.[16] And although greater than 90% of sports-related concussions among children are not associated with an LOC, it is important to inquire about LOC to rule out other injuries.[17,18] Symptoms after the first 4 weeks after injury are considered those the initial concussion, and those after 4 weeks are considered postconcussion syndrome (PCS),

which can last anywhere from weeks to several months. It is therefore important to obtain pertinent history from both the initial injury and at follow-up to determine is any new or different symptoms are present and if they are part of normal recovery. A large majority (80% to 90%) of concussions resolve in 7 to 10 days; however, full recovery can vary, particularly in children and adolescents.[8]

Physical Exam

An onsite licensed health care provider should initially ensure that the athlete is medically stable and has an open airway, adequate breathing, and circulation (ABCs). The health care provider must then determine the appropriate method of removing the player from the field and address any first aid issues such as active bleeding. After this, one should observe the injured player for immediate clinical symptoms and physical signs such as LOC, headache, dizziness, drowsiness, confusion, and seizure. Physicians, if possible, should also assess gait, balance, cranial nerve function, and coordination as part of a comprehensive neurologic examination. If the athlete displays an altered mental status or LOC, he or she should be immediately transferred to a hospital with neurosurgical services.

To assess a potentially concussive injury, one can use a sideline assessment tool such as the third edition of the Sport Concussion Assessment Tool (SCAT3).[19] The SCAT3 is a standardized checklist for evaluating injured athletes for concussion, incorporating the Glasgow Coma Scale, Maddocks Score, scaled score of physical symptoms, cognitive assessment, neck examination, balance examination, and coordination examination. After initial assessment, the player should be monitored for increasing severity of initial symptoms or emergence of new symptoms. Those diagnosed with concussion should not be allowed to return to play (RTP) on the day of injury.[8]

Imaging

As mentioned previously, concussions do not result in structural damage to the brain and therefore cannot be distinguished with CT or MRI. However, if there is a suspected intracranial hemorrhage from athletic injury, CT should be used. It is important for on-field medical staff and personnel to understand the general characteristics of the four basic types of hematomas: epidural, subdural, subarachnoid, and intracerebral.

Epidural hematomas are typically, but not always, characterized by a brief LOC. Individuals might present with a lucid interval where there is marked improvement before rapid decline in mental status. The athlete may regain consciousness before the subsequent deterioration and headache. This occurs due to blood from meningeal arteries building up between the dura mater and the skull. As a result a convex collection of blood is noted on imaging. Bleeding usually occurs on the same side of injury, and players who sustain epidural hematomas should be removed from the field and escorted to a hospital with neurosurgical services. There, the hematoma must be evacuated and a full recovery is expected if treated promptly.[20]

A subdural hematoma is the most common fatal athletic head injury. Injured players experience LOC and do not usually regain consciousness. They should be sent immediately for neurosurgical evaluation. Blood escapes from torn bridging veins in the subdural space and builds between the dura mater and arachnoid mater, ultimately resulting in a concave collection of blood expanding past suture lines.[21] Although a smaller subdural hematoma is self-limiting and requires only small catheter drill for evacuation, a craniotomy is needed to access a larger subdural hematoma. The risk of complications is dependent on the size and rate of change of the subdural hematoma, but the prognosis is poor because of direct damage to the brain.[22]

A subarachnoid hemorrhage (SAH) consist of bleeding into the subarachnoid space, an area that houses CSF on the surface of the brain. A player who suffers an SAH from head trauma will likely present with rapid onset, severe headache ("worst headache ever"), pulsating towards the back of the head. Some patients will have neck stiffness, vomiting, seizures, and a decrease or LOC. Players should be taken to a hospital for a neurosurgical evaluation with CT scan. There they will receive treatment to reduce bleeding and prevent vasopasm.[23] Surgery is likely not required if no vascular ruptures are present and the bleeding is contained superficially.[24]

An intracerebral hemorrhage involves bleeding of the brain tissue itself. After the initial traumatic head injury, an athlete with cerebral bleeding will often present with severe headache and vomiting. This injury is commonly confused with SAH. Players should be referred to neurosurgical services. The mortality rate is between 35% and 52% and is even higher when the brainstem is affected; only 20% of survivors of survivors are expected to have a full recovery at 6 months.[25]

Decision-Making Principles

As with all head injuries, players should be initially assessed for airway, breathing, and circulation and have their cervical spine stabilized. Athletes should be immediately removed from play if a concussion is suspected. The diagnosis of a concussion should be made using a multidisciplinary approach involving clinical symptoms, physical signs, cognitive impairment, neurobehavioral features, and sleep disturbance.[8] It might be necessary to gather information from families, coaches, and teammates if a player is unable to provide enough details of the injury. Furthermore, clinical assessment tools such as Standardized Assessment of Concussion (SAC), Balance Error Scoring System (BESS), and SCAT3[19] can be used but should not supplant a clinician's judgment in assessing an athlete for a concussion. Because concussions are the result of functional but not structural damage to the brain, neuroimaging contributes little to the diagnosis and should only be used to rule out intracranial bleeding. Thus clinicians should avoid ordering a brain CT or brain MRI unless there is concern for a skull fracture, progressive neurologic symptoms, or focal neurologic findings.[26]

Treatment Options

The only proven treatments for concussions are cognitive and physical rest. Cognitive rest entails avoiding concentration-driven activities such as school work, video games, and even leisurely reading. Players diagnosed with concussions should not RTP on the same day of injury; however, there is no broad consensus on the appropriate guidelines for returning players. It is widely agreed

that players should not RTP until they are asymptomatic,[8,16,27] and during this recovery period, players should not take analgesic or sedative medications to mask postconcussion symptoms.[28] The latest (2016) Zurich International Consensus Statement on Concussion[8] in Sport and the American Medical Society for Sports Medicine[16] both endorse a stepwise progression in physically demanding activity for players who previously suffered from concussion and are subsequently asymptomatic off medicine. The steps of the Zurich Statement progress in the following order: symptom-limited activity, light aerobic exercise, sport-specific exercise, noncontact training drills, full-contact practice, and finally RTP. Each of these steps must be separated by at least 24 hours of asymptomatic activity before the athlete may progress to the next step after a brief initial period of rest (24–48 hours). Finally, it is generally recommended that children suffering from concussions be treated more conservatively than adults.[8,27] Athletes with concussions should be monitored for symptoms while in the rest and recovery period. Individuals who suffer concussions are at increased risk of suffering subsequent concussions.[29–31]

⚑ Authors' Preferred Technique

Players with suspected concussions should be immediately removed from play and assessed by a licensed health care professional for clinical symptoms and physical signs of the injury. If the player shows signs characteristic of intracranial bleeding, he or she should be quickly sent to a hospital with neurologic services and there undergo appropriate neuroimaging and surgery, if necessary. Individuals suffering only a concussion should be given time for physical and cognitive rest until symptoms resolve before returning to light aerobic physical activity. They can then graduate in a stepwise fashion to full-contact play if they remain asymptomatic while off medications.

Results

As mentioned previously, the overwhelming majority (80% to 90%) of concussions will resolve spontaneously in 7 to 10 days. Those with symptoms persisting past 10 days should be evaluated for coexisting pathologies through conventional neuroimaging and neuropsychological testing. Although there is no effective drug treatment for concussion itself, symptoms of concussions and PCS that persist can be treated with antidepressants and analgesics, as well as cognitive, vestibular, physical, and psychological therapy.[32]

Complications

Postconcussion Syndrome

PCS is a set of symptoms that lasts more than 4 weeks after the initial concussion. Common symptoms include headache, dizziness, insomnia, fatigue, irritability, poor concentration, poor memory, depression, and photophobia. There is a correlation between severity of symptoms and severity of neurologic impairment.[33] Diagnosis of PCS is difficult because of the great overlap of symptoms may be observed in conditions such as chronic pain (CP).[34] PCS usually resolves within 1 month, but the syndrome can last from months to years and possibly cause permanent damage or disability.[35] Persistent postconcussive syndrome (PPCS) is used to define a set of symptoms lasting 3 or more months after the injury. Although there is no treatment for PCS, symptoms of PCS can be treated with antidepressants or nonsteroidal analgesics. In addition, some 40% of patients with PCS are referred to psychological consultations.[32] Furthermore, earlier intervention by specialists was correlated with reduced severity of postconcussion symptoms.[36] However, there is no reliable way to treat PCS when it persists.

Future Considerations

Despite the wide prevalence of concussions, the research on its treatment is lacking. Further inquiry is required to understand the optimal time and type of rest for recovery. Moreover, although it is thought that some low-level exercise might be of benefit for those slow to recover from concussions, the optimal timing and intensity of activity have not been established.[8] Studies are also needed to investigate pharmacologic interventions in managing symptoms of concussions that last greater than 10 days. Finally, further research is needed into concussions as a predictor of chronic neurobehavioral impairment.[37]

SPINE

Introduction

The human spinal column is made up of 33 vertebrae. Each vertebra, composed of bone and hyaline cartilage, consists of a vertebral body and vertebral arch, formed by laminae and pedicles. The spine functions to provide support the body and protect the spinal cord within the vertebral foramen. Spinal nerves exit and enter through intervertebral foramina for the spine to serve as the bridge between the central and peripheral nervous systems.

Approximately 9% of spinal cord injuries (SCIs) in the United States are caused by sporting accidents, making them the fourth leading cause of SCI, behind motor vehicle accidents, falls, and violence.[38–40] Common spine injuries include muscle spasms, avulsion fractures, compression fractures, disc herniations, and strains. More severe, although less common, are catastrophic cervical spine injuries (CCSIs), which are defined as injuries that cause structural damage to the cervical spine and are associated with actual or potential damage to the spinal cord. CCSIs include unstable fractures or dislocations, intervertebral disc herniations, and cervical cord neuropraxia (CCN). This chapter will focus on the most common mild sports spine injury, muscle strains and ligamentous sprain, and the most frequent CCSI, unstable fractures and dislocations.[41]

UNSTABLE FRACTURES AND DISLOCATIONS OF THE CERVICAL SPINE

A fracture and/or dislocation is defined as unstable if, when placed under a physiologic load, the spine is unable to maintain the same preinjury motions to prevent major deformities, debilitating pain, or damage to the spinal cord and nerve roots.[42] The historical radiographic criteria for unstable fractures and dislocations are 11 degrees of angular displacement or 3.5 mm of horizontal displacement between adjacent vertebrae.[43] Unstable fractures and dislocations of the cervical spine typically result in permanent neurologic damage. These injuries usually occur in the lower cervical spine, where the spinal cord occupies nearly 75%

of the cross-sectional area of the spinal canal.[44] In high-contact sports such as hockey and football, the injury most frequently associated with cervical spine injury is compression. In its neutral position, the cervical spine forms a protective lordotic curve, which allows the energy impacts on cervical spine to dissipate across intervertebral discs and paravertebral muscles. However, when the head is tilted forward and flexed during impact on the top of the head, forces are transmitted down an aligned cervical spine in a process known as axial loading. If pushed passed its maximal load, the cervical spine will fail, leading to fracture, dislocation, or subluxation.

History

Obtaining a comprehensive history is important in diagnosing problems from pain in the neck and back. Firstly, identify the events surrounding the pain; high-impact injuries such as collisions or falls would be characteristic of disruptions in bones or ligaments, whereas overuse would be indicative of muscle strains or spasms. Physicians should distinguish the location of pain, the pain severity, onset and frequency of symptoms, modifying factors, and whether or not the pain radiates. Furthermore, it is necessary to conduct a thorough neurologic examination by checking for headache, impaired vision, impaired fine motor control, imbalance, impaired gait, or tingling and numbness in the extremities.

Physical Examination

It is especially important that when dealing with players with cervical spine injuries that the leading on-staff health personnel address ABCs while simultaneously immobilizing the cervical spine through manual traction or cervical orthosis. After the cervical spine has been immobilized, the injured athlete should place onto a spine board with extreme prudence. It is recommended that a player's shoulder pads and helmet should be left on until the player is moved to a hospital setting so as to minimize movement of the cervical spine.[45,46] Exceptions to this rule includes instances where the helmet is not properly fitted to prevent independent movement of the head and helmet or if the head equipment prevents neutral alignment of the cervical spine.[46] Moreover, the helmet and shoulder pads in the cases of American football and ice hockey should not be independently removed because this will disrupt spinal alignment. Removal of the facemask, however, is recommended and considered to be much less compromising than removal of the helmet. In cases where the airway is disrupted, jaw thrusts or head tilts can be performed. If a player's headwear in any way prevents the process of opening the airway, both the helmet and shoulder pads should be removed while maintaining cervical alignment.[47] Players with suspected cervical spine injuries should be immediately transferred to a hospital with spine trauma services.

Imaging

Indication of advanced imaging in cases of sustained blunt cervical spine trauma can be determined using the National Emergency X-Ray Utilization Study (NEXUS) clinical criteria: no midline cervical tenderness, no focal neurologic deficits, normal cognition, no intoxication, and no painful, distracting injuries. If all five of these criteria are met, the patient has almost certainly not sustained a cervical spine injury, and further imaging is contraindicated.[48,49] If any of the criteria are not met, x-ray films first should be taken from the lateral view so that all seven cervical vertebrae and the C7-T1 junction can be visualized. Further imaging from the lateral view with the patient's arm extended over the head (swimmer's view) might be necessary to visualize the C7-T1 junction. If there are no obvious fractures from the lateral views, physicians should proceed with anteroposterior and open-mouth odontoid views. If no fractures are observed, lateral flexion and extension views can also be taken when there is a suspected instability. If any fractures are observed in radiographs or the patient presents with neurologic deficits, CT and MRI are recommended. CT scans in the sagittal, coronal, or axial plane can provide a more detail to identify spinal fractures or dislocations (Fig. 123.2). MRIs can be used to identify damage to the spinal cord, intervertebral discs, or posterior ligamentous complex.

Decision-Making Principles

Most cervical injuries will include ligamentous sprain and/or muscle strain without osseous or neurologic injury. Players will present with pain localized on the cervical spine, reduced range of motion (ROM), and tenderness to palpitation. In these cases the injury is usually self-limited and players should be able to RTP if he or she has full ROM, full-strength in the neck, and no pain in the neck upon axial loading.[50] However, ligamentous injury can result in cervical spine instability. Severe forms of ligamentous instability in the cervical spines of young athletes are often masked by youthful ligamentous laxity, as well as through cervical muscle spasms.[50] Thus whenever subluxation of the

cervical spine is observed in imaging, that player should wear a cervical collar for 2 to 4 weeks before repeated imaging. Athletes should then be allowed to RTP only if there is a normal return to function without pain and no evidence of progression.

Those patients who are conscious, responsive, and not intoxicated, with suspected unstable cervical spine fractures and dislocations should be reduced as soon as possible and stabilized with a halo ring device. An MRI or contrast-enhanced CT scan can then be used to rule out the presence of retropulsed intervertebral disc material, which is implicated in the neurologic deterioration of patients undergoing reduction of the cervical spine. Athletes who sustain unstable lower cervical spine fractures or dislocations can present with a spectrum of neurologic dysfunction, with the most severe case being complete quadriplegia, whereas there is rarely spinal cord damage due to fractures or dislocations of the upper cervical spine because there is proportionally greater space within the spinal canal compared with lower segments. Furthermore, unstable cervical fractures/dislocations do not always result in upper motor neuron lesions. Under some circumstances, there will only be lower motor neuron dysfunction.

Treatment Options

Musculoligamentous sprain and strain are typically self-limited and relived by rest, although icing and nonsteroidal antiinflammatory drugs (NSAIDs) can help to reduce pain.[51] Treatment of cervical spine injury is dependent on the degree of instability and/or neurologic impairment. Unstable fractures are treated surgically with an anterior decompression and fusion or posterior spinal fusion. However, posterior stabilization and fusion was found to lead to unsuccessful outcomes in nearly half of cases of rotationally unstable cervical due to late kyphosis caused by disc collapse or inability of the midline stabilization procedure to control rotational instability.[52] However, the anterior fusion procedure was not associated with residual deformity, and even those with incomplete spinal cord lesions and radiculopathy showed improvement in spinal cord function.[52]

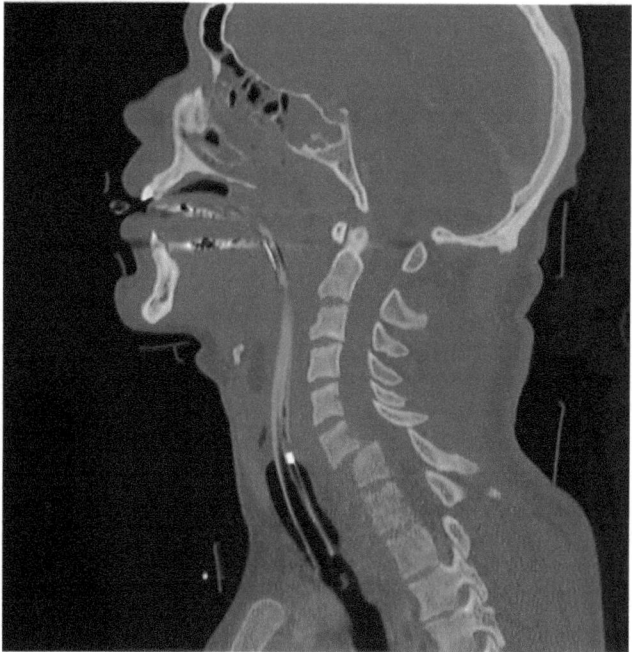

Fig. 123.2 Sagittal computed tomography demonstrating a cervical fracture and dislocation at the level of C6-C7. (By Frank Gaillard [CC BY-SA 3.0 (https://creativecommons.org/licenses/by-sa/3.0)], via Wikimedia Commons.)

🏃 Authors' Preferred Technique

Players who sustain musculoligamentous sprain and/or strain should be removed from play and treated conservatively with rest, icing, and NSAIDs until asymptomatic. It is imperative to perform a comprehensive physical exam and history so as to rule out more serious osseous or neurologic injures. Most sprains and strains are self-limiting, and players should be able to return to competition if they are free of neck pain upon axial loading, have a full ROM, and normal neck strength.

Athletes who sustain cervical spine fractures should at the very least be deferred from playing until the facture has healed. If the fracture is stable, it should resolve without the need for surgical intervention and the player should be able to return by the next season. Those with unstable fractures who require a halo vest or surgical stabilization may be unable to safely return to contact sports. Moreover, those with previous cervical spine fractures are at increased risk for subsequent fractures due to their altered spinous biomechanics. Although there is a high frequency of cervical spine injuries in contact sports, there is no universal agreement of standard guidelines for returning to pre-injury activity levels.[53,54] Despite a lack of consensus on specific measures, it is agreed that before returning to play, athletes should be asymptomatic, pain free, neurologically intact, and have full strength and ROM.[50,54]

Postoperative Management

Players with only musculoligamentous pain and/or strain should be monitored for deterioration of structural and neurologic function and should not engage in sporting activity until asymptomatic. Those with unstable cervical fractures and/or dislocations that require anterior surgical fusion should be monitored for degeneration of intervertebral discs adjacent to the spot of fusion.[55] Moreover, it might be necessary to stabilize the cervical spine with a cervical orthosis or halo ring device until the neck has regained its support.

Results

Ultimately, most athletes with neck or back pain have a self-limiting musculoligamentous injury that will resolve with rest and treatment with NSAIDs and icing. Athletes who sustain unstable cervical fractures and/or dislocations can lead to a wide range of results depending on severity and location. Injuries can vary from transient radiculopathies to permanent, complete SCI. The most common pattern is pronounced weakness in the upper extremities and less pronounced weakness in the lower extremities, a phenomenon known as central cord syndrome.[38]

Complications
Disc Degeneration

Several clinical studies have pointed to increased rates of disc degeneration adjacent to the levels of anterior cervical spinal fusion.[55–57] This is caused by the shift of load from fused spinal segment to adjacent levels, causing earlier disc degeneration. Moreover, significant increases in intradiscal pressure and segmental motion occurs at levels adjacent to disc fusion during normal ranges of motion.[55]

Future Considerations

Unstable cervical spine fractures, although rare, are among the most disabling injuries in contact sports. Further research is needed into developing better protective equipment, as well as educating players, coaches, and sporting administrators into preventing maneuvers that put the cervical spines of athletes at risk. Finally, more scientific inquiries should be made into the variety of surgical treatments for unstable cervical spine fractures, particularly comparisons between anterior and posterior approaches to stabilization and fusion.

For a complete list of references, go to ExpertConsult.com.

SELECTED READINGS

Citation:
McCrory P, et al. Consensus statement on concussion in sport: the 4th International Conference on Concussion in Sport held in Zurich, 2012. Br J Sports Med. 2013;47(5):250–258.

Level of Evidence:
IV

Summary:
This paper revises and updates the consensus formed in the first three symposia on concussion in sport. It is intended for use by health care professionals in dealing with patients suffering from sports-related concussions. The document addresses issues such as the definition of concussion, concussion management, return-to-play protocols, and injury prevention. Finally, it incorporates the SCAT3 assessment tool.

Citation:
Harmon KG, et al. American Medical Society for Sports Medicine position statement: concussion in sport. Br J Sports Med. 2013;47(1):15–26.

Level of Evidence:
IV

Summary:
This document is presented as a tool for physicians to evaluate and manage sports-related concussions. It includes discussions of the definition, pathophysiology, incidence, diagnosis, education, prevention, and legislation of concussions in the United States.

Citation:
Cantu RC, et al. Return to play after cervical spine injury in sports. Curr Sports Med Rep. 2013;12(1):14–17.

Level of Evidence:
III

Summary:
The authors of this paper present detailed descriptions on a variety of cervical spine injuries in sports. It includes discussions and return to play protocols for burners or stingers, spear tackler's spine, muscular sprain and ligamentous strain, cervical spine fractures, spinal stenosis, and transient quadriplegia.

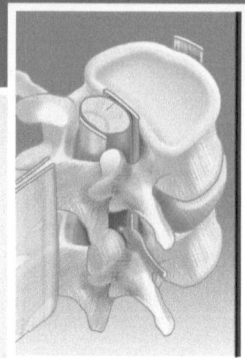

124

Imaging of the Spine

Adil Samad, M. Farooq Usmani, A. Jay Khanna

Along with a comprehensive history and physical examination, imaging is essential for the evaluation of the patient who presents with suspected or known spine pathology. It facilitates preoperative assessment of a patient, generation of a differential diagnosis, selection of the most likely diagnosis, postoperative evaluation, and monitoring of disease progression. Unlike radiologists, most orthopaedic surgeons have little, if any, formal training in the systematic evaluation and interpretation of imaging studies. On the other hand, the orthopaedic surgeon has access to information that the radiologist does not, such as a patient's history and physical examination, which can affect diagnosis and surgical decision-making. Experience may help the clinician decide which imaging modality is best for a patient, evaluate imaging studies effectively, determine the most likely diagnosis, and use the imaging studies in conjunction with clinical findings to guide surgical decision-making. We suggest that a team approach in conjunction with a radiologist will help the surgeon systematically evaluate each imaging study, correlate studies with the clinical information more accurately, reduce the incidence of unnecessary imaging, and increase the likelihood of making the correct and clinically relevant diagnosis and treatment decisions.

The purpose of this chapter is to review the imaging modalities currently used for evaluation of the spine in terms of evolving technique, image quality, speed, cost, availability, and safety, with a specific focus on the evaluation of degenerative diseases of the spine.

IMAGING MODALITIES

Radiographs

Radiographs involve the use of ionizing radiation and a radiation detector. Radiography can be discussed in detail based on the medium used as a radiation detector. In conventional radiography (CR), a film is used as a radiation detector. The film undergoes chemical processing after radiation exposure before the final image appears on the film and can be viewed against a bright light to illuminate the target anatomy. In digital radiography (DR), a digital detector is exposed to radiation transmitted through the patient. The imaging plate and image processor are used to convert radiation energy to light energy and eventually to a digital image, which can be stored and viewed on a computer. DR has been further subclassified into different forms based on

the type of detector used. Computed radiography, the initial type of DR developed in the early 1990s, uses a photo-stimulable phosphor plate, whereas direct radiography, developed in the late 1990s to early 2000s, uses semiconductor-based sensors, such as selenium, or selenium and cesium iodode.[1] The images created via DR can be directly transferred to picture archiving and communication system (PACS). PACS has a wide range of functions from image acquisition, digital display windows, storage of image, and generation of hard copies.

Until as late as the 1990s, a conventional film cassette was the primary method of acquiring radiographic images of the bones, but digital image acquisition has replaced the cassette method at almost all institutions. Advantages of DR include improved image quality, speed, accessibility, less radiation exposure, availability of postimaging processing and quality optimization, lower cost, and ease of image storage and retrieval.

Radiography (conventional or digital) is a widely available and cost-effective modality for the initial evaluation of the spine; it is valuable for trauma assessment, determination of coronal and sagittal deformity, identification of spondylosis and spondylolisthesis (and their progression), and detection of osteolytic and osteoblastic lesions suggestive of malignancy. Initial evaluation often begins with anteroposterior (AP) and lateral views of the area of interest (Fig. 124.1). The need for additional studies, such as oblique, flexion, or extension views, is determined by the clinical situation; for example, stress radiographs may be obtained to evaluate instability, which may be seen in patients with ligamentous injuries, or tension radiographs would be recommended in the evaluation of scoliosis. Radiographs can be used to determine the level of abnormality preoperatively and intraoperatively, and to provide a rapid evaluation of hardware placement and deformity correction intraoperatively and postoperatively.

Although radiography provides a relatively effective assessment of the osseous structures and their alignment, it is limited in its ability to visualize soft tissues, the spinal cord, the occipitocervical and cervicothoracic junctions, and bone marrow involvement. Furthermore, reductions in bone mass are evident on radiographs only after a 30% to 50% decrease in bone mineral density.[2,3] Therefore radiography is not the most sensitive technique for the evaluation of bone pathologies, such as osteoporosis, which are due to decrease bone density.

EOS 2D/3D X-Ray Imaging System

EOS is a biplane x-ray imaging system manufactured by EOS imaging. It uses slot-scanning technology in which the radiation source and detector move in different planes during image acquisition. The slot-scanning technology can image the full length of the body up to 175 cm, and thus remove the need to manually join images. The quality of images is similar in nature to CR.[4] It can take posteroanterior (PA) and lateral images simultaneously and construct a three-dimensional (3D) mode, which can allow analysis of vertebral rotation, flexion, translation, or rotation of scoliotic curve. The current software is effective for imaging patients of all ages, but 3D constructions cannot be made for children younger than 6 years of age.[5] Indications for the use of EOS are in diseases that change under load, such as scoliosis, lordosis, or kyphosis. It is increasingly being used for spine, pelvis, lower limb, and gait analysis imaging, and is considered a good technique for assessing global spinal sagittal balance and its relationships with the pelvis and lower limbs (Fig. 124.2).[6]

EOS produces high-quality images with less radiation than CR. Studies comparing EOS with conventional x-rays showed that image quality was comparable or slightly better with EOS. EOS images were superior or equivalent to computed radiography in image quality and structure visibility in 97.2% and 94.3% of images, respectively.[7] Additionally, radiation dose was significantly

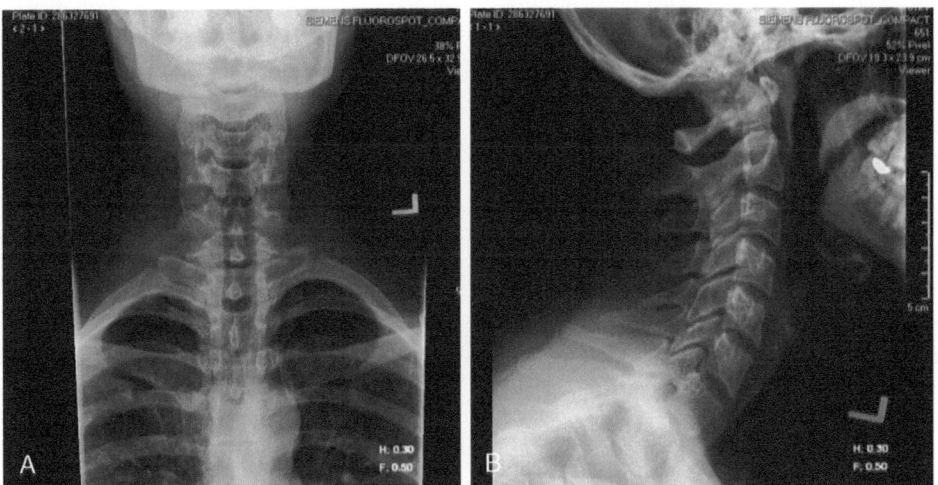

Fig. 124.1 Anteroposterior (A) and lateral (B) radiographs of the C spine at a neutral position showing normal lordosis.

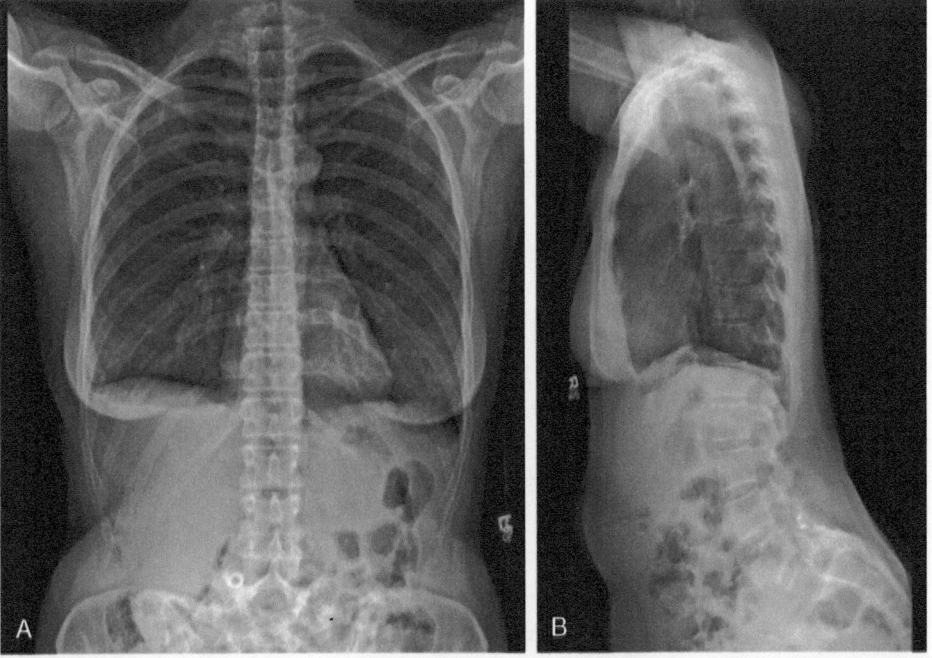

Fig. 124.2 EOS 2D/3D can produce complete anteroposterior (A) and lateral (B) images of the axial skeleton with one shot. Note that compared to the image quality of x-ray images in Fig. 124.1, EOS 2D/3D images are very similar.

lower with EOS than with x-rays. In one study, the mean surface dose with EOS for PA spine was 0.23 milligray (mGy) compared with 1.2 mGy for x-ray. In lateral images, the mean dose was 0.37 mGy compared with 2.3 mGy with x-ray.[8] Recently, EOS imaging has launched a micro-dose protocol that reduces patient dose by a factor of 5.5.[5] Even though absolute radiation dose is decreased, the lifetime health benefits of reduced radiation dose from EOS are small. The EOS system is costly and its cost effectiveness is limited by the number of patients it is used for in a given time period. Thus far, EOS has not shown to be cost effective relative to x-ray.[5,9]

Similar to CR, the EOS system is a tool for the imaging of the skeleton only. EOS images can be acquired within 10 to 30 seconds and can be done while the patient is standing in an upright position. 3D images can be constructed within 15 minutes. EOS software helps with 3D modeling of the spine based on anatomical landmarks defined by the reader and the defined clinical parameters. Luminosity and contrast can be adjusted on the software to help with identification of anatomical landmarks.[10] Even though 3D images can be constructed from EOS, the 3D images are not comparable to the 3D images obtained from computed tomography (CT) as it does not provide information on soft tissues such as muscles, spinal cord, nerves, and viscera. EOS, therefore, is a not a good imaging technique for the degenerative spine. In one study, anterior and posterior margins of intervertebral disks were visible in 22% and 64% of cases with EOS, respectively, compared with 84% and 97% with magnetic resonance imaging (MRI).[11]

Computed Tomography

Like CR, CT uses ionizing radiation, but the radiation doses tend to be very high relative to radiographs. Unlike radiography, this modality acquires images in the axial plane, produces cross-sectional images, and allows for sagittal and coronal 3D reconstructions via post image acquisition processing. Multidetector row CT can acquire all the necessary data for a chest and abdomen study during a single-breath hold, or 15 seconds. CT is the examination of choice for assessing the bony structures of the spine, but the soft tissue assessment is often limited and requires augmentation with a contrast medium. CT is usually part of trauma and tumor staging protocol because it is relatively fast to acquire images, and it is usually not limited by patient medical conditions. Trauma protocols usually image the whole spine including the skull. CT is the imaging of choice for tumor assessment. In tumor protocol, usually the thoracic, lumbar, and sacral spine are imaged as part of the CT of chest, abdomen, and pelvis.[12]

For CT imaging, the patient is usually in a supine position to ensure limited movement of the spine associated with breathing. CT is sensitive to motion and distorts images due to metal implants. Therefore these two factors can be a limiting factor in obtaining imaging. Since metal implants in the spine are usually made of titanium, routine CT protocols are usually sufficient to obtain good-quality images in the presence of the implants. CT is sensitive for reactive bone change in infection. However, because of the high radiation dose associated, when feasible, MRI should be considered for better assessment of soft tissue abnormalities.[12] The radiation dose for a chest abdomen and pelvis CT is about 20 mSv compared to about 1.5 mSv for a PA spine x-ray. It is unclear what amount of radiation dose increases the risk of cancers, but the range is placed above 200 mSv.[13]

High-contrast resolution and multiplanar reconstruction—the most important advantages of CT—permit an excellent evaluation of the spine for accurate characterization of the osseous details of a lesion, the degree of bony destruction, and spinal alignment (Fig. 124.3). 3D reconstructions can assist in careful fracture evaluation, preoperative planning, and the examination of complex deformity.[14,15] Although CT is effective for bony degenerative change, it is not the optimal imaging choice for degenerative disk disease. Intravenous contrast can enhance the diagnosis of disc herniation by providing improved delineation of the soft tissue. Finally, CT plays an important role in myelography for demonstrating the outline of nerve roots, and cauda equina (see below). CT-guided interventions, such as biopsies of various lesions, nerve root, facet joint blocks, epidural injection, and even screw placement in spinal surgery, is an integral utility of the technology.

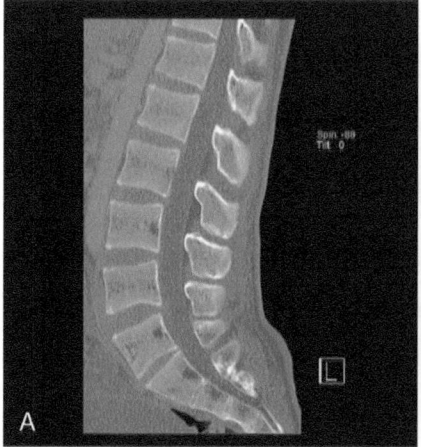
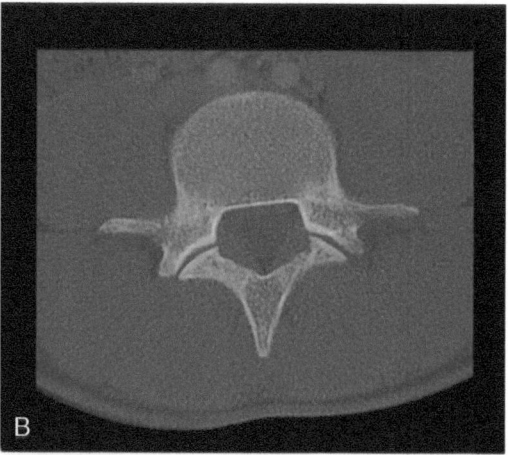

Fig. 124.3 Sagittal reconstructed (A) and axial computed tomography (B) images through L-Spine. The soft tissue is poorly differentiated but bony structures are visualized with great detail.

Magnetic Resonance Imaging

MRI generates multiplanar images that have excellent anatomic and spatial resolution but, unlike CR and CT, it does not involve ionizing radiation. MRI relies on the response of hydrogen nuclei in intracellular and extracellular fluids to a magnetic field generated by the machine. MRI starts by generating an artificial magnetic field to orient the atomic nuclei in one direction. Radiofrequency pulses are then applied to change the direction in which the nuclei are pointing. When the pulse is removed, the nuclei shift back to their steady-state position. Nuclei from fluids of different cells revert to steady state at different rates, ranging from tens of milliseconds to seconds. The translation of the released energy creates discrete regions of varying signal intensities or brightness on the images. The differences in relaxation timing allow the system to distinguish between tissues. The intensity of the signal depends on the number of protons within different tissues, that is, the water content of those tissues. The tissues release the absorbed energy at different rates, which are distinguished as T1 or T2.[16] T1 images reflect the time it takes for nuclei to return to realign with the main magnetic field after the radiofrequency pulse is stopped. T2 reflects the time it takes for nuclei that are spinning to lose their excitation.

An MRI sequence is the combination of radiofrequency pulses, various pre-determined parameters, and magnetic gradients that produce an image with a particular intensity of each tissue type. For the orthopedic surgeon, understanding T1-weighted, T2-weighted, and proton density (PD)-weighted images are the most critical MRI sequences. T1-weighted images, also referred to as T1WI, can be thought of as the most anatomical of images; these images most closely resemble the color gradients of tissue macroscopically. In T1-weighted image (T1WI), fat is bright and the cerebrospinal fluid (CSF) cortex, tendons, and ligaments are dark. It is useful for focusing on anatomical details because the dark CSF, tendons, ligaments, and cortex are surrounded by the bright fat. These are most useful for hemorrhage, marrow replacing masses, or identifying lipoma lesions. Edema and fluid are not well characterized on T1WI.[16] T2-weighted images are best suited for the analysis of pathology related to soft tissue,

bone, ligaments, tendons, joints, bursa, synovium, and muscle. In T2-weighted images, CSF, edema, synovial fluid, fluid cyst, and fresh blood appear bright. On the other hand, old blood, bone, muscle, tendons, white matter, appear dark to gray.[17] Finally, PD-weighted images are the third type of MRI sequence that are essential for an orthopaedic surgeon. PD is an intermediate sequence with some aspects of T1 and others of T2. PD is the ideal sequence for the assessment of joints because it can distinguish between fluid, hyaline cartilage, and fibro cartilage. Fluid (CSF, joint fluid) and fat appear white while muscle, cartilage appear gray to dark. PD was found to be superior to T2-weighted images for detecting lesions in the cervical spinal cord.[18]

The fundamental advantage of MRI is its ability to provide a high-resolution depiction of osseous and soft-tissue structures. With respect to the spine, MRI provides excellent visualization of the vertebral body, intervertebral discs, spinal canal, posterior elements, ligaments, paraspinal muscles, nerve roots, and the spinal cord (Fig. 124.4). With multiplanar imaging and the use of various pulse sequences, MRI facilitates abnormality characterization and has been shown to have high sensitivity and specificity for the detection of various disease processes (e.g., 93% and 94%, respectively, for vertebral osteomyelitis[19]). MRI has also proved invaluable in the assessment of neoplasms of the spine, with a greater accuracy than CT.[20] With regard to the degenerative spine, MRI allows for excellent evaluation of the degree of central and foraminal stenosis as well as the degree of other degenerative changes such as facet arthropathy and degenerative disc disease.

The disadvantages of using MRI include the inability to scan patients with cardiac pacemakers or other embedded ferromagnetic material.[21] However, new technology is underway to produce implants and pacemakers that are MRI compatible.[22] MRI can produce a limited quality image for patients with instrumentation because of metal artifact, even with less ferromagnetic metals (such as titanium) that produce less artifact.[23] Additionally, there are often problems in obtaining a scan in patients with claustrophobia and, compared with CT, MRI has an inferior ability to assess the detail of osseous or calcified structures. Relative contraindications to MRI include the first trimester of pregnancy.

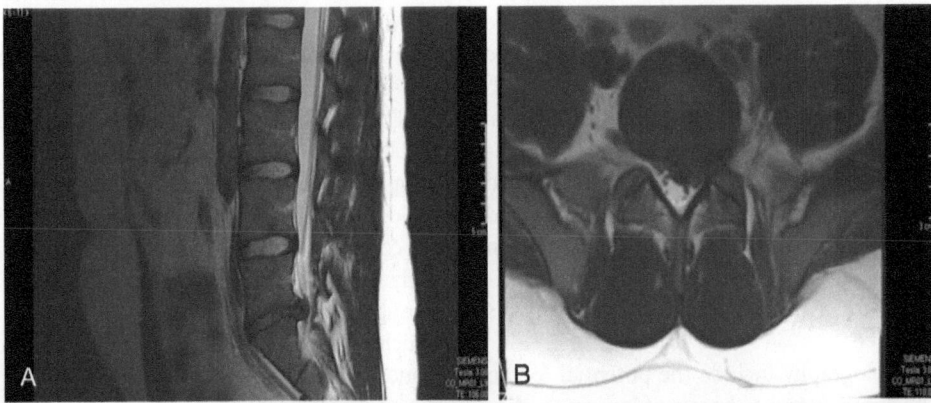

Fig. 124.4 Sagittal (A) and axial (B) T2 magnetic resonance imaging images show the soft tissue structures in the lumbar spine. Notably, disc herniation can be appreciated at the L5-S1 disc. The axial image shows that the disc herniates more towards the right than the left.

Myelography

Myelography is radiography of the spine after injection of a nonionic contrast material into the subarachnoid space, via a lumbar or cervical puncture. The major indications for its use include the imaging of a patient for whom MRI is contraindicated (because of claustrophobia, the presence of pacemaker, etc.), the degradation of image quality in the presence of spinal hardware or cases where kyphoscoliosis makes MRI acquisition challenging and interpretation difficult. Even with the above noted disadvantages of MRI, except for those situations in which metal artifact is a factor, MRI is superior to myelography for the evaluation of spinal abnormality, and has been shown to have a substantially greater accuracy in the detection of herniated disks and a lower false-positive rate.[24-26] Myelography was the diagnostic test of choice in the 1980s and over time it was superseded by MRI. Between 1999 and 2009, its use declined by almost half, largely owing to the accessibility, availability, and comprehensive imaging obtainable via an MRI.[27] Studies have shown the superiority of myelography for the evaluation of some diagnoses such as nerve root compression. In one series of surgically confirmed patients with nerve root compression, MRI underestimated the compression by about 30% compared to only 5% to 7% by myelography.[28] Similarly, myelography can be more reliable when deciding the levels for decompressive lumbar surgery, and MRI can underestimate spinal canal and the foramina width.[29]

In myelography, a water-soluble nonionic contrast agent, such as iohexol (Omnipaque) and iopamidol (Isovue), is injected usually at L2/L3 level under real-time CR, which is called fluoroscopy. Using fluoroscopy allows the identification and correction of an accidental injection into the epidural space and to check whether contrast is obstructed. The fluoroscopy is then used to obtain images. Alternatively, in most cases, CT images are obtained. These images are evaluated for evidence of compression of the CSF column, disc herniation or compression, bony osteophytes, spinal stenosis, intramedullary tumors, nerve root compression, or meningitis.[27,30] Myelography, in conjunction with CT, affords an excellent evaluation of foraminal stenosis and stenosis adjacent to spinal instrumentation such as pedicle screws.

In the degenerative lumbar and cervical spine, it is important to carefully trace the pathway of each nerve root sleeve to evaluate for foraminal stenosis and to carefully examine the axial CT images to evaluate for central stenosis. Compared with MRI, the use of myelography is not as common. For this reason, less experienced clinicians may not be familiar with the evaluation of these imaging studies. Nevertheless, all clinicians should attempt to evaluate the postmyelography imaging studies and then correlate their impressions with the radiology reports. In patients for whom spinal surgery is being considered, a clinician may also consult with a radiologist experienced in this technique.

Disadvantages of myelography include the potential for an allergic reaction to the contrast agent, the use of ionizing radiation, a lower seizure threshold, bleeding, risk of infection, headache, nausea, the invasiveness of and pain associated with the examination, the time and expertise needed to perform the study, the risk of neural damage, and the inability to determine areas of compression below the blocks in contrast flow.[31-34] The primary contraindication to myelography is allergy to the nonionic contrast agent. Relative contraindications include seizure disorder, bleeding disorders, concurrent use of anticoagulants, infection or skin disease over the site of injection, and pregnancy.

Nuclear Scintigraphy

Nuclear scintigraphy is a quick, relatively inexpensive, widely available, and sensitive test used for the evaluation of musculoskeletal pathology. Unlike the previously mentioned imaging modalities, nuclear scintigraphy (also termed radionuclide bone scan) provides anatomic and physiologic information via the administration of a radiopharmaceutical compound, usually technetium-99m-labeled diphosphonates, into a patient's venous system. The radioisotope is preferentially deposited in regions of increased bone remodeling or activity. It usually takes 2 to 6 hours after injection for 50% of the dose to be deposited in the skeletal system.[35] The deposition of the radioisotope allows areas of increased or decreased bone turnover to be differentiated by a scintillation camera that detects and localizes the gamma radiation emitted by the injected agent. The radiotracer uptake depends on blood flow and the rate of new bone formation. Depending on the purpose of the bone scan, different imaging protocols are used.

The commonly used "three-phase" radionuclide bone scan acquires images at different postinjection times. In phase 1 (blood-flow phase), 2- to 5-second images are obtained during the first minute after injection. This demonstrates the perfusion characteristics and the quality of blood flow to a certain area. For phase 2 (blood-pool or soft-tissue phase), images are obtained 5 to 10 minutes after injection aimed at understanding the pooling of blood since inflammation can increase blood collection in the infected area. In phase 3 (delayed or static bone phase), the radiotracer usually deposits into bone mineral, and images are generally taken 2 to 3 hours post-injection. The degree of uptake depends on the blood flow and the rate of new bone formation. In some cases, a phase 4 static image is taken after 24 hours to assess for overall distribution of the radiotracer (Fig. 124.5). In osteomyelitis, for example, there is focal hyperperfusion, focal hyperemia, and focally increased bone uptake. The sensitivity for detection of osteomyelitis by nuclear scintigraphy ranges from 70% to 100% when increased uptake is noted on all three phases.[36-39]

This modality is particularly useful for the evaluation of metabolic bone disorders, stress fractures, primary and metastatic neoplasms, infections, and degenerative disorders.[39-43] Other major advantages of nuclear scintigraphy are that it can evaluate the complete skeleton in one study, and can detect osseous lesions early because of its high sensitivity. These characteristics make scintigraphy ideal for surveying the skeleton for metastatic disease, which is one of the most common indications for this modality. Bone scans are extremely sensitive—more sensitive than CR—for detecting skeletal abnormalities due to metastatic disease. In 75% of patients with malignancy and bone pain, a bone scan is usually abnormal.[35] Nuclear scintigraphy also can be used in

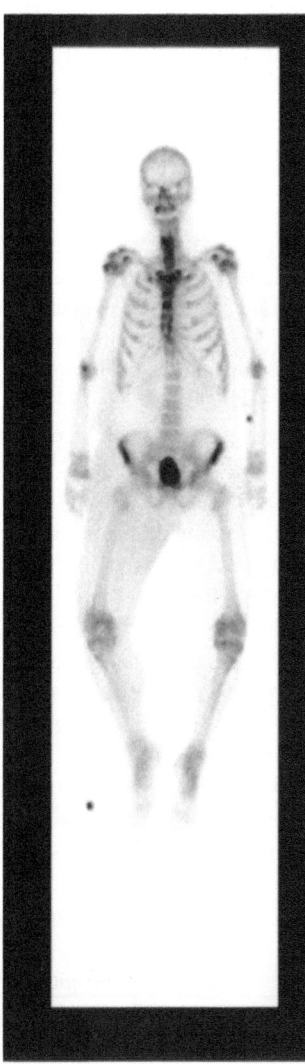

Fig. 124.5 DEXA scan in a 52-year-old male shows the increased signal intensity in regions with higher uptake of the radioisotope, notably the pelvic rim, physeal plate of the distal femur, proximal radius, and shoulder region. The radioisotope is cleared by the kidneys and hence the increased uptake in the bladder.

lieu of MRI to help determine the age of vertebral compression fractures.

Nuclear scintigraphy has several disadvantages. Most importantly, it is relatively nonspecific; any condition that causes increased bone turnover will appear similar. Furthermore, aggressive lesions that do not allow time for remodeling, or osteoblastic lesions with a low metabolic rate, can generate a falsely negative study.[41] It also requires a substantial length of time to complete the study and has poor spatial resolution. However, single-photon emission computed tomography (SPECT) can improve the spatial resolution of nuclear scintigraphy because it helps to detect osseous lesions in more complex anatomical regions, such as the spine and pelvis. SPECT (see below) has improved the ability to detect vertebral metastases and to localize lesions within different areas of the vertebra, including the pars intra-articularis in patients with suspected or known isthmic spondylolisthesis.[44,45]

Functional Metabolic Imaging

Functional metabolic imaging is an imaging technique that aims to assess the physiologic activity in the bone or soft tissue by measuring changes in blood flow, chemical composition, uptake of glucose, or changes in metabolism. Unlike the imaging techniques discussed earlier, functional imaging focuses on exploring the physiologic activity of a tissue rather than elucidating the anatomical details of a structure. Positron emission tomography (PET) is another form of nuclear medicine imaging modality and is a type of functional metabolic imaging that is used in the evaluation of physiologic changes in various tissues. In its most common form, 18-F-labeled 2-fluoro-2-deoxyglocose (FDG) is used as the positron-emitting radionuclide tracer that emits gamma radiation at levels proportional to intracellular glucose metabolism.[46] The concentration of FDG is proportional to the level of metabolic activity of the tissue. FDG usually takes about 30 minutes to 1 hour for systemic incorporation into the various body tissues.[47] Therefore a scan is done usually 30 minutes after injection. Increasingly, PET is combined with a CT in the same machine, and the patient gets a PET and CT in one visit. CT allows the reconstruction of a 3D image series that provides anatomical detail, whereas PET collects data on metabolic information. As a result, one image series is used for anatomical and metabolic assessment of the patients.[48-50]

The primary indications for this modality are the detection of primary and metastatic neoplasms and the evaluation of tumor response to treatment. Because neoplasms often have higher rates of metabolic activity than normal surrounding tissue, a PET scan can identify tissue with higher metabolic activity. The applications of PET scanning for musculoskeletal conditions continue to grow: differentiation between osteoporotic and pathologic vertebral fractures, between aseptic loosening and infection in knee and hip arthroplasty, and between benign and metastatic spinal metastases.[51,52] The principal disadvantages of a PET scan are its limited availability and high cost.

Single Photon Emission Computed Tomography

SPECT/CT is another form of functional metabolic imaging that relies on a radionuclide for imaging of the spine. SPECT uses a gamma ray camera detector to capture gamma rays released by an injected radioisotope material. PET and SPECT have some differences that make SPECT a more suitable imagining technique for many different imaging needs.[53] SPECT is cheaper relative to PET partially because it can use longer lived and easily obtainable radioisotopes. SPECT uses technetium-99m, iodine-123, or iodine-131 radioisotopes as opposed to the flourine-18 isotope used in PET. Relative to PET, SPECT has a lower contrast and spatial resolution (maximum resolution of about 1 cm). Similar to a PET, SPECT can be combined with a CT, (SPECT/CT) to provide functional information from the SPECT and anatomic information from the CT. Combining the CT is helpful because it can also improve the attenuation and the quality of the photon emission data.[54,55] As a result, a single imaging technique can be used to acquire high-quality functional and anatomical information.

SPECT/CT has numerous uses in the evaluation of orthopaedic pathologies, such as fractures in the spine, compression fractures of the vertebra, evaluation of malignancies, infections, bone trauma, and identifying degenerative changes. For example, using SPECT/CT fractures of pars interarticularis can be distinguished from areas of increased activity such as facet joint arthritis.[56] There is strong evidence for the higher sensitivity of SPECT/CT compared to SPECT alone or nuclear scintigraphy for the detection of bone tumor. In one study, SPECT/CT had a sensitivity of 100% for the detection of cancerous lesions in the spine compared with 64% for nuclear scintigraphy and 86% for SPECT alone.[57,58]

Interventional Radiology Techniques

Interventional radiology (IR) is a subspecialty of radiology in which fluoroscopy, CT, or MRI are used to guide a wide range of percutaneous treatments throughout the body, including the musculoskeletal system. Under image guidance, tissue samples can be obtained that can lead to diagnosis and, in turn, can guide or directly assist with therapeutic intervention, for example, image-guided biopsies and aspirations, radiofrequency ablation (RFA), vertebroplasty, kyphoplasty, and angiography.

IR has played an increasingly dominant role in the management of previously surgically treated diseases. Image-guided RFA is used to treat benign and metastatic bone lesions. Advantages of RFA over surgery include short procedures, the possibility of outpatient treatment, lower morbidity, and decreased cost. In vertebroplasty and kyphoplasty, fluoroscopy, or CT guidance can facilitate an accurate transpedicular approach and guide cement placement for treatment of painful lesions of the spine.[59] Angiography, which is often used for the evaluation of vascular tumors, can be combined with embolization before surgical intervention. Angiography and embolization are especially useful for hypervascular tumors, such as aneurysmal bone cyst, giant cell tumor, and angiosarcoma. Preoperative arterial embolization improves visibility during surgery, and permits safer and faster surgery.[60] In some cases, IR is a safer and more effective procedure than surgical intervention. Osteoid osteoma was historically removed with wide resection to excise the small nidus. Surgery was found to be associated with a higher risk of fracture and longer immobilization. In the last 10 years, percutaneous CT-guided ablation has become increasingly popular because of the high success rate and the low morbidity. CT-guided ablation can be used in many parts of the skeleton, except when the osteoma is close to neurovascular structures.[61]

IMAGING OF THE DEGENERATIVE SPINE

The primary reasons for presentation to a spine care specialist are conditions such as low back pain, neck pain, numbness and tingling in legs, and limited mobility in the spine. Degenerative diseases of the spine are one of the most common presenting diagnoses for patients. Such patients often present with neck pain (alone or in conjunction with radicular arm pain), back pain (alone or in conjunction with radicular leg pain), signs and symptoms of myelopathy, or signs and symptoms of neurogenic claudication.

For patients with benign neck or back pain, 70% to 90% show improvement in symptoms within 1 month after initial presentation.[62,63] Therefore imaging in the form of conventional radiographs is usually delayed for 6 weeks after initial presentation in the absence of "red flags" (e.g., fever, chills, trauma, night or rest pain, weight loss, history of malignancy, or neurologic deficit). However, because patients frequently present initially to their primary care physician or to the emergency department, 6 weeks often can elapse by the time they are evaluated by a spine specialist. For this reason, many specialists obtain conventional radiographs on an initial evaluation.

For a patient with degenerative changes of the cervical or lumbar spine, initial radiographs should be scrutinized for the presence of degenerative changes. Evidence of spondylosis is seen in most spines of elderly patients.[64-66] After conventional radiographs have been evaluated, the patient is often referred for nonoperative treatment, including antiinflammatory medications, physical therapy, and interventional pain management as needed. MRI studies are not usually indicated as one of the initial studies, but may be considered if the symptoms persist. As described above, MRI is the imaging modality of choice for the degenerative spine because it provides excellent multiplanar (axial, sagittal, and coronal) evaluation and facilitates careful evaluation of spinal alignment and morphology of the vertebral bodies and disc. Most importantly, with regard to the degenerative spine, this imaging modality helps evaluate for the presence or absence of spinal stenosis.

An MRI imaging study of the spine is best evaluated by using a systematic approach. One such approach is described here[67]:
1. Determine which pulse sequences and specialized MRI imaging studies are available for review. This includes identifying whether it is a T1-weighted image, a conventional T2-weighted image, or PD. Usually, MRI of the spine includes images in the sagittal and axial planes.
2. Evaluate T2-weighted (often sagittal plane) images for recognition of areas of increased T2-weighted signal that are not physiologic or expected. Disc herniation can be identified by following the bright high-intensity signal of the CSF.
3. Evaluate T1-weighted images for improved detection of anatomic detail and the correlation of the disturbance in local and regional anatomy on the T1-weighted images with areas of increased signal intensity on the T2-weighted images.
4. Evaluate specialized MRI pulse sequences that may be specific to the region or the disease process of interest such as PD or fat-suppressed T2-weighted images. The pulse sequences will be selected based on the pathology being evaluated.
5. Correlate the above imaging information with the patient's history, physical examination, and laboratory study results to determine the most likely differential diagnostic considerations.

For the evaluation of degenerative disc disease, the degree of stenosis should be evaluated on the MRI study. Although there are several objective measures of stenosis, most clinicians tend to use the words "mild," "moderate," and "severe" based on their own criteria. More objective measures of stenosis include a definition for the lumbar spine as a cross-sectional area less than

100 mm^2.[68] On CR, relative stenosis in the cervical spine is defined as an AP canal diameter of less than 13 mm, and absolute stenosis is defined as an AP canal diameter of less than 10 mm.[69] Although less experienced clinicians tend to evaluate stenosis only on the sagittal images, we suggest the additional use of axial T2-weighted images to help evaluate for stenosis in the central canal, the lateral recess, and the neural foramina.

Degenerative disc changes of the spine are common with up to 70% to 80% of the population showing evidence of disc degeneration by the time they are 50. The elderly have especially high rates of degenerative changes of the spine, although many patients with such degenerative changes may be asymptomatic.[70-72] For example, Boden et al. found that 28% of 67 asymptomatic patients had abnormal MRI findings suggestive of a herniated nucleus pulposus or lumbar stenosis. Additionally, those who were more than 60 years old had a higher incidence of degenerative findings. Of the 60- to 80-year-old age group, 93% had MRI evidence of degenerated discs: 79% with bulging discs and 36% with disc herniations.[70] In a similar study of the cervical spine, Boden et al. found that 28% of 63 asymptomatic patients older than 40 years had abnormal MRI findings (disc herniations, bulging discs, and foraminal stenosis). When evaluating for disc space narrowing or signs of degeneration, nearly 60% of 63 asymptomatic patients older than 40 years had positive findings.[71]

IMAGING STUDY INTERPRETATION

As with all diagnostic studies, there are several limitations with regard to imaging the spine that should be considered. These limitations can be divided into the following broad categories: (1) lack of correlation of the imaging findings with the patient's history and physical examination; (2) lack of correlation of imaging findings with findings on other imaging modalities; (3) poor understanding of normal anatomic variance; and (4) abnormal anatomic and physiologic findings that are common in asymptomatic patients.

Other potential limitations relate to the practice of clinicians providing the formal readings for imaging studies. It is important to note that there is a tendency for specialists to focus on their area of interest when evaluating various imaging studies. For example, an orthopaedic surgeon evaluating AP and lateral radiographs of the lumbar spine may focus on the spine, which could result in missing other findings such as bowel obstruction, nephrolithiasis, gallstones, or a lytic lesion of the ileum. If the clinician is solely responsible for evaluating the imaging studies, then he or she must completely evaluate all images and all aspects of the images for musculoskeletal and nonmusculoskeletal-related diagnoses. In such cases, the clinician must carefully and critically evaluate all imaging studies using a systematic approach. For example, instead of selecting a few radiographs from the jacket or a few images on the workstation to make the diagnosis of L4-L5 grade-1 spondylolisthesis with moderate stenosis, the clinician must evaluate all pulse sequences and every single image to rule out additional findings. Reading such films in detail requires additional time on the part of the clinician, but the team approach that combines the expertise of a trained radiologist with clinical patient information provided by the clinician can help ensure an accurate diagnosis and can guide treatment.

CONCLUSION

Conventional and advanced imaging studies, along with a comprehensive history and physical examination, are essential in the diagnosis and treatment of patients with known or suspected spine pathology. There are a wide variety of available imaging techniques with which the surgeon should be familiar, which include conventional radiographs, EOS 2D/3D, CT, MRI, myelography, nuclear scintigraphy, PET/CT, and SPECT/CT. As these techniques evolve with time, and as new imaging modalities are introduced, it is important for surgeons to stay current with the changing capabilities and limitations of each technique. Because of the increasing sophistication and complexity of the imaging modalities, it is important for the clinician to actively collaborate with their radiologist colleagues to understand all the details and nuances of a particular technique. The interpretation of imaging studies in consultation with colleagues in radiology, when needed, is crucial. Such consultation, and a team approach, helps ensure that accurate and complete information is obtained from the imaging studies, which can be correlated with each patient's individual clinical profile.

FUTURE CONSIDERATIONS

One of the primary areas for advancement in spine surgery is the use of intraoperative imaging, especially in conjunction with minimally invasive procedures, or for patients with advanced deformity.

Currently, several types of imaging studies can be obtained in the operating room. The existing modality of choice is fluoroscopy, which provides real-time image acquisition. However, it involves a substantial amount of radiation and does not provide imaging in the axial plane. Several systems now offer the acquisition of CT images, which provide axial imaging, reconstructed sagittal and coronal imaging, and 3D volumetric imaging. Intraoperative MRI and MRI-compatible operating room suites are also available in selected centers in the United States. Although the use of advanced imaging modalities in the operating room may improve outcomes and patient safety, there remains room for the optimization of current-generation systems in terms of ease and efficiency of incorporation into operating room workflow and overall quality, resolution, and accuracy of the images.

As with any technology, imaging systems will continue to evolve and improve. Other potential developments that will affect future imaging of the spine include the increased speed of CT and MRI with newer generations of these systems, multiple-access imaging, decreased cost, and improved image resolution (especially MRI, with the introduction of 3.0-T systems). The clinician will continue to be responsible for keeping abreast of these new technologies, critically evaluating the clinical efficacy and cost effectiveness of imaging, and safely incorporating the modalities into clinical practice.

For a complete list of references, go to ExpertConsult.com.

SELECTED READINGS

Citation:

Hartley KG, Damon BM, Patterson GT, et al. MRI techniques: a review and update for the orthopaedic surgeon. *J Am Acad Orthop Surg.* 2012;20(12):775–787.

Level of Evidence:

IIIa

Summary:

MRI is one of the most important imaging techniques at the disposal of orthopaedic surgeons. This article provides an excellent summary of the various sequences used in MRI and the application of these sequences. The authors discuss the appropriate skills needed for the evaluation of pathologies with MRI and the analysis of MRI images.

Citation:

Melhem E, Assi A, El Rachkidi R, et al. EOS((R)) biplanar x-ray imaging: concept, developments, benefits, and limitations. *J Child Orthop.* 2016;10(1):1–14.

Level of Evidence:

IIIa

Summary:

EOS is new tool that is competing with conventional radiograph for the evaluation of spine disease. In this article, Melhem et al. discuss the potential applications of EOS in various musculoskeletal disorders and compare them against conventional radiographs on different parameters (radiation dose, cost, accessibility, image quality).

Citation:

Saha S, Burke C, Desai A, et al. SPECT-CT: applications in musculoskeletal radiology. *Br J Radiol.* 2013;86(1031): 20120519.

Level of Evidence:

IIa

Summary:

SPECT/CT is a technology with significant potential. The article by Saha et al. reviews the technique, basic principles, and applications of SPECT/CT. The authors provide guidance on the analysis of SPECT/CT from different regions of the skeleton and provide case series and examples to illustrate their points.

Citation:

Bastiaannet E, Groen H, Jager PL, et al. The value of FDG-PET in the detection, grading and response to therapy of soft tissue and bone sarcomas: a systematic review and meta-analysis. *Cancer Treat Rev.* 2004;30(1):83–101.

Level of Evidence:

IIa

Summary:

PET/CT uptake is commonly used for the evaluation of metabolic activity of malignancies. This systematic review evaluated the evidence for the uptake of FDG in soft tissue and bone sarcomas. The study is significant in highlighting the parameters needed to evaluate when assessing PET/CT studies.

Citation:

Love C, Din AS, Tomas MB, et al. Radionuclide bone imaging: an illustrative review. *Radiographics.* 2003;23(2):341–358.

Level of Evidence:

IIc

Summary:

Bone scintigraphy continues to play an important role in the evaluation of bone density and various pathologic conditions. Love et al. provide a comprehensive review on the evaluation of bone scans and focus on pathologies related to multiple joints. In this article, they include an excellent collection of normal and pathologic images obtained through bone scintigraphy.

Citation:

Ozdoba C, Gralla J, Rieke A, et al. Myelography in the age of MRI: why we do it, and how we do it. *Radiol Res Pract.* 2011;329017.

Level of Evidence:

V

Summary:

The authors provide a comprehensive overview of the current uses of myelography. The focus is on the details of obtaining optimal myographic studies and they discuss the current applications in the era of more advanced imaging techniques. This article provides appropriate guidelines on the analysis of myelographic images.

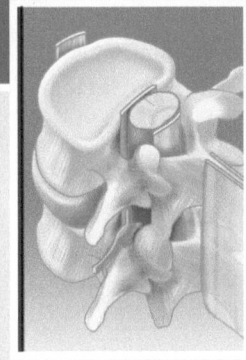

125

Emergency and Field-Side Management of the Spine-Injured Athlete

Korin Hudson, Michael Antonis, William Brady

Spine injuries in athletic events are uncommon, representing only 9% of the total spine injuries presenting to trauma centers.[1] Spine injuries are potentially catastrophic events for the participants; these injuries can lead to significant morbidity and can alter a life permanently. Although thoracolumbar injuries do occur in athletics, the vast majority are less serious and usually involve repetitive and overuse mechanisms. This chapter will focus on the acute management of cervical spine injuries that present more acutely, requiring immediate skilled intervention and appropriate care at every step to prevent any increase in morbidity.

EPIDEMIOLOGY

Athletic spine injuries represent only a small proportion of all spine injuries presenting to trauma centers, and cervical spine injuries make up only a small fraction of all athletic event–related injuries. Despite the relatively low incidence, the potential for permanent disability or complete loss of function from these injuries requires a heightened sense of awareness. A number of databases and scoring systems have been developed over the past several years in an attempt to better quantify and classify the number and types of injuries that occur and the outcomes that result.

In the United States, American football players are at the highest risk for severe cervical spine injuries, averaging approximately eight catastrophic cervical spine injuries each year. These cervical spine injuries can result in incomplete recovery, and approximately six of these eight injuries result in quadriplegia.[2,3] Other high-risk sports include ice hockey, gymnastics, rugby, diving, and cheerleading.[4-6] So-called extreme sports and motor sports convey a risk of spine injuries similar to those commonly associated with vehicular trauma and less like those associated with other sports; this includes an increased risk of acute thoracic and lumbar spine injuries. Skiing and snowboarding are also high-risk sports with the potential increased risk for fractures of the thoracic or lumbar spine.[7,8]

FIELD MANAGEMENT

Pre-Event Planning

The management of any athlete with a suspected spine injury begins before the event, with pre-event meetings and the development a site-specific emergency action plan (EAP). Team physicians or event physicians for large tournaments should be involved in all stages of planning. These plans must include athletic training staff, emergency medical services (EMS), athletic directors, and event coordinators, as well as any other key participants. The plan should include specific role delineation for equipment management and spinal motion control (see later), with a clear decision pathway and chain of command for transport decisions. Local officials should designate hospitals in the area that have capabilities to manage acute spinal cord injuries. The capabilities include, but are not limited to, advanced radiology imaging, orthopaedic and/or neurosurgical care, and trauma care capability for participants of all ages. Any athletes with potentially serious injuries should be preferentially transported to these predetermined emergency departments (EDs), if needed, with a prearrival call by the event physician.

Pre-event planning also includes the outfitting of athletes in proper protective equipment. Protective equipment varies sport to sport but may include helmets, shoulder pads, protective eyewear, and mouth guards. All members of the medical team should be familiar with the protective equipment that they may encounter and should be familiar with the removal of the equipment in an emergency situation.

Furthermore, pre-event planning can include injury prevention strategies. Examples of such strategies include the following: teaching athletes how to tackle properly in American football, proper checking techniques in ice hockey and lacrosse, proper heading techniques in soccer, and teaching athletes how to minimize the risk of serious injury from falls in gymnastics and cheerleading. The elimination of spear tackling in football—a maneuver that places the cervical spine of the tackler at risk due to a slightly flexed position (a significant axial load)—in 1976 by a National Collegiate Athletic Association (NCAA) rule represented a significant change directed at player safety. So-called heads-up football tackling has led to a significant reduction in the number of cervical spine injuries in the years since the spear-tackling technique was banned.[9-11] Finally, athletes and coaches should be instructed on what to do if an injury does occur, including not moving a potentially spinal-injured athlete and how to summon assistance from the medical teams in an emergency.

As noted previously, injuries in extreme sports and motor sports tend to mimic vehicular trauma rather than other athletic injuries. For this reason, physicians and other health care professionals providing care at motor sport events should be prepared for this type of traumatic injury. These injuries are best managed according to the basic and advanced trauma life support (BTLS/ATLS) guidelines, with consideration of local trauma center protocols.[12,13]

When considering the pre-event planning for potential spine injury, roles should be assigned in advance; a chain of command and decision pathways should be established allowing for efficient and effective management when an injury occurs.[14] The specific roles will be outlined later but may need to be adapted for different settings and different numbers of providers. Collegiate and professional teams may have a fully staffed ambulance, several athletic trainers, and several team physicians available, whereas a rural high school team may have none of these resources on site when an injury occurs. An EAP needs to be specific to the team, site, and availability of resources.

In addition to an EAP, an "emergency toolkit" can be prepared and available at all times during practice and competition. The toolkit will vary depending on the sport and site but should include the necessary equipment to remove protective athletic equipment (i.e., facemask) quickly without disruption to spine immobilization and allow for emergent airway intervention or the performance of cardiopulmonary resuscitation (CPR). These tools will be described in further detail later, but it is critical that medical professionals have more than one device available and are familiar with the safety equipment used by their team/league so the providers have the appropriate removal devices immediately available. In addition, splints and equipment for spinal motion control, including a cervical collar, vacuum splint, and/or long spine board, should also be available. If the listed equipment is not present on the sidelines for all practices and competitions, the medical staff, coaches, etc. need to know where to access a first aid kit, automatic external defibrillator, and additional emergency equipment. Most importantly, all staff should be aware of the procedure for activating EMS and must be able to properly provide a dispatcher with information including the practice or competition location; this requires immediate access to a phone to call 911 or other appropriate local EMS resources.

Approaching the Injured Athlete on the Field

On-field emergencies fall into several categories, and often it is best to think in terms of a flowchart (Fig. 125.1). Consider first the immediate threats to life and assess the athlete's vital functions, using the airway, breathing, circulation, and disabilities (ABCDs) approach to evaluation. This evaluation can be accomplished with a quick assessment of level of consciousness—the awake, alert athlete who is answering questions appropriately meets all criteria and the sideline physician can move on to the next phase of the exam. The Glasgow Coma Scale (GCS; Fig. 125.2) is often used in trauma assessment, with lower scores suggesting a higher risk of serious injury.[15] A simpler system, such as the AVPU scale, may be more useful in emergency situations. In this system, the patient's mental status is divided into one of four categories based on their response to stimulation: A—alert; V—verbal, responds to verbal stimuli; P—pain, responds

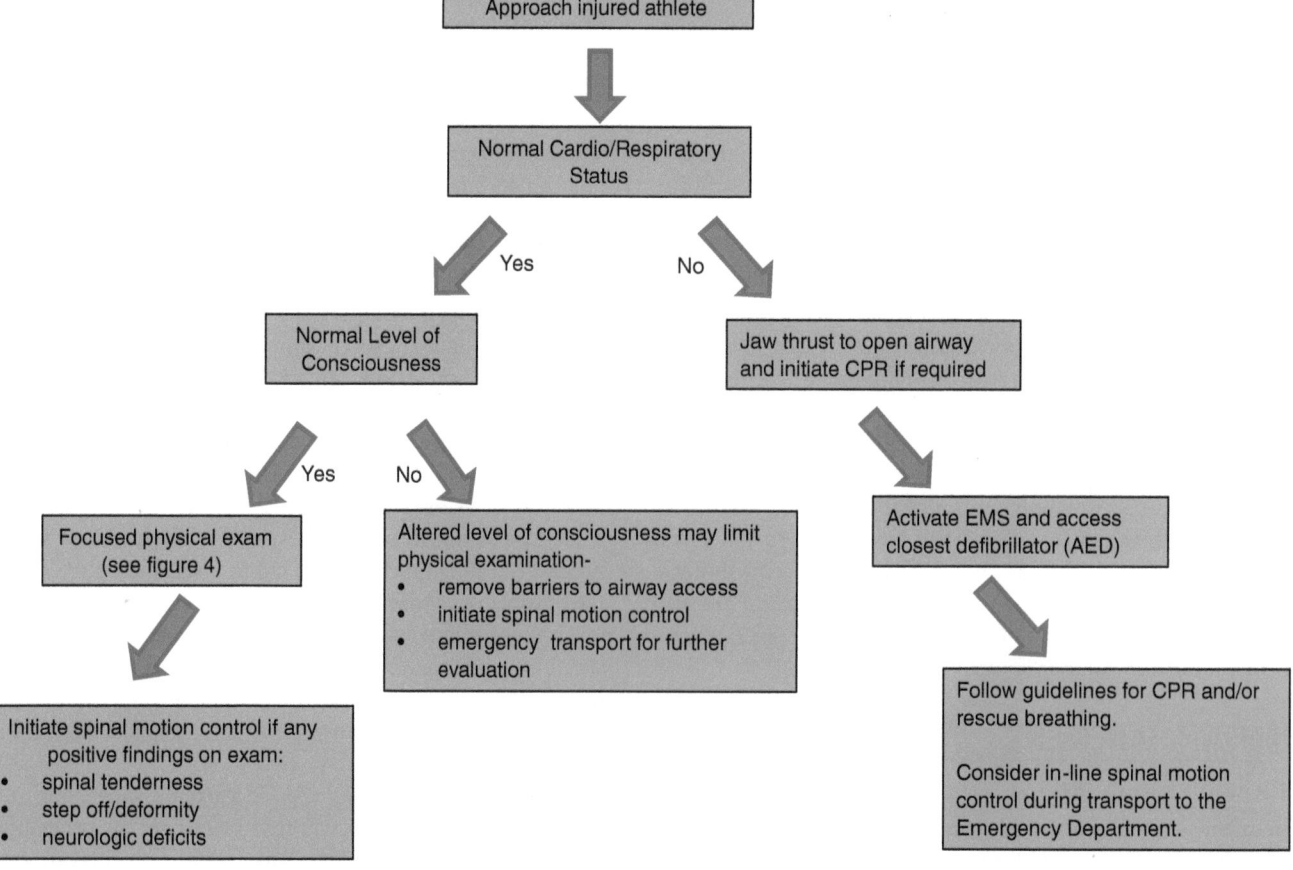

Fig. 125.1 Approach to the injured athlete. *AED,* Automated External defibrillator.

Eye	Verbal	Motor
4- Spontaneous eye opening	5- Oriented	6- Obedient/Follows Commands
3- Eyes open to voice	4- Confused/Disoriented	5- Purposeful
2- Eyes open to pain	3- Inappropriate	4- Withdraws to painful stimuli
1- No response	2- Incomprehensible/Moaning	3- Flexion response to pain
	1- No response	2- Extension response to pain
		1- No response

Fig. 125.2 Glasgow Coma Scale.

to painful stimuli; and U—unresponsive or unconscious.[16] The AVPU scale is easier to apply in emergency settings while still providing important information about a patient's mental status and medical condition.

For the unconscious athlete, a pulse check should be performed and adequacy of respirations should be assessed. If either is found to be inadequate, immediately remove any accessory intraoral devices (i.e., mouthguard). However, the clinician should be cautious with the routine removal of other protective equipment without further clinical examination. A jaw thrust should be used to open the airway; the jaw thrust maneuver and placement of an oropharyngeal airway have less effect on cervical spine alignment than does the performance of a "head tilt" maneuver that places the cervical spine in extension.[17,18] Appropriate ventilation may be maintained with the use of a bag-valve mask ventilation as needed. Additional airway maneuvers and/or CPR should also be initiated immediately if indicated. Protective chest equipment may be removed by cutting through the laces or elastic straps either in the axilla or over the sternum to expose the chest. With these cut, the pads can be opened, allowing access to the chest for compressions and/or the application of cardiac defibrillator pads.

Choosing the optimal technique for definitive emergency airway management is often perceived as a clinical dilemma, and many clinicians believe that orotracheal intubation is hazardous in the presence of a known or potential cervical spine injury.[19] However, several studies have shown that operator skill and comfort in performing a specific airway technique should guide the selection of a particular method. Several authors have concluded that orotracheal intubation is safe and effective when performed with in-line cervical stabilization.[17,20-23] Using a cadaver model, Gerling et al.[24] showed no significant vertebral body movement during orotracheal intubation with manual in-line stabilization. With the relatively recent advent of video-assisted laryngoscopy (VAL), many have questioned whether this technique improves patient safety versus direct laryngoscopy. There appears to be general consensus that VAL does provide significantly better glottic visualization. Turkstra et al.[25] also found that cervical spine motion was reduced by 50% at the C2–C5 levels when VAL was used. These findings were opposed by Robitaille et al.,[26] who concluded that there was no significant difference found between direct laryngoscopy and VAL at any cervical level in regard to motion. The use of a supraglottic airway device may also be considered, because these may be placed with minimal movement of the cervical spine and provide an airway for less-advanced providers. Supraglottic devices are not considered definitive airway protection.[27] The current ATLS guidelines[13] state orotracheal intubation with in-line manual cervical spine stabilization is the definitive airway procedure in the apneic patient. Finally, physicians must be prepared to perform a surgical airway in trauma patients with potential cervical spine injuries who cannot be intubated orally or nasally.

In athletes wearing protective equipment with facemasks, the facemask will need to be removed prior to invasive airway maneuvers. In fact, the facemask should be removed regardless of whether airway maneuvers are required at the time of initial evaluation on the field. This is performed for the purposes of ongoing monitoring of the airway and allows for immediate interventions if deterioration occurs. Athletic trainers and physicians who work with athletes in sports that use protective equipment (hockey, lacrosse, football, motorsports, etc.) should be familiar with the brand/type of equipment worn by their athletes and should possess the necessary tools to assist in the removal of equipment in an emergent case. The facemask is generally attached by several retention clips. These clips are typically made of soft plastic material and fastened to the helmet by screws or spring-loaded fasteners. In the latter case, special devices are provided by the manufacturer that depress the center of the clip, activating the spring and causing the clip to fall apart, releasing the bar of the facemask. In facemask equipment where the clips are connected with screws, a manual or electric-powered screwdriver may be used to remove the screw. In studies, a power screwdriver has proven to be faster and easier to use than devices designed to cut through the plastic clips. The electric drivers deliver the least force and movement to the head during helmet removal.[28,29] Manual screw drivers may be used as a "back-up" method. Tools that cut through the plastic clips themselves, while producing somewhat more force and movement, are also an alternate method of accessing the airway if electronic and manual methods fail (Fig. 125.3).

If the ABCs are intact and the patient is awake and answering questions appropriately, then the clinician may move on to a focused physical examination (Fig. 125.4). The examination should include an assessment for pain and/or tenderness, as well as strength, sensation, and reflexes. Examination findings that suggest spine injury may include: midline neck pain, step-offs, palpable deformities, tenderness on palpation, weakness in the extremities, or persistent and/or bilateral numbness and tingling.

- In many cases, the face mask is affixed to the helmet using a plastic clip and a standard screw.
  - A cordless or battery operated screwdriver can remove the screw allowing the clips to be opened and the facemask to be removed with minimal force on the cervical spine.
  - A manual screwdriver may also be used but may increase the chance of head/neck movement and requires additional time.

- Special shears may be used to cut through the plastic clips
  - 2 cuts should be made through each clip, on either side of the facemask bar
  - The resulting small piece of plastic clip may be discarded allowing the facemask to be removed.
  - Caution should be used as this method may require additional force which could be transmitted to the spine.

- Some helmets have spring loaded clips that attach the facemask to the helmet and a special device to open the clips.

- In many case the facemask may not need to be removed completely, but instead only the lower clips must be removed, allowing the facemask to swing up as if on a hinge across the forehead. This allows for access to the airway without removing all of the fasteners.

- More than one removal device should be available to use in the event that the primary device/method fails

Fig. 125.3 Steps for appropriate facemask removal.

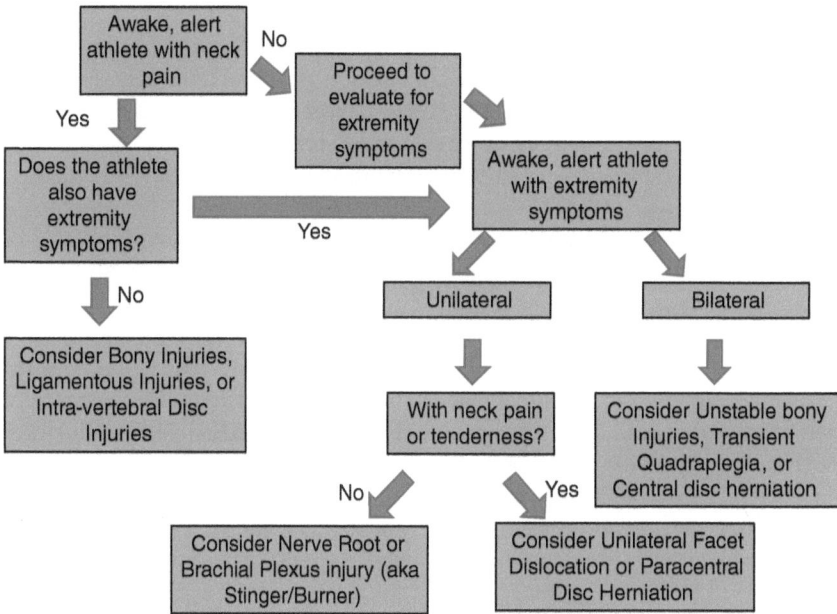

Fig. 125.4 Focused physical exam. (Modified from Zahir U, Ludwig SC. Sports-related cervical spine injuries: on-field assessment and management. *Sems Spine Surg.* 2010;22[4]:173–180.)

When these signs/symptoms are present, care should be taken to minimize the movement of the spine while preparing the athlete for transport for definitive care (Fig. 125.5). In the absence of neck pain, evaluation of active and passive range of motion (ROM) should be performed. Serial examinations are important to assess for progression or resolution of symptoms.

Preparing for Transport

When preparing the athlete for transport, the clinician must start the assessment with a high regard to the initial positioning in which the athlete is found at the end of the play. Athletes generally either land prone, supine, or side-laying. Fig. 125.6 depicts the key steps for management of athletes in each position. Depending on the sport, conditions such as weather, surface (ice hockey or ski slopes), barricades or walls (ice hockey, arena football), and other hazards (motocross motorcycle racing) must also be considered when attempting extrication of the athlete.

After manual in-line stabilization of the cervical spine has been achieved by a single clinician (usually the first clinician to reach the injured athlete) and the airway secured, as previously described if needed, attention should be turned toward managing equipment. In a 2001 position statement, the Inter-Association Task Force for the Care of the Spine Injured Athlete[30] published recommendations stating that football helmets and shoulder pads should remain in place (with the facemasks removed) during transport to the hospital. These guidelines recommend limiting spinal motion with a rigid immobilization device and suggest that protective equipment may be removed in the hospital. However, it should be noted that equipment in other sports such as hockey, lacrosse, and motor sports may not keep the spine in a neutral

position and may need to be removed or padded in a way to maintain neutral spinal alignment during transport. Furthermore, the guidelines from the Inter-Association Task Force are under revision at the time of the writing of this text, and there may be a move to offer clinicians in the field the discretion to consider the removal of equipment prior to transport. Athletic trainers and team physicians have more familiarity with athletic equipment and with the proper equipment removal procedures that require a number of trained providers and several specific deliberate steps (Fig. 125.7).

Once the decision has been made to transport, with or without equipment in place, a coordinated response between team medical staff and EMS is required. The term "spinal immobilization" is somewhat of a misnomer because it is impossible to completely immobilize all the spinal levels during transport. It is still reasonable and appropriate to attempt to minimize any and all spinal motion during evaluation and transport. The awake, alert athlete with pain and without significant motor deficits may be able to "self-splint," allowing for transport on a stretcher in a semirecumbent position. For athletes with neurologic deficits, a greater level of protection is obviously required. Although their value in minimizing movement and further injury has not been proven, the application of a rigid cervical collar may help to minimize movement of the cervical spine during transport, especially in the athlete with altered mental status. However, a cervical collar may not fit on an athlete wearing certain protective equipment. In these cases, foam head blocks and tape or

---

Criteria for Spinal Motion Restriction With Cervical Collar and Rigid Spine Board

- Blunt trauma with altered level of consciousness
- Spinal Pain or Tenderness
- Anatomic Deformity of the Spine
- Neurologic complaint or deficits (weakness, numbness, or paresthesia)
- High energy mechanism of injury associated with:
  - Intoxication
  - Inability to communicate
  - Distracting injury

Fig. 125.5 Criteria for spinal motion restriction (SMR). (Modified from NATA consensus statement [6/2015] and ACEP policy statement [1/2015].)

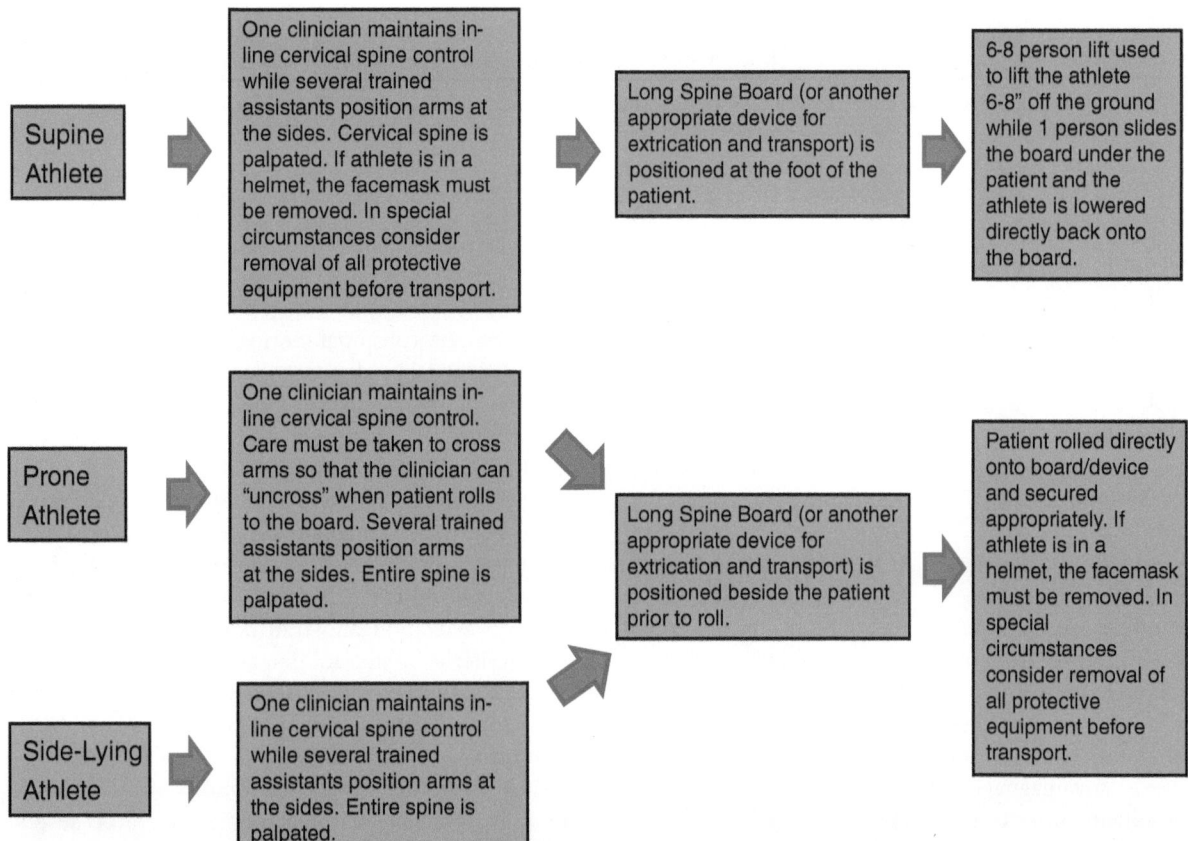

Fig. 125.6 Steps for spinal motion control and preparation for transport.

Steps for Removal of Protective Equipment

- The most trained provider should take control of the cervical spine, maintaining in-line stabilization.

- If found in a prone or side-lying position, the patient should be log rolled (arms at the side) into a supine position.

  - If a long spine board will be used for immobilization, it should be positioned beneath the patient during the log roll process to minimize the number of times the patient will be moved.

- If immediate airway access is required, consider removing the facemask using the appropriate method for the specific helmet.

- Simultaneously, a second provider can expose the chest and prepare the pads for removal by cutting the jersey and through the midline over the sternum through any laces, ties, elastic or soft plastic that holds the pads in place.

  - Any additional equipment (neck roll, rib pads, etc) should also be fastened in the midline with laces or straps that can be cut in a similar fashion.

  - Any shirt or compression garment can also be cut if direct access to the chest is required, i.e. for AED pad placement.

- Remove the chin strap and consider deflating air bladder (if present) and removing cheek pads if needed for remove the helmet.

  - Caution should be used in removing the cheek pads as force is required to unfasten the snaps that hold them in place. This force may be transmitted to the cervical spine causing movement and the provider in charge of maintaining control of the cervical spine must be prepared.

- A second responder should assume cervical spine control from a caudal direction, using their hands behind the occiput and around the jaw bilaterally. The providers forearms should rest on the patient's chest for further stability.

- 3-4 responders on each side of the patient should kneel beside the patient with hands/forearms under the patient. A coordinated lift may be performed, 3-4 inches off the ground to allow a long spine board to be slid in from the feet towards the head of the patient.

- The provider at the head may use the ear holes to pull laterally on the helmet shell, rotating the helmet forwards slightly to gently remove the helmet. The provider holding the head should be prepared because once the helmet is removed, there is a tendency for the head to drop, extending the neck. It is critical the provider maintains in-line control of the cervical spine during this crucial step.

- The 2 halves of the shoulder pads may be pulled apart and the pads can be removed by sliding out in a cephalad direction over the head. A coordinated lower may be performed to lay the patient onto the immobilization device.

- If there is any remaining space between the occiput and the spine board, a folded towel or foam pad may be placed to minimize extension of the neck during the remainder of the immobilization process.

- A rigid cervical collar should be applied and the provider at the head should resume control of the cervical spine.

Fig. 125.7 Steps for removal of protective athletic equipment. (Modified from Kleiner DM, Almquist JL, Bailes J, et al. *Prehospital Care of the Spine-Injured Athlete: A Document from the Inter-Association Task Force for Appropriate Care of the Spine-Injured Athlete.* Dallas: National Athletic Trainers' Association; 2001.)

similar devices may be used to minimize head movement during transport. A scoop stretcher, full-body vacuum splint, or rigid spine board all may be appropriate devices for spinal motion control. These devices should be used for extrication from the field of play and, depending on local protocols and transport times, may be continued during transport to the ED.

EMERGENCY DEPARTMENT EVALUATION

In the hemodynamically unstable patient, ED evaluation should proceed according to appropriate trauma guidelines. The ED specialist must first prioritize acute life threats while protecting the spine.[13] Some studies have shown that protective athletic equipment interferes with adequate imaging and should be removed before any imaging is obtained.[31,32] In the hemodynamically stable patient, protective equipment may be removed using the systematic process outlined previously. In addition to the method described in the figure, Horodyski et al. reported

decreased cervical spinal motion while removing equipment in a cadaver model by elevating the torso approximately 30 degrees prior to the removal of shoulder pads.[33] However, this method requires an additional provider and may exacerbate thoracic and lumbar injuries if present.[34]

The National Emergency X-Radiography Utilization Group criteria and the Canadian C-spine rules (Fig. 125.8) provide a clinical decision support tool for the evidence-based requisite for imaging.[35,36] Athletes who have already met criteria for EMS activation and transport to the ED will often meet these criteria. Standard diagnostic imaging has historically included plain radiographs including anteroposterior, lateral, and odontoid views. Particular attention should be directed to the odontoid-C1 and the C7-T1 junctions. However, many centers are moving towards computed tomography (CT) as the primary mode for imaging of the spine in trauma because it is more efficient and has a higher sensitivity and specificity compared with plain radiographs.[37-39] Providers are cautioned to exercise

Clinical Decision Rules for Cervical Spine Imaging

- NEXUS Criteria
  - Cervical spine radiography is indicated for patients with traumatic injury unless they meet ALL of the following criteria:
    - No posterior, midline spinal tenderness
    - No intoxication
    - Normal level of alertness
    - No neurologic deficits
    - No painful distracting injuries

- Canadian C-Spine Rule
  - For alert (GCS = 15), stable trauma patients with potential cervical spine injury, ALL of the following conditions must be met or radiographs should be obtained.
    - No high risk factors (ANY of the following require imaging)
      - Age ≥ 65 yo
      - Dangerous mechanism of injury (fall from ≥ 3 ft, axial load to head/neck speed motor vehicle accident, ejection, or rollover, accidents involving motorized recreational vehicles, bicycle collision)
    - In low-risk patients, allows assessment of range of motion (a "no" to any of the following requires imaging)
      - Simple, rear-end motor vehicle accident
      - Seated position in the ED
      - Ambulatory at any time since traumatic incident
      - Delayed onset of neck pain
      - Absence of cervical spine tenderness
    - The patient must be able to actively rotate their neck 45 deg right and left, if they are unable to do so, radiographs should be obtained

Fig. 125.8 Clinical decision rules for cervical spine imaging. (Modified from Hoffman JR, Mower WR, Wolfwon AB, et al. Validity of a set of clinical criteria to rule out injury to the cervical spine in patients with blunt trauma. *N Engl J Med.* 2000;343[2]:94–99; and Stiell IG, Wells GA, Vandemheen KL, et al. The Canadian C-spine rule for radiography in alter and stable trauma patients. *JAMA.* 2001;286[15]:1841–1848.)

conservative clinical judgment when considering the possibility of a spine (or other significant) injury; the clinical decision tools assist with decision-making but do not make decisions for the clinician.

CT and plain-film radiographs are the best imaging modalities for evaluating bony injuries. Magnetic resonance imaging (MRI) is a superior modality when evaluating soft tissue injuries and is the only imaging modality that evaluates the spinal cord directly. MRI can be used to evaluate ligamentous and disk pathology, as well as to provide evaluation of marrow edema within bony structures. Selective use of MRI is appropriate in certain cases, such as persistent neurologic deficit or when vascular or nerve root injuries are suspected.[37] However, MRI is time consuming, not ubiquitously available, resource intensive, and expensive. These considerations make MRI imaging impractical for most athletes and trauma patients.

A condition known as spinal cord injury without radiography abnormality, or SCIWORA, is used in older literature to describe persistent neurologic deficits in cases where bony and ligamentous injuries were not found on plain radiographs or CT scans.[40,41] Due to the increasing use of MRI, the incidence of SCIWORA has decreased because it is now possible to identify more soft tissue etiologies for symptoms. The term SCIWORA is still used to describe a patient with a neurologic injury pattern that is suspicious for spinal cord injury but in whom plain radiographs

and CT scan do not identify an etiology. MRI is the next logical step in the evaluation and treatment of such injuries.[42]

COMMON ACUTE SPINAL INJURIES

Acute spinal injuries are separated into several broad categories, including bony injuries, disc herniations, stingers/burners, and transient quadriplegia; bony injuries and disc herniations can occur with and without neurologic compromise.

Bony injuries related to acute fractures and dislocations are among the most common and potentially catastrophic of spinal cord injuries in athletes, along with concomitant soft tissue injuries.[43] Injuries to the high cervical spine are rare in sports but may be seen with high-energy mechanisms or diving injuries. In the lower cervical spine, C5 is the most commonly injured vertebrae, with C5 on C6 as the most common site of spinal subluxation. A narrower diameter of the cervical cord in the lower cervical spine may lead to an increased incidence of neurologic injury at these levels.[44] See Fig. 125.9 for a list of common bony injuries of the cervical spine.

Transient tetraplegia, also called spinal cord neurapraxia or cervical cord neurapraxia, is a term describing a spectrum of injuries. The spectrum of transient tetraplegia ranges from simple weakness to brief, self-limited paralysis without abnormalities on routine imaging, including MRI.[45] This injury most often

Injury	Description	Characteristics
Flexion Injuries:		
• Wedge Fracture	• Compression fracture of the vertebral body	• Typically stable and without neurologic sequelae
• Teardrop Fracture	• Small triangular fragment at the antero-inferior aspect of the vertebral body	• Often associated with an injury to intervertebral disk and a severe ligament injury; an unstable fracture often associated with neurologic injury, treated with reduction and surgical fixation
• Unilateral Facet Dislocation	• Combined flexion & rotation causes displaced facet to become wedged into the intervertebral foramen	• Typically a stable injury; may present with signs/symptoms of associated nerve root injury. Treatment is closed reduction and halo-vest immobilization
• Bilateral Facet Dislocation	• Involves 50% anterior translation of the vertebral body	• Extremely unstable injury; often associated with severe spinal cord injury and injury or occlusion of the vertebral artery; requires reduction and surgical stabilization
Extension Injuries		
• Hangman's Fracture	• Bilateral spondylolysis of the axis (C2); rare in sports but may occur in diving accidents	• Very unstable injury, though the majority are managed non-operatively
Compression/Axial Load Injuries		
• Jefferson Fracture	• Burst fractures of the posterior elements of C1	• Unstable, but co-existent neurologic injuries are rare; up to 40% associated with C2 fractures
• Burst Fractures	• Comminuted fracture of the vertebral body may displace fracture fragments into the spinal canal leading to spinal cord injury	• Extremely unstable and often requires surgical stabilization
Other Mechanisms		
• Clay Shoveler's Fracture	• Due to a direct blow to the spinous process, such as when a weight lifter drops a loaded weight bar onto their neck from overhead	• Stable and is not typically associated with neurologic deficits
• Dens Fractures	• May occur with falls or high energy trauma. Classified by what part of the Dens is fractured: Type I-tip of the Dens; Type II waist of the Dens; Type III-base and into the ring of C2	• Treatment of dens fractures varies by type of fracture.

Fig. 125.9 Osseous cervical spine injuries seen in athletes. (Modified from Kanwar, R, Delasobera, BE, Hudson, KB, Frohna, W. Emergency department evaluation and treatment of cervical spine injuries. *Emerg Med Clin North Am.* 2015;33[2]:241–282.)

occurs after a mechanism that combines slight neck flexion with axial loading. Athletes with transient neurapraxia often present with motor weakness and sensory changes without neck pain or tenderness. These athletes will maintain full ROM on examination. The neurologic deficits and dangerous mechanism warrant radiographic imaging to rule out more serious injury.

Stingers/burners are common injuries in contact and collision athletic events. Approximately half of NCAA college football players report experiencing this type of injury each year.[45] Stingers/burners are the result of compression of the neural foramen with associated stretch on the contra lateral brachial plexus and/or nerve roots. The mechanism involves forced lateral neck flexion associated with mild extension.[46] These forces result in transient unilateral dysesthesias and numbness in the affected limb that may also be associated with some degree of motor weakness. These athletes usually have full ROM and no neck pain or spinal tenderness. The injury is usually self-limited with symptoms resolving in 24 to 48 hours and do not require imaging. Persistent symptoms beyond 48 hours should necessitate further diagnostic studies.[47]

Acute traumatic disc herniations may also occur in athletics. These injuries may lead to a range of symptoms, including pain, paresthesias, and/or weakness in a dermatomal distribution. The motor/sensory dermatome will guide imaging recommendations for the level of neuroforaminal stenosis. In the acute setting, neurologic deficits indicate a need for urgent imaging, with MRI clearly the modality of choice.[34]

CONCLUSION

Appropriate care of any athlete with a spine injury begins long before the athletic competition. All involved personnel should participate in the development and frequent review of an EAP. Physicians and athletic trainers need to be aware of the most common injury mechanisms and be able to identify common injury patterns. When injuries occur, teamwork on the part of medical personnel is imperative. Care must be taken to protect the athlete against further injury, minimize movement, and properly manage protective equipment during transport to an appropriate medical facility for further evaluation and care.

For a complete list of references, go to ExpertConsult.com.

SELECTED READINGS

Citation:

Swartz EE, Boden BP, Courson RW, et al. National Athletic Trainers' Association position statement: acute management of the cervical spine injured athlete. *J Athl Train.* 2009;44(3):306–331.

Level of Evidence:

V

Summary:

A consensus statement of the on-field management of the athlete with a cervical spine injury

Citation:

Stiell IG, Wells GA, Vandemheen KL, et al. The Canadian C-Spine Rule for radiography in alert and stable trauma patients. *JAMA.* 2001;286(15):1841–1848.

Level of Evidence:

II

Summary:

The Canadian C-Spine Rule, a highly sensitive decision rule for use of C-spine radiography in alert and stable trauma patients, was elucidated from 10 large community and academic centers that allowed for 100% sensitivity of clinically significant C-spine injury, with an overall reduction of radiographic ordering by half during the 3-year study period.

Citation:

Kanwar R, Delasobera BE, Hudson KB, et al. Emergency department evaluation and treatment of cervical spine injuries. *Emerg Med Clin North Am.* 2015;33(2):241–282.

Level of Evidence:

V

Summary:

This chapter provides a review of the current concepts and trends in the emergency department evaluation and imaging protocols.

Citation:

National Spinal Cord Statistical Center. Spinal cord injury facts and figures at a glance: 2016. https://www.nscisc.uab.edu/Public/Facts%202016.pdf. Accessed April 23, 2017.

Level of Evidence:

II

Summary:

An analysis of data from the NSCSC that depicts the incidence, prevalence, race, age, life expectancy, and use of services by patients suffering spinal cord injury in the United States.

126

Concussion and Brain Injury

David P. Trofa, Jon-Michael E. Caldwell, Xudong Joshua Li

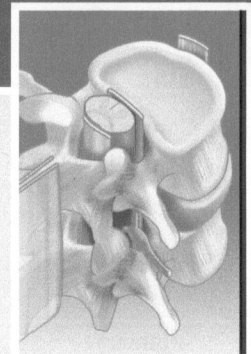

Among the wide range of injuries that occur in the sports arena, traumatic brain injury (TBI) is a health problem that has garnered increasing public awareness during recent years. This heightened interest has been largely driven by intense media exposure, as well as the retirement of prominent professional athletes with cognitive and behavioral dysfunction purportedly representing lingering sequelae of brain injury. Player safety concerns have become an area of special focus for professional leagues, such as the National Football League (NFL) and National Hockey League (NHL), as well as organizations such as the International Olympic Committee and the National Collegiate Athletic Association (NCAA), with a resulting impact on collegiate, high school, and recreational sports.

Key to a discussion of sports brain injury is an understanding of the terminology applied to the topic. *TBI* is an umbrella term that encompasses a range of clinical labels that vary based on severity. Mild traumatic brain injury (mTBI) involves an impact to or acceleration/deceleration of the head resulting in at least a temporary alteration in consciousness or loss of consciousness (LOC) of less than 20 minutes, a Glasgow Coma Scale score of 13 to 15, and no findings on neuroimaging.[1] mTBI is alternately referred to as *mild head injury, minor head injury,* and *concussion.* The vast majority of brain injuries sustained by athletes are mild events that would be considered concussions[2]; moderate, severe, and penetrating traumatic brain injuries are less common. For practical purposes, in this chapter mTBI, mild head injury, and concussion are considered synonymous, and the term *concussion* is used throughout this chapter.

The intent of this chapter is to provide a resource for the clinician on the diagnosis and management of sports concussion. A brief historical context for the issue of sports concussion, relevant definitions, and epidemiology are presented; the clinical presentations that can occur after a concussive blow are also reviewed, and a clear concussion management and return-to-play (RTP) decision-making process is given.

BACKGROUND

Concussion is not a modern phenomenon. Numerous references to cranial injury can be found in ancient medical reports and mythological literature by such figures as Hippocrates and Homer. The recognition of concussion as a separate entity from more severe head injuries was made as far back as the first century AD by Rhazes, an Arabian physician who described concussion as an abnormal physiologic state lacking gross traumatic brain lesions. Modern-day literature, however, has predominately focused on moderate to severe brain injuries, with relatively little attention given to mild brain injuries, whether sports-related or not.

The topic of concussion began to be taken seriously by medical science in the 1980s, when clinical and epidemiologic studies received media attention in a *Wall Street Journal* article, "Silent Epidemic: Head Injuries Often Difficult to Diagnose, Get Rising Attention." The growing consensus that mild head injury was in fact not innocuous was based on the identification of neuropsychological deficits in problem solving, attention, and memory lasting up to 3 months after a trauma was sustained.[3] In addition, primate studies documented histologic evidence of axonal shear and strain during experimentally induced acceleration-deceleration mild head injury.[4,5]

Because the study of concussion does not lend itself to randomized controlled trials, significant strides were made when Barth and colleagues[3,6] turned to the collegiate sports arena to address the problem of finding adequate control subjects and accounting for the effects of premorbid functioning in the study of concussion. The sporting venue provided a large number of potential participants who were likely to experience mild acceleration-deceleration head trauma. Data from 10 universities showed that athletes who sustained a concussion had neurocognitive deficits at 24 hours and 5 days after concussion but recovered by the 10th day, a recovery curve that has been replicated by other studies.[7,8] This seminal study set the methodologic standard for baseline and serial neuropsychological testing as the best way to determine the effect of concussion, and this approach of using individual athletes as their own controls and as a model for understanding brain injury in general was termed the Sports as a Laboratory Assessment Model (SLAM).[9] The SLAM approach helped establish concussion as a sports medicine issue with broader implications for mTBI in other areas (e.g., motor vehicle accidents).

Definition of Concussion

As noted at the outset of this chapter, a widely varying set of terms and defining parameters exist for the topic of sport related concussion (SRC), and this lack of clarity and consistency has hampered the study of concussion to a significant degree. The two most common definitions used in sports concussion research are from the American Academy of Neurology (AAN) Practice Parameters and the Concussion in Sports Group (CISG;

commonly referred to as the Vienna, Prague, Zurich, and Berlin Conferences). In 1997 the AAN defined concussion as an altered mental state that may or may not include LOC.[10] Four years later, the CISG group proposed that concussion is a "complex pathophysiologic process affecting the brain, induced by traumatic biomechanical forces," and included common features of concussion that incorporate clinical, pathologic, and biomechanical constructs to supplement the definition.[11] This definition was updated in 2017 to state "Sport related concussion is a traumatic brain injury induced by biomechanical forces," with common features including "1. SRC may be caused either by a direct blow to the head, face, neck, or elsewhere on the body with an 'impulsive' force transmitted to the head; 2. SRC typically results in the rapid onset of short-lived impairment of neurologic function that resolves spontaneously. However, in some cases, signs and symptoms evolve over a number of minutes to hours; 3. SRC may result in neuropathologic changes, but the acute clinical signs and symptoms largely reflect a functional disturbance rather than a structural injury and, as such, no abnormality is seen on standard structural neuroimaging studies; 4. SRC results in a range of clinical signs and symptoms that may not involve loss of consciousness. Resolution of the clinical and cognitive features typically follows a sequential course. However, in some cases symptoms may be prolonged."[12]

This definition largely reaffirms that established by the prior Consensus Conferences in Zurich[11,13] and reflects the current trend toward emphasizing the biomechanical force, time course of symptoms, and the functional nature of the injury, as opposed to the structural emphasis used in more severe forms of TBI.

Epidemiology

The Centers for Disease Control and Prevention estimates that approximately 1.6 to 3.0 million sports-related concussions among high school students will be reported each year in the United States, and during the past decade, emergency department visits for sports concussions among children and adolescents increased by 60%.[14-16] Such estimates likely underestimate the actual occurrence, given that many leagues lack the medical oversight to identify concussions.[17] Recent studies suggest that 8.9% of all high school athletic injuries were concussions,[18] and estimates for collegiate sports range from 5% to 18%, with more than 52,000 concussions reported between the academic years beginning in 2009–2013.[19,20] The incidence of sports concussion is expected to continue to rise in part because of the increase in sports participation by both male and female athletes at the collegiate and high school levels, but also because of increased knowledge, detection, and reporting of the injury, including the adoption of sports injury surveillance systems.[21]

Pathophysiology

A full discussion of the pathophysiology underlying concussion is beyond the scope of this chapter. The interested reader is referred to the work of Giza and Hovda for a thorough understanding of the topic.[22,23] In brief, concussion occurs as a result of linear and rotational accelerations and decelerations to the brain and is thought to cause a multifactorial neurometabolic cascade of physiologic changes. This process begins with cell body expulsion

of sodium and potassium into the intracellular space and an influx of calcium, as well as mild edema and a resultant decrease in cerebral blood flow in the setting of initial hyperglycolysis. As glucose is consumed and blood flow is limited, a state of hypoglycolysis ensues, which slows the neurochemical return to homeostasis. This dysautoregulation in addition to axonal injury, impaired neurotransmission, and protease activation leading to cell death explain how clinical signs of brain dysfunction can be observed in the absence of readily detectable physical damage.[23] This cascade begins within minutes of the injury and can be active for several weeks.[23]

Clinical Presentation

When the question is raised as to why concussion in sports represents an important problem that must be identified, the answer lies in the known consequences demonstrated by concussed athletes, who may present with acute, catastrophic, lingering, or long-term sequelae.

Although it is controversial and rare, a potentially catastrophic outcome from concussion termed *second impact syndrome* (SIS) is sometimes manifested. This most severe consequence of concussion was part of the initial impetus for a formalized approach to concussion management and RTP criteria. First described in detail in 1984,[24] the syndrome is said to occur when a second concussion is sustained before the symptoms of the first have fully resolved. The second impact may appear minor and may not occur on the same day. The athlete may not initially appear injured but may collapse and lose consciousness shortly after the event, with respiratory failure, coma, and even death possibly ensuing. Underlying the SIS phenomena is the notion that the brain appears to have a decreased threshold for sustaining a concussion of any severity with each subsequent trauma.[25] The pathophysiology behind SIS is not fully understood, but it has been suggested that the subclinical edema and increased intracranial pressure from the first concussive impact make the brain successively more vulnerable to the second impact through autodysregulation and subsequent vascular engorgement. This condition manifests as malignant cerebral edema and herniation of the uncus or the cerebellar tonsils through the foramen magnum, resulting in brainstem failure.[24] However, recent systematic reviews of the literature regarding this syndrome found a dearth of high quality literature, unclear actual mortality rates (though nearly all studies said the rate was "high"), and "severe lack of definitive structure" as to what signs and symptoms are associated with it, leading the authors to conclude "SIS is not a credible, literature supported diagnosis."[26,27]

Persistent symptoms (also known as postconcussive syndrome or PCS) may remain after a sports concussion is sustained and reflect a failure of normal clinical recovery.[12] Most concussed athletes demonstrate gradual, spontaneous recovery, generally within 2 to 10 days after injury,[6,7,11,28] consistent with laboratory animal studies showing short-lived effects of concussion,[22,23] and with meta-analytic studies demonstrating no evidence of impairment beyond 3 months.[29,30] However, the fact that some people experience persistent sequelae has been recognized for quite some time. For example, at 3-month follow-up, 34% of an mTBI clinical (nonsports) sample had not yet returned to work, and 24%

demonstrated measurable neurocognitive deficits.[3] The Fourth International Conference of Concussion in Sport defined prolonged recovery as symptom persistence greater than 10 to 14 days from injury for adults and greater than 4 weeks in children; however, the definitions used in the literature vary from 10 days to more than 2 months.[13,31,32] Persistent symptoms can include neurologic symptoms such as headache, dizziness, and nausea; cognitive deficits, such as impaired attention, slowed mental processing, and memory dysfunction; and emotional or psychological disruption, including depression or irritability. It is important to note that the presence of one or more of these symptoms after a concussion is sustained in an athlete is not diagnostic of delayed recovery, since such symptoms are extremely common in a host of other conditions. For example, PCS type symptomatology has been demonstrated in 81% of subjects in a chronic pain sample with no history of concussion.[33] As such, the clinician may find the identification of persistent symptoms difficult. One challenge is that the athlete may present with vague, subjective symptoms that are nonspecific. Issues of effort and secondary gain may also be a contributing factor in some cases. Furthermore, the differential diagnosis often includes mood and anxiety disorders, as well as sleep disruption, which can lead to or mimic PCS symptoms. Neuropsychological assessment can be quite useful in this situation, because objective evaluation can help parse out the factors contributing to the athlete's atypical presentation. Structural imaging (MRI and CT) are of limited value in evaluation of these patients and advanced techniques such as fMRI, diffusion tensor imaging, MR spectroscopy, and quantitative EEG have unclear clinical significance.[31,34]

In addition to the clinical presentations of SIS and PCS, a third potential clinical presentation known as chronic traumatic encephalopathy (CTE) can occur after multiple concussions.[35] This outcome appears to be dose-related long-term response of repeated concussions and subconcussive blows and has been studied in groups of retired football, rugby, and boxing athletes.[36–39] The combination of repetitive sports head injury–related damage with that of age-related neuronal loss[40] may result in the development of clinical signs of CTE, often appearing years after the end of the athlete's career.[41] Though the diagnosis of CTE is based on neuropathologic evidence collected postmortem, its clinical course can be characterized by long-term deficits in executive functioning, processing speed, verbal learning, and visual memory; motor impairments, including impaired coordination, spasticity, and parkinsonism; as well as behavioral problems such as emotional dysregulation and disinhibition.[37,42,43] Referred to as "dementia pugilistica" in early literature,[44] CTE in its advanced stage can be clinically indistinguishable from other advanced dementias. Neuropathologically, CTE is a progressive tauopathy with gliosis and neurofibrillary tangles, as well as common gross elements of reduced brain weight, enlarged ventricles, volume loss in the corpus callosum, cavum septum pellucidum, and scarring and neuronal loss of the cerebellar tonsils.[45] The pathology of CTE has been most frequently demonstrated in the brains of professional athletes[46] and can be widespread throughout the brain given the nonfocal nature of repeated head trauma. Similarly, elevated tau protein levels have been detected in the plasma of both injured and noninjured

contact athletes relative to non-athlete controls with increased tau levels corresponding to delayed return to sport.[43,47] Although long-term deficits in the form of persistent symptoms can manifest after a single concussive blow, it is generally assumed that a concussed athlete can expect a favorable prognosis if the injury is safely managed. The risk of outcomes such as SIS, persistent symptoms, and CTE can be significantly reduced with proper concussion identification, examination, and intervention.

EXAMINATION

The goal of sports concussion examination is to identify the concussion, assess the injury, determine its effects, and devise appropriate interventions. The traditional approach to this task involved simply gauging the signs and symptoms of the concussion and their resolution over time. Many different classification schemes for concussion exist, and definitions and criteria continue to evolve. Historically, the two most widely used systems for grading concussion were those proposed by the AAN in 1997 and Cantu in 2001. These systems used three grades to represent mild, moderate, and severe concussion based on the clinical presentation of the athlete and placed considerable emphasis on LOC (AAN) or posttraumatic amnesia (PTA; Cantu) as severity indicators. Despite early TBI literature showing that coma duration is an important predictor of outcome,[48] more recent studies have found that the relationship between LOC and injury outcome in the realm of mTBI and sports concussion is less certain.[49] Concussion grading systems are now considered obsolete, and an individualized approach to concussion diagnosis and management is favored, consistent with the CISG guidelines.

Although monitoring subjective symptoms is an important aspect of concussion management, it cannot be the sole means of gauging effect and recovery. It is now understood that fewer than half of concussed athletes spontaneously report their symptoms,[50] citing doubt that the injury was severe, not wanting to leave the game, or general lack of awareness about concussion as reasons for not reporting. For these and other reasons, the modern model for concussion examination, outlined by the CISG Conferences, emphasizes an individualized approach that incorporates neurocognitive evaluation. Several computer-administered measures (outlined later) are validated for the assessment of concussion sequelae. The standard practice has evolved to include such standardized tools in both preseason and postinjury assessment. Current guidelines recommend that athletes not resume a gradual progression of activity until their concussion symptoms have remitted. Thus neurocognitive testing has become a valuable tool in identifying subtle cognitive symptoms and their resolution.

Baseline (Preseason) Assessment

Baseline neuropsychological assessments have been advocated by some authors and increased in popularity with the development of computerized tests in the 1990s. Advocates of preseason testing point out the results of any evaluation vary based on many factors other than the actual injury, including intelligence and cultural background, learning disabilities, and previous concussion history.[51] This situation applies to neurologic findings as well; for example, up to 20% of athletes normally experience a headache while in the midst of competition,[52] and approximately 3% of the healthy population exhibit pupillary asymmetry.[53] Erroneous conclusions about the cognitive and neurologic state of an athlete may be drawn without an awareness of these baseline characteristics. However, other authors have shown these tests may have poor test-retest reliability, vary between group and individual administration or alternate forms, suffer from measurement errors, and may not offer an improvement over postinjury testing alone (when compared with normative data as opposed to individualized preseason baseline).[54–56] Routine mandatory preseason baseline neurocognitive testing is not recommended by either the Berlin conference or the American Medical Society of Sports Medicine guidelines.[12,57]

Neurocognitive baselines may be obtained for athletes with the use of computerized methods in an individual or group setting with a trained examiner. Several tools are available for the specific purpose of assessing concussion severity and resolution. These tools include the Automated Neuropsychological Assessment Metrics[58]; the Immediate Post-concussion Assessment and Cognitive Testing (ImPACT Applications Inc., Pittsburgh, PA)[8,59]; the Concussion Resolution Index (HeadMinder Inc., New York, NY)[60]; and the Computerized Cognitive Assessment Tool (Axon Sports [formerly CogSport], Wausau, WI).[61] The Automated Neuropsychological Assessment Metrics measures processing speed, resistance to interference, and working memory. The Immediate Post-concussion Assessment and Cognitive Testing tool was developed specifically for athletes, and assesses reaction time and a range of attentional and memory skills, accompanied by a self-report postconcussion scale. The Concussion Resolution Index is a web-based set of cognitive tasks that measure simple and complex reaction time, attention, memory, and cognitive processing speed. Axon is also an Internet-based system and includes eight tasks designed to sample a range of cognitive functions.

Sideline Assessment

The first step in the assessment of concussion is to recognize that a concussion may have occurred. It is important to remember that signs and symptoms may be delayed or rapidly changing in the acute phase, and injured athletes may exhibit no obvious indications that they are concussed. Therefore sideline assessment is warranted for any athlete who has received a significant blow to the head or an athlete who does not appear to "be him or herself" in response to a lesser degree of contact.[62] This assessment involves evaluation of the athlete both on the field, or more commonly on the sideline, as well as in a controlled environment such as the locker room, and usually is conducted by a physician or a certified athletic trainer with expertise in concussion evaluation and management.

An obvious goal of the sideline assessment is to determine if the athlete has signs that signal the presence of severe intracranial or spinal cord injury and whether transport to a medical facility is required.[63] Once this determination is made, any individual should be removed from the field for further assessment. Classic signs such as LOC, retrograde amnesia, or frank neurologic deficit may be helpful but are absent in a minority of injured athletes.[64]

In general, the sideline evaluation should assess for signs of confusion, loss of balance, headache, dizziness, and slowed responding, in addition to informal cranial nerve, motor, sensory, and reflex testing[65] and, importantly, cognitive screening. For athletes with no obvious acute symptoms, physical maneuvers such as push-ups or jumping jacks can help determine whether concussive signs or symptoms develop with exertion and resultant increased intracranial pressure.[63] Sideline assessment should also incorporate a mental status examination that targets orientation, concentration, and memory. Notably, standard orientation questions (time, place, person) have been shown to be unreliable following a sports injury relative to memory assessment.[12,66] Concentration may be gauged by tasks such as repeating strings of three to five digits both forward and backward, serial subtraction of numbers, or repeating a well-known verbal sequence such as months of the year or days of the week backward. Memory can be informally and qualitatively assessed by recall of three items at different intervals after the injury or repeating assignments of a number of previous plays.[49,65]

Although these informal methods of sideline assessment are helpful, a standardized approach is preferable.[67] A number of standardized methods for determining the severity of a concussion and the initial symptoms have been developed for use in the sideline evaluation of athletes. The Concussion Recognition Tool 5 (CRT5) was developed by the CISG as a pocket guide for nonmedically trained personnel to identify SRC as well as guide removal from play decisions.[68] The Standardized Assessment of Concussion (SAC) is a 5-minute measure administered by a trained physician or athletic trainer and includes five orientation questions, a five-word learning test, reciting digits backward, reciting the months of the year in reverse, and delayed word recall.[69] The SAC provides a 30-point composite score to gauge neurocognitive function and also includes a standard neurologic screening, exertional maneuvers, and means of assessing LOC and PTA. Normative data for comparison are also available.[70] The SAC is available in paper form and a pocket-card format, and has been adapted for use with smartphone technology. The Balance Error Scoring System is an objective measure of postural stability for use on the sideline.[71] The 5-minute procedure requires the injured athlete to maintain three stances (double, single, and tandem) for 20 seconds with the eyes closed and both hands on his or her hips. Scoring is based on six types of errors over six test trials. The Standardized Concussion Assessment Tool (SCAT5) is another standardized tool that incorporates elements of the aforementioned SAC and a graded rating of common physical and cognitive signs and symptoms.[72] Recently revised to the fifth version, the test battery takes 10 minutes to administer and updates the widely used SCAT3. This test has also been developed into a pediatric version (Child SCAT5) for use in children age 5 to 12.[73] The Berlin Conference recommended use of the SCAT5 and Child SCAT5 for sideline concussion assessment.[12] The tool is easily accessible online and may be freely copied for distribution to individuals, teams, groups, and organizations.

After a sideline evaluation, any athlete considered to have sustained a concussion should be removed from the sporting environment and undergo a multimodal medical evaluation with a more detailed neuropsychological assessment. The concussed player should not be allowed to return to play (RTP) the day of injury. Serial exams should be conducted over the first few hours after injury to monitor for signs of deterioration. Finally, to provide an objective basis for detecting the effects of the concussion, the athlete should undergo postinjury neurocognitive assessment. This brief repeat evaluation can occur within 24 to 48 hours after the suspected concussion if the athlete appears to be symptom free. This aspect of concussion management may provide increased sensitivity for identifying cognitive impairment resulting from concussion when physical symptoms are limited or resolved.[74] However, conducting the brief repeat evaluation 7 days after the injury has been found to provide more unique information regarding impairment than routine assessment conducted relatively close in time to the sideline assessment.[75]

Comprehensive Assessment

In the case of a single uncomplicated concussion or subconcussive event, it is generally anticipated that the athlete will experience full resolution of symptoms within the 2- to 14-day natural recovery curve. In cases with an atypical presentation, a more comprehensive evaluation may be necessary. Athletes with preexisting or comorbid conditions (e.g., learning or attention disorders, depression, or substance abuse), those who report or demonstrate a slower than expected recovery, or those who have sustained multiple previous concussions should be considered for expanded assessment. In these situations, a referral for comprehensive outpatient neuropsychological evaluation is indicated, which includes a clinical interview, record review, and objective testing of aptitude and cognitive functioning, and provides individualized recommendations for the athlete and relevant treatment providers. In addition, further medical assessment may be warranted for atypical concussion cases (e.g., neuroophthalmology).

Imaging

Acute evaluation of concussion may incorporate at least one form of brain imaging. Computed tomography is an appropriate choice to rule out the presence of intracranial hemorrhage and skull fracture, and is the imaging option of choice for concussion evaluation in most emergency departments. Magnetic resonance imaging (MRI) with an angiogram can be obtained if carotid dissection or stroke is suspected, and MRI studies may also identify a diffuse injury such as axonal shearing.

It is important to emphasize that most concussions are unlikely to produce observable signs upon testing with these traditional radiologic techniques. Advanced diagnostics such as functional MRI, diffusion tensor imaging, MR spectroscopy, fluid biomarkers, and genetic testing are, at present, only practical and widely available in the research setting and are of uncertain clinical utility.[12] Although structural neuroimaging continues to rule out the presence of serious pathology that would be beyond that of a mild concussive injury, brain imaging is less relevant in the context of typical concussion management.

MANAGEMENT

The cornerstone of acute management of concussion is both physical and cognitive rest. It is theorized that rest may aid recovery by reducing immediate postconcussive symptoms and decreasing brain metabolic demand.[12] However, there is likely no benefit to continuing strict prescribed rest beyond the acute phase (1 to 2 days) after injury, and most athletes should begin a gradual resumption of activity as tolerated, followed by a graduated protocol to RTP.[76–78]

An athlete who experiences one concussive event is three times more likely to sustain another concussion in the same season, usually within 10 days of the first injury.[79] As previously outlined, the athlete is at heightened risk for severe sequelae of repeated concussions, particularly during the acute stage when the brain is more susceptible to subsequent insult. The prolonged recovery of multiply concussed athletes has been demonstrated with lingering cognitive and gait stability deficits.[25,80] Players who sustain a concussion are more likely to experience LOC with the next injury.[25,81] Furthermore, the force threshold for concussive injury may be far less for a second impact[79]; therefore subconcussive events must be considered as possible risk factors when discussing concussion outcome and management. A subconcussive blow is an apparent brain insult with insufficient force to cause the hallmark symptoms of concussion.[82] These more minor events conceivably occur at a high rate during both competitive play and practice. Investigation with use of the Head Impact Telemetry System to record the frequency, magnitude, and location of head impacts found that a group of college football players sustained on average 1000 subconcussive impacts over the course of a single season.[83] The notion that repetitive blows may cause equivalent, if not greater, damage than a single mild concussion has been suggested previously.[84]

It is possible that the number of concussions sustained plays a more important role in long-term outcomes than the severity of the concussions. The animal experimental literature has shown that two or more concussive blows produce greater deficits than predicted by single blows and that repeated blows can accelerate the deposition of β-amyloid.[85] The heightened risks of repeat concussive injury have also been extended to human studies.[79,86] Contact athletes with a history of multiple concussions have an increased risk of depression and cognitive deficits later in life (though, notably, the majority of former players assess their functional status as normal).[87] What is unknown is "how many is too many," and this number will vary for individual athletes.

Different groups and individuals are more susceptible than others, and the nature of their symptoms and deficits may vary. For example, younger athletes appear to be particularly vulnerable to negative outcomes, with greater susceptibility to SIS and longer recoveries.[88] Compared with their college counterparts, high school athletes may be more vulnerable to concussion, exhibit a more protracted recovery, and have longer lasting cognitive deficits.[8,89] However, the literature is insufficient at present to distinguish between the presentation, management, or prognosis between children, adolescents, and adults. Differences by gender may also exist, with some evidence that females experience a higher incidence of persistent symptoms compared with their male counterparts, although this literature is still equivocal.[90,91]

Given the well-documented risks involved in returning an athlete to play, the potential for delayed onset of symptoms; variable symptom reporting; the nonlinear, individualized nature of recovery; and the known long-term risks for such consequences as CTE, the accepted standard for concussion management is that concussed athletes are held from competition until they are completely asymptomatic at rest and during exertion (which involves either physical or cognitive activities). When the previously outlined examination process is followed, the clinician is equipped with appropriate data with which to approach an RTP determination.

Return to Play

The primary focus of concussion management revolves around the appropriate implementation of RTP guidelines. Historically many different classification systems have been used to guide RTP decisions. The AAN published multiple guidelines and classification systems for concussion management from 1990 to 2005, all of which were based on clinical experience and expert opinion. The Cantu system of concussion grading was also revised to guide RTP decisions, and the Colorado Medical Society is another frequently referenced model for RTP.[92,93] These models added much to the field of sports concussion but were criticized for lack of empirical basis and standardization, and for being overly restrictive.

Newer approaches have replaced the use of grading systems of acute symptoms with more emphasis on the individual's path of symptom resolution rather than preconceived timelines. This process has been guided by recommendations of the CISG, which produced a series of consensus documents that evolved from the first summary statement in 2001 (Vienna Conference) to a second statement in 2004 (Prague Conference), the third and fourth iterations following the Zurich Conferences in 2009[11] and 2013,[13] and the Berlin conference in 2016.[12]

The consensus models a graduated recovery and rehabilitation strategy. The current Berlin protocol (Table 126.1), like its predecessor, calls for immediate removal from practice or play after a suspected concussion, standardized sideline assessment, and no RTP on the day of injury. The protocol then follows a stepwise process that progresses through six graduated steps that take 24 hours each. If any postconcussion symptoms occur within a step, the athlete is returned to the previous asymptomatic level for another 24 hours until resuming the graded process. It should be noted that cognitive rest and restriction from cognitive exertion (e.g., schoolwork, video gaming, and texting) is as equally important as physical rest and restriction from physical exertion during the course of recovery. Clinicians involved in the care of athletes should be well versed in the guidelines and should engage in a dynamic approach to RTP that takes into account the individual's history with careful attention to age, number of previous concussions, severity of concussion, and comorbidities such as other health issues, mood or psychiatric history, and substance use. The Berlin consensus statement recommends that children and adolescents not return to sports until they have successfully returned to academics with the caveat that early introduction of symptom-limited activity is appropriate.[12] The 2013 AAN guidelines suggest a conservative approach to RTP for children and further recommend no RTP for any concussed athlete until he or she is assessed by a licensed health care professional trained in concussion management.[94]

Retiring an Athlete

One of the most challenging aspects of sports concussion management is the issue of when to retire an athlete from play. In the face of limited empirical data on the topic and the great variability in both immediate symptoms and long-term effects that individual athletes demonstrate after sustaining single or multiple concussions, no clearly defined method exists to guide the clinician or team.[95] At the collegiate and professional level, the financial, social, and legal implications also weigh into such decisions. However, several important factors clearly must be taken into consideration to make a reasoned decision, including age, sex, medical and concussion history, sport, position and level of play, and concussion specific symptoms and testing results.[96] When an athlete begins to demonstrate a longer period of recovery from symptoms, experiences concussive symptoms from forces that are increasingly mild, or does not return to baseline neurocognitive functioning, then it may be time for the athlete to stop playing.[97] In addition, the athlete's functioning in multiple settings should be considered; for example, problems at school or home or behavioral problems can signal the need to consider retirement from play. A particularly conservative approach is recommended with children, where the decision must be based solely on the future health of the patient.[96]

INTERVENTIONS

Sport concussion interventions are targeted in three main areas. The most critical means of intervention is education. Concerted

Rehabilitation Stage	Functional Exercise at Each Stage of Rehabilitation	Objective of Each Stage
1. Symptom-limited activity	Daily activities that do not provoke symptoms	Gradual reintroduction of work/school activities
2. Light aerobic exercise	Walking, swimming, or stationary cycling at slow to medium pace. No resistance training	Increase heart rate
3. Sport-specific exercise	Running or skating drills; no head impact activities	Add movement
4. Noncontact training drills	Harder training drills (e.g., passing drills). May start progressive resistance training	Exercise, coordination, and increased thinking
5. Full contact practice	After medical clearance, participate in normal training activities	Restore confidence and assess functional skills by coaching staff
6. Return to play	Normal game play	

TABLE 126.1 **Concussion in Sports Group Graduated Return-to-Sport Protocol**

From McCrory P, Meeuwisse W, Dvorak J, et al. Consensus statement on concussion in sport—the 5th International Conference on Concussion in Sport held in Berlin, October 2016. *Br J Sports Med.* 2017;bjsports-2017-097699. doi:10.1136/bjsports-2017-097699..

efforts must be made to improve concussion awareness for athletes, their parents, coaches, athletic trainers, and school and league administrators. A basic understanding of what constitutes a concussion, the signs to look for, the importance of removing the athlete from further concussion risk, and the need to obtain an appropriate examination will go a long way toward improving outcomes. The need for education is highlighted by actions such as the passage of the Lystedt Law, named for Zackery Lystedt, who sustained a TBI when he returned to a middle school football game after experiencing a concussion. The legislation, passed in 2009, aims to protect athletes by mandating that athletes, parents, and coaches be educated about the dangers of concussions each year, that a player suspected of having a concussion be removed from play, and that a licensed health care professional clear the athlete for RTP.[98] "Lystedt laws" are being enacted nationwide to outline educational requirements and the need for clearance by a qualified professional any time a concussion is suspected.

A second area of intervention is, of course, prevention. The data on protective equipment are somewhat mixed with regard to whether headgear and helmets actually reduce concussion incidence. It has been suggested that such equipment has little ability to stop concussion, because helmets are not able to prevent deceleration and rotation forces on the brain.[99] The most powerful means of prevention may be rule changes within the sport, and a clear precedent exists for organizational changes. For example, the NFL made the tackling method of using one's head or helmet to hit another player ("spearing") an illegal technique in an effort to curb serious injury. Likewise, disallowing body checking in ice hockey for children under 13 has resulted in a significant reduction in concussion rate among these players.[100,101] Attention should be directed to both game time and practice activity, since the incidence of concussion in each phase is roughly similar.[20] Rules such as limiting helmet-to-helmet contact by enacting penalties or other consequences would have beneficial effects for athlete protection and brain health. Furthermore, fair play and the distinction between aggressive play and violence should be emphasized within sporting organizations.

CONCLUSION

The neuroscience and clinical study of sports concussion remains a developing area that has increasingly become the focus of both laypeople and researchers alike in light of the knowledge that concussions can exert meaningful effects on the athlete both in the short and long term. Given the number of variables that can influence concussion symptoms and length of recovery, individualized multimodal clinical management of concussed athletes guided by a clearly defined concussion evaluation process is paramount. The challenge for the future is to delineate factors that contribute to individual susceptibility to concussive blows, the variables that influence prognosis, and methods of preventing catastrophic, prolonged, and long-term outcomes, as well as to increase the awareness of sport concussion in players, their families, sporting organizations, treatment providers, and the general public.

For a complete list of references, go to ExpertConsult.com.

SELECTED READINGS

Citation:

Belanger HG, Vanderploeg RD. The neuropsychological impact of sports-related concussion: a meta-analysis. *J Int Neuropsychol Soc.* 2005;11(4):345–357.

Level of Evidence:

II

Summary:

This meta-analysis of 21 studies involving 790 cases of concussion and 2014 control cases was conducted to determine the impact of sports-related concussion across six cognitive domains. Results provide compelling evidence that sports-related concussion has no significant effect on neuropsychological function by 7 to 10 days after injury in the athletic population at large, although long-term participation in sports involving head contact may be associated with small, adverse sequelae.

Citation:

Echemendia RJ, Cantu RC, et al. Return to play following brain injury. In: Lovell M, Echemendia R, Collins M, eds. *Traumatic Brain Injury in Sports: an International Neuropsychological Perspective.* Lisse, The Netherlands: Swets and Zeitlinger; 2004.

Level of Evidence:

V

Summary:

The authors propose a model for return-to-play decision-making that takes into account the complexity of multiple factors and variables. Informed decision-making involves consideration of data from many different sources.

Citation:

Giza CC, Hovda DA. The neurometabolic cascade of concussion. *J Athl Train.* 2001;36(3):228–235.

Level of Evidence:

II

Summary:

The authors use more than 100 articles from both basic science and clinical literature to review the underlying pathophysiologic processes of concussive brain injury and relate these neurometabolic changes to clinical sports-related issues such as injury to the developing brain, overuse injury, and repeated concussion.

Citation:

Gysland SM, Mihalik JP, Register-Mihalik JK, et al. The relationship between subconcussive impacts and concussion history on clinical measures of neurologic function in collegiate football players. *Ann Biomed Eng.* 2011;40(1):14–22.

Level of Evidence:

II

Summary:

This study is the first to investigate the relationship between repetitive subconcussive head impacts and clinical measures of neurologic impairment while monitoring sustained impacts throughout the course of a single collegiate football season. The methodologies presented could help establish a foundation for future longitudinal study aimed at answering questions about the possible relationship of recurrent subclinical blows and later depression, early-onset dementia, and chronic traumatic encephalopathy.

Citation:

McCrory P, Meeuwisse W, Dvorak J, et al. Consensus statement on concussion in sport—the 5th International Conference on Concussion in Sport held in Berlin, October 2016. *Br J Sports Med.* 2017;bjsports-2017-097699. doi:10.1136/bjsports-2017-097699.

Level of Evidence:

V

Summary:

These guidelines improved on those previously presented by the same conference in Vienna, Prague, and Zurich, and constitute the most widely used protocol for our current understanding of and approach to sport concussion.

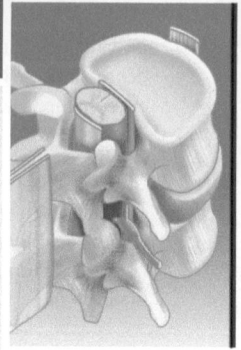

127

Stingers

Sandip P. Tarpada, Woojin Cho

INTRODUCTION

The terms "*stinger*" and "*burner*" are synonymous, and together represent a range of brachial nerve plexopathies. Initially described by Chrisman et al.,[1] stingers are almost invariably trauma-mediated, unilateral, reversible injuries of the upper extremity. While stingers are among the most commonly cited injuries of the cervical region, they are solely pathology of peripheral nerves. Most often, traction secondary to trauma will cause burning and paresthesia along a C5–C6 motor and sensory distribution, resulting in transient weakness and numbness[2-4] The vast majority of cases resolve within minutes. However, in rare cases, symptoms may persist for weeks to months, resulting in significant impairment to quality of life.[4]

Contact sports, particularly American football and rugby, are among the most commonly cited settings for stingers. Indeed, over half of all contact-sport athletes will develop a stinger during their career. While previous studies have found that up to 65% of football players report at least one stinger injury, recent work suggests a lower incidence of about 20% to 30%.[5,6] Defensive ends/linebackers and offensive linemen appear to be at the highest risk. Similar estimates have been made among rugby players and wrestlers.[5-7] However, some have called into question the accuracy of these figures, as stingers have traditionally been underreported.[6] Recurrence is common, accounting for nearly one in five stinger injuries.[6] Recurrent injury increases the risk of permanent nerve damage, which underscores the importance of proper athlete education and injury prevention. The purpose of this chapter is to review the history, exam, imaging, decision, and treatment options for the management of stingers. The authors will also discuss their preferred approach, return to play (RTP), and future considerations.

HISTORY

The most common setting of a stinger injury in the athlete is during play. Compressive trauma or traction occurs to an athlete whose neck is rotated contralateral to the blow. Such trauma may also depress the ipsilateral shoulder, increasing brachial plexus strain. Depending on the extent of injury, the patient may instinctually "shake out" the affected extremity, support it with the unaffected contralateral extremity, or report generalized pain in the area of the supraclavicular fossa.[8] Compression, traction, and hyperextension injury are thus the three major

mechanisms of stinger injury, and will be discussed with greater detail in a further section.

Pain from a stinger injury, true to its namesake, is frequently described as a burning paresthesia, with associated numbness and heaviness of the affected extremity. While the C5–C6 distributions are most commonly involved, circumferential rather than dermatomal radiation of pain down the extremity is not uncommon. Sensorimotor deficits, when present, typically rectify within several minutes. However, fewer than 1 in 10 patients may have residual symptoms lasting several weeks[3]

PHYSICAL EXAMINATION

A physical examination is warranted in any athlete with a suspected injury to the brachial plexus, as it can provide crucial details for further management. Evaluation initially begins with a focused cervical spine exam, followed by the characterization of musculoskeletal or neurologic abnormalities. Specific clinical exam techniques may then be used to identify the lesion location.

In the setting of apparent trauma to the neck, loss of consciousness, or gross deformity, the patient's cervical spine should be empirically immobilized until further imaging can be performed. Additionally, tenderness to direct palpation of the cervical spine in the presence of any trauma, even in the absence of obvious trauma, warrants application of a hard cervical collar. After the exclusion of cervical instability, basic evaluation of neck and extremity range of motion (ROM) and sensation should follow. It is important to note that stinger injuries are rarely bilateral, and do not affect the lower extremities; such signs point towards a more sinister pathology of the cervical spine.

Sensorimotor anomalies may be quickly and efficiently screened for on the field. Weakness of the deltoid and diminished wrist extension suggests C5 and C6 motor deficits, respectively.[9] These findings, along with a reduction in lateral upper extremity and forearm sensation, represent the most common presentation of stinger injuries. Triceps weakness and reduced wrist flexion suggest C7 pathology, while weakness in finger flexion or medial forearm sensation suggests involvement of C8. A T1 abnormality, though rare, presents with loss or diminished sensation to the medial arm, and weakness of the intrinsic muscles of the hand (Fig. 127.1 and Table 127.1).

Evaluation of the native anatomy of the patient may also provide clinical information. The upper trunk of the brachial plexus runs superficially approximately 2 cm above the clavicle at the level of the C6 vertebral body. Known as the Erb point, this location describes the convergence of the C5 and C6 nerve roots. Direct palpation of the Erb point may elicit a Tinel sign—reproduction of numbness and tingling in the distal extremity along a C5–C6 distribution.[9,10] The Tinel sign has both variable sensitivity (45% to 75%) and specificity (55% to 75%).[10,11]

The Spurling test while traditionally used to evaluate for cervical spine radiculopathy, may also be positive in a stinger injury. A positive Spurling test involves the reproduction of paresthesia down the affected extremity upon turning the patients neck toward the side of the suspected lesion, extending the neck, and applying compression of forehead contralaterally. It is thought that the traction applied during a Spurling maneuver may reproduce the mechanism of the stinger injury, thereby also reproducing the symptoms of a stinger. The Spurling test appears to show 30% to 100% sensitivity and 75% to 99% specificity in the literature.[10] Despite the question of variable sensitivity and intraobserver reliability, these examinations may provide useful evidence to an otherwise complicated clinical picture.

The supraspinatus and infraspinatus, along with the biceps and deltoid, appear to be most often involved in stinger injuries.

In cases where a lesion of C5 or C6 nerve roots must be distinguished from an upper trunk lesion, a clinician may test for a long thoracic nerve or dorsal scapular nerve palsy. Involvement of either nerve may result in scapular winging, though long thoracic nerve palsy would result in medial winging during a Serratus wall test, while dorsal scapular nerve lesions exhibit lateral winging and rhomboid weakness.[11]

IMAGING

Torg et al. first described the Torg ratio in 1986, a metric that is currently used to characterize cervical spinal stenosis.[19] Originally, it was developed to radiographically predict the risk of developing chronic stinger syndrome in the otherwise healthy athlete. On lateral radiograph, the Torg ratio may be calculated by measuring the diameter of the spinal canal (distance from the midpoint of the superior and inferior endplates of the posterior aspect of the vertebral body to the corresponding point on the spinolaminar line). This distance is then divided by the anteroposterior (AP) vertebral body diameter to form the Torg ratio (Fig. 127.2). Initially, a number of studies suggested that a

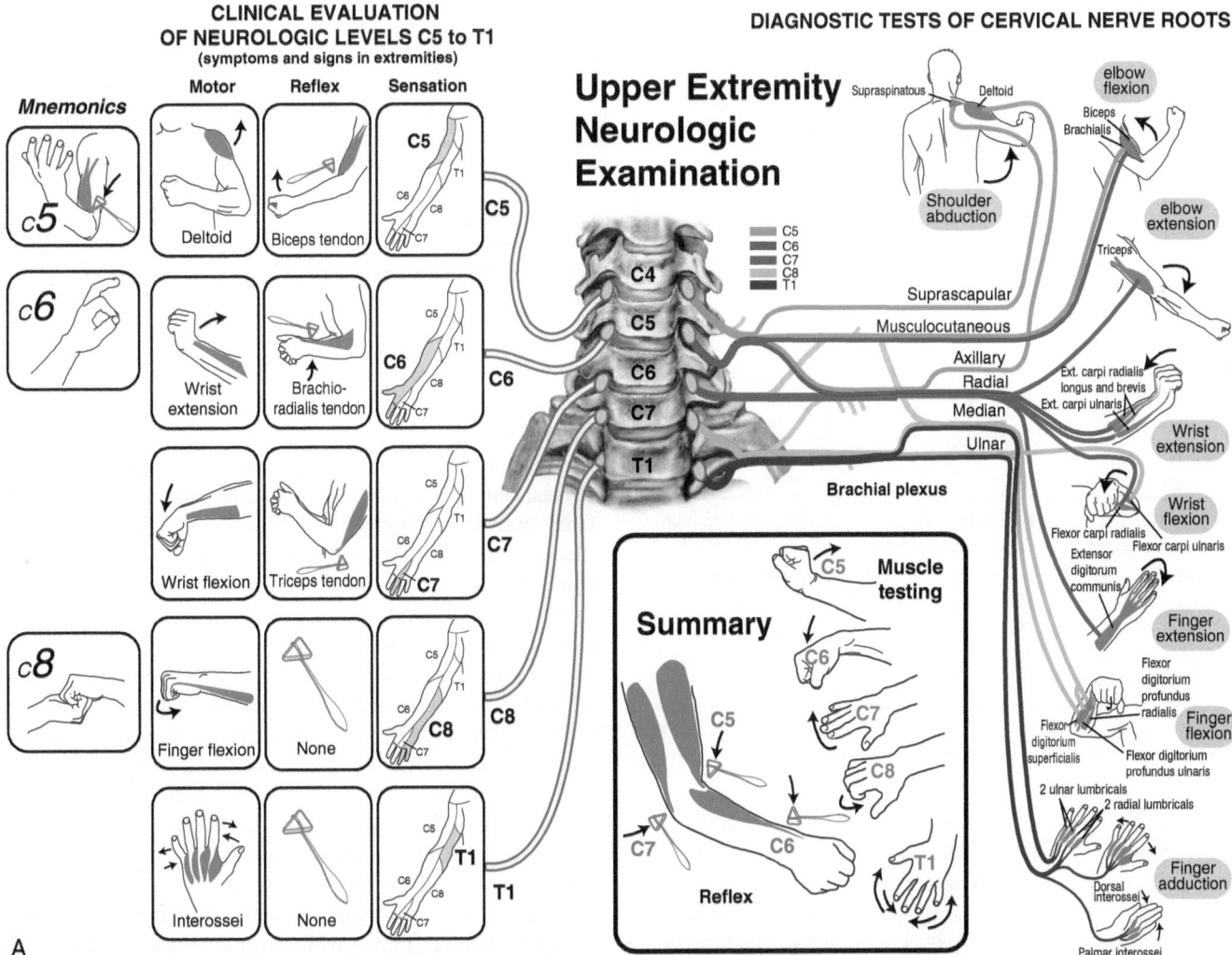

Fig. 127.1 (A and B) Examination of the upper extremity for strength, sensation, and reflexes. (From Miller MD, Thompson SR, Hart JA. *Review of Orthopaedics*. Philadelphia: Elsevier; 2012.)

Continued

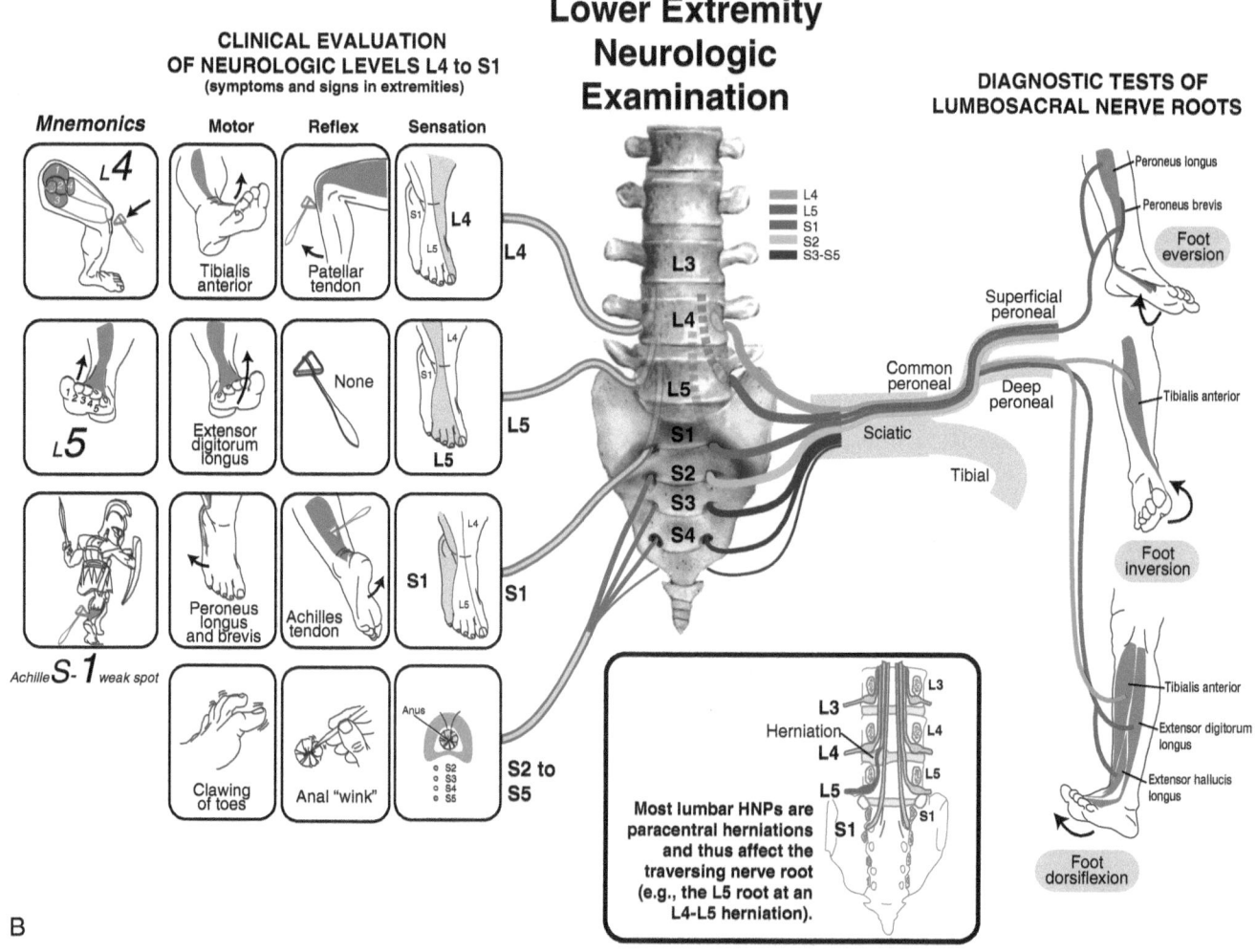

Fig. 127.1, cont'd

TABLE 127.1   Evaluation of Motor Function in Burners and Other Brachial Plexus Injuries

Muscle	Innervation	Clinical Test
Deltoid	Axillary (C5, C6)	Shoulder abduction
Supraspinatus	Suprascapular (C5, C6)	"Full can" abduction
Infraspinatus	Suprascapular (C5, C6)	External rotation
Biceps brachii	Musculocutaneous (C5, C6)	Elbow flexion
Pronator teres	Median (C6, C7)	Forearm pronation
Triceps brachii	Radial (C7, C8)	Elbow extension
Abductor digiti minimi	Ulnar (C8, T1)	Fifth digit abduction

From Kuhlman G, McKeag D. The "burner": a common nerve injury in contact sports. *Am Fam Physician.* 1999;60(7):2.

Torg ratio below 0.7 to 0.8 indicated substantial spinal stenosis and increased risk of a future stinger during contact sports, with lower value corresponding to higher risk. Since the Torg ratio was first described, a number of subsequent studies have found it to have high sensitivity, but relatively poor predictive value and high user dependency.[20,21] Although the Torg ratio is no longer widely used in the setting of stinger injuries, it nevertheless remains an important metric for the classification of cervical stenosis.

More recent literature has explored a novel method of predicting the risk for future stinger injury in the athlete. The mean subaxial cervical space available for the cord (MSCSAC) index—a measurement determined by averaging the difference between sagittal spinal cord diameter and sagittal spinal canal diameter from levels C3 through C6—appears to show some promise in this setting. In theory, any injury mechanism (e.g., hyperextension) that would diminish the MSCSAC would cause undue compression of the underlying cord, predisposing to recurrent stinger injury. In 2009, Presciutti et al. performed a comparison of 103 NFL athletes and 43 age-matched nonathlete controls. After obtaining cervical magnetic resonance imaging (MRI) and radiographs, the Torg ratio and the MSCSAC index were calculated for each subject. They found that MSCSAC was significantly different among athletes with and without chronic stingers, and among athletes and nonathlete controls. Furthermore, an MSCSAC index of less than 4.3 predicted a 13-fold increased risk of chronic stinger development, with 80% sensitivity and 96% specificity.[20] A recent case study describing a Division 1 collegiate football player with chronic stinger syndrome also demonstrated findings consistent with those of Presciutti et al.[21] While the effectiveness of the MSCSAC index as a predictive tool remains promising, further rigorous research in the form

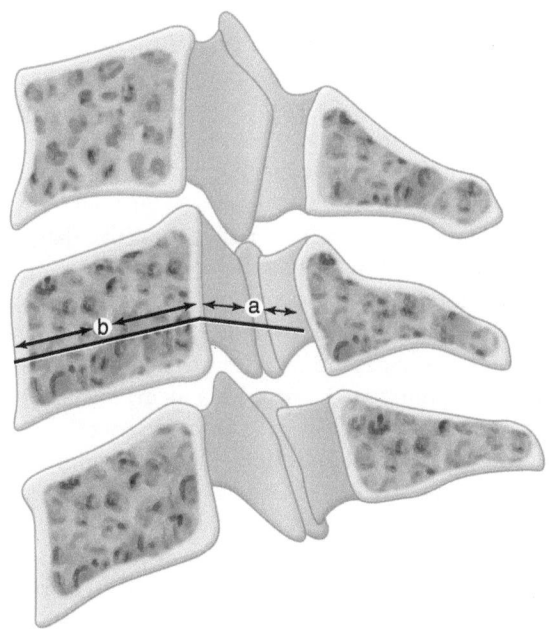

Fig. 127.2 The ratio method defined by Torg and colleagues uses a cervical spine lateral radiograph to predict an athlete's risk of sustaining a stinger. The Torg ratio is defined as the canal diameter *(a)* divided by the vertebral body diameter *(b)*. (Modified from Torg J, Pavlov H, Genuario S, et al. Neurapraxia of the cervical spinal cord with transient quadriplegia. *J Bone Joint Surg.* 1986;68:1354–1370.)

of prospective studies and clinical trials must be undertaken before the use of this method becomes widespread.

While imaging studies are not necessarily required in athletes with a suspected stinger injury, they may be critical for ruling out serious cervical pathology, particularly in those with prolonged, bilateral, or severe symptoms. In the past, lateral flexion and extension radiographs were often used to evaluate the cervical spine. Recently, however, a growing body of literature has supported the replacement of radiographs with computer tomography (CT). In a 2009 prospective study of 1505 patients brought to a level 1 trauma center, traditional radiographs were found to have poor sensitivity for cervical pathology (36%) when compared to CT (100%).[12] When patients were stratified by low, medium, and high risk, based on mechanism of injury, this divide was even more pronounced in low-risk patients. Since then a number of studies, including large randomized trials, have found screening CT to exhibit superior sensitivity, specificity, interobserver, and intraobserver reliability when compared to radiograph, in both obtunded and nonobtunded patients.[13-15] Furthermore, current research suggests that newer techniques of CT imaging, such as adaptive statistical iterative reconstruction (ASiR), may further increase the beneficial value of CT in this setting through reduction in radiation exposure by up to 36%.[16] MRI may be used instead of CT when evaluating stingers in both adult and pediatric populations.[17,18] In general, the acuity and severity of symptomatology should guide the decision to use MRI, which should be based on the individual patient's entire clinical picture.

Electromyography (EMG) has shown some utility in the evaluation of a stinger injury. In addition to differentiating preganglionic and postganglionic lesions, EMG can aid in determining lesion severity.[22] Although the process of wallerian degeneration begins as early as 24 to 36 hours following injury, nerve segment distal to the lesion may continue to propagate normal signal pattern for up to 2 to 3 weeks. For this reason, EMG is indicated only for those patients with persistent symptoms for a minimum of 2 weeks. EMG findings may be variable, but commonly include normal to increased insertional activity, fibrillations and positive sharp waves at rest, and an incomplete interference pattern.[22,23] Depending on the severity of nerve damage, postganglionic injuries do not appear to preclude spontaneous resolution, whereas preganglionic injuries or nerve root avulsions have little chance for recovery without surgical intervention.

CLASSIFICATION AND DECISION-MAKING PRINCIPLES

Clinical decision-making, in the context of a stinger injury, necessarily relies on the mechanism of injury. To date, three mechanisms of injury have been explored in the literature These include direct compression of the Erb point, lateral traction of the brachial plexus, and cervical spine hyperextension (Fig. 127.3). Each of these mechanisms can occur independently, or concomitantly with one another.

Compression of the superficial nerves at the Erb point is a frequently cited mechanism of stinger injury in the football player. During a direct tackle, the superomedial margin of the scapula can be forced towards a player's shoulder pad, or vice versa. The resultant compressive forces are then transmitted to the upper trunk of the brachial plexus that intervenes between these structures.[24,25] Compressive injury also may occur as a result of any action that forcibly diminishes the diameter of the cervical foramina such as rapid head rotation or pre-existing cervical stenosis.

Brachial plexus traction is a common mechanism of injury in football players, but can also affect wrestlers, rugby players, bicyclists, and skiers. Injury occurs when the athlete head is forcibly bent contralateral to the affected side, and the ipsilateral shoulder is depressed. This can be the result of a direct tackle in the case of contact sports, or landing onto the side of an athlete's helmet following a high-speed fall (cyclists, skiers, etc.).[24]

Hyperextension injuries can occur as a result of a head-on blow to the athlete, often with the force vector facing posteriorly. Here, rapid neck extension compresses the cervical nerve root through brief cervical foramen collapse, resulting in motor and/or sensory deficits. Athletes with degenerative disease of the cervical spine, such as stenosis or disk disease, are more prone to nerve root compression subsequently following a hyperextension event.[25]

Besides the above mentioned three major mechanisms, in young athletes, stinger injuries may be associated with high magnitude acceleration of the head. In one study, Campolettano et al. analyzed 6813 impacts among 34 youth football players. They found that 6.0% of these impacts met the definition of "high magnitude" with head acceleration exceeding 40 g. Overall, the authors found that tackling drills during practice, rather than in-game injury, were responsible for up to 50% of high-magnitude impact exposures among young football players. Furthermore, specific tackling drills, such as the "King of the hill" drill, were strongly associated with head acceleration over 60 g.[26]

Sir Herbert Seddon was among the first to describe injuries to the peripheral nervous system in 1942. Today, his classification scheme remains largely utilized to describe the severity of brachial plexus injuries. Stinger injuries are stratified into grade I, II, and III, with each grade describing varying levels of severity (Table 127.2). Grade I injuries represent neuropraxia, in which conduction across a nerve is interrupted despite the presence of full axonal continuity. Although neuropraxias themselves can vary in severity, a key feature is that there is no violation of the epineurium, the perineurium, or the endoneurium of the affected nerve. Wallerian degeneration does not occur, and thus complete recovery is expected within days to weeks of the injury. On EMG, the patient may exhibit conduction block, positive sharp waves, and lack of fibrillation potentials.[2,9,27]

Axonotmesis describes a peripheral nerve injury in which there is axonal disruption, and is indicative of a grade II stinger injury. Grade II stingers are more severe than grade I, but are fortunately less common. Because the epineurium and perineurium are preserved, grade II stingers, axonal regeneration remains possible without surgical intervention. Following injury, nerve conjunction transiently ceases, leading to significant sensorimotor deficits on the affected side. Wallerian degeneration then follows. At 3 weeks post injury, EMG may show some recovery of nerve conduction with fibrillation potentials and positive sharp waves.[2,9] While symptoms may persist for weeks to months, full recovery can take over a year.

Grade III stingers exhibit neurotmesis and are thus the most severe. Neurotmesis involves complete or partial transection of the nerve, including endoneurium, perineurium, epineurium, and any myelinating cells in proximity to the injury. Conduction studies are variable, but can be similar to those found in grade II injuries if the affected nerve is only partially destroyed. Grade III injuries are accompanied by wallerian degeneration, severe sensorimotor, and/or autonomic dysfunction, and require prompt surgical intervention.[27]

TREATMENT OPTIONS

The initial treatment of a stinger injury centers on patient stabilization and removal from play. A thorough history and physical examination should be obtained as described in previous sections of this chapter. A high index of suspicion should be used when evaluating any injured player, as the patient may not immediately alert athletic trainers, especially when symptoms are transient.[24]

Athletes with transient symptoms lasting only seconds, with complete resolution and benign physical exam findings, likely experienced a grade I, mild neuropraxia. Such patients can be managed symptomatically, and may be permitted to immediately RTP at the discretion of the athletic and coaching staff. Any player experiencing symptoms longer than a few seconds likely have a grade I, moderate neuropraxia, and should be removed from play for the remainder of the competition.

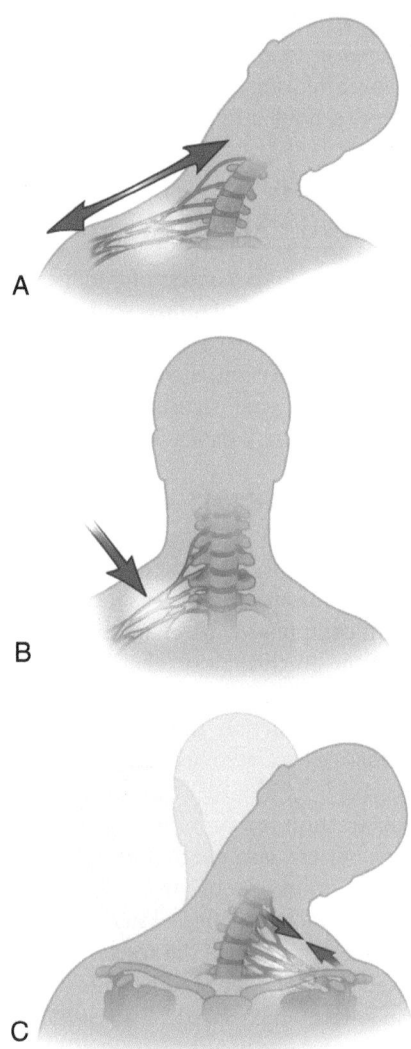

Fig. 127.3 Mechanisms of stingers. (A) Traction to the brachial plexus from ipsilateral shoulder depression and contralateral lateral neck flexion. (B) A direct blow to the supraclavicular fossa at the Erb point. (C) Compression of the cervical roots or brachial plexus from ipsilateral lateral flexion and hyperextension. (From Kuhlman G, McKeag D. The "burner": a common nerve injury in contact sports. *Am Fam Physician*. 1999;60[7]: 2035–2040.)

Grade	Nerve Injury	Electromyographic Findings	Prognosis
1	Neurapraxia	Normal	Most resolve within minutes
2	Axonotmesis	Positive waves with fibrillation	Recovery in 12–18 months
3	Neurotmesis	Acute denervation	Variable; possible complete loss of function

TABLE 127.2 Classification of Stinger Injury Defined by Nerve Injury, Electromyographic Findings, and Prognosis for Recovery

Physical exam should be performed at the time of injury, at the end of play, and at 24 hours after injury for these individuals. The patient should also undergo cervical radiography, particularly if strength, ROM, and sensation has not returned to baseline. Treatment grade I, severe neuropraxia incorporates all of the above steps, and additionally includes repeated physical examination of the patient up to 2 weeks following injury.[24,28] Additional imaging such as MRI or CT may be considered on a per-patient basis.

Serial examination and cervical imaging are also warranted in patients with grade II stingers. These patients should be closely followed for up to 2 weeks after initial injury, in a similar fashion to those with severe neuropraxia. Cervical imaging options include standard AP, lateral, and odontoid view radiographs, as well as MRI; CT also may be used if the patient develops symptoms suspicious of a cervical fracture.[24,28]

Patients with grade III injury will exhibit severe weakness and sensorimotor dysfunction lasting more than 2 to 3 weeks. For these individuals, nerve conduction studies, such as EMG, are valuable for establishing nerve function and monitoring rehabilitation. MRI and conduction study findings should guide clinical decision-making, and surgical consultation is indicated for severe irreparable nerve damage.[24,28,29]

Symptomatic treatment of nerve injury-related pain is indicated in all patients regardless of injury grade. First-line treatment includes the application of ice and the use of nonsteroidal antiinflammatory drugs (NSAIDs) to address local inflammation. Physical therapy is of value to those with symptoms that limit ranging of the cervical spine and the affected extremity. In this situation, an emphasis should be placed on regaining active and passive neck ROM, and improving the strength of musculature surrounding the site of injury. While the use of high-dose steroids remains contraindicated in patients with peripheral nerve injuries, a short course of low-dose oral steroids in patients with severe symptoms is generally accepted among most physicians.[28,29] Similarly, cortisone injection near the site of nerve injury also may provide some symptomatic relief, though there are currently no concrete guidelines surrounding this. Muscle relaxants may be judiciously used in the patient with pain secondary to spasm of the musculature surrounding the injury.[30]

🔖 Authors' Preferred Technique

Given the prevalence of stingers, the potential for life-altering complications and comorbid injuries, and the high propensity of underreporting observed throughout the literature, the authors advocate for the evaluation of all athletes exhibiting neurologic symptoms following in-game trauma. Any athlete sustaining symptoms that persist during sideline evaluation should be removed from competition and reevaluated after the game and 24 hours after injury. Unstable cervical injury should be managed according to local protocol; usually cervical CT should be obtained in patients exhibiting signs suggestive of fracture such as focal cervical tenderness. We find that initial CT imaging provides definitive information regarding cervical injury, and is generally appropriate for most injury patterns we encounter. Radiographs are an appropriate alternative if CT imaging is not available. If symptoms persist after 3 days, an MRI should be obtained. Serial imaging studies and exams are performed for 2–3 weeks following injury, until symptoms show improvement. If symptoms do not resolve at this time, EMG studies are obtained. We do not routinely use cortisone injections, oral steroids, or muscle relaxants, but do encourage rest, ice, the use of NSAIDs, and physical therapy when appropriate. Patients may be allowed to RTP following (1) complete resolution of pain, numbness, and tingling, (2) achievement of baseline muscle strength and ROM, and (3) subjective feeling of "readiness" to return to sport (Fig. 127.4). The patient should be cautioned that recurrence of injury is common, and should be encouraged to use protective equipment in the future.

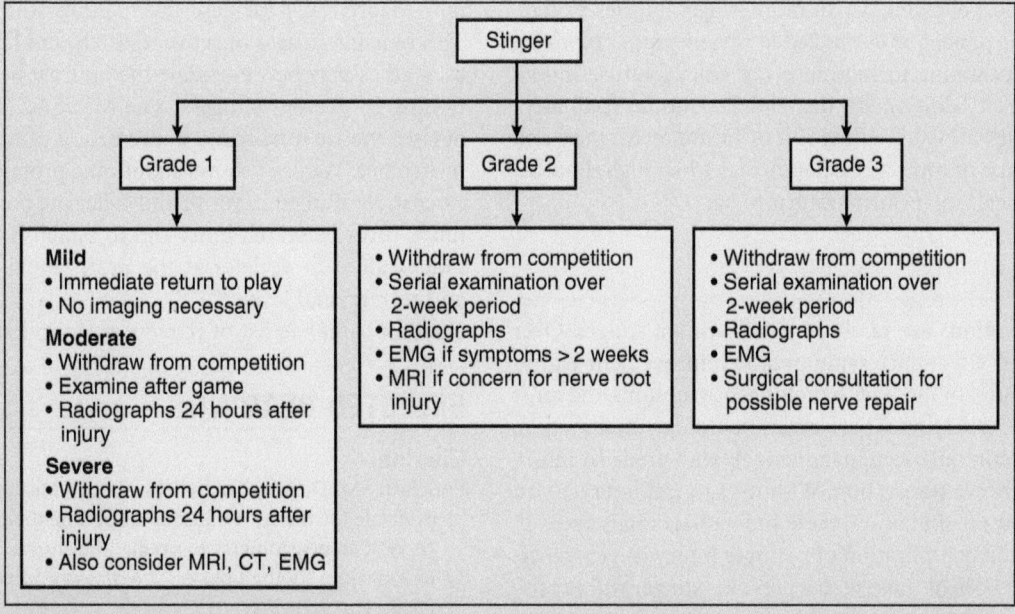

Fig. 127.4 Management of stingers based on grade of injury. *CT,* Computed tomography; *EMG,* electromyography; *MRI,* magnetic resonance imaging.

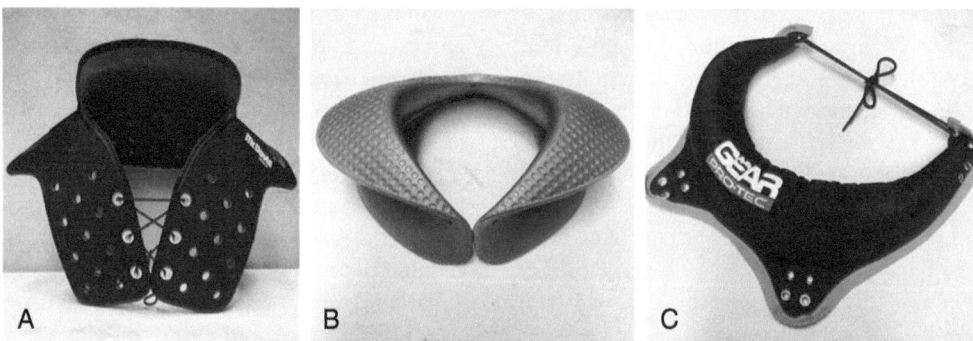

Fig. 127.5 Examples of protective and preventative equipment. (A) Anterior view of the Cowboy Collar, typically worn under the athlete's shoulder pads. (B) The Kerr Collar, a protective collar that reduces axial load and prevents neck hyperextension. (C) The Cervical Neck Roll, worn under protective padding, also prevents excessive neck motion.

RETURN TO PLAY

The exact criteria for RTP among athletes with a stinger injury remains controversial. Still, the vast majority of physicians agree that complete resolution of symptoms, the return of preinjury motor strength and ROM, and the ruling out of other serious pathology on imaging, are all prerequisites to RTP.[24,31] Typically, fulfillment of these criteria within a few minutes of injury, in a patient that has had no prior stingers, is sufficient for immediate RTP. In the past, Weinstein has recommended that athletes with moderate fibrillation potentials on EMG, and function deficits 2 weeks after injury should not be allowed to RTP, though the relationship between EMG results and recovery is not entirely clear.[32] Cantu has suggested that a history of 3 or more previous stingers should be a relative contraindication to RTP. Kepler has added that patients with recurrent stingers, particularly within the same season, should be radiographically cleared to RTP following each episode. Following two or more stinger injuries, experts suggest that the patient be counseled to review proper blocking and tackling technique to minimize the risk of future injury, prior to return.[28] Additionally, the clinician should facilitate a thorough conversation about the risk of future recurrence, and encourage the use of protective equipment, such as high shoulder pads or a cervical roll, prior to return to sport.[29]

SEQUELA

Severe complications are rarely seen following a stinger. Over 90% of patients experience symptomatic improvement within 24 hours of injury. In those with prolonged symptoms, the most life-altering complication is permanent neurologic dysfunction. This is most commonly seen in individuals with grade III injury and complete nerve transection. Without surgical intervention and subsequent rehabilitation, these individuals rarely recover. A more common complication of a stinger injury is recurrence. Indeed, 50% to 60% of those with a previous stinger will experience one or more later episodes.[33] Levitz et al. were among the first to describe the chronic stinger syndrome, and suggested that cervical foraminal stenosis and degenerative disk disease may be associated with an increased risk of future recurrence.[33] As mentioned in previous sections of this text, the Torg ratio has historically been used as a quantitative metric to predict the risk for the development of chronic stinger syndrome.[19] More recently, the MSCSAC index has been proposed to better serve this purpose, with promising evidence supporting its predictive value.[20,21]

FUTURE CONSIDERATIONS

The prevention of initial injury and injury recurrence remains a target of future research. Recent literature has suggested that the use of the "Kerr Collar" minimizes head acceleration and force transmission better than the use of the "Cowboy" or "Bullock Collars" do, although all of these collars have significant protective value.[34] (Fig. 127.5). However, Concannon et al. have cautioned that equipment that excessively limits head extension may theoretically increase the risk for other cervical injury.[35] This remains an area of active research, and further biomechanical studies may best elucidate the optimal head and neck positioning to prevent stingers. The MSCSAC index is a recently devised metric used to aid in prediction of future stinger injury recurrence. While it shows significant promise, it has not been extensively studied in youth and collegiate populations. Furthermore, future research must aim to establish baseline MSCSAC index values in athletes at the professional, semiprofessional, and recreational levels.[20,36,37]

For a complete list of references, go to ExpertConsult.com.

SELECTED READINGS

Citation:
Presciutti SM, Deluca P, Marchetto P, et al. Mean subaxial space available for the cord index as a novel method of measuring cervical spine geometry to predict the chronic stinger syndrome in American football players. *J Neurosurg Spine.* 2009;11(3):264–271.

Level of Evidence:
II

Summary:
Presciutti et al. propose and evaluate the use of the mean subaxial space available for the cord (MSCSAC) index as an alternative quantitative parameter to the Torg ratio for predicting the risk of recurrent stingers. The authors retrospectively reviewed cervical magnetic resonance imaging from 103 male NFL athletes and 43 age-matched controls. Torg ratio and MSCSAC index were calculated, and receiver operator curves were obtained for each of the modalities. An MSCSAC index value of 5.0 mm produced a sensitivity of 80% and a negative likelihood ratio of 0.23 for predicting chronic stingers. The authors concluded that MSCSAC index measurement may be an appropriate screening test in at-risk patients.

Citation:
Huang P, Anissipour A, Mcgee W, et al. Return-to-play recommendations after cervical, thoracic, and lumbar spine injuries. *Sports Health*. 2016;8(1):19–25.

Level of Evidence:
IV

Summary:
Huang et al. provide a comprehensive review and discussion of return to play guidelines for a wide range of cervical injuries. Their work provides useful references to both the current literature and expert opinion pertaining to the management of athletes with stingers and other trauma-mediated injury. They conclude that, at a minimum, individuals with cervical injuries should have complete symptomatic relief and return to baseline strength and range of movement prior to return to play. Finally, they cover injury-specific nuances in management of the injured athlete

Citation:
Green J, Zuckerman SL, Dalton SL, et al. A 6-year surveillance study of "Stingers" in NCAA American Football. *Res Sports Med*. 2016;25(1):26–36.

Level of Evidence:
II

Summary:
In this retrospective review of prospectively collected data, Green et al. report on the prevalence of stingers reported among 57 NCAA football teams over the course of 6 years. They found an injury rate of 2.04 per 10,000 athlete exposures. Stingers were reported primarily in the preseason (80.3%) and 18.8% of injuries were recurrent. The most high-risk positions for injury were defensive ends/linebackers (25.8%) and offensive linemen (23.6%). The authors conclude that stingers may be less common than previously reported in the literature within the collegiate football population.

128

Traumatic Injuries of the Cervical Spine in the Athlete

Adam L. Shimer, Bayan Aghdasi

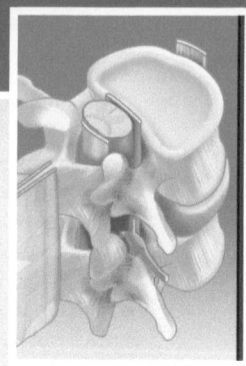

This chapter provides an evidence-based approach to history and physical examination, initial stabilization and triage, diagnosis and imaging, treatment, and outcomes for cervical spine injuries in athletes. Cervical spine injury ranges from neuropraxias, to herniated discs, to complete spinal cord injury. The latter is rare but devastating and warrants a high index of suspicion and familiarity with spine immobilization protocols when suspected. On-field catastrophic neurologic injury has decreased over the past 30 years[1]; nevertheless, providers must maintain a high index of suspicion, especially in cases of high-velocity axial loading, which is the most common implicated mechanism of injury.[2] This information is important for team physicians and trainers.

HISTORY

Football, diving, rugby,[3,4] and other sports constitute the second most common cause (10%) of catastrophic cervical spine injuries (10,000 annually), after motor vehicle collision (MVC).[5,6] Football is the most researched of these, with 7 decades of Annual Survey of Football Injury Research (ASFIR) data culminating in a reduction of traumatic quadriplegia incidence from 10 to 1 per 100,000 football participants since outlawing spear tackling in 1976.[7]

First responders to an on-field injury should perform primary and secondary surveys, immobilizing the head while ruling out spine injury and assessing airway, breathing, and circulation. Cardiac defibrillation, neurologic exam, equipment removal, and transport are then performed.[8,9] The neurologic exam should assess level of consciousness, sensation, and strength.

Immobilization in a cervical collar and rigid spine board is an established historical precedent for transport.[10] New recommendations emphasize limited spinal manipulation.[11] Spine board immobilization is recommended for palpable step-off or spine tenderness, focal neurologic deficit, altered consciousness, or distracting injury.[12] Medication list, allergies, and time of latest oral intake should be communicated.

PHYSICAL EXAMINATION/ON-FIELD EVALUATION

On-field response requires preparation, planning, equipment, and an organized chain of command. First priorities include assessing scene safety and airway patency. Maintain in-line cervical immobilization while assessing airway, breathing, circulation (ABCs). Note airway obstructions, tracheal deviation, and subcutaneous emphysema. Check pulses, and apply pressure over active bleeding. Measure heart rate and blood pressure. Assign level of consciousness (alert, responsive to verbal vs. painful stimuli, unresponsive) or Glasgow Coma Scale. Remove clothing to visualize surface anatomy, noting any deformity, crepitus, abrasions, penetrating trauma, burns, tenderness, lacerations, and swelling.

Spine boarding and equipment removal should be decided upon prior to transport.[13] Some studies support leaving equipment in place until after transport.[14,15] Even perfect execution engenders a risk of injury.[16] If the helmet or shoulder pads need to be removed, both should be removed to avoid flexion/extension of the cervical spine. Jaw thrust and not head tilt is the appropriate airway access maneuver.[17] Log rolling remains the appropriate technique for prone athletes, to position the spine board beneath them, but fewer cases of iatrogenic neurodeterioration have been documented with newer techniques.[18]

To remove equipment, the team leader stands over the head and stabilizes the C-spine while another provider straddles the patient and cuts down the jersey/shoulder pads and under-arm straps.[19] This also facilitates defibrillator pad placement.[20] Roles are then reversed, holding C-spine from below while two providers pull off the helmet. If three trained providers are not present, facemask removal is an alternative.[21] If quick-release mechanisms are not built-in, cordless screwdrivers or heavy shears may prove instrumental in making bilateral cuts or removing the two screws in the plastic clip affixing the facemask.[22] Chin strap and cheek pad removal facilitate helmet removal while towels are temporarily placed beneath the head to prevent C-spine extension.[23] Shoulder pads can then slide over the head allowing application of a rigid cervical collar.

The sports medicine team may escalate care via emergency medical transport services and communicate injury mechanism, developments, and interventions during on-field management. Intracranial pressure should be monitored by serial neurologic examination.[13] Acuity and resource availability should factor into destination selection for transport. Computed tomography (CT), magnetic resonance imaging (MRI), and spine surgeon availability are important destination determinants. Advanced verbal notice to the receiving facility is helpful.

IMAGING

Cervical spine x-rays are important unless the patient is pain-free throughout a full range of motion (ROM), is nontender to palpation, is alert and oriented with no distracting injuries or inebriation, and has no neurodeficits.[24] With 30,000 patients, the National Emergency X-Ray Utilization Study trial demonstrated 99.8% negative predictive value and 99% sensitivity using these criteria, which reduces unnecessary radiation. Advanced age or high-energy mechanism merit cervical spine x-rays including anteroposterior (AP), lateral, and odontoid views, adding swimmer's view if C7 to T1 is inadequately visualized. Unremarkable radiographic and clinical exam may be followed by flexion/extension views to rule out dynamic instability.

Regular postinjury reevaluation for neurologic weakness or signs of intracranial pressure allows prompt acquisition of advanced imaging.[25] This helps to rule out skull fracture, subdural or epidural hematoma, hemorrhage, or edema. However, concussion has no structural findings on imaging.[26]

Three-dimensional (3D) reconstruction with fine cuts in sagittal, axial, and coronal planes is indicated if clinical exam or x-rays are abnormal. CT scan rapidly identifies injury even without equipment removal,[27] with 90% to 100% sensitivity and specificity,[28] respectively. Speed, power, subtlety, and cervicothoracic visibility have led CT to replace plain films as first line imaging. Maintenance of spinal precautions during transfers is imperative. C-collar should remain in place until clearance of the C-spine.

MRI is indicated[29] for neurodeficits and soft tissue characterization of posterior ligamentous complex (PLC), herniated nucleus pulposus (HNP), and spinal cord injury or if spinal cord injury without radiographic abnormality (SCIWORA) is suspected. Neurodeficits or radiographic injury merit spine surgery consultation.

CT head should be acquired in cases of open, depressed, or basilar skull fracture, persistent headache or vomiting, high-energy mechanism, anterograde amnesia, or evidence of supraclavicular trauma.[30] Delayed electromyography provides baseline and prognostic information about preganglionic versus postganglionic brachial plexopathies, with isolated motor (poor) versus combined motor and sensory (favorable) potential loss, respectively.[31]

DECISION-MAKING PRINCIPLES OF DIAGNOSIS AND TREATMENT

Cervical sprain/strain is a diagnosis of exclusion, characterized by unremarkable plain radiographs in the context of mild neck tenderness and stiffness devoid of paresthesias or neurodeficit. It can be monitored closely and managed expectantly with rest and a low threshold for CT scan. Stingers or burners are transient upper extremity weakness (often C5 or 6 root) often accompanied by paresthesias with negative imaging findings and approximately 50% likelihood of lifetime recurrence.[32] They result from traction injuries to nerve roots[33] or the brachial plexus.[34] Another neuropraxia, burning hands syndrome, is a central cord variant without permanent deficit characterized by bilateral weakness and/or dysesthesias of the hands corresponding to spinothalamic/corticospinal tract injury without imaging findings.[35] This too is self-limiting. Transient quadriplegia (also known as spinal cord concussion) is an acute, traumatic, self-limited total paralysis lasting minutes to hours with an incidence of 7 per 10,000 football players. It may result from a pincer mechanism[36] without predisposition to recurrent neurologic symptoms.[37]

Herniated cervical intervertebral disc or HNP can occasionally be an acute traumatic entity with central and/or neuroforaminal stenosis experienced as axial/periscapular neck pain with upper extremity dermatomal myeloradiculopathy, paresthesias, weakness, gait ataxia, or loss of manual dexterity, and sometimes bowel/bladder dysfunction with quadriplegia. Neurologic deficit is an indication for urgent MRI and surgical decompression.[2] Surgery includes anterior cervical discectomy and fusion (ACDF) for central compression or posterior foraminotomy for foraminal HNP.

Spinous and transverse process and vertebral body fractures with less than 20% height loss often are stable nonoperative injuries, demonstrating less than 3.5 mm or 11 degrees of translational or angular instability, respectively, on flexion/extension radiographs.[38] Atlantoaxial instability is often the result of transverse alar ligament (TAL) injury, which manifests in atlantodens interval (ADI) widening beyond 3 mm on midsagittal CT.[39] TAL injury in Jefferson C1 ring fractures[40] are unstable when the combined bilateral overhang of C1 over C2 lateral masses on odontoid view or coronal CT exceeds 7 mm. Atlantoaxial instability is treated with C1/2 fusion.

Anderson and D'Alonzo classify C2 dens fractures[41] into alar ligament tip avulsions (type 1), treated in C-collar; watershed area fracture through dens waist (type 2), treated with fusion/osteosynthesis in cases of risk factors for nonunion; and base of dens fracture through cancellous body of axis (type 3), which go on to union with collar immobilization.

Traumatic spondylolisthesis of C2 (hangman's fractures) are classified by Levine and Edwards[42] into minimally displaced (type 1), treated with rigid orthosis; angulated (type 2A), treated with halo vest; angulated and translated (type 2B), treated with traction and halo vest; and bilateral pars fractures with subaxial facet dislocation (type 3), treated with posterior arthrodesis.

Single column compression fractures of the subaxial cervical spine[43] can be treated in a C-collar. Unstable[38] two-column burst injuries are treated with anterior or posterior arthrodesis and possible corpectomy. Anterior-inferior teardrop fractures require CT evaluation of coronal and sagittal plane injury and surgical stabilization due to a high incidence of quadriplegia.[44]

Hyperflexion injuries can cause unshingling and unilateral or bilateral facet dislocation visible on x-ray (25% or 50% intersegmental subluxation, respectively) or CT imaging and should be reduced using cervical tongs and traction in the awake and oriented patient. Any change in neurologic status or failed reduction prompts MRI to rule out HNP prior to emergent open reduction.[45] Bilateral versus unilateral facet dislocation has a much higher rate of quadriplegia.

Cervical stenosis is defined as canal AP diameter less than 14 mm on lateral x-ray or Torg ratio (AP diameter of canal divided by vertebral body) less than 0.8[46] and may predispose to spinal cord injury. Complete spinal cord injury has an incidence of 0.33 in high school and 1.33 in college athletes, with 11,000 cases and $9.7 billion cost annually. It is a devastating and irreversible injury encountered most often in professional football players making a defensive tackle.[47] Emergent decompression and stabilization is indicated.

Central cord syndrome is an incomplete hyperextension injury in elderly congenitally narrowed canals producing upper and distal more than lower and proximal musculature weakness. This is the most common and least devastating incomplete injury.[48] Brown-Séquard is a penetrating trauma-induced cord hemisection syndrome characterized by ipsilateral corticospinal tract motor paralysis and contralateral pain and temperature sensation disruption. Its prognosis is also favorable. Anterior cord syndrome, the most devastating incomplete injury, can be the result of ischemic or compressive injury to the anterior two-thirds of the cord from anterior spinal artery stroke or HNP/hyperflexion disrupting all but the dorsal columns. Rarely, one sees isolated posterior artery stroke of the dorsal columns and isolated loss of proprioceptive and vibratory sense in posterior cord syndrome.

Sprains and strains are treated with activity modification and cautious gameplay to tolerance until resolution of pain, stiffness, and tenderness. Neuropraxias are treated with withdrawal from game play and rest until resolution of all paresthesias, weakness, and pain with ROM.[49] Recurrent neuropraxia warrants equipment modification and physical therapy for shoulder girdle strengthening. Thereafter gameplay may resume. Symptomatic HNP without weakness or deficit can be treated nonoperatively. Single-level ACDF procedure is compatible with return to competitive sports,[3] and return to play (RTP) can be gradually initiated after radiographic evidence of fusion. Fractures and unstable injuries of the cervical spine should be evaluated by a spine surgeon to determine treatment options.

RETURN TO PLAY

Spine precautions should be maintained until full compliance with neurologic exam is possible. C-collar necessity can be reevaluated 1 to 2 weeks after injury in clinic with flexion/extension radiographs. RTP requires physical/cognitive rest until asymptomatic prior to return to school[50] and neurologic and musculoskeletal exam and concussion reassessment prior to clearance.[51] Twenty-four-hour cycles of light aerobic activity, mildly elevated heart rate, sport-specific and noncontact drills and medical clearance prior to full-contact practice are recommended.[52]

After cervical sprain, athletes may return to sport when full painless ROM has been reestablished without tenderness to palpation. After neuropraxic injury, strength, as well as pain-free ROM of the C-spine and extremities and complete resolution of paresthesias, numbness, and tingling, are necessary prior to returning to competitive play. Players with stingers that resolve completely or transient quadriplegia that lasts less than 24 hours without any residual deficits may also RTP without contraindication, provided this was the patient's first episode. Three episodes of stingers, prolonged symptoms, or transient quadriplegia lasting more than 24 hours are considered relative contraindications to return to competitive contact sport. Absolute contraindications include multiple episodes of transient quadriplegia, clinical or MRI evidence of cervical myelopathy, and cervical pain or neurologic deficits.

After an athlete has sustained a neuropraxia, he or she may RTP if the previous criteria are met and the Torg ratio is greater

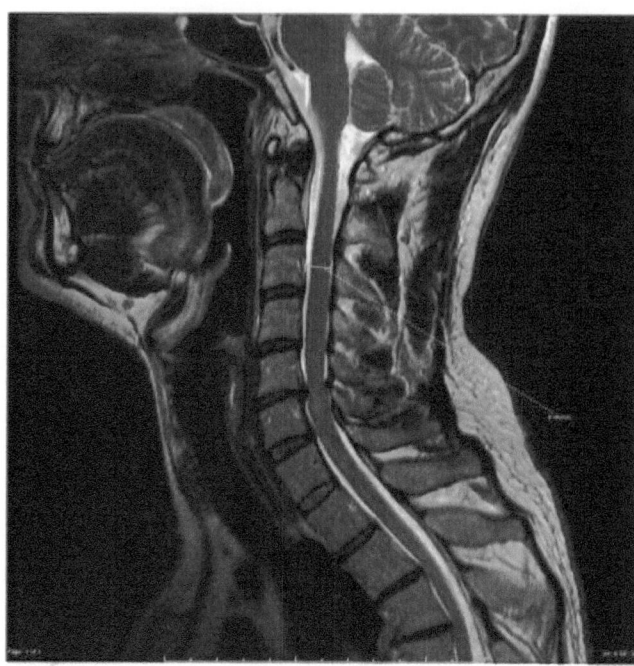

Fig. 128.1 Congenital cervical stenosis. Torg ratio: Anteroposterior (AP) diameter of spinal canal divided by AP diameter of corresponding vertebral body: greater than 0.8 normal, less than 0.8 congenital stenosis, and increased risk of neurologic injury.

than 0.8, defined as the ratio of the AP diameter of the canal divided by that of the vertebral body. Torg ratio less than 0.8 is consistent with a diagnosis of congenital cervical stenosis (Fig. 128.1), which places the athlete at increased risk of neurologic injury. Imaging evidence of intervertebral disk herniation, degenerative change, or cord deformation on MRI in this context is considered a relative contraindication for RTP. If there is MRI evidence of cord injury, defect, edema, or myelomalacia in the context of prior neuropraxic episode the athlete should be absolutely contraindicated from return to competitive contact sports. Likewise, evidence of ligamentous instability, prolonged symptoms greater than 36 hours, or multiple neuropraxic episodes should constitute an absolute contraindication. Numerous reports of professional-level elite contact and power sport athletes safely returning to same level of play after single level ACDF surgery have been published. Therefore evidence suggests that short-segment fixation in the cervical spine is not a contraindication for competitive sport. Individualized assessment of severity of pathology and surgical complexity will determine the ultimate competitive potential and timeline for RTP in these cases.

Spear tackler's spine is another absolute contraindication to competitive sport that risks axially loading a vulnerable cervical spine. A subset of football players demonstrate this condition, which includes findings of congenital stenosis, loss of physiologic lordosis (Fig. 128.2), posttraumatic changes on imaging of the cervical spine, and/or behavioral history of spear tackling techniques during gameplay. Players demonstrating these characteristics should be barred from competitive football or other contact sports. Coaching regarding proper tackling technique (Fig. 128.3)

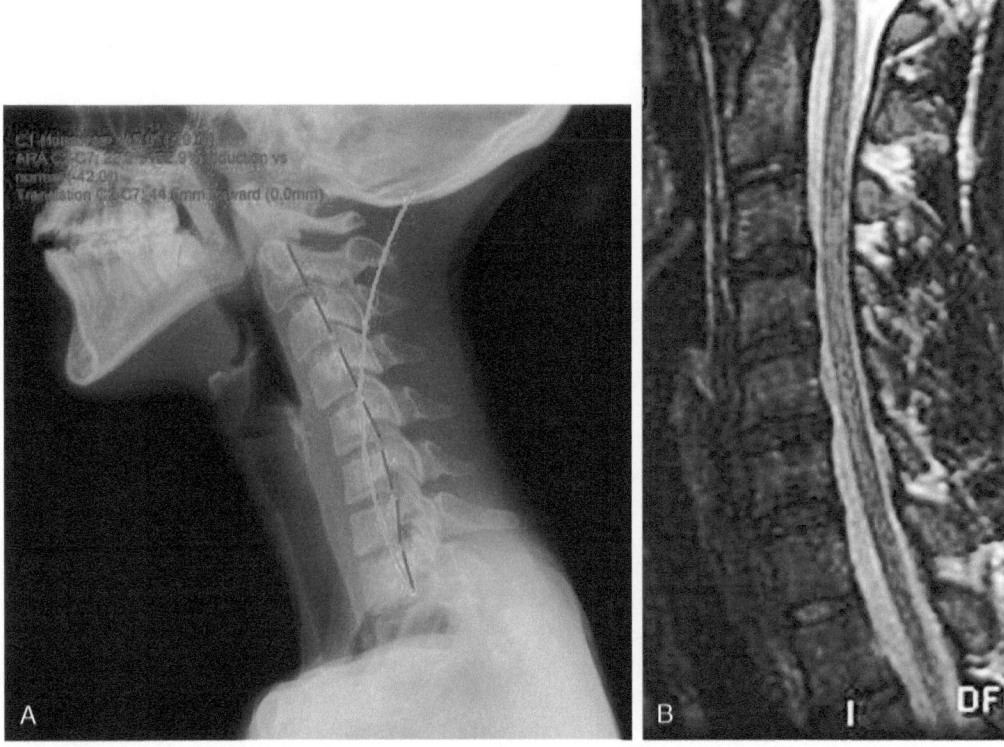

Fig. 128.2 Spear tackler's spine. (A) Loss of the normal lordosis of the cervical spine (standing neutral x-ray), (B) congenital stenosis of the central canal (recumbent sagittal magnetic resonance imaging), posttraumatic changes resembling spondylosis of multilevel disc bulge and ligamentous hypertrophy.

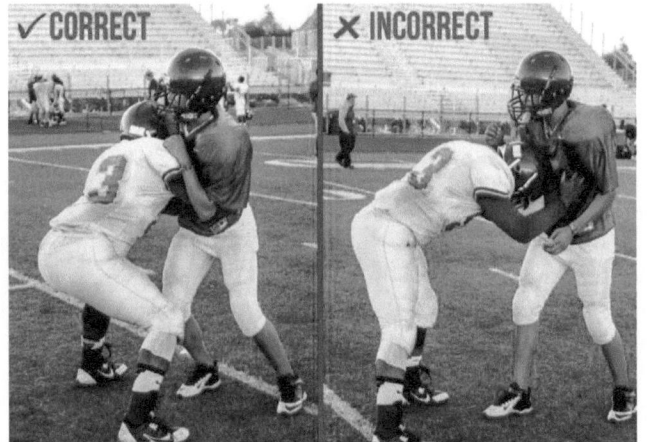

Fig. 128.3 Proper tackling technique involves a low center of gravity, directing the shoulder at the ball-carrier's beltline. Crucially, the tackler keeps his/her head up at all times and wraps up the ball-carrier's legs, so he/she falls to his or her side, taking both players to the ground together.

is crucial to avoid catastrophic neurologic injury from axially loading the cervical spine during spear tackling.

CONCLUSIONS

Physician, trainer, emergency medical services (EMS), and others are part of a team-based approach to sports medicine.[53] Team preparation should be performed annually and before each practice/game. Communication is critical between trainers and teachers for customized student-athlete care.[54] This is also important for post–return to sport monitoring.

For a complete list of references, go to ExpertConsult.com.

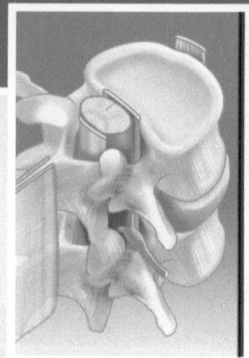

129

Traumatic Injuries of the Thoracolumbar Spine in the Athlete

Nourbakhsh Ali, Anuj Singla

Trauma to the thoracolumbar spine in athletes is common and can vary from minor sprain to major spinal fracture. Severe and potentially unstable spinal injuries are uncommon in sports-related trauma, but may be seen in athletes participating in contact sports or high velocity accidents. In addition to the contact and collision sports, athletes participating in certain noncontact sports like gymnastics, diving and weight lifting are also at risk for back trauma. Treatment of the injury and the recovery thereafter also varies widely depending on the pathology.

Irrespective of the underlying pathology, acute back pain is the most common symptom related to back trauma in athletes. The incidence of low back pain in athletes has been reported to be as high as 30%, and it can affect all athletes regardless of the position or the intensity of play.[1] Internal disc disruption is the most common cause of low back pain in young athletes. Lumbar disc disruption can cause a variety of symptoms, including back pain to radicular leg pain.[2–7] Some specific spine injuries are more common in certain sports (Table 129.1). Spondylolysis is more common in adolescent athletes, whereas internal disc disruption is more common between the ages of 18 and 50, and facet joints as well as sacroiliac (SI) joints more commonly caused back pain after the age of 50.[8] This chapter will cover the risk factors, history, examination, and imaging in the diagnosis of traumatic thoracolumbar spine injuries, and review the decision-making process and return-to-play (RTP) consideration in these athletes.

Risk Factors

During growth spurt the rate of bone growth surpasses the pace of muscle and ligaments growth, which leads to muscle imbalance and inflexibility.[9] Overuse injuries are more common during this period.[10] Avulsion of the ring apophyses as a secondary ossification center can happen due to repetitive flexion exercises. Disc can also herniate through the ring apophysis. Spina bifida or dysplasia of the posterior elements is a risk factor for spondylolysis.[11] Less skeletally mature children are at increased risk of spine injury when playing contact sports with physically larger players.[12]

Hyperlordosis of the lumbar spine due to hip flexor or hamstring tightness, genu recurvatum, increased femoral anteversion, abdominal muscle weakness, or increased thoracic kyphosis can also exert extra stress on the posterior spinal elements.[10] Other risk factors include malalignment of the lower extremities and pelvis, weak lower abdominal muscles, and abnormal pelvis and

sacral morphology.[13,14] Increased pelvis incidence increases to a shear forces across the L5 pars interarticularis. Decreased pelvis incidence can also damage the L5 pars through the nutcracker mechanism. Both situations can result in spondylolysis and progress to spondylolisthesis. Sex-specific spine injury and pathologies are summarized in Table 129.2.

HISTORY

A complete history of the injury that led to the onset of back pain, the mechanism of injury, location and radiation of pain, exacerbating or alleviating activities, the type of sport(s) that the athlete has been involved in, the training regimen, any recent increase in the volume or intensity of training, the position played, diet, menstrual history, previous injuries, and treatments should be obtained.[10] Red flags include constitutional symptoms, history of infection, or cancer, weight loss, night sweats, fevers, chronic cough, immunocompromised patients, intravenous drug use, recent infection, and nonmechanical back pain worse at night. Urinary or stool incontinence should raise the concern about myelopathy or cauda equina syndrome. Cauda equina syndrome might also include lower extremity weakness/numbness, saddle anesthesia, and sexual dysfunction. Myelopathy can be caused by vertebrae fracture, epidural hematoma and retropulsion, or disc herniation at the level of the cervical or thoracic spine. The symptoms include ataxia, motor weakness, and in cases of cervical spinal cord impingement, the patient will have problems with the coordination of the hands.[15] Performance-enhancing steroids might compromise immune system and increase the propensity to infection. Wheelchair-bound athletes might also develop spine infections as a result of decubitus ulcer or recurrent urinary tract infection.[16]

PHYSICAL EXAMINATION

Physical exam should start with inspection of the back and extremities, palpation of the spine, and evaluation of the gait and range of motion (ROM) of the spine. Neurologic exam includes testing the strength, sensation, and reflexes. Nerve root impingement will cause radicular pain, possible sensory loss, weakness, or diminished reflexes.[17] Looking at the level of the shoulders and pelvis as well as the Adam forward bending test can help identify scoliosis. Skin abnormalities such as hemangiomas, café-au-lait spots, skin dimples, or hairy patches may

TABLE 129.1	Specific Spine Injuries in Certain Sports	
Sports		**Spine Injury/Pathology**
Rowers, and male football players, offensive and defensive linemen		Disc herniation
Baseball players and swimmers, gymnasts, weightlifters		Lumbar disc degeneration
Linemen, gymnasts, weightlifters, track and field athletes, and soccer players, dance, figure skating		Isthmic spondylolisthesis, spondylolysis
Gymnastics, wrestling, volleyball, and weight lifting		Vertebral body apophyseal avulsion fracture
Joggers		Stress fracture of the lamina
Ballet dancers		Fracture of the pedicle
Ballerina		Facet stress fractures
Classic ballet, rhythmic gymnastics, swimming, throwing, and serving, single arm throwing sports		Minor spine curves, scoliosis

TABLE 129.2 Spine Injuries in Males Versus Females	
Male	**Female**
Scheuermann kyphosis	Spondylolysis in ballet, figure skating, and gymnastics
	Spondylolisthesis (higher in children of European descent than in those of African descent)
	Scoliosis
	Sacral stress fractures in long-distance runners

be associated with underlying spine abnormalities.[12] The positive straight leg raise (SLR) test is the provocation of radicular pain after 30 to 60 degrees of hip flexion while the patient is in the supine or sitting position.[18]

Pain with spine flexion can suggest injury to the anterior elements of the spine, including vertebrae fractures or muscle strain or disc disruption. Limitation of the spine forward flexion might be due to tight hamstrings. Pain with extension might indicate injury to the posterior spinal elements or SI joint.[11]

IMAGING

In the absence of red flag signs and after a thorough history and physical exam, the treatment of the athlete can be started without obtaining spine images, especially in cases of nonspecific acute low back pain.[19–22] It is very important to avoid any unnecessary radiation to young athletes.[23] Spine imaging is more appropriate when there is a history of trauma, and history of spine abnormalities or spondylolysis, or if the low back pain failed to respond to nonoperative management for 6 weeks or more.[24] Magnetic resonance imaging (MRI) is indicated in the presence of red flag signs, positive neurologic findings, history of infection or metastases, symptoms refractory to nonoperative management, and planning interventional procedures.[19,23]

DECISION-MAKING PRINCIPLES

Thoracolumbar Fractures

Thoracolumbar junction is the most common site for thoracic and lumbar spinal trauma. The most common primary force vectors responsible for spinal fractures include axial compression, lateral compression, flexion, extension, distraction, shear,

and rotation. These individual vectors or their combinations can explain most of the commonly seen spinal injuries.

Spinal Stability

Spinal stability is one of the most important treatment determining factors in case of spinal trauma. It is described in terms of mechanical spinal stability and neurologic stability. Mechanical spinal stability defines the structural integrity of the spine and its ability to resist deforming forces. The Dennis classification system[24] for three column theory is commonly used for mechanical spinal stability. Anterior column is composed of the anterior longitudinal ligament (ALL), anterior vertebral body, and anterior annulus. The middle column comprises the posterior vertebral body, posterior annulus, and posterior longitudinal ligament (PLL), while the ligamentum flavum, neural arch, facet joints/capsule, and posterior ligamentous complex constitute posterior column. Involvement of two or more columns is considered mechanically unstable and may warrant stabilization. The presence or absence of neurologic deficit defines the neurologic stability of the spine.

The Thoracolumbar Injury Classification and Severity Score (TLICS)[25] is one of the commonly used classification systems that incorporates concepts of both mechanical and neurologic stability to help guide surgical versus conservative management of spinal fractures. Three injury characteristics, including (1) morphology of injury determined by radiographic appearance, (2) integrity of the posterior ligamentous complex, and (3) neurologic status of the patient, are analyzed and scored. A total score of 5 or more is considered an indication for surgical spinal stabilization (Table 129.3).

Compression Fractures

Compression fractures, though common in the general aging population, are relatively rare in young athletes. These fractures result from axial compression force with the resultant anterior column failure. It may involve superior/inferior or both end plates or anterior cortex buckling (Fig. 129.1). These fractures are usually mechanically stable and rarely neurologically involved. Plain radiographs/CT imaging is generally sufficient, and MRI is indicated only in suspected posterior complex/neurologic involvement. The prognosis is usually favorable and may be treated with observation/bracing. Surgical stabilization may be considered only in case of severe height loss (more than 50%) and significant kyphosis (more than 30 degrees), which is suggestive of potential posterior ligamentous complex involvement and possible spinal instability.[26]

Burst Fractures

Burst fractures are a type of compression fracture related to high-energy axial loading spinal trauma that results in disruption of the posterior vertebral body cortex with retropulsion into the spinal canal (Fig. 129.2). Distinction between compression and burst fractures may be difficult on plain radiographs and CT scan can help. MRI can provide substantial information on the involvement of the posterior ligamentous complex.

These fractures may be stable or unstable and can have varying degree of neurologic involvement.[27] Considerations for surgery include neurologic and mechanical instability. Neurologic involvement may require surgical decompression and stabilization. These fractures may be amenable to bracing/surgical stabilization, depending on the stability of spinal column.

TABLE 129.3	Thoracolumbar Injury Classification and Severity Score	
Type	**Qualifiers**	**Points**
Injury Morphology		
Compression		1
Burst		2
Translational/rotational		3
Distraction		4
Integrity of Posterior Ligamentous Complex		
Intact		0
Indeterminate		2
Injured		3
Neurologic Status		
Intact		0
Nerve root		2
Cord/conus	Complete	2
	Incomplete	3
Cauda equine		3

Chance Fractures

Chance fractures are caused by flexion-distraction force vectors and involve axial compression of anterior column with transverse/distraction injury to middle/posterior columns (Fig. 129.3). Posterior column involvement could be bony or ligamentous. Ligament injuries may be evident by widening of facet joints/interspinous space on radiographs/CT. MRI is usually indicated and can identify the ligamentous involvement. These injuries are common with restrained car lap seatbelts (seatbelt fractures) and commonly associated with intra-abdominal injuries. Bony Chance fractures may be considered for bracing, while ligamentous involvement of posterior column may usually require surgical stabilization.

Fracture-Dislocations

These are highly unstable injuries caused by combination of various force vectors commonly seen in high energy trauma. All three spinal columns are involved with resultant spinal instability (Fig. 129.4). Facet joint disruption (fracture/dislocation) is associated with vertebral body translation. Spinal cord/conus with neurologic injuries is involved in 50% to 60% of these injuries. These injuries are typically both neurologically and mechanically unstable and require surgical intervention.

Extension/Extension-Distraction Injuries

These are relatively uncommon injuries and are usually seen in ankylosed spine associated with ankylosing spondylitis (AS) or diffuse idiopathic skeletal hyperostosis (DISH).

Stress Fractures

In addition to traumatic acute fractures, sudden unaccustomed increase in the training volume can cause stress fractures. Stress fractures of the spine represent 0.4% to 0.6% of all the stress fractures. Risk factors for stress fractures among athletes include low body mass index, endurance running, increase in the training intensity, and low bone mineral density.[16] Pedicle stress fracture or "pediculolysis" can happen in association with a contralateral spondylolysis.[28–30] Stress facet fractures have been reported with repetitive hyperextension activities, including gymnastics and

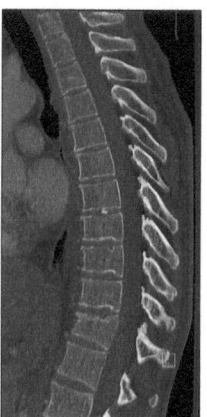

Fig. 129.1 Compression fracture.

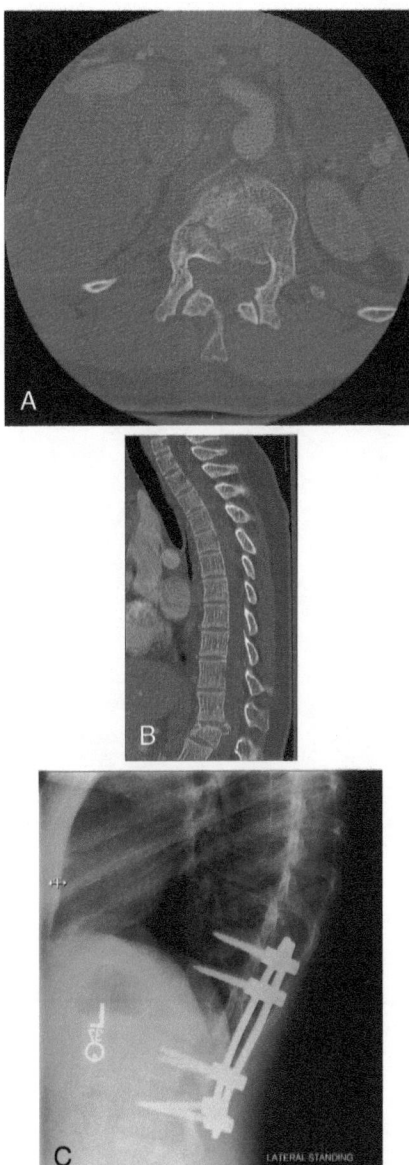

Fig. 129.2 Burst fracture. (A) and (B) Sagittal and axial computed tomography showing Burst fracture at T12. (C) Post spinal stabilization.

ballet dancing, and can usually be treated nonoperatively with rest and bracing.[16,31]

Vertebral Body Apophyseal Avulsion Fracture

Apophyseal ring fractures or limbus fractures are exclusively seen in skeletally immature adolescents. The apophyseal ring ossifies at the age of 4 to 6 and fuses to the body of the vertebrae at the age of 18. It is firmly attached to the annulus fibrosis, which is stronger than the osteocartilaginous junction. Following a compression or traction force, the apophyseal ring can be avulsed and retropulsed into the spinal canal. Apophyseal ring fractures happen at L4-L5 in more than 90% of cases.[32,33] Injuries to the apophyseal ring might happen during repetitive flexion and extension exercises. There is usually no neurologic deficit.

The flexion and extension of the spine is limited; there is paraspinal muscle spasm. Computed tomography can better delineate the retropulsed bony fragments compared with MRI. Management usually starts with rest and anti-inflammatories. In case of significant neurologic deficit, the fragment needs to be excised surgically.[12]

Strains, Sprains, and Contusions

Strains, sprains, and contusions are the diagnosis of exclusion. Sprains happen due to the stretching of the ligaments beyond their elastic limit, and strains are muscle tears due to concentric or eccentric loading. Blunt impact to the soft tissues causes contusion and might result in hematoma formation and pain. This can cause spasm and localized tenderness. Hematoma or edema

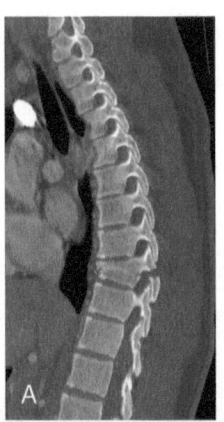

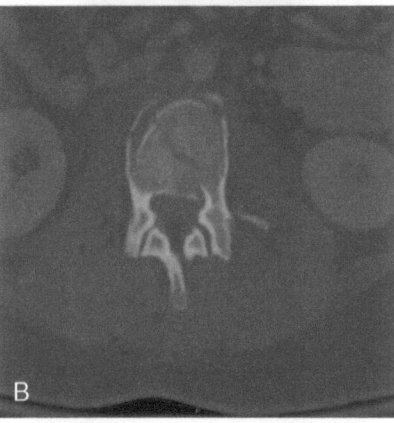

Fig. 129.3 Chance fracture. (A) and (B) Sagittal and axial views showing 3 column flexion distraction fracture.

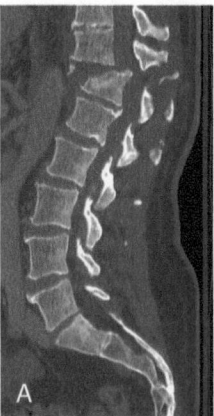

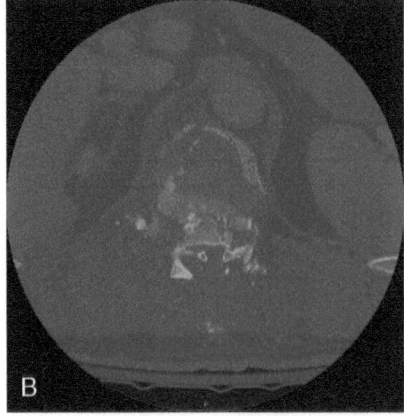

Fig. 129.4 Fracture dislocation. (A) and (B) Sagittal and axial images of fracture dislocation with severe spinal canal stenosis.

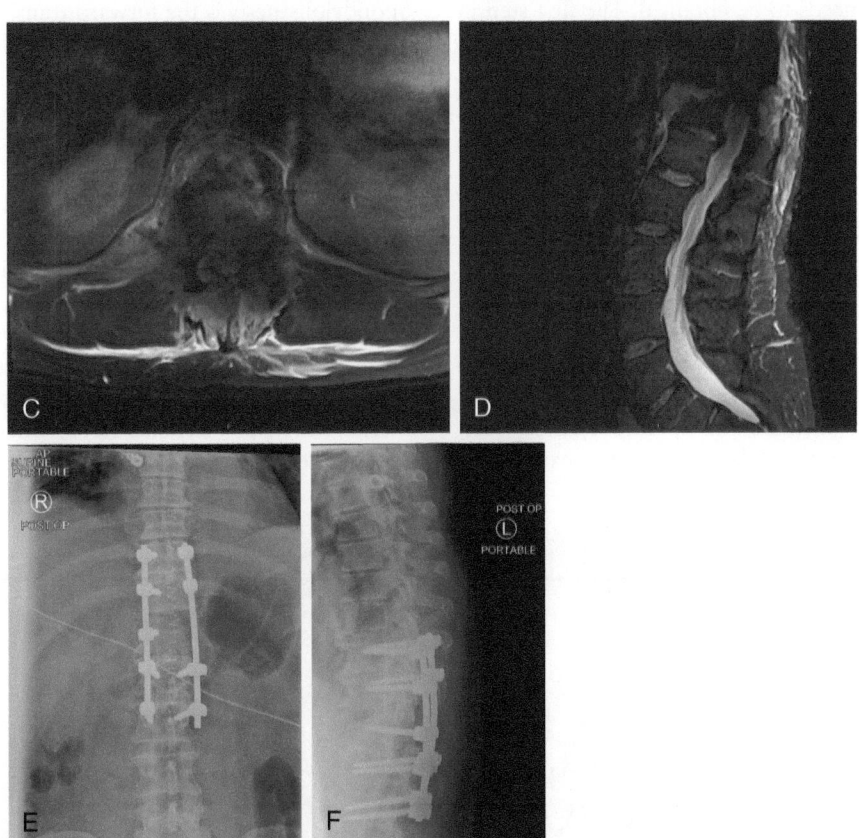

Fig. 129.4, cont'd (C) and (D) Magnetic resonance imaging images showing severe cord contusion. (E) and (F) Post spinal decompression and stabilization.

can be seen on the MRI scan. Management should start with nonsteroidal antiinflammatory drugs (NSAIDs), activity modification, and icing followed by progressive rehabilitation.[32]

Disc Herniation

Herniation of disc and subsequent impingement of the nerve roots in the lateral recess or the neural foramen can cause back pain with varying degree of radicular pain. Symptomatic disc herniations are located at L4-L5 and L5-S1 in 90% of cases.[34,35] Valsalva maneuver and coughing can increase pain. SLR can aid the diagnosis. As previously mentioned, MRI is not necessary in the acute phase of radicular symptoms with stable exam without neurologic deficit. If the symptoms are progressive or refractory, MRI needs to be obtained. The first step in treatment includes physical therapy and extension-based stabilization program, NSAIDs, and occasionally epidural steroid injections. Surgery is indicated in cases of progressive neurologic deficit, refractory pain, and cauda equina syndrome (Fig. 129.5). After regaining the full pain-free ROM of the lumbar spine, full strength in the lower extremities, and completion of a sports specific therapy, athletes may return to their previous activity.[12]

Spondylolysis

Spondylolysis (Fig. 129.6) is a defect in the pars interarticularis, which may be caused by repetitive torsion and extension of the spine and less commonly acute trauma. Spondylolysis has been seen in up to 47% of young athletes with back pain, more commonly at L5 on the left side.[8,36] Spondylolysis has equal prevalence among boys and girls; however, historically it was thought to be more common in boys.[14,37] It is more common in gymnasts and football linebackers due to repetitive hyperextension of the lumbar spine.[16]

Most common presenting symptoms include chronic refractory back pain, especially on repetitive activity and spinal extension. Neurologic symptoms including radiculopathy are not usual in the absence of associated spondylolisthesis. Incidental radiographic finding of pars defect in a completely asymptomatic athlete is also not uncommon.

Spondylolisthesis

Spondylolisthesis is the forward translation of rostral over the caudal vertebrae (Fig. 129.7). Spondylolisthesis can be classified as: dysplastic (I), isthmic (II), degenerative (III), traumatic (IV), and pathologic (V). The dysplastic type, though less common, has 32% chance of progression compared with 4% in the isthmic type.[38]

Symptoms include extension-related low back pain and pain with impact, such as during jumping. There is also decreased hamstring flexibility.[10] If spondylolisthesis causes neuroforaminal stenosis, the athlete may also complain of radicular symptoms and signs. Examination might reveal hyperlordosis of the lumbar spine, muscle spasm, hamstring tightness, and pain with extension of the spine and single-legged hyperextension test, which localizes the side of spondylolysis when the patient stands on the ipsilateral leg.[10]

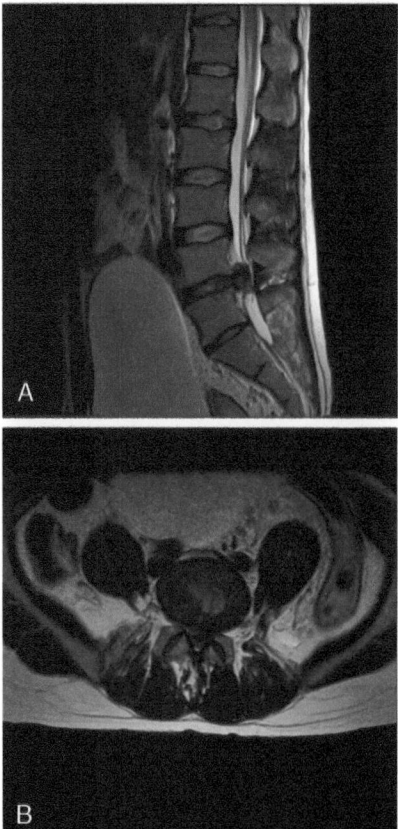

Fig. 129.5 Lumbar disc herniation. (A) and (B) L5-S1 disc herniation with severe central canal stenosis.

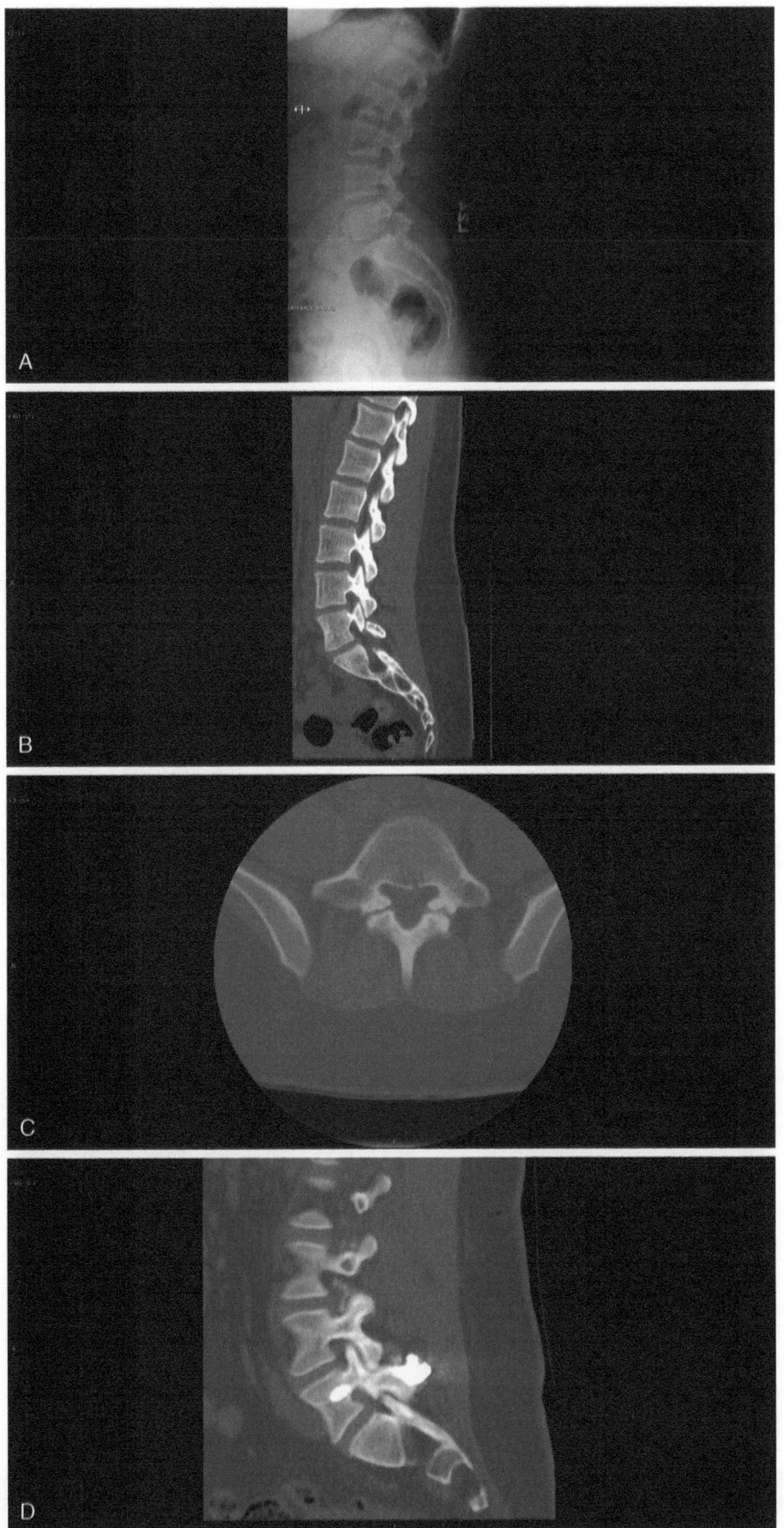

Fig. 129.6 Spondylolysis. (A) and (B) Lateral radiograph and Sagittal computed tomography (CT) images showing L5 pars defect. (C) Axial CT image. (D) Sagittal and (E) axial CT images showing healed pars defect.

Continued

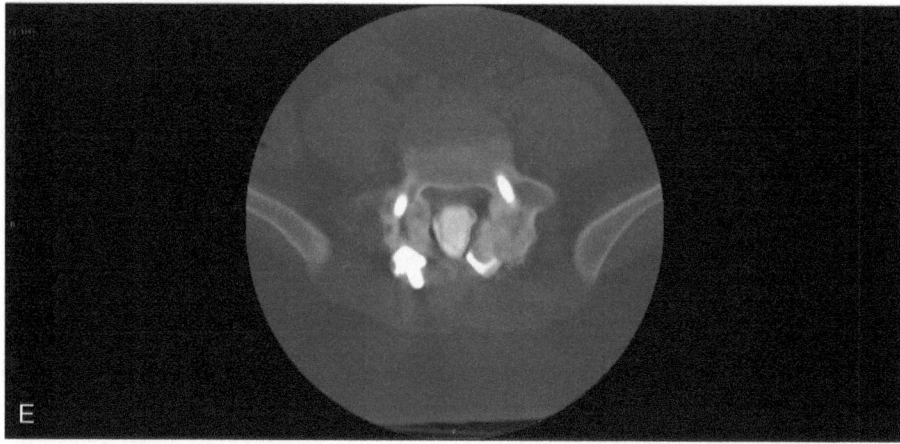

Fig. 129.6, cont'd

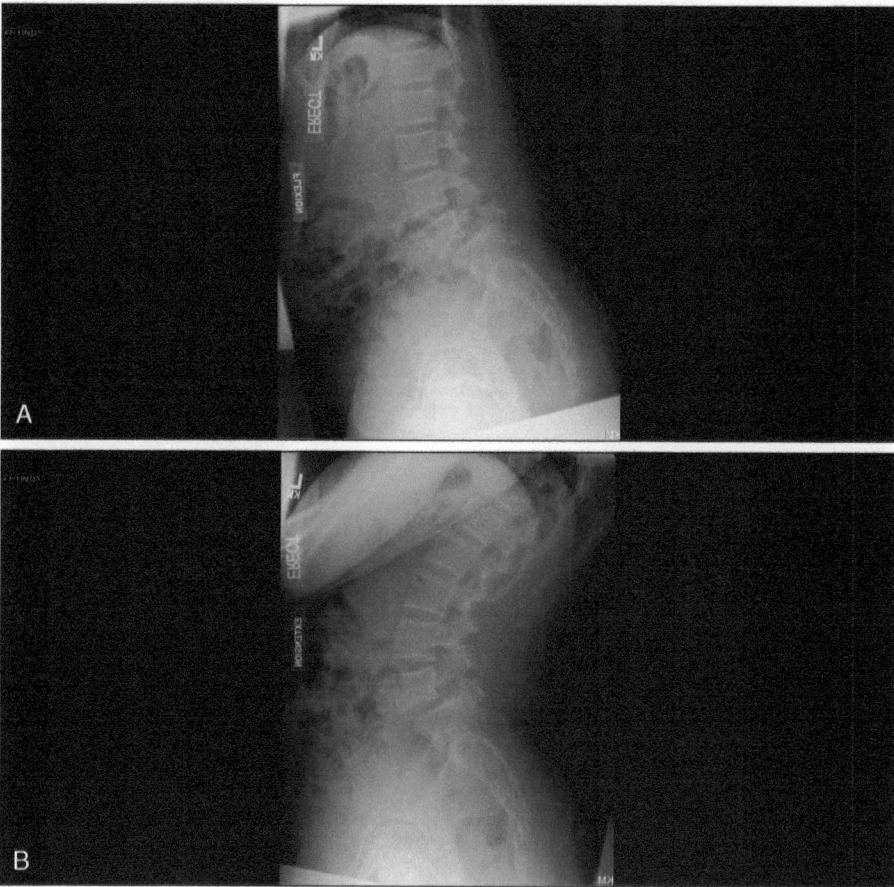

Fig. 129.7 Spondylolisthesis. (A) and (B) Flexion and extension stress images showing L5 pars defect and spondylolisthesis.

The AP view of the lumbar spine might show developmental defects such as spina bifida. The lateral view might show the lytic lesion in the pars interarticularis (see Fig. 129.6) or spondylolisthesis. The "neck of the Scottie dog" lesion is a stress reaction of the pars interarticularis on the oblique views. Because of the high amount of radiation dose, many institutions discourage the routine use of oblique views. Only one-third of the stress fractures can be seen on plain x-rays.[2] On the single-photon emission computed tomography (SPECT) bone scan, active bony lesions over shows up as an area with increased uptake. Computed tomography confirms the presence of pars interarticularis stress fracture and also can be used to monitor the healing process.[9]

Posterior Element Overuse Syndrome

Repeated extension and rotation of the spine can cause posterior element overuse syndrome, which involves musculotendinous junction, ligaments, and facet joints. It is also called *hyperlordotic low back pain*. This is the most common cause of low back pain in adolescents after spondylolysis.[2] The symptoms include pain with extension of the spine, paraspinal muscle tenderness.

Management consists of antiinflammatories and icing. Rehabilitation should start with pain-free activities, and preventing hyperextension, abdominal strengthening, antilordotic exercises, thoracolumbar, and hamstring stretches should be included in the rehabilitation regimen.[10]

Sacroiliac Joint

The SI joint pain can be a cause of low back pain in athletes, and it might radiate to the lower extremity with variable patterns. It is more commonly seen in cross-country skiers and rowers and in athletes who perform single leg stance activities like gymnastics, skating, and bowling. It can result from axial loading and rotation, direct trauma shearing forces across the joint, enthesopathy, and ligamentous injuries, scoliosis, and leg length discrepancy. SI joint pain can be due to infection, inflammation such as seronegative spondyloarthropathy, or Crohn disease. Stress fracture of the sacrum can also cause SI joint pain.[10] There are no definitive exacerbating or relieving movements that can be specifically attributed to SI joint pain. Patients usually complain of a midline back pain.[2] On exam, pain is localized to the buttock or lumbar region and worsens with spine extension. If inflammation or infection is suspected, erythrocyte sedimentation rate, C-reactive protein, rheumatoid factor, antinuclear antibody, and HLA-B27 can be obtained.[10]

Treatment Options

The myriad spinal conditions, injuries, and surgical options highlight the need to evaluate spine injuries according to each specific injury and its respective treatment modality. Activity should be limited till complete evaluation of any serious underlying injury. In the absence of red flags, unstable spine, or major trauma, most athletes respond favorably to conservative treatment. The natural course of acute low back pain is usually favorable, and the athlete should be encouraged to remain active. This will increase the likelihood of quicker recovery when compared with bedrest.[24] Most episodes of low back pain resolve in 2 to 4 weeks.[39] Biomechanical studies have shown that effective control of multifidus and transversus abdominus can increase the segmental stability of the spine. Core muscle strengthening can prevent the recurrence of low back pain.[40] This has been shown to be more effective than education and medical management for the treatment of low back pain.[39,41] Short-term outcomes have been reported from epidural steroid injections for discogenic back pain.[42,43]

The use of lumbar corsets, braces, and traction as treatment options for low back pain is not supported in the literature.[3,44] If the patient fails to respond to nonoperative management for 6 weeks, further imaging and possibly more invasive procedures like epidural injections are recommended. If surgery is delayed, it does not result in worse neurologic outcomes.[45] The recurrence rates of low back pain has been reported to be between 50% and 84% in the general population.[46–48]

Sacroiliac Joint

Treatment starts with rest, antiinflammatories, and physical therapy, as well as manipulation. Rehabilitation should target core strengthening and the lumbosacral, pelvis, and gluteal regions.[2] In case of sacral stress fracture, protected weight bearing is recommended until the pain resolves.[10] If the improvement reaches a plateau, SI joint injections can be therapeutic as well as diagnostic.[2]

Spondylolysis and Spondylolisthesis

The first line of treatment includes activity modification, physical therapy, or bracing for 3 to 6 months. The goal of physical therapy is to decrease lumbar lordosis, along with core muscle strengthening and hamstring stretching. Activities that cause pain should be avoided—especially extension activities. Strengthening of the hip flexors, hamstring, and abdominal muscles are recommended. A lumbar brace can decrease the amount of lordosis and decrease the pressure on the pars interarticularis. An example of this is the Boston brace, which is molded in 0 to 15 degrees of flexion.

RTP after nonoperative management is allowed when the patient achieves pain-free ROM of the lumbar spine. The activity needs to be gradually increased as the patient goes back to sports. If bracing was used, it should be continued until the athlete resumes full painless activity. At that point, the brace can be weaned off gradually. Nonoperative management has been shown to be successful in providing good to excellent clinical results in 78% of patients, and up to 89% of patients return to sports.[16,49–53] Unilateral lesions and half of bilateral lesions are reported to heal better; however, healing rarely occurs in chronic lesions and dysplastic spondylolisthesis. In most patients, fibrous union can provide acceptable stability.[32,54,55]

When the patient resumes full painless activity out of the brace, the spondylolysis/spondylolisthesis is considered clinically healed. The athlete should be followed every 4 to 6 months with standing lateral films on until skeletal maturity to monitor the amount of slip progression. Surgical stabilization is considered when there is more than 50% of slip, in the presence of neurologic symptoms, or in cases of persistent pain.[9] Surgical procedures include pedicle screw and hook technique, the Buck technique with translaminar screws, and spinous process or transverse process wiring.

Fractures

The guidelines for treatment of stable or unstable spine fractures in athletes are the same as nonathletes. In general, a treatment plan needs to be individualized for any spinal fracture. Immediate goals of treatment include stabilizing the spine (observation/bracing vs. surgical stabilization) while the fracture heals. Surgical indications for spine fractures include neurologic compromise due to herniated disc, hematoma or fracture fragments, or mechanical instability, including fracture dislocations.[32] For most stable fractures, after the resolution of pain and evidence of radiologic union and a period of rehabilitation, athletes can return to sports activities.[56] For incomplete cord injuries, surgical intervention in the first 24 to 72 hours provides better neurologic outcomes compared with delayed surgery.[57,58]

Compression fractures, spinous process fractures, and transverse process fractures can usually be treated with bracing/observation, and the athletes can return to full activity after complete resolution of symptoms.[59]

POSTOPERATIVE MANAGEMENT AND RETURN TO PLAY

Despite a lack of consensus and specific recommendations, there is universal agreement that athletes should be pain free, completely neurologically intact, and have full strength and ROM before returning to play after spinal injury.[59,60] Gradual resumption of activity and extended conditioning is universally recommended. Allowing the athletes to return to contact sports is an even more difficult decision.

Athletes with stable fractures can usually return to full activity after complete healing. Spinal fusions that bypass transition zones in thoracolumbar region are an absolute contraindication to participation in contact sports.[60,61] Similarly, fusions that terminate at these transition zones represent a contraindication for RTP. However, players may RTP if a fusion does not cross transitional levels and they meet general criteria.[60,61] Successful conservative or surgical treatment of lumbar disk herniation is generally well accepted for return to full contact sports. A very high successful RTP rate (up to 81%)[62] has been reported for athletes with disc herniation. RTP after 2 to 6 months is plausible for contact sports after percutaneous discectomy and microdiscectomy and 4 to 8 weeks for lighter activities such as golf.[60]

RTP after surgical treatment of spondylolysis is controversial, and formal criteria are lacking. Guidelines do not recommend return to contact sports after fusion of spondylolysis and spondylolisthesis.[60]

For a complete list of references, go to ExpertConsult.com.

SELECTED READINGS

Citation:
Huang P, Anissipour A, McGee W, et al. Return-to-play recommendations after cervical, thoracic, and lumbar spine injuries: a comprehensive review. *Sports Health.* 2016;8(1):19–25.

Level of Evidence:
IV

Summary:
Despite a lack of consensus and specific recommendations, there is universal agreement that athletes should be pain free, completely neurologically intact, and have full strength and range of motion before returning to play after spinal injury.

Citation:
Haus BM, Micheli LJ. Back pain in the pediatric and adolescent athlete. *Clin Sports Med.* 2012;31(3):423–440. doi:10.1016/j.csm.2012.03.011.

Level of Evidence:
IV

Summary:
Acute trauma or chronic overuse can contribute to the development of pain in athletes. The differential diagnosis of acute pain includes thoracolumbar fractures, acute disc herniation, muscular sprains, and apophyseal ring injuries. The overuse injuries include spondylolisthesis and spondylolysis, hyperlordotic mechanical back, and degenerative disc disease.

Citation:
Mautner KR, Huggins MJ. The young adult spine in sports. *Clin Sports Med.* 2012;31(3):453–472. doi:10.1016/j.csm.2012.03.007.

Level of Evidence:
IV

Summary:
Internal disc disruption is the most common cause of low back pain in young athletes. The natural course of acute low back pain is favorable in athletes. The focus of rehabilitation should be on core stability and strengthening of the hip girdle. Epidural steroid injections and more invasive procedures can be considered if the athlete does not respond to nonoperative management.

Citation:
Lawrence JP, Greene HS, Grauer JN. Back pain in athletes. *J Am Acad Orthop Surg.* 2006;14(13):726–735.

Level of Evidence:
IV

Summary:
Self-limiting symptoms, as opposed to persistent or recurrent symptoms, should be differentiated in athletes. Different kinds of sports place different loads on the spine and result in specific spinal pathologies. Physical conditioning can help avoid spine injuries in recreational athletes.

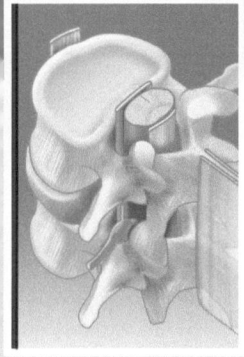

130

Degenerative Conditions of the Cervical and Thoracolumbar Spine

Gregory Grabowski, Todd M. Gilbert, Evan P. Larson, Chris A. Cornett

Degenerative conditions of the cervical, thoracic, and lumbar spine are encountered at all levels of medical referral. Because of their prevalence, all practitioners, from primary care providers to spine specialists, should possess a basic understanding of the epidemiology, pathophysiology, diagnosis, and treatment principles of these conditions. The aim of this chapter is to provide an overview of the conditions most frequently encountered by primary care and specialty physicians alike. With an understanding of these conditions, informed decisions may be made regarding their appropriate diagnosis, management, and specialty referral.

DEGENERATIVE CERVICAL SPINE

Axial Neck Pain

Cause and Epidemiology

Axial neck pain affects a significant portion of the US population. Its incidence increases with age, and multiple studies have shown a linear progression of its prevalence between the ages of 20 and 60. By the age of 65, as many as 95% of US adults suffer from some form of neck pain; in up to 10% of patients, the neck pain is severe.[1,2]

Numerous biomechanical and biochemical factors appear to contribute to the complex interplay that results in the sensation of axial neck pain. Examples include cumulative trauma, repetitive stress, and repetitive injury. Radiographic evidence of degenerative cervical spinal disease appears to contribute to neck pain, but the presence of such degeneration on imaging does not necessarily guarantee that a given patient will complain of neck pain.[3]

Cervical Motion Segment

The cervical motion segment is the basic functional unit of the cervical spine. It is composed of two adjacent cervical vertebral bodies and the intervertebral disc between them. Several soft tissue structures stabilize the cervical motion segment, including the anterior longitudinal ligament (ALL), posterior longitudinal ligament (PLL), interspinous ligament, ligamentum flavum, and the synovial capsules of the facet joints that flank the posterolateral aspect of the spinal canal bilaterally.[4]

The ALL is a strong band of the ligamentous tissue that runs along the anterior aspect of the vertebral bodies and intervertebral discs from the base of the skull to the sacrum. It functions as a primary stabilizer of the spine.[5] The PLL runs from the body of the C2 vertebra to the posterior surface of the sacrum. Its fibers coalesce with the ligamentum flavum anteriorly and the supraspinous ligament posteriorly. The multiple cervical motion segments work together to allow complex movement.[5]

Intervertebral Disks

The intervertebral discs are crucial to the normal function of the spinal unit. They are composed of a soft central nucleus pulposus, a tough, fibrous circumferential annulus fibrosus, and the two adjacent vertebral end plates on the proximal and distal aspects of the structure. Thus the disc unit provides a cushion between the two vertebrae it separates and facilitates motion between them. There are 6 cervical, 12 thoracic, and 5 lumbar intervertebral discs. The nucleus pulposus is composed of randomly oriented collagen fibrils and the proteoglycans that they bind. These molecules are hydrophilic, and the structure is composed primarily of water. Deforming forces on the structure cause it to disperse outward in various directions.[6] The annulus fibrosus is a tough, fibrous, circumferential structure. It is composed of layered collagen fibers organized in alternating directions that buffer the spinal column from complex multidirectional motions. The annulus prevents extrusion of the nucleus from between the vertebral end plates when compressive forces are applied. When prevention fails, such extrusion leads to the clinical phenomenon of a herniated intervertebral disc. The vertebral end plates are composed of hyaline cartilage and form a physical buffer between the intervertebral discs and vertebral bodies in the spinal column. Together the components of the intervertebral disc allow a complex host of movements, including axial compression, distraction, axial rotation, and lateral flexion.[6,7]

Facets

The spinal facet joints, otherwise known as apophyseal or zygapophyseal joints, are formed by the articulation between the superior articular facet of the inferior vertebra with the inferior articular facet of the superior vertebra; they are surrounded by robust synovial capsules. Each spinal motion segment contains two facet joints located between the pedicle and lamina of each respective vertebrae.[8] With their corresponding intervertebral discs, the facet joints serve a crucial role in the posterior and rotatory stability of the spinal column. As dictated by the three-column model of spinal stability, the spine is composed of three interrelated columns that form the overall structure. The anterior column is composed of the ALL and anterior two-thirds of the intervertebral discs. The middle column is composed of the posterior third of the vertebral body and disc and the PLL. The posterior column is composed of all structures posterior to the PLL. Facet joint orientation gradually transitions from coronal to sagittal alignment with progression towards the lumbar spine. Cervical facet joints are oriented at 45-degree angles in relation to the coronal plane and allow flexion, extension, lateral flexion, and rotation. Thoracic facet joints are situated at 60 degrees from the coronal plane and allow only lateral flexion and rotation. Lumbar facet joints are situated perpendicular to the coronal plane and thus allow only flexion and extension.[8]

Uncovertebral Joints

The uncovertebral joints, or Luscka joints, are found in the cervical spine between the C3 and C7 vertebrae. These joints form as a consequence of the normal degenerative changes associated with aging. The uncinate processes are superior projections found on the lateral aspect of the vertebral bodies.[9] As intervertebral joint space narrowing occurs with age, the lateral aspect of the proximal vertebral body gradually comes into contact with its corresponding uncinate process and the joint is formed. These joints are thought to serve multiple functions.[9] Because of their posterolateral location relative to the vertebral body, they provide a buffer in this region and protect adjacent structures that are at risk for disc herniation. Through a similar effect, they prevent posterior translation of the proximal vertebra relative to the distal vertebra and the associated neural injury that could ensue were this to occur.[9] Osteophytes that form as a result of uncovertebral arthrosis can have clinical implications secondary to compression of the cervical spinal nerve roots and vertebral arteries.[9]

Cervical Spondylosis
Epidemiology

Disc degeneration in the region of the cervical spine is referred to as cervical spondylosis, and it is a prevalent cause of neck pain in the aging population. It ultimately leads to a degenerative cascade that can compromise the space within the spinal canal and intervertebral foramina, and age is a strong predictor of the condition. Some 90% of men over 50 and women over 60 have evidence of cervical spinal degenerative changes on radiographic imaging (Figs. 130.1 and 130.2).[10] There is an increase in the annual incidence of degenerative changes between the cervical spinal levels of C3 and C7 up to age 50 as well as hyperosteogenesis and spinal stenosis up to age 60. After these age points the annual incidence appears to decrease. Cervical spondylosis in younger populations is generally due to prior trauma to the cervical spine.[10]

Pathoanatomy

The development of cervical spondylosis progresses in a stepwise fashion. It arises from a characteristic degenerative cycle that begins with intervertebral disc degradation. This generally leads to joint degradation, which in turn causes ligamentous changes. They then give rise to deformity and resulting kyphosis secondary to loss of disc height, with resulting load transfer to the facet joints and uncovertebral joints. This load transfer precipitates the formation of uncinate spurs and facet joint arthrosis. The

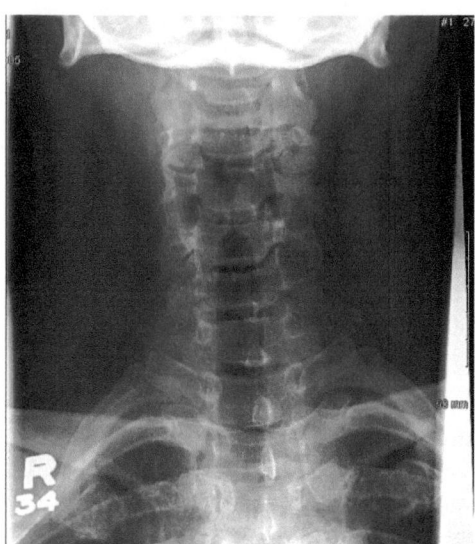

Fig. 130.1 Anteroposterior x-ray of cervical degenerative disc disease.

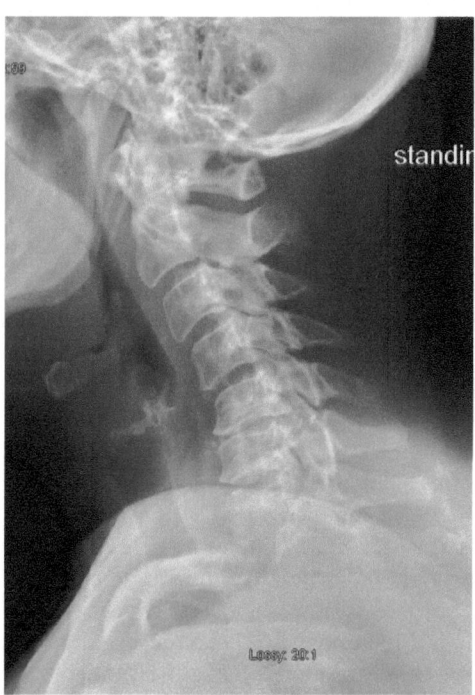

Fig. 130.2 Lateral x-ray of cervical degenerative disc disease.

cumulative effect of these actions is compression of the spinal cord and exiting nerve roots.[11]

Discogenic Pain

Discogenic pain is multifactorial. The sinuvertebral nerve, a branch of the ventral ramus, innervates the spinal meninges, intervertebral disc, and PLL, and facet joint arthrosis stimulates the dorsal primary ramus, serving as another source of pain.[12] The pain of cervical spondylosis is similar to that reported with infection or tumor but lacks concurrent constitutional symptoms such as fever, sweats, weight loss, and chills. The pain associated with infection or tumor also tends to intensify with time and lacks specific patient-reported aggravating or relieving factors.[13]

Degenerative disc disease causes pain that is worsened by physical activity and relieved by rest. It may wax and wane intermittently, but for the most part it does not become markedly worse or better over long time periods. Symptoms such as extreme unremitting pain, extremity weakness or clumsiness, and inability to perform activities of daily living are concerning for infection or tumor and should not be overlooked.[13]

Cervical Disc Herniation, Foraminal Stenosis, and Cervical Radiculopathy

There are three types of cervical disc herniation. In the first type, bulging nucleus, the annulus remains intact and the herniating nucleus pulposus merely forms an outpouching as it presses against the annulus. In the case of the extruded disc type, the nucleus pulposus herniates through the annulus but is prevented from further herniation by a competent PLL. In the sequestered type, the material of the pulposus herniates through both the annulus fibrosus and nucleus pulposus and is free within spinal canal. Classification of herniated nucleus pulposus (HNP) based on location includes central, posterolateral, and lateral disc herniation. Disc herniation can cause compression of exiting spinal nerve roots and leads to foraminal stenosis and resultant cervical radiculopathy.[18]

Stenosis within the intervertebral foramina, formed laterally by the confluence of the superior and inferior vertebrae in the cervical spine, produces a symptom complex referred to as radiculopathy. Radicular pain is commonly defined as shooting pain that travels down an affected upper or lower extremity with compression of a spinal nerve root. When present in the cervical spine, it is typically described as shooting pain that originates in the neck and travels down the arm. When the history of radicular pain is being obtained, it is crucial to determine the distribution of the pain relative to the spinal nerve root affected, as pain and weakness typically follow a dermatomal distribution.[19]

For assessment of degenerative disk disease of the spine and spinal cord or nerve root compression, x-ray and magnetic resonance imaging (MRI) are the studies of choice.[13] Although their visualization of soft tissues is limited, x-rays should always serve as the first-line imaging studies. MRI should then be obtained to better visualize the soft tissue structures associated with the spinal cord and nerve roots, and this is usually sufficient alone when operative management of degenerative cervical spinal pathology is being planned. Plain radiographs are the primary imaging studies obtained during the initial evaluation of acute symptoms, when the examiner is not necessarily considering surgery. Unless there is a history of trauma, tumor, or infection, they do not necessarily need to be ordered at the first onset of pain. Radiographs provide general information characteristic of or related to cervical spondylosis as well as indications regarding osteophyte formation, bone quality of the cervical vertebrae, and the presence of osteophytes.[13]

Computed tomography (CT) scanning of the cervical spine provides additional information regarding the bony architecture and offers better resolution of osseous structures and landmarks than MRI. It is not, however, typically required as part of an imaging workup in a patient who has failed nonsurgical management of radiculopathy.[20]

Electrophysiologic studies are used primarily in the differentiation of radicular neck pain from other neuropathies of the upper extremity. Peripheral neuropathy can exist independently or concurrently in the setting of radiculopathy and is best distinguished and characterized using these studies. In the setting of concurrent neck pain, conditions such as carpal tunnel syndrome, brachial plexitis, and ulnar neuropathy can also masquerade as radicular pain from foraminal stenosis. Electrophysiologic diagnostic studies can also aid in the diagnosis of a patient with nonspecific upper extremity complaints that do not fit clearly with findings demonstrated on other imaging studies or with expected clinical syndromes.[13]

Central Stenosis and Cervical Myelopathy

Central cervical spinal stenosis, or the narrowing of the canal through which the cervical spinal cord travels in the cervical spine, causes the clinical presentation of cervical myelopathy.[14] Central cervical stenosis can arise anteriorly through the disc, with space-occupying herniation, disc calcification encroaching upon the volume of the spinal canal, or the formation of osteophytes (Fig. 130.3). It can also arise posteriorly, with hypertrophy of the posterior longitudinal ligament or facet joints bilaterally. A combination of these phenomena, leading to circumferential narrowing and compromise of the spinal canal, also commonly occurs.[14]

Central spinal canal narrowing, if sufficiently severe, causes myelopathy. The most common myelopathic presenting symptoms include neck pain, occipital headache, extremity weakness, paresthesias, and/or clumsiness. Gait and urinary disturbances are late findings and less reliable.[15] On imaging, patients with cervical myelopathy often display bony spurs of the intervertebral disc and vertebral body end plate, kyphotic cervical spine deformity, loss of disc space height, and anterior compression secondary to

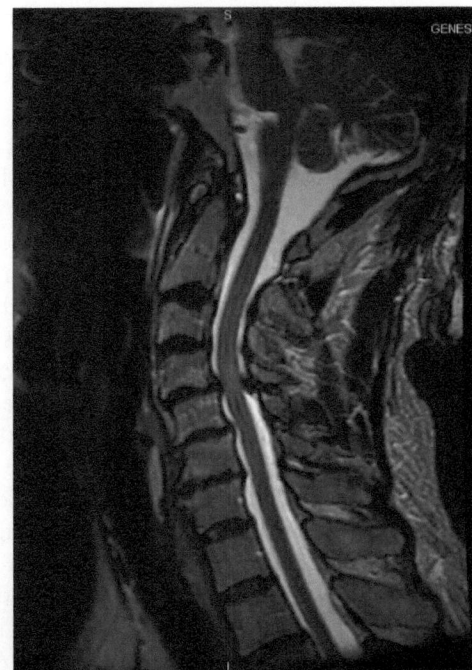

Fig. 130.3 Magnetic resonance image of cervical spinal stenosis.

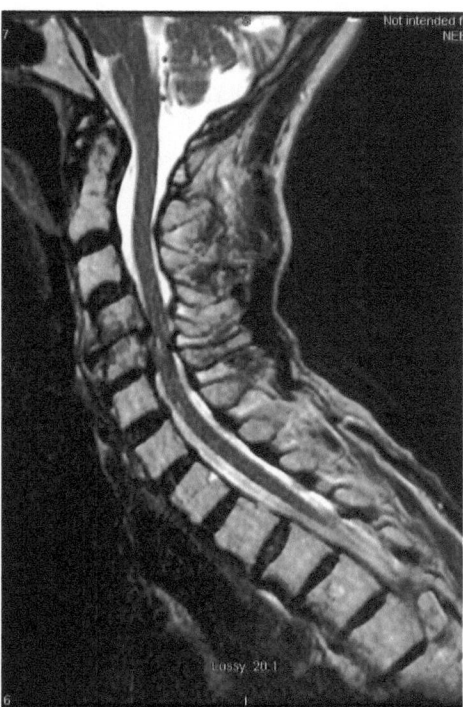

Fig. 130.4 Lateral magnetic resonance image of cervical spinal stenosis.

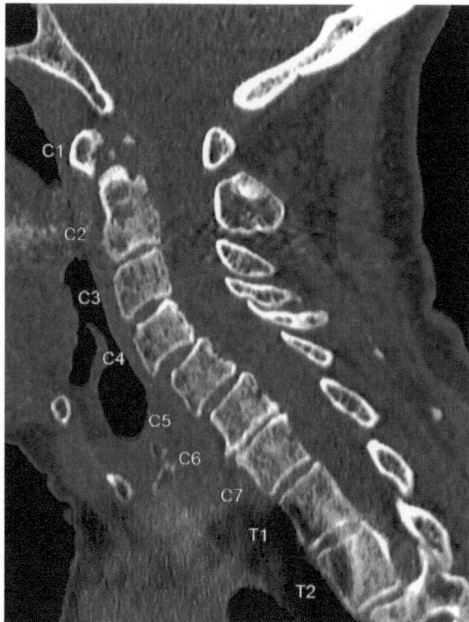

Fig. 130.5 Computed tomography image of the cervical spine.

osteophytes.[15] These changes lead not only to narrowing of the spinal canal but also to mechanical compromise of the functional spinal unit. If the unit becomes sufficiently compromised, the resulting mechanical changes can lead to ischemia and further compromise of spinal cord function (Fig. 130.4).[15]

The utilization of imaging studies is central to the diagnosis of cervical myelopathy. In the presence of clinical signs suggestive of myelopathy, imaging studies generally demonstrate a narrowed, compressed spinal canal. Sagittal canal diameter less than 10 to 13 mm, a cord compression ratio less than 0.40, and a Torg ratio of less than 0.75 are all predictive of elevated risk for presence or development of cervical spondylotic myelopathy.[16,17]

Rheumatoid Cervical Spondylitis

Rheumatoid cervical spondylitis presents in the vast majority of patients with rheumatoid arthritis (RA) and involves three patterns of instability: atlantoaxial subluxation, basilar invagination, and subaxial subluxation. Rheumatoid cervical spondylitis presents with signs and symptoms that are similar to those found in cervical myelopathy, including neck pain and stiffness, occipital headaches, and a gradual onset of weakness and loss of sensation in the extremities.[21] Physical examination of the patient with rheumatoid cervical spondylitis reveals the presence of hyperreflexia, weakness of the upper and lower extremities, and ataxia.[21] Flexion-extension radiographs are the primary imaging study obtained in the diagnosis of rheumatoid cervical spondylitis. CT imaging is obtained if surgery is being considered so as to better delineate bony anatomy, and MRI is used to evaluate the degree of spinal cord compression and identify insult to the cord.[21] Rheumatoid cervical spondylitis is treated first with nonoperative pharmacologic therapy for RA. Recent advances in the pharmacologic management of RA have led to

a decrease in the operative management of rheumatoid cervical spondylitis, but in the event that nonoperative management fails and surgical intervention becomes necessary, spinal decompression and stabilization is used to prevent further progression of neurologic deficits. Patients should be counseled prior to surgery that operative intervention may not reverse existing neurologic deficits that were present before the decompression operation was performed.[21]

Atlantoaxial subluxation is present in 50% to 80% of patients with RA and most commonly occurs as anterior subluxation of C1 on C2 (Fig. 130.5). It results when pannus formation between the dens and the ring of C1 causes destruction of the transverse ligament and dens, leading to subluxation. Posterior C1-C2 fusion is indicated if the anterior atlanto-dens interval, measured on lateral flexion-extension radiographs, is greater than 10 mm, the posterior atlanto-dens interval (space available for cord) is less than 14 mm, or there is the progressive myelopathy on clinical presentation. Occiput-C2 fusion of the posterior C1 arch is indicated when atlantoaxial subluxation is combined with basilar invagination. Resection of the C1 posterior arch may be required in this operation if the atlantoaxial subluxation is not reducible.[21]

Basilar invagination, otherwise known as superior migration of the odontoid, or SMO, occurs when the tip of the dens migrates superiorly through the foramen magnum due to erosion and bone loss between the occiput and C1/C2. It is present in 40% of RA patients and commonly presents in combination with fixed atlantoaxial subluxation. Operative fusion of C2 to the occiput is indicated with progressive cervical migration greater than 5 mm, neurologic compromise, or a cephalomedullary angle less than 135 degrees on MRI.[21]

Subaxial subluxation is present in 40% of patients with RA and, unlike atlantoaxial subluxation and basilar invagination, it commonly occurs at multiple levels within the cervical and lumbar spine. Subaxial subluxation occurs due to pannus formation and soft tissue instability of the facet joints and Luschka joints. Subluxation greater than 4 mm or 20% is often consistent with cord compression. Cervical height index, a measure of body height/width of less than 2.0 mm, is an extremely sensitive and specific value in the prediction of impending neurologic compromise. Operative posterior fusion and wiring is indicated with subaxial subluxation greater than 4 mm or 20% in the presence of persistent pain and progressive neurologic compromise.[21]

Ossified Posterior Longitudinal Ligament

Ossified posterior longitudinal ligament (OPLL) is multifactorial in etiology. It commonly occurs in patients of Southeast Asian descent, affects men more than women, and most commonly presents between C4 and C6 in the cervical spine. Factors thought to contribute to the condition include diabetes, obesity, a high-salt diet, poor calcium absorption, and mechanical stress placed on the PLL. OPLL is often asymptomatic but can commonly present with symptoms of dysphasia. Less commonly, symptoms of myelopathy may be present. Radiographs of the lateral cervical spine demonstrate OPLL, MRI demonstrates soft tissue anatomy and cord compromise, and CT demonstrates features of the cervical bony anatomy (Fig. 130.6). Nonoperative observation is indicated only in patients with mild symptoms or those who are too medically unstable to undergo surgery. In patients presenting with dynamic myelopathy, interbody fusion without decompression is indicated. In patients whose kyphotic cervical spine precludes posterior decompression, anterior corpectomy with possible OPLL resection is indicated. In patients with a lordotic spine, in which the spinal cord is allowed to separate itself from the anterior compression caused by the OPLL, posterior

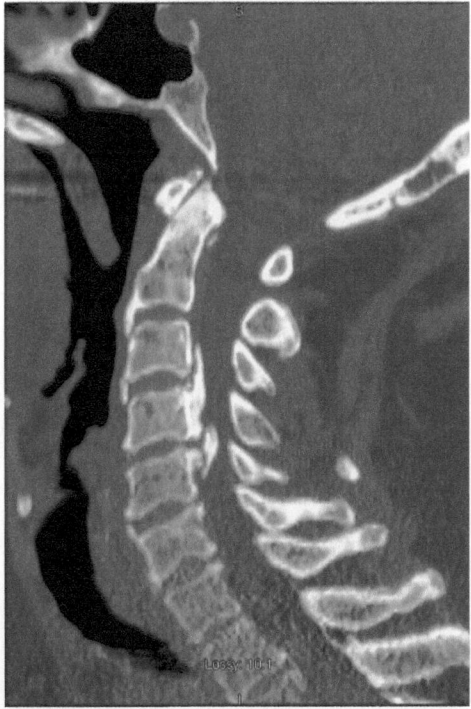

Fig. 130.6 Lateral computed tomography of an ossified posterior longitudinal ligament.

laminoplasty or laminectomy with fusion may serve to treat the condition.[22]

DEGENERATIVE THORACOLUMBAR SPINE

Degenerative Thoracic Spine

Anatomic features of the thoracic spine differ significantly from those found in the cervical spine. Vertebral body size increases progressively from T1 to T12. The diameter of the spinal canal varies considerably in this region and is most narrow at T2 and T10. The zygapophyseal joints of the thoracic spine are oriented at approximately 60 degrees from the coronal plane and allow some rotation and minimal flexion and extension to protect the ribs.[18] The pedicle walls in the thoracic spine are twice as thick medially as they are laterally; their length decreases from T1 to T4 and then increases with each more distal vertebra. The shortest pedicle, located on T4, has an average length of only 14 mm.[18,23] Thoracic spinal nerves exit the spinal column laterally through intervertebral foramina and supply sensory and motor innervation to the chest and abdominal walls; degenerative changes in this region are less likely to be clinically significant.[23]

As in the cervical spine, pathologic entities including discogenic pain, disc herniation, foraminal stenosis, radiculopathy, spinal stenosis, and myelopathy can all present in the thoracic spine as well. Owing to the presence of the chest wall and articulations with the ribs, however, the thoracic spine is inherently more stable, and the majority of these conditions present only very rarely. Of the foregoing list, only thoracic disc herniation is sufficiently clinically relevant to warrant discussion in this chapter. Although it is the most common degenerative condition of the thoracic spine, thoracic disc herniation is a somewhat unusual condition overall, accounting for only 1% of all HNP events. It most commonly presents between the fourth and sixth decades of life because, with continued desiccation, the aging disc becomes progressively less likely to herniate through the surrounding annulus fibrosis. The herniation usually involves levels of the thoracic spine from the middle region to the lower levels, with 75% of all thoracic disc herniations occurring between T8 and T12.[18]

Thoracic degenerative disc herniation has a variable presentation. Although patients most commonly report a history of axial back or chest pain, band-like thoracic or abdominal radicular pain along the course of the affected intercostal nerve is also frequently reported. With a herniation between the T2 and T5 vertebral spinal levels, arm pain is a presenting symptom. Bowel or bladder changes are present in 15% to 20% of patients with thoracic disc herniation. Symptoms of numbness, paresthesias, sensory changes, myelopathy, and paraparesis distal to the level of the lesion as well as sexual dysfunction have also been reported. Physical examination of the patient with thoracic disc herniation reveals localized midline and paraspinal tenderness, paresthesias, and dysesthesia in the affected dermatomal distribution. With resultant cord compression, symptoms of myelopathy such as weakness, hyperreflexia, clonus, and presence of a Babinski sign can be noted.[18]

Diagnostic imaging of the affected spinal region is essential. Lateral thoracic spinal radiographs may be significant for disc space narrowing and osteophyte formation, but MRI more clearly delineates the soft tissue anatomy and is thus a more useful method of imaging thoracic degenerative disc herniation. The disadvantage of MRI scanning is, ironically, its image resolution. Because of MRI's high resolution, there is an inherently high false-positive rate as well. When the majority of asymptomatic patients are imaged using MRI, thoracic disc abnormalities are noted, with frank disc herniations and cord compression present in a smaller but significant portion of those imaged. Although these findings are most certainly structurally accurate, the imaging findings are not clinically relevant in the absence of corroborating symptoms as described previously.[24,25]

As with all cases of disc herniation, regardless of presenting spinal level, a trial of nonoperative therapy is first indicated. Interventions such as activity modification and physical therapy, as well as immobilization, short-term rest, analgesia, and thoracic spinal injections may be employed; these are successful in relieving symptoms in the majority of cases. Operative discectomy, which may include possible hemicorpectomy or fusion, is indicated in the setting of an acute disc herniation and in severe cases causing stenosis severe enough to lead to myelopathy on clinical history and physical exam. In contrast to myelopathy originating from the cervical spinal levels, myelopathic signs caused by thoracic spinal pathology appear only in the lower extremities. If there is obvious progressive neurologic deterioration, the need for surgery becomes much more pressing.[18]

Degenerative Lumbar Spine
Overview of Low Back Pain

Low back pain is an extremely common problem, with a lifetime prevalence of between 50% and 80% frequently reported in the literature. Because of this, the economic and social burden of the condition in developed countries is enormous. However, despite its prevalence, the true etiologic and pathogenic factors contributing to low back pain, especially mechanical low back pain, remain poorly understood. The most common cause of low back pain is a muscle strain.[26] Other common causes include overactivity, which can cause stretching and microinjury of muscular and ligamentous fibers, or acute injury to the intervertebral discs. Risk factors for low back pain are numerous and highly variable, including obesity and smoking, lifestyle factors such as prolonged or heavy lifting or prolonged sitting, or the presence of job dissatisfaction in the clinical history.[26,27] The astute clinician should not miss red flags for a more serious cause of the condition. The use of intravenous drugs with a history of fever and chills is concerning for an infectious etiology.[27] A prior diagnosis of cancer elsewhere in the body can be indicative of vertebral metastatic disease. A history of trauma, such as a motor vehicle accident or a fall from significant height, should arouse clinical suspicion for acute fracture and prompt the appropriate diagnostic workup. Finally, a history of bowel and bladder symptoms in conjunction with numbness and tingling in the saddle region should lead to prompt evaluation with appropriate imaging modalities and subsequent decompressive surgery if the condition is diagnosed. Despite these serious causes of low back pain, the vast majority of cases are caused by non–life

threatening mechanical factors, and resolve without formal treatment within 1 year.

Lumbar Spine Anatomy

The anatomy of the lumbar region of the spine differs from that of the cervical and thoracic regions. In its normal nonpathologic alignment, an average of 60 degrees of lumbar lordosis is observed, ranging from approximately 20 to 80 degrees. The disc spaces account for the majority of this lordosis, and the L3 vertebra is the most prominent anteriorly in the lordotic curve.[28,29] The lumbar vertebral bodies are the largest in the axial spine and are accompanied by posterior arches; these are formed by pedicles and lamina, spinous processes, transverse processes, and the pars interticularis. The pars is a mass of bone unique to the superior and inferior articular facets and is the site at which spondylolysis occurs. The lumbar vertebral bodies receive their blood supply from segmental arteries, the dorsal branches of which also supply blood to the dura and posterior elements.[28,29]

Unlike those of the cervical spine, lumbar spinal nerve roots are matched to their corresponding vertebrae. Whereas a mismatch exists in the cervical spine (C6 nerve root travels under the C5 pedicle), in the lumbar spine the numbered nerve roots are matched and travel under their respective pedicles (L5 nerve root under L5 pedicle). The orientation of the nerve roots also serves to affect the clinical presentation produced when nerve roots are compressed by disc herniation.[30] Whereas the horizontal orientation of exiting cervical nerve roots leads to identical presentations with paracentral and foraminal disc herniations, the vertical orientation of lumbar spinal nerve roots produces distinct presentations depending on how far from the midline the disc herniation occurs. The spinal cord terminates in the filum terminale at approximately the level of T12; thus there is no true cord below this level. Neural impulses are instead transmitted via the cauda equina, which begins at L1 and traverses the remaining length of the spinal canal. Compression of these nerve roots, termed *cauda equina syndrome*, is a potentially devastating condition that, when discovered, warrants emergent surgical decompression and stabilization. Presenting symptoms of cauda equina syndrome include bilateral leg pain, saddle anesthesia, lower extremity sensorimotor changes, and bowel/bladder dysfunction.[30]

Discogenic Low Back Pain

Lumbar intervertebral discs are the main source of discogenic spinal pain in humans. Discogenic low back pain is a controversial condition that has only recently begun to become more widely accepted as a cause of idiopathic axial back pain. It is thought to originate from injury and resultant repair of the annulus fibrosus, and pathologic examination of discs of patients with discogenic low back pain demonstrates fissures in the annulus as well as abundant granulation tissue within these fissures that is extensively innervated.[26] Contrary to other tissue types, because of their avascular nature, the healing of intervertebral discs proceeds from the outside to the inside. With the exception of its posterior region, the normal disc is poorly innervated.[26] The posterior region of the disc receives innervation from both the sinuvertebral nerve and direct branches from the ramus communicans or the ventral ramus. Branches from the gray ramus communicans supply the lateral regions of the disc, and the anterior region is supplied by anterior discal nerves arising from the sympathetic plexus, which supplies the ALL. Sympathetic afferent fibers convey pain impulses.[26,27] A phenomenon referred to as *peripheral sensitization* occurs when mechanical stimuli that normally exert little effect on disc nociceptors can, under certain circumstances, generate a pain response that is amplified. Because of this, some damaged discs cause pain clinically and some do not.

The diagnosis of discogenic low back pain is based on clinical history and imaging modalities, which include x-ray, MRI, and provocative discography. Only about 20% of patients with low back pain have a defined pathologic or anatomic etiology that can be definitively identified. Lumbar spine radiographs are generally the first diagnostic imaging studies ordered; they may show findings consistent with disc degeneration and disc space narrowing. MRI demonstrates these findings in greater detail, showing degenerative discs without findings of stenosis or herniation.[31] Studies have shown that although provocative discography can aid in making the diagnosis, it can lead to the acceleration of disc degeneration as an increased likelihood of disc herniation, changes in the vertebral end plates, and loss of disc height over time.[32]

A trial of nonoperative management is indicated as a first-line therapeutic modality in the treatment of discogenic low back pain. Pharmacologic treatment, including analgesics, nonsteroidal antiinflammatory drugs (NSAIDs), and muscle relaxants are commonly employed, but evidence for their efficacy is lacking. Long-term treatment with narcotics is generally avoided, although there is limited evidence of its ability to allow for a small improvement in pain and function.[26] Exercise therapy via the McKenzie method is popular among physical therapists and has been shown to be slightly more effective than manipulation and as effective as strength training. If pharmacologic therapy, lifestyle modification, and exercise fail to improve symptoms, epidural steroid injections are commonly performed. Although there has been significant debate regarding the effectiveness of these injections and indication for their use, recent systematic reviews have shown that the alleviation of pain and functional relief of symptoms experienced by patients who received them were at least fair.[26] Although their mechanism of action is not completely understood, it is believed to be secondary to the generation of a neural blockade that interrupts nociceptive input, the reflexive mechanism of the afferent fibers, and the self-sustaining central pattern of pain-generating neurons. Corticosteroids also reduce inflammation by inhibiting the release of numerous inflammatory mediators and in doing so produce a local anesthetic effect. Although some authors advocate lumbar spinal fusion as a potential option for refractory discogenic low back pain, this procedure should be approached with caution, as the reported results vary considerably among studies and the rate of complications following these operations is not negligible.[26]

Lumbar Disc Herniation and Radiculopathy

The topic of lumbar disc herniation and resultant radiculopathy is enormous and large enough to compose an entire chapter or even textbook alone. The purpose of this section is not to provide an exhaustive review of the topic but rather to outline major principles of the pathophysiology, epidemiology, diagnosis, and treatment of the condition. As in the cervical and thoracolumbar regions of the spine, lumbar disc herniation occurs when the central region of the intervertebral disc, the nucleus pulposus, extrudes through the annulus fibrosus. Resultant irritation and compression of the dural sac or lumbar nerve roots leads to the clinical symptoms of lumbar radiculopathy, which is the most common reason for the performance of spinal surgery. Moreover, rates of surgical intervention have increased owing to the higher prevalence of advanced imaging and the improved safety of surgical procedures. Disc herniation occurs in all age groups but is most commonly reported in the fourth and fifth decades of life. No obvious risk factors for the development of lumbar radiculopathy have been identified, and although smoking and bearing repetitive and vibratory loads both lead to an increase in incidence of the condition, the difference they produce is small.[33]

The sciatic pain of lumbar radiculopathy is multifactorial but probably most closely related to mechanical compression of the lumbar nerve roots as a result of disc herniation, which occurs secondary to degenerative changes within the involved structures, thus weakening them and predisposing them to failure. The resultant ischemia sensitizes the nerve roots and their dural coverings to pain, and symptoms of sciatica are generated.[34] Extruded disc herniations, in which the material of the pulposus pierces through the annulus, produce higher levels of inflammatory cell infiltration. These inflammatory cells are thought to originate from the peripheral vasculature and are important for the generation of sciatic pain. Since this phenomenon is less apparent in nonextruded (contained) disc herniation, the predominant effect in contained herniation is that of simple mechanical compression. In extruded herniation, the dominant effect is that of inflammatory cell activity.[34,35]

As with most conditions of the lumbar spine, the clinical presentation of lumbar disc herniation is variable. The typical presentation begins as an initial period of low back pain that progresses to leg symptoms after approximately a week and sometimes persists further to only involve the legs. Since lumbar radiculopathy usually occurs secondary to a focal area of disc herniation, symptoms usually present unilaterally. Because of the somewhat more complex course of lumbar spinal nerves as they exit the canal, the position of lumbar disc herniation has implications for the symptom complex observed. Central (midline posterior) herniation is commonly associated only with back pain; it may, however, be associated with symptoms of cauda equina syndrome and constitute a surgical emergency.[36] Paracentral (posterolateral) herniation causes symptoms in the distribution of the distal spinal nerve root as it descends to its point of exit through the intervertebral foramen. For example, a herniation of the L4/L5 disc in this position causes symptoms in the L5 distribution. Conversely, far lateral (foraminal) herniation causes symptoms in the distribution of the proximal nerve root as it exits the foramen. In this scenario, a herniation of the L4/L5 disc causes symptoms in the L4 distribution. Physical examination must include thorough testing of all lumbar nerve root distributions for weakness and reflex abnormalities.[36]

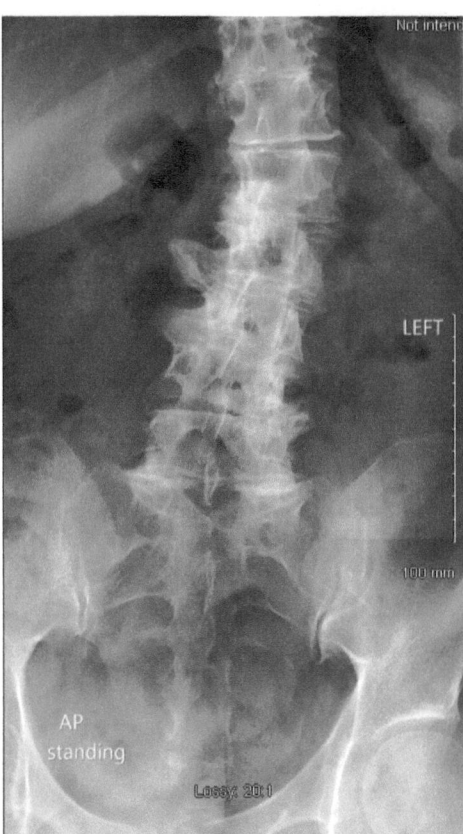

Fig. 130.7 Anteroposterior x-ray of lumbar degenerative joint disease.

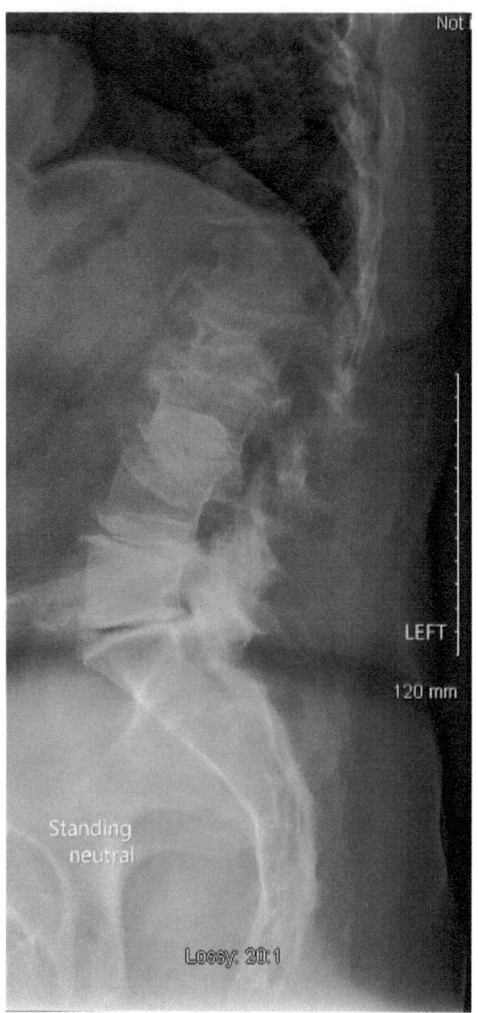

Fig. 130.8 Lateral x-ray of lumbar degenerative joint disease.

Since obtaining plain radiographs of the lumbar spine is inexpensive, radiography should be performed in all cases that require evaluation for the condition (Figs. 130.7 and 130.8). Although plain radiographs are not useful in evaluating the soft tissue elements affected by lumbar radiculopathy, they have utility in excluding other conditions that could be contributory. The primary imaging modality utilized in the evaluation of lumbar disc herniation is MRI, and the thorough assessment of the soft tissues it allows renders it indispensable in the diagnostic algorithm (Figs. 130.9 and 130.10). Lumbar disc herniations are classified on MRI according to shape. A disc herniation whose base is wider than its height from the margin of the disc is referred to as a *protrusion*, which may be focal or broad and concentric. A herniation whose base is narrower than its height is an *extrusion*. A herniation whose pulposus material has lost continuity with the disc is referred to as a *sequestration*.[37]

Because the natural history of lumbar disc herniation includes relief of symptoms over a period of 4 to 6 weeks, with 90% of patients' symptoms resolving by 3 months, the mainstay of initial therapy is conservative treatment. Conservative therapeutic modalities focus on relieving pain, increasing physical activity levels, and avoiding rest. NSAIDs are the primary medical therapy administered owing to their antiinflammatory activity. Analgesics may also be used to assist the activity of NSAIDs if patients report persistent pain.[38] Transforaminal injection of anesthetics and corticosteroids has been shown to be a safe and effective alternative to oral therapy secondary to lumbar disc herniation. In addition to analgesic and antiinflammatory medications, physiotherapy that includes gentle exercise and stretching is essential to the conservative treatment algorithm.[39]

Although most cases of lumbar disc herniation with resultant radiculopathy resolve spontaneously with conservative therapy alone, absolute and relative indications for operative management of the condition do exist. As with many conditions affecting the spinal cord, absolute indications for urgent surgical management include symptoms of cauda equina syndrome or substantial paresis on exam.[36] Relative indications for operative management include sciatica that is unresponsive to conservative therapy for at least 6 weeks or motor deficit greater than grade 3 on physical examination. Recently advocates for early surgical intervention in the literature have cited the faster return to function despite equivalent outcomes of operative management of lumbar radiculopathy and the economic favorability of surgical management due to faster return to work. Operative management of lumbar radiculopathy generally involves some form of a discectomy. Although traditional discectomy is still utilized by some surgeons, microdiscectomy and minimally invasive procedures have gained favor in recent years. Owing to the favorable results associated with microdiscectomy, both during the operation and in the long term, it is the preferred surgical technique. Aggressive removal of lumbar disc material

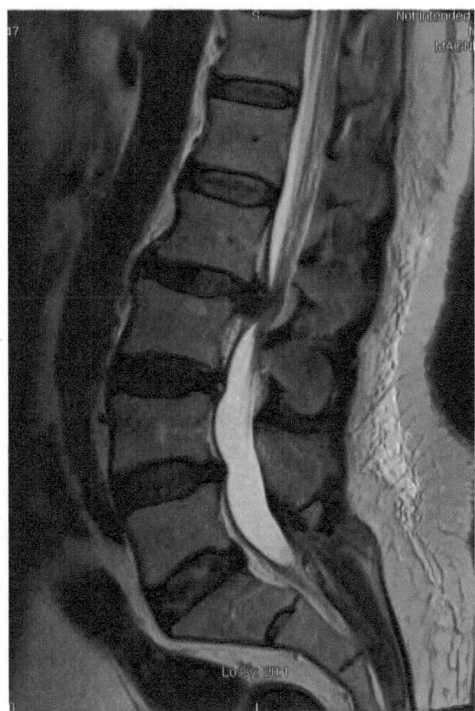

Fig. 130.9 Lumbar herniation, sagittal T2 image.

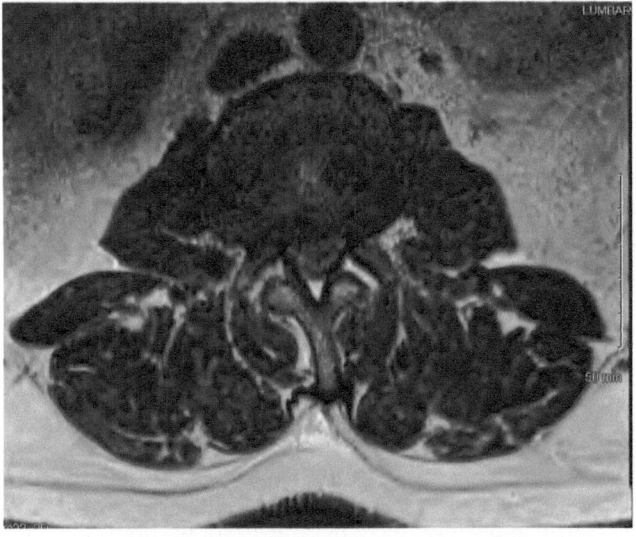

Fig. 130.10 Lumbar herniation, axial T2 image.

has been associated with a greater incidence of lumbar pain and greater acceleration of degenerative changes in the lumbar spine. Because the ligamentum flavum provides a barrier between the nerve roots, the dura mater, and the epidural fat, its preservation during the operation is thought to result in a favorable prognosis and effective formation of epidural fibrosis following the operation.[40] Arthrodesis or arthroplasty do not have a clear role in the typical operative management of disc herniation.[36]

Synovial Facet Cysts

The etiology of synovial facet cysts, cystic formations arising from the synovial lining of the posterolateral synovial joint capsules, remains unclear, but factors including spinal instability,

facet joint arthropathy, and degenerative spondylolisthesis (DS) are associated with the formation of spinal cysts. Synovial facet cysts occur predominantly in the lumbar spine. Patients with lumbar synovial facet cysts generally present in their 60s, but such cysts have been discovered in patients ranging from 28 to 94 years of age. Female:male ratios of between 1:1 and 4:1 have been reported in the literature.[41] Although the epidural growth of synovial cysts in the spinal canal and the resulting compression of neural structure causes the clinical symptoms associated with synovial facet cysts, they may also be asymptomatic incidental findings. The clinical presentation of synovial facet cysts depends on their size and relation to surrounding neural structures. In patients who do present with clinical symptoms, low back pain is the most common symptom, followed by radicular pain, sensory deficits, motor deficits, and reflex abnormalities.[42] A small minority of patients present with cauda equina, lateral recess, or spinal stenosis syndrome. Synovial cysts are lined internally with cuboid or pseudostratified columnar epithelial cells and filled with clear or straw-colored fluid. They can rarely hemorrhage and bleed into surrounding soft tissues, causing mass effect and resultant spinal cord compression.[43]

The diagnosis of symptomatic synovial facet cysts is based on clinical presentation and imaging modalities. Plain radiographic imaging does not contribute significantly to the diagnosis of synovial facet cysts, but it is important in the exclusion of other conditions such as DS and metastatic spinal disease. CT and MRI are both used routinely to characterize synovial facet cysts and to plan for their operative management. On MRI, synovial cysts appear as smooth, well-circumscribed extradural cystic masses located in close proximity to the facet joints. Because of its excellent visualization of the soft tissue elements of the lumbar spine, MRI is the diagnostic imaging modality of choice in the workup of a presumed synovial facet cyst. The appearance of synovial cysts on CT is dependent on its content and factors such as calcification, blood, inflammatory activity, and osseous structure involvement can all affect the appearance of the cyst with this modality.[44]

Owing to its mobility, the L4/L5 vertebral level is the site of presentation of a majority of synovial facet cysts. L5-S1 is considered the second most common site of development of these cystic masses, followed by L3-L4 and L2-L3. The development of synovial cysts is independent of laterality, and cysts are found equally in left- and right-sided facet joints of the lumbar spine.[42] Numerous factors have been associated with the development of these cysts, including degenerative spondylosis, spinal instability, spinal trauma, facet arthropathy, and hypermobile facet joints. DS appears to be strongly associated.[42]

Management of synovial facet cysts begins with a trial of conservative therapy. Observation, oral analgesics, physical therapy, and bracing have all been reported in the literature. After failure of conservative modalities, CT-guided needle aspiration, cyst punctures, and intra-articular corticosteroid injection may be employed. Although direct puncture of cysts by means of translaminar CT can be an effective means of temporary relief, most cysts managed by this method will recur within 6 to 12 months.[45] Steroid injections, first reported in 1985, typically yield short-term improvement in symptoms or no improvement at all, but a few series have reported acceptable long-term results.[46] In cases of intractable pain or residual neurologic deficits, surgical treatment is indicated. The specific style of surgical management depends primarily on the location, size, and involvement of surrounding structures. Surgical management involves removal of the offending cyst followed by additional spinal fusion procedures as indicated for resultant or preexisting spinal instability, listhesis, or spondylosis.[47] Outcomes following surgical management of synovial facet cysts for intractable clinical symptoms have generally been favorable, and operative management of the condition must be tailored to each individual patient based on the clinical presentation and imaging findings.[47]

Degenerative Lumbar Spinal Stenosis

Degenerative lumbar spinal stenosis (LSS) is by definition a secondary, or acquired, stenosis resulting from the cumulative effect of lumbar degenerative changes. The canal stenosis associated with the condition may result from narrowing in multiple dimensions in the axial plane, including the anteroposterior, transverse, or combined diameter.[48] Structures whose pathology can contribute to degenerative LSS include the intervertebral disc, facet joints, and ligamentum flavum. Hypertrophy of the ligamentum flavum occurs secondary to cumulative mechanical stress, most notably along the structure's dorsal aspect. Decreased disc height and facet joint hypertrophy also contribute to this process, and the cumulative effect of these processes serves to narrow the central spinal canal.[48] In addition to the slow progression of these degenerative changes, acute changes in lumbar spinal position lead to changes in the volume available for the contained neural structures. With axial loading and extension in the sagittal plane, the space within the lumbar spinal canal decreases (Fig. 130.11). Conversely, with axial distraction and flexion in the

sagittal plane, the space within the canal increases. The effects of these acute changes in position have important clinical implications in the evaluation of LSS, and questions regarding these effects should always be posed to the patient during his or her evaluation.[48]

Evaluation of a patient with presumed LSS begins with the history and physical examination. Neurogenic claudication is most commonly reported; it causes shooting pain radiating from the low back to the buttock, posterior thigh, and posterior leg. Symptoms can also include involvement of the groin and anterior thigh as well as fatigue, heaviness, weakness, and paresthesias.[49] Symptoms are most commonly reported bilaterally but can less commonly present unilaterally, and leg pain is usually the most troublesome symptom.[49]

In neurogenic claudication, flexion increases available space within the spinal canal and reduces symptoms, whereas extension reduces space and increases symptoms. Patients will typically report exacerbation of symptoms with lying flat and alleviation with lying on their side or going up stairs, which flexes the spine. They walk with a typical "simian stance," which involves slight knee and hip flexion, allowing slight flexion of the spinal canal. In vascular claudication, spinal position has no effect on symptoms, and the distance patients can walk before developing symptoms is shorter. Descending stairs does not cause pain, and pulse examination is abnormal.[50]

Radiologic imaging is helpful in the diagnosis of degenerative LSS, but it is important that the findings be correlated with the clinical history. Although there is no universally accepted definition of central, lateral recess, and foraminal stenosis, the values most commonly cited are relative spinal stenosis at a diameter of 10 to 12 mm and absolute spinal stenosis at a diameter less than 10 mm.[51] Criticisms of this method include its inability to consider the trefoil shape of the spinal canal and intrusive behavior of the ligamentum flavum and disc material in degenerative spinal stenosis.[52] Another view, proposed by Schonstrom et al., is that constrictions in cross-sectional area that leave 70 to 80 mm^2 of the spinal canal's area unconstructed would be unlikely to cause clinical symptoms consistent with cauda equina syndrome. Any degree of stenosis, however, can lead to nonurgent symptoms of nerve root compression.[53]

The treatment of degenerative LSS begins conservatively, with treatment modalities including medications, physical therapy, exercises and bracing, and epidural injections. Although conservative treatment modalities are almost always employed as the first-line therapy for this condition, there is little evidence that in the literature to guide their utilization. Commonly used medications include analgesics, NSAIDs, muscle relaxants, and opioids, each posing unique risks and challenges to their administration.[48] A course of physical therapy with comprehensive rehabilitation including manual therapy, stretching, and strengthening of the lumbar spinal musculature and hips is frequently utilized, with an emphasis on endurance exercises. Although courses involving these modalities are extremely prevalent early in the treatment course of degenerative LSS, few prospective randomized trials have evaluated their effectiveness. When medical therapy, physical therapy, and endurance training fail to alleviate symptoms, epidural corticosteroid injections are commonly employed. Although

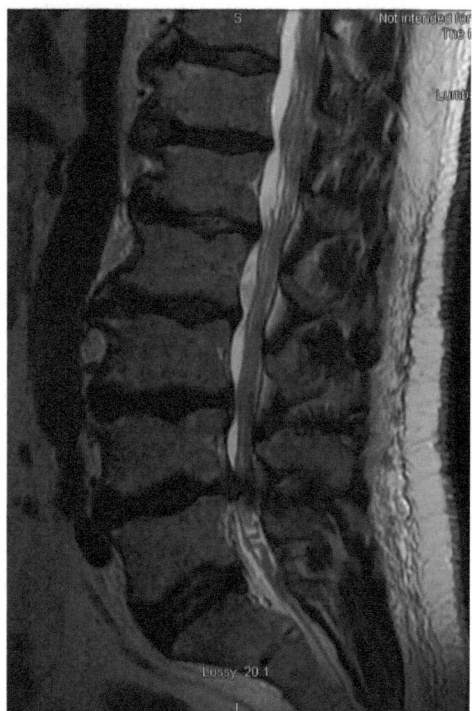

Fig. 130.11 Magnetic resonance image of lumbar spinal stenosis.

30% of epidural corticosteroid injections are performed for LSS, there are few data to support their efficacy.[48]

When conservative treatment modalities fail to relieve the pain and disability associated with degenerative LSS, surgery may be considered as a treatment option. Surgical management of LSS typically involves a decompressive laminectomy with or without concomitant fusion to address the instability thought by some surgeons to be generated during posterior element removal and canal decompression.[54] The long-term success rates of decompressive laminectomy are generally favorable, depending on the cited endpoint, ranging from 45% to 72%; two recent major studies found improvement in pain and pain/function for surgery versus nonoperative treatment, respectively.[54] When they compared unilateral laminotomy, bilateral laminotomy, and laminectomy, Thomé et al. found bilateral laminotomy to provide superior relief of back and leg pain both at rest and while walking. However, walking distance without symptom development was improved in all three groups.[55] Although serious complications and death are very rare with surgical management of degenerative LSS, they can occur. Thus as with any surgical procedure, the patient must be counseled thoroughly prior to consenting to the procedure. The true complication rate of the procedure remains largely unknown, since few large studies have reported complication rates associated with surgical management. Shared decision-making is an important component of preoperative planning, and patients must be active members of the process. Overall the outcomes of surgical management of degenerative LSS are excellent, with improvements in quality of life similar to those experienced by patients undergoing total knee arthroplasty.[54]

Degenerative Spondylolisthesis

DS is a condition in which degenerative changes in the lumbar spine cause a proximal vertebral body to slip anteriorly or posteriorly relative to the vertebral body distal to it.[56] Symptoms in DS generally develop in patients over the age of 40, and the condition causes a variable clinical presentation. In one study, a mean slip of 14% was reported, highlighting the mild degree to which DS causes anterior translation of the proximal vertebral body relative to the distal.[57] Because the neural arch remains intact, however, even a small degree of slip can generate a shear force that is substantial enough to cause cauda equina syndrome. Although the precise cause of DS is unknown, the factors most intimately related probably include (1) facet joint arthritis, leading to a loss in normal structural support; (2) stabilizing ligament malfunction, most likely secondary to hyperlaxity; and (3) poor muscular control, leading to a lack of effective secondary stabilization. These factors in concert are thought to lead to sagittal instability and resultant DS.[56] With progression of the slip, the facet joint capsules hypertrophy, the ligamentum flavum buckles, and the intervertebral discs bulge forward, further contributing to the slip. Risk factors for DS include age greater than 50, multiparity, sagittally oriented facet joints, African American ethnicity, hyperlordosis, and elevated pelvic incidence. DS occurs at L4/L5 at a rate 6 to 9 times greater than at other levels owing to the strength of the iliolumbar ligaments, which hold L5 firmly in place without stabilizing L4.[56]

As with many conditions affecting the lumbar spine, the main complaint of the patient with DS is back pain.[58] Patients typically describe the pain as intermittent and a recurring pattern of symptoms that may occur over many years. Pain is generally worse with physical activity or changes in position of the lumbar spine, and commonly worsens throughout the day. Symptoms in the legs also occur frequently and are commonly the reason patients ultimately become concerned and seek formal evaluation. Leg pain typically presents diffusely in the lower extremities, involving the distribution of the L5 and/or L4 nerve roots. A history of alternation of leg pain between the legs is a common complaint and strongly suggestive of DS.[58] When radiculopathy presents unilaterally, it is usually due to L5 compression at the level of the lateral recess. Extreme stenosis can result from DS; when it occurs, it can lead to symptoms of cauda equine syndrome. In contrast to the acute, sometimes devastating bowel and bladder symptoms caused by lumbar disc herniation, symptoms in DS are often insidious and subtle. As with all stenotic conditions of the lumbar spine, adoption of a position of flexion increases the anteroposterior diameter of the spinal canal and alleviates symptoms.[58]

The diagnosis of DS is confirmed with imaging studies. Although plain radiographs are typically sufficient to diagnose DS (Fig. 130.12), advanced imaging studies are required for preoperative planning. The essential finding on the lateral radiographic view is anterior displacement of L4 on L5 or less commonly L5 on S1 or L3 on L4, with an intact neural arch noted posteriorly.[59] Because of the intact pars interarticularis, spinous processes are visualized translated anteriorly with their

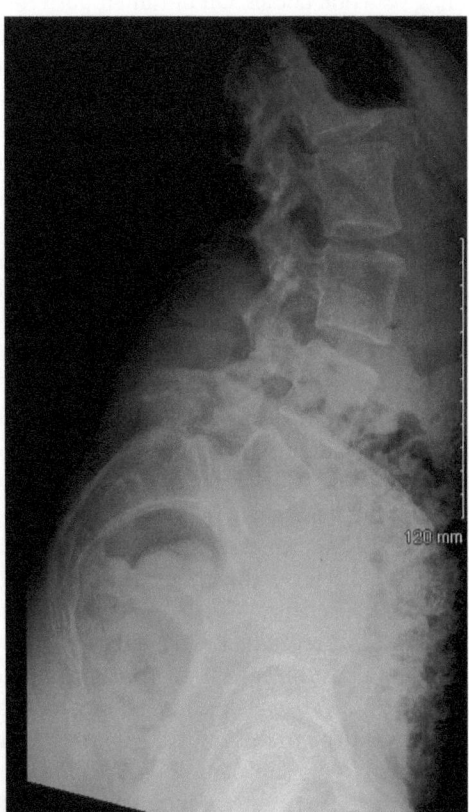

Fig. 130.12 Lumbar spondylolisthesis.

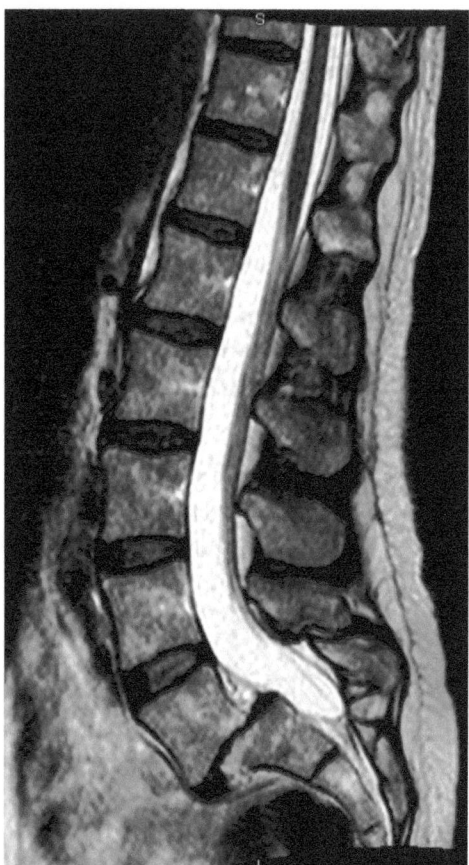

Fig. 130.13 Magnetic resonance image of lumbar spondylolisthesis.

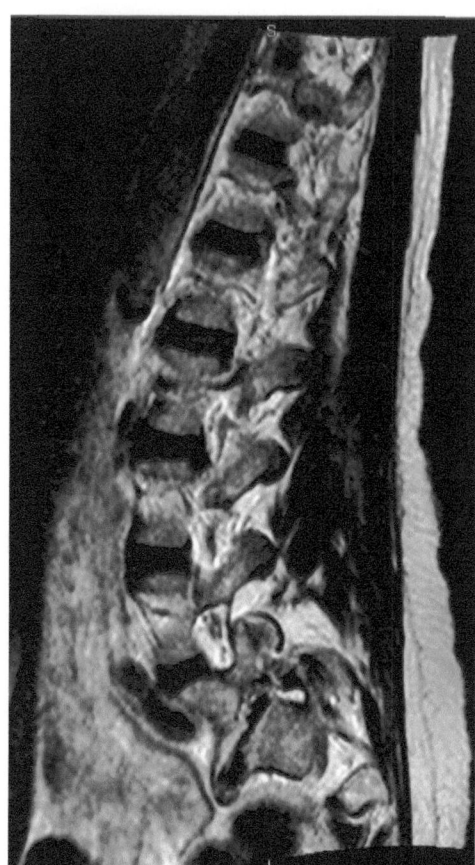

Fig. 130.14 Magnetic resonance image of spondylolisthesis foraminal stenosis.

corresponding vertebral bodies. On the anteroposterior lumbar radiograph, hemisacralization of L5 is typically noted. Generalized findings of a degenerative lumbar spinal disease are also noted, including narrowing of the disc spaces, sclerosis of the vertebral end plates, marginal peridiscal osteophytes, and hypertrophy and sclerosis of the facet joints.[59] MRI further characterizes the osseous features of DS and also demonstrates the degree to which the neural and dural soft tissues are affected (Figs. 130.13 and 130.14). MRI should be ordered for diagnostic confirmation in all but the most obvious plain radiographic cases and should always be obtained when surgical management of DS is being considered.[59]

Two methods are used to grade spondylolisthesis. The first, proposed by Meyerding, divides the superior aspect of the distal vertebra into four quadrants and grades slips I to IV based on the position of the posterior cortex of the proximal vertebral body on lateral/sagittal imaging. The second method, proposed by Taillard, is similar but expresses the slip of the proximal vertebral body on the distal vertebral body as a percentage of the total anteroposterior diameter.[60] Taillard's method is more widely accepted because of its reproducibility.[59]

The treatment algorithm of DS is similar to that of most degenerative conditions affecting the lumbar spine. Conservative treatment can usually be trialed initially. Approximately three-quarters of patients who are neurologically intact on initial presentation do not deteriorate over time; if this is the case, conservative treatment is appropriate.[61] If patients describe a

history of neurogenic claudication or have bowel or bladder symptoms on initial presentation, conservative therapy should be bypassed in favor of primary surgical management owing to poor outcomes when these patients are treated nonsurgically. Even in the presence of nonclaudicatory neurologic symptoms, a patient with low back pain and DS should be managed nonoperatively.[61] No optimal protocol has been definitively established in the literature, and although many have been proposed, most share the same basic elements. Vibert et al. described a typical protocol as 1 to 2 days of rest, a short course of antiinflammatory medications to follow, and referral to physical therapy if symptoms persist longer than 1 to 2 weeks.[62]

A complete discussion of the operative management of DS is beyond the scope of this chapter. In general, however, indications for surgical treatment of DS include (1) persistent/recurrent low back pain, leg pain, or neurogenic claudication, causing a significant diminution in quality of life and persisting despite at least 3 months of nonsurgical treatment; (2) a progressive neurologic deficit of any kind; and (3) bowel or bladder symptoms of any kind.[63] When any of these are present, surgical treatment is indicated and should be performed expeditiously. Operative management of DS generally involves posterior decompression with posterolateral fusion.[64] Reduction of the listhesis is generally deferred in favor of laminectomy, wide decompression, and foraminotomy.[64]

For a complete list of references, go to ExpertConsult.com.

Pediatric Sports Medicine

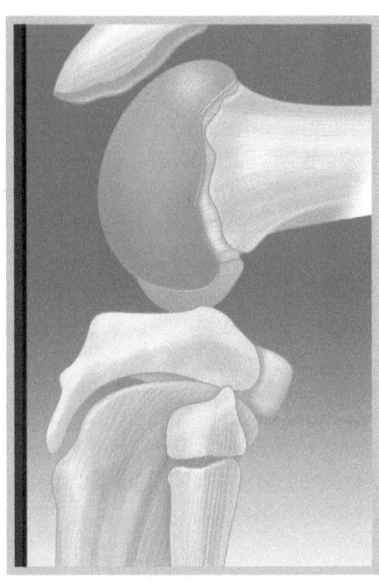

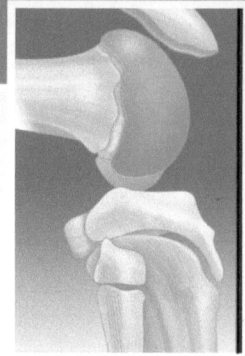

131

The Young Athlete

Benton E. Heyworth, Mininder S. Kocher

Sports injuries in pediatric and adolescent athletes are being seen with increasing frequency, due to a variety of factors, including increased participation in higher levels of intensity and competition at younger ages, increased recognition of injuries in this age group, and the advent of arthroscopy and magnetic resonance imaging (MRI). The pediatric athlete differs from the adult athlete in terms of physiology, growth, psychology, and skills. Injury patterns are specific to the age of the athlete and the sport he or she plays. An understanding of the special considerations of pediatric athletes and common injury patterns in this population is necessary for the successful management of their sports injuries.

EPIDEMIOLOGY

Pediatric Sports Participation

During the past 30 years, the number of children and adolescents participating in physical activity and team sports has significantly increased, with the largest increase among female adolescents.[1] The overall trend has shifted from the largely unstructured, unsupervised "free play" of the early 20th century to the evolution of organized and highly structured youth sports activities.[2] It is estimated that currently up to 30 million children and adolescents participate in an organized sport in the United States. In 1995, reports indicated that 15 million 5- to 14-year-olds played baseball in the United States.[3]

The Youth Risk Behavior Survey (YRBS) was a large population-based study performed throughout the 1990s that enabled accurate assessment of emerging trends in youth sports participation. Results from the 1997 survey indicated that 62% of US high school students participated in one or more sports teams, with the majority playing in a combination of both school and non-school teams.[4]

The YRBS study highlighted a number of significant demographic differences when results were compared for age, gender, and ethnicity. Although the number of girls participating in sports teams has increased fivefold during the past 30 years, a disparity continues to exist between genders according to the 1997 YRBS study.[1] Although almost 70% of male high school students participate in sports, only 53% of similarly aged female high school students exhibit the same level of sporting interest.[1,4] This gender disparity was even more dramatic among ethnic minorities, with only 40% of Hispanic and African-American girls participating compared with 62% and 71% for boys, respectively.[4]

Furthermore, progression into adolescence was also associated with a reduction in the involvement of both boys and girls in vigorous sporting activities.[1,4] In boys, participation in vigorous exercise (defined as activity causing shortness of breath, lasting at least 20 minutes, 3 days a week) reduced from 81% in grade 9 to only 67% by grade 12.[1] As expected, this trend was even more pronounced in girls, with 61% of female ninth graders participating in vigorous exercise compared with only 41% by 12th grade.[1]

The growth and increasing popularity of school and community youth sports programs have become an integral part of American youth culture and have the potential to enhance the long-term physical and psychosocial health of children and adolescents who participate in these programs.[4]

Pediatric Sports Injury

Increased youth participation in sports and physical activities and specialization in particular sports (and positions) at an earlier age have resulted in an increase in sports-related injuries as a result of trauma and overuse.[2] The annual incidence of sports injuries within the United States is estimated to be approximately 3 million, with up to 70% of those injuries resulting from youth sports activities.[3] High school athletics account for more than 2 million injuries annually, including 500,000 doctor visits and 30,000 hospitalizations.[5] More than 3.5 million children younger than the age of 14 years are treated annually for sports injuries.[5] The financial costs of managing these injuries in 1996 was well in excess of $1 billion.[3]

Pediatric sports injuries are often unique, not only in terms of the underlying pathologic findings but also with regard to the challenges in managing these injuries. Many patients participate in several teams during a given season, the rest periods between seasons are short if not nonexistent, and the demand for sporting success from parents, schools, and sporting establishments is increasing.[6]

Pediatric sports injuries can be classified according to the age of the athlete, the type of injury, and the type of sport/activity being played when the injury occurred.[7] From an epidemiologic standpoint, these classifications assist in identifying potential risk factors for injury and implementing prevention strategies and rehabilitation plans that are appropriate for the age of the patient and the sport being played.

Several studies have identified a correlation between an increased risk of sports-related injury and the increased age of the pediatric athlete.[7] A number of explanations for these findings have been postulated, including a greater opportunity for injury in the adolescent athlete because of longer game times, along with more frequent and intense practices.[7] The provision of medical assistance at many high school and college games allows increased reporting of injuries.[7] It appears that anatomic factors, such as the increased size of the athletes and the resultant increased force and speed of collisions, play an insignificant role, because the same trend was noted for both contact and noncontact sports.[7]

Sports injuries can be broadly divided into acute traumatic and overuse-type injuries according to their pathophysiologic characteristics.[7] Although many acute traumatic injuries are the result of random events, overuse injuries are often the result of entrenched training errors and therefore have greater potential for prevention.[7] The difficulty lies in identifying these overuse injuries because initially they can be only subtly disabling when compared with an immediate fall to the ground after a sprain, for example.

It is important that an injury be viewed in the context of the sport in which it occurred because an injury that may be functionally disabling for one sport may have no relevance in another sport.[7] Furthermore, it is important for physicians to recognize that time lost from sports participation is often more of a concern to athletes, their families, and their coaches than the nature of the injury itself.[7] These perceived differences in injury severity inevitably affect management programs.

Among school athletes, football has the highest rate of injury, with wrestling not far behind.[3] The rate of injury in both males and females at the high school and college levels is comparable, with the exception of knee injuries, which occur at a slightly greater rate in females at the college level.[8] Fortunately, fatal sports injuries are rare. Mueller and Cantu[9] reported 160 nontraumatic deaths in high school and college athletes in the United States between 1983 and 1993, with the primary cause being heart related; only a small number of the injuries were heat related. These investigators also reported 53 traumatic deaths from 1982 to 1992 in football players, resulting primarily from head and neck trauma.[9]

OVERUSE INJURIES AND SPORTS SPECIALIZATION

In the past several years, increased attention has been paid towards the role of sports specialization among youth athletes and the reported increase in pediatric overuse injuries. A number of overuse injuries that are unique to adolescents and preadolescents, such as apophysitis, apophyseal avulsion injuries, and physeal stress injuries, have been reported in higher numbers.[74-75] In response to such trends, the American Medical Society for Sports Medicine (AMSSM) published a position statement in 2014, in which the authors articulated modern definitions of overuse injuries, provided an evidence-based review of trends adversely affecting the musculoskeletal health of young athletes, and delineating the risk factors for pediatric sports injuries and the phenomenon of "burnout."[76] Importantly, "sports specialization" was defined as intensive, year-round training in a single sport at the exclusion of other sports. Although a systematic review of the literature related to youth sports specialization in 2016

demonstrated that historical evidence for this phenomenon was scarce, studies are rapidly emerging elucidating its adverse effects.[77] Bell and McGuine, in a series of studies on high school athletes, demonstrated a clear association between specialization and increased injury risk in adolescents.[78-80] Moreover, although specialization was shown to increase over the career of high school athletes who progressed to division 1 college athletics, early specialization was *not* shown to be a requirement for progressing to this higher level of athletic success.[81] Myer et al. described the risk factors for injury in young athletes to be year-round single-sport training, participation in more competition, decreased age-appropriate play, and involvement in individual sports that require early development of technical skills.[82]

Youth Sports Injury Prevention

With recent evidence more firmly establishing the association between injury and specialization, the focus of many authors has shifted towards identification of factors reducing injury rates.[83] For example, physicians, coaches, and parents have been targeted as critical figures in the encouragement of young athletes towards greater consideration of cross-training, engagement of multiple sports through the course of a given year, and longer periods of physical rest from specific activities. Not only will this provide for critical healing of tissues stressed by repetitive activities but also aids in the development of a greater diversity of motor skills. Periodic intervals of strength and conditioning, in place of active competition, and neuromuscular training programs are emphasized as important principles for injury prevention in the growing musculoskeletal system. For example, a number of different simple neuromuscular training programs, such as the FIFA-11 program an injury prevention program developed by a panel of international experts, with the support of the Federation Internationale de Football Association (FIFA), and other anterior cruciate ligament injury prevention programs, have been shown to decrease lower extremity injury rates and optimize performance.[84-85] Continued study on the various factors that may decrease youth injury risks—from improved equipment to thoughtfully structured approaches to training—will be essential in keeping young athletes on the field and out of physicians' offices. The STOP Sports Injuries program, a public outreach campaign sponsored by the American Orthopaedic Society for Sports Medicine (AOSSM) and designed to facilitate prevention of youth sports injuries, is emblematic of the larger transition from treatment towards avoidance of overuse-related conditions before they arise, many of which are highly preventable.[86]

EXERCISE PHYSIOLOGY

Endurance Training

The increased popularity of endurance sports such as swimming, running, rowing, and cycling among children and adolescents has heightened awareness of aerobic training as a means of maximizing performance.[10,11] The beneficial effect of aerobic training in adults is now well established, with increases in maximal oxygen uptake (Vo_2max) of up to 15% to 20% reported in the literature.[11] However, the ability to enhance the aerobic capacity of children and adolescents through endurance training remains controversial because many of the studies to date have been methodologically flawed and largely neglected adolescents.[10-14]

Although several physiologic parameters may be used to measure aerobic fitness, Vo_2max is the most commonly used in studies involving adult endurance.[10,11] The usefulness of this parameter in children has been questioned because most children fail to ever reach the plateau consistent with Vo_2max.[10,11] As a result, Vo_2max has been replaced with peak Vo_2 in pediatric endurance studies, which instead measures the highest Vo_2 level achieved prior to the point of voluntary exhaustion.[10,11]

Despite the traditional view that prepubescent children are incapable of improving their aerobic capacity through endurance training, evidence to the contrary is now emerging in the literature.[10,11] A review of 22 studies by Baquet et al.[10] demonstrated that a 5% to 6% increase in peak Vo_2 among both children and adolescents is possible with appropriate aerobic training. The ability to achieve these increases is influenced by several factors, including baseline peak Vo_2 levels, program design, maturity level, and genetics.[10,11]

The role of pubertal status on a child's ability to enhance aerobic capacity through endurance training remains unclear because of a lack of quality longitudinal data.[10,11] Early research indicated that for the same relative training intensity, greater gains in peak Vo_2 were demonstrated for circumpubertal relative to prepubertal subjects.[10,11] Two theories have been used to explain this finding: first, the existence of a so-called *maturational threshold* below which training-induced adaptations in aerobic fitness were physiologically limited, and second, the fact that the greater level of habitual activity among children maintained their Vo_2 closer to its maximum potential, making additional increases in peak Vo_2 more difficult to achieve.[10,11] Although data are limited, evidence is slowly emerging to contradict these theories as a better understanding is gained of the role of genetic, environmental, and endocrine influences.[10,11,14] High-quality longitudinal studies that document not only chronologic age but also maturity status are essential.[11]

Designing a program that incorporates appropriate levels of training duration, frequency, and intensity is essential to achieving the desired increase in aerobic capacity.[10,11,14] In their literature review, Baquet et al.[10] found that three to four 30- to 60-minute sessions per week was optimal. Interestingly, no clear relationship was found between the length of training program and peak Vo_2 improvement.[10] Training intensity is generally defined in terms of the percentage of maximal heart rate.[10,11] Several studies have confirmed that a heart rate that exceeds 80% of maximum is required to obtain significant increases in peak Vo_2.[10]

Comparison between continuous and interval training and the effect on peak Vo_2 is limited to prepubertal children.[10,14] Nine of the 16 studies reviewed by Baquet et al.[10] demonstrated a significant increase in peak Vo_2 after continuous training. However, only 3 of the 16 studies showed improvement when the heart rate was less than or equal to 80% of the maximum.[10] The implementation of continuous training among children poses difficulties with regard to compliance and motivation.[14] Interval training is not only easier to put into practice but has more consistently positive results. Programs that combine continuous and intermittent exercises make interpretation of results difficult.[10]

The increasingly competitive nature of sports has resulted in reluctance by athletes to take adequate breaks from training and performing.[15] The damaging effects of prolonged endurance training on skeletal muscle and function are well documented in the literature, as is the huge capacity of human skeletal muscle for repair and adaptation, given adequate recovery time.[15] A study by Grobler et al.[15] demonstrated that, although minor exercise-induced muscle damage is a precursor for adaptation, the reparative capacity of skeletal muscle is limited and the cumulative effects of repetitive trauma and injury to skeletal muscle may lead to reduced performance, especially in long-distance runners. Further research is needed to investigate the limits of skeletal muscle regenerative capacity after a chronic injury.[15]

Flexibility

Extremes of joint and ligament laxity have important implications for the pediatric athlete because of the increased risk of both acute traumatic and overuse-type sporting injuries, in addition to a number of degenerative orthopaedic conditions, many of which have long-term implications for sports participation and performance.[16,17]

Childhood is associated with a gradual reduction in flexibility, with the greatest loss occurring around puberty as a result of a growth-induced muscle-tendon imbalance.[18] This loss of flexibility is less pronounced in females.[18] Excessive tightness during this time of rapid growth is thought to play a major role in both acute and overuse-type injuries affecting in particular the lower back, pelvis, and knee.[17] Slight improvements in flexibility are observed after the pubertal growth spurt in both males and females until early adulthood, at which point it plateaus and then starts to decline once again.[18]

Although only 4% to 7% of the general population meets all the criteria for generalized ligament laxity, evaluation of flexibility remains an essential component of the clinical assessment of a young athlete because it enables identification of the persons at increased risk, in addition to providing invaluable information for injury prevention and rehabilitation programs.[17,19] Studies performed by Marshall and colleagues in 1980 demonstrated that increased flexibility was associated with a greater risk of sports-related injuries, particularly in sports requiring rapid change of direction or acceleration.[17]

Although several instrumented tests are available to test the flexibility of individual joints, simple screening tests such as the modified Marshall test devised in 1978 are more commonly used as a routine part of the clinical assessment of the young athlete.[17] By measuring thumb to forearm apposition, the modified Marshall test can quickly identify extremes of flexibility that warrant further, more in-depth investigation and assessment that is relevant to the athlete's given sporting interest.[17]

Strength Training

Traditionally, strength training was discouraged among the pediatric population because of the perceived risk of growth disturbances and other injuries.[16] However, research during the past 20 years has demonstrated that not only can strength training be a safe and effective component of any comprehensive fitness program, but it can also provide clear health benefits to the pediatric age group.[20-23] These benefits include improved athletic performance as a result of increased coordination, muscle strength, and power, in addition to enhancement of long-term health as a result of increased cardiorespiratory fitness, reduced risk of injury, and improved bone mineral density and blood lipid profile.[21,22,24]

Research shows that expertly tailored strength-training programs in children and adolescents are associated with increased muscle strength and performance advantages in sports such as football and weightlifting.[24] Increases in strength of 50% to 65% above baseline have been reported in the prepubescent athlete over a 2- to 3-month training period.[25] However, in the preadolescent child, this increased strength occurs in the absence of muscle hypertrophy, highlighting the role of neurogenic adaptation as the likely cause. Neurogenic adaptation refers to the recruitment of increased motor neurons that can fire with each muscle contraction.[24] Moreover, the loss of benefits after the program is discontinued for 6 weeks provides further evidence for this hypothesis.[22] In contrast, strength training during and after puberty is further enhanced by the hormonally induced increase in muscle growth that occurs in both males and females.[24]

Although the risk of injury associated with strength training is real, research shows that it is no greater than in any other sport when adult supervision is available to ensure use of proper technique and implementation of safety precautions.[22,24] Data obtained by the National Electronic Injury Surveillance System between 1991 and 1996 were used to estimate that strength training was responsible for more than 20,000 injuries annually in the group of athletes who were younger than 21 years.[26] However, the usefulness of these results is limited by the lack of distinction between competitive and recreational injuries or comments regarding the quality of the equipment being used or the presence of adult supervision.[24] Of note, 40% to 70% of the injuries were attributable to muscle strains, primarily within the lumbar area.[24] Case reports indicate that children and adolescents participating in strength training may be at risk of specific lumbar injuries, including herniated intervertebral disks, paraspinous muscle sprains, spondylolisthesis, and pars interarticularis stress fractures.[22]

Thermoregulation and Heat-Related Injuries

Even though heat-related illnesses are preventable,[27] heat stroke remains the third most common cause of exercise-related death among high school athletes in the United States after head injuries and cardiac disorders.[28]

Several physiologic characteristics unique to the pediatric population contribute to the thermoregulatory disadvantage they face in extreme climatic conditions, including increased surface area to body mass ratio, reduced sweating capacity, greater generation of metabolic heat per mass unit, and a slower rate of heat acclimatization.[27,29] A large surface area to body mass ratio is advantageous in mild to moderate climates because of the increased convective surface it provides.[28] However, in hot, humid weather, this large ratio provides a larger area for heat influx, thereby raising the core temperature and increasing the risk of heat-induced illnesses.[28] Conversely, in cold climates, enhanced

metabolic heat production and cutaneous vasoconstriction are often insufficient to overcome the heat lost from their vast surface area, particularly in cold water.[30]

Sweat glands play a central role in the pediatric athlete's ability to thermoregulate. By 3 years of age, the number of sweat glands a person shall possess is fixed.[28] Despite having a greater density of sweat glands per skin area than adults, the sweating capacity in children is restricted because of a lower sweating rate and a higher sweating threshold.[31] As a result, the ability of children to dissipate body heat by evaporation is reduced until the transition is made to an adult sweating pattern in late puberty.[27,29]

The reluctance of children to drink while engaging in prolonged exercise further exacerbates this thermoregulatory disadvantage.[32] The American Academy of Pediatrics recommends prehydration, in addition to enforced periodic drinking during the course of prolonged exercise.[27,33] Although water is readily available, flavored drinks are often easier for children to tolerate.[27] Moreover, because the risk of dehydration is even greater in children with certain diseases or conditions such as cystic fibrosis, diabetes, and anorexia, the need for optimal fluid intake during exercise is essential.[27]

PSYCHOSOCIAL ASPECTS OF SPORTS PARTICIPATION

Psychosocial Development

Participation in sports activity is associated with a large number of health benefits that can influence both physical and psychosocial well-being. The social interaction associated with sports participation is instrumental in a child's psychosocial development, including character development, self-discipline, emotion control, cooperation, empathy, and leadership skills.[31] The acquisition of new skills aids in building confidence and self-esteem.[31] It also allows children to experiment with success and failure in a low-risk environment.[34]

The YRBS study mentioned earlier in this chapter was a nationally representative study conducted throughout the 1990s by the Centers for Disease Control and Prevention. It evaluated the new trends in sports participation, with a particular focus on health behaviors.[4] The study revealed a strong positive trend between sports participation and several types of positive health behaviors in white males and females, including consumption of fruit and vegetables as part of a healthy diet, reduced levels of smoking or illegal drug use, and a reduced risk of suicide.[4] However, this trend was not found among ethnic minorities, and among Hispanics and African Americans, the risk of negative health behaviors actually increased with sports participation.[4]

Readiness for Sport

Knowledge of cognitive and motor developmental milestones and the factors that motivate children and adolescents to participate in sports is essential when designing sports activities that are both rewarding and beneficial.[31,34] Motor development is a sequential process like any other developmental milestone, and the rate of progression varies among children.[35] Participation in most sports requires fundamental motor skills such as kicking, throwing, running, jumping, and catching.[35] Most children acquire these skills through informal "play," but mastery often requires more formal instruction and repetition.[35] Although this process of acquisition and mastery can potentially be accelerated through intensive instruction and practice, research shows that it rarely speeds up motor development or leads to enhanced athletic performance.[35]

The principal motivating factors for young children to participate in sports activities are fun and enjoyment.[31] For an activity to be viewed as enjoyable, it must include a certain level of excitement but ultimately a sense of personal achievement associated with the improvement or mastery of specific skills.[31] We must acknowledge that, although virtually all children have the ability to acquire new motor skills, the ease of acquisition and degree of mastery may vary among children.[34] Research has shown that children who feel less competent with one particular skill are less likely to continue with that sport in the long term.[34] Therefore it is important that young children be exposed to a range of sports that challenge and enable them to acquire a variety of fundamental motor skills.[34]

Progression into adolescence is not only associated with a number of physical changes resulting from the pubertal growth spurt but also a shift in the motivational factors influencing sports participation.[31,34] Cognitive and motor development is now sufficient to allow for the incorporation of strategy into sports such as football or basketball.[35] The need for fun and excitement is overtaken by social factors such as interaction with friends and physical appearance, although mastery of skills remains important.[31,35] Differing rates of progression through puberty can result in inequality within and between genders.[35] Persons who experience earlier growth spurts may be temporarily taller, heavier, and stronger, which often leads to unrealistic expectations because of the erroneous conclusion that they are destined to become better athletes than their less mature peers.[35]

Adult Involvement

The level of adult involvement has increased significantly with the evolution of organized youth sports. Although the traditional role of "supervisor" still exists, the nature of adult involvement in youth sports has also evolved. An increased level of sophistication has developed as a result of the advent of specialized coaches, sports psychologists, nutritionists, and personal trainers, all of which undoubtedly affect the psychosocial development of the young athlete.

Adults are vital for the enforcement of rules and the creation of a safe, controlled environment in which to impart their knowledge and assist children and adolescents in the acquisition of new skills and the development of appropriate attitudes regarding sports.[27,28] However, the involvement of adults in sports activities can also have a detrimental impact on psychosocial development through the expression of negative and unsportsmanlike behavior, negative reinforcement, and the enforcement of demands and expectations that exceed the child's abilities.[31,34,87]

In the early years of life, parental influence is instrumental in the development of lifelong core values and attitudes.[31] By 12 years of age, a child's attitudes to winning are already well established and often directly reflect the values held by their parents.[31] These values and attitudes are often acquired through observation of parental behavior, and although extreme parental behavior is rare, the use of negative comments or reinforcements is frequent.[31] Variation was found between sporting codes, with the greatest incidence of extreme parental behavior occurring in soccer and rugby.[31] Children of relaxed and supportive parents who positively reinforce their child's performance are not only more self-confident but are more likely to be successful athletes.[31,34]

As the child progresses to adolescence, the role of parents starts to diminish as the role of the coach increases.[31] Through the provision of feedback and reinforcement, coaches have a large impact on the confidence and self-perception of the young athlete.[31]

The increasingly competitive nature of sports has led to a shift in goals that are largely adult-oriented and focus on winning at any cost.[3] Competitive behaviors start to emerge at 3 to 4 years of age, and the potential exists to either enhance or exploit this trait through the use of sports.[31] The danger arises when the demands and expectations placed on young athletes by their parents or coaches exceed their abilities.[31] This phenomenon can result in the development of unhealthy competitive behavior with serious antisocial interpersonal consequences or even problems such as burnout and chronic stress.[31,36]

NUTRITION

The nutritional concerns of the pediatric athlete are complex and unique compared with those of their adult counterparts because they involve the interaction between normal growth and development and the optimization of athletic performance.[37,38]

During the 1980s it was erroneously believed that leanness correlated with enhanced athletic performance as a result of studies that demonstrated a positive correlation between running performance and percentage of body fat.[39] Not only is scientific evidence lacking to prove that weight reduction alone improves athletic performance, but in fact deliberate caloric restriction in children and adolescents is likely to have detrimental implications, not only for their athletic performance but also for their growth and development and general health.[39] Unfortunately, these erroneous beliefs are often perpetuated nowadays by coaches who have little or usually no training in nutrition for athletes.[39] The employment of school-based coaches is often dependent on the success of their teams, and controlling an athlete's weight is often the easiest parameter by which a coach can try to ensure athletic success.[39] In fact, by reducing fat in the diet, it is possible that essential sources of protein and minerals and vitamins such as calcium, magnesium iron, zinc, B$_{12}$, and other fat-soluble vitamins that are critical for growth also may be eliminated from the diet.[38]

Diet should play an integral role in any comprehensive training program, with specific attention to energy requirements, including appropriate combinations of protein, carbohydrates, fat, vitamins, and minerals.[38] These requirements are often subject to large interindividual variation not only between sporting codes but often within a given sport.[38]

Results of the YRBS study in the 1990s confirmed that children and adolescents involved in regular sporting activities not only maintain healthier diets including greater amounts of fruit and vegetables but are often less concerned with caloric intake and energy balance.[4] For young athletes, the energy requirements must be sufficient to ensure normal growth and development but must also provide the additional calories to account for physical training.[38] The recommendations for estimated energy requirements in young athletes set by the Food and Nutrition Board are based on age, height, weight, and physical activity classification.[38]

Protein is an essential part of a young athlete's diet because it is required to build amino acids necessary for the growth and development of lean body mass and healthy bones but also as an alternative to carbohydrates as a source of energy.[38] Research is lacking regarding the recommended daily protein intake for young athletes.[38] Twelve percent to 15% of the dietary energy of adults should come from protein; however, the energy demands of children are greater, especially when they are involved in competitive, intensive training during periods of rapid growth.[38]

Research shows that children and adolescents up to the age of 13 to 15 years have restricted glycolytic capacity, which calls into question the role of high-carbohydrate diets for younger children.[38] Regardless, nutritionists recommend that at least 50% of a young athlete's diet consist of carbohydrate because of the importance of this energy source during high-intensity training.[39] A significant amount of research is needed with regard to the optimal nutrition of the pediatric athlete.

PERFORMANCE-ENHANCING SUBSTANCES

The use of performance-enhancing substances is increasing among children and adolescents as a result of media exposure, the availability of so-called *natural supplements*, the absence of formal drug testing in schools, and the increasingly competitive nature of youth sports.[40] Pediatric athletes are at high risk because of increased susceptibility to societal pressures at a time where they are often dealing with complex developmental and psychosocial changes.

The term *ergogenic* is derived from the Greek "to make work" and refers to the inherent ability of many substances to enhance athletic power and/or endurance.[40] In many cases, the ergogenic effects of a substance are actually secondary to their intended use.[40] It is therefore essential that physicians dealing with athletes, especially those competing in high-level sports, have a working knowledge of substances that contain ergogenic properties, because inappropriate prescribing/counseling may result in the disqualification of an athlete from a competition.[41]

Anabolic-Androgenic Steroids

Although a wide range of performance-enhancing substances are available in the United States, anabolic-androgenic steroids are by far the most publicized and intensely studied. Anabolic-androgenic steroids are a synthetic analog of the male hormone testosterone, and their use in the pediatric athlete for both performance and enhancement of the physique has been documented in the medical literature for well over 20 years.[40] The use of androgenic steroids is widespread; an estimated 4% to 12% of male adolescents and 0.5% to 2% of female adolescents used anabolic-androgenic steroids in the 1990s even though they were banned by almost every major athletic governing body.[41,88]

As the name suggests, anabolic-androgenic steroids have both masculinizing and tissue-building effects, and thus when they are used in conjunction with adequate strength training and proper diet, they have the ability to increase muscle size and strength, enabling high-intensity workouts and possibly even a reduced recovery time after workouts.[40] As a result, athletes who are attracted to the substance tend to be those whose sport requires strength (such as weightlifters, throwers, and football players) or frequent, high-intensity workouts (such as swimmers and runners).[40]

Research conducted by Kindlundh et al.[90] in 1999 demonstrated a significant correlation between the use of anabolic-androgenic steroids in adolescents and the abuse of other common drugs such as alcohol, tobacco, cannabis, and opioids.

Although the perceived performance-enhancing benefits appear high, the adverse effects of using anabolic-androgenic steroids are extensive and often irreversible.[40] In addition to the personality changes and psychological problems that are associated with steroid use, premature closure of epiphyseal plates with subsequent linear growth arrest, irreversible alopecia, gynecomastia, and acne and irreversible masculinization of secondary sexual characteristics in females are just a few of the more dramatic and often psychologically devastating adverse effects of anabolic-androgenic steroids.[40,42]

Regulation of Performance-Enhancing Substances

Drug testing is both time consuming and expensive, making the widespread testing of young athletes virtually impossible.[32] Nonetheless, many schools and youth organizations have implemented voluntary drug testing, which has a dual benefit of identifying and assisting athletes with abuse problems and reducing the peer pressure to use drugs.[30]

With the introduction of the Dietary Supplement Health and Education Act in 1994, the role of the Food and Drug Administration in regulating "natural supplements" was eliminated.[15] Since that time, "natural agents" such as creatinine, androstenedione, and dehydroepiandrosterone (DHEA) have been widely accessible via health stores and the internet.[15] This accessibility results in an erroneous perception that these substances are "safe," even though the absence of regulatory control eliminates any legal requirement of manufacturers to declare all active ingredients and potential interactions and fully test their products for short- and long-term effects.[30]

The use of performance-enhancing drugs among athletes of any age is unethical, unhealthy, and potentially life threatening.[32] As physicians we have a responsibility to acquire and impart factual knowledge to young athletes who are contemplating the use of these substances. Although the effectiveness of using scare tactics that emphasize the negative effects of substance use has been questioned, a clear role exists for positive counseling with regard to healthy alternatives such as strength training and conditioning, nutrition, and skill acquisition through coaching and camps.[32]

ARTHROSCOPY IN CHILDREN

The use of arthroscopy in the pediatric and adolescent population has dramatically expanded during the past decade as a result of increased youth participation in sport and the subsequent rise in sports-related injuries.[6] With the advent of smaller, more sophisticated arthroscopic instruments during the past decade, the major obstacle to the application of arthroscopy in children was overcome.[6] In fact, after extensive experience, Gross[43] noted that despite the difference in joint size, basic techniques of arthroscopy are largely the same in both children and adults. At present, arthroscopy is indicated in the management of shoulder, elbow, wrist, hip, knee, and ankle injuries within the pediatric population.[6] Advantages of arthroscopy in this population include reduced postoperative morbidity, smaller incisions, more rapid return to activities, decreased inflammatory response, and improved visualization of joint structures.[6]

Shoulder injuries in the pediatric athlete include acute fractures, overuse injuries such as little league shoulder (Fig. 131.1), and shoulder instability (Fig. 131.2). Most major shoulder injuries requiring arthroscopy are related to instability and can be divided into two descriptive groups: traumatic anterior instability and multidirectional instability.[4,6,38-41,43-51]

The incidence of elbow injuries continues to increase as a result of the growing popularity of youth sports. Many of the elbow injuries are repetitive, overuse-type injuries, such as osteochondritis dissecans (OCD), which is prevalent in athletes who participate in baseball, racket sports, and gymnastics.[52] In fact, "little league elbow" is now an accepted term for a common overuse injury in young throwing athletes, with etiologies including a fragmented medial epicondyle (Fig. 131.3), OCD (Figs. 131.4 and 131.5), ulnar hypertrophy, and medial epicondylitis.[49,52-54]

Wrist arthroscopy is not a commonly practiced treatment modality among pediatric and adolescent patients because many injuries achieve successful healing nonoperatively and because of the restricted size of the joint space.[54] Kocher et al.[55] noted an increasing incidence of repetitive use–type injuries such as triangular fibrocartilage injuries (Fig. 131.6), and they believe that arthroscopy is indicated for débridement or determination

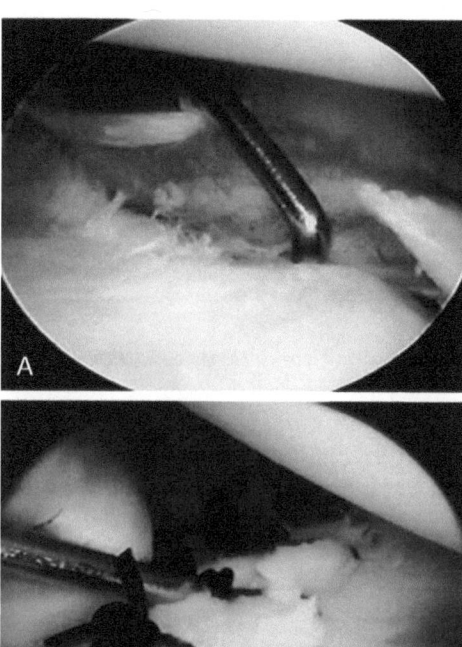

Fig. 131.2 Traumatic anterior shoulder instability. (A) Bankart lesion. (B) Repair of a Bankart lesion.

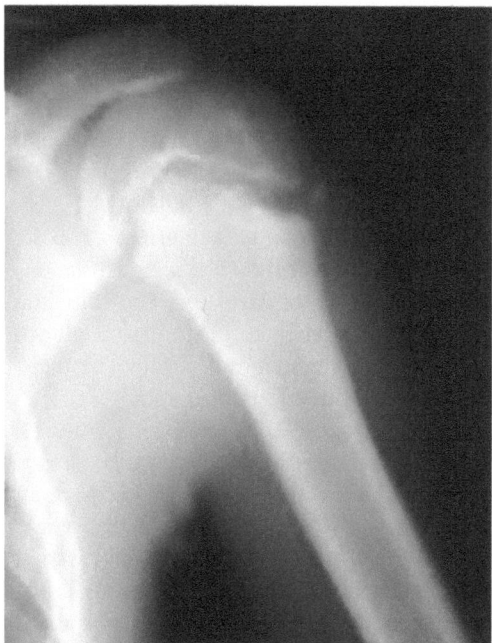

Fig. 131.1 An example of "little league shoulder," which is associated with widening of the proximal humeral physis as a result of repetitive overuse.

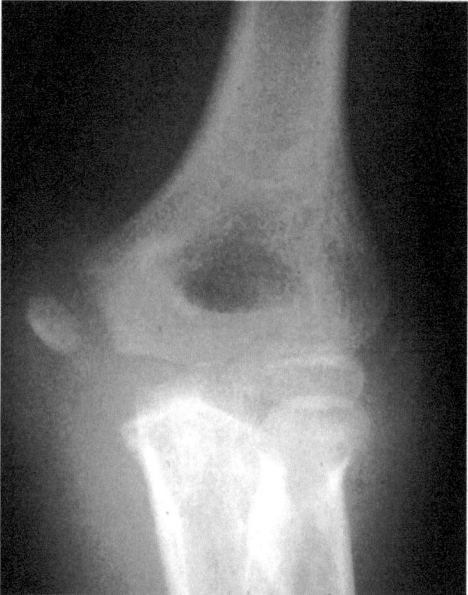

Fig. 131.3 Medial epicondyle widening associated with "little league elbow."

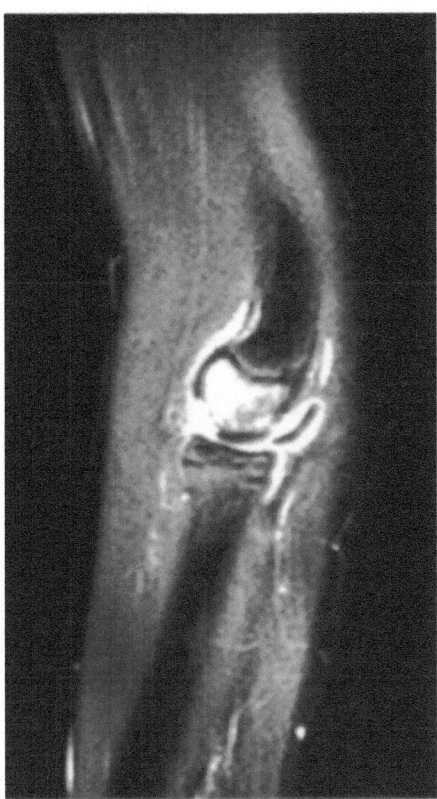

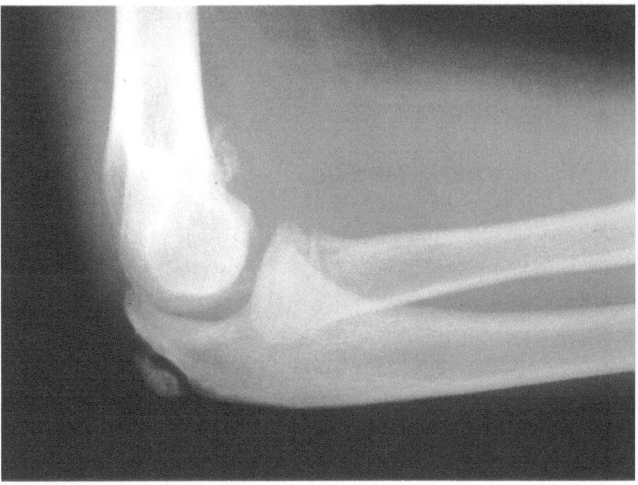

Fig. 131.5 A lateral radiograph of the elbow demonstrating a loose body in the anterior elbow.

Fig. 131.4 A sagittal magnetic resonance imaging scan of the elbow demonstrating a chondral defect of the capitellum associated with osteochondritis dissecans.

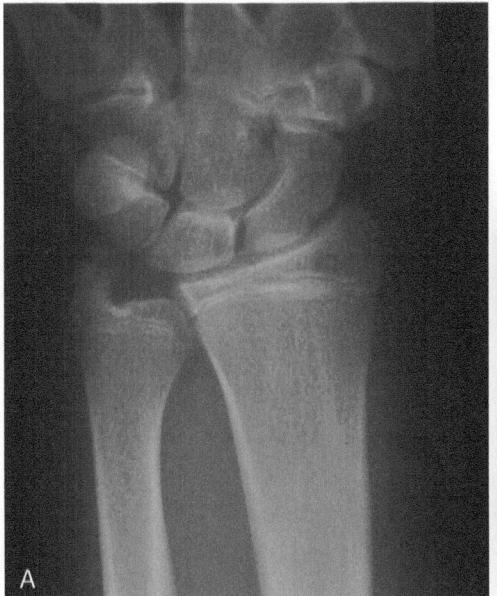

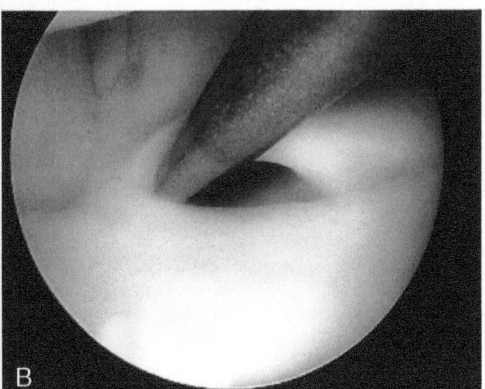

Fig. 131.6 An ulnar styloid fracture (A) associated with a triangular fibrocartilage tear (B).

of the extent of ligamentous injury in patients who fail to respond to nonoperative therapies.[55,56]

Although hip arthroscopy is a commonly used diagnostic and treatment modality for pathologic conditions of the hip in the adult population, its application in the pediatric population is just beginning to increase. Indications in the pediatric population include isolated labral tears (Fig. 131.7), loose bodies, chondral injuries, and internal derangement associated with Perthes disease and epiphyseal dysplasias.[57-60] The risk of complications, although small, does exist and includes pudendal nerve irritation and recurrent injury.[6]

Currently the largest application of arthroscopy in the pediatric and adolescent population is in the treatment of knee disease and is directly attributable to increased athletic activity.[43] Key indications for knee arthroscopy include OCD (Figs. 131.8 and 131.9), discoid meniscus, tibial spine fractures (Figs. 131.10 and 131.11), and partial and complete anterior cruciate ligament tears.[61-69]

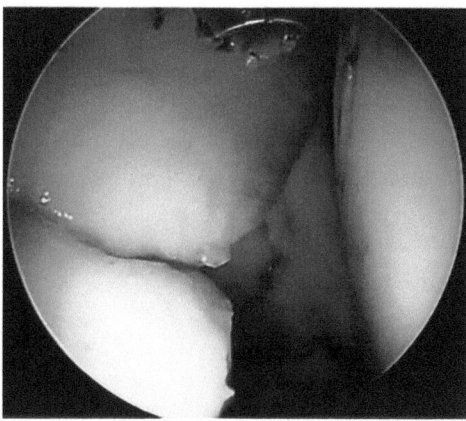

Fig. 131.7 A radial labral tear of the hip.

As more knee arthroscopy procedures are being performed on children and adolescents, additional investigations into the safety of such procedures have been performed. For example, venous thromboembolic events (VTEs), such as deep venous thrombosis (DVT) and pulmonary embolus (PE), which were previously thought to be exceedingly rare, have recently been reported in small series. One study from a high-volume pediatric hospital described a series of seven adolescent patients who developed symptomatic VTEs.[89] Interestingly, all patients had one or more risk factor, such as oral contraceptive use, smoking, obesity, or a concomitant open procedure at the time of arthroscopy, suggesting that perhaps select adolescents should undergo some form of DVT prophylaxis in the perioperative period. Given the rising volume of pediatric sports medicine surgeries, this remains an important area of future research to facilitate more definitive guidelines or recommendations.

Currently, the use of ankle arthroscopy in the pediatric population is restricted to a small number of conditions, including OCD, loose body removal, and triplane fracture repair, because of technical challenges resulting from the size of the joint and the risk of neurovascular damage.[43,70-73]

CONCLUSIONS

Pediatric sports injuries are being seen with increased frequency. Just as the child is not a "little adult," the pediatric athlete is not a "little adult athlete." An understanding of the unique considerations of the pediatric athlete with respect to epidemiologic factors, endurance, flexibility, strength, thermoregulation, psychology, and nutrition is important background knowledge. Recognition of common injury patterns of the shoulder, elbow, wrist, hip, knee, and ankle is essential to effective management.

For a complete list of references, go to ExpertConsult.com.

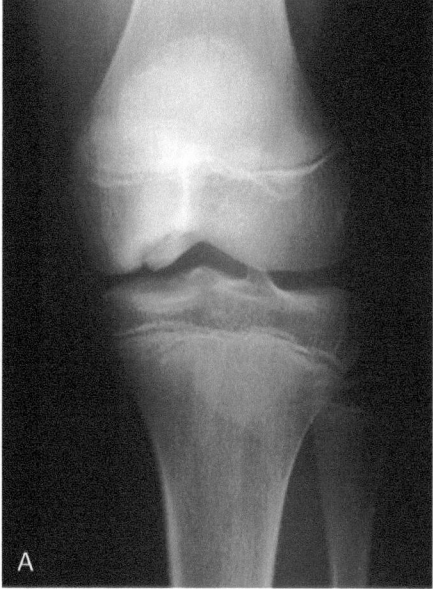
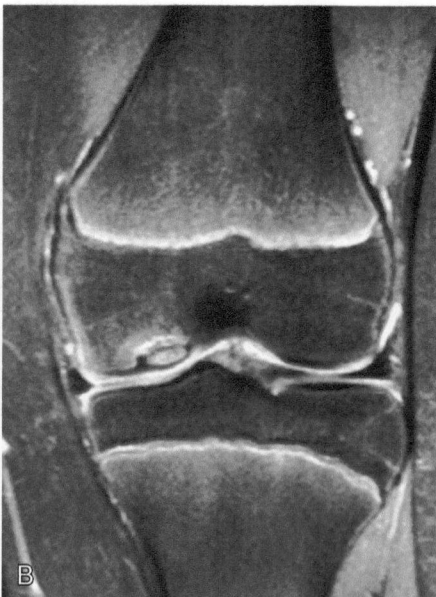

Fig. 131.8 Osteochondritis dissecans of the knee. (A) An anteroposterior radiograph. (B) A corresponding coronal magnetic resonance image.

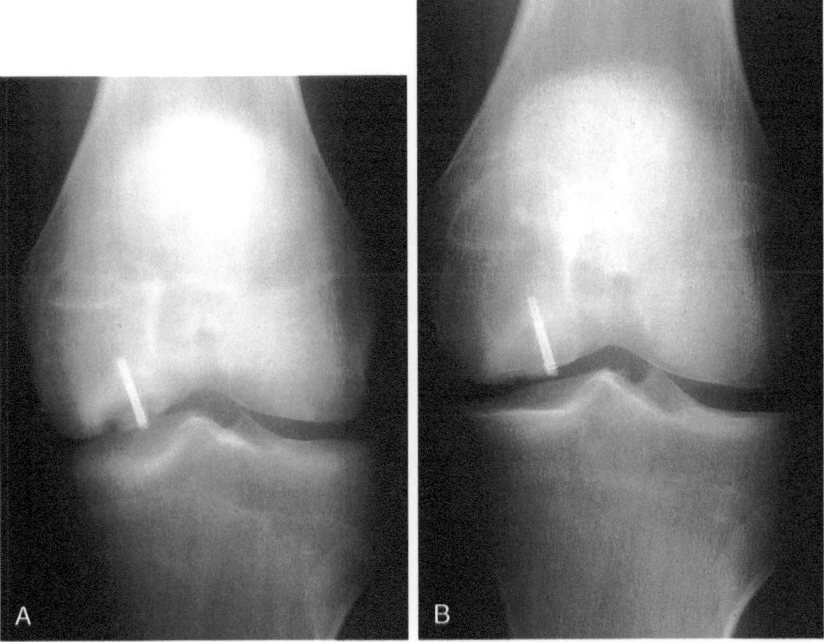

Fig. 131.9 Fixation of an unstable osteochondritis dissecans lesion of the knee. (A) An anteroposterior radiograph obtained immediately after the operation. (B) A radiograph obtained 3 months after the operation demonstrating healing of the lesion.

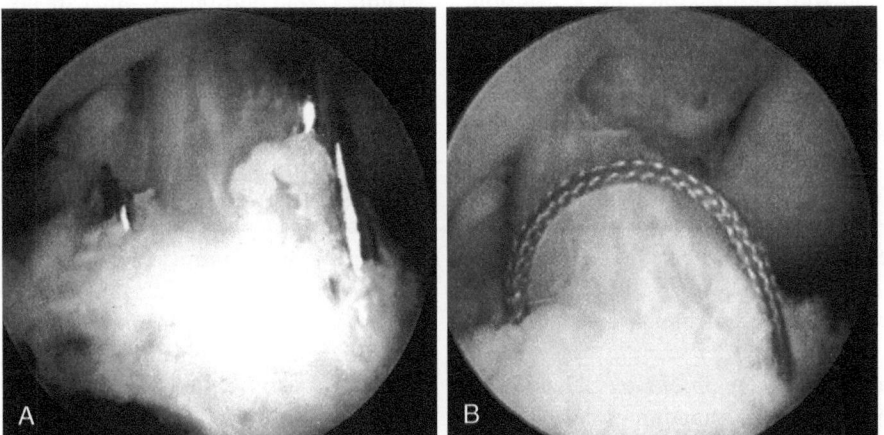

Fig. 131.10 Suture fixation of a tibial spine fracture. (A) Guidewires brought through the tibial spine fragment. (B) Suture fixation.

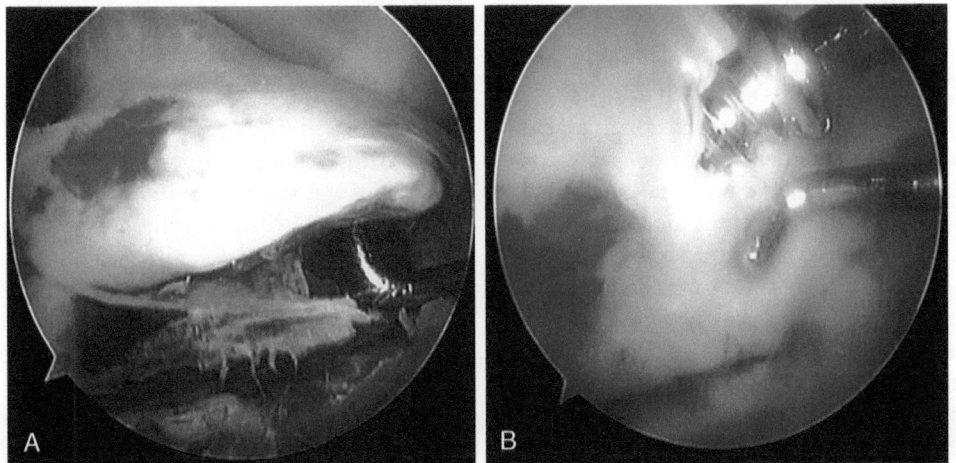

Fig. 131.11 Epiphyseal cannulated screw fixation of a tibial spine fracture. (A) A displaced fracture. (B) Screw fixation.

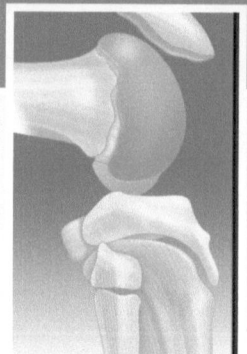

132

Imaging Considerations in Skeletally Immature Athletes

Andrew M. Zbojniewicz

An increasing number of injuries are being seen in young, skeletally immature patients, which may be due to a decrease in free play combined with an increase in participation in competitive organized sports, sport specialization, and a general lack of physical preparedness.[1] In this population, unique injuries are encountered related to the presence of an open growth plate, which is often the "weak link" between tendon and bone. An injury may be related to a single acute event or to overuse, with approximately 50% of all injuries seen in pediatric sports medicine practices being attributed to overuse.[1]

Single acute traumatic events consist primarily of fractures through bone, dislocation with ligamentous injury, avulsion fractures, or a combination of these processes. Overuse injuries primarily relate to chronic stress of the growth plates, fatigue-type stress fractures of bone, and less commonly tendinosis.

An evaluation of sports injuries in young children versus adolescents found that children 5 to 12 years of age most often had acute traumatic bony injuries to the upper extremity, whereas overuse injuries to bone, such as apophysitis and osteochondritis dissecans, predominated in the lower extremities.[1] Patients 13 to 17 years of age were more likely to have soft tissue than bony injuries, including anterior cruciate ligament injuries and meniscal tears.[1]

This chapter emphasizes common conditions encountered in the course of imaging the skeletally immature athlete. A brief review of the pathophysiology common to many injuries seen in this group of patients is followed by a region-based review of specific conditions in this population.

PATHOPHYSIOLOGY COMMON TO INJURIES IN THE SKELETALLY IMMATURE ATHLETE

The weakest part of the developing skeleton is the cartilage at the growth plates of the epiphyses and apophyses, with ligamentous structures shown to be two to five times stronger that open growth plates.[2,3] Compared with adults, in whom acute tensile forces most commonly result in injury to the myotendinous junction, injury in skeletally immature patients most commonly occurs at or near osteochondral interfaces.[4] It is because of the relatively weak cartilage present at the growth plates of apophyseal sites that avulsion fractures are more common in skeletally immature patients. When the tensile force overcomes the resistance of the cartilage at the growth plate, an acute avulsion fracture will occur.

Chronic repetitive stress, on the other hand, can lead to abnormal widening of the growth plates and may be seen clinically with pain or growth disturbance. Different mechanisms may exist depending on whether the applied stress is a repetitive compressive force or a traction force.

Pathophysiologically, the newly formed bone adjacent to the growth plates within the metaphyses is relatively fragile, with poor resistance to the compressive forces that can occur with repetitive weight-bearing stress in sporting activities.[5] This repetitive microtrauma can disrupt the metaphyseal blood supply, thus limiting the delivery of necessary nutrients—such as calcium, vitamin D, and phosphates—that are needed for osteogenesis in endochondral ossification.[5] Consequently, long columns of hypertrophic cartilage cells from the physis extend into the metaphysis.[5] It is this extension of unmineralized cartilage that results in the characteristic widening of the growth plates in conditions such as gymnast's wrist. With traction forces, a chronic repetitive musculotendinous pull at the apophyseal site can outpace the ability of the body to repair the injury, resulting in the proliferation or hypertrophy of chondrocytes, microfractures, and inflammatory cells that has been termed *apophysitis*.[6] This manifests as apparent physeal widening and a pattern of adjacent bone marrow and muscle edema on magnetic resonance imaging (MRI).

When repetitive stress is applied to bone, it responds by increasing the rate of cortical resorption and remodeling of the haversion system, ultimately leading to weakened cortical bone.[3] When the rate of osteoclastic activity outpaces the rate of osteoblastic activity and persistent stress is applied through the weakened bone, fracture may occur.[3]

SHOULDER

Development

The proximal humeral growth plate begins to close at around 14 years of age, starting centrally, and concluding posterolaterally at around 17 years.[7] Additional growth plates are present at the scapula, related to secondary ossification centers. These are important because they can be confused for fractures and can act as a point of weakness through which fractures may occur. The subcoracoid secondary ossification center forms within the superior glenoid with a bipolar growth plate present anteriorly at the base of the coracoid and posteriorly at the scapula. This ossification center contributes to growth of the superior third of the glenoid and starts to ossify between 8 and 10 years of age, completing typically by 16 to 17 years.[7] The inferior glenoid secondary ossification center forms from multiple centers, resulting in a horseshoe-shaped epiphysis at the lower two-thirds of the glenoid that typically appears around 14 to 15 years of age and closes by 17 to 18 years[7] (Fig. 132.1A and B).

At the clavicle, the medial cartilaginous epiphysis begins to ossify at 18 years of age, closing between 22 and 25 years.[2] The lateral end of the clavicle can also have a secondary ossification center, but much less consistently. When present, it was thought to develop around 19 to 20 years of age and then to close quickly within a few months.[8] However, more recent evidence based on a study using MRI identified this secondary ossification center in patients between 11 and 15 years of age.[8] Owing to the rarity of this finding, its presence could result in an erroneous diagnosis of fracture.

The acromion forms from multiple ossification centers and is traditionally reported to reach complete closure between 18 and 25 years of age. However, the same MRI study also found that secondary ossification centers within the acromion can begin to ossify as early as 10 years of age and often close by 16 years.[8] This is clinically relevant because it means that a symptomatic os acromiale may be seen in adolescent patients and is not only an adult problem.

Acute Injuries

Acute injuries are typically found in contact sports such as football, hockey, and wrestling, although other high-velocity sports such as snow and water skiing can result in fractures due to direct impact when falls occur.

Midshaft clavicular fractures can occur in all age groups; however, a fracture unique to the immature skeleton that is typically seen in patients less than 13 years of age is the distal clavicular periosteal sleeve fracture.[2] This fracture can mimic an acromioclavicular joint injury owing to displacement of the clavicle, although characteristically the acromioclavicular and coracoclavicular ligaments are intact. Fracture may occur either through the distal clavicular physis and be radiographically occult or may occur through the metaphysis and be visible on radiographs. Either way, subsequent stripping of the periosteal sleeve occurs, which often results in clavicular elevation and apparent disruption of the coracoclavicular ligaments, which are in fact uninjured and still attached to the periosteum (Fig. 132.2). Unlike some grade 3 acromioclavicular joint injuries, these injuries are typically treated conservatively, with eventual ossification seen along the stripped periosteum. Similarly, injuries to the medial clavicle in the skeletally immature patient are more likely to represent a Salter 1 or 2 fracture than true dislocation, which may have an impact on treatment (Fig. 132.3).

Another unique fracture to the skeletally immature athlete is a fracture through the base of the coracoid, which typically involves the growth plate at the base of the coracoid (Fig. 132.4A and B). Salter-Harris 2 fractures and greater tuberosity avulsion fractures are other fractures that also may occasionally be encountered (Fig. 132.5).

Acute injuries can also affect the soft tissue constraints of the shoulder. The glenohumeral joint is particularly prone to soft tissue injury due to its large range of motion (ROM) and the glenohumeral articulation, which provides negligible osseous stability, relying almost entirely on static and dynamic soft tissue stabilizers. It is not a surprise then, that shoulder dislocations may be seen in young athletes participating in contact sports. In addition to labral and capsuloligamentous injuries, shoulder dislocations can result in osseous fractures to the glenoid and humerus, known as Bankart and Hill-Sachs lesions, respectively, although in younger patients, care should be taken not to call the normal inferior glenoid ossification centers a fracture (see Fig. 132.1). Rotator cuff tears can also uncommonly be seen in young athletes following a single traumatic event; when present, they are often also associated with labral injury.[9] Although these

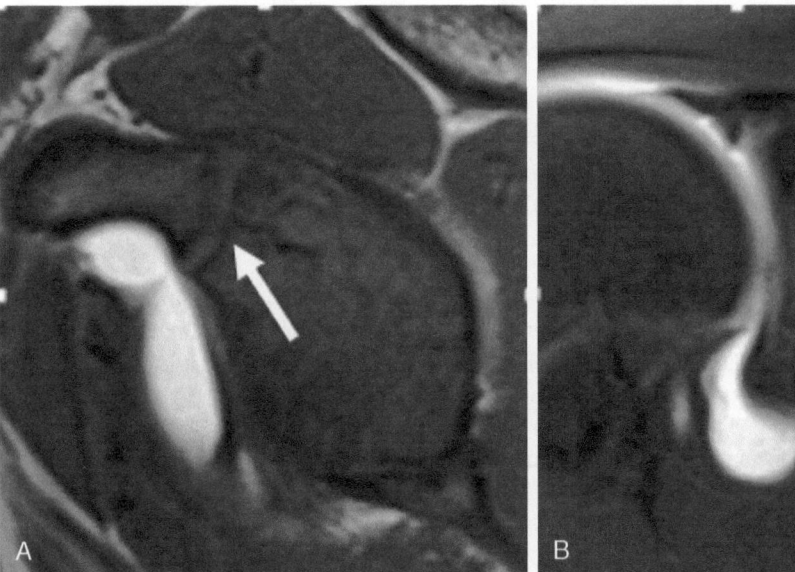

Fig. 132.1 (A) Sagittal T1 image shows the normal growth plate at the base of the coracoid *(arrow)*. (B) Coronal T1 fat-suppressed image shows the growth plate for the subcoracoid secondary ossification center *(superior arrow)* and inferior glenoid secondary ossification center *(inferior arrow)*. This should not be confused with a fracture following trauma.

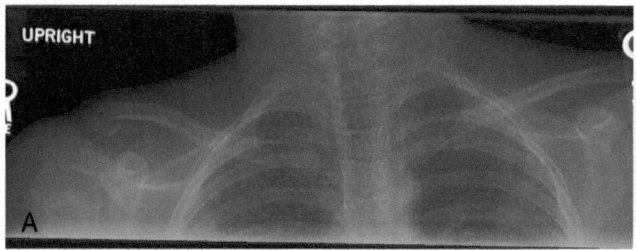
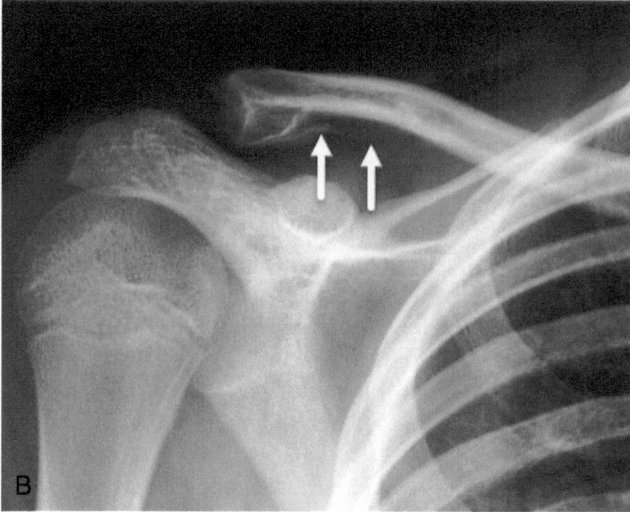

Fig. 132.2 (A) Anteroposterior radiograph of the bilateral clavicles shows a fracture of the distal right clavicle with widening of the coracoclavicular space. (B) Follow-up radiograph shows early periosteal new bone *(arrows)* related to the stripping of the periosteum, causing the elevated clavicle. The coracoclavicular ligaments are intact.

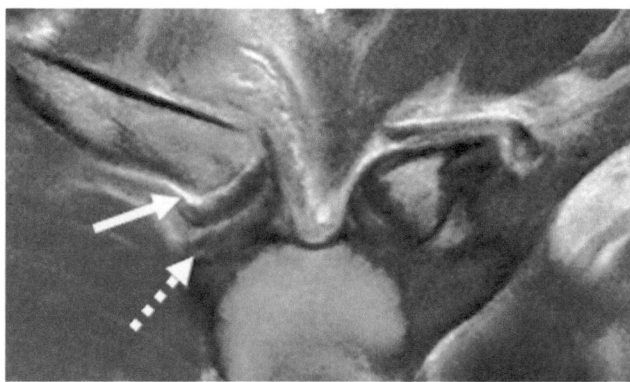

Fig. 132.3 Images from a 15-year-old boy injured playing football. Coronal non–fat-suppressed fluid-sensitive sequence demonstrates a fracture through the medial clavicular growth plate separating the metaphysis from the epiphysis, consistent with a Salter 1 fracture *(arrow)*. The fibrocartilaginous disk within the sternoclavicular joint *(dashed arrow)* and capsule remains intact.

injuries may be seen in skeletally immature patients, they are not typical for this population.

Overuse Injuries

The quintessential overuse injury of the shoulder in the skeletally immature athlete is referred to as "Little Leaguer shoulder," which is not a Salter 1 fracture but rather a chronic stress injury to the growth plate, which, as discussed previously, disrupts normal endochondral ossification and results in widening and irregularity of the growth plate on radiographs (Fig. 132.6A–C). The posterolateral growth plate in the proximal humerus is last to close and should not be confused with a chronic stress injury. If findings are equivocal, a contralateral view of the shoulder with the humerus in external rotation can be performed. Performance of a complete radiographic series for comparison purposes is unnecessary and exposes the patient to unnecessary

radiation. On MRI, growth plate widening can be seen on the ubiquitous fat-suppressed fluid-sensitive sequences often performed when joints are being imaged, but they are particularly well visualized on non–fat-suppressed images.

Another overuse injury that can be seen is the symptomatic os acromiale. Although an os acromiale has historically been considered to represent failure to incorporate the ossification centers of the acromion after 25 years of age, more recent literature has found that os acromiale can occur between 11 and 15 years, as discussed previously.[8] Differentiation of normal acromial ossification centers from an os acromiale lies in evaluating the shape of the interface between the centers and the acromion; an arched shape is characteristic of a normal developmental ossification center, whereas a transverse interface perpendicular to the long axis of the acromion suggests os acromiale (Fig. 132.7).[10] When this finding is being evaluated on MRI, fluid at the interface and a surrounding marrow edema pattern present on fluid-sensitive sequences in the context of an os acromiale suggests instability and motion of the ossicle (Fig. 132.8).[10]

Glenohumeral instability—including anterior, posterior, or multidirectional instability—can occur related to the cumulative stress applied during sport activities such as baseball, football, tennis, swimming, or volleyball.[11] Imaging findings related to overuse can be subtler than those related to a single traumatic event, and although labral pathology may be seen, MRI studies including MR arthrography can also be normal or show only a redundant capsule. Instability can also lead to pathologic internal impingement with subsequent labral or rotator cuff pathology, which is typically readily visible on MRI examinations, although these injuries are not unique to this population. However, it is important to remember that just the fact that a patient is young and has open growth plates does not mean that he or she cannot present with adult-type pathology. Indeed, a complete knowledge of adult pathology is also required when studies in skeletally immature patients are being interpreted (Fig. 132.9).

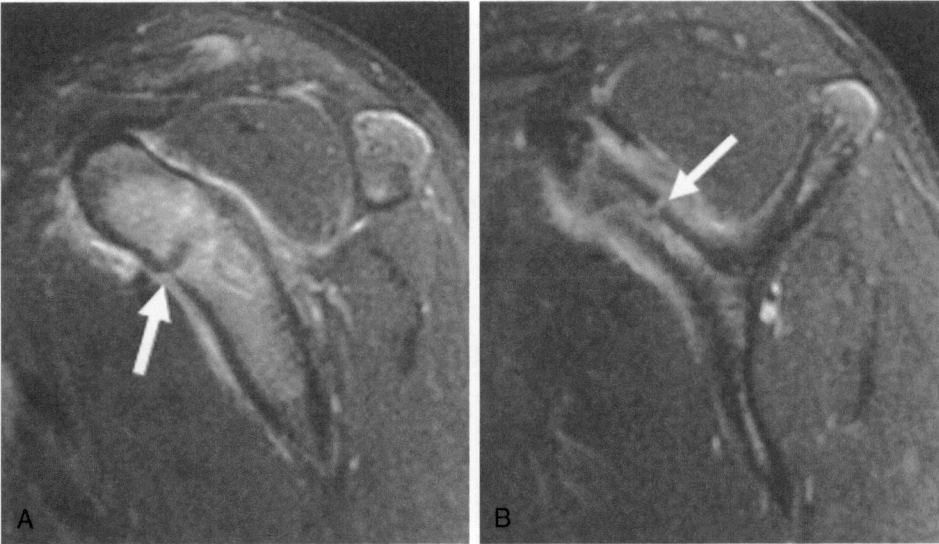

Fig. 132.4 (A) Sagittal fat-suppressed fluid-sensitive T2-weighted sequence shows abnormal bone marrow and soft tissue edema pattern associated with fracture through the growth plate medial to the coracoid *(arrow)*. (B) More medial images from the same sequence show propagation of the fracture into the scapular body *(arrow)*.

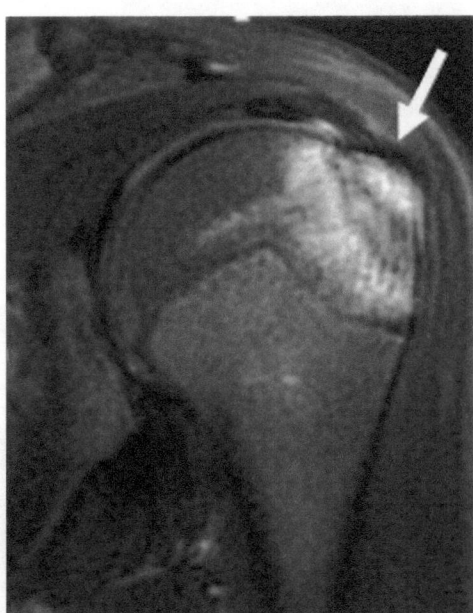

Fig. 132.5 Coronal fat-suppressed fluid-sensitive T2-weighted sequence shows an avulsion fracture *(arrow)* of the greater tuberosity in this skeletally immature patient. The bright signal within marrow relates to hemorrhage and edema associated with the fracture.

ELBOW

Development

A common mnemonic used to remember the normal pattern of development of the ossification centers of the distal elbow is CRITOE, which stands for Capitellum, Radial head, Internal (medial) epicondyle, Trochlea, Olecranon, and External (lateral) epicondyle. These ossification centers typically arise at 1, 5, 7, 10, and 11 years, respectively, with ossification centers in girls

typically appearing 6 to 12 months earlier than those in boys.[2] Absence of an ossification center at an age when it should already be seen should raise concern for a displaced avulsion fracture. If there is a question of whether the observed findings are pathologic or normal, imaging of the contralateral elbow may be useful.

Acute Injuries

Acute fractures about the elbow are commonly seen in young active children, two of the most common being supracondylar and lateral condylar fractures. Supracondylar fractures typically occur following a hyperextension mechanism after a fall on an outstretched hand, whereas lateral condylar fractures occur when a varus force is applied to an extended elbow with the forearm supinated.[2] A common fracture seen in the older child athlete, typically 9 to 14 years of age, is an acute medial epicondyle avulsion fracture. This fracture accounts for approximately 20% of all pediatric elbow fractures and can be seen associated with overhead throwers due to the valgus stress applied with the throwing motion, but it can also be seen with falls on an outstretched hand (Fig. 132.10).[2] This fracture is also commonly associated with elbow dislocations, which may be seen in young athletes, particularly gymnasts. Careful assessment of the ossification centers is advised in the context of an elbow dislocation so as not to miss a displaced medial epicondyle into the humeroulnar joint.[2]

Overuse Injuries

Little Leaguer elbow comprises a constellation of findings related to overuse, which are seen as a result of the stress placed on the elbow in the skeletally immature athlete. This entity has classically involved young baseball players, although the spectrum of injuries may involve other overhead athletes such as tennis players or javelin throwers. Injuries are caused by either the tension

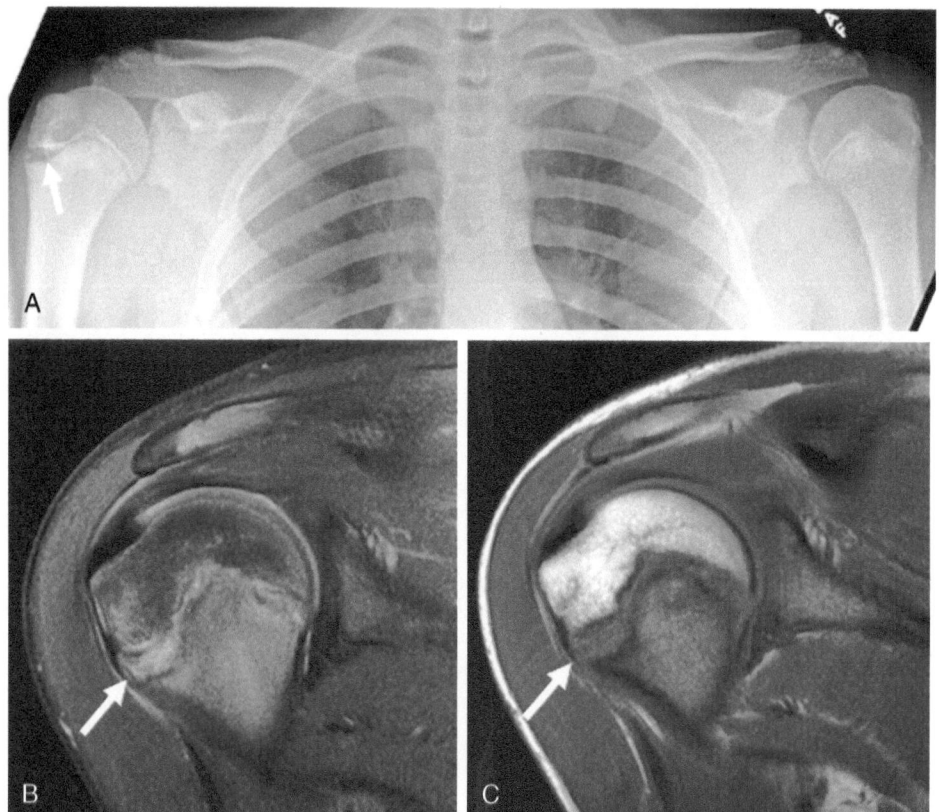

Fig. 132.6 (A) Anteroposterior radiograph of both shoulders shows widening of the right proximal humeral growth plate characteristic of "Little Leaguer shoulder." (B) Widening of the growth plate *(arrows)* seen on a fat-suppressed fluid-sensitive sequence and (C) a non–fat-suppressed T1-weighted sequence.

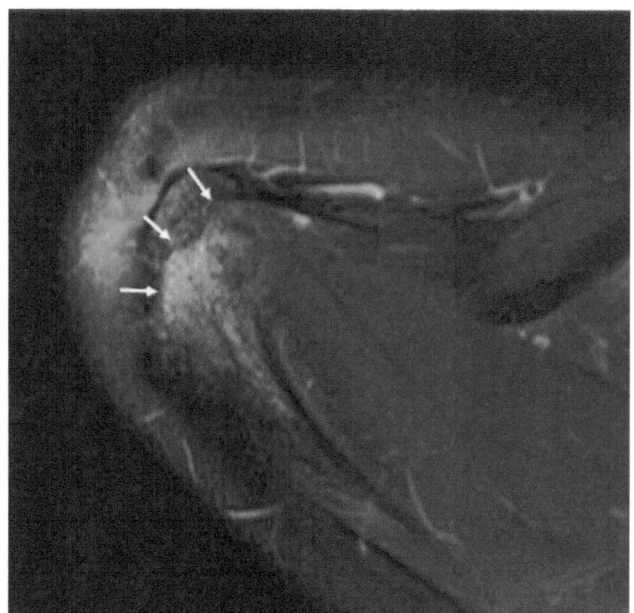

Fig. 132.7 Axial T2-weighted fluid-sensitive sequence from a 13-year-old patient demonstrates the normal arched configuration *(arrows)* of the distal acromial ossification center. Note the normal increased signal at the metaphysis, which is related to red marrow.

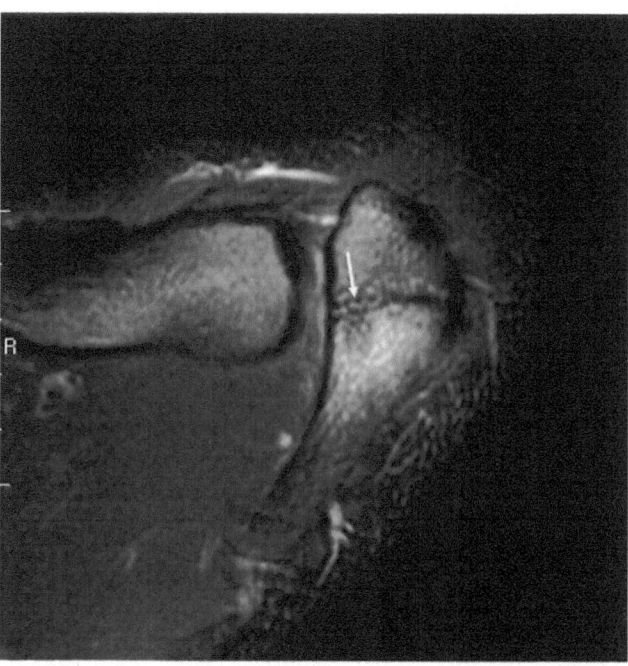

Fig. 132.8 Axial T2-weighted fluid-sensitive sequence from a 16-year-old patient shows a transverse interface perpendicular to the long axis of the acromion consistent with an os acromiale. Fluid signal *(arrow)* at the interface suggests instability of the ossicle and symptomatic os acromiale.

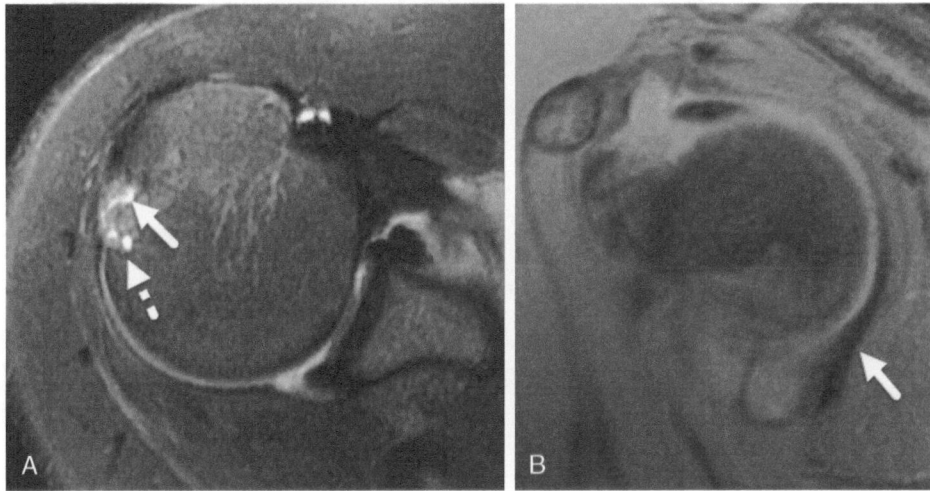

Fig. 132.9 Pathologic internal impingement. (A) Axial T2-weighted fluid-sensitive sequence from a 14-year-old boy shows a small articular side insertional tear of the infraspinatus tendon *(arrow)* as well as small cystic foci at the posterolateral humerus *(dashed arrow)* near the bare area. (B) Sagittal proton-density fat-suppressed sequence shows abnormal thickening of the posterior band of the inferior glenohumeral ligament *(arrow)*, which can be associated with a glenohumeral internal rotation deficit.

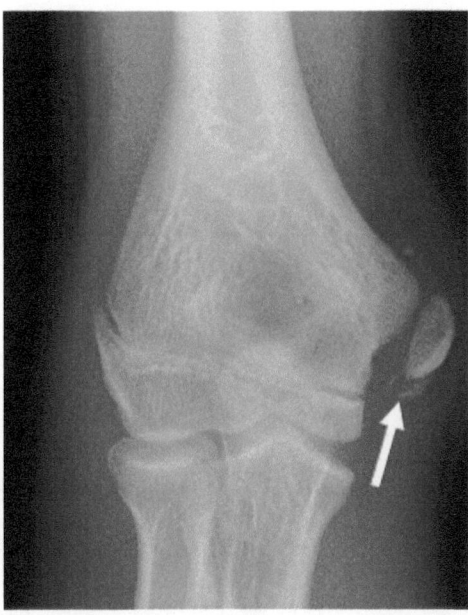

Fig. 132.10 Anteroposterior radiograph from a 13-year-old boy who felt a pop while throwing a baseball shows a medial epicondylar avulsion fracture. Note also the irregular ossification *(arrow)* inferior to the ossification center, which likely relates to chronic repetitive microtrauma to the developing center subsequent to chronic valgus stress on the ulnar collateral ligament in this thrower.

applied to the medial epicondyle, common flexor tendon, and ulnar collateral ligament at the medial elbow or the compressive forces applied to the radial side of the elbow. Posteromedial shear forces can also affect the posterior articular surface.[2] Younger children with wider growth plates are at greater risk of injury at the bone-cartilage interface, whereas adolescents are at greater risk of injury to soft tissue structures such as the ulnar collateral ligament.

Little Leaguer Elbow

Repeated tension to the medial elbow in young skeletally immature athletes can result in chronic repetitive traction injury to the medial epicondylar apophyseal growth plate, also called traction apophysitis. These patients may have normal radiographs in as many as 85% of cases.[2] When abnormal, radiographs may reveal widening and irregularity of the growth plate, irregular ossification, fragmentation, or sclerosis, whereas MRI findings will consist of growth plate widening, adjacent bone marrow edema pattern, and sometimes soft tissue edema pattern (Figs. 132.11 and 132.12). A severe marrow edema pattern may result in replacement of the normal hyperintense white marrow signal on T1-weighted imaging. If there is doubt as to whether a growth plate is actually widened on radiographs, a single view of the contralateral side can be obtained for comparison.

Chronic stress to the posterior elbow at the olecranon can be seen in gymnasts and throwers as well as football and hockey players; it results in identical findings of a traction apophysitis as described previously at the medial epicondyle but instead involves the olecranon (Fig. 132.13). In older patients the posteromedial shear forces that occur with throwing can result in findings of valgus extension overload, including loss of cartilage and osteophytes. Injury to the ulnar collateral ligament can also occur in the adolescent athlete.

Compressive injury to the lateral elbow can result in Panner disease and osteochondritis dissecans involving the capitellum. Similar to injury of the growth plates, these entities are felt to relate to disruption of the blood supply to the capitellum.

Panner disease affects a younger age group, typically children less than 12 years of age, and has a better prognosis, generally healing without consequence. On imaging, Panner disease tends to affect the entire capitellum.[2] Radiographs may show subtle demineralization with corresponding lucency early in the disease

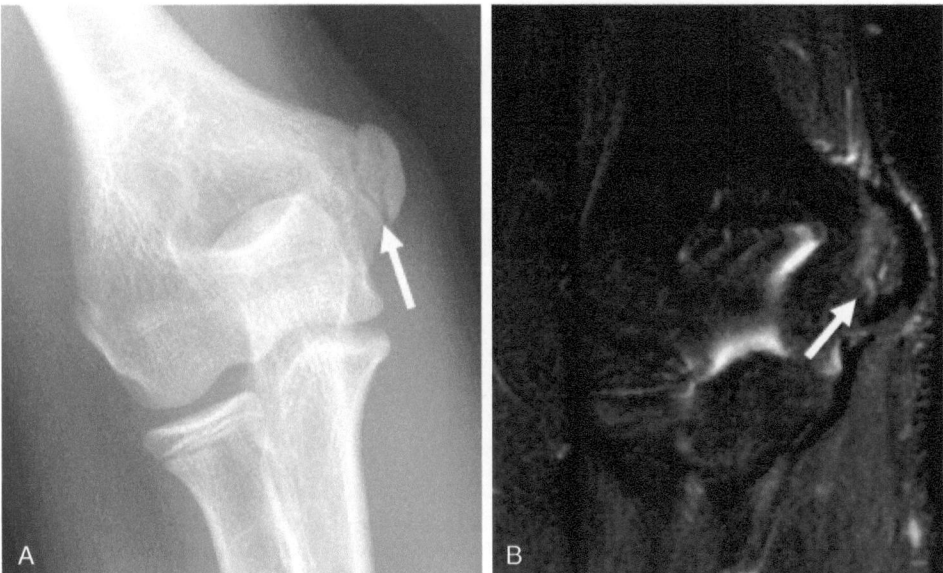

Fig. 132.11 A 13-year-old boy with shooting pain for 2 years while throwing a baseball. (A) Anteroposterior radiograph demonstrates a normal appearance of the growth plate *(arrow)*. (B) Coronal T2-weighted fluid-sensitive sequence shows abnormal marrow edema pattern *(arrow)* about the growth plate as well as small fluid signal within the growth plate consistent with traction apophysitis.

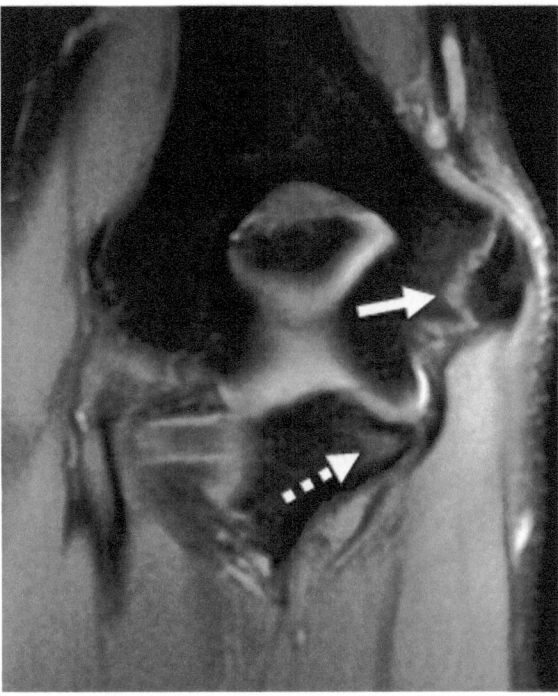

Fig. 132.12 A 14-year-old baseball player with medial elbow pain. Coronal proton-density (PD) fat-suppressed sequence shows widening and irregularity of the growth plate of the medial epicondylar ossification center *(arrow)*. There is also a subtle marrow edema pattern within the ulna *(dashed arrow)* near the insertion of the ulnar collateral ligament (UCL) due to repetitive stress and adaptive thickening of the UCL.

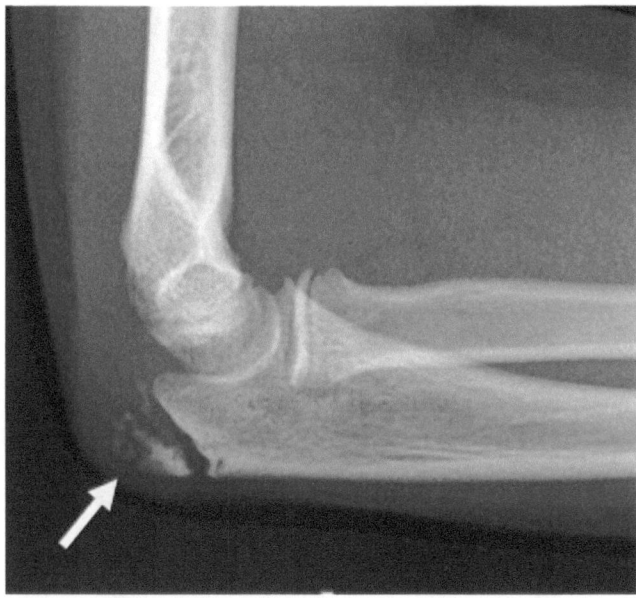

Fig. 132.13 A 10-year-old gymnast with posterior elbow pain. Lateral radiograph shows irregularity of the olecranon ossification center *(arrow)* consistent with chronic repetitive traction injury.

process, later progressing to sclerosis and fragmentation.[2] On MRI, there can be loss of the normal white hyperintense signal representative of fat within marrow on T1-weighted images with variable signal on T2-weighted images, which can range from diffusely hyperintense to heterogeneous with areas of decreased signal when sclerosis is present. Articular cartilage should be intact and intra-articular bodies are not seen.

Osteochondritis dissecans (OCD) is a more severe manifestation of the compressive forces at the lateral elbow and typically occurs after the age of 11 years.[2] OCD tends to have more focal involvement of the anterior and lateral epiphysis and findings can be radiographically occult. Early manifestations on radiographs consist of subtle subchondral lucency with later findings consisting of sclerosis, fragmentation, and flattening (Fig. 132.14).

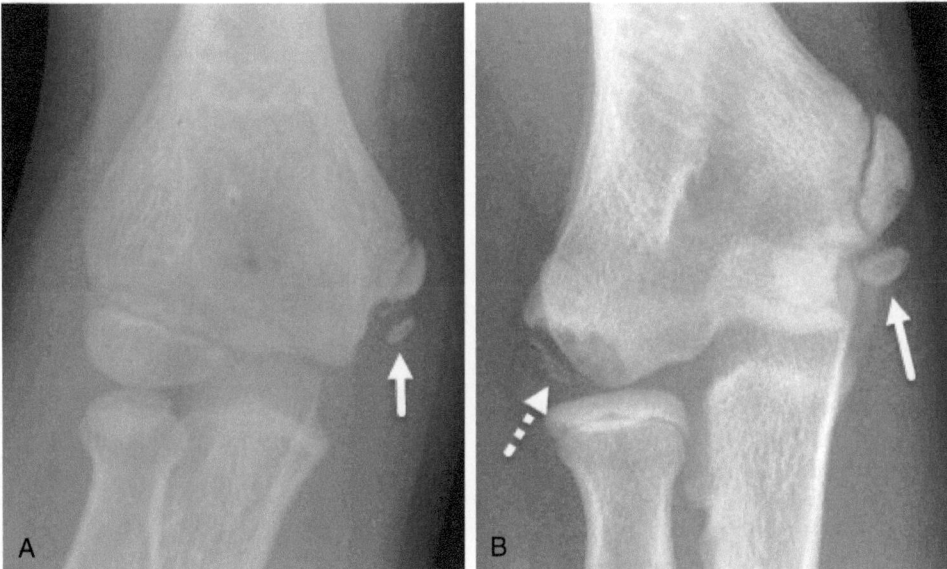

Fig. 132.14 (A) Anteroposterior radiograph from a 14-year-old baseball player with medial elbow pain shows fragmentation *(arrow)* of the medial epicondylar apophysis consistent with chronic repetitive traction injury. (B) The same patient shows a persistent ossicle at the medial elbow *(arrow)* as a sequela of prior traction apophysitis with interval development of fragmentation and lucency at the capitellum *(dashed arrow)* consistent with osteochondritis dissecans.

MRI is useful as it can help to stage the severity of the lesion by evaluating the integrity of the overlying cartilage and can identify displaced intra-articular bodies, which may have an impact on treatment.

Although Little Leaguer elbow is a common cause of medial pain at the elbow in young athletes, other conditions such as ulnar nerve instability and ulnar neuropathy can be present and diagnosed on imaging studies, including MRI and ultrasound. These conditions are not exclusive to the skeletally immature athlete; however, they can be a cause of medial elbow pain. Briefly, ulnar neuropathy can occur either due to repetitive irritation in the context of ulnar nerve instability or because of repeated compression within the confined space of the cubital tunnel. Ulnar nerve instability can consist of pure dislocation of the ulnar nerve, or it may be combined with dislocation of the medial head of the triceps. These entities can easily be differentiated with ultrasound, which is important, as the surgical approach may differ.[12] It should be noted that 16% of the population may have an asymptomatic ulnar nerve dislocation, and its mere presence does not alone indicate that it is a symptom generator.[12]

WRIST

Acute Injuries

Fractures of the distal radius are commonly associated with sports injuries, with soccer being the most common sport in which such fractures occur.[2] They tend to occur where there is a transition of dense lamellar bone at the diaphysis to porous bone at the metaphysis.[2] This transition occurs more distally in older patients; therefore fractures in older children occur closer to the growth plate, often consisting of Salter 2 fractures.[2] Patients with Salter 2 fractures must be followed over time in order to identify

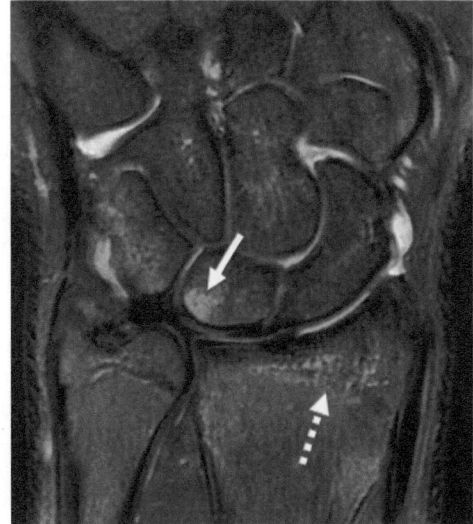

Fig. 132.15 Coronal T2-weighted fat-suppressed fluid-sensitive sequence shows premature closure of the distal radial growth plate *(dashed arrow)* with ulnar positive variance. A bone marrow edema pattern at the ulnar aspect of the lunate bone is present, associated with ulnar abutment *(arrow)*.

the formation of a premature pathologic bone bridge at the growth plate, which, if undetected can result in ulnar positive variance and potentially ulnar abutment (Fig. 132.15). Distal radial fractures are also commonly associated with ulnar styloid fracture and injuries of the triangular fibrocartilage complex (TFCC). Isolated TFCC injuries can also occur, although imaging features will be identical to those described in adults.

Scaphoid fractures are also frequently encountered, typically in athletes between the ages of 13 and 15 years and rarely in those before 10 years of age.[13] These fractures can occur in addition to a fracture of the distal radius, so it is important to continue looking for additional fractures after one abnormality is seen on a radiograph so as to avoid missing another important finding; this is known as a "satisfaction of search." Both a standard posteroanterior (PA) radiograph as well as a PA view with ulnar deviation is recommended when there is concern for a scaphoid fracture. MRI can be useful in detecting radiographically occult fractures. Follow-up radiographs after conservative management can also be used to help identify a radiographically occult fracture that is healing, although it is important to note that in adolescents it may take up to 7 weeks to identify healing changes on radiographs.[13]

Scapholunate ligament injuries can also occur in skeletally immature patients and are difficult to diagnose on radiographs owing to the presence of unossified cartilage. The scapholunate distance on radiographs does not reach the normal adult value of 2 mm until at least 12 years of age.[13] MRI or MR arthrography may be useful for diagnosis. More severe injuries can result in carpal dislocation, including perilunate or lunate dislocation, which may occur with or without coexisting carpal bone and radial styloid fractures.

Overuse Injuries

Overuse injuries at the wrist are commonly seen in gymnasts, particularly female gymnasts who experience repeated hyperextension and axial loading on the wrists in many of their activities. This compressive force affects the distal radius, resulting in abnormal widening and irregularity of the growth plates, referred to as "gymnast's wrists" (Fig. 132.16A–C). Treatment consists of rest; however, if such patients continue their gymnastic activities, growth at the level of the distal radial growth plate can be impaired, resulting in relative overgrowth of the ulna and ulnar positive variance. The latter can lead to ulnar abutment, which is a pathologic process resulting from repetitive impact of the ulna on the TFCC and ulnar aspect of the proximal carpal row. This can manifest as chondral degeneration and a pattern of bone marrow edema at the ulnar aspect of the lunate on

MRI as well as pathology of the lunotriquetral ligament and TFCC, specifically injuries to the articular disk of the TFCC (Fig. 132.17). Severe cases of gymnast's wrist can result in hypertrophic bone at the dorsal margins of the metaphysis. This hypertrophic bone can result in repetitive irritation of the overlying tendons and subsequent tendinopathy, tears, and tenosynovitis (Fig. 132.18).

Other findings that can be seen in the young gymnast include dorsal carpal impingement, an overuse condition that can lead to dorsal wrist pain and is related to repetitive hyperextension

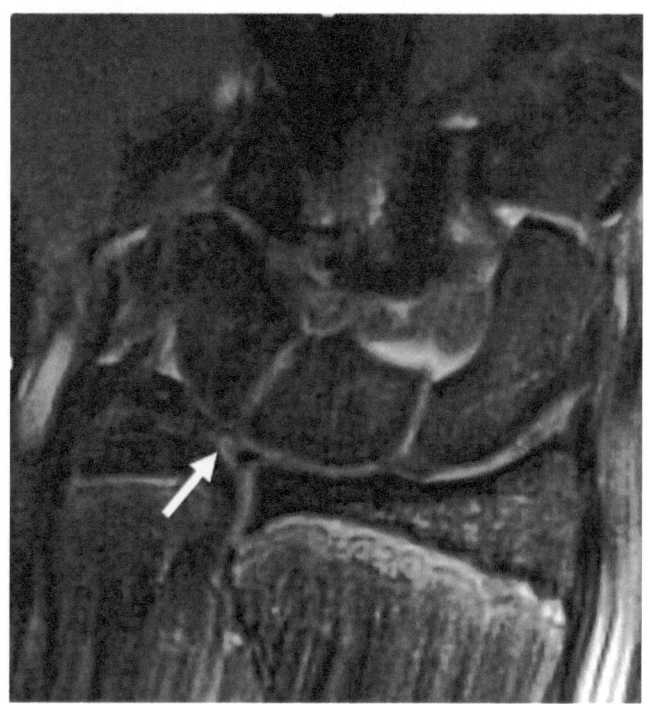

Fig. 132.17 Skeletally immature patient with history of chronic physeal stress to the distal radial growth plate (not shown) shows ulnar positive variance with a tear at the articular disk of the triangular fibrocartilage complex *(arrow)*.

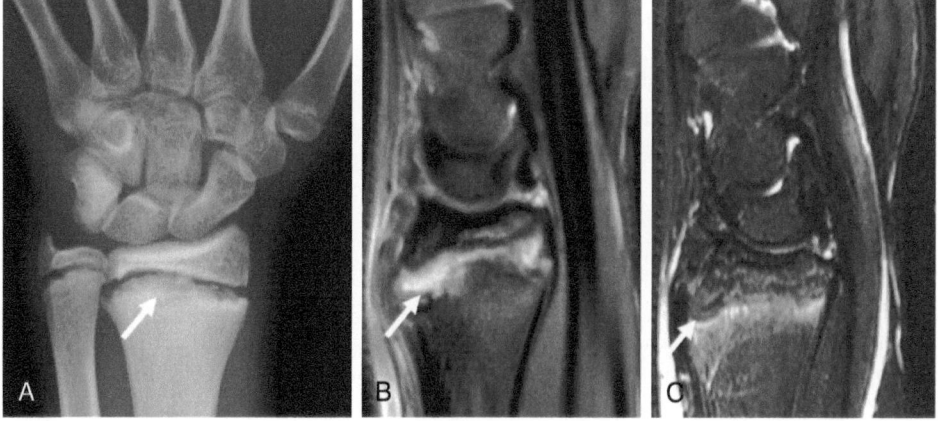

Fig. 132.16 (A) Anteroposterior radiograph shows abnormal widening and irregularity of the distal radial growth plate *(arrow)* consistent with chronic physeal stress, also called gymnast's wrist. (B) Sagittal T2-weighted fat-suppressed fluid-sensitive image shows abnormal widening and increased signal in the growth plate *(arrow)*. (C) The same sequence in the same patient 8 months later, after rest, shows resolution of the abnormal signal at the level of the growth plate *(arrow)*. Residual hyperintense signal in the metaphysis relates to red marrow.

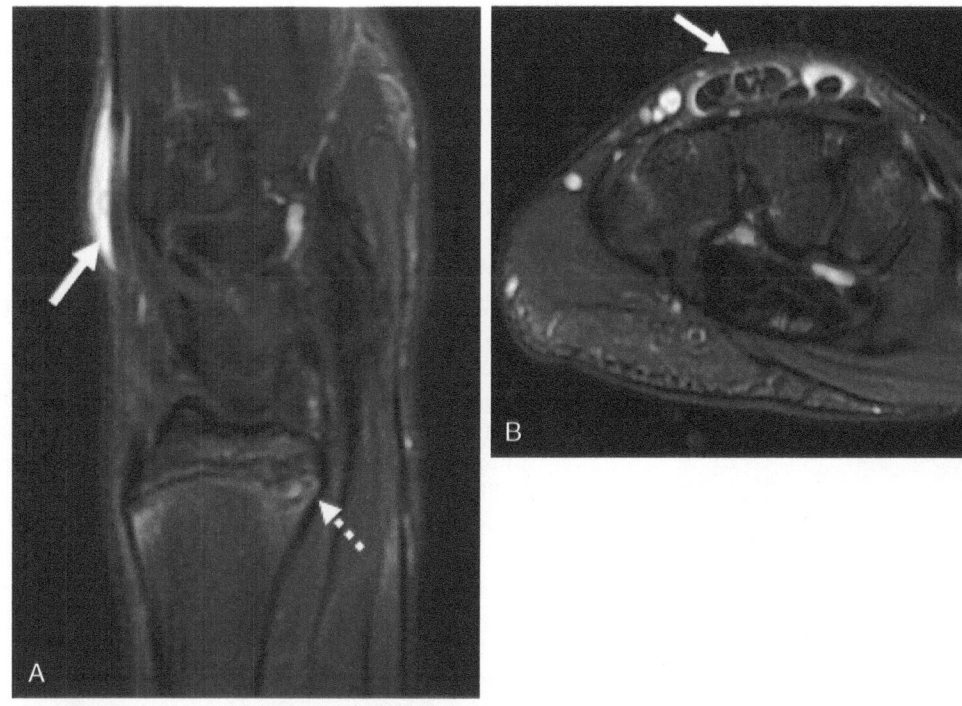

Fig. 132.18 A 14-year-old female gymnast presenting with a palpable mass at the dorsal wrist and pain with wrist extension and weight bearing. (A) Sagittal T2-weighted fat-suppressed fluid-sensitive sequence shows irregularity of the distal radial growth plate *(dashed arrow)* with abnormal fluid within the dorsal extensor tendon sheath *(arrow)* indicative of tenosynovitis. (B) Axial T2-weighted fat-suppressed sequence shows extensor tendinopathy, longitudinal tears, and tenosynovitis *(arrow)* within the fourth compartment compartment related to repetitive irritation within the narrowed fibro-osseous tunnel at the dorsal wrist following development of hypertrophic bone subsequent to chronic physeal stress.

of the wrist (Fig. 132.19). Dorsal wrist impingement can also affect young athletes who frequently perform push-ups or bench-press activities and results from development of dorsal radiocarpal synovitis with subsequent impingement.[13]

HIP

Acute Injuries

Femoral fractures and hip dislocations may occur, particularly in high-impact sports such as football, but they are not exclusive to skeletally immature athletes and are not seen with near the frequency of fractures in the upper extremity.

Apophyseal avulsion fractures are acute injuries commonly seen in the lower extremity in skeletally immature patients. Apophyseal avulsion fractures most frequently occur at the pelvis, which may relate to the large number of apophyses and the strength of the muscles that attach to them.[14] Most apophyseal avulsion fractures are readily diagnosed on radiographs, typically manifested by a curved thin piece of bone separated from the origin and asymmetric to the contralateral side, and usually do not require advanced imaging. When performed, MRI will typically demonstrate displacement of the apophysis, a linear fluid signal at the junction between the apophysis and growth plate, and a soft tissue edema-like signal. Occasionally chronic avulsion fractures may be associated with bone formation that may mimic a neoplasm, and MRI or CT may be useful for clarification.[14]

The most common site of avulsion is the ischial tuberosity; this can be caused by extreme active contraction of the hamstrings in runners or with excessive passive lengthening in cheerleaders or dancers.[15] The second most common site of involvement is the anterior superior iliac spine (ASIS), which is the site of origin of the sartorius and tensor fascia lata; these fractures can be seen associated with forceful extension of the hip in runners (Fig. 132.20A and B).[15] Avulsions of the anterior inferior iliac spine (AIIS) can be subtler and occur at the site of origin of the rectus femoris; they are less common than ASIS avulsions.[15] These fractures are thought to relate to rapid high-energy knee extension combined with hip extension in sports involving kicking, such as soccer.[16] Fracture malunion associated with inferior displacement of the apophyseal fragment can result in a bony protrusion sometimes referred to as a "pelvic digit" or "iliac rib." A small subset of patients may have associated limited ROM and pain with flexion, referred to as sub-spine impingement (Fig. 132.21).[16] Other less common avulsion fractures can occur at the iliac crest apophysis, the pubic body involving the symphysis pubis, as well as the lesser and greater trochanters.

Although most avulsion fractures about the pelvis can be diagnosed on radiographs, in younger patients apophyseal avulsion fractures can be radiographically occult. This has been described at the ischial apophysis but it may occur at other sites.[17] The ischial apophysis begins to ossify between 13 and 15 years of age and closes between 16 and 25 years.[18] Avulsion fractures that occur prior to the onset of ossification will not be seen on radiographs and require MRI for diagnosis.

Overuse Injuries

Chronic repetitive microtrauma to the apophysis—also referred to as chronic repetitive stress injury to the apophysis, traction apophysitis, or simply apophysitis—is also frequently encountered at the pelvis and can affect the same apophyseal sites. On

radiographs, findings may consist of irregularity or fragmentation of the apophysis and widening of the growth plate. On MRI, such widening will frequently be present in addition to a pattern of bone marrow and soft tissue edema pattern. Linear fluid signal at the interface between the apophysis and displacement of the apophysis suggest an acute avulsion fracture, which can be superimposed on chronic injury or may represent a de novo acute event. It is important to note that findings of chronic repetitive microtrauma to the apophysis can be seen incidentally and may not actually be the reason for the presenting pain (Fig. 132.22A–C).

Labral tears can occur following a single acute event, although frequently they may be associated with femoroacetabular impingement or adolescent hip dysplasia. Femoroacetabular impingement is not exclusive to the skeletally immature athlete and imaging findings will be similar to those seen in adults. Although femoroacetabular impingement has become a popular topic in hip imaging as a potential etiology for hip pain, adolescent hip dysplasia can be easily overlooked but is also important because it can be a source of pain and can lead to chondral and labral

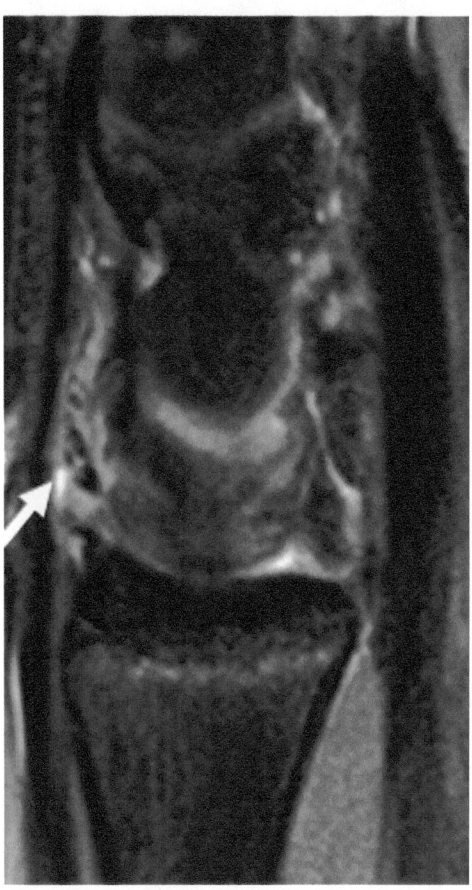

Fig. 132.19 Sagittal T2-weighted image in a 14-year-old gymnast with dorsal wrist pain shows abnormal hyperintense T2 signal material *(arrow)* surrounding the dorsal extrinsic ligaments related to synovitis and eventually requiring surgical débridement.

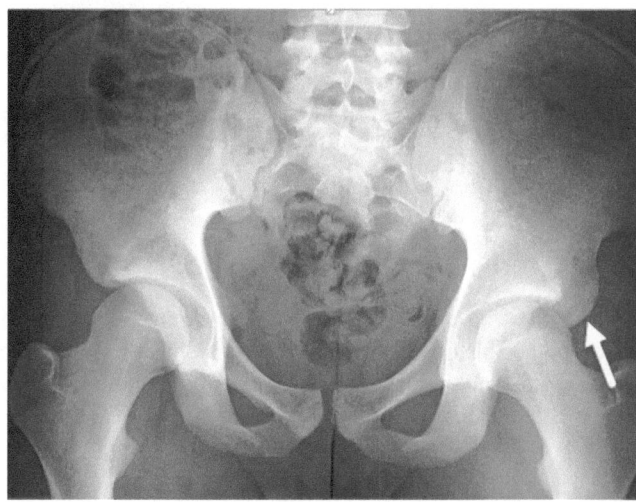

Fig. 132.21 Anteroposterior radiograph of the pelvis shows a prominent osseous protuberance *(arrow)* from the left anterior inferior iliac spine related to chronic healing of a prior avulsion fracture. This configuration can be associated with subspine impingement.

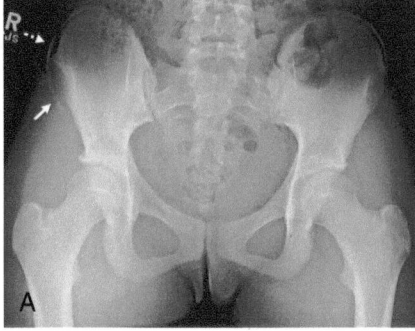
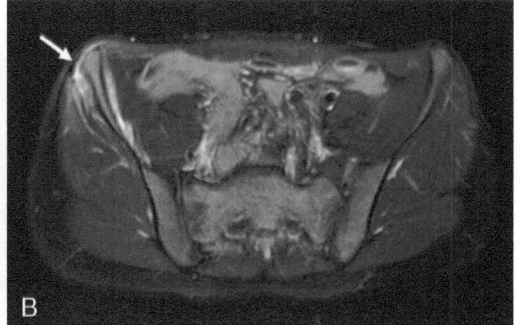

Fig. 132.20 A 16-year-old male runner with right hip pain. (A) Curvilinear bone fragment at the anterior superior iliac spine *(arrow)* extending to involve the anterior iliac crest apophysis *(dashed arrow)*. (B) Axial T2-weighted sequence shows a hypointense mildly displaced apophyseal avulsion fragment *(arrow)*. Fluid signal is present at the level of the growth plate between the fragment and the ileum and there is edema-like signal in the adjacent soft tissues relating to edema and hemorrhage in this acute injury.

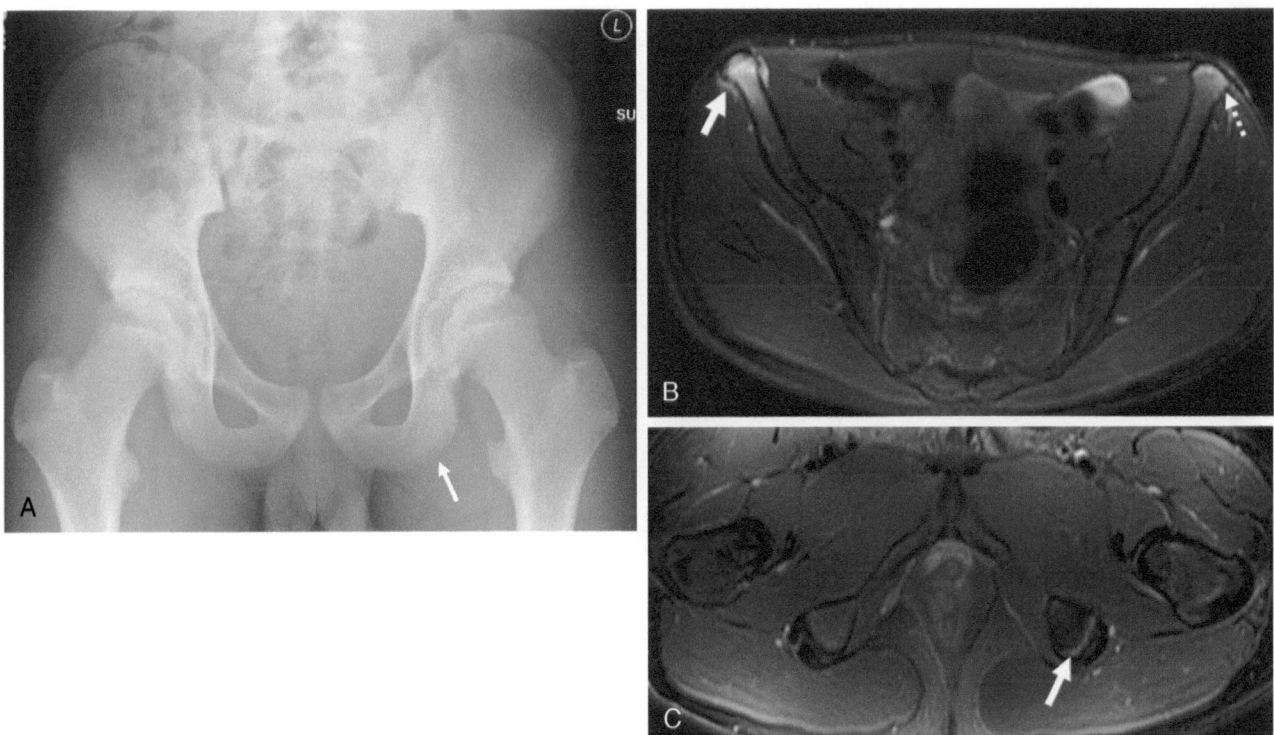

Fig. 132.22 Right hip pain. (A) Anteroposterior radiograph of the pelvis shows irregularity and widening of the growth plate at the left ischial tuberosity *(arrow)*. (B) Axial T2-weighted fluid-sensitive sequence shows asymmetric bone marrow and soft tissue edema pattern at the right anterior superior iliac spine *(arrow)* consistent with repetitive microtrauma. Note that the apophysis is not displaced. Growth plate widening and irregularity is also seen on the left, although it is asymptomatic. (C) Similarly, asymmetric growth plate widening and irregularity is seen at the left ischial tuberosity *(arrow)*, corresponding to findings on the radiograph but with no clinical symptoms.

damage and subsequent premature osteoarthritis.[19] Findings can be subtle, particularly on MRI and even on radiographs if one is not accustomed to looking for this entity. All MRI examinations for hip pain should be interpreted with accompanying radiographs. A standard radiographic examination of hip pain in adolescents should include at a minimum a well-positioned single anteroposterior (AP) view of the pelvis, which can be used to evaluate the degree of acetabular coverage, as well as a frog-leg lateral view to evaluate for slipped capital femoral epiphysis in patients whose growth plates are still open. Careful attention to technique is strongly advised, as a poorly performed study can lead to spurious findings.

The AP view of the pelvis should be obtained with the patient supine, both lower extremities at 15 degrees of internal rotation (to maximize the length of the femoral neck), tube oriented perpendicular to the table, and the crosshairs of the beam centered on a point midway between the superior border of the pubic symphysis and a line connecting the two anterior superior iliac spines.[20] A false profile view should also be performed if there is concern for hip dysplasia as it allows assessment of the degree of anterior coverage of the acetabulum. This view is performed with the patient standing and the affected hip against the cassette, foot parallel to the cassette, pelvis rotated 65 degrees in relation to the bucky wall stand, and beam centered at the femoral head.[20]

The AP view of the pelvis can be used to assess the degree of acetabular inclination via the Tönnis angle, created by drawing a reference line, which can be drawn between the centers of the femoral heads, the inferior aspect of the teardrops, or at the ischial tuberosities. The angle between this reference line and a line connecting the inferior and lateral aspects of the sourcil (sclerotic weight-bearing zone of the acetabulum) is the Tönnis angle. Normal values lie between 0 and 10 degrees.[20] Values greater than 10 degrees suggest dysplasia, with patients at risk for structural instability, whereas with values less than 0 degrees, patients are at risk for pincer-type femoroacetabular impingement.[20] The lateral center edge angle of Wiberg is used to assess adequate coverage of the superolateral femoral head by the acetabulum. This angle is obtained by drawing a line superior from the center of the femoral head, perpendicular to the transverse axis of the pelvis (using a reference line discussed previously), and a second line from the center of the femoral head to the lateral aspect of the sourcil.[20] A similar angle drawn on the false profile view is the anterior center-edge angle of Lequesne, formed by a vertical line from the center of the femoral head and an additional line from the center of the femoral head to the anterior aspect of the sourcil (Fig. 132.23A–C).[20] A lateral center edge angle less than 25 degrees may indicate inadequate coverage of the femoral head, whereas an anterior center edge angle of less than 20 degrees can be indicative of structural instability.[20]

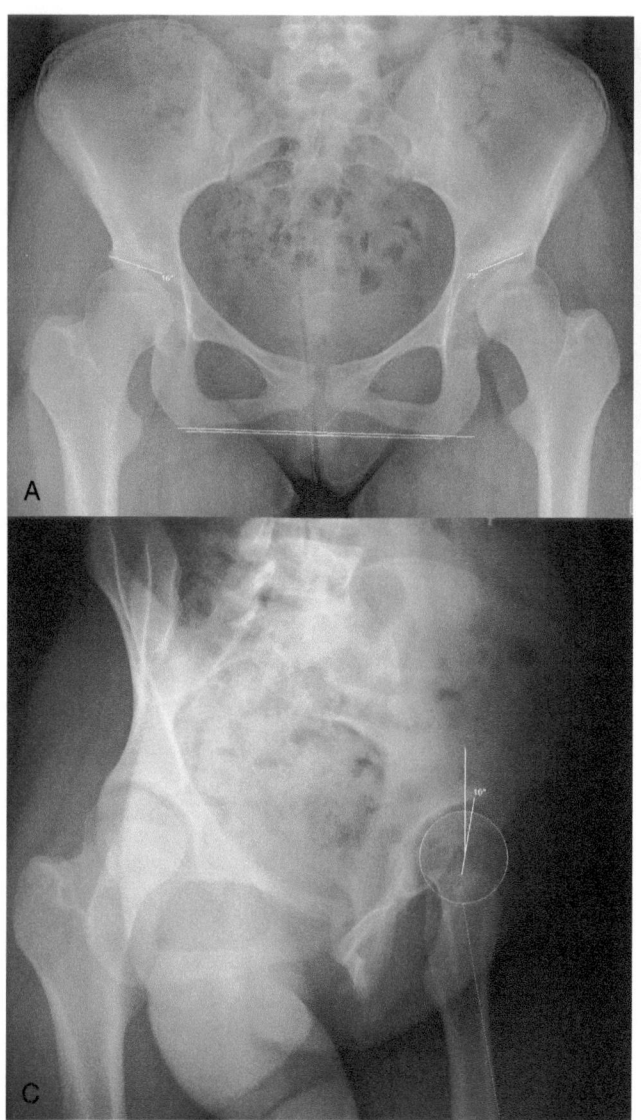

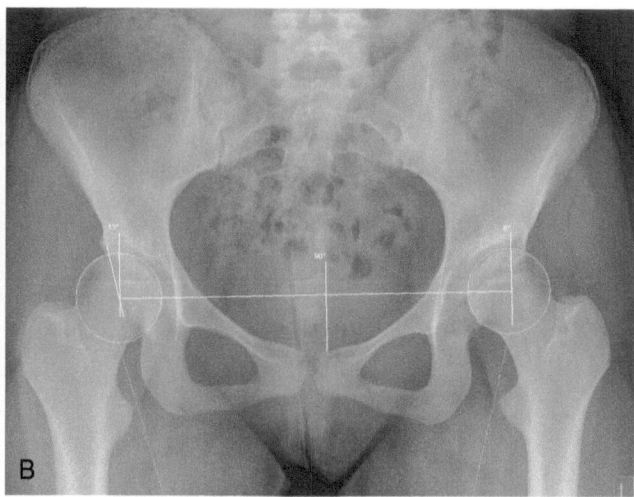

Fig. 132.23 A 17-year-old female with hip dysplasia, left more severe than the right. (A) Tönnis angle. (B) Lateral center edge angle. (C) Anterior center edge angle.

Ischiofemoral impingement, internal/external snapping hip, and femoral neck stress fractures may also be a cause for hip pain in the adolescent athlete, although they are not exclusive to the skeletally immature athlete. Ischiofemoral impingement and stress fractures are easily diagnosed on MRI, whereas internal and external snapping hip is best diagnosed with dynamic ultrasound.

KNEE

Acute Injuries

Distal femoral fractures involving the physis are not common, accounting for only 1% of all physeal fractures. When present, however, they can represent important injuries, as they may be associated with a significant growth disturbance resulting in leg-length discrepancy.[14] A high index of suspicion must be present in adolescent patients with knee pain following trauma as these fractures may be radiographically occult. Sometimes the only finding present on radiographs will be medial soft tissue

swelling, which may relate to hemorrhage or subperiosteal hematoma. MRI findings can be surprisingly subtle, with subtle fluid signal at the level of the physis, entrapped periosteum within the distal femoral physis, or subperiosteal hematoma. Sometimes entrapped periosteum within the fracture site may be the only sign of a fracture.

Adolescents are more vulnerable to avulsion fractures than younger children owing to their greater muscle strength and the relative weakness of the osteocartilaginous interfaces.[4] Avulsion fractures about the knee can involve the cruciate ligaments, collateral ligaments and supporting tendons, extensor mechanism, or retinacula.

Avulsion fractures associated with the extensor mechanism, which are exclusive to the immature skeleton, include tibial tubercle avulsion fractures and the patellar sleeve fracture. Tibial tubercle avulsion fractures typically occur in males between the ages of 13 and 17 years when the normal fibrocartilage present at the proximal tibial physis deep to the ossifying tibial tubercle apophysis is replaced by weaker hyaline cartilage.[4] These fractures are typically associated with jumping (e.g., quadriceps contraction with extension) or landing (e.g., rapid flexion against a contracted quadriceps).[4] Fractures can involve only the growth plate or can extend into the metaphysis (Salter 2), epiphysis (Salter 3), or both (Salter 4).[4] Entrapment of adjacent tissue can occur, which can be incidental or may prevent adequate closed reduction (Fig. 132.24A and B).[4]

Avulsion fractures of the extensor mechanism in the skeletally immature patient can also involve a sleeve of unossified patellar cartilage often with small osseous fragments; these are referred to as patellar sleeve fractures.[4] They are most commonly seen involving the patellar tendon at the distal pole but can also involve the quadriceps tendon at the proximal pole. The mechanism of injury relates to resistance against forceful quadriceps extension.[4] Radiographs will often show a displaced ossific fragment associated with the proximal or distal pole of the patella; if there is substantial displacement, it will be known as patella baja or alta, respectively. Joint effusion may be present if there is substantial involvement of the articular cartilage. MRI is typically performed to evaluate the integrity of the articular cartilage at the patella, which may result in the need of operative fixation.[4]

Preexisting Osgood-Schlatter disease or Sinding-Larsen-Johansson disease may predispose to tibial tubercle or patellar avulsion fractures. In the absence of obvious displacement, a nondisplaced acute avulsion fracture superimposed on chronic changes of chronic repetitive microtrauma is typically differentiated by the clinical history of an acute event. MRI may show fluid at the osteochondral interface and a pattern of increased soft tissue or bone marrow edema pattern.

Injuries to the anterior cruciate ligament are commonly found in young athletes approaching skeletal maturity or skeletally mature patients, but also can occur in skeletally immature patients. The imaging findings of anterior cruciate ligament (ACL) tears and associated pathology are similar to those seen in adults. However, MRI has been shown to be less accurate for the diagnosis of ACL tears in the pediatric age group (ages 4 to 14), and there are age-related differences in the appearance of the ACL in children.[21] Specifically, the ACL has a more horizontal orientation both in the sagittal and coronal planes and the bundles are often less well defined, with intermediate signal on fluid-sensitive sequences, which should not be mistaken for a tear.[22] In the acute setting, secondary findings of ACL injury, such as pivot shift bone contusions, can be helpful in supporting a diagnosis of ACL injury, but diagnosis can be more complicated in the subacute or chronic setting. Awareness of the differences in the appearance of the ACL in young children, evaluating for presence of the ACL in all three imaging planes, or thin section imaging with three-dimensional isotropic sequences can all be useful in obtaining the correct diagnosis.

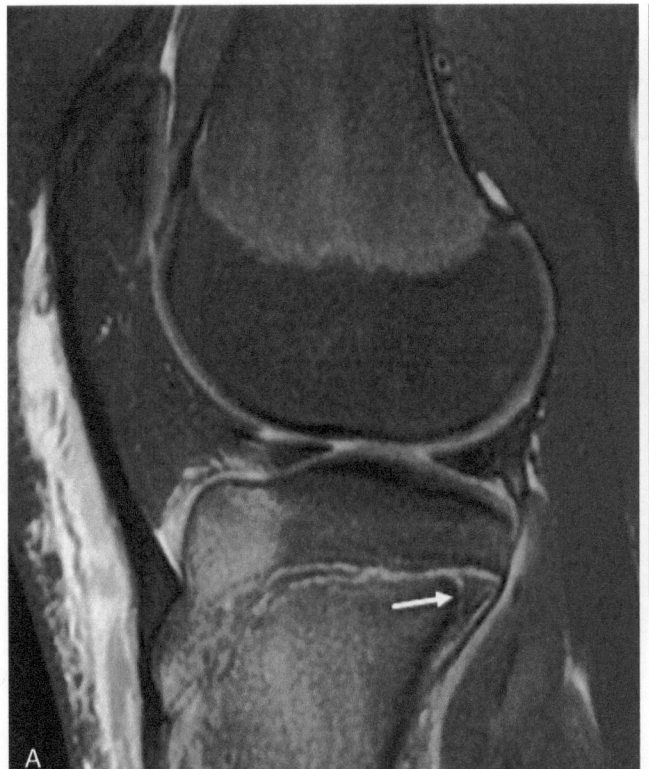
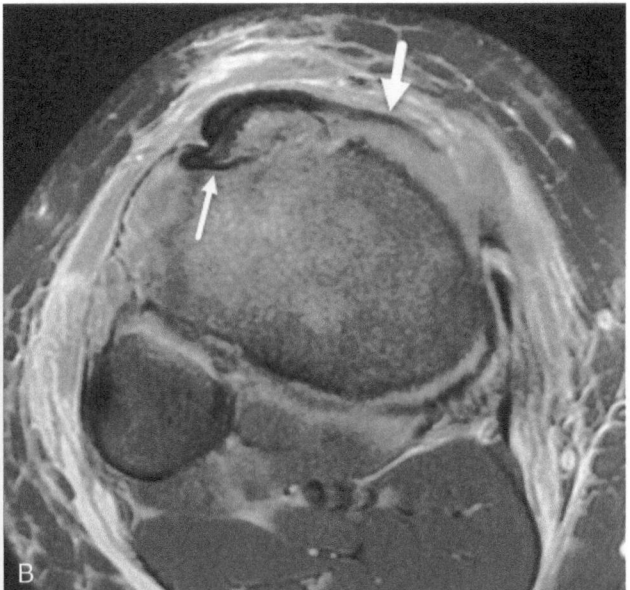

Fig. 132.24 A 14-year-old male with an avulsion fracture of the tibial tubercle with a Salter 2 pattern. (A) Sagittal T2-weighted fat-suppressed fluid-sensitive sequence shows edema and hemorrhage in the anterior soft tissues, an extensive bone marrow edema pattern within the proximal tibia with hyperintense signal within the physis, and a subtle posterior metaphyseal fracture line (arrow). The lack of displacement can make this fracture radiographically occult. (B) Axial T2-weighted fat-suppressed image demonstrates entrapped periosteum within the lateral fracture site (thin arrow) and elevated periosteum medially (thick arrow).

Following ACL injury, a determination of skeletal maturity is often required in order to decide on the treatment approach, since open growth plates can interfere with traditional ACL reconstruction techniques. Although many systems exist, the skeletal bone age is most commonly evaluated using a single PA view of the left hand with correlation to a book of age-related male and female standards compiled by Greulich and Pyle.[23] A skeletal age is determined based on the assessment of multiple variables when the patient's degree of skeletal maturity is compared with age- and gender-specific standards. In determining the patient's skeletal age, greater reliance is traditionally placed on the growth centers of the phalanges as opposed to the growth centers of the carpal bones. The sesamoids at the thumb metacarpophalangeal (MCP) joint, when present, are useful in determining the skeletal age. However, a shorthand bone age method has been developed for clinicians as a simpler, more efficient method using only a single criterion for each age; it has been shown to be comparable in accuracy to traditional methods.[24]

In addition to purely ligamentous injuries to the ACL in skeletally immature patients, the same mechanism of injury can result in an avulsion fracture of the tibial eminence due to the weaker immature unossified epiphyseal cartilage.[4,14] These fractures typically involve boys 8 to 14 years of age.[4] The Meyers and McKeever classification is frequently used in relation to these fractures and consists of a type 1 nondisplaced fracture, type 2 fracture with elevated but posteriorly hinged fragment, type 3 fracture with displaced fragment, or type 4 fracture when comminuted.[4] Entrapped tissue can prevent nonoperative closed reduction and may require surgical reduction; it is more common in type 2 and 3 fractures.[4,25] Entrapped tissue involves either the transverse intermeniscal ligament or the anterior horns of the menisci (Fig. 132.25A and B).

Avulsion fractures can occur from the medial patella in the context of a patellar dislocation-relocation injury, which is a common injury in the adolescent athlete. Imaging findings are similar to those seen in adults. Briefly, tensile and shear forces on the patella during dislocation and compressive and shear forces between the patella and lateral femoral condyle with relocation can result in osteochondral injury.[26] Radiographs typically show a large joint effusion, sometimes with avulsion fracture from the medial patella seen on sunrise or Merchant views or a crescentic piece of bone related to a displaced osteochondral fracture fragment. MRI is typically performed to evaluate for large osteochondral fractures and displaced intra-articular bodies that may require surgical treatment, although MRI can also assess the integrity of the medial retinaculum (including the medial patellofemoral ligament), check for the presence of trochlear dysplasia, and evaluate the tibial tuberosity-trochlear groove distance, which can affect treatment.[26] Beware of blood clot that may fill the site of a full-thickness cartilage injury, particularly at the medial patella, which may obscure the donor site related to an obvious displaced osteochondral fragment.

Overuse Injuries

Chronic repetitive microtrauma or apophysitis at the knee occurs at the distal pole of the patella and tibial tubercle and has been given the eponyms Sinding-Larsen-Johansson and Osgood-Schlatter disease, respectively. Osgood-Schlatter disease is common in adolescents, particularly with "jumping sports," and occurs at an earlier stage of ossification than avulsion fractures of the tibial tubercle, although preexisting Osgood-Schlatter disease may predispose to avulsion fractures. The condition is often bilateral (20%–30% of cases) and is typically diagnosed clinically.[14] Characteristic radiographic findings consist of fragmentation of the tibial tubercle, thickening of the distal patellar tendon, and increased density of the prepatellar soft tissues and deep infrapatellar fat pad. Similar findings are seen on MRI in addition to a bone marrow edema pattern in the apophysis and adjacent tibial epiphysis;

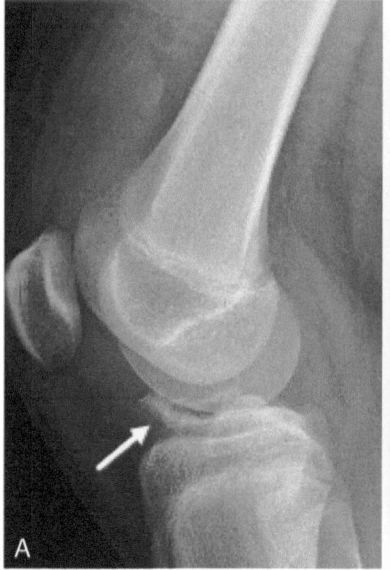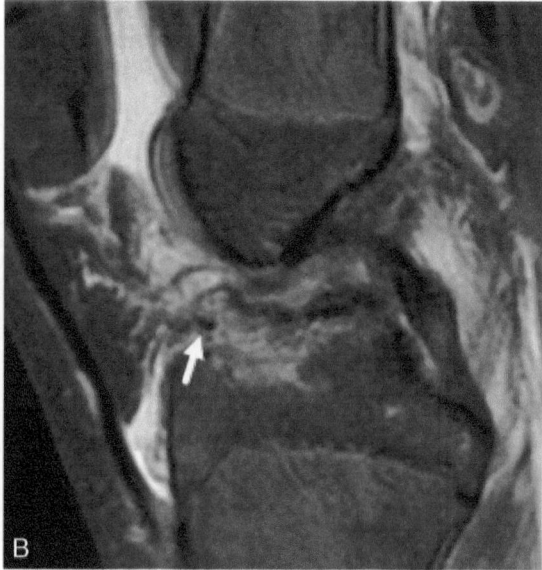

Fig. 132.25 A 13-year-old boy with a fracture of the tibial eminence. (A) Lateral radiographs show a displaced fracture of the tibial eminence *(arrow)*. (B) Sagittal T2-weighted fat-suppressed fluid-sensitive sequence shows an entrapped transverse intermeniscal ligament *(arrow)* beneath the displaced fragment, which may prevent non-operative closed reduction.

intermediate signal and thickening of the tendon, reflective of a tendinopathy; as well as abnormal fluid in the deep infrapatellar bursa, reflective of bursitis. Ultrasound is not commonly performed, although it does an excellent job in highlighting the findings (Fig. 132.26A and B). It should be noted that fragmentation of the tibial tubercle in and of itself is not diagnostic of Osgood-Schlatter disease and may be seen in asymptomatic patients. Chronic changes of Osgood-Schlatter disease on MRI typically show absence of the tendinopathy, infrapatellar bursitis, and bone marrow edema pattern.

Sinding-Larsen-Johansson disease is also typically diagnosed clinically, although radiographic findings consist of fragmentation of the inferior pole of the patella and thickening of the proximal patellar tendon. MRI will also demonstrate a bone marrow edema pattern at the lower pole of the patella as well as edema in the adjacent soft tissues.

A similar entity in the skeletally mature young athlete is proximal patellar tendinopathy, also known as "jumper's knee," which can be a chronically debilitating condition, often refractory to conservative management. Instead of the fragmentation seen at the inferior pole of the patella in a skeletally immature patient, these patients will have closed growth plates and abnormal thickening of the proximal tendon with or without edema in the adjacent Hoffa fat pad and irregularity at the osseous enthesis. On MRI this will consist of thickening and abnormal intermediate-signal tissue on fluid-sensitive sequences, typically within the deep central portion of the proximal tendon. On ultrasound there will be thickening with decreased echogenicity and loss of the normal packed fibrillar pattern of the tendon as well as increased blood flow with color or power Doppler imaging, representative of neovascularity within the abnormal tendon tissue. Increasing evidence has shown that patients with proximal patellar tendinosis refractory to conservative treatment may benefit from a minimally invasive intervention such as tendon fenestration (also known as dry needling) with

or without platelet-rich plasma injections, which is preferably performed using ultrasound guidance in order to direct the treatment specifically to the abnormal tissue while sparing normal tissue.[27,28]

OCD can be a source of chronic pain in the young athlete and is considered juvenile OCD when the growth plates are still open or adult OCD when the growth plates are closed. The Research in Osteochondritis Dissecans of the Knee (ROCK) group has defined OCD as "a focal, idiopathic alteration of subchondral bone with risk for instability and disruption of adjacent articular cartilage that may result in premature osteoarthritis."[29] Over 70% of cases are found at the lateral aspect of the medial femoral condyle and radiographs will typically show a faint well-defined or ill-defined lucency within subchondral bone, sometimes associated with peripheral sclerosis or a well-defined osseous fragment within the bed of the OCD site.[14] A compete knee radiographic series for evaluation of OCD will typically include an AP view, tunnel view, lateral view, and sunrise or Merchant view. Some cases of OCD will be seen only on the tunnel view, which better profiles the posterior aspect of the condyle, or the sunrise or Merchant view for the less common patellar or trochlear OCD.

A possible conundrum when radiographs in young athletes are being evaluated is differentiating an ossification variant from OCD. Unlike with OCD, patients with what has been termed an "ossification variant" do not have clinical symptoms, do not progress to unstable OCD lesions, and resolve spontaneously. Ossification variants do not occur in girls greater than 10 years old or in boys greater than 13 years old; they tend to occur in the posterior third of the femoral condyle, have spiculated borders or a puzzle-piece configuration, extend deeper into the subchondral bone with a lesional angle less than 105 degrees, and have no adjacent marrow edema pattern on MRI. OCD tends to be centered within the middle third of the condyle and is flatter with lesional angle greater than 105 degrees. On T2-weighted

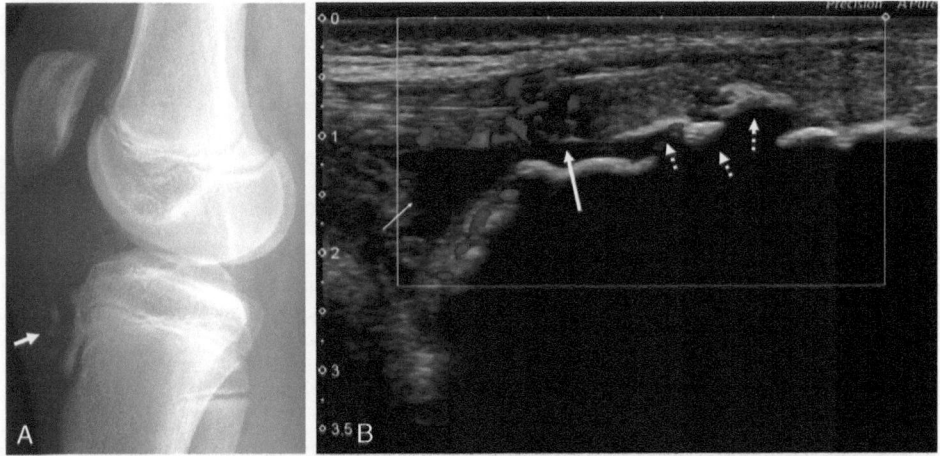

Fig. 132.26 Osgood Schlatter disease. (A) Anteroposterior radiograph shows fragmentation at the tibial tubercle *(arrow)*, thickening of the patellar tendon, and soft tissue swelling. (B) Long axis sonographic image with color Doppler shows the white echogenic bony acoustic landmarks of the fragmented tibial tubercle apophysis *(dashed arrows)*, increased color flow related to neovascularity within tendinosis *(arrow)*, and deep infrapatellar bursitis *(thin arrow)*.

MRI sequences, OCD lesions will have a marrow edema pattern within subchondral bone, bands of hyperintense signal either within subchondral bone or at the cartilage-bone interface, or cyst-like foci within subchondral bone.

Currently the primary role of MRI in the context of OCD is to confirm presence of an OCD and to evaluate the likelihood of stability in order to help guide appropriate treatment. However, multi-institutional studies are under way in the hope of providing a more robust treatment algorithm based on a variety of imaging and clinical features. Juvenile OCD has greater healing potential than adult OCD and also has different imaging features suggestive of instability.[30,31] In adults, DeSmet's refined criteria for determining instability in the knee and ankle based on several features on T2-weighted sequences are often used and consist of (1) a well-defined or ill-defined line of hyperintense signal equal to joint fluid at the femur-fragment interface measuring 5 mm or more in length, (2) a discrete round focus of hyperintense signal deep to the OCD lesion measuring 5 mm or more, (3) a focal defect in articular cartilage that measures greater than 5 mm in width, and (4) hyperintense signal equal to joint fluid traversing the articular cartilage and subchondral bone plate into the lesion.[32] However, more recent studies by the same group have found different criteria for determining juvenile OCD instability at the knee, namely (1) rim-like hyperintense signal equal to joint fluid in addition to a deeper linear margin of hypointense signal plus multiple sites of discontinuity in the subchondral bone plate or (2) multiple cyst-like foci or a single cyst-like focus greater than or equal to 5 mm (Fig. 132.27).[30] An ill-defined confluent band of hyperintense signal within subchondral bone and a single small cyst-like focus measuring less than 5 mm can be seen in stable juvenile OCD lesions (Fig. 132.28).

A zone of focal periphyseal edema (FOPE) will occasionally be encountered on MRI examinations performed for knee pain in adolescent patients and can be a potential etiology for pain when no other abnormality is seen to explain pain on the MRI examination. The etiology of this finding is felt to relate to normal physiologic physeal closure.[33] Beyond its potential as a source of pain in the young athlete, it is important not to confuse this finding with another etiology, such as osteomyelitis or neoplasm. It is important to note that this finding should be seen around the time of physiologic growth plate closure, typically in girls 11 to 14 years old and boys 13 to 14 years old. Radiographs should demonstrate narrowing of the growth plates related to early growth plate closure. On MRI there will be characteristic patterns of bone marrow edema, sometimes with a "bowtie" configuration within both the epiphysis and metaphysis, centered at the growth plate of the distal femur or proximal tibia; however, anecdotally this finding has also been seen in the fibula as well as in the proximal humerus and femur (Fig. 132.29). A marrow edema pattern centered around the growth plate in a younger age group without evidence of physiologic growth plate closure should prompt thoughts of another etiology.

Imaging features of a synovial impingement syndrome are frequently found in the young athlete. In particular, fat pad impingement involving the superolateral Hoffa fat pad, also known as patellar tendon–lateral femoral condyle friction syndrome, can be a cause of anterior knee pain in athletes and is

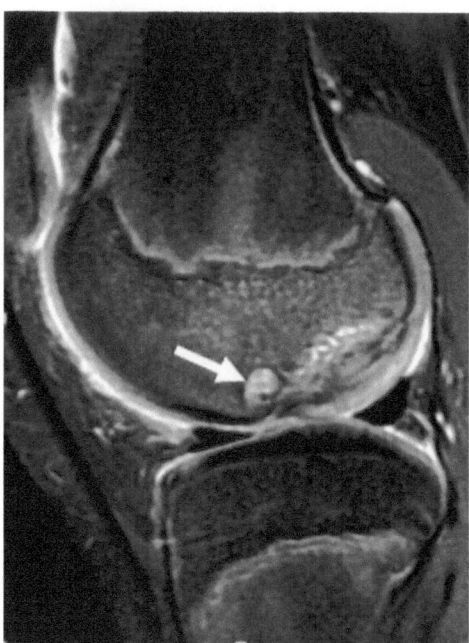

Fig. 132.27 Unstable juvenile osteochondritis dissecans (OCD). Sagittal T2-weighted fat-suppressed fluid-sensitive sequence shows a single 6-mm cyst-like lesion *(arrow)* at the anterior aspect of the OCD site, multiple sites of discontinuity in the subchondral bone plate, and irregularity of contour at the articular surface.

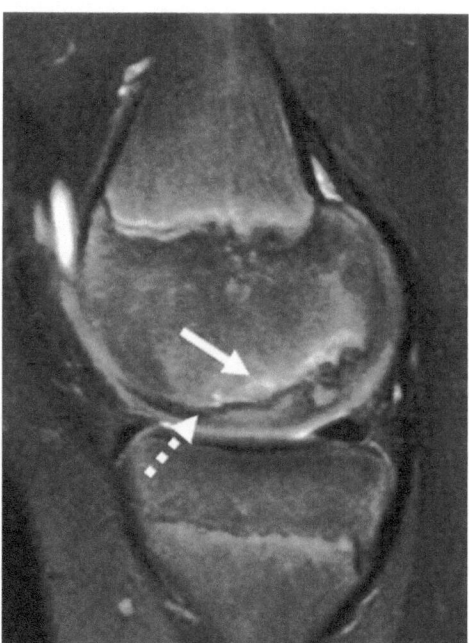

Fig. 132.28 Stable juvenile osteochondritis dissecans (OCD). Sagittal T2-weighted fat-suppressed fluid-sensitive sequence shows an ill-defined confluent band of hyperintense signal within subchondral bone *(arrow)*, a tiny cyst-like lesion at the anterior aspect of the OCD site, and a continuous subchondral bone plate *(dashed arrow)*.

frequently seen in both symptomatic and asymptomatic patients; it has been associated with patellar maltracking. Plica can also be a cause of pain in young athletes, typically associated with the medial patellar plica and can mimic a medial meniscal tear. MRI findings suggestive of a symptomatic plica can include a

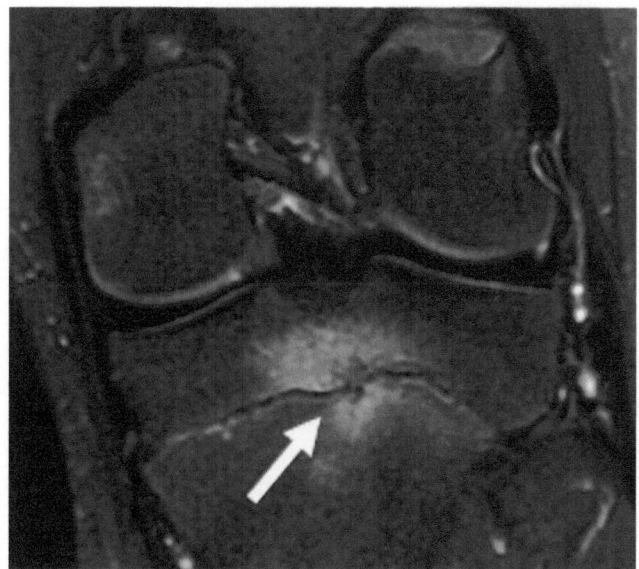

Fig. 132.29 Coronal T2-weighted fat-suppressed fluid-sensitive sequence shows a typical zone of focal periphyseal edema centered about the growth plate *(arrow)*.

thickened plica, hyperintense signal within articular cartilage suggesting softening in the adjacent medial patellar facet, or localized intermediate signal material surrounding the plica on fluid-sensitive sequences consistent with thickened synovial tissue/synovitis. Ultrasound has also been shown to be useful in the diagnosis of medial patellar plica syndrome and can be diagnosed in the presence of three criteria: (1) continuous band-like echo representing the plica anterior to the medial femoral condyle, (2) movement of the plica under the patella with the patella pushed medially by approximately 1 cm, and (3) pain or discomfort at the medial knee with the examination.[34]

LOWER LEG/ANKLE/FOOT

Acute Injuries

Triplane and Tillaux fractures can be termed transitional fractures due to their occurrence between the ages of 14 and 16 years, when the growth plates are closing.[14] The lateral aspect of the tibial growth plate is susceptible to fracture because it is the last region to close.[14] A fracture isolated to the anterolateral aspect of the tibial epiphysis is termed a juvenile Tillaux fracture, whereas a similar fracture pattern but with additional extension into the metaphysis with a coronal plane is termed a triplane fracture. CT is typically performed following the diagnosis of these fractures on radiographs because studies have shown substantial changes in treatment decisions and surgical planning when CT is performed in the context of distal tibial fractures involving the articular surface.[14] The amount of gap/distraction at the articular surface and the degree of articular surface step-off are important findings to guide treatment. Since these fractures occur close to skeletal maturity, when there is little further growth potential, they should not present a risk for growth disturbance but rather the potential for premature

osteoarthrosis if not properly reduced. However, Salter 2 fractures occurring at the distal tibia in younger athletes should be followed closely with radiographs to evaluate for a pathologic bone bridge at the growth plate, which can result in growth disturbance.

Ankle sprains are common injuries also in the skeletally immature athlete; however, in general the imaging findings are similar to those in adults. Radiographs will often show lateral soft tissue swelling and an ankle joint effusion. Nondisplaced Salter Harris 1 or 2 fractures can frequently be present, involving the distal fibular growth plate in the setting of an ankle sprain, and they can be radiographically occult in the acute setting. When the swelling on radiographs appears to be centered over the growth plate rather than distal to the malleolus, an occult fracture can be suspected. Conservative management and follow-up imaging in 10 to 14 days can be useful to evaluate for periosteal new bone in the context of a healing radiographically occult fracture. In very young patients, avulsion fractures can occur through the unossified epiphyseal cartilage and be occult on radiographs or can involve a small crescent of bone. Normal variant accessory ossicles are common at the medial malleolus, although lateral ossicles, sometimes referred to as os subfibulare, are likely most often related to prior trauma. Chronic ununited avulsion fractures can result in a painful syndrome referred to as a symptomatic os subfibulare.[35] A bone marrow edema pattern surrounding the site of nonunion on MRI and corresponding pain confirms the diagnosis (Fig. 132.30A and B).

Similar to adults, young athletes can develop impingement syndromes about the ankle either related to prior ankle sprain or congenital variation such as an os trigonum or a prominent posterolateral talar tubercle, also called a Stieda process. However, the imaging appearance is the same as in adults.

Overuse Injuries

In children and adolescents, stress fractures are most commonly encountered in the lower extremity, with the tibia accounting for 50%, fibula 20%, and metatarsal or tarsal bones approximately 7% of cases (Fig. 132.31).[14] Radiographs should be the first imaging study ordered if there is concern for stress fracture, although they will be negative in up to 90% of cases.[14] Follow-up radiographs in 10 days may subsequently show evidence of healing with periosteal reaction.[14] Although bone scan was traditionally used to evaluate for stress fractures when radiographs were negative, MRI is currently the preferred modality due to its increased specificity and lack of ionizing radiation. With MRI, tibial stress injuries can be graded based on severity, with grade 1 consisting of only periosteal edema. Grade 2 consists of marrow edema pattern on fluid-sensitive sequences but normal signal on T1-weighted images, whereas grade 3 will have hypointense signal on T1-weighted images, in addition to the marrow edema pattern on fluid-sensitive sequences. A discrete fracture line will be present in grade 4 stress injury.[14]

Chronic repetitive stress injury is also seen involving apophyses at the feet. The eponym for involvement of the calcaneal apophysis is Sever disease, whereas involvement of the apophysis at the base of the fifth metatarsal is Iselin disease. Sever disease is the most common cause of heel pain in athletes 5 to 11 years

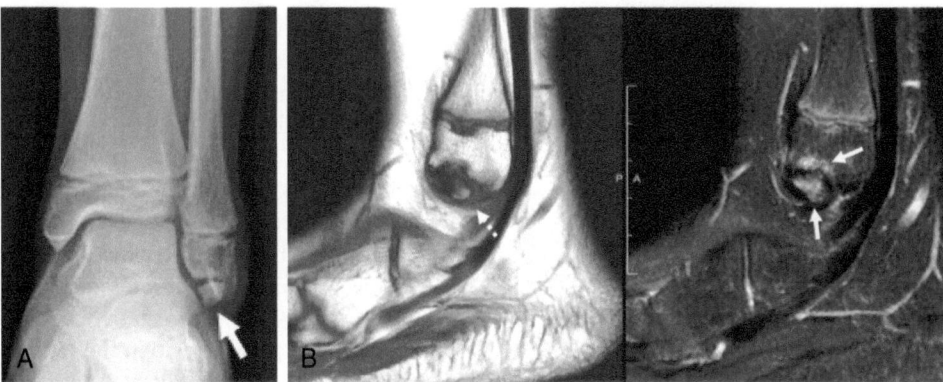

Fig. 132.30 (A) Anteroposterior radiograph showing an ossific fragment at the tip of the fibula *(arrow)*. (B). Sagittal T1- and corresponding T2-weighted fat-suppressed fluid-sensitive sequence shows the ossific fragment on T1 *(dashed arrow)* with an associated bone marrow edema pattern both within the ossicle and the adjacent fibula on the T2-weighted images *(arrows)*, suggesting a symptomatic ossicle.

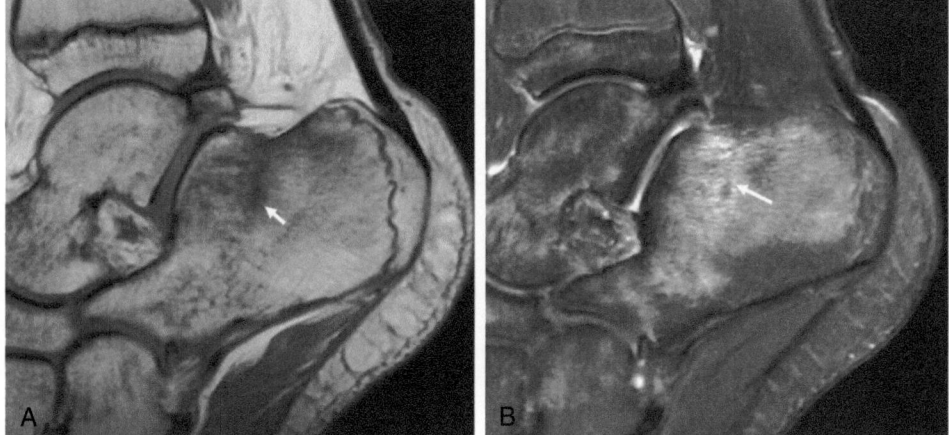

Fig. 132.31 (A) Sagittal T1-weighted image shows a linear band of decreased signal *(arrow)* within the body of the calcaneus oriented perpendicular to the trabecula, characteristic of a stress fracture. Note the more vague decreased signal within the marrow surrounding the fracture site. (B) Sagittal T2-weighted fat-suppressed fluid-sensitive sequence also shows the linear band of decreased signal *(arrow)* with surrounding hyperintense marrow edema pattern.

old.[14] This diagnosis is usually made clinically with radiographs performed to exclude other etiologies such as a stress fracture. Fragmentation and sclerosis, findings sometimes associated with chronic repetitive stress elsewhere in the body, is frequently seen normally at the calcaneal apophysis and is not specific for Sever disease. A bone marrow edema pattern within the apophysis, sometimes with adjacent soft tissue edema, is suggestive of the diagnosis on MRI. MRI findings of Iselin disease are similar to other sites of chronic repetitive stress around the body, as discussed previously.

OCD can also affect the ankle joint, typically involving the talar dome, although because many of the osteochondral abnormalities seen in the ankle have a direct relation to prior trauma, the more generic term *osteochondral lesion* is often used. Multiple staging systems have been described based on radiography, arthroscopy, CT, and MRI; a discussion of all of these systems is beyond the scope of this chapter.[36] On CT, subchondral cyst-like foci, fragment detachment, fragmentation, and displaced fragments suggest instability.[36] DeSmet's previously discussed

MRI criteria were also demonstrated to be applicable to the ankle and are often used to determine instability, but in practice a thorough description of the findings is recommended in order to apply findings to a chosen staging system if desired.

Repetitive stress in the setting of a tarsal coalition can result in pain in the young athlete. Tarsal coalitions can also contribute to recurrent ankle sprains. Coalitions result from failure in segmentation of two ossification centers in utero and can be purely osseous or fibrocartilaginous. The calcaneonavicular or talonavicular joints are most frequently involved and coalitions can be bilateral in up to 50% of patients.[14] Foot radiographs are often diagnostic for calcaneonavicular coalition either showing an elongated anterior process on the lateral radiograph, the so-called anteater nose sign, or direct visualization of the abnormal articulation on the oblique foot radiograph either showing complete osseous coalition or close approximation of the bones with irregularity and sclerosis at the articulation. Talonavicular coalitions can be more difficult to appreciate on radiographs; when present, they are usually identified on a lateral radiograph as a "continuous C sign" between the sustentaculum tali of the calcaneus and the talus. CT is often performed to evaluate for coalition, although MRI can readily diagnose coalition and can also evaluate for an associated stress reaction or ligamentous pathology.

A symptomatic accessory navicular is another commonly encountered condition in the young athlete related to instability between the accessory ossicle at the navicular tuberosity and the navicular. Accessory navicular bones can be classified based on their appearance; type 1 has small, round, smooth margins; it is found within the posterior tibialis tendon and typically not symptomatic. Type 2 is larger, with irregular margins between the ossicle and the navicular at the site of the fibrocartilaginous bridge and is most frequently symptomatic. Type 3 is also called a cornuate navicular; this variant consists of complete osseous fusion of the ossicle to the navicular and is less commonly symptomatic. On radiographs, the presence of a type 2 navicular and symptoms centered at this region is suggestive of a symptomatic accessory navicular, also called accessory navicular syndrome. This can be confirmed on MRI by showing a bone marrow edema pattern within the ossicle and adjacent navicular bone as well as adjacent reactive soft tissue edema on fluid-sensitive sequences.

Intrasheath subluxation is a condition that can result in pain and a snapping sensation of the ankle; it may be confused with peroneal tendon dislocation and superior peroneal retinacular injury. In and of itself this condition is unlikely to be symptomatic and simple reassurance may be enough, although with repetitive irritation, inflammation may occur, resulting in pain.[37] This condition is not diagnosed on MRI and relies on dynamic ultrasound if the clinical history and physical examination findings are indeterminate.

SPINE

Low back pain is relatively common, occurring in 40% of children and adolescents prior to adulthood; however, a structural cause is found in only 12% to 26% of cases.[38] Spondylolysis is the most common structural cause of low back pain in this population, although studies using single photon emission computed tomography (SPECT) in the evaluation of low back pain have found other abnormalities in up to 40% of positive cases.[38] Other abnormalities can include interspinous bursitis, endplate-apophyseal injuries, facet hypertrophy, transitional vertebrae (also known as Bertolotti syndrome), sacral stress fractures, and sacroiliac joint syndrome.[38] An MRI study performed on elite-level female gymnasts demonstrated anterior ring apophyseal injuries and degenerative disc disease most commonly followed by spondylolysis.[39]

Interspinous bursitis can occur subsequent to repetitive flexion and extension of the spine, particularly in gymnasts. This can strain the interspinous ligaments and cause adjacent spinous processes to touch each other. Bursa may subsequently form, with bursitis leading to low back pain.[40] This mechanism of interspinous bursitis may be the adolescent equivalent of Baastrup disease, also known as kissing spine syndrome, which occurs in an older population related to abnormal contact of spinous

processes but due to chronic degenerative changes. Spinous process apophysitis has also been described and can mimic spondylolysis clinically. However, it is important to differentiate this entity because the length of treatment and long-term sequelae are different.[41] Spinous process apophysitis occurs through a similar mechanism as interspinous bursitis and indeed, may be related and coexist.

Imaging evaluation of low back pain is primarily based on history and physical examination. Patients with neurologic symptoms will typically obtain a more urgent workup with MRI, whereas other patients without "red flags" will typically obtain radiographs, CT, MRI, or SPECT.[38] Radiography is typically the first imaging test performed. Although oblique views were traditionally performed in the workup of low back pain in adolescents, more recent studies show no significant difference in sensitivity or specificity between a two-view or four-view radiographic study. Owing to the substantially increased radiation burden delivered, a four-view radiographic series should be avoided.[42,43] Radiographs, CT, and MRI may show defects within the pars interarticularis, although SPECT and MRI can identify a stress reaction or nondisplaced stress fracture without lysis. In the case of stress reaction or nondisplaced stress fracture at the pars interarticularis, SPECT will show symmetric or asymmetric increased radiotracer uptake localized to the pars interarticularis with or without sclerosis on the CT portion of the study.[38] MRI will demonstrate a bone marrow edema pattern with or without a band of decreased T1 and T2 signal corresponding with sclerosis on CT (Fig. 132.32A).[38] Interspinous bursitis will demonstrate increased signal on fluid-sensitive sequences at the level of the interspinous ligaments of the lower lumbar spine, which may also be seen in conjunction with

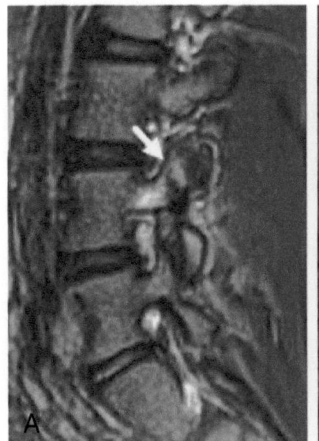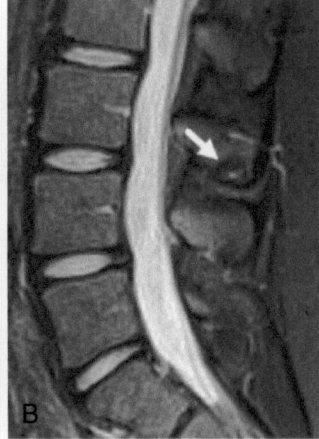

Fig. 132.32 A 14-year-old with chronic low back pain over 2 months. (A) Sagittal short tau inversion recovery (STIR) sequence shows a marrow edema pattern within the posterior elements of L4 centered about a band of hypointense T2 signal *(arrow)*, indicative of a nondisplaced stress fracture at the pars interarticularis. (B) Sagittal STIR image shows irregularity at the inferior spinous process *(arrow)* and increased signal at the level of the interspinous ligaments, which suggests coexisting traction apophysitis and interspinous bursitis.

irregularity of the posteroinferior spinous processes, consistent with repetitive traction injury/apophysitis in the young athlete (see Fig. 132.32B).

MISCELLANEOUS

Although the majority of patients presenting with pain or limitation in activity to a sports medicine practitioner will have an acute or overuse injury, it must be remembered that at times other things, such as a neoplasm, juvenile idiopathic arthritis, or infection, may cause the symptoms. However, a complete discussion of these topics is beyond the scope of this chapter.

For a complete list of references, go to ExpertConsult.com.

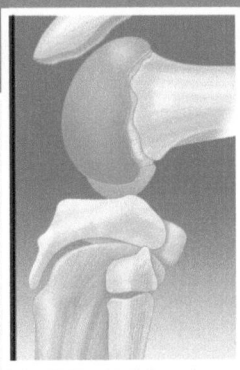

133

Shoulder Injuries in the Young Athlete

Andrew T. Pennock, Eric W. Edmonds

ANATOMY

Skeletally immature bone contains growth plates, or physes, that represent the primary site of longitudinal bone growth. This area of rapidly growing cartilage transitions to bone by a process called endochondral ossification. Due to the nature of this rapid development, physes have much less tensile strength than the surrounding bony epiphysis and metaphysis, thereby rendering the physis more vulnerable to injury as a result of compressive and shearing forces. Injuries to the growth plate are characterized by rapid healing and remodeling but also have the potential for growth arrest or disturbance.[7]

Clavicle

The clavicle forms by intramembranous ossification during the fifth gestational week from two different ossification centers in the diaphysis of the bone. The medial physis of the clavicle is the most important, providing up to 80% of the longitudinal growth of this bone. The medial epiphysis is one of the last in the body to ossify, appearing between 12 and 19 years of age and fusing to the shaft of the clavicle at age 22 to 25 years. The lateral clavicular epiphysis is rarely visualized radiographically, ossifying and fusing during a period of a few months at approximately 19 years of age (Fig. 133.1).[7,8]

Scapula

The four primary anatomic components of the scapula are the body, glenoid, acromion, and coracoid. The body of the scapula is oriented at a 30- to 45-degree angle to the coronal plane of the body, and it forms by intramembranous ossification through multiple ossification centers that are highly variable in terms of number and position. The glenoid has an average of 5 degrees of superior tilt and retroversion of 3 to 9 degrees in relationship to the long axis of the scapula.[9,10] The base of the coracoid and upper glenoid develop from a common physis that ossified at approximately 10 years of age. A variable ossification center can appear at puberty at the tip of the coracoid and may be mistaken as an avulsion fracture. The acromion ossifies through several centers that appear by puberty and fuse by the age of 22 years. Failure of fusion of one of the acromial physes can result in an unfused os acromiale, which may have future clinical implications (Fig. 133.2).[11,12]

Proximal Humerus

The humerus is completely ossified throughout its diaphyseal and metaphyseal portions at birth, with the secondary ossification center for the head appearing 6 months after birth. The secondary ossification center for the greater tuberosity appears by age 3 years, followed by the secondary center for the lesser tuberosity approximately 2 years later. By age 5 to 7 years, the three proximal ossification centers of the humeral head, greater tuberosity, and lesser tuberosity coalesce to become a single proximal ossification center. The proximal humeral physis usually closes between 18 and 22 years of age and accounts for approximately 80% of longitudinal growth of the humerus.[8] The head forms an upward head shaft angle between 130 and 140 degrees and is in 25 to 30 degrees of retroversion as it relates to the humeral epicondyles (Fig. 133.3).[13]

CLAVICLE FRACTURES

Clavicle fractures account for 8% to 15% of all skeletal injuries in children.[14] Despite these injuries being extremely common, little historical attention in the literature had been focused on this topic. The principal reason for this was the belief of Rang and others that "if the two ends of a clavicle fracture are in the same room they will heal and remodel adequately."[15] These fractures can be classified as either lateral, midshaft, or medial, with midshaft fractures occurring most frequently.

Midshaft Clavicle Fractures

Over the past 10 years, a renewed interest in the clavicle has occurred, largely driven by several clinical trials showing the benefits of surgical stabilization of displaced clavicle fractures in adults.[16] As a result, many have begun to apply these principles to adolescent and even pediatric patients. Two recent studies have shown a more than doubling of pediatric clavicle fractures being fixed surgically over the past 10 years.[17,18] This trend is likely occurring as a result of several factors, including the lack of literature in this younger patient population, fear that a mismanaged clavicle fracture may lead to a less satisfactory functional outcome, parental and patient pressure to return young athletes to the sports field quickly, and differing reimbursement regimens for nonoperative versus operative management.

AP View

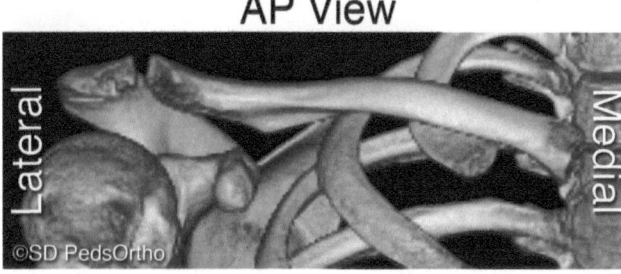

Superior View

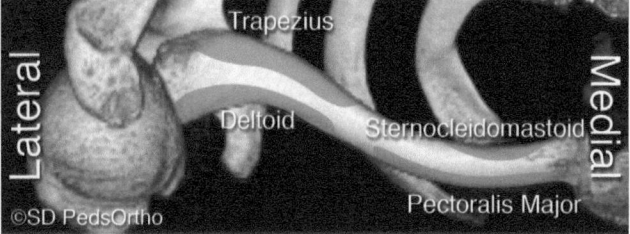

Inferior View

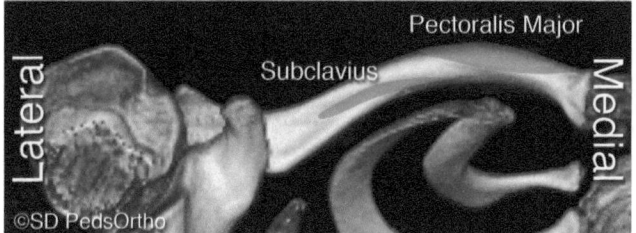

Fig. 133.1 Muscle attachments to the clavicle. *AP,* Anteroposterior.

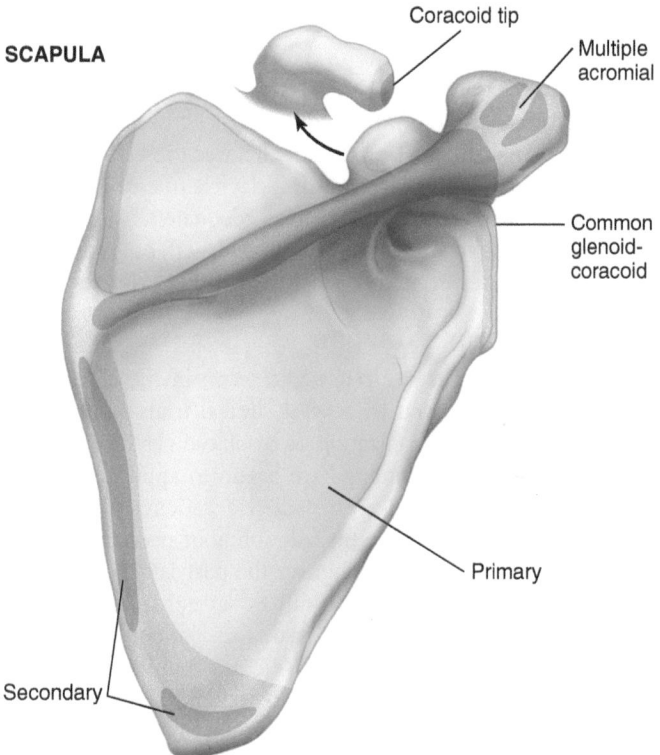

Fig. 133.2 Scapular ossification centers.

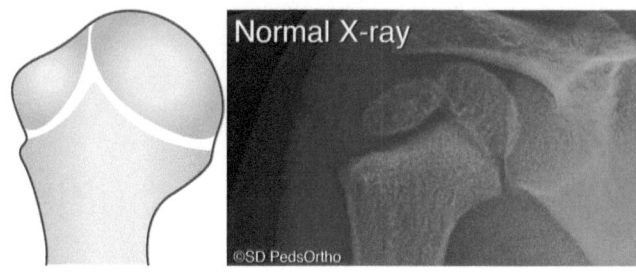

Fig. 133.3 Proximal humerus ossification centers.

History

Most clavicle fractures occur as a result of a direct fall on the shoulder with the arm at the side, but less commonly a fracture may occur as a result of a direct blow or a fall on an outstretched hand. Sports participation, especially contact sports including football, rugby, wrestling, and hockey, are responsible for the largest percentage of these fractures in adolescence. However, with our nation's increased interest in extreme sports such as bike motocross (BMX), motorcycle racing, and mixed martial arts (MMA), these higher-energy fractures are being seen more frequently.

Physical Examination

The examination of a child or adolescent with a clavicle fracture is relatively straightforward given the superficial nature of the bone. Typically, the patient will present with the arm being held in an adducted position close to the body with the opposite hand supporting the injured extremity. The skin should be inspected for an open fracture or significant tenting which has the rare chance to erode through the skin with severe angulation. Limb- and life-threatening concerns, although extremely rare, can occur and need to be identified immediately. These include vascular injuries (subclavian vessels), neurologic injuries (brachial plexus), and injuries to the mediastinal structures (esophagus, trachea, pleura, lung) by angulated or displaced fragments.

Imaging

Almost all midshaft clavicle fractures can be adequately identified with a single anteroposterior (AP) view. Typically, a second view, such as an apical lordotic view or 30-degree cephalic tilt view, is obtained, which can provide further information as to the fracture's displacement, shortening, or comminution (Fig. 133.4).

Treatment Options

Nonoperative treatment. Nearly all mildly displaced clavicle fractures can be treated with either a sling or a figure-of-eight brace. A theoretical advantage of the figure-of-eight brace is that it potentially pulls the shoulders back, minimizing fracture fragment overlap. A practical advantage is that it frees the extremity, making simple daily tasks such as computing easier. In contrast, practical advantages of the sling include its ease of use, its ubiquitous availability, and its cost effectiveness. Two clinical trials failed to show significant outcome differences between slings and figure-of-eight braces.[19,20] As a result, there is a bias with most surgeons preferring slings. When a nonoperative approach

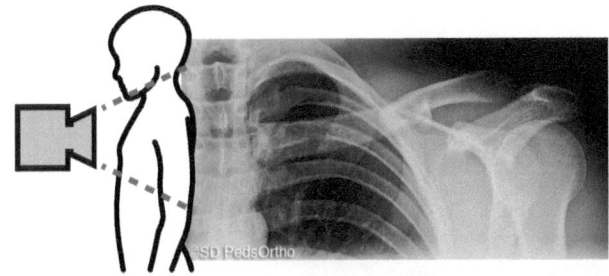

Standard AP
Allows good visualization of the superior/inferior displacement of shaft fractures.

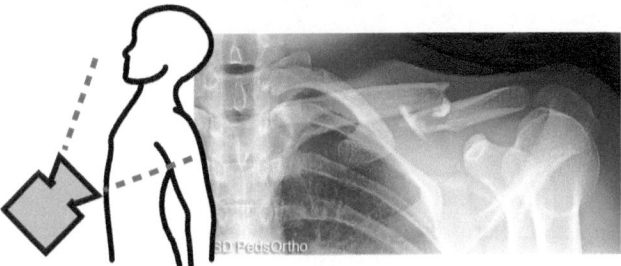

Apical Lordotic View
Tube angled 40-45° – Patient arching/leaning back
Allows better visualization of anterior/posterior translation of the fracture fragments and visualization of the medial clavicle without overlap of the sternum.

Fig. **133.4** Anteroposterior *(AP)* and apical lordotic views of the clavicle.

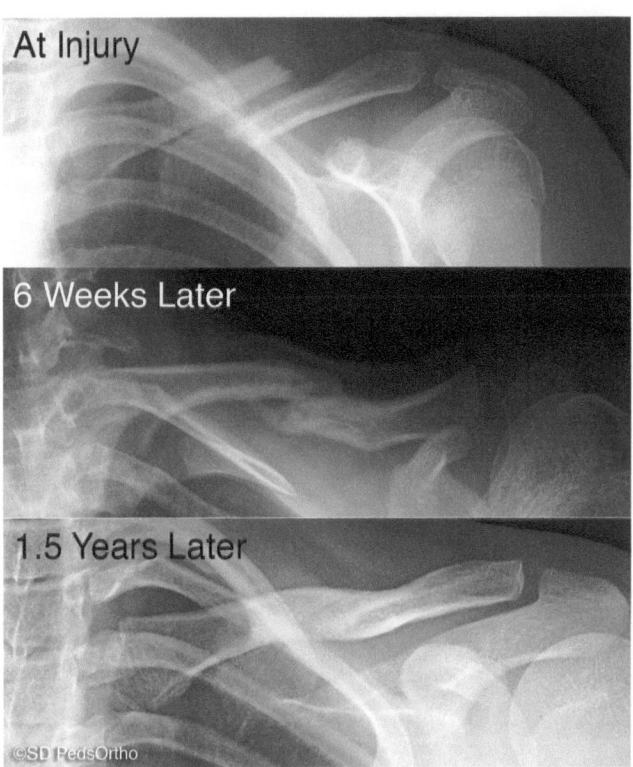

Fig. **133.5** Shortened midshaft clavicle fracture in a teenager demonstrating the remodeling potential of these fractures.

is used, the fracture is protected for 4 to 6 weeks, with contact sports avoided for another 6 weeks. As in most injuries, half the treatment consists of educating the parents about the normal course: An unsightly lump may appear with fracture healing (callus) and will potentially persist for a year while remodeling progresses (Fig. 133.5).

Operative treatment. For the rare midshaft clavicle fracture requiring surgery, fixation can be achieved with a precontoured plate or an intramedullary device. To date, no study has compared the results of these two implants in the pediatric population, but there are case series reporting good outcomes with both approaches (Fig. 133.6).[21] Theoretical advantages of plate fixation are that it can be used with all fracture patterns (even severe comminution), and it creates a rigid construct enabling early mobilization and rapid return to sports. The primary advantages of intramedullary devices are that they potentially minimize the scar length, lessen any infraclavicular numbness, and are potentially less prominent and symptomatic. When plate fixation is selected, the use of a precontoured plate may lessen the need for implant removal.[22] After surgery, a sling is used for comfort for 1 to 2 weeks, allowing early hand, elbow, and shoulder motion exercises. Strengthening exercises are initiated at approximately 6 weeks, when interval healing is appreciated on radiographs. For noncontact sports, it is reasonable to return patients as early as 6 weeks if the patient has no pain, full range of motion (ROM), and good strength. For higher-risk sports and activities, a longer period upwards of 3 months may be necessary to minimize the chance of a refracture. Anecdotally, we have found that patients with displaced fractures undergoing surgical fixation can return

to sports faster, but certainly, we do not want to advocate that this as justification for operative intervention.[23] Implants are routinely left in place but may need to be removed in as many as 40% of cases.[24]

Results

Historic data examining pediatric and adolescent patients with midshaft fractures would suggest that these fractures heal reliably with few residual symptoms.[25,26] However, these studies did not take into account the amount of fracture shortening or displacement and did not look at patient-reported outcomes or formal strength testing. Two current studies have examined functional outcomes and strength testing in patients with displaced midshaft clavicle fractures, and good outcomes were achieved with nonoperative treatment, with no major functional deficits.[26,27] However, a separate study by Vander Have et al. showed that symptomatic malunions can occur in adolescent patients and may be as high as 20%.[23] Currently, optimal surgical indications in this patient population have yet to be clarified. When surgical intervention is pursued, good outcomes have been almost uniformly reported.[27-30]

Complications

Complications are uncommon but can occur both with operative and nonoperative treatment. The most common complications of nonoperative treatment include symptomatic malunions, refracture (especially fractures with residual angulation), and the rare nonunion (<15 having been reported in the literature) (Fig. 133.7). The most common complications of surgical intervention are implant related (10% to 40%), but nonunions,

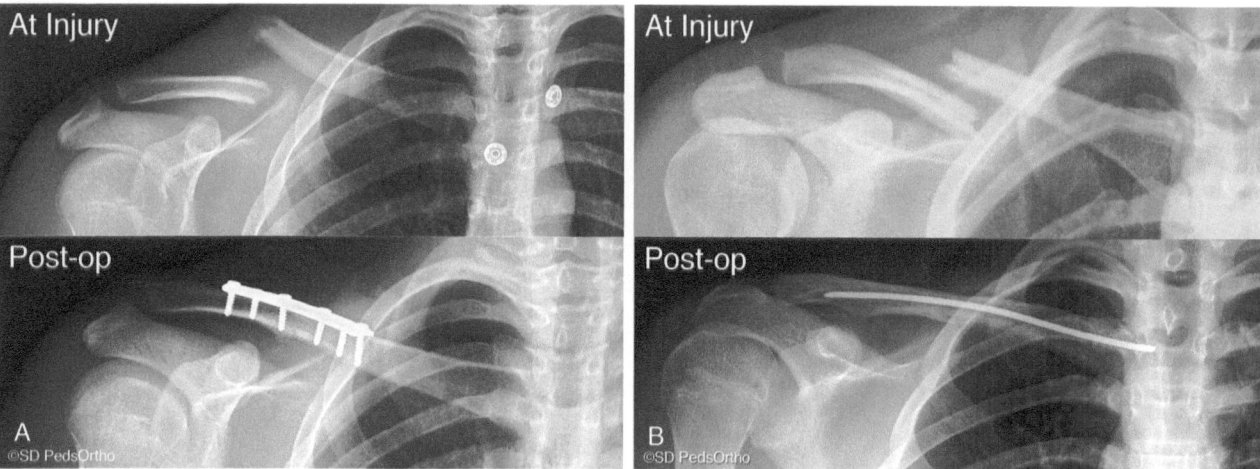

Fig. 133.6 (A) Displaced midshaft clavicle fracture fixed with a precontoured superior plate. (B) Similar fracture treated with an intramedullary device.

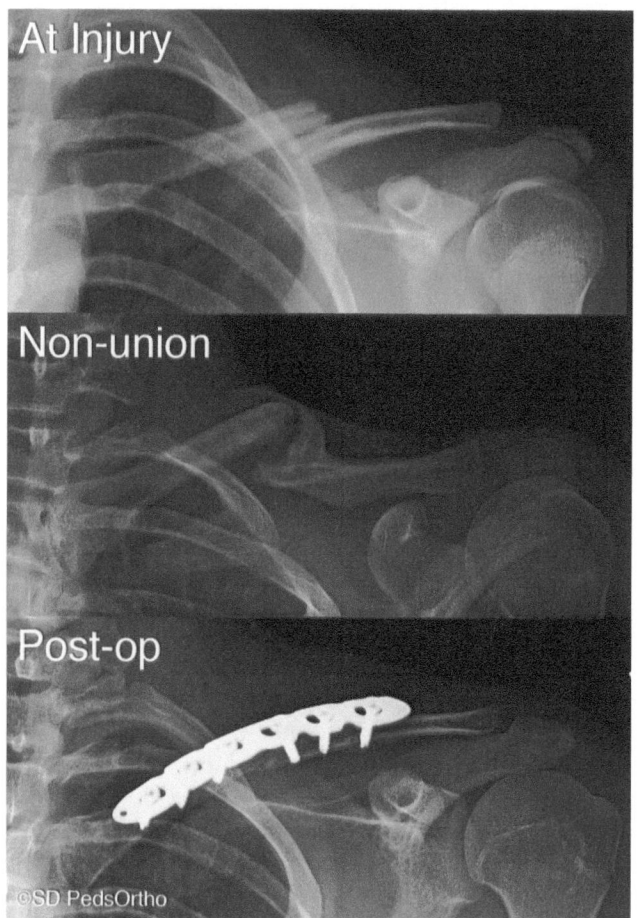

Fig. 133.7 Although rare, clavicle nonunions can occur in adolescents.

refractures, infections, and neurovascular injuries have also been reported.[23-31]

Lateral Clavicle Physeal Fractures

Although injuries to the distal clavicle in children are similar in many ways to the adult acromioclavicular (AC) joint injury, the distinct differences are a reflection of the developmental anatomy of the distal clavicle. The distal clavicle is surrounded by a thick periosteal sleeve that is continuous laterally with the AC joint capsule and inferiorly with the coracoclavicular ligaments. The physis of the distal clavicle lies within the periosteal sleeve medial to the attachment of the AC joint capsule. The epiphysis, which is rarely apparent radiographically, is tightly bound to the AC joint; failure in the skeletally immature athlete therefore usually occurs through the physis as opposed to an adultlike dislocation through the AC joint. Classification of distal clavicle injuries is based on the degree of disruption of the periosteal sleeve and the direction and degree of displacement of the shaft fragment (see Fig. 133.8).[32]

History

Typically, the athlete has a history of a fall on the point of the shoulder. The blow directed to the top of the scapula can lead to disruption of the periosteal sleeve and fracture through the physis. There is immediate pain, and the athlete may relate a feeling of instability. Transient symptoms of numbness or dysesthesia are occasionally experienced, similar to that of a brachial plexus stinger or burner.[33,34] The injury may occur with an indirect mechanism, such as a fall on an outstretched, adducted arm that drives the humeral head into the acromion.[33,34]

Physical Examination

On inspection, the amount of deformity relates to the degree of injury. Mild type I and type II injuries may demonstrate only localized swelling, whereas type III and type V injuries are characterized by clinically significant deformity caused by the displaced distal clavicle shaft. Type II and III injuries may appear fairly benign when visualized from the front, but, when inspected from above, the deformity of the displaced clavicle posterior into the trapezius can be recognized. The athlete often supports the affected arm with the opposite hand and resists shoulder ROM. Tenderness to palpation over the distal clavicle is uniformly present. Acutely, muscle strength testing is limited by pain. Neurologic testing should be performed to rule out brachial plexus involvement. In less severe cases, the cross-arm adduction test is usually positive. This test is performed by positioning the shoulder into flexion of 90 degrees followed by bringing the arm

Dameron and Rockwood lateral clavicle fracture classification
(the epiphgysis and periosteum typically remain in place and the shaft displaces)

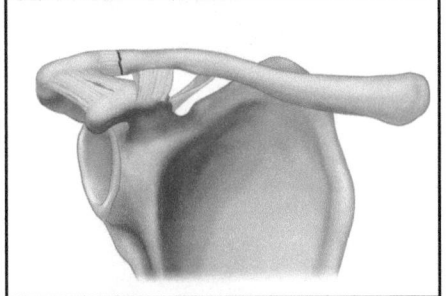

1) No significant displacement

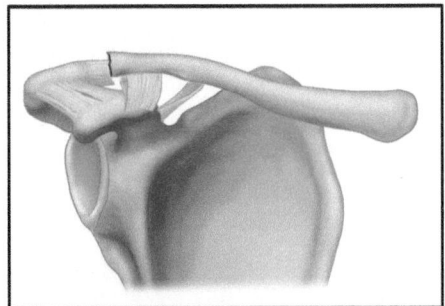

2) Mild displacement (<25%)

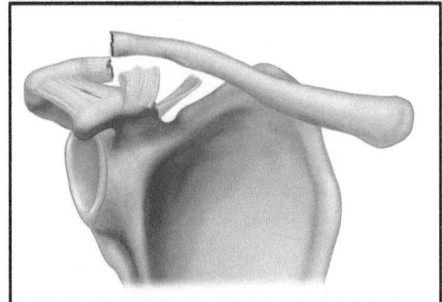

3) Superior displacement (25–100%)

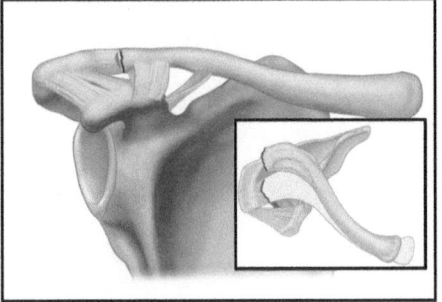

4) Posterior displacement

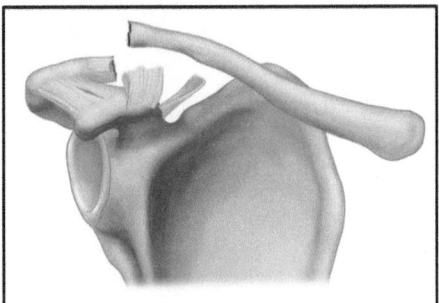

5) Superior displacement (>100%)

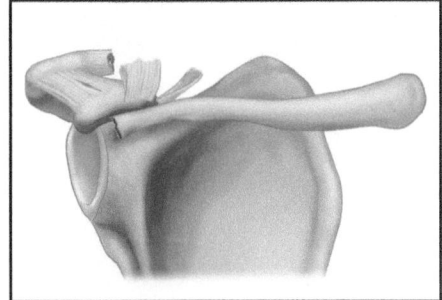

6) Inferior displacement

Fig. 133.8 Dameron and Rockwood classification of pediatric distal (lateral) clavicle fractures.

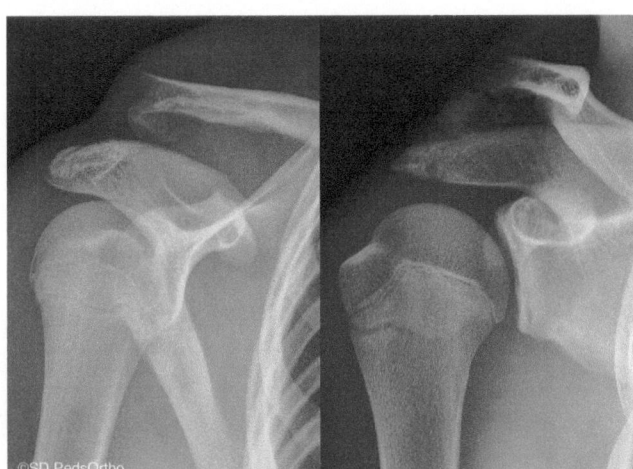

Fig. 133.9 Anteroposterior and Zanca views of the distal clavicle.

across the chest into adduction. Pain referable to the AC joint region is a positive test finding.[33-35]

Imaging

In the case of injury to the distal clavicular physis, routine AP views may be overpenetrated; a special Zanca view may therefore be indicated (Fig. 133.9).[36] This view is performed by angling the beam 10 to 15 degrees toward the head and using only 50% of the standard AP shoulder penetration. The distal clavicular epiphysis is rarely visualized on plain films because it appears and fuses over a short period at approximately 19 years of age. Distal physeal injury is therefore inferred by the degree of shaft

displacement in relation to the acromion and coracoid. Comparison views of the opposite shoulder can often be useful, particularly when trying to determine the normal coracoclavicular distance. The axillary lateral view is important to differentiate a type IV injury by demonstrating the posterior position of the shaft fragment in relation to the acromion. Stress views of the shoulder are not necessary in assessing distal clavicular physeal injury.[33]

Treatment Options

Nonoperative treatment. Injuries to the distal clavicular physis represent Salter-Harris type I injuries, and healing is virtually always the rule. The periosteal sleeve remains in continuity with the AC joint capsule and the coracoclavicular ligaments; stability is achieved when the periosteal sleeve fills with healing new bone. Even in cases with large degrees of displacement, remodeling potential in this injury is significant and residual deformity is unusual. Nonoperative treatment is therefore acceptable in most type I, II, and III cases of distal clavicular physeal fracture.[33,34,37-40] In younger patients with greater degrees of remodeling potential, even cases of type V injury should be considered for nonoperative treatment. Nonoperative treatment includes a short period of immobilization and supportive care with ice and analgesics followed by a progressive rehabilitation and return to play (RTP) program. Type I or II injuries may be able to return as early as 1 to 2 weeks but typically take 4 to 6 weeks, whereas type III and type V injuries treated nonoperatively will normally take 6 weeks or longer.

Operative treatment. Surgical treatment for fractures of the distal clavicular physis is reserved for type IV injuries, type VI

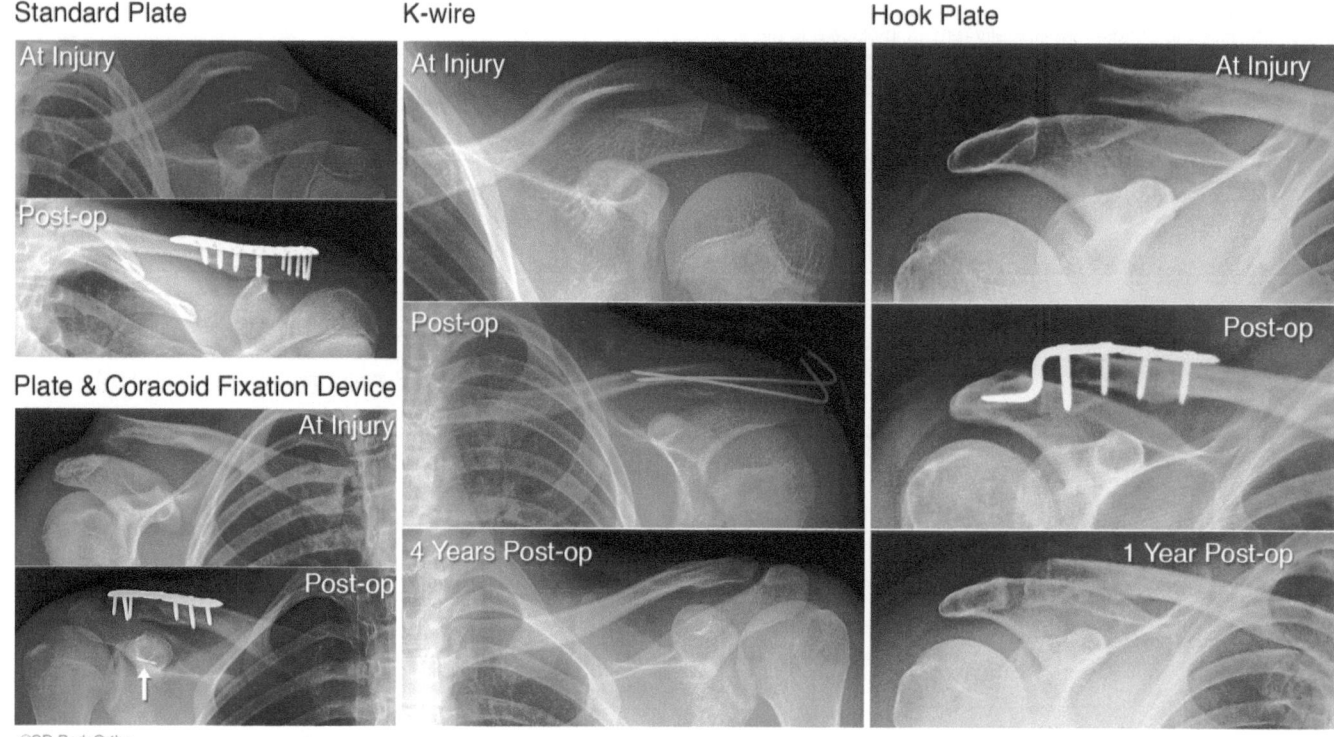

Fig. 133.10 Surgical options for lateral clavicle fractures.

injuries, and type V injuries in adolescents who have less remodeling capability. The procedure includes reduction of the displaced shaft fragment and repair of the periosteal sleeve versus fixation with plates and screws, Kirschner wires, or coracoclavicular fixation devices (Fig. 133.10).[33,34,39,41-43] After surgery a sling is used for 2 weeks, allowing early hand and elbow motion and shoulder pendulum exercises. Between 2 and 6 weeks gentle shoulder motion progresses, but lifting is not allowed. Progressive strengthening and functional activities are then initiated as tolerated. After surgical treatment, RTP follows complete radiographic healing and rehabilitation, which may require 10 to 12 weeks.

Results

Because of the great potential for healing and remodeling of this fracture in this age group, results for treatment of an injury to the distal clavicular physis are almost uniformly good. Several reports in the literature for both surgical and nonoperative treatment demonstrate good results.[39,40,43,44]

Complications

Although most distal clavicle fractures heal uneventfully with nonoperative treatment, occasionally a nonunion will be identified, especially in an older adolescent patient with a type IV or V fracture that is button-holed through the trapezius muscle. The primary complication of surgical treatment is related to the implants either being symptomatic given the superficial nature of the distal clavicle or inadequate fixation resulting in loss of reduction, which is not uncommon given the small size of the lateral fracture fragment.

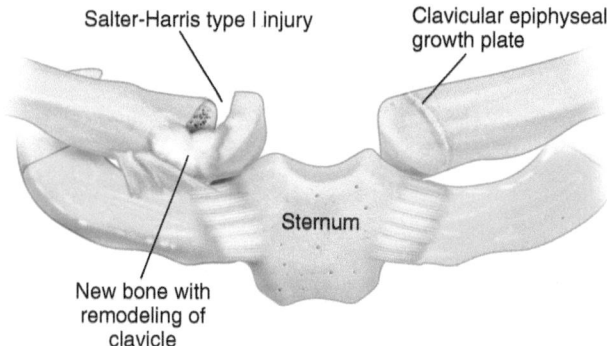

Fig. 133.11 Salter-Harris I fracture of the medial clavicle with anterior displacement.

Medial Clavicle Physeal Fractures

Injuries to the medial end of the clavicle represent between 1% and 6% of all clavicular injuries in skeletally immature patients.[45-50] These fractures are classified according to the anatomic position of the shaft fragment in relation to the epiphysis and sternum. The shaft can be displaced either anteriorly or posteriorly as it penetrates the periosteal sleeve that remains attached medially to the epiphysis and joint capsule. Although anterior displacement is the most common type of injury, posterior displacement is the most important to recognize because of potential impingement of structures within the mediastinum. Most of these physeal fractures are characterized as Salter-Harris type I and II injuries (Fig. 133.11).[51]

History

Injury to the medial clavicle can occur as a result of either direct or indirect forces, with the indirect mechanism being most common. A typical history given by the athlete includes a fall with the athlete's opposite shoulder on the ground while several other players pile on top of the shoulder, applying significant compressive force directly to the medial clavicle. The less common direct mechanism may occur when a force is applied directly to the anteromedial aspect of the clavicle during contact sports, resulting in a fracture through the physis. If displacement results, the shaft fragment would penetrate the periosteal tube posteriorly and potentially become retrosternal, with possible injury to structures within the mediastinum. Most athletes with medial clavicular physeal fracture have immediate pain with a specific traumatic episode. It is important to elicit any symptoms of impingement on mediastinal structures if a posterior displacement is suspected. Symptoms of shortness of breath, choking, difficulty swallowing, or any neurologic or vascular symptoms should be of concern to the examiner.

Physical Examination

In a nondisplaced injury to the medial physis, the ligaments of the joint and periosteal sleeve are intact. The patient reports pain with ROM of the upper extremity. The area is typically swollen and tender to palpation, but instability and crepitus are absent. In a more severe injury to the physis with displacement of the shaft fragment, swelling, and severe pain with any movement of the arm are common. The injured arm is often supported with the normal arm, and the head may be tilted toward the side of the dislocated joint because of spasm of the surrounding musculature. Swelling may be substantial, disguising the position of the displaced shaft fragment. Careful palpation of the shaft in relation to the epiphysis and sternum should be performed in an attempt to discern anterior versus posterior displacement. In suspected posterior displacement, careful examination of the upper extremity should document neurologic status and adequacy of pulses or any venous congestion that may be present. Breathing difficulties, voice changes, or a choking sensation should be noted. If the patient demonstrates some or all of these signs and symptoms of mediastinal impingement, treatment becomes a relative emergency and should be promptly instituted.

Imaging

Plain radiographs of the medial clavicle, including the AP and lateral views, can be difficult to interpret because of overlap with other structures, including sternum, ribs, and spine. A special oblique view, known as the serendipity view, has proven to be the most valuable plain radiographic technique. With the patient supine in the center of the x-ray table, the tube is tilted at a 40-degree angle off the vertical, centered directly on the sternum. This view demonstrates a side-to-side comparison of the medial clavicle and sternoclavicular joint and allows evaluation of potential displacement or fracture.[52] In cases with suspected posterior displacement, a computed tomography (CT) scan may be necessary to confirm the fracture/dislocation and the degree and location of displacement (Fig. 133.12).

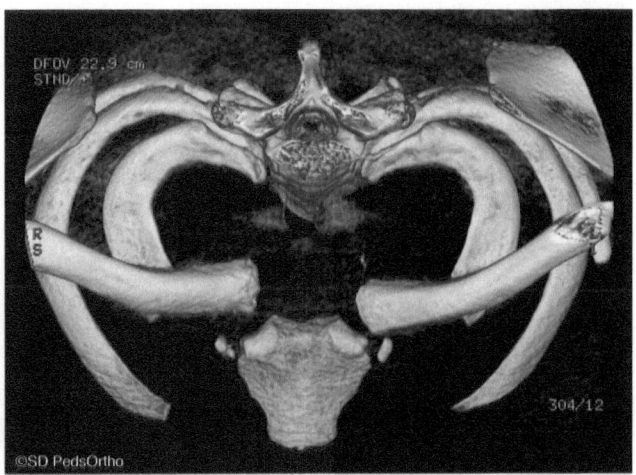

Fig. 133.12 Computed tomography three-dimensional reconstruction of a posteriorly displaced medial clavicle fracture.

Treatment Options

As is the case of all fractures involving physes, the expectation for rapid healing and significant remodeling in fractures of the medial clavicle is the rule. With this in mind, treatment of these fractures will be generally more conservative than in cases of sternoclavicular joint dislocation. Conclusive data regarding recognition, treatment, and specific outcomes are limited to case reports and small series, but results of treatment for this injury are generally good by whatever means.[45-49,53] Treatment is based on both the degree and direction of displacement of the shaft fragment, with special attention to cases with posterior position of the shaft fragment that may result in impingement of mediastinal structures.[54-58] In physeal fractures with mild to moderate displacement in either direction, treatment is always by observation and supportive care. If significant anterior displacement of the medial physeal injury is recognized, closed reduction can be considered. If attempted, closed reduction should be performed with the patient under general anesthesia and positioned supine with a pad between the shoulders. While applying lateral traction on the arm, direct pressure is applied to the anteriorly displaced clavicle while the shoulder is pushed posteriorly. The reduction is maintained by placing the patient in a figure-of-eight splint for 2 to 4 weeks. If the clavicle fracture is unstable, the deformity is accepted, and healing and remodeling of the fracture will usually correct any residual deformity. Some clinicians suggest that benign neglect can be successful for all fractures with anterior displacement.[59]

In athletes who demonstrate posterior displacement of the medial physeal fracture, closed reduction should be performed with the patient under general anesthesia (Fig. 133.13). Of note, many surgeons prefer to have a general surgeon or cardiothoracic surgeon available for these procedures. With the patient in the supine position and a pad placed between the shoulders, traction is applied to the abducted arm, which is then slowly brought into extension. It may be necessary to apply lateral and anterior traction to the medial clavicle either manually or with a percutaneous towel clip to accomplish reduction. The reduction is usually stable, with the shoulders held back in a figure-of-eight

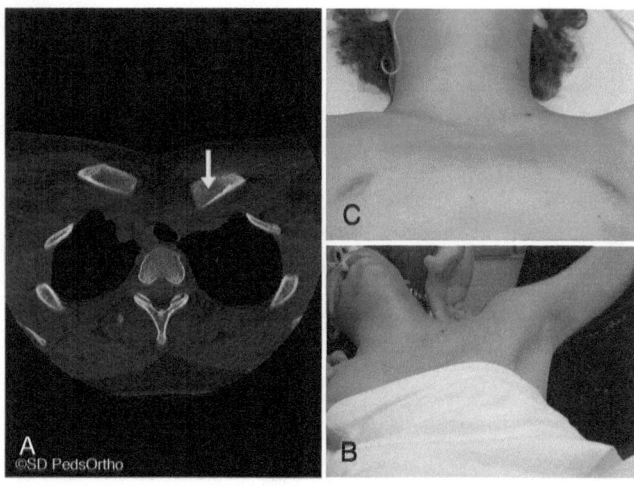

Fig. 133.13 A 14-year-old male who sustained a posteriorly displaced medial clavicle fracture. (A) A computed tomography scan confirms posterior displacement *(arrow)*. (B) In thin patients, the clavicle can sometimes be reduced using manual manipulation with traction on the arm. (C) Closed reduction was successful in this patient. He was then placed into a figure-of-eight brace.

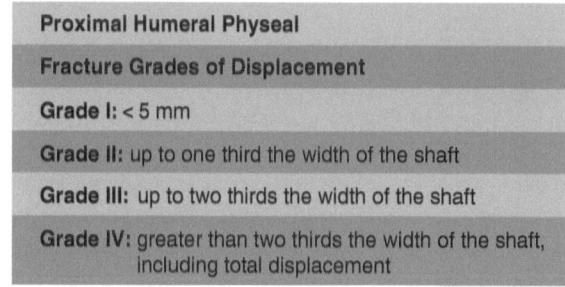

Proximal Humeral Physeal
Fracture Grades of Displacement
Grade I: < 5 mm
Grade II: up to one third the width of the shaft
Grade III: up to two thirds the width of the shaft
Grade IV: greater than two thirds the width of the shaft, including total displacement

Fig. 133.14 Proximal humeral physeal fracture grades of displacement.

dressing or strap. If the posterior physeal injury cannot be easily reduced closed, and if the patient has no symptoms of impingement of the mediastinal structures, the injury can be treated expectantly. Healing and remodeling commonly result in a stable clavicle with no long-term sequelae.[60] Open reduction of a medial clavicular physeal injury is indicated for cases of irreducible posterior displacement in a patient with signs and symptoms of compression of the mediastinal structures. Reduction performed through an open approach is usually accomplished without difficulty. Reduction is maintained by repairing the thick periosteal tube and maintaining the patient in a figure-of-eight brace as for closed reduction. Successful results for the open treatment of posteriorly displaced medial clavicular physeal fractures in young athletes have been reported.[61-63]

Complications

Acute complications associated with medial clavicular physeal fracture are primarily limited to impingement of mediastinal structures. Long-term issues related to malunion are unusual in the skeletally immature patient because of the great propensity for remodeling of the physeal fracture with time. Many complications have been previously reported with the use of metallic implants for fixation of fractures and dislocations in this area. Pin breakage and migration have led most authors to recommend that metal not be used in the medial clavicle and sternoclavicular joint.[52,64-67]

PROXIMAL HUMERUS FRACTURES

Although fractures involving the upper extremities are the most common injuries in young athletes, the incidence of proximal humeral physeal injuries has been reported to range between 2% and 7%.[68-70] Despite this relatively low incidence, these injuries can be serious in terms of time lost from participation.[71] Fractures involving the proximal humeral physis usually occur as a

result of high-energy sports such as football, soccer, hockey, skiing, skateboarding, and BMX riding. Fractures of the proximal humeral physis can be classified by location and the degree of displacement (Fig. 133.14). In addition, fracture stability is important in the treatment algorithm and depends on the degree of initial displacement and the degree of initial trauma. When the physis is involved, these fractures can also be described using the Salter-Harris outlined in Fig. 133.15.

History

Fractures through the proximal humeral physis typically occur in adolescent males as they near skeletal maturity.[72] Salter-Harris type I fractures are less common and tend to occur in athletes younger than 12 years of age. In adolescent athletes 12 years and older, most fractures are Salter-Harris type II fractures.[73] These fractures tend to occur as the result of direct or indirect mechanisms.[74] Falls directly onto the shoulder or a blunt force or strike are responsible for most direct mechanisms, whereas indirect trauma tends to result from a fall on an outstretched hand with the arm abducted and externally rotated.[75]

Physical Examination

Athletes with nondisplaced fractures often present with only minimal swelling and tenderness localized over the proximal humerus. Motion and resisted rotation are limited because of pain. When greater degrees of physeal displacement are present, considerable bleeding into the soft tissues can produce marked swelling. The athlete reports pain with any motion and usually holds the extremity adducted to the chest, supported at the elbow and forearm with the opposite hand. The neurologic and vascular status of the upper extremity must be assessed to rule out injury to any peripheral nerves, the brachial plexus, or vascular structures.[76]

Imaging

Routine radiographs of the shoulder, including the AP view and axillary lateral view, should be obtained if possible. Frequently, an axillary lateral view is challenging in these situations because the patient is unable to elevate the arm secondary to pain. In such cases a transthoracic lateral, a scapular Y view, or a clear view may be helpful to properly and safely evaluate the shoulder (Fig. 133.16). Occasionally, a CT scan will be necessary to better evaluate an intra-articular fracture, to identify a lesser tuberosity fracture, or to better identify the degree of displacement or comminution if present. All radiographs should be scrutinized for

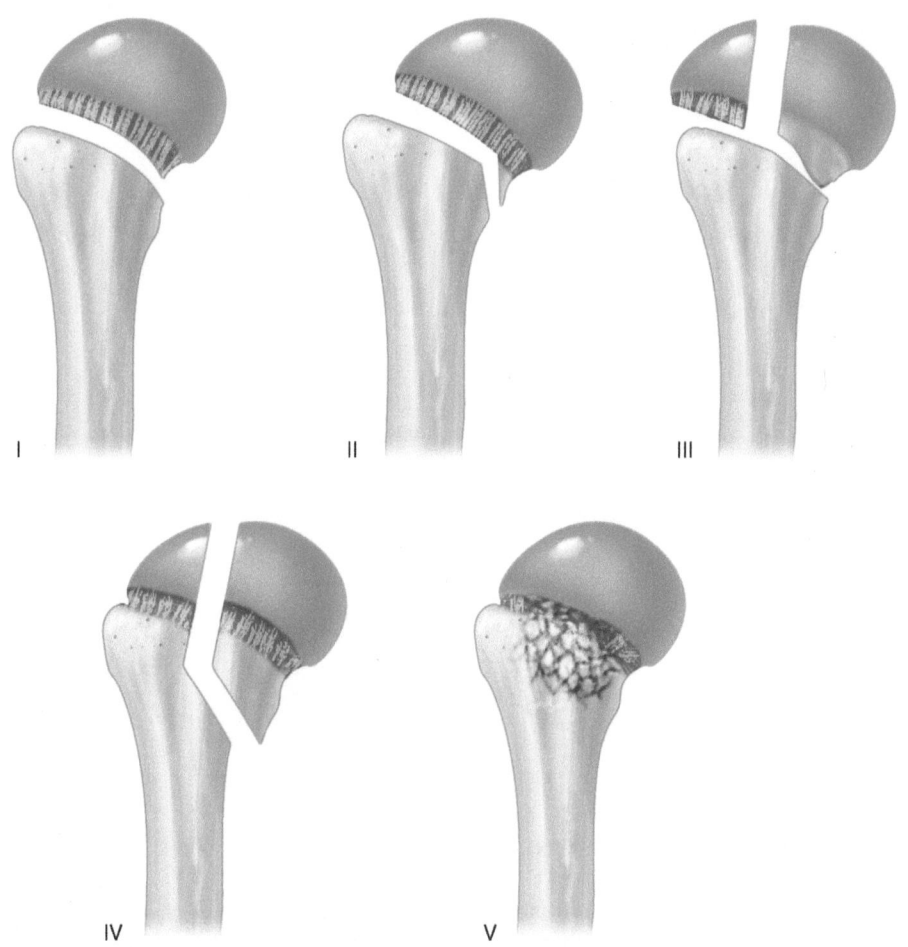

Fig. 133.15 Salter-Harris classification in proximal humerus fractures. Type I: fracture through the physis only. Type II: fracture involving the physis with a metaphyseal fragment. Type III: fracture involving the physis with intra-articular extension. Type IV: physeal fracture with intra-articular and metaphyseal extension. Type V: crush injury to the physis.

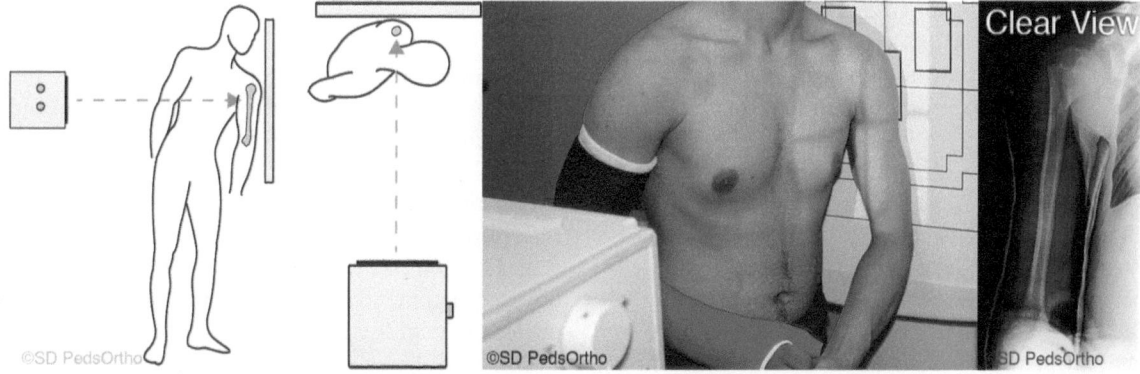

Fig. 133.16 The "clear view" may be performed orthogonal to the anteroposterior view. It allows accurate visualization with decreased radiation compared to the transthoracic view.

a pathologic fracture because unicameral and aneurysmal bone cysts (UBCs and ABCs, respectively) are not infrequent in this patient group (Fig. 133.17).

Treatment

The proximal humeral physis contributes approximately 80% of the longitudinal growth of the humerus, thus allowing great potential for remodeling after fracture. The younger the athlete, the greater the potential for remodeling, and the need for anatomic alignment is less important. However, in the adolescent athlete with less growth remaining, adequate time to remodel the deformity may not remain. The dilemma for the treating physician then becomes when to use aggressive treatment for these fractures. Although no absolute criteria exist in the literature

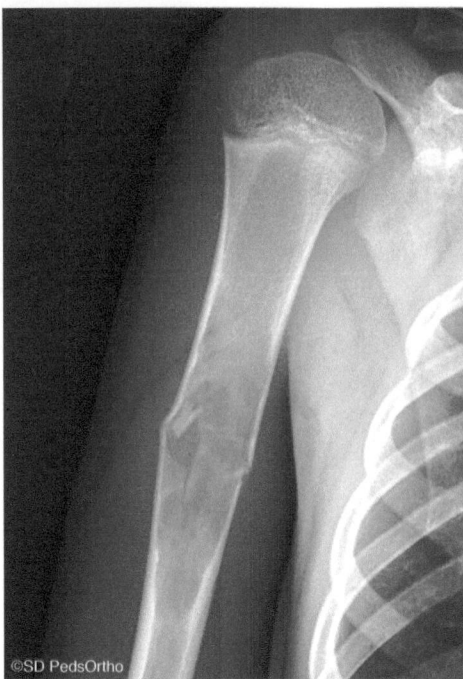

Fig. 133.17 Unicameral bone cyst (UBC) with a pathologic fracture through the humerus. The "fallen leaf" sign is pathognomonic for a UBC.

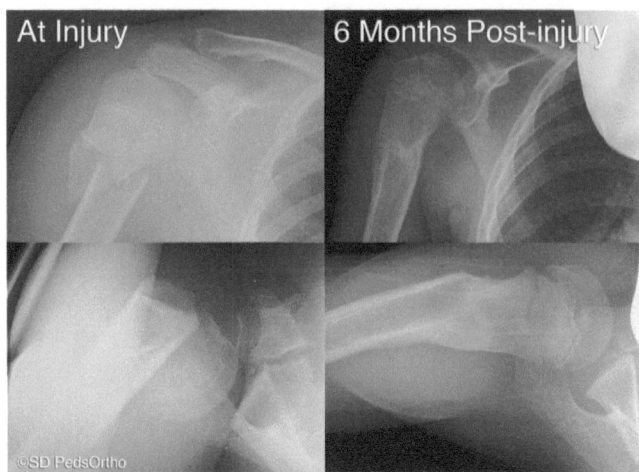

Fig. 133.18 Significant remodeling can occur in skeletally immature patients with proximal humerus fractures as can be seen in these 6-month postinjury films.

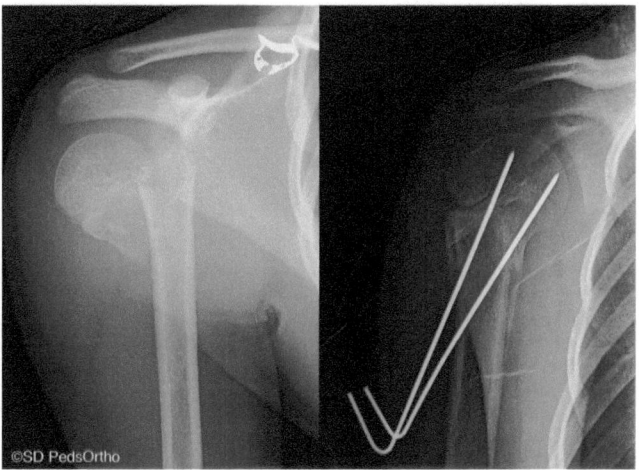

Fig. 133.19 With unstable displaced fractures, retrograde Kirschner wires may be necessary to stabilize the fracture reduction.

as to what amount of displacement or angulation can be tolerated before closed reduction or surgical intervention is necessary, several authors have made recommendations. Some have suggested surgery for fractures with angulation greater than 40 degrees or 50% displacement regardless of age.[80,81] Others have suggested that the patient's age should be factored into decision-making, with angulation up to 75, 60, and 45 degrees being acceptable in patients younger than 7 years, 8 to 11 years, and 12 years or older, respectively.[82]

Nonoperative Treatment

In cases of nondisplaced to mildly displaced or angulated fractures, treatment is usually successful without attempting reduction of the fracture (Fig. 133.18). Initial protection in a sling or shoulder immobilizer followed by rehabilitation is usually all that is necessary to obtain a good result. Most authors reserve attempts at closed reduction for displaced fractures.[83] The argument for reduction of the fragments is that it decreases the degree of shortening and varus deformity that develops if the malalignment is allowed to persist. Various closed methods have been advocated to realign the fracture fragments into a more anatomic position. Closed reduction can be performed under anesthesia by bringing the distal shaft fragment into flexion with some abduction and external rotation to align it with the flexed, abducted, and externally rotated proximal epiphyseal fragment.[77] After closed reduction, options to maintain position without internal fixation include a sling, brace, cast, or olecranon pin skeletal traction, but this a treatment more of historical interest.

Operative Treatment

Indications for operative treatment include inability to gain an adequate closed reduction or inability to maintain anatomic

closed reduction. Most authors prefer a closed technique when possible, followed by percutaneous pin fixation under fluoroscopic control. This has been shown to be a highly effective method of maintaining an unstable reduction.[79,84-88] Typically two to three smooth or threaded tip pins are passed from the metaphysis retrograde across the fracture into the humeral head (Fig. 133.19). This technique has the advantage of maintaining fracture alignment with the arm in the normal position, supported only with a sling or brace. The pins can be removed within 2 to 4 weeks due to the rapid healing of the physeal fracture. Retrograde nailing with elastic nails has gained popularity, particularly in fractures involving the metaphysis.[89-91] On occasion, an open reduction is necessary when a satisfactory reduction cannot be obtained by a closed manipulation or in cases of open fractures or vascular injuries. Failure to obtain adequate closed reduction is more common in Salter-Harris type III and IV injuries and occasionally in cases of Salter-Harris I and II fractures in which the periosteum or the biceps tendon has become interposed in the fracture site. Fixation after open reduction can include smooth or threaded tip pins, screws, retrograde nails, or contoured plate fixation. Screws and plate fixation would only be used in athletes very near skeletal maturity. Many reports have cited the success of open reduction and fixation in these difficult cases, with most patients returning to sports without limitations typically at approximately 12 weeks.[90,91]

Complications

Acute complications associated with proximal humeral fractures in young athletes are rare but include neurologic and vascular injuries that occasionally require intervention.[76,77] Major skeletal complications include growth arrest, malunion, and avascular necrosis of the humeral head. Growth arrest after fracture is very unusual, although varus deformity and shortening from malunion are common but well tolerated. In the adolescent nearing skeletal maturity, fracture deformity can occasionally produce a disabling loss of motion for an overhead athlete.[78,79] Avascular necrosis of the humeral head is rare in the skeletally immature athlete. Most case reports describe transient symptoms with little long-term disability.[78,92] Complications associated with percutaneous pinning include pin tract infections, pin migration, and osteomyelitis. Close observation of any percutaneous placed pin should be performed until they can be removed, and, if prolonged stabilization may be necessary, consideration should be given to burying the wires. Although osteomyelitis is uncommon, it is a potentially severe complication that may require multiple débridements and antibiotics to eradicate.[93]

LESSER TUBEROSITY FRACTURES

Fracture of the lesser tuberosity of the proximal humeral physis is a rare injury and is frequently associated with other trauma around the shoulder.[94-98] This injury represents an avulsion of the tuberosity by a violent contraction involving the subscapularis tendon. These fractures are difficult to diagnose in the acute situation, possibly because of the challenges in obtaining adequate radiographic visualization of the fracture and a lack of specific clinical findings. Up to 50% of cases of lesser tuberosity fracture in the skeletally immature athlete have been reported to be missed on initial presentation.[99,100]

History

The athlete usually gives a history of a traumatic injury during a contact sport involving an external rotation force applied to the arm in a leveraged position.[77] Acutely the patient has mild swelling, limited ROM, and pain. Weakness of internal rotation may be noted by the patient. Many of these patients present several weeks after injury with persistent shoulder pain and weakness.

Physical Examination

If the athlete presents acutely, the shoulder is diffusely tender and guarded. Mild swelling may be present. Motion is limited by pain and strength testing is limited. If the presentation is delayed, the ROM has usually improved but weakness and pain are noted with resisted internal rotation. The lift-off test and the belly-press test may be positive.

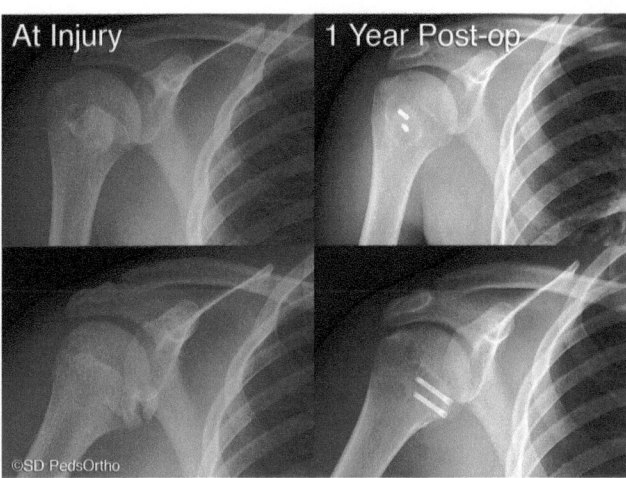

Fig. 133.20 *Left image:* lesser tuberosity nonunion. *Right image:* six-week postoperative films after a nonunion repair.

Imaging

Standard radiographs, including AP and axillary lateral views, should be performed in all patients, but they may fail to demonstrate the fracture.[77] CT scans will confirm the fracture if needed, and magnetic resonance imaging (MRI) may be used to assess the shoulder for other soft tissue injuries.

Treatment Options

If the fracture is nondisplaced, it can be successfully treated with nonoperative management. A sling is used for protection for 4 to 6 weeks followed by rehabilitation. Displaced fractures and nondisplaced fractures with a delay in treatment are commonly treated surgically (Fig. 133.20).[101,102] Some authors recommend surgical treatment for all lesser tuberosity avulsion fractures in throwing athletes because malunion may lead to decreased overhead sports function.[77,99] Surgical repair of the lesser tuberosity fracture can be accomplished with heavy suture through drill holes, suture anchors, or screw fixation. Results with surgical treatment have been reported as good in terms of full return to athletic function.[101-104]

Complications

Both nonunion and malunion of fractures of the lesser tuberosity have been reported.[99,101] Nonunited fractures are usually painful, and malunited fragments often lead to bony impingement anteriorly, which can limit motion. This can be disabling for the athlete who uses his shoulder for overhand sports activities.

GLENOHUMERAL INSTABILITY

The anatomy of the glenohumeral joint allows a high degree of functional mobility but with a sacrifice of inherent stability. The incidence of shoulder instability in the young athlete varies by age and gender, with older adolescent males having the highest rate of instability and patients younger than 13 years having a considerably lower rate of dislocation but a higher rate of proximal humeral physeal fractures.[105-107] Reports of glenohumeral dislocation due to trauma in children younger than 10 years of age are limited to very small numbers and case studies.[108,109]

ANTERIOR INSTABILITY

History

Anterior instability is the most common type of traumatic instability, representing the majority of dislocations in all age groups. These dislocations are frequently seen in contact and collision sports, with a mechanism of forced shoulder abduction and external rotation. As a result of this force, the humeral head is translated anteriorly, causing damage to the anterior-inferior glenohumeral ligaments and labrum, eventually resulting in joint subluxation or dislocation. When evaluating a young athlete with instability, important considerations include arm dominance, primary sport with a focus on collision sports and/or throwing sports, patient age, number of episodes of instability, previous treatment, and direction of instability. For example, patients with a history of dozens of instability events or instability while sleeping are clinical clues that there may be significant glenoid bone loss, a large Hill-Sachs lesion, or significant shoulder laxity that can be seen in patients with collagen abnormalities or multidirectional instability. Recurrent instability of the shoulder is the most common complication associated with nonoperative treatment of a first-time dislocation.

Physical Examination

Acutely, patients with a traumatic anterior glenohumeral dislocation present with pain and an obvious deformity from the anteroinferiorly displaced humeral head and relatively prominent acromion. The affected arm is usually supported by the opposite hand and held in a slightly abducted and externally rotated position. Motion is limited by pain. The athlete who presents after a subluxation episode or after dislocation with spontaneous reduction demonstrates tenderness with guarding but no deformity. Careful examination of the neurologic and vascular status is mandatory. The axillary nerve is the most commonly injured neurologic structure after dislocation and may occur in 5% to 35% of patients who sustain a first-time shoulder dislocations.[106]

Sensory examination of the axillary nerve can be accomplished by testing the sensory distribution of the nerve along the upper lateral arm by light touch or pinprick, whereas the motor innervation of the nerve can be assessed by examining the deltoid by having the patient abduct the shoulder (Fig. 133.22). The presence of both the radial and ulnar pulses should be noted. Absence of the pulses or swelling with a rapidly expanding hematoma suggests a rare vascular injury.[115]

Patients presenting subacutely or with recurrent instability will typically have full ROM and symmetric or near-symmetric strength. Provocative tests for anterior instability include the anterior apprehension test and the relocation test.[116] The anterior apprehension test can be performed with the patient standing, sitting, or supine on the examination table (Fig. 133.23). While the scapula is stabilized, the patient's arm is brought into abduction and external rotation. The result is positive when the test elicits a feeling of apprehension or instability with or without pain. If positive, a relocation test can then be performed by applying a posteriorly directed force to the anterior shoulder, helping to stabilize the glenohumeral joint. A resultant decrease in apprehension with this maneuver represents a positive test.

Imaging

Acute and recurrent traumatic instability of the shoulder is best evaluated initially with routine radiography. The trauma series for the shoulder includes a minimum of two views taken at right angles to each other. The AP view and axillary lateral view are the most important views to confirm that the glenohumeral joint is reduced, but a transscapular Y view is occasionally used as an alternative to the axillary lateral view (Fig. 131.21). Postreduction films in both planes are important to confirm reduction and assess for fractures that may be difficult to visualize on the initial injury films. The postreduction films often reveal a posterolateral humeral head impaction fracture (Hill-Sachs lesion) but can also reveal fractures involving the anterior glenoid rim (bony Bankart lesion). The anterior glenoid rim is best evaluated for fracture or deficiency on an axillary lateral or modified axillary lateral view (West Point view).[119] The size and position of the glenoid

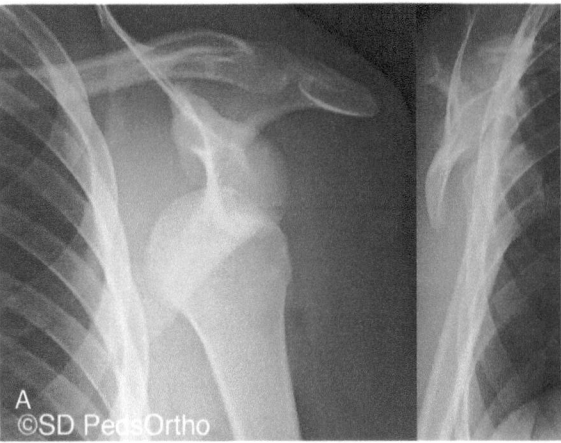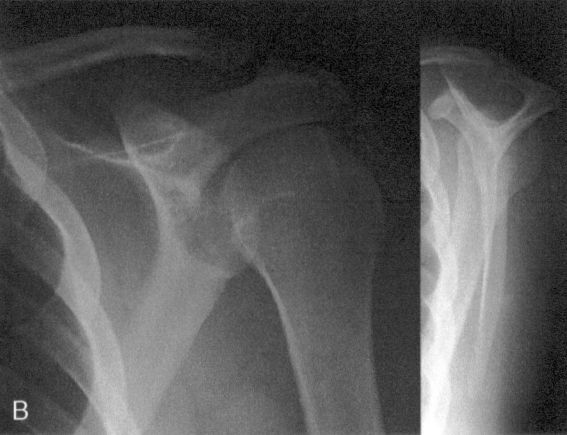

Fig. 133.21 (A) Anterior shoulder dislocation in a 15-year-old male football player. (B) Postreduction film demonstrating a large Hill-Sachs deformity.

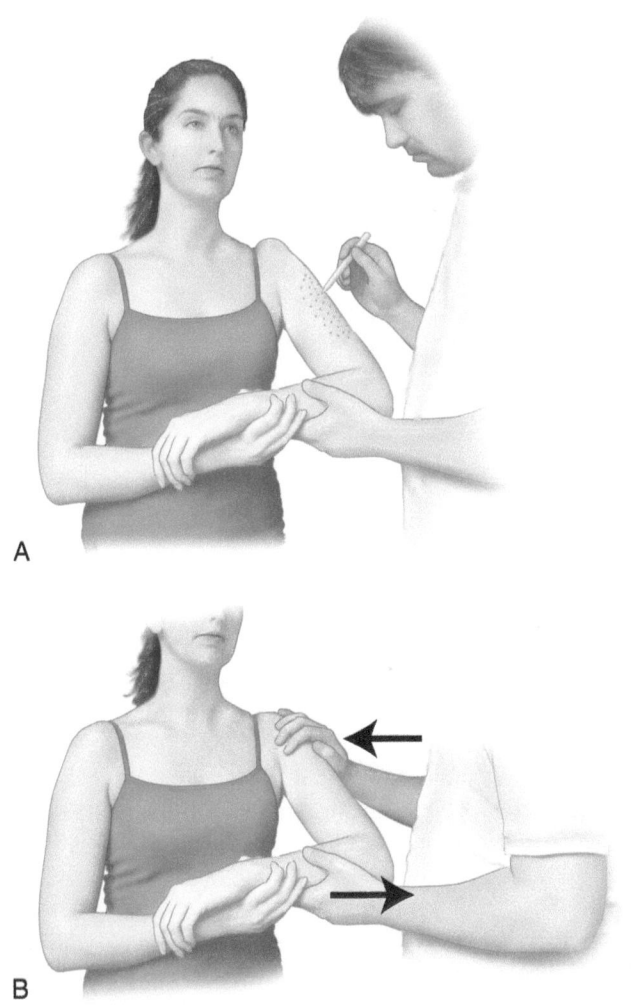

A

B

Fig. 133.22 (A) Clinical evaluation of the axillary nerve during initial assessment of a patient with anterior dislocation. Sensory distribution can be tested to light touch on the upper lateral arm. (B) Motor testing is accomplished by palpating contraction of the deltoid muscle during resisted abduction.

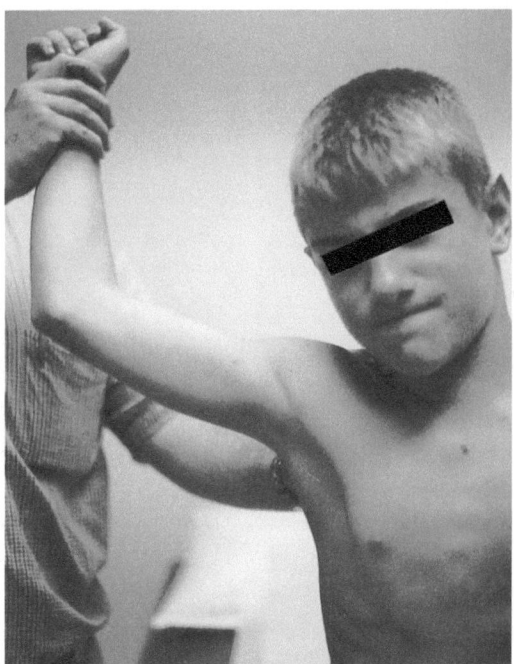

Fig. 133.23 A positive anterior apprehension test in a young athlete with recurrent anterior instability.

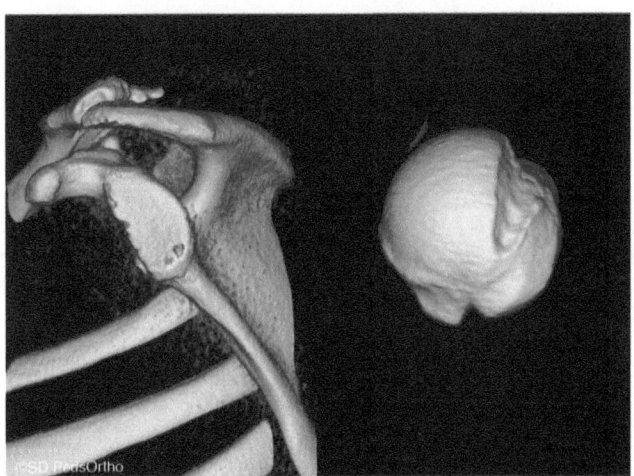

Fig. 133.24 *Left image:* computed tomography (CT) three-dimensional reconstruction view with digital subtraction of the humeral head demonstrating the anteroinferior glenoid bone loss. *Right image:* CT images showing size and orientation of the posterior humeral head impaction fracture, Hill-Sachs deformity.

rim fracture and the Hill-Sachs deformity have been reported to affect the odds of recurrent instability, as well as the success of surgical treatment. Bone loss is not uncommon in adolescent patients with instability, with 48% of patients having at least mild bone loss and 13% having bone loss involving more than 20% of the glenoid.[120] Quantitative assessment of bone loss can be performed with either MRI or CT (Fig. 133.24). In patients with significant bone loss, three-dimensional (3D) reconstructions using a CT scan may provide the physician with a better understanding of glenoid deficiency or the size and orientation of the Hill-Sachs deformity. MRI remains the standard for the evaluation of soft tissue pathology associated with shoulder instability (Fig. 133.25). MRI is commonly combined with arthrography to evaluate injury to capsular and labral structures, articular surfaces, and tendons. Damage to these soft tissue structures can be successfully visualized in a high percentage of cases including more subtle pathology like a humeral avulsion of the glenohumeral ligament (HAGL lesion).[121]

Treatment Options
Nonoperative Treatment
The initial treatment for a dislocated shoulder, whether acute or recurrent, is accomplished by closed reduction. A careful assessment of the neurovascular status should be performed both before and after reduction, with particular attention to axillary nerve function. Early reduction can often be accomplished without anesthesia, but if significant pain and muscle spasm limit success, then appropriate intra-articular anesthesia or intravenous analgesia and sedation are used.[122,123] Closed reduction of a suspected dislocation in the athlete younger than 14 years before radiographic confirmation is certainly more hazardous than in an adolescent or adult due to the higher frequency of

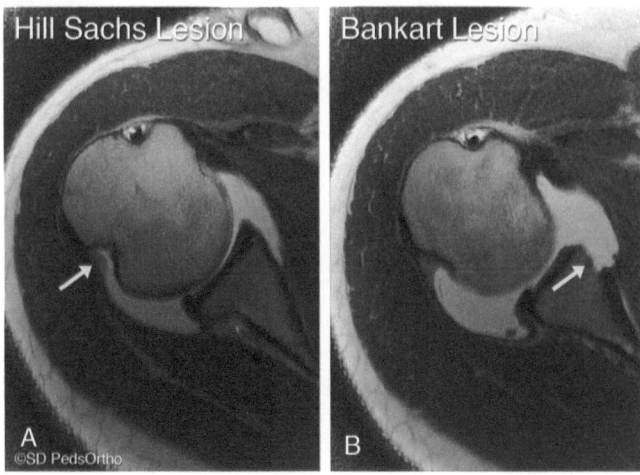

Fig. 133.25 (A) Hill-Sachs deformity (arrow) involving the posterior humeral head. (B) Arthroscopic images depicting a Bankart lesion anteriorly with stripping of the labrum from the glenoid (arrow).

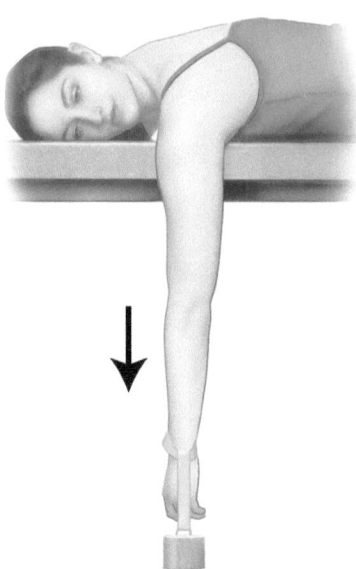

Fig. 133.27 Stimson technique for reduction of anterior dislocation of the shoulder.

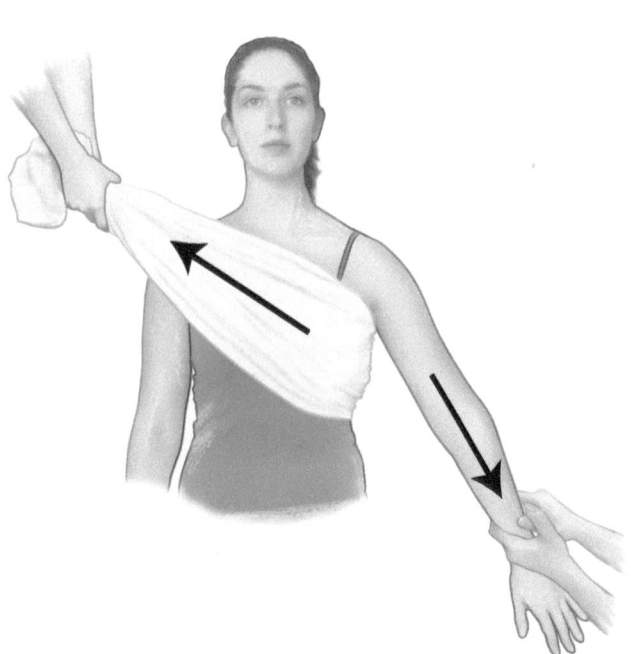

Fig. 133.26 The traction/countertraction technique for reduction of anterior dislocation of the shoulder.

proximal humeral physeal fracture in this age group.[117,118] If possible, radiographs should be taken before reduction.

The traction/countertraction technique for reduction of anterior shoulder dislocation is performed with the patient in the supine position (Fig. 133.26). Longitudinal traction is applied to the arm on a continuous basis while countertraction is applied to the thorax with a sheet passed around the patient's trunk through the axilla. Reduction is accomplished by loosening the humeral head from its locked position on the anterior glenoid rim by overcoming muscle spasm through the longitudinally applied traction. Once the head is disimpacted, spontaneous reduction occurs. In the Stimson maneuver for closed reduction, the patient is placed prone on an examination table. The

dislocated arm is allowed to hang off the edge of the table while a weight of 10 to 15 pounds is suspended from the patient's wrist (Fig. 133.27). Spontaneous reduction of the humeral head occurs as the shoulder musculature is relaxed by the gravity-assisted traction. This technique is particularly useful in situations of a single person attempting the reduction. The abduction maneuver for reduction is performed with the patient in the supine position. The arm is supported by the examiner with the elbow flexed. The shoulder is gently abducted and externally rotated into the overhead position, thus reproducing the mechanism of injury. Reduction occurs as the arm is then brought to the side with extension, adduction, and gentle internal rotation. After closed reduction, appropriate radiographs are obtained to confirm the position of the humeral head and to rule out associated fracture. The arm is immobilized in a sling for comfort and protection. The duration of immobilization is controversial, with two studies demonstrating lower recurrence rates in young, at-risk patients treated with 4 to 6 weeks of immobilization and a 3- to 6-month delay in return to athletic activities.[124,125] However, other reports suggest that neither the length of immobilization nor the type or duration of rehabilitation alters the natural history of recurrence.[126,127] Itoi et al. showed that immobilization of the arm in external rotation helped anatomically reduce the labrum and lowered the rates of future instability.[128] However, subsequent studies have failed to validate these results. Therefore most practitioners have not incorporated this practice because immobilization in external rotation is more challenging for both the patient and the practitioner.[129] A rehabilitation program focusing on rotator cuff and periscapular strengthening is begun as soon as comfort allows in an attempt to prevent recurrent instability. The single most common complication of treatment for acute anterior shoulder instability in the skeletally immature is recurrent instability, with rates ranging from 48% to 100%.[130,131] In the athlete with recurrent anterior instability of the shoulder, nonoperative treatment has had limited success in preventing further recurrence. Although aggressive rehabilitation programs and bracing have been used to decrease frequency, these methods are a temporizing measure before definitive surgical treatment is performed.

Operative Treatment

Historically, the vast majority of first-time shoulder dislocators were treated nonoperatively and surgery was reserved for patients with recurrent instability.[110–114,132–136] Over the past decade, there has been a general movement towards arthroscopic stabilization for a first-time dislocator, especially in athletes participating in collision and contact sports.[105,127,136] The rationale is that acute surgical stabilization reduces the rate of recurrence, potentially provides better clinical outcomes, and may lower rates of future arthritis. To date, limited prospective comparative studies have been performed in the adolescent or pediatric population looking at the results of nonoperative treatment compared with surgical stabilization for first-time dislocators. Two studies have shown lower rates of recurrence with acute stabilization in this young patient population.[137,138]

The preferred treatment for patients with recurrent instability with no significant bone loss is either an open or arthroscopic labral repair and capsulorrhaphy. In the past 20 years, there has been a major shift in the sports medicine community, with most surgeons favoring arthroscopic stabilization. Although an arthroscopic approach provides a more cosmetic approach and better access to the superior and posterior labrum compared with an open approach, no study to date has shown superior outcomes or lower recurrence rates with arthroscopy. Although outcomes are typically good after arthroscopic or open stabilization, recent data strictly focusing on younger patients with longer follow-up have shown relatively high recurrence rates between 30% and 50%.[139,140]

When patients have significant glenoid bone loss (>20%) or when they have failed either an open or arthroscopic labral repair or capsulorrhaphy, a coracoid bone transfer may be indicated. A Bristow procedure involves transferring just the tip of the coracoid including the coracobrachialis and short head of the biceps attachment to the anteroinferior glenoid. A Latarjet involves the transfer of a larger segment of the coracoid, enabling the bony reconstruction of the deficient glenoid rim (Fig. 133.28). In the pediatric and adolescent population, results of these techniques are limited, but promising outcomes have been reported.[141] Major concerns about these procedures include loss of external rotation, implant-related complications, and poststabilization arthritis.[142-146]

Complications

The most frequent complication associated with surgical treatment is recurrence of instability, which can range from 10% to 50% depending of the sport of participation, the patient's age, and the amount of bone loss. Mild loss of external rotation is not uncommon and is fortunately well tolerated in most athletes, but it can be detrimental particularly to overhead-throwing athletes. Loss of external rotation is more common with bony reconstructions such as the Latarjet, as well as posterior-based procedures such as the Remplissage. Other complications such as neurologic injury and infections have been reported but are rare.

Authors' Preferred Technique

Arthroscopic stabilization can be performed in either the beach chair or lateral decubitus position. We prefer the lateral decubitus position because it provides better access to the posterior labrum, capsule, and humeral head. We routinely use an anterosuperior portal (placed through the rotator interval), a midanterior portal (placed just superior to the subscapularis tendon), and a posterior portal (placed just lateral to a standard posterior portal approximately 2 cm below the tip of the acromion to facilitate posterior anchor placement and instrumentation if necessary). If the anterior labral tear extends posteroinferiorly, we routinely establish a percutaneous posterolateral portal to facilitate anchor placement posteriorly between the 6 and 9 o'clock positions. Once the labral tear is identified, it is liberated from the glenoid, where it is typically scarred medially on the glenoid neck. After the labrum is mobilized and reduced back to its anatomic position on the glenoid, we routinely place a minimum of three anchors between the 3 and 6 o'clock position anteriorly. Starting with the most inferior anchor, a capsulorrhaphy is performed with capsular bites measuring approximately 1 cm. The amount of capsular plication is titrated based on the patient's laxity and primary sport. Be careful not to overtighten an overhead thrower's dominant arm or he or she may have difficulty regaining full external rotation and return to throwing. At our institution, we use both knotless and knotted anchors. With improvements in anchor technology, we do not believe there are substantial differences in anchor performance, and this decision may be left to the surgeon's preference. When a bony Bankart lesion is encountered, we prefer fixing or incorporating the bony glenoid fragment into the labral repair. If the fragment is small, we will place the anchors in a standard fashion and loop the sutures around the bony fragment. If the fragment is larger, we will perform a suture bridge technique with one anchor placed medially to the fracture fragment in the glenoid neck and a second anchor placed on the glenoid face. The sutures from the medial anchor will then be placed around the fracture fragment, labrum, and capsule and secured to the glenoid face using the second anchor. In cases where a large engaging Hill-Sach lesion is encountered, we will routinely add in a Remplissage procedure or tenodesis of the infraspinatus. We typically perform this supplemental procedure prior to the anterior labral repair and capsulorrhaphy. For most Hill-Sachs lesions, two anchors placed in the nadir of the Hill-Sachs deformity with the sutures pulled through the infraspinatus with a suture passing device and tied in the subacromial space is enough to "fill" the bony defect. Postoperatively, the shoulder is protected in an immobilization device for 6 weeks while gentle ROM is allowed. At 6 weeks, rotator cuff– and scapular-strengthening exercises are commenced. At 12 weeks, the athlete is started on general weightlifting activities and proprioception retraining. Contact sports are avoided for 6 months.

POSTERIOR INSTABILITY

Historically, traumatic posterior instability of the shoulder has been reported to be much less common than anterior instability, representing only 4% of traumatic dislocations. However, several recent studies seem to indicate that posterior instability is actually more common than once recognized. These findings may be attributable to improved imaging techniques and greater awareness of the problem.

History

Posterior shoulder instability may be the result of an acute traumatic event or the cumulative effect of repetitive microtrauma.[152] Posterior dislocations of the shoulder can be secondary either to a direct blow to the anterior shoulder or to indirect trauma with the shoulder in flexion, internal rotation, and adduction,

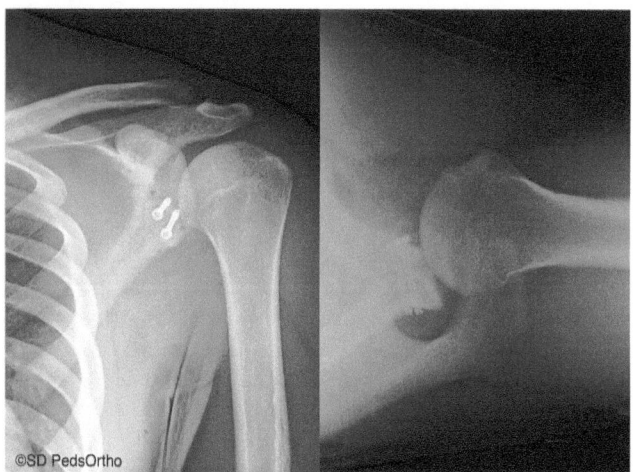

Fig. 133.28 Latarjet procedure performed on a 16-year-old male who had failed a previous attempt at arthroscopic stabilization with significant glenoid bone loss.

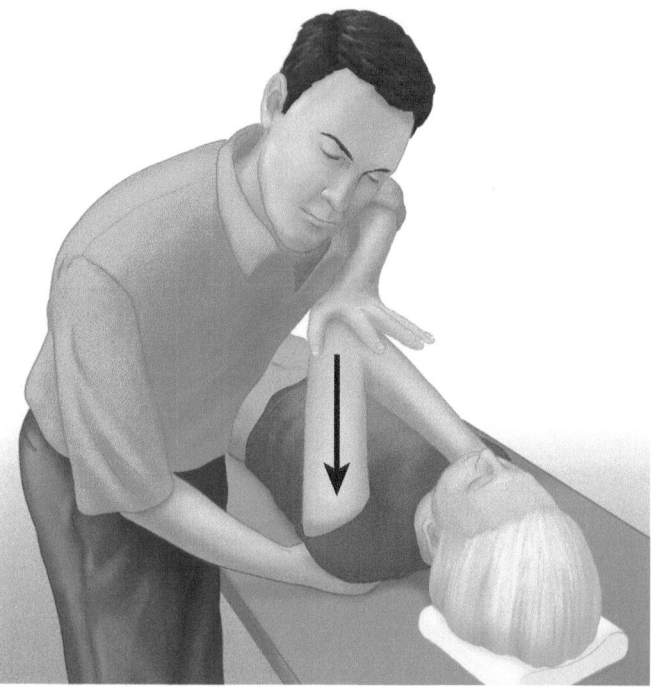

Fig. 133.29 Posterior stress test. A posterior force is applied axially through the humerus. The test is positive if there is palpable crepitus or subluxation of the humeral head. The test often elicits pain, but this is not as specific a finding as crepitus or subluxation.

as can be seen during seizures or in cases of electric shock. The more common recurrent posterior subluxation of the shoulder may result from repetitive microtrauma to the posterior capsule, leading to attenuation of the capsular tissue. Persons who engage in repetitive pushing/blocking motions, such as football lineman, overhead-throwing athletes, tennis players, and swimmers, are at particular risk for recurrent posterior subluxation.[153-154] A subset of ball throwers with glenohumeral internal rotation deficit (GIRD) may experience repetitive microtrauma after release of the ball, resulting in progressive tearing of the posteroinferior labrum of the glenoid.

Clinically, patients with posterior instability of the shoulder report pain and limited ability to move the arm. In cases with complete dislocation, patients are usually aware that the shoulder is out of place but may not be able to describe the direction of the dislocation. Subluxation is much more common than dislocation in athletes. When subluxation occurs, the prominent report is pain, with only half of patients reporting a sensation of instability.

Physical Examination

An acute posterior dislocation of the shoulder is extremely rare and is less apparent on clinical examination when compared with the more common anterior dislocation. The arm is usually held across the abdomen with the shoulder internally rotated and adducted. The shoulder is tender to palpation, and the patient avoids motion. Only on close inspection by visualizing the shoulder from above can the clinician visualize flattening of the anterior aspect of the shoulder with prominence of the coracoid and a fullness posteriorly created by the dislocated humeral head. The hallmark of the diagnosis is a lack of shoulder external rotation and inability to supinate the forearm. These examination findings are subtle and sometimes difficult to elicit in the acute situation and may result in the examiner missing the diagnosis. Examination of the athlete with chronic posterior instability is usually relatively normal on clinical inspection. The shoulder may demonstrate tenderness at the posterior joint line, mild

swelling, and decreased ROM. The posterior stress test is typically positive and may be performed with the patient in either the supine or upright position (Fig. 133.29). The arm is flexed to 90 degrees and internally rotated. The examiner then loads the humerus axially against the glenoid by pushing the arm posteriorly with the patient's scapula either stabilized by the examination table or the clinician's hand. The test is positive when subluxation of the humeral head over the glenoid rim is palpated or observed. The jerk test is similar to the posterior stress test in terms of position. The examiner puts the arm into the horizontally adducted position and attempts to subluxate the shoulder posteriorly. When the arm is then moved rapidly into a horizontally abducted position, the shoulder is reduced with a palpable and often visible jerk. The jerk test may be positive for crepitus and a catch when the arm is taken from the adducted to the abducted position.

Imaging

The radiographic evaluation of posterior instability is similar to that of anterior instability. Often, radiographs are normal, but they may reveal a reverse Hill-Sachs lesion, a posterior bony Bankart lesion, a fracture of the lesser tuberosity of the humerus, glenoid retroversion, or glenoid hypoplasia. MRI has become the standard in evaluating posterior instability of the shoulder (Fig. 133.30). Combined with arthrography, MRI provides details about the soft tissue injuries associated with posterior instability including labral, chondral, and tendinous pathology. In addition, both the size of the reverse Hill-Sachs lesion and the degree of posterior glenoid bone loss can be quantified, which may influence treatment decision-making.

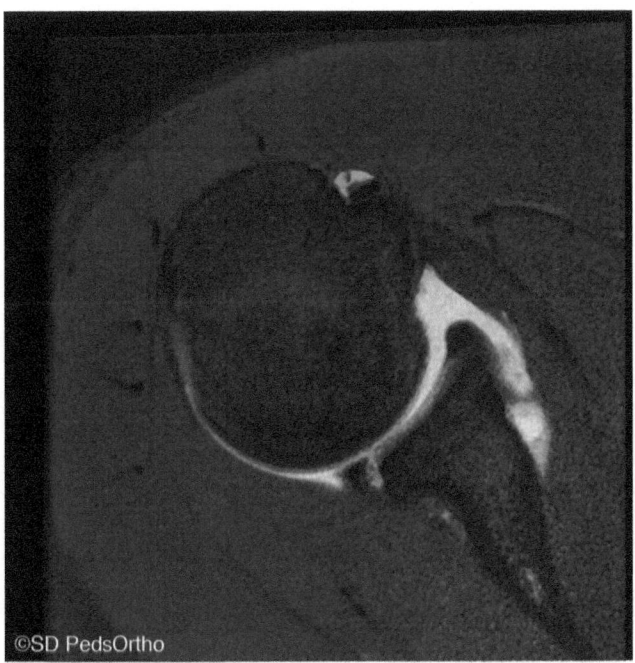

Fig. 133.30 Magnetic resonance imaging axial image demonstrating a posterior labral tear and posterior subluxation of the humeral head in a football lineman.

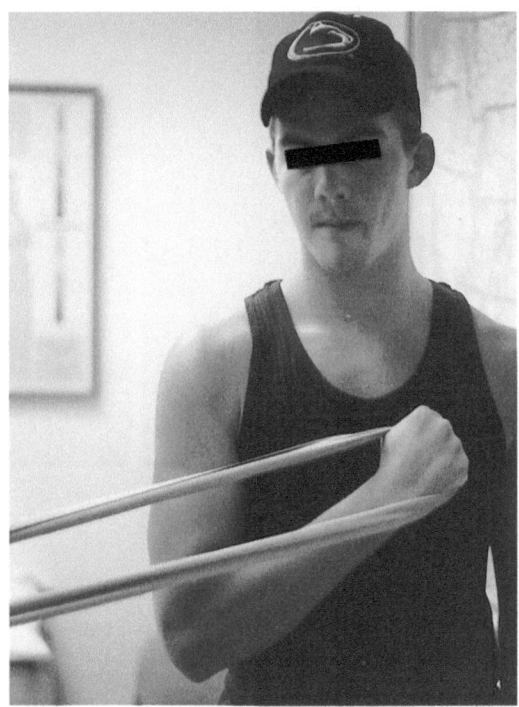

Fig. 133.31 Rehabilitation of the rotator cuff to improve dynamic stability of the shoulder.

Treatment Options
Nonoperative Treatment

Nonsurgical modalities are the first line of treatment for any patient with recurrent posterior shoulder instability. For most patients, surgery can be avoided with a focused course of physical therapy, in which reported success rates approach 80%.[155-157] The aim of physical therapy is to strengthen the dynamic muscular stabilizers of the shoulder, including the posterior deltoid, the internal rotators, and the periscapular muscles, to compensate for the damaged or deficient static stabilizers (Fig. 133.31). These exercises may be used in conjunction with modification of activity and biofeedback. In general, nonsurgical treatment should be pursued for 3 to 6 months. If this conservative approach fails, surgical stabilization should be considered and may consist of an open or arthroscopic soft tissue procedure or an intra-articular or extra-articular bone procedure.

Operative Treatment

Historically, the open posteroinferior shift has been the most popular surgical treatment for posterior shoulder instability. Although this procedure has been increasingly replaced by arthroscopic procedures, there is still a role for open stabilization of the shoulder, especially in cases with glenoid bone loss or dysplasia. The procedure is performed through a posterior approach that either splits or incises the infraspinatus muscle or develops a plane between the infraspinatus and teres minor muscles. When splitting the infraspinatus, care should be taken in dividing the muscle at a distance of more than 1.5 cm medial to the glenoid to avoid damaging the branches of the supra-scapular nerve.[158,159] A T-shaped capsulotomy is performed that permits inspection of the joint and allows the repair of any

posterior labral injury. Bone augmentation can then be performed as necessary. Superior advancement and plication of the posterior capsule is performed with the arm in 20 degree of abduction and neutral rotation. If the capsular tissue is attenuated it can be reinforced with the infraspinatus tendon.

As arthroscopic techniques and instrumentation have improved, there has been a trend toward the arthroscopic as opposed to open treatment of posterior shoulder instability. The arthroscopic approach has several advantages over open surgery, including less disruption of normal shoulder anatomy; less postoperative pain; better visualization and assessment of intra-articular pathology and landmarks; the ability to perform concomitant procedures, such as repairs of superior labrum anterior to posterior (SLAP) tears; addressing rotator cuff pathology; repairs of capsular rents; and better cosmesis. Most arthroscopic techniques use a posterior capsular plication with a posterior Bankart repair if a labral lesion is identified (Fig. 133.32).

Surgical outcomes with an arthroscopic approach to posterior shoulder instability have been promising. Multiple authors have reported success rates exceeding 90%, with good subjectively assessed outcomes and low recurrence rates of instability.[147-151,160-165] However, to date, few studies have compared an open approach with an arthroscopic approach for treating posterior shoulder instability. Bottoni et al. conducted a retrospective study of arthroscopically treated shoulders as compared with 12 shoulders treated with an open procedure.[166] Overall, they noted improvements in both groups, with similar rates of recurrent instability, but better subjectively reported outcomes and lower rates of disability in the arthroscopically treated group.

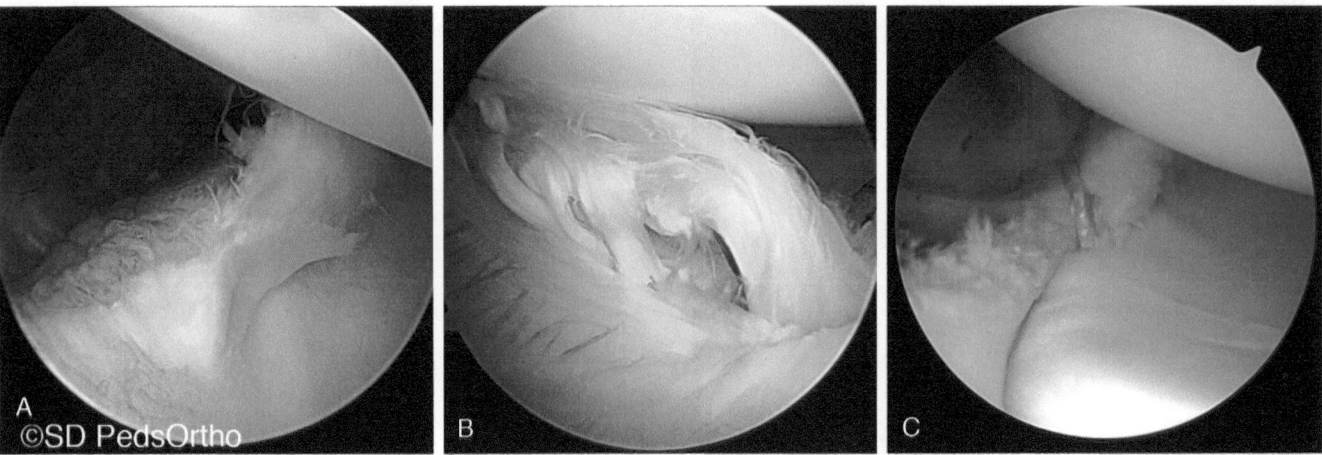

Fig. 133.32 (A) Arthroscopic view as seen from the anterior portal of a posterior labral tear. (B) Unstable labral tear as viewed from the posterior portal. (C) Labrum after repair and débridement.

ATRAUMATIC INSTABILITY/ MULTIDIRECTIONAL INSTABILITY

Atraumatic instability of the glenohumeral joint in the skeletally immature athlete is frequently encountered in individuals with generalized ligamentous laxity participating in overhead sports. If the direction of instability occurs in more than one direction (anterior, posterior, and/or inferior), the term multidirectional instability is appropriate. Atraumatic instability is characterized by redundancy and hyperelasticity of the capsule with increased intra-articular volume, resulting in multidirectional laxity of the shoulder. This multidirectional laxity is not always symptomatic but is a prerequisite for pathologic atraumatic instability.[167]

History

Atraumatic instability can be categorized as voluntary or involuntary depending on the degree of conscious control the patient exerts on the shoulder during the instability episode. A shoulder "dislocation" in a child or adolescent without a clear, significant history of trauma suggests an instance of atraumatic instability. Episodes of instability may occur with activities such as throwing, hitting an overhead serve in tennis and volleyball, or swimming. Atraumatic instability associated with secondary impingement symptoms is a common cause of shoulder pain in the young athlete involved in sports that require repetitive overhand motion. These patients rarely report instability but instead report pain exacerbated by repetitive sports activity. Most of these individuals do not recognize their own inherent multidirectional laxity; it is therefore difficult from the patient's history to determine that instability is truly the primary underlying pathology. Voluntary instability is accomplished by patients with multidirectional laxity through conscious firing of certain muscle groups and inhibition of their antagonists while combining these muscle manipulations with certain arm positions that lead to subluxation of the glenohumeral joint. The most notable finding in cases of voluntary instability is the lack of pain associated with the subluxation or dislocation episode. Pathologic voluntary instability is rarely recognized as such by the individual and is often associated with psychological or emotional instability.[168-170]

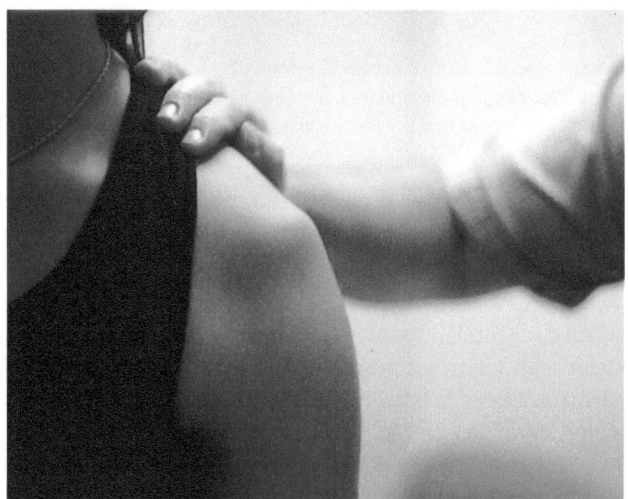

Fig. 133.33 The sulcus sign commonly associated with multidirectional laxity of the shoulder.

Physical Examination

On examination, the shoulder ROM is typically normal or increased and specific tenderness is usually absent. Signs of multidirectional laxity at the shoulder are always present. A positive sulcus sign is recognized as a dimpling of the skin or sulcus noted below the acromion when manual longitudinal traction is applied to the arm (Fig. 133.33). This is a result of inferior subluxation of the humeral head within the glenohumeral joint. Significant humeral head translation can also be elicited with the load and shift testing performed with the patient in the lateral decubitus position. Most patients will also demonstrate evidence of ligamentous hyperlaxity in other joints, including hyperextension at the elbows, knees, and metacarpophalangeal joints. The Beighton-Horan scale may be used to evaluate patients with joint laxity. Skin hyperelasticity with striae may also be present and may suggest the presence of an underlying collagen abnormality. Some athletes present with secondary impingement findings, and in these situations it is not uncommon to observe

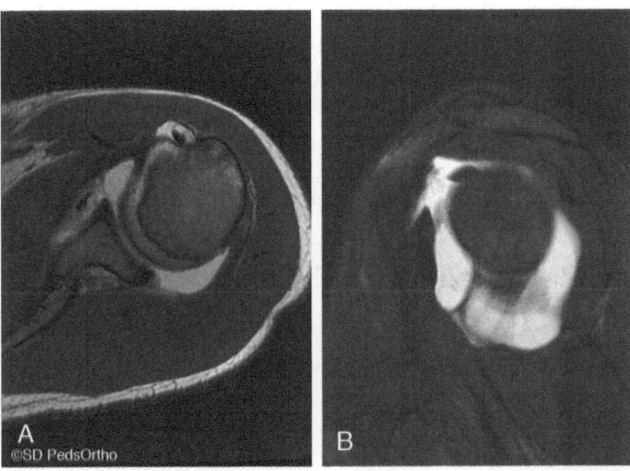

Fig. 133.34 (A) Magnetic resonance imaging (MRI) axial image in a patient with atraumatic instability with a capacious capsule but no labral tear. (B) MRI sagittal image demonstrating increased intra-articular volume of the shoulder joint.

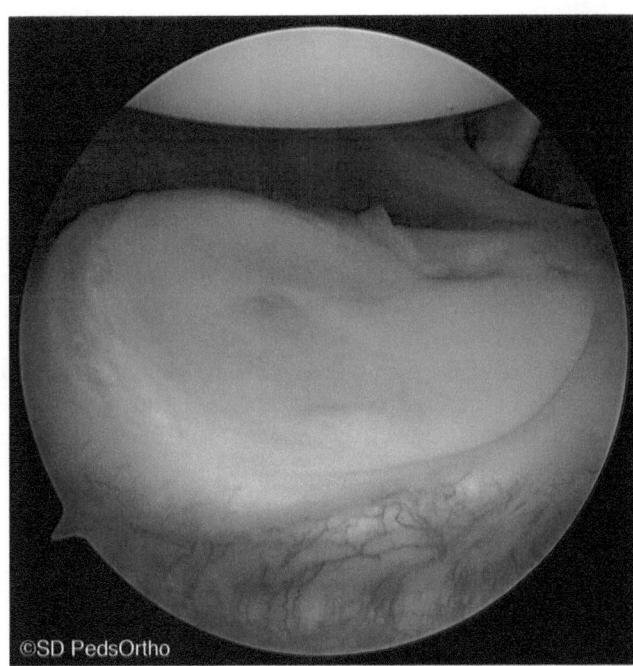

Fig. 133.35 Arthroscopic view seen from the posterior portal of a patient with atraumatic instability with a "drive through sign" from a large capacious capsule.

restricted motion from pain, impingement findings, and painful resisted external rotation and forward elevation.

Imaging

The radiographic examination in athletes with atraumatic instability is normal. Stress radiographs can be used to supplement the clinical examination to demonstrate instability in the anterior, posterior, and inferior directions but is usually unnecessary. Findings such as the Hill-Sachs lesion of the humeral head or glenoid rim fracture are not characteristic of atraumatic instability and may suggest a traumatic etiology. Magnetic resonance arthrography commonly demonstrates an abnormally patulous, redundant capsule with a large intra-articular volume and occasional inflammation without structural damage (Fig. 133.34).

Treatment Options
Nonoperative Treatment

A nonoperative approach is indicated as the initial treatment in every case of atraumatic instability. This nonoperative treatment emphasizes a vigorous rehabilitation program involving strengthening of the dynamic stabilizers, improvement of proprioception, and avoidance of provocative activities. Most patients with atraumatic instability improve their symptomatic shoulder instability with this program. Burkhead and Rockwood reported an 80% success rate in the treatment of atraumatic instability with a vigorous rehabilitation program.[125] Neer and Foster, in the classic description of multidirectional laxity, restricted surgical intervention to patients who did not respond to a 12-month rehabilitation program.[171] For athletes who demonstrate voluntary atraumatic instability, the same conservative program is indicated and surgery is typically avoided because studies have shown failure rates ranging from 43% to 100% in this population.[172,173]

Operative Treatment

Historically, an open inferior capsular shift was the procedure of choice for patients with symptomatic multidirectional atraumatic

instability who did not improve after a thorough rehabilitation program. This procedure has been reported to have good outcomes even in younger patient groups.[171,174] More recently, surgeons have moved towards arthroscopic stabilization with a combination of anterior and posterior capsular plications typically performed with suture anchors (Fig. 133.35).[175,176] Results of this procedure have been promising with good clinical outcomes, relatively high rates of return to sport, and low rates of recurrence.[177,178] Patients who undergo either an open or an arthroscopic capsular shift are treated with a very slow and controlled postoperative program. Immobilization in a sling continues for 6 weeks after surgery. At that time, a gentle ROM program is begun along with a rotator cuff and scapular muscle strengthening program. Ballistic training and heavier weightlifting activities are deferred for at least 4 months. Return to full activities requires 6 to 9 months.

OVERUSE INJURIES

Proximal Humerus Epiphysiolysis (Little League Shoulder)

Little league shoulder represents failure or stress fracture through the proximal humeral physeal plate as a result of repetitive microtrauma. The most common cause is the application of repetitive rotational forces applied to the proximal humerus in the immature athlete during the throwing motion. The forces generated in the upper extremity during the throwing motion and overhand sports motion are considerable both in rotation and compression at the shoulder. When these types of repetitive forces are applied to the physis over time, it is easy to understand how injury could occur. Currently, more and more skeletally immature athletes are participating in year-round overhand sports with substantial increased exposure. As would be expected, the increased exposure has led to an increase in the incidence of proximal humeral stress injury. For this reason, strict pitching limits have been developed by many organizations governing youth baseball.[179]

History

Most patients with a proximal humeral stress fracture are between the ages of 11 and 14 years and are involved in throwing or repetitive overhand sports.[179-184] The majority of these athletes are boys who participate in baseball, but athletes involved in volleyball and softball can also be affected. Pain is usually gradual in onset over weeks to months, with a superimposed subacute episode that brings the problem to attention. Often a short trial of rest has been attempted, with improvement followed by recurrent symptoms upon return to throwing.

Physical Examination

Physical examination is normal, without swelling, deformity, or discoloration. There is localized tenderness to palpation over the proximal humerus. Restricted ROM can be present secondary to pain, but many of these athletes will also have selective loss of internal rotation of their dominant throwing arm, also known as GIRD. Pain can usually be elicited with resisted external rotation and abduction.

Imaging

On plain radiographs, widening of the proximal humeral physeal plate is the hallmark finding. This widening usually begins laterally and extends across the physis as the stress lesion progresses. Comparison views are helpful in early cases to distinguish subtle physeal changes (Fig. 133.36). MRI and bone scan studies are unnecessary for diagnosis in most cases and do not add information that would alter treatment protocols.

Treatment

Rest is the primary treatment for this stress injury. The athlete should refrain from throwing and all other upper extremity activities, including lifting, hitting, or contact, until there are no

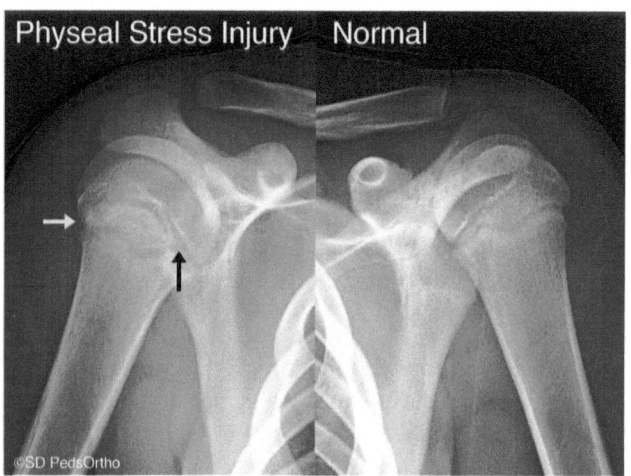

Fig. 133.36 Proximal humerus physeal epiphysiolysis or "little league shoulder" demonstrating widening of the physis. A contralateral film may be helpful to confirm the diagnosis.

symptoms with daily activity for 6 weeks. At that stage, rehabilitation is started, including shoulder stretching and strengthening of the rotator cuff and scapular stabilizers. Return to overhead athletics is allowed when the athlete is asymptomatic and rehabilitation is completed. This usually requires 8 to 12 weeks. It is not uncommon for the physis on the x-rays to remain persistently wide until the patient has reached skeletal maturity. For this reason, we do not routinely use serial radiographs to determine when the patient may return to sport. A throwing protocol is often used, focusing on gradually increasing the amount of pitching along with frequency and velocity, with a special focus on core and lower extremity strengthening and stability. The athlete's pitching technique and frequency should be addressed before return to pitching is considered.[179]

Complications

Although rare, displacement of the proximal humeral physis with continued throwing in the clinical setting of stress fracture has been documented.[179] Treatment after displacement may require reduction and internal fixation. Avascular necrosis of the epiphysis has also been reported.[92] All these cases occurred in high-performance male pitchers who were 11 to 13 years old.

Rotator Cuff Tears

Although rotator cuff tears are a frequent cause of shoulder pain in adults, they have been reported to be rare injuries in pediatric patients, representing less than 1% of all rotator cuff tears.[185] This pathology is being increasingly recognized in adolescent athletes as a result of greater physician awareness, improved MRI techniques, and increased utilization of arthroscopy. An MRI study evaluating a consecutive series of pediatric patients undergoing a shoulder MRI revealed that 12% of patients had a rotator cuff tear.[186]

History

Most rotator cuff pathology in adolescents is a result of repetitive overuse injuries in the overhead athlete, but occasionally a single traumatic event may be the cause. The most common tendon involved is the supraspinatous in 68% of cases, and most tears are partial-thickness articular sided tears (72%), with less than 10% representing full-thickness tears (Fig. 133.37).[186] Approximately 30% to 50% of patients will have associated labral pathology, and it is not clear what percentage of these rotator cuff tears are asymptomatic and represent only incidental findings on an MRI. Screening studies in asymptomatic collegiate and professional swimmers and baseball players have shown that a large percentage will have abnormalities to the rotator cuff.[187-189]

Physical Examination

Examination is similar to the adult patient focusing on range-of-motion and strength testing of the supraspinatus, infraspinatus, and subscapularis. In particular, throwing athletes with shoulder pain frequently have selective loss of internal rotation (GIRD). Given the high association with other shoulder joint pathology, the examination should also include tests focusing on the labrum, scapula, and AC joint. Deficiencies in core stability and postural

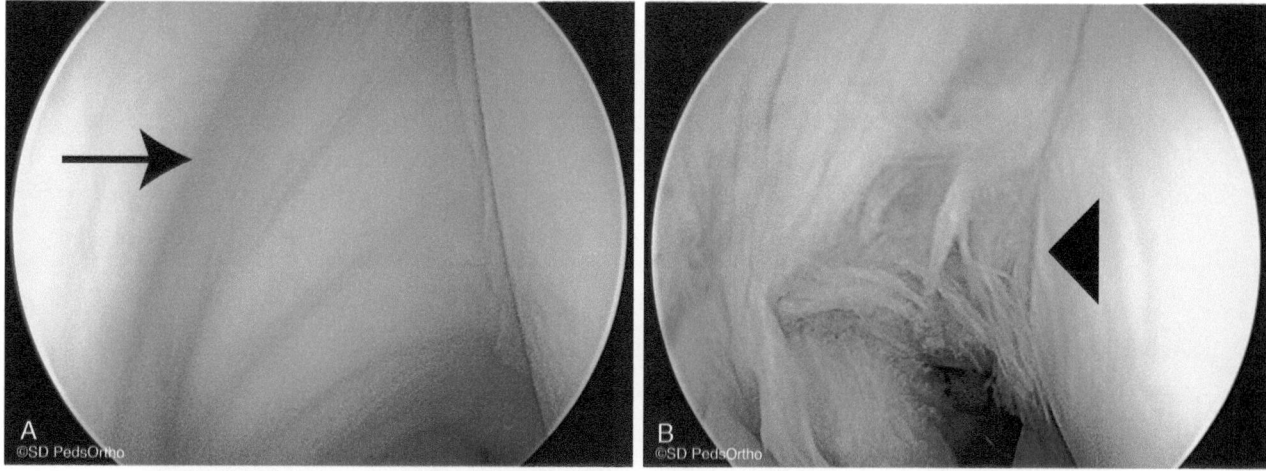

Fig. 133.37 (A) Arthroscopic appearance of a normal supraspinatus tendon *(arrow)* viewed from the posterior portal. (B) Partial-thickness rotator cuff tear involving the supraspinatus *(arrow)* frequently seen in athletes participating in overhead sports.

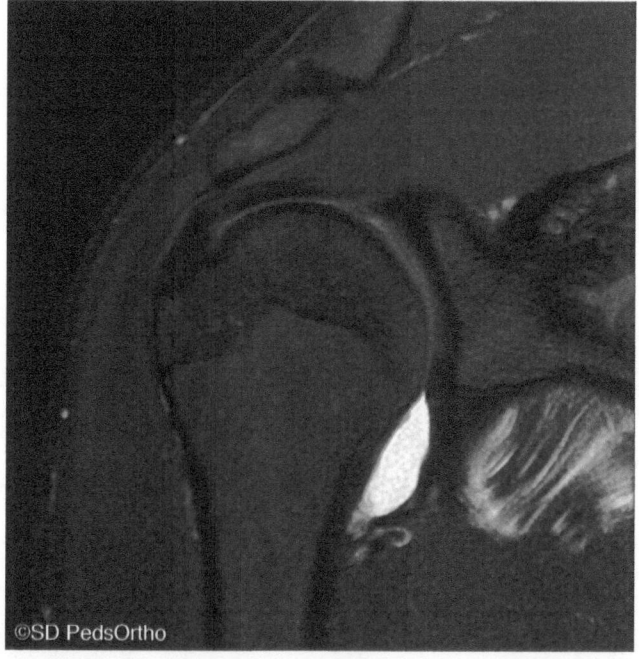

Fig. 133.38 Magnetic resonance imaging coronal image depicting a partial-thickness tear of the supraspinatus.

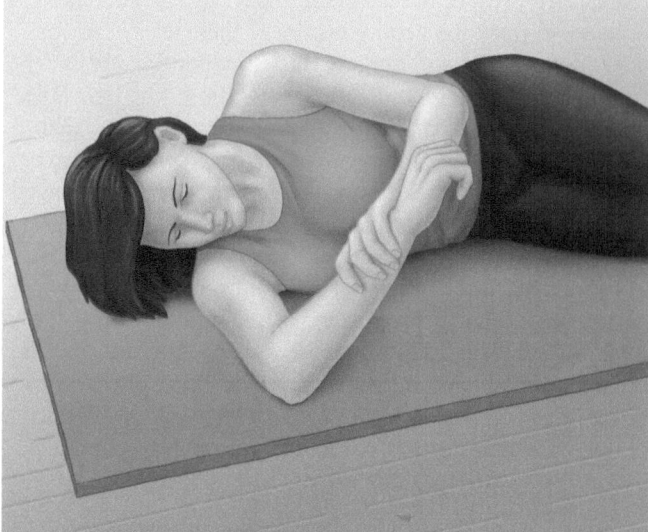

Fig. 133.39 Sleeper stretch for glenohumeral internal rotation deficit or posterior capsular tightness.

control may also predispose to cuff pathology and should also be evaluated.

Imaging

MRI remains the standard tool for the evaluation of the rotator cuff, but many centers are using ultrasound as a more dynamic and cost-effective means to evaluate the cuff. Many institutions (like ours) still prefer MR arthrography because it optimizes visualization of subtle articular sided cuff tears (Fig. 133.38).

Treatment

Nonoperative treatment. Nonoperative treatment of cuff pathology in adolescent patients is similar to that in adults, including a period of rest and activity modification followed by

ROM exercises and a progressive strengthening program focusing on the rotator cuff and periscapular musculature. In addition, stretching exercises focusing on the posterior capsule, such as the sleeper stretch, are initiated (Fig. 133.39). In overhead athletes, a core-strengthening program addressing the entire kinetic chain may be fundamental for long-term success. Working with the athlete's coaching staff to optimize technique, training regimens, and competition schedules is also very helpful in safely returning the athlete to sport. We place an emphasis on avoiding playing a single overhead sport year-round and recommend that throwers in particular have 3 to 4 months a year with no throwing. A nonoperative approach to adolescent patients with rotator cuff tears has been shown to be successful in 68% of patients.[186] Although the natural history of a partial-thickness tear in an adult tends to not heal or progress to a full-thickness tear, it is not clear if these tears suffer the same fate in this younger patient population.[190] It is possible that, with appropriate rest

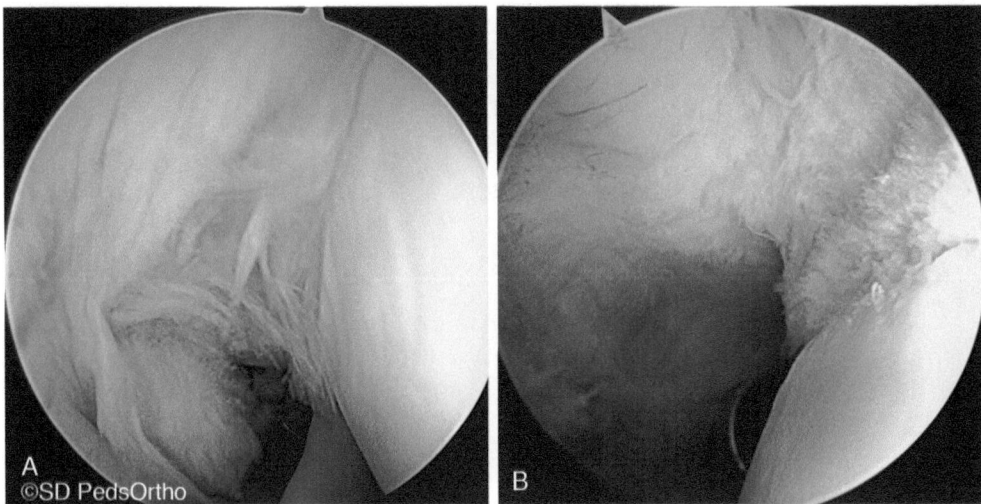

Fig. 133.40 (A) Arthroscopic view of a partial-thickness supraspinatus tear. (B) Appearance after débridement.

and rehabilitation, some of these partial tears will spontaneously heal. Future prospective ultrasound and MRI studies will be necessary to track the natural history of these tears.

Operative treatment. Surgery is reserved for the rare patient with a full-thickness rotator cuff tear and those who have failed a prolonged course of nonoperative treatment greater than 3 months' duration. When a nonoperative approach fails, partial tears (<50% of the thickness of the tendon) may be managed with arthroscopic débridement, whereas more full-thickness tears require surgical repair that can typically be performed arthroscopically (Fig. 133.40). Few case series have been published in the pediatric and adolescent population on the surgical management of rotator cuff tears. The largest series to date evaluating the outcomes of 53 adolescent patients age 9 to 19, all of whom had partial rotator cuff tears, showed that 43% could be managed nonoperatively. Outcomes in the surgical cohort were reasonable, but only 70% of athletes returned to their preoperative level of competition.[191]

Snapping Scapula

Snapping scapula is an uncommon condition of the shoulder that results in painful crepitation and snapping around the scapula with shoulder motion. It is caused by either structural (osteochondroma, Luschka tubercle, or a hooked superomedial border of the scapula) or nonstructural anatomic pathology (scapular dyskinesia, pectoralis muscle tightness, and/or rhomboid weakness) within the scapulothoracic joint that interferes with the normal gliding of the scapula along the chest wall.

History

In young athletes, more than 90% of cases of snapping scapula will have overuse as the major contributing factor, particularly in overheard sports such as swimming, tennis, and baseball.[192] This is different than in adult series, where 70% of cases have reported trauma as the initial leading cause.[193]

Physical Examination

Snapping scapula is confirmed with physical examination. Typically, the patient can recreate the snapping by taking the shoulder

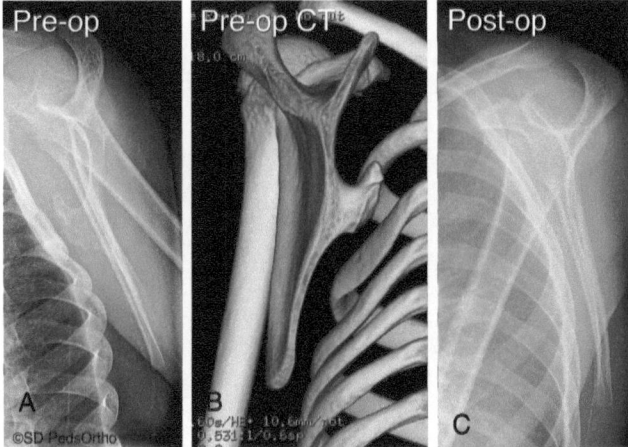

Fig. 133.41 (A) Scapular Y view showing an osteochondroma on the ventral surface of the scapula. (B) Computed tomography *(CT)* three-dimensional reconstruction showing the location, size, and orientation of the osteochondroma. Note the compensatory change of the ribs. (C) Postresection radiograph taken 3 years after surgery.

through a ROM or shrugging the joint. It is important to evaluate the patient for any obvious osteochondroma, as well as any scapular dyskinesia or winging.

Imaging

Standard shoulder radiographs including an AP, axillary lateral, and scapular-Y view are obtained, but these will rarely reveal a structural abnormality. In cases where a structural abnormality such as an osteochondroma are suspected, a CT scan may be performed. The use of 3D reconstructions with the CT scan has been shown to be the most sensitive test for subtle osteochondromas or incongruities of the superomedial border of the scapula (Fig. 133.41).[194,195]

Treatment

Nonoperative treatment. For nonstructural pathology, therapy is directed at relieving inflammation and bursitis and reducing fibrosis with a focused stretching program that targets the pectoralis muscles, as well as a strengthening program targeting the rhomboids and trapezius muscles. This approach, combined with rest and activity modification, should be pursued for a minimum of 3 months. A nonoperative approach has been shown to be successful at alleviating symptoms and returning athletes to sport in 75% of cases, but athletes and their families should be counseled that one-third will continue to experience snapping.[192]

Operative treatment. For the relatively uncommon structural causes of snapping scapula, surgical intervention is focused on excising the osteochondroma, the prominent Luschka tubercle, or the hooked superomedial of the scapula. For the more common nonstructural causes, some surgeons favor an arthroscopic isolated lysis of adhesions and bursectomy, whereas others favor either an open or arthroscopic superomedial corner resection of the scapula. To date, there are little data to guide treatment in the adolescent population with a nonstructural cause of snapping. In the only series to date on the topic, Haus et al. found that superomedial corner resection with a mini-open approach provided more consistent results than an arthroscopic lysis of adhesions.[192]

Scapular Dyskinesia

Scapular winging is abnormal scapulothoracic posture and motion, resulting from numerous underlying causes. Primary winging occurs when muscular weakness disrupts the normal balance of the scapulothoracic joint. This typically occurs with weakness of the serratus anterior, trapezius, or rhomboids (Fig. 133.42). Secondary winging occurs when pathology of the glenohumeral joint disrupts the coordinated motion of the scapula.[196]

History

The most common cause of scapular winging is paralysis of the serratus anterior muscle secondary to an injury to the long thoracic nerve.[197] This tends to be a stretch injury to the nerve after blunt trauma to the lateral chest wall that can occur in collision athletes, such as football players, wrestlers, or hockey players, or from repetitive activities that involve the head tilting away from the nerve and the arm extending overhead, as occurs in baseball pitching, javelin throwing, and tennis serving. Paralysis of the

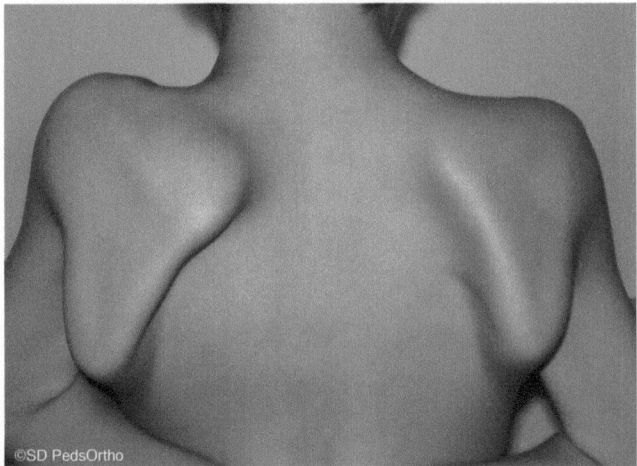

Fig. 133.42 Clinical photograph of serratus anterior muscle palsy with medial winging. Note the prominence of the medial scapular border.

trapezius muscle in athletes typically occurs from blunt trauma or a stretch injury to the spinal accessory nerve as it courses down the neck. This may be seen in football players or wrestlers from a direct blow during a tackle or a check in a lacrosse or hockey player from an aberrant stick.[198] Secondary causes of scapular winging in the young athlete frequently occur as the result of shoulder instability, particularly posterior instability. Electromyography (EMG) studies have shown that painful subluxation of the shoulder deactivates the serratus anterior muscle, resulting in winging.[199]

Physical Examination

Examination of the patient from behind with full visualization of both scapulae is essential for the proper evaluation of scapular winging. Dysfunction of the serratus anterior muscle results in medial winging with the scapula migrating superiorly and the inferior pole rotating medially. These patients will also have difficulty with active forward elevation beyond 120 degrees. Dysfunction of the trapezius results in lateral winging, with the scapula migrating inferiorly and the inferior pole rotating laterally. These patients will have difficulty with shrugging the affected shoulder.

Imaging

Initial imaging should include radiographs of the cervical spine, shoulder, and scapula to help rule out cervical spine disease, a fracture malunion, an accessory rib, or an osteochondroma. Advanced imaging typically is not necessary. In cases of scapular winging that fail to resolve over 6 weeks, a nerve conduction study and EMG are valuable in distinguishing neuromuscular causes of winging.

Treatment

Nonoperative treatment. Because most cases of scapular winging are the result of neuropraxic injury, they typically resolve over 6 to 9 months. Initial treatment consists of activity modification, analgesics including antiinflammatory drugs, and physical therapy.

Operative treatment. In recalcitrant cases where there is no evidence of nerve recovery after 12 to 24 months, a muscle transfer may be indicated. For chronic dysfunction of the serratus anterior, most surgeons will advocate transfer of the pectoralis major muscle that may require augmentation with autograft or allograft. For a trapezius muscle palsy that does not recover with time, an Eden-Lange muscle transfer, involving lateralization of the rhomboids and the levator scapulae, has been shown to provide improved shoulder function and muscle strength.[196]

For a complete list of references, go to ExpertConsult.com.

SELECTED READINGS

Citation:
Pandya NK, Namdari S. Shoulder arthroscopy in children and adolescents. *J Am Acad Orthop Surg.* 2013;21(7):389–397.

Level of Evidence:
Review

Summary:
This article summarizes the various pediatric shoulder pathologies that can be managed with an arthroscope with a focus on anatomy, anesthetic considerations, patient positioning, and technical pearls.

Citation:
Chen FS, Diaz VA, Loebenberg M, et al. Shoulder and elbow injuries in the skeletally immature athlete. *J Am Acad Orthop Surg.* 2005;13(3):172–185.

Level of Evidence:
Review

Summary:
Children participating in recreational and organized sports are particularly susceptible to a broad spectrum of shoulder and elbow injuries involving both osseous and soft tissue structure. This article discusses common pediatric injuries specific to the shoulder and appropriate treatment.

Citation:
Pandya NK, Namdari S, Hosalkar HS. Displaced clavicle fractures in adolescents: facts, controversies, and current trends. *J Am Acad Orthop Surg.* 2012;20(8):498–505.

Level of Evidence:
Review

Summary:
This review article summarizes the controversial nature of the management of adolescent clavicle fractures, with both a historical perspective and a focus on recent literature demonstrating a surgical trend.

Citation:
Popkin CA, Levine WN, Ahmad CS. Evaluation and management of pediatric proximal humerus fractures. *J Am Acad Orthop Surg.* 2015;23(2):77–86.

Level of Evidence:
Review

Summary:
This review article summarizes the anatomy, classification, radiographic imaging, and treatment options of pediatric patients with proximal humerus fractures.

Citation:
Longo UG, van der Linde JA, Loppini M, et al. Surgical versus nonoperative treatment in patients up to 18 years old with traumatic shoulder instability: a systematic review and quantitative synthesis of the literature. *Arthroscopy.* 2016;32(5): 944–952.

Level of Evidence:
Review

Summary:
Systemic review evaluating the outcomes of surgical and nonoperative treatment in patients aged 18 years or younger with traumatic shoulder instability.

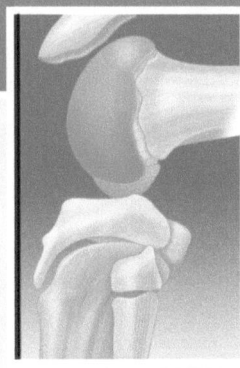

134

Elbow Injuries in Pediatric and Adolescent Athletes

James P. Bradley, Luke S. Austin, Alexander B. Kreines, Fotios P. Tjoumakaris

RELEVANT ANATOMY AND BIOMECHANICS

Osteology

Skeletal growth around the elbow typically follows a characteristic development process. The elbow joint consists of the articulation of the distal humerus with the ulna (the ulnohumeral joint), the articulation of the distal humerus with the radial head (the radiocapitellar joint), and the proximal articulation of the radius and ulna (the proximal radioulnar joint). Skeletal maturation occurs from the primary ossification centers of the humerus, radius, and ulna, along with six secondary ossification centers. The sequence of ossification is the capitellum, proximal radius, medial epicondyle, trochlea, olecranon, and lateral epicondyle.[1-3] When evaluating radiographs, variation can occur in the appearance of the ossification centers as distinct structures, and correlation with the contralateral extremity can help determine disease in questionable cases.

The ossification of the distal humerus extends to the condyles at birth and progresses through the secondary centers at various stages of development. The lateral condyle and capitellum appear in the second year of life.[4] On a normal lateral radiograph of the elbow, the anterior humeral line intersects the anterior third of the capitellar ossific nucleus (Fig. 134.1). This line is helpful in characterizing supracondylar fracture displacement in children. In the third year of life, the proximal radius ossific nucleus begins to ossify and is typically present in most children by age 4 years. Notches or clefts in the proximal radius metaphysis can sometimes be seen and are considered part of the normal variability of maturation.[5,6] The medial epicondylar ossific nucleus begins to ossify between the ages of 5 and 6 years; however, fusion of the epiphysis does not occur until 15 to 16 years of age, placing this physis under stress during the throwing motion well into adolescence.[7] The secondary ossification center of the olecranon process appears around age 7 to 9 years, whereas the trochlear ossific nucleus appears around age 9 to 10 years.[8] The last center to appear is the lateral epicondyle, usually after age 10 years, and this center rapidly fuses to the lateral condyle shortly after being visible on radiographs. A thorough understanding of the stages of ossification and the appearance of the centers of ossification is critical for clinicians who treat pediatric elbow injuries (Fig. 134.2). Any heterogeneous appearance to the nuclei or differences relative to the contralateral extremity in terms of size, density, position, or fragmentation could indicate abnormal development

and may be the result of repetitive stress to the elbow, inducing vascular changes with resultant alterations in the maturation process. A failure to appreciate the normal progression of growth at the elbow could result in misdiagnosis, improper treatment, and progressive developmental abnormality.

The osseous anatomy surrounding the elbow contributes significantly to stability of the elbow joint. Approximately 50% of elbow stability arises from the congruity of the ulnohumeral articulation.[9] In serial olecranon excision studies, progressive loss of the proximal olecranon resulted in linear decreases in elbow stability at 0 and 90 degrees of elbow motion.[10] The radial head provides 15% to 30% of valgus stability to the elbow joint, and may be more important in the throwing athlete for providing valgus stability through the midrange of motion.[9] Studies evaluating the load transmission across the elbow joint have shown that forces of up to three times body weight can be seen, and forces that are generated during throwing may be even higher.[11,12] Thus it is not surprising that a small deficiency in the elaborate stability-controlling mechanisms of the elbow may have a significant and cumulative effect on elbow function.

Ligaments and Soft Tissue

Whereas 50% of the stability of the elbow joint arises from the osseous anatomy, the remaining 50% is derived from the ligamentous and soft tissue attachments (e.g., the anterior capsule, the medial or ulnar collateral ligament [UCL], and the lateral radial collateral ligament).[9] With regard to the muscular attachment sites around the elbow, laterally the common extensor origin is located at the lateral epicondyle and can be a common source of pathologic findings in persons who participate in racquet sport and repetitive motion activities. This source is perhaps more prominent in the adult population, with abnormalities classically located within the extensor carpi radialis brevis (lateral epicondylitis). Anteriorly, the brachialis and biceps serve as a powerful flexor and supinator of the elbow, respectively. Posteriorly, the triceps attachment on the proximal aspect of the olecranon serves as the main extensor to the elbow and can be injured in young athletes who have an eccentric contractile injury. Although injury or strain of these muscle groups can occur, this pathologic condition is less often seen in the pediatric population. Medially, the flexor and pronator attachment sites serve as powerful medial stabilizers to the elbow, particularly in the athlete

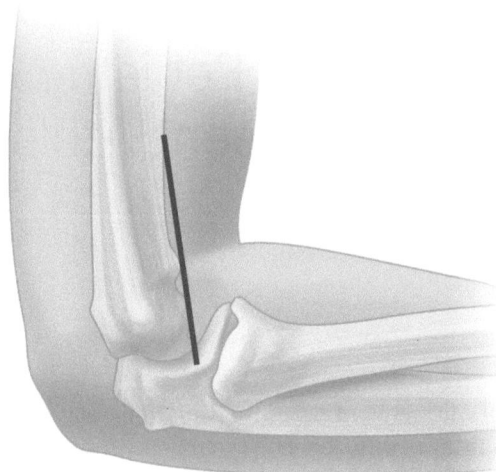

Fig. 134.1 On a normal lateral radiograph of the pediatric elbow, the anterior humeral line intersects the anterior third of the capitellum and is helpful in characterizing displacement in supracondylar humerus fractures.

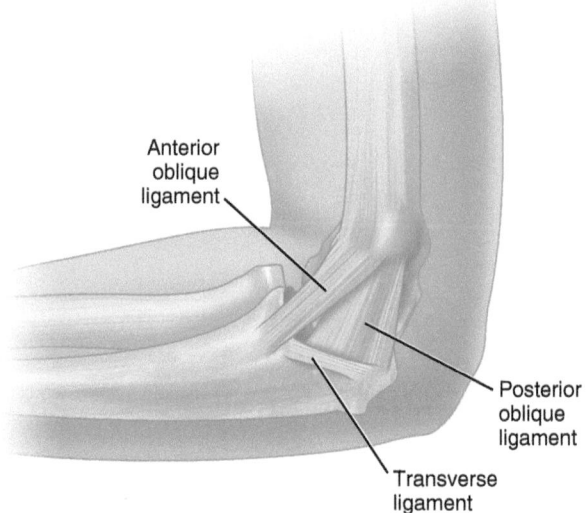

Fig. 134.3 The ulnar collateral ligament of the elbow consists of the anterior oblique bundle, the intermediate bundle, and the posterior oblique bundle.

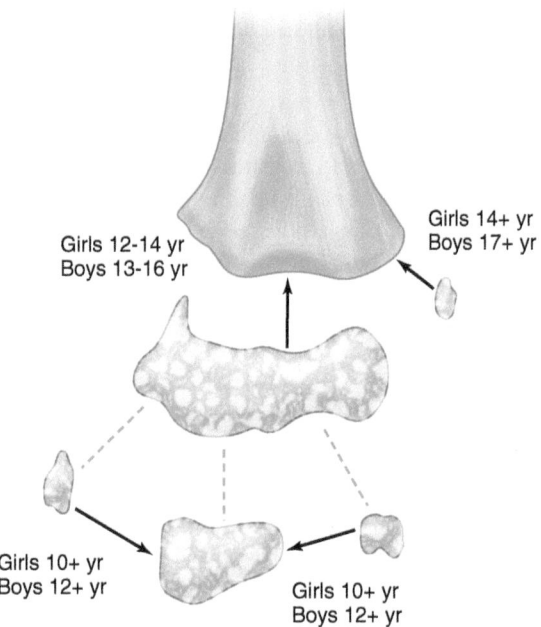

Fig. 134.2 The usual ages at which the ossific centers fuse to each other and to the distal humerus in boys and girls.

whose sport entails throwing. Repetitive strain at this site can be seen in the throwing population or, alternatively, in golfers, in whom it can manifest as medial epicondylitis.

The UCL complex of the elbow is a broad ligament on the medial side of the elbow that provides restraint to valgus stress (Fig. 134.3).[13] The ligament consists of three portions: the anterior oblique bundle, the posterior oblique bundle, and the transverse ligament or intermediate bundle. The anterior oblique bundle is the main medial stabilizer to the elbow and arises from the medial epicondyle with an insertion to the medial aspect of the

coronoid process. This ligament becomes more important during high-velocity throwing, when a large valgus force is placed on the medial elbow structures. Both the anterior and posterior bundles of the ligament provide stability during the full arc of motion, with the anterior band having a larger burden in extension and the posterior band having a more important role in flexion. The lateral collateral ligament provides varus stability to the elbow, and in recent years its role as a major contributor to posterolateral rotatory elbow stability has been more extensively studied.[14] The lateral collateral (or radial collateral) ligament complex is composed of three main parts: the lateral UCL, the radial collateral ligament, and the accessory lateral collateral ligament (Fig. 134.4). The radial collateral ligament courses from the lateral epicondyle to the annular ligament of the proximal radioulnar joint. The lateral UCL courses from the posterior lateral epicondyle, travels across the annular ligament, and attaches on the crista supinatoris of the ulna. This ligament is the primary restraint to posterolateral elbow stability. The accessory lateral collateral ligament originates from the inferior aspect of the annular ligament and attaches to the tubercle of the supinator. The lateral ligamentous complex is classically injured or disrupted during an elbow dislocation or iatrogenically during surgery around the posterolateral aspect of the elbow. These ligaments, combined with the anconeus muscle, form a lateral elbow complex that provides both dynamic and static restraint to elbow instability in both varus and rotation. The lateral ligament complex is rarely injured in children as a result of repetitive use or microtrauma; however, the medical literature includes case reports that describe reconstruction or repair of this complex when persistent instability exists.[15,16] The diagnosis is often challenging because children may describe vague pain and soreness with certain activities, but without the characteristic instability that is the hallmark of this clinical entity in adults.

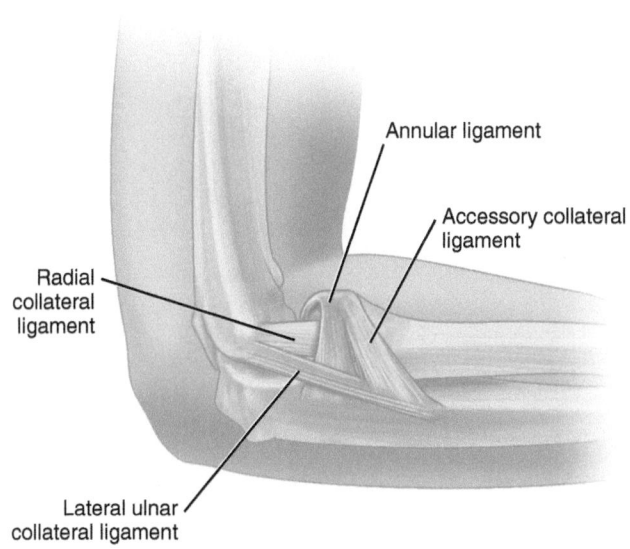

Fig. 134.4 The lateral collateral ligament complex of the elbow is demonstrated, including the lateral ulnar collateral ligament, the radial collateral ligament, and the accessory collateral ligament.

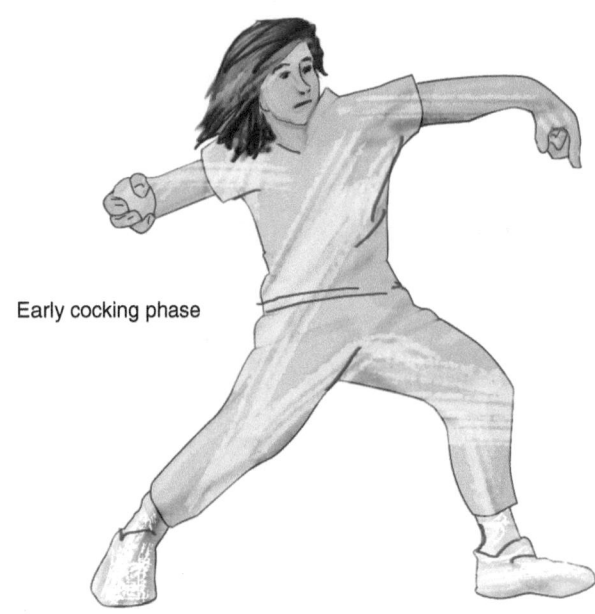

Fig. 134.6 The early cocking phase of throwing.

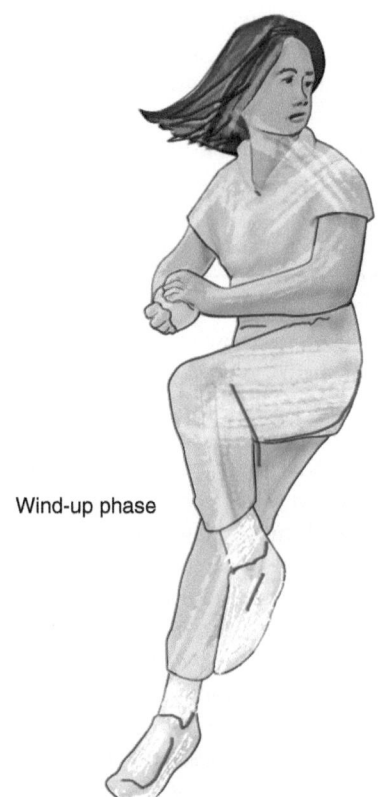

Fig. 134.5 The wind-up phase of throwing.

Biomechanics in Throwing Sports
Throwing Motion

The throwing motion is common in many sports played by children and adolescents. Football, baseball, and overhead racquet sports such as tennis are the characteristic activities that demonstrate the biomechanics of the elbow during throwing and

are most common in this age group. The pitching motion has been analyzed extensively in the adult and pediatric sports medicine literature. Repetitive valgus and distraction forces of the medial pediatric elbow have been observed during pitching and are thought to be the etiology in the development of medial UCL disease, medial epicondylitis, and epicondyle avulsions. The pitch has been divided into five stages[17–19]:

1. Wind-up (ends when the ball leaves the nonthrowing hand; Fig. 134.5)
2. Cocking
   a. Early cocking (shoulder abduction and rotation; ends when the forward foot hits the ground; Fig. 134.6)
   b. Late cocking (maximum shoulder external rotation is achieved; Fig. 134.7)
3. Acceleration (begins with internal rotation of the humerus and ends with ball release; Fig. 134.8)
4. Deceleration (eccentric contraction of all muscles; center of gravity moves over plantar foot)
5. Follow-through (ends when all motion is complete; Fig. 134.9)

One of the fundamental concepts in understanding the throwing motion as it relates to pitching is the "kinetic chain."[20] The kinetic chain of throwing refers to the role that core and proximal musculature play into the development of force required for throwing. Proximal muscle activation results in postural adjustments that allow the body to balance the forces that are required for throwing.[21] These muscle activations create force moments, which are a product of adjacent segment motion and position. The moments occur at proximal segments and are important for generating force delivered to distal motion segments, such as the elbow.[22] One investigation demonstrated that younger pitchers may not produce as much force generation from their lower core segments, which may place larger demands on the upper extremities of youths who pitch and can ultimately cause

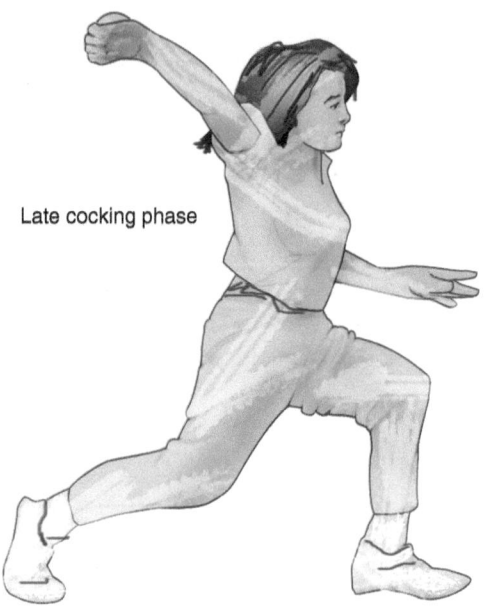

Late cocking phase

Fig. 134.7 The late cocking phase of throwing.

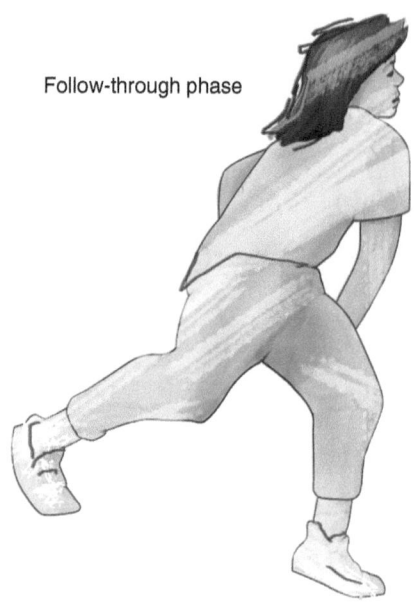

Follow-through phase

Fig. 134.9 The follow-through phase of throwing.

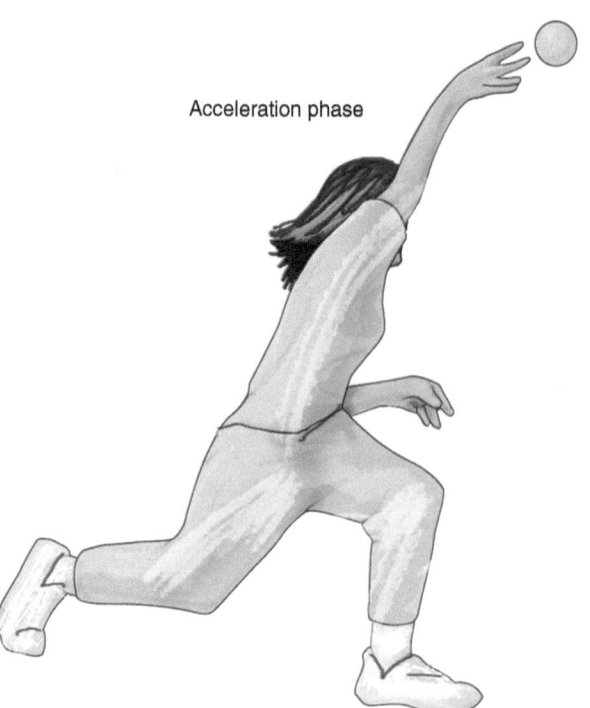

Acceleration phase

Fig. 134.8 The acceleration phase of throwing.

pain and disability.[23] Other investigations have documented that youths who pitch and adults who pitch have similar kinematics, while also demonstrating that youth pitchers who are deficient in their mechanics on key parameters are less efficient, place higher valgus loads across their elbows, and demonstrate higher humeral internal rotation torque.[24,25] Lack of proximal force production may cause the elbow to be lower than the shoulder during the acceleration phase of throwing (as a result of a lack

of elbow elevation and extension prior to shoulder rotation), which places increased tensile forces on the medial elbow.[20] In the ideal motion, maximal elbow extension occurs prior to maximum shoulder rotation, which couples internal rotation of the shoulder to pronation about the elbow, preventing medial tensile or valgus overload. Teaching proper throwing mechanics in youth sports and limiting the opportunities of young throwers to "overuse" their arms is critical in preventing pathologic conditions of the elbow.

Forces around the elbow during throwing. During the early and late cocking phases of throwing, significant distraction forces are placed on the medial elbow structures. This tensile force is transmitted to the medial UCL and medial epicondyle. In the pediatric population, the most vulnerable area of injury is the medial epicondylar physis, which can be avulsed with repetitive injury. In addition, the UCL can become stretched or incompetent, the flexor pronator mass can become strained, and the ulnar nerve can be stretched, resulting in neurologic symptoms. Whereas distraction forces are applied on the medial elbow, compressive forces are encountered on the lateral elbow structures during the early and late cocking phases.[17–19] Sequelae of this repetitive compression of the radial head against the capitellum can result in growth disturbances, osteochondral fractures and loose bodies, and altered growth of the radial head.[17,18]

During the acceleration phase of throwing, extreme pronation of the forearm results in a tension force on the lateral and posterolateral elbow structures. Lateral epicondylitis may result from repetitive overuse and strain of these muscles during this phase of throwing. During follow-through, hyperextension of the elbow places strain on the olecranon process and the anterior capsule. In late adolescence and into young adulthood, this stress can manifest as posteromedial elbow spurs, posterior/triceps spurs, and traction spurs of the coronoid process. Classic overload symptoms of the elbow result from forces generated during the throwing motion and are helpful in determining pathologic findings: tensile overload of the medial restraints, compression overload of the lateral elbow, shear forces of the posteromedial elbow, and extension overload of the lateral restraints.[18,26]

OVERVIEW OF PATHOLOGIES

Little Leaguer's Elbow

Little leaguer's elbow, or medial apophysitis, is a broad term used to describe a spectrum of pathologic conditions that can occur in the young baseball player or thrower. Although we typically associate this spectrum of injury with baseball, a wide range of throwing or overhead sports, including javelin, tennis, and football, can present in a similar fashion. The throwing motion in the developing athlete is associated with significant force across the medial elbow.[18] During the throwing motion, and particularly in the late cocking phase of throwing, a valgus traction force is created on the medial elbow structures (i.e., the medial epicondyle, epicondylar apophysis, and medial ligament complex), whereas a compressive force is transmitted to the lateral side of the elbow (radial head and capitellum). With repetitive stress to the medial elbow, microtrauma and potentially degeneration of these structures may occur.[27] The subsequent tissue breakdown can cause the characteristic spectrum of disease: delayed or accelerated growth of the medial epicondyle, traction apophysitis and fragmentation of the medial epicondyle, medial epicondylitis, osteochondritis of the capitellum, hypertrophy of the ulna, osteochondral injury to the radial head, and olecranon apophysitis with delayed physeal closure.

Aside from overuse and repetitive stress to the medial elbow, young pitchers are believed to have altered mechanics relative to older athletes. Younger pitchers may initiate trunk rotation earlier in the throwing motion, which causes hyperangulation at the shoulder and increased torque along the longitudinal axis of the humerus during late cocking, predisposing them to elbow and shoulder pathology.[27] Early trunk rotation occurs before the scapula and humerus are properly positioned in space. The resultant increase in horizontal abduction of the shoulder during stride results in excessive angulation of the shoulder throughout the cocking phase, which can predispose the athlete to anterior shoulder instability and an elevation in the horizontal adduction force applied to the humerus. When obtaining the history, a focus on the athlete's prior education regarding proper throwing mechanics, initiation of pitch counts with rest periods, and supervision for manifesting symptoms are all helpful in determining the prevention strategies that were in place for the athlete prior to the development of symptoms and can help guide treatment. Young athletes may not present in a typical fashion, and the symptoms may range from medial elbow pain and decreased throwing effectiveness to decreased throwing distance.

History

Obtaining a thorough history in pediatric and adolescent patients can often be challenging. The clinician must assess the overall

affect of the child, as well as the importance of the sport in his or her daily life. Some children may underreport their symptoms, so they may continue playing, whereas other children may overreport their symptoms in situations in which they feel pressured to compete by family or friends or pressured by the requirements of the daily routine. The age of the patient is important because it may provide a clue to the potential diagnosis. Patients in their early childhood and in whom the secondary ossification centers have yet to appear are more likely to report pain originating from the medial elbow as a result of repetitive injury to the ossification center and apophysis.[18] Throwing forces may impede the characteristic appearance and growth of these ossification centers. In adolescence (which terminates with the fusion of the secondary centers of ossification with their respective long bones), muscle mass and force generation during throwing dramatically increase. In this age group, avulsion of the medial epicondyle can occur with resulting fracture displacement (Fig. 134.10). Incomplete avulsions are more common near the end of adolescence as fusion of the medial epicondyle occurs. With repetitive stress to the medial epicondyle, nonunions and delayed unions may occur and cause continued pain into young adulthood. When the patient enters young adulthood (after fusion of all the secondary ossification centers), injuries to the muscles and soft tissue attachments of the elbow are more common. Injury to the UCL and strain of the flexor/pronator mass are characteristically seen as overuse syndromes in this patient cohort.

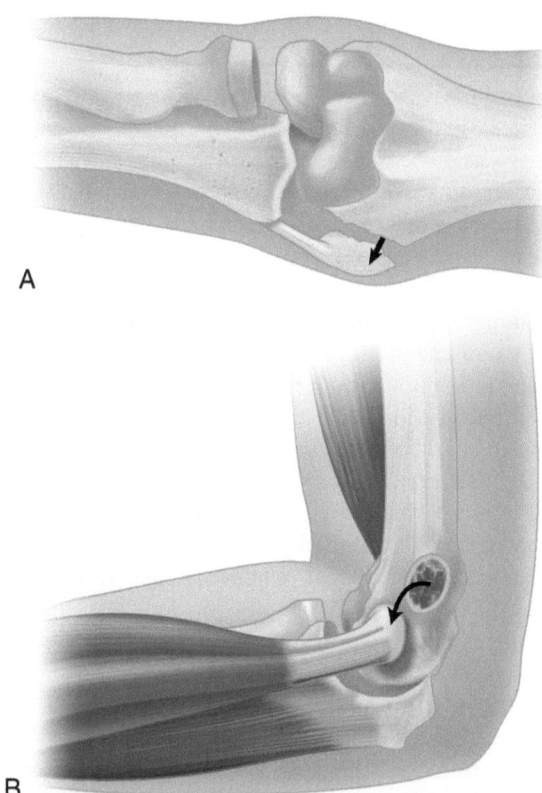

Fig. 134.10 (A and B) An avulsion fracture through the medial epicondyle, with attached ulnar collateral ligament and flexor/pronator mass.

In addition to age, the position of the throwing athlete should be elicited. Pitchers and quarterbacks place the most strain on their arms within their respective sports relative to other position players. In baseball, the likelihood of injury is more prevalent in pitchers and less likely in infielders, catchers, and outfielders, in decreasing order.[17] Athletes who engage in throwing often injure themselves as a result of repetitive overuse rather than direct trauma, making hand dominance an important factor in determining injury.

In addition to this demographic information, the clinician should inquire about pain, which is often the presenting complaint. The onset, character, duration, intensity, location, persistence, and temporal association (e.g., night, day, or with activity) of the pain are important in both diagnosis and formulating a treatment plan. The onset of the pain can be gradual with an overuse injury pattern or more sudden if an avulsion fracture of the medial epicondyle is encountered. The pain may be dull or aching in patients with chronic injuries, or sharp and severe when a more identifiable, acute episode is the culprit.

The duration of the pain is important in determining prognosis. Short episodes of soreness are distinguished from pain that is present before, during, and after throwing, which is a more worrisome finding that could represent chronic overuse and portend a poorer prognosis. The location of the pain can help determine which structures are at risk. The temporal association of the pain is important in determining the most likely site of pathologic findings. Pain during the throwing motion in the late cocking phase typically implies medial overload or instability in a young adult or adolescent patient. Pain at rest or at night could indicate another underlying cause, and a neoplastic process should be ruled out in these instances.

In addition to pain, other symptoms may be present. Decreased ROM, swelling, decrease in velocity or control, and paresthesias or dysesthesias into the upper extremity, particularly the ulnar nerve, can also occur and should be evaluated. Decreased internal rotation of the shoulder has been associated with an increase in humeral retrotorsion seen in overhead throwing athletes, specifically those involved in baseball.[28] Increased humeral retrotorsion has been demonstrated in dominant throwing arms in youth and adult populations when directly compared with nondominant arms.[28,29] In an adult pitching population, increased retrotorsion was shown to be a preventive adaptation for injury in the shoulder but a contributor for injury to the elbow.[30] Further studies regarding humeral retrotorsion and internal rotation deficits are needed to asses for the true effect on injury patterns in youth and adolescent throwers. After the symptoms have been elicited, a more detailed athletic history should also be obtained. The number of innings pitched, pitch count, type of pitches thrown, pitching rotation schedule, and training schedule can help determine if the athlete is placing his or her arm at risk for injury. Identifying a strain prior to ligament incompetence or growth plate disturbance is important to optimize treatment and prognosis. Associated injuries should also be evaluated, as well as any downstream (wrist/hand) or upstream (shoulder/neck) symptoms that could compromise successful treatment.

The surgical history of the elbow and shoulder should also be evaluated because altered biomechanics of both joints can place increased strain on the elbow during throwing. A thorough medical and family history should also be elicited for all patients with particular attention to any history of osteochondritis, Perthes disease, Kohler disease, and Osgood-Schlatter disease. When patients with any of these diseases participate in sports that increase the articular cartilage demand around the elbow, the likelihood of abnormal epiphyseal development is increased.[17] In addition, a history of delayed skeletal maturation could cause a young child to throw on an age-determined team beyond his or her physiologic tolerance, which could lead to elbow abnormalities.

Physical Examination

The physical examination is first focused on the overall demeanor and affect of the young athlete. The examination should proceed in a fairly systematic fashion to decrease the risk of missing associated injuries. A complete examination of the cervical neck for range of motion (ROM), tenderness, and associated provocative tests (e.g., the Spurling test) can help determine cervical spine pathology. Both shoulders should be examined for strength, ROM, and stability. Abnormalities of the scapulothoracic joint, including scapular dyskinesia, should be sought, as should any evidence of internal rotation contracture of the glenohumeral joint, which can contribute to pathologic conditions of the elbow.[20,30] Both elbows should first be inspected and evaluated for any asymmetry, deformity, or hypertrophy. Throwers often have hypertrophy of the muscles of their dominant arm or an alteration of the carrying angle. ROM of the elbows is assessed in flexion and extension, along with pronation and supination. The medial, lateral, and posterior elbow structures are palpated to elicit any tenderness. Because of the relative subcutaneous position of the osseous structures around the elbow, the medial epicondyle, lateral epicondyle, radial head, olecranon process, and collateral ligaments are readily identified and palpated to specifically identify any areas of discomfort. Patients with medial apophysitis typically demonstrate a flexion contracture greater than 15 degrees with point tenderness over the medial epicondyle.[31]

Palpation of the ulnar nerve is also performed in flexion and extension to evaluate for tenderness and subluxation. With slight flexion, the olecranon fossa can be examined, and gentle pressure can indicate pain over the posteromedial or posterolateral portion of the olecranon fossa. In slight flexion of 25 to 35 degrees, the olecranon is "unlocked" and the ligamentous stability of the elbow can be assessed. The lateral ligaments are assessed with slight varus and internal rotation stress applied to the arm, whereas the medial ligaments are assessed with valgus and external rotation stress applied to the arm.[32] With the elbow flexed 90 degrees and the patient actively supinating, the distal biceps tendon can also be palpated in the antecubital fossa. The insertion of the triceps muscle is also easily identified on the olecranon process, and both of these muscles can be actively tested with flexion/supination and extension, respectively. Comparison is made to the contralateral extremity for any subtle differences that could indicate elbow instability or weakness. The examination concludes with a detailed neurovascular examination of the distal extremity.

Imaging

Routine radiographs are an essential part of the evaluation of children and adolescents with elbow pain. Anteroposterior (AP), lateral, reverse axial, and comparison views are often obtained to rule out any osseous injury or irregularity of the growth centers. When injury to the ligaments is suspected, stress views can be obtained; however, a normal stress view does not rule out the presence of a significant ligamentous injury. Within the spectrum of little leaguer's elbow, a variety of pathologic conditions can be seen on radiographs. Fragmentation, enlargement, or fracture of the medial epicondyle can sometimes be appreciated.[33] Laterally, osteochondritis dissecans (OCD) can be appreciated as a lucency in the capitellum on oblique radiographs, or in advanced cases, degenerative arthritis and loose bodies may be visualized. Posteriorly, hypertrophy of the ulna may be present, which can impinge in the olecranon fossa of the distal humerus. With repetitive impingement, osteophytes and loose bodies may be visualized in the posterior compartment. Occasionally stress fractures of the ulna or olecranon apophysis can occur, in addition to delayed union at these sites. Classic findings of medial apophysitis include fragmentation and widening of the medial epiphyseal lines relative to the contralateral elbow.

Although most diagnoses can be confirmed with a thorough history, physical examination, and review of radiographs, other imaging modalities have been shown to increase sensitivity and the specificity of diagnosis. Ultrasound has been investigated as a potential imaging modality for evaluating OCD lesions of the capitellum and fragmentation of the medial epicondyle.[34] Bone scans can help determine areas of increased activity in persons with overuse injuries, and computed tomography (CT) scans can help better identify osseous anatomy in instances of fractures and loose bodies with osteophyte formation. Perhaps the most sensitive imaging modality is magnetic resonance imaging (MRI). MRI is helpful in evaluating the soft tissue structures of the elbow (UCL, biceps, triceps, and extensor/flexor tendon attachment sites), the articular cartilage (OCD, loose bodies, and avascular necrosis), and epiphyseal development (apophysis and epiphysis).[35,36] In addition, in cases of OCD, MRI can help in decision-making with regard to surgical intervention. MRI often demonstrates more positive findings in patients with little leaguer's elbow than do traditional radiographs; however, these findings rarely alter clinical management of these patients.[18]

Decision-Making Principles

No hallmark sign accompanies the diagnosis of little leaguer's elbow; often it is the constellation of symptoms, physical signs, and confirmatory findings on radiographs or MRI that leads to the diagnosis. A high index of suspicion is warranted when any child presents with elbow pain and is involved in competitive sports that entail throwing. With prompt diagnosis and treatment, patients can often avoid more serious and long-term sequelae that are associated with this spectrum of injury. Perhaps equally as important is recognizing the variability

and normal findings that exist in this population. Hypertrophy of the throwing arm, valgus alignment of the extremity, and flexion contractures are fairly common in this patient population and by themselves rarely warrant treatment in asymptomatic patients.[37]

Treatment Options

Treatment of little leaguer's elbow is tailored toward the specific diagnosis that is causing the pain or disability. Because this diagnosis can present along a continuum of injury, from a strain of the medial epicondyle to fracture and incompetence of the UCL, treatment is dependent on a multitude of factors: the injury severity, acuity, level of disability, and age. In patients who do not require acute surgical intervention and who have the capacity to heal, a period of rest is often warranted. In most cases, abstinence from throwing for 4 to 6 weeks results in the cessation of symptoms. The use of ice and nonsteroidal antiinflammatory medications has been shown to be beneficial in the acute stages. Currently no role exists for the use of injected corticosteroids in the management of medial apophysitis. In more severe cases, use of a removable posterior splint with immobilization may be warranted. After 6 weeks of rest, ROM is restored with gentle exercises and strengthening is begun. After 8 weeks, a throwing program is generally begun. Beyond rest, proper instruction on throwing mechanics may reduce the incidence of elbow injuries in these patients. In one investigation, it was found that youth who pitched with better pitching mechanics produced lower humeral internal rotation torque, lower elbow valgus load, and more efficiency during throwing.[24] This study has implications for the prevention of injury through better instruction. With regard to the frequency of pitching and the types of pitches thrown, a prior report demonstrated that the slider was associated with an 86% risk of elbow pain in youth who pitch, and a strong association was found between shoulder and elbow injuries and the number of games played and pitches thrown.[38] Development of the curve ball in youth baseball has been a controversial topic over the past few years. Initially it was thought to place significant stress across the medial elbow leaving athletes prone to injury.[39,40] Several studies have since refuted this notion and have shown that the forces across the medial elbow are highest in the fastball.[41-43] Currently the US Baseball Medical & Safety Advisory Committee (USAB-MAC) advises against teaching the curveball before the age of 14, and the American Sports Medicine Institute (ASMI) identifies the curveball and slider as a potential injury risk in inexperienced pitchers.[44,45] Perhaps the best treatment strategy known is prevention. Preventing excessive pitching in youth sports, enforcing rest days in between outings, discouraging year-round play, and watching for signs of fatigue will likely have a positive impact on the young pitcher's medial elbow. Fatigue has been shown to be a prominent risk factor for injury, and a recent study has shown that a loss of hip to shoulder separation is an early sign in adolescent pitchers.[46] Current guidelines have been developed for pitch counts in youth baseball as well, with the recommendation of pitches based on age. In 2010, Little League Baseball revised the previous guidelines set in 2007 that are in place today. Youths age 7 to 8 are allowed 50 pitches per day, which increases to 75 pitches per day at age 9 to 10. This amount can be increased by intervals of 10 for every 2 years of chronologic age up to age 18. Pitchers 14 years and under are required to rest 1 day for up to 35 pitches thrown with a 1-day rest increase for every 15 pitches thrown thereafter. Ages 15 to 18 require 1 day of rest up to 45 pitches thrown with a 1-day rest increase for every 15 pitches thrown thereafter.[47,48]

Results

Most patients with medial apophysitis return to sport at their preinjury level of competition with conservative treatment. No large-scale results of conservative management of this entity have been published. Because this diagnosis encompasses such a wide range of pathologic conditions, each distinct clinical entity has a varying prognosis with treatment.

Complications

With repetitive injury, after return to sport, the athlete is at risk for the development of growth disturbances around the elbow, persistent pain, avulsion fractures, OCD, and valgus instability after physeal closure.

Osteochondritis Dissecans and Panner Disease (Osteochondrosis)

OCD is a focal lesion of the capitellum that typically occurs in adolescents between 13 and 16 years of age. Theories regarding the origination of this pathologic process vary, with some authors believing that the compressive forces from throwing result in valgus overload and contribute significantly to its development. Other investigations have pointed to the biomechanical mismatch between the capitellum and radial head as a causative mechanism. The etiology of this disease is multifactorial and likely results from microtrauma in the setting of cartilage mismatch and joint susceptibility.[49] Histology from patients who underwent surgery for OCD of the capitellum demonstrated damage to the articular cartilage surface as a result of repetitive stress after a degenerative and reparative process of articular and subchondral fracture.[50] Separation of the fragment occurs on the cartilage surface and may proceed to the subchondral bone in advanced stages.[50]

Panner disease is a clinical entity that is distinct from OCD and is more common in younger patients. This clinical entity is a reversible, degenerative process of the capitellum that begins earlier in childhood, typically between the ages of 7 and 10 years, and involves the secondary ossification center of the capitellum. The hallmark of Panner disease is a process of degeneration followed by regeneration and recalcification.[34,51] Potential causes of Panner disease have been attributed to endocrine disorders, fat embolism, congenital and hereditary factors, the tenuous blood supply of the capitellum, and repetitive trauma. In the child, the most common cause of lateral elbow pain is Panner disease; however, by adolescence OCD becomes the most common source of this pain. Panner disease has a rather acute onset, with fragmentation of the entire capitellar ossific nucleus.

History

Patients with OCD most commonly report elbow pain with decreased ability to throw and may localize their symptoms on the lateral side of the elbow. The onset is typically insidious, and as the process progresses, loose bodies may form, which can cause the sensation of a "locking elbow." Patients report joint stiffness and lack of ROM and may report catching within the joint. Patients with Panner disease may have difficulty describing their symptoms; however, it is usually an aching lateral-sided elbow pain that may be accompanied by swelling. Patients may report an inability to throw a ball or achieve terminal extension of the elbow. Most patients with either condition do not report a traumatic injury or other inciting event. It is important to identify causative mechanisms such as repetitive throwing, endocrine disorders, or family history that could implicate the diagnosis.

Physical Examination

In persons with Panner disease, the dominant arm is typically affected. On physical examination, patients may report tenderness over the lateral elbow and capitellum with slight effusion and synovial thickening. ROM is typically affected, with a lack of terminal extension of 20 to 30 degrees.[52] Also noticeable may be a slight lack of pronation or supination with tenderness while attempting this movement.[49]

In patients with OCD, the elbow may not demonstrate significant swelling. Because this clinical entity is commonly associated with little leaguer's elbow, many of the clinical manifestations are similar. Tenderness and laxity of the medial elbow, tenderness over the lateral epicondyle and capitellum, and clicking of the joint may be evident. In most patients, the pain may be difficult to localize because of the spectrum of pathologic conditions that is characteristic in these patients. Patients typically have diminished ROM, and in the setting of loose bodies, they may have acute, sharp pain with certain movements.

Imaging

In the setting of Panner disease, radiographs in the early stages of the disease demonstrate irregularity of the capitellum with areas of radiolucency and sclerosis, particularly near the physis. After several months, radiographs show enlarged areas of radiolucency with reconstitution of the bony epiphysis. After a period of 1 to 2 years, the epiphysis returns to a normal configuration without flattening. A recent meta-analysis showed no correlation between radiographic parameters and symptoms.[53] In some patients, the adjacent radial head may undergo early maturation compared with the contralateral elbow.

In the setting of OCD, supplemental radiographs such as oblique views or 45-degree flexed views can help better visualize the lesion in suspected cases. The classic finding in pediatric and adolescent OCD is a focal area in the anterolateral capitellum with rarefaction and irregularity of the articular surface. Sclerotic bone may surround the lesion, and loose bodies may be seen when the articular lesion becomes detached.[34] Healing of the lesion can take months to years and is visualized on radiographs as ossification of this radiolucent lesion. CT with or without arthrography may help better delineate the osseous anatomy and articular surface. MRI is the most sensitive test and may detect lesions prior to their appearance on radiographs. In lesions that appear early in the disease process, T1-weighted sequences may detect decreased signal intensity within the lesion, with a normal appearance on T2-weighted sequences. Fat suppressed T2-weighted images are sensitive for detecting OCD lesions on the capitellum but maintain low specificity. Suspicious lesions detected on T2 fat suppressed sequencing can be further correlated on T1.[54] In more advanced cases, high signal intensity and cyst formation around the lesion could indicate impending detachment and loose body formation (Fig. 134.11).[55] More advanced MRI techniques with gadolinium may help define fragment stability and determine staging and prognosis.[56]

Decision-Making Principles

In persons with Panner disease, the key to optimal management is proper diagnosis and recognition. When the clinician recognizes that Panner disease is usually a self-limited condition that disappears by adolescence, proper care and instruction can be provided to both the patient and family.[53] With OCD, several factors determine proper management and treatment. Classification systems of OCD have been devised to help standardize reporting and define treatment. In one of the first classification systems based on AP radiographs, the authors outlined three grades of OCD.[57] In grade I, radiographs demonstrated a translucent cystic shadow in the middle or lateral capitellum. In grade II, a clear zone or split line between the lesion and the adjacent subchondral bone is evident. In grade III, loose bodies are present.[57] This classification was shown to be the most reliable based on CT and radiography.[58] The International Cartilage Repair Society (ICRS) developed the following classification system for defining OCD lesions intraoperatively. ICRS OCD I indicates a stable lesion with a continuous but softened area covered by intact cartilage; ICRS OCD II, a lesion with partial discontinuity that is stable when probed; ICRS OCD III, a lesion with a complete discontinuity that is not yet dislocated; and ICRS OCD IV, an empty defect as well as a defect with a dislocated fragment or a loose fragment lying within the bed.[59] A

recent MRI grading system utilizing T2-weighted imaging was proposed that accurately estimates the stability of an OCD lesion compared with intraoperative ICRS grading.[56] Treatment for these lesions is based on stability and is dependent on the ability of the lesion to heal based on the physiologic condition of the elbow (Table 134.1).[60] Based on this classification system, lesions deemed stable heal to completion with nonsurgical management, whereas unstable lesions demonstrate improved results with surgery.[60] As the characterization of capitellar lesions evolves, it will become increasingly important to use this information to predict prognosis and guide treatment. Management of OCD of the elbow is primarily determined by the integrity of the articular cartilage and the stability of the lesion. Unstable lesions are typically managed with surgical intervention, whereas stable lesions demonstrate more intrinsic ability for healing.

Treatment

In general, Panner disease is self-limited and treatment is largely symptomatic. Activity modification, rest, and antiinflammatories have been reported treatment options, with a majority of patients obtaining resolution of symptoms without morbidity.

In the early stages of OCD, treatment is largely nonoperative. Early-grade, stable lesions in patients with open physes are typically managed with a period of rest and cessation of sports participation. The amount of time that the patient refrains from participating in sports is determined by the length of time that symptoms persist. The typical duration is 3 to 6 weeks, followed by a 3- to 6-month period of progressive strengthening and ROM until full participation is achieved. Bracing and the use of nonsteroidal antiinflammatory medication may have a role; however, these treatments are largely supportive and have not been shown to provide tremendous benefit in the literature.[60,61] In a small series, low-intensity pulsed ultrasound has been shown to shorten the repair period in nonoperatively treated patients.[62]

Surgery for OCD of the elbow is typically reserved for patients who have closed physes, loose bodies, mechanical symptoms, unstable lesions on radiographs or MRI, or who have failed to respond to nonoperative management after 6 months and have a stable lesion. The best surgical procedure for patients with OCD of the elbow is a topic of considerable debate. Surgical options include open or arthroscopic fragment excision (with or without abrasion arthroplasty, drilling, or microfracture), fixation of the unstable or displaced lesion, bone grafting,

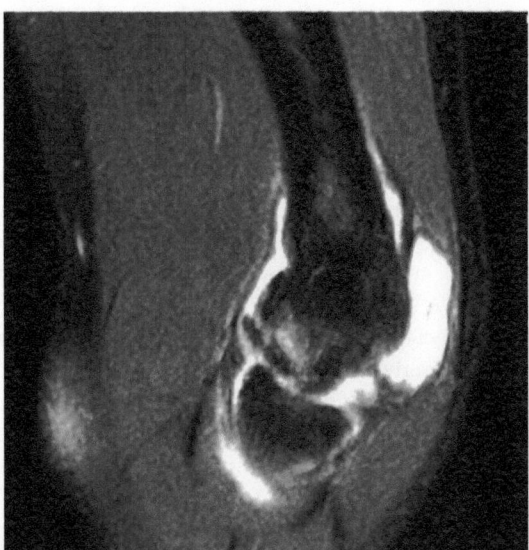

Fig. 134.11 A T2-weighted sagittal magnetic resonance imaging scan of a detached or semidetached osteochondritis dissecans lesion in a 12-year-old male adolescent.

TABLE 134.1	Characteristics of Osteochondritis Dissecans Lesions Based on Stability	
Classification	**Capitellar Growth Plate**	**Range of Motion**
Stable	Open	Normal
Unstable	Closed	Restricted

Data from Ruchelsman DE, Hall MP, Youm T. Osteochondritis of the capitellum: current concepts. *J Am Acad Orthop Surg.* 2010;18(9):557–567.

osteotomy, and osteochondral autograft transplantation (the OAT procedure). Our preference is fixation of these fragments when they are larger and when adequate purchase can be obtained with a 3.0-mm headed cannulated screw. Screw removal is typically necessary 3 months after fixation and healing. When smaller lesions are present, loose body removal and microfracture of the defect is a good surgical option.

Results

The spontaneous healing rates of patients with OCD are varied, and the results in the literature vary from excellent to poor. Mihara et al.[49] found that 25 of 30 early-stage lesions healed at final follow-up, whereas only 1 of 9 late-stage lesions had healed. A significant correlation of healing with open physes compared with closed physes was noted. In another study with longer follow-up, the authors found that more than 50% of the patients with stable lesions treated nonsurgically had mild discomfort at a mean follow-up of 13.6 years.[61] In a different study, 50% of patients treated nonsurgically had persistent elbow symptoms with activities of daily living and also demonstrated radiographic evidence of osteoarthritis at 12.6-year follow-up.[63] These results demonstrate the variability in the outcomes of these patients; however, proper assessment of the stability of the lesion may be the reason for the discrepancy in the data.

For surgical treatment, the results may depend on the technique used, the stage of the lesion, and the length of follow-up of the patients. For open excision of the fragment and débridement, Bauer et al.[64] demonstrated poor results at long-term follow-up, with 40% of patients reporting recurrence of symptoms and loss of elbow extension. These patients all had advanced lesions at the time of surgery. Other studies have demonstrated more encouraging results, with nearly 50% of patients returning to athletics.[60] Short- and midterm results of patients who have undergone arthroscopic débridement and marrow stimulation techniques such as drilling or microfracture are encouraging.[65–67] A recent meta-analysis in adolescents demonstrated an average return to sport of 87%.[68] In one report, the authors studied three elite gymnasts who underwent arthroscopic débridement and microfracture after failure of an initial trial of nonoperative management. They found full ROM and return to sport in all three patients at 1-year follow-up with hyaline-like cartilage on postoperative MRI.[69] Improvements in Disabilities of the Arm, Shoulder, and Hand scores and symptoms were shown in another study; however, many of the patients demonstrated decreased ability to participate in some sports because of their elbow.[70] Lewine et al.,[71] in a more recent study, was able to demonstrate resolution of clinical or radiographical findings in 15 of 21 patients. Seven of these patients were unable to return to their primary sport. In a large retrospective review of fragment fixation versus excision, the authors compared 12 patients who underwent fixation with 55 patients who underwent excision of the unstable lesion. The authors found that fragment fixation performed better than removal, and they recommended bone grafting for higher grade lesions.[60] A recent retrospective review demonstrated healing in 20 of 26 elbows with younger patient age and smaller lesions demonstrating superior results.[72] Several other studies show improved outcomes using fragment fixation

with an average return to sport of 68%.[72–75] Osteotomy is a surgical option in the management of these patients, but it is rarely performed in the United States. In Japan, one study demonstrated good outcomes in baseball pitchers, with six of seven returning to sports, and all seven demonstrated remodeling of the capitellum at 6 months with a mean increase in ROM of 12 degrees.[76] OAT has gained much attention as a treatment option for OCD due to the growing body of evidence over the past decade. Indications include lesions that engage the radial head, larger lesions, higher grade lesions, and laterally based lesions on the capitellum. Recent literature has suggested that larger and more lateral based lesions often perform poorly without aggressive surgical treatment.[77,78] The short-term results of the OAT procedure in the literature are promising, with more than 90% of patients in most series returning to their preinjury level of function without radiographic degenerative changes.[79–81] A recent retrospective review of highly competitive adolescent athletes undergoing OAT for unstable capitellar OCD lesions demonstrated a return to play (RTP) of 100% as well as an increase in ROM and reported outcomes. Osteochondral fragment fixation was compared with the OAT procedure demonstrating similar results with regards to ROM, outcome scores, and RTP; however there was a 50% reoperation rate in the fragment fixation group. All patients in the reoperation group had large widespread lesions, leading the authors to conclude that OAT may provide better stability in those lesions.[73]

Complications

Patients with Panner disease have relatively few complications. Most patients demonstrate the natural history of the condition with progression to healing. A few may experience worsening symptoms, loose body formation, and progression to an OCD clinical scenario. With OCD, most complications arise from incomplete healing of the lesion. Progression to loose body formation, osteoarthritis, limited ROM, and disability can occur, and athletes should be counseled on the possibility of not returning to their preinjury level of sport. Surgical complications can include infection, stiffness, hardware failure, neurologic injury (affecting the ulnar nerve), and failure to restore normal congruity to the elbow.

Medial Epicondyle Avulsion Fractures

Medial epicondyle fractures are common fractures in children and adolescents, accounting for 11% to 20% of all elbow fractures in this patient population.[82] In many instances, this fracture pattern is associated with elbow dislocation; however, in the throwing athlete, this situation is rarely the case, and it is more commonly associated with repetitive overuse and traction on the medial epicondyle from the flexor/pronator mass.[83] Alternatively, a valgus force on the elbow while falling on an outstretched hand can also cause this injury pattern. These fractures most commonly occur in boys, with a peak incidence in age of 11 to 12 years.[82–85]

History

Patients who sustain this injury likely report acute, sudden pain in their elbow localized over the medial epicondyle. Patients may have reported a subluxation event or feeling a pop in their elbow that precipitated the swelling and discomfort. The history of pain may include sudden elbow pain in the setting of chronic elbow symptoms. A thorough and detailed athletic history is warranted to associate the pathologic condition with the throwing motion, and the constellation of findings seen in little leaguer's elbow should be sought.

Physical Examination

Physical examination typically demonstrates swelling in the area of the elbow, loss of a normal elbow contour (in cases of dislocation), and crepitus with ROM. Diminished ROM is present, and associated neurologic symptoms may occur because the ulnar nerve lies in close proximity to the posterior aspect of the medial epicondyle. In patients who require surgery, elbow stability can be assessed with the gravity-assisted valgus stress test (Fig. 134.12).[86]

Imaging

The diagnosis is typically made with standard AP, lateral, and oblique radiographs of the elbow. Evaluating displacement on the AP radiograph may be the most accurate method of diagnosis; however, several studies have demonstrated the difficulty of and low interobserver agreement with the assessment of displacement.[87] Recently, a distal humerus axial view was proposed, which is obtained by centering the beam on the distal humerus, 15 to 25 degrees from the long axis of the humerus above the shoulder. In a cadaveric study, the authors were able to demonstrate increased accuracy and reliability of true displacement when compared with AP, lateral, and internal rotation radiographs.[88] CT can be used to more accurately assess displacement in patients with these fractures; one study demonstrated that in cases in which the fracture was thought to be minimally displaced on radiographs, significant displacement was encountered on CT.[89]

Decision-Making Principles

The management of medial epicondyle fractures is controversial. Traditionally, this injury has been managed conservatively, and good results have been reported.[90–93] The decision to treat the fracture surgically is typically reserved for open fractures and injuries in which fracture fragments are incarcerated within the joint space. Surgical fixation may be indicated for severely displaced fragments, cases in which valgus instability is present in the athlete who places a high demand on the elbow, and when the ulnar nerve is compromised. With regard to fracture displacement as an indication for surgery, some authors advocate fixation for fragments with as little as 2 mm of displacement, whereas other authors recommend this treatment for fragments demonstrating greater than 15 mm of displacement.[91–93] Currently there is no consensus on the amount of displacement required to necessitate surgical fixation, nor are there studies correlating the amount of displacement to clinical outcomes. Operative and nonoperative treatment in the setting of acute avulsion fractures among adolescent pitchers demonstrated equivalent outcomes and RTP.[94] Integrating the clinical history, examination, radiographs, and demands of the patient are all important in selecting the proper treatment for patients in this setting.

Treatment

Our preferred nonoperative treatment consists of immobilization in a long-arm cast with the elbow flexed to 90 degrees for 4 weeks. After removal of the cast, a splint can be applied with progressive ROM and return to sport after union is achieved. Surgical techniques for fractures meeting surgical criteria include suture repair, Kirschner wire fixation, screw fixation, and excision of the fragment with suturing of the soft tissue to the medial periosteum.[95,96] Recent literature has described the use of resorbable devices and suture anchor fixation.[97,98] Goals of surgery are to recreate the normal stability and mechanics of the elbow, and to create an epiphysiodesis of the medial epicondyle. Rigid internal fixation with screws (3.0, 3.5, or 4.0 mm, depending on the size of the epicondyle fragment) allows for earlier mobilization and may provide optimum stability.[90] Postoperatively, patients can be managed with a posterior splint, gentle exercises, and RTP once union is achieved and symptoms resolve.

Results

Reported results of nonoperative and operative management have generally been acceptable in the medical literature, even when fibrous union is achieved.[90–93] Up to a 90% nonunion rate has been reported with nonoperative management; however, these are largely asymptomatic.[99] A shift toward operative treatment in recent years is likely due to the emerging concept of medial elbow stability in throwing and overhead athletes. If bony union is the primary outcome variable, surgical fixation provides better results in this regard, with a systematic review demonstrating 92% union in the surgically treated group and 50% union in the group managed without surgery.[100] Despite the higher union rates with screw or wire fixation, the patients managed without surgery achieved pain levels comparable with those of the surgical treatment group, with a trend toward less pain in the conservatively managed cohort. Functional outcome studies have demonstrated relative favorability for both treatment modalities, with some reports demonstrating improved functional results in patients managed without surgery. In a cohort of adolescent athletes including pitchers, 2-year follow-up data showed excellent outcome scores and a RTP rate of 100% in both the operative and nonoperatively treated groups.[101] Although substantial valgus deformity occurs in fewer than 10% of patients, one study reported cubitus valgus as high as 35% after treatment.[102] Some

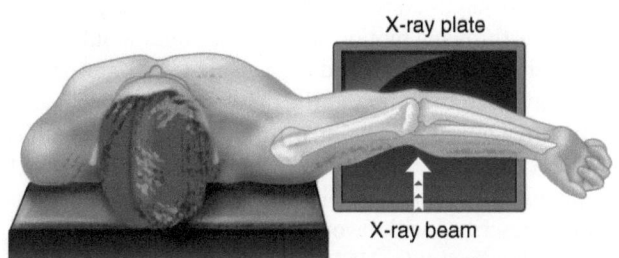

X-ray plate

X-ray beam

Fig. 134.12 The gravity stress test is shown. The arm is placed in full external rotation, permitting the weight of the forearm to deliver a valgus stress to the elbow.

studies have also demonstrated loss of ROM after both surgical and nonsurgical treatment (37 degrees and 15 degrees, respectively).[83] Many studies lack power due to insufficient sample size.

Complications

Complications from either treatment modality include loss of ROM, nonunion, and cubitus valgus. Two studies have obtained successful treatment of symptomatic nonunions, with one using open reduction internal fixation with cannulated screws and the other a tension band construct with bone grafting.[103,104] Surgical complications include myositis ossificans, septic arthritis, pin tract or wound infections, and radial nerve injury.[105]

Medial Collateral Ligament Injury

Injuries to the UCL, although uncommon in children and adolescents, have an increasing incidence as muscle mass and force increase in young adults. UCL injuries occur more commonly in adults but have been seen and treated in young adults and adolescents. Recently, the overall incidence of ulnar collateral reconstruction has risen, especially in the young athlete.[106,107] Multifactorial reasons for this rise include increased participation in year-round athletics and lack of adherence to established guidelines. A recent survey of more than 750 young male pitchers found that despite the ASMI guidelines; 45% participated in a league with no pitch count or limits.[40] This spectrum of injury is closely associated with little leaguer's elbow and is part of the spectrum of injury that can be seen with valgus stress placed on the elbow during sports that entail throwing, particularly pitching.

History

Most patients have an insidious progression of discomfort and report pain over the medial elbow for months or even years before the ligament is definitively torn. Ruptures of the ligament occur as a sudden traumatic event, after which the elbow is painful enough to warrant cessation of throwing. Often patients report preexisting problems with elbow pain prior to this catastrophic event. Patients with overuse or attenuation of the ligament report medial elbow pain that is exacerbated by throwing, particularly in the late cocking and acceleration phases of throwing.[108]

Physical Examination

On physical examination, patients demonstrate tenderness along the course of the UCL, from the medial epicondyle to the sublime tubercle. Subtle findings of instability are often present, demonstrated by flexing the elbow to 25 degrees to unlock the olecranon from its fossa and gently stressing the medial side of the elbow. This test assesses the competency of the anterior band of the UCL, as does the moving valgus stress test.[108] The posterior band of the ligament is tested with the milking maneuver, which is performed by pulling the patient's thumb with the forearm supinated, shoulder extended, and elbow flexed more than 90 degrees. Typically, pain with these maneuvers can be indicative of subtle instability and is deemed a positive finding. UCL injuries can commonly be associated with existing elbow or shoulder pathology including apophysitis and tendonitis, so a thorough evaluation of both joints is necessary.

Imaging

Plain radiographs are typically normal, except in cases of chronic injuries where the findings of valgus extension overload are found, such as posterior spurring and osteophyte formation. In patients with chronic valgus instability, excessive forces are placed on the posteromedial elbow during terminal elbow extension, which can result in degenerative changes of the posteromedial compartment, manifesting as spurring and joint space narrowing on routine radiographs. Stress views can be obtained, and relative widening of greater than 2 mm (compared with the contralateral extremity) can be considered a positive finding and indicative of instability. Comparison views may be necessary to more accurately determine pathology. A recent retrospective study found that patients diagnosed with a UCL injury had a significantly varus carrying angle and valgus distal humeral articular surface angle when compared with the control group.[109] Stress ultrasonography has been utilized to demonstrated progressive thickening of the UCL as years of professional pitching increase; however, these findings are limited in adolescent pitchers.[110,111] MRI is the most sensitive test to evaluate the UCL and also helps delineate concomitant pathologic conditions in the area of the elbow. MRI and MRI arthrography may demonstrate thickening of the ligament in many asymptomatic patients. In patients with instability, the ligament may demonstrate attenuation or a tear from either the medial epicondyle or the sublime tubercle. Chondromalacia of the posteromedial compartment could indicate chronic valgus instability and may also be detected on MRI.[112,113]

Decision-Making Principles

When considering surgical versus nonsurgical treatment, many factors go into determining the optimum strategy. Patients are likely surgical candidates when they have experienced an acute rupture, have signs of chronic instability, and have failed to respond to conservative treatment. Surgical treatment is best reserved for patients who wish to continue participating in sports that place a high demand on the medial elbow, including sports that entail throwing and gymnastics.[108,114]

Treatment

In most instances, conservative treatment is warranted, which consists of rest, immobilization, use of nonsteroidal antiinflammatory medication, and physical therapy to restore strength, flexibility, and stability. The flexor and pronator muscle groups should be targeted because they are important secondary dynamic stabilizers to valgus stress around the elbow.[115] Targeted evaluation of the throwing motion and biomechanics should be instituted by the coaching staff and trainers to identify any problems that could be contributing to the development of UCL abnormalities. In a mixed population of adult and adolescent athletes, treatment of partial tears of the UCL with autologous platelet-rich-plasma (PRP) injection followed by a targeted rehab protocol has been described with favorable results.[116,117]

Surgical treatment for UCL insufficiency is offered after failure of a trial of 6 months of conservative management with persistent symptoms in the older athlete whose sport entails throwing. Complete tears of the ligament in young athletes typically require surgical intervention. In select cases, direct surgical repair of the ligament can be attempted when direct avulsions off the medial epicondyle occur and the native ligament appears to be of good quality. In a study comprised of adolescent and college aged athletes, the authors showed a 97% return to sport rate with a failure rate of 6.7% with direct repair.[118] Reconstruction of the ligament with a palmaris or gracilis tendon autograft is a better option when a tenuous ligament repair is imminent.[119] Surgical reconstruction with a tendon graft is also indicated in the following circumstances: acute ruptures in throwers who lack enough remaining tissue ligament for a primary repair, the need to reestablish valgus stability in the presence of symptomatic chronic laxity, after débridement of calcific tendonitis in athletes if insufficient tissue is available to effect a primary repair, and when multiple episodes of recurring pain with throwing occur after periods of conservative care.[120–122] Figure of eight tendon reconstruction, as advocated by Jobe et al.,[114] or the docking technique, as advocated by Altcheck, are good options, and good results have been reported in the literature (Fig. 134.13).[114,123,124]

Results

Many young patients respond favorably to a trial of conservative treatment. In one study of athletes that outlined the treatment of UCL insufficiency with conservative treatment, 42% of patients returned to sport;[125] however, no randomized prospective studies have been performed to compare this treatment method with surgical reconstruction. Early results of PRP injection for partial UCL tears show improved outcomes over conservative management alone; however, studies are limited.[116,117] Prospective and retrospective studies evaluating the outcome of UCL reconstruction have demonstrated favorable results, with the majority of athletes returning to their preinjury level of participation. In one study evaluating the results in high school baseball pitchers, 74% of athletes were able to return to high-level throwing, which is comparable with the results seen in more mature athletes.[126] Jones et al.[127] performed UCL reconstruction utilizing the docking technique in a large group of adolescent athletes. Overall 87% of patients achieved an excellent result with inferior results noted in patients with concomitant OCD lesions. In a systematic review of UCL reconstructions, the authors found favorable results overall with success rates improved with use of a muscle-splitting approach, less handling of the ulnar nerve, and use of the docking technique. Lower complication rates were found, and increased RTP was found using the docking technique over the remaining

fixation techniques.[128,129] Both the docking and double docking techniques have shown equivalent outcomes in recent studies, with no outcome differences in graft selection.[130] Overall, reconstruction results range from a 70% to 90% successful return to sport at the preinjury level.[114,124,126,128,131]

Complications

Complications of surgical reconstruction include infection, fracture of the medial epicondyle and proximal ulna, ulnar nerve injury, and persistent pain and instability.

Posterior Elbow Pathologic Conditions (Posteromedial Impingement and Olecranon Osteochondrosis)

Injuries to the posterior compartment of the elbow are rare injuries in children and adolescents (Fig. 134.14). These injury patterns typically develop as late sequelae of chronic overuse syndromes (e.g., little leaguer's elbow and valgus extension overload). Pathologic conditions of the posterior elbow develop in response to chronic and repetitive extension overload from repetitive triceps contraction during the deceleration and follow-through phases of throwing. Posteromedial impingement is a term that denotes abutment of the medial aspect of the olecranon against the olecranon fossa as a result of valgus stress during terminal extension. Childhood injuries are more characteristically olecranon apophysitis and osteochondrosis with irregular ossification. In athletes approaching adolescence and young adulthood, these injuries are more commonly stress fractures or avulsion injuries of the olecranon apophysis with physeal widening, delayed fusion, or fragmentation.[132,133] In young adults and after skeletal maturity, this spectrum of injury presents as posteromedial elbow impingement as a result of valgus extension overload, with osteophytes, loose bodies, and persistent elbow pain.[108] Recently it has been postulated that the result of repetitive posteromedial impingent in adolescents results in olecranon tip fractures as opposed to osteophyte formation seen in adult populations.[134]

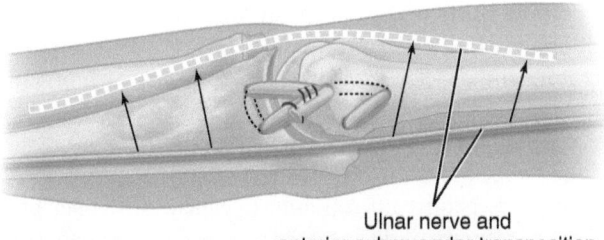

Ulnar nerve and
anterior submuscular transposition

Fig. 134.13 An example of a medial collateral ligament reconstruction with anterior submuscular transposition of the ulnar nerve.

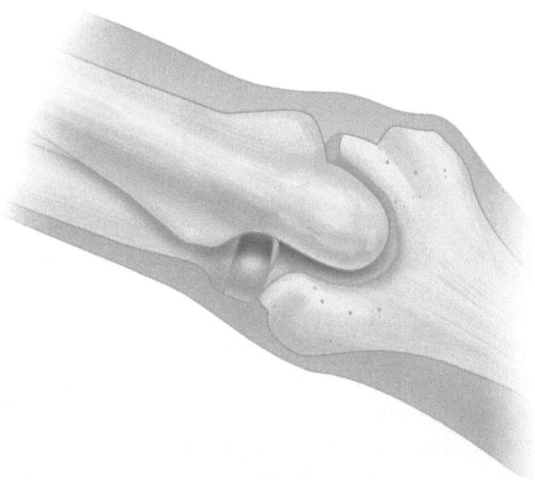

Fig. 134.14 The posterior compartment of the elbow.

History

Patients with pathologic conditions of the posterior elbow typically report pain in the posterior compartment of the elbow. This pain may be most noticeable, as the elbow is taken into extension or during the follow-through phase of throwing. Symptoms of locking or catching within the elbow joint could be a result of the presence of loose bodies.

Physical Examination

Physical examination shows pain in terminal extension, and patients may have tenderness to palpation over the posteromedial elbow and olecranon fossa. Because this injury can be the result of chronic valgus instability, assessment of the UCL should also be performed with stress testing as previously described. Tenderness over the proximal olecranon apophysis could indicate a stress fracture in this region, and distal triceps pain or pain with resisted elbow extension may indicate pathologic conditions within the extensor mechanism.

Imaging

Routine radiographs may demonstrate the presence of stress fractures or widening of the olecranon apophysis. These radiographs should be inspected for fragmentation, avulsions, or delayed fusion, which could indicate pathologic findings at this site. In cases in which injury is suspected, comparison views of the contralateral elbow can be obtained. With posteromedial impingement, osteophytes of the posteromedial olecranon may be visualized, along with loose bodies within the posterior compartment. Traction spurs of the proximal olecranon and triceps attachment are seen best on the lateral projection.[135–137] MRI can be used to evaluate for concomitant pathologic conditions such as UCL tears, osteochondral lesions, and stress reactions, and can help locate loose bodies within the joint space.

Decision-Making Principles

Posterior elbow abnormalities are best managed based on the presenting diagnosis. The age of the patient often determines the most likely diagnosis in this setting. Younger patients are more likely to respond to conservative treatment, particularly when chronic insufficiency of the UCL has yet to develop. In older patients, avulsions of the proximal olecranon and triceps attachment and other injuries that denote chronicity may require surgical management.

Treatment

Treatment is tailored to the individual according to the age of the patient and the diagnosis. Osteochondrosis and stress fractures in younger patients usually respond to a period of rest (with or without immobilization), with progression to ROM and strengthening exercises after symptoms resolve. When returning to play, throwers are typically advanced with a rehabilitation program focusing on proper throwing mechanics and neuromuscular control, with progression to dynamic control and improvement of power. Avulsion[138] fractures with less than 2 mm of displacement can usually be treated conservatively with splint immobilization followed by functional ROM and strengthening exercises. Small apophyseal fragments that do not compromise the extensor mechanism can be excised in patients who fail to respond to conservative treatment. Large avulsion fragments can be surgically treated with screw or suture fixation. In patients who have stress fracture nonunions or delayed union of the olecranon physis, open reduction and internal fixation with bone grafting is a viable option when a protracted period of conservative treatment fails.[135] In a cohort of adolescent overhead throwing athletes, two unique patterns of olecranon physeal nonunions were identified and treated successfully with internal fixation and autografting.[139] Removal of loose bodies and posteromedial osteophytes can also be performed for more mature patients who have persistent posteromedial elbow symptoms. A minimally invasive arthroscopic approach should be instituted in these cases to possibly optimize function and decrease morbidity. Posterior olecranon spur resection should be performed with care, because increasing bone resection creates more strain in the UCL with valgus load.

Results

The results of nonsurgical treatment are generally favorable, with most patients returning to sports after a trial of conservative treatment. Results of stress fracture and delayed physeal closure with surgical fixation have been reported in the literature in small case series with favorable outcomes in nearly all patients.[135,139] Excision of spurs and loose bodies can provide symptomatic relief in most patients; however, addressing the underlying valgus instability through physical therapy or medial ligament reconstruction may be necessary to prevent further episodes. In a recent 2-year follow-up looking at arthroscopic resection of olecranon tip fractures, the authors found a good to excellent result in 85% of patients, with inferior results occurring in patients with undergoing concomitant UCL reconstruction.[134] The pediatric literature has a paucity of data regarding this treatment because most reports focus on adult athletes.

Complications

Complications can include nonunion, persistent pain, progression of posterior compartment osteoarthritis, and disability. Surgical complications include infection, wound complications, persistent nonunion, and progression of instability or iatrogenic instability as a result of surgical treatment.

Medial/Lateral Epicondylitis

A common anatomic location for pain in pediatric tennis players is the elbow, with 25% of 16- to 18-year-old boys and girls reporting previous or current elbow pain in survey data from the US Tennis Association.[140] Medial epicondylitis, lateral epicondylitis, or apophysitis of either epicondyles can be seen in skeletally immature and developing tennis athletes. Racquet sports place significant demand on the developing elbow as a result of repetitive eccentric contraction of the wrist extensors.[141] This demand can also be seen in throwers during the follow-through phase of throwing.[142] Repetitive microtrauma in patients with open physes can lead to apophysitis during childhood and the early adolescent period, with transition to epicondylitis in the late adolescent and young adult patient populations. Lateral epicondylitis has been associated with equipment issues used in racquet sports, including grip size, metal racquets, tightly strung racquets, and racquets with increased vibration.[143,144] Poor mechanics related to the backhand technique have also been associated with lateral epicondylitis. Proper[145] equipment sizing and instruction on proper mechanics of play are paramount in preventing this injury from developing and becoming a persistent problem for the young athlete. Anatomic studies examining the extensor carpi radialis brevis, which is implicated in lateral epicondylitis, have shown a unique anatomic location that makes its undersurface vulnerable to abrasion against the lateral edge of the capitellum during elbow motion.[146] Medial epicondylitis, although not as common as lateral epicondylitis, can be seen more commonly in baseball pitchers, golfers, and athletes who create significant valgus force at the elbow.[147] Valgus force created at the elbow can place increased strain on secondary stabilizers such as the flexor and pronator muscles, which arise from the medial epicondyle.[148] Poor technique with improper warm-up and fatigue can lead to injury and inflammation of the flexor/pronator mass. Implicated muscles of this muscle group are the flexor carpi radialis and pronator teres. In a prior study, the authors found macroscopic tearing of the flexor/pronator group in all of the patients who underwent surgical treatment for medial epicondylitis.[149] Just as with lateral epicondylitis, medial epicondylitis can be treated and hopefully prevented with appropriate equipment sizing, proper mechanics, warm-up, and stretching, so that symptoms do not persist into adulthood.

History

Patients with lateral epicondylitis typically report a burning-like pain on the lateral side of the elbow. Initially the pain is primarily activity related, and activities involving wrist extension may precipitate the pain. This injury is common in patients who play racquet sports, and this history should be elicited. Medial epicondylitis is similar in presentation to lateral epicondylitis, with symptoms arising from the medial elbow. Patients should be asked about exacerbating sports and activities for both conditions and if any associated neurologic symptoms are present, such as numbness and tingling, to rule out compression neuropathies.

Physical Examination

In persons with lateral epicondylitis, physical examination usually demonstrates pain and tenderness to palpation over the common extensor origin of the lateral epicondyle. Patients have pain with resisted wrist extension referred to the lateral side of the elbow. ROM is usually not affected. Persons with medial epicondylitis present with pain and tenderness to palpation over the medial elbow and may demonstrate increased pain with resisted wrist flexion. Pain may be associated with valgus stress testing of the elbow, which could indicate underlying valgus laxity as the cause of the pain.

Imaging

Routine radiographs are usually normal; however, in some cases, calcification may be present at the tendon origin. In younger patients, widening and fragmentation of the apophysis may be seen. MRI evaluation may prove useful in instances in which

there is a question of diagnosis. MRI may demonstrate increased signal on T2-weighted imaging or partial tearing of the tendon attachment of the lateral epicondyle. The reliability of MRI in detecting pathologic conditions was demonstrated to be excellent in a recent study, with good interobserver agreement; however, no correlation of MRI findings with symptoms was found in the patients studied.[150]

Decision-Making Principles

Most young patients with medial and lateral epicondylitis are managed nonoperatively. Surgery is rarely indicated in this patient population. Most patients respond to conservative treatment measures and modification of activity with a short period of cessation of sports participation.

Treatment

Conservative treatment is mostly supportive for epicondylitis and apophysitis in the pediatric and adolescent patient populations. Cessation of sports participation and inciting activity is begun with or without a course of antiinflammatory medication and physical therapy. Therapy is aimed at restoring ROM, stretching the offending muscle group, and strengthening the muscles surrounding the elbow. Counterforce straps and wrist braces may offer additional relief from symptoms in patients who are not responding to other conservative measures. Additional therapies such as shock wave treatment, ultrasound, and light wave therapy are investigational and have shown variable results in the literature.[151,152] Corticosteroid injections may be offered to young adults, although their utility in treating this condition has been questioned. A level I study in adults comparing autologous blood, corticosteroid therapy, and placebo saline solution injection for the treatment of lateral epicondylitis demonstrated no advantage of one treatment over the other.[153] A recent meta-analysis of randomized control trials showed no difference between corticosteroid injection and placebo injection.[154] The role of platelet-rich plasma is currently being intensely investigated, with some studies demonstrating improvement in patients with lateral epicondylitis.[155,156] Surgery is rarely indicated in this patient population but can consist of débridement of the extensor or flexor tendon in refractory cases. Surgery can be performed with a percutaneous, arthroscopic, or open technique.

Results

Results of conservative treatment are generally favorable with both lateral and medial epicondylitis. In a systematic review evaluating the different types of therapy for lateral epicondylitis, the authors found that all types of therapy substantially improved the outcomes of patients, with eccentric strengthening being the most exhaustively studied.[151,157] Eccentric strengthening exercises have demonstrated benefit in the literature; however, whether this treatment is better than stretching alone or stretching with concentric strengthening is unclear.[152,158] A recent randomized study showed significant improvement with eccentric strengthening when compared with concentric strengthening with short-term follow-up.[159] Nonsteroidal antiinflammatory medications (both topical and oral) are routinely prescribed for persons with epicondylitis; however, studies have shown both positive benefit and no benefit when compared with placebo.[160,161] Current use of this modality is based on physician preference and the ability of the patient to tolerate treatment. Corticosteroid injections are still routinely used in practice for alleviating the pain of lateral epicondylitis. Although studies have shown acute benefit, most investigations that report long-term outcomes demonstrate no advantage to the use of corticosteroid for this condition.[156,162–166] Surgical treatment, although rarely offered to young patients, has shown good results in the literature, regardless of the technique used, with one study showing improvement in outcomes in more than 90% of patients.[149,167–172] Recently, arthroscopic techniques such as extensor carpi radialis brevis release have been studied and may provide small improved outcomes when compared to open techniques.[173] The treatment of medial epicondylitis mirrors the outcomes of lateral epicondylitis, with most patients responding favorably to nonsurgical management and good to excellent results in most patients who are ultimately candidates for surgical intervention.[174,175]

Complications

Complications from conservative treatment are rare. Antiinflammatory medications may cause impaired renal function and gastrointestinal adverse effects, although in younger patients these effects are usually self-limiting. Corticosteroids may cause pigmentation changes of the skin and fat atrophy with a low risk of tendon rupture.[176] Three or greater corticosteroid injections prior to surgery have been shown to be most significant risk factor for revision surgery.[177] Surgical treatment complications include infection, iatrogenic elbow instability from excessive release, nerve injury, and heterotopic ossification.[149,176,178,179]

SUMMARY

The treatment of elbow maladies in children and adolescents requires a thorough understanding of developing skeletal anatomy, biomechanics of sport, and a multitude of pathologic conditions that are characteristic in this patient population. With thorough history-gathering techniques, a comprehensive physical examination, and judicious use of musculoskeletal imaging, the diagnosis is usually readily delineated. Treatment is largely nonoperative in this patient population; however, understanding the need for surgery in select cases can help optimize the outcome.

For a complete list of references, go to ExpertConsult.com.

SELECTED READINGS

Citation:
An KN, Morrey BF. Biomechanics of the elbow. In: Morrey, ed. *The Elbow and Its Disorders*. Philadelphia: WB Saunders; 1985.

Level of Evidence:
Book chapter

Summary:
This chapter focuses on the biomechanics of the elbow as it relates to anatomy, range of motion, and stability.

Citation:
Jobe FW, Stark H, Lombardo SL. Reconstruction of the ulnar collateral ligament in athletes. *J Bone Joint Surg Am.* 1986;68A:1158–1163.

Level of Evidence:
IV

Summary:
The authors of this case series outline the results of ulnar collateral ligament reconstruction in 16 athletes (most of whom were in sports entailing throwing). After surgery, 10 of the 16 athletes returned to their previous level of competition.

Citation:
Yadao MA, Field LD, Savoie FH III. Osteochondritis dissecans of the elbow. *Instr Course Lec.* 2004;53:599–606.

Level of Evidence:
Book chapter/instructional course lecture

Summary:
The authors of this comprehensive review outline the pathophysiology, diagnosis, and treatment of osteochondritis dissecans of the elbow joint. The article is a very good review of current concepts regarding this topic.

Citation:
Chen FS, Diaz V, Loebenberg M, et al. Shoulder and elbow injuries in the skeletally immature athlete. *J Am Acad Orthop Surg.* 2005;13:172–185.

Level of Evidence:
Review article

Summary:
The authors of this review article provide an overview of common shoulder and elbow maladies in pediatric and adolescent patients. little leaguer's elbow, osteochondritis dissecans, epicondylitis, and other pathologic conditions are comprehensively reviewed.

Citation:
Nirschl RP, Pettrone FA. Tennis elbow: the surgical treatment of lateral epicondylitis. *J Bone Joint Surg Am.* 1979;61A:832–839.

Level of Evidence:
IV

Summary:
Tennis elbow surgery was performed for eight elbows in one of the first reports of this technique. An overall improvement rate of 97.7% was reported, with 85% of patients returning to rigorous activity.

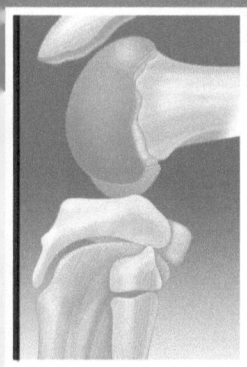

135

Wrist and Hand Injuries in the Adolescent Athlete

Sonia Chaudhry

The incidence of hand injuries increases 20-fold after age 10, with sports being the most common mechanism of injury.[1] High impact sports such as football tend to produce injuries from single traumatic events, whereas repetitive overuse injuries are more common in sports such as gymnastics, golf, and tennis. We have focused on conditions and treatment considerations unique to the adolescent population.

One of the most challenging conditions is pain of unclear etiology. To minimize frustration in patients, parents, coaches, and physicians, it is important to have a clear treatment algorithm for these situations. Patients with neurologic-type symptoms in a nonanatomic distribution should be examined for neural tension signs more proximally, and nerve gliding exercises may be the key to achieving return to sport. Nonspecific wrist pain is common due to ligamentous laxity and muscular immaturity. A neuromuscular training program emphasizing resistive strengthening relieves symptoms in most patients.[2] A baseline therapy evaluation for grip and pinch strength is followed by a 6-week exercise program while concomitantly protecting the wrist joint and modifying activities. Patients who fail to improve their strength should continue exercises. If their pain is ongoing despite improved strength, MRI evaluation is undertaken. As always, it is important to validate symptoms and tailor treatment to patient goals.

FINGER FRACTURES

Fractures account for two-thirds of hand injuries in the under 16 age group.[1] Skeletally immature patients are vulnerable to unique patterns of injuries, as the weak points in their anatomy are the growth plate and subcapital region of the phalanges. The Seymour fracture is an open fracture of the distal phalanx through the physis that can present similar to a mallet injury, with about half occurring during sports.[3] Subcapital fractures of the phalangeal neck appear deceptively benign and therefore often have a delayed presentation. Phalangeal base fractures are most commonly seen in the small finger proximal phalanx, 22 of 34 fingers in one series,[4] where they carry the eponym "extra octave fracture" due to ulnar dorsal angulation giving the appearance of the small finger trying to reach further on piano keys. Metacarpal fractures can occur in any age group, but are most common in 10- to 19-year-olds involved in basketball, football, or bicycling.[5]

History

Seymour fractures often occur with hyperflexion of the distal interphalangeal (DIP) joint similar to a mallet finger, though many describe a "crushing" component to their mechanism. Bleeding at the time of injury distinguishes an open fracture from a closed nailbed or distal tuft injury. Prior antibiotic treatment should be determined.

Subcapital fractures also occur after crush injuries in sports, with immediate pain and swelling. Bruising may be minimal in this relatively avascular region. Motion, specifically flexion, is limited. With restricted motion, patients can be relatively painless, often leading to delayed presentation.

Phalangeal base fractures occur most commonly with a dorsal ulnar pull on the digit, resulting in immediate pain and deformity. Reduction may or may not have been attempted on the field. Boxer's fractures occur after direct impact of the dorsal 5th metacarpal head. True boxing is a rare cause, as punching should axially load the 2nd and 3rd metacarpal heads. Patients will notice decreased prominence of the knuckle. If patients complain of repetitive snapping or popping, one should suspect a "boxer's knuckle," or sagittal band rupture allowing subluxation of the extensor tendon.

Physical Examination

Swelling, integrity of the nail and nailfold, ecchymosis, and resting position should be noted. A Seymour fracture may have been splinted in extension with the proximal nail resting superficial to the eponychial fold. This can give the subtle appearance of a longer nail. There will be an extension lag at the DIP joint. Dried blood should be noted, as well as any signs of infection in late presenting cases. As with any injury, concomitant injuries should be looked for, with the most common being additional finger fractures.[3]

Phalangeal neck fractures will present with a swollen proximal interphalangeal (PIP) or DIP joint, depending on whether the fracture is in the proximal or middle phalanx, respectively. Tenderness to palpation is important, as this indicates the fracture is mobile and more amenable to percutaneous reduction. Flexion is limited due to pain and angulation. Coronal plane angulation is examined in extension, while malrotation is best assessed for with flexed digits to demonstrate under- or overlapping. In patients unable to flex due to pain, passively extending the wrist will utilize the tenodesis effect to flex the digits (Fig. 135.1). This

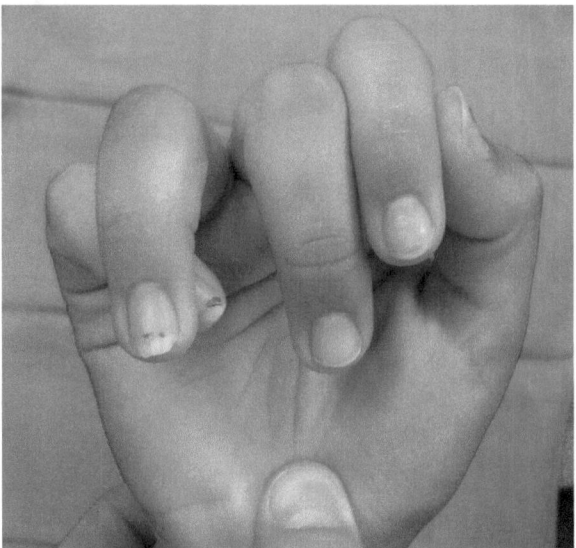

Fig. 135.1 Wrist extension utilizing tenodesis effect to flex digits, revealing digit scissoring, or overlapping, from malrotation deformity.

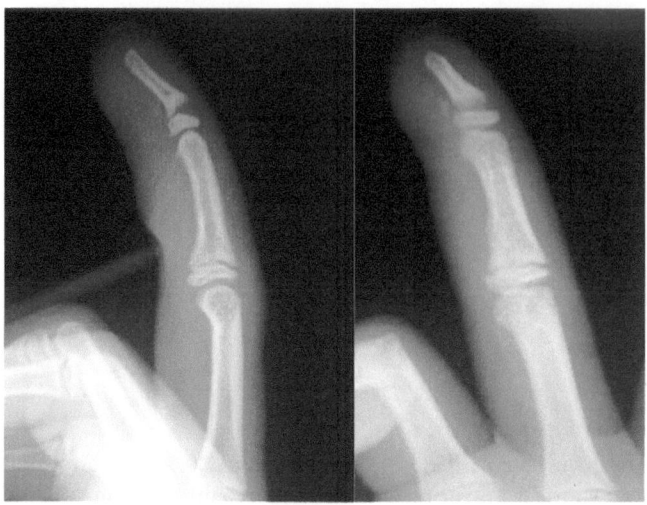

Fig. 135.2 Lateral and oblique radiographs demonstrating an open fracture through the physis of the distal phalanx, or Seymour fracture, in the typical posture of flexion.

can be done while palpating the scaphoid tubercle, as all digit tips should point toward the tubercle in flexion.

Phalangeal base fractures will have obvious hyperextension and ulnar angulation around the metacarpophalangeal (MCP) joint. Making a full fist may be still possible due to composite flexion. Boxer's fractures demonstrate a depressed knuckle. Rarely the apex dorsal angulation will cause skin tenting, threatening open injury due to thin skin and tendon covering.[6] Malrotation is uncommon but crucial to assess for. Contralateral comparison is important, as there are varying degrees of baseline digit angulation.

Imaging

Anteroposterior (AP), lateral, and oblique radiographs of the digit should be obtained for all finger injuries, as there will be less digital overlap on the lateral and oblique views compared with hand radiographs, which are more appropriate for metacarpal fractures. Resting position and soft tissue swelling are important to note in addition to the fracture. Seymour fractures will show flexion through the distal phalangeal physis (Fig. 135.2). If held in extension, however, the injury can be subtle with widening of the physis alone.

Subcapital fractures are often missed on the AP view, as hyperextension causes bony overlap. If not familiar with skeletally immature radiographs, the interpreter may mistake the transverse fracture line for a physis. Physes should be proximal in the phalanges instead of the distal neck region. One should check for intra-articular extension, as intercondylar fractures tend to be more unstable and will often flex and shorten, even when initially nondisplaced. The lateral view will typically demonstrate extension of the distal fragment. Malrotation can be a subtle "double bump" of the condyles of the phalangeal head on a true lateral where adjacent condyles are collinear (Fig. 135.3A).

Phalangeal base and metacarpal fractures are best assessed on oblique views of the finger and hand, respectively, as other views minimize apparent angulation. These fractures likely involve

the physis in a Salter Harris II pattern. Angulation is typically dorso-ulnar in the small finger proximal phalanx (Fig. 135.4A) and palmar-radial in the metacarpal neck.

Decision-Making Principles

Hand fractures will often present late, as athletes are able to continue playing, and fear of restrictions may lead patients to downplay their injury. Radiographs should be obtained with any history of trauma and immediate swelling. Juxta-articular soft tissue injuries and unstable finger fractures have acute presentations too similar to distinguish accurately by clinical exam alone. Examination under digital block is poorly tolerated in the adolescent patient.

Both Seymour and subcapital fractures are inherently unstable; therefore operative stabilization is indicated in all but absolutely nondisplaced fractures. Phalangeal base and metacarpal neck fractures are close to both the physis and the 5th MCP joint with multiplanar motion. This allows for remodeling as well as better tolerance of angulation.[7]

Treatment Options

Nailbed injuries with underlying closed distal tuft fractures are stabilized by the nail itself and managed nonoperatively. Due to instability, Seymour fractures are operative injuries involving a combination of antibiotics, nailbed repair, fracture reduction, and stabilization. One study recommended oral antibiotics be given immediately and continued 4 days postoperatively in any case treated over 6 hours after presentation.[3] Nailbed repair was traditionally employed with a fine absorbable suture such as 6.0 chromic; however, a randomized control trial (RCT) demonstrated faster repair time and similar results using 2-octylcyanoacrylate (Dermabond; Ethicon Inc, Somerville, NJ).[8] Fracture stabilization produces a more favorable environment for soft tissue healing and theoretically minimizes infection in Seymour fractures. Splinting alone risks late displacement; therefore pinning is often employed.

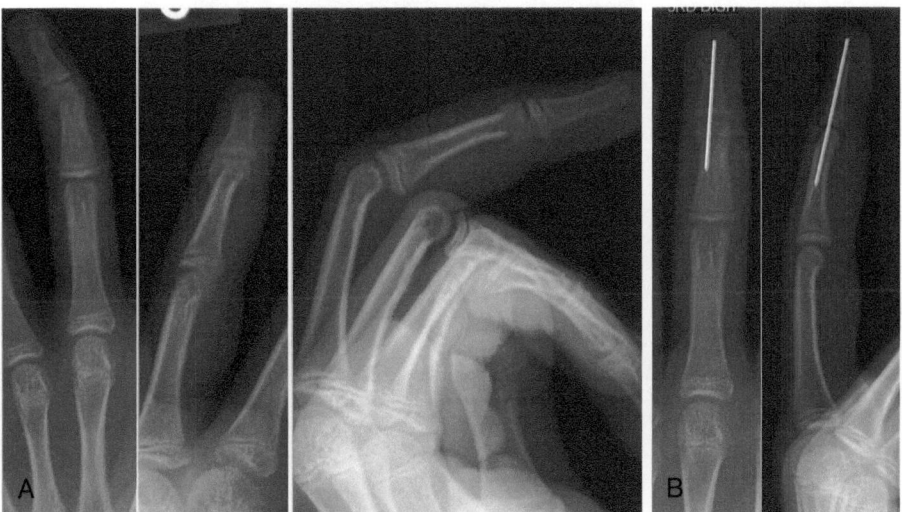

Fig. 135.3 Radiographs of a 12-year-old patient's finger (A) demonstrating a middle phalangeal neck fracture in ulnar deviation, extension, and malrotation. The degree of malrotation is such that the lateral view of the digit shows both the condyles, as it is an anteroposterior (AP) of the fracture fragment. AP and lateral after closed reduction and pinning (B) show restoration of anatomic alignment and stabilization with a buried intrafocal pin. Note the lateral demonstrating overlap of the condyles of both the proximal and middle phalanges, confirming correction of malrotation, as this is difficult to assess clinically once an interphalangeal joint is pinned in extension.

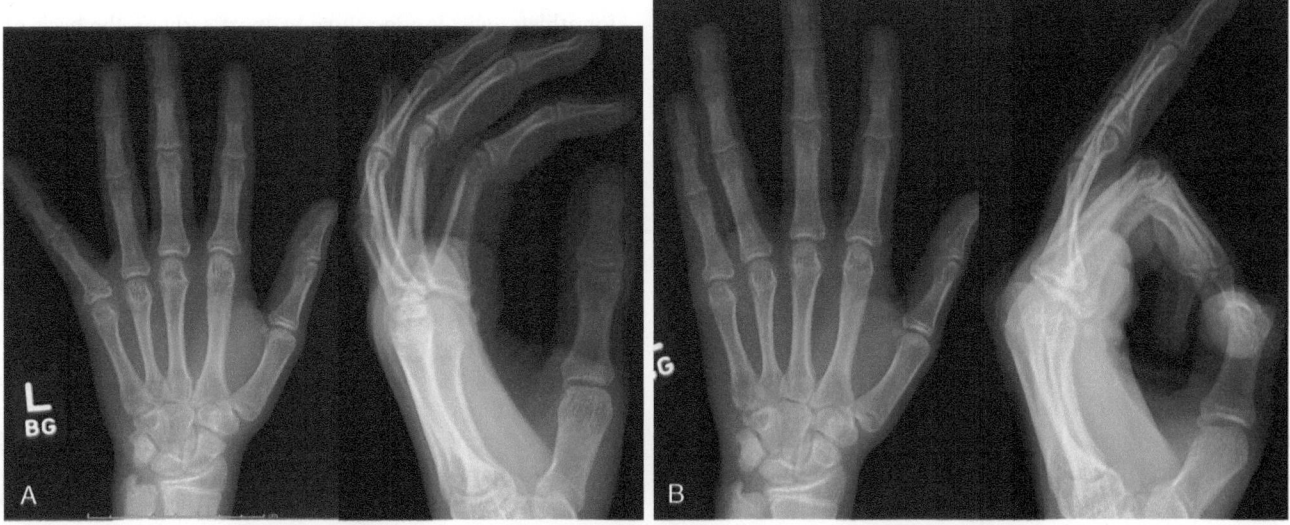

Fig. 135.4 Anteroposterior and lateral radiographs in a 16-year-old show a small finger proximal phalangeal base Salter Harris II fracture in the typical position of extension and ulnar deviation (A). Closed reduction under digital nerve block was followed by buddy strapping and post reduction radiographs (B) showing improved alignment.

Nonoperative management is rarely indicated for subcapital fractures. Nondisplaced fractures can be immobilized in extension with weekly radiographs for the first 3 weeks to ensure maintained alignment. While splinting is not ideal in this often-noncompliant age group, it allows for better lateral radiographs. Digital overlap will obscure a good lateral if casted. Displaced fractures are ideally close reduced and percutaneously pinned (see Fig. 135.3B). Phalangeal neck fractures over 3 weeks from injury may be difficult to reduce closed. Percutaneous osteoclasis can be attempted; however, open reduction should be undertaken with caution, as the tenuous blood supply of the mostly articular

distal fragment through the collaterals can be disrupted. Internal fixation with headless screws can be considered to allow early postoperative motion, as the PIP joint is prone to stiffness.

Phalangeal base fractures are mostly amenable to nonoperative management. Within the first 2 weeks, fracture site mobility should allow closed reduction with ligamentotaxis with or without digital nerve block (see Fig. 135.4B). The broad fracture surface across the physis and metaphysis lends it to be relatively stable. Acutely irreducible fracture has been reported with entrapped tendon and is a rare indication for open reduction. If operative reduction is undertaken, Kirschner wire (K-wire) stabilization

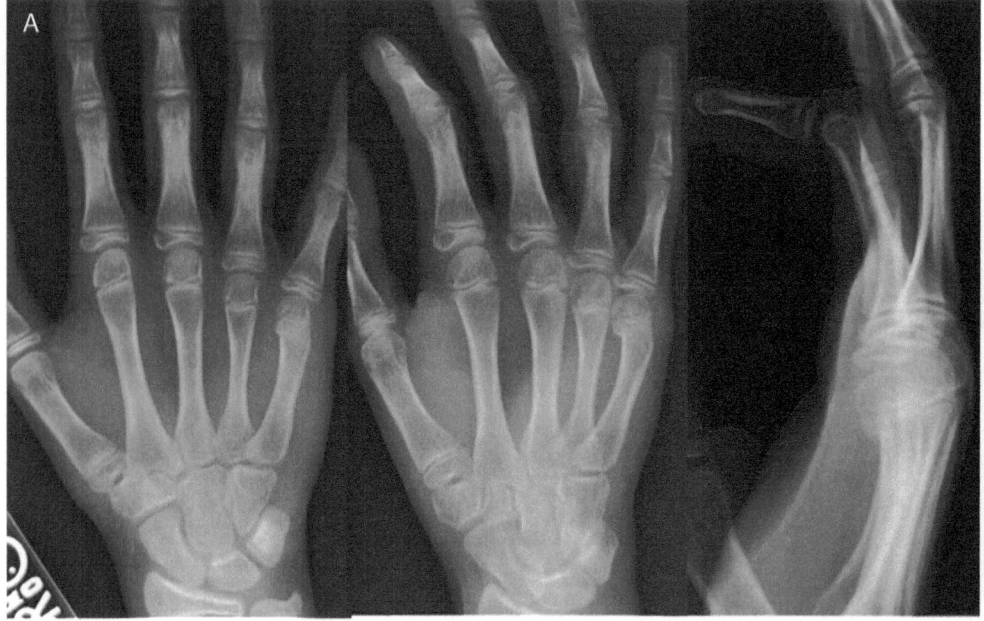
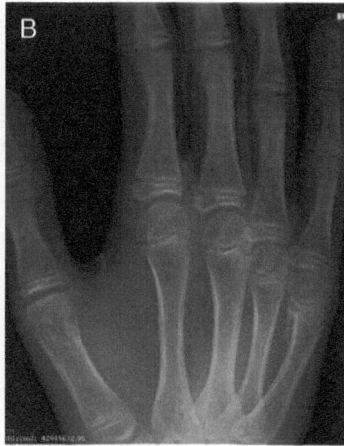

Fig. 135.5 Radiographs of the hand (A) demonstrate a Salter Harris II 5th metacarpal neck fracture, known as a boxer's fracture. Maximum angulation is noted on the oblique view in the typical palmar radial direction. Oblique view 2 weeks postinjury (B) demonstrates maintained alignment and callus formation in a patient managed with buddy strapping.

is performed by entering the head of the proximal phalanx and driving the pin across the flexed MCP joint, leaving the PIP free.[4] In late presenting injuries that cannot be close reduced, it is prudent to allow healing and consider later corrective osteotomy. This allows remodeling and minimizes the risk of iatrogenic damage to the physis.

Boxer's fractures, though relatively unstable, are also amenable to nonoperative treatment in most cases (Fig. 135.5). If reduction is performed, the ring and small fingers are traditionally casted in the intrinsic plus position (MCP flexion and PIP/DIP extension) for 4 weeks. Casting in MCP joint extension up to the PIP joints has been shown to be well tolerated with better range of motion (ROM) and grip strength without any difference in fracture angulation compared with traditional intrinsic plus positioning in a RCT.[9] Operative indications include open injuries, multiple fractures, malrotation, shortening causing pseudoclawing, and strong patient/parent preference. Multiple percutaneous pin configuration options have been described. Internal fixation options exist, such as a condylar blade plate, but involve crossing the physis in adolescents and may become stress risers for additional fractures with subsequent trauma.

Postoperative Management

Patients with K-wires are splinted or casted for protection of the fracture and hardware. Pins left percutaneously out of the skin are removed in the clinic around 4 weeks postinjury (later in cases where osteoclasis was required), after checking radiographs to confirm provisional healing. Buried pins that do not prevent PIP motion, such as those crossing only the DIP joint, can be left longer and removed after injection of local anesthetic. Removable splints allowing early ROM are employed until fractures are fully consolidated around 6 weeks postinjury. Protocols are modified

for athletes wishing to return to sport early on the basis of the individual and the sport's rules on playing with braces.

Results

Seymour fractures generally do well, with one series showing 23 of 24 patients regaining full motion with good satisfaction and no cases of infection.[3] Phalangeal neck fractures treated with percutaneous pinning were recently shown to have 92% good to excellent results.[15] No patients had open reduction, as percutaneous osteoclasis was successfully performed up to 36 days after injury.

Phalangeal base and boxer's fractures have similar outcomes. In a series of 34 phalangeal base fractures, all but two severely displaced fractures healed without complications or residual deformity with full ROM.[4] For boxer's fractures, a prospective study of fractures angulated up to 75 degrees treated with Coban self-adherent wrap (3M, St. Paul, MN) and buddy tape showed all patients to be satisfied and functionally unimpaired with no loss of grip strength.[16] A RCT demonstrated final fracture alignment to be no different with this soft wrap method compared with reduction and casting.[17]

Complications

One series of Seymour fractures reported complications in half of patients, though the majority were minor, such as nail and subtle distal phalanx growth disturbances. Secondary fracture displacement can occur if stabilization is not performed.[3]

Subcapital fracture nonunion is reported, usually in thumbs managed nonoperatively, while malunion is more common in the digits.[18]

Phalangeal base fractures treated with open reduction or late osteotomy carry a risk of stiffness from tendon adhesions

---

✏ Author's Preferred Technique

Seymour fractures, when possible, have antibiotics and tetanus prophylaxis administered acutely. Under finger tourniquet control, the nail plate is removed, as it blocks reduction and cleansing of the open fracture. The Betadine-cleansed nail or a piece of Xeroform dressing is placed under the eponychial fold to splint it open, and the fracture is reduced with a combination of extension and volar directed translational pressure. It is important to hold this reduction, as the fracture is unstable, and multiple reductions can damage the physis. A K-wire, usually 0.045 in adolescents, is inserted into the digit tip and driven across the physis and distal interphalangeal (DIP) joint to rest in the middle phalanx. The K-wire is cut and left buried. Dermabond is used to repair the nailbed, secure the nail plate, and cover the pin site, except in cases with concern for infection, as drainage should be allowed. I do not routinely prescribe antibiotics postoperatively, and instead reserve it for cases that appear contaminated.

Displaced, angulated, or rotated proximal phalangeal neck fractures are managed with closed reduction and intrafocal pinning when possible. I utilize a technique of proximal interphalangeal flexion and rotation to obtain reduction, followed by K-wire insertion through the head of the proximal phalanx. The wire is driven out through the base of the proximal phalanx, holding the MCP joint in full flexion and pulled proximally until it rests just subchondral in the proximal phalanx head. The PIP joint is extended to allow the wire to be driven into the middle phalanx for additional fixation.[10] One 0.045 K-wire will typically hold the digit in the intrinsic plus position and incur sufficient stability; however, this can be supplemented with an additional wire for rotational control as needed. Pins are left percutaneous, and a protective overlying cast is placed.

Middle phalangeal neck fractures are managed similarly,[11] with the difference that slight angulation and flexion deficits are better tolerated near the DIP joint. For subacute fractures that are still tender, I will perform dorsolateral percutaneous osteoclasis with a K-wire. I do not risk avascular necrosis (AVN) with open

reduction. Some sagittal remodeling may occur[12,13] through the growth plate under the cartilage cap. For limitation of flexion alone, volar bone spike can be removed to clear the subcondylar fossa and tends to improve motion.[12] For malrotation or angulation, corrective osteotomy can be performed in a safer region more proximally in the shaft.

Phalangeal base fractures are best managed with closed reduction under digital nerve block. Entry into the ulnar aspect of the palmodigital crease allows lidocaine infiltration proximally about both radial and ulnar digital nerves, as well as dorsally for a complete block. This is better tolerated than a needlestick into the sensitive palm. For the small finger, a fulcrum such as a thin pen is placed into the 4th webspace. The small finger is brought over this fulcrum into hyperflexion and maximum radial deviation. A palpable reduction is typically appreciated. Postreduction radiographs are obtained, though clinical appearance and ROM determine acceptable alignment.

Boxer's fractures are managed nonoperatively with the exceptions noted previously. Closed reduction is with the Jahss maneuver, flexing the MCP joint and extending the PIP joint to push the metacarpal head dorsal while relaxing the intrinsic muscles. When no reduction is desired, my preference is for buddy taping as soon as comfort allows. Some patients will request higher degrees of immobilization, in which case various prefabricated boxer's fracture braces are commercially available and stocked in the clinic. Athletes can return to sports as soon as pain and mobility allow,[14] often within 2 weeks once the fracture has stabilized with provisional callus. Operative management is with closed or percutaneous reduction when possible. With a Kapandji technique, a K-wire inserted into the fracture site dorsolaterally can lever on the intramedullary canal of distal fragment as needed. Stabilization is performed with 2 K-wires, typically 0.045 or 0.054, inserted into the dorsal metacarpal head from ulnar and radial and driven to the base of the metacarpal, left percutaneous.

---

requiring tenolysis. Malunion in hyperextension for phalangeal base fractures or hyperflexion for boxer's fractures may cause a pseudo-claw deformity from extensor shortening.[4]

Future Considerations

Studies of Seymour fractures and all nailbed and open distal phalanx fractures are needed to guide appropriate antibiotic use. Subcapital fractures are increasingly studied; however, specific factors associated with delayed presentation remain unknown. For phalangeal base and metacarpal fractures that remain angulated, it is difficult to rely on remodeling when there is limited growth potential remaining, as is often the case in adolescent athletes. Further study into the rate of angular correction in various planes for hand injuries would help guide treatment.

JAMMED FINGER

Soft tissue injuries account for one-third of hand trauma in patients under 16 years,[1] and the PIP is the most common location of digital injury in sports. Common injuries affecting the PIP joint include contusion or rupture of the volar plate, radial and ulnar collateral ligaments (RCL and UCL), and central slip. The volar plate injury is the second most common injury in softball, second to mallet fractures.[19]

History

Patients may report a specific hyperextension mechanism or only remember the finger was "jammed," typically by a ball

impacting the fingertip. A history of joint dislocation or deformity at the time of injury should be elicited along with any appreciation of a "pop" at the time. Predictable injury patterns occur depending on the direction of dislocation. Dorsal dislocation injures the volar plate, lateral dislocation affects the collaterals, and volar dislocation is associated with central slip tear. Central slip injury is also caused by direct dorsal impact or forced PIP flexion.

The chronicity of the injury and type and length of immobilization should be clarified. In addition, patients should be asked about pain, limitation of function/ROM, or both. The differential diagnosis for a flexed digit includes pulley rupture, damage to extensor tendon, fracture, and dislocation.[20] Less common is the extended digit, which may be due to flexor rupture or a volar dislocation. Rapid forced flexion or volar dislocation will result in central slip disruption with or without a dorsal middle phalanx fracture.

Physical Examination

Bruising and swelling can persist long after tenderness has resolved. Resting position and ROM should be checked. Normal PIP ROM is from 0 to 110 degrees. Passive PIP extension may cause discomfort or demonstrate lack of a firm endpoint with volar plate injury. Contracture of the injured volar plate leads to pseudo-boutonnière deformity, or PIP joint flexion contracture without DIP deformity.

Boutonnière deformity will be present if the central slip and triangular ligament both tear and allow the lateral bands

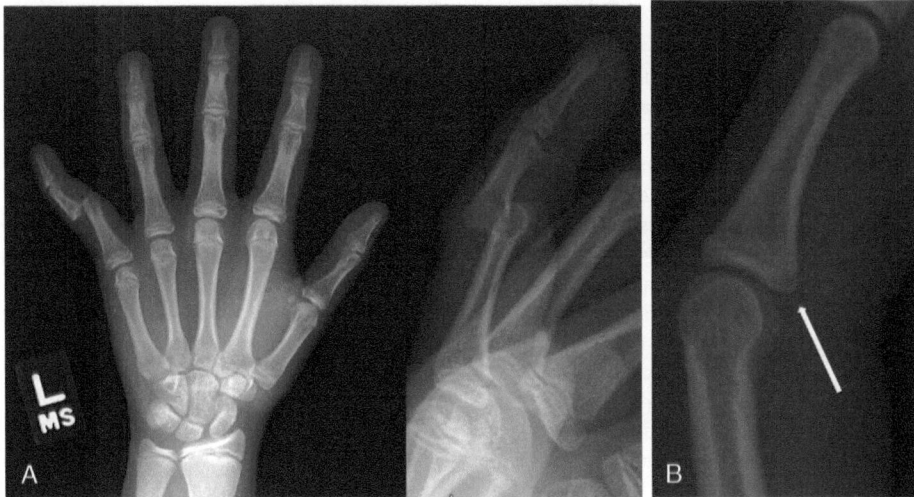

Fig. 135.6 Posterolateral dislocation of the small finger proximal interphalangeal joint is seen on anteroposterior and lateral radiographs (A). A close-up of the postreduction lateral radiograph (B) demonstrates a minimally displaced Salter Harris II fracture of the volar middle phalanx base *(arrow)*, which represents a stable avulsion fracture of the volar plate.

to subluxate volar to the PIP joint. As this is not always present acutely, a high degree of suspicion for central slip injury is necessary and should be evaluated with the Elson test, with digital block for pain as needed. When the PIP joint is flexed, the DIP is normally unable to be actively extended due to slack in the lateral bands. DIP hyperextension via lateral bands during resisted extension of the flexed PIP indicates central slip injury.

Varus and valgus stress of the PIP joint in full extension and 30 degrees of flexion tests the accessory and proper collaterals, respectively. While the index finger RCL is most commonly injured, it is more common to have a combination RCL and UCL injury.

Imaging

Finger radiographs are examined for joint congruency, resting position, and any fractures. With volar plate injuries, an avulsion fracture from the middle phalangeal base may be seen, present in 38% of injuries in one study.[19] In skeletally immature patients, this may be a Salter Harris III or IV pattern involving the physis with an epiphyseal component with or without a metaphyseal component (Fig. 135.6). Dorsal fracture may be present with volar dislocation or central slip avulsion. Collateral ligament injury may be accompanied by avulsion fracture in the subcondylar fossa of the proximal phalanx. Stress radiographs can reveal joint widening but are usually not tolerated acutely and are unnecessary with chronic injury, as physical exam is diagnostic. Advanced imaging with high resolution MRI can demonstrate further detail but is rarely necessary.

Decision-Making Principles

Painless full ROM with a stable joint is the goal. This is achieved with brief periods of immobilization to allow soft tissue healing followed by mobilization to prevent contracture. Unstable joints must be stabilized prior to allowing ROM.

Treatment Options

Dorsal or lateral dislocations are generally able to be close reduced. Volar dislocation may have soft tissue interposition or a rotatory component with the lateral condyle buttonholed between the collateral ligament and lateral band. MCP and PIP flexion may allow the digit to be rotated back into place; otherwise open reduction is indicated. Postreduction, the digit should be examined for stability, rigidly immobilized, and radiographed.

Most soft tissue injuries and small bony avulsions can be mobilized early and buddy strapped. Sports can be continued with protection, though use of the rigid splint may compromise glove fit and grip strength. In rare cases, primary repair of soft tissues such as collateral ligaments is indicated if interposed into the joint and requiring open removal, though stiffness is common following this repair.[20]

The exception to early motion is acute central slip injury, which is treated with 6 weeks of full time extension splinting of the PIP joint followed by nighttime splinting for an additional 6 weeks to prevent late boutonnière deformity. DIP motion is encouraged while splinting to draw lateral bands into the dorsal position.[21] Open injuries and large dorsal fractures are operative.

⚲ Author's Preferred Technique

Acute nonoperative management is as above. Patients that present subacutely with proximal interphalangeal (PIP) stiffness undergo static progressive splinting. To achieve extension, the splint includes a point of counterforce on the palmar aspect of the metacarpal head to prevent MCP joint hyperextension while working on PIP motion.

An associated fracture of the middle phalanx involving more than 30% of the articular surface with associated PIP instability is an indication for operative stabilization. Similar to adults, percutaneous pinning, dynamic traction,[22] or internal fixation with mini-fragment screws can be employed. Hemi hamate arthroplasty for volar fractures and suture anchor repair of central slip dorsal avulsion are also considered.[23,24]

Postoperative Management

Motion exercises are started 2 weeks postoperatively for most injuries, or until percutaneous pins are removed. Early return to play (RTP) with the PIP joint protected in a rigid cast can be considered for certain sports; however, if PIP extension will hinder function or splinting is not allowed, the athlete will be restricted for a minimum of 6 weeks.

Results

Children with PIP hyperextension injuries have better outcomes than adults. An RCT showed buddy strapping for a week to produce better resolution of edema and pain compared with a group treated with a week of Alumafoam extension blocking orthosis.[25] Full motion was regained in 65% at 1 week and 91% at 2 weeks.

Collateral ligament injuries of the PIP joint treated with buddy taping for an average of 3 weeks demonstrate 77% recovery of grip strength and 84% recovery of ROM at 6 months. Increased disability is associated with delayed treatment, female gender, and radial digit injury at 3 months.[26]

Complications

Untreated injuries can lead to pain, deformity, instability, and degenerative joint disease.[20] Boutonnière deformity can develop within 2 to 3 weeks after central slip tear. PIP flexion contractures not responding to progressive splinting may need open release.

DISTAL RADIAL PHYSEAL STRESS REACTION

More than half of gymnasts experience wrist pain, usually with more than 6 months of duration.[27] Ninety percent of those with wrist pain still have it a year later. The differential includes both bony conditions (distal radial physeal stress, impaction syndromes, scaphoid stress fracture, carpal chondromalacia, avascular necrosis [AVN] of the capitate) and soft tissue abnormalities (dorsal impingement, triangular fibrocartilage complex [TFCC] tears, ganglia, carpal, or distal radial ulnar joint [DRUJ] instability).

The skeletally immature population tends to have negative ulnar variance that becomes more negative with maturation, as the distal ulna physis closes before that of the distal radius. The more ulnar negative the wrist, however, the more an axial load is borne by the distal radial physis. Gymnasts, by contrast, are relatively ulnar positive, and become more so with increasing years of practice and higher body weight.[28] While this theoretically protects the distal radial physis, pathologic dynamic loading of the wrist in ligamentously lax gymnasts can still occur. The mechanism of "gymnast's wrist," or physeal stress injury, is likely a combination of vascular insufficiency and mechanical growth inhibition in accordance with the Hueter-Volkmann law.[2] In addition, ulnar positive wrists are more likely to demonstrate TFCC pathology and dynamic ulnocarpal impaction.

History

The history is the key to diagnosis. Patients often complain of achy dorsocentral wrist pain during or after loaded extension activities. Specific gymnastic risk factors include soft mats that lend to increased wrist dorsiflexion, twisting vault routines that produce dorsiflexion with ulnar deviation, and beam activities with locked forearms that transmit rotational moments to the wrist.[27] The physis is most vulnerable during rapid growth, occurring on average around years 10 to 14.

Physical Examination

Distal radial physeal tenderness is often present, especially dorsally. The push-up test, loading the wrist in extension as when pushing up out of a chair, may reproduce radial or ulnar pain from distal radial physeal loading or dynamic ulnar carpal impaction, respectively. There may be a subtle loss of wrist extension and grip strength. These findings are also present with occult ganglia and dorsal impingement; therefore location of tenderness is a key feature. Long-standing cases with physeal growth disturbance may have a prominent ulnar styloid from relative overgrowth. The DRUJ should be examined for stability and compared with the contralateral side, as ulnar overgrowth may lead to an incongruent articulation with the sigmoid notch.

Imaging

Stress-related distal radial physeal changes are present on radiographs in 10% of gymnasts.[28] Findings include widening of the physis, irregular borders, radial-sided cystic changes, a beaked epiphysis, and haziness within the physis. Ulnar variance should be measured on an AP taken in neutral rotation. The Hafner method of measuring ulnar variance involves comparing the most proximal and distal extents of the distal radial and ulnar physes (Fig. 135.7).[29] The distal extent of epiphyseal ossification is not as reliable as the thickness of the unossified portion of the distal radius and ulnar are not known. Late-stage deformity

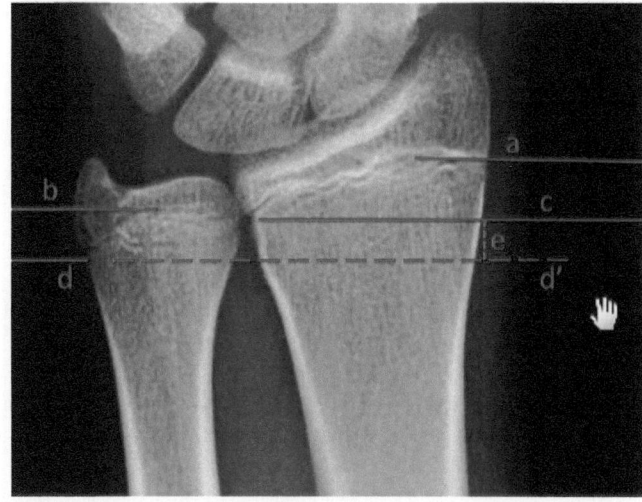

Fig. 135.7 Ulnar variance in a skeletally immature wrist is best assessed on an anteroposterior taken in neutral rotation, with the shoulder abducted 45 degrees and the elbow flexed to 90 degrees. The vertical distances between lines tangential most distal (*a* to *b*) and proximal (*c* to *d*) portions of the distal radial and ulnar metaphyses are measured. the line from the most proximal ulnar metaphysis portion (*d*) has been extended (*d'*) to demonstrate how to measure the variance (*e*).

can involve a Madelung-like deformity with a volar and ulnar directed distal radial articular surface.

MRI has not been shown to be a useful prognostic tool.[30] All asymptomatic college gymnasts show MRI changes in the wrist ligaments, tendons, and cartilage.[31] Eighty percent also show bony changes and cysts/fluid collections, despite remaining asymptomatic for several years.

Decision-Making Principles

Three stages have been described to guide treatment, with the mainstay being activity restriction. Stage 1 is a clinical diagnosis without radiographic changes, and management is gradual return to sport after symptoms cease with complete rest. Stage 2 is when radiographic changes are present, and return to sport averages 2 to 4 months. Stage 3 demonstrates characteristic radiographic changes along with positive ulnar variance. It is unclear how reversible the injury is once growth disturbance has occurred.

Treatment Options

While prevention of repetitive wrist loading would be the best treatment for the general health of the wrist, this is often not an option for elite athletes. An initial cessation from weight bearing on the wrist is recommended until symptoms resolve. Despite a lack of evidence, bracing is often employed upon return to sport, with restrictions implemented again if symptoms recur. Recommendations from Waters and Bae include cyclic progressive training cycles, alternating loading (pushing activities 1 day, pulling the next), bracing such as tiger/lion paws, and a regimen of 6 weeks of rest followed by 6 weeks of closed chain exercises prior to resuming open chain activities.[2] They emphasize that restrictions should be guided by soreness rather than absolute time periods.

Radiographic follow-up of the wrist is prudent to assess for ongoing growth disturbance. Progression of ulnar positive variance is an indication for epiphysiodesis of the distal ulna with ulnar shortening as needed.

✒ Author's Preferred Technique

Due to high rates of noncompliance with elite athletes, specifically gymnasts, I initially institute a period of short arm casting for 4 weeks to ensure rest. This is followed by continued restriction of loaded extension activities while initiating ROM and grip strengthening exercises. While radiographs rarely show resolution of physeal changes, follow-up radiographs are obtained around 8 weeks to check for progression of any positive findings. In the absence of progressive changes, the athlete is gradually returned to sport with brace protection when possible and instructions to cease loading if symptoms recur.

Indications for distal ulnar epiphysiodesis include an open physis with progressively positive ulnar variance or symptomatic ulnocarpal impingement, and in the latter case this is combined with ulnar shortening osteotomy. Epiphysiodesis is performed with a direct ulnar approach and drilling the physis in all directions. Systematic spherical curettage is then performed until the soft feel of the physis has given way to the rough scraping of cancellous bone. The distal ulnar epiphysis is notorious for incomplete epiphysiodesis, and therefore this is performed quite meticulously.[32,33] In the case of suspected TFCC pathology, wrist arthroscopy is concomitantly performed.

Postoperative Management

Epiphysiodesis is followed by 2 weeks of splint protection and early mobilization with protected lifting for an additional 4 weeks. Ulnar shortening osteotomy is followed by lifting restrictions until radiographic healing—typically 8 weeks.

Results

No studies have demonstrated specific outcomes of treatment; however, symptomatic relief is reported with activity restriction.

Complications

Growth arrest has been reported; however, the incidence and preventability is unknown.

FUTURE CONSIDERATIONS

Prospective studies to quantify the "dose" of loading that leads to this injury would be helpful in guiding training.[27] As with pitch counts in baseball, injury may be prevented by limiting the quantity of high impact wrist activities that gymnasts undertake in a particular competition or training season.

SCAPHOID FRACTURE

Scaphoid fractures in children and adolescents are increasing owing to increased sports participation. While radiographs are reported to miss the fracture in 2% to 6% of adult cases, misdiagnosis is more common in children due to its relative rarity in children, accounting for only 3% of hand and wrist fracture, and difficulty interpreting skeletally immature radiographs.[34]

History

The most common mechanism is a fall onto the outstretched radially deviated and pronated hand. There is immediate pain and swelling, though many continue their sport. Radial-sided pain persists, and patients may complain of a weak wrist with limited motion. Timing of injury is relevant, as one-third of pediatric scaphoid fractures present late with chronic nonunion.[35] Reasons for delayed presentation including moderate symptoms and fear of losing one's position on the team.[34]

Physical Examination

Classic tenderness is in the anatomic snuffbox between the abductor pollicis longus and the extensor pollicis brevis, corresponding to the scaphoid waist. Volar pain (over the distal tubercle), pain with radial deviation, and pain with active wrist motion are associated with higher likelihood of fracture in children.[36] Non-acute injuries should have assessment of ROM and carpal stability.

Imaging

In addition to the standard three wrist views, specialized clenched fist and ulnar deviation views will dorsally rotate the scaphoid in order to orient the fracture line more parallel to the radiograph beam.[37] Seventy-one percent of fractures in adolescents are of the waist.[35] If the distal pole is flexed, it will demonstrate the "cortical ring sign," which is the tubercle seen on fos. The proximal fragment should be examined for sclerosis, especially in late presenting injuries and proximal pole fractures, as this may indicate AVN. The significance of this finding as it correlates to clinical healing is unclear. In addition, one should be aware of the rare bipartite scaphoid, as this can mimic scaphoid fracture, though some believe this to represent asymptomatic pseudarthrosis of the scaphoid.[34]

The scapholunate interval should also be examined for widening. While 2 mm is typical in adults, skeletally immature patients have a wider interval averaging 9 mm at age 7. Contralateral comparison should be made, though carpal ossification may not be symmetric.[34] Lateral radiographs should be examined for carpal alignment. Lines along the axes of the scaphoid and capitate, as well as the perpendicular to the lunate, are used to measure the scapholunate angle, normally 30 to 60 degrees.[37] Both displaced scaphoid fractures and dorsal intercalated segment instability secondary to scapholunate ligament injury will have an increased scapholunate angle from flexion of the distal scaphoid pole and extension of the lunate.

MRI is cost effective for suspected fracture in the face of negative radiographs. It will reveal low signal fracture line surrounded by marrow edema. It can also demonstrate other causes of pain, such as additional carpal fractures, bone contusions, or soft tissue injuries.[37] One study of early MRI within a few days of injury for all suspected scaphoid fractures in children demonstrated 22% to have scaphoid fractures. Other injuries included other carpal fractures in 19%, distal radius fracture in 7%, and no distinct injury in 23%.[38] MRI is the current gold standard for advanced imaging, though ultrasound and CT can also be utilized.

Decision-Making Principles

Considerations for treatment include fracture orientation, location, displacement, angulation, chronicity, proximal pole radiographic appearance, and patient factors such as tolerance of immobilization.

Treatment Options

As initial radiographs may not clearly demonstrate a fracture line, it is recommend that all clinically suspected scaphoid fractures in children be immobilized with repeat radiographs in 2 weeks, where 30% of radiographically occult fractures become evident.[36] Early MRI can be considered for earlier definitive diagnosis. Proximal pole and displaced, angulated, or unstable waist fractures are managed operatively similar to adults.

Nondisplaced waist fractures are amenable to either nonoperative or operative management. Comparison of long and short arm casting in a RCT demonstrated similar union rates but faster healing with the former.[39] A higher extent of union on CT was seen at 10 weeks post-casting, with short arm casts that excluded the thumb.[39] Subacute fractures, up to 6 months postinjury, have also been shown to have 96% union rates with delayed casting.[40] RTP is safe 4 weeks after injury in a playing cast for nonoperative fractures.[14] Operative management is with headless cannulated compression screw often placed percutaneously from a volar or dorsal approach, which can be arthroscopically assisted (Fig. 135.8).

Author's Preferred Technique

Short arm casting excluding the thumb is applied for clinically suspected scaphoid fracture regardless of radiographic confirmation, as even in the absence of fracture, this assists in recovery of the contusion and/or soft tissue injury. Occult injuries have repeat radiographs performed out of cast in 2 weeks if tenderness persists. A low threshold for MRI is employed for patients desiring return to sport out of cast.

Nonoperative treatment consists of casting for 6 to 12 weeks, depending on when union is apparent on radiographs. A limited-cut CT is often performed to confirm bridging bone around 8 weeks postinjury if radiographs are not definitive. This regimen is applied to all nondisplaced distal pole and incomplete waist fractures, along with select nondisplaced waist fractures. All displaced waist and proximal pole fractures along with a subset of nondisplaced waist fractures are managed with headless cannulated compression screws. My preference is to perform percutaneous reduction when possible from either a dorsal or volar approach, the latter with the technique detailed nicely by Zlotlow.[41] Fractures requiring open reduction are approached from the dorsal side for reduction and fixation. Chronic injuries and nonunions are supplemented with bone graft placed through the drilled screw tract prior to hardware application. Pedicled bone grafting is reserved for cases with high suspicion of avascular necrosis based on MRI appearance of the proximal pole or intraoperative assessment of bone quality. My preference is for a 1 to 2 intercompartmental supraretinacular artery graft fixed with K-wires.

Postoperative Management

A short arm volar splint is placed for 2 weeks postoperatively, followed by prefabricated removable brace application to protect the fracture during healing while allowing removal for ROM exercises. RTP varies from 2 weeks postoperatively in a playing cast for noncontact sports to 8 to 12 weeks or until CT-proven union for other sports such as wrestling and gymnastics.[14]

Results

A retrospective review of 351 fractures in patient under 18 years found union rates of 90% and 96.5% in nonoperative and operative fractures, respectively.[35] Children that go on to union have excellent functional outcomes regardless of operative or nonoperative management at long-term follow-up.[42] A meta-analysis of RCTs comparing operative and nonoperative treatment in adults demonstrated operative treatment to produce better functional outcomes, patient satisfaction, grip strength, time to union, and time off work, despite higher complication rates.[43] There was no difference in pain, ROM, cost, or malunion/nonunion rates.

Lower union rates are found with casting alone for chronic, displaced, and proximal fractures in children.[35] Late presentation and osteonecrosis are each independent predictors of worse outcome in children.[42] One series of 13 nonunions in children, 75% from sports injuries, demonstrated all to unite after operative stabilization, usually with concomitant bone grafting.[44]

Complications

Scaphotrapezial arthritis occurs more commonly with operatively managed fractures in adults,[43] though it is unclear if this is also true of adolescents. There is a small incidence of nonunion, malunion, and proximal pole AVN with any treatment method.

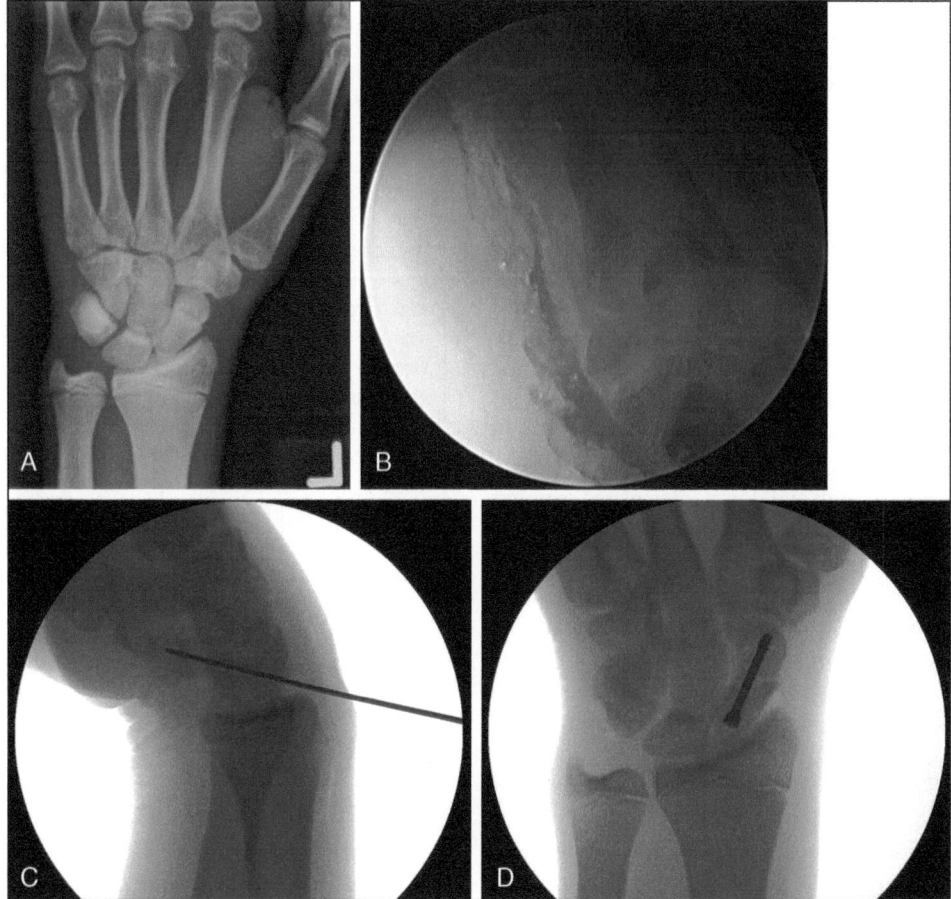

Fig. 135.8 A minimally displaced scaphoid fracture in an adolescent basketball player is demonstrated on anteroposterior radiograph (A). Arthroscopic view of the fracture confirms reduction of the fracture (B). Stabilization is performed with dorsal percutaneous guidewire placement (C) followed by cannulated headless compression screw placement (D).

Future Considerations

Various methods of judging fracture stability and proximal pole vascularity on imaging have been studied,[45] but the clinical significance of this is unclear. Studies to better predict which fractures go on to nonunion and avascular necrosis would help guide treatment.

For a complete list of references, go to ExpertConsult.com.

SELECTED READINGS

Citation:

Carruthers KH, Skie M, Jain M. Jam injuries of the finger: diagnosis and management of injuries to the interphalangeal joints across multiple sports and levels of experience. *Sports Health.* 2016;8(5):469–478.

Level of Evidence:

V

Summary:

A clinical review of the "jammed" finger is presented and covers pathology at both the PIP and DIP joints. Topics include collateral ligament injuries, pulley ruptures, volar plate injuries, central slip injuries, and finger fractures and dislocations.

Citation:

Lin JD, Strauch RJ. Closed soft tissue extensor mechanism injuries (mallet, boutonniere, and sagittal band). *J Hand Surg Am.* 2014;39(5):1005–1011.

Level of Evidence:

V

Summary:

The authors present a review of the following three traumatic extensor tendon problems: Mallet, boutonnière, and sagittal band injuries. Anatomy, presentation, and treatment are reviewed.

Citation:

Gholson JJ, Bae DS, Zurakowski D, et al. Scaphoid fractures in children and adolescents: contemporary injury patterns and factors influencing time to union. *J Bone Joint Surg Am.* 2011;93(13):1210–1219.

Level of Evidence:

III

Summary:

A retrospective analysis of 351 scaphoid fractures in patients under 18 years demonstrated the most common fracture location to be the scaphoid waist. Nonoperative management led to union in 90%. One-third of patients presented late with chronic nonunion.

Citation:
Matzon JL, Cornwall R. A stepwise algorithm for surgical treatment of type II displaced pediatric phalangeal neck fractures. *J Hand Surg Am.* 2014;39(3):467–473.

Level of Evidence:
IV

Summary:
A series of 61 phalangeal neck fractures treated with closed or percutaneous reduction and pinning are presented. Full functional recovery was achieved in 53 patients. Open reduction was not necessary in any patient, even up to 36 days postinjury.

Citation:
Rettig AC. Athletic injuries of the wrist and hand. Part I: traumatic injuries of the wrist. *Am J Sports Med.* 2003;31(6):1038–1048.

Citation:
Rettig AC. Athletic injuries of the wrist and hand. Part II: overuse injuries of the wrist and traumatic injuries to the hand. *Am J Sports Med.* 2004;32(1):262–273.

Level of Evidence:
V

Summary:
Athletic injuries of the hand and wrist are reviewed in this two-part paper divided into traumatic and overuse conditions. Scaphoid, hamate, lunate, and pisiform fractures are discussed. Ligamentous injuries of the wrist covered include scapholunate and lunotriquetral injuries, along with midcarpal instability. DRUJ and TFCC injuries are also covered. Overuse injuries of the wrist with different tendinopathies are reviewed. Lastly, finger injuries ranging from fractures to soft tissue injuries are detailed.

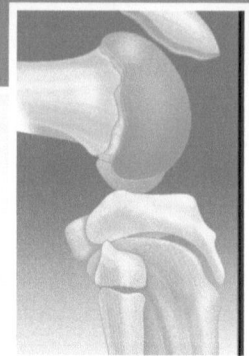

136

Pediatric and Adolescent Hip Injuries

Yi-Meng Yen, Mininder S. Kocher

Almost a decade ago it was estimated that over 30 million children participated in organized sports programs, with a third of them suffering an injury yearly that required evaluation by a nurse or physician.[1] There are physical and physiologic differences between the adolescent and adult athlete that may cause the younger athlete to be more vulnerable to injury. Children may not have as much coordination and musculoskeletal balance, as limb mass increases faster than limb length.[61] Muscle tendon growth lags behind bone growth and growing cartilage is more susceptible to stress and injury. These sports injuries are partly due to children's increased participation in sports and the propensity for children to focus on a single sport, leading to an increased risk of overuse injuries. More recently it has been reported that up to 2.6 million young athletes each year have injuries that warrant a visit to the emergency room, costing almost $2 billion yearly.[55]

Injuries to the hip and pelvis in pediatric and adolescent patients have been reported in the past several decades,[68,82,90,91,144,179] but are now receiving increasing interest because of advances in arthroscopic treatment and magnetic resonance imaging (MRI). Injuries around the hip can be caused by a single traumatic event or repetitive microtrauma. The majority of injuries around the hip in children are soft tissue, apophyseal, or bony injuries that require supportive management, with the minority of injuries requiring surgical intervention. There is likely an effect of sex and age on hip injuries due to sports, with females sustaining more chronic overuse and soft tissue injuries compared with males.[171] This chapter offers an overview of common injuries around the hip in the pediatric and adolescent athlete.

BONY INJURIES

Avulsion Fractures

Apophyseal avulsion fractures of the pelvis are injuries that occur almost exclusively in adolescence. For example, a sudden, violent, unbalanced muscle contraction is applied through the musculotendinous units during sporting activities. The cartilaginous growth plate at the apophysis fails, resulting in an avulsion fracture of the pelvis.[118] Once the injury has occurred, the bony displacement is limited by the periosteum and the surrounding muscle fascia. Sports such as soccer, rugby, ice hockey, gymnastics, and sprinting that involve kicking, rapid acceleration and deceleration, and jumping are commonly associated with avulsion fractures. Intensive training exposes the epiphyseal plate to repeated

tensile stress while overstrengthening the muscles around the joint. The inherent weakness of the epiphyseal plate combined with the increased demand on the musculature predispose the adolescent athlete to avulsion injury.

The sites for apophyseal injury around the hip include the ischium (hamstring attachment), anteroinferior iliac spine (AIIS; rectus femoris), anterosuperior iliac spine (ASIS; sartorius), iliac crest (abdominal musculature), lesser trochanter (iliopsoas) (Fig. 136.1), and greater trochanter (abductors). In the two largest studies of avulsion fractures, the most common location of such fractures were the AIIS in 33%, ASIS in 28%, and the ischial tuberosity (IT) in 30%, affecting males predominantly (75%).[153,158] The clinical presentation typically follows a traumatic incident with an acute onset of localized pain and the description of a "pop." Palpation and passive stretching of the muscle is typically quite painful, and patients will assume a position that places the least tension on the involved muscle. Although clinical presentation is often diagnostic, radiographic imaging is useful to determine the location, size, and degree of bony displacement.

Initial management of the majority of avulsion fractures is usually conservative, including rest and ice, followed by protected weight bearing with crutches until symptoms resolve.[71] Light isometric stretching, full weight bearing, and strengthening exercises are started when the patient is free of pain. Return to sports occurs after full pain-free range of motion (ROM) and full strength are achieved, which can take anywhere from 8 weeks to 6 months. A recent meta-analysis found that patients undergoing surgery had a higher overall success rate and return to sports compared with those treated conservatively.[41] However, there is usually a need for surgical intervention in avulsion fractures where the fragment has displaced more than 1.5 cm and there is loss of function or painful nonunion. In the case of the IT avulsion fracture, several reports have advocated repair if the bony fragment is greater than 2 cm; otherwise the fibrous nonunion can lead to chronic buttock pain, decreased hamstring strength, or potentially symptoms affecting the sciatic nerve.[31,54,71,159,184] Although it is generally agreed that large displaced fragments (>2 cm) may require surgical fixation, the optimal timing of surgery still remains unclear (Fig. 136.2).

Stress Fractures

Stress fractures of the femoral neck are most commonly seen in distance runners and young people enlisted in the military; the incidence is as high as 21% to 31% among these groups.[13,51,122]

Similarly, the incidence of stress fractures of the femoral neck in young female athletes has been reported to be up to 20%.[22] Such fractures can also occur in children younger than 10 years of age.[19] Stress fractures originate from either abnormal forces on normal bone (fatigue fractures) or normal forces on abnormal bone (insufficiency fractures).[145] These overuse injuries result from repetitive microtrauma on the bone and occur when the extent of damage exceeds the remodeling process. The most common sites of stress fractures in the hip area are in the femur, pubic rami, iliac crest, and sacroiliac joints.[110] Stress fractures of the femoral neck are particularly important because they often go untreated or unrecognized and can lead to the potentially devastating consequence of an acute femoral neck fracture.[83,143] Female athletes are more likely to develop stress fractures because of the classic female athlete triad: amenorrhea, eating disorders, and low bone density.[59,143,151] Additional risk factors include chronic glucocorticord use, smoking, hyperparathyroidism, hyperthyroidism, malabsorption syndromes, and calcium deficiencies.[14,34,36,48,57,60,117,125,127,129,134,178]

Stress fractures of the hip often present with only subtle clinical symptoms, making the diagnosis difficult. Hip pain associated with these stress fractures presents with an insidious onset of vague groin discomfort that is worse with activity and alleviated by rest. Patients often provide a history of a recent increase in their running or activity. As the fracture worsens, pain may occur earlier or even at rest. On physical examination, pain may be reproduced at the extremes of ROM, particularly with internal rotation.[21] A positive Trendelenburg test, inability to do a straight leg raise against resistance, and inability to hop on the affected side should raise suspicion of a stress fracture.[137] Plain radiographs are often negative in the acute setting; therefore advanced imaging may be required. Bone scan or MRI can be more helpful for diagnosing a stress fracture and should be considered if plain films are not diagnostic (Fig. 136.3).

The management of hip stress fractures is based on location, chronicity, and causative factors.[144] Femoral neck fractures occur in two different patterns, tension versus compression.[38] Tension-sided stress fractures are located on the superolateral femoral neck, more commonly in adults, and they may become displaced. Management of these types of fractures should be with percutaneous cannulated screws placed up the femoral neck. Tension-sided compression fractures are at higher risk for nonunion, deformity, and avascular necrosis. Compression-sided fractures occur in the inferomedial neck; they rarely displace but can cause a mild varus deformity. Younger patients typically present with compression-sided femoral neck stress fractures, which can be managed conservatively.[107,168] In most adolescents, conservative treatment includes non-weight bearing on the affected leg until radiographic union, nonsteroidal antiinflammatory drugs (NSAIDs), gentle ROM exercises, and regional muscular strengthening can be initiated. If healing does not occur within 6 to 8 weeks, use of a bone stimulator may be tried. Return to play should be allowed only after complete healing on clinical and radiographic examination. Treatment of any

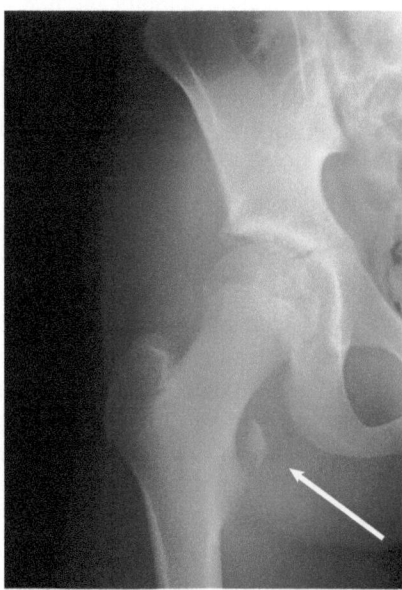

Fig. 136.1 Avulsion fracture of the lesser tuberosity in a skeletally immature patient. The *white arrow* denotes the site of avulsion.

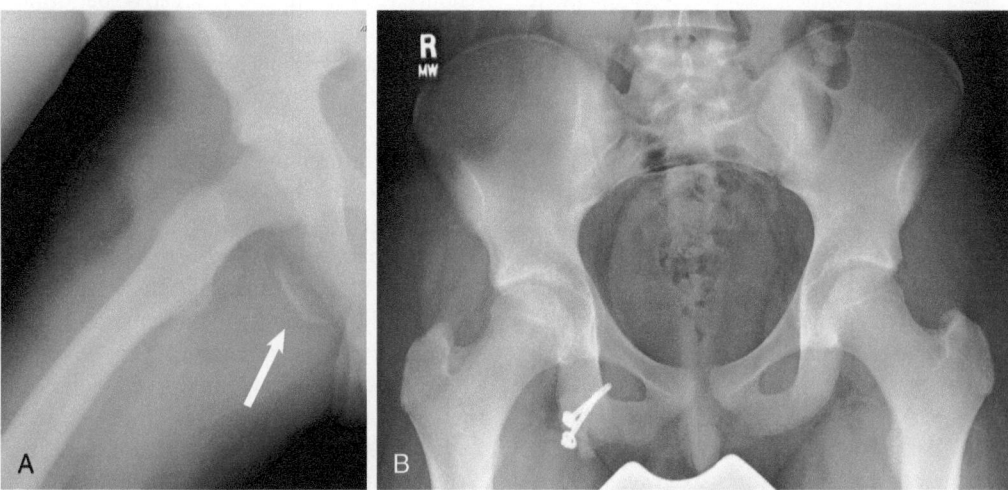

Fig. 136.2 (A) Avulsion fracture of the ischial tuberosity. The *white arrow* denotes a large fragment of ischium. (B) The same patient after open reduction and internal fixation

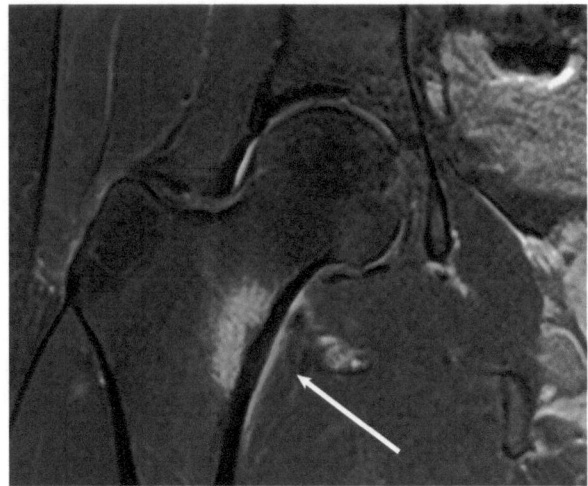

Fig. 136.3 Magnetic resonance image of a stress fracture of the inter-trochanteric region of the hip in an adolescent female. The *white arrow* denotes an area of edema due to the stress fracture.

underlying endocrine or other disorder is paramount to prevent recurrence.

Fractures

Fractures around the hip are relatively rare in the adolescent and pediatric population, accounting for less than 1% of fractures. These fractures usually result from high-energy trauma or a fall from a height rather than from participation in sports. Fractures can occur in the femoral head and femoral neck, the subtrochanteric region of the femur, and around the pelvic ring. Fractures around the pelvis can occur as single breaks due to the elasticity of the child's pelvis and can injure the triradiate cartilage, leading to growth disturbances of the acetabulum.[27,63,64] Radiographs of the pelvis and orthogonal views of the hip are usually diagnostic, but computed tomography (CT) can be useful in many cases.

Fractures of the acetabulum are generally treated nonoperatively in cases of minimal displacement, disruption of a small fragment, stable fracture patterns, or Salter-Harris I or II fractures of the triradiate. Operative intervention has been recommended in communited, open, and unstable fracture patterns; however, long-term results have not been encouraging.[27,62–64]

Fractures of the femoral head and neck are classified by the method of Delbet, comprising type 1 (transphyseal), type II (transcervical), type III (cervicotrochanteric), and type IV (inter-trochanteric) fractures.[32] Type I fractures are the least common but have the highest rate of osteonecrosis (38%–100%, depending on the presence of femoral head dislocation).[126,144] Irreducible fractures require open reduction and internal fixation.[160] Types II and III should be treated with anatomic reduction and internal fixation[160]; they are the most commonly encountered femoral neck fracture in children. Type II fractures have approximately twice the risk of avascular necrosis of type III fractures.[126,144] There may be some role for decompression of the capsular hematoma associated with femoral neck fractures, as lower rates of avascular necrosis were seen in patients who had a capsular decompression.[136] Type IV fractures and subtrochanteric femoral

fractures are extracapsular and have the most favorable prognosis. These fractures should be treated with anatomic reduction and internal fixation with blade plate fixation or screw side plate fixation.[2,18,84,106] In some cases intramedullary nailing or a dynamic hip screw can be used for subtrochanteric femoral fractures.[169] Postoperatively these patients are generally instructed to ambulate with crutches and protected weight bearing.

Dislocation

Hip dislocation is relatively uncommon in the adolescent population, accounting for less than 5% of all traumatic hip dislocations. Traumatic hip dislocation in children differs from the same in adults in that it is classified as a low-energy injury in the majority of patients when it results from a sports injury or fall from a relatively low height.[116,159,176,189] This difference is due to increased joint laxity in children, making dislocation possible with relatively minor trauma. Proximal femoral deformity has also been postulated to cause instability and may contribute to posterior hip dislocation.[109,138]

Although the femoral head in children may dislocate in any direction, posterior dislocations occur more frequently, accounting for over 90% of all hip dislocations.[10,93,116,176] The hip is usually held in flexion, adduction, and internal rotation with a posterior dislocation. The neurovascular status must be documented thoroughly and blunt trauma to the ipsilateral knee should be noted. Diagnosis can be made by history and physical examination. The femoral head can sometimes be palpated posteriorly. Radiographs, which should include a view of the entire pelvis and orthogonal views of the affected hip, are usually diagnostic. Radiographs should be examined carefully in order to evaluate for ipsilateral physeal injury or an associated femoral neck fracture. A CT scan can be useful to detect bony fragments within the joint as well as concomitant injury; however, MRI may becoming the modality of choice.[111]

The treatment for a traumatic hip dislocation is an emergent closed reduction within the first 6 hours of the time of injury so as to minimize the risk of avascular necrosis. The incidence of avascular necrosis is about 5% to 15% of all patients, but it increases by as much as 20-fold if the time to reduction is after 6 hours.[93,116] Closed reduction can be performed in the emergency room, but we prefer reduction in the operating room with general anesthesia and imaging (Fig. 136.4). Open reduction is performed only if the hip is irreducible after two to three reduction attempts or if soft tissue or bony fragments are interposed between the head and the acetabulum. The approach should be the same as the direction of the dislocation—that is, a posterior approach for a posterior dislocation. The acetabulum should be cleared of any debris, osteochondral fragments fixed if large enough, and the soft tissue repaired if possible.

The major complication after a dislocated hip is avascular necrosis of the femoral head.[11,116,141,176] When a traumatic dislocation is associated with femoral epiphysiolysis, the risk of avascular necrosis is almost 100%.[10,66,86,140] A patient who has had a delayed reduction should undergo MRI to assess for avascular necrosis 3 to 6 months after the injury. An alternative algorithm has been proposed to obtain an MRI 6 weeks after injury. If there is normal marrow signal, no further imaging is necessary; if abnormal

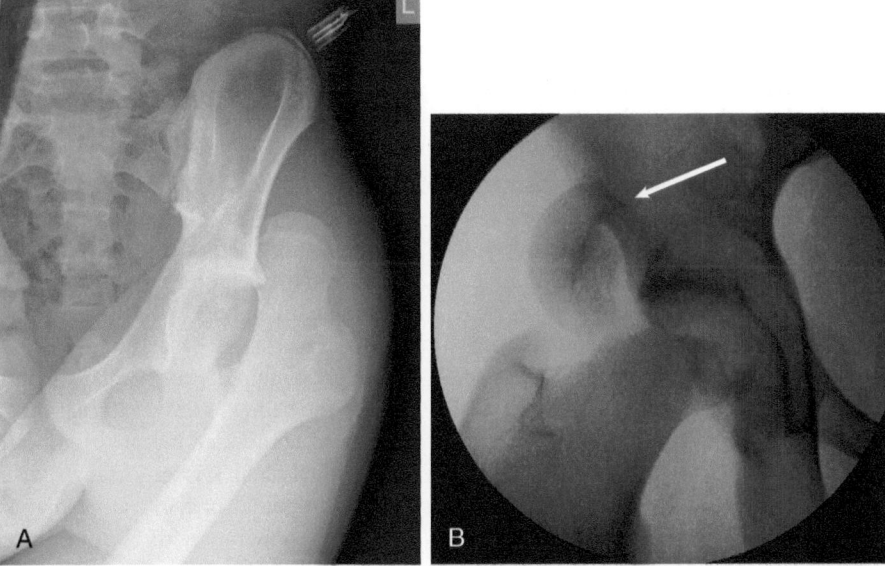

Fig. 136.4 (A) Posterior dislocation of the hip in a skeletally immature patient. (B) Epiphysiolysis during reduction of a dislocated hip. Open reduction and internal fixation of the epiphysis was necessary

signal is noted, a follow-up scan should be performed at 3 months.[150] Other complications include sciatic nerve injury, late posttraumatic osteoarthritis, coxa magna, heterotopic ossification, and recurrent dislocation.[189]

There have been some studies on intra-articular pathology evaluation by hip arthroscopy following hip dislocation,[77,147] which have been corroborated by an open surgical approach.[138] In all patients, there was documentation of intra-articular pathology, including chondral damage, labral tears, ligamentum teres tears, and adhesions.[154] Hip arthroscopy in the acute setting may be difficult because of fluid extravasation and should be considered only in the most experienced hands.

Pathologic Lesions

Very rarely both benign and malignant lesions may be found when the patient with hip pain is being evaluated. The most common benign lesions are simple bone cysts and osteoid osteomas, whereas the most common malignant tumors are osteosarcoma and Ewing sarcoma.[155] Radiographs and advanced imaging (CT and/or MRI) should be obtained to evaluate the lesion's location and size and to check for the presence of fracture as well as soft tissue extension and metastatic manifestations. Some simple benign lesions heal or regress spontaneously and need only close observation, whereas others, if quite large, may need surgical intervention. If malignancy is suspected, referral to orthopaedic oncology is advisable, as adjunctive and wide resection surgery may be indicated.

SOFT TISSUE INJURIES

Muscle Injury

Muscle strains and contusions are common in the young athlete.[49] Muscle strains are associated with improper warm-up, previous injury, fatigue, weather conditions, and uneven surfaces among other factors.[15,16] A muscle strain occurs in the hip area when muscle is functioning eccentrically—that is, the muscle is contracting while being lengthened. The most susceptible muscles involved are those that cross two joints, in particular the rectus femoris, hamstrings, and adductors.[16] A fall or direct blow causes a muscle contusion, which is commonly seen in contact sports.

The diagnosis of a muscle strain or contusion is typically straightforward. For a muscle strain, a high-velocity activity is usually being performed and the patient reports a sudden and intense pain in the affected muscle. There is usually localized pain and tenderness of the affected muscle with varying degrees of ecchymosis. The patient is usually unable to continue the activity and to use the muscle immediately. A contusion can be distinguished from a muscle rupture by the fact that with a contusion or strain the ability to continue using the muscle remains; the distinction can also be made by the mechanism of injury. Nonsurgical treatment varies, but all approaches involve the same principles. An early compression wrap and icing will help to control edema, bleeding, and swelling. NSAIDs are used for the first several days. Immobilization and partial weight bearing can help to provide comfort and muscle protection in the early period. Early ROM should comprise gentle stretching with progression to strengthening when muscle pain has resolved. Functional activities can start once strength has returned. Surgical intervention is rarely indicated.

Myositis ossificans can occur after moderate or severe injuries.[15] The vastus intermedius of the quadriceps is most commonly affected in this condition. It is usually diagnosed clinically by persistent soft tissue swelling, particularly with a muscle that is warm and tender to the touch. A radiograph will become evident, with heterotopic bone formation around 2 to 4 weeks after the injury. The size of the myositis ossificans usually stabilizes by 6 months but can cause continued pain and may delay rehabilitation.[180] Surgery is usually not indicated.

Bursitis

Bursitis occurs at two major areas around the hip, the iliopsoas bursa and the greater trochanteric bursa. The iliopsoas bursa is the largest synovial bursa in the body and is located between the iliopsoas tendon and the lesser trochanter, extending upward into the iliac fossa beneath the iliacus muscle.[24] The greater trochanteric bursa is located on the lateral side of the greater trochanter and cushions the gluteal tendons, iliotibial band, and tensor fascia latae.[161] A smaller, less common bursa is the iliopectineal bursa, which is situated between the iliopsoas muscle belly and the femoral head. Causes of bursitis include chronic microtrauma, arthritis, regional muscle dysfunction, overuse, and acute injury.[56,161] Hip bursitis is commonly caused by repetitive motion of the hip during cycling or running or a direct injury to the hip such as by a fall or a tackle onto the greater trochanter.

Clinical presentation depends on which bursa is affected. Iliopsoas bursitis causes pain the anterior groin, tenderness to palpation over the lesser trochanter, and pain with resisted hip flexion (Stinchfield test).[114] Symptoms of trochanteric bursitis include pain on the lateral aspect of the hip and thigh, pain from sitting to standing, and pain on walking up stairs. Having the patient lie on his or her side and reproduce the motion of riding a bike can elicit tenderness. In both cases, erythema, swelling, and warmth may be present over the front or side of the hip. Diagnosis is usually clinical and imaging is often unnecessary. Plain films can sometimes show round calcifications that are isolated around the greater trochanter in the case of trochanteric bursitis.[161] Ultrasound or MRI can be used to localize areas of inflammation.

Treatment of bursitis is almost always conservative, including rest, ice, NSAIDs, gentle stretching, and physical therapy. Ultrasound-guided steroid injections may help to alleviate the painful symptoms of bursitis. In recalcitrant cases, surgical bursectomy or tendon release may be helpful (open or arthroscopic).[17,75,166,188]

Athletic Pubalgia

Athletic pubalgia has unfortunately become a term referring to pain around the groin, which can encompass osteitis pubis, adductor dysfunction, sports hernia, or other pelvic/abdominal muscular injuries. However, most clinicians regard athletic pubalgia as meaning a sports or "sportsman's" hernia,[120,124,162] although there is no universally accepted definition Adductor dysfunction causes tenderness localized to the adductor longus insertion; on examination there is pain with adduction against resistance and with stretch in abduction. This is usually managed nonoperatively, with measures including rest and physical therapy. Occasionally, the use of injected corticosteroids can give relief,[157] and adductor tenotomy has been shown to provide long-term relief in recalcitrant cases.[4,108]

Osteitis pubis causes tenderness to palpation at the pubic symphysis. Chronic osteitis pubis can cause chronic changes that induce inappropriate osteoclastic activity and osseous resorption on plain radiographs[112,115] as well as the "secondary cleft sign" on MRI[20]; edema is seen around the pubis on MRI in acute cases.[128,175] Osteitis pubis is treated normally with rest and physical therapy,[69] with injections,[70,139] and with surgical intervention[130,182] in recalcitrant cases.

Athletic pubalgia is a syndrome resulting from weakness of the posterior wall of the inguinal canal causing nerve irritation and disruption and instability of the muscular attachments.[3,102,120,132,172] Athletic pubalgia can be thought of as an overuse injury[7,58] in which the muscular attachments of the pelvis are unbalanced, which leads to a loss of postural control and an increase in the shear forces across the pelvis. Most patients report insidious unilateral, dull, achy pain in the groin that is significantly exacerbated by activities such as running, cutting, or twisting. Coughing, sneezing, and Valsalva-type maneuvers usually worsen the pain. Physical examination can show tenderness over conjoined tendon, adductor origin, distal rectus insertion, and the inguinal canal. It is important to distinguish athletic pubalgia from an inguinal or femoral hernia. Newer MRI imaging can be useful, showing rectus abdominis tendon injury and subtle abnormalities of the myofascial layers of the abdominal wall.[5,187] Prevention with measures to improve core and hip stability and flexibility is paramount in decreasing the incidence of athletic pubalgia.[121] Nonoperative measures include rest, antiinflammatories, strengthening of the core musculature, and postural control.[39,94] Surgical exploration should be considered if nonoperative treatment has failed after 3 to 6 months and other diagnoses have been excluded. Surgical measures include primary pelvic floor repair without mesh,[119,131] open anterior mesh repair,[65,81] and laparoscopic mesh repair.[42] Surgical repairs should be referred to an appropriate surgeon.

Snapping Hip (Coxa Saltans)

A snapping hip is characterized by an audible or visible popping or snapping sound when the hip is brought through a certain ROM. It can be painful and is often exacerbated by sporting activities, particularly with running up and down a hill. Three typical types of snapping hip have been described: lateral or external (iliotibial band), internal or medial (psoas), and intraarticular.[6] The external type is the most common and involves the posterior border of the iliotibial band or the anterior border of the gluteus maximus tendon snapping over the greater trochanter when the hip is flexed from an extended position or with internal and external rotation while the hip is extended.[156] The external snapping is often visible as the iliotibial band clunks over the greater trochanter. The internal snapping hip is the iliopsoas tendon snapping over the iliopectineal eminence or the femoral head; it is often painful and audible.[40] The intraarticular snapping can be caused by a loose body, chondral flap, labral tear, or synovial plica.[8,113]

The history and physical is usually diagnostic for the location and cause of the snapping hip. Patients with external snapping hip can often reproduce the symptoms voluntarily. Internal snapping hip occurs when the hip is moved from a flexed and abducted position to an extended and adducted position; this can often be seen by ultrasonography. MRI is indicated if intra-articular pathology is suspected. Initial management of coxa saltans externa or interna includes physical therapy for stretching of the iliotibial band or iliopsoas. Antiinflammatory medications, rest, and bursal injections can also be effective. If conservative management does not relieve the symptoms, surgical intervention may be considered. Open surgical approaches involving fractional lengthening or release have been performed,[44,173,181] although few reports have been described in adolescents.[40] Recently arthroscopic treatment has been described with good short-term success for both coxa saltans interna and externa.[75,76,78,80,177]

LABRAL TEARS

The acetabular labrum is a ring of fibrocartilage that almost encircles the acetabulum of the hip joint and is believed to deepen the acetabulum, enhance joint stability, and provide a fluid seal for the articulating femoral head and acetabulum.[45-47] Injuries to the labrum occur during sports because of mechanical stresses or twisting in sports such as football, soccer ballet, ice hockey, and others. The patient may complain of hip or groin pain and experience catching or locking of the hip during certain maneuvers. Disorders such as hip dysplasia and femoroacetabular impingement increase the risk of labral tears. Tears can occur in any part of the labrum but are more common in the anterosuperior portion of the acetabulum, perhaps due to the higher stresses in this region.[101] Radiographic imaging of the pelvis and hip can demonstrate a dysplasia, femoroacetabular impingement, or other abnormality, but an MR arthrogram is the most commonly used modality for diagnosing labral tears.[23,85]

Arthroscopy has become the standard for diagnosing and treating acetabular labral tears. Conservative management may alleviate pain, but surgical repair or débridement is the most definitive treatment (Fig. 136.5). Several studies have shown good long-term results and return to sports after labral treatment in both adults and adolescents.[26,74,89,165] When irreparable tears are encountered in the adolescent athlete, the labral sealing mechanism can be reestablished by performing a reconstruction of the labrum using graft tissue (autograft or allograft hamstring, iliotibial band, tibialis anterior, or posterior or ligamentum).[9]

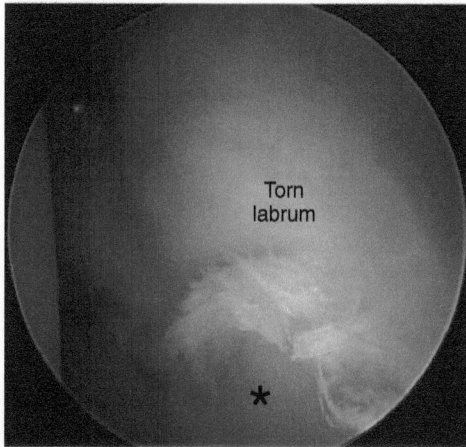

Fig. 136.5 Arthroscopic picture of a left hip depicting a large tear in the labrum. The *black asterisk* denotes the articular surface of the acetabulum.

ACQUIRED DISEASE

Femoroacetabular Impingement

Femoroacetabular impingement has been gaining increasing attention as a common etiology of hip pain in athletes.[52,53] Anatomically, the concept of femoroacetabular impingement is that certain minor morphologic alterations to the hip joint combined with repetitive abutment of the femoral head-neck junction against the anterior rim of the acetabulum lead to chondrolabral dysfunction and eventual early degeneration of the hip joint. The morphologic alterations may be either on the acetabular side (pincer impingement) or the femoral head-neck side (cam impingement) or both.[95] FAI is now being recognized as a significant cause of hip pain in the adolescent population.[163]

Patients often present with an insidious onset of groin pain that is made worse with sporting activity. There may be an associated labral tear and patients often describe their pain with a hand cupped over the anterolateral hip with the thumb and forefinger in the shape of a "C."[25] Impingement can be detected with decreased hip flexion and limited internal rotation and a positive impingement (flexion, adduction, and internal rotation) test. Radiographic imaging should include an anteroposterior (AP) view of the pelvis and orthogonal views of the hips.[30] A bony prominence at the head-neck junction is indicative of a cam lesion, whereas acetabular overcoverage or retroversion on the radiograph is termed a pincer. Additional MRI imaging can be helpful for evaluation of the soft tissues of the joint, including the cartilage and labrum.[99]

Treatment goals include improving hip muscle flexibility, pelvic tilt, strength, and posture. Progression of arthritic changes from impingement can be gradual but if left untreated can cause severe permanent injury to the articular surfaces of the joint. Refractory pain should be managed by either open surgical dislocation or arthroscopic treatment.[52,92] Good results have been achieved in the adolescent population with arthroscopic intervention[33,43,148,149] even in revision cases.[135]

Legg-Calve-Perthes

Legg-Calve-Perthes disease is an idiopathic self-limiting condition involving avascular necrosis of the femoral epiphysis. The exact etiology of the disease is largely unknown, although a number of vascular causes have been proposed. In the 100 years since this disease was first described there has been little insight into its etiology and pathophysiology. It typically presents within the first decade of life predominantly among males 4 to 8 years of age.[87] Bilateral involvement is uncommon, occurring about 15% of the time, but is almost never simultaneous. The pathogenesis is complex and passes through multiple stages, initially avascular necrosis, fragmentation, resorption, and collapse and then reossification. The Catterall[28] and Herring[67] classifications are the two most common systems used to give a prognosis depending on the location of necrosis and percent of femoral head involvement. The natural history of the disease is variable, largely dependent on age at the time of diagnosis and degree of involvement of the femoral head. Age less than 9 years and less than 50% of involved femoral head are predictive factors for a good prognosis.[67] The younger the child is at the time of the

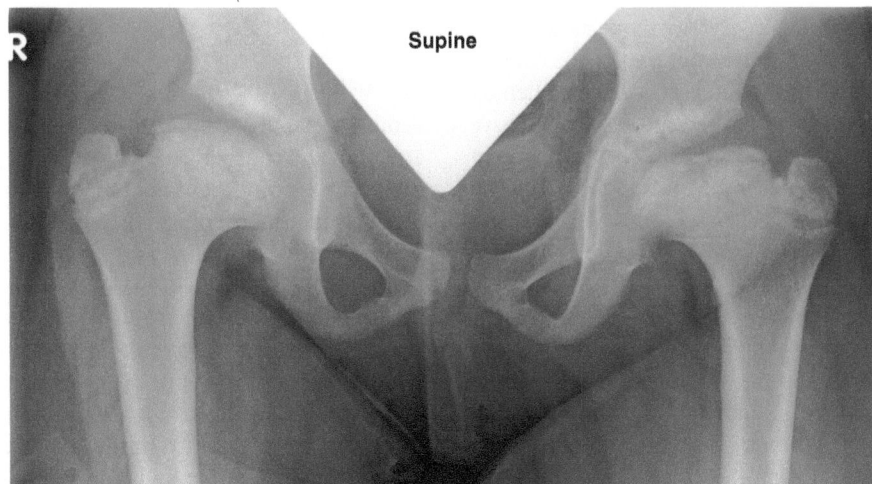

Fig. 136.6 Bilateral Legg-Calve-Perthes disease. The right side of the femoral head is in the reossification stage while the left side is in the fragmentation stage.

onset of disease, the greater the time there is for subsequent growth and remodeling. Fifty percent of patients who had childhood Perthes disease who did not receive treatment developed osteoarthritis in the fifth decade of life.[123]

Perthes disease is specific to the hip joint and typically presents as an insidious unilateral painless limp. If pain is present it is usually mild, exacerbated by activity and commonly referred to the knee. The most common physical examination findings include decreased internal rotation and abduction of the hip. AP and lateral radiographs are diagnostic (Fig. 136.6). The goal of treatment is to try to contain the femoral head within the acetabulum, which can be performed by traction, casting, abduction bracing, tendon releases, or osteotomies of the femur or acetabulum. At present there is little conclusive information in the literature regarding one treatment method over the other. In patients with severe disease, surgical intervention appears to be preferable compared with nonoperative treatment. Patients over the age of 8 classified as B or B/C according to the Herring classification have a better outcome with surgical intervention.[67] Adolescents who have had a history of Legg-Calve-Perthes disease may present later in life with an abnormally shaped femoral head that predisposes them to FAI. Arthroscopic treatment of residual cam deformity from Perthes patients showed restoration of hip geometry and good short-term results.[50,79]

Slipped Capital Femoral Epiphysis

Slipped capital femoral epiphysis (SCFE) involves the posterior displacement of the proximal femoral epiphysis with concomitant extension and external rotation of the femoral neck and shaft. It is a common hip disorder of adolescence, occurring most often in obese African American males between 10 and 16 years of age.[146] SCFE is usually associated with pubertal growth but may be due to trauma, endocrine disorders, or inflammatory disorders. Increased body mass index is also a significant risk factor.[104] Bilateral involvement can occur in up to 60% of cases.[103] The classification of SCFE has been traditionally based on the acuity of symptoms and severity of the slip; however, a greater emphasis is now being placed upon mechanical stability of the

slip due to a greater prognostic value. A mechanically stable slip is such that the patient can bear weight with or without crutches, whereas a patient with an unstable slip is unable to bear weight because of pain.[105] An unstable slip typically represents an acute physeal fracture with displacement.

Accurate, early diagnosis of SCFE is important to prevent short- and long-term complications, including chondrolysis of the joint and avascular necrosis of the femoral head. The average duration of symptoms is 5 months for stable slips. The complaints are often insidious and ambiguous, with activity related hip, thigh, or knee pain.[91] The delayed onset of significant pain and dysfunction may allow for progression of a stable to an unstable slip, which has major implications on long-term prognosis.[88] Physical examination shows obligate external rotation of the affected side; AP and frog-leg lateral radiographs are diagnostic. If a slip is suspected and is negative on plain films, an MRI should be obtained (Fig. 136.7). Treatment is always operative, with the gold standard now involving in situ pinning with a single screw crossing the physis. Severe slips with significant deformity have recently been treated with a modified Dunn osteotomy through a surgical dislocation approach.[73,100,167,186] However, there is a clear relationship between stability and severity of the slip and the postoperative risk of avascular necrosis. Additionally, a cam lesion can develop at the time of the SCFE. Although remodeling can occur,[35,37] damage to the acetabular labrum and cartilage has been noted with both open and arthroscopic approaches.[96,98,164] Multiple reports have detailed good results with arthroscopic resection of the resulting cam deformity from the SCFE along with screw removal.[12,29,72,96,98,174,185] Additionally, a recent report on arthroscopic subcapital realignment osteotomy appears promising.[152]

CONCLUSION

Although there are a multitude of injuries that can occur around the hip and pelvis, some occur as a result of a disease process whereas most occur as the result of trauma. The prevention of such injuries in the adolescent and pediatric population is

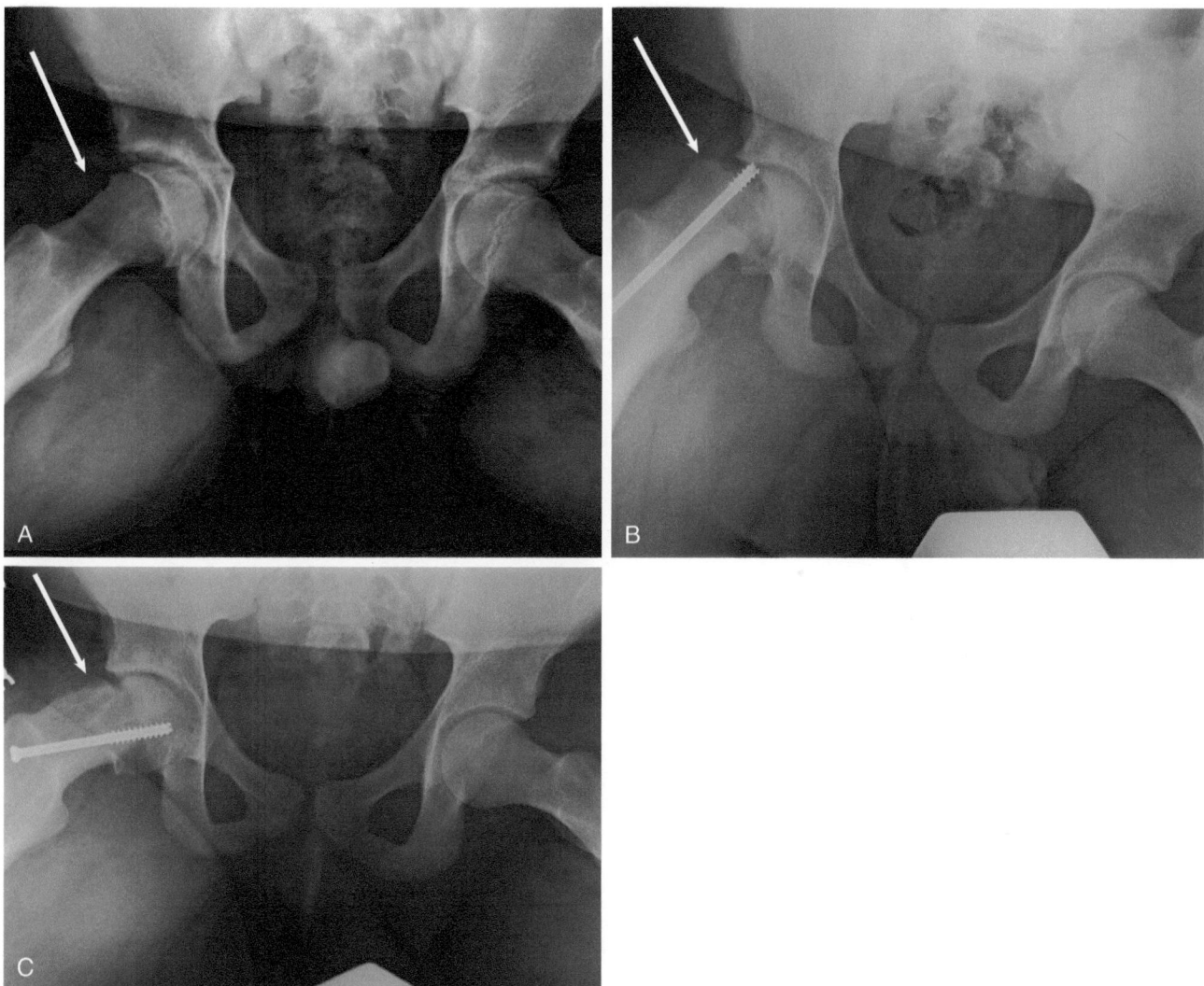

Fig. 136.7 (A) Mild slipped capital femoral epiphysis on the right hip that underwent in situ pinning with a single cannulated screw. The *white arrow* depicts the slip. (B) In the same patient the epiphysis grew off the screw and continued to slip. The *white arrow* shows the increase in the metaphyseal bump. (C) After repinning of the slipped capital femoral epiphysis with fusion of the physis. The *white arrow* shows the residual femoroacetabular impingement.

immensely important. Almost all sports involve the use of the lower extremity and core stability. A number of studies have linked the lack of core stability with the development of hip and pelvic injuries.[97,133,142,170,183] These studies underscore the importance of developing, strengthening and maintaining the flexibility of the core muscle group. Improvement to the core muscle group can help to decrease the likelihood and/or severity of hip and pelvic injury in the adolescent athlete. Further research and programs to develop and improve strategies to prevent injury are warranted.

For a complete list of references, go to ExpertConsult.com.

SELECTED READINGS

Citation:

Eberbach H, Hohloch L, Feucht MJ, et al. Operative versus conservative treatment of apophyseal avulsion fractures of the pelvis in the adolescents: a systematical review with meta-analysis of clinical outcome and return to sports. *BMC Musculoskelet Disord.* 2017;18(1):162.

Level of Evidence:

V

Summary:

This meta-analysis of 596 patients with avulsion fractures of the pelvis provides evidence for operative versus nonoperative treatment.

Citation:

Ganz R, Parvizi J, Beck M, et al. Femoroacetabular impingement: a cause for osteoarthritis of the hip. *Clin Orthop Relat Res.* 2003;417:112–120.

Level of Evidence:

IV

Summary:

This article is the sentinel paper on femoroacetabular impingement. It has significantly influenced the understanding of hip pathology and subsequent treatment regimens.

Citation:

Millis MB, Lewis CL, Schoenecker PL, et al. Legg-Calve-Perthes disease and slipped capital femoral epiphysis: major developmental causes of femoroacetabular impingement. *J Am Acad Orthop Surg.* 2013;21(suppl 1):S59–S63.

Level of Evidence:

V

Summary:

An excellent review of childhood hip disorders causing femoroacetabular impingement. this article underscores the development of irreversible chondral damage and advocates early treatment.

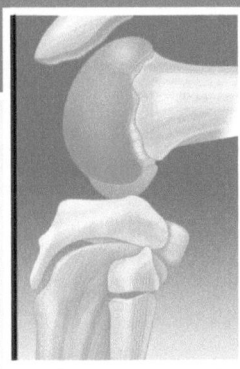

137

Knee Injuries in Skeletally Immature Athletes

Matthew D. Milewski, James Wylie, Carl W. Nissen, Tricia R. Prokop

ANTERIOR CRUCIATE LIGAMENT INJURIES

Injuries to the anterior cruciate ligament (ACL) in skeletally immature athletes were traditionally thought to be rare. Historically, the incidence of ACL rupture in this population was reported as 1% to 3.4%.[1-4] Avulsion of the tibial spine was reported to be more common than ACL rupture.[3] However, as awareness of these injuries has increased, and with improvements in diagnostic modalities, especially MRI, ACL rupture is increasingly recognized in skeletally immature athletes who present with a knee injury. Injuries to the ACL have been reported in children as young as 4 years of age.[5] In patients presenting with a hemarthrosis, the incidence of ACL rupture has been reported to be between 26% and 65%.[6-9] It is now believed that the rate of ACL rupture in patients with open physes may exceed the rate of tibial spine fractures.[10] Whether a young athlete sustains an ACL rupture or a tibial spine fracture may depend on the loading rate at the time of injury and the morphology of the intercondylar notch.[11-13]

History and Physical Examination

Skeletally immature athletes who have sustained an ACL rupture present very similarly to more mature athletes with similar injuries. As stated previously, the rate of ACL injury in a patient presenting with a hemarthrosis approaches 70%.[14] Patients often state that during a pivoting or cutting activity they heard a "pop," felt immediate pain and swelling in the knee, and were unable to return to full activity. As with other populations, the skeletally immature athlete may sustain an ACL rupture after a contact injury, but noncontact injuries are more common. After such an injury, athletes may describe continued instability with cutting or pivoting activities or can often have symptoms even with activities of daily living.

On examination, skeletally immature athletes should be assessed for the presence of an effusion, range of motion (ROM), a neurovascular examination, and standard knee ligament and hip and ankle assessments. Special attention should be directed to the Lachman, anterior drawer, and varus/valgus laxity tests both on the affected and contralateral knees because skeletally immature athletes can often have increased global laxity, and asymmetry in their examinations is an important diagnostic criterion. Patients with a suspected ACL rupture should also be closely examined for pathologic meniscal findings, with an assessment of joint line tenderness, flexion pinch, and McMurray tests. An assessment of patellar instability is also crucial in this population of young athletes who present with a painful effusion, because this diagnosis can often mimic an ACL injury.

Especially crucial to the examination of a skeletally immature patient with a potential ACL rupture is an assessment of physical maturity. Several methods may be used to assess physical maturity in adolescents. Tanner and Whitehouse[15] correlated physiologic development signs with height, weight, height velocity, and weight velocity. Tanner staging is the most common means of assessing physical maturity on physical examination. Although many pediatricians are familiar and comfortable with this staging assessment, many sports medicine physicians may be unfamiliar or uncomfortable with this process. Self-Tanner staging, intraoperative Tanner staging, and growth relative to family members can be used to supplement the physical examination.[16]

Imaging

Standard sports-oriented radiographs of the knee should be obtained for skeletally immature athletes presenting with a suspected ACL injury. These radiographs include a standing anteroposterior (AP), standing notch or tunnel view, and lateral and sunrise views to assess for associated injuries such as osteochondritis dissecans (OCD; seen best on the notch view), patellar subluxation (seen best on the Merchant view), tibial spine fracture (seen best on the lateral view), and physeal injuries. In cases in which surgical intervention is likely, a mechanical axis radiograph for limb length and a standardized posteroanterior radiograph of the left hand is recommended to determine bone age using the Greulich and Pyle atlas. Further mention of bone age in this chapter refers to this technique.[17] A simplified version of determining bone age has been recently developed.[18] Often, contralateral knee views are necessary to better assess any asymmetry in the physes if a distal femoral or proximal tibial physeal injury is suspected. A Segond fracture or lateral capsular avulsion adjacent to the proximal tibia can be seen and is highly correlated with an ACL injury. This likely represents an avulsion of the anterolateral complex of the knee.[19] The anterolateral complex/anterolateral ligament (ALL) is currently a hotly debated topic in ACL reconstruction at this time, and further study is needed to determine its importance, especially in the pediatric and adolescent patient with an ACL tear, because recent studies have shown variable anatomy in pediatric knees.[20,21]

MRI has increasingly become the modality of choice for imaging the ACL. Direct evidence of ACL injury on MRI includes discontinuity of ACL fibers in any three imaging planes and the "empty notch sign," in which fluid signal instead of ACL signal is seen at the proximal attachment site; this finding is best observed on T2-weighted images. In the acute setting, the injured or ruptured ACL can appear as an edematous mass with increased T2-weighted signal and abnormal morphologic features. In the subacute setting, it can appear discontinuous and less edematous with a more linear fragmented appearance, or it may even be completely absent in the chronic setting.[22,23] In some cases a nearly normal ACL can be seen on the sagittal images when the ACL has scarred down to the posterior cruciate ligament (PCL). The axial and coronal images can be helpful, especially in evaluating the femoral footprint.[24] The proximal ACL avulsion that scars to the PCL can be a point of confusion at the time of arthroscopy because the distal portion of the ACL can appear normal and can also create a pseudo–end point on examination.

Indirect evidence on MRI of an ACL injury can include a hemarthrosis and a pivot shift bone contusion, which is usually seen on the lateral femoral condyle and posterolateral tibial plateau. In addition, evidence of a deepened sulcus sign may be seen with an irregular-appearing lateral femoral condyle sulcus with a depth greater than 2 mm. Other indirect evidence of ACL injury on MRI includes a visible Segond fracture, the anterior drawer sign (i.e., increased anterior tibial translation), or buckling of the PCL, which may be nonspecific.[25]

Decision-Making Principles

The decision to proceed with operative treatment of the ACL-deficient knee in a skeletally immature athlete is challenging and currently evolving for athletes, parents, and providers. The rationale for operative treatment of ACL injuries in skeletally immature patients is based on studies documenting the increased risk of meniscal damage, chondral damage, chronic instability, and inability to return to sports in these athletes.[26] These risks must be balanced against the potential complications associated with ACL reconstruction in this population, which include growth arrest with resulting angular deformity or leg length discrepancy.

The risk of growth disturbance has been examined in numerous animals, with use of a transphyseal reconstruction technique across open physes.[27–30] Guzzanti et al.[27] first demonstrated this risk in a rabbit model. Houle et al.[29] and Edwards and Grana[30] also showed significant risk of deformity with soft tissue grafts placed under tension across both canine and rabbit physes. Stadelmaier et al.[28] showed no evidence of physeal arrest when tension was not applied to soft tissue grafts.

Several clinical studies have reported growth disturbances associated with ACL reconstruction in the skeletally immature athlete.[3,31,32] Risk factors associated with growth disturbances and angular deformities include transphyseal hardware fixation or bone plugs and lateral extra-articular tenodesis. A meta-analysis

reported a 1.8% overall risk of growth disturbance in skeletally immature athletes undergoing ACL reconstruction.[33]

Prevention

ACL injuries in all athletes can have serious short- and long-term consequences, especially in the youngest populations. Strategies to prevent these injuries have been developed and are becoming increasingly refined and important both on an individual and public health level.[34] These programs focus on education, stretching, proprioceptive training, plyometrics, sports-specific agility, jump and landing training, and progressive resistance weight training for the lower extremities.[35–39] Sports medicine providers may want to consider implementing these preventive training programs, especially for high school athletes. A recent meta-analysis reporting on 24 studies and more than 1000 patients found that these programs are efficacious at preventing both knee injuries and specifically ACL tears.[40] It is still unclear if pre–high school–aged patient populations are able to comply and take advantage of the benefits of these training programs.

Conservative Treatment

Traditional recommendations for the treatment of the ACL-deficient knee in the skeletally immature athlete included delayed surgical treatment until skeletal maturity with interim functional bracing, physical therapy, and activity modification.[4,41–44] Certain circumstances may dictate conservative treatment or a delay in surgical intervention, such as personal or medical reasons that would increase the risk of surgery or in the setting of an incomplete ACL tear without a secondary injury.

Treatment of Partial Anterior Cruciate Ligament Tears

Treatment of partial ACL tears in the skeletally immature athlete entails decision-making principles similar to those used in athletes with complete ACL tears. If the clinical examination and the patient's symptoms are consistent with instability with activities and the inability to return to sport, or the patient has associated injuries such as meniscal tears or chondral damage indicative of an ACL-deficient knee or recurrent effusions are present, a partial ACL tear should be considered functionally incompetent. If the young athlete's symptoms and examination findings are not indicative of instability, then conservative treatment with functional bracing, physical therapy, and activity modification could be considered.

Treatment Algorithm for Anterior Cruciate Ligament Reconstruction Based on Skeletal Maturity

Milewski et al.[16] have described an algorithm for deciding the operative surgical technique in skeletally immature athletes (Figs. 137.1 and 137.2). After appropriate decision-making and conservative treatment has been considered, skeletal age is determined by bone age using radiographs of the hand.[18]

For prepubescent adolescents (i.e., those with a skeletal age <7 years), the physeal-sparing combined intra-articular and extra-articular reconstruction technique with an iliotibial band

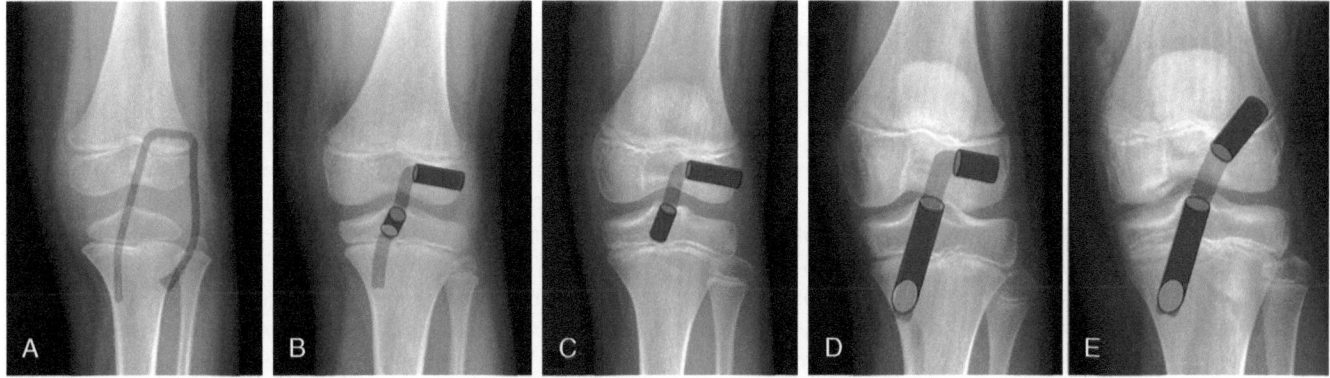

Fig. 137.1 Radiographs revealing representative images of patients with bone ages of 6 to 14 years. (A) Bone age of 6 years: Micheli-Kocher intra-articular extra-articular procedure. (B) Bone age of 8 years: Anderson all-epiphyseal procedure, which has been modified. (C) Bone age of 10 years: Ganley-Lawrence all-epiphyseal docking procedure. (D) Bone age of 12 years: Hybrid all-epiphyseal femoral transphyseal tibial procedure. (E) Bone age of 14 years: Transphyseal femoral and tibial reconstruction with soft tissue only at the level of the physis. (From Milewski MD, Beck NA, Lawrence JT, et al. Anterior cruciate ligament reconstruction in the young athlete: a treatment algorithm for the skeletally immature. *Clin Sports Med.* 2011;30[4]:801–810.)

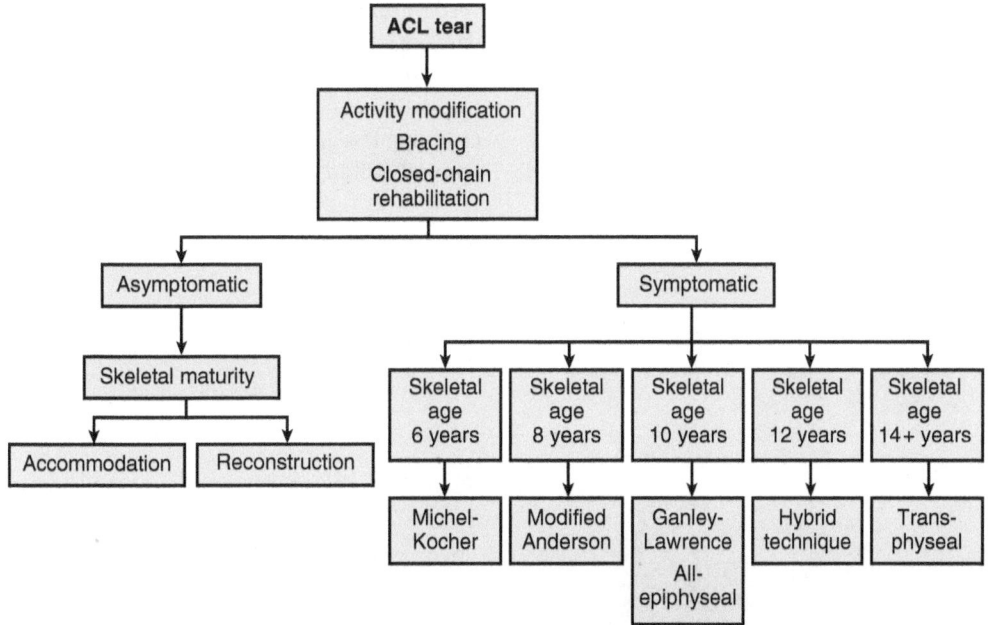

Fig. 137.2 A treatment algorithm for patients with a ruptured anterior cruciate ligament *(ACL)*. After a trial of activity modification, bracing, and closed-chain rehabilitation, symptomatic patients are candidates for surgical reconstruction. Prepubescent patients are at greatest risk for growth disturbances, and physeal-sparing techniques such as an all-epiphyseal or combined intra-articular and extra-articular reconstruction are used. Soft tissue transphyseal reconstruction is performed on older/postpubescent patients. (From Milewski MD, Beck NA, Lawrence JT, et al. Anterior cruciate ligament reconstruction in the young athlete: a treatment algorithm for the skeletally immature. *Clin Sports Med.* 2011;30[4]:801–810.)

described by Kocher et al.[45] is recommended. Older children with a small lateral femoral condyle may also be appropriate candidates for this technique.

For athletes with a skeletal age of 7 to 12 years, an all-epiphyseal reconstruction as described by Lawrence et al.[46] is advocated. Ganley has recommended a modification to this technique, and the technique is described by Anderson[47] for use in

adolescents who have less than 20 mm of epiphyseal length. In these patients, cortical button fixation is used on both the femur and tibia for an all-epiphyseal tunnel procedure with a hamstring autograft.

For 13-year-old female athletes and 13- to 14-year-old male athletes, transphyseal reconstruction with a quadrupled hamstring autograft is recommended. This procedure can be modified using the hybrid anatomic technique with an all-epiphyseal femoral tunnel and a transphyseal tibial tunnel if a significant amount of growth is believed to remain and if the surgeon prefers to use the newer anatomic ACL techniques of centering the tunnels within the anatomic footprint.

Treatment

Anterior Cruciate Ligament Reconstruction Techniques

After operative treatment of an ACL-deficient knee is elected, it must be decided whether to use a physeal-sparing or physeal-respecting technique or a traditional technique for ACL reconstruction. Physeal-sparing techniques for ACL reconstruction were initially described with use of patellar tendon grafts without drill holes by DeLee and Curtis[2] and using hamstring tendon grafts by Brief[48] and Parker et al.[49]

Kocher et al.[45] have described and advocated use of a physeal-sparing combined intra-articular and extra-articular reconstruction with an autogenous iliotibial band in prepubescent children who are at Tanner stage 1 or 2. This reconstruction technique has no bone tunnels and incorporates a lateral extra-articular iliotibial band reconstruction to help control rotation as described by Losee et al.[50] (Fig. 137.3).

Anderson,[47] as well as Guzzanti et al.,[51] have described physeal-sparing hamstring graft reconstruction techniques. Both techniques require extraosseous tensioning of the graft across the tibial physis. Anderson's reconstruction technique uses a hamstring graft tensioned across epiphyseal tunnels in the femur and tibia

with the graft extending out of the tibial tunnel and across the tibial physis and attached with a screw and post construct in the tibial metaphysis.

Lawrence and colleagues at Children's Hospital of Philadelphia have recently described an all-epiphyseal ACL technique using femoral and tibial epiphyseal tunnels confirmed with intraoperative computed tomography (CT).[46] Use of an intraoperative CT scan or fluoroscopy is necessary to avoid the physes (see Fig. 137.1C).

More traditional transphyseal reconstruction techniques have also been used in skeletally immature athletes.[52,53] These techniques become more appropriate as the patient approaches skeletal maturity. Aronowitz et al.[52] and Kocher et al.[54] have shown that Tanner stage 3 athletes have little risk of angular deformity or leg length discrepancy. Shea et al.[55] used MRI of children's knees to show that drill holes could ideally affect less than 5% of the total volume of both the tibial and femoral physes and was central in the tibia but more peripheral in the femur, which was hypothesized to increase the risk of growth arrest.

Investigators in many older series relied on traditional transtibial tunnel drilling for transphyseal reconstructions. The more vertical tunnels used in these techniques may minimize physeal damage by producing a hole of a smaller aperture in the physis. However, the vertical graft position may not fully restore the normal kinematics of the knee and may be less "anatomic" by centering less graft in the anatomic ACL footprint. Independent femoral drilling techniques such as those using an accessory

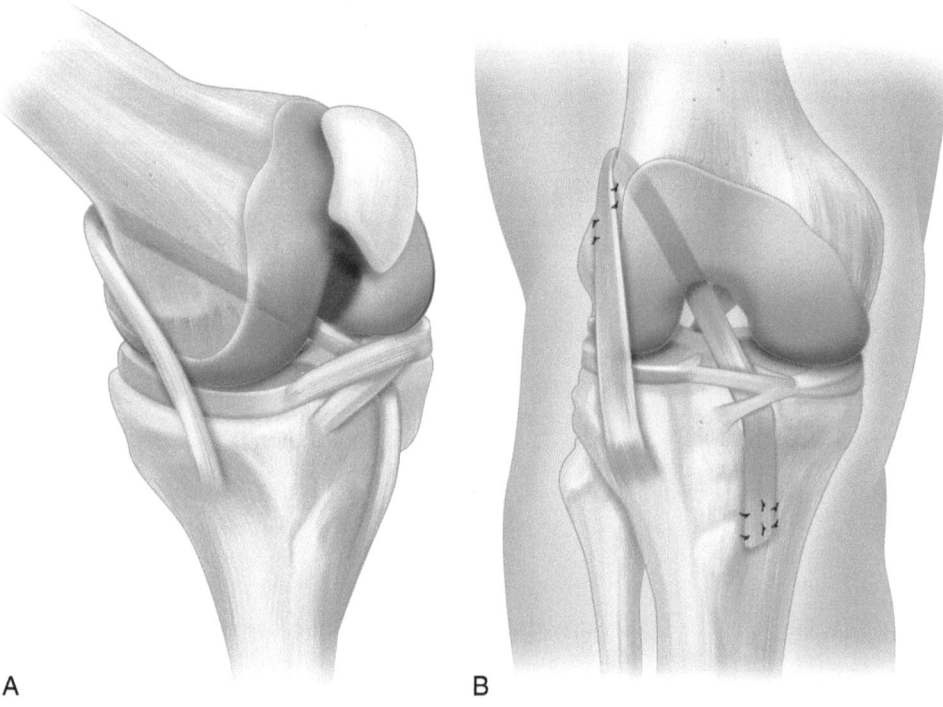

A   B

Fig. 137.3 (A and B) The iliotibial band graft is passed over the top of the lateral femoral condyle, through the knee, under the intermeniscal ligament, and into the groove in the proximal tibia. The graft is sutured to the lateral femoral condyle with the knee in 90 degrees of flexion and 15 degrees of external rotation. It is then sutured to the periosteum of the proximal tibia with the knee in 20 degrees of flexion. (From Scott WN, ed. *Insall and Scott Surgery of the Knee.* 5th ed. New York: Elsevier; 2012.)

medial portal, a two-incision technique, or a retrograde drilling outside-in technique have been advocated to place the femoral tunnel within the anatomic footprint.[56] In skeletally immature athletes with open physes, Nelson and Miller[57] have shown that the femoral tunnel produced by these drilling techniques crosses the lateral femoral physis obliquely and eccentrically and would potentially damage a much larger area of physis and perichondral ring than a more vertical, less anatomic tunnel. Given the increased risk of growth disturbance with these newer anatomic reconstruction techniques, an all-epiphyseal femoral tunnel combined with a traditional transphyseal tibial tunnel hybrid technique may be used (Fig. 137.4).[16,57] Recent anatomic studies have described anatomic and radiograph techniques for safer all epiphyseal femoral tunnel drilling.[58,59] Specifically, radiographic landmarks have been obtained to guide avoidance of the lateral collateral ligament complex on the lateral aspect of the femur using a lateral radiograph of the knee (Fig. 137.5).

Postoperative Management and Rehabilitation

Postoperative rehabilitation after ACL reconstruction in the skeletally immature athlete is similar to the approaches used in more mature athletes. It is generally recommended that postoperative rehabilitation be divided into phases with specific criteria for progression. Emphasis on attainment of these goals rather than a precise postoperative time frame allows adaptations to be made as needed for the skeletally immature athlete.

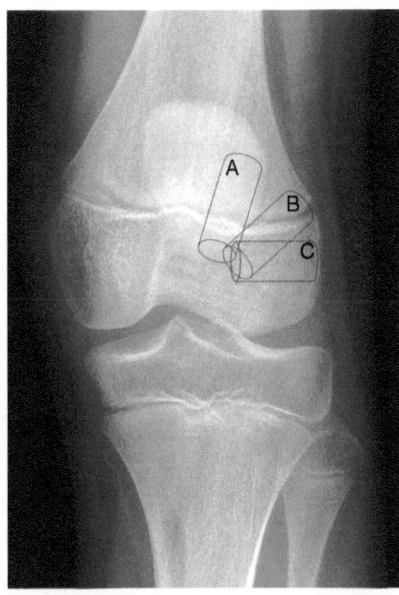

Fig. 137.4 Amount and location of femoral physis affected using different operative techniques. (A) The location of a vertically orientated tunnel, which affects less of the femoral physis but is typically outside the native anterior cruciate ligament (ACL) footprint. (B) The location of a classic anatomic accessory medial portal, or outside-in technique, that places the tunnel anatomically in the ACL footprint but affects a large portion of the distal femoral physis. (C) The location of a femoral tunnel, which is in the anatomic center of the ACL footprint within the epiphysis in a trajectory. It avoids the femoral physis. (From Milewski MD, Beck NA, Lawrence JT, et al. Anterior cruciate ligament reconstruction in the young athlete: a treatment algorithm for the skeletally immature. *Clin Sports Med.* 2011;30[4]:801–810.)

Authors' Preferred Technique

Anterior Cruciate Ligament Reconstruction

- Given the increased incidence of secondary injuries and less optimal outcomes with conservative or delayed reconstructive procedures in skeletally immature athletes, we attempt to schedule ACL reconstruction within the first 3–5 weeks after the injury.
- Elimination of effusion and regaining full ROM are preferred.
- Inability to gain full, painless ROM often denotes displaced meniscal fragments. In this case, earlier intervention is appropriate.
- Patients should be encouraged to use crutches until ambulation without a limp is achieved.
- Crutch use after ambulation without a limp is preferred to prevent meniscal injury.
- Our graft choice is uniformly hamstring autografts in these primary ACL reconstructions.
- Grafts smaller than 8 mm have been shown to have an increased rate of failure[60] and should be measured after pretensioning[61]; it is still controversial as to the minimum graft diameter in a skeletally immature population. Augmentation with allograft was popular but may have an increased failure rate.[62] Consideration for contralateral harvest or alternative graft sources (quadriceps vs. contralateral hamstring augmentation) can be considered.
- The determination of which physeal-respecting approach we use depends on the skeletal age of the patient and relative remaining growth as determined by a posteroanterior radiograph of the left hand.
- Our approach for prepubescent athletes is to perform an all-epiphyseal reconstruction with fixation performed with cortical button fixation. Combined intra-articular and extra-articular reconstruction that spares the physes can also be used in this population, especially if the patient's skeleton is very immature or the epiphysis is insufficient for adequate tunnel lengths.

- Use of fluoroscopy or an intraoperative CT scan is essential to ensure that femoral and tibial tunnels appropriately respect the femoral and tibial physes.
- Setting up the C-arm or intraoperative CT scanner before beginning the operation is helpful so that "real time" drilling with guidance can be performed.
- The proximal tibial epiphyseal tunnel should generally be at least 20 mm to attempt an all-epiphyseal ACL reconstruction to ensure an adequate length of graft in the tunnel for fixation and incorporation.
- Tibial and femoral drilling can be performed with a retrograde drill such as the FlipCutter, (Arthrex, Naples, FL) using fluoroscopic guidance.
- Placing a small-diameter Kirschner wire prior to drilling with the retrograde drill is useful to ensure that tunnel placement successfully avoids the physes. These drill systems are not cannulated, and thus the guidewire is removed prior to drilling.
- Fixation can be performed with interference screws as initially described or with loop fixation for both the femoral and tibial portions.[46]
- In pubescent patients, we perform a hybrid fixation with epiphyseal fixation on the femur and transphyseal drilling on the tibia and fixation distal to the tibial physis and apophysis.
- Fluoroscopy is again key to successfully avoiding the femoral physis. It can also be used to measure the distance from the tibial aperture to the tibial physis for appropriate tibial screw length.
- Tibial tunnel placement should be made as vertical as possible to minimize the aperture created in the physis.
- In late pubescent patients, fixation is performed with loop fixation on the femur and expansion devices on the tibia.
- Transphyseal femoral tunnels, when used, should attempt to cross the femoral physis as centrally as possible without jeopardizing the femoral tunnel footprint to lessen the possibility of differential physeal growth.

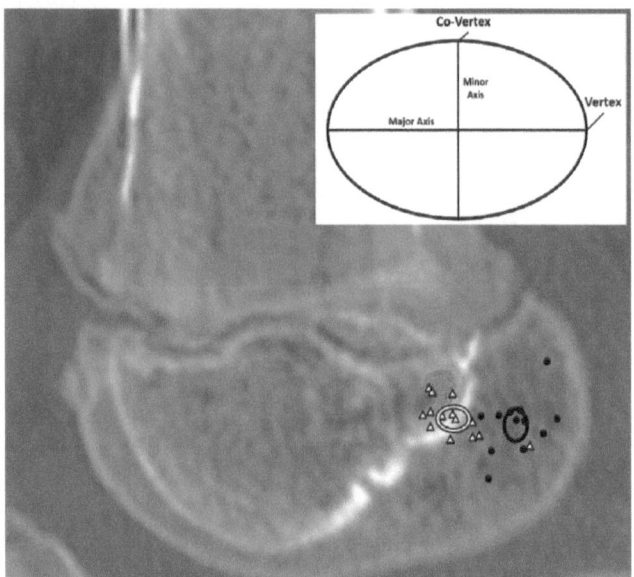

Fig. 137.5 The 95% confidence intervals and distribution of individual lateral collateral ligament *(white triangles)* and anterior cruciate ligament *(black circles)* origins. The inset shows the elliptical footprint orientation and terminology reference. (From Shea KG, Cannamela PC, Fabricant PD, et al. Lateral radiographic landmarks for ACL and LCL footprint origins during all-epiphyseal femoral drilling in skeletally immature knees. *J Bone Joint Surg Am.* 2017;99:506–511.)

The focus of the first phase of rehabilitation is to decrease postoperative impairments while protecting the patient and the surgical intervention. The value of postoperative bracing has been debated in the literature. Some benefits may include less pain, fewer complications due to postoperative effusion, and prevention of knee flexion contractions during the early phases of rehabilitation; however, no long-term benefits have been demonstrated with regard to ROM, joint laxity, patient-reported outcomes, or functional outcomes.[63,64] During this phase, immediate ROM with an emphasis on knee extension is recommended to decrease pain, minimize patellofemoral complications, and reduce arthrofibrosis.[65] A review by Beynnon et al.[63] suggests that immediate weight bearing after ACL reconstruction is not detrimental to the graft and may decrease anterior knee pain. Goals for this phase are to decrease pain and joint effusion, obtain full knee extension and 90 degrees of knee flexion, and restore patella mobility and volitional quadriceps activation.[66,67] Attainment of these goals indicates the athlete is ready to progress to the next phase of rehabilitation.

The goals of the second postoperative phase are to eliminate pain and effusion, progress toward full knee flexion, restore normal ambulation, improve proprioception, and progress strengthening of quadriceps and hamstrings.[66,67] To obtain significant improvements in knee strength and overall function, strengthening exercises should be performed both in the open and closed kinetic chain position.[68] Multiple studies have supported that open kinetic chain knee extension exercises initiated early on in the rehabilitation program increase strength and minimize patellofemoral joint stress while allowing for protection of the graft when performed isotonically between the range of 90 and 40 degrees of knee flexion and isometrically at 90, 60, or 0 degrees of knee flexion.[65,69–75]

Closed kinetic chain strengthening exercises should be implemented as dictated by weight-bearing status, pain level, and available ROM. Closed kinetic chain exercises not only assist in strengthening but are functional and emphasize cocontraction and neuromuscular control. Early on in the rehabilitation program, knee flexion ROM should be limited to between 0 and 60 degrees during closed chain strengthening, to decrease stress placed on the ACL graft and patellofemoral joint.[65,71,73] After postoperative week 9 the knee flexion ROM for both open and closed chain strengthening can progress due to increased tensile strength of the graft.[65]

Postoperative rehabilitation should incorporate strengthening and neuromuscular control to allow the patient to initiate running and plyometric training during the third phase.[66,67] Emphasis should be placed on strengthening and neuromuscular training of the hip and core of athletes after ACL reconstruction. Impairments in transverse plane hip motions, frontal plane knee motions, and trunk displacement have been attributed to increased risk of ACL injury, especially in female athletes.[76–80] Injury prevention training with a focus on strengthening and lower extremity alignment has demonstrated improvements in hip and knee kinematics in female athletes.[81]

Return to play (RTP) is not based on one specific criterion but instead on a constellation of criteria including ROM, proprioception, functional strength, and knee/graft stability.[82] In the adult population, it is recommended that athletes return to sport when hop tests and strength of hamstrings and quadriceps are 85% of the noninvolved limb and when the calculated hamstring to quadriceps ratio is less than 15% compared with the noninvolved limb.[65,83] Passing specific functional return to sport criteria decreases the risk of graft rupture after return to sport.[84] In general, most skeletally immature athletes are able to return to sports approximately 6 to 12 months after undergoing their reconstruction. Although there is no convincing evidence to support the use of functional bracing for return to sport following ACL reconstruction, some authors have advocated for the benefit of bracing after combined extra-articular and intra-articular iliotibial extraphyseal reconstruction has been performed.[63,85]

Complications

The most serious complications of ACL injuries and reconstructions in skeletally immature patients are those associated with growth disturbances. Findings of animal studies and anecdotal reports of human growth disturbances demonstrate that these concerns are valid. The possibility of growth disturbance, including the possibility of angular deformity, leg length discrepancy, and overgrowth, needs to be fully disclosed and discussed with patients and their families. The appropriate approach then needs to chosen given the patient's skeletal age, and long-term follow-up is necessary to watch for the earliest signs of any growth disturbance, including use of long leg mechanical axis radiographs until skeletal maturity is achieved.

Future Direction

The increased incidence of ACL injuries in skeletally immature athletes has increased the need to look deeper into the issues surrounding this devastating injury. The most important questions that need to be studied and answered are the long-term outcome with regard to function and arthritic conditions of the different techniques.

MENISCAL INJURIES

The incidence of meniscal tears in skeletally immature athletes has been increasing,[86] likely because of improved awareness by sports medicine providers, increased youth sports participation, and increased use of advanced imaging such as MRI. Identifying and treating these meniscal injuries in young athletes is crucial to maintaining normal joint mechanics and preserving and protecting articular cartilage. Preserving as much of the meniscus as possible is crucial, especially in the adolescent athlete, because of the long-term consequences of aggressive débridement.[87]

Development

The meniscus forms by 8 weeks of embryologic development (Fig. 137.6). By week 14 it has a normal anatomic appearance.[88] The entire meniscus is vascularized during the fetal period, but this vascularization gradually recedes by age 9 months, with the central third already avascular at this point in development.[89] By 10 years of age, the meniscus has developed its adult structure, with only the peripheral 10% to 30% of the medial meniscus and only the peripheral 10% to 25% of the lateral meniscus receiving a direct vascular supply.[90]

Anatomy

The meniscus consists of type I collagen fibers that are arranged in a circumferential pattern parallel to its long axis with radial,

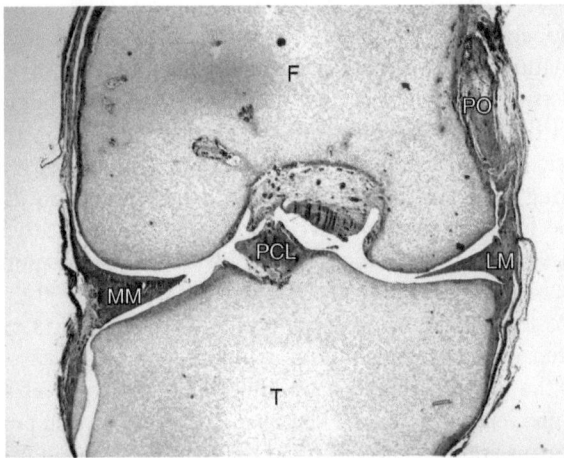

Fig. 137.6 Fetus HK24F, 12.5 weeks old, frontal section (see text). *F*, Femur; *LM*, lateral meniscus; *MM*, medial meniscus; *PCL*, posterior cruciate ligament; *PO*, popliteus muscle; *T*, tibia. (Goldner, ×20.) (From Scott WN, ed. *Insall and Scott Surgery of the Knee.* 5th ed. New York: Elsevier; 2012.)

oblique, and vertical fibers that reduce hoop stresses.[91] Inferior meniscal surfaces are flat, whereas the superior surfaces are concave. This shape allows for conformity of the femoral condyles with the tibial plateau surfaces. The meniscus is thus able to increase contact area and congruency, thereby reducing contact stresses and aiding in shock absorption. The medial meniscus is C-shaped; it covers approximately 50% of the medial tibial plateau and attaches to the medial joint capsule by the meniscotibial and coronary ligaments. It is able to translate approximately 2.5 mm posteriorly with femoral rollback during knee flexion. The lateral meniscus is circular, covering approximately 70% of the lateral tibial plateau. There are no attachments to the capsule at the popliteal hiatus, and the lateral meniscus translates 9 to 11 mm with knee flexion.[91,92] The ligaments of Humphrey and Wrisberg are accessory meniscofemoral ligaments that are present in up to 84% of people.[93]

History and Physical Examination

In adolescents, nondiscoid meniscus injuries are usually a result of trauma during sports and typically involve a twisting injury or directional change. Pain is usually the chief complaint, but effusion, giving way, and mechanical symptoms such as snapping, catching, and locking also may be present. In one study, meniscal tears were found in 47% of preadolescents (aged 7 to 12 years) and 45% of adolescents (aged 13 to 18 years) with an acute traumatic knee hemathrosis.[8] In both age groups the authors found that the medial meniscus was most commonly injured (70% in preadolescents and 88% in adolescents). A possible ACL tear should always be suspected in this population because 36% of the adolescents in this series with meniscal injuries also had an ACL tear.

On examination, effusion is usually indicative of intra-articular pathologic conditions in this age group. Skeletally immature athletes with meniscal injuries often have joint line tenderness on palpation. It is sometimes difficult to examine children with a painful knee, and they might not tolerate full ROM. One option is to use a modified McMurray maneuver, which involves pain with rotational varus or valgus stress at 30 to 40 degrees of knee flexion. It is always important to check ACL integrity with a Lachman test and compare it with the contralateral side because a high correlation exists with meniscus disease. The Lachman test is a reliable indicator of ACL injury. KT-1000 measurements were found to be increased in younger patients when measuring anterior tibial translation.[94] When physical examination was performed by experienced examiners, Kocher et al.[95] found that it was 62% sensitive and 81% specific for medial meniscus tears and 50% sensitive and 89% specific for lateral meniscus tears.

Imaging

Initial workup should include standard AP, lateral, tunnel, and sunrise radiographic views. These views are helpful in detecting patellar dislocation, osteochondral fractures, physeal fractures, and loose bodies. The tunnel view is included to evaluate for OCD. The sunrise view may show patellar subluxation.

When the history and physical examination are suggestive of a meniscal tear and radiographs are normal, an MRI is usually ordered. Compared with adults, MRI in children has lower sensitivity and specificity in assessing meniscus tears because of the higher vascularity of a child's meniscus, which appears as intrameniscal enhancement, resembling meniscal tears.[96] Children younger than 12 years were found to have 62% sensitivity and 78% specificity compared with 90% sensitivity and 96% specificity in children between the ages of 12 and 16 years.[95] When evaluating an MRI for a meniscal tear, one should look for the enhancement to extend to the superior or inferior articular surfaces of the meniscus.

Decision-Making Principles

The basic principle in the treatment of meniscal injuries in children and adolescents is to preserve as much meniscal tissue as possible to minimize subsequent articular cartilage degeneration. The developing meniscus has an increased potential for healing because of its increased vascularity. When the history, physical examination, and imaging are consistent with meniscal injury and appropriate conservative options have been tried or considered, then surgery can be recommended in the skeletally immature patient.

Treatment Options

Nonoperative

After a meniscal injury is confirmed, initial management with conservative treatment including rest, activity modification, physical therapy for strengthening, and possible bracing can be considered. This approach is usually recommended for patients without mechanical symptoms or with imaging findings that are inconclusive or indeterminate. If the patient remains asymptomatic, then initial nonsurgical management can be continued.

Operative

Symptomatic meniscal tears in children and adolescents that have failed to respond to conservative treatment are usually treated surgically. Longitudinal tears in the red-red zone that measure 10 mm or less and are manually displaceable less than 3 mm may heal without repair.[97] Arthroscopic partial meniscectomy is most commonly performed but does produce increased contact stresses. Cadaver studies showed a 65% increase in contact stress when removing small bucket-handle medial meniscus tears. Débridement of the posterior horn of the medial meniscus can increase contact stresses almost to the level of a total meniscectomy, which is 235% of normal.[98] Authors of one study with a 5.5-year follow-up in 20 patients, with an average age of 15 years old, who underwent partial or total meniscectomy found that 75% were still symptomatic, 80% had radiographic evidence of osteoarthritis, and 60% were dissatisfied with their results.[87] At 10- to 20-year follow-up, 50% of patients who underwent a total meniscectomy had evidence of osteoarthritis based on radiographic evidence, symptoms, and functional loss.[99] Current indications for a partial meniscectomy in the skeletally immature athlete include irreparable meniscal tears such as radial tears, horizontal cleavage tears, and a complex degenerative tear in the white-white zone. It is preferred that as limited a partial meniscectomy as possible be performed for a damaged, unstable meniscus. A total meniscectomy is contraindicated.

Many meniscus tears in skeletally immature patients can be repaired. The types of tears most amenable to repair include longitudinal tears in the red-red zone or red-white zone, bucket-handle tears without significant injury to the bucket-handle fragment, and lateral meniscus posterior horn tears, which have a good vascular supply. All techniques first require débridement of loose degenerative edges and rasping of the perimeniscal synovial edges or trephination into the peripheral zone to promote vascular inflow to the repair site. The inside-out vertical mattress suture technique is still considered the "gold standard." It uses absorbable or nonabsorbable suture with flexible needles that are placed through the meniscus in vertical or horizontal fashion and are tied down over the capsule through a separate incision. When repairing posterior horn tears, a posterolateral or posteromedial approach must be made to protect the posterior neurovascular structures with retractors. An outside-in technique is often helpful for isolated anterior horn tears or anterior portions of bucket-handle tears. If needed, open repairs can be performed through either posterolateral or posteromedial incisions for peripheral tears and are useful for posterior horn medial meniscal tears in patients with tight medial compartments.[100] All-inside techniques have gained popularity again. Previously, these techniques included use of devices such as darts, arrows, and screws to anchor the meniscal tear to the capsule or peripheral meniscus. Unfortunately, they did not have the ability to compress across the tear site. A recent meta-analysis suggests a higher failure rate of all-inside devices compared with traditional inside-out repairs in the setting of ACL reconstruction.[101] Newer repair systems are suture based and provide the ability to compress at the tear site. More contemporary data will be needed to compare these newer generation devices with inside out repairs at mid to long term.

Postoperative Management

Postoperative management after meniscal surgery in skeletally immature patients is similar to management in adults, with the understanding that both the young athlete and his or her family must be thoroughly informed of the expectations for activity restriction and rehabilitation after surgery. If bracing, weight-bearing restrictions, or specific rehabilitation protocols will need to be followed postoperatively, improved compliance will be achieved if both the patient and family are counseled appropriately before surgery.

Postoperative protocols are typically separated into meniscal repair and transplantation or meniscectomy. It is essential that the physical therapist be informed of the type of surgical intervention performed because variations in postoperative protocols are made according to the type, location, and size of the meniscal injury.[102] Concomitant procedures such as ligamentous reconstructions or comorbidities such as articular cartilage damage also affect the potential for rehabilitation and the plan of care.[102]

Following partial meniscectomies, most surgeons allow immediate weight bearing as tolerated with the use of axillary crutches, due to the postoperative sequelae of effusion and quadriceps inhibition. Rehabilitation after a meniscectomy can progress as tolerated with the initial goals of eliminating pain and effusion, attaining knee ROM of 0 to 90 degrees with good patellar mobility, ambulating without an antalgic gait, and regaining volitional neuromuscular control of the lower extremity. Full and painless knee ROM should be obtained approximately 6 weeks after the operation.[102] Ongoing rehabilitation should emphasize strengthening of the lower extremities while progressing toward return to the previous level of function by the third postoperative month.

Depending upon the surgical technique and location of isolated meniscal repairs, many surgeons restrict weight bearing for 4 to 8 weeks and restrict ROM using a hinged knee brace for 4 to 6 weeks to minimize joint compressive and shear forces.[102] The initial phases of rehabilitation emphasize decreasing pain and swelling, improving ROM, and regaining volitional quadriceps activation while protecting the surgical repair. Therapeutic exercises and neuromuscular training should progress in a manner consistent with postoperative ROM and weight-bearing guidelines. The range of knee excursion for open and closed kinetic chain exercises will be restricted to minimize stress to the meniscal repair and the patellofemoral joint.

Return to sport after isolated meniscal repair is generally allowed 4 to 6 months after the operation if the young athlete has regained full ROM and adequate strength and remains asymptomatic during functional activities.[102] Regardless of the type of surgical intervention, patients should be monitored for pain in the tibiofemoral compartment, painful clicking at the knee, lack of progress with ROM, decreased patellar mobility, or persistent joint effusion.[102]

Results

The results of partial or total meniscectomies in children and adolescents are poor, with early onset of osteoarthritis.[87,98] Although increased success rates are associated with meniscal repairs in younger patients, few long-term outcome studies have been performed regarding meniscal repair in this age group. In one series of 29 arthroscopic meniscal repairs in 26 patients with a mean age of 15.3 years, no meniscal symptoms were noted at an average of 5 years of follow-up, and 24 of 26 patients returned to their preinjury level of sports activity. Of note, 15 of 26 patients had a simultaneous ACL reconstruction, all the tears were in the posterior horn of either the medial or lateral meniscus, and 22 of the 29 tears were in the red-red zone. The mean time between injury and surgery was 6.7 months. Twenty-five repairs were performed with the inside-out technique, and four were performed with an all-inside technique.[103] In another series of 71 meniscal repairs in adolescents with a mean age of 16 years, clinical healing was seen in 75% at a mean 51-month follow-up. All tears extended into the avascular white-white zone and were repaired with use of an inside-out technique. In patients undergoing a simultaneous ACL reconstruction, the success rate was even higher at 87%. Given the increased healing rate of meniscal tears in the setting of ACL reconstruction, many advocate for

marrow stimulation techniques in the setting of an isolated meniscal repair to augment healing.[104] Failure rates in patients with marrow stimulation to augment their isolated meniscal repairs are similar to those undergoing concomitant ACL reconstruction.[104]

Complications

Complications from arthroscopic partial or total meniscectomy or meniscal repair are rare but may include painful neuroma, arthrofibrosis, complex regional pain syndrome, and iatrogenic chondral injury from the surgery or from a protruding implant.

Future Considerations

Although short-term and midterm results are encouraging for meniscal repair, especially in the setting of simultaneous ACL reconstruction, long-term results are needed to determine if newer techniques for meniscal preservation are successful in decreasing the risk of osteoarthritis in the future for these skeletally immature athletes.

DISCOID MENISCUS

The discoid meniscus was first described by Young in 1887 after cadaveric dissection. It is almost exclusively found in the lateral meniscus and, in some studies, has been shown to have a higher prevalence of approximately 15% in Asian populations; however, it has a prevalence of only 3% to 5% in the US population.[105] Approximately 20% of patients with a discoid meniscus have bilateral discoid menisci. The true prevalence of discoid menisci is unknown because many discoid menisci are asymptomatic.

Discoid menisci generally occupy greater than normal coverage of the lateral tibial plateau and are uniformly thickened. They can represent a spectrum of meniscal morphologic features and stability. Discoid menisci are thought to be a congenital anomaly because menisci are not discoid shaped during development. Increased meniscal thickness and width may also be due to compensatory changes for an unstable meniscus during development.[106]

Classification

The Watanabe classification system is most commonly used (Fig. 137.7).[107] This classification system describes three types of discoid meniscus based on arthroscopic appearance and stability of the meniscus. Type I (stable, complete) menisci are stable to probing and complete; the meniscus is block shaped and covers the entire lateral tibial plateau. Type II (stable, incomplete) menisci cover 80% or less of the tibial plateau. Type III menisci, also known as the Wrisberg variant (unstable), have a thickened posterior horn but otherwise appear normal. They lack posterior meniscal attachments with the exception of the meniscofemoral ligament of Wrisberg, which causes the lateral meniscus to have posterior horn hypermobility. When the knee goes into extension, the posterior horn can be pulled into the intercondylar notch and can result in snapping knee syndrome. Klingele et al.[108] examined peripheral rim instability patterns of

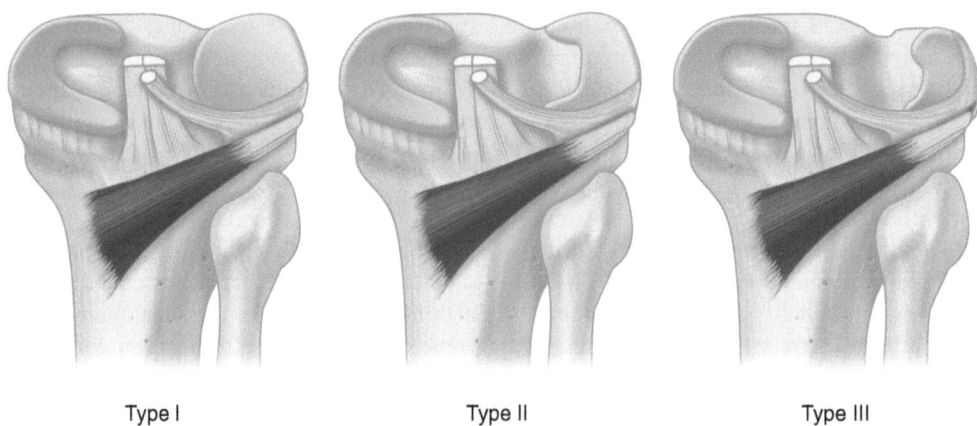

Type I   Type II   Type III

Fig. 137.7 Watanabe classification of discoid lateral meniscus. Type I is a complete variant, type II is a partial variant, and type III is a Wrisberg variant. (From Scott WN, ed. *Insall and Scott Surgery of the Knee*. 5th ed. New York: Elsevier; 2012.)

128 discoid menisci. They found that 62.1% were complete and 37.9% were incomplete. Peripheral rim instability was found in 28.1%, of which 47.2% occurred in the anterior horn, 38.9% in the posterior horn, and 11.1% in the middle third. Peripheral instability was more common in younger patients, with a mean age of 8.2 years, and in patients with complete discoid lateral menisci.

History and Physical Examination

The clinical presentation of a discoid meniscus may vary. Stable discoid menisci usually are first noticed in older children who present with mechanical knee symptoms similar to those of a meniscal tear. These stable menisci are prone to tearing because of increased thickness and abnormal vascularity.[89] Compared with normal menisci, discoid menisci have also been shown on transmission electron microscopy to have a decreased number of collagen fibers with a more disorganized pattern.[109] Discoid menisci without an associated tear are often asymptomatic and are often found incidentally on MRI or during knee arthroscopy.

Children with unstable discoid menisci often present with intermittent snapping and popping within the knee. This phenomenon is called "snapping knee syndrome" and usually occurs when the knee is brought from flexion to extension; it may cause pain and apprehension.[110] Unstable discoid menisci are usually found in younger patients with a Wrisberg type I discoid-appearing morphology, in which the meniscus is a solid block covering the entire tibial plateau.[108]

Physical examination findings can include joint effusion, limited motion, terminal extension discomfort, a lateral joint line bulge, joint line tenderness to palpation, and pain or popping during the McMurray test. This popping during the McMurray test is a result of subluxation of the unstable lateral meniscus. Very often a lack of terminal extension mimicking a knee flexion contracture is present in children with discoid menisci. It is always important to examine and assess the symptom history of the contralateral knee as well because of the high rate of bilateral discoid menisci.

Imaging

Standard knee radiographs are normal in most children with discoid menisci, but some radiographs occasionally indicate subtle findings, such as squaring of the lateral femoral condyle, a widened lateral joint line, cupping of the lateral tibial plateau, and mild hypoplasia of the tibial spine.

MRI is the radiographic study of choice for diagnosing a discoid meniscus. The diagnosis is made if the transverse meniscal diameter is greater than 15 mm or 20% of the tibial width on coronal views, or if continuity of the anterior and posterior horns of the lateral meniscus is seen on three or more consecutive sagittal images of 5-mm thickness.[111,112] Types II (incomplete) and III (Wrisberg variant) discoid menisci may appear normal on MRI. However, type III discoid menisci may appear to have some minimal posterior horn anterior subluxation or have a high signal on T2-weighted images between the lateral meniscus and joint capsule, resembling a peripheral tear appearance.[113] MRI has been shown to have low sensitivity (38.9%) in diagnosing a discoid lateral meniscus in children compared with an 88.9% sensitivity of physical examination.[114]

Decision-Making Principles

If a discoid meniscus is asymptomatic and found incidentally, it should be treated with observation. The knee is functioning well and may have adapted to this abnormal anatomy. Surgery is indicated in patients with symptomatic discoid menisci for whom conservative management has failed, similar to the management of normal meniscal tears. This surgical indication includes discoid menisci with or without an associated tear as defined on MRI.

Treatment Options

After it has been decided that a symptomatic discoid meniscus will be managed arthroscopically, the first issue to address is the size. This issue is addressed with a partial meniscectomy, also called *saucerization*. Saucerization is performed to create a stable and functional remaining meniscus that will provide adequate shock absorption. A minimum of 6 to 8 mm of the peripheral rim is left intact. Larger peripheral rims have been shown to have higher repeat tear rates.[115] This remnant peripheral rim may be thicker than a normal meniscus and may require an undersurface débridement to recreate a more normal structure.

If peripheral instability occurs after saucerization, meniscal repair to the capsule is performed. Meniscal tears after saucerization are repaired in the same fashion as a nondiscoid meniscus tear. Remaining tears that cannot be repaired undergo débridement to a stable rim. If a horizontal cleavage tear remains, the unstable leaflet is usually débrided.

A total meniscectomy is rarely performed in children and adolescents; it is generally reserved for only the most difficult of unsalvageable cases.

Postoperative Management

Postoperative management is similar to that of other pathologic meniscal conditions. Following saucerization alone, immediate weight bearing and ROM are allowed as tolerated.[116] It is crucial to work on extension exercises immediately because many of these patients have long-standing terminal extension limitations from their chronic discoid meniscus. Patients who undergo saucerization and meniscal repair are placed in a hinged knee brace with restricted ROM between 0 and 90 degrees and limited weight bearing for 6 weeks.[116] Return to sports is generally allowed approximately 4 months after the surgical procedure is performed.

Results

A total meniscectomy was traditionally used for the treatment of symptomatic discoid menisci, and although this approach is no longer recommended, the long-term results have been reported with mixed findings. Habata et al.[117] and Okazaki et al.[118] found excellent functional scores with minimal radiographic changes after a total meniscectomy at 14- to 16-year follow-up. It has been suggested that young patients adapt to increased articular cartilage stress after meniscectomy. Authors of another study examined 17 knees in children with a mean age of 9 years who were treated with a total meniscectomy.[119] They found that 10 knees had clinical symptoms and radiographic changes of lateral compartment arthritis at 19.8-year follow-up. Two of the knees had lateral femoral condyle OCD lesions. Authors of another study compared long-term clinical and radiographic outcomes in a series of 125 complete and incomplete discoid menisci managed with partial or total meniscectomy.[120] They found better radiographic results at 5-year follow-up with partial meniscectomy. The long-term prognosis was based on the volume of removed meniscus.

Saucerization has become more accepted as standard treatment for discoid menisci. Short-term and midterm results of this treatment have been reported. In a retrospective review, authors looked at 11 knees in children with a mean age of 11.5 years who were treated with arthroscopic saucerization for their discoid menisci.[121] At 4.5-year follow-up, all patients had good to excellent clinical results with no radiographic degenerative changes. Authors of another study looked at 27 consecutive discoid menisci in children with a mean age of 10.1 years who were treated with saucerization and repair.[122] Prior to repair, they found that 77% of the discoid menisci were unstable, with anterior horn instability being most common. At 3.1-year follow-up, 21 patients had excellent clinical results and 3 patients reported residual knee pain. In patients undergoing saucerization, smaller meniscal width (<5 mm) and the amount of meniscal extrusion postoperatively are correlated with degenerative change at a mean 39 months postoperatively.[123] Although midterm results are encouraging, long-term results to demonstrate whether saucerization can prevent the development of clinical and radiographic osteoarthritis are still lacking.

Patients who have undergone a total meniscectomy may be candidates for meniscal transplantation. In a cadaveric study of nondiscoid knees, a total lateral meniscectomy was found to decrease the total contact area by 45% to 50% and increase peak local contact pressure by 235% to 335%.[124] Even though the discoid knee has some anatomic and biomechanical differences compared with the nondiscoid knee, these changes are quite significant and should be considered when contemplating meniscal transplantation after a total meniscectomy. A meniscal transplantation may increase the total contact area and decrease the peak local contact pressure. In a study of 14 patients who underwent meniscal allograft transplantation after a previous total meniscectomy for a torn discoid lateral meniscus, Lysholm knee scores improved from 71.4 to 91.4 at a mean 4.8-year follow-up.[125] Only one allograft tear was observed in six second-look arthroscopies. Similarly, in 36 patients aged 12 to 16, meniscal transplantation improved patients' subjective knee symptoms and had only a 6% reoperation rate for meniscal intervention, with no transplant failures.[126] These midterm results are encouraging.

Complications

Complications related to arthroscopic treatment of discoid menisci are similar to those of normal menisci. Perhaps most concerning are the risks of late arthritis, especially in patients with total or subtotal meniscectomies. A higher rate of retearing of the abnormal discoid meniscus tissue may be expected compared with normal menisci. In addition, an association of lateral femoral condyle OCD lesions has been reported with discoid menisci after meniscectomy.

Although it is not a complication, sports medicine providers should be aware of the high rate of bilateral discoid menisci. Patel et al.[127] recently reported on children with symptomatic bilateral discoid menisci compared with children who had bilateral discoid menisci, only one of which was symptomatic. They found that patients younger than 12 years and those with complete or Wrisberg-type menisci were more likely to have symptoms and require surgical treatment for their contralateral discoid menisci.

Future Considerations

The increasing understanding of the pathogenesis of the discoid meniscus has led to debate regarding the treatment of stable asymptomatic discoid menisci. Traditionally these menisci are managed with observation; however, prophylactic débridement may possibly prevent symptoms, instability, or future tears. In addition, long-term results are needed to address the risks of arthritis in the lateral compartment when counseling patients who have undergone meniscal saucerization with or without repair.

PATELLAR INSTABILITY

Patellar instability affects approximately 43 of 100,000 children.[128] It has been generally accepted that it is easier to return to sport after a patellar instability episode compared with other knee ligamentous injuries or instability in other joints such as the glenohumeral joint. However, Atkin et al.[129] demonstrated that only 66% of athletes were able to return to sport after patellar instability and 50% had some degree of limitation at 6-month follow-up. The rate of redislocation is high in pediatric and adolescent populations. Buchner et al.[130] showed that patients younger than 15 years had a 52% redislocation rate versus a 25% rate for the entire cohort. Cash and Hughston[131] found a 60% redislocation rate in younger adolescents aged 11 to 14 years versus a 33% rate for older adolescents aged 15 to 18 years. Authors of one study found a higher dislocation rate in women, but subsequent meta-analysis has shown no real sex predilection.[132] A family history of patellar instability has been shown to be a major risk factor for repeat dislocation in patients with a previous dislocation.[129,133] In a recent long-term follow-up study, patients with patellar instability had a 50% incidence of patella femoral arthritis at 25 years follow-up, which was worse in patients with recurrent dislocations and chondral injuries.[134] This suggests that prevention of recurrent instability may be important for the long-term health of the joint.

Embryology

The patella develops during the seventh week of gestation but does not begin to ossify until age 4 to 6 years.[135] The patellar facets and trochlear sulcus are well formed in neonates but become more evident as the cartilage thins with age on both the patella and trochlea. The cartilaginous sulcus has been shown to measure between 134 and 155 degrees and remain consistent through development, but the osseous sulcus angle is inversely proportional to age (Fig. 137.8).[128]

Pathoanatomy and Risk Factors

Multiple anatomic factors and potential genetic predilection can lead to the risk for recurrent patellar instability in young athletes. These factors include family history; patellar alta; trochlear dysplasia; increased anatomic Q angle; increased tibial tubercle–trochlear groove distance; medial patellofemoral ligament (MPFL) insufficiency; vastus medialis oblique (VMO) hypoplasia; contractures of the lateral knee structures, including the lateral retinaculum, iliotibial band, and rectus and vastus lateralis; femoral anteversion; tibial external torsion; genu valgum; and possibly excessive foot pronation.

History and Physical Examination

Young patients who have had an episode (or episodes) of patellar instability often provide a more vague description of their symptoms than do adult patients. Very often, young patients report

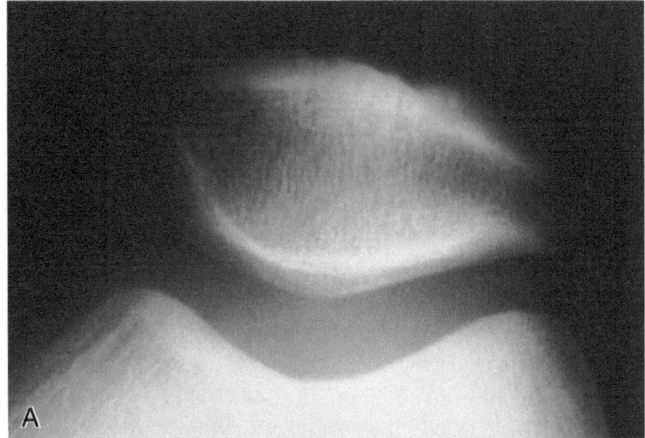

Fig. 137.8 Sunrise view of the patellofemoral joint in an adult man (A) and an 8-year-old boy (B). (From Hinton RY, Sharma KM. Acute and recurrent patellar instability in the young athlete. *Orthop Clin North Am.* 2003;34:385–396.)

that "my knee dislocated" or provide a history very similar to that of an ACL injury, reporting that they twisted, heard or felt a "pop," and had immediate pain and swelling. If they report a true patellar dislocation on a field of play, it is important to ask if a reduction was required or performed on the field or at a local emergency department. It is also important to assess if they have a history of patellar subluxation or dislocation or if a family history of this entity exists. Mechanical symptoms after such an event including locking, popping, and catching can be indicative of a loose body. A history of prior knee pain is especially important to consider, including anterior knee pain and pain when using stairs and squatting, for example. These young athletes should also be assessed for contralateral knee pain or instability symptoms. Awareness of a history of joint hyperlaxity is useful when assessing these patients.

When examining a young athlete either after a frank patellar dislocation or when chronic patellar instability is present, it is important to assess for signs of an effusion or hemarthrosis. Quadriceps girth or size should be assessed compared with the contralateral side, especially in the area of the VMO. A full knee examination as previously outlined should be performed to check for associated ligament injury, joint line tenderness, and meniscal signs. Specific to assessment of the patellofemoral joint, a patellar apprehension test should be performed to assess for subjective instability. Patellar glide and tilt tests should be performed to assess for increased lateral translation and increased lateral retinacular tightness, respectively. As knee ROM is assessed, patellar tracking should also be assessed. The presence of a J-sign is indicative of patellar instability. The patient's overall lower extremity alignment should also be assessed specifically for the Q angle and for femoral anteversion, external tibial torsion, and pes planovalgus.

Imaging

Standard radiographs should be obtained, including standing AP, lateral, notch, and Merchant views. The lateral radiograph should be assessed for patellar alta, which is a risk factor for patellar instability. The Insall-Salvati ratio is difficult to use in pediatric patients because portions of the patella and tibial tubercle are still cartilaginous. Instead, the Blackburn-Peel method can be used, or the Koshino method can be used in pediatric patients to assess patellar height (Fig. 137.9).[136,137] AP, lateral, and Merchant views can be assessed for signs of patellar fracture, sleeve avulsions, or patellar or femoral osteochondral fracture. However, radiographs have been shown to detect only 23% of osteochondral injuries.[138]

MRI is useful in assessing patients after a patellar instability episode for several reasons. It has been shown to be 85% sensitive and 70% accurate in detecting an MPFL injury.[139,140] MRI can determine the location and extent of an osteochondral injury, along with the site of MPFL disruption. A typical bone bruise pattern can be seen after patellar dislocation with edema under the medial patellar facet and along the midportion of the lateral femoral condyle.

Decision-Making Principles

Patellar instability can be a tremendously challenging problem for skeletally immature athletes, parents, and sports medicine providers. First, the scope of the patient's patellar instability needs to be assessed, and it should be determined whether the instability is acute and traumatic or chronic and atraumatic. Second, the presence of an osteochondral fracture or cartilaginous loose body should be assessed both by the history of mechanical symptoms, physical examination, and potentially advanced imaging. In skeletally immature first-time patellar dislocations, there is more commonly a patellar chondral injury and patellar-sided MPFL injury.[141] The presence of a loose body might necessitate earlier surgical intervention. In addition to assessing the knee for signs of patellar instability, the entire patient needs to be considered in terms of risk factors for patellar instability, including patella alta, a shallow trochlear groove and trochlear dysplasia, MPFL injury, patellar tilt, valgus knee alignment, femoral anteversion, external tibial torsion, pes planovalgus, and hypoplastic tibial tubercles. A recent economic model reported that both initial nonoperative and initial operative management were cost effective in the treatment of adolescent first-time dislocators but initial operative management led to the greatest increase in quality-adjusted life years at 10 years after injury.[142]

Treatment Options
Nonoperative Management

Conservative treatment of a first-time patellar dislocation without mechanical symptoms indicative of a loose body is standard. Some controversy exists regarding the issue of whether immobilization should be used immediately after a dislocation. Maenpaa and

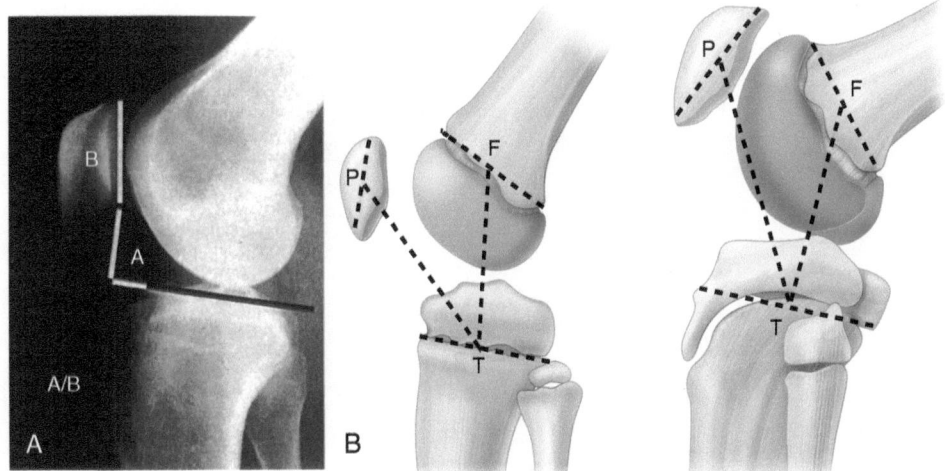

Fig. 137.9 (A) The Blackburne-Peel ratio *(A/B)* compares the perpendicular distance from the lower articular margin of the patella to the tibial plateau *(A)* and the length of the articular surface of the patella *(B)*. (B) The Koshino index *(PT/FT)* compares the patellar-tibial *(PT)* distance between the midpoint of the patella *(P)* and the midpoint of the proximal tibia at the physis *(T)* with the femoral-tibial *(FT)* distance between the midpoint of the femur at the physis *(F)* and the midpoint of the proximal tibia at the physis *(T)*. ([A] From Blackburne JS, Peel TE. A new method of measuring patellar height. *J Bone Joint Surg Br.* 1977;59:241–242; and Scott WN, ed. *Insall and Scott Surgery of the Knee.* 5th ed. New York: Elsevier; 2012. [B] From Koshino T, Sigimoto K. New measurement of patellar height in the knees of children using the epiphyseal line midpoint. *J Pediatr Orthop.* 1989;9:216–218.)

Lehto[143] reported a dislocation rate that was three times higher with immediate mobilization compared with initial immobilization. In general, most sports medicine providers immobilize the knee for several weeks followed by gradual mobilization. A hinged knee brace, often with a lateral buttress for patellar stabilization, can be used until full painless ROM is possible. Physical therapy is recommended to assist initially with regaining ROM, soft tissue swelling mobilization, quadriceps strengthening (especially focusing on the VMO), electrical stimulation for VMO activation, and patellar taping. McConnell taping has been shown to decrease pain and increase quadriceps activity during rehabilitation, despite perhaps not truly medializing the patella.[144,145] In addition, functional exercise incorporating the entire lower extremity kinetic chain including core and hip stability should be integrated in the rehabilitation program because these forces may be important in controlling patellofemoral stability and pain.[146] Later stages of rehabilitation focus on continued quadriceps strengthening, gait training, closed chain exercises, proprioceptive training, and sports-specific training before allowing a full return to activities. RTP is usually allowed after full ROM is restored without pain, swelling, or instability symptoms. Some providers may choose to allow RTP once strength is 80% to 85% compared with the contralateral side, along with a satisfactory single-leg hop test and two-legged hop test.

Operative Treatment

In first-time acute patellar dislocations in skeletally immature patients, immediate operative intervention is generally reserved for patients who have a displaced osteochondral fracture or lesion. Open reduction and fixation of osteochondral lesions is generally reserved for lesions greater than 1 cm in diameter with bone attached to the fragment. Smaller lesions or lesions without bone attached are generally treated with removal of the loose body. The osteochondral lesion can be treated with chondroplasty or microfracture initially. Larger lesions may require further treatment, which can include osteochondral autograft transplantation (OATS), matrix-assisted autologous chondrocyte implantation (MACI), or osteochondral allograft treatment.

The MPFL is the primary ligamentous restraint to lateral dislocation. After surgical treatment is determined to be necessary, reestablishing the integrity of the MPFL is crucial to restoring patellar stability. Acutely, the MPFL can be repaired, but such repair has shown mixed long-term results.[147–150] The MPFL can be reconstructed with either autograft or allograft in skeletally immature athletes. It is crucial for the graft to be of sufficient length, especially if a loop-type construct that is doubled back is used (Fig. 137.10). In skeletally immature patients with open distal femoral physes, the anatomic MPFL femoral attachment

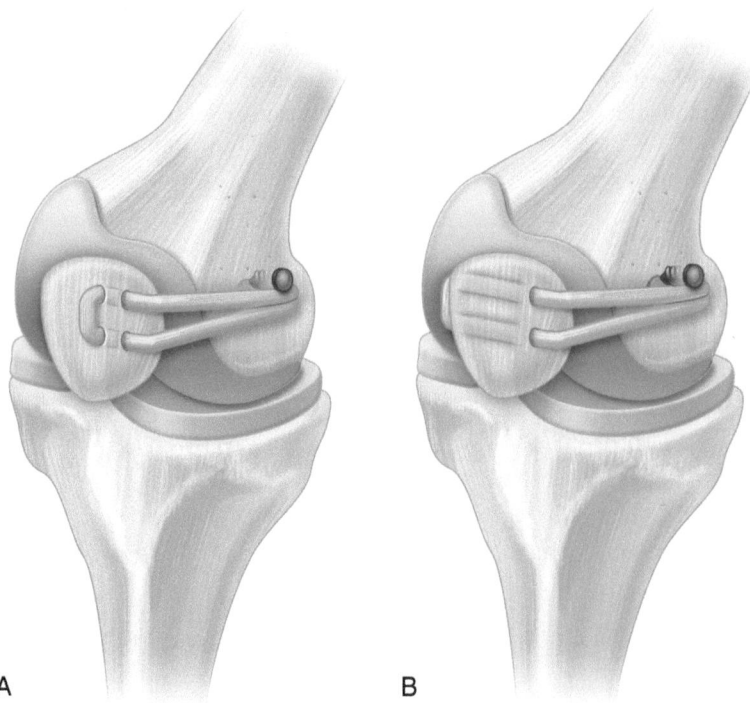

A   B

Fig. 137.10 (A) Medial patellofemoral ligament (MPFL) reconstruction using a gracilis tendon that is looped through two tunnels in the medial half of the patella. The tunnels exit in the midline of the patella, avoiding tunnels that pass across the full width of the bone. The femoral fixation at the adductor tubercle is by means of an interference screw. (B) MPFL reconstruction using a free gracilis tendon that is passed through two transverse tunnels in the proximal part of the patella. The femoral fixation at the adductor tubercle is by means of an interference screw. ([A] From Scott WN, ed. *Insall and Scott Surgery of the Knee.* 5th ed. New York: Elsevier; 2012; courtesy M. Lind. [B] From Christiansen SE, Jacobsen BW, Lund B, et al. Reconstruction of the medial patellofemoral ligament with gracilis tendon autograft in transverse patellar drill holes. *Arthroscopy.* 2008;24:82.)

point, which is just posterior to the medial epicondyle, is very close to the physis. The graft fixation or graft tunneling procedures performed in more mature patients would risk a growth disturbance or arrest, and thus it is often necessary to place the femoral attachment point in a nonanatomic position to avoid the physis. This position is generally just anterior and proximal to the medial epicondyle and 4 to 5 mm distal to the growth plate.[151] However, this position is somewhat controversial, with other surgeons suggesting that the femoral tunnel or attachment point be placed just proximal to the physis. Patellar fixation can be performed with a single or double tunnel. Screw fixation can be used in the patella, or a loop can be used through the patella without hardware. The application of appropriate tension to the graft in MPFL reconstruction is always crucial, but especially in skeletally immature patients in whom the femoral fixation point also needs to avoid the physis. According to Wall and Romanowski, tension of between 30 and 60 degrees of flexion should be placed on the MPFL graft.[151] If the patella tracks medially in flexion, the pin is moved distally. If the patella tracks medially in extension, the pin is moved proximally. If the pin is too anterior, it tightens in terminal extension and flexion. If the pin is too posterior, it loosens in terminal extension and flexion.

Skeletally immature athletes, and in particular especially young children with patellar instability, present a unique challenge to sports medicine care providers. Surgical options such as tibial tubercle osteotomies are not possible in young patients who have open tibial physes. A number of "nonanatomic" reconstruction procedures have been used both historically and in patients with particularly difficult and challenging cases of patellar instability, such as athletes with congenital patellar dislocations, collagen disorders, neuromuscular and metabolic syndromes, and mechanical alignment issues.

The isolated lateral release is rarely used or indicated in patients with traumatic instability but often is needed in combination with other procedures in patients with long-standing chronic patellar dislocations or congenital dislocations.

The Galeazzi procedure involves use of the semitendinosus as a restraint to lateral subluxation. The semitendinosus is harvested proximally with an open-ended tendon harvester, leaving the distal portion attached. The patella is exposed, and often a lateral release is performed. A patellar tunnel is made from proximal lateral to distal medial. The semitendinosus tendon is passed retrograde and folded over the anterior surface of the patella and secured there with suture. Tension is applied to the graft at 45 to 60 degrees of flexion.

The Roux-Goldthwaite procedure is another nonanatomic reconstruction procedure that has been used in skeletally immature patients.[152–154] This procedure involves splitting the patellar tendon and detaching the distal end of the lateral half, which is then passed posterior to the medial half and reattached medially into the pes anserinus. Although tension is also applied at 45 to 60 degrees of flexion in this procedure, it is difficult to achieve appropriate tension in both limbs of the patellar tendon, which is one of the criticisms of this technique. This patellar tendon rerouting procedure is generally combined with a medial retinacular plication.

Multiple tibial tubercle osteotomies are available for realignment in the surgical treatment of patellar instability but require that the tibial tubercle physis be closed. Premature closure of the tibial tubercle portion of the tibial physis can result in a recurvatum deformity. After the tibial tubercle physis has closed, the most popular option is currently the anteromedial tibial tuberosity transfer popularized by Fulkerson.[155,156] Earlier versions include the Hauser osteotomy, which included a distal medial transfer of the tibial tubercle combined with a lateral retinaculum release and medial imbrication along with the Elmslie-Trillat osteotomy, which involved only medialization, and the Maquet osteotomy, which involved only anterior elevation of the tubercle.

Postoperative Management

Rehabilitation after MPFL reconstruction should emphasize lower limb alignment in all phases of rehabilitation to avoid dynamic hip internal rotation and knee valgus, which can lead to stress on the healing reconstruction.[157] A skeletally immature athlete often wears a hinged patellar stabilizing brace for approximately 6 weeks. The brace should be locked in full extension during the first postoperative week and can be unlocked during the second week, based upon the patient's available ROM, but should not exceed 45 degrees. During postoperative weeks 2 through 6, the brace can be opened approximately 10 degrees per week, depending upon the patient's available ROM. Younger patients undergoing more extensive patellar realignment procedures, especially nonanatomic reconstructions, may require a longer immobilization period and a slower rate of mobilization

Partial weight bearing is generally allowed immediately unless a simultaneous microfracture or osteotomy was performed. Weight bearing may progress from ambulation with crutches and a knee brace locked in extension to ambulation with crutches and the brace unlocked. Use of crutches and the brace may be discontinued after postoperative week 6, when the patient demonstrates sufficient strength and control of the limb to protect the knee from transverse and frontal plane stress.[157]

Initial phases of rehabilitation emphasize quadriceps activation and ROM with the goal of attaining full knee extension by week 2 and 90 degrees of knee flexion by 6 weeks after the operation to prevent adhesions.[157] Manual therapy should be incorporated to treat postoperative swelling, scar formation, and joint mobility. Care should be taken to avoid lateral patellar glides until after the sixth postoperative week, to allow for tissue healing. Rehabilitation should continue to progress with strengthening, ROM, and proprioception training until the patient is ready to return to unrestricted sports at approximately 6 months after surgery, depending on the patient's function and symptoms.[157]

Results

Medial imbrication or repair has led to marginal results long term.[147–150] MPFL reconstruction has been associated with excellent results in terms of preventing recurrent patellar instability. In two series combined, only 5 of 170 patients who had undergone MPFL reconstruction experienced repeat subluxation or dislocations.[158,159] Failed MPFL reconstruction may be associated with trochlear or patellar dysplasia.[160] In the skeletally mature patient, the tibial tubercle osteotomy can be a powerful tool to address patellar instability and lead to low recurrence rates and high patient satisfaction.[161] Nonanatomic reconstruction techniques have good results in select patients but should be recommended with caution in skeletally immature athletes who do not have congenital patellar dislocations, collagen disorders, neuromuscular and metabolic syndromes, and mechanical alignment issues.

Complications

The surgical treatment of patellar instability has multiple potential pitfalls and complications. Potentially the most disheartening complication is recurrent instability. As previously mentioned, failure of MPFL reconstruction with recurrent instability is usually due to unrecognized trochlear or patellar dysplasia. Arthrofibrosis is another potential complication of any surgical treatment of the knee. In the skeletally immature athlete, potential growth arrest after a ligament reconstruction with or without an osteotomy is a particular concern, and careful preoperative planning and intraoperative attention should minimize this risk. Patellar fracture is a recognized complication after MPFL reconstruction.[162] Minimizing the size and number of tunnels and related hardware within the patella can help to reduce this risk. Due to this, some have advocated for medial reconstruction in the quadriceps tendon to spare the patella.[163] Patellofemoral arthrosis is a particularly concerning complication after patellar instability surgery and is difficult to quantify in this population. It can certainly be part of the natural history of articular cartilage damage caused by recurrent patellar instability.[134] It can also be a potential complication of overtension of an MPFL reconstruction, improper femoral tunnel placement, or overloading of the patellofemoral joint with improper translation of the tibial tubercle osteotomy.

Future Considerations

As the sports medicine community advances the ligament reconstruction of the MPFL, techniques for skeletally immature athletes will need to focus on reconstructions that are anatomic, spare the physes, decrease the risk of patellar fracture, minimize the risk of dislocation, and reduce the risk of applying too much tension. In addition, the use of concurrent bony procedures and their contribution to patellofemoral stability and long-term development of arthrosis will need to be further quantified. With a recent study showing a 50% incidence of arthrosis 25 years after patellar dislocation, long-term follow-up studies will be needed to determine whether stabilization decreases this incidence.

OSTEOCHONDRITIS DISSECANS

OCD is an acquired potentially reversible lesion of subchondral bone that often results in delamination of the articular surface and sequestration of subchondral bone. The term was originally coined by Konig in 1887, who recognized at that time that it was a potential cause of loose bodies and degenerative changes.[164]

The peak prevalence of OCD diagnosis is noted during the preteen years; OCD is thought to be rare among children younger than 10 years and less common after skeletal maturity. The estimated incidence of adolescent OCD is between 0.2% and 0.3% based on knee radiographs and 1.2% based on knee arthroscopy studies.[165] The male/female ratios have been quoted as being between 2:1 and 5:3, although the incidence of OCD diagnoses in females is on the rise.

Etiology

Several theories have been proposed regarding the etiology of juvenile OCD, including both single and repetitive trauma. Green[166] reported a 40% rate of trauma prior to diagnosis of OCD in 1966. Since then, authors have found an increased incidence in young, very active athletes, with a statistically significant association between OCD and increased involvement in sports. In Sweden it was found that 55% to 60% of patients with OCD participated in high-level sports.[165,167,168] In 1933 Fairbanks concluded that the OCD lesion on the medial femoral condyle was caused by repetitive contact on the tibial spine, a conclusion later supported by other authors.[169,170] However, Cahill has refuted some of these claims by showing no history of trauma in 204 cases of OCD; he postulated a stress reaction or fracture as the cause of the lesion.[171]

Inflammation has also been proposed as a possible causative factor in the formation of the OCD lesion and, in fact, was Konig's original hypothesis. Other investigators have postulated that a genetic predisposition exists for OCD lesions.[172-175] This theory was refuted by Petrie[176] but supported by the association of OCD with other diseases such as familial epiphyseal dysplasia, Legg-Calvé-Perthes disease, and Stickler syndrome.[168]

Regardless of the etiology, ischemia or avascular necrosis has been proposed as the first event in the formation of juvenile OCD.[177,178] In 1978 Milgram showed that revascularization occurred in partially attached lesions. Limited uptake of radionuclide and labeled tetracycline has also been shown in these lesions.[179] However, in 1950 Rogers and Gladstone[180] disagreed with the idea of ischemia as a cause by showing vascular anastomoses in more than 200 specimens, and Yonetani et al.[181] showed no osseous necrosis in their samples of OCD.

History and Physical Examination

The skeletally immature athlete with an OCD lesion often presents with the insidious onset of knee pain that is worse with participation in high-energy sports. As the lesion progresses, symptoms occur with minimal activity and eventually at rest. At more advanced stages of disease, patients have pain, swelling, effusions, and mechanical symptoms such as locking, popping, and catching if a loose body is present. Ligamentous stability and a lack of meniscal disease are usually found. The Wilson maneuver or sign involves pain elicited by extension of the knee from 90 degrees of flexion to 30 degrees of flexion while internally rotating the tibia. Pain should be relieved by external rotation in the same arc, which is obviously specific for lesions involving the medial femoral condyle in the classic location and has been found to have poor reliability as a specific test for OCD lesions (Fig. 137.11).[182]

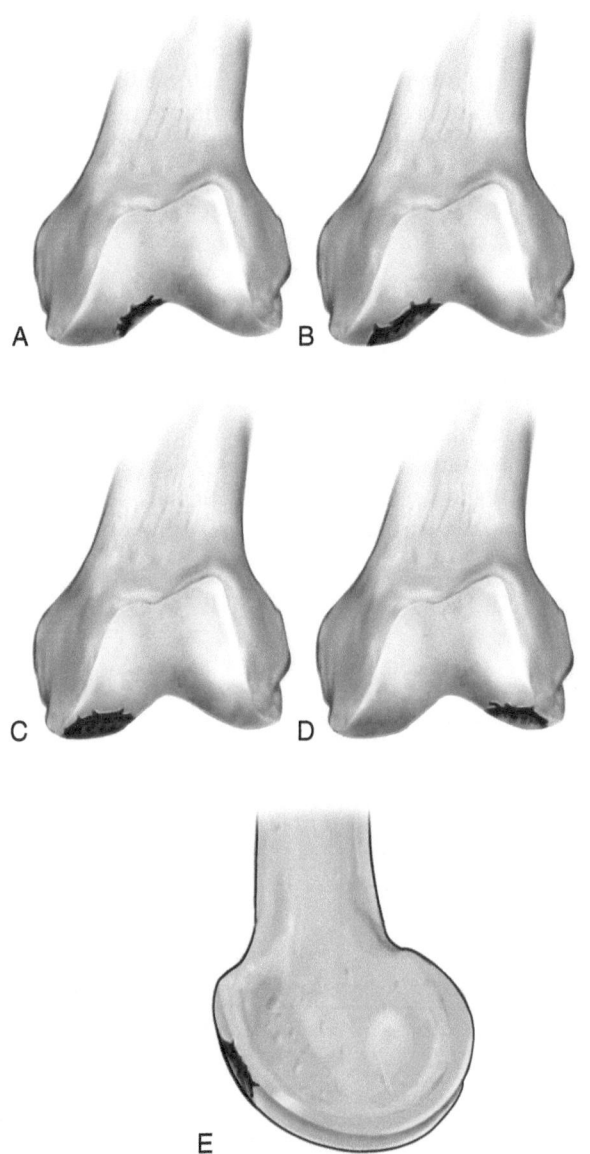

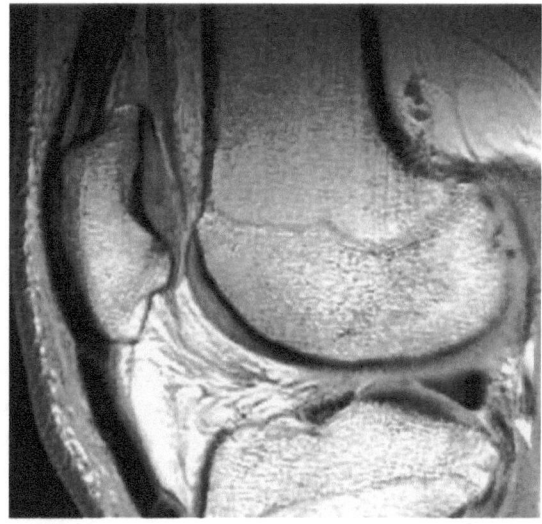

Fig. 137.12 Osteochondritis dissecans of the patella.

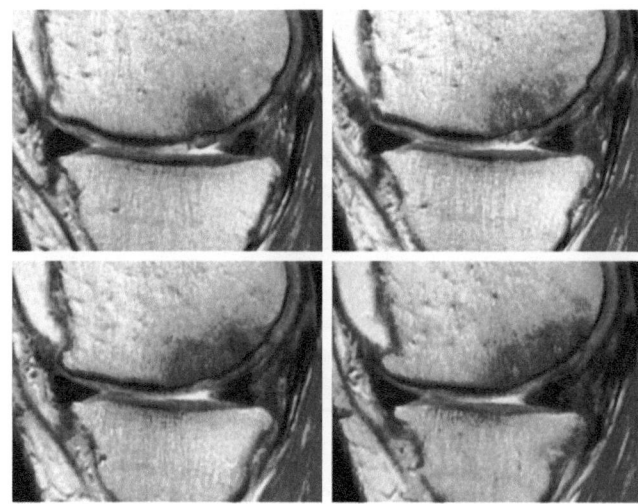

Fig. 137.13 Osteochondritis dissecans of the femur.

Fig. 137.11 Location of osteochondritis dissecans of the femoral condyles. Medial condyle: classic, 69% (A); extended classic, 6% (B); inferocentral, 10% (C). Lateral condyle: inferocentral, 13% (D); anterior, 2% (E). (Modified from Aichroth P. Osteochondritis dissecans of the knee. *J Bone Joint Surg Br.* 1971;53:440–447.)

Radiographs

Standard radiographic evaluation includes an AP, lateral, sunrise, and a notch or tunnel view for a patient with a suspected OCD lesion of the knee. Of these views, the notch view is often the most revealing and specific. Many medial femoral condyle OCD lesions can be missed on a standard AP view and are better seen on the notch view.

CT scans have been used in the past, but because of radiation concerns and improvements in technology, MRI has now largely replaced the use of CT scans for OCD evaluation. Bone scans were used in the past and were shown to be useful for classifying OCD lesions by Cahill and Berg when compared with radiographs.[183] This grading system had five stages based on radiograph

and bone scan activity but was later reported to have limited correlation with lesion stability and the future need for surgery.[184] Paletta et al.[185] were able to show that in four of five patients with open physes and increased uptake on a bone scan, their OCD lesions healed without surgery.

MRI has become a standard higher-level imaging modality to assess OCD lesions in skeletally immature patients. DeSmet et al.[186,187] defined the criteria on MRI for instability in adult OCD lesions. They found that a high signal line beneath the lesion was the most predictive. Other signs of instability included a focal defect or fracture in the articular cartilage along with the presence of subchondral cysts. Kijowski et al.[188] found that the criteria cited by DeSmet et al. was 100% sensitive and specific for adult OCD but not for juvenile OCD, for which it was only 11% specific for instability. They found that secondary criteria with a high signal rim could increase specificity to 100%. These secondary criteria were multiple breaks in the subchondral bone plate, outer rim of low T2-weighted signal intensity, and a rim of fluid signal intensity (Figs. 137.12 and 137.13).

Unfortunately, no valid or reliable criteria currently exist with which to grade or prognosticate juvenile OCD. This problem is being addressed by a multidisciplinary, multicentered national group referred to as ROCK (Research in Osteochondritis of the Knee). Currently the ROCK group has established the radiographic features of OCD lesions that are reliable between readers and have shown that judging fragment healing has good interrater and intrarater reliability.[189,190] Radiographic and arthroscopic grading scales have shown them to be valid and reliable.[191] The ROCK arthroscopic grading classification can be useful in defining the OCD morphology intraoperatively (Fig. 137.14). An MRI system is being developed and will be evaluated soon to help providers not only in the diagnosis of juvenile OCD but also guide the treatment and future prognosis of these lesions.

Decision-Making Principles

In the treatment of juvenile OCD lesions, determining the stability of the lesion at presentation and trying to predict which lesions may become unstable over time is paramount.[192,193] Although deciding whether a lesion is stable is difficult, in this skeletally immature population, some authors have shown that conservative treatment works well for stable lesions and leads to good outcomes.[192,193] In an effort to better define stable lesions, Wall et al.[193] developed a nomogram to predict the potential for healing of an OCD lesion. This predictive tool took into account aspects of the lesion, including the relative size, location, and symptoms, and has been used effectively for stable lesions.

In a multicenter trial of the European Pediatric Orthopaedic Society it was also found that stability was associated with a good prognosis.[168] In this trial it was also found that smaller lesions, lesions in the most common location (i.e., the lateral edge of the medial femoral condyle), a lack of sclerosis on radiographs, and lesions in younger patients did better overall. Unfortunately, it was also shown that pain, swelling, radiographs, and CT scans were not good predictors for dissection of the lesion. However, when a separation between the native

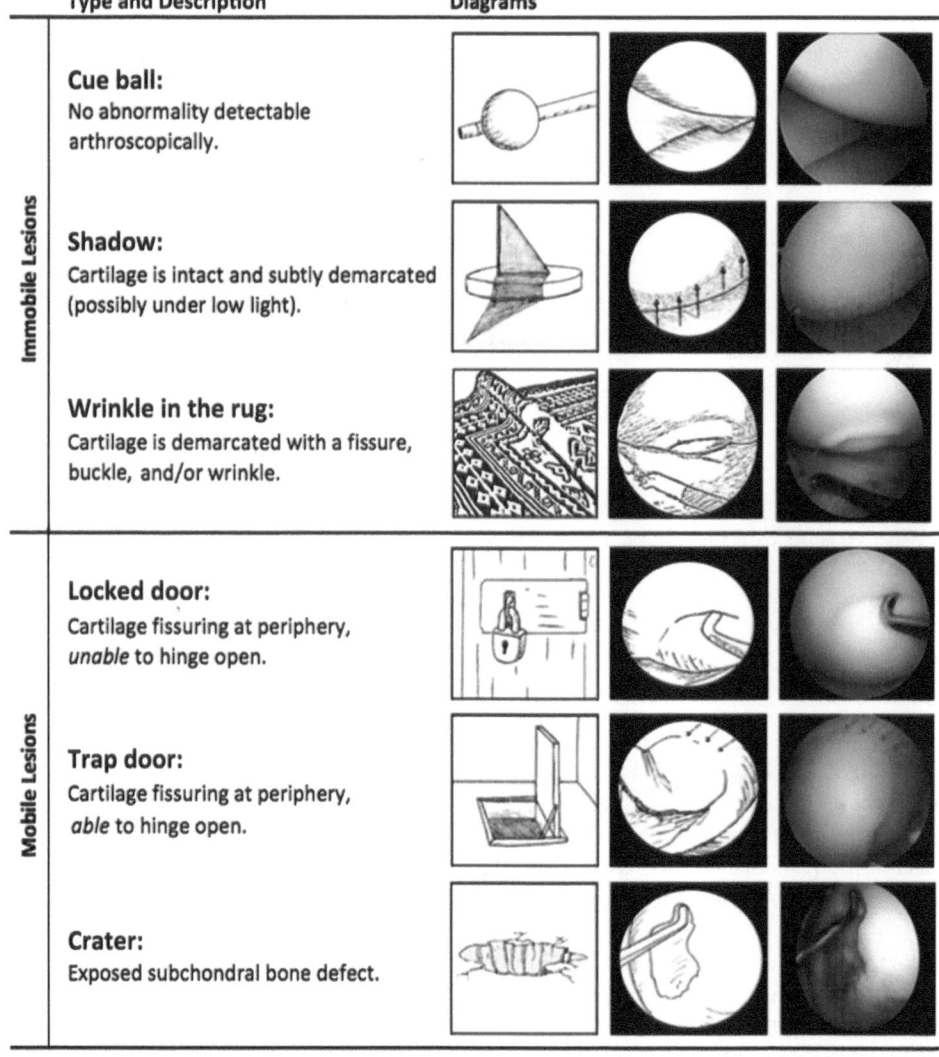

Fig. 137.14 The Research in Osteochondritis of the Knee (ROCK) study group arthroscopic classification system for osteochondritis dissecans lesions. (From Carey JL, Wall EJ, Grimm NL, et al. Novel Arthroscopic Classification of Osteochondritis Dissecans of the Knee. *Am J Sports Med.* 2016;44:1694–1698.)

and progeny bone existed, surgical intervention led to improved results.

During the past several years, many medical organizations have begun to emphasize and produce clinical practice guidelines (CPGs). The American Academy of Orthopaedic Surgeons (AAOS), as a part of this process, has recently put together a CPG for the treatment of OCD.[194,195] The AAOS was able to make only a few recommendations to help guide the diagnosis and care of OCD in adults or adolescents in this CPG but did describe and propose the research necessary to improve the care of persons with these lesions.

The treatment of juvenile OCD is in a stage of evolution. The study and long-term evaluation of current treatment techniques is underway at many centers; the multicentered ROCK group is part of this effort. As these centers and groups compile data to help direct care, the decision process will become clearer and evidence based. However, to a great extent, only level IV and V evidence is available at this point.

A developing trend is the increasingly aggressive care that is being promoted. This trend is driven by two somewhat obvious but underappreciated issues. First, the chance for achieving an excellent outcome is better when the OCD is in the early stages of the continuum of its progression. The second issue is the significantly poor results that occur once the progeny bone/lesion becomes loose or free.

Treatment Options

The initial step in the algorithm of the treatment of juvenile OCD depends on the stability of the lesion. Nonoperative treatment focuses on off-loading the lesion.[192] Off-loading traditionally was achieved with a long leg cast but has now evolved to include the use of crutches, braces, unloader braces, and more permanent steps such as osteotomies. Although they are not standardized, most unloading protocols recommend at least 6 weeks of care, with some protocols extending to as long as 6 months.[193,196,197]

Preoperative examination and radiographic findings may suggest the extent of the lesion, but the final determination of the full extent of the lesion is assessed arthroscopically and occasionally by mini-arthrotomy. As many investigators have shown, preoperative evaluations are often found to be incomplete at the time of arthroscopy, and thus equipment and time must be available for all potential treatment options.

In lesions that were determined to be stable at initial presentation but have failed to progress toward healing or are determined to be stable but have a risk for progression, care is directed toward stimulating healing of the lesion. These lesions are determined to be stable (cueball, shadow, and wrinkle in the rug) on the ROCK arthroscopic classification (see Fig. 137.14). This stimulation is often accomplished by drilling of the lesion to stimulate the reestablishment of a vascular supply, which is performed either in a transarticular or extra-articular fashion. This technique is generally reserved for lesions in situ, with the decision of which method of drilling to perform being dependent on the condition of the articular cartilage and the location of the lesion. Some investigators advocate transarticular drilling, which allows visualization of the lesion arthroscopically and treatment of the entire lesion. The

drawback to this technique of drilling is that the articular cartilage surface is violated by the drilling.[198,199] Extra-articular drilling avoids the penetration of the articular cartilage but requires another means of determining complete treatment of the lesion. This determination can be achieved with the use of fluoroscopy intraoperatively.[200] Both methods have produced good results in appropriate patients.

The other branch of the algorithm in juvenile OCD involves the treatment of unstable lesions. These lesions are the mobile lesions in the ROCK classification (see Fig. 137.14). The decision to attempt fixation of the lesion is dependent on several factors, including the age of the patient, the size and depth of the lesion, the presence or lack of bone on the progeny fragment, sclerosis of the bone, and the condition of the articular cartilage. If the progeny fragment remains in situ or is partially attached with a bony fragment on it, then fixation of the lesion is generally recommended. Many fixation methods are available, including bioabsorbable screws,[201–203] metal screws,[199,204–207] pins or darts, and bone pegs (Fig. 137.15).[200,208–210] The bioabsorbable screws have the advantages of not interfering with MRI and not needing to be removed, but they are more fragile, and multiple reports have been made of hardware failure with use of these devices.[211] Other investigators have used biologic fixation for these lesions with use of OATS. This technique is technically demanding and requires a donor site with requisite donor site morbidity. However, it offers a biologic fixation method without the need for hardware or eventual hardware removal. Longer-term studies and comparison studies are needed to examine these fixation techniques.

More involved lesions, including those that are completely loose or hinged, similar to a trap door, may require more extensive steps to improve the chance of healing. If the lesion is hinged, it is generally recommended that the sclerotic bone beneath the lesion be removed to allow better bleeding bone surfaces for healing. Some authors suggest bone grafting or use of bone graft substitutes during this process.[212,213] Once the lesion has been prepared and reduced either arthroscopically or through a mini open approach, the previously noted fixation devices can be used.

For lesions that are not salvageable at the time of arthroscopic examination, OCD treatment options are similar to those used for other articular cartilage salvage and reconstruction options. Removal of the loose fragments alone has resulted in poor outcomes in long-term follow-up.[214–217] Lesions in which the loose OCD lesion has fragmented into smaller pieces and lesions that no longer have bone stock on the articular cartilage lesion are not considered salvageable. In addition to providing biologic fixation, OATS plug transfers can provide autograft articular cartilage to fill a full-thickness defect. Other options for larger lesions include MACI and fresh osteochondral allograft transplantation.

Results

Results of OCD treatment vary greatly according to the qualities of the lesion at the time of treatment, as well as the associated comorbidities that exist. However, most authors note that symptomatic stable lesions, when treated appropriately both technically and during their rehabilitation, do very well; this has been our experience as well. In these situations, once long-term healing

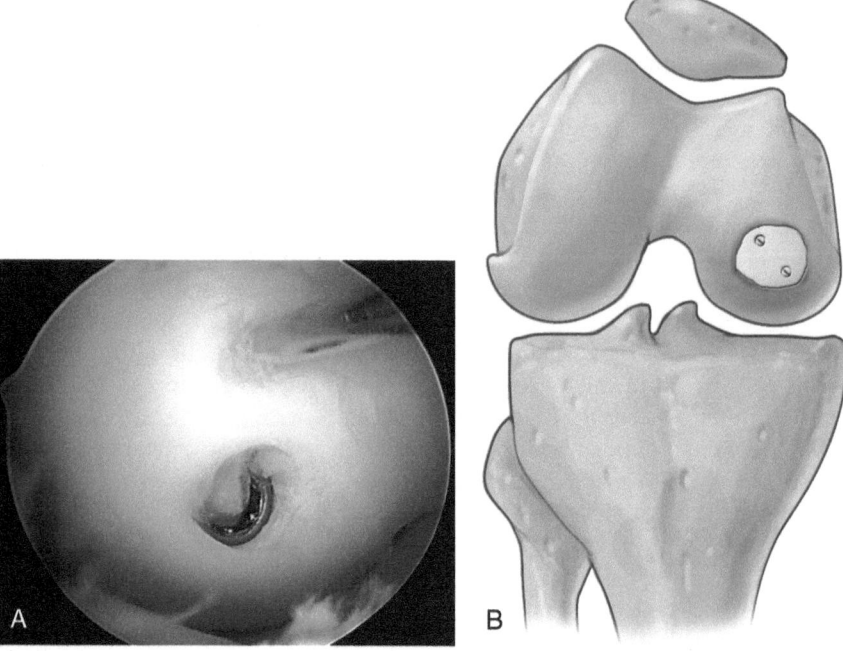

Fig. 137.15 (A and B) Screw fixation of an osteochondritis dissecans lesion (OCD). Note that the screw is seated below the articular cartilage surface to reduce injury to the tibial articular surface (A). (B) A typical appearance of medial femoral condyle OCD fixation. (From Miller MD, Cole BJ, Cosgarea A, et al, eds. *Operative Techniques: Sports Knee Surgery.* Philadelphia: Elsevier; 2008.)

Authors' Preferred Technique

Osteochondritis Dissecans Lesions

- It is our bias that symptomatic knee OCD lesions should undergo arthroscopic evaluation with treatment at an early stage.
- This bias is based on the fact that less chance of progeny bone/lesion displacement exists earlier in treatment. This view is certainly controversial, because many surgeons have reported satisfactory healing of OCD lesions with extended periods of conservative treatment.
- Arthroscopic management should include:
  - Probing of the lesion helps to determine stability. Probing is followed by drilling if the lesion is stable or fixation with bioabsorbable or metal screws, bone plugs, or dowels if any element of instability is noted.
  - Drilling can be performed transarticularly or extra-articularly using smooth, small-diameter (0.045 or 0.062) Kirschner wires.
  - Transarticular drilling should be performed with direct visualization arthroscopically.
  - Extra-articular drilling should be performed with fluoroscopic guidance to ensure that the pins are engaging the lesion in both the AP and lateral projections. We often use the Micro Vector drill guide system (Smith & Nephew, Andover, MA) to assist with placement of the initial pin.
- It is also necessary to ensure that the articular cartilage is not violated with the pin.
- Extra-articular drilling, to ensure adequate penetration of the lesion, is performed eight times per square centimeter.[200]
- When or if the lesion has begun to fragment, we attempt to save the progeny fragment by débriding the base of the lesion either arthroscopically or via an open procedure. The base is then grafted with bone as needed and fixed with appropriate screws or bone plugs.
- If the OCD fragment is not salvageable, we will débride the lesion to a stable cartilage rim and perform marrow stimulation at the base of the lesion. Isolated fragment removal is avoided due to poor long-term outcomes.
- If symptoms continue, we recommend that the lesion be treated with a cartilage reparative procedure (such as MACI) if the depth of bone loss is less than 4 mm or with OATS or a fresh osteochondral allograft if the patient has greater bone loss.

has occurred, patients have normally functioning knees and often forget that their problem ever existed. Unstable lesions, although more variable, can also have excellent outcomes. The key to their prognosis is the recreation and reestablishment of a smooth cartilage surface with a solid subchondral bone foundation. A retrospective natural history study showed that patients who underwent fragment excision had higher rates of osteoarthritis at long-term follow-up compared with patients undergoing fragment fixation or resurfacing.[217] Even larger, initially unsalvageable lesions can have excellent outcomes with the use of osteochondral

allografts when the lesion is treated appropriately.[218] A concern with the use of allografts includes reports of midterm failures when, for unknown reasons, the allograft fragment fails. This outcome has been reported by some investigators after 4 years of an otherwise excellent course.[219]

Complications

Few complications occur in the treatment of juvenile OCD. Intraoperative concerns include improper placement of fixation devices or breakage of drill pins and screws. Nontechnical complications revolve primarily around the failure of healing of the lesions and the cartilage degeneration that can result.

Future Considerations

The treatment of juvenile OCD is evolving. As the lesions become better recognized and evaluated, better care decisions and presumably better long-term outcomes will occur. As the AAOS pointed out in its CPG, a substantial need exists for better-designed studies that look at all of the issues surrounding OCD diagnosis and care. As mentioned, many of these studies are being completed or are underway.

OSTEOCHONDROSES OF THE KNEE

Disordered endochondral ossification of a previously developing epiphysis results in osteochondrosis.[220] The stresses of repetitive activity can lead to changes within the apophysis, a primary area of development in the young athlete. As the skeleton matures, changes in the bone and cartilage of the apophysis can cause the symptoms that lead to the diagnosis of tendinopathy. Advanced radiographic findings are consistently found within the tendon in mature individuals; however, in young athletes, radiographic findings show changes only in the bone and cartilage. Classically, young athletes with osteochondrosis present with pain localized to the origin or insertion of a tendinous insertion.

Osgood-Schlatter Disease

In the early 1900s two separate clinicians, Osgood and Schlatter, first reported osteochondrosis of the tibial tubercle. They described pain over the tibial tubercle with running and jumping in active adolescents. The disease occurs in children who are undergoing rapid growth when stress is placed on the developing tubercle through patellar tendon force. Osgood and Schlatter stressed that this condition is due to repetitive loading in the area causing a traction apophysitis of the tibial tubercle, not an avulsion fracture.

Osgood-Schlatter disease is now one of the most well-known overuse syndromes. It was originally reported to be more common in boys than in girls.[221,222] The prevalence in girls is on the rise because of the increasing number of female athletes. Girls typically experience the condition between the ages of 10 and 13 years, and boys experience it between the ages of 12 and 14 years, coinciding with their growth spurts. Its incidence was found to be 21% in athletic adolescents compared with 4.5% of nonathletic adolescents.[221] Osgood-Schlatter disease is found bilaterally in 20% to 30% of affected persons.

This condition develops most commonly in boys who participate in the sports of running, basketball, and hockey, whereas it develops most commonly in girls who participate in the sports of gymnastics, volleyball, and figure skating. These sports involve running and jumping, which require repeated loading of the knee in flexion and forced extension of the knee by eccentric quadriceps contraction. The force of the quadriceps extensor mechanism is magnified by the patellar mechanism and transferred to the immature tibial tubercle.

The exact cause of Osgood-Schlatter disease has yet to be identified, but it is universally found in adolescents who undergo

a rapid period of growth. During this time an imbalance occurs between bone and muscle growth, which may lead to susceptibility of the apophysis to overuse injury. Several studies have attempted to identify a relationship between patella alta, Osgood-Schlatter disease, and tibial tubercle avulsion fractures.[221,223,224] None of these studies has found a link between any of these three entities. Repetitive microtrauma appears to be an integral part of the development of Osgood-Schlatter disease because there is a much lower prevalence in nonactive persons.[221]

Patients usually present with pain and swelling over the tibial tubercle. These active adolescents may report increased pain with running, jumping, or kneeling. The pain is usually gradual in onset. Parents often report that they notice an antalgic gait. Tenderness to palpation, swelling, and prominence of the tibial tubercle are often found on physical examination. The distal half of the patella tendon may be tender to palpation. Quadriceps and hamstring tightness may be appreciated. Pain can also be reproduced with resisted knee extension. Bone irregularities can often be palpated in chronic cases. The differential diagnosis of Osgood-Schlatter disease includes avulsion fracture of the tibial tuberosity, patellofemoral stress syndrome, pes anserinus bursitis, Sinding-Larsen-Johansson disease, and infection.

To further evaluate the tibial tuberosity, plain radiographs of the affected knee are ordered. The lateral radiograph is the most helpful in assessing the extensor mechanism (Fig. 137.16). Patients with Osgood-Schlatter disease may have separation or fragmentation of the tibial tubercle apophysis. The tibial tubercle may also be enlarged. Radiographs are also important for excluding other diagnoses such as cysts, tumors, or infection.

The natural history of Osgood-Schlatter disease has been evaluated.[221,225,226] Krause et al.[225] looked at 50 patients with Osgood-Schlatter disease. Half of the patients were treated with a form of nonoperative treatment, and half of the patients received no treatment. When followed up to adulthood, most patients in both groups had no residual symptoms. Treatment usually entails activity modification, ice, stretching, and strengthening

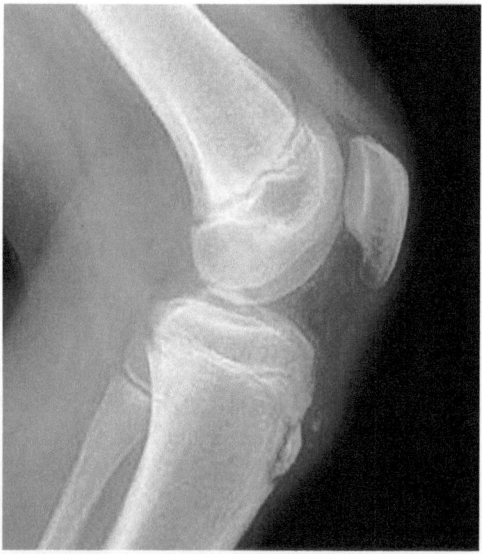

Fig. 137.16 Osgood-Schlatter disease of the tibial apophysis.

exercises. Stretching should focus on the quadriceps, hamstrings, and iliotibial band. Occasionally immobilization in a splint or brace is needed to control pain. The splint or brace should be removed daily for exercises to maintain knee ROM. Although symptoms are usually self-limited, pain may persist until the apophysis closes. Some of these patients may continue to have pain as adults because of the formation of a separate ossicle. Surgical excision of the ossicle is required in the rare cases in which nonsurgical treatment fails to treat this pain.[227] Pihlajamaki et al.,[228] in a long-term follow-up study of military recruits who underwent surgery for the treatment of unresolved Osgood-Schlatter disease, reported that 87% had no restrictions of daily activity and 75% returned to their preoperative activity level.

Sinding-Larson-Johansson Disease

Sinding-Larson-Johansson disease is an osteochondrosis of the inferior pole of the patella. It is predominantly seen in active adolescent boys between the ages of 11 and 13 years. No reports have been made yet of an increased prevalence in females associated with increased young female athletic activity. Sinding-Larson-Johansson disease traditionally presents in slightly younger patients compared with those with Osgood-Schlatter disease because the maturation of the inferior pole of the patella occurs before that of the tibial tuberosity. Rarely, the diagnoses of both of these conditions at the same time have been reported.[229,230]

Patients with Sinding-Larson-Johansson disease report pain at the patella–patella tendon junction associated with running, jumping, and ascending or descending stairs. The pain improves with rest. On physical examination, patients have tenderness to palpation at the patella–patella tendon junction, and they occasionally have swelling. The examination should also look for other possible causes of activity-related anterior knee pain. A palpable defect at this junction and an extensor lag or inability to perform a straight-leg raise should raise concern for a patellar sleeve fracture.

AP, lateral, and Merchant radiographic views of both knees should be obtained. At the inferior pole of the patella, calcification or ossification can often be identified (Fig. 137.17). These radiographs can also aid in the diagnoses of other entities, including patella sleeve fractures, Osgood-Schlatter disease, bipartite patella, patella alta, and patella baja.

Sinding-Larson-Johansson disease is a self-limited condition with resolution of symptoms after full maturation of the inferior pole of the patella, which is usually a 12- to 18-month period. Treatment is similar to the treatment for Osgood-Schlatter disease. The emphasis of treatment is on decreasing pain and inflammation with activity modification and use of ice and antiinflammatory medications. Physical therapy programs emphasize an eccentric quadriceps-loading program and lower extremity stretching.[231] Sports participation should be limited until symptoms improve. Few late sequelae of the disease occur, with one report of a fracture through a previously united ossicle.[232] Remaining symptomatic separate ossicles are rare. Excision could be considered in adults who have pain when nonoperative management fails.

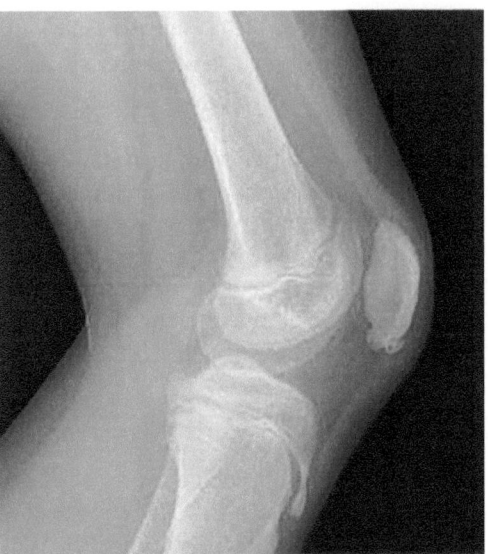

Fig. 137.17 Sinding-Larsen-Johansson disease.

Superior Pole Osteochondrosis

Similar to Osgood-Schlatter and Sinding-Larson-Johansson diseases, superior pole osteochondrosis is a traction apophysitis. Very few reports of superior pole osteochondrosis have been made.[233–235] It can be distinguished from Osgood-Schlatter and Sinding-Larson-Johansson diseases by clinical examination and radiographic findings. It is most commonly found in active boys between the ages of 10 and 11 years. Patients report anterior knee pain that is poorly localized by the patient. Palpation of the superior patella-quadriceps junction reproduces pain. Radiographs show various stages of fragmentation and ossification based on chronicity of symptoms. Tyler and McCarthy[233] found osteonecrosis and reparative changes on histologic examination in patients with superior pole osteochondrosis. These findings are similar to those seen in persons with Osgood-Schlatter and Sinding-Larson-Johansson disease.[236] Like these other entities, superior pole osteochondrosis is a self-limited process. Treatment consists of activity modification, use of ice and antiinflammatory medication, and therapy.

PHYSEAL FRACTURES IN THE AREA OF THE KNEE

Skeletally immature athletes are at risk for unique injuries in the area of the knee involving their open physes. These injuries usually require significant trauma but have been associated with a variety of sporting activities. Their diagnosis and treatment involve special consideration. Distal femoral physeal fractures represent fewer than 1% of all fractures in children and between 6% and 9% of physeal fractures.[237,238] However, they are associated with a 20% to 90% complication rate.[239–245] Most commonly, they are associated with a growth disturbance or angular deformity. The distal femoral physis produces approximately 70% of the growth of the femur or a length of approximately 9 to 10 mm/year. The physis is more undulating than other long bone physes, and therefore fractures often extend through multiple layers of the physis. Tibial spine fracture is another unique injury in the skeletally immature athlete. It involves an avulsion of the ACL chondroepiphyseal attachment. It has a similar pattern of injury as ACL injury but in a younger population. These injuries have been associated with a variety of meniscal and chondral damage intra-articularly. Kocher et al.[246] found the incidence of meniscal tears with these fractures to be 3.8%. Other unique proximal tibial physeal injuries include tibial tubercle avulsions and proximal tibial physeal fractures. Because the proximal tibial physis is more stable than the distal femur, these injuries represent fewer than 1% of all physeal separations. However, these injuries require significant force and trauma, and therefore associated injuries are common and need to be closely followed. Tethering of the popliteal artery to the posterior tibia occurs that places it and its branches at risk during these physeal injuries. Distal swelling and compartment syndrome can be associated with these injuries. The tibial tuberosity may avulse in adolescents, especially during jumping or eccentric loading landing patterns, which can cause contraction of the quadriceps against the fixed tibia or passive flexion of the knee against a contracted quadriceps.

History and Physical Examination

Distal femoral physeal fractures in skeletally immature athletes are most commonly the result of torsional or valgus stress against the knee. Bright et al.[247] have shown in an animal model that the prepubescent male is less resistant to physeal separation and that the physis is weakest in torsion. The mechanism of injury can also dictate the fracture and physeal injury pattern.[247] Bending causes physeal separation on the tension side of the fracture, whereas the Salter-Harris II metaphyseal fragment usually occurs on the compression side. This fragment, referred to as the *Thurston-Holland fragment,* represents a portion of the metaphysis that has fractured, whereas the physis remaining attached to this segment is not separated. The Salter-Harris type II fracture pattern is the most common fracture pattern for displaced distal femoral physeal fractures. In addition, Salter-Harris type III fractures can occur when the medial condyle fractures off both through the physis medially and extending through the intracondylar notch with valgus stress. The medial collateral ligament (MCL) remains attached to the condylar fracture during valgus stress and can occur as the physis begins to close because this physis generally closes centrally first. Many of these physeal fractures in the area of the knee are present with a pronounced hemarthrosis, particularly the tibial spine fractures. Affected patients often report hearing a "pop" and having instability after an awkward landing or during a cutting activity. Patients with a tibial tubercle avulsion or proximal tibial physeal fracture often had a hyperextension injury. Because the metaphysis is often posteriorly displaced, the popliteal artery may stretch in the area of the trifurcation. A series of vascular examinations is needed if proximal tibial physeal injury is suspected.

On examination, patients with a distal femoral physeal fracture may exhibit abnormal laxity on varus or valgus stress that can mimic an MCL or lateral collateral ligament/posterolateral corner injury. They have been associated with residual ligamentous laxity

after healing (8% in one series) that may represent stretch injury to the ligament in addition to the physeal fracture.[240] Salter-Harris type III fractures of the medial femoral condyle are highly associated with cruciate ligament injuries. In addition to a thorough examination of knee stability, it is crucial to document the neurovascular status distally. As mentioned previously, these fractures can be associated with vascular compromise in some cases. In addition, varus stress injuries may result in peroneal nerve stretch and neurapraxia. Patellar height should also be measured and compared with the contralateral knee because patella alta can be seen in tibial tubercle avulsions along with patellar sleeve avulsion fractures. When examining the tibial tubercle, it is important to distinguish a chronic condition such as Osgood-Schlatter disease from an acute tibial tubercle fracture or avulsion. Both a history of symptoms and their severity, along with physical examination findings such as knee effusion, patellar height difference, and inability to perform a straight-leg raise, help to distinguish these two entities.

Imaging

In addition to standard radiographs, stress views were traditionally recommended to evaluate a patient for a suspected distal femoral or tibial physeal fracture. However, given the risk of further damage to the physis and improvement in MRI, MRI may be a better means of evaluating potential physeal injuries that are not clear on radiographs or when compared with contralateral films. A CT scan can be used for evaluating intra-articular extension, especially in the cases of Salter-Harris type III and IV fractures of the distal femur, tibial spine, and tibial tubercle fractures.

Tibial spine fractures are often classified by the Meyers and McKeever classification system (Fig. 137.18).[248] Type I fractures are minimally displaced; type II fractures are hinged anteriorly with an intact posterior portion; and type III fractures are completely separated (Figs. 137.19 and 137.20). Type IV fractures were added to the classification system later and are also completely displaced and rotated.[249]

Tibial tubercle and proximal tibial physeal fractures are also best evaluated on the lateral view or in the sagittal plane. A CT scan is sometimes needed to evaluate for intra-articular extension or displacement. A modified Watson-Jones classification system of tibial tubercle fractures has been developed. Type I fractures are a physeal separation through the tubercle apophysis but distal to the junction of the ossification centers of the tubercle and the epiphysis. Type II fractures are a physeal separation through the junction of the tubercle and epiphysis. Type III fractures extend through the proximal tibial epiphysis intraarticularly. Type IV fractures extend posteriorly through the physis. Type V fractures involve an avulsion of the periosteal attachment of the patellar tendon.

Decision-Making Principles
Treatment Options

Distal femoral physeal fractures can be treated both conservatively and operatively, with the amount of initial displacement generally dictating the treatment plan. Closed reduction and immobilization are best for a nondisplaced or minimally displaced

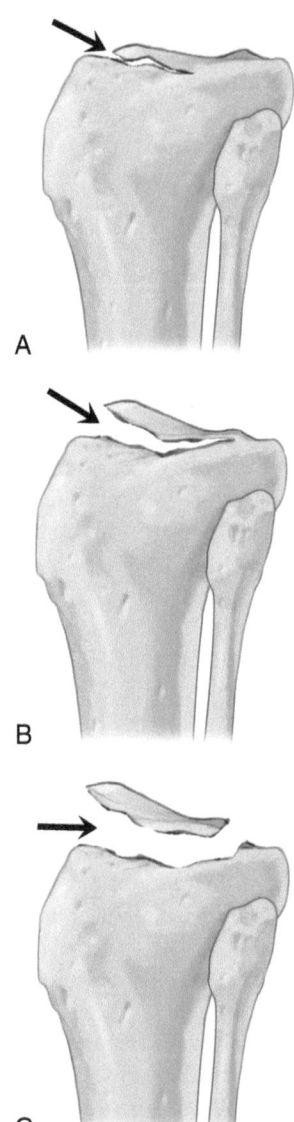

Fig. 137.18 Meyers and McKeever classification of tibial eminence fractures in children. (A) Type I is a nondisplaced fracture. (B) Type II is a displaced fracture that is hinged posteriorly. (C) Type III fractures are completely displaced.

fracture. Closed reduction and percutaneous pinning versus screw fixation is appropriate for displaced Salter-Harris type I and II fractures that reduce anatomically with closed reduction. If screw fixation is used, the Salter-Harris type II fragment must be large enough for adequate screw purchase (if the screw is placed proximal and parallel to the physis). In general, rigid immobilization or supplemental pin fixation is often needed in addition to fixation of the Thurston-Holland fragment, given the large lever arm distal to the fracture fixation. Open reduction and internal fixation are advocated for irreducible Salter-Harris type I and II fractures and all displaced Salter-Harris type III and IV fractures of the distal femur (Fig. 137.21).

Tibial spine fractures that are nondisplaced or reduce anatomically with closed reduction using hyperextension and casting can be treated in a closed fashion with immobilization. In general, the

knee must be kept in full extension or slight hyperextension to maintain reduction, and casting or brace immobilization needs to continue for 4 to 6 weeks, depending on the radiographic progression of healing. For tibial spine fractures that do not respond to closed reduction, multiple techniques are available for reduction and fixation. Traditionally, open reduction using a parapatellar arthrotomy approach and screw fixation was used. Screws are generally kept within the epiphysis to avoid damage to the physis. Arthroscopic reduction and internal fixation techniques are also available. Lateral and medial meniscal tears have been described in conjunction with tibial spine fractures, and arthroscopic examination allows for diagnosis and treatment of these lesions. Meniscal tears and the intermeniscal ligament have been described as blocks to reduction and often need to be addressed to allow an anatomic reduction (Fig. 137.22). Once reduction is achieved arthroscopically, either percutaneous screw fixation or suture fixation can be performed. Suture fixation involves passing sutures through the chondroepiphyseal portion of the tibial spine avulsion or the distal aspect of the native ACL and bringing these sutures down across the physis; tension can be applied, and they can be tied across a metaphyseal bone bridge or the sutures can be fixed with anchors (Fig. 137.23). Suture fixation with a number five ultra–high-molecular-weight polyethylene core has better failure characteristics and stiffness than screw or epiphyseal suture anchor fixation.[250,251] Multiple different suture configurations have shown excellent failure properties in biomechanical testing.[252] Number five Vicryl suture has similar time zero biomechanical properties but loses 50% of its strength by 3 weeks in vivo, so may not be an optimal fixation method give the possibility of delayed failure.[253] Similarly, biomechanical studies favor ultra–high-molecular-weight polyethylene suture over absorbable polydioxanone suture (PDS-II).[254]

Nondisplaced proximal tibial physeal fractures can also be treated with immobilization with a cast and eventually a brace. Minimally displaced fractures can be treated with closed reduction and smooth pin or screw fixation. Depending on the age of the athlete, smooth pin fixation may be more appropriate for younger patients with wide-open physes. Open reduction and internal fixation is reserved for fractures that fail to respond to closed reduction, are widely displaced, have intra-articular step-off, or have associated neurovascular issues that need to be addressed simultaneously. Tibial tubercle fractures follow a similar decision-making algorithm. Some persons have advocated the use of arthroscopy to evaluate and assist in the treatment of intra-articular fractures. However, this technique should be undertaken with caution because these patients are already at risk for increased swelling distally given the risk of vascular injury, and the added fluid extravasation from arthroscopy can increase the risk of compartment syndrome.

Complications

Each physeal fracture pattern around the knee has been associated with complications. The major complications include nonunion, malunion, neurovascular compromise (particularly with proximal tibial physeal fractures), compartment syndrome, growth arrest and/or angular deformity (particularly with distal femoral

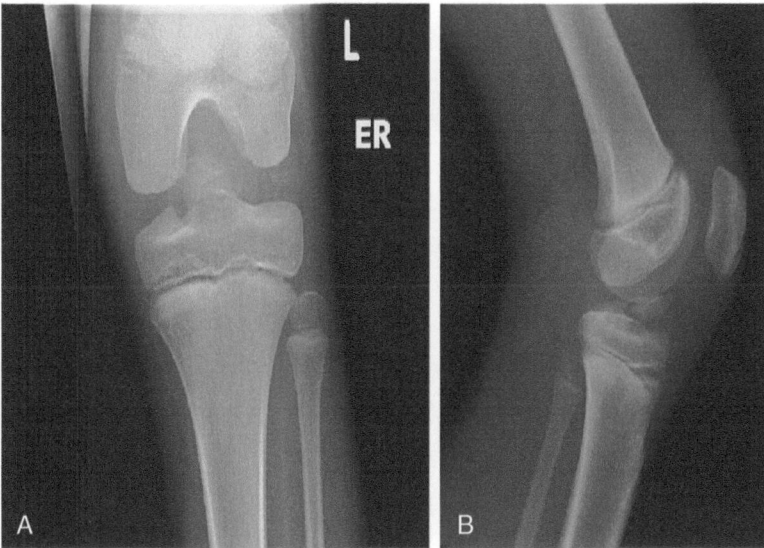

Fig. 137.19 Anteroposterior (A) and lateral (B) radiographs of a type III tibial eminence fracture.

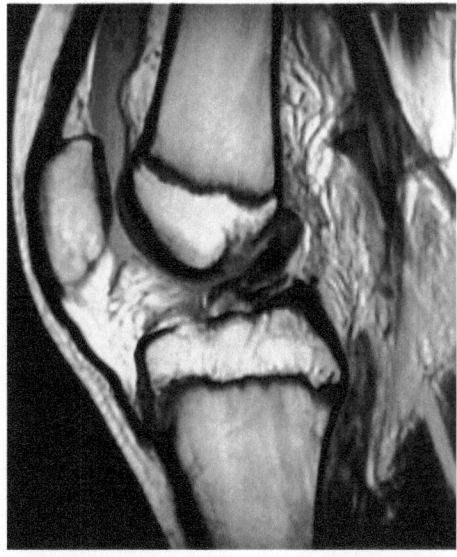

Fig. 137.20 Sagittal magnetic resonance imaging section showing a type III tibial eminence fracture.

physeal fractures), associated ligamentous injury or residual laxity (particularly with tibial spine fractures and intraarticular distal femoral physeal fractures), and stiffness/arthrofibrosis.[238–245,254–264] Particular attention should be given to the difficult situation of arthrofibrosis after physeal or tibial spine fractures. Vander Have et al.[265] reported a 12.5% risk of distal femoral physeal fracture and subsequent growth arrest after manipulation following tibial eminence fracture treatment complicated by arthrofibrosis.

For a complete list of references, go to ExpertConsult.com.

SELECTED READINGS

Citation:

Anderson AF. Transepiphyseal replacement of the anterior cruciate ligament in skeletally immature patients. A preliminary report. *J Bone Joint Surg Am.* 2003;85A(7):1255–1263.

Level of Evidence:

IV

Summary:

Anderson reports one of the first case series of transepiphyseal anterior cruciate ligament reconstruction with use of quadruple hamstring autograft. This article includes an excellent technical description of the procedure along with relevant figures and fluoroscopic images.

Citation:

Kocher MS, Garg S, Micheli LJ. Physeal sparing reconstruction of the anterior cruciate ligament in skeletally immature prepubescent children and adolescents. *J Bone Joint Surg Am.* 2005;87A(11): 2371–2379.

Level of Evidence:

IV

Summary:

The authors of this classic article describe physeal-sparing, combined intra-articular and extra-articular reconstruction of the anterior cruciate ligament, and provide a minimum of 2-year follow-up data. An excellent technical description of the procedure accompanies results that show a low revision rate and minimal risk of growth disturbance.

Citation:

Lawrence JT, Argawal N, Ganley TJ. Degeneration of the knee joint in skeletally immature patients with a diagnosis of an anterior cruciate ligament tear: is there harm in delay of treatment? *Am J Sports Med.* 2011;39(12):2582–2587.

Level of Evidence:

III

Summary:

The authors of this excellent cohort study show that increased time from injury to anterior cruciate ligament reconstruction in children younger than 14 years of age was associated with an increased risk of medial meniscal tears and lateral compartment chondral injury.

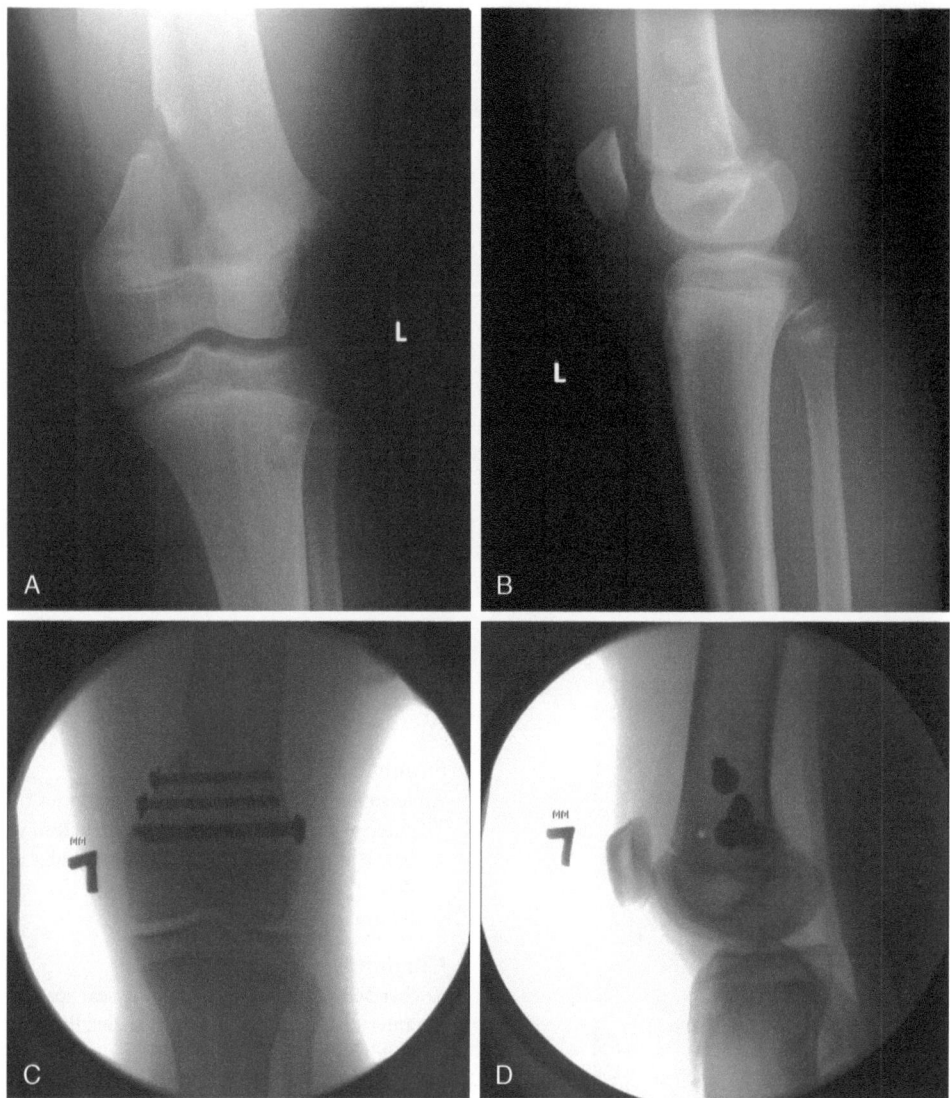

Fig. 137.21 (A) An anteroposterior (AP) radiograph of distal femoral physeal fracture. (B) A lateral radiograph of a distal femoral physeal fracture. (C) An AP radiograph after closed reduction internal fixation of a distal femur physeal fracture. (D) A lateral radiograph after closed reduction internal fixation of a distal femoral physeal fracture. (Courtesy Children's Orthopedic Center. From Scott WN, ed. *Insall and Scott Surgery of the Knee.* 5th ed. New York: Elsevier; 2012.)

Citation:
Lawrence JT, et al. All-epiphyseal anterior cruciate ligament reconstruction in skeletally immature patients. *Clin Orthop Relat Res.* 2010;468(7):1971–1977.

Level of Evidence:
IV

Summary:
The authors of this case series describe an anatomic all-epiphyseal anterior cruciate ligament reconstruction technique for skeletally immature patients. Fluoroscopic or intraoperative computed tomography scan image guidance is necessary for tunnel placement.

Citation:
Kocher MS, Klingele K, Rassman SO. Meniscal disorders: normal, discoid, and cysts. *Orthop Clin North Am.* 2003;34(3):329–340.

Level of Evidence:
V

Summary:
The authors provide an excellent review of meniscal disease in pediatric and adolescent patients. Topics include meniscal tears, discoid meniscus, and meniscal cysts.

Citation:
Palmu S, et al. Acute patellar dislocation in children and adolescents: a randomized clinical trial. *J Bone Joint Surg Am.* 2008;90A(3): 463–470.

Level of Evidence:
II

Summary:
In this prospective study, nonoperative and acute surgical repair is compared for first-time patellar dislocations in children younger

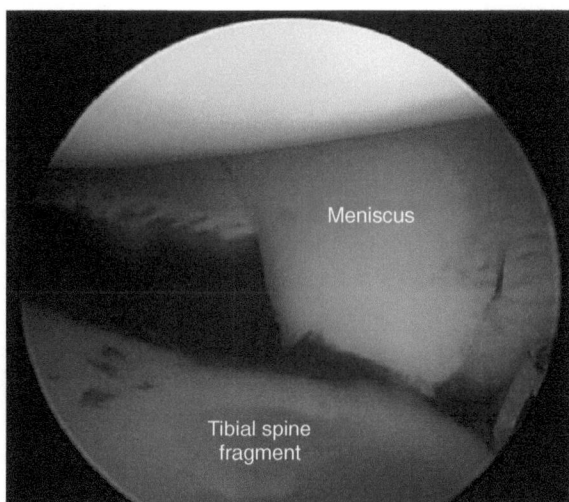

Fig. 137.22 Anterior horn of the medial meniscus entrapped under the tibial spine fragment. (From Scott WN, ed. *Insall and Scott Surgery of the Knee.* 5th ed, New York: Elsevier; 2012.)

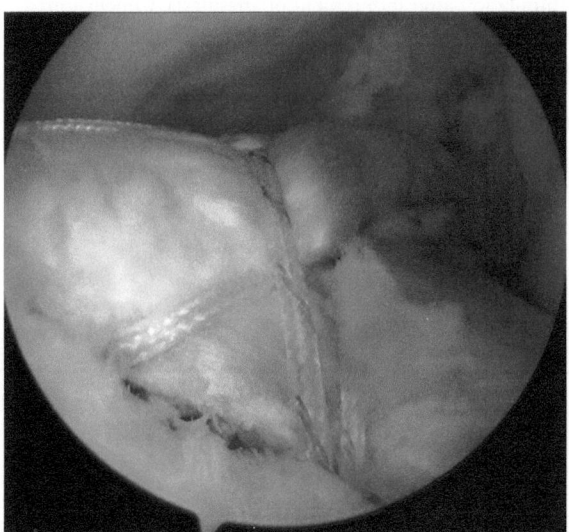

Fig. 137.23 Picture of final fixation of a type three tibial spine avulsion fracture in a 9 year-old male after sustaining the injury during a skiing accident. Fixation was achieved with two Ultra-high-molecular-weight polyethylene (UHMWPE) sutures (#2 Ultrabraid, Smith & Nephew, Andover, MA) passed through the distal aspect of the anterior cruciate ligament and then through two drill tunnels with fixation distally within the metaphysis.

than 16 years. Long-term follow-up showed a high rate of recurrent instability in both cohorts but similar subjective outcomes. Initial surgical treatment was not recommended in this population. A family history of patellar instability was shown to be a significant predictor for recurrence.

Citation:

Paterno MV, Schmitt LC, Ford KR, et al. Biomechanical measures during landing and postural stability predict second anterior cruciate ligament injury after anterior cruciate ligament reconstruction and return to sport. *Am J Sports Med.* 2010;38(10):1968–1978.

Level of Evidence:

II

Summary:

This prospective study of 56 athletes post ACL reconstruction provides biomechanical reasoning that poor neuromuscular control of the hip and knee during a jumping task is predictive of a second ACL injury.

Citation:

Escamilla RF, MacLeod TD, Wilk KE, et al. Anterior cruciate ligament strain and tensile forces for weight-bearing and non-weight-bearing exercises: a guide to exercise selection. *J Orthop Sports Phys Ther.* 2012;42(3):208–220.

Level of Evidence:

V

Summary:

This nonsystematic review of the literature is a thorough summary of the biomechanical evidence regarding exercise prescription of open- versus closed-kinetic chain therapeutic exercises with respect to graft tension for patients post ACL reconstruction.

Citation:

Noyes FR, Heckmann TP, Barber-Westin SD. Meniscus repair and transplantation: a comprehensive update. *J Orthop Sports Phys Ther.* 2012;42(3):274–290.

Level of Evidence:

V

Summary:

Noyes and colleagues provide an excellent update regarding the clinical examination, surgical interventions, postoperative rehabilitation, and clinical outcomes for patients with meniscal pathologies.

Citation:

Fithian DC, Powers CM, Khan N. Rehabilitation of the knee after medial patellofemoral ligament reconstruction. *Clin Sports Med.* 2010;29(2):283–290.

Level of Evidence:

V

Summary:

Fithian and colleagues provide an evidence-based approach to postoperative rehabilitation for patients following medial patellofemoral ligament reconstruction.

Citation:

Sanders TL, et al. High rate of osteoarthritis after osteochondritis dissecans fragment excision compared with surgical restoration at a mean 16-year follow-up. *Am J Sports Med.* 2017;Epub ahead of print.

Level of Evidence:

III

Summary:

A natural history study of OCD of the knee showing high rates of osteoarthritis and knee arthroplasty with isolated fragment excision and lower rates with fragment fixation or chondral defect grafting.

Citation:

Chambers HG, et al. Diagnosis and treatment of osteochondritis dissecans. *J Am Acad Orthop Surg.* 2011;19(5):297–306.

Level of Evidence:
IV

Summary:
In this clinical practice guideline, recommendations are outlined based on a systematic review of the published literature on osteochondritis dissecans treatment. Although the recommendations are graded as mostly weak or inclusive, this review will help to shape future research.

Citation:
Wall EJ, et al. The healing potential of stable juvenile osteochondritis dissecans knee lesions. *J Bone Joint Surg Am.* 2008;90A(12): 2655–2664.

Level of Evidence:
II

Summary:
In this excellent study of stable osteochondritis dissecans lesions in skeletally immature patients, lesions with an increased size, associated swelling, and/or mechanical symptoms are shown to be less likely to heal. A nomogram is produced from their data to predict healing based on normalized height/weight and symptoms.

Citation:
Kocher MS, et al. Tibial eminence fractures in children: prevalence of meniscal entrapment. *Am J Sports Med.* 2003;31(3):404–407.

Level of Evidence:
IV

Summary:
In this large case series of operatively treated type II and III tibial eminence fractures, a high rate of meniscal entrapment is shown under displaced fractures. The anterior horn of the medial meniscus was most commonly entrapped. Operative treatment was recommended for all type III eminence fractures and type II fractures that did not reduce in extension.

Citation:
Vander Have KL, et al. Arthrofibrosis after surgical fixation of tibial eminence fractures in children and adolescents. *Am J Sports Med.* 2010;38(2):298–301.

Level of Evidence:
IV

Summary:
Case series from four institutions show a high rate of arthrofibrosis after operative treatment of tibial eminence fractures. The series also show an increased risk of iatrogenic physeal fracture from manipulation after inducement of anesthesia. Conclusions include focusing on sufficient stabilization at the time of the initial surgery to allow early postoperative rehabilitation and performing subsequent manipulation only upon inducement of anesthesia in conjunction with a lysis of adhesions.

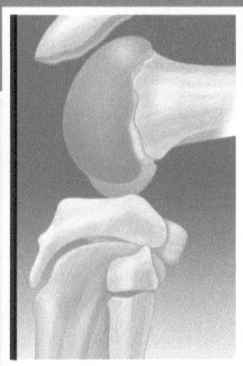

138

Foot and Ankle Injuries in the Adolescent Athlete

J. Andy Sullivan, James R. Gregory

Most of the injuries that occur in the ankle and foot of the pediatric athlete are not unique to athletic participation but occur normally during childhood. However, some injuries occur with greater frequency in the athlete. The conditions covered in this chapter occur in childhood and may present in the athlete, raising the question of whether the athlete should be allowed to participate in sports activities. As a general rule, in all of these conditions, if a patient has an injury or an operation, we allow return to play (RTP) when he or she has full range of motion (ROM) and the strength and ability to perform all the activities involved in the sport without pain.

VARIATIONS OF NORMAL ANATOMY

Tarsal Coalition

Tarsal coalition is a bony or fibrous or cartilaginous connection of two or more of the tarsal bones. The cause is unknown, but it has been established that the condition results from failure of differentiation and segmentation of the primitive mesenchyme.[1,2] The overall clinical incidence is 1% to 3%.[1,3,4] The incidence of osseous, cartilaginous, or fibrous coalition was 13% in a cadaver study, suggesting that many coalitions are asymptomatic.[5] The most common coalitions are the calcaneonavicular and talocalcaneal types, which are bilateral in approximately 60% and 50% of cases, respectively.[1,3,4] More than one type of coalition can exist in one foot. A review of 60 cases of tarsal coalition[6] found that 6 of 30 patients had multiple coalitions in the same foot. The exact mode of inheritance is unknown, but it is postulated to be autosomal dominant with variable penetrance.[3]

Most patients seek medical care during early adolescence, at a time when the coalition is ossifying. The pain is vague in nature and insidious in onset. The patient may have a history of frequent ankle sprains or precipitating trauma. Sports participation or running over uneven ground may accentuate the pain. The pain is thought to be due to microfractures in the coalition.[7] Physical findings include pain on palpation over the subtalar joint, limited subtalar motion, and at times pes planus and ankle valgus. The peroneal muscles may be tight and resist inversion, but true muscle spasm occurs rarely (Fig. 138.1). Any condition that injures the subtalar joint can produce similar symptoms.

The clinical diagnosis can be confirmed by radiographic imaging. Plain radiographs, especially the 45-degree oblique view (Fig. 138.2), usually demonstrate the calcaneonavicular coalition and other less common coalitions, such as the calcaneocuboid. The talocalcaneal coalition (TCC) is difficult to visualize on plain radiographs, but secondary changes, which may suggest the need for other studies (Fig. 138.3), include beaking and shortening of the talar neck, a middle subtalar facet that cannot be seen, elongation of the lateral process of the calcaneus, a ball-and-socket ankle joint, and the C-sign (see Fig. 138.3).

Crim and Kjeldsberg[8,9] studied two groups of 30 patients with tarsal coalition and 17 control subjects. A second group of patients with 150 weight-bearing radiographs for nontraumatic foot pain were reviewed for cases of undetected tarsal coalition. These investigators identified several previously undescribed plain radiographic signs for coalitions. For calcaneonavicular coalitions, these signs were altered navicular structure and visualization of the bar on the anteroposterior (AP) radiograph. For TCCs, the changes were a dysmorphic sustentaculum tali, nonvisualization of the middle subtalar facet, and shortening of the talar neck. When these criteria were used in the 150 prospective cases, three previously undetected coalitions were diagnosed and then confirmed by computed tomography (CT), with no false-positive results.

If a calcaneonavicular coalition is present on plain radiographs, a CT scan should be obtained to ensure that no other coalitions exist, which is necessary for surgical planning (see Fig. 138.2). A CT or magnetic resonance imaging (MRI) scan can also be performed if a coalition is suspected clinically but none is identified on plain films. CT is easily performed, delineates bony anatomy quite well, and can be formatted into a three-dimensional (3D) image that is useful when planning surgery. MRI has the advantage of demonstrating fibrous or cartilaginous lesions, as well as bony lesions. MRI avoids radiation but at greater cost than CT.

El Rassi and colleagues reviewed 19 patients with symptoms and signs consistent with tarsal coalition and normal imaging studies.[10] These investigators used technetium-99m scintigraphy and found slightly increased uptake in the middle facet. They obtained good or fair results in all patients after resection of hypervascular capsule and synovium, which had produced arthrofibrosis.

The initial treatment of these conditions should include conservative measures aimed at relieving the pain. These measures are empirical and include casting and the use of various shoe

inserts and orthotics. The main indication for surgical resection is persistent pain. For calcaneonavicular coalition, resection of the bar with interposition of the extensor digitorum brevis is usually associated with good results. Studies by Cowell[3] and Jayakumar and Cowell[11] indicated that 23 of 26 feet treated in this manner became symptom free.

TCC historically was more difficult to recognize, and its surgical management is less certain.[12] Before the advent of CT, the diagnosis was often confirmed at the time of surgery. Jayakumar and Cowell[11] reported that up to one-third of their patients responded to conservative treatment, and they believed that few indications for resection exist. This conclusion was based on evidence from family studies indicating that many adults with tarsal coalition were asymptomatic. The surgical alternatives include resection of the bar with interposition of fat or tendon, calcaneal osteotomy, and triple arthrodesis.

Scranton[11,13] reviewed 14 patients with 23 symptomatic TCCs. Five feet (in three patients) were treated successfully with casts. Four feet were treated with triple arthrodesis. Eight patients with 13 coalitions that had been resected had a good result. The review was performed at a mean of 3.9 years after surgery. In Scranton's series, approximately half of the joint surface was removed in

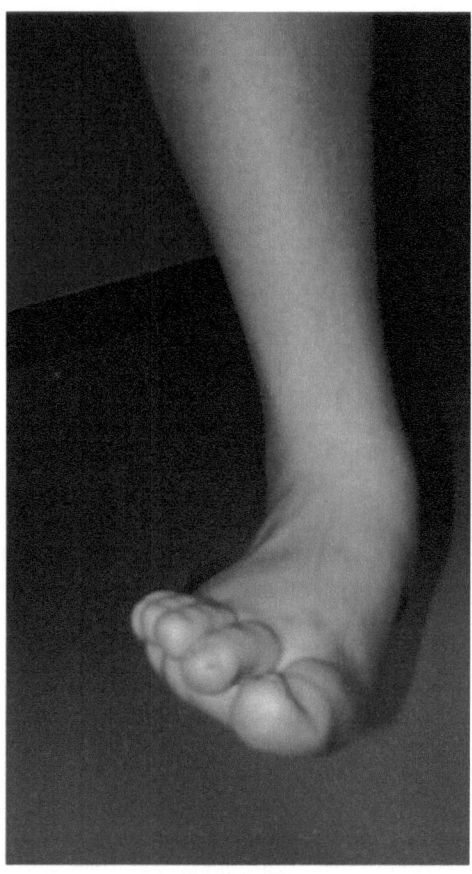

Fig. 138.1 This patient had a tarsal coalition in the right foot. Note that the foot is held in an everted position. Attempted inversion caused pain and resistance.

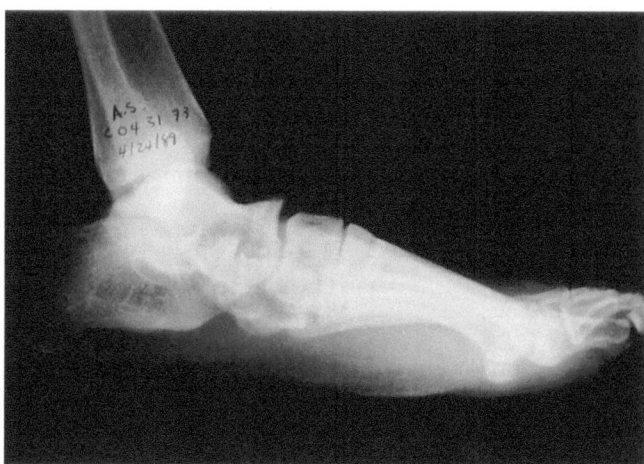

Fig. 138.3 A lateral radiograph of the foot. Note the beaking of the talus and the widening of the talonavicular joint. The subtalar joint is narrowed, and there is a C-sign. This is a dense line originating with the dome of the talus, continuing posteriorly, and ending with the sustentaculum talus.

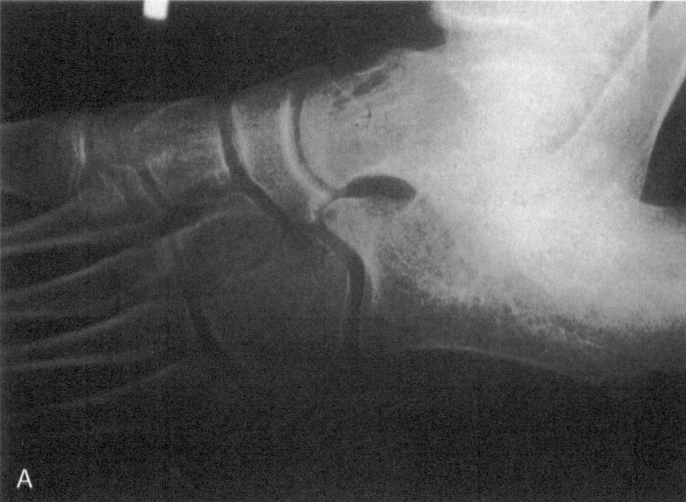
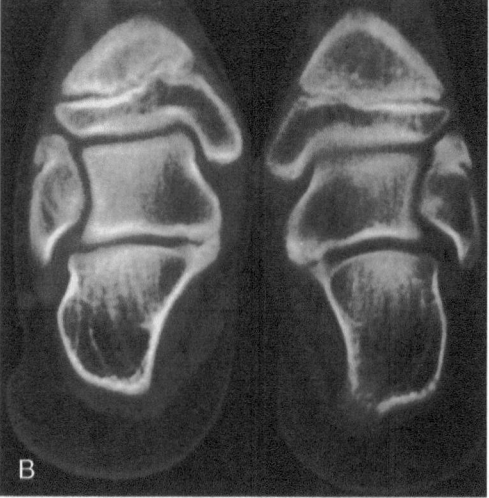

Fig. 138.2 Plain radiography (A) and a computed tomographic scan (B) showing calcaneonavicular and talocalcaneal coalitions, which occurred bilaterally in this patient. The patient presented with a painful, rigid foot and was having difficulty playing tennis.

some patients.[13] In the series reported by Swiontkowski and associates,[14] 10 patients were treated for TCC—four by resection of the bar, and the remainder with some type of arthrodesis. This article stressed that the talar beak is not a true degenerative sign and therefore is not a contraindication to resection of the bar. Olney and Asher[15] evaluated nine patients with persistent pain from 10 middle-facet TCCs who were treated with resection of the bar and an autogenous fat graft. At an average follow-up of 42 months, the results were rated excellent in five patients, good in three patients, fair in one patient, and poor in one patient. In one patient who underwent a repeat operation, the fat graft had been replaced by fibrous tissue.

Luhmann and Schoenecker[16] used CT to evaluate TCC in 25 feet. They quantified heel valgus and the size of the coalition relative to the posterior facet. The ratio of mean TCC cross-sectional area to the posterior facet was 53.4%. Mean hindfoot valgus was 17.8 degrees. Statistical analysis determined a significant association between TCC greater than 50% the size of the posterior facet and poor outcome ($P = .014$). Heel valgus greater than 21 degrees was also associated with poor outcome ($P = .014$). However, good results were obtained in some patients with a TCC greater than 50% and in patients with heel valgus greater than 21 degrees.

Comfort and Johnson[17] reviewed resection of 20 TCCs at an average of 29 months of follow-up. They found good or excellent results with resections involving less than one-third of the total joint surface. They did not find increasing age to be a contradiction to the procedure. Gantsoudes et al.[18] have provided an excellent review of outcomes with use of interpositional fat. In 49 feet with a minimum follow-up of 12 months (and an average follow-up of 42.6 months), an average score of 90/100 (excellent) was achieved with use of the American Orthopedic Foot and Ankle Society Hindfoot scale. Eleven patients (34%) required subsequent surgery to correct foot alignment. Good to excellent results were achieved in 85% of patients.[18]

The management of these coalitions is still controversial and awaits the results of larger series with longer follow-up. Patients with persistent symptoms who do not have degenerative findings have the option of continued conservative care, resection of the coalition, or arthrodesis. Talar beaking is not necessarily a degenerative sign. Factors to consider are the size of the coalition and the age of the patient. Severe malalignment of the foot is a contraindication to resection alone. Although a triple arthrodesis was considered a treatment for failed resections and continued pain, other options should be considered to balance or realign the foot. A sliding osteotomy or medial closing wedge as described by Cain and Hyman can be used to realign the foot.[19] Mosca has written that correction of the valgus deformity and any equinus contracture appears to be as important as resection of the coalition. He recommends calcaneal lengthening osteotomy with gastrocnemius or Achilles tendon lengthening as effective in these cases for correcting deformity and relieving pain in these rigid flat feet.[20]

Adolescent Bunion

The cause of adolescent bunion is unknown. Fifty percent to 60% of patients have a positive family history.[21] Patients with

this condition have an increased intermetatarsal angle (the angle between the first and second metatarsals, normally 10 degrees) and an increased first metatarsal–phalangeal angle (normally 20 degrees). Many patients also have a relaxed flatfoot and a long first metatarsal ray. None of these conditions is known to be the cause of adolescent bunion. Footwear has been implicated, but because bunions occur in cultures in which shoes are not worn, this theory seems unlikely.

Patients with adolescent bunion report pain, prominence, and difficulty associated with footwear. On examination, lateral deviation of the toe is found, along with a medial prominence and a wide forefoot. The bursa that is a prominent part of the adult deformity may be present but is usually less impressive. Arthritis and decreased ROM are also less common. The patient should be evaluated with AP and lateral weight-bearing radiographs. The joint space is usually maintained. The sesamoids may be laterally displaced in advanced cases. The medial eminence of the metatarsal head is prominent, and a sagittal groove may be present medially.

Children should be treated nonsurgically whenever possible. Alteration or stretching of footwear may alleviate symptoms. Although some series have claimed a success rate of 80% to 95%, this high rate of success has not been the universal experience. Factors implicated in these complications included failure to correct the abnormal deviation of the first metatarsal, failure to correct the soft tissues, weight bearing that was begun too early, inadequate immobilization, and osteotomy performed distal to the open physis. Patients with a hypermobile flatfoot or a long first ray also seemed to be more prone to recurrence.

Indications for surgery include pain that is not responsive to conservative measures and severe deformity. The goals of surgery should include realignment of the first ray and of the metatarsophalangeal joint, cosmesis, and prevention of arthritis. Arthrodesis and resection have no place in the normal child. In general, the most common procedures are distal soft tissue realignment, a distal osteotomy such as the Mitchell or chevron technique, or a proximal realignment or Scarf osteotomy combined with soft tissue procedures. In some cases, both distal and proximal osteotomies are required to align the metatarsal and correct the joint alignment. Phalangeal osteotomies may be indicated to correct alignment of the metatarsophalangeal joint. In the senior author's experience, it is not unusual for a female athlete to present with a bunion, usually bilateral. Often these athletes are basketball or soccer players and have increased intermetatarsal and metatarsophalangeal angles. In these patients the most common procedure the senior author now performs is a bunionectomy, release of the abductor hallucis, a Scarf osteotomy, and capsular imbrication. Most patients have returned to sport in 3 to 6 months. Postoperatively the senior author has the patient wear a toe spica cast for 3 to 6 weeks, and then the wearing of regular shoes is gradually resumed.

Accessory Navicular

Numerous accessory ossicles can occur in the foot, and awareness of these accessory ossicles is necessary to avoid confusing them with an acute fracture. The most common accessory ossicles are the os trigonum posterior to the talus and the os vesalianum at the base of the fifth metatarsal. The accessory navicular is a separate ossification center of the navicular. It may be completely separate or joined by a synchondrosis. It may also present as a large or cornuate (horn-shaped) prominence on the medial side of the navicular (Fig. 138.4). We now know that only a small slip of the tendon inserts into this ossicle and that these patients are no more likely to have flatfoot than are those with a normal navicular.[22]

Many of these patients are asymptomatic. Symptomatic patients experience pain directly over the prominence, usually from footwear over the prominence. If the shoes are stretched or altered over this prominence, symptoms may be relieved. Other patients experience pain when the posterior tibial tendon is stretched or placed under tension. In persons with persistent pain, simple excision of the ossicle without rerouting of the tendon is usually successful.[19,20]

Cavus Foot

Cavus is defined as an increase in the height of the longitudinal arch of the foot. A variety of other modifiers, such as cavovarus and calcaneocavus, are used to further describe the position of the heel. Often the patient has claw toes or hammertoes and metatarsal head calluses. The presenting complaint can be pain or abnormal wear of the shoe. A cavus foot is usually the result of muscle imbalance that is caused by an underlying neurologic disorder. The patient should undergo a meticulous neurologic examination so that evidence of disorders such as Charcot-Marie-Tooth disease, spinal dysraphism, or a spinal tumor can be detected. Nerve conduction studies may be indicated to diagnose the varieties of peripheral neuropathies. Initial radiographic evaluation should include weight-bearing views of the feet and at least an AP view of the entire spine in search of an occult spinal anomaly. An MRI of the entire spine and a neurologic consult are indicted if any question exists of an underlying neurologic disorder.

SOFT TISSUE INJURIES

The ligaments of the ankle insert on the epiphyses distal to the physeal line (Fig. 138.5). Because the physis is the weakest link in this bone-tendon-bone interface, it is usually the part that gives way when significant force is applied to the ankle. High-grade ankle sprains are unusual in the skeletally immature athlete. Physeal fractures that do occur are discussed in the next section. Minor ankle sprains occur and are diagnosed by a history of inversion or eversion strain with findings of tenderness over the anterior talofibular or deltoid ligament. Treatment consists of the usual conservative means of rest, ice, compression, elevation, and immobilization. Formal rehabilitation is rarely necessary but may be beneficial for the competitive athlete. Continued pain or disability should provoke a search for other more serious injury.

Recurrent subluxation of peroneal tendons can occur in the adolescent athlete. Usually, a history of injury is followed by recurrent episodes of a snapping sensation and pain. The subluxation can be provoked by forceful dorsiflexion with

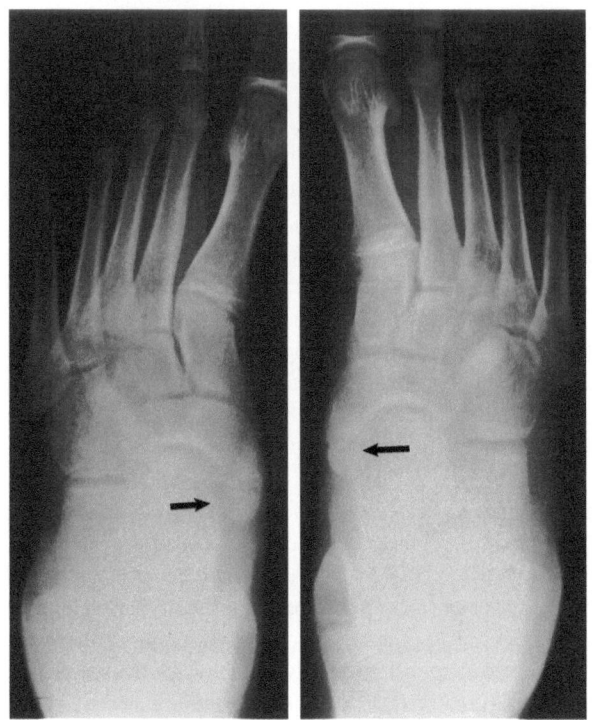

Fig. 138.4 Large bilateral cornuate prominent accessory naviculars *(arrows)*. They are joined by a synchondrosis to the navicular.

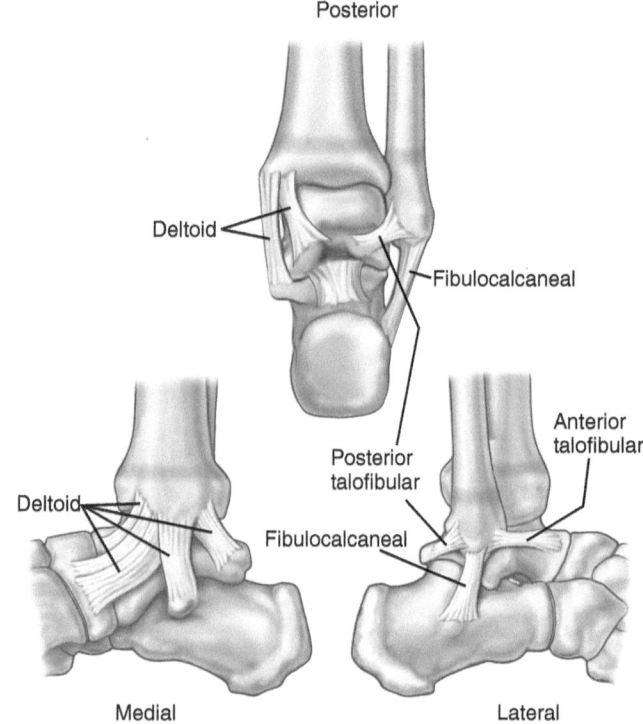

Fig. 138.5 Posterior, medial, and lateral views of the ligaments of the ankle.

the foot everted. In patients whose symptoms are sufficiently severe, surgical correction may be indicated. Surgical alternatives include deepening the groove on the fibula, creating a bony block, and reconstructing the superior peroneal retinaculum. The first two are rarely useful in treatment of the pediatric athlete because the physis is still open. Poll and Dui-jfjes reviewed nine patients aged 15 to 45 years (average age, 25 years) who underwent reconstruction with the posterior calcaneofibular ligament attached to a bone block.[23] Good results were reported.

Contusions on the foot are treated in the same way as those on any other area. Blisters are a frequent problem and require alleviation of the stress, which is usually provided by a new shoe and protection until healing occurs. Tinea pedis (athlete's foot) usually responds to a regimen of antifungal medication, along with education about the need to change socks frequently and to use antifungal powders.

FRACTURES AROUND THE ANKLE

There are two excellent reviews on this topic.[24,25] The one by Wuerz is the most recent. Numerous systems have been proposed to classify ankle injuries. All of these classification systems take into account the position of the foot at the time of injury and the force applied. The Salter-Harris classification[26] is based on the mechanism of injury and the pathoanatomy of the fracture pattern through the physis, as interpreted on plain radiographs and is the system most commonly used. The authors described types I through V. Type V, a crush injury, has been added to the original classification. It is difficult to recognize on plain radiographs at the time of injury; it is the result of a high-energy crush and is not discussed in this chapter (Fig. 138.6).

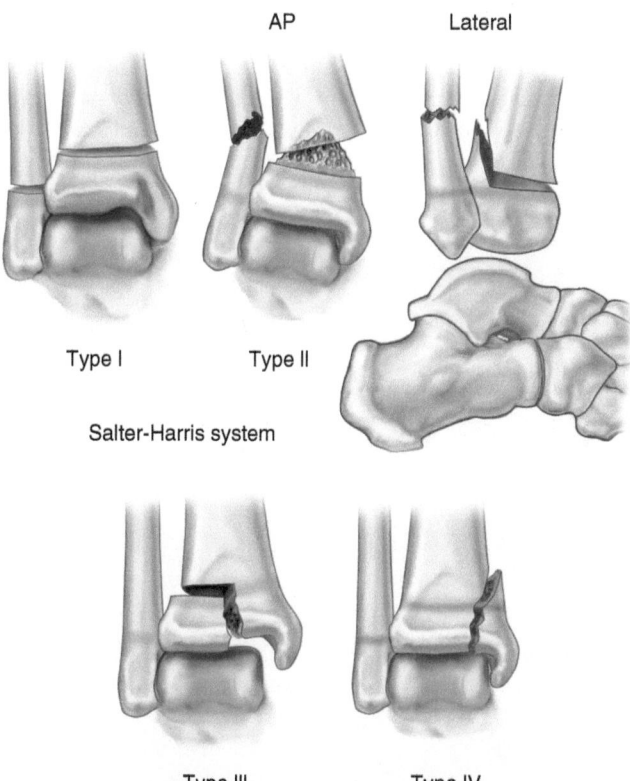

AP   **Lateral**

Type I   **Type II**

Salter-Harris system

Type III   **Type IV**

Fig. 138.6 Fracture patterns of the distal tibial and fibular physes classified by the Salter-Harris system. *AP*, Anteroposterior.

In the skeletally immature patient, the tibiotalar joint surface is rarely disturbed. The injury pattern changes in adolescence as the physis begins to close. Closure is usually complete by age 14 in females and age 16 in males. The outcome of the injury depends on the type of physeal injury and its management. Tension injuries usually produce Salter-Harris type I and II injuries of the physis. Compression forces can produce Salter-Harris type III and IV injuries. Podeszwa and Mubarak[24] state that the incidence of accessory centers of ossification is 20% in the medial malleolus and 1% in the lateral malleolus. These must be considered when looking at unusual fracture patterns. Rohmiller and colleagues have recently used the Lauge-Hansen system to look at the mechanism of injury in Salter-Harris type II distal tibial fractures.[27] This topic is discussed later in this chapter.

Clinical Evaluation

The mechanism of injury and the time elapsed since the accident should be noted. The neurovascular status of the foot should be carefully documented. The amount of swelling and the status of the skin are important. Gentle examination should be carried out to seek areas of point tenderness, especially over the physis. This examination may be more useful than radiographs in diagnosing Salter I fractures of the distal fibula. Plain radiography should include AP, lateral, and mortise views. CT and MRI are valuable techniques in assessing and classifying some fractures not clearly seen on plain radiographs, especially those that are intra-articular, because they allow more accurate evaluation of the fragments. CT is easily performed and less expensive than MRI and does not require sedation in the young child. Carey and associates[65] performed a study of plain films and MRI in 14 patients with acute injuries. The direct visualization of cartilage afforded by MRI improved evaluation of growth plate injury in each case. MRI changed Salter-Harris classification or staging in two of nine patients for whom fractures were visualized on conventional radiographs, allowed the detection of radiographically occult fractures in 5 of 14 cases, and resulted in a physical change in management for 5 of the 14 patients studied. MRI has an important role in the evaluation of acute pediatric growth plate injury, particularly when diagnostic uncertainty persists after the evaluation of conventional radiographs. MRI allows detection of occult fractures, may alter Salter-Harris staging, and may lead to a change in patient management. CT and MRI are particularly useful in the juvenile fracture of Tillaux and in triplane fractures.

Because treatment and prognosis depend on the Salter-Harris classification, the fractures are discussed according to fracture type. Podeszwa and Mubarak recommend open reduction in all physeal fractures with a gap of 3 mm or more.[24,28] They found entrapped periosteum as the main offender in causing the gap. Trapped periosteum has been implicated in an increased incidence of premature physeal closure (PPC).[29] Removal of epiphyseal metallic implants has been recommended when used in Salter type III and IV fractures of the tibia because the contact pressures as measured in cadavers are increased by the presence of epiphyseal screws. They mention the alternative use of bioabsorbable screws to obviate the need for removal.[28,30] As a general rule, any metallic fixation crossing the physis when growth potential remains should be removed to lessen the risk of physeal closure. Whenever possible, fixation should not cross the physis, and, if necessary, smooth pins should be used and then removed as soon as early healing has occurred.

Salter-Harris Type I

Salter-Harris I fractures of the distal fibula are very common in young children and may be misdiagnosed as a sprain and go untreated. They are diagnosed by swelling and tenderness on exam and slight widening of the physis on radiographs. Immobilization in a cast or boot for 3 to 4 weeks is sufficient. In 40 years of practice, the senior author has never seen a closure of the distal fibula with a Salter I fracture. Salter-Harris I fractures of the distal tibia can be missed as well. Careful clinical exam and scrutiny of the radiographs reveal widening of the physis in the area of tenderness and swelling.

Salter-Harris Type II

The Salter-Harris type II injury is uncommon or is frequently unrecognized in the fibula. Salter-Harris type II injury of the distal tibia combined with a fracture of the distal fibula is one of the most common injuries of the ankle, accounting for 47.3% of cases in the series compiled by Peterson and Cass.[31]

Rohmiller and colleagues studied 91 Salter-Harris type I and II fractures of the distal tibia. No distinction was made between types I and II.[27] Treatment options include no reduction and use of a cast, closed reduction and use of a cast, closed reduction and use of percutaneous pins and a cast, and open reduction with internal fixation. They found a 39.6% incidence of PPC. Using the Lauge-Hansen classification system, they found a significant increased incidence of PPC in pronation-abduction injuries (54%) compared with supination–external rotation injuries (35%). The most important determinant of PPC was the amount of fracture displacement after reduction. In some cases, periosteum was trapped in the fracture site medially, blocking reduction. These investigators thought that operative treatment might decrease the incidence of PPC. They recommended obtaining less than 2 mm of displacement in a child with 2 years of growth remaining to decrease the risk for PPC.

Traditional closed treatment consists of wearing a long-leg bent-knee cast for 2 to 3 weeks followed by a short-leg walking cast for 4 weeks. Dugan and coworkers reviewed 56 patients with this injury who were treated with a long-leg weight-bearing cast for 4 weeks.[32] There were no nonunions and no angular deformities. There was one case of clinically insignificant premature closure of the growth plate. Use of a long-leg weight-bearing cast for 4 weeks appears to be the treatment of choice because it allows early healing, low morbidity, and rapid rehabilitation. A boot can be used after 4 weeks to begin ROM.

Salter-Harris Type III

In adolescents, a Salter-Harris type III injury is also known as the *juvenile fracture of Tillaux*. The distal tibial physis closes first in the central region and then from the medial side toward the

fibula. An external rotation force applied to the partially closed physis applies traction on the physis through the anterior inferior talofibular ligament. This process avulses a fragment of the lateral physis, which remains attached to the ligament (Fig. 138.7). Closed reduction with use of an anesthetic should be attempted. The injury can be treated in a closed manner if the fragment is not displaced more than 2 mm, or if it can be reduced in a closed manner and percutaneously fixed. A smooth wire or a guidewire can be used in an attempt to satisfactorily reduce the fragment and pin it percutaneously. Most of these injuries require open reduction and fixation of the fragment with a pin or cancellous screw.

Fractures of the medial malleolus can be either type III or IV injuries. If displaced less than 2 mm, they may be treated in a closed manner, paying close attention to the medial joint space. Initially this treatment should consist of a long-leg non–weight-bearing cast for 3 weeks, followed by wearing a short-leg walking cast for 3 weeks. In open reduction cases if the Thurston-Holland fragment is large enough, it can be attached to the metaphysis to avoid crossing the physis. If it is not large enough to gain sufficient fixation, the pins should cross the physis. These injuries are the most unpredictable of ankle epiphyseal injuries. Near-anatomic reduction must be obtained.[33]

Salter-Harris Type IV

The Salter-Harris type IV group includes some of the medial malleolar fractures and the triplane fractures. The triplane fracture, first described by Marmor, is so named because the fracture lines extend from the physis into the transverse, sagittal, and coronal planes (see Fig. 138.7).[34-36] This type of fracture may be mistaken for a Salter-Harris type II injury if the radiographs are not carefully scrutinized.

Many authors have described this fracture and have argued about the number of fragments involved.[35-37] Most of these studies were based on plain radiography. Fig. 138.7 illustrates the

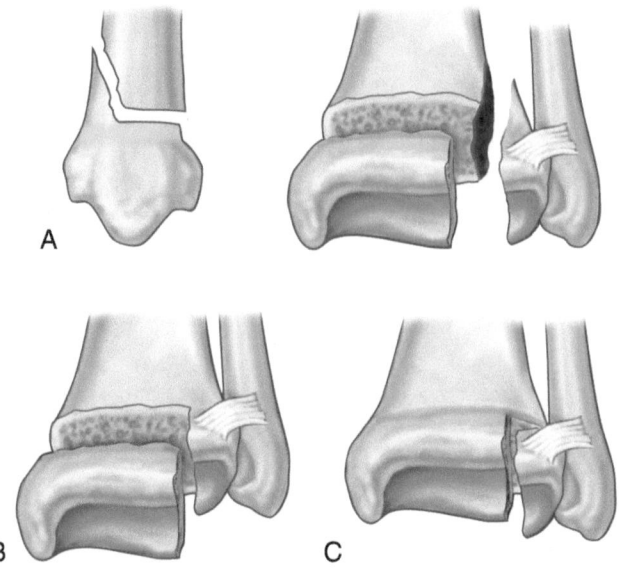

Fig. 138.7 (A) and (B) The triplane fracture can consist of two or more fragments. (C) The juvenile fracture of Tillaux.

possibilities. In the two-part fracture, the main fragment is the tibial shaft, including the medial malleolus and a portion of the medial epiphysis. The second fragment is the remaining epiphysis, which is attached to the fibula. In the three-part injury, the third fragment is usually an anterior free epiphyseal fragment. Brown and colleagues studied 51 children with tibial triplane fractures.[2] By evaluating them with CT with multiplanar reconstructions, these authors have used the best radiographic evaluation possible to define the number of fragments. The classic two-fragment type with medial epiphyseal extension was most frequent (occurring in 33 of 51 children). All three-fragment types (occurring in 8 of 51 children) had a separate anterolateral fragment. Extension to the medial malleolus was common (occurring in 12 of 51 children). None of the four reported fracture types involving anteromedial extension was seen.

Karrholm reviewed the literature on this injury.[38] Triplane fracture made up 7% of physeal injuries in girls and 15% in boys. Of the injuries, 35% were treated closed without manipulation, 30% by manipulation and casting, and 35% by open reduction and internal fixation.

If this injury can be reduced to within 2 mm, it may be treated in a closed manner. In the series reported by Cooperman,[34] 13 of 15 fractures were treated in a closed manner, and in the series reported by Dias and Giergerich five of eight were treated in this way.[35] In the series by Ertl,[36] residual displacement of more than 2 mm was associated with a high incidence of late symptoms. Obtaining a reduction of less than 2 mm by either closed or open means did not ensure an excellent result. Poor results may be related to damage done to the articular surface or to the amount of displacement. Fractures outside the weight-bearing area did not show this tendency toward poor results.

Evaluation of the adequacy of reduction in this injury is difficult, and because most authors recommend manipulation after induction of general anesthesia, the only radiographic means of diagnosis available is plain radiography. Our preferred method is manipulation, after the patient is sedated, by internal rotation of the foot; this manipulation is usually performed in the emergency department. If any question exists about the adequacy of reduction on plain radiographs, CT or plain tomography is used to evaluate the articular surface and the reduction (Fig. 138.8). If displacement is greater than 2 mm, open reduction with internal fixation is performed, which may require two incisions. The first is an anterolateral incision, which permits identification of the anterolateral fragment. Usually, it is first necessary to reduce and fix the posterior fragment. If this procedure cannot be performed in a closed manner, a second posteromedial approach is used to reduce the fragment under direct vision. Fixation is achieved with cannulated screws, cancellous screws, or pins. These injuries require the patient to wear a cast for 6 weeks.

Prediction of Outcome

The prognosis for an ankle fracture in a skeletally immature patient depends on the following factors:

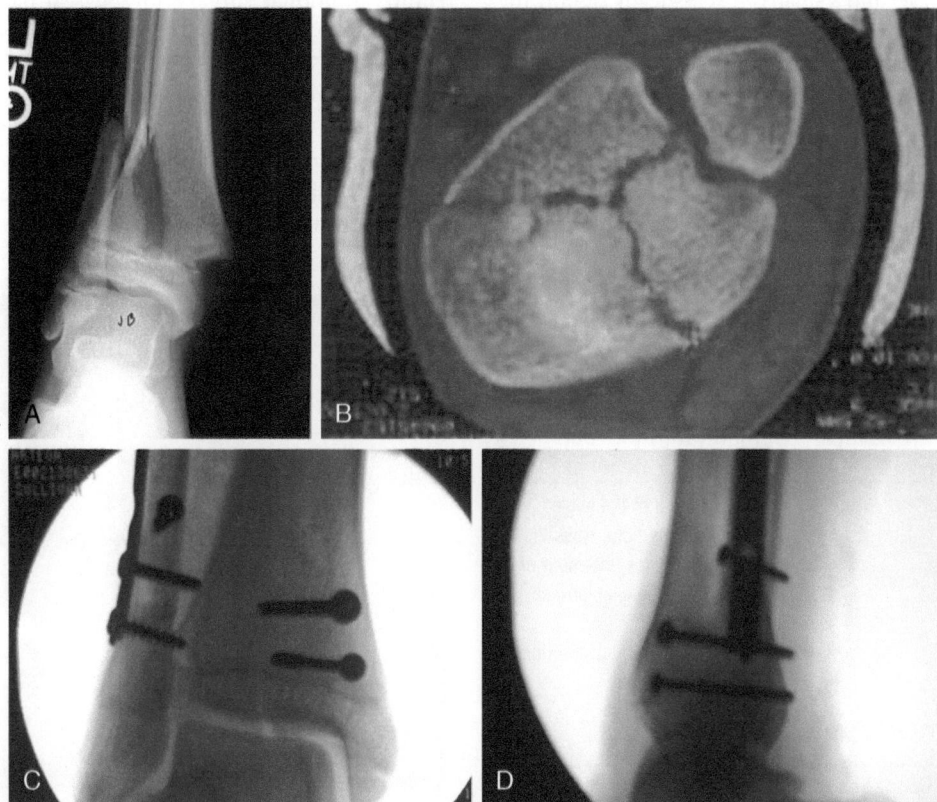

Fig. 138.8 (A) Anteroposterior view of a triplane and (B) computed tomography scan showing multiple fragments (C), (D). The position achieved by open reduction. (D) The position retained after hardware removal.

1. Mechanism of injury
2. Salter-Harris classification
3. Quality of the reduction
4. State of skeletal maturity
5. Amount of displacement
6. Miscellaneous modifiers (e.g., open fracture, vascular injury, infection, systemic illness, and interposed periosteum)

Spiegel[37] retrospectively studied a series of closed distal tibial physeal injuries; 184 patients (of 237) were followed up for an average of 28 months. The authors looked specifically at the complications of angular deformity of greater than 5 degrees and shortening of more than 1 cm, joint incongruity, or asymmetric closure of the physis. These complications appeared to correlate with the Salter-Harris type, the amount of displacement or comminution, and the adequacy of reduction. The patients were divided into the groups shown in Table 138.1.

The overall complication rate was 14.1% for the 184 patients. Salter-Harris II injuries of the tibia appeared to be the least predictable because the incidence of complications remained approximately the same, regardless of the amount of displacement. Displacement is not always mentioned as one of the factors involved in prediction of outcome, but it is intuitive that greater displacement implies greater force, with damage more likely to the articular cartilage, the circulation, and the soft tissues important in healing. Karrholm thought the good results were based on the adequacy of the reduction.[38]

Near-anatomic reduction of type II injuries of the tibia is desirable. Gruber and associates have shown in an animal model that interposed periosteum in an intact physis produces a spectrum of changes at the tissue level and a small but statistically significant leg-length discrepancy compared with fracture alone.[39] Because this is a spectrum, it may explain the unpredictable nature of these injuries and support the need to remove interposed periosteum (Fig. 138.9). Residual displacement after attempted closed reduction may be a result of this interposition.

The patient in Fig. 138.10A was treated by closed manipulation and casting. He had residual medial displacement (see Fig. 138.10B and C). Follow-up radiographs show the development of a defect in the medial cortex. A valgus ankle deformity subsequently developed (see Fig. 138.10D), which would indicate that the medial physis and suspected interposed periosteum grew more than the lateral side. He required a varus tibial osteotomy and physeal closure. Although some patients experience normal growth despite the medial cortical defect, the unpredictability and high frequency in the article by Rohmiller and colleagues support a near-anatomic reduction with less than 2 mm of displacement in a child with more than 2 years of growth remaining.[27] These injuries must be followed up until the patient attains skeletal maturity or a normal growth pattern is ensured because some patients will experience premature closure and an angular deformity.[33]

The juvenile fracture of Tillaux and the triplane fracture result from incomplete closure of the physis. Because growth is nearing an end, angular deformity and shortening are uncommon. In these patients, the tibiotalar joint surface is disturbed and must be restored to as near normal as possible to prevent incongruity and subsequent traumatic arthritis. In the series by Cooperman and colleagues, triplane fractures were reduced by internally rotating the foot while the patient was in a state of general anesthesia.[34] The adequacy of reduction was determined by plain tomography. Dias and Giergerich reported on nine Tillaux and triplane fractures that were followed up for an average of 18 months, and all patients did well.[35]

Peterson and Cass reviewed all Salter-Harris type IV distal tibial injuries seen at the Mayo Clinic, with particular attention given to injuries of the medial malleolus.[31] Nine of 18 patients with these injuries experienced PPC of a sufficient degree to require additional surgery for physeal bar resection, angular deformity, or leg-length discrepancy. Thirteen of these patients received their care at the Mayo Clinic, and of these, 11 had closed injuries. Six patients were treated with closed reduction and a short-leg cast. Five patients underwent open reduction and internal fixation. Five additional patients in the study had been referred to the clinic because of complications of a closed injury that had been treated in a closed manner. The investigators concluded

TABLE 138.1	Complications of Ankle Fractures	
Group	Complication Rate (%)	Salter-Harris Group and Bone Involved
Low risk (89 patients)	6.7	Types I and II of the fibula, type I of the tibia, types III and IV with displacement of less than 2 mm, epiphyseal avulsion injuries
High risk (28 patients)	32	Types III, IV, and V of the tibia Tillaux and triplane
Unpredictable (66 patients)	16.7	Type II of the tibia

Data from Spiegel PG, Cooperman DR, Laros GS. Epiphyseal fractures of the distal ends of the tibia and fibula. A retrospective study of two hundred and thirty-seven cases in children. *J Bone Joint Surg Am.* 1978;60(8):1046–1050.

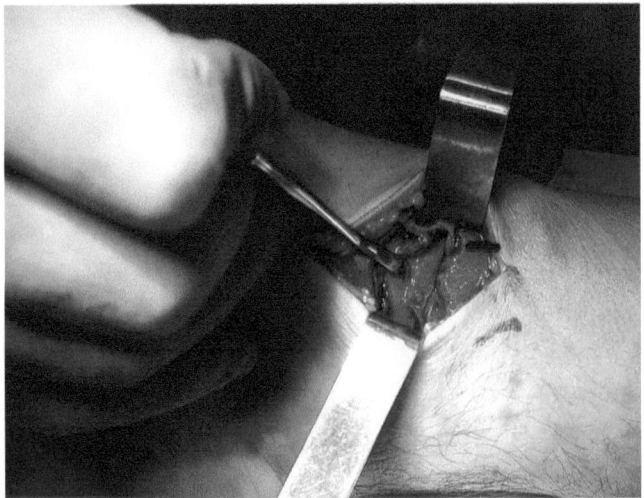

Fig. 138.9 The Freer elevator is on the metaphyseal periosteum that is inverted into the physeal fracture site. The black mark is on the epiphyseal fragment.

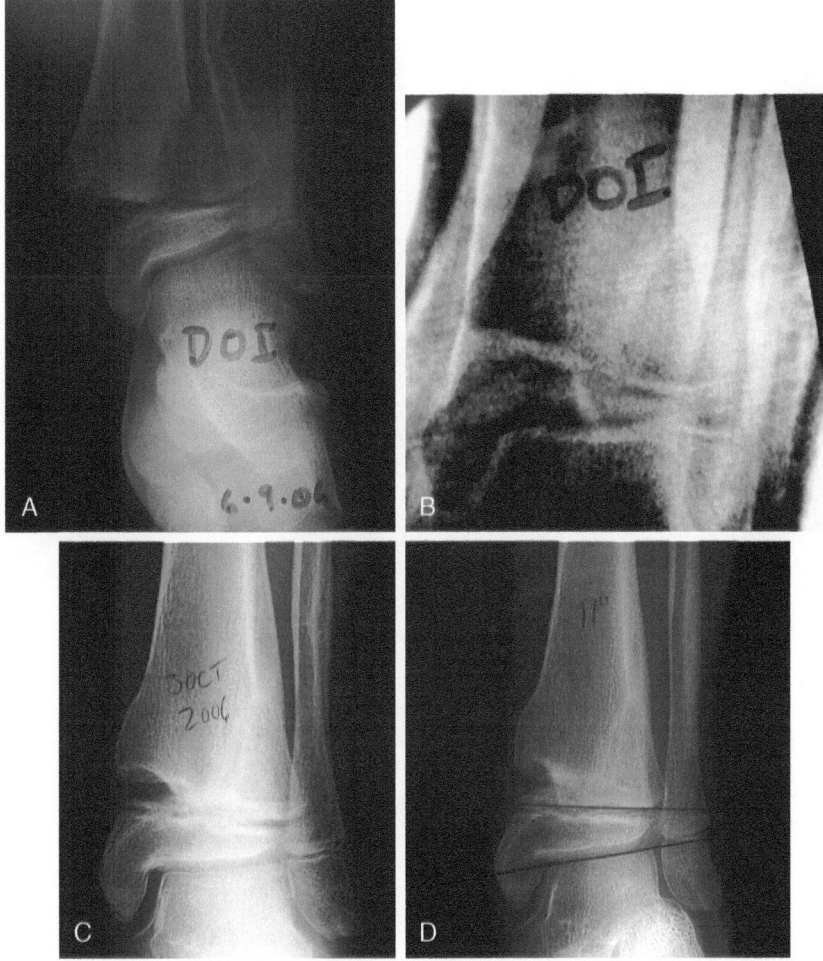

Fig. 138.10 (A) An anteroposterior (AP) radiograph on the day of injury of this Salter-Harris type II tibial fracture. (B) A postreduction AP radiograph. (C) An AP radiograph at 4 months. (D) An AP radiograph at 2 years.

that oblique radiographs are necessary to ensure an accurate diagnosis and to confirm the adequacy of the reduction. Some injuries that resemble type III injuries are actually type IV injuries. The authors also found that partial arrest that results in angular deformity was more common than complete arrest. They concluded that three patterns of medial malleolar injury exist and that type IV injuries constitute the most common and most dangerous pattern because they usually occur in a patient who has remaining growth potential (Fig. 138.11). The authors also concluded that the medial malleolus requires anatomic reduction, which often necessitates open reduction and internal fixation.

In any patient with an open physis, it is preferable to avoid crossing the physis with a fixation device. This goal can usually be achieved by placing smooth pins from metaphysis to metaphysis or from epiphysis to epiphysis. At times, crossing the physis cannot be avoided. Smooth pins can be used, and care should be taken that they do not cross within the physis. Patients need to be followed up until skeletal maturity is achieved or until one is certain that a normal growth pattern is occurring. An asymmetric Harris growth arrest line may be the earliest clue to an abnormal growth pattern (see Fig. 138.11).

FRACTURES IN THE FOOT

Fractures of the foot resulting from participation in sports are unusual in children. Fractures of the metatarsals can result from direct trauma (Fig. 138.12) and can be treated by immobilization in a short-leg walking cast. The most controversial fracture in the foot may be an avulsion injury at the base of the fifth metatarsal.

Fractures of the fifth metatarsal in children can be divided into distal physeal fractures, fractures of the proximal diaphysis, and avulsion fractures of the apophysis. The fifth metatarsal has its epiphysis distally and an apophysis proximally. The tendon of the peroneus brevis is inserted into the apophysis. With inversion stress, the apophysis can be avulsed. Findings include tenderness at the base of the fifth metatarsal and radiographic confirmation of widening of the apophysis. Treatment should be symptomatic with compression and partial weight bearing until the pain subsides. Use of crutches and an elastic bandage may be sufficient. Two to 3 weeks in a short-leg cast or boot also yields good results.

Fracture of the proximal diaphysis of the fifth metatarsal (Jones fracture) is less common in skeletally immature patients

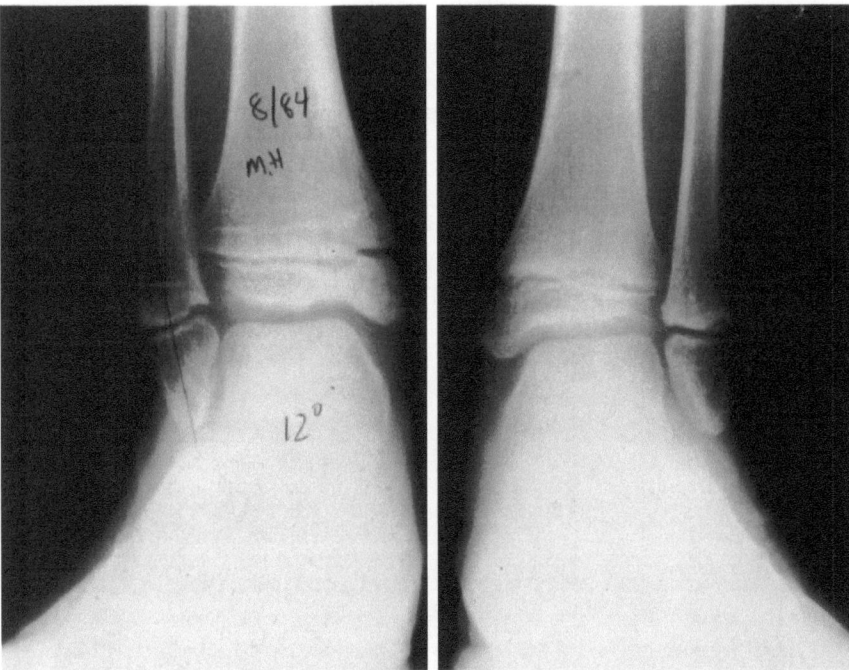

Fig. 138.11 This patient sustained a Salter-Harris type IV medial malleolar fracture, which was treated in a closed manner. The patient was referred 6 months after injury, at which time she had trouble remembering which ankle had been injured. These radiographs were taken 18 months after the injury. Resection of a bony bridge and interposition were required. She resumed growth, and the fibular angular deformity had been corrected. Note the irregular Harris growth arrest lines.

and usually occurs in the 15- to 20-year age range.[40] When such fractures occur, a trial of immobilization in a short-leg walking cast is indicated because many acute fractures heal. Even fractures with delayed union may heal if they are treated conservatively.[40] Early operative intervention in highly competitive athletes has been advocated by some investigators, but others have shown that each patient needs to be treated individually because some of these fractures will heal if treated conservatively, allowing early return to athletics.[40-42] Early operative intervention in the pediatric athlete is rarely if ever indicated. Patients with established nonunion require operative treatment that includes reopening of the medullary canal, bone grafting, and internal fixation (Fig. 138.13).

Fractures of the toes are unusual in athletes. Buddy taping a fractured toe to the adjacent toe or wearing appropriate shoes for a few weeks and avoiding participation in sports until the toe is asymptomatic is the approach used to treat most phalangeal fractures. Articular fractures are even more rare. The only one that may merit consideration of operative management is an intra-articular physeal fracture of the great toe. These fractures should be reduced to as near-anatomic alignment as possible by whatever means necessary (Fig. 138.14).

Stress fractures are less common among children than adults but cannot be entirely dismissed. Some children participate in marathons and other sporting events that can result in stress fractures. Basketball, soccer, and other team sports have tournaments that may require considerable running. The stress fracture shown in Fig. 138.15 resulted from a tournament and was thought to be a sprain. Stress fractures are also common in high school cross-country athletes. Given that it is a stress reaction and requires

rest and/or immobilization before resumption of activity, a stress fracture is often a season-ending event for runners.

Yngve found 131 pediatric stress fractures in 23 references in the literature.[43] Two of the 131 reports documented metatarsal fractures—two of the tarsal navicular and one of the medial sesamoid. The primary training error was "too much too soon." Other factors that should be considered are a change in training surface or equipment (shoes), an overlap of two sports, and a sudden change in intensity of training (tournaments). Diagnosis depends on an appropriate history, a high index of suspicion, and the presence of localized tenderness and edema at times. The differential diagnosis includes contusion, tendinitis, and sprains.

The initial radiograph may be normal but should be diagnostic in half of cases. One should look for cortical thickening or a translucent fracture line. A bone scan may be diagnostic at this stage and may be particularly helpful if the diagnosis is in question and one wishes to avoid immobilization. A bone scan may be indicated when the diagnosis is in doubt and the athlete wishes to RTP. MRI has also been used to identify occult stress fractures. Conversely, immobilization for 2 weeks in a cast is usually diagnostic in that pain is relieved; repeat radiographs are then positive, making a bone scan unnecessary. Although some of these fractures heal without use of a cast, the athlete should be immobilized for protection from himself or herself, as well as from well-meaning parents and coaches.

Osteochondral Lesions of the Talus

The term osteochondral lesions of the talus (OLT) encompasses two main pathologies: osteochondritis dissecans (OCD) and

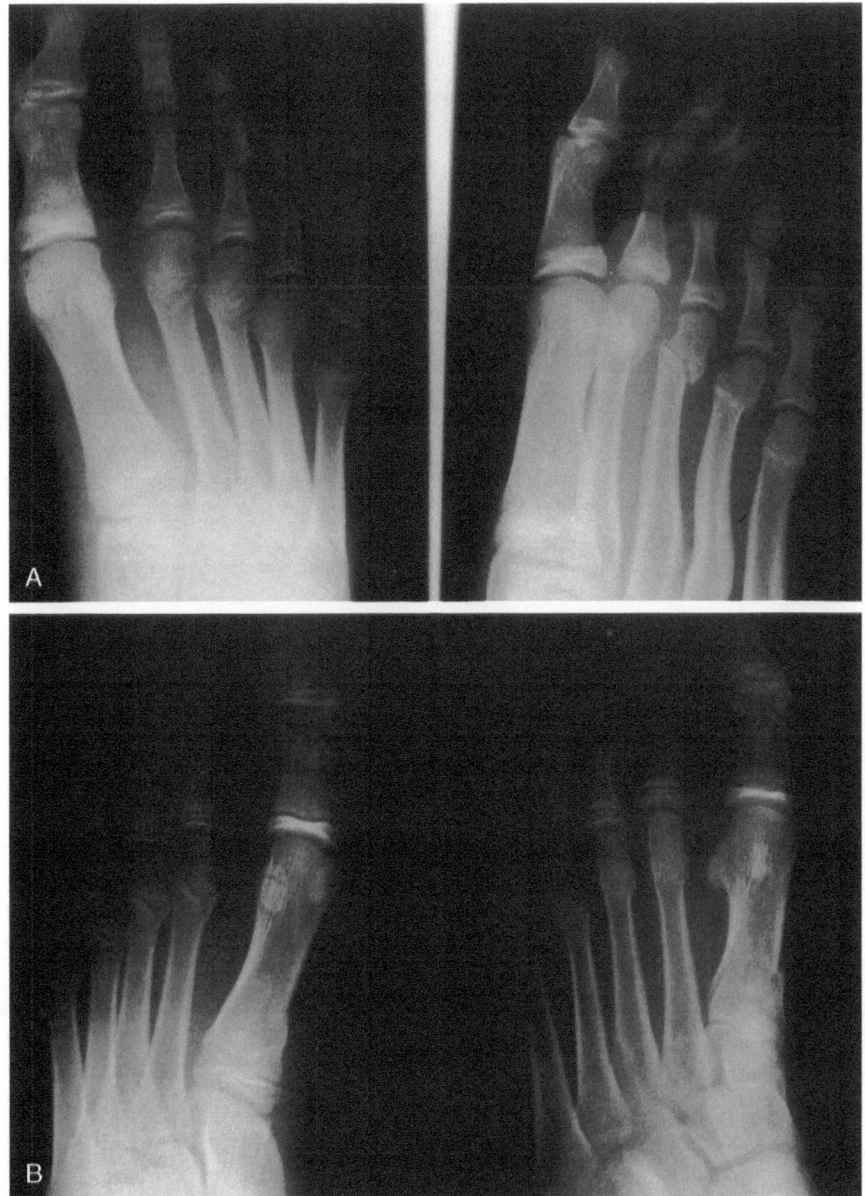

Fig. 138.12 (A) This patient sustained fractures of the lateral four metatarsal necks when he caught his foot on a base while sliding. (B) This patient sustained a fracture of his first metatarsal when he was stepped on during a football game.

osteochondral fractures. OLT is the more commonly used term, as opposed to delineating between the two. Prevalence of OLT has increased with the advent of more sensitive imaging modalities to identify these lesions.[44-46] True OCD lesions are classically attributed to a vascular insult, but there is more evidence supporting trauma as the initial insult, especially ankle instability events.[47-51] OLT was classically described as anterolateral and posteromedial in location. With the advent of better 3D imaging, we now appreciate that centromedial lesions are more common, followed by centrolateral.[52,53]

Berndt and Harty[48] developed a classification system based on the amount of damage and the degree of displacement involved. This system, in a slightly modified form, is still in use:

Stage I: Localized trabecular compression
Stage II: Incompletely separated fragment

Stage IIA: Formation of a subchondral cyst
Stage III: Undetached, undisplaced fragment
Stage IV: Displaced or inverted fragment

Most series consist predominantly of adults; however, 21 of 29 patients studied by Canale and Belding experienced onset of symptoms during the second decade.[49] CT and MRI can reveal lesions not seen on plain films and also make staging more accurate. These techniques may reveal that this disorder is more common among adolescents than was previously suspected. Hao et al.[50] compared conventional MRI with 3D MRI (fast spoiled gradient recalled acquisition in the steady state [FSPGR]) in a group of 21 patients with suspected cartilage lesions. All lesions were confirmed by arthroscopy. The investigators concluded that T1-weighted 3D fat-suppressed FSPGR MRI is more sensitive than is conventional MRI in detecting defects of articular cartilage

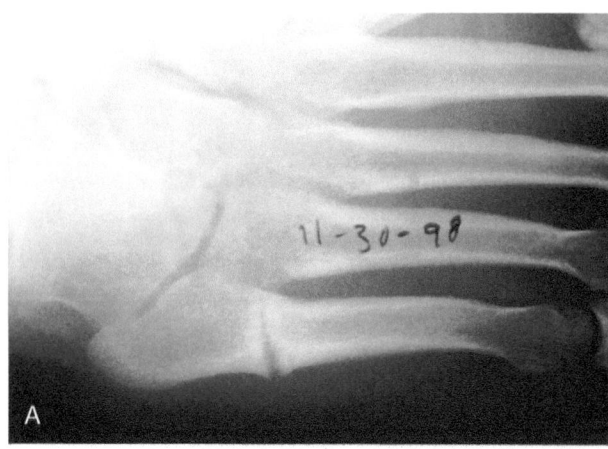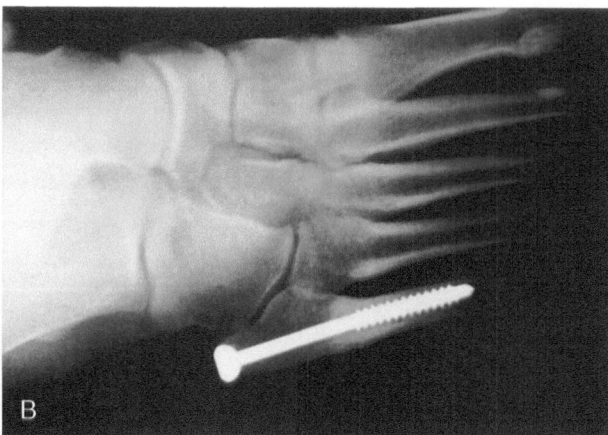

Fig. 138.13 (A) This patient sustained a fracture of the diaphysis of the fifth metatarsal. This radiograph was obtained 2 months after treatment with a cast. The metatarsal was tender to palpation, and the patient walked with a limp. (B) This radiograph was obtained after treatment with internal fixation and a local bone graft from the calcaneus.

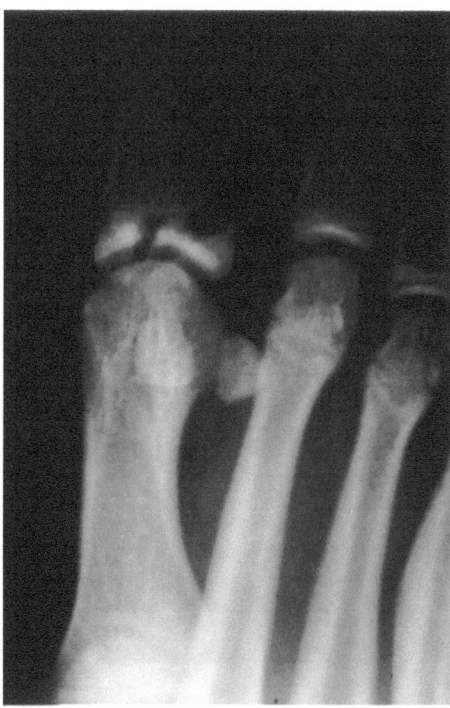

Fig. 138.14 This intra-articular fracture was treated with closed reduction and percutaneous pinning.

covering OLT. Proper treatment depends on identification of the lesion and accurate staging.

Canale and Belding suggested that nonoperative treatment by immobilization of all stage I, stage II, and medial stage III (Berndt and Harty classification) lesions would result in a high percentage of good clinical results and delayed development of arthrosis.[49] Persistent symptoms after conservative treatment were an indication for operative treatment by excision and curettage. These investigators further recommended that all stage III lateral lesions and all stage IV lesions be treated by immediate excision and curettage of the lesion. Anderson and associates

recommended immobilization for 6 weeks for patients with stage I and II fractures, but they cautioned that these patients need to be followed up for a prolonged time so that delayed development of arthrosis can be detected.[47] Operative treatment was recommended for patients with stage IIA, III, and IV lesions.

Letts and colleagues reviewed 24 children treated since 1983 for OCD of either the medial or lateral dome of the talus (two were bilateral).[51] The average age at presentation was 13 years, 4 months. Nonoperative treatment included activity restriction, physiotherapy, and immobilization. Surgical intervention was required in 15 ankles (58%). Surgical treatment included arthroscopy (1), arthrotomy and drilling of the defect (9), drilling with excision of the lesion (3), excision of the lesion (2), and pinning of the fragment (1). Most recent follow-up revealed resolution or decreased symptoms in 25 patients (96%) and no change in one patient. MRI was useful in preoperative assessment in six cases. In this series, a slight female preponderance was noted (58%). Higuera and coworkers reported good to excellent results in 94.8% of children.[54] Cuttica et al. reported favorable results with marrow stimulation techniques such as drilling or microfracture in contained lesions measuring less than 1.5 cm.[55] For larger uncontained lesions, they recommend consideration of a more extensive initial procedure.

Kramer et al. reviewed 109 ankles in 100 patients over a 10-year period. Multiple different interventions were included. They showed a high reoperation rate, at 27%, usually for postoperative images that looked the same or worse. Despite that, they had a high overall satisfaction and return to sport, 82% and 84%, respectively. Female sex and higher body mass index favored a worse outcome.

Perumal and colleagues retrospectively reviewed 31 subjects with a mean age of 11.9 years treated nonoperatively with 6 to 8 weeks weight-bearing cast followed by lace-up ankle brace.[56] They had 6 months of sports and activity restriction. All had repeat radiographs at the end of the 6 months: 16% of subjects had complete clinical and radiologic improvement, and 77% had persistent radiographic lesions. Another 6 months of activity

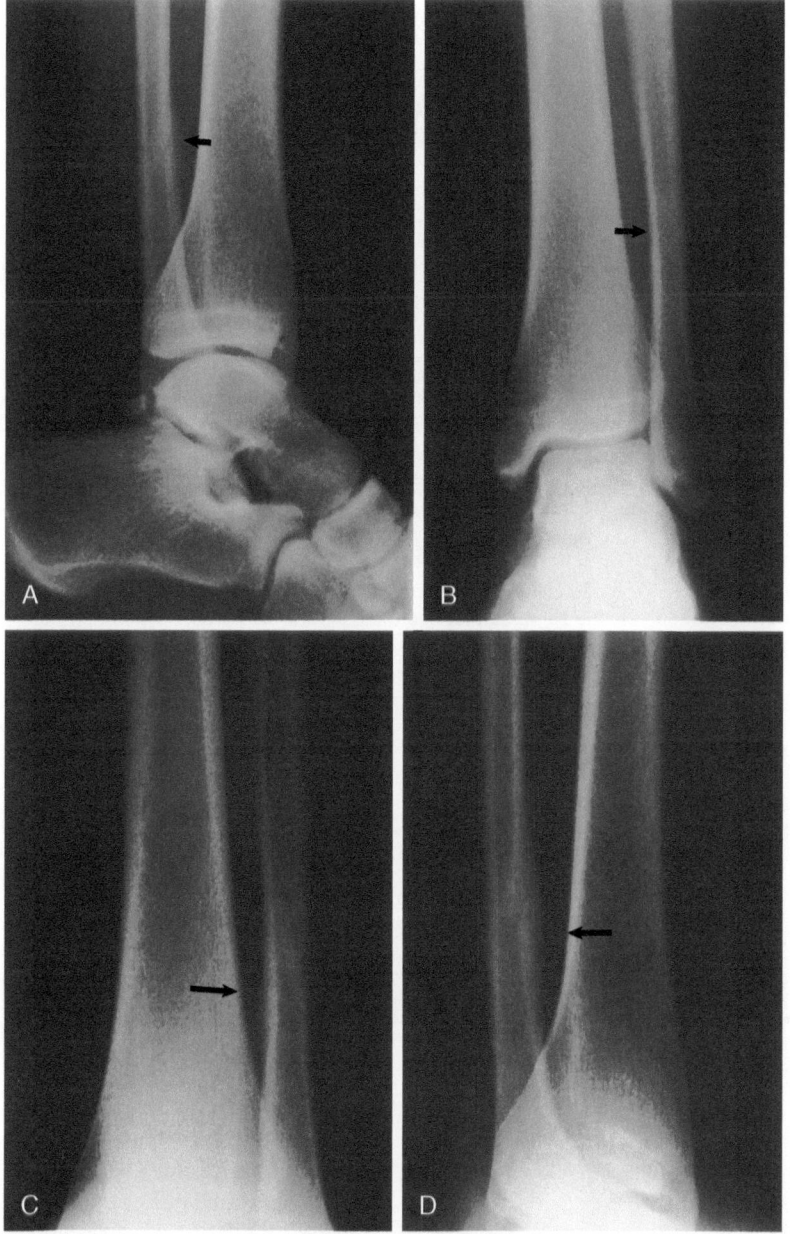

Fig. 138.15 This patient presented with localized tenderness just above the ankle. After being injured in a basketball tournament, she continued to play with a presumptive diagnosis of a sprained ankle. The initial radiographs (A and B) showed periosteal elevation *(arrows)*. Follow-up radiographs (C and D) taken after 2 weeks of treatment with a short-leg walking cast illustrate new bone formation *(arrows)*.

modification was implemented for those with persistent OCD lesions, 46% of these went on to have no symptoms, despite persistent lesions on radiographs, and 42% of these underwent subsequent surgery for unhealed painful lesions.

For those who fail nonoperative management, multiple operative interventions have been described. Microfracture/bone marrow stimulation with or without fixation,[57-59] osteochondral autograft or allograft,[60] and chondrocyte implantation are all options and depends on the size, depth, location, and stability of the lesion. As arthroscopic techniques have advanced, so has the ability to address these lesions via a scope and avoid the additional morbidity of a medial malleolar osteotomy.

Osteochondroses in the Foot

The osteochondroses are a group of conditions of unknown origin. Suggested causes have included endocrinopathies, vascular phenomena, infection, and trauma.[61] Many of these conditions are now known to represent radiographic variations of normal ossification of the epiphysis. Most are named for the person or persons who originally described them. They all include a pattern of clinical symptoms coupled with a radiograph that suggests that the epiphysis or apophysis is undergoing necrosis. In the foot, the most commonly described conditions are Kohler syndrome and Freiberg infarction.

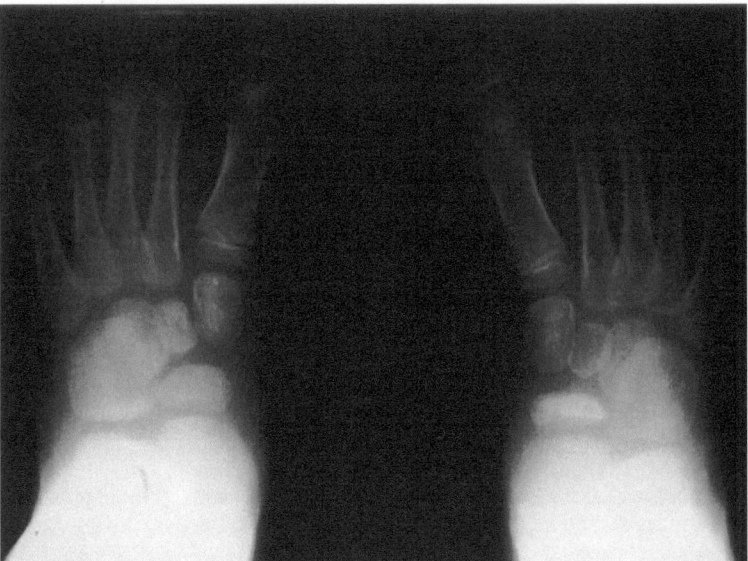

Fig. 138.16 This patient presented with undisplaced fractures of the metatarsals. The condensed, narrowed appearance of the navicular is the same as that seen in patients with Kohler syndrome, but it was an incidental finding in this patient.

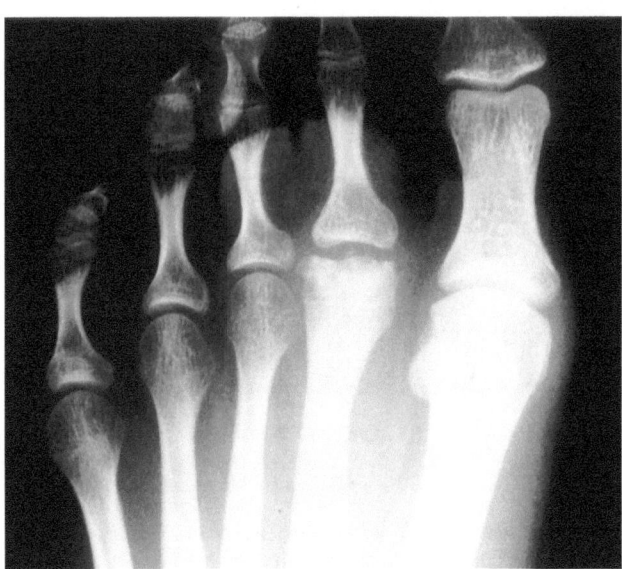

Fig. 138.17 This anteroposterior radiograph of the foot shows irregularity and collapse of the second metatarsal head.

Kohler syndrome is a clinical syndrome consisting of pain in the midfoot coupled with a finding of localized tenderness over the navicular. Radiographs demonstrate increased density and narrowing of the tarsal navicular. Irregular ossification in this bone may be the rule rather than the exception, and thus the existence of this condition is in question (Fig. 138.16). Williams and Cowell reviewed a series of patients with the following findings.[62] Thirty percent of males and 20% of females demonstrated irregular ossification in the tarsal navicular. Most patients appeared to respond to 6 weeks of immobilization in a cast. All 23 patients eventually became asymptomatic, and the navicular became normal. The authors believed that patients treated in a cast became asymptomatic sooner than did those treated with

shoe inserts. Regardless of treatment, no long-term problems were associated with this condition, again raising the question of whether it is a distinct pathologic condition.

Freiberg disease is a condition of condensation and collapse of the second metatarsal head and articular surface. It commonly occurs during the second decade of life while the epiphysis is still present.[63] It is of unknown cause and is more common among females. Many causes have been proposed, but repetitive trauma probably plays a role. The lesion occurs most commonly in the second or third metatarsal (Fig. 138.17), which are the longest and least mobile of the metatarsals.[61] The patient presents with pain on weight bearing and has localized tenderness over the metatarsal head. Radiographs reveal collapse of the articular surface (see Fig. 138.17). Conservative treatment with a cast or orthotic device that minimizes weight bearing over the involved head is often successful in relieving the pain. Surgical treatment consisting of removal of loose bodies or bone grafting has been reported for persistent symptoms. A dorsiflexion osteotomy to relieve weight bearing has also been reported to work well. Removal of the metatarsal head should be avoided because this procedure results in transfer of weight bearing to the adjacent metatarsal heads. Prosthetic replacement has also been tried but is not indicated in children. In most instances, the disease runs its course and the head reossifies within 2 to 3 years.

Sever disease is a term used to refer to a nonarticular osteochondrosis or a traction apophysitis (Fig. 138.18). The real question is whether a distinct syndrome exists and, if it does, whether the apophysis has anything to do with it. The calcaneal apophysis appears and develops in the 5- to 12-year age range and is typically irregular. Often, a child with heel pain and an irregular apophysis has the same radiographic finding in the opposite asymptomatic heel. Rachel et al. recently reported a 5% rate of diagnosis of another lesion on lateral radiographic images of children with heel pain and presumed calcaneal apophysitis.[64]

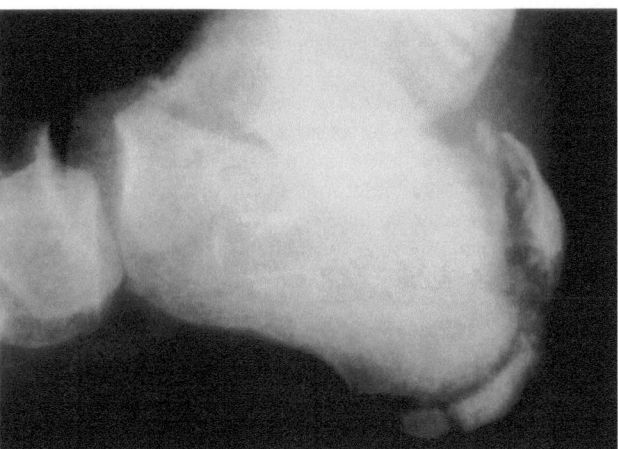

Fig. 138.18 A lateral radiograph of the calcaneus. Note the irregularity, especially in the superior part of the apophysis. Fragmentation and increased density are common occurrences in the calcaneal apophysis.

In response, they recommend routine lateral radiographs of children presenting with insidious onset of heel pain to rule out other potentially more aggressive diagnoses. These children are usually in the 9- to 12-year age range and are active in sports. They may have a tight heel cord. The calcaneus serves as the insertion of the powerful gastrocnemius-soleus muscle and the origin of the plantar fascia. Traction or overuse can strain these structures, producing pain. Stretching may be beneficial. Symptomatic treatment by avoidance of the offending exercise is usually curative. Shock-absorbing inserts or a heel cup may be advantageous. A heel lift to relieve some of the pull of the gastrocnemius-soleus or at times an arch support for a child with a high arch may also provide symptomatic relief. Heel cord–stretching exercises may be tried. In addition, splinting at night and/or short-term immobilization in a controlled ankle movement walker boot or weight-bearing cast may provide symptom relief. One must carefully search for the point of maximal tenderness and seek its cause rather than implicating an irregular apophysis, which is probably not the source of the pain. The exact time frame for resolution of symptoms in children with heel pain is unknown and at times can be vexing. If we believe that the child has complied with the previous conservative measures and is no better after 2 to 3 months, we proceed with further workup, such as a bone scan and other studies, to seek more occult sources of the pain.

SYSTEMIC ILLNESS

Systemic illness can present with foot pain and must be considered in the pediatric and adolescent athlete. Rheumatoid arthritis or hemophilia can involve the subtalar joint. Osteomyelitis can involve the foot but is unusual unless the patient has a history of a puncture wound. Acute lymphocytic leukemia is a great masquerader and can infiltrate the bones of the foot. Although they are rare, these types of diseases must be considered. One cannot develop tunnel vision and believe that all pain in an athlete is of a traumatic origin.

SHOES AND ORTHOTICS

The athletic shoe business is lucrative, as is shown by the intense marketing, endorsement, and competition for the introduction of new technology and an edge in the marketplace. Little scientific evidence supports the hype associated with shoe sales. Most often, the advertisements depict current sports heroes wearing shoes from the high end of the price scale, and they tell us little about the shoes themselves. Athletic shoes should fit adequately in both width and length. The models and range of widths available are more limited for children. The material should be reasonably soft. Too often, children's athletic shoes are made of stiff, unyielding, synthetic material and are poorly padded around the heel counter. Multisport shoes with small-diameter, evenly spaced cleats that distribute weight bearing more evenly are preferable to cleated or studded shoes. Padding over the heel counter and ankle may increase comfort. Most shoes now come with a built-in arch support that has little scientific basis but may give some support to children with a well-developed arch. Children with flatter feet may actually find it necessary to remove the pad. Barefoot running or running in toe shoes is a hot, controversial topic for which no literature relating to children is available, and the senior author would not recommend it.

Orthotics is another area of controversy. An asymptomatic flexible flatfoot should be left alone. No evidence exists to support the idea that an orthotic will bring about any structural change in such a foot. A painful flatfoot should prompt a thorough search for its cause, such as a tarsal coalition. Orthotics may be tried in a patient with aching feet or shins and a flexible flatfoot. Heel cups may be beneficial in the symptomatic treatment of heel pain. Little if any scientific information is available about the use of sports orthotics in children.

For a complete list of references, go to ExpertConsult.com.

SELECTED READINGS

Citation:
Wuerz TH, Gurd DP. Pediatric physeal ankle fracture. *J Am Acad Orthop Surg.* 2013;21(4):234-244.

Level of Evidence:
IV

Summary:
This is a comprehensive review of current diagnosis and management of pediatric physeal ankle fractures.

Citation:
Vincent KA. Tarsal coalition and painful flatfoot. *J Am Acad Orthop Surg.* 1998;6(5):274–281.

Level of Evidence:
V

Summary:
Vincent provides a comprehensive review of the types of tarsal coalition and their diagnosis and management.

Citation:
Letts M, Davidson D, Ahmer A. Osteochondritis dissecans of the talus in children. *J Pediatr Orthop.* 2003;23(5):617–625.

Level of Evidence:
IV

Summary:
Since 1983, 24 children treated for osteochondritis dissecans of the talus at a major Canadian pediatric referral center were followed up. Two children had bilateral involvement, for a total of 26 lesions. The patients included 10 boys and 14 girls. The lesion involved the medial aspect of the talus in 19 patients, the lateral aspect in 5 patients, and the central talar dome in 3 patients. Magnetic resonance imaging was very useful in preoperative assessment in six cases. Surgical intervention was required in 15 ankles (58%). Results at the most recent follow-up revealed resolution or decreased symptoms in 25 patients (96%) and no change in 1 patient (4%).

Citation:
Podeszwa DA, Mubarak SJ. Physeal fractures of the distal tibia and fibula (Salter-Harris type I, II, III, and IV fractures). *J Pediatr Orthop.* 2012;32(Suppl 1):S62–S68.

Level of Evidence:
V Review Article

Summary:
The authors provide an excellent up-to-date review of physeal fractures of the distal tibia and fibula.

Citation:
Gantsoudes GD, Roocroft JH, Mubarak SJ. Treatment of talocalcaneal coalitions. *J Pediatr Orthop.* 2012;32(3):301–307.

Level of Evidence:
IV

Summary:
A retrospective review was performed for all patients who underwent surgical treatment for a symptomatic talocalcaneal coalition over a 13-year period. Ninety-three feet were treated with excision and fat graft interposition by six surgeons. The authors concluded that a symptomatic talocalcaneal coalition can be treated with excision and fat graft interposition and that good to excellent results can be achieved in 85% of patients. Patients should be counseled that a subset may require further surgery to correct malalignment.

Citation:
Cuttica DJ, Smith WB, Hyer CF, et al. Osteochondral lesions of the talus: predictors of clinical outcome. *Foot Ankle Int.* 2011;32(11):1045–1051.

Level of Evidence:
IV

Summary:
A retrospective review of a group of patients treated operatively for osteochondral lesions of the talus was performed to determine factors that may have affected outcome. The treatment of osteochondral lesions of the talus remains a challenge for the foot and ankle surgeon. Arthroscopic débridement and drilling often provide satisfactory results. However, larger lesions and uncontained lesions are often associated with inferior functional outcomes and may require a more extensive initial procedure.

Citation:
Perumal V, Wall E, Babekir N. Juvenile osteochondritis of the talus. *J Pediatr Orthop.* 2007;27(7):821–825.s

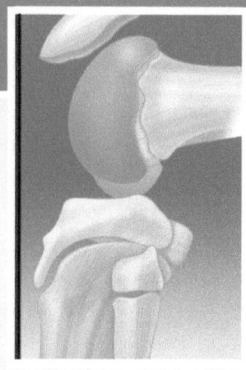

139

Head Injuries in Skeletally Immature Athletes

Tracy Zaslow

The incidence of sports- and recreation-related traumatic brain injuries (TBIs) has continued to increase during the past decade.[1] The two most common athletic activities associated with emergency department treatment for TBI are bicycling and football.[2] Risk for TBI is inherent to participation in sports and recreation activities, and compared with adults, children and adolescents have an increased risk for TBIs, with increased severity and prolonged recovery.[2] TBI is a term that encompasses a broad range of head injuries and includes concussion, skull fracture, epidural hematoma, subdural hematoma, intracerebral hematoma, and subarachnoid hemorrhage.

CONCUSSION

Concussion is defined as a complex, transient, pathophysiologic process that affects the brain and is induced by traumatic biomechanical forces.[3] Concussions occur with rapid onset and involve short-lived neurologic impairment that typically resolves spontaneously. *Acute clinical presentation reflects a functional disturbance rather than structural injury.* Injury occurs on a biochemical level without significant detectable gross anatomic changes, which supports the understanding that the changes are based on temporary neuronal dysfunction, not cell death.[4] Biochemical neuronal dysfunction occurs as a result of a combination of shifts in ion balance, altered glucose metabolism, impaired connectivity, and changes in neurotransmission. This biochemical dysfunction presents clinically in patients with a constellation of symptoms that may include any combination of one of more of the following: headache, dizziness, confusion, disorientation, hearing/visual disturbances, and/or loss of consciousness. It is important to understand that this range of clinical symptoms may or may not involve loss of consciousness. Historically, athletes referred to concussive episodes as a "ding" or "getting your bell rung"; these terms may describe the disorientation experienced by the athletes and are suspicious, if not defining, for a concussive injury. Results of neuroimaging studies (i.e., skull radiographs and head computed tomography [CT] or magnetic resonance imaging [MRI]) are typically normal, further supporting the understanding that concussion is a functional disturbance without true gross structural abnormality.

Biomechanics and Pathophysiology

When rotational or angular acceleration forces are applied to the brain, a shear strain occurs on the neural elements, leading to a neurometabolic cascade and the clinical features of concussion. The biomechanical injury to the brain causes an immediate release of excitatory neurotransmitters (Fig. 139.1).

The binding of the excitatory neurotransmitters, such as glutamate, lead to further neuronal depolarization with further destabilization of the ionic equilibrium, including influx of calcium and efflux of potassium (Fig. 139.2).[5]

To restore the ionic homeostasis, neuronal membrane potential energy (adenosine triphosphate) is required to enable operation of the sodium-potassium pump. This increased glucose demand ("hypermetabolism") occurs in the face of decreased cerebral blood flow. Metabolic supply/demand mismatch leads to cell dysfunction and increased vulnerability of the cell to a second insult (Fig. 139.3).

After the initial period of "hypermetabolism," a period of decreased metabolism occurs in the concussed brain. Calcium levels may remain elevated and impair mitochondrial oxidative metabolism, further worsening the energy deficits. In addition, neurofilament and microtubule function is disrupted by intra-axonal calcium flux, impairing posttraumatic neural connectivity.

On average, these biochemical changes take 7 to 10 days to normalize in adults (see Fig. 139.2), but normalization can take longer in the growing brain of a child and adolescent. Interestingly, the clinical recovery parallels this biochemical normalization. Changes in cerebral blood flow may also occur with concomitant impairment of vascular autoregulation, which can result in cerebral edema and may persist beyond the acute phase.

Epidemiology

Twenty-one percent of all TBIs among children in the United States are associated with sports participation.[6] Although death from a sports injury is rare, the leading cause of death from a sports-related injury is a brain injury. Football, gymnastics, and ice hockey reported the highest number of sports-related fatalities from 1982 to 2014 according to the 33rd annual report of the National Center for Catastrophic Sport Injury Research.[7]

Concussions occur commonly in sports in which helmets are and are not worn. The rates of sports-related concussion are estimated at 1.6 to 3.8 million sports-related concussions per year[8]; however, only 8% to 19% of concussions are associated with a loss of consciousness.[9,10] The rate in high school athletes is 0.14 to 3.66 injuries per 100 player seasons at the high school level, accounting for 3% to 5% of injuries in all sports.[11,12] At the collegiate level, the exposure rate is 0.5 to 3.0 injuries per

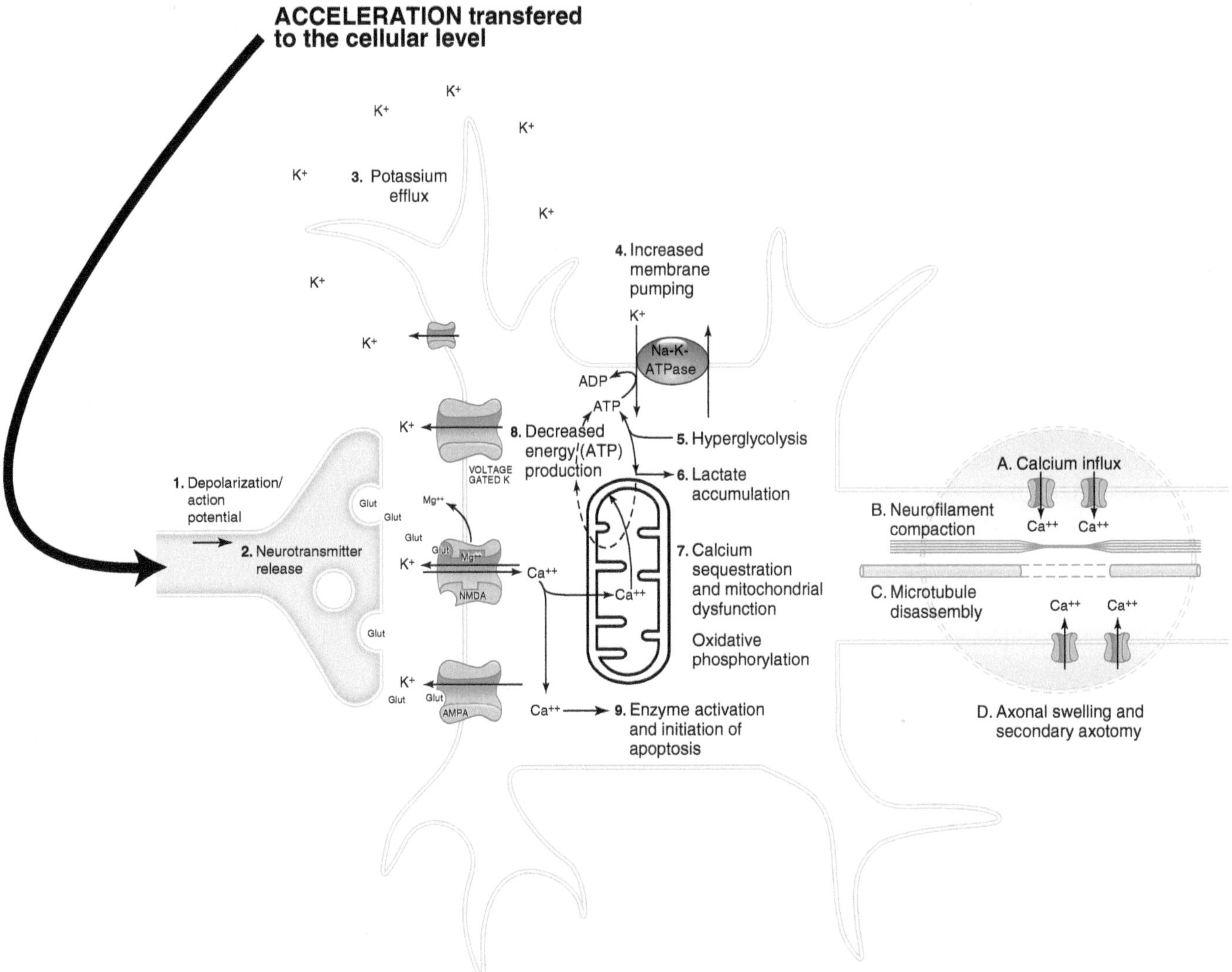

**ACCELERATION transfered
to the cellular level**

K+

K+

K+

3. Potassium
efflux

K+

K+

K+

4. Increased
membrane
pumping

K+

Na-K-
ATPase

ADP

ATP

8. Decreased
energy (ATP)
production

5. Hyperglycolysis

VOLTAGE
GATED K

K+

6. Lactate
accumulation

1. Depolarization/
action
potential

Glut

Glut

Glut

Mg++

2. Neurotransmitter
release

Glut

Mg++

K+

NMDA

Ca++

Ca++

7. Calcium
sequestration
and mitochondrial
dysfunction

Oxidative
phosphorylation

K+

Glut

Glut

AMPA

Ca++

9. Enzyme activation
and initiation of
apoptosis

A. Calcium influx

Ca++   Ca++

B. Neurofilament
compaction

C. Microtubule
disassembly

Ca++   Ca++

D. Axonal swelling and
secondary axotomy

Fig. 139.1 The biochemical changes that occur in the neuron with concussion. *ADP,* Adenosine diphosphate; *ATP,* adenosine triphosphate; *ATPase,* adenosine triphosphatase. (Modified from Giza CC, Hovda DA. Ionic and metabolic consequences of concussion. In: Cantu RC, Cantu RI, eds. *Neurologic Athletic and Spine Injuries.* Philadelphia: WB Saunders; 2000.)

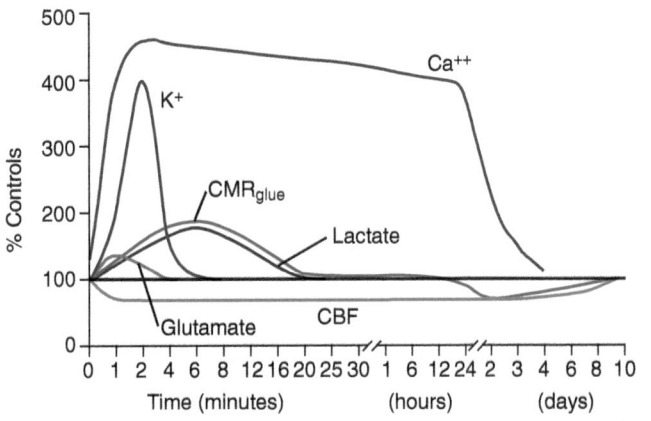

Fig. 139.2 Ionic and metabolic consequences of concussion. *CBF,* Cerebral blood flow; *CMR,* cerebral metabolic rate. (From Giza CC, Hovda DA. Ionic and metabolic consequences of concussion. In: Cantu RC, Cantu RI, eds. *Neurologic Athletic and Spine Injuries.* Philadelphia: WB Saunders; 2000.)

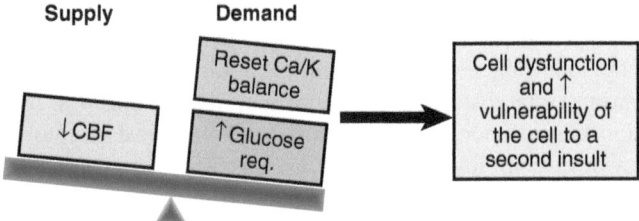

Fig. 139.3 Metabolic supply/demand mismatch in the neuron after concussion. *CBF,* Cerebral blood flow.

1000 athlete exposures.[12] Trends have shown a significant (60%) increase in concussion rates in young athletes (<19 years old) during the past decade.

Although sports participation overall is increased, this increase is likely related to better reporting, recognition, and diagnosis of concussion. Historically, concussion reporting rates have been poor. In a survey of 1532 varsity football athletes, 47% of players who sustained concussions continued to play without reporting their injuries to anyone. The most common reason athletes did not share the presence of symptoms was that the athletes did not believe the concussion was serious enough to report. Other reasons for underreporting were that athletes did not want to leave the game, did not realize a concussion was sustained, and did not want to let their teammates down.[13] Another study reported that 70.4% of football players and 62.7% of soccer players experienced symptoms of concussion within one season,[14] further supporting the understanding that the current reported concussion rates are likely much lower than actual rates because of unrecognized concussions.

Concussion can occur in any sport, from football to basketball to cheerleading; different studies have shown differing incident rates. A recent systematic review and meta-analysis showed the three sports with the highest incidence rates of sports-related concussion were rugby, hockey, and American football, with 4.18, 1.20, and 0.53 per 1000 athletic exposures (AEs), respectively,[15] whereas another meta-analysis indicated the highest incident rates for tae kwon do (8.77 per 1000 athlete exposures), rugby (9.05 per 1000 player games), amateur boxing (7.9 per 1000 athlete exposures), and boys' high school ice hockey (3.6 per 1000 athlete exposures).[11] When specifically looking at rates of sports-related concussion in the high school population, another study showed that boys' sports accounted for 53% of athlete exposures and 75% of all concussions. Football had the highest incident rate and accounted for the majority of concussions (53.1%), followed by boys' lacrosse (9.2%). Among girls' sports, soccer had the highest rate of concussions and was the second highest of the 12 high school sports studied.[16]

History

Concussions can present seconds, minutes, or hours after an indirect or direct force to the head. The signs and symptoms of concussion fall into four main categories: physical, cognitive, emotional, and sleep (Table 139.1).[17,18]

The self-reported Post-concussion Symptom Scale is a useful tool for initial assessment and also serves to facilitate follow-up. The scale is a 7-point Likert scale graded from 0 (no symptoms) to 6 (severe symptoms); multiple scales are available with a range of symptoms included. Although no specific scale has been assessed for reliability, self-reported postconcussive symptoms are associated with ongoing cerebral hemodynamic abnormalities and mild cognitive impairments.[19] Headache is the most frequently reported symptom.[20] Loss of consciousness occurs in only 8% to 19% of concussions[9,10] and is not a defining feature of concussion; however, when prolonged loss of consciousness (>30 seconds) occurs, further evaluation may be necessary. The strongest and most consistent predictor of slower recovery from sports-related concussion is severity of symptoms in the first day, or initial days, after injury; conversely, a low level of initial symptoms is a favorable prognostic indicator.[3] Understanding the presence of preexisting medical and mental health disorders, including migraine headaches, depression, anxiety, learning disabilities, cognitive delays, and attention-deficit disorders, is important because concussion may cause an exacerbation of underlying symptoms; in addition, athletes with preexisting mental health problems or migraine headaches may have a more prolonged recovery course, more than 1 month.[3] However, although those with attention-deficit disorder or learning disabilities may require more extensive educational support in returning to school, they do not appear to be at greater risk for prolonged symptoms.[3] Athletes with preinjury depression, sleep disturbances, and/or attention-deficit/hyperactivity disorder may not have a baseline (preinjury) symptom score of zero and thus are not expected to have a symptom score of zero prior to considering return to play (RTP).

Recognizing concussion may be difficult in athletes for a number of reasons. Athletes may not recognize symptoms as serious and thus not report them. Symptoms may be delayed and not appear until several hours after a concussive event occurs.[21] In addition, athletes may not volunteer their symptoms to avoid restriction from play and because they fear they will let down their teammates.[13]

Physical Examination

Initial assessment on the sidelines follows the protocol of all acute head and neck injuries and begins with assessment of the airway, breathing, and circulation (ABCs) and stabilization

TABLE 139.1	Signs and Symptoms of Concussion		
Physical	**Cognitive**	**Emotional**	**Sleep**
Headache	Feeling "foggy"	Irritability	Drowsiness
Nausea	Feeling slowed down	Sadness	Sleeping more or less than usual
Vomiting	Difficulty concentrating	Anxiety	Difficulty falling asleep
Balance problems	Amnesia	Emotional lability	
Visual problems	Confusion	Depression	
Sensitivity to light	Slow response to questions		
Sensitivity to noise	Repeating questions		
Fatigue	Difficulty with schoolwork		
Dazed/stunned affect	Loss of consciousness		
Seizure			

of the cervical spine. If an athlete is unconscious after head or neck trauma, a cervical spine injury is assumed until neurologic function in all four limbs is determined to be intact and the athlete reports no neck pain or cervical spine tenderness on palpation. Immediate emergency transport with cervical precautions is essential if this evaluation is unable to be completed; if the athlete is wearing a helmet and pads, the gear should not be removed for transport, but the facemask should be removed to provide access to the airway. For athletes in whom cervical spine injuries are not suspected, evaluation can be performed on the sidelines.

When concussion is suspected, the athlete should be removed from the sporting environment and undergo a standardized multimodal assessment. Sideline assessment includes review of the athlete's symptoms, neurologic evaluation, and cognitive and balance testing. Initial neurologic testing should begin with evaluation of eye response, verbal response, and motor response as per the Glasgow Coma Scale. The next steps included further evaluation of neurologic status with examination of pupil size and symmetry, vision, reflexes, sensation, and strength. When the athlete appears stable, testing of memory, coordination, concentration, and gait/balance can ensue. Numerous sideline assessment tools are available to facilitate expedient and standardized assessments, both as printable forms and smartphone applications, including Maddocks questions,[22] Standardized Assessment of Concussion,[23] Balance Error Scoring System (BESS),[24] and the Sport Concussion Assessment Tool version 5 (i.e., SCAT 5 or Child SCAT5). The SCAT5 and the Child SCAT 5 provide a comprehensive protocol ideal for sideline assessment.[3] The SCAT 5 was released as part of the Consensus Statement on Concussion in Sport. The Child SCAT5 is designed for children 5 to 12 years old and has a symptom assessment for parent/teacher/coach/caregiver and children to report symptoms; in addition, portions of the examination, including neurologic screen and balance testing, are tailored to the younger athlete.[3] In all of these tests, individualized baseline information is useful.

The Maddocks questions are a set of sport-specific questions designed to evaluate orientation, short-term memory, and long-term memory; these questions may provide more accurate responses than the usual orientation to time, day, date, and location. Examples of Maddocks questions are "Who scored last in the match?" and "Did your team win the last game?" These questions are useful only on the sidelines (not in a clinic setting) and are included in the comprehensive SCAT5.

Balance is an important part of the assessment after head trauma. Historically, the Romberg test has been used to assess balance subjectively. However, the BESS provides a quantifiable balance test that is straightforward to perform and objectively assesses postural stability. The BESS may be performed on the sidelines or in a clinic setting.[25-27] The BESS test has been shown to be a valid and reliable tool.[28,29] The BESS test is performed with the patient in three positions, first on a firm surface and then on a less-stable surface, a 10-cm-thick piece of foam. The three positions, which are well described in the SCAT5, include (1) standing flat on both feet with the hands placed on the iliac crest; (2) standing on a single leg on the nondominant foot; and (3) standing in tandem stance, heel-to-toe, with the nondominant

---

BOX 139.1   Balance Testing Errors

Hands lifted off the iliac crest
Opening eyes
Step, stumble, or fall
Moving the hip to >30 degrees of abduction
Lifting the forefoot or heel
Remaining out of the test position for >5 seconds

---

foot in back of the other. The athlete is instructed to hold each position, to the best of his or her ability, for 20 seconds while the examiner observes the athlete for errors (Box 139.1). The examiner scores the test by adding the number of errors (one error point for each error during each 20-second test). For the 5- to 9-year-old athlete, the single leg stance can be omitted to accommodate for normal developmental skillset. Because fatigue and setting have an effect on the test, it is recommended that the test be completed 15 minutes after cessation of exercise and in the same setting where the follow-up testing will be performed.[30,31] Ideally, athletes will have a baseline evaluation that includes the BESS test prior to the start of the season so that comparison of postinjury and baseline testing may be incorporated to most reliably incorporate balance testing results into the RTP plan.

Although basic neurocognitive assessments are included as part of the Standardized Assessment of Concussion/SCAT5, more in-depth testing may be helpful to determine a player's readiness for safe RTP, especially in cases with chronic symptoms and questions of the athlete's truthfulness. Neuropsychological testing can be performed in one of two ways—with pencil-and-paper testing administered by a neuropsychologist or with computerized neuropsychological testing. Accessibility, time, and cost often limit the practical implication of the pencil-and-paper testing, but it can be extremely useful in cases complicated by prolonged symptoms and difficulty returning to school. Computerized testing is currently used more widely because of the ease of use and short testing times (30 to 45 minutes). Ideally, baseline neuropsychological testing is performed prior to injury to enable it to be used most effectively. Schools and teams have begun to offer and administer tests proctored by school personnel, usually athletic trainers.

Imaging

Results of conventional neuroimaging (i.e., skull radiographs and head CT/MRI scans) are usually normal in persons who have had a concussion; however, prudent use of neuroimaging must be considered if an intracranial structural injury is suspected. The signs and symptoms that increase concern for a more serious injury include a worsening severe headache, seizures, focal neurologic signs, and circulatory changes (Box 139.2).

Other considerations to help determine when neuroimaging is appropriate are prolonged loss of consciousness (>30 seconds) and persistently worsening symptoms. A CT scan is the first-line testing modality recommended to evaluate for intracranial hemorrhage and skull fractures during the first 24 to 48 hours after injury.[32] Performing a CT scan is absolutely

BOX 139.2   Red Flags for Intracranial Structural Injury

Severe, worsening headache
Seizures
Focal neurologic findings
Repeated emesis
Significant drowsiness/difficulty awakening
Slurred speech
Poor orientation/significant confusion
Significant irritability
Slowed pulse
Increased systolic blood pressure with decreased diastolic blood pressure
Pupil irregularity
Loss of consciousness >1 minute

not recommended for all concussed athletes, especially children, because of a small increased risk of brain cancer and leukemia as a result of radiation exposure.[33] MRI is most effectively used in cases of prolonged symptoms (>3 weeks) and is primarily performed to rule out underlying structural pathology such as Arnold-Chiari malformation or arteriovenous malformation, which may cause a prolonged recovery from a concussive injury. Emerging MRI and functional imaging modalities including diffusion tensor imaging, magnetic resonance spectroscopy, single photon emission CT, and cerebral angiography may facilitate the diagnosis of concussion and assist in making RTP decisions.

Decision-Making Principles

The differential diagnosis of concussion includes epidural hematoma, subdural hematoma, intracerebral hematoma, and subarachnoid hemorrhage.

Epidural hematoma is a rapidly progressing intracranial hematoma that occurs from a tear of the middle meningeal artery that normally supplies the dura (the outermost covering of the brain). A fracture of the temporal bone often precipitates this hematoma. Blood accumulates between the skull and the dura and can rapidly reach a fatal size within 30 to 60 minutes. The classic clinical presentation is an athlete who sustains a blow to the head with immediate loss of consciousness followed by a lucid interval. However, the presentation can vary; sometimes the athlete may not lose consciousness, or he or she may regain consciousness with symptoms of severe, progressing headache followed by a decline in the level of consciousness. These worsening symptoms occur because the clot accumulation is causing increased intracranial pressure. If the diagnosis is an epidural hematoma, it is often obvious within the first 1 to 2 hours after injury. Treatment is emergent evacuation of the hematoma because, if the pressure is removed and no further bleeding occurs, a significant recovery can be made. However, if it is not treated expediently, an epidural hematoma can rapidly lead to death. All athletes who sustain a head injury must be monitored closely and frequently for the first 24 to 48 hours with direct access to full neurosurgical services in the event of emergency.

A *subdural hematoma* occurs as a result of bleeding between the brain surface and the dura; it is considered the most common fatal head injury in athletes.[34] A subdural hematoma may occur as a result of one of a few different mechanisms, including a tear in a vein(s) running from the surface of the brain to the dura; diffuse injury to the surface of the brain; a torn venous sinus; or, less commonly, a torn small artery on the surface of the brain. Subdural hematomas are associated with brain tissue injury and thus are associated with a greater morbidity because even if the clot is evacuated early, underlying brain tissue injury has already occurred.

An *intracerebral hematoma* occurs from intracranial hemorrhage from bleeding into the brain substance itself, usually from a torn artery or congenital vascular lesion such as an aneurysm or arteriovenous malformation. Clinically, athletes present with rapidly progressive neurologic deterioration after a head trauma. Immediate medical attention is essential, but death occasionally occurs before the athlete is even transported to a medical facility. A full autopsy is recommended in these cases to establish the potential underlying anatomic malformation and to clarify the causative factors.

A *subarachnoid hemorrhage* is intracranial bleeding within the cerebrospinal fluid space along the surface of the brain. Bleeding occurs most commonly after head trauma from disruption of the tiny surface brain blood vessels. However, it can also result from a ruptured cerebral aneurysm or arteriovenous malformation. Brain swelling may be associated and may require a decompressive craniectomy, but surgery is not required for the hemorrhage itself.

Treatment Options

Treatment of concussion is entirely nonoperative. The goal of managing an athlete with concussion is to facilitate expedient resolution of symptoms and safe RTP. Initial treatment involves physical and cognitive rest and requires comprehensive education of the patient and his or her caregivers so they understand the management plan. Management practices are based on the 5th International Conference on Concussion in Sports,[3] which is the current standard of care. Previously many grading systems were used for concussions; however, all of the recent guidelines now focus on symptoms and returning to play. Regardless of the severity of the injury, an athlete is not allowed to RTP as long as symptoms are present.

Relative rest is an important part of the concussion management plan. This restriction is based on the pathophysiologic principle that in the setting of a metabolic imbalance and energy crisis within the brain, any increased energy demand in the brain from physical activity may worsen symptoms and delay recovery[36] and concerns for repeat head injury during sports participation. However, limited early physical activity has been shown to be safe, effective, and better than rest alone after a brief period of rest during the acute phase (24 to 48 hours) after injury.[3,37-43]

Cognitive rest is also essential to minimize symptoms and maximize recovery. After sustaining a concussion, athletes often report difficulty attending school, taking tests, and keeping up with assignments. Cognition is "exercise" for the brain and requires increased energy demand in the face of the postconcussion energy crisis in the brain and thus should be avoided until symptoms subside. Cognitive rest may involve staying home from school, attending only a few classes, decreased schoolwork load, allowance of extra time to complete coursework and tests, avoiding standardized testing, and taking rest breaks during the day. In addition, all activities that require concentration or offer stimulus to the brain must be avoided as part of cognitive rest, including playing video games, using the computer, watching television (especially intense, dramatic, violent programming), listening to loud music, and exposure to bright lights. Development of an individualized return to learn program with appropriate school accommodations is recommended to facilitate recovery. Lastly, because of slowed reaction times, licensed drivers with a concussion should avoid driving until they are cleared for activity.

Treatment should be individualized and specifically targeted at the symptom profile identified on assessment. In addition to symptom-limited aerobic exercise programs, targeted physical therapy programs addressing neck strain and vestibular dysfunction and cognitive behavioral therapy to address mood disturbances may be implemented as needed. If pharmacotherapy is prescribed, health care providers must recognize that pharmacologic agents may mask or modify symptoms of concussion.

Return to Play

After a concussion, athletes should not RTP on the day of injury, especially for the pediatric or adolescent athlete. Legislation in all 50 states in the United States requires all athletes with a suspected concussion to be removed from any sports participation until they are given clearance to RTP from a licensed health care professional. Although most athletes display resolution of symptoms within 7 to 10 days, the recovery time frame may be longer in children and adolescents.[21]

For deciding when to RTP, asymptomatic athletes are directed to follow a medically supervised stepwise process, based on the summary and agreement statement of the 5th International Conference on Concussion in Sports.[3] The patient should never return to contact play while symptomatic; however, athletes are encouraged to become gradually more active while staying below their cognitive and physical symptom-exacerbation thresholds. All RTP programs must be individualized because every athlete recovers at a different pace. In addition, concussed athletes should be free from concussion-related symptoms and not using any pharmacologic agents that may mask or modify symptoms; decisions regarding RTP while still on such medication must be considered carefully by the treating clinician.[3] The following protocol is recommended by the 5th International Conference on Concussion as a guideline to be completed with appropriate supervision (Table 139.2):

Each level requires at least 24 hours, and a minimum of 5 days is required to progress through the protocol to be cleared for full participation. However, any return or increase of symptoms at any stage of the protocol is indication that concussion recovery is inadequate. If any postconcussion symptoms reoccur or worsen the patient should drop back to the previous asymptomatic level and try to progress again after 24 hours. If an athlete completes all

TABLE 139.2   Gradual Return-to-Play Protocol

Level	Activity
1	Symptom-limited activity (daily activities that do not provoke symptoms)
2	Light aerobic exercise (e.g., walking, stationary cycling)
3	Sport-specific training (e.g., skating for hockey, running for soccer)
4	Noncontact training drills (e.g., passing drills, progressive resistance training)
5	Full-contact training after medical clearance
6	Return to sport/normal game play

levels with minimum of 24 hours between levels, tolerates noncontact training activities without symptom, the athlete is considered cleared to advance to contact practice and ultimately full game play if asymptomatic with practice. While athletes may advance through the RTP protocol with symptoms, they cannot advance beyond noncontact activity until at preconcussion baseline, ideally symptom free. Athletes with a history of multiple concussions or prolonged postconcussion syndrome may require longer intervals as they progress through each level of recovery.

Athletes who have sustained traumatic intracranial bleeding may begin the gradual RTP protocol for noncontact sports after a minimum of 6 weeks to enable the bone flap to heal after a craniotomy; however, after traumatic intracranial bleeding, decisions regarding return to activity and ultimate potential return to contact sport are determined by the neurosurgery team.

Complications

Although the large majority of concussions self-resolve within 7 to 10 days in adults and 3 to 4 weeks in children, complications may occur, including postconcussion syndrome (PCS), second-impact syndrome, long-term effects, and chronic traumatic encephalopathy (CTE).

PCS refers to the presence of symptoms beyond the normal duration of recovery. Many variations exist in the specifics of the PCS definition, and no set of criteria is universally accepted. PCS is commonly defined as the persistent presence of three or more symptoms with the duration loosely defined and broadly variable between sources. The two most commonly applied definitions are proposed by the World Health Organization International Statistical Classification of Diseases and Related Health Problems (ICD)-10 and the *Diagnostic and Statistical Manual of Mental Disorders,* fourth edition (DSM-IV) (Table 139.3). However, the DSM-V significantly changed the specific defining criteria, and now classifies PCS within major or mild neurocognitive disorder due to TBI.

Second-impact syndrome is a debated term that applies to the pathophysiology that occurs when an athlete sustains a second head trauma prior to complete symptom resolution after an initial head injury. Second impact syndrome results in cerebral vascular congestion that progresses to diffuse cerebral swelling and is associated with a high mortality rate. This second hit occurs during the period of enhanced vulnerability characterized by an increased brain cell demand for glucose in the face of

TABLE 139.3 WHO and DSM-IV Postconcussion Syndrome Definitions

	Who ICD-10	DSM-IV
Minimum duration of symptoms	na	3 months
Number of symptoms	3	3
Defining symptoms	Headache	Fatigue
	Dizziness/vertigo	Disordered sleep
	Easily fatigued/easily tired	Headache
	Irritability	Vertigo/dizziness
	Poor concentration	Anxiety
	Forgetfulness	Depression
	Sleep disturbance	Personality changes
	Depression	Apathy
	Anxiety	

DSM-IV, Diagnostic and Statistical Manual of Mental Disorders, 4th edition; *ICD-10,* International Statistical Classification of Diseases and Related Health Problems; *na,* not applicable; *WHO,* World Health Organization.
(Modified from Kashluba S, Casey JE, Paniak C. Evaluating the utility of ICD-10 diagnostic criteria for postconcussion syndrome following traumatic brain injury. *J Int Neuropsychol Soc.* 2006;12:111–118; and American Psychiatric Association. *Diagnostic and Statistical Manual of Mental Disorders.* 4th ed. Washington, DC: American Psychiatric Association; 2000.)

reduced cerebral blood flow and impaired cerebral vascular autoregulation. Because pediatric and adolescent athletes have demonstrated longer recovery times from the initial decreased cerebral blood flow,[44] these younger athletes are at higher risk of second impact syndrome.

The long-term effects of one or multiple concussions are inconsistent and largely unknown because minimal large-scale scientific investigation of the long-term consequences of brain injury in athletes has been performed. Studies of amateur boxers reveal similar chronic neurocognitive effects[47]; however, professional boxers show much more significant long-term neurocognitive effects, with older studies showing that 17% of retired boxers demonstrate CTE.[48] A genetic predisposition to CTE may exist. More recent studies accounting for the reduction in exposure to repetitive head trauma and increasing medical monitoring of boxers predict a lower incidence in the future.[36,47,48] A recent systematic review looking at original research of retired athletes 10 or more years after injury found that some former athletes have depression and cognitive deficits later in life, and there is an association between these deficits and multiple prior concussions.[49] Former athletes are not at increased risk for death by suicide.[49-51] Former high school American football players do not appear to be at increased risk for later life neurodegenerative diseases; in two medical record linkage studies of former high school football players, the rates of dementia, mild cognitive impairment, and parkinsonism did not differ in comparison with control subjects.[49,52,53] National Football League (NFL) retirees with a history of three or more concussions show a threefold increase in the risk of depression and memory problems and a fivefold increased prevalence of mild cognitive impairment (e.g.,

memory, concentration, and speech) when compared with retirees without a history of concussion.[54,55] However, in a study of retired NFL players, mortality and suicide rates *are lower* than the general population.[50] Further study is necessary to better understand long-term sequelae from concussion.

CTE is described as a progressive neurodegenerative disease that is associated with repetitive head trauma. CTE can only be diagnosed by neuropathologic examination of the brain. Consensus criteria that provide a standardized approach for the neuropathology of CTE have been developed by the US National Institutes of Neurological Disease and Stroke (NINDS) and the National Institute of Biomedical Imaging and Bioengineering (NIBIB). Trauma is hypothesized as a trigger of progressive brain cell degeneration, leading to an accumulation of an abnormal protein called tau; however, no direct cause-effect relationship has been demonstrated yet between CTE and sports-related concussion or exposure to contact sports. CTE presents clinically with symptoms of headaches, memory loss, disorientation, impaired judgment, impulse control problems, aggression, depression, tremors, abnormal gait/speech, and ultimately dementia and sometimes suicide; symptoms may develop months, years, and decades after the traumatic events and often the diagnosis is made postmortem at autopsy. Further prospective, longitudinal, population-based, blinded neuropathologic studies evaluating athletes involved in high- and low-impact sports are needed to further understand this pathology.

Future Considerations

Currently, concussion is a diagnosis made subjectively based on history and supported by neurocognitive and balance testing; however, no diagnostic test is available to facilitate an objective diagnosis. Future research and medical advances will likely further elucidate the underlying disease and improve the diagnosis and management of concussive injuries.

For a complete list of references, go to ExpertConsult.com.

SELECTED READINGS

Citation:
McCrory P, Meeuwisse W, Dvorak J, et al. Consensus statement on concussion in sport: the 5th International Conference on Concussion in Sport held in Berlin, October 2016. *Br J Sports Med.* 2017;51:838–847.

Level of Evidence:
III

Summary:
Although evidence-based recommendations are limited, the authors of this article review consensus based on a systemic review of current medical literature and expert opinion for diagnosis and management of concussion.

Citation:
Halstead ME, Walter KD. The council on Sports Medicine and Fitness. Clinical report: sports-related concussion in children and adolescents. *Pediatrics.* 2010;126(3):597–615.

Level of Evidence:
III

Summary:
Although evidence-based recommendations are limited, the authors of this review provide a summary of current medical literature, which is a helpful tool for the management of concussion in children.

Citation:
Giza CC. The neurometabolic cascade of concussion. *J Athl Train.* 2001;36(3):228–235.

Level of Evidence:
III

Summary:
This article is an excellent review of the underlying neuropathophysiologic processes of concussive brain injury and the associated neurometabolic changes in relation to clinical sports-related issues. Results from more than 100 articles of basic science and clinical medical literature are summarized.

Citation:
Maugans TA, Farley C, Altaye M, et al. Pediatric sports-related concussion produces cerebral blood flow alterations. *Pediatrics.* 2012;129:28–37.

Level of Evidence:
III

Summary:
The authors report a small study in which 12 children who experienced sports-related concussion were evaluated with use of multiple modalities, including ImPACT neurocognitive testing, T1- and susceptibility-weighted magnetic resonance imaging, diffusion tensor imaging, proton magnetic resonance spectroscopy, and phase-contrast angiography.

Citation:
Guskiewicz KM. Balance assessment in the management of sport-related concussion. *Clin Sports Med.* 2011;30(1):89–102.

Level of Evidence:
III

Summary:
The authors of this study investigate the efficacy of a clinical balance testing procedure for the detection of acute postural stability disruptions after sports-related concussion.

Citation:
Manley G, Gardner AJ, Schneider KJ, et al. A systematic review of potential long-term effects of sport-related concussion. *Br J Sports Med.* 2017;51:969–977.

Level of Evidence:
III

Summary:
Systematic review of original research focused on potential long-term effects, 10 or more years after injury of sports-related concussion in retired athletes.

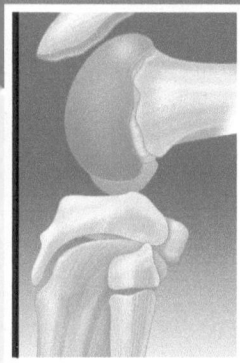

140

Spine Issues in Skeletally Immature Athletes

Lindsay M. Andras, David L. Skaggs

There are many challenges facing the sports physician in the care of the spine in pediatric athletes. They may be asked to evaluate a child or adolescent with a known condition and assess whether he or she can safely participate in athletic activities. Second, when an acute traumatic event has occurred, sports physicians may be asked to evaluate and provide initial management for the injured athlete. In addition, sports physicians manage and treat conditions that create chronic pain or deformity and may have an impact on sports participation.

The anatomic differences between the mature and growing spine can make these varied roles more complicated. In addition to injuries that are observed in both children and adults, the growing spine leads to injuries that are unique to the pediatric and adolescent populations. This chapter describes the relevant anatomy and related injuries observed in the young athlete, as well as key components in the evaluation of these spine conditions and their management. In addition, guidelines for both restriction from sports and timing of return to athletic activities are provided.

ANATOMY

Fracture patterns and biomechanics, particularly in the cervical spine, differ for children based on age. In younger children, the fulcrum is at C2-C3 because of their proportionally large skulls. Consequently, for children younger than 8 years, 87% of cervical spine injuries occur at or above C3 and 50% are associated with head injuries.[1] Older children have fracture patterns similar to those of adults, with the subaxial spine most commonly affected.

Diagnosis of cervical spine injuries in the child can be challenging, particularly in the younger age groups, because much of the cervical spine has not yet ossified. The anterior ring of C1 does not ossify until after the age of 1 year, making detection of injury in this region especially challenging (Fig. 140.1). Between the ages of 3 and 6 years, fusion of the dens to the neural arches and anterior body occurs, which can be mistaken for a fracture at the base of the odontoid. By age 6 years, the spinal canal of the cervical spine has reached adult dimensions. Lateral radiographs show a progressively increasing facet angle from birth to 8 years of age that allows motion through flexion and extension and contributes to the appearance of pseudosubluxation often seen at C2-C3 and C3-C4. Pseudosubluxation can be differentiated from true subluxation on plain radiographs

by the maintenance of the Swischuk line, which is a straight line drawn along the spinolaminar line (the anterior edge of the posterior neural arch; Fig. 140.2). However, care should be taken as while pseudosubluxation is a normal finding and does not require treatment, injuries can also occur at this level (Figs. 140.3A and B). In addition, incomplete ossification often gives the appearance of wedging of the cervical vertebral bodies on lateral radiographs until age 10 years. The atlantodens interval (ADI) may be increased in children. As opposed to adults, in whom a normal ADI is less than 3 mm, in young children the ADI may be up to 4.5 mm without signifying injury.

Additional considerations also exist in the pediatric thoracolumbar spine compared with the adult spine. The ring apophysis that extends peripherally around the vertebral body is adherent to the annulus of the intervertebral disk and can be at risk for injury. These injuries may be mistaken both clinically and radiographically for a pediatric disk herniation.

GENERAL HISTORY AND PHYSICAL EXAMINATION FOR EVALUATION OF THE PEDIATRIC SPINE

The sports physician may be evaluating the spine of a pediatric patient in preparation for participation in athletic activities, after an acute event that occurs while participating in a sport, or when the patient has chronic pain. It is important to differentiate the more common generalized aches and pains that accompany both athletic training and adolescence from more serious causes of pain. Atypical pain may be indicative of a more serious injury, a tumor, infection, or another more severe clinical entity. Box 140.1 outlines key elements in the history that can guide the clinician in making this distinction.

In evaluating spinal injuries, the mechanism and impact can alert the clinician to more critical conditions. In acute scenarios in which a potentially unstable spine injury is suspected, proper immobilization of the spine is necessary to prevent worsening of the injury. For children younger than 8 years, a pediatric backboard with a recess should be used to accommodate their proportionally large head size and prevent additional injury from the acute flexion that can be caused by a traditional backboard.

The physical examination is critical but also challenging in the child with suspected spinal injury. In cases in which spinal instability is not suspected, the focused neurologic examination outlined (Box 140.2) provides an efficient assessment and can be performed even in young children.

SPONDYLOLYSIS/SPONDYLOLISTHESIS

Spondylolysis is a defect in the pars interarticularis and is most commonly found at the L5 level. It is by far the most common cause of back pain, accounting for up to 47% of cases in the adolescent population in some series.[2] The prevalence of spondylolysis is approximately 6% among the general population.[3] Approximately 80% of cases are bilateral, whereas 20% of cases are unilateral. When a patient has an associated slippage of a vertebra in relation to the adjacent vertebra, the term "spondylolisthesis" is used.

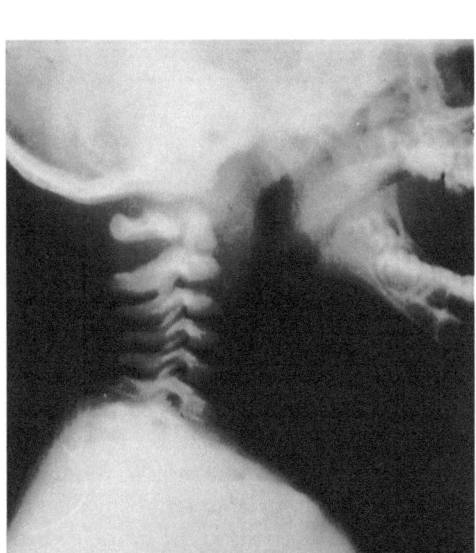

Fig. 140.1 Detection of cervical spine injuries or abnormalities in the young child can be challenging, because much of the cervical spine has not yet ossified. The anterior ring of C1 does not ossify until after the age of 1 year and is not visible on plain radiographs at that age, as depicted here.

BOX 140.1   Pediatric Back Pain Red Flags

The following pain characteristics are not associated with typical muscular back pain and warrant further investigation.

- Night pain
- Pain in young children, especially if they stop playing
- Frequent pain at rest, not including sitting (pain with prolonged sitting in school is extremely common in teens with mechanical low back pain)
- Back pain associated with an abnormal gait, limp, unsteadiness on feet, and so on.
- With associated constitutional symptoms (e.g., fever, lethargy, weight loss, loss of appetite)
- Atypical location, especially thoracic rather than lumbar pain (although pain in the trapezius/periscapular muscles is often due to backpacks)
- History of worsening pain
- With neurologic symptoms or physical findings (cavus foot, etc.)
- Kyphosis
- With important cutaneous findings (e.g., high and deep dimple, hairy patch, café-au-lait spots suggestive of neurofibromatosis)
- Positive finger test (child localizes pain to area the size of a fingertip)
- Positive coin test (have child keep the back straight when picking something up)
- Listing to side on Adams forward bend
- Tight hamstrings (popliteal angle >50 degrees)

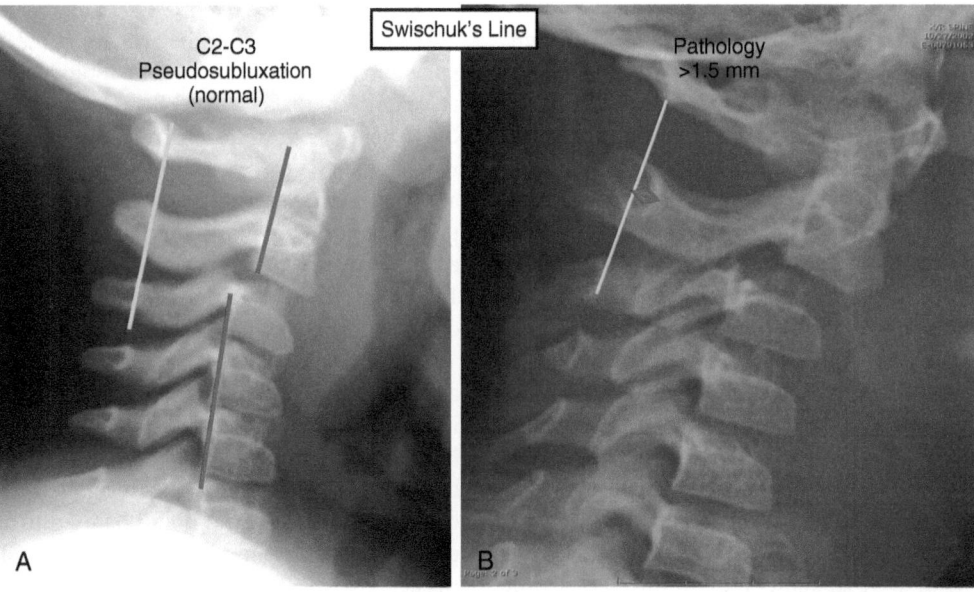

Fig. 140.2 Pseudo-subluxation can be differentiated from true subluxation on plain radiographs by the maintenance of the Swischuk line (green), which is a straight line drawn along the anterior edge of the posterior neural arch. (A) The patient has no acute injury, which is confirmed by the maintenance of this line. (B) The patient has a change in the relation of the posterior elements to this line, which represents true subluxation. (Courtesy Children's Orthopedic Center, Los Angeles, CA.)

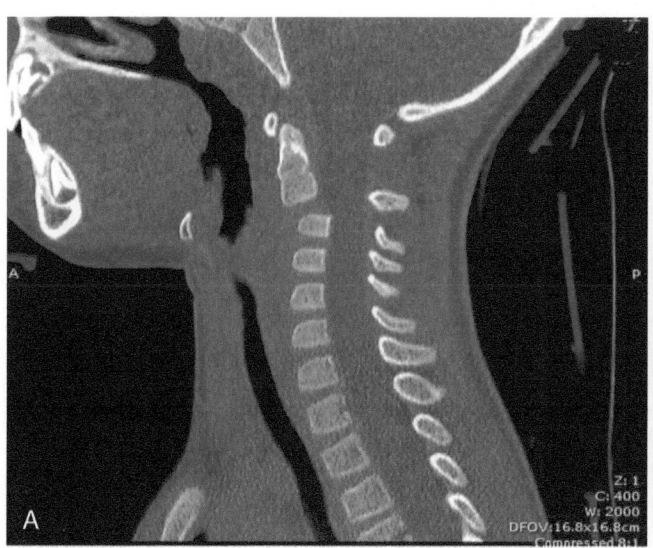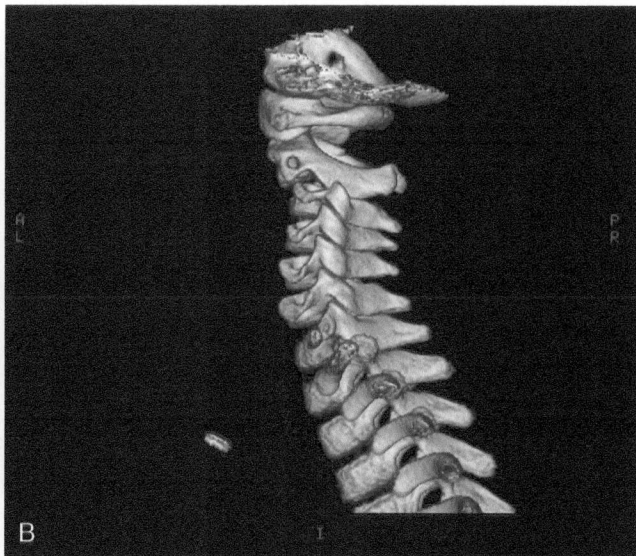

Fig. 140.3 (A and B) Although pseudosubluxation is a normal finding that does not require treatment, true injuries can also occur at this level. Sagittal and 3D computed tomography scan images of a 3-year-old involved in a high-speed motor vehicle collision demonstrate jumped facets at C2-C3. Magnetic resonance imaging confirmed extensive associated ligamentous injury.

BOX 140.2 60-Second Neurologic Examination

Hop on each foot, one at a time
Walk on heels
Reflexes
Foot inspection
Ankle dorsiflexion to assess muscle tone and clonus
Sensation
Popliteal angle

From Skaggs DL, Flynn JM. *Staying Out of Trouble in Pediatric Orthopaedics*. Philadelphia: Lippincott Williams & Wilkins; 2005.

Classification

Spondylolisthesis can be classified on the basis of either the type of the spondylolisthesis or the degree of displacement. The five types of spondylolisthesis are dysplastic, isthmic, degenerative, traumatic, and pathologic.[4,5] Of these, dysplastic (in which facet joints allow anterior translation) and isthmic (associated with a lesion of the pars interarticularis) types are most commonly encountered in children. Spondylolisthesis can also be classified by the degree of displacement in relation to the adjacent vertebra with use of the Meyerding grading system (shown in Fig. 140.4, with an example of a grade 3 spondylolisthesis), where 1% to 24% = 1, 25% to 49% = 2, 50% to 74% = 3, and 75% to 100% = 4. Cases in which the amount of displacement exceeds 100% are referred to as *spondyloptosis*.

History and Physical Examination

Spondylolysis is associated with sports such as gymnastics, volleyball, football, diving, and pole vaulting, in which repetitive hyperextension occurs, but can be seen in essentially any sport. A typical history is one of activity-related back pain that is well localized to the lower spine, with radiating pain in the buttocks or legs in some cases. Approximately 40% of patients recall a traumatic event at the onset of pain.[6]

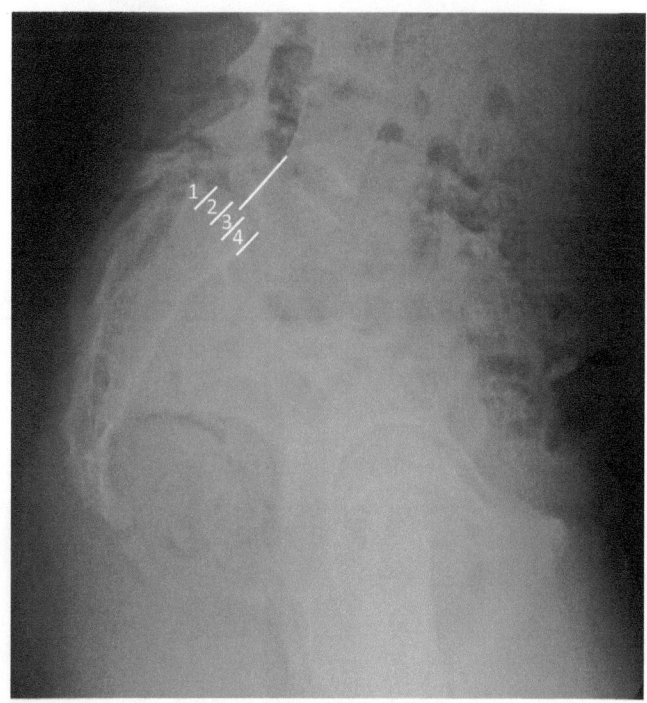

Fig. 140.4 An example of grade 3 spondylolisthesis using the Meyerding grading system. This system describes the percentage of translation of the superior vertebral body relative to the inferior vertebral body. Grade 1 = 1% to 24%; grade 2 = 25% to 49%; grade 3 = 50% to 74%; and grade 4 = 75% to 100%. Cases in which the amount of displacement exceeds 100% are referred to as spondyloptosis. (Courtesy Children's Orthopedic Center, Los Angeles, CA.)

On physical examination, patients may have lumbar hyperlordosis. Conversely, they may have flattening through the lumbar region in cases of severe pain or a high-grade spondylolisthesis.[7] The classic physical exam finding is pain with standing spine hyperextension, especially during single-leg stance or with concomitant twisting. Hamstring contractures are commonly associated with spondylolysis/spondylolisthesis. In some severe cases, this condition leads to the abnormal gait pattern described by Phalen and Dickson,[8] consisting of crouching, a short stride, and an incomplete swing phase.

Imaging

A great deal of controversy exists regarding the optimal imaging modality for evaluation of spondylolysis. Although the characteristic "collar of the Scottie dog" observed on oblique radiographs is often difficult to appreciate, plain radiographs are commonly used as first-line imaging (Fig. 140.5). In some series, more than half of spondylolysis lesions (53%) can be missed on plain films alone.[9] A single photon emission computed tomographic (CT) bone scan is more sensitive for detecting defects of the pars but is nonspecific and thus is positive for other pathologic conditions, including infection, osteoid osteomas, and neoplasms.[10] Single photon emission CT may also miss older, "cold" lesions. Consequently, our practice is to obtain a spot lateral of L5-S1 and then move directly to a limited CT if the signs and symptoms are consistent with a spondylolysis.

Since the advent and development of CT, many studies have verified that CT is more sensitive than plain radiographs in detecting early spondylolytic lesions.[11] In addition, even in patients with radiographs that demonstrate spondylolysis, a CT scan may be helpful for treatment planning to assess the acuity of the spondylolytic lesion.[12] MRI has been suggested as another imaging modality for evaluation of spondylolysis, but the reported sensitivity ranges from 25% to 86%.[13–15] In our own series, we found that up to 64% of spondylolysis cases in symptomatic patients can be missed if MRI is the only diagnostic imaging study performed.[16] Consequently, it is standard protocol at our institution to obtain a limited CT scan when presented with a patient whose history and physical examination are suggestive of spondylolysis and an MRI scan that appears "normal."

Treatment

Most children have resolution of symptoms with conservative treatment consisting of activity modification and bracing. In acute cases, an attempt at achieving bony union is made and activity is restricted. Although reports in the literature are variable, an estimated 75% to 100% of acute unilateral lesions and 50% of acute bilateral lesions heal (Fig. 140.6), whereas essentially no chronic defects heal.[7] Approximately 90% of athletes return to their prior level of sports participation at an average of 5 to 6 months,[17] which suggests that in many cases a fibrous union is sufficient for symptomatic improvement because the rates of returning to sport exceed the rate of achieving bony union.[7]

No consensus has been reached regarding the type of bracing or protocol for wear. The Boston thoracolumbar sacral orthosis, an antilordotic brace, and braces with a thigh cuff have all been

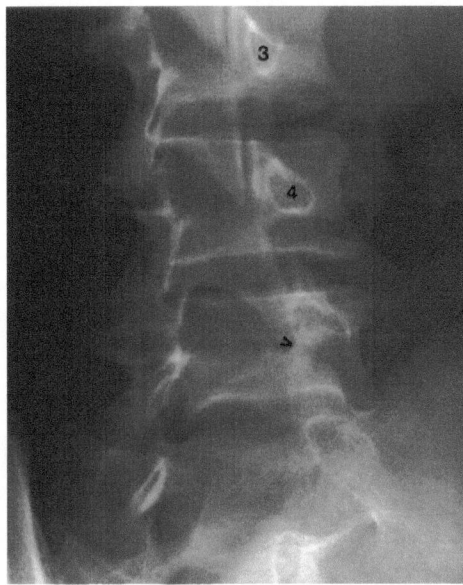

Fig. 140.5 The characteristic "collar of the Scottie dog" observed on oblique radiograph. (Courtesy Children's Orthopedic Center, Los Angeles, CA.)

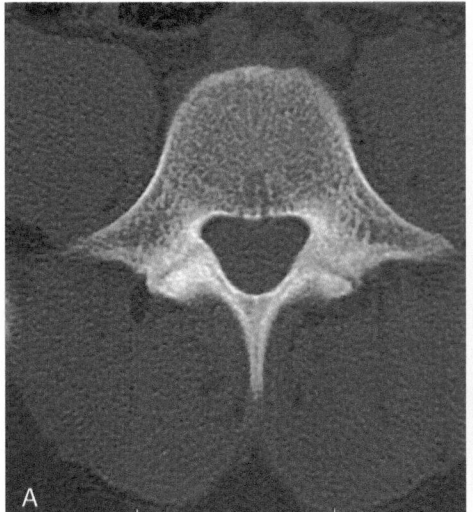
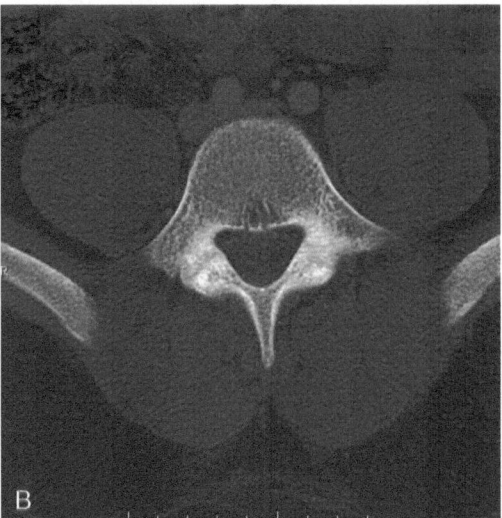

Fig. 140.6 (A) The presence of a bilateral pars defect on a noncontrast computed tomography (CT) scan consistent with a diagnosis of acute spondylolysis. (B) A subsequent CT scan with contrast-confirmed healing of the defect after successful conservative treatment. (Courtesy Children's Orthopedic Center, Los Angeles, CA.)

used. Some authors suggest that braces be worn for 23 hours a day for 4 to 6 months.[18] In general, when we are attempting to heal the fracture, our preferred treatment of patients with acute spondylolysis is to begin with an antilordotic brace worn any time the patient is weight bearing, including a thigh cuff if tolerated, for the first month. A lumbosacral orthosis without a thigh cuff provides very little immobilization to L5-S1. In acute cases, bracing is continued for approximately 3 months, and a limited CT scan is then performed to evaluate for bony healing prior to return to sport.

In chronic cases in which the bone does not heal, conservative treatment is based on symptoms. A variety of braces prevent excessive hyperextension of the lumbar spine. In some cases, patients can return to their prior level of activity while using such a brace. Core strengthening may play a role in long-term prevention of symptoms.

In cases in which the patient has unresolved pain after more than 6 months of conservative treatment, intolerance of conservative treatment, a greater than 50% slip of the spondylolisthesis, or neurologic symptoms, surgical intervention is considered. Numerous techniques have been described both for direct repair and for fusion of the involved segment. A direct repair should not be considered in cases of spondylolisthesis. Techniques for direct repair include the Buck technique of direct screw fixation across the pars defect, wiring between the transverse and spinous process, and pedicle screws with an attached sublaminar hook described by Kakiuchi.[19–21] Prior to consideration of a direct repair, an MRI scan should be obtained to evaluate the integrity of the intervertebral disk. If the intervertebral disk is abnormal, a fusion is preferred. Fusion may consist of a posterior only approach, with or without a transforaminal lumbar interbody fusion. Another option for fusion is an anterior and posterior fusion for additional stability. A great deal of controversy continues to exist with regard to in situ fusion versus reduction of the spondylolisthesis. The increased neurologic risks of reduction must be weighed against the risks of implant failure, slip progression, and pseudarthrosis associated with in situ fusion.[22,23] See Fig. 140.7 for our treatment algorithm for spondylolysis/spondylolisthesis.

Results

Rates of return to sports participation after surgical treatment are high, ranging from 80% to 100%.[24] Nevertheless, it is an area of high stress, and implant complications are frequently observed, with posterior fusion techniques resulting in a high reoperation rate, up to 47% in one series, with many of these presenting several years after the initial procedure.[25] This may reflect that the population of patients pursuing operative management often represents a subset of very competitive athletes who return to a high level of activity. For this reason, in many of these cases, our center and others have begun favoring the more aggressive approach of a combined anterior and posterior fusion. Fig. 140.8A and B shows an example of a patient treated with fusion who returned to a high level of sports participation.

APOPHYSEAL RING FRACTURES

The vertebral ring apophysis appears at the age of 6 years and fuses to the vertebral body at approximately the age of 17 years.[26]

Mechanical stress on the apophyseal ring can lead to a fracture of the vertebral growth plate, resulting in an apophyseal ring fracture. This clinical entity, unique to the immature pediatric spine, causes pain similar to that of a disk herniation.

History and Physical Examination

Pain is usually described as acute in onset and is often severe. Radicular pain is less common than in adult disk herniations because the injury is less likely to have a lateral component. A straight-leg raise test may be positive.

Imaging

This injury is often difficult to appreciate on plain radiographs, although such radiographs are generally obtained as an initial step in evaluating the patient with back pain. A CT scan allows accurate characterization of the osseous injury (Fig. 140.9). MRI is generally obtained as well in these cases to allow for evaluation of the adjacent intervertebral disk and nerve roots. However, MRI scans frequently miss this injury or are misread as a disk herniation because the thin bony component of the apophysis may not be appreciated (see Fig. 140.9).

Treatment

In contrast to herniated disk material, the posterior endplate lesion is typically not absorbed. Although injuries with very small osseous fragments may be treated conservatively, such treatment usually results in continued pain. The mainstay of treatment is surgical excision of the protruding fragment. A recent report by Higashino et al.[27] supports favorable long-term outcomes in patients with these injuries.

CHANCE FRACTURES

Chance fractures consist of a flexion-distraction injury with failure of both the anterior elements in flexion and the posterior elements in distraction. They were described by Chance as a traumatic horizontal splitting of the spine.[28] Chance fractures are often unstable and require surgical management. Consequently, differentiating between a stable compression fracture and a three-column Chance fracture is imperative for proper management of these injuries. Our institution has reported on several patients whom we cared for with unstable Chance fractures that were initially misdiagnosed as compression fractures, with a mean delay in treatment of 3 months.[29]

History and Physical Examination

Sports injuries are one of the most common mechanisms of injury for pediatric Chance fractures, alongside motor vehicle accidents and falls. These injuries are accompanied by the acute onset of pain and a high incidence of neurologic injury. Arkader et al. reported a 43% incidence of neurologic injury in a multicenter series of pediatric patients with Chance fractures. Of those with neurologic deficits, only 53% made a full recovery.[30] Consequently, a thorough neurologic exam is imperative. In addition, as these injuries may be misdiagnosed as compression fractures, it is important to have a high index of suspicion for possible Chance fractures when evaluating patients with a known

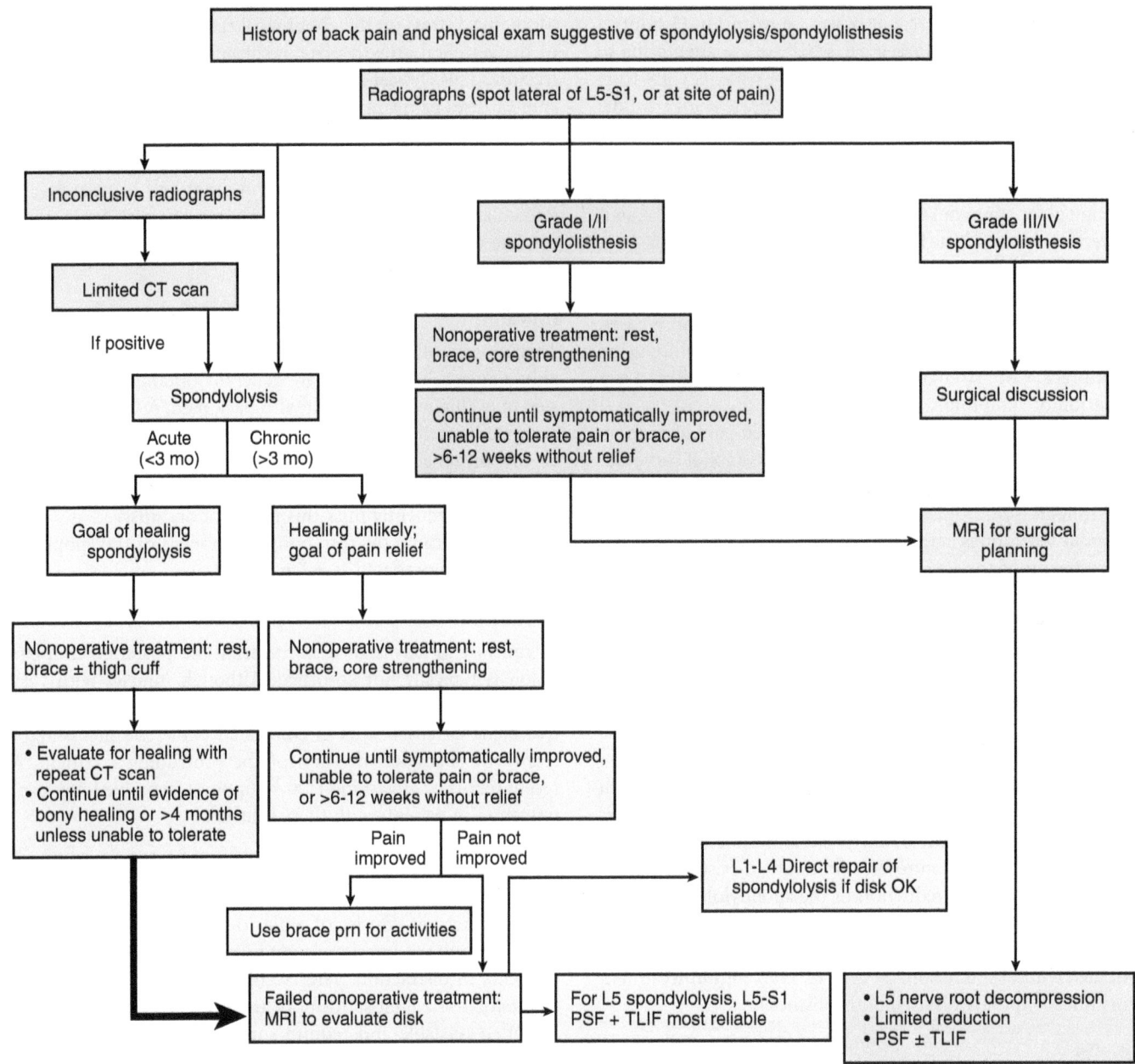

Fig. 140.7 A treatment algorithm for spondylolysis/spondylolisthesis. *CT*, Computed tomography; *MRI*, magnetic resonance imaging; *prn*, as needed; *PSF*, posterior spinal fusion; *TLIF*, transforaminal lumbar interbody fusion.

flexion injury of the anterior column. Clinical concern should be raised if there is tenderness to palpation posteriorly or any swelling or step-off to suggest involvement of the posterior elements with a three-column injury. In addition, there may be a kyphotic deformity at the level of the injury. This may be present initially, depending on the magnitude of the injury, or may develop in cases that are misdiagnosed in a more delayed fashion.

Imaging

The initial evaluation of spine trauma through the thoracolumbar region typically consists of an anteroposterior (AP) and lateral radiograph of the thoracolumbar spine. In cases where a neurologic deficit is present, an MRI of the spine is also obtained. This will reveal the extent of the ligamentous injury. A CT scan is often helpful to define the extent of the osseous injury and

differentiate a purely ligamentous Chance fracture from one with a significant osseous component.

Treatment

Arkader et al. showed improved outcomes in operatively managed pediatric Chance fractures when compared with those treated nonoperatively. In their series, 45% of patients had a good outcome (defined as no chronic pain or neurologic deficit) in the nonoperative group compared with 84% in the operative group.[30] Nevertheless, in a neurologically intact patient where there is an osseous rather than a ligamentous injury posteriorly, successful treatment may be possible with a thoracolumbar brace that is fitted so that it provides support at the level of injury to prevent development of kyphosis. In operatively managed patients, treatment typically consists of a level 1 or 2 fusion at the level

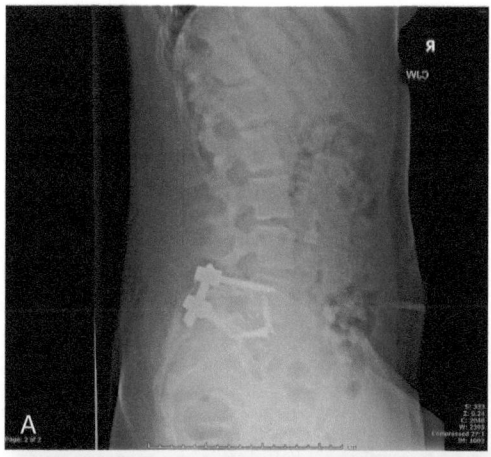

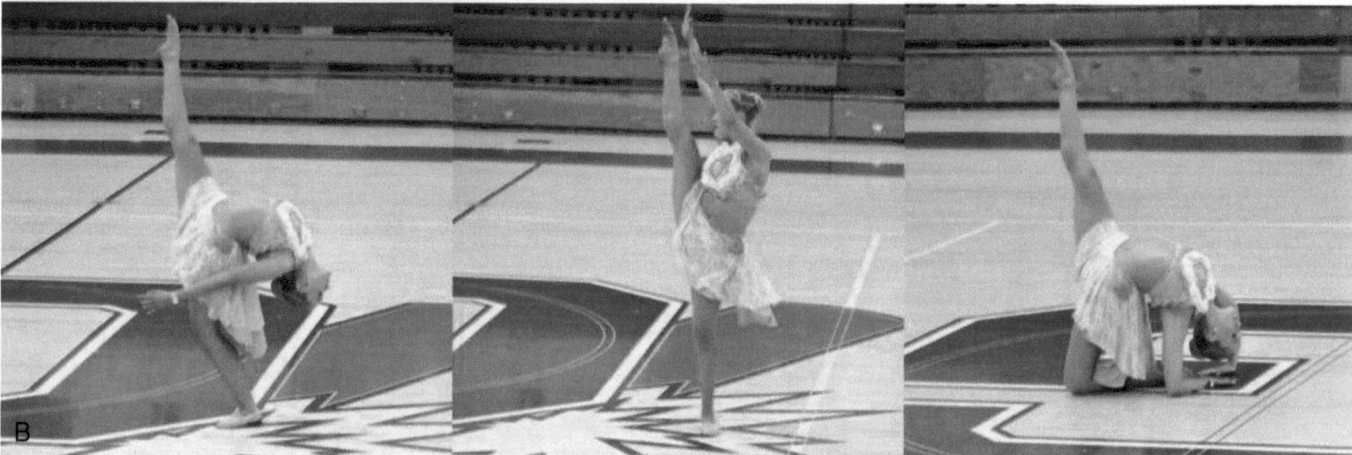

Fig. 140.8 (A and B) This 17-year-old female with an L5 spondylolysis was in severe pain despite months of conservative management. Following a successful anterior and posterior spinal fusion of L5-S1, she returned to competitive dance. Clinical photos demonstrate that she maintained excellent flexibility and range of motion following this one-level fusion.

of injury, though more levels may need to be included in cases where significant kyphotic deformity is present.

SACRAL FACET FRACTURES

Sacral facet fractures are a rare injury but an important diagnosis to recognize. They should be considered in the young athlete who has localized back pain with extension. This diagnosis may be easily missed on plain radiographs, bone scans, and MRI, which are frequently negative in these cases.[31,32] CT is the imaging modality of choice in cases in which this diagnosis is suspected. An example is shown in Fig. 140.10. Authors of a recent case series of elite athletes reported on treatment with removal of the intra-articular fracture fragments by a minimally invasive muscle-sparing approach. In cases where the fragment is removed early, resolution of pain and return to full sports is anticipated, while if long-standing there may be degenerative changes to the facet joint that develop leading to a more negative outcome.[32]

SCOLIOSIS

Scoliosis is defined as curvature of the spine of greater than 10 degrees. Although most cases of scoliosis are idiopathic, idiopathic scoliosis is a diagnosis of exclusion. The clinician should be careful to consider other diagnosis such as neurofibromatosis, Marfan syndrome, or Ehlers-Danlos syndrome, with which the scoliosis may be associated. Many patients with adolescent idiopathic scoliosis—which has a prevalence of nearly 3%—participate in sports.[33] Once other potential concomitant conditions have been eliminated, idiopathic scoliosis is not a contraindication to participation in sports.

History and Physical Examination

At presentation, approximately 20% of patients with scoliosis have back pain, which is similar to the percentage of adolescents who have back pain in general.[34] For back pain that is localized, constant, progressive, predominantly occurs at night, or limits activities, further evaluation with MRI is warranted. The clinician should also ask about constitutional symptoms and any bowel or bladder issues. These atypical symptoms necessitate further evaluation for other causes and for spinal cord compression.

Physical examination can be divided into three components: (1) assessment of the curve, (2) evaluation for any neurologic concerns, and (3) examination for any stigmata that suggest a cause that is not idiopathic. The Adams forward bend test then allows assessment of the rotation. Prominence should be noted on the same side as the convexity of the curve. In cases in which a lumbar prominence is noted on the concavity, a leg length

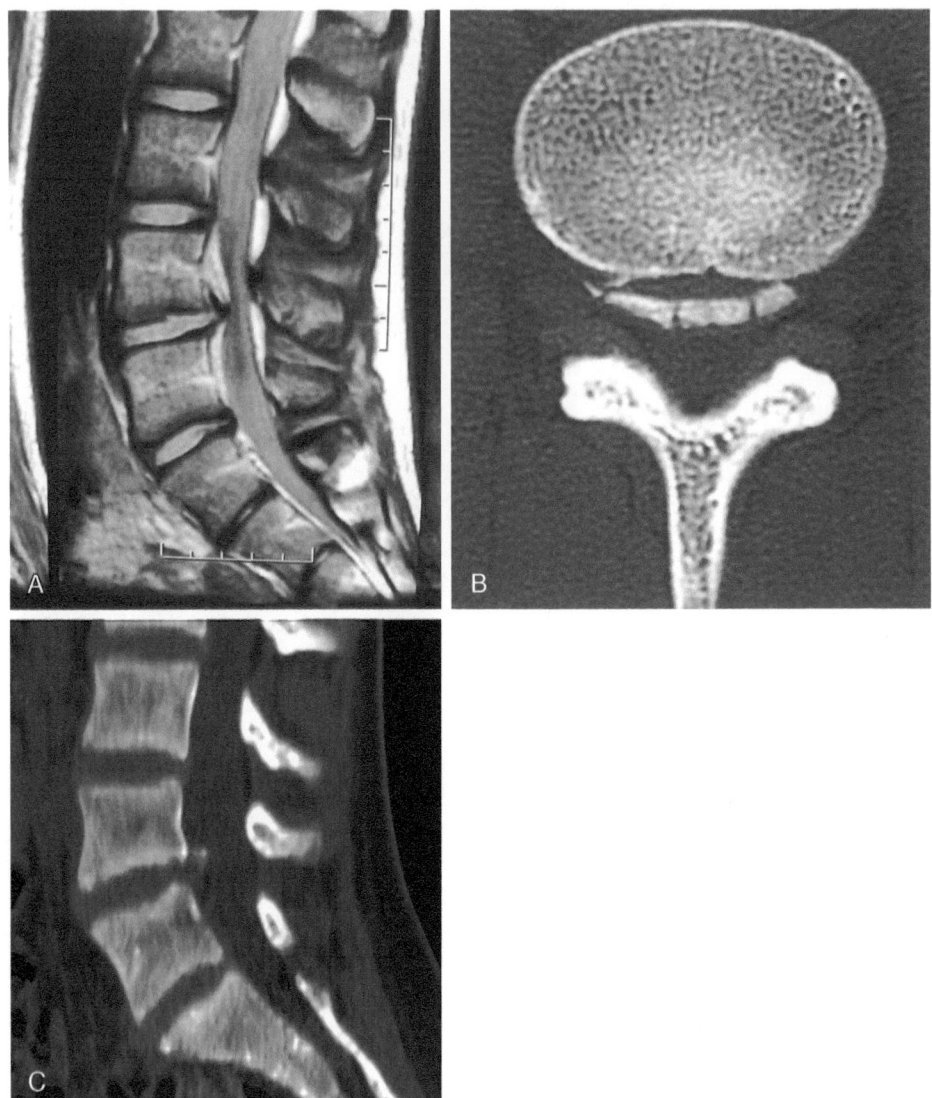

Fig. 140.9 Magnetic resonance imaging (A) gives the appearance of a disk herniation, but a computed tomography scan (B and C) clearly shows that it is in fact an apophyseal ring fracture. (Courtesy Children's Orthopedic Center, Los Angeles, CA.)

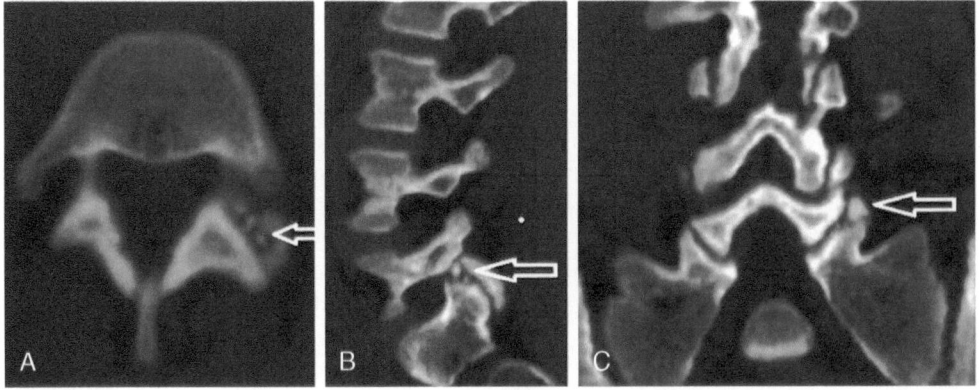

Fig. 140.10 Magnetic resonance imaging scan (A) and A computed tomography scans (B and C) depicting a sacral facet fracture *(arrows)*. (Courtesy Children's Orthopedic Center, Los Angeles, CA.)

discrepancy should be suspected, and the curve may be compensatory. With the patient bent forward, scoliometer readings can be obtained. Although highly variable, a reading of 7 degrees on a scoliometer is considered an indication to obtain a radiograph and correlates to an approximately 20-degree curve.[35]

After assessment of the curve, a focused neurologic evaluation should be performed (see Box 140.2). Any change in sensation or strength, gait abnormality, foot deformity, unequal reflexes, or sustained clonus suggests a cause that is not idiopathic. Cutaneous findings of axillary freckles, more than three café-au-lait spots, or neurofibromas suggest neurofibromatosis. A high-arched palate, ligamentous laxity, and pectus deformities warrant consideration of Marfan syndrome.

Imaging

If the clinical examination suggests the possibility of scoliosis, then initial radiographic evaluation consists of a standing posteroanterior and lateral radiograph of the thoracolumbar spine. This radiograph ideally includes the pelvis and is not collimated to allow for evaluation of closure of the triradiate cartilage and the Risser sign, which are important components in assessing the growth remaining and the risk of progression. Care should be taken to evaluate for concomitant pathologic conditions on the lateral radiograph. In particular, in persons with symptomatic spondylolysis/spondylolisthesis, an associated scoliosis is present in 25% to 40% of cases, but it may be easily overlooked if the focus is entirely on the spinal curvature.[36]

Attention should also be directed to the sagittal contour of the patient with idiopathic scoliosis. Due to the three-dimensional nature of scoliosis, rotation and resultant hypokyphosis are generally observed through the thoracic region. If this area is instead kyphotic, one should suspect other etiologies. In cases in which a cause other than idiopathic scoliosis is suspected, an MRI should be obtained. Although recommendations vary, indications for an MRI include (1) neurologic abnormality (weakness/abnormal reflexes), (2) severe pain, (3) young patients (younger than 11 years) with curves greater than 20 degrees, (4) atypical patterns (i.e., a left-sided thoracic curve, congenital scoliosis, short angular curves, or a severe deformity >70 degrees), and (5) rapid progression (i.e., >1 degree per month).[37]

In cases where there is a question as to the amount of growth remaining, a radiograph of the hand may be obtained to better assess skeletal maturity. Evaluation of this radiograph with a modified classification described by Sanders et al. has been found to be a more accurate predictor of risk of progression than Risser staging or Greulich and Pyle bone age.[38]

Treatment

Treatment is based on the risk of curve progression. The two major components in the evaluation are curve magnitude and skeletal maturity (i.e., the amount of growth remaining). Lonstein and Carlson have reported that if the condition is not treated, 68% of patients who are at Risser level 0 to 1 with a 20- to 29-degree curve will progress, whereas only 23% of patients who are at Risser level 2 to 4 with a curve of the same magnitude will show signs of progression.[39] Currently none of the genetic testing available reliably allows identification of the curves that will progress, as opposed to curves that will not progress.

Nonoperative treatment consists predominantly of bracing. Protocols and indications vary with much of the debate centering around the contradictory evidence with regard to bracing, which has been complicated by compliance issues. In 2010, Katz et al.[40] reported on 82% of patients who wore a brace more than 12 hours a day did not have a progression of their curve, compared with 31% who did not progress with brace wear of fewer than 7 hours per day.[40] Another landmark article was published in 2013 in the *New England Journal of Medicine* by Dolan and Weinstein reporting the results of the BRAIST trial.[41] In this multicenter, randomized prospective study between observation and bracing, the success rate was 72% in the braced group compared with 48% in the observation group.[41] In general, bracing with a thoracolumbosacral orthosis (Boston or Rigo Cheneau brace) can be considered for curves of 25 to 40 degrees, with substantial growth remaining (Risser level 3 or less; though more accurately assessed by Sanders staging) and a curve apex below T7.

For curves that reach 50 degrees, surgical intervention is generally recommended. This recommendation is based on the high rate of progression of curves with that magnitude even after skeletal maturity and the ultimately significant cardiopulmonary effects.[33] Currently posterior spinal fusion with pedicle screw fixation is the most common surgical treatment for idiopathic scoliosis. Complications include ileus (6%), early infection (1% to 2%), late infection (up to 5%), pseudarthrosis (3%), and neurologic deficit (0.4% to 0.7%).[37]

Scoliosis and Sports Participation

Numerous studies have demonstrated that exercise is not sufficient to inhibit the progression of idiopathic scoliosis. Although it may not alter the natural history, swimming has been shown to help maintain flexibility of the spine, as well as strength and endurance.[42] Although it is widely recognized that scoliosis should not present a contraindication to sports participation, many questions remain about when it is appropriate for patients to return to sports in cases in which athletes have undergone surgical treatment. Survey responses from 261 pediatric spine surgeons indicate that the majority of these surgeons allow children to return to noncontact sports participation between 6 months and 1 year after spinal fusion for adolescent idiopathic scoliosis.[43] Even more variable was the timing for return to contact sports. In most cases of uncomplicated posterior spinal fusion for idiopathic scoliosis, we allow return to sports as tolerated, including contact sports, at around 3 months after the operation. However, this return is dependent on the understanding of both the patient and parent that some very small increase in the risk of a catastrophic spinal injury may exist, along with the agreement to undertake this shared risk.

Varying reports have been made regarding the long-term impact of surgical treatment for scoliosis on sports participation. In 2002, a survey of patients with scoliosis who were treated both operatively and nonoperatively reported no significant difference in sports participation, but both groups had decreased participation compared with control subjects.[44] More recently, Fabricant et al.[45] reported a correlation between the distal level of the fusion and return to sports after posterior spinal fusion. In their study, only 59% returned to their preoperative level of athletic activity at an average of 5.5 years of follow-up.[45] Their study did not include a nonoperatively treated group for comparison. Selective posterior spinal fusions, more stable constructs with pedicle screws, and postoperative protocols with earlier return to physical activity may help improve outcomes, but as of yet, data on this topic are limited.

ATLANTOAXIAL INSTABILITY

Atlantoaxial instability may be either acute, as a result of a traumatic event, or chronic. Acute atlantoaxial instability may occur as a result of severe flexion of the cervical spine. An ADI of 5 mm or more in children in the setting of an acute injury may signify that the transverse ligament has been injured and that instability is present. Magnetic resonance imaging (MRI) can further elucidate the extent of the injury. If the transverse ligament is injured, posterior spinal fusion of C1 and C2 is usually necessary to prevent further compromise to the spinal cord.

ATLANTOAXIAL INSTABILITY IN DOWN SYNDROME

More commonly the physician is faced with management of chronic atlantoaxial instability in patients with Down syndrome. This instability may be either symptomatic or asymptomatic. The estimated incidence of asymptomatic atlantoaxial instability in persons with Down syndrome is up to 22%, whereas only 2% to 3% of persons with Down syndrome have symptomatic atlantoaxial instability.[46] The literature currently does not include any reports of children with Down syndrome without preceding neurologic symptoms who have had a traumatic injury with sports participation that resulted in progression to symptomatic instability. The history and physical examination are especially important in the evaluation of these patients, as even patients with normal cervical spine radiographs may develop instability over time.[47]

History and Physical Examination

The history is key in this patient population because the physical examination may be challenging. The revised American Academy of Pediatrics 2011 guidelines mark a shift away from routine radiographic screening and emphasize the need for a physical exam and parental counseling to monitor for development of any symptoms on a biannual basis.[48] Symptoms to inquire about include neck pain, fatigability, difficulty walking, abnormal gait, and worsening coordination/clumsiness or change in bowel or bladder habits. Physical examination should include evaluation of neck range of motion (ROM), gait, strength, spasticity, hyperreflexia, and clonus.

Imaging

Both the screening and management of atlantoaxial instability in persons with Down syndrome have become extremely controversial. The American Academy of Pediatrics has retracted its recommendation for assessment of potential atlantoaxial

instability and currently advises against imaging in asymptomatic persons.[48] In 2014, the Special Olympics also modified their requirements and no longer require routine radiographs for athletes. Instead they now rely on the completion of a medical form that includes a review of symptoms for adverse neurologic effects, including those that could result from spinal cord compression or symptomatic atlantoaxial instability. These forms are to be completed a minimum of every 3 years, though many programs require them on a more frequent basis. Radiographs should be obtained if there are any symptoms suspicious for this. The guidelines established by Special Olympics state that an ADI of greater than 4.5 mm is considered to be atlantoaxial instability.[49] Other authors have suggested that measurement of the space available for the cord (spinal canal width) of less than 14 mm is a more relevant predictor of neurologic injury, though this remains controversial in younger age groups. Nakamura et al. reported on use of the C1 to C4 ratio of space available for the cord (SAC), which had a high inter and intrarater reliability and can account for change with age and growth.[50] They reviewed more than 250 children with Down syndrome and found that a C1/C4 SAC of less than 0.8 was associated with a high chance of developing myelopathy.[50] If either an abnormal space available for the cord or an abnormal ADI is detected, further evaluation by a pediatric spine surgeon is warranted. In cases in which the ADI is greater than 10 mm or the child is symptomatic, an MRI scan may be helpful in the evaluation.

A similar issue for pediatric athletes with Down syndrome is the consideration of atlantooccipital hypermobility. Atlantooccipital instability has been underappreciated and should be considered when evaluating radiographs in this population.[51] A Power ratio of greater than 1.0 signifies anterior instability.[52] In addition, posterior instability has also been described, but the clinical significance of this instability is as yet unclear.[53]

Decision-Making Principles

Activity restriction on the basis of asymptomatic atlantoaxial instability is a topic of great controversy. Opponents argue that no cases have been reported of patients with isolated radiographic atlantoaxial instability who sustained a neurologic injury as a result of sports participation.[54] In addition, no cases have been reported of asymptomatic atlantoaxial instability progressing to symptomatic atlantoaxial instability as a result of a sports-related injury.[55] Based on their own internal review, the Special Olympics committee has consequently transitioned from routine screening radiographs to a medical form that emphasizes a history and review of symptoms to check for any evidence of spinal cord compression that could be due to atlantoaxial instability. If any of those symptoms are present, a flexion extension lateral cervical spine radiograph is obtained. For patients with an ADI of greater than 10 mm, spinal fusion is generally recommended. Fig. 140.11 shows our preferred treatment in the screening and management of asymptomatic persons with Down syndrome.

Currently no recommendations exist regarding atlantooccipital hypermobility in terms of clearance for the Special Olympics or other sporting activities in the young athlete with Down syndrome, but it should be considered when monitoring for the more common atlantoaxial instability.[51]

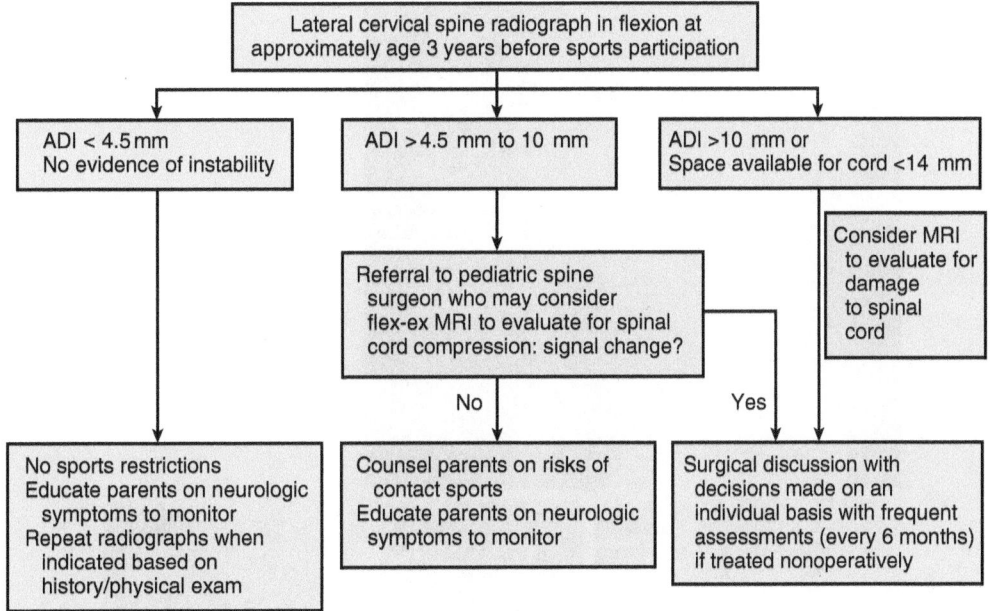

Fig. 140.11 The authors' screening protocol for asymptomatic patients with Down syndrome. *ADI*, Atlanto-dens interval; *flex-ex*, flexion-extension; *MRI*, magnetic resonance imaging.

Treatment

Aside from activity restrictions, no other nonoperative treatments are available for atlantoaxial instability. Operative management consists of posterior arthrodesis. Prior to fusion, particular attention needs to be given to the occipitocervical articulation. If there is evidence of instability observed at this level, in cases where the C1/C2 alignment is irreducible, or where decompression is needed of that region is required, the occiput is generally included in the fusion. Many techniques for atlantoaxial fusion have been described, including the use of wires, plates, and transarticular screws with either a rib or iliac crest graft. For smaller children, two commonly used techniques are the Mah modified Gallie technique and the Brooks technique. In the Mah modified Gallie technique, a wire is passed under the posterior arch of C1, looped over a threaded Kirschner wire that is placed in the spinous process of C2, and then tightened to secure a rectangle of corticocancellous autograft in position.[56] In the Brooks technique, two sublaminar wires are passed under both C1 and C2 and used to secure two trapezoids of the iliac crest graft that are wedged between C1 and C2.[57] Halo vest immobilization is required until bony fusion has been achieved. Screw fixation has also been utilized, particularly in older children. In cases where the occiput needs to be included, the authors preference is fixation with a plate. An important distinction is the cases of instability that are reducible, which can be positioned in extension to restore normal anatomic alignment, thus providing adequate space for the cord, and those that are not reduced by positioning in extension. In the latter cases, a concomitant decompression is often needed (Fig. 140.12A–C).

Results

Fusion rates in the setting of atlantoaxial instability in persons with Down syndrome have historically been poor and range from 40% to 80%.[58] An improvement in these results has been reported by Menezes and Ryken[59] by incorporating the occiput when indicated and implementing prolonged immobilization with a halo postoperatively, with recommendations of 4 months for C1-C2 fusion and 6 months when the occiput is included. Complication rates are high for this procedure. Segal et al.[60] have reported a 100% complication rate and an 18% mortality rate.

ROTATORY ATLANTOAXIAL SUBLUXATION

A common cause of acute torticollis is rotatory atlantoaxial subluxation, which occurs when the lateral mass of the atlas locks behind the ipsilateral lateral mass of the axis. It is most often traumatic in nature in healthy children, although other possible causes exist, such as Grisel or Sandifer syndrome. Rotatory atlantoaxial subluxation may occur after even minor trauma during sports participation or even with coughing episodes. It also may be associated with conditions that feature ligamentous laxity in this region, including Down syndrome, Marfan syndrome, or rheumatoid arthritis.

History and Physical Examination

On presentation, patients have a "cock robin" torticollis with their head tilted toward one shoulder and their chin rotated in the opposite direction. Patients may report neck pain and occasionally occipital neuralgia or symptoms of vertebrobasilar insufficiency. This condition is differentiated from muscular torticollis both by the acuity and by the absence of a palpable sternocleidomastoid on the shortened side. Conversely, the lengthened sternocleidomastoid may feel tight from being stretched. Most affected children are neurologically intact, but a thorough neurologic examination should be performed.

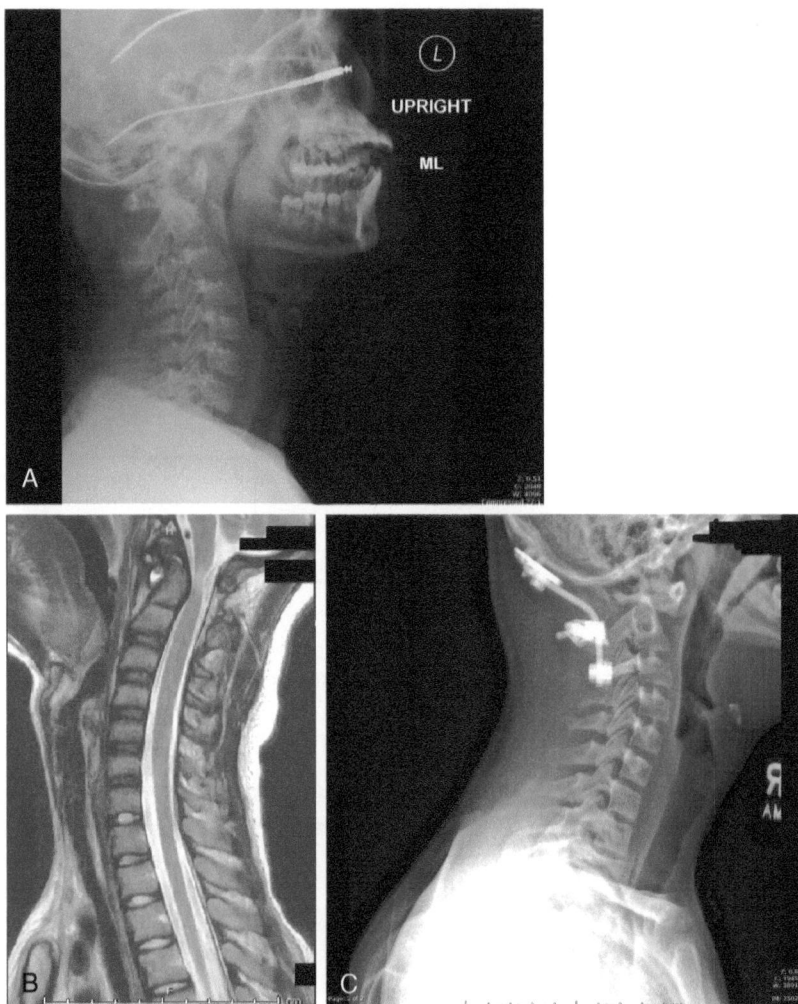

Fig. 140.12 (A-C) A 14-year-old male with Down syndrome who presented after several months of worsening gait instability and weakness. (A) Lateral radiograph showed marked anterior displacement of C1 on C2 which did not reduce. (B) Magnetic resonance imaging demonstrated compression and cord signal change at the level of the C1. The patient underwent decompression and occipitocervical fusion, after which he made a full neurologic recovery.

Imaging

Radiographic evaluation should include an open-mouth AP and lateral radiograph of the cervical spine. The technician should take the image as a true lateral view of the skull, which results in images that are more easily interpreted and show a true lateral view of the axis and rotation of the remainder of the spine. For further evaluation or if the diagnosis is unclear, a CT scan can provide additional clarity (Fig. 140.13). Dynamic CT scans allow for a more complete assessment of this area and avoid an ambiguous test result due to positioning, but should be limited to the upper cervical spine (occiput to C3) to minimize radiation.

Treatment

Treatment is time dependent because the subluxation becomes more difficult to reduce with the passage of time. In addition, persistent subluxation may damage the transverse ligament and result in subsequent instability or recurrence if a reduction is obtained.[61] In general, if the diagnosis is made and treatment starts 1 month or less from the time of the injury, then nonoperative management with either a cervical collar or head halter traction

is often sufficient. In patients in whom treatment is initiated less than 1 week after the onset of symptoms, immobilization in a soft collar for a few days is often sufficient to both obtain and maintain a reduction. For patients who begin treatment 1 to 4 weeks after the onset of symptoms, head halter traction can be used. If reduction is attempted with head halter traction, the position can be maintained with the use of a noninvasive halo. If these measures fail or if the injury occurred more than 4 weeks prior to the beginning of treatment, closed reduction with a noninvasive halo may be attempted, with reduction likely once the head is rotated past midline. A CT scan confirms the reduction. Use of the noninvasive halo may be continued for 4 to 6 weeks to allow scarring and maintenance of the reduction.[62] If instability or loss of reduction occurs, then repeat reduction with the noninvasive halo followed by surgical stabilization with posterior atlantoaxial fusion is indicated. Although it was once thought that late presentation of rotatory atlantoaxial instability frequently resulted in irreducible or recurrent subluxation and fusion was frequently needed, two recent series have challenged this assertion. Glotzbecker et al. reported a 73% success rate in patients treated nonoperatively with a mean delay of presentation

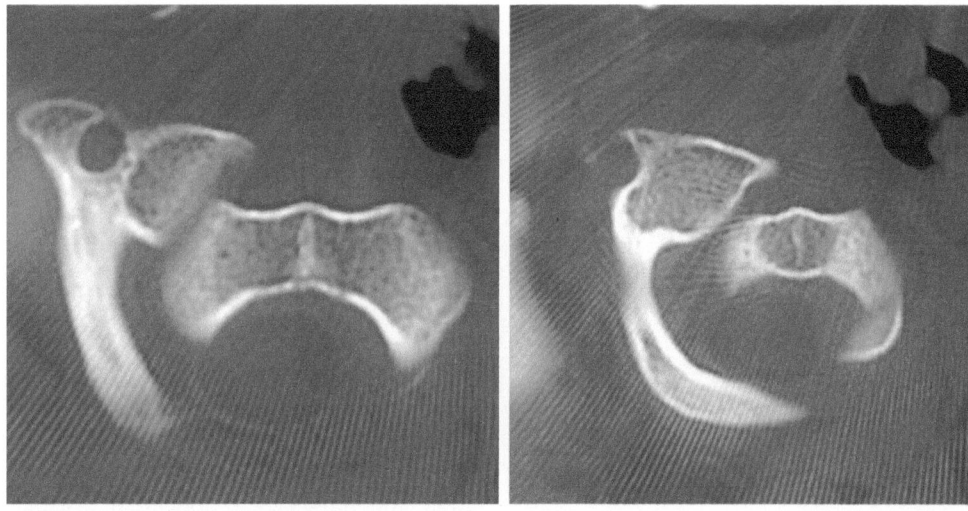

Fig. 140.13 A computed tomography scan showing that C1 is subluxated on C2 with the lateral mass of the atlas locked behind the ipsilateral lateral mass of the axis. (Courtesy Children's Orthopedic Center, Los Angeles, CA.)

of 18 weeks.[63] Chechik et al. reported a 100% success rate with patients treated nonoperatively with a mean delay of 11 weeks to presentation.[64] Although the authors recommend that this condition be treated promptly to optimize results, it appears that even in cases of delayed presentation, a trial of conservative therapy is warranted.

ODONTOID FRACTURES

Odontoid fractures account for 10% of all cervical spine injuries in children and the majority of pediatric cervical spine fractures.[65] In children younger than 7 years, the fracture occurs through the synchondrosis at the base of the dens. This position can make the diagnosis more challenging because the synchondrosis may be mistaken for a fracture or, conversely, the fracture may be assumed to be the synchondrosis and overlooked (see Fig. 140.14).

Classification

Odontoid fractures in children are described with use of the adult classification system of Anderson and D'Alonzo. Type I is an avulsion fracture of the tip of the dens. Type II is the most common and is through the base of the dens. In type III, the fracture extends into the vertebral body.

History and Physical Examination

Odontoid fractures occur more commonly from flexion mechanisms but have also been described from forced hyperextension. Although most authors have reported that pediatric odontoid fractures are not associated with neurologic injury, one series reported neurologic injury in 8 of 15 children younger than 6 years who had odontoid fractures.[66] A thorough physical examination should be performed to evaluate for this possibility. Typically these children have neck pain and decreased ROM. Direct point tenderness is not necessarily present.

Imaging

The synchondrosis at the base of the dens should be fused by age 6 years. After this age, any evidence of a radiographic abnormality

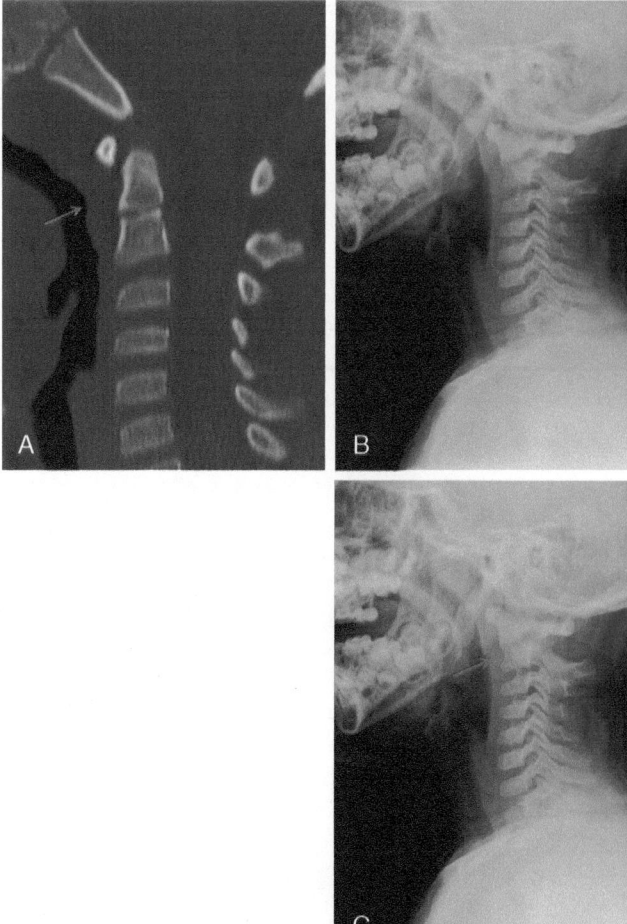

Fig. 140.14 A 4-year-old male who had sustained a fall on his head had an initial computed tomography scan (A) and radiograph (B) that were read as negative. The odontoid fracture *(arrows)* was missed because it was assumed to be just his normal physis despite the associated swelling. He presented 2 weeks later to his primary care physician with neck pain; a lateral radiograph taken at that time (C) shows significant displacement through the fracture site. Treatment consisted of closed reduction and halo placement. (Courtesy Children's Orthopedic Center, Los Angeles, CA.)

in this region suggests a fracture. In children younger than 7 years, great care must be taken to not mistake normal anatomy for an acute injury or conversely to neglect a fracture by attributing it to normal development. Assessment for swelling in the retropharyngeal space can be helpful in this differentiation. Nevertheless, the clinician should keep in mind that if the patient is crying, the child will have an apparent increase in the width of the retropharyngeal space. In situations in which the diagnosis is unclear and clinical suspicion is high, an MRI may be obtained for further evaluation. Fig. 140.14 shows the initial CT scan of a 4-year-old boy who fell on his head and whose odontoid fracture was missed because this fracture was assumed to be just his normal physis despite the associated swelling. He presented to his primary care physician with neck pain 2 weeks later, and a lateral radiograph showed significant displacement through the fracture site.

Treatment

Most of these injuries can be treated by stabilization in a halo vest. The alignment of the fracture is generally improved with the head positioned in slight extension. The amount of acceptable angulation and the potential for remodeling varies with age and remains controversial, although one report of patients younger than 3 years with angulation of greater than 30 degrees showed that remodeling led to a normal structure with no associated sequelae.[67] In children 7 years of age or older, the fractures behave more like adult fractures and are treated accordingly. Cases of nonunion of type II odontoid fractures in this group have been reported and can be treated with a screw placed via a direct anterior approach.[68] Consideration should also be given to the possibility of additional ligamentous injury causing instability, which necessitates C1-C2 fusion.

CONGENITAL ANOMALIES OF THE CERVICAL SPINE

Congenital anomalies may involve either failure of formation or segmentation of vertebrae. Numerous anomalies exist, and each case warrants evaluation for concomitant stenosis or instability. Evidence of instability may warrant surgical management and at the very least avoidance of sporting activities. One such clinical entity is os odontoideum. In this condition, the dens is not fused to the body of the C2 vertebrae. Another commonly encountered congenital anomaly is that of Klippel-Feil, the term given to a congenital fusion (or failure of segmentation) of two or more cervical vertebrae.

Classification

Klippel-Feil anomalies are divided into two types. Type I is a multilevel deformity in which a large fusion mass is present, and type II is a fusion of either one or two levels.

History and Physical Examination

Although os odontoideum was once believed to be exclusively a congenital condition, more recently a posttraumatic cause has also been proposed.[69] Evidence supports both posttraumatic and congenital causes, and in reality, two separate clinical entities may exist.[70] The clinician may be evaluating a patient because

of an incidental radiographic finding or because pain or neurologic symptoms are present.

Patients with Klippel-Feil syndrome may have the classic triad of a low hairline, a short neck, and decreased cervical ROM, but these findings are present in fewer than 50% of cases.[71] These patients may also have an associated Sprengel deformity due to failure of the scapula to descend. Evaluation of a person with Klippel-Feil syndrome also may be in response to an incidental radiographic finding. In all cases, a thorough evaluation for any neurologic symptoms or physical findings must be performed.

Imaging

At a minimum, imaging consists of AP, lateral, and flexion extension radiographs of the cervical spine. In cases of odontoid abnormalities, improved visualization is obtained with an open-mouth odontoid view. If evidence of instability or concern about instability is present on the basis of neurologic abnormalities, an MRI of the spine is warranted. A flexion-extension MRI is preferred in many cases to evaluate for any subtle changes indicative of dynamic cord compression. Prior to performing the flexion component of the MRI, it is advisable to obtain a neutral MRI and confirm that there isn't already cord signal change that would suggest flexion for the MRI may cause neurologic trauma.

It is also important to differentiate a persistent ossiculum terminale from an os odontoideum. These clinical entities differ in that the os terminale is small in size and located above the transverse atlantal ligament. Consequently, this condition is generally not associated with instability, although there are case reports of this occurring when associated with other syndromes.[72]

An additional consideration in the patient with congenital anomalies of the spine is the increased incidence of genitourinary issues and congenital heart disease in this patient population. Given the concomitant incidence, it is recommended that these patients should have a cardiac evaluation and renal ultrasound prior to consideration of sports participation. For example, the presence of renal abnormalities, such as a solitary kidney, may pose additional risks with sports participation.[73] Although recommendations vary, a diagnosis and discussion of the risks prior to sports participation are warranted.[74]

Treatment

In cases of os odontoideum in which the patient has neurologic symptoms and evidence of radiographic instability, a cervical fusion of the first and second cervical vertebrae is indicated. In cases of asymptomatic instability, the treatment is controversial, and both radiographic surveillance and surgical management have been recommended. Little evidence supports either decision. In persons with os odontoideum, as well as odontoid agenesis or hypoplasia, participation in contact sports is usually contraindicated. The literature includes multiple reports of injury to patients with previously undiagnosed os odontoideum that resulted in a neurologic injury, including respiratory-dependent quadriplegia.[75]

In persons with Klippel-Feil syndrome, the potential for spinal cord injury is due to the abnormal motion of the adjacent unfused segments. Pizzutillo has reported that more than 90 cases of neurologic injury have occurred in patients with Klippel-Feil syndrome because of associated occipitocervical anomalies, chronic instability, disk disease, or degenerative joint disease.[76] More than two-thirds of these cases were associated with a single-level fusion of the upper cervical spine.[77] Although no consensus has been achieved on this topic, a congenital fusion at level C3 or higher is sometimes considered a relative contraindication to participation in collision sports and warrants evaluation by a pediatric spine surgeon. Conversely, patients with a one-level fusion below the level of C3, a normal neck ROM, the absence of occipitocervical abnormalities, and the absence of instability do not have any contraindication to sports participation.[75]

SPINAL CORD INJURY WITHOUT RADIOGRAPHIC ABNORMALITY

The acronym SCIWORA was coined by Pang and Wilberger[78] to describe a spinal cord injury with motor, sensory, or combined deficits in the absence of any vertebral fracture or malalignment on plain radiographs or a CT scan. Although SCIWORA has been described in persons of all ages, it is most commonly observed in the pediatric population and accounts for an estimated 19% to 34% of all spinal cord injuries.[78–80] A great deal of controversy surrounds this condition, including its definition, diagnosis, and optimal management. In many cases, the term is a misnomer because clear evidence of the neurologic injury is observed on MRI. In some series, such as the one reported by Bosch et al.,[81] 50 of the 60 MRI scans obtained were interpreted as normal.[32] Conversely, a recently published meta-analysis found that of the 392 cases identified, every patient with a diagnosis of SCIWORA with an MRI scan had evidence of either intraneural or extra-neural injury.[82] In a series by Hamilton and Myles,[83] the onset of neurologic symptoms was delayed in 23% of cases (range, 6 to 72 hours).

History and Physical Examination

Patients with SCIWORA have sustained a traumatic event and have a subsequent neurologic deficit. Most cases of SCIWORA involve the cervical spine, but cases involving the thoracic and lumbar spine have also been described.[84] Motor vehicle accidents, falls, and sports are frequent mechanisms, though a 2012 review of a national database reported sports as the most common, accounting for 40% of the injuries. SCIWORA is most commonly associated with a flexion injury, but distraction and extension injuries have also been described with this diagnosis.[85] The severity of the neurologic injury is highly variable, ranging from isolated nerve root involvement to complete quadriplegia. The spine is usually tender with the presence of significant local swelling or a hematoma.

Imaging

By definition, the absence of any vertebral fracture or malalignment on plain radiographs or a CT scan must be observed to assign the diagnosis of SCIWORA. MRI scans of the brain and spine are also obtained for persons with this condition to evaluate for evidence of spinal cord injury and any other central nervous system abnormality in the differential. Several anatomic explanations for the more frequent occurrence of SCIWORA in

the pediatric cervical spine have been proposed, including a more horizontal orientation of the facet joints, anterior wedging of the vertebral bodies, and increased elasticity of the ligaments and joint capsules. A sentinel finding on MRI of a ligamentous Chance fracture that may be missed on plain films is significant, as evidenced by a subcutaneous hematoma around the failed posterior elements and/or an increased T2-weighted signal at the interspinous ligament.

Treatment

A wide spectrum of severity is found in this condition, ranging from deficits localized to one nerve root to complete paralysis. Because of the variation in clinical presentations, the appropriate management is difficult to determine. Uses of corticosteroids, mannitol, hyperbaric oxygen, and bracing have all been described.[81] The variable treatment protocols instituted from one institution to the next have further confounded this analysis and made it impossible with the currently available data to ascertain if steroids are of true benefit. Some authors have also argued against bracing or immobilization; they believe it is not indicated based on a lack of associated instability. Other authors, including Launay et al.,[82] have recommended treatment with immobilization. In their study, they compared a subgroup of 93 patients treated with immobilization only (with no use of steroids or other medications) and divided them into groups who were immobilized for 8 weeks and for 12 weeks. These investigators observed complete recovery in 42% of the patients immobilized for 12 weeks, but in only 34% of the patients immobilized for 8 weeks.[82]

At our institution, the following protocol is used in the management of persons with SCIWORA: In cases in which evidence of spinal instability exists (i.e., ligamentous injury, including ligamentous Chance fractures), we believe that spinal fusion with instrumentation is the most reliable treatment to protect the patient from further injury and allow early rehabilitation. If no evidence exists of an occult injury that may be associated with instability, then we do not routinely immobilize these patients.

CONCLUSION

Evaluation of the growing spine is associated with unique challenges and concerns. Nevertheless, with appropriate treatment, successful return to sport can often be achieved in pediatric and adolescent athletes.

For a complete list of references, go to ExpertConsult.com.

SELECTED READINGS

Citation:
Jackson RS, Banit DM, Rhyne AL, et al. Upper cervical spine injuries. *J Am Acad Orthop Surg.* 2002;10:271–280.

Level of Evidence:
III

Summary:
The authors describe the unique anatomy of the upper cervical spine, mechanisms of injury, and injury patterns, and review nonoperative and operative treatment of these injuries.

Citation:

Bull MJ. Clinical report: health supervision for children with down syndrome. *Pediatrics*. 2011;128:393–406.

Level of Evidence:

V

Summary:

This article includes guidelines from the American Academy of Pediatrics on caring for patients with Down syndrome and managing associated conditions.

Citation:

Tokunaga S, Ishii Y, Aizawa T, et al. Remodeling capacity of malunited odontoid process fractures in kyphotic angulation in infancy. *Spine*. 2011;36:E1515–E1518.

Level of Evidence:

III

Summary:

The authors performed a retrospective study of odontoid fractures that occurred in children younger than 3 years of age with a minimum of 20-year follow-up; they compared these patients with 127 patients who did not have a history of cervical spine trauma. At final follow-up, patients who had sustained odontoid fractures did not demonstrate a difference in odontoid process tilt angle compared with control subjects.

Citation:

Sankar WN, Wills BP, Dormans JP, et al. Os odontoideum revisited: the case for a multifactorial etiology. *Spine*. 2006;31:979–984.

Level of Evidence:

IV

Summary:

The authors reviewed 519 cervical spine radiographs for cases of os odontoideum. A history of trauma was reported in only 8 of 16 cases, supporting the theory that two separate etiologies may exist for the os odontoideum: posttraumatic and congenital.

Citation:

Grinsell MM, Showalter S, Gordon KA, et al. Single kidney and sports participation: perception versus reality. *Pediatrics*. 2006;118(3):1019–1027.

Level of Evidence:

III/V

Summary:

The authors report a combination of a survey of 135 American Society of Pediatric Nephrology members (level of evidence: V) and a review of literature on sports-related kidney injuries (38 articles; level of evidence: III). Although only one article reported one injury to a single kidney that was managed conservatively without sequelae, 62% of respondents said they would not allow sports participation by patients with a single kidney.

Citation:

Launay F, Leet AI, Sponseller PD. Pediatric spinal cord injury without radiographic abnormality. *Clin Orthop Relat Res*. 2005;433:166–170.

Level of Evidence:

III

Summary:

The authors provide a meta-analysis of 392 published cases of spinal cord injuries without radiographic abnormalities and evaluation of the mechanism of injury, risk factors, treatment, and prognosis.

Citation:

Weinstein SL, Zavala DC, Ponseti IV. Idiopathic scoliosis: long-term follow-up and prognosis in untreated patients. *J Bone Joint Surg Am*. 1981;63A:702–712.

Level of Evidence:

III

Summary:

The authors provide a classic article on the prognosis of persons with idiopathic scoliosis that is untreated with an average follow-up of 39 years.

Citation:

Fabricant PD, Admoni SH, Green DW, et al. Return to athletic activity after posterior spinal fusion for adolescent idiopathic scoliosis: analysis of independent predictors. *J Pediatr Orthop*. 2012;32(3):259–265.

Level of Evidence:

II

Summary:

The authors performed a retrospective cohort study of patients with adolescent idiopathic scoliosis in which 60% returned to sports at an equal or higher level of physical activity after surgery. A distal level of fusion, Lenke classification, and postoperative SRS-22 scores were each independent predictors of rate of return to the preoperative level of activity.

Citation:

Hu S, Tribus CB, Diab M, et al. Spondylolisthesis and spondylolysis. *J Bone Joint Surg Am*. 2008;90A:656–671.

Level of Evidence:

Instructional course lecture

Summary:

The authors provide a review on nonoperative and operative management, and prognosis of patients with spondylolisthesis and spondylolysis.

Citation:

Higashino K, Sairyo K, Katoh S, et al. Long term outcomes of lumbar posterior apophyseal end plate lesions in children and adolescents. *J Bone Joint Surg Am*. 2012;94A:e74.

Level of Evidence:

III

Summary:

This study demonstrated a favorable outcome for pediatric patients with posterior endplate lesions in both operatively and nonoperatively managed cases with a mean follow-up of 14 years.

INDEX

Page numbers followed by "*f*" indicate figures, "*t*" indicate tables, and "*b*" indicate boxes.

A

Abductor testing, 933
Abductors, of hip, 917
Abrasions, 253–254
  synovial, 1148
Abscess, skin, 203–204, 203*f*
Acceleration, 17–19, 17*t*, 18*f*
Accessory navicular, 1727–1728, 1728*f*
Accessory obturator nerve, of hip, 916
Accessory portal, 711, 951, 951*f*
Acetabulum
  cup depth, 938
  depth of, 908
  development, 907, 908*f*
  inclination, 938
  labrum, 313, 911, 911*f*–912*f*
  version, 907–908, 938
  volume of, 908
Acetaminophen, perioperative pharmacology, 338
Achilles tendon
  imaging, 1381–1383, 1382*f*–1383*f*
  injuries, 1476–1482
    complications, 1482
    decision-making principles, 1478–1479
    future considerations, 1482
    history, 1476
    imaging, 1477–1478, 1478*f*
    physical examination, 1477, 1477*f*
    postoperative management, 1480–1481
    results, 1481–1482
    treatment options, 1479–1480, 1479*t*,
      1480*b*–1481*b*, 1480*f*
  repair, platelet-rich plasma for, 54
ACL. *See* Anterior cruciate ligament
ACL-Return to Sport After Injury (ACL-RSI)
  scale, 387–389
Acne mechanica, 254–255, 255*f*
Acoustic shadowing, in ultrasonography, 79–80,
  80*f*
Acquired disease, hip, 1693–1694
Acromioclavicular (AC) joint, 397
  injuries, 645–678
    anatomy, 646*f*–647*f*, 646*t*
    classification, 645, 648*f*
    complications, 664
    decision-making principles, 653–655, 653*t*
    future considerations, 677
    history, 647–648, 649*f*
    imaging, 651–653, 652*f*, 654*f*–655*f*
    physical examination, 648–651, 650*t*, 651*f*
    postoperative management, 663–664
    results, 664, 665*t*–666*t*
    return-to-play guidelines, 663–664
    treatment, 655–659, 656*f*–658*f*
      anatomic coracoclavicular reconstruction,
        659*b*–663*b*, 659*f*–663*f*
  pathologies, 406
Acromion, imaging, 414–415, 414*f*–415*f*
  magnetic resonance imaging, 415–417, 416*f*,
    418*f*
Actifit implant, 42
Action plan, emergency, 150, 151*b*
Action-reaction, 19, 19*f*–20*f*
Acute bronchitis, 209
Acute compartment syndrome (ACS), 154
Acute kidney injury, 229

Acute mountain sickness (AMS), 242–243, 243*b*
Acute otitis externa, 213–214
Acute pneumonia, 209–210
Acute rotator cuff trauma, 548
Adaptive sports equipment
  amputee athlete, 317
  cerebral palsy, 321
  intellectually disabled athletes, 323
  visually impaired athletes, 323
  wheelchair athlete, 320
Adductor
  anatomy, 1007–1008, 1008*f*
  hip, 920
  pathology, 1007–1017
  strains, 1011–1012, 1050–1051
    complications, 1051
    decision-making principles, 1051
    future considerations, 1051
    history, 1050
    imaging, 1050, 1050*f*
    nonoperative management, 1011
    operative management, 1011–1012
    physical examination, 1050
    results, 1051
    return to play, 1051
    treatment options, 1013*b*, 1013*f*, 1050–1051,
      1051*b*
  tenotomy, 1016
Adductor canal nerve block, 333, 333*f*
Adenovirus, waterborne diseases, 212–213
Adhesive capsulitis, 407, 424, 425*b*, 426*f*
  in female athlete, 310–312, 311*t*
  idiopathic, 581–582
Adipose-derived stem cells (ADSCs), 57–58, 58*f*
Adolescent bunion, 1727
Adrenal hormones, 69*t*, 70
Adson test, 636–638, 637*f*
Adult involvement, in pediatric sports, 1610
Age/aging
  anterior cruciate ligament injuries, 1188–1189
  anterior shoulder instability, 452
  articular cartilage lesions, 1164
  articular cartilage repair, 12
  skeletal muscle and, 68
Alcohol, 290–291
Allergic contact dermatitis, 258
Allergies
  anesthesia, 339
  preparticipation physical evaluation, 149
Allograft, 31–32
  augmentation of, 32
  autograft *vs.*, healing of, 32–33
  meniscal, transplantation, 1142
  osteochondral, 1166, 1173*f*–1174*f*, 1176
  particulated juvenile cartilage, 1165–1166,
    1172*f*, 1176
Alpha angle, 938
Altitude sickness. *See* Acute mountain sickness
American football injuries. *See* Football injuries
Amputation, traumatic, 154
Amputee athletes, 316–317
  adaptive sports equipment, 317
  exercise, 316, 316*t*
  medical considerations, 316–317
    bone spurs, 317
    dermatologic conditions, 316–317

Amputee athletes (*Continued*)
    heterotopic ossification, 317
    musculoskeletal injuries, 316
    neuroma, 317
AMS. *See* Acute mountain sickness
Amylin analog therapy, 221
Anabolic-androgenic steroids, 284–287, 1611
  adverse effects, 285–287
    cardiovascular, 286
    hepatic, 286
    musculoskeletal, 286
    psychiatric, 286–287
  athletic performance considerations, 285
  physiologic considerations, 284–285
Analgesic medications, for knee arthritis, 1279
Anaphylaxis, 153
Anatomic coordinate system, 16
Anatomic coracoclavicular reconstruction,
    659*b*–663*b*, 659*f*–663*f*
Anatomic reconstructions, for lateral and
    posterolateral corner injuries of knee,
    1255–1256
Androstenedione, 287
Anemia, 196. *See also* Red blood cells, disorders of
Anesthesia
  arthroscopy
    elbow, 708
    principles, 110, 110*f*
    synovectomy, 1129
  intraoperative care, 327–329. *See also* Regional
      anesthesia
    positioning, 329
    tourniquets, 328–329
  neuraxial, 329
  perioperative complications, 339–340
    allergic reactions, 339
    Parsonage-Turner syndrome, 339–340
  perioperative medicine and, 325–340
    cardiac considerations, 326–327
    diabetes mellitus, 327
    respiratory considerations, 325–326, 326*f*
  perioperative pharmacology, 335–339
    acetaminophen, 338
    buprenorphine, 337–338
    dexmedetomidine, 338–339
    ketamine, 338
    methadone, 337
    nonsteroidal antiinflammatory drugs, 338
    opioids, 337
    propofol, 338
  regional, 328
    arm, 330
    benefits, 328
    complications, 328
    contraindications, 328
    elbow, 330–332
    femur, 332–333
    forearm, 330–332
    hand, 330–332
    hip, 332–333
    intravenous, 334
    knee, 332–333
    neuraxial anesthesia, 329
    orthopaedic surgeries and, 327
    patient characteristics, 327
    peripheral nerve block, 329–330

Anesthesia (Continued)
  shoulder, 330
  techniques, 329–335
  thigh, 332–333
Angiography, of popliteal artery entrapment
    syndrome, 1353–1354, 1354f
Angular kinematics, 22
Ankle
  arthrodesis, 1427b, 1427f
  arthroscopy, 1421–1435, 1422f
    calcaneoplasty, 1433–1435
    endoscopic Haglund resection, 1433–1435
    soft tissue conditions, 1421–1428, 1422f
    subtalar arthroscopy, 1428–1433
  biomechanics, 1359–1369
  decision-making, 1370–1379
  diagnosis, 1370–1379
  forefoot, 1515–1526
    hallux rigidus, 1523–1526
    metatarsalgia, 1519–1522
    sesamoid dysfunction, 1516–1519,
      1517b–1518b
    turf toe, 1515–1516, 1516b
  history, 1372–1379, 1373f–1378f
  imaging, 1380–1392
    computed tomography, 1380
    ligaments, 1387–1388, 1388f
    magnetic resonance imaging, 1380–1381
    nerve entrapment, 1389–1391
    osteochondral lesions, 1388–1389, 1389f
    plantar fasciitis, 1391, 1391f
    radiographs, 1380, 1381f
    tendons, 1381–1386, 1381f
    ultrasound, 1380
  injuries
    in adolescent athlete, 1725–1740
      fractures, 1729–1733, 1729f, 1732f–1734f,
        1732t
      orthotics, 1739
      shoes, 1739
      soft tissue, 1728–1729, 1728f
      systemic illness, 1739
      variations of normal anatomy, 1725–1728
    articular cartilage, 1484–1503
    in female athlete, 305–306
    figure skating, 117–118
    lacrosse, 122
    ligamentous, 1444–1461
    tendons, 1462–1483
    volleyball, 127
  joint, biomechanics, 1360–1363, 1361f–1362f
  lateral ligament, reconstruction, 1426b
  pathologies, 1370–1371
  pediatric, 1633–1635
    acute injuries, 1633, 1634f
    overuse injuries, 1633–1635, 1634f
  peripheral nerve entrapment around,
      1402–1420
    deep peroneal nerve, 1415–1416, 1415f
    interdigital neuralgia (Morton neuroma),
      1416–1419
    lateral plantar nerve, 1411–1412
    medial plantar nerve, 1412–1413
    saphenous nerve, 1405–1407, 1405f–1406f
    superficial peroneal nerve, 1413–1415, 1413f
    sural nerve, 1402–1405, 1403f
    tarsal tunnel syndrome, 1407–1411, 1407f
  physical examination, 1371–1372
  plantar fasciitis, 1509–1513
    complications, 1513
    decision-making principles, 1510
    future considerations, 1513
    history, 1509
    imaging, 1509, 1509f
    physical examination, 1509
    postoperative management, 1511

Ankle (Continued)
    results, 1511–1513
    treatment options, 1510–1511, 1510f, 1511b,
      1512f
  posterior heel pain, 1504–1508, 1505f
    complications, 1508
    decision-making principles, 1505–1506
    future considerations, 1508
    history, 1504
    imaging, 1504–1505, 1505f–1506f
    physical examination, 1504, 1505f
    postoperative management, 1508
    results, 1508
    treatment options, 1506–1507
  sprains, 115, 371, 380–381
    balance, 381, 382f–383f
    bracing, 380–381
    coordination, 381
    dorsiflexion range of motion, 381
    education of risk, 381
    hypomobility issues, 381
    lateral, 1444–1450, 1445f
    medial, 1450–1453
    strength training, 381
    taping, 369, 369f–370f, 380–381
Ankle block, 333–334
Ankle-brachial index (ABI) testing, 1395
Anomalous coronary artery, 168
Anterior arthroscopic débridement, 1425b
Anterior center edge angles, 937–938
Anterior compartment
    arthroscopic synovectomy, of knee, 1129, 1130t
    release, 1399
Anterior cruciate ligament (ACL)
    anatomy, 1069, 1070f, 1185–1186, 1186f
    basic science, 1186–1187
    biology, 1187
    biomechanics, 1185–1186, 1186f
    chronic insufficiency, 1284, 1284f
    injuries, 1185–1198
      biofeedback, 1196
      clinical history, 1187
      complications, 1197–1198
      decision-making principles, 1188–1190
      electrical stimulation, 1196
      epidemiology, 1187, 1199
      in female athlete, 307, 308t–309t, 309f
      functional training, 1196–1197
      future considerations, 1198
      graft type, 1197
      history, 1185
      imaging, 1188, 1188f
      muscle training, 1195–1196, 1196f
      pediatrics, 1697–1703
        complications, 1702
        decision-making principles, 1698
        future direction, 1703
        history, 1697
        imaging, 1697–1698
        partial tears, 1698
        physical examination, 1697
        postoperative management, 1701–1702
        reconstruction, 1700–1701, 1700f–1702f,
          1701b
        rehabilitation, 1701–1702
        treatment, 1698–1700, 1699f
      physical examination, 1187–1188
      postoperative management, 1192–1197
      proprioception, 1196
      reconstruction, 1193b–1195b, 1193f–1195f
        causes of failure, 1202–1203
        in female athlete, 310
        primary graft choice, 1203
        results, 1197–1198
        two-stage, 1207
      rehabilitation, 1192–1195, 1197

Anterior cruciate ligament (ACL) (Continued)
    return to play, 389t, 1197
    revision, 1189–1190, 1192, 1199–1210, 1208b
      advanced imaging, 1202, 1202f
      complications in, 1209
      decision-making principles, 1202–1204
      future considerations, 1209
      history, 1199–1200
      imaging, 1200–1202, 1200f
      multiple, 1209
      physical exam, 1200
      postoperative management, 1207–1209
      results, 1209
      treatment options, 1204–1207
    single vs. double bundle, 1197
    surgery, platelet-rich plasma for, 54–55
    tear, 377–380, 378f–379f
    treatment options, 1190–1192
  microanatomy, 1186
  MRI, 1110–1111, 1111f–1112f
  multiligament knee injuries and, 1267–1268
  partial tear, 1189
Anterior drawer test, 1377–1379, 1444, 1446f
Anterior interosseous nerve neuropathy, 899f
Anterior interosseous syndrome (AIN), 694,
    746–747
  complications, 747
  decision-making principles, 746
  history, 746
  physical examination, 746
  postoperative management, 747
  results, 747
  return-to-play guidelines, 747
  treatment, 746
Anterior intramuscular transposition, 750, 751f
Anterior shoulder instability, 440–462
  anatomy, 440–441, 441f–442f
  decision-making principles, 450–454
    age, 452
    associated injuries, 453–454
    contact sports, 453
    first-time vs. recurrent instability, 452–453
    in-season management, 453
    synthesis, 454, 454t
  future considerations, 461–462
  history, 447
  imaging, 448–450, 450f–452f
  pathoanatomy, 441–447, 443f–444f, 443t, 446f
  physical examination, 447–448, 448f–449f
  treatment options, 454–461
    complications, 461
    emergency department, 455
    nonoperative sling immobilization, 455
    on-field management, 454–455
    rehabilitation, 455
    results, 461
    surgical management, 455–461, 456b
Anterior subcutaneous transposition, 750, 750f
Anterior submuscular transposition, 750–751, 751f
Anterior tibial tendons, 1386, 1387f
  injuries, 1462–1464
    complications, 1464
    decision-making principles, 1462
    history, 1462
    imaging, 1462
    physical examination, 1462, 1463f
    postoperative management, 1463
    results, 1463–1464
    treatment options, 1462–1463, 1463b–1464b,
      1464f
  translation of, 1247–1248
Anteroinferior iliac spine, 908
Anterolateral ligament, of knee, 1070–1071, 1071f
Anterolateral portal, 778–779, 950–951, 950f
Anteromedial portal, 777–778
Anteroposterior view, 408, 409f

Antiepileptic drug (AED), 231
Apophyseal ring fractures, 1753, 1756f
Appositional ossification, 14
"Apprehension test", 404
Arachnoid mater, 1528
Arch taping, 368–369
Arcuate ligament complex, 1246
Arm. See also Entrapment neuropathies
    radial nerve, 752
    regional anesthesia, 330
Arrhythmias, 172–173
    atrial fibrillation, 172
    catecholamine polymorphic ventricular
        tachycardia (CPVT), 172–173, 173f
    channelopathies, 172–173
    Wolff-Parkinson-White syndrome, 172
Arrhythmogenic right ventricular cardiomyopathy
    (ARVC), 168
Arthritis
    glenohumeral, 592–608
        classification, 592–595
        complications, 606, 607t
        decision-making principles, 603–604
        epidemiology, 592
        future considerations, 607
        history, 595
        physical examination, 595–596
        postoperative management, 605–606, 606t
        presentation, 595
        prior operative notes, 596
        return-to-play guidelines, 606
        treatment, 596–603, 604b, 604f–605f
    hip, 1053–1060
        complications, 1060
        decision-making principles, 1057
        future direction, 1060
        history, 1053
        imaging, 1055–1057, 1055f–1056f, 1055t
        physical examination, 1053–1055
        postoperative management in, 1059
        results, 1059–1060
        surgical treatment, 1058–1059
        treatment options, 1057, 1060b
    knee, 1277–1292
        decision-making principles, 1283–1284
        history, 1277, 1278t
        imaging, 1277–1279, 1278f–1279f
        postoperative management, 1289, 1289t
        results, 1289, 1290t
        treatment options, 1279–1283, 1280f, 1284f
            nonoperative, 1279–1280
            not recommended, 1280
            operative, 1280–1283
    rheumatoid, 594–595, 594f
Arthrodesis
    ankle, 1427b, 1427f
    arthroscopic ankle, 1427b, 1427f
    metatarsophalangeal, 1525, 1525f
Arthrography, 76–77, 76f–77f
    computed tomography, 87, 87f
    magnetic resonance imaging, 415–417, 416f
    rotator cuff, 417–422
    shoulder, 410–411, 410f
Arthropathy
    capsulorrhaphy, 593, 593f
    dislocation, 593
    instability, 592–595
        chondrolysis, 593–594
        osteonecrosis, 595, 595f, 595t
        rheumatoid arthritis, 594–595, 594f
Arthroplasty, 605–606
    for knee arthritis, 1283
    return to sport after, 1283
    total hip, 1059

Arthroscope, 105–107, 106f
Arthroscopic ankle arthrodesis, 1427b, 1427f
Arthroscopic biceps tenodesis, 532
Arthroscopic bursal resection, 617b–619b,
    617f–619f
Arthroscopic capsular release, 585–586
Arthroscopic plication, 481
Arthroscopic portals, 110, 817–819, 818f–819f
    accessory, 711
    hip, 950–952
        anterolateral, 950–951, 950f
        distal anterolateral accessory, 951, 951f
        modified mid-anterior, 951, 951f
        posterolateral, 951–952
    posterolateral, 951–952
Arthroscopic posterior shoulder stabilization,
    470b–472b, 470f–472f
Arthroscopic probe, 107
Arthroscopic subtalar arthrodesis, 1430b–1431b
Arthroscopic subtalar débridement, 1429b–1430b,
    1429f–1430f
Arthroscopic suprapectoral biceps tenodesis,
    533b, 533f–534f
Arthroscopic synovectomy, of knee, 1127–1131
    anesthesia, 1129
    complications, 1130
    decision-making principles, 1128–1130,
        1128f–1129f
    future direction, 1130–1131
    history, 1127
    imaging, 1127–1128
    physical examination, 1127
    positioning, 1129
    postoperative management, 1130
    results, 1130
    surgical steps, 1129–1130
        anterior compartments, 1129, 1130t
        posterior compartments, 1129–1130
    treatment options, 1128–1129, 1129b
Arthroscopy, 105–113
    anesthesia, 110, 110f
    ankle, 1421–1435, 1422f
        calcaneoplasty, 1433–1435
        endoscopic Haglund resection, 1433–1435
        soft tissue conditions, 1421–1428, 1422f
    applications of, 105
    for calcaneal fractures, 1431b
    complications, 110–112
    diagnostic, 110
    elbow, 707–719, 767b, 767f–768f
        complications, 718
        decision-making principles, 707–712
        fluid management, 708–709
        future considerations, 718
        history, 707
        imaging, 707
        instrumentation, 708–709, 709f
        physical examination, 707
        portal placement, 709–711, 709t
        postoperative management, 718
        return-to-play guidelines, 718
        treatment, 707–712, 717b
    equipment in, 105–109, 106f
        arthroscope, 105–107, 106f
        arthroscopic probe in, 107
        basket forceps in, 107–108, 108f
        cannulas in, 108
        electrocautery in, 108–109
        fluid pump, 107
        grasping forceps in, 108
        instruments and, 107
        knives in, 108
        motorized shavers in, 107–108
        radiofrequency instruments and, 108–109

Arthroscopy (Continued)
        scissors in, 108
        switching sticks in, 108
    hip, 947–956, 1058–1059, 1058f
        contraindications, 947
        femoroacetabular impingement, 965–967,
            966f, 966t
        indications, 947–948
        learning curve for, 948
        operating room set-up, 948–950
        positioning for, 948–950
        procedure for, 950–955
    knee, 1121–1126, 1280–1281
        complications, 1125–1126
        diagnostic, 1123–1125, 1125f
        indications, 1121
        instrumentation, 1125
        lateral and posterolateral corner injuries,
            1254, 1254f
        portal placement, 1121–1123, 1122f–1124f
        positioning, 1121, 1122f
        postoperative care, 1125
        preoperative evaluation, 1121
    lateral epicondylitis, 724
    for meniscal injuries, 1140
    motion, loss, in elbow, 776–781, 777f–781f
        anterolateral portal, 778–779
        anteromedial portal, 777–778
    pediatric, 1612–1614, 1612f–1615f
    posterior hindfoot, 1470b, 1471f
    principles, 109–110
        anesthesia, 110, 110f
        arthroscopic portals in, 110
        diagnostic arthroscopy, 110
        patient positioning, 109–110, 109f–110f
        preoperative, 109
        preparation, 109–110, 109f–110f
        surgical technique, 109
    reduction, 824b–825b, 824f–825f
    scaphoid nonunions, reduction of, 824–825,
        825t
    shoulder, 433–439
        anatomy, 435–436
        background, 433
        complications, 438–439
        contraindications, 433
        diagnostic examination, 436–438,
            437f–438f
        indications, 433
        open procedures vs., 433
        portal placement, 435–436, 436f
        positioning, 434–435, 434f
        preoperative imaging, 433–434
        setup, 435
        visualization, 435
    subtalar, 1428–1433
        complications, 1432–1433
        decision-making principles, 1429
        history, 1429
        imaging, 1429
        physical examination, 1429
        postoperative management, 1431
        results, 1431–1432
    triangular fibrocartilage complex, 828, 828t
    wrist, 817–834
        anatomy, 819–820, 820f–821f
        carpal instability, 821–824, 821t, 822f–823f
        class I traumatic injuries, 829–832,
            829f–831f
        class II degenerative injuries, 832
        complications, 833
        fracture, 824–828
        future considerations, 833
        ganglionectomy, 832–833, 832f

Arthroscopy (Continued)
  management, 829–832, 829f–831f
  set-up, 817–819, 818f–819f
  triangular fibrocartilage complex, 828, 828t
Articular cartilage, 9–12
  cell-matrix interactions, 11
  clinical relevance and further developments in, 12
  defects, 1179f
    depth, 12
    size, 12
    surgical management, 1178–1184
      palliative, 1179
      reparative, 1179–1181, 1180f–1181f
      restorative, 1181–1184, 1182f
      treatment, 1178–1184
  extracellular matrix, 11
  hip, 913–914
  injuries, 1484–1503. See also Osteochondral lesions
    revision anterior cruciate ligament injuries and, 1203–1204
  lesions (ACL), 1161–1177
    anatomy, 1161–1162
    biomechanics, 1161–1162
    classification, 1162, 1162t
    complications, 1176
    decision-making principles, 1163–1164
    future considerations, 1176–1177
    history, 1162–1163
    imaging, 1163
    physical examination, 1163
    postoperative management, 1166–1167
    results, 1174–1176
    return to play, 1167
    treatment options, 1164–1166, 1167b–1173b, 1168f
  repair, 11–12
  structure and composition, 10–11, 10f
  zones of, 10–11, 10f
Articular hyaline cartilage, restoration of, 1488
Articular surfaces, 431–432, 431f–432f
Articulation, scapulothoracic, 398
Artifacts, magnetic resonance, 98–99
ARVC. See Arrhythmogenic right ventricular cardiomyopathy
Aseptic meningitis, 214
  waterborne diseases, 212–213
Aspirin, 191–192
Asthma, 190, 325
Athlete. See also Elite athlete
  amputee, 316–317
    adaptive sports equipment, 317
    exercise physiology, 316
    medical considerations, 316–317, 316t
  with cerebral palsy, 320–321
    adaptive equipment, 321
    exercise, 320–321, 320b
    medical considerations, 321
  collegiate, 155
  in contact sports, 453
  with diabetes, 218–226. See also Diabetes
    diagnosis, 218–219
    epidemiology, 218
    exercise, physiologic changes of, 221–223, 221f, 222t
    management, 223–225, 223f
    treatment, 219–221
  exercise-induced bronchoconstriction, risk for, 175
  female. See Female athlete
  gastrointestinal medicine in, 189–195
  genitourinary trauma in, 227–229
  hematologic medicine, in, 196–200
  high school, 155
  infectious diseases in, 201–217

Athlete (Continued)
  injured, approach to, 1554–1556, 1554f
  intellectually disabled, 321–323
    adaptive equipment, 323
    exercise physiology, 322
    medical considerations, 322–323
  posterior cruciate ligament injuries, 1211–1212, 1212f
  professional, 155
  with special needs, 150
  visually impaired, 323
  wheelchair, 317–320
    adaptive, 320
    exercise, 317–318
    medical considerations, 318–320
"Athlete's foot" (tinea pedis), 249, 250f
Athlete's nodules (collagenomas), 255, 255f
Athletic heart syndrome, 326
Athletic pubalgia, 1007–1017
  anatomy, 1007–1008, 1008f
  complications, 1016
  decision-making principles, 1011
  future considerations, 1016
  historical background, 1008
  history, 1009
  imaging, 1010–1011
    dynamic ultrasonography, 1010–1011
    magnetic resonance imaging, 1010, 1010f–1011f
    radiographic analysis, 1010, 1010f
  pediatrics, 1692
  physical examination, 1009, 1009f
    diagnostic injections, 1009
  treatment options, 1011–1016, 1014b
    adductor strain, 1011–1012, 1013b, 1013f
    osteitis pubis, 1014–1016, 1016b
    sports hernia, 1012–1014, 1014b, 1014f
Athletic trainer, 342–346
  education, 342–343, 343b, 343t
  regulation, 343, 344t
  scope of practice, 344–346
    clinical diagnosis, 344, 345f
    emergent care, 344–345
    health care administration, 346
    health promotion, 344
    immediate care, 344
    injury prevention, 344
    psychosocial strategies, 345–346
    referral, 345–346
    therapeutic interventions, 345, 345f
  working relationship, 344
Athletic training, 342, 343b. See also Training
Atlantoaxial instability, 1758
  in Down syndrome, 1758–1759
    decision-making principles, 1758, 1759f
    history, 1758
    imaging, 1758
    physical examination, 1758
    results, 1759
    treatment, 1759, 1760f
Atlas, spine, 1533
Atraumatic hip microinstability, 977–978
Atraumatic instability, 1654–1655
  history, 1654
  imaging, 1655, 1655f
  physical examination, 1654–1655, 1654f
  treatment options, 1655, 1655f
Atria, 160–161
Atrial fibrillation, 172
Augmentation
  allograft, 32
  autograft, 30–31
  ligament, 5–7
  meniscal repair, 9
  tendon, 5–7

Auto racing injuries, 117
Autogenous cancellous bone grafting, 1491
Autograft, 30
  allograft vs., 32–33
  augmented, 30–31
  bone-tendon-bone, 30
  osteochondral, 1165, 1167b–1173b, 1169f–1171f, 1175
  semitendinosus, 31
  soft tissue, 31
Autologous chondrocyte implantation, 42–43, 1165, 1167b–1173b, 1171f, 1175–1176, 1489
Autologous matric induced chondrogenesis (AMIC), 1489
Autonomic dysreflexia, 319–320
AVPU scale, for injured athlete, 1554–1555
Avulsion fractures, 928, 1052, 1688, 1689f
Axial neck pain, 1593–1594
Axillary brachial plexus block, 332
Axillary lateral view, 408, 409f
Axillary nerve compression, 630b
Axillary nerve palsy, 629–630
  anatomy, 629
  biomechanics, 629
  clinical evaluation, 629–630
  decision-making principles, 630
  diagnostic studies, 630
  results, 630

B

Back. See also Spine
  injuries, 118–121, 126
  pain, 128, 1598
Bacterial infections, 246–249
  cellulitis/erysipelas, 247–248, 248f
  erythrasma, 248–249, 249f
  folliculocentric infections, 246, 247f
  impetigo, 246–247, 247f
  pitted keratolysis, 248, 248f
  pseudomonal folliculitis (hot tub folliculitis), 249, 249f
  skin, 203–205
    definition, 203
    diagnosis, 203–204, 203f–204f
    epidemiology, 203
    pathobiology, 203
    prevention, 204
    return-to-play guidelines, 204–205
    treatment, 204
Balance, 381, 382f–383f
Balance Error Scoring System (BESS), 1744, 1744b
Bankart repair, arthroscopic, 457b–459b, 458f, 461
Baseball injuries, 114–115
  elbow, 115
  lower extremity, 115
  pediatric, 115
  shoulder, 114–115
  sliding, 115
Basketball injuries, 115–116
  ankle sprains, 115
  concussion, 116
  dental, 116
  facial, 116
  finger, 116
  hand, 116
  knee, 115–116
  sudden death, 116
  tendinitis, 116
Basket forceps, 107–108, 108f
"Baxter's nerve", 1411
Beach chair position, 329
Bear-hug test, 404, 559
Beighton scoring method, 1446t
Belly-press test, 404, 559

Biceps
    distal
        tendinitis, 725–728
            complications, 727
            decision-making principles, 725–726
            future considerations, 727–728
            history, 725
            imaging, 725, 726f
            physical examination, 725, 725f
            postoperative management, 727
            results, 726
            return-to-play guidelines, 727
            treatment, 726, 726b
        tendon rupture, 731–741
            anatomy, 731, 732f–733f
            biomechanics, 731–732
            classification, 732, 732b
            complications, 736–737
            decision-making principles, 735
            epidemiology, 731
            history, 732–733
            imaging, 733–734, 734f
            physical examination, 733, 733f
            postoperative management, 735
            results, 735–736
            treatment, 734–735, 735t, 736b, 736f
    imaging, 422–424, 425f
    tendon, long head of, 424–427, 427f
    tenodesis, 524, 532, 1254–1255
    tenosynovitis, 548
    tenotomy, 531–532
Biceps femoris muscle, 1245–1246
    long head of, 1245–1246
    short head of, 1246
Biceps pulley, 422–424, 425f
Bicuspid aortic valve, 168–169, 170f–171f
Bier block, 334
Bifurcate ligament sprain, 1456–1457
    complications, 1458
    decision-making principles, 1457
    history, 1457
    imaging, 1457
    physical examination, 1457
    postoperative management, 1457
    results, 1457–1458
    treatment, 1457, 1457b
Bioabsorbable implants, 1204
BioCart II, 44
Biofeedback, 1196
Biologic augmentation, repair with, 571
Biologic stimulation, 1147–1150
Biomechanics, 16–29
    ankle, 1359–1369
        joints, 1360–1363, 1361f–1362f
    anterior cruciate ligament, 1185–1186,
        1186f
    articular cartilage lesions, 1161–1162
    axillary nerve palsy, 629
    basic concepts, 16–19
        coordinate systems, 16
        degrees of freedom, 16–17, 18f
        Newton's laws, 17–19, 17t
        scalars, 16
        units of measure, 16, 17t
        vectors, 16, 18f
    distal biceps tendon rupture, 731–732
    distal triceps tendon rupture, 737
    dynamics, 22–23
        joint motions in, 22–23, 23f
        kinematics, 22
        kinetics, 23
        relative motion, 22
    elbow, 681–685
    extensor mechanism injuries, 1319, 1320f

Biomechanics (Continued)
    factors affecting properties, 27
    foot, 1359–1369
    head, 1535, 1535f
        injuries, 1538, 1539f
    hip, 907–924
        gait cycle in, 921–922
        joint, forces around, 922–923
        motions in, 921
        spine and, relationship of, 923–924,
            923f
        stability in, 921
    knee, 1072–1073, 1073f
        joint, 1077–1080
        lateral and posterolateral corner injuries,
            1246, 1247f
        ligament, 1075–1077, 1076f
        meniscal, 1080–1082
        patellofemoral joint, 1082–1087
        techniques, 1073–1074, 1074f
        tibiofemoral joint, 1074–1080
    lateral corner injuries, 1246, 1247f
    long thoracic nerve palsy, 625, 625f
    mechanics, classes of, 23–24
        fluid mechanics, 23–24
        rigid body mechanics, 23
        viscoelasticity and, 24, 24f–25f
    meniscus, 1134–1135
    methods, 24–29
        functional tissue engineering, 28–29
        improving performance, 28
        injury prevention, 28
        mechanical properties, 25–27, 26f–27f
        practical application, 27–29
        stiffness vs. flexibility testing, 27
        structural properties, 24–25, 25f–26f
        surgical reconstruction, 28
    patellofemoral joint, 1082–1087
    pediatrics
        concussion, 1741, 1742f
        throwing, 1663–1665
    rotator cuff and impingement lesions, 542–543
        biceps function, 542, 543f
        function, 542, 542f
        scapular function, 543
        static stabilizers, 542–543
    spinal accessory nerve palsy, 627–628
    spine, 1535, 1535f
    statics in, 19–22
        force vectors, 21
        free-body diagrams, 20f, 21
        ligament and joint contact forces in, 21–22
        moment/torque vectors, 21
    subtalar joint, 1363–1365, 1363t, 1364f–1366f
    suprascapular nerve palsy, 621–622, 622f
    throwing, 1663–1665
    transverse tarsal joints, 1365, 1367f
    wrist, 789–790, 790f, 835
BioSeed-C, 44
Birth control, in female athlete, 301, 301t
Bladder
    injuries, 227
    neurogenic, 319
Blisters, friction, 254
Blood-borne infections, 210
BMAC. See Bone marrow aspirate concentrate
        (BMAC)
Bone, 12–15
    appositional ossification, 14
    cellular biology, 13
    circulation, 13
    formation, 14
    fracture healing in, biology, 14–15, 14t–15t
    injuries, hip, 925–926

Bone (Continued)
    matrix, 13
    pediatrics, 1688–1691
    realignment of, procedures for, 1300–1301
    remodeling, 13
    tissue surrounding, 13–14
    types, 12–13, 12f
Bone grafting, 715b–716b, 1204
Bone marrow aspirate (BMA), 1489
Bone marrow aspirate concentrate (BMAC), 57,
        57f
Bone scans, 88–89, 89f
    meniscal transplantation, 1155
    posterior cruciate ligament injuries, 1214
Bone-tendon-bone autograft, 30
Bony anatomy
    hip, 907–911
    pertinent, patellar instability, 1294, 1294f
Borderline dysplasia, 977
Bowel, neurogenic, 319
Boxing
    injuries, 116–117
        facial, 116–117
        neurologic, 117
        upper extremity, 117
    professional vs. amateur, 116
Braces
    ankle sprains, 380–381
    knee arthritis, 1279–1280
Brachial plexus, 330, 331f
Brain, 1528–1529
    injury, 1562–1569
        background, 1562–1564
        clinical presentation, 1563–1564
        definition, 1562–1563
        epidemiology, 1563
        imaging, 1566
        interventions, 1567–1568
        management, 1566–1567
        pathophysiology, 1563
        physical examination, 1564–1566
        retiring athlete, 1567
        return-to-play, 1567, 1567t
Brainstem, 1528–1529
Bronchitis, acute, 209
Bronchodilators, for exercise-induced
        bronchoconstriction, 177
BST-CarGel, 44
Bunion, adolescent, 1727
Buprenorphine, perioperative pharmacology,
        337–338
Burners, 406, 1579
Burning hands syndrome, 1579
Bursae
    around hip joint, 920–921
    iliopsoas, 921
    knee, 1068–1069
    trochanteric, 920–921
Bursitis
    iliopsoas, 980
    olecranon, 728–730, 728f
        complications, 730
        decision-making principles, 728–729
        future considerations, 730
        history, 728, 728f
        imaging, 728, 729f
        physical examination, 728
        postoperative care, 730
        results, 730
        treatment, 729, 729b, 729f
    pediatrics, 1692
    trochanteric, 1001–1002, 1002b
Burst fractures, of thoracolumbar spine, 1584,
        1585f

C

C sign, 929–930, 930f
Caffeine, 290
  historical perspectives, 290
  mechanism of action, 290
  side effects, 290
Calcaneoplasty, 1433–1435
  complications, 1435
  decision-making principles, 1433
  history, 1433
  imaging, 1433
  physical examination, 1433
  postoperative management, 1434
  results, 1434
Calcaneum fracture, 1456–1457
  arthroscopically assisted treatment, 1431b
Calcified cartilage zone, 11
Calcium, 279
Calluses, 254
Cam impingement, 927–928, 957, 958f
Cancellous bone, 12f, 13
Cannulas, in arthroscopy, 108
Capacity, to exercise, 71–73, 71f
Capitate carpal injuries, 843–845, 844b, 844f
Capitate fracture, 809
Capsule
  innervation, 914–916
    accessory obturator nerve, 916
    femoral nerve, 916
    inferior gluteal nerve, 916
    obturator nerve, 916
    quadratus femoris, nerve to, 916
    sciatic nerve, 916
    superior gluteal nerve, 916
  joint
    capsular ligaments, 914
    safe zone, 916, 916f
    zona orbicularis in, 914
  structure, 427–431
    anatomy, 427–428
    anterior, 428–429, 429f–430f
    instability, 426f, 428
    multidirectional, 430, 430f
    posterior, 429, 430b, 430f
  vascularization, 916, 917f
Capsuloligamentous restraints, 680–681, 682f
Capsulorrhaphy arthropathy, 593, 593f
Carbohydrates, 277–278, 278t
Carbuncles, 246, 247f
Cardiac arrest, 153
Cardiorespiratory response, to exercise, 72, 72f, 72t
Cardiovascular system
  abnormalities, in intellectually disabled
      athletes, 322–323
  elite athlete
    electrocardiogram and electrophysiologic
        adaptations, 161, 161f
    rigorous athletic training and, 160–161
    screening, 162–166, 163b
    structural adaptations, 160–161
  preoperative care, 326–327
    athletic heart syndrome, 326
    hypertrophic cardiomyopathy, 326–327
    preparticipation physical evaluation, 145–147,
        145b–146b
Carpal tunnel release, 903b, 903f
Carpals
  fractures, 807–809
    capitate, 809
    hamate, 809
    imaging, 807–809
    scaphoid, 807–808, 807f–808f
    trapezium, 808–809, 809f
  injuries, 835–856
    anatomy, 835
    biomechanics, 835

Carpals (Continued)
    capitate, 843–845, 844b, 844f
    future considerations, 854–855
    hamate, 840–843, 840f–843f, 843b
    instability, 848–851, 848f–850f, 850b
    Kienböck disease, 846–847
    ligament, anatomy and mechanics, 848–851,
        848f–850f, 850b
    lunate, 845–847, 846f, 847b
    lunotriquetral injuries, 848
    perilunate instability, 851–854, 851f–855f,
        853b
    pisiform, 847–848, 847f, 848b
    scaphoid, 835–836, 837b, 837f
    scapholunate injuries, 848
    trapezium, 838–840, 838f–840f, 840b
    trapezoid, 845, 845b
    triquetrum, 836–838, 838b, 838f
  instability, 821–824, 821t, 822f–823f
Cartiform, 1183–1184
Cartilage
  articular, 9–12, 913–914
    cell-matrix interactions, 11
    clinical relevance and further developments
        in, 12
    defect
      depth, 12
      size, 12
    extracellular matrix, 11
    repair, 11–12
    structure and composition, 10–11, 10f
    zones of, 10–11, 10f
  knee, 1116–1118, 1118f–1119f
  repair, 42–45, 59–60
  restoration
    indications, 1163
    platelet-rich plasma, 55
Cartilage Autograft Implantation System (CAIS),
    44
Cartilage Regeneration System (CaReS), 43
CartiONE, 1182
Cartistem, 1181–1182
Cartiva, 44
Catecholamine polymorphic ventricular
    tachycardia (CPVT), 172–173, 173f
Causalgia, 902
Cavus foot, 1728
Celiac disease, 194–195
Cell-matrix interactions, 11
Cellulitis, 203–204, 203f, 247–248, 248f
Central compartment
  femoroacetabular impingement, 967
  hip arthroscopy, 952–954, 952f–953f
Cerebellum, 1528–1529
Cerebral edema, high-altitude, 242–243
Cerebral palsy, 320–321
  adaptive equipment, 321
  exercise, 320–321, 320b
  medical considerations, 321
    epilepsy/seizures, 321
    medications, 321
    musculoskeletal injuries, 321
    spasticity, 321
Cerebrum, 1528–1529
Cervical disc herniation, 405–406
Cervical motion segment, 1593
Cervical spine, 1533
  congenital anomalies of, 1762–1763
  degenerative, 1593–1604
    axial neck pain, 1593–1594
    cervical spondylosis, 1594–1596,
        1594f–1596f
    ossified posterior longitudinal ligament,
        1597, 1597f
    rheumatoid cervical spondylitis, 1596–1597,
        1596f

Cervical spine (Continued)
    uncovertebral joints, 1594
  injuries, 1578–1581
    decision-making principles, 1579–1580
    diagnosis, 1579–1580
    history, 1578
    imaging, 1578–1579
    on-field emergencies, 152–153
    on-field evaluation, 1578
    physical examination, 1578
    return to play, 1580–1581, 1580f–1581f
    sprain, 1579
    strain, 1579
    treatment, 1579–1580
  unstable fractures and dislocations
    decision-making principles, 1542
  unstable fractures and dislocations of,
      1541–1543
    complications, 1543
    future considerations, 1543
    history, 1541
    imaging, 1541–1542, 1542f
    physical examination, 1541
    postoperative management, 1543
    results, 1543
    treatment options, 1542–1543, 1542b
Cervical spondylosis, 405
Cervical stenosis, 405
Cervical strain, 405
Chance fractures, 1584, 1586f, 1753–1755
Channelopathies, 172–173
Cheilectomy, 1524, 1524f
Cheiralgia paresthetica, 902
Chilblains (perniosis), 257, 258f
Children. See Pediatrics
Chondral injuries, 942, 943f, 967
Chondrocytes, 11
Chondrofix, 1183
Chondrolysis, 593–594
ChondroMimetic, 43
Chronic anterior cruciate ligamentous
    insufficiency, 1284, 1284f
Chronic pain, in stiff shoulder, 580, 580b
Chronic peroneal tendon dislocation, 1474f,
    1475b
Chronic proximal hamstring tendinopathy, 1041
Chronic rotator cuff disease, 548
Chronic traumatic encephalopathy (CTE), 1747
Circulation, bone, 13
Class II degenerative injuries, 832
Class I traumatic injuries, 829–832, 829f–831f
Clavicle
  anatomy, 1637, 1638f
  fractures, 139, 139f
  medial, excision, 675
  midshaft fractures, 1637–1640, 1639f–1640f
  physeal fractures, 1637–1644
    lateral, 1640–1642, 1641f–1642f
    medial, 1642–1644, 1642f–1644f
Clinical Decision Rules for Cervical Spine
    Imaging, 1559f
Clinical diagnosis, 344, 345f. See also Physical
    examination
Closed boutonnière (central slip rupture),
    875–877, 875f–877f
Closed kinetic chain, 1195–1196, 1196f
Coaches, disagreements with, 157
Cocaine, 292
Coils, in magnetic resonance imaging, 99–100,
    100f
Cold injury, 240–242
  frostbite, 241–242
  hypothermia, 240–241
Cold water immersion, 358
Collagen meniscus implant (CMI), 41–42
Collagenomas, 255, 255f

Collapsed athlete, 151–152, 151t
Collateral ligament
    assessment, posterior cruciate ligament injuries, 1213–1214
    injury, 700–702
        imaging, 700–702, 701f
        lateral, 702, 703f
        ulnar, 701–702, 701f–702f
    knee, 1069–1071
    multiligament knee injuries, 1267
Collegiate athletics, ethical/legal issues with, 155
Colonic ischemia, 194
Combined impingement, 927–928
Common warts, 251–252, 252f
Commotio cordis, 173
Compact bone, 12–13, 12f
Compartment testing, 1397–1398, 1397t
Competition, diabetic athlete, 223
Complex lacerations, 262–263, 264f
Complex regional pain syndrome, 1316
Compression, 624
    intermittent, 362, 362f
    radial sensory nerve, 756, 756f
Compression fractures, of thoracolumbar spine, 1583–1584, 1584f
Compression neuropathies, elbow, 691–694
    median nerve, 693–694
    radial nerve, 692–693
    ulnar nerve, 691–692, 691f–692f
Computed tomographic angiography (CTA), 1353, 1353f
Computed tomography (CT), 85–88
    advantages, 87, 87f–88f
    ankle, 1380
    arthrography, 87, 87f
    disadvantages, 87–88, 88f
    elbow, 697–698
    femoroacetabular impingement, 964, 965f
    foot, 1380
    glenohumeral joint, 411, 411f
    hip, 938–939
    knee, 1105f
    medial clavicle physeal fractures, 1643, 1643f
    patellar instability, 1298, 1299f
    popliteal artery entrapment syndrome, 1353, 1353f
    positron emission tomography, 90, 93f
    scapulothoracic disorders, 614
    single photon emission, 88, 89f
    spine, 1546, 1546f
    technical considerations, 85–87, 86f–87f
Concomitant injury, 1249
Concomitant intra-articular pathology, revision anterior cruciate ligament injuries and, 1203
Concussion, 1530–1531, 1562–1569
    background, 1562–1564
    basketball, 116
    clinical presentation, 1563–1564
    definition, 1562–1563
    epidemiology, 1563
    in female athlete, 303–304, 304t
    imaging, 1566
    interventions, 1567–1568
    lacrosse, 122
    management, 1566–1567
    pathophysiology, 1563
    physical examination, 1564–1566
        baseline (preseason) assessment, 1564–1565
        comprehensive assessment, 1566
        sideline assessment, 1565–1566
    retiring athlete, 1567
    return-to-play, 1567, 1567t

Concussion (Continued)
    in skeletally immature athletes, 1741–1747
        biomechanics, 1741, 1742f
        complications, 1746–1747, 1747t
        decision-making principles, 1745
        epidemiology, 1741–1743
        future considerations, 1747
        history, 1743, 1743t
        imaging, 1744–1745, 1745b
        pathophysiology, 1741, 1742f
        physical examination, 1743–1744
        return to play, 1746, 1746t
        treatment options, 1745–1746
    soccer, 125–126
    volleyball, 128
Conditioning, in female athlete, 294–296, 296t
Confidentiality, 155
Congenital disease, in elite athlete, 166–169
Contact sports, athletes in, 453
Continuous catheter techniques, 334
Contra coup contusion, 1112
Contractions, of skeletal muscle
    physiology, 62–64, 64f
    types, 65
Contrast agents, 99, 99f
Contrast tissue, 95, 95f–96f, 96t
Contusions, 1043–1052
    groin, 1047, 1047f
    iliac crest, 1043–1044, 1044f
        complications, 1044
        history, 1043
        imaging, 1043, 1044f
        physical examination, 1043
        results, 1044
        return to play, 1044
        treatment options, 1043, 1043b
    quadriceps, 1044–1047, 1044t
        complications, 1047
        decision-making principles, 1046
        future considerations, 1047
        history, 1044–1045
        imaging, 1045, 1045f
        physical examination, 1045
        results, 1046
        return to play, 1046
        treatment options, 1045–1046, 1046b
    thoracolumbar spine, 1585–1588
Conventional radiography, 74–78
    advantages, 77
    arthrography, 76–77, 76f–77f
    disadvantages, 77–78, 78f
    fluoroscopy, 75–76, 75f–76f
    technical considerations, 74–75, 75f
Coordinate systems, 16
Coordination training, 381
Coracoclavicular reconstruction, anatomic, 659b–663b, 659f–663f
Core muscle injury, 1007–1017
Core strength, 69
Corneal abrasion, 269
Corns, 254
Coronary artery disease (CAD), 169
Coronoid process, 683, 683f
Cortical bone, 12–13, 12f
Corticosteroids
    exercise-induced bronchoconstriction, 177
    knee arthritis, 1280
    platelet-rich plasma vs., 53
Costoclavicular maneuver, 636–638, 637f
Countercoup injury, 1538, 1539f
Coup injury, 1538, 1539f
Coxa saltans, 925, 996–1001, 1692–1693
    external, 999–1001
    internal, 996–997

CPVT. See Catecholamine polymorphic ventricular tachycardia
Cranial meninges, 1528
Cranial nerve (CN), 1529
Cranium, 1528, 1529f
Creatine, 288–289
    adverse effects, 289
    historical perspectives, 288
    physiology, 288–289
Crepitus, 581, 609, 611b, 611f, 611t, 614–615, 616f–617f
Criteria for Spinal Motion Restriction (SMR), 1557f
Critical limb ischemia (CLI), 1351
Cross-table lateral view, 935, 936f
Cruciate ligaments
    anterior, 1069, 1070f
    in joint biomechanics, 1077–1079
    knee, 1069
    posterior, 1069, 1070f
    reconstruction, for multiligament knee injuries, 1267
Cryotherapy, for pain, 358–359
Cryptosporidiosis, 211–212
CT. See Computed tomography
CTA. See Computed tomographic angiography
Cubital tunnel syndrome, 691–692, 691f–692f, 747–752, 748f
    complications, 752
    decision-making principles, 749
    history, 749
    physical examination, 749
    postoperative management, 752
    results, 752
    return-to-play guidelines, 752
    treatment, 749–751
        anterior intramuscular transposition, 750, 751f
        anterior subcutaneous transposition, 750, 750f
        anterior submuscular transposition, 750–751, 751f
        medial epicondylectomy, 751
        in situ decompression, 749–750, 750f
        technique, 751–752
Curettage, 1487–1488
Cutaneous infections, 246–253
    bacterial infections, 246–249
    fungal infections, 249–250
    mycobacterial infections, 252
    parasitic infections, 252–253
    viral infections, 250–252
Cutaneous larva migrans, 253, 253f
Cytokine, in meniscal injuries, 1149

D
Dashboard injury, posterior cruciate ligament injuries and, 1211
Débridement
    Achilles tendon rupture, 1480b–1481b, 1480f
    anterior arthroscopic, 1425b
    arthroscopic subtalar, 1429b–1430b, 1429f–1430f
    lateral epicondylitis, 716b, 717f
    osteochondral lesions, 1487–1488
    osteochondritis dissecans, 714b–715b, 714f
    posterior tibial tendon injury, 1467b–1468b, 1467f
    revision rotator cuff repair, 569
    SLAP tear, 524
Decision-making principles
    acromioclavicular joint, 653–655, 653t
    adductor strains, 1051

Decision-making principles (Continued)
AIN syndrome, 746
ankle, 1370–1379
anterior cruciate ligament injuries, 1188–1190
age, 1188–1189
associated injuries, 1189
gender, 1189
operative vs. nonoperative treatment, 1188
partial tear, 1189
revision, 1189–1190
anterior shoulder instability, 450–454
age, 452
associated injuries, 453–454
contact sports, 453
first-time vs. recurrent instability, 452–453
in-season management, 453
synthesis, 454, 454t
articular cartilage lesions, 1163–1164
age, 1164
cartilage restoration, 1163
contraindications, 1163
defect chronicity, 1164
osteochondritis dissecans lesions, 1164
treatment algorithm, 1164
athletic pubalgia, 1011
atlantoaxial instability, 1758, 1759f
atraumatic hip microinstability, 977–978
axillary nerve palsy, 630
borderline dysplasia, 977
calcaneoplasty, 1433
cervical spine
dislocations, 1542
injuries, 1579–1580
unstable fractures and dislocations, 1542
cubital tunnel syndrome, 749
distal biceps tendinitis, 725–726
distal biceps tendon rupture, 735
distal triceps tendon rupture, 738, 738b
elbow, 687–696
history, 687–689, 688f
motion, loss, 774–776, 775f
pathologies, 687
physical examination, 689–691
throwing injuries, 760–761
entrapment neuropathies, 743
exertional compartment syndromes, 1396–
1397, 1396t–1397t
extensor mechanism injuries, 1327
external coxa saltans, 999, 1000b
flexor hallucis longus injuries, 1470
foot, 1370–1379
glenohumeral arthritis, 603–604, 604b,
604f–605f
gluteus medius and minimus tears, 990, 991b
Haglund resection, 1433
hallux rigidus, 1523–1524
hamstring injuries, 1037
hand, 793–805
head injuries, 1540
hip, 925–934
arthritis, 1057
dysplasia, 975–978, 975f–976f
interdigital neuralgia, 1418
internal coxa saltans, 997, 997b
ischiofemoral impingement, 1004, 1005b, 1005f
knee, 1089–1103, 1101f–1102f
arthritis, 1283–1284
arthroscopic synovectomy, 1128–1130,
1128f–1129f
lateral and posterolateral corner injuries,
1253
motion, loss of, 1337–1338, 1337t, 1338f
lateral epicondylitis, 722
lateral plantar nerve entrapment, 1411
leg, 1370–1379
pain, 1396–1397, 1396t–1397t

Decision-making principles (Continued)
long thoracic nerve palsy, 627
medial collateral ligament and posterior medial
corner injuries, 1234–1235
medial epicondylitis, 722
medial plantar nerve entrapment, 1413
meniscal injuries, 1142–1147
metatarsalgia, 1520
Morton neuroma, 1418
multidirectional instability, 479–480
multiligament knee injuries, 1266–1267
olecranon bursitis, 728–729
olecranon osteochondrosis, 1674
osteochondral lesions, 1486, 1486f–1487f
osteochondritis dissecans, 1669, 1669t
patellar instability, 1299–1301
pediatrics
anterior cruciate ligament (ACL) injuries,
1698
concussion, 1745
discoid meniscus, 1706
distal radial physeal stress reaction, 1684
finger fractures, 1678
jammed finger, 1682
lateral epicondylitis, 1675
Little League elbow, 1667
medial collateral ligament injury, 1672
medial epicondyle avulsion fractures, 1671
medial epicondylitis, 1675
meniscal injuries, 1703
osteochondritis dissecans, 1669, 1669t,
1714–1715
Panner disease, 1669, 1669t
patellar instability, 1709
physeal fractures, 1719–1720
posterior elbow pathologic conditions, 1674
scaphoid fracture, 1685
PIN syndrome, 755
piriformis syndrome, 1003, 1003b
plantar fasciitis, 1510
posterior heel pain, 1505–1506
posterior medial corner injuries, 1234–1235,
1235f
posterior shoulder instability, 468
posterolateral corner injuries, 1253
posteromedial impingement, 1674
pronator syndrome, 745
quadriceps contusion, 1046
quadriceps strains, 1049
radial tunnel syndrome, 752–755
revision anterior cruciate ligament injuries,
1202–1204
revision rotator cuff repair, 568–569, 569t,
570f
revision shoulder instability, 493–494
rotator cuff and impingement lesions, 547–548
acute rotator cuff trauma, 548
chronic rotator cuff disease, 548
subacromial impingement and biceps
tenosynovitis, 548
scapulothoracic disorders, 614–615
crepitus, 614–615
injection, 615, 615f
pain, 614–615
pathologies, 615
treatment, 615
sesamoid dysfunction, 1517
soft tissue conditions, ankle arthroscopy, 1424
spinal accessory nerve palsy, 629
sternoclavicular joint, 668, 673f
stiff shoulder, 585
subscapularis injury, 559–560
subtalar arthroscopy, 1429
superficial peroneal nerve entrapment, 1414
superior labrum anterior to posterior (SLAP)
tears, 505–506, 506f

Decision-making principles (Continued)
suprascapular nerve palsy, 624
tarsal tunnel syndrome, 1408
thoracic outlet syndrome, 639–640
thoracolumbar spine injuries, 1583–1591
triceps tendinitis, 725–726
trochanteric bursitis, 1002, 1002b
turf toe, 1515–1516
wrist, 793–805
Decompression
endoscopic, for posterior hip pain, 1027–1030,
1028t–1029t, 1029f–1030f
in situ, 749–750, 750f
spinoglenoid notch, 625
suprascapular notch, 625
Deep bursae, 920
Deep gluteal syndrome, 1020–1024
anatomy, 1020–1021, 1021f
etiology, 1021–1024, 1021f–1023f
operative treatment, 1027–1030
physical examination, 1024–1026,
1024f–1026f
preoperative and postoperative rehabilitation,
1027–1030, 1027f–1028f
Deep peroneal nerve entrapment, 1415–1416,
1415f
history, 1415
imaging, 1416
physical examination, 1415–1416
postoperative management, 1416
results, 1416
treatment options, 1416, 1416b
Deep venous thrombosis (DVT), 180–188
clinical manifestations, 182–184
diagnosis, 182–184
imaging, 182–184, 185f–186f
laboratory findings, 182–184
normal physiology, 180, 181f
return to play, 185–186
risk factors, preoperative, 180–181
sports issues in, 185–186
thromboembolic prophylaxis, 182, 183t–185t
travel and, 185–186
treatment, 184–185, 187t
Deep zone, of articular cartilage, 11
Degenerative arthritis, in female athlete, 303
Degenerative cervical spine, 1593–1604
axial neck pain, 1593–1594
cervical spondylosis, 1594–1596, 1594f–1596f
imaging, 1550–1551
ossified posterior longitudinal ligament, 1597,
1597f
rheumatoid cervical spondylitis, 1596–1597,
1596f
uncovertebral joints, 1594
Degenerative joint disease, of hip, 926, 927f
Degenerative thoracolumbar spine, 1597–1604
discogenic low back pain, 1598–1599
low back pain, 1598
lumbar disc herniation, 1599–1601, 1601f
lumbar spinal stenosis, 1602–1603, 1602f
lumbar spine, 1598–1604
radiculopathy, 1599–1601, 1600f
spondylolisthesis, 1603–1604, 1603f–1604f
synovial facet cysts, 1601–1602
thoracic spine, 1597–1598
Degrees of freedom, 16–17, 18f
Dehydroepiandrosterone (DHEA), 287
Delayed gadolinium, for magnetic resonance
imaging, 101
Delayed-onset muscle soreness, 68
Deltoid ligament injury. See Medial ankle sprains
DeNovo Natural Tissue, 1182
Dental injuries, 269–270. See also Teeth
basketball, 116
fractured teeth, 270

Dental injuries (Continued)
 handball, 122
 periodontal/displacement injuries (loose teeth),
  270
 primary vs. permanent teeth, 269, 270f
Dephasing, in magnetic resonance imaging, 95
De Quervain tenosynovitis, 859–860, 859f
 postoperative management and return to
  sports, 860
 treatment options, 859, 859b, 860f
Dermatology, 149
 amputee athletes and, 316–317
Dermatophytoses, 249–250, 250f
Dermatoses, 246–259
 cutaneous infections, 246–253
  bacterial infections, 246–249
  fungal infections, 249–250
  mycobacterial infections, 252
  parasitic infections, 252–253
  viral infections, 250–252
 environmental dermatoses, 256–257
  aquatic dermatoses, 256
  irritant contact dermatitis, 256–257
  photodermatoses, 256
  thermal damage, 257, 257f
 mechanical dermatoses, 253–256
  abrasions/lacerations, 253–254
  acne mechanica, 254–255, 255f
  athlete's nodules (collagenomas), 255, 255f
  calluses and corns, 254
  friction blisters, 254
  hemorrhage, 254, 254f–255f
  hidradenitis suppurativa, 255–256, 256f
  striae, 254, 255f
 urticaria, anaphylaxis, and immunologic
  disorders, 257–258
Dexmedetomidine, perioperative pharmacology,
  338–339
dGEMRIC MRI, 101
DHEA. See Dehydroepiandrosterone
Diabetes
 athlete with, 218–226
  definition, 218
  diagnosis, 218–219
   morning after, 219
  epidemiology, 218
  exercise, physiologic changes of, 221–223,
   221f, 222t
  management, 223–225, 223f
  treatment, 219–221
   amylin analog therapy, 221
   incretin, 221
   insulin, 220, 221t
   insulin analogs, 220
   medical nutrition therapy, 219–220
   oral hypoglycemic agents, 220
 gestational, 218
 overt, 218
 prediabetes, 218
 type 1, 218, 221, 221f
  management, 224–225
 type 2, 218
  management, 225
Diabetes mellitus, 218, 327
 pathophysiologic responses to exercise,
  222–223
Diagnosis, 344, 345f
Diagnostic arthroscopy, 110, 1123–1125,
  1125f
 lateral and posterolateral corner injuries of
  knee, 1254, 1254f
 meniscal insufficiency, 1157
 proximal biceps tendon pathology, 531–532
Dial test, 932, 1213, 1250, 1250f

Diarrhea, 192–194, 212
Dietary Supplement Health and Education Act in
  1994, 1611
Diffusion weighted imaging, 100, 100f
Digits, 801. See also Fingers
 distal interphalangeal joint, 801–802, 803f
 flexor pulley injury, 804
 fractures and dislocations, 883–897
  ligamentous injuries and dislocations,
   883–892
  osseous and soft tissue injuries of thumb,
   892–896
 metacarpophalangeal joint, 803–804
 proximal interphalangeal joint, 802–803, 804f
 ulnar collateral ligament, 804, 804f
DIP joint. See Distal interphalangeal (DIP) joint
Disagreements, with coaches, 157
Disc degeneration, 1543
Disc herniation
 cervical, 405–406, 1595
 lumbar, 1599–1601, 1601f
 thoracolumbar spine, 1588, 1588f
Discogenic pain
 cervical spondylosis, 1594–1595
 low back, 1598–1599
Discoid meniscus, 1140–1142, 1141f–1142f,
  1705–1708
 classification, 1705–1706, 1706f
 complications, 1707
 decision-making principles, 1706
 future considerations, 1707–1708
 history, 1706
 imaging, 1706
 physical examination, 1706
 postoperative management, 1707
 results, 1707
 treatment options, 1706–1707
Dislocation
 arthropathy, 593
 cervical spine, 1541–1543
  complications, 1543
  decision-making principles, 1542
  future considerations, 1543
  history, 1541
  imaging, 1541–1542, 1542f
  physical examination, 1541
  postoperative management, 1543
  results, 1543
  treatment options, 1542–1543, 1542b
 chronic peroneal tendon, 1474f, 1475b
 distal interphalangeal joint, 888–890
 elbow, 699
 hip, 942, 944f–945f, 1690–1691, 1691f
 knee, 154, 1345–1349, 1346f
  anterior, 1345
  clinical presentation, 1346–1347, 1346t,
   1347f
  complications, 1349
  imaging, 1348
  physical examination and testing of,
   1347–1348, 1347f
  popliteal artery repair, 1349b
  posterior, 1345–1346
  postoperative management, 1349
  treatment options, 1348–1349
  vascular injury, 1346
 metacarpophalangeal, 892–894
 patellar, 1293
 perilunate, 809–810, 810f
 proximal interphalangeal joint, 885–888,
  885f–890f
 sternoclavicular joint, 673, 674f–676f
 transscaphoid perilunate fracture, 825–826,
  826f

Displacement injuries (loose teeth), 270
Distal anterolateral accessory portal (DALA), in
  hip arthroscopy, 951, 951f
Distal biceps tendon
 rupture, 695, 703–704, 704f, 731–741
  anatomy, 731, 732f–733f
  biomechanics, 731–732
  classification, 732, 732b
  complications, 736–737
  decision-making principles, 735
  epidemiology, 731
  history, 732–733
  imaging, 733–734, 734f
  physical examination, 733, 733f
  postoperative management, 735
  results, 735–736
  treatment, 734–735, 735t, 736b, 736f
 tendinitis, 725–728
  complications, 727
  conservative, 726
  decision-making principles, 725–726
  future considerations, 727–728
  history, 725
  imaging, 725, 726f
  operative, 726, 727f
  physical examination, 725, 725f
  postoperative management, 727
  results, 726
  return-to-play guidelines, 727
  treatment, 726, 726b
Distal femoral osteotomy, 1282
Distal humerus, anatomy, 683
Distal interphalangeal (DIP) joint, 789, 801–802,
  803f
 dislocations, 888–890
Distal radial physeal stress reaction, pediatrics,
  1683–1684
 complications in, 1684
 decision-making principles, 1684
 future consideration in, 1684
 history, 1683
 imaging, 1683–1684, 1683f
 physical examination, 1683
 postoperative management, 1684
 results, 1684
 treatment options, 1684, 1684b
Distal radioulnar joint, disorders of, 865–872
 anatomy, 865–866, 866f–867f
  blood supply, 866
 complications, 870–871
 history, 867, 867t
 imaging, 868–870
  computed tomography, 868
  magnetic resonance imaging, 868, 869f
  radiographs, 868, 868f
  treatment, 868–870, 870f
 physical examination, 867–868
 postoperative management, 870, 871f
 triangular fibrocartilage complex tears,
  866–867
  class 1 tears (traumatic), 866
  class 2 tears (degenerative), 866–867
  Palmer Classification, 867t
Distal radius fractures, 806–807, 826–827
Distal tibial plafond, osteochondral lesions of,
  1500–1501, 1500f–1501f
Distal triceps tendon rupture, 737–740
 anatomy, 737, 737f
 biomechanics, 737
 classification, 737
 complications, 740
 decision-making principles, 738, 738b
 epidemiology, 737, 737b
 future considerations, 740

Distal triceps tendon rupture *(Continued)*
history, 738
imaging, 738
physical examination, 738
postoperative management, 740
results, 740
treatment, 738–739
nonoperative, 738
operative, 739, 739*f*
technique, 740*b*, 740*f*
Dominant deep bursa, 920
DOMS. *See* Delayed-onset muscle soreness
Doping, 283–293
erythropoietin, 287–288
historical perspectives, 287
mechanism of action, 288
side effects, 288
testing, 288
Dorsal quadrant, 794*t*, 796–798, 797*f*–798*f*
Dorsiflexion range of motion, 381
Double-bundle reconstruction
posterior cruciate ligament injuries, 1218–1219,
1218*f*, 1225–1229
in revision setting, 1206–1207
Down syndrome, atlantoaxial instability in,
1758–1759
decision-making principles, 1758, 1759*f*
history, 1758
imaging, 1758
physical examination, 1758
results, 1759
treatment, 1759, 1760*f*
Draping, hip arthroscopy, 949–950, 950*f*
Drilling, 1487–1488
Drugs. *See also* Medications; Medicine
ergogenic, 283–290
anabolic-androgenic steroids, 284–287
caffeine, 290
creatine, 288–289
doping, 287–288
growth hormone, 289–290
steroid supplements, 287
testosterone, historical perspectives, 283–284
recreational, 290–293
alcohol, 290–291
cocaine, 292
inhalants, 293
marijuana, 291–292
tobacco, 292
using, 156
Dunn view, 935, 937*f*
Duplex ultrasonography, of popliteal artery
entrapment syndrome, 1352, 1352*f*
Dura mater, 1528
DVT. *See* Deep venous thrombosis
Dynamic contrast enhancement, in MRI,
101–103
Dynamic imaging, in forces, of hip joint, 923
Dynamics, in biomechanics, 22–23
joint motions in, 22–23, 23*f*
kinematics, 22
kinetics, 23
relative motion, 22
Dynamometer, 386, 386*f*
Dyspepsia, 191–192
Dysphagia, 192
Dysplasia, hip, 971–978
decision-making, 975–978
atraumatic hip microinstability, 977–978
borderline dysplasia, 977
dysplasia, 975–978, 975*f*–976*f*
history, 973
imaging, 974–975, 975*f*
pathologies, 971–973
dysplasia and, 971–973, 972*f*–973*f*
physical examination, 973–974

E

EAMC. *See* Exercise-associated muscle cramps
Ears, preparticipation physical evaluation, 145
Echo
gradient, 96–97, 97*f*
sequence, ultrashort time to, 100–101
spin, 96, 97*f*
time, 95
train, 96
Education, for athletic trainer, 342–343, 343*b*,
343*t*
EHS. *See* Exertional heat stroke
EIB. *See* Exercise-induced bronchoconstriction
Elastin, 3
Elastography, ultrasound, 83–84, 83*f*
Elbow, 680–686, 720–730. *See also* Entrapment
neuropathies
anatomy, 680–681
capsuloligamentous restraints, 680–681, 682*f*
elbow musculature, 681
osseous, 680, 681*f*
anterior
history, 688
palpation, 690
arthroscopy, 707–719
complications, 718
decision-making principles, 707–712
fluid management, 708–709
future considerations, 718
history, 707
imaging, 707
instrumentation, 708–709, 709*f*
physical examination, 707
portal placement, 709–711, 709*t*
postoperative management, 718
return-to-play guidelines, 718
treatment, 707–712, 717*b*
biomechanics, 681–685
compression neuropathies, 691–694
decision-making principles, 687–696
diagnosis, 687–696
distal biceps tendinitis, 725–728
decision-making principles, 725–726
history, 725
imaging, 725, 726*f*
physical examination, 725, 725*f*
postoperative management, 727
results, 726
treatment, 726, 726*b*
history, 687–689, 688*f*
imaging, 697–706, 698*f*
collateral ligament injury, 700–702, 701*f*
computed tomography, 697–698
conventional radiographs, 697
lateral epicondylitis, 702–704, 703*f*
loose bodies, 700
magnetic resonance arthrography, 699
magnetic resonance imaging, 698–699
medial epicondylitis, 702–704
tendon ruptures, 703–704, 704*f*
trauma, 699–700
ulnar neuropathy, 704, 705*f*
ultrasound, 699
injuries
baseball, 115
golf, 119–120
throwing, 757–771
inspection, 689
joints, stability, 694–695
lateral
history, 687–688
palpation, 689
lateral epicondylitis, 720–725
decision-making principles, 722
history, 720, 721*t*
imaging, 721, 721*f*–722*f*

Elbow *(Continued)*
physical examination, 720, 721*f*
postoperative management, 724
treatment, 721*f*, 722–724
Little League, 1612, 1612*f*
medial
history, 688
palpation, 689–690
medial epicondylitis, 720–725
decision-making principles, 722
history, 720, 721*t*
imaging, 721, 721*f*–722*f*
physical examination, 720, 721*f*
postoperative management, 724
treatment, 721*f*, 722–724
motion, 681–683, 772–784
complications, 782–783
decision-making principles, 774–776, 775*f*
follow-up, 782
history, 772–773
imaging, 774, 774*f*
physical examination, 773–774
postoperative management, 782
rehabilitation, 782
results, 782–783, 783*t*
return-to-play guidelines, 782
surgery, 776–782, 777*f*
treatment, 774–776, 775*f*
musculature, 681
olecranon bursitis, 728–730, 728*f*
complications, 730
decision-making principles, 728–729
future considerations, 730
history, 728, 728*f*
imaging, 728, 729*f*
physical examination, 728
postoperative care, 730
results, 730
treatment, 729, 729*b*, 729*f*
palpation, 689–690
pathologies, 687
pediatrics, 1619–1623
acute injuries, 1619, 1621*f*
development, 1619
injuries, 1661–1676
Little League, 1621–1623, 1622*f*–1623*f*,
1665–1668
overuse injuries, 1619–1623
physical examination, 689–691
posterior
history, 688–689
palpation, 690
pediatrics, 1673–1674, 1673*f*
regional anesthesia, 330–332
stability, 683–685
trauma, 699–700
fracture, 699
occult, 699, 700*f*
stress, 700
triceps tendinitis, 725–728
decision-making principles, 725–726
history, 725
imaging, 725, 726*f*
physical examination, 725, 725*f*
postoperative management, 727
results, 726
treatment, 726, 726*b*
Electrical stimulation, 359, 1196
Electrocardiogram, 161, 161*f*, 163–164, 164*f*
Electrocautery, 108–109
Electromyography, 614
Electrophysiology, 161, 161*f*, 742–743
Elite athlete, 158–174
acquired cardiovascular conditions, 169–173
arrhythmias, 172–173
atrial fibrillation, 172

Elite athlete (Continued)
  catecholamine polymorphic ventricular
    tachycardia (CPVT), 172–173, 173f
  channelopathies, 172–173
  commotio cordis, 173
  coronary artery disease (CAD), 169
  hyperlipidemia, 172
  hypertension, 169–172
  myocarditis, 169, 171f
  postural orthostatic tachycardia syndrome
    (POTS), 173
  syncope, 173
  Wolff-Parkinson-White syndrome, 172
  cardiovascular care
    electrocardiogram and electrophysiologic
      adaptations, 161, 161f
    rigorous athletic training and, 160–161
    screening, 162–166, 163b
    structural adaptations, 160–161
  future, 173–174
  gender, 161–162, 162f
  genetics, 161–162, 162f
  historical perspective, 158–159
  medical home of, 159–160
  race, 161–162, 162f
  structural/congenital disease, 166–169
    arrhythmogenic right ventricular
      cardiomyopathy, 168
    bicuspid aortic valve, 168–169, 170f–171f
    congenital anomalous coronary artery, 168
    hypertrophic cardiomyopathy, 167
    Marfan syndrome, 169, 171f
Elson test, 875, 876f
Emergencies
  action plan, 150, 151b, 1553
  on-field, 150–155
    anaphylaxis, 153
    cardiac arrest, 153
    cervical spine injury, 152–153
    collapsed athlete, 151–152, 151t
    emergency action plan, 150, 151b
    environmental factors, 154
    head injury, 152
    limb-threatening injuries, 154
    tension pneumothorax, 153
  spine injuries, 1553–1561, 1559f
    common acute, 1559–1560, 1560f
    emergency management, 1553–1561, 1559f
    field-side management, 1553–1561,
      1554f–1558f
Emergency department, 455
Emergency medical services (EMS), 1553
Emergent care, 344–345
Encephalitis, 214–215
Endochondral bone formation, 14
Endocrine system, preparticipation physical
  evaluation, 149
Endoscopic Haglund resection, 1433–1435
  complications, 1435
  decision-making principles, 1433
  history, 1433
  imaging, 1433
  physical examination, 1433
  postoperative management, 1434
  results, 1434
  treatment, 1433b–1434b, 1434f
Endoscopy, for hamstring injuries, 1037–1039,
  1038f
Endotenon, 2, 3f
Endothelial damage, 180
Endurance training, 1607–1608
Energy metabolism, of skeletal muscle, 65–66,
  65f
Enthesis, fibrocartilaginous, 2–3

Entrapment neuropathies, 742–756
  complications, 743
  decision-making principles, 743
  history, 742
  imaging, 742
  median nerve, 743–745, 744f
  physical examination, 742
  postoperative management, 743
  radial nerve, 752, 753f
  testing, 742–743
  treatment, 743
  ulnar nerve, 747, 748f. See also Cubital tunnel
    syndrome
Environmental dermatoses, 256–257
  aquatic dermatoses, 256
    hair discoloration, 256
    swimmer's itch and seabather's eruption,
      256, 257f
  irritant contact dermatitis, 256–257
  photodermatoses, 256
    skin cancer, 256
    sunburn, 256
  thermal damage, 257, 257f
Environmental factors, during on-field
  emergencies, 154
Environmental illness, 235–245
  cold injury, 240–242
    frostbite, 241–242
    hypothermia, 240–241
  exertional heat illness
    definition, 235
    epidemiology, 235
    exercise-associated collapse, 237
    exercise-associated hyponatremia, 239–240
    exercise-associated muscle cramps, 236–237
    exertional heat exhaustion, 235–236
    exertional heat stroke, 236
    exertional rhabdomyolysis, 237–238
    exertional sickling collapse, 238–239
    heat syncope, 237
  high-altitude illness, 242, 244t
    acute mountain sickness, 242–243
    high-altitude cerebral edema, 242–243
    high-altitude headache, 242–243
    high-altitude pulmonary edema, 243–245
EOS 2D/3D x-ray imaging system, of spine,
  1545–1546, 1545f
Epicondylectomy, medial, 751
Epicondylitis
  lateral, 687, 702–704, 703f, 720–725
    complications, 725
    decision-making principles, 722
    future considerations, 725
    history, 720, 721t
    imaging, 721, 721f–722f
    physical examination, 720, 721f
    postoperative management, 724
    results, 724–725
    return-to-play guidelines, 724
    splinting, 722
    treatment, 721f, 722–724
  medial, 688, 702–704, 720–725
    complications, 725
    decision-making principles, 722
    future considerations, 725
    history, 720, 721t
    imaging, 721, 721f–722f
    physical examination, 720, 721f
    postoperative management, 724
    results, 724–725
    return-to-play guidelines, 724
    splinting, 722
    treatment, 721f, 722–724
  surgical management, 724

Epidural hematoma, 1745
Epilepsy, 230–234. See also Seizure
  cerebral palsy, 321
  classification, 230
  diagnosis, 230–231
  evaluation, 230–231
  intellectually disabled athletes, 322
  safety considerations of, 232–234, 233b
  terminology of, 230
  treatment, 231
Epilepsy syndrome, 230
Epimysium, 62, 63f
Epitenon, 2, 3f
EPO. See Erythropoietin
Equipment. See also Instruments
  adaptive sports
    amputee athlete, 317
    cerebral palsy, 321
    intellectually disabled athletes, 323
    visually impaired athletes, 323
    wheelchair athlete, 320
  arthroscopic, 105–109, 106f
    arthroscope, 105–107, 106f
    arthroscopic probe in, 107
    basket forceps in, 107–108, 108f
    cannulas in, 108
    electrocautery in, 108–109
    fluid pump, 107
    grasping forceps in, 108
    instruments and, 107
    knives in, 108
    motorized shavers in, 107–108
    radiofrequency instruments and, 108–109
    scissors in, 108
    switching sticks in, 108
Ergogenic drugs, 283–290
  anabolic-androgenic steroids, 284–287
  caffeine, 290
  creatine, 288–289
  doping, 287–288
  growth hormone, 289–290
  steroid supplements, 287
  testosterone, historical perspectives, 283–284
Erysipelas, 247–248, 248f
Erythrasma, 248–249, 249f
Erythropoietin (EPO), 197, 287–288
Ethical/legal issues, in sports medicine, 155–157
  collegiate athletics, 155
  confidentiality, 155
  disagreements with coaches, 157
  drug use, 156
  high school athletics, 155
  informed consent, 156, 156t
  professional athletics, 155
Eucapnic voluntary hyperventilation (EVH),
  176–177
Exacerbating factors, for stiff shoulder, 580–581
Excision, 1487–1488
Exercise
  amputee athletes and, 316, 316t
  capacity, 71–73, 71f
  cardiorespiratory response to, 72, 72f, 72t
  cerebral palsy, 320–321, 320b
  core strength, 69
  diabetic athlete, physiologic changes of,
    221–223, 221f, 222t
  hormonal adaptation to, 69–71, 69t
    adrenal hormones, 69t, 70
    gonadal hormones, 69t, 70–71
    pancreatic hormones, 69t, 71
    pituitary, 69–70, 69t
  immune system, 201–202, 202f
  intellectually disabled athletes, 322
  low-impact, for knee arthritis, 1279

Exercise (Continued)
  muscle during
    delayed-onset soreness of, 68
    fatigue, 67
  neuromuscular adaptation to, 67–68
  pediatrics, 1607–1609
    endurance training, 1607–1608
    heat-related injuries, 1609
    strength training, 1608–1609
    thermoregulation, 1609
  physiology, 62–73
  respiratory response to, 72–73
  seizure and, 231–232
  visually impaired athletes, 323
  wheelchair athletes, 317–320
Exercise-associated collapse (EAC), 237
Exercise-associated hyponatremia (EAH),
    239–240
Exercise-associated muscle cramps (EAMC),
    236–237
Exercise-induced anaphylaxis, 257–258
"Exercise-induced arterial hypoxemia", 73
Exercise-induced bronchoconstriction (EIB),
    175–179
  athletic populations at risk, 175
  clinical presentation, 175–176, 176b
  complications, 178–179
  definition, 175
  diagnosis, 176–177
    differential, 176, 176b
    history, 176
    objective testing, 176–177
  prevalence of, 175, 176t
  return to play, 179, 179f
  sideline management, 178, 178b, 179f
  treatment options, 177
    nonpharmacologic therapy, 177
    pharmacologic therapy, 177, 177t
    technique, 178b, 178f
Exertional compartment syndromes, 1393–1401,
    1394t
  anatomy, 1393–1394, 1394f, 1394t
  classification, 1394–1395
  compartment testing, 1397–1398, 1397t
  complications, 1400
  decision-making principles, 1396–1397,
    1396t–1397t
  diagnostics/imaging, 1395–1396, 1396f
  epidemiology, 1393
  history, 1395
  pathophysiology, 1394
  physical examination, 1395
  postoperative care, 1398
  results, 1400
  return to play, 1400
  treatment options, 1398
Exertional heat exhaustion (EHE), 235–236
  diagnosis, 235
  prevention, 236
  return to play, 235–236, 236b
  treatment, 235
Exertional heat illness (EHI)
  definition, 235
  epidemiology, 235
  exercise-associated collapse, 237
  exercise-associated hyponatremia, 239–240
  exercise-associated muscle cramps, 236–237
  exertional heat exhaustion, 235–236
  exertional heat stroke, 236
  exertional rhabdomyolysis, 237–238
  exertional sickling collapse, 238–239
  heat syncope, 237
Exertional heat stroke (EHS), 236, 236b
Exertional rhabdomyolysis (ER), 237–238,
    238b
Exertional sickling collapse, 238–239, 238t

Extension/extension-distraction injuries, of
    thoracolumbar spine, 1584–1585
Extensor carpi ulnaris tendinopathy,
    861–862
Extensor mechanism, 1113–1116, 1115f–1117f
  injuries, 1318–1334, 1330b
    anatomy, 1318–1319, 1319f
    biomechanics, 1319, 1320f
    clinical outcomes, 1331–1333
    complications, 1333
    decision-making principles, 1327
    future considerations, 1333
    history, 1322–1323
    imaging, 1324–1326
    patella, 1318–1319
    patellar and quadriceps tendon structure in,
      1320, 1320f–1321f
    patient evaluation, 1322–1326
    physical examination, 1323–1324
    postoperative management, 1330–1331
    quadriceps tendon, 1318
    treatment options, 1327–1330
Extensor tendons, 790–791, 790f–791f
Extensors, of hip, 919–920
External coxa saltans, 999–1001
  complications, 1000
  decision-making principles, 999, 1000b
  future considerations, 1000–1001
  history, 999
  imaging, 999
  physical examination, 999, 999f
  postoperative management, 1000
  results, 1000, 1001t
  techniques, 1000b, 1000f–1001f
  treatment options, 999–1000
External rotation, 1247
  recurvatum test, 1250, 1250f
External rotators, of hip, 920
Extra-articular augmentation, 1192
Extracellular matrix
  articular cartilage, 11
  bone, 13
  cell-matrix interactions, 11
  ligaments, 3
  meniscus, 8
  tendons, 3
Eyes
  injuries, 269
    corneal abrasion, 269
    hyphema, 269
    iridodialysis, 269
    retinal detachment, 269
    ruptured globe, 269
  preparticipation physical evaluation, 145

F
Fabellofibular ligament, 1246
Face
  fractures, 264–268
    evaluation, 264–266, 266b
    frontal sinus fractures, 268
    mandible fractures, 267, 267f
    midface fractures, 267–268
    nasal fractures, 266–267, 266f–267f
    orbital fractures, 268, 268f
  injuries
    basketball, 116
    boxing, 116–117
    handball, 122
  soft tissue injuries to, 260–263, 262f
    general considerations, 260–262
      anesthesia, 260
      antibiotics, 261
      choice of closure, 261
      cleaning, 260–261

Face (Continued)
      postclosure wound care, 261–262
      timing of repair, 260
    management, 262–263
      complex lacerations, 262–263, 264f
      intraoral/tongue lacerations, 263
      lateral face lacerations, 263, 265f
      lip lacerations, 263, 264f
      periorbital lacerations, 263
      simple lacerations, 262, 262f–263f
      soft tissue ear injuries, 263
Facemask removal, in athlete, 1555, 1556f
Facets, 1593–1594
False-profile view, 936, 937f
Fasciotomy, 1398
Fast spin-echo, 96, 97f
Fat, 277–278, 278t
  suppression, 98, 99f
Fatigue, muscle, 67
Fatty infiltration, 422, 423f
Fecally derived recreational water-related illness,
    211
  non-, 213–214
    acute otitis externa, 213–214
    hot tub folliculitis, 213
    Pseudomonas infections, 213
  other, 212–213
Female athlete, 294–314
  anterior cruciate ligament tears, 377–380,
    378f–379f
  general considerations, 294–304
    birth control, 301, 301t
    concussion, 303–304, 304t
    conditioning, 294–296, 296t
    degenerative arthritis, 303
    female athlete triad, 298–299, 298f, 299t
    hydration, 296–298
    nutrition, 296–298, 297t–298t
    osteopenia, 299–301, 300f, 300t
    osteoporosis, 299–301, 300f, 300t
    pregnancy, 301–302, 302t
    psychological issues, 302–303
  importance and recognition of, 294, 295t
  orthopaedic injuries, 304–314
    acetabular labral injuries, 313
    ankle, 305–306
    anterior cruciate ligament injuries, 307,
      308t–309t, 309f
    anterior cruciate ligament reconstruction,
      310
    epidemiology, 304–305
    femoroacetabular impingement, 313
    foot, 305–306, 305t, 306f
    frozen shoulder/adhesive capsulitis, 310–312,
      311t
    idiopathic scoliosis, 313–314
    noncontact anterior cruciate ligament injury,
      307–309, 308f, 310f
    patellofemoral pain syndrome, 306–307,
      306t
    shoulder instability, 312–313, 312f
    stress fractures, 314
  triad, 298–299, 298f, 299t
Femoral neck stress fractures, 132–133, 132f–133f
Femoral nerve, of hip, 916
Femoral nerve block, 332–333, 333f
Femoral nerve stretch test, 933
Femoral osteotomy, 1301
Femoral tunnel, for revision anterior cruciate
    ligament injuries, 1205–1206, 1206f
Femoroacetabular impingement (FAI), 313,
    957–970, 958f
  complications, 969
  diagnosis, 960–965
    computed tomography, 964, 965f
    magnetic resonance arthrography, 964

Femoroacetabular impingement (FAI)
  (Continued)
    magnetic resonance imaging, 963–964,
      963f–964f
    plain radiographs, 960–963, 961f–963f
    ultrasonography, 964–965
  history, 958–959, 959f
  imaging, 942, 944f
  intra-articular injection, 965–969
  management, 965–969
    hip arthroscopy, 965–967, 966f, 966t
    nonoperative, 965
    open surgical dislocation, 965
    operative, 965
    outcomes, 969
    rehabilitation, 967–969
  pediatrics, 1693
  physical examination, 959–960, 959t, 960f
Femur
  anatomy, 1064–1065, 1065f
  head-neck junction of, 909–910
  neck
    internal bony architecture of, 910, 910f
    version, 909
  proximal, development, 908–909
  regional anesthesia, 332–333
Fibrin clot augmentation, 1148
Fibroblasts, tendon-specialized. See Tenocytes
Fibrocartilaginous enthesis, 2–3
Fibula-based reconstruction, 1256
Fibular collateral ligament, 1070, 1071f, 1113,
  1244–1245
Field-side management, of spine injuries,
  1553–1561, 1554f–1558f
Figure-of-eight reconstruction, 675, 675b, 676f
Figure skating injuries, 117–118
Fingers. See also Digits
  fractures, pediatrics, 1677–1681
    complications, 1680–1681
    decision-making principles, 1678
    future considerations, 1681
    history, 1677
    imaging, 1678, 1678f–1679f
    physical examination, 1677–1678, 1678f
    postoperative management, 1680
    results, 1680
    treatment options, 1678–1680, 1680f, 1681b
  injuries
    basketball, 116
    volleyball, 127–128
  jammed, 1681–1683
    complications, 1683
    decision-making principles, 1682
    history, 1681
    imaging, 1682, 1682f
    physical examination, 1681–1682
    postoperative management, 1683
    results, 1683
    treatment options, 1682, 1682b
  jersey, 878–880, 878f–880f
  mallet, 873–875, 874f
  metacarpophalangeal joints, 787–788
Fixation
  for posterior cruciate ligament injuries, 1219
  for revision anterior cruciate ligament injuries,
    1204, 1204f
Flexibility testing, stiffness testing vs., 27
Flexion, abduction, and external rotation
  (FABER) test, 932
Flexion-extension, elbow, 681, 683f
Flexors
  hip, 917–919
  pulley injury, 804
  wrist, 791

Flexor carpi radialis tendinopathy, 862
Flexor carpi ulnaris tendinopathy, 862–863, 862b,
  862f–863f
Flexor digitorum longus tendon transfer
  for Achilles tendon rupture, 1480b–1481b
  for posterior tibial tendon injury, 1467b–1468b
Flexor hallucis longus, 1384–1385, 1385f
  injuries, 1469–1472
    complications, 1471–1472
    decision-making principles, 1470
    future considerations, 1472
    history, 1469
    imaging, 1469, 1470f
    physical examination, 1469
    postoperative management, 1471
    results, 1471
    treatment options, 1470, 1470b, 1471f
Flexor retinaculum reconstruction, for posterior
  tibial tendon injury, 1467b–1468b
Flight dysrhythmia, 323
Flip angle, in magnetic resonance imaging, 94
Fluid mechanics, 23–24
Fluid pump, 107
Fluoroscopy, 75–76, 75f–76f
Focal seizures, 230
Foot
  biomechanics, 1359–1369
  decision-making, 1370–1379
  diagnosis, 1370–1379
  forefoot, 1515–1526
    hallux rigidus, 1523–1526
    metatarsalgia, 1519–1522
    sesamoid dysfunction, 1516–1519,
      1517b–1518b
    turf toe, 1515–1516, 1516b
  imaging, 1380–1392
    computed tomography, 1380
    ligaments, 1387–1388, 1388f
    magnetic resonance imaging, 1380–1381
    nerve entrapment, 1389–1391
    osteochondral lesions, 1388–1389, 1389f
    plantar fasciitis, 1391, 1391f
    radiographs, 1380, 1381f
    of tendons, 1381–1386, 1381f
    ultrasound, 1380
  injuries, 117
    in adolescent athlete, 1725–1740
      fractures, 1733–1739, 1735f–1737f
      orthotics and, 1739
      shoes and, 1739
      soft tissue injuries of, 1728–1729, 1728f
      systemic illness and, 1739
    articular cartilage, 1484–1503
    in female athlete, 305–306, 305t, 306f
    ligamentous, 1444–1461
    tendons, 1462–1483
  metatarsal break in, 1365–1367, 1367f–1368f
  orthoses, 1436–1439
    clinical application, 1437–1439, 1438t–1439t,
      1440f
    research in, 1436–1437, 1437f
  orthotics, 372–374
  osteochondroses in, 1737–1739, 1738f–1739f
  pathologies, 1370–1371
  pediatric, 1633–1635
    acute injuries, 1633, 1634f
    cavus, 1728
    overuse injuries, 1633–1635, 1634f
  peripheral nerve entrapment around,
    1402–1420
    deep peroneal nerve, 1415–1416, 1415f
    interdigital neuralgia (Morton neuroma),
      1416–1419
    lateral plantar nerve, 1411–1412

Foot (Continued)
    medial plantar nerve, 1412–1413
    saphenous nerve, 1405–1407, 1405f–1406f
    superficial peroneal nerve, 1413–1415,
      1413f
    sural nerve, 1402–1405, 1403f
    tarsal tunnel syndrome, 1407–1411, 1407f
  physical examination, 1372–1379, 1373f–1378f
  plantar fasciitis, 1509–1513
    complications, 1513
    decision-making principles, 1510
    future considerations, 1513
    history, 1509
    imaging, 1509, 1509f
    physical examination, 1509
    postoperative management, 1511
    results, 1511–1513
    treatment options, 1510–1511, 1510f, 1511b,
      1512f
  posterior heel pain, 1504–1508, 1505f
    complications, 1508
    decision-making principles, 1505–1506
    future considerations, 1508
    history, 1504
    imaging, 1504–1505, 1505f–1506f
    physical examination, 1504, 1505f
    postoperative management, 1508
    results, 1508
    treatment options, 1506–1507
  shoes, 1439–1442
    anatomy, 1440, 1441f
    insole, 1441
    midsole, 1440–1441
    outsole, 1440
    selection and fitting of, 1442, 1442t
    upper, 1441–1442
  taping, 368–372, 369f
  variations of normal anatomy, 1725–1728
  windlass mechanism, 1365–1367, 1367f–1368f
Foot-strike hemoglobinuria, 196
Football injuries, 118–119
  head, 118
  lower extremity, 118–119
  neck, 118
  upper extremity, 118
Foraminal stenosis, cervical, 1595
Force
  around hip joint, 922–923
  ground reaction, 19
  joint contact, 21–22
  joint reaction, 19, 19f–20f
  production of skeletal muscle, 64–65
  vectors, 21
Forced flexion, adduction, and internal rotation
  of hip (FADIR), 932
Forearm. See also Entrapment neuropathies
  contracture, 773
  regional anesthesia, 330–332
Forefoot, 1515–1526
  hallux rigidus, 1523–1526
    complications, 1526
    decision-making principles, 1523–1524
    examination of, 1523, 1523f
    history, 1523
    imaging, 1523
    results, 1525
    treatment options, 1524–1525
  metatarsalgia, 1519–1522
    complications, 1522
    decision-making principles, 1520
    future considerations of, 1522
    history, 1519
    imaging, 1520
    physical examination, 1519–1520

Forefoot (Continued)
  postoperative management, 1521–1522
  results, 1522
  treatment options, 1520–1521, 1521f–1522f, 1522b
 sesamoid dysfunction, 1516–1519, 1516b
  complications, 1519
  decision-making principles, 1517
  history, 1517
  imaging, 1517, 1518f
  physical examination, 1517
  postoperative management, 1518–1519
  results, 1519
  treatment options, 1517–1518, 1518b, 1519f
 turf toe, 1515–1516
  anatomic classification, 1518t
  complications, 1516
  decision-making principles, 1515–1516
  history, 1515
  imaging, 1515, 1516b
  physical examination, 1515
  postoperative management, 1516
  results, 1516
  treatment options, 1516, 1517b, 1517f
45-degree Dunn view, 935, 937f
Fracture-dislocations, of thoracolumbar spine, 1584, 1586f–1587f
Fractures, 131–142, 1690
 ankle, 1729–1733, 1729f, 1732f–1734f, 1732t
 calcaneum, 1456–1457
 capitate, 809
 carpal, 807–809
 cervical spine injuries, 1579
 clavicle, 139, 139f
 distal radius, 826–827
 elbow, 699
  occult, 699, 700f
  stress, 700
 in foot, 1733–1739, 1735f–1737f
 hamate, 809
 imaging, 807–809
 metacarpals, 814–815, 815f
 patellar, 1322, 1322b
  clinical outcomes, 1332–1333
  complications, 1333
  decision-making principles, 1327
  history, 1323
  imaging, 1326, 1326f
  nonoperative treatment, 1327–1328, 1328f
  operative treatment, 1329–1330
  physical examination, 1324
  postoperative management, 1331
 pediatrics
  apophyseal ring, 1753, 1756f
  avulsion, 1688, 1689f
  Chance, 1753–1755
  clavicle physeal, 1637–1644
  finger, 1677–1681
  hip, 1690
  lesser tuberosity, 1647
  medial epicondyle avulsion, 1670–1672
  physeal, 1718–1721
  proximal humerus, 1644–1647
  sacral facet, 1755, 1756f
  scaphoid, 1684–1686
  stress, 1688–1690, 1690f
 repair, 14–15
 return to sport, 139–142, 140f–141f
 rib, 137–139
 Salter-Harris
  type I, 1729f, 1730
  type II, 1729f, 1730, 1733f
  type III, 1729f, 1730
  type IV, 1729f–1731f, 1730–1731

Fractures (Continued)
  scaphoid, 807–808, 807f–808f, 824
  stress, 131–139
   biomechanical factors of, 131–132
   classification, 132t
   elbow, 700
   fatigue and training errors causing, 132
   in female athlete triad, 131
   femoral neck, 132–133, 132f–133f
   genetic factors, 132
   metatarsal, 135–136
   navicular, 136, 137f
   nutrition and, 132
   olecranon, 764–765, 764f–765f
   pars, 136–137, 138f
   proximal fifth metatarsal, 134–135, 135f–136f
   tibial, 133–134, 134f–135f
   teeth, 270
   thoracolumbar, 1583
    burst, 1584, 1585f
    Chance, 1584, 1586f
    compression, 1583–1584, 1584f
    stress, 1584–1585
    vertebral body apophyseal avulsion, 1585
   transscaphoid perilunate, 825–826, 826f
   trapezium, 808–809, 809f
   wrist arthroscopy, 824–828
    arthroscopic reduction, 824b–825b, 824f–825f
    scaphoid nonunions, 824–825, 825t
    technique, 827–828, 827f
Free-body diagrams, 20f, 21
Freiberg disease, 1738, 1738f
Frequency selective fat saturation, 98
Fresh-frozen allografting, 1488–1489
Friction blisters, 254
Frog-leg lateral view, 935, 937f
Froment sign, 900f
Frontal sinus fractures, 268
Frostbite, 241–242
  diagnosis, 241
  laboratory, 241
  pathophysiology, 241
  prevention, 242
  treatment, 241–242
Frozen shoulder, 310–312, 311t, 581
FTE. See Functional tissue engineering
Functional heartburn, 191
Functional leg lengths, 936
Functional metabolic imaging, of spine, 1549
Functional tissue engineering, 28–29
Functional training, 1196–1197
Fungal infections, 249–250
  dermatophytoses, 249–250, 250f
  Malassezia, 250, 251f
  skin, 205–206
Furuncles, 246, 247f

G
Gadolinium, delayed, 101
Gait
  alignment of, posterior cruciate ligament and, 1214
  cycle, 921–922, 1359, 1360f
  examination of
   lateral and posterolateral corner injuries of knee, 1251
   medial collateral ligament and posterior medial corner injuries, 1231
   multiligament knee injuries, 1265
   patellar instability, 1296
  kinetics, 1359–1360, 1360f
Gallium scans, 90, 92f–93f
Ganglionectomy, 832–833, 832f

Gastrocnemius tendon, lateral, 1246
Gastroesophageal reflux disease (GERD), 190–191
Gastrointestinal system
 medicine
  in athlete, 189–195
   lower gastrointestinal tract conditions, 192–195, 193t
   pathophysiology, 189
   upper gastrointestinal tract conditions, 189–192
  preparticipation physical evaluation, 148
Gastrointestinal tract ischemia, 189
Geissler technique, 824–825
Gender
 anterior cruciate ligament injuries, 1189
 of elite athlete, 161–162, 162f
Generalized seizures, 230
Genetics, of elite athlete, 161–162, 162f
Genitourinary system
 preparticipation physical evaluation, 148
 trauma, 227–229
  classification, 227, 228t
  definition, 227, 228t
  diagnosis, 227–228
  epidemiology, 227
  pathobiology, 227
  pathophysiology, 227
  return-to-play guidelines, 229
  treatment, 228–229
GERD. See Gastroesophageal reflux disease
Gestational diabetes, 218
GIRD. See Glenohumeral internal rotation deficit
Glasgow Coma Scale, to injured athlete, 1554–1555, 1555f
Glenohumeral arthritis, 407
Glenohumeral internal rotation deficit (GIRD), 431
 pathophysiology, 514
 treatment options, 518
Glenohumeral joint, 395–396, 395f–396f
 arthritis, 592–608
  classification, 592–595
  complications, 606, 607t
  decision-making principles, 603–604
  epidemiology, 592
  future considerations, 607
  history, 595
  physical examination, 595–596
   arthroscopic images, 596
   imaging, 596, 597f–598f
  presentation, 595
  prior operative notes, 596
  return-to-play guidelines, 606
  treatment, 596–603, 604b, 604f–605f
 capsule, 396–397
 imaging, 408–432
  abnormalities, 414–432
  arthrography, 410–411, 410f
  computed tomography, 411, 411f
  conventional radiography, 408–410, 409b
  magnetic resonance imaging, 412–414, 413f, 413t
  ultrasonography, 411–412, 412f, 412t
 instability, 1647–1648
Glucose, 221, 221f, 222t
Gluteal nerves, superior and inferior, 1032–1033, 1032f, 1032t
Gluteus maximus, 920
Gluteus medius, 917
 tears, 990–996
  complications, 996
  decision-making principles, 990, 991b
  future considerations, 996
  history, 990
  imaging, 990, 991f

Gluteus medius (Continued)
  physical examination, 990
  postoperative management, 995
  results, 995, 996t
  techniques, 991b–992b, 992f–995f
  treatment options, 990
Gluteus minimus, 917
  tears, 990–996
    complications, 996
    decision-making principles, 990, 991b
    future considerations, 996
    history, 990
    imaging, 990, 991f
    physical examination, 990
    postoperative management, 995
    results, 995, 996t
    techniques, 991b–992b, 992f–995f
    treatment options, 990
Glycolytic energy system, 65–66
Godfrey test, for posterior cruciate ligament
    injuries, 1212–1213, 1213f
Golf injuries, 119–120
  elbow, 119–120
  forearm, 119–120
  hand, 120
  lower back, 119
  shoulder, 120
  wrist, 120
Gonadal hormones, 69t, 70–71
Gore-Tex implant, 39
Gradient echo, 96–97, 97f
Graft/grafting
  bone, 715b–716b
  harvest, 1191
  healing, 1192
  for multiligament knee injuries, 1267
  for posterior cruciate ligament injuries, 1219
  for revision anterior cruciate ligament injuries,
    1207
  selection, 1190–1191
  tension and fixation, 1191–1192
  timing, 1190–1192
  tissue, 30–34
    allograft, 31–32
    autograft, 30
    future direction, 33
  type, 1197
Granuloma, swimming pool/fish tank, 252, 252f
Grasping forceps, 108
Great arteries, 161
Great veins, 161
Greater trochanter, 910, 910f
Greater trochanteric pain syndrome (GTPS), 925
Groin contusions, 1047
Ground reaction force, 19
Growth factor modulation, in meniscal injuries,
    1149
Growth hormone, 289–290
  adverse effects, 289–290
  historical perspectives, 289
  mechanism of action, 289
GTPS. See Greater trochanteric pain syndrome
Guyon canal release, 903b, 903f
Gymnastics injuries, 120–121

H
HACE. See High-altitude cerebral edema
Haglund deformity, 1477
Haglund resection, endoscopic, 1433–1435
  complications, 1435
  decision-making principles, 1433
  history, 1433
  imaging, 1433

Haglund resection, endoscopic (Continued)
  physical examination, 1433
  postoperative management, 1434
  results, 1434
  treatment, 1433b–1434b, 1434f
Hair discoloration, 256
Hallux rigidus, 1523–1526
  complications, 1526
  decision-making principles, 1523–1524
  examination of, 1523, 1523f
  history, 1523
  imaging, 1523
  results, 1525
  treatment options, 1524–1525
    nonoperative, 1524
    operative, 1524–1525, 1524f–1525f
    technique, 1526b
Hamate carpal injuries, 840–843, 840f–843f, 843b
Hamate fracture, 809
Hamstring injuries
  open surgery, 1037, 1038f
Hamstrings, 919–920, 919f
  injuries, 1034–1042, 1035f
    complications, 1041–1042
    decision-making principles, 1037
    future considerations, 1042
    history, 1034–1035
    imaging, 1036–1037, 1036f–1037f
    physical examination, 1035–1036
    postoperative management, 1039–1040
      rehabilitation in, 1039–1040
    results, 1040–1041
    treatment options, 1037–1039
      nonoperative, 1037
      surgical, 1037–1039
      techniques, 1039b, 1039f–1040f
  strains, 376
    causes, 376
    preventing, 377, 377f, 377t
    risk factors, 376–377
Hand, 785–792
  decision-making principles, 793–805
  diagnosis, 793–805
  extensor tendons of, 790–791, 790f–791f
  history, 793–794
  imaging, 806–816
    metacarpal fracture, 814–815, 815f
    pulley injuries, 814
    thumb ulnar collateral ligament injury, 814,
      815f
  injuries. See also Wrist/hand injuries
    basketball, 116
    golf, 120
  joints, 787–789
    distal interphalangeal, 789, 789f
    metacarpophalangeal, of fingers, 787–788
    proximal interphalangeal, 788–789
    thumb, 789
  muscles, 785–787, 788f
  nerves, 785, 787f
  neuropathies, 898–905
    decision-making principles, 901
    future considerations, 904
    history, 898
    imaging, 900–901, 900f, 901t
    physical examination, 898–900, 899f–900f
    postoperative management and return to
      play, 902–903, 903b, 903f
    results, 903–904
    treatment options, 901–902
  physical examination, 793–794, 794f
  quadrants
    dorsal, 794t, 796–798, 797f–798f
    radial, 794–796, 794t, 795f–796f

Hand (Continued)
    ulnar, 794t, 798–800, 799f
    volar, 794t, 800–801, 800f, 802f–803f
  regional anesthesia, 330–332
  skin, 785, 786f
  tendons, 785–787, 788f
Handball injuries, 121–122
Hardware complications, of subscapularis injury,
    565
Hawkins test, 404, 545f
HBV. See Hepatitis B virus
HCM. See Hypertrophic cardiomyopathy
HCV. See Hepatitis C virus
Head
  anatomy, 1528, 1529f
    brain, 1528–1529
    intervertebral disk, 1534
    ligaments, 1534
    muscles, 1534
    neurologic tissues, 1534–1535, 1534f
    skull (cranium), 1528, 1529f
    spine, 1531–1533, 1532f–1533f
  biomechanics, 1535, 1535f
  brain injury, 1562–1569
    background, 1562–1564
    clinical presentation, 1563–1564
    definition, 1562–1563
    epidemiology, 1563
    imaging, 1566
    interventions, 1567–1568
    management, 1566–1567
    pathophysiology, 1563
    physical examination, 1564–1566
    retiring athlete, 1567
    return-to-play, 1567, 1567t
  concussion, 1530–1531, 1562–1569
    background, 1562–1564
    clinical presentation, 1563–1564
    definition, 1562–1563
    epidemiology, 1563
    imaging, 1566
    interventions, 1567–1568
    management, 1566–1567
    pathophysiology, 1563
    physical examination, 1564–1566
    retiring athlete, 1567
    return-to-play, 1567, 1567t
  injuries, 1529–1530, 1530f–1531f, 1538–1541
    anatomy, 1538
    biomechanics, 1538, 1539f
    complications, 1540–1541
    decision-making principles, 1540
    football, 118
    future considerations, 1541
    history, 1539
    ice hockey, 121
    imaging, 1539–1540
    on-field emergencies, 152
    pathophysiology, 1538–1539
    physical exam, 1539
    results, 1540
    in skeletally immature athletes, 1741–1748.
      See also Concussion
    treatment options, 1540, 1540b
  preparticipation physical evaluation, 145
  stingers, 1570–1577
    classification, 1573–1574, 1574t
    decision-making principles, 1573–1574
    future considerations, 1576, 1576f
    history, 1570
    imaging, 1571–1573, 1573f
    mechanism of, 1573, 1574f
    physical examination, 1570–1571, 1571f–
      1572f, 1572t

Head (Continued)
return to play criteria, 1576
sequela, 1576
treatment options, 1574–1575, 1575b, 1575f
Head-neck offset, 938
Head sphericity, 938
Headache, high-altitude, 242–243
Healing. See also Repair
autograft vs. allograft, 32–33
bone, biology, 14–15, 14t–15t
graft, 1192
tendon and ligament
factors affecting, 5, 6t
methods for augmentation of, 5–7
Health promotion, 344
Heartburn, functional, 191
Heat
balance, 240
exertional illness
definition, 235
epidemiology, 235
exercise-associated collapse, 237
exercise-associated hyponatremia, 239–240
exercise-associated muscle cramps, 236–237
exertional heat exhaustion, 235–236
exertional heat stroke, 236
exertional rhabdomyolysis, 237–238
exertional sickling collapse, 238–239
heat syncope, 237
illness, 149–150
loss, 240
production, 240
related injuries, 1609
stroke, exertional, 236, 236b
Heat syncope (HS), 237
Heel pain, posterior, 1504–1508, 1505f
complications, 1508
decision-making principles, 1505–1506
future considerations, 1508
history, 1504
imaging, 1504–1505, 1505f–1506f
physical examination, 1504, 1505f
postoperative management, 1508
results, 1508
treatment options, 1506–1507
nonoperative therapy, 1506–1507
operative therapy, 1507
technique, 1507b, 1507f
Heel strike, 932
Hematologic disease, preparticipation physical evaluation, 148–149
Hematologic medicine, in athlete, 196–200
hemostasis disorders, 198–200
red blood cells disorders, 196–198
Hematuria, exercise-induced, 228
Hemispheres, brain, 1528–1529
Hemoglobin S, 197
Hemoglobinopathies, 196
Hemophilia, 199
Hemorrhage, 254, 254f–255f
Hemostasis, disorders of, 198–200
definition, 198–199, 199f
diagnosis, 199–200
epidemiology, 199
pathophysiology, 199
return-to-play guidelines, 200
treatment, 200
Hepatitis A, waterborne diseases, 212
Hepatitis B virus (HBV), 210
Hepatitis C virus (HCV), 210
Hepcidin, 197
Hernia, sports, 1007, 1012–1014, 1014b, 1014f
Herniation, disk, 1579
Herpes gladiatorum, 251f
Herpes simplex, 250–251, 251f

Herpes simplex virus (HSV), 205
definition, 205
diagnosis, 205
epidemiology, 205
pathobiology, 205
return-to-play guidelines, 205, 205t
treatment, 205
Heterotopic ossification (HO), 317, 319, 718
Hidradenitis suppurativa, 255–256, 256f
High-altitude cerebral edema (HACE), 242–243
High-altitude headache (HAH), 242–243
High-altitude illness (HAI), 242, 244t
acute mountain sickness, 242–243
high-altitude cerebral edema, 242–243
high-altitude headache, 242–243
high-altitude pulmonary edema, 243–245
High-altitude pulmonary edema (HAPE), 243–245
High school athletics, ethical/legal issues with, 155
High tibial osteotomy, for chronic PCL injuries, 1219–1220
Hilton's law, 929
Hindfoot conditions, 1504–1514
plantar fasciitis, 1509–1513
posterior heel pain, 1504–1508, 1505f
Hip
anatomy, 907–924
bony, 907–911
arthritis, 1053–1060
arthroscopy, 1058–1059, 1058f
complications, 1060
decision-making principles, 1057
future direction, 1060
history, 1053
imaging, 1055–1057, 1055f–1056f, 1055t
physical examination, 1053–1055
postoperative management in, 1059
results, 1059–1060
resurfacing for, 1058
surgical treatment, 1058–1059
techniques, 1060b
treatment options, 1057
arthroscopy, 947–956
contraindications, 947
femoroacetabular impingement, 965–967, 966f, 966t
indications, 947–948
learning curve for, 948
operating room set-up, 948–950
positioning for, 948–950
procedure for, 950–955
biomechanics, 907–924
gait cycle in, 921–922
joint, forces around, 922–923
motions in, 921
spine and, relationship of, 923–924, 923f
stability in, 921
bone injuries, 925–926
center position, 938
contusions, 1043–1052
groin, 1047, 1047f
iliac crest, 1043–1044, 1044f
quadriceps, 1044–1047, 1044t
decision-making, 925–934
degenerative joint disease in, 926, 927f
diagnosis, 925–934
dysplasia and instability
decision-making, 975–978, 975f–976f
atraumatic hip microinstability, 977–978
borderline dysplasia, 977
dysplasia and instability of, 971–978
history, 973
imaging, 974–975, 975f
pathologies, 971–973, 972f–973f
physical examination, 973–974

Hip (Continued)
history, 928–929, 928f, 929b
imaging, 935–946
computed tomography, 938–939
magnetic resonance evaluation, 939–946
plain radiographic images, interpretation, 936–938
radiographic techniques, 935–936
ultrasound, 946
infection, 928
injuries, 118
inspection, 929
instability, 926, 971–978
decision-making, 975–978, 975f–976f
atraumatic hip microinstability, 977–978
borderline dysplasia, 977
history, 973
imaging, 974–975, 975f
pathologies, 971–973, 972f–973f
physical examination, 973–974
intra-articular, 911–914
acetabular labrum, 911, 911f–912f
articular cartilage, 913–914
ligamentum teres, 912, 913f
pathology, 927–928
joint
bursae around, 920–921
capsule, 914–916
muscles around, 916–920, 918t
prenatal, development, 907
kinematics of, 921–924
gait cycle in, 921–922
joint, forces around, 922–923
motions in, 921
spine and, relationship of, 923–924, 923f
stability in, 921
ligamentous laxity, evaluation, 932
measurements of, 930–931
nerve entrapment injuries, 927
pain, posterior, 1018–1033
pathologies, 925–928, 926b
pediatrics, 928, 1625–1628, 1688–1696
acute injuries, 1625–1626, 1626f
overuse injuries, 1626–1628, 1627f–1628f
physical examination, 929–933
range of motion of, 930–931, 931t
regional anesthesia, 332–333
soft tissue injuries, 925
special maneuvers, 932–933
sprain and dislocation, 942, 944f–945f
strains, 1043–1052
adductor, 1050–1051
classification, 1047, 1047t
quadriceps, 1047–1050
symptom localization, 929–930, 930f–931f
History of patient
Achilles tendon injuries, 1476
acromioclavicular joint injuries, 647–648, 649f
adductor strains, 1050
AIN syndrome, 746–747
anterior cruciate ligament injuries, 1185
anterior shoulder instability, 447
arthroscopic synovectomy, of knee, 1127
articular cartilage lesions, 1162–1163
athletic pubalgia, 1009
calcaneoplasty, 1433
cervical spine
injuries, 1578
unstable fractures and dislocations of, 1541
cubital tunnel syndrome, 749
deep peroneal nerve entrapment, 1415
distal biceps tendinitis, 725
distal biceps tendon rupture, 732–733
distal triceps tendon rupture, 738

History of patient (*Continued*)
elbow, 687–689, 688f, 757–758, 758f, 772–773
endoscopic Haglund resection, 1433
entrapment neuropathies, 742
exercise-induced bronchoconstriction, 176
exertional compartment syndromes, 1395
extensor mechanism injuries, 1322–1326
external coxa saltans, 999
femoroacetabular impingement, 958–959, 959f
flexor hallucis longus injuries, 1469
glenohumeral arthritis, 595
gluteus medius and minimus tears, 990
hallux rigidus, 1523
hamstring injuries, 1034–1035
hand, 793–794
head injuries, 1539
hip, 928–929, 928f, 929b
  arthritis, 1053
  arthroscopy, 947
  dysplasia and instability, 973
iliac crest contusion, 1043
iliopsoas pathology, 982
interdigital neuralgia, 1417
internal coxa saltans, 996
ischiofemoral impingement, 1003–1004, 1004f
knee, 1089–1091, 1090t
  arthritis, 1277, 1278t
  lateral and posterolateral corner injuries,
    1248–1249
  motion loss, 1335–1336
lateral epicondylitis, 720, 721t
lateral plantar nerve entrapment, 1411
leg pain, 1395
medial epicondylitis, 720, 721t
medial plantar nerve entrapment, 1412
meniscus, 1132, 1137
metatarsalgia, 1519
Morton neuroma, 1417
multidirectional instability, 477
multiligament knee injury, 1264
olecranon bursitis, 728, 728f
osteochondral lesions, 1484
patellar instability, 1293, 1294f
patellofemoral pain, 1309–1310
pediatrics, 1052
  anterior cruciate ligament (ACL) injuries,
    1697
  apophyseal ring fractures, 1753
  atraumatic instability, 1654
  cervical spine, 1762
  concussion, 1743, 1743t
  discoid meniscus, 1706
  distal radial physeal stress reaction, 1683
  Down syndrome, atlantoaxial instability in,
    1758
  finger fractures, 1677
  jammed finger, 1681
  lateral clavicle physeal fractures, 1640
  lateral epicondylitis, 1675
  lesser tuberosity fractures, 1647
  Little League elbow, 1665–1666, 1665f
  medial clavicle physeal fractures, 1643
  medial collateral ligament injury, 1672
  medial epicondyle avulsion fractures,
    1670–1671
  medial epicondylitis, 1675
  meniscal injuries, 1703
  odontoid fractures, 1761
  osteochondritis dissecans, 1668, 1712, 1713f
  osteochondrosis, 1668
  Panner disease, 1668
  patellar instability, 1708–1709
  physeal fractures, 1719
  posterior elbow pathologic conditions, 1674

History of patient (*Continued*)
  proximal humerus epiphysiolysis, 1656
  proximal humerus fracture, 1644
  rotatory atlantoaxial subluxation, 1759
  scaphoid fracture, 1684
  scoliosis, 1755–1757
  spinal cord injury without radiographic
    abnormality, 1763
  spinal injuries, 1749–1750, 1750b
  spondylolisthesis, 1751–1752
  spondylolysis, 1751–1752
  traumatic anterior instability, 1648, 1648f
  traumatic posterior instability, 1651–1652
peroneal tendon injuries, 1472–1476
PIN syndrome, 755
piriformis syndrome, 1002
plantar fasciitis, 1509
popliteal artery entrapment syndrome, 1350
posterior heel pain, 1504
posterior shoulder instability, 465
preparticipation physical examination,
  145–150
pronator syndrome, 745
quadriceps contusion, 1044–1045
quadriceps strains, 1048
radial tunnel syndrome, 754
revision shoulder instability, 489
saphenous nerve entrapment, 1405
scapulothoracic disorders, 609–611
sesamoid dysfunction, 1517
soft tissue, ankle arthroscopy, 1423
sprains
  ankle, 1444–1446, 1450–1451
  bifurcate ligament, 1457
  Lisfranc, 1458
  syndesmosis, 1453–1454
sternoclavicular joint injuries, 664
stiff shoulder, 579–583
  crepitus, 581
  exacerbating factors, 580–581
  pain, 579–581, 580b
  relieving factors, 580–581
  stiffness, 581
  weakness, 581
stingers, 1570
subscapularis injury, 558–559, 558f
subtalar arthroscopy, 1429
superficial peroneal nerve entrapment, 1413
superior labrum anterior to posterior (SLAP)
  tears, 502
sural nerve entrapment, 1402
tarsal tunnel syndrome, 1408
thoracic outlet syndrome, 636
thoracolumbar spine injuries, 1582
triceps tendinitis, 725
trochanteric bursitis, 1001–1002
turf toe, 1515
wrist, 793–794, 857–858
HIV. *See* Human immunodeficiency virus
Hook of hamate fractures, 900f
Hop tests, 388f
Hormones
  adaptation to exercise of, 69–71, 69t
  adrenal, 69t, 70
  gonadal, 69t, 70–71
  pancreatic, 69t, 71
  pituitary, 69–70, 69t
Hot tub folliculitis, 213
HSV. *See* Herpes simplex virus
Hueter-Volkmann law, in bone remodeling, 13
Human immunodeficiency virus (HIV), 210
Humerus, proximal, 1637, 1638f
Hyalofast, 1181
Hyalograft C, 43–44

Hydration, 278–279, 279t
  considerations, 278
  gastrointestinal tract conditions, 189
  monitoring, 278–279
Hydrodilatation, 585
Hygiene, for preventing infectious disease, 202
Hypercoagulability, 180
Hyperlipidemia, 172
Hypertension, 169–172
Hypertrophic cardiomyopathy (HCM), 167,
  326–327
Hyphema, 269
Hypomobility issues, 381
Hyponatremia, 229
  exercise-associated, 239–240
Hypothalamic-pituitary-testicular (HPT) axis, 70
Hypothermia, 240–241
  diagnosis, 240–241
  heat balance, 240
  pathophysiology, 240
  prevention, 241
  thermal balance, 240
  treatment, 241

I

IBS. *See* Irritable bowel syndrome
Ice hockey injuries, 121
Idiopathic adhesive capsulitis, 581–582
Idiopathic anterior knee pain, 1314–1315
Idiopathic scoliosis, 313–314
Idiopathic thrombocytopenic purpura (ITP), 199
IFI. *See* Ischiofemoral impingement
ILFL. *See* Iliofemoral ligament
Iliac crest contusion, 1043–1044, 1044f
  complications, 1044
  history, 1043
  imaging, 1043, 1044f
  physical examination, 1043
  results, 1044
  return to play, 1044
  techniques, 1043b
  treatment options, 1043
Iliocapsularis muscle, 919
Iliofemoral ligament (ILFL), 914, 915f
Iliopsoas, 917–919
  anatomy, 979–980, 980f–981f
  bursa, 921
  bursitis, 980
  complications, 987–988
  function of, 979–980, 980f–981f
  history, 982
  imaging, 983–984
  impingement, 980–983, 982f, 986–987
  pathology, 979–989
  physical exam, 982–983
  postoperative management, 984
  results, 984–987
  snapping, 980, 981f, 982, 983f, 984–986
  techniques, 986b–987b, 987f
  tendonitis, 980
  treatment options, 984, 984f–986f
Iliotibial band, 1244
Imaging, 74–104. *See also specific imaging
  modalities*
  acromioclavicular joint injuries, 651–653, 652f,
    654f–655f
  adductor strains, 1050, 1050f
  ankle, 1380–1392
    computed tomography, 1380
    ligaments, 1387–1388, 1388f
    magnetic resonance imaging, 1380–1381
    nerve entrapment, 1389–1391
    osteochondral lesions, 1388–1389, 1389f

Imaging (Continued)
plantar fasciitis, 1391
radiographs, 1380, 1381f
tendons, 1381–1386, 1381f
ultrasound, 1380
anterior cruciate ligament injuries, revision, 1200–1202, 1200f
anterior shoulder instability, 448–450, 450f–452f
apophyseal ring fractures, 1753, 1756f
arthroscopic synovectomy, of knee, 1127–1128
articular cartilage lesions, 1163
athletic pubalgia, 1010–1011
dynamic ultrasonography, 1010–1011
magnetic resonance imaging, 1010, 1010f–1011f
radiographic analysis, 1010, 1010f
brain injury, 1566
calcaneoplasty, 1433
cervical spine
congenital anomalies of, 1762
injuries, 1578–1579
unstable fractures and dislocations of, 1541–1542, 1542f
collateral ligament injury, 700–702, 701f
computed tomography, 85–88
advantages, 87, 87f–88f
disadvantages, 87–88, 88f
technical considerations, 85–87, 86f–87f
concussion, 1566
conventional radiography, 74–78, 1104, 1105f
advantages, 77
arthrography, 76–77, 76f–77f
disadvantages, 77–78, 78f
fluoroscopy, 75–76, 75f–76f
technical considerations, 74–75, 75f
deep venous thrombosis, 182–184, 185f–186f
diffusion weighted, 100, 100f
distal biceps tendon rupture, 733–734, 734f
distal triceps tendon rupture, 738
Down syndrome, atlantoaxial instability in, 1758
elbow, 697–706, 698f
collateral ligament injury, 700–702, 701f
computed tomography, 697–698
conventional radiographs, 697
distal biceps, 725, 726f
lateral epicondylitis, 702–704, 703f, 721, 721f–722f
loose bodies, 700
magnetic resonance arthrography, 699
magnetic resonance imaging, 698–699
medial epicondylitis, 702–704, 721, 721f–722f
motion, loss, 774, 774f
olecranon bursitis, 728, 729f
tendon ruptures, 703–704, 704f
throwing injuries, 760, 761f
trauma, 699–700
triceps tendinitis, 725, 726f
ulnar neuropathy, 704, 705f
ultrasound, 699
endoscopic Haglund resection, 1433
exertional compartment syndromes, 1395–1396, 1396f
extensor mechanism, 1113–1116, 1115f–1117f
injuries, 1324–1326
external coxa saltans, 999
femoroacetabular impingement
computed tomography, 964, 965f
magnetic resonance arthrography, 964
magnetic resonance imaging, 963–964, 963f–964f
plain radiographs, 960–963, 961f–963f
ultrasonography, 964–965

Imaging (Continued)
foot, 1380–1392
computed tomography, 1380
ligaments, 1387–1388, 1388f
magnetic resonance imaging, 1380–1381
nerve entrapment, 1389–1391
osteochondral lesions, 1388–1389, 1389f
plantar fasciitis, 1391
radiographs, 1380, 1381f
tendons, 1381–1386, 1381f
ultrasound, 1380
genitourinary trauma, 228
glenohumeral arthritis, 596, 597f–598f
gluteus medius and minimus tears, 990, 991f
hallux rigidus, 1523
hamstring injuries, 1036–1037, 1036f–1037f
hand, 806–816
metacarpal fracture, 814–815, 815f
pulley injuries, 814
thumb ulnar collateral ligament injury, 814, 815f
head injuries, 1539–1540
hip, 935–946
arthritis, 1055–1057, 1055f–1056f, 1055t
computed tomography, 938–939
dysplasia and instability, 974–975, 975f
magnetic resonance evaluation, 939–946
plain radiographic images, interpretation, 936–938
radiographic techniques, 935–936
ultrasound, 946
iliac crest contusion, 1043, 1044f
iliopsoas, 983–984
interdigital neuralgia, 1417–1418
internal coxa saltans, 996–997
ischiofemoral impingement, 1004
key points, 104
knee, 1104–1120
arthritis, 1277–1279, 1278f–1279f
background, 1104
cartilage, 1116–1118, 1118f–1119f
computed tomography, 1105f
dislocation in, 1348
ligaments, 1110–1113, 1111f–1115f
magnetic resonance imaging, 1105–1106
motion, loss, 1336–1337, 1337f
musculotendinous structures, 1110, 1111f
osseous structures, 1116–1118, 1118f–1119f
pitfalls, 1109–1110, 1110f
lateral and posterolateral corner injuries of knee, 1251–1253
magnetic resonance imaging, 1251–1253, 1252f
radiographs, 1251, 1251f
ultrasound, 1253
latissimus dorsi injuries, 576, 577f
leg pain, 1395–1396, 1396f
magnetic resonance, 92–100
advantages, 102
contraindications, 102–103
delayed gadolinium for, 101
Dgemric, 101
diffusion weighted imaging, 100, 100f
disadvantages, 102, 102f
dynamic contrast enhancement in, 101–103
image formation of, 94–95
image quality in, 100
protocols for, 93, 94f
proton density in, 95, 96f, 96t
pulse sequences, 95–98
T1, 95, 95f, 96t
T2, 95, 96t
technical considerations of, 93–100
ultrashort time to echo sequence for, 100–101

Imaging (Continued)
medial collateral ligament and posterior medial corner injuries, 1232–1234, 1233f–1235f
meniscus, 1106–1109, 1106f–1109f
injuries, 1138–1139, 1138f
metatarsalgia, 1520
Morton neuroma, 1416–1419
multiligament knee injuries, 1265–1266, 1265f–1266f
nerve entrapment
deep peroneal nerve, 1416
lateral plantar nerve, 1411
medial plantar nerve, 1413
saphenous nerve, 1406
superficial peroneal nerve, 1414
sural nerve, 1403–1404
nuclear medicine, 88–92
advantages, 90, 93f
bone scans in, 88–89, 89f
disadvantages, 90–92, 94f
gallium scans in, 90, 92f–93f
labeled white blood cell scans in, 89–90, 91f
PET/CT scans, 90, 93f
planar imaging, 88, 89f
SPECT/CT imaging, 88, 89f
technical considerations, 88
odontoid fractures, 1761–1762, 1761f
patella
fractures, 1326, 1326f
instability, 1297–1299, 1298f–1299f
tendinopathy, 1324–1325, 1324f–1325f
tendon ruptures, 1325–1326, 1325f–1326f
pectoralis major muscle injuries, 575
pediatrics, 1052
anterior cruciate ligament (ACL) injuries, 1697–1698
atraumatic instability, 1655, 1655f
concussion, 1744–1745, 1745b
discoid meniscus, 1706
distal radial physeal stress reaction, 1683–1684, 1683f
finger fractures, 1678, 1678f–1679f
jammed finger, 1682, 1682f
lateral clavicle physeal fractures, 1641
lateral epicondylitis, 1675
lesser tuberosity fractures, 1647
Little League elbow, 1667
medial clavicle physeal fractures, 1643, 1643f
medial collateral ligament injury, 1672
medial epicondyle avulsion fractures, 1671
medial epicondylitis, 1675
meniscal injuries, 1703–1704
osteochondritis dissecans, 1668–1669, 1669f
osteochondrosis, 1668–1669, 1669f
Panner disease, 1668–1669, 1669f
patellar instability, 1709, 1709f
physeal fractures, 1719, 1720f–1721f
posterior elbow pathologic conditions, 1674
proximal humerus epiphysiolysis, 1656, 1656f
proximal humerus fractures, 1644–1645, 1645f–1646f
scaphoid fracture, 1684–1685
traumatic anterior instability, 1648–1649, 1649f–1650f
traumatic posterior instability, 1652, 1653f
piriformis syndrome, 1003
plantar fasciitis, 1509, 1509f
popliteal artery entrapment syndrome, 1352–1354
angiography, 1353–1354, 1354f
computed tomography and computed tomographic angiography, 1353, 1353f
duplex ultrasonography, 1352, 1352f

Imaging *(Continued)*
    magnetic resonance angiography, 1352–1353, 1353*f*
    magnetic resonance imaging, 1352–1353, 1353*f*
    posterior heel pain, 1504–1505, 1505*f*–1506*f*
    posterior shoulder instability, 467–468, 467*f*–468*f*, 468*t*
    postoperative, 1118–1120, 1119*f*–1120*f*
    preoperative, 433–434
    quadriceps contusion, 1045, 1045*f*
    quadriceps strains, 1048, 1048*f*
    radiation exposure in, 103–104, 103*t*
    revision rotator cuff repair, 568
    revision shoulder instability, 490–493, 491*f*–492*f*
    rotator cuff and impingement lesions, 547
        magnetic resonance imaging, 547, 547*f*
        plain radiographs, 547
        ultrasonography, 547
    rotatory atlantoaxial subluxation, 1760, 1761*f*
    scapulothoracic disorders, 614
        computed tomography, 614
        electromyography, 614
        magnetic resonance imaging, 614
        radiographs, 614
        ultrasound, 614, 614*f*–615*f*
    scoliosis, 1757
    sesamoid dysfunction, 1517, 1518*f*
    soft tissue, ankle arthroscopy, 1423–1424
    spinal cord injury without radiographic abnormality, 1763
    spine, 1544–1552
        computed tomography, 1546, 1546*f*
        degenerative, 1550–1551
        EOS 2D/3D x-ray imaging system, 1545–1546, 1545*f*
        functional metabolic imaging, 1549
        future considerations, 1551
        interventional radiology, 1550
        magnetic resonance imaging, 1547, 1547*f*
        myelography, 1548
        nuclear scintigraphy, 1548–1549, 1549*f*
        radiographs, 1544, 1545*f*
        single photon emission computed tomography, 1549–1550
        study interpretation, 1551
    spondylolisthesis, 1752, 1752*f*
    spondylolysis, 1752, 1752*f*
    sternoclavicular joint injuries, 667–668, 670*f*–672*f*
    stiff shoulder, 584–585
    stingers, 1571–1573, 1573*f*
    subscapularis injury, 559, 559*f*
    subtalar arthroscopy, 1429
    superior labrum anterior to posterior (SLAP) tears, 503–504, 505*f*
    tarsal tunnel syndrome, 1408
    techniques, 74–103
    tendons, ruptures, 703–704, 704*f*
    thoracic outlet syndrome, 638–639, 638*f*–639*f*
    thoracolumbar spine injuries, 1583
    3D acquisitions in, 98, 98*f*
    thrower's shoulder, 515–516, 516*f*
    trochanteric bursitis, 1002
    turf toe, 1515, 1516*b*
    2D acquisitions in, 98, 98*f*
    ulnar neuropathy, 704, 705*f*
    ultrasonography, 78–85, 1104–1105, 1106*f*
        advantages, 84
        disadvantages, 84–85, 85*f*
        dynamic, 84, 84*f*
        elastography, 83–84, 83*f*
        musculoskeletal, 79–83, 80*f*–83*f*
        technical considerations, 78–79, 79*f*

Imaging *(Continued)*
    wrist, 806–816, 807*f*
        carpal fractures, 807–809
        distal radius fractures, 806–807
        intrinsic carpal ligament injury, 810–812, 811*f*
        Kienböck disease, 810
        perilunate dislocation, 809–810, 810*f*
        tendinopathies, 858–859, 858*f*
        tendon injuries, 812–813, 812*f*–813*f*
        triangular fibrocartilage complex injury, 813–814, 813*f*–814*f*
        ulnar impaction syndrome, 810
Immature bone, 12, 12*f*
Immediate care, 344
Immune system, exercise and, 201–202, 202*f*
Immunizations, 149, 202
Impairment-based rehabilitation programs, 355–357, 356*f*
Impetigo, 246–247, 247*f*
Impingement. *See also* Rotator cuff and impingement lesions
    cam, 957, 958*f*
    femoroacetabular, 942, 944*f*, 957–970, 958*f*, 1693
        complications, 969
        diagnosis, 960–965
        history, 958–959, 959*f*
        intra-articular injection, 965–969
        management, 965–969
        physical examination, 959–960, 959*t*, 960*f*
    iliopsoas, 980–983, 982*f*, 986–987
    ischiofemoral, 1003–1006
        complications for, 1006
        decision-making principles, 1004, 1005*b*, 1005*f*
        future considerations, 1006
        history, 1003–1004, 1004*f*
        imaging, 1004
        physical examination, 1004
        results, 1006
        treatment options, 1004–1006
    pincer, 958*f*, 967
    posterior, 1426*b*, 1426*f*
    posteromedial, 1673–1674, 1673*f*
        complications, 1674
        decision-making principles, 1674
        history, 1674
        imaging, 1674
        physical examination, 1674
        results, 1674
        treatment, 1674
    syndrome, 406
    test, 614, 614*f*, 933
Implants, 35–49
    cartilage repair, 42–45
    ligament reconstruction, 38–41
    meniscus repair, 41–42
    osteochondral repair, 42–45
    suture anchors for, 46–47
    sutures for, 45–46
    tendon repair, 35–38
In-season management, of anterior shoulder instability, 453
In silico studies, in forces, of hip joint, 922, 923*f*
In situ decompression, 749–750, 750*f*
Incretin, 221
Inertia, 17, 17*t*, 18*f*
Infections
    bacterial skin, 203–205
    blood-borne, 210
    elbow arthroscopy, 718
    fungal skin, 205–206

Infections *(Continued)*
    hip, 928
    lower respiratory tract, 209–210
    neurologic, 214–215
    Pseudomonas, 213
    skin and soft tissue, 203–206
    unusual, 215–216
    upper respiratory tract, 206–209
Infectious diarrhea, 212
Infectious diseases, 201–217
    blood-borne infections, 210
        hepatitis B virus, 210
        hepatitis C virus, 210
        human immunodeficiency virus, 210
    epidemiology, 201
    exercise and immune system, 201–202, 202*f*
    lower respiratory tract infections, 209–210
        acute bronchitis, 209
        acute pneumonia, 209–210
    neurologic infections, 214–215
        encephalitis, 214–215
        meningitis, 214–215
    preparticipation physical evaluation, 148–149
    prevention, 202–203
    skin and soft tissue infections, 203–206
        bacterial skin infections, 203–205
        fungal skin infections, 205–206
        herpes simplex virus, 205
    unusual infections, 215–216
        leptospirosis, 215
        Naegleria fowleri, 215–216
        schistosomiasis, 216
    upper respiratory tract infections, 206–209
        infectious mononucleosis, 207–208
        measles, 208–209
    waterborne diseases and recreational water-related illness, 210–213
        cryptosporidiosis, 211–212
        fecally derived, 211
        infectious diarrhea, 212
        nonfecally derived, 213–214
Infectious mononucleosis (IM), 207–208
Inferior gluteal nerve, 916, 1032–1033, 1032*f*, 1032*t*
Inflammatory phase, of tendon and ligament repair, 4
Informed consent, 156, 156*t*
Infraclavicular block, 332
Inhalants, 293
Injections
    diagnostic, for athletic pubalgia, 1009
    knee arthritis, 1280
    lateral epicondylitis, 721*f*, 723
    medial epicondylitis, 721*f*, 723
    scapulothoracic disorders, 615, 615*f*
Injuries, 114–130
    acetabular labral, 313
    Achilles tendon, 1476–1482
        complications, 1482
        decision-making principles, 1478–1479
        future considerations, 1482
        history, 1476
        imaging, 1477–1478, 1478*f*
        physical examination, 1477, 1477*f*
        postoperative management, 1480–1481
        results, 1481–1482
        treatment options, 1479–1480, 1479*t*, 1480*b*–1481*b*, 1480*f*
    acromioclavicular joint, 645–678
        anatomy, 646*f*–647*f*, 646*t*
        classification, 645, 648*f*
        complications, 664

Injuries *(Continued)*
    decision-making principles, 653–655, 653*t*
    future considerations, 677
    history, 647–648, 649*f*
    imaging, 651–653, 652*f*, 654*f*–655*f*
    physical examination, 648–651, 650*t*, 651*f*
    postoperative management, 663–664
    results, 664, 665*t*–666*t*
    return-to-play guidelines, 663–664
    treatment, 655–659, 656*f*–658*f*
  ankle, in adolescent athlete, 1725–1740
  anterior cruciate ligament
    in female athlete, 307, 308*t*–309*t*, 309*f*
    knee, 1185–1198
  anterior tibial tendon, 1462–1464
    complications, 1464
    decision-making principles, 1462
    history, 1462
    imaging, 1462
    physical examination, 1462, 1463*f*
    postoperative management, 1463
    results, 1463–1464
    treatment options, 1462–1463, 1463*b*–1464*b*,
        1464*f*
  articular cartilage, 1484–1503
  back, 118–121, 126
  bone, 925–926
  brain, 1562–1569
    background, 1562–1564
    clinical presentation, 1563–1564
    definition, 1562–1563
    epidemiology, 1563
    imaging, 1566
    interventions, 1567–1568
    management, 1566–1567
    pathophysiology, 1563
    physical examination, 1564–1566
    retiring athlete, 1567
    return-to-play, 1567, 1567*t*
  carpal, 835–856
    anatomy, 835
    biomechanics, 835
    capitate, 843–845, 844*b*, 844*f*
    carpal instability, 848–851, 848*f*–850*f*, 850*b*
    future considerations, 854–855
    hamate, 840–843, 840*f*–843*f*, 843*b*
    Kienböck disease, 846–847
    ligament, anatomy and mechanics, 848–851,
        848*f*–850*f*, 850*b*
    lunate, 845–847, 846*f*, 847*b*
    lunotriquetral injuries, 848
    perilunate instability, 851–854, 851*f*–855*f*,
        853*b*
    pisiform, 847–848, 847*f*, 848*b*
    scaphoid, 835–836, 837*b*, 837*f*
    scapholunate injuries, 848
    trapezium, 838–840, 838*f*–840*f*, 840*b*
    trapezoid, 845, 845*b*
    triquetrum, 836–838, 838*b*, 838*f*
  cervical spine, 1578–1581
  chest, 123
  cold, 240–242
    frostbite, 241–242
    hypothermia, 240–241
  collateral ligament, 700–702
    imaging, 700–702, 701*f*
    lateral, 702, 703*f*
    ulnar, 701–702, 701*f*–702*f*
  concomitant, 1249
  dental, 269–270
    basketball, 116
    fractured teeth, 270
    handball, 122
    periodontal/displacement injuries (loose
        teeth), 270
    primary *vs.* permanent teeth, 269, 270*f*

Injuries *(Continued)*
  elbow
    baseball, 115
    golf, 119–120
    throwing, 757–771
  extensor mechanism, 1318–1334, 1330*b*
    anatomy, 1318–1319, 1319*f*
    biomechanics, 1319, 1320*f*
    clinical outcomes, 1331–1333
    complications, 1333
    decision-making principles, 1327
    future considerations, 1333
    history, 1322–1323
    imaging, 1324–1326
    patella, 1318–1319
    patellar and quadriceps tendon structure in,
        1320, 1320*f*–1321*f*
    patient evaluation, 1322–1326
    physical examination, 1323–1324
    postoperative management, 1330–1331
    quadriceps tendon, 1318
    treatment options, 1327–1330
  eyes, 269
    corneal abrasion, 269
    hyphema, 269
    iridodialysis, 269
    retinal detachment, 269
    ruptured globe, 269
  facial
    basketball, 116
    boxing, 116–117
    handball, 122
  finger
    basketball, 116
    volleyball, 127–128
  flexor hallucis longus, 1469–1472
    complications, 1471–1472
    decision-making principles, 1470
    future considerations, 1472
    history, 1469
    imaging, 1469, 1470*f*
    physical examination, 1469
    postoperative management, 1471
    results, 1471
    treatment options, 1470, 1470*b*, 1471*f*
  flexor pulley, 804
  foot, 1725–1740
  hamstrings, 1034–1042, 1035*f*
    complications, 1041–1042
    decision-making principles, 1037
    future considerations, 1042
    history, 1034–1035
    imaging, 1036–1037, 1036*f*–1037*f*
    physical examination, 1035–1036
    postoperative management, 1039–1040
        rehabilitation in, 1039–1040
    results, 1040–1041
    treatment options, 1037–1039
        nonoperative, 1037
        surgical, 1037–1039
        techniques, 1039*b*, 1039*f*–1040*f*
  hand
    basketball, 116
    golf, 120
  head
    football, 118
    ice hockey, 121
    on-field emergencies, 152
    in skeletally immature athletes, 1741–1748
  heat-related, 1609
  intrinsic carpal ligament, 810–812, 811*f*
  knee
    basketball, 115–116
    figure skating, 118
    lacrosse, 122
    rowing, 123

Injuries *(Continued)*
    skiing, 124
    swimming, 126
    volleyball, 127
  lateral corner, 1244–1263
  latissimus dorsi muscle, 576–578
    anatomy, 576
    classification, 576
    imaging, 576, 577*f*
    mechanisms of, 576
    physical examination, 576, 577*f*
    teres major, 578
    treatment, 576–578, 578*f*
  ligaments, 3–4
    collateral ligament injuries of
        metacarpophalangeal joint, 894–896,
        894*f*–896*f*
    distal interphalangeal joint, 888–890
    metacarpophalangeal joint, 883–885, 884*f*
    phalangeal fractures, 890–892, 891*f*–893*f*
    platelet-rich plasma for, 53–54
    proximal interphalangeal joint, 885–888,
        885*f*–890*f*
  limb-threatening, 154
    acute compartment syndrome, 154
    knee dislocation, 154
    traumatic amputation, 154
  lower back, 119
  lower extremity
    basketball, 115
    football, 118–119
    gymnastics, 120
    ice hockey, 121
    snowboarding, 125
    soccer, 125
    tennis, 126–127
  lumbar spine, 123
  lunotriquetral, 848
  medial collateral ligament, 1231–1243,
        1672–1673
  meniscal, 1703–1705
    anatomy, 1703
    complications, 1705
    decision-making principles, 1704
    development, 1703, 1703*f*
    future considerations, 1705
    history, 1703
    imaging, 1703–1704
    physical examination, 1703
    postoperative management, 1704–1705
    results, 1705
    treatment options, 1704
  muscle, 574–578
    latissimus dorsi, 576–578
    other, 574–578
    pectoralis major, 574–576
    platelet-rich plasma for, 56
  musculoskeletal, 128–129
    amputee athletes, 316
    cerebral palsy, 321
    intellectually disabled athletes, 322
    visually impaired athletes, 323
  neck, 118
  neurologic, 117, 718
  pectoralis major, 574–576
    anatomy, 574
    classification, 574–575
    imaging, 575
    mechanisms of, 574
    physical examination, 575
    treatment, 575–576, 576*f*
  pediatric. *See* Pediatrics
  peroneal tendon, 1472–1476
    complications, 1476
    decision-making principles, 1473–1474
    future considerations, 1476

Injuries (*Continued*)
  history, 1472
  imaging, 1473, 1473*f*
  physical examination, 1472–1473, 1472*f*
  postoperative management, 1475
  results, 1475–1476
  treatment options, 1474–1475, 1474*f*–1475*f*,
    1475*b*
  posterior cruciate ligament, 1211–1230,
    1220*b*–1222*b*, 1221*f*–1223*f*
  posterior medial corner, 1231–1243
    complications in, 1242
    decision-making principles, 1234–1235,
      1235*f*
    future considerations, 1243
    history, 1231
    imaging, 1232–1234, 1233*f*–1235*f*
    physical exam, 1231–1232
    postoperative management, 1239–1240
    results, 1240–1242
    return-to-play guidelines, 1240*b*
    treatment options, 1235–1236
  posterolateral corner, 1244–1263
  prevention, 344, 376–384
    ankle sprains, 380–381
    anterior cruciate ligament tears, 377–380,
      378*f*–379*f*
    biomechanics, 28
    hamstring muscle strains, 376
    taping for, 371
      ankle sprains, 371
      patellofemoral pain, 371
      plantar fasciitis, 371
      plantar fasciosis, 371
  psychological adjustment to, 272–276
    complications, 275
    decision-making principles, 273
    future considerations, 275
    historical perspective and evolution, 272–273
    postinjury management and outcome, 275
    preparticipation screening, 273
    treatment options, 274*b*
  pulley, 814
  return to activity and sport after, 385–391
  scapholunate, 848
  shoulder
    anterior instability, 453–454
    baseball, 114–115
    golf, 120
    handball, 122
    skiing, 124
    swimming, 126
    volleyball, 128
  soft tissue
    foot and ankle, 1728–1729, 1728*f*
    hip, 1691–1693
    wrestling, 129
  spine
    common acute, 1559–1560, 1560*f*
    emergency management, 1553–1561, 1559*f*
    epidemiology, 1553
    field-side management, 1553–1561,
      1554*f*–1558*f*
  sport-specific, 114–130. *See also* specific sports
    auto racing, 117
    baseball, 114–115
    basketball, 115–116
    boxing, 116–117
    figure skating, 117–118
    football, 118–119
    golf, 119–120
    gymnastics, 120–121
    handball, 121–122
    ice hockey, 121

Injuries (*Continued*)
    lacrosse, 122
    rowing, 123
    rugby, 123–124
    running, 124
    skiing, 124–125
    snowboarding, 124–125
    soccer, 125–126
    swimming, 126
    tennis, 126–127
    volleyball, 127–128
    wrestling, 128–129
  sternoclavicular joint, 664–677
    anatomy, 667, 667*f*–670*f*
    complications, 677
    decision-making principles, 668, 673*f*
    future considerations, 677
    history, 664
    imaging, 667–668, 670*f*–672*f*
    physical examination, 664–667
    postoperative management, 677
    results, 677
    return-to-play guidelines, 677
    treatment, 673
  stress, 942–944, 945*f*
  subscapularis, 556–566, 557*f*
    anatomy, 556–557
    classification, 558
    decision-making principles, 559–560
    function of, 557
    future considerations of, 565–566
    history, 558–559
    imaging, 559, 559*f*
    mechanism of, 557–558
    physical examination, 558–559, 558*f*
    treatment options, 560–565, 561*f*–562*f*
  tendon, 3–4, 873–882, 874*f*
    closed boutonnière (central slip rupture),
      875–877, 875*f*–877*f*
    complications, 881–882
    future considerations, 882
    Jersey finger, 878–880, 878*f*–880*f*
    mallet finger, 873–875, 874*f*
    platelet-rich plasma for, 53–54
    pulley injury, 880–881, 880*f*–881*f*
    sagittal band rupture, 877–878, 877*f*
  throwing, 757–771
    complications, 770
    decision-making principles, 760–761
    future considerations, 770
    history, 757–758, 758*f*
    imaging, 760, 761*f*
    physical examination, 758–760, 759*f*–760*f*
    postoperative management, 768
    results, 768–770
    return to play, 768
    treatment, 761–765
  thumb, 124
  triangular fibrocartilage complex, 813–814,
    813*f*–814*f*
  ulnar collateral ligament, 700–702
  upper extremity
    figure skating, 118
    football, 118
    gymnastics, 120
    ice hockey, 121
    rowing, 123
    snowboarding, 124–125
    soccer, 125
    tennis, 127
  weight-loss-related, 129
  wrist
    class I traumatic, 829–832, 829*f*–831*f*
    class II degenerative, 832

Injuries (*Continued*)
    golf, 120
    tendons, 812–813, 812*f*–813*f*
    volleyball, 127–128
  Innervation, of knee, 1072
  Insole, 1441
  Inspection
    elbow, 689
    hip, 929
    knee, 1091–1092, 1091*b*, 1091*f*–1092*f*
    patellofemoral pain, 1310–1311,
      1311*f*–1312*f*
    scapulothoracic disorders, 611–612
  Instability arthropathy, 592–595
    capsulorrhaphy arthropathy, 593, 593*f*
    chondrolysis, 593–594
    dislocation arthropathy, 593
    osteonecrosis, 595, 595*f*, 595*t*
    rheumatoid arthritis, 594–595, 594*f*
  Instruments. *See also* Equipment
    arthroscopic, 107
    hip arthroscopy, 948, 948*f*–949*f*
    knee arthroscopy, 1125
    radiofrequency, 108–109
    wrist arthroscopy, 817, 818*f*
  Insulin, 220, 221*t*
  Insulin analogs, 220
  Intellectually disabled athletes, 321–323
    adaptive equipment, 323
    exercise, 322
    medical considerations, 322–323
      cardiac abnormalities, 322–323
      epilepsy/seizures, 322
      musculoskeletal injuries, 322
      visual impairment, 322
  Interdigital nerve, magnetic resonance imaging,
    1389–1390, 1390*f*
  Interdigital neuralgia, 1416–1419
    complications, 1418–1419
    decision-making principles, 1418
    etiologies of, 1417
    history, 1417
    imaging, 1417–1418
    pathomechanism of, 1417
    physical examination, 1417
    postoperative management, 1418
    results, 1418
    treatment options, 1418, 1419*b*, 1419*f*
  Intermittent compression, 362, 362*f*
  Internal coxa saltans, 996–997
    author's preferred techniques, 998*b*, 998*f*
    complications, 997
    decision-making principles, 997, 997*b*
    history, 996
    imaging, 996–997
    physical examination, 996, 997*f*
    postoperative management, 997
    results, 997, 998*t*
    treatment options, 997
  Internal fixation, 1488, 1488*f*
  Internal impingement
    pathophysiology, 513, 513*f*
    treatment options, 517
  Internal rotators, of hip, 917
  Interscalene block, 330, 332*f*
  Intersection syndrome, 860–861, 860*f*
    return to sports, 861
    treatment options, 860–861, 861*b*
  Interventional radiology (IR), of spine,
    1550
  Intervertebral disks, 1534, 1593
  Intra-articular pathology, of hip, 927–928
  Intracerebral hematoma, 1745
  Intramembranous bone formation, 14

Intraoperative care, during anesthesia, 327–329.
    See also Regional anesthesia
  positioning, 329
  tourniquets, 328–329
Intraoral/tongue lacerations, 263
Intraosseous hypertension, of patella, 1316
Intravascular hemolysis, 196
Intrinsic carpal ligament injury, 810–812, 811*f*
Inversion recovery, 97–98, 97*f*
Iontophoresis, 360–361
Iridodialysis, 269
Iron, 279
Irritable bowel syndrome (IBS), 194
Ischemic conditions, of lower gastrointestinal
    tract, 194
Ischiofemoral distance (IFD), 911
Ischiofemoral impingement (IFI), 1003–1006
  complications for, 1006
  decision-making principles, 1004, 1005*b*, 1005*f*
  future considerations, 1006
  history, 1003–1004, 1004*f*
  imaging, 1004
  physical examination, 1004
  results, 1006
  treatment options, 1004–1006
Ischiofemoral ligament (ISFL), 914
Isokinetic strength testing, 386, 387*f*
Isolated structure reconstruction, 1255–1256
ITP. *See* Idiopathic thrombocytopenic purpura

J
Jammed finger, 1681–1683
  complications, 1683
  decision-making principles, 1682
  history, 1681
  imaging, 1682, 1682*f*
  physical examination, 1681–1682
  postoperative management, 1683
  results, 1683
  treatment options, 1682, 1682*b*
Jersey finger, 878–880, 878*f*–880*f*
Jobe's test, 546*f*
"Jock itch" (tinea cruris), 249, 250*f*
Jogger's foot, 1412
Joints
  biomechanics
    ankle, 1360–1363, 1361*f*–1362*f*
    cruciate ligaments, 1077–1079
    medial and lateral collateral ligaments,
        1079–1080
    patellofemoral, 1082–1087
    tibiofemoral, 1074–1080
  capsule
    hip, 914–916
    knee, 1071–1072, 1072*f*
  contact forces, ligament and, 21–22
  distal interphalangeal, 801–802, 803*f*
  elbow
    motion, 681–683
    stability, 683–685
  glenohumeral, 395–396, 395*f*–396*f*, 408–432
  hand, 787–789
    distal interphalangeal, 789, 789*f*
    metacarpophalangeal, of fingers, 787–788
    proximal interphalangeal, 788–789
    thumb, 789
  hip
    bursae around, 920–921
    muscles around, 916–920, 918*t*
    prenatal, development, 907
  metacarpophalangeal, 803–804
  metatarsophalangeal, 1365–1367, 1367*f*–1368*f*
  motions, 22–23, 23*f*
  proximal interphalangeal, 788–789, 802–803,
      804*f*

Joints *(Continued)*
  reaction force, 19, 19*f*–20*f*
  resurfacing techniques, 599–603, 600*f*–601*f*
  shoulder, 395–398
    acromioclavicular joint, 397
    glenohumeral, 395–396, 395*f*–396*f*
    glenohumeral joint capsule, 396–397
    scapulothoracic articulation, 398
    sternoclavicular joint, 397, 397*f*
  stability, 694–695, 1081–1082
  sternoclavicular, 664–677
    anatomy, 667, 667*f*–670*f*
    complications, 677
    decision-making principles, 668, 673*f*
    future considerations, 677
    history, 664
    imaging, 667–668, 670*f*–672*f*
    physical examination, 664–667
    postoperative management, 677
    results, 677
    return-to-play guidelines, 677
    treatment, 673
  subtalar, biomechanics, 1363–1365, 1363*t*,
      1364*f*–1366*f*
  transverse tarsal, 1365
Joint cryotherapy, 366
Joint loading, in articular cartilage repair, 11–12
Joint mobility, 350
Joint reactive forces, muscular contributions and,
    684–685, 685*f*
Joint space width, 938
Joint-sparing techniques, 598–599, 599*f*
J sign, dynamic change in, patellar instability and,
    1296, 1296*f*

K
Ketamine, perioperative pharmacology, 338
Kienböck disease, 810, 832–833, 832*t*, 833*f*,
    846–847
Kinematics, 22
  ankle joint, 1360–1363
  hip, 921–924
    gait cycle in, 921–922
    joint, forces around, 922–923
    motions in, 921
    spine and, relationship of, 923–924, 923*f*
    stability in, 921
  subtalar joint, 1363–1365, 1363*t*, 1364*f*–1366*f*
  transverse tarsal joints, 1365, 1367*f*
Kinetic chain, 1195–1196, 1196*f*
Kinetics, 23, 1359–1360, 1360*f*
Klippel-Feil syndrome, 1762
Knee
  anatomy, 1062–1063
    bursae, 1068–1069
    joint capsule, 1071–1072, 1072*f*
    ligaments, 1069–1071
    muscular, 1065–1068, 1066*f*
    neurovascular, 1072
    osseous, 1063–1065, 1064*f*
    superficial, 1062–1063, 1063*f*
    synovial membrane, 1071–1072, 1072*f*
  arthritis, 1277–1292
    decision-making principles, 1283–1284
    history, 1277, 1278*t*
    imaging, 1277–1279, 1278*f*–1279*f*
    nonoperative treatment, 1279–1280
    operative options for, 1280–1283
    postoperative management, 1289, 1289*t*
    results, 1289, 1290*t*
    treatment not recommended, 1280
    treatment options, 1279–1283, 1280*f*, 1284*f*
  arthroscopic synovectomy of, 1127–1131
    anesthesia, 1129
    complications, 1130

Knee *(Continued)*
    decision-making principles, 1128–1130,
        1128*f*–1129*f*
    future direction, 1130–1131
    history, 1127
    imaging, 1127–1128
    physical examination, 1127
    positioning, 1129
    postoperative management, 1130
    results, 1130
    surgical steps, 1129–1130
    technique, 1129*b*
    treatment options, 1128–1129
  arthroscopy, 1121–1126
    complications, 1125–1126
    diagnostic, 1123–1125, 1125*f*
    indications, 1121
    instrumentation, 1125
    portal placement, 1121–1123, 1122*f*–1124*f*
    positioning, 1121, 1122*f*
    postoperative care, 1125
    preoperative evaluation, 1121
  articular cartilage lesions, 1161–1177
    anatomy, 1161–1162
    biomechanics, 1161–1162
    classification, 1162, 1162*t*
    complications, 1176
    decision-making principles, 1163–1164
    future considerations, 1176–1177
    history, 1162–1163
    imaging, 1163
    physical examination, 1163
    postoperative management, 1166–1167
    results, 1174–1176
    return to play, 1167
    treatment options, 1164–1166, 1167*b*–1173*b*,
        1168*f*
  biomechanics, 1072–1073, 1073*f*
    joint, 1077–1080
    ligament, 1075–1077, 1076*f*
    meniscal, 1080–1082
    patellofemoral joint, 1082–1087
    techniques, 1073–1074, 1074*f*
    tibiofemoral joint, 1074–1080
  decision-making, 1089–1103, 1101*f*–1102*f*
  diagnosis, 1089–1103
  dislocation, 154, 1345–1349, 1346*f*
    anterior, 1345
    clinical presentation, 1346–1347, 1346*t*,
        1347*f*
    complications, 1349
    imaging, 1348
    physical examination and testing of,
        1347–1348, 1347*f*
    popliteal artery repair, 1349*b*
    posterior, 1345–1346
    postoperative management, 1349
    treatment options, 1348–1349
    vascular injury, 1346
  history, 1089–1091, 1090*t*
  imaging, 1104–1120
    background, 1104
    cartilage, 1116–1118, 1118*f*–1119*f*
    computed tomography, 1105*f*
    extensor mechanism, 1113–1116,
        1115*f*–1117*f*
    ligaments, 1110–1113, 1111*f*–1115*f*
    magnetic resonance imaging, 1105–1106
    menisci in, 1106–1109, 1106*f*–1109*f*
    musculotendinous structures, 1110, 1111*f*
    osseous structures, 1116–1118,
        1118*f*–1119*f*
    pitfalls, 1109–1110, 1110*f*
    postoperative, 1118–1120, 1119*f*–1120*f*
    radiographs, 1104, 1105*f*
    ultrasound, 1104–1105, 1106*f*

Knee *(Continued)*
  injuries
    basketball, 115–116
    figure skating, 118
    lacrosse, 122
    rowing, 123
    skiing, 124
    swimming, 126
    volleyball, 127
  inspection, 1091–1092, 1091*b*, 1091*f*–1092*f*
  instability, 1282
  lateral and posterolateral corner injuries,
      1244–1263
    anatomy, 1244–1248
    classification, 1248, 1248*t*
    complications in, 1260–1261, 1262*f*
    decision-making principles, 1253
    future considerations, 1262
    history, 1248–1249
    imaging, 1251–1253, 1251*f*–1252*f*
    layers of lateral side of, 1244
    nonoperative management, 1253
    pediatric, 1262
    physical examination, 1249–1251,
        1249*f*–1250*f*
    postoperative management, 1256–1260,
        1259*t*
    repair *vs.* reconstruction, 1253
    results, 1260, 1260*t*–1261*t*
    return to play, 1260
    structures, 1244–1246, 1245*f*
    surgical considerations, 1254–1256
    techniques, 1257*b*, 1257*f*–1258*f*
    timing of diagnosis, 1253
    treatment options, 1253–1256
  ligamentous stability in, 1097–1101,
      1098*f*–1101*f*
  meniscus, 1096–1097, 1097*f*
    injuries, 1132–1153
      arthroscopy, 1140
      biologic stimulation, 1147–1150
      classification, 1136–1137, 1136*f*–1137*f*
      complications, 1151–1152
      critical points in, 1152
      decision-making principles, 1142–1147
      future considerations, 1152
      history, 1137
      imaging, 1138–1139, 1138*f*
      physical examination, 1137–1138
      postoperative management, 1150–1151
      results, 1151
      return to play, 1151
      surgery for, 1139–1140, 1143–1147
      treatment options, 1139–1142
  motion, loss of, 1335–1344
    complications, 1342
    decision-making principles, 1337–1338,
        1337*t*, 1338*f*
    future considerations, 1343
    history, 1335–1336
    imaging, 1336–1337, 1337*f*
    physical examination, 1336, 1336*f*
    postoperative management, 1340–1342,
        1340*f*–1341*f*
    results, 1342
    return to sports and, 1342
    treatment options, 1338–1339, 1339*b*–1340*b*,
        1339*f*–1340*f*
  multiligament injuries, 1264–1276, 1269*b*–
      1273*b*, 1269*f*–1273*f*
    acute management, 1267
    complications, 1274
    decision-making principles, 1266–1267
    future considerations, 1274–1276

Knee *(Continued)*
    history, 1264
    imaging, 1265–1266, 1265*f*–1266*f*
    nonoperative treatment, 1266
    operative treatment, 1266
    physical examination, 1264–1265
    postoperative management, 1273–1274
    results, 1274, 1275*t*
    special considerations, 1267
    surgical timing of, 1266
    treatment options, 1267–1269
  palpation, 1092–1094, 1093*f*
  patella, 1095–1096, 1095*f*–1096*f*
  patellofemoral pain, 371, 1308–1317
  pediatrics, 1628–1633
    acute injuries, 1628–1630, 1629*f*–1630*f*
    injuries, 1697–1724
    osteochondroses, 1717–1718
    overuse injuries, 1630–1633, 1631*f*–1633*f*
  physical examination, 1091
  popliteal artery entrapment syndrome in,
      1349–1356
    classification, 1350–1351, 1350*f*
    clinical presentation, 1351
    complications, 1356
    criteria for return to play, 1356
    history, 1350
    imaging, 1352–1354, 1352*f*–1353*f*
    physical examination and testing of,
        1351–1352
    postoperative management, 1356
    treatment options, 1354–1356, 1355*f*,
        1356*b*
  range of motion of, 1094–1095, 1094*f*–1095*f*
  regional anesthesia, 332–333
  stability, 369–370, 370*f*
  strength testing, 1094–1095, 1094*f*–1095*f*
  synthesis in, 1101–1102, 1101*f*–1102*f*
  taping, 369–370
  vascular problems, 1345–1357
    dislocations of, 1345–1349, 1346*f*
    vascular problems of, 1345–1357
Knives, in arthroscopy, 108
Kohler syndrome, 1738, 1738*f*
Kyphotic thoracic spine, 1533

L

Labeled white blood cell scans, 89–90, 91*f*
Labrum, 427–431
  conditions, 939
  injuries, 967, 967*f*
  superior labrum, anterior, and posterior
      (SLAP) tears, 430–431, 430*f*, 431*t*
  tears, 941–942, 942*f*
    hip, 1614, 1614*f*
    pediatrics, 1693, 1693*f*
  variant, 939, 939*f*–941*f*
Lacerations
  face
    complex, 262–263, 264*f*
    lateral, 263, 265*f*
    intraoral/tongue, 263
    lip, 263, 264*f*
    mechanical dermatoses, 253–254
    periorbital, 263
Lacrosse injuries, 122
Lactate, 66
Lag signs, 404
Laryngopharyngeal reflux disease (LPRD), 190
Laser, 361–362
Latarjet-Patte coracoid transfer, 459*b*–461*b*, 460*f*,
    461
Lateral ankle ligament reconstruction, 1426*b*

Lateral ankle sprain, 1444–1450, 1445*f*
  classification, 1447*t*
  complications, 1450
  decision-making principles, 1447
  history, 1444–1446
  imaging, 1446–1447, 1447*f*
  physical examination, 1444–1446, 1446*f*, 1446*t*
  postoperative management, 1450
  results, 1450
  treatment, 1447–1449
    conservative, 1447–1448
    surgical, 1448–1449, 1448*f*
    technique, 1449*b*, 1449*f*
Lateral capsular ligament, mid-third, 1246
Lateral center edge angles, 937
Lateral clavicle physeal fractures, 1640–1642,
    1641*f*
  complications, 1642
  history, 1640
  imaging, 1641
  physical examination, 1640–1641
  results, 1642
  treatment options, 1641–1642, 1642*f*
Lateral closing wedge high tibial osteotomy, 1281,
    1282*t*
Lateral collateral ligaments, 684, 685*f*, 694,
    1079–1080
Lateral compartment osteoarthritis, 1284, 1284*f*
  osteotomy for, 1282
Lateral compartment release, 1399
Lateral corner injuries, 1244–1263
  anatomy, 1244–1248
  biomechanics, 1246, 1247*f*
  classification, 1248, 1248*t*
  complications in, 1260–1261, 1262*f*
  decision-making principles, 1253
  future considerations, 1262
  history, 1248–1249
  imaging, 1251–1253, 1251*f*–1252*f*
    magnetic resonance imaging, 1251–1253,
        1252*f*
    radiographs, 1251, 1251*f*
    ultrasound, 1253
  layers of lateral side of, 1244
  neurovascular structures, 1246
  nonoperative management, 1253
    grade I injuries, 1253
    grade II injuries, 1253
    grade III injuries, 1253
  pediatric, 1262
  physical examination, 1249–1251, 1249*f*–1250*f*
  postoperative management, 1256–1260,
      1259*t*
  repair *vs.* reconstruction, 1253
  results, 1260, 1260*t*–1261*t*
  return to play, 1260
  structures, 1244–1246, 1245*f*
    arcuate ligament complex, 1246
    biceps femoris muscle, 1245–1246
    biomechanics, 1246, 1247*f*
    fabellofibular ligament, 1246
    fibular collateral ligament, 1244–1245
    iliotibial band, 1244
    lateral gastrocnemius tendon, 1246
    mid-third lateral capsular ligament, 1246
    neurovascular, 1246
    popliteus tendon complex, 1245
  surgical considerations, 1254–1256
    diagnostic arthroscopy, 1254, 1254*f*
    primary repair, 1254, 1254*f*
    reconstruction techniques, 1254–1255
  techniques, 1257*b*, 1257*f*–1258*f*
  timing of diagnosis, 1253
  treatment options, 1253–1256

Lateral epicondylitis, 687, 702–704, 703f, 720–725, 1674–1676
  arthroscopy, 724
  complications, 725, 1676
  decision-making principles, 722, 1675
  future considerations, 725
  history, 720, 721t, 1675
  imaging, 721, 721f–722f, 1675
  physical examination, 720, 721f, 1675
  postoperative management, 724
  results, 724–725, 1675–1676
  return-to-play guidelines, 724
  splinting, 722
  treatment, 721f, 722–724, 1675
    injections, 721f, 723
    management, 724b
    splinting, 722
    surgery, 723–724, 723f
    therapy, 722–723
Lateral face lacerations, 263, 265f
Lateral gastrocnemius tendon, 1246
Lateral impingement test, 932
Lateral meniscus, 1069, 1069f
Lateral patella compression syndrome, 1316
Lateral plantar nerve entrapment, 1411–1412
  complications, 1412
  decision-making principles, 1411
  history, 1411
  imaging, 1411
  physical examination, 1411
  postoperative management, 1412
  results, 1412
  treatment options, 1411–1412, 1412b, 1412f
Lateral position, 933
Latissimus dorsi muscle, injuries to, 576–578
  anatomy, 576
  classification, 576
  imaging, 576, 577f
  mechanisms of, 576
  physical examination, 576, 577f
  teres major, 578
  treatment, 576–578, 578f
Lavage, 1487–1488
LCPD. See Legg-Calvé-Perthes disease
Left ventricle, 160
Leg
  decision-making, 1370–1379
  diagnosis, 1370–1379
  exertional compartment syndromes, 1393–1401, 1394t
    anatomy, 1393–1394, 1394f, 1394t
    classification, 1394–1395
    compartment testing, 1397–1398, 1397t
    complications, 1400
    decision-making principles, 1396–1397, 1396t–1397t
    diagnostics/imaging, 1395–1396, 1396f
    epidemiology, 1393
    history, 1395
    pathophysiology, 1394
    physical examination, 1395
    postoperative care, 1398
    results, 1400
    return to play, 1400
    treatment options, 1398
  history, 1372–1379, 1373f–1378f
  pain, 1393–1401, 1394t
    anatomy, 1393–1394, 1394f, 1394t
    classification, 1394–1395
    compartment testing, 1397–1398, 1397t
    complications, 1400
    decision-making principles, 1396–1397, 1396t–1397t
    diagnostics/imaging, 1395–1396, 1396f
    epidemiology, 1393
    history, 1395

Leg (Continued)
    pathophysiology, 1394
    physical examination, 1395
    postoperative care, 1398
    results, 1400
    return to play, 1400
    treatment options, 1398
  pathologies, 1370–1371
  physical examination, 1371–1372
Legg-Calvé-Perthes disease (LCPD), 928, 1693–1694, 1694f
Leptospirosis, 215
Les Autres group, 323
Lesions. See also specific lesions
  articular cartilage, 1161–1177
  osteochondral, 1388–1389, 1389f. See also Talus, osteochondral lesions of
  pathologic, 1691
Lesser trochanter, 911
Lesser tuberosity fractures, 1647
  complications, 1647
  history, 1647
  imaging, 1647
  physical examination, 1647
  treatment options, 1647, 1647f
Leukotriene modifiers, for exercise-induced bronchoconstriction, 177
Lift-off test, 404, 546f, 558–559
Ligaments, 2–7
  ankle, 1387–1388, 1388f
  anterior cruciate
    MRI, 1110–1111, 1111f–1112f
    partial tear, 1189
    revision, 1189–1190, 1192
  arcuate, 1246
  bifurcate, sprain, 1456–1457
    complications, 1458
    decision-making principles, 1457
    history, 1457
    imaging, 1457
    physical examination, 1457
    postoperative management, 1457
    results, 1457–1458
    treatment, 1457, 1457b
  biomechanics, 1075–1077, 1076f
  capsular, 914
  carpal injuries, 848–851, 848f–850f, 850b
  collateral, 1069–1071, 1079–1080
  cruciate, 1069, 1077–1079
    anterior, 1069, 1070f
    in joint biomechanics, 1077–1079
    posterior, 1069, 1070f
  fabellofibular, 1246
  fibular collateral, 1113, 1244–1245
  foot, 1387–1388, 1388f
  force measurement of, 1074–1075
  head, 1534
  healing
    factors affecting, 5, 6t
    methods for augmentation of, 5–7
  iliofemoral, 914, 915f
  imaging, 1110–1113, 1111f, 1115f
  injuries, 3–4
    ankle, 1444–1461
    collateral ligament injuries of metacarpophalangeal joint, 894–896, 894f–896f
    distal interphalangeal joint, 888–890
    foot, 1444–1461
    metacarpophalangeal joint, 883–885, 884f
    phalangeal fractures, 890–892, 891f–893f
    platelet-rich plasma for, 53–54
    proximal interphalangeal joint, 885–888, 885f–890f
  intrinsic carpal, 810–812, 811f
  ischiofemoral, 914, 915f

Ligaments (Continued)
  joint contact forces and, 21–22
  knee, 1069–1071
  lateral ankle, reconstruction, 1426b
  laxity, 1187–1188
    evaluation, 932
    untreated, revision anterior cruciate ligament injuries and, 1203
  medial collateral, MRI in, 1113, 1114f
  mid-third lateral capsular, 1246
  pediatrics, 1661–1662, 1662f–1663f, 1697–1703
  posterior cruciate, 1112
  pubofemoral, 914, 915f
  reconstruction, implants for, 38–41
  repair, 4–5
    platelet-rich plasma for, 53–55
  spine, 1534
  stability, in knee, 1097–1101, 1098f–1101f
  strain measurement of, 1075
  structure of, 2–3
  ulnar collateral, 701–702, 701f–702f, 804, 804f
    injuries, 814, 815f
Ligamentum teres, 912, 913f, 932–933
Lightning, 154
Limb-threatening injuries, 154
  acute compartment syndrome, 154
  knee dislocation, 154
  traumatic amputation, 154
Linear kinematics, 22
Lip lacerations, 263, 264f
Lisfranc sprains, 1458–1460
  complications, 1460
  decision-making principles, 1459
  history, 1458
  imaging, 1458–1459, 1459f
  physical examination, 1458
  postoperative management, 1459–1460
  results, 1460
  treatment, 1459, 1460b, 1460f
Little League elbow, 1612, 1612f, 1621–1623, 1622f–1623f, 1665–1668
  complications, 1668
  decision-making principles, 1667
  history, 1665–1666, 1665f
  imaging, 1667
  physical examination, 1666–1667
  results, 1668
  treatment options, 1667–1668
Little League shoulder, 1612, 1612f, 1655–1656
  complications, 1656
  history, 1656
  imaging, 1656, 1656f
  physical examination, 1656
  treatment, 1656
"Load and shift test", 405
Load transmission, 1080–1081
Local anesthetic agents, 334–335
  systemic toxicity, 334–335, 335t
Localization pain, 580, 580b
Log roll test, 932
Long thoracic nerve palsy, 625–627
  anatomy, 625, 625f
  biomechanics, 625, 625f
  clinical evaluation, 625–627, 626f
  decision-making principles, 627
  diagnostic studies, 627
  results, 627
  technique, 627b
Loose bodies, 700, 763–764
  removal, 712b, 712f–713f
Low-impact exercise, for knee arthritis, 1279
Lower back injuries, 119
Lower extremity
  injuries
    basketball, 115
    football, 118–119

Lower extremity (Continued)
  gymnastics, 120
  ice hockey, 121
  snowboarding, 125
  soccer, 125
  tennis, 126–127
  innervation, 332
  strength, restoration of, 386, 386f–387f
Lower gastrointestinal tract conditions, 192–195,
    193t
  celiac disease, 194–195
  diarrhea, 192–194
  irritable bowel syndrome, 194
  ischemic conditions, 194
  lower gastrointestinal bleeding, 194
Lower respiratory tract infections, 209–210
  acute bronchitis, 209
  acute pneumonia, 209–210
Lumbar disc herniation, 1599–1601, 1601f
Lumbar spine
  anatomy, 1598
  degenerative, 1598–1604
  injuries, 123
  stenosis, 1602–1603, 1602f
Lunate carpal injuries, 845–847, 846f, 847b
Lunotriquetral injuries, 848

M

Maddocks questions, 1744
Magnetic field strength, 99
Magnetic resonance angiography (MRA)
  elbow, 699
  popliteal artery entrapment syndrome,
    1352–1353, 1353f
Magnetic resonance arthrography, 99, 99f
  femoroacetabular impingement, 964
  hip dysplasia and instability, 974
  revision rotator cuff repair, 568
Magnetic resonance imaging (MRI), 92–100
  advantages, 102
  ankle, 1380–1381
    ligaments, 1387–1388, 1388f
  anterior tibial tendons, 1386, 1387f
  athletic pubalgia, 1010, 1010f–1011f
  contraindications, 102–103
  delayed gadolinium for, 101
  Dgemric, 101
  diffusion weighted imaging, 100, 100f
  disadvantages, 102, 102f
  dynamic contrast enhancement in, 101–103
  elbow, 698–699
  entrapment neuropathies, 742
  femoroacetabular impingement, 963–964,
    963f–964f
  flexor hallucis longus, 1384–1385, 1385f
  foot, 1380–1381
    ligaments, 1387–1388, 1388f
  glenohumeral joint, 412–414, 413f, 413t
    acromion, 415–417, 416f–418f, 417b
    osseous outlet, 415–417, 416f–418f, 417b
    rotator cuff, 419–422, 420f–424f, 423b
  hip, 939–946
    chondral injury, 942, 943f
    dysplasia and instability, 974
    femoroacetabular impingement, 942,
      944f
    hip sprain and dislocation, 942, 944f–945f
    labral conditions, 939
    labral variant, 939, 939f–941f
    labrum tear, 941–942, 942f
    stress injuries, 942–944, 945f
  iliopsoas, 979, 983–984
  interdigital nerve, 1389–1390, 1390f

Magnetic resonance imaging (MRI) (Continued)
  knee, 1105–1106
    arthritis, 1278–1279
    lateral and posterolateral corner injuries of
      knee, 1251–1253, 1252f
    medial collateral ligament and posterior medial
      corner injuries, 1232–1234, 1234f
    meniscal transplantation, 1155, 1155f
    multiligament knee injuries, 1265, 1266f
    osteochondral lesions, 1388–1389, 1389f
    patellar instability, 1298–1299, 1299f
    patellofemoral pain, 1313–1314, 1315f
  pediatrics
    of traumatic anterior instability, 1648–1649,
      1650f
    of traumatic posterior instability, 1652, 1653f
  peroneal tendon, 1385–1386, 1385f–1386f
  popliteal artery entrapment syndrome,
    1352–1353, 1353f
  posterior cruciate ligament injuries, 1214
  posterior tibial tendon, 1383–1384
  revision rotator cuff repair, 568
  scapulothoracic disorders, 614
  spine, 1547, 1547f
  technical considerations, 93–100
    artifacts, 98–99
    coils, 99–100, 100f
    contrast agents, 99, 99f
    fat suppression, 98, 99f
    image formation, 94–95
    image quality, 100
    imaging protocols, 93, 94f
    magnetic field strength, 99
    proton density, 95, 96f, 96t
    pulse sequences, 95–98
    T1, 95, 95f, 96t
    T2, 95, 96t
    tissue contrast, 95, 95f–96f, 96t
    ultrashort time to echo sequence for, 100–101
Malassezia, 250, 251f
Mallet finger, 873–875, 874f
Mandible fractures, 267, 267f
Manipulation, 363
  under anesthesia (MUA), 585–586
Manual therapy, 354–355, 355f, 356t
  for pain, 357, 358t
March hemoglobinuria, 196
Marfan syndrome, 169, 171f
Marijuana, 291–292
Marrow stimulation, 1164–1165, 1167b–1173b,
    1169f, 1174–1175
Mast cell stabilizers, for exercise-induced
    bronchoconstriction, 177
Matrix
  bone, 13
  extracellular, 11
    cell-matrix interactions, 11
    meniscus, 8
    tendons and ligaments, 3
Matrix-assisted chondrocyte implantation
    (MACI), 43
Maximum oxygen uptake (Vo₂ max)
  adrenal hormones and, 70
  in exercise capacity, 71
McCarthy test, 932
MCP joint. See Metacarpophalangeal (MCP)
    joints
MDI. See Multidirectional instability
Measles, 208–209
Measure, units of, 16, 17t
Mechanical dermatoses, 253–256
  abrasions/lacerations, 253–254
  acne mechanica, 254–255, 255f
  athlete's nodules (collagenomas), 255, 255f

Mechanical dermatoses (Continued)
  calluses and corns, 254
  friction blisters, 254
  hemorrhage, 254, 254f–255f
  hidradenitis suppurativa, 255–256, 256f
  striae, 254, 255f
Mechanics
  classes, 23–24
  fluid, 23–24
  rigid body, 23
  viscoelasticity and, 24, 24f–25f
Medial ankle sprains, 1450–1453
  complications, 1452–1453, 1453f
  decision-making principles, 1451
  history, 1450–1451
  imaging, 1451, 1451f
  physical examination, 1450–1451
  results, 1452
  treatment, 1452, 1452b
Medial clavicle
  excision, 675
  physeal fractures, 1642–1644, 1642f
    complications, 1644
    history, 1643
    imaging, 1643, 1643f
    physical examination, 1643
    treatment options, 1643–1644, 1644f
Medial collateral ligament (MCL), 694–695,
    694f–695f
  injuries, 1231–1243, 1672–1673
    complications, 1242, 1673
    decision-making principles, 1234–1235,
      1235f, 1672
    future considerations, 1243
    history, 1231, 1672
    imaging, 1232–1234, 1233f–1235f, 1672
    physical exam, 1231–1232, 1233f, 1233t
    physical examination, 1672
    postoperative management, 1239–1240,
      1239t
    results, 1240–1242, 1673
    return-to-play guidelines, 1240b
    treatment options, 1235–1236, 1236b–1238b,
      1236f–1238f, 1672–1673, 1673f
  joint biomechanics, 1079–1080
  knee, 1069–1070, 1070f
  MRI, 1113, 1114f
Medial collateral osteoarthritis, 1284b
Medial compartment osteoarthritis, 1283,
    1283t
  arthroplasty for, 1283
  osteotomy for, 1281, 1281f
Medial displacement calcaneal osteotomy, for
    posterior tibial tendon injury, 1467b–1468b
Medial epicondyle avulsion fractures, 1670–1672
  complications, 1672
  decision-making principles, 1671
  history, 1670–1671
  imaging, 1671
  physical examination, 1671, 1671f
  results, 1671–1672
  treatment, 1671
Medial epicondylitis, 688, 720–725, 751,
    1674–1676
  complications, 725, 1676
  decision-making principles, 722, 1675
  future considerations, 725
  history, 720, 721t, 1675
  imaging, 721, 721f–722f, 1675
  physical examination, 720, 721f, 1675
  postoperative management, 724
  results, 724–725, 1675–1676
  return-to-play guidelines, 724
  splinting, 722

Medial epicondylitis *(Continued)*
   treatment, 721*f*, 722–724, 1675
      injections, 721*f*, 723
      management, 724*b*
      splinting, 722
      surgery, 722–724, 723*f*
Medial meniscus, 1068
Medial opening wedge high tibial osteotomy,
   1281, 1282*t*, 1285*b*–1288*b*, 1285*f*–1288*f*
Medial patellofemoral reconstruction, 1301*b*–
   1302*b*, 1302*f*–1303*f*
Medial plantar nerve entrapment, 1412–1413
   decision-making principles, 1413
   history, 1412
   imaging, 1413
   physical examination, 1412
   postoperative management, 1413
   treatment options, 1413
Medial tibial stress syndrome (MTSS), 1393
Median nerve, 743–745, 744*f*
   AIN syndrome, 746–747
      complications, 747
      decision-making principles, 746
      history, 746
      physical examination, 746
      postoperative management, 747
      results, 747
      return-to-play guidelines, 747
      treatment, 746
   pronator syndrome, 745–746
      complications, 746
      decision-making principles, 745
      history, 745
      physical examination, 745
      postoperative management, 745–746
      results, 746
      return-to-play guidelines, 745–746
      technique, 746*f*
      treatment, 745
Median nerve compression, elbow, 693–694
Medical home, of elite athlete, 159–160
Medical nutrition therapy, 219–220
Medications. *See also* Drugs
   cerebral palsy, 321
   preparticipation physical evaluation, 149
Medicine. *See also* Medications; Nuclear medicine
   gastrointestinal, 189–195
      lower gastrointestinal tract conditions,
         192–195, 193*t*
      pathophysiology, 189
      upper gastrointestinal tract conditions,
         189–192
   hematologic, 196–200
      hemostasis disorders, 198–200
      red blood cells disorders, 196–198
Meningitis, 214–215
   aseptic, waterborne diseases, 212–213
   classification, 214
   definition, 214
   diagnosis, 214–215
   epidemiology, 214
   pathobiology, 214
   prevention, 215
   return-to-play guidelines, 215
   treatment, 215
Meningoencephalitis, 214
Meniscal insufficiency
   history, 1154
   physical examination, 1154–1155, 1155*f*
   treatment options, 1156–1158, 1157*b*
      bone plug and trough, 1158
      diagnostic arthroscopy, 1157
      nonoperative management, 1156
      operative management, 1156
      positioning, 1157
Meniscal regeneration, 9

Meniscal transplantation, 1154–1160
   complications, 1159–1160
   contraindications, 1156
   contributing factors, 1156, 1156*f*
   decision-making principles, 1155–1156
   future considerations, 1160
   imaging, 1155
   indications, 1155–1156
   lateral, 1157, 1157*f*
   medial, 1157–1158, 1158*f*
   pathophysiology, 1155–1156
   postoperative management, 1159
   results, 1159
Meniscectomy, 1143–1144, 1144*f*
Meniscus, 7–9, 1068–1069, 1068*f*
   allograft transplantation, 1142
   anatomy, 1132–1134, 1133*f*–1134*f*
   biomechanics, 1080–1082, 1134–1135, 1135*f*
   cysts, 1140
   discoid, 1140–1142, 1141*f*–1142*f*
   epidemiology, 1135–1136
   extracellular matrix, 8
   function of, 1134–1135, 1135*f*
   history, 1132
   injuries, 8–9, 1132–1153, 1703–1705
      anatomy, 1703
      arthroscopy, 1140
      biologic stimulation, 1147–1150
      classification, 1136–1137, 1136*f*–1137*f*
      complications, 1151–1152, 1705
      critical points in, 1152
      decision-making principles, 1142–1147,
         1704
      development, 1703, 1703*f*
      future considerations, 1152, 1705
      history, 1137, 1703
      imaging, 1138–1139, 1138*f*, 1703–1704
      physical examination, 1137–1138, 1703
      postoperative management, 1150–1151,
         1704–1705
      results, 1151, 1705
      return to play, 1151
      revision anterior cruciate ligament injuries,
         1203
      surgery for, 1139–1140, 1143–1147
      treatment options, 1139–1142, 1704
   in joint stability, 1081–1082
   knee, 1096–1097, 1097*f*, 1106–1109,
      1106*f*–1109*f*
   lateral, 1069, 1069*f*
      fascicular tears, 1140
   load transmission, 1080–1081
   medial, 1068
   pediatrics
      anatomy, 1703
      discoid, 1705–1708
      injuries, 1703–1705
   repair, 9
      all-inside, 1147, 1148*f*
      augmentation in, 9
      in avascular portions, 9
      basics of, 1144
      cell-based approaches, 1149
      factors affecting, 9
      implants for, 41–42
      inside-out, 1144–1146, 1145*f*–1146*f*
      outside-in, 1146–1147, 1147*f*
      platelet-rich plasma, 55–56
      scaffolds for, 9, 1149–1150
      stem cell-based therapy, 60
      techniques, 1143*b*, 1143*f*
      in vascular regions, 9
   root tears, 1140
   structure of, 7–8, 7*f*, 1132–1134, 1133*f*–1134*f*
   variants, 1140–1142, 1141*f*–1142*f*
Meralgia paresthetica, 927

Mesenchymal stem cells (MSCs)
   in allograft, 32
   silk-based scaffold and, 39
   three-dimensional matrices, 1181–1182
Metabolism, energy, 65–66, 65*f*
Metacarpal fracture, 814–815, 815*f*
Metacarpophalangeal (MCP) joints, 803–804
   collateral ligament injuries of, 894–896,
      894*f*–896*f*
   fingers, 787–788
   ligamentous injuries and dislocations, 883–885,
      884*f*
Metatarsal
   break, 1365–1367, 1367*f*–1368*f*
   first, osteochondral lesions of, 1501, 1502*f*
   stress fractures, 135–136
Metatarsalgia, 1519–1522
   complications, 1522
   decision-making principles, 1520
   future considerations of, 1522
   history, 1519
   imaging, 1520
   physical examination, 1519–1520
   postoperative management, 1521–1522
   results, 1522
   treatment options, 1520–1521
      nonoperative, 1520–1521
      operative, 1521, 1521*f*
      technique, 1522*b*, 1522*f*
Metatarsophalangeal arthrodesis, 1525, 1525*f*
Metatarsophalangeal joint, 1365–1367,
   1367*f*–1368*f*
Methadone, perioperative pharmacology, 337
Methicillin-resistant *Staphylococcus aureus*
   (MRSA), skin infections, 203–204, 204*f*
Microfracture, 1164–1165, 1487–1488
Microinstability, atraumatic hip, 977–978
Mid-anterior portal, modified, in hip arthroscopy,
   951, 951*f*
Midface fractures, 267–268
Midsole, 1440–1441
Minced cartilage techniques, 1182, 1183*f*
Mineralization, endochondral bone formation
   and, 14
Mitochondrial respiration, 66
Mobilization, 363, 364*f*–365*f*
   with movement, 363–365, 365*f*
Modalities. *See* Imaging
Modified mid-anterior portal, in hip arthroscopy,
   951, 951*f*
Modified Thomas test, 933
Molluscum contagiosum, 252, 252*f*
Moment/torque vectors, 21
Montelukast, for exercise-induced
   bronchoconstriction, 177
Morton neuroma, 1416–1419
   complications, 1418–1419
   decision-making principles, 1418
   etiologies of, 1417
   history, 1417
   imaging, 1417–1418
   pathomechanism of, 1417
   physical examination, 1417
   postoperative management, 1418
   results, 1418
   treatment options, 1418, 1419*b*, 1419*f*
Mosaicplasty, 1488
Motion. *See also* Range of motion
   dorsiflexion range of, 381
   elbow, 681–683, 690, 772–784
      arthroscopy, 776–781, 777*f*–781*f*
      complications, 782–783
      decision-making principles, 774–776, 775*f*
      follow-up, 782
      history, 772–773
      imaging, 774, 774*f*

Motion *(Continued)*
  physical examination, 773–774
  postoperative management, 782
  rehabilitation, 782
  results, 782–783, 783*t*
  return-to-play guidelines, 782
  surgery, 776–782, 777*f*
  treatment, 774–776, 775*f*
 hip, 921
 joint, 22–23, 23*f*
  mobility, 350
 loss, knee, 1335–1344
  complications, 1342
  decision-making principles, 1337–1338,
    1337*t*, 1338*f*
  future considerations, 1343
  history, 1335–1336
  imaging, 1336–1337, 1337*f*
  physical examination, 1336, 1336*f*
  postoperative management, 1340–1342,
    1340*f*–1341*f*
  results, 1342
  return to sports and, 1342
  treatment options, 1338–1339, 1339*b*–1340*b*,
    1339*f*–1340*f*
 maintenance of, 349–350
 relative, 22
 restoration of, 349–350
 rolling, 22–23, 23*f*
 sliding, 22–23, 23*f*
 spinning, 22–23, 23*f*
 throwing, 1663–1665, 1663*f*–1664*f*
 varus, 1246–1247
Motion-sparing procedures, in advanced
  degeneration, 1525
Motor testing, for ankle, foot, and leg,
  1374–1375
Motor unit, 62
Motorized shavers, 107–108
MRA. *See* Magnetic resonance angiography
MRI. *See* Magnetic resonance imaging
MSCs. *See* Mesenchymal stem cells (MSCs)
Multibody dynamics, 922, 922*f*
Multidirectional instability (MDI), 476–488, 482*b*,
  482*f*, 1654–1655
 decision-making principles, 479–480
 future considerations, 480–481
 history, 477, 1654
 imaging, 479, 479*f*, 1655, 1655*f*
 physical examination, 477–479, 477*t*–478*t*, 478*f*,
  1654–1655, 1654*f*
 postoperative management, 481–483, 483*f*
 results, 483–487, 484*t*–485*t*
  complications, 486–487
  return to sport, 485–486, 486*t*
 treatment options, 480–481, 1655, 1655*f*
  arthroscopic plication, 481
  open inferior capsular shift, 480–481, 480*f*
Multiligament knee injuries, 1264–1276,
  1269*b*–1273*b*, 1269*f*–1273*f*
 acute management, 1267
 complications, 1274
 decision-making principles, 1266–1267
 future considerations, 1274–1276
 history, 1264
 imaging, 1265–1266, 1265*f*–1266*f*
 nonoperative treatment, 1266
 operative treatment, 1266
 physical examination, 1264–1265
 postoperative management, 1273–1274
 results, 1274, 1275*t*
 special considerations, 1267
 surgical timing of, 1266
 treatment options, 1267–1269

Muscles
 balance of, patellar instability and, 1296–1297,
  1297*f*
 biceps femoris, 1245–1246
  long head of, 1245–1246
  short head of, 1246
 cramps, exercise-associated, 236–237
 delayed-onset soreness of, 68
 elbow, 681
 energy technique, 366–367
 fatigue, 67
 fibers, classification, 62, 63*t*
 hand, 785–787, 788*f*
 head, 1534
 hip joint, 916–920, 918*t*
  abductors, 917
  adductors, 920
  extensors, 919–920
  external rotators, 920
  flexors, 917–919
  internal rotators, 917
 injuries
  latissimus dorsi, 576–578
  other, 574–578
  pectoralis major, 574–576
 knee, 1065–1068, 1066*f*
  anterior, 1066
  lateral, 1068
  medial, 1067–1068, 1067*f*
  posterior, 1066–1067, 1067*f*
 pediatrics, 1691
 performance
  restoration of, 350–351
   hypertrophy *vs.* motor learning, 350–351
   inhibition/activation, 350
 shoulder
  rotator cuff, 398–399, 398*f*
  scapular muscles, 399
 spine, 1534
 training, 66–67, 1195–1196, 1196*f*
Musculoskeletal system
 injuries, 128–129
  amputee athletes, 316
  cerebral palsy, 321
  intellectually disabled athletes, 322
  visually impaired athletes, 323
  wheelchair athletes, 318
 preparticipation physical evaluation, 148, 148*b*
 tissues
  articular cartilage, 9–12
  bone, 12–15
  meniscus, 7–9
  physiology pathophysiology, 2–15
  tendon and ligament in, 2–7
 ultrasound, 79–83, 80*f*–83*f*
Mycobacterial infections, 252
Mycobacterium marinum (swimming pool or fish
  tank granuloma), 252, 252*f*
Myelography, of spine, 1548
Myelopathy, cervical, 1595–1596
Myocarditis, 169, 171*f*
myofascial release, 367
Myositis ossificans, 1046–1047, 1046*f*

N

Naegleria fowleri, 215–216
Nanofiber scaffolds, 37–38
Nasal fractures, 266–267, 266*f*–267*f*
Natural supplements, 1611
Nausea, 192
Navicular stress fractures, 136, 137*f*
Neck shaft angle, 909, 936–937
Neer test, 404, 545*f*

Nerve entrapment, 621–631
 ankle, 1389–1391, 1390*f*–1391*f*
 axillary nerve palsy, 629–630
  anatomy, 629
  biomechanics, 629
  clinical evaluation, 629–630
  decision-making principles, 630
  diagnostic studies, 630
  results, 630
 deep peroneal nerve, 1415–1416, 1415*f*
  history, 1415
  imaging, 1416
  physical examination, 1415–1416
  postoperative management, 1416
  results, 1416
  treatment options, 1416, 1416*b*
 foot, 1389–1391, 1390*f*–1391*f*
 hip, 927
 interdigital neuralgia (Morton neuroma),
  1416–1419
  complications, 1418–1419
  decision-making principles, 1418
  etiologies of, 1417
  history, 1417
  imaging, 1417–1418
  pathomechanism of, 1417
  physical examination, 1417
  postoperative management, 1418
  results, 1418
  treatment options, 1418, 1419*b*, 1419*f*
 lateral plantar nerve, 1411–1412
  complications, 1412
  decision-making principles, 1411
  history, 1411
  imaging, 1411
  physical examination, 1411
  postoperative management, 1412
  results, 1412
  treatment options, 1411–1412, 1412*b*,
   1412*f*
 long thoracic nerve palsy, 625–627
  anatomy, 625, 625*f*
  biomechanics, 625, 625*f*
  clinical evaluation, 625–627, 626*f*
  decision-making principles, 627
  diagnostic studies, 627
  results, 627
  technique, 627*b*
 medial plantar nerve, 1412–1413
  decision-making principles, 1413
  history, 1412
  imaging, 1413
  physical examination, 1412
  postoperative management, 1413
  treatment options, 1413
 peripheral, 1402–1419
 saphenous nerve, 1405–1407, 1405*f*–1406*f*
  history, 1405
  imaging, 1406
  physical examination, 1405–1406
  results, 1406–1407
  treatment options, 1406
 shoulder, 621
 spinal accessory nerve palsy, 627–629
  anatomy, 627–628
  biomechanics, 627–628
  clinical evaluation, 628–629, 628*f*
  decision-making principles, 629
  diagnostic studies, 629
  results, 629
  technique, 629*b*
 superficial peroneal nerve, 1413–1415, 1413*f*
  decision-making principles, 1414
  history, 1413

Nerve entrapment (Continued)
   imaging, 1414
   physical examination, 1413–1414
   postoperative management, 1415
   results, 1415
   treatment options, 1414–1415, 1414b, 1414f
   suprascapular nerve palsy, 621–625
      anatomy, 621–622, 622f
      biomechanics, 621–622, 622f
      clinical evaluation, 622–623, 623f
      decision-making principles, 624
      diagnostic studies, 623–624, 623f
      results, 624–625
   sural nerve, 1402–1405, 1403f
      history, 1402
      imaging, 1403–1404
      physical examination, 1402–1403
      postoperative management, 1405
      results, 1405
      treatment options, 1404, 1404b, 1404f
Nerves. See also Neuropathies
   accessory obturator, 916
   capsular innervation, 914–916
      accessory obturator nerve, 916
      femoral nerve, 916
      inferior gluteal nerve, 916
      obturator nerve, 916
      quadratus femoris, nerve to, 916
      sciatic nerve, 916
      superior gluteal nerve, 916
   femoral, 916
   hand, 785, 787f
   inferior gluteal, 1032–1033, 1032f, 1032t
   median, 743–745, 744f
      AIN syndrome, 746–747
      pronator syndrome, 745–746
   obturator, 916
   quadratus femoris, 916
   radial, 752
      PIN syndrome, 755–756
      radial tunnel syndrome, 752–755, 753f
   sciatic, 1018–1020, 1019f–1020f
   superior gluteal, 1032–1033, 1032f, 1032t
   ulnar, 747, 748f. See also Cubital tunnel
      syndrome
Neuraxial anesthesia, 329
Neurologic infections, 214–215
   encephalitis, 214–215
   meningitis, 214–215
Neurologic system
   assessment, 690–691, 691f
   injuries, 117, 718
   preparticipation physical evaluation, 148
   tissues, 1534–1535, 1534f
Neuroma, 317
   Morton, 1416–1419
      complications, 1418–1419
      decision-making principles, 1418
      etiologies of, 1417
      history, 1417
      imaging, 1417–1418
      pathomechanism of, 1417
      physical examination, 1417
      postoperative management, 1418
      results, 1418
      treatment options, 1418, 1419b, 1419f
Neuromuscular electrical stimulation, 366
Neuromuscular training, 69
Neuropathies
   entrapment, 742–756
      complications, 743
      decision-making principles, 743
      history, 742
      imaging, 742
      median nerve, 743–745, 744f
      physical examination, 742

Neuropathies (Continued)
      postoperative management, 743
      radial nerve, 752, 753f
      testing, 742–743
      treatment, 743
      ulnar nerve, 747, 748f. See also Cubital
         tunnel syndrome
   wrist and hand, 898–905
      decision-making principles, 901
      future considerations, 904
      history, 898
      imaging, 900–901, 900f, 901t
      physical examination, 898–900, 899f–900f
      postoperative management and return to
         play, 902–903, 903b, 903f
      results, 903–904
         complications, 904
      treatment options, 901–902
Neurovascular anatomy, of knee, 1072
Neutral Ober test, 933
Newton's laws, 17–19, 17t
   first law (inertia), 17, 17t, 18f
   second law (acceleration), 17–19, 17t, 18f
   third law (action-reaction), 19, 19f–20f
Night pain, in stiff shoulder, 580, 580b
90-degree Dunn view, 935, 937f
Noncontact anterior cruciate ligament injury, in
   female athlete, 307–309, 308f, 310f
Nonfecally derived waterborne diseases, 213–214
   acute otitis externa, 213–214
   hot tub folliculitis, 213
   Pseudomonas infections, 213
Nonoperative sling immobilization, 455
Nonsteroidal antiinflammatory drugs (NSAIDs)
   dyspepsia, 191–192
   knee arthritis, 1279
   perioperative pharmacology, 338
Nonthermal ultrasound treatments, 360–363
   compression, 362, 362f
   iontophoresis, 360–361
   laser, 361–362
   phonophoresis, 360
   range of motion, 362
   stress fracture healing, 360, 361f
   superficial heat, 362–363
Nose, preparticipation physical evaluation, 145
NSAIDs. See Nonsteroidal antiinflammatory
   drugs
Nuclear medicine, 88–92
   advantages, 90, 93f
   bone scans in, 88–89, 89f
   disadvantages, 90–92, 94f
   gallium scans in, 90, 92f–93f
   labeled white blood cell scans in, 89–90, 91f
   PECT/CT scans, 90, 93f
   planar imaging, 88, 89f
   SPECT/CT imaging, 88, 89f
   technical considerations, 88
Nuclear scintigraphy, of spine, 1548–1549, 1549f
Nutrition
   carbohydrates, 277–278, 278t
   fat, 277–278, 278t
   gastrointestinal tract conditions, 189
   hydration, 278–279, 279t
      considerations, 278
      in female athlete, 296–298, 297t–298t
      gastrointestinal tract conditions, 189
      monitoring, 278–279
   pediatrics, 1610–1611

O
Ober testing, 933
Obstructive sleep apnea (OSA), 325–326, 326f
Obturator nerve, of hip, 916
Occult fracture, 699, 700f

OCD. See Osteochondritis dissecans (OCD)
OCLs. See Osteochondral lesions
Odontoid fractures, 1761–1762
   classification, 1761
   history, 1761
   imaging, 1761–1762, 1761f
   physical examination, 1761
   treatment, 1762
Off-the-shelf surface allograft transplantation,
   1182–1184, 1183f
OHAs. See Oral hypoglycemic agents
Olecranon bursitis, 728–730, 728f
   complications, 730
   decision-making principles, 728–729
   future considerations, 730
   history, 728, 728f
   imaging, 728, 729f
   physical examination, 728
   postoperative care, 730
   results, 730
   treatment, 729, 729b, 729f
Olecranon osteochondrosis, 1673–1674, 1673f
   complications, 1674
   decision-making principles, 1674
   history, 1674
   imaging, 1674
   physical examination, 1674
   results, 1674
   treatment, 1674
Olecranon process, 684, 684f
Olecranon stress fracture, 764–765, 764f–765f
On-field emergencies, 150–155
   anaphylaxis, 153
   anterior shoulder instability, 454–455
   cardiac arrest, 153
   cervical spine injuries, 152–153, 1578
   for collapsed athlete, 151–152, 151t
   emergency action plan, 150, 151b
   environmental factors, 154
   head injury, 152
   limb-threatening injuries, 154
      acute compartment syndrome, 154
      knee dislocation, 154
      traumatic amputation, 154
   tension pneumothorax, 153
Open biceps tenodesis, 532
Open inferior capsular shift, 480–481, 480f
Open kinetic chain, 1195–1196, 1196f
Operating room set-up, in hip arthroscopy,
   948–950
Opioids, perioperative pharmacology, 337
Oral hypoglycemic agents (OHAs), 220
Orbital fractures, 268, 268f
Orthobiologics, 50–61
   platelet-rich plasma
      in cartilage restoration, 55
      composition, 50–53, 52f, 52t
      definitions, 50
      growth factors, 51, 53t
      ligament-related disorders/repair, 53–55
      in meniscal repair, 55–56
      for muscle injuries, 56
      preparation, 50–53, 52f, 52t
      properties of, 50
      sports medicine and, 50–53, 51f
      tendon-related disorders/repair, 53–55
   stem cell-based therapy
      application, 58
      in cartilage repair, 59–60
      definitions, 56–58, 57f–58f
      in meniscal repair, 60
      preparations, 56–58, 57f–58f
      in sports medicine, 56–58, 57f
Orthopaedic injuries, in female athlete, 304–314
   acetabular labral injuries, 313
   ankle, 305–306

Orthopaedic injuries, in female athlete (*Continued*)
  anterior cruciate ligament
    injuries, 307, 308t–309t, 309f
    reconstruction, 310
  epidemiology, 304–305
  femoroacetabular impingement, 313
  foot, 305–306, 305t, 306f
  frozen shoulder/adhesive capsulitis, 310–312, 311t
  idiopathic scoliosis, 313–314
  noncontact anterior cruciate ligament injury, 307–309, 308f, 310f
  patellofemoral pain syndrome, 306–307, 306t
  shoulder instability, 312–313, 312f
  stress fractures, 314
Orthopaedic surgeries, 327
Orthoses, foot, 1436–1439
  clinical application, 1437–1439, 1438t–1439t, 1440f
  research in, 1436–1437, 1437f
Orthotics, 372–374, 1739
  foot evaluation, 372
  materials, 373, 373f
  overuse issues, 373–374
  types, 373, 373f
OSA. *See* Obstructive sleep apnea
Osgood-Schlatter disease, 1717–1718, 1717f
Osseous, 680, 681f
  knee, 1063–1065, 1064f, 1116–1118, 1118f–1119f
    femur, 1064–1065, 1065f
    patella, 1065, 1065f–1066f
    tibia, 1065
  outlet, 415–417, 416f–418f, 417b
    imaging, 414–415, 414f
Ossification
  appositional, 14
  heterotopic, 317, 319, 718
Ossified posterior longitudinal ligament (OPLL), 1597, 1597f
Osteitis pubis, 1007, 1014–1016
  complications, 1016
  nonoperative management, 1014–1015
  operative management, 1015–1016
  treatment, 1016b
Osteoarthritis
  lateral compartment, 1284, 1284f
  medial collateral, 1284b
  medial compartment, 1283, 1283t
    arthroplasty for, 1283
    osteotomy for, 1281, 1281f
  primary, 592
  tricompartmental, arthroplasty for, 1283
Osteoarticular stability, elbow, 683–684, 683f–684f
Osteoblasts, 13
Osteochondral allografts, 1488–1489
  transplantation, 1166, 1173f–1174f, 1176
Osteochondral autografts, 1488–1489
  transfer, 1165, 1167b–1173b, 1169f–1171f, 1175
Osteochondral lesions (OCLs)
  distal tibial plafond, 1500–1501, 1500f–1501f
  first metatarsal, 1501, 1502f
  imaging, 1388–1389, 1389f
  talus, 1484–1500, 1734–1737
    decision-making principles, 1486, 1486f–1487f
    diagnosis, 1484–1486
    history, 1484
    imaging, 1484–1486, 1485f
    physical examination, 1484
    postoperative management, 1500
    results, 1490–1493, 1490b

Osteochondral lesions (OCLs) (*Continued*)
    return to play, 1500
    treatment options, 1486–1490
Osteochondral repair, implants for, 42–45
Osteochondritis dissecans (OCD), 1668–1670
  complications, 1670
  débridement, 714b–715b, 714f
  decision-making principles, 1669, 1669t
  history, 1668
  imaging, 1668–1669, 1669f
  knee, 1614f–1615f
  lesions, 1164
  pediatrics, 1712–1717
    complications, 1716–1717
    decision-making principles, 1714–1715
    etiology, 1712
    future considerations, 1717
    history, 1712, 1713f
    physical examination, 1712, 1713f
    radiographs, 1713–1714, 1713f–1714f
    results, 1715–1716
    treatment options, 1715, 1716b, 1716f
  physical examination, 1668
  results, 1670
  suture fixation, 715b–716b
  treatment, 1669–1670
Osteochondrosis, 1668–1670
  complications, 1670
  decision-making principles, 1669, 1669t
  in foot, 1737–1739, 1738f–1739f
  history, 1668
  imaging, 1668–1669, 1669f
  knee, 1717–1718, 1717f–1718f
  olecranon, 1673–1674, 1673f
    complications, 1674
    decision-making principles, 1674
    history, 1674
    imaging, 1674
    physical examination, 1674
    results, 1674
    treatment, 1674
  physical examination, 1668
  results, 1670
  superior pole, 1718
  treatment, 1669–1670
Osteoclasts, 13
Osteocytes, 13
Osteology, 1661, 1662f
Osteonecrosis, 595, 595f, 595t
Osteopenia, 299–301, 300f, 300t
Osteoperiosteal bone graft, 1489
Osteoporosis, 299–301, 300f, 300t
Osteotomy, 1524–1525
  distal femoral, 1282
  femoral, 1301
  high tibial
    for chronic PCL injuries, 1219–1220
    lateral closing wedge, 1281, 1282t
    medial opening wedge, 1281, 1282t, 1285b–1288b, 1285f–1288f
    patient satisfaction after, 1283
  hip arthritis, 1058
  knee arthritis, 1281–1283, 1281b
  lateral compartment osteoarthritis, 1282
  medial displacement calcaneal, for posterior tibial tendon injury, 1467b–1468b
  proximal tibial, 1255, 1255f, 1259b, 1259f, 1282
  return to sport after, 1283
  tibial tuberosity, 1300–1301, 1305b
Outsole, 1440
Overt diabetes, 218
Overuse injuries, pediatrics, 1655–1659
Oxidative system, 66

P
PAES. *See* Popliteal artery entrapment syndrome
Paget-Schroetter syndrome, 633
Pain
  back, 128, 1598
  chronic, 580, 580b
  combined with instability
    arthroplasty for, 1283
    osteotomy for, 1282–1283
  leg, 1393–1401, 1394f
    anatomy, 1393–1394, 1394f, 1394t
    classification, 1394–1395
    compartment testing, 1397–1398, 1397t
    complications, 1400
    decision-making principles, 1396–1397, 1396t–1397t
    diagnostics/imaging, 1395–1396, 1396f
    epidemiology, 1393
    history, 1395
    pathophysiology, 1394
    physical examination, 1395
    postoperative care, 1398
    results, 1400
    return to play, 1400
    treatment options, 1398
  localization, 580, 580b
  modulation, 357, 357t
  night, 580, 580b
  patellofemoral, 371, 1308–1317
    anatomy, 1308–1309, 1309f
    diagnostic studies, 1313–1314, 1314f–1315f
    differential diagnosis, 1310t
    history, 1309–1310
    inspection, 1310–1311, 1311f–1312f
    palpation, 1311
    patient evaluation, 1309–1314
    physical examination, 1310–1311
    provocative tests, 1312–1313, 1312f–1313f
    range of motion and strength in, 1311–1312
    specific conditions, 1314–1316
      complex regional pain syndrome, 1316
      idiopathic anterior knee pain/patellofemoral pain syndrome, 1314–1315
      intraosseous hypertension of patella, 1316
      lateral patella compression syndrome and, 1316
      synovial impingement syndromes, 1315–1316, 1316f
  posterior heel, 1504–1508, 1505f
    complications, 1508
    decision-making principles, 1505–1506
    future considerations, 1508
    history, 1504
    imaging, 1504–1505, 1505f–1506f
    physical examination, 1504, 1505f
    postoperative management, 1508
    results, 1508
    treatment options, 1506–1507
  posterior hip, 1018–1033
    deep gluteal syndrome in, 1020–1024
    operative treatment, 1027–1030
    physical examination, 1024–1026, 1024f–1026f
    preoperative and postoperative rehabilitation, 1027–1030, 1027f–1028f
    pudendal nerve entrapment in, 1030–1032, 1031f–1032f, 1031t
    sciatic nerve
      characteristics, 1018–1020, 1019f–1020f
      entrapment, 1020–1024
    superior and inferior gluteal nerves in, 1032–1033, 1032f, 1032t
  scapulothoracic disorders, 614–615
  stiff shoulder, 579–581, 580b

Pain *(Continued)*
  treatments, 357–360
    cryotherapy, 358–359
    edema/inflammation, 359
    electrical stimulation, 359
    manual therapy, 357, 358t
    transcutaneous electrical nerve stimulation, 359
    ultrasound, 359–360
Palpation
  elbow, 689–690
  knee, 1092–1094, 1093f
  patellofemoral pain, 1311
  scapulothoracic disorders, 612–613
  stiff shoulder, 583–584
Palsy. *See also* Cerebral palsy
  axillary nerve, 629–630
    anatomy, 629
    biomechanics, 629
    clinical evaluation, 629–630
    decision-making principles, 630
    diagnostic studies, 630
    results, 630
  long thoracic nerve, 625–627
    anatomy, 625, 625f
    biomechanics, 625, 625f
    clinical evaluation, 625–627, 626f
    decision-making principles, 627
    diagnostic studies, 627
    results, 627
    technique, 627b
  spinal accessory nerve, 627–629
    anatomy, 627–628
    biomechanics, 627–628
    clinical evaluation, 628–629, 628f
    decision-making principles, 629
    diagnostic studies, 629
    results, 629
    technique, 629b
  suprascapular nerve, 621–625
    anatomy, 621–622, 622f
    biomechanics, 621–622, 622f
    clinical evaluation, 622–623, 623f
    decision-making principles, 624
    diagnostic studies, 623–624, 623f
    results, 624–625
Pancreatic hormones, 69t, 71
Panner disease, 1668–1670
  complications, 1670
  decision-making principles, 1669, 1669t
  history, 1668
  imaging, 1668–1669, 1669f
  physical examination, 1668
  results, 1670
  treatment, 1669–1670
Para-athlete, 315–324
  amputee athlete, 316–317
    adaptive sports equipment, 317
    exercise physiology, 316
    medical considerations, 316–317, 316t
  cerebral palsy, 320–321
    adaptive equipment, 321
    exercise, 320–321, 320b
    medical considerations, 321
  classification, 315
  intellectually disabled athlete, 321–323
    adaptive equipment, 323
    exercise physiology, 322
    medical considerations, 322–323
  Les Autres group, 323
  visually impaired athletes, 323
  wheelchair athlete, 317–320
    adaptive equipment, 320
    exercise, 317–318
    medical considerations, 318–320

Parasitic infections, 252–253
  cutaneous larva migrans, 253, 253f
  pediculosis capitis, 252–253
  scabies, 253, 253f
Paratenon, 2, 3f
Paratenonitis, 1320–1321
Paresthesias, 688
Pars stress fractures, 136–137, 138f
Parsonage-Turner syndrome, 339–340
Partial anterior cruciate ligament tears, 1189
Particulated juvenile cartilage allograft, 1165–1166, 1172f, 1176, 1489, 1490f
Patella, 1095–1096, 1095f–1096f, 1318–1319
  anatomy, 1065, 1065f–1066f
  fractures
    decision-making principles, 1327
  fractures of, 1322, 1322b
    clinical outcomes, 1332–1333
    complications, 1333
    history, 1323
    imaging, 1326, 1326f
    nonoperative treatment, 1327–1328, 1328f
    operative treatment, 1329–1330
    physical examination, 1324
    postoperative management, 1331
  instability, 1293–1307, 1708–1712
    complications, 1304–1306, 1304b, 1304f
    decision-making principles, 1299–1301, 1709
    embryology, 1708, 1708f
    episode of
      acute, 1295–1296, 1299–1300
      subacute, first-time, 1300–1301
      subacute, recurrent, 1300–1301
    examination overview for, 1295–1297
    future considerations, 1306, 1712
    history, 1293, 1294f, 1708–1709
    imaging, 1297–1299, 1298f–1299f, 1709, 1709f
    pathoanatomy, 1708
    physical examination, 1294–1295, 1708–1709
    postoperative management, 1304–1306, 1711
    prone examination of, 1297
    results, 1304, 1306, 1711–1712
    risk factors for, 1708
    sitting examination, 1296, 1296f
    static standing and gait examination of, 1296
    supine examination of, 1296–1297, 1297f
    treatment options, 1299–1301, 1709–1711, 1710f
  intraosseous hypertension of, 1316
  rupture, 1321–1322
    clinical outcomes, 1332
    complications, 1333
    decision-making principles, 1327
    history, 1323
    imaging, 1325–1326, 1325f–1326f
    nonoperative treatment, 1327
    operative treatment, 1328–1329, 1329f
    physical examination, 1324, 1324f
    postoperative management, 1330–1331
  structure of, 1320, 1320f–1321f
  tendinopathy, 1320–1321
    clinical outcomes, 1331–1332, 1332f
    complications, 1333
    history, 1322–1323
    imaging, 1324–1325, 1324f–1325f
    physical examination, 1323–1324, 1323t
    postoperative management, 1330
Patellar apprehension test, 1297
Patellar ballottement test, 1277
Patellar glide test, 1296–1297, 1297f
Patellar tilt test, 1296, 1297f
Patellofemoral joint
  biomechanics, 1082–1087
  contact area, 1082–1084, 1083f
  force transmission, 1084–1087, 1084f–1086f

Patellofemoral pain, 370–371, 1308–1317
  anatomy, 1308–1309, 1309f
  diagnostic studies, 1313–1314, 1314f–1315f
  differential diagnosis, 1310t
  history, 1309–1310
  inspection, 1310–1311, 1311f–1312f
  palpation, 1311
  patient evaluation, 1309–1314
  physical examination, 1310–1311
  provocative tests, 1312–1313, 1312f–1313f
  range of motion and strength in, 1311–1312
  specific conditions, 1314–1316
    complex regional pain syndrome, 1316
    idiopathic anterior knee pain/patellofemoral pain syndrome, 1314–1315
    intraosseous hypertension of patella, 1316
    lateral patella compression syndrome and, 1316
    synovial impingement syndromes, 1315–1316, 1316f
  taping, 370, 370f
Patellofemoral pain syndrome (PFPS), 306–307, 306t, 1314–1315
Pathologic bone, 12, 12f
Pathologic lesions, 1691
Pathologies
  adductor, 1007–1017
  ankle, 1370–1379
  elbow, 687
  foot, 1370–1379
  hip dysplasia and instability, 971–973, 972f–973f
  iliopsoas, 979–989
  leg, 1370–1379
  proximal biceps tendon, 526–539
  scapulothoracic disorders, 615
Patient, satisfaction of, after high tibial osteotomy, 1283
Patient history. *See* History of patient
Patrick test, 932
Patterned electrical nerve stimulation, 366, 366f
Pectineus, 919
Pectoralis major muscle, injuries to, 574–576
  anatomy, 574
  classification, 574–575
  imaging, 575
  mechanisms of, 574
  physical examination, 575
  treatment, 575–576, 576f
Pediatrics, 1606–1614
  ankle injuries, 1633–1635, 1725–1740
    acute, 1633, 1634f
    fractures, 1729–1733, 1729f, 1732f–1734f, 1732t
    normal anatomy, 1725–1728
    orthotics and, 1739
    overuse, 1633–1635, 1634f
    shoes and, 1739
    soft tissue injuries of, 1728–1729, 1728f
    systemic illness and, 1739
  arthroscopy, 1612–1614, 1612f–1615f
  baseball injuries, 115
  concussion, 1741–1747
    biomechanics, 1741, 1742f
    complications, 1746–1747, 1747t
    decision-making principles, 1745
    epidemiology, 1741–1743
    future considerations, 1747
    history, 1743, 1743t
    imaging, 1744–1745, 1745b
    pathophysiology, 1741, 1742f
    physical examination, 1743–1744
    return to play, 1746, 1746t
    treatment options, 1745–1746
  elbow injuries, 1619–1623, 1661–1676
    acute, 1619, 1621f
    anatomy, 1661–1665

Pediatrics (Continued)
  biomechanics, 1661–1665
  development, 1619
  lateral epicondylitis, 1674–1676
  ligaments, 1661–1662, 1662f–1663f
  Little League, 1621–1623, 1622f–1623f, 1665–1668
  medial collateral ligament injury, 1672–1673
  medial epicondyle avulsion fractures, 1670–1672
  medial epicondylitis, 1674–1676
  osteochondritis dissecans, 1668–1670
  osteology, 1661, 1662f
  overuse, 1619–1623
  Panner disease, 1668–1670
  pathologies, 1665–1676
  soft-tissue, 1661–1662, 1662f–1663f
epidemiology, 1606–1607
exercise, 1607–1609
foot injuries, 1633–1635, 1725–1740
  acute, 1633, 1634f
  fractures, 1733–1739, 1735f–1737f
  orthotics and, 1739
  overuse, 1633–1635, 1634f
  shoes and, 1739
  soft tissue injuries of, 1728–1729, 1728f
  systemic illness and, 1739
fractures
  avulsion, 1688, 1689f
  hip, 1690
  lesser tuberosity, 1647
  proximal humerus, 1644–1647
  stress, 1688–1690, 1690f
head injuries, 1741–1748
hip, 1625–1628
  conditions, 928
  injuries, 1688–1696
    acute, 1625–1626, 1626f
    overuse, 1626–1628, 1627f–1628f
injury, 1606–1607
knee injuries, 1628–1633, 1697–1724
  acute, 1628–1630, 1629f–1630f
  anterior cruciate ligament (ACL) injuries, 1697–1703
  discoid meniscus, 1705–1708
  meniscal injuries, 1703–1705
  osteochondritis dissecans, 1712–1717
  osteochondroses, 1717–1718
  overuse, 1630–1633, 1631f–1633f
  patellar instability, 1708–1712
  physeal fractures, 1718–1721
lower leg, 1633–1635
  acute injuries, 1633, 1634f
  overuse injuries, 1633–1635, 1634f
nutrition, 1610–1611
pathophysiology, 1616
performance-enhancing substances, 1611
shoulder, 1616–1618, 1637–1660
  acute injuries, 1617–1618, 1618f–1619f
  development, 1616–1617, 1617f
  overuse injuries, 1618, 1620f–1621f
soccer injuries, 126
spine issues in, 1635–1636, 1635f, 1749–1764
  apophyseal ring fractures, 1753
  atlantoaxial instability, 1758
  Down syndrome, atlantoaxial instability in, 1758–1759
  rotatory atlantoaxial subluxation, 1759–1761
  sacral facet fractures, 1755
  scoliosis, 1755–1758
  spinal cord injury without radiographic abnormality (SCIWORA), 1763
  spondylolisthesis, 1750–1753
  spondylolysis, 1750–1753

Pediatrics (Continued)
  sports participation, 1606
  strength training in, 68
  wrist and hand injuries, 1623–1625, 1677–1687
    acute, 1623–1624, 1623f
    distal radial physeal stress reaction, 1683–1684
    finger fractures, 1677–1681
      complications, 1680–1681
      decision-making principles, 1678
      future considerations, 1681
      history, 1677
      imaging, 1678, 1678f–1679f
      physical examination, 1677–1678, 1678f
      postoperative management, 1680
      results, 1680
      treatment options, 1678–1680, 1680f, 1681b
    jammed finger, 1681–1683
      complications, 1683
      decision-making principles, 1682
      history, 1681
      imaging, 1682, 1682f
      physical examination, 1681–1682
      postoperative management, 1683
      results, 1683
      treatment options, 1682, 1682b
    overuse, 1624–1625, 1624f–1626f
    scaphoid fracture, 1684–1686
      complications, 1685
      decision-making principles, 1685
      future considerations, 1686
      history, 1684
      imaging, 1684–1685
      physical examination, 1684
      postoperative management, 1685
      results, 1685
      treatment options, 1685, 1685b, 1686f
Pediculosis capitis, 252–253
Pedowitz criteria, for chronic exertional compartment syndrome, 1396, 1396t–1397t
Pelvis injuries
  figure skating, 118
  gymnastics, 120–121
Performance, biomechanics for improving, 28
Performance-enhancing substances, 1611
Performance enhancing supplements (PES), 280, 281t
Periacetabular osteotomy (PAO), 971
Perilunate dislocation, 809–810, 810f
Perilunate instability, 851–854, 851f–855f, 853b
Perimysium, 62, 63f
Periodontal/displacement injuries (loose teeth), 270
Perioperative complications, with anesthesia, 339–340
  allergic reactions, 339
  Parsonage-Turner syndrome, 339–340
Perioperative pain management, 335
Perioperative pharmacology, 335–339
  acetaminophen, 338
  buprenorphine, 337–338
  dexmedetomidine, 338–339
  ketamine, 338
  methadone, 337
  nonsteroidal antiinflammatory drugs, 338
  opioids, 337
  perioperative pain management, 335, 336t–337t
  propofol, 338
Periorbital lacerations, 263
Periosteum, 13–14
Peripheral compartment
  femoroacetabular impingement, 967, 968f
  hip arthroscopy, 954–955, 954f–955f

Peripheral nerve entrapment, 319, 1402–1420
  deep peroneal nerve, 1415–1416, 1415f
    history, 1415
    imaging, 1416
    physical examination, 1415–1416
    postoperative management, 1416
    results, 1416
    treatment options, 1416, 1416b
  interdigital neuralgia (Morton neuroma), 1416–1419
    complications, 1418–1419
    decision-making principles, 1418
    etiologies of, 1417
    history, 1417
    imaging, 1417–1418
    pathomechanism of, 1417
    physical examination, 1417
    postoperative management, 1418
    results, 1418
    treatment options, 1418, 1419b, 1419f
  lateral plantar nerve, 1411–1412
    complications, 1412
    decision-making principles, 1411
    history, 1411
    imaging, 1411
    physical examination, 1411
    postoperative management, 1412
    results, 1412
    treatment options, 1411–1412, 1412b, 1412f
  medial plantar nerve, 1412–1413
    decision-making principles, 1413
    history, 1412
    imaging, 1413
    physical examination, 1412
    postoperative management, 1413
    treatment options, 1413
  saphenous nerve, 1405–1407, 1405f–1406f
    history, 1405
    imaging, 1406
    physical examination, 1405–1406
    results, 1406–1407
    treatment options, 1406
  superficial peroneal nerve, 1413–1415, 1413f
    decision-making principles, 1414
    history, 1413
    imaging, 1414
    physical examination, 1413–1414
    postoperative management, 1415
    results, 1415
    treatment options, 1414–1415, 1414b, 1414f
  sural nerve, 1402–1405, 1403f
    history, 1402
    imaging, 1403–1404
    physical examination, 1402–1403
    postoperative management, 1405
    results, 1405
    treatment options, 1404, 1404b, 1404f
  tarsal tunnel syndrome, 1407–1411, 1407f
    decision-making principles, 1408
    electrodiagnostic studies, 1408
    etiologies of, 1407–1408, 1407t
    history, 1408
    imaging, 1408
    physical examination, 1408
    postoperative management, 1410
    results, 1410–1411
    treatment options, 1408–1409, 1409b–1410b, 1409f–1410f
Peritenon, 2
Peritrochanteric disorders, 990–1006
  coxa saltans, 996–1001
  gluteus medius and minimus tears, 990–996
  ischiofemoral impingement, 1003–1006

Peritrochanteric disorders (Continued)
  piriformis syndrome, 1002–1003
  trochanteric bursitis, 1001–1002
Peroneal nerve entrapment
  deep, 1415–1416, 1415f
    history, 1415
    imaging, 1416
    physical examination, 1415–1416
    postoperative management, 1416
    results, 1416
    treatment options, 1416, 1416b
  superficial, 1413–1415, 1413f
    decision-making principles, 1414
    history, 1413
    imaging, 1414
    physical examination, 1413–1414
    postoperative management, 1415
    results, 1415
    treatment options, 1414–1415, 1414b, 1414f
Peroneal tendons, 1385–1386, 1385f–1386f
  injuries, 1472–1476
    complications, 1476
    decision-making principles, 1473–1474
    future considerations, 1476
    history, 1472
    imaging, 1473, 1473f
    physical examination, 1472–1473, 1472f
    postoperative management, 1475
    results, 1475–1476
    treatment options, 1474–1475, 1474f–1475f, 1475b
Pertinent bony shoulder, 393–395, 394f
PET/CT scans. See Positron emission tomography/computed tomography scans
PFPS. See Patellofemoral pain syndrome
Phalangeal fractures, 890–892, 891f–893f
Phonophoresis, 360
Phosphagen energy system, 65
Physeal fractures, 1718–1721
  complications, 1720–1721
  decision-making principles, 1719–1720
  history, 1719
  imaging, 1719, 1720f–1721f
  lesser tuberosity fractures, 1647
    complications, 1647
    history, 1647
    imaging, 1647
    physical examination, 1647
    treatment options, 1647, 1647f
  physical examination, 1719
  proximal humerus fractures, 1644–1647, 1644f–1645f
    complications, 1647
    history, 1644
    imaging, 1644–1645, 1645f–1646f
    physical examination, 1644
    treatment, 1645–1646, 1646f
  treatment options, 1719–1720, 1722f–1723f
Physical examination
  Achilles tendon injuries, 1477, 1477f
  acromioclavicular joint, 648–651, 650t, 651f
  for adductor strains, 1050
  AIN syndrome, 746
  ankle, 1372–1379, 1373f–1378f
  anterior cruciate ligament injuries, 1187–1188
  anterior shoulder instability, 447–448, 448f–449f
  articular cartilage lesions, 1163
  athletic pubalgia, 1009, 1009f
  brain injury, 1564–1566
  calcaneoplasty, 1433
  cervical spine
    injuries, 1578
    unstable fractures and dislocations of, 1541
  concussion, 1564–1566
  cubital tunnel syndrome, 749

Physical examination (Continued)
  digits, 801
  distal biceps, 725, 725f, 733, 733f
  distal triceps, 738
  elbow, 689–691
    inspection, 689
    joint stability, 694–695
    maneuvers, 695
    motion, loss, 773–774
    neurologic assessment, 690–691, 691f
    palpation, 689–690
    throwing injuries, 758–760, 759f–760f
  endoscopic Haglund resection, 1433
  exertional compartment syndromes, 1395
  extensor mechanism injuries, 1323–1324
  external coxa saltans, 999, 999f
  femoroacetabular impingement, 959–960, 959t, 960f
  flexor hallucis longus injuries, 1469
  foot, 1372–1379, 1373f–1378f
  glenohumeral arthritis, 595–596
    arthroscopic images, 596
    history, 595
    imaging, 596, 597f–598f
    presentation, 595
    prior operative notes, 596
  gluteus medius and minimus tears, 990
  of hallux rigidus, 1523, 1523f
  hamstring injuries, 1035–1036
  hand, 793–794, 794f
  head injuries, 1539
  hip, 929–933
    arthritis, 1053–1055
    dysplasia and instability, 973–974
    inspection, 929
    ligamentous laxity, evaluation, 932
    measurements in, 930–931
    range of motion, 930–931, 931t
    special maneuvers, 932–933
    symptom localization, 929–930, 930f–931f
  iliac crest contusion, 1043
  iliopsoas, 982–983
  interdigital neuralgia, 1417
  internal coxa saltans, 996, 997f
  ischiofemoral impingement, 1004
  knee, 1091
    arthroscopic synovectomy of, 1127
    dislocation, 1347–1348, 1347f
    lateral and posterolateral corner injuries, 1249–1251, 1249f–1250f
    loss of motion, 1336, 1336f
    popliteal artery entrapment syndrome in, 1351–1352
  lateral epicondylitis, 720–725
  latissimus dorsi muscle, 576, 577f
  leg, 1372–1379, 1373f–1378f
    pain, 1395
  medial collateral ligament and posterior medial corner injuries, 1231–1232, 1233f, 1233t
  medial epicondylitis, 720
  meniscal injuries, 1137–1138
  metatarsalgia, 1519–1520
  Morton neuroma, 1417
  multidirectional instability, 477–479, 477t–478t, 478f
  multiligament knee injuries, 1264–1265
  nerve entrapment
    deep peroneal, 1415–1416
    lateral plantar, 1411
    medial plantar, 1412
    of saphenous, 1405–1406
    superficial peroneal, 1413–1414
    sural, 1402–1403
  olecranon bursitis, 728
  osteochondral lesions, 1484

Physical examination (Continued)
  patella
    instability, 1294–1295
      pertinent bony anatomy, 1294, 1294f
      pertinent soft tissue anatomy, 1294–1295, 1295f
    tendinopathy, 1323–1324, 1323t
    tendon ruptures, 1324, 1324f
  patellofemoral pain, 1310–1311
  pectoralis major muscle, 575
  pediatrics, 1052
    anterior cruciate ligament (ACL) injuries, 1697
    apophyseal ring fractures, 1753
    atraumatic instability, 1654–1655, 1654f
    cervical spine, congenital anomalies of, 1762
    concussion, 1743–1744
    discoid meniscus, 1706
    distal radial physeal stress reaction, 1683
    Down syndrome, atlantoaxial instability in, 1758
    finger fractures, 1677–1678, 1678f
    jammed finger, 1681–1682
    lateral clavicle physeal fractures, 1640–1641
    lateral epicondylitis, 1675
    lesser tuberosity fractures, 1647
    Little League elbow, 1666–1667
    medial clavicle physeal fractures, 1643
    medial collateral ligament injury, 1672
    medial epicondyle avulsion fractures, 1671, 1671f
    medial epicondylitis, 1675
    meniscal injuries, 1703
    odontoid fractures, 1761
    osteochondritis dissecans, 1668, 1712, 1713f
    osteochondrosis, 1668
    Panner disease, 1668
    patellar instability, 1708–1709
    physeal fractures, 1719
    posterior elbow pathologic conditions, 1674
    proximal humerus epiphysiolysis, 1656
    proximal humerus fractures, 1644
    rotatory atlantoaxial subluxation, 1759
    scaphoid fracture, 1684
    scoliosis, 1755–1757
    spinal cord injury without radiographic abnormality, 1763
    spine, 1749–1750, 1751b
    spondylolisthesis, 1751–1752
    spondylolysis, 1751–1752
    traumatic anterior instability, 1648, 1649f
    traumatic posterior instability, 1652, 1652f
  peroneal tendon injuries, 1472–1473, 1472f
  PIN syndrome, 755
  piriformis syndrome, 1002–1003
  plantar fasciitis, 1509
  posterior cruciate ligament injuries, 1212–1214
    collateral ligament assessment, 1213–1214
    external rotation of tibia (Dial test) in, 1213
    gait and limb alignment in, 1214
    posterior drawer test, 1212, 1213f
    posterior sag test (Godfrey test) in, 1212–1213, 1213f
    quadriceps active test, 1212–1213
    reverse pivot-shift test, 1213
  posterior heel pain, 1504, 1505f
  posterior hip pain, 1024–1026, 1024f–1026f
  posterior shoulder instability, 465–467, 466f, 466t
  preparticipation, 144–150
    allergies, 149
    athletes with special needs, 150
    cardiovascular system, 145–147, 145b–146b
    dermatology, 149
    ears, 145
    endocrine system, 149

Physical examination (Continued)
eyes, 145
gastrointestinal system, 148
genitourinary system, 148
goals, 144
head, 145
heat illness, 149–150
hematologic disease, 148–149
history, 145–150
immunizations, 149
infectious disease, 148–149
medications, 149
musculoskeletal system, 148, 148b
neurologic system, 148
nose, 145
objectives, 144
organization, 144–145
physical examination, 145–150
pulmonary system, 147–148
setting, 144–145, 145t
throat, 145
timing, 144–145
pronator syndrome, 745
quadriceps contusion, 1045
quadriceps strains, 1048
radial tunnel syndrome, 754
revision anterior cruciate ligament injuries,
1200
revision rotator cuff repair, 568
revision shoulder instability, 489–490, 490f
rotator cuff and impingement lesions, 543–547,
544f–546f
scapulothoracic disorders, 611–614
inspection, 611–612
palpation, 612–613
range of motion, 613
strength, 613
testing, 613–614
sesamoid dysfunction, 1517
soft tissue, ankle arthroscopy, 1423
sprains
ankle, 1444–1446, 1446f, 1446t, 1450–1451
bifurcate ligament, 1457
Lisfranc, 1458
syndesmosis, 1453–1454
sternoclavicular joint, 664–677
stingers, 1570–1571, 1571f–1572f, 1572t
subscapularis injury, 558–559, 558f
subtalar arthroscopy, 1429
superior labrum anterior to posterior (SLAP)
tears, 502–503, 504t
tarsal tunnel syndrome, 1408
thoracic outlet syndrome, 636–638, 637f–638f
thoracolumbar spine injuries, 1582–1583
thrower's shoulder, 514–515
triceps tendinitis, 725, 725f
trochanteric bursitis, 1002
turf toe, 1515
wrist, 793–794, 794f
tendinopathies, 858
Physical therapy, for knee arthritis, 1280
Pia mater, 1528
Pill esophagitis, 192
PIN syndrome. See Posterior interosseous nerve
(PIN) syndrome
Pincer impingement, 927–928, 957–958, 958f, 967
Piriformis syndrome, 1002–1003, 1003b
Pisiform carpal injuries, 847–848, 847f, 848b
Pitted keratolysis, 248, 248f
Pituitary hormones, 69–70, 69t
Pityrosporum folliculitis, 251f
Plain radiography
femoroacetabular impingement, 960–963,
961f–963f

Plain radiography (Continued)
interpretation, 936–938
acetabular cup depth, 938
acetabular inclination, 938
acetabular version, 938
alpha angle, 938
anterior center edge angles, 937–938
functional leg lengths, 936
head-neck offset, 938
head sphericity, 938
hip center position, 938
joint space width, 938
lateral center edge angles, 937
neck shaft angle, 936–937
trabecular pattern, 937
rotator cuff and impingement lesions, 547
Planar imaging, 88, 89f
Plantar fascia, 368–369
Plantar fasciitis, 371, 1391, 1391f, 1509–1513
complications, 1513
decision-making principles, 1510
future considerations, 1513
history, 1509
imaging, 1509, 1509f
physical examination, 1509
postoperative management, 1511
results, 1511–1513
treatment options, 1510–1511, 1510f, 1511b,
1512f
Plantar fasciosis, 371
Plantar midfoot ecchymosis, 1373, 1373f
Plantar nerve entrapment
lateral, 1411–1412
complications, 1412
decision-making principles, 1411
history, 1411
imaging, 1411
physical examination, 1411
postoperative management, 1412
results, 1412
treatment options, 1411–1412, 1412b, 1412f
medial, 1412–1413
decision-making principles, 1413
history, 1412
imaging, 1413
physical examination, 1412
postoperative management, 1413
treatment options, 1413
Platelet-rich plasma, 1148–1149
in cartilage restoration, 55
composition, 50–53, 52f, 52t
definitions, 50
growth factors, 51, 53t
for knee arthritis, 1280
ligament-related disorders/repair, 53–55
in meniscal repair, 55–56
for muscle injuries, 56
preparation, 50–53, 52f, 52t
properties of, 50
sports medicine and, 50–53, 51f
tendon and ligament-related disorders/repair,
53–55
Achilles tendon repair, 54
anterior cruciate ligament surgery and,
54–55
ligament injuries, 53–54
rotator cuff repair, 54
tendon injuries, 53–54
Pneumonia, acute, 209–210
Pneumothorax, tension, 153
Polyetheretherketone (PEEK), as suture anchors,
47
Polymethylmethacrylate (PMMA), for bone
fixation, 39

Polytetrafluoroethylene (PTFE), for ACL
reconstruction, 39
Popliteal artery entrapment syndrome (PAES),
1349–1356
classification, 1350–1351, 1350f
clinical presentation, 1351
complications, 1356
criteria for return to play, 1356
history, 1350
imaging, 1352–1354, 1352f–1353f
angiography, 1353–1354, 1354f
computed tomography and computed
tomographic angiography, 1353, 1353f
duplex ultrasonography, 1352, 1352f
magnetic resonance angiography, 1352–1353,
1353f
magnetic resonance imaging, 1352–1353,
1353f
physical examination and testing of, 1351–1352
postoperative management, 1356
treatment options, 1354–1356, 1355f, 1356b
Popliteal artery repair, in knee dislocation,
1349b
Popliteus tendon complex, 1245
Portal placement
arthroscopic, 110
elbow arthroscopy, 709–711, 709t
accessory portal, 711
order of, 712
posterior radiocapitellar portal, 711
proximal anterolateral portal, 711
proximal anteromedial portal, 710–711
proximal posterolateral portal, 711
standard anterolateral portal, 711
standard anteromedial portal, 709, 710f
straight posterior portal, 711
hip arthroscopy, 950–952
anterolateral, 950–951, 950f
distal anterolateral accessory, 951, 951f
modified mid-anterior, 951, 951f
posterolateral, 951–952
knee arthroscopy, 1121–1123, 1122f–1124f
shoulder arthroscopy, 435–436, 436f
wrist arthroscopy, 817–819, 818f–819f
Position/positioning
arthroscopic synovectomy, of knee, 1129
during arthroscopy, 109–110, 109f–110f
beach chair, 329
elbow arthroscopy, 708, 708f
hip arthroscopy, 948–950
hip center, 938
knee arthroscopy, 1121, 1122f
shoulder arthroscopy, 434–435, 434f
Positron emission tomography/computed
tomography scans, 90, 93f
Postclosure wound care, for face facial injuries,
261–262
Postconcussion syndrome (PCS), 1540–1541,
1746, 1747t
Posterior apprehension test, 404–405, 932
Posterior compartment release, 1399, 1399f
Posterior compartments, in arthroscopic
synovectomy, of knee, 1129–1130
Posterior cruciate ligament
injuries, 1211–1230, 1220b–1222b, 1221f–1223f
complications in, 1229
decision-making, 1214–1216
future considerations, 1229
history, 1211–1212
imaging, 1214
bone scan and, 1214
magnetic resonance imaging, 1214
radiography, 1214
isolated, 1224–1225, 1227t

Posterior cruciate ligament (Continued)
    nonoperative treatment, 1216
        decision-making, 1215–1216
    operative treatment, 1216–1217
        results, 1224–1229
    physical examination, 1212–1214
        collateral ligament assessment, 1213–1214
        external rotation of tibia (Dial test) in, 1213
        gait and limb alignment in, 1214
        posterior drawer test, 1212, 1213f
        posterior sag test (Godfrey test) in, 1212–1213, 1213f
        quadriceps active test, 1212–1213
        reverse pivot-shift test, 1213
    postoperative management, 1224, 1224b
    treatment options, 1216–1220, 1216f–1217f
        graft choice and fixation, 1219
        high tibial osteotomy in, 1219–1220
        single-bundle vs. double-bundle reconstruction, 1218–1219, 1218f, 1225–1229
        transtibial tunnel vs. tibial inlay techniques, 1217–1218, 1225, 1228t
    knee, 1069, 1070f
    MRI, 1112
    multiligament knee injuries, 1268
Posterior drawer test, for posterior cruciate ligament injuries, 1212, 1213f
Posterior elbow pathologic conditions, 1673–1674, 1673f
    complications, 1674
    decision-making principles, 1674
    history, 1674
    imaging, 1674
    physical examination, 1674
    results, 1674
    treatment, 1674
Posterior heel pain, 1504–1508, 1505f
    complications, 1508
    decision-making principles, 1505–1506
    future considerations, 1508
    history, 1504
    imaging, 1504–1505, 1505f–1506f
    physical examination, 1504, 1505f
    postoperative management, 1508
    results, 1508
    treatment options, 1506–1507
        nonoperative therapy, 1506–1507
        operative therapy, 1507
        technique, 1507b, 1507f
Posterior hindfoot arthroscopy, 1470b, 1471f
Posterior hip pain, 1018–1033
    deep gluteal syndrome in, 1020–1024
    operative treatment, 1027–1030
        endoscopic decompression in, 1027–1030, 1028t–1029t, 1029f–1030f
    physical examination, 1024–1026, 1024f–1026f
    preoperative and postoperative rehabilitation, 1027–1030, 1027f–1028f
    pudendal nerve entrapment in, 1030–1032, 1031f–1032f, 1031t
    sciatic nerve
        characteristics, 1018–1020, 1019f–1020f
        entrapment, 1020–1024
    superior and inferior gluteal nerves in, 1032–1033, 1032f, 1032t
Posterior impingement, 431, 1426b, 1426f
Posterior interosseous nerve (PIN) syndrome, 687–688, 693, 755–756
    complications, 756
    decision-making principles, 755
    history, 755
    postoperative management, 755
    results, 755–756
    return-to-play guidelines, 755

Posterior interosseous nerve (PIN) syndrome (Continued)
    technique, 755
    treatment, 755
Posterior medial corner injuries, 1231–1243
    complications in, 1242
    decision-making principles, 1234–1235, 1235f
    future considerations, 1243
    history, 1231
    imaging, 1232–1234, 1233f–1235f
    physical exam, 1231–1232
    postoperative management, 1239–1240
    results, 1240–1242
    return-to-play guidelines, 1240b
    treatment options, 1235–1236
Posterior radiocapitellar portal, 711
Posterior sag test (Godfrey test), for posterior cruciate ligament injuries, 1212–1213, 1213f
Posterior shoulder instability, 463–475
    arthroscopic posterior shoulder stabilization for, 470b–472b, 470f–472f
    background, 463
    complications, 474–475
    decision-making principles and, 468
    future considerations, 475
    history, 465
    imaging, 467–468, 467f–468f, 468t
    pathogenesis of, 463–465, 464f–465f
    physical examination, 465–467, 466f, 466t
    postoperative management, 469–473
    results, 473–474
    treatment options, 468–469
        contraindications, 469
        indications, 469
Posterior tibia
    tendon, 1383–1384, 1383f–1384f
    tendon, injuries, 1464–1469
        complications, 1469
        decision-making principles, 1466
        future considerations, 1469
        history, 1465
        imaging, 1465–1466, 1465f
        physical examination, 1465, 1465f
        postoperative management, 1468
        results, 1468–1469
        treatment options, 1466–1467, 1466f–1467f, 1467b–1468b
    translation of, 1247–1248
Posterolateral corner injuries, 1244–1263
    anatomy, 1244–1248
    classification, 1248, 1248t
    complications in, 1260–1261, 1262f
    decision-making principles, 1253
    future considerations, 1262
    history, 1248–1249
    imaging, 1251–1253
        magnetic resonance imaging, 1251–1253, 1252f
        radiographs, 1251, 1251f
        ultrasound, 1253
    layers of lateral side of, 1244
    nonoperative management, 1253
        grade I injuries, 1253
        grade II injuries, 1253
        grade III injuries, 1253
    pediatric, 1262
    physical examination, 1249–1251, 1249f–1250f
    postoperative management, 1256–1260, 1259t
    repair vs. reconstruction, 1253
    results, 1260, 1260t–1261t
    return to play, 1260
    structures, 1244–1246, 1245f
        anterior/posterior tibial translation, 1247–1248
        arcuate ligament complex, 1246
        biceps femoris muscle, 1245–1246

Posterolateral corner injuries (Continued)
    biomechanics, 1246, 1247f
    external rotation, 1247
    fabellofibular ligament, 1246
    fibular collateral ligament, 1244–1245
    iliotibial band, 1244
    lateral gastrocnemius tendon, 1246
    mid-third lateral capsular ligament, 1246
    neurovascular, 1246
    popliteus tendon complex, 1245
    varus motion, 1246–1247
    surgical considerations, 1254–1256
        diagnostic arthroscopy, 1254, 1254f
        primary repair, 1254, 1254f
        reconstruction techniques, 1254–1255
    techniques, 1257b, 1257f–1258f
    timing of diagnosis, 1253
    treatment options, 1253–1256
Posterolateral corner sling procedure, 1255
Posterolateral drawer test, 1249, 1249f–1250f
Posterolateral portal, in hip arthroscopy, 951–952
Posteromedial impingement, 1673–1674, 1673f
    complications, 1674
    decision-making principles, 1674
    history, 1674
    imaging, 1674
    physical examination, 1674
    results, 1674
    treatment, 1674
Postoperative rehabilitation, for posterior hip pain, 1027–1030, 1027f–1028f
Postural orthostatic tachycardia syndrome (POTS), 173
Power stroke, 63
Pre-event planning, in spine injuries, 1553–1554
Prediabetes, 218
Pregnancy, in female athlete, 301–302, 302t
Preoperative arthroscopy, 109
Preoperative imaging, 433–434
Preoperative rehabilitation, for posterior hip pain, 1027–1030, 1027f–1028f
Preparticipation physical evaluation, 144–150
    allergies, 149
    athletes with special needs, 150
    cardiovascular system, 145–147, 145b–146b
    dermatology, 149
    ears, 145
    endocrine system, 149
    eyes, 145
    gastrointestinal system, 148
    genitourinary system, 148
    goals, 144
    head, 145
    heat illness, 149–150
    hematologic disease, 148–149
    history, 145–150
    immunizations, 149
    infectious disease, 148–149
    medical home, 159–160
    medications, 149
    musculoskeletal system, 148, 148b
    neurologic system, 148
    nose, 145
    objectives, 144
    organization, 144–145
    physical examination, 145–150
    pulmonary system, 147–148
    setting, 144–145, 145t
    throat, 145
    timing, 144–145
Pressure sores, 319
Primary anterior cruciate ligament reconstruction, 1193b–1195b, 1193f–1195f
Primary osteoarthritis, 592
Primary vs. permanent teeth, 269, 270f
Probe, arthroscopic, 107

ProChondrix, 1183
Professional athletics, ethical/legal issues with, 155
Progression, criterion-based, principles, 351–352
  key criteria for rehabilitation protocols and
      progression
    balance, 352, 352f
    movement quality, 352
    muscle performance, 351–352
    outcome measures, 351
    pain, 351
    range of motion, 351
  return-to-sport considerations, 352
Progressive loading, 389, 390f–391f
Pronation-supination, elbow, 681–683
Pronator syndrome, 688, 693–694, 745–746
  complications, 746
  decision-making principles, 745
  history, 745
  physical examination, 745
  postoperative management, 745–746
  results, 746
  return-to-play guidelines, 745–746
  technique, 746f
  treatment, 745
Prone examination
  hip, 933
  patellar instability, 1297
Prophylaxis, thromboembolic, 182, 183t–185t
Propofol, perioperative pharmacology, 338
Proprioception, anterior cruciate ligament
    injuries, 1196
Protective equipment, removal of, in injured
    athlete, 1558f
Protein, 277–278, 278t
Protocols
  in magnetic resonance imaging, 93, 94f
  in rehabilitation, 1208–1209
Proton density, 95, 96f, 96t
Provocative tests, for patellofemoral pain,
    1312–1313, 1312f–1313f
Proximal anteromedial portal, 710–711
Proximal biceps tendon pathology, 526–539
  complications, 538
  decision-making principles, 529–530, 530f
  future considerations, 538
  history, 526
  imaging, 528–529, 529f
  introduction, 526
  physical examination, 526–528, 527t, 528f
  postoperative management, 534–538
    biceps tenodesis rehabilitation protocol,
        534–535
    biceps tenotomy rehabilitation protocol, 534
    phase I: protective phase (day 1 to week 6),
        535
    phase II: moderate protection phase (weeks
        7 to 12), 535–538
    phase III: minimum protection phase (weeks
        13 to 20), 538
    phase IV: advanced strengthening phase
        (weeks 21 to 26), 538
  results, 537t, 538
  treatment options, 530–534
    nonoperative management, 530
    open subpectoral biceps tenodesis, 534, 535f
    surgical management, 530–532, 531f
Proximal femur, development, 908–909
Proximal fifth metatarsal stress fractures,
    134–135, 135f–136f
Proximal hamstring tendinopathy, chronic, 1041
Proximal humerus, 1637, 1638f
  epiphysiolysis, 1655–1656
    complications, 1656
    history, 1656

Proximal humerus (Continued)
    imaging, 1656, 1656f
    physical examination, 1656
    treatment, 1656
  fractures, 1644–1647, 1644f–1645f
    complications, 1647
    history, 1644
    imaging, 1644–1645, 1645f–1646f
    physical examination, 1644
    treatment, 1645–1646, 1646f
Proximal interphalangeal joint, 788–789, 802–803,
    804f
  ligamentous injuries and dislocations, 885–888,
      885f–890f
Proximal posterolateral portal, 711
Proximal tibial osteotomy, 1255, 1255f, 1259b,
    1259f, 1282
Proximal tibiofibular joint instability, 1259b, 1259f
Pseudoanemia, 196
Pseudomonal folliculitis (hot tub folliculitis), 249,
    249f
Pseudomonas infections, 213
Psoas minor, 979
Psychological adjustment, to athletic injury,
    272–276
  complications, 275
  decision-making principles, 273
  future considerations, 275
  historical perspective and evolution, 272–273
  postinjury management and outcome, 275
  preparticipation screening, 273
  treatment options, 274b
Psychological issues, in female athlete, 302–303
Psychosocial strategies, 345–346
Pubofemoral ligament (PFL), 914
Pudendal nerve entrapment, 1030–1032,
    1031f–1032f, 1031t
Pulley injuries, 814, 880–881, 880f–881f
Pulmonary edema, high-altitude, 243–245
Pulmonary embolism, 180–188
  clinical manifestations, 182–184
  diagnosis, 182–184
  imaging, 182–184, 185f–186f
  laboratory findings, 182–184
  normal physiology, 180, 181f
  return to play, 185–186
  risk factors, preoperative, 180–181
  sports issues in, 185–186
  thromboembolic prophylaxis, 182, 183t–185t
  travel and, 185–186
  treatment, 184–185, 187t
Pulmonary system, preparticipation physical
    evaluation, 147–148
Pulse check, in unconscious athlete, 1555
Pulse sequences, in magnetic resonance imaging,
    95–98
  2D acquisitions, 98, 98f
  3D acquisitions, 98, 98f
  gradient echo, 96–97, 97f
  inversion recovery, 97–98, 97f
  spin echo, 96, 97f

Q

Quadrants, of hand/wrist
  dorsal, 794t, 796–798, 797f–798f
  radial, 794–796, 794t, 795f–796f
  ulnar, 794t, 798–800, 799f
  volar, 794t, 800–801, 800f, 802f–803f
Quadratus femoris, nerve to, 916
Quadriceps
  contusion, 1044–1047, 1044t
    complications, 1047
    decision-making principles, 1046

Quadriceps (Continued)
    future considerations, 1047
    history, 1044–1045
    imaging, 1045, 1045f
    physical examination, 1045
    results, 1046
    return to play, 1046
    techniques, 1046b
    treatment options, 1045–1046
  strains, 1047–1050
    complications, 1049
    decision-making principles, 1049
    future considerations, 1050
    history, 1048
    imaging, 1048, 1048f
    physical examination, 1048
    results, 1049, 1049f
    return to play, 1049
    techniques, 1049b
    treatment options, 1048–1049, 1048t,
        1049f
  tendinopathy
    decision-making principles, 1327
  tendinopathy of, 1320–1321
    clinical outcomes, 1331–1332, 1332f
    history, 1322–1323
    imaging, 1324–1325, 1324f–1325f
    physical examination, 1323–1324, 1323t
  tendon rupture, 1321–1322
    clinical outcomes, 1332
    complications, 1333
    history, 1323
    imaging, 1325–1326, 1325f–1326f
    nonoperative treatment, 1327
    operative treatment, 1328–1329, 1329f
    physical examination, 1324, 1324f
    postoperative management, 1330–1331
  tendon structure of, 1320, 1320f–1321f
Quadriceps active test, for posterior cruciate
    ligament injuries, 1212–1213
Quadriceps angle
  patellar instability and, 1296, 1296f
  patellofemoral pain and, 1310–1311
Quadrilateral space syndrome (QSS), 629–630
Quadriplegia, transient, 1579

R

Race, of elite athlete, 161–162, 162f
Radial head, elbow, 683–684, 684f
Radial nerve, 752
  compression neuropathies, 692–693
  PIN syndrome, 755–756
    complications, 756
    decision-making principles, 755
    history, 755
    postoperative management, 755
    results, 755–756
    return-to-play guidelines, 755
    technique, 755
    treatment, 755
  radial tunnel syndrome, 752–755, 753f
    complications, 755
    decision-making principles, 754
    history, 754
    physical examination, 754
    postoperative management, 755
    results, 755
    return-to-play guidelines, 755
    technique, 754–755
    treatment, 754
Radial quadrant, 794–796, 794t, 795f–796f
Radial sensory nerve compression, 756,
    756f

Radial tunnel syndrome (RTS), 687–688,
    692–693, 693f, 752–755, 753f
  complications, 755
  decision-making principles, 754
  history, 754
  physical examination, 754
  postoperative management, 755
  results, 755
  return-to-play guidelines, 755
  technique, 754–755
  treatment, 754
    anterolateral approach, 754, 754f
    posterior approach, 754
Radiation exposure, in imaging, 103–104,
    103t
Radiculopathy
  cervical, 1595
  lumbar, 1599–1601, 1600f
Radiofrequency excitation pulse, in magnetic
    resonance imaging, 94
Radiofrequency instruments, for arthroscopy,
    108–109
Radiographic densities, 75, 75f
Radiographic tunnel positioning, for revision
    anterior cruciate ligament injuries,
    1200–1202, 1201f
Radiography. See also Plain radiography
  ankle, 1380, 1381f
  athletic pubalgia, 1010, 1010f
  conventional, 74–78
    advantages, 77
    arthrography, 76–77, 76f–77f
    disadvantages, 77–78, 78f
    fluoroscopy, 75–76, 75f–76f
    technical considerations, 74–75, 75f
  elbow, 697
  foot, 1380, 1381f
  glenohumeral joint, 408–410, 409b
    acromioclavicular articulation views, 410
    anteroposterior view, 408, 409f
    axillary lateral view, 408, 409f
    Grashey view, 408
    scapular Y view, 408–409, 409f
    Stryker notch view, 409–410
  hip, 935–936
    cross-table lateral view, 935, 936f
    dysplasia and instability, 974
    false-profile view, 936, 937f
    45-degree Dunn view, 935, 937f
    frog-leg lateral view, 935, 937f
    90-degree Dunn view, 935, 937f
    standing anteroposterior pelvic view, 935,
        936f
  iliopsoas, 983–984
  knee, 1104, 1105f
    arthritis, 1277–1278, 1278f–1279f
    lateral and posterolateral corner injuries,
        1251, 1251f
    medial collateral ligament and posterior medial
        corner injuries, 1232, 1233f
    meniscal transplantation, 1155
    multiligament knee injuries, 1265, 1265f
    patellar instability, 1297–1298, 1297t, 1298f
    patellofemoral pain, 1313, 1313f–1314f
    pediatrics
      of medial clavicle physeal fractures, 1643
      of osteochondritis dissecans, 1713–1714,
          1713f–1714f
      of traumatic anterior instability, 1648–1649
      of traumatic posterior instability, 1652
    posterior cruciate ligament, 1214
    scapulothoracic disorders, 614
    spine, 1544, 1545f
Range of motion (ROM), 349–350, 362
  active, 350
  ankle, 1375

Range of motion (ROM) (Continued)
  elbow, 683, 690
  hip, 930–931, 931t
  immobilization and, 350
  knee, 1094–1095, 1094f–1095f
  passive, 350
  patellofemoral pain, 1311–1312
  restoration, 385–386, 386f
  scapulothoracic disorders, 613
  stiff shoulder, 583, 584b
Readiness for sport, 1609–1610
Reconstruction
  anatomic coracoclavicular, 659b–663b,
      659f–663f
  anterior cruciate ligament, 1193b–1195b,
      1193f–1195f, 1700–1701, 1700f–1702f,
      1701b
    causes of failure, 1202–1203
    primary graft choice, 1203
    treatment options, 1204–1207
    two-stage, 1207
  figure-of-eight, 675, 675b, 676f
  flexor retinaculum, for posterior tibial tendon
      injury, 1467b–1468b
  for lateral and posterolateral corner injuries of
      knee, 1254–1255
    anatomic, 1255–1256
    biceps tenodesis, 1254–1255
    fibula-based, 1256
    posterolateral corner sling procedure in,
        1255
    proximal tibial osteotomy, 1255, 1255f,
        1259b, 1259f
    split biceps tendon transfer, 1255
  lateral ankle ligament, 1426b
  ligament, implants for, 38–41
  surgical, 28
Recreational drug use, 290–293
  alcohol, 290–291
  cocaine, 292
  inhalants, 293
  marijuana, 291–292
  tobacco, 292
Recreational water-related illness, 210–213
  cryptosporidiosis, 211–212
  fecally derived, 211
    non, 213–214
    other, 212–213
  infectious diarrhea, 212
Rectus femoris, 919
Recurrent instability
  anterior cruciate ligament injuries, 1199
  anterior shoulder instability, 452–453
Red blood cells, disorders of, 196–198
  definition, 196
  diagnosis, 197–198, 197f
  epidemiology, 196
  pathophysiology, 196–197, 197t
  return-to-play guidelines, 198
  treatment, 198
Referral, 345–346
Referred pain
  intrathoracic source, 406
  the neck, 405–406
Regional anesthesia, 328
  arm, 330
  benefits, 328
  complications, 328
  contraindications, 328
  elbow, 330–332
  femur, 332–333
  forearm, 330–332
  hand, 330–332
  hip, 332–333
  intravenous, 334
  knee, 332–333

Regional anesthesia (Continued)
  neuraxial anesthesia, 329
  orthopaedic surgeries and, 327
  patient characteristics, 327
  peripheral nerve block, 329–330
  shoulder, 330
  techniques, 329–335
  thigh, 332–333
Regional pain syndrome, complex, 1316
Regulation, of athletic trainer, 343, 344t
Rehabilitation, 345–346
  anterior cruciate ligament injuries, 1192–1195,
      1197
  anterior shoulder instability, 455
  femoroacetabular impingement, 967–969
  glenohumeral arthritis, 605–606
  hamstring injuries, 1039–1040
  motion, loss in elbow, 782
  posterior hip pain, 1027–1030, 1027f–1028f
  principles, 347–353, 1207–1208
    chronic workload ratio, 347–348, 348f
    envelope of function and, 347, 348f
    matched dosing of internal and external
        load, 348, 348f
    patient modifiers, 349
    tissue healing considerations,
        348–349
    tissue-specific considerations, 349
      articular cartilage, 349
      bone, 349
      labral/meniscal, 349
      ligament, 349
      tendon, 349
    protocol for, 1208–1209
Relative motion, 22
Relieving factors, for stiff shoulder,
    580–581
"Relocation test", 404
Remodeling phase
  of fracture repair, 14
  of tendon and ligament repair, 5
Renal medicine, 227–229
Renal sports medicine, metabolic problems in,
    229
Repair. See also Healing
  Achilles tendon, platelet-rich plasma for, 54
  articular cartilage, 11–12
  cartilage, 42–45
    stem cell-based therapy, 59–60
  fracture, 14–15
  for lateral and posterolateral corner injury of
      knee, 1254, 1254f
  ligament, 4–5
    platelet-rich plasma for, 53–55
  meniscal, 9, 41–42
    all-inside, 1147, 1148f
    augmentation in, 9
    in avascular portions, 9
    basics of, 1144
    factors affecting, 9
    inside-out, 1144–1146, 1145f–1146f
    outside-in, 1146–1147, 1147f
    platelet-rich plasma, 55–56
    scaffolds for, 9
    stem cell-based therapy, 60
    techniques, 1143b, 1143f
    in vascular regions, 9
  osteochondral, 42–45
  rotator cuff, platelet-rich plasma for, 54
  tendon, 35–38
    platelet-rich plasma for, 53–55
Reparative phase, of tendon and ligament repair,
    5
Repetition time, in magnetic resonance imaging,
    95
Resistance exercises, for subscapularis injury, 564

Resisted internal rotation test, 933
Resonant frequency, in magnetic resonance
    imaging, 94
Respiration, mitochondrial, 66
Respiratory considerations, preoperative care,
    325–326
  asthma, 325
  obstructive sleep apnea, 325–326, 326f
Respiratory response, to exercise, 72–73
Respiratory tract infections
  lower, 209–210
    acute bronchitis, 209
    acute pneumonia, 209–210
  upper, 206–209
    diagnosis, 207
    epidemiology, 206
    infectious mononucleosis, 207–208
    measles, 208–209
    pathobiology, 206–207
    prevention, 207
    return-to-play guidelines, 207
    treatment, 207
Retinal detachment, 269
Retiring, 1567
Return to play
  acromioclavicular joint, 663–664
  acute bronchitis, 209
  acute otitis externa, 214
  acute pneumonia, 210
  adductor strains, 1051
  after arthroplasty, 1283
  after osteotomy, 1283
  AIN syndrome, 747
  anterior cruciate ligament injuries, 1197
  articular cartilage lesions, 1167
  bacterial skin infections, 204–205
  brain injury, 1567, 1567t
  concussion, 1567, 1567t, 1746, 1746t
  cryptosporidiosis, 212
  cubital tunnel syndrome, 752
  deep venous thrombosis, 185–186
  distal biceps, 727
  elbow, 718, 768
  encephalitis, 215
  exercise-associated collapse, 237
  exercise-associated hyponatremia, 239
  exercise-associated muscle cramps, 237
  exercise-induced bronchoconstriction, 179,
    179f
  exertional heat exhaustion, 235–236, 236b
  exertional heat stroke, 236, 236b
  exertional rhabdomyolysis, 238b
  fractures, 139–142, 140f–141f
  fungal skin infections, 206
  genitourinary trauma, 229
  glenohumeral arthritis, 606
  heat syncope, 237
  hemostasis disorders, 200
  herpes simplex virus, 205, 205t
  iliac crest contusion, 1044
  infectious diarrhea, 212
  infectious disease prevention, 202–203
  infectious mononucleosis, 208
  lateral epicondylitis, 724
  loss of knee motion, 1342
  measles, 209
  medial collateral ligament and posterior medial
    corner injuries, 1240b
  medial epicondylitis, 724
  meningitis, 215
  meniscal injuries, 1151
  motion, loss in elbow, 782
  osteochondral lesions, 1500
  PIN syndrome, 755

Return to play (Continued)
  popliteal artery entrapment syndrome, 1356
  pronator syndrome, 745–746
  quadriceps contusion, 1046
  quadriceps strains, 1049
  radial tunnel syndrome, 755
  red blood cells disorders, 198
  scapulothoracic disorders, 619
  seizure, 232–234
  sternoclavicular joint, 677
  stingers, 1576
  thoracolumbar spine injuries, 1592
  triceps tendinitis, 727
  upper respiratory tract infections, 207
Reverse pivot-shift test, 1213, 1251
Revision anterior cruciate ligament, 1189–1190,
    1192
  injuries, 1199–1210, 1208b
    advanced imaging, 1202, 1202f
    complications in, 1209
    decision-making principles, 1202–1204
    future considerations, 1209
    history, 1199–1200
    imaging, 1200–1202, 1200f
    multiple, 1209
    physical exam, 1200
    postoperative management, 1207–1209
    results, 1209
Revision rotator cuff repair, 567–573
  complications, 571–573, 572t–573t
  decision-making principles, 568–569, 569t,
    570f
  future considerations of, 573
  history patient with, 567–568
  imaging, 568
  noncuff tear etiologies of, 568t
  physical examination, 568
  postoperative management, 571
  results, 571–573, 572t–573t
  treatment options, 569–571
    with biologic augmentation, 571
    débridement alone, 569
    nonoperative, 569
    revision repair, 569–571
    technique, 571b, 572f
Revision shoulder instability, 489–501
  complications, 499–500
  decision-making principles, 493–494
  future considerations, 500, 500f
  history, 489
  imaging, 490–493, 491f–492f
  physical exam, 489–490, 490f
  postoperative management, 498–499
  preferred surgical technique, 495–498,
    496f–499f
  results, 499
  treatment options, 494–495, 494f
Rhabdomyolysis, 229
  exertional, 237–238, 238b
Rheumatoid arthritis, 594–595, 594f
Rheumatoid cervical spondylitis, 1596–1597,
    1596f
Rib, fractures, 137–139
Right ventricle, 160
Rigid body mechanics, 23
Rigorous athletic training, cardiovascular
    adaptations and, 160–161
"Ringworm" (tinea corporis), 249
"Roller-wringer effect", 557
Rolling motion, 22–23, 23f
ROM. See Range of motion
Roos elevated arm test, 636–638, 638f
Rosenberg view, knee arthritis and, 1278,
    1278f–1279f

Rotator cuff, 35–36, 398–399, 398f, 417–422
  débridement, 522–523
  magnetic resonance imaging, 419–422,
    419f–424f, 419t, 423b
  pathology, 406–407
  repair, 523–524
    platelet-rich plasma for, 54
  revision, 567–573
    complications, 571–573, 572t–573t
    decision-making principles, 568–569, 569t,
      570f
    future considerations of, 573
    history patient with, 567–568
    imaging, 568
    noncuff tear etiologies of, 568t
    physical examination, 568
    postoperative management, 571
    results, 571–573, 572t–573t
    treatment options, 569–571
      with biologic augmentation, 571
      débridement alone, 569
      nonoperative, 569
      revision repair, 569–571
      technique, 571b, 572f
  tears, 406, 1656–1658, 1657f–1658f
Rotator cuff and impingement lesions, 540–555
  anatomy, 540–542, 541f
  biomechanics, 542–543
    biceps function, 542, 543f
    function, 542, 542f
    scapular function, 543
    static stabilizers, 542–543
  decision-making principles, 547–548
    acute rotator cuff trauma, 548
    chronic rotator cuff disease, 548
    subacromial impingement and biceps
      tenosynovitis, 548
  future considerations, 554
  historical perspective, 540
  history, 543
  imaging, 547
    magnetic resonance imaging, 547, 547f
    plain radiographs, 547
    ultrasonography, 547
  physical examination, 543–547, 544f–546f
    impingement test, 546–547
  treatment options, 548–554
    complications, 554
    nonoperative, 549–550
    operative, 550–554, 550b–553b, 551f–552f
    preventive, 548–549, 549f
Rotator interval, 422–424, 425f
Rotatory atlantoaxial subluxation, 1759–1761
  history, 1759
  imaging, 1760, 1761f
  physical examination, 1759
  treatment, 1760–1761
Rowing injuries, 123
  chest, 123
  knee, 123
  lumbar spine, 123
  upper extremity, 123
Rugby injuries, 123–124
Runner's diarrhea, 193
"Runner's trots", 193
Running injuries, 124
Ruptured globe, 269

S

Sacral facet fractures, 1755, 1756f
Sacral stress fracture, 926
Sacroiliac joint, injuries of, thoracolumbar spine
    and, 1591

Sagittal band rupture, 877–878, 877f
Salter-Harris fracture
    type I, 1729f, 1730
    type II, 1729f, 1730, 1733f
    type III, 1729f, 1730
    type IV, 1729f–1731f, 1730–1731
Saphenous nerve block, 333
Saphenous nerve entrapment, 1405–1407,
    1405f–1406f
    history, 1405
    imaging, 1406
    physical examination, 1405–1406
    results, 1406–1407
    treatment options, 1406
Sarcomeres, 62, 63f
Sarcopenia, 68
Sartorius, 919
Scabies, 253, 253f
Scaffolds
    meniscal, 1149–1150
    for meniscal repair, 9
Scalars, 16
Scaphoid
    carpal injuries, 835–836, 837b, 837f
    fractures, 807–808, 807f–808f, 824, 1684–1686
        complications, 1685
        decision-making principles, 1685
        future considerations, 1686
        history, 1684
        imaging, 1684–1685
        physical examination, 1684
        postoperative management, 1685
        results, 1685
        treatment options, 1685, 1685b, 1686f
    nonunions, 824–825, 825t
Scapholunate injuries, 848
Scapula, 1637, 1638f
Scapular bursitis, 609, 611b, 611f, 611t, 616–617,
    616f–617f
Scapular dyskinesia, 619
    pediatrics, 1659, 1659f
Scapular dyskinesis, 609, 612f–613f, 616t
Scapular lag, 543
Scapular muscles, 399
Scapular retraction test, 614
Scapular winging, 609, 612f–613f, 612t, 619
Scapular Y view, 408–409, 409f
Scapulothoracic articulation, 398
Scapulothoracic disorders, 609–620, 610f, 610t
    complications, 620
    crepitus, 609, 611b, 611f, 611t
    decision-making principles, 614–615
        crepitus, 614–615
        injection, 615, 615f
        pain, 614–615
        pathologies, 615
        treatment, 615
    future considerations, 620
    history, 609–611
    imaging, 614
        computed tomography, 614
        electromyography, 614
        magnetic resonance imaging, 614
        radiographs, 614
        ultrasound, 614, 614f–615f
    physical examination, 611–614
        inspection, 611–612
        palpation, 612–613
        range of motion, 613
        strength, 613
        testing, 613–614
    postoperative management, 619
    results, 619–620
    return-to-play guidelines, 619
    scapular bursitis, 609, 611b, 611f, 611t
    scapular dyskinesis, 609, 612f–613f, 616t

Scapulothoracic disorders (Continued)
    scapular winging, 609, 612f–613f, 612t
    treatment, 615–619
        arthroscopic bursal resection, 617b–619b,
            617f–619f
        nonoperative, 615–616
        operative, 616–619
Schistosomiasis, 216
Sciatic nerve
    characteristics, 1018–1020, 1019f–1020f
    of hip, 916
Sciatic nerve block, 333
Sciatic nerve entrapment, 1020–1024
    anatomy, 1020–1021, 1021f
    etiology, 1021–1024, 1021f–1023f
    operative treatment, 1027–1030
    physical examination, 1024–1026, 1024f–1026f
    preoperative and postoperative rehabilitation,
        1027–1030, 1027f–1028f
Scintigraphy, nuclear, 1548–1549, 1549f
Scissors, in arthroscopy, 108
Scoliosis, 1755–1758
    history, 1755–1757
    idiopathic, 313–314
    imaging, 1757
    physical examination, 1755–1757
    sports participation, 1757–1758
    treatment, 1757
Scour test, 932
Scratch collapse test, 691–692
Screening, for cardiovascular system, 162–166,
    163b
    electrocardiogram, 163–164, 164f
    transthoracic echocardiography, 164–166,
        165f–167f
SCT. See Sickle cell trait
Seabather's eruption, 256, 257f
Second-impact syndrome, 1746–1747
Secondary deep bursa, 920
Sedation, in orthopedic patient, 339, 339t
Seizure, 230. See also Epilepsy
    acute management, 232
    exercise and, 231–232
    return-to-activity guidelines of, 232–234
Semitendinosus autograft, 31
Septic arthritis, of hip, 928
Septic meningitis, 214
Sesamoid dysfunction, 1516–1519, 1516b
    complications, 1519
    decision-making principles, 1517
    history, 1517
    imaging, 1517, 1518f
    physical examination, 1517
    postoperative management, 1518–1519
    results, 1519
    treatment options, 1517–1518
        nonoperative, 1517
        operative, 1518, 1519f
        technique, 1518b
Sever disease, 1738–1739, 1739f
Shavers, motorized, 107
Shoes, 1739
    sports, 1439–1442
        anatomy, 1440, 1441f
        insole, 1441
        midsole, 1440–1441
        outsole, 1440
        selection and fitting of, 1442, 1442t
        upper, 1441–1442
Short external rotators, 920
Short tau inversion recovery (STIR), 97–98
Shoulder, 393–401
    anatomy, 393–395, 394f
    anterior instability, 440–462
        anatomy, 440–441, 441f–442f
        decision-making principles, 450–454

Shoulder (Continued)
    future considerations, 461–462
    history, 447
    imaging, 448–450, 450f–452f
    pathoanatomy, 441–447, 443f–444f, 443t,
        446f
    physical examination, 447–448, 448f–449f
    treatment options, 454–461
        complications, 461
        emergency department, 455
        nonoperative sling immobilization, 455
        on-field management, 454–455
        rehabilitation, 455
        results, 461
        surgical management, 455–461, 456b
    arthrography, 410–411, 410f
    arthroscopy, 433–439
        anatomy, 435–436
        background, 433
        complications, 438–439
        contraindications, 433
        diagnostic examination, 436–438, 437f–438f
        indications, 433
        open procedures vs., 433
        portal placement, 435–436, 436f
        positioning, 434–435, 434f
        preoperative imaging, 433–434
        setup, 435
        visualization, 435
    biomechanics, 400
    complex, 399–400
    decision-making, 402–407
    diagnosis, 402–407
    examination of, 568
    history, 402–403
    imaging
        abnormalities, 402
        glenohumeral joint, 408–432
    injuries
        baseball, 114–115
        golf, 120
        handball, 122
        pediatrics, 1637–1660
        skiing, 124
        snowboarding, 124–125
        swimming, 126
        volleyball, 128
    instability, 406–407
    joints, 395–398
        acromioclavicular joint, 397
        glenohumeral, 395–396, 395f–396f
        glenohumeral joint capsule, 396–397
        scapulothoracic articulation, 398
        sternoclavicular joint, 397, 397f
    kinetics, 400
    little league, 1612, 1612f
    multidirectional instability, 476–488, 482b, 482f
        decision-making principles, 479–480
        future considerations, 480–481
        history, 477
        imaging, 479, 479f
        physical examination, 477–479, 477t–478t, 478f
        postoperative management, 481–483, 483f
        results, 483–487, 484t–485t
            complications, 486–487
            return to sport, 485–486, 486t
        treatment options, 480–481
            arthroscopic plication, 481
            open inferior capsular shift, 480–481, 480f
    muscles, 398–400
        rotator cuff, 398–399, 398f
        scapular muscles, 399
    nerve entrapment, 621
    pathologies, 406–407
        acromioclavicular joint, 406
        rotator cuff, 406–407

Shoulder (Continued)
  pediatric, 1616–1618
    acute injuries, 1617–1618, 1618f–1619f
    development, 1616–1617, 1617f
    overuse injuries, 1618, 1620f–1621f
  pertinent bony, 393–395, 394f
  physical examination, 403–405
  posterior instability, 463–475
    arthroscopic posterior shoulder stabilization, 470b–472b, 470f–472f
    background, 463
    complications, 474–475
    decision-making principles, 468
    future considerations, 475
    history, 465
    imaging, 467–468, 467f–468f, 468t
    pathogenesis, 463–465, 464f–465f
    physical examination, 465–467, 466f, 466t
    postoperative management, 469–473
    results, 473–474
    treatment options, 468–469
      contraindications, 469
      indications, 469
  regional anesthesia, 330
  stiff, 579–591
    acquired causes, 582–583
    anatomy, 579
    complications, 589–590
    decision-making principles, 585
    future considerations, 590
    history, 579–583
    idiopathic adhesive capsulitis, 581–582
    imaging, 584–585
    pain, 579–581, 580b
    pathologies causing, 581b
    physical examination, 583–584
    postoperative management, 586–589
    primary causes, 581–582
    results, 589, 589t
    secondary causes, 582–583
    treatment options, 585–586, 586b
Shoulder instability, 1612, 1612f
  in female athlete, 312–313, 312f
  revision, 489–501
    complications, 499–500
    decision-making principles, 493–494
    future considerations, 500, 500f
    history, 489
    imaging, 490–493, 491f–492f
    physical exam, 489–490, 490f
    postoperative management, 498–499
    preferred surgical technique, 495–498, 496f–499f
    results, 499
    treatment options, 494–495, 494f
Sickle cell trait (SCT), 196, 238
Silk-based scaffold, 39
Simple lacerations, 262, 262f–263f
Sinding-Larsen-Johansson disease, 1718, 1718f
Single-bundle reconstruction, for posterior cruciate ligament injuries, 1218–1219, 1218f, 1225–1229
Single photon emission computed tomography, 88, 89f
  of spine, 1549–1550
Single photon emission computed tomography/computed tomography imaging, 88, 89f
Sitting examination, of patellar instability, 1296, 1296f
Skeletal muscle
  aging effects on, 68
  contractions
    physiology, 62–64, 64f
    types, 65

Skeletal muscle (Continued)
    energy metabolism, 65–66, 65f
    force production, 64–65
    physiology, 62–66, 63t
    structure, 62, 63f
Skeletally immature athletes, 1616–1636
Skiing injuries, 124–125
Skin
  cancer, 256
  of hand, 785, 786f
  in medial collateral ligament and posterior medial corner injuries, 1231–1232
  soft tissue infections, 203–206
    bacterial skin infections, 203–205
    fungal skin infections, 205–206
    herpes simplex virus, 205
Skull, 1528, 1529f
SLAP tears. See Superior labrum anterior to posterior (SLAP) tears
"Sliding filament theory", 62–63
Sliding injuries, 115
Sliding motion, 22–23, 23f
Slipped capital femoral epiphysis, 928, 1694, 1695f
Snapping, iliopsoas, 980, 981f, 982, 983f, 984–986
Snapping hip syndrome, 925
  pediatrics, 1692–1693
Snapping scapula, pediatrics, 1658–1659, 1658f
Snowboarding injuries, 124–125
Soccer injuries, 125–126
"Soft spot" portal, 711
Soft tissue
  anatomy, patellar instability, 1294–1295, 1295f
  ankle arthroscopy, conditions amenable to, 1421–1428, 1422f
    complications, 1428
    decision-making principles, 1424
    future considerations, 1428
    history, 1423
    imaging, 1423–1424
    nonoperative management, 1424
    physical examination, 1423
    postoperative management, 1427
    results, 1427–1428
    surgical technique, 1424–1426, 1425f
  autograft, 31
  elbow, stability of, 684–685, 685f
  injuries
    ear, 263
    foot and ankle, 1728–1729, 1728f
    hip, 925, 1691–1693
    pediatrics, 1661–1662, 1662f–1663f
Soreness, delayed-onset muscle, 68
Spasticity, 319, 321
Special needs, athletes with, 150
Special tests, patellar instability and, 1296–1297, 1297f
SPECT. See Single photon emission computed tomography
SPECT/CT imaging. See Single photon emission computed tomography/computed tomography imaging
Speed test, 405
Spin echo, 96, 97f
Spin lattice relaxation, 95
Spin-spin relaxation, 95
Spinal accessory nerve palsy, 627–629
  anatomy, 627–628
  biomechanics, 627–628
  clinical evaluation, 628–629, 628f
  decision-making principles, 629
  diagnostic studies, 629
  results, 629
  technique, 629b
Spinal cord injury, 1559

Spinal cord injury without radiographic abnormality (SCIWORA), 1763
Spinal stability, in thoracolumbar spine injuries, 1583
Spinal stenosis, cervical, 1595–1596, 1595f–1596f
Spine, 1531–1533, 1532f–1533f. See also Back
  anatomy, 1528, 1529f
    brain, 1528–1529
    intervertebral disk, 1534
    ligaments, 1534
    muscles, 1534
    neurologic tissues, 1534–1535, 1534f
    skull (cranium), 1528, 1529f
  biomechanics, 1535, 1535f
  cervical
    congenital anomalies of, 1762–1763
    injuries, 152–153, 1578–1581
  hip and, 923–924, 923f
  imaging, 1544–1552
    computed tomography, 1546, 1546f
    degenerative, 1550–1551
    EOS 2D/3D x-ray imaging system, 1545–1546, 1545f
    functional metabolic imaging, 1549
    future considerations, 1551
    interventional radiology, 1550
    magnetic resonance imaging, 1547, 1547f
    myelography, 1548
    nuclear scintigraphy, 1548–1549, 1549f
    radiographs, 1544, 1545f
    single photon emission computed tomography, 1549–1550
    study interpretation, 1551
  injuries, 1541
    common acute, 1559–1560, 1560f
    emergency management, 1553–1561, 1559f
    epidemiology, 1553
    field-side management, 1553–1561, 1554f–1558f
    issues, in skeletally immature athletes, 1749–1764
      anatomy, 1749, 1750f–1751f
      history, 1749–1750, 1750b
      physical examination, 1749–1750, 1751b
    pediatric, 1635–1636, 1635f
Spinning motion, 22–23, 23f
Spinoglenoid notch compression, 624
Spinoglenoid notch decompression, 625
Splinting, 722
Split biceps tendon transfer, 1255
Spondylolisthesis, 1750–1753
  classification, 1751, 1751f
  degenerative, 1603–1604, 1603f–1604f
  history, 1751–1752
  imaging, 1752, 1752f
  physical examination, 1751–1752
  results, 1753, 1755f
  thoracolumbar spine, 1588–1591, 1590f
  treatment, 1752–1753, 1752f, 1754f
Spondylolysis, 1750–1753
  classification, 1751, 1751f
  history, 1751–1752
  imaging, 1752, 1752f
  physical examination, 1751–1752
  results, 1753, 1755f
  thoracolumbar spine, 1588, 1589f–1590f, 1591
  treatment, 1752–1753, 1752f, 1754f
Spondylosis, cervical, 405, 1594–1596
  disc herniation, 1595
  discogenic pain, 1594–1595
  epidemiology, 1594, 1594f
  foraminal stenosis, 1595
  myelopathy, 1595–1596
  pathoanatomy, 1594

Spondylosis, cervical (Continued)
  radiculopathy, 1595
  rheumatoid, 1596–1597, 1596f
  spinal stenosis, 1595–1596, 1595f–1596f
Spontaneous osteonecrosis, 1117
Sport Concussion Assessment Tool version 5
  (SCAT5), 1744
Sport-specific injuries, 114–130. See also specific
  sports
  auto racing, 117
  baseball, 114–115
  basketball, 115–116
  boxing, 116–117
  figure skating, 117–118
  football, 118–119
  golf, 119–120
  gymnastics, 120–121
  handball, 121–122
  ice hockey, 121
  lacrosse, 122
  rowing, 123
  rugby, 123–124
  running, 124
  skiing, 124–125
  snowboarding, 124–125
  soccer, 125–126
  swimming, 126
  tennis, 126–127
  volleyball, 127–128
  wrestling, 128–129
Sports
  epilepsy and, 230–234
  forefoot problems in, 1515–1526
  shoes and orthoses, 1436–1443
Sports equipment. See Equipment
Sports hernia, 1007, 1012–1014, 1014b, 1014f
Sports medicine rehabilitation, 354–367
  impairment-based rehabilitation programs,
    355–357
  joint cryotherapy, 366
  manipulation, 363
  manual therapy, 354–355, 356t
  mobilization, 363, 364f–365f
    with movement, 363–365, 365f
  modalities, 354, 355f
  muscle dysfunction, 365–366
  muscle energy technique, 366–367
  myofascial release, 367
  neuromuscular electrical stimulation, 366
  nonthermal ultrasound treatments, 360–363
    compression, 362, 362f
    iontophoresis, 360–361
    laser, 361–362
    phonophoresis, 360
    range of motion, 362
    stress fracture healing, 360, 361f
    superficial heat, 362–363
  pain modulation, 357
  patterned electrical nerve stimulation, 366, 366f
  thermal effects of ultrasound, 363
  treatments for pain, 357–360
    cryotherapy, 358–359
    edema/inflammation, 359
    electrical stimulation, 359
    manual therapy, 357, 358t
    transcutaneous electrical nerve stimulation,
      359
    ultrasound, 359–360
  trigger point therapy, 367, 367f
Sports nutrition, 277–282
  carbohydrate, 277–278, 278t
  energy balance, 277
  fat, 277–278, 278t
  hydration, 278–279, 279t
    considerations, 278
    monitoring, 278–279

Sports nutrition (Continued)
  minerals, 279–280
  nutrient timing, 280, 280t
  protein, 277–278, 278t
  sports supplementation, 280, 281t
  vitamins, 279–280
Sports participation, in pediatrics, 1606
  adult involvement, 1610
  psychosocial development, 1609
  readiness for sport, 1609–1610
Sports pharmacology
  ergogenic drugs, 283–290
    anabolic-androgenic steroids, 284–287
    caffeine, 290
    creatine, 288–289
    doping, 287–288
    growth hormone, 289–290
    steroid supplements, 287
    testosterone, historical perspectives, 283–284
  recreational drug use, 290–293
    alcohol, 290–291
    cocaine, 292
    inhalants, 293
    marijuana, 291–292
    tobacco, 292
Sprains
  ankle, 115, 371, 380–381
    balance, 381, 382f–383f
    bracing, 380–381
    coordination, 381
    dorsiflexion range of motion, 381
    education of risk, 381
    hypomobility issues, 381
    lateral, 1444–1450, 1445f
    medial, 1450–1453
    strength training, 381
    taping, 380–381
  bifurcate ligament, 1456–1457
    complications, 1458
    decision-making principles, 1457
    history, 1457
    imaging, 1457
    physical examination, 1457
    postoperative management, 1457
    results, 1457–1458
    treatment, 1457, 1457b
  cervical spine injuries, 1579
  hip, 942, 944f–945f
  Lisfranc, 1458–1460
    complications, 1460
    decision-making principles, 1459
    history, 1458
    imaging, 1458–1459, 1459f
    physical examination, 1458
    postoperative management, 1459–1460
    results, 1460
    treatment, 1459, 1460b, 1460f
  sternoclavicular joint, 673
  syndesmosis, 1453–1456
    complications, 1456
    decision-making principles, 1454
    history, 1453–1454
    imaging, 1454, 1455f
    physical examination, 1453–1454
    postoperative management, 1456
    results, 1456
    treatment, 1454–1456, 1456b
  of thoracolumbar spine, 1585–1588
Standard anterolateral portal, 711
Standard anteromedial portal, 709, 710f
Standing anteroposterior pelvic view, 935,
  936f
Standing apprehension test, 1250–1251, 1250f
Stasis, 180
Static standing, examination of, for patellar
  instability, 1296

Statics, 19–22
  force vectors, 21
  free-body diagrams, 20f, 21
  ligament and joint contact forces,
    21–22
  moment/torque vectors, 21
Stem cell-based therapy
  application, 58
  cartilage repair, 59–60
  definitions, 56–58, 57f–58f
  meniscal repair, 60
  preparations, 56–58, 57f–58f
  sports medicine, 56–58, 57f
Stem cells, for knee arthritis, 1280
Stenosis, cervical, 405
Sternoclavicular joint, 397, 397f
  injuries, 664–677
    anatomy, 667, 667f–670f
    complications, 677
    decision-making principles, 668, 673f
    future considerations, 677
    history, 664
    imaging, 667–668, 670f–672f
    physical examination, 664–667
    postoperative management, 677
    results, 677
    return-to-play guidelines, 677
    treatment, 673
Steroids, anabolic-androgenic, 1611
Stiff shoulder, 579–591
  acquired causes, 582–583
  anatomy, 579
  complications, 589–590
  decision-making principles, 585
  future considerations, 590
  history, 579–583
    crepitus, 581
    exacerbating factors, 580–581
    pain, 579–581, 580b
    relieving factors, 580–581
    stiffness, 581
    weakness, 581
  idiopathic adhesive capsulitis,
    581–582
  imaging, 584–585
  pathologies causing, 581b
  physical examination, 583–584
    inspection, 583, 583f
    motion, 584, 584b
    special testing, 584, 584b
    strength, 584, 584b
  postoperative management, 586–589
  primary causes, 581–582
  results, 589, 589t
  secondary causes, 582–583
  treatment options, 585–586, 586b
  technique, 586b–588b, 586f–588f
Stiffness, flexibility testing vs., 27
Stimulation, electrical, for pain, 359
Stinchfield test, 932
Stingers, 406, 1570–1577, 1579
  classification, 1573–1574, 1574t
  decision-making principles, 1573–1574
  future considerations, 1576, 1576f
  history, 1570
  imaging, 1571–1573, 1573f
  mechanism of, 1573, 1574f
  physical examination, 1570–1571, 1571f–1572f,
    1572t
  return to play criteria, 1576
  sequela, 1576
  treatment options, 1574–1575, 1575b,
    1575f
Straight-leg raise (SLR) test, 932
Straight posterior portal, 711
Strain energy density, 26

Strains, 25–26, 26f, 1043–1052
  adductor, 1011–1012, 1050–1051
    complications, 1051
    decision-making principles, 1051
    future considerations, 1051
    history, 1050
    imaging, 1050, 1050f
    physical examination, 1050
    results, 1051
    return to play, 1051
    technique, 1051b
    treatment options, 1050–1051
  cervical, 405
    spine injuries, 1579
  hamstring, 376
    causes, 376
    preventing, 377, 377f, 377t
    risk factors, 376–377
  quadriceps, 1047–1050
    complications, 1049
    decision-making principles, 1049
    future considerations, 1050
    history, 1048
    imaging, 1048, 1048f
    physical examination, 1048
    results, 1049, 1049f
    return to play, 1049
    technique, 1049b
    treatment options, 1048–1049, 1048t, 1049f
  of thoracolumbar spine, 1585–1588
Strength testing
  in knee, 1094–1095, 1094f–1095f
  shoulder, 404
Strength training, 381
  muscular response to, 66–67
  pediatrics, 1608–1609
  in young athletes, 68
Stress, 25–26, 26f
Stress fractures, 131–139
  biomechanical factors, 131–132
  classification system, 132t
  elbow, 700
  fatigue and training errors causing, 132
  in female athlete, 131, 314
  femoral neck, 132–133, 132f–133f
  genetic factors, 132
  healing, 360, 361f
  metatarsal, 135–136
  navicular, 136, 137f
  nutrition and, 132
  olecranon, 764–765, 764f–765f
  pars, 136–137, 138f
  pediatrics, 1688–1690, 1690f
  proximal fifth metatarsal, 134–135, 135f–136f
  in thoracolumbar spine, 1584–1585
  tibial, 133–134, 134f–135f
Stress injuries, 942–944, 945f
Striae, 254, 255f
Structural disease, in elite athlete, 166–169
Stryker Intra-Compartmental Pressure Monitor,
    for compartment pressure measurement,
    1397
Subacromial decompression and rotator cuff
    repair, 550
Subacromial impingement, 548
Subarachnoid hemorrhage, 1745
Subdural hematoma, 1745
Subscapularis injury, 556–566, 557f
  anatomy, 556–557
  classification, 558
  decision-making principles, 559–560
  function, 557
  future considerations, 565–566
  history, 558–559, 558f

Subscapularis injury (Continued)
  imaging, 559, 559f
  mechanism, 557–558
  physical examination, 558–559, 558f
  treatment options, 560–565, 561f–562f
    complications, 565
    postoperative rehab, 562–564
    results, 564–565
    technique, 563b–564b, 563f–564f
Substances, performance-enhancing, 1611
Subtalar arthroscopy, 1428–1433
  complications, 1432–1433
  decision-making principles, 1429
  history, 1429
  imaging, 1429
  physical examination, 1429
  postoperative management, 1431
  results, 1431–1432
Subtalar joint, biomechanics, 1363–1365, 1363t,
    1364f–1366f
Sudden death, 116
"Sulcus sign", 405
Sunburn, 256
Superficial anatomy, of knee, 1062–1063, 1063f
Superficial bursa, 920
Superficial heat, 362–363
Superficial peroneal nerve entrapment, 1413–
    1415, 1413f
  decision-making principles, 1414
  history, 1413
  imaging, 1414
  physical examination, 1413–1414
  postoperative management, 1415
  results, 1415
  treatment options, 1414–1415, 1414b, 1414f
Superficial zone, of articular cartilage, 10, 10f
Superior gluteal nerve, 1032–1033, 1032f, 1032t
  of hip, 916
Superior labrum anterior to posterior (SLAP)
    tears, 407, 502–510, 503f–504f, 507b–508b,
    507f–508f
  débridement, 524
  decision-making principles, 505–506, 506f
  future considerations, 509
  history, 502
  imaging, 503–504, 505f
  physical examination, 502–503, 504t
  repair, 524
  treatment options, 506–509, 507f
    complications, 509
    postoperative management, 508
    results, 508–509
Superior pole osteochondrosis, 1718
Supine position, 932–933
  hip arthroscopy, 948
Supraclavicular block, 330–332, 332f
Supraclavicular pressure test, 636–638, 637f
Suprascapular block, 330
Suprascapular nerve palsy, 621–625
  anatomy, 621–622, 622f
  biomechanics, 621–622, 622f
  clinical evaluation, 622–623, 623f
  decision-making principles, 624
  diagnostic studies, 623–624, 623f
  results, 624–625
Suprascapular notch compression, 624b
Suprascapular notch decompression, 625
Sural nerve entrapment, 1402–1405, 1403f
  history, 1402
  imaging, 1403–1404
  physical examination, 1402–1403
  postoperative management, 1405
  results, 1405
  treatment options, 1404, 1404b, 1404f

Surface landmarks, in hip arthroscopy, 950
Surgery
  arthroscopic synovectomy, of knee, 1129–1130
    anterior compartments, 1129, 1130t
    posterior compartments, 1129–1130
  hamstring injuries, 1037–1039
  hip arthritis, 1058–1059
  lateral epicondylitis, 722–723, 723f
  medial epicondylitis, 722–723, 723f
  meniscal injuries
    indications, 1139–1140
    techniques, 1143–1147, 1144f
  meniscectomy, 1143–1144, 1144f
  motion, loss in elbow, 776–782, 777f
    arthroscopy, 776–781, 777f–781f
    open release, 781–782
  multiligament knee injuries, timing of, 1266
  orthopaedic, 327
  shoulder, 455–461, 456b
Surgical considerations, for lateral and
    posterolateral corner injuries of knee,
    1254–1256
  diagnostic arthroscopy, 1254, 1254f
  primary repair, 1254, 1254f
  reconstruction techniques, 1254–1255
Suture anchors, 46–47
Sutures
  anchors, 46–47
  for implants, 45–46
Sweat rate measurement, 240b
Swimmer's itch, 256
Swimming injuries, 126
  back, 126
  knee, 126
  shoulder, 126
Swipe test, 1277
Switching sticks, in arthroscopy, 108
Symptom localization, of hip, 929–930, 930f–931f
Syncope, 173
Syndesmosis sprain, 1453–1456
  complications, 1456
  decision-making principles, 1454
  history, 1453–1454
  imaging, 1454, 1455f
  physical examination, 1453–1454
  postoperative management, 1456
  results, 1456
  treatment, 1454–1456, 1456b
Synovial abrasion, 1148
Synovial facet cysts, 1601–1602
Synovial impingement syndrome, 1315–1316,
    1316f
Synovial joints, 9. See also Articular cartilage
Synovial membrane, of knee, 1071–1072, 1072f
Synthesis, in knee, 1101–1102, 1101f–1102f
Systemic illness, foot pain and, 1739

T
T1 magnetic resonance imaging, 95, 95f, 96t
T2 magnetic resonance imaging, 95, 96t
Talar tilt test, for lateral ankle sprain, 1445–1446,
    1446f
Talon noir, 254, 254f
Talus, osteochondral lesions of, 1484–1500
  complications, 1501–1502
  decision-making principles, 1486, 1486f–1487f
  diagnosis, 1484–1486
  history, 1484
  imaging, 1484–1486, 1485f
  physical examination, 1484
  postoperative management, 1500
  results, 1490–1493, 1490b
  return to play, 1500

Talus, osteochondral lesions of *(Continued)*
  treatment options, 1486–1490
    nonoperative, 1486–1487
    operative, 1487–1490, 1487*b*, 1488*f*
    technique, 1493*b*–1498*b*, 1494*f*–1498*f*, 1499*t*
Taping, 368
  ankle sprains, 380–381
  arch, 368–369
  cost effectiveness, 372
  effectiveness, 370–371
  injury prevention, 371
    ankle sprains, 371
    patellofemoral pain, 371
    plantar fasciitis, 371
    plantar fasciosis, 371
  length of effectiveness, 372
  summary, 372
  techniques
    ankle, 369, 369*f*–370*f*
    criticisms of, 371–372
    foot, 368–372, 369*f*
    knee, 369–370
    toe, 369
Tarsal coalition, 1725–1727, 1726*f*
Tarsal tunnel, magnetic resonance imaging,
    1390–1391, 1390*f*–1391*f*
Tarsal tunnel syndrome, 1407–1411, 1407*f*
  decision-making principles, 1408
  electrodiagnostic studies, 1408
  etiologies, 1407–1408, 1407*t*
  etiologies of, 1407–1408, 1407*t*
  history, 1408
  imaging, 1408
  physical examination, 1408
  postoperative management, 1410
  results, 1410–1411
  treatment options, 1408–1409, 1409*b*–1410*b*,
    1409*f*–1410*f*
Team medical coverage, 144–157
  ethical/legal issues in sports medicine, 155–157
    collegiate athletics, 155
    confidentiality, 155
    disagreements with coaches, 157
    drug use, 156
    high school athletics, 155
    informed consent, 156, 156*t*
    professional athletics, 155
  on-field emergencies, 150–155
    anaphylaxis, 153
    cardiac arrest, 153
    cervical spine injury, 152–153
    for collapsed athlete, 151–152, 151*t*
    emergency action plan, 150, 151*b*
    environmental factors, 154
    head injury, 152
    limb-threatening injuries, 154
    tension pneumothorax, 153
  preparticipation physical evaluation, 144–150
    allergies, 149
    athletes with special needs, 150
    cardiovascular system, 145–147, 145*b*–146*b*
    dermatology, 149
    ears, 145
    endocrine system, 149
    eyes, 145
    gastrointestinal system, 148
    genitourinary system, 148
    goals, 144
    head, 145
    heat illness, 149–150
    hematologic disease, 148–149
    history, 145–150
    immunizations, 149
    infectious disease, 148–149
    medications, 149
    musculoskeletal system, 148, 148*b*

Team medical coverage *(Continued)*
    neurologic system, 148
    nose, 145
    objectives, 144
    organization, 144–145
    physical examination, 145–150
    pulmonary system, 147–148
    setting, 144–145, 145*t*
    throat, 145
    timing, 144–145
Teeth
  fractures, 270
  primary *vs.* permanent, 269, 270*f*
Tendinitis, 4, 1320–1321
  triceps, 725–728
    complications, 727
    decision-making principles, 725–726
    future considerations, 727–728
    imaging, 725, 726*f*
    physical examination, 725, 725*f*
    postoperative management, 727
    results, 726
    return-to-play guidelines, 727
    treatment, 726, 726*b*
Tendinopathies, 4, 761–762
  chronic proximal hamstring, 1041
  elbow, 720–730
  patellar and quadriceps, 1320–1321
    clinical outcomes, 1331–1332, 1332*f*
    complications, 1333
    decision-making principles, 1327
    history, 1322–1323
    nonoperative treatment, 1327
    operative treatment, 1328
    physical examination, 1323–1324, 1323*t*
    postoperative management, 1330
Tendon mobilization, of subscapularis injury,
    560
Tendon repair, implants for, 35–38
Tendonitis, iliopsoas, 980
Tendons, 2–7. *See also* Ligaments
  Achilles, 1381–1383, 1382*f*–1383*f*
  ankle, 1381–1386
  anterior tibial, 1386, 1387*f*
  distal biceps rupture, 731–741
    anatomy, 731, 732*f*–733*f*
    biomechanics, 731–732
    classification, 732, 732*b*
    complications, 736–737
    decision-making principles, 735
    epidemiology, 731
    history, 732–733
    imaging, 733–734, 734*f*
    physical examination, 733, 733*f*
    postoperative management, 735
    results, 735–736
    treatment, 734–735, 735*t*, 736*b*, 736*f*
  distal triceps rupture, 737–740
    anatomy, 737, 737*f*
    biomechanics, 737
    classification, 737
    complications, 740
    decision-making principles, 738, 738*b*
    epidemiology, 737, 737*b*
    future considerations, 740
    history, 738
    imaging, 738
    physical examination, 738
    postoperative management, 740
    results, 740
    treatment, 738–739
  extensor
    hand, 790–791, 790*f*–791*f*
    wrist, 790–791, 790*f*–791*f*
  extracellular matrix, 3
  foot, 1381–1386

Tendons *(Continued)*
  gastrocnemius, 1246
  hand, 785–787, 788*f*
  healing
    factors affecting, 5, 6*t*
    methods for augmentation of, 5–7
  injuries, 3–4
    imaging, 812–813, 812*f*–813*f*
    platelet-rich plasma for, 53–54
    wrist, 812–813, 812*f*–813*f*
  long head of biceps, 424–427, 427*f*–428*f*
  peroneal, 1385–1386, 1385*f*–1386*f*
  popliteus, 1245
  posterior tibial, 1383–1384, 1383*f*–1384*f*
  quadriceps, 1318
    rupture, 1321–1322
    structure, 1320, 1320*f*–1321*f*
    tendinopathy, 1320–1321
  repair, 4–5
    platelet-rich plasma for, 53–55
  ruptures, 703–704, 704*f*
    distal biceps tendon, 703–704, 704*f*
  structure of, 2–3, 3*f*
  tibia
    anterior, 1386, 1387*f*
    injuries, 1462–1464
    posterior, 1383–1384, 1383*f*–1384*f*
Tendoscopy, for posterior tibial tendon injury,
    1467*b*–1468*b*, 1467*f*
Tennis injuries, 126–127
Tenocytes, 3
Tenosynovectomy, for posterior tibial tendon
    injury, 1467*b*–1468*b*
Tenosynovium, 2
Tenovagina, 2
Tension pneumothorax, 153
Tensor fascia lata, 917
Testes, injuries, 227
Testing rate, 27
Thalassemia, 196
Therapeutic interventions, 345, 345*f*
Thermal balance, 240
Thermogenesis, 240
Thermoregulation, 319, 1609
Thigh
  contusions, 1043–1052
    groin, 1047, 1047*f*
    iliac crest, 1043–1044, 1044*f*
    quadriceps, 1044–1047, 1044*t*
  regional anesthesia, 332–333
  strains, 1043–1052
    adductor, 1050–1051
    classification, 1047, 1047*t*
    quadriceps, 1047–1050
Thomas test, 932
Thompson test, for Achilles tendon injuries, 1477,
    1477*f*
Thoracic outlet syndrome (TOS), 633*b*
  anatomy, 634–636, 634*f*–635*f*
  classification, 632–633
  complications, 642
  decision-making principles, 639–640
  history, 636
  imaging, 638–639, 638*f*–639*f*
  physical examination, 636–638, 637*f*–638*f*
  postoperative management, 642–643
  results, 641–642
  treatment, 640–641, 641*f*–642*f*
  vascular problems and, 632–644
Thoracic spine, degenerative, 1597–1598
Thoracolumbar spine
  degenerative, 1597–1604
    discogenic low back pain, 1598–1599
    low back pain, 1598
    lumbar disc herniation, 1599–1601, 1601*f*
    lumbar spinal stenosis, 1602–1603, 1602*f*

Thoracolumbar spine (Continued)
    lumbar spine, 1598–1604
    radiculopathy, 1599–1601, 1600f
    spondylolisthesis, 1603–1604, 1603f–1604f
    synovial facet cysts, 1601–1602
    thoracic spine, 1597–1598
    injuries, 1582–1592
        burst fractures, 1584, 1585f
        Chance fractures, 1584, 1586f
        classification and severity, 1584t
        compression fractures, 1583–1584, 1584f
        contusions, 1585–1588
        decision-making principles, 1583–1591
        disc herniation, 1588, 1588f
        extension/extension-distraction,
            1584–1585
        fracture-dislocations, 1584, 1586f–1587f
        history, 1582
        imaging, 1583
        physical examination, 1582–1583
        postoperative management, 1592
        return to play, 1592
        risk factors, 1582, 1583t
        sacroiliac joint, 1591
        spinal stability, 1583
        spondylolisthesis, 1588–1591, 1590f
        spondylolysis, 1588, 1589f–1590f, 1591
        sprains, 1585–1588
        strains, 1585–1588
        stress fractures, 1584–1585
        thoracolumbar fractures, 1583
        treatment options, 1591
        vertebral body apophyseal avulsion fracture,
            1585
3D acquisitions, in magnetic resonance imaging,
    98, 98f
Throat, preparticipation physical evaluation, 145
Thromboembolic prophylaxis, 182, 183t–185t
Thromboembolism, 180
Thrombophilia, 180
Thrombosis, 180
Thrower's shoulder, 511–525
    adaptations to, 511–512
    biomechanics throwing, 512–513, 512f
    complications, 524
    decision-making principles, 516–517, 516f
    future considerations, 524–525
    history, 514
    imaging, 515–516, 516f
    pathophysiology, 513–514
        dynamic shoulder and scapular stability,
            513–514
        glenohumeral internal rotation deficit,
            514
        internal impingement, 513, 513f
    physical examination, 514–515
    results, 521–524
    treatment options, 517–518, 518b–521b,
        518f–520f
        biceps tenodesis, 518
        glenohumeral internal rotation deficit,
            518
        internal impingement, 517
        interval throwing program, 522t
        partial-thickness rotator cuff tears, 517
        pitching program, 523t
        posterior capsular contracture, 518
        SLAP tear, 517–518
Throwing
    biomechanics, 1663–1665
    injuries, 757–771
        complications, 770
        decision-making principles, 760–761
        future considerations, 770

Throwing (Continued)
        history, 757–758, 758f
        imaging, 760, 761f
        physical examination, 758–760, 759f–760f
        postoperative management, 768
        results, 768–770
        return to play guidelines, 768
        treatment, 761–765
    motion, 1663–1665, 1663f–1664f
Throwing cycle, 685
Thumb
    distal interphalangeal joints, 789
    injuries, 124
    ulnar collateral ligament injury, 804, 804f, 814,
        815f
Tibia
    anatomy, 1065
    proximal osteotomy, 1255, 1255f, 1259b,
        1259f
    stress fractures, 133–134, 134f–135f
    tendons
        anterior, 1386, 1387f
        injuries, 1462–1464
        posterior, 1383–1384, 1383f–1384f
    translation of, anterior/posterior, 1247–1248
Tibial inlay techniques, for posterior cruciate
    ligament injuries, 1217–1218, 1225, 1228t
Tibial slope, role of, 1192
Tibial spine fracture, 1615f
Tibial tendons
    anterior, 1386, 1387f
    posterior, 1383–1384, 1383f–1384f
Tibial tuberosity osteotomy (TTO), 1300–1301,
    1305b
Tibial tunnel, for revision anterior cruciate
    ligament injuries, 1206
Tibiofemoral joint
    biomechanics, 1074–1080
    ligaments
        biomechanics, 1075–1077, 1076f
        cruciate, 1077–1079
        force measurement of, 1074–1075
        lateral collateral, 1079–1080
        medial collateral, 1079–1080
        strain measurement of, 1075
Tillaux fractures, juvenile, 1730, 1730f
Tinea versicolor, 250f
Tinel test, 691, 691f
Tissue contrast, in MRI, 95, 95f–96f, 96t
Tissue engineering
    polymer fibers in, 38
    scaffolds in, 35
TissueMend implant, for tendon repair, 36
Tissues
    engineering, functional, 28–29
    graft, 30–34
        allograft, 31–32
        autograft, 30
        future direction, 33
    musculoskeletal
        articular cartilage, 9–12
        bone, 12–15
        meniscus, 7–9
        physiology pathophysiology, 2–15
        tendon and ligament in, 2–7
    neurologic, 1534–1535, 1534f
    storage, 27
Titin, 64
Tobacco, 292
Toe
    taping, 369
    turf, 1515–1516
        anatomic classification, 1518f
        complications, 1516

Toe (Continued)
        decision-making principles, 1515–1516
        history, 1515
        imaging, 1515, 1516b
        physical examination, 1515
        postoperative management, 1516
        results, 1516
        treatment options, 1516, 1517b, 1517f
Tonnis angle, 938
Torque vectors, 21
Total hip arthroplasty, hip arthritis, 1059
Tourniquets, 328–329
Trabecular pattern, 937
Traction, hip arthroscopy, 948–949
Training
    athletic, 342, 343b
    coordination, 381, 382f–383f
    diabetic athlete, 223
    endurance, 1607–1608
    functional, 1196–1197
    muscle, 1195–1196, 1196f
    muscular response to, 66–67
    neuromuscular, 69
    strength, 381, 1608–1609
    strength, in young athletes, 68
Transient quadriplegia, 1579
Transitional zone, of articular cartilage, 10, 10f
Transplantation, meniscal allograft, 1142
Transport, of injured athlete, 1556–1558,
    1557f
Transposition
    anterior intramuscular, 750, 751f
    anterior subcutaneous, 750, 750f
    anterior submuscular, 750–751, 751f
Transthoracic echocardiography (TTE), 164–166,
    165f–167f
Transtibial tunnel, for posterior cruciate ligament
    injuries, 1217–1218, 1225, 1228t
Transtriceps portal, 711
Transverse tarsal joints, kinematics and
    biomechanics, 1365, 1367f
Trapezium carpal injuries, 838–840, 838f–840f,
    840b
Trapezium fracture, 808–809, 809f
Trapezoid carpal injuries, 845, 845b
Trauma
    elbow, 699–700
    genitourinary, in athlete, 227–229
        classification, 227, 228t
        definition, 227, 228t
        diagnosis, 227–228
        epidemiology, 227
        pathobiology, 227
        pathophysiology, 227
        return-to-play guidelines, 229
        treatment, 228–229
    imaging, 699–700
Traumatic anterior instability, 1648–1651
    complications, 1651
    history, 1648, 1648f
    imaging, 1648–1649, 1649f–1650f
    physical examination, 1648, 1649f
    treatment options, 1649–1651, 1650f, 1651b,
        1652f
Traumatic posterior instability, 1651–1653
    history, 1651–1652
    imaging, 1652, 1653f
    physical examination, 1652, 1652f
    treatment options, 1653, 1653f–1654f
Trendelenburg gait, 929
Trephination, 1147–1148
Triangular fibrocartilage complex (TFCC)
    injuries, 813–814, 813f–814f
    arthroscopy, 828, 828t

Triangular fibrocartilage complex tears, 866–867
  class 1 tears (traumatic), 866
  class 2 tears (degenerative), 866–867
  Palmer classification, 867t
Triceps
  distal rupture, 737–740
    anatomy, 737, 737f
    biomechanics, 737
    classification, 737
    complications, 740
    decision-making principles, 738, 738b
    epidemiology, 737, 737b
    future considerations, 740
    history, 738
    imaging, 738
    physical examination, 738
    postoperative management, 740
    results, 740
    treatment, 738–739
  strength test, 690, 691f
  tendinitis, 725–728
    complications, 727
    decision-making principles, 725–726
    future considerations, 727–728
    history, 725
    imaging, 725, 726f
    physical examination, 725, 725f
    postoperative management, 727
    results, 726
    return-to-play guidelines, 727
    treatment, 726, 726b
      conservative, 726
      operative, 726, 727f
Tricompartmental osteoarthritis, arthroplasty for,
    1283
Trigger point therapy, 367, 367f
Triquetrum carpal injuries, 836–838, 838b,
    838f
Trochanteric bursae, 920–921
Trochanteric bursitis, 1001–1002, 1002b
Trochleoplasty, 1301
TruFit CB plug, 44
Tunnel grafting, 1204–1205, 1205f
Tunnel malpositioning, 1203
  correction of, 1204, 1204f
Turf toe, 1515–1516
  anatomic classification, 1518t
  complications, 1516
  decision-making principles, 1515–1516
  history, 1515
  imaging, 1515, 1516b
  injuries, 1367
  physical examination, 1515
  postoperative management, 1516
  results, 1516
  treatment options, 1516
    nonoperative, 1516
    operative, 1516
    technique, 1517b, 1517f
2D acquisitions, in magnetic resonance imaging,
    98, 98f
Type 1 diabetes, 218, 221, 221f
  management, 224–225
Type 2 diabetes, 218
  management, 225

U

Ulnar collateral ligament, 684
Ulnar collateral ligament (UCL) injuries,
    701–702, 701f–702f, 762–763, 762f–763f,
    765b–766b, 766f, 768–770, 769f
  reconstruction, 763f
  thumb, 804, 804f, 814, 815f
Ulnar impaction syndrome, 810
Ulnar nerve, 747, 748f

Ulnar nerve compression, 691–692, 691f–692f
Ulnar neuritis, 765, 765f, 770
Ulnar neuropathy, 704, 705f. See also Cubital
    tunnel syndrome
Ulnar quadrant, 794t, 798–800, 799f
Ulnar styloid fracture, 1613f
Ultimate load, in biomechanics, 24–25
Ultrashort time to echo sequence, 100–101
Ultrasonography, 78–85, 946
  advantages, 84
  ankle, 1380
  disadvantages, 84–85, 85f
  dynamic, 84, 84f
    in athletic pubalgia, 1010–1011
  elastography, 83–84, 83f
  femoroacetabular impingement, 964–965
  foot, 1380
  glenohumeral joint, 411–412, 412f, 412t
  iliopsoas, 979, 983–984
  knee, 1104–1105, 1106f
  lateral and posterolateral corner injuries of
      knee, 1253
  musculoskeletal, 79–83, 80f–83f
  revision rotator cuff repair, 568
  scapulothoracic disorders, 614, 614f–615f
  technical considerations, 78–79, 79f
  thermal effects, 363
Uncovertebral joints, 1594
Units of measure, 16, 17t
Unstable fractures, of cervical spine, 1541–1543
  complications, 1543
  decision-making principles, 1542
  future considerations, 1543
  history, 1541
  imaging, 1541–1542, 1542f
  physical examination, 1541
  postoperative management, 1543
  results, 1543
  treatment options, 1542–1543, 1542b
Upper extremity
  injuries
    figure skating, 118
    football, 118
    gymnastics, 120
    ice hockey, 121
    rowing, 123
    snowboarding, 124–125
    soccer, 125
    tennis, 127
  innervation, 330
Upper gastrointestinal tract conditions, 189–192
  dyspepsia, 191–192
  dysphagia, 192
  functional heartburn, 191
  gastroesophageal reflux disease, 190–191
  nausea, 192
  vomiting, 192
Upper respiratory tract infections (URTIs),
    206–209
  diagnosis, 207
  epidemiology, 206
  infectious mononucleosis, 207–208
  measles, 208–209
  pathobiology, 206–207
  prevention, 207
  return-to-play guidelines, 207
  treatment, 207
Urticaria, 257, 258f
URTIs. See Upper respiratory tract infections

V

Vail Sport Test, 387
Valgus extension overload (VEO), 763–764, 770
Valgus stress testing, in medial collateral ligament
    and posterior medial corner injuries, 1232

Varus motion, 1246–1247
Varus talar tilt test, 1377–1379
Vascular system, thoracic outlet syndrome,
    632–644
Vascular tendons, 2
Vascularization
  capsule, 916, 917f
  knee, 1072
Vectors, 16, 18f
  force, 19f–20f, 21
  moment/torque, 21
Velocity, 22
Venous thromboembolism (VTE), 180–181
Ventilator anaerobic threshold, 71–72
VEO. See Valgus extension overload
Verruca vulgaris (common warts), 251–252, 252f
Vertebral body apophyseal avulsion fracture, 1585
Vincula, 2
Viral infections, 250–252
  herpes simplex, 250–251, 251f
  molluscum contagiosum, 252, 252f
  verruca vulgaris (common warts), 251–252,
      252f
Virchow triad, 180
Viscoelasticity, 24, 24f–25f
Viscosupplementation, for knee arthritis, 1280
Visually impaired athletes, 323
  adaptive equipment, 323
  exercise, 323
  medical considerations, 323
    flight dysrhythmia, 323
    musculoskeletal injuries, 323
Vitamin D, 279–280
Vitamins, 279–280
Volar quadrant, 794t, 800–801, 800f, 802f–803f
Volleyball injuries, 127–128
  ankle, 127
  back pain, 128
  concussion, 128
  finger, 127–128
  knee, 127
  shoulder, 128
  wrist, 127–128
Vomiting, 192
von Willebrand disease (vWD), 199
VTE. See Venous thromboembolism

W

Wall push-up, 613
Wartenberg syndrome, 902
Warts, common, 251–252, 252f
Waterborne diseases, 210–213
  cryptosporidiosis, 211–212
  fecally derived, 211
    non, 213–214
    other, 212–213
  infectious diarrhea, 212
Weight loss, knee arthritis and, 1279
Weight-loss-related injuries, 129
Wheelchair athletes, 317–320
  adaptive equipment, 320
  exercise physiology, 317–318
  medical considerations, 318–320
    autonomic dysreflexia, 319–320
    heterotopic ossification, 319
    musculoskeletal injuries, 318
    neurogenic bladder and bowel, 319
    peripheral nerve entrapment, 319
    pressure sores/ulcers, 319
    spasticity, 319
    thermoregulation, 319
Whiplash injury, 405
White blood cell scans, labeled, 89–90, 91f
Windlass mechanism, 1365–1367, 1367f–1368f
Wolff-Parkinson-White (WPW) syndrome, 172

Women. *See Female athlete*
WPW. *See* Wolff-Parkinson-White (WPW)
    syndrome
Wrestling injuries, 128–129
    musculoskeletal, 128–129
    skin infections, 129
    soft tissue, 129
    weight-loss-related issues, 129
Wright test, 636–638, 637*f*
Wrist, 785–792
    anatomy, 789–790, 790*f*, 792*f*
    arthroscopy, 817–834
        anatomy, 819–820, 820*f*–821*f*
        carpal instability, 821–824, 821*t*, 822*f*–823*f*
        class I traumatic injuries, 829–832, 829*f*–831*f*
        class II degenerative injuries, 832
        complications, 833
        fracture, 824–828
        future considerations, 833
        ganglionectomy, 832–833, 832*f*
        management, 829–832, 829*f*–831*f*
        set-up, 817–819, 818*f*–819*f*
        triangular fibrocartilage complex, 828, 828*t*
    biomechanics, 789–790, 790*f*, 835
    carpal injuries, 835–848
    decision-making principles, 793–805
    diagnosis, 793–805
    extensor tendons, 790–791, 790*f*–791*f*
    flexors, 791
    history, 793–794
    imaging, 806–816, 807*f*
        carpal fractures, 807–809
        distal radius fractures, 806–807
        intrinsic carpal ligament injury, 810–812, 811*f*
        Kienböck disease, 810
        perilunate dislocation, 809–810, 810*f*

Wrist *(Continued)*
        tendon injuries, 812–813, 812*f*–813*f*
        triangular fibrocartilage complex injury,
            813–814, 813*f*–814*f*
        ulnar impaction syndrome, 810
    injuries
        golf, 120
        rowing, 123
        tendons, 812–813, 812*f*–813*f*
        volleyball, 127–128
    neuropathies, 898–905
        decision-making principles, 901
        future considerations, 904
        history, 898
        imaging, 900–901, 900*f*, 901*t*
        physical examination, 898–900, 899*f*–900*f*
        postoperative management and return to
            play, 902–903, 903*b*, 903*f*
        results, 903–904
        treatment options, 901–902
    pediatric, 1623–1625
        acute injuries, 1623–1624, 1623*f*
        overuse injuries, 1624–1625, 1624*f*–1626*f*
    physical examination, 793–794, 794*f*
    quadrants
        dorsal, 794*t*, 796–798, 797*f*–798*f*
        radial, 794–796, 794*t*, 795*f*–796*f*
        ulnar, 794*t*, 798–800, 799*f*
        volar, 794*t*, 800–801, 800*f*, 802*f*–803*f*
Wrist/hand injuries
    pediatrics, 1677–1687
        distal radial physeal stress reaction,
            1683–1684
        finger fractures, 1677–1681
        future considerations, 1684
        jammed finger, 1681–1683
        scaphoid fracture, 1684–1686

Wrist tendinopathies, 857–864
    complications, 863
    De Quervain tenosynovitis, 859–860, 859*f*
        postoperative management and return to
            sports, 860
        treatment options, 859, 859*b*, 860*f*
    extensor carpi ulnaris tendinopathy, 861–862
        classification, 861
        criteria for return to sports, 861–862
        special tests, 861
        treatment options, 861
    flexor carpi radialis tendinopathy, 862
    flexor carpi ulnaris tendinopathy, 862–863,
        862*b*, 862*f*–863*f*
    future considerations, 863–864
    history, 857–858
    imaging, 858–859, 858*f*
    intersection syndrome, 860–861, 860*f*
        return to sports, 861
        treatment options, 860–861, 861*b*
    physical examination, 858
    results, 863, 863*f*

Y

Y-balance test, 387, 388*f*
Yergason test, 405
Young athlete, 1606–1614. *See also* Pediatrics

Z

Zimmer Collagen Repair Patch, 36–37
Zona orbicularis, 914